SEXUALLY TRANSMITTED DISEASES

NOTICE

SEXUALLY TRANSMITTED DISEASES

THIRD EDITION

Editors

King K. Holmes, MD, PhD
Professor of Medicine, Adjunct Professor, Microbiology, Epidemiology; Director, Center for AIDS and STD, University of Washington; Head, Infectious Diseases, Harborview Medical Center, Seattle, Washington

P. Frederick Sparling, MD
Professor and Chairman, Department of Medicine, University of North Carolina, Chapel Hill, North Carolina

Per-Anders Mårdh, MD, PhD
Director of Uppsala University, Centre for STD Research, Uppsala, Sweden

Stanley M. Lemon, MD
Professor and Chair, Department of Microbiology and Immunology, University of Texas Medical Branch at Galveston, Galveston, Texas

Walter E. Stamm, MD
Professor of Medicine, Head, Division of Allergy and Infectious Diseases, University of Washington, Seattle, Washington

Peter Piot, MD, PhD
Executive Director, Joint UN Programme on HIV/AIDS, Geneva, Switzerland

Judith N. Wasserheit, MD, MPH
Director, Division of STD Prevention, National Center for HIV, STD, and TB Prevention, Centers for Disease Control and Prevention, Atlanta, Georgia

ORTHO

McGraw-Hill
HEALTH PROFESSIONS DIVISION

New York St. Louis San Francisco Colorado Springs Auckland Bogotá
Caracas Hamburg Lisbon London Madrid Mexico Milan Montreal
New Delhi Paris San Juan São Paulo Singapore Sydney Tokyo Toronto

McGraw-Hill

A Division of The McGraw-Hill Companies

SEXUALLY TRANSMITTED DISEASES, Third Edition

1 2 3 4 5 6 7 8 9 0 QPK QPK 9 9 8 8

ISBN 0-07-135982-6 NON RETURNABLE

This book was set in Sabon Roman by Progressive Information Technologies, Inc. The editors were J. Dereck Jeffers and Pamela Hanley; the production supervisor was Richard Ruzycka; the cover designer was Edward Schultheis. Quebecor Printing/Kingsport was printer and binder.

This book is printed on acid-free paper.

Library of Congress Cataloging in Publication Data

Sexually transmitted diseases / editors, King K. Holmes . . . [et al.].
—3rd ed.
p. cm.
Includes bibliographical references and index.
ISBN 0-07-029688-X
1. Sexually transmitted diseases. I. Holmes, King K.
[DNLM: 1. Sexually Transmitted Diseases. WC 140 S5174 1999]
RC200.S49 1999
616.95′1—dc21
DNLM/DLC
for Library of Congress

98-31523
CIP

CONTENTS

Part VI SEXUALLY TRANSMITTED PATHOGENS

Section 1: Overview of Host Immunity and Molecular Pathogenesis and STD

Section 2: HIV and Other Primate Retroviruses

Section 3: Herpesviruses, Human Papillomavirus, Hepatitis B Virus, Molluscum Contagiosum

Section 4: Bacteria

Section 5: Protozoa and Fungi

Section 6: Ectoparasites

Part VII STD CARE MANAGEMENT

A. Overview

Section 2: Management of STD Syndromes in Women

Section 3: Management of STD Syndromes in Men

Section 4: Management of Dermatologic and Extragenital Manifestations of STD/HIV

Part IX PREVENTION AND CONTROL OF STD/HIV

Section 1: Public Health Program Perspectives

Section 2: Special Aspects of STD/HIV Prevention and Control in Developing Countries and Resource Poor Settings in Industrialized Countries

Part X SPECIAL MEDICAL/LEGAL/SOCIAL ISSUES

CONTRIBUTORS*

Jonathan G. Ainsworth [40]
The Jeffris Wing, St Mary's Hospital, Paddington, London, United Kingdom

William Albritton [38]
St Boniface Hospital, Winnipeg, Canada

John Alderete, PhD [43]
Professor of Microbiology, Department of Microbiology, University of Texas Health Science Center, San Antonio, Texas

Miriam J. Alter, PhD [26]
Chief, Epidemiology Section, Hepatitis Branch, Centers for Disease Control, Atlanta, Georgia

John Ambroziak, Ph.D. [18]
Division of Hematology/Oncology, Cancer Research Institute and Department of Medicine, University of California at San Francisco, San Francisco, California

Deborah J. Anderson, PhD [13]
Associate Professor of Obstetrics, Gynecology and Reproductive Biology, Director, Fearing Laboratory, Brigham and Women's Hospital, Harvard Medical School, Boston, Massachusetts

Roy M. Anderson, FRS [3]
Linacre Chair & Head, Department of Zoology, University of Oxford, Oxford, United Kingdom

Sevgi O. Aral, PhD [4,88,93]
Associate Director for Science, Division of STD Prevention, Centers for Disease Control, Atlanta, Georgia

Ronald C. Ballard, PhD, M.I. Biology [64]
Associate Professor and Head, National Reference Centre for STD, Department of Medical Microbiology, South Africa Institute for Medical Research and University of Witwatersrand, Johannesburg, South Africa

Michael P. Bates, MD [22]
Acting Instructor Medicine, Allergy and Infectious Diseases, Fred Hutchinson Cancer Research Center, University of Washington, Seattle, Washington

Ronald Bayer, MD [107]
Professor, Columbia University School of Public Health, New York, New York

Consuelo M. Beck-Sague, MD, FAAP [53,105]
Associate Director, Minority and Women's Health, NCID, Centers for Disease Control and Prevention, Atlanta, Georgia

*The numbers in brackets following the contributor name refer to chapter(s) authored or co-authored by the contributor.

Richard E. Berger, MD [61]
Professor of Urology, University of Washington, Seattle, Washington

Stuart M. Berman, MD [9]
Chief, Adolescent Activities Unit, Division of STD Prevention, National Center for HIV/STD and TB Prevention, Centers for Disease Control, Atlanta, Georgia

Stephen A. Billstein, MD, MPH [46]
Senior Associate Director of Clinical Operations, Sandoz Pharmaceutical Company, East Hanover, New Jersey

William A. Blattner, MD [19]
Head, Epidemiology and Prevention Studies, Institute of Human Virology, University of Maryland, Baltimore, Maryland

Gail Bolan, MD [8]
Director, STD Prevention and Control, San Francisco Department of Public Health, San Francisco, California

William R. Bowie, MD [60]
Professor of Medicine, Faculty of Medicine, Division of Infectious Diseases, University of British Columbia, Vancouver, British Columbia, Canada

Alan M. Brandt, MD [2]
Professor Department of Social Medicine, Harvard Medical School, Boston, Massachusetts

Donald C. Bross, JD, PhD [106]
Professor & Councel, The C. Henry Kempe Center, Denver, Colorado

Robert C. Brunham, MD [79,80]
Professor and Head, Department of Medical Microbiology, University of Manitoba Basic Sciences Building, Winnipeg, Manitoba, Canada

Susan Buchbinder, MD [70]
Chief, Research Branch, San Francisco AIDS Office, and San Francisco Department of Public Health, San Francisco, California

Willard Cates, Jr, MD [78,79]
President, Family Health Institute, Family Health International, Durham, North Carolina

Connie Celum, MD, MPH [70]
Associate Professor, Director STD Clinic, Department of Medicine, University of Washington, Seattle, Washington

John W. Chandler, MD [66]
Department of Opthamology, University of Wisconsin Medical School, Madison, Wisconsin

Max A. Chernesky, PhD [92]
Chief of Medical Microbiology, Professor of Pediatrics and Pathology, Chair, Medical Microbiology, McMaster University, St. Joseph's Hospital, Regional Virology and Chlamydia Laboratory, Hamilton, Ontario, Canada

Margaret A. Chesney, PhD [72]
Professor of Medicine, Co-Director, Center for AIDS Prevention Studies, University of California–San Francisco Center for AIDS Prevention Studies, San Francisco, California

Diane Civic, PhD [6]
University of Washington School of Social Work, Seattle, Washington

Peggy Clarke, MPH [56]
Vice President, World Health Communications, New York, New York

Farley Cleghorn, MD, MPH [19]
Institute of Human Virology, University of Maryland, Baltimore, Maryland

Myron Cohen, MD [13]
Professor of Medicine, Microbiology, and Immunology; Chief, Division of Infectious Diseases, The University of North Carolina, Chapel Hill, North Carolina

Roy Colven, MD [63]
Assistant Professor, Department of Dermatology, University of Washington, Seattle, Washington

Robert W. Coombs, MD, PhD [71]
Associate Professor Laboratory Medicine and Medicine, Director of Retrovirus Laboratory, University of Washington, Seattle, Washington

Lawrence Corey, MD [21]
Professor of Laboratory Medicine, University of Washington, and Head, Program in Infectious Diseases, Fred Hutchinson Cancer Research Center, Seattle, Washington

Raoul A. Coutinho, MD, PhD [10]
Head, Department of Public Health and Environment, Municipal Health Service, Amsterdam, The Netherlands

J. Randall Curtis, MD [49]
Assistant Professor Department of Medicine, University of Washington, Seattle, Washington

Gina A. Dallabetta, MD [100]
Technical Support Director HIV/AIDS Programs, Family Health International, Arlington, Virginia

Jacqueline E. Darroch, PhD [91]
Senior Vice President and Vice President for Research, The Alan Guttmacher Institute

Kevin M. De Cock, MD, FRCP, DTM&H [101]
Chief, Division of HIV/AID Prevention, Surveillance and Epidemiology, Centers for Disease Control and Prevention, Atlanta, Georgia

Lynda S. Doll, PhD [11,54]
Chief, Behavioral Intervention Research Branch, Centers for Disease Control and Prevention, Atlanta, Georgia

John M. Douglas, Jr, MD [27]
Associate Director, Denver Disease Control Services, Associate Professor of Medicine and Preventive Medicine, University of Colorado Health Sciences Center, Denver, Colorado

W. Lawrence Drew, MD, PhD [22]
Professor, Laboratory Medicine, University of California San Francisco; Director, Clinical Microbiology, Mt Zion Medical Center, San Francisco, California

Libby Edwards, MD [65]
Chief of Dermatology, Department of Internal Medicine, Carolinas Medical Center, Charlotte, North Carolina

Anke A. Ehrhardt, PhD [8]
Director, HIV Center, Columbia University, NYS Psychiatric Institute, New York, New York

Joseph J. Eron, Jr, MD [74]
Associate Professor of Medicine, Division of Infectious Diseases, University of North Carolina at Chapel Hill, Chapel Hill, North Carolina

David Eschenbach, MD [58]
Professor, Chief of Division of Obstetrics and Gynecology, Department of Obstetrics and Gynecology, University of Washington, Seattle, Washington

Anthony Fauci, MD [17]
Director, National Institute of Allergy and Infectious Diseases, National Institutes of Health, Bethesda, Maryland

Martin Fishbein, PhD [54]
Professor, Annenberg School for Communications, Public Policy Center, University of Pennsylvania, Philadelphia, Pennsylvania

Susan Folkman, MD [72]
Professor of Medicine, Co-Director, Center for AIDS Prevention Studies, University of California at San Francisco, San Francisco, California

Denise Galloway, PhD [24]
Research Professor, Microbiology; University of Washington; Fred Hutchinson Cancer Research Center, Seattle, Washington

Mary Rogers Gillmore, PhD [6]
Associate Dean for Research, Professor, School of Social Work, University of Washington, Seattle, Washington

Daniel O. Graney, PhD [50,51]
Associate Professor, Biological Structure, School of Medicine, University of Washington, Seattle, Washington

Judith B. Greenberg, PhD [56]
Health Scientist, Disease Prevention, Centers for Disease Control, Division of Sexually Transmitted Diseases, Atlanta, Georgia

Joel R. Greenspan, MD, MPH [97]
Centers for Disease Control and Disease Prevention, Atlanta, Georgia

Ian Grimm, MD [67]
Associate Professor of Medicine, Division of Digestive Diseases, University of North Carolina, Chapel Hill, North Carolina

Richard L. Guerrant, MD [44]
Professor, Chief, Division of Geographic and International Medicine, Department of Medicine, University of Virginia Health Sciences Center, Charlottesville, Virginia

Laura T. Gutman, MD [82,87]
Associate Professor Pediatrics and Pharmacology, Director, Duke Pediatric STD Program, Duke University, Durham, North Carolina

Margaret R. Hammerschlag, MD [83]
Professor of Pediatrics and Medicine, Children's Medical Center of Brooklyn, Kings County Hospital Center, University Hospital of Brooklyn, Long Island College Hospital, Brooklyn, New York

H. Hunter Handsfield, MD [32,52]
Professor of Medicine, University of Washington; Director, Seattle-King County Sexually Transmitted Diseases Control Program, Harborview Medical Center, Seattle, Washington

Bernadine P. Healy, MD [36]
Dean, College of Medicine and Public Health, The Ohio State University, Columbus, Ohio

Karen Hein, MD [9]
Executive Officer, Institute of Medicine, National Academy of Sciences, Washington, D.C.

Sharon L. Hillier, PhD [14,42]
Associate Professor, Department of Obstetrics and Gynecology, Director, Reproductive Infectious Disease Research, University of Pittsburgh/Magee Women's Hospital, Pittsburgh, Pennsylvania

Martin S. Hirsch, MD [74]
Professor of Medicine, Harvard University; Infectious Disease Unit, Massachusetts General Hospital, Boston, Massachusetts

King K. Holmes, MD, PhD [4,42,48,57,88,89]
Professor of Medicine, Director, Center for AIDS and STDs, University of Washington, Head, Infectious Diseases, Harborview Medical Center, Seattle, Washington

David R. Holtgrave, PhD [95]
Associate Professor of Psychiatry and Behavioral Medicine, Centers for AIDs Intervention Research, Director of Cost Effectiveness Studies Core Associate, Director for Programs, Medical College of Wisconsin, Milwaukee, Wisconsin; Centers for Disease Control and Prevention AIDS/STD/TB Center, Atlanta, Georgia

Edward W. Hook, III, MD [32,91]
Professor of Medicine, University of Alabama at Birmingham, Birmingham, Alabama

Robert Hornick, PhD [96]
Professor, Annenberg School for Communication, University of Pennsylvania, Philadelphia, Pennsylvania

Monir Islam, MD, MPH [104]
Division of Research and Intervention Development, World Health Organization, Geneva, Switzerland

Carole Jenny, MD, MBA [105]
Associate Professor of Pediatrics, Brown University School of Medicine, Rhode Island Hospital, Providence, Rhode Island

David Shumway Jones, MA [2]
Department of the History of Science, Harvard University, Boston, Massachusetts

Haskins Kashima, MD [86]
Professor of Otolaryngolo/Oncology, Head and Neck Surgery, Johns Hopkins University School of Medicine, The Johns Hopkins Hospital, Baltimore, Maryland

William J. Kassler, MD [98]
Branch Chief, Program Evaluation and Preventive Health Services Research Branch, Division of STD Prevention National Center for HIV, STD, Centers for Disease Control and Prevention, Atlanta, Georgia

Elly T. Katabira, MB, ChB [101]
Department of Medicine, Mulago Hospital, Makerere University Medical School, Kampala, Uganda, Africa

Jeffrey A. Kelly, PhD [95]
Professor of Psychiatry and Behavioral Medicine, Director, Center for AIDs Intervention Research, Medical College of Wisconsin, Milwaukee, Wisconsin

Gerald Keusch, PhD [41]
Director, Fogarty International Center, Tufts New England Medical Center, Division of Geological Medicine, Boston, Massachusetts

Nancy B. Kiviat, MD [25,59]
Professor of Pathology, University of Washington, Seattle, Washington

Barbara Klencke [76]
AIDS Division, University of California at San Francisco, San Francisco, California

Scott Koenig, MD, PhD [17]
Vice President, Research MedImmune, Inc, Gaithersburg, Maryland

Laura A. Koutsky, PhD [25,59]
Associate Professor, Department of Epidemiology, HPV Research Group, University of Washington, Seattle, Washington

John N. Krieger, MD [43,51,62]
Professor of Urology, University of Washington, Seattle, Washington

Marie Laga, MD, MSc, PhD [102]
Institute voor Tropsiche Geneeskunde, Antwerpen, Belgium

David J. Landry, MS [91]
Senior Research Associate, The Alan Guttmacher Institute, New York, New York

Stanley M. Lemon, MD [15,26,67]
Professor and Chair, Department of Microbiology and Immunology, University of Texas Medical Branch, Galveston, Texas

Jay A. Levy, MD [18]
Professor of Medicine, Division of Hematology/Oncology, Cancer Research Institute and Department of Medicine, University of California at San Francisco, San Francisco, California

Wilma Lim, MD [81]
Clinical Assistant Professor, Department of Pediatrics, University of North Carolina, Chapel Hill, North Carolina

David Mabey, MD [91]
Clinical Sciences, London School of Hygiene and Tropical Medicine, University of London, London, United Kingdom

Per-Anders Mårdh, MD, PhD [53]
Director, Uppsala University, Centre for STD Research, Uppsala, Sweden

Christina M. Marra, MD [77]
Assistant Professor, University of Washington, Department of Neurology, Seattle, Washington

David H. Martin, MD [60]
Harry E. Bascomb MD, Professor of Medicine, School of Medicine, Louisiana State University Medical Center, New Orleans, Louisiana

Henry Masur, MD [75]
Chief, Critical Care Medicine, National Institute of Health, Bethesda, Maryland

Nyssa Matson, LCSW [87]
Clinician, Duke University/Pediatric Social Work Department, Medical Center, Durham, North Carolina

William M. McCormack [40]
The Jeffris Wing, St Mary's Hospital, Paddington, London, United Kingdom

Andre Meheus, PhD [37]
Professor, Epidemiology and Community Medicine, University of Antwerp, Antwerpen, Belgium

Thierry E. Mertens, MD [98]
Director, Office of HIV/AIDS and STDs, WHO, Geneva, Switzerland

Stephen A. Morse, MSPH, PhD [53]
Associate Director Science Division, AIDS/STDs and Tuberculosis Lab Research, Centers for Disease Control, Atlanta, Georgia; Adjunct Professor of Microbiology and Immunology, Emory School of Medicine, Georgia and University of Alabama at Birmingham

Stephen Moses, PhD [10]
Associate Professor, University of Manitoba, Medical Microbiology, Winnepeg, Manitoba, Canada; Department of Community Health, University of Nairobi, Nairobi, Kenya

Phoebe Mounts, PhD [86]
Associate Professor, School of Hygiene and Public Health, The Johns Hopkins Medical Institute, Baltimore, Maryland

F. Kevin Murphy, MD, FACP [84]
Clinical Associate Professor, Internal Medicine, University of Texas Southwestern Medical Center, Dallas, Texas

Daniel M. Musher, MD [35,36]
Professor of Medicine and Microbiology/Immunology, Baylor College of Medicine, Chief of Infectious Diseases, Veteran's Affairs Medical Center, Houston, Texas

Elizabeth N. Ngugi, RN, PhD [10]
Senior Lecturer, Department of Community Health, University of Nairobi, Nairobi, Kenya

Nigel O'Farrell, MD, MRCP [39]
Communicable Diseases Epidemiology, London School of Hygiene and Tropical Medicine, London, United Kingdom

Kevin O'Reilly, PhD [104]
Division of Research and Intervention Development, World Health Organization, Geneva, Switzerland

David G. Ostrow, MD [11]
Associate Professor, Department of Psychiatry and Behavioral Medicine, Medical College of Wisconsin, Center for AIDS Intervention Research, Milwaukee, Wisconsin

Mead Over [1]
The World Bank, Washington, D.C.

Jorma Paavonen, MD [59]
Professor of Obstetrics/Gynecology, University Central Hospital, Haartmaninkatu, Helsinki, Finland

Nancy S. Padian, PhD [88]
Associate Professor, Department of Obstetrics/Gynecology and Reproductive Sciences, University of California, San Francisco, California

Peter Perine, MD [30]
University of Washington, Seattle, Washington

Peter Pertel, MD [20]
Clinical Instructor, Department of Microbiology/Immunology and Department of Medicine, Northwestern University Medical School, Chicago, Illinois

Peter Piot, MD, PhD [1,5,100]
Executive Director, Joint United Nations Programme on HIV/AIDS, Geneva, Switzerland

Thomas A.E. Platts-Mills, MD [47]
Professor of Medicine, Microbiology, Head of Asthma and Allergic Disease Center, Allergy Division, University of Virginia Health Center, Charlottesville, Virginia

Francis A. Plummer, MD [10]
Professor of Medicine and Medical Microbiology, Department of Microbiology, University of Manitoba, Winnipeg, Manitoba, Canada

John J. Potterat [55]
Director, STD/HIV Programs, El Paso County Department of Health and Environment, Colorado Springs, Colorado

Thomas C. Quinn, MD [69]
Division of Infectious Diseases, The Johns Hopkins University, Baltimore, Maryland

Justin D. Radolf, MD [33,84]
Professor of Internal Medicine and Microbiology, Department of Medicine/ID Division, University of Texas Southwest, Dallas, Texas

Jonathan I. Ravdin, MD [44]
Professor, Department of Medicine, University of Minnesota, Minneapolis, Minnesota

Michael F. Rein, MD [47]
Professor of Internal Medicine, Associate Chair for Undergraduate Medical Education, University of Virginia Health Center, Charlottesville, Virginia

Edward P. Richards, JD, MPH [106]
Professor, University of Missouri Law School at Kansas City, Kansas City, Missouri

Peter A. Rice, MD [68]
Professor of Medicine, Director, STD Clinic and Director, Maxwell Finland Laboratory, ID Section, Boston Medical Center, Boston City Hospital, Boston, Massachusetts

Martha Rogers, MD [81]
Division of HIV/AIDS Prevention, Centers for Disease Control and Prevention, Atlanta, Georgia

Allan Ronald, MD [38]
St Boniface Hospital, Winnipeg, Manitoba, Canada

Michael W. Ross, MA, PhD, MPH [7]
Professor, Public Health, School of Public Health/CHPD, University of Texas Health Sciences Center, Houston, Texas

Richard B. Rothenberg, MD, MPH [55]
Professor, Department of Family and Preventive Medicine, Emory University School of Medicine, Atlanta, Georgia

Caroline A. Ryan, MD, MPH [48]
Associate Director for International Activities, Division of STD Prevention, Centers for Disease Control and Prevention, Atlanta, Georgia

Pablo J. Sanchez, MD [84]
Associate Professor of Pediatrics, Division of Pediatric ID, University of Texas Southwestern Medical Center, Dallas, Texas

Julius Schachter, PhD [28]
Professor of Laboratory Medicine, Epidemiology, and Biostatistics, University of California at San Francisco, Chlamydia Research Laboratory, San Francisco, California

Kenneth F. Schulz, PhD, MBA [84]
Clinical Professor, Department of OB/Gyn, University of North Carolina, Chapel Hill, Director of HIV Prevention Trials Division, Family Health International, Chapel Hill, North Carolina

Bernard Schwartländer [5]
Center for International Research, United States Bureau of the Census, Washington, D.C.

Pepper Schwartz, PhD [6]
Professor of Sociology, University of Washington, Seattle, Washington

Cynthia Sears, MD [44]
Associate Professor, Johns Hopkins University School of Medicine, Division of ID & Gastro-enterology, Baltimore, Maryland

Keerti Shah, MD, DrPH [86]
Professor of Molecular Microbiology and Immunology Director of STD CRC, The Johns Hopkins School of Public Health, Baltimore, Maryland

Nicholas Shaheen, MD [67]
Assistant Professor of Medicine, Division of Digestive Diseases, University of North Carolina, Chapel Hill, North Carolina

Joanna E. Siegel, ScD [99]
Assistant Professor, Department of Maternal and Child Health, Harvard School of Public Health, Boston, Massachusetts

Kathleen J. Sikkema, PhD [95]
Assistant Professor, Center for AIDs Intervention Research, Medical College of Wisconsin, Milwaukee, Wisconsin

Werasit Sittitrai, PhD [104]
Center for International Research, United States Bureau of the Census, Washington, D.C.

John Sixbey, MD [23]
Professor, Department of Microbiology and Immunology, Feist-Willer-LSUMC Cancer Center, Louisiana State University Medical Center, Shreveport, Louisiana

Karen S. Slobod, MD [23]
St Jude's Children's Research Hospital, Division of Infectious Diseases, Memphis, Tennessee

William A. Smith, EdD [96]
Executive Vice President, Academy for Educational Development, Washington, D.C.

Jack Sobel, MD [45]
Professor of Medicine, Chief, Division of Infectious Diseases, Wayne State University, Department of Medicine, Detroit Medical Center, Detroit, Michigan

David H. Spach, MD [73]
Associate Professor of Medicine, Division of Infectious Diseases, University of Washington Harborview Medical Center Madison Clinic, Seattle, Washington

P. Frederick Sparling, MD [15,31,34]
Professor and Chairman, Department of Medicine, University of North Carolina, Chapel Hill, North Carolina

Patricia G. Spear, PhD [20]
Department of Microbiology/Immunology, Guy and Anne Youmans, Professor and Chairman, Northwestern University Medical School, Chicago, Illinois

Katherine M. Spooner, MD [75]
Critical Care Medicine, National Institute of Health, Bethesda, Maryland

Michael E. St. Louis, MD [89]
Chief, Epidemiology and Surveillance Branch, Division of STD Prevention, Centers for Disease Control and Prevention, Atlanta, Georgia

Sergio Stagno, MD [85]
Katherine Reynolds Ireland, Professor and Chairman, Department of Pediatrics, The University of Alabama at Birmingham, School of Medicine, Birmingham, Alabama

Lola V. Stamm, MD [33]
Associate Professor Epidemiology, School of Public Health, Department of Epidemiology, University of North Carolina at Chapel Hill, Chapel Hill, North Carolina

Walter E. Stamm, MD [29,30]
Professor of Medicine, Head, Division of Allergy and Infectious Disease, School of Medicine, University of Washington, Seattle, Washington

Katherine M. Stone, MD [94]
Medical Epidemiologist, Division of STD Prevention, National Center for HIV, STDs, and TB Prevention, Centers for Disease Control and Prevention, Atlanta, Georgia

Morton Swartz, MD [36]
Massachusetts General Hospital, Department of Medicine, Division of Infectious Disease, Boston, Massachusetts

Ronald Swanstrom, PhD [16]
Professor, Department of Biochemistry and Biophysics, University of North Carolina at Chapel Hill, Chapel Hill, North Carolina

Milton R. Tam, PhD [103]
Technical Director, Diagnostics Development, PATH, Seattle, Washington

David Taylor-Robinson, MD, MRCP, FRC Palt [40]
The Jeffris Wing, St Mary's Hospital, Paddington, London, United Kingdom

Elizabeth L. Thomas, MPH [94]
Consultant, Population Services International, Washington, D.C.

Celeste Thorpe [41]
Instructor of Medicine, Tufts University School of Medicine, Boston, Massachusetts

Eugeni Tikhomirov, MD, PhD [37]
Medical Officer, Division of Emerging and Other Communicable Diseases Surveillance and Control, World Health Organization, Geneva, Switzerland

Judith Timyan, PhD [94]
Vice President, Director of Health Programs, Population Services International, Washington, D.C.

Ronald O. Valdiserri, MD, MPH [90]
Deputy Director, National Center for HIV, STDs, and TB Prevention, Centers for Disease Control and Prevention, Atlanta, Georgia

C. Johannes van Dam, MD, MSc [100]
Senior Program Associate and Deputy Director, Horizons Project, The Population Council, Washington, D.C.

Anneke van den Hoek, MD [12]
Coordinator, AIDSA Research, Municipal Health Service, Amsterdam, Netherlands

Janice R. Verley [69]
Division of Infectious Diseases, The Johns Hopkins University, Baltimore, Maryland

Paul Volberding, MD [76]
Professor of Medicine, Director, AIDS Division, University of California at San Francisco, San Francisco, California

Louis A. Vontver, MD [50]
Professor, Director, Division of Medical Education, Department of Obstetrics and Gynecology, University of Washington, Seattle, Washington

Bea Vuylsteke, MD, MSc [102]
Institute of Tropical Medicine, Department of Infection and Immunity, Division of Microbiology, Antwerpen, Belgium

Anna Wald, MD, MPH [21]
Assistant Professor, Department of Medicine and Epidemiology; Medical Director, Virology Research Clinic, University of Washington, Seattle, Washington

John W. Ward, MD [97]
Editor, MMWR Series, Director, Office of Scientific and Health Communications Epidemiology Program Office, National Centers for Disease Control and Prevention, Atlanta, Georgia

Judith N. Wasserheit, MD, MPH [8,90,93]
Director, Division of STD Prevention, Centers for Disease Control and Prevention, Atlanta, Georgia

D. Heather Watts, MD [80]
Director of Obstetrical and Gynecological Research, Pediatric Adolescent and Maternal AIDs Branch, National Institute of Child Health and Human Development, NIH, Bethesda, Maryland

Peter O. Way, MD [5]
Center for International Research, United States Bureau of the Census, Washington, D.C.

Robert D. Weber [13]
University of North Carolina at Chapel Hill, School of Medicine, Chapel Hill, North Carolina

Robert Wehbie, MD, PhD [16]
Boice-Willis Clinic, Rocky Mountain, North Carolina

Lars Weström, MD, DMS [58]
Associate Professor of OB/Gyn, University Hospital, Lund, Sweden

Richard J. Whitley, MD [85]
Loeb Eminent Scholar Chair in Pediatrics, Professor of Pediatrics, Microbiology, and Medicine, University of Alabama at Birmingham, Children's Hospital, Birmingham, Alabama

Richard J. Wolitski, MA [54]
Leader, Individual and Small Group Interventions Team; Behavioral Intervention Research Branch, Division of HIV/AIDS Prevention, CDC, Atlanta, Georgia

Robert W. Wood, MD [90]
Director, AIDS Control Program, Seattle-King County, Department of Public Health, Associate Professor of Medicine, University of Washington, Seattle, Washington

INTRODUCTION

STD AS EMERGING INFECTIONS

Since 1975 when planning for the first edition of this book began, at least 12 new sexually transmitted pathogens have been identified (Table 1). Some were discovered through use of new diagnostics tests, and some, like HIV-1, HIV-2, and HIV subtype O, appeared as truly new infections, emerging because of changing socioeconomic forces leading to changes in sexual behavior. A host of other pathogens—e.g., cytomegalovirus (CMV), several hepatitis viruses (HAV, HBV, HCV), several intestinal bacterial and parasitic pathogens—have also become newly recognized as sexually transmissible through clinical epidemiological studies.

EVOLUTION OF TERMINOLOGY: VD, STD, STI, AND RTI

The terminology used to refer to the topic addressed by this book has also evolved from the older term venereal diseases, which in the US is still defined narrowly in some state law and regulations as consisting only of those diseases recognized as sexually transmitted when the laws were written, i.e., syphilis, gonorrhea, chancroid, lymphogranuloma venereum and granuloma inguinale. Evolution to the term sexually transmitted diseases reflects recognition of the increasing number of infections or conditions that are sexually transmissible.

What are the distinctions between sexually transmitted diseases (STD), infections (STI), or pathogens; sexually *transmissible* diseases, infections, or pathogens; and reproductive tract infections (RTI, not to be confused with respiratory tract infections, also called RTI by pulmonologists). These terms all are used throughout this book. Some distinctions are evident: a pathogen causes infection, which may result in disease; a pathogen may not qualify as a full-fledged sexually *transmitted* pathogen, but could be a sexually *transmissible* pathogen when non-sexual routes of transmission predominate. Viruses like CMV and HBV may qualify as predominately sexually transmitted pathogens in adults but not in children; for CMV this may have been especially true in the 70s and 80s when the sexual revolution was in full swing, but probably not in the early part of the century when most children probably acquired the virus from other children without having sex, and perhaps not in the 90s when intimate nonsexual contact between children in preschool day care centers has increasingly led to children acquiring CMV, with subsequent transmission back to their mothers. The term RTI is preferred by some in the reproductive health field to encompass conditions like bacterial vaginosis, for which the designation as an STD is debated; and to attempt to destigmatize the detection and treatment of those infections which are sexually transmitted.

STD PATHOGENS AND SYNDROMES

The total number of distinct sexually transmitted or transmissible pathogens now exceeds 30 (Table 2). Many of these can be further categorized into multiple types and subtypes that may have differing clinical manifestations. For a few of these pathogens, sexual transmission is not yet well-defined, but seems quite likely on the basis of indirect clinical epidemiologic evidence. Many of clinical syndromes caused by infections with these pathogens are summarized in Table 3. These can appear in every subspecialty of medicine, in every health care setting. With the advent of phosphodiesterase-5 inhibitors for treatment of impotence, even geriatrics can become increasingly involved in this field.

THIS BOOK IS DESIGNED FOR SPECIALISTS AS WELL AS FOR PRIMARY CARE CLINICIANS

The past quarter century has also seen extraordinary improvement in the quality of the science, and growth in the overall quantity of new information concerning STDs. Fortunately, the qualifications and enthusiasm of professionals now entering the field are also higher than ever, as STD clinical, research, and teaching activities have reentered the academic mainstream after a long separation, pulled increasingly by the epidemic of sexually transmitted HIV/AIDS, and by increasing recognition of both the magnitude of the problem and of the availability of effective new tools and new disease prevention models to deal with STDs, and the increasing concern about STD/HIV in the reproductive health field. The organization of the academic discipline and of medical services for STD differ markedly across the world. In the UK, consultants in genitourinary medicine deal with STD, ambulatory care for HIV infection, and related genitourinary diseases. In much of Europe, including Eastern Europe, Africa, as well as in Latin America, and Asia, a varying proportion (small in Western Europe) of "dermatovenereologists" devote much of their time to clinical care, teaching, and research on STD. In Australia and New Zealand, the University of Sydney offers a Master of Health degree and a Diploma of Medicine in Sexual Health, and specialists are certified by an Australian College. In North America, clinicians, microbiologists, and allied health workers from many disciplines specialize in clinical care or research related to STD and HIV-fields which still tend to be separate in terms of interest and practice in parts of North America. In contrast, in most developing countries, where STD and HIV are rampant and 90% of the world's STD and HIV infections occur, and increasingly in Eastern Europe, the primary care clinician has the major role in providing services for STD and HIV care.

At a policy and practice level, the field of STD has also become a more integral part of efforts to improve reproductive health both in developing countries and in the industrialized world. The explosion of new information on the impact of STD/HIV on reproductive health makes comprehensive knowledge of STD and HIV essential for reproductive health specialists. In many parts of the developing world, pharmacists or alternative care providers provide much of the frontline care, and specialists tend to see treatment failures or referrals, although special STD clinics may provide efficient care to a large proportion of the male population.

Paradoxically, in industrialized countries, as STD comes under better control, and outbreaks of imported STD emerge as the major problem, the relative importance of the STD specialist will increase in public health settings best equipped to contain outbreaks of infection. Similarly, as the HIV epidemic comes under better control, and care becomes more complex, the role of the HIV clinical specialist is again increasing, even in the context of managed care.

CHANGES IN THE THIRD EDITION

This 3rd edition of Sexually Transmitted Diseases aims to provide comprehensive and authoritative information on the clinical, microbiological, and public health aspects of STD including HIV infection, as an essential reference for the specialist as well as for

Table 1. Sexually Transmissible Pathogens Newly Identified or Newly Emergent Since 1975. Although Sexual Transmission Has Not Yet Been Formally Proven for Several of These Pathogens, the Clinical Epidemiologic Context Makes This Likely.

Pathogen	Year identified
Human papilloma viruses (>25 genital types)	1976–present
HTLV-types I and II	1980, 1982
Mycoplasma genitalium	1981
Mobiluncus curtisii, M. mulieris	1981
Helicobacter fenneliae, H. cinaedi	1985
HIV type 1, type 2, subtype 0	1983, 1986, 1990
Hepatitis C virus	1989
Human herpes virus type 8	1995

Modified from Eng TR, Butler WT (eds). The hidden epidemic: Confronting sexually transmitted diseases. Institute of Medicine, Washington DC, National Academy Press, 1997.

the primary health care clinician. This edition welcomes new editors Judith Wasserheit, who has organized a new section on prevention and control of STDs; and Peter Piot, who has introduced new sections on the global epidemiology of HIV and AIDS, and on special aspects of STD/HIV prevention and control in developing countries. Overall, nearly half of the 107 chapters are completely new, and nearly all those with continuing authors have been largely rewritten. The 8-plus year gestation since the last edition helps account for the extensive changes required and the overall "weight" of the evidence presented in this edition.

The Editors wish to particularly thank Ronald A. Nelson for his indispensible editorial contribution. This edition would not have been completed without him.

Table 2. Sexually Transmissible Pathogens and Associated Disease Syndromes

Pathogen	Associated disease or syndrome
Bacteria	
Neisseria gonorrhoeae	Urethritis, epididymitis, proctitis, cervicitis, endometritis, salpingitis, perihepatitis, barholinitis, pharyngitis, conjunctivitis, prepubertal vaginitis, prostatitis (?), accessory gland infection, disseminated gonococcal infection (DGI), chorio-amnionitis, premature rupture of membranes, premature delivery, amniotic infection syndrome
Chlamydia trachomatis	All of the above except DGI, plus otitis media, rhinitis, and pneumonia in infants, and Reiter's syndrome
Mycoplasma hominis	Postpartum fever, salpingitis (?)
Ureaplasma urealyticum	Nongonococcal urethritis
Mycoplasma genitalium	(?) Nongonococcal urethritis
Treponema pallidum	Syphilis
Gardnerella vaginalis	Bacterial ("nonspecific") vaginosis (in conjunction with *Mycoplasma hominis* and vaginal anaerobes, such as *Mobiluncus spp*)
Mobiluncus curtisii	Bacterial vaginosis
Mobiluncus mulieris	Bacterial vaginosis
Haemophilus ducreyi	Chancroid
Calymmatobacterium granulomatis	Donovanosis (granuloma inguinale)
Shigella spp	Shigellosis in men who have sex with men (MSM)
Campylobacter spp	Enteritis, proctocolitis in MSM
Helicobacter cinaedi	?Proctocolitis; dermatitis, bacteremia in AIDS
Helicobacter fenneliae	?Proctocolitis; dermatitis, bacteremia in AIDS
Viruses	
Human immunodeficiency virus, types 1 and 2, and subtype 0	HIV disease, AIDS
Herpes simplex virus	Initial and recurrent genital herpes, aseptic meningitis, neonatal herpes
Human papillomavirus	Condyloma acuminata, laryngeal papilloma, intraepithelial neoplasia and carcinoma of the cervix, vagina, vulva, anus, penis
Hepatitis A virus	Acute hepatitis A
Hepatitis B virus	Acute hepatitis B, chronic hepatitis B, hepatocellular carcinoma, polyarteritis nodosa, chronic membranous glomerulonephritis, mixed cryoglobulinemia (?), polymyalgia rheumatica (?)
Hepatitis C virus	Acute hepatitis C, chronic hepatitis C, hepatocellular carcinoma, mixed cryoglobulinemia, chronic glomerulonephritis
Cytomegalovirus	Heterophil-negative infectious mononucleosis; congenital CMV infection with gross birth defects and infant mortality, cognitive impairment (e.g., mental retardation, sensorineural deafness); protean manifestations in the immunosuppressed host
Molluscum contagiosum virus	Genital molluscum contagiosum
Human T-cell lymphotrophic virus, types I and II	Human T-cell leukemia or lymphoma, tropical spastic paraparesis, other
Human herpes virus type 8	Kaposi's sarcoma, body cavity lymphoma, multicentric Castleman's disease, ?multiple myeloma
Protozoa	
Trichomonas vaginalis	Vaginal trichomoniasis, NGU
Entamoeba histolytica	Amebiasis in men who have sex with men (MSM)
Giardia lamblia	Giardiasis in MSM
Fungi	
Candida albicans	Vulvovaginitis, balanitis
Ectoparasites	
Phthirus pubis	Pubic lice infestation
Sarcoptes scabiei	Scabies

Table 3. Selected Syndromes and Complications of Sexually Transmitted Pathogens

Syndrome or complication	Associated sexually transmitted pathogen
In men	
AIDS	Human immunodeficiency virus, types 1 and 2
Urethritis	*Neisseria gonorrhoeae*, *Chlamydia trachomatis*, herpes simplex virus, *Ureaplasma urealyticum*, ?*Mycoplasma genitalium*, *T. vaginalis*
Epididymitis	*C. trachomatis*, *N. gonorrhoeae*
Intestinal infections	
Proctitis	*N. gonorrhoeae*, herpes simplex virus, *C. trachomatis*
Proctocolitis or enterocolitis	*Campylobacter spp*, *Shigella spp*, *Entamoeba histolytica*, ?Helicobacter sp.
Enteritis	*Giardia lamblia*
In women	
AIDS	Human immunodeficiency virus, types 1 and 2
Lower genitourinary tract infection	
Vulvitis	*Candida albicans*, herpes simplex virus
Vaginitis	*Trichomonas vaginalis*, *C. albicans*
Vaginosis	*Gardnerella vaginalis*, *Mobiluncus spp*, other anaerobes, *Mycoplasma hominis*
Cervicitis	*N. gonorrhoeae*, *C. trachomatis*, herpes simplex virus
Pelvic inflammatory disease	*N. gonorrhoeae*, *C. trachomatis*, *M. hominis*, anaerobes, Group B streptococcus
Infertility	
Postsalpingitis, postobstetrical, postabortion	*N. gonorrhoeae*, *C. trachomatis*, *M. hominis* (?)
Pregnancy morbidity	Several STDs have been implicated in one or more of these conditions
Chorioamnionitis, amniotic fluid infection, prematurity, premature rupture of membranes, preterm delivery, postpartum endometritis, ectopic pregnancy	
In men and women	
Neoplasia	Human papillomavirus
Cervical, vulvar, vaginal, anal, and penile, intrepithelial neoplasia, carcinoma	
Hepatocellular carcinoma	Hepatitis B virus, hepatitis C virus
Kaposi's sarcoma, body cavity lymphoma, multicentric Castleman's disease, ?multiple myeloma	Human herpes virus type 8
T-cell lymphoma/leukemia	HTLV-I
Genital ulceration	Herpes simplex virus, *T. pallidum*, *Haemophilus ducreyi*, *Calymmatobacterium granulomatis*, *C. trachomatis* (LGV strains)
Acute arthritis with urogenital or intestinal infection	*N. gonorrhoeae*, *C. trachomatis*, *Shigella spp*, *Campylobacter spp*
Hepatitis	Hepatitis A, B, and C viruses, cytomegalovirus, *Treponema pallidum*
Genital warts	Human papillomavirus
Molluscum contagiosum	Molluscum contagiosum virus
Ectoparasite infestations	*Sarcoptes scabiei*, *Phthirus pubis*
Heterophil-negative mononucleosis	Cytomegalovirus, Epstein-Barr virus (some evidence for sexual transmission)
Tropical spastic paraparesis	Human T-cell lymphotrophic virus, type I
In neonates and infants	
Neonatal systemic infection, with potential cognitive impairment, deafness, death	Cytomegalovirus, herpes simplex virus, *T. pallidum*, HIV
Conjunctivitis	*C. trachomatis*, *N. gonorrhoeae*
Pneumonia, ?chronic pulmonary disease	*C. trachomatis*, *U. urealyticum* (?)
Otitis media	*C. trachomatis*
Sepsis, meningitis	Group B streptococcus
Laryngeal papillomatosis	HPV

NOTE: For each of the above syndromes, some cases cannot yet be ascribed to any cause and must currently be considered idiopathic. "?" indicates a possible associated syndrome.

Sources for Tables 2 & 3: Cates W Jr, Holmes KK. Sexually transmitted diseases. In: Last JM, Wallace RB, eds. Maxcy-Rosenau-Last Public Health and Preventive Medicine. 14th ed. Norwalk, CT: Appleton & Lange, 1998:137–155. Holmes KK, Handsfield HH. Sexually transmitted diseases: Overview and clinical approach. In: Fauci A, et al. (eds). Harrison's principles of internal medicine. 14th ed. New York: McGraw-Hill, Inc., pp 801–812, 1998.

PART I SOCIOECONOMIC IMPACT OF SEXUALLY TRANSMITTED DISEASES/HIV

Chapter 1

The public interest in a private disease: An economic perspective on the government role in STD and HIV control*

Mead Over

Sexually transmitted diseases are painful and sometimes deadly. However, the same is true of many other diseases and also of pollution, crime, poverty, traffic accidents, and armed conflict. Governments in all countries, and especially in the poorest countries of the world, must struggle to fulfill a multitude of important roles with extremely limited resources. Should the prevention and control of sexually transmitted diseases be one of the short list of activities that are part of the irreducible core of government responsibility?

Some people would argue that sexually transmitted diseases (STDs) should not be on the short list. Starting from the premise that sexual activity is almost always a voluntary activity subject to individual control, many would argue that the individual should take responsibility for his or her own actions and should pay the penalty in health cost if poor luck leads to an STD. This chapter takes the contrary view. It shows how individual choices made with full information about risks and consequences can nevertheless lead to a socially undesirable outcome. The implication is that some government intervention to prevent and control STDs is socially desirable.

THE ECONOMIC FRAMEWORK FOR EVALUATING GOVERNMENT INTERVENTIONS

Government intervention in any realm is justified only if it improves social welfare relative to the situation that would obtain in the absence of such intervention. This statement is obvious, but difficult to apply to actual public expenditure decisions. One of the principal difficulties is that different observers can legitimately have different views of the proper definition of social welfare. The standard way to avoid paralysis by this difficulty in economics is to divide the problem of improving social welfare into two steps: first, the maximization of total national well-being (efficiency); second, the distribution of that well-being among social groups (equity). If government intervention net of its costs increases total national well-being, the intervention is said to enhance the efficiency of the economy. If the intervention also furthers equity by improving the distribution of social rewards or reducing poverty, so much the better. If the intervention worsens equity, then society must judge whether the increase in total welfare is large enough to justify the associated reduction in the equity with which it is distributed. A mixed policy that uses some of the extra social product owing to the intervention to improve the well-being of the poorest citizens or, alternatively, of those who lose most from the policy intervention, might be preferred.

In addition to the difficulty of defining social welfare, a second important difficulty in evaluating a given intervention is properly characterizing the situation that would exist in the absence of the intervention. There are two aspects of this problem: defining the counter-factual and measuring the opportunity cost of the resources used in the intervention. In the case of sexually transmitted diseases, identifying what would happen in the absence of government intervention, the counter-factual, is often difficult. Ideally, governments should be able to draw on a body of scientific research that compares the rate of new sexually transmitted infection in a group that has benefited from a given intervention to that in an otherwise comparable group that has not received such an intervention. In fact, such controlled trials are all too rare.

The opportunity costs of an intervention are defined as the value of the resources in their next best use. Identifying the opportunity cost of the government resources is not difficult in theory, but often is in practice. For example, suppose that the next best use of resources spent on STDs is to use them instead to vaccinate children against measles. In theory, the opportunity cost of the resources is the value of the lives of the children who would have been saved by the measles vaccination program. However, comparing the lives of children saved from measles to the lives of adults saved from AIDS is not easy to do. In practice, attempts to compare the value of different lives by converting them all to a common metric such as the disability-adjusted life-year (or DALY) have met with less than universal acceptance, because of the inescapable arbitrariness of any proposed adjustment factors.

EFFICIENCY ARGUMENTS FOR GOVERNMENT INTERVENTION

This section and the box present several reasons that government should intervene to slow the spread of the AIDS epidemic despite the fact that it is primarily spread by private sexual acts between two consenting individuals.

THE CONVENTIONAL ARGUMENT FOR INTERVENTION

It is well accepted that government interventions that subsidize the prevention or treatment of airborne or waterborne infectious diseases or the prevention of vector-borne parasitic infections can enhance efficiency. To what degree do these arguments generalize directly to the case of sexually transmitted diseases, including HIV?

Starting from the premise that well-functioning markets will allocate social resources to maximize national output, economists have typically argued that specific market failures prevent people from reaching an efficient allocation of resources to treat or prevent infectious or vector-borne diseases. These market imperfections are "externalities" in the case of the infectious diseases and "public goods" in the case of the vector-borne diseases.

An "externality" occurs when a market transaction between two parties creates an unpriced effect on a third party. An example of such an unpriced effect is the beneficial impact on one's neighbor's health of one's own decision to seek treatment for an air- or waterborne infectious disease. The existence of an externality causes the market (in this case, the market for treatment of the disease) to fail because it prevents the individuals involved in the transaction from incorporating all of the social costs and benefits of their transaction. The health care provider may be considering all of his costs, including the opportunity costs of his workers, equipment and of his own time, when he decides the price he wishes to receive for the treatment. However, the patient does not take into account the benefits to his neighbor—and to his neighbor's neighbor—of his treatment, and so is willing to pay less for

*This chapter draws on Kremer[1] and Hammer[2] and on discussions with Martha Ainsworth, David Bloom, Paul Gertler, and Chris Jones.

treatment than the total worth of the treatment to him and his neighbor and his neighbor's neighbor. Because of the market failure, the patient will consume less than the socially optimal quantity of the treatment in question.

A pure "public good" is a good that has two specific attributes. It is "nonrivalrous" in consumption, meaning that its consumption by one person does not reduce its availability for consumption by another; and it is "nonexcludable" in consumption, meaning that if one person in a community consumes it, no other person in the same community can be feasibly excluded from consuming it also. Economic terminology distinguishes a "public good" from a "merit good," the latter being defined as a good that society prefers the poor to consume. For example, although food is a private, not a public, good, many societies guarantee a minimum amount of it to everyone on the grounds that it is a "basic need" or "merit good." (See later in this chapter for a discussion of health care as a merit good.) The eradication of a disease vector, like the anopheles mosquito, which transmits malaria, is a pure public good by this definition. Markets fail to produce the socially optimum amount of a public good, because each individual hopes that others will pay for it and he can "free-ride" on the others' largesse. Because of this market failure, the public good may not be produced at all unless the government intervenes and taxes everyone in order to finance its production.

EXTENDING THE ARGUMENT TO SEXUALLY TRANSMITTED DISEASES

In order to consider extending these arguments to STDs, reflect on an artificial example relating to an airborne infectious disease, tuberculosis (TB). Suppose that a person, B, rides to and from work every day in a carpool with person A and both know that A has TB. Suppose that both A and B live and work alone, so there is no risk of either infecting anyone else. B asks A if he is planning to seek treatment, but B responds that he has neither the time nor the money for doctors right now, especially since TB treatment is costly and time-consuming. Should the government be involved by, for example, subsidizing the TB treatment for A?

Leaving aside equity issues that might arise if A were poor (to be considered in the next section), there is no reason for the government to be involved in this case. It's true that A's condition imposes costs on B. In response to these costs, B can choose to abandon the convenient carpool arrangement or, alternatively, offer to help A pay for treatment. A and B will negotiate an agreement to share the costs of the doctor visit. The share of costs between them will be determined by their relative bargaining power in the relationship, so that either might end up paying much less for the treatment than he would have been willing to pay. If B is not sure whether A will comply with treatment, B can accompany A to the treatment sessions. The end result, however, will be an efficient outcome, as the two parties "internalize" the externality by their negotiated settlement.

But what if a third person is involved? Suppose the uninfected member of the two-person carpool, B, rides home in a different carpool at the end of the day with another uninfected person, C. That third person will clearly place some value on the continued non-infectious status of B. If C can be convinced that B is threatened by infection that could be prevented by paying for A's treatment, and again if the search costs of finding another evening carpool partner are significant, the probability of infection is high enough and the treatment cost is low enough, then C will be willing to contribute to the cost of curing A's TB. The willingness of C to contribute will increase the offer that B can make to A and enable treatment to occur when it otherwise might not have for lack of a sufficient offer by B.

The problem, and the reason that government intervention might be efficiency enhancing even in this example of two-person carpools, is that person B may have no way to demonstrate to C that B has contributed to A's cure. In the absence of a reliable monitoring technique available to C, C will not be willing to offer as much to B as B's contribution to A's cure is really worth to C. This is the problem of asymmetric information and would be a reason that a government subsidy for TB treatment could enhance efficiency even in the absence of the free-rider problem appealed to in the preceding section.

To what degree do the two arguments for government intervention in the case of airborne infectious diseases, the public good and the asymmetric information arguments, also apply to an STD? An STD is typically transmitted in the course of a sexual contact between two individuals, not between one individual and an entire group. In the carpool example, the uninfected member had an incentive to contribute to the cure of the infected member. Thus, the free-rider problem does not arise with STDs in the same way as with air- or waterborne diseases. The straightforward public good justification for subsidizing treatment is not applicable. (However, the public good justification applies indirectly to HIV, through its exacerbating effect on the spread of air- and waterborne infectious diseases.)

Now consider the argument based on asymmetric information. Just as person B in the carpool example had no way of convincingly demonstrating to person C that B had protected himself by subsidizing A's treatment, a person who uses a condom in a sexual contact has no way of convincingly demonstrating this fact to another sexual partner in order to be compensated for it. To extend the analogy, suppose that person A is a sex worker, person B is a client of A, and person C is the client's regular sexual partner or "girlfriend." (In this example, the points can be made even more dramatically by reversing the genders of A, B, and C. However, data show that fewer wives than husbands have extramarital sexual relations.) If the girlfriend knew in advance that her partner frequents sex workers and could reliably monitor his condom use with the sex worker, she would be willing to compensate him in some way for using them and her willingness to compensate him would increase his willingness to use the condom with the sex worker. For example, she might be more willing to remain in the relationship with him or to have sex with him without a condom, if he could prove that he has used a condom with his other partners. Thus, it is the unavailability to C of a reliable way of monitoring B's condom use that produces the externality and the potential for efficiency enhancing government intervention.

However, the inability of a woman to monitor her partner's condom use with other partners is exacerbated by two additional considerations. First, in most societies a woman will be unaware that her regular partner is having sex with other women and would feel threatened by the knowledge. Indeed, a husband's announcement that he is having sex with other women would in many cultures be interpreted by the wife as a signal that he wants to dissolve the marriage. To imagine that she would compensate him for using condoms with other women requires imagining that she would remain in the relationship given his announcement that he is having sex with other women. Even supposing that she would remain, as in many cultures she would be required to do, the compensation she would be willing to pay would be reduced by the reduction in the utility of the relationship owing to the knowledge of the extramarital affairs. Since it is impossible to convey to the wife the utility *enhancing* message that her husband uses condoms with other women without simultaneously conveying the utility *reducing* message that her husband is having sex with those women, the man cannot be compensated for the true difference in the utility to his wife of condom use.

A second and more important reason that the market failure engendered by asymmetric information can be quite large in this case is related to the epidemiological dynamics of an STD epidemic. The sex worker, person A, does not typically restrict her services to a single man, B. She serves a series of people, with each of whom she has a relationship similar to her relationship to B. Whether or not she uses a condom with B will affect not only B and C, but also all of her other clients and their marriage partners. In all of these linked relationships a monitoring problem will arise that is similar to that among A, B, and C. Because of the dynamic chain of sexual relationships, an increase in condom use by A and B lowers the probability of infection not only of C, but also of all the other people in the chain. Because of the asymmetric information, the prevalence rate of STDs, including HIV, will be higher and condom use lower than in the absence of all of these externalities. This result is inefficient, because all of the interacting persons would prefer the situation with lower STD prevalence and more condom use, but none of them, individually or jointly, has the power to make the trades that bring about this situation.

The degree to which the dynamics of an STD epidemic magnifies the positive externalities of a government intervention depends critically on how the intervention is targeted. For example, if person A, the sex worker in the preceding example, has relatively few partners and those partners are otherwise monogamous, strengthening her resolve to bargain for condom use will have a relatively small impact on the STD prevalence rate. On the other hand, if she has a great many partners, each of whom also has many partners, her condom use will have a large multiplicative effect on the epidemic.[1,3,5,7] The greater the reduction in STD prevalence from the condom subsidy, the greater the efficiency gain from the intervention.

A diagram can help to show clearly how a government subsidy to condom use can improve the welfare of all parties involved, including the man who dislikes condoms, his regular partner (whom we call his wife) with whom he does not use a condom, and his casual partner (whom we call his "extramarital" partner).

The box figure displays the husband's utility from extramarital sex, H, as a function of the prevalence rate of HIV infection, P, in the upper half of the figure and the wife's utility (or rather her disutility) of the husband's extramarital sex, W, in the bottom half of the figure. The utility of the husband's extramarital partner is not shown in the figure, but is introduced in the discussion that follows.

Both husband and wife assume that condoms are perfectly protective, so both the husband's utility of extramarital sex with a condom, H_c, and the wife's disutility of his extramarital sex with a condom, $W_c < 0$, are horizontal lines, unaffected by the probability that the husband's partner is infected, P. In order to account for the fact that many men choose not to use condoms even when they know that their partners might be infected, the husband's utility from sex without a condom, H_n, is drawn as superior to his utility of sex with a condom, H_c, up until a relatively high prevalence rate.[1] However, the wife has no such preference regarding her husband's pleasure from sex without a condom. In fact, she would prefer he use a condom even in the absence of risk of an STD, in order to prevent his impregnating another woman. Therefore, her dislike of his sex without a condom is greater than her dislike of his sex with a condom even at zero prevalence rate.

Given that the probability of the husband's casual partner being infected with HIV is P_1, the husband will prefer not to use a condom and will derive utility H_1 from the extramarital encounter. Assuming she is aware of his encounter, the wife derives disutility W_1 from it. As we argued in the preceding, the fact that the wife cannot monitor the husband's condom use means that she cannot offer him the trade of $W_c - W_1$ in exchange for his use of a condom.

If most of the husband's casual partners have many other casual partners and believe themselves to be uninfected with HIV, they would prefer to use condoms to protect themselves from STDs, including HIV, and also from pregnancy, if they had the knowledge and bargaining power to impose their preferences. Now suppose that a government intervention changes the bargaining power between the husband and his casual partners so that one quarter of them succeed in insisting on a condom during intercourse. The immediate result will be to reduce the husband's utility from each encounter to a weighted average of H_n and H_c, which is illustrated by H_2 in box Fig. 1-1. However, the wife's utility will increase, from W_1 to W_2, partially or perhaps completely offsetting her husband's utility loss. Depending on the relative magnitudes of the two utility changes and the cost of the government intervention, the intervention may have already increased total social welfare. Since this change involves an increase in two people's utility at the expense of a decrease in another's, it is not a move to greater efficiency, but rather a redistribution of welfare from the husband to the wife and his casual partner.

The longer-term effect of the government intervention can improve the welfare of the husband as well as of the women and the casual partners and thus be unequivocally efficiency enhancing. By intervening such that one-quarter of all encounters are protected by condoms, the prevalence rate will be reduced from P_1 to some smaller number such as P_2. This change will improve the utility of both the husband and the wife, with the husband attaining H_3 and the wife W_3 and will clearly improve the utility of the casual partners. If the prevalence rate drops far enough, as drawn in the box figure, the husband's utility will be increased even above his preintervention utility level of H_1.

Since the husband's welfare is greater at H_3 with prevalence rate P_2 than at H_1 with prevalence rate P_1, why was government intervention necessary to move him from zero to 25 percent condom use? The reason is that sexual partners do not have equal information about each others practices with others, i.e., asymmetric information. If all sexual partners could prove to subsequent partners that they had previously used a condom, then condom use would be adequately rewarded and the epidemic would naturally evolve from P_1 down to the lower level, P_2. However, in the absence of a method for proving to subsequent partners that one has used condoms in the past, no partner faces the appropriate incentives for condom use. This is a genuine case of market failure, since the husband and all men like him would like to trade 25 percent condom use for a move from H_1 to H_3. However, they can neither be compensated by their casual sexual partners nor by their wives for doing so. Owing to market failure, trades that would benefit all parties are not available.

How likely is it that an intervention that subsidizes an increase in condom use in extramarital sexual contacts will actually produce an efficiency gain? Or, in terms of the box figure, how likely is it that P_2 will be far enough below P_1 for H_3 to be above H_1? The answer depends on the number of extramarital partners the husband has and the number of partners each of his partners has. The greater the sexual activity of the husband and his partners, the larger the reduction in seroprevalence that will result from any given increase in the percentage of condom use. Thus, if the population of husbands and extramarital partners is heterogeneous, with some of them having more partners than others, a public intervention to facilitate condom use in these relationships will have the most positive externalities if it is targeted to the higher activity groups.

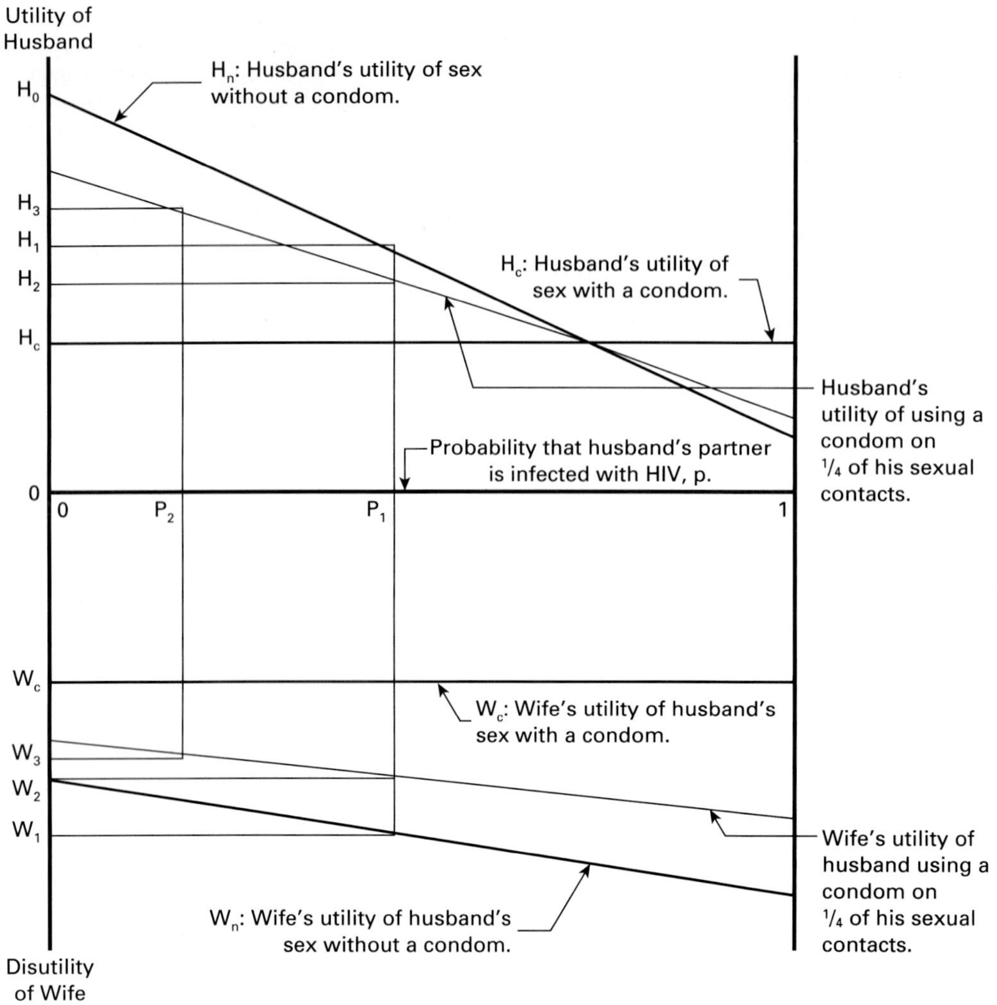

Box Fig. 1-1. The effect of the husband's extramarital sex on his utility and on his wife's disutility as a function of husband's condom use and the prevalence of HIV.

THE IMPLICATIONS OF HIV TESTING FOR GOVERNMENT INTERVENTION

HIV testing and the market for condoms

The discussion to this point has ignored the existence of blood tests for HIV infection and the fact that the cost of testing the blood or saliva of one's prospective partner for antibodies to HIV is rapidly decreasing. In a few years saliva tests will be available that cost only a few dollars, can be administered by anyone, and require only a few minutes. Soon thereafter it may even be possible to administer a test to one's prospective partner without his or her knowledge by, for example, obtaining a sample of bodily fluids on a piece of "litmus" paper. How will the availability of such technology affect the public economics of the HIV epidemic?

Given current technology, it is extremely difficult to test one's partner without his or her knowledge and the cost of testing is high relative to purchasing power in most developing countries. Thus, the availability of testing makes it possible, at substantial cost, for one to ascertain one's own infection status without informing one's partner. In this situation, individuals can use testing as a means of increasing the asymmetry of information between themselves and others in society, whether they be sexual partners, employers, or insurance companies. Such increased asymmetry has the potential of worsening the market failure problems described in the preceding section.

A government policy that would marginally reduce the asymmetry of information in some relationships would be to subsidize testing of people only in pairs. For example, whether the government allowed private firms to offer blood testing services or offered such services itself, it would mandate that two people who declare themselves to be current or prospective sexual partners can be jointly tested and jointly informed of each others' results for the same price otherwise charged to individuals. Although there would be some leakage owing to misrepresentation by individuals who pretend to be partners in order to receive tests at half price, on balance such a policy would tend to improve the symmetry of information between sexual partners.

One possible negative result of such "partner-observed" testing has been stressed by Philipson and Posner. The demand for such testing would originate in peoples' desire to have sex without a condom. Suppose that a woman insists on observing the test of her prospective husband. If the man agrees, and tests negative, she will agree to marry him and he will have access to unprotected sex with her. However, if she is actually infected, then he may also become so. On the other hand, if he tests positive, she will refuse him and he will subsequently agree to unprotected sex with people whose lifestyle suggests a high probability that they are infected. If some of those are uninfected, he may infect them. Thus, "[i]n either case he substitutes potentially infecting sex for safe sex," thus generating a negative externality and potentially exacerbating the spread of the epidemic.[6]

The proposed policy avoids one prong of this dilemma by subsidizing only partner-observed joint testing. Thus, in the example, the partnership would have proceeded to marriage and the use of unprotected sex only if both had tested negative, removing the possibility that the woman would subsequently infect the man owing to her current, unexpectedly positive, infection status. The other prong of the dilemma cannot be so easily avoided, but is less significant for the epidemic because the high-risk uninfected partner is likely to become infected soon whatever the behavior of the man under discussion.

As the advance of technology lowers the cost of testing and makes one's partner's infection status more easily available, the information asymmetries attributable to HIV, and therefore the public stake in its control, will decline. However, this decline will be slow in developed countries and even slower in developing ones. Substantial asymmetries are likely to remain for several decades, justifying continued government intervention to facilitate protected sexual intercourse.

HIV testing by employers of employees

In addition to the individual demand for HIV testing, there is a demand by some employers to test the blood of applicants or of current employees. Such employers apparently believe that, by identifying and excluding the HIV-positive candidates, they will reduce their health care and attrition costs and thus improve their profitability.

Regardless of the empirical validity of the employer's belief, the policy of screening workers and excluding or dismissing those who test positive, imposes negative externalities on the rest of society. First, since HIV infection is not related to current productivity, the practice of excluding workers by infection status effectively discriminates among workers based on their expected future decline in productivity or increase in health care expenditures. This practice could logically apply to workers over 50 years old, or female workers who might have children. Discrimination against workers based on attributes unrelated to their current productivity is inefficient, because it deprives society of the contribution that these groups could make to the economy. Furthermore, each firm that evades its share of the responsibility for the health care costs of HIV infected workers, forces these costs onto society at large. In a society where 10 or 20 percent of the prime-age work force is HIV infected, employer policies that discriminate against these workers will result in substantial social costs.

An additional reason to discourage employer discrimination is the possibility that employers who do not discriminate will have a greater incentive to sponsor workplace information and condom distribution programs, because they will bear some of the costs of HIV sickness. Governments throughout the world should encourage private firms to adopt a socially responsible approach to the HIV/AIDS epidemic, including workplace education programs and a refusal to screen workers for HIV.

HIV testing by health insurers

Potential purchasers of health insurance have information about the health risks they face that is unavailable to the insurance company. Those who believe themselves at greater risk are willing to pay more for health insurance and are more likely to buy it at any given premium than those who consider themselves healthy. The result is that the people who hold health insurance are typically more likely to be sick than those who do not, raising the cost of the health insurance premium over what it would be if everyone contributed. Although individual insurers can attempt to protect themselves from this "adverse selection" problem in a variety of ways, the only systematic solution to the problem, and arguably the most efficient one, is universal health insurance coverage financed by tax revenue. However, universal coverage is an expensive option and beyond the reach of the poorest countries. By offering universal coverage, but restricting it to catastrophic problems only, a government can dramatically reduce the danger of adverse selection while limiting its own costs and stimulating the private health insurance market.

The HIV epidemic has doubly exacerbated the potential information asymmetry between the insurer and the insured. First, the insured has information about his or her own sexual behavior that the insurer does not have and that information has new pertinence for future health care costs. Second, the insured can have a blood test giving absolute knowledge of HIV status that is unavailable to the insurance company. Because it is possible to spend a great deal on medical care for HIV/AIDS, these two problems can destroy the health insurance industry, or prevent its establishment, in countries with even small seroprevalence rates. Since the health insurance industry provides a valuable product, this destruction would be a serious market failure.

Of course, the blood test for HIV can also be used by insurers to partially redress the imbalance of information between them and the insured. Use of the test enables insurers to limit the tendency of people to apply for insurance when they find out, or suspect, that they are HIV infected. Although one can empathize with individuals in this position, allowing them to buy insurance without revealing their HIV status would result in massive efficiency losses. In countries that have, or are launching, private health insurance industries, government should establish guidelines that protect the rights of infected persons while enabling the health insurers to protect themselves. A market-based approach that deserves further study is the creation of special insurance policies specifically for people who are HIV-infected, as has occurred in South Africa, for example.

SEXUALLY ACTIVE PEOPLE MAY HAVE INSUFFICIENT KNOWLEDGE OF THE RISKS AND HOW TO AVOID THEM

At the beginning of the HIV epidemic, when the disease was unknown, individuals making the decision to enter a sexual relationship or to provide commercial sex services did so with some knowledge, however incomplete, of the existing sexually transmitted diseases.

In the past 15 years, sexual behavior has become much more dangerous, yet the evidence suggests that people's knowledge has not kept abreast of the changes. For example, as late as 1993 surveys of sex workers in 13 states of India found that fewer than 50 percent had ever heard of AIDS in all but one state. And even in Africa, where infection rates are highest, up to 50 percent of women with a casual partner did not know that condoms could protect against AIDS.

To the extent that sexually active people are ignorant of the danger of unprotected sex and are not able to find the information they need to protect themselves, there is an argument for public intervention in the dissemination of information. However, since information is not a pure public good (it is nonrivalrous, but excludable), public dissemination is potentially justified only if private channels of information are not already doing an adequate job of supplying information to each risk group in accordance with the social benefits from that group's knowledge. In countries with active, unfettered press and radio markets, the profit motive is likely to encourage the dissemination of large amounts of information to the general public about anything related to human sexuality. For the general public, the main functions of the government can be to feed accurate information to the press, to provide "corrections" when the press appears to be giving misinformation and, as an example to the public, to advertise its inclusion of persons known to be living with HIV or AIDS in the battle against AIDS and also in other high-profile community events. In countries where the HIV epidemic is just beginning and private sector media are reluctant, the government might take the initiative by an initial model information campaign and then withdraw funding from this activity while sending the signal that it encourages private sector dissemination efforts in the same vein.

However, the preceding argument that intervention efforts should be targeted to the most sexually active applies equally to public information about STDs and AIDS. Although more sexually active people have a greater self-interest in learning about STDs, the positive externalities associated with their knowledge suggest that they will nevertheless value such information at less than the social benefits of their acquiring it. Thus, there is a possible government role in subsidizing acquisition by the most sexually active of timely and accurate information about STDs and about protective strategies.

In addition to the basic facts about the transmission and health effects of HIV, sexually active people need to know the riskiness of unprotected sex in their own milieu. For example, the rational behavior modeled in the box presupposes knowledge by all parties of the prevalence rate of HIV infection in various population groups. Therefore, there is an important government role in facilitating and, if necessary, subsidizing disease surveillance efforts. To be as relevant as possible to individual decision making, surveillance data should be collected and publicized that is specific to each of the major urban centers in a country. If the prevalence rate can be collected for different risk groups within each urban center, it will be even more useful.

HIV TRANSMISSION EXACERBATION BY INFECTION WITH OTHER STDs

The preceding argument for the positive externalities associated with condom use applies equally to HIV and to the other STDs, although the consequences of infection and therefore the weight of the argument are stronger for the former. However, the fact that STDs have now been found in two important studies to substantially exacerbate the transmission of HIV means that all of the market failures that apply to HIV also affect the other STDs.[4,5] Furthermore, STDs can be cured as well as prevented. Therefore, the epidemiological interaction between the HIV and the other STDs greatly strengthens the argument for subsidizing the treatment of the classic STDs.[3]

HIV TRANSMISSION AMONG DRUG USERS

The economic analysis of the externalities associated with using contaminated needles is identical to that of unprotected sex (e.g., in the box, the dangerous activity of the husband outside the household could be sharing needles with a fellow drug user, instead of extramarital sex). The reasons why the wife of a drug user can not sufficiently compensate her husband for using clean needles are identical to the reasons why she can not adequately compensate him for condom use. The policy conclusion is the same, also: Provided that it can be accomplished at sufficiently low cost, government subsidy of clean needles can enhance efficiency.

HIV AND EQUITY

The preceding sections establish that the HIV epidemic engenders several market failures and that government intervention could increase social welfare, making many people better off. However, the HIV epidemic also creates or exacerbates several social inequities that many governments will also want to redress through government intervention.

PREVENTIVE INTERVENTIONS

One possible inequity relates directly to the preceding discussion of the efficiency gains from the man's condom use with nonregular sexual partners. That discussion made clear that the woman's ability to compensate the man for outside condom use could, subject to limitations on her ability to monitor his condom use, help to internalize the external costs of unprotected sex. However, in many societies the wife has little or no bargaining power in the relationship. If she has been unable to retain any of the benefits (i.e., the "gains from trade") accruing to their marriage, then she has no discretionary resources with which to compensate her husband, even if she wishes to do so. In particular, she may not have the power to refuse to have sex without a condom in sexual relations with her husband, or to refuse him his favorite meal or the repair of his favorite shirt, and thus may not be able to offer these compensations in exchange for his assurances of condom use outside. Although it is difficult to provide wives with more bargaining power in their current marriages, a government intervention that subsidizes the husband's condom use with outside partners (or taxes unprotected sex with those partners) will immediately redistribute welfare from the husband to the wife (see the box). For some societies, this may be reason enough for such interventions.

The preceding discussion has paid insufficient attention to the perspective of person A, the outside person in the triangular relationship, whether she is a sex worker or a noncommercial extramarital partner. (The feminine pronoun is used for clarity of exposition. The outside partner might, of course, be male.) If she has multiple partners and is well-informed, she is aware of being at high risk of HIV infection and is likely to prefer protected to unprotected sex. A government intervention that facilitates her access to condoms, increases her skill at negotiating condom use or, through persuasive public health messages targeted at her partners, reduces their resistance to condom use, will redistribute well-being toward her in the short run. This will be true whether or not the long-run benefit of reduced seroprevalence is enough to make her clients better off as modeled in the box. Redistribution from her client to her is likely to correspond to a transfer from a higher to a lower end of the income distribution. Such transfers would be consistent with a progressive policy toward income redistribution.

MITIGATION INTERVENTIONS

Orphaned children are a social problem whatever their cause, especially if they lose their parents when they are young. Since a high prevalence of HIV infection among reproductive age adults greatly increases the number of orphaned children, the epidemic is the occasion for increased attention to the plight of orphans. However, there is no obvious reason to single out AIDS orphans for special attention. In particular, some AIDS orphans are not poor or reside in households that are not poor, and therefore would absorb resources that could be better spent elsewhere on poverty relief. A concern for equity, properly construed, will target assistance efforts to the poorest orphans, regardless of the cause of their parents' death. To the extent that poor orphans can be identified, they can be a particularly useful target group for antipoverty safety net policies or for policies designed to mitigate the impact of the epidemic.

In popular use, the term "equity" is typically applied to issues of income distribution and redistribution. The discussion in this chapter has adopted the broader view that any redistribution of welfare from the better off to the worse off is equity enhancing. Thus, it is appropriate to consider the impact of public policy on the distribution of well-being between those who are free of infection and the HIV infected. On this dimension, at least, the former are better off than the latter and therefore might be the target of equity-motivated redistributive policies. Relevant policies include health sector policies that affect access to treatment and other policies that affect access to employment, housing, and so on.

Societies differ in their willingness to subsidize curative health care. Some societies argue that health care is a "basic need" or "merit good," and therefore that the government should assure access to basic health care for all citizens regardless of ability to pay. Other societies are skeptical of the claim that health care is different from many other goods and services with claims to being basic needs. These include not only education and basic nutritional requirements, but also roads, housing, and telephone service, for example. However, whatever the views of a specific society regarding the degree to which health care should be subsidized, a guiding principle for fair and compassionate treatment of HIV-infected people in the health care system should be comparability with the treatment accorded those suffering from other equally serious and difficult to treat illnesses.

Thus, a government that decides to provide antiretroviral medication, at a cost of thousands of dollars a year per patient, should be prepared to provide chemotherapy for cancer patients, heart surgery for heart disease patients, kidney dialysis and transplant for end-stage renal disease patients, and so on. Similarly, if opportunistic illnesses of the HIV-infected are treated at a subsidized rate, then the same subsidy should apply to the treatment of other infectious diseases. Once a government has accepted the argument that fairness for AIDS patients means fairness for cancer patients also, any proposed subsidy policy for all these similar diseases must be evaluated relative to the opportunity cost of the resources. The consequence will be that a poor country will cover a smaller share of costs for the average patient than a rich country with the same views on the degree to which health care is a merit good.

Unless a society is able to afford a 100 percent subsidy rate for treating all patients with AIDS or a similar expensive adult chronic condition, some patients will be unable to pay their portion of the cost of care. An equitable health care policy will make allowance for these patients by providing greater subsidies for the most indigent. However, the system of subsidies should be organized so that it benefits the poorest patients, regardless of the disease from which they suffer.

Government policies that oppose employment discrimination by HIV status have the advantage of enhancing efficiency as well as equity, and therefore are good candidates for implementation, provided that their cost is low. On the other hand, discrimination by health insurers according to the HIV status of the applicant reduces the asymmetry of information between the contracting parties and hence enhances efficiency. As discussed, such discrimination should be impeded only in countries with universal health insurance coverage.

RESOURCES FOR STDs NOW AND IN THE FUTURE

This last section of the chapter sums up the discussion and adds some final remarks in several areas. First, the section shows that the argument for government intervention in the cases of STD/HIV programs is at least as strong as the more traditional argument in favor of government control of TB. The section concludes by considering two kinds of interaction between culture and the HIV epidemic. On the one hand, the epidemic is likely to affect cultural practices, especially sexual practices and some of these changes are likely to slow the epidemic. On the other hand, in the short run cultural preferences to avoid the subject of sexuality may impede HIV control to the great detriment of the populations concerned.

A COMPARISON OF STDS AND TB

Although the argument for subsidizing the treatment and prevention of TB is firmly based on the theory of public goods, that for STDs lacks that support, except indirectly through the disease's effect on other communicable diseases, especially including TB. On the other hand, as argued in the text and demonstrated in the box, the asymmetry in information between sexual partners produces a clear efficiency argument in favor of government intervention to control STDs, and particularly HIV. Furthermore, the more heterogeneous the sexual behavior of the population and the easier it is to target the most sexually active with STD treatment and with subsidies and persuasion to use condoms, the larger the efficiency gains from government intervention to control STDs and AIDS. Thus, in practice the allocation of resources between TB and STD/HIV control on efficiency grounds should depend on the costs of government interventions and the number of (both primary and secondary) infections that can be prevented.

Figure 1-1 shows conceptually how resources should be allocated between the two sets of interventions. Suppose that a given amount of budget is available that a health ministry must allocate between TB and STDs/HIV. The length of the horizontal axis AD in the figure represents that fixed budget. Then any point on the line in the figure, such as point B, represents a division of these resources between the programs. Measuring the dollars spent on STD/HIV control from the left of the figure, line MB_{HIV} represents the marginal benefit, measured in deaths averted, of every additional dollar spent on those programs. By ranking the STD/HIV programs from left to right according to the size of their benefit per dollar, the line MB_{HIV} can be drawn as downward sloping from left to right. Then construct a similar line labeled MB_{TB}, which slopes downward from the right axis of the figure. The point where the two lines cross will represent the most efficient division of resources between the two programs.

The division of resources between the two programs will clearly depend on the specifics of the country situation. Figure 1-1 shows the outcome in two situations in which the budget is the same and the prevalence and threat of TB are the same, but the prevalence rate of HIV infection differs. In a country with a low prevalence rate of HIV infection, the number of cases that can be prevented by a highly targeted program can be enormous, but expansion of that program beyond the small group of people who are most at risk has rapidly diminishing value. The result is that point B will be the most efficient allocation of resources between the two programs, with amount AB going to the STD/HIV program and BD going to TB control. In contrast, in a country where the infection rate among those with the largest number of partners is already high, the value of the first and most targeted dollar of STD/HIV control will be smaller. However, in the high-prevalence country the fact that STDs and particularly HIV are more widespread means that there can be substantial benefits from expanding the program to people who are less sexually active. In the high-prevalence country, this logic leads to the amount AC being spent on STD/HIV control, whereas the smaller amount CD is spent on TB control. (This discussion ignores the fact that HIV control will also slow the spread of tuberculosis.)

Once resources are optimally divided between the two programs, which in the high-prevalence country would be at point C,

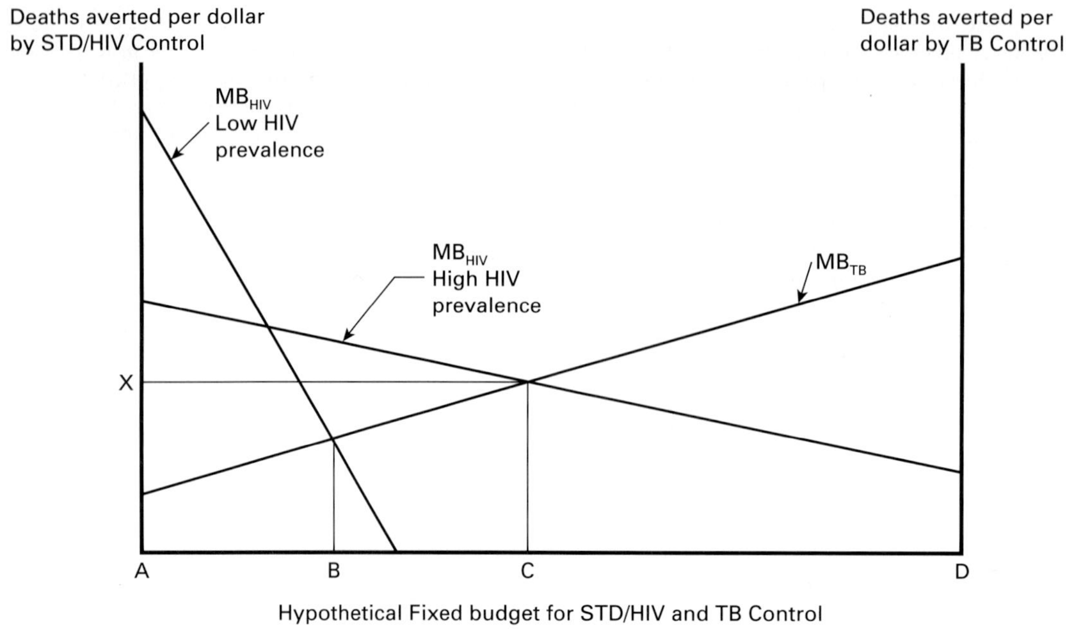

Fig. 1-1. Optimal division of fixed budget between STD/HIV and TB control in a low- and high-prevalence country.

the common marginal benefit of the two programs is given by X, which is the number of additional deaths the country could avert if the budget of the entire STD/HIV and TB program were expanded by one dollar. If this number is large in relation to similar values from other diseases and taking into account everything that individuals would do in the absence of government intervention, then the program manager can argue that the country should expand his budget for both TB and STD/HIV programs. Indeed a large value of X suggests that expanded allocations to health in general would improve overall social welfare.

How do STD/HIV programs and TB programs compare on equity grounds? Expenditures to prevent and control TB are broadly redistributive, because poverty is a risk factor for that disease. The correlation between socioeconomic status and risk of HIV is less clear, but there are strong redistributive arguments for intervention against HIV as a policy to redistribute social welfare toward the spouses and children of sexually active, multipartner adults.

Thus, in the abstract it is impossible to say whether the argument for government intervention is stronger for HIV or for TB. The answer depends partly on the current incidence rates of the two diseases in the country in question, on the actions that private individuals and firms would take in the absence of government intervention,[2] on the cost and managerial efficiency of the various disease prevention programs, and on the equity considerations in both programs. However, at least potentially, the public economics argument for prevention and control of HIV is as strong as that for TB.

LONGER-TERM SOCIAL ADJUSTMENTS TO HIV/AIDS

In view of the danger of the HIV epidemic and the clear market failures described in the preceding, it would be surprising if societies that have learned through hard experience that AIDS is fatal and sexually transmitted did not evolve mechanisms to internalize some of these externalities. Obvious areas for welfare-enhancing social innovation include the nature of the marriage contract and the degree of social acceptance accorded to condoms in extramarital and even in marital sexual relations.

In casual sexual relations, sex workers and others with multiple sexual partners will prefer condom use as long as they are uninfected. As time passes and new uninfected cohorts enter the commercial and casual sex markets knowing of the threat of AIDS, the proportion of such workers who are uninfected, and will demand risk premiums for sex without a condom in order to remain that way, will grow. The risk premium for sex without a condom will be higher in areas where infection rates are higher and will fluctuate over time in a countercyclical pattern to infection rate.[6] However, in general, it can be expected that the trend toward increased acceptability of condom use will continue both in casual and marital sexual relations.

The existence of the HIV epidemic has dramatically increased the significance of past sexual experience and the potential costs of future marital infidelity and is thus likely to substantially change the bargaining process leading to marriage in societies where HIV prevalence is high. In such societies, new marriages may be based on implicit contracts that allow for more monitoring and less tolerance of extramarital affairs than did the marriages of the past. Even existing marriage contracts may be implicitly renegotiated, at least by spouses with the power to do so. However, these new more tightly monitored marriages will be even more subject to one of these sources of market failure than were the old, because with reinforced monitoring the spouse who is apprised of infidelity will be even more surprised than under the lax system of the past. Hence, the possibility of compensation by the spouse for condom use outside the marriage will be even more remote. As long as condom protection entails reduced utility to one partner in the sexual encounter and HIV remains a serious threat, there will be a role for government intervention to subsidize its use.

CULTURAL VALUE SYSTEMS AND THE EVALUATION OF HIV/AIDS POLICIES

This separation of the evaluation of a government intervention into efficiency and equity components ignores an important and influential feature of the HIV epidemic that affects all governments' decisions regarding the control of HIV: the fact that the disease is primarily spread by behavior that most societies condemn or at least deplore. In most societies some behavioral responses that would slow the spread of AIDS (e.g., abstinence from extramarital sexual relations or intravenous drug use) are viewed as morally correct, and others (e.g., the use of condoms during extramarital relations or of clean needles to inject drugs) as facilitating immoral activity. Such societies are likely to attach more value to a government intervention that encourages abstinence than to one that subsidizes the use of condoms or clean needles, even if they have identical implications for economic efficiency and equity. Such social preferences are valid on their own terms and arguably may themselves be justifiable as efficiency and equity enhancing. However, to the extent that the policy of promoting abstinence rather than condoms or needles entails substantial losses of efficiency and equity as conventionally measured, societies and their governments must be aware of these costs before rejecting the more efficient and/or equitable policy options.

Governments have the option to ignore AIDS or to intervene only with messages that exhort people to be monogamous. Indeed, one way of eliminating the market failures described in the preceding would be for people to change their preferences away from multipartner and toward monogamous sexual relations. In view of the overwhelming evidence that a large minority of men and a smaller minority of women in most societies have many sexual partners over their lifetime, and the more limited evidence that AIDS is an insufficient threat to radically change this behavior, such exhortation is unlikely to correct the market failures or to slow the epidemic. Societies that choose to condemn extramarital sex rather than to subsidize and facilitate protected sex are likely to pay large costs in terms of excess numbers of AIDS cases and reduced utility from sex both within and outside marital relationships.

References

1 Kremer M. Integrating behavioral choice into epidemiological models of AIDS. *Quarterly Journal of Economics.* 1996; 111–2, pp. 549–73.

2 Hammer J. Economic analysis for health projects. *World Bank Res Observ* 1997;12:47.

3 Over M, Piot P. HIV infection and sexually transmitted diseases. In: DT Jamison DT et al. (eds). *Disease control priorities in developing countries.* New York: Oxford University Press, 1993.

4 Grosskurth H et al. Impact of improved treatment of sexually transmitted diseases or HIV infection in rural Tanzania: Randomised controlled trial. *Lancet* 1995;346:530.

5 Laga M et al. Condom promotion, sexually transmitted diseases treatment and declining incidence of HIV-1 infection in female Zairian sex workers. *Lancet* 1994;344:246.

6 Philipson TJ, Posner RA. *Private choices and public health: The AIDS epidemic in an economic perspective.* Cambridge: Harvard University Press, 1993.

7 World Bank. *Confronting AIDS: Public Priorities in a Global Epidemic.* New York, Oxford University Press, 1997.

PART II HISTORY OF STD

Chapter 2

Historical perspectives on sexually transmitted diseases: challenges for prevention and control

Allan M. Brandt
David Shumway Jones

It is a basic and tragic irony of human life that intimate physical relations entail the risk of infectious disease. The very nature of sexual contact offers obvious opportunities for the movement of microorganisms—some of which cause disease—from one individual to another. Such sexually transmitted diseases have, in all likelihood, always been present. This relationship makes the history of STDs both long and complex.

It is a similarly tragic irony that despite medical efforts against sexually transmitted diseases and the existence, since the 1940s, of powerful treatments for them, these diseases persist, even thrive, in the 1990s.[1] Historical analysis can reveal the substantial obstacles that have prevented successful management of these epidemics. For instance, the cultural meanings associated with sexual relations have often been transferred to the diseases transmitted by those relations. STDs thus become not just biological and medical problems, but also social and political problems. Both medical and public health interventions fail to address the full complexity of these social diseases.

The recent emergence of HIV/AIDS has added new relevance to the history of STDs. In a remarkably short period of time, AIDS has become a dominant issue in both medical and social discussion of health. This has led historians to ask new questions specific to the history of HIV as well as to return to the earlier history of STDs with new questions: Do past problems and solutions give us any guidance for managing HIV in the present? Does our knowledge of HIV change our understanding of how other STDs have been interpreted and managed? Furthermore, the history of HIV itself reinforces ideas about the complexity of STDs as both medical and cultural entities. Painfully reminding us of the ties between sex and disease, HIV confirms that STDs will remain as much a problem for the twenty-first century as they have been for past centuries.

In this chapter we show how knowledge of the history of STDs informs our present understanding of STDs. We cannot provide a comprehensive overview of the subject. Instead, we will discuss three crucial issues. First, we will examine the category of "sexually transmitted" diseases. As history and current practice have shown, this collection of diseases is neither constant nor easily defined. Moreover, labeling a disease as sexually transmitted has tremendous implications for efforts to control that disease. Second, we will review some classic approaches to the history of STDs. These include questions of the origin and specificity of different STDs, as well as biomedical and public health efforts to manage STDs.

Finally, we will focus on selected issues brought to special relevance by the emergence of HIV/AIDS. Specifically, we hope to illustrate the need for a complex model of these diseases. Understanding how the mode of transmission and the attached cultural attitudes can be of critical importance in both clinical and public health approaches to STDs, and recognizing that STDs require an integrated model of medical, ecological, social, and political influences on disease, are crucial if we are to produce realistic strategies for managing sexually transmitted diseases in both national and international contexts.

THE PROBLEM OF SEXUAL TRANSMISSION

Since the sixteenth century, observers have recognized the sexual transmission of syphilis, identified it as a "venereal disease," and stigmatized its victims. Despite episodic concern with casual transmission, the category of venereal disease remained unproblematic for centuries. The emergence of HIV, however, as well as new understanding of other old and new diseases, has challenged the naturalness of the category of "sexually transmitted" diseases. At the same time, it has reinforced the tremendous cultural burden of diseases associated with sexual contact.

THE PROBLEMATIC CATEGORY OF "SEXUALLY TRANSMITTED DISEASES"

At first glimpse, the category of STDs seems obvious enough. After all, this is a textbook about sexually transmitted diseases, and the table of contents reveals the expected cast of characters: HIV, herpes, HPV, chlamydia, gonorrhea, syphilis, and pubic lice. The recent Institute of Medicine (IOM) report on the "hidden epidemic" of STDs includes a similar list.[1] However, if the category is examined in more detail, it is readily exposed as a problematic category: it is not completely clear which diseases belong in the category of STDs, nor is it clear whether the diseases really have enough in common to be considered a meaningful group.

It might seem simple enough to define sexually transmitted diseases as those infections that can be acquired through sexual contact. After all, contact of mucus membranes allows easy transmission of many microorganisms. This seems clear enough for STDs such as gonorrhea and chlamydia. However, some agents, especially HIV, have significant nonsexual transmission: Is it correct to characterize someone who received HIV by intravenous drug use as suffering from a sexually transmitted disease? Similarly, as discussed in both this textbook and in the IOM report, other diseases that are not typically sexually transmitted, such as hepatitis B or various enteric pathogens, can be transmitted in that fashion. Intimate sexual contact also facilitates the transmission of a variety of nongenital infections, such as respiratory tuberculosis and even the common cold. Finally, some diseases that are not sexually transmitted can be associated with the frequency of sexual contact, as with urinary tract infections in women.[1–3]

Even when STDs can be defined by a common mode of transmission, the diseases vary enormously in their manifestations. Some, like oral herpes or vaginal yeast infections, are often little more than nuisances—although their psychological manifestations may be chronic and severe. HIV, in contrast, has become a leading cause of death among young adults. Some diseases, like pelvic inflammatory disease, have dramatic acute courses, as well as long-term health consequences. Others, like cervical cancer secondary to Human Papilloma Virus, or the varied manifestations of AIDS, can appear decades after the moment of transmission. It is not clear that the sometime shared mode of transmission imposes a meaningful natural category over such a diverse range of disease courses and outcomes.

Finally, the group of STDs shifts over time. Three hundred years ago, physicians and the public had an undifferentiated notion of venereal disease; in retrospect this included syphilis and gonorrhea, and probably many other diseases. Today physicians recognize dozens of diseases that can be sexually transmitted; some of these, including HPV and HIV have only been identified in the past two decades. Although some diseases have probably been around for centuries and just unrecognized, others, possibly HIV, might truly be new to this century. Meanwhile, the prevalence of existing STDs varies widely over time, reflecting changes in sexual mores and practices as well as the impact of public health efforts and biomedical intervention. The HIV epidemic, for instance, began at a moment of relative complacency concerning infectious disease. The Western, developed world had experienced a health transition from the predominance of infectious to chronic disease and had come to focus its resources and attention on systemic, noninfectious disease. Physicians had been confident that penicillin and other antibiotics would eliminate the problem of STDs. STDs had largely vanished from cultural concern. The HIV epidemic fractured this widely held belief in medical security.

THE SIGNIFICANCE OF THE MODE OF TRANSMISSION

Regardless of the complications surrounding the category of STDs, this group of diseases does share, to varying extents, a common mode of transmission. Taken together, STDs make explicit the significance vested in particular modes of transmission of infectious organisms. In this sense, the meaning and ultimate epidemiological significance of this set of infections is fundamentally tied to the changing historical nature of human sexual relations. Since sexual ethics and practices vary widely over time and across cultures, the meaning and significance of sexually transmitted diseases has also been highly variable. These diseases suggest the powerful relationships of biological, medical, cultural, and political variables as they effect patterns of disease. In the case of STDs, the stigmas associated with sexual behavior are often transferred to the diseases transmitted by that behavior, often resulting in denial and clinical awkwardness. Thus social pathology is superimposed on top of the clinical pathology of the disease.

For instance, in many cases the presence of a sexually transmitted disease exposes the implicit presence of a certain sexual behavior. The victims of that disease then fall victims to the stigmas of that behavior. This was most striking with the emergence of HIV/AIDS in the United States during the early 1980s. As the disease spread through the homosexual community, it often generated not sympathy but scorn from observers. Some saw the fatal disease as just punishment for an immoral behavior. Others thought that victims should be identified and isolated to prevent them from spreading it to others. Some religious groups used the epidemic as an occasion to reiterate their moral views about sexual behavior, drug use, sin, and disease; AIDS was seen as "proof" of their moral order. Although not all reactions were this extreme, the hostile conservative climate did not facilitate effective public health education and intervention.[4–6]

Meanwhile, as had happened with the earlier epidemics of syphilis, not all victims were treated equally. Some victims were perceived as the "guilty perpetrators" of the epidemic, obtaining their infections from high-risk, morally condemnable behaviors. Others, who had received their infections through blood transfusions or perinatally, were seen as the "innocent victims." This tendency to seek blameworthy individuals and groups has gone hand in hand with the stigmatization of STDs. People tend to seek the origins of the disease and blame the people who introduced it to them. During the syphilis epidemic of the 1490s and early 1500s, the disease was typically blamed on foreign countries. For instance, the French called it the Italian disease, the Italians the French disease.[7] Similarly, the early years of the HIV epidemic were characterized by blaming geographic locales, as happened with Haiti, or Africa and the Kinshasa highway.[5,8] Sometimes this has gone so far as to point the finger at a single person, the so-called "patient zero" of an epidemic.[4]

The stigma produced by the mode of transmission can have strongly negative effects on efforts to contain the disease. A society that can only discuss sex awkwardly and in hushed tones will have trouble discussing STDs prevention and treatment. In the 1934, for instance, Thomas Parran, then New York State commissioner of public health, was censored for using the words "syphilis" and "gonorrhea" on a CBS radio broadcast; Parran decried this "conspiracy of silence," which prevented frank discussion of STDs.[9] In extreme cases, when a society has a notion that the disease is a just punishment for immoral behavior and thus a disincentive against that behavior, then there can be ambivalence or even hostility against prevention and treatment. For instance, during World War I, U.S. Army officials feared that distributing condoms to the soldiers would only promote sexual activity. During the 1950s, some doctors expressed concerns about the widespread use of penicillin to treat syphilis, suggesting that it could lead to moral degeneracy.[9] Most recently, condom and needle distributions, which have been shown to reduce incidence of HIV, have met with substantial political resistance.[10–12]

As these last examples show, the state has often taken an active interest in STD control and prevention. This public concern with individual illness occurs for many reasons, but all relate to the issue of sexual transmission: the contagious nature of the diseases, their moral associations, and the desire to protect the "innocent victims." In the nineteenth century, for instance, bureaucratic interventions against STDs, as with regulation of prostitution, were based on the rationale that these diseases had powerful deleterious consequences not only for the wayward individual, but for the family and society as well. Given the rising concerns about the impact of these diseases in an increasingly ordered and industrialized world, no longer would the State leave those infected to their own designs. Venereal diseases became a primary vehicle for expanding and defining the police powers of the State in the sphere of public health.

State efforts against STDs have typically swung between two essential modes of action. The first, articulated by Prince Morrow and the social hygiene movement of the Progressive Era, contended that the best way to prevent infection was by adherence to a sexual ethic that made it impossible to acquire a STD. Essentially this meant restricting all sexual relationships to marriage; the principal means of achieving this goal was through education to encourage abstinence and the repression of prostitution, assumed to be the central locus of infection. This view dominated efforts made by the U.S. Army during World War I to prevent the use of prostitutes by soldiers of the Allied Expeditionary Force. The alternative view, instrumental in orientation, sought to sever the problem of sexually transmitted diseases from any particular sexual ethic. According to this position, individuals should be provided with means of preventing infection and, if infected, appropriate treatment. This view is typified by the Army's approach during World War II, which acknowledged that use of prostitutes was inevitable and began a program of condom distribution.[13]

These two longstanding approaches have been widely voiced since the onset of the AIDS epidemic. Adherents of the moral approach argue that the instrumentalists actually encourage infection by unwittingly promoting risky sexual behavior—according to this argument good morals and good health go hand in hand. In this view, STDs function in the social order by making sexual encounters more dangerous, thus encouraging "appropriate" behaviors. They advocate prevention through abstinence from "dangerous" sexual behaviors. On the other side, advocates of the instrumental orientation counter that the moralists promote infection by restricting access to explicit education and preventive techniques. They encourage frank discussion of sexuality and HIV as well as widespread distribution of condoms. Believing sexual contact to be inevitable, they seek to make it safe. Both approaches reflect implicit social values about sexuality, medicine, and disease.

Finally, as states have acted on their interests in preventing STDs, they have frequently come into conflict over civil liberties. Attempts to protect U.S. soldiers from prostitutes led to the incarceration of thousands of women. In a more recent example, the federal government has recently (May 1996) mandated that states reduce the rates of perinatal transmission of HIV by 50 to 95 percent by the year 2000. This will likely require mandatory, or at least strongly recommended, testing of pregnant women for HIV and mandatory treatment of those found to be infected. Such policies are likely to generate serious controversy, as states balance their interest in protecting the health of (future) children against the rights of women to refuse testing and treatment.[14]

MAJOR THEMES IN THE HISTORY OF STDs

Perhaps because of their complex relations with morality and politics, sexually transmitted diseases have attracted historical inquiry for centuries. Since syphilis and gonorrhea have traditionally been the most widely recognized STDs, most of the historical accounts have focused on them. Many examples could be given of historians' attempts to understand both the diseases themselves and the social responses to them. To provide a representative cross section, we discuss: (1) the debates over the origin of syphilis; (2) the history of medical understanding of syphilis and gonorrhea; (3) "magic bullets" and the biomedical model of disease; and (4) the history of public health campaigns against syphilis.

THE ORIGINS OF SYPHILIS

One of the leading questions in the history of medicine, for nearly 500 years, has been the origins of syphilis. It is clear that in the last years of the fifteenth century a devastating epidemic of infectious syphilis swept Western Europe.[7] Observers quickly recognized that the disease, characterized by skin ulcers and eruptions, often causing systemic illness and death, was spread through sexual contact. The intensity of the epidemic led to considerable speculation among physicians and lay people concerning its origins. The sudden onset of the epidemic led many observers to conclude that this was a new disease, brought back from the Americas by Columbus' crew in 1493. The virulence of the epidemic, according to this argument, suggests that a new organism had been introduced for which Europeans had no previous exposure, and thus, no immunity. And indeed, there is considerable historical, archeological, and paleopathological evidence that this is the case.[15] This would make syphilis the counterpart of the dozens of diseases that swept from Europe and Africa to the Americas, devastating the Native American populations.[16]

Many competing explanations, however, have been given for the origin of syphilis. Some have argued that syphilis had been in Europe prior to the fifteenth century, but had never been distinguished from leprosy, which can have similar dermatologic symptoms. According to such theories, treponemal infections (pinta, yaws, endemic, and venereal syphilis) had previously been common, mild, and chronic. Changes in European standards of living and in environmental conditions, however, made casual spread of treponemal infections less common. Better hygiene, for instance, reduced skin-to-skin transmission; as a consequence, people were no longer routinely infected during childhood. By the time of Columbus' voyages, only the hardier, sexually transmitted strains survived in Europe, producing the appearance of a new epidemic disease.[17,18]

THE SPECIFICITY OF SYPHILIS AND GONORRHEA

In addition to investigating the origins of the diseases, historians have documented the processes by which the diseases were recognized by physicians as distinct entities. For instance, from the sixteenth century until well into the nineteenth, most doctors assumed gonorrhea and syphilis were manifestations of the same disease. Both were viewed as different forms of inoculation with the same poison or "virus." By the mid-eighteenth century, however, a vigorous debate had been generated between dualists, arguing for specificity of the two conditions, and unicists, claiming a single affliction. In a classic episode in this debate, John Hunter (1728–1793), the renowned British surgeon and experimental pathologist, reportedly inoculated his own penis with pus from a patient with gonorrhea. When he subsequently developed a syphilitic chancre, he concluded that the two diseases were really one, as he had long argued. He had not suspected, however, that this patient was infected with both syphilis and gonorrhea, a not uncommon situation.[19]

During the nineteenth century the question was slowly resolved. French venereologist Philippe Ricord (1799–1889) established the specificity of the two infections through a series of experimental inoculations; he also differentiated the primary, secondary, and tertiary stages of syphilis infection.[20] Researchers, such as Rudolf Virchow (1821–1902), a leading figure in the development of modern pathology, documented the range of systemic manifestations that syphilis and gonorrhea can produce. The isolation of the distinct causative organisms for gonorrhea by Albert Neisser (1855–1916) in 1879, and for syphilis by protozoologist Fritz Schaudinn (1871–1906), and syphilologist Erich Hoffmann (1868–1959) in 1905, provided the final evidence in the debates.[21]

"MAGIC BULLETS" AND THE BIOMEDICAL MODEL

The identification of the causative organisms in these and other infectious diseases opened the door for a new biomedical model of disease. Researchers realized that they might be able to discover a specific therapy for each specific disease. They hoped that these "magic bullets" would then allow for the successful treatment and eradication of these diseases.

The first step, the development of a diagnostic test, followed soon after the discovery of the slender, spiral *Treponema pallidum*. August Wassermann (1866–1925) and his colleagues Neisser and Bruck applied the complement fixation reaction discovered by Jules Bordet (1870–1961) and Octave Genou (1875–1957) to the spirochete.[22] The resulting blood test could detect syphilis in even asymptomatic patients. Then, in 1909, Nobel laureate immunologist Paul Ehrlich (1854–1915) announced the discovery of the arsenic compound Salvarsan, a chemotherapeutic cure for syphilis. Ehrlich's discovery, based on a combination of serendipity, persistence, and brilliance, marked a fundamental breakthrough in the history of modern medical science: For the first time, a specific chemical compound had been demonstrated to kill a specific microorganism. Ehrlich called the substance—the 606th arsenical he had synthesized—a "magic bullet," a drug that would seek out and destroy its mark. He posited that the world of twentieth century bioscience would be the elucidation of magic bullets to cure disease.[23]

These three major discoveries, the organism, the test, and the treatment, appeared to fulfill the promise of the biomedical revolution of the late nineteenth century. Salvarsan was heralded as the dawn of the modern age of clinical medicine. Physicians throughout the world wrote to Ehrlich eagerly seeking supplies of the drug. They triumphantly reported miraculous recoveries from the greatly feared disease. However, the triumph did not last. Salvarsan was toxic, difficult to administer, and required an extensive regimen of treatment, sometimes for as long as 2 years. Only 25 percent of all treated patients apparently received the full complement of treatment.[24] New compounds, the neoarsphenamines, improved the situation only slightly.

The discovery, in 1943, of the efficacy of penicillin against syphilis renewed hope that the biomedical model of specific disease and specific treatment would lead to triumph over syphilis. Unlike Salvarsan, Penicillin truly was a "wonder drug." With a single shot, the scourge of disease would be avoided. Incidence of syphilis fell dramatically, and in the last years of the 1950s, rates of infection in the United States reached all-time lows. It appeared that the venereal diseases would join the ranks of other infectious diseases that had come under the control of modern medicine.[25]

Despite the widespread availability of antibiotics, however, rates of syphilis and other STDs began to climb again in the nations of Western Europe, the United States, as well as the developing world in the early 1960s. Although many public health officials and physicians attributed this increase to changes in sexual mores in the wake of the growing availability of contraceptives, the rise also correlates with a substantial fall in funding for public venereal disease programs. By the late 1950s much of the machinery, especially procedures for public education, case-finding, tracing, and diagnostics, had been cut back.[26]

The bitter irony of syphilis and the other STDs is that the "magic bullet" did not eliminate them. Currently, five of the ten most commonly reported infections, and 87 percent of the cases, are STDs.[1] Even in the face of highly effective treatments, the infections have endured, marking a crucial paradox of modern medicine. The issue is not merely the development of effective treatments, but the process by which they are deployed, the means by which they move from laboratory to full allocation to those affected. Effective treatments without adequate public education, counseling, and timely access to clinical services may not affect the relative incidence of disease. And although effective treatments exist for a number of highly prevalent bacterial infections such as syphilis and gonorrhea, for other viral STDs there are no curative treatments. This explains, in part, the dramatic rise in numbers of cases of herpes simplex virus during the 1970s and 1980s. This worldwide resurgence of STDs is particularly worrisome in the current context because it appears likely that individuals with sexually transmitted infection are at increased risk for infection with the AIDS virus.[27]

PUBLIC HEALTH CAMPAIGNS AGAINST STDs

Historians have not limited themselves to the study of physicians and diseases. Much has been written about societal attempts to minimize or eradicate STDs. Officials in the United States have often tried to limit the spread of syphilis by repressing prostitution and criminalizing commercial sex. For instance, concern over prostitution and commercial sex reached unprecedented heights by the time of World War I, touching off a comprehensive and vigorous antivenereal disease campaign. Although the U.S. military devised a program of vigorous exercise and explicit sexual education to protect the troops, the campaign centered on the problem of prostitution. Specifically, the military tried to shut down the red-light districts that invariably sprang up near military camps. Posters, films, and other educational materials repeatedly warned the soldiers, "A German bullet is cleaner than a whore."[28,13] The U.S. Congress supported these measures by passing the Chamberlain-Kahn Act in 1918, which allowed the quarantining and incarceration of thousands of women suspected as prostitutes.[29,30] When the U.S. troops arrived in France, these American efforts to ban prostitution came into conflict with French efforts to allow regulated prostitution.

Such vigorous campaigns have not been limited to the military. Civilian public health officials have tried a series of techniques, most notably premarital screening and contact tracing. For instance, starting with Connecticut in 1935, virtually every state attempted premarital syphilis screening of prospective brides and grooms. It was hoped that these programs would protect people from being unwittingly infected by an infected fiancee. However, premarital screening did not perform as desired. Diagnostic tests have had significant problems with oversensitivity; for instance, as many as 25 percent of positive results with the Wasserman test were false positives.[31] Similarly, since the population being tested has had a low prevalence of syphilis, widespread screening programs, which have been estimated to cost \$80 million annually, detect few cases (premarital screening accounted for only 1.27% of all detected cases of syphilis) and therefore have high costs per case found—as much as \$240,000 per case.[32,33] Similar problems have been encountered in evaluating premarital screening for HIV.[34]

In the 1930s, as states began premarital screening, public health officials also began contact tracing and case finding. By identifying a patient's sexual contacts, these individuals could be apprised of the possibility of infection, tested, and, if need be, treated. Only in this way, officials argued, could the geometric progression of infection be stopped. Syphilitic patients, however, often did not wish to reveal the names of their sexual contacts. Moreover, actually finding the contacts has required time-consuming "shoe-leather epidemiology." The impact of case-finding remains difficult to evaluate. The search for infections required sensitive and difficult probing; it demanded that an individual discuss intimacies with strangers, secrets that could wreck havoc in the infected person's life. Contact epidemiology clearly brought many unsuspecting individuals into treatment before they could spread their infections to others. But the knowledge that information regarding contacts would be sought by public health professionals also had the effect of encouraging some individuals to seek the aid of practitioners who guaranteed absolute confidentiality, interfering with essential processes of case-reporting.[13] Such problems were even more acute with efforts at contact tracing with the HIV epidemic in the 1980s.[4]

Other efforts against STDs operated at different levels. Physicians, for instance, often publicized the damage that syphilis could do to families, the "innocent victims" of a man's transgressions. The train of family tragedy was a frequent cultural theme in these years. In 1913 a play by French playwright Eugene Brieux, *Les Avaries*—performed before packed theaters in Paris and New York—told the story of a young man about to be married who contracts syphilis from a prostitute. Though warned by his physician not to marry, he disregards this advice only to spread the infection to his wife; soon after, she bears a congenitally infected child. The story was told and retold, and it revealed deep cultural values about science, social responsibility, and the limits of medicine.[35,36] The knowledge that profligate men "visited" their sins on their wives and children led to a dramatic change in professional attitudes. Syphilis was redefined from "carnal scourge" to "family poison." The notion of "innocent" infections had the effect of dividing victims; some deserved attention, sympathy, and medical support, others did not. This promoted stigmatization and victim-blaming of those who were considered culpable for the epidemic.

Finally, historians have shown how these efforts to protect public health have often exposed cultural prejudice and anxieties. Concerns about venereal disease also reflected a pervasive fear of the urban masses, the growth of the cities, and the changing nature of familial relationships.[13] As concerns about eugenics and race heightened on both sides of the Atlantic, these diseases were typically associated with so-called "degenerative stocks." Rates of infection were cited as an index of sexual immorality and a failure to exercise individual control. By the early twentieth century, these infections had become, pre-eminently, a marker of sexual transgression and moral degeneracy. Such attitudes fostered an environment that allowed the Tuskegee Syphilis Study, in which effective treatment for syphilis was withheld from a group of black men for four decades in order to study the so-called natural history of syphilis.[37,38] This study, loosely based on the Oslo Study of untreated syphilis (1890–1910), was not halted until 1972 following extensive negative exposure in the press.

THE NEED FOR COMPLEX MODELS OF DISEASE

The historical examples discussed so far, from the origins of syphilis to the stigma attached because of the mode of transmission and the debates over the state role in protecting public health, all demonstrate the great complexity of the problem of sexually transmitted diseases, both as disease entities and as societal responses. The emergence of HIV and AIDS has only added to the complexity. Many new questions have been asked specific to HIV: Where did HIV come from and how did it spread? How has the initial localization of HIV/AIDS in stigmatized groups interfered with efforts to manage the disease? How did HIV/AIDS acquire the varied cultural meanings it now carries? Although HIV has raised many new questions for historians, it also reveals many parallels with the earlier histories of other STDs. Some aspects of the social history of HIV bear striking resemblance to the history of syphilis. For instance, in both epidemics certain groups were blamed and stigmatized for spreading the disease. Societal prudishness prevented frank discussion of sexuality and STDs, hindering public health efforts. Some effective interventions, such as the widespread distribution of condoms, were not implemented out of fear of promoting sexual licentiousness.

Both types of historical studies—new questions and old parallels—have much to teach both physicians and policy experts. Taken as a whole, however, such historical inquiry illustrates one fundamental point: Sexually transmitted diseases—complex ecological, moral, social, and political constructs—require complex models of disease. Single-minded efforts, either to prevent STDs through education and behavior modification, or to eradicate diseases by producing "magic bullets," are doomed to fail. In this last section, we will review the obstacles encountered by both public health and biomedical efforts against STDs, and show how these problems become further complicated when seen in international perspective. We will conclude with a vision for a complex model of STDs that will enable integrated, multimodal campaigns against STDs.

LIMITS OF PUBLIC HEALTH AND BIOMEDICAL EFFORTS TO CONTROL STDs

As described herein, a wide variety of public health interventions have been attempted against STDs. Whether preaching abstinence, regulating prostitutes, distributing condoms, or screening couples before marriage, public health officials have used both moral and instrumental approaches to prevent STDs. These efforts been hindered by both entanglement with moral debates and limitations of the approaches themselves.

For instance, public health officials have orchestrated major efforts at education, hoping that informed people would make wise behavioral decisions to protect themselves from STDs. In the first half of this century, syphilis education campaigns failed in the face of many obstacles. Some programs were censored by the federal government because of "obscene" references to syphilis. Others only contributed to pervasive fears of infection, to the stigma associated with the diseases, and to the discrimination against its victims. Current efforts at AIDS education face similar obstacles. To be effective, AIDS education must be explicit, focused, and appropriately targeted to a range of at-risk social groups. This challenge remains unmet.

During the course of the twentieth century, more radical and intrusive compulsory measures to control STDs, such as quarantine, also have been attempted. These, too, have failed. During World War I, as hysteria about the impact of STDs rose, Congress passed legislation that allowed the quarantine of anyone suspected of harboring a venereal disease and spreading infection. Although more than 20,000 women were detained during the war, the program had no apparent impact on the rates of infection, which actually climbed during the war. In the case of AIDS, where there is no medical intervention to render individuals permanently noninfectious, quarantine is totally impractical because it would require lifelong incarceration of the infected.[31] Thus the nature of the diseases, the limits of the interventions, and the need to balance public good and individual rights have combined to pose serious obstacles to public health interventions.

Biomedical efforts to prevent and control STDs have run into similar obstacles. As discussed earlier, 50 years of effective treatments have not eradicated syphilis and gonorrhea; in fact, over recent years the incidence of these diseases has actually increased. For some other STDs, such as herpes and human papilloma virus, no curative treatments have yet been found.

Recently, biomedical efforts against HIV have received the most attention. Initial disappointment over the value of AZT and other nucleotide analogs has given way to tremendous excitement over chemokines, protease inhibitors, and various combination therapies. At the 11th International Conference on AIDS in Vancouver in July 1996, Peter Piot, head of the United Nations Programme on HIV/AIDS declared that "Nobody can call AIDS an inevitably incurable disease any more."[39] This "elation" has dominated media coverage of HIV, from *Time* magazine's "Man of the Year" or *Science* magazine's "Breakthrough of the Year" to the declaration in *The New York Times Magazine* of "The End of AIDS."[40–43] Case reports of patients who have miraculously cleared the virus from their blood, increased their CD4 counts, and reduced their burden of opportunistic infections, are complemented by a CDC report showing that the annual number of deaths from AIDS has fallen for the first time since the epidemic began.[44,45]

However, many problems persist. The triple therapy regimens are immensely complicated, requiring some patients to take dozens of pills at different times throughout the day; for fear of fostering drug resistance, some doctors have considered withholding such treatment from patients who will be unable to follow the regimen properly.[46] Some patients are unable to tolerate the drugs' many side effects. Although the drugs seem highly effective, data on long-term outcomes has not yet been collected, and HIV has already shown a remarkable ability to develop resistance to many drugs. Even if the drugs do prove to be successful, their costs—between $15,000 and $20,000 per patient per year—might be prohibitive for widespread distribution; and although many patients show improvement, death remains the endpoint in many trials.[47]

But even if protease inhibitors and combination therapies do prove to be the "magic bullet" against HIV, they might still be of limited value. After all, penicillin, which is cheap, requires only a single dose, and is uniformly effective, has not "conquered" syphilis and gonorrhea. It is unclear what impact the new HIV drugs—expensive, complex dosing, unknown effectiveness—will have.

INTERNATIONAL PERSPECTIVES

These issues become especially acute in developing countries. Now home to over 90 percent of the 22.6 million cases of HIV infection, few of these countries can afford to provide the expensive regimens now being developed in the United States.[43] Nor do many of the countries have the resources for elaborate education and prevention campaigns. These problems are exacerbated in many cases by demographic, economic, and political unrest; these conditions, with the associated poverty, displacement, and marginalization, provide fertile ground for epidemics of HIV and other STDs.[48,49]

Moreover, international comparisons have shown that the epidemiology of HIV differs greatly in different countries. Early in the epidemic, observers defined three patterns of HIV epidemics: pattern I, typically seen in developed countries such as the United States, in which most of the cases are from homosexual transmission or intravenous drug users; pattern II, seen in developing countries in subsaharan Africa and Latin America, in which most cases are from heterosexual transmission; and pattern III, countries with few cases of HIV.[48] These differences reflected variations in both cultural practices and viral characteristics, and had significant impacts on public health programs. Recently a new pattern has emerged: In parts of Asia, such as Thailand, the epidemic has grown explosively over the past 5 years, spreading from injection drug users and female sex workers to their clients, who in turn infect their wives. Now, in cities across southeast and south Asia, as many as 2 percent of all pregnant women are infected. In Thailand, this explosive growth has been marked by viral specialization, with different strains segregated into different risk groups.[50]

Finally, studies of heterosexual transmission in different countries have highlighted the symbiotic relationship of comorbidities of HIV and other STDs. At the biomedical level, researchers have recognized that the genital ulcers of chancroid, syphilis, and herpes, as well as the nonulcerating genital mucosal infections such as gonorrhea and chlamydia, all facilitate the transmission of HIV; meanwhile, HIV-induced immunosuppression alters and exacerbates the course of these diseases.[51] At the social level, many of the underlying risk factors for infection with one STD—from poverty to gender inequality—are the same risk factors for others. These factors combine to create a complex epidemic of multiple, interrelated infections.

THE NEED FOR INTEGRATED APPROACHES

These examples, from the limits of biomedical and public health approaches to the complexities of STDs in international perspective, show that STDs are not just a simple problem to be managed by individual patients and their physicians. Instead, STDs illustrate the complex interactions of bioecology, medicine, culture, and politics. Just as syphilis had revealed basic social conflicts regarding the nature of sexuality and responsibility for disease at earlier historical moments, in the last decades of the twentieth century, HIV disease became the focus of these debates. The AIDS epidemic, appearing suddenly and globally, shattered expectation of a relatively stable world of infectious disease. AIDS, like syphilis in the past, engenders powerful social conflicts about the meaning, nature, and risks of sexuality; the nature and role of the State in protecting and promoting public health; the significance of individual rights in regard to communal good; the nature of the doctor–patient relationship and social responsibility in times of epidemic disease.

AIDS also has clearly demonstrated the relationship of biological and behavioral forces in determining patterns of health and disease. The lifelong infectiousness of carriers; the private, biopsychosocial nature of sexual behavior and drug use; the fact that those at greatest risk are already stigmatized, have all made effective public policy interventions even more difficult. Meanwhile, the very nature of the virus itself, its complex and mutagenic nature, its different manifestations in different cultural environments, makes the success of both short-term technological breakthroughs—"magic bullets"—and long-term public health programs unlikely. Altering the course of the epidemic by human design thus has proven to be no easy matter.

The long history of syphilis and the short history of HIV both clearly show the limits of specific interventions implemented individually. Penicillin—cheap, easy to give, extremely effective, and without many significant side-effects—did not meet its expected promise. Now, after billions of dollar have been spent searching for a magic bullet for HIV, optimism over protease inhibitors is tempered by knowledge of their limitations. Prospects of a biomedical triumph over the HIV epidemic seem slim. Meanwhile, attempts at social engineering have had little success. For syphilis and HIV, attempts at either moralizing or education have had limited impact: either individuals are willing to make choices they know to be dangerous, or they have lost control over their actions.

The limits of magic bullets and public health initiatives for syphilis illustrate that narrow-focused efforts against STDs have little effectiveness on their own—STDs reveal limitations of both the biomedical model of disease as well as traditional public health interventions. No doubt, effective treatments for specific disease are a critical component in their control, but they are not a panacea. No doubt, education and condom distribution can decrease the rates of transmission. But infectious diseases constitute complex bioecological problems in which host, parasite, and a range of social and environmental forces interact. No single medical or social intervention thus can adequately address the problem. Efforts against STDs must reflect the diversity of their causes and their associations. They must address microbiology, ecology, culture, and politics. The varied knowledge we now have of STDs must produce varied actions.

The history of sexually transmitted diseases is indicative of the complex relationship of human behavior to health. Behavior is subject to a range of influences, biological and cultural, economic and political. In this fundamental respect, sexual relations are likely to remain a mode for the transmission of infectious diseases. The nature of these diseases, their medical and public meanings, as well as their epidemiologic patterns will necessarily be shaped by their particular historical, social, and cultural contexts.

References

1 Institute of Medicine: *The Hidden Epidemic: Confronting Sexually Transmitted Diseases.* Washington, D.C., National Academy Press, 1996.

2 Holmes KK et al: *Sexually Transmitted Diseases,* 3rd ed. New York, McGraw-Hill, 1998.

3 Hooton TM et al: A Prospective Study of Risk Factors for Symptomatic Urinary Tract Infection in Young Women. *New Engl J Med* 335: 468, 1996.

4 Shilts R: *And the Band Played On.* New York, St. Martin's Press, 1987.

5 Watney S: *Practices of Freedom.* Durham, Duke University Press, 1994.

6 Treichler P: AIDS, Homophobia and Biomedical Discourse: An Epidemic of Signification. *October* 43:31, 1987.

7 Quetel C: *History of Syphilis.* Baltimore, Johns Hopkins Press, 1990.

8 Farmer P: *AIDS and Accusation: Haiti and the Geography of Blame.* Berkeley, University of California Press, 1992.

9 Brandt AM: The Syphilis Epidemic and its Relation to AIDS. *Science* 239:375, 1988.

10 Des Jarlais DC et al: HIV incidence among injecting drug users in New York City syringe-exchange programmes. *Lancet* 348:987, 1996.

11 Stimson GV: AIDS and injecting drug use in the United Kingdom, 1987–1993: the policy response and the prevention of the epidemic. *Social Sci Med* 41:699, 1995.

12 Anderson W: The New York Needle Trial: the politics of public health in the age of AIDS. *Am J Pub Health* 84:1506, 1991.

13 Brandt AM: *No Magic Bullet: A Social History of Venereal Disease in the United States since 1880.* New York, Oxford University Press, 1987.

14 Wilfert CM: Beginning to Make Progress Against HIV. *N Engl J Med* 335:1678, 1996.

15 Baker BJ et al: The Origin and Antiquity of Syphilis. *Cur Anthropol* 29:703, 1988.

16 Crosby AW: *The Columbian Exchange: Biological and Cultural Consequences of 1492.* Westport, CT, Greenwood, 1972.

17 Cockburn TA: The Origin of the Treponematoses. *Bull WHO* 24:221, 1961.

18 Hudson EH: Christopher Columbus and the History of Syphilis. *Acta Tropica* 25:1, 1968.

19 Flegal KF: Changing Concepts of the Nosology of Gonorrhea and Syphilis. *Bull Hist Med* 48:571, 1974.

20 Crissey JT et al: *The Dermatology and Syphilology of the Nineteenth Century.* New York, Praeger, 1981.

21 Pusey WA: *Syphilis as a Modern Problem.* Chicago, American Medical Association, 1915, pp. 31–35.

22 Wassermann A et al: *Eine serodiagnostische Reaktion bei Syphilis.* Leipzig, George Thieme, 1906.

23 Marquardt M: *Paul Ehrlich.* New York, Henry Schuman, 1951.

24 Ward PS: The American Reception of Salvarsan. *J Hist Med* 36:59, 1981.

25 Brown WJ et al: *Syphilis and Other Venereal Diseases.* Cambridge, Harvard University Press, 1970.

26 Anderson OW: *Syphilis and Society.* Chicago, Center for Health Administration Studies, 22, 1965.

27 Centers for Disease Control and Prevention: *Morbid Mortal Wkly Rept* 36:393, 1987.

28 Colonel Care Poster Series (n.d. 1918?) in American Social Hygiene Association Papers, Folder 113:6, University of Minnesota.

29 US Interdepartmental Social Hygiene Board: *Program of Protective Social Measures.* Washington, D.C., Government Printing Office, 1920.

30 Dietzler MM: *Detention Houses and Reformatories.* US Interdepartamental Social Hygiene Board. Washington, D.C., Government Printing Office, 1922.

31 Brandt AM: AIDS in Historical Perspective: Four Lessons from the History of Sexually Transmitted Diseases. *Am J Pub Health* 78:367, 1988.

32 Felman Y: Repeal of mandated premarital tests for syphilis: A survey of state health officers. *Am J Pub Health* 71:155, 1981.

33 Haskell RJ: A cost benefit analysis of California's mandatory premarital screening program for syphilis. *W J Med* 141:538, 1984.

34 Cleary PD et al: Compulsory premarital screening for the human immunodeficiency virus. *JAMA* 258:1757, 1987.

35 Brieux E: *Damaged Goods* (translated by John Pollack). New York, Brentanos (printed for the Connecticut Society of Social Hygiene), 1912.

36 Rosenkrantz BG: Damaged Goods: Dilemmas of Responsibility for Risk. *Milbank Quart* 57:1, 1979.

37 Brandt AM: Racism and Research: The Case of the Tuskegee Syphilis Study. *Hastings Ctr Rept* 8:21, 1978.

38 Jones JH: *Bad Blood: The Tuskegee Syphilis Experiment.* New York, The Free Press, 1981.

39 Piot P, quoted in Cohen J: Chemokines Share Center Stage with Drug Therapies. *Science* 273:302, 1996.

40 Cowley G et al: New AIDS Optimism: Can a blend of three drugs collar the virus? *Newsweek* (July 22):68, 1996.

41 Sullivan, A: When plagues end: notes on the twilight of an epidemic: *The New York Times Magazine* (November 10):52, 1996.

42 Man of the Year. *Time* 148 (December 20):52, 1996.

43 Breakthrough of the Year: New Hope in HIV Disease. *Science* 274: 1988, 1996.

44 CDC: Update: Trends in AIDS Incidence, Deaths, and Prevalence—United States, 1996. *MMWR* 46:165, 1997.

45 Altman LK: U.S. Reporting Sharp Decrease in AIDS Deaths. *The New York Times* (February 28):1, 1997.

46 Sontag D et al: Doctors Withhold H.I.V. Pill Regimen from Some, Fearing Stronger H.I.V. *The New York Times* (March 2):1, 1997.

47 Corey L et al: Therapy for Human Immunodeficiency Virus Infection—What Have We Learned? *N Engl J Med* 335:1143, 1996.

48 Mann JM et al: The International Epidemiology of AIDS. *Sci Am* 259 (October):82, 1988.

49 Farmer P et al: Women, Poverty and AIDS: An Introduction. *Culture, Med Psychiat* 17:387, 1993.

50 Weniger BG et al: The March of AIDS through Asia. *New Engl J Med* 335:343, 1996.

51 Aral SO et al: Sexually Transmitted Diseases in the AIDS Era. *Sci Am* 264 (February):62, 1991.

PART III EPIDEMIOLOGY

Chapter 3

Transmission dynamics of sexually transmitted infections

Roy M. Anderson

This chapter describes how an understanding of the transmission dynamics of sexually transmitted infectious disease agents can help in interpreting observed epidemiological trends, in guiding the collection of data toward further understanding, and in designing programs for the control of infection and disease in the community. A major goal is to sharpen understanding of the interplay between the variables that determine the typical course of infection within an individual and the variables that control the pattern of infection and associated disease within communities of people.

Mathematical models that mirror biological processes are a key tool in developing an understanding of the transmission dynamics of an infectious agent. When combined with good surveillance, carefully designed cross-sectional and longitudinal epidemiologic studies of the pattern of infection and disease in defined populations, and clinical epidemiological studies, mathematical models provide a template that facilitates the interpretation of observed patterns and the collection and analysis of data.[1] Sensibly used, mathematical models are no more, and no less, than tools for thinking about things in a precise manner.

Most sexually transmitted diseases (STDs) possess characteristics that differ somewhat from those of infections such as measles or malaria, which have received the greatest attention in the literature on transmission dynamics. First, for infections such as human immunodeficiency virus (HIV) and hepatitis B, the communities or populations at risk for infection tend to be some fraction of the total community (e.g., sexually active adults, intravenous drug users, homosexual or bisexual men, or newborn infants). The groups at risk and the interrelationships between them require careful definition. Second, in contrast with many directly transmitted respiratory viral or bacterial infections, the intensity of transmission is not obviously related to population density. Among the sexually active segment of a population, the prevalence or incidence of infection is related to the distribution of various types of sexual activity that facilitate transmission Third, the carrier phenomenon, in which certain individuals harbor asymptomatic infection, perhaps for long periods, is important in determining the net rate of transmission. This is the case for many women infected with gonorrhea and is especially important in the spread of HIV, in which infected persons may be asymptomatic but infectious to their sexual partners for many years. Fourth, many STDs induce little or no acquired immunity, such that if recovery occurs (perhaps resulting from chemotherapeutic treatment), individuals are susceptible to reinfection. In other cases, such as HIV or herpes-virus infection, the infectious agent persists within the host and is able to evade the immunological defenses that aim to eliminate the infection, perhaps for the entire life of the host. This seems to be the case in the majority of people infected with HIV or the genital herpes-virus. The reasons for persistence are not clearly understood, but genetic variability in the infectious agent population within the host (HIV) and the occupancy of immunologically privileged sites (herpes-virus) are important factors. Fifth, great variability in the course of infection (particularly the incubation period between first infection and the diagnosis of symptoms of disease) is typically observed in groups of infected persons. Genetic variability in both host and infectious agent populations is often a significant factor in the observed heterogeneity in the typical course of infection in an individual patient. For example, a recent study of cohorts of individuals repeatedly exposed to HIV-1 in the United States suggests that people homozygous for a 32-base-pair deletion allele of the structural gene that encodes for a chemokine receptor on CD4+ T cells (CCR5–coreceptor for HIV strains that predominate in early stages of infection) are resistant to infection, whereas heterozygotes can acquire infection but have a slow rate of progression to acquired immunodeficiency syndrome (AIDS) by comparison with homozygous individuals with no deletion in the gene.[2] Similar studies of rates of progression to AIDS after infection also suggest that the presence of a particular phenotype of clade B HIV-1 (syncytial-inducing viral forms) typically results in more rapid progression to disease by comparison with patients who do not harbor this phenotype.[2] Sixth and finally, patterns of STD infections in communities are characterized by great heterogeneity in transmission rates within and between different populations. Such variability is directly related to differences in sexual behavior. This aspect of human behavior appears to be much more heterogeneous in defined populations than the behaviors that influence the transmission of many other types of infectious agents.

This brief review of the biological and behavioral factors that determine the transmission dynamics of STDs focuses on identifying the major components of the transmission rate, on how these components vary in human communities, and on how each component influences epidemiological pattern. Simple mathematical models are employed to provide a framework for the analyses, but technical details are omitted, with the emphasis placed on what theory tells us about both the interpretation of observed patterns and what needs to be measured via epidemiological study to facilitate understanding. In this latter context, special attention is paid to the behavioral component of transmission.

DETERMINANTS OF THE RATE OF TRANSMISSION

Many parameters and processes influence the net rate at which transmission occurs within a defined community. A composition measure of their influence is provided by the basic reproductive number of an infection R_0, which represents the average number of secondary cases generated by one primary case in a defined population of sexually active individuals. For most STDs, it is convenient to divide the sexually active population into compartments representing susceptible people, infected persons who are not yet infectious to their sexual contacts, and infectious individuals. Reproductive or transmission success therefore can be defined in terms of the generation of secondary cases of infection without reference to the number or density of infectious organisms transmitted between hosts.

The measurement of reproductive success is not straightforward, particularly when many sources of heterogeneity influence the host and infectious agent parameters that contribute to the magnitude of R_0. This is especially true in the case of STDs, since much variability exists in the sexual habits that facilitate transmission. However, the derivation of the composite measure R_0 and its estimation from data are important because its value determines both the shape and magnitude of an epidemic and the endemic prevalence or incidence of infection.

To start, let us consider the simplest possible case, namely, a single risk group that mixes homogeneously (chooses sexual partners at random). This will form the template for sequential re-

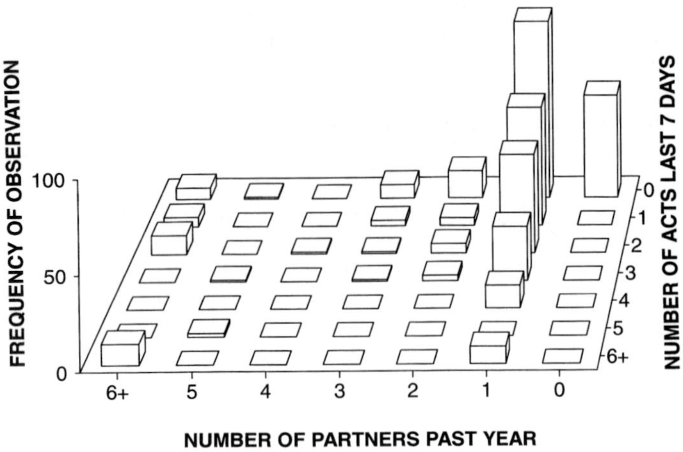

Fig. 3-1 Numbers of different sex partners in the past plotted as a bivariate frequency distribution by year and sex acts (penile-vaginal sex) in the past 7 days recorded in the U.K. survey of sexual attitudes and lifestyles (Johnson et al., 1994).

finements associated with recorded heterogeneities in the component parameters that determine the magnitude of R_0. For the simple case,

$$R_0 = \beta D c \tag{1}$$

where β is the average probability of transmission per partner sexual contact, D is the average duration of infectiousness of an infected person, and c is the average number of sexual partnerships formed per unit of time. What is meant exactly by average is not straightforward, since epidemiological studies reveal much variability between and within specific populations. It is therefore necessary to take into account the underlying distributional properties of each parameter (β, D, and c) if R_0 is to be defined precisely.

When an STD is introduced into a naive population, the infectious agent will spread and persist provided $R_0 \geq 1$. Otherwise, after the generation of a few secondary cases, the chain of infection will stutter to extinction. If an epidemic occurs, its rate of growth in the early stages (when most sexual contacts are susceptible) is determined by the magnitude of R_0, where the doubling time t_d (average time period for the doubling of reported cases) is given by

$$t_d = (D ln2)/(R_0 - 1) \tag{2}$$

As the infection spreads, more and more contacts are with those already infected, and hence the generation of secondary cases declines and the incidence of infection will decline after its epidemic peak to an endemic state where the prevalence y is given by

$$y = 1 - 1/R_0 \tag{3}$$

and the effective reproductive number R is equal to unity (i.e., each primary case generates exactly one secondary case).

THE TRANSMISSION COEFFICIENT β

In our simple definition of R_0, the transmission coefficient is defined per sexual partner contact per unit of time. However, within sexual partnerships or relationships, the number of sex acts per unit of time that create the opportunity for transmission will vary among different individuals. The term β can be reformulated to take account of such detail. If, on average, there is some constant probability δ per sexual act (of a defined type) of transmission, and if these probabilities compound independently where sex act numbers are randomly distributed, then

$$\beta \sim [1 - \exp(-\delta n)] \tag{4}$$

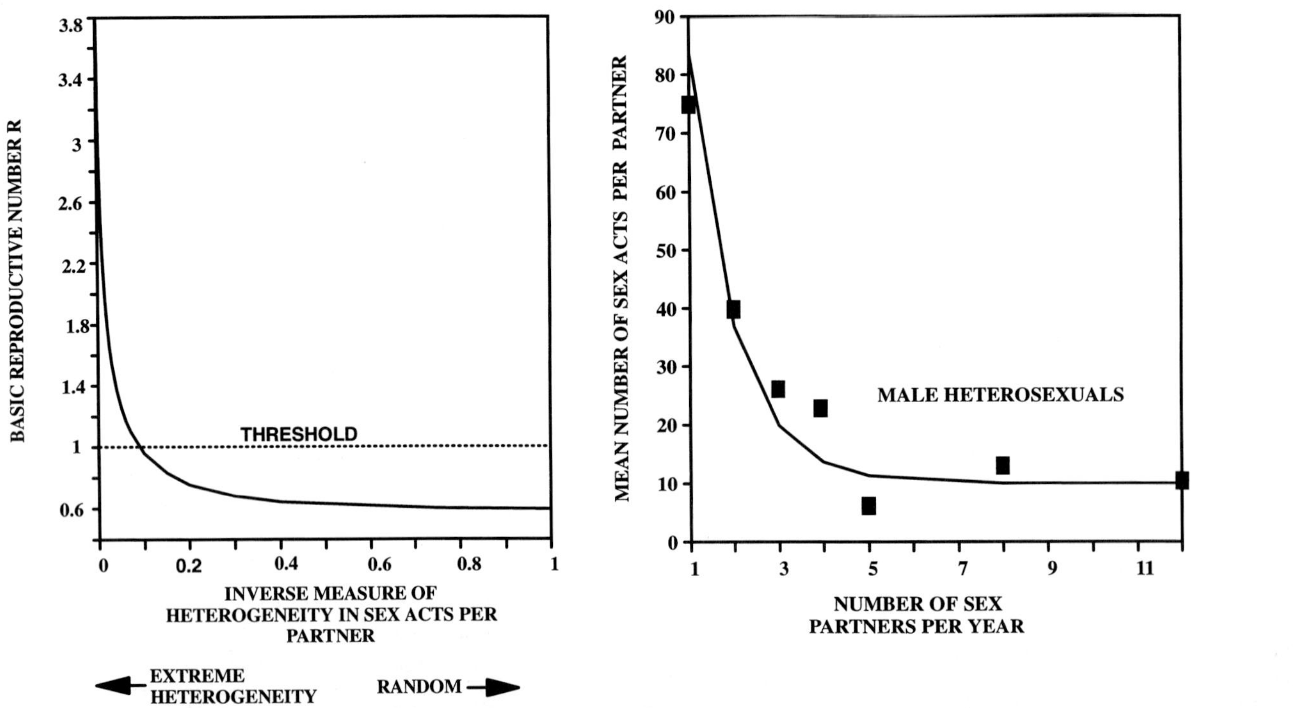

Fig. 3-2 (a) Predicted relationship between the magnitude of the case reproductive number R_0 and an inverse measure of the degree of heterogeneity in the distribution of sex acts per partner (Anderson, 1994). Reported acts per partner reveal much heterogeneity, where a few report many acts per unit of time and most report few. (b) Observed relationship between mean number of sex acts per partner and number of sex partners in the past year (data from the U.K. survey of sexual attitudes and lifestyles; see Anderson, 1994).

Table 3-1. Transmission Probabilities and Durations of Infectiousness.

Infectious agent	Disease	Transmission probability (per partnership)	Mean duration of infectiousness D (untreated) in years
Neisseria gonorrhoeae	Gonorrhoea	0.5	0.5
Chlamydia trachomatis	Urethritis/ Salpingitis	0.2	1.0
Treponema pallidum	Syphilis	0.6	0.5
Haemophilus ducreyi	Genital ulcer	0.8	0.08
HIV-1	AIDS	0.05–0.15	8–12

where n is the average number of acts per unit time. However, this method of estimation omits much detail, since we also need to take into account the variability in n within the population and variation in the value of δ according to a number of factors such as type of sex act (e.g., penile-vaginal, oral-penile, or anal sex) and the phenotypes of the transmitting infectious agents and the recipient host. Furthermore, we also need to take into account the heterogeneity in the distribution of sex acts within the sexually active population under study. Surveys of sexual behavior reveal aggregated or nonrandom distributions of reported sex acts per unit of time (Fig. 3-1). Furthermore, such studies also hint at correlations between different measures of sexual activity such as reported sex acts and reported sex partners per unit period of time.[3] Both factors act to enhance the magnitude of R_0 (given a fixed mean number of acts for the population.[4]) They therefore enhance the likelihood of the infection persisting in a given population (Fig. 3-2). In brief, many heterogeneities influence the magnitude of β. Thus measures of its average value via discordant partner or contact tracing studies must be interpreted with caution because the degree of variability around the average, and its source, can influence both the magnitude of R_0 and the prevalence and incidence of infection.

Tables 3-1 through 3-4 record a series of estimates of the magnitude of β for different STDs. Recorded estimates of the magnitude of β range from a very high likelihood of transmission for infections such as gonorrhea and syphilis to a low probability for infections such as HIV and Chlamydia. In the case of HIV, the magnitude of β also varies by viral type, where, for example, HIV-1 has a greater probability of transmission via heterosexual contact than HIV-2. In this particular case, transmissibility appears

Table 3-2. Per-partner HIV-1 Transmission Probabilities from Heterosexual Couples (=proportion of partners positive) [Mastro and de Vincenzi (1996)].

Country	Male index case	Female index case
USA	14/28 – 50%	12/71 – 71%
USA	10/55 – 18%	2/25 – 8%
USA	61/307 – 20%	1/72 – 1%
USA	21/201 – 10%	—
USA	73/142 – 51%	7/11 – 64%
USA	7/32 – 22%	0/14 – 0%
Europe	10/148 – 7%	—
Europe	15/78 – 19%	1/18 – 6%
Europe	82/404 – 20%	19/159 – 12%
Europe	156/524 – 30%	21/206 – 10%
Thailand	108/250 – 43%	—
Average	23.4%	12.1%

Table 3-3. Estimates of Per-Sex-Act HIV-1 Transmission Probabilities (Mastro and de Vincenzi, 1996).

Study population	Country	Transmission route	Per-sex-act transmission probability
Heterosexual couples	USA	Penile-vaginal male to female	0.0014
	USA	Penile-vaginal male to female	0.0008–0.001
	USA	Penile-vaginal both	0.001
	Europe	Penile-vaginal male to female	0.0005–0.001
	Thailand	Penile-vaginal male to female	0.002
Heterosexual men	Kenya	Penile-vaginal female CSW to male	0.13
	Thailand	Penile-vaginal female CSW to male	0.031–0.056
Homosexual men	USA	Receptive penile-anal	0.005–0.03

to be positively associated with pathogenicity.[5] Whether or not different clades of HIV-1 differ in their respective transmissibilities remains uncertain at present.[5]

THE INFECTIOUS PERIOD D

The typical duration and degree of infectiousness of an infected person are also subject to variation. Within the incubation period of a defined disease, infectiousness may vary widely at different times after infection. In the case of HIV, for example, infectiousness (whether in the context of horizontal or vertical transmission) is thought to be closely associated with viral load in the patient, typically being high in the few months after infection, low for a long and variable period (often of many years), and high again as serious disease develops (Fig. 3-3). If we split the incubation period of AIDS up into three phases, of durations t_1, t_2, and t_3, with infectiousness in each period mirrored by different values for the transmission coefficient (β_1, β_2, and β_3), then R_0 is defined as

$$R_0 = c(\beta_1 t_1 + \beta_2 t_2 + \beta_3 t_3) \quad (5)$$

where $D = t_1 + t_2 + t_3$. The magnitudes of β_1 and t_1 (early infectiousness) determine the rate at which an epidemic grows in its early phase, whereas the overall magnitude of R_0 determines the size of the epidemic and the stable endemic prevalence of infection.[6] The overall duration of the incubation period of STDs often varies widely between individuals, and Weibull or gamma probability distributions can be used to describe such variability. Figure 3-4 displays some of the observed incubation period distributions for AIDS. For a fixed mean of the incubation period D, any epidemic will grow more quickly if the variance around this mean is low than if it is large.

The duration of infectiousness can be influenced by interventions such as chemotherapy. Drug treatment therefore helps not

Table 3-4. Epidemiological Characteristics of HIV-1 and HIV-2 (Anderson and May, 1996).

Property	HIV-1	HIV-2
Mean incubation period	5–10 Yrs	>20 Yrs?
Vertical transmission rate (%)	11%–35%	0.5%–3%
Horizontal transmission probability (act)	0.001	0.0002–0.0001

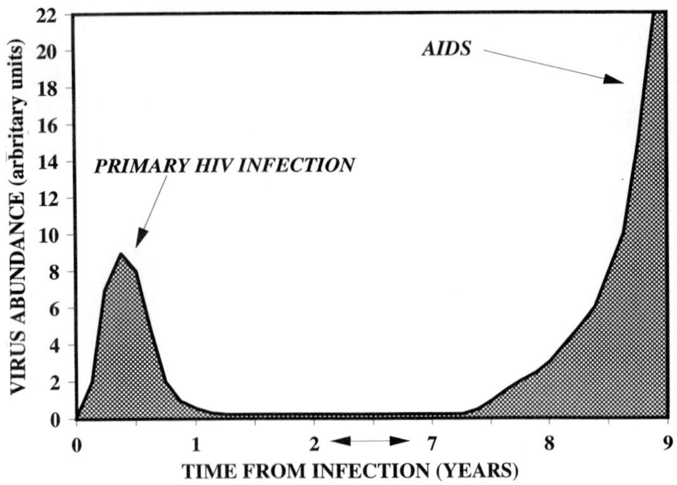

Fig. 3-3 Diagramatic representation of typical changes in HIV viral burden over the incubation period of AIDS.

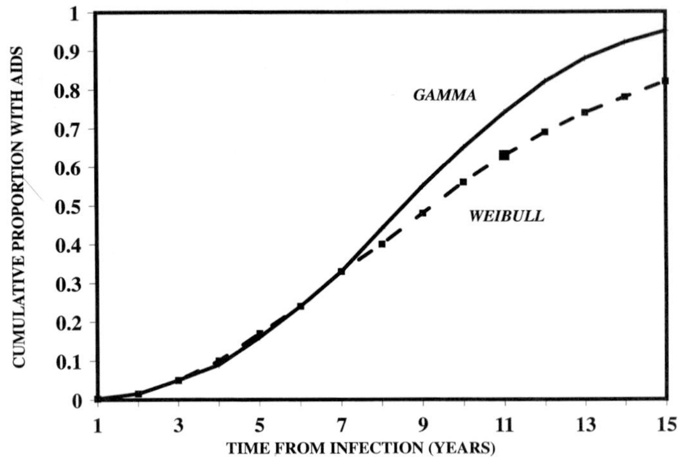

Fig. 3-4 Observed (up to year 7) and predicted cumulative distribution of those with AIDS as a function of time after infection in patients not treated with chemotherapeutic agents (predictions for years 7 to 15 based on either the Weibull or gamma distribution; see Hendriks et al., 1993).

only the individuals treated but also the community via its action in reducing the value of R_0 in proportion to the fraction treated successfully. Early diagnosis and treatment obviously maximize impact.

THE RATE OF NEW SEXUAL PARTNER ACQUISITION C

The most important measure of sexual behavior is the rate of new sexual partner acquisition per unit of time. Other factors are also of importance, such as the frequency and types of sex acts within a partnership and the distribution of these properties within the sexually active population, the frequency of concurrent partnerships, and the patterns of mixing between different segments or strata of the sexually active population. All are important determinants of the transmission success, but sex partner change rate occupies a central position in determining the generation of secondary cases.

Rates of sexual partner change vary greatly within and between societies. They are associated with a wide range of demographic and socioeconomic factors such as age, gender, educational attainment, and income. In broad terms, surveys reveal much het-

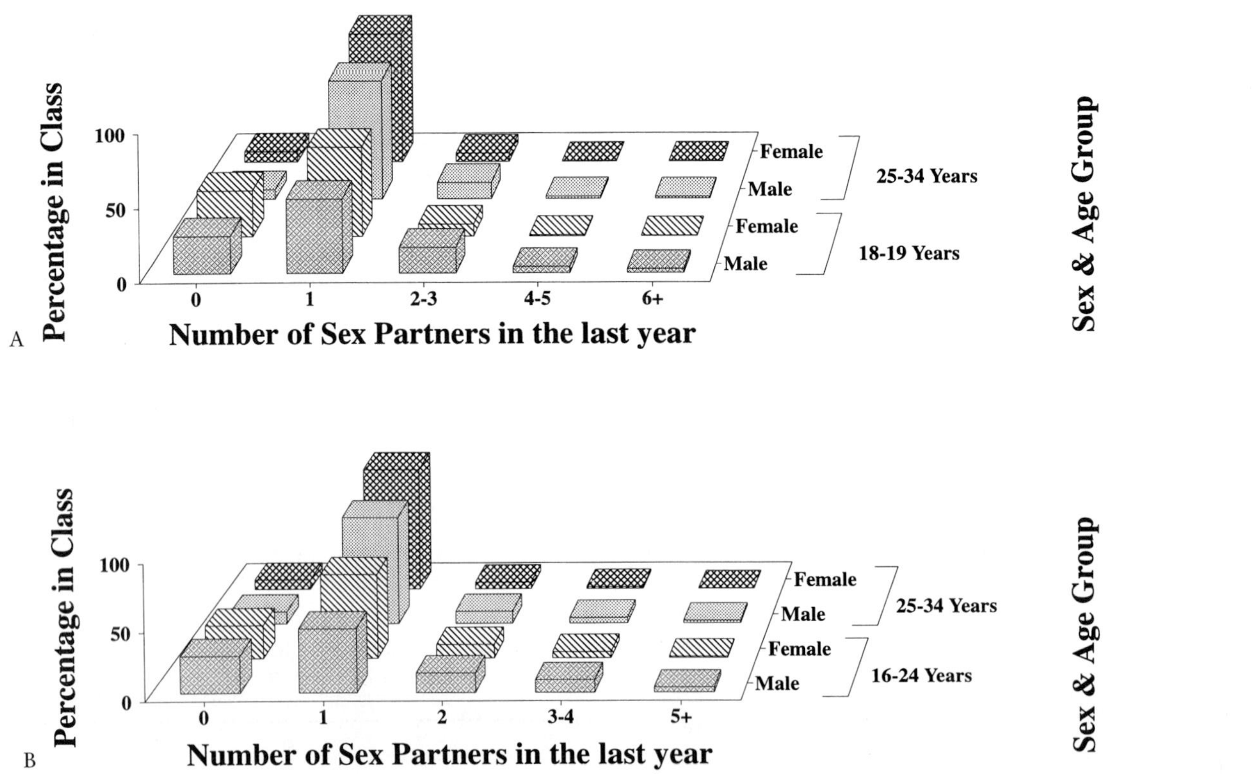

Fig. 3-5 Frequency distributions of reported sex partners in the past year in the U.K. and French surveys of sexual behavior (Johnson et al., 1994; ACSF, 1994), stratified by age and sex. The data are for heterosexuals.

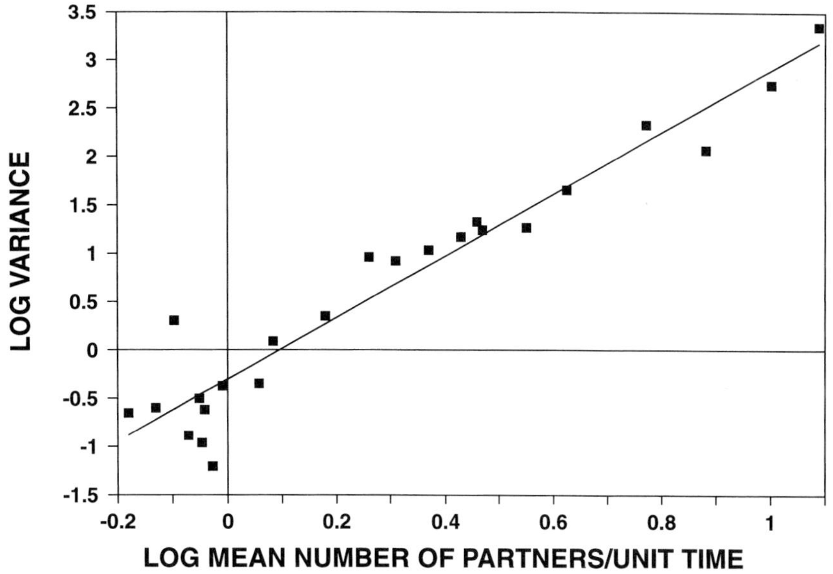

Fig. 3-6 Relationship between the logarithm of the variance in reported sex partner numbers per unit of time and the logarithm of the mean (U.K. survey; see Anderson and May, 1988).

erogeneity, with most people reporting few partners and a few reporting many, as illustrated in Fig. 3-5. These distributions are skewed or aggregated in form, where the variance exceeds the mean in value, in all societies and all stratifications of defined populations. Interestingly, plots of the logarithm of the variance (σ^2) in reported numbers of sex partners (over a defined time period such as 1 year or lifetime) versus the logarithm of the mean (m) reveal a straight line with a slope of approximately 3 independent of country, study population (i.e., homosexual or heterosexual), or method of survey. Those few who report very high numbers of different sex partners are a major influence on this pattern[7] (Fig. 3-6).

The definition of R_0 (see Eq. 3.1) is changed once heterogeneity in sex partner numbers is taken into account. The new definition is

$$R_0 = \beta(m + \sigma^2/m)D \qquad (6)$$

where β and D are as before and m and σ^2 are the mean and variance of new sex partner numbers per unit time. This expression makes clear the role of heterogeneity in STD persistence in communities where most have too few different sexual partners to ensure that the chains of transmission continue. Even when the mean m is small, a high variance σ^2 created by a core group of highly sexually active individuals will ensure that R_0 exceeds unity in value.

Heterogeneity in sexual activity also has a major influence on the endemic prevalence or incidence of infection. A simple illustration of this is provided by its influence on a closed epidemic in a population of fixed size. It is possible to calculate the fraction infected during the epidemic for various values of R_0 and the variance in sexual partner change rate.[8] As illustrated in Fig. 3-7, if variability is high (for a fixed mean of one new partner per year), the fraction infected is low, and vice versa. Thus, paradoxically, high variability enhances the likelihood that the sexually transmitted infectious agent will persist over time in the community while at the same time restricting infection to a small core of highly sexually active individuals. The concept of a core group of people who play the major role in STD persistence in the wider population is of major importance in the design of policies for the control of infection and disease.

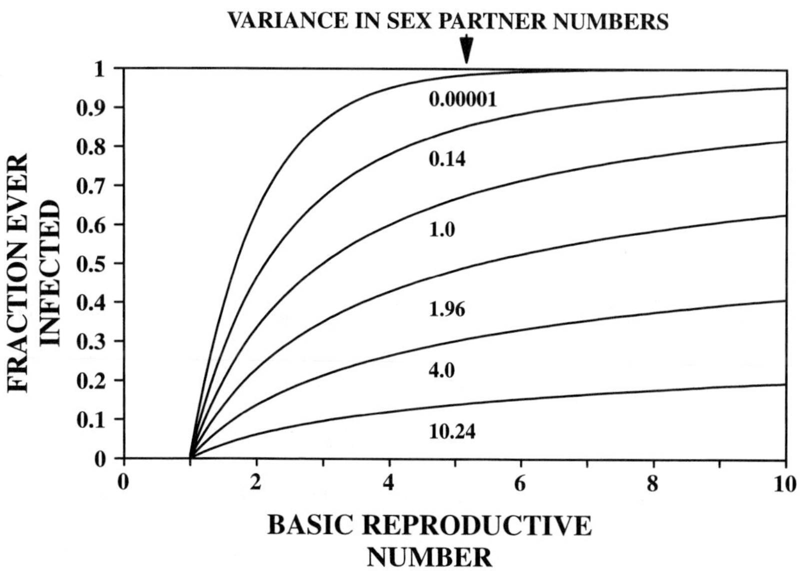

Fig. 3-7 The fraction infected in an epidemic of an STD in a closed population as a function of the case reproductive number and the variance in the rate of acquisition of new sexual partners.

Much detail has been omitted in the preceding discussion, and more complications are introduced in the following section. However, before leaving sex partner acquisition rate, it is important to note the relevance of behavioral surveys designed to record such information in sufficient detail to calculate means and variances. There are, of course, many problems associated with the collection of such data and in ascertaining the veracity of responses. Furthermore, the rate of acquisition of new partners is one facet of a series of behaviors relevant to STD transmission.

MIXING WITHIN AND BETWEEN RISK GROUPS

Mixing within and between risk groups (i.e., who has sexual contact with whom) is an important component of the transmission of STDs. Mixing within a population may be studied at a variety of levels, depending on the stratification of the population. The latter may be based on spatial residence location, ethnic background, socioeconomic factors, age, or indeed sexual behavior (Fig. 3-8). All these factors are important determinants of observed epidemiological pattern, but one is of particular importance and transcends other stratifications, namely, sexual activity as recorded by the rate of new sexual partner acquisition. If we divide the frequency distribution of reported sex partner numbers per defined period of time (see Fig. 3–5) into n groups (with constant or variable intervals on the horizontal axis), then we can define an n by n mixing matrix whose elements p_{ij} define the proportion of the sexual partnerships of someone in group i formed with an individual of the same (homosexual relationships) or opposite (heterosexual relationships) sex in group j. There is a set of important constraints on the values of the elements, namely,

$$\sum_{t=1}^{n} p_{ij} = 1,\ 1 > p_j > 0,\ p_{ij}P_ic_i = p_{ji}P_jc_j$$

where P_j is the proportion of the population in group j and c_j is the mean rate of new sexual partner acquisition in this group. In verbal terms, these constraints simply state that the sum of the proportions of contacts with other and with the defining group must equal unity, the proportions must lie between 0 and 1, and the total number of partnerships formed by individuals in group i with people in group j must equal the total number of partnerships formed by individuals in group j with people in group i. The latter constraint simply ensures that supply matches demand. In most sexually active populations, the supply and demand issue is a very dynamic one where the elements of the mixing matrix will change as the social and behavioral process governing the interplay alter. This may be very complex in the case of lethal diseases such as AIDS, where mortality may have a disproportionate effect on the number of people in the highest sexual activity class.[9]

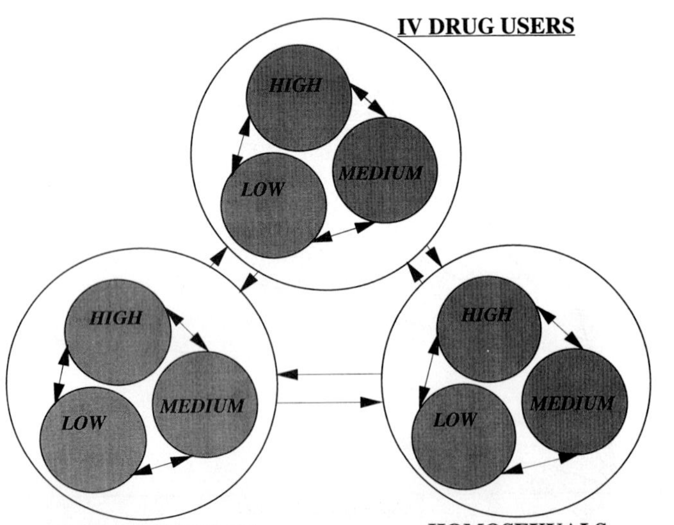

Fig. 3-8 Schematic diagram of the linkages between different risk groups and within different risk strata in each group.

Once the population is stratified into risk groups on the basis of the prime route by which infection is acquired (i.e., in the case of HIV, intravenous drug use, sexual contact) and by the definition of classes of sexual activity (based on high, medium, or low rates of sexual partner change), the definition of R_0 must be based on mixing between classes or broader strata (Fig. 3–7). More precisely, we need to define a basic reproductive number $R(0)_{ij}$ for the secondary cases of infection generated by contacts of infected persons in group j with susceptibilities in group i, where

$$R(0)_{ij} = c_j p_{ij} \beta D \tag{7}$$

In other words, there is a matrix of reproductive numbers, and the STD could persist in the total population even when only some subset of these values exceeds unity. More precisely, the core group of high sexual activity individuals is likely to have an $R(0)_{ij}$ value well in excess of unity, whereas other groups may have values less than unity. What happens overall in the population depends critically on the pattern of mixing between high- and low-activity groups. If mixing is like with like, or assortative, then an infectious person in the high-activity group is likely to pass it on to a person who is likely to have sufficient new sexual partners to yet again ensure that the chain of transmission continues. Alternatively, if mixing is like with unlike, or disassortative, then the high-activity infected wastes his or her contacts with a person in a low sexual activity class because the latter is unlikely to continue the chain of transmission. In other words, assortative mixing promotes the persistence of infection in the core group of high sexual activity, but via less frequent contacts outside the core group, it ensures the persistence of infection in the population as a whole.

Theory has outstripped data in this important area, but recently, a number of epidemiological and behavioral surveys have begun to measure the magnitudes of the elements of the mixing matrix via contact tracing studies that include an interview on sexual habits of both index cases and contacts.[10] Such studies reveal moderate degrees of assortative mixing for the criteria of sexual activity, spatial location of residence, and other socioeconomic plus educational attainment indicators, as recorded in Fig. 3-9.[11]

Patterns of mixing between age classes of the two sexes also can be an important determinant of epidemiological pattern. For example, in many societies men typically form sexual relationships with women who are younger than themselves. In the case of a lethal disease such as AIDS, this can act to focus infection and disease in younger women in the peak reproductive age classes. It obviously acts to influence the age-related distribution of infection in the two genders, as well illustrated by HIV-1 infection in many societies (Fig. 3-10).

GENDER

In heterosexual transmission of STDs, the typical course of infection and infectiousness may vary between males and females. For example, the probability of transmission of HIV-1 is typically greater from infected male to susceptible female than vice versa. In such cases there will be different R_0 values for male-to-female and female-to-male transmission, although there will be a composite R_0 for heterosexual transmission, where in the simple case of random mixing

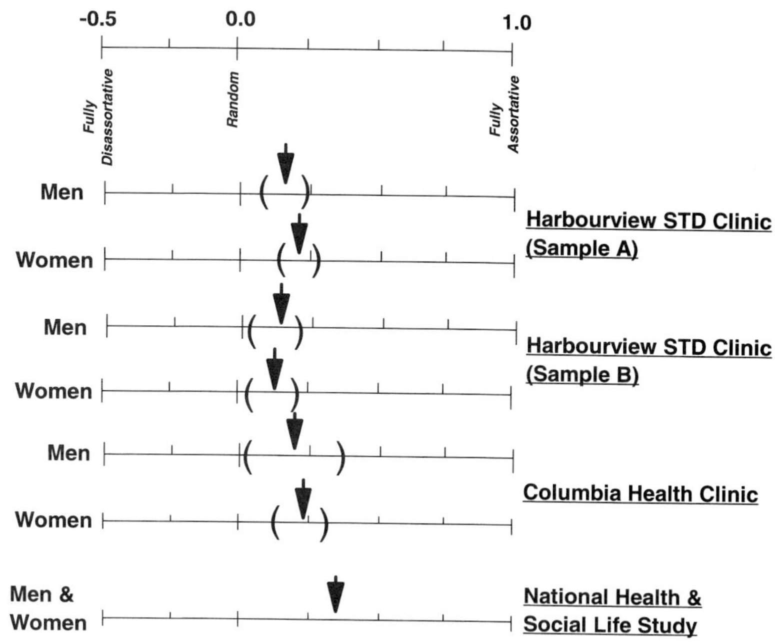

Fig. 3-9 Measures of the degree of assortativeness in mixing between sexual activity classes in four studies of sexual behavior in the United States, three of which were based on contact tracing in STD clinics. The measure presented, Q, varies from a value of 1.0 for fully assortative (no between-group mixing), to a value of 0 for random mixing, to a value of −0.5 for fully disassortative mixing (Garnett et al., 1996).

$$R_0 = (\beta_1 c_1 \beta_2 c_2)^{1/2} D \tag{8}$$

assuming that only the β and c values differ between the sexes with the subscript 1 denoting females and subscript 2 denoting males. The ratio r of the incidence of infection in males to that in females is approximately given by

$$r = (\beta_2 c_2 / \beta_1 c_1)^{1/2} \tag{9}$$

This equation shows clearly that there is no reason to assume a 1 : 1 ratio if the male-to-female transmission probability (β_1) is significantly different from that for female-to-male transmission (β_2), as is the case for HIV-1. However, to counteract this trend, which is apparent for other STDs as well as HIV, the variance in sex partner change ($c = m + \sigma^2/m$; see Eq. 3.6) is often significantly higher for females than for males by virtue of a cadre of female prostitutes who preserve the overall balance in supply and demand of sexual partnerships between the sexes in populations where males tend to be more promiscuous than the typical female. If this is so, then we could have c_2 significantly larger than c_1, which will act to counterbalance any tendency for β_1 to exceed β_2 and result in case ratios of roughly 1 : 1 for the two sexes.

CONCURRENT PARTNERSHIPS

The duration of a sexual partnership plays a significant role in the transmission dynamics of STDs. Its significance is related to the typical duration of infectiousness of a given infection. For short durations of infectiousness (i.e., gonorrhea), the core group of highly sexually active individuals who change sexual partnerships frequently plays a very key role in maintaining transmission within defined communities. For long durations of infectiousness (i.e., HIV and hepatitis B), those who change sexual partners infrequently may still play an important role in generating secondary cases of infection. In both instances, however, individuals with

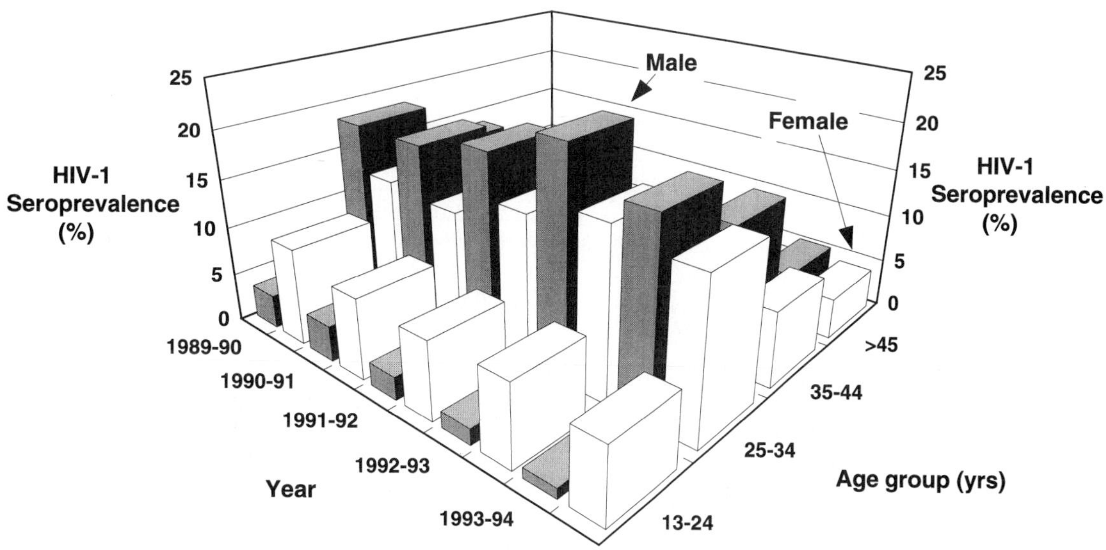

Fig. 3-10 Longitudinal and cross-sectional trends in HIV-1 seroprevalence, stratified by sex, in a rural community in Uganda (Mulder et al., 1994).

two or more simultaneous (i.e., concurrent) partners can play a central role in the spread of infection. Indeed, an individual with concurrent partners can in principle acquire infection from one partner and pass it on to another without gaining any new partners. As such, our earlier definition of R_0 needs revision, since in its simplest form transmission success was assumed to be dependent on the rate of acquisition of new sexual partners.

The frequency of reporting concurrent sexual partners is often high in both developed and developing countries. In both cases, the reported frequency is higher for males than for females. Once this factor is taken into account, the expression for the case reproductive number R_0 is modified[12] to

$$R_0 = R_0{}^1 + P_0 \quad (10)$$

where $R_0{}^1$ is our original definition (Eq. 3.1) for a homogeneously mixing population, and $P_0 = \beta c\Gamma$, where β and c are as defined in Eq. (3.1) and Γ is the average partnership duration. As such, $c\Gamma$ is therefore the average number of partners an individual has at any instant in time. The new case reproductive number represents the two components, of transmission to new partners ($R_0{}^1$) and transmission to existing partners. The inclusion of transmission arising from concurrent partners provides important new insights into the interpretation of observed epidemiological pattern.[13] Most important, its presence at levels recorded in behavioral studies in Table 3-5 helps explain the very rapid spread of STDs such as HIV when initially introduced into a high-risk group. Observed trends in HIV incidence over time, in high-risk communities such as gay men in urban centres in Europe and North America, reveals a very rapid spread of infection. Such patterns are difficult to explain unless unrealistically high average rates of sexual partner acquisition are assumed. The inclusion of transmission arising from concurrent partners as well as new partners alters the situation such that more rapid growth of the epidemic can occur via networks of sexual contact in the space of a few years where concurrency exists in the partnership structure of individuals in the network of sexual relationships. The relative contribution of concurrency partnership transmission to overall transmission success is defined by the ratio of the average duration of partnerships to the average duration of infectiousness, whether the transmission probability is defined per partnership or period of time. The existence of a high prevalence of concurrent partners among the sexually active population is of particular importance in ensuring the persistance of infection in low-risk groups. If infectiousness is high early in the incubation period, the importance of concurrent parties to overall transmission success is increased.[14]

Table 3-5. Reported Concurrent Sexual Partners (Parker and Anderson, 1997).

Country	Sample size	Inclusion criteria	Reported concurrent partners
Zimbabwe	711	Married men	40% (past year)
Kenya	2960	Age 15–59, M+F	M:25%, F:4% (past year)
Cote d'Ivoire	2433	Age 15+, M+F	M:44%, F:11% (past year)
Zaire	6625	M:20–59, F:15–49	M:23%, F:1% (past 6 months)
Thailand	2374	Ever had sex, M+F	M:28%, F:1% (past 6 months)
UK	18000+	All ages, M+F	M:15%, F:8% (past 5 years)
USA	1600+	All ages, married	M:<25%, F:<10% (ever)

VERTICAL TRANSMISSION

Many STDs are transmitted vertically from mother to infant either before birth, during birth, or near to birth. HIV-1 is an example where high rates of vertical transmission (on the order of 15 to 30 percent) prevail in many developing countries. This route of transmission is a cause of much morbidity and, in the case of HIV, mortality, but in general it contributes little, if anything, to the long-term reproductive success of the pathogen.

EPIDEMIOLOGICAL PATTERN

The components that contribute to transmission success influence epidemiological pattern in different ways. This section outlines some of the key effects in longitudinal trends in the incidence or prevalence of infection.

THE SIMPLE EPIDEMIC

In susceptible populations previously unexposed to a sexually transmitted infectious agent, the spread of infection will give rise to an epidemic provided $R_0 \geq 1$. For the case of random or homogeneous mixing, prevalence will rise to a stable endemic state y whose magnitude is given by

$$y = 1 - 1/R_0 \quad (11)$$

If the disease is a cause of morbidity or R_0 is high in magnitude, the prevalence may rise and then fall as it approaches the endemic stable state. At the same time, the incidence of infection will rise rapidly and then fall dramatically to the stable state where each primary case gives rise to exactly one secondary case. This concept is illustrated in Fig. 3-11, where prevalence and incidence are plotted over time for an epidemic in a virgin population (where the parameters are set to mimic the spread of HIV in a male homosexual community). If the magnitude of R_0 is high, spread will be rapid, whereas if it is low, spread will take place over many decades before the endemic equilibrium is reached (Fig. 3-12).

Understanding the pattern of a simple epidemic is essential in the context of interpreting the impact of interventions to control the spread of an STD. As recorded in Fig. 3-11, an epidemic in a virgin population is bell shaped, where incidence decays from its peak in the absence of any intervention or change in behavior. This arises from changes in the magnitude of the effective reproductive number R over the course of the epidemic as more and more sexual contacts are made with those already infected. This saturation effect progressively reduces the magnitude of R until it attains unity at the endemic state. Saturation may occur at a low prevalence of infection if marked heterogeneity in sexual activity pertains in the population (see Fig. 3-7). To measure the impact of any intervention on the incidence of infection is not easy in the absence of either comparison with a control community in which interventions are absent or detailed data on behavior. Once the infection has attained the endemic state (stable incidence), then the impact of an intervention is simply reflected by the decline in prevalence or incidence.

VARIABLE INFECTIOUSNESS

Variation in infectiousness to sexual partners over the incubation period of an STD in the index case can have a marked influence on epidermiological pattern. HIV infection is an example where infectiousness appears to be closely correlated with viremia. This

Fig. 3-11 Predicted longitudinal trends in the prevalence and incidence of an epidemic of HIV-1 in a gay male community based on a simple model of viral spread.

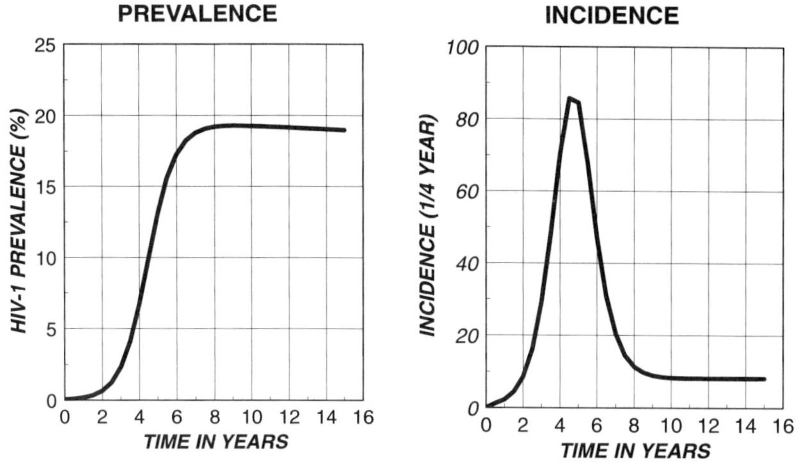

varies from high early after infection to low for most of the long incubation period to high again once symptoms of serious immunodeficiency appear. The pattern varies widely between patients such that in some individuals who progress rapidly to full-blown AIDS, viremia remains high for most of the short incubation period. Recent epidemiological studies suggest that the early infection phase in the incubation period of AIDS is the most important in terms of transmission to susceptible sexual contacts. The influence of this on the course of an epidemic is illustrated in Fig. 3-13, where three examples are plotted, one in which infectiousness is high early in the incubation period, one in which it is high early, low in the middle, and high late, and one in which it is high only in the late phase. The average infectiousness over the total incubation period is the same in all three cases, such that the endemic prevalence of infection is constant. Early high infectiousness leads to a much more rapidly developing epidemic, with late infectiousness leading to a very slow rise in the incidence of disease.[6]

WHO MIXES WITH WHOM

The structure of the mixing matrix that captures the details of a sexual partner network has a very profound influence on the pattern of an epidemic. An illustration of this point is presented in Fig. 3-14, which depicts the course of three epidemics in a susceptible sexually active community with the case reproductive number held constant for all three cases. The only factor varied is the degree of assortativeness (like with like) in mixing between different sexual activity classes (defined on the basis of the rate of acquisition of new sexual partners). When mixing is highly or moderately assortative, where those who are highly sexually active tend to choose most of their sexual partners from within their own activity class, the epidemic spreads quickly and may exhibit multiple peaks as the epidemic passes in waves through the high, medium, and low classes. Highly assortative mixing therefore leads to a rapid epidemic, but the endemic prevalence of infection is much lower than would be the case if mixing where random.[15,16] Empirical studies of mixing patterns tend to reveal moderate assortativeness, and hence these multiple peaked epidemics are of considerable practical significance. For example, the incidence of HIV may peak and then decline before rising again as the infection spreads from the high- to the lower-risk groups. The latter are much greater in size than the former, and hence

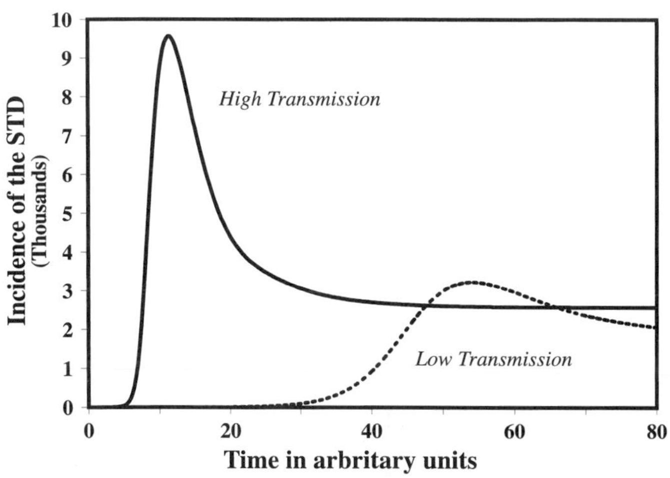

Fig 3-12 Influence of the magnitude of the case reproductive number R_0 on the incidence of an STD over time (parameters chosen to reflect the spread of HIV-1).

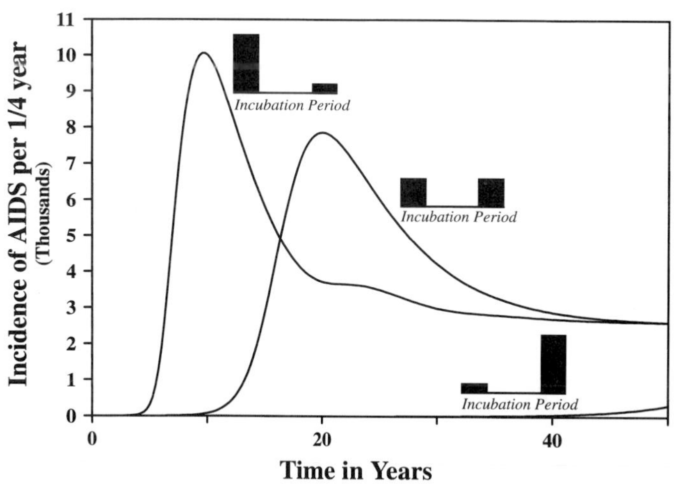

Fig. 3-13. The influence of variation in infectiousness over the course of the incubation period of AIDS on epidemic pattern. Three examples are plotted, one in which infectiousness is high in the early phase, one in which it is high early on, one in which it is low in the middle of the incubation period, and one in which it is high only in the late phase. The overall average infectiousness over the total incubation period is held constant.

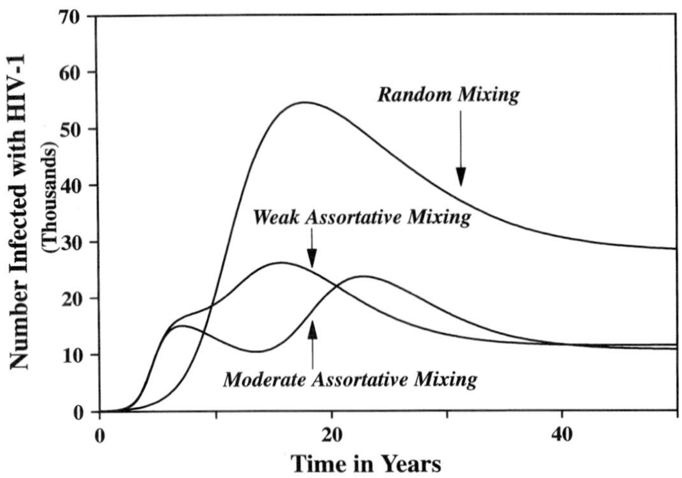

Fig 3-14 Influence of the pattern of mixing between sexual activity classes (defined on the basis of the rate of new sexual partner acquisition) on the pattern of an HIV-1 epidemic.

even though at less risk, the number of cases of infection may be greater in medium- as opposed to high-risk groups. In the absence of an understanding of the effects of different mixing patterns, a rise in the incidence of infection after the early peak could be interpreted as an increase in risky behavior within a defined community. This, of course, may be true, but a simpler interpretation is provided by the epidemic moving in waves via the high- to medium- to low-risk groups, where within-group mixing is much more frequent than between-group sexual contact. A possible illustration of this effect is presented in Fig. 3-15, which records temporal trends in the incidence of HIV-1 infection in a cohort of gay men in Amsterdam.[17] Past the early peak, incidence rises again more than 10 years after the start of the epidemic. However, caution must be exercised in the interpretation of such trends in the absence of detailed data on temporal trends in sexual behavior.

The impact of different mixing patterns on the likelihood that a given STD can persist in a defined community, and the endemic prevalence resulting if persistence is possible, are complex and depend on the precise quantitive detail of the degree of within and between sexual activity class contact and the prevaling rates of sexual partner change in each activity class. In heterosexual communities in sub-Sahara Africa, where HIV has spread extensively, the degree of assortativeness in mixing has a major influence on the pattern of the epidemic. An illustration of this is presented in Fig. 3-16, which records the longitudinal trends in prevalence for three different degrees of assortative mixing. For high within activity class mixing, HIV prevalence settles to around 25 percent in sexually active women. This figure is similar to that recorded in many urban communities, although whether this is a consequence of highly assortative mixing cannot be assessed at present due to the absence of empirical studies in developing countries of the kind presented in Fig. 3-9.

In many developing countries the persistence of STDs such as gonorrhea, syphilis, and HIV in low-risk heterosexual communities is thought to be due to the activities of a small core of highly sexually active individuals who change partners frequently. Theoretical studies support this conclusion. They indicate that even if mixing is assortative with the basic reproductive number less than unity in the majority of the population (the lower/medium sexual activity classes), a small degree of mixing with the core group (in which $R_0 \gg 1$) is sufficient to ensure endemic persistence in the entire sexually active population. This point is illustrated in Fig. 3-17, which records a simulated epidemic of HIV-1 in a population in which 10 percent are in the core group and 90 percent are in the low risk group. Despite the fact that the R_0 for the majority group is less than unity, a small degree of mixing with the core group maintains the infection in both. The prevalence in the low-activity group is less than 0.5 percent, whereas that in the core group is on the order of 40 percent. In this particular example, AIDS-induced mortality acts to reduce the portion in the core group as the epidemic develops.

COFACTORS THAT ENHANCE TRANSMISSION

An individual infected with one STD is sometimes more likely to acquire a different infection due to damage to the epithelial surfaces of the genital organs that appears to enhance the likelihood of transmission during sexual contact. For example, a variety of STD infections have been shown to be important cofactors enhancing the likelihood of HIV-1 infection, as recorded in Table 3-6. Analyses of the importance of cofactors, based on models of the transmission dynamics of two STDs circulating in the same community,[9] reveal that the doubling time t_d of an epidemic of an invading STD into a community where the cofactor STD is already endemic is given by

$$t_d = D[ln(2)]/[R_0 a^2 y - 1] \tag{12}$$

where R_0 is the case reproductive number of the invader, D is its average duration of infectiousness, and y is the endemic prevalence of the cofactor STD. The term a denotes the degree to which the transmission probability of the invader is enhanced by the

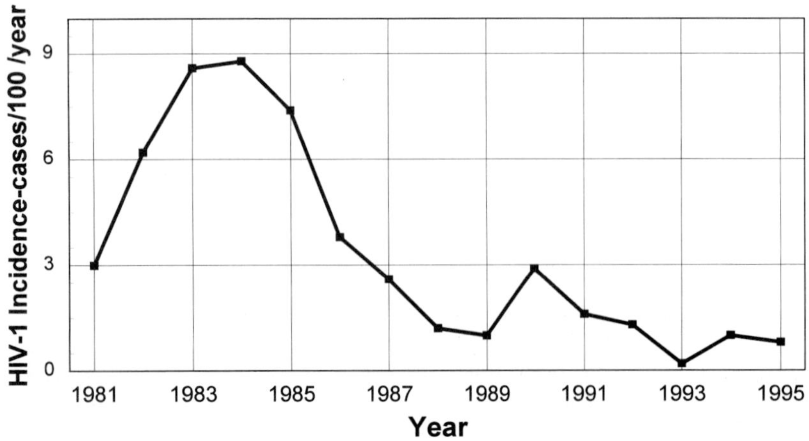

Fig. 3-15 Observed trends in the incidence of HIV-1 infection in a cohort of gay men in Amsterdam, Holland, over the period 1981–1995 (Coutinho et al., 1996).

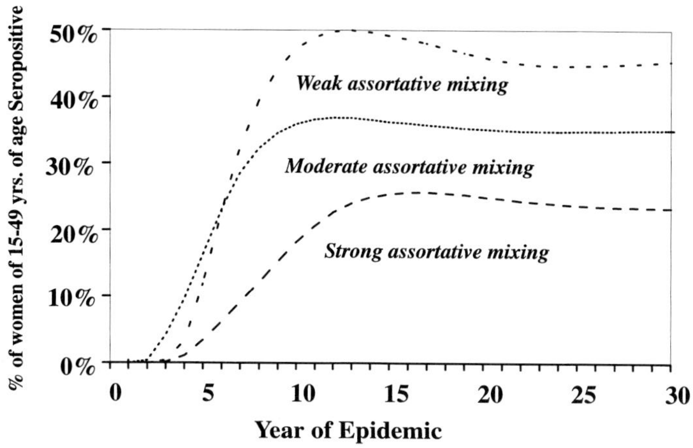

Fig. 3-16 Influence of the degree of assortative mixing on the pattern of an HIV-1 epidemic in a sub-Saharan African country within sexually active women (Garnett and Anderson, 1996).

presence of the cofactor STD. The assumption is that the transmission of the invader is enhanced by factor a if either party has the cofactor and by factor a^2 if both are infected with the cofactor. The term a measures the relative risk and a^2y is the attributable risk in a given population. Clearly, if a is greater than unity and y is on the order of 10 percent or so, the doubling time is greatly enhanced by the presence of the cofactor. This is one explanation

Table 3-6. STDs Patterns and Cofactors that Increase Transmission.

Reference	Study group	Site	STD	Factor by which HIV transmission increased
Plummer et al (1991)	Female sex workers	Nairobi, Kenya	GUD	3.3
			Chancroid	2.7
Laga et al (1993)	Female sex workers	Kinshassa, Zaire	Gonorrhea	4.8
			Chlamydia	3.6
			Trichomoniasis	1.9

of why HIV-1 has spread so quickly in poor communities in developing countries where other STDs such as chancroid and gonorrhea are very prevalent. With respect to control, Eq. (3.12) makes clear the advantages of reducing the prevalence of the cofactor in attempting to control the spread of HIV. Recent epidemiologic studies based on treating cofactor STDs have provided evidence of the benefits of this form of intervention.[18]

CONTROL

An understanding of the transmission dynamics of STDs provides a good template for the design and interpretation of intervention

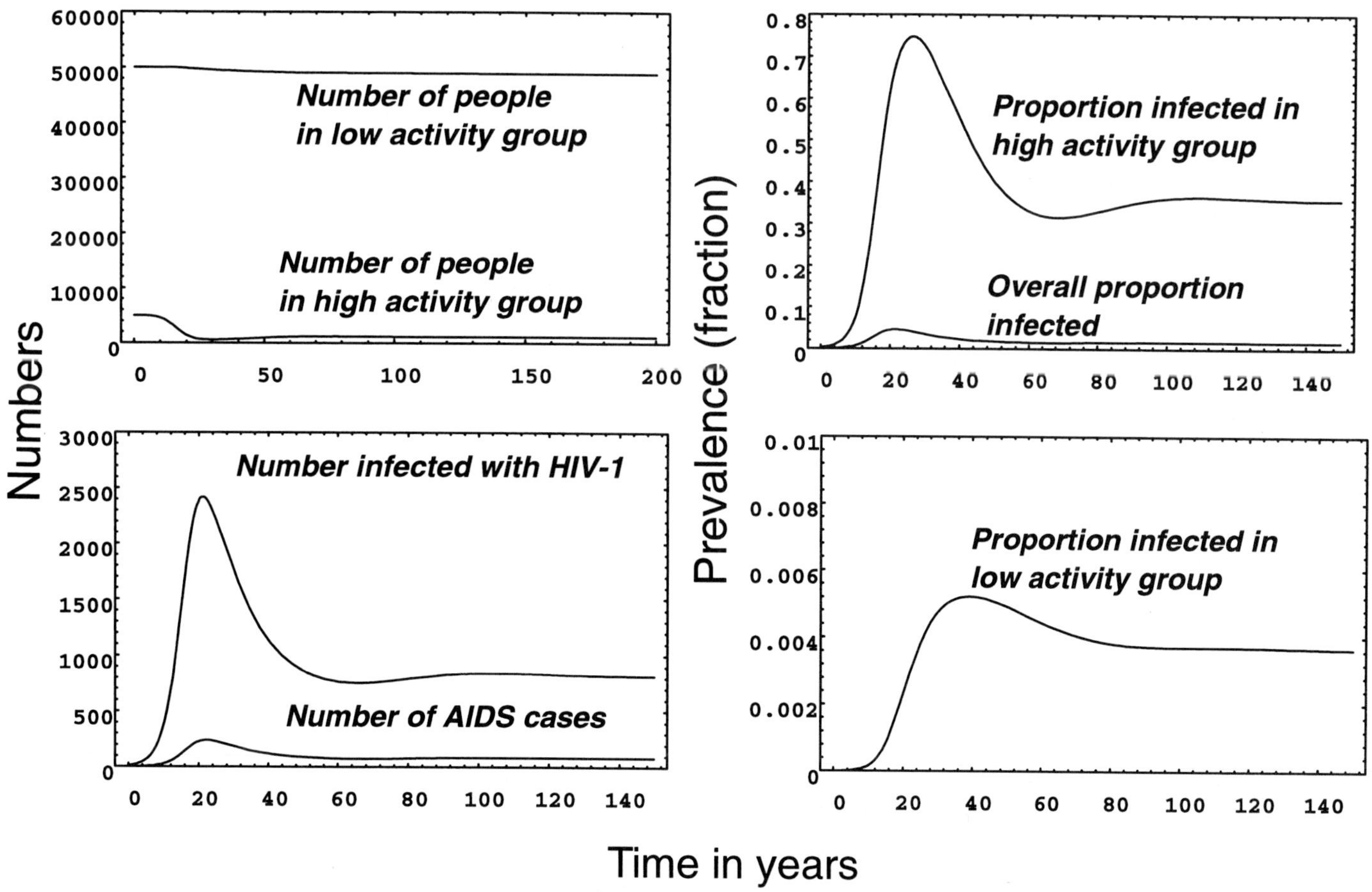

Fig. 3-17 Longitudinal trends in HIV-1 seroprevalence in a heterosexual population stratified into high- and low-risk groups where mixing is moderately assortative. In the low-risk group the case reproductive number is less than unity in value, but infection is maintained in this group via infrequent contact with individuals in the high-risk group, where the case reproductive number is greatly in excess of unity.

studies. The simple expressions for the case reproductive number R_0 provide insights into how different interventions are likely to influence transmission success and consequently the prevalence of infection ($y = 1 - 1/R_0$) in defined populations. Options include education to promote condom use (a reduction in the transmission probability β), reductions in sex partner acquisition rates (c), chemotherapy (a reduction in the duration or degree of infectiousness D) and in some cases (hepatitis B), vaccination (a reduction in the supply of susceptibles). More complex models that incorporate other facets of sexual behavior, such as heterogeneity in rates of sexual partner acquisition (σ^2), concurrent partners, and mixing patterns, provide further insights of practical relevance. For example, education aimed at the core group of highly sexually active individuals to promote condom use or reduce new partner numbers will have a dispropotionate effect on the net rate of transmission.

Similarly, a reduction in the frequency of concurrent partnerships also will have a major impact. In both cases, who changes behavior is more important than the average change in a community. For example, in the simulation recorded in Fig. 3-17, a reduction in partner acquisition rates in the core group will act to reduce prevalence in core and noncore groups. Overall, however, the degree of reduction in the prevalence of infection in the population will depend on the degree to which the magnitude of R_0 is decreased. Changes near to the boundary of persistance (R_0 just greater than unity in value) will have a much greater impact than similar changes when R_0 is large.[10,22]

Well-formulated frameworks for the study of transmission dynamics also provide a means by which costs and benefits of different intervention programs can be compared. This is of particular importance in developing countries, where resources for intervention are limited, and in the context of the possible development and introduction of new vaccines. For example, in the case of HIV-1, concern has been expressed over the appropriateness of developing vaccine candidates that may have low efficiency.[19] However, analyses based on the transmission dynamics of the virus suggest that such products can be of considerable value in areas where HIV-1 has spread extensively.[20] A different example is provided by hepatitis B and the desirability of introducing mass vaccination in low-prevalence countries such as the United Kingdom. In this case, the key issue is what type of program to introduce, namely, either mass vaccination of adolescents, targeted vaccination at STD clinic attendees, or mass infant immunization. Recent analyses suggest that, for the United Kingdom, the most cost-effective approach (number of carriers of infection prevented per vaccine dose) is vaccination of infants born to infected mothers after antenatal screening. However, they also reveal that benefits accrue slowly over time and depend sensitively on the vaccine coverage achieved. Mass vaccination of young adolescents is predicted to be much more beneficial in the shorter term because of the short delay before they become sexually active. The benefit of targeting infants born to infected mothers only appears in the longer term due to the long delay before they attain sexual maturity. Screening and immunization of STD clinic attendees have the most immediate effect. These results clearly indicate that interpretation of cost and benefit must be based on a clear definition of the time period on which assessment is to be based.[21]

A further question related to assessment of cost and benefit is that of the desirability of using multiple interventions at the same time to reduce the prevalence of a particular STD. In the case of gonorrhea, these might include education, screening, contact tracing, and treatment. At present, few analyses have been undertaken, but there is an urgent need to understand more about this issue, particularly in developing countries where resources are limited. Preliminary assessments of this problem reveal much complexity, where whether or not two interventions are synergistic, additive, or antagonistic depends cricitally on the details of the prevailing patterns of sexual behavior in the target community and the overall magnitude of R_0. However, in general, when R_0 is high prior to the introduction of interventions, analyses suggest that synergism is the most likely outcome. In other words, combining different methods of control will be cost-beneficial.[3,22]

CONCLUSIONS

Many factors control the rate of spread of STDs. They include those which determine the typical course of infection in an individual and those which determine transmission between people. The study of these factors within a unified framework provides the basis for understanding the transmission dynamics of any given STD, for interpreting the observed epidemiological pattern, and for the design and evaluation of control interventions. The past two decades have seen the development of theoretical frameworks to aid in this process, and today they provide an increasingly robust template for interpretation and prediction.

Although not addressed in this brief review, these templates are also beginning to shed insights into the generation and persistence of strain structure in infectious agent populations.[23] This aspect is of increasing importance with the recognition, via molecular epidemiological studies, that populations of infectious agents, including many STDs, contain many distinct antigenic variants or serotypes. In the study of pathogenesis, immunity, and vaccine design, antigenic variability is of major importance.

Perhaps the most important facet of STD epidemiology is the prevailing pattern of sexual behavior that determines transmission in defined populations. Many aspects of behavior are important, including rates of partner acquisition, concurrent partnerships, and type of sexual activity. In all cases, the most striking feature of behavioral surveys, independent of study community, is the great heterogeneity that pertains. Understanding the causes and consequences of this variability is key, both to the interpretation of epidemiological pattern and in the design of programs to control infection and disease.

References

1 Anderson RM, May RM: *Infectious Diseases of Humans: Dynamics and Control.* Oxford, Oxford University Press, 1991.

2 Dean M et al: Genetic restrictions of HIV-1 infection and progression to AIDS by a deletion allele of the CKR5 structural gene. *Science* 273: 1856–1862, 1996.

3 Garnett GP, Anderson RM: Sexually transmitted diseases and sexual behavior: Insights from mathematical models. *J Infect Dis* 174(2): S150–Sl6l, 1996.

4 Anderson RM: The Croonian Lecture. Populations, infectious disease and immunity: A very nonlinear world. *Philos Trans R Soc Lond [B]* 346:457–505, 1994.

5 Anderson RM, May RM: The population biology of the interaction between HIV-1 and HIV-2: Coexistence or competitive exclusion? *AIDS* 10:1663–1673, 1996.

6 Anderson RM: Epidemiology of HIV infection: Variable incubation plus infectious periods and heterogeneity in sexual activity. *J R Stat Soc [A]* 151:66–93, 1988.

7 Anderson RM, May RM: Epidemiological parameters of HIV transmission. *Nature* 333:514–519, 1988.

8 May RM, Anderson RM: Transmission dynamics of HIV infection. *Nature* 326:137–142, 1987.

9 Boily M-C, Anderson RM: Human immunodeficiency virus transmission and the role of other sexually transmitted diseases: measures of association and study design. *Sexually Transmitted Diseases* 23:313–332, 1996.

10 Garnett GP et al: Sexual mixing patterns of patients attending STD clinics. *J Sex Transm Dis* 23:248–257, 1996.

11 Aral SO et al: Demographic and behavioral concordance between sex partners: Effects of demographic and partnership characteristics, sexual behavior and infection status. *Sex Transm Dis* (in press).

12 Watts CH, May RM: The influence of concurrent partnerships on the dynamics of HIV/AIDS. *Math Biosci* 108:89–104, 1992.

13 Parker CG, Anderson RM: Concurrent sexual partnerships: Mathematical models of the transmission dynamics of HIV and the case reproductive number. *IMA J Math Appl Med Biol* (in press).

14 Parker CG, Anderson RM: Concurrent sexual partnerships: The significance of heterogeneities in the transmission probability of HIV. *AIDS* (in press).

15 Jacquez JA et al. Modeling and analyzing HIV transmission: The effect of contact patterns. *Math Biosci* 92:119–199, 1988.

16 Gupta S et al: Networks of sexual contacts: Implications for the pattern of spread of HIV. *AIDS* 3:807–817, 1989.

17 Coutinho RA et al: *The Amsterdam Cohort Studies on HIV Infection and AIDS.* Amsterdam, University of Amsterdam, 1996.

18 Grosskurth H et al: Impact of improved treatment of sexually transmitted diseases on HIV infection in rural Tanzania: Randomised controlled trial. *Lancet* 346:530–536, 1995.

19 Moore J, Anderson RM: The WHO and why of HIV vaccine trials. *Nature* 372:313–314, 1994.

20 Anderson RM, Garnett GP: Low-efficacy HIV vaccines: Potential for community-based intervention programmes. *Lancet* 348:1010–1014, 1996.

21 Williams JR et al: The transmission dynamics of hepatitis B in the U.K.: A mathematical model for evaluating costs and effectiveness of immunization programmes. *Epidemiol Infect* 116:71–89, 1996.

22 Garnett GP, Anderson RM: Strategies for limiting the spread of HIV in developing countries: Conclusions based on studies of the transmission dynamics of the virus. *J AIDS* 9:500–513, 1994.

23 Gupta S et al. The maintenance of strain structure in populations of recombining infectious agents. *Nature Med* 2:437–442, 1996.

Bibliography

Hendriks JCM, Medley GF, van Griensven GJP, Coutinho RA, Heisterkamp SM, & van Druten HAM. 1993. The treatment-free incubation period of AIDS in a cohort of homosexual men. *AIDS* 7:231–239.

Jacquez JA, Simon CP, Koopman J, Saftenspiel L, & Perry T. 1988. Modelling and analyzing HIV transmission: the effect of contact patterns. *Mathematical Biosciences* 92:119–199.

Johnson AM, Wadsworth J, Wellings K, & Field J. 1994. *Sexual Attitudes and Lifestyles.* Oxford:Blackwell Scientific Publications.

Laga M, Manoka A, Kivuvu M et al. 1993. Non-ulcerative sexually transmitted diseases as risk-factor for HIV-1 transmission in women. Results from a cohort study. *AIDS* 7:95–102.

Laumann EO, Gagnon JH, Michael RT, & Michaels S. 1994. *The social organization of sexuality: Sexual practices in the United States–Chicago.* The University of Chicago Press.

Mastro T & de Vincenzi I. 1996. Probabilities of sexual HIV-1 transmission. *AID* (suppl A): S75–S82.

May RM & Anderson RM. 1987. Transmission dynamics of HIV infection. *Nature* 326 (or 342):137–142.

Moore J & Anderson RM. 1994. The WHO and why of HIV vaccine trials. *Nature* 372:313–314.

Mulder DW, Nunn AJ, Wagner H-U, Kamali A, & Kengeya-Kayondo JF. 1994. HIV-incidence and HIV-1-associated mortality in a rural Ugandan population cohort. *AIDS* 8:87–92.

Parker CG & Anderson RM. 1997. Concurrent sexual partnerships: mathematical models of the transmission dynamics of HIV and the case reproductive number. *IMA Journal Mathematics Applied to Medicine & Biology.* (in press).

Parker CG & Anderson RM. 1997. Concurrent sexual partnerships: the significance of heterogeneities in the transmission probability of HIV. *AIDS* (in press).

Plummer FA, Simonsen JN, Ngugi EN et al. 1991. Cofactors in male-female sexual transmission of human immunodeficiency virus type 1. *Journal of Immunodeficiency* 163:233–239.

Watts CH & May RM. 1992. The influence of concurrent partnerships on the dynamics of HIV/AIDS. *Mathematical Biosciences* 108:89–104.

Williams JR, Nokes DJ, Medley GF, & Anderson RM. 1996. The transmission dynamics of Hepatitis B in the UK: a mathematical model for evaluating costs and effectiveness of immunization programmes. *Epidemiology and Infection* 116:71–89.

Chapter 4

Social and behavioral determinants of the epidemiology of STDs: Industrialized and developing countries

Sevgi O. Aral
King K. Holmes

INTRODUCTION

Dynamically changing demographic, economic, and cultural forces underlie the behaviors that directly determine the spread of STDs. In most industrialized countries, particularly those with strong economic and social welfare and health care infrastructures, the incidence of curable STDs such as gonorrhea and syphilis declined rapidly during the AIDS era among educated middle and upper classes. AIDS programs promoting behavior change and risk reduction, when combined with adequate access to services for early detection and treatment of STDs, have apparently been sufficient to control the curable STDs, if not the viral STDs. Some of these countries have eliminated endemic transmission of gonorrhea and syphilis in large areas, and now must focus on containing periodic reintroduction from higher prevalence areas within the country, or from other countries. In the United States, incidences of the same STDs have declined much more slowly, with large geographic regions and most large cities still experiencing high rates of endemic transmission of these infections among urban, poor, and minority populations, and with highest rates among sexually active adolescent females; local outbreaks of less common STD, such as chancroid, still occur within selected population groups of lower socioeconomic status, perhaps among those least likely to modify behaviors. During the 1990s, AIDS has increasingly shifted to these populations, as predicted by the National Academy of Sciences.[1] The relatively new phenomenon of sex in exchange for drugs has contributed to epidemics of gonorrhea, syphilis, chancroid, and HIV infection; and parenteral transmission of several STD pathogens (e.g., HIV, HBV) is closely linked to subsequent sexual transmission of these pathogens in the United States since the mid-1980s. In several industrialized or semi-industrialized countries, especially those of the former USSR, commercial sex has emerged as a major factor in STD transmission. In many of the developing countries, additional social problems—such as rampant population growth, rural to urban migration, work-related travel, growing economic inequity between the rich and the poor, low education and low status of women, political instability and wars—all result in behaviors that fuel the hyperendemic transmission of STDs, with continuing epidemic spread of the newest STDs, HIV infection.

EVOLVING CONCEPTS IN STD EPIDEMIOLOGY

Understanding of the epidemiology of STDs has continued to evolve rapidly since the second version of this chapter was prepared in the late 1980s. Increasingly, attention has focused on underlying socioeconomic and cultural determinants of STDs in entire populations, and on dynamic patterns of the spread of infection through sexual networks and through populations. As discussed in Chapter 3, the three direct determinants of the rate of spread of each sexually transmissible pathogen are: (1) probability of exposure of susceptible to infectious persons; (2) the mean efficiency of sexual transmission when such exposures occur; and (3) the mean duration of infectiousness of individuals who become infected. Increasingly, efforts to understand the dynamics of transmission have focused on the factors that influence these three component determinants of transmission.

EXPOSURE OF SUSCEPTIBLE TO INFECTED PERSONS

National surveys of sexual behavior in the United Kingdom, France, and the United States have revealed that, at any point in time, the great majority of the population does not engage in high-risk sexual behaviors, even though many individuals go through life stages during which they do.[2–4] These surveys also showed considerable variation in sexual behaviors across local populations. A recent comparison of the British and American surveys revealed similarities in mean numbers of sexual partners, but greater polarization of sexual behaviors and attitudes in the United States.[5] The proportion reporting a large number of partners and few or no partners was greater in the United States than in the United Kingdom. The authors hypothesized that those with the highest number of partners accounted for higher incidence rates of STDs and HIV in the United States, where the polarization of sexual behaviors was associated with polarization in attitudes towards sexuality that impeded STD/AIDS prevention efforts.

Surveys of sexual behaviors in developing countries undertaken by the World Health Organization, and by the Demographic and Health Surveys, show widely differing patterns of sexual behavior in different regions of the world.[6,7] Other population-based studies including those in San Francisco, Uganda, and Thailand, have indicated, respectively, patterns of sexual mixing to be potential risk factors for HIV infection, concurrent partnerships (as opposed to sequential "serial monogamy") to increase the rate of spread of sexually transmitted infections, and bridge populations to spread infection from high to low prevalence subgroups within a population.[8–11] Models of STD transmission dynamics, population-based sexual behavior data, and findings of earlier STDs and HIV partner notification studies all highlight the importance of sexual mixing patterns (or networks), and of the "high" extreme of the sexual activity distribution (so-called "tails" of the distribution, representing those with largest numbers of partners) in determining the epidemiology of STDs.[5] These developments are consistent with the importance of "core groups," in maintaining endemic and epidemic transmission of curable STDs, which has been central to the conceptual framework for the epidemiology of STD transmission. The sexual networks that both fuel and channel the spread of STDs, and the social networks through which risk-enhancing or preventive behaviors diffuse, presumably undergo changes, both separately and in their interaction with each other, as STD epidemics progress through different phases.

EFFICIENCY OF TRANSMISSION PER EXPOSURE

Determinants of efficiency of sexual transmission include host susceptibility, the infectious virulence of the pathogen (e.g., the 50 percent infection dose, or ID_{50}, assuming host susceptibility is held constant), and the amount or concentration of pathogens shed in semen or genital fluids, which in turn is related to the natural history of infection. The type of sexual exposure (i.e., sexual practices), also indirectly influence susceptibility, operating through host susceptibility, which varies according to the anatomic site exposed. Similarly, the "infectivity" of the infected person, operates through the inoculum size delivered and the infectious virulence of the pathogen, both of which may vary in different stages of infection.

DURATION OF INFECTIVITY

The duration of infectivity is also based on the natural history of each type of infection, as well as on the intrinsic efficacy and use-effectiveness (including population coverage, uptake, and adherence with the required dosage schedule) of chemotherapeutic or immunity-enhancing approaches to shortening this duration.

Prevention interventions can operate on more than one of the preceding determinants of transmission. For example, vaccines or acquired immunity can produce absolute immunity to infection, thereby decreasing the number of susceptibles in the population and decreasing exposure of susceptibles to infecteds; can create partial immunity to infection, thereby decreasing the efficiency of transmission, especially for low inoculum exposures; or could simply attenuate infection, allowing infection to occur on exposure, but shortening the duration of infectivity, and perhaps decreasing the inoculum size and efficiency of subsequent transmission to a new partner.

TIMING, INTENSITY, AND TARGETING OF PREVENTIVE INTERVENTIONS

Increasingly, changes in STD rates and their determinants are understood within a framework of time-dependent mutual interaction between the spread of a specific STD and the efforts developed to prevent it. Very small but early beginnings can have large scale impact both in the spread of STDs and in their prevention. Because of the product of the three determinants of transmission must reach a critical threshold before an STD pathogen can spread within a population, even a trivial reduction in one or more of the determinants could, in theory, drop the reproductive rate of spread below that threshold, and ultimately eliminate the pathogen from the population. In the infected individual, the antimicrobial susceptibility of the pathogen, the rate at which the pathogen replicates itself, and the activity and half-life of the antibiotic, determine the choice, dose, and timing of antibiotic therapy. Similarly, in preventing spread of STDs in populations, the mean duration and mean efficiency of transmission of the infection, the density of affected sexual networks, and the effectiveness of preventive interventions, determine the intensity, mix, schedule, and target of preventive interventions required. Cost-effectiveness modeling repeatedly indicates that compared to interventions for the general population, targeted interventions that focus on core groups have greater impact and are most cost-effective.[12–15]

The general inadequacy of STD health care services in the United States, suggests the contribution of inadequate STD services to STD morbidity in populations.[16] Data now accumulating on STD related health care-seeking indicate the role of health behaviors on duration of infectiousness, and hence, on STD epidemiology (see Chap. 93).

DIFFERENCES AND SIMILARITIES IN THE EPIDEMIOLOGY OF BACTERIAL AND VIRAL STDs

Our understanding of the epidemiology of viral STDs had changed markedly from the mid-1970s to the mid-1980s. Epidemic increases in clinically apparent symptomatic genital herpes and genital warts and in sexually transmitted hepatitis B virus infection in industrialized countries preceded the current HIV epidemic. During the 1980s, improved tests for type-specific serum antibody to HSV-2; detection of type-specific HPV DNA and antibody to HPV; application of tests for HIV antibody, for quantitating HIV viral load, and for differentiating HIV subtypes have led to clinical epidemiologic studies that disclose a greatly expanded scope of infections with these incurable viral STDs. Such studies are beginning to give a clearer picture of the distribution and determinants of these infections. Research on the natural history of these three infections over the past several years has improved our understanding of their epidemiology (see Chaps. 21 and 25), and now permits comparison with the natural history and epidemiology of the major bacterial STDs.

Sexual transmission also contributes substantially to the overall transmission of cytomegalovirus, and HTLV-1, and also may contribute to the transmission of hepatitis C virus, human herpes virus type-8, and HTLV-II, but much more extensive research on the natural history and epidemiology of these as sexually transmitted pathogens is required. Specific chapters in this book consider the epidemiology of these pathogens.

The natural history of infection for the bacterial and viral STDs shows some general differences, as well as similarities. Strategies employed by various bacterial and viral STD pathogens to evade the human immune response must be especially important (see Chaps. 13 and 15). Because these pathogens require intimate personal contact for transmission, and often depend on core groups of heavily exposed individuals to sustain their propagation, they could not survive if they induced solid long-lasting immunity in a large proportion of core group members. Two of the bacterial STD pathogens *(N. gonorrhoeae, C. trachomatis),* have evolved into multiple antigenic variants, each can eventually be eliminated by a host immune response, but without inducing immunity to other antigenic variants, so that even heavily exposed individuals (e.g., sex workers), remain highly susceptible to variants they have not yet encountered. Mechanisms used by *H. ducreyi* and *T. pallidum* to persist in the population, and by *T. pallidum* to persist in the individual, are not yet well understood. Most viral STD pathogens (e.g., HSV, HIV, HBV, HTLV, HPV, CMV) have developed strategies for very prolonged persistence in a varying proportion of infected hosts, giving a long duration of potential infectivity. Current research aims to develop vaccines against *N. gonorrhoeae* and *C. trachomatis* that can prevent infection with all or most antigenic variants of these organisms; and also aims to better understand and prevent or eliminate the chronic persistence of viral STD pathogens.

The emergence of viral STDs has prompted reappraisal of the relative importance of sexual behavior, use of contraceptives (or barrier prophylaxis), and health behaviors, in the epidemiology of STDs. In particular, until recently, health care-seeking behaviors, and early diagnosis and treatment, have been important determinants only of the incidence of the curable STDs. In the future, more effective antiviral regimens may become potentially important in preventing transmission of viral STDs, such as HIV and HSV; and vaccination should eventually have a greater impact on sexual transmission of HBV.

The efficiency of transmission of most if not all bacterial and viral STDs peaks in the early stages of infection, because genital shedding and infectivity are at peak levels (teleologically, this is a survival strategy for the pathogens). The rate of transmission is high early in infection for another reason: To the extent that rapid partner change occurs only intermittently during the lifecycle of an individual, those periods when individuals acquire an STD are also periods when they are most likely to transmit—so that rates of exposure to other susceptible people tend to be relatively high for those who are newly infected. Thus, although strategies for control of viral STDs have largely depended on societal efforts at changing sexual and protective behaviors through health education and changing behavioral norms of the general public, and through individualized counseling of the clinically infected carrier, a new perspective also emphasizes the importance of early detection and treatment of viral STDs where resources allow, together with vaccine development and promotion, and research on ways to interrupt chronic infection.

Essentially, there is a continuum from those STDs that are most preventable by biomedical interventions because of availability of vaccine (hepatitis B), to those most readily controlled by early detection and treatment (e.g., chancroid and syphilis); to those containable by curative treatment only where resources for detection are also available (e.g., gonorrhea, chlamydia), to those that potentially may become less transmissible when resources are available both for early detection and for suppressive therapy (e.g., HSV and possibly HIV), to those for which currently available medical interventions offer little promise in preventing transmission, and the major hope for prevention lies in vaccine development (e.g., HPV).

Similarly, there is a continuum in the extent to which spread of various STDs requires very high rates of partner change and unprotected exposure to new partners, and therefore in the relative susceptibility of various STDs to decreases in rates of partner change or to condom use within core groups. Those that appear very dependent on high rates of partner change include chancroid, syphilis, and HIV; although those that appear not to require high rates of partner change, and that may therefore be slower to respond to behavioral interventions targeting core groups, include HSV, and HPV. At the present time these two viral STDs are less concentrated in core groups and more widely spread across a variety of socioeconomic and racial–ethnic categories in populations. Thus, in developing countries, the absence of resources needed for diagnosis of chlamydial infection or gonorrhea in women makes these diseases more analogous to the incurable viral STDs, and prevention of most STDs in such countries has largely depended on societal efforts at health education and behavior change.

HISTORY OF STD EPIDEMIOLOGY AND THE EVOLVING LEVEL OF EVIDENCE

As indicated above, our understanding of the epidemiology of STDs has evolved steadily during the past half century (Fig. 4-1). As data accumulated, approaches to study design changed, and the nature of the major hypotheses reflected these changes. In addition, the multifactorial nature of the STD problem increasingly necessitated multidisciplinary approaches. Essentially, the field of STD epidemiology evolved from careful clinical observations and case studies of microbial etiology, and descriptions of prevalence and distribution of morbidity based on surveillance data (descriptive epidemiology) throughout the 1950s; to studies of risk factors associated with specific diseases and their complications in individuals (analytic epidemiology), particularly since the early 1970s; to studies of population transmission dynamics and cost-effectiveness analyses, particularly since the early 1980s; and to prevention trials including randomized controlled trials (RCTs) of prevention first at the individual, and later at the community level, during the 1990s. The CONSORT statement for improving the quality of reporting results of randomized controlled trials is now influencing not only the reporting, but also the design and conduct of such trials.[17] Interestingly, early intervention trials focused first almost exclusively on vaccines or on behavioral interventions, for both individuals and communities, and most of the behavioral trials did not emphasize changing the behaviors of those already infected with chronic STDs, or changing health care-seeking behavior, and few addressed changing the behaviors of health care professionals. However, as more biomedical interventions become available, attention has shifted to RCTs of biomedical interventions at both individual and community levels, and to improving health care-seeking behaviors and the behaviors of care providers.

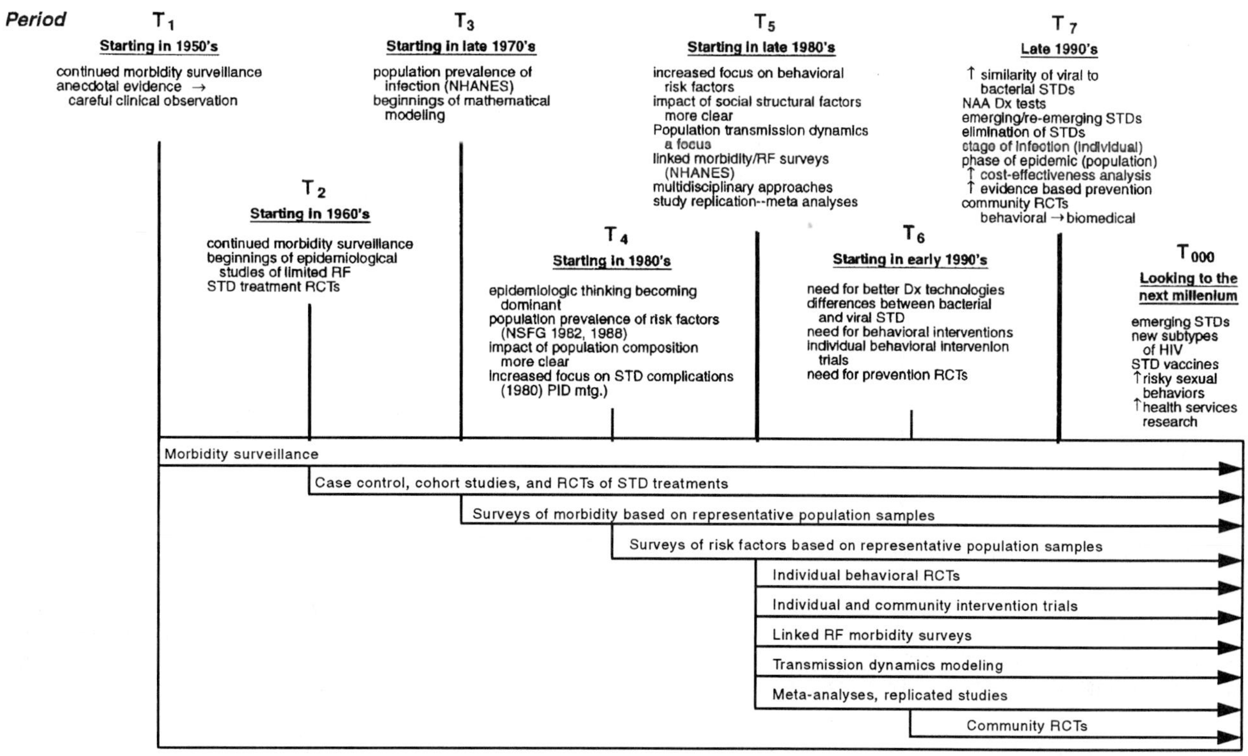

Fig. 4-1. History of STDs epidemiology and the evolving level of evidence.

Table 4-1. Estimated Number of New STDs (in Millions) in 1995 in Adults between Ages of 15 and 49, for All Regions of the World

	Syphilis		Gonorrhea		Chlamydia		Trichomoniasis	
	Males	Females	Males	Females	Males	Females	Males	Females
North America	0.072	0.072	0.83	0.92	1.64	2.34	3.78	4.23
Western Europe	0.10	0.10	0.60	0.63	2.30	3.20	5.30	5.76
Australasia	0.005	0.005	0.063	0.069	0.12	0.17	0.29	0.32
Latin America and the Caribbean	0.56	0.70	3.45	3.67	5.01	5.12	8.52	9.10
Sub-Saharan Africa	1.56	1.97	7.30	8.38	6.96	8.44	15.07	15.35
North Africa and Middle East	0.28	0.33	0.77	0.77	1.67	1.28	2.32	2.22
Eastern Europe and Central Asia	0.050	0.050	1.17	1.16	2.15	2.92	4.9	5.17
East Asia and Pacific	0.26	0.30	1.80	1.47	2.70	2.63	4.83	4.53
South and South East Asia	2.66	3.13	14.56	14.55	20.2	20.28	39.59	35.87
Overall	5.55	6.66	30.54	31.62	42.75	46.38	84.60	82.55

FROM: Gerbase AC et al: Global prevalence and incidence estimates of selected curable STDs. *Sex Transm Infect* 74(Suppl 1):S15.

As methodology evolved, awareness of the importance of study replication has increased; with the appearance of meta-analyses of the STD literature, and existing or newly planned Cochran Collaboration Groups for infectious diseases, AIDS, and STDs, demand for stronger evidence of efficacy of preventive interventions has also accelerated.[18]

The rest of this chapter is organized along the lines of this evolution of understanding of STD epidemiology and the level of evidence; then explores trends in the social and demographic correlates and determinants of STDs; and concludes with a discussion of implications for the future.

DESCRIPTIVE EPIDEMIOLOGY OF SELECTED STDS AND SEXUALLY TRANSMITTED INFECTIONS

Subsequent chapters of this book describe the epidemiology of the various STDs and STD pathogens in detail. This chapter focuses on cross-cutting comparisons, that illustrate general or differing aspects of STD epidemiology. Not all STDs are reportable, and even reportable diseases are seldom reported completely. Data from most of the world are sketchy, occasionally based on prospective cohort studies of incidence, or on serially repeated prevalence surveys, but more often based on sporadic prevalence surveys, or solely on anecdotes. Populations sampled in developing societies most often have included STD clinic patients or family planning clinic patients, who are not representative of the total population; and less often prenatal or primary care clinics or other more representative population samples. Prenatal samples generally best represent fertile married women of reproductive age who seek prenatal care; they often underrepresent the single women who are at highest risk, and underrepresent women rendered infertile or sub-fertile by past or present STDs, including HIV infection and they underrepresent women without access to acceptable hospital-based care. Thus, a detailed review of the descriptive epidemiology of STDs in individual developing countries is beyond the scope of this chapter. A good source for several recent studies of the prevalence of STDs in various populations in developing countries is provided in the supplement on Syndromic Management of STDs, published in *Sexually Transmitted Infections* (74[Suppl 1]: S1-S178, 1998). Also from that volume is an update from the World Health Organization on the estimated number of cases and annual incidence of syphilis, gonorrhea, chlamydial infections, and trichomoniasis, based on the prevalence of STDs from various populations in clinical surveys, and the estimated mean duration (D) of infection for each of these STDs with incidence = [prevalence/(1-prevalence)] × (1/D). (Tables 4-1 and 4-2). The overall estimated number of new cases of these four STDs per year for males and females ages 15 to 49 totaled 333 million, with 12.2 million cases of syphilis, 62.2 million of gonorrhea, 89.1 million of chlamydial infections, and 167.2 million cases of trichomoniasis. These estimates suggest that 90 percent of these STDs are in developing countries.

In general, data on reported STDs from North America and many countries of Europe, as well as from Australia and New Zealand showed steady increases in the incidence of all STDs during the 1960s, with leveling off or decline of most of the bacterial STDs but continual increases in viral STDs and genital chlamydial infections during the 1970s and 1980s. The incidence of gonorrhea and syphilis began to decline at different times, and declined

Table 4-2. Estimated Annual Incidence Rate of New STDs (per 1000) in Adults between the Ages of 15 and 49*

	Syphilis		Gonorrhea		Chlamydia		Trichomoniasis	
	Males	Females	Males	Females	Males	Females	Males	Females
North America	0.094	0.094	10.85	12.04	21.46	30.73	49.36	55.42
Western Europe	0.94	0.94	5.59	6.01	21.46	30.73	49.36	55.42
Australasia	0.94	0.94	10.85	12.04	21.46	30.73	49.36	55.42
Latin America and the Caribbean	4.48	5.59	27.56	29.23	40.03	40.77	68.05	72.45
Sub-Saharan Africa	12.33	15.39	57.71	65.47	55.04	65.95	119.18	119.91
North Africa and Middle East	3.37	4.24	9.15	9.76	19.93	16.29	27.59	28.20
Eastern Europe and Central Asia	0.63	0.63	14.83	14.67	27.29	37.09	62.13	65.66
East Asia and Pacific	0.63	0.78	4.35	3.79	6.53	6.75	11.68	11.65
South and South East Asia	5.48	6.85	30.03	31.80	41.65	44.32	81.63	78.41

*For all regions of the world.

FROM: Gerbase AC et al: Global prevalence and incidence estimates of selected curable STDs. *Sex Transm Infect* 1998 74(Suppl 1):S15.

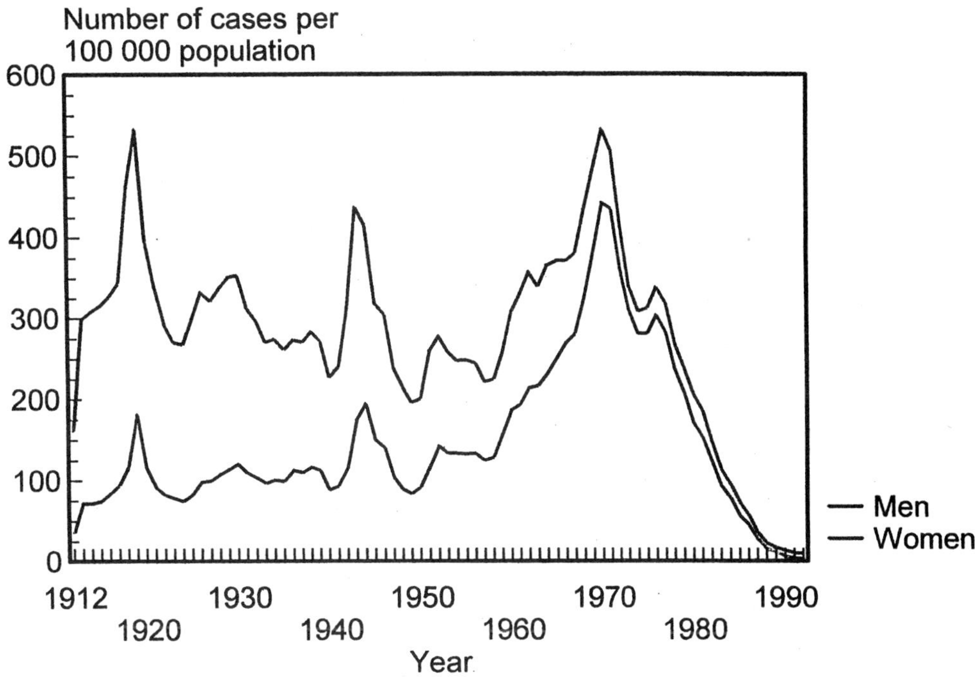

Fig. 4-2. Trends in incidence of gonorrhea in Sweden by gender 1912–1995. Note the steady decline in the ratio of male : female cases during most of this period, and the precipitous drop in incidence in both sexes, beginning in 1970 (data provided by D. Danielsson).

at differing rates, in these industrialized countries. The sex ratio of males to females with bacterial STDs has declined for several decades. Gonorrhea and syphilis have continued to decline during the 1990s, and chlamydial infections have begun declining in Nordic countries, and in those areas of the United States and Canada and elsewhere where chlamydia control programs have been initiated. In the Southern Hemisphere, a few regions doing relatively well economically (e.g., Costa Rica, Thailand, and Harare, Zimbabwe) have experienced declining rates of bacterial STDs during the 1990s. In contrast, some countries are experiencing explosive epidemics of bacterial STDs (e.g., China, Mongolia, and Russia and the Newly Independent States of the former USSR), and many countries in Eastern Europe, Southern Africa, and Asia continue to experience epidemic increases in HIV infection.[19–21]

GONORRHEA

Trends in industrialized countries

The major bacterial STDs include gonorrhea, chlamydial infection, syphilis, and in many developing countries, chancroid. In Sweden (Fig. 4-2), where long-term data are available, several periods of increased gonorrhea rates coincided roughly with World Wars I and II, and with the "sexual revolution" of the 1960s and

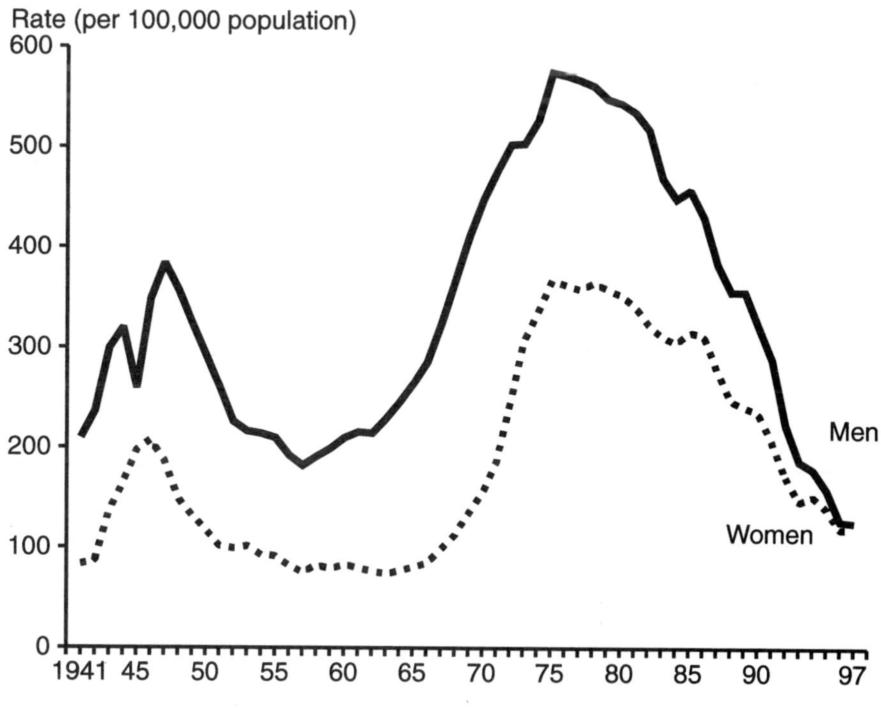

Fig. 4-3. Trends in incidence of reported gonorrhea by gender, United States, 1941–1997 (provided by R. Roegner, CDC).

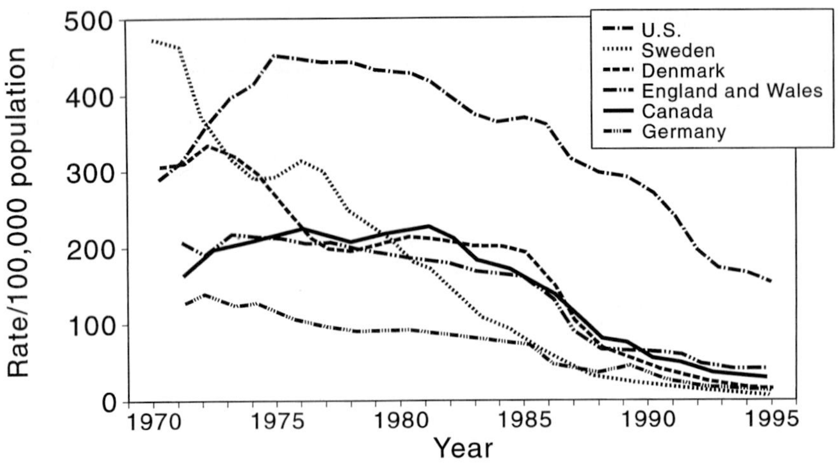

Fig. 4-4. Comparisons of trends in the number of cases of reported gonorrhea in industrialized countries, 1970–1995.

1970s. An extraordinary decline in the incidence of reported gonorrhea per 100,000 population then followed—from an all time peak of 974 cases in 1970 to 62 cases in 1987 to four cases in 1996. Gonorrhea has become a rare and largely imported disease in Sweden. The male : female sex ratio for gonorrhea also declined throughout much of this century, but accelerated in the 1960s and 1970s with the use of selective culture media for isolation of *Neisseria gonorrhoeae* and with partner notification, both of which led to increasing detection of infected women during the 1960s and 1970s. This occurred simultaneously with the "sexual liberation" of women coinciding with the advent of oral contraception in the 1960s; and with decreasing rates of STDs in homosexual men during the AIDS era.

In the United States (Fig. 4-3), the incidence of reported gonorrhea increased during World War II, peaked in 1946, then decreased until 1957, and subsequently increased again for nearly two decades. From 1962 through 1975, the incidence increased steadily at about 15 percent per year, peaking at 473 per 100,000 in 1975, then declining at an accelerating pace to 324 per 100,000 in 1987, 247 per 100,000 in 1991, 149 per 100,000 in 1995, and 124 in 1996—the lowest ever since the beginning of World War II.[22] In 1987, the number of cases reported from public STD clinics (526,000) was over twice as high as the number reported by private providers (255,000). The proportion reported from STD clinics has been declining somewhat in recent years, with only 51.6 percent reported from STD clinics in 1996; for women nearly two-thirds of gonorrhea cases were reported from non-STD clinic sources. The male : female ratio of reported incidence initially increased to over 3 : 1 by 1966, then declined rapidly to about 1.5 : 1 by 1973, and remained rather constant at that level through 1987. By 1992 the male to female ratio had dropped to 1.3 and by 1996 it was 1.1.

Comparisons of trends in the incidence of gonorrhea in industrialized countries are shown in Fig. 4-4. Gonorrhea incidence per 100,000 population had fallen to 31.5 by 1994 in the United Kingdom; and to 18.6 in Canada by 1995. Overall rates of reported gonorrhea in the United States in 1995 were 22.4 times those in Sweden, 7.8 times those in Canada, and 4.6 times those of the United Kingdom. This under-estimates the true differences in rates, because smaller proportions—perhaps only about half of the cases of gonorrhea occurring in the United States—are reported.

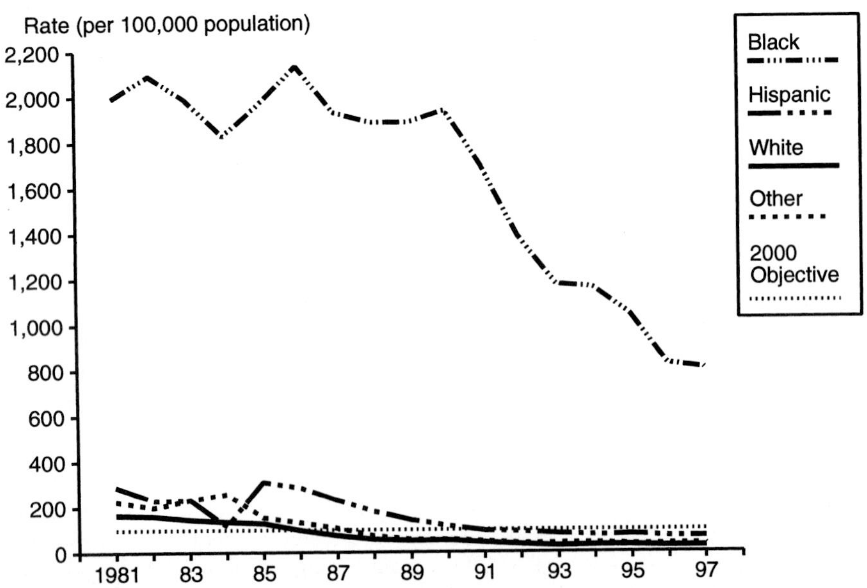

Note: "Other" includes Asian/Pacific Islander and American Indian/Alaska Native populations. Georgia was excluded in 1994.

Fig. 4-5. Trends in reported gonorrhea per 100,000 population by race and ethnicity, United States, 1981–1997. Trends in reported cases in part reflect trends in reporting. Because reporting by private sources is incomplete, shifts in health care utilization from public to private sources may mask increases or exaggerate apparent decreases in disease incidence (provided by R. Roegner, CDC).

Influence of sociodemographic factors on gonorrhea morbidity in the United States

The incidence and trends in incidence of reported gonorrhea cases in the United States differ by racial group. Between 1975 and 1984, the annual incidence of reported gonorrhea declined less among white women (8.9 percent decline) and white men (13.6 percent) than among men and women of other races (19.2 and 18.3 percent, respectively). Trends after 1984 reversed this picture; the race differential between whites and blacks grew between 1984 and 1987 (Fig. 4-5). In 1996, the incidence of reported gonorrhea per 100,000 was 826 among black non-Hispanics, 106 among American Indian/Alaskan Natives, 69 among Hispanics, 26 among white non-Hispanics, and 18.6 among Asian/Pacific Islanders. Among 15- to 19-year-old African-American non-Hispanics, the 1996 reported gonorrhea incidence was 3,791 per 100,000—the highest age, gender, and race ethnicity-adjusted rates in the United States.[22]

In the United States gonorrhea incidence has also been strongly associated with socioeconomic status (SES) and residence. For example, in 1986 and 1987 in Seattle, Washington, census tracts representing the lowest SES quartile accounted for 58 percent of reported gonorrhea.[23] Data from the Gonococcal Isolate Surveillance Project (GISP) in the United States suggests a further concentration of morbidity among core transmitters as rates decline.[24] As rates of gonorrhea and pelvic inflammatory disease decline in many local areas, morbidity becomes concentrated in low SES core groups residing in low SES areas.[25] A recent analysis of gonorrhea morbidity in United States cities with greater than 200,000 population showed that six factors accounted for 75 percent of the variation in gonorrhea morbidity in these cities: population density, percent households with female heads, city government general expenditure per capita, violent crime rate, percent of families below poverty level, and percent of births to mothers younger than 20.[26]

Gonorrhea incidence among men who have sex with men (MSM), which had declined remarkably in response to the HIV epidemic, has started increasing in discrete local areas in the recent past. Between 1993 and 1996 the annual number of patients with urethral, pharyngeal, and/or rectal gonorrhea increased by 82 percent from 74 to 139, at a clinic serving MSM in Washington, D.C. At the same clinic the percent of gonorrhea patients tested for HIV who were HIV-positive increased from 23 to 43 percent.[27] In addition the GISP surveillance data show that urethral gonorrhea among MSM has been increasing in several cities on the West Coast and in Denver.[28]

Recent trends in antimicrobial resistance in *N. gonorrhoeae*

In the United States, beta-lactamase-producing strains of *N. gonorrhoeae* were first isolated in 1976. Initially, the reported numbers of such strains remained stable at less than 100 cases per year, and most cases were linked to overseas travel or military importation. In 1980, however, beta-lactamase-producing strains started to increase; the total number of reported cases exceeded 4500 by 1982. This early increase may have reflected the spread of such strains in developing countries, and continued importation from endemic areas such as Korea, the Philippines, and Africa. Eventually, however, beta-lactamase-producing gonococci became entrenched in some communities, and the number of reported cases began to increase sharply after 1984.[29] In retrospect, this might have been partly attributable to adaptive stabilization of beta-lactamase plasmids in *N. gonorrhoeae*. By 1987 the number of reported beta-lactamase-positive isolates had reached 16,608 per year, and accounted for 1.8 percent of all reported gonorrhea: 64 percent of cases occurred in the three areas previously identified as hyperendemic: Florida, New York City, and Los Angeles.[30,31] As the incidence of infections with beta-lactamase-producing strains of *N. gonorrhoeae* increased, the epidemiology changed: overseas travel and contact with female sex workers (FSWs) were identified as important risk factors in early outbreaks; but once beta-lactamase-producing gonococci became endemic, their distribution came to parallel that of endemic, antibiotic-sensitive gonorrhea, predominantly involving inner-city residents, members of ethnic minority groups, and heterosexuals.[31,32] For example, in an outbreak of approximately 200 cases of gonorrhea caused by a unique beta-lactamase-positive strain of *N. gonorrhoeae* in Seattle, the first cases predominantly involved Caucasian and Hispanic men with a history of contact with female sex workers; after a few months, most cases occurred in heterosexual black men and women, most of whom gave histories of commercial sex or illegal drug use.[33] Even though homosexual men are at high risk for gonococcal infections, outbreaks of beta-lactamase-producing strains among homosexual men have been rare.

During the 1990s, levels of gonococcal antimicrobial resistance in the United States have been generally stable, with about one-third of isolates resistant to penicillin or tetracycline, higher than in some other industrialized countries.[34] The recent emergence of reduced susceptibility to ciprofloxacin has been a new concern. Among men attending one clinic in Cleveland, Ohio, reduced susceptibility to ciprofloxacin increased from 2 percent in 1991 to 16 percent in 1994.[35] The overall proportion of gonococci isolated in the GISP with intermediate susceptibility (minimal inhibiting concentration .125 to 0.5 mg ciprofloxacin/mL) or resistance (MIC^{3} 1.0 mg/ml) declined somewhat during 1995 to 1997, although strains with high-level fluoroquinolone resistance have been isolated sporadically.[36] Fluoroquinolone-resistant strains remain uncommon in Latin America, Africa, and Europe as well, at least up to the late 1990s. However, in southeast Asia and the western Pacific, gonococcal fluoroquinolone resistance has rapidly emerged as a major problem. For example, in the Philippines, high level resistance (MIC^{3} 4 mg ciprofloxacin/mL) appeared during 1996 in a high proportion of isolates from FSW, and was associated with a high rate of failure to respond to a single oral dose of ciprofloxacin 500 mg.[37] A history of self-initiated antimicrobial prophylaxis was found associated with infection with ciprofloxacin-resistant gonococci.[38]

SYPHILIS

Trends in industrialized countries

Syphilis may fluctuate in incidence more dramatically than gonorrhea as sexual behaviors change. For example, the incidence of primary and secondary syphilis rose sharply in both sexes in Sweden during World Wars I and II (Fig. 4-6). Following World War I, the incidence of syphilis fell rapidly, coinciding with the increased availability of improved diagnostic tests and the arsenicals. After a brief rise in incidence during World War II, the incidence fell again, coinciding with the introduction of penicillin. The incidence rose again during the sexual revolution of the early 1960s, and unlike gonorrhea, continued to increase after 1970, with epidemic spread among MSM until the recognition of AIDS in 1981. The incidence of syphilis per 100,000 population in Sweden then fell to 0.8 in 1995. The decline in the male : female ratio from the early 1900s, from a range of about 2.5 : 1 in the early 1900s to a range of about 1.5 to 1 from the mid-1940s to the mid-1950s, was less dramatic for syphilis than for gonorrhea.

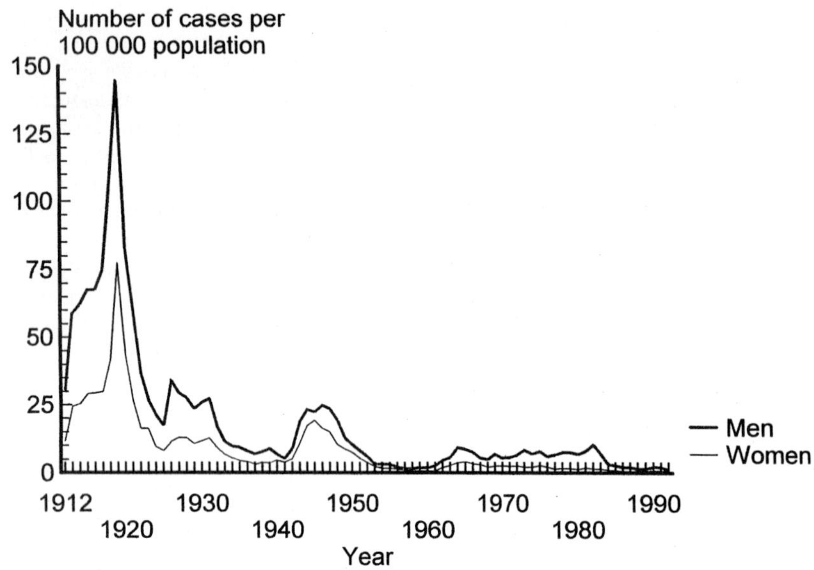

Fig. 4-6. Trends in the incidence of reported primary and secondary syphilis by gender in Sweden, 1912–1995 (data provided by D. Danielsson).

Thereafter, a dramatic reversal of this trend occurred, reaching a peak male : female ratio of 6.5 : 1 in 1982, then falling sharply again after recognition of the AIDS epidemic, and adoption of safer sex practices by MSM.

In the United States, the incidence of primary and secondary syphilis rose during World War II, reaching a peak of 76 cases per 100,000 in 1947, then (as in Sweden) fell to a nadir of about four per 100,000 for 1955 to 1958 (Fig. 4-7). In 1959 the trend reversed, and the incidence rose rapidly in men and women, to 12 per 100,000 in 1965, triple the level of a decade earlier. Factors considered responsible at the time included declining federal, state, and local appropriations for venereal disease control (federal dollar expenditures alone dropped from 17 million to 3 million annually in 1955); a de-emphasis on syphilis in medical teaching (e.g., in 1955, the phrase "and syphilology" was dropped from the *"AMA Archives of Dermatology and Syphilology")*; and a shift in management of syphilis from the public health clinic to the private office, with the availability of penicillin. From 1965 through 1982 the ratio of male : female cases increased steadily.

From 1982 through 1986, reflecting AIDS-related behavior change among homosexual and bisexual men, the reported national primary and secondary syphilis incidence in men dropped steadily from 22.5 cases per 100,000 to 16.2 per 100,000, whereas rates in females changed little. However, from 1985 to 1990, unlike the situation in Sweden, the incidence of primary and secondary syphilis increased sharply and unexpectedly in both men and women in the United States. A sharp rise in the number of reported cases of primary and secondary syphilis among black men and women accounted for most of this increase, with sporadic, local syphilis outbreaks contributing substantially to this national morbidity. Interestingly, these outbreaks occurred in areas where earlier outbreaks of chancroid had occurred, and where heterosexual HIV seropositivity rates were highest, such as New York, Los Angeles, some areas in Texas, and in south Florida, all areas where crack-cocaine use and exchange of sex for drugs had become common.

Levels of primary and secondary syphilis morbidity per 100,000 in the United States have subsequently fallen dramatically, from 23.5 in men and 17.3 in women in 1990 to 3.6 among men and 2.9 among women in 1997. Even in the south, which has con-

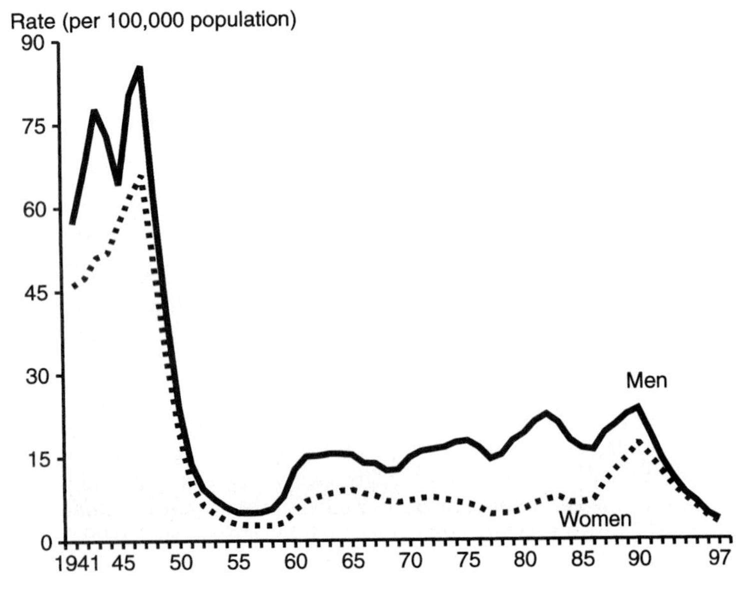

Fig. 4-7. Trends in incidence of reported primary and secondary syphilis by gender, United States, 1941–1997 (provided by R. Roegner, CDC).

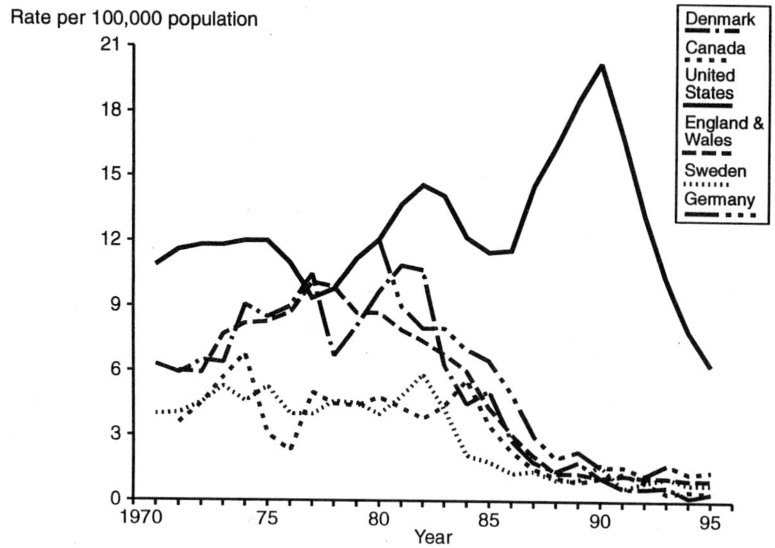

Fig. 4-8. Comparisons of trends in the number of cases of reported primary and secondary syphilis in industrialized countries, 1970–1995.

sistently reported greater morbidity than other regions, from 1990 to 1995 the syphilis rate decline by 80 percent. The male to female ratio of syphilis cases has been approaching 1.0.

Comparison of recent primary and secondary syphilis trends in selected industrialized countries from 1970 through 1995 are shown in Fig. 4-8. Trends in Canada have paralleled those observed in Sweden, with peak rates in 1980, and a continuous fall since then, and no transient increase in the late 1980s when the crack cocaine epidemic was essentially limited to the United States. As of 1995, primary and secondary syphilis rates per 100,000 population were 4.4 per 100,000 in the United States, 1.4 in Germany, 1.0 in England and Wales, 0.8 in Sweden, 0.4 in Denmark, and 0.4 in Canada.

Eastern Europe has experienced an explosive outbreak of STDs, including HIV infection, since the fall of the "iron curtain" in 1990. This is best documented for syphilis. For example, in the Russian Federation, the annual number of reported cases of syphilis increased steadily from 7911 in 1990 to 392,616 in 1997, a 50-fold increase (Fig. 4-9)! The number of cases of congenital syphilis in the Russian Federation increased from 15 in 1990 to 470 in 1996. although these data could be influenced by changes in the numbers of people tested, or in the numbers reported, ongoing surveillance of seven occupational groups also documented striking increases in the prevalence of syphilis seroreactivity (Fig. 4-10). The test used in the occupational screening program is known in Russia as the "express test"—a cardiolipin test analogous to the VDRL; positive reactions are confirmed by FTA tests. Large syphilis epidemics have also been seen in the Baltic States, and are ongoing in Belarus, the Republic of Moldova, Ukraine, and several Central Asian countries, especially Kazakhystan and Kyrgyzstan.

With the resurgence of syphilis in eastern Europe and migration of sex workers across borders into western Europe, syphilis has increasingly become an imported disease in western Europe. For example, in Finland, during 1997, 85 percent of 147 early syphilis cases were imported from Russia, and 10 percent from Latvia.

Influence of sociodemographic factors on syphilis morbidity in the United States

Data on sex preference, available on a national basis only through 1982, showed that the proportion of U.S. men with primary and secondary syphilis who named other men as sex partners had increased from 23 percent in 1969 to 42 percent in 1982. In the state of Washington, the proportion of men with primary and

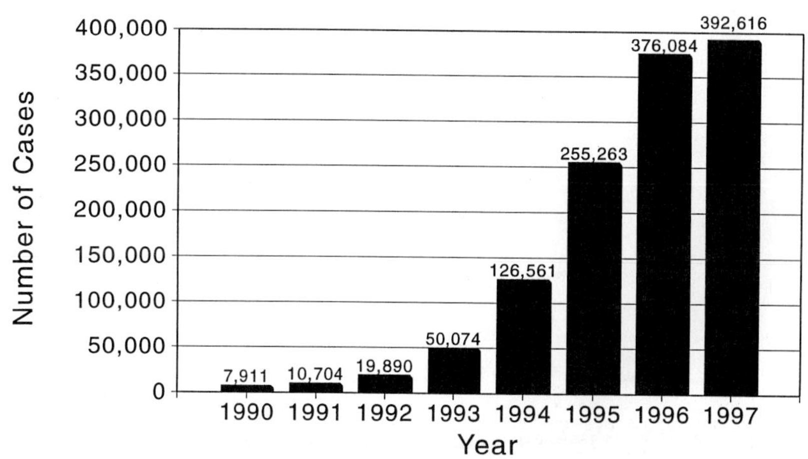

Fig. 4-9. Trends in annual number of reported cases of syphilis in the Russian Federation, 1990–1997.

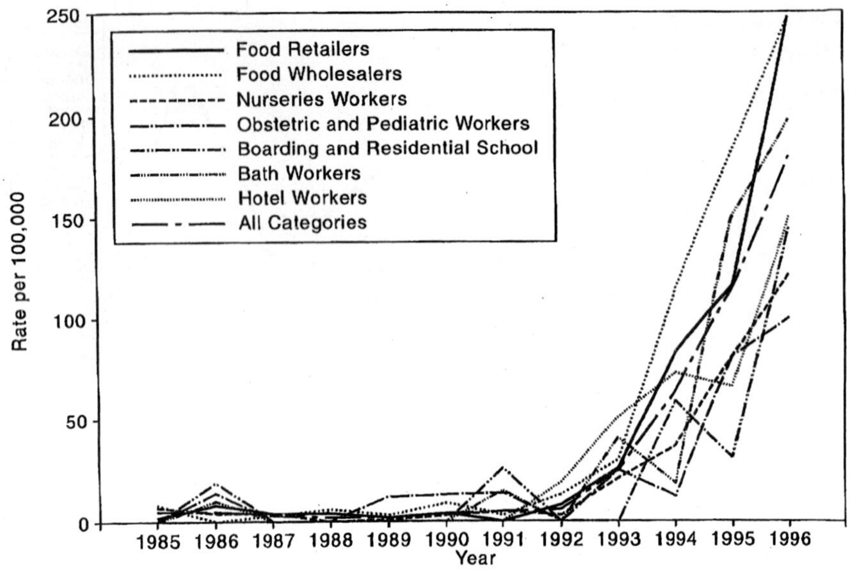

Fig. 4-10. Trends in prevalence of positive serologic tests for syphilis in seven occupational groups, Russian Federation (data kindly provided by Adrian Renton, Imperial College School of Medicine and Tatiana Shuvalova, Chief Dermatol Venereologist, Moscow Region).

secondary syphilis who named men as sex partners increased from 31 percent in 1960 to about 81 percent by 1973.[39] After the advent of the HIV/AIDS epidemic, this percentage fell drastically to 8 percent of cases in men in 1988, even as the overall number of cases of primary and secondary syphilis plummeted. However, more recently MSM accounted for 13 (65 percent) of 20 cases of primary or secondary syphilis in men during 1997 and the first half of 1998, representing both an absolute and relative increase in syphilis among MSM.

Nationally, the abrupt rise in primary and secondary syphilis in African-Americans beginning in 1986 coincided with the crack cocaine epidemic, and continued through 1990, after which rates began to fall equally rapidly (Fig. 4-11). During 1997, the incidence of primary and secondary syphilis per 100,000 in the United States was 22.0 among blacks, 1.6 for hispanics, 0.5 for whites, and 0.6 for other groups. In 1990 58 percent of all U.S. counties reported no cases of primary or secondary syphilis. By 1997 this percentage was up to 75 percent, with 31 (1 percent) of 3115 counties reporting 50 percent of all primary and secondary syphilis cases, and 186 (6 percent) of the countries reporting 85 percent of all cases. Highest rates occurred in the south. In addition, outbreaks of primary and secondary syphilis still occur. For example, the number of primary and secondary syphilis cases reported in Baltimore City has increased steadily by 4.6-fold, from 144 in 1993 to 669 in 1997. The outbreak has been attributed to use of crack cocaine and the exchange for drugs for sex but may be even more related to withdrawal of resources for public STD services in Baltimore, and to forced relocation of low income persons to new areas of the city. Outreach to persons in prisons or juvenile detention, drug treatment programs, and youth enrolled into Job Corps training programs has disclosed high seroprevalence of syphilis in all such settings, as discussed in the following.

A most interesting and concerning pattern in P&S syphilis morbidity is its overlap with seroprevalence of HIV among childbearing women, and with the incidence of gonorrhea, particularly in Southeastern United States (Fig. 4-12). The most recent data available on prenatal HIV seroprevalence were for 1994, after which national antenatal HIV seroprevalence surveys were arbitrarily stopped by the U.S. Congress.

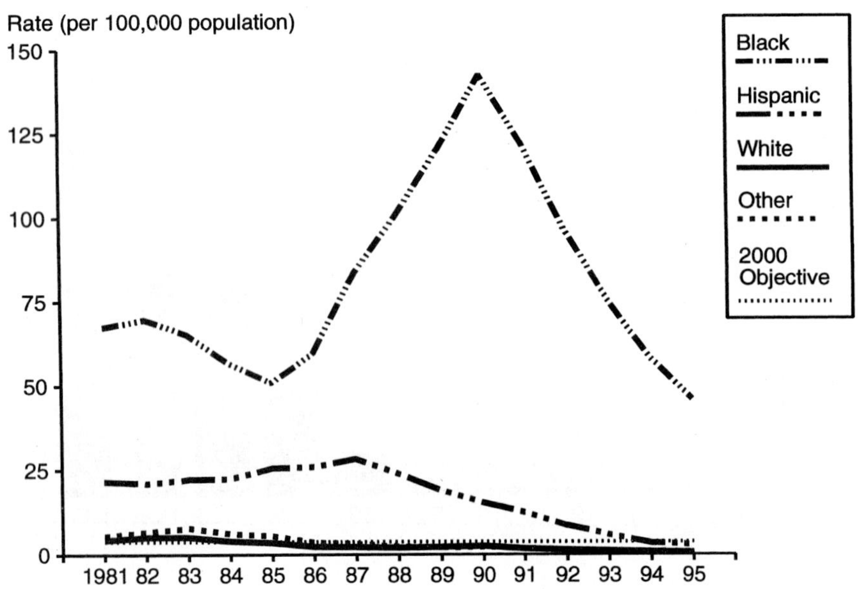

Fig. 4-11. Trends in reported primary and secondary syphilis per 100,000 population by race and ethnicity, United States 1981–1997 (provided by R. Roegner, CDC).

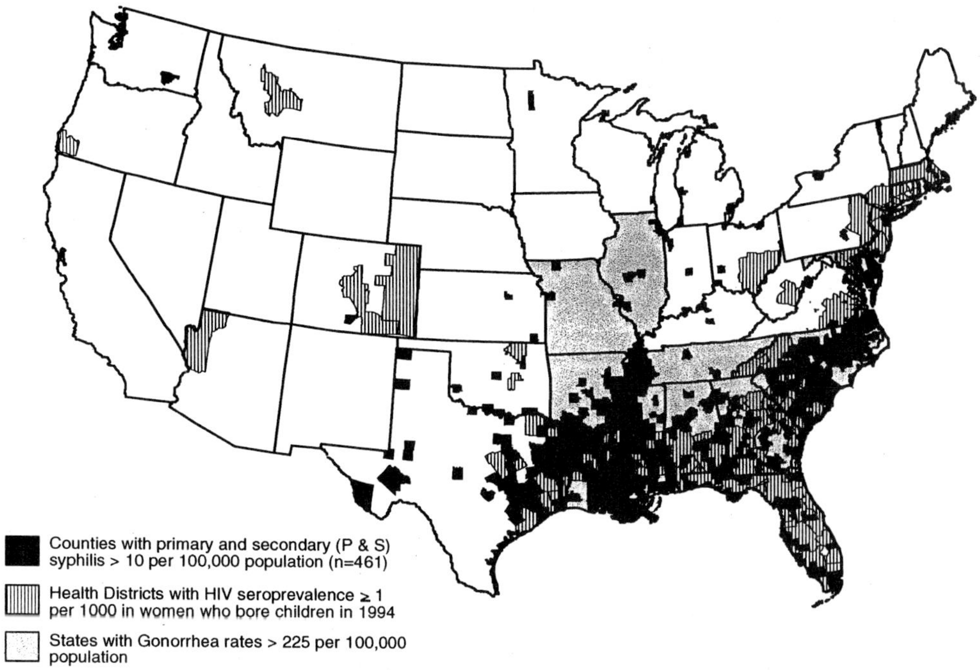

Fig. 4-12. Health districts in the United States with the highest HIV seroprevalence in women who bore children in 1994, counties reporting the highest primary and secondary syphilis rates (1993), and states reporting the highest gonorrhea rates (1993).

Prospects for elimination of syphilis

With 75 percent of counties in the United States reporting no syphilis cases during 1997, a syphilis elimination program has begun. As in western Europe, the focus is now shifting away from screening large numbers of people to detect endemic cases, toward rapid control of outbreaks to contain imported syphilis, and syphilis reemerging in groups previously at high risk (e.g., homosexual men).

CHLAMYDIA TRACHOMATIS INFECTIONS

Chlamydia trachomatis has become the most prevalent sexually transmitted bacterial infection in North America and Europe.[22] The number of cases of chlamydial infections has fallen steadily in Sweden, in association with implementation of routine screening for infection in women, and with strengthened partner notification (Fig. 4-13).

In the United States, indirect estimates based on the incidence of syndromes associated with *C. trachomatis* as determined by visits to private physicians, or on the case ratio of *C. trachomatis* to *N. gonorrhoeae* infections, indicated over 4 million infections per year as of 1986.[41] The annual number of infections among women (2.6 million) was estimated to be greater than the number of infections among men (1.8 million).[41,42] The distribution of chlamydia to gonorrhea ratios across population subgroups indicated a higher proportion of chlamydial infection, relative to gonorrhea, among whites, the young, and women using oral contraceptives, and individuals of higher socioeconomic status.

Accurate national time trends in incidence of proven *C. trachomatis* infections cannot yet be defined because of changes in reporting and increasing laboratory surveillance. Trends of nongon-

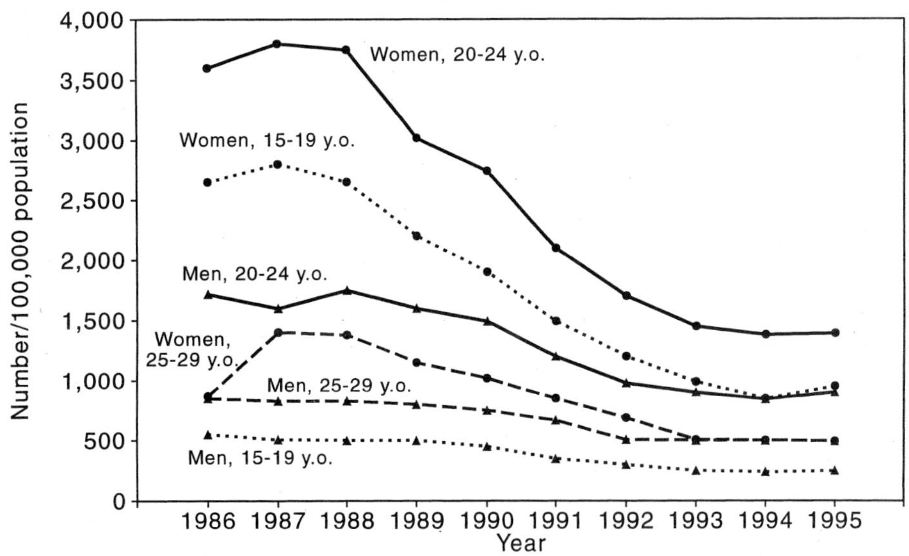

Fig. 4-13. Number of cases of chlamydial infection diagnosed in Sweden per 100,000 population by 5-year age groups and by gender, 1986–1995.

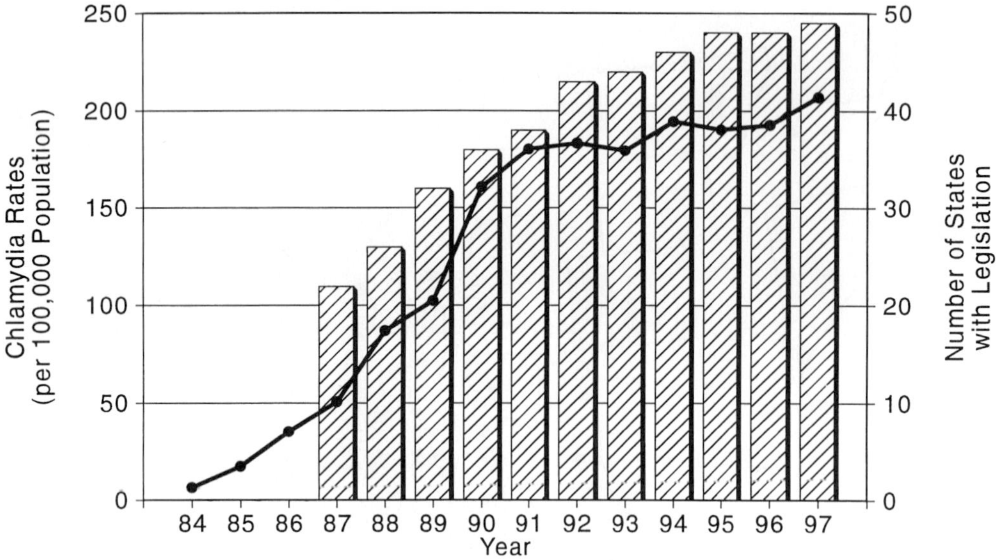

Fig. 4-14. Number of states with reporting laws for *Chlamydia trachomatis* infections and reported rates, United States, 1987–1997 (provided by R. Roegner, CDC).

ococcal urethritis (NGU) incidence in men provided a reasonable approximation, in the past, when the proportion of NGU cases attributable to *C. trachomatis* remained fairly consistent at about 40 percent between the early 1970s and the end of the 1980s.[42,43] Based on the number of visits by men to private physicians' offices, NGU increased between the mid-1960s and the end of the 1980s in the United States as well as in the United Kingdom. In 1972 in the United States, the number of visits to private physicians' offices for NGU surpassed the number for gonococcal urethritis for the first time, and by 1987 NGU was more than twice as common as gonococcal urethritis. The increase in office visits for NGU relative to office visits for gonococcal urethritis was owing mainly to a decline in gonorrhea after 1971, rather than an increase in NGU. However, in England and Wales, and other developed countries the reported number of cases of NGU continued to increase steadily, even as the reported number of cases of gonococcal urethritis declined. In recent years in the United States, a declining proportion of NGU has been attributable to chlamydial infection in some studies, making trends in NGU no longer a useful surrogate for trends in *C. trachomatis* infection. Similarly, other indicators for the incidence of chlamydial infection, such as mucopurulent cervicitis,[44] or pelvic inflammatory disease (PID), do not provide useful surrogates for trends in genital chlamydial infections.[44]

Starting in the late 1980s efforts for early detection and treatment of chlamydial infection now results in more disease notifications to state health departments and CDC than any other infectious disease (Fig. 4-14).

During 1996, state-specific chlamydia positivity rates (among 15- to 24-year-old women test population) again reflect testing bias. The prevalence of chlamydia test positivity dropped by almost two-thirds during the first 7 years of implementation of federally funded chlamydia screening in Pacific Northwest family planning clinics, after which rates have leveled off. Adolescents continue to have the highest rates of disease. More recently initiated chlamydia screening programs in other regions of the country are also showing declines in prevalence, demonstrating that serial monitoring of prevalence in family planning clinics, like serial monitoring in prenatal clinics, represents a useful approach to monitoring the impact of screening programs (Fig. 4-15).

A higher prevalence of infection has been found among 16- to

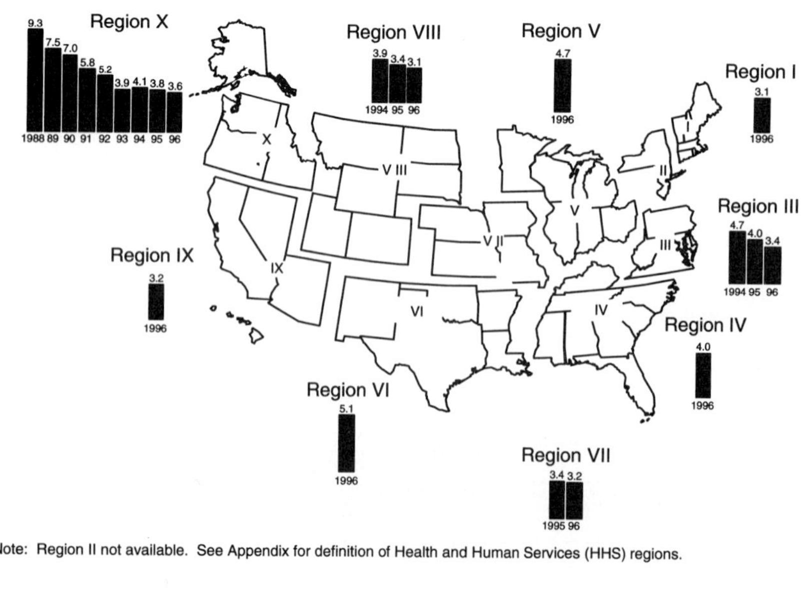

Note: Region II not available. See Appendix for definition of Health and Human Services (HHS) regions.

Fig. 4-15. Serial monitoring of the prevalence of *C. trachomatis* infection among women tested in family planning clinics, by region, in the United States (provided by R. Roegner, CDC).

Fig. 4-16. Reported cases of chancroid, United States, 1981–1997 (provided by R. Roegner, CDC).

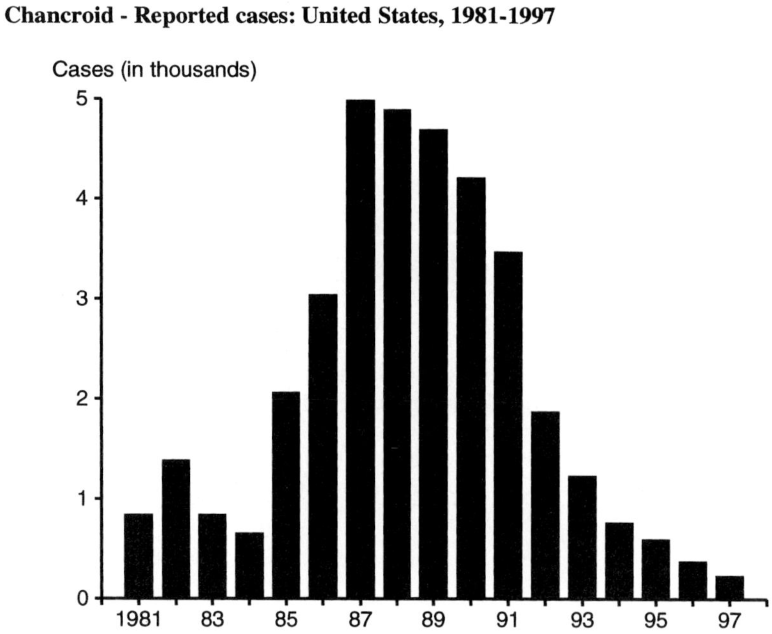

24-year-old female entrants into the U.S. Job Corps; in 1995 this population had a mean prevalence of 11.6 percent, with state-specific prevalences ranges from 4.2 percent to 17.1 percent.[45] Non-STD clinic-based surveys of chlamydial infection using urine-based DNA-amplification testing in San Francisco, Seattle, and other parts of the world document high prevalence of infection among teenagers and young adults from the general population.[46,47] High rates of urethral infection have also been found by screening young men, supporting extension of selective screening to young men as well.[47]

In summary, teenagers and young adults of both genders in the United States have high prevalence rates of chlamydial infection—particularly in high-risk populations. Low incidence of chlamydial infection reported from those states and counties with high rates of chlamydial prevalence indicate weak chlamydia control efforts.

CHANCROID

In the 1970s and 1980s most reported cases of chancroid in the United States occurred in sporadic outbreaks, in Los Angeles, Dallas, Boston, New York City, and several Florida cities, leading to an extraordinary increase from 850 cases in 1981 to 4986 cases of chancroid in the United States by 1987 (Fig. 4-16). Because chancroid may facilitate HIV transmission and because recent U.S. outbreaks of chancroid were in metropolitan areas and heterosexual populations of high HIV prevalence, this increased incidence was considered to be of great public health importance.[48,49] Chancroid is recognized far more frequently among men than women. For example, in the United States during 1987, the male : female sex ratio was 5.8 : 1 for reported cases of chancroid, compared with 0.94 : 1 for genital herpes. The link between lack of circum-

Fig. 4-17. Initial visits to physicians' offices for trichomonal and other vaginal infections, United States, 1966–1997 (source IMS America).

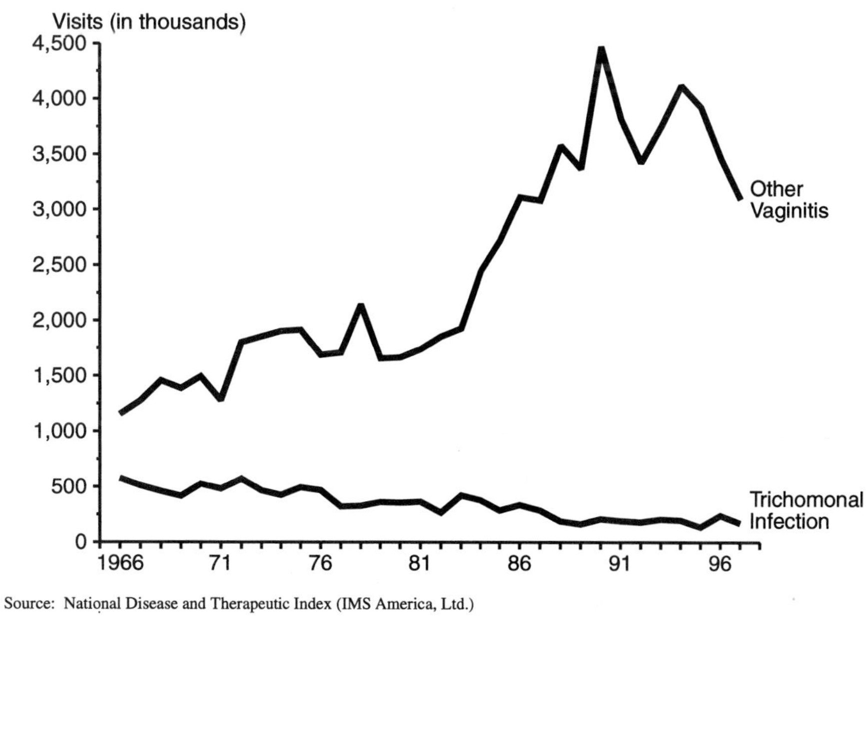

cision and STDs is best established for chancroid, and cultural circumcision practices probably also have an important influence on the incidence of chancroid in different ethnic groups.[50]

Patterns of commercial sex help to explain high male:female sex ratios, not only in recent U.S. outbreaks but in many developing countries of Africa, Asia, and Latin America where chancroid is endemic. For example, the prevalence of genital ulcers in sex workers in a poor neighborhood of Nairobi, Kenya, was an extraordinary 42 percent in the early 1980s, and the majority were culture-positive for *Hemophilus ducreyi*.[51]

Since 1987, reported cases of chancroid have declined steadily in the United States to 243 cases in 1997.[22] However, the accuracy of the data early in the U.S. chancroid epidemic were questionable because of the lack of a readily available diagnostic test for *H. ducreyi*.[52,53] In Jackson, Mississippi in 1994 to 1995, use of a multiplex polymerase chain reaction assay for *H. ducreyi* identified chancroid as the major cause of genital ulcers.[53] In two outbreaks, in New Orleans and Jackson, chancroid was associated with crack cocaine use, exchange of sex for drugs, and delayed health care seeking.[52,53]

VAGINAL TRICHOMONIASIS AND OTHER VAGINAL INFECTIONS

The NDTI survey in the United States indicates a decline in initial visits to physicians' offices for vaginal trichomoniasis from an estimated 579,000 in 1966 to 190,000 in 1988, with relatively unchanged rates since then (175,000 in 1997) (Fig. 4-17). During this same period, initial visits for other vaginal infections (etiology not defined) increased from an estimated 1,155,000 in 1966 to 4,474,000 in 1989, then declined irregularly to 3,100,000 in 1997.

GENITAL HERPES

Genital herpes simplex virus infection spread rapidly from the mid-1960s until the onset of the AIDS epidemic (see Chap. 21). The annual number of patient consultations with private physicians in office practice for newly diagnosed symptomatic genital herpes in the United States increased 12.5-fold, from 18,000 in 1966 to over 225,000 visits in 1990, then declined irregularly to 167,000 in 1997 (Fig. 4-18). People 20 to 29 years of age had more office visits than other age groups. Women outnumbered men in genital herpes-related physician consultations, reflecting either true gender differentials in genital herpes incidence, or differences in health care-seeking behavior.

During the 1970s and 1980s media attention may have increased both physicians' and patients' awareness of the signs and symptoms of genital herpes, increasing the proportions of patients with genital herpes who sought physician consultations and received a correct diagnosis.[42] However, based on the percentage of adults with serum antibody, the true annual incidence of new HSV-2 infections in the United States clearly exceeds the number of physician consultations for newly diagnosed symptomatic genital infections by several-fold.

The most recent data on HSV-2 seroprevalence in the United States were collected in a stratified random sample of the U.S. population through the National Health and Nutrition Examination Survey (NHANES) III (1988 to 1994) (Fig. 4-19). According to these findings, in 1991 (midpoint of the survey), HSV-2 seroprevalence in persons 12 years of age and older was 21.9 percent, corresponding to 44.9 million infected persons. Seroprevalence was greater in women (25.6 percent) than in men (17.8 percent), and was greater in blacks (45.9 percent) than in whites (17.6 percent). Independent predictors of HSV-2 seropositivity included gender, race/ethnicity, age, education, poverty, cocaine use, and lifetime number of sex partners.[54] Only 9.2 percent of seropositive people reported a history of genital herpes. Between 1978 and 1991 age-adjusted HSV-2 seroprevalence increased 30 percent. The increase in seroprevalence was five-fold among 12- to 19-year-old whites. Increases among blacks and older whites were smaller.[57]

In Sweden a cohort study of 839 girls 14 to 15 years of age begun in 1972 has shown an increase in prevalence of antibodies to HSV-2 from 0.4 percent at ages 14 to 15 to 22 percent by the end of the study.[55] The calculated yearly hazard rate was 0.005 for the time interval 1972 to 1976, increasing to 0.024 for 1976 to 1980 and 0.023 for 1980 to 1987.

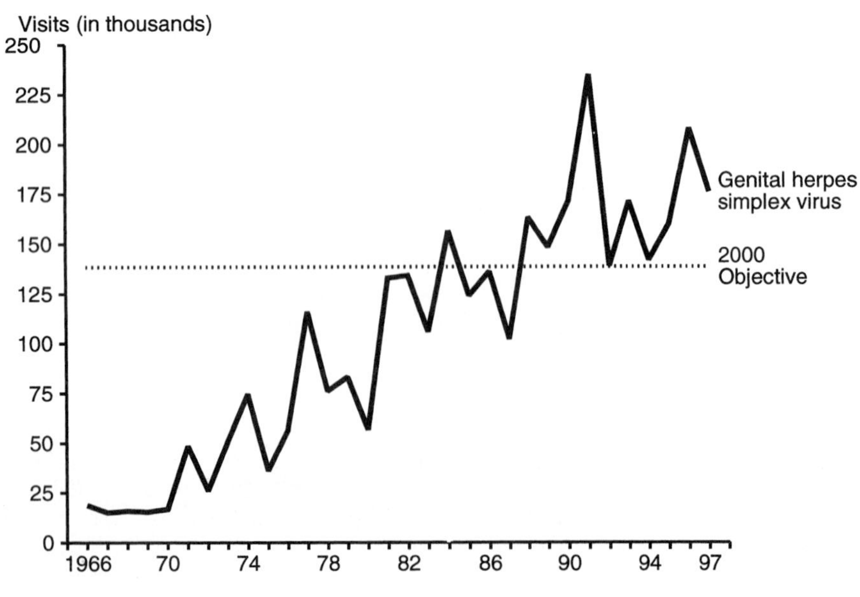

Fig. 4-18. Genital herpes simplex virus infections: Initial visits to physicians' offices, United States, 1966–1997 (source: IMS, America).

Fig. 4-19. HSV-2 seroprevalence among whites, blacks, and Mexican Americans, by age group and gender, NHANES III (1988–1994) (ref 54, with permission from The New England Journal of Medicine).

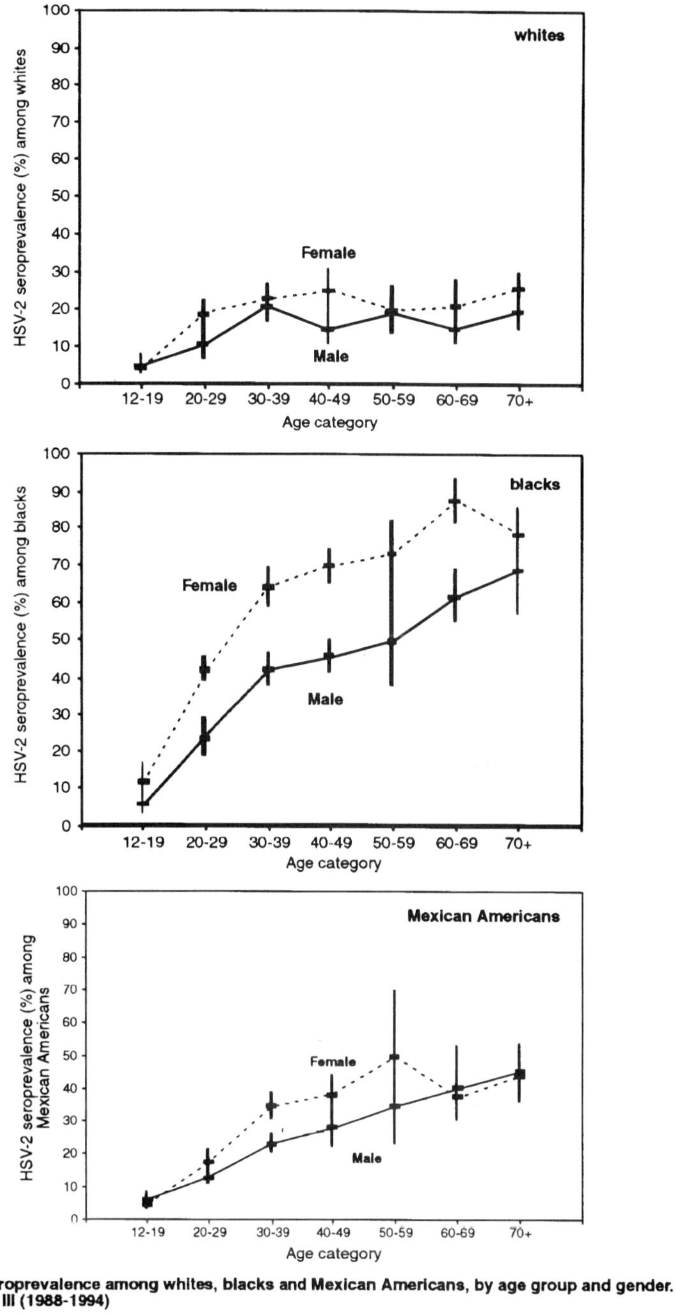

GENITAL HUMAN PAPILLOMAVIRUS INFECTIONS

The associations between certain types of HPV and precancerous or invasive lesions of the cervix, vagina, vulva, anus, and penis have been clearly documented, and as a result, interest in and physician awareness of genital HPV infections have increased (see Chap. 25). Presently, genital and anal HPV and HSV infections appear to be the most prevalent STDs in the United States. As with genital HSV infections, HPV infections are far more often subclinical than they are associated with lesions recognized by the infected individual. By screening for HPV DNA every 3 months, using PCR amplification tests, the cumulative incidence of genital HPV infections in one study was 43 percent over a 3-year period among sexually active female University students.[56] Serologic tests for antibody to those types of HPV found in the genital tract are now helping to further define the epidemiology of genital HPV infection in the same way that serologic tests have elucidated the epidemiology of HSV-2 infection.

Because external genital warts are mostly caused by type 6 or 11 HPV, physician–patient consultations for this condition provide the best available indicator of trends in the incidence of genital infections by HPV types 6 or 11. Initial visits to physician offices for genital warts increased from 55,695 in 1966 to over 351,370 in 1987; from 1987 to 1997, initial visits to physicians' offices declined to around 145,000 (Fig. 4-20). The extent to which this rise and fall represents the natural history of the spread of the epidemic of HPV 6 and 11 through the U.S. population, versus changes in health care-seeking or diagnosis versus a rise and fall in risk taking behaviors, remains undefined.

Among sexually active women, the prevalence of cervical HPV

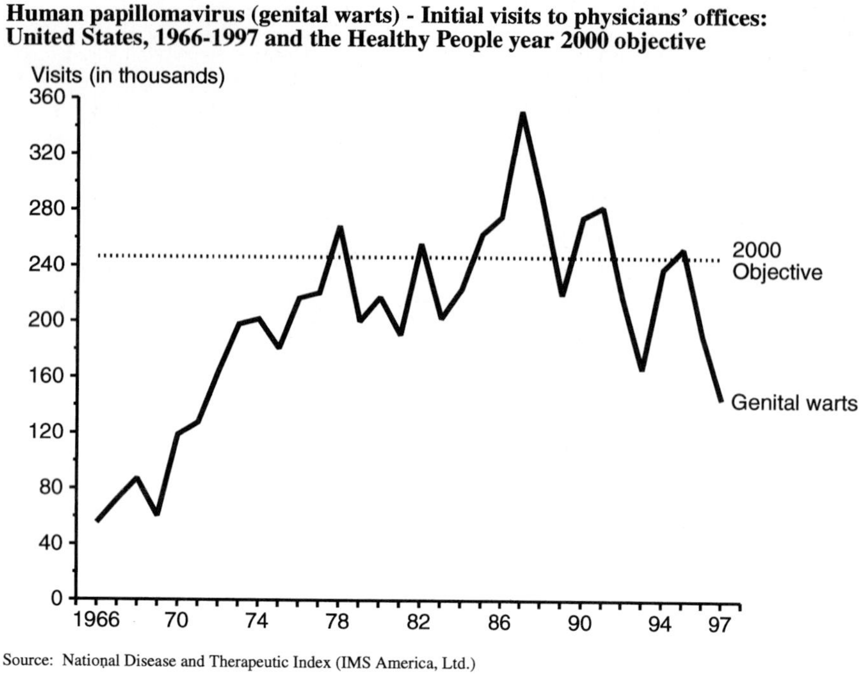

Fig. 4-20. Genital warts. Number of initial visits to private physicians' offices, United States, 1966–1997 (source: IMS, America).

Table 4-3. Characteristics of Persons Aged ≥13 Years with HIV, by Disease Status at Initial Diagnosis in the United States* (25 states†, January 1994–June 1997)

	Disease Status at Initial HIV Diagnosis				
	HIV		AIDS		
Characteristic	No.§	(%¶)	No.§	(%¶)	Total
Sex					
Male	37,996	(72)	16,866	(83)	54,862
Female	14,689	(28)	3,348	(17)	18,037
Race/Ethnicity**					
White, non-Hispanic	17,929	(34)	9,171	(45)	27,100
Black, non-Hispanic	30,229	(57)	9,127	(45)	39,356
Hispanic	3,581	(7)	1,660	(8)	5,241
Other/Unknown	949	(2)	256	(1)	1,205
Risk/Exposure category					
Men having sex with men	17,098	(32)	8,866	(44)	25,964
Injecting-drug user	9,671	(18)	3,959	(20)	13,630
Men having sex with men/ Injecting-drug user	2,088	(4)	843	(4)	2,931
Heterosexual contact	9,279	(18)	2,428	(12)	11,707
Other/Unreported	14,552	(28)	4,116	(20)	18,668
Age group (yrs)					
13–24	7,200	(14)	653	(3)	7,853
25–29	9,384	(18)	2,239	(11)	11,623
30–34	11,916	(23)	4,503	(22)	16,419
35–39	10,030	(19)	4,608	(23)	14,638
≥40	14,159	(27)	8,210	(41)	22,369
Total††	52,690		20,215		72,905

*For persons who had not had an HIV diagnosis before being diagnosed with AIDS, their AIDS diagnosis date is considered their earliest HIV diagnosis date; for persons initially reported with HIV who subsequently had AIDS diagnosed and reported, they are presented by the earliest diagnosis date, which is their HIV diagnosis.

†Alabama, Arizona, Arkansas, Colorado, Idaho, Indiana, Louisiana, Michigan, Minnesota, Mississippi, Missouri, Nevada, New Jersey, North Carolina, North Dakota, Ohio, Oklahoma, South Carolina, South Dakota, Tennessee, Utah, Virginia, West Virginia, Wisconsin, and Wyoming.

§Numbers are estimates after adjustments for reporting delays. Point estimates are presented for reproducibility of the data.

¶Percentages may not total 100 because of rounding.

**Persons of races other than black and white were included under "other/unknown" because estimates were too small for meaningful analysis.

††Column totals include missing/other for some categories (e.g., missing sex). Persons infected through receipt of blood or blood products are included under other/unreported risk.

DNA has been highest for teenagers and those in the early twenties, and lower for older women (see Chap. 25). The natural history of genital HPV infection in men remains largely undefined, although the short-term natural history of incident genital infection by various HPV types is being defined in women by serial cervicovaginal PCR testing, and cervical cytology, and by serologic studies. It appears that the median duration is for HPV-16 (about 1 ½ years); and the shortest duration is for HPV 6 and 11 (about 5 to 6 months).[56] Type specific serum antibody detectable by current assays develops slowly over several months in the majority of infected women. The longer duration of HPV-16 shedding may help explain its relatively high incidence in the population.

Based on these preliminary findings from cohort studies, and together with data from national surveys of sexual behavior (see the following), it is not unlikely that the majority of adults in the United States, perhaps three-quarters, have been infected with one or more types of genital HPV.

HIV infection

Global perspectives on the epidemiology and surveillance of HIV infection are provided in Chapters 5 and 97. In the United States and Western Europe, the impact of improved antiretroviral therapy on delaying progression of HIV infection to AIDS, and in prolonging survival of those who have developed AIDS, has made surveillance of AIDS alone a poor indicator for the incidence of HIV infection, and for the movement of the epidemic through subpopulations. A 1998 report compared data on initial diagnoses of HIV infections in persons ≥13 years of age versus AIDS surveillance data for the 25 states that conducted name-based HIV reporting during January 1994 to June 1997 (Table 4-3). During this period in these states, the initial diagnosis was HIV infection in 52,690 cases (72 percent) and was AIDS in 20,215 (28 percent). Over the 2½-year period, declines in numbers of cases with AIDS at initial diagnosis were somewhat greater than declines in numbers with diagnosis of HIV infection at diagnosis, as expected;

Table 4-4. Number of Women 15 to 44 Years of Age and Percent Distribution by Lifetime Number of Male Sexual Partners*

	Number of Male Partners								
	0	1	2	3	4	5	6–9	10 or More	
All women	11.2	24.6	12.6	10.3	8.9	8.1	11.7	12.7	(15.5)†
Age at interview									
15–19 years	49.9	18.3	11.1	7.3	3.5	2.7	4.8	2.6	(3.7)
20–24 years	12.3	23.2	13.7	12.7	8.8	7.7	11.5	10.5	(13.9)
25–29 years	4.5	23.6	14.0	10.4	10.4	9.7	13.7	13.7	(16.9)
30–34 years	2.8	24.2	12.6	10.2	11.6	10.2	13.1	15.4	(18.0)
35–39 years	1.6	25.8	11.6	10.5	9.2	9.5	13.9	18.0	(20.5)
40–44 years	1.6	31.5	12.7	10.7	8.9	8.2	12.0	14.4	(17.7)
Marital status									
Currently married	—§	36.9	14.2	10.1	9.3	8.1	10.6	10.9	(13.2)
All unmarried	22.0	12.6	11.0	10.5	8.5	8.2	12.7	14.5	(17.7)
Never married	29.4	13.7	11.3	10.0	7.5	6.8	10.5	25.5	(13.6)
Formally married	0.1	9.5	10.1	11.9	11.5	12.2	19.2	25.5	(29.8)
Age at first intercourse									
Under 16 years	—	11.6	12.1	11.3	9.7	10.7	19.1	24.6	(29.0)
16 Years	—	20.1	13.7	13.7	10.9	10.8	15.0	15.7	(18.8)
17 Years	—	19.8	14.5	13.0	13.5	11.2	13.4	14.5	(18.8)
18 Years	—	28.0	14.4	11.8	11.4	9.1	12.4	12.9	(14.9)
19 Years	—	39.2	14.8	11.6	8.4	8.6	9.4	7.6	(9.2)
20 Years	—	55.3	16.1	8.8	6.4	4.2	5.4	3.3	(4.6)
Education at interview**									
No high school diploma or GED 3	0.6	28.3	15.3	12.7	8.2	9.5	13.1	12.4	(15.8)
High school diploma or GED 3	2.1	25.8	13.6	11.6	10.2	9.0	13.3	14.4	(17.1)
Some college, no bachelor's degree	4.9	24.2	10.5	9.7	10.9	10.6	13.0	16.3	(19.9)
Bachelor's degree of higher	4.9	26.6	12.2	9.4	9.6	7.8	13.3	16.2	(18.9)
Poverty level income at interview**									
0–149 percent	3.6	22.9	14.0	11.9	10.6	9.7	12.6	14.6	(17.7)
0–99 percent	3.7	22.8	14.1	11.7	11.1	10.5	11.9	14.3	(17.6)
150–299 percent	3.7	28.4	13.4	10.1	9.8	8.6	11.6	14.4	(17.6)
300 percent or higher	3.1	25.5	11.6	10.5	9.8	9.3	14.5	15.8	(18.7)
Race and Hispanic origin									
Hispanic	12.3	39.2	16.0	9.4	5.1	5.9	5.6	6.7	(8.5)
Non-Hispanic black	9.4	14.0	12.4	14.0	11.4	11.5	12.7	14.5	(18.8)
Non-Hispanic white	10.6	23.5	12.1	10.0	9.2	8.1	12.8	13.8	(16.4)
Non-Hispanic other	22.4	36.3	12.6	6.4	5.1	4.8	6.2	6.2	(7.8)

*Based on responses from interviewer-administered questionnaire: United States, 1995.

†Data in parenthesis show percent reported 10 or more partners on the Audio Computer-assisted self interview. Note higher percentage of respondents reported 10 or more partners by Audio CASI than by interviewer-administered questionnaire.

§Category not applicable.

**Limited to women 22–44 years at interview.

3/GED is general equivalency to diploma.

From the National Survey of Family Growth, ref 57.

NOTE: percents may not add to 100 due to rounding.

and as shown in the table, cases detected among those diagnosed with HIV infection were more likely than those diagnosed with AIDS to be blacks, women, young, and infected through heterosexual contact. Surveillance of HIV infection, though subject to testing bias, provides the best information on the progress of the epidemic, and on the impact of and needs for preventive interventions.

These differences in distribution of those with HIV infection versus those with the late sequelae of HIV (AIDS) may prove heuristic in planning and interpreting surveillance of other STIs and their sequelae [e.g., HPV and the HPV-related genital or anal cancers; HBV and hepatocellular carcinoma; HTLV-1 and neurologic sequelae; cervical infection and infertility].

PELVIC INFLAMMATORY DISEASE, ECTOPIC PREGNANCY, AND OTHER STD COMPLICATIONS

The major complications of sexually transmitted infections include AIDS; cancer (cervix, vagina, vulva, anus, penis, liver, Kaposi's sarcoma, forms of body cavity and lymphoma T-cell leukemia); PID and related sequelae; complications of pregnancy and the puerperium; congenital, perinatal, and postnatal infections of the fetus/infant; various neurologic syndromes, and a variety of other diseases. Selected aspects of the epidemiology of these complications are discussed in the following.

Pelvic inflammatory disease

Trends in pelvic inflammatory disease (PID) reflect not only trends in incidence, but also changing diagnostic criteria, and changing management practices, which recently have involved decreasing rates of hospitalization. The U.S. National Survey of Family Growth (NSFG), performs repeated surveys of reproductive age women living in the United States, providing data on trends in PID.[57] In 1995, 8 percent of women reported past treatment for PID, including 8 percent of Hispanic women, 7 percent of non-Hispanic white women, and 11 percent of black women.[57–59] PID was twice as common among women who reported vaginal douching regularly (12 percent) than among those who did not douche (6 percent). PID was also twice as common among those with 10 or more sex partners in their lifetimes (14 percent) as among women who had had two or three partners (7 percent). Although the distribution of PID across population groups was

Table 4-5. Number of Women 15 to 44 Years of Age and Percent Distribution by Number of Male Sexual Partners in the last 12 Months*

	Number of Male Partners					
	0	1	2	3	4 or more	
All women	34.5	47.0	11.2	11.2	4.1	(8.6)†
Age at interview						
15–19 Years	55.8	28.6	8.2	3.7	3.7	(7.4)
20–24 Years	23.1	52.3	14.9	5.2	4.6	(11.2)
25–29 Years	20.4	58.0	13.7	4.6	2.9	(9.0)
30–34 Years	24.0	55.8	12.7	4.6	2.9	(8.7)
35–39 Years	30.6	52.0	11.5	3.3	2.7	(8.3)
40–44 Years	37.9	53.4	5.4	2.0	1.2	(5.7)
Marital status						
Never married	39.4	43.7	10.0	3.8	3.2	(8.2)
Formally married	20.3	56.7	14.5	4.9	3.7	(9.6)
Age at first intercourse						
Under 16 years	10.6	57.6	17.4	7.3	7.1	(17.5)
16 Years	12.3	64.7	14.9	4.8	3.6	(9.3)
17 Years	14.0	65.1	13.5	4.2	3.3	(9.4)
18 Years	18.0	60.7	13.8	5.1	2.4	(7.7)
19 Years	25.5	58.8	10.0	4.0	1.7	(4.3)
20 Years or older	37.7	51.0	8.0	2.0	1.3	(3.3)
Education at interview§						
No high school diploma or GED**	19.2	63.6	10.6	3.6	3.1	(15.2)
High school diploma or GED	21.1	58.0	12.5	5.1	3.2	(9.8)
Some college, no bachelor's degree	28.6	51.8	13.3	3.6	2.7	(7.3)
Bachelor's degree or higher	33.5	49.9	11.1	3.4	2.2	(5.3)
Poverty level income at interview§						
0–149 Percent	22.3	56.0	14.0	5.2	2.6	(13.1)
0–99 Percent	21.4	57.5	12.9	5.3	2.9	(15.2)
150–299 Percent	27.2	53.0	12.1	4.7	3.0	(7.7)
300 Percent or higher	28.0	56.3	10.4	2.6	2.8	(5.9)
Race and Hispanic origin						
Hispanic	41.2	45.7	6.9	2.5	3.6	(6.8)
Non-Hispanic black	23.7	52.5	14.7	6.0	3.1	(13.1)
Non-Hispanic white	35.1	46.5	11.1	3.9	3.4	(7.5)
Non-Hispanic other	56.1	32.6	7.0	2.4	1.9	(7.5)

*Based on responses from interviewer-administered questionnaire; United States, 1995.

†Responses given in the Audio CASI indicate 4 or more partners reported by higher percentage of respondents by Audio CASI than by interviewer-administered questionnaire.

§Limited to women 22–44 years at interview.

**GED is general equivalency to diploma.

(ref 60).

NOTE: percents may not add to 100 owing to rounding.

similar in 1982, 1988, and 1995, the prevalence of PID apparently declined during this time from 14 percent in 1982 to 11 percent in 1988, and 8 percent in 1995.[57–59]

Ectopic pregnancy

Ectopic pregnancy is the leading cause of pregnancy-related death during the first trimester, responsible for 9 percent of all pregnancy-related deaths in the United States in 1992. Women who have one ectopic pregnancy are at increased risk for another such pregnancy and for future infertility. In the United States, the reported number of hospitalizations for ectopic pregnancy increased from 17,800 in 1970 to 88,400 in 1989.[60] Based on the National Hospital Discharge Survey (NHDS), the estimated number of hospitalizations for ectopic pregnancy was 64,400 in 1990, 55,600 in 1991, and 58,200 in 1992, (95 percent CI = 48,600 to 67,700) for a rate of 10.6 per 1,000 reported pregnancies (i.e., ectopic, legal abortions, and live births).

This analysis of the estimated number of ectopic pregnancies, based only on hospitalizations, indicates a decline since the late 1980s. However, in part this decline reflects the shift toward treating ectopic pregnancy in an outpatient setting. When data from NHDS are combined with data from the National Hospital Ambulatory Medical Care Survey (NHAMCS), the estimated total number of ectopic pregnancies in 1992 was 108,800—nearly double the estimated number of hospitalized cases.[60]

Thus, combining data for hospitalized and ambulatory cases suggests that the incidence of ectopic pregnancy, instead of declining in the late 1980s, may have increased steadily since 1970.[60] To what extent this represents increased ascertainment is uncertain. Outpatient management of ectopic pregnancy—first reported in 1987—has increased together with the earlier detection of unruptured ectopic pregnancies as the result of sensitive radioimmunoassays for human chorionic gonadotropin and high-resolution transvaginal ultrasound. Outpatient management may include laparoscopic salpingectomy or salpingostomy, or methotrexate therapy. In particular, outpatient pharmacologic treatment of ectopic pregnancy with methotrexate has resulted in decreased patient morbidity, a preservation of reproductive capability, and, when compared with inpatient surgical treatment, an estimated cost savings of $10,000 per case.

Surveillance data on ectopic pregnancy are not available for the period after 1992. However, estimates based on pregnancy outcome data collected in 1995 by the NSFG continue to indicate that ectopic pregnancies constituted 2 percent of all pregnancies during the 1987 to 1990 period and during the 1991 to 1994 period. The estimated yearly averages were 105,180 and 110,880 ectopic pregnancies for the two periods, respectively (Anjari Chandra, personal communication).

The increase in ectopic pregnancies over the past three decades was not confined to the United States. From the mid-1970s through the mid-1980s, the incidence of ectopic pregnancy more than doubled in many countries of the Western world, including Sweden, Norway, Ireland, Canada, and Finland, even as the incidence of gonorrhea was declining.[61] Suggested explanations include the effects of changes in the management of infertility, and ectopic pregnancy (leading to recurrent ectopic pregnancies), and an increasing incidence of silent or subclinical PID.

Adverse outcomes of pregnancy

Although data are not available on trends of every type of AOP, recent studies provide estimates of the magnitude of the problem, which is covered in detail in Chapter 80.[62] Approximately 400,000 infants are born prematurely each year in the United States, and of these more than 20,000 die in the fetal or neonatal period and another 20,000 end up with long-term neurologic sequelae. As many as 100,000 of these preterm births and 5000 or more deaths, as well as a similar number of major disabilities, may be associated with maternal STDs. The greatest potential for achieving improvement in adverse outcomes of pregnancy associated with sexually transmitted diseases may lie in reducing the excess number of preterm births, many apparently associated with antenatal bacterial vaginosis.

Cervical cancer

In the past, health care behavior has been less important in the epidemiology of incurable viral STDs than in the epidemiology of curable bacterial STDs, as discussed in the following. One exception is cervical carcinoma, a complication of cervical HPV infection. Regular cervical cytologic screening does allow early detection and treatment of cervical dysplasia, preventing progression to invasive cervical carcinoma. The incidence of cervical cancer is exceptionally high in developing countries that lack programs for preventing cervical cancer; and has been rising in some countries where the recommended frequency for cytology screening is relatively low. The higher incidence of cervical cancer in blacks than in whites in the United States could be attributable either to more frequent cervical HPV infection or to less frequent cytology screening or to both factors. Similarly, because early diagnosis and treatment of invasive cancer predicts better prognoses, the higher mortality rate for cervical cancer in black women than in white women could also reflect differences in health care behavior.

STDS IN SPECIAL POPULATIONS

Special populations are disproportionately affected by STD morbidity in most countries all over the world. In the United States, sex workers, homeless persons, adolescents and adults in detention, and migrant workers are among special populations with high STD morbidity. The Institute of Medicine report on STDs emphasized the importance of outreach to these special populations for STD control.[63] In general, the prevalence of cervical infection is highest during the first few years after beginning sex work, and declines with age and immunity; whereas serologic evidence of past STDs or chronic viral STDs increases with increasing duration of sex work, reflecting cumulative acquisition of infection (see Chap. 10). A protective effect of consistent condom use against many of these infections has been found among sex workers in cross-sectional studies and cohort studies, although commercial sex in areas of high STD endemicity unfortunately leads to high cumulative rates of STDs, including HIV, even among women reporting consistent condom use.[64–66] In industrialized countries, rates of STDs among female sex workers are currently highest among those using illicit drugs, such as heroine or cocaine. Very high rates of some of these STDs, sometimes including HIV infection, have been reported among sex workers in the United States.[67]

In Chicago, 26 percent of homeless women seeking gynecological care had trichomoniasis, 6 percent had gonorrhea, and 5 percent had pelvic inflammatory disease.[68] In Baltimore, 8 percent of homeless men and 11 percent of homeless women had positive gonorrhea or syphilis tests, and nearly one-third reported a prior STD.[69]

Adolescents and adults in detention facilities (juvenile detention, local jails incarcerating persons with short-term sentences or awaiting trial, and state or federal prisons) also have remarkably high levels of STD morbidity. In 1994, gonorrhea rates among male adolescents in detention were 152 times greater than those among male adolescents in the general population; the gonorrhea rate among female adolescents in detention was 42 times higher than the rate among female adolescents in the general population.[70] In juvenile detention centers, the prevalence of various bacterial STDs among those entering the facilities was nearly one-third among females in Seattle in the mid-1980s; and during the 1990s, 15 percent of males in San Francisco, and 12 percent of males in Alabama.[71–73]

In the main jail facility for men in Los Angeles County, the rate of infectious syphilis was 507 cases for 100,000 persons—more than 11 times the rate in the general population.[74] At the Cook County Jail in 1996, RPR screening of women arrestees identified 176 (22 percent) of Chicago's 803 early syphilis cases in women.[75] Between 1993 and 1994, routine STD testing indicated that up to 17 percent of inmates in U.S. correctional facilities were infected with syphilis, up to 32.5 percent were positive for gonorrhea, and up to 4.4 percent were positive for chlamydia.[77] In a 1988 sample of female inmates at Riker's Island in New York, 35 percent were positive for genital HPV infection; 27 percent had positive cultures for chlamydia; 16 percent were syphilis seroreactive; and 8 percent had positive cultures for gonorrhea.[78] Among incarcerated women in recent studies, 35 percent were syphilis seroreactive, 27 percent had chlamydial infection, and 8 percent had gonorrhea.[79–80] In anonymous serosurveys of inmates throughout the United States, the prevalence of HIV-1 seropositivity ranges from less than 1 percent to as high as 25.6 percent; female inmates often had higher rates than men.[77]

Finally, STDs including HIV infection, are major health problems among migrant workers (see Chap. 12).[81,82] Limited access to health care, language and cultural barriers, and limited economic resources, combined with sexual behaviors that expose migrant workers to high-risk partners tend to perpetuate high levels of STD morbidity among this group.[83,84]

DIRECT AND INDIRECT DETERMINANTS OF POPULATION TRANSMISSION DYNAMICS

Each of the three direct determinants of the rate of spread of STDs in a population—rate of exposure, efficiency of transmission per exposure, and duration of infectivity—are driven by a complex set of factors.

DETERMINANTS OF EXPOSURE: TRENDS AND PATTERNS OF SEXUAL BEHAVIOR

Our understanding of the relevant components of sexual behavior that influence risk of STDs, including HIV infection, has changed considerably over the past few decades. A better understanding of the epidemiology of specific STDs, and the greater need for preventive interventions to change sexual behavior in the context of increasing viral STDs, initiated such changes in the early 1980s. The AIDS epidemic has been the single most important factor to both highlight the need for more systematic information on sexual behavior and facilitate an unprecedented increase in infection-related studies of sexual behavior.

The term "sexual behavior" involves many components: sexual experience and activity, age at sexual debut or "coitarche," current and lifetime number of sex partners, frequency of sexual intercourse, consistency of sexual activity, mode of recruitment of sexual partners and duration of sexual unions, and types of sexual practice.[85] Although the conjoint distribution of the component variables in the population determines aggregate exposure to the risk of STDs, the specific relationship between each of these variables and the risk of various STDs with differing natural histories, and the distribution of these variables across population subgroups, have by no means been fully defined.

The population at risk for STDs has been very simply defined in terms of age groups, often assuming those between ages 15 and 45 may engage in sexual intercourse with new partners. Further refinements of this concept have included in the population at risk only the sexually experienced, defined as persons who have ever had sexual intercourse.[86] However, current sexual activity, rather than sexual experience per se, is a more accurate measure of current exposure to the risk of STDs.[87]

Trends in sexual behavior in the United States

The most recent data on the sexual behavior of reproductive age American women indicate that trends toward earlier and more liberal sexual behavior may have recently come to a halt, or even reversed.[57] About 50 percent of teenagers (15 to 19 years of age) reported in 1995 that they had ever had sexual intercourse, compared with 53 percent in 1988 and 47 percent in 1982. The percent of teens 15 to 17 who ever had intercourse was 33 percent in 1982, 38 percent in 1988, and 38 percent in 1995. For teens 18 to 19, these figures were 64 percent in 1982, 74 percent in 1988, and 70 percent in 1995. It appears that one of the principal changes between 1988 and 1995 was a postponement of intercourse for women 18 to 19 years of age.

In 1995, for 8 percent of women aged 15 to 44 years who had had intercourse, their *first* intercourse was not voluntary. For those whose first intercourse occurred at age 15 or younger, that first intercourse was non-voluntary for 16 percent, compared with 7 percent or less at age 16 or older. The percent whose first intercourse was involuntary appears to have dropped from nearly 10 percent before 1975 to about 6 percent in the 1990s.[57]

One of the most frequently used risk markers in STDs research is age at first sexual intercourse. This variable has often been employed to describe sexual activity levels of populations and to monitor the so-called sexual revolutions and evolutions. Age at sexual debut has two epidemiological functions: first as a true risk factor, causally related to disease outcome, and second as an indicator of other aspects of sexual activity. Etiologically, age at sexual debut has been independently associated with the development of cervical cancer in some studies, and in other studies with *C. trachomatis* antibody prevalence and with HIV infection, perhaps owing to the biological development of the female cervix during the teenage years.[88] As a risk indicator, age at sexual debut is correlated with sociodemographic factors such as race and socioeconomic status, sexual behavior variables, number of sex partners, and specific STDs. Age at sexual debut together with age at first marriage has been the primary variable documenting the sexual revolution of the 1970s.[89]

Risk of exposure to an STD is directly associated not only with number of infected sex partners, but also with the prevalence of STDs within one's pool of potential choice of sex partner(s). The number of sex partners within a specific time period, often 1 or 3 months, has been shown to be a risk factor for having gonorrhea, chlamydia, genital herpes, and human papillomavirus infections.[90–93] Lifetime number of sex partners is associated with the risk of cervical and other genital cancers, as well as with the prevalence of serum antibody reflecting past exposure to various STDs. (This is essentially true for all STD pathogens for which serologic tests are available.) However, the relationship between number of sex partners and STD risk is not simple; it is of course influenced by the partner's sexual behavior, and the varying infectiousness of infected partners.

The most recent data on lifetime number of sex partners of reproductive age American women was collected in 1995 by the National Survey of Family Growth (see Table 4-4).[57] The greatest percentage of women 15 to 44 years of age (24.6 percent) had had only one lifetime partner, but 12.7 percent reported 10 or more partners. Moreover, a comparison of responses to the interviewers with responses to the computer-assisted self interview (CASI) indicate that the sensitive data collected by interviewers tend to yield underestimates of high-risk behaviors, an observation recently confirmed by Turner et al.[94]

About 38 percent of women 15 to 44 years of age had never been married when interviewed the last 12 months, while 3.3 percent reported four or more partners (Table 4-5). Again these responses apparently were underestimates, since 8.6 percent reported four or more partners over the past year during the audio CASI.

Some individuals are at risk for acquiring STDs because of their own risky sexual behaviors; with multiple partners, these persons have a relatively high likelihood not only of being infected but also of transmitting the infection, and have been termed "high-frequency transmitters." Poor health care behavior (e.g., failure to seek treatment while remaining sexually active with symptoms of STDs) is another common feature of high-frequency transmitters of the curable STDs. Other individuals are at risk for STDs solely because of the sexual behaviors of their partners; their likelihood of infecting others is relatively low. This second category can be described as "receivers." Although all infected persons are by definition, receivers, it appears, without much systematically collected data, that a higher proportion of women than of men are only receivers.

Some studies have shown a nonlinear increase in risk of certain STDs with increasing numbers of sex partners.[95–97] The marginal increase in STD risk suddenly multiplied as the number of sex partners reached certain threshold levels. In general, for many STDs, with further increases in numbers of partners, the risk then begins to level off, most likely this is largely owing to acquired immunity. The nonlinear relationship between increasing number of sex partners and increasing STD risk points to the importance of two other dimensions of sexual behavior: choice of partners and contact with core groups of high STD risk individuals.

Exposure to an STD transmitter depends on how one chooses one's sex partners and on the prevalence of STD in the pool of available partners. Both in the general population and among STD clinic attendees, marked gender differentials exist in the recruitment of sex partners. Compared with men, women tend to report meeting their potential partners through less casual associations, and to know them better and for longer periods of time prior to becoming sexually involved with them.[88,98,99] A nondiscriminating approach to sex partner recruitment increases the probability of sexual contact with members of high-risk core groups and thus of exposure to STDs. Better understanding of patterns of partner recruitment in population subgroups helps to explain some of the variability in STD risk.

The 1995 NSFG sheds some light on the age distribution of sex partners of young women.[57] About two-thirds (66 percent) of women who had their first *voluntary* intercourse before age 16 had first partners under 18 years of age; 21 percent had first partners aged 18 to 19; 7 percent had first partners aged 20 to 22; 2 percent had first partners 23 to 24 years of age, and 4 percent had first partners aged 25 or older. Only 3 percent of women had their first intercourse with a man they just met, 61 percent were "going steady" or "going together" with the man they had intercourse with their first time, and about one in five were engaged or married to him. Among women aged 40 to 44 (born in 1951 to 1955), 23 percent were married to their partner at first intercourse, whereas only 5 percent of women aged 15 to 19 (born 1971 to 1975) were married to their first partner. Women who lived with both of their parents throughout their childhood were more likely than other women to have been married to their partner at first intercourse.

About 69 percent of those first married in 1965 to 1974 had their first intercourse before marriage, compared with 89 percent of those first married in the 1990s. Only 2 percent of those first married in 1965 to 1974 had their first intercourse 5 years or more before marriage, compared with 55 percent of those first married in the 1990s.

Despite interference from Congress in funding of research involving surveys of sexual behavior, several other methodologically sound surveys have been conducted in the United States. Zelnik and Kantner studied adolescent sexual behavior in national probability samples in 1971, 1976, and 1979, documenting steadily increasing rates of premarital intercourse by teenaged females throughout the 1970s.[100] The National Survey of Adolescent Males found that from 1988 to 1991, 17.5 to 19.0-year-old males experienced a significantly younger mean age of first intercourse and a significant increase, from 2.0 to 2.6, in the mean number of sexual partners over the past 12 months, with no increase in frequency of condom use.[101,102] The 1973, 1976, 1982, and 1988 cycles of the National Survey on Family Growth showed a continuing increase in the proportion of female teenagers 15 to 19 years old who were sexually experienced, from 28.6 percent in 1970 to 51.5 percent in 1988, including an increase among white teenagers from 44.1 percent to 51.5 percent during the early AIDS era from 1985 to 1988.[103] Similarly, the General Social Survey collected limited data annually from 1988 to 1990 on sexual behaviors of the U.S. adults, providing perhaps the best comparison yet available of recent sexual behaviors of males and females, with data stratified by age, race, and marital status.[104] Results help explain age and race disparities in rates of STDs in the United States, and suggest that more than 22.5 million U.S. adults had two or more sex partners during the preceding year, with an estimated 4.8 million having had five or more partners. The 1990 National AIDS Behavioral Surveys also assessed HIV-related sexual risk behaviors.[105] The 1990 National Survey of Men, provided data on sexual behaviors of men 20 to 39 years of age, on and race/ethnicity differences in numbers of sexual partners; these data paralleled the General Social Survey results and help explain race/ethnicity disparities in bacterial STD rates in the United States.

Overall, sexual attitudes and behaviors became steadily more liberal in the United States throughout the 20th century. With oral contraception in the early 1960s came partial elimination of the double standard of sexual behavior of men and women. The sexual revolution extended to homosexual and bisexual men at the same time. During the 1970s and 1980s, an increasing percentage of young women had premarital intercourse, and recent birth cohorts have had more partners than earlier birth cohorts. During the AIDS era, gay men decreased risky sexual behaviors, but some young gay men now resume such behaviors. Surveys through 1990 to 1991 do not suggest dramatic reduction in multipartner, casual, or risky sex among heterosexuals. Cocaine-associated risky sexual behavior has emerged since 1985 as a major factor in the spread of STDs.

Demography as destiny?

Previous reviews have emphasized the impact on STD incidence of growth in the absolute and relative size of the population belonging to the adolescent or young adult age groups.[110] In the United States, the post–World War II "baby-boom" generation began to reach late adolescence in the early 1960s, ushering in epidemic increases not only of STDs, but also of teen pregnancy and juvenile crime, including homicide. The decline in STD rates and in crime caused by teens and young adults that began around 1980 (interrupted in the late 80s by the crack cocaine epidemic, see the following), has continued through the 1990s. However, the children of the "baby-boom" generation are now reaching adolescence. The size of the teenage population is again expected to increase by 20 percent in the decade from 1996 through 2005, with greatest increases in African-American and Hispanic populations, creating a new wave of demographic pressure for STD transmission.

Impact of the crack cocaine epidemic in the United States

The epidemic of freebase (later crack) cocaine use appeared as early as 1982 New York, and also in the Bahamas where it was temporarily and epidemiologically associated with major epidemic of HIV and genital ulcer disease, including chancroid, syphilis, and lymphogranuloma venereum, caused by the L2 strain of *C. trachomatis*. Crack use spread throughout the United States and the Caribbean during the early and mid-1980s. Thus far, use of crack cocaine has not spread as extensively in other parts of the world. Although the estimated number of current cocaine users dropped from a peak of 5.8 million in 1985 *to 1.3 million in 1992,* the number of weekly users has not fallen since 1985.[111] It is crack use by adolescents and young adults that has been of greatest interest to those concerned about the impact of cocaine on STDs, as well as the impact on crime. The estimated number of emergency room encounters for cocaine use by smoking (crack use in recent years) increased rapidly, from 1983 to 1989. After an encouraging decline in 1990, the numbers shot up again through 1995 (Fig. 4-21). These encounters presumably reflect those cocaine users getting into greatest physiological difficulties with the drug. The percentage of cocaine users seen in emergency rooms who acknowledged use by smoking increased from 41 percent in 1990 to 53 percent in 1992, then declined to 34 percent in 1995. Because the "purity" of street cocaine rose from 58 percent in 1990 to 74 percent in 1992, the number of emergency room encounters for cocaine overdose may not provide the best measure for trends in use of crack cocaine. The Drug Use Forecasting (DUF) program (now known as the ADAM program) of the National Institute of Justice has provided an alternative surveillance tool.[113] This program tests for cocaine metabolized in urine from newly "booked" arrestees in 24 large cities in the United States. Most of those with cocaine in the urine are thought to be crack users. Although the DUF survey showed marked geographic variation in the stages of the crack epidemic, as of 1996 the epidemic was in decline in young people in 17 of 24 DUF locations, including all nine locations on East and West Coasts.[112] For example, the rate of detected cocaine in urine among 18- to 20-year-old arrestees decreased from 70 percent in 1989 to 22 percent in 1996 in Manhattan; and from 46 percent in 1988 to 25 percent in 1990 (where it remained through 1996) in Los Angeles. The perspective of those monitoring the crack cocaine epidemic provides a very intriguing paradigm not dissimilar from our perspective on STD epidemics. As Golub and Johnson noted:

> "A subgroup of hard-core (sic) users of other drugs are the first users of cocaine in a local area (the incubation phase), followed by a rapid expansion of use among their more numerous friends and associates (during the expansion phase). When the drug becomes popular, it is adopted by youths coming of age (around 18). At this time the epidemic is well established (defining a plateau phase). When new young people coming of age no longer see crack as the drug of choice, the decline phase sets in.

The DUF data suggest a decline in juvenile crack use as a precursor to a more general decline; and indicates that the epidemic is in the decline phase on the East and West Coasts, but still in the plateau phase (as of 1996) in the interior of the country, for example, in Atlanta, St. Louis, and Phoenix. The similarity to the concepts of core groups and the "dynamic topology" of STD epidemics is striking.[195]

The epidemics of teenage antisocial behaviors and crack use clearly promote the epidemic spread of STDs. In juvenile detention populations, the combined prevalence of gonorrhea and chlamydial infection typically averages about 20 percent in girls. Gonorrhea is now linked to membership in street gangs.[112] Crack use is directly related to syphilis, gonorrhea, and chancroid, as well as HIV infection.[113] Crack use leads to several STD risk behaviors, including exchange of sex for drugs or money.[117]

Trends in sexual behavior in developing countries

Sociodemographic data and ethnographic research suggest progressive liberalization of sexual behavior during the 19th and 20th centuries, as a result of colonial and economic development, urbanization, population growth, and other factors discussed in the following.[116,117] These changes probably best explain the subsequent epidemic spread of HIV and other STDs.[121] The HIV epidemic has led to qualitative behavioral research and formal sexual behavioral surveys in many developing countries. None approach the size of the sexual behavior surveys recently completed in the United Kingdom, France, or the United States, but generalizations are possible.[2–4] Invariably the reported rate of change of sex part-

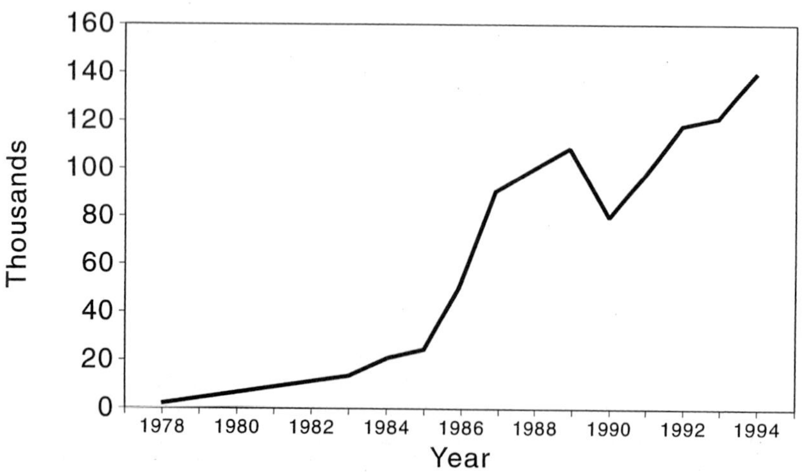

Fig. 4-21. Emergency room encounters for cocaine use by smoking, 1983–1995. Drug Abuse Warning Network, 1998 (US Substance Abuse and Mental Health Administration).

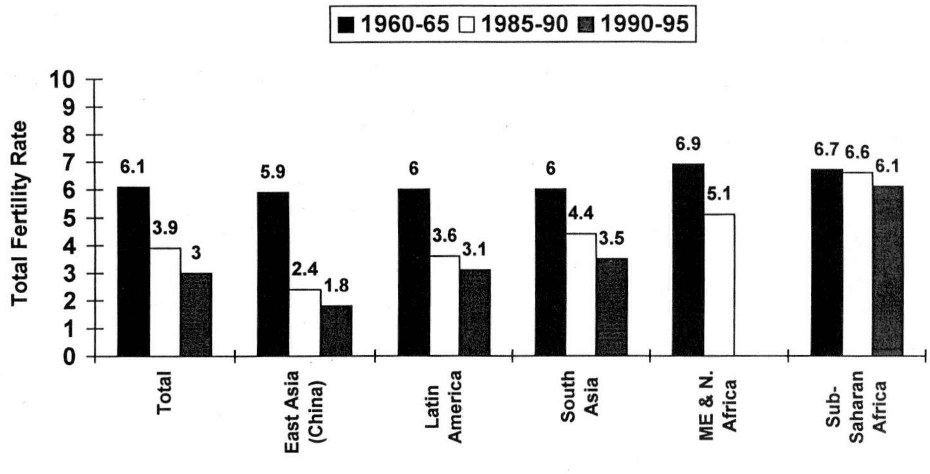

Fig. 4-22. Fertility trends in the developing world, by regions. From United Nations 1991 and 1996 World Population Sheet.

[1] Source: United Nations, 1991 and 1996 World Population Data Sheet

ners for men exceeds that for women. In six African countries surveyed in 1988 to 1990, the percentage of respondents who had engaged in casual or commercial sex in the last 12 months ranged from 8 to 44 percent for men, and 2 to 17 percent for women, with the percent of men engaging in such behavior two to four times higher than the percent of women in five of the countries.[6] In Asia and Latin America, scattered general population surveys indicate even higher differences in proportions of men and women engaging in casual or commercial sex. These gender differences in sexual behaviors in Asia and Latin America also exceed gender differences in the industrialized countries.

A series of studies of risk behaviors and STD/HIV infection in men having sex with other men in the Dominican Republic, Peru, and Nicaragua disclosed similar distinctive typologies of self-identification among MSM (transvestites, homosexual, bisexual, and heterosexual), with substantially higher rates of receptive anorectal sex and of HIV infection and other STI among those who self-identify as transvestite or homosexual.[118] Data on long-term trends in these patterns of same sex behavior are needed but largely lacking at present.

Similarly, prototypic patterns of heterosexual behavior have been postulated by Van Vliet et al., and shown in mathematical modeling to have markedly different impacts on transmission of HIV.[15] Examples of the rapid emergence of commercial sex and of the growing problem of trafficking in women from Central and Eastern to Western Europe, illustrate the importance of changing patterns of sexual behavior on the epidemiology of STDs; however, long-term analyses of trends in patterns of sexual behavior in the developing countries are not available.

Role of sexual mixing, sexual networks, and partner concurrency

Some of the most exciting developments in our understanding of the role of sexual behavior in determining the probability of exposure between infected and uninfected persons (and thus the rate of spread of STDs in the population), in the 1990s have been in the areas of patterns of partner mixing, sexual networks, and partner concurrency.[119–125] Deterministic mathematical modeling has been used to describe how patterns of sex partner mixing, such as random, assortative (like with like), or disassortative, can influence the course of an HIV epidemic.[123] Empirical data on patterns of mixing have been collected from surveys conducted in Uganda, Thailand, the United Kingdom, France, and the United States as well as a few smaller studies.[2–4,9,10,119,120,126,127] Concurrent partnerships, existence of "bridge" persons, who have sex both with members of high- and low-risk groups or with groups specifically found to have high STD prevalence and with groups with low STD prevalence.[11,125–129] High density of sexual networks (i.e., a large number of sexual connections among all members of a group), variance in a population's distribution of number of sex partners, and the extent to which so called "core groups" are embedded in the general population are all, in theory, associated with faster spread of sexually transmitted infections in the population, and higher STD rates.[121]

Two specific questions have interested STD epidemiologists in recent years. One is: Why are STD rates in the United States much higher than those in European countries, even though sexual behavior as measured by the usual parameters, including mean number of partners, is similar across these populations? The second question is: Why do African Americans in the United States have higher infection rates for most bacterial STDs, even after attempts to control on all relevant risk factors? To a great extent, the differences in access to STD services between the United States and European countries, and between African and white Americans within the United States, resulting in larger durations of infectiousness (D) for Americans in general, and African-Americans in particular, provide answers to both of these questions. However, differences in sexual behavior not reflected in means, medians, or other measures of central tendency and characteristics of sexual networks may also contribute to these differences, as discussed in the following.

Comparison of sexual behaviors in the United States and United Kingdom

Sexual behaviors of Americans and the British show both striking similarities and striking differences.[5] Similarities include age at sexual debut, rates of homosexual experience (3.8 percent in the United Kingdom versus 3.9 percent in the United States), rates of extramarital sex reported by men and women (4.7 and 1.9 percent in the United Kingdom versus 4.8 and 1.6 percent in the United States), rates of condom use in men and women (22.5 and 17.1 percent in the United Kingdom versus 17.5 and 15.3 percent in the United States), gender differences in sexual behavior, age pattern of sexual behavior, declining rates of virginity at marriage, and the age pattern of reported multiple sex partners. On the other hand, important differences between the sexual behavior of Americans and the British include: higher rates of virginity at marriage in the United States, and a larger percent of men in the United States, especially older men, reporting excess of 20 sex partners over their lifetime.

The United States apparently has greater variation than the United Kingdom in several dimensions of sexual behavior—a fact that gets overlooked when attention is focused on means, medians, and other measures of central tendency. First, both tails of the distribution of the onset of partnered sexual activity are bigger in the United States, where a larger proportion begin partnered sexual activity earlier and a larger proportion are abstinent prior to marriage. Second, both tails of the distribution of the number of partners within the past year are bigger in the United States, where larger proportions of men and women report having no sex partner (11.0 percent and 11.7 percent in the United Kingdom versus 11.3 percent and 13.2 percent in the United States) and larger proportions report having 5 or more sex partners (1.5 percent and 0.3 percent in the United Kingdom versus 3.2 and 1.6 percent in the United States). Third, tails of the distribution of number of lifetime partners are bigger in the United States, where larger proportions tend to report having no sex partners (4.2 percent and 3.2 percent in the United Kingdom versus 5.7 percent and 5.4 percent in the United States) and larger proportions report having more than 21 partners (7.8 percent and 1.2 percent in the United Kingdom versus 12.7 percent and 2.4 percent in the United States).[5] This greater variation in sexual behavior in the United States is associated with two to three times higher self-reported history of STDs. The new cases of STDs, as seen by the National Health Services in the United Kingdom and as reported to the Centers for Disease Control and Prevention in the United States were, respectively, 3.0 cases per 1000 population in 1989 and 3.5 cases per 1000 population in 1990. This latter figure is clearly an underestimate given less complete reporting of STDs in the United States.

The association between higher STD incidence and greater variance in numbers of sex partners is consistent with predictions based on a model of STD transmission dynamics.[121] In addition, it may relate to the difficulty faced in the United States in the formulation of effective and efficient public health policy in the area of STD prevention.[5] The greater variation in sexual behaviors in the United States is associated with and perhaps contributes to, greater polarization of attitudes toward risky sexual behaviors in the United States, where risky behavior is more often rejected as unacceptable or wrong. In matters of opinion about sexual matters, British men and women in every age group are consistently more liberal in terms of premarital sex (8.1 percent and 10.7 percent in the United Kingdom think it is wrong versus 24 and 32.7 percent in the United States); extramarital sex (76.4 percent and 82.6 percent think it is wrong in the United Kingdom versus 88.9 percent and 93.5 percent in the United States); and homosexual sex (67.4 percent and 53.6 percent think it is wrong in the United Kingdom versus 74.7 percent and 69.3 percent in the United States). Those who reject risky behaviors as wrong also may be more likely to reject the needed health policy decisions, blocking their formulation and implementation.

In comparing sexual behaviors of African Americans and white Americans, available data from the National Health & Social Life Survey (NHSLS)[4] indicated infection may spread more extensively among African Americans because the African-American core group (defined as those who have had four or more sex partners in the past twelve months, some concurrently) is significantly more likely to have contacts with its adjacent group (defined as those who had one or two partners in the past months, who were concurrent or who had been paid for sex, those who had three partners who may have been concurrent or not, and those who had four or more partners, none of whom were concurrent), than the white or Hispanic core groups do with their respective adjacent groups.[4,129] In addition, the percentage belonging to core and adjacent subgroups are higher for the African-American subpopulation, (11 and 25 percent, respectively) than for the white subpopulation (5 and 14 percent, respectively). Of three racial/ethnic American subpopulations (white non-Hispanic, Hispanic, and African), African Americans have the highest levels of assortative mixing, regardless of their level of sexual activity. Whites also express strong self-selection for their own racial/ethnic group, but the strength of this preference is weaker than it is for African Americans. On the other hand the more sexually active whites tend to be the more race/ethnicity exclusive in their partner choice. Thus, in terms of transmission of infection, the two racial/ethnic groups tend to be somewhat isolated from each other; Hispanic Americans appear to contribute disproportionately to bridging between them.

The sexual mixing patterns by race/ethnicity and by region also suggest an explanation for the regional pattern of STD morbidity in the United States. The Southern region of the United States has the highest rates of infection for syphilis and gonorrhea.[22] According to the NHSLS 1992 data, in the Southern region, which includes Arkansas, Tennessee, North Carolina, South Carolina, Georgia, Alabama, Mississippi, and Louisiana, the African-American core group, perhaps because of its greater likelihood of rural residence, has a stronger tendency to have sexual partnerships outside of the core group than African-American core groups in other census regions.[4]

DETERMINANTS OF TRANSMISSION EFFICIENCY

Following the emergence of the AIDS epidemic, many studies have focused on the determinants of HIV transmission efficiency. Results of these studies also shed new light on our understanding of transmission efficiency of other STDs.

Susceptibility of the uninfected host

Host susceptibility to invasive STD pathogens depends on entry of the pathogen into cells through one or more surface receptors. Factors linked to inflammation or immune activation may influence susceptibility by altering number of susceptible target cells or the receptivity of these cells.[130] Microscopic erosions may allow the pathogen to enter the bloodstream directly. Factors that interfere with or facilitate the survival of the pathogenic organism on the genital skin or the genital, rectal, or oral mucosa may decrease or increase susceptibility (see Chaps. 3 and 13). For example, the vaginal pH may affect the survival of HIV under some conditions; vaginal ecology, specifically, the absence of H_2O_2-producing lactobacilli has been associated with vaginal infections, as well as with acquisition of HIV infection (see Chap. 14).[131]

Epidemiologic and molecular biologic data suggest that some hosts may have acquired immunity to HIV-1 infection.[132–133] In addition, mutations or deletions in chemokine-receptor genes, which serve as co-receptors (with CD4) for HIV-1, have been associated with inherited resistance to transmission or progression of HIV-1 infection.[134] Various related potential mechanisms for this type of resistance to infection include lack of expression of the abnormal co-receptor on the T-cell surface; in CCR5/CCR5Δ32 heterozygotes, decreased expression of the normal CCR5 receptor on the cell surface; and upregulation of C-C β chemokines (RANTES, MIP-1α, and MIP-1β), which could inhibit viral attachment.[135] How host genetics plays a role in determining susceptibility to other STDs remains largely undefined. Pre- or post-exposure prophylaxis may potentially decrease susceptibility to STDs. The effect on susceptibility to infection of administering antiviral agents immediately after sexual exposure to HIV is not known although zidovudine administered following needle-stick injuries is associated with decreased risk of HIV infection.[136] Commercial sex workers in many areas use continuous antibiotic therapy as prophylaxis against bacterial STDs. Whether or not this practice reduces susceptibility of the individual, it increases the likelihood of the emergence of resistant gonococci.[38]

Several studies have given evidence that reproductive tract infections with other sexually transmitted pathogens increase both acquisition and transmission of HIV; and through similar mechanisms, a given STD may increase susceptibility to other STDs as well.

Conversely, prior HSV-1 infection decreases susceptibility to acquisition of HSV-2 infection (see Chap. 21). Acquired specific immunity to several STDs pathogens also occurs. Strain-specific immunity to *C. trachomatis* and *N. gonorrhoeae* may be conferred by prior infection with antigenically related strains.[137,138] Finally, specific immunity to HBV can of course be induced by hepatitis B immunoglobulin and hepatitis B vaccine.

Anatomical determinants of efficiency of transmission: male circumcision and cervical ectopy

The weight of evidence indicates that male circumcision decreases host susceptibility to several STDs, particularly including chancroid, and HIV.[50,139] The prevalence of HIV infection is 1.7 to 8.2 times as high in men with foreskins as in circumcised men, and the incidence of infection is eight times as high. Ecological comparisons have shown a striking geographic association between HIV seroprevalence and usual male circumcision practice in Africa (Fig. 4-23).[50] Given the striking association between lack of penile circumcision and HIV infection in case control studies and in ecologic studies in Africa, it seems inescapable that this is one of the most neglected risk factors in the HIV epidemic in developing countries (where lack of circumcision is also a risk factor for chancroid, as discussed in the following); and more attention to this issue in prevention efforts, perhaps in prevention trials, is urgently needed.

A recent survey based on a national random sample of the U.S. population found no relationship of circumcision to STDs, but evidence for STDs was based only on self-reported history of STDs, rather than proven STDs.[140] Several studies have found a correlation of lack of circumcision with chancroid (or with undifferentiated genital ulcers in chancroid-endemic areas). Lack of circumcision has also been held to be a risk factor for penile cancer.[50,141–143] Finally, both candida and nonspecific balanitis occur more commonly among uncircumcised men, and uncircumcised boys have an increased risk of urinary tract infection. Opponents of male circumcision cite the risk of surgical trauma and infection, selective anecdotal data suggesting circumcision decreases sexual pleasure in the male, and the possibility that circumcision of the infant lowers the threshold for subsequent pain tolerance.[50,144]

Biologically plausible hypotheses might explain the associations of STDs and HIV with having a foreskin. The recesses of the preputial sac are said to be "nonkeratinized" (i.e., like the vaginal and buccal epithelium, not covered by a layer of nonnucleated, keratin-dense squamous cells) that might predispose to secondary physical trauma or microbial infection.[50,144] Similarly, balanitis per se might predispose to invasion by microbial pathogens. The preputial sac might serve as a reservoir for STDs pathogens acquired during intercourse, from which invasion of the urethra or squamous epithelium might proceed. Clinical manifestations of urethritis, warts, or genital ulcers might go undetected longer in an uncircumcised man, which could increase transmission or complications of STDs.

However, circumcision practices are clearly related to religion, ethnicity and tribal culture, and economic status, all factors that are also strongly correlated with sexual behavior and STD risk,

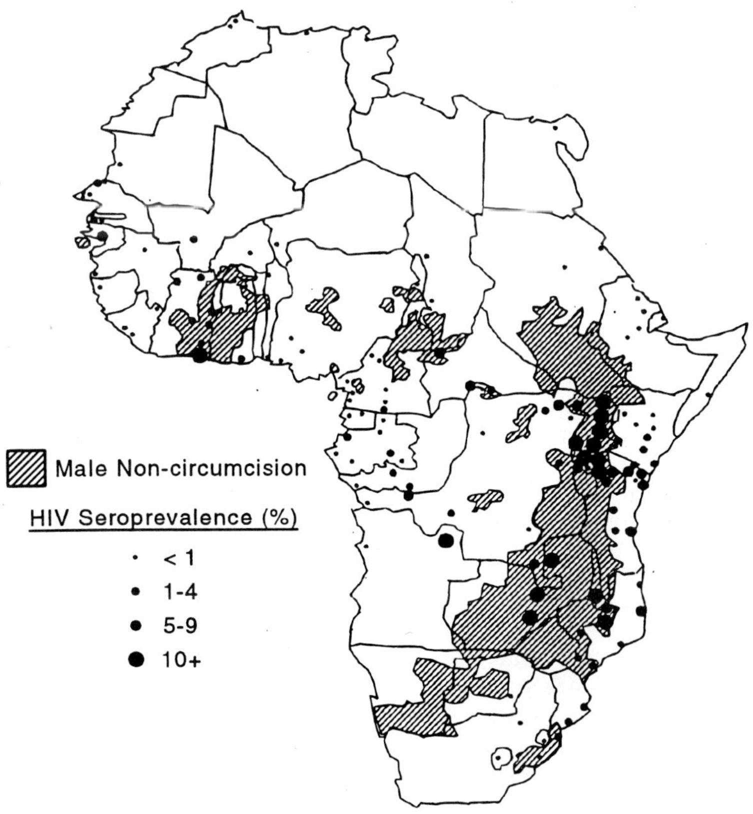

Fig. 4-23. Map of Africa showing political barriers and usual male circumcision practice, with point estimates of general adult population HIV seroprevalence superimposed (ref 50, with permission from Sexually Transmitted Infections).

and therefore could confound studies of the relationship of circumcision to HIV infection and other specific STDs.

Cervical ectopy (the presence on the exposed face of the cervix of a single layer of columnar cells that are typically found inside the os) increases susceptibility to chlamydial infection, perhaps to gonorrhea, and to HIV infection.[50,110,145–147] Cervical ectopy decreases with increasing age and smoking, and increases with hormonal contraceptive use, and may partly mediate the association of early age at sexual debut and hormonal contraceptive use with increased risk for cervical infection, and perhaps the link seen in some studies between early sexual debut and cervical cancer.[145] The increased risk for STDs, including HIV infection in young women because of cervical ectopy represents a powerful rationale for delaying sexual debut, and for use of condoms for some time after sexual debut.

Contraceptives, barrier methods, and microbicides

Condoms, used consistently and correctly, obviously protect both sexes against HIV and other STDs (see Chap. 78).[148,149] Barrier methods such as the diaphragm used with spermicide probably also offer some protection, particularly against organisms transmitted mainly between the male urethra and the cervix (e.g., *C. trachomatis, N. gonorrhoeae*). Condoms, used properly probably offer good protection against organisms, such as *C. trachomatis* and *N. gonorrhoeae;* but because male condoms may not completely prevent contact between the epithelium of the penis and the vulva, probably offer less protection against those which commonly infect stratified squamous epithelium such as herpes simplex virus and human papilloma virus (see Chaps. 78 and 94).

Spermicides containing nonoxynol-9 appear to offer modest protection against some STDs, even though most studies demonstrating this protective effect failed to reach statistical significance. Data from cross-sectional studies suggested protection against HIV as well, but two completed randomized controlled trials-one using the N-9 containing sponge, one using N-9 containing film-showed no protection against HIV (see Chap. 78).[150,151]

Data on the effects of hormonal contraceptives on susceptibility to STDs including HIV are mixed (see Chap. 78). Oral contraceptive usage has been associated with decreased risk of severe PID, with increased risk of cervical infection with *C. trachomatis,* and possibly with increased risk of cervical infection with *N. gonorrhoeae.*[110,145,152,153] Some studies report a protective effect of hormonal contraceptives to HIV infection while others report increased risk, possibly due to cervical ectopy and thinning of the vaginal wall. However, the two studies with statistically significant results suggest that hormonal contraceptive use increases susceptibility to HIV infection.[153,154] Of four studies that examined effects of injectable hormones on susceptibility to HIV, two reported statistically significant results, both suggesting increased risk.[154,155] A metaanalysis of the effects of hormonal contraception on risk of acquisition of HIV suggests a small but significantly increased risk.

Thus, trends in STD and HIV infection may be influenced by changing patterns of contraceptive use, which may influence not only sexual behavior, but also efficiency of transmission of STDs. Contraceptive attitudes and usage patterns certainly have been changing, at least in the United States. As of 1995, the major contraceptive methods used in the United States were female sterilization (18 percent) and the oral contraceptive pill (17 percent), followed by the male condom (13 percent), and male sterilization (7 percent).[57] The pill was the leading method used by women under age 30. Among women ages 30 to 44, female sterilization was the leading method. Nearly 30 percent of women who used the pill as their only method of contraception reported inconsistent use. Of the 9.7 million women using only coitus-dependent contraceptive methods at sometime in the 3 months before the interview, almost 33 percent, used them inconsistently, that is, not at every act of intercourse.

Between 1982 and 1988, condom use remained steady among married women, at about 15 percent, whereas among the unmarried it increased markedly, from 9 to 16 percent. In 1995, condom use by partners of unmarried women was 14 percent. Fifty-four percent of women who had sexual intercourse for the first time during the 1990s had used condoms. This figure had been 36 percent in the 1980s, and only 18 percent in the 1970s.[57]

Patterns of knowledge and use of condoms in most other parts of the world are less well known. During the 1970s in developed countries, the proportion of currently married females of childbearing age who reported current use of condoms ranged from a low of 2 to 3 percent in Yugoslavia, Bulgaria, and Romania to a high of 50 percent in Japan; this percentage was 32 in Finland, 25 in Denmark, 18 in the United Kingdom, 16 in Norway, and 13 in Italy.

Survey data from around the developing world on prevalence of knowledge and use of condoms among reproductive-age women were compiled in 1989.[156] These data revealed a wide range in knowledge of condoms, with the least knowledge in sub-Saharan Africa, including those countries with high HIV prevalence. Knowledge of condoms was most widespread in Latin America and the Caribbean, where over 80 percent of currently married women of reproductive age were familiar with condoms. Countries in Asia tended to report lower levels of knowledge of condoms. In the Middle East and North Africa, the proportion of women reporting knowledge of condoms ranged from 26 to 61 percent. Least knowledge of condoms was reported for Nigeria, Benin, and Mali.

Among developing countries, those in and around the Caribbean had highest rates of reported condom use: Costa Rica (13 percent), Trinidad and Tobago (12 percent), Jamaica (8 percent), and Barbados and Venezuela (5 percent). Prevalence of reported condom use was 2 to 4 percent in India, Bangladesh, Mexico, Brazil, Malaysia, Turkey, and Tunisia. In a majority of developing countries with available data, less than 1 percent of couples reported condom use. This pattern was observed in all of mainland sub-Saharan Africa, including countries such as Zimbabwe and Botswana, which have relatively high overall contraceptive prevalence; in most of North Africa and the Middle East; and in some Caribbean and Latin American nations, such as Haiti, El Salvador, Honduras, and Bolivia.

More recent surveys on knowledge and current use of condoms among reproductive age married women revealed more encouraging findings (Leo Morris, personal communication) (Table 4-6). In 1993 and 1994, in sub-Saharan Africa, 85 to 95 percent of women were familiar with condoms, but only 1 to 2 percent reported use of condoms. In Asia and the Near East, knowledge of condoms by married women was somewhat lower. In China in 1992, only 1 percent of married women used condoms. In Latin America and the Caribbean, knowledge of condoms ranged from 51 percent in Bolivia to 99 percent in Jamaica and Costa Rica; reported use of condoms ranged from 1 percent in the Dominican Republic to 17 percent in Jamaica.

Among unmarried women between 15 and 49 years of age, data collected between 1993 and 1996 showed that the percent with knowledge of condoms ranged from 87 percent in Mali in 1996 to 100 percent in Brazil in 1996, and the percent currently using condoms ranged from 8 percent in Mali in 1996 to 36 percent in Jamaica in 1996.

Past efforts by family planning groups have emphasized condom use for contraception, rather than for STD prophylaxis. Some family planning workers now express concern that condom promotion for disease prophylaxis may stigmatize condom use and undo the results of past efforts to promote condom accept-

Table 4-6. Percentage of Sexually Active Married and Unmarried Women 15 to 49 with Knowledge of Condoms and Using Condoms National Surveys, 1993–1996

Country	Year of Survey	Percentage with Knowledge	Currently Using Condoms
Married women			
Kenya	1994	85	1
Zimbabwe	1994	95	2
China	1992	—	1
Egypt	1995	52	1
India	1993	58	3
Indonesia	1994	67	1
Philippines	1993	94	1
Turkey	1993	81	7
Costa Rica	1993	99	16
Jamaica	1993	99	17
Paraguay	1996	93	6
Peru	1996	88	4
Columbia	1995	98	4
Ecuador	1994	70	3
El Salvador	1993	93	2
Guatemala	1995	52	2
Bolivia	1994	51	1
Dominican Republic	1996	98	1
Unmarried women			
Ivory Coast	1994	92	11
Mali	1996	87	8
Uganda	1995	94	15
Zimbabwe	1994	98	14
Brazil	1996	100	17
Jamaica	1993	99*	36

*All women.

Leo Morris, personal communication.

ability. Nonetheless, current global public health efforts to increase condom use to prevent transmission of STDs, including HIV, are directed to essentially all sexually active individuals who do not use condoms, particularly in developing countries. Interest is growing in more targeted promotion of condom use for those at highest risk of STDs (e.g., sex workers, clients of sex workers, and those engaging in casual sex), which may be a more practical, realistic, and cost-effective approach to STD prevention.

Sexual practices

Clearly, unprotected anorectal sex is a risk for acquiring HIV infection not only for men, but also for women, and for acquiring hepatitis B virus infection.[96,157] During vaginal intercourse, women appear to be at somewhat higher risk than men of acquiring HIV infection and several other STDs as well; probably including HSV-2 infection, gonorrhea, chlamydia, and others. Sex during menstruation may increase a woman's risk of acquiring HIV infection.[158] Whether susceptibility to other STDs also increase during menstruation is not known.

Inoculum size: A determinant of the level of infectiousness of the infected host

From the standpoint of the pathogen, production of epithelial lesions and inflammatory exudates or diarrhea, and initially unfettered growth of the organism to high concentrations in genital fluids, represent strategies for transmission to new hosts and hence for self-propagation and persistence in the population. Thus, infections with HIV, like those with hepatitis B, HSV, *C. trachomatis, N. gonorrhoeae, T. pallidum,* and many other STD pathogens are probably most infectious in the early stage of infection, with infectivity increasing as the concentration of the organism in the genital tract increases, and decreasing as the pathogen-specific host immune response suppresses concentrations of the pathogen.[159–162] To the extent that STDs are acquired during periods of rapid partner change, the pathogen benefits by achieving an early peak in transmissibility. Data on viral concentration in blood and semen generally support the association between stage of infection and transmission of HIV.[163–165] However, some studies found no relation.[166,167]

Therapy

Even for the incurable STDs, antiviral drugs may decrease the infectivity of the host by decreasing the concentrations of virus in genital secretions. Highly active antiretroviral therapy (HAART) clearly reduces the concentration of HIV-1 RNA in plasma, and data on the impact of HAART on viral RNA and DNA in semen, cervicovaginal fluid, and anorectal secretions are just beginning to emerge, and are generally suggesting a beneficial effect on viral shedding, thereby potentially decreasing infectiousness (T. Lampinen, personal communication). Similarly, with genital HSV infection, suppressive antiviral therapy decreases clinical recurrences and antiviral shedding; randomized controlled trials of suppressive therapy would be required to definitively prove that suppressive therapy prevents transmission of infection to HSV seronegative partners.

Inflammation and other reproductive tract infections

Inflammation and immune activation may affect the production of virus or bacteria and increase or decrease the level of infectiousness of the infected host.[139] Similarly, factors that inhibit or facilitate survival of the pathogenic organism in or on the oral, genital, or rectal mucosae may effect infectiousness of the infected host. For example, in theory, vaginal ecology may affect the concentration of a pathogen in the vagina of an infected host just as it affects susceptibility among the uninfected. Presence of other STDs increases HIV infectiousness. Seminal leukocytosis,[168] gonococcal urethritis,[169,170] and shedding of cytomegalovirus in semen[171] are associated with increased detection of HIV in semen or urethral swab specimens. Treatment of urethritis diminishes detection of HIV in the urethra and the concentration of HIV in the semen.[169,170] For women data are more limited but consistent with an influence of cervical infection on cervical shedding of HIV.[172,173] Similar data on the impact of genital inflammation or reproductive tract infection on shedding of other STDs are inconclusive.

Other determinants of level of infectivity

Partners of uncircumcised men are more likely than partners of circumcised men to be infected with HIV. This suggests either that lack of circumcision may increase level of infectiousness, or that uncircumcised men are simply more likely to have HIV infection in a particular ecologic setting, or both hypotheses may be true.[139,174]

Shedding of HIV may be increased during menstruation, pregnancy, and hormonal contraception. Men who have sex with HIV infected women during menstruation are over threefold more likely to have HIV infection as those who do not.[175] Some data suggest that during pregnancy HIV infected women were two or three times more likely to have HIV detected in genital secretions.[146,176,177]

One recent study also demonstrated an association of hormonal contraception with increased cervical shedding of HIV, suggesting a possible impact on transmission from female to male.[173]

DETERMINANTS OF DURATION OF INFECTIOUSNESS

As discussed in the preceding, the primary determinant of duration of infectivity of any specific sexually transmitted infection is the natural history of that infection. Access to effective treatment has become the most important factor in reducing the duration of infectiousness (and infection) of bacterial STDs. In some developing countries, inadequate clinical, laboratory, pharmacy, and public health infrastructure allows the duration of infectiousness for even the curable STDs to approach that of the natural history of infection. In the industrialized countries, antiviral therapies now may also influence the level of infectiousness of some of the viral STDs, making this parameter now relevant to both bacterial and viral STDs. Health care seeking behaviors of the population, behaviors of health care providers and properties of the health care system all influence the duration of infectiousness (and infection).

Even in the United States, the existing infrastructure for provision of STD care is woefully inadequate. The public STD clinics are unable to provide sufficient access to all persons seeking health care; and have generally not made hepatitis B vaccination available to high risk groups to reduce spread of the first vaccine preventable STDs; or played a major role until recently in diagnostic testing and partner notification for *Chlamydia trachomatis* infection.[16,63,178] The inadequacy of the STD health service infrastructure and the resulting preventable increment in duration of infectiousness is a major reason why the United States has the highest rates of STDs among developed countries (see Chap. 93).

DETERMINANTS OF COMPLICATIONS AND SEQUELAE OF STDS

The many complications of bacterial STDs result from poor health care access, quality, and utilization. Many other behaviors also influence complications. Just one example, pelvic inflammatory disease, has been associated with vaginal douching, which is more common among black women, and may contribute to the increased rates of pelvic inflammatory disease and its sequelae in black women.[179,180] Conversely, oral contraception use seems to decrease the risk of clinically overt pelvic inflammatory disease among women with cervical chlamydial infection.[152]

In 1988, 37 percent of U.S. women 15 to 44 reported douching regularly. In 1995, this proportion had declined to 27 percent. Douching remained more common than average among Hispanic women (34 percent), black women (55 percent), women who did not finish high school (53 percent), and those who have had PID (41 percent). Black college graduates were more likely to douche regularly than white college graduates (40 percent versus 9 percent).[58,181]

HIV infection and immunosuppression increase the frequency, severity, and chronicity of recurrent genital and anal HSV infections, and predispose to acyclovir resistance during therapy of recurrences. HIV infection also predisposes to increased rates of external genital warts, genital and anorectal HPV shedding, and anal and cervical dysplasia, and perhaps to invasive genital and anal cancers. HIV infection predisposes to opportunistic CMV complications, and also may influence the risk and severity of pelvic inflammatory disease among women with cervical or vaginal infection.[182]

Finally, variation in the STD pathogens themselves influences disease manifestations. For example, strains of *N. gonorrhoeae* that require arginine, hypoxanthine, and uracil for growth accounted for a high proportion of cases of gonorrhea in the United States and Europe during the 1960s and 1970s and caused most cases of gonococcal bacteremia, but had reduced propensity to cause pelvic inflammatory disease.[183] Non-prototype variants of HPV-16 are more likely than prototypic strains, to produce moderate to severe cervical dysplasia.[185]

RISK MARKERS AND RISK FACTORS FOR STDS

In STD epidemiology the terms risk factor, risk marker (or risk indicator), and risk determinant have been used interchangeably without much attention to the existence of a *causal* link between the relevant attribute or exposure and the disease or disease outcome. Similarly, little differentiation has been made between modifiable and nonmodifiable risk factors, an important distinction within the context of prevention.

Many of the traditional STD risk factors appear to be correlates of the probability of encountering an infected partner, whereas others may influence the probability of infection if exposed, or the probability of disease if infected. Although the causal link between demographic variables and STDs can probably be explained in terms of coincidental differences in sexual behavior or disease prevalence, such variables may be most accurately referred to as risk markers or risk indicators. For example, single marital status and inner-city residence fall into this category.

Other variables, such as sexual behaviors and health care behaviors, are directly related to the probability of exposure to STDs, to infection following exposure, or to complications if infected, and can be referred to as true risk factors.

Of the major sexual behavioral risk factors for STDs discussed earlier, all but specific sexual practices really represent attempts to measure the probability of exposure to an infected partner.

Health care behaviors that can reduce the risk of acquiring STDs or prevent complications include use of condoms for prophylaxis, early consultation for diagnosis and treatment, compliance with therapy, and partner referral (see Chap. 93). Absence of such behaviors can be regarded as risk factors for STDs. As noted, douching, although undertaken for "feminine hygiene," may actually increase the risk of PID and its sequelae.[179,180]

Several other variables could function both as risk markers and risk factors, or are difficult to classify as one or the other at present. For example, young age and gender are certainly risk indicators, indirectly related to risk of STDs as correlates of sexual behavior and of disease prevalence in sex partners. However, age and gender may also directly influence host susceptibility. For example, the higher prevalence of cervical ectopy in young women may influence susceptibility to certain STD pathogens such as *C. trachomatis,* and older individuals may have acquired immunity to STD pathogens, resulting in fewer infections per exposure. Regarding gender-specific risk, the risk of infection per exposure during vaginal intercourse may be greater for the female than for the male with respect to several STD pathogens such as *N. gonorrhoeae, C. trachomatis,* hepatitis B virus, herpes simplex virus, and HIV, although available evidence remains inconclusive.[185–188] Some behavioral factors, such as smoking and young age at sexual debut, generally assumed to be indicators of risk rather than causally related to disease outcome, have been linked to specific infections or related syndromes such as cancer of the cervix even when other risk indicators and sexual behaviors are adjusted for in statistical analyses. Further empirical evidence is needed to conclusively determine whether these variables and others like them operate as true causal risk factors or are simply coincidental markers of high-risk sexual behaviors. Epidemiologic studies of putative risk factors, such as smoking can attempt to adjust for high-risk sexual behaviors, such as lifetime numbers of sex partners, but all partners are not alike, and it is difficult to control adequately for choice of riskier partners. Alcohol and drug abuse can perhaps be referred to as "risk modifiers," since they produce situational modification of sexual behavior or health care behavior.

COMMERCIAL SEX AS A RISK FACTOR FOR STDS

The contribution of sex work to the spread of STDs has been assessed by monitoring the incidence or prevalence of STDs in female sex workers (FSW) and the proportion of male patients with STDs who acknowledge recent sex with a FSW (see Chap. 10). Studies have focused on specific outbreaks of syphilis, chancroid, and resistant gonorrhea, as well as HIV infection. The sociodemography of the men involved in these outbreaks has often (but not always) involved some form of transiency, as in the case of foreigners, servicemen, and migrant laborers. Transient populations are by definition not integrated into the community; their only sexual, and sometimes social, interaction with the main community may be through FSW contact. The gender-selective nature of most international migration (especially initially), and of temporary unskilled and semiskilled labor reinforce, through the unavailability of women, the demand for FSW contact. Women who migrate or become refugees are also at increased risk of STDs, as they may lack other means of support and become sex workers (see Chap. 12).[84] The social profiles of both the men and women involved in some STD outbreaks in migrants and travelers have involved the exchange of drugs for sex and vice versa.

The recent pattern in the United States reflects trends in use of crack cocaine. In a 1986 to 1987 Seattle outbreak of a unique strain of PPNG, within a few months after the strain had been introduced into the community, approximately 80 percent of infections with this strain occurred in individuals who had had sex with FSWs or were themselves FSWs, or who had used illicit drugs around the time that infection occurred.[33] On a global basis, commercial sex has been most common in settings characterized by poverty, social disintegration, and a double standard of sexual behavior (e.g., Latin American countries). Where many of these factors coincide, commercial sex is most prevalent.[189,190] Commercial sex and FSW contact are clearly major factors in the epidemiology of HIV and other STDs in many developing countries of Africa, Asia, and Latin America.[11,88,90,92,192] In such settings, the great majority of STD clinic attendees are male, and the majority of those with gonorrhea, syphilis, or chancroid identify the suspected source contact as a FSW. The role of sex with FSWs in the epidemiology of these STDs now requires close attention not only in developing countries, but also in the former Soviet Union and in the United States, where occurrence of bacterial STDs is contracting around an expanding core of inner-city minority populations.

PREVENTION TRIALS

Prevention trials targeting particular risk factors for STDs can help confirm the role of the risk factor, as swell as guide preventive interventions that directly influence the epidemiology of STDs. The search for conclusive results in the evaluation of interventions to prevent STDs, including HIV, has resulted in increasing numbers of controlled prevention trials in the past decade. Such trials are generally classified either as behavioral or biomedical intervention trials, although in reality, even those based on a biomedical intervention require supportive behavioral intervention components (e.g., to motivate vaccine acceptance and compliance, and prevent relapse to riskier behaviors by those who might otherwise feel safe after vaccination); and as discussed in the following, behavioral interventions benefit from biomedical outcome measures.

BEHAVIORAL PREVENTIVE INTERVENTION TRIALS

In the past behavioral interventions were usually for chronic disease prevention. The best prevention trials have been related to cardiovascular disease prevention. These have included both individual and community level interventions and were evaluated at both individual and community levels.[193]

In STDs and HIV prevention several specific issues need to be considered. First, the behaviors targeted for change (e.g., sexual behaviors) are difficult to measure objectively. Dependence on self-reports of behavior creates additional problems in that interventions may change reports of behavior without changing the behavior itself.[193] Second, individuals who change one risk behavior often change other risk behaviors in a countervailing direction, necessitating use of summary measures that reflect the net effects of these changes.[194] Third, the transmission dynamics of STDs are influence not only by sexual behavior but also by additional factors, such as phase of the epidemic, population prevalence, transmission probability, duration of infectiousness, and specific characteristics of transmission networks, resulting in different trends in the incidence of various STDs in the same populations.[195,196] Fourth, the nature of the relationship between sexual behavior and STD incidence varies across the phases of the epidemic.[195] At the individual level, the magnitude of risk associated with particular behaviors depends on the infectiousness of the infected partner. Finally, as eloquently stated recently, whereas adjustment for confounding factors may be feasible in epidemiologic studies of etiologic factors, bias in adoption of behavior change (or in intervention assignment) is inherently part of the practice of medicine and public health, and the idea that such bias can be simply adjusted away may be wishful thinking.[197] In this context it is interesting to note that data sets from randomized controlled trials with null findings, when analyzed in the same manner as cohort studies with adjustment for confounding, can misleadingly indicate that the intervention was effective (Ward Cates and Ron Roddy, personal communication). This observation is congruent with earlier conclusions that the many advantages provided by randomization when subgroups are defined by baseline characteristics are lost when follow-up responses are used to define patient subgroups.[198]

In the light of all these considerations, it is increasingly obvious that in evaluating behavioral interventions to prevent STDs, and HIV, data from randomized controlled trials are particularly important, the choice of outcome measure is critical, and the outcome measure of choice is the appropriate biomedical measure of the STD or STDs of interest.[193,199]

Most evaluations of behavioral interventions to date have employed less rigorous study designs and behavioral outcome measures. A systematic review of computerized abstracts from International AIDS conferences between 1989 and 1992 showed that only 10 of 15,946 abstracts reported on randomized controlled trials of behavioral interventions.[193] Two more recent critical reviews of behavioral interventions in general and behavioral interventions for young people reported similar findings.[200,201] These reviews also indicated that many behavioral intervention studies focused only on determinants of behavior such as knowledge, beliefs, and attitudes as outcome measures.

Although the majority of behavioral intervention studies do not employ randomized controlled designs or biomedical outcome measures, some remarkably important studies have been completed recently. Among the most important of these, in terms of public health implications, is Project RESPECT. This project was designed to specifically evaluate the efficacy of individual HIV prevention counseling in changing high risk behaviors and preventing new STDs. This study of high-risk heterosexuals is among the first randomized trials of HIV/STD prevention counseling.[202] The study, conducted among HIV negative, heterosexual STD clinic patients enrolled from five U.S. inner-city STD clinics (Baltimore, Denver, Long Beach, Newark, San Francisco), compared: (1) Enhanced Counseling (a four-session counseling intervention, each session of 1 hour duration) based on theories of behavioral science, social cognitive theory, and the theory of reasoned action, and aimed at changing attitudes, self-efficacy, and perception of risk regarding consistent condom use with all sex partners); (2) Client-Centered HIV Prevention Counseling (two sessions of 20 minutes each), an intervention based on CDC's client-centered counseling model recommended for use with HIV testing, and aimed at increasing clients' perceptions of personal risk, exploring barriers, and facilitators around risk reduction, and negotiating an incremental risk reduction plan that emphasized consistent condom use with all sex partners); and (3) HIV Education (the control intervention that was purely informational, using two brief, didactic messages about HIV and STDs prevention that encouraged consistent condom use with all sex partners, similar to the type of prevention messages given at most STD clinics). The Enhanced Counseling and Client-Centered Counseling interventions were significantly more effective than the HIV education intervention at decreasing high-risk behaviors and preventing new STDs. These findings were consistent across study sites and gender. Most of the STD reduction occurred in the first 6 months. At 12 months there were no differences across intervention and control groups in condom use, but a 20 percent reduction in new STDs for counseling interventions remained significant (although the 12-month difference was attributable to the reductions achieved during the first 6 months). The amount and duration of the effect of counseling in Project RESPECT were modest, but from the population perspective even modest changes in behaviors of high risk STD clinic patients could have a substantial impact on STD and HIV transmission.

Another multisite randomized HIV prevention trial, coordinated by the National Institute of Mental Health, developed and evaluated a seven-session intervention targeting sexual behavior change among low-income individuals at high risk for HIV infection.[203,204] Participants were largely recruited from STD clinics, with a smaller number from primary health care settings. The intervention group experienced significant reductions in reported unprotected sexual exposures and lower rates of gonococcal infection in men (based on chart review), but urine LCR tests at 12 months showed no difference in prevalence of gonococcal or chlamydial infections. Taken together, Project RESPECT and the NIMH trial suggest an impact on behavior with transient reduction in bacterial STD incidence. The feasibility is lower for wide scale implementation in public health settings of the seven-session intervention employed in the NIMH trial than for the two-session Project RESPECT intervention. The impact of the latter two-session intervention was especially encouraging, but the need for "booster" counseling sessions to achieve more persistent effects requires more study.

A third randomized controlled study, a culture- and gender-specific risk-reduction intervention targeting African-American and Hispanic STD clinic patients in San Antonio, Texas, reduced reinfection rates with gonorrhea and chlamydia among high risk minority women, and these effects apparently persisted for 12 months.[205]

The behavioral intervention trials mentioned in the preceding randomized individuals across intervention and control conditions. Behavioral intervention trials that randomize groups or larger units are even fewer in number. A study in Zimbabwe randomized work-sites to an HIV-prevention health education intervention, women at the work-sites that received the intervention reportedly experienced a subsequent significant reduction in HIV incidence, compared with the control work-sites.[206]

A recently completed study randomized 180 randomly selected pharmacies in Lima Peru to intervention and control conditions.[207] The intervention consisted of education on STD recognition, management, and prevention counseling. Intervention significantly improved the amount of STD counseling provided by pharmacies, but did not influence STD recognition or management in pharmacies.[208] In another effort researchers in the United Kingdom have conducted a four-school randomized trial to assess the feasibility of a large randomized controlled trial of peer-led sex education in schools.[206] The findings suggest that evaluation of peer-led sex education through a randomized controlled trial is acceptable to schools, pupils, and parents. In general, pupils who received peer-led sex education responded more positively than those in control schools.

BIOMEDICAL PREVENTIVE INTERVENTION TRIALS

A randomized controlled trial provided empirical evidence for the effectiveness of screening for cervical chlamydial infection followed by timely and appropriate treatment has emerged as the key strategy for the prevention of pelvic inflammatory disease. Participants were unmarried female health maintenance organization enrollees 18 to 34 years of age with risk factors for chlamydial infection. They were randomized to receive chlamydia screening or routine care. In this study, cervical chlamydia screening led to a 56 percent reduction in the incidence of pelvic inflammatory disease during 1 year of follow-up.[209]

Another intervention trial assessed the effect of nonoxynol-9 (N-9) film on the rates of gonococcal and chlaymdial infections and HIV infection in a cohort of sex workers.[210] A two-year triple-masked multi-clinic randomized controlled trial was conducted among 1292 HIV-negative non-pregnant sex workers between the ages of 18 to 45 in Cameroon. Women were randomized to use condoms and N-9 film or condoms and placebo film, were counseled monthly to use both at every coital act, and were examined monthly for a mean of 14 months. The study found no additional effect of N-9 over that of condoms on the rate of cervical infection or HIV infection in this population of sex workers. Although they reported high rates of condom use, the rate of new gonorrhea infections was 31.1 infections per 100 woman-years in the placebo group and 33.3 per 100 woman-years in the N-9 group (RR = 1.07, 95 percent C.I. 0.83 to 1.39). The rate of chlamydial infections was 22.2 per 100 woman-years for placebo users and 20.6 per 100 woman years for N-9 users (RR = 0.93, 95 percent C.I. 0.68 to 1.26). These results are consistent with an earlier randomized controlled trial of N-9 containing cervical sponges, showing no reduction in HIV acquisition among Nairobi sex workers.[211] Some previous trials had shown modest efficacy of N9 in preventing gonococcal or chlamydial infection in women (see Chap. 78).

A landmark HIV prevention trial randomized communities to biomedical intervention and control conditions to assess the effect of the community level intervention. This community randomized trial conducted in the Mwanza region of Tanzania was the first randomized trial to demonstrate an impact of a preventive intervention on HIV incidence in a general population. It showed that improved syndromic management of STDs at the primary health care level reduced HIV incidence by about 40 percent.[212] HIV incidence was compared in six intervention communities and six pair-matched comparison communities. A random cohort of 1000 adults, 15 to 54 years of age, from each community was surveyed at baseline and at follow-up 2 years later. The intervention included establishment of an STD reference clinic, staff training in syndromic management, regular supervisory visits to health facilities, and provision of antimicrobials, and general population health education about STDs and health-care-seeking for STD symptoms.

A subsequent HIV-prevention trial in the Rakai district of Uganda randomized clusters of villages to mass treatment of STDs every 10 months versus antiparasitic treatment alone. Serologic screening and treatment for syphilis, and syndromic management for STDs, were offered both to intervention and control villages. The study showed no effect on HIV incidence, but significant improvements in pregnancy outcomes.[213,214] The differences in outcome of the Mwanza and Rakai studies are intriguing. The Mwanza study focused on treatment of symptomatic STDs only; whereas the Rakai study provided antimicrobials to the entire population, some of whom had prevalent STDs. In the Mwanza trial, the intervention villages achieved a lower rate of seroconversion to active syphilis, and of symptomatic urethritis in men. The Rakai study offered serologic screening and treatment for syphilis, and syndromic management for STDs both in the intervention and the control communities. Thus, at the point the Rakai study was terminated, absolute differences between intervention and control groups in prevalence of STDs (other than trichomoniasis and syphilis seroreactivity) were small: by the end of the study, there were no significant differences between intervention and control clusters in prevalence of gonorrhea, chlamydial infection, or bacterial vaginosis, or in frequency of reported genital ulcer disease, or in proportion seeking care for STD symptoms. The impact of systemic antimicrobial therapy on normal flora in uninfected individuals (e.g., transient suppression of potentially protective H_2O_2-producing lactobacilli or increasing vulvovaginal candidiasis, both potential risk factors for HIV acquisition), represent possible confounders of any beneficial impact of reduced STD prevalence.[155] Differences in the relative prevalence of STDs and HIV in the Mwanza and Rakai districts (higher prevalence of HIV infection in Rakai) and basic differences in study design and in the nature of the interventions also may account for the differences in outcome. A recent paper provided a useful methodologic overview of community randomization trials of STD/HIV preventive interventions.[215]

ASSESSING EFFECTIVENESS OF POLICY INTERVENTIONS

Randomized controlled intervention trials at individual, group, or community levels provide the best empirical evidence for the effectiveness of preventive measures. However, preventive measures with the greatest impact include so called structured interventions, often based on policy changes. Use of randomized controlled trials to assess the effects of policy interventions is usually not feasible; more creative approaches are needed for this purpose.

One well-known strategy is to combine information from many sources and check for consistency across data sets. This is the approach employed in assessing the effects of the policies adopted by the Thai HIV/AIDS Control Program, which required 100 percent condom use in commercial sex. Evaluation is based on reductions in STD cases in government clinics, and declines in HIV/STDs observed through surveys of men and commercial sex workers. More recently, a comparison of two cohorts of military conscripts showed a decline in HIV incidence from 2.48 per 100 person-years between 1991 to 1993 to 0.55 per 100 person-years between 1993 and 1995. STD incidence declined even more, with an overall ten-fold decrease between 1991 to 1993 and 1993 to 1995.[216] The most recent analysis of trends in prevalence of HIV infection among young men conscripted into the military during May or November each year show that the prevalence peaked in 1992 to 1993 and has been declining since, with possible leveling off in the most recent group of conscripts (Fig. 4-24).

Another approach has been used in demonstrating the effectiveness of alcohol taxation on reducing STD rates among youth.[217] Between 1982 and 1994 there were 34 instances of a state beer tax increase in the United States. The investigators conducted a non-parametric quasi-experiment comparing the proportional changes in STD rates in states with and without a tax increase over the same period, and employed a time series econometric analysis, evaluating the effect of the level of beer taxation on the proportional changes in STD rates, controlling for legal minimum drinking age, per capita income, and state and year differences. The results showed that in 26 (77 percent) of the states with an increase in beer tax, there was a greater proportional decrease in gonorrhea rates among males in both the 15 to 19 and

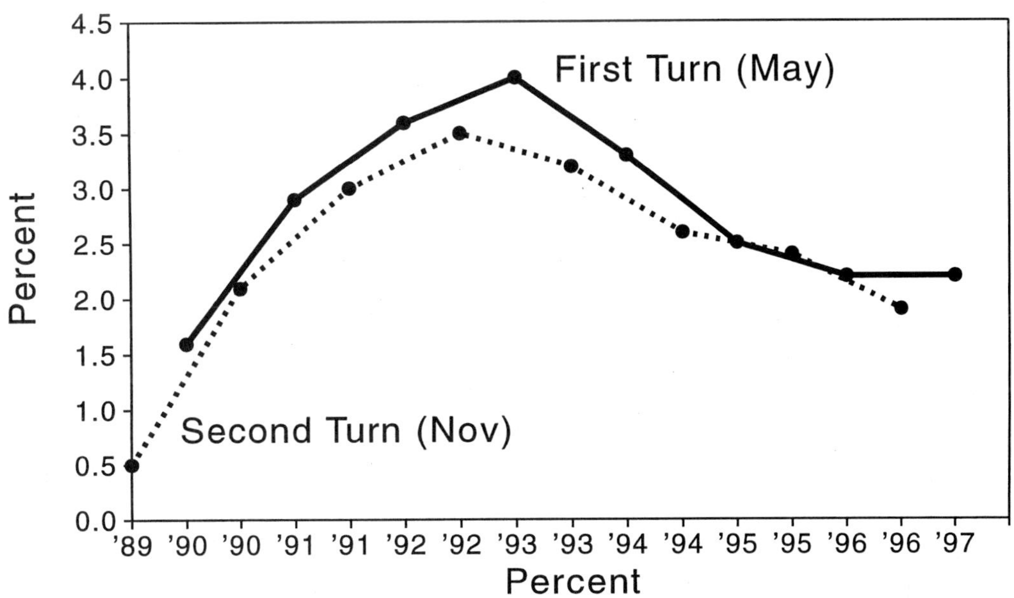

Fig. 4-24. Trends in prevalence of HIV seropositivity in Thai Army conscripts entering service in May or November, 1989–1997 (source: Armed Forces Research Institute of Medical Sciences, Thailand. Kindly provided by Dr. Suporu Koetsawang).

the 20 to 24 age groups as compared to the proportional change among the states without a tax increase. Similar patterns were observed for females. It was estimated that a $0.15 tax increase on a six-pack of beer would reduce gonorrhea incidence rates by roughly 10 percent among the 15 to 19 year age group. The feasibility, non-invasive nature, and relatively low cost of this study is remarkable, and of course its findings, not having been based on sample data, are completely generalizable to the study population. Non-obtrusive measures to assess the effectiveness of policy interventions to reduce STDs, including HIV, warrant further evaluation.

As indicated by a recent comparison of sexual lifestyles in the United States and the United Kingdom, the greater dispersion in sexual behavior in the United States than in the United Kingdom implies a need for strong public health policy, but that the same dispersion creates strong opinions about inappropriate sexual behavior that make implementation and evaluation of strong health policy decisions difficult.[5]

SOCIOECONOMIC AND DEMOGRAPHIC CORRELATES OF STDS

As the end of the 20th century approaches, the world's population finds itself in the midst of major demographic, economic, social, and political change creating remarkable social instability. These changes and the resulting instability greatly increase the chances of sexual mixing among all groups and categories of people, including mixing between individuals who are infected with STDs and those who are not. Dramatic examples in recent times of the influence of such instability on STDs include: (1) the epidemic spread of STDs in China after opening its borders, with increasing internal migration of men to urban settings for work, and reintroduction of sex work; (2) the epidemic spread of STDs within the former USSR, and from the former USSR to adjacent European countries after the fall of communism; (3) rapid spread of HIV to and within South Africa, associated with massive migration to and within that country after elimination of apartheid; and (4) the rapid spread of HIV and STDs in Cambodia during the mid-1990s, after the devastation wrought by the Khmer Rouge, followed by continuing political instability.[19] The impact of social instability leading to explosive increases in the spread of both bacterial and viral STDs can be limited through health promotion resulting in adoption of preventive behaviors by individuals, and through provision of adequate health services resulting in early detection and treatment of bacterial and viral STDs. Unfortunately, the powerful social forces that bring about increased sexual mixing also result in circumstances that make effective health promotion and adequate provision of health services difficult.

The social conditions in most developing societies are already fueling the spread of STDs. Despite a few success stories, in most of the developing world effective health promotion and health service provision are hard to achieve. In most of the developed countries the spread of STDs appear to be under control; however, political, and economic conditions of the 1990s may well lead to situations that challenge the established favorable balance between the social forces that spread STDs and those that limit their spread even in these societies. In the following, we discuss the demographic, economic, social, and political trends of the late 1990s, that have direct or indirect effects on patterns of sexual mixing, health promotion, and health service provision. Some of these have recently been highlighted by Thurow.[218]

First, the global demographic trends exert tremendous pressures that foster STDs transmission. The World Bank projects an increase in the world's population from 5.7 billion in 1994 to 8.5 billion by 2030, and 2 billion of these people will be born in countries where daily earnings are less than $2. In addition, the volume of geographic mobility has reached unprecedented levels, with tens of millions of people moving across countries, in response to the push of very difficult economic, social, and political conditions at home and the pull of higher standards abroad. In the 1980s 7.9 million people legally moved into the United States and 7.3 million people legally moved into the rest of the first world. Within the third world, millions of people move from somewhat poorer to somewhat richer countries, or from countries marked by political strife to countries that are relatively more peaceful. Falling standards of living in developing countries increase the volume of migration. More than 2 million people move per year in Asia. Over 100 million people in the world live outside of the country where they were born, 23 million as refugees.[219] Current examples include movements from Mexico to the United States, from North Africa to Europe, and from Eastern and Central Europe to Western Europe. These large-volume migration streams often consist of low-wage unskilled workers, who have an important impact on the wages of unskilled workers in the receiving countries. Hostility directed at those coming in has important social, economic, and political implications relevant to public health in general and STDs in particular.

Second, changes in technology, transportation, communication, and ideology reinforce development of a global economy. Goods tend to be produced where it is cheapest to produce them, and sold all over the world, resulting in continuously declining earnings for the majority of workers. The rate of growth of world economy declined from 5.0 percent per year (corrected for inflation) during the decade of the 1960s, to 3.6 percent per year in the 1970s, and to 2.8 percent per year in the 1980s. During the first half of the 1990s the growth rate was only 2.0 percent per year.[218] The most developed countries in the world are experiencing economic difficulties in the mid-1990s; unemployment rates are high in Europe (10.8 percent in 1995), economic growth apparently stopped in Japan.

In the United States, where the real per capita gross domestic product (GDP) rose 36 percent from 1973 to 1995, the real hourly wages of non-supervisory workers (a vast majority of the work force) declined 14 percent during the same period.[218] Declines in earning capacity have been particularly sharp for the young. Despite increases in average educational attainment, real earnings of those 25 to 34 years of age fell by 25 percent. Among those 18 to 24, the percentage earning less than $12,195 rose from 18 percent in 1979 to 40 percent in 1989. If current trends continue, by the turn of the century real wages of non-supervisory workers will be below 1950 levels. During the decade of the 1980s all earning gains accrued to the top 20 percent of the workforce, with 64 percent of the gains going to the top 1 percent of the workforce.

During periods of economic development levels of inequality rise, thus increasing inequality is expected in developing countries. However, current trends indicate rapidly rising inequality even in the most developed societies. In the United States inequality has been rising since 1968, at an accelerated pace. By the 1990s, both between and within groups, inequality was rising in every industrial, occupational, educational, demographic, and geographic group. Men were the most sharply affected group, and among them earnings inequalities doubled from the early 1970s to the early 1990s.[218] Corporate downsizing, with outsourcing, makes it possible to increase productivity while reducing real wages; this increases inequality. In the United States, many people who are downsized exit the labor force while others remain unemployed for extended periods of time, and almost two-thirds of those who are re-employed experience wage cuts.

In addition, the most advanced economies also appear to be producing a group of people whose potential productivity is so low that they are not wanted by the private economy at any wage rate, the so-called "lumpen proletariat."[218] This group includes the homeless, those who have dropped out of (or been dropped from) the work-force, and those in jail or on probation. In 1994 in the United States, men in jail or on probation outnumbered men who were unemployed. Increasing inequality, declining real wages or increasing unemployment, corporate downsizing, and the creation of a lumpen proletariat are trends which have started in the United States but have spread to Europe and the rest of the developed world.

Third, the end of communism has already led to significant social and economic changes and will most probably lead to many more. The collapse of the Union of Soviet Socialist Republics (USSR) has created major economic and population movements, within the area that used to be USSR, across the neighboring countries, and, to a lesser extent, all over the world. As would be expected during such periods of major social upheaval, exchange of goods, services, favors of all kinds, including sex, accompany these movements. It is likely that, in the long run, the processes set into motion by the end of communism will further reinforce the population movements, inequalities, declining earnings, and the emergence of the lumpen proletariat, as discussed above.

Fourth, the rise of religious fundamentalism and ethnic separatism is creating major social upheaval and violent confrontation within and between national units, all over the world. Since both of these phenomena tend to expand during periods of economic uncertainty, their rise may continue for some time.

Fifth, in most of the world the development of human resources is largely neglected. Growing capitalist economies tend not to invest in the educational system, the environment, public health, and infrastructure development in general. As a result in many developing countries these systems function poorly. Even in the developed countries, governments tend to increase consumption in the present, at the cost of decreasing investment in the future; systems of education, health, and human resource development in general suffer. To the extent that the education and training of human resources lag behind the demands of the evolving technology and the economic system, the ranks of the lumpen proletariat, the unemployed, and the minimally skilled-minimally paid workers tend to grow. This may create a growing problem during an era in which the dominant industries increasingly require high levels of education and skill.

Sixth, in most of the world, perhaps with the exception of Western Europe, public health functions tend to be endangered by the increasing tensions between the public and the private sector, one example of this phenomenon being the evolving relationship between managed care and public health in the United States. Activities that limit the spread of infectious disease in the society as a whole are clearly in the public health domain.

Seventh, the vacuum created by the lack of fit between the demands of the economic system and the inadequate development of the human resources in a society tend to be filled by processes that provide alternative sources of money and power, such as trading in the black market, trading in firearms or drugs, gang activities, and exchange of sex for money and other goods. Often these activities are clustered, with illicit exchanges in one type of good leading to exchanges for other illicit goods. The recent crack epidemic in the United States has been associated with epidemics of crime, violence, syphilis, chancroid, gonorrhea, and HIV.

Against this background of global trends, since the end of the 1980s, the inner city, minority populations of developed countries, particularly the United States, appear to have profiles resembling populations of developing countries (particularly their urban populations) appear to have similar profiles with respect to several demographic, economic, and sociopolitical characteristics that are associated with high levels of STD incidence. Both developing countries and inner-city, minor populations have a youthful population, composed of relatively high and increasing proportions of sexually active adolescents and young adults. Both developing countries and inner-city minority populations undergo rapid demographic change. Developing countries in general have high rates of urbanization, and population movement of all types, including permanent or temporary rural–rural migration, rural–urban migration, or urban–urban migration.[220] Inner-city urban populations of developed countries also exhibit high physical mobility.[221,222] Rapid economic change similarly marks the diverse populations of inner cities of the developed world and whole societies of the underdeveloped world. The transition from agricultural self-sufficiency to dependence on income from wage labor, which properly describes the economic state of most underdeveloped countries, is one of the best known periods of rapid economic change in society; it involves structural transformations of the most basic kind.[223] The changes being introduced into the inner-city minority communities of the United States through the sale of drugs, especially crack cocaine, are described by observers in similar terms. Large sums of money change hands very rapidly in the course of drug trade; are suddenly introduced into the daily lives of inner-city communities, often through very young teenagers, radically altering the existing social structure of these communities.

Developing countries and inner-city minority populations both have unstable power hierarchies and are thus marked by rapid political change. The frequency of civil wars, coups, and border disturbances, and the extensive need for police and military presence to assure peace in everyday life, are indicators of lack of political stability in many countries of the third world. Similarly, more frequent violence in inner-city communities in the United States indicates the tentative nature of power hierarchies existing in these communities. The disruptive effects of drug use and drug trade on the stability of these communities are visible.

The rapid demographic, economic, and political changes in these populations result in a high level of transience and marginality; the normative structure is destabilized, and social disintegration reigns.[223] In these social systems, the basic patterning of dependency and of opportunity reinforce inequality-based social exchanges. Institutions such as commercial sex and drug trade actually emerge as adaptive responses to the existing sociopolitical structures and function as social factors that enhance the spread of STDs.

SUMMARY AND IMPLICATIONS FOR THE FUTURE

Although efforts at individual and societal behavior change may seem inconsequential in the face of the preceding macro-societal issues, the evidence for changing sexual behaviors of homosexual men after 1982, at least in the industrialized countries, stands as testimony to the actual power of efforts to change these behaviors. The epidemic spread of syphilis in homosexual men, beginning in the mid-1960s and culminating in 1982, undoubtedly reflect a real but poorly documented increase in high-risk sexual behaviors—both increasing rates of partner change, and perhaps increasing numbers practicing both insertive and receptive anorectal sex—that contributed to, and may have been solely responsible for, the epidemic sexual spread of HIV infection within that population. Perhaps the epidemic increase of syphilis among gay men during the seventies, and the less well documented epidemic increases of other infectious causes of epidemic proctitis during the same period, also served to increase the efficiency of transmission concurrently with the increase in the frequency of encountering new partners.

The steady decrease in incidence of gonorrhea and syphilis among adult white heterosexuals in the United States and other industrialized countries is consistent with effective public health control measures, and with a decrease in unsafe sexual behaviors in this group, as in homosexual men. However, in the United States, we saw transient reemergence of syphilis, chancroid, and gonorrhea in some communities of young, black, and Hispanic inner-city poor populations, in association with a reemergence of commercial sex, and exchange of sex for drugs in the United States during the late 1980s, and in Russia today. We are now seeing a striking reemergence of these diseases in China and parts of the former USSR. These increases, coupled with the continuing increase in incidence of viral STDs, decreased the relative accessibility of public health care for STDs. Persons who could afford them utilized private sources for STD care. Among poor populations with increasing exposure related in part to increased commercial sex or sex for drugs, and delay of treatment because of inability to afford private care, bacterial STDs have spread at epidemic rates. How will this pattern play out in various parts of the world? Will the underlying changes of sexual behavior, together with the emerging epidemic of other STDs in such inner-city populations, be sufficient to sustain an epidemic of heterosexual spread of HIV, analogous to what has been seen in much of Africa? In the United States, a new campaign for syphilis elimination endorses the premise that effective health promotion and other preventive intervention, if adequately supported, can overcome these pressures for continued transmission, at least for this one STD.

However, as the reservoir of bacterial STDs retrenches to specific high-risk heterosexual populations—so-called core groups—in industrialized countries, innovative programs are needed to focus traditional STD control efforts on these groups. Such efforts not only could contain the spread of bacterial STDs but could be highly effective in limiting the spread of HIV. However, traditional efforts involving diagnosis, treatment, and partner notification are less effective for the incurable viral STDs and, in some developing countries, have limited effectiveness even for certain of the bacterial STDs that re hard to diagnose, such as gonorrhea and chlamydial infection. Here, behavioral interventions are relatively more important.

Thus, we are optimistic about the growing efficacy of the tools and interventions becoming available to prevent STD, including HIV infection; these tools and interventions must be deployed on the basis of a clear understanding of the epidemiology of the diseases to be prevented. However, realistic projections about the future must be tempered by awareness of powerful underlying socioeconomic forces that drive transmission of HIV and other STDs in many parts of the world.

References

1 "Social Impact of AIDS in the United States," National Research Council. National Academy Press, Washington DC, 1993.

2 Johnson AM et al: Sexual lifestyles and HIV risk. *Nature* 360(6403): 410–412, 1992.

3 AIDS and sexual behaviour in France. ACSF investigators. *Nature* 360(6403):407–409, 1992.

4 Laumann EO et al: *The social organization of sexuality*. Chicago, University of Chicago Press, 1994.

5 Michael RT et al: Private sexual behavior, public opinion, and public health policy related to sexually transmitted diseases: A U.S.-British comparison. *Am J Public Health* 88(5):749–54, 1998.

6 Caraël M et al: Overview and selected findings of sexual behaviour surveys. *AIDS* 5:S65, 1991.

7 Cleeland J, Terry B: *Sexual behavior and AIDS in the developing world*. Taylor & Frances Ltd, London, 1995.

8 Siegel D, et al: Prevalence and correlates of herpes simplex infections: the population-based AIDS in Multiethnic Neighborhoods study. *JAMA* 268:1702–1708, 1992.

9 Morris M et al: Concurrent partnerships and HIV transmission in Uganda. Abstract (#Tu.D.473) presented at the XI International Conference on AIDS, Vancouver, July 7–12, 1996.

10 Morris M et al: Bridge populations in the spread of HIV/AIDS in Thailand. *AIDS* 10(11):1265–1271, 1996.

11 Gorbach et al: Bridging between high and low risk groups in Cambodia: Potential importance in the spread of STDS/HIV. Population Association of America 1998 Annual Meeting, Chicago, IL April 2–4, 1998, Abstract #10120.

12 Over M, Ainsworth M: *Confronting AIDS: Public priorities in a global epidemic*. Washington DC, The World Bank, 1997.

13 World Bank: World Development Report, 1993: Investing in Health. Oxford, UK, Oxford University Press, 1993.

14 Over M, Piot P: Human immunodeficiency virus infection and other sexually transmitted diseases in developing countries: Public health importance and priorities for resource allocation. *J Infect Dis* 174(suppl 2):S162–175, 1996.

15 Van Vliet C et al: Effectiveness of HIV prevention strategies under alternative epidemiological scenarios: Evaluation with the model STDSIM (unpublished data).

16 Landry DJ, Forrest JD: Public health departments providing sexually transmitted disease services. *Fam Plann Perspect* 28(6):261–266, 1996.

17 Begg C et al: Improving the quality of reporting in randomized controlled trials. The CONSORT statement. *JAMA* 276:637–639, 1996.

18 Cochran Collaborations for Infectious Diseases, AIDS, STDS. Cochran Library, Website addresses: ⟨http://www.cochrane.co.uk⟩ or ⟨http://hiru.mcmaster.ca/cochrane/default.htm⟩, 1998.

19 Cohen M et al: Successful eradication of sexually transmitted diseases in the People's Republic of China: Implications for the 21st century. *J Infect Dis* 174(suppl 2):S223–229, 1996.

20 Purevdawa E et al: Rise in sexually transmitted diseases during democratization and economic crisis in Mongolia. *Int J STDS AIDS* 8(6):398–401, 1997.

21 Tichonova L et al: Epidemics of syphilis in the Russian Federation: Trends, origins, and priorities for control. *Lancet* 350(9072):210–213, 1997.

22 Division of STDS Prevention. Sexually Transmitted Disease Surveillance, 1996. U.S. Department of Health and Human Services, Public Health Service. Atlanta: Centers for Disease Control and Prevention, September 1997.

23 Rice RJ et al: Sociodemographic distribution of gonorrhea incidence: Implications for prevention and behavioral research. *Am J Public Health* 81:1252, 1991.

24 Fox KK et al: Changing epidemiology of gonorrhea: findings from a sentinel system. Abstract presented at the 12th Meeting of the International Society for STDS Research. Seville, Spain, October 1922, 1997.

25 Aral SO et al: Social and behavioral correlates of pelvic inflammatory disease. *Sex Trans Dis* 25:378–385, 1998.

26 Zaidi AA et al: Socio-demographic factors associated with gonorrhea rates in the United States: An ecologic analysis. Abstract presented at the 12th Meeting of the International Society for STDS Research. Seville, Spain, October 1922, 1997.

27 Barrow RY et al: Increase in gonorrhea and HIV co-infection among men who have sex with men, Washington, D.C. Abstract presented at the 12th Meeting of the International Society for STDS Research. Seville, Spain, October 1922, 1997.

28 Centers for Disease Control and Prevention: Gonorrhea among men who have sex with men: Selected sexually transmitted diseases clinics, 1993–1996. *MMWR* 46(38):889–892, 1997.

29 Handsfield HH et al: Epidemiology of penicillinase-producing *Neisseria gonorrhoeae* infections: Analysis by auxotyping and serotyping. *N Engl J Med* 306:950, 1982.

30 Centers for Disease Control: Penicillinase-producing *Neisseria gonorrhoeae*-United States, Florida. *MMWR* 35:12, 1986.

31 Centers for Disease Control: Penicillinase-producing *Neisseria gonorrhoeae*—United States, 1986. *MMWR* 36:107, 1987.

32 Jaffe HW et al: Infections due to penicillinase-producing *Neisseria gonorrhoeae* in the United States: 1976–1980. *J Infect Dis* 144: 19-1, 1981.

33 Handsfield HH et al: Localized outbreak of penicillinase-producing *Neisseria gonorrhoeae:* A paradigm for introduction and spread of gonorrhea in a community. *JAMA* 1989;261:2357–2361.
34 Fox KK et al: Sentinel surveillance for antimicrobial resistance in *Neisseria gonorrhoeae.* Abstract presented at the 12th Meeting of the International Society for STDS Research. Seville, Spain, October 1922, 1997 [Abstract no. O150].
35 Gordon SM et al: The emergence of *Neisseria gonorrhoeae* with decreased susceptibility to ciprofloxacin in Cleveland, Ohio: Epidemiology and risk factors. *Ann Intern Med* 125:465, 1996.
36 Centers for Disease Control and Prevention: Fluoroquinolone-resistant *N. gonorrhoeae,* San Diego, California, 1997. *MMWR* 47:405–408, 1993.
37 Aplasca MR et al: High rates of failure after treatment with ciprofloxacin: Are fluoroquinolones no longer useful for gonorrhea treatment: in Abstracts of the 4th International congress on AIDS in Asia and the Pacific; October 1997, Manila, Philippines. [Abstract].
38 Klausner J et al: Predictors of gonococcal infection and of antimicrobial-resistant *Neisseria gonorrhoeae* among female sex workers, Republic of the Philippines, 1996–1997. (Submitted)
39 Blount JH, Holmes KK: Epidemiology of syphilis and the nonvenereal treponematoses, in *The Biology of the Parasitic Spirochetes.* Johnson RC (ed). New York, Academic Press, 1976, pp. 157–176.
40 Centers for Disease Control and Prevention: Outbreak of primary and secondary syphilis: Baltimore City, Maryland, 1995. *MMWR* 45(8):166–169, 1996.
41 Washington AE et al: Incidence of *Chlamydia trachomatis* infections in the United States: Using reported *Neisseria gonorrhoeae* as surrogate, in *Chlamydial Infections.* D Oriel et al (eds). Cambridge, England, Cambridge University Press, 1986, p 487.
42 Cates W Jr: Epidemiology and control of sexually transmitted diseases: Strategic evolution, in *Infectious Disease Clinics of North America,* 1987, vol 1, no 1, p 1.
43 Judson FN: Epidemiology and control of nongonococcal urethritis and genital chlamydial infections: A review. *Sex Transm Dis* 8(Suppl):117, 1981.
44 Brunham RC et al: Mucopurulent cervicitis: The ignored counterpart in women of urethritis in men. *N Engl J Med* 311:1, 1984.
45 Centers for Disease Control and Prevention: *Chlamydia trachomatis* genital infections United States, 1995. *MMWR* 46(9):193–198, 1997.
46 Klausner JD et al: An update III. Knock-knock: Door-to-door population based survey of risk behavior and *Chlamydia trachomatis* prevalence in young women living in low income neighborhoods in the San Francisco Bay Area. 125th Meeting of the American Public Health Association, November 9–13, 1997, Indianapolis, IN.
47 Marrazzo JM et al: Community-based urine screening for Chlamydia trachomatis with a ligase chain reaction assay. *Ann Intern Med* 127(9):796–803, 1997.
48 Plummer FA et al: Detection of human immunodeficiency virus type 1 (HIV-1) in genital ulcer exudate of HIV-1 infected men by culture and gene amplification. *J Infect Dis* 161(4):810–811, 1990.
49 Hayes RJ et al: The cofactor effect of genital ulcers on the per-exposure risk of HIV transmission in sub-Saharan Africa. *J Trop Med Hyg* 98(1):1–8, 1995.
50 Moses S et al: Male circumcision: assessment of health benefits and risks. *Sex Transm Infect* 1998, in press.
51 Kreiss JK et al: AIDS virus infection in Nairobi prostitutes. Spread of the epidemic to East Africa. *N Engl J Med* 314(7):414–418, 1986.
52 DiCarlo RP et al: Chancroid epidemiology in New Orleans men. *J Infect Dis* 172(2):446–452, 1995.
53 Morse SA et al: Comparison of clinical diagnosis and standard laboratory and molecular methods for the diagnosis of genital ulcer disease in Lesotho: Association with human immunodeficiency virus infection. *J Infect Dis* 175(3):583–589, 1997.
54 Fleming DT et al: Herpes simplex virus type 2 in the United States, 1976 to 1994. *N Engl J Med* 337:1105–11, 1997.
55 Christenson B et al: A 15-year surveillance study of antibodies to herpes simplex virus types 1 and 2 in a cohort of young girls. *J Infect* 25(2):147–154, 1992.
56 Ho GY et al: Natural history of cervicovaginal papillomavirus infection in young women. *N Engl J Med* 338(7):423–428, 1998.
57 National Center for Health Statistics: Vital and health statistics. Fertility, family planning, and women's health: New data from the 1995 national survey of family growth. Series 23: Data from the national survey of growth, no. 19. Hyattsville, MD, February 1997.
58 Aral SO et al: Declining prevalence of pelvic inflammatory disease (PID) and vaginal douching among reproductive age US women: 1995. Abstract presented at the 12th Meeting of the International Society for STDS Research. Seville, Spain, October 19–22, 1997.
59 Aral SO et al: Social and behavioral correlates of pelvic inflammatory disease. *Sex Trans Dis,* 25(7):1–8, 1998.
60 Centers for Disease Control and Prevention: Ectopic Pregnancy: United States, 1990–1992. *MMWR* 44:46, 1995.
61 Skjeldestad FE et al: Increasing incidence of ectopic pregnancy in one Norwegian county: A population based study, 1970–1993. *Acta Obstet Gynecol Scand* 76:159, 1997.
62 Goldenberg RL et al: Sexually transmitted diseases and adverse outcomes of pregnancy. *Infect Perinatol* 24:23, 1997.
63 Committee on Prevention and Control of Sexually Transmitted Diseases: Institute of Medicine: *The hidden epidemic: Confronting sexually transmitted diseases.* Washington DC, National Academy Press, 1997.
64 Sanchez J et al: Sexually transmitted infections in female sex workers: Reduced by condom use but not by a limited periodic examination program. *Sex Transm Dis* 1998;25(2):82–89.
65 Plummer FA et al: The importance of core groups in the epidemiology and control of HIV-1 infection. *AIDS* 5 (Suppl 1):S169–S176, 1991.
66 Laga M et al: Condom promotion, sexually transmitted diseases treatment, and declining incidence of HIV-1 infection in female Zairian sex workers. *Lancet* 344(8917):246–248, 1994.
67 Darrow WW: Assessing targeted AIDS prevention in male and female prostitutes and their clients, in *Assessing AIDS Prevention,* Paccaud F et al (eds). Basel, Switzerland, Birkhäuser Verlag, 1992, pp 215–231.
68 Johnstone H et al: Incidence of sexually transmitted diseases and Pap smear results in female homeless clients from the Chicago Health Outreach Project. *Health Care Women Int* 14(3):293–299, 1993.
69 Breakey WR et al: Health problems of homeless men and women in Baltimore. *JAMA* 262:1352, 1989.
70 CDC: *Juvenile detention.* Atlanta, 1996.
71 Bell TA et al: Sexually transmitted diseases in females in a juvenile detention center. *Sex Transm Dis* 12(3):140–144, 1985.
72 Shafer MA: Sexual behavior and sexually transmitted diseases among male adolescents in detention. [Editorial] *Sex Transm Dis* 21:181–182, 1994.
73 Oh MK et al: Sexual behavior and sexually transmitted diseases among male adolescents in detention. *Sex Transm Dis* 21:127–132, 1994.
74 Cohen D et al: The potential role of custody facilities in controlling sexually transmitted diseases [published erratum appears in *Am J Public Health* 82:684, 1992]. *Am J Public Health* 82:552–556, 1992.
75 Center for Disease Control and Prevention: Syphilis screening among women arrestees at the Cook County jail: Chicago, 1996. *MMWR* 47:432–433, 1998.
76 Hammet TM et al: 1994 Update: HIV/AIDS and STDs in correctional facilities. Washington, D.C.: U.S. Department of Justice, Office of Justice Programs, National Institute of Justice/US Department of Health and Human Services, Public Health Service, CDC, December 1995.
77 Bickell NA et al: Human papillomavirus, gonorrhea, syphilis, and cervical dysplasia in jailed women. *Am J Public Health* 81:1318, 1991.
78 Holmes MD et al: Chlamydial cervical infection in jailed women. *Am J Public Health* 83(4):551–555, 1993.

79 Blank S et al: Incident syphilis among women admitted to a New York City women's correctional facility. Abstract presented at Twelfth Meeting of the International Society for STDS Research. Seville, Spain, October 19–22, 1997 [Abstract no. P822].

80 Centers for Disease Control and Prevention: Assessment of sexually transmitted diseases services in city and county jails: United States, 1997. *MMWR* 47:429–431, 1998.

81 Centers for Disease Control and Prevention: HIV infection, syphilis, and tuberculosis screening among migrant farm workers: Florida, 1992. *MMWR* 41:723, 1992.

82 Jones et al: HIV-related characteristics of migrant workers in rural South Carolina. *So Med J* 84:1088, 1991.

83 Bechtel GA et al: Family, culture, and health practices among migrant farm workers. *J Commun Health Nurs* 12:15, 1995.

84 Brewer T et al: Migration, ethnicity and environment: HIV risk factors for women on the sugar cane plantations (bateyes) of the Dominican Republic. *AIDS* 12(14):1879–87, 1998.

85 Aral SO, Cates W Jr: The multiple dimensions of sexual behavior as risk factor for sexually transmitted disease: The sexually experienced are not necessarily sexually active. *Sex Transm Dis* 16(4):173–177, 1989.

86 Bell TA, Holmes KK: Age-specific risks of syphilis, gonorrhea, and hospitalized pelvic inflammatory disease in sexually experienced US women. *Sex Transm Dis* 22:291, 1984.

87 Aral SO et al: Gonorrhea rates: What denominator is most appropriate? *Am J Public Health* 78:702, 1988.

88 Sanchez J et al: Gender differences in sexual practices and seroprevalence of sexually transmitted infections. *Am J Public Health* 86: 1098–1107, 1996.

89 Hofferth SL et al: Premarital sexual activity among U.S. teenage women over the past three decades. *Fam Plann Perspect* 19:46, 1987.

90 D'Costa LJ et al: Prostitutes are a major reservoir of sexually transmitted diseases in Nairobi, Kenya. *Sex Transm Dis* 12:64, 1985.

91 Handsfield HH et al: Criteria for selective screening for *Chlamydia trachomatis* infection in women attending family planning clinics. *JAMA* 255:1730, 1986.

92 Schachter J et al: Screening for chlamydial infections in women attending family planning clinics. *West J Med* 1387:375, 1983.

93 Syrjanen K et al: Sexual behavior of women with human papillomavirus (HPV) lesions of the uterine cervix. *Br J Vener Dis* 60:243, 1984.

94 Turner CF et al: Adolescent sexual behavior, drug use, and violence: Increased reporting with computer survey technology. *Science* 280(5365):867–873, 1998.

95 Schreeder MT et al: Hepatitis B in homosexual men: Prevalence of infection and factors related to transmission. *J Infect Dis* 146:7, 1982.

96 Alter MJ et al: Hepatitis B virus transmission between heterosexuals. *JAMA* 256:1307, 1986.

97 Dan B: Sex and the singles whirl: The quantum dynamics of hepatitis B. *JAMA* 256:1344, 1986.

98 Research and Forecasts, Inc: *The Abbott Report: STDs and Sexual Mores in the 1980s*. New York, July 14, 1987.

99 Aral SO et al: Unpublished data.

100 Zelnik M, Kantner JF: Sexual activity, contraceptive use and pregnancy among metropolitan-area teenagers: 1971–1979. *Fam Plann Perspect* 12(5):230–231, 1980.

101 Sonenstein FL et al: Sexual activity, condom use and AIDS awareness among adolescent males. *Fam Plann Perspect* 21:152, 1989.

102 Ku L et al: Young men's risk behaviors for HIV infection and sexually transmitted diseases, 1988 through 1991. *Am J Public Health* 83: 1609, 1993.

103 Centers for Disease Control: Current trends: Premarital sexual experience among adolescent women: United States, 1970–1988. *MMWR* 39(51–52):929–932, 1991.

104 Anderson JE, Dahlberg LL: High-risk sexual behavior in the general population. Results from a national survey, 1988–1990. *Sex Transm Dis* 19:320, 1992.

105 Catania JA et al: Prevalence of AIDS-related risk factors and condom use in the United States. *Science* 258:1101, 1992.

106 Billy JO et al: The sexual behavior of men in the United States. *Fam Plann Perspect* 25(2):52–60, 1993.

107 Tanfer K et al: Condom use among U.S. men, 1991. *Fam Plann Perspect* 25(2):61–66, 1993.

108 Grady WR et al: Condom characteristics: the perceptions and preferences of men in the United States. *Fam Plann Perspect* 25(2):67–73, 1993.

109 Klepinger DH et al: Perceptions of AIDS risk and severity and their association with risk-related behavior among U.S. men. *Fam Plann Perspect* 25(2):74–82, 1993.

110 Holmes KK: Human ecology and behavior and sexually transmitted bacterial infections. *Proc Natl Acad Sci USA* 91:2448–2455, 1994.

111 Substance Abuse and Mental Health Services Administration: *Preliminary Results from the 1996 National Household Survey on Drug Abuse* and from the 1996 Drug Abuse Warning Network. Department of Health and Human Services, Washington, DC, 1997.

112 Golub AL, Johnson BD: Crack's decline: Some surprises across U.S. cities. National Institute of Justice, 1997.

113 Centers for Disease Control: Gang-related outbreak of penicillinase-producing Neisseria gonorrhoeae and other sexually transmitted diseases: Colorado Springs, Colorado, 1989–1991. *MMWR 42(2):25–28, 1993.*

114 Marx R et al: Crack, sex, and STDs. *Sex Transm Dis* 18:92, 1991.

115 Greenberg J et al: Behaviors of crack cocaine users and their impact on early syphilis intervention. *Sex Transm Dis* 19:346, 1992.

116 Caldwell J, Caldwell P: High fertility in sub-Saharan Africa. *Sci Am* 262: 118, 1990.

117 Caldwell JC, Caldwell P: The demographic evidence for the incidence and cause of abnormally low fertility in tropical Africa. *World Health Stat Q* 36:2, 1983.

118 Tabet SR et al: Sexual behaviors and risk factors for HIV infection among men who have sex with men in the Dominican Republic. *AIDS* 10(2):201–206, 1996.

119 Garnett GP, Anderson RM: Contact tracing and the estimation of sexual mixing patterns: The epidemiology of gonococcal infections. *Sex Transm Dis* 20:181–191, 1993.

120 Garnett GP et al: Sexual mixing pattern of patients attending STD clinics. *Sex Transm Dis* 23(3):248–257, 1996.

121 Anderson RM et al: The significance of sexual partner contact networks for the transmission dynamics of HIV. *J Acq Immun Def Synd* 3:417–429, 1990.

122 Ghani AC et al: The role of sexual partnership networks in the epidemiology of gonorrhea. *Sex Transm Dis* 24(1):45–54, 1997.

123 Gupta S et al: Networks of sexual contacts: implications for the pattern of spread in HIV. *AIDS* 3:807–817, 1989.

124 Klovdakel AS: Social networks and the spread of infectious diseases: The AIDS example. *Soc Sci Med* 21:1203–1216, 1985.

125 Morris M, Kretzschmar M: Concurrent partnerships and the spread of HIV. *AIDS* 11(5):641–648, 1997.

126 Stoner BP et al: Comparative epidemiology of gonococcal and chlamydial network membership: Implications for transmission patterns (in press).

127 Aral SO et al: Sexual mixing patterns including linking and bridge populations, in spread of gonococcal and chlamydial infections. *AJPH,* 1998, in press.

128 Kretzschmar M, Morris M: Measures of concurrency in networks and the spread of infectious disease. *Math Biosci* 133(2):165–195, 1996.

129 Laumann EO, Youm Y: Social, attitudinal and behavioral determinants of sexually transmitted infections: In search of the core, in *The Social Organization of Sexuality: Further Studies*. Laumann EO, Michael RT (eds). Chicago, University of Chicago Press, Chap 10, in press.

130 Royce RA: Sexual transmission of HIV. *N Engl J Med* 336:1072, 1997.

131 O'Connor TJ et al: The activity of candidate virucidal agents, low

pH and genital secretions against HIV-1 in vitro. *Int J STDS AIDS* 6(4):267–272, 1995.
132 Shearer GM, Clerici M: Protective immunity against HIV infection: has nature done the experiment for us? *Immunol Today* 17:21, 1995.
133 Dragic T et al: HIV-1 entry into CD4+ cells is mediated by the chemokine receptor CC-CCKR-5. *Nature* 38:667, 1996.
134 Paxton WA et al: The HIV type 1 coreceptor CCR5: Its role in viral transmission and disease progression. *AIDS Res Hum Retroviruses* 14(Suppl 1):S89–S92, 1998.
135 Jeang KT: Mechanism of transdominant inhibition of CCR5-mediated HIV-1 infection by CCR5Δ32. 12th World AIDS Conference, Geneva, Switzerland, June 1998 [Abstract no. 54/111a5].
136 Centers for Disease Control and Prevention: Case-control study of HIV seroconversion in health-care workers after percutaneous exposure to HIV-infected blood: France, United Kingdom, and United States, January 1988–August 1994. *MMWR* 44:929, 1995.
137 Brunham RC et al: The epidemiology of *Chlamydia trachomatis* within a sexually transmitted diseases core group. *J Infect Dis* 173(4): 950–956, 1996.
138 Plummer FA et al: Epidemiologic evidence for the development of serovar-specific immunity after gonococcal infection. *J Clin Invest* 83(5):1472–1476, 1989.
139 Royce R: Does male circumcision prevent HIV infection? in *AIDS in the World*. Mann JM et al (eds). Cambridge, Harvard University Press, 1992, pp. 645–652.
140 Laumann EO et al: Circumcision in the United States: Prevalence, prophylactic effects, and sexual practice. *JAMA* 277:1052, 1997.
141 Dodge OG, Kavati JN: Male circumcision among the peoples of East Africa and the incidence of genital cancer. *East Afr Med J* 42:98, 1965.
142 Boczko S, Freed S: Penile carcinoma in circumcised males. *NY St J Med*, November 1979:1903.
143 Hosze K, McClirdy S: Circumcision and the risk of cancer of the penis. *Am J Dis Child* 134:484, 1980.
144 Fink AJ: *Circumcision: A parent's decision for life*. Mountain View, CA, Kavanah Publishing Co., 1988.
145 Critchlow CW et al: Determinants of cervical ectopia and of cervicitis: Age, oral contraception, specific cervical infection, smoking, and douching. *Am J Obstet Gynecol* 173(2):534–543, 1995.
146 Clemetson DB et al: Detection of HIV DNA in cervical and vaginal secretions: prevalence and correlates among women in Nairobi, Kenya. *JAMA* 269:2860, 1993.
147 Plourde PJ et al: Human immunodeficiency virus type 1 seroconversion in women with genital ulcers. *J Infect Dis* 170:313, 1994.
148 de Vincenzi I: A longitudinal study of human immunodeficiency virus transmission by heterosexual partners. *N Engl J Med* 331:341, 1994.
149 Fischl MA et al: Evaluation of heterosexual partners, children, and household contacts of adults with AIDS. *JAMA* 257:640, 1987.
150 Feldblum P et al: The effectiveness of barrier methods of contraception in preventing the spread of HIV. *AIDS* 9:S85, 1995.
151 Daly CC et al: Contraceptive methods and the transmission of HIV: implications for family planning. *Genitourin Med* 70:1110, 1994.
152 Wølner-Hanssen P et al: Decreased risk of symptomatic chlamydial pelvic inflammatory disease associated with oral contraceptive use. *JAMA* 263:54, 1990.
153 Gertig DM et al: Risk factors for sexually transmitted diseases among women attending family planning clinics in Dar-es-Salaam, Tanzania. *Genitourin Med* 73:39–43, 1997.
154 Plummer FA et al: Cofactors in male-female sexual transmission of human immunodeficiency virus type 1. *J Infect Dis* 163(2):233–239, 1991.
155 Martin HL et al: Hormonal contraception, sexually transmitted diseases, and risk of heterosexual transmission of human immunodeficiency virus type-1. *J Infect Dis* 178(4): 1053–1059, 1998.
156 Ungchusak K et al: Determinants of HIV infection among female commercial sex workers in Northeastern Thailand: Results from a longitudinal study. *J Acquir Immune Defic Syndr Hum Retrovirol* 12(5):500–507, 1996.
157 Goldberg HI et al: Knowledge about condoms and their use in less developed countries during a period of rising AIDS prevalence. *Bull World Health Organ* 67(1):85–91, 1989.
158 Padian NS et al: Risk factors for postcoital bleeding among women with or at risk for infection with human immunodeficiency virus. *J Infect Dis* 172(4):1084–1087, 1995.
159 Ahlgren DJ et al: Model-based optimization of infectivity parameters: A study of the early epidemic in San Francisco. *J Acquir Immune Defic Syndr* 3:631, 1990.
160 Anderson RM, May RM: *Infectious diseases of humans: Dynamics and control*. Oxford, England, Oxford University Press, 1991.
161 Jacquez JA et al: Role of the primary infection in epidemics of HIV infection in gay cohorts. *J Acquir Immune Defic Syndr* 7:1169, 1994.
162 Koopman J: Emerging objectives and methods in epidemiology. *Am J Public Health* 86:630, 1996.
163 Mellors J et al: Prognosis in HIV-1 infection predicted by the quantity of virus in plasma. *Science* 272:1167, 1996.
164 Liuzzi G et al: Analysis of HIV-1 load in blood, semen and saliva: Evidence for different viral compartments in cross-sectional and longitudinal study. *AIDS* 10:F51–F56, 1996.
165 Vernazza PL et al: Detection and biologic characterization of infectious HIV-1 in semen of seropositive men. *AIDS* 8:1325, 1994.
166 Krieger JN et al: Intermittent shedding of human immunodeficiency virus in semen: Implications for sexual transmission. *J Urol* 154: 1035, 1995.
167 Rasheed S et al: Presence of cell-free human immunodeficiency virus in cervicovaginal secretions is independent of viral load in the blood of human immunodeficiency virus-infected women. *Am J Obstet Gynecol* 175:122, 1996.
168 Muller CH et al: Effects of clinical stage and immunological status on semen analysis: Results in human immunodeficiency virus type 1-seropositive men. *Andrologia* 30(Suppl 1):15–22, 1998.
169 Moss GB et al: Human immunodeficiency virus DNA in urethral secretions in men: Association with gonococcal urethritis and CD4 cell depletion. *J Infect Dis* 172:1469, 1995.
170 Cohen MS et al: Reduction of concentration of HIV-1 in semen after treatment of urethritis: Implications for prevention of sexual transmission of HIV-1. AIDSCAP Malawi Research Group. *Lancet* 349(9069):1868–1873, 1997.
171 Atkins MC et al: Fluctuations of HIV load in semen of HIV positive patients with newly acquired sexually transmitted diseases. *Br Med J* 313:341, 1996.
172 Ghys PD et al: The associations between cervicovaginal HIV shedding, sexually transmitted diseases and immunosuppression in female sex workers in Abidjan, Cote d'Ivoire. *AIDS* 11(12):F85–F93, 1997.
173 Mostad S et al: Hormonal contraception, vitamin A deficiency, and other risk factors for shedding of HIV-1 infected cells from the cervix and vagina. *Lancet* 350:922–927, 1997.
174 Hunter D: AIDS in sub-Saharan Africa: The epidemiology of heterosexual transmission and the prospects for prevention. *Epidemiology* 4:63, 1993.
175 European Study Group on Heterosexual Transmission of HIV: Comparison of female to male and male to female transmission of HIV in 563 stable couples. *Br Med J* 304:809, 1992.
176 Henin Y et al: Virus excretion in the cervicovaginal secretions of pregnant and nonpregnant HIV-infected women. *J Acquir Immune Defic Syndr* 6:72, 1993.
177 Kreiss J et al: Association between cervical inflammation and cervical shedding of human immunodeficiency virus DNA. *J Infect Dis* 170: 1597, 1994.
178 Aral SO et al: Sexually transmitted diseases in the AIDS era. *Sci Am* 264:62–69, 1991.
179 Wølner-Hanssen P et al: Association between vaginal douching and pelvic inflammatory disease. *JAMA* 263:1936–1941, 1990.
180 Chow WH et al: Vaginal douching as a potential risk factor for tubal ectopic pregnancy. *Am J Obstet Gynecol* 153:727, 1985.

181 Aral et al: Vaginal douching among women of reproductive age in the United States: 1988. *Am J Public Health* 82:210, 1992.

182 Cohen C et al: Effect of HIV-1 infection upon acute salpingitis: a laparoscopic study, *J Infect Dis* 1998, in press.

183 Holmes KK et al: Salpingitis: Overview of etiology and epidemiology. *Am J Obstet Gynecol* 138:893–900, 1980.

184 Xi LF et al: Analysis of human papillomavirus type 16 variants indicates establishment of persistent infection. *J Infect Dis* 172:747–755, 1995.

185 Hooper RR et al: Cohort study of venereal disease: I: The risk of gonorrhea transmission from infected women to men. *Am J Epidemiol* 108:136, 1978.

186 Lycke E et al: The risk of transmission of genital *Chlamydia trachomatis* infection is less than that of genital *Neisseria gonorrhoeae* infection. *Sex Transm Dis* 7:6, 1980.

187 Peterman T et al: Risk of HIV transmission from heterosexual adults with transfusion-associated infections. *JAMA* 259:55, 1988.

188 Holmes KK et al: Heterosexual transmission of human immunodeficiency virus: overview of a neglected aspect of the AIDS epidemic. *J Acq Immun Def Synd* 1:602–610, 1988.

189 Day S: Prostitute women and AIDS. Antropology. *AIDS* 2:421, 1988.

190 Padian NS: Prostitute women and AIDS: Epidemiology. *AIDS* 2:413, 1988.

191 Holmes KK et al: Impact of a gonorrhea control program, including selective mass treatment, in female sex workers. *J Infect Dis* 174(Supp 2):S230–S239, 1996.

192 Ryan CA et al: Explosive spread of HIV-1 and sexually transmitted diseases in Cambodia. *Lancet* 1998;351:1175.

193 Aral S, Peterman T: Defining behavioral methods to prevent sexually transmitted diseases through intervention research, in *Infectious disease clinics of North America: Sexually transmitted diseases in the AIDS era: Part I.* Cohen MS et al. 1993, pp. 861–873.

194 Peterman TA et al: Association between behavior change and STDS incidence? Abstract presented at 12th Meeting of the International Society for STDS Research. Seville, Spain, October 19–22, 1997 [Abstract no. P603].

195 Wasserheit JN, Aral SO: The dynamic topology of sexually transmitted disease epidemics: Implications for prevention strategies. *J Infect Dis* 174(Suppl 2):S201, 1996.

196 Hamers FF et al: Syphilis and gonorrhea in Miami: Similar clustering, different trends. *Am J Public Health* 85:1104, 1995.

197 Green S: Editorial: The eating patterns study—the importance of practical randomized trials in communities. *Am J Public Health* 87: 541, 1997.

198 Koepsell TD et al: Invited commentary: Symposium on community intervention trials. *Am J Epidemiol* 142(6):594–595, 1995.

199 O'Leary A et al: Reflections on the design and reporting of STDS/HIV behavioral intervention research. *AIDS Education and Prevention* 9:1, 1997.

200 Oakley A et al: Behavioral interventions for HIV/AIDS prevention. *Curr Sci* 9:479, 1995.

201 Oakley A et al: Sexual health education interventions for young people: A methodological review. *Br Med J* 310:158, 1995.

202 Kamb ML et al: Efficacy of risk-reduction counseling to prevent human immunodeficiency virus and sexually transmitted diseases: a randomized controlled trial. Project RESPECT Study Group. *JAMA* 280: 1161–7, 1998.

203 Fishbein M, Coutinho R (eds). NIMH Multisite HIV Prevention Trial *AIDS* 11 Suppl 2:S1–S63, 1997.

204 The NIMH multisite HIV prevention trial: Reducing HIV sexual risk behavior. The National Institute of Mental Health (NIMH) Multisite HIV Prevention Trial Group. *Science* 280(5371):1889–1894, 1998.

205 Shain RN et al: A controlled randomized trial of a risk-reduction intervention: Behaviors contributing to reduced rates at 12 months' follow-up. Abstract presented at the 12th Meeting of the International Society for STDS Research. Seville, Spain, October 19–22, 1997.

206 Machekano R et al: A peer education intervention reduces HIV infection among factory workers in Zimbabwe. Abstract presented at the 5th Conference on Retroviruses and Opportunistic Infections, Chicago, Illinois, USA, February 1–5, 1997 [Abstract: Session 6, no. 15].

207 Garcia PJ et al: Syndromic management of STDs in pharmacies: evaluation and randomized intervention trial. *Sex Transm Infect* 74(Suppl 1):S153–S158, 1998.

208 Stephenson J et al: Can sexual health intervention in schools be evidence-based? Abstract presented at the 12th Meeting of the International Society for STDS Research. Seville, Spain, October 19–22, 1997.

209 Scholes D et al: Prevention of pelvic inflammatory disease by screening for cervical chlamydia infection. *NEJM* 334:1362, 1996.

210 Ryan K: An RCT to measure the effect of nonoxynol-9 film use on cervical gonorrheal and chlamydial infections. Abstract presented at the 12th Meeting of the International Society for STDS Research. Seville, Spain, October 19–22, 1997.

211 Kreiss J et al: Efficacy of nonoxynol 9 contraceptive sponge use in preventing heterosexual acquisition of HIV in Nairobi prostitutes. *JAMA* 268:477–482, 1992.

212 Grosskurth H et al: Impact of improved treatment of sexually transmitted diseases on HIV infection in rural Tanzania: Randomized controlled trial. *Lancet* 346:530, 1995.

213 Wawer MJ, Gray RH, Sewankambo NK et al: Results of a randomized community trial of STD mass treatment for AIDS prevention, Rakai District, Uganda. Laurel. In press.

214 Grey RH et al: A randomized trial of STDS control during pregnancy in Rakai, Uganda: Impact on maternal and infant health. 12th World AIDS Conference, Geneva, Switzerland, July 1998 [Abstract no 23276].

215 Hayes R et al: Randomized trials of STDS treatment for HIV prevention: report of an international workshop. HIV/STDS Trials Workshop Group. *Genitourin Med* 73(6):432–443, 1997.

216 Celentano DD et al: Decreasing incidence of HIV and sexually transmitted diseases in young Thai men: Evidence for success of the HIV/AIDS control and prevention program. *AIDS* 12(5):F29–F36, 1998.

217 Chesson H, Harrison P: Alcohol and risky sex: the effect of beer taxes on sexually transmitted disease rates among youth. Abstract presented at the 12th Meeting of the International Society for STDS Research. Seville, Spain, October 19–22, 1997 [Abstract no. 0203].

218 Thurow L: *The future of capitalism: how today's economic forces shape tomorrow's world.* Boston, Morrow, 1996.

219 Office of Technology Assessment of US Congress: *Multinationals and the National Interest.* Washington, DC, 1995.

220 Danziger S, Gottschalk P (eds): *Uneven Tides.* New York, Russell Sage, 1993, p. 7.

221 Sly DF: Lifetime migration patterns in Kenya, 1963, in *Advancing Agricultural Production in Africa.* Nairobi, Heinemann Educational Books, 1984, p. 68.

222 Wallace R: A synergism of plagues: "Planned shrinkage" contagious housing destruction and AIDS in the Bronx. *Environ Res* 47:1, 1988.

223 Harris FR, Wilkins RW: *Quiet Riots: Race and Poverty in the United States.* New York, Pantheon, 1988.

Chapter 5

The global epidemiology of HIV and AIDS

Peter O. Way
Bernhard Schwartländer
Peter Piot

BACKGROUND

At the middle of the second decade of the AIDS pandemic, there still remains much uncertainty about the extent of HIV infection in many countries; the past, current, and future incidence of AIDS; and the demographic, social, and economic impacts of this pandemic on populations around the world. This uncertainty is caused by weak surveillance systems, lack of access to appropriate medical care, deficiencies in the diagnosis and reporting of AIDS cases, and the lack of adequate vital registration systems.

However real and important these uncertainties, there is a tremendous amount that we do know about HIV and AIDS around the world. Scientifically designed seroprevalence studies of particular populations and sentinel surveillance systems aimed at monitoring HIV prevalence levels in antenatal women or STD clinic patients, for example, have contributed enormously to our understanding of current levels and trends of HIV infection among those populations. A variety of epidemiological models, ranging from simple spreadsheet models to complex multisectoral deterministic and stochastic models have helped us to look both forward and backward in time, even though our view remains obscured. Such models have provided valuable insights into the dynamics of these epidemics.

This chapter focuses on several broad themes. First, we present a number of concepts and perspectives that frame our approach. Second, we look at regional trends in HIV infection in various population groups worldwide. Third, we examine the implications of these trends in terms of population impacts. Finally, we look toward the future based on emerging trends.

SOURCES OF DATA

Our knowledge of HIV seroprevalence in populations in countries around the world has been increasing exponentially, both in quality and quantity. However, our sources of information remain generally the same as they were at the beginning of the AIDS pandemic. These are: (1) reported AIDS cases; (2) HIV seroprevalence data based on sentinel surveillance systems; and (3) HIV prevalence data from other studies targeting selected populations.

AIDS CASES

AIDS cases are reported by individual countries to the World Health Organization (WHO). These data are compiled and are widely cited, but they are known to have huge reporting problems relating both to reporting delays and to underreporting of cases. Through November 20, 1997, over 1.7 million cases of AIDS had been reported to the WHO from 197 countries or areas. Data by region show the concentration of reported AIDS cases in Africa and the Americas (Fig. 5-1). However, based on estimates of the HIV-infected population by country, the WHO and the Joint United Nations Programme on HIV/AIDS (UNAIDS) and WHO estimate that, in fact, 12.9 million adult and pediatric AIDS cases had occurred through 1997.[1]

FOCUS ON HIV

Because of the incubation period between initial HIV infection and the development of AIDS, case data for AIDS, even if complete, can only reflect the situation several years in the past. Ideally, data on HIV incidence, including information on risk and sociodemagraphic indicators, should be included in a monitoring system for HIV/AIDS. This information, however, is not available in all countries in the world. Many of those who are infected do not know about their HIV infection (probably more than 90% globally), and even of those who do the test, the date of infection is usually unknown or was many years before the test. Thus, in order to understand the current status of HIV infection, we need to focus on HIV seroprevalence data. These data are collected in a variety of settings, using nonstandard protocols, so there are often serious problems of comparability. Even so, these data represent our best opportunity to track the level and trends in HIV infection in various population groups in countries around the world.

SENTINEL SURVEILLANCE

In recent years, countries have increasingly established routine sentinel surveillance systems for tracking HIV infection in selected populations such as women attending antenatal clinics and sexually transmitted disease clinic attenders. These data provide extremely valuable data, since they track infection in relatively fixed populations and geographic areas over time. They do not, however, reflect patterns and trends in true population cohorts; and the populations they access may not be representative of the general population.[2]

Tracking these data represents a serious challenge because of the multiple venues in which this information is presented. Many reports from seroprevalence studies are presented at major international and regional conferences. Some of these reports will eventually be published in scientific journals, whereas others will not have this opportunity. In order to maximize access to this important information, much of these data have been compiled into a database for use by researchers and international organizations. The *HIV/AIDS Surveillance Database*, maintained since 1987 at the International Programs Center (U.S. Bureau of the Census), contains over 36,600 pieces of aggregate data from seroprevalence surveys drawn from over 4000 publications and presentations. Increasingly, these surveys sample representative populations or are part of a sentinel surveillance system. Data from these sources document the rapid and continuing increases in HIV seroprevalence in populations in developing countries. They also highlight the patterns of HIV infection among populations classified by demographic factors such as age and sex, as well as the geographic dispersion of infection within a country. These levels and patterns determine, to a large extent, the severity and the age pattern of the subsequent mortality impact of the AIDS epidemics.

UNAIDS ESTIMATES

The Joint United Nations Programme on HIV/AIDS (UNAIDS) has released revised estimates of the prevalence of HIV infection

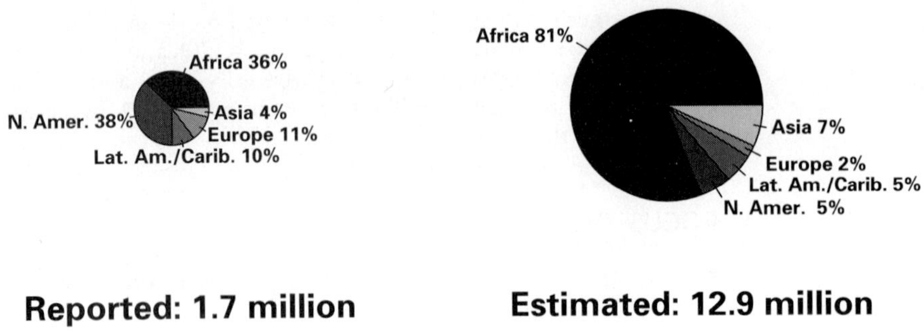

Fig. 5-1. Reported and estimated AIDS cases in adults and children through 1997.

by region. These data were derived from the seroprevalence data described in the preceding, in consultation with researchers and epidemiologists. Based on those figures, at the end of 1997, an estimated 30.6 million people were living with HIV worldwide. Two-thirds of these were estimated to be in Africa, with Asia accounting for nearly another one-fourth of the total (Fig. 5-2).[3] These data will be periodically updated to reflect current understanding of HIV/AIDS epidemics worldwide.

MODES OF TRANSMISSION

The majority of HIV transmission worldwide today is heterosexual. In Africa, this has always been the predominant mode. Of course, with heterosexual transmission there is an increase in vertical transmission (i.e., mother to child). In Latin America, initial epidemics were largely caused by infections in injecting drug users and those with homosexual contacts, but that situation has been changing over the past decade, with an increasing role for heterosexual transmission.[4] In Asia, HIV infection appears to be moving rapidly into the general population from those at highest risk of infection. Again, in this region, heterosexual transmission predominates.[5] In the United States and Western Europe, transmission has been predominantly among those with homosexual contact and injecting drug users.[6] Infection levels among heterosexuals in these countries has increased only slowly, and in recent years may be relatively stable in some countries.

MULTIPLE EPIDEMICS AND VARIATION IN RISK

The understanding of variations in levels of risk in populations is central to the understanding of how HIV infection spreads. A national HIV/AIDS epidemic can be seen as a series of separate epidemics, affecting different populations—those with different levels of risk—each with a differing level of HIV infection and resulting impact. Here, the "core group" concept has been useful in understanding the dynamics of epidemics.[7] However, it must be recognized that this important epidemiological concept may be difficult to translate directly into operational programs and targeted prevention messages. Keys to the speed of spread of HIV through the population may include specific risk behaviors, patterns of interaction, and the presence of cofactors (e.g., other STDs) that may facilitate the transmission of HIV, and the impact of prevention programs in various parts of the population.

HIV/AIDS IN AFRICA

OVERVIEW

According to UNAIDS estimates, 20.8 million people were living with HIV in Africa at the end of 1996. Although the number of reported AIDS cases from the region numbers only 617,000, the actual number is acknowledged to be much greater, with an estimated 10.4 million AIDS cases since the beginning of the pandemic. Patterns of HIV infection in the region show a great deal of variation, with some countries (or at least major urban areas) beginning to show signs of stabilization, while other countries are experiencing rapid growth in infection levels. At this point in the pandemic, the high levels of HIV infection suggest that the demographic, social, and economic impacts of HIV/AIDS will be greater in this region than in any other world region.

HIV-2 is found only in a few countries predominantly in West Africa and in the former Portuguese colonies of Angola and Mozambique. The routes of transmission and risk factors for HIV-1 and HIV-2 are similar and both result in AIDS.[8] However, the latency period for HIV-2 appears to be longer, and vertical transmission (from mother to child) is rare.[9] For this reason the following discussion will primarily focus on HIV-1.

PREGNANT WOMEN

The inroads HIV has made into the general population can be seen in the levels and trends of HIV infection among pregnant women in urban settings in Africa. Much information has been gathered on pregnant women. Since many pregnant women will attend an antenatal clinic at some point during their pregnancy, this population is relatively easy to monitor over time. Research has shown that women in traditional marriages and regular partnerships rarely exhibit risky sexual behaviors.[10] However, UNAIDS estimates that worldwide more than 40 percent of all new HIV infections are in women, and in sub-Saharan Africa the share is around 50 percent.[11] A study of HIV positive Baganda women in Uganda suggested that the husband's behavior put the women at risk since most of these women had no sexual partners outside of marriage.[12] In another study in Kigali, Rwanda, 24 percent of women who thought they were in mutually monogamous relationships were HIV positive.[13] Even among women who had only one lifetime partner—their husband—21 percent were infected. Although little or no information is available for the partners of these women, these findings imply that HIV seroprevalence among the men is at least as high if not higher.

Among urban women attending antenatal clinics, infection rates are lower than in more vulnerable populations such as sexworkers, but in nearly half of the countries in sub-Saharan Africa, infection rates for these urban populations exceed 5 percent (Fig. 5-3). Among these women, higher HIV-1 seroprevalence levels are found in in urban centers along the Rift Valley and extending from Kenya to South Africa. In fact, in several of these countries, HIV-1 seroprevalence levels among this "low-risk" population in major cities are around 25 percent. In West Africa, the apparent epicenter for HIV-1 is Abidjan, Côte d'Ivoire, where infections levels are between 10 and 20 percent. In Northern Africa, in contrast,

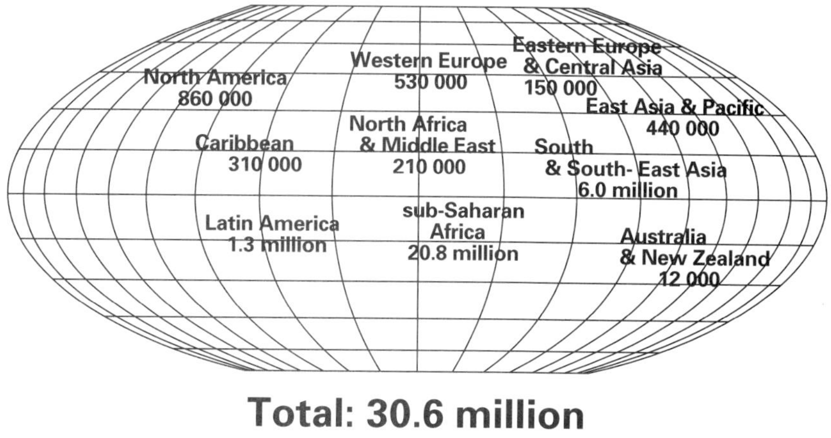

Fig. 5-2. Adults and children estimated to be living with HIV/AIDS as of end 1997.

some infection has been documented in most countries, but current levels of HIV are much less than 1 percent of pregnant women.

Thus far, we have examined primarily patterns and trends in urban epidemics. In Africa, data tend to show a pattern of differential infection levels between urban and rural areas within a country. Large differentials in HIV infection levels between urban and rural areas of a country have been found in many sub-Saharan countries. In Burundi, for example, 20 percent of sampled pregnant women in Bujumbura were HIV seropositive in 1992, whereas 5 percent of pregnant women in semiurban areas and 2 percent of pregnant women in rural areas were infected. In Malawi, 33 percent of urban pregnant women tested were HIV positive compared to 12 percent of rural pregnant women (1993). Similar patterns have been seen from studies conducted in Côte d'Ivoire, Rwanda, Tanzania, and Uganda.

A variety of studies of pregnant women have been conducted in African countries over the past 10 or more years (Fig. 5-4). In Uganda, Zambia, and Malawi these studies show a consistent and rapid increase in HIV infection levels among pregnant women in major cities of these countries. By 1990, more than 20 percent of the samples of pregnant women in those areas were infected. Kigali, Rwanda (not shown in Fig. 5-4), with a reported infection rate of over 30 percent since 1989, is another major urban area with high levels of infection. In the neighboring country of Burundi, 20 percent of pregnant women attending prenatal clinics in Bujumbura were HIV positive in 1992.

On the other hand, seroprevalence levels among pregnant women in Kinshasa, Democratic Republic of the Congo (former Zaire), have been relatively stable at fairly low levels over the past several years. Researchers, however, suspect that these reported stable seroprevalence levels may be masking increasing incidence levels among younger age groups.[14]

In contrast to this pattern, alarming increases in levels of HIV infection have been recently recorded among pregnant women in several countries in Southern Africa. In Francistown, Botswana, HIV seroprevalence increased from less than 10 percent in 1991 to over 40 percent in 1997, and in Gaborone, HIV seroprevalence

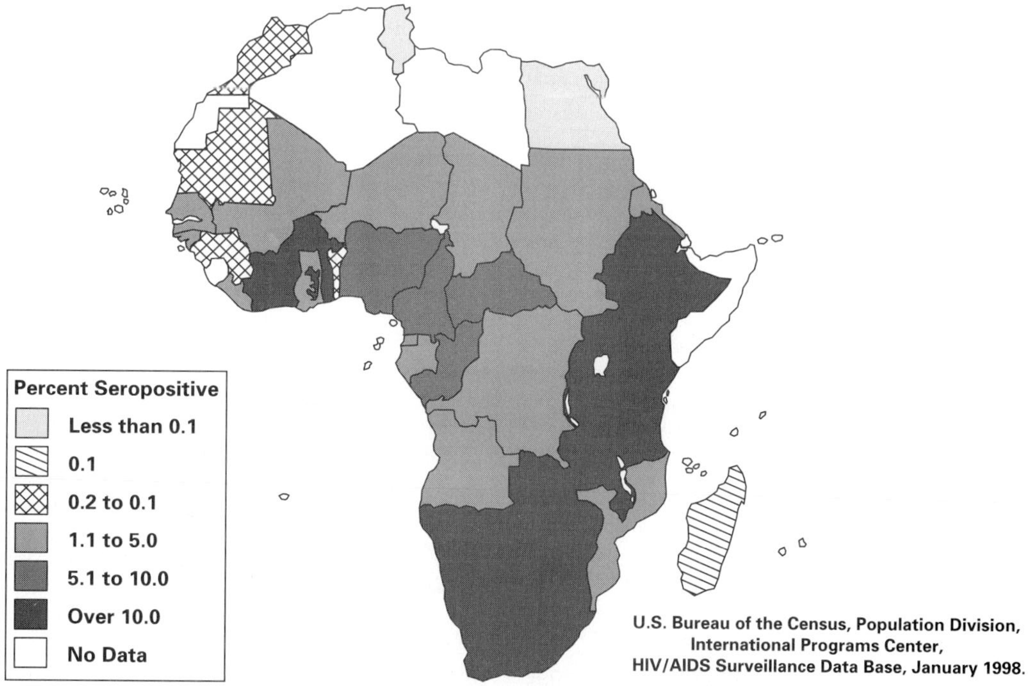

Fig. 5-3. African HIV-1 seroprevalence for pregnant women in urban populations.

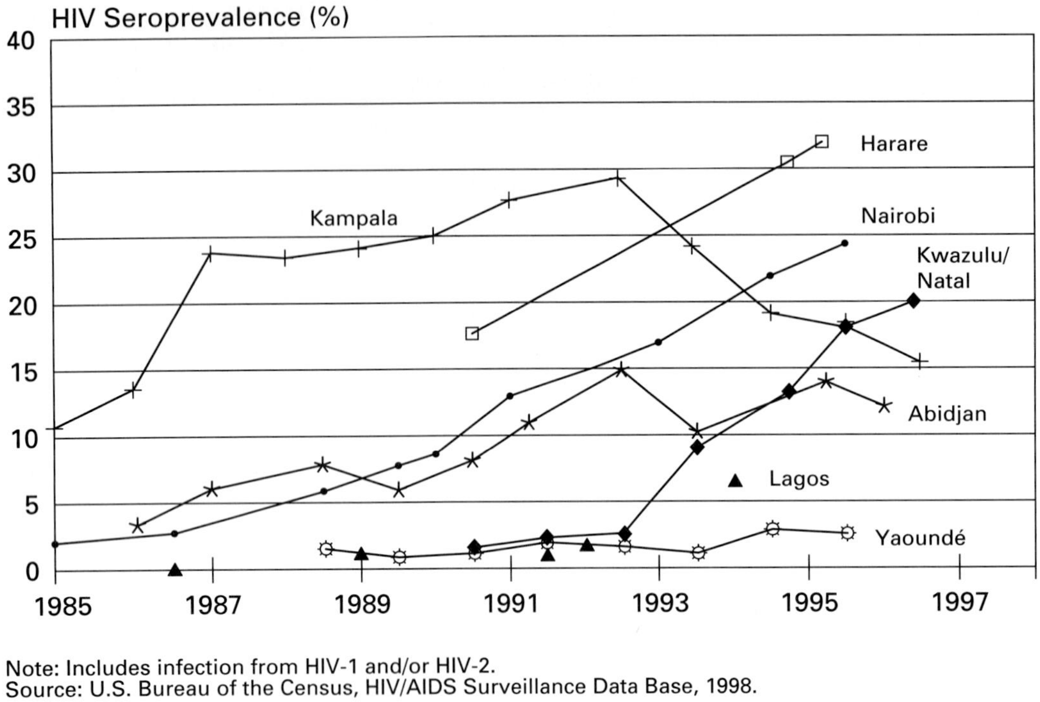

Fig. 5-4. HIV seroprevalence for pregnant women in selected urban areas of Africa: 1985–1987.

rose from 6 percent in 1990 to 34 percent in 1997. Another recent study showed 1995 infection rates among pregnant women in Harare, Zimbabwe, at 32 percent.[15] And in Kwazulu/Natal province in South Africa, infection rates for pregnant women have increased from under 2 percent in 1990 to nearly 20 percent in 1996 (see Fig. 5-4).

OTHER VULNERABLE POPULATIONS

Earlier, the concept of separate epidemics within a country was discussed, corresponding to variations in levels of risk. In data from Nairobi, this variation is reflected in levels and trends in HIV infection data spanning nearly a decade and a half (Fig. 5-5). Following the introduction of the virus to Kenya, HIV infection in sex workers increased early and quickly, reaching over 80 percent in some recent studies. Males attending STD clinics represent another high-risk population, since most of this group have had multiple partners and many are clients of sex workers. A recent study found HIV infection over 30 percent in this population. Finally, we can see the spread of HIV infection to a lower-risk population; women attending antenatal clinics. Until the mid-1980s very little infection was detected in this population, but 17 percent tested positive in a study conducted in 1993.

Patients attending STD clinics can be considered a sample of the population with frequent casual sexual contact, since they or their partners are likely to have had sexual contact with others. They are at elevated risk both owing to the presence of multiple partners as well as the potentially enhanced risk of HIV infection among those with various other STDs.[16]

Studies of STD patients in several African countries have documented HIV infection levels over 50 percent (Fig. 5-6). Patterns of sex differentials in HIV infection are now becoming more consistent. In all of the cases shown here, females have higher HIV infection levels than males. Although the majority of those attending STD clinics in Africa are men, women who attend are typically more likely to test positive for HIV. This reflects the greater vulnerability of women to HIV infection and the extent to which HIV has reached into the general population in Africa.

In studies of STD patients in the capital cities of Tanzania,

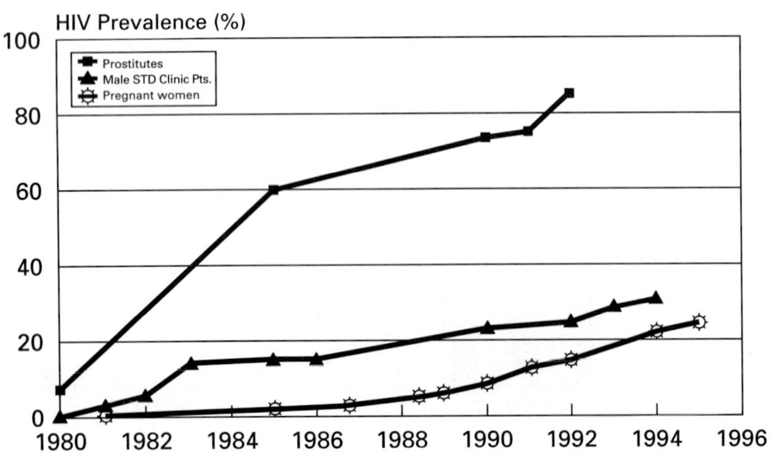

Fig. 5-5. HIV epidemics in Nairobi by risk group: 1980–1995.

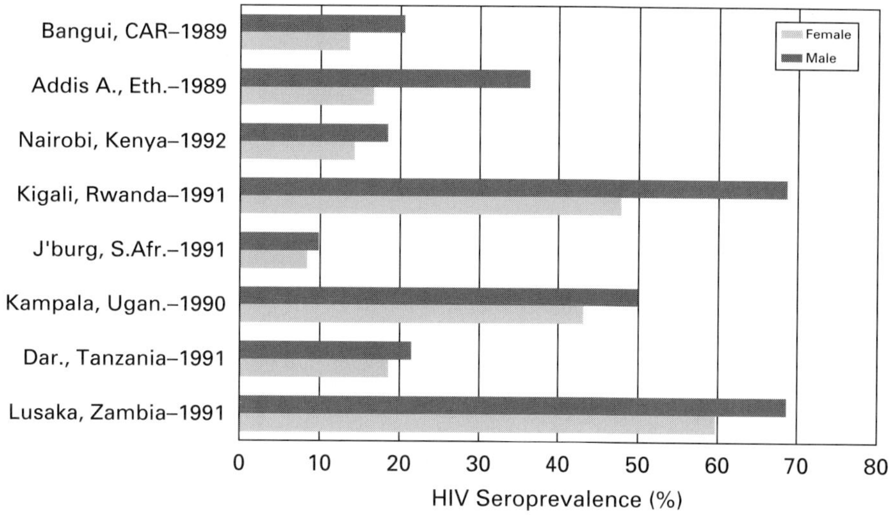

Fig. 5-6. HIV seroprevalence for STD patients by sex in selected African countries.

Note: Includes infection from HIV-1 and/or HIV-2.

Kenya, Côte d'Ivoire, and most recently in South Africa (black females) infection levels had reached over 20 percent. Recent data from Botswana also indicate high levels of HIV seroprevalence in STD clinic patients, reaching as high as 39 percent in Gaborone, 49 percent in Lobatse district, and 60 percent in Francistown.[17]

Available data from several behavioral studies from African countries suggest that a differential in sexual behavior exists, with males more likely to engage in casual sexual contacts than females.[19] These surveys also showed significantly different sexual behavior among countries.

PATTERNS BY AGE AND SEX

Because of variation in the introduction of the virus, differentials in sexual behavior by age, the growth of the epidemic, and mortality owing to AIDS, there tends to be a consistent age pattern of HIV infection in heterosexual epidemics. Peak infection levels tend to occur in the 20s and early 30s, with decreasing levels after those ages. Age patterns by sex are influenced by the tendency for males to choose a younger female as a spouse (as well as a casual sexual partner). This behavior results in higher HIV infection levels in younger females than males in the same age cohort, whereas older males tend to have higher infection levels than females of the same age. This pattern is shown in Fig. 5-7 for Masaka, Uganda.[18] The high levels of HIV infection noted in this figure for those under age 20 should serve to underscore the need for prevention programs aimed at this extremely vulnerable age group.

MATURING EPIDEMICS

Recent data on urban populations in some African settings suggest the possibility that these epidemics are plateauing and may not increase much further. Examples for such a situation are Zambia and Malawi, where prevalence rates seem to stabilize after substantial increases over the past years (see Fig. 5-4). This situation is not new or unique—stable prevalence at lower levels has characterized the situation in Kinshasa since the mid-1980s.

Such stabilization is a natural part of the epidemic process, and occurs as a natural result of a dynamic balance between new infections and deaths. An underlying high incidence of new HIV infections among the young may therefore be masked by high numbers of deaths removing those dying of AIDS or other HIV disease. For example, in Rakai district in Uganda between 1990 and 1992, an observed decrease in the prevalence among pregnant

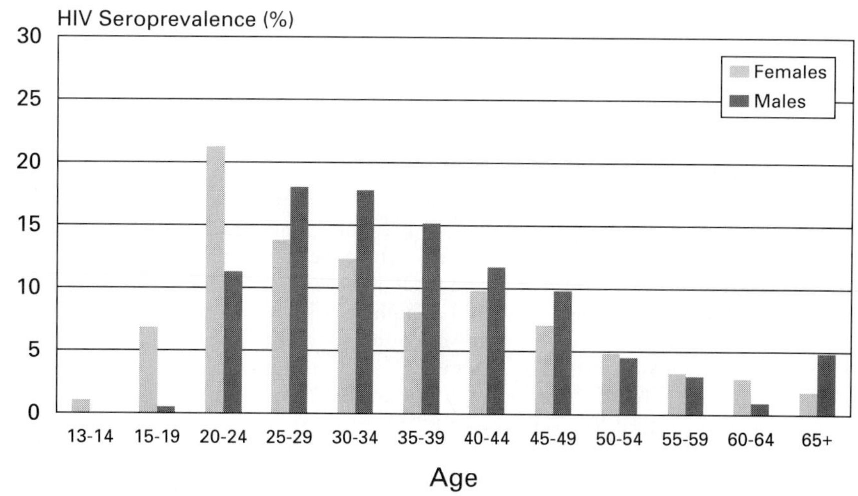

Fig. 5-7. HIV seroprevalence of adult population Masaka, Uganda by age and sex: 1980–1990.

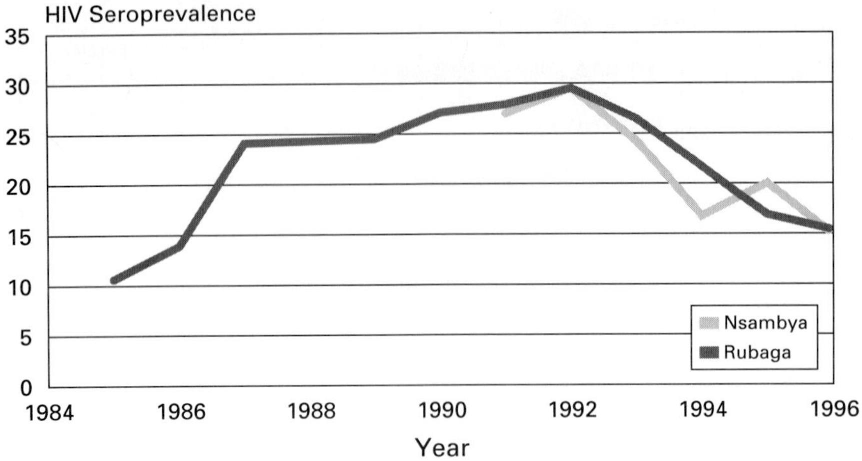

Fig. 5-8. HIV seroprevalence for pregnant women in two sentinel sites, Kampala, Uganda: 1985–1996.

women of 2.0 percentage points resulted from a decrease of 4.3 percent owing to mortality and net outmigration, and an increase of 2.3 percent owing to new infections.[20] Therefore, to conclude from stabilizing or even declining prevalence rates either that the epidemic will wane by itself in the absence of interventions, or that prevention efforts are no longer necessary, would have tragic consequences for future generations.

Another major transformation that occurs as epidemics mature is the shifting of new infections to the young. Although new HIV/AIDS epidemics are characterized by high levels of new infections across a wide age spectrum, in mature epidemics new infections shift to younger cohorts just beginning sexual activity and risk taking.

A unique development for Africa is seen in Uganda. This country was among the first to be heavily hit by HIV, with dramatic rates of HIV infection already in the late 1980s. However, rates for some urban centers started to decrease since the early 1990s (Fig. 5-8). During the same period major changes in individual risk behavior could be documented, namely, a later onset of sexual activity, fewer partners, and increased condom use.[21] This clearly shows that prevention works and it should be taken as an encouraging example of best practice and as a model for other countries in the region.

The preceding discussion highlights the importance of continued efforts to monitor epidemic trends, implement effective behavior change interventions, and evaluate the impact of such interventions on the actual behaviors of the populations at risk.

HIV/AIDS IN LATIN AMERICA AND THE CARIBBEAN

OVERVIEW

The HIV pandemic continues to spread throughout Latin America and the Caribbean region. However, HIV prevalence studies document great variation in HIV infection rates between populations and countries. Sexual transmission, including homosexual, bisexual, and heterosexual transmission, continues to be the main mode of transmission in all of the countries. HIV infection has been detected both in populations considered at highest risk, as well as in populations at lower risk in a number of countries in both Latin America and the Caribbean. The situation is still unfolding and HIV continues to spread, revealing itself in one country after another, indicating a need for continued preventive measures.

The initial spread of HIV infection and resulting AIDS cases in the Latin America and Caribbean region was predominantly among injecting drug users and Men having Sex with Men (MSM). However, as these epidemics have matured, heterosexual transmission has increased along with perinatal transmission. By the end of 1997, a total of 212,000 AIDS cases had been reported to WHO from the Americas excluding the United States and Canada, whereas the estimate of the total number of persons with HIV for 1997 in this area was over 1.6 million.

PREGNANT WOMEN

HIV infection among pregnant women is still relatively rare in a number of Latin America and Caribbean settings. In Latin America, studies in only four countries have found HIV infection levels above 1 percent (Fig. 5-9). Haiti, with studies showing infection levels of 6 and 8 percent, has by far the highest HIV prevalence levels in the region.

In the Caribbean, HIV epidemics have spread more widely. In five countries, various studies document HIV infection over 1 percent among pregnant women. Among those countries reporting data, HIV infection has been detected among pregnant women in all but two countries; Cayman Islands and Grenada.

OTHER VULNERABLE POPULATIONS

Injecting drug use is a worldwide phenomenon, from Asia, Europe, and North America to Latin America and the Caribbean. In the last several years, HIV has spread among injecting drug users in a greatly increased number of countries, often very rapidly. This rapid increase may be associated with the lack of awareness of the HIV/AIDS threat and the common use of drug injecting equipment not only among friends, but also among the larger "community" of injecting drug users.[22] Although published data on HIV seroprevalence among IDU in Latin America and the Caribbean are very limited, significant levels of HIV infection have been found among sampled populations. In a study conducted in Buenos Aires, Argentina, in 1993, for example, 52 percent of IDU were HIV positive (Fig. 5-10). Other studies from 1990 to 1992 in Mexico and Brazil reported HIV levels ranging from 9 to 31 percent. In addition, HIV infection has been found among drug users (those who may or may not be using a needle) in other countries. In one such study, 13 percent were infected in a survey of 224 "crack" cocaine users in the Bahamas in 1990 to 1991. Another study conducted in Montevideo, Uruguay, found 52 percent of drug users tested to be HIV positive.

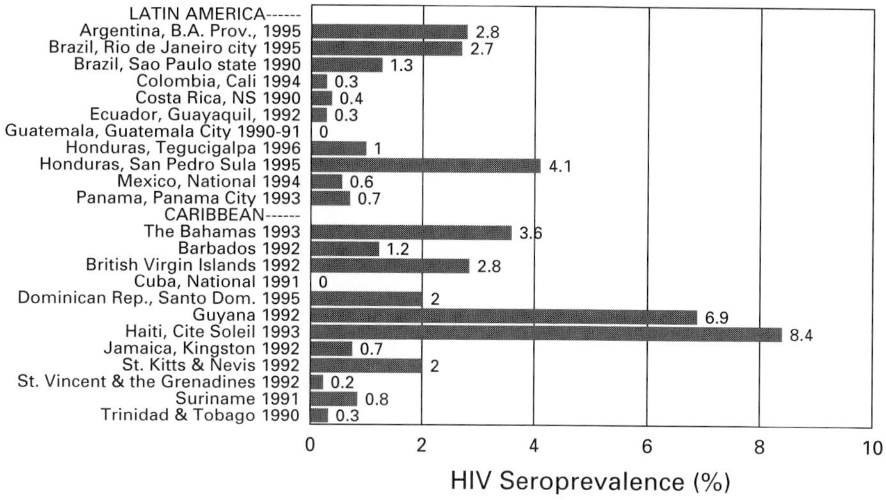

*Location not specified for all countries

Fig. 5-9. HIV seroprevalence for pregnant women in Latin America and the Caribbean: 1990–1996.

HIV infection among sex workers has been detected in a number of countries within all six subregions of Latin America. In the Andean, Southern Cone, Central America Isthmus subregions, and in Mexico, studies indicate HIV infection levels among this population are below 10 percent (Fig. 5-11). Meanwhile, several areas in Latin Caribbean and Brazil have reported HIV seroprevalence over 10 percent.

In the Caribbean, available data from sex worker populations show considerable variation in HIV infection levels. Relatively high levels of infection were detected in studies conducted in Trinidad and Tobago, Jamaica, and Guyana, with one-fourth of tested sex workers HIV positive in Guyana. Lower infection levels were reported in Antigua, Barbuda, and Suriname.

Data on HIV infection among STD clinic patients are available for five of the six subregions of Latin America. In three subregions, HIV infection levels were over 7 percent for locations in one or more countries. These countries include Argentina, Honduras, Dominican Republic, and Haiti. Reports from several of the remaining countries note HIV infection levels under 1 percent among STD patients.

In the Caribbean, studies conducted among STD patients in several countries reported HIV infection levels over 10 percent. These countries include the Bahamas, Guyana, Trinidad, and Tobago. Most other countries in the Caribbean reported some HIV infection among STD patients.

HIV infection levels for STD patients by gender are available for a limited number of countries. In contrast to the pattern observed in Africa, male STD patients in this region appear to be at higher risk than female patients, at least at the present stage of the epidemic. These data show a consistent pattern of higher infection levels for males than for females (Fig. 5-12). In four out of the five sites, males were approximately twice or more as likely to be infected than were females.

Various studies clearly document the spread of HIV infection among homosexual/bisexual men since 1984. In all the countries for which data are now available, moderate to high levels of HIV infection have been detected among members of the populations tested. In Latin America, male homosexual and bisexual contact continues to be the predominant mode of HIV transmission for Brazil, Mexico, Central American Isthmus, and Andean area subregions.

Studies conducted in many of the capital cities in Latin America among MSM reported prevalence rates ranging from 3 percent in Costa Rica in 1992 to over 40 percent in Mexico City in 1992

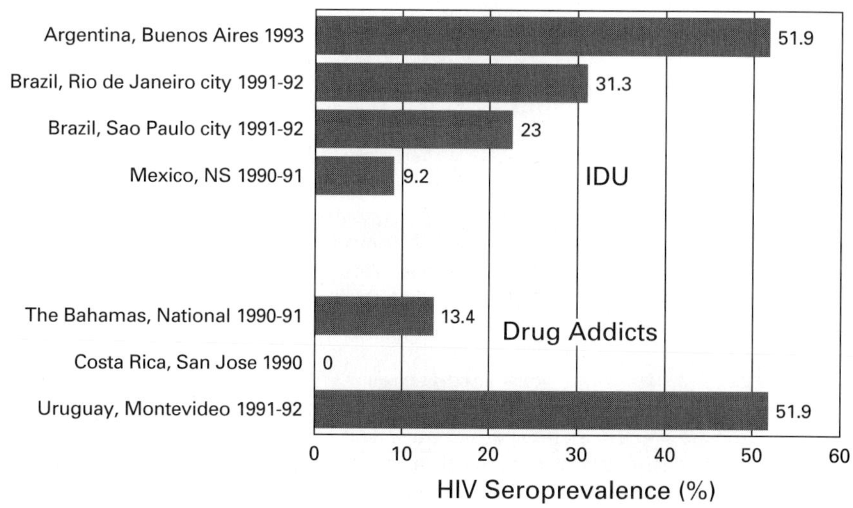

NS = Location not specified

Fig. 5-10. HIV seroprevalence for injecting drug users and drug addicts, Latin America and the Caribbean: 1990–1993.

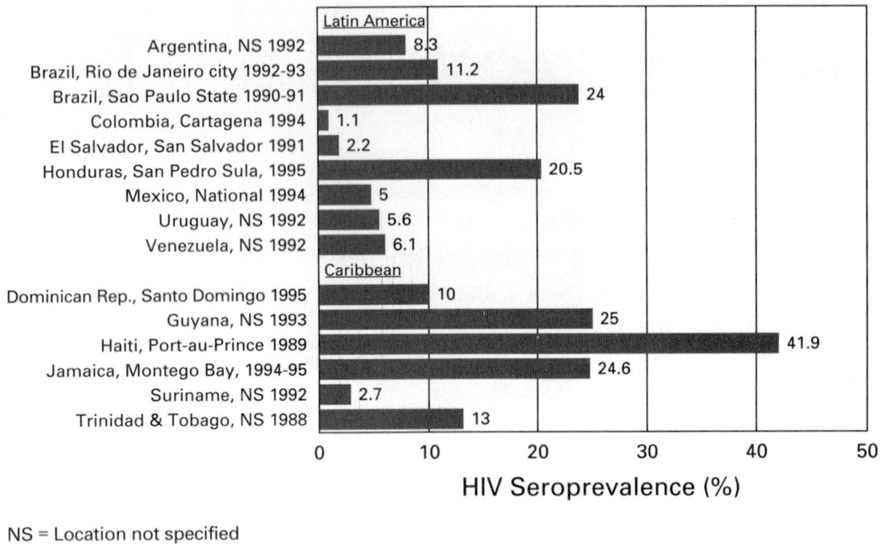

Fig. 5-11. HIV seroprevalence for sex workers in Latin America and the Caribbean: 1988–1995.

(Fig. 5-13). In the Andean subregion, HIV infection ranges from 5 to 6 percent in Colombia and Peru to over 30 percent in Venezuela. A recent study of MSM in Rio de Janeiro city found nearly one in four to be HIV positive. Of the 14 countries in the region for which data are available, four reported infection levels of over 20 percent; in five other countries, various studies noted HIV seroprevalence between 10 and 20 percent; whereas studies in the remaining five countries reported that between 2 and 10 percent of homosexuals and/or bisexuals tested were HIV positive.

HIV/AIDS IN ASIA

OVERVIEW

In the mid- to late 1980s, there was speculation that somehow Asian populations might be spared the threat of the spread of HIV and AIDS. This hope was fueled by the fact that until the late 1980s little evidence of epidemic spread of HIV was available. We now know that this was a futile hope. In high-risk populations throughout the population, levels of HIV infection are increasing rapidly. Especially worrying is the fact that HIV epidemics in some Asian countries are also reaching quickly into the population at lower risk of infection. The spread of HIV infection in Thailand and India have received considerable attention, but infection also appears to be increasing rapidly in a number of other Asian countries, especially in Southeast Asia.

As of the end of 1997, WHO had received reports of only 74,000 AIDS cases in the region—about one-eighth of the number reported from Africa. However, by the end of 1997, UNAIDS and WHO estimated that 6.4 million Asians were living with HIV. This represents more than one out of five infections globally—only a few year into the epidemic in most of the countries in the region.

MULTIPLE EPIDEMICS

As typical for early epidemics, HIV in Asia is spreading most rapidly among those at highest risk—which for this region tends to be injecting drug users. Infection in other populations follows, but will likely not reach the levels of those at higher risk. This phe-

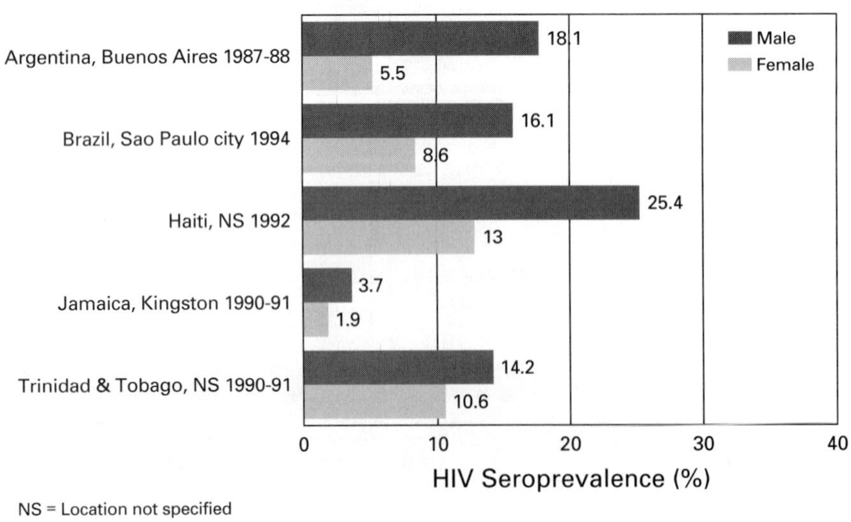

Fig. 5-12. HIV seroprevalence for STD clinic patients, by sex, in Latin America and the Caribbean: 1987–1994.

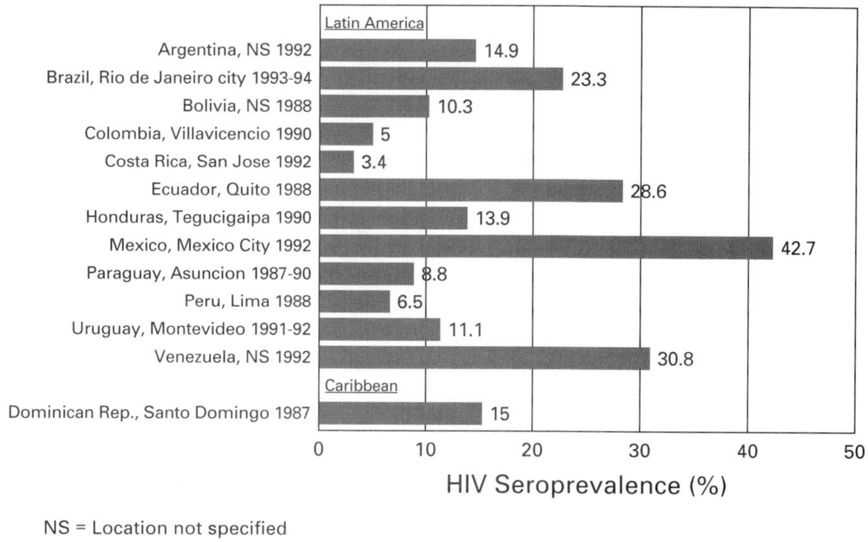

Fig. 5-13. HIV seroprevalence for male homosexuals and bisexuals in Latin America and the Caribbean: 1987–1992.

nomenon is illustrated for Asia in the several epidemics in Bangkok (Fig. 5-14). Note the explosion of infection among injecting drug users in the late 1980s, followed by increases in infection among sex workers, and then STD patients. After 1990, infection among pregnant women grew, reaching nearly 2 percent in 1995 and 1996. Recent decreases in young military recruits are the result of intensive intervention programs, mainly the 100 percent condom use program in the Thai sex industry, which was introduced in the early 1990s (Fig. 5-15).

ANTENATAL WOMEN

HIV infection among pregnant women in Asia has reached several percent in some areas. For India as well as for other countries in the region, a critical question is how fast HIV will spread to the densely populated rural areas from the cities that are now showing signs of infection in the general population. In Thailand, HIV infection among pregnant women is about three times as high in the North as in Bangkok, and in Myanmar HIV has reached some level of infection even in secondary cities (Fig. 5-16).

The potential for rapid spread of HIV infection even among the general population is illustrated by Fig. 5-17 A and B, which show infection levels for Thailand by province in 1990 and 1996.

In 1990, HIV was only present in samples of antenatal women in 13 of the 73 provinces reporting—provinces reported no positive test results (Fig. 5-17A). However, by 1996 only five provinces reported no infections among antenatal women tested, and 27 provinces reported infection levels of over 2 percent (Fig. 5-17B).

OTHER VULNERABLE POPULATIONS

In addition to the epidemic among injecting drug users in Thailand already noted, in other parts of Asia, HIV infection among injecting drug users has also risen rapidly. By the early 1990s prevalence had reached two-thirds or more of some samples of drug users in Myanmar and in China's "golden triangle" area (Fig. 5-18). In Vietnam, nearly one-third of injecting drug users were reported HIV positive.

India's vast population and diverse regions make for similarly diverse regional epidemics. Some areas in India have very HIV prevalence rates, whereas others exhibit much lower rates of in-

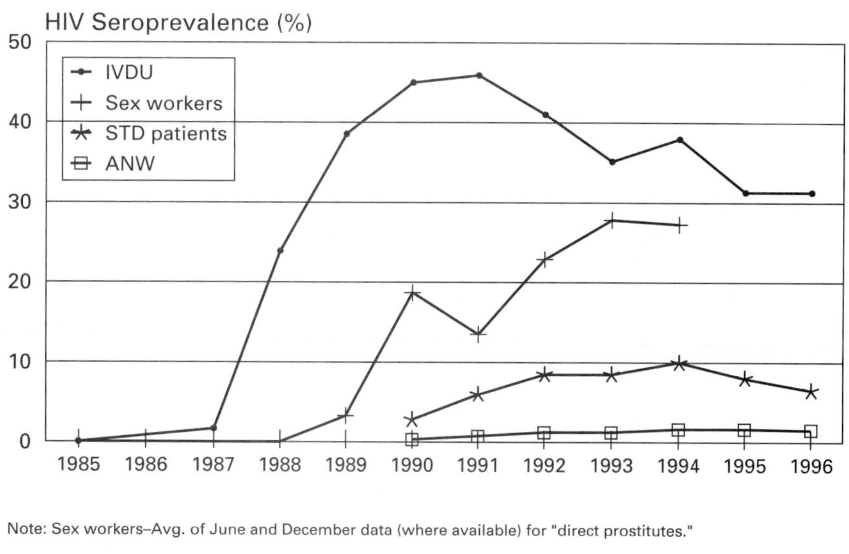

Fig. 5-14. HIV seroprevalence for selected populations in Bangkok, Thailand: 1985–1996.

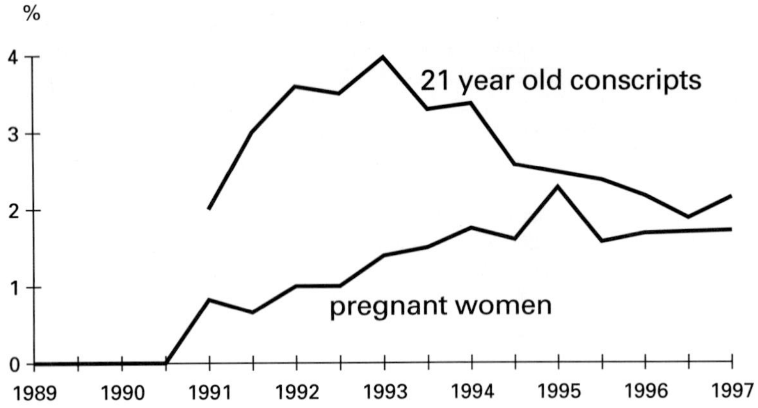

Fig. 5-15. HIV prevalence in pregnant women and 21-year-old military conscripts, Thailand.

fection. A 1991 national estimate for injecting drug users placed the HIV prevalence rate at 38 percent.

SEX WORKERS

HIV infection has been reported among populations of sex workers through the Asian region. Most countries in Southeast Asia report at least some infection in these population (Fig. 5-19). In this regard, data from Myanmar, Cambodia, and Thailand are particularly worrisome, with prevalence reaching one-fourth to one-third of the tested population in several settings. These rates indicate continued high levels of exposure to the risk of infection. Because of the large numbers of clients for each sex worker within a given period of time, studies among this population have noted the difficulty in avoiding HIV infection once the virus has been introduced into the population.

A number of other countries in Southeast Asia have detected some HIV infection among this population, even though HIV has not, as yet, made major inroads into the general population. Such infection trends have important implications for the future spread of HIV in the region, and should serve as warning signals for stepped-up intervention efforts.

In India, HIV prevalence for sex workers has already reached high levels in many areas. One-quarter or more of the sex workers tested in several major cities in the early 1990s were HIV positive. Low levels of HIV infection in the other areas shown should not be a signal for complacence, as variation in the timing of the introduction of HIV to these particular sites may explain their apparent lag.

For several cities in India, we can construct a time series of data, illustrating the spread of HIV among sex workers. Data for six sites show the ability of HIV to spread rapidly once it is introduced (Fig. 5-20). In Bombay and Pune, in particular, HIV increased from under 10 percent of sex workers to over 40 percent within a 4-year period. Noteworthy is the continuing low level of HIV infection among sex workers in Calcutta, which has had a very active and comprehensive HIV prevention program for several years.

STD CLINIC PATIENTS

In a number of sites in Southeast Asia, HIV infection rates among STD patients range from 4 to 10 percent. Myanmar and Thailand stand out for their high levels of infection in this population. Cambodia stands out as a country with a nascent HIV/AIDS epidemic that appears to be growing rapidly. Several other countries in the region have rates below 1 percent. In East Asia and Sri Lanka, rates are also relatively low, based on studies through the early 1990s. In India, data for seven of the 13 available sites show HIV infection levels for STD patients above 8 percent. One out of every five STD patients tested positive for HIV in samples in Hubli and Pune.

In summary, HIV prevalence studies in Asia show wide differences in infection rates between populations. However, with the exception of Myanmar, India, and Thailand, in most of the Asian

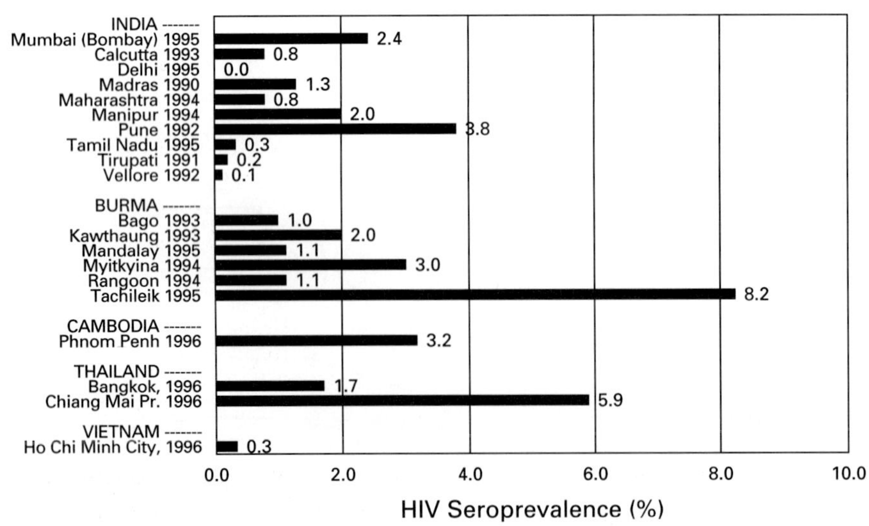

Fig. 5-16. HIV seroprevalence for pregnant women in Asia: 1990–1996.

region it is difficult to show the extent of HIV infection and to determine trends because of the limited nature of the data available. Although HIV was introduced into Asia at later date than much of the rest of the world, the virus has already been detected in the general population of many of the countries of the region, and the potential for its continued spread is great.

WESTERN AND EASTERN EUROPE

Through November 1997, over 197,000 AIDS cases had been reported from the 46 countries of the WHO European region. The distribution of modes of transmission in Europe differs considerably from that reported from Africa, Latin America, and Asia discussed in the preceding. Based on AIDS cases reported through early 1997, 35 percent were attributed to homosexual/bisexual contact, 40 percent injecting drug use, 15 percent heterosexual contact, and 10 percent other sources.[23]

However, the modes of transmission of HIV have been changing over time. Before 1990, most AIDS cases had occurred among men who had sex with men. Since that time, the predominant transmission category has been injecting drug users, whereas male homosexual/bisexual transmission has been declining (Fig. 5-21). Over this period, however, heterosexual transmission has been

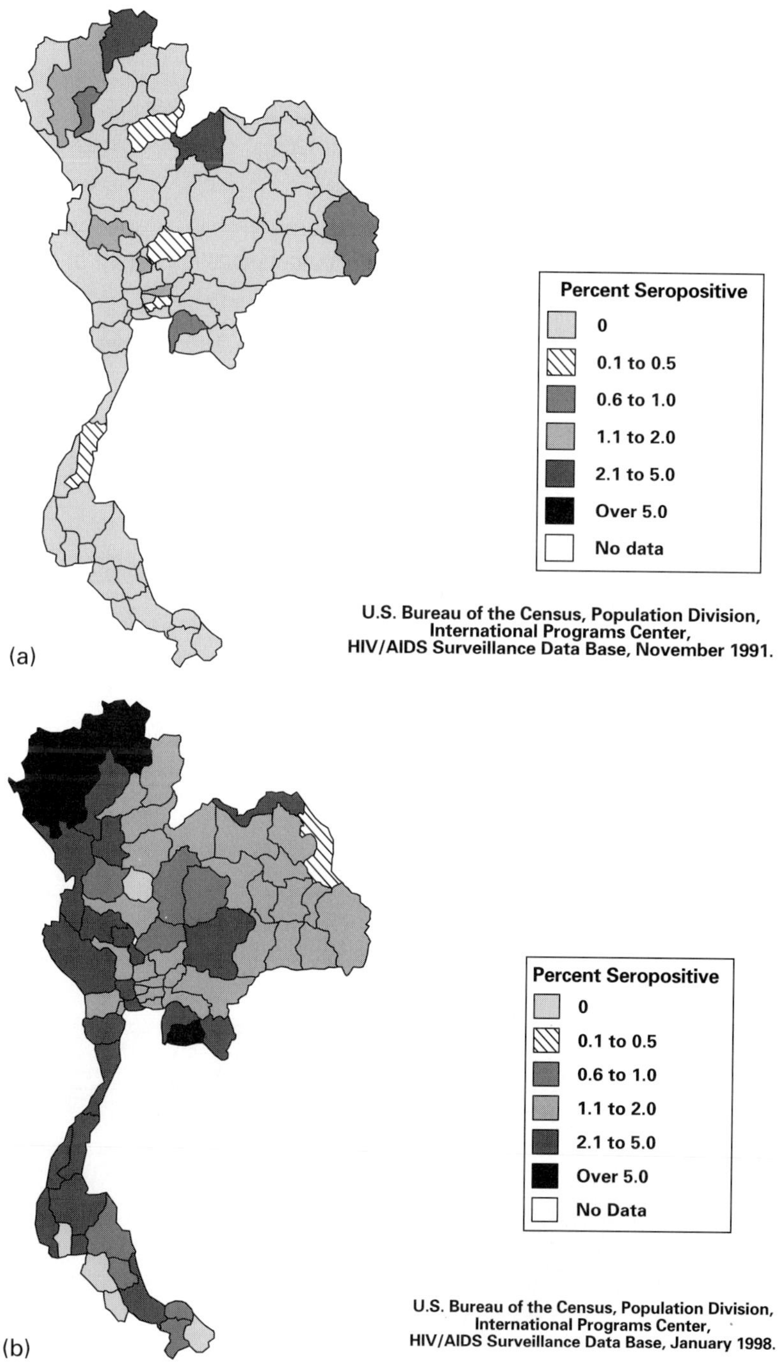

Fig. 5-17*A*. HIV seroprevalence among pregnant women, Thailand: June 1990. *B*. HIV seroprevalence among pregnant women, Thailand: June 1996.

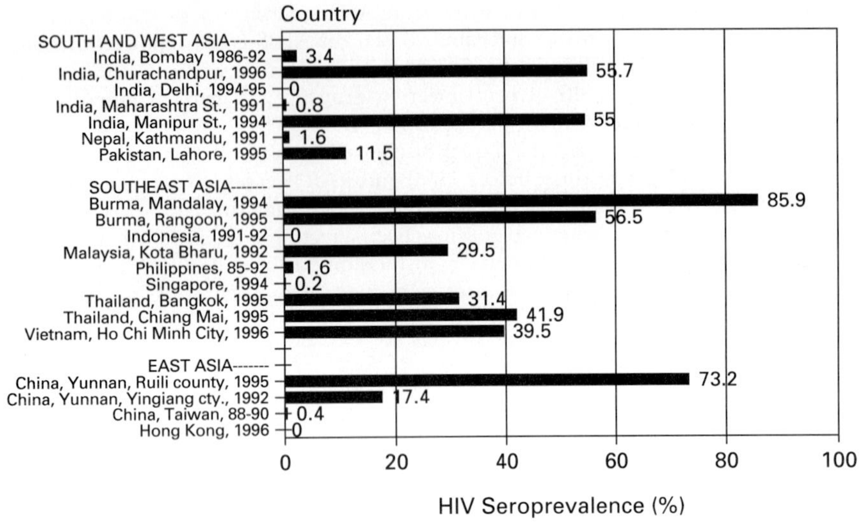

Fig. 5-18. HIV seroprevalence for injecting drug users in Asia: 1986–1996.

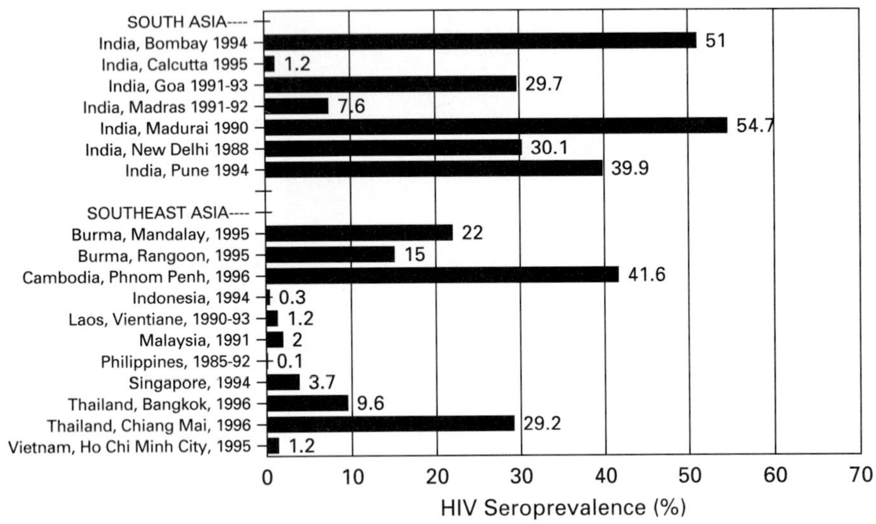

Fig. 5-19. HIV seroprevalence for sex workers in Asia: 1985–1996.

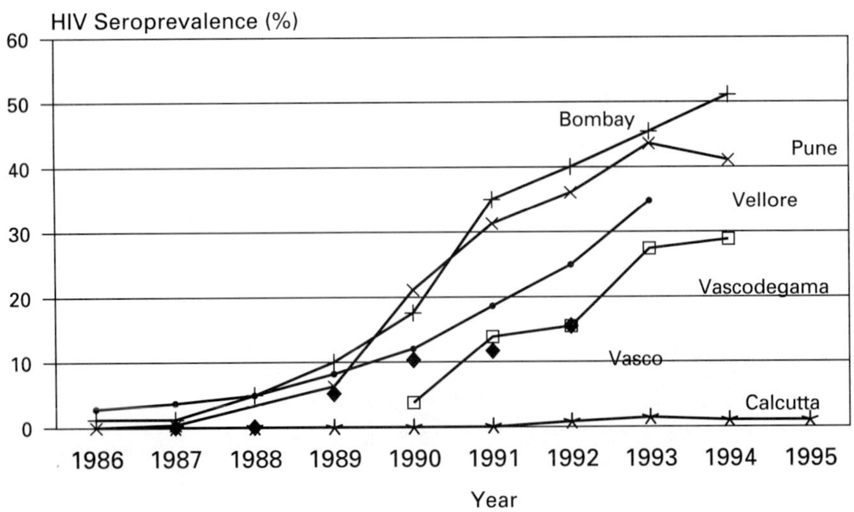

Fig. 5-20. HIV seroprevalence for sex workers in India: 1986–1995.

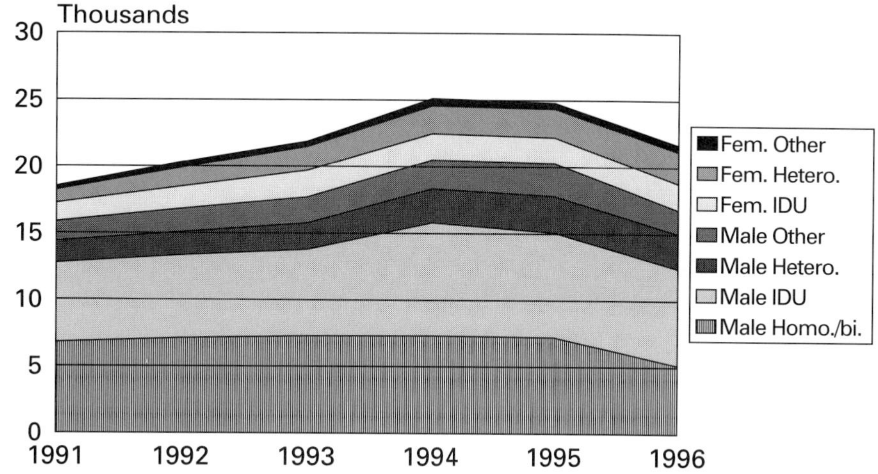

Fig. 5-21. Reported adult AIDS cases in the WHO European region by mode of transmission and sex: 1991–1996.

Source: European Centre for the Epidemiological Monitoring of AIDS, 1997, "HIV/AIDS Surveillance in Europe," First Quarter, Saint-Maurice, France.

increasing, as have AIDS cases among women. Annual AIDS cases in Europe appear to have peaked in 1994 and 1995, with decline reported by many countries in 1996. At least a portion of the decline has to be attributed to more efficient treatment of those HIV positive, whereas reductions in the incidence of new HIV infections in some populations in the since the mid- to late 1980s following effective prevention activities targeted at the most vulnerable groups and the general population are also contributing to the observed decline.

Drug injection is behind the dramatic surge in HIV infection in several Eastern European nations, accounting for the majority of the 100,000 new infections estimated to have occurred in 1997. In Ukraine, where approximately 70 percent of infections have been in drug users over the last 3 years, 25,000 cases of HIV infection have been reported so far, half of them in 1997. It is possible that a similar pattern will be seen elsewhere in the region. Russian officials estimate there are about 350,000 regular drug users in the country, many of them sharing injecting equipment.

The potential for sexual spread also exists. In Russia, Belarus, and Moldova, new cases of syphilis rocketed from very low levels in the late 1980s to well above 2 per 1000 population by 1996, with continuously increasing trends (Fig. 5-22). An untreated sexually transmitted disease not only makes HIV (when present) spread much more easily from one partner to the other but is important as a marker of potential HIV spread because it has the same transmission route—unprotected sex (intercourse without a condom).

IMPLICATIONS

POPULATION IMPACTS

Based on the magnitude of HIV epidemics in some countries and the demographic and geographic characteristics of those epidemics, we can draw a number of implications relating to the potential demographic impact of such epidemics. The age pattern of infection and the heterosexual nature of these epidemics will result in mortality increases both for middle-aged adults and infants and children. Since women, even if they are infected at a young age, will typically live until their late 20s, the fertility impact is not clear. Many HIV-infected women will bear several children. Depending on the severity of the epidemic, population growth rates will be reduced. But the potential for negative population growth will depend on levels of fertility and the extent to which HIV epidemics reach substantial proportions in the rural areas of countries, particularly in Africa and Asia.

A well-estalished measure of demographic impact is life expectancy at birth. Today AIDS is systematically cutting down life expectancy in the countries where the disease is most common. The gains achieved over the last few decades in much of the developing world will be canceled out in some places by HIV. Life expectancy in Botswana rose from under 43 years in 1955 to 61 years in 1990. Now, with between 25 and 30 percent of the adult population infected with HIV, life expectancy is expected to drop back to levels last seen in the late 1960s (Fig. 5-23). By the end of

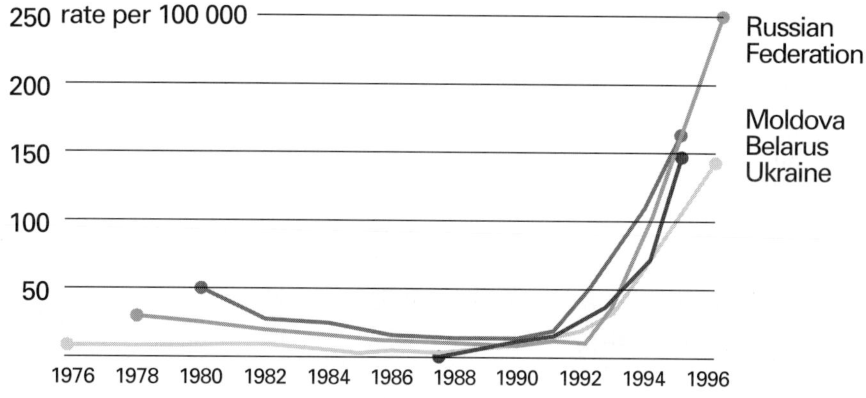

Fig. 5-22. Number of new syphilis cases in Belarus, Moldova, Russian federation, and Ukraine.

Source: National AIDS Control Programmes, 1997

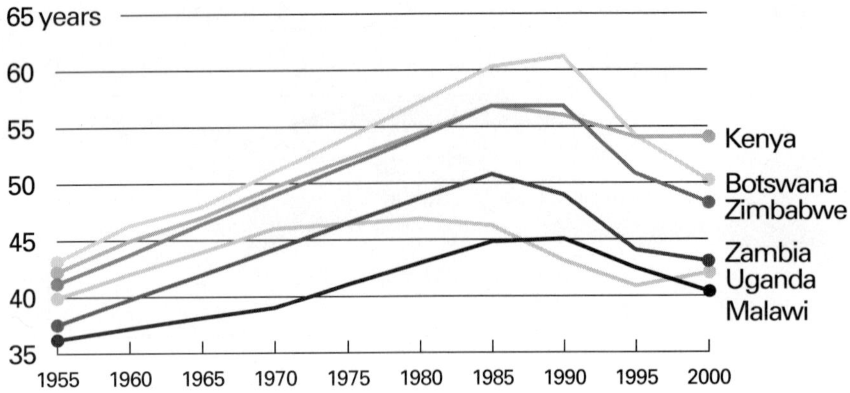

Fig. 5-23. Impact of HIV/AIDS epidemic on projected life expectancy at birth—selected sub-Saharan countries.

Source: World Population Prospects: The 1996 revision, *United Nations Population Division, 1996*

the decade, Zimbabwe will see 10 years wiped off the life expectancy of a child born in 1990. In Uganda, one study in a rural area measured the lifespan of the population as a whole and compared it with that of the people who were not HIV-infected. It concluded that where 8 percent of the population was HIV-positive, the presence of AIDS in the community cut overall life expectancy by 16 years.

The high mortality owing to HIV/AIDS also has major impacts on families. It is estimated that since the beginning of the epidemic more than 8 million children have lost their mothers to AIDS when they were less than 15 years old—and many of these also lost their fathers. It is estimated that this figure will almost double by the year 2000.

The worst is still to come. Since the beginning of the epidemic, it is estimated that 11.7 million people around the world have died of AIDS and HIV-related causes. That is just one-third of the number currently infected. Indeed, half as many people were infected this year alone as have died in the whole epidemic to date. Because the vast majority of people living with HIV are in the developing world, access to antiretrovirals is often difficult or impossible. Also, these drugs do not constitute a cure: They are not effective in everyone, and at this point it is impossible to say how long their effects will last. Thus, many if not most of the 30 million people currently infected may well die in the relatively near future, perhaps within the next decade.

Developing nations have made great strides in increasing infant and child survival in recent decades. These gains, too, are threatened by HIV. Already, one-quarter more babies under 12 months old in Zimbabwe and Zambia are dying than would be the case if there were no HIV. By 2010, Zimbabwe's infant mortality rate is expected to rise by 138 percent because of AIDS, and its under-five mortality rate by 109 percent (Fig. 5-24). In Côte d'Ivoire, child mortality will rise by over two-thirds.

CONCLUSION

There is a growing gap between the developed and the developing world—not only with respect to the scale of HIV spread but also morbidity and mortality from AIDS. In North America, Western Europe, Australia, and New Zealand, newly available antiretroviral drugs are reducing the speed at which HIV-infected people develop AIDS. In most of these countries substantial decreases in AIDS incidence have been observed since 1996. In addition, early and targeted prevention programs were successful in reducing the number of HIV infections—especially in the high-risk groups—in the mid- to late 1980s, further limiting the impact of the disease.

The picture in the less developed world is very different. The number of new infections has reached dramatic levels and is still increasing in many regions. However, because of the long latency period between infection and the development of HIV-related diseases, the major impact of the disease is still to come—even if new infections could be reduced in the near future. Different than many other diseases HIV has caused an invisible pandemic. Because of the lack of resources and awareness, nine out of 10 HIV-infected persons do not know about their HIV infection and very often

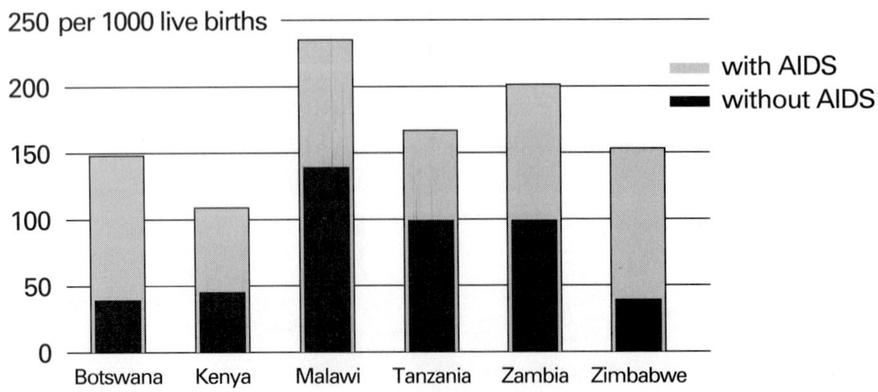

Fig. 5-24. Estimated impact of AIDS on under-5-year-old child mortality rates—selected African countries: 2010.

Source: *US Bureau of the Census*

also do not have a chance to learn about it even if they would like to. This fact further complicates the implementation of effective prevention programs.

However, there are some very encouraging signs of success:

- In Uganda decreases in HIV prevalence in some urban sites have been reported. In parallel, substantial decreases in risk behavior have shown that prevention can work in developing countries with severe epidemics.
- In neighboring Tanzania, a program of aggressive treatment of STDs resulted in a reduction of 42 percent in the incidence of new HIV infections compared with communities without such a program.
- Throughout Africa, condom sales have taken off, although not nearly enough condoms are being used.
- In Thailand, a relatively grim picture of only a few years ago has become more hopeful as a result of widespread condom use and decreasing levels of STDs.

Although it is clear that in the absence of a widely available cure and effective vaccines HIV/AIDS is not a transient phenomenon, these findings should encourage all parts of societies, including researchers, policy makers, and donors as well as NGOs and community-based organizations, to help develop enabling environments that will deliver care and support to those being affected and opportunities to prevent the further spread by increased knowledge and availability of preventive technologies.

References

1 WHO, UNAIDS: HIV/AIDS. The current global situation of the HIV/AIDS pandemic. *Weekly Epidemiol Rec* 1997;72:357–358.
2 UNAIDS. Case study: Reaching regional consensus on improved behavioral and sero-surveillance for HIV. *Best Pract Collect Draft,* 1997.
3 WHO, UNAIDS: HIV/AIDS. The current global situation of the HIV/AIDS pandemic. *Weekly Epidemiol Rec* 1997;72:357–358.
4 Pan American Health Organization. *AIDS surveillance in the Americas: Quarterly report.* Washington, DC: Regional Program on AIDS/STD, Division of Disease Prevention and Control, 1996.
5 Weniger BG, Brown T. The march of AIDS through Asia. *N Engl J Med* 1996;335:343–345.
6 European Centre for the Epidemiological Monitoring of AIDS. *HIV/AIDS Surveillance in Europe.* Saint-Maurice, France: First quarter report, 1997.
7 Yorke JA, Hethcote HW, Nold A. 1978, Dynamics and control of the transmission of gonorrhea. *Sex Trans Dis* 1978;5:51–56.
8 DeCock KM, Brun-Veginet F. Epidemiology of HIV-2. *AIDS* 1989; 3(suppl):S89–S95.
9 Andreasson P-A, Dias F, Naucler A, et al. A prospective study of vertical transmission of HIV-2 in Bissau, Guinea-Bissau. *AIDS* 1993;7: 989–993.
10 Cleland J, Ferry B. *Sexual Behaviour and AIDS in the Developing World.* Geneva: World Health Organization, 1995.
11 UNAIDS, WHO: *Report on the Global HIV/AIDS Epidemic,* 1997.
12 Rwabukwali C, McGrath JW, Schumann DA, et al. *Socioeconomic determinants of sexual risk behavior among Baganda women in Kampala, Uganda.* Florence, Italy: VII International Conference on AIDS, 1991.
13 Allen S, Lindan C, Serufilira A, et al. Human immunodeficiency virus infection in urban Rwanda. *JAMA* 1991;266:1657–1663.
14 Batter V, Matela B, Nsuami M, et al. High HIV-1 incidence in young Women masked by stable overall seroprevalence among childbearing women in Kinshasa, Zaire: Estimating incidence from serial seroprevalence data. *AIDS* 1994;8:811–818.
15 Latif AS. A report on a study to determine the aetiology and pattern of STD amongst men and women presenting to health centres in Harare, Zimbabwe, and to determine risk factors for cervicitis among symptomatic and asymptomatic women, unpublished, 1995.
16 Wasserheit JN, Aral SO, Holmes KK. *Research Issues in Human Behavior and Sexually Transmitted Diseases in the AIDS Era.* Washington, DC: American Society for Microbiology, 1991.
17 Botswana National AIDS Control Programme, Ministry of Public Health. *Sentinel Surveillance 1997 Results,* unpublished, 1997.
18 Nunn AJ, Kengeya-Kayondo JF, Malaba SS, et al. Risk factors for HIV-1 infection in adults in a rural Ugandan community: A population study. *AIDS* 1994;8:81–86.
19 Cleland J, Ferry B. *Sexual Behaviour and AIDS in the Developing World.* Geneva: World Health Organization, 1995.
20 Serwadda D, Gray RH, Wawer MJ, et al. *HIV-1 Incidence and Prevalence among Pregnant Women in a Population-Based Rural Cohort, Rakai District, Uganda.* Vancouver: XI International Conference on AIDS, 1996.
21 Asiimwe-Okiror G, Opio AA, Musinguzi J, et al. Change in sexual behaviour and decline in HIV infection among young pregnant women in Urban Uganda. *AIDS* 1997;11:1757–1763.
22 Des Jarlais DC, Friedman SR, et al. International epidemiology of HIV and AIDS among injecting drug users. *AIDS* 1992;6:1053–1068.
23 European Centre for the Epidemiological Monitoring of AIDS. *HIV/AIDS Surveillance in Europe.* Saint-Maurice, France: First quarterly report, 1997.

PART IV SOCIAL AND PSYCHOLOGICAL DETERMINANTS OF SEXUALITY

Chapter 6

The social context of sexuality: the case of the United States

Mary Rogers Gillmore
Pepper Schwartz
Diane Civic

Sociologists, though mindful of our biological heritage, maintain that human behavior cannot be understood without reference to the cultural, historical, and social context in which individual lives are enacted. We assume that as social history changes, people change. That is why Barzum and Graff (quoted in C. Wright Mills) remarked that: "The title of Dr. Kinsey's famous book *Sexual Behavior in the Human Male* is a striking instance of a hidden—and in this case false—assumption: the book is not about human males, but about men in the United States in the mid-twentieth century."[1] The social circumstances which affect sexual behavior may vary from large-scale socioeconomic conditions, such as the greatly increasing numbers of women in the labor force, to intimate interactions between two people. In the final analysis, sociologists assert not only that human *behavior* is socially patterned but that human character, personality, identity—indeed, human thought—are affected by the same social forces that affect behavior. A sociological analysis seeks to identify the social factors which produce variation in sexual behavior and to explain why and how these factors influence sexual behavior.

We begin this chapter with an examination of postwar social trends and suggest how these social changes affected sexuality. We then describe current patterns of sexual behavior for heterosexuals: teenagers, single adults, and married adults. Next we look at patterns of sexual behavior among gay men and lesbians. Although we have not included a separate section on bisexuality, we have incorporated findings on bisexuals in each of the major sections below. This choice reflects two facts: there is a paucity of research on bisexuals, and many studies purporting to focus on homosexuals have included respondents who also engage in heterosexual activities. The chapter concludes with some speculation about future trends in sexual behavior based on current trends in the social and sexual scene. But even as we write, patterns of sexual behavior are changing in response to changing social forces in our society and in response to the AIDS threat.

POSTWAR SOCIAL AND SEXUAL TRENDS: EVOLUTION AND REVOLUTION

The trends in sexual behavior that troubled Americans in the late sixties and early seventies were not apparent in 1945, although they had probably been slowly evolving throughout much of the century. These changes in sexual behavior were accompanied by and related to other social changes that were also occurring during the postwar period. Divorce rates, which had been rising very slowly since the turn of the century, briefly zoomed upward toward the end of the war but soon dropped to rates only slightly higher than prewar figures. Young men and women were marrying at the youngest ages on record, and rates of first marriage were the highest ever as young men returned from the service. As a consequence, women were having their first babies at a younger age than during the war years and having larger families (typically four children) than would have been predicted on the basis of the decline in fertility rates that had occurred during the first half of the century. These postwar changes fostered the baby boom, but the dramatic consequences of this seemingly innocuous "population bulge" would not become apparent until much later.

The Kinsey studies, published in this postwar era, suggested not only that Americans were engaging in a wider variety of sexual activities both in and outside of marital relationships than would be expected on the basis of the prevailing moral attitudes of the time, but also that such behaviors were increasing.[2,3] Three of Kinsey's findings were deeply disturbing to the public: the frequent use of prostitutes by men, both married (10 to 20 percent) and unmarried (70 percent); the prevalence of homosexual activities (Kinsey estimated that 37 percent of American males and 13 percent of females had had at least one homosexual experience); and the substantial rate of extramarital affairs.

These data suggest that significant changes in sexual behavior had been happening at least since World War II and perhaps even since the turn of the century. What the sixties ushered in was not a *revolution* in sexual behavior but rather an acceleration in rates of changes which were already occurring. Given the dramatic increase in the adolescent population in the sixties due to the baby boom, along with the trend toward increased premarital sexuality among teenagers that had been occurring for quite some time, it is not surprising that Americans leapt to the conclusion that society was in moral decay. What were the major social trends that occurred after World War II, and how might they have influenced sexual behavior?

There was a movement of large numbers of young (predominately white middle-class) Americans into colleges, which produced dramatic changes in the lives of many young men and women. As young people began to delay marriage in order to pursue education, they were removed from the direct supervision of their families. The rising age at first marriage left more years between puberty and marriage. These changes meant that larger numbers of young unmarried men and women had more time and freedom to explore their sexuality.

At the same time, dramatic changes were occurring in female labor-force participation. Although poor women had always been in the labor force, and though the rate of female participation had been slowly creeping up since the 1920s, when it was 23.7 percent, a dramatic increase occurred in the two decades between 1960 and 1980. By 1986, a majority of women with children under the age of six—over half the married and separated women and 74 percent of the divorced women—were in the labor force.[4] This transition from homemaking to paid labor-force participation greatly increased women's autonomy and provided opportunities for sexual liaisons that had not existed previously for the majority of American women. During this two-decade period of rapid change, the divorce rate made a quantum leap, placing a large number of sexually experienced but newly single persons in the sexual marketplace. That they continued to be sexually active though no longer married is hardly surprising.

Most people did not remain unmarried for long, however. Although the divorce rate soared, remarriage was also commonplace. About four out of five divorced men and three out of four divorced women remarried within three years. This fostered the appearance that the institution of marriage had been reaffirmed, but it had changed radically in two important ways. First, the permanence of the marital union could no longer be taken for granted. This became more apparent as divorce rates for second marriages proved to be even higher than for first marriages. Second, not everyone remarried—the proportion of unmarried persons in the population was rising[5]—and this small but significant trend produced profound changes in the sexual choices of men and women.

These same social trends gave impetus to the women's liberation movement, and with it a revised ideology about female sexuality. A new literature articulated women's concerns, differentiated female from male sexual needs, and called for a redefinition of sexuality which took both men's and women's preferences into account.[6] The marriage literature became more focused on sexual problems in marriage and courtship that were caused by *male* rather than female inadequacies, and guides to better lovemaking such as *The Joy of Sex* became best sellers. The pressure on men to become competent lovers, for women to be orgasmic and assertive in their sexual desires, changed the meaning and experience of sex for both men and women. This new ideology was accompanied by increasingly more permissive attitudes about sexuality.[7,8] The emergence of women as sexually independent actors and the liberalization of attitudes about female sexuality represent a truly new phase of American sexual history.

The sixties were the culmination of this sexual evolution. Trends in sexual behavior which had been occurring for decades became more prominent as a result of the sheer numbers of the baby boom generation. In a period of just three decades the lives of American women and the meaning of marriage and family had been inexorably altered, especially for those who were white and middle class. This, and not changes in sexual behavior, is the real "revolution" in American society.

THE 1980S AND 1990S: A NEW CONSERVATISM?

After a period of at least two decades in which Americans experienced marked changes in marriage and divorce patterns, in labor force participation by women, and in social attitudes, some stabilization of these trends has been evident in the 1980s and 1990s. The divorce rate, after two decades of rapid increase, remained nearly flat throughout the 1980s and into the 1990s and appears to have stabilized, although it remains at the highest level ever recorded.[5,9,10] It appears that the aging of the baby boom cohort has naturally flattened the divorce rate, but the high divorce rate is not just an artifact of that cohort's unique instability. Census experts estimate that approximately 50 percent of all marriages now taking place will end in divorce. The rate of first marriage, which had been declining since World War II, remained fairly stable throughout the 1980s, and the rate of remarriage, which had been declining since the mid-1960s, appears to have stabilized in recent years.[5,10]

Other social changes appear to be continuing. The median age at first marriage, which has been rising since the mid-1950s, has increased sharply since the mid-1980s.[10] For women, the median age at first marriage in 1990 (23.9) was at the highest level recorded since the census first began collecting such data in 1890. For men, the median age at first marriage (26.1) equals the 1890 all-time high. This recent rise in age at first marriage is partly a continuation of the post-war trend toward increasing proportions of young men and women delaying marriage to seek a college education;[11] however, it probably has more to do with the current economic outlook for young people. Relative to the mid-1970's, a higher percentage of American women in 1990 have never married, and this is especially so among African American women.[5] Whereas in 1960 only 28 percent of women ages 20 to 24 had never married, by 1990, 63 percent of women in this age group had not yet married.[10] Although the difference is not as dramatic for men, the proportion of never-married young men in this age group has risen from 53 percent in 1960 to 79 percent in 1990. Moreover, about three-fourths of the women who divorced in the past remarried, but current trends suggest that the rate is dramatically lower today.[5,9,10]

As might be expected, given these trends in marriage, the rate of premarital births has been increasing.[10] In the early 1960s, only 8.5 percent of non-Hispanic white women had ever experienced a premarital birth, but by the late 1980s that figure had risen to over 20 percent. Similar trends are evident for women of color: the rate of premarital births for African American women has risen from 42 percent in the early 1960s to 70 percent in the late 1980s, and it has risen from 19 percent to 38 percent for Latina women during this same period. These birth rates suggest that the delay in first marriages, coupled with a growing number of single previously married individuals in the population, has not been accompanied by sexual abstinence among the unmarried. Based on the findings of a recent national survey that showed that only 10 percent of men and 6.2 percent of women ages 18 to 24 report that they have never had vaginal intercourse[12] (and no doubt some of these have had other forms of sexual intercourse), it is clear that the vast majority of young unmarried men and women are sexually experienced. Even into the 1990s, age at first intercourse continues to decline. Since age at first marriage is increasing, we can predict that the lifetime number of sexual partners will increase. Zelnik et al. have shown that the longer the interval between first intercourse and first marriage, the more partners a sexually active woman has,[13] and we assume the same to be true for men.

The AIDS epidemic also appears to have influenced sexual behavior, at least in the case of gay men. However, heterosexuals appear to be slow to change their behavior, perhaps because they mistakenly define AIDS as a disease of gay men or because AIDS has not been perceived as a significant threat. Although contraceptive use is more prevalent than ever among adult heterosexuals—75 percent of females in their twenties who were queried in a national survey reported using a contraceptive at last intercourse—condoms, which reduce the risk of contracting AIDS as well as the risk of unwanted pregnancies, are not the contraceptive of choice.[14] A recent national study showed that only 24 percent of unmarried noncohabiting adults always use condoms with a primary partner and only 36 percent always use them with a secondary partner.[12] Moreover, teenagers, especially younger ones, are much less likely to use contraceptives of any type.[13] However, there is evidence that condom use is increasing among teenage males.[15]

RESEARCH ON SEXUAL BEHAVIOR: A CAUTION

While the U.S. census has provided regular population-based information on a number of social factors such as marriage and divorce for more than a century, there has not been regular population-based survey of adult sexual behavior which employed representative sampling.[16] Instead, we have been relying on the Kinsey data to inform us about the sexual behavior of Americans. In addition to being dated, the Kinsey studies—which were based on volunteer samples—have well-known biases. Until very recently, nationally representative information about adult sexual behavior has come from studies (such as the General Social Surveys and the National Surveys of Family Growth) that primarily were focused on other topics and did not collect in-depth information on sexual behaviors. In 1983, Tanfer obtained more extensive information on the sexual behaviors (mostly contraceptive use) of young adult women ages 20 to 29,[14] but it was not until the 1990s that more extensive information on adult sexual behaviors based on nationally representative surveys was available. In 1991, Billy and colleagues at Battelle Institute in Seattle conducted a national survey of the sexual behaviors of adult men ages 20 to 39 (the National Survey of Men, or NSM),[17] and in 1992 Laumann and colleagues at National Opinion Research Center (NORC) conducted the most comprehensive survey based on a national probability sample of adult sexual behavior to date, the National Health and Social Life Survey (NHSLS).[12]

Nationally representative surveys of adolescent sexual behavior were conducted somewhat earlier. In 1971, 1976, and 1979 Zelnik and Kantner surveyed urban female adolescents ages 15 to 19 about pregnancy-related behaviors.[13,18] In 1979 they included young men ages 17 to 21. In 1988 Sonenstein, Peck, and Ku surveyed a national probability sample of young men ages 15 to 19 about their sexual behaviors, reinterviewing the young men in 1991.[19,20] As is true for adult behavior, some information about adolescent sexual behavior has been obtained from national studies designed for other purposes (for example, Leigh et al., 1994).[21]

These nationally representative studies are extremely important for providing population-based estimates of sexual behaviors that are relevant to the transmission of AIDS and other sexually transmitted diseases. It is regrettable that such studies were not conducted earlier, so that efforts to stem the transmission of AIDS could have been based on representative data about what Americans are doing sexually and the effects of AIDS on their sexual behavior. In an unprecedented intrusion of politics into science, both the Laumann, et al., study of adult sexual behavior and a study of adolescent sexual behaviors that was to have been conducted by the another research center were denied funding by Congress, even though both had been reviewed very highly by NIH and would have been funded under the normal scientific review process. Laumann and his colleagues were able to obtain funding from the private sector in order to conduct their study (see Laumann et al. for details).[22]

Earlier studies of sexuality were based on convenience samples. The volunteer respondents in such studies tended to be white and middle class, as well as younger, better educated, and from somewhat higher socioeconomic levels than the general population. Refusal rates were sometimes very high (70 to 90 percent nonresponse rates were not unusual), adding another source of possible bias. Further, several major studies of sexual behavior were conducted at different periods in American history, leaving us in a quandary as to whether differences in findings are due to the uniqueness of the particular (nonrepresentative) sample or whether they represent changes over time in sexual behavior. We suspect, however, that when the data show a consistent pattern (for example, increasing prevalence of premarital intercourse), the general trend is probably accurately charted, although the exact figures may not be accurate. (See References 12 and 23–25 for reviews of these earlier studies of sexual behavior.)

Additional caution is warranted because much of the literature on sexuality classifies individuals as either homosexual or heterosexual. This classification implicitly assumes that behavior and sexual orientations are congruent and that sexual orientations, like biological sex, are discrete categories. There are ample data to show that these assumptions are false. From the early studies of Kinsey et al.[2,3] to the more recent research on sexuality,[15–17] the clear and consistent message is that few people are exclusively homosexual or heterosexual—in either sexual orientation or behavior—throughout their lives. Moreover, some people define themselves as exclusively homosexual even though they have never had even a single sexual contact with a member of the same sex.[28] Analogously, some people (for example, "swingers" or incarcerated men and women) may define themselves as exclusively heterosexual, even though they have sexual relations with members of the same sex. Some of the recent studies have avoided this dilemma by analyzing sexual behaviors without reference to the sexual orientation of the individual.

Because much existing research on sexuality classifies people into discrete categories, we have used these categories in organizing this chapter. However, we think it is in the scientific community's best interest to keep in mind that actors—single, married, divorced, heterosexual, and homosexual—may inhabit more than one category in their lifetimes and that the aware observer will keep the complications of human sexual behavior in mind.

SEXUAL BEHAVIOR OF HETEROSEXUALS

PREMARITAL SEX AMONG TEENAGERS

According to the 1992 NHSLS, nearly 80 percent of U.S. adults between the ages of 18 and 59 believe that teenage sex is always or nearly always wrong.[12] Nevertheless, perhaps no trend in sexual behavior has been better documented than the increase over time in premarital intercourse, especially among teenagers. Data from the Kinsey studies suggest that this trend may have been occurring since the turn of the century,[3,29] and recent data suggest that the trend is continuing.

Zelnick and Kantner's data from national probability samples of metropolitan women ages 15 to 19 show a consistent increase over time in the prevalence of premarital intercourse among teenagers throughout the 1970s.[18] Recent data from the National Survey of Family Growth suggest that this pattern persists;[30] for example, the percentage of teenage women who are sexually experienced increased from 44.1 percent in 1985 to 51.5 percent in 1988. Although a higher percentage of African American than white teens are sexually experienced, this gap has narrowed over time as more white teenagers become sexually active. In 1988, 59 percent of African American women and 51 percent of white women ages 15 to 19 had had premarital intercourse.

Even though the data are sparser for teenage males, studies consistently show that sexual experience is more prevalent among teen males than among teen females. Zelnick and Kantner's 1979 survey of metropolitan teenagers, their first survey to include males, showed that 70 percent of white males and 75 percent of African American males ages 17 to 21 had experienced premarital intercourse.[18] In 1988, data from the National Survey of Adolescent Males indicated that by age 19, 96 percent of African American, 76 percent of white, and 81 percent of Hispanic never-married males were sexually experienced.[19] These race and sex differences in premarital intercourse have been found by others as well.[2,3,26] Taken as a whole, the available data on premarital intercourse suggest that over half of today's teenage women and four-fifths or more of teenage men in the United States are sexually experienced. Thus, the political conservatism that is growing in this country does not seem to be affecting the sexual behaviors of teenagers as yet.

Zelnik and Kantner's data indicate that age at first intercourse for females, both African American and white, declined during the 1970s.[18] Their 1979 data show that age at first intercourse was lower for males and for African Americans. More recent data suggest that the age at first intercourse is continuing to decrease slightly.[12,19,21] A recent national study found evidence of a sharp increase in initiation of sexual intercourse at age 14 for boys, but this did not happen for girls until age 15.[21] Only 3 percent of 14-year-old girls in this study were sexually experienced, compared with 37 percent of the 15-year-old girls, whereas for boys, 6 percent of 13-year-olds but 24 percent of 14-year-olds were sexually experienced. By age 16, however, the percentages were similar (about 48 percent of both sexes were sexually experienced).

Racial and ethnic differences in teen sexual activity have been found consistently in national surveys, with African Americans reporting a higher incidence of premarital sex and sex at a younger age than other races.[11,19,21,31] In their recent national study, Sonenstein et al. found that African American males were about two years ahead of white and Hispanic teens in the proportion having had intercourse by a given age.[19] However, compared to young white men, African American young men are more likely to have first ejaculated in activity with a heterosexual partner and less likely to have masturbated by age 15, suggesting that sexuality may be expressed differently by teenagers of different racial and ethnic backgrounds.[32]

The number of years teenagers are sexually active is the strongest correlate of their lifetime number of sexual partners. Of teenage women who had been sexually active for less than one year in 1976 only 12 percent had more than one premarital sexual partner, compared with 80 percent of teen women who had been sexually active for four or more years.[13] In a multivariate analysis of 1988 data on teenage males, years since first intercourse was a robust predictor of both the number of lifetime partners and number of partners in the past 12 months.[19]

Contrary to popular stereotypes, sexually experienced teens are not highly sexually active. One recent national survey found that unmarried sexually experienced teenage males had an average of six months in the past year in which they had no sexual partner.[19] In another national study, sexually active teens reported having had intercourse a mean of 11 times in the past year—less than once a month. Moreover, 42 percent of sexually active teen males and 37 percent of sexually active teen females had not had sexual intercourse in the month prior to the study.[21]

In conclusion, premarital intercourse is more prevalent than ever among teenagers; adolescents are initiating sex at younger ages than previously; and adolescents have a greater number of partners in their lifetimes than previously, owing to the delay between first intercourse and first marriage. Nevertheless, teenagers are not very sexually active compared with single adults. This difference underscores the importance of social factors in predicting sexual activities. Most teenagers are still ensconced in their families and in other social institutions which exert a conservative influence on their social (including sexual) behaviors. The real problem teenagers pose, in terms of social and public health concerns, is their failure to protect themselves against unwanted pregnancies and sexually transmitted diseases. The sporadic nature of teen sexual behavior, the apparent unwillingness of teenagers to plan for sexual activities, and their ambivalence about pregnancy present barriers to effective contraception and STD protection.

SEXUALITY AMONG SINGLE (NONCOHABITING) ADULTS

In the late 1940s and early 1950s Kinsey et al. found that 71 percent of males but only 33 percent of females had experienced premarital intercourse by the age of 25.[2,3] By 1974, virtually all the men and two-thirds of the women Hunt[26] studied were sexually experienced by this age.[15] In 1992, when Laumann et al. conducted the NHSLS, 88 percent of men and 94 percent of women ages 18 to 24 said that they had had vaginal intercourse.[12] Because of low marriage rates at these ages, most of this represents premarital sex. This figure for men is comparable to that obtained in the 1991 NSM, in which 90 percent of 20-to-24-year-old men said that they had had sex.[17] Data from the NHSLS show that, regardless of marital status, only 5 percent of U.S. men and 3 percent of U.S. women ages 18 to 59 report never having had vaginal intercourse.[12] Thus, married or not, the vast majority of the U.S. population are sexually experienced by their mid-twenties.

The NHSLS study also asked about frequency of intercourse.[12] Among never-married adults ages 18 to 59, most of whom are in the younger age groups, men report having vaginal intercourse 5.6 times a month and women report a frequency of 5.3 times a month, just slightly lower than that reported by men. These rates of vaginal intercourse are similar to those reported by formerly married adults. Relative to persons in other marital statuses, unmarried noncohabiting respondents in the study reported the lowest frequency of sex, which Laumann et al. attribute to lowered access to a regular partner. Only about one-fourth reported sex two or more times a week.

Although data on other forms of sexual intercourse are sparse, several recent studies using nationally representative samples have asked adults about both oral and anal intercourse. Among never-married respondents in the 1992 NHSLS, about two-thirds of men and 60 percent of women report having experienced oral sex.[12] Rates of oral sex were comparable for formerly married women and somewhat higher for formerly married men. However, oral sex was more common in shorter-term relationships. The NSM found higher rates of oral sex among white (nearly 80 percent) than among African American (43 percent) respondents.[17] Thus, oral sex is a relatively common feature of sexual interactions between men and women, but there are gender, marital status, and racial/ethnic variations in the prevalence of this form of sexual expression.

There is a paucity of data on anal sex from the pre-AIDS era, but recent national surveys of sexual behavior have asked about this form of sexual intercourse. Results of these studies suggest that anal sex is far less common than oral sex among single heterosexuals, but it is not as rare as is commonly believed. Approximately 23 percent of single men and 20 percent of single women report having had heterosexual anal sex at some time in their lives, and about 10 percent of single men and women reported having anal sex with an opposite-sex partner in the past year.[12] In their NSM, Billy et al. also found that about 20 percent of men reported ever having had anal sex.[17] More never-married than formerly married men (13.8 percent vs. 8.1 percent) reported anal sex in the past month; this is as would be expected, since the never-married category included gay men. As with oral sex, Billy et al. found that white men were more likely to report anal sex than African American men (21 percent vs. 13.6 percent, respectively). Rates of anal sex were highest among those who identified themselves as Hispanic, especially for recent anal sex. Almost one-quarter of Hispanics, compared to fewer than 10 percent of non-Hispanics reported anal sex in the last month. There has been some suggestion that heterosexual anal sex among persons of Hispanic origin may be used as a means of contraception and for Hispanic women it may be a way to remain a "technical virgin," although this explanation requires further investigation.[33] Men in the NSM who reported anal sex appear to have initiated this behavior at a much later age than vaginal intercourse (the mean age of first anal intercourse was 22).[17] The data reported in this study were not broken down by marital status; thus, these figures include both married and single adult men.

Although these data show that heterosexual anal sex among single adults in the US is far less common than oral sex, they also show that it is not a rare event. Even if only 10 percent of adult men and women have recently had heterosexual anal intercourse, this represents a large number of adults potentially at risk of contracting HIV and other rectally transmitted STDs. As with other forms of sexual intercourse, the rates of heterosexual anal intercourse vary by gender, race/ethnicity, and marital status. Because anal sex has been assumed to be rare among heterosexuals, public health messages about the risk of HIV from anal intercourse have been aimed primarily at gay men. The data suggest that such messages should be targeted to heterosexuals as well. Because women are the receptive partners in anal sex, they are at especially high risk should their partner be infected. Effective AIDS prevention among heterosexuals is especially challenging because those most at risk often have the least say in sexual encounters.

It has been found consistently that single adult men have more sexual partners on average than single adult women. Data from a national survey conducted in 1991 showed that among adults ages 18 to 25, 76 percent of whom were unmarried, about 34 percent of men but only 15 percent of women had two or more sexual partners in the past year.[34] About two-thirds of the women surveyed reported having had only one sexual partner during that time. Only 16 percent of respondents identifying as Hispanic reported multiple sex partners in the past year, whereas about one-fourth of white men and African American men and women reported two or more partners during this time.

In the NHSLS, men reported a median of six sex partners since age 18 compared to a median of two partners for women (all marital statuses combined).[12] In this study, Laumann et al. found that young unmarried men were the group most likely to have had five or more sex partners in the past five years. They also found for the sample as a whole that as the number of sex partners in the past 12 months increased, the likelihood that a person was having a sexual relationship with more than one person at a time also increased, as did the likelihood of having sex only once with a person. Their data suggest that after the mid-1960s people were likely to have more sex partners than prior to this time, but that the onset of the AIDS epidemic in 1980 may have flattened this trend for the youngest birth cohort.

Although some studies suggest that divorced men and women are more sexually active than sexually experienced never-marrieds, data from recent studies do not support this contention. Hunt's data showed that divorced men had a median frequency of intercourse of more than twice a week, and the rate was almost as high for divorced women.[26] Similar findings were obtained by Spanier and Thompson.[35] These frequencies are about the same as those reported by married respondents. Moreover, Hunt's data indicated that divorced males typically had sex with eight partners per year, while divorced women had a median of four partners per year, and that the overwhelming majority of both had engaged in oral sex during the past year.[26] Based on such data, Hunt concluded that the divorced tend to be sexually liberated, not only relative to the previously married of Kinsey's day, but also relative to sexually active never-married adults. However, data from the recent NHSLS suggest that never-married adults have sex at about the same rate as those who are divorced, widowed, or separated.[12] Whether there has been a real change in sexual behaviors of previously married individuals, perhaps in response to the AIDS epidemic, cannot be determined from the data because, as noted earlier, no regular nationally representative surveys of adult sexual behavior have been conducted and the earlier studies were based on convenience samples, making it difficult to draw general conclusions.

There is some evidence, however, that American adults may be changing their behavior in response to the AIDS epidemic. In a 1989 survey of 1,600 young urban heterosexual men and women, almost 50 percent reported that they had made some change in their sexual behavior in response to the AIDS epidemic.[36] African Americans were more likely than white individuals to have altered their sexual behavior. The most common change reported was a reduction in the number of sexual partners and choosing partners more carefully. Somewhat less common was using condoms more frequently.

SEXUALITY AMONG UNMARRIED COHABITING COUPLES

Although exact rates of cohabitation are not available, there is consensus among researchers that a dramatic rise in cohabitation rates occurred after 1960, and this increase became especially noticeable in the late 1970s.[37–41] In 1970 the number of cohabiting couples was estimated to be 523,000; in 1978 it had risen to 1.1 million.[38] Census experts project that the rate will continue to rise dramatically into the 1990s,[9] and data from the recent NHSLS suggest that this trend indeed is occurring.[12]

The increased prevalence of cohabitation has been attributed to several factors, including the liberalization of attitudes about alternative lifestyles; the increase in age at first marriage; an increase in sexual freedom, so that marriage is not as necessary a prerequisite to gaining access to a sexual partner; and more honesty in reporting as the social disapproval of such arrangements declines. Laumann et al. point out that, by and large, adult men and women in the United States ". . . overwhelmingly continue to form long-term social and sexual live-in partnerships, as they have for decades" (Ref. 12, p. 476). What has changed is that fewer of these live-in relationships are marriages than was previously the case.

In their NHSLS, Laumann et al. found that cohabitation was more likely among men and women who had had sex before the age of 18.[12] Men who formed live-in partnerships at younger ages were more likely to form a cohabitational union than marriage. Among women, cohabitation was more common among African Americans than among whites. Rates of cohabitation were also higher for previously married persons than for the never-married.[40] Both Croake et al. and Johnson found that cohabiting couples were more permissive and more sexually active than the general population.[42,43] Ninety-four percent of the males and 86 percent of the females in the Croake et al. study had been sexually experienced by the age of 18. These rates are higher than those reported for teenagers as a whole. Similarly, Newcomb, comparing cohabiting couples with noncohabitors, found that cohabitors had had earlier and greater sexual experience than did noncohabiting single persons.[44] Data from the NHSLS likewise suggest that cohabiting couples are more sexually active than persons in other relationship statuses.[12] Among cohabitors, 56 percent of men and 60 percent of women had sex two or more times a week in the past year. In contrast, about 40 percent of married persons reported a similar level of sexual activity. Laumann et al. suggest, however, that the difference in sexual activity between cohabitors and married persons is largely attributable to age, since sexual frequency declines somewhat with age and cohabitors are likely to be younger than married persons.

According to the NHSLS, cohabiting persons report a greater number of sexual partners in the past year than do married persons but not as many partners as single noncohabiting individuals.[12] For example, 23 percent of single women ages 18 to 29 who were cohabiting at the time of the survey reported two or more partners in the past year, compared to only 4 percent of married women. However, 34 percent of single noncohabiting women reported having two or more partners during this time. Men in this age group have a similar pattern: 33 percent of those cohabiting reported two or more partners, but only 8 percent of married men reported two or more partners, compared to 48 percent of single noncohabiting men. Whether these sexual relationships were occurring simultaneously (that is, the cohabitor was having sexual liaisons outside the relationship) or serially cannot be discerned.

Blumstein and Schwartz found that in the early 1980s both male and female cohabitors were much more likely than married couples to engage in sex outside of their relationships.[45] Consistent with findings from other studies, male cohabitors were slightly more likely than females cohabitors to have sex outside the relationship, but the difference was small (33 versus 30 percent). The modal number of partners outside the relationship varied from two to five for male cohabitors, while the mode was only one for female cohabitors. A significant minority of female cohabitors (41 percent), however, reported that they had from two to five outside partners. Although Laumann et al. did not report data specific to concurrent relationships among cohabitors, they attempted to estimate the likelihood of simultaneous sexual relationships for their sample as a whole (that is, without regard to relationship status).[12] They found that approximately half of those who reported two partners in the past year had these partners concurrently, while 61 percent of those with three partners, 75 percent of those with four partners, and over 80 percent of those with five or more partners had some of these sexual relationships concurrently rather than serially. Thus, as the number of recent sexual partners increases, the likelihood that some of these relationships are occurring at the same time also increases.

Taken as a whole, the data on cohabiting heterosexuals suggest that cohabitors have sex more frequently than either single noncohabiting or married individuals, that they became sexually experienced at a younger age, and that they are more likely to have sexual partners outside of the relationship than married persons. As with other forms of sexual behavior, there are both race and gender differences in these patterns.

In conclusion, there appear to have been five significant changes in the sexual behavior of heterosexual single persons since Kinsey's day. The prevalence of premarital intercourse has greatly increased, the age at first intercourse has declined, and the lifetime number of sexual partners appears to have increased. In addition, the tremendous growth of cohabitation among heterosexuals since the 1970s, especially among middle-class whites, represents an arrangement in which premarital and nonmarital sex is explicit, indeed taken for granted. Finally, the growth of the divorce rate has resulted in a population of sexually experienced but single persons who continue to be sexually active despite the loss of a regular partner. The implication is that there is a large and growing segment of the adult heterosexual population who are not married but nevertheless are sexually active, many of whom have more than one partner in a year's time. Further, since the proportion of divorced persons who remarry is declining, we expect both the prevalence of nonmarital sex and the number of sexual partners single persons have over the course of their lives to increase. On the other hand, it appears that in the 1990s people are not as sexually active as popular myth would have us believe. Data from the 1992 NHSLS, for example, suggest that about 83 percent of the population had either just one sexual partner or no sexual partners in the past 12 months.[12]

SEXUALITY OF MARRIED PERSONS

Sex within the marital relationship

Data from the recent NHSLS by Laumann et al. suggest that vaginal intercourse is the most common form of sexual expression among married couples; 80 percent said that they always have vaginal intercourse when they have sex.[12] The frequency of intercourse among married couples depends on a number of factors, including age, social class, and duration of marriage. Laumann et al. found that although a little over one-third of married individuals reported having sex two to three times a week, the most common pattern was for married persons to have sex a few times a month. Surprisingly, about the same proportion of never-married cohabitors as married persons reported sex two to three times a week, although previously married cohabiting individuals were more likely than either married or never-married cohabiting persons to have sex this often. As noted above, single persons who are not cohabiting reported even less frequent sex. Studies consistently show an inverse relationship between the frequency of intercourse within the marital relation and duration of marriage.[2,3,12,26,45–48] The data also indicate that the frequency of marital intercourse declines with age of the partners, though Blumstein and Schwartz's data suggest that marital duration is the more important factor.[45] We suspect that the decline in rates of intercourse over time in a marriage are a function of both familiarity and the exigencies of child rearing.

Although both Hunt and Westoff claimed that the frequency of marital coitus has increased over time,[26,46] we find remarkably similar rates across studies (see the study by Greenblat).[47] What may have changed for married couples, if anything, is the prevalence of sexual activities other than intercourse. Oral sex, for example, has become a more common part of marital sexuality.[26,45,49] In the NHSLS study, 25 percent of married men and 17 percent of married women said that active oral sex was part of their most recent sexual encounter, and 23 percent of men and 17 percent of women report receptive oral sex during their most recent episode of sex.[12] Anal sex among married couples is less commonly reported, though it does not appear to be rare. Hunt indicated that about 25 percent of the married respondents in his study had tried anal sex at some time in their lives, though few performed it regularly.[26] Similarly, Tavris and Sadd found that 43 percent of the married women who responded to the Redbook survey had tried anal sex, but only 2 percent engaged in it regularly.[49] The recent NHSLS study indicated that while 27 percent of married men have had anal sex sometime in their lives, only 2 percent engaged in anal sex in their last sexual encounter.[12] Similarly, 21 percent of women reported having had anal sex at some time in their lives, but only 1 percent had had anal sex at the last event. These data suggest that while vaginal sex is the single most common form of sexual intercourse among married couples, as is true among single heterosexuals, oral sex has become a common part of marital sexuality. Although experiencing anal sex at some point in a life cycle does not appear to be a rare event among heterosexuals, anal sex as a regular part of married sexuality remains relatively rare.

Nonmonogomy among married couples

Rates of nonmonogamy among married persons vary somewhat from study to study. Kinsey et al. found somewhat higher rates of nonmonogamy among the better educated, women over age 25, and persons from "white-collar" backgrounds.[2,3] Although the overall rates of nonmonogamy appear unchanged since Kinsey's day,[26] nonmonogamy appears to have increased among younger persons. Data presented by Hunt, by Blumstein and Schwartz, and by Leigh et al. suggest that younger married persons have higher rates of nonmonogamy than do older persons.[26,45,50] Moreover, we suspect that rates of nonmonogamy have increased for women, although reliable data do not exist regarding such a trend. We think this is likely because of increasing premarital sexuality, increased opportunities, the availability of contraceptives, and the acceptance by women and the larger society of the notion that women have sexual needs and rights similar to men's. Nonetheless, when married persons are asked about their sexual relationships, their replies indicate that nonmonogamy rates are relatively low. For example, approximately 90 percent of women and 75 percent of men in each of the four birth cohorts examined in the NHSLS reported being completely monogamous over the entire course of their marriages.[12] Similar rates were reported in the 1991 General Social Survey.[51] As these data show, nonmonogamy among married persons is much more likely to be practiced by men. Younger respondents (under age 40) and African-American respondents report higher rates of nonmonogamy than other groups.[50]

Although the overall rate of nonmonogamy among married couples may not be increasing, it occurs in a sizable minority of couples, and that fact should signal concern about STDs among married persons. Given that somewhere around one-quarter of married men report extramarital affairs, and assuming that most of these are unknown to their wives, wives may be at greater risk of STDs than they or their clinicians expect. Further, as others have also pointed out (see review by Thompson),[52] reported rates are likely to underestimate the true incidence, since nonmonogamy is still widely disapproved despite the liberalization of attitudes toward premarital sex.

Mate swapping, group sex, and "swinging"

Only a few studies have examined other forms of nonmonogamy among married persons, such as group sex, "swinging" (mate swapping), and none have been based on representative sampling. Those that have asked about these behaviors report similar incidences of about 1 to 3 percent of married couples who have ever tried it and a much lower proportion who are regular participants.[26,49,53] Studies suggest that married couples who participate in swinging or group sex are typically white-collar, college-educated couples in their thirties who appear to be quite conventional, even conservative, in other areas of their lives.[53–57]

Although sexual contact between females is usually acceptable among swingers, sexual contact among males is forbidden, and gay men are typically excluded from such groups. Anecdotal evidence suggests that this is especially true since AIDS has become well publicized. Indeed, many swinging groups allegedly require evidence that members are seronegative. Despite the outbreak of AIDS, there is no evidence to suggest that these forms of nonmonogamy have begun to disappear, but the available data on this activity are sparse and are not based on nationally representative sampling.

Same-sex contacts by married persons

Laud Humphries shocked both researchers and lay people with his report in 1970 that 54 percent of the respondents he observed in homosexual encounters in "tearooms" (public restrooms) were married and leading double lives.[58] More recent studies, however, suggest that while many homosexual men and women have had heterosexual contacts at some point in their lives, only a tiny proportion of married men and women also engage in homosexual contacts. Saghir and Robins found that although 18 percent of the 89 gay men they studied had been married, only 2 percent were currently married,[59] a figure similar to that reported in the Kinsey studies.[2] Data from the recent NHSLS showed that only 1.7 percent of men and 0.8 percent of women who were married reported any same-gender contact in the last five years.[12] These figures suggest that most extramarital affairs among married individuals occur with opposite sex partners.

Studies based on nonprobability sampling suggest that a substantial minority of gay men have been married at some time during their lives. The range typically reported is 17 to 20 percent, although rates are higher among individuals who identify as bisexuals.[6,27,60,61] Further, an even greater proportion have engaged in heterosexual sex after puberty. For example, three-quarters of the men in the 156 gay male couples studied by McWhirter and Mattison had sexual experience with women beyond puberty.[62] In a recent national survey it was found that among the small number of men who identified themselves as homosexual or bisexual, 42 percent were married and living with their wives.[63] These married gay or bisexual men were more likely than their unmarried counterparts to be members of ethnic minorities and to have less than a high-school education, suggesting that this survey may have reached men who are underrepresented in the usual surveys. A substantial proportion of gay men and lesbians have had heterosexual sex, which in some cases represents changes over time in their sexual identities. Of those respondents in the NHSLS who reported any same-gender sexual activities, irrespective of their sexual identities, over half of both men and women reported sex with both genders in the last five years.[12] This finding has implications for the spread of STDs between heterosexual and homosexual populations.

Lesbians have been studied far less than gay men. Perhaps as a result, the prevalence rates for marriages in this group varies more from study to study than does the rate for gay males. Bell and Weinberg reported that about 35 percent of the lesbians they studied had had at least one marriage,[27] whereas Schaefer reported a marriage rate of only 14 percent.[64] Gundlach and Reiss found a 29 percent marriage rate among the lesbians they studied.[65] Lesbians report much more heterosexual intercourse than do gay men. For example, Peplau et al. reported that 80 percent of the 127 lesbians they studied had had sexual intercourse with a man at some time in their lives.[66] In fact, the median number of men with whom these respondents engaged in sex was five. Similar rates of heterosexual coitus were reported by Schaefer.[64] These figures suggest that clinicians should not assume that lesbians have little or no risk for STDs.

Clearly, many gay men and lesbian women have had sex, sometimes a substantial amount, with members of the opposite sex. Similarly, members of married couples—how many it is impossible to say—have had extramarital sexual relations with members of their own sex. These persons are not necessarily "closeted" homosexuals—they simply may not define the experience of sex with a person of the same sex as homosexuality. This may be true, for example, of "swingers" or of bisexuals (see studies by Blumstein and Schwartz).[67,68] Thus, it is not safe to assume that a person who defines him- or herself as exclusively heterosexual is in fact behaviorally exclusively heterosexual.

In conclusion, the data on sexuality among married couples have two important implications. First, a significant minority of married persons engage in extramarital sexual relations, and most, although not all, do so without their spouse's consent. Second, in a small proportion of these extramarital sexual relations, how many it is difficult to say, the spouse's extramarital partner may be a member of the same sex. These findings suggest not only that the clinician would be wise to ask about behavior rather than sexual orientation, but also that some married persons will perceive themselves to be at no (or low) risk of STDs when in fact their spouse's extramarital sexual activities may place them at risk.

SEXUAL BEHAVIOR OF GAY MEN AND LESBIANS

Most studies conducted before the outbreak of AIDS in this country found higher rates of sexual activity among gay men than among heterosexual men.[59,60] Bell and Weinberg reported that the modal frequency of sex among both African American and white homosexual men was two to three times a week, although overall African Americans reported higher frequencies than did whites.[27] Weinberg and Williams reported that 50 percent of male homosexuals had sex at least once a week,[60] while about two-thirds of Bell and Weinberg's respondents reported this frequency. About 20 percent of the white female homosexual respondents studied by Bell and Weinberg reported engaging in sex about once a week, while the majority of African-American homosexual women engaged in sex two or more times a week. However, this racial difference disappeared when age was controlled. These rates of sexual frequency for lesbians are similar to those reported by others.[66]

Gay men, prior to the outbreak of AIDS, had on average more sexual partners during their lifetimes than heterosexual males.[59,69] Bell and Weinberg found that over 40 percent of white men and one-third of African American men had at least 500 partners during their homosexual careers, and an additional one-fourth of the men surveyed reported between 100 and 500 partners.[27] Further, over 90 percent of the homosexual male respondents reported having had at least 25 partners. Most of the whites, and fewer but still a majority of African-Americans, said that more than half of their partners had been strangers before the sexual encounters. A higher proportion of whites than African Americans had sex only once with a given partner. In sharp contrast to gay men, the majority of lesbians studied by Bell and Weinberg reported fewer than five partners in the past year. Few of these sexual partners were strangers; in fact, 62 percent of the lesbians reported that they had never engaged in sex with strangers. In a survey conducted in 1985 in New York City, gay men were asked about their sexual behavior before the AIDS outbreak and afterwards. The median frequency of sexual episodes in a one-year period had increased from 30 pre-AIDS episodes to 36 post-AIDS episodes; however, the median number of partners had decreased from 5 to 3 during that period. These data suggest that gay men are reducing their number of sexual partners, not the frequency of their sexual activities, as a means of reducing their risk of contracting HIV.

As is true of heterosexuals, oral sex is very common among gay men and lesbians, both African American and white; males have higher rates than females. The majority of both African American and white men in Bell and Weinberg's study reported engaging in oral sex at least once a week, but just 28 percent of the white women and 42 percent of the African-American women reported this frequency.[27] In the recent NHSLS, a higher proportion of men identifying as homosexual or bisexual reported having oral sex, both active and receptive, than men in the general population (90 percent compared to 75-80 percent).[12] These data showed that men who had any same-gender partners in the last five years were about as likely as men who did not engage in oral sex. (It is important to note that the number of participants in the NHSLS who have sex with same-sex partners was very small.)

Among both African-American and white gay men in Bell and Weinberg's study, fellatio was the most commonly reported sexual activity.[27] For white men, mutual masturbation was the second most common activity, whereas for African-Americans it was anal sex. In Hunt's sample of gay men, only 20 percent had performed anal sex and even fewer (18 percent) had engaged in receptive anal intercourse.[26] Among lesbians, mutual masturbation was the most frequently reported sexual activity, followed by oral sex.[27] Both men with a gay identity and those with same-sex partners in the recent NHSLS were over twice as likely as men in the entire sample to have had insertive anal sex.[12] In the cohort of gay men followed in the San Francisco Men's Health Study, continuously monogamous men were more likely than nonmonogamous men to report unprotected anal sex in both 1984 and 1988.[70] They were also more likely than nonmonogamous men to report in 1984 that unprotected anal sex was their favorite sexual activity. These data suggest that gay men may be choosing monogamy as a form of protection against contracting AIDS.

Studies consistently show age differences in the sexual activities of gay men. Younger men have more partners, a greater frequency of sex, "cruise" more, and have shorter relationships than older men,[27,59,60,71] while older men are more likely to pay for sex.[27] A 1989 study of San Francisco gay men showed that gay men under age 30 were over twice as likely to have had unprotected anal intercourse in the past year as those over 30.[72]

Several ongoing research projects are focusing on the changes in sexual behaviors of gay and bisexual men in response to the AIDS threat. These studies have consistently shown decreases in both the overall number of sexual partners and the number of partners not previously known (anonymous partners) reported by gay men.[73–76] The evidence also suggests that receptive anal intercourse without a condom and oral sex in which semen is swallowed have also declined.[74–76] For example, the rate of unprotected anal sex for the San Francisco cohort was 50 percent in 1984 and only 12 percent in 1988.[70] However, as Ostrow et al. point out, consistent condom use and avoidance of receptive anal sex are behaviors highly susceptible to relapse.[77] Furthermore, a significant minority of gay men continue to engage in high-risk sexual activities despite knowledge of the risks involved.[78,79] Because some gay men are resuming risky sex while others are changing their behaviors toward safer sex, Ostrow et al. point out the limitations of studying sexual behavior change at the aggregate level.[77] Studies of gay men's behavior change in response to the AIDS threat have another limitation: they tend to include only men who identify as gay or bisexual, and such studies may not be reaching men who have sex with men but who are not gay or bisexual identified.

COUPLED HOMOSEXUALS

Although the data suggest that gay men tend to have more partners, somewhat greater frequency of sex, and relationships of shorter duration than heterosexuals, many gay men have long-term relationships with a primary partner—perhaps as many as 50 percent.[80] In the pre-AIDS era, monogamy appears to have been the exception rather than the rule in such relationships.[27,45,59,80,81] In contrast, lesbian couples tend to be monogamous.[45,66,82] The incidence of nonmonogamy for homosexual couples varies somewhat from study to study. Blumstein and Schwartz found in their pre-AIDS study that over 80 percent of the gay male couples but only 28 percent of the lesbian couples they studied in the pre-AIDS era had been nonmonogamous,[45] rates similar to those reported by others. Celibacy rates for gay men have not changed much between 1984 and 1990—generally about 11 to 18 percent—suggesting that this is not the preferred mode of protection against contracting AIDS.[70,77]

Of those respondents who had been nonmonogamous at some time during the course of their relationships, Blumstein and Schwartz found that the majority of lesbians (53 percent) had had sex with only one other partner.[45] In marked contrast, 43 percent of the gay men studied had more than 20 partners outside their primary relationship, and an additional 30 percent had 6 to 20 outside partners. The incidence of nonmonogamy among both lesbian and gay couples increased with relationship duration, especially after the first few years.

In the initial stages of their relationships, gay male couples have sex far more frequently than do heterosexual or lesbian couples, but they experience a sharper decline in sexual frequency over time relative to married couples.[45] This apparent decline in frequency must be interpreted in the light of the nonmonogamy rates for gay males, which suggest that interest in sex has not declined over time. Blumstein and Schwartz found not only that lesbian couples had a lower frequency of sex than any other couple type but also that the women apparently were not compensating for this with outside partners.

Oral sex is a common and accepted sexual activity for gay male and lesbian couples, but it is considerably less common for lesbians. Both Blumstein and Schwartz[45] and McWhirter and Mattison[62] found oral sex to be more common than anal sex among gay couples. For example, of the gay men Blumstein and Schwartz studied only 4 percent rarely or never engaged in oral sex with their partners, while 30 percent said that they rarely or never have anal sex. This does indicate, however, that over two-thirds of the gay men engaged in anal sex regularly.

In conclusion, pre-AIDS studies of gay men consistently showed that gay men had greater intensity of sexual activities (greater frequency, greater number of partners, more nonmonogamy), regardless of whether they were single or in a relationship, than men of other sexual orientations. However, as noted above, the sexual activities of gay men have changed in response to the AIDS threat; whether the changes will persist we do not know. Compared with gay men, lesbians engage in sex less frequently, have fewer partners, engage in casual sex less often, and have longer relationships with lower rates of nonmonogamy. These gender differences in sexual activities of gay men and lesbians are mirrored in the sexual activities of heterosexual men and women.

The recent national studies[12,17,19,21,50] have made a very valuable contribution to our understanding of sexuality. However, they did not oversample gay men, lesbians, and bisexual individuals, whose numbers in these studies are therefore very small. Therefore, we must be cautious about generalizing the findings to these groups.

CONCLUSIONS AND A LOOK AT THE FUTURE

By organizing this chapter by sexual orientation and by single versus coupled persons, we have implicitly suggested two social factors that are related to the prevalence and intensity of sexual behaviors. But even within types of relationships there is considerable variation. Marriages, for example, can be either monogamous or nonmonogamous. Perhaps even more dramatic is the strong effect of gender on sexual behavior. The sexual behaviors of heterosexual and homosexual men look more similar than different when compared with the sexual behaviors of women, whether homosexual or heterosexual. Men become sexually active earlier, have a greater prevalence of premarital sex, have more partners, have a greater frequency of sex, are more likely to engage in casual sex, and are more likely to be nonmonogamous than are women. While many researchers would claim that this difference is inherent in the "beast," we are less confident that such differences can be so easily attributed to biology. As Ford and Beach have pointed out,[83] there is considerable variation cross-culturally in the sexual behaviors of men and women. Moreover, the sexual behaviors of men and women in our culture are becoming more and more alike over time.

We also see systematic differences in sexual behavior by socioeconomic status and by race or ethnicity. What these differences imply is that one's social location (for example, one's class and race) carries with it a set of meanings and expectations regarding sexual activities, just as it shapes speech, values, attitudes, and a host of other social behaviors. However, one caution is warranted when interpreting race and ethnicity effects. Few studies have controlled for socioeconomic status when examining racial and ethnic differences in sexual behavior. Because members of racial and ethnic minorities are overrepresented among those of lower socioeconomic status, what is interpreted as a race or ethnicity effect could be a class effect.

We have attempted to give the reader an overview of sexual behavior in the last 20 years, but even as we write society is changing. The rise in premarital sexual activity that has been occurring at least since World War II and probably since the turn of the century was enabled in part by the technological advances of birth control; by the development of the modern women's liberation movement; and by the social conditions and ideologies that promoted later marriage, women's entry into the labor force, and a high divorce rate. There is no reason to believe that all the present sexual practices and beliefs would stay in place if society changed drastically. Indeed, there is evidence of dramatic change in the behavior of gay men in the AIDS epicenters of the country. However, there is also evidence that young gay men are taking sexual risks and that some gay men have found it hard to maintain the changes in sexual behavior that they made in response to the AIDS epidemic.

At present we are hearing about the worries of the sexually active heterosexual population, but changes in behavior appear to be modest. Continuing late age at first marriage and the recycling of divorced people back into dating at various times in their lives mean that sex outside of marriage is likely to continue long into the foreseeable future. On the other hand, there is no indication that values about extramarital sex are becoming more permissive, and so whatever nonmonogamy occurs will probably continue to be clandestine. A serious disease such as AIDS confronting nonmonogamous married men and women might motivate them to take precautions, but until AIDS becomes even more common among heterosexuals it is unlikely that much change will be evident. Whether this will remain true for married homosexuals and bisexuals, we cannot say. Since homosexual desires cannot be satisfied within marriage, the impetus for concealed, discreet sexual contact will continue unless AIDS proves to be a more powerful deterrent than it has heretofore. However, it is possible that married homosexuals and bisexuals may be increasing their use of protection in their extramarital liaisons as concern about AIDS continues to spread.

The very nature of teenage sexuality—erratic and ambivalent—indicates continued, if irregular, sexual activity. It seems as if the consequences must be more likely and more immediate to produce major changes in teenagers' sexual risk taking. While an education campaign has been mounted virtually nationwide to tell children and adolescents about AIDS, education alone does not appear sufficient to produce major behavioral changes toward safer sex. Education and other prevention efforts among teenagers have been hampered by conservatives who feel that any discussion of sexuality except to give a strong abstinence message is wrong. The argument appears to be based on the misguided notion that talking about sexuality will encourage it among teenagers. However, the evidence overwhelmingly suggests that this does not occur.

One caveat here is that older heterosexual women of the baby boom generation are disadvantaged demographically (having fewer men available the older they become) and thus may have a less active sex life than would be expected given the sexually liberated attitudes and behaviors they display. On the other hand, to the extent that marriage (or remarriage after the loss of a spouse through death or divorce) appears unlikely for many in this cohort, the only sex available is out of wedlock. We expect, therefore, that a certain percentage will accept serendipitous sexual encounters or affairs with married men because it may be their only opportunity for physical intimacy. Given that at least 8 percent of women are expected to be single throughout the life cycle, that 28 percent of all households are presently headed by single women, and that the majority of women will be single for at least several years in adulthood, it seems that sex outside of marriage will be a continuing part of the American way of life.

But just because our society has removed the necessity of having sex within the confines of marriage it does not follow that we are sexually "sophisticated" or terribly sexually liberated. Data from both the recent NSM and NHSLS studies suggest that, as a whole, Americans are not as sexually liberal as appeared to be the case in the 1970s.[17,12] Whether this represents change over time or whether Americans were never as sexually liberated as was thought cannot be deduced from the available data because, as noted at the beginning of this chapter, until recently there were no data about adult sexual behavior based on nationally representative samples. Men and women—gay or straight, married or single—still do not easily discuss or plan their sexual conduct with one another. Ultimately we must recognize the limits of people's ability to approach their sexuality in a rational manner.

The "social accounting"—prevalence, incidence, frequency

etc.—that we have presented is, we believe, a necessary first step toward understanding human sexual behavior. But it is no more than a point of departure. In order to make further inroads we need to understand how the conditions of people's lives structure the choices that they make. There are reasons for the differences in sexual behavior between African-Americans and whites, the young and the old, gays and straights, males and females, upper and lower classes. Once we have a better understanding of the factors that predict these differences in sexual behaviors, we will be in a much better position as individuals, practitioners, and public policy makers, to design and implement more effective strategies in the interest of public health.

References

1 Mills CW: *The Sociological Imagination*. New York, Oxford University Press, 1959.
2 Kinsey AC et al: *Sexual Behavior in the Human Male*. Philadelphia, Saunders, 1948.
3 Kinsey AC et al: *Sexual Behavior in the Human Female*. Philadelphia, Saunders, 1953.
4 U.S. Department of Commerce. *Statistical Abstracts of U.S.*, 107th ed, 1987.
5 Norton AJ, Moorman JE: Current trends in marriage and divorce among American women. *J Marriage Fam* 49:3, 1987.
6 Masters WH, Johnson VE: *Human Sexual Response*. Boston, Little Brown, 1966.
7 Reiss IL: *Premarital Sexual Standards in America*. New York, Free Press, 1960.
8 Glenn ND, Weaver CN: Attitudes toward premarital, extramarital, and homosexual relations in the U.S. in the 1970s. *J Sex Res* 15:108, 1979.
9 Glick PC: Marriage, divorce, and living arrangements: prospective changes. *J Fam Issues* 5:7, 1984.
10 Lugaila T: Households, Families, and Children: A 30-year Perspective. Current Population Reports, U.S. Department of Commerce, 1992, pp 23–181.
11 Rodgers WL, Thornton A: Changing patterns of first marriage in the United States. *Demography* 22:265, 1985.
12 Laumann EO et al: *The Social Organization of Sexuality: Sexual Practices in the United States*. Chicago, The University of Chicago Press, 1994.
13 Zelnik M et al: *Sex and Pregnancy in Adolescence*. Beverly Hills, Sage, 1981.
14 Tanfer K, Horn MC: Contraceptive use, pregnancy, and fertility planning among single women in their twenties. *Fam Plann Perspect* 17: 10, 1985.
15 Jones EF et al: *Teenage Pregnancy in Industrialized Countries*. New Haven, Yale University Press, 1986.
16 Institute of Medicine: *Confronting AIDS: Directions for Public Health, Health Care, and Research*. Washington, DC, National Academy Press, 1986.
17 Billy JOG et al: The sexual behavior of men in the United States. *Family Plann Perspect* 24:52, 1993.
18 Zelnik M, Kantner J: Sexual activity, contraceptive use, and pregnancy among metropolitan-area teenagers: 1971–1979. *Fam Plann Perspect* 12:230, 1980.
19 Sonenstein FL et al: Levels of sexual activity among adolescent males in the United States. *Fam Plann Perspect* 23:162, 1991.
20 Ku LC et al: Young men's risk behaviors for HIV infection and sexually transmitted diseases, 1988 through 1991. *Am J Public Health* 83:1609, 1993.
21 Leigh BC et al: Sexual behavior of American adolescents: results from a U.S. national survey. *J Adol Health* 15:117, 1994.
22 Laumann EO et al: A political history of the National Sex Survey of Adults. *Fam Plann Perspect* 26:34, 1994.
23 Turner CF et al (eds): *AIDS: Sexual Behavior, and Intraveneous Drug Use*. Washington, DC, National Academy Press, 1989.
24 Miller, HG et al (eds): *AIDS: The Second Decade*. Washington, DC, National Academy Press, 1990.
25 McKinney K, Sprecher, S: *Human Sexuality: The Societal and Personal Context*. Norwood, NJ, Ablex, 1989.
26 Hunt M: *Sexual Behavior in the 1970s*. Chicago, Playboy Press, 1974.
27 Bell AP, Weinberg MS: *Homosexualities*. New York, Simon and Shuster, 1978.
28 Ponse B: *Identities in the Lesbian World: The Social Construction of Self*. Westport, CT, Greenwood, 1978.
29 Downy L: Intergenerational changes in sex behavior: a belated look at Kinsey's males. *Arch Sex Behav* 9:267, 1980.
30 Pratt WF et al: Understanding U.S. fertility: Findings from the national survey of family growth, cycle III. *Popul Bull* 39(5), 1984.
31 Furstenberg FF et al: Race differences in the timing of adolescent intercourse. *Am Sociol Rev* 52:511, 1987.
32 Weinberg MS, Williams CJ: Black sexuality: a test of two theories. *J Sex Res* 26:197, 1988.
33 Maurin, Barbara, personal communication, University of California, San Fransisco, May, 1995.
34 Binson D et al: IV. Multiple sexual partners among young adults in high-risk cities. *Fam Plann Perspec* 25(6):268, 1993.
35 Spanier GB, Thompson L: *Parting: the aftermath of separation and divorce*. Beverly Hills, Sage, 1984.
36 Melnick SL et al: Changes in sexual behavior by young urban heterosexual adults in response to the AIDS epidemic. *Pub Health Rep* 108: 582, 1993.
37 Macklin ED: Nonmarital heterosexual cohabitation. *Marriage Fam Rev* 12:1, 1978.
38 Glick PC, Spanier GB: Married and unmarried cohabitation in the United States today. *J Marriage Fam* 42:19, 1980.
39 Glick PC, Norton RJ: Marrying, divorcing, and living together in the United States today. *Popul Bull*, 32:36, 1977.
40 Clayton RR, Voss HL: Shacking up: cohabitation in the 1970s. *J Marriage Fam* 39: 273, 1977.
41 Bower DW, Christopherson V: University student cohabitation: a regional comparison of selected attitudes and behavior. *J Marriage Fam* 39: 447, 1977.
42 Croake JW et al: *Unmarrieds Living Together: It's Not all Gravy!* Dubuque, Iowa, Kendall/Hunt, 1974.
43 Johnson P: Courtship and Commitment: A Study of Cohabitation on a University Campus. Master's thesis, University of Iowa, 1969.
44 Newcomb MD: Sexual behavior of cohabitors: a comparison of three independent samples. *J Sex Res* 22: 492, 1986.
45 Blumstein P, Schwartz P: *American Couples*. New York, Morrow, 1983.
46 Westoff CF: Coital frequency and contraception. *Fam Plann Perspect* 6:135, 1974.
47 Greenblat CS: The salience of sexuality in the early years of marriage. *J Marriage Fam* 45:289, 1983.
48 Udry JR: Changes in the frequency of marital intercourse from panel data. *Arch Sex Behav* 9: 319, 1980.
49 Tavris C, Sadd S: *Redbook Report on Female Sexuality*. New York, Dell, 1977.
50 Leigh BC et al: The sexual behavior of U.S. adults: results from a national survey. *Am J Public Health* 83:1400, 1993.
51 Greeley AM et al: Americans and their sexual partners. *Society* 27(5): 36–42, 1990.
52 Thompson AP: Extramarital sex: a review of the research literature. *J Sex Res* 19:1, 1983.
53 Gilmartin B: *The Gilmartin Report*. Secaucus, NJ, Citadel Press, 1978.
54 Jenks RJ: Swinging: a test of two theories and a proposed new model. *Arch Sex Behav* 14:517, 1985.
55 O'Neill G, O'Neill N: Patterns in group sexual activity. *J of Sex Res* 6:101, 1970.
56 Smith JR, Smith LG: Co-marital sex and the sexual freedom movement. *J Sex Res* 6:131, 1970.
57 Varni CA: An exploratory study of spouse swapping, in *Beyond Monogamy*, JR Smith, LG Smith (eds). Baltimore, Johns Hopkins University Press, 1974, p 246.
58 Humphreys L: *Tearoom Trade*. Chicago, Aldine, 1970.

59 Saghir MT, Robins E: *Male and Female Homosexuality: A Comprehensive Investigation*. Baltimore, Williams and Wilkins, 1973.
60 Weinberg MS, Williams CJ: *Male Homosexuals*. London, Oxford University, 1974.
61 Harry J: *Gay Couples*. New York, Praeger, 1984.
62 McWhirter DP, Mattison AM: *The Male Couple*. Englewood Cliffs, NJ, Prentice-Hall, 1984.
63 Harry J: A probability sample of gay males. *J Homosex* 19:89, 1990.
64 Schaefer S: Sexual and social problems of lesbians. *J Sex Res* 12:50, 1976.
65 Gundlach R, Reiss BF: Self and sexual identity in the female, in *New Directions in Mental Health*, BF Reiss (ed). New York, Grune and Stratton, 1968.
66 Peplau LA et al: Loving women: attachment and autonomy in lesbian relationships. *J Soc Issues* 34:7, 1978.
67 Blumstein P, Schwartz P: Bisexuality: some social psychological issues. *J Soc Issues* 33:30, 1977.
68 Blumstein PW, Schwartz P: Bisexuality in women. *Arch Sex Behav* 5: 171, 1976.
69 Schofield MG: *Sociological Aspects of Homosexuality: A Comparative Study of Three Types of Homosexuals*. Boston, Little, Brown, 1965.
70 McKusick L et al: Longitudinal predictors of reductions in unprotected anal intercourse among gay men in San Francisco: the AIDS Behavioral Research Project. *Am J Public Health* 80:978, 1990.
71 Harry J, DeVall, WB: *The Social Organization of Gay Males*. New York, Praeger, 1978.
72 Stall R et al: A comparison of younger and older gay men's HIV risk-taking behaviors: the communication technologies 1989 cross-sectional study. *J Acquir Immune Defic Syndr* 5:682, 1992.
73 Ostrow DG et al: Sexual behavior change and persistence in homosexual men. Paper presented at the International Conference on AIDS, Atlanta, GA, Apr 14–17, 1985.
74 Siegel K, Hirsch DA: Modifications in sexual practices among asymptomatic gay men in New York City. Paper presented at the International Conference on AIDS, Atlanta, GA, Apr 14–17, 1985.
75 Martin JL: The impact of AIDS on New York City gay men: changes in sexual behavior patterns. Paper presented at the 113th annual meeting of the American Public Health Association, Washington, DC, Nov 21, 1985.
76 McKusick L et al: Reported changes in the sexual behavior of men at risk for AIDS, San Francisco, 1982–1984. *Public Health Rep* 22, 1985.
77 Ostrow DG et al: Sexual behavior research on a cohort of gay men, 1984–1990: can we predict how men will respond to interventions? *Arch Sex Behav* 23:531, 1994.
78 Coates TJ et al: AIDS: a psychosocial research agenda. *Ann Behav Med* 9:21, 1987.
79 Roffman R et al: AIDS risk reduction project: a report to the King County Department of Public Health. Seattle, WA, June, 1987.
80 Peplau LA, Gordon SL: The intimate relations of lesbians and gay men, in *Gender Roles and Gender Behavior*, ER Allgeier, NB McCormick (eds). Palo Alto, CA, Mayfield, 1983.
81 Peplau LA, Cochran S: Value orientations in the intimate relationships of gay men. *J Homosex* 6:1, 1981.
82 Cotton WI: Social and sexual relationships of lesbians. *J Sex Res* 11: 139, 1975.
83 Ford CS, Beach FA: *Patterns of Sexual Behavior*. New York, Harper and Row, 1951.

Chapter 7

Psychological perspectives on sexuality and sexually transmitted diseases

Michael W. Ross

Psychological variables are closely associated with sexually transmitted diseases (STDs) in both immediate (social psychology of situational pressures to engage in sex that may lead to higher risk of infection) and more distant (personality styles or attitudes toward sex and sexuality that may put an individual at greater risk of STD infection) senses. This chapter focuses on psychological aspects of sexuality as they may affect both risk of STD infection and presentation for and response to treatment. A third area of psychology associated with human immune-deficiency virus (HIV) disease and other STDs such as genital herpes is that of clinical psychology or psychiatry, in which maladaptive or psychopathologic responses to infection (or fear of infection) may occur. A brief review of theories of sexual behavior precedes these observations.

PSYCHOLOGICAL THEORIES OF HUMAN SEXUALITY

Sexual behavior is considered an inborn drive in humans: Even infants show signs of sexual behavior. Sex drive may be markedly modified by cultural, social, and interpersonal factors. Freud termed the energy of sex the *libido* and believed that, along with hostility and aggression, it accounted for most of the motivation behind human behavior. Freud postulated that the individual was born potentially able to respond to any individual sexually but that socialization through a series of stages directed the sexual urge toward heterosexual contact. Freud's stages included the oral stage, the anal stage, the genital stage, the latency stage, and the reawakening of sexual impulses at puberty. Major studies of children's sexual thinking[1] show that sexual understanding follows three Piagetian stages of nonsexual, transitional sexual, and fully sexual stages of cognition rather than Freud's stages, and these depend strongly on the cultural and educational information on sexuality available to children and adolescents.

There is general agreement that a fundamental propensity to act sexually exists but that it may be modified by learning. Ford and Beach[2] note that cultural conditioning accounts for the extent and type of sexual expression but falls short of accounting for what is biologically possible in humans. The psychological process of molding sexual expression is through conditioning. Modeling, in which individuals learn roles or behaviors through observing the behavior of others, is also involved.[3] Nevertheless, little is understood about the specific development of heterosexual or homosexual behavior, which probably results from the interaction of biologic and social factors. Sexuality has a number of different aspects and meanings depending on variation in person, time, culture, age, and situation. Ross[4] has noted (Table 7-1) that multiple meanings of sexual expression are learned. Sexuality is not a unitary phenomenon but part of social interaction and best explained by contingencies of reinforcement acting on a basic biologic drive. For people in all cultures, sex is multidetermined but most commonly associated with seeking comfort, finding pleasure, and survival.[5]

PSYCHOLOGICAL VARIABLES ASSOCIATED WITH RISK OF SEXUALLY TRANSMITTED INFECTION

The psychological variables associated with increased risk of contracting STDs include those which are associated with behaviors that carry an increased risk of infection. In addition to specific behaviors such as high partner numbers, specific sexual practices (including condom use), and the context in which the sex occurs, this chapter generally reviews the variables that have been associated with STD infection. Where psychosocial factors are associated with risk of STD infection, this provides a possibility of modifying such factors to decrease the probability of infection as well as to develop information on which intervention strategies may be based.

PERSONALITY AND ATTITUDINAL VARIABLES

Hart[6] has argued not only that there is increasing recognition of venereal disease as a behavioral disease but also that sociologic variables implicated in venereal disease may be related primarily to the personality of the individual. He reported for his heterosexual sample that an increase in extroversion and, to a lesser extent, neuroticism, as measured by the Eysenck Personality Inventory,[7] was associated with increased STD infection. Similar findings are reported by other researchers: Eysenck[8] found that extroverts will have intercourse earlier, more frequently, with more different partners, and in more different positions than introverts; they also will engage in more varied sexual behavior outside intercourse and engage in longer foreplay. Measuring attitudes on Eysenck's Sexual Attitudes Inventory (ESAI), Fulford et al.[9] found STD clinic subjects to be less interested than Eysenck's controls in physical sex and pornography and to have less sexual excitement and greater prudishness, sexual disgust, and neurotic sexual attitudes. Homosexual patients did not differ from heterosexual patients, and bisexual patients accounted for most of the differences that were found. Familial variables also have been implicated: Hart[10] has reported soldiers coming from large (four or more children) families as significantly more at risk for STD infection, and Ross[11,12] reported that the extremes of rejecting and overly supportive parental relationships were among the significant predictors of multiple STD infections in the four Western countries he studied.

Personality and attitudinal variables may be associated with increased risk of STD infection in men. Ross[13] found that beliefs about the meaning of sexuality and its social and political implications predicted sexual behavior in Swedish homosexual men. Eysenck[8] found that high psychoticism scorers (those who tend to be isolated, affectless, and aggressive) also were more sexually curious, more accepting of premarital sex, more promiscuous, and more hostile. Extroverts scored high on the promiscuity scales and low on the nervousness scale (more promiscuous and less sexually nervous), while high scorers on the neuroticism scale had significantly lower scores on sexual satisfaction and significantly higher scores on excitement, nervousness, sexual hostility, sexual guilt, and sexual inhibition. High neuroticism scores are also closely associated with venereoneurosis.[5]

Fulford et al.[9] used the ESAI and found that while neuroticism correlated positively with syphilis and gonorrhea infections, extroversion correlated negatively with the diagnosis of syphilis. Ross[13] refactored the ESAI after rewording it to make it appropriate for homosexual men and derived nine interpretable dimen-

Table 7-1. Theoretical Aspects and Meanings of Sexual Relationships

Aspects	Meanings
Reproduction	Continuation of species
Religious	Symbolic of union
Emotional	Extension of love for partner
Release of sexual urge	Release of frustration or libido
Financial	Prostitution
Duty	Socially expected, as in some marriages
Antisocial statement	Rejection of parental/social values
Ritual	During particular ceremonies, symbolic
Hedonistic (recreational)	Enjoyment
Experimental	Exploration of sexual feelings and behaviors
Relational	As part of wider social and attitudinal affinities
Dominance	Rape, expression of difference in relative power
Peer-sanctioned	Normative, status-associated
Forbidden or taboo	Associated with guilt or punishment
Dynastic	Cementing relations between families or groups
Mentor	Teaching sexuality to younger individuals

SOURCE: From Ross.[4]

sions. He found that, as anticipated, sexual attitudes did underlie sexual behaviors. In fact, six of the nine scales were predictors of partner numbers, five were predictors of particular sexual practices, and six were predictors of places of partner contact. All these scales were related in a curvilinear rather than linear fashion to partner numbers, with those with zero and high partner numbers having greater sexual prudishness and fear of sexual relationships and lower interest in pornography, degree of sexual excitability, and sexual permissiveness. Those with higher partner numbers were highest on the scale measuring lack of control of libido.

Sensation seeking has been implicated more recently in STD (including HIV) risk behaviors. Kalichman et al.[14] found that sensation seeking predicted HIV risk behavior in homosexual men, and even with substance use controlled for, sexual adventurism and sensation seeking were major predictors of unsafe sexual behavior. This also has been confirmed in heterosexual men: Bogaert and Fisher[15] were able to predict a significant proportion of the variance of partner numbers using sensation-seeking measures. It appears that there is a constellation of disinhibition, including Eysenck's psychoticism and extroversion, as well as sensation seeking, significantly related both to safety and partner numbers.

PSYCHOSOCIAL VARIABLES

The environmental stresses of war and immigration produce behavior patterns that many would not otherwise experience.[5,16] Half the men with gonorrhea in the United Kingdom in the 1960s were immigrants. Single migrants may have numerous sexual encounters until they settle into their new cultural backgrounds.[17] This also holds for non-Western societies: Hart[18] reported that in single laborers and married immigrants in Papua New Guinea, recourse to prostitutes and, to a lesser extent, homosexual behavior is more common and that venereal disease is a prominent sequel. STD incidence rates in immigrants and soldiers are increased markedly (in comparison with baseline rates prior to immigration or war), and instability and insecurity are associated with lack of discrimination and increase in frequency of sexual contacts. However, Kelus[19] took random samples of STD clinic attenders and inhabitants in a Polish town and found no differences between inhabitants and patients apart from a tendency for patients to be more urbanized and less religious. Hooker[20] has suggested that for some, the seeking of sexual contacts is an activity that is isolated from all other aspects of their lives. We cannot assume that psychological factors that influence sexual contacts will be obvious in other areas of the individual's life.

PSYCHOLOGICAL CONCOMITANTS OF PARTNER NUMBERS

Partner numbers are an important determinant of STD infection, since they can increase (depending on prevalence) the probability of infection. If sexual practices that do not transfer body fluids are utilized, partner numbers are immaterial, and if all partners are mutually monogamous and uninfected, there is no risk. Ross[21] found that partner numbers were not invariably associated with risk of STD infection in homosexual men, although this also will depend on disease prevalence. Schofield[22] reports that there is little if any evidence that individuals with high partner numbers have personality defects, are emotionally damaged, or come from a less than adequate social milieu. Goode and Troiden[23] found that homosexual men with higher partner numbers tended to prefer emotionally superficial sex and were less well educated. Partner numbers can be depressed during dysphoric mood states (confusion, fatigue, and distress).[13] High partner numbers also may protect from psychological decompensation through their effect on increasing self-esteem. Depression increased in homosexual men who reduced their risk of contracting HIV,[24] which suggests that there is some association between mood and partner numbers.

Bogaert and Fisher[15] found that number of sexual partners in heterosexual men was best predicted by hypermasculinity and sensation seeking. A personality construct they labeled "disinhibition" (sensation seeking, hypermasculinity, Eysenck's psychoticism,[8] and erotophilia) accounted for a substantial proportion of variance in partner numbers. The homosexual male with high partner numbers sees himself as conventionally masculine, prefers a more feminine partner, and has high alcohol consumption. He may have had a more negative parental rearing pattern and be under less stress than men with low partner numbers, be more involved in the homosexual subculture, see his homosexuality as more central to his lifestyle, and have had more STD infections.[13] These data illustrate the multifactorial nature of the variables associated with high partner numbers in white, Western cultures.

PSYCHOLOGICAL CONCOMITANTS OF PARTICULAR SEXUAL PRACTICES

Practices that involve the transmission of body fluids, including unprotected anal or vaginal intercourse, brachioproctic ("fist fornication") activities, and fellatio may transmit pathogens; mutual masturbation and frottage (rubbing bodies together) will not. Haist and Hewitt[25] noted that homosexual men who preferred the anal insertee role also tended to prefer the oral insertee role in fellatio. However, Hooker[26] reported no relationship between sexual activity preferences and sex role. Ross[13] found that homosexual men who preferred oral activities, including both fellatio and analingus, appear to be differentiated from those with no such preference by negative maternal rearing patterns and euphoric mood states, suggesting that such behaviors may be related both to gratification of oral dependency needs and to hedonism. Preference for insertor and insertee roles in both fellatio and anal intercourse appeared to be strongly related to conventional masculine and feminine sex roles, and activities such as full-body contact and mutual masturbation appear not to be related to sex role.

These last two activities appear to occur when there is emphasis on emotional as well as physical closeness, and they are associated with decreased frequencies of STD infection. Ross's data also suggest that sexual socialization into homosexual subcultures and, to a lesser extent, parental and peer models have a major influence on the type of sexual activities indulged in: Increased time and degree of socialization into the homosexual subculture increase preference for specific roles, as does degree of organization of the homosexual subculture within which that socialization occurs. Preference for particular practices does appear to be more a function of increasing sexual experience, although the influence of masculine and feminine sex roles is significant. There is no literature on heterosexual concomitants of particular sexual practices.

Safe (or safer) sex involves protection by use of male or female condoms. Psychological characteristics associated with use of condoms include more assertive personality styles and lower depression and dysphoric mood in both cross-sectional and longitudinal studies.[27,28]

PSYCHOLOGICAL CONCOMITANTS OF PARTNER ANONYMITY AND PLACES OF SEXUAL CONTACT

Partner anonymity and place of sexual contact play an important part in STD infection; the links are threefold. First, the possibility of partner notification of anonymous partners is virtually impossible. Second, in some places of anonymous contact such as gay bathhouses, there are opportunities for multiple contacts with multiple partners within a short time span. Third, such places may generate their own demands, which may lead to person-situation interactions in which the effect of being in the situation is significant. Apart from the classic study of Humphreys,[29] which classified men using public conveniences as places for sexual gratification into four groups ("trade," ambisexuals, gays, and closet queens), and the work of Lewis and Ross[30] on sex and drug use at gay dance parties, there are few data on places of sexual contact. Humphreys' "trade" group comprised working-class married men. Two-thirds took an insertor role in fellatio in sexual encounters. Ambisexuals were married men with high income: Two-thirds of this group were insertees in fellatio and saw themselves as bisexual. The gay group was comprised of individuals who were unmarried, had no preference for sexual roles, and had independent occupations, whereas the "closet queens" also were unmarried but in lower-middle-class occupations in which they were dependent on others for employment, and they avoided the homosexual subculture. They preferred to play the insertor role, at least until they lost their attractiveness.

Ross[13] noted few differences between those preferring particular places of meeting sexual partners. Those meeting partners through "cruising" have more positive mood states and higher self-esteem than others and were markedly different from those who frequented bathhouses, who appear to be more depressed, avoiding close emotional contacts, probably as a result of much more negative parental relationship models. It appears that psychological variables, particularly mood states, are strongly associated with the drive for partners and the context in which they are sought, with a relationship between mood and partner seeking.

PSYCHOLOGICAL CONCOMITANTS OF CONDOM USE

Several studies have noted psychological variables associated with condom use. Personality variables associated with increased condom use in homosexual men include increased scores on the dominance and aggression scales of the Adjective Check List and decreased scores on the abasement and deference scales.[27] Longitudinally, mood states (as measured by the Profile of Mood States) associated with a move to safer sex included those with lower depression, anger and hostility, fatigue, confusion, and total dysphoric mood scores.[28] These data suggest that assertiveness and lack of dysphoric mood are both associated with increased condom use. In a comparative study in heterosexual and homosexual men, Treffke et al.[31] found that attitudes toward condoms were strongly associated with both general assertiveness and condom assertiveness in heterosexual men but that there was no association in homosexual men. Psychological data on psychological concomitants of condom use may not be generalized across sexual orientation and probably not across gender.

THE PSYCHOLOGY OF SEXUALLY TRANSMITTED INFECTIONS

The second area of importance in considering psychological aspects of STDs is the psychological aspects of infection, such as reactions and abnormal behavior in those infected. This section considers the presentation and management of the psychosocial manifestations and psychopathology of STDs. Psychological sequelae to STD exposure are poorly understood, frequently unrecognized, and inadequately managed, despite being among the most common conditions encountered in STD practice.[5] Psychological and psychiatric problems in STD practice may be divided into three categories: the normal range of psychological reactions to STDs, abnormal reactions to STD infection (or belief in infection), and sexual dysfunctions that may become apparent in the course of consultation or present initially to STD clinics.

PSYCHOSOCIAL RESPONSES TO SEXUALLY TRANSMITTED INFECTION

Over 40 percent of patients attending public STD clinics have been classified as psychiatric cases on the basis of screening tests.[32] A subsequent study noted that the anxiety caused by the presenting problem probably was the cause of such a high figure, since less than 5 percent had a sufficiently abnormal level of distress to justify calling it psychopathologic.[33] Another study reported that less than 5 percent of STD patients required psychiatric referral,[34] although Barczak et al.[35] reported that 31 percent had anxiety and depression not affected by the physical symptoms of STDs and that these were significantly more prevalent in females. Significant life events in the past 6 months were related to presence of physical symptoms, and if there were no life events in this time frame, a psychiatric diagnosis was more likely (this relationship may be related to increase in sexual activity following traumatic life events). It is therefore important to differentiate the normal range of reactions to STD infection from psychopathologic ones.

Ross[13] has postulated a model of the meaning of STDs to the individual that explains the beliefs underlying psychological reactions to STDs and the reasons for psychopathology when it occurs. In discussing the meaning of STDs to the individual, there are at least four separate attributions.

1. STDs are a deserved outcome of indiscriminate sexual behavior and punishment for sexual sins.
2. STDs are a consequence of individual inadequacy that leads to sexually indiscriminate behavior.
3. STDs are a consequence of a breakdown in traditional social values and rapid social change.
4. STDs are solely the result of an individual coming into intimate contact with a virulent pathogen.

There is a hierarchy of decreasing blame from attributions 1 to 4 and a similar hierarchy of the degree to which individuals see themselves responsible for the infection. The degree to which there is a psychological investment in sexual behavior is also important. The meaning of STDs to the patient and, to a lesser degree, to the attending health professional will affect not only the compliance with treatment but also the psychological sequelae and the subsequent risks of exposure to STDs the individual takes. The interaction between patients and physicians who hold conflicting attributions for STDs may lead to tension, anger, transference and countertransference issues, and resistance to taking advice or treatment, particularly where more divergent attributions are held. One should ascertain one's own position and make some estimate of the position of one's patient before seeking to educate or to modify risky behaviors.

Abnormal reactions to STD infection may arise from any of the four attitudes toward STDs noted above. These reactions may be further classified into *abnormal illness behavior* and *venereoneuroses.* Psychotic reactions that are either triggered by an STD or have major venereologic components are recognizable by such classic psychotic features as delusional thought patterns and the inability of patients to be convinced by rational discussion. Such patients with psychotic reactions generally also will have a history of psychotic illness.

ABNORMAL ILLNESS BEHAVIOR

Abnormal illness behavior has important implications for treatment. In the case of individuals with an erroneous conviction that they have an STD, there is abnormal illness behavior in terms of both general hypochondriasis and a strong disease conviction without demonstrable pathology. There also may be an indication that patients believe they "deserve" the infection, as noted above. Perhaps more common is the refusal to see an STD as an illness but perhaps only as a minor nonsignificant risk of a particular lifestyle. In the case of the absence of any illness behavior, patients frequently may compromise treatment by discontinuing medication after symptoms have resolved, continuing sexual activity after symptom resolution but before clearance, or not returning for proof of cure. Thus both extreme illness behavior and lack of illness behavior can be abnormal and may have implications for the management of STDs.

Ross[36] found that it was the repeated STD clinic attenders rather than the first attenders who displayed the greatest anxiety and hypochondriasis over STD infection. Those with higher previous numbers of infections also tended to deny life stresses more and attribute their problems solely to the episode of illness. Such individuals also displayed significantly higher disease conviction and symptom preoccupation and higher levels of symptom exaggeration. In comparison, first attenders tended to deny that an STD was an illness (denial of acquisition of a stigmatizing illness). Compared with other illnesses, in which there may be substantial secondary gain through sympathy, illness behavior would appear to be different in STDs and to develop as a function of repeated infections. STD infection tends to be seen as a chance event until after several infections, when it is then seen not only as an illness but also as a result of particular behaviors. Ross also found that there were few differences in illness behavior with STD infections between heterosexual and homosexual men, apart from the fact that there is a less negative reaction to STD infection among gay men. The STD clinic population was closer in illness behavior scores to a psychiatric outpatient population than a general practice one. It is unclear whether the disturbance was a function of having a stigmatized illness such as an STD or inherent in STD clinic attenders.

Ross[37] also found that admission of homosexuality in STD clinics varied significantly between countries (20 to 52 percent of homosexually active men did not admit to being homosexual), although not between private and public clinics. The variables predictive of whether the respondent reveals his homosexual orientation when presenting to a STD clinic or medical practitioner are coherent. Nonadmitters are likely to conceal their homosexuality from most people, to expect the most negative social reaction to their homosexuality from significant others and society in general, and to believe in much more rigid and conservative sex roles for men and women. Compared with those who admit to homosexual contact, nonadmitters are more likely to report themselves as being more bisexual than exclusively homosexual, to have had no previous STD, and to have had poor relationships with their mother during adolescence. They are also more likely to be unassertive.

The lack of previous sexually transmitted infections in nonadmitters suggests that the clinic situation will be a new and potentially frightening one, in which condemnation is expected: In subsequent visits to a clinic, the patient will tend to be more open if the clinician's approach has been nonjudgmental. When clinicians take histories in a manner that implies that any sexual contact was a heterosexual one, the patient may not have the courage to make a correction. These data do suggest that there are significant and consistent psychological factors operating to prevent some homosexual men from revealing same-sex contacts in the context of STD clinics. However, these psychological factors clearly will operate in interaction with environmental factors such as the clinic, the clinician, and the legal and social climate regarding homosexuality. The imposition of shame and guilt on sexual interactions by religious and other traditional moralities is the single most important cause of psychological problems in STD treatment, and if the physician is able to assess and deal with this early in the treatment process, many difficulties may be prevented or minimized. To fail to do so may even introduce or reinforce shame or guilt and produce an iatrogenically strengthened psychopathology. A high index of suspicion for psychosocial problems attendant on STD infection or reported infection is mandatory to ensure maximal compliance with treatment, partner notification, and preventive education, and the possible contribution of psychosocial factors to relapse or reinfection should not be underestimated.

COMMON RESPONSES TO SEXUALLY TRANSMITTED INFECTIONS

There is a large literature on the response to genital herpes infection, reviewed by Longo and Koehn.[38] They note that much of the research on the impact of genital herpes is neither longitudinal in comparison with the premorbid psychological state nor comparative with other curable STDs. Nevertheless, there are elements of response that are common across studies. For people who have had genital herpes for less than a year, negative life events, depression, anxiety, anger, and social alienation predict herpes simplex virus (HSV) recurrences; for over a year, high levels of depression and low self-esteem are consistently associated with more frequent HSV recurrences. It is important to note that *responses* to infection may lead to these states, thus setting up a cycle of response and recurrence. Stronks et al.[39] compared people with genital herpes to both a control group with gonorrhea and to their reported premorbid adjustment and found that while there was no difference in outcome for those with HSV or gonorrhea, both had significantly increased anxiety, sexual inhibition, bitterness toward sexual partners, and increased psychological complaints compared with a no-STD control group. There was a significant interaction between premorbid state and morbid change, however, with the HSV group increasing markedly in psychological complaints and the gonorrhea group increasing minimally. Carney et al.,[40] in a longitudinal study, found that the first episode of genital herpes had a significantly negative psychological impact, with over 60 percent meeting screening criteria for being a psychiatric case, as measured by the General Health Questionnaire. However, two-thirds of these became noncases if there was no recurrence of disease. If there were recurrences, the level of psychiatric case classification stayed high. A clinical study[41] found that the majority of people with genital HSV report that infection made them less capable of physical warmth and intimacy and less able to enjoy sex and made them feel less sexually desirable. This extended outside sexual contacts: All reported that work performance also was hampered. A majority reported disturbance of affect, feeling that genital HSV is incompatible with happiness, and being pessimistic about the future course of the illness. Depression also was reported by 84 percent. Sexual dysfunctions including reduced interest, reduced ability to achieve orgasm, avoidance of intimacy, and reduced enjoyment of sex, as well as feeling repugnant to others (over 30 percent of Americans say they would not associate with someone who has HSV[42]) were reported.

VENEREONEUROSES

Venereoneuroses may be divided into those neuroses which manifest with exposure to infection, including overreaction to infection, venereophobias, and abnormal disease convictions, and factitious STDs and AIDS.

Venereal overreaction and hypochondriasis

Hart[5] notes that individuals may be abnormally preoccupied with bodily processes, manifesting as a genitally focused hypochondriasis. Irrational concern is focused on urethral, anal, or vaginal discharge or the appearance and sensations of the genitalia. There may be an obsessional element to these or compulsive genital examination, which may itself cause irritation or discharge. Acceptance of these symptoms (or the patient's description of these symptoms) without objective evidence of infection or relapse may promote venereoneurosis and aggravation of the neurotic tendencies of the patient. Hart[5] also has reported that penile manipulation to produce discharge (often including the vigorous squeezing of the glans and shaft, in contrast to the more usual cautious manipulation) is a feature of such patients. In other manifestations, abnormal attention may be paid to irregularities in pigmentation or skin surface, skin tags, sebaceous cysts and hair follicles, and pearly penile papules. Demands for treatment, in the absence of demonstrable infection or pathology, are one indication of the presence of venereoneurosis, and Hart believes that such patients tend to be more severely disturbed.

Miller et al.[43] have reported that in the case of HIV infection, individuals will focus on the nonspecific nature of the symptoms of HIV infection and attend for minor changes in skin pigmentation that they believe is Kaposi's sarcoma or for minor changes in respiratory function that they believe indicative of an opportunistic pulmonary infection. In some cases, obsessional palpation of cervical and axillary lymph nodes will lead to local irritation that may be interpreted as lymphadenopathy. Management involves discussing the patient's specific anxieties, and an opportunity to talk about these may in itself provide considerable relief. In the case of concern over acquired immune-deficiency syndrome (AIDS) in those who have been infected with HIV, it is important to focus on the patient's specific concerns, including fear of exposure, stigmatization, pain, death, and the uncertainty associated with the diagnosis of HIV infection and the likelihood of progression.

Venereophobias

Venereophobias have been recognized for most of this century, with syphilophobia as the earliest manifestation reported.[44] At present, AIDS phobias are reported more commonly,[45] probably because of the increase in publicity surrounding AIDS and the mortality and morbidity associated with it. In syphilo- and AIDS phobias, inividuals at no or low risk of contracting the disease believe that they are infected. While more accurately described as an abnormal disease conviction than a phobia, in some cases there also will be irrational precautions to avoid catching AIDS and fear or avoidance of situations in which there is a perceived risk of catching AIDS. AIDS-phobic patients differ from venereoneurotics in that symptoms usually are not genitally focused and often cannot be traced to a specific sexual episode. Ross[45] also has reported that underlying conflicts and life stresses are likely to be major contributors and that such presentations usually are associated with guilt over sexual behavior (commonly sexual activity outside a primary relationship or bisexual or homosexual contact). The trigger is usually life stresses, often relationship related, or media publicity on AIDS. The belief in infection sometimes may be near delusional in quality, with patients refusing to believe the results of HIV tests or going from clinic to clinic in search of a test result that confirms their worst fears.

Management of venereophobias must encompass more than just reassurance of noninfection, which the patient may interpret as not being taken seriously. Excessive physical intervention, beyond that necessary to exclude disease, reinforces the patient's belief in the existence of disease. Taking a brief sexual history and a history of current concerns and stresses and recent conflicts frequently will bring out the underlying issues of guilt or concern over moral self-image or sexual orientation. Brief interpretive counseling focusing on the conflicts underlying the phobia and on the stresses that promote such conflicts, with emphasis on giving patients a degree of insight into the processes that lead them to present with an abnormal disease conviction, often will resolve the problem. However, referral to appropriate mental health professionals should be considered and not delayed if resolution does not occur.

Symptoms but no objective microbiologic evidence of infection in women presenting at gynecology or STD clinics were not associated with any evidence of differences between them and women with microbiologic evidence of disease, or neither symptoms nor abnormal microbiologic findings, on life stress, sex guilt, or global personality function. However, these symptomatic but microbiologically normal women indicated significantly lower marital satisfaction and thought that their relationship was less sexually satisfying to their partner. McGuire et al.[46] suggested that preoccupation with vaginal symptomatology might reconcile for these women the difference between the objective and subjective evaluations of their sexual relationships.

Factitious illness

Several cases of factitious AIDS have been reported.[47–49] The individual may present stating that he or she has been diagnosed as having full AIDS at another center, but findings on examination do not accord with this. Immediate professional consultation with the center of previous treatment usually confirms that the claim of illness is incorrect. Individuals who have been confirmed to have factitious AIDS may be either seeking the secondary gain of sympathy and hospitalization or seeking to come to terms with the death of a significant other from AIDS. In the few cases reported, individuals usually strongly deny the diagnosis of factitious illness (Munchausen's syndrome) and may present in the future with other factitious illnesses with substituted symptoms.

Such individuals frequently are quite medically sophisticated and may present plausible histories. Referral for psychiatric assessment is strongly recommended in such cases.

ACQUIRED IMMUNE DEFICIENCY SYNDROME AND HIV INFECTION

Reactions to HIV infection may be more extreme than reactions to other STDs for four reasons. First, the fully developed disease is fatal. Second, in Western societies AIDS is commonly associated with stigmatized minority groups (homosexual and bisexual men, illicit injecting drug users, and prostitutes), and a substantial component of attitudes toward AIDS comprises antihomosexual and antiminority beliefs and attribution of blame.[50] Third, such attitudes may be internalized in those infected and may lead to guilt and self-blame. Fourth, medical attendants also may contribute to stigmatization through overprecautions or avoidance of contact.[51] Consequently, the emotional impact on the patients upon informing them that they are infected with HIV is not significantly different from the news they have AIDS-related symptoms or full AIDS.[52]

Psychological complications of HIV infection may be exogenous or endogenous. Exogenous complications arise from the psychosocial stresses resulting from negative societal and interpersonal reactions to AIDS. Faulstich[53] notes that the "worried well" (whether infected or not) may exhibit generalized anxiety and panic attacks, along with excessive somatic preoccupation and fear of the disease. On diagnosis of HIV infection or AIDS, individuals may exhibit disbelief and denial, followed by depressive and anxiety symptoms. Emotional distress commonly may lead to adjustment disorders with depressed mood or major depression. Recurrent psychological themes include uncertainty about disease progression, social isolation (imposed or adopted), dealing with terminal illness, and guilt or blame over lifestyle. Suicidal ideation may be present.

Endogenous complications result from the neuropsychiatric sequelae of HIV infection, either from the direct effect of HIV neural infection, opportunistic central nervous system (CNS) infections, or CNS neoplasia. Up to half of patients with AIDS present signs and symptoms of CNS infection, including subacute encephalitis characterized by malaise, social withdrawal, lethargy and reduced sexual drive (these also may be signs and symptoms of depressed mood). Subsequently, signs of progressive dementia may appear. Neuropsychiatric deficits typically may involve impaired language, memory, and integrative abilities and occasionally depressed mood, and their insidious onset makes it important to maintain a high index of suspicion that psychological symptoms may indicate onset of neurologic involvement.

The potential for depressive reactions, sexual acting out, and further discrimination, stigmatization, and loss of social supports makes informed consent and adequate pre- and post-HIV test counseling mandatory.[54] Where individuals are infected with HIV, frequent psychological support (or referral to appropriate agencies) and attention to patient's genuine fears of exposure, pain, discrimination, abandonment, and death are indicated, rather than general reassurance, which may be interpreted as being dismissive. In cases of chronic depressed mood, pharmacotherapy or referral for psychotheraputic treatment is indicated.

PSYCHOSEXUAL PROBLEMS

Studies in Europe and India[32,55] and clinical experience in Africa have noted that sexual dysfunctions may present to STD clinics or be detected in STD clinics. In some countries, the clinical specialty of andrology serves men with STDs and psychosexual problems, as well as infertility and various urologic disorders. Over 13 percent of STD clinic presentations are for sexual dysfunctions in India, compared with only 4 percent in psychiatric clinics. Of these, over 80 percent are males with concerns over the effect of masturbation, erectile dysfunction, and premature ejaculation. Generally, presenting dysfunctions in males will include premature ejaculation, retarded ejaculation, and erectile dysfunction ("impotence"); in females, anorgasmia, general dysfunction ("frigidity"), and rarely, vaginismus (spasm of the muscles of the vaginal introitus preventing penetration). Psychosexual problems usually occur in STD patients secondary to pain from infection or trauma or from fear of infection, reinfection, or of infecting others. Patients or clinicians also sometimes may ascribe sexual dysfunction to STDs in the absence of objective evidence of an STD, and some clinicians may inappropriately offer therapy for a nonexistent STD in an effort to relieve sexual dysfunction.

In the case of mild or transient dysfunctions, the STD clinician can provide reassurance that such transient dysfunctions are not unusual and often are limited to particular partners, situations, and times, and information or education to correct misapprehensions that affect sexual performance is appropriate. However, chronic psychosexual problems that are not a result of physical pathology warrant referral to sex therapists. It is not uncommon to detect psychosexual dysfunctions in the course of history taking or treatment, and for some individuals, the STD clinic will be the first point of consultation for this problem. While the majority of sexual dysfunctions probably are mild and transient and may resolve with adequate information and encouragement, the major dysfunctions in males and females listed above require more specific therapy from specialists in psychosexual dysfunctions.

In summary, psychological variables may be determinants of STD infection, and psychological problems are commonly associated with acquisition of STDs. The physician should be aware of the range, nature, and presentations of these disorders, which may adversely affect attendance, compliance, and treatment, as well as the psychological state of the individual.

References

1 Goldman R, Goldman J: *Children's Sexual Thinking*. London, Routledge & Kegan Paul, 1984.

2 Ford, CS, Beach FA: *Patterns of Sexual Behavior*. New York, Harper & Row, 1951.

3 Shope DF: *Interpersonal Sexuality*. Philadelphia, Saunders, 1975.

4 Ross MW: A theory of normal homosexuality, in *Male and Female Homosexuality: Psychological Approaches,* L Diamant (ed). New York, Hemisphere, pp 237–259, 1987.

5 Raffaelli M et al: Sexual practices and attitudes of street youth in Belo Horizonte, Brazil. *Soc Sci Med* 37:661–670, 1993.

6 Hart G: *Sexual Maladjustment and Disease: An Introduction to Modern Venereology*. Chicago, Nelson-Hall, 1977.

7 Eysenck HJ, Eysenck SBG: *Manual of the EPI*. London, London University Press, 1964.

8 Eysenck HJ: *Sex and Personality*. London, Abacus, 1978.

9 Fulford KWM et al: Social and psychological factors in the distribution of STDs in male clinic attenders: II. Personality disorders, psychiatric illness and abnormal sexual attitudes. *Br J Vener Dis* 59:381–385, 1983.

10 Hart G: Factors influencing venereal infection in a war environment. *Br J Vener Dis* 50:68–72, 1974.

11 Ross MW: Sexually transmitted diseases in homosexual men: A study of four societies. *Br J Vener Dis* 60:52–55, 1984.

12 Ross MW: Sociological and psychological predictors of STD infection in homosexual men. *Br J Vener Dis* 60:110–113, 1984.
13 Ross MW: *Psychovenereology: Personality and Lifestyle Factors in Sexually Transmitted Diseases in Homosexual Men*. New York, Praeger, 1986.
14 Kalichman SC et al: Sexual sensation seeking: Scale development and predicting AIDS-related behavior among homosexually active men. *J Pers Assess* 62:385–397, 1994.
15 Bogaert AF, Fisher WA: Predictors of university men's number of sexual partners. *J Sex Res* 32:119–130, 1995.
16 Armytage WHG: Changing incidence and patterns of sexually transmitted diseases, in *Proceedings of the 15th Annual Symposium of the Eugenics Society*, London: Academic Press, 1981, pp 159–170, 1980.
17 Oriel JD: The global pattern of sexually transmitted diseases. *S Afr Med J* 61:993–998, 1982.
18 Hart G: Social and psychological aspects of venereal disease in Papua New Guinea. *Br J Vener Dis* 50:453–458, 1974.
19 Kelus J: Social and behavioral aspects of venereal disease. *Br J Vener Dis* 49:167–170, 1973.
20 Hooker E: Male homosexual lifestyles and venereal disease, in *Proceedings of the World Forum on Syphilis and Other Treponemotoses*. Public Health Service Publication 977. Washington, U.S. Government Printing Office, 1964.
21 Ross MW: Predictors of partner numbers in homosexual men: Psychosocial factors in four societies. *Sex Transm Dis* 11:119–122, 1984.
22 Schofield M: *Promiscuity*. London: Victor Gollancz, 1976.
23 Goode E, Troiden RR: Correlates and accompaniments of promiscuous sex among male homosexuals. *Psychiatry* 43:51–59, 1980.
24 McKusick L et al: Longitudinal predictors of reductions in unprotected anal intercourse among gay men in San Francisco: The AIDS Behavioral Research Project. *Am J Public Health* 80:978–983, 1990.
25 Haist M, Hewitt J: The butch-fem dichotomy in male homosexual behavior. *J Sex Res* 10:68–75, 1974.
26 Hooker E: An empirical study of some relations between sexual patterns and gender identity in male homosexuals, in *Sex Research: New Developments*, J. Money (ed). New York, Holt, Rinehart & Winston, pp 24–52, 1965.
27 Ross MW: Personality factors which differentiate homosexual men with positive and negative attitudes toward condom use. *NY State J Med* 88:626–628, 1988.
28 Ross MW: Psychological determinants of increased condom use and safer sex in homosexual men: A longitudinal study. *Int J STD AIDS* 1:98–101, 1990.
29 Humphreys RAL: *Tearoom Trade: A Study of Impersonal Sex in Public Places*. London: Duckworth, 1970.
30 Lewis LA, Ross MW: *A Select Body: The Gay Dance Party Subculture and the HIV/AIDS Pandemic*. London: Cassell, 1995.
31 Treffke H et al: The relationship between attitude, assertiveness and condom use. *Psychol Health* 6:45–52, 1992.
32 Catalan J et al: Sexual dysfunction and psychiatric morbidity in patients attending a clinic for sexually transmitted diseases. *Br J Psychiatry* 138:292–296, 1981.
33 Fitzpatrick R et al: Survey of psychological disturbance in patients attending a sexually transmitted diseases clinic. *Genitourin Med* 62: 111–115, 1986.
34 Bhanji S, Mahony JDH: The value of a psychiatric service within the venereal disease clinic. *Br J Vener Dis* 54:566–568, 1978.
35 Barczak P et al: Patterns of psychiatric morbidity in a genitourinary clinic. *Br J Psychiatry* 152:698–700, 1988.
36 Ross MW: Illness behavior among patients attending a sexually transmitted disease clinic. *Sex Transm Dis* 14:174–179, 1987.
37 Ross MW: Psychosocial factors in admitting to homosexuality in sexually transmitted disease clinics. *Sex Transm Dis* 12:83–86, 1985.
38 Longo D, Koehn K: Psychosocial factors and recurrent genital herpes: A review of prediction and psychiatric treatment studies. *Int J Psychiatry Med* 23:99–117, 1993.
39 Stronks DL et al: Psychological consequences of genital herpes: An exploratory study with a gonorrhea control group. *Psychol Rep* 73: 395–400, 1993.
40 Carney O et al: A prospective study of the psychological impact on patients with a first episode of genital herpes. *Genitourin Med* 70:40–45, 1994.
41 Drob S et al: Genital herpes: The psychological consequences. *Br J Med Psychol* 58:307–315, 1985.
42 Aral SO et al: Genital herpes: Does knowledge lead to action? *Am J Public Health* 75:69–71, 1985.
43 Miller JD et al: A "pseudo-AIDS" syndrome following from fear of AIDS. *Br J Psychiatry* 146:550–551, 1985.
44 MacAlpine I: Syphilophobia. *Br J Vener Dis* 33:92–99, 1957.
45 Ross MW: AIDS phobias: A study of four cases. *Psychopathology* 21: 26–30, 1988.
46 McGuire LS et al: Psychosexual functioning in symptomatic and asymptomatic women with and without signs of vaginitis. *Am J Obstet Gynecol* 137:600–603, 1980.
47 Miller F et al: Two cases of factitious acquired immune deficiency syndrome. *Am J Psychiatry* 143:1483, 1986.
48 Robinson EN, Latham RH: A factitious case of acquired immune deficiency syndrome. *Sex Transm Dis* 14:54–57, 1987.
49 Taylor S, Hyler SE: Update on factitious disorders. *Int J Psychiatry Med* 23:81–94, 1993.
50 Ross MW: Measuring attitudes toward AIDS: Their structure and interactions. *Hosp Commun Psychiatry* 39:1306–1308, 1988.
51 Amchin J, Polan HJ: A longitudinal account of staff adaptation to AIDS patients on a psychiatric ward. *Hosp Commun Psychiatry* 37: 1235–1238, 1986.
52 Rosser BRS, Ross MW: Perceived emotional and life change impact of AIDS on homosexual men in two countries. *Psychol Health* 2:301–317, 1988.
53 Faulstich ME: Psychiatric aspects of AIDS. *Am J Psychiatry* 144:551–556, 1987.
54 Ross MW, Channon-Little LD: *Discussing Sexuality: A Guide for Health Practitioners*. Sydney, Australia, MacLennan & Petty, 1991.
55 Rao RVR: Prevalence of psychosexual problems in patients attending the STD clinic. *Ind J Sex Transm Dis* 7:67–69, 1986.

PART V PROFILES OF GROUPS AND BEHAVIORS WITH HIGH PRIORITY FOR INTERVENTION

Chapter 8

Gender perspectives and STDs

Gail Bolan
Anke A. Ehrhardt
Judith N. Wasserheit

INTRODUCTION

Gender influences sexual behaviors and sexually transmitted disease (STD) susceptibility, which together affect the efficiency of STD transmission. Gender also affects the likelihood that STD care will be sought, the ease with which infection is detected, the type of health care received, how partners are managed, and the long-term reproductive health consequences of sexually transmitted infections. The magnitude of these differences varies depending on a number of other factors, such as age, socioeconomic status, cultural norms, education, and marital status, and must be considered when designing strategies for STD prevention and management.

GENDER DIFFERENCES IN SEXUAL BEHAVIOR

Sexual behavior varies from individual to individual, by social context, and within different societies. One of the critical categories of differentiation is gender. Girls, boys, women, and men not only have different bodies, they are also socialized into different gender roles that significantly influence their sexual behavior. Thus, gender influences physical characteristics and social roles that, in turn, affect the expression of sexual behavior patterns. Furthermore, gender differences in sexual behavior may change with one's age, social contacts, or cultural norms.[1] Prevention and treatment of sexually transmitted diseases require sexual negotiation and cooperation between partners. In the case of heterosexual encounters, women's and men's gender roles are clearly important modifiers of negotiation about sexual practices and means of protection.

It has been suggested that the strong early effects of gender on social behaviors of young children are the roots for some of the sexual interactions that occur among adolescents and subsequently among adults.[2] For example, in studies of children in same or mixed gender groups who were asked to set up a cooperative system, all groups managed to achieve cooperation. However, the techniques used were different and one child in each group emerged as the dominant one. In the boys' group, dominant boys tended to use physical force, whereas dominant girls used verbal persuasion. The same experiment on mixed groups of two boys and two girls resulted in the boys achieving the dominant role and the girls occupying helping positions. The verbal persuasion that worked for girls with other girls was not effective with boys, and girls' attempts to influence boys often were not very effective even at the early age of 33 months.[3]

The development of sexuality also starts long before puberty. Both boys and girls masturbate long before puberty and engage in playful sexual behavior with each other throughout the first decade. Although sexual activities in childhood are exploratory and sporadic, in adolescence sexual concerns and behavior become a major part of everyday life and become linked to falling in love, erotic imagery, and involvement with another person.[4]

From the earliest manifestations of sexual behavior, gender differences between adolescent boys and girls are apparent. Although most adolescents begin having intercourse in their mid to late teens, boys tend to initiate sexual intercourse at an earlier age than young women. Different surveys are consistent in reporting that approximately 70 percent of young men and about 50 percent of young women have experienced sexual intercourse by age 18.[5] Data from the 1995 National Survey of Family Growth suggest a slight decrease in young women between the ages of 15 to 19 years who report sexual intercourse, 50 percent in 1995 compared to 55 percent in 1990.[6]

In addition to initiating sexual activity earlier, young men also report more partners than young women; for example, 17 percent reported five or more partners before age 18 compared to 5.5 percent of women.[7] Young women often experience their first sexual intercourse with a sexual partner who is older than they are. In 1995, about two-thirds of women who had their first voluntary intercourse before they were 16 had had a first partner who was under the age of 18; however, one-third had had first partners who were at least 18 to 19 years of age.[6]

It is believed that earlier age of onset of intercourse is associated with higher total numbers of lifetime sexual partners. However, definitive evidence is lacking in this regard. Kinsey et al. documented for adolescent males who started sexual behavior early, a lifetime pattern of greater sexual activity than for their peers who initiated sexual activity at a later age.[8] In this report, however, sexual activity may have been either within a single long-term relationship or with numerous partners. Since the Kinsey report, other data from adolescents confirm that, in comparison with females in the same age group, adolescent males have a higher number of partners during adolescence. In one study, the proportion of males aged 18 to 19 with multiple partners was 50 percent, compared to 34 percent of females in the same age group.[9] However, age of onset of intercourse was not included in the analyses and longitudinal information was not available to indicate whether this pattern was sustained beyond the adolescent period to result in higher numbers of lifetime partners among men.

Other important gender differences are related to the context of sexual intercourse during adolescence. More young men state that they wanted their first intercourse to happen than young women, who reported more often being forced or coerced. For instance, in 1995 about 8 percent of women 15 to 44 years of age report that their first intercourse was not voluntary.[6] If voluntarily engaging in sex, women and men differ in their reasons to do so. Young women more often cite affection and love for their partner, whereas young men are more likely to be motivated by curiosity about sex.[7]

In addition to the number of partners, gender differences are also seen in rate of sex partner change, another important factor in disease transmission and especially in sustaining STDs in a population. When people live in a coupled relationship (marriage or cohabitation), the rate of partner change drops and many restrict their sexual activity to the primary partner relationship, at least for a while. Both men and women have fewer partners with age. However, men report more partners than women, a pattern that persists over the life course. The group with the highest proportion having had five or more partners within the past year is young, unmarried men.[7] These data suggest that males have more high-risk sexual behaviors as defined by age of first intercourse, number of partners, and rate of sexual partner change. Thus, risk reduction prevention efforts that emphasize partner numbers and rate

Sections of this chapter are an updated version of the chapter entitled Age, Gender, and Sexual Risk Behaviors for Sexually Transmitted Diseases in the United States by Ehrhardt and Wasserheit in *Research Issues in Human Behavior and Sexually Transmitted Diseases in the AIDS Era*. Washington D.C., ASM, 1191 (reference 1).

of sex partner change may often be more appropriate for males than females.

Risk for STD is not only determined by partner number and rate of sex partner change, but also by sexual practice within a hierarchy of risk from receptive anal intercourse and penile-vaginal intercourse as high risk for infection (depending on the STD) to oral sex as relatively lower risk. Vaginal intercourse as a lifetime incidence is almost universally practiced by women (97%) and men (95%).[7] However, vaginal intercourse with an infected partner puts a woman at greater risk for infection with HIV and other STDs than a man.

Oral sex is not as commonly practiced as vaginal sex and more men report receiving or performing oral sex at last sexual encounter than women. However, lifetime incidence of oral sex is similar among men and women, approaching three-quarters.[7] Women and men who practice oral sex vary by race, education, and religion. Generally, whites report higher rates than all other racial or ethnic groups, and men and women with higher education more frequently experience oral sex. Finally, religion is also associated with lifetime incidence of oral sex. Its effect is minimal, however, and is confounded by other factors, such as education.[7]

Unlike oral sex, anal sex is not part of the repertoire of regular sexual practices for most women and men in the United States. Approximately, 25 percent of men and 20 percent of women have experienced anal intercourse at least once, but only about 10 percent report it over the last year.[7] Receptive anal intercourse puts women and men at much greater risk for HIV infection and several other STDs than the insertive male partner.

Perceptions regarding condom use and barriers to use, two factors that influence condom behaviors, also differ by gender. In the 1991 study of American men, involving several thousand African-American and white American men, ages 20 to 39, 27 percent of sexually active men reported using a condom in the 4 weeks before the interview.[10] The same survey assessed perceptions regarding consequences of condom use. From a psychological and interpersonal perspective, men most frequently stated that a condom "shows that you are a concerned and caring person." However, the same men usually agreed that using a condom sends unwanted messages to the sexual partner, such as it "makes your partner think that you have AIDS" or "shows that you think your partner has AIDS." Other important obstacles included embarrassment when buying condoms and concerns that condom use results in reduced sexual sensation, that care must be taken during sex to prevent condom breakage, and that quick withdrawal after sex is required or the condom may come off.

Women, on the other hand, are much more concerned about their male partners' reactions if they introduce condom use. Issues of trust and commitment to the relationship are barriers coupled with a strong wish for the availability of a repertoire of methods that are independent of partner negotiations.[11,12] Since men have more control over condom use than women do, effective interventions to increase condom use should be designed specifically for men.

Our knowledge of sexual behavior among older men and women, in general, is lacking because of prejudice and a societal focus on youth and young adults. With increasing age, both men and women undergo sociological and physiological changes that may affect their sexual behaviors. In a classic study of 100 women between the ages of 43 and 53, Neugarten reported that two-thirds of the women described no effect of menopause on sexuality, with the other one-third being split, half attributing a positive effect to the end of pregnancy concerns and the other half judging sexuality as less important.[13]

Middle-aged men also experience hormonal changes, especially a decrease in testosterone.[14] It may take them longer to achieve erections, because of these changes or medications for other health problems. They may also experience sporadic impotence, which may produce so much anxiety that some men begin to reduce or avoid sexual behavior. Others may continue a very active sex life. However, condom use may be avoided by some because it is seen as an additional impediment to erectile performance and thus becomes an important issue for STD and HIV prevention in older adults.

Our knowledge about sexuality in the elderly is even more fragmentary. One of the isolated studies on sexual behaviors in the elderly collected data on 102 women and 100 men between the ages of 80 and 102.[15] Both men and women were considered to be in good physical and mental health and gender differences were found. Seventy percent of women compared with 38 percent of the men did not have sexual intercourse. More men than women still masturbated. More men than women who had sexual intercourse enjoyed it, whereas there had not been any difference regarding sexual enjoyment reported between men and women when they were younger.

These gender differences in sexual behaviors identified at all ages make it imperative that we tailor our prevention strategies for STDs and HIV infection to the different patterns among men and women, and are cognizant of the fact that to be effective we need specific programs for men and women that are aimed at the specific risk behaviors we want to change. One can not attribute changes in sexual behavior to any one main factor; rather they have to be seen as the result of an interplay of different factors, some physiological and some sociological, that vary by gender.

GENDER DIFFERENCES IN COMMUNICATION AND NEGOTIATIONS

Gender roles obviously are important modifiers in how sexual encounters are negotiated and who determines which sexual practices will prevail. Women and men often follow a specific gender script when they engage in sexual behavior with each other. For instance, it is currently still the expected norm that men more frequently initiate sexual behavior within a new relationship and that they have greater power in determining whether condoms are used or not.[16] Thus, it is essential for the design of effective interventions to be gender specific.

Currently, it is well accepted that realistic strategies for protection for women are embedded in the social and gender-specific contexts of their relationships with men. The importance of gender-specific interventions aiming at behavior change for women and for men is also borne out in recent reviews of the effectiveness of interventions for women at risk for HIV and STDs.[17,18] A review of 47 studies revealed that there were 30, which showed some impact on sexual risk behavior. The impact varied by intervention type, session duration, and whether studies included women alone or both men and women. The review classified 16 studies that provided the reader with enough detail and methodological rigor to be included in a more detailed analysis and discussion (Table 8-1).[18–37] The review concluded that HIV prevention programs can be effective in changing sexual risk behavior among women, particularly when targeted directly to women and focused on the relevant behavioral skills of empowerment, negotiation, and refusal. Thus, prevention for women needs to focus on negotiation and refusal skills rather than simply on condom enhancement.

It is important to stress that negotiation in sexual encounters is not only straightforward verbal persuasion, but can be indirect, using behavioral signals and circuitous reasoning. For instance, in a recent study, women were asked to describe their communication patterns with men around safer sex.[38] Although many women initiate talking about risk of unprotected sexual intercourse in a

Table 8–1. Review of HIV Interventions for At-Risk Women in the US, Puerto Rico, and Canada 1980–1996*

Intervention Type Authors	Age of Women Participants	Gender Specific?	# of Sessions[1]	Significant?	Outcomes[2]	Follow-up Period
Informational						
Kalichman et al., 19	M = 32.1	Yes	1	Yes	*HIV testing; condom request*	2 Weeks
Kalichman and Coley, 20	M = 26.8 (s.d. = 8.1)	Yes	1	Yes	*HIV testing;* condom use	2 Weeks
Condom/spermicide skills						
Calsyn et al., 21, 22	M = 39.1	No	1	No	Condom use; number of partners	4 and 18 months
HIV counseling and testing						
Ickovics et al., 23	M = 30.8 (range = 18–61)	Yes	1	No	Condom use	2 Weeks and 3 months
Enhanced HIV counseling and testing						
Nyamathi et al., 24	Group Means = 32.3, 33.3	Yes	1	Yes[3]	*Number of partners*	2 Weeks
Nyamathi et al., 25	M = 31.3 (s.d. = 9.5)	Yes	1	Yes[3]	*Number of partners*	2 Weeks
Relational skills						
Schilling et al., 26; El-Bassel and Schilling, 27	90% 21–42	Yes	5	Yes	*Condom use and acquisition;* number of partners	2 Weeks and 15 months
Cohen et al., 28	M = 26.6	No	1	No	STD reinfection rate	6–9 months
Cohen et al., 29	most early to late 30s	No	1	No	STD reinfection rate	6–9 months
McCusker et al., 30	53% from 25 to 34	No	7	No	Condom use; number of partners	Median 48 weeks
Smith and Dickson, 31	M = 18.8	Yes	1	No	Condom use	2 Months
Hobfoll et al., 32	M = 21 (range 16–29)	Yes	5	Yes	*Condom use and acquisition; spermicide use;* spermicide acquisition	6 Months
Kelly et al., 33	M = 29	Yes	5	Yes	*Condom use; unprotected vaginal intercourse;* number of partners	3 Months
El-Bassel et al., 34	M = 32.8 (range 18–55)	Yes	16	Yes	*Safer sex improvement or maintenance*	1 Month
Community						
Tross et al., 35, 36	not reported	Yes	—	Yes	*Condom use*	8–16 months
Santelli et al., 37	range = 17–35	Yes	—	Yes	*Condom use*	1 Year

*This table was previously published as *Table IX Studies Meeting Minimal Methodological Criteria* in Exner, Seal and Ehrhardt, 1997 (reference 18).
[1]Number of sessions of significant intervention or greatest number of sessions among nonsignificant interventions.
[2]Significant variables are italicized.
[3]Both an information-enhanced and a relational skills-enhanced HIV counseling intervention yielded significant reductions in partner numbers. There was not a no treatment control; thus, this may be a cohort effect.

new relationship and may suggest condom use, most of them dramatically change their approach if their partner is unwilling and introduces issues of lack of trust. In response, women tend to reassure their partner and deflect the issues. They often switch to pregnancy prevention or other reasons for safer sex that are more acceptable to both their partner and themselves. At the same time, many women admit to remaining concerned and worried about STDs and HIV, but are unable to insist on safer sex with an unwilling partner. One is reminded of the early childhood studies, described in the preceding, which demonstrated that girls and boys use gender-specific styles of negotiation around cooperation and dominance and which showed that girls in early childhood tend to use verbal persuasion, which is effective with other girls but not with boys.[3]

GENDER DIFFERENCES IN STD SUSCEPTIBILITY

Just as gender differences in sexual behavior may affect transmission of STDs (including HIV infection) and development of sequelae, physiological changes in the genital tract also influence these outcomes, particularly in females. (Table 8-2) In adolescent girls, these behavioral and biomedical factors act synergistically

Table 8–2. Gender Differences Affecting STDs Clinical and Epidemiological Factors

STD transmission and manifestations	
Susceptibility	F ≫ M (HIV Infection) F > M (discharge syndromes) F ~ M (genital ulcers)
Infectiousness	No gender-specific data
Symptoms	More common and specific in M
Signs	More common and specific in M
STD complications	
Upper tract infection	F ≫ M
Infertility	F only
Genital cancer	F ≫ M
Adverse outcomes of pregnancy Fetal wastage, low birth weight, prematurity, congenital or neonatal infection)	F only
Increased HIV transmission	F and M

F = females
M = males

to dramatically increase the risk of sexually transmitted infections and their complications. Subsequently, however, these factors often contribute differentially; in women during the reproductive years, sexual and health behaviors may outweigh biological factors as determinants of disease incidence, whereas in postmenopausal women, physiological changes with the potential to facilitate transmission of STDs, including HIV, are usually offset by behavioral patterns that are relatively protective.

In the female, susceptibility to STDs and their sequelae is a function of a number of physiological factors, including the type of epithelial lining in the lower genital tract; the resident flora and acidity (pH) of the vagina; the characteristics of the cervical mucus; the patency of the endocervical canal; the phase of the menstrual cycle; and the immunological repertoire of the individual.[39,40] During the cascade of developmental events that stretches from birth through adolescence, there are significant alterations in each of these.

The striking changes that occur in cellular morphology in the vagina and the cervix have a direct effect on the spectrum of STDs found at each stage of development. In the first several weeks of life, because of the residual effect of maternal estrogen, the vagina of the neonate is lined by stratified squamous epithelium similar to that of adults.[41,42] These cells are resistant to chlamydial and gonococcal infection but are susceptible to trichomoniasis and candidiasis. From about 1 month of age until menarche, the squamous epithelium is replaced by thin, atrophic columnar epithelium that supports chlamydial and gonococcal growth. Beginning with the estrogen stimulation associated with puberty, thicker, glycogen-containing stratified squamous epithelium again covers the vaginal vault and columnar epithelium is limited to the cervix.

The interface between these two types of epithelium is called the squamocolumnar junction, and age-related changes in its location may also influence susceptibility to STDs. During adolescence, this junction is often exposed on the surface of the cervix (ectocervix). With aging, it usually migrates into the endocervical canal. Ectocervical columnar epithelium is referred to as the zone of ectopy, and because of the affinity of gonococci and chlamydiae for columnar cells, its size is believed to correlate with risk of cervical infection.[42–44]

From infancy to adolescence, vaginal ecology shifts from a normal or endogenous flora dominated by enteric organisms to one in which lactobacilli are the most common species.[45,46] Over this same period, probably because of lactic acid production by the lactobacilli, vaginal fluid becomes more acidic, with a fall in pH from about 7.0 during childhood to the 4.0 to 4.5 range after puberty. This shift, together with lactobacillus production of hydrogen peroxide and other antibacterial products, inhibits the growth of some genital tract pathogens in vitro.[40,47,48] However, the clinical relevance of resident flora in susceptibility to STDs remains unclear. Gonococcal infection rates in women exposed to men with gonorrhea, for example, do not appear to vary with patterns of cervicovaginal flora.[40] More recently, it has been hypothesized, based on in vitro studies, that lactobacilli and lower pH, may have a protective effect on HIV transmission; however, to date studies have been inconclusive.[49]

Cervical mucus production, the third potential defense against infection, also fluctuates in response to hormonal changes from birth to adolescence. Paralleling the epithelial changes described in the preceding, cervical mucus is abundant through the first month of life and then relatively scant until puberty.[50] Around puberty, high levels of estrogen stimulate copious mucus secretion, but in contrast to mucus of older adolescents or adult women, this mucus is easily penetrable by organisms, as well as by sperm. After menarche, a monthly cycle of mucus production is established, with maximal secretion and minimal viscosity during the periovulatory phase (midcycle).[51]

These changes in cervical mucus may affect transmission of STDs or development of sequelae in several ways. Perhaps most important, cervical mucus provides a functional barrier both against attachment of pathogens to epithelial surfaces and against ascent of organisms into the uterus and fallopian tubes. The former is probably facilitated by the lubricating effect of the mucus, and by binding of organisms to carbohydrate complexes in the mucus matrix.[39] Mucus also appears to provide support for other defenses against infection, such as antibacterial enzymes, antibodies, and leukocytes.[39,40,51]

Patency or opening of the endocervical canal occurs at approximately 9 or 10 years of age and explains the dramatically increased risk of upper tract infection (pelvic inflammatory disease, or PID) observed in peripubertal girls with cervical infection compared with younger children.[52] The penetrability of peripubertal cervical mucus mentioned in the preceding and immunological naiveté are probably the major biological reasons for the higher incidence of PID in this group than in older adolescents and adult women.

In women, during the adult reproductive years, physiological changes that affect risk of STDs are related primarily to the menstrual cycle, pregnancy, and contraceptive use. The menstrual cycle appears to influence risk of upper tract infection in women. Several studies suggest that symptomatic gonococcal or chlamydial PID occurs most frequently during the first week of the cycle.[53,54] The reasons for this are poorly understood but may include the relative penetrability of the cervical mucus plug during menses and the reflux of potentially contaminated blood into the fallopian tubes, a phenomenon that often accompanies menstrual uterine contractions. In gonococcal infection, two other factors may be important. Iron, which is abundant in menstrual blood, may promote gonococcal growth. In addition, the type of gonococcus that causes tubal infection (transparent phenotype) proliferates at the cervix during menstruation.[55,56]

Pregnancy is associated with immunological, anatomical, and microbiological changes that affect risk of STDs and their sequelae.[57–59] Host defenses, for example, are normally suppressed during pregnancy, probably as a maternal adaptation to avoid immunological rejection of the fetus as a foreign body. This immune suppression often affects the course of genital tract infections. It is thought to be responsible for the accelerated progression or expression of human papillomavirus, the augmented frequency and severity of recurrences of genital herpes (herpes simplex virus), and the relatively benign course of syphilis observed during pregnancy.[60–64]

Gestational changes may increase susceptibility to cervicitis but tend to protect the upper tract from infection. Cervical infection may be facilitated by hormone-driven increases in the size of the zone of ectopy.[65] Simultaneously, decreased penetrability of the cervical mucus plug and obliteration of the uterine cavity by the growing fetus decrease the risk of PID.[51] After week 16 of pregnancy, however, the fetal membranes rest over the internal cervical opening, and infection of these membranes (chorioamnionitis) increases in frequency.

The microbiological changes that occur during pregnancy may have evolved primarily to provide a safe cervicovaginal environment for the infant during delivery, but may also protect the woman from acquisition of some STDs. In the lower genital tract, changes such as decreased pH, increased glycogen stores, and increased vascularity facilitate growth of lactobacilli and suppress growth of several other bacterial species, particularly anaerobes. As discussed, products of lactobacilli inhibit growth of pathogens such as gonococci in vitro.[48]

Finally, contraceptives are often important factors in altering risk of STDs during the reproductive years.[66–69] Condoms and diaphragms serve as mechanical barriers to attachment of genital pathogens.[68] Laboratory testing of spermicides indicates that compounds such as nonoxynol-9 can kill most sexually transmitted organisms, including gonococci, chlamydia, treponemes, trichomonads, herpes simplex virus, and HIV.[66,70] Clinical studies of the efficacy of spermicides in prevention of STDs support these findings with respect to gonorrhea and chlamydia, but have been inconclusive with respect to HIV.[70–75] One issue may be that with very frequent use, spermicides may cause local inflammation and genital ulceration, possibly offsetting the decreased number of viable organisms with an increased likelihood of infection per organism.

Intrauterine devices and hormonal contraceptives influence risk of STDs and their sequelae principally via effects on host defenses.[66] Users of intrauterine devices run a 1.5- to twofold increased risk of PID compared with women who are not using contraceptives.[76,77] This risk appears to be greatest around the time of insertion and is due to contamination of the uterine cavity with cervicovaginal flora.[78] Intrauterine devices may also impair uterine clearance mechanisms when organisms do breach the cervical barrier. Oral contraceptive pills may increase risk of cervical chlamydial infection by increasing the size of zone of ectopy.[44,79–82] Oral contraceptive pills, however, appear to decrease both the frequency and severity of PID.[83–87] Possible mechanisms for these protective effects include reduced penetrability of cervical mucus, reduced uterine contractions during menses, and alteration of immunological responses. The impact of injectable hormonal agents on STDs has not been examined systematically.

With aging beyond the reproductive years, hormonal changes in women and waning immune defenses in both sexes predispose to increased incidence and severity of genital tract infections. These increases are, however, largely theoretical and generally have not been reflected in studies of older populations. Probably the most important reason for this is that the sexual behaviors discussed in the preceding section on gender differences in sexual behavior generally place individuals over 50 years of age at low risk of exposure to STD pathogens. The tendency of health care providers to omit testing for STDs in geriatric patients and the small number of studies of STDs in this age group may also contribute to this impression.

At menopause, a sharp decline in estrogen levels heralds atrophic changes in the vagina, with thinning of the epithelium, reduced lubrication, and narrowing and shortening of the vaginal canal.[42,88] These changes may be less pronounced in postmenopausal women who continue to be sexually active, but it is not clear whether level of sexual activity is modulated by discomfort secondary to senescent changes or whether degree of atrophy is modulated by sexual activity.[89] Decreases in vascularity and glycogen content in the lower genital tract have been postulated to result in alterations of cervicovaginal flora in postmenopausal women, but most studies have failed to confirm major shifts.[42,90]

Unfortunately, little is known about analogous physiological changes in the male that might affect an individual's risk of STDs or their sequelae. For example, although the epithelial lining of the male urethra has been well characterized, we could find no data on changes with age.[91] Similarly, although a few investigators have examined the normal urethral flora in adolescent males, little information is available on normal flora at earlier or older ages or on the role of these organisms in protection against STDs.[92] Finally, there is evidence that seminal and prostatic fluids contain factors with marked antibacterial activity, but no understanding of when or how boys begin to exhibit significant levels of these factors in genital secretions.[93–96] The dearth of data on changes in the anus and rectum also limits discussion of biological risk factors for STDs associated with anal intercourse in men having sex with men and in heterosexual women.

One factor that does appear to alter risk of acquisition of STDs in males is circumcision. Most studies have not controlled for potentially confounding behavioral variables and therefore cannot be considered definitive. However, both in industrialized countries and in the developing world, lack of circumcision has been linked repeatedly to an increased risk of a broad spectrum of STDs inducing chancroid, syphilis, gonorrhea, and HIV infection.[97–102] Recent studies that adjusted for potentially confounding demographic, behavioral, and clinical factors have identified an association between uncircumcised status and syphilis or gonorrhea in the United States, and HIV or urethritis in Africa.[101,102] The biological mechanisms for these associations are not well understood, but may include the tendency of the foreskin to serve as a reservoir for STD pathogens and the susceptibility of the nonkeratinized foreskin to trauma and secondary microbial invasion. The presence of a foreskin may also decrease detection of STDs, thereby increasing the likelihood both of complications and additional transmission. It is likely that part of the STD risk associated with lack of circumcision can be circumvented by careful genital hygiene and self-examination. Yet the weight of the evidence suggests that foreskin is also a site of biological vulnerability to STDs and that in communities in which there is a high population prevalence of infection, circumcision may have significant personal and public health benefits.

GENDER DIFFERENCES IN TRANSMISSION OF STDS

Rigorous studies of STD transmission are scarce because they are difficult to perform both logistically and ethically. Available data, which are not definitive, have suggested that transmission of STD pathogens that cause a discharge or reside in genital secretions (e.g., HIV, Hepatitis B, gonococci, chlamydiae) are generally more efficient from male-to-female than from female-to-male.[103–111] For example, male-to-female transmission of HIV may be at least 20 times as efficient as female-to-male transmission.[105] Although, in general, transmission of gonorrhea or chlamydia is more efficient than HIV, the gender difference in efficiency of transmission may not be as great.[112,113] Transmission of STD pathogens that cause genital ulcers or lesions (e.g., herpes simplex virus, treponemes, and *Haemophilus ducreyi*, the causative organism of chancroid) has appeared to be roughly equally efficient between genders but definitive data are lacking.[98,114] The absence of differential transmission in the case of herpes, syphilis, and chancroid may be owing to the facts that genital ulcer pathogens depend on small breaks in the epithelium to establish infection and that microtrauma probably occurs in both partners during vigorous sexual intercourse. However, more recent studies suggest male-to-female transmission of herpes simplex virus is more efficient than female-to-male. In a study of discordant couples, the annual risk of genital herpes transmission was 19 percent from men to women but only 5 percent from women to men.[115] Herpes simplex virus seroprevalence studies have also demonstrated that women are more likely than men to be infected with HSV-2, a finding that could be explained by differences in sexual behavior or more efficient male-to-female transmission.[116]

In the case of STD pathogens that cause discharge, the more efficient transmission from male to female may be partly due to more extended contact with pathogens after sexual exposure among women with infected male partners than among men with infected female partners. If the male partner has one of these STDs, infected semen is deposited in the vagina and remains there following intercourse; in contrast, if the female partner is infected, the male's exposure to organisms is largely limited to the duration of coitus. It is also possible that the cervix is more easily infected than the urethra of the male. However, in one recent study using DNA amplification tests to detect chlamydia, rates of infection in sexual partnerships were nearly identical.[113] These data suggest that after multiple episodes of sexual intercourse the cumulative risk of infection may not differ by gender. Additional studies of infection rates by gender using more sensitive diagnostic methods are needed to better define gender differences in transmission efficiency of gonorrhea and chlamydia, both following a single exposure and following multiple sexual contacts.

GENDER DIFFERENCES IN HEALTH CARE-SEEKING BEHAVIORS AND HEALTH CARE SERVICES

Although overall, women are more likely than men to seek health care, care for STDs appears to be an important exception for several reasons.[117–119] Women infected with STDs are far more likely than men to be asymptomatic or minimally symptomatic. For example, approximately 75 percent of chlamydia-infected women are asymptomatic compared with about 50 percent of men. Furthermore, for anatomical reasons, both abnormal discharge and painless genital lesions may be more likely to go unnoticed in women than men. When symptoms of STDs do occur, these are generally less clearly attributable to STDs in women than men and may be mistakenly diagnosed as other infectious processes, including urinary tract and vaginal infections in women. In addition, even traditionally painful syndromes such as chancroid are frequently associated with milder symptoms in women.[120] Even among infected women who do interpret symptoms as potential cues to action, presentation to a public STD clinic may be so stigma-laden that it is not considered a viable option. In many societies around the world, contracting an STD is considered a rite of passage to manhood for an adolescent boy or an insignificant nuisance for an older man, but an extremely shameful occurrence for a young girl and her whole family.

Women also have health care alternatives that are not available to men. Many women who can afford to do so consult gynecologists for symptoms of STDs. Too often in the past, these providers have had limited STD expertise and laboratory capabilities and have failed to provide adequate sexual history taking, diagnosis, treatment, counseling, or partner management.[121–123]

Health care systems have added to the gender differences in access to STD care. Until recently, family planning programs have focused on reducing fertility and ignored closely related reproductive health problems such as STDs. These programs also failed to address the needs of male partners. Conversely, STD clinics have traditionally served men well, but were less sensitive to the needs of women.[123]

STD care also depends, in part, on the quality of the physician–patient relationship. Gender related difficulties have been reported by lesbian, bisexual, and heterosexual women as well as gay men and transgender people.[124–127] Physician attitudes, prejudices, and assumptions about sexual practices adversely affect the provision of STD care by gender. One example has been the failure to identify HIV infections in women compared with men because of a different threshold of suspicion by providers.[128]

Another alternative to seeking medical care has been use of over-the-counter douches, vaginal yeast products, or other intravaginal preparations as home remedies for symptoms of STDs. Women are more likely than men to self-treat and unfortunately, their use often masks, rather than cures infection.[129] Since no specific diagnosis is made, treatment is often incorrect and partners are not notified and treated appropriately.[129] Recent studies also suggest that douching is linked to an increased incidence of upper tract infection and ectopic pregnancy, either because of incomplete eradication of pathogens or because organisms are forced up into the uterus by the pressure with which the douche is applied.[130–132]

GENDER DIFFERENCES IN DETECTION OF STDS

Even when women do seek STD care, detection of STDs is frequently more difficult in women than in men. Gender differences in the predictive value of clinical symptoms, signs, and of laboratory tests present problems.[133] Although clinical diagnosis in the absence of laboratory testing can be useful in men with STDs, the two most common syndromes in women, vaginitis and cervicitis, cannot be used to reliably diagnose STDs on clinical criteria alone. The low sensitivity and specificity of clinical signs and symptoms of nonulcerative STDs in women have necessitated the use of laboratory tests that have traditionally required speculum examination and more expensive, technically sophisticated diagnostic procedures. Furthermore, the large number and variety of cells and bacteria that are normally present in the vaginal vault reduce the sensitivity and specificity of methods such as Gram staining and fluorescent monoclonal antibody staining of lower tract specimens. Cultures of cervicovaginal secretions are also more likely than cultures of the male urethra to be uninterpretable because of contamination by resident nonpathogenic organisms. In addition, the presence of inhibitors such as blood, that interfere with DNA amplification tests and result in false negative tests may be more common in cervical specimens than specimens from the male urethra.[134] Last, specimen collection from the endocervix in females may be hampered by cervical mucus and a small cervical os. On the other hand, accurate diagnosis of STDs in men is usually relatively simple and inexpensive, with the exceptions of trichomoniasis and chlamydia detection, for which urethral columnar epithilium has been needed for adequate specimen collection.

The recent advent of urine-based testing for chlamydia and gonorrhea using more sensitive nucleic acid amplification techniques should reduce these detection problems in the future for both sexes. The preceding factors of contamination and decreased sensitivity owing to vaginal flora do not appear to compromise the test performance characteristics of these new, urine-based nucleic acid amplification tests. These urine-based tests provide a unique opportunity to expand screening beyond the traditional clinic-based setting; women no longer have to undergo an invasive pelvic examination and men no longer need experience a painful urethral swab to be tested. Future STD detection options for women include patient-collected vaginal swabs, which are currently under investigation for chlamydia detection and appear promising.

Although STDs in women are more difficult to diagnosis than those in men, the recommended STD treatment regimens appear to be equally efficacious in women and men.[135]

GENDER DIFFERENCES IN PARTNER MANAGEMENT

An essential component in managing STDs at both the individual and community level is to ensure adequate treatment of sexual partners before resuming sexual activity. In addition, it is important for individuals to protect themselves from future infections. Gender differences in relationships are multifactorial and widespread. Violence against women, often in the context of sexuality and reproduction, double standards of sexual behavior, and the imbalance of power in many sexual relationships, frequently limit women's capacity to protect themselves, even when they have the information and knowledge to do so.[136]

If women have difficulty protecting themselves from STDs, then treatment of partners exposed to STDs may also be problematic. Studies have suggested that one risk factor associated with recurrent STDs among women is continued sexual contact with a partner who failed to be treated.[137] Another contributory factor may be that male partners fail to inform other partners about the need for treatment. Without treatment of all parties involved, recurrent infections will occur among those treated, unless barrier methods are being used consistently. Traditionally, it is only for some STDs, such as syphilis, that health department staff assist in locating partners and ensuring that they receive adequate treatment; for other STDs, such as chlamydia, client-initiated partner notification is the rule. Even with health department assistance, many partners are never found and some individuals, especially women, may fail to disclose partners for fear of abuse or termination of relationships. Thus, innovative models, such as patient-delivered partner therapy, are currently being evaluated.

GENDER DIFFERENCES IN ADVERSE OUTCOMES OF STDS

Women infected with STD pathogens and infants born to infected women bear a disproportionate burden of STDs-related complications. Adverse outcomes of STDs are more severe and frequent among women than men for a number of reasons. As discussed, women are more biologically susceptible if exposed and more likely to go unrecognized or untreated. These untreated infections are more likely to lead to complications and result in a variety of short- and long-term health consequences that disproportionately affect women.

Women infected with *Neisseria gonorrhoeae* or *Chlamydia trachomatis* frequently develop upper genital tract infection. If not adequately treated, 10 to 45 percent of women infected with gonorrhea and 10 to 30 percent of women infected with chlamydia develop pelvic inflammatory disease.[138–141] Some cases of pelvic inflammatory disease required surgical intervention. Over 25 percent of women with acute pelvic inflammatory disease will have long-term sequelae; one in five will become infertile and one in 10 will have a tubal pregnancy.[142–144] Ectopic pregnancy is the leading cause of first-trimester deaths among American women in the United States.[145] Another 20 percent of women with pelvic inflammatory disease will experience chronic pelvic pain and pain during intercourse from scarring in the pelvis.[142,143] In contrast, infertility caused by gonorrhea or chlamydia is a very rare complication in men.[146,147]

Certain types of human papilloma virus are associated with the development of cervical, vulvar, vaginal, and anal cancers in women.[148] Heterosexual men infected with human papilloma virus, however, are at risk only for cancer of the penis, which is relatively rare. These malignancies are common, particularly cervical cancer, which is the second most common cancer in women worldwide and was responsible for approximately 5000 deaths in American women in 1997. Cervical infection with the oncogenic types of human papilloma virus is associated with 90 percent of invasive cervical cancer.[149]

Pregnant women and their infants are particularly vulnerable to complications of STDs.[58] Active infection with STDs during pregnancy may result in a range of serious health problems, including spontaneous abortions, stillbirths, premature rupture of membranes, and preterm delivery. Severe central nervous system damage is of particular concern with several STDs in the fetus or infant. In addition, eye infections (which can lead to blindness), and pneumonia (which may be associated with chronic lung disease), can result when infants of women with cervical infections are exposed during delivery.

Last, HIV infection, one of the most deadly sexually transmitted diseases, may be considered a complication of other STDs because of the increased HIV transmission that is associated with other STDs.[150] Both in this sense and in terms of HIV complications, themselves, HIV is more symmetric in the gender distribution of complications. However, efficiency of transmission is greater from men to women than women to men and thus, the potential for gender differences in HIV prevalence in some populations is very real.

TRANSGENDER ISSUES

By the age of 3 or 4 years, most children have firmly established a gender identity that is continuously solidified and reinforced throughout childhood and adolescence. Once gender identity is established, it becomes an integral part of a person's personality. In most cases, gender assignment at birth is congruent with prenatal biological development. However, even in children with prenatal genetic or hormonal anomalies, gender identity is strongly depended on postnatal rearing, demonstrating the strong effects of learning and social reinforcement.[151,152]

Women and men who are unable to identify with their assigned gender at birth may be given a diagnosis of Gender Identity Disorder or classify themselves as transgender individuals.[153] The diagnosis of Gender Identity Disorder requires two personality manifestations: strong and persistent cross-gender identification, and evidence of persistent discomfort about one's assigned gender. Women and men who meet criteria of Gender Identity Disorder or identify as a transgender person often assume the desired gender role and may seek hormonal and surgical sex reassignment.[154,155]

Postoperative male-to-female transgender individuals are also at risk for STDs. Following penile inversion gender reassignment, the neovagina is lined with stratified squamous epithelium, which is normally resistant to infection with *Neisseria gonorrhoeae*.[156] However, feminizing hormonal replacement therapy may increase the susceptibility of the neovagina to STDs. In addition, gonococcal and chlamydial vaginitis reported in prepubertal females and postmenopausal women, respectively, raises concerns about these types of infection in the neovagina. Although the urethra in a postoperative male-to-female transgender individual is the most likely site of gonococcal and chlamydial infection and both symptomatic and asymptomatic cases have been reported, gonococcal infection of the neovagina has also been reported anecdotally.[157–159] The literature is devoid of information on STDs in the pre- and postoperative female-to-male transgender individuals, but the potential for STDs in this group is also plausible.

HIV is another STD disproportionately affecting the transgender community, possibly because of intravenous drug use and because a disproportionate number of transgender individuals, especially postoperative male-to-females, work in the commercial sex industry.[160]

CONCLUSIONS

Risk factors for and adverse outcomes of STDs vary by gender with women being disproportionately affected. Differences in vulnerability and sequelae result because of biologic factors and behavioral patterns including sexual practices, communication and negotiation, and health care seeking and access. These factors may be compensatory (low behavioral risk and high physiological risk) or synergistic (high behavioral risk and high physiologic risk). Therefore, it is essential that intervention strategies of risk reduction, prevention, and health care be tailored and targeted with regards to these gender perspectives to have the highest probability of impact. Lastly, gender specific interventions, to be most effective, must be interdisciplinary and should focus on the interplay among sexual behavior, health care behavior and biomedical factors that determine the host-pathogen interaction.

References

1 Ehrhardt AA et al: Age, gender, and sexual risk behaviors for sexually transmitted diseases in the United States, in *Research Issues in Human Behavior and Sexually Transmitted Diseases in the AIDS Era.* Wasserheit JN et al (eds). Washington, DC, American Society for Microbiology, 1991, pp. 97–121.

2 Maccoby EE: Gender as a social category. *Dev Psychol* 24:755–765, 1988.

3 Jacklin CN et al: Social behavior at 33 months in same-sex and mixed-sex dyads. *Child Dev* 49:557–569, 1978.

4 Meyer-Bahlburg HFL: Sexuality in early adolescence, in *Handbook of Human Sexuality,* Wolman BB et al (eds). Englewood Cliffs, NJ, Prentice-Hall, Inc. 1980, pp. 61–82.

5 *Facts in Brief: Teen Sex and Pregnancy.* New York, The Alan Guttmacher Institute, 1996.

6 *Fertility, Family Planning and Women's Health: New data from the 1995 National Survey of Family Growth. Series 23: Data from the National Survey of Family Growth No. 19.* DHHS Publication No. (PHS) 97–1995.

7 Laumann EO et al: *The Social Organization of Sexuality: Sexual Practices in the United States.* Chicago and London, The University of Chicago Press, 1994.

8 Kinsey AC et al: *Sexual Behavior in the Human Male.* Philadelphia, Saunders, 1948.

9 Centers for Disease Control. Premarital sexual experience among adolescent women—United States, 1970–1988. *Morbid Mortal Wkly Rep* 39: 929–932, 1991.

10 Tanfer K et al: Condom characteristics: The perceptions and preferences of men in the United States. *Fam Plan Perspec* 25:67–73, 1993.

11 Ehrhardt AA et al: Prevention of heterosexual transmission of HIV: Barriers for women. *J Psychol Hum Sex* 5:1/2:37–67, 1992.

12 Stein ZA: HIV prevention: The need for methods women can use. *Am J Public Health* 80:460–462, 1990.

13 Neugarten BL: Women's attitudes towards the menopause. *Vita Hum* 6:140–153, 1963.

14 Davidson HP et al: Hormonal changes and sexual functioning in aging men. *J Clin Endocrinol Metab* 57:71–77, 1983.

15 Bretschneider JG et al: Sexual interest and behavior in healthy 80-102 year olds. *Archives of Sexual Behavior,* 17, 109–129, 1988.

16 Ehrhardt AA: Sex, Love and Gender Scripts. Presented at the International Academy of Sex Research, Provincetown, MA, September 21, 1995.

17 Ehrhardt AA et al: A review of HIV interventions for at-risk women, Office of Technology Assessment; The Effectiveness of AIDS Prevention Efforts. Washington, DC, U.S. Congress, 1995.

18 Exner TM et al: A review of HIV interventions for at-risk women. *AIDS Behav* 1:93–124, 1997.

19 Kalichman SC et al: Culturally tailored HIV-AIDS risk-reduction messages targeted to African-American urban women: Impact on risk sensitization and risk reduction. *J Consult Clin Psychol* 61:291–295, 1993.

20 Kalichman SC et al: Context framing to enhance HIV-antibody-testing messages targeted to African-American women. *Health Psychol* 14:247–254, 1995.

21 Calsyn DA et al: Ineffectiveness of AIDS education and HIV antibody testing in reducing high-risk behaviors among injection drug users. *Am J Public Health* 82:573–575, 1992.

22 Calsyn DA et al: Longitudinal sexual behavior changes in injecting drug users. *AIDS* 6:1207–1211, 1992.

23 Ickovics JR et al: Limited effects of HIV counseling and testing for women. *JAMA* 272:443–448, 1994.

24 Nyamathi AM et al: Outcomes of specialized and traditional AIDS counseling programs for impoverished women of color. *Res Nurs Health* 16:11–21, 1993.

25 Nyamathi AM et al: Evaluation of two AIDS education programs for impoverished Latina women. *AIDS Educ Prev* 6:296–309, 1994.

26 Schilling RF et al: Building skills of recovering women drug users to reduce heterosexual AIDS transmission. *Pub Health Rept* 106:297–304, 1991.

27 El-Bassel N et al: 15-month follow-up of women methadone patients taught skills to reduce heterosexual HIV transmission. *Pub Health Rept* 107:500–504, 1992.

28 Cohen DA et al: Condoms for men, not women: Results of brief promotion programs. *Sex Trans Dis* 19:245–251, 1992.

29 Cohen DA et al: Group counseling at STD clinics to promote use of condoms. *Pub Health Rept* 107:727–731, 1992.

30 McCusker J et al: Behavioral outcomes of AIDS educational interventions for drug users in short term treatment. *Am J Pub Health* 83: 1463–1466, 1993.

31 Smith EA et al: The impact of a condom desensitization program on female college students. *Health Values* 17:21–31, 1993.

32 Hobfoll SE et al: Reducing inner-city women's AIDS risk-activities: A study of single, pregnant women. *Health Psychol* 13:397–403, 1994.

33 Kelly JA et al: HIV/AIDS prevention for women seen in urban primary care clinics: Effects of intervention to change high-risk sexual behavior patterns. *Am J Pub Health* 84:1918–1922, 1994.

34 El-Bassel N et al: Preventing HIV/AIDS in drug-abusing incarcerated women through skills building and social support enhancement, Preliminary outcomes. *Soc Work Res* 19:131–141, 1995.

35 Tross S et al: Evaluation of a peer outreach HIV prevention program for female partners of injecting drug users (IDUs) in New York City (NYC). *IX Int Conf AIDS* 9:840, abstract no. PO-D13-3737, 1993.

36 Tross S et al: Changing consistent condom use norms among inner city female partners of injection drug users: The companera program HIV prevention newsletter distribution/peer outreach project. Unpublished manuscript, 1995.

37 Santelli JS et al: Interim outcomes for a community-based program to prevent perinatal HIV transmission. *AIDS Educ Prev* 7:210–220, 1995.

38 Williams SP et al: Woman's negotiations. Strategies for safer sex with their male partners. In preparation.

39 Cohen MS et al: Host defenses and the vaginal mucosa. *Scand J Nephrol* 86:13–22, 1985.

40 Cohen MS: Genitourinary mucosal defenses, in *Sexually Transmitted Diseases,* 3rd Ed, Holmes KK et al (eds). New York, McGraw-Hill, 117–127, 1998.

41 Singleton AF: Vaginal discharge in children and adolescents. *Clin Pediatr* 19:799-804, 1990.

42 Holmes KK: Lower genital tract infection in women: Urethral, cervical and vaginal infections, in *Sexually Transmitted Diseases*, 3rd Ed, Holmes KK et al (eds). New York, McGraw-Hill, 527–546, 1998.

43 Draper DL et al: Scanning electron microscopy of attachment of *Neisseria gonorrhoeae* colony phenotypes to surfaces of human genital epithelia. *Am J Obstet Gynecol* 138:818–826, 1980.

44 Harrison HR et al: Cervical *Chlamydia trachomatis* infection in university women: relationship to history, contraception, ectopy, and cervicitis. *Am J Obstet Gynecol* 153:244–251, 1985.

45 Cruickshank R et al: The biology of the vagina in the human subject II. The bacterial flora and secretion of the vagina at various age-periods and their relation to glycogen in the vaginal epithelium. *J Obstet Gynaecol Br Emp* 41:208–226, 1934.

46 Hammerschlag MR et al: Microbiology of the vagina in children: Normal and potentially pathogenic organisms. *Pediatrics* 62:57–62, 1978.

47 Mardh PA et al: In vitro interactions between lactobacilli and other microorganisms occurring in vaginal flora. *Scand J Infect Dis Suppl* 40:47–51, 1983.

48 Saigh JH et al: Inhibition of *Neisseria gonorrhoeae* by aerobic and facultatively anaerobic components of the endocervical flora: Evidence for a protective effect against infection. *Infect Immunol* 19: 704–710, 1978.

49 O'Connor T et al: The activity of candidate virucidal agents, low pH and genital secretions against HIV-1 in vitro. *Int J STD AIDS* 6:267–272, 1995.

50 Madile BM: The cervical epithelium from fetal age to adolescence. *Obstet Gynecol* 47:536–539, 1976.

51 Vickery BH et al: The cervix and its secretion in mammals. *Physiol Rev* 48:135–154, 1968.

52 Gutman LT: Gonococcal disease in infants and children, in *Sexually Transmitted Diseases,* 3rd Ed, Holmes KK et al (eds). New York, McGraw-Hill, 803–810, 1998.

53 Eschenback DA et al: Pathogenesis of acute pelvic inflammatory disease: Role of contraception and other risk factors. *Am J Obstet Gynecol* 128:838–850, 1977.

54 Sweet RL et al: The occurrence of chlamydial and gonococcal salpingitis during the menstrual cycle. *JAMA* 255:2062–2064, 1986.

55 Sparling PF: Biology of *N. gonorrhoeae*, in *Sexually Transmitted Diseases,* 3rd Ed, Holmes KK et al (eds). New York, McGraw-Hill, 131–148, 1998.

56 Plummer FA: Antibodies to opacity proteins (Opa) correlate with a reduced risk of gonococcal salpingitis. *J Clin Invest* 93:1748, 1994.

57 Brunham RC et al: Depression of the lymphocyte transformation response to microbial antigens and to phytohemagglutinin during pregnancy. *J Clin Invest* 72:1629–1638, 1983.

58 Watts H et al: Sexually transmitted diseases including HIV infection in pregnancy, *Sexually Transmitted Diseases,* 3rd Ed, Holmes KK et al (eds). New York, McGraw-Hill, 1998.

59 Sabahi F et al: Qualitative and quantitative analysis of T lymphocytes during normal human pregnancy. *Am J Reprod Immunol* 33:381–93, 1995.

60 Rando RF et al: Increased frequency of detection of human papillomavirus deoxyribonucleic acid in exfoliated cervical cells during pregnancy. *Am J Obstet Gynecol* 161:50–55, 1989.

61 Schneider A et al: Increased prevalence of human papillomaviruses in the lower genital tract of pregnant women. *Int J Cancer* 40:198–201, 1987.

62 Brown ZA et al: Genital herpes in pregnancy: risk factors associated with recurrences and asymptomatic shedding. *Am J Obstet Gynecol* 153:24–30, 1985.

63 Vontver LA et al: Recurrent genital herpes simplex virus infection in pregnancy: infant outcome and frequency as asymptomatic recurrences. *Am J Obstet Gynecol* 143:75–84, 1982.

64 Moore JE: Studies on the influence of pregnancy in syphilis. I. The course of syphilitic infection in pregnant women. *Johns Hopkins Med Bull* 34:89–99, 1923.

65 Singer A: The uterine cervix from adolescence to the menopause. *Br J Obstet Gynaecol* 82:81–99, 1975.

66 Cates W Jr: Contraception, Contraceptive technology, and STD, in *Sexually Transmitted Diseases,* 3rd Ed, Holmes KK et al (eds). New York, McGraw-Hill, 1998.

67 Carlin EM et al: Women, contraceptives and STDs including HIV. *Int J STD AIDS* 6:373–386, 1995.

68 Timyan J et al: Barrier methods for the prevention of sexually transmitted diseases, in *Sexually Transmitted Diseases,* 3rd Ed, Holmes KK et al (eds). New York, McGraw-Hill, 1998.

69 Hatcher R et al: *Contraceptive Technology.* New York, Irvington Publishers, 1994.

70 Feldblum PJ et al: The protective effect of nonoxynol-9 against HIV infection. *Am J Public Health* 84:1032–1034, 1994.

71 Niruthisard S et al: Use of nonoxynol-9 and reduction in rate of gonococcal and chlamydial cervical infections. *Lancet* 339:1371–1375, 1992.

72 Weir SS et al: The use of nonoxynol-9 for protection against cervical gonorrhea. *Am J Public Health* 84:910, 1994.

73 Kreiss J et al: Efficacy of nonoxynol-9 contraceptive sponge use in prevention of heterosexual acquisition of HIV in Nairobi prostitutes. *JAMA* 268:477–482, 1992.

74 Weir SS et al: Nonoxynl-9 use, genital ulcers, and HIV infection in a cohort of sex workers. *Genitourin Med* 71:78, 1995.

75 Ward H et al: Nonoxynol-9 in lubricated condoms: Results of a study in female prostitutes. *Sex Trans Dis* 23:413, 1996.

76 Grimes DA: Intrauterine devices and pelvic inflammatory disease: Recent developments. *Contraception* 36:97–109, 1987.

77 Buchan H et al: Epidemiology of pelvic inflammatory disease in parous women with special reference to intrauterine device use. *Br J Obstet Gynaecol* 97:780–788, 1990.

78 Lee NC et al: Type of intrauterine device and the risk of pelvic inflammatory disease. *Obstet Gynecol* 62:1–6, 1983.

79 Washington AE et al: Oral contraceptives, *Chlamydia trachomatis* infection and pelvic inflammatory disease. *JAMA* 253:2246–2250, 1985.

80 Park BJ et al: Contraceptive methods and the risk of *Chlamydia trachomatis* infection in young women. *Am J Epidemiol* 142(7) 771–778, 1995.

81 Critchlow CW et al: Determinants of cervical ectopia and of cervicitis: age, oral contraception, specific cervical infection, smoking, and douching. *Am J Obstet Gynecol* 173:534–543, 1995.

82 Cottingham J et al: *Chlamydia trachomatis* and oral contraceptive use: A quantitative review. *Genitourin Med* 68:209–216, 1992.

83 Rubin GL et al: Oral contraceptives and pelvic inflammatory disease. *Am J Obstet Gynecol* 144:630–635, 1982.

84 Panser LA et al: Type of oral contraceptive in relation to acute, initial episodes of pelvic inflammatory disease. *Contraception* 93:91–99, 1991.

85 Svensson L et al: Contraceptives and acute salpingitis. *JAMA* 251: 2554–2555, 1984.

86 Wolner-Hanssen P et al: Decreased risk of symptomatic chlamydial Pelvic Inflammatory Disease associated with oral contraceptive use. *JAMA* 263:54–59, 1990.

87 Westrom L et al: in *Sexually Transmitted Diseases,* 3rd Ed, Holmes KK et al (eds). New York, McGraw-Hill, 1998.

88 Mooradian AD et al: Sexuality in older women. Arch Intern Med 150:1033–1038, 1990.

89 Leiblum S et al: Vaginal atrophy in the postmenopausal woman: The importance of sexual activity and hormones. *JAMA* 249:2195–2198, 1983.

90 Osborne NG et al: Genital bacteriology: A comparative study of premenopausal women with postmenopausal women. *Am J Obstet Gynecol* 135:195–198, 1979.

91 Colleen SL: The human urethral mucosa: an experimental study with emphasis on microbial attachment. *Scand J Urol Nephrol Suppl* 68: 4–55, 1982.

92 Chambers CV et al: Microflora of urethra in adolescent boys: relationship to sexual activity and nongonococcal urethritis. *J Pediatr* 110:314–321, 1987.

93 Colleen S et al: Magnesium and zinc in seminal fluid of healthy males and patients with non-acute prostatitis with and without gonorrhoea. *Scand J Urol Nephrol* 9:192–197, 1975.

94 Fair WR et al: Prostatic antibacterial factor. *Urology* 7:169–177, 1976.

95 Krieger JN et al: Canine prostatic secretions kill *Trichomonas vaginalis. Infect Immunol* 37:77–81, 1982.

96 Mardh PA et al: Inhibitory effect on the formation of chlamydia inclusions in McCoy cells by seminal fluid and some of its components. *Invest Urol* 17:510–513, 1980.

97 American Academy of Pediatrics, Report of the Task Force on circumcision. *Pediatrics* 84:388–391, 1989.

98 Aral SO et al: Epidemiolgy and social/behavior determinants of STD: Industralized and developing countries, in *Sexually Transmitted Diseases,* 3rd Ed, Holmes KK et al (eds). New York, McGraw-Hill, 1998.

99 Moses S et al: The association between lack of male circumcision and risk for HIV infection: A review of the epidemiological data. *Sex Trans Dis* 21(4):201–210, 1994.

100 Kreiss JK et al: The association between circumcision status and human immunodeficiency virus infection among homosexual men. *J Infect Dis* 168:1404–1408, 1993.

101 Cook LS et al: Circumcision and sexually transmitted diseases. *Am J Pub Health* 84:197–201, 1994.

102 Tyndall MW et al: Increased risk of infection with human immunodeficiency virus type 1 among uncircumcised men presenting with genital ulcer disease in Kenya. *Clin Infect Dis* 23:449–453, 1996.

103 Peterman TA et al: Risk of human immunodeficiency virus transmission from heterosexual adults with transfusion-associated infections. *JAMA* 259:55–58, 1988.

104 Royce RA et al: Sexual transmission of HIV. *N Engl J Med* 336: 1072–1078, 1997.

105 Padian NS: The heterosexual transmission of human immunodeficiency virus (HIV) in northern California: results from a ten-year study. *Am J Epidemiol* 146 (4):350–357, 1997.

106 Alter MJ et al: Hepatitis B virus transmission between heterosexuals. *JAMA* 256:1307–1310, 1986.

107 Rosenblum LS et al: Heterosexual transmission of hepatitis B virus in Belle Glade, Florida. *J Infect Dis* 161:407–411, 1990.

108 Hooper RR: Cohort study of venereal disease: I. The risk of gonorrhea transmission from infected women to men. *Am J Epidemiol* 108: 136–144, 1978.

109 Holmes KK: An estimate of the risk of men acquiring gonorrhea by sexual contact with infected females. *Am J Epidemiol* 91:170–174, 1970.

110 Lycke E et al: The risk of transmission of genital Chl*amydia trachomatis* infection is less than that of genital *Neisseria gonorrhoeae* infection. *Sex Transm Dis* 7:6–10, 1980.

111 Worm AM et al: Transmission of chlamydial infections to sexual partners. *Genitourin Med* 63:19–21, 1987.

112 Viscidi RP et al: Transmission of *Chlamydia trachomatis* among sex partners assessed by polymerase chain reaction. *J Infect Dis* 168:488–492, 1993.

113 Quinn TC et al: Epidemiologic and microbiologic correlates of *Chlamydia trachomatis* infection in sexual partnerships. *JAMA* 276: 1737–1742, 1996.

114 Nahmias AJ et al: *Genital and Neonatal Herpes*. London: John Wiley, 1996, pp. 93–108.

115 Mertz GJ et al: Risk factors for sexual transmission of genital herpes. *Ann Intern Med* 116:197–202, 1992.

116 Fleming DT et al: Herpes simplex virus type 2 in the United States, 1976–1994. *N Engl J Med* 3337:1105–1111, 1997.

117 Hibbard JH et al: Gender roles, illness orientation and use of medical services. *Soc Sci Med* 17:129–137, 1983.

118 Neighbors HW et al: Sex differences in professional help seeking among adult Black Americans. *Am J Commun Psychol* 15:403–417, 1987.

119 Amaro H et al: Health care utilization for sexually transmitted diseases: Influence of patient and provider characteristics, in *Research Issues in Human Behavior and Sexually Transmitted Diseases in the AIDS Era*. Washington, DC, American Society for Microbiology, 1991, pp. 140–160.

120 Ballard R et al: Chancroid, in *Atlas of Sexually Transmitted Diseases and AIDS*, Morse SA et al (eds). London, Mosby-Wolf, 1996, pp. 47–64.

121 Laurence L: How OB-GYNs are failing women. *Glamour* 292–296, 1997.

122 Gibbs RS et al: A survey of practices in infectious diseases by obstetrician-gynecologists. *Obstet Gynecol* 83:631–636, 1994.

123 Institute of Medicine: *The Hidden Epidemic: Confronting Sexually Transmitted Diseases*. Washington, DC, National Academy Press, 1997.

124 Smith EM et al: Health care attitudes and experiences during gynecologic care among lesbians and bisexuals. *Am J Public Health* 75: 1085–1087, 1995.

125 Weiss L et al: Women's attitudes toward gynecologic practices. *Obstet Gynecol* 54:110–114, 1979.

126 Pauly IB et al: Physicians' attitudes in treating male homosexuals. *Hum Sex* 4:27–45, 1970.

127 Dardick L et al: Openness between gay persons and health professionals. *Ann Intern Med* 93:115–119, 1980.

128 Wortley PM et al: AIDS in women in the United States. Recent Trends. *JAMA* 278:911–916, 1997.

129 Irwin DE et al: Self-treatment patterns among clients attending sexually transmitted clinics and the effect of self-treatment on STD symptom duration. *Sex Trans Dis* 24:372–377, 1997.

130 Wolner-Hanssen P et al: Association between vaginal douching and acute pelvic inflammatory disease. *JAMA* 263:1036–1941, 1990.

131 Kendrick JS et al: Vaginal douching and the risk of ectopic pregnancy among black women. *Am J Obstet Gynecol* 176:991–997, 1997.

132 Daling JR et al: Vaginal douching and the risk of tubal pregnancy. *Epidemiology* 2:40, 1991.

133 Morse S et al: Issues in the laboratory diagnosis of STDs, in *Sexually Transmitted Diseases*, 3rd Ed, Holmes KK et al (eds). New York, McGraw-Hill, 1998.

134 Bauwens JE et al: Diagnosis of *Chlamydia trachomatis* endocervical infections by a commercial polymerase chain reaction assay. *J Clin Microbiol* 31:3023–3027, 1993.

135 Centers for Disease Control. 1998 Guidelines for Treatment of Sexually Transmitted Diseases. *Morbid Mortal Weekly Rep* 47, 1997.

136 Plichta SB et al: Violence and gynecologic health in women <50 years old. *Am J Obstet Gynecol* 174:903–907, 1996.

137 Fortenberry JD et al: Recurrent sexually transmitted infections (STI) among adolescent females (Abstract no. 172). Eleventh Meeting of the International Society for STD Research. New Orleans, LA, August 30, 1995.

138 Westrom L: Incidence, prevalence, and trends of acute pelvic inflammatory disease and its consequences in industrialized countries. *Am J Obstet Gynecol* 138;880, 1980.

139 Platt R et al: Risk of acquiring gonorrhea and prevalence of abnormal adnexal findings among women recently exposed to gonorrhea. *JAMA* 250:3205–3209, 1983.

140 Westrom L: Chlamydial and gonococcal infection in a defined population of women. *Scand J Inf Dis* 32 (suppl):157S, 1982.

141 Stamm WE et al: Effect of treatment regimens for *Neisseria gonorrhoeae* on simultaneous infection with *Chlamydia trachomatis. N Engl J Med* 310:545–549, 1984.

142 Westrom L et al: Pelvic inflammatory disease and infertility. A cohort study of 1,844 women with laproscopically verified disease and 657 control women with normal laproscopic findings. *Sex Transm Dis* 19:185, 1992.

143 Kani J et al: Epidemiology of pelvic inflammatory disease, in *Pelvic Inflammatory Disease*, Berger GS et al (eds). New York, Raven Press, 1992, p. 7.

144 Cates W et al: Sexually transmitted diseases, pelvic inflammatory disease, and infertility: An epidemiologic update. *Epidemiol Rev* 12;199, 1990.

145 Centers for Disease Control: Ectopic pregnancy—United States, 1990–1992. *MMWR* 44:46, 1995.

146 Hook EW III et al: Gonococcal infection in the adult, in *Sexually Transmitted Diseases*, 3rd Ed, Holmes KK et al (eds). New York, McGraw-Hill, 1998.

147 Stamm WE: *C. trachomatis* infection in the adult, in *Sexually Transmitted Diseases*, 3rd Ed, Holmes KK et al (eds). New York, McGraw-Hill, 1998.

148 Koutsky L et al: Genital HPV infection, in *Sexually Transmitted Diseases*, 3rd Ed, Holmes KK et al (eds). New York, McGraw-Hill, 1998.

149 Koutsky L: Epidemiology of genital human papillomavirus infection. *Am J Med* 102:3–8, 1997.

150 Fleming DT et al: The contribution of other sexually transmitted diseases to sexual transmission of HIV infection: From epidemiological synergy to public health policy. Genitourinary Med, invited review, submitted.

151 Ehrhardt AA: Gender differences: A biosocial perspective. *Psychol Gender* 32:37–57, 1985.

152 Money J et al: Man and woman, boy and girl: The differentiation and dimorphism of gender identity from conception to maturity. Baltimore, The Johns Hopkins University Press, 1972.

153 Diagnostic and Statistical Manual of Mental Disorders, 4th Ed, DSMV-IV, Washington, DC., *American Psychiatric Association*, 1994.
154 Gilbert DA et al: Transsexual surgery in the genetic female. *Clinics in Plastic Surgery* 15:471–487, 1988.
155 Rubin SO: Sex-reassignment surgery male-to-female. Review, own results and report of a new technique using the glans penis as a pseudoclitoris. *Scand J Urol Nephrol* Suppl 154:1–28, 1993.
156 Eldh J: Construction of a neovagina with preservation of the glans penis as a clitoris in male transsexuals. *Plast Reconstr Surg* 91:895–900, 1993.
157 Fiumara NJ et al: Gonorrhoea and condyloma accuminata in a male transsexual. *Br J Vener Dis* 49:478–479, 1973.
158 Fiumara NJ et al: Asymptomatic gonococcal urethritis in a male transsexual female. *Br J Vener Dis* 54:130–131, 1978.
159 Bodsworth NJ et al: Gonococcal infection of the neovagina in a male-to-female transsexual. *Sex Transm Dis* 21:211–212, 1994.
160 Modan et al: Prevalence of HIV antibodies in transsexual and female prostitutes. *Am J Public Health* 82:590–592, 1992.

Chapter 9
Adolescents and STDs*

Stuart M. Berman
Karen Hein

Making the transition from childhood to being healthy sexual adults is one of the major tasks and challenges facing young people. A successful transition implies forming intimate relationships while avoiding the acquisition of sexually transmitted diseases. Yet it is apparent from the current data that around the world, for a combination of reasons involving biology, psychology, ambient culture, and changing mores, adolescents who have had sexual intercourse have the highest rates of STDs—including HIV in some locales—of any age group. As stated by one researcher, "the challenge lies in getting teenagers to view their relationships in a more realistic light without destroying the positive ways in which these (relationships) may also add to their lives."[1] This chapter describes the magnitude of the STD problem among adolescents, the factors that contribute to their risk of infection, and the STD prevention activities which are effective among these young people.

EXTENT OF THE RISK

Most population-based rates of sexually transmitted disease underestimate the risk of STD for sexually active adolescents because the rate is inappropriately expressed as cases of disease divided by the number of individuals in this age group. Yet only those who have had intercourse are at risk for STDs. *For rates to reflect risk among those who are sexually experienced, appropriate denominators should include only the number of individuals in the demographic group who have had sexual intercourse.* Whereas nearly all 20- to 24-year-olds have had sexual intercourse, this is true of only 50 percent of women 15 to 19 years old.[2] This underestimation of rates is greatest among the youngest adolescents, since only a small proportion of them have had sex. In general, when rates are corrected for the percentage in the group who are sexually active, the youngest adolescents have the highest STD rates of any age group.[3]

CHLAMYDIA

Chlamydia trachomatis infection is the STD most strongly associated with adolescents. Numerous clinic-based studies have demonstrated that prevalence of cervical chlamydia is greatest among sexually active individuals under 20 years of age, being approximately twice that found among older individuals.[4–11] A recent study among 16- to 24-year-old female enrollees in the Job Corps (a national training program for disadvantaged and out-of-school youth) demonstrates high prevalence among these sexually active young people in all regions of the country (Fig. 9-1), with prevalence somewhat higher among those 16 to 19 years of age and among minority populations (15 percent, 11 percent, and 9 percent among African Americans, Hispanics, and whites, respectively).[12]

Although the majority of studies have been performed among females, tests performed on urine specimens, among other tests, have been used recently to evaluate prevalence among males. The findings are similar to those for females, with prevalence of chlamydia being greatest among those under 25 years of age (the data are too limited to permit comparison between those under 20 and over 25 years of age), and somewhat greater among minority youth. Prevalence among males has usually been found to be 5 to 10 percent,[13–17] somewhat less than among females. This is consistent with mathematical models that assume the likelihood of symptomatic infection is greater and the duration shorter among males.[18]

The DNA amplification tests for chlamydia, which can be performed on urine, have permitted adolescents to be tested in community settings outside health care facilities.[17] A study in Denver found that 11 percent (25/226) of adolescents accessed on inner-city streets were infected.[19] In New Orleans, screening conducted in 3 junior/senior high schools identified infection in 9.7 percent of females and 4.0 percent of males tested without regard to sexual experience.[20]

Recurrent infection may be particularly worrisome, since there is evidence that such infections are more likely to be associated with development of significant tissue damage (for example, to the fallopian tubes) than is primary infection. The risk of recurrent infection is twice as high among adolescents as among older women,[21] as shown in Table 9-1. Many recurrent infections are associated with the continuing presence of a sex partner who has remained untreated.[22,23]

A population-based evaluation of chlamydia prevalence among males has recently been performed in the United States. Preliminary analyses indicate that among males 15 to 25 years old the prevalence ranges from 2 to 6 percent and is slightly higher among men over 20 years of age and among African Americans.[24] Comparable data for women are not available. However, among female adolescents tested at least twice in family planning clinics in Washington, Oregon, Idaho, and Alaska from 1988 through 1991, 22 percent were found to be infected on at least one visit.[25] Similar findings were produced by a population-based study in Umea, Sweden, which evaluated cumulative risk of chlamydia by serologic tests.[26] The prevalence of *C. trachomatis,* identified by culture among 19-year-old women was 5.5 percent (3/55).[27] However, 29.1 percent of these women and 18.0 percent of 21-year-old women ($n = 139$) showed serologic evidence of previous chlamydial infection.[26]

When age-specific data are available from other countries, chlamydia prevalence has been found to be greatest among adolescents.[28,29] Although chlamydia prevalence has not been extensively studied in most other countries, the data that are available indicate that prevalence is at least as high as that found in the United States, except for locales such as Scandinavia with extensive chlamydia testing programs.[30,31]

GONORRHEA

Although overall rates of gonorrhea have been decreasing for 20 years in the United States, with rates falling by almost 65 percent from the peak of 467 cases per 100,000 in 1975, the decrease among adolescents has not kept pace. For example, from 1981 through 1991, although the overall rate of gonorrhea among males declined 46 percent, the rate among males 15 to 19 years old did not decline at all. From 1985 to 1995, whereas the overall rate among females decreased 53 percent, rates among females 15 to 19 years old decreased by 39 percent.[11] As a result there has

*(From Holmes KK et al: *Sexually Transmitted Diseases,* 3rd ed. New York: McGraw-Hill, Inc. (In press.) Used with permission.)

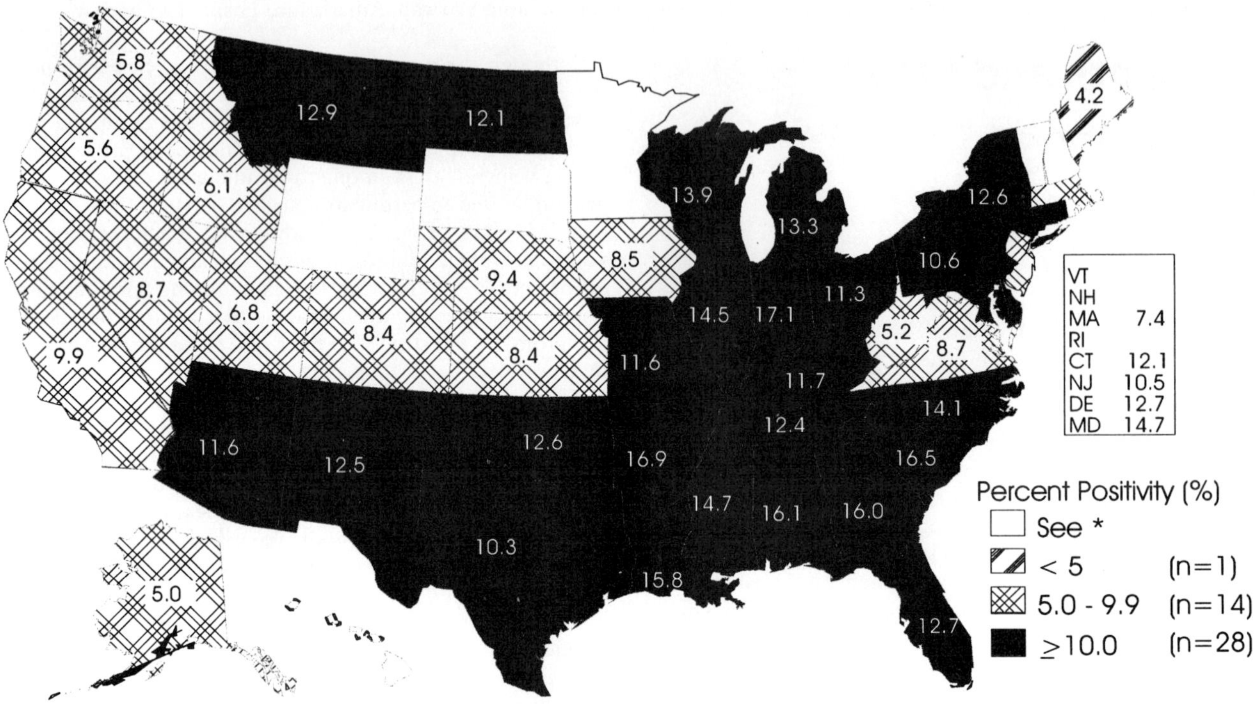

Fig. 9-1. Chlamydia infection: percent positivity among 16- to 24-year-old women entering the U.S. Job Corps, by state of residence, 1995.

been a growing difference between the rate among older females and the rate among females 15 to 19 years of age, which has been the highest of any age group since 1984. Since only about half of the women in this age group have had intercourse, actual rates among females 15 to 19 years old who are sexually experienced are probably twice as high. This pattern, in which the rate of gonorrhea is found to decline least among adolescents, has also been observed in the United Kingdom.[31]

In the United States, rates of reported gonorrhea among African American adolescents are over 25-fold higher than among their white counterparts. In the past decade, the disparity has increased slightly. The reasons for this inequality are not known. Data from San Francisco, adjusted for socioeconomic status and occupation, document persistent racial differentials, with rates among African American youth 28.7 times higher than those among whites.[32] Contributing factors may include lack of access to care, since gonorrhea is easily diagnosed and treated.

Rates of gonorrhea in much of the industrialized world are significantly lower than in the United States. In Germany and Sweden endemic gonorrhea has nearly been eliminated.[33,34] However, in much of the developing world rates are still very high, as shown by the prevalence of the disease (up to 22 percent) in antenatal or family planning clinics and village surveys.[31,35] When age-specific data are reported, prevalence is usually found to be highest among adolescents.[30,36]

Table 9-1. Risk for Recurrent Chlamydial Infection

Site	Age	Risk
Wisconsin[21]	<15	54%
	15–19	30%
	20–29	15%
Indianapolis[23]	(Adolescent clinic)	38%
Northwest states[25]	15–19	18%

SYPHILIS

Syphilis is still endemic in the United States, although almost eliminated in much of the developed world. In the United States, rates of primary and secondary syphilis are highest among 20- to 24-year-olds—a pattern similar to that in developing countries.[30] Rates among 15- to 19-year-olds appear to be approximately half those in the older group,[11] but these reports overestimate the differential because they have not been corrected for sexual experience. During the U.S. syphilis epidemic of 1986 to 1990, while rates of syphilis among males of all ages rose 45.5 percent, rates among males 15 to 19 years old increased 41.4 percent; similarly, rates among women of all ages increased 138 percent compared to 130 percent among females 15 to 19 years old. A recent study in Houston found not only that adolescents had the highest rate of syphilis but also that the increase in their syphilis rate was temporally associated with a sharp increase in HIV seroprevalence, from 1.6 to 3.8 percent, among adolescents attending STD clinics.[37]

Syphilis is quite prevalent in the developing world (2 to 16 percent among antenatal attendees; up to 30 percent in other clinic-based evaluations).[31,38] A population-based evaluation in Tanzania revealed that the prevalence of TPHA seropositivity among 15- to 24-year-olds across 12 villages ranged from 9 to 17 percent.[39] A population-based survey in rural Nigeria found 2.6 percent of sexually active teenagers (under 20 years old) to have syphilis.[29]

HUMAN PAPILLOMAVIRUS

Studies demonstrate that prevalence of human papillomavirus (HPV) is highest among adolescents and young adults.[40] Investigators report rates of infection of approximately 25 to 50 percent when testing with Southern blot or polymerase chain reaction (PCR) (Table 9-2). Prevalence of genital HPV

Table 9-2. Prevalence of Human Papillomavirus Infection among Adolescent and Young Adult Females

Author	Setting and population	Specimen	Test	Prevalence by site, age, or lifetime number of partners	Percent infections with high-risk types (types 16 and 18, with or without other types)
Rosenfield[153] (n = 249)	Adolescent clinic 13–21 years	Cervicovaginal lavage	Southern blot	Overall: 38.2% 1 partner: 31% (34/107)	Type 16: 16% Type 18: 15%
Moscicki[154] (n = 661)	Family planning clinic 13–19 years	Cervical swab	ViraPap	Overall: 15.4% 1–3 partners; 10% (39/393)	Type 16/18: 46%
Bauer[155] (n = 467)	University health center Mean age 22.9 years	Vulvar swab Cervical swab	PCR	46% any site 33% cervix 43% vulva	Type 16: 19% Type 18: 11%
			ViraPap	11% any site 7% cervix 8% vulva	
Bauer[156] (n = 453)	HMO ob-gyn 16–18 years (16–24 years: n = 81)	Cervicovaginal lavage	PCR	16–24 years: 32.1% 16–29 years 1 partner: 3.8% 2–5 partners: 37.9%	Type 16: 15% (40 contained 16, 18, 31, 33, 35, 39, 45, 51, 56, 58)
Hildesheim[157] (n = 404)	Inner city ob-gyn hospital clinics 16–72 years (16–24 years: n = 163)	Cervicovaginal lavage	PCR	16–24 yr olds: 39%	
Wheeler[158] (n = 357)	University health center 18–47 years Median age 23 years (18–20 years: n = 79, 21–25 years: n = 152)	Cervical swab	PCR	18–20 yr olds Overall: 43.0% ≤2 partners: 22.2% 21–25 yr olds Overall: 48.7% ≤2 partners: 31.3%	Type 16: 18% Any cancer associated type (16, 18, 31, 33, 35, 39, 45, 51, 52): 47%
Karlsson[159] (n = 602)	Population-based survey among 19-, 21-, 23-, and 25-year-olds	Cervical swab	PCR	Overall: 1 partner: 5.9% 2–3 partners: 20.8% 19-yr-olds: 20.0% 21-yr-olds: 17.3% 23-yr-olds: 19.0% 25-yr-olds: 33.1%	Any cancer associated type (16, 18, 31, 33, 35, 39, 45, 56): 54%
Fisher[160] (n = 107)	Suburban adolescent clinic Mean age: 18.5 yrs	Cervicovaginal lavage	Southern blot	Overall: 32% ≤2 partners: 21% (10/47)	Any cancer associated type (16, 18, 31, 33, 45, 56): 42%
Jamison[161] (n = 634)	3 urban adolescent clinics 12–18 yrs	Cervical swab	ViraPap	Overall: 15.6% ≤1 partner: 8.3% (18/217)	Type 16/18: 46% (31, 33, 35: in an additional 4.9)

PCR = polymerase chain reaction.

infection among adolescent females with only one or two partners is consistently above 10 percent and is often as high as 25 percent or more. These HPV prevalences may well reflect a vulnerability of the immature cervix to infection. Women with persistent infection are at particular risk for cervical dysplasia.[41]

HERPES SIMPLEX

Few individuals with *Herpes simplex* type 2 (HSV-2) infection have recognized symptoms or signs.[42] However, population-based serologic data are available from analyses of specimens obtained in the years 1976 to 1980 and 1988 to 1994 from nationally representative samples of the U.S. population for the National Health and Nutrition Examination Surveys (NHANES). These analyses demonstrated that cumulative risk for HSV-2 infection rises with age.[43] In general, seroprevalence was higher among females than males (OR = 1.6) and higher among African Americans than among whites (OR = 5.7). The data among 12- to 19-year-olds followed a similar pattern but indicated that prevalence of HSV-2 increased substantially among adolescents from 1978 to 1991. Increases were disproportionately greater among whites than among African Americans, perhaps reflecting changes in sexual behavior (Table 9-3).[44]

PELVIC INFLAMMATORY DISEASE

Since pelvic inflammatory disease (PID) is usually caused by either gonorrhea or chlamydia, and since these infections are most prevalent among sexually active adolescent females, this group is also at substantial risk for PID. In 1980 the estimated risk of PID among sexually active 15-year-olds in Sweden was 12.5 percent, and among sexually active 16-year-olds it was 10 percent, with progressive decreases with increasing age.[45] The investigators calculated that the risk of developing salpingitis for those with chlamydial infection was approximately 70 percent greater among women between 15 and 19 than among women between 20 and 24 years old; among those with gonorrhea, the risk for 15- to 19-year-olds was about 20 percent less than among the 20- to 24-year-olds.[46]

Although most women with PID are treated on an ambulatory

Table 9-3. HSV-2 Seroprevalence among 12- to 19-Year-Olds in the United States

	1979	1991
Males:		
Whites	0.5%	4.6%
Blacks	3.4%	5.7%
Females:		
Whites	1.3%	4.3%
Blacks	7.5%	11.7%

Source: National Health and Nutrition Examination Surveys (NHANES).[44]

basis, available data do not permit accurate assessment of rates of ambulatory treatment among adolescents. Therefore, incidence of PID among adolescents can be estimated best by analyzing rates of hospitalization. A recent evaluation found that rates of hospitalization for acute PID decreased over the decade of the 1980s.[47] However, the decline in rate of hospitalization was least among 15- to 19-year-olds, so that by 1988 these adolescent women had the highest rate of hospitalization. If rates were based only upon those adolescents who had intercourse, the risk for hospitalization with PID among sexually active 15- to 19-year-olds would be approximately twice as high as among sexually active 20- to 24-year-olds. These data should be interpreted with caution since changes in clinical management of patients with PID could bias the result: by the end of the 1980s hospitalization was recommended for adolescents with PID,[48] while ambulatory management may have become more widely accepted for older women. Nevertheless, the age-specific differences are striking

A study in Philadelphia found that adolescent females diagnosed with PID sought care an average of 7.8 days after the onset of symptoms compared with 5.6 days for adults.[49] Such behavior is of particular importance given the finding that the risk of impaired fertility or ectopic pregnancy increases significantly with increasing delay between onset of symptoms and receipt of care.[50]

HUMAN IMMUNODEFICIENCY VIRUS (HIV)

Recent reports from around the world indicate that sexually active adolescents are at substantial risk for HIV infection, experiencing some of the highest rates of HIV acquisition, particularly among females. Furthermore, the high rate among adolescents of STDs such as gonorrhea and chlamydia suggests added vulnerability for these young people, since these infections can increase the risk of HIV transmission.[51,52] In the United States the number of AIDS cases diagnosed in individuals under 20 years of age is a small percentage of all AIDS cases, especially when cases associated with hemophilia or perinatal transmission are excluded. However, this analysis is deceptive, since the average time from acquisition of HIV infection to diagnosis of AIDS is approximately 10 years and is probably greater among those who acquire infection in their teenage years.[53] Even with such qualifiers, the number of cases of AIDS among 15- to 19-year-olds diagnosed in the years 1993 to 1995 was 177 percent greater than the number diagnosed from 1988 to 1992, whereas cases diagnosed among older individuals increased 122 percent.[54]

Studies in the United States have demonstrated that prevalence of HIV infection is appreciable in several populations of adolescents. Prevalence has frequently exceeded 1 percent among adolescents seen at STD clinics, among those at shelters for homeless and runaway youth, and among those in correctional facilities (Table 9-4). Many of these young people have had sex in exchange for drugs, shelter, or food ("survival sex"). Infection has been associated with use of crack cocaine, injection drug use, and exchange of sex for money. Although rates are substantial among young men who have sex with other men,[55] overall the data indicate that a large proportion of cases among adolescents are attributable to heterosexual transmission.[56] For example, the prevalence in New York City from 1987 to 1990 among childbearing women under 20 years of age was 0.58 percent, with African American and Hispanic teenagers being at increased risk (0.68 and 0.57 percent, respectively).[55] Studies from 1988 to 1993 among Job Corps entrants 16 to 21 years old found that slightly fewer than 0.3 percent were HIV infected.[55] African American youth

Table 9-4. Summary of HIV Seroprevalence Data from Adolescent Clinics by Clinic Setting and Sex, 1993

Clinic setting and client gender	Total centers[a]	Total specimens tested[b]	Centers analyzed[c,d]	Percent positive	
				Median[e]	Range[f]
Adolescent medicine clinics					
Males	31	2,969	10	0.0	(0.0–3.4)
Females	31	10,224	29	0.0	(0.0–3.1)
Total	31	13,193	31	0.0	(0.0–3.2)
Homeless and runaway youth clinics					
Males	3	752	3	1.9	(0.0–2.9)
Females	3	971	3	1.1	(0.6–1.5)
Total	3	1,723	3	1.6	(0.4–2.0)
Juvenile detention centers					
Males	7	3,461	6	0.0	(0.0–3.6)
Females	4	363	3	2.8	(0.7–5.0)
Total	7	3,824	6	0.1	(0.0–3.9)

Source: CDC, National HIV Serosurveillance Summary Update, 1993.

[a] Includes centers funded to conduct unlinked surveys in 1993.
[b] Includes all specimens tested in 1993.
[c] Includes only clinics reporting at least 50 specimens collected and tested according to CDC protocol.
[d] Gender analyzed for centers reporting at least 50 specimens per group.
[e] The median rate for centers in each category.
[f] Range is from lowest to highest rates of centers in each category.

Fig. 9-2. HIV seroprevalence in Job Corps entrants, by sex and date of entrance,* January 1988–December 1993. *Annual prevalences adjusted for differences in age, race/ethnicity, region, and MSA.

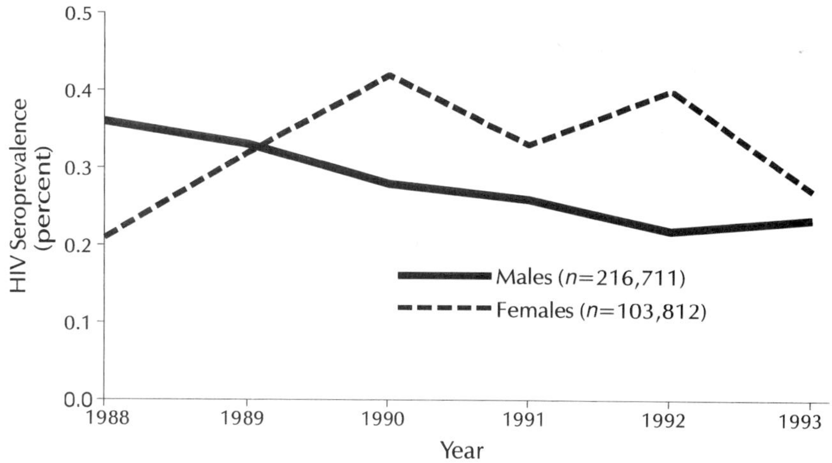

were at greater risk of infection, and although prevalence decreased among males during this period, it increased slightly among women from 0.2 to 0.3 percent (Figure 9-2).

Young men who have sex with men are at very substantial risk for HIV infection. In San Francisco from 1992 to 1993, 9.4 percent of such young men under 22 years of age, accessed in public settings near gay-associated sites, had HIV infection[57]; similar findings have been demonstrated elsewhere.[58] The risk of HIV that these young men confront is consistent with recent observations that young gay males are less likely to practice safe sex than older individuals.[59]

Estimates of the total number of people with AIDS who were infected as adolescents have been calculated recently. Back-calculations revealed that during the period 1987 to 1991 an estimated 25 percent of HIV infections were acquired before the age of 22.[60] Furthermore, a clinic-based study found that risk of HIV among STD clinic attendees was highest for those aged 15 to 19; the seroconversion rate was 7.1 per 100 person-years among these adolescents and 5.0 or less for all older age groups.[61]

Cross-sectional studies of HIV prevalence (Table 9-5) and longitudinal studies of HIV incidence (Table 9-6) conducted in developing countries have also demonstrated that young females are at high risk.

Table 9-5. HIV Prevalence among Adolescents and Young Adults in Developing Countries

Setting, age, and sex	Percent HIV+	Country	Author
Antenatal clinics			
<20 years (F) (n = 875)	10.0	Tanzania	Kigadye[162]
<20 years (F) (n = 276)	11.2	Rwanda	Chao[163]
<21 years (F) (n = 1851)	24.0	Malawi	Dallabetta[164]
Community surveys			
15–24 years (M) (n = 2097)	1.8	Tanzania	Grosskurth[165]
15–24 years (F) (n = 2545)	4.1		
15–19 years (M) (n = 1104)	0.9	Uganda	Wawer[166]
15–19 years (F) (n = 1337)	5.7		

DETERMINANTS OF STD/HIV RISK AMONG ADOLESCENTS

Adolescence is a unique time of life, when societal, biologic, behavioral, and developmental factors all act in concert to increase the likelihood of STD acquisition.

BIOLOGICAL FACTORS

Several aspects of physical development may be relevant to the high risk of STDs among adolescents. The histology of the cervix and vagina undergo dramatic changes from childhood through puberty and into adulthood. Newborns show effects of exposure to maternal estrogen, which produces the squamous epithelium lining of the vagina as seen in adults. Soon after birth these squamous cells are replaced with columnar epithelium. At puberty, estrogen exposure causes the vaginal lining to thicken again with layers of squamous epithelium. Such epithelial changes may be particularly important at the cervix, since the persistence of cervical columnar epithelium in young women appears to significantly increase their vulnerability to STDs. Although cervical columnar epithelium eventually recedes completely, to be replaced with squamous epithelium, this replacement is a gradual process, continuing well into adulthood. Typically, the cervix in the adolescent still displays areas of exposed columnar epithelium,[62] a

Table 9-6. HIV Incidence over Two Years among Adolescents and Young Adults in Developing Countries

Age and sex		HIV Sero-conversion	Country	Author
Antenatal clinic				
<20 yrs		10.5%	Rwanda	Bulterys[70]
20–22 yrs		4.1%		
23–25 yrs		2.2%		
26–30 yrs		0.8%		
Community survey				
15–19 yrs	(M)	0.6%	Tanzania	Grosskurth[141]
	(F)	3.9%		
20–24 yr	(M)	1.7%		
	(F)	1.6%		
25–34 yr	(M)	2.7%		
	(F)	1.8%		

condition often referred to as *ectopy*. This is significant because *Chlamydia trachomatis* infects columnar, not squamous, epithelium.

The presence of ectopy has repeatedly been associated with chlamydial infection, even after adjusting for sexual behavior and other confounders.[63,64] Although it may be that chlamydial infection causes the appearance of columnar epithelium on the cervix,[62] longitudinal studies have demonstrated that ectopy is associated with increased risk of subsequent infection.[65,66]

The presence of ectopy also appears to increase the risk for other STDs and their adverse outcomes. *Neisseria gonorrhoeae* attaches preferentially to columnar epithelium rather than squamous tissue. In addition, there is growing evidence that ectopy may contribute to HIV acquisition[67,68] and HIV shedding.[69] Ectopy may therefore partially account for the high incidence of HIV among adolescent women[70] by increasing both infectivity and susceptibility.[69] The vasculature found with the columnar epithelium associated with ectopy is more superficial and more easily traumatized than that of squamous epithelium, theoretically permitting HIV-infected cellular elements from the circulation to gain access to the mucosal surface, and infected monocytes and lymphocytes to reach the circulation.

The vaginal flora also changes during puberty. The appearance of *Lactobacillus* spp. results in reduction of the high vaginal pH levels of childhood to the more acidic pH associated with adulthood. The higher vaginal pH of early adolescence may be associated with a lower prevalence of hydrogen-peroxide-producing organisms. However, causal links between these anatomic or physiologic changes and STD acquisition have not yet been demonstrated.

Changes in mucosal anatomy produce changes in mucus production, which is minimal in childhood. Mucus production is greatly increased in early puberty, but the mucus is thinner than that found in older adolescents or adult women. Thinner mucus may permit organisms to penetrate more easily and to attach to mucosal sites or gain access to the upper tract.

Unfortunately, there is very little information about how development in males affects their risk of STD acquisition or transmission.

PSYCHOLOGICAL AND COGNITIVE DEVELOPMENT

The stages of adolescence have been arbitrarily categorized as "early," "middle," and "late" and have been considered in terms of psychologic, physiologic, and social development (Table 9–7). Development in each of these areas is not necessarily parallel. Individuals are often advanced in some categories but slower than their age-matched peers in others. Furthermore, growth in some of the cognitive areas is strongly influenced by the quality of teaching or role modeling they experience.[71] This is particularly relevant for STD prevention, where adults may use indirect methods of educating or rely on "scare tactics" rather than utilize skills training. Several characteristics of adolescents, particularly in early or middle stages of development may have important implications for STD risk and prevention. Younger adolescents frequently use a concrete style of reasoning, focusing on the present time, and are unable to conceptualize the long-term impact that current actions may have until they reach middle or late adolescence. Since some STDs (for example, HIV or chlamydia) may have adverse effects that are not experienced for a decade or more, it should not be surprising that younger adolescents may not take actions needed to avoid such consequences. Furthermore, adolescents may have difficulty correctly implementing complex tasks (such as condom use) involving a series of steps that must be accomplished in a certain sequence to be effective. Finally, many parents, educators, and health care workers do not teach about STD risk or even details of pubertal development until long after many adolescents are at risk for STDs. Therefore, these youths do not have even the basic information to make informed choices.

SEXUAL BEHAVIOR

Over the last century, sociocultural and behavioral changes have combined with changes in aspects of the developmental physiology of adolescents to increase the risk of STDs among these young people. Biologically, the average age at menarche has decreased (although it has been stable over the last generation). At the same time, societal changes have resulted in increases in the average age at which young men and women marry. As a result, whereas 100 years ago young men in the United States spent approximately 7 years between maturation and marriage, today the interval is 13 years; for young women, the interval between menarche and marriage has increased from 8 years to 14. For this reason alone, it should be expected that premarital sex in the United States has increased.[72]

Changes in sexual behavior have placed adolescents at increased risk of STDs, with the trend to earlier age at first intercourse occurring worldwide.[73–76] In the United States, several ongoing, population-based surveys provide information about the sexual behavior of adolescents. They show that during the past

Table 9-7. Highlights of Adolescent Development Stages

Early Adolescence: Females ages 9–13 Males ages 11–15	Middle Adolescence: Females ages 12–16 Males ages 14–17	Late Adolescence: Females ages 16 and older Males ages 17 and older
• Puberty as hallmark	• Increased independence from family	• Autonomy nearly secured
• Adjusting to puberty such as secondary sexual characteristics	• Increased importance of peer group	• Body image and gender role definition nearly secured
• Concern with body image	• Experimentation with relationships and sexual behaviors	• Empathetic relationships
• Beginning of separation from family, increased parent-child conflict	• Increased abstract thinking	• Attainment of abstract thinking
• Presence of social group cliques		• Defining of adult roles
• Concentration on relationships with peers		• Transition to adult roles
• Concrete thinking but beginning of exploration of new ability to abstract		• Greater intimacy skills
		• Sexual orientation nearly secured

Source: Report of the National Commission on Adolescent Sexual Health, 1995.[167]

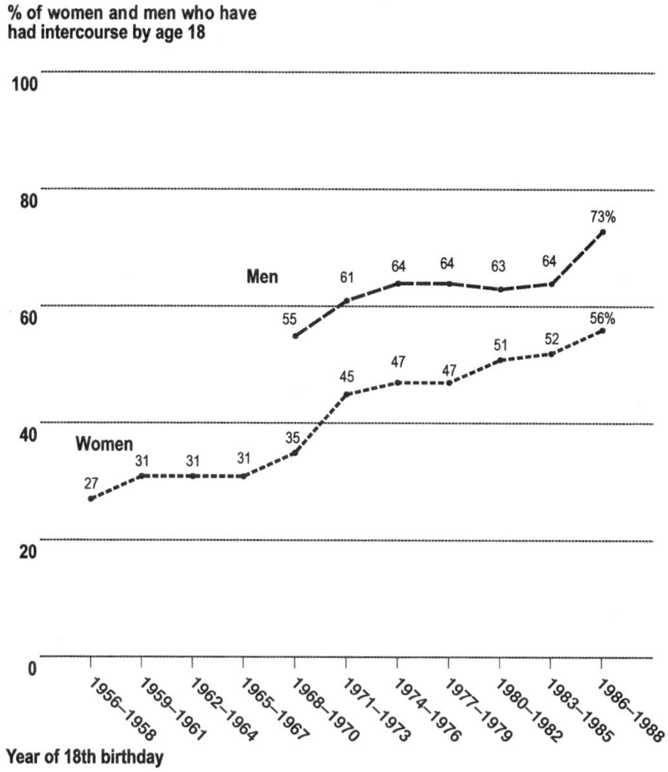

Fig. 9-3. Sex in the teen years is increasingly common. Over the past three decades, growing proportions of women and men have become sexually active in their teens. Today 56% of women and 73% of men have had intercourse before their 18th birthday. (Data obtained from Alan Guttmacher Institute: *Sex and America's Teenagers, 1994.*)

several decades the proportion of teenagers who have experienced premarital sexual intercourse has steadily increased (Fig. 9-3), and that age of first intercourse has steadily decreased (Figs. 9-4 and 9-5), although recent data indicate that this trend has leveled off in the United States over the half-decade through 1995.[77–79a] These trends have occurred despite concern about HIV infection. As a result, in the late 1980s, 56 percent of 18-year-old females and 73 percent of 18-year-old males had had sex. Of particular note, in 1970 only 5 percent of women in the United States had had premarital intercourse by age 15, whereas in 1988, 26 percent had engaged in intercourse by this age.[80] At each age a greater percentage of males than females have been sexually active; in general, the percentage of males who have had sexual intercourse is approximately equal to that of females 1 year older.

In addition, younger age of sexual "debut" is associated with a greater number of sexual partners, an important determinant of STD risk.[81] In 1988, among American women 15 to 24 years of age who were sexually active for the same length of time (less than 24 months), over 40 percent of 15- to 19-year-olds had had two or more partners, compared with only 26 percent of women 20 years of age or older.[80] Younger age of sexual debut (below age 18) is also associated with ongoing sexual risk among unmarried women, with an increased likelihood of having two or more recent partners.[82] Nevertheless, partner acquisition tends to follow a pattern of serial monogamy, with fewer than 10 percent of sexually active adolescents having more than one partner within a 3-month period.[81]

Population-based data demonstrate that condom use has increased substantially, but also that use is not consistent. Surveys indicate that more adolescents are using condoms. In the United States between 1983 and 1988, 65 percent of females used contraception at first intercourse, compared with 47 percent of females in the period 1975 to 1979; this increase was entirely a result of increased use of condoms.[83] Comparison data over time are also available for adolescent males. In 1979, 21 percent of never-married urban males 17 to 19 years old reported using condoms at last intercourse, compared with 58 percent in 1988. Reported use was greatest among African American males.[84] However, follow-up data indicate that as males get older and as the duration of the existing relationship increases, condoms are less likely to be used, while forms of contraception that offer less protection against STDs are used more, particularly oral contraceptives.[85] This pattern has also been reported from other countries, such as Australia,[86] Canada,[87] and New Zealand.[88] It is noteworthy that the combined effect of serial monogamy and diminishing use of condoms over the duration of a relationship may be particularly important in exposure to and ongoing transmission of organisms such as HSV-2, chlamydia, HPV, and HIV, which are associated with chronic and often asymptomatic infection.

Fig. 9-4. Percentage of females who have had intercourse by each age; 1958–1960 and 1985–1987 cohorts. (Reproduced with permission from Moore KA et al: *Adolescent Sex, Contraception, and Child bearing: A Review of Recent Research.* Washington, DC, Child Trends, Inc. 1995.)

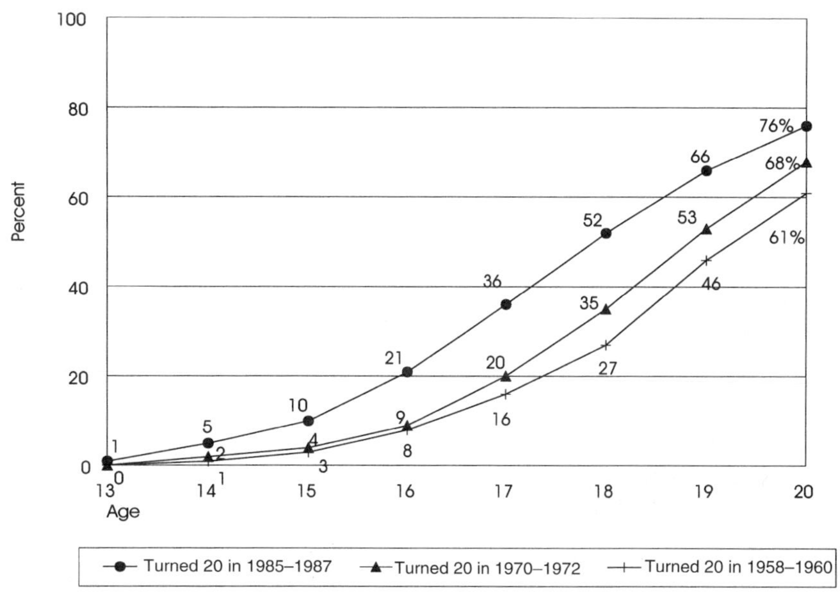

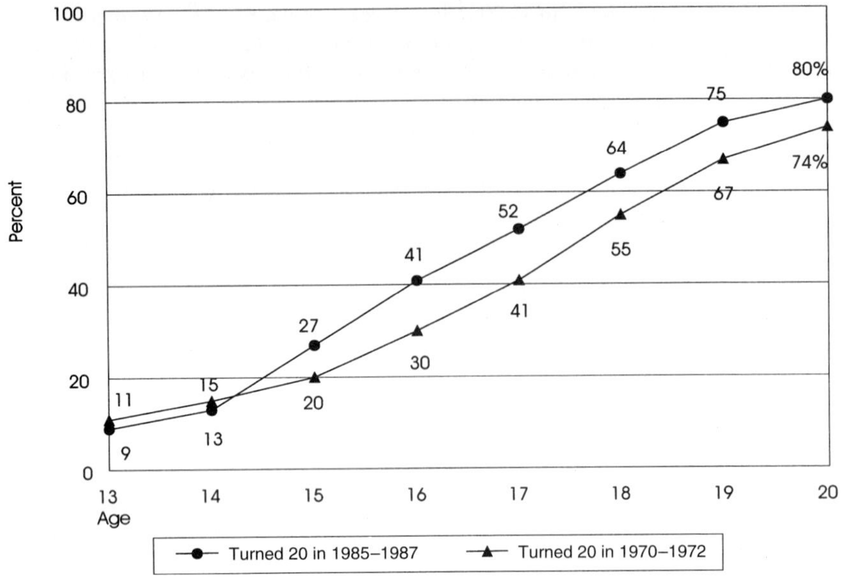

Fig. 9-5. Percent of males who have had intercourse by each age; 1970–1972 and 1985–1987 cohorts. (Reproduced with permission from Moore KA et al: *Adolescent Sex, Contraception, and Childbearing: A Review of Recent Research*. Washington, DC, Child Trends, Inc. 1995.)

Although more people are using condoms, few people, including adolescents, use them consistently. Among unmarried women in the United States, 59 percent of 15- to 19-year-olds reported using condoms for at least 1 month during the 4 years before interview, but only 31 percent of these women's partners used condoms consistently.[89] Furthermore, the young people most at risk for STDs appear to use condoms least.[90] A survey among adolescent males indicated that those who were substance abusers or had paid for sex were among the least likely to have used condoms at last intercourse.[84] Young males were less likely than older males to use condoms at first intercourse with partners they perceived to be at higher STD risk.[85] Among young people with two or more partners, individuals with greater numbers of partners were less likely to use condoms consistently with either primary or secondary partners.[91] A similar pattern has been observed in other countries.[92]

Use of condoms is a complex behavior, but we can make some generalizations about determinants of condom use upon which to base prevention strategies. Many studies,[93,94] but not all,[95,96] indicate that use is associated with perceived risk of HIV infection. Youths who think their peers use condoms are more likely to use them,[95,97–99] as are adolescents who feel that their partner would support their use.[90,100,101] Adolescents are often mistaken about what their partners believe, however, with females overestimating the resistance and negative attitudes that males have about condom use.[102]

Studies have noted that self-efficacy, perceived risk, and partner support are important factors in increased condom use.[99,103] For example, many young females who feel confident that they could get their partner to use condoms or could discuss condom use with them are not using condoms.[1,104] An important factor appears to be the extent to which young people underestimate their partners' risk of infection. Young homosexual males[59] believe that they are safe if they have sex with younger partners. Heterosexual females often feel that they have little or no risk of acquiring HIV from their male partners and believe in their boyfriends' statements of fidelity, often despite having a history of STD themselves.[1] A major concern, however, is the belief that their partners, particularly their steady partners, would view the request to use a condom as indicating a lack of trust. Conversely, if the request for use is made by the male, the female may assume he is dating outside the relationship. Approaches to reconciling these issues are complex and require skillful and practiced communication, as well as interventions suitable for sexually active adolescents who are in the formative phases of social skill development. Other barriers to condom use that are unique to adolescents include lack of ready availability.[94] Embarrassment about purchasing condoms may be a particular obstacle for girls.[104]

LEGAL AND ETHICAL ISSUES

Adolescents have unique legal status with regard to the provision of health care. Legally they are accorded more rights than children, but in some matters they may have rights that differ from those of adults. However, in all states of the United States, adolescents can be diagnosed and treated for STDs without parental consent or knowledge, and some states have specific provisions regarding testing for and treating HIV infection. Beyond STD diagnosis and treatment, there are three basic issues providers confront in dealing with adolescents[105]:

1. Does the adolescent have the authority to consent to care without parental involvement?
2. Does the adolescent have the authority to release or prevent release of confidential information (particularly to parents)?
3. Is the adolescent or another source responsible for payment for services rendered? Can adolescents insist that parents not be contacted?

In the United States the answers vary by state.[106,107] However, some generalizations are possible. First, it should be noted that in most states the age of majority is 18, but in three states (Alabama, Nebraska, and Wyoming) it is 19. Parents usually have the responsibility for medical care for their minor children and are liable for the costs of their care. However, as stated, all states either have specific statues or otherwise permit the diagnosis and treatment of "venereal disease" (the usual terminology) without parental consent.

Consent

Although all states permit a minor to consent to STD care without parental consent, some states identify an age criterion. As of 1994, in five states (Alabama, California, Delaware, Illinois, and Vermont) minors must be at least 12 years old to consent to STD-related care, and in five states (Hawaii, Idaho, New Hampshire, North Dakota, and Washington) they must be 14 years old.

Parental notification

In general, providers are obligated to maintain confidentiality, although communication with parents is sometimes addressed specifically. However, as of 1994 in only two states (Connecticut and Florida) are providers specifically prohibited from notifying parents of a minor who seeks STD-related care. All other states either permit the provider to notify parents or do not address the issue.

Liability

Most states have not specifically addressed this issue. However, in six states (Connecticut, District of Columbia, Hawaii, Minnesota, Montana, and Oklahoma), the minor who seeks STD care is liable for costs. In many others it is stated that the parents are *not* liable, so cost recovery would not be a reason to contact them.

The specific issue of a minor consenting to HIV testing and treatment has been addressed by some states.[108] Many states have statutes that permit emancipated minors in "special circumstances"—for example, who are married, are themselves parents of children, or are living apart from their parents—to consent to care, including diagnosis and treatment of HIV infection. In addition, many states have laws specifically authorizing minors to give consent for HIV testing. Furthermore, several other states indirectly authorize minors to consent to diagnosis and treatment of HIV infection by either: (1) stating that HIV/AIDS is a sexually transmitted disease and permitting minors to consent to diagnosis and treatment of STDs; or (2) stating that HIV/AIDS is a reportable, infectious, or communicable disease, and that minors are authorized to give consent for the diagnosis and treatment of such conditions. As a result, adolescents in well over half of the states can consent to diagnosis and treatment of HIV infection.

Clinicians caring for adolescents should know the laws regarding medical treatment of minors in their locale. Some health care workers may feel a conflict between the desire to honor a minor's right to confidentiality and the desire to involve a parent or other adult. In addition to being aware of laws supporting an adolescent's right to confidential care for STDs, providers should realize that by disclosing confidential information they may undermine the ability of any provider to care for the adolescent in the future, particularly with regard to these sensitive issues.

HEALTH CARE UTILIZATION AND COMPLIANCE

The data suggest that adolescents in the United States obtain health care for all types of problems less often than older or younger individuals. In 1985, U.S. adolescents 10 to 18 years of age made an average of 1.6 visits to private, office-based physicians, compared with the national average of 2.7 for all ages.[109] Barriers to care relate to adolescents' stage of development. They may wish to arrange care on their own but lack knowledge of or transportation to available services. Since their parents usually have the insurance or Medicaid information, adolescents may be unable to document coverage, and they usually cannot pay for their care themselves. They may be put off by child-oriented waiting rooms or feel unwelcome in facilities that are geared to adults. When adolescents do obtain care, they may be seen by clinicians poorly trained in adolescent issues. From the adolescents' perspective, information about services or the services themselves may be unavailable.

Obtaining STD-related health care presents even more problems for young people. Over 37 percent of tenth-grade students did not know where to get treated for STDs and over 40 percent would be embarrassed to ask a doctor about symptoms related to the genitourinary tract.[110] Adolescents are very concerned about confidentiality and claim they would not seek care for problems relating to sexuality if they believed their parents would find out.[111] However, over one-third of tenth-graders in a national survey thought that the health department would inform parents about STDs and that most clinics required parental consent to treat STDs.[110]

Either because they are not sufficiently trained or because they are unaware of or unwilling to address the needs and desires of their young clients, physicians frequently are not useful sources of STD information for adolescents. Although many young people are concerned about STDs[112] and would like more information from their doctors, a survey among college freshmen found that 79 percent had never received counseling about STDs.[113]

In many countries STD treatment for females is seen in the most stigmatizing terms,[114] and unmarried young women are too ashamed to access care, such as family planning services, where needed treatment can be obtained. Despite the attention and education concerning HIV infection, adolescents, particularly females, are not informed about STD symptoms. A population-based study in Ethiopia found that 90 percent of young females had untreated symptoms such as discharge and irritation that warranted care but which the women accepted as normal.[29]

In the United States, improvement in STD and HIV services for adolescents may require that managed care organizations take into consideration the unique situations posed by and facing young people. There is concern that with fewer categorical services, perhaps affecting categorical STD care, there may be fewer options for services. Fee-for-service providers or primary care providers who function as the "gateway" to the system may not be well-attuned to the needs of adolescents. The advent of managed care has put the funding and perhaps the very existence of some school-based clinics in question. Currently those school-based clinics with a full range of services are among the few sources of accessible, affordable, and comprehensive care for adolescents.[115] Many such clinics provide reproductive health services that include counseling, gynecologic exams, and the diagnosis and treatment of STDs.

Contrary to "conventional wisdom," young people and adults adhere to prescribed regimens equally well.[116] Adherence is often dependent upon provider behavior. Clinicians can improve adherence among adolescents by explaining the rationale for the treatment. Efforts should be made to address the circumstances adolescents face. Providers tend to underestimate adolescents' knowledge and the obstacles that adolescents face in implementing medical instructions. Recent studies suggest that extra efforts on the part of providers can greatly improve compliance.[117]

Having convenient, effective treatment regimens can help. The availability of azithromycin, which permits single-dose treatment of chlamydia, offers promise of facilitating improved compliance for treatment of adolescent patients and partners.[118] Although an individual course of treatment is expensive, studies indicate that such therapy can be cost-effective: by resulting in improved compliance among patients and partners it may decrease rates of complications.[119] In addition, new diagnostic techniques may provide access to adolescents through an expanded range of settings. As mentioned, DNA amplification tests for chlamydia can be performed on urine, allowing specimens to be obtained in street settings,[19] in school clinics,[20] and at other community locations.[17]

CURRENT AND FUTURE DIRECTIONS FOR STD PREVENTION AMONG ADOLESCENTS

Effective STD prevention for adolescents requires involvement by numerous individuals and institutions that have contact with young people, and it should include activities implemented in several different settings. Despite the many challenges facing prevention of STDs among adolescents, there are encouraging findings from interventions based in schools or in the community, implemented in clinics or via mass media, or resulting from policy decisions.

There is evidence that the best school-based programs can be effective in postponing age of first intercourse and in decreasing rates of unprotected intercourse,[120] but the curricula in many schools need to be strengthened. School-based programs have been controversial, despite having the support of over 90 percent of parents in the United States[121] and despite studies documenting that sex education has not increased the percentage of young people becoming sexually active.[122] Since 95 percent of 5- to 17-year-olds in the United States are enrolled in school,[123] school-based programs can reach the vast majority of children and younger adolescents. In 1994 in the United States, HIV-prevention education was required in 78.7 percent of states and 83 percent of school districts and was taught in a required course in 85.6 percent of all middle school/junior high and senior high schools. STD education was required in 65 percent of states and 80.9 percent of school districts and was included as a topic in a required course in 84.1 percent of middle school/junior high and senior high schools. However, the programs need to be strengthened, since only 15.6 percent of teachers received training in STD prevention in the prior 2 years, and only 37 percent of teachers discussed the correct use of condoms.[124] Furthermore, greater emphasis on STD knowledge is needed. In 1995 a survey found that 42 percent of adolescents could not name an STD other than HIV/AIDS and only 3 percent named chlamydia,[125] the most common bacterial STD in the United States.

Effective educational interventions have also been developed for nonschool settings, where youth who are not in school but at greater risk[126] can be accessed. These interventions, which were tested in randomized trials, were effective in reducing risk among African American youth accessed in clinic-based settings or in the community[127–129] and among runaway youth in shelters.[130] A consistent finding is that information alone does not facilitate such behavior change. These studies are limited in number of study participants and duration of follow-up, but they have demonstrated reductions in self-reported risk behavior, although not in infection rates. This is important, since reductions in self-reported risk may not be accompanied by decreases in infection rate.[131]

These effective risk-reduction education programs, whether school-based or not, share nine characteristics. They have: (1) a narrow focus on reducing specific risky behaviors, (2) a theoretical grounding in social learning theory, social influence theory, or theories of reasoned action, (3) at least 14 h of instruction or, if less, instruction in small groups, (4) a variety of interactive teaching methods designed to encourage the participants to personalize the information, (5) activities to convey the risks of unprotected sex and how to avoid them, (6) instruction on social pressures and how to deal with them, (7) clear reinforcement of individual values and group norms appropriate to the age and experience of the pupils (staying abstinent or avoiding unprotected sex), (8) opportunities to practice communication and negotiation skills to increase confidence, and (9) effective training for individuals implementing the program.[122]

Peer facilitators have much to contribute in implementation of such interventions. They have been effective in programs to delay age of sexual debut[132] and in programs to prevent smoking[133] or decrease use of alcohol or marijuana.[134] Peers can teach social skills, model health-promoting behaviors, and serve as credible models. The last is particularly important, since the perception that peers support using condoms is strongly associated with their use.[99] Furthermore, peer facilitators have been shown to be as effective as adult facilitators, are preferred by adolescents,[135] and derive important personal benefit from performing prevention activities.

Some schools have tried to overcome the barriers adolescents encounter in obtaining condoms. In the United States over 400 schools have condom availability programs.[136] In this controversial approach,[137] most of these schools make condoms available through school personnel. Only a few make condoms available through peers, baskets, bowls, or vending machines, although these approaches are more effective for increasing availability.[136] Studies are still needed to evaluate the effect these programs have on sexual risk behavior.

Clinic-based services to diagnose and treat STDs can make a significant difference in the prevalence of these diseases. As a pilot project for the national program to prevent STD-related infertility, screening for cervical *Chlamydia trachomatis* was implemented in 160 family planning clinics in the northwestern United States (Alaska, Idaho, Oregon, and Washington), with treatment, education, and partner referral for those found to be infected. Prevalence of chlamydia among females 15 to 19 years old decreased from 10.5 percent in 1989 to 4.7 percent in 1995.[11] Reductions in chlamydia rates have previously been reported with implementation of widespread chlamydia screening, most notably in Sweden,[138] where several measures were enacted to address chlamydia, including mandated testing and partner notification. Such studies, and others from Wisconsin[139] and Columbus, Ohio,[140] clearly demonstrate that with widespread access to diagnosis and treatment—for example, through screening at family planning, prenatal care, and youth clinics—the prevalence of chlamydial infection among young, sexually active females can be substantially decreased. In some instances, however, the percentage decline has been less among adolescents than among older populations, despite greater coverage.[140] This suggests that additional activities are needed to reach other populations of young people, such as young males, for testing. Approaches to accessing such populations in nonclinic-based settings are now feasible and can have a substantial yield.[17,19]

The importance of providing effective treatment for STDs was also demonstrated in a population-based randomized controlled trial from Tanzania, which evaluated the effect of improved STD diagnosis and treatment on HIV incidence in six matched pairs of villages. The rationale for the intervention was the impressive evidence that sexually transmitted diseases markedly increase the probability of HIV transmission.[141] Overall, HIV incidence was 40 percent lower among subjects in the intervention communities than among those in control communities, a finding that was consistent across the community pairs. It is important to note the unpublished finding that among females 15 to 19 years old, 1.2 percent (2/167) of those in intervention communities and 3.9 percent (7/178) in comparison sites seroconverted; the results among males 15 to 19 years old were 1.0 percent (2/180) and 0.6 percent (1/174) for intervention and comparison communities, respectively. *Therefore, the intervention appeared effective among young women, the group at greatest risk for incident HIV and for whom the barriers to care are usually greatest.* The implications for the United States are important, since the rates of most STDs are highest among adolescents—and since U.S. adolescents face formidable barriers to care.

In Thailand, implementation and legal enforcement of a policy to promote safer sex practices in commercial sex establishments—the "100 percent condom campaign"[142]—was effective in reducing the prevalence of HIV among 21-year-old males selected by lottery for the military. In the cohorts conscripted in 1991 and 1993 the prevalence of HIV was 10.4 to 12.5 percent, but it was 6.7 percent in the 1995 cohort. This decrease was associated not only with an increase in the men's reported use of condoms with sex workers but also with a decrease (from 81.4 to 63.8 percent) in the proportion of men who reported having sexual relations with a sex worker.[143] However, the young men's use of condoms with girlfriends did not increase, so additional approaches are clearly needed to protect young people of both sexes.

The use of mass media has been effective in disseminating information and, in at least one instance, promoting a specific sexual behavior change among young people. In countries such as Zaire and Ghana, mass media campaigns were associated with increases among adolescents in knowledge and awareness of HIV,[144] and a Swiss multimedia campaign significantly increased condom use among adolescents and young adults,[145] although neither the number of partners reported nor the percentage of adolescents who reported being sexually active decreased. To further focus prevention efforts, some health information campaigns have utilized principles from social marketing, which recognizes that the audience is not a monolithic group and that messages must be tailored to specific, relatively homogeneous audiences.[146] In the United States several projects targeting adolescents are utilizing such an approach,[147] but they have not yet been evaluated.[148,149]

These strategies have not usually been coordinated with other effective approaches and they have usually been limited in scope; they have not been associated with widespread reductions in either sexual risk behavior or disease levels. By recent reports, Uganda stands an exception: in that country HIV prevalence among pregnant females 15 to 19 years old fell from 17 percent in the years 1990 through 1993 to 11 percent in the years 1994–1995. This decline was accompanied by reports of increases in condom use, decreases in numbers of sex partners, and increases in age of sexual debut.[150] Although a range of approaches has been implemented in Uganda, what specifically is responsible for this improvement is not yet known.[151]

In summary, there are effective strategies which, if coordinated and implemented broadly, should result in healthier behavior and lower rates of STDs among adolescents. Health education messages found to be effective can be provided with consistency across the different levels of social context of adolescents' lives,[152] and educational and health service activities can be systematically linked across schools, media, community organizations, and health care settings. Clinicians can be trained in effective techniques for dealing with young people; providers, together with adolescents, can conduct a meaningful assessment of risk of STDs and provide appropriate counseling and treatment. Prevention and care for adolescents must be accessible, affordable, and comprehensive, and it must be provided by professionals who are knowledgeable and committed to caring for young people, in communities and cultures attentive to young people's needs.

References

1 Overby KJ, Kegeles SM: The impact of AIDS on an urban population of high-risk female minority adolescents: implications for intervention. *J Adolesc Health* 15:216, 1994.

2 Marx R, Aral SO: Gonorrhea rates: what denominator is most appropriate? *Am J Public Health* 79:1057, 1989.

3 Bell TA, Holmes KK: Age-specific risks of syphilis, gonorrhea, and hospitalized pelvic inflammatory disease in sexually experienced U.S. women. *Sex Transm Dis* 11:291, 1984.

4 Bagshaw SN, Edwards D: Risk factors for *Chlamydia trachomatis* infection of the cervix: a prospective study of 2000 patients at a family planning clinic. *NZ Med J* 100:401, 1987.

5 Addiss DG et al: Selective screening for *Chlamydia trachomatis* infection in nonurban family planning clinics in Wisconsin. *Fam Plann Perspect* 19:252, 1987.

6 Malotte CK et al: Screening for chlamydial cervicitis in a sexually active university population. *Am J Public Health* 80:469, 1990.

7 Campbell WF, Dodson MG: Clindamycin therapy for *Chlamydia trachomatis* in women. *Am J Obstet Gynecol* 162:343, 1990.

8 Barnes RC et al: Quantitative culture of endocervical *Chlamydia trachomatis*. *J Clin Microbiol* 28:774, 1990.

9 Handsfield HH et al: Criteria for selective screening for *Chlamydia trachomatis* infection in women attending family planning clinics. *JAMA* 255:1730, 1986.

10 Schachter J et al: Screening for chlamydial infections in women attending family planning clinics. *West J Med* 138:375, 1983.

11 Centers for Disease Control and Prevention, Division of STD Prevention: *Sexually Transmitted Disease Surveillance, 1995*. Atlanta, U.S. Department of Health and Human Services, Public Health Service, 1996.

12 Shakarishvili A et al: *Chlamydia trachomatis* Infection in Disadvantaged Young Women across the United States: Findings from the U.S. Job Corps. The 11th Meeting of the International Society for STD Research, abstr 023, 1995.

13 Werner MJ, Biro FM: Urinary leukocyte esterase screening for asymptomatic sexually transmitted disease in adolescent males. *J Adolesc Health* 12:326, 1991.

14 Shafer MA et al: Urinary leukocyte esterase screening test for asymptomatic chlamydial and gonococcal infections in males. *JAMA* 262: 2562, 1989.

15 Shafer MA et al: Evaluation of urine-based screening strategies to detect *Chlamydia trachomatis* among sexually active asymptomatic young males. *JAMA* 270:2065, 1993.

16 Leonardi GP et al: Evaluation of three immunoassays for detection of *Chlamydia trachomatis* in urine specimens from asymptomatic males. *J Clin Microbiol* 30:2793, 1992.

17 Marrazzo JM et al: Community-based urine screening for *Chlamydia trachomatis* infection with a ligase chain reaction assay. *Ann Intern Med* 127:796, 1997.

18 Kretzschmar M et al: Modeling prevention strategies for gonorrhea and chlamydia using stochastic network simulations. *Ann Epidemiol* 144:306, 1996.

19 Reitmeijer CA et al: Feasibility and yield of screening urine for *Chlamydia trachomatis* by PCR among high-risk male youth in field-based and other nonclinic settings. *Sex Transm Dis* 24:429, 1997.

20 Farley T et al: Screening High School Students for *Chlamydia trachomatis* Using a Urine Ligase Chain Reaction Test. The 34th Annual Meeting of the Infectious Diseases Society of America, 1996.

21 Hillis SD et al: Risk factors for recurrent *Chlamydia trachomatis* infections in women. *Am J Obstetr Gynecol* 170:801, 1994.

22 Fortenberry JD, Evans DL: Routine screening for genital *Chlamydia trachomatis* in adolescent females. *Sex Transm Dis* 16:168, 1989.

23 Blythe MJ et al: Recurrent genitourinary chlamydial infections in sexually active female adolescents. *J Pediatr* 121:487, 1992.

24 St. Louis ME: (Division of STD Prevention, CDC) Personal communication, 1997.

25 Mosure DJ et al: Predictors of *Chlamydia trachomatis* infection among female adolescents: a longitudinal analysis. *Am J Epidemiol* 144:997, 1996.

26 Jonsson M et al: The influence of sexual and social factors on the risk of *Chlamydia trachomatis* infections, a population-based serologic study. *Sex Transm Dis* 22:355, 1995.

27 Jonsson M et al: The silent suffering women—a population-based study on the association between reported symptoms and past and present infections of the lower genital tract. *Genitour Med* 71:158, 1995.

28 Behets FM et al: Control of sexually transmitted diseases in Haiti: results and implications of a baseline study among pregnant women living in Cité Soleil Shantytowns. *J Infec Dis* 172:764, 1995.

29 Brabin L et al: Reproductive tract infections and abortion among adolescent girls in rural Nigeria. *Lancet* 345:300, 1995.

30 Adolescent Health Program: Sexually Transmitted Diseases amongst Adolescents in the Developing World. WHO/ADH/93.1, 1993.

31 De Schryver A, Meheus A: Epidemiology of sexually transmitted diseases: the global picture. *Bull WHO* 68:639, 1990.

32 Ellen JM et al: Socioeconomic differences in sexually transmitted disease rates among black and white adolescents, San Francisco, 1990 to 1992. *Am J Public Health* 85:1546, 1995.

33 Piot P, Islam MQ: Sexually transmitted diseases in the 1990s. Global epidemiology and challenges for control. *Sex Transm Dis* (suppl) 21: S7, 1994.

34 Kohl PK: Epidemiology of sexually transmitted diseases. What does it tell us? *Sex Transm Dis* (suppl) 21:S81, 1994.

35 Berkley S: The public health significance of sexually transmitted diseases for HIV infection in Africa, in *AIDS and Women's Reproductive Health,* LC Chen, JS Amor (eds). New York, Plenum Press, 1990, pp 73–84.

36 Daly CC et al: Risk factors for gonorrhoea, syphilis, and trichomonas infections among women attending family planning clinics in Nairobi, Kenya. *Genitour Med* 70:155, 1994.

37 Levine WD et al: Dual Epidemics of Syphilis and HIV Infection among Adolescent African-American Women in Houston, 1988–1993. The 11th Meeting of the International Society for STD Research, abstr 051, 1995.

38 Meheus A et al: Genital infections in prenatal and family planning attendants in Swaziland. *East Afr Med J* 57:212, 1980.

39 Mosha F et al: A population-based study of syphilis and sexually transmitted disease syndromes in north-western Tanzania: 1. Prevalence and incidence. *Genitour Med* 69:415, 1993.

40 Burk RD et al: Declining prevalence of cervicovaginal human papillomavirus infection with age is independent of other risk factors. *Sex Transm Dis* 23:333, 1996.

41 Ho GYF et al: Persistent genital human papillomavirus infection as a risk factor for persistent cervical dysplasia. *J Nat Cancer Inst* 87: 1365, 1995.

42 Koutsky LA et al: Underdiagnosis of genital herpes by current clinical and viral-isolation procedures. *New Engl J Med* 326:1533, 1992.

43 Johnson RE et al: A seroepidemiologic survey of the prevalence of herpes simplex virus type 2 infection in the United States. *New Engl J Med* 321:7, 1989.

44 Fleming DT: Herpes simplex virus type 2 in the United States, 1976 to 1994. *N Engl J Med* 337:1105, 1997.

45 Westrom L: Incidence, prevalence, and trends of acute pelvic inflammatory disease and its consequences in industrialized countries. *Am J Obstetr Gynecol* 138:880, 1980.

46 Westrom L et al: Chlamydial and gonococcal infections in a defined population of women. *Scand J Infec Dis* (suppl) 32:157, 1982.

47 Rolfs RT et al: Pelvic inflammatory disease: trends in hospitalizations and office visits, 1979 through 1988. *Am J Obstetr Gynecol* 166:983, 1992.

48 Shafer MA, Sweet RL: Pelvic inflammatory disease in adolescent females. Epidemiology, pathogenesis, diagnosis, treatment, and sequelae. *Pediatr Clin North Amer* 36:513, 1989.

49 Spence MR et al: Pelvic inflammatory disease in the adolescent. *J Adolesc Health Care* 11:304, 1990.

50 Hillis SD et al: Delayed care of pelvic inflammatory disease as a risk factor for impaired fertility. *Am J Obstetr Gynecol* 168:1503, 1993.

51 Laga M et al: Non-ulcerative sexually transmitted diseases as risk factors for *HIV*-1 transmission in women: results from a cohort study. *AIDS* 7:95, 1993.

52 Wasserheit JN: Epidemiological synergy: interrelationships between human immunodeficiency virus infection and other sexually transmitted diseases. *Sex Transm Dis* 19:61, 1992.

53 Goedert JJ et al: A prospective study of human immunodeficiency virus type 1 infection and the development of AIDS in subjects with hemophilia. *New Engl J Med* 321:1141, 1989.

54 Centers for Disease Control and Prevention: First 500,000 AIDS cases—United States, 1995. *MMWR* 44:849, 1995.

55 Lindegren ML et al: Epidemiology of human immunodeficiency virus infection in adolescents, United States. *Pediatr Infec Dis J* 13:525, 1994.

56 Hein K et al: Comparison of HIV+ and HIV− adolescents—risk factors and psychosocial determinants. *Pediatrics* 95:96, 1995.

57 Lemp GF et al: Seroprevalence of HIV and risk behaviors among young homosexual and bisexual men: the San Francisco/Berkeley young men's survey. *JAMA* 272:449, 1994.

58 Valleroy LA et al: HIV and risk behaviour prevalence among young men who have sex with men sampled in six urban counties in the USA. The 11th Conference on AIDS, abstr 2407, 1996.

59 Hays RB et al: High HIV risk-taking among young gay men. *AIDS* 4:901, 1990.

60 Rosenberg PS et al: Declining age at HIV infection in the United States. *New Engl J Med* 330:89, 1994.

61 Otten MW et al: High rate of HIV seroconversion among patients attending urban sexually transmitted disease clinics. *AIDS* 8:549, 1994.

62 Critchlow CW et al: Determinants of cervical ectopia and of cervicitis—age, oral contraception, specific cervical infection, smoking, and douching. *Am J Obstetr Gynecol* 173:534, 1995.

63 Stergachis A et al: Selective screening for *Chlamydia trachomatis* infection in a primary care population of women. *Am J Epidemiol* 138: 143, 1993.

64 Johnson BA et al: Derivation and validation of a clinical diagnostic model for chlamydial cervical infection in university women. *JAMA* 265:3161, 1990.

65 Louv WC et al: Oral contraceptive use and the risk of chlamydial and gonococcal infections. *Am J Obstet Gynecol* 160:396, 1989.

66 Rahm VA et al: *Chlamydia trachomatis* in sexually active teenage girls. Factors related to genital chlamydial infection: a prospective study. *Genitour Med* 67:317, 1991.

67 Moss GB et al: Association of cervical ectopy with heterosexual transmission of human immunodeficiency virus: results of a study of couples in Nairobi, Kenya. *J Infec Dis* 164:588, 1991.

68 Plourde PJ et al: Human immunodeficiency virus type 1 seroconversion in women with genital ulcers. *J Infec Dis* 170:313, 1994.

69 Clemetson DB et al: Detection of HIV DNA in cervical and vaginal secretions: prevalence and correlates among women in Nairobi, Kenya. *JAMA* 269:2860, 1993.

70 Bulterys M et al: Incident HIV-1 infection in a cohort of young women in Butare, Rwanda. *AIDS* 8:1585, 1994.

71 Gilligan C, Wiggins G: The origins of morality in early childhood relationships, in *The Emergence of Morality in Young Children,* Jerome Kagan, Sharon Lamb (eds). Chicago, University of Chicago Press, 1987, pp 277–305.

72 Forrest JD: Timing of reproductive life stages. *Obstetr and Gynecol* 82:105, 1993.

73 Friedman HL: Changing patterns of adolescent sexual behavior: consequences for health and development. *J Adolesc Health* 13:345, 1992.

74 Graham CA: AIDS and the adolescent. *Internat J STD AIDS* 5:305, 1994.

75 Oakley A et al: Sexual health education interventions for young people: a methodological review. *BMJ* 310:158, 1995.

76 Caraël M et al: Overview and selected findings of sexual behaviour surveys. *AIDS* 5:S65, 1991.

77 Centers for Disease Control and Prevention: Trends in sexual risk behavior among high school students—United States, 1990, 1991, and 1993. *MMWR* 44:124, 1995.

78 Sonnenstein FL et al: Changes in sexual behavior and condom use among teenaged males: 1988 to 1995. *Am J Pub Health* 88:956, 1998.

79 Centers for Disease Control and Prevention: CDC surveillance summaries. *MMWR* 45 (no.SS-4), 1996.

79a Abma JC et al: Fertility, family planning, and women's health: new data from the 1995 National Survey of Family Growth. National Center for Health Statistics. *Vital Health Stat* 23(19), 1997.

80 Centers for Disease Control and Prevention: Premarital sexual experience among adolescent women—United States, 1970–1988. *MMWR* 39:929, 1991.

81 Kost K, Forrest JD: American women's sexual behavior and exposure to risk of sexually transmitted diseases. *Fam Plann Perspect* 24:244, 1992.

82 Seidman SN et al: Predictors of high-risk behavior in unmarried American women: adolescent environment as risk factor. *J Adolesc Health* 15:126, 1994.
83 Mosher WD, McNally JW: Contraceptive use at first premarital intercourse: United States, 1965–1988. *Fam Plann Perspect* 23:108, 1991.
84 Sonnenstein FL et al: Sexual activity, condom use, and AIDS awareness among adolescent males. *Fam Plann Perspect* 21:152, 1989.
85 Ku L et al: The dynamics of young men's condom use during and across relationships. *Fam Plann Perspect* 26:246, 1994.
86 Dunne MP et al: Age-related increase in sexual behaviours and decrease in regular condom use among adolescents in Australia. *Internat J STD AIDS* 5:41, 1994.
87 Nguyet NT et al: Sexual behaviors and condom use: a study of suburban male adolescents. *Adolescence* 29:37, 1994.
88 Fergusson DM et al: AIDS knowledge and condom use in a birth cohort of 16-year-olds. *NZ Med J* 107:480, 1994.
89 Potter LB, Anderson JE: Patterns of condom use and sexual behavior among never-married women. *Sex Transm Dis* 20:201, 1993.
90 Weisman CS et al: Consistency of condom use for disease prevention among adolescent users of oral contraceptives. *Fam Plann Perspect* 23:71, 1991.
91 Binson D et al: Data from the National AIDS Behavioral Surveys: IV. Multiple sexual partners among young adults in high-risk cities. *Fam Plann Perspect* 25:268, 1993.
92 MacDonald NE et al: High-risk STD/HIV behavior among college students. *JAMA* 263:3155, 1990.
93 Hingson RW et al: Beliefs about AIDS, use of alcohol and drugs, and unprotected sex among Massachusetts adolescents. *Am J Public Health* 80:295, 1990.
94 Donald M: Determinants of condom use by Australian secondary school students. *J Adolesc Health* 15:503, 1994.
95 Brown LK et al: Predictors of condom use in sexually active adolescents. *J Adolesc Health* 13:651, 1992.
96 Weisman CS et al: AIDS knowledge, perceived risk, and prevention among adolescent clients of a family planning clinic. *Fam Plann Perspect* 21:213, 1989.
97 Romer D et al: Social influences on the sexual behavior of youth at risk for HIV exposure. *Am J Public Health* 84:977, 1994.
98 Shafer MA, Boyer CB: Psychosocial and behavioral factors associated with risk of sexually transmitted diseases, including human immunodeficiency virus infection, among urban high school students. *J Pediatr* 119:826–833, 1991.
99 DiClemente RJ et al: African-American adolescents residing in high-risk urban environments do use condoms—correlates and predictors of condom use among adolescents in public housing developments. *Pediatrics* 98:269, 1996.
100 Pendergrast RA Jr. et al: Attitudinal and behavioral correlates of condom use in urban adolescent males. *J Adolesc Health* 13:133, 1992.
101 Plichta SB et al: Partner-specific condom use among adolescent women clients of a family planning clinic. *J Adolesc Health* 13:506, 1992.
102 Kegeles SM et al: Sexually active adolescents and condoms: changes over one year in knowledge, attitudes, and use. *Am J Public Health* 78:460, 1988.
103 Joffe A: Adolescents and condom use. *Am J Dis Childr* 147:746, 1993.
104 Guttmacher S et al: Gender differences in attitudes and use of condom availability programs among sexually active students in New York City public high schools. *J Am Med Wom Assoc* 50:99, 1995.
105 English A: Legal and Ethical Concerns, in *Textbook of Adolescent Medicine,* ER McAnarney (ed). Philadelphia, Saunders, 1992:95–99.
106 Paradise E, Horowitz R: Minor's Consent To Treatment for STD/Venereal Disease, in *Runaway and Homeless Youth: A Survey of State Law,* Appendix F. American Bar Association, Washington DC, 1994.
107 English A et al: *State Minor Consent Statutes: A Summary.* Center for Continuing Education in Adolescent Health, Cincinnati OH, 1995.
108 English A: Adolescents and HIV: Legal and Ethical Questions, in *The HIV Challenge. Prevention Education for Young People,* M Quackenbush et al (eds). Santa Cruz, CA, ETR Associates, 1995, pp 259–285.
109 U.S.Congress, Office of Technical Assessment: *Adolescent Health, Vol. 3: Crosscutting Issues in the Delivery of Health and Related Services.* OTA-H-467, 1991.
110 American School Health Association: *The National Adolescent Student Health Survey,* Oakland, CA, Third Party Publishing, 1989.
111 Marks A et al: Assessment of health needs and willingness to utilize health care resources of adolescents in a suburban population. *J Pediatr* 102:456, 1983.
112 Malus M et al: Priorities in adolescent health care: the teenager's viewpoint. *J Fam Pract* 25:159, 1987.
113 Joffe A et al: Health counseling for adolescents: what they want, what they get, and who gives it. *Pediatrics* 82:481, 1988.
114 Laga M: STD control for HIV prevention—it works. *Lancet* 346:518, 1995.
115 U.S.General Accounting Office: *School-Based Health Centers Can Promote Access to Care.* GAO/HEHS-94-166, 1994.
116 Litt IF, Cuskey WR: Compliance with medical regimens during adolescence. *Pediatr Clin North Amer* 27:3, 1980.
117 Friedman IM, Litt IF: Adolescents' compliance with therapeutic regimens. Psychological and social aspects and intervention. *J Adolesc Health Care* 8:52, 1987.
118 Hammerschlag MR et al: Single dose of azithromycin for the treatment of genital chlamydial infections in adolescents. *J Pediatr* 122:961, 1993.
119 Haddix AC et al: The cost-effectiveness of azithromycin for *Chlamydia trachomatis* infections in women. *Sex Transm Dis* 22:274, 1995.
120 Kirby D et al: School-based programs to reduce sexual risk behaviors: a review of effectiveness. *Public Health Reports* 109:339, 1994.
121 Gallup A: The 19th annual Gallup Polls of the public's attitudes toward the public school. *Gallup Poll* 69,1987.
122 Kirby D: Sex and HIV/AIDS education in schools. *BMJ* 311:403, 1995.
123 National Center for Education Statistics: *Digest of Education Statistics, 1993.* Washington, D.C. Publisher: U.S. Dept of Education 1993.
124 Centers for Disease Control and Prevention: School-based HIV prevention education—United States, 1994. *MMWR* 45:760, 1996.
125 American Social Health Association: Teenagers know more than adults about STDs, but knowledge among both groups is low. *STD News* 3, 1996.
126 Centers for Disease Control and Prevention: Health risk behaviors among adolescents who do and do not attend school—United States, 1992. *MMWR* 43:129, 1994.
127 Jemmott JB et al: Reductions in HIV risk-associated sexual behaviors among black male adolescents: effects of an AIDS prevention intervention. *Am J Public Health* 82:372, 1992.
128 St. Lawrence JS et al: Cognitive-behavioral intervention to reduce African-American adolescents' risk for HIV infection. *J Consult and Clin Psychol* 63:221, 1995.
129 DiClemente RJ, Wingood GM: A randomized controlled trial of an HIV sexual risk-reduction intervention for young African-American women. *JAMA* 274:1271, 1995.
130 Rotheram-Borus MJ et al: Reducing HIV sexual risk behaviors among runaway adolescents. *JAMA* 266:1237, 1991.
131 Orr DP et al: Behavioral intervention to increase condom use among high-risk female adolescents. *J Pediatr* 128:288, 1996.
132 Howard M, McCabe JB: Helping teenagers postpone sexual involvement. *Fam Plann Perspect* 22:21, 1990.
133 Telch MJ et al: Social influences approach to smoking prevention: the effects of videotape delivery with and without same-age peer leader participation. *Addict Behav* 5:21, 1990.
134 Perry CL: Prevention of alcohol use and abuse in adolescence: teacher- vs. peer-led intervention. (Special Issue: Preventive Interventions in Adolescence.) *Crisis* 10:52, 1989.

135 Jemmott JB et al: Abstinence and safer sex HIV risk-reduction interventions for African American adolescents: a randomized controlled trial. *JAMA* 279:1529, 1998.
136 Brener ND et al: School Condom Availability Programs in the United States. The 11th Conference on AIDS, abstr 2818, 1996.
137 English A: Condom distribution in the schools. *J Adolesc Health* 14: 562, 1993.
138 Ripa T: Epidemiologic control of genital *Chlamydia trachomatis* infections. *Scand J Infect Dis,* suppl 69:157, 1990.
139 Addiss DG et al: History and features of the Wisconsin *Chlamydia trachomatis* control program. *Fam Plann Perspect* 26:83, 1994.
140 Mertz KJ et al: Trends in the prevalence of chlamydial infections: The impact of community-wide testing. *Sex Transm Dis* 24:169, 1997.
141 Grosskurth H et al: Impact of improved treatment of sexually transmitted diseases on HIV infection in rural Tanzania—randomised controlled trial. *Lancet* 346:530, 1995.
142 Rojanapithayakorn W, Hanenberg R: The 100-percent condom program in Thailand. *AIDS* 10:1, 1996.
143 Nelson KE et al: Changes in sexual behavior and a decline in HIV infection among young men in Thailand. *New Engl J Med* 335:297, 1996.
144 McCauley AP, Salter C: Meeting the needs of young adults. *Population Reports,* Series J, 1995.
145 Hausser D, Michaud PA: Does a condom-promoting strategy (the Swiss Stop-AIDS campaign) modify sexual behavior among adolescents? *Pediatrics* 93:580, 1994.
146 Flora JA et al: Communication Campaigns for HIV Prevention: Using Mass Media in the Next Decade, in *Assessing the Social and Behavioral Science Base for HIV/AIDS Prevention and Intervention. Background Papers,* Institute of Medicine (ed). Washington DC, National Academy Press, 1995, pp 129–154.
147 Convisser J: Lessons from Africa: Condom Social Marketing for U.S. Teens. International Conference on AIDS, abstr PC0492, 1994.
148 Rugg D et al: Evaluating the Contributions of Social Marketing to HIV Prevention in Five U.S. Communities. The 11th Conference on AIDS, abstr 2880, 1996.
149 Convisser J et al: Community-Based Social Marketing Replicating the Project Action HIV Prevention Project for Teenagers in the United States. The 11th Conference on AIDS, abstr 4365, 1996.
150 Asiimwe-Okiror G et al: Declines in the HIV Prevalence in Ugandan Pregnant Women and Its Relationship to HIV Incidence and Risk Reduction. The 11th Conference on AIDS, abstr 905, 1996.
151 Mulder D et al: Decreasing HIV-1 seroprevalence in young adults in a rural Ugandan cohort. *BMJ* 311:833, 1995.
152 Hamburg DA et al: Adolescent Health Promotion in the Twenty-First Century: Current Frontiers and Future Directions, in *Promoting the Health of Adolescents,* SG Millstein et al (eds). New York, Oxford University Press, 1993, pp 375–388.
153 Rosenfeld WD et al: High prevalence rate of human papillomavirus infection and association with abnormal papanicolaou smears in sexually active adolescents. *Am J Dis Childr* 143:1443, 1989.
154 Moscicki AB et al: Human papillomavirus infection in sexually active adolescent females: prevalence and risk factors. *Pediatr Research* 28: 507, 1990.
155 Bauer HM et al: Genital human papillomavirus infection in female university students as determined by a PCR-based method. *JAMA* 265:472, 1991.
156 Bauer HM et al: Determinants of genital human papillomavirus infection in low-risk women in Portland, Oregon. *Sex Transm Dis* 20: 274, 1993.
157 Hildesheim A et al: Determinants of genital human papillomavirus infection in low-income women in Washington DC. *Sex Transm Dis* 20:279, 1993.
158 Wheeler CM et al: Determinants of genital human papillomavirus infection among cytologically normal women attending the University of New Mexico student health center. *Sex Transm Dis* 20:286, 1993.
159 Karlsson R et al: Lifetime number of partners as the only independent risk factor for human papillomavirus infection—a population-based study. *Sex Transm Dis* 22:119, 1995.
160 Fisher M et al: Cervicovaginal human papillomavirus infection in suburban adolescents and young adults. *J Pediatr* 119:821, 1991.
161 Jamison JH et al: Spectrum of genital human papillomavirus infection in a female adolescent population. *Sexually Transmitted Diseases* 22: 236, 1995.
162 Kigadye RM et al: Sentinel surveillance for HIV-1 among pregnant women in a developing country: three years' experience and comparison with a population serosurvey. *AIDS* 7:849, 1993.
163 Chao A et al: Risk factors associated with prevalent HIV-1 infection among pregnant women in Rwanda. *Internat J Epidemiol* 23:371, 1994.
164 Dallabetta GA et al: High socioeconomic status is a risk factor for human immunodeficiency virus type 1 (HIV-1) infection but not for sexually transmitted diseases in women in Malawi: implications for HIV-1 control. *J Infect Dis* 167:36, 1993.
165 Grosskurth H et al: A community trial of the impact of improved sexually transmitted disease treatment on the HIV epidemic in rural Tanzania: 2. Baseline survey results. *AIDS* 9:927, 1995.
166 Wawer MJ: Baseline survey data, Rakai project. Personal communication, 1996.
167 Haffner DW: Facing Facts: Sexual Health for America's Adolescents. Report of the National Commission on Adolescent Sexual Health, 1995.

Chapter 10

Sex workers and their clients in the epidemiology and control of sexually transmitted diseases

Francis A. Plummer
Roel A. Coutinho
Elizabeth N. Ngugi
Stephen Moses

For a communicable disease to be maintained in a population, an infected individual must infect on average more than one new susceptible, resulting in a basic reproductive rate for the disease of one or greater. For sexually transmitted diseases the basic reproductive rate is the product of the transmission efficiency of the disease pathogen, the effective rate of partner change in the population, and the average duration of infectiousness.[1] Since most members of a population are monogamous over at least short periods of time, STD transmission is in general maintained in populations through limited numbers of individuals having multiple partners. Groups of such individuals, whose members are at highest risk of acquiring and transmitting a sexually transmitted disease, are sometimes called "core groups."[2] Given their central role in the epidemiology of STDs, including HIV infection, these groups must also be a major focus of STD control efforts.

Sex workers, or prostitutes, together with their clients form one such group. In this chapter we consider prostitution in the context of the epidemiology and control of sexually transmitted diseases. Several authoritative discussions on the history, sociology, and dynamics of prostitution are available,[3-6] so these topics are discussed here only where relevant to the epidemiology and control of STDs.

DEFINITION OF SEX WORK

Society offers many definitions of sex work, or prostitution, none of which is entirely satisfactory. It is difficult to define adequately an activity which takes so many forms in so many different parts of the world. The pejorative connotation of the term *prostitute* also causes some to take exception to any definition. The definition used here is a person (woman, man, or child) who exchanges sexual services for an immediate cash or in-kind return. In this chapter it is not our intent to cast blame on one side or other of the prostitute-client relationship, but rather to discuss the importance of sex work in the epidemiology of STDs and how focused interventions directed at sex workers and their clients might contribute to STD control.

DYNAMICS OF SEX WORK

Until the beginning of this century STDs were generally considered to spread almost exclusively through prostitution, and consequently the control of STDs was synonymous with the control and often repression of sex work. By the eighteenth century, in some European countries such as France, prostitution was officially regulated. Prostitutes had to register with the police, and registered prostitutes were regularly checked by a medical doctor. Due to the limitations of medical knowledge at that time and the absence of effective therapy for sexually transmitted infections, the impact of these medical check-ups was probably negligible. In any case, most prostitutes did not register with the police. Regulation may even have contributed to the spread of STDs, as some prostitutes, especially those who were found to be ill and therefore not allowed to work, traveled from place to place to avoid police registration. In the second half of the nineteenth century the movement to repress prostitution grew in strength in both Europe and the United States. Consequently, by the end of the century many countries had adopted laws making prostitution illegal.

Sex work at the present time takes many forms in different social strata, societies, and nations, encompassing New York call girls, Nairobi slum prostitutes, and Japanese geishas. The common denominator of these groups is the sale of sex, but reasons for selling sex may differ considerably. For an impoverished woman living in an urban slum in Africa, selling sex may be seen as the only means of economic survival for herself and her family; for an impoverished family in rural Thailand, sending a young daughter to a city to sell sex may also be viewed as the only means for the family's economic survival. In other settings, some women may sell sex to support a drug habit; for other women, selling sex may be a means of achieving an income sufficient to meet expectations; and for still others, it may be a part-time occupation, a source of supplemental income.[7] It is important to understand these motivations in developing approaches to STD control. A relatively educated woman who has another profession to turn to, or one who has a family to consider, may be more receptive to an STD prevention program than one who sells sex to pay for drugs. Sex workers who are involved in other legally proscribed activities, such as drug use, may be difficult to reach through programs involving figures of authority.[8,9]

Although few data are available, it seems likely that the sale of sex is analogous to the sale of other commodities and is subject to the laws of supply and demand. When sex is difficult to obtain it becomes a valuable commodity, and when the demand for sex or a particular type of sexual encounter is unmet prostitution flourishes.[3] Relative scarcity of sex existed in North America and Europe prior to the "sexual revolution" of the mid-twentieth century, continues to exist in many parts of the developing world,[10] and exists generally in populations in which the number of unattached males greatly exceeds the number of females. This commonly occurs, for example, in seaports and around military bases, in African and Asian cities as a result of selective male migration to urban areas,[7] and during armed conflicts. In Nairobi, for example, clients of prostitutes often comprise single men, or married men whose wives reside in rural areas or are pregnant.[11] The phenomenon of a small number of women having sex with a large number of men is extremely important in STD epidemiology.

In Western countries at the present time, the purchase of sex does not appear in general to be a frequently occurring phenomenon. In a study on sexual behavior in Great Britain, it was found that only 3.6 percent of men reported ever having paid a female sex worker for sex.[12] In a telephone survey conducted among a representative sample of 20,000 persons in France, 3.3 percent of men reported buying sex from a female prostitute in the five years preceding the interview.[13] Similar data have been published from other industrialized countries. There is evidence, however, that in less developed countries men purchase sex from female prostitutes more frequently. A study by the World Health Organization found that in the Ivory Coast, Lesotho, Togo, and Kenya from 8 to 13 percent of sexually active men in the general population reported purchasing sex from a female sex worker in the previous year.[14] Among some groups, such as long-distance truck drivers, commercial sex is reported much more frequently.[15] A study among a general population group of 1,100 young men in northern Thailand indicated that three-quarters of them had paid for sex from a female sex worker at some time.[16]

In one of the few studies on the sexual behavior of male clients of female sex workers it was found that about one-half of 559 male clients interviewed by telephone in the Netherlands had restricted themselves to only one type of prostitution (such as sex club, home, or street prostitution) and that 90 percent of them reported consistently using condoms during vaginal sex.[17] Links between different kinds of prostitution were rare: only 3 percent of clients used more than one type. As the female sex workers themselves did not frequently report moving from one kind of prostitution to another, it may be inferred from this study that prostitutes should not be considered as one single entity but as a number of perhaps sparsely connected groups. The low level of contact between groups coupled with the high levels of condom use could explain, in part, the slow spread of HIV infection among heterosexuals in industrialized countries. The situation is quite different in many developing countries, where prostitution has likely played an important role in the spread of HIV.

The sale of homosexual sex occurs in industrialized and some developing countries, but it seems to be a much more limited phenomenon than the sale of heterosexual sex. In some industrialized country settings, male injecting-drug users may sell sex to men in exchange for money or drugs. The role of male-male prostitution in the spread at least of HIV infection seems to be limited, since anal intercourse appears to be rather infrequent in this context and since, when it does occur, condoms are often used.[18,19] The following discussion will focus on female prostitution, since most available data come from studies of women.

SEX WORK AND THE EPIDEMIOLOGY OF SPECIFIC SEXUALLY TRANSMITTED DISEASES

The relative role of sex-worker or client core groups in the epidemiology of a particular STD depends upon the frequency and nature of commercial sex transactions and upon the transmission dynamics of the STD. When a large segment of the male population has sex with prostitutes, the role will generally be large. This appears to be the case, for example, in Nairobi, where in one study, almost 15 percent of a sample of men residing in an urban slum reported having purchased sex from a female sex worker at least once during the previous three months.[11]

It has been noted that in the absence of effective treatment and prevention programs the transmission efficiency and duration of infectivity are relatively stable characteristics of STD pathogens.[20] The frequency of interaction between an infected individual and a new susceptible is therefore the critical determinant of the reproductive rates of STDs. As indicated previously, core groups such as sex workers and their clients, because of their high rates of partner change, are important in the transmission dynamics of all STDs. Some diseases, however, such as chancroid and syphilis, are characteristically associated with sex work because the average duration of infectiousness of these STDs is relatively short, requiring high rates of partner change to maintain transmission in populations. Sex work therefore is particularly important for their persistence. It has been suggested that as STD treatment and prevention programs improve in quality and expand in scope, the duration of infectiousness and perhaps transmission efficiency of the targeted STDs decrease.[21] As a result, these STDs as well will increasingly become concentrated in core groups such as sex workers and their clients. Furthermore, because members of many core groups experience stigmatization, discrimination, and marginalization, their access to STD-related health care may be relatively low, resulting in increased durations of infectiousness. In addition, they may be less likely to adopt measures to reduce transmission efficiency, such as increased use of condoms and other safer-sex practices. These additional behavioral factors also contribute to higher reproductive rates.

GONOCOCCAL AND CHLAMYDIAL INFECTIONS

In 1959 Rosenthal and Vandow, finding a decline in the prevalence of gonorrhea among prostitutes arrested for soliciting in New York City (from 23.6 percent in 1946 to 5.2 percent in 1956), stated that "the prostitute is no longer the major vector of venereal disease" and that "the promiscuous amateur" was filling the role.[22] In fact, the prevalences of *Neisseria gonorrhoeae* and *Chlamydia trachomatis* infection among sex workers have been found to be highly variable (Table 10-1) and to depend, among other things, upon the frequency and nature of sexual encounters, characteristics of clients, levels of condom use, and frequency of medical examinations.[23–35] Low prevalences of gonorrhea (under 1 percent) have, for example, been reported from registered prostitutes in Vienna,[28] while among lower-social-stratum prostitutes in Kenya and Rwanda, gonorrhea prevalences in the order of 50 percent have been found.[23,29]

The incidence of infection is also variable. Very high incidences have been reported from developing countries in prostitutes of lower socioeconomic strata: for example, in Nairobi an 11 percent weekly incidence of gonococcal cervicitis[23] and in Bangkok 31.7 new gonococcal infections and 43.1 new *C. trachomatis* infections per 100 woman-months of observation.[36] In Sheffield, England during the years 1969 to 1972, it was estimated that between 24

Table 10-1. Prevalence of *N. gonorrhoeae* and *C. trachomatis* Infections in Populations of Prostitutes

City	Year	Prevalence, %	Reference number
***N. Gonorrhoeae* infections**			
Industrialized countries			
Fresno, California, USA	1979	22	24
Colorado Springs, Colorado, USA	1979	22	25
Atlanta, Georgia, USA	1981	17	26
Groningen, Netherlands	1988	10	27
Vienna, Austria			
registered	1989	0.3	28
nonregistered	1989	7	28
Developing countries			
Nairobi, Kenya			
upper social stratum	1985	16	23
middle social stratum	1985	28	23
lower social stratum	1985	46	23
Butare, Rwanda	1974	51	29
Philippines	1969	15	30
Singapore	1977	9	31
Kinshasa, Zaire	1991	23	32
***C. Trachomatis* infections**			
Industrialized countries			
Vienna, Austria			
registered	1989	2	28
nonregistered	1989	10	28
Oviedo, Spain	1990	32	33
Developing countries			
Kinshasa, Zaire	1991	13	32
Tegucigalpa, Honduras	1989	31	34
Dakar, Senegal	1992	14	35

and 75 percent of male gonococcal infections were directly acquired from prostitutes.[37] A case-control study among predominantly African American gonorrhea patients in San Francisco in 1988 found that 32 percent of the female patients and none of the controls had received money or drugs in exchange for sex.[38] In Fresno, California[24] and Colorado Springs, Colorado[25] programs of screening or mass treatment for gonococcal infection in prostitutes resulted in declines in the incidence of gonococcal infections in the general community. These data suggest that in some areas of the world and in certain subgroups, sizable fractions of gonococcal and chlamydial transmission are attributable to sex workers and their clients. Since, in addition, many nonprostitute-acquired infections are likely secondary to prostitute-acquired infections, successful intervention in sex-worker/client core groups is crucial to gonorrhea and chlamydia control.

Sex workers using prophylactic antibiotics have played and possibly continue to play an important role in the development of *N. gonorrhoeae* resistant to antimicrobial agents. The practice of taking prophylactic penicillin[39,40] seems to have selected for a higher prevalence of penicillinase-producing *N. gonorrhoeae* (PPNG) in prostitutes in the Far East during the initial phase of the PPNG pandemic.[41] Sexual contact by travelers with PPNG-infected sex workers in other countries may have led to importation of PPNG into the United States.[42] In the Netherlands the first PPNG strain was described in 1977, and by 1981, 18 percent of the *N. gonorrhoeae* strains isolated at the public health laboratory in Amsterdam were PPNG. Prostitution was found to have played an important role in the spread of both the African and Asian plasmid types.[43]

SYPHILIS

Syphilis and prostitution have long been associated. At the height of the U.S. syphilis epidemic in the early twentieth century, 25 percent of all cases of syphilis were estimated to have been transmitted through commercial sex.[44] A recent rise in the number of reported cases of syphilis in the United States has been attributed to increased heterosexual transmission, especially among African Americans and Hispanics.[45] At least part of this increase is due to prostitution linked with crack cocaine use.[46] North American epidemics of syphilis in heterosexuals have been described in Fresno, California[24]; Winnipeg, Manitoba[47]; Edmonton, Alberta[48]; and Baltimore, Maryland.[49] Each of these outbreaks has been associated with prostitution in urban core areas. In Amsterdam, prostitutes who use "hard" drugs have been identified as being at high risk for syphilis.[50] Since the prevalence of syphilis in the general heterosexual population is extremely low, it seems plausible that a large proportion of syphilis cases among heterosexuals in North America and Europe is attributable to female sex workers and their clients.

Syphilis is also highly prevalent among prostitutes in developing countries. In Tegucigalpa, Honduras, 50 percent of a group of female prostitutes had specific treponemal antibodies,[51] and in a large group of over 3000 female sex workers in Mexico City the prevalence of latent asymptomatic syphilis was 8.2 percent.[52] These data suggest that in developing countries as well, commercial sex likely plays an important role in the spread of syphilis.

CHANCROID

Chancroid has been highly associated with sex workers and their clients, particularly those in lower socioeconomic strata, in virtually every major North American outbreak that has been reported. In several modern epidemics of chancroid (Winnipeg, Manitoba[53]; Orange County, California[54]; south Florida[55]; New York City[56]; and New Orleans[57]), sex work has been linked with much of chancroid transmission, often in association with drug use and the sale of sex for drugs. In Nairobi, an area of high chancroid endemicity, 66 percent of men with chancroid attending an STD clinic reported a paid sex partner as the source contact.[58] In a study among one group of Nairobi prostitutes, the prevalence of culture-proven chancroid was 13 percent.[59]

The reasons for the association between chancroid and lower-socioeconomic-stratum prostitution are not entirely clear. As the epidemiology of chancroid is currently understood, most female transmitters of *Haemophilus ducreyi* have clinical genital ulceration.[58] It may be that poor women, in need of income and with restricted access to health care, ignore ulcer symptoms rather than forgo income for several days. Certainly in the Nairobi prostitute cohorts women continue to have sex, at times in spite of severe genital ulceration. In addition, as has been alluded to above, it has been postulated that because of chancroid's relatively short duration of infectivity (compared to other STDs), chancroid epidemics can only be maintained in populations that have very high rates of partner change,[60] such as those seen typically among lower-socioeconomic-stratum female sex workers.

Control of some urban North American epidemics of chancroid, such as those in Winnipeg and in Orange County, has been achieved primarily by identifying and treating the affected populations of prostitutes.[53,54] Control has proven more difficult, however, in areas such as New York City, southern Florida, and New Orleans, where prostitution and drug use are intimately linked.[61]

HUMAN IMMUNODEFICIENCY VIRUS INFECTION

Human immunodeficiency virus infection is the most important STD associated with sex work. Sex workers and their clients are major groups at risk of acquiring and transmitting HIV.

The first hint that sex workers were at risk for HIV infection came from a study reporting lymphadenopathy and altered T-cell subset ratios in New York City prostitutes.[62] Female sex workers in Africa were first identified as a risk group for HIV infection in the mid-1980s, when several studies found an extremely high prevalence of HIV infection in women selling sex. Prostitutes in an early study in Kigali, Rwanda had an HIV prevalence of 88 percent.[63] In Nairobi the prevalence of HIV infection was 66 percent among 64 lower-socioeconomic-stratum prostitutes and 31 percent among 26 higher-socioeconomic-stratum prostitutes.[64] Subsequent studies in Uganda and Zaire yielded similar results.[65,66] Prostitutes in Africa also have an extremely high incidence of HIV infection. In a prospective 30-month study of HIV-negative prostitutes in Kenya, the cumulative HIV incidence was 67 percent.[67] High prevalences and incidences of HIV infection have also been observed in some Asian countries. In the national HIV surveillance round conducted in Thailand in 1993, the median HIV prevalence among female sex workers was approximately 30 percent.[68] The annual HIV incidence among female sex workers in Thailand is also very high, ranging from 24 to 29 percent.[69]

In Africa, Thailand, and other developing regions, commercial sex is also important in HIV transmission. The concentration of HIV infection in urban areas and along major overland trucking and trade routes indirectly implicates sex work in the spread of HIV through East Africa.[70,71] In a Kenyan study, male STD clinic patients in Nairobi who reported frequent prostitute contact as well as past and current genital ulcer disease (both of which are highly prostitute-associated) were more likely to be HIV infected.[72] In the same population an HIV incidence of 8 percent was estimated to have followed a single sexual encounter with an

HIV-infected prostitute.[73] Another study in Nairobi estimated that 3750 men per day are exposed to HIV through sexual contact with one group of prostitutes.[74]

The high prevalence among female sex workers of other sexually transmitted diseases is an important factor facilitating HIV transmission. Genital tract infections and inflammation probably increase HIV shedding in the female genital tract, rendering a woman more infectious to a sexual partner.[75–78] Thus, prostitutes are likely more efficient transmitters of HIV because of their high prevalence of genital ulcers and perhaps other STDs.[79] Additional factors serving to amplify transmission are that an immunosuppressed individual is likely more susceptible to acquiring genital ulcers, and the ulcers are more refractory to treatment than in an individual with a normal immune system.[80,81]

The prevalence of HIV infection has also been studied in North American and European female sex workers. Early studies from the mid-1980s in London, Paris, and Nuremberg found that none of 50, 56, and 399 prostitutes respectively were infected with HIV.[82–84] In Athens, 6 percent of 200 prostitutes who did not use intravenous drugs were found to be HIV positive.[85] More recent studies have also found low HIV prevalence rates.[86–88] The prevalence of HIV infection is higher, however, among intravenous-drug-using prostitutes. Ten of 14 such women in a study in Paderome, Italy and 14 of 18 in Zurich, Switzerland were found to be HIV infected.[89,90] In a large study of registered prostitutes in then West Germany, half of 17 HIV-positive women among 2000 tested were intravenous drug users.[91] HIV prevalences of over 50 percent were found among intravenous as well as nonintravenous (crack cocaine) drug-using prostitutes in New York and New Jersey.[92] In Amsterdam, 30 percent of drug-using prostitutes were found to be infected with HIV, and other STDs were also highly prevalent in this group.[93] Although a high proportion of prostitutes reported practicing safe sex, the high frequency of STDs suggests that there is potential for HIV transmission to their clients.

It appears, then, that in European countries most prostitutes acquire HIV infection primarily through intravenous drug use or from intravenous-drug-using sex partners.[94] This also occurs in North America, but the crack cocaine epidemic, with its accompanying sex-for-drugs phenomenon, is probably responsible as well for a large proportion of sex-work-associated HIV infection.[95] The substantial number of prostitutes infected with HIV creates considerable potential for transmission of the virus to the general heterosexual population. That this has not already occurred to a greater extent may be a result of high levels of condom use, the use of nonpenetrative sex, or the relative absence of other cofactors such as genital ulcer disease.

INTERVENTIONS

Given the importance of sex workers and their clients in STD epidemiology, a key component of STD/HIV control strategies should be to intervene among these groups.[96] Two general approaches to intervention are possible (Table 10-2). First, strategies may focus on sex work itself by (1) criminalizing the practice of prostitution, (2) penalizing clients of prostitutes, (3) regulating legalized prostitution, (4) reducing the willingness of women to become prostitutes, and (5) reducing the demand of men for sexual services. Second, they may concentrate on STDs by (1) reducing STD prevalence in prostitutes, and (2) reducing STD transmission from sex workers to clients and from clients to sex workers.

Table 10-2. Intervention Strategies to Control STDs among Sex Workers and Their Clients

Directed at sex work:
Criminalizing prostitution
Penalizing clients of prostitutes
Regulating legalized prostitution
Reducing the supply of prostitutes
Reducing the demand for prostitutes
Directed at reducing STD transmission:
Decreasing STD prevalence in sex workers
Decreasing STD transmission from sex workers to clients and from clients to sex workers

INTERVENTIONS DIRECTED AT SEX WORK

The first three strategies listed in Table 10-2 under "interventions directed at sex work" involve legal approaches and assume that prostitution is an undesirable activity. Moral stances or the association of prostitution with other crimes is often the motivation for the legal approach, which has generally proven to be ineffective. Modern efforts to control prostitution by legal means began with the social reform movements in the nineteenth and twentieth centuries.[3,6] In North America these efforts have gradually lapsed into an attitude of partial unofficial tolerance of prostitution despite its continued illegality. Periodic crusades against prostitutes probably do little to control STDs.[8,9] Prostitution is officially illegal in most developing countries but flourishes because of social and economic realities. Again, a situation of unofficial tolerance with periodic "swoops" to arrest prostitutes has evolved.

Some European countries have developed systems of regulation of prostitution, whereby sex work is partly legal and prostitutes must submit to periodic examination and testing for STDs. These systems may have some effect on controlling STDs, but many sex workers do not wish to be registered, and a requirement to do so may make them more refractory to seeking care within the health system.

Interventions may also be directed at the supply side of the sex-worker-client equation. Two broad kinds of strategies can be envisioned: reducing the economic necessity to sell sex, and reducing women's willingness to sell sex. The first strategy addresses the root causes of poverty and marginalization and can ultimately only be effected through significant societal change. In the shorter term, special programs to identify and promote alternative economic opportunities for female sex workers have been advocated, and to a limited extent undertaken, in some developing countries. These programs tend to be labor-intensive, and while they may be of benefit to individual women, the impact on the overall supply of sex workers is unknown. This is particularly problematic in many developing countries, where a virtually unlimited supply of poor women is available to replace women exiting sex work. The second strategy relies upon identifying motivations for not selling sex which are stronger than those for selling sex. One such motivation may be the health risks of STDs. Pelvic inflammatory disease, infertility, cancer of the cervix, and AIDS are good reasons for women to reduce their risk behavior. However, in many developing-country settings, economic necessity often overrides such considerations.

On the demand side, interventions may be directed at the clients of prostitutes. One can work to decrease the willingness of men to purchase sex through education regarding the health risks involved. The impact of this approach is uncertain, but some successful efforts in this regard have been reported from Africa.[97,98]

INTERVENTIONS DIRECTED AT REDUCING STD TRANSMISSION

Interventions directed at reducing STD transmission have consisted of two main approaches: decreasing STD prevalence in sex workers, and reducing transmission from sex workers to clients and from clients to sex workers. A number of programs have attempted to reduce the prevalence of different bacterial STDs in prostitutes. This is essentially the approach that was taken in controlling chancroid and syphilis outbreaks in Fresno, Winnipeg, and Orange County.[24,53,54] Other programs have attempted to control gonococcal infections in this way.[23,25]

This strategy is directed at eradicating or at least dramatically reducing the prevalence of STDs in the sex worker half of the sex-worker-client interaction through active case finding and early treatment. It has worked well for controlling some chancroid and syphilis outbreaks in North American cities, presumably because the outbreaks were confined to relatively small and discrete core groups. The impact of such programs on other bacterial STDs, such as gonorrhea, is less well documented.[99] Gonorrhea has a much wider core group, and the rates of reinfection may be extremely high. In Nairobi, in a prospective study of gonococcal infection in prostitutes, the mean time to reinfection was 12 days.[23] Although screening and treatment undoubtedly resulted in fewer secondary cases of gonococcal infection and a lowering of gonococcal morbidity among sex workers, the time to reinfection was so short that a screening program would need to employ extremely frequent visits to be effective.

Therefore, where STD incidence is high, and for viral STDs in particular, an additional STD control strategy must be considered: preventing sex workers from becoming infected by their clients, and preventing clients in turn from becoming infected by sex workers. A comprehensive approach combining health education, individual and group empowerment, promotion of condom use, screening and treatment for bacterial STDs, and the promotion of economic alternatives for female sex workers is the one that is advocated.

Such programs have been developed from the mid-1980s in several African countries, including Kenya,[100] Zimbabwe,[101] Zaire,[102] Nigeria,[103] and Ghana.[104] They are essentially community health programs, involving the community of sex workers and clients in program organization and decision making. Program specifics vary, but all successful programs involve an initial establishment of trust with the community followed by community mobilization and empowerment, using a peer-mediated educational approach with the sex workers themselves providing leadership and support for their peers.[100] Peer educators serve as links to the community, as health educators, and as distributors of condoms. They promote risk reduction strategies, including increased condom use and reduction in numbers of sex partners, and in some programs they provide information about expanding economic opportunities for female sex workers. They also encourage women to seek medical care promptly if they experience STD-related symptoms. Other important program features include an unlimited provision of free condoms, and ensuring unstigmatized access to good quality STD-related health services, either by setting up dedicated health clinics for sex workers or by strengthening existing health facilities. Some programs also address the client side of the sex-worker/client interaction, through interventions in workplaces and other locales where men can be accessed. Populations involved have included long-distance truck drivers in Tanzania,[105] fishermen in Zimbabwe,[106] military recruits in Rwanda,[107] and factory workers in Uganda.[108]

Most female-sex-worker programs have successfully increased reported condom use, from virtually zero to over 80 percent of reported sexual contacts,[74,100–104] and some have documented declines in STD and/or HIV prevalence and incidence.[74,101,102] The ultimate effect of such programs on HIV transmission may be large, primarily because they lead to reduced transmission to the sex workers' male clients and thus from the clients to their other female sex partners. Using a simple model, and assuming 80 percent condom use and an average HIV female-to-male transmission efficiency of 1 percent, it has been estimated that over 10,000 new cases of HIV infection are prevented annually by a sex worker intervention program in the Pumwani area of Nairobi (Table 10-3).[109] This program involves only about 500 sex workers resident in the area at any given time. Even with more conservative estimates of levels of condom use and of average transmission efficiency, the estimated number of new cases of HIV infection prevented annually still runs into the thousands. Such programs probably have an effect beyond a direct reduction in HIV transmission, by decreasing the prevalence and incidence of other STDs which act as cofactors to enhance HIV transmission.[110]

Another model for reducing STD transmission from sex workers to clients and from clients to sex workers is one which has been adopted in Thailand, where a heterosexual HIV epidemic began in the late 1980s. The epidemic spread very rapidly, fueled to a large extent by commercial sex. At that time condom use was uncommon. In 1991, after some pilot projects, the government began to strongly promote the use of condoms among sex workers and their clients. In most sex establishments in Thailand having sex with a condom became the norm. Most brothel owners and prostitutes participated in the "100 percent condom" policy, and there was a threat of sanctions if they did not. As part of the program the government provided condoms free of charge, and at the same time undertook a media campaign to promote condom use. As a result of this program, reported condom use between sex workers and their clients increased dramatically, from 14 percent in 1989 to 94 percent in 1993, according to surveys among sex workers. At the same time the number of nationally reported cases of syphilis, gonorrhea, chancroid, lymphogranuloma venereum, and nongonococcal urethritis declined. For example, syphilis declined from 11,855 cases in 1987 to 3,645 in 1993, gonorrhea from 109,289 cases in 1987 to 14,750 in 1993, and chancroid from 38,754 cases in 1987 to 1,990 in 1993. HIV incidence also appears to have declined.[111]

DEVELOPMENT OF PROGRAMS

No single blueprint exists for the development of programs for STD control among sex workers and their clients. Of necessity, the approach will vary with the country, society, culture, legal system, dynamics of sex work, and resources available. Programs involving women in western countries who sell sex to support a drug habit will differ from programs involving women in developing countries who sell sex for economic survival. However, some general principles derived from experiences in Africa and elsewhere can be outlined. Sex workers themselves should be in-

Table 10-3. Estimated New Primary and Secondary Cases of HIV Infection Prevented Annually among Clients of Prostitutes by the STD/HIV Control Program in Pumwani, Nairobi

HIV transmission efficiency	Cases	New cases with no intervention	Cases prevented with 80% condom use	Cases prevented with 50% condom use
1%	Primary	5,250	3,400	2,150
	Secondary	10,500	6,800	4,300
	Total	15,750	10,200	6,450
0.2%	Primary	1,050	675	425
	Secondary	2,100	1,350	850
	Total	3,150	2,025	1,275
2%	Primary	10,500	6,800	4,250
	Secondary	21,000	13,600	8,500
	Total	31,500	20,400	12,750

From Moses et al,[109] used with permission.

volved from the early stages in program development. A primary health care approach should be used, involving communities in their own health care, as people are better motivated when they feel that they are acting for themselves rather than in response to external authority. Program participants should also have convenient and unstigmatized access to health care.

Programs must be implemented in a nonjudgmental and humane manner. If people feel stigmatized by participation in a program, it will fail. Constant communication with participants (listening to their concerns and informing them of program results) is also crucial to continued success.

One of the first difficulties encountered in program implementation may be convincing decision makers of the need. Such programs are often viewed by authorities as operating mainly for the benefit of prostitutes, and because prostitutes have a limited constituency they are easy to ignore. Sustained political lobbying may be necessary, with emphasis on the potential cost-effectiveness of STD control activities directed toward sex workers and their clients.

Another difficulty is in identifying sex workers and clients and gaining their confidence. Women and men involved in an activity which is so stigmatized, usually illegal, and frequently associated with other illegal activities are often distrustful of authority. The initial approach must be carefully thought out. In some situations it may mean working with bar or brothel management. Where no formal organization of prostitutes exists, initial efforts may consist of trying to reach individual women in bars or on streets and then attempting to develop group identity and solidarity.

Maintaining a program may present problems related to continued funding, rifts within the sex worker community, and pressure from outside groups. Dealing with such problems requires commitment from program staff and good management skills. Continuing political and financial support and effective program planning, management, monitoring, and evaluation skills are all critical to program sustainability and success.[101]

SUMMARY AND CONCLUSIONS

Sex workers and their clients are one of the major core groups for STD transmission, but their relative contribution to STD transmission in a given setting will vary. Their overall importance is probably greatest in many developing countries, where poverty, lack of opportunities for women, selective male migration to cities, generally low levels of condom use, and insufficient health resources create both a high occurrence of prostitution and high rates of STD transmission. However, outbreaks of certain STDs (such as chancroid, syphilis, PPNG, and in some situations HIV infection) have been associated with sex work in industrialized countries, so even there sex workers and their clients may be important in STD epidemiology.

Interventions directed at core groups are critical in controlling sexually transmitted diseases. STD control programs developed in conjunction with sex workers and their clients, focusing on preventing them from becoming infected and on promptly detecting and treating sexually transmitted infections when they do occur, can be an effective means of reducing STD transmission in the population as a whole.

References

1 May RM, Anderson RM: Transmission dynamics of HIV infection. *Nature* 326:137, 1987.

2 Yorke JA et al: Dynamics and control of the transmission of gonorrhea. *Sex Transm Dis* 5:51, 1978.

3 Hart G: *Sexual Maladjustment and Disease.* Chicago, Nelson Hall, 1977.

4 James J: Prostitutes and Prostitution, in *Deviants: Voluntary Actors in a Hostile World*, E Sagarin, F Montanino (eds). Morristown NJ, General Learning Press, 1977, p 368.

5 Bess BE, James SS: Prostitution, in *The Sexual Experience*, BJ Sadock et al (eds). Baltimore, Williams and Wilkins, 1976, p 594.

6 White L: Prostitutes, reformers, and historians. *Crim Just Hist* 4:201, 1985.

7 Muga E: *Studies in Prostitution (East, West, and South Africa, Zaire, and Nevada).* Nairobi, Kenya Literature Bureau, 1980.

8 Barton SE et al: Female prostitutes and sexually transmitted diseases. *Br J Hosp Med* 38:34, 1987.

9 Rosenberg MJ, Weiner JM: Prostitutes and AIDS: A health department priority? *Am J Publ Hlth* 78:418, 1988.

10 Skegg DCG et al: Importance of the male factor in cancer of the cervix. *Lancet* 2:581, 1982.

11 Moses S et al: Sexual behaviour in Kenya: implications for sexually transmitted disease transmission and control. *Soc Sci Med* 39:1649, 1994.

12 Johnson AM et al: A pilot study of sexual lifestyle in a random sample of the population of Great Britain. *AIDS* 3:135, 1989.

13 Analyse des Comportements Sexuels en France (ACSF) Investigators: AIDS and sexual behavior in France. *Nature* 360:407, 1992.

14 Caraël M et al: Overview and selected findings of sexual behaviour surveys. *AIDS* 5(suppl 1):S65, 1991.

15 Carswell JW et al: Prevalence of HIV-1 in East African lorry drivers. *AIDS* 3:759, 1989.

16 Nopkesorn T et al: HIV-1 infection in young men in northern Thailand. *AIDS* 7:1233, 1993.

17 de Graaf R et al: Segmentation of heterosexual prostitution into various forms: a barrier to the potential transmission of HIV. AIDs Care 8:417, 1996.

18 Coutinho RA et al: Role of male prostitutes in the spread of sexually transmitted diseases and HIV. *Genitourin Med* 64:207, 1988.

19 de Graaf R et al: Homosexual prostitution and the potential spread of HIV in the Netherlands [letter]. *J Acq Immunodef Syndrome* 7: 526, 1993.

20 Brunham RC, Plummer FA: A general model of sexually transmitted disease epidemiology and its implications for control. *Med Clin N Amer* 74:1339, 1990.

21 Wasserheit JN, Aral SO: The dynamic topology of sexually transmitted disease epidemics: implications for prevention strategies. *J Infect Dis* 174(suppl 2):S201, 1996.

22 Rosenthal T, Vandow J: Prevalence of venereal disease in prostitutes. *Br J Vener Dis* 34:94, 1959.

23 D'Costa LJ et al: Prostitutes are a major reservoir of sexually transmitted diseases in Nairobi, Kenya. *Sex Transm Dis* 12:64, 1985.

24 Jaffe HW et al: Selective mass treatment in a venereal disease control program. *Am J Publ Hlth* 69:1181, 1979.

25 Potterat JJ et al: Gonorrhea in street prostitutes: epidemiologic and legal implications. *Sex Transm Dis* 6:58, 1979.

26 Conrad GL et al: Sexually transmitted diseases among prostitutes and other sexual offenders. *Sex Transm Dis* 8:241, 1981.

27 Ruijs GJ et al: Prevalence, incidence, and risk of acquiring urogenital gonococcal or chlamydial infection in prostitutes working in brothels. *Genitourin Med* 64:49, 1988.

28 Stary A et al: Medical health care for Viennese prostitutes. *Sex Transm Dis* 18:159, 1991.

29 Meheus A et al: Prevalence of gonorrhoea in prostitutes in a central African town. *Br J Vener Dis* 58:50, 1974.

30 Johnson DW et al: An evaluation of gonorrhea case finding in the chronically infected female. *Am J Epidemiol* 90:438, 1969.

31 Khoo R et al: A study of sexually transmitted diseases in 200 prostitutes in Singapore. *Asian J Infect Dis* 1:77, 1977.

32 Vuylsteke B et al: Clinical algorithms for the screening of women for gonococcal and chlamydial infection: evaluation of pregnant women and prostitutes in Zaire. *Clin Infect Dis* 17:82, 1993.

33 Vázquez F et al: Gonorrhea in women prostitutes: clinical data and auxotypes, serovars, plasmid contents of PPNG, and susceptibility profiles. *Sex Transm Dis* 18:5, 1991.

34 Venegas VS et al: Gonorrhoea and urogenital chlamydial infection in female prostitutes in Tegucigalpa, Honduras. *Intl J STD AIDS* 2:195, 1991.

35 Van Dyck et al: Accuracy of two enzyme immunoassays and cell culture in the detection of *Chlamydia trachomatis* in low and high risk populations in Senegal. *Eur J Clin Microbiol Infect Dis* 11:527, 1992.

36 Bonhomme MG et al: Incidence of sexually transmitted diseases among massage parlour employees in Bangkok, Thailand. *Intl J STD AIDS* 5:214, 1994.

37 Turner EB, Morton RS: Prostitution in Sheffield. *Br J Vener Dis* 52: 197, 1976.

38 Schwarcz SK et al: Crack cocaine and the exchange of sex for money or drugs. Risk factors for gonorrhea among black adolescents in San Francisco. *Sex Transm Dis* 19:7, 1992.

39 Perine PL et al: Epidemiology and treatment of penicillinase-producing *Neisseria gonorrhoeae* . *Sex Transm Dis* 6:152, 1979.

40 Rajan VS et al: Epidemiology of penicillinase-producing *Neisseria gonorrhoeae* in Singapore. *Br J Vener Dis* 57:158, 1981.

41 Goh CL et al: Chemoprophylaxis and gonococcal infections in prostitutes. *Int J Epidemiol* 13:3446, 1984.

42 Handsfield HH et al: Epidemiology of penicillinase-producing *Neisseria gonorrhoeae* infections. Analysis by auxotyping and serogrouping. *N Engl J Med* 306:950, 1982.

43 Ansink-Schipper MC et al: Epidemiology of PPNG infections in Amsterdam: analysis by auxanographic typing and plasmid characterisation. *Br J Vener Dis* 60:23, 1984.

44 Parran T: *Shadow on the Land: Syphilis.* New York, Regnal and Hitchcock, 1937.

45 Centers for Disease Control: Continuing increase in infectious syphilis—United States. *MMWR* 37:35, 1988.

46 Rolfs RT et al: Risk factors for syphilis: cocaine use and prostitution. *Am J Publ Hlth* 80:853, 1990.

47 Lee C et al: Epidemiology of an outbreak of infectious syphilis in Manitoba. *Am J Epidemiol* 125:277, 1987.

48 Romanowski B et al: Epidemiology of an outbreak of infectious syphilis in Alberta. *Intl J STD AIDS* 2:424, 1991.

49 Beilenson P et al: Outbreak of primary and secondary syphilis—Baltimore City, Maryland, 1995. *MMWR* 45:166, 1996.

50 Coutinho RA et al: Influence of special surveillance programmes and AIDS on declining incidence of syphilis in Amsterdam. *Genitourin Med* 63:210, 1987.

51 Venegas VS et al: Human immunodeficiency virus infection and syphilis in Honduran female prostitutes. *Intl J STD AIDS* 2:110, 1991.

52 Calderon-Jaimes E et al: Prevalence of antitreponemal antibodies in 3,098 female prostitutes in Mexico City. *Clin Infect Dis* 46:431, 1994.

53 Hammond GW et al: Epidemiologic, clinical, laboratory, and therapeutic features of an urban outbreak of chancroid in North America. *Rev Infect Dis* 2:867, 1980.

54 Blackmore CA et al: An outbreak of chancroid in Orange County, California: descriptive epidemiology and disease control measures. *J Infect Dis* 151:840, 1985.

55 Becker TM et al: *Haemophilus ducreyi* infection in south Florida: a rare disease on the rise? *South Med J* 80:182, 1987.

56 Centers for Disease Control. Chancroid—New York City, Dallas. *MMWR* 34(suppl 4):75S, 1985.

57 DiCarlo RP et al: Chancroid epidemiology in New Orleans men. *J Infect Dis* 172:446, 1995.

58 Plummer FA et al: Epidemiology of chancroid and *Haemophilus ducreyi* in Nairobi, Kenya. *Lancet* 2:1293, 1983.

59 Simonsen JN et al: HIV infection among lower socioeconomic strata prostitutes in Nairobi. *AIDS* 4:139, 1990.

60 Boily MC, Brunham RC. The impact of HIV and other STDs on human populations. Are predictions possible? *Infect Dis Clin N Amer* 7:771, 1993.

61 Martin DH, DiCarlo RP: Recent changes in the epidemiology of genital ulcer disease in the United States. The crack cocaine connection [Review]. *Sex Transm Dis* 21(suppl 2):S76, 1994.

62 Wallace JI et al: T-cell ratios in New York City prostitutes [Letter]. *Lancet* 1:58, 1983.

63 Van de Perre P et al: Female prostitutes: a risk group for infection with human T-cell lymphotropic virus type III. *Lancet* 2:524, 1985.

64 Kreiss JK et al: AIDS virus infection in Nairobi prostitutes: extension of the epidemic to East Africa. *N Engl J Med* 314:414, 1986.

65 Carswell JW: HIV infection in healthy persons in Uganda. *AIDS* 1: 223, 1987.

66 Mann JM et al: HIV infection and associated risk factors in female prostitutes in Kinshasa, Zaire. *AIDS* 2:249, 1988.

67 Plummer FA et al: Co-factors in male-female sexual transmission of human immunodeficiency virus type 1. *J Infect Dis* 163:233, 1991.

68 Brown T et al: The recent epidemiology of HIV and AIDS in Thailand. *AIDS* 8(suppl 2):S131, 1994.

69 Weniger BG: Experience from HIV incidence cohorts in Thailand: implications for HIV vaccine efficacy trials. *AIDS* 8:1007, 1994.

70 Piot P et al: Retrospective seroepidemiology of AIDS virus infection in Nairobi populations. *J Infect Dis* 155:1108, 1987.

71 Bwayo J et al: Human immunodeficiency virus infection in long-distance truck drivers in East Africa. *Arch Intern Med* 154:1391, 1994.

72 Simonsen JN: Human immunodeficiency virus infection among men with sexually transmitted diseases. Experience from a center of Africa. *N Engl J Med* 319:274, 1988.

73 Cameron DW et al: Female to male transmission of human immunodeficiency virus type 1: risk factors for seroconversion in men. *Lancet* 2:403, 1989.

74 Ngugi EN et al: Prevention of HIV transmission in Africa: the effectiveness of condom promotion and health education among high risk prostitutes. *Lancet* 2:887, 1988.

75 Kreiss JK et al: Association between cervical inflammation and cervical shedding of human immunodeficiency virus DNA. *J Infect Dis* 170:1597, 1994.

76 Mostad S et al: Cervical and Vaginal HIV-1 DNA Shedding in Female STD Clinic Attenders, in *Abstracts, Vol 2,* Eleventh International Conference on AIDS, Vancouver, Canada, July 7–12, 1996, abstr We.C.333.

77 Ghys PD et al: Genital Ulcers Increase Cervical-Vaginal Shedding of HIV-1 in Female Sex Workers in Abidjan, Côte d'Ivoire. *Final Program and Abstract Book*, Ninth International Conference on AIDS and STD in Africa, Kampala, Uganda, December 10–14, 1995, abstr TuA 094.

78 Ghys PD et al: The Associations Between Cervico-Vaginal HIV-1 Shedding and Sexually Transmitted Diseases, Immunosuppression, and Serum HIV-1 Viral Load in Female Sex Workers in Abidjan, Côte d'Ivoire, in *Abstracts, Vol 2,* Eleventh International Conference on AIDS, Vancouver, Canada, July 7–12, 1996, abstr We.C.332.

79 Laga M et al: Non-ulcerative sexually transmitted diseases as risk factors for HIV-1 transmission in women: results from a cohort study. *AIDS* 7:95, 1993.

80 Ghys PD et al: Genital ulcers associated with human immunodeficiency virus-related immunosuppression in female sex workers in Abidjan, Ivory Coast. *J Infect Dis* 172:1371, 1995.

81 Tyndall M et al: Ceftriaxone no longer predictably cures chancroid in Kenya. *J Infect Dis* 167:469, 1993.

82 Barton SE et al: HTLV-III antibody in prostitutes [Letter]. *Lancet* 2:1424, 1985.

83 Brenky-Faudeux D, Fribourg-Blanc A: HTLV-III antibody in prostitutes [Letter]. *Lancet* 2:1424, 1985.

84 Smith GL, Smith KF. Lack of HIV infection and condom use in licensed prostitutes[Letter]. *Lancet* 2:1392, 1986.

85 Papaevangelou G et al: LAV/HTLV-III infection in female prostitutes [Letter]. *Lancet* 2:1018, 1985.

86 van Haastrecht HJ et al: HIV prevalence and risk behaviour among prostitutes and clients in Amsterdam: migrants at increased risk for HIV infection. *Genitourin Med* 69:251, 1993.

87 Scott GR et al: Outreach STD clinics for prostitutes in Edinburgh. *Intl J STD AIDS* 6:197, 1995.

88 Alary M et al: Risk behaviours for HIV infection and sexually transmitted diseases among female sex workers from Copenhagen. *Int J STD AIDS* 5:365, 1994.

89 Tirelli U et al: HTLV-III antibodies in drug-addicted prostitutes used by US soldiers in Italy [Letter]. *JAMA* 256:711, 1986.

90 Luthy R et al: Prevalence of HIV antibodies among prostitutes in Zurich, Switzerland. *Klin Wochenschr* 65:287, 1987.

91 Schultz S et al: Female-to-male transmission of HTLV-III [Letter]. *JAMA* 255:1703, 1986.

92 Sterk C: Cocaine and HIV seropositivity [Letter]. *Lancet* 1:1052, 1988.

93 Van den Hoek JAR et al: HIV infection and STD in drug addicted prostitutes in Amsterdam: potential for HIV heterosexual transmission. *Genitourin Med* 65:146, 1989.

94 Estebanez P et al: HIV and female sex workers [Review]. *Bull WHO* 71:397, 1993.

95 Cohen et al: High-risk behaviors for HIV: a comparison between crack-abusing and opioid-abusing African-American women. *Journal of Psychoactive Drugs* 26:233, 1994.

96 Plummer FA et al: The importance of core groups in the epidemiology and control of HIV-1 infection. *AIDS* 5(suppl 1):S169, 1991.

97 Omari MA et al: Changes in Behaviour and the Incidence of HIV and Other Sexually Transmitted Diseases in Truck Drivers from East Africa, in *Poster Abstracts*, Seventh International Conference on AIDS, Florence, Italy, June 16–21, 1991, abstr W.C.3118.

98 Mandaliya K et al: Behavior Intervention in Trucking Workers in Mombasa: Decreased Incidence of STDs and Risk Behavior, in *Final Program and Abstract Book*, Ninth International Conference on AIDS and STD in Africa, Kampala, Uganda, December 10–14, 1995, abstr TuC 124.

99 Holmes KK, et al: Impact of a gonorrhea control program, including selective mass treatment, in female sex workers. *J Infec Dis* 174(suppl 2): S230, 1996.

100 Ngugi EN, Plummer FA: Health outreach and control of HIV infection in Kenya. *J Acq Immunodef Syndrome* 1:566, 1988.

101 Ngugi EN et al: Focused peer-mediated educational programs among female sex workers to reduce sexually transmitted disease and human immunodeficiency virus transmission in Kenya and Zimbabwe. *J Infect Dis* 174(suppl 2):S240, 1996.

102 Laga M et al: Condom promotion, sexually transmitted diseases treatment, and declining incidence of HIV-1 infection in female Zairian sex workers. *Lancet* 344:246, 1994.

103 Williams E et al: Implementation of an AIDS prevention program among prostitutes in the Cross River State of Nigeria [Letter]. *AIDS* 6:229, 1992.

104 Asamoah-Adu A: Evaluation of a targeted AIDS prevention intervention to increase condom use among prostitutes in Ghana. *AIDS* 8: 239, 1994.

105 Mwizarubi B: HIV/AIDS Education and Condom Promotion for Truck Drivers, Their Assistants and Sex Partners in the United Republic of Tanzania, in *Effective Approaches to AIDS Prevention, Report of a Meeting*. Geneva, World Health Organization, 1993, publ WHO/GPA/AIDS/93.1.

106 Wilson D et al: Using Public and Private Infrastructure for Cost-Effective Intervention among Inaccessible Fishermen in Rural Zimbabwe, in *Poster Abstracts*, Eighth International Conference on AIDS, Amsterdam, Netherlands, July 19–24, 1992, abstr PoC 4527.

107 Karita E: STD/HIV Prevention, Education and Promotion of Condom Use among Military Recruits in Rwanda, in *Effective Approaches to AIDS Prevention, Report of a Meeting*. Geneva, World Health Organization, 1993, publ WHO/GPA/AIDS/93.1.

108 McCombie S: Evaluation of a Workplace-Based Peer Education Program in Uganda, in *Poster Abstracts*, Eighth International Conference on AIDS, Amsterdam, Netherlands, July 19–24, 1992, abstr PoD 5765.

109 Moses S et al: Controlling HIV in Africa: effectiveness and cost of an intervention in a high-frequency STD transmitter core group. *AIDS* 5:407, 1991.

110 Plummer FA et al: Sexual Transmission of HIVs and the Role of Sexually Transmitted Diseases, in *AIDS in Africa*, M Essex et al (eds). New York, Raven Press, 1994, p 195.

111 Hanenberg RS et al: Impact of Thailand's HIV-control programme as indicated by the decline of sexually transmitted diseases. *Lancet* 344:243, 1994.

Chapter 11

Homosexual and bisexual behavior

Lynda S. Doll
David G. Ostrow

Since identification of the first cases of acquired immunodeficiency syndrome (AIDS), the highest cumulative number of AIDS cases in the United States has occurred among men who engage in same-sex behavior (males who have sex with males, or MSMs).[1] Numerous community-based organizations, in collaboration with state and local health departments and universities, have mounted intervention programs to assist MSMs to initiate and maintain safer sexual behaviors. In this chapter we examine the success of these programs by reviewing trends in rates of sexually transmitted diseases (STDs), including HIV infection, and in self-reported sexual risk behaviors and their determinants for this population. We also review a range of intervention models that have been developed for MSMs in the United States, including available evaluation data.

Three additional populations are covered in our review of infection rates and intervention models: bisexual men, and homosexual and bisexual women. Because of assumptions about lower risk levels among these populations, as well as the tendency to aggregate bisexual and exclusively homosexual populations, research and intervention programs for these men and women have developed more slowly. Hence, our understanding of the public health risks of these populations and of how to intervene appropriately are still emerging.

MEN WHO HAVE SEX WITH MEN

The highly diverse population of men who have sex exclusively with men may include men who self-identify as gay, bisexual, or heterosexual. Since the primary goal of this chapter is to assess continued STD risk levels and relevant prevention efforts among homosexual and bisexual populations, we describe trends—in this and in other sections—according to the behavior of individuals (either exclusively same-sex or bisexual sexual contact) rather than on their self-identity. While some research described in this section included bisexual men in the samples, the major focus of these studies was on gay men whose recent sexual contact was exclusively with other men.

Estimation of the prevalence of male same-sex behaviors is among the most difficult and controversial topics in contemporary behavioral research. In their preamble to the chapter on homosexuality in the scientific report on the 1994 National Health and Sexual Life Survey (NHSLS), Laumann and colleagues state that "estimating a single number for the prevalence of homosexuality is a futile exercise because it presupposes assumptions that are patently false: that homosexuality is a uniform attribute across individuals, that it is stable over time, and that it can be easily measured."[2]

Among the most vexing problems in these estimations is the lack of uniform and consistent definitions for homosexual behaviors, separate from same-sex object preferences and relationships. Depending on whether one asks about sexual behaviors in the past month, year, multiyear period, or since puberty, and whether the question specifies oral or anal intercourse, the occurrence of orgasm, mutual masturbation, or just sexual arousal by or with members of the same sex, recent estimates of prevalence rates for homosexual behaviors range from approximately 1 percent to over 10 percent of the adult U.S. male population.[2–7] Estimates of current homosexual behavior (for example, within the past year) usually range from 3 to 7 percent of adult males.[2–7] Demographic differences in prevalence rates are particularly difficult to estimate because of small sample sizes. However, results recently published from six national probability surveys showed higher rates of homosexual behavior in the last five years among white men, men living in urban areas, and men with higher levels of education.[6] With such a wide range of estimates and strong barriers to obtaining better data on homosexual behavior, particularly among men of color, it is difficult to assess infection rates or service needs among homosexual men. Efforts currently underway to conduct a national probability survey of gay and bisexual men may result in more precise estimates.[8]

STD RATES

National data on STDs are not routinely reported by sexual orientation in the United States. However, data on MSMs are available for several large urban areas and suggest dramatic declines over the past decade in rates of rectal gonorrhea in men, perhaps the most sensitive indicator of male-to-male transmission (Figure 11-1).[9] For example, the numbers of cases of rectal gonorrhea reported in New York City declined from 1,673 cases in 1982 to 50 in 1994. In the much smaller city of Denver, the decline was from a peak of 1,861 cases of gonorrhea and 163 cases of syphilis in 1981 to 63 and 13 cases respectively in 1993. Similar declines were reported in San Francisco, Los Angeles County, Boston, and King County (Seattle).[9] San Francisco has since noted a small but significant increase in rectal gonorrhea proctitis rates in the past one or two years.[10] Preliminary data from a clinic serving primarily MSMs in Washington, D.C. showed an approximately 50 percent increase in gonorrhea from 1993 to 1995.[11] It is too early to tell if these represent the beginning of new outbreaks of STDs among homosexual men.

The extent to which these rates reflect trends in nonurban areas or among subpopulations such as men of color are unclear. An assessment of STD rates among MSMs attending STD clinics in Washington, D.C. and Denver reinforces the need for further targeted STD prevention efforts. In 1996 about 60 percent of MSMs diagnosed with gonorrhea at the previously mentioned clinic in Washington, D.C. were African American.[11] In Denver, from 1987 through 1994, the highest prevalence of gonorrhea among MSMs occurred among African American men and among men 19 years old and younger. HIV seropositive men were also more likely than currently seronegative men to have been diagnosed with gonorrhea, early syphilis, recurrent genital herpes, and genital warts.[12] While it might be informative to compare these rates among specific subgroups of MSMs with changes over the same period of time among heterosexual men, the lack of systematic data collection on the sexual orientation of STD clinic patients and on specimen site for gonococcal and other STD tests prevent such comparisons. More systematic recording of STD data, including data on viral STDs, needs to be encouraged to help us understand which populations are at continued high risk of STDs and HIV infection.

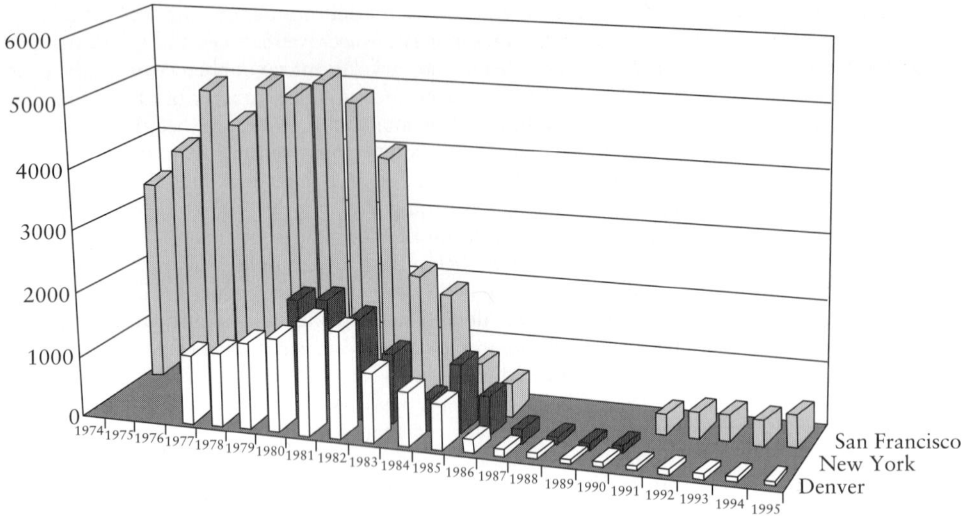

Fig. 11-1. Annual rates of rectal GC (GC proctitis) in men reported in three U.S. cities, 1974-1995. Figures for New York are the total numbers of all GC proctitis cases reported to the City Health Department in each year; figures for San Francisco represent only cases diagnosed at the San Francisco City Clinic; figures for Denver represent the total number of all GC cases diagnosed in gay men. *(Sources of data: Denver Department of Health and Hospitals, Frank Judson, M.D. and Susan Dias, M.D.; New York City Department of Health, Bureau of Sexually Transmitted Diseases, Isaac B. Weisfuse, M.D., M.P.H.; San Francisco Health Department, STD Control Division, Bob Kohn, M.P.H.)*

RATES OF HIV INFECTION AND AIDS

Through 1996, 59 percent of all adult cases of AIDS (287,576 of 488,300 cases) have occurred among MSMs. While the number of cases reported in 1996 among MSMs (27,316 cases) represented a decline in the rate of increase in this population, MSMs continued to constitute the largest single transmission category in 1996 (50 percent).

Most striking in AIDS surveillance data on MSMs are differential rates of increase when examined by race/ethnicity, age, or geographic location.[1] Comparing 1989 with 1994, rates were highest among African American MSMs during each year (20.8 and 37.3 per 100,000 adult men, respectively), with the largest proportionate increase also occurring in this population (79 percent). This compared with a 61 percent increase for Hispanic MSMs, a 77 percent increase for American Indian/Alaskan Native MSMs, and 14 percent for white MSMs. Among men in the youngest age group (13 to 24 years), rates increased 31 percent for African American MSMs and 39 percent for Hispanic MSMs but decreased 31 percent for white MSMs. Other important differences between 1989 and 1994 included greater increases in cases among MSMs in rural and medium sized Metropolitan Statistical Areas (MSAs) compared to MSAs with greater than 2.5 million. While the highest rates for MSMs in 1994 were still reported from New York (44.4 per hundred thousand), Los Angeles (34.9 per hundred thousand), and San Francisco (127.7 per hundred thousand), these cities all reported significant decreases among white MSMs while the rates for African American MSMs increased approximately 50 percent.

Data on HIV infection prevalence and incidence rates among homosexual men are spotty at best. Such data come from cohort studies of seroincidence rates conducted among primarily white gay men and from HIV seroprevalence studies conducted in sentinel STD clinics. In general, cohort studies have reported annual HIV infection rates of 2 to 4 percent among both younger and older men in larger MSAs.[13–16] The sentinel STD clinic studies have revealed high but gradually declining overall seroprevalence rates for gay men (average, 33 percent for 1988 through 1992; range, 5 to 52 percent for the same period).[17] The highest seroprevalence rates have been found among white gay men from clinics in larger urban areas. The overall decrease in seropositivity rates for gay men (from 45 percent in 1988 to 29 percent in 1992) are attributed primarily to decreases among younger white MSMs (under 30 years old), and among Hispanic and "other" race/ethnicity subgroups of MSMs.

While the sentinel clinic data on younger gay men are promising, data from San Francisco indicate that rates of new infections among younger gay men may still be extremely high in some cities. In samples of younger gay men in that epicenter, seroprevalence rates have ranged from 9 percent for 17-to-22 year olds[18] to 29 percent for 27-to-29 year olds,[13] with estimated yearly seroincidence rates of 2.5 to 4.4 percent for these age groups.[19] Thus, while there has been an overall stabilization in the numbers of newly diagnosed AIDS cases among MSMs, these statistics may mask continuing high rates of HIV infections and STDs, particularly among specific subpopulations defined by race/ethnicity, geographic location, and age cohort. A significant minority of MSMs may continue to engage knowingly or unknowingly in unsafe sexual practices. As discussed below, current trends indicating continued high risk activities among subgroups of MSMs may reflect, at least in part, a return to unsafe practices among men who had previously discontinued unprotected anal sex. These men may have relapsed in the context of "safer-sex burnout" or other psychological factors associated with the ongoing impact of the AIDS epidemic on gay men. Anecdotal information also suggests that the availability of new treatments for HIV, such as protease inhibitors, may have reduced the fear associated with acquiring HIV among some men and in some cases facilitated unsafe practices. The extent of such beliefs and their association with risk behaviors is unclear and deserves attention from clinicians and public health staff working with MSMs.

CONTROVERSY OVER WHAT CONSTITUTES SAFER SEX

A key question related to understanding the multiple ongoing epidemics of HIV infection and other STDs among MSMs is whether or not the transmission risk factors have changed for this population during the first decade of the epidemic. A number of modeling and case-control studies utilizing the same long-term observational cohorts mentioned above have consistently demonstrated that unprotected anal intercourse continues to be the predominant route of HIV transmission among gay men.[15] However, considerable controversy exists over the role of alternative forms of intercourse, such as protected anal intercourse and unprotected oral intercourse, usually labeled as "safer sex" in educational materials for MSMs. Controversy over the former type of safer sex primarily concerns the failure rate of condoms during anal sex. For example, the multisite vaccine feasibility cohort study conducted in Denver, San Francisco, and Chicago reported an overall seroincidence rate of 2.4 per 100 person-years during the first 18 months of observation.[16] Independent predictors of HIV seroconversion in that study were (1) having a known HIV seropositive sexual partner, (2) injection drug use, (3) urethritis, (4) condom failure (which ranged from 10 to 25 percent among seroconverting men), (5) age less than 25 years, and (6) unprotected receptive anal sex. While that particular study did not explore the reasons for reported high rates of condom breakage, previous studies have indicated that use of improper lubricants (for example, oil-based rather than the recommended water-soluble lubricants) and improper handling of condoms account for the majority of condom breaks.[20] In addition, it may be considerably more socially acceptable to report condom breakage than failure to use a condom.

Possible HIV transmission through oral sex among MSMs has been the subject of several anecdotal reports[21,22] as well as a case-control study based on HIV seroconverters from three different San Francisco prospective studies.[23] In contrast, a case-control study based on 76 seroconverters participating in both the Chicago Multisite AIDS Cohort Study (MACS) and the Coping and Change Study (CCS) between 1984 and 1992 indicated that oral sex could not account for a detectable portion of seroconversions in that cohort.[15] These studies have focused debate on the lack of definitive data on (1) the relative risk of HIV transmission through unprotected oral sex, and (2) the role various cofactors, such as oral pathology in the receptive partner and stage of infection of the insertive partner, may play in modifying that risk. Nevertheless, there is consensus among experts that unprotected oral sex without ejaculation is a much safer sexual practice than unprotected anal intercourse. Given that both unprotected anal intercourse and prevalent HIV infections continue to occur among subgroups of gay men, the remainder of this section of the chapter will focus on these important findings and on HIV prevention efforts among MSMs.

TRENDS IN RISK BEHAVIORS

Almost since the beginning of the AIDS epidemic among MSMs, there have been reports of dramatic changes in sexual behavior among men practicing unprotected anal intercourse (UAI). UAI has been the focus of most behavior change studies of MSMs because of its clear-cut association with AIDS,[24] prevalent HIV infections,[25] and HIV seroconversion in prospective study cohorts.[26,27] Early safer-sex educational materials produced for MSMs emphasized the need to decrease the number of sexual partners with whom one had UAI and to substitute safer (protected anal sex or oral sex) and safe (mutual masturbation and frottage) activities.

Data on national trends on changes in unsafe sexual behaviors are not available for men who report sex with men. However, one recent probability survey provides national, cross-sectional data. The National AIDS Behavior Survey, a 1992 telephone survey of persons living in selected urban areas, assessed a limited number of risk behaviors among men who reported a history of same-sex behaviors.[6] In this sample (N = 192), 24 percent reported no sex partners, 41 percent reported one partner, and 35 percent reported two or more partners in the last year. Almost 70 percent of the men reported consistent (100 percent) condom use in the last six months.

Data on trends in unsafe sexual behaviors are available from prospective observational cohort studies initiated early in the epidemic. These studies demonstrated rapid declines in rates of UAI and numbers of anal sex partners among men in San Francisco,[28] Chicago,[29] and New York.[30] For example, among men in the Chicago MACS/CCS cohort the proportion of unprotected anal sex acts dropped from initial rates of 88 percent in 1984 to 21 percent in 1988, with parallel decreases in annualized seroincidence rates of from 9 percent to less than 1 percent.[31] Similar declines were observed in the other MACS cities,[19] as well as in reports from both smaller cities and rural areas.[32]

Since 1990 it has been increasingly recognized that continued unsafe sex is largely occurring among men who have already made substantial changes toward safer sex but have difficulty maintaining those changes indefinitely.[33,34] Whether this phenomenon is labeled "safe-sex burnout" or "relapse," it is important to note that whenever behavior change occurs in response to a long-term health threat on the scale that has been observed among MSMs, lapses to previously enjoyed behaviors are inevitable. In addition, some observers have noted that UAI under specific circumstances, such as in the context of a committed long-term relationship, may not be considered risky sex by the participants, but may rather be part of a negotiated form of safer sex for that couple.[35] Thus, the dilemma for behavioral researchers has been to avoid labels and absolutes while finding effective interventions that significantly decrease the risk of HIV transmission. Toward this end, a large number of studies have looked at psychosocial, relationship, and environmental factors predictive of change to safer sex or lapses to unsafe sex, in hopes of identifying factors which can be the basis of behavioral interventions for MSMs.

PSYCHOSOCIAL PREDICTORS OF SEXUAL BEHAVIOR CHANGE

Several excellent reviews have summarized the large number of psychosocial studies of sexual behavior change among MSMs.[36–39] What strikes anyone trying to organize this large and growing literature conceptually are two concerns. First, as was originally pointed out by Becker and Joseph,[36] few observational studies have employed theoretical models of health behavior change, and those that have usually ignore some of the unique aspects of sexual behavior change made by MSMs in the midst of a highly stigmatized epidemic. Second, the definition of risky sex used and the sampling of the particular subpopulation of MSMs within a community may in themselves be major determinants of both the behavior changes observed and their psychosocial correlates. Thus, it is difficult to organize this literature concisely and in a way that will be useful to the researcher or interventionist in search of consistent observations across multiple subpopulations of MSMs. However, when a staged model of behavior change, such as the Stages of Change Model of Prochaska and DiClemente[40] or the AIDS Risk Reduction Model[41] is used to organize research findings, some trends emerge across study populations. As Prochaska and colleagues stated in their review of behavior change findings in studies of gay men at risk of HIV:

> Discussing the difficulties of modifying problem behaviors, Mark Twain said, "Habit is habit, and not to be flung out of the window, but coaxed downstairs a step at a time." The past decade of research has led us to similar conclusions: Cessation of problem behaviors or adoption of more healthful ones does not occur automatically through one trial learning. Change requires movement through discrete motivational stages over time, the active use of different processes of change at different stages, and modification of cognitions, affect and behaviors.[37]

For the rest of this section and in Table 11-1 we use a modified hierarchical classification based on the AIDS Risk Reduction Model ("ARRM Model")[41] that itself is based on the Stages of

Change Model to organize the current state of knowledge of psychosocial, relationship, and environmental factors predictive of risk behavior change among MSMs. We omit discussion of what Prochaska calls the "precontemplators" (persons with no intention of changing their behavior), as MSMs still engaging in risky sex in the 1990s uniformly report at least awareness of the need to consider some forms of behavioral modification.[42] We include Prochaska's "contemplators" with the "initiators of change." As for men who have stopped trying to attain safe sex, they fall off any current staged model of sexual behavior change. Some researchers may include them in the "precontemplation" stage of the Stages of Change Model[42] as men with awareness of the need to change but no intentions of doing so. For purposes of examining psychosocial predictors of behavior change, however, we do not feel that these men should be lumped with men who are not yet aware of the need to adopt safer sexual pactices. The largely psychological issues of survivor guilt, hopelessness, fatalism, and loss of self-efficacy that men who have stopped trying experience do not seem to fall into any of the stages of either the ARRM or our modified staged model of change. If this group of MSMs does indeed turn out to represent a significant portion of gay men continuing to have unsafe sex, and if these men are not reached by standard HIV prevention models, then we would suggest adding a fifth stage.

Thus, we suggest four major stages of sexual behavior change within which to organize the current state of knowledge on predictors of change: (1) *Initiation*, wherein an individual contemplates the problem, becomes ready to change, and begins to take steps to reduce HIV risk, although these changes may not be consistent or large enough to substantially reduce the level of risk; (2) *Consolidation,* in which the person reaches a level of sexual behavior change where HIV risk is reduced to zero or near zero; (3) *Maintenance,* wherein the individual sustains the changes made in the previous two stages over a sufficient period—usually 6 months or longer—to feel comfortable with the new behavioral repertoire; and (4) *Relapse,* a period of sustained return to risky sex, often accompanied by feelings of guilt, shame, and loss of personal efficacy to maintain sexual safety.

While the four stages used here are presented as a linear progression, individuals may enter the change cycle at any point and may lapse or relapse to an earlier stage at any time. In fact, multiple lapses occurring throughout the experience of changing highly reinforced behaviors, such as sexual behavior, smoking, and eating habits, are considered the norm.[43] When lapses occur repetitively and in a pattern that diminishes an individual's sense of self-efficacy, resumption of habitual high-risk sexual activity and return to an earlier stage of behavior change may occur.[44] Thus, it is critical that any intervention program stress the inevitability of lapses and the acquisition of skills to prevent such lapses from developing into full-fledged relapses. Long-term research such as the Chicago MACS/CCS cohort studies emphasizes the practical importance of preventing relapse to sustained UAI among MSMs: seroconversion rates for men progressing from the initiation to maintenance stages dropped from approximately 4 per 100 person-years of observation to 0.5 per 100 person-years but then rose to 3 per 100 person-years for men relapsing to UAI for one year or longer.[34]

While much of the available data on predictors are limited to cross-sectional samples or to long-term cohort studies of more narrowly defined subpopulations, a picture of the most salient predictors of behavior change at each stage of this four-stage model has emerged (see Table 11-1). Perhaps most consistent across studies and subpopulations of MSMs are (1) the positive associations between sexual behavior change and self-efficacy, skills, and positive coping styles; and (2) the negative associations of sexual behavior change with low self-efficacy, denial/fatalistic coping styles, and substance use.[45] It is no surprise then, that most current intervention programs for MSMs emphasize these aspects.[38] In contrast, some factors may have inconsistent associations, depending upon the subpopulation or type of predictor variables under study. Other factors, such as substance use and preference for UAI, may be both barriers to the initiation of change and correlates of behavioral relapse. Thus, while the factors listed in Table 11–1 can serve as a menu for psychosocial and intervention research in this area, they cannot be taken as dogma and must be assessed for any specific subpopulation of MSMs prior to undertaking educational or other interventions with that group.

Studies of young MSMs provide an illustration of research with apparent contradictory findings. For example, younger age is frequently cited in studies as predicting higher rates of UAI at baseline, difficulty progressing to the maintenance of safety, and higher rates of relapse to unsafe sex in the long term.[46–48] However,

Table 11-1. Predictors of Stages of Sexual Behavior Change among Gay/Bisexual Men

	Stage of Change		
Initiation	Consolidation	Maintenance	Relapse
	Increasing self-efficacy		Reduced self-efficacy
Knowledge of AIDS and HIV risks	Supportive peer norms for safer sex		Conflict with social network
Recognition of own risk vulnerability	Rewards and reinforcement of changes		Extreme affective states
			Depression, hypomania
			Extreme sexual arousal
			Extreme sense of intimacy
Availability of condoms	Increased ability to use condoms		Preference for UAI
	Increased enjoyment of condom use or substitute safe behaviors		Impulsivity, sensation seeking, distraction, coping styles
Partner(s) acceptance of behavior change	Partner(s) support for behavior change		Change in partnership status
Strength of behavior change intentions		Confidence in reduced HIV risk resulting from change	Fatalism about becoming HIV+
Sexual assertiveness, negotiation and communications skills			Sense of futility, safer-sex burnout
Higher age and educational level			Substance use, especially poppers, cocaine or crack, Ecstacy or amphetamines
Learning one's HIV serostatus			

whether this will be true for younger men who have disclosed their sexual orientation since 1985 and whose homosexual behavior patterns are still being established in the AIDS era is yet to be demonstrated. A second example of the sometimes contradictory effects can be seen in data on social and sexual network integration in this same population. In an ongoing study of New York City MSMs aged 18 to 24,[30] approximately one-third of the men engaged in receptive UAI with a single partner. These men were more likely to be in a coupled relationship, know their partner's HIV status, and be more integrated into the gay community than men who did not practice receptive UAI. However, a small proportion of the men (6 percent) engaged in receptive UAI with multiple partners. These particularly high risk men differed from the first group on multiple psychosocial measures: they reported multiple mental health problems, including more drug use, higher levels of internalized homophobia, and AIDS-related distress. The investigators suggest that for this small group of very high risk young men, receptive UAI with multiple partners may be part of their coping response to the internal and external stressors of being gay in the time of AIDS. Obviously, different intervention strategies must be employed with these very different subpopulations of young gay men.

Perhaps even more important are the inconsistent effects of gay community integration and of exposure to peer norms concerning sexual safety. In the majority of published studies, increased gay community integration and agreement with peer norms is associated with lower rates of UAI.[49] However, if an individual finds himself in conflict with his social network regarding safer-sex norms, or is integrated into a social network that engages in UAI and/or substance use with sexual partners, those peer norm influences may be substantial barriers to the attainment and maintenance of consistent safer sexual practices.[50] For behaviorally bisexual men in particular, gay community integration may not act as a buffer against sexual risk.[51]

MSMs who use psychoactive substances such as "poppers," cocaine, amphetamines, or the "designer drugs" (Ecstasy and Special K), are both more likely to engage in receptive UAI[52] and more likely to become infected than those who do not use these drugs. This is found even when studies are controlled for number of partners or number of anal exposures.[15] Studies suggest that both episodic substance use and risky sex among MSMs may reflect, at least in part, underlying risk or sensation-seeking personality dispositions.[53,54] Again, interventions may differ depending on the type of drug(s) used, whether or not this use is episodic or habitual, and whether or not injection drug use is involved.

The picture becomes even more complicated when nonwhite populations of MSMs are studied. We have discussed the disproportionate rates of newly diagnosed AIDS cases and, presumably, recently acquired HIV infections among African American and Hispanic MSMs.[1] Additional studies have shown continued rates of risky sexual behavior among samples of African American,[55] Hispanic,[56] and Asian[57] gay men. Studies attempting to understand the underlying predictors and most effective intervention strategies for minority MSMs are just beginning to provide some preliminary answers, and most of these studies are with African American urban men.[58–60] In general, there appear to be at least three major areas in which sexual risk behavior correlates for African American men differ from the picture described above based on white men: (1) cultural factors related to the meanings of sexual behavior and sexual identification; (2) socioeconomic differences which limit the availability of information, social support, and other resources predictive of sexual behavior change; and (3) differences in identity with and participation in gay communities, which may provide limited HIV prevention information and intervention programs for minority MSMs. These various factors often coexist, producing significant barriers to sexual behavior change among minority MSMs. For example, African American MSMs are often bisexual, have little or no gay community identification, may not recognize the HIV infection risk of their homosexual behaviors, and may not even be aware of the various behavior change education programs available for minority MSMs.

INTERVENTION MODELS

This section emphasizes the growing body of literature on HIV-related behavioral intervention trials. To date, little research has been reported on intervention trials focusing on the prevention of other STDs among gay men. New research examining the role of health-care seeking and partner notification in the prevention of STDs may provide important information for programs targeting this population.[61] Given the influence of the presence of other STDs on the transmission of HIV, assessing the role of various STD intervention or control programs in preventing HIV among gay men may also be a critical area of new research.

While the majority of controlled HIV intervention trials have been conducted among MSMs, even these have been quite limited in both number and approach.[62–66] Overall, interventions for MSMs that have been systematically studied and described include brief counseling and testing, limited small-group interventions, ongoing relapse-prevention programs, and community-based norm-changing and dissemination projects. This section will briefly review that cumulative experience and make recommendations for future prevention efforts.

By now it is generally agreed that brief, standardized counseling and testing (C and T) produces little if any behavior change among seronegative gay men but can be an important factor in reducing risky sex among seropositive men.[67,68] However, counseling and testing is most important as a behavior-change tool when it is viewed as the entry point for ongoing case management and more intensive behavioral interventions.[69] Recently there has been increasing interest in behavioral case management for seronegative as well as seropositive men. For example, the Gay Men's Health Crisis (GMHC) campaign, "Staying negative—it's not automatic," has utilized these approaches.[70]

Most small-group interventions for at-risk MSMs have been based on cognitive-behavioral[64] and social learning[71] principles. These approaches posit that individuals can be assisted in affecting behavior change by (1) encouraging change readiness through accurate perception of personal vulnerability and understanding of risk reduction steps; (2) teaching the cognitive and behavioral skills needed to implement risk reduction; (3) promoting the application of these skills in real-life situations; and (4) encouraging social, relationship, and other activity changes that serve to reinforce ongoing change maintenance. Valdiserri and colleagues[72] randomly assigned gay men to attend either an AIDS education program or a day-long workshop that combined risk education with skills training in areas such as condom use and safer-sex negotiation. Men who attended the skills training workshop exhibited increased condom use and decreased rates of high-risk behavior relative to those in the comparison intervention. Kelly and his colleagues[73,74] examined the impact of a multiple session cognitive-behavioral group intervention on the risk behavior levels of MSMs. In an intervention comprised of six or twelve 90-minute group sessions that focused on risk education, skills training, and reinforcement of change efforts, participants achieved substantial reductions in high-risk sexual practices relative to men assigned to a control condition. For example, receptive UAI decreased to near-zero levels, and condom use increased from about 20 percent at baseline to about 75 percent at three month follow-up. Recently Peterson and colleagues extended this model, demonstrating that a series of three cognitive-behavioral and skills-development workshops that were culturally tailored for African American MSMs could produce significant reductions in HIV risk behaviors at 12 and 18 months of follow-up compared to a control group receiving information only.[75]

While these small-group interventions produced substantial reductions in high-risk sexual behavior, longer term follow-up of cohorts revealed significant levels of relapse. For example, two-year follow-up of participants in the 12-session intervention program revealed that approximately 40 percent of the men had resumed having receptive UAI.[76] Higher levels of recreational drug use, younger age, higher number of receptive UAI partners, and preference for receptive UAI prior to participation in the intervention were all predictive of relapse in the Kelly studies.

In addition to the face-to-face group interventions described above, there have been several reports of successful community-level behavior change trials focused on MSMs. Kelly and colleagues[77,78] have described the effects of a community-level intervention that recruited and trained popular opinion leaders among the gay population of small cities to disseminate behavior-change recommendations and safer-sex normative messages. Evaluation of this community-level intervention model indicated that it is possible to produce downward shifts in the overall sexual-risk behavior patterns of MSMs in smaller, easily defined communities by exposing population members to repeated messages delivered by popular opinion leaders endorsing condom use.

The AIDS Community Demonstration Project is a second example of research testing a community-level intervention targeting MSMs. This study utilized intervention and control communities of MSMs to study the impact of peer outreach and small media such as pamphlets or newsletters. The media included theory-based role-model stories that described behavior-change efforts by peers. In the intervention community, consistent condom use (100 percent use of condoms in the past 30 days) increased significantly, from 52 to 65 percent with nonprimary male partners and from 10 to 15 percent for vaginal intercourse with primary female partners.[79]

Approaches similar to those used by Kelly and colleagues and the Community Demonstration Projects have been implemented by community-based organizations in larger and more diverse cities. These include STOP AIDS in San Francisco and the previously mentioned GMHC project. However, other controlled evaluations of community-level approaches in major epicenters have either not been undertaken or have revealed changes in attitudes and intentions but not in behaviors.[80]

A multidimensional, targeted intervention program has recently been evaluated for young MSMs.[81] This pilot study utilized a two-city intervention-control comparison, with the intervention program consisting of peer leadership training and outreach, peer-led small-group interventions, and a city-wide publicity campaign. Independently recruited cohorts in Eugene, Oregon and in the comparison city (Santa Barbara, California) provided evidence of significant reductions in UAI in the intervention city over a two-year period. GMHC has utilized a similar multi-dimensional, targeted intervention program for MSMs who use substances in New York City. This program combines peer-led outreach activities, small-group interventions led by gay substance abuse counselors, and community-wide publicity programs that focus on the links between the use of substances and high risk sex.[82]

The studies described in this section reveal several promising intervention approaches for MSMs. Overall, the research suggests that no single intervention strategy is likely to be effective in promoting and maintaining broadscale risk reduction among MSMs. A combination of intensive targeted small-group interventions, long-term relapse prevention elements such as monthly small-group booster sessions, and community-wide norm changing campaigns may produce the most widespread and greatest reductions in the sexual risk behaviors of MSMs. These efforts would need to be sustained for long periods of time, perhaps indefinitely, for levels of high risk behavior to stay below the threshold for continued epidemic level HIV transmission among MSMs.

MEN WHO HAVE SEX WITH MEN AND WOMEN

Data on the population of men who report bisexual contact are scarce, and interpretation is limited by the fact that the cultural meanings associated with sexual behavior and identity are not clearly understood for this population. Interpretation of risk levels is also difficult, because researchers have used different convenience samples and usually select study participants based on sexual identification rather than behavior.

Estimates of the prevalence of bisexual contact share the same limitations as those reported for exclusively homosexual men. Standardized definitions of what constitutes bisexuality have not been agreed upon. Hence, prevalence data are reported across studies for differing time periods, using a variety of sexual behaviors. Estimates of lifetime incidence range from approximately 1 to 7 percent of men, depending upon the questions used by the survey and whether bisexual contact has been measured since puberty, age 18, or the last 5 or 10 years.[2,4,5,6,83] More consensus has been reached on estimates of bisexual contact in the last year, with most surveys showing fewer than 1 percent of men reporting such recent behavior.[2,5] Few data on demographic differences have been published, and existing findings should be viewed with caution given the small sample size in most analyses. However, a recent synthesis of results from six national probability surveys showed that compared to exclusively homosexual men, bisexual men were more likely to be younger, African American, married, and less educated.[6]

STD RATES

Despite apparent declining rates of rectal gonorrhea among MSMs,[9] the number of incident cases of STDs among bisexual men, specifically, is unknown. Indeed, preliminary results from at least two studies suggest the need for further investigation. Data from a minority, inner-city STD clinic population in New York City[84] showed that bisexual men had higher rates of both syphilis and HIV than did exclusively heterosexual clinic patients. Data from a representative sample of approximately 16,000 active-duty, male military enlistees also showed bisexual men reported higher rates of STDs in the previous 24 months (15.4 percent) than did gay (11.3 percent) or heterosexual men (9.1 percent).[85] It is unclear how generalizable these data are to the larger population of bisexual men. However, three factors suggest reduced STD rates among the majority of gay men may not reflect trends among bisexual men: (1) higher reported rates of STDs in minority populations overall,[86] (2) higher reported prevalences of bisexual behavior among minority men, [6,60] and (3) higher reported rates of sexual risk among minority bisexual men.[60, 87, 88]

HIV INFECTION AND AIDS RATES

The prevalence of HIV infection among bisexual men in the United States is unknown. Through December 1996, the CDC received reports of AIDS in 76,075 men with a history of bisexual behavior since 1977. This represented 21 percent of the cumulative total of AIDS cases among men reporting sex with men. Both AIDS case reports and other research suggest that bisexual contact among persons with AIDS is more likely to be reported by African American and Hispanic men than by white men.[89] These same data show that bisexual men with AIDS are twice as likely as exclusively homosexual men with AIDS to report injection drug use.

The role of male bisexual behavior in the transmission of HIV to female partners is uncertain. Between 1989 and 1993 the annual incidence rates of AIDS in women reporting a male bisexual partner rose from 2.8 to 6.8 per 1,000,000 among African American women, from 1.8 to 3.59 per 1,000,000 among Hispanic women, and from 0.06 to 0.98 per 1,000,000 among white women. Additional research suggests potential heightened risk for female partners. Higher rates of anal sex with female partners have been reported among bisexual men than among exclusively heterosexual men.[90,91] Also, fewer than half of bisexual men may inform female partners of their male sexual contacts.[92–94] However, despite these data, AIDS case reports show that fewer than 8 percent of women infected through heterosexual contact have had sexual contact with a bisexual man. Hence, at this point in the epidemic widespread transmission from bisexual men to heterosexual women has probably not occurred or been detected.

TRENDS IN RISK BEHAVIORS

Few quantitative studies of male bisexual behavior are available, and of those that are, few examine risk behaviors. Data from national probability samples or from longitudinal surveys addressing the extent of behavior change among bisexual men are lacking. Similarly, predictors of risk behaviors in this population have been inadequately examined.

A diverse group of cross-sectional studies have examined sexual risk behaviors with male partners among bisexual men. Overall, this research suggests two trends. First, many bisexual men may engage in relatively high rates of unprotected anal sex with male partners (for example, approximately 33 percent of bisexual men recruited in recent studies using community[87] and bar samples[95]). Below we note four contexts of bisexual behavior in which we believe rates of these sexual risk behaviors with male partners may be particularly high. Second, bisexual men probably engage in relatively fewer episodes of sexual behavior with male partners than do exclusively homosexual men; thus, the risk of sexual transmission from a male partner may be lower among bisexual men.[96–99] HIV seroprevalence data from Seattle provide partial support for this hypothesis. Among 5,480 men recruited for a prevention study, seroprevalence was highest among self-identified gay men (27 percent), followed by bisexually identified (12 percent) and heterosexually identified (8 percent) men who reported sex with men.[100] While these figures may largely reflect the high infection rates in the communities in which these men find sex partners, they may also suggest higher rates of risk behaviors in gay-identified men.

A second group of studies describes lower levels of sexual risk behaviors with male than with female partners.[87,101–103] In a cohort of over 500 African American and white bisexual men,[87] 31 percent reported unprotected anal sex with a man and 42 percent reported unprotected vaginal sex with a woman in the last six months. No racial differences were found in rates of unprotected anal sex with male partners, though African American men were more likely to report both unprotected vaginal sex and unprotected penetrative sex with *both* a man and a woman. Among men recruited from public "cruising" areas in southern Los Angeles County, 56 percent of nongay-identified men (the majority of whom were bisexual) reported condom use every time during anal sex with main male partners and 71 percent with casual male partners. In contrast, only 33 percent reported consistent condom use during vaginal sex with main partners and 25 percent with casual partners.[102]

In addition to these studies assessing the prevalence of risk behaviors, Doll and Beeker[60] identified four contexts in which bisexual behavior is both more likely to occur and likely to be associated with greater HIV risk: (1) male prostitution,[104–107] (2) injection drug use,[108, 109] (3) sexual identity exploration,[110–112] and (4) culturally specific gender roles and norms that may characterize some African American and Hispanic communities in the United States.[88,113,114] The data reviewed by Doll and Beeker suggest that men who sell sex to men engage in high rates of sexual risk with male and female paying and nonpaying partners, often in conjunction with injection drug use. As noted earlier, HIV seroprevalence rates have been found to be disturbingly high among younger gay men. Many of these younger men may engage in sex with both men and women. During this period of sexual identity exploration, little emotional support and few role models are available to help youth negotiate complex choices about sexual behaviors and risk. Finally, an accumulating body of evidence suggests that African American and Hispanic men may engage in higher rates of bisexual contact than do white men. As we have noted, seroprevalence data also highlight the disproportionate risk of exposure to HIV infection and STDs in communities of color. Several cultural explanations have been proposed for high rates of bisexuality, including homophobia, strong ties to family and ethnic identity, gender role expectations, and attitudes about masculinity. However further research is needed to clarify the role of each of these and other potential explanations in the observed infection rates.

INTERVENTION MODELS

In this section we review several intervention models for bisexual men. To date, no data have been published on the effectiveness of existing programs or the extent of exposure of bisexual men to them. Hence we provide only descriptions of potentially effective HIV risk-reduction programs, first for bisexually active men generally, and then for bisexual men within the four high-risk contexts that Doll and Beeker identified.[60] No programs specifically targeting bisexual men who are at risk for or have been exposed to other STDs have been described.

Mass and specialized media may play a critical role in targeting bisexual men. Programs such as one developed by the Health Education Authority in the United Kingdom[115] strive to increase public awareness about bisexual behavior and HIV risk and to direct individuals to hot lines or other access points for information and services.

Education and support for risk reduction, particularly for populations where homosexual behavior is covert, may be provided by health and social service providers or by community outreach to locations where men live, work, socialize, and have sex.[116,117] Mobile vans, street corners, and storefront drop-in centers may be appropriate venues for person-to-person outreach. For example, in programs such as "Wake Up My Brother," heterosexually identified men conduct outreach in parks and bars where nongay-identified men who have sex with men may meet one another.[118]

To sustain risk reduction behaviors in this population may require the support of bisexuality-oriented organizations or groups where men can meet, learn to talk about sex, and define realistic sexual options.[119] Gay communities have also been encouraged to diversify their programs for a range of MSMs, including married men, hustlers, youth, and gay men of color.

In addition to these more generic programs, a limited number of intervention models have been developed for each of the four high-risk subpopulations we have identified. Interventions for male prostitutes have typically used peer educators to distribute condoms and materials, provide social support, and refer men to services.[120] Other intervention components that may be critical for this population are vocational training, drug and alcohol treatment, and training in negotiation skills to increase the man's control over his commercial sex transactions.[107]

Facilities for needle exchange, methadone maintenance, and drug and alcohol treatment are important access points for bisexual men who inject drugs. Interventions in these sites must effectively address both drug and sexual risk with both male and female partners. Other important venues for community outreach and distribution of condoms may include liquor stores and bars, barber shops, video arcades, and commercial or public cruising areas.

Expanded services, including counseling, outreach, and shelter programs, are needed for youth and other men exploring their sexual identity, in order to promote self-acceptance and to encourage individuals to access relevant social networks. Youth support groups offering a sense of shared community, gay-identified positive role models, and emotional support for the "coming out" process may be provided through gay-identified community organizations.[121,122] However, for youth who are bisexually identified or from cultures where homosexual behavior is particularly stigmatized, the emphasis on gay-identified groups may be inappropriate.[121] Anonymous venues may be critical to reach such youth. Anonymous individual and group-based HIV risk-reduction counseling may be provided by telephone.[123] Additional programs are also needed for homeless and runaway youth, many of whom engage in "survival sex" with male partners.[124]

Finally, intervention strategies for bisexual men of color must be developed by men in their communities to assure that such programs are compatible with community language, values, and norms. Social intolerance of homosexuality may need to be addressed by promoting legal and policy reform. Also needed are training programs for health and social service providers and for staff of religious and other community-based organizations, to facilitate greater comfort and skill in working with persons with diverse sexual preferences. Since male bisexual behavior is often linked to poverty, substance use, and commercial sex work, especially in communities of color, any effort to change sexual behavior must take into account the social and economic context in which such behavior is embedded.[125]

WOMEN

The small literature on STD and HIV risk among lesbian and bisexual women is even more limited than that for bisexual men. Again, there is almost no foundation of basic sexuality research on this diverse population to clarify the cultural meanings associated with the sexual behavior and identity of these women. There is also a lack of data describing STD and HIV prevalence rates as well as transmission dynamics in these populations.

Data on the prevalence of same-gender contact among women in the United States has received almost no attention in published reports of national probability surveys of sexual behavior. Two recent reports, however, provide initial figures. Turner, Danella, and Rogers[7] analyzed data from eight national probability surveys conducted from 1970 through 1991. Lifetime prevalence of same-gender contact increased by birth cohort, with fewer than 2 percent of women born before or during the 1930s, compared to 7.1 percent of women born in the 1960s, reporting same-gender contact. Same-gender contact during the last year has been estimated to range from less than 1 percent to 1.5 percent.[2,7] Both studies show that the majority of women reporting same-gender contact also reported sexual contact with men.

STD RATES

Data on STD rates among lesbian and bisexual women are limited, largely originating from urban samples. Higher STD rates are often reported among bisexual women. A 1993 study of lesbian and bisexual women recruited from public venues in San Francisco and Berkeley, California showed 2.2 percent of women had a lifetime history of STDs, 5.4 percent had markers for hepatitis B, and 0.4 percent had markers for syphilis.[126] Using a convenience sample of lesbian and bisexual women attending music festivals, Johnson and colleagues found a higher frequency of self-reported gynecologic infections, including STDs, among bisexual than among lesbian women.[127] Similarly, Marrazzo and her colleagues identified human papilloma virus (HPV) through polymerase chain reaction (PCR) among 54 percent of an STD clinic sample of women who had had sexual contact with both men and women in the last year, 34 percent of women with lifetime bisexual sexual contact but no male contact in the last year, and 29 percent of exclusively homosexual women.[128] Finally, in a survey of female attendees of a New York City STD clinic, women with same-sex partners (93 percent of whom also had male partners) reported nearly twice the rates of HIV, syphilis, any genital ulcer disease, and any STD as exclusively heterosexual women.[129]

HIV INFECTION AND AIDS RATES

Sexual transmission of HIV from an infected woman to her female partner is possible but rare.[130–135] Transmission through other routes, such as the exchange of menstrual blood during sexual activity and exposure to infected semen during artificial insemination, is also possible but unlikely to pose significant risks in practice.[136] Indeed, research to date suggests that the major risk factors for HIV infection among women who have sex with women are injection drug use and sex with an infected man.[126,129,137,138] Examination of AIDS cases reported to CDC through June 1991 showed that 0.9 percent of adult women with AIDS were women reporting sexual contact with another woman since 1978. Of these 164 women, 152 (93 percent) reported having injected drugs; the remainder had received a blood transfusion before 1985.[137] A second study of 1,122 women reported with HIV or AIDS between January 1990 and September 1993 found 55 women reported bisexual contact and 10 exclusively homosexual contact during the previous five years.[134] Among the 10 exclusively homosexual women, 8 reported injection drug use and one had received a blood transfusion before 1985. One exclusively homosexual woman, who reported several drug-using female partners and at least one partner diagnosed with AIDS, was the lone possible case of woman-to-woman transmission.

Prevalence of HIV infection among lesbian and bisexual women in the United States is unknown. In the only systematic study of HIV seroprevalence in this population, six of 550 women (1.2 percent) recruited from public venues in San Francisco and Berkeley were found to be HIV infected, with all reporting a history of injection drug use or sexual contact with men.[126]

TRENDS IN RISK BEHAVIORS

Studies assessing HIV risk behaviors in women who have sex with women are still few in number and largely based on convenience samples, from which definitive conclusions may not be drawn. Data from national probability surveys are unavailable. Among the existing studies it is possible to piece together a picture of potentially high rates of sexual and drug-related behaviors, particularly among bisexual women. With regard to sexual risk, research from several San Francisco samples has shown 82 to 98 percent of lesbian and bisexual women reported sex in the last three years with a male partner and 16 to 34 percent with a bisexual male partner.[136] A survey of 1,086 women from East Coast locales also showed 13 percent to 42 percent of lesbian and bisexual women reporting sex with a bisexual man since 1978.[139] Only 10 percent of women in this latter study reported consistent condom use with bisexual male partners and 4 percent with injection-drug-using male partners. Additionally, only 18 percent of those reporting injection drug use and 9 percent of those who had previously engaged in any high-risk sexual behavior practiced what they considered to be safer sex with their female partners. With regard to drug-related risk, several studies report 2 to 3 percent of homosexual and bisexual women reporting injection drug use in the last three years and 2 to 10 percent since 1978.[136,139] Research has also found that women with female sex partners were more likely than exclusively heterosexual women to inject with used syringes and to exchange sex for drugs or money.[140,141]

INTERVENTION MODELS

Only one published study has described an intervention targeting women who have sex with women. Conducted in San Francisco bars, dance clubs, and sex clubs, the intervention utilized a peer outreach model that included individual interviews and group presentations at the various venues.[142] While quantitative data were not collected, qualitative data provide insights on important messages that should be included in future interventions for this population.

These data emphasize that to be effective, interventions must be culturally and community specific, emphasizing themes related to gender, race/ethnicity, and sexual orientation as they target lesbian and bisexual women. Among lesbian or bisexual women who inject drugs or have sex with men, the risk for HIV may be similar to that of heterosexual women. However, lesbian and bisexual women frequently do not perceive themselves to be at risk for HIV.[141] Thus, interventions for these populations must address women's personal perception of vulnerability for HIV and, in particular, biases about risk based on risk-group category or sexual identity rather than behavior. Interventions must also address (1) the range of risk-reduction activities women may engage in, such as reduction in number of partners, HIV testing, and condom use; (2) drug use; (3) partner selection; and (4) intimacy, trust, and communication within relationships.[142,143] Finally, and as important as these psychosocial issues, there is a critical need to assure that condoms or other effective barriers are available to and used appropriately by at-risk women.

CONCLUSIONS

This chapter provides mixed conclusions for those evaluating prevention efforts for homosexual or bisexual men and women. AIDS cases are declining among some MSMs. But rates are increasing among younger men, men of color, and men living in nonurban settings. Promising intervention models have been identified through research, particularly for white gay men, and these models are currently being tested with other populations of gay men. However, few controlled trials of theory-based interventions are underway for bisexual men or for lesbian or bisexual women. Indeed, our understanding of risk behaviors and their psychosocial determinants remains inadequate for these three populations.

The data reveal other important gaps in our knowledge and practice. We continue to lack important information on (1) national and local trends in STD and HIV infection rates among all three populations; (2) cultural beliefs and practices related to sexual behavior and sexual identity; (3) age- and gender-related differences in the development of sexual identity and risk seeking; (4) the role of homophobia, of the stigma associated with HIV infection and other STDs, and of other community attitudes and beliefs as barriers to individual risk reduction and effective interventions for these populations; and (5) the extent to which effective intervention models are being implemented outside research settings. A critical challenge of the future will be to evaluate interventions arising "naturally" within communities. Equally important will be efforts to translate and then diffuse models found to be effective through controlled trials to prevention programs.

Research also suggests several emerging trends in prevention efforts for these three populations and others. First, the emphasis on community interventions reflects the growing trend away from interventions being implemented *for* others to a model of collaboration among community members, program developers, and researchers to facilitate implementation of high-quality interventions *by community members*. Where the community structure is weak or just emerging, the intervention may need to address community cohesiveness and behavior change simultaneously. Second, the emphasis on helping sexually active men and women to initiate and *maintain* risk-reduction activities is clearly reflected in the importance now attributed to case management (in association with repeated counseling and testing) and to comprehensive, multistrategy prevention approaches. Both themes sadly reflect the recognition that prevention efforts will probably need to be maintained throughout the lifetime of homosexual and bisexual men and women.

Finally, it is important to note the changing climate for conducting intervention research and programs among the populations we have described in this chapter. Gay and bisexual men have experienced profound personal loss because of the AIDS epidemic. Individuals, care givers, friendship networks, leaders responsible for conducting prevention programs—all aspects of gay communities—have suffered profound losses. While there have been fewer losses in lesbian communities, many women from these communities have volunteered tirelessly in AIDS-related programs. Understanding and addressing the stress and burnout that such a situation guarantees will be critical to the success of primary prevention programs for these populations.

References

1 Centers for Disease Control: Update: Trends in AIDS among men who have sex with men—United States, 1989–1994. *MMWR* 44: 401, 1995.

2 Laumann EO et al: *The Social Organization of Sexuality*. Chicago, The University of Chicago Press, 1994.

3 Fay RE et al: Prevalence and patterns of same-gender sexual contact among men. *Science* 243:338, 1989.

4 Smith TW: Adult sexual behavior in 1989: Number of partners, frequency of intercourse, and risk of AIDS. *Fam Plann Perspect* 23:102, 1991.

5 Rogers SM, Turner CF: Male-male sexual contact in the U.S.A.: Findings from five samples, 1970–1990. *J Sex Res* 28:491, 1991.

6 Binson D et al: Prevalence and social distribution of men who have sex with men: United States and its urban centers. *J Sex Res* 32:245, 1995.

7 Turner CF et al: Sexual behavior in the United States, 1930–1990: Trends and methodological problems. *Sex Transm Dis* 22:173, 1995.

8 Catania J: Personal communication. Center for AIDS Prevention Studies, San Francisco, September 1995.

9 Coates TJ et al: *Does HIV Prevention Work for Men Who Have Sex with Men (MSM)?* Washington DC, Office of Technology Assessment, 1995.

10 Kohn R: Personal communication. San Francisco Health Department, STD Control Division, May, 1996.
11 Barrow R: Personal Communication. Centers for Disease Control and Prevention, Atlanta GA, January 1997.
12 Dias SP et al: Rates of Sexually Transmitted Diseases (STD) in Gay Men in the AIDS Era. Presented at the Annual Meeting of the Infectious Disease Society of America, San Francisco, September, 1995.
13 Osmond DH et al: HIV infection in homosexual and bisexual men 18–29 years of age—The San Francisco Young Men's Health Study. *Am J Public Health* 84:1933, 1994.
14 Meyer I et al: Patterns of sexual behavior and risk taking among young New York City gay men. *AIDS Educ Prev* 7:13, 1995.
15 Ostrow DG et al: A case-control study of human immunodeficiency virus type 1 seroconversion and risk-related behaviors in the Chicago MACS/CCS cohort, 1984–1992. *Am J Epidemiol* 142:875, 1995.
16 Buchbinder SP et al: Feasibility of human immunodeficiency virus vaccine trials in homosexual men in the United States: risk behavior, seroincidence, and willingness to participate. *J Infect Dis* 174:954, 1996.
17 Weinstock HS et al: Trends in HIV seroprevalence among persons attending sexually transmitted disease clinics in the United States, 1988–1992. *J Acquir Immune Defic Syndr* 9:514, 1995.
18 Lemp GF et al: Seroprevalence of HIV among young homosexual and bisexual men. The San Francisco/Berkeley Young Men's Survey. *JAMA* 272:449, 1994.
19 Kingsley LA et al: Temporal trends in human immunodeficiency virus type 1 seroconversion 1984–1989. A report from the Multicenter AIDS Cohort Study (MACS). *Am J Epidemiol* 134:331, 1991.
20 Martin DJ: Inappropriate lubricant use with condoms by homosexual men. *Public Health Rep* 107:468, 1992.
21 Mayer K et al: Human immunodeficiency virus and oral intercourse. *Ann Intern Med* 107:428, 1987.
22 Grutzmeier S et al: HIV Transmission in Gay Men in Stockholm, 1990–1992; Six Cases of HIV Infection Through Oral Sex. Presented at the Eleventh International Conference on AIDS, Berlin, June 1993.
23 Samuel MC et al: Factors associated with human immunodeficiency virus seroconversion in homosexual men in three San Francisco cohort studies. *J Acquir Immune Defic Syndr* 6:303, 1993.
24 Jaffe HW et al: National case-control study of Kaposi's sarcoma and pneumocystis carinii pneumonia in homosexual men: Part 1. Epidemiologic results. *Ann Intern Med* 99:145, 1983.
25 Darrow WW et al: Risk factors for human immunodeficiency virus (HIV) infections in homosexual men. *Am J Public Health* 77:479, 1987
26 Kingsley J et al: Risk factors for seroconversion to human immunodeficiency virus among male homosexuals. Results from the Multicenter AIDS Cohort Study. *Lancet* 1:345, 1987.
27 Schecter MT et al: The Vancouver Lymphadenopathy-AIDS Study: 6. HIV seroconversion in a cohort of homosexual men. *Can Med Assoc J* 135:1355, 1986.
28 McKusick L et al: Reported changes in the sexual behavior of men at risk for AIDS, San Francisco, 1982–1984. The AIDS Behavioral Research Project. *Public Health Rep* 100:622, 1985.
29 Joseph J et al: Magnitude and determinants of behavioral risk reduction: Longitudinal analysis of a cohort at risk for AIDS. *Psychol Health* 1:73, 1987.
30 Martin JL: The impact of AIDS on gay male sexual behavior patterns in New York City. *Amer J Public Health* 77:578, 1987.
31 Ostrow DG: Risk reduction for transmission of human immunodeficiency virus in high-risk communities. *Psychiatr Med* 7:79, 1989.
32 Kelly JA et al: AIDS risk behavior patterns among gay men in small southern cities. *Amer J Public Health* 80:416, 1990.
33 Ekstrand ML et al: Maintenance of safer sexual behaviors and predictors of risky sex: The San Francisco Men's Health Study. *Amer J Public Health* 80:973, 1990.
34 Adib MS et al: Stages of sexual behavior change to reduce the risk of HIV/AIDS: The Chicago MACS/CCS cohort. *J Psychol and Human Sexuality*, 7:121, 1995.
35 Kippax S et al: Sustaining safe sex in homosexually active men. *National AIDS Bulletin* (Australia) 6:38, 1992.
36 Becker MH et al: AIDS and behavioral change to reduce risk [Review]. *Amer J Public Health* 78:394, 1988.
37 Prochaska et al: The transtheoretical model of change and HIV prevention [Review]. *Health Educ Q* 21:471, 1994.
38 Kelly JA: Advances in HIV/AIDS Education and Prevention. *Fam Relations* 44:345, 1995.
39 Hospers HJ et al: Determinants of safe and risk-taking sexual behavior among gay men [Review]. *AIDS Educ Prev* 7:74, 1995.
40 Prochaska JO et al: Toward a Comprehensive Model of Change, in *Treating Addictive Behaviors,* HN Miller (ed). New York, Plenum Press, 1986, pp 3–27.
41 Catania J et al: Towards an understanding of risk behavior: An AIDS risk reduction model (ARRM). *Health Educ Q* 17:381, 1990.
42 Gold R: Why We Need to Rethink AIDS Education for Gay Men. Presented at the Second International Conference on AIDS' Impact: Biopsychosocial Aspects of HIV Infection, Brighton, England, July, 1994.
43 Marlatt GA et al: *Relapse Prevention: Maintenance Strategies in the Treatment of Addictive Behaviors.* New York, Guilford Press, 1985.
44 Bandura A: Self-efficacy: Toward a unifying theory of behavior change. *Psychol Rev* 84:191, 1977.
45 Hays RB et al: HIV prevention for gay and bisexual men in metropolitan cities, in *Preventing AIDS. Theories and Methods of Behavioral Interventions*, RJ DiClemente, JL Peterson (eds). New York, Plenum Press, 1994, pp 267–296.
46 McCusker J et al: Predictors of AIDS-preventive behavior among homosexually active men: A longitudinal study. *AIDS* 3:443, 1989.
47 Johnson RW et al: Education strategies for prevention of sexual transmission of HIV, in *Behavioral Aspects of AIDS,* DG Ostrow (ed). New York, Plenum Press, 1990, pp 43–74.
48 Remafedi G: Predictors of unprotected intercourse among gay and bisexual youth: knowledge, beliefs, and behavior. *Pediatrics* 94:163, 1994.
49 Seibt AC et al: Relationship between safe sex and acculturation into the gay subculture. *AIDS Care* 7 (suppl 1):87, 1995.
50 Ostrow DG: AIDS prevention through effective education. *Daedalus* 118:229, 1993.
51 McKirnan DJ et al: HIV-risk sexual behavior among bisexually active men: The role of gay identification and social norms. Unpublished manuscript, University of Illinois at Chicago 1995.
52 Stall R et al: Alcohol and drug use during sexual activity and compliance with safe sex guidelines for AIDS: The AIDS Behavioral Research Project. *Health Educ Q* 13:359, 1986.
53 Kalichman SC et al: Sexual sensation seeking. Scale development and predicting AIDS-related behavior among homosexually active men. *J Personality Assess* 62:385, 1994.
54 Ostrow DG et al: Sexual Adventurism Mediates the Substance Use-Risky Sex Relationship among Gay Men. Abstracts NIDA Conference on AIDS and Drug Abuse, Scottsdale AZ, June, 1995b, B-4:4.
55 Peterson JL et al: High-risk sexual behavior and condom use among gay and bisexual African American men. *Amer J Public Health* 82: 1490, 1992.
56 Diaz RM: HIV Risk in Latino Gay/Bisexual Men: A Review of Behavioral Research, in *Latino Gay Men and HIV: The Cultural Meaning of High-Risk Behavior*, RM Diaz. New York, Routledge, 1997.
57 Choi KH et al: High HIV risk among gay Asian and Pacific Islander men in San Francisco. *AIDS* 9:306, 1995.
58 Mays VM et al: The language of black gay men's sexual behavior: implications for AIDS risk reduction. *J Sex Res* 29:425, 1992.
59 Peterson JL: AIDS-Related Risks and Same-Sex Behaviors among African American Men, in *AIDS, Identity and Community,* GM Herek, B Greene (eds). Thousand Oaks CA, Sage, 1995, pp 85–104.
60 Doll LS et al: Male bisexual behavior and HIV risk in the United States: synthesis of research with implications for behavioral interventions. *AIDS Educ Prev* 8:205, 1996.
61 Fishbein M: Personal communication. Centers for Disease Control and Prevention, Atlanta GA, September, 1995.

62 Kelly JA et al: Psychological interventions to prevent HIV infection are urgently needed. New priorities for behavioral research in the second decade of AIDS. *Amer Psychol* 48:1023, 1993.
63 Holtgrave DR et al: An overview of the effectiveness and efficiency of HIV prevention programs. *Public Health Rep* 110:134, 1995.
64 Kelly, JA: *Changing HIV Risk Behavior: Practical Strategies.* New York, Guilford Press, 1995.
65 Oakley A et al: Behavioral interventions for HIV/AIDS prevention. *AIDS* 9:479, 1995.
66 Stryker J et al: Prevention of HIV infection: Looking back, looking ahead. *JAMA* 273:1143, 1995.
67 Higgins DL et al: Evidence for the effects of HIV antibody counseling and testing on risk behaviors. *JAMA* 266:2419, 1991.
68 Doll LS et al: HIV Counseling and Testing, in *AIDS Testing,* 2nd ed, Schochetman G, George JR (eds). New York, Springer-Verlag, 1994, pp 302–319.
69 Beltran ED et al: Predictors of sexual behavior change among men requesting their HIV-1 antibody status: The Chicago MACS/CCS cohort of homosexual/bisexual men, 1985–1986. *AIDS Educ Prev* 5: 185, 1993.
70 Nimmons D: Personal communication. Gay Men's Health Crisis, New York, December, 1995.
71 Bandura A: *Social Foundations of Thought and Action: A Social Cognitive Theory.* Englewood Cliffs NJ, Prentice-Hall, 1986.
72 Valdiserri RO et al: AIDS prevention in homosexual and bisexual men: results of a randomized trial evaluating two risk reduction interventions. *AIDS* 3:21, 1989.
73 Kelly JA et al: Behavioral intervention to reduce AIDS risk activities. *J Consult Clin Psychol* 57:60, 1989.
74 Kelly JA et al: A skills training group intervention model to assist persons in reducing risk behaviors for HIV infection. *AIDS Educ Prev* 2:24, 1990.
75 Peterson J et al: Evaluation of an HIV intervention strategy among African American homosexual and bisexual men. *AIDS,* 10:319, 1996.
76 Kelly JA et al: Predictors of vulnerability to AIDS risk behavior relapse. *J Consult Clin Psychol* 59:163, 1991.
77 Kelly JA et al: HIV risk behavior reduction following intervention with key opinion leaders of population: an experimental analysis. *Amer J Public Health* 81:168, 1991.
78 Kelly JA et al: Community AIDS/HIV risk reduction: the effects of endorsements by popular people in three cities. *Amer J Public Health* 82:1483, 1992.
79 Johnson W: Personal communication. Centers for Disease Control and Prevention, Atlanta GA, August 1995.
80 Miller RL: Assisting gay men to maintain safer sex: an evaluation of an AIDS service organization's safer sex maintenance program. *AIDS Educ Prev* 7:48, 1995.
81 Kegeles SM et al: The Mpowerment Project: A community-level prevention intervention for young gay and bisexual men. *Amer J Public Health* 86:1129, 1996.
82 Elovich R: *Harm Reduction and Steps Toward Change. The Role of Counseling: Working with Ambivalence and Building Motivation for Change. A Training Source Book.* New York, Gay Men's Health Crisis, 1995.
83 Billy JOG et al: The sexual behavior of men in the United States. *Fam Plann Perspect* 25:52, 1993.
84 Bevier P et al: The Role of Bisexual Men in a "Heterosexual" Syphilis/ HIV Core Group in New York City. Presented at the Eleventh International Conference on AIDS, Berlin, 1993.
85 Temoshok LR: HIV exposure risk in the U.S. Army vs. general civilian populations. Under review.
86 Hahn RA et al: Race and the prevalence of syphilis seroreactivity in the United States population: a national sero-epidemiologic study. *Amer J Public Health* 79:467, 1989.
87 McKirnan D et al: Bisexually active men: social characteristics and sexual behavior. *J Sex Res* 32:64, 1994.
88 Stokes JP et al: Ethnic differences in sexual behavior, condom use, and psychosocial variables among black and white men who have sex with men. *J Sex Res* 33:373, 1996.
89 Diaz T et al: Sociodemographics and HIV risk behaviors of bisexual men with AIDS: results from a multistate interview project. *AIDS* 7:1227, 1993.
90 Padian N et al: Male-to-female transmission of human immunodeficiency virus. *JAMA* 258:788, 1987.
91 Beeker C et al: Bisexuality, Drug Use, and Prostitution among Men Intercepted an Urban Neighborhoods with High IDU Prevalence. Presented at the Ninth International Conference on AIDS, Berlin, 1993.
92 Freeman AC et al: Gay, Bisexual, and Straight Men Who Have Sex with Men: HIV Risk And Disclosure. Presented at the Eighth International Conference on AIDS, Amsterdam, 1992.
93 Wolitski RJ: Bisexual Men's Disclosure of Same-Sex Activity to Female Partners. Unpublished manuscript, 1994.
94 Stokes J et al: Female sexual partners of bisexual men: what they don't know might hurt them. *Psychol Women's Quart* 20:267, 1996.
95 Heckman TG et al: Differences in HIV risk characteristics between bisexual and exclusively gay men. *AIDS Educ Prev,* 7:504, 1995.
96 Centers for Disease Control and Prevention: Condom use among men who have sex with men and the relationship to sexual identity—Dallas 1991. *MMWR* 42:7, 1993.
97 Doll LS et al: Homosexually and nonhomosexually identified men who have sex with men: a behavioral comparison. *J Sex Res* 29:1, 1992.
98 Lever J et al: *Behavioral patterns and sexual identity of bisexual males.* Santa Monica, CA, Rand Corporation, 1992.
99 Stokes JP et al: Bisexual men, sexual behavior, and HIV/AIDS, in *Bisexuality: The Psychology and Politics of an Invisible Minority,* B Firestein (ed). Thousand Oaks, CA. 1996, pp 149–168.
100 Wood RW et al: HIV transmission: Women's risk from bisexual men. *Amer J Public Health* 3:1757, 1993.
101 Stokes JP et al: Sexual behavior, condom use, disclosure of sexuality, and stability of sexual orientation in bisexual men. *J Sex Res* 30:1, 1993.
102 Wolitski RJ: HIV Risk Practices of Gay-Identified and Nongay Identified Men Who Have Sex with Men. Presented at the annual meeting of the American Public Health Association, San Francisco, 1993.
103 Ekstrand ML et al: Bisexual men in San Francisco are not a common vector for spreading HIV infection to women: The San Francisco Men's Health Study. *Amer J Public Health* 84:915, 1994.
104 Morse EV et al: The male street prostitute: A vector for transmission of HIV infection into the heterosexual world. *Soc Sci Med* 32:535, 1991.
105 Morse EV et al: Sexual behavior patterns of customers of male street prostitutes. *Arch Sex Behav* 21:347, 1992.
106 Elifson KW et al: Risk factors associated with HIV infection among male prostitutes. *Amer J Public Health* 83:79, 1993.
107 Simon PM et al: Barriers to human immunodeficiency virus related risk reduction among male street prostitutes. *Health Educ Q* 20:261, 1993.
108 Lewis DK et al: Sexual behavior and sexual identity in male injection drug users. *J AIDS* 7:190, 1994.
109 Centers for Disease Control and Prevention: HIV risk factors of male injecting-drug users who have sex with men—Dallas, Denver, and Long Beach, 1991–1994. *MMWR* 44:767, 1995.
110 Hays RB et al: High HIV risk-taking among young gay men. *AIDS* 4:901, 1990.
111 Reinisch JM et al: Sexual behavior and AIDS: lessons from art and sex research, in *AIDS and Sex,* B Voeller et al (eds). New York, Oxford University Press, 1990, pp 37–80.
112 Lemp GF et al: HIV seroprevalence and risk behaviors among young gay and bisexual men: The San Francisco/Berkeley Young Men's Survey. *JAMA* 272:449, 1994.
113 Peterson JL: Black men and their same-sex desires and behaviors, in *Gay Culture in America: Essays From the Field,* G Herdt (ed). Boston, Beacon Press, 1992, pp 147–164.
114 Wright JW: African American male sexual behavior and the risk for HIV infection. *Hum Org* 52:421, 1993.
115 Stevens C: Personal communication. Geneva, Switzerland, 1992.

116 Beckstein D: AIDS Prevention in Public Sex Environments: Outreach and Training Manual. Santa Cruz CA, Santa Cruz AIDS Project, 1990.

117 Beeker C: Final Report on Hispanic Nongay-Identified Men Who Have Sex with Other Men: A Formative Research Study. Atlanta GA, Centers for Disease Control and Prevention, 1993.

118 U.S. Conference of Mayors: Assessing the HIV-Prevention Needs of Gay and Bisexual Men of Color. Washington DC, 1994.

119 Rubenstein M et al: A profile of the San Francisco bisexual center. *J Homosex* 11:227, 1985.

120 Miller R: Gay Men's Health Crisis (GMHC) Hustler Peer Education Project. Presented at the Hustler Network Peer Education Conference, San Francisco, October, 1993.

121 Martin AD et al: The stigmatization of the gay and lesbian adolescent. *J Homosex* 17:163, 1988.

122 Herdt G et al: *Children of Horizons*. Boston, Beacon Press, 1993.

123 Roffman RA et al: Continuing unsafe sex: assessing the need for AIDS prevention counseling. *Public Health Rep* 105:202, 1990.

124 Elie R: Hetrick-Martin Institute's Project First Step. Presented at the Hustler Network Peer Education Conference, San Francisco, October, 1993.

125 Schilling RF et al: Developing strategies for AIDS prevention research with black and Hispanic drug users. *Public Health Rep* 104:2, 1989.

126 Lemp GF et al: HIV seroprevalence and risk behaviors among lesbians and bisexual women in San Francisco and Berkeley, California. *Amer J Public Health* 85:1549, 1995.

127 Johnson SR et al: Comparison of gynecologic health care problems between lesbians and bisexual women: a survey of 2,345 women. *J Reprod Med* 32:805, 1987.

128 Marrazzo J: Personal communication. Seattle-King County Department of Public Health, January 1997.

129 Bevier PJ et al: Women at a sexually transmitted disease clinic who reported same-sex contact: their HIV seroprevalence and risk behaviors. *Amer J Public Health* 85:1366, 1995.

130 Marmor M et al: Possible female-to-female transmission of human immunodeficiency virus. *Ann Intern Med* 105:969, 1986.

131 Chu SY et al: Epidemiology of reported cases of AIDS in lesbians, United States 1980–89. *Amer J Public Health* 80:1380, 1990.

132 Petersen LR et al: No evidence for female-to-female HIV transmission among 960,000 female blood donors. *J Acquir Immune Defic Syndr* 5:853, 1992.

133 Cohen H et al: Risk assessment of HIV transmission among lesbians. *J Acquir Immune Defic Syndr* 6:1173, 1993.

134 Chu SY et al: Female-to-female sexual contact and HIV transmission. *JAMA* 272:433, 1994.

135 Raiter R et al: No HIV-1 transmission through lesbian sex. *Lancet* 344:270, 1994.

136 Kennedy MB et al: Assessing HIV risk among women who have sex with women: scientific and communication issues. *JAMWA* 50:103, 1995.

137 Chu SY et al: Update: epidemiology of reported cases of AIDS in women who report sex only with other women, United States, 1990–1991. *AIDS* 6:518, 1992.

138 McCombs S et al: Epidemiology of HIV-1 infection in bisexual women. *J Acquir Immune Defic Syndr* 5:850, 1992.

139 Einhorn L et al: HIV-risk behavior among lesbians and bisexual women. *AIDS Educ Prev* 6:514, 1994.

140 Young M et al: Assessing risk in the absence of information: HIV risk among women injection drug users who have sex with women. *AIDS Public Policy* 7:175, 1992.

141 Gomez CA: Lesbians at Risk for HIV: The Unresolved Debate, in *AIDS, Identity, and Community*, GM Herek, B Greene (eds). Thousand Oaks, CA, Sage, 1995, pp 19–31.

142 Stevens PE: HIV prevention education for lesbians and bisexual women: a cultural analysis of a community intervention. *Soc Sci Med* 39:1565, 1994.

143 Morrow KM: Lesbian Women and HIV/AIDS: An Appeal for Inclusion, in *Women at Risk: Issues in the Primary Prevention of AIDS*, A O'Leary, LS Jemmott (eds). New York, Plenum Press, 1995, pp 237–257.

CHAPTER 12

STDs, HIV/AIDS, ethnicity, and migrant populations

Anneke van den Hoek

INTRODUCTION

Migration and travel have always played an important role in the spread of infectious diseases, including STDs. For more than five centuries travelers such as sailors and soldiers have been blamed for the spread of STDs. A well-known example is Christopher Columbus and his sailors bringing syphilis from the New World to Spain. Some of the returning sailors enlisted in the army of the French king Charles VIII, who recruited soldiers from all European countries. When all these soldiers eventually returned home, syphilis broke out all over Europe.[1] The French called the disease the Italian disease, and the Italians called it the French disease.

The spread of penicillinase-producing *Neisseria gonorrhoeae* (PPNG) is a more recent example of the distances and speeds at which STD pathogens may travel. In 1975 the first cases of PPNG emerged in the Far East and in western Africa. In early 1976 the first cases of PPNG were identified in the United States in men who had had sexual contacts in East Asia.[2] In the Netherlands the first PPNG infection was diagnosed in late 1976, in an air hostess who was infected by a colleague from the Philippines.[3]

Another new infectious disease, acquired immunodeficiency syndrome, or AIDS, was described shortly thereafter. First identified in homosexual men, hemophiliacs, and injecting drug users, the disease was also very soon seen in recent immigrants to the United States from Haiti, among central African immigrants in Belgium,[4,5] and among whites who had traveled and had heterosexual contacts in Africa.[6]

RISK GROUPS FOR STDS AND SEXUALLY ACQUIRED HIV INFECTION

Risk groups for STDs and sexually acquired HIV infection (STD/HIV) are defined by the presence of determinants of risky sexual behavior. Important determinants include the number of sexual partners, rates of partner change, specific sexual practices, and the use of condoms. The prevalence of STD/HIV in the population from which one chooses sexual partners also determines risk for acquiring STD/HIV.

Various demographic factors have also been related to the acquisition of STD/HIV. These include age, gender, and marital status, as well as ethnicity, migration status, socioeconomic status, and education. These last four factors are, of course, strongly interrelated. Demographic factors may have a direct relation to sexual behavior and health practices (for example, to condom use and to health-care-seeking behavior), as well as an impact on the social environment from which one chooses partners.[7]

Epidemics of STD/HIV are frequently seen in men who temporarily have to stay away from their families. The heterogeneity of economic growth rates has led to high levels of geographic mobility.[7–9] In particular, the combination of the migrant labor system with long familial separations has resulted in a disintegration of long established marital and sexual patterns. The unequal sex ratio in towns men migrate into encourages prostitution. Both migrant labor and prostitution have led to epidemics of STD/HIV among these populations all over the world.[7–9]

The migratory labor system has been regarded as essential in the transmission of HIV in eastern, central, and southern Africa.[8] Also, long-distance truck drivers—particularly in Africa and more recently in Asia—play an important role in the spread of STD/HIV. Drivers and their assistants are frequent clients of prostitutes in the towns along the main trucking routes.[9] Military service men and sailors are also traditionally viewed as risk groups for STD, because of their frequent sexual contacts with prostitutes. Currently, airplane crews and travelers, including so-called sex tourists (men and women who travel long distances for sexual contacts), may be regarded as groups with potentially increased risk for STD/HIV. Prostitutes also travel long distances to offer their sexual services elsewhere. This international migration of prostitutes has now become an important part of the sex industry.[10]

That people at risk for STD/HIV have traveled or are still traveling can be illustrated by the number of nationalities of visitors to the STD clinics of the Municipal Health Service in Amsterdam (Figure 12-1). In 1995 about 9,000 men and women visited the STD clinic for a new consultation; 31 percent of the men and 29 percent of the women were non-Dutch. Altogether, 108 nationalities were counted, 97 among the men and 77 among the women.

MIGRANT PROSTITUTION IN EUROPE

Migrant prostitution, also called mobile prostitution, is occurring on a large scale within Europe. Women come to Europe from all over the world: from Latin America, West Africa, Asia, and increasingly during the past few years from eastern Europe. The underlying reason that these women migrate and work as prostitutes is the miserable economic conditions in their own countries. A study in the Dominican Republic of 80 women who had worked as prostitutes outside the country showed that they had worked in 27 countries, including 8 European countries.[10]

Information on numbers of migrant prostitutes are in general not available. In Amsterdam, it is estimated that approximately 40 percent of the sex workers come from developing countries, mainly from Latin America. After a few months of working in one European country, migrant prostitutes may move to another country. Fieldwork among migrant prostitutes in Amsterdam in 1992 through 1993 showed that one-third of them had arrived in the country during the previous three months.[11]

A study in Germany showed that migrant prostitutes come there from all over the world (33 different countries) but that prostitutes of different nationalities work in different parts of the country. In northern and eastern Germany, migrant prostitutes were mainly from eastern Europe; in Frankfurt, mainly from Latin America; in Duisburg, from Africa; and in Essen, from France. In Berlin, the largest number of migrant prostitutes were from eastern Europe, the next largest number from Thailand.[12] Migrant prostitutes in general are low-class prostitutes, meaning they are seldom found in sex clubs, but rather solicit their clients on the streets, in brothels, or from behind windows (so-called window prostitutes). In the Netherlands and Germany migrant laborers form the main group of clients of migrant prostitutes, and this may be the case in other countries as well.[12,13]

In what follows, recent data on the relationship of race, ethnicity, and nationality and of migration and travel to the spread of STD/HIV will be presented and discussed.

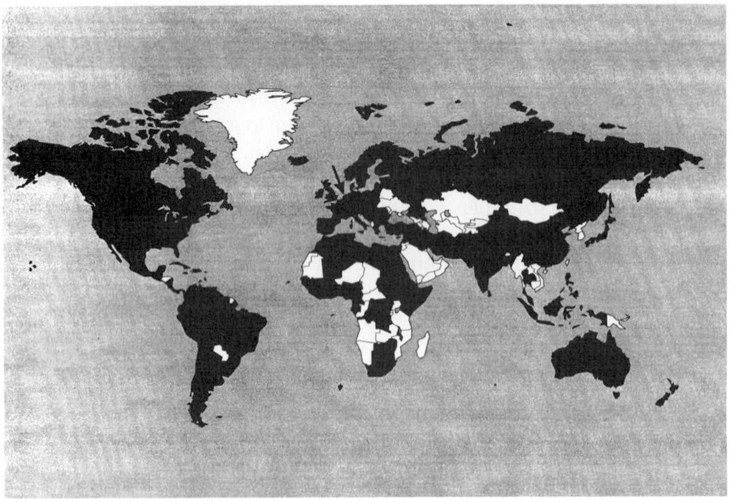

Fig. 12-1 Depicted in dark gray are the nationalities of visitors to the STD clinic in Amsterdam, Netherlands in 1995. One hundred eight nationalities were counted among the 8,895 visitors. Thirty-one percent of the male and 29 percent of the female visitors were of non-Dutch nationality.

RELATION OF ETHNICITY/NATIONALITY AND MIGRATION/TRAVEL TO STD/HIV IN EUROPE

SEXUALLY TRANSMITTED DISEASES IN EUROPE

In the early eighties, before the beginning of the AIDS epidemic, the number of cases of gonorrhea started to decline throughout Europe. In the mid-eighties a further and steeper decline occurred. The first decline has been attributed to improved case management (including improved STD diagnostics, treatment, health education, and partner notification), and the second to a decline in risky sexual behavior, particularly among homosexual men. This trend was seen all over Europe, although the onset of the decline varied. In Sweden the gonorrhea incidence started to drop in 1971, and except in 1974 to 1976 this decrease continued through the 1970s and 1980s.[14] The incidence of syphilis also declined during the eighties in Europe. The decline began in 1983 in Sweden and Denmark and in 1985 in the Netherlands. In England and Wales the incidence has fallen consistently since 1978.[15] Chancroid, the third classic STD, is a rare disease in Europe.

Extensive spread of HIV began in the late 1970s and early 1980s. As in the United States and Australia, the primary groups affected by the disease in western Europe were homosexual men and injecting drug users. Heterosexual spread of HIV, though increasing, accounts for a relatively small proportion of new infections.

In Europe only scarce data exist on the impact of nationality/ethnicity and migration/travel on the risk for STD/HIV. Not all countries have a reporting system for classic STDs, and of those that do, only a few report by nationality/ethnicity. The Scandinavian countries have some data on the country of acquisition of an STD. In Denmark in 1990 it appeared that of the 56 reported cases of syphilis, 68 percent of the men and 57 percent of the women had acquired the disease outside Denmark (mainly in Africa and Southeast Asia).[16] It is unknown whether these percentages represent mainly foreigners (for example, asylum seekers who carry an STD from the country of origin) or Danes who became infected outside their country—for example, during holidays. In Sweden in the same year 76 percent of the 143 reported syphilis cases were diagnosed in foreigners.[17]

In England and Wales, place of acquisition is known only for PPNG infections. Of the 124 cases of PPNG infections reported in 1993, 39 had been acquired abroad, including 12 in the Far East, 15 in Africa, 8 in other European countries, and 2 in other areas.[18] In Switzerland, of all STDs reported in 1990 and 1991, 25 percent and 22 percent, respectively, were imported from abroad; and of the PPNG infections reported during these 2 years, 60 percent were imported. Of the imported STD cases, 26 percent in 1990 and 31.5 percent in 1991 were imported from Asia.[19]

In the Netherlands specific studies have dealt with nationality and migrant status as risk markers for STDs. In Amsterdam the annual number of infections with PPNG strains remained more or less stable from 1983 until 1990, while the number of non-PPNG infections declined dramatically. A cross-sectional study was conducted in 1989 and 1990 to assess determinants of PPNG infections among heterosexuals diagnosed with gonorrhea. It appeared that PPNG infections were especially common among Central and South American window prostitutes and their clients, who were predominantly Turkish men.[20] Apparently these populations of migrant prostitutes and migrant clients—among whom PPNG infections predominantly circulate, showing a stable trend—reduced their risky sexual behaviors less than the general Dutch population.

A study of a cohort of heterosexuals with multiple partners attending the STD clinic in Amsterdam showed—after controlling for sexual behavior—that those born outside the Netherlands were more likely to be STD-infected at entry into the study.[21] However, for acquisition of STD during this longitudinal study, ethnicity proved not to be an independent risk factor except for the acquisition of chlamydial infection in women.[13] Differential health-care-seeking behavior may therefore underlie ethnicity as a risk factor for higher STD prevalence. However, additional studies have shown that migrant men and women have indeed reduced their risky sexual behavior less than the indigenous population. In 1991 groups of prostitutes and clients of prostitutes (both groups without a history of injection drug use) were studied to determine HIV prevalence and correlates of inconsistent condom use. Half of the participants were recruited at the STD clinic in Amsterdam and half at prostitute work sites. HIV prevalence appeared to be fairly low (1.5 percent among the prostitutes and 0.5 percent among the clients), but inconsistent condom use was found to be relatively high among prostitutes who had migrated from Latin America and among migrant clients of prostitutes.[22] Another study at the STD clinic in Amsterdam showed that from 1982 through 1989 heterosexuals turned to safer sexual practices but that notable exceptions were Turkish men and foreign prostitutes.[23]

HIV/AIDS IN EUROPE

In England, Wales, and Northern Ireland the majority of heterosexually acquired HIV infections have been attributable to sexual contact in countries where heterosexual transmission is the main transmission route (mainly in sub-Saharan Africa). By the end of 1991, 79 percent of the 417 heterosexually acquired AIDS cases and 74 percent of the 1438 heterosexually acquired HIV infections had been acquired abroad.[24] In Denmark about half of the persons with heterosexually acquired HIV infection, notified between August 1990 through January 1993, had been infected outside Denmark.[25] The majority of these persons had grown up outside Denmark, mainly in Africa. In Sweden, of the 230 cases of heterosexually acquired HIV infections reported in 1993, 194 (84 percent) had been diagnosed in foreigners. Of the remaining 36 heterosexually acquired HIV infections in Swedes, 18 had been acquired outside Sweden.[26] In Norway, through December 31, 1990, a total of 115 (12 percent) of HIV-positive subjects had a history of sexual contact with prostitutes, of whom 58 percent had had contact abroad.[27] In Amsterdam HIV surveillance among pregnant women has shown a stable low HIV prevalence (0.12 percent) since 1988, and here also the majority of the heterosexually acquired HIV infections have involved women coming from AIDS-endemic areas.[28]

In Belgium, 1365 asylum seekers arriving between November 1988 and January 1989 were studied for prevalence of HIV infection. Of the Africans, mainly coming from central Africa, 3.7 percent were HIV-seropositive; of the Asians, mainly coming from central and southeast Asia, only 0.2 percent were seropositive; and among the Europeans, mainly coming from southeastern Europe, none had HIV antibodies.[29]

A multicenter study among prostitutes in nine European countries in 1990 through 1991 showed that among noninjecting women the HIV prevalence was 1.5 percent; low education and origin from sub-Saharan Africa were associated with HIV infection independent of other risk factors.[30] Research conducted in 1989 through 1990 in Andalusia (Spain) among more than 500 noninjecting prostitutes who were recruited at their workplaces showed that 2.3 percent of them were infected with HIV. HIV infection was associated with having sexual contacts with clients originating from Africa as well as with a history of genital ulcers and anal intercourse.[31]

RELATION OF RACE AND MIGRATION TO STDS AND HIV/AIDS IN THE UNITED STATES

SEXUALLY TRANSMITTED DISEASES IN THE UNITED STATES

In the United States, race and ethnicity are strongly associated with incidence of STD/HIV, which is much higher in the African-American and Hispanic populations than in whites. These racial and ethnic differences in STD rates vary for different diseases.[32] Complications such as pelvic inflammatory disease and ectopic pregnancy, and death due to these complications, are also more common in nonwhite women than in white women.[36,37]

In contrast to trends in Europe, in the United States the number of syphilis cases increased from 1985 through 1990 by more than 50 percent. The increase was seen in men as well as women, but mainly among African-Americans and in low income areas, both urban and rural. The number of reported gonorrhea cases began to decline in the early eighties in both men and women and in all ethnic groups. However, the incidence was much higher in African-Americans than in Hispanics and whites. In 1988, African-Americans made up 11.5 percent of the population but accounted for 76 percent of reported primary and secondary syphilis cases and 78 percent of reported gonorrhea cases. Hispanics made up 6.4 percent of the population, but accounted for 12 percent of reported syphilis cases and 5 percent of reported cases of gonorrhea. Whites represented 80 percent of the population but accounted for 12 percent of reported syphilis and 16 percent of reported gonorrhea cases.[32]

Beginning in 1984, numerous outbreaks of chancroid have occurred in the United States, mainly among African-Americans and Hispanics. Prostitutes appeared to be important in disease transmission, as were individuals who had traveled from outbreak areas or from outside the United States.[33]

Data on the prevalence and incidence of chlamydial infections in the United States are not comprehensive, because no national surveillance system exists for chlamydia. Therefore, data on the relative frequency of genital chlamydial infections in different racial groups are limited. In San Diego County, California, women attending family planning services are routinely screened for chlamydia. From July 1989 through June 1993 the prevalence of chlamydia among African-American women was 8.5 percent, more than 1.5 times that among Hispanic women (5.3 percent) and white women (4.5 percent). During this 4-year period, the prevalence declined minimally among African-American women and steadily among white and Hispanic women.[34] A study conducted in Colorado Springs, Colorado, in which gonorrhea cases were compared with chlamydia cases, showed that the latter cases were more likely to involve individuals who were white and younger than the gonorrhea patients.[35]

Genital herpes infections are also more common in African-Americans than in whites. A seroepidemiologic survey conducted from 1976 to 1980 showed a prevalence of HSV-2 antibodies of 20 percent in whites and 65 percent in African-Americans. Among African-Americans in all age groups, but not in whites, higher rates were found in women than in men. The racial difference remained after controlling for other demographic factors, including socioeconomic status.[38]

HIV/AIDS IN THE UNITED STATES

As STDs enhance the transmission of HIV, racial and ethnic differences in STD incidence have important consequences for the HIV/AIDS epidemic.[39,40] The epidemic of AIDS has paralleled the epidemics of syphilis and chancroid. For example, Florida, which has experienced large epidemics of syphilis and chancroid, also has one of the highest incidences of AIDS.[41] Indeed, racial and ethnic minorities bear a disproportionate share of the burden of AIDS. In 1990, AIDS cases in African-Americans reached a rate of 42 per 100,000 population and in Hispanics 32 per 100,000, compared to 12 per 100,000 in whites. In 1993, racial and ethnic minorities accounted for 45,039 of 89,165 AIDS cases (51 percent) reported among adult and adolescent males. The AIDS rate per 100,000 population was among African-American females (73) approximately 15 times greater than the number among white females (5), and the number of cases among African-American males (266) was nearly 5 times greater than that among white males (57).[42]

A longitudinal study conducted from 1987 through 1989 among active-duty personnel in the military confirm the reported data on AIDS cited above: the overall HIV incidence rate for African-Americans was substantially higher than for whites. During the study period the incidence rate declined in whites but increased in African-Americans.[43]

MIGRANT WORKERS IN THE UNITED STATES

In 1986, an estimated 2.7 to 4.0 million persons in the United States were classified as migrant and seasonal farm workers.[44] Among migrant farm workers in Florida screened in 1992, 8 percent had reactive serologic tests for syphilis and 5 percent were HIV-1 antibody–seropositive.[45] Positive syphilis serology was associated with use of crack cocaine, and HIV-1 seropositivity was associated with having had more than two partners during the last 6 months, a history of syphilis, and (among men) having ever paid for sex. Injecting drug use and homosexual contacts were rarely reported. No data were given on the race or ethnicity of the migrant workers. The 8 percent prevalence of positive syphilis serology was much higher than the 0.8 percent prevalence reported in a national serologic survey.[46]

EXPLANATIONS FOR THE DIFFERENTIAL RATES OF STD/HIV/AIDS IN THE UNITED STATES

Some of the differences in the rates of STDs and HIV/AIDS between whites and nonwhites may be due to reporting bias, as African-Americans and Hispanics are more likely to visit public clinics, where reporting is thought to be more complete than in private clinics. Recent data from a national survey on levels of STD experience showed that race/ethnicity was independently associated with reported gonorrhea experience, but less strongly than expected from the surveillance data.[47] African-American respondents were 2.6 times as likely as others to report having had gonorrhea, whereas in the national surveillance data the gonorrhea rate of African-Americans was 24 times that of whites. These results suggest that the surveillance data do partly reflect underreporting of STDs among higher socioeconomic groups with access to private health care.

Although further explanations for higher rates of STDs and HIV/AIDS among African-Americans in the United States are not fully explored, race may be a marker strongly associated with risk factors for STDs, such as low socioeconomic status, access to health care, health-care-seeking behavior, illicit drug use, and residence (and sexual contacts) in communities with high prevalences of STDs. In addition, the age-specific prevalence of many STD risk behaviors is higher among minority populations of lower socioeconomic status. Among those 15 to 19 years of age, the percentage with sexual experience was higher for minority than for nonminority populations. However, age at sexual debut declined among whites and the nonpoor during the eighties, resulting in diminishing racial/ethnic differences.[48] A larger subset of African-American men than white men practices a high rate of partner change,[49] and condoms may be used less by minorities than by whites.[50]

The increase in syphilis in the eighties has been attributed to several factors: an increase in the use of hard drugs (crack cocaine), an increase in the form of prostitution in which drugs are exchanged for sex, and increasingly limited access to health care. In the eighties an epidemic of crack cocaine use occurred in the United States. Lifetime, past year, and past month crack use was at least twice as high among African-Americans and Hispanics as among whites in 1988.[51] The increase in the use of crack resulted in increasing exchange of sex for drugs. Among adolescent crack smokers, HIV prevalence appeared to be considerably higher than among noncrack smokers (15.7 percent versus 5.2 percent, all noninjecting drug users), and high-risk sexual behavior accounted for the higher prevalence of HIV infection among the crack smokers. After controlling for sexual behavior, the association of HIV infection with crack smoking disappeared.[52]

Sexual behavior is only one behavioral component of the elevated STD incidence among African-Americans. Health behaviors (such as vaginal douching) that are more prevalent among African-Americans may also enhance susceptibility to acquiring an STD or to developing complications of STDs. Less access to and less use of health facilities also probably contribute to a higher prevalence of STDs and a higher incidence of STD complications among certain minority populations. Because of the many ecologic factors contributing to the higher prevalence of STDs among these populations, minority individuals who live and form sexual partnerships in some minority communities have a higher risk of becoming infected with STDs irrespective of their own individual sexual or health behaviors.

As stated by other authors: "little is known about the sexual behavior of Americans in general, and less about sexual behavior differences among racial and ethnic groups. In particular, almost nothing is known about partner choice, an aspect of sexual behavior that is a most important determinant of STD risk."[32]

RELATION OF RACE/ETHNICITY AND MIGRATION/TRAVELING TO STDS AND HIV/AIDS IN AFRICA, AUSTRALIA, AND ASIA

AFRICA

A seroepidemiologic study in Ethiopian women showed high rates of exposure to genital chlamydia infection, which was related to ethnic group, religion, very early age of sexual debut and of first marriage, and drift into prostitution.[53] In the republic of Djibouti, HIV prevalence data and predominance of Ethiopian nationality among prostitutes suggested importation of HIV from Ethiopia via prostitutes and their clients.[54] In Kenya in the early 1980s, HIV infection in prostitutes was associated with having had sex with men traveling from Central Africa.[55] In men attending the STD clinic in Nairobi, travel outside Kenya and frequent sexual contacts with prostitutes were among the risk factors associated with HIV seropositivity.[56]

The role of truck drivers and their assistants in the spread of STDs and HIV is shown in studies conducted among truck drivers in East Africa and Nigeria. Both study populations reported many casual partners (only 5 percent of Nigerian truck drivers reported no sex partners besides their wife) and had a high frequency of STD/HIV.[9,57,58]

In eastern, central, and southern Africa the migratory labor system has been of major importance in the transmission of STDs and HIV infection.[8] In western Africa, expatriates and migrant workers also appear to play a major role in the spread of HIV. For example, a study of persons in rural Senegal who had traveled and worked in another African country for more than 6 months in the last 10 years demonstrated HIV seropositivity in 27 percent of the men and 11 percent of the women, compared with 0.5 percent in the control group.[59]

In a recent longitudinal cohort study in a rural Ugandan population, information was collected for all adults on change of residence over a 3-year period and its association with HIV-1 status. Almost all who entered the area had moved from similar rural areas, and only a small proportion came from the city of Kampala, where rates are known to be high. Nonetheless, change of residence (even within the rural area) appeared to be strongly associated with an increased risk of HIV-1 infection in this rural population. This increased risk is probably the result of more risky sexual behavior among those who moved.[60]

AUSTRALIA

In Australia it was found that Aboriginal women attending the STD clinic were at increased risk for both gonococcal and chlamydial infection. However, as this was a cross-sectional study, the increased risk may reflect differences in health-seeking behavior. In other words, a higher proportion of Aboriginal women may attend the clinic only for severe complaints, and fewer of them may be among the "worried well."[61]

Of the heterosexual male cases of gonorrhea diagnosed in Sydney but acquired outside Australia, 89 percent were acquired in Southeast Asia, mainly in the Philippines and Thailand. Beginning as early as 1982 there was a marked decline in the number of cases of gonorrhea acquired heterosexually within Australia, but no such decline was seen in the number of cases acquired outside Australia, though the number of these cases was small.[62]

A study[82] conducted in Sydney among sex workers attending a public STD clinic for the first time between June 1991 and May 1993, showed that international sex workers (predominantly from Thailand, Malaysia, and China) reported less condom use and had significantly higher prevalences of chlamydia, gonorrhea, and clinical herpes compared to local sex workers.

ASIA

In Thailand there are marked variations in HIV prevalence both geographically and by socioeconomic status. The highest levels of HIV infection have been recorded in the north of Thailand and among lower-class prostitutes.[63,64] A study among 800 female commercial sex workers in northern and southern Thailand showed that the nationality of clients may also be a risk factor for HIV infection. In prostitutes, having predominantly Thai customers (in comparison with foreign, mainly Malaysian, customers) increased the risk for HIV infection independently.[64] This example runs counter to many cited in this chapter, in which sex with foreigners carried a higher risk of HIV.

In the sixties and early seventies STDs in China had essentially been eliminated, but in the eighties and nineties they have again become a public health problem. In addition to a growing number of travelers from other countries, China has a large population of Chinese migrant workers within the country and faces a reemergence of prostitution where these workers congregate in the large cities. Heterosexually acquired cases of AIDS and HIV infection have so far been found mainly in coastal areas and large municipalities. In coastal areas, AIDS and HIV infection have been diagnosed mainly in people who have traveled abroad to visit relatives, whereas in the cities AIDS and HIV have generally been seen in populations practicing high-risk behaviors within the country. Infection among workers who have worked overseas predominates inland.[65]

SEXUAL BEHAVIOR WHILE ABROAD

There are only a few studies that have addressed people's sexual behavior while they are abroad. In Copenhagen in 1987, guests at an inn were interviewed as to whether they carried condoms with them in their luggage while traveling, whether they had engaged in any sexual relationship during their stay in Copenhagen, and if so, whether their contacts were Danes or foreigners and whether they had used a condom. Participants, with a mean age of 22.5 years, were from 55 different countries, and many of them had stayed in Copenhagen only 1 or 2 days. Of the men, 21 percent reported always carrying condoms while traveling, while 43 percent never did so; of the women, 6 percent always and 79 percent never did so. Ninety-seven of the men (13 percent) and 42 of the women (9 percent) had had sexual contacts in Copenhagen. Consistent condom use in these sexual contacts appeared to be infrequent.[66]

Danes were also interviewed as to their HIV risk behaviors when they travel to Greenland, because the population of Greenland has behavioral characteristics that may predict a high risk of HIV spread once HIV is introduced into the population. It appeared that the median lifetime number of sexual partners was more than twice as high among male travelers (median, 12 partners) as among nontravelers (median, 5 partners). A significantly higher percentage of male travelers than nontravelers reported prostitute contact and a history of STDs. Travelers to Greenland were also more likely to have visited other places outside Europe, including HIV-endemic areas.[67]

In the United Kingdom it was estimated that U.K. residents made 31.2 million visits abroad in 1990. To describe sexual behavior and risk taking in U.K. travelers abroad, a study was conducted in Nottingham in a random sample of 978 adult patients of a general clinical practice. Each was sent an anonymous postal questionnaire, and 56 percent responded. Sixty-six percent reported travel abroad in the past year. Of the 354 travelers, 30 (8 percent) had had a "romantic or sexual relationship" with a new partner during their last trip, 17 (4.8 percent) had had sexual intercourse; 9 of these 17 had used condoms, of whom 5 had always used them.[68]

In London, in 1991 to 1992, a study was done on the sexual behavior of persons who visited the hospital for tropical diseases for a checkup after spending less than 3 months in a tropical country. Of 782 people invited to participate in the study, 97 percent agreed to do so. The mean age of the men was 32 and of the women 28.5 years. Sixteen (2.2 percent) of the 757 were HIV-antibody-positive; 141 (18.6 percent) reported sexual contacts with new partners during their most recent trip, of whom 73 (52 percent) reported only one partner. Condoms were used infrequently or never by 64 percent.[69]

Among STD clinic patients in Bergen, Norway in 1989, 41 percent reported having had sexual contact(s) with a new partner abroad in the 5 years preceding the interview. These contacts were mainly in Europe, particularly in Spain, Denmark, and Greece. Sexual contacts outside Europe were most frequently reported from the United States, Brazil, and Thailand. The highest proportion reporting sexual contacts abroad was found among male clients of prostitutes. Consistent condom use was low, particularly after use of alcohol.[27]

In the Netherlands, Dutch expatriates and their family members returning from at least 6 months in sub-Saharan Africa were asked to complete a questionnaire on sexual, occupational, and other risk factors and to undergo HIV testing. Overall, 1968 (86 percent) agreed to participate. Four (0.4 percent) of the 1122 men and 1 (0.1 percent) of the 846 women were HIV-seropositive. Eighty-nine men (7.9 percent) and 18 women (2.1 percent) had lived with an African partner; an additional 344 men (30.7 percent) and 111 women (13.1 percent) had had heterosexual contacts with other partners. Fewer than a quarter of the men and women who had had African partners had used condoms consistently.[70] Researchers in Antwerp, Belgium studied European expatriates working in Central Africa. Of the HIV-seronegatives, 51 percent reported extramarital sex with a local woman and 31 percent with a prostitute.[71]

A recent study by Adams et al.[72] showed that military personnel can still be regarded as a risk group for STDs. British troops spending short periods of time in a tropical environment were significantly more likely to acquire an STD than men in the same age groups in England and Wales. Thirty-nine percent of STD cases reported prostitute contact as a source of disease. Of patients questioned about condom use, 70 percent reported that they did not normally use a condom. However, a study in a stable European British force showed a pattern and incidence of STDs comparable to that of the U.K. population.[73]

A study was conducted among Dutch marines and naval personnel serving 6 months on a United Nations mission in Cambodia to determine sexual risk behavior and incidence of STDs. All personnel received extra education on STD prevention prior to deployment, and condoms were freely available. Forty-five percent reported having had sexual contacts with prostitutes or the local population. Young age and single marital status were independent risk markers for having such contact. Consistent condom use was reported by 89 percent, inconsistent use by 10 percent, and no use at all by 1 percent. Risk factors for inconsistent use and nonuse were being 40 years of age or older and having had a higher number of contacts. In the total population of 2289 persons, 43 cases of STD were diagnosed.[74]

HIV infections contracted during peacekeeping activities in Cambodia have been documented in military personnel from Indonesia and Uruguay. These infections appeared to be with HIV-1 subtype E, which at that time was uncommon in the infected individuals' home countries.[80,81] This finding illustrates clearly the global dispersion of HIV-1 linked to the movement of people.

Kleiber and Wilke did an interesting study on sex tourism. In 1990 they interviewed German male sex tourists in Thailand with respect to demographic data and use of condoms. The majority of these tourists were between 30 and 40 years old (range 20 to 76 years) and single and had a well-paid job. More than two-thirds had previously traveled outside Europe during the past 5 years, of whom half also had had sexual contact with indigenous women in Germany. The countries most frequently mentioned as destinations, after Thailand, were the Philippines, Kenya, and Brazil. As the authors say, an important risk factor for unsafe sex was "liebe" (love). The majority of the men, did not see their Thai girlfriends as prostitutes but more as intimate friends, with whom they felt no necessity to use condoms. These men did not regard themselves as sex tourists but more as caring and loving partners. There were, of course, also men who went to Thailand for sex only; these men used condoms more often than the "caring" men, but their condom use was still rather infrequent. Of all the men studied, between 30 percent and 40 percent used condoms consistently, depending on where the sexual contact took place (the percentage was lower if the sexual contact took place in the hotel where the tourist resided).[75]

Swiss residents made a total of 7,450,000 trips abroad in 1988, of which 10 percent were to developing countries. It is said that in spite of intensive anti-AIDS campaigns, 30 percent of Swiss tourists have casual contacts abroad. In a group of single Swiss tourists who had traveled mainly to Brazil and Kenya, 60 percent had had casual contacts, of whom 27 percent never or infrequently used condoms.[19]

Among 282 U.S. Peace Corps volunteers serving in Zaire between 1985 and 1988, no seroconversions to HIV were documented. All volunteers received extensive education and counseling during their stay in Zaire. During the study period, the rate of all STDs among Peace Corps volunteers in Africa decreased from 131 to 68 per 1000 study population per year.[76]

Australian researchers studied the planned sexual behavior of young Australian visitors to Thailand. Persons seeking medical advice before traveling to Thailand without a spouse or partner were interviewed using a self-administered questionnaire. Only 34 percent of the sample reported a definite intention not to have sex in Thailand. Twenty-four percent more men than women said they would have sex with a Thai national; 13.7 percent of men said they would have sex with a "bar girl"; and 82 percent of the sample reported they would use condoms 100 percent of the time.[77] In 1991, researchers studied a group of Australian men who had had sex in Southeast Asia in the 3 months prior to visiting an STD clinic. Sixty percent of these men had had sexual activity with identified prostitutes during their trip, and 25 percent reported having had sex with five or more partners. Only 28 percent of the men who had had sex with casual partners and/or prostitutes claimed to have consistently used condoms.[78]

DISCUSSION AND CONCLUSION

Comprehensive, clear data on the relationship of STDs and HIV/AIDS to race and ethnicity are available only from the United States. Explanations for the relationships found are less clear. Higher rates among nonwhites may be partly explained by reporting bias, since nonwhites are more likely to use public health facilities, which have a better reporting system than private ones. However, behavioral risk factors for STDs, including HIV/AIDS (high partner change rate and low condom use), are more prevalent in minority populations, particularly among those with a low socioeconomic status. In addition, the crack epidemic of the eighties and early nineties, which occurred particularly among African-Americans, resulted in an increase in prostitution in which drugs are exchanged for sex. This crack epidemic has also paralleled an increase in syphilis, chancroid, and gonorrhea among African-Americans. Differences in health and health-seeking behavior may also account for some of the differences in the prevalence rates. To what extent race and ethnicity simply reflect poverty, less education, and migrant status—all long established and accepted risk markers—is not clear.

In Europe, no data are available on the relation of race/ethnicity to STD/HIV/AIDS, but some countries, mainly in northern Europe, do report the nationality of persons with STD/HIV/AIDS. The number of reported cases of syphilis and gonorrhea has strongly declined during the past decade, and particularly in the Nordic countries, relatively few cases of the classic STDs still occur. The relative contribution of foreigners to the residual number of reported cases of STDs has increased. What is not always clear is whether the infection has been acquired outside the country or whether foreigners are at greater risk of acquiring an STD inside the country. Migrant prostitution is occurring on a large scale all over Europe. Migrant prostitutes are in general very mobile, moving within one country and from one country to another, often on a tourist visa. Relatively new is the migration of women from eastern to western Europe to work in prostitution. Foreigners, including migrant laborers, are to a large extent the clients of migrant prostitutes, forming a separate network in which STD/HIV may spread rapidly. Some studies have shown that foreigners have reduced their risky sexual behavior less than the indigenous population.

The associations found between nationality and rates of STDs, including HIV/AIDS, most probably are explained by the relationship of foreign nationality to low socioeconomic status and migrant status. Barriers to effective prevention programs in these groups are the many languages spoken, the differences in cultural background, and the mobility itself. Heterosexually acquired HIV infection in Europe is mainly seen in persons from AIDS-endemic countries or in persons having sex with persons from AIDS-endemic countries.

Although existing data are scarce, travel and sexual contacts abroad, including (unsafe) sexual contacts of the so-called sex tourists, appear to be of increasing importance in the epidemiology of STD/HIV in Europe and Australia. In Africa and Asia, migrant labor and prostitution play an important role in the STD and HIV epidemics, as does long-distance truck driving. Migration, not only to high-prevalence cities but also within rural areas, is associated with increased risk for STD/HIV.

In conclusion, the relative contribution of minority and migrant populations in the spread of heterosexually acquired STDs and HIV infection has been increasing. The great mobility of people (for whatever reason), the distances and the speed with which they travel, the resulting import and export of STDs and HIV everywhere in the world—from one area to another, from one country to another, and from one continent to another—show that STD and HIV control is no longer solely of national concern. All data emphasize the need for a global STD and AIDS control program. Only if we recognize the necessity of international collaboration, both in STD/HIV prevention efforts and in STD case management, may we begin to contemplate real control of these diseases.

References

1 Waugh MA: History of Clinical Developments in Sexually Transmitted Diseases, in *Sexually Transmitted Diseases,* KK Holmes et al (eds). New York, McGraw-Hill, 1990.

2 Adler MW: Epidemiology and Treatment of Penicillinase-Producing *Neisseria gonorrhoeae,* in *Recent Advances in Sexually Transmitted Diseases,* JD Oriel, JRW Harris (eds). Edinburgh, Churchill-Livingstone, 1986.

3 Stolz E: Mede in naam van de werkgroep voor gonorroebestrijding: Penicillinasevormende gonokokkenstam geïsoleerd in Rotterdam. *Nederlands Tijdschrift voor Geneeskunde* 121:620–622, 1977.

4 Centers for Disease Control: Opportunistic infections and Kaposi's sarcoma among Haitians in the United States. MMWR 31:353–361, 1982.

5 Clumeck N et al: Acquired immunodeficiency syndrome in African patients. *N Engl J Med* 310:492–497, 1984.

6 Vittecoq D et al: Acquired immunodeficiency syndrome after travelling in Africa: an epidemiological study in seventeen Caucasian patients. *Lancet* 1:612–614, 1987.

7 Aral SO et al: Demographic and Societal Factors Influencing Risk Behaviors, in *Research Issues in Human Behavior and Sexually Transmitted Diseases in the AIDS Era,* JN Wasserheit et al (eds). Washington DC, American Society for Microbiology, 1991.

8 Hunt CW: Migrant labor and sexually transmitted disease: AIDS in Africa. *J Health and Social Behav* 30:353–373, 1989.

9 Carswell JW et al: Prevalence of HIV-1 in East African lorry drivers. *AIDS* 3:759–761, 1989.

10 Koenig ER: International prostitutes and transmission of HIV. *Lancet* 1:782–783, 1989.

11 van der Helm TCM: Annual Report 1992–1993. Amsterdam, *Gemeentelÿke Geneeskundige en Gezondheidsdients,* 1994.

12 Hornle R: Prostitutionstourismus nach Deutschland. *Gesundheitswesen,* 56:204–207, 1994.

13 Prins M et al: Incidence and risk factors for acquisition of sexually transmitted diseases in heterosexuals with multiple partners. *Sex Transm Dis* 21:258–267, 1994.

14 Centers for Disease Control: *Sexually Transmitted Diseases, 1991.* Atlanta, U.S. Department of Health and Human Service, Public Health Service, Division of STD/HIV Prevention, July 1992.

15 de Schrijver A, Meheus A: Epidemiology of sexually transmitted diseases: the global picture. *Bull WHO* 68:639–654, 1990.

16 World Health Organization: *Wkly Epidemiol Rec* no 24, 1991.

17 Renton A, Whitaker L: Using STD Occurrence to Monitor AIDS Prevention: Final Report Assessing AIDS Prevention, EC Concerted Action on Assessment of AIDS/HIV Preventive Strategies. Lausanne, Institut Universitaire de Médicine Sociale et Préventive, 1991.

18 Catchpole MA: Personal communication. London, Public Health Laboratory Service, Gonococcal Reference Laboratory, 1995.

19 Eichmann A: Sexuell übertragbare Krankheiten nach Reisen in tropische Länder. *Schweizerische Medizinische Wochenschrit Journal* 123:1250–1255, 1993.

20 Prins M et al: Determinants of penicillinase-producing *Neisseria gonorrhoeae* infections in heterosexuals in Amsterdam. *Genitourin Med* 70:247–252, 1994.

21 Hooykaas C et al: The importance of ethnicity as a risk factor for STDs and sexual behaviour among heterosexuals. *Genitourin Med* 67:378–383, 1991.

22 van Haastrecht HJA et al: HIV prevalence and risk behaviour among prostitutes and clients in Amsterdam: migrants at increased risk for HIV infection. *Genitourin Med* 69:251–256, 1993.

23 van Haastrecht HJA et al: Evidence for a change in behaviour among heterosexuals in Amsterdam under the influence of AIDS. *Genitourin Med* 67:199–206, 1991.

24 Evans BG et al: Heterosexually acquired HIV-1 infection: cases reported in England, Wales and Northern Ireland, 1985 to 1991. *Communicable Disease Report* 2:R49–55, 1992.

25 Smith E: Mandatory anonymous HIV surveillance in Denmark: the first results of a new system. *Am J Public Health* 84:1929–1932, 1994.

26 Swedish Institute for Infectious Disease Control: Annual Report 1993, Stockholm, Smittskyddsinstitutet, 1994.

27 Tveit KS et al: Casual sexual experience abroad in patients attending an STD clinic and at high risk for HIV infection. *Genitourin Med* 70: 12–14, 1994.

28 Bindels PJE et al: The HIV prevalence among pregnant women in the Amsterdam region (1988–1991). *Eur J Epidemiol* 10:331–338, 1994.

29 Vranckx R, Coenjarts A: Politieke vluchtingen: een groot risicogroep voor AIDS en hepatitis B? *Archives Belges de Médecine Sociale Hygiène Médecine du Travail et de Médecine Lègale* 47:34–37, 1989.

30 European Working Group on HIV Infection in Female Prostitutes: HIV infection in European female sex workers: epidemiological link with use of petroleum-based lubricants. *AIDS* 7:401–408, 1993.

31 Pineda JA et al: HIV-1 infection among non-intravenous drug user female prostitutes in Spain. No evidence of evolution to pattern II. *AIDS* 6:1365–1369, 1992.

32 Moran JS et al: The impact of sexually transmitted diseases on minority populations in the United States. *Pub Health Rep* 104:560–565, 1989.

33 Schmid GP et al: Chancroid in the United States: re-establishment of an old disease. *JAMA* 258:3265–3268, 1987.

34 Centers for Disease Control: Chlamydia prevalence and screening practices—San Diego County, California, 1993. *MMWR* 43:366–375, 1994.

35 Zimmerman HL et al: Epidemiological differences between chlamydia and gonorrhea. *Am J Public Health* 80:1338–1342, 1990.

36 Grodstein F, Rothman KJ: Epidemiology of pelvic inflammatory disease. *Epidemiology* 5:234–242, 1994.

37 Goldner TE et al: Surveillance for ectopic pregnancy—United States, 1970–1989. *MMWR* 42:73–85, 1993.

38 Johnson RE et al: A seroepidemiologic survey of the prevalence of herpes simplex virus type 2 infection in the United States. *N Engl J Med* 321:7–12, 1989.

39 Wasserheit JN: Epidemiological synergy interrelationships between human immunodeficiency virus infection and other STD. *Sex Transm Dis* 61–77, 1992.

40 Laga M et al: Non-ulcerative sexually transmitted diseases as risk factor for HIV-1 transmission in women: results from a cohort study. *AIDS* 7:95–102, 1993.

41 Grey MR: Syphilis and AIDS in Belle Glade, Florida, 1942 and 1992. *Ann Intern Med* 116:329–334, 1992.

42 Centers for Disease Control: AIDS among racial/ethnic minorities—United States, 1993. *MMWR* 43:644–655, 1994.

43 DiClemente RJ: Epidemiology of AIDS, HIV prevalence, and HIV incidence among adolescents. *J School Health* 62:325–330, 1992.

44 Farmworkers Justice Fund: Farmworker Demographics, in *The Occupational Health of Migrant and Seasonal Farmworkers in The United States.* Washington DC, 1986.

45 Centers for Disease Control: HIV infection, syphilis, and tuberculosis screening among migrant farm workers—Florida, 1992. *MMWR* 41: 723–725, 1992.

46 Hahn RA et al: Race and prevalence of syphilis seroreactivity in the United States population: a national seroepidemiologic study. *Am J Public Health* 79:467–470, 1989.

47 Anderson JE et al: Factors associated with self-reported STDs: data from a national survey. *Sex Transm Dis* 21:303–308, 1994.

48 Aral SO: Sexual behavior in sexually transmitted disease research, an overview. *Sex Transm Dis* 21(2 Suppl):S59-S64, 1994.

49 Seidman SN, Aral SO: Subpopulation differentials in STD transmission. *Am J Public Health* 82:1297, 1992
50 Centers for Disease Control: Heterosexual behaviors and factors that influence condom use among patients attending a sexually transmitted disease clinic—San Francisco. *MMWR* 39:685–689, 1990.
51 National Institute on Drug Abuse: National Household Survey on Drug Abuse: Population Estimates 1988. Department of Health and Human Services publ (ADM) 89:1636.
52 Edlin BR et al: Intersecting epidemics—crack cocaine use and HIV infection among inner-city young adults. Multicenter Crack Cocaine and HIV Infection Study Team. *N Engl J Med* 331:1422–1427, 1994.
53 Duncan ME et al: Seroepidemiological and socioeconomic studies of genital chlamydial infection in Ethiopian women. *Genitourin Med* 68: 221–227, 1992.
54 Rodier G et al: L'infection par le virus de l'immunodéficience humaine en République de Djibouti: révue de la littérature et données régionales. *Médecine Tropicale* 53:61–67, 1993.
55 Kreiss JK et al: AIDS virus in Nairobi prostitutes: spread of the epidemic to East Africa. *N Engl J Med* 314:414–418, 1986.
56 Simonsen JN et al: Human immunodeficiency virus infection among men with sexually transmitted diseases. *N Engl J Med* 319:274–278, 1988.
57 Orubuloye IO et al: The role of high-risk occupations in the spread of AIDS: truck drivers and itinerant market women in Nigeria. *Internat Fam Plann Perspect* 19:43–48, 1993.
58 Bwayo J et al: Human immunodeficiency virus infection in long-distance truck drivers in East Africa. *Arch Intern Med* 154:1391–1396, 1994.
59 Kane F et al: Temporary expatriation is related to HIV-1 infection in rural Senegal. *AIDS* 7:1261–1265, 1993.
60 Nunn AJ et al: Migration and HIV-1 seroprevalence in a rural Ugandan population. *AIDS* 9:503–506, 1995.
61 Hart G: Factors associated with genital chlamydial and gonococcal infection in females. *Genitourin Med* 68:217–220, 1992.
62 Donovan B et al: Heterosexual gonorrhoea in central Sydney: implications for HIV control. *Med J Austr* 154:175–180, 1991.
63 Siraprapasiri T et al: Risk factors for HIV among prostitutes in Chiangmai, Thailand. *AIDS* 5:579–582, 1991.
64 Limanonda B et al: Condom use and risk factors for HIV-1 infection among female commercial sex workers in Thailand [letter]. *Am J Public Health* 84:2026–2027, 1994.
65 Xinhua S et al: AIDS and HIV infection in China. *AIDS* 8:S55-S59, 1994.
66 Worm AM, Lillelund H: Condoms and sexual behaviour of young tourists in Copenhagen. *AIDS Care* 1:93–96, 1989.
67 Melbye M, Biggar RJ: A profile of HIV-risk behaviours among travellers—a population-based study of Danes visiting Greenland. *Scand J Social Med* 22:204–208, 1994.
68 Gillies P: HIV related risk behaviour in UK holiday makers. *AIDS* 6: 339–340, 1992.
69 Hawkes S et al: Risk behaviour and HIV prevalence in international travellers. *AIDS* 8:247–252, 1994.
70 Houweling H, Coutinho RA: Risk of HIV infection among Dutch expatriates in sub-Saharan Africa. *Internat J STD AIDS* 2:252–257, 1991.
71 Bonneux L et al: Risk factors for infection with human immunodeficiency virus among European expatriates in Africa. *Br Med J* 297:581–584, 1988.
72 Adams EJ: Sexually transmitted diseases in transient British forces in the tropics. *Genitourin Med* 70:94–96, 1994.
73 Masterton RG, Strike PW: Sexually transmitted diseases in a British military force in peacetime Europe, 1970–1983. *Genitourin Med* 64: 54–58, 1988.
74 Hopperus Buma APCC et al: Sexual behavior and sexually transmitted diseases in Dutch marines and naval personnel on an United Nations mission to Cambodia. *Genitourin Med* 71:172–175, 1995.
75 Kleiber D, Wilke M: AIDS-bezogenes risikoverhalten von (sex-)touristen in Thailand, in *Sexualverhalten in Zeiten von AIDS,* W Heckmann, MA Koch (eds). Berlin, Sigma Rainer Bohn Verlag, 1994.
76 Cappello M et al: Human immunodeficiency virus infection among Peace Corps volunteers in Zaire. *Arch Int Med* 151:1328–1330, 1991.
77 Mulhall BP et al: Planned sexual behaviour of young Australian visitors to Thailand. *Med J Austr* 158:530–535, 1993.
78 Rowbottom J: Risks taken by Australian men having sex in South East Asia. *Venereology* 4:56–59, 1991.
79 Quinn TC: Population migration and the spread of types 1 and 2 human immunodeficiency viruses. *Proc National Acad Sci* 91:2407–2414, 1994.
80 Soeprapto W et al: HIV and peacekeeping operations in Cambodia. *Lancet* 346:1304–1305, 1995.
81 Artenstein AW et al: Multiple introductions of HIV-1 subtype E into the western hemisphere. *Lancet* 346:1197–1198, 1995.
82 O'Connor CC et al: Sexual health and use of condoms among local and international sex workers in Sydney. *Genitourin Med* 72:47–51, 1996.

PART VI SEXUALLY TRANSMITTED PATHOGENS

Chapter 13

Genitourinary mucosal defenses

Myron S. Cohen
Deborah J. Anderson

Many sexually transmitted disease pathogens initiate infections at mucosal surfaces. In this chapter we discuss the interaction between microbial pathogens and the host surfaces. This discussion also includes: (1) a brief review of mucosal histology; (2) microbial adherence to the mucosa and possible microbial penetration of epidermis; (3) the interaction between microorganisms at the mucosal surface; (4) nonspecific mucosal defense mechanisms that help to prevent infection; and (5) humoral and cellular immunity at the mucosal surface, with emphasis on specializations of the mucosal immune compartment. This information leads to consideration of mucosal vaccines.

THE STRUCTURE OF MUCOSA

The epidermis and mucosal surfaces provide protection from invading pathogens. These tissues include an epithelial layer resting on a basement membrane (the basal lamina) and underlying connective tissue (the lamina propria). Mucosal tissues vary in morphology depending on their location and function. Mucosal epithelium can consist of one or numerous levels, and may include glands that project deep into the lamina propria. In contrast to the epidermis, mucosal surfaces are devoid of hair follicles.

In the epidermis a layer of basal germinative cells undergo mitosis and exit toward the surface. During their migration these cells undergo changes in shape, and they extrude their nuclei (cornification) to form an outer horny layer (stratum corneum and granulosum); the formation of the stratum corneum is termed keratinization.[1,2] Whereas the epidermis maintains an irregular, hard surface by virtue of the formation of the horny layer, the mucosal epithelium is shiny and smooth. Moisture is provided to the mucosa in two ways. First, a hydrophilic surface layer of glycoproteins and glycolipids is formed by epithelial cells, called the glycocalyx.[3] Second, goblet-shaped epithelial cells secrete a thick hydrophilic glycoprotein gel (mucus). Both the glycocalyx and mucus act as mucosal barriers, and may play a variety of important physiological functions as well.

Mucosa can be further defined by the morphology of the outermost layer (apical) cells and by the orientation of these cells.[2] Epithelial cells can have squamous, cuboidal or columnar shape, and are arranged in either a single (simple) or stratified layer. Simple columnar epithelium can also appear "pseudostratified," as the mucosa is folded during contraction and distention. Transitional epithelium is intermediate between and contains both simple and columnar cells. The thickness of the mucosa in the female is maintained by estrogen in the menstruating female and hormonal replacement in the postmenopausal woman.[4] Prepubertal and postmenopausal women have a thin (estrogen-deficient) epithelial lining.

The mucosa of the male and female urethra and of the female endocervix is composed of simple columnar epithelium, whereas the vagina and the ectocervix are composed of stratified squamous epithelium.[4,5] Cornification of some cells occurs in the vaginal epithelium in response to maternal or postpubertal hormones. The area where the endocervix meets squamous epithelium of the ectocervix is termed the squamocolumnar junction, and this effectively connects the upper and lower genital tract. In adolescent or pregnant women and women using oral contraception, the squamocolumnar junction extends beyond the external cervical os, creating a physiologic eversion known as ectopy. Increased availability of receptive cells in this area may favor the growth of some mucosal pathogens.

ACQUISITION OF MICROBIAL FLORA IN THE GENITAL TRACT

ADHERENCE

Many microorganisms recovered from the genitourinary mucosal surface are transient and do not attach to the underlying tissue. Adherence of organisms to the mucosa represents a critical point of interaction. Organisms that are unable to attach and are swept away by mucociliary activity (e.g., in the cervix) and the mucus stream will generally not be able to efficiently damage underlying structures. Attachment may be followed by bacterial division without evidence of inflammation (colonization); this process leads to the formation of "normal," indigenous, or autochthonous microflora.[7,8] Alternatively, attachment of microorganisms may be associated with tissue damage and local inflammatory response (e.g., uncomplicated chlamydial and gonococcal infections) or disseminated disease (e.g., syphilis, disseminated gonococcal infection). Studies of human male and female urethral mucosa have demonstrated a very skewed distribution in bacterial attachment. That is, only a minority of urethral mucosal cells carry attached bacteria, but multiple bacteria attach to individual mucosal cells.[7] Differences in adherence to microscopically indistinguishable cells have been observed.[9] This suggests subtle differences in surface characteristics of urogenital mucosal cells.

The process by which bacteria attach to the mucosa can be summarized as follows. First, it is likely that microbes "sense" chemoattractant stimuli that lead them to bind to epithelial tissue.[10] At this point the organisms must find a suitable environment for the formation of flagellae and/or surface factors (adhesins) that will ultimately enhance their attachment. There is increasing evidence that some bacteria have genetic mechanisms that allow rapid adaptation to different environments. For example, fimbriated (piliated) *Escherichia coli* attach efficiently to mucosa (see the following), but nonfimbriated cells are better adapted to disseminated disease, perhaps because they are less likely to attach to neutrophils.[11,12] Pathogenic *E. coli* are programmed to undergo a frequent switch between the fimbriated and nonfimbriated states, which allows survival of the fittest organisms.[13] Gonococcal attachment to epithelial cells may depend on dynamic pili and outer membrane proteins.[14] The molecular adhesins of several bacterial fimbriae have been described.[15,16]

Subsequent to achieving the proper morphological state, a pathogen must overcome repelling physicochemical forces and penetrate the mucous gel that overlies the epithelium.[17] The physical characteristics of this gel vary dramatically in response to hormones as well as to other pharmacological stimuli.[18–20] The mucous gel may act as a comfortable environment (rich in nutrients to support bacterial growth) or may harbor specific and nonspecific defense mechanisms, compounds with antimicrobial activity produced by organisms colonizing the mucosal surfaces, and other factors that could impede the ability of the pathogen to reach the mucosa.[21] The antipathogenic activity of mucus will be discussed in more detail below.

BIOPHYSICAL FACTORS THAT AFFECT ADHERENCE

A wide variety of pathogens that have the ability to adhere to isolated epithelial cells or to intact mucosal tissue in vitro have been identified. The physicochemical characteristics that allow adherence of *Enterobacteriaceae*, different Gram-positive cocci (e.g., *Staphylococcus epidermidis* and *saprophyticus*), and *Neisseria gonorrhoeae* have received attention.[14,22–24] For the purposes of this discussion, the gonococcus—a common and important STD pathogen—will be used as a primary example.

It has been suggested that adherence depends on the outcome of specific and nonspecific interactions that must take place over both long and short distances.[17,23] Epithelial cells as well as bacterial pathogens have a net negative charge that results in an electrostatic repulsive force and therefore acts to prevent adherence. The eukaryotic cell surface charge is regulated by the ionized carboxylic groups of N-acetylneuraminic acid (which constitutes the bulk of the glycocalyx) as well as other anionic groups, including alkaline phosphatase and ribonuclease-susceptible phosphate groups, and the beta- and gamma-carboxy groups of aspartic and glutamic acid, and heparin sulfate.[17,23,24] The surface charge of bacteria is affected by the characteristics of the cell envelope and the formation of fimbriae or other adhesins.[23] The surface charge is also affected by compounds in the microenvironment. Heparin-like molecules may serve as cell surface receptors, and exogenous heparin may block binding of gonococci to epithelial cells.[24]

A theoretical explanation for the adherence of species that should be frankly repulsive is essential. One hypothesis that has gained attention is the notion of long-range attraction (at distances greater than 4 Å) between bacteria and mucosal cells. In the early 1940s, Derjaquin, Landau, Verwey, and Ovherbeek advanced a theory, the DLVO hypothesis, to explain the paradoxical attraction between negatively charged hydrophobic colloid particles.[25] Experimental evidence provided by these investigators showed that the attraction or repulsion of particles is dependent on the distance at which this interaction is evaluated. Because repulsive energy decreases more rapidly than attractive force, a curve can be drawn that indicates a distance where bacterial-cell adhesion might actually be favored. Evidence to support this interaction has been summarized by Watt and Ward.[26] Furthermore, surface charge becomes less negative as pH is reduced because of a decrease in the dissociation of charged groups at anionic sites. Not surprisingly, if binding of bacteria to vaginal cells is measured at a reduced pH, a dramatic increase in binding can be documented.[27] In addition, if surface charge is raised by blocking anionic sites with compounds such as 1-ethyl-3-(dimethyl-aminopropyl) carbodilimide, a similar increase in binding of bacteria can be shown.[28]

These electrochemical forces are nonspecific. Another nonspecific variable is the hydrophobic-hydrophilic interaction between the pathogen and the cell; this interaction seems most important at close distances (short-range interaction).[22] Several groups have reported that those *Enterobacteriaceae* that are more hydrophobic display increased adherence to tissue culture cells relative to organisms that are less hydrophobic.[29–31] The importance of the hydrophobic interaction is less clear for the binding of gonococci.[26] Van Oss has suggested that a hydrophobic interaction may also be important for the binding of organisms to neutrophils (see the following).[32]

BACTERIAL ADHESINS

Once close interaction becomes possible, one or more bacterial cell surface characteristics (adhesins) probably mediate binding to specific cell receptors.[7,21,23] Ofek, Beachey, and several of their coworkers demonstrated that a mannose-binding (type I pilus) protein in many strains of *E. coli* allows the attachment of such organisms to buccal epithelial cells.[11,12,23,33,34] It seems more than likely that this bacterial ligand is located in fimbriae.[10,11,35–37] A mannose resistant, type II, "P-fimbria" also allows attachment to uroepithelial cells glycolipid receptors that share the disaccharide gal-alpha-1–4-gal-beta, and a unique helper region at the tip of this pilus has recently been described.[38,39] Attachment to epithelial cell receptors has a major impact on the pathogenesis of urinary tract infections.[40,41] P pili are critical to pyelonephritis.[41] Type 1 pili appear to play a role in cystitis.[42] In very recent work Langermann and coworkers provided compelling evidence that the FimH adhesin presented in type 1 pili are required for bladder infection.[16] Passive and active immunity directed against FimH prevented infection in a model of murine cystitis.[16]

A clear advantage in binding to human cells exfoliated from the urogenital tract and human cells in tissue cell culture including fallopian tube explants can be demonstrated among piliated gonococci.[26,43,44] The precise nature of the mucosal receptor(s) for binding of gonococcal pili is still under investigation, but carbohydrates may be involved.[26] A specific gonococcal pilin ligand (pilC) has been described.[15] Nonfimbriated gonococci are also able to bind to eukaryotic cells, although less efficiently. Several investigators have described outer membrane protein(s) (in the Opa group) that increase attachment of gonococci to mucosal cells, as well as polymorphonuclear neutrophils (PMN).[24,45–47] In addition, opacity mediated binding may depend on a unique epithelial cell antigen blocked by monoclonal antibodies directed against carcinoembryonic antigen.[48]

Binding of gonococci is influenced by the ionic concentration, pH, growth conditions, and temperature of the experimental medium.[26] Most recently it has been demonstrated that gonococcal attachment and invasion of epithelial cells are affected by heparin-like molecules, whereas sialylation of lipoligosaccharides appears to effect invasion of epithelial cells.[24,47] Energy metabolism may also play a role in bacterial adherence.

Attachment of the bacterial species that do not form fimbriae deserves special attention. Gram-positive cocci may associate by virtue of surface lipoteichoic acids.[23] An attachment protein of mycoplasmas has been described that allows the binding of this organism to tracheal epithelium.[49]

With regard to *Candida albicans*, person-to-person variation in the ability of the yeast to adhere to vaginal and buccal epithelial cells has been described.[50] Although little variation between epithelial cell types has been demonstrated, *C. albicans* cells adhere in greater number per cell than other *Candida* species less often encountered as vaginal pathogens.[51] *Candida* do not adhere better to vaginal cells from patients with recurrent vulvovaginal candidiasis than to cells from healthy subjects.[52]

Microbial interaction may be important to keep *Candida* spp. in the vagina at a low number. When the indigenous vaginal flora are disturbed by therapy with broad-spectrum antibiotics, fungi may increase dramatically in number.[53] It is thought that the disappearance of antifungal compounds produced by bacteria of normal vaginal flora may contribute to the expanding yeast flora.

Attachment of pathogens can be cell specific: Gonococci and chlamydia attach to columnar epithelial cells; trichomonas and Human Papilloma Virus (HPV) attach to squamous epithelium; *T. pallidum* infects squamous and columnar epithelial cells.[54–58] HIV appears to infect Langerhans' cells found in the mucosa.[59] The attachment and penetration of HIV has been extensively studied and is discussed in detail elsewhere in this book.[59]

NORMAL FLORA OF THE GENITAL TRACT

Organisms that cause an inflammatory response are pathogens; those that merely colonize the mucosa of normal hosts are designated normal flora.[8] The normal flora play a significant role in defense against infection by genital pathogens. The composition of the normal flora of the genital tract has been studied in great detail and will be reviewed elsewhere in this book. In males, the urethra normally contains comparatively few microorganisms (e.g., *S. epidermidis*, alpha-streptococci, corynebacteria). On the other hand, the female genital tract, especially the vaginal secretions, contains 10^8 to 10^9 bacteria per gram of fluid examined.[60] Both facultative (e.g., *S. epidermidis*, streptococci, and *E. coli*) and anaerobic (e.g., peptococci, lactobacilli, and *Bacteroides* spp.) bacteria can be isolated.[61–63] Facultative aerobic bacteria decrease in number in premenstrual specimens, whereas anaerobes tend to remain constant.[61–63] *Ureaplasma urealyticum* is often found in the genital tract of both males and females.[64] Mycoplasma hominis occurs in a proportion of healthy women. Although *M. hominis* is more commonly found in women with genital infections, its etiologic role in vaginitis and cervicitis is uncertain.[65] A co-occurrence of *M. hominis* and bacteria associated with bacterial vaginosis can be demonstrated.[66] Acquisition of *U. urealyticum* and *M. hominis* is directly related to sexual activity. Neither chlamydiae nor viruses are considered part of the normal vaginal flora.[67,68] On the other hand, it is clear that chlamydia, HSV, CMV, and HPV can frequently be recovered from asymptomatic men and women.[67,68a–d]

The normal flora of the vagina are highly susceptible to the local environment and hormonal influence. The most traditional and well-studied view implies that glycogen is deposited in the vaginal epithelium in response to estrogenic hormones, and that glycogen is an optimal substrate for the growth of lactobacilli.[69] The vaginal flora is believed to be restricted to those organisms that do well in an acidic environment.[69] Lactobacilli may produce substrates and enzymes that interact with other organisms in the female genital tract.[70,71] Production of hydrogen peroxide by lactobacilli may be particularly important.[72]

L(+)-lactate, generated by lactobacilli or human cells including phagocytes, appears to be a particularly important substrate for *N. gonorrhoeae*.[73,74] Metabolism of L(+)-lactate by gonococci leads to more aggressive utilization of molecular oxygen than metabolism of other carbohydrates, allowing gonococci to "steal" oxygen from phagocytes, limiting production of microbicidal free radicals.[73] Small concentrations of L(+)-lactate lead to accelerated sialylation of gonococci, allowing gonococci greater resistance to serum, and altering attachment to cellular targets.[74,74a]

The low level of lactobacilli in the vagina during menopause cannot be attributed to glycogen deficiency.[75] Experiments in rats indicate that release of nutrients during vaginal epithelial proliferation and exfoliation has the most profound effects on the vaginal flora.[76]

It has also been suggested that estrogen per se (independent of the deposition of glycogen) may have a direct effect on the number of organisms and composition of the bacterial flora.[77,78] Gonococci possess steroid receptors and progesterone suppresses their energy metabolism; L(+)-lactate metabolism is least susceptible to the effects of progesterone (Lysko and Morse, unpublished data).[78]

Staphylococcal species recovered from the vagina can also become important pathogens. *S. saprophyticus* is a common cause of urinary tract infections in both males and females.[79,80] *S. saprophyticus* adhere to epithelial cells and epithelial cell casts recovered from urine sediments. When high-absorbency tampons are used during menses, vaginal *S. aureus* may proliferate and produce a toxin(s) responsible for some or all of the manifestations of the toxic shock syndrome.[81–83]

In addition, the genital tract represents an area of special concern because of its obvious importance to the fetus, which must pass through during birth. Group B streptococci, chlamydiae, HIV, viruses of the herpes group (herpes simplex virus types 1 and 2, cytomegalovirus) are major sources of disease for neonates;[84,85] isolation of these pathogens in the genital tract deserves special attention, even when the host suffers no immediate adverse consequences.

MICROBIAL INTERACTIONS

There is a complicated interaction between pathogenic organisms and the indigenous bacterial flora as well as between organisms of these two categories.[8] This interaction may result in either synergy or antagonism of the genital pathogen. Vaginal lactobacilli in vitro can inhibit the growth of a wide variety of bacterial species that can grow on the genital mucosal surfaces, including genital pathogens.[70–72] Lactobacilli produce a number of compounds with antibacterial activity, including lactocidin, acidolin, acidophilin, and lactacin B as well as lactic acid and hydrogen peroxide.[70–72] Hydrogen peroxide produced by lactobacilli inhibits the growth of gonococci and HIV in vitro.[86,87] On the other hand, some of these organisms can inhibit lactobacilli. Growth of gonococci is inhibited in vitro, for example, by *Aeromonas* spp., lactobacilli, staphylococci, streptococci, vibrios, a variety of Gram-negative rods, and *Candida* spp.[88–91]

The contribution of the microflora to defense of the gastrointestinal tract mucosa in vivo is obvious, particularly in patients with severe neutropenia.[92] The clinical relevance of microbial interaction in the genital tract is far less certain and is an area that requires further evaluation. The rate of gonorrhea in women exposed to men infected with *N. gonorrhoeae* was not noticeably affected by the quantity or quality of the cervical-vaginal flora.[93] Superinfection of cervical explants with gonococci markedly increased formation of chlamydial inclusions.[94] This is nicely correlated with coinfection observed clinically.[66,95] Although gonococci have generally been considered aerobic, they are able to use nitrite as a terminal electron acceptor.[96,97] Gonococci grown under anaerobic conditions express new outer membrane proteins recognized by antibodies from patients recovering from PID or DGI.[97] Serum and L(+)-lactate metabolism greatly enhances gonococcal O_2 consumption, and could facilitate the anaerobic microenvironment of the vagina.[73,98]

Interactions between staphylococci and other genital flora have also been studied. As early as 1899, Grosz and Kraus showed that staphylococci inhibited the growth of gonococci, presumably through the production of extracellular antibacterial substances such as beta-acetylglucosaminidase or lysostaphin.[99] Coagulase-negative staphylococci, which are normal genital flora, also excrete inhibitory substances limiting growth of a variety of Gram-negative (e.g., gonococci) and Gram-positive competitors.[100–102] Some of these antibacterial products are most active at pH 5.5 to 6.5, consistent with the vaginal environment.

PROTECTION FROM INFECTION: NONSPECIFIC FACTORS

MUCUS

Once mucus has been secreted onto an epithelial surface, it provides a variety of functions, certainly the most important of which include lubrication and selective separation from exogenous macromolecules.[18,103–105] Human semen and vaginal secretions are rich in mucus.[18,105] Mucus in the female genital tract is derived primarily from goblet-shaped epithelial cells in the cervix.[105] Endocervical cells express 5 mucin genes (MUC1, 4, 5AC, 5B, and 6); ectocervical and vaginal cells express MUC 1 and 4.[106] The secretion and structure of mucus are susceptible to a variety of pharmacological stimuli. Mucus in the female genital tract is quite clearly under hormonal control, and dramatic changes in viscosity can be demonstrated during the menstrual cycle.[18,105] Interestingly, these rheological changes are associated with very minor alterations in protein structure.[18]

Mucus in the genital tract is of paramount importance to conception, and it may also play a role in host defenses in a variety of ways.[18,19,105] First, mucus may act to exclude a variety of pathogens or antigens. The altered flora and increased inflammation that are associated with atrophic vaginitis (where mucus content is decreased for a variety of reasons) may be viewed as a clue to the importance of this secretion. Second, since mucus is rich in carbohydrates, it has been suggested that one or more sugar moieties may be offered to the invading pathogen and occupy a critical bacterial ligand, thereby interfering with the adherence of the pathogen to the epithelial layer.[19,107] Mucins may also serve for attachment of immunoglobulins, cytokines, and other biologically active substances in the genital tract. Carbohydrate residues in mucus may also act as receptors for the bacteria constituting the indigenous flora.[107]

Mucus plays an indirect role in host defenses by providing an appropriate support medium for other defenses (e.g., lactoferrin, lysozyme, antibody) or by providing an appropriate environment in which phagocytic cells can engulf and kill invading pathogens. Leukocytes are capable of rapidly migrating through cervical mucus. The hypothesis that mucus may contribute to immunological defense is supported by the observation that oral presentation of antigen-antibody complexes in the rodent gut directly stimulates the secretion of mucus by epithelial cells in response to a specific antigen challenge.[108] Alternatively, it is possible that mucus or one of its components interferes with host defenses.[109,110]

Other antimicrobial secretions

Both lysozyme and lactoferrin have been detected in genital secretions. Lysozyme hydrolyzes beta-1,4 linkages of microorganisms in which this enzymatic site is available, and thereby allows osmotic lysis or the formation of spheroplasts in vivo.[111] It has also been suggested that lysozyme may inhibit bacterial adherence by stearic hindrance. In cell cultures lysozyme had no inhibitory effect on chlamydiae, and at certain concentrations it actually stimulated the formation of intracytoplasmic chlamydial inclusions.[112] Lysozyme may act most effectively in concert with other antimicrobial defenses.[111,112]

Lactoferrin is an iron-binding protein that may slow bacterial growth by competing for this essential element, or by direct microbicidal action.[113–115] Payne and colleagues have suggested that bacterial strains (e.g., *N. gonorrhoeae*) that produce uncomplicated mucosal infections are relatively poor in their ability to obtain iron in competition with the host, whereas those strains that produce disseminated infection have an enhanced ability to acquire iron.[116] Mickelsen et al. have reported that gonococcal auxotrophs that are most commonly associated with asymptomatic infection (Arg-Hyx-Ura-strains) are poor in their ability to acquire iron from lactoferrin relative to other strains.[117] It was suggested that these strains might fail to produce local disease because they do not multiply effectively when forced to compete with lactoferrin for iron. Under these circumstances the inception of disseminated gonococcal infection with menses might be owing in part to the provision of iron in the form of hemin and transferrin, which would then abolish the limitations imposed by lactoferrin at the mucosal surface. It should be noted, however, that work with experimental urethral gonorrhea has demonstrated that gonococci unable to gain iron from lactoferrin can establish infection, in sharp contrast to organisms unable to use transferrin as an iron source, which cannot cause infection.[118] Little, if any, information is available regarding the iron utilization of other genital pathogens. The lactoferrin concentration in vaginal secretions ranges between 3.8 and 218 g/mg of protein, and the concentration can increase during inflammation as neutrophils release their lactoferrin.[119–121] Lactoferrin concentration is greatest just after menses, and falls off sharply during the latter (secretory) phase of the menstrual cycle. Women receiving estrogen/progesterone oral contraceptive pills were found to have persistently low levels of lactoferrin, emphasizing the hormonal regulation of this compound. Lactoferrin can also work to limit the inflammatory response, as discussed below.[113,122]

Defensins may also contribute to innate immune defenses in the genital tract. Defensins are small (29-42aa), cationic, antimicrobial peptides with a broad spectrum of activity that includes bacteria, fungi, and enveloped viruses.[123] These peptides have six cysteine residues that form three disulfide bonds, and dependent on the spacing of the cysteines are classified into the α-defensins and the β-defensins.[123] Defensins are found in neutrophils and selected epithelia, and human beta defensin-1 (HBD-1) is the major antimicrobial activity in airway surface fluid.[124] HBD-1 and the α-defensin human defensin-5 (HD-5) have both recently been identified in female reproductive tract epithelia and cervicovaginal secretions, and expression of HD-5 appears to be influenced by the menstrual cycle and inflammation.[125a,b]

Another element that may play an important role at the mucosal surface is zinc.[126–129] Zinc is found in high concentration in prostatic tissue and secretions, and it is believed to be the active ingredient of "prostatic antibacterial factor" described by Fair and coworkers.[126,128] Zinc inhibits the growth of a variety of urinary pathogens, including *Chlamydia trachomatis*, *Candida* spp., herpes simplex, and *Trichomonas vaginalis*.[126–131]

Although patients with prostatic disease generally have a depressed concentration of zinc, the concentrations encountered are generally higher than those required to inhibit most pathogens that have been examined.[126] The concentration of zinc in vaginal mucus ranges between 7.95 and 62 mg/mg of protein.[132] Other metal ions, for example, Cu^{2+}, inhibit the formation of chlamydial inclusions in tissue cell cultures.[114]

Polyamines, such as spermine, found in high concentrations in prostatic fluid have a cidal effect on many bacteria. Spermidine and spermine also have been demonstrated to interfere with *C. trachomatis* in tissue cell culture.[114] On the other hand, these same polyamines may facilitate the growth of HIV.[133]

SPECIFIC IMMUNE MECHANISMS AT THE MUCOSAL SITES

THE COMMON MUCOSAL IMMUNE SYSTEM

General issues

Antibodies produced in response to parenteral (systemic) immunization are detectable in mucosal secretions, but usually in relatively low titer. Recent studies have shown that mucosal immunization generally achieves a superior antibody response in mucosal secretions. The mucosal immune response depends on inductive sites within mucosal tissues where antigens are sampled and host defenses committed (Fig. 13-1). The best studied inductive sites include Peyer's patches in the small intestine (i.e., gut-associated lymphoreticular tissue), bronchus and nasal tissue; all

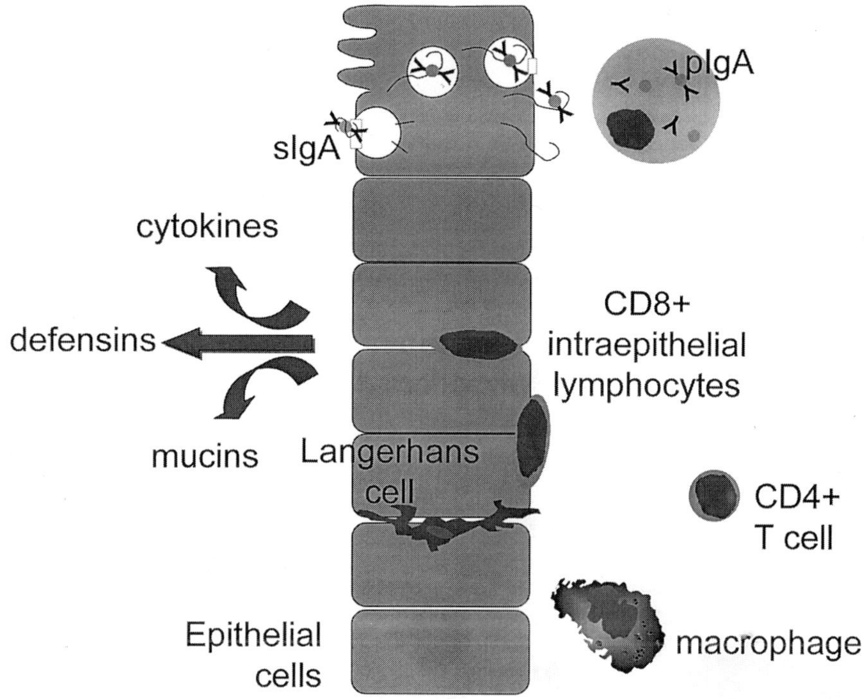

Fig. 13-1. Schematic representation of immunologic mediators associated with lower genital tract mucosal epithelium.

the mucosal inductive sites are believed to function in consort in a mucosal associated lymphoreticular tissue network.[134]

Antigens encountered by lymphoid cells, macrophages and dendritic cells or specialized (microfold) M cells are sampled. The turnover and function of these cells can be affected by hormones.[4,20] Intraepithelial dendritic cells (called Langerhan's cells) and macrophages may migrate after antigen sampling, and this could lead to dissemination of infecting pathogens such as HIV.[59] The M cells play a unique role.[135] Many areas of mucosa are represented by a single epithelial cell layer sealed by tight junctions that exclude peptides and macromolecules. In some areas (e.g., bronchial epithelium) lymphoid follicles with an overlaying follicle associated epithelium (FAE) include unique M cells that provide functional openings to the epithelium. The biology and function of the M cell have been recently reviewed.[135]

Antigens presented to specific T and B cells lead to their activation, and these cells leave the inductive site through the lymphatics, circulate in the blood, and "home" to tissues committed to antigen specific response, where effector responses can transpire. The Th1 cells are important in systemic cell-mediated immune responses, and are particularly important for macrophage activation. The Th2 cells are critical for immunoglobulin formation, and the B-cell help/cytokines generated determine the class of immunoglobulins formed.

Lymphocytes are characterized by their surface markers, their expression of receptors, and their production of differing cytokines.[134] Antigen presenting and effector cells have been identified in the male and female genital mucosa.[153] Indeed, Langerhans' cells and macrophages may serve as the initial target of HIV infection.[59] Effector functions conducted at mucosal surfaces can be broadly divided into humoral and cellular.

T cell homing to mucosal sites

Some of the receptors involved in T-lymphocyte homing to and localization within mucosal tissue have been characterized. The integrin $\alpha 4\beta 7$ [LPAM-1] that is expressed on most naive murine [CD45RA+] T cells and a subset of memory [CD45RO+] T cells, mediates binding to Peyer's patch high endothelial venules [HEV], but not peripheral lymph node HEV.[136] The ligand for LPAM-1 is the immunoglobulin superfamily adhesion molecule MAD-CAM-1 that is expressed on mucosal venules, and the interaction between the two is thought to play an important role in lymphocyte homing to mucosal sites.[137] In both humans and mouse an integrin has been identified that is almost exclusively expressed by T cells residing in the mucosa. This is also a $\beta 7$ integrin, but it is co-expressed with an as yet unidentified α chain. In the mouse it is known as the $\beta 7\alpha$M290 integrin and in humans as the HML-1 antigen or $\beta 7\alpha$e integrin.[138–140] Murine studies suggest that this molecule is induced after mucosal localization.[141] The in vitro addition of transforming-growth factor beta [TGFβ] to stimulated lymph node cells increases expression of the $\beta 7$ subunit, and changes the associated $\alpha 4$ subunit to αM290; this has been hypothesized to be the possible mechanism of induction of this receptor at mucosal surfaces, as mucosal epithelial cells produce TGF-β.[142] The ligand for the $\beta 7\alpha$e mucosal-associated antigen is E-cadherin, an adhesion molecule expressed by epithelial cells.[143] Based on this information, it appears likely that the $\beta 7\alpha$e integrin plays a role in adhesion, modulating and focusing effector cell activity in the mucosal epithelium. It is likely that this mechanism also plays a role in localization of T cells in the genital tract mucosal since T lymphocytes in human genital tract mucosae express HML-1, and genital tract epithelial cells express TGF-β and E-cadherin.

FEMALE GENITAL TRACT

The female genital tract was defined as part of the common mucosal immune system in the early 1960s through adoptive transfer studies in which murine mesenteric lymph node cells (primarily IgA phenotype) homed to the nodes and gut as well as the cervix, vagina, uterus, and mammary glands of the mouse; in contrast, peripheral lymph node cells homed to the peripheral nodes and produced IgG.[144] The components of the mucosal defenses of the female genital tract have been characterized (Fig. 13-2,

Immunological Mediators in the Human Genital Tract

A. Female

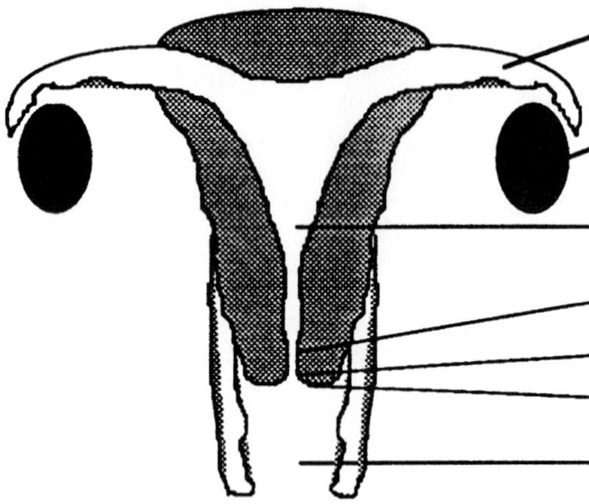

	Cellular			Humoral	
	T	Mϕ	LC	PC	pIgR
Fallopian Tube	+	+	-	+	+
Ovary	+	+++	-	-	-
Endometrium	++	++	-	±	+
Endocervix	++	++	-	++	+
Transformation Zone	+++	+++	++	+++	+++
Ectocervix	++	++	++	++	±
Vagina	+	++	++	+	-

B. Male

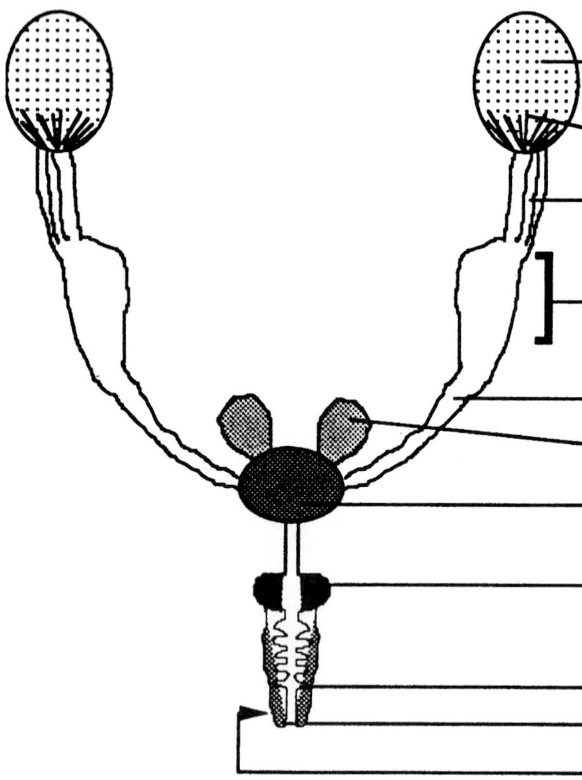

	Cellular			Humoral	
	T	Mϕ	LC	PC	pIgR
Testis	±	++	-	-	-
Rete Testis	+	++	-	-	+*
Efferent Ducts	+	++	-	-	+*
Epididymis	++	+++	-	-	+*
Vas Deferens	++	+++	-	-	+*
Seminal Vesicles	++	+++	-	-	+*
Prostate	++	+++	-	+	+
Bulbourethral Glands	++	++	?	?	?
Penile Urethra	+++	+++	-	++	++
Fossa navicularis	++	+	++	+	-
Foreskin	+	+	++	-	-

***Patchy**

Fig. 13-2. Regional localization of immune cells in the human genital tract epithelium. T = T lymphocytes, M∅ = macrophage, LC = Langerhan's cell, PC = plasma cell, pIgR = polymeric immunoglogulin receptor-positive epithelial cells.

Table 13-1).[145] Plasma cells are concentrated in the subepithelial layers of the human endocervix, but substantial numbers are also found in the ectocervix, vagina, and fallopian tubes. Plasma cells are rarely detected in the human ovary, endometrium, or myometrium. The T-cell population of the human and primate female reproductive tract varies considerably from tissue to tissue. In the normal human endometrium, T cells are rarely seen in the proliferative phase of the menstrual cycle, but increase in number in the secretory phase, often forming small aggregates.[146] The majority of these endometrial T cells express the CD8 antigen, particularly those found in the lymphoid aggregates and within the epithelium.[146,147] A population of phenotypically unusual (CD2+, CD3-, CD4-, CD8-, CD56+) lymphocytes are seen in the endometrial stroma in the secretory phase of the menstrual cycle and early pregnancy.[146] CD8 positive T lymphocytes are numerous within the epithelium of the ectocervix, vagina, and transformation zone.[147–149] Substantial infiltrates of CD8 and CD4 positive cells are seen in the stroma of the transformation zone, often in lymphoid aggregates, but T cells are relatively sparse in the stroma of the ectocervix and vagina.[150] The particularly high numbers of T lymphocytes in the transformation zone of the cervix has led some researchers to speculate that this is a particularly immunologically dynamic region.[148] There are no apparent differences in the numbers of intraepithelial T cells in the lower genital tract at different stages of the menstrual cycle, although potential functional differences have not as yet been addressed (Pudney et al, unpublished).

In the endometrium and endocervix, the predominant classical antigen presenting cells are macrophages; in the vagina and ectocervix, Langerhans' cells are also present.[59,148,151] These are potent antigen presenting cells that are found throughout the epidermis and nonkeratinized squamous epithelia. After activation, these cells migrate from the epithelium to draining lymph nodes, where they present antigens to T lymphocytes, thereby initiating an immune response. Langerhan's cells in the epithelium express a phenotype that is characteristically CD1a, MHC class II, Fcγ, CD3, and CD4 positive; following activation they also express a variety of adhesion molecules, including ICAM-1 (CD54) and LFA-3 (CD58).[152] Langerhans' cells show marked variation in their distribution within the lower genital tract, with the highest numbers found in the vulva and ectocervix, and the lowest numbers in the vagina.[148] A recent study in rats demonstrated that antigen presentation within the female reproductive tract may vary with different stages of the menstrual cycle, with less efficient antigen presentation by vaginal macrophages and dendritic cells occurring immediately prior to ovulation.[153] This observation has implications for local vaccine delivery as well as for better understanding of the immunological events associated with reproductive processes.

Table 13-1. Cytokines Produced by Human Genital Tract Epithelial Cells*

A. Proinflammatory cytokines		
IL-1α		
IL-1β		
IL-6		
GM-CSF		
TNF-α		
B. Chemokines		
	C-X-C Family:	IL-8
		Gro-α
		Gro-β
		Gro-γ
		Rantes
	C-C Family:	MCP-1
		MIP-1α
		MIP-1β
C. Downregulatory cytokines		
TGF-β		

* No evidence for production of Il-2, IL-4, Il-5, IFN-γ

Cervical and vaginal epithelial cells are a primary source of cytokines including Il-8, Il-6, Il-1α, Il-1β, G,M-CSF, M-CSF, TGF-β, MIP1α, MIP1β, and RANTES; many of these cytokines have been harvested from cervicovaginal secretions (Table 13-1).[154a] Cytokine concentrations differ between HIV+ and control subjects, and some cytokines may promote the replication of HIV.[154a–d,155a] Other infections known to affect vaginal cytokine levels include BV, HPV, and chlamydia.[155b,c,155c]

As no organized inductive sites such as Peyer's patches have been identified in the female reproductive tract, local immune responses are thought to be less efficient than at other sites. Considerable effort is being spent on the development of improved methods to effect immune responses in the genital tract. There are essentially two schools of thought: The first contends that induction must occur in the gut or bronchus, with boosting and subsequent migration of sensitized cells to the genital tract mucosa; the second proposes that novel adjuvants or technologies can be developed to effectively stimulate and maintain local genital tract immunity.[156]

MALE GENITAL TRACT

Formal proof that the male urogenital tract is part of the common mucosal immune system was provided by elegant lymphocyte transfer and homing studies performed by Husband and colleagues.[157] T lymphocytes are not usually detected in the healthy human testis, but are seen in the rete testis, epididymis, vas deferens, and urethra, with CD8+ cells predominating within the epithelial cell layer.[5,158,159] A majority of the intraepithelial lymphocytes (IEL) in the urethra are positive for the integrin $\alpha^E\beta7$ (mucosal-associated antigen). T lymphocytes have been cloned out of human semen and urethral secretions, and have been demonstrated to have cytolytic and helper cell functions.[160] Macrophages are abundant in the human and primate urogenital tract: in the testicular interstitium, the epididymis, the epithelium and connective tissue of the excurrent ducts and accessory glands, and in the penile urethra.[5,158,159,161,162] Testicular macrophages actively secrete a variety of cytokines that have been implicated in Leydig cell endocrine function as well as spermiogenesis. Unlike the female lower urogenital tract, Langerhans' cells are rarely detected in the penile urethra but are abundant in the epithelium of the foreskin, and the fossa navicularis.[5,163] Unique innate defense mechanisms of the male reproductive tract include the presence of high concentrations of zinc, polyamines, and prostaglandins.[126–133,164]

Humoral immunity

Antibody is readily detected in mucosal secretions.[164–171] Antibody molecules can act directly to interfere with attachment of bacteria or to neutralize viruses; they can act in concert with complement components to exert bactericidal activity; or, with the help of complement, they can opsonize pathogens to enhance their interaction with phagocytic cells or make them more susceptible to intracellular lysis.

The concentration of IgA may exceed the concentration of IgG or IgM in cervical mucus and urethral secretions, whereas in other genital tract secretions (i.e., semen, vaginal fluid) IgG isotype antibodies often predominate.[134,170–172] Antibody is produced locally by plasma cells in the submucosal tissue, which lie in close proximity to the epithelium.[171a] B cells expressing IgD and M on their surface must be switched to IgA expression, which depends on switch T lymphocyte (TSW) and exposure to interleukins, including IL-4.[170] Bacterial lipopolysaccharides and environmental antigens may also play a role.[170] Interleukins 5 and 6 are important for B-cell proliferation, differentiation, and IgA secretion.[170] After commitment to IgA production B cells migrate to the appropriate submucosal sites, directed in part by recognition of receptors on high endothelial venules.[170,171] IgA producing plasma cells have been detected in the endo- and ectocervix, and also the male urethra (Fig. 13-1).[5,171a]

More than 40 mg/kg of mucosal IgA is generated each day.[134] The IgA found in mucosal secretions (sIgA) is different from serum IgA (see Fig. 13-2). It is composed of 10-S dimer (300,000 daltons) and a J chain. The J chain is made by plasma cells and appears to polymerize 7-sIgA monomers (the IgA normally found in serum) into 10-S dimers. A polymeric Ig receptor (p-IgR) expressed by certain mucosal epithelial cells binds polymeric immunoglobulin (IgA, IgM), which can then be transported through the cell to the mucosal surface; after their secretion, IgA and IgM retain a portion of the receptor called secretory component that provides resistance to proteolytic substances found in genital secretions. Secretory component is generated by rough endoplasmic reticulum. The production of secretory component is regulated by cytokines. For example, interferon gamma and tumor necrosis factor upregulate the intracellular pool of the p-IgR.[173]

IgA consists of two subclasses (IgA1 and 2) that can be identified on the basis of structural and antigenic differences.[174] In many mucosal secretions, the IgA subclass predominates. Studies related to the concentration of IgA1 and 2 in genital secretions are in progress. An equal number of plasma cells committed to IgA1 and 2 can be detected in the female genital mucosa.[171a]

IgG, IgM, and IgA subclass antibodies including sIgA have been detected in semen and sterile prostatic fluid from healthy men.[164,175–178] Pathogen-specific secretory IgA has been detected in the semen of men infected with *Chlamydia trachomatis, Escherichia coli,* and *Neisseria gonorrhoeae.*[156,177–179] Levels of all immunoglobulin types are approximately ten times higher in prostatic fluid than semen, suggesting that a large proportion of immunoglobulin may be derived from the prostate.[164,176] However, few plasma cells are detected in normal human prostates, and recent studies suggest that the penile urethra may be the primary source of sIgA in semen from normal men.[158] In normal penile urethral tissue, epithelial cells stain strongly for secretory component, and numerous IgA-and J chain-positive plasma cells are detectable in the submucosa. Furthermore, high concentrations of sIgA are detectable in pre-ejaculatory fluid, suggesting that there is local urethral production and transport of IgA (Haimovici and Anderson, unpublished).

The formation and secretion of IgA is clearly susceptible to external stimuli. IgA directed at specific gonococcal antigens can be detected after infection and lasts for at least several weeks.[180,181] Furthermore, McChesney and colleagues have shown that systemic (intramuscular) presentation of antigen (gonococcal pilin) leads to an increased concentration of antibody in vaginal or urethral secretions.[181] This antibody may arise by the migration of responsive immunocytes to target tissues or by leakage of serum antibodies. The former theory is favored because a disproportionately high concentration of secretory IgA (sIgA) relative to IgG or IgM recovered from genital secretions examined.[180] In a recent study of IgA levels in cervicovaginal secretions from HIV-infected women, high IgA levels were associated with genital tract inflammation, suggesting that inflammatory cytokines may enhance the recruitment, differentiation and function of IgA+ plasma cells at this site.[180a]

A variety of specific biological functions for sIgA have been demonstrated. Using gut mucosa, Walker and colleagues were able to show that sIgA interfered with absorption of some antigens.[182] Antigen-sIgA complexes stimulate mucus production, which may then impede the access of pathogens to the mucosa.[108] The ability of s-IGA to interfere with the adherence of a wide variety of bacteria to mucosal surfaces has been repeatedly demonstrated.[166] Tramont and his colleagues have shown that both IgG and IgA inhibit the attachment of *N. gonorrhoeae* to epithelial cells and that antibodies isolated in genital secretions subsequent to natural infection are strain-specific and last for several weeks.[180] Binding of sIgA to different gram-negative rods alters the bacteria to make them hydrophilic, which might then interfere with their attachment to epithelial cells; paradoxically, however, sIgA reduces net negative surface charge which might be expected to make the bacteria less "repulsive" to the cell surface layer.[183] Furthermore, in general no advantage in phagocytosis by neutrophils can be demonstrated when bacteria are opsonized with IgA.[184–186] Bisno and coworkers, however, reported enhanced phagocytosis of virulent gonococci opsonized by serum IgA isolated from a patient recovering from a disseminated gonococcal infection.[185]

Although sIgA antibodies are able to agglutinate bacteria, they do not have innate bactericidal activity.[187] sIgA antibody may activate the alternative pathway of complement and thereby stimulate a lytic complex.[188] Several groups have suggested that the combination of lysozyme, sIgA, and complement may form a bactericidal defense.[186,187] At present the complement concentration of genital secretions is not well appreciated, although Price and Boettcher have reported that the hemolytic complement levels of cervical mucus are 11.5 percent of those of serum, and women with HIV may have even higher levels.[154,189] The biological relevance of the bactericidal activity of secretory antibody is not known. Several bacterial species (including gonococci) have evolved mechanisms to evade the bactericidal activity of serum (Fig. 13-3).[190–192] Joiner et al. showed that blocking immunoglobulin G directed against the porin (*Por*) protein competes with bactericidal antibody for binding to gonococci.[192] There was enhanced complement activation but decreased killing in the presence of this antibody.[192] Gonococci demonstrate other mechanisms to resist serum killing.[193,193a] The observation that many gonococci isolated in mucosal surfaces are sensitive to the complement-mediated action of serum raises serious doubt about the importance of the complement-mediated bactericidal mechanism as a mucosal defense.[194] sIgA could play a role in defense against *Chlamydia trachomatis.*[156,195,195a]

Secretory antibodies are of undoubted importance in defense against a variety of viruses, as demonstrated by the ablation of the mucosal carriage of poliovirus after oral (Sabin) vaccine and the clear protection offered against certain rhinoviruses by nasal immunization capable of eliciting sIgA.[196,197] The interaction between HIV and sIgA is of particular importance in vaccine development. Serum IgA antibodies and sIgA induced by vaccination are able to neutralize some strains of HIV in vitro.[198] In a recent study of women exposed to HIV but uninfected, high levels of IgA directed against HIV were detected in cervicovaginal secretions.[181a] Women with HIV infection may have decreased concentrations of cervicovaginal sIgA, which may be increased by inflammation.[154,199]

Finally, sIgA could play unexpected biological roles. Neisserial IgA1 protease cleaves lysosomal/late endosome associated membrane protein (LAMP1) in vitro.[199a–c] An IgA protease mutant was impaired in growth in epithelial cells, and LAMP 1 was degraded at a slower rate in cells infected with mutant compared to control bacteria. Most recently, Pohlner and coworkers reported that an IgA encoded peptide is capable of acting is an intranuclear transcription factor.[199c]

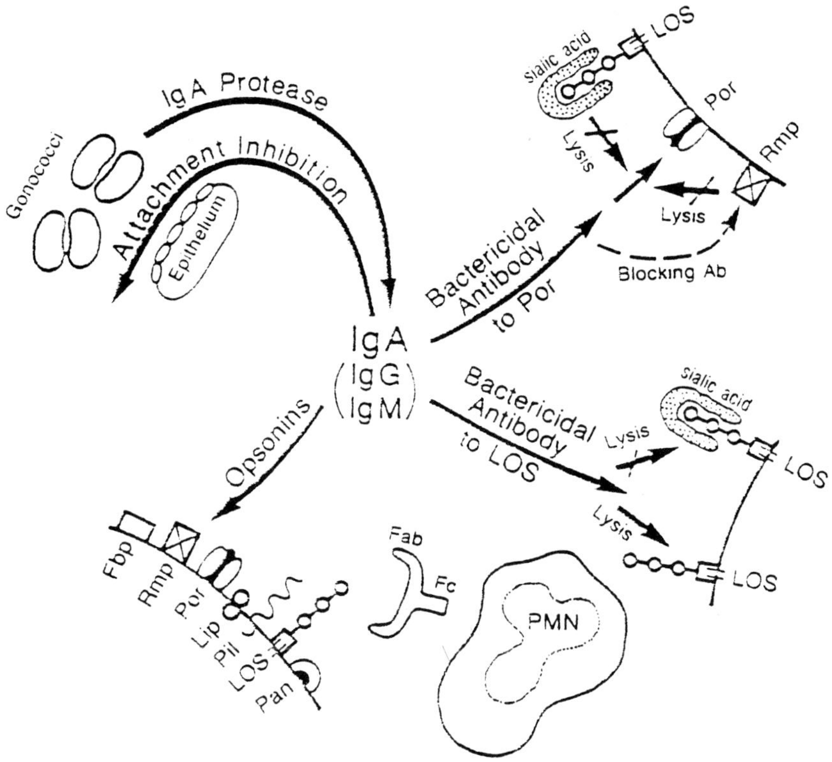

Fig. 13-3. Gonococci resist serum-mediated defenses.[153] Secretory IgA may block gonococcal attachment, but a gonococcal protease degrades IgA_1. IgG and IgM directed against porin (Por) and/or LOS lead to complement-mediated gonococcal lysis. However, blocking antibodies directed against Protein III (Rmp) or sialylation of LOS may inhibit serum killing, most likely by interfering with complement fixation.[193a] IgG and IgM could also opsonize gonococci and facilitate their uptake by phagocytes. Sialylation of LOS may interfere with opsonization.

A variety of microorganisms elaborate a protease that cleaves IgA at the hinge, thereby rendering sIgA subclass I inactive.[200,201] Mulks and Plaut have reported that only pathogenic species of *Neisseria* produce IgA protease, implying that the protease is a major virulence factor in gonococcal infection.[202] The relative importance, however, of sIgA in defense against gonococci remains poorly understood; the presence of sIgA in urethral secretion does not seem to prevent recurrent infection.[179,203] On the other hand, sIgA may help to prevent symptomatic salpingitis in patients who develop local endocervical gonococcal infection.[204] Most recently, it has been possible to show that IgA protease is not required for gonococcal urethral infection (Johannsen et al., unpublished observations).

Cellular immune responses

Phagocytic Cells. Professional phagocytic cells (PMNs and monocytes) are critical for survival and most probably play an important defensive role at the mucosal surface. During granulocytic inflammation mucosal secretions are enriched with granulocyte proteins (e.g., lactoferrin, defensins) and these proteins can be used to monitor the degree of inflammation.[121] The interaction between PMNs and gonorrhea, chlamydiae, group B streptococci, trichomonads, H. ducreyi, and viruses, including HIV-1 have been studied.[205–210]

Neutrophils are responsible for the inflammation associated with some of these infections. A discussion of this subject is most easily divided according to the essential functions of the phagocytic cell (Fig. 13-4).[113,211]

Chemotaxis and Adherence. Phagocytic cells must be signaled to migrate to areas of bacterial invasion. The necessary signals may emanate from the microbial pathogen involved, by the generation of complement components (C5a) when the pathogen is allowed to interact with serum, or by chemokines produced by activated or injured epithelial cells (Table 13-1). Most recently, it has become clear that cell-derived chemokines represent the most potent neutrophil chemoattractants.[211] There is disagreement about whether gonococci release soluble chemoattractants into the culture supernatant.[212,213] Densen and coworkers have provided evidence that gonococci isolated from mucosal surfaces (in uncomplicated infections) generate complement-derived chemoattractants significantly more rapidly than gonococci isolated from patients with disseminated infection, implying that a rapid inflammatory response may help to prevent invasion or dissemination of gonococci.[214] The cytokines responsible for the inflammatory response during gonococcal urethritis have been examined and IL-8 is of particular importance.[215] No information is available to explain the absence of an inflammatory response in the urethra of men who harbor gonococci in the absence of symptoms, although it is possible to induce asymptomatic gonococcal infection using molecular mutants of gonorrhoeae such as a pilin deletion (Cannon et al., unpublished observation). As part of the mobilization and homing process phagocytes attach to blood vessels in a fashion similar to lymphocytes. Neutrophils bind to endothelial cells through attachment to a variety of receptors, which are likely modified by cytokines generated as part of the inflammatory response (Fig. 13-4).

Attachment and Ingestion. Attachment of bacteria to phagocytic cells results from nonspecific factors, ligand-receptor interactions, and opsonization with serum-derived immunoglobulin and complement. All three components of this system are probably important. As stated, NgA is a poor opsonin. Neutrophils express two different receptors for immunoglobulin (FcRII and III) that serve distinct functions. Immunoglobulin bound to FcRII receptors mediates release of lysosomal enzymes, whereas FcRII stimulates release of such enzymes as well as reactive oxygen intermediates. There is strong evidence that one or more surface factors (perhaps outer-membrane proteins) of the gonococcus mediate attachment to neutrophils in the absence of serum.[205] Alter-

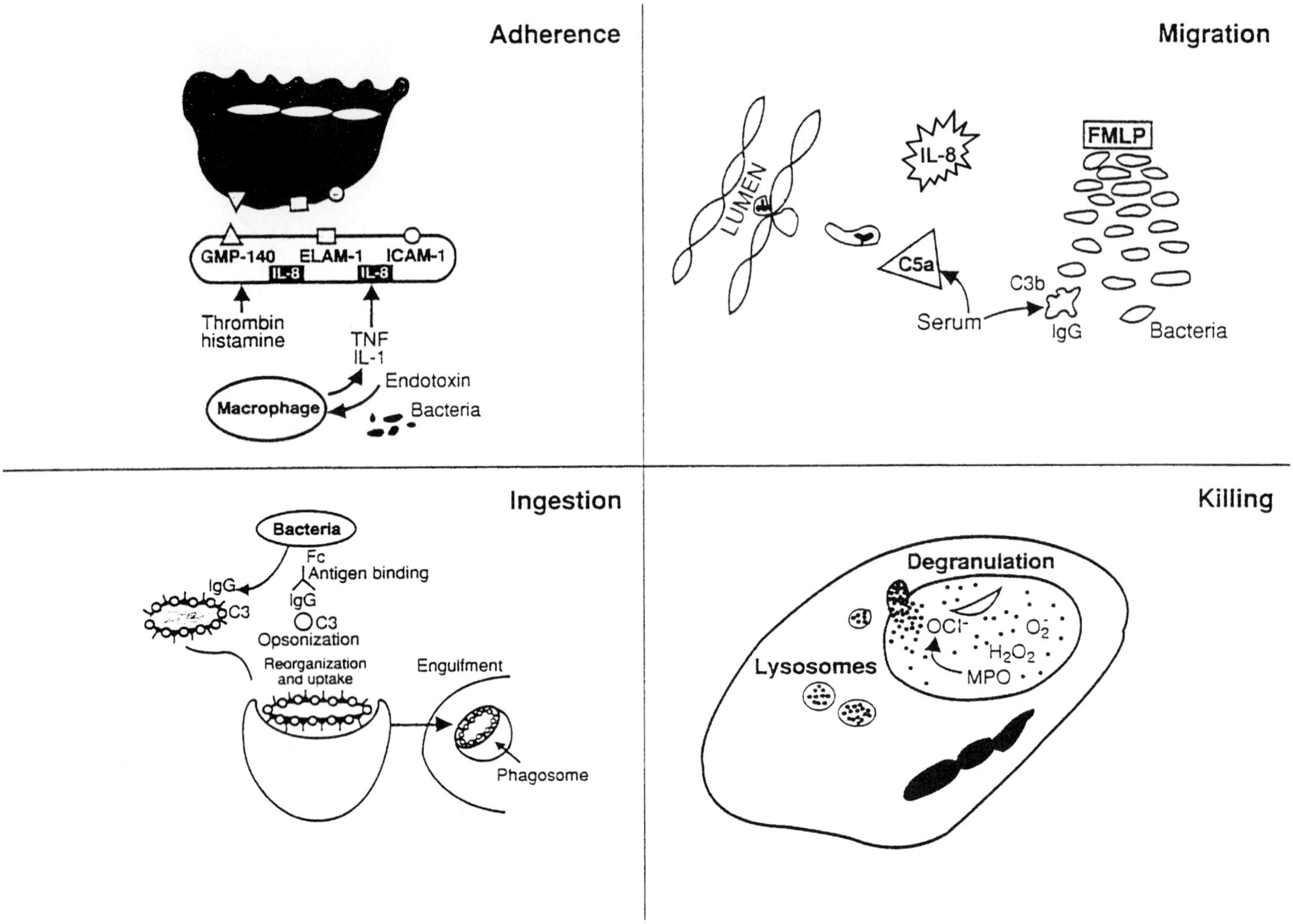

Fig. 13-4. A series of coordinate behaviors lead to the optimal function of neutrophils. These activities include a adherence to blood vessel walls, migration into the tissues, phagocytosis, and microbial killing. *Upper left:* The expression of neutrophils of a group of receptors recognized by endothelial cell counterreceptors allows adherence to blood vessels and diapedesis. Receptors and counterreceptors are modulated by a variety of cytokines and environmental stimuli. GMP-140 is a granule-bound E selectin. ELAM-1 is endothelial cell adhesion molecule (another E selectin), and ICAM-1 is a member of the immunoglobulin supergene family; all three are endothelial cell counterreceptors. Homing receptors that recognize counterreceptors include the selectin LAM-1 and the integrin LFA-1. TNF = tumor necrosis factor; IL-1 = interleukin 1; and IL-8 = interleukin 8. *Upper right:* Neutrophils migrate into the tissues in response to chemoattractants, including the fifth component of complement (C5a) and formylated bacterial peptides such as N-formyl-methionyl-leucyl-phenylalanine (FMLP). *Lower left:* Coating of invading microbes by complement and immunoglobulin allows the recognition of the organisms by neutrophils. Neutrophils bind to these substances with specific receptors and "zipper" microbes into a phagosome. *Lower right:* Microbial killing results from the complementary actions of reactive oxygen species and microbicidal proteins released from degranulating lysosomes. MPO = myeloperoxidase.

natively, studies using both visual and metabolic assays support the notion that serum may enhance the cellular association of some types of gonococci. Bacterial energy metabolism is also required for maximal attachment of gonococci to phagocytic cells, presumably by interfering with charge derived from the proton motive force.[216] Also, growth of gonococci in physiologic media such as serum allows expression of new outer membrane proteins and decreases attachment to polymorphonuclear leukocytes, perhaps in part owing to sialylation in vivo of gonococcal lipoligosaccharides.[74a,217] Attachment to phagocytic cells must be carefully separated from ingestion, but a variety of methodological problems make experimentation in this area difficult. Studies designed to investigate the ingestion of gonococci have found that fimbriae as well as other surface factors may be antiphagocytic.[205,218,219]

Whereas cellular association with phagocytic cells is generally looked on as a distinct disadvantage to the pathogen, special mention should be made of situations in which phagocytic cells may act as a reservoir of infection. Cytomegalovirus is associated with blood leukocytes and it is possible that cellular association may also be found with other herpes viruses as well.[220] After ingestion of chlamydiae by monocytic phagocytes (see the following), the chlamydiae inhibit the fusion of lysosomes with the phagocytic vacuole and are then able to resist intracellular killing.[221] The tropism of some variants of HIV-1 for macrophages and Langerhans' cells has been well-documented and depends on utilization of unique chemokine (i.e., CCR5) and CD4 receptors.[22,223,224]

Microbicidal Metabolism. Neutrophilic phagocytes have unique ability to kill microbial pathogens using oxygen and glucose metabolism (the respiratory burst) to make toxic oxygen-reduction products such as superoxide and hydrogen peroxide and prepackaged bactericidal granule enzymes.[113] Microbicidal metabolism is triggered by the perturbation of the phagocyte membrane, regardless of whether or not ingestion actually occurs. The components of microbicidal metabolism have been reviewed extensively.[113] The neutrophil oxidase system allows formation of superoxide anion, and "downstream" formation of other reactive oxygen species. *N. gonorrhoea, C. trachomatis, T. vaginalis* are sensitive to reactive oxygen species, *H. ducreyi* appears to be partially resistant to neutrophils.[209] As discussed, neutrophil microbicidal proteins recovered from vaginal secretions also play a role.[113,115,121,122,123,205]

Both oxygen-dependent and oxygen-independent mechanisms can kill chlamydiae in vitro.[225–227] Interestingly, several authors have noted that phagocytic cells infected with viruses are impaired in their ability to use oxygen, form oxygen-reduction products, and kill bacterial pathogens.[228,229]

Available evidence supports the concepts that PMNs and monocytes are competent to kill ingested gonococci, although some authors have suggested that gonococci are capable of intracellular survival, perhaps related to unique resistance proteins.[205,230] Chlamydia also generate heat shock proteins during stress and phagocytosis, which may play a role in resistance or act as chronic immunogens.[231] Ross and Densen reported that serum-sensitive gonococcal isolates are more susceptible to neutrophil killing than are serum-resistant organisms, perhaps because of enhanced opsonization by the early components of complement.[232]

The specific mechanisms employed by PMNs to kill gonococci have been the subject of intense investigation. Rest and coworkers reported that neutrophils incapable of using molecular oxygen (cells from patients with chronic granulomatous disease) were competent to kill gonococci.[205] Daly and coworkers observed that gonococcal isolates differ in their susceptibility to nonoxidative killing by azurophilic PMN granule contents; these differences seem to be based on minor variations in peptidoglycan cross-linking.[233] Strains of gonococci that are likely to cause gonococcal bacteremia (penicillin-sensitive isolates) seem to be more resistant to killing by PMN granules than penicillin-resistant strains, which rarely cause gonococcal bacteremia. Gonococci in the presence of serum or phagocytic cells demonstrate enhanced metabolism, which can be ascribed to L(+)-lactate oxidation.[73] Under some conditions serum-stimulated bacterial respiration can completely eliminate the formation of reactive oxygen derivatives by neutrophils.[217]

Less is known about the mechanisms employed by phagocytic cells to kill other sexually transmitted pathogens. PMNs are competent to kill trichomonads by oxygen-dependent mechanisms.[208] In fascinating phase-contrast microscopy of these events, Rein and coworkers showed that neutrophils surround, attack, and fragment the trichomonads, and that the trichomonad can subsequently be ingested in pieces.[208] *H. ducreyi* stimulates neutrophil oxygen metabolism, which may in part lead to death of the bacteria. Using a pig model for chancroid,[233a] Kawula et al. have demonstrated formation of ulcers in neutropenic animals, with recovery of a larger number than organisms possible in controls (personal communication). These results demonstrate that the organism itself can lead to ulcer formation, and that granulocytes suppress growth of bacteria in vivo.

Monocytic phagocytes

Monocytic phagocytes include peripheral blood monocyte, and tissue macrophages. Monocytic phagocytes employ similar (but not identical) microbicidal mechanisms as neutrophils. Monocytic phagocytes are activated by one or more cytokines toward optimal microbicidal activity. The most important cytokine appears to be interferon gamma.[234] It has been demonstrated, for example, that chlamydiae can grow well in resident monocytic phagocytes, but can be killed by interferon-gamma-activated macrophages.[234] The mechanism by which chlamydiae are killed by such macrophages appears to involve a unique handling of tryptophan metabolism after activation of indoleamine-2,3-dioxygenase, which degrades tryptophan to kynurenine. Activation of this enzyme limits tryptophan concentration to a level below that required for chlamydial growth.[235] Chlamydiae are inhibited by tumor necrosis factor by a similar mechanism, although interferon beta may act as an intracellular intermediate.[236] Interferon gamma can be recovered in endocervical secretions, and it is found in increased concentrations in secretions from patients infected with *C. trachomatis*.[237]

Cell-mediated immunity and delayed type hypersensitivity

Lymphocyte transformation of blood leukocytes in response to a variety of pathogens, including *N. gonorrhoeae*, chlamydial infection, *T. pallidum*, and viruses of the herpes group has been demonstrated.[238–242] In general, patients who have experienced one or more of these infections can be expected to have a lymphocytic response in vitro, although these responses may be susceptible to a variety of factors and generally are not protective against recurrent infection. These responses may be particularly susceptible to hormonal regulation. When all the components of cell-mediated immunity (lymphocytes, macrophages, cytokines) function properly, the host can be expected to demonstrate a competent effector response, including macrophage activation, enhanced function of natural killer (NK) cells and cytotoxic lymphocytes (CTL), with further regulation of sIgA (see Fig. 13-5). The molecular basis for these events has been recently reviewed.[134] Cells capable of cell-mediated cytotoxicity, antibody-dependent cytotoxicity, and natural killer *Cell* activity have all been harvested from mucosal tissue.[134]

Delayed-type hypersensitivity (DTH) resulting from cell-mediated immunity develops after cutaneous injection of antigens. In the guinea pig conjunctival inclusion model, disruption of DTH leads to persistent, nonlethal infection, suggesting that humoral and cell-mediated immunity are involved in defense against this pathogen.[243] Human papillomavirus (HPV) produces more severe infection in patients receiving immunosuppressive therapy and in pregnant women.[244] Protection from recurrence of herpes simplex virus (HSV) infection is closely correlated with the generation of interleukin-2 and enhanced function of NK cells.[245]

The immune response can be destructive rather than protective. Cell-mediated immune response by antigens of microbes no longer cultivatable could be responsible for the pathogenesis of a variety of infectious and immunologic diseases. This hypothesis has become extremely important in chlamydial disease. Working with *C. trachomatis*, Morrison et al. demonstrated that a genus-specific 57- to 60-kD protein elicited immune-mediated ocular sensitivity in guinea pigs.[231] This protein is identical to the *E. coli* heat shock protein GroEL. The 57-kD protein initiates trachoma-like disease in the guinea pig. Expression of many heat-shock proteins can be evoked by stressful environmental conditions and/or oxygen free radicals generated during the attack of phagocytes, suggesting a mechanism for the formation of these proteins in vivo. These observations provide an attractive explanation for some of the chronic, destructive aspects of chlamydia infection.

Sexually transmitted disease (STD) pathogens can adversely affect the cell-mediated immune response. This is of greatest importance in HIV disease. The acquired immunodeficiency syndrome (AIDS) is characterized by a decline in the CD4 helper cell population that predisposes to a broad variety of opportunistic infections and neoplasms. The frequency of mucosal infections and difficulty of treatment of some STD pathogens in patients with HIV suggests compromise to mucosal defenses, although this has been incompletely characterized.

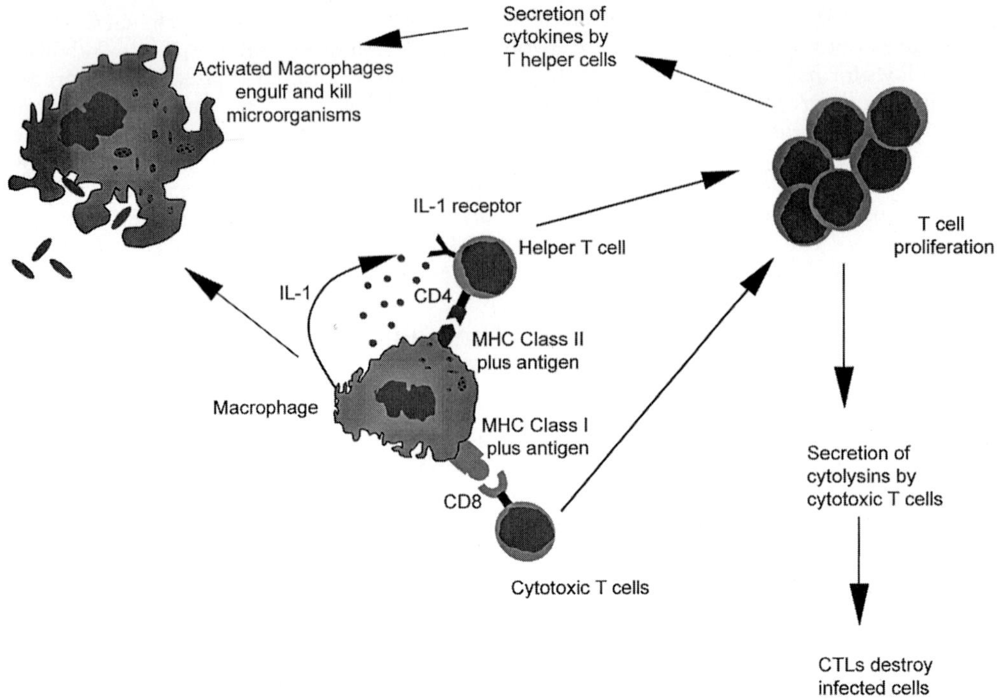

Fig. 13-5. Cell mediated immunity as determined by the interaction between lymphocytes, macrophages and cytokines. Through the function of this system, activated macrophages are expected to engulf and kill microorganisms and cytotoxic T cells and natural killer cells are generated which would defend against other pathogens present in the mucosa through the influence of the appropriate inflammatory cells.

Mucosal Defenses and STD Vaccines. Whereas systemic immunization may induce a weak immune response at mucosal sites, there is considerable recent evidence indicating that mucosal vaccination strategies are needed for prevention of STDs. Mucosal immunity might enable sIgA or other Ig isotypes to reduce colonization of potential pathogens, or facilitate their elimination. Such immunity might allow activated T cells or macrophages to clear local infections and prevent sytemic invasion of a pathogen. In addition, a preexisting immune response might reduce the concentration of a pathogen shed in the genital secretions by an infected host during initial infection, thereby reducing the efficiency of transmission to susceptible patients. Preventive vaccines for *N. gonorrhoeae*, chlamydia, HSV, HPV, CMV, and HIV-1 are in development.[246,247] Therapeutic vaccines for HPV are also in development.[248] Successful STD vaccines will have to capitalize on modulation of the mucosal immune system. Truly massive amounts of information directed toward the development of such vaccines are now available.[249] Mucosal vaccines might work best through site-specific mucosal delivery; there is accumulating evidence that vaginal and rectal mucosal immunization is more effective in inducing vaginal antibody titers than immunization at other mucosal sites.[250–251] Progress in mucosal delivery has been rapid.[249–252] Mucosal immunization is still limited by requirements for repeated exposure, high antigen dosage, and the use of adjuvants. Further immunomodulation has been used to force switching of local nodes to a mucosal (Th2) response, and conocommitant increased secretion of sIgA.[253] On the down side, development of STD vaccine is limited by experimental failures (i.e., a glycoprotein vaccine for HSV, a therapeutic vaccine for HIV), limited appropriate animal models, and a serious concern that a vaccine directed against one STD pathogen (i.e., HIV) might encourage (promiscuous) behavior, worsening the overall burden of STDs in a population. These concerns notwithstanding, it seem likely that one or more successful STD vaccines will surface in the second millennium. These vaccines will be developed and evolve directly from our knowledge of mucosal immunity.

References

1 Holbrook KA, Wolff K: Structure and development of the skin. In: Dermatology in General Medicine, TB Fitzpatrick et al (eds). New York, McGraw-Hill, 1987, 4th Edition.
2 Lever WF, Schaumberg-Lever G: Histopathology of the Skin. Philadelphia, Lippincott, 1975, p 13.
3 Bennett HS: Morphological aspects of extracellular polysaccharides. *J Histochem Cytochem* 11:14, 1963.
4 Young WG, Newcomb GM, Hosking AR: The effect of atrophy, hyperplasia, and keratinization accompanying the estrous cycle on Langerhans cells in mouse vaginal epithelium. *Am J Anat* 174: 173, 1985.
5 Pudney J, Anderson DJ: Immunobiology of the human penile urethra. *Am J Pathol* 147: 155, 1995.
6 Jackson SM, Elias PM: The skin as an organ of protection against the external environment. In: Dermatology in General Medicine, TB Fitzpatrick et al (eds). New York, McGraw-Hill, 1987, 4th Edition.
7 Colleen S et al: Bacterial colonization of human urethral mucosa. 1: Scanning electron microscopy. *Scand J Urol Nephrol* 24 14:9, 1980.
8 Savage DC: Adherence of normal flora to mucosal surfaces. In: Bacterial Adherence, EH Beachey (ed). London, Chapman & Hall, 1980, p 33.
9 Gibbons RJ, van Houte J: Bacterial adherence in oral microbial ecology. *Annu Rev Microbiol* 24 29:19, 1975.
10 Adler J et al: Chemotaxis toward sugars in *Escherichia coli. J Bacteriol* 115:824, 1973.
11 Ofek L, Beachey EH: Mannose binding and epithelial cell adherence of *Escherichia coli. Infect Immun* 22:247, 1978.
12 Bar-Shavit Z et al: Mannose residues on phagocytes as receptors for the attachment of *Escherichia coli* and *Salmonella typhi. Biochem Biophys Res Comm* 78:455, 1977.
13 Eisenstein B: Phase variation of type 1 fimbriae in *Escherichia coli* is under transcriptional control. *Science* 214:337, 1981.
14 Meyer TF: Pathogenic neisseriae-a model of bacterial virulence and genetic flexibility. *Int J Med Microbiol* 274:135, 1990.
15 Rudel T et al: Interaction of two variable proteins (PilE and PilC)

required for pilus-mediated adherence of *Neisseria gonorrhoeae* to human epithelial cells. *Mol Microbiol* 6: 3439, 1992.

16 Langerman S et al: Prevention of mucosal *Escherichia coli* infection by FimH-adhesion-based systemic vaccination. *Science* 276:607, 1997.

17 Colleen S: The human urethral mucosa: An experimental study with emphasis on microbial attachment. *Scand J Urol Nephrol* (suppl) 68:14, 1982.

18 Gibbons RA: Mucus of the mammalian genital tract. *Br Med Bull* 34:34, 1978.

19 Parke DV: Pharmacology of mucus. *Br Med Bull* 34:89, 1978.

20 Wira CR, Richardson J, Prabhala R (1994). Endocrine regulation of mucosal immunity: Effect of sex hormones and cytokines on the afferent and efferent arms of the immune system in the female reproduction tract. In "Handbook of Mucosal Immunology" (PL Ogra, J Mestecky, ME Lamm, W Strober, JR McGhee, and J Bienenstock, eds.) Pp. 705–718. Academic Press, San Diego.

21 Freter R: Prospects for preventing the association of harmful bacteria with host mucosal surfaces. In: Bacterial Adherence, EH Beachey (ed). London, Chapman & Hall, 1980, p 441.

22 Colleen S et al: Physics--chemical properties of *Staphylococcus epidermidis* and *Staphylococcus saprophyticus* as studied by aqueous polymer two-phase systems. *Scand J Infect Dis*, 24:165, 1980.

23 Beachey EH: Bacterial adherence in animals and man, in Bacterial Adherence, EH Beachey (ed). London, Chapman & Hall, 1980, p 3.

24 Chen T et al: Adherence of pilus-opa+ gonococci to epithelial cells in vitro involves heparan sulfate. *J Exp Med* 182:511, 1995.

25 Verwey EJW, Ovherbeek TG: The Theory of Stability of Lymphophobic Colloids. Amsterdam, Elsevier, 1948.

26 Watt PU, Ward ME: Adherence of *Neisseria gonorrhoeae* and other *Neisseria* species to mammalian cells. In: Bacterial Adherence, EH Beachey (ed). London, Chapman & Hall, 1980, p 253.

27 Mardh P-A, Westrim L: Adherence of bacteria to vaginal epithelial cells. *Infect Immun* 13:661, 1976.

28 Heckels JE et al: The influence of surface change on the attachment of *Neisseria gonorrhoeae* to human cells. *Gen Microbiol* 96:359, 1976.

29 Perers L et al: Association of some enterobacteria with the intestinal mucosa of mouse in relation to their partition in aqueous polymer two-phase systems. *Acta Pathol Microbiol Scand* 85B:308, 1977.

30 Smythe CJ et al: Differences in hydrophobic surface characteristics of porcine enteropathogenic *Escherichia coli* with or without K88 antigen as revealed by hydrophobic interaction chromatography. *Infect Immun* 22:462, 1978.

31 Kihlstrom E, Edebo L: Association of viable and inactivated *Salmonella typhimurium* MS and MR 10 with HeLa cells. *Infect Immun* 14:851, 1976.

32 Van Oss CJ, Gillman CF: Phagocytosis as a surface phenomenon: Contact angles and phagocytosis of encapsulated bacteria before and after opsonization by specific antiserum and complement. *Reticuloendothel Soc* 12:492, 1972.

33 Ofek I et al: Adherence of *Escherichia coli* to human mucosal cells mediated by mannose receptors. *Nature* 265:623, 1977.

34 Ofek I et al: Surface sugars of animal cells as determinants of recognition in bacterial adherence. *Trends Biochem Sci* 3:159, 1978.

35 Salit IE, Gotschlich EC: Hemagglutination by purified type I *Escherichia coli* pili. J Exp Med 146:1169, 1977.

36 Salit IE, Gotschlich EC: Type I *Escherichia coli* pili: Characterization of binding to monkey kidney cells. *J Exp Med* 146:1182, 1977.

37 Issacson RE et al: In vitro adhesion of *Escherichia coli* to porcine small intestinal epithelial cells: Pili as adhesive factors. *Infect Immun* 21:392, 1978.

38 Lomberg H et al: Influence of blood group on the availability or receptors for attaching *E. coli. Infect Immun* 51:9, 1986.

39 Lindberg F et al: Localization of the receptor-binding protein adhesin at the tip of the bacterial pilus. *Nature* 328:84, 1987.

40 Lomberg H, Svanborg-Eden C: Density of mucosal receptors for attaching *Escherichia coli. Monographs in Allergy* 24:35, 1988.

41 Roberts JA et al: The Gal (alpha 1–4) Gal-specific tip adhesin of *Escherichia coli* P-fimbriae is needed for pyelonephritis to occur in the normal urinary tract. *Proc Nat Acad Sci* 91:189, 1994.

42 Hultgren SJ et al: Regulation of production of type 1 pili among urinary tract isolates of *Escherichia coli. Infect Immun* 54:613, 1986.

43 Swanson J: Studies on gonococcus infection. IV: Pili: Their role in attachment of gonococci to tissue culture cells. *J Exp Med* 137:571, 1973.

44 Mardh P-A et al: Attachment of bacteria to exfoliated cells from the urogenital cells. *Invest Urol* 16:322, 1979.

45 Lambden PR et al: Variations in surface protein composition associated with virulence proteins in opacity types of *Neisseria gonorrhoeae. J Gen Microbiol* 114:305, 1979.

46 Swanson J: Adhesion and entry of bacteria into cells: A model for the pathogenesis of gonorrhoea. In: The Molecular Basis of Microbial Pathogenicity, H Smith et al (eds). Weinheim, Verlag Chemie, 1980 p 17.

47 Gorby G, Simon D, Rest RF: *Escherichia coli* that express *Neisseria gonorrhoeae* opacity-associated proteins attach to and invade human fallopian tube epithelium. *Ann NY Acad Sci* 730:286–288, 1994.

48 Virji M et al: Carcinoembryonic antigens (CD66) on epithelial cells and neutrophils are receptors for Opa proteins of pathogenic neisseriae. *Mol Micro* 22:941 1996.

49 Hu PC et al: *Mycoplasma pneumoniae* infections: Role of a surface protein in the attachment organelle. *Science* 216:313, 1982.

50 Sobel JD et al: *C. albicans* adherence to vaginal epithelial cells. *J Infect Dis* 143:76, 1981.

51 King RD et al: Adherence of *C. albicans* and other *Candida* species to mucosal epithelial cells. *Infect Immun* 27:667, 1980.

52 Hoist E et al: Bacterial vaginosis: Microbiology and clinical findings. *Eur J Clin Bacteriol* 6:536, 1987.

53 Fleury FJ: Adult vaginitis. *Clin Obstet Gynecol* 24:407, 1981.

54 McGee ZA et al: The evolutionary watershed of susceptibility to gonococcal infection. *Microb Pathogen* 9:131, 1990.

55 Byrne GL. Host cell relationships. In: Barron AL [ed.] Microbiology of Chlamydia, Boca Raton, FL: CRC Press, 1988; 135–150.

56 Nielsen MH, Nielsen R: Electron microscopy of *Trichomonas vaginalis donne*: interaction with vaginal epithelium in human trichomoniasis. *Acta Pathol Microbiol Scand* [B] 83:305, 1975.

57 Oriel D. Genital human papillomavirus infection. In: Holmes KK, Mardh PA, Sparling PF, Wiesner PJ, Cates W Jr., Lemon SM, Stamm WE, eds. Sexually Transmitted Diseases, 2nd ed. New York: McGraw-Hill, 1990, 433–441.

58 Repesh LA et al: Scanning electron microscopy of the attachment of *Treponema pallidum* to nerve cells *in vitro. Br J Vener Dis* 58: 211, 1982.

59 Spira AI et al: Cellular targets of infection and route of viral dissemination after an intravaginal inoculation of simian immunodeficiency virus into rhesus macaques. *J Exp Med* 183:215, 1996.

60 Bartlett JG et al: Quantitative bacteriology of the vaginal flora. *Infect Dis* 136:271, 1977.

61 Ohm MJ, Galask RP: Bacterial flora of the cervix from 100 prehysterectomy patients. *Am J Obstet Gynecol* 122:683, 1975.

62 Pfau A, Jacks T: The bacterial flora of the vaginal vestibule, urethra, and vagina in the normal premenopausal woman. *J Urol* 118:292, 1976.

63 Fair WR et al: Bacteriologic and hormonal observations of the urethra and vaginal vestibule in normal, premenopausal women. *J Urol* 104:426, 1970.

64 Mardh P-A, Westrom L: T-mycoplasmas in the genito-urinary tract of the female. *Acta Pathol Microbiol Scand* [B] 78:367, 1970.

65 McCormack WR, Taylor-Robinson D: Genital mycoplasmas. *N Engl J Med* 302:1003, 1980.

66 Soper, DE. Pelvic Inflammatory Disease. In: Infectious Disease Clinics of North America II, MS Cohen, EW Hook III and PJ Hitchcock (eds.) Philadelphia, W.B. Saunders Company, Pp. 821–840, 1994.

67 Schachter J: Chlamydial infections. *N Eng J Med* 298:428, 1978.

68 Rawis WE, Campione-Piccardo J: Epidemiology of herpes simplex virus type I and type II infections. In: The Human Herpesviruses: An Interdisciplinary Perspective, AJ Nahmias et al (eds). New York, Elsevier, 1980, p 32.

68a Quinn TC et al: Epidemiologic and microbiologic correlates of *Chlamydia trachomatis* infection in sexual partnerships. *JAMA* 276: 21, 1996.

68b Wald A et al: Frequent genital herpes simplex virus 2 shedding in immunocompetent women. Effect of acyclovir treatment. *J Clin Invest* 99:1092, 1997.

68c Krieger JN et al: Seminal shedding of human immunodeficiency virus type 1 and human cytomegalovirus: Evidence for different immunologic controls: *J Infect Dis* 171:1018, 1995.

68d Anderson DJ. The effect of genital tract infection and inflammation on male infertility. In: Infertility in the Male. 3rd ed. L. Lipshultz and S. Howard, eds. Mosby 1996, Pp. 326–335.

69 Cruickshank R, Sharman A: The biology of the vagina in the human subject II: The bacterial flora and secretion of the vagina in relation to glycogen in the vaginal epithelium. *J Obstet Gynecol Br Emp* 41: 208, 1939.

70 Mårdh P-A, Soltesz LV: In vitro interactions between lactobacilli and other microorganisms occurring in the vaginal flora. *Scand J Infect Dis* Suppl 40:47, 1983.

71 Metha AM et al: Isolation and purification of an inhibitory protein from *Lactobacillus acidophilus. AC Microbes* 37:37, 1983.

72 Hughes VL, Hillier SL: Microbiologic characteristics of *Lactobacillus* products used for colonization of the vagina. *Obstet Gynecol* 75:244, 1990.

73 Britigan BE et al: Neutrophil derived lactate stimulates the metabolism of *Neisseria gonorrhoeae*: An unappreciated aspect of the phagocytic respiratory burst. *J Clin Invest* 88:318, 1988.

74 Parsons NJ et al: Lactic acid is the factor in blood cell extracts which enhances the ability of CMP-NANA to sialylate gonococcal lipopolysaccharide and induce serum resistance. *Microb Pathog* 20:87, 1996.

74a McGee DJ, Chen GC, Rest RF: Expression of sialyltransferase is not required for interaction of *Neisseria gonorrhoeae* with human epithelial cells and human neutrophils. *Infect Immun* 64:4129, 1996.

75 Gregoire AT et al: The glycogen content of the human vaginal epithelial tissue. *Fertil Steril* 22:64, 1971.

76 Larsen B, Galask RP: Vaginal microbial flora: Practical and theoretic relevance. *Obstet Gynecol* 55:1005, 1980.

77 Larsen B et al: Role of estrogen in controlling the genital microflora of female rats. *Appl Environ Microbiol* 34:534, 1977.

78 Morse SA, Fitzgerald TJ: Effect of progesterone on *Neisseria gonorrhoeae. Infect Immun* 10:1370, 1974.

79 Stamey TA: Pathogenesis and treatment of urinary tract infections: Some observations of the pathogenesis of recurrent bacteriuria in women and children. Baltimore, Williams & Wilkins, 1980, p 219.

80 Hovelius B et al: *Staphylococcus saprophyticus* in the aetiology of nongonococcal urethritis. *Br J Vener Dis* 55:369, 1979.

81 Schlievert PM et al: Identification and characterization of an exotoxin from *Staphylococcus aureus* associated with toxic shock syndrome. *J Infect Dis* 143:569, 1981.

82 Bergdoll MS et al: A new staphylococcal enterotoxin, enterotoxin F, associated with toxic-shock syndrome *Staphylococcus aureus* isolates. *Lancet* 1:1017, 1981.

83 Todd JK: Toxic shock syndrome: A perspective through the looking glass. *Ann Intern Med* 96:839, 1982.

84 Remington JS, Klein JO: Infectious Diseases of the Fetus and Newborn Infant. Philadelphia, Saunders, 1995, 4th Edition.

85 Tovo PA, de Martino M, Gabiano C, et al. Mode of delivery and gestational age influence perinatal HIV-1 transmission. *J Acquir Immune Defic Syndr Hum Retrovirol* 11:88, 1996.

86 Zheng H, Alcorn TM, and Cohen MS: Effects of H2O2-producing lactobacilli on *Neisseria gonorrhoeae* growth and catalase activity. *J Infect Dis* 170:1209, 1994.

87 Klebanoff SJ, Coombs RW: Viricidal effect of *Lactobacillus acidophilus* on human immunodeficiency virus type 1: possible role in heterosexual transmission. *J Exp Med* 174:289, 1991.

88 Kave D, Levinson ME: In vitro inhibition of growth of *Neisseria gonorrhoeae* by genital microorganisms. *Sex Transm Dis* 4:1, 1977.

89 Hipp SS et al: Inhibition of *Neisseria gonorrhoeae* by a factor produced by *Candida albicans. Appl Microbiol* 27:192, 1974.

90 Shtibel R: Inhibition of growth of *Neisseria gonorrhoeae* by bacterial interference. *Can J Microbiol* 22:1430, 1976.

91 Saig JH et al: Inhibition of *Neisseria gonorrhoeae* by aerobic and facultatively anaerobic components of the endocervical flora. Evidence for a protective effect against infection. *Infect Immun* 19:704, 1978.

92 Schimpff SC et al: Origin of infection in acute nonlymphocytic leukemia: Significance of hospital acquisition of potential pathogens. *Ann Intern Med* 77:707, 1972.

93 Meck L, Sparling PF: Personal communication.

94 Moorman DR, Sixbey JW, Wyrick PB: Interaction of *Chlamydia trachomatis* with human genital epithelium in culture. *J Gen Micro* 132:1055, 1986.

95 Sweet RL et al: The occurrence of chlamydial and gonococcal salpingitis during the menstrual cycle. *JAMA* 255:2062, 1986.

96 Clark VL et al: Induction of and repression of outer membrane proteins by anaerobic growth of *Neisseria gonorrhoeae. Infect Immun* 55:1359, 1987.

97 Clark VL et al: Presence of antibodies to the major anaerobically induced gonococcal outer membrane protein in sera from patients with gonococcal infections. *Microb Pathog* 5:381, 1988.

98 Britigan BE, Cohen MS: Effects of human serum on bacterial competition for molecular oxygen. *Infect Immun* 52:657, 1986.

99 Grosz S, Kraus R: Bacteriologische Studien uber den Gonococcus. *Arch Dermatol Syph Wien* 45:329, 1899.

100 Loeb LJ et al: An antibiotic produced by *Micrococcus epiderimitis. Can f Res (E)* 28:212, 1950.

101 Soltesz LV, Mardh P-A: Antibiosis caused by bacteriolytic enzymes of coagulase-negative staphylococci with special reference to *Staphylococcus saprophyticus*, in Coagulase-negative Staphylococci, P-A Mardh, KH Schleiffer (eds). Almquist & Wiksell International, Stockholm, 1986, p 59.

102 Soltez LV, Mardh P-A: Lethal effect of *Staphylococcus aureus* in embryonated hen's eggs inhibited by coagulase-negative staphylococci. In: Coagulase-negative Staphylococci, P-A Mardh, KH Schleifer (eds). Almquist & Wiksell International Stockholm, 1986, p 75.

103 Reid L, Clamp JR: The biochemical and histochemical nomenclature of mucus. *Br Med Bull* 34:5, 1978.

104 Edward PAW: Is mucus a selective barrier to macromolecules? *Br Med Bull* 39:55, 1978.

105 Elstein M: Functions and physical properties of mucus in the female genital tract. *Br Med Bull* 34:83, 1978.

106 Gipson IK, Ho SB, Spurr-Michaud SJ, Tisdale AS, Zhan Q, Torlakovic E, Pudney J, Anderson DJ, Toribara NW, Hill JA. Mucin genes expressed by human female reproductive tract epithelia. *Biol Reprod* 56:999–1011, 1997.

107 Williams RC, Gibbons RJ: Inhibition of streptococcal attachment to receptors on human buccal epithelial cells by antigenically similar salivary glycoproteins. *Infect Immun* 11:711, 1975.

108 Lake AM et al: intestinal goblet cell mucus release. II: In vivo stimulation by antigen in the immunized rat. *J Immunol* 122:834, 1979.

109 Corbeil LB et al: Disseminated gonococcal infection in mice. *Infect Immun* 26:984, 1979.

110 Brooks GF et al: Human seminal plasma inhibition of antibody complement-mediated killing and opsonization of *Neisseria gonorrhoeae* and other gram-negative organisms. *J Clin Invest* 67:1523, 1981.

111 Strominger JL, Ghuysen JM: Mechanisms of enzymatic bacteriolysis. *Science* 156:213, 1967.

112 Mårdh PA et al: Inhibitory effect on the formation of chlamydial inclusions in McCoy cells by seminal fluid and some of its components. *Invest Urol* 17:510, 1980.

113 Cohen MS: Molecular events in the activation of human neutrophils for microbial killing. *Clin Infect Dis* 18:S170, 1994.
114 Oram JD, Reiter B: Inhibition of bacteria by lactoferrin and other iron-chelating agents. *Biochem Biophys Acta* 170:351, 1968.
115 Yamauchi K et al: Antibacterial activity of lactoferrin and a pepsin-derived lactoferrin peptide fragment. *Infect Immun* 61:719, 1993.
116 Payne SM, Finkelstein RA: The critical role of iron in host bacterial interactions. *J Clin Invest* 61:1428, 1978.
117 Mickelsen PA et al: Ability of *Neisseria gonorrhoeae, Neisseria meningitidis*, and comitensal *Neisseria* species to obtain iron from lactoferrin. *Infect Immun* 35:915, 1982.
118 Cornelissen CN et al: The gonococcal transferrin receptor is required for human infection (submitted).
119 Cohen MS et al: Preliminary observations on lactoferrin secretion in human vaginal mucus: Variation during the menstrual cycle and evidence of hormonal regulation, and implications for infection with *N. gonorrhoeae. Am J Obstet Gynecol* 157:122, 1987.
120 Heine RP, Wiesenfeld H, Dibiasi F, et al. Cervical lactoferrin levels are elevated in women with sexually transmitted diseases (STD). 35th ICAAC, San Francisco, September 17–22 1995: Abstract.
121 Rein MF et al: Use of a lactoferrin assay in the differential diagnosis of female genital tract infections and implications for the pathophysiology of bacterial vaginos. *Sex Trans Dis* 23:517, 1996.
122 Rosen GM et al: Free radicals and phagocytic cells. *FASEB J* 9:200, 1995.
123 Lehrer RI, Lichtenstein AK, Ganz T. Defensins: Antimicrobial and cytotoxic peptides of mammalian cells. *Annu Rev Imunol* 11:105, 1993.
124 Goldman MJ, Anderson GM, Stolzemberg ED, Kart UP, Zasloff M, Wilson JM: Human β defensin-1 is a salt-sensitive antibiotic in lung that is inactivated in cystic fibrosis. *Cell* 88:553, 1997.
125a Valore EV, Park CH, Quayle AJ, Wiles KR, McCray PB, Ganz T: Human β defensin-1, an antimicrobial peptide of urogenital tissues. *J Clin Invest* 101:1633, 1998.
125b Quayle AJ, Porter EM, Nussbaum AA, Wang YM, Brabec C, Yip KP and Mok SC. Gene expression, immunolocalization and secretion of human defensin-5 in female reproductive tract. *Am J Pathol* 152:1247, 1998.
126 Fair WR et al: Prostatic antibacterial factor: Identity and significance. *Urology* 7:169, 1976.
127 Mardh P-A, Colleen S: Antimicrobial activity of human semen. *Scand J Urol Nephrol* 9:17, 1975.
128 Colleen S et al: Magnesium and zinc in seminal fluid of healthy males and patients with non-acute prostatitis with and without gonorrhoeae. *Scand J Urol Nephrol* 9:192, 1975.
129 Soll DR et al: Zinc and regulation of growth and phenotype in the infectious yeast *Candida albicans*. *Infect Immun* 32:139 1981.
130 Fridlender B et al: Selective inhibition of Herpes simplex virus type I DNA polymerase by zinc ions. *Virology*, 89:551, 1978.
131 Krieger IN, Rein MF: Canine prostatic secretions kill *Trichomonas vaginalis*. *Infect Immun* 37:77, 1982.
132 Cohen MS et al: Host defenses and vaginal mucosa: A reevaluation. *Scand J Urol Nephrol* 86:13, 1985.
133 Zhang H, Dornadula G, Pomerantz RJ: Endogenous reverse transcription of human immunodeficiency virus type 1 in physiological microenvironments: An important stage for viral infection of nondividing cells. *J Virol* 70:2809, 1996.
134 Staats, HF and McGhee, JR: Application of basic principles of mucosal immunity to vaccine development. In: Mucosal Vaccines, H. Kiyono, P.L. Ogra, and J.R. McGhee (eds.) New York, Academic Press, 1996, Pp. 17–33.
135 Neutra, MR and Kraehenbuhl, JP: Antigen uptake by M cells for effective mucosal vaccines. In: Mucosal Vaccines, H. Kiyono, P.L. Ogra, and J.R. McGhee (eds.) NewYork, Academic Press, 1996, Pp. 41–51.
136 Berlin C, Berg EL, Briskin MJ et al: cr4,B7 integrin mediates lymphocyte binding to the mucosal vascular addressin MAdCAM-1. *Cell* 74:185, 1993.
137 Kilshaw PJ, Murant SJ. Expression and regulation of (7 β) integrins on mouse lymphocytes: Relevance to the mucosal immune system. *Eur J Immunol* 21:2591, 1991.
138 Cerf-Benussan N, Begue B, Gagnon J et al: The human intraepithelial lymphocyte marker HML-1 is an integrin consisting of a (7 subunit associated with a distinctive a chain, *Eur J Immunol* 22:273, 1992.
139 Parker CM, Cepek KL, Russell GJ et al.: A family of (7 integrins on human mucosal lymphocytes. *PNAS* 8989:1924, 1992
140 Kilshaw PJ, Murant SJ: A new surface antigen on intraepithelial lymphocytes in the intestine. *Eur J Immunol* 20:2201, 1990.
141 Moro I et al: Expression of SC, IL-6 and TGF-(in epithelial cell lines. *Adv Exp Med Biol* 371(A):175, 1995.
142 Cepek KL et al: Integrin (E7 mediates adhesions of T lymphocytes to epithelial cells. *J Immunol* 150:3459, 1993.
143 Cepek KL et al: Adhesion between epithelial cells and T lymphocytes mediated by E-cadherin and the alpha E Beta 7 integrin. *Nature* 372: 190, 1994.
144 McDermott MR, Bienenstock J: Evidence for a common mucosal system. 1. Migration of B immunoblasts into intestinal, respiratory and genital tissues. *J Immunol* 122:1892, 1979.
145 Kutteh WH, Mestecky J. Secretory immunity in the female reproductive tract. *Am J Reprod Immunol* 31:40, 1994.
146 Bulmer JN, Lunny DP, Hagin SV: Immunohistochemical characterization of stromal leukocytes in nonpregnant human endometrium. *Am J Reprod Immunol* 17:83, 1988.
147 Kamat BR, Isaacson PG: The immunocytochemical distribution of leukocytic subpopulations in human endometrium. *Am J Pathol* 127:66, 1986.
148 Edwards JNT, Morris HB: Langerhans' cells and lymphocyte subsets in the female genital tract. *Brit J Obstet Gynecol* 92:974, 1985.
149 Miller CJ, Vogel P, Alexander NJ et al: Localization of SIV in the genital tract of chronically infected female rhesus monkeys. *Am J Pathol* 141:655, 1992.
150 Edwards JNT, Morris HB: Langerhans' cells and lymphocyte subsets in the female genital tract. *Brit J Obstet Gynecol* 92:974, 1985.
151 Bjereke S, Scott H, Braathen LR et al: HLA-DR expressing Langerhans-like cells in vaginal and cervical epithelium. *Acta Obstet Gynecol Scand* 585–589, 1983.
152 deGraaf JJ et al: Expression of cellular adhesion molecules in Langerhan's cell Histiocytosis and normal Langerhans' cells. *Am J Pathol* 147:1161, 1983.
153 Wira CR, Rossoll RM: Antigen-presenting cells in the female reproductive tract: Influence of sex hormones on antigen presentation in the vagina. *Immunology* 84:505, 1995.
154a Fichorova RN, Anderson DJ. Cytokines in the cervical vaginal environment. In: Cytokines in Reproduction. ed: JA Hill. Springer-Verlag (In Press.)
154b Sha BE et al: Evaluation of immunologic markers in cervicovaginal fluid of HIV-infected and uninfected women: Implications for the immunologic response to HIV in the female genital tract. *J AIDS* 16:161, 1997.
154c Belec L, Gherardi R, Payan C, Prazuck T, Malkin J-E, Benissan CT, Pilot J. Proinflammatory cytokine expression in cervicovaginal secretions of normal and HIV-infected women. *Cytokine* 1995; 7: 568–574.
154d Anderson DJ, Politch JA, Tucker LD, Fichorova R, Haimovici F, Tuomala RE, Mayer KH. Quantitation of mediators of inflammation and immunity in genital tract secretions and their relevance to HIV type-1 transmission. *AIDS Research and Human Retroviruses* 14(51)543–549, 1998.
155a Spear GT et al: A potent activator of HIV-1 replication is present in the genital tract of a subset of HIV-1 infected and uninfected women. *J AIDS*, 1997.
155b Platz-Christensen JJ, Mattsby-Baltzer I, Thomsen P, Wiqvist N. Endotoxin and interleukin 1-α in the cervical mucus and vaginal fluid of pregnant women with bacterial vaginosis. *Am J Obstet Gynecol* 1993; 169:1161–1166.
155c Clerici M, Merola M, Ferrario E, Trabattoni D, Villa MC. Cytokine production patterns in cervical intraepithelial neoplasia: association

with human papillomavirus infection. *J Nat Cancer Inst* 1997; 89: 245–250.

155d Rasmussen SJ, Eckman L, Quayle AJ, Shen L, Zhang Y-X, Anderson DJ, Flere J, Stephens RS, Kagnoff MF. Secretion of proinflammatory cytokines by epithelial cells in response to Chlamydia infection suggests a central role for epithial cells in chlamydia pathogenesis. *J Clin Invest* 1997; 99:77–87.

156 Anderson DJ. The importance of mucosal immunology to problems in human reproduction. *J Reprod Immunol* 31:3–19, 1996.

157 Husband AJ, Clifton VL: Role of intestinal immunization in urinary tract defense. *Immunol Cell Biol* 67:371, 1989.

158 Pudney JA, Anderson DJ: Organization of immunocompetent cells and their function in the male reproductive tract. In: WHO Symposium on Local Immunity in Reproductive Tract Tissues. PD Griffin and PM Johnson (eds.) Oxford Univ. press, pp. 131–146, 1993.

159 El-Demiry MIM, James K: Lymphocyte subsets and macrophages in the male genital tract in health and disease. *Eur J Urol* 14:226, 1988.

160 Quayle AJ,Coston WMP, Trocha A, Kalams S, Mayer KH, Anderson DJ. Detection of HIV-1 specific cytotoxic T lymphocytes in the semen of HIV-infected individuals. *J Immunol* (In Press)

161 Wang YE, Holstein AF: Intraepithelial lymphocytes in the human epididymis. *Cell Tissue Res* 233:517, 1983.

162 Miller CJ, Vogel P, Alexander, NJ et al: Pathology and localization of SIV in the reproductive tract of chronically infected male rhesus macaques. *Lab Invest* 70:255, 1994.

163 Hussain A, Lehner, T: Comparative investigation of Langerhans' cells and potential receptors for HIV in oral, genitourinary and rectal epithelia. *Immunology* 85:475, 1995.

164 Alexander NJ, Anderson DJ: Immunology of Semen (Modern Trends). *Fertil Steril* 47: 192, 1987.

165 Hulka IF, Omran K: The uterine cervix as a potential local antibody secreter. *Am J Obstet Gynecol* 104:440, 1969.

166 McNabb PC, Tomasi TB: Host defense mechanisms at mucosal surfaces. *Annu Rev Microbiol* 35:477, 1981.

167 Tomasi TB, Grey HM: Structure and function of immunoglobulin A. *Prog Allergy* 16:136, 1972.

168 Tomasi TB: Secretions, in The Immune System of Secretions, AG Osler, L Weiss (eds). Englewood Cliffs, N.J., Prentice-Hall, 1976.

169 Strober W et al: Recent Advances in Mucosal Immunity. New York, Raven Press, 1982.

170 McGhee JR et al: Regulation of IgA synthesis and immune response by T cells and interleukins. *J Clin Immunol* 9:175, 1989.

171 Russell MW, Mestecky J: Induction of the mucosal immune response. *Rev Infect Dis* 10:S440, 1988.

171a Mestecky J, Kutteh W, Jackson S: Mucosal immunity in the female genital tract: Relevance to vaccination efforts against the human immunodeficiency virus. *AIDS Res Human Retroviruses* 10:S2, 1994.

172 Chipperfield EJ, Evans BA: Effect of local infection and oral contraception on immunoglobulin levels in cervical mucus. *Infect Immun* 11:215, 1975.

173 Brandtzaeg P: Overview of the mucosal immune system. *Curr Top Microbiol Immunol* 146:13, 1989.

174 Verman JP, Heremans JF: Subclasses of human immunoglobulin A based on differences in the alpha polypeptide chain. *Science* 153: 647, 1966.

175 Fowler JE, Kaiser DL, Mariano M: Immunologic response of the prostate to bacteriuria and bacterial prostatitis: Part I. Immunoglobulin concentrations in prostatic fluid. *J Urol* 128:158, 1982.

176 Fowler JE, Mariano M: Immunoglobulin in seminal fluid of fertile, infertile, vasectomy and vasectomy reversal patients. *J Urol* 129: 869, 1983.

177 Fowler JE, Mariano M: Immunologic response of the prostate to bacteriuria and bacterial prostatitis. II. Antigen specific immunoglobulin in prostatic fluid. *J Urol* 128:165, 1982.

178 Kojima H, Wang SP, Kuo CC et al. Local antibody in semen for rapid diagnosis of *Chlamydia trachomatis epididym. J Immunol* 140:528, 1988.

179 McMillan A, McNeillage G, Young H: Antibodies to *Neisseria gonorrhoeae*: a study of the urethral exudates of 232 men. *J Infect Dis* 140:899, 1979.

180 Tramont EC: Inhibition of adherence of *Neisseria gonorrhoeae* by human genital secretions. *J Clin Invest* 59:117, 1977.

180a Haimovici F, Mayer KH, Anderson DJ. Quantitation of HIV-1 specific IgG, IgA and IgM antibodies in human genital tract secretions. *J AIDS* 15:185–191, 1997.

181 McChesney D et al: Genital antibody response to a parenteral gonococcal pilus vaccine. *Infect Immun* 36:1006, 1982.

181a Mazzoli S et al: HIV-specific mucosal and cellular immunity in HIV-seronegative partners of HIV-seropositive individuals. *Nature Med* 3:1250, 1997.

182 Walker WA et al: intestinal uptake of macromolecules: Effect of oral immunization. *Science* 177:608, 1972.

183 Magnusson K-E et al: Reduction of phagocytosis, surface hydrophobicity and charge of *Salmonella typhimurium* MR10 by reaction with secretory IgA (SIgA) *Immunology* 36:439, 1979.

184 Qui PG et al: Phagocytosis in subacute bacterial endocarditis: Localization of the primary opsonic site to Fc fragment. *J Exp Med* 128:553, 1968.

185 Bisno AL et al: Human immunity to *Neisseria gonorrhoeae* acquired serum opsonic antibodies. *J Lab Clin Med* 86:221, 1975.

186 Adinolfi M et al: Serological properties of A antibodies to *Escherichia coli* present in human colostrum. *Immunology* 10:517, 1966.

187 Hill IR, Porter P: Studies of bactericidal antibody to *Escherichia coli* of porcine serum and colostral immunoglobulins and the role of lysozyme with secretory IgA. *Immunology* 26:1239, 1974.

188 Goize 0, Muller-Eberhard HJ: The C3-activator system: An alternate pathway of complement activation. *J Exp Med* 134:90S, 1971.

189 Price RJ, Boettcher B: The presence of complement in human cervical mucus and its possible relevance to infertility in women with complement-dependent sperm immobilizing antibodies. *Fertil Steril* 32:61, 1979.

190 McCutchan JA et al: Role of blocking antibody in disseminated gonococcal infection. *J Immunol* 121:1884, 1978.

191 Shafer WM et al: Serum sensitivity of *Neisseria gonorrhoeae*: Role of lipopolysaccharide. *J Infect Dis* 149:175, 1984.

192 Joiner KA et al: Mechanism of action of blocking immunoglobulin G for *Neisseria gonorrhoeae. J Clin Invest* 76:1765, 1985.

193 Cohen MS, Sparling PF. Mucosal infection with *Neisseria gonorrhoeae. J Clin Invest* 89:1699, 1992.

193a Ram S, Sharma AK, Simpson SD, Gulati S, McQuillen DP, Pangburn MK, Rice PA. The Maxwell Finland Laboratory for Infectious Disease, Boston Medical Center, Boston, Massachusetts 02118, USA. sram:bu.edu A novel sialic acid binding site on factor H mediates serum resistance of sialylated *Neisseria gonorrhoeae. J Exp Med* 187(5):743–752, 1998.

194 Brooks GF, Ingwer I: Studies on the relationships between serum bactericidal activity and uncomplicated genital infections due to *Neisseria gonorrhoeae. J Infect Dis* 138:333, 1978.

195 McComb DE et al: *Chlamydia trachomatis* in women: Antibody in cervical secretions as a possible indicator of genital infection. *J Infect Dis* 139:628, 1979.

195a Brunham RC et al: Correlation of host immune response with quantitative recovery of *Chlamydia trachomatis* from the human endocervix. *Infect Immun* 39:1491, 1983.

196 Ogra PL et al: Immunoglobulin response in serum and secretions after immunization with live and inactivated polio vaccine and natural infection. *N Engl J Med* 279:893, 1968.

197 Perkins JC et al: Evidence for protective effect of an inactivated rhinovirus vaccine administered by the nasal route. *Ant J Epidemiol* 90:319, 1969.

198 Staats HF, McGhee JR: Mucosal immunity in HIV infection. In: Immunology of HIV Infection, S. Gupta (ed.) New York, Plenum Press, pp. 387–416, 1996.

199 Belec L, Meillet D, Gaillard O, Prazuck T, Michel E, Ekome JN, Pillot J. Decreased cervicovaginal production of both IgA1 and IgA2 subclasses in women with AIDS. *Clin Exp Immunol* 101:100, 1995.

199a Lin L et al: The *Neisseria* type 2 IgAi protease cleaves LAMP1 and promotes survival of bacteria within epithelial cells. *Mol Micro* 24: 1083, 1997.
199b Hauck CR, Meyer TF: The lysosomal/phagosomal membrane protein h-lamp-1 is a target of the IgA1 protease of *Neisseria gonorrhoeae. FEBS Letters* 405:86, 1997.
199c Pohlner J et al: Uptake and nuclear transport of *Neisseria* IgA1 protease associated a-proteins in human cells. *Mol Micr* 17:1073, 1995.
200 Plaut AG et al: Differential susceptibility of human IgA immunoglobulins to streptococcal IgA protease. *J Clin Invest* 54:1295, 1974.
201 Plaut AG et al: *Neisseria gonorrhoeae* and *Neisseria meningiditis*. Extracellular enzyme cleaves human immunoglobulin A. *Science* 190:1103, 1975.
202 Mulks MH, Plaut AG: IgA protease production as a characteristic distinguishing pathogenic from harmless Neisseriaceae. *N Engl J Med* 299:973, 1978.
203 Kearns DH et al: Paradox of the immune response to uncomplicated gonococcal urethritis. *N Engl J Med* 289:1170, 1973.
204 O'Reilly RJ et al: Secretory IgA antibody responses to *Neisseria gonorrhoeae* in the genital secretions of infected females. *J Infect Dis* 133:113, 1976.
205 Shafer WM, Rest RF. Interactions of gonococci with phagocytic cells. *Annu Rev Microbiol* 43:121, 1989.
206 Wyrick PB, Brownridge EA: Growth of *Chlamydia psittaci* in macrophages. *Infect Immun* 19:1054, 1978.
207 Anderson DC et al: Luminol-enhanced chemiluminescence for evaluation of type III group B streptococcal opsonins in human sera. *J Infect Dis* 141:320, 1980.
208 Rein MF et al: Trichomonacidal activity of human polymorphonuclear neutrophils: Killing by disruption and fragmentation. *J Infect Dis* 142:575, 1980.
209 Lagergard T et al: Serum bactericidal activity and phagocytosis in host defense against Haemophilus ducreyi. *Microbi Pathog* 18:37, 1995.
210 Elbim C et al: Polymorphonuclear neutrophils from human immunodeficiency virus-infected patients show enhanced activation, diminished fMLP-induced L-selectin shedding, and an impaired oxidative burst after cytokine priming. *Blood* 84:2579, 1994.
211 Luster AD: Chemokines–chemotactic cytokines that mediate inflammation. *NEJM* 338:436, 1998.
212 James AN, Williams RP: Chemotactic factor(s) of *Neisseria gonorrhoeae. Curr Microbiol* 241:341, 1978.
213 Watt PJ, Medlen AR: Generation of chemotaxins by gonococci, in: Immunobiology of Neisseria Gonorrhoeae, GF Brooks et al (eds) Washington, DC, American Society for Microbiology, 1978, p 239.
214 Densen P et al: Gonococci causing uncomplicated gonorrhea or disseminated gonococcal infection differ in stimulation of neutrophil chemotaxis and phagocytosis, in Genetics and Immunobiology, of Pathogenic Neisseria, S Normark, D Danielsson (eds). Hemavan, Sweden, EMBO Workshop, 1980.
215 Ramsey KH et al: Inflammatory cytokines produced in response to experimental human gonorrhea. *J Infect Dis* 172:186, 1995.
216 Weber RD et al: Energy is required for adherence of *Neisseria gonorrhoeae* to phagocytic and non-phagocytic cells. *Infect Immun* 57: 785, 1989.
217 Britigan BE et al: Effects of human serum on the growth and metabolism of *Neisseria gonorrhoeae: An alternative view of serum. Infect Immun* 50:738, 1985.
218 Punsalang AP Jr., Sawyer WD: Role of pili in the virulence of *Neisseria gonorrhoeae. Infect Immun* 8:255, 1973.
219 Rosenthal RS et al: Ethylenediaminetetraacetic acid-sensitive antiphagocytic activity of *Neisseria gonorrhoeae. Infect Immun* 15:817, 1977.
220 Winston DJ et al: Prophylactic granulocyte transfusions during human bone marrow transplantation. *Am J Med* 68:893, 1980.
221 Eisenberg LG, Wyrick PB: Inhibition of phagolysosome fusion is localized to *Chlamydia psittaci-* laden vacuoles. *Infect Immun* 32: 889 1981.
222 Stevenson M, Gendelman HE: Cellular and viral determinants that regulate HIV-1 infection in macrophages. *J Leuk Biol* 5693:278, 1994.
223 Baldwin GC et al: Human immunodeficiency virus causes mononuclear phagocyte dysfunction. *Proc Nat Acad Sci* USA. 87:3933, 1990.
224 Huang Y et al: The role of a mutant CCR5 allele in HIV-1 transmission and disease progression. *Nature Med* 2:1240, 1996.
225 Yong EC et al: Toxic effect of human polymorphonuclear leukocytes on *Chlamydia trachomatis. Infect Immun* 37:422, 1982.
226 Yong EC, Chi EY et al: Degradation of *Chlamydia trachomatis* in human polymorphonuclear leukocytes: An ultrastructural study peroxidase-positive phagolysosomes. *Infect Immun* 53:427, 1986.
227 Register KB et al: Nonoxidative antimicrobial effects of human polymorphonuclear leukocyte granule proteins on *Chlamydia spp. vitro. Infect Immun* 55:2420, 1987.
228 Sawyer WD: Interaction of influenza virus with leukocytes and its effect on phagocytosis. *J Infect Dis* 119:541, 1969.
229 Faden H et al: Effect of viruses on luminol dependent chemiluminescence of human neutrophils. *Infect Immun* 24:673, 1979.
230 Parsons NJ et al: A determinant of resistance of *Neisseria gonorrhoeae* to killing by human phagocytes: An outer membrane lipoprotein of about 20 kDa with a high content of glutamic acid. *J Gen Microbiol* 1323:3277, 1986.
231 Morrison RP, Lyng K, Caldwell HD: Chlamydial disease pathogenesis. Ocular hypersensitivity elicited by a genus-specific 57-kd protein. *J Exp Med* 169:663, 1989.
232 Ross SG, Densen P: Local and disseminated gonococcal isolates differ in opsonic requirements and efficiency of phagocytosis by neutrophils. *Clin Res* 30:378A, 1982.
233 Daly JA et al: Gonococci with mutations to low-level penicillin resistance exhibit increased sensitivity to the oxygen-independent bactericidal activity of polymorphonuclear leukocyte granule extracts. *Infect Immun* 35:826, 1982.
233a Hobbs MM et al: Swine model of *Haemophilus ducreyi* infection. *Infect Immun* 63:3094, 1995.
234 Nathan CF, Murray HW, Wiebe ME, Rubin BY. Identification of interferon-gamma as the lymphokine that activates human macrophage oxidative metabolism and antimicrobial activity. *J Exp Med* 158(3):670–689, 1983 Sep 1.
235 Moulder JW. Interaction of *chlamydiae* and host cells *in vitro. Microbiol Rev* 55:143, 1991.
236 Shemer-Avni Y, Wallach D, Sarov I: Reversion of the antichlamydial effect of tumor necrosis factor by tryptophan and antibodies to beta interferon. *Infect Immun* 57:3484, 1989.
237 Arno JN et al: Interferon gamma in endocervical secretions of women infected with *Chlamydia trachomatis. J Infect Dis* 162: 1385, 1990.
238 Kraus SJ et al: Lymphocyte transformation in repeated gonococcal urethritis. *Infect Immun* 2:655 1970.
239 Hanna L et al: Human cell-mediated immune response to chlamydial antigens. *Infect Immun* 23:412, 1979.
240 Haliberg T et al: Pelvic inflammatory disease in patients, infected with *Chlamydia trachomatis*: *In vitro* cell mediated immune response to chlamydial antigens. *Genitourin Med* 61:247, 1985.
241 Pavia CS et al: Selective *in vitro* response of thymus-derived lymphocytes from *Treponema pallidum*-infected rabbits. *Infect Immun* 18:603, 1977.
242 Shore SL, Feorino PM: Immunology of primary herpes virus infection in humans. in: The Human Herpesviruses: An Interdisciplinary Perspective, AJ Nahmias et al (eds.) New York, Elsevier, 1980, p.267.
243 Rank RG, Barron AL: Effect of antithymocyte serum on the course of chlamydial genital infection in female guinea pigs. *Infect Immun* 41:846, 1983.
244 Ferenezy A: Treating genital condyloma during pregnancy with the carbon dioxide laser. *Am J Obstet Gynecol* 148:9, 1984.
245 Weinberg A, Basham TY, Merigan TC: Regulation of guinea pig immune functions by interleukin 2: Critical role of natural killer activity in acute HSV-2 genital infection. *J Immunol* 37:3310, 1986.

246 Sparling PF, Elkins C, Wyrick PB, Cohen MS. Vaccines for bacterial sexually transmitted infections: A realistic goal? *Proc Natl Acad Sci* USA 91:2456, 1994.

247 Adimora AA, Sparling PF, Cohen MS. Vaccines for classic sexually transmitted diseases. In: *Sexually Transmitted Diseases in the AIDS Era: Part II.* Infect Dis Clinics N Am. Cohen MS, Hook EW, Hitchcock PJ (eds.) vol. 8, 1994.

248 Schiller JT: Papillomavirus vaccines: current status and future prospects. Advances in Dermatology, 11:355, 1996.

249 Ogra PL, Kiyono H, McGhee JR. Mucosal Vaccines. Academic Press, New York, 1996.

250 Kozlowski PA, Cu-uvin S, Seutra MR, Flanigan TP. Comparison of the oral, rectal and vaginal immunization routes for induction of antibodies in rectal and genital tract secretions of women. *Infect Immun* 65:1387.

251 Crowley-Nowick PA, Bell MC, Brockwell R, Edwards RP, Chen S, Partridge EE, Mestecky J. Rectal immunization for induction of specific antibody in the genital tract of women. *J Clin Immunol* 17: 370–379, 1997.

252 Livingston JB, Lu S, Robinson H, Anderson DJ. DNA immunization of the female genital tract. *Infect Immun* 66:322.

253 Daynes RA, Enioutina EY, Butler S, Mu HH, McGee ZA, Araneo BA. Department of Pathology, University of Utah, Salt Lake City, 84132, USA. Induction of common mucosal immunity by hormonally immunomodulated peripheral immunization. *Infection and Immunity* 64(4):1100–1109. 1996 Apr.

Chapter 14
Normal vaginal flora

Sharon L. Hillier

If we regard the vaginal microflora in its totality as a flexible population occupying a particular ecologic niche and acting as a barrier to the establishment of other organisms, then the degree of acute stress tolerated by this microflora must have defined limits. . . . If the acute stress is either too large or too long, the flexibility of the microflora may not accommodate this degree of change. The microflora may then collapse as a functional entity, providing a less protective environment against pathogenic microorganisms that are capable of rapid proliferation.

Andrew Onderdonk, 1992[1]

INTRODUCTION

Most women who become infected by sexually acquired diseases acquire them during heterosexual intercourse. For women, transmission of STDs occurs predominantly within the vaginal ecosystem. Although the routine use of condoms can prevent many STDs by blocking the entry of infectious particles into this ecosystem, many women are not aware that their sexual partners are infected.

Although partners studies have demonstrated that susceptibility to gonorrhea in women may be associated with the microbial flora, our knowledge of the importance of the normal genital flora in conferring resistance to STDs has not been well defined.[2] However, recent studies suggest that a decrease in vaginal lactobacilli may increase a woman's susceptibility to heterosexually acquired HIV.[3–5] With the worldwide recognition that HIV is spread predominantly through heterosexual contact, there has been an increased recognition of the need for topical microbicides that could be applied intravaginally to decrease transmission of STDs and HIV.[6,7] However, any products that have adequate activity against STDs and HIV may also have deleterious effects on the normal vaginal ecosystem. This chapter on the human vaginal ecosystem summarizes the microbial components of the vagina, the effects of contraceptive methods and sexual intercourse on this ecosystem, and how topical microbicides effect this flora. Further, the association between the vaginal flora and susceptibility to infections are summarized.

HISTORY OF VAGINAL FLORA STUDIES

The first definitive study of the vaginal flora was published by Döderlein in 1894.[8] The earliest studies led to the view that the normal vaginal flora consisted predominantly of the acid-producing Gram-positive rods now referred to as *Lactobacillus* spp. It was Döderlein who first reported on the use of *Lactobacillus* in treating gonorrhea among prostitutes in 1892, and was a real visionary in his early recognition of the normal vaginal microflora as a deterrent to infection.[8]

As summarized by Larson and Galask, the early studies of the vaginal microflora revealed that many other organisms in addition to lactobacilli had to be considered part of the normal vaginal microflora.[9] As early as 1928, Harris and Brown reported that 26 of 30 normal women had anaerobes present in the vaginal flora postpartum.[10] In 1938, Weinstein reported that 93 percent of pregnant women and 90 percent of nonpregnant women had anaerobes present as part of the vaginal flora.[11] The importance of estrogen in stimulating the disposition of glycogen in the vaginal epithelial tissue, and its subsequent effect on vaginal colonization by lactobacilli was described by investigators in the 1930s.[12,13]

Even though Hite et al. and others had firmly established the importance of anaerobes in the vaginal flora by the middle 1940s, many studies evaluating the etiology of vaginitis failed to include techniques for the detection of obligate anaerobes.[14] As discussed in Chapter 42, the failure to perform careful culture techniques for obligate anaerobes led to the erroneous conclusion that *Haemophilus vaginalis*, now known as *Gardnerella vaginalis*, was the sole etiologic agent of bacterial vaginosis in 1955.[15]

In the 1970s with the advent of newer methods for the culture and identification of anaerobes, several studies were published that more carefully described the vaginal or cervical microflora.[16–19]

Genital mycoplasmas were first recognized to be part of the vaginal ecosystem over 50 years ago, and their possible association with vaginitis syndromes was first suggested in 1958.[20] *Ureaplasma urealyticum* has also long been recognized as a part of the normal vaginal microflora of pregnant and nonpregnant women, but most studies do not suggest a pathogenic role for this organism in the lower genital tract.[21] A study published in the early 1980s supported the role of *Mycoplasma hominis* in bacterial vaginosis.[22]

THE NORMAL VAGINAL ECOSYSTEM OF REPRODUCTIVE AGE WOMEN

The vaginal microflora is best described using frequencies of common vaginal microbes, as well as their relative concentration in the vaginal fluid. As shown in Table 14-1, the frequency and concentration of many facultative organisms is dependent on whether the woman has bacterial vaginosis (BV) or normal, *Lactobacillus*-predominant microflora.[23] However, even if "normal" vaginal microflora is restricted to those women having a *Lactobacillus*-dominant flora as defined by Gram stain, 46 percent of women are colonized *by G. vaginalis*, 78 percent are colonized by *U. urealyticum,* and 31 percent are colonized by *Candida albicans*.[23]

The frequency and species of anaerobic members of the vaginal microflora are summarized in Table 14-2. Nearly all women are vaginally colonized by obligately anaerobic Gram-negative rods and *Peptostreptococcus* spp.[23] Although some species of anaerobes are present at higher frequencies or concentrations among women with BV, it is clear that the microbial flora is complex and cannot be defined simply by the presence or absence of lactobacilli, *Gardnerella*, mycoplasmas, and anaerobes.

VAGINAL MICROFLORA OF PREPUBERTAL GIRLS AND POST-MENOPAUSAL WOMEN

Lactobacilli produce lactic acid from glucose, keeping the vagina at an acidic pH. In premenarchal girls there is little glycogen or glucose present in the vaginal fluid. After puberty, glycogen is deposited on the vaginal epithelium under estrogenic control.[12] Glycogen is metabolized by vaginal epithelial cells to glucose, which then serves as a substrate for *Lactobacillus* to convert glucose to lactic acid. Any women with sufficient estrogen to have glycogen deposition on the vaginal epithelium have enough glucose to furnish adequate nutrients for the growth of *Lactobacillus* in the vagina.

Table 14-1. Frequency and Concentration of Facultative Microorganisms in the Vaginal Flora of 171 Pregnant Women, Stratified by Vaginal Flora Pattern (as Assessed by Gram Staining)[23]

Organism(s)	Frequency* among women with indicated pattern (cfu/mL†)			
	Normal (n = 85)	Intermediate (n = 47)	BV (n = 39)	p‡
Lactobacillus spp.				
Total	96 ($10^{7.0}$)	85 ($10^{6.6}$)	67 ($10^{6.3}$)	<0.001
H_2O_2-positive	61 ($10^{7.2}$)	40 ($10^{6.5}$)	5 (—)	<0.001
Gardnerella vaginalis	46 ($10^{6.0}$)	79 ($10^{6.8}$)	92 ($10^{7.7}$)	<0.001
Diphtheroids	72 ($10^{3.8}$)	89 ($10^{3.9}$)	76 ($10^{4.4}$)	0.15
Bacillus spp.	4 (—)	4 (—)	0 (—)	0.28
Staphylococcus aureus	5 (—)	9 (—)	3 (—)	0.64
Coagulase-negative staphylococci	89 ($10^{4.0}$)	81 ($10^{4.4}$)	67 ($10^{4.0}$)	0.02
Viridans streptococci	55 ($10^{4.7}$)	66 ($10^{4.0}$)	72 ($10^{5.2}$)	0.03
Enterococcus spp.	39 ($10^{5.1}$)	30 ($10^{5.4}$)	13 ($10^{4.2}$)	0.003
Group B streptococci	15 ($10^{4.2}$)	17 ($10^{4.1}$)	21 ($10^{5.8}$)	0.20
Escherichia coli	17 ($10^{4.1}$)	15 ($10^{3.0}$)	21 ($10^{4.6}$)	0.59
Klebsiella spp.	2 (—)	2 (—)	5 (—)	0.40
Haemophilus influenzae	1 (—)	0 (—)	3 (—)	0.52
Mycoplasma hominis	15 ($10^{3.5}$)	38 ($10^{4.8}$)	61 ($10^{5.2}$)	<0.001
Ureaplasma urealyticum	78 ($10^{5.0}$)	91 ($10^{5.0}$)	92 ($10^{5.0}$)	0.01
Candida albicans	31 (—)	17 (—)	21 (—)	0.41

*As a percentage.
†Mean number of cfu/mL of vaginal fluid for women who were culture-positive for the organism. Mean concentrations were not calculated for *C. albicans* or for those organism of which fewer than five isolates were obtained.
‡Mantel-Haenszel linear association (for frequencies).

The vaginal microflora of women is also directly related to levels of estrogen. The vaginal microflora of a newborn female is thought to be obtained from the mother at the time of delivery. Therefore, it is generally thought that vaginal microflora of newborn females is similar to that of the mother, although the data to support this are scant. As the maternally derived estrogen is reduced and girls enter their premenarchal period, the vaginal flora is comprised predominantly of anaerobic rods and cocci.[24] In a study of 19 prepubertal girls who had not been sexually abused, 89 percent were reported to have anaerobic Gram-negative rods in the vagina, and 89 percent were colonized by *Peptostreptococcus* spp.

Prepubertal girls have low frequencies of lactobacilli, *G. vaginalis, Prevotella bivia,* genital mycoplasmas, and yeast (Table 14-3).[24] In contrast, women of reproductive age without vaginal infections are usually colonized by lactobacilli (92 percent) and over half women will be vaginally colonized by *G. vaginalis*.[23] In postmenopausal women who have not received estrogen replacement therapy, only about half remain colonized by lactobacilli and the frequencies of *G. vaginalis*, *Prevotella bivia*, and the genital mycoplasmas are also decreased.[25] Other members of the vaginal microflora do not appear to be under estrogen control. As shown in the table, the frequency of coliforms such as *E. coli, Enterococcus*, viridans streptococci and staphylococci are relatively constant among women regardless of estrogen status. *E. coli* may in fact be somewhat less frequent women having adequate levels of estrogen, but the role of estrogen versus sexual activity and colonization with *E. coli* has not been fully described.

The complex interactions between vaginal pH and *Lactobacillus* is suggested by studies evaluating the effect of estrogen replacement therapy on the vaginal microflora of postmenopausal women. In two studies, the frequency of vaginal lactobacilli increased among women receiving estrogen replacement therapy.[26,27] In a study following a group of women before and after estrogen replacement therapy, it was found that the mean vaginal pH after estrogen therapy in lactobacilli-positive subjects was 4.4 $\pm$ 0.4, compared with 5.2 $\pm$ 0.3 in lactobacilli-negative subjects (p = 0.02).[27] Prior to estrogen therapy, there was no difference in vaginal pH for women with or without lactobacilli, suggesting that both the presence of estrogen and lactobacilli are needed to achieve an optimal vaginal pH.

THE ROLE OF H_2O_2-PRODUCING *LACTOBACILLUS* IN THE VAGINA

In addition to producing acid, some species of lactobacilli produce hydrogen peroxide (H_2O_2).[28,29,30] H_2O_2 is toxic to a wide variety of microorganisms at levels of 0.75 to 5 μg/mL, a concentration attainable in the vaginal fluid of women with vaginal lactobacilli. H_2O_2 of microbial origin interacts with peroxidases produced by the host along with halide ion. The product of this reaction is a potent oxidant that is toxic to many bacteria.[31] Over the past 5 years a number of studies have been published that have evaluated the prevalence of H_2O_2-producing *Lactobacillus* in the vaginal flora of women (Table 14-4). In studies of women between the ages of 16 and 45, the prevalence of H_2O_2-producing *Lactobacillus* has varied from 42 to 74 percent.[23,32–34] Comparatively, premenarchal girls aged 1 to 6 are unlikely to be colonized with H_2O_2-producing lactobacilli, whereas postmenopausal women have an intermediate prevalence of H_2O_2-producing lactobacilli.[24,25]

The ability of H_2O_2-positive, but not H_2O_2-negative strains, of lactobacilli to kill HIV in vitro was first documented in 1991.[35] Likewise, the in vitro activity of H_2O_2-positive strains of lactobacilli against the bacterial vaginosis-associated microorganisms, *G. vaginalis* and *Bacteroides bivus*, was established by the same investigators.[30] The specific importance of H_2O_2 as the toxic molecule produce by lactobacilli was shown by demonstrating that the microbicidal activity of lactobacilli was destroyed when catalase, an enzyme that degrades H_2O_2, was added.[30] These data suggested that the H_2O_2 produced by lactobacilli may play an important role in acting as a natural microbicide within the vaginal ecosystem.

Four clinical studies conducted in populations of pregnant and nonpregnant women in the United States and Japan have shown that the prevalence of bacterial vaginosis in low (4 percent) among women colonized with H_2O_2-producing strains of lactobacilli (Ta-

Table 14-2. Frequency and Concentration of Anaerobic Microorganisms in the Vaginal Flora of 171 Pregnant Women, Stratified by Vaginal Flora Pattern (as Assessed by Gram Staining)[23]

	Frequency* among women with indicated pattern (cfu/mL†)			
Organism(s)	Normal (n = 85)	Intermediate (n = 47)	BV (n = 39)	p‡
Anaerobic gram-negative rods				
Any number	91 ($10^{4.3}$)	89 ($10^{5.0}$)	100 ($10^{6.0}$)	0.11
>10^5 cfu/mL	33 (—)	45 (—)	62 (—)	0.002
Prevotella bivia/disiens§				
Any number	61 ($10^{4.1}$)	68 ($10^{4.6}$)	77 ($10^{5.5}$)	0.11
>10^5 cfu/mL	15 (—)	21 (—)	39 (—)	0.005
Prevotella intermedia	7 ($10^{4.0}$)	13 ($10^{4.4}$)	10 ($10^{4.4}$)	0.55
Prevotella corporis/Bacteroides levii‖	21 ($10^{4.0}$)	28 ($10^{2.5}$)	39 ($10^{5.0}$)	0.05
Prevotella melaninogenica	4 ($10^{3.4}$)	6 ($10^{3.5}$)	5 ($10^{3.6}$)	0.75
Prevotella loeschii	2 (—)	0 (—)	5 (—)	0.29
Prevotella spp.	14 ($10^{3.4}$)	13 ($10^{4.2}$)	15 ($10^{3.6}$)	0.90
Porphyromonas asaccharolytica	31 ($10^{3.0}$)	40 ($10^{3.7}$)	36 ($10^{3.7}$)	0.44
Bacteroides fragilis group#	9 ($10^{3.5}$)	19 ($10^{3.6}$)	15 ($10^{3.7}$)	0.29
Bacteroides ureolyticus	36 ($10^{3.0}$)	40 ($10^{3.5}$)	59 ($10^{4.0}$)	0.01
Fusobacterium nucleatum	8 ($10^{3.3}$)	19 ($10^{2.9}$)	21 ($10^{3.8}$)	0.05
Mobiluncus spp.	5 (—)	13 (—)	28 (—)	0.004
Lactobacillus spp.	17 ($10^{5.2}$)	11 ($10^{5.3}$)	21 ($10^{6.0}$)	0.58
Clostridium spp.	7 (—)	2 (—)	15 (—)	0.11
Actinomyces spp.	6 ($10^{2.1}$)	13 ($10^{3.0}$)	15 ($10^{4.0}$)	0.09
Propionibacterium acnes	22 ($10^{4.2}$)	13 ($10^{4.0}$)	8 ($10^{4.1}$)	0.04
Bifidobacterium species	4 (—)	2 (—)		0.48
Peptostreptococcus (any)				
Any number	92 ($10^{4.2}$)	91 ($10^{4.9}$)	90 ($10^{5.3}$)	0.73
>10^5 cfu/mL	26 (—)	47 (—)	59 (—)	0.002
Peptostreptococcus prevotti	32 ($10^{3.0}$)	27 ($10^{4.0}$)	49 ($10^{5.0}$)	0.02
Peptostreptococcus tetradius				
Any number	21 ($10^{3.7}$)	36 ($10^{4.3}$)	41 ($10^{5.0}$)	0.05
>10^4 cfu/mL	6 (—)	19 (—)	28 (—)	0.007
Peptostreptococcus anaerobius	1 (—)	2 (—)	8 (—)	0.05
Peptostreptococcus magnus	53 ($10^{4.2}$)	34 ($10^{4.8}$)	49 ($10^{4.1}$)	0.67
Peptostreptococcus asaccharolyticus	88 ($10^{4.0}$)	66 ($10^{4.3}$)	72 ($10^{4.5}$)	0.14
Peptococcus niger	20 ($10^{2.7}$)	30 ($10^{3.2}$)	31 ($10^{2.8}$)	0.18
Veillonella species	14 ($10^{3.5}$)	11 ($10^{3.2}$)	13 ($10^{3.6}$)	0.83

*As a percentage.

†Mean number of cfu/mL of vaginal fluid for women who were culture-positive for the organisms. Mean concentrations were not calculated for *C. albicans* or for those organisms of which fewer than five isolates were obtained.

‡Mantel-Haenszel linear association (for frequencies).

§Includes 106 isolates designated *P. bivia* and 24 designated *P. disiens.*

‖Includes 32 isolates designated *P. corporis* and 14 designated *B. levii.*

#The 32 isolates from 23 women included *B. fragilis* (6), *B. bulgatus* (5), *B. ovatus* (7), *B. distasonis* (4), *B. uniformis* (2), *B. caccae* (3), and *B. multiacidus* (5).

ble 14-5). By comparison, approximately one-third of women who are vaginally colonized by *Lactobacillus* that do not produce H_2O_2 have bacterial vaginosis.[23,32–34] Surprisingly, not all women lacking *Lactobacillus* by culture have bacterial vaginosis. As shown in Table 14-5, 56 percent of 114 women having no lactobacilli by culture were found to have bacterial vaginosis. These data suggest that the absence of *Lactobacillus* is not synonymous with the presence of bacterial vaginosis. Further, the consistency of the findings among pregnant and nonpregnant women, and the similarity of the findings among women enrolled in the United States and Japan, suggests that the production of the H_2O_2 by lactobacilli may play a crucial role in protecting against the overgrowth of pathogens in the vagina.

The identity of the species of *Lactobacillus* of importance in the vagina has been the subject of several studies.[29,36,37] Older studies using conventional identification methods such as sugar fermentation and other biochemical assays have identified *Lactobacillus acidophilus* and *Lactobacillus fermentum* as the primary species of importance in the vagina. However, several investigators have since questioned the reliability and reproducibility of these methods for the species identification of *Lactobacillus*. The taxonomy of *Lactobacillus* underwent revision based on DNA homology.[38] When DNA homology methods were employed in evaluating the lactobacilli recovered from 27 healthy women, Giorgi et al., identified *Lactobacillus crispatus* and *Lactobacillus jensenii* as the predominant vaginal *Lactobacillus* species that colonize asymptomatic women.[37] This has been confirmed in additional cross-sectional studies using DNA-based methods to identify species of lactobacilli (Hillier, unpublished data).

OTHER ANTIMICROBIAL PRODUCTS PRODUCED BY LACTOBACILLI

Lactic acid is the principal component responsible for vaginal acidity. Both vaginal and cervical epithelial cells have the capacity to convert glycogen to glucose, which is further metabolized to lactic acid through cellular glycolysis. The resident glucose can be converted to lactic acid by lactic acid bacteria that may be present in the vaginal microflora as well. Therefore, vaginal acidity is de-

Table 14-3. A Comparison of the Vaginal Microflora of Prepubertal Girls, Women of Child-Bearing Age, and Postmenopausal Women[25]

Isolate	Percentage of women with indicated isolate (mean concentration)* Prepubertal (n = 19)	Pregnant (n = 132)	Postmenopausal (n = 73)
Facultative lactobacilli	11 (ND)	92 ($10^{6.8}$)	49 ($10^{5.7}$)
Gardnerella vaginalis	0	58 ($10^{6.4}$)	27 ($10^{5.3}$)
Coryneforms	42 ($10^{5.2}$)	78 ($10^{3.8}$)	58 ($10^{4.0}$)
Yeasts	0	26 (ND)	1 (ND)
Coliforms	32 ($10^{5.3}$)	16 ($10^{3.7}$)	41 ($10^{4.8}$)
Anaerobic Gram-negative rods	89 ($10^{6.9}$)	90 ($10^{4.5}$)	89 ($10^{4.1}$)
Prevotella bivia	11 (ND)	61 ($10^{4.3}$)	33 ($10^{3.8}$)
Fusobacterium spp.	26 ($10^{5.7}$)	12 ($10^{3.1}$)	7 (ND)
Peptostreptococcus	89 ($10^{6.9}$)	92 ($10^{4.5}$)	88 ($10^{4.5}$)
Staphylococci	68 ($10^{5.3}$)	86 ($10^{4.1}$)	59 ($10^{3.1}$)
Viridans streptococci	42 ($10^{6.1}$)	59 ($10^{4.4}$)	74 ($10^{4.2}$)
Group B *Streptococcus*	0	16 ($10^{4.2}$)	23 ($10^{5.6}$)
Enterococcus	32 (ND)	33 ($10^{5.2}$)	38 ($10^{4.4}$)
Mycoplasma hominis	0	23 ($10^{4.3}$)	0
Ureaplasma urealyticum	20 (ND)	82 ($10^{5.0}$)	13 ($10^{4.6}$)
Actinomyces	32 ($10^{6.8}$)	8 ($10^{2.5}$)	15 ($10^{5.1}$)

*Data in parentheses are cfu/g; mean concentration calculated for those categories in which five or more subjects were positive.

pendent on having adequate levels of estrogen as well as the presence of lactic acid-producing bacteria such as lactobacilli. Concentrations of lactobacilli are probably important determinants of vaginal pH as well. In prepubertal females, lactobacilli are generally present at concentrations of less than 100,000 colony forming CFU/G of vaginal fluid, whereas in women of reproductive age, the median concentration of lactobacilli in vaginal fluid is between 10 and 100 million CFU/g of vaginal fluid.[23,24] The increased concentration of lactic acid-producing bacteria in the vaginal fluid may result in a lower pH determining decreased susceptibility to infection.

Some authors have suggested that vaginal pH by itself is an important marker for bacterial pathogens and menopausal status. In 55 premenopausal patients who were evaluated and assessed for the presence of pathogens, Caillouette et al. described that women with normal flora or yeast colonization had statistically significantly lower vaginal pH levels to compared to women colonized by β-hemolytic streptococci, *G. vaginalis*, or mixed organisms.[39] Among postmenopausal women who had not received hormone replacement therapy, they reported that 55 of 64 women had vaginal pH levels above 4.5. By contrast 80 of 88 postmenopausal women who had received HRT had a vaginal pH of $\leq$4.5. Further, these investigators noted that vaginal pH was a marker for the serum estradiol level. Although the study was small, the authors suggested that use of vaginal pH assessment could be a powerful screening tool to assess estradiol levels and, in effect, to establish proper estrogen dosing.[39]

Some investigators have suggested that there is racial variation in vaginal pH among sexually active young women.[40] In one study of 273 sexually active adolescents in Denver, vaginal pH was measured through the use of pH paper. Women with lower genital tract infections such as bacterial vaginosis, were excluded. These authors reported that the mean vaginal pH among African-American women was 5.3 $\pm$ 0.7, whereas women of other races had a mean pH of 4.7 $\pm$ 0.6. Some recent studies have also documented that African-American women are less likely to be vaginally colonized by lactobacilli compared to Caucasian women.[41] This finding may explain the increased vaginal pH in African-American women, but studies are needed to clarify the association of race and vaginal pH.

The other antibacterial activities of human lactobacilli strains have been evaluated in a number of ways. Coconnier et al. recently evaluated the antibacterial properties of *L. acidophilus* using spent cultures supernatants.[42] They demonstrated that culture supernatants of human strains of *L. acidophilus* had in vitro activity against Gram-negative and -positive pathogens as well as enteroinvasive pathogens. They also tested the activity of these supernatants in a *Salmonella typhimurium* mouse model and demonstrated the in vivo protective effect of this *Lactobacillus* metabolite. These authors speculated that the antimicrobial activity produced by *L. acidophilus* could be owing to an unusual acidic amino acid present in a novel peptide agent.[42] Other investigators have reported that *Lactobacillus* does not inhibit common genital pathogens such as *G. vaginalis* and anaerobic Gram-negative rods.[43] However, the testing was performed at pH of 6.0 to 6.5, a vaginal pH not frequently found in estrogenized women. These investigators speculated that antagonistic properties between lactobacilli and other species in the ecosystem were probably owing to bacteriocins. Lactacin B is one such bacteriocin produced by *L. acidophilus*. Barefoot and Klaenhammer described bacteriocins produced by 52 vaginal strains of *L. acidophilus*.[44] These investigators reported that there was no broad spectrum inhibitory activity of *acidophilus* against other organisms when the effects of H_2O_2 and other organic acids were elim-

Table 14-4. Prevalence of H_2O_2-Producing Lactobacilli (LB+) in the Vaginal Flora of Different Populations of Women

Author	Year	Pregnant	Age	No. Women	Prevalence of LB+ (%)
Hillier[32]	1992	Yes	16–42	275	46
Hillier[23]	1993	Yes	16–40	170	42
Hawes[33]	1996	No	16–45	182	65
Puapermopoonsiri[34]	1996	Yes	21–37	118	74
Hill[24]	1995	No	1–6	19	11
Hillier[25]	1997	No	55–79	73	38

Table 14-5. The Prevalence of Bacterial Vaginosis among Women Colonized Vaginally by H_2O_2-Producing Lactobacilli (LB+) or Lactobacilli that Do Not Produce H_2O_2 (LB−)

Author	Year	Prevalence of Bacterial Vaginosis			
		LB+	LB−	No LB	*P*
Hillier[32]	1992	10/127 (8%)	29/86 (34%)	37/62 (60%)	<0.001
Hillier[23]	1993	2/71 (3%)	23/74 (31%)	14/25 (56%)	<0.001
Hawes[33]	1996	3/118 (3%)	10/40 (25%)	11/24 (46%)	<0.001
Puapermopoonsiri[34]	1996	3/87 (3%)	11/28 (39%)	2/3 (66%)	<0.001
Composite		18/403 (4%)	73/228 (32%)	64/114 (56%)	<0.001

*Compared to women having no vaginal lactobacilli (No LB).

inated. Although lactacin B was identified as a bacteriocin produced by *L. acidophilus*, its activity was limited to other lactobacilli. These investigators did not confirm earlier reports that a second bacteriocin called lactocidin was produced by lactobacilli.[45] This study by Barefoot and Klaenhammer confirms that production of bacteriocins occurs, but that the antagonism of lactobacilli against other pathogens is not owing to these products.

FLUCTUATIONS IN THE NORMAL VAGINAL FLORA

The normal vaginal flora is complex and dynamic. By definition, this means that fluctuations in the vaginal microbial ecosystem will occur day-to-day. One method to assess daily fluctuations in vaginal microflora is through the use of Gram-stained vaginal smears.[46] In one such study, Schwebke et al. used self-obtained vaginal smears from 18 women to assess vaginal flora patterns over a 30-day period.[47] They reported that among women with a *Lactobacillus*-predominant vaginal flora, two patterns were observed. The first pattern was one in which *Lactobacillus* persisted at high levels throughout the 30-day period. A second pattern consisted of intermittent predominant lactobacilli interspersed with days in which *Gardnerella* and *Bacteroides* morphotypes appeared along with normal or reduced numbers of *Lactobacillus* morphotypes. Three of seven women who initially had *Lactobacillus*-predominant flora achieved vaginal scores as high as 7 or 8, indicative of bacterial vaginosis, but these alterations persisted for only 1 to 2 days. They noted that the increase in *Gardnerella* and *Bacteriodes* morphotypes was most concentrated around the time of menses, but that there were sporadic variations that also occurred throughout the cycle for some women. These authors suggested that alterations in vaginal microflora around the time of menses may represent a "critical period" during which exogenous factors could tip the ecology balance in favor of bacterial vaginosis.[47]

A similar study assessing fluctuations in normal vaginal flora was published by Priestley et al.[48] In this study 26 subjects were followed over an 8-week period. Sampling was conducted two to seven times weekly and women completed diary cards reporting sexual and other behaviors. In addition, vaginal swabs were obtained for culture of *Candida*, *G. vaginalis*, anaerobes, *M. hominis*, and *U. urealyticum*. These authors reported that only four of the 26 subjects had normal vaginal microbiology throughout the study period. One woman who was not sexually active had bacterial vaginosis throughout the 8-week period of follow-up, and nine (35 percent) developed intermittent BV. Although some women developed symptoms during the study period, symptoms correlated very poorly with microbiologic findings. These authors concluded that bacterial vaginosis and candidiasis can occur intermittently at high frequencies and that acquisition of BV occurred more commonly among women having unprotected sex.[48]

A third study using vaginal smears to assess vaginal microflora over the menstrual cycle was conducted in 22 volunteers.[49] These authors reported that one-half of the women had normal flora throughout the cycle and an additional one-third had basically normal flora that transitioned to intermediate flora or bacterial vaginosis. As in the other studies, these authors reported that most of the changes occurred near the time of menses. Taken together these three studies, along with previously published studies using vaginal cultures to assess alterations in the vaginal microflora, suggest that the vaginal ecosystem is dynamic.[50–52] These studies all suggest that alterations in the vaginal microflora most frequently occur around the time of menses and following intercourse. One limitation of the published studies is that they are relatively small in size and short in duration.

Two longitudinal cohort studies have been published assessing the transitions in vaginal microflora in nonpregnant women. As noted in Chapter 42, similar studies have been published assessing the fluctuations in vaginal flora in pregnant women. One study was conducted in 163 women with paired cultures 4 months apart.[33] *Lactobacillus* cultures and assessment of H_2O_2 production was assessed at each of the two visits. As shown in Table 14-6, 79 percent of 107 women initially colonized by H_2O_2-producing *Lactobacillus* were persistently colonized by H_2O_2-producing strains 4 months later. By contrast fewer than one-half of women initially colonized by H_2O_2-negative strains of lactobacilli remained persistently colonized by those strains 4 months later. Finally, 40 percent of 20 women initially lacking lactobacilli remained negative for lactobacilli, whereas only 25 percent of women spontaneously acquired vaginal colonization by an H_2O_2-producing strain.

Another study assessing alterations in vaginal lactobacilli in a population of 60 commercial sex workers in Africa.[53] From these 60 women, 224 vaginal *Lactobacillus* culture results were obtained at baseline and follow-up visits. These authors calculated transition probabilities for changes in lactobacilli after 2 weeks of nonoxynol-9 or placebo use. These authors also found that H_2O_2-negative strains of lactobacilli were more likely to be lost than were H_2O_2-producing strains of lactobacilli whether women used the nonoxynol-9 or placebo gels. Women with H_2O_2-producing strains of *Lactobacillus* who used nonoxynol-9 were almost twice as likely to retain H_2O_2-producing strains compared to women who used placebos.[53] Taken together these data suggest that the amount of fluctuation in vaginal colonization by *Lactobacillus* and other organisms could relate to sexual behavior, use of intra-

Table 14-6. Correlation between Results of First and Second Vaginal *Lactobacillus* Cultures

Lactobacillus status at second visit	*Lactobacillus* status at baseline		
	None (n = 20)	H_2O_2− (n = 36)	H_2O_2+ (n = 107)
No lactobacilli	8 (40)	2 (22)	15 (14)
H_2O_2−	7 (35)	16 (44)	8 (7)
H_2O_2+	5 (25)	12 (33)	84 (79)

NOTE: Data are no. (%) of subjects. +, positive; −, negative.

vaginal products, hormonal status, menstruation, and the type of *Lactobacillus* initially colonizing the vagina.

EFFECT OF MENSES AND INTERCOURSE ON THE VAGINAL MICROFLORA

As noted in the preceding, longitudinal studies in which vaginal flora has been assessed using Gram strains, suggests that the vaginal microflora becomes less *Lactobacillus*-predominant during menses and intercourse, two times when vaginal pH is elevated owing to menstrual blood or semen. Adherence of vaginal isolates to exfoliated vaginal epithelial cells was assessed in 10 healthy sexually active young women over two menstrual cycles.[54] These authors reported that there was no significant difference in the adherence of *Lactobacillus* species, *G. vaginalis*, or *E. coli* to vaginal epithelial cells over the menstrual cycle. This suggested the alterations in the vaginal microflora observed over the menstrual cycle probably do not relate to changes in binding of organisms to epithelial cells that are hormonally related. However, our understanding of the mechanism by which lactobacilli from the human vagina bind to epithelial cells is not well understood. One study evaluating the binding of *Lactobacillus* to fibronectin found that binding was increased at pH 4.0 and many strains of lactobacilli were unable to bind at pH 7.2.[55] Therefore, some of the alterations in the vaginal microflora during the menstrual period may relate to the decreased capacity of lactobacilli to bind at higher vaginal pHs.

A large number of studies have evaluated the effects of various catamenial products on the vaginal microflora during menses. In one such study, the effect of tampon usage on the vaginal microflora of 35 healthy women was determined following the random assignments of these women to either tampon or sanitary napkins usage for three consecutive menstrual cycles.[56] These authors determined that colonization by coagulase negative staphylococci increased significantly among tampon users compared to napkin users, but the shifts in microflora occurred only during menstruation and not at other sampling times. A summary of two such studies are presented in Table 14-7. As shown, women were evaluated prior to menses and then on days 2 to 4 during menses. As shown, there was a trend towards decreased colonization by *Lactobacillus* species during menses compared to the premenstrual sample, although the numbers of women evaluated in these studies were to small to achieve statistical significance. In one study there was an increase in the prevalence of anaerobic Gram-negative rods during menses compared to the premenstrual sample.[57] However, in the second study no such increase in anaerobes was observed.[58] Both studies showed an increase in colonization by *E. coli* during menses, although it was statistically significant in only one of these.[57]

Table 14-7. Effect of Menses on the Vaginal Microflora

	Published studies			
	Larsen*		Onderdonk†	
Microorganism	−	+	−	+
GBS	16%	26%	NS	NS
Enterococcus	19%	52%	NS	NS
E. coli	13%	29%	37%	58%
Candida	16%	16%	NS	NS
Lactobacillus	87%	74%	91%	84%
G. vaginalis	26%	19%	13%	21%
Bacteroides	7%	23%	91%	84%
Staph aureus	0%	9%	NS	NS

*31 women: 20 tampons, 11 pad; day 2–3 menses.[57]
†18 women: All tampon users; day 4 menses.[58]
NS = Not specified.

Table 14-8. Effect of Sexual Intercourse on the Vaginal Flora

		Post intercourse	
Organism	Pre (%) $n = 33$	Next Am (%) $n = 33$	36 hours post (%) $n = 33$
Lactobacillus	94	100	97
H_2O_2+	79	76	76
G. vaginalis	58	36	38
Anaerobic Gram-negative rods	42	48	61
E. coli	18	64*	48*
Enterococcus	21	52*	39*
GBS	9	15	24

*Statistically different from baseline.
Ref: Hillier, Stamm, Hooten, unpublished. Adapted from data presented in ref 59.

The effect of sexual intercourse on the vaginal microflora has usually been evaluated in the context of evaluating how various contraceptive methods might impact the vaginal microbial ecosystem.[59] As shown in Table 14-8, vaginal intercourse appears to have little effect on the frequency of lactobacilli. However, there was a significant increase in vaginal colonization by both *Enterococcus* and *E. coli* following intercourse. There was also a trend toward increased colonization by group B *Streptococcus* following intercourse. These three groups of organisms colonize the perineum. It is likely that the act of heterosexual intercourse introduces these organisms into the vaginal ecosystem, and that the increased vaginal pH occurring during intercourse may increase survival of these organisms.

EFFECT OF NONOXYNOL-9 AND OTHER BIRTH CONTROL METHODS ON THE VAGINAL FLORA

Many young women use vaginal products including lubricants, contraceptives, antifungals, and douches. Each of these products can alter the vaginal ecosystem by changing vaginal pH, altering the vaginal fluid by direct dilution or by altering the capacity of organisms to bind to the vaginal epithelium. Nonoxynol-9 is the most commonly used vaginal contraceptive, and it is available in the form of gels, foams, suppositories, or creams. In vitro, nonoxynol-9 has activity against lactobacilli, but there are little data to suggest that routine use of nonoxynol-9 decreases colonization by *Lactobacillus*.[59–61] In one study women were evaluated prior to intercourse, the next morning following intercourse, and 24 hours later for alterations in the vaginal flora.[59] There were three groups of women, one of which used an nonoxynol-9 foam with a condom, one group who used spermicidal gel with a diaphragm and a third group who used oral contraceptives. In this study, the concentration and frequency of lactobacilli did not decrease following N-9 use. In another recent study conducted among commercial sex workers, use of nonoxynol-9 containing gel was actually associated with increased colonization by H_2O_2-producing lactobacilli compared to women using placebo gel.[53] As noted in the following, nonoxynol-9 is being evaluated as a topical microbicide in human and animal studies. During its evaluation in animal studies, nonoxynol-9 was shown to have no activity against lactobacilli in the monkey model.[61a] Nevertheless, decreases in colonization by lactobacilli have been reported in nine of 16 women using nonoxynol-9 gels in another study.[61b] Prophylactic use of a 3 percent nonoxynol gel during vaginal intercourse during a 6-month study did not result in an increased incidence of bacterial vaginosis, trichomoniasis, or yeast vaginitis, suggesting that routine use of nonoxynol-9 does not cause pathologic changes in the vaginal ecosystem.[62]

The effects of nonoxynol-9 contraceptives on the vaginal epithelium probably relate to exposure frequency and dosage. Use of sponges containing 1000 mg of nonoxynol-9 was associated with an increased frequency of genital ulcers, but daily application of a gel containing 52.5 mg of nonoxynol-9 did not result in epithelial disruption among commercial sex workers.[63,64] However, in another study evaluating suppositories containing 150 mg of nonoxynol-9, disruption of the vaginal or cervical epithelium occurred twice to four times as frequently when women used nonoxynol-9 one to four times daily as compared to women who used nonoxynol-9 suppositories every other day.[65] The effects of vaginal irritation on induction of inflammatory medicators, and their possible effect on the vaginal microflora has not been evaluated.

The effects of other birth control methods on the vaginal microflora are less well understood. As noted in Chapter 42, use of intrauterine contraceptive devices is associated with an increased incidence of bacterial vaginosis. However, studies published in the 1980s also suggest that women who use oral contraceptives or intrauterine contraceptive devices are more likely to have obligately anaerobic organisms colonizing the cervix compared to women using barrier methods of contraception.[66] In our experience, the vaginal microflora of women using oral contraceptives, barrier methods, or no contraception are remarkably similar after accounting for sexual and douching behavior.

THE EFFECT OF DOUCHE PRODUCTS AND "DRY-SEX" ON THE VAGINAL ECOSYSTEM

Douching is a common practice in women throughout the world. Douching may alter a woman's susceptibility to infection by altering the vaginal microflora, removing protective components from the vagina or cervix, or by promoting ascension of microorganisms from the lower to the upper reproductive tract. Douching is more frequent among low income women and ethnic minorities in the United States.[67] Routine douching for hygiene has been shown to double the risk of acquiring bacterial vaginosis.[33] A cross-sectional study of African women showed an increased prevalence of vaginal yeast among women who used douche products containing antiseptics.[68] In this study, women who douched using noncommercial preparations were 70 percent more likely to have HIV, whereas women douched with commercial antiseptics had a 40 percent decreased frequency of HIV.[68]

In one study evaluating the effects of a single use of a douche product on the vaginal microflora, Onderdonk reported that nonmedicated douches has a more transient effect on the vaginal microflora compared to those containing antimicrobial agents such as iodine.[1] However, he noted that even nonantiseptic douches had an effect on the vaginal microbial ecosystem and that persistent use could alter the microflora and collapse the capacity of the vaginal ecosystem to resist change. A better understanding of how different douche products effect young women's susceptibility to infection are urgently needed so that women can be counseled appropriately regarding the health risks associated with douching.

The thick, glycogen-rich vaginal epithelium is one of the primary structural defenses mechanisms of the female reproductive tract. In premenarchal girls and postmenopausal women, the lack of estrogen results in a thinning of the vaginal epithelium. There is a decreased cell division on the basal and parabasal levels of the vaginal epithelium.[69] In postmenopausal women elastic fibers of the lamina propria are replaced with nonelastic collagen. The decreased thickness of the epithelium, combined with loss of elastic structure, renders the vagina more susceptible to damage during sexual activity. In some cultures, the use of drying or astringent agents is common in order to heighten a sense of "tightness" during sex.[70] The practice of "dry sex" acts to remove the lubricating vaginal fluid and may increase the susceptibility of the genital tract to infection. Dryness during sex has been associated with pain during intercourse, which is linked to postcoital bleeding.[71] Postcoital bleeding increases the risk of male-to-female transmission of HIV three- to fivefold.[72,73] Whether the use of traditional vaginal agents for "dry sex" is linked to postcoital bleeding has not been studied extensively, but the use of these agents has been linked to increased HIV in some populations.[74]

THE EFFECT OF ANTIBIOTICS USED TO TREAT GENITAL INFECTIONS ON THE VAGINAL MICROFLORA

Antimicrobial agents used to treat nongenital and genital infections can adversely effect the vaginal microbial ecosystem. Lactobacilli are susceptible to beta lactam antibiotics such as amoxicillin as well as cephalosporins that are frequently used to treat genital tract infections.[75–77] By contrast doxycycline appears to be inactive against lactobacilli owing to the high prevalence of transposable tetracycline resistance genes in lactobacilli.[77] In some cases the activity of systemic or local antibiotics on the vaginal ecosystem is hard to predict because they have effects not only on lactobacilli but other organisms present within the same ecosystem. For example, ampicillin has activity against lactobacilli and its use initially leads to a decrease in vaginal colonization by lactobacilli among women with bacterial vaginosis (Table 14-9). However, because ampicillin presumably has activity against some of the other organisms present in the vagina that compete in that some ecosystem, ampicillin usage was found to have a net beneficial impact on vaginal colonization by lactobacilli 1 month after therapy.[78] Not surprisingly, antibiotics such as metronidazole, applied either topically or orally had no negative activity against lactobacilli, but lead to a net increase in vaginal colonization by this organism.[78] Clindamycin cream used for the treatment of bacterial vaginosis and applied locally lead to an initial decrease in colonization by lactobacilli but, like ampicillin, lead to an increase in *Lactobacillus* colonization 1 month post-therapy.

Agents used for the treatment of chlamydial cervicitis such as azithromycin and doxycycline had limited, if any, activity against *Lactobacillus* as might be expected.[78] Effect of short-term cephalosporin and quinolone use again lactobacilli has not been well investigated. However, use of antifungals for treatment of yeast vaginitis do not appear to adversely effect colonization by lactobacilli (see Table 14-9).

TOPICAL MICROBICIDES FOR PREVENTION OF STDS/HIV

Vaginal microbicides are products for vaginal administration of compounds that could be used to prevent the spread of sexually transmitted disease, including HIV.[6,7] The ideal vaginal microbicide would be safe and effective as well as tasteless, odorless, nontoxic, stable in most climates, and affordable. Topical microbicides would be used chronically with every act of intercourse. Topical microbicides differ substantially from traditional antimicrobics in that they would be expected to kill on contact much like disinfectants. Topical microbicides optimally have activity against common bacterial STDs, including chlamydia and gonorrhea, as well as *T. vaginalis* and viral STDs, including herpes and HIV.

A number of in vitro and clinical studies have been devised to

Table 14-9. Effect of Treatments for Vaginitis and Cervicitis on Vaginal Colonization by Lactobacilli (LB)

Treatment	No. of women		Visit		
			Pretreatment (%)	1 week (%)	>1 month (%)
Cervicitis					
Doxycycline	43	All LB	81	72	78
		LB+*	60	49	59
		LB−†	21	23	19
Azithromycin	17	All LB	65	ND‡	71
		LB−	53	ND‡	47
		LB−	24	ND‡	24
Bacterial vaginosis					
Metronidazole oral	27	All LB	41	81	91
		LB+	4	48	43
		LB−	37	48	61
Vaginal	18	All LB	67	83	94
		LB+	22	61	59
		LB−	56	67	71
Clindamycin vaginal	28	All LB	50	25	87
		LB+	29	11	57
		LB−	25	21	17
Ampicillin	32	All LB	47	47	61
		LB+	6	13	23
		LB−	41	41	45
Yeast vaginitis					
Fluconazole	8	All LB	100	100	100
		LB+	75	88	63
		LB−	38	13	38
Clotrimazole	7	All LB	100	86	100
		LB+	29	43	40
		LB−	71	43	60

*Women having H_2O_2-positive lactobacilli exclusively or in addition to H_2O_2-negative lactobacilli.
†Women having H_2O_2-negative lactobacilli exclusively or in addition to H_2O_2-positive lactobacilli.
‡ND = not determined.
Adapted from ref 78.

assess the activity of potential vaginal microbicides. The types of compounds being evaluated as topical microbicides include chemically modified proteins, bioengineered molecules, surfactants, acid buffering agents, and some natural products.[6,7] A number of antiseptics have activity against lactobacilli, and in vitro testing suggests that chronic use of these products may have an adverse effect on the vaginal microbial ecosystem.[79] Chlorhexidine gluconate at a concentration of 0.05 percent has been evaluated for its activity on the vaginal microflora in the monkey model. Use of chlorhexidine gluconate at that concentration had no apparent activity against colonization by lactobacilli, viridians streptococci, anaerobic Gram-negative rods or cocci.[80] By contrast, use of benzalkonium chloride in the same monkey model resulted in loss of lactobacilli and a decrease in colonization by anaerobic Gram-negative rods.[80] The use of chlorhexidine gluconate as a microbicide has been evaluated owing to its activity against HIV as well as *C. trachomatis*.[81,82]

Intravaginal dextrin sulfate has been assessed for its impact on the vaginal microflora in a limited number of patients and it was reported that there was no impact on vaginal colonization by *Lactobacillus* after introduction of a gel containing dextrin sulfate into the vagina.[83] However, a later publication by the same group of authors suggested that there may be a two-log reduction in the concentration of vaginal lactobacilli following introduction of dextrin sulfate into the vagina.[61]

Perhaps the most well investigated microbicide is nonoxynol-9. As noted in the preceding, nonoxynol-9 was reported to have activity against lactobacilli in vitro. However, a number of clinical studies have suggested that chronic use of nonoxynol-9 does not lead to a decrease in colonization by vaginal lactobacilli, but does lead to increase colonization by both *Enterococcus* and *E. coli*. However, some authors have concluded that nonoxynol-9 has a inappreciable protective effect against both gonorrhea and chlamydial infection, whereas others have argued that there are few data that suggest that nonoxynol-9 offers protection from infection.[84,85] The potential activity of nonoxynol-9 for prevention of STDs and HIV has been mixed and studies are still underway to evaluate whether use of nonoxynol-9 can decrease the spread of HIV.

ASSOCIATION BETWEEN THE VAGINAL MICROFLORA AND STDS

In addition to playing a role in determining whether microbial flora are conductive to the development of bacterial vaginosis, H_2O_2-producing lactobacilli may also confer protection on exposure to sexually transmitted disease. The concept that the vaginal microflora plays a role in resistance to gonorrhea was investigated widely in the 1970s. Kraus and Ellison initially speculated that the urethral flora of the male might protect against acquisition of gonorrhea.[86] In 1976, Shtibel published in vitro studies that suggested that *Neisseria gonorrhoeae* could be inhibited by some components of the normal microflora, including staphylococci and diphtheroids.[87] McBride et al. evaluated the qualitative and quantitative differences in *Lactobacillus* among women who were contacts of male partners with *N. gonorrhoeae* compared to 20 women attending the private practice clinic.[88] They reported that only one of 15 patients exposed to *N. gonorrhoeae* was vaginally colonized by *Lactobacillus*, and that this patient failed to become infected, whereas more than one-half of the private patients were vaginally colonized by *Lactobacillus*. Perhaps the best study to assess the role of vaginal microflora to susceptibility of infection in women was published by Saigh et al.[2] They reported that women vaginally lacking lactobacilli were less likely to become infected following sexual intercourse with a male infected by *N. gonorrhoeae* compared to women colonized by lactobacilli.

In a study of 127 women with H_2O_2-producing lactobacilli, 86 women with H_2O_2 negative lactobacilli and 62 without vaginal lactobacilli, women with H_2O_2-producing lactobacilli were the least likely to have *Chlamydia trachomatis, T. vaginalis,* and symptomatic *Candida*.[32] In another larger study from the Vaginal Infections and Prematurity cohort of pregnant women, the prevalence of *N. gonorrhoeae, C. trachomatis,* and *T. vaginalis* were significantly lower in women with predominant vaginal lactobacilli compared to women with reduced or no lactobacilli.[89] In a large cross-sectional study of rural Uganda women, similar trends were found.[4] Women with predominant vaginal lactobacilli had a decreased prevalence of gonorrhea, chlamydia, syphilis, and trichomoniasis.[4]

Little is understood about how lactobacilli could prevent these infections. However, in one recent study suggests that H_2O_2-producing lactobacilli directly inhibits the growth and catalase activity of *N. gonorrhoeae* by producing the combination of acid, peroxide, and protein inhibitor of catalase activity.[90]

THE RELATIONSHIP BETWEEN THE VAGINAL ECOSYSTEM AND HIV

The relationship between the vaginal microbial flora and susceptibility to HIV has recently been reviewed.[91] After a laboratory study was published showing that H_2O_2-producing lactobacilli were cidal to HIV, the first clinical data suggesting that the presence of vaginal lactobacilli may protect against heterosexual transmission of HIV was published by Cohen and coworkers.[3] In this study 144 commercial sex workers in Thailand, women with bacterial vaginosis and women lacking vaginal lactobacilli as assessed by Gram stain had an increased risk of HIV. In a recently published study of 4718 women in rural Uganda, a similar finding was observed.[4] Women with *Lactobacillus*-predominant vaginal flora as assessed by Gram-stained vaginal smears, had a 14 percent prevalence of HIV. Women with reduced *Lactobacillus* as assessed by vaginal smear, had a 40 percent increase in the seroprevalence of HIV.[3] Women with severe bacterial vaginosis had a 90 percent increased risk of HIV. Taking together, women with a vaginal flora characterized by lack of predominant vaginal lactobacilli had a 50 percent increase in HIV prevalence. A third cross-sectional study of women in Zimbabwe showed a strong correlation between absence of lactobacilli by gram stain and HIV seropositivity (odds ratio [OR] = 2.0, $p < 0.05$).[92] In a fourth cross-sectional study of 6667 pregnant women in Malawi, the prevalence of HIV increased from 12 percent in those with normal vaginal flora to 30 percent among those with severe bacterial vaginosis (OR = 2.5, 95 percent confidence interval), and seroconversion was higher among those with more markers for abnormal vaginal ecosystem.[5] Finally, one preliminary report from a longitudinal study reported by Martin and colleagues showed that female sex workers in Kenya who are vaginally colonized by *Lactobacillus* had a trend toward decreased incidence of both gonorrhea and HIV.[93]

Additional studies are needed to confirm the relationship between an altered vaginal microflora and acquisition of HIV. In addition, studies are urgently needed to better identify the biologic basis explaining why women with an altered vaginal system are at increased risk of HIV. Nevertheless, these five studies show a consistent link between increased prevalence of HIV and a decrease in the levels of vaginal lactobacilli.

THE NORMAL VAGINAL ECOLOGY OF PREGNANCY

The vaginal ecology of pregnant women does not differ substantially from that of nonpregnant women. However, studies conducted over the last decade have established that most of the organisms causing amniotic fluid infection or chorioamnionitis originate in the lower genital tract. In addition, recent studies have established that some organisms that are considered to be part of the normal vaginal microflora are associated with an increased risk of preterm or low birth weight delivery when they are present at high density concentrations in the vaginal fluid. Both Group B *Streptococcus* and *E. coli* have been linked with preterm or low birth weight delivery, and are known to directly invade the chorioamnion and cause chorioamnionitis.[94–98] Other vaginal microorganisms which are part of the normal flora, including those associated with bacterial vaginosis, have been linked to a increased risk of preterm birth, amniotic fluid infection, and chorioamnionitis, as discussed in Chapter 42. In contrast, high-density vaginal colonization by *Lactobacillus* species has been linked with a decreased risk of most adverse outcomes of pregnancy.[99–102] Thus, the constituents of the normal vaginal ecosystem play a role in establishing the risks of preterm or low birth weight delivery, amnionitis, chorioamnionitis, and postpartum infections during pregnancy. The vaginal microbial flora of pregnant women are described in Tables 14–1 and 14-2.

In the past it was widely postulated that during pregnancy the vaginal flora changed to become more *Lactobacillus*-predominant as gestational age increased. In one study, women were evaluated at different points in pregnancy and postpartum.[103] Different women were evaluated at each time period such that the study was a series of cross-sectional studies of women at different stages of pregnancy, rather than a longitudinal study of a defined group of pregnant women. They reported that 85 percent of women were positive for lactobacilli at 8 to 13 weeks of pregnancy, 97 percent were positive at 34 to 40 weeks' gestation, compared to only 64 percent at 6 weeks postpartum. However, since different groups of women were studied at different intervals, the changes in *Lactobacillus* frequency over pregnancy may have reflected differences in the patient population at the different study intervals. More recent data derived from a cohort of pregnant women evaluated at three time points (23 to 26, 30 to 33, and 34 to 36 weeks' gestation) has shown that the frequency of lactobacilli remains relatively constant over the second and third trimesters of pregnancy.[104]

Ethnicity has been reported to have an impact on the vaginal microflora of pregnant women. The vagina microflora of women of different ethnic groups was evaluated in the Vaginal Infections and Prematurity study that included over 13,000 women.[41] In this study, it was found that black women were more likely to be colonized by Group B *Streptococcus*, anaerobic Gram-negative rods, *M. hominis*, and *U. urealyticum* as compared with white or Hispanic women. Black women were also significantly more likely to have bacterial vaginosis, *T. vaginalis, C. trachomatis*, and *N. gonorrhoeae* compared to white women. In contrast, Hispanic women were more likely than white women to be colonized by Group B *Streptococcus*, but were otherwise very similar to white women with respect to the frequency of genital microorganisms. Asian women had comparatively lower frequency of all genital pathogens, and had significantly less *U. urealyticum* compared to white women.

In a smaller study from the United Kingdom, African and

Caribbean women were found to have higher levels of abnormal vaginal flora and bacterial vaginosis compared to white women, whereas Asian women were found to have lower frequencies of bacterial vaginosis and abnormal vaginal flora than white women.[101] It has been noted that when black and white women of similar incomes are compared, there is still a twofold or greater discrepancy in the rate of preterm delivery among black women.[41] Hispanic women, on the other hand, have one of the lowest rates of low birth weight in the United States, even though the Hispanic women included in studies have usually had modest income levels. Some authors have postulated that the disparity of preterm low birth weight among black versus white women may relate to the substantial ethnic differences in the rates of genital tract infections that may lead to preterm birth.[41]

As noted, sexual activity is thought to have an impact on the vaginal ecosystem. Frequency of sexual intercourse during pregnancy was evaluated in the Vaginal Infections and Prematurity Study.[105] These investigators interviewed women at 23 the 26 weeks' gestation, at two time periods in the third trimester and again at delivery. Not surprisingly, they found that 61 percent of the pregnant women reported having vaginal intercourse one or more times weekly in the second trimester of pregnancy, whereas only 28 percent of women reported this frequency of intercourse in the last month of pregnancy. These authors reported that women positive for *G. vaginalis* or *M. hominis* who engaged in frequent sexual intercourse during pregnancy were at higher risk of preterm delivery, compared to women colonized by these organisms who did not have frequent intercourse. The authors speculated that frequent sexual intercourse may introduce organisms from the vagina into the cervix that could begin the process of upper tract infection leading to preterm birth. What emerged from this study was that intercourse itself was not a risk factor for preterm birth, but rather frequent intercourse among women with certain lower genital tract infections.

Although many constituents of the normal flora have been linked with adverse outcomes of pregnancy, there is a substantial body of data that suggests that vaginal colonization by lactobacilli may protect against adverse outcomes of pregnancy. If lactobacilli protect against pregnancy complications, it is likely related to the concentration of lactobacilli in the vagina and whether they are the predominant members of the vaginal microflora. It may also be related to hydrogen peroxide production by lactobacilli. In 1988, Martius et al. reported that women having vaginal lactobacilli as detected by culture were less likely to deliver preterm compared to women lacking vaginal lactobacilli.[106] In 1991, Krohn et al. published a study of 211 women who were evaluated during preterm labor at less than 34 weeks' gestation. Quantitative vaginal cultures were performed from the women. She reported that those women having greater than 1077 colony forming units of facultative *Lactobacillus* per gram of vaginal fluid had a 40 percent reduction in the incidence of preterm birth (rate ratio = 0.6, 95 percent confidence interval, 0.4 to 0.9).[107] Holst performed a small case-control study of 87 women in which she reported that only 18 percent of women delivering preterm were vaginally colonized by H_2O_2-producing lactobacilli, compared to 78 percent of women delivering at term ($p < 0.001$).[100] By contrast, lactobacilli that did not produce hydrogen peroxide were recovered equally often from those delivering preterm and at term suggesting that H_2O_2-producing lactobacilli were more protective against pregnancy complications than strains that were negative for hydrogen peroxide.

In some cases, detection of lactobacilli in the vagina is performed by direct examination of a Gram-stained vaginal smear rather than by culture of vaginal fluid. In these cases, the *Lactobacillus* morphotypes are visualized and their relative quantity compared to small Gram-negative or Gram-variable rods is evaluated.[46] In one such study conducted in the United Kingdom, it was reported that women having *Lactobacillus*-predominant vaginal flora had a rate of pregnancy loss between 16 to 24 weeks' gestation of only 1 percent, compared to a 5 percent incidence among those with reduced lactobacilli, and an incidence of pregnancy loss of 7 percent in those women lacking vaginal lactobacilli.[101] A follow-up cross-sectional study compared the history of second trimester pregnancy loss among women with *Lactobacillus*-predominant flora, women with reduced lactobacilli, and bacterial vaginosis. The authors reported that women with *Lactobacillus*-predominant vaginal flora were significantly less likely to have a history of a second trimester pregnancy loss compared to women with reduced or no lactobacilli detected by direct Gram stain.[108] In the Vaginal Infections and Prematurity Study, women with *Lactobacillus* detected by culture or by vaginal Gram stain were significantly less likely to deliver preterm and low birth weight.[99] Another data analysis from this same group of women showed that these having vaginal *Lactobacillus* were also less likely to deliver an infant who was small for gestational age.[102]

The mechanism by which lactobacilli could protect against adverse outcomes of pregnancy probably relates to their effect against other genital pathogens, including those associated with bacterial vaginosis. It is clear that many women treated for bacterial vaginosis do not become recolonized with *Lactobacillus* that produce hydrogen peroxide.[78] Thus, additional strategies for reconstituting the vaginal microflora of women following treatment of bacterial vaginosis are needed in order to prevent these adverse outcomes of pregnancy.

MICROBIAL INTERACTIONS IN THE VAGINAL ECOSYSTEM

The complex nature of the microbial interactions in the vaginal ecosystem have been often studied but little understood. Perhaps the most frequently discussed example of this misunderstanding relates to the perception that vaginal lactobacilli decrease yeast vaginitis. In vitro studies demonstrate that *Candida albicans* is inhibited by culture supernatants of *Lactobacillus acidophilus*.[109] Further, H_2O_2-produced by lactobacilli in combination with myeloperoxidase also have antifungal effects.[110] *Lactobacillus acidophilus* in various forms have been used to treat yeast vaginitis.[111] Some investigators have gone so far as to suggest that ingestion of yogurt containing *Lactobacillus acidophilus* prevents recurrent Candida vaginitis.[112] Nevertheless, clinical studies of women with acute recurrent vulvovaginitis have demonstrated that women who have recurrent yeast vaginitis have the same frequency and concentration of *Lactobacillus* as women without recurrent infections.[113] This is in agreement with large studies conducted in pregnant women, which have confirmed that vaginal colonization by *Lactobacillus* is positively associated with yeast colonization.[104] The same observation was made by Hawes et al. in their longitudinal study showing that women who were vaginally colonized by lactobacilli had a somewhat increased risk of acquisition of yeast vaginitis compared to women without lactobacilli.[33] Nevertheless, many women who seek medical care for chronic vaginal symptoms report using *Lactobacillus*-containing products orally or vaginally to restore the vaginal microflora in the mistaken belief that this will prevent recurrent vaginitis.[114]

Our knowledge and understanding of the microbial interactions in the vagina and their effects on susceptibility to infection are clearly inadequate. Recent studies have suggested that the microbial interactions in the vagina are much more complex than has been appreciated in the past. For example, Pybus and Onderdonk have recently published data establishing that there is a commensal, symbiotic relationship between *Gardnerella vaginalis* and *Pre-*

votella bivia involving ammonia. *Gardnerella vaginalis* produces amino acids that are in turn utilized by *Prevotella bivia*. *Prevotella bivia* produces ammonia that stimulates the growth of *Gardnerella vaginalis*. The symbiosis between *Prevotella bivia* and *Gardnerella vaginalis* may explain the increased frequency of these organisms in bacterial vaginosis and the fact that they appear to increase in concert among women with abnormal vaginal flora.

Another example of microbial interactions in the vagina comes from Sturm, who described the inhibition of the chemotactic response by granulocytes by obligate anaerobes.[116] Coincubation of *G. vaginalis* with *Mobiluncus mulieris* or *Bacteroides ureolyticus* significantly reduced the chemotactic response of granulocytes compared to *G. vaginalis* alone. Culture filtrates of *Prophyromonas asaccharolytica* similarly decreased the chemotactic response of granulocytes to both *G. vaginalis* and *E. coli*.[116] These data were interpreted as showing that the presence of succinate-producing anaerobes in the vagina could inhibit chemotaxis of white blood cells, which may play a role in inhibiting the immune response to these pathogens. This mechanism of inhibition of immune function has been described in the abscess, where anaerobes play an etiologic role.[117]

Trichomonas vaginalis produces a number of cysteine proteases that are thought to play an important role in the virulence of this protozoan.[118] The cysteine proteases must be activated by disulfide reducing reagents in order to be functional. Alderete evaluated the vaginal washes from 48 patients and found vaginal fluid has a reducing environment adequate for activation for trichomonad proteases. Importantly, H_2O_2 reversibly neutralizes these trichomonad proteases. This could suggest that *Trichomonas vaginalis* may be carried as a commensal among women with H_2O_2-producing *Lactobacillus* because of its inability to express its primary virulence determinant. This is possible only if sufficient amounts of H_2O_2 are produced, but this observation does raise other questions. For example, could the increased prevalence of trichomoniasis in African-American women be related to a greater reducing level (higher pH) in the vaginal fluid, perhaps owing to lower levels of lactobacilli?

Another manner in which vaginal microorganisms may interact is through their adherence to vaginal epithelial cells, or their competition with other organisms for attachment sites. In a recent study by Boris et al., vaginal strains of *Lactobacillus* from healthy premenopausal women were shown to self-aggregate and adhere to vaginal epithelial cells, displacing other vaginal pathogens such as *Gardnerella vaginalis*.[119] The surface components of lactobacilli that were involved in self-aggregation appear to be proteins for *Lactobacillus gasseri* and lipoproteins for *Lactobacillus acidophilus* and *L. jensenii*. These authors suggested that the vaginal epithelial cell receptors for lactobacilli were glycolipids that act as the targets for the competition between lactobacilli and other pathogenic microbes. It is possible that lactobacilli in the vagina may protect the vaginal epithelium by self-aggregating and adhering to vaginal epithelial cells, or by interfering with colonization through binding of common receptors to those of potential pathogens.

BACTERIAL FLORA OF THE SIGMOID NEOVAGINA

A sigmoid neovagina is sometimes created for female patients who are congenitally missing a vagina and for male transsexuals in whom a vagina is desired. The sigmoid neovagina is created surgically from an isolated segment of the colorectum. One study describing the microflora of a sigmoid neovagina reported that the average pH of a neovagina is 8 (range 7 to 9), in contrast to a pH of 4.0 to 5.5 among estrogenized females.[120] This was not surprising given the lack of estrogen in these subjects. The microflora found in a neovagina is quite distinct from that of normal vagina in that the predominant species appear to be facultative Gram-negative rods such as *E. coli*, which are found in concentrations of 10^8 to 10^{11} CFU/g of discharge. Lactobacilli were recovered from 10 of the 15 patients, but usually at lower concentrations than are observed in natural vaginas. Not surprisingly, the anaerobic Gram-negative rods, usually found in the colon (*Bacteroides fragilis* group) were also common inhabitants of the neovagina. The authors concluded that the flora of the neovagina probably represents a remnant of the flora present at the time of its surgical formation of the vagina from the colorectum. Although these investigators attempted to isolate genital mycoplasmas, *Trichomonas vaginalis, Candida, Neisseria gonorrhoeae, and Chlamydial trachomatis,* none of these organisms were recovered.

References

1 Onderdonk AB et al: Quantitative and qualitative effects of douche preparations on vaginal microflora. *Obstet Gynecol* 80:333–338, 1992.

2 Saigh JH et al: Inhibition of *Neisseria gonorrhoeae* by aerobic and facultatively anaerobic components of the endocervical flora: Evidence for protective effect against infection. *Infect Immunol* 19:704–710, 1978.

3 Cohen CR et al: Bacterial vaginosis and HIV seroprevalence among female commercial sex workers in Chiang Mai, Thailand. *AIDS* 9: 1093–1097, 1995.

4 Sewankambo N et al: HIV-1 infection associated with abnormal vaginal flora morphology and bacterial vaginosis. *Lancet* 350:546–550, 1997.

5 Taha TE et al: Bacterial vaginosis and disturbances of vaginal flora: Association with increased acquisition of HIV. *AIDS* 12:1699–1706, 1998.

6 International Working Group on Vaginal Microbicides: Recommendations for the development of vaginal microbicides. *AIDS* 10:1–6, 1996.

7 Elias CJ, Coggins C: Female-controlled methods to prevent sexual transmission of HIV. *AIDS* 10 (Suppl 3):S43–S51, 1996.

8 Döderlein A: Die scheidensekretunterschugen. *Zentralbl Gynakol* 18: 10–14, 1894.

9 Larsen B, Galask RP: Vaginal microbial flora: Practical and theoretical relevance. *Obstet Gynecol* 55:1005–1135, 1980.

10 Harris JW, Brown JH: The bacterial content of the vagina and uterus on the fifth day of the normal puerperium. *Bull Johns Hopkins Hosp* 43:190–200, 1928.

11 Weinstein L: The bacterial flora of the human vagina. *Yale J Biol Med* 10:247–260, 1938.

12 Cruickshank R, Sharman A: The biology of the vagina in human subject. II. The bacterial flora and secretion of the vagina at various age periods and their relation to glycogen in the vaginal epithelium. *J Obstet Gyaecol Br Empire* 41:208–226, 1934.

13 Weinstein L, Howard JH: The effect of estrogenic hormone on the H-ion concentration and the bacterial content of the human vagina, with special emphasis to the Döderlein bacillus. *Am J Obstet Gynecol* 37:698–703, 1939.

14 Hite KE et al: A study of the bacterial flora of the normal and pathologic vagina and uterus. *Am J Obstet Gynecol* 53:233–238, 1947.

15 Gardner HL, Dukes CD: *Haemophilus vaginalis* vaginitis. *Am J Obstet Gynecol* 69:962–972, 1955.

16 Gorbach SL et al: Anaerobic microflora of the cervix in healthy women. *Am J Obstet Gynecol* 117:1053–1055, 1973.

17 Ohm MJ, Galask RP: Bacterial flora of the cervix from 100 prehysterectomy patients. *Am J Obstet Gynecol* 122:683–687, 1975.

18 Goplerud CP et al: Aerobic and anaerobic flora of the cervix during pregnancy and the puerperium. *Am J Obstet Gynecol* 126:858–868, 1976.

19 Hammerschlag MR et al: Anaerobic microflora of the vagina in children. *Am J Obstet Gynecol* 131:853–856, 1978.
20 Hunter CA, Long KR: A study of the microbiological flora of the vagina. *Am J Obstet Gynecol* 75:865–869, 1958.
21 Taylor-Robinson D, McCormack WM: The genital mycoplasmas. I. *N Engl J Med* 302:1003–1010, 1980.
22 Paavonen J et al: *Mycoplasma hominis* in nonspecific vaginitis. *Sex Transm Dis* 10:271–274, 1983.
23 Hillier SL et al: The normal vaginal flora, H_2O_2-producing lactobacilli, and bacterial vaginosis in pregnant women. *Clin Infect Dis* 16(Suppl 4):S273–281, 1993.
24 Hill GB et al: Anaerobes predominate among the vaginal microflora of prepubertal girls. *Clin Infect Dis* 20(Suppl 2):S269–270, 1995.
25 Hillier SL, Lau RJ: Vaginal microflora in postmenopausal women who have not received estrogen replacement therapy. *Clin Infect Dis* (Suppl 2):S123–126, 1997.
26 Larsen B et al: Effect of estrogen treatment on the genital tract flora of post-menopausal women. *Obstet Gynecol* 60:20–24, 1980.
27 Ginkel PD et al: The vaginal flora in postmenopausal women: The effect of estrogen replacement. *Infect Dis Obstet Gynecol* 1:94–97, 1993.
28 Whittenbury R: Hydrogen peroxide formation and catalase activity in the lactic acid bacteria. *J Gen Microbiol* 35:13–26, 1964.
29 Eschenbach DA et al: Prevalence of hydrogen peroxide-producing *Lactobacillus* species in normal women and women with bacterial vaginosis. *J Clin Microbiol* 27:251–256, 1989.
30 Klebanoff et al: Control of the microbial flora of the vagina by H_2O_2-generating lactobacilli. *J Infect Dis* 164:94–100, 1991.
31 Klebanoff SJ: Myeloperoxidase-medicated antimicrobial systems and their role in leukocyte function, in *Biochemistry of the phagocytic process,* Schultz J (ed). Amsterdam, North Holland, 1970, pp. 89–110.
32 Hillier SL et al: The relationship of hydrogen peroxide-producing lactobacilli to bacterial vaginosis and genital microflora in pregnant women. *Obstet Gynecol* 79:369–373, 1992.
33 Hawes SE et al: H_2O_2-producing lactobacilli and acquisition of vaginal infections. *J Infect Dis* 174:1058–1063, 1996.
34 Puapermpoonsiri S et al: Vaginal microflora associated with bacterial vaginosis in Japanese and Thai pregnant women. *Clin Infect Dis* 23: 748–752, 1996.
35 Klebanoff SJ, Coombs RW: Viricidal effect of *Lactobacillus acidophilus* on human immunodeficiency virus type-1: Possible role in heterosexual transmission. *J Exp Med* 174:289–292, 1991.
36 Ragosa M, Sharpe M: Species differentiation of human vaginal lactobacilli. *J Gen Microbiol* 23:197–201, 1960.
37 Giorgi A et al: Identification of vaginal lactobacilli from asymptomatic women. *Microbiologia* 10:377–384, 1987.
38 Johnson JL et al: Taxonomy of the *Lactobacillus acidophilus* group. *Int J Syst Bact* 30:53–68, 1980.
39 Caillouette JC et al: Vaginal pH as a marker for bacterial pathogens and menopausal status. *Am J Obstet Gynecol* 176:1270–1277, 1997.
40 Stevens-Simon C et al: Racial variation in vaginal pH among healthy sexually active adolescents. *Sex Transm Dis* 21:168–172, 1994.
41 Goldenberg RL et al: Bacterial colonization of the vagina during pregnancy in four ethnic groups. *Am J Obstet Gynecol* 174:1618–1621, 1996.
42 Coconnier MH et al: Antibacterial effect of the adhering human *Lactobacillus acidophilus* strain LB. *Antimicrob Agents Chemother* 41: 1046–1051, 1997.
43 Nagy E et al: Antibiosis between bacteria isolated from the vagina of women with and without signs of bacterial vaginosis. *APMIS* 99: 739–744, 1991.
44 Barefoot SF, Klaenhammer TR: Detection and activity of lactacin B, a bacteriocin produced by *Lactobacillus acidophilus. Appl Environ Microbiol* 45:1808–1815, 1983.
45 Upreti GC, Hinsdill RD: Production and mode of action of lactocin 27: Bacteriocin from a homofermentative *Lactobacillus. Antimicrob Agents Chemother* 7:139–145, 1975.
46 Nugent RP et al: Reliability of diagnosing bacterial vaginosis is improved by a standardized method of Gram stain interpretation. *J Clin Microbiol* 29:297–301, 1991.
47 Schwebke JR et al: The use of sequential self-obtained vaginal smears for detecting changes in the vaginal flora. *Sex Trans Dis* 24:236–239, 1997.
48 Priestley CJF et al: What is normal vaginal flora? *Genitourin Med* 73:23–28, 1997.
49 Keane FE et al: A longitudinal study of the vaginal flora over a menstrual cycle. *Int J STD AIDS* 8:489–494, 1997.
50 Brown WJ: Variations in the vaginal bacterial flora. *Ann Intern Med* 96:931–934, 1982.
51 Johnson SR et al: Qualitative and quantitative changes of the vaginal microbial flora during the menstrual cycle. *Am J Reprod Immunol Microbiol* 9:1–5, 1985.
52 Sautter RL, Brown WJ: Sequential vaginal cultures from normal young women. *J Clin Microbiol* 11:479–484, 1980.
53 Richardson BA et al: Use of nonoxynol-9 and changes in vaginal lactobacilli. *JID* 178:441–445, 1998.
54 Sobel JD et al: Adherence of bacteria to vaginal eipthelial cells at various times in the menstrual cycle. *Infect Immunol* 32:194–197, 1981.
55 Nagy E et al: Fibronectin binding of *Lactobacillus* species isolated from women with and without bacterial vaginosis. *J Med Microbiol* 37:38–42, 1992.
56 Chow AW, Barlett KH: Sequential assessment of vaginal microflora in healthy women randomly assigned to tampon or napkin use. *Rev Infect Dis* 11:S68–S73, 1989.
57 Larsen B, Galask RP: Vaginal microbial flora: Composition and influences of host physiology. *Ann Intern Med* 96:926–930, 1982.
58 Onderdonk AB et al: Quantitative assessment of vaginal microflora during use of tampons of various compositions. *Enviorn Microbiol* 53:2772–2778, 1987.
59 Hooton TM et al: *Escherichia coli* bacteriuria and contraceptive method. *JAMA* 265:64–69, 1991.
60 McGroarty JA et al: Hydrogen peroxide production by *Lactobacillus* species: Correlation with susceptibility to the spermicidal agent nonoxynol-9. *J Infect Dis* 165:1142–1144, 1992.
61 Hooton TM et al: Nonoxynol-9: Differential antibacterial activity and enhancement of bacterial adherence to vaginal epithelial cells. *J Infect Dis* 164:1216–1219, 1991.
61a Patton DL et al: Effects of nonoxynol-9 on vaginal microflora and chlamydial infection in a monkey model. *Sex Transm Dis* 23:461–464, 1996.
61b Rosenstein IJ et al: Effect of normal vaginal flora of three intravaginal microbicidal agents potentially active against human immunodeficiency virus type 1. *J Infect Dis* 177:1386–1390, 1998.
62 Barbone F et al: A follow-up study of contraception, sexual activity, and rates of trichomoniasis, candidiasis, and bacterial vaginosis. *Am J Obstet Gynecol* 163:510–514, 1990.
63 Kreiss J et al: Efficacy of nonoxynol-9 contraceptive sponge use in preventing heterosexual acquisition of HIV in Nairobi prostitutes. *JAMA* 268:477–482, 1992.
64 Martin HL et al: Safety of a nonoxynol-9 vaginal gel in Kenyan prostitutes: A randomized clinical trial. *Sex Transm Dis* 24:279–283, 1997.
65 Roddy RE et al: A dosing study of nonoxynol-9 and genital irritation. *Int J STD AIDS* 4:165–170, 1993.
66 Haukkamaa M et al: Bacterial flora of the cervix in women using different methods of contraception. *Am J Obstet Gynecol* 154:520–524, 1986.
67 Aral SO et al: Vaginal douching among women of reproductive age in the United States: 1988. *Am J Obstet Gynecol* 82:210–214, 1992.
68 Gresenquet G et al: HIV infection and vaginal douching in central Africa. *AIDS* 11:101–106, 1997.
69 Steger RW, Hafez ESE: Age-associated changes in the vagina, in *The human vagina,* Hafez ESE, Evans TN (eds). Amsterdam, Elsevier/North-Holland, 1978, pp. 95–106.
70 Runganga A et al: The use of herbal and other agents to enhance sexual experience. *Soc Sci Med* 35:1037–1042, 1992.
71 Padian NS et al: Risk factors for post-coital bleeding among women with or at risk for infection with human immunodeficiency virus. *J Infect Dis* 172:1084–1087, 1995.

72 Padian N et al: Female-to-male transmission of human immunodeficiency virus. *JAMA* 266:1664–1667, 1991.
73 Seidlin M et al: Heterosexual transmission of HIV in a cohort of couples in New York City. *AIDS* 7:1247–1254, 1993.
74 Dallabeta GA et al: Traditional vaginal agents use and association with HIV infection in Malawian women. *AIDS* 9:293–297, 1995.
75 Hamilton Miller JM, Shah S: Susceptibility patterns of vaginal lactobacilli to eleven oral antibiotics. *J Antimicrob Chemother* 33:1059–1060, 1994.
76 Herra CM et al: The in vitro susceptibilities of vaginal lactobacilli to four broad-spectrum antibiotics, as determined by the agar dilution and E test methods. *J Antimicrobial Chemother* 35:775–783, 1995.
77 Roberts MC, Hillier SL: Genetic basis of tetracycline resistance in urogenital bacteria. *Antimicrobiol Agents Chemother* 34:261–264, 1990.
78 Agnew KJ, Hillier SL: The effect of treatment regimens for vaginitis and cervicitis on vaginal colonization by lactobacilli. *Sex Transm Dis* 22:269–273, 1995.
79 Juliano C et al: In vitro antibacterial activity of antiseptics against vaginal lactobacilli. *Eur J Clin Microbiol* 11:1166–1169, 1992.
80 Patton DL et al: The vaginal microflora of pig-tailed macaques and the effects of chlorhexidine and benzalkonium on this ecosystem. *Sex Transm Dis* 23:489–493, 1996.
81 Harbison MA, Hammer SM: Inactivation of human immunodeficiency virus by Betadine products and chlorhexidine. *J Acq Immun Defic Synd* 2:16–20, 1989.
82 Lyons JM, Ito JI: Reducing the risk of *Chlamydia trachomatis* genital tract infection by evaluating the prophylactic potential of vaginally applied chemicals. *Clin Infect Dis* 21(Suppl 2):S174–177, 1995.
83 Stafford MK et al: A placebo-controlled, double-blind prospective study in healthy female volunteers of dextrin sulphate gel. *J Acq Immun Def Synd Hum Retrov* 14:213–218, 1997.
84 Cook RL, Rosenberg MJ: Do spermicides containing nonoxynol-9 prevent sexually transmitted infections? A meta-analysis. *Sex Transm Dis* 25:144–150, 1998.
85 Roddy RE et al: Microbicides, meta-analysis, and the N-9 question. Where's the research? *Sex Transm Dis* 25:151–153, 1998.
86 Kraus SJ, Ellison N: Resistance to gonorrhea possibly medicated by bacterial interference. *Appl Microbiol* 27:1014–1016, 1974.
87 Shitibel R: Inhibition of growth of *N. gonorrhoeae* by bacterial interference. *Can J Microbiol* 22:1430–1436, 1976.
88 McBride ME et al: Method for studying the role of indigenous cervical flora in colonization by *Neisseria gonorrhoeae*. *Br J Ven Dis* 54:386–393, 1978.
89 Hillier SL et al: Characteristics of three vaginal flora patterns assessed by gram stain among pregnant women. *Am J Obstet Gynecol* 166: 938–944, 1992.
90 Zheng H et al: Effects of H_2O_2-producing lactobacilli on *Neisseria gonorrhoeae* growth and catalase activity. *J Infect Dis* 170:1209–1215, 1994.
91 Hillier SL: The vaginal microbial ecosystem and resistance to HIV. *AIDS Res Human Retrovir* 14(Suppl 1):S1–S5, 1998.
92 Gwanzura L et al: Vaginal lactobacilli and HIV transmission in African women. Abstr. XI Intl. Conf. AIDS, No. C. 4509.
93 Martin H et al: Association between presence of vaginal lactobacilli and acquisition of HIV and STDs. Abstr. XI Intl. Conf. AIDS, No. C. 2692.
94 Alger LS et al: The association of *Chlamydia trachomatis, Neisseria gonorrhoeae*, and group B streptococci with preterm rupture of the membranes and pregnancy outcome. *Am J Obstet Gynecol* 159:397–404, 1988.
95 Regan JA et al: Colonization with group B streptococci in pregnancy and adverse outcome. *Am J Obstet Gynecol* 174:1354–1360, 1996.
96 Krohn MA et al: Vaginal colonization by *Escherichia coli* as a risk factor for very low birth weight delivery and other perinatal complications. *J Infect Dis* 175:606–610, 1997.
97 McDonald HM et al: Vaginal infection and preterm labour. *Br J Obstet Gynecol* 98:427–435, 1991.
98 Hillier SL et al: Microbial etiology and neonatal outcomes associated with chorioamnion infection. *Am J Obstet Gynecol* 165:955–960, 1991.
99 Hillier SL et al: Association between bacterial vaginosis and preterm delivery of a low-birth-weight infant. *N Engl J Med* 333:1737–1742, 1995.
100 Holst E et al: Bacterial vaginosis and vaginal microorganisms in idiopathic premature labor and association with pregnancy outcome. *J Clin Microbiol* 32:176–186, 1994.
101 Hay PE et al: Abnormal bacterial colonization of the genital tract and subsequent preterm delivery and late miscarriage. *Br Med J* 308:295–298, 1994.
102 Germain M et al: The genital flora in pregnancy and its association with intrauterine growth retardation. *J Clin Microbiol* 32:2162–2168, 1994.
103 Goplerud CP et al: Aerobic and anaerobic flora of the cervix during pregnancy and the puerperium. *Am J Obstet Gynecol* 126:858–868, 1976.
104 Cotch MF et al: Epidemiology and outcomes associated with moderate to heavy *Candida* colonization during pregnancy. *Am J Obstet Gynecol* 178:374–380, 1998.
105 Read JS, Klebanoff MA. Sexual intercourse during pregnancy and preterm delivery: Effects of vaginal microorganisms. *Am J Obstet Gynecol* 186:514–519, 1993.
106 Martius J et al: Relationships of vaginal *Lactobacillus* species, cervical *Chlamydia trachomatis*, and bacterial vaginosis to preterm birth. *Obstet Gynecol* 71:89–95, 1988.
107 Krohn MA et al: Vaginal *Bacteroides* species are associated with an increased rate of preterm delivery among women in preterm labor. *J Infect Dis* 164:88–93, 1991.
108 Lahli-Camp JM et al: Association of bacterial vaginosis with history of second trimester miscarriage. *Hum Reprod* 11:1575–1578, 1996.
109 Collins EB, Hardt P: Inhibition of *Candida albicans* by *Lactobacillus acidophilus*. *J Dairy Sci* 63:830–832, 1979.
110 Lehrer RI: Antifungal effects of peroxidase systems. *J Bacteriol* 99: 361–365, 1969.
111 Friedlander A et al: *Lactobacillus acidophilus* and vitamin B complex in the treatment of vaginal infection. *Panminerva Medica* 28:51–53, 1986.
112 Hilton E et al: Ingestion of yogurt containing *Lactobacillus acidophilus* as prophylaxis for candidal vaginitis. *Ann Int Med* 116:353–357, 1992.
113 Sobel JD, Chaim W: Vaginal microbiology of women with acute recurrent vulvovaginal candidiasis. *J Clin Microbiol* 34:2497–2499, 1996.
114 Nyirjesy P et al: Over-the-counter and alternative medicines in the treatment of chronic vaginal symptoms. *Obstet Gynecol* 90:50–53, 1997.
115 Pybus V, Onderdonk AB: Evidence for a commensal, symbiotic relationship between *Gardnerella vaginalis* and *Prevotella bivia* involving ammonia: Potential significance for bacterial vaginosis. *J Infect Dis* 175:406–413, 1997.
116 Sturm AW: Chemotaxis inhibition by *Gardnerella vaginalis* and succinate producing vaginal anaerobes: Composition of vaginal discharge associated with *G. vaginalis*. *Genitourin Med* 65:109–112, 1989.
117 Rotstein OD et al: Succinic acid, a metabolic by-product of *Bacteroides* species, inhibits polymorphonuclear leukocyte function. *Infect Immun* 48:402–405, 1985.
118 Alderete JF, Provenzano D: The vagina has reducing environment sufficient for activation of *Trichomonas vaginalis* cysteine proteinases. *Genitourin Med* 73:291–296, 1997.
119 Boris S, Barbes C: Adherence of human vaginal lactobacilli to vaginal epithelial cells and interaction with uropathogens. *Infect Immun* 66: 1985–1989, 1998.
120 Toon A et al: Bacterial flora of the sigmoid neovagina. *J Clin Microbiol* 31:3314–3316, 1993.

Chapter 15

Pathogenesis of sexually transmitted viral and bacterial infections

S.M. Lemon
P.F. Sparling

INTRODUCTION

Viruses and bacteria represent fundamentally different life forms. Although, like viruses, many bacterial species are obligate intracellular parasites, bacterial cells generally contain most if not all of the elements of an energy-generating system required for life (chlamydia are an exception). Viruses, on the other hand, derive their energy sources exclusively from those available within the host cell. Thus, viruses are usually much smaller and biochemically much simpler pathogens. Unlike bacteria, viruses generally contain only a single species of nucleic acid, either RNA or DNA, and follow biochemical processes of transcription and translation that are based on eucaryotic biology. Thus, viruses and bacteria differ fundamentally in their strategies for multiplication. Viruses dissociate into their constituent biochemical components following entry into host cells, then reassemble after replication of their genomes and expression of their protein components. Bacteria maintain their integrity throughout the multiplication cycle, even if they are obligate intracellular parasites.

Despite these basic differences in their biology, pathogenic viruses and bacteria have evolved remarkably similar strategies for invasion of and persistence within their human hosts. These common strategies include general mechanisms by which pathogens attach to and enter specific host cell types, cause disease, and attempt to evade host immune responses.

The production of disease by invading bacteria or viruses results ultimately from the tendency of these infectious agents to evolve toward species with enhanced capacity for survival within human populations. However, whether disease occurs or not is irrelevant to the infectious agent as long as its capacity to spread and persist among humans is maximized. This overriding Darwinian principle applies to all infectious agents and has resulted in many different microbial survival strategies. Some infectious agents have evolved strategies that maximize their replication within the infected host, such that large quantities of virus or bacteria may be shed acutely into the environment and result in new human infections. A good example of such a pathogen is influenza virus. More commonly, however, infectious agents have evolved strategies that result in long-term colonization or persistence of infection, usually with lesser quantities of virus or bacteria present within secretions or shed into the environment. Long-term persistence results in repetitive opportunities for transmission of the agent between individuals, ensuring its survival within human populations. Thus, the ability to establish persistent infection is a common and important determinant of the pathogenicity of many bacteria and viruses. This is particularly true for sexually transmitted pathogens.

CELLULAR ATTACHMENT AND ENTRY

Cellular attachment and penetration represent the first two steps in the replication cycle of any virus. Similarly, virtually all bacteria must attach to cells to cause infection. Attachment generally is achieved through a highly specific interaction between surface features of the infectious virion or bacterium, and one or more molecules expressed on the cell surface that represent the cellular receptor or accessory coreceptor molecules. In the case of viruses, binding to the cellular receptor molecule brings the virion into close proximity with the cell surface, but secondary interactions with coreceptors are often required to facilitate penetration of the cell by the virus. In the absence of either receptor or coreceptor, there is no infection. These interactions are important determinants of the pathogenicity of individual viruses and bacteria, as they often play an important role in determining cellular tropisms and host range.

The human immunodeficiency virus type 1 (HIV-1) represents a good example of such specific interactions among sexually transmitted viruses. HIV-1 usually initiates infection of certain lymphocyte subsets, monocytes, and macrophages via binding of its surface envelope glycoprotein (env) with the cellular CD4 molecule. Although this interaction is generally necessary for infection of a cell by HIV-1, it is not sufficient, as further interactions between the virus and additional surface molecules are essential for viral penetration. T-cell adapted laboratory strains of HIV-1 require a seven-transmembrane, G protein-coupled receptor, fusin or CXCR4, to mediate penetration.[1] Fusin enables the env protein of HIV-1 to mediate cell fusion, and in CD4-negative cells it can also serve as a primary receptor for these strains of HIV-1.[2] In the case of nonsyncytium-inducing virus strains that have a predilection to infect monocyte/macrophages, the viral coreceptor is the cellular beta chemokine receptor, CC-CKR-5.[3,4] These molecular interactions have important clinical consequences. Caucasian individuals who are homozygous for a 32-basepair deletion that abrogates expression of functional CC-CKR-5 appear to be resistant to infection with macrophage-tropic or dual-tropic strains of HIV-1.[5] This mutant allele is present with a high frequency in Caucasian populations, but absent in the black populations of Western and Central Africa. Population-based studies have also shown that the frequency of heterozygotes is 35 percent lower among HIV-1 infected persons than in the general population, suggesting that persons with a single mutant allele have quantitatively lower expression of CC-CKR-5 leading to relative resistance against the infection.

There are numerous other examples where specific interactions of viruses with their receptors and accessory coreceptor molecules play an important role in defining the host range and thus pathogenicity of viruses. For many viruses, however, the identity of cellular receptor is not known. In other cases, the cellular receptor may be expressed in a ubiquitous fashion, and therefore plays little or no role in determining the types of cells that can be infected with the virus. This may be the case with human cytomegalovirus, as its surface glycoprotein B is capable of interacting with surface heparin sulfate proteoglycans from a wide variety of cell types.[6] Similarly, herpes simplex virus (HSV) is able to infect a wide variety of different cell types. The envelope glycoprotein D of HSV binds directly to a member of the tumor necrosis factor receptor superfamily. The expression of this protein in chinese hamster ovary cells (one of few cell types resistant to HSV penetration and infection) renders these cells permissive for infection.[7]

In the case of sexually transmitted bacteria, tissue and species tropisms are also determined, at least in part, by the specificity of interactions between attachment ligands and host receptors. For example, gonococcal pili initiate attachment but the appropriate receptor is found only on human cells.[8] Although a variety of other factors undoubtedly contribute to host specificity (e.g., gonococci can only use human transferrin as an obligate iron source), ligand–receptor interactions in attachment are crucial. Some bacteria use multiple attachment ligands for binding to host cells; for example, gonococci also use opacity (Opa) proteins and probably Lipooligosaccharide (LOS) to bind tightly to host cells (see Chap. 31). High-frequency phase and antigenic variation of attachment ligands may prepare the bacterium for attachment to different cells (which may have different receptor specificities), both on different organs in the same person, and on the same tissues in different persons.[2–18] At least, this is the inferred basis for the very rapid (1–2 days) in vivo selection of different pili and opacity proteins that has been noted during experimental gonococcal infection of male volunteers.[19,20] These variants emerge too quickly for *de novo* immune responses to select such variants.

Many bacteria also invade host epithelial cells. Such bacteria include supposedly extracellular pathogens such as the gonococcus.[21,23] Others apparently do not invade cells, but slip between cells during systemic infection. *T. pallidum* is an example of the latter. Mechanisms are unclear in both pathogens, especially *T. pallidum*. Recent work suggests there are several coordinated steps involved in invasion of epithelial cells by gonococci, including expression of a particular Opa variant; a switch from the piliated to a nonpiliated state; and a switch from a sialylated LOS to nonsialylated LOS.[22,23] With the apparent assistance of porin protein, the epithelial cell membrane is functionally penetrated, and at least a measure of intracellular growth ensues before gonococci egress from the basal surface, gaining access to the subepithelial space and to the bloodstream.[21]

OTHER DETERMINANTS OF TISSUE TROPISM

In addition to specific receptor interactions, other features of cellular physiology may define the host range and tropisms of viruses as well as bacteria. Although they are known to exist, in many cases, the specific nature of these cellular "host factors" remain poorly defined. In the case of DNA viruses, it is likely that in many cases such host factors are differentiation-specific cellular transcription factors. This is where the general dependence of viruses on eucaryotic regulatory mechanisms becomes very important, as viruses may contain tissue-specific promoter-enhancer elements.[25,26] For example, human papillomaviruses (HPVs) replicate only within suprabasal cells of the epithelium. These viruses cannot be propagated in conventional cell cultures, reflecting the absence of differentiated cellular function(s) required for their replication. In vivo, the expression of RNA transcripts from the DNA genomes of HPV type 16 and 18 (HPV16 and HPV18) is generally restricted to differentiated suprabasal cells, and there is little evidence that these DNAs are transcriptionally active within undifferentiated basal cells. This distribution matches the tissue distribution of the differentiation-specific transcriptional activator Epoc-1/Skn-1a, and it has been shown that this transactivator specifically stimulates the E6/E7 promoters of HPV16 and HPV18.[27] Transient transfection assays and DNA-binding studies similarly indicate that Skn-1a also specifically transactivates the viral transcriptional control region of HPV1a.[28] This positive interplay between differentiation-dependent, epidermis-specific transactivators and viral enhancer elements is likely to play an important role in restricting the replication of HPVs to differentiated epithelial cells.

Similarly, the liver-specific tropism of human hepatitis B virus (HBV) may be related at least in part to a requirement for liver-specific transcriptional transactivators. Candidate transcriptional factors include hepatic nuclear factor 3 (hnf-3) and the CCAAT/enhancer binding protein (C/EBP). These have been shown to bind to, and in the case of C/EBP transactivate, the HBV enhancer element.[29,30] In the case of HBV, however, it is likely that cellular receptor interactions also play a role in restricting the replication of the virus, since the HBV enhancer element is very active in rat hepatoma cells that do not otherwise support replication of the virus.[31] Thus, there may be both receptor restriction and postreceptor–penetration restrictions on the ability of this virus to replicate in any particular cell type. Liver cells do not maintain their differentiated functions for long periods of time in tissue culture systems, and this is why HBV cannot be grown in any type of continuous cell culture in vitro. Hepatitis C virus (HCV) also appears to be highly hepatotropic. Unlike HBV and HPV, however, HCV is a positive-strand RNA virus and does not replicate its genome via a DNA intermediate (see Chap. 26). Host cell-specific factors clearly exist for these types of viruses and they contribute to their specific cell tropisms. However, they have never been satisfactorily characterized.

Some bacterial cell tropisms may have similar underlying mechanisms. Recently, *Haemophilus ducreyi* were found to grow preferentially in the deepest cell layers of the subepithelial dermis. In addition, chlamydia are requisite intracellular pathogens because they cannot synthesize their own ATP. As a consequence, they have evolved to scavenge intracellular mitochondrial supplies of ATP. Although there is no evidence that chlamydial tissue tropisms are driven by cellular differences in availability of energy, it is possible that this may contribute to the apparent preference of chlamydia for mucosal epithelium.

MECHANISMS OF DISEASE PRODUCTION

DIRECT VERSUS IMMUNOPATHOLOGIC EFFECTS ON THE INTEGRITY OF TISSUES

As indicated in the preceding, cellular tropism and host range are important determinants of the pathogenicity of both viruses and bacteria. Equally important, however, is the impact of the virus or bacteria on the biology of the infected cell. At the simplest level, infection of a cell by a virus or bacterium may lead to cell death. In the case of viruses, this may result from one or more specific mechanisms. Many viruses express specific proteins that have as their major function the induction of a blockade in normal host cell metabolism (cellular translation and transcription) such that the metabolic machinery of the cell is subverted preferentially to viral replication. For obvious reasons, the expression of such proteins is usually highly toxic to the cell. Cellular destruction or "direct cytopathic effect" is considered to be responsible for the disease manifestations of many lytic viruses, including, for example, herpes simplex virus (HSV). On the other hand, many cells may respond to the presence of an invading virus by the induction of apoptosis and the initiation of programmed cell death. Some viruses appear to have evolved mechanisms to prevent or delay apoptosis, thus potentially prolonging productive infection and maximizing replication. For example, recent work has shown that HSV-1 induces apoptosis at multiple metabolic checkpoints, but has also evolved mechanisms to block apoptosis at each point.[32] The inhibition of apoptosis by HSV-1 also prevents apoptosis induced by virus-specific cytotoxic T lymphocytes, thereby conferring on the infected cell a certain measure of resistance to the host's cell-mediated immune responses.[33]

However, many viruses are not intrinsically cytopathic. HBV is a prime example, as many infected HBsAg carriers are asymptomatic and without overt evidence of active liver disease. Despite this, such carriers may be very infectious, with a high titer of virus in their blood, semen, saliva, and genital secretions (see Chap. 26). Available data suggest that the presence or absence of liver disease is largely determined by the immunologic response to the virus.[34] Thus, chronic hepatitis B results from a relatively vigorous but unsuccessful attempt on the part of the host to eliminate the infection. HLA-restricted, CD8-positive lymphocyte responses play a critical role in this process, initiating an inflammatory cascade that involves the elaboration of soluble cytokines, including interferon-γ, and the recruitment of other types of inflammatory cells to the liver. In some instances, this immunologic response ultimately results in elimination of the infection. However, in many HBsAg carriers, these responses result in the immune destruction of hepatocytes and the activation of stellate cells that produce an abnormal matrix, the hallmark of cirrhosis. Oxidative stress accompanies this process and may lead to mutations in cellular DNA that result in the malignant transformation of hepatocytes. Thus, chronic liver inflammation and the occurrence of hepatocellular carcinoma reflect the immune response to the virus, rather than specific virus effects. Similar indirect mechanisms may contribute to the progressive immune destruction of infected CD4-positive lymphocytes in patients with HIV-1 infection.

Some bacterial disease processes may also be owing largely to immunopathologic responses. For instance, there is substantial evidence that complications of genital chlamydia infections (salpingitis, Reiter's syndrome) are correlated with and may be owing to stimulation of antibodies against a heat-shock protein (hsp60).[35,36] In principle, such antibodies can crossreact with human homologs, which are antigenically similar to chlamydia hsp60. Further evidence for an immune mechanism underlying tissue damage in chlamydia infections is the association of salpingitis with particular HLA haplotypes in primates and women.[37,38] Pathology associated with *T. pallidum* infections may also be owing to immune mechanisms. The paucity of organisms in spinal cord samples from patients with tabes dorsales suggests a possible immunopathogenic process. In experimental inoculations of humans, gummas occurred only in those subjects who had a history of earlier syphilis, strongly suggesting that hypersensivity contributed to the development of the granulomatous lesions.[39]

In contrast, gonococcal tissue damage appears to be caused by the direct toxic effects of lipid A and peptidoglycan fragments, although each of these endotoxins triggers a complex cascade of inflammatory mediators, including cytokines, which are integral to normal host immune defenses such as interleukin-1, tumor necrosis factor (TNF), and others.[40,41] However, this is not immunopathology in the usual sense of the word. Cytokines and chemokines may also play important roles in viral infections. For example, the HSV-1 envelope glycoprotein D inhibits the interaction of LIGHT, a new member of the TNF family, with the herpes virus entry mediator, which is an orphan member of the TNF receptor family.[7,42] LIGHT may interfere with the ability of HSV-1 to enter cells, whereas the binding of glycoprotein D to this receptor seems likely to alter normal signal transduction processes. This is clearly the case with HIV-1, as the replication of this virus is significantly influenced by a complex network of inhibitory and stimulatory cytokines and chemokines.[43] Macrophage-tropic strains of HIV-1 induce a signal when the HIV env glycoprotein binds to the CCR5 chemokine receptor (see the preceding).[44] This signal may promote the replication of the virus by activating the infected cell, increasing the number of infected cells by induced chemotaxis of activated CD4-positive cells to the site of virus replication.

PRODUCTION OF TOXINS BY BACTERIA AND VIRUSES

Despite similarities in mechanisms of disease production by viruses and bacteria, there are important differences. The elaboration of extracellular toxins plays an important role in the pathogenesis of many bacterial infections, both purulent and nonpurulent. *H. ducreyi* is a prime example, since it produces two cytotoxins, which probably are crucial to the tissue-destructive, ulcer-generating pathology that characterizes chancroid.[45,46] In contrast, virus infections generally have not been associated with production of specific toxins. Recently, however, the nonstructural glycoprotein 4 (NSP4) of rotavirus has been shown to induce diarrhea in mice in an age- and dose-dependent fashion.[47] Rotavirus NSP4 enhances chloride secretion through a calcium-dependent signal transduction pathway, and thus it acts as a true enterotoxin.

ALTERED CELLULAR GROWTH AND DIFFERENTIATION

Some viruses are capable of altering differentiated cellular functions, resulting in the production of disease by mechanisms that do not exist among bacteria. A prime example is the altered cellular growth that follows infections by molluscum contagiosum virus (MCV), leading to the distinctive cutaneous lesions of molluscum. A more extreme example is the proliferation of epithelial cells that is induced by infection with HPVs. HPV-related epithelial malignancies and cellular transformation appear to be related to the expression of two specific HPV proteins, the E6 and E7 oncoproteins, by high-risk HPV subtypes.[48] The Kaposi's sarcoma-associated herpesvirus (KSHV) also expresses several transforming proteins. When expressed in rodent fibroblasts, the KSHV K1 gene product results in deregulation of cell growth, with changes in the cellular morphology that are indicative of transformation.[49] Similarly, the KSHV K9 protein is an oncogene which inhibits the interferon signaling pathway and which is capable of transforming cells such that they grow to form colonies in soft agar.[50]

On the other hand, the altered cell growth that results in the hepatocellular cancer that complicates chronic hepatitis C is likely to have an alternative explanation. Since HCV is an RNA virus that does not replicate within the nucleus but only the cytoplasm of infected hepatocytes, it is likely that the root cause of these tumors is chronic inflammation, as is the case in chronic hepatitis B.[34] Nonetheless, at least two HCV proteins have been suggested to have cellular transforming activities.[51,52] The biological significance of these data remain in question.

Finally, in the case of viruses, disease may also be caused by destruction of specific subsets of cells that express essential and highly specific differentiated functions. A classic example is the development of the acquired immunodeficiency syndrome following HIV-1 mediated depletion of the CD4 lymphocyte population.

EVASION OF HOST IMMUNE RESPONSES

Persistence of an infecting agent almost always involves a mechanism to evade or otherwise foil the host immune response. In the case of viruses, this involves three general strategies: latency, antigenic variation, and specific inhibition of immune effector mechanisms. Bacteria use fundamentally similar strategies, with the exception of latency that, strictly defined, is specific to viruses.

LATENT INFECTIONS

The induction of latent infection by herpesviruses such as HSV represents a uniquely effective mechanism of evading the host immune response. During latent infection only a very small number of viral proteins are actively expressed, providing few targets for the immune system. Major structural antigens of the virus are not synthesized, and there is no production of infectious virus. There is no cytopathic effect, and the viral genome is maintained through cell divisions largely by the cellular metabolic machinery. However, latency is periodically reversed, with reactivation of the infection leading to the production of infectious virions. Thus, latent infections clearly contribute to the overall survival of herpesviruses within human populations. This general strategy is not available to bacteria (and most other types of viruses) because of fundamental differences in replication strategies.

However, certain bacteria can persist for prolonged periods with little evident replication: mycobacteria are one example, and *T. pallidum* may be another. *T. pallidum* can be reactivated by corticosteriod therapy after a long period of dormancy in rabbits, and a similar phenomenon may underlie the long periods in which there is no disease activity (clinical "latency") before the onset of late syphilis. There also is some evidence that chlamydia can persist in eukaryotic cells without overt replication and release of infectious particles, which is latency by most definitions.[27] Unlike latent viral infection, however, there is little evidence that latency of chlamydia is clinically important.

ANTIGENIC VARIATION

Antigenic variation is a second and generally more common strategy by which infectious agents foster persistence. Mechanisms exist among all classes of infectious agents, viruses, prokaryotes, and eukaryotes, for altering the sequence of key epitopes of the pathogen that are recognized by both cellular and humoral arms of the host immune system.

The simplest mechanism for antigenic variation is that which is found among the RNA viruses and lentiviruses including HIV-1. The polymerases expressed by these viruses, whether RNA-dependent RNA polymerase or reverse transcriptase, lack the 3′–5′ exonuclease activity associated with the proof-reading function of DNA polymerases. This results in a high error rate during transcription of the viral genome, leading to impressive mutational rates among these viruses. The extent to which antigenic variation actually occurs is dependent on the ability of the viral protein to sustain mutations without loss of critical function, and the strength and type of selective forces applied by the host immune response.

Prime examples of this phenomenon include antigenic variation within hypervariable regions of the envelope glycoproteins of HIV-1 and HCV. Antigenic variation in the V3 loop of HIV reduces the ability of pre-existing antibodies to bind to the newly mutated peptide sequences in the loop. Thus, these mutations cause a reduction in the ability of these antibodies to neutralize virus infectivity.[54] Thus, variation in the envelope glycoproteins is likely to contribute to B cell escape and viral persistence. Cytotoxic T-cell escape may follow a mutational event within short sequential peptide sequences that serve as T-cell epitopes. Similar mechanisms account for the extensive "quasispecies" variation seen with many persistent RNA viruses such as HCV, and also result in the rapid emergence of resistance of HIV-1 to reverse transcriptase or protease inhibitors. The best defense against the latter phenomenon is to severely limit viral replication with a cocktail of antiviral drugs, as replication of the virus and transcription of its genome are essential to the generation of new quasispecies variants.

Antigenic variation is also common in many pathogenic bacteria. Among the sexually transmitted bacteria, the gonococcus is the most completely studied. The dominant theme that emerges from these studies is the complexity and elegance of the strategies for rapid alteration in expression of cell surface antigens (on–off), and for variation in the primary sequence (and thus antigenicity) of many of these antigens. Pili and opacity proteins each undergo phase variation (expression alternating with nonexpression) and antigenic variation (variations in antigenic structure of the expressed protein) at rates approximating 1×10^{-3} to 1×10^{-4} per cell per generation (Figs. 15-1 and 15-2). Interestingly, these rates closely approximate the frequency of base misincorporation by the RNA polymerases of RNA viruses. In the case of *pili*, the fundamental mechanism is crudely analogous to those used in antibody variations. Recombination between one of many variant incomplete *pil* loci (*pilS*, for silent) and a pilin expression locus, *pilE* results either in a different pilin protein (antigenic variation), or a faulty one that cannot be secreted and assembled into a pilus (phase variation).[9–11] *Opa* proteins vary by a totally different mechanism involving slipped-strand mispairing of a pentameric CTCTT repeat element in the opa gene, leading to translational frame shifts. An *opa* gene is "off" when out of translational frame, and "on" when in frame. Since there are about 12 complete *opa* genes, each of which is slightly different, the random high frequency shifting in each *opa* gene results in a constantly shifting mosaic of expressed Opa proteins.[12,13] Similar mechanisms underlie

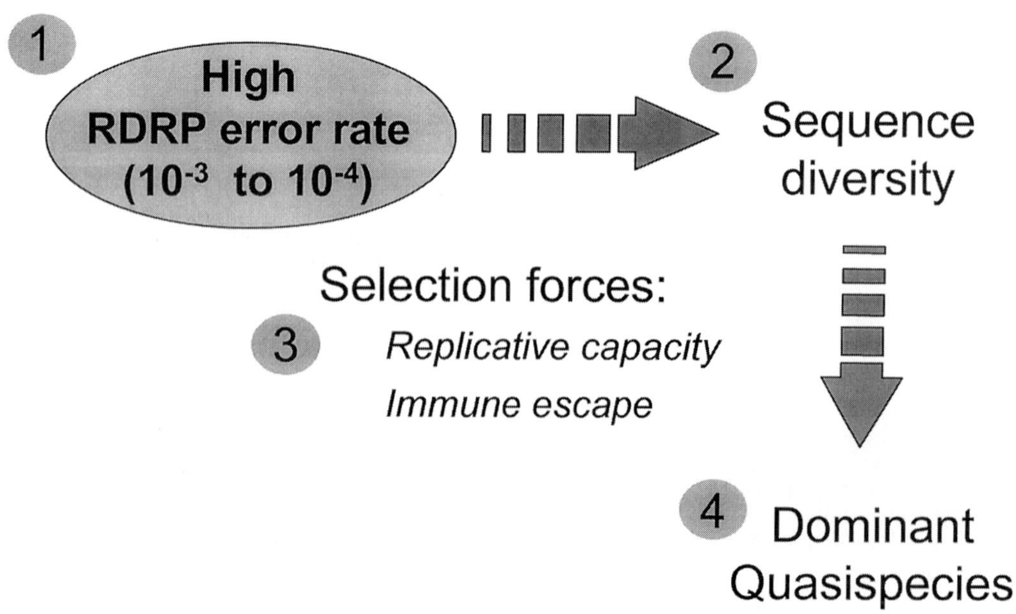

Fig. 15-1. Mechanism accounting for antigenic variation among viruses such as hepatitis C virus and HIV-1 which replicate through an RNA intermediate. RDRP represents "RNA-dependent RNA polymerase" (or reverse transcriptase, in the case of HIV-1).

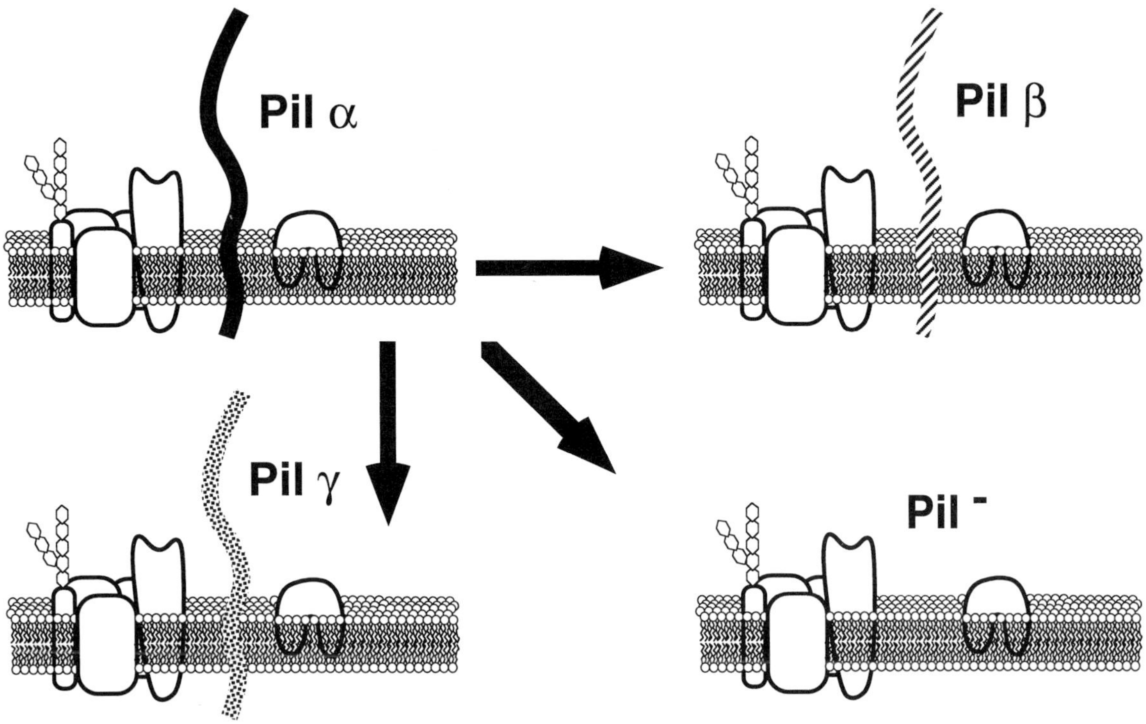

Fig. 15-2. Phase and antigenic variation in gonococcal pilin. Recombination between variant incomplete *pilS* genes and *pilE* (the pilin expression locus) result in either antigenic variations (Pil$\alpha \rightarrow$ Pilβ or Pilγ), or phase variation (Pil$\alpha \rightarrow$ Pil$^-$). The Pil$^-$ phenotype sometimes reverts to Pil$^+$ when recombination with another for *pilS* gene restores the ability of *pilE* to produce functional pili.

the high frequency variations in expressed length of the core LOS polysaccharide chain (Fig. 15-3).[16,55]

The result is that any population of $>10^6$ gonococci is quite heterogeneous, with multiple variants expressing a bewildering mixture of pili, Opa and LOS antigens. This prepares the organism for specific immune evasion from antibodies aimed at epitopes on one of these antigens, and for binding to different receptors on different cells on different tissues and/or people. Truly, gonococci always "have their bags packed ready to travel."

Other bacterial antigens undergo slower evolution, by relatively rare missense mutations that slowly alter antigenic structure (e.g., gonococcal porin, chlamydia major outer membrane protein, or MOMP). Recently, however, it has been recognized that gonococci can exchange blocks of chromosomal DNA between different strains in nature, resulting in mosaic genes that have altered structure, function, and antigenicity.[56–59] Indeed horizontal DNA exchange of this sort appears crucial to evolution of gonococcal IgA1 protease, altered penicillin binding protein 1, and probably porin protein (M. Hobbs et al., personal communication).[56,58]

IMMUNE DISRUPTION

Yet a third general mechanism by which viruses may evade host immune responses involves the direct disruption of host immune mechanisms. Herpesviruses such as HSV and cytomegalovirus (CMV) express proteins (ICP47 in the case of HSV, and US6 in the case of cytomegalovirus) that block the normal peptide transporter (TAP) function required for presentation of viral peptide fragments to MHC Class I restricted T cells.[60,61] ICP47 binds to TAP within the cytosol, preventing the transport of peptide fragments into the endoplasmic reticulum, whereas the CMV US6 is a secreted glycoprotein that interacts with TAP within the lumen of the endoplasmic reticulum. Disruption of transporter protein function by CMV and HSV may lessen the extent to which the infection is recognized by the host immune system. Variola virus, a poxvirus, expresses a large number of proteins that interfere specifically with various arms of the immune system, including one protein that blocks activation of the classical complement pathway.[62] However, the related poxvirus responsible for molluscum contagiosum, MCV, lacks many of these proteins that suppress the host immune response.

Bacterial strategies for immune disruption appear to be limited to production of enzymes that cleave immunoglobulins, such as the gonococcal IgA1 protease. This cleaves IgA1 at the hinge region, thereby largely inactivating it, which may help to evade specific immune responses on mucosal surfaces. The importance of IgA1 protease is uncertain, however, since human responses at genital surfaces appear to be made up of 50% sIgA1 and 50% sIgA2. The latter lacks the hinge structures required for cleavage by the gonococcal IgA1 protease, and thus is protease resistant. Moreover, there are considerable quantities of IgG at the site of mucosal infections that is also not susceptible to IgA1 protease.

MOLECULAR MIMICRY

Another mechanism of pathogenesis involves the expression of proteins that are able to mimic specific host cell molecules in either structure or function. This strategy is particularly evident among viruses with larger genomes that are capable of expressing a wider variety of proteins. KSHV is an excellent example, as its genome encodes a number of proteins with sequences or motifs similar to those encoded by the human genome. These viral proteins resemble cellular cyclins and growth factors and are likely to control cellular growth and differentiation in a manner that is favorable to virus survival.[50,63] Other human homologs expressed by KSHV include macrophage inflammatory protein (MIP) chemokines, interleukin-6, and interferon regulatory factor.[50,63] The poxvirus MCV encodes a large number of similar proteins that interfere with normal functions of the immune system.[65] These include proteins that block chemotactic responses to the chemokine MIP1-a,

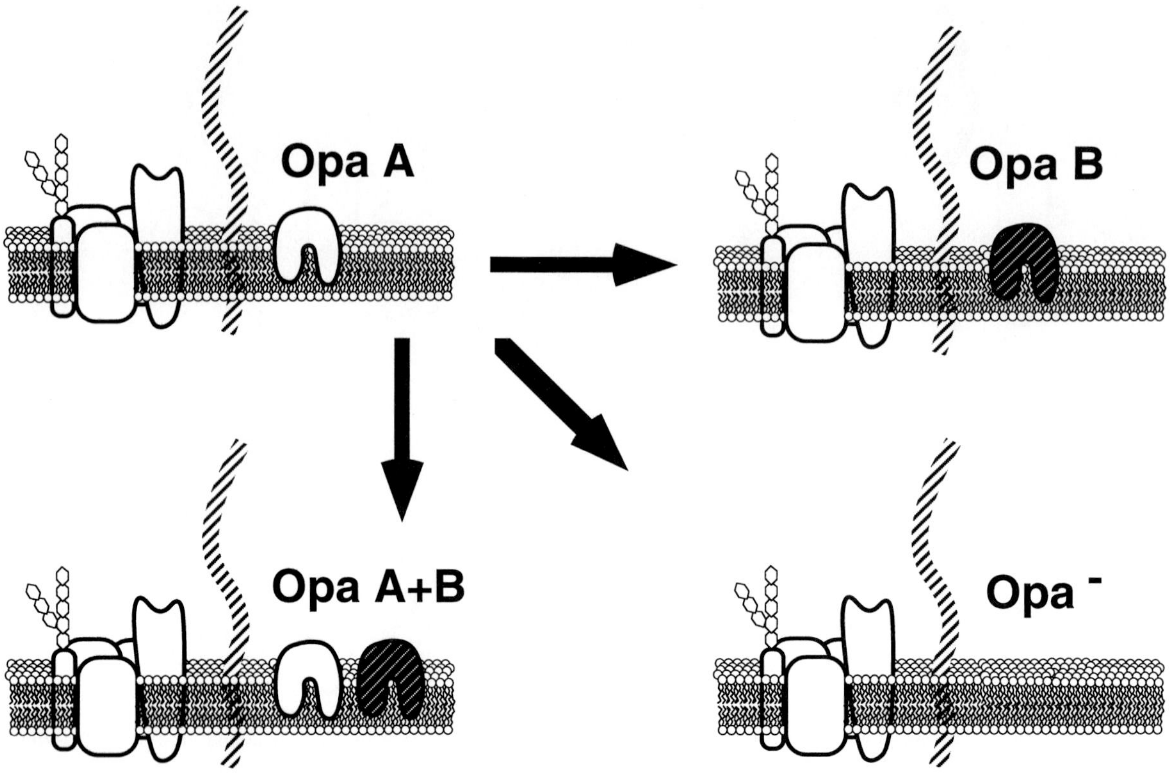

Fig. 15-3. Phase and antigenic variation in the gonococcal opacity protein family. Gonococci possess multiple (up to 12) complete *opa* genes, each of which is transcribed but only some of which are translated. Successful translation depends on the number of [CTCTT} repeats in the *opa* genes; when N = 3, 6, 9, 12, 15, etc., Opa is expressed, but all other variations in the number {CTCTT} repeats throws the gene out of translational frame and no Opa is expressed. Slipped-strand errors during DNA replication frequently alters the number of the [CTCTT] repeats, resulting in spontaneous on-off switching in each *opa* gene. Since the product of each *opa* gene is somewhat different, this also results in antigenic variation.

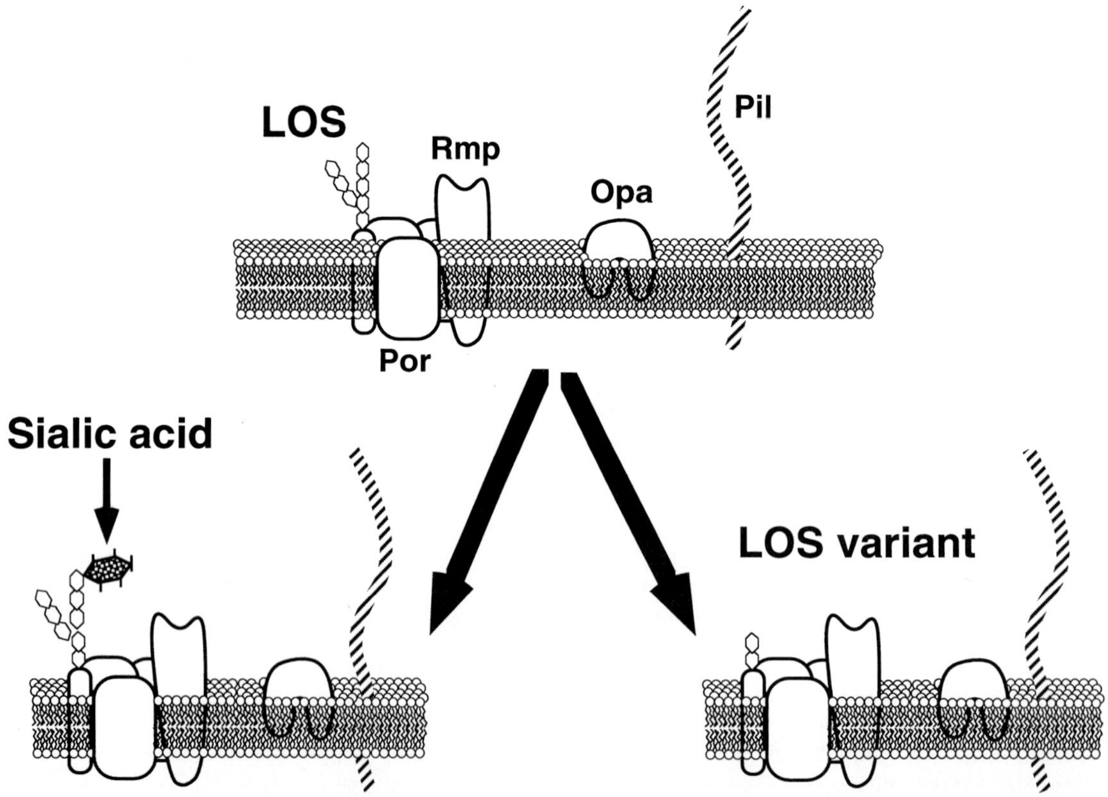

Fig. 15-4. Masking due to sialylation of gonococcal LOS, and the effects of phase variation in LOS on sialylation. Gonococci phase—vary the length and structure of the LOS core polysaccharide by slipped strand mispairing changes in short polypyrimidine repeats within genes that are involved in core polysaccharide synthesis. Full length LOS can be sialylated, but truncated LOS cannot be sialylated. When LOS is sialylated, anti-porin antibodies cannot reach their target, and porin is "masked."

as well as MHC-Class I, chemokine, and glutathione peroxidase homologs.[65,66] MCV also expresses a selenoprotein that may help to protect the infected cell from oxidative stress.[67] Bacterial mimicry also occurs, as for example the identity between host glycolipids and the terminal epitope on gonococcal LOS, and meningococcal group B sialic acid capsule and brain sialic acids of identical structure.[68]

MASKING

By "masking," we mean "covering up," as for instance one raises an umbrella to ward off rain. In a sense, all intracellular pathogens are "masked" because antibody and complement cannot follow them inside the cell. However, in this usage we refer particularly to production of specific structures that physically block access of host defenses to the cell surface of the pathogen. Bacterial capsules may play such a role, but none is important for any of the bacterial STD pathogens. Although gonococci do not make a true capsule, they clearly display masking when they add neuraminic acid (sialic acid) to their LOS polysaccharide chain.[69,70] (This is done by use of a gonococcal sialyltransferase and host-derived CMP-N-acetyl neuraminic acid.) Sialylation creates a sort of molecular umbrella, effectively covering up both LOS and neighboring porin protein from attack by complement fixing antibodies, rendering the organism resistant to bactericidal antibodies.[71,72] The extensive glycosylation of the HIV env protein and the HCV E1 and E2 envelope proteins (which results in an approximate doubling of molecular mass of each of the proteins) may also serve to mask the exterior surface of the viral envelope from antibody recognition.

BLOCKING ANTIGENS

Production of so-called "blocking antigens" is yet another mechanism that bacteria have evolved to evade otherwise effective antibody defenses. In the case of the gonococcus, a constant (invariant) antigen designated reduction modifiable protein (Rmp) strongly elicits host production of non–complement fixing IgG antibodies. On binding to Rmp, these antibodies prevent the proper conformational deposition of complement-fixing antiporin antibodies onto the closely juxtaposed porin molecule, thus blocking the antiporin bactericidal attack.[73,74] The presence of blocking antibodies helps to render gonococci resistant to killing by normal human serum, and promotes infection between sexual partners.[75] A somewhat similar masking strategy may also exist among viruses. Recent crystallographic studies suggest that the V3 loop of the HIV-1 envelope protein may act to mask the cellular receptor interaction site on the assembled HIV envelope from antibody attack. This would be a clever trick, because the CD4 interaction site must be relatively conserved in structure if it is to function effectively. According to this hypothesis, the CD4 receptor-binding site is unmasked by a conformational rearrangement of the *env* protein that flips the V3 away and precedes docking of the envelope protein to the CD4 molecule.

OTHER MECHANISMS OF IMMUNE EVASION

Although no term has been coined yet to aptly describe the phenomenon, *T. pallidum* is thought to evade host defenses in part by presenting very few antigenic proteins on its phospholipid rich outer envelope.[76] Thus, proteins on the *T. pallidum* cell envelope are termed TROMP, for treponemal rare outer membrane protein. By analogy to relative radar invisibility of airplanes with certain shapes and compositions, this microbial strategy might be termed "stealth."[77]

CONCLUSION

Clearly, many STD pathogens are masters of immune evasion. This explains, at least in part, why herpesviruses, papillomaviruses, HIV, and *T. pallidum* persist so long in human hosts, and why gonococci are so adept at causing repeat infectious. These concepts also help to understand how gonococci, chlamydia, and others persist in the host in the face of an apparently vigorous immune response. Details of the strategies are discussed further in the respective chapters that follow. We can appreciate how difficult is the task of designing vaccines for these infections agents. Most have evolved over a very long time in humans, and it is no surprise that these pathogens are survivors.

References

1 Feng Y et al: HIV-1 entry cofactor: functional cDNA cloning of seven-transmembrane, G protein-coupled receptor [see comments]. *Science* 272:872, 1996.

2 Endres MJ et al: CD4-independent infection by HIV-2 is mediated by fusin/CXCR4. *Cell* 87:745, 1996.

3 Deng H: Identification of a major co-receptor for primary isolates of HIV-1 [see comments]. *Nature* 381:661, 1996.

4 Alkhatib G et al: CC CKR5: a RANTES, MIP1alpha, MIP1beta receptor as a fusion cofactor for macrophage-tropic HIV-1. *Science* 272: 1955, 1996.

5 Samson M et al: Resistance to HIV-1 infection in caucasion individuals bearing mutant alleles of the CCR-5 chemokine receptor gene [see comments]. *Nature* 382:722 and 668, 1996.

6 Boyle KA et al: Receptor-binding properties of a soluble form of human cytomegalovirus glycoprotein B. *J Virol* 72:1826, 1998.

7 Whitbeck JC et al: Glycoprotein D of herpes simplex virus (HSV) binds directly to HVEM, a member of the tumor necrosis factor receptor superfamily and a mediator of HSV entry. *J Virol* 71:6083, 1997.

8 Pearce WA: Attachment role of the gonococcal pili: Optimum conditions and quantitation of adherence of isolated pili to human cells in vitro. *J Clin Invest* 61:931, 1978.

9 Hagblom P et al: Intragenic recombination leads to pilus antigenic variation in *Neisseria gonorrhoeae. Nature* 315:156, 1985.

10 Haas R et al: Release of soluble poilin antigen coupled with gene conversion in *Neisseria gonorrhoeae. Proc Natl Acad Sci USA* 84:9079–9083, 1987.

11 Swanson J et al: Gene conversion variations generate structurally distinct pilin polypeptides in *Neisseria gonorrhoeae. J Exp Med* 165: 1016, 1987.

12 Stern A et al: Opacity genes in *Neisseria gonorrhoeae*: Control of phase and antigenic variation. *Cell* 47:61, 1986.

13 Stern A et al: Common mechanism controlling phase and antigenic variation in pathogenic *Neisseria. Mol Microbiol* 1:15, 1987.

14 Demarco de Hormaeche R et al: Gonococcal variants selected by growth in vivo or in vitro have antigenically different LPS. *Microbial Pathogen* 4:289, 1988.

15 Griffiss JM et al: Physical heterogeneity of neisserial lipooligosaccharides reflects oligosaccharides that differ in apparent molecular weight, chemical composition, and antigenic expression. *Infect Immunol* 55: 1792, 1987.

16 van Putten JPM et al: Molecular mechanisms and implications of infection of lipopolysaccharide variation in *Neisseria. Mol Microbiol* 16: 847, 1995.

17 Gray-Owen SD et al: Differential *Opa* specificities for CD66 receptors influence tissue interactions and cellular response to *Neisseria gonorrhoeae. Mol Microbiol* 26:971, 1997.

18 Jonsson AB et al: Sequence changes in the pilus subunit lead to tropism variation of *Neisseria gonorrhoeae* to human tissue. *Mol Microbiol* 13:403, 1994.
19 Seifert HS et al: Multiple gonococcal pilin antigenic variants are produced during experimental human infections. *J Clin Invest* 93:2744–2749, 1994.
20 Jerse AE et al: Multiple gonococcal opacity proteins occurs during experimental urethral infection in the male. *J Exp Med* 179:911, 1994.
21 Lin L et al: The *Neisseria* Type 2 Iga1 protease cleaves LAMP1 and promotes survival or bacteria within epithelial cells. *Mol Microbiol* 24:1083, 1997.
22 van Putten JPM: Phase variation of lipopolysaccharide directs interconversion of invasive and immunoresistant phenotypes of *Neisseria gonorrhoeae*. *EMBO J* 12:4043, 1993.
23 Bessen D et al: Interactions of gonococci with HeLa cells: Attachment, detachment, replication, penetration, and the role of protein 11. *Infect Immunol* 54:154, 1986.
24 Ilver D et al: Transcellular passage of *Neisseria gonorrhoeae* involves pilus phase variation. *Infect Immunol* 66:469, 1998.
25 Kenney S et al: JC virus enhancer-promoter active in human brain cells. *Science* 226:1337, 1984.
26 Cripe TP et al: Transcriptional regulation of the human papillomavirus-16 E6-E7 promoter by a keratinocyte-dependent enhancer, and by viral E2 trans-activator and repressor gene products: implications for cervical carcinogenesis. *EMBO J* 6:3745, 1987.
27 Yukawa K et al: Regulation of human papillomavirus transcription by the differentiation-dependent epithelial factor Epoc-1/skn-1a. *J Virol* 70:10, 1996.
28 Andersen B et al: Characterization of Skn-1a/i POU domain factors and linkage of papillomavirus gene expression. *J Biol Chem* 272: 15905, 1997.
29 Lopez-Cabrera M et al: Transcriptional factor C/EBP binds to and transactivates the enhancer element II of the hepatitis B virus. *Virology* 183:825, 1991.
30 Ori A et al: Hepatitis B virus enhancer binds and is activated by the hepatocyte nuclear factor 3. *Virology* 207:98, 1995.
31 Shih CH et al: In vitro propagation of human hepatitis B virus in a rat hepatoma cell line. *Proc Natl Acad Sci USA* 86:6323, 1989.
32 Galvan V et al: Herpes simplex virus 1 induces and blocks apoptosis at multiple steps during infection and protects cells from exogenous inducers in a cell-type-dependent manner. *Proc Natl Acad Sci USA* 95: 3931, 1998.
33 Jerome KR et al: Herpes simplex virus type 1 renders infected cells resistant to cytotoxic T-lymphocyte-induced apoptosis. *J Virol* 72:436, 1998.
34 Chisari FV et al: Hepatitis B virus immunopathogenesis. *Ann Rev Microbiol* 13:29, 1995.
35 Peeling RW et al: Antibody to chlamydia hsp60 predicts an increased risk for chlamydia pelvic inflammatory disease. *J Infect Dis* 175:1153, 1997.
36 Eckert LO et al: Prevalence and correlates of antibody to chlamydia heat shock protein in women attending sexually transmitted disease clinics and women with confirmed pelvic inflammatory disease. *J Infect Dis* 175:1453, 1997.
37 Lichtenwalner, AB et al: Evidence of genetic susceptibility to *Chlamydia trachomatis*-inducted pelvic inflammatory disease in the pig-tailed macaque. *Inf Immunol* 65:2250, 1997.
38 Kimani J et al: Risk factors for *Chlamydia trachomatis* pelvic inflammatory disease among sex workers in Nairobi, Kenya. *J Infect Dis* 173:1437, 1996.
39 Magnuson HT et al: Inoculation syphilis in human volunteers. *Medicine* 35:33, 1956.
40 Gregg CR et al: Toxic activity of purified lipopolysaccharide of *Neisseria gonorrhoeae* for human fallopian tube mucosa. *J Infect Dis* 143: 532, 1981.
41 Melly MA et al: Ability of monomeric peptidoglycan fragments from *Neisseria gonorrhoeae* to damage human fallopian-tube mucosa. *J Infect Dis* 149:378, 1984.
42 Mauri DN et al: LIGHT, a new member of the TNF superfamily, and lymphotoxin alpha area ligands of herpesvirus entry mediator. *Immunity* 8:21, 1998.
43 Fauci AS: Host factors and the pathogenesis of HIV-induced disease. *Nature* 384:529, 1996.
44 Weissman D et al: Macrophage-tropic HIV and SIV envelope proteins induce a signal through the CCR5 chemokine receptor. *Nature* 389: 981, 1997.
45 Palmer KL et al: An isogenic haemolysin-deficient mutant of *Haemophilus ducreyi* lacks the ability to produce cytopathic effects on human foreskin fibroblasts. *Mol Microbiol* 21:13, 1996.
46 Cope LD et al: A diffusible cytotoxin of *Haemophilus ducreyi*. *Proc Natl Acad Sci USA*, 94:4056, 1997.
47 Ball JM et al: Age-dependent diarrhea induced by a rotaviral nonstructural glycoprotein. *Science* 272:101, 1996.
48 Alani RM et al: Human papillomaviruses and associated malignancies. *J Clin Oncol* 16:330, 1998.
49 Lee H et al: Deregulation of cell growth by the K1 gene of Kaposi's sarcoma-associated herpesvirus. *Nat Med* 4:435, 1998.
50 Gao SJ et al: KSHV ORF K9 (vIRF) is an oncogene which inhibits the interferon signaling pathway. *Oncogene* 15:1979, 1997.
51 Ray RB et al: Hepatitis C virus core protein cooperates with *ras* and transforms primary rat embryo fibroblasts to tumorigenic phenotype. *J Virol* 70:4438, 1996.
52 Sakamuro D et al: Hepatitis C virus nonstructural protein NS3 transforms NIH 3T3 cells. *J Virol* 69:3893, 1995.
53 Beatty WL et al: Reactivation of persistent *Chlamydia trachomatis* infection in cell culture. *Infec Immunol* 63:199, 1995.
54 Nara PL et al: Emergence of viruses resistant to neutralization by V3-specific antibodies in experimental human immunodeficiency virus type 1 IIIB infection of chimpanzees. *J Virol* 64:3779, 1990.
55 Gotschlich EC: Genetic locus for the biosynthesis of the variable portion of *Neisseria gonorrhoeae* lipooligosaccharide. *J Exp Med* 180: 2181, 1994.
56 Sarubbi FA et al: Transfer of antibiotic resistance in mixed cultures of *Neisseria gonorrhoeae*. *J Infect Dis* 130:660, 1974.
57 Spratt BG: Hybrid penicillin-binding proteins in penicillin-resistant strains of *Neisseria gonorrhoeae*. *Nature* 332:173, 1988.
58 Lomholt H et al: Comparative characterization of the iga gene encoding IgA1 protease in *Neisseria meningitidis*, *Neisseria gonorrhoeae* and *Haemophilus influenzae*. *Mol Microbiol* 15:495, 1995.
59 Zhou J et al: Interspecies recombination, and phylogenetic distortions, within the glutamine synthetase and shikimate dehydrogenase genes of *Neisseria meningitidis* and commensal *Neisseria* species. *Mol Microbiol* 23:799, 1997
60 Fruh K et al: A viral inhibitor of peptide transporter of antigen presentation. *Nature* 375:415, 1995.
61 Hill A et al: Herpes simplex virus turns off the TAP to evade host immunity. *Nature* 375:411, 1995.
62 Buller RM et al: Poxvirus pathogenesis. *Microbiol Rev* 55:80, 1991.
63 Godden-Kent D et al: The cyclin encoded by Kaposi's sarcoma-associated herpes virus stimulates cdk6 to phosphorylate the retinoblastoma protein and histone H1. *J Virol* 71:4193, 1997.
64 Moore PS et al: Molecular mimicry of human cytokine and cytokine response pathway genes by KSHV. *Science* 274:1739, 1996.
65 Bugert JJ et al: Recent advances in molluscum contagiosum virus research. *Arch Virol Suppl* 13:35, 1997.
66 Krathwohl MD et al: Functional characterization of the C—C chemokine-like molecules encoded by molluscum contagiosum virus types 1 and 2. *Proc Natl Acad Sci U.S.A.* 94:9875, 1997.
67 Shisler JL et al: Ultraviolet-induced cell death blocked by a selenoprotein from a human dermatotropic poxvirus. *Science* 279:102, 1998.
68 Mandrell RE et al: Lipo-oligosaccharides (LOS) of mucosal pathogens: molecular mimicry and host modification of LOS. *Immunobiology* 187:382, 1993.
69 Parsons JN et al: Sialylation of lipopolysaccharide and loss of absorption of bacterial antibody during conversion of gonococci to serum resistance by cytidine 5- monophospho-N-acetyl neuraminic acid. *Microbiol Pathogen* 7:63, 1989.
70 Smith H et al: Sialylation of *Neisserial* lipopolysaccharide: A major influence on pathogenecity. *Microbiol Pathogen* 19:365, 1995.

71 Bramley J et al: A serum-sensitive, sialytransferase-deficient mutant of *Neisseria gonorrhoeae* defective in conversion to serum resistance by CMP-NANA or blood cell extracts. *Microbial Pathogen* 18:187, 1995.
72 Elkins C et al: Antibodies to N-terminal peptides of gonococcal porin are bactericidal when gonococcal lipopolysaccharide is not sialylated. *Mol Microbiol* 5:2617, 1992.
73 Rice PA et al: Characterization of serum resistance of *Neisseria gonorrhoeae* that disseminate: Roles of blocking antibody and gonococcal outer membrane proteins. *J Clin Invest* 70:157, 1982.
74 Rice PA et al: Immunoglobulin G antibodies directed against protein III block killing of serum-resistant *Neisseria gonorrhoeae* by immune serum. *J Exp Med* 164:1735, 1986.
75 Rice PA et al: Serum resistance of *Neisseria gonorrhoeae*. Does it thwart the inflammatory response and facilitate the transmission of infection? *Ann NY Acad Sci* 730:714, 1994.
76 Radolf JD: Treponema pallidum and the quest for outer membrane proteins. *Mol Microbiol* 16:1067, 1995.
77 Finlay BB et al: Common themes in microbial pathogenicity revisited. Micro Molec Biol Rev, 61:137, 1997.

Chapter 16

The biology of HIV, SIV, and other lentiviruses

Ronald Swanstrom
Robert Wehbie

TAXONOMY AND CLASSIFICATION

Retroviruses are named for an unusual step in their life cycle, the synthesis of DNA from an RNA template. In most biological systems genetic information flows from DNA to DNA or from DNA to RNA. The reverse flow of genetic information that characterizes retroviruses is not unique to retroviruses but rather identifies a widely dispersed set of genetic entities. Most of these entities share the feature of encoding the enzyme responsible for DNA synthesis utilizing an RNA template, reverse transcriptase (RT), first discovered in retrovirus particles in 1970.[1,2]

Many organisms carry mobile DNA elements that duplicate themselves at new positions in the host genome by reverse transcribing an RNA copy of the element into DNA and inserting the DNA copy at a new location in the host chromosome. In excess of 10 percent of our own genomes consist of thousands of copies of two such elements, called L1 and alu. These elements are still active in transposition as evidenced by the appearance of new germline mutations revealed by insertions into important genes.[3] At present three families of viruses are known to utilize a reverse transcription strategy: the plant virus family of caulimoviruses (with cauliflower mosaic virus as the best known example), the hepadnavirus family (found in birds and mammals with human hepatitis B virus, HBV, as a well known example), and retroviruses.

Retroviruses are currently divided into seven distinct genera (Fig. 16-1) and humans have been infected by viruses representing at least several of these genera. One of these genera is represented by lentiviruses, which include the human immunodeficiency virus type 1 (HIV-1) and HIV-2.[4,5] Another important human pathogen is human T-cell leukemia virus type 1 (HTLV-1).[6] This virus was isolated from tumor cells derived from patients with adult T-cell leukemia (ATL) shortly after it was appreciated that ATL showed geographic clustering suggestive of an infectious agent.[7] HTLV-1 is the causative agent of ATL and another syndrome called HTLV-associated myelopathy (HAM). HTLV-1 and HTLV-2, which is possibly associated with a form of hairy cell leukemia, are genetically distinct from the lentivirus group of retroviruses and are more similar to a retrovirus that causes leukemia in cows (bovine leukemia virus, BLV) (see Fig. 16-1).[8] These viruses are classified in the BLV-HTLV genus.

The other examples of human retroviruses are more unusual. One is called human foamy virus, a member of the spumavirus lineage (see Fig. 16-1). Viruses of this class have been isolated from cultured cells from a number of mammalian species. They are not known to cause any disease; the human origin of the human foamy virus is still debated since it is widely found in chimpanzees but not in humans.[9,10] A new human retrovirus, related to the type-B and -D retroviruses, has recently been described, and the previous descriptions of other human retroviruses are reviewed therein.[11] Finally, the remnants of infections of ancestral primates can be found in our genomes in the form of defective copies of integrated viral DNA that were genetically fixed after infection of germ cells or early embryos (human endogenous retrovirus, HERV) (see Fig. 16-1). None of these endogenous retroviruses is known to be active in humans today. More information about the number of infections of nonhuman primates and humans, and the historical timing of those infections will become available as the human genome project progresses.

HISTORICAL PERSPECTIVE

THE DISCOVERY OF RETROVIRUSES AS ONCOGENIC AGENTS

Most histories of retroviruses start with the dramatic discovery by Peyton Rous in 1911 that a virus, Rous sarcoma virus (RSV) could cause cancer.[12] Rous showed that a cell-free extract of a chicken sarcoma could be passed through a filter and the filtrate used to induce sarcomas in new chickens. The work of Rous was preceded by that of Ellermann and Bang, who described the transmission of chicken leukemia using cell-free extracts (avian leukosis virus, ALV).[13] However, the neoplastic nature of leukemia was not appreciated at the time and their observations received much less attention.

The isolation of other tumor-causing retroviruses followed the early work of Ellermann and Bang and of Rous. As these and other agents were discovered it became clear that there were two broad classes of agents: One class of viruses causes cancer after a long latency period (e.g., ALV, mouse mammary tumor virus [MMTV], and murine leukemia virus [MLV]), whereas the other class gives rise to cancer rapidly (e.g., RSV). The origin of this difference was shown to be the presence of an additional gene (oncogene) in the acutely transforming viruses that is not present in the slowly transforming viruses.[14] Subsequently it was shown that the oncogene is derived from the host cell and represents a normal host gene (proto-oncogene) that has the potential to become a transforming gene.[15] The mechanism of tumor induction by the slowly transforming retroviruses is distinct from but related to that of the acutely transforming retroviruses; in the former case, the chance integration of viral DNA next to a cellular proto-oncogene in its chromosomal location activates inappropriate expression of the proto-oncogene (insertional activation). Our understanding of the mechanism of transformation by the acutely and slowly transforming retroviruses provided our first view of cellular proto-oncogenes, an important group of genes that now numbers close to two hundred.

DISCOVERY OF LENTIVIRUSES

The first description of a retrovirus was in retrospect that of an animal lentivirus (EIAV), and involved the demonstration of transmission of equine infectious anemia by a cell-free extract of blood from an infected horse.[16] However, the conceptual framework that has led to our understanding of the lentivirus family came from later work with a lentivirus of sheep.

There are two fundamental differences between lentiviruses and most other retroviruses: Lentiviruses do not cause cancer, and they do establish chronic infections that result in a long incubation followed by a chronic symptomatic disease. The "slow" (*lenti* is Latin for slow), chronic nature of these infections was first appreciated for a disease of sheep called maedi-visna (*maedi* = labored

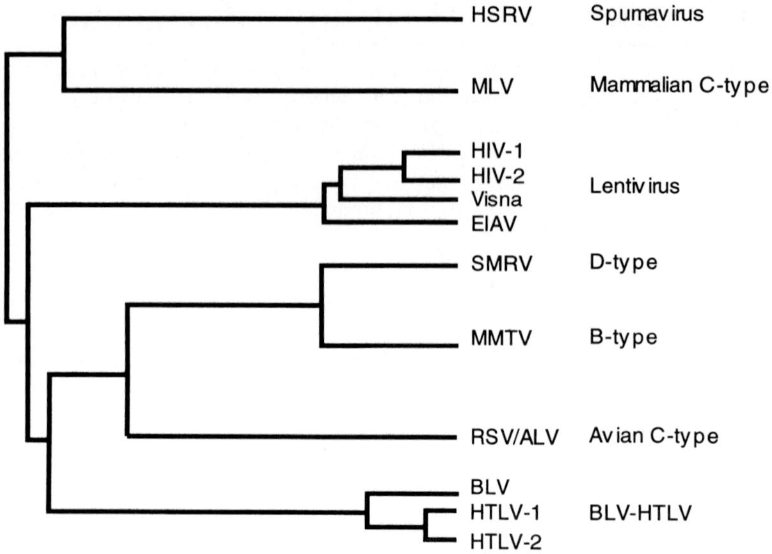

Fig. 16-1. Phylogeny of retroviruses based on a comparison of nucleotide sequences. The phylogenetic relationship of retroviruses is shown for selected retroviruses. The seven recognized genera of retroviruses are shown by name on the right. Additional genera are likely to be added as new retroviruses are identified, especially from nonmammalian species. Adapted from refs. 113 and 202.

breathing, *visna* = paralysis and wasting in Icelandic sheep).[17] Lentiviruses take their name from this distinctive feature of the infection. The appreciation of this disease in Icelandic sheep flocks likely was the result of their previous prolonged isolation and the subsequent introduction of visna virus with the importation of European sheep.[18]

Diseases subsequently recognized as owing to lentiviruses were noted quite early, with descriptions of equine relapsing anemia in 1843 and a progressive pneumonia in South African sheep in 1915.[19,20] As previously referred to, such disease in sheep would later be associated with neurological disease in Icelandic sheep (visna) and attributed by Sigurdsson in 1954 to a "slow virus."[17] Two decades later, a bovine lentivirus (BIV) was discovered, and in 1974 investigations of epizootic leukoencephalopathy in kid goats disclosed another lentivirus.[21,22] This caprine encephalitis lentivirus would subsequently be associated with a chronic arthritis and named CAEV.[23–25] The description of HIV-1 in 1983 was followed by discovery of the simian immunodeficiency viruses (SIVs).[4,26] More recently, a feline lentivirus (FIV) and a second bovine lentivirus (Jembrana disease virus) have been identified.[27,28]

BIOLOGICAL LESSONS FROM ANIMAL LENTIVIRUSES

Animal lentiviruses infect a range of animals from sheep to chimpanzees with a spectrum of manifestations ranging from asymptomatic infection to frank immunodeficiencies. Despite this apparent diversity, the interactions of these viruses with their respective hosts follow common pathways. Following the discovery of HIV-1, interest in the nonhuman lentivirus markedly increased with the goal of applying this knowledge to the treatment and prevention of AIDS in humans. In this section, the pathophysiology of animal lentivirus infections will be briefly reviewed in regard to the insights this knowledge provides for the understanding of HIV-1 infection.

THE CLINICAL MANIFESTATIONS OF LENTIVIRAL INFECTION VARY AMONG HOSTS

As has become evident with HIV infection in humans, responses to lentiviral infection vary among individual hosts. At one extreme, the lentiviruses of some species appear to be nonpathogenic. In contrast, some animals within a species are more prone to disease, and cross-species transmission of a previously nonpathogenic lentivirus may result in severe disease in a naive population. For example, a high percentage of Sooty Mangabey macaques are infected in the wild by SIV (SIV_{smm}) and show no sign of disease.[29–33] Yet, cross-species transmission of this SIV to Rhesus macaques in captivity resulted in an AIDS-like illness.[34–38] As will be discussed in a later section, HIV-2 and probably HIV-1 entered the human population by cross-species transmission. Interestingly, indigenous lentiviruses have not been reported for new-world monkeys. This suggests that old world monkey ancestors became infected by a lentivirus, and coevolved with the virus into a relationship without disease, at a time after early African anthropoids colonized the continent of South America approximately 40 million years ago.

In a situation analogous to nonpathogenic SIV in old-world monkeys, certain breeds of sheep are infected with visna virus (or ovine lentivirus, OvLV) and do not develop disease. Other breeds, such as Icelandic, Border Leicester, and Texel sheep, are particularly susceptible to lentiviral disease.[39] Moreover, infected lambs often suffer from more pronounced symptoms and have an accelerated disease course.[40,41] In fact, the young of all susceptible species and breeds (including human infants) are more prone to lentiviral disease and often manifest degrees of disease that do not occur in adults. As will be discussed, acute HIV encephalitis and a lentiviral lymphoid interstitial pneumonitis (LIP) are common in the pediatric AIDS population, but infrequently occur in adult AIDS patients. The molecular determinants of these differing species, intrabreed, and age susceptibilities to lentiviral disease are poorly defined.

MONOCYTE LINEAGE CELLS PLAY A CENTRAL ROLE IN ALL LENTIVIRAL INFECTIONS

In contrast to the ability of HIV to infect both lymphocytes and macrophages, the lentiviruses of sheep, goats, and horses have a cell range predominantly limited to macrophages.[42–46] However, despite the clear association of these animal lentiviruses with disease, the roles of the macrophage in HIV infection are less well defined. Nonetheless, the many similarities existing between human and animal lentiviral diseases and the growing knowledge of macrophage–HIV interaction suggest that macrophages are likely to be intimately involved in dissemination of HIV throughout the body, in viral persistence and in the end-organ diseases in humans that are believed to be owing principally to HIV replication.

Monocytes differentiate into a variety of tissue macrophages and share a common lineage with dendritic cells.[47] In addition, some studies suggest that dendritic cells differentiate from monocytes.[48] The fact that macrophage-tropic lentivirus predominates in transmission and that dendritic cells are preferentially infected by virus with this phenotype indicates that macrophages and/or dendritic cells are likely the initial targets of infection by the lentiviruses.[49,50] As an illustration of this point, intravaginal inoculation of SIV_{mac} in rhesus macaques and subsequent localization of the virus by in situ polymerase chain reaction (PCR) in serially sacrificed animals has revealed an initial infection of submucosal dendritic cells and subsequent systemic spread of the virus through draining lymph nodes.[51]

It has been proposed that macrophages are a significant reservoir for HIV and the major cell pool responsible for viral persistence.[52–55] Although human studies as yet do not support this proposal, inferences from animal lentivirus biology, studies of monocytes/macrophages in vitro, and the slow biphasic decay of HIV in the blood following drug inhibition of HIV replication are suggestive of a slow-to-turn-over source of HIV within the macrophage cell pool.

Lentiviral infections of sheep, goats, and horses often pass through periods in which there is little apparent viral replication followed by disease in selected organs characterized by intense viral replication within the macrophages of these tissues.[42–44,46,56–58] Although it is not clear whether viral replication in the affected tissues results from heightened replication in previously infected macrophages of the tissue, or from new infection of these tissue macrophages by virus produced at another site, the restricted macrophage tropism of these animal viruses suggests that events occur that induce lentiviral replication within a macrophage subpopulation and also likely enhance the ability of selected tissue macrophages to support this viral replication. Interestingly, monocytes present in the blood of humans and animals are resistant to infection in vitro by the lentiviruses from these species.[42,58,59] Yet, on maturation in culture these cells develop an increasingly heightened susceptibility to infection by the appropriate lentivirus, and viral replication may be further enhanced as the cells become terminally mature and/or are activated.[46,58,60,61] Thus, infected macrophages may disseminate HIV through the body and across tissue planes on their migration/maturation, although they harbor the virus at a relatively lower rate of viral replication until the cells are terminally differentiated or activated by some stimulus. Such stimuli may include lipopolysaccharides of bacteria, cytokines such as TNF-α, and complement.[61]

THE CELL TROPISM OF THE LENTIVIRUS DICTATES THE DISEASE MANIFESTATIONS

In general, lentiviral infections are characterized by an initial period of intense viral replication occasionally associated with acute disease followed by viral persistence and often chronic or late diseases. In addition to an acute retroviral syndrome and the lymphadenopathy that occur with infection by many of the lentiviruses and in a significant number of HIV-infected humans, lentiviral replication within a given tissue may result in tissue-specific disease. The diseases induced by the ungulate lentiviruses typify this situation.

The disease manifestations of lentivirus infection are largely governed by cell and tissue tropisms of the virus or viral subspecies. As previously referred to, the tropism of the ungulate lentiviruses is for cells of the monocyte/macrophage lineage with resulting clinical disorders being largely a reflection of active viral replication in these cells. Likewise, the lentiviruses of felids, monkeys, and humans infect monocyte/macrophage lineage cells and produce primary disease. However, these latter lentiviruses are also tropic for lymphocytes and the immunosuppression that results is often the principal clinical manifestation of these viral infections. Thus, the study of ungulate lentiviral diseases has allowed a view of HIV infection apart from the disease manifestations resulting from lymphocyte depletion.

Central nervous system disease

All lentiviral species are neurotropic and potentially neurovirulent. In humans, a significant fraction of those infected with HIV develop neurological disease as a primary consequence of their HIV infection with resulting encephalitis, motor/sensory abnormalities, or dementia.[62] As previously referred to, the young of many host species are particularly prone to development of a severe lentiviral encephalitis; implying that the immature nervous system is more susceptible to infection and/or more prone to the damage resulting from this infection. Adult hosts also develop neurological symptoms of lentivirus infection. However, unlike their young, neurological disease in the adult tends to be gradually progressive in nature, and with feline, simian, and human lentiviral infection, is often associated with the late, immunosuppression phase of infection.

Although sheep and caprine lentiviruses have been known for decades to induce neurologic diseases, the means by which the lentiviruses gain access to the CNS and the pathogenesis of the resulting neuronal damage remain ill-defined. Virus must enter the CNS either as cell-free virus via a breach in the blood–brain barrier or as cell-associated virus during diapedesis. In addition, the possibility exists that lentiviral infection of CNS endothelial cells provides both a portal and means of viral spread in the CNS. The ungulate lentiviruses, SIV, and HIV all replicate in primary CNS endothelial cultures and lentiviral CNS lesions are in part characterized by perivascular inflammation.[63–67] However, macrophages are often a key component of these perivascular infiltrates and infected microglial cells are uniformly found in the brains of affected individuals.[63] These pathological findings together with the observation that SIV isolated from the brains of macaques infected with lymphocyte-tropic virus had evolved the *env* determinants of macrophage-tropism, indicate a pivotal role of the macrophage in lentiviral CNS disease.[68,69]

The hallmark of lentiviral CNS disease is neuronal dysfunction, but neurons are not infected by these viruses and pathological changes in the brain may be minor in the face of significant clinical symptoms. Thus, neurons are likely damaged secondarily to lentiviral replication within other cells, such as microglial cells and perivascular macrophages. The mechanism(s) of neuronal damage has been the subject of much debate and research. Lentiviral products (i.e., Tat, gp41) or factors released from infected macrophages have been implicated with proposed mechanisms of neuronal damage including roles for cytokines, nitric oxide, and other substances.[62,70,71]

Pulmonary disease

Human infants infected with HIV often suffer from a pulmonary disorder termed lymphoid interstitial pneumonia (LIP), which is characterized pathologically by alveolitis and lymphoid peribronchovascular infiltrates.[72–74] The prototypical lentiviral disease of sheep, maedi, closely resembles LIP.[41,74,75] The pulmonary lesions in these animals are similar to LIP in humans.[75,76] Although this animal disease was described almost 50 years ago, the pathogenesis of the lentiviral pulmonary diseases has not been defined. However, the strong similarities between LIP and maedi suggest that LIP is mediated largely by HIV replication in alveolar macrophages. Macaques infected with macrophage-tropic SIV develop an interstitial pneumonia with a rich intra-alveolar macrophage infiltrate, in addition to neurological disease.[77]

As with CNS disease, lung damage by the lentiviruses is likely secondary to macrophage infection and may be mediated via macrophage released products (i.e., cytokines) and by lymphocytes responding to viral antigens presented by infected macrophages.[74–78] Lentiviral infections of several species have been shown to upregulate the expression of MHC class II genes in macrophages.[46,79–82]

Blood dyscrasias

Lentiviral infection often is accompanied by abnormal blood counts, although these abnormalities may not be clinically noted as disease. However, with HIV infection these abnormalities may result in severe clinical disease, and in horses infected with EIAV, such abnormalities are the main manifestation of the infection. As such, the pathogenesis of the blood dyscrasias induced by EIAV have been extensively studied and are likely analogous to those in humans resulting from HIV. The anemia of EIAV appears to be multifactorial, with proposed mechanisms being suppression of erythroid progenitors secondary to bone marrow macrophage infection, autoimmune hemolytic anemia, and diminished available iron.[18,83,84] In addition, as with human HIV infection, EIAV infection of horses may also result in immune thrombocytopenia.[85]

Gastrointestinal and hepatic diseases

Gastrointestinal and hepatic diseases are common in HIV infection, but are usually attributable to opportunistic infections. However, acute HIV infection may be associated with diarrhea, and evidence is emerging that HIV can directly result in GI disease later in the course of infection. Animal lentiviral infections clearly highlight the potential of the lentiviral damage resulting from tissue macrophage or regional lymphoid tissue involvement. Extreme examples of the virulent potential of the lentiviruses in the GI tract are the fulminant hepatic necrosis occasionally occurring with acute EIAV infection in horses and the fatal enteropathy in macaques following infection by SIV_{smm}PBj14.[86,87] This SIV strain induces a rapidly fatal enteropathy as a result of massive infection of intestinal lymphoid follicles.[86–89] Fortunately, such virulence does not occur with HIV, but by analogy to SIV, the potential does exist.

MODES OF ANIMAL LENTIVIRUS TRANSMISSION PARALLEL THAT OF HIV

Lentiviruses are transmitted exclusively via body fluids. With the fortunate exception of EIAV transmission by insect vectors, the modes of HIV transmission can be viewed as a composite of the routes by which other lentiviruses are spread. Animal lentiviruses are transmitted mainly through lactation and injuries from fighting, with sexual and maternal-to-fetal routes of transmission being relatively less frequent. By comparison, worldwide HIV is largely transmitted through vaginal intercourse. In addition, maternal-to-fetal transmission is common, but infection by the virus through human milk is infrequent. Despite these quantitative differences in the routes of transmission between HIV and the animal lentiviruses, transmission mechanisms of animal lentiviruses have proven to be useful as models of HIV transmission.

Maternal-to-infant transmission of HIV may occur antepartum or during delivery on exposure of the neonate to HIV-infected fluids. Details of these transmissions have been difficult to discern from human studies alone. Although intrauterine/perinatal transmission of SIV does not appear to occur in the wild, transmission to fetal and newborn rhesus macaques has been achieved experimentally.[90] Ultrasound-guided inoculation of SIV_{mac} into the amniotic fluid and oral administration of this virus to Rhesus monkey neonates resulted in a high rate of transmission.[91–94] Intravenous inoculation of pregnant macaques with SIV during midgestation also resulted in a high rate of both maternal and fetal infection.[95] In this animal system, although the mothers developed a genetically diverse virus population by parturition, all infants were infected with only macrophage-tropic virus. Taken together, these studies indicate that maternal-to-fetus or infant transmission of lentiviruses can occur across mucous membranes and that macrophages may have a central role in fetal infection in utero.

Inflammatory lesions either directly owing to lentiviral replication or resulting from a different process may augment lentivirus transmission. For example, the major route of ovine and caprine lentivirus transmission is via excretion of macrophage-borne virus in milk, and this transmission is enhanced by a lentivirus-induced mastitis.[96] By analogy, fairly strong evidence suggests that macrophage-tropic HIV is the predominant phenotype transmitted sexually, and other sexually transmitted diseases that cause inflammation enhance this transmission.[97–99] Although the inflammatory mechanisms enhancing viral transmission in these situations differ, these examples highlight the common pathways of transmission the lentiviruses employ and again emphasize the important role of the macrophage-tropic virus in lentivirus biology.

SIV INFECTION OF RHESUS MACAQUES AS A MODEL OF HIV-1 INFECTION

Studies of the nonprimate animal lentiviruses have provided invaluable insights into the pathophysiology of HIV infection. In certain instances, these animal systems are valid models of human and HIV interactions. However, the close phylogenetic relationship of humans and macaques, the close relatedness of SIV and HIV, and the striking clinical similarities of human HIV infection with the disease caused by SIV_{mac} and SIV_{smm} in the Rhesus macaque, clearly establish these SIV-infected animals as the system of choice for modeling HIV infection in humans.

As in humans, SIV infection of Rhesus macaques results in CD4+ lymphocyte depletion, immunosuppression, secondary malignancies, the direct end-organ damages of lentiviral infection previously discussed, and opportunistic infections. Many of the opportunistic infections occurring in these infected macaques are by the same pathogens associated with human AIDS, including *Toxoplasma gondii, Pneumocystis carinii, Salmonella* spp., *Cryptosporidium, Candida,* and cytomegalovirus.[39,77] The lymphomas occurring in these animals often result from the simian equivalent of EBV and possibly HHV-8, and as such parallel the pathogenesis of these malignancies in human AIDS.[100,101]

The rhesus macaque has been employed as a model of heterosexual and perinatal human HIV transmission. Intravaginal inoculation of these animals with SIV_{mac}251 with subsequent localization of the virus by in situ PCR in serially sacrificed animals has revealed an initial infection of submucosal dendritic cells and subsequent systemic spread of the virus through draining lymph nodes.[51] Other studies have highlighted the usefulness of the SIV/macaque model for studies of genital HIV shedding.[102–104]

Genetic manipulation of SIV has permitted a powerful means of testing the viral determinants of disease and has allowed the SIV-Rhesus macaque system to model more closely HIV infection.

In order to investigate specific HIV gene products in treatment or vaccination programs using macaques, SIV/HIV-1 hybrid viruses (SHIV) have been constructed that contain the HIV-1 gene of interest (i.e., *env* or the reverse transcriptase coding domain of *pol*) in place of the SIV equivalent.[105–107] Likewise, manipulation of the *env* gene has allowed the testing of cell tropisms and the role of macrophage-tropic SIV in AIDS.[68,108,109] As will be discussed, deletion of the SIV *nef* gene results in decreased virulence. Similar deletion strategies in SIV have been employed to investigate the roles of the other regulatory genes.[110]

Finally, the highly virulent simian lentivirus SIV_{smm}PBj14 further highlights how lentiviral genomic changes can impact on virulence. The pathogenesis of SIV_{smm}PBj14 is due to its ability to replicate in resting peripheral blood mononuclear cells, to activate lymphocytes, and to induce lymphocyte proliferation.[87,89] Changes in the U3 region of the viral LTR appear to be responsible at least in part for this phenotype.[111] Specific mutations within the *nef* gene have also been implicated in this rapid progression phenotype.[112] Although an HIV equivalent of SIV_{smm}PBj14 has not emerged, the availability of a strain of SIV that induces rapid onset of disease and death may facilitate an understanding of the pathogenic mechanisms of acute lentiviral infections and provide an animal system for the rapid in vivo testing of antiretroviral drugs.

MORPHOLOGY OF THE RETROVIRUS PARTICLE

Retroviruses are enveloped viruses with two identical copies of viral genomic RNA condensed in a nucleocapsid core (Fig. 16-2). The viral envelope is derived from the plasma membrane of the host cell during virus budding. Inserted in the envelope is a virus-encoded glycoprotein Env, the gene product of the *env* gene. Underlying the envelope is the viral matrix protein (MA), which is initially derived from the Gag (group-specific antigen) polyprotein precursor, the product of the *gag* gene. The nucleocapsid core consists of two other proteins derived from the Gag precursor, the capsid protein (CA) and the nucleocapsid protein (NC). NC binds viral RNA in the core, which is surrounded by CA. The core can have a variety of forms depending on the retrovirus, ranging from essentially spherical to cylindrical. In the case of HIV-1 and other lentiviruses, the core is cone-shaped (see Fig. 16-2). Several viral enzymes, encoded in the *pro* and *pol* genes and including RT, are associated with the nucleocapsid core.

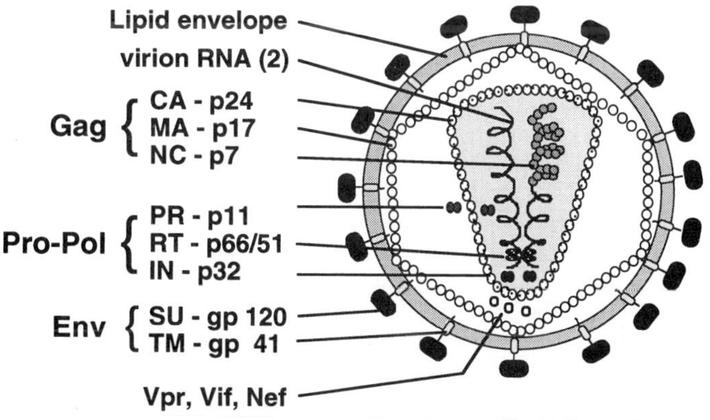

Fig. 16-2. Virion structure. A diagram showing a model of the arrangement of the major components of the HIV-1 particle. The arrangement shown is based on limited experimental work using thin section electron microscopy and the fractionation of subviral components. The accessory proteins Vpr, Vif, and Nef have recently been detected in virus particles. Viral proteins are identified by size (e.g., p24 is a 24-kDa protein), by a two-letter identifier (e.g., CA for capsid), and as part of the gene product from which they are derived (e.g., CA from the Gag precursor).

STRUCTURE OF THE RETROVIRAL GENOME

The viral genome as found in virus particles consists of two identical strands of single-stranded RNA. The RNA has features of a eukaryotic mRNA in that it has a 5′ cap, a 3′ poly A tail, and is of the coding or positive sense. The two RNAs are weakly held together near their 5′ ends in a poorly characterized structure called the dimer linkage structure. The lengths of the monomeric RNA for retroviruses with the smallest genomes are on the order of 7000 nucleotides long; the lentiviruses encode more gene products than retroviruses with simpler genomes and as a result have a longer genome, on the order of 10,000 nucleotides long.

All retrovirus genomes encode four primary replicative genes: *gag*, *pro*, *pol*, and *env*. *gag* encodes the structural proteins of the capsid, *pro* encodes the viral protease responsible for cleaving precursor proteins, *pol* encodes RT and the viral integrase (IN), and *env* encodes the envelope glycoprotein. These genes always appear in this order on the viral genome starting near the 5′ end (Fig. 16-3).

More complex retroviruses encode additional genes beyond the four primary replicative genes; these are referred to as auxiliary or accessory genes, although in many cases their functions are as indispensable as the replicative genes. HIV-1 encodes six accessory genes within the 3′ half of its genome: *vif*, *vpr*, *vpu*, *tat*, *rev*, and *nef* (see Fig. 16-3).

Cis-acting replication sequences are those that function as part of the genome either to identify it as the viral genome or to participate directly in expression or replication of the genome. For retroviruses the genome exists in an RNA and a DNA state at different times during the virus life cycle, and as a result *cis*-acting sequences are present in the genome that function within the context of DNA or RNA (see Fig. 16-3). As RNA the genome must be packaged and dimerized; the sequence that identifies viral RNA for packaging is called the packaging signal (**Ψ**). In general both **Ψ** and the dimer linkage structure lie near the 5′ end of the genome, although for HIV-1 the sequences involved in these functions are incompletely defined. The RNA has a short direct repeat at the 5′ end and at the 3′ end just inside of the poly A tail (called R) that functions during viral DNA synthesis. Also located near the 5′ end and the 3′ end are the positions of the primers for the first and second strand of viral DNA synthesis. Near the 5′ end is a sequence that is complementary to the 3′-terminal 20 nucleotides of a cellular tRNA. A tRNA bound to this site (called the primer binding site, or PBS) primes the first strand of viral DNA synthesis. A stretch of purines near the 3′ end (called the polypurine tract, or PPT) serves as primer for the second strand of viral DNA. For the lentiviruses an additional PPT is present in the middle of the genome to allow the second strand of DNA to be synthesized in two segments, presumably to increase the rate of synthesis. The RNA also encodes signals for splicing and polyadenylation, functions that are carried out by the host machinery. Finally, two regions of HIV-1 RNA interact with two viral gene products: the TAR region interacts with Tat to upregulate the expression of viral RNA, and the RRE interacts with Rev to enhance the nuclear export of the singly spliced and unspliced viral RNAs.

A different set of sequences function at the DNA level. During viral DNA synthesis part of the sequences in the RNA form of the genome (U5 and U3) are duplicated to make the DNA product longer than its RNA template. This generates direct repeats at the

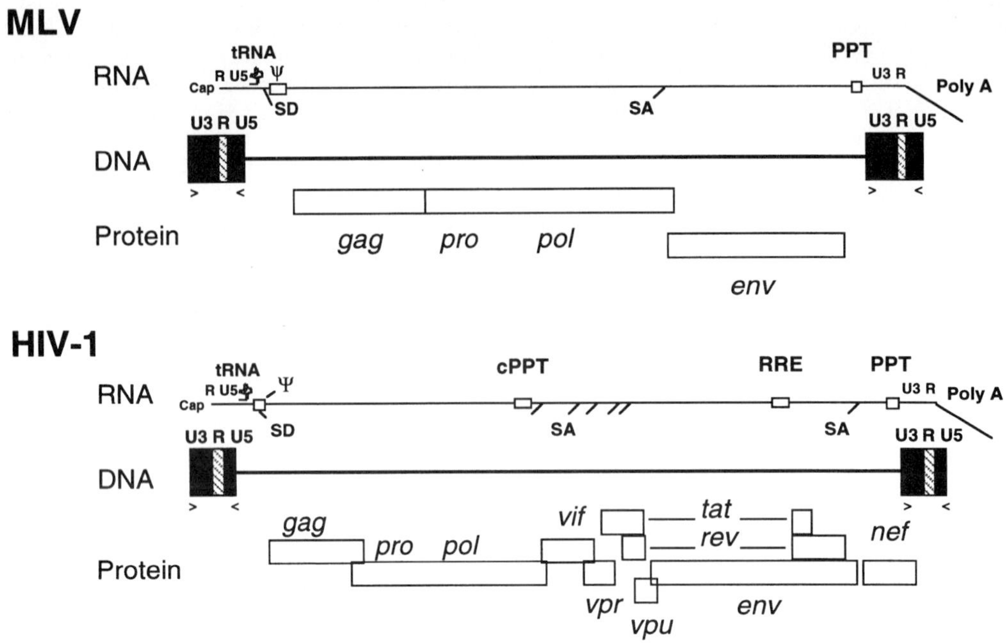

Fig. 16-3. The viral genome. The genetic organization of MLV and HIV-1. The structure of viral genomic RNA, linear viral DNA, and the encoded protein reading frames are shown for both MLV (a simple retrovirus) and HIV-1 (a complex retrovirus). The RNAs are capped at the 5′ end and have a poly A tail at the 3′ end. In the RNA form, the genome is bounded by the small R sequence that is a short direct repeat that participates in the early steps of viral DNA synthesis. The position of the genome-bound tRNA is shown bounding the U5 sequence. The major splice donor site is shown (SD) with a tick mark below the line. In MLV there is a single splice acceptor site (SA) for the expression of the *env* gene. HIV-1 has a major splice donor site near the 5′ end of the genome and several splice acceptor sites for the expression of the multiple accessory genes in addition to *env* (which is expressed as part of a *vpu-env* bicistronic mRNA). The splice sites for the *tat-rev* intron are shown above the line. The packaging sequence (Ψ) is located near the 5′ end of the genome. For HIV-1, the RRE element is shown in the *tat-rev* intron. Both viruses have a polypurine tract (PPT) bounding the U3 sequence; HIV-1 has an additional central PPT near the middle of the genome. The DNA is colinear with the RNA but contains a direct repeat of the U3RU5 sequence motif forming the LTR. The LTR is bounded by a short inverted repeat that is important in the integration reaction. For MLV *gag* and *pro-pol* are in the same reading frame and are joined at low frequency during protein synthesis by readthrough suppression in which the termination codon is read as a coding triplet and translation proceeds from *gag* into *pro-pol*, allowing synthesis of the Gag-Pro-Pol precursor. For HIV-1, *gag* and *pro-pol* are in different reading frames and are joined at a low frequency by translational frameshifting.

ends of the DNA that were not present in the RNA (Fig. 16–3). These direct repeats are called the long terminal repeat, or LTR. Within the LTR are sequences that function as promoter and enhancer for the expression of viral RNA, and these sequences are selectively active within the upstream LTR. Also, the LTRs are themselves bounded by short inverted repeats that function at the ends of the DNA during the integration reaction. Details and references covering retrovirus replication and genome organization are reviewed elsewhere.[113]

RETROVIRUS LIFE CYCLE

DISCRETE STEPS IN RETROVIRUS REPLICATION

Receptor specificity

Retroviruses share the general aspects of their life cycle with all viruses: binding to the cell surface, entry into the cell, replication and expression of the viral genome, virus assembly, and exit from the cell. Viruses use a diverse group of surface molecules as receptors to bind to the target cell. Only very similar retroviruses share receptor specificity, as can be inferred from the few cases where the receptor is known. Thus, although the receptor for HIV-1 and HIV-2 is known while the receptors for the other lentiviruses are not known, it is likely that the receptor specificity varies even among lentiviruses. The receptor for HIV-1 and HIV-2 is the CD4 molecule, a surface protein that marks the T-helper subset of T lymphocytes.[114] This protein is also expressed on macrophages, which may be another target of replicating virus in the body.

Entry into the cell

Binding to CD4 occurs through an interaction with the Env surface glycoprotein complex, gp120/gp41. The binding of CD4 to gp120 juxtaposes the virus particle to the target cell and is believed to initiate a conformational change within the gp120/gp41 oligomeric complex that leads to fusion of the viral and cellular membranes. The influenza virus HA protein provides a model for a mechanism of glycoprotein-mediated membrane fusion. By analogy with HA, the hydrophobic amino terminus of gp41 becomes exposed after the binding of gp120 to CD4. This hydrophobic region, called the fusion peptide, inserts into the host cell membrane, bringing the viral and cellular membranes close enough in proximity that the lipid bilayers realign into one. The joining of the membranes transfers the viral nucleocapsid core to the inside of the cell.

Fusion of HIV-1 with the cell membrane requires a coreceptor in addition to CD4. Although HIV-1 will bind to CD4 on the surface of the cell, a member of the chemokine receptor family must also be present to mediate the fusion step.[115] As discussed in the following, HIV-1 can change its tropism among CD4-expressing cells by evolving to use different coreceptors, and such evolution may contribute to an accelerated disease course.

Viral DNA synthesis

Reverse transcriptase that was packaged during virion formation mediates the synthesis of viral DNA in the next round of replication. DNA synthesis takes place in the cytoplasm of the newly infected cell. The template for DNA synthesis is the single-stranded RNA genome that is converted to a linear double-stranded DNA product. The components of DNA synthesis are the viral DNA polymerase (RT), its associated RNase H activity that degrades the RNA template after it is converted into an RNA/DNA hybrid, a cell-derived tRNA primer annealed near the 5′ end of the viral genome that serves as the primer for the first strand of DNA synthesis, and one or more polypurine tracts (PPT) in the RNA template that are left by RNase H to prime the synthesis of the second strand of DNA.

The synthesis of viral DNA follows an elegant and complex pathway.[116] There are several aspects of this process that make it especially distinctive. First, during the course of DNA synthesis three breaks in the template must be negotiated. The first comes shortly after the initiation of DNA synthesis (using the tRNA primer) when the growing DNA chain reaches the 5′ end of the template. The presence of the short repeat at the ends of the RNA (R) allows the newly synthesized DNA to pair its complementary copy of the R sequence with the copy of R at the 3′ end of the genome, allowing DNA synthesis to continue along the length of the genome. The other discontinuities appear when the first strand completes copying the RNA template, and when a short second strand synthesized near the right (5′) end of the first DNA strand copies to the end of its template. At this point the 3′ end of each of the two DNA strands represents the sequences present at the position where the original tRNA primer was bound (PBS), with one of these copies being the complement of the other. This allows the sequences at the 3′ end of each DNA strand to base pair. DNA synthesis now goes to completion with each strand positioned to use the other as template that, when copied to the end, results in a linear duplex DNA.

The second distinctive feature of DNA synthesis is that the DNA product is longer than the RNA template.[117,118] There are no new sequences in the DNA but some of the sequences in the RNA are duplicated and rearranged during DNA synthesis so that the DNA product has several features that were not present in the RNA template. Where the RNA template had a short terminal repeat R, the DNA has a long terminal repeat (LTR). Because of the jumping of template breaks during DNA synthesis, the U5 and U3 sequences in the RNA are brought together, separated by a copy of the R sequence, in a new arrangement that makes up the LTR. The duplication of these rearranged sequences both makes the DNA product longer and results in the terminal duplication. Knowledge of reverse transcriptase as an essential viral protein involved in virus replication identified it as a target for antiviral therapy.

Integration of viral DNA

The linear DNA product moves to the nucleus, where it undergoes integration into the host chromosomal DNA. This reaction is mediated by the viral integrase protein (IN) that, like RT, is brought into the cell as part of the infecting nucleoprotein complex.[119] The integration reaction actually starts in the cytoplasm as each 3′ end of the linear viral DNA is shortened by removal of the two terminal nucleotides that are adjacent to a canonical CA dinucleotide.[120] A short inverted repeat is also a feature of the LTR boundaries that plays a role in integrase specificity. In the nucleus IN makes a staggered cleavage in host DNA and joins the shortened strands of the linear viral DNA to the cleaved host DNA. Repair synthesis results in integrated viral DNA that is shortened by two base pairs relative to the product of DNA synthesis, and a short duplication of host DNA flanking the inserted viral DNA. In the integrated state the viral DNA is referred to as the provirus or proviral DNA. A fraction of the unintegrated linear viral DNA in the nucleus is circularized in a dead-end reaction.[121]

Transcription of integrated DNA

Integrated DNA is transcribed into RNA by the host RNA polymerase II, and the RNA transcript has the features of a cellular mRNA (5′ cap and 3′ poly A tail). Transcription starts within the upstream LTR and ends just downstream of the corresponding position in the downstream LTR (creating the R repeat in the RNA) (see Fig. 16-3). Viral DNA sequences upstream of the RNA start site, a region referred to as U3, function as enhancers and promoter for transcription, utilizing host factors for these functions for the most part. Many retroviruses encode transcription activators that increase the level of transcription. In the case of HIV-1 the Tat protein binds to a stem-loop structure called TAR that forms near the 5′ end of the newly synthesized RNA. The binding of Tat to TAR results in the increased synthesis of viral RNA.[122]

Splicing and transport of viral RNA

Newly synthesized HIV-1 RNA has one of four fates. (1) It can be multiply spliced, which removes several introns to generate small transcripts that encode *tat*, *rev*, and *nef*. (2) It can be singly spliced, which removes a single intron spanning *gag* and *pol* to express *env* and several other small proteins. (3) It can remain unspliced and used as mRNA for *gag*, *pro*, and *pol*. (4) Finally, it can remain unspliced and serve as genomic RNA in the assembly of new virions. The singly spliced and unspliced RNAs require the presence of Rev protein interacting with a region of RNA structure called the RRE (Rev Response Element, located within the *env* gene and in the *tat/rev* intron) for export from the nucleus.[123]

Synthesis of viral proteins

Most of the viral proteins are synthesized in the cytoplasm of the infected cell. The exceptions are integral membrane proteins that are synthesized by ER-bound ribosomes, with the protein being transported into the lumen of the ER (e.g., the Env protein and the Vpu protein). Most of the RNAs encode a single protein. Viral mRNAs for *vif*, *vpr*, *tat*, *rev*, and *nef* are expressed from separate spliced RNAs. However, HIV-1 uses two different strategies to translate two proteins from each of two different mRNAs. First, the full-length RNA transcript is translated using the 5′ most open reading frame to synthesize the Gag protein. Approximately 5 percent of the time a frameshifting event occurs near the right end of the *gag* reading frame that leaves the translation machinery in the −1 reading frame, which encodes the *pro* and *pol* genes. Translation continues, generating a Gag-Pro-Pol fusion protein that is present at 5 percent the concentration of the Gag precursor. In contrast, a small open reading frame for *vpu* is present upstream of the *env* reading frame. Both the Vpu and Env proteins are synthesized from a single bicistronic mRNA.[124]

Assembly of virus particles

The major components of assembly of the retroviral particle are the Gag and Gag-Pro-Pol precursors, the Env protein precursor, and genomic RNA. For HIV-1 the Gag and Gag-Pro-Pol precursors are directed to the inner face of the plasma membrane of the cell by signals at the N terminus of Gag, this includes the N-terminal modification of myristylation and the presence of basic residues that interact with the negatively charged lipid head groups. Gag selectively packages full-length viral RNA during the assembly process. Multimeric Gag–Gag interactions occur (presumably also with the less abundant Gag-Pro-Pol precursor) at the plasma membrane to effect a bud from the cell. The other two major components of the assembling particle are the viral RNA, two copies of which are specifically packaged through interactions with Gag, and the Env protein. The Env precursor, gp160, is secreted into the ER during its synthesis. A stop transfer signal near its C terminus anchors Env in the membrane, leaving a C terminal cytoplasmic tail with the majority of Env in the lumen of the ER where glycosylation occurs. The Env protein is transported through the Golgi, presumably after forming a homotrimer, and in the late Golgi the Env precursor is cleaved by a cellular furin-like protease to generate the gp120 and gp41 mature products that stay associated. These are anchored in the plasma membrane on the surface of the cell, and a specific interaction between the cytoplasmic tail of gp41 and the MA domain of Gag brings the oligomeric gp41/gp120 complex into the virus particle.[124]

Proteolytic processing

An integral part of the assembly process is the proteolytic processing of the Gag and Gag-Pro-Pol precursors by the *pro*-encoded viral protease (PR). The protease is activated during the assembly process and mediates the cleavage of these precursors to their mature components (for HIV-1 Gag: MA, CA, NC, and p6; for Pro: PR; and for Pol: RT, and IN). The enzymes gain full activity only after being released from the precursor, and the virion undergoes a dramatic morphological change from an open immature state to a condensed nucleocapsid core with the processing of the Gag precursor (Fig. 16-4). These processing steps are required for infectivity, and for this reason the viral protease has become an important target for the development of anti-HIV inhibitors.[124]

Accessory proteins

Some retroviruses encode only the *gag*, *pro*, *pol*, and *env* genes, and the entire replication scheme of a retrovirus can be understood with only the function of those proteins. Thus, the existence of additional gene products encoded by more complex retroviruses such as HIV-1 presents a challenge to understand their role either within the context of replication or in virus–host interactions. HIV-1 encodes six accessory proteins: Vif, Vpr, Vpu, Tat, Rev, and Nef. Vif enhances the efficiency of DNA synthesis during the subsequent round of replication by an unknown mechanism.[125,126] Vpr appears to be bifunctional in that it arrests cells in G2 of the cell cycle and also plays a role in the transport of the nucleocapsid replication complex to the nucleus in nondividing cells.[127–129] Vpu is also bifunctional in that it increases the efficiency of particle release from the cell and helps dissociate newly made gp160 from premature interactions with newly made CD4 in the ER.[130–132] Tat functions as a transactivator of transcription, and Rev directs the nuclear to cytoplasmic transport of unspliced and singly spliced viral RNAs.[133–136] Finally, Nef is involved in the removal of surface CD4 from the infected cell and also plays a poorly defined role in enhancing virus infectivity.[137–141]

Infection of quiescent cells

Simple retroviruses such as murine leukemia virus require dividing cells to integrate their DNA.[142] This need is thought to reflect a requirement for a breakdown of the nuclear membrane to allow the integration complex access to chromosomal DNA. In contrast, lentiviruses appear to have the capacity to infect nondividing cells such as macrophages, and this ability may be an important feature of both their ability to establish a chronic infection and their pathogenicity. Simple retroviruses synthesize only a small amount of DNA when they infect a nondividing cell. Lentiviruses must overcome this block to viral DNA synthesis, although the basis for this is not known. Vpr, which has a nuclear localization signal, appears to play an important role in the transport of the replication complex into the nucleus of nondividing cells, although it is dispensable in dividing cells.[129] Although it is clear that other lentiviruses such as EIAV are able to infect nondividing macrophages, it is not known if the basis for doing this is the same as for HIV-1. However, among the primate lentiviruses (HIV-1, HIV-2, and SIVs), the *vpr* gene is conserved.

REPLICATION RATES, ERROR RATES, AND RECOMBINATION: IMPLICATIONS FOR ANTIVIRAL THERAPY AND THE EVOLUTION OF RESISTANCE

Turnover of HIV-infected cells in the body is on the order of 2 days.[143,144] This observation suggests that the virus is undergoing active and continuous replication in the body, perhaps on the order of 300 replication cycles per year. There are on the order of one billion infectious events per day, as measured by the turnover of infected cells. This large number of replication cycles in an infected person provides the virus with the opportunity to develop genetic diversity as its primary defense against immune and antiviral suppression of replication.

The viral DNA polymerase is error prone, incorporating about one mismatched nucleotide per genome per round of replica-

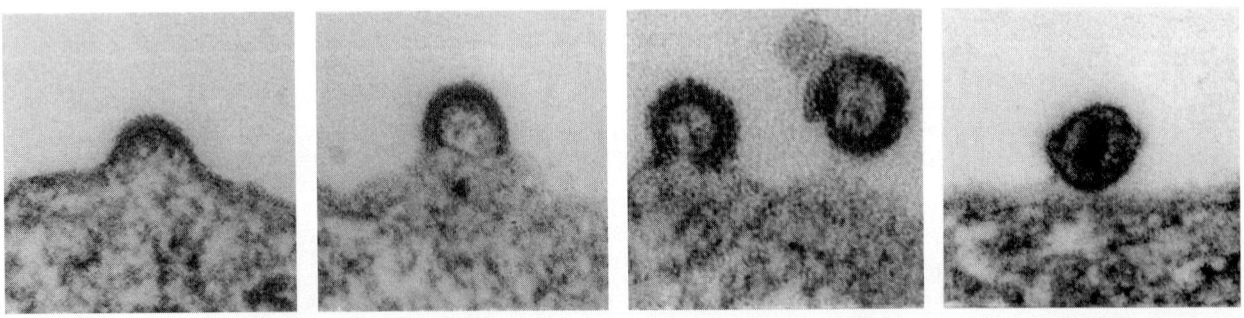

Fig. 16-4. Virus assembly and budding. Electron micrographs of HIV-1 budding through the plasma membrane of the cell. The first two panels show Gag proteins oligomerizing beneath the cell membrane forcing a bud. Panel three shows an immature virion form at a late stage of budding and a budded virion that has retained the immature form. The fourth panel shows the typical condensed core associated with a mature infectious virus particle. Taken from ref 203 with permission.

tion.[145,146] Given the amount of replication that occurs, the virus establishes a pool of genetic variants that has been called a swarm or quasispecies. Variants are maintained based on fitness, although even modestly unfit variants are maintained at a low level.[147] As the selective pressure changes either through changes in the immune system or as the result of drug selection, variants in the pool that have a growth advantage in the presence of the selective pressure are enriched. In the extreme case, selection for resistance to a potent non-nucleoside RT inhibitor, which requires a single coding change to give high level resistance, is complete within 2 weeks.[148,149] The appearance of resistance is considerably slower if the selective pressure is less, as in the case of AZT, or if the selective pressure is sufficiently high to slow the amount of virus replication.[150,151] In the extreme case of completely suppressive therapy there is no virus replication and therefore no chance to evolve mutations. This strategy is unlikely to work if a single mutation can confer resistance since it is likely that most single mutations pre-exist in the virus population. However, treatment strategies that require multiple mutations to give high level resistance have the potential to suppress completely virus replication.

One confounding feature of the biology of HIV-1 is that although virus turnover is rapid the previous genetic complexity is not lost. Viral DNA is present in peripheral blood cells, and to a large extent is not expressed and turns over slowly. Actively replicating virus must be present in this pool of DNA but it makes up only a fraction of the DNA that is present. The rest of the DNA represents sequences that were actively replicating over the previous months.[152] The existence of these sequences means that one cannot reverse selective pressure in the hopes of repeating some previous selective success—the previous winners in that selection still exist genetically in the form of this DNA. Thus, drug resistance markers can persist in the genetic pool even after removal of drug and the reappearance of wild-type virus. The genetically silent sequences can reappear when the previous selection is reapplied, either by stochastic re-expression of the integrated DNA or perhaps through superinfection followed by recombination with an actively replicating virus. High rates of recombination are a feature of retroviruses in general, and the potential for recombination to impact the evolution of drug resistance has been demonstrated in the laboratory.[153-156]

MOLECULAR DETERMINANTS OF PATHOGENESIS

VIRAL LOAD

The workhorse of the clinical assessment of HIV-1 disease progression has been the level of CD4+ T cells in the blood. The level is normally in the range of 1000/uL but during the course of an HIV-1 infection can drop to undetectable levels. Most patients survive at least until CD4+ T cells drop to 50/uL, and the chances of dying from AIDS increases as the CD4+ T cell level drops (see Chapters 17 and 18). However, another measure of HIV-1 infection can predict the time course of disease progression.

Virus replication results in the release of virus from the infected cells. Some of this virus circulates in the blood as free virus particles. These particles turn over rapidly, on the order of 6 hours.[157] The rapid turnover of these particles makes their presence a sensitive measure of ongoing virus replication. The higher the level of virus in the plasma the higher the level of virus replication. A direct measure of virus in the plasma (viral load) is made by quantitating the amount of viral RNA. High levels of viral RNA in the plasma are correlated with more rapid disease progression, whereas lower levels indicate a slower progression.[158] The RNA levels have predictive value up to 10 years ahead. In most cases differences in viral load between infected people are probably owing to differences in the ability of the immune system to limit active virus replication, although the details of these differences are poorly understood.

NSI AND SI

All isolates of HIV-1 use the CD4 molecule as the receptor on target cells. However, different isolates vary in their use of members of the chemokine receptor family as coreceptors. The most common form of HIV-1 uses CCR5 as a coreceptor and is able to infect both macrophages and CD4+ T helper cells.[159-163] This form does not grow in transformed T-cell lines and is referred to as macrophage-tropic and nonsyncytium-inducing (NSI). A common variant uses the CXCR4 coreceptor, is unable to infect macrophages but can infect CD4+ T helper cells and transformed T-cell lines where it causes syncytium.[164,165] This variant is referred to as T-cell-line-tropic and syncytium-inducing (SI).

Transmission occurs almost exclusively with NSI variants, and in about one-half of infected people only NSI variants are ever detected during the course of the infection.[97,98] However, in the other half of infected people SI variants appear as CD4+ T cells drop below 400/uL.[97] The SI variants evolve de novo in each person from the NSI variants. When these SI variants appear the rate of loss of CD4+ T cells increases and the disease course is accelerated.[166-168]

The major determinant of the SI phenotype is found at a region designated as variable region 3, or V3.[169-173] The change in the use of coreceptors suggests a change in the population of cells that are supporting replication. Thus SI variants may be evolving to replicate in a new (but as yet undefined) niche in the body, a niche, such as a new tissue or cell type, that is distinct from the one that supports the replication of the NSI variants. Alternatively, the use of a different coreceptor may simply support more rapid replication.

ROLE OF ACCESSORY GENES

Transmission rates for HIV-1 can be low, suggesting that in these cases the infecting inoculum is small. Under these circumstances it is possible to have a defective virus transmitted. This appears to be the case with several examples of people who were infected with a virus deleted in the *nef* gene.[174-176] Such viruses grow well in cell culture. However, work in the SIV model system showed that *nef*-deleted viruses are maintained only at very low levels in infected monkeys.[177] People who have been fortuitously infected with *nef*-deleted virus have similar low virus loads and no evidence of disease progression. These observations point to an important role for *nef* in vivo and suggest that at least some of the variability in virus load and disease progression seen between different infected people may be owing to infection with defective but still replication competent virus.

HIV-1 AND HIV-2

The human immunodeficiency viruses can be broadly divided into two groups: HIV-1 and HIV-2. Both of these viruses cause AIDS. However, it appears that the pace of disease progression is slower with HIV-2 than it is with HIV-1.[178] It may be that HIV-2 grows less well in humans, giving lower viral loads and slower disease progression. There is strong evidence that HIV-2 infection of humans is the result of an interspecies transfer of this virus from the primate sooty mangabey (see the following). Interspecies transfers of viruses have unpredictable outcomes so it is not surprising that two related but distinct viruses would replicate to different levels in a common heterologous host.

VACCINATION AGAINST LENTIVIRUS INFECTION

Development of an effective HIV vaccine has proven to be a formidable task. Fortunately, scattered successes with lentivirus vaccines in animals together with experiments of nature that highlight the potential of an attenuated HIV vaccine provide hope. Inactivated vaccines appear effective against infection by FIV and some promising results have been obtained for such vaccine preparations in models of EIAV, and the ovine/caprine lentiviruses infection.[179–181] In contrast, some subunit ungulate vaccines appear to potentiate infection.[180,182–184] The most promising evidence for the potential of vaccination against HIV infection comes from the effectiveness of a live attenuated (*nef*-deleted) vaccine in adult Rhesus macaques.[185] Although an attenuated version of HIV-1 poses obvious concerns, there is a lack of disease progression in humans infected from a common source by HIV-1 containing an analogous deletion within the *nef* gene suggesting the potential of this approach.[176,186]

ORIGIN OF HIV

PHYLOGENETIC ANALYSIS

Sequence analysis and comparison allows one to compare the extent of relatedness between different lentiviruses. Viruses frequently cluster in this analysis, suggesting a more recent shared ancestor of the members comprising the cluster. Primate lentivi-

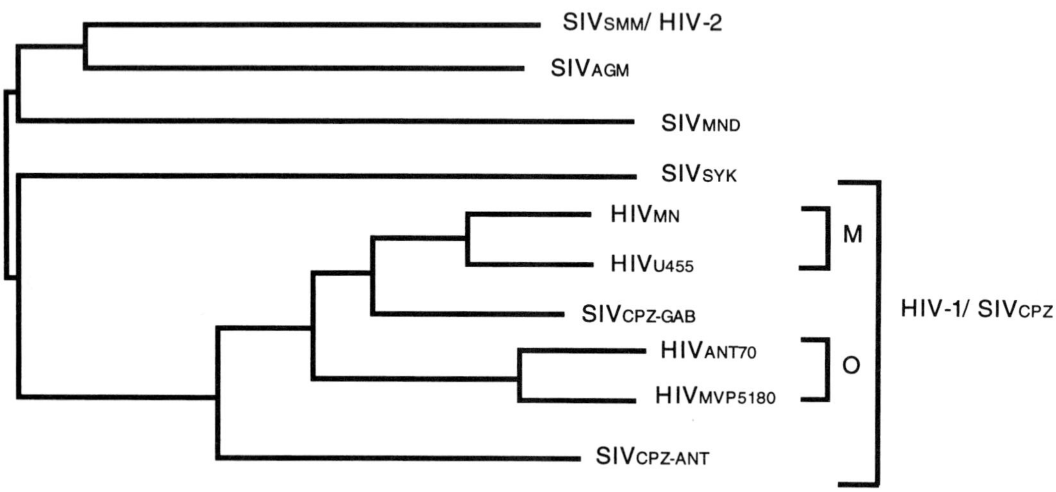

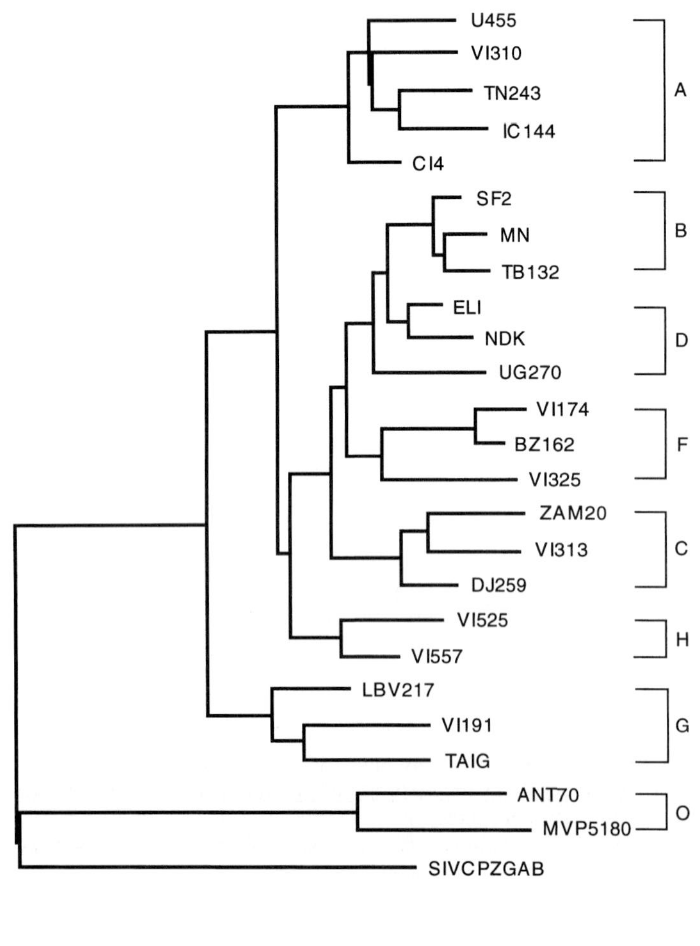

Fig. 16-5. Phylogenetic relationships of primate lentiviruses. *A.* Lineages of primate lentiviruses. Adapted from ref. 200. The five major lineages of primate lentiviruses are shown (SIV_{smm}/HIV-2, SIV_{agm}, SIV_{mnd}, SIV_{syk}, and HIV-1/SIV_{cpz}). Examples of HIV-1 main group (M) and outliers (O) are also shown interspersed with different SIV_{cpz} isolates. SIV_{smm} and HIV-2 are shown together. They are not identical but rather different isolates of each interspersed with different isolates of the other.[187] *B.* Subtypes of HIV-1. Adapted from ref. 188. Several examples of each main group subtype of are shown for subtypes A through H, except E, which is a recombinant with a subtype A virus. Also shown are two examples of the outlier group (O) and SIV_{cpzgab}.

ruses can be viewed as comprising at least five distinct lineages represented by infection of different nonhuman primate species: sooty mangabeys, mandrils, African green monkeys, Sykes monkeys, and chimpanzees (Fig. 16-5A). HIV-2 clearly overlaps in this analysis with viruses isolated from the primate sooty mangaby, and the initial range of HIV-2 in western Africa overlaps the range of sooty mangabys.[187] This type of evidence strongly suggests the presence of HIV-2 in humans represents an interspecies transfer of SIV_{smm} to humans. Furthermore, different HIV-2 isolates show distinct lineages within the SIV_{smm} cluster, suggesting multiple introductions of SIV_{smm} into humans.[187] The similarity of SIV_{smm} to SIV_{mac} suggests further spread of SIV_{smm} among other primates in captivity.

Within the HIV-1 group of viruses, isolates cluster into distinct lineages that have been termed subtypes (Fig. 16-5B).[188,189] Most of the subtypes coexist in sub-Saharan Africa. However, the foci of infections that have occurred as the epidemic has spread worldwide have frequently been established with virus from a single subtype. One example is the virus that is found in western Europe and in the United States is almost exclusively of subtype B. In a few cases viruses from two separate subtypes can been found cocirculating in a population. One example of this is in Thailand where both subtype B and E viruses are found.[190–192] These viruses are found in different populations, E in the group where infections are spread through heterosexual contact (especially through commercial sex workers) and B among IV drug users. It has been suggested that these viruses have adapted to their different modes of transmission.[193] However, this seems unlikely as the distribution of the two subtypes is changing in Thailand as the epidemic progresses.[194] The subtype E virus found in Thailand represents a recombinant virus consisting of a subtype A virus with a new *env* gene derived from an unknown HIV-1-like parent.[195] It has recently been appreciated that many HIV-1 isolates represent recombinants between viruses of two different subtypes.[196,197]

The case for interspecies transfer as the origin of HIV-1 is less clear by comparison with HIV-2 but still suggestive. HIV-1 is most similar to the SIV from chimpanzees (SIV_{cpz}), and several HIV-1 isolates (the "Outlier Group") are as distant from the bulk of HIV-1 sequences (the "Main Group") as are the SIV_{cpz} isolates (Fig. 16-5B).[198–200] However, most HIV-1 isolates are less similar to SIV_{cpz} than is seen in the HIV-2/SIV_{smm} comparison. Also, SIV_{cpz} has been isolated from only a few animals, leaving open the question of whether chimpanzees are the natural host for this virus.[201] Nonetheless, HIV-1 and SIV_{cpz} sequences form a cluster that is distinct from the other lineages of primate lentiviruses but no more distinct than the other lineages are among themselves. Thus, the human lentiviruses are phylogenetically embedded within a larger family of widely dispersed lentiviruses of old world primates.

RECENT IMPACT OF URBANIZATION AND TRANSPORTATION

As noted, the transmission of SIV_{smm} to humans as HIV-2 is strongly supported by phylogenetic analysis. The evidence also suggests that such transmissions have occurred more than once. It is possible that interspecies transmission of HIV-1 has occurred multiple times as has HIV-2, and perhaps these transmissions have occurred over an extended period of time (as happens with many viruses). In this view what has changed in recent times is the opportunities for transmission within the human population. When interspecies transmission occurs in a rural population the infection may remain local and even die out. However, when chronically infected persons have access to large population centers and the opportunity to have multiple sex partners, and these population centers are connected by transportation corridors, then the opportunity to establish the virus more widely in the human population exists.

ACKNOWLEDGMENTS

The work of the authors is supported by the National Institutes of Health. Steve Pettit and David Irlbeck provided invaluable assistance in preparing the figures.

References

1 Temin HM et al: RNA-dependent DNA polymerase in virions of Rous sarcoma virus. *Nature* 226:1211–1213, 1970.

2 Baltimore D: RNA-dependent DNA polymerase in virions of RNA tumour viruses. *Nature* 226:1209–1211, 1970.

3 Kazazian HJ et al: Haemophilia A resulting from de novo insertion of L1 sequences represents a novel mechanism for mutation in man. *Nature* 332:164–166, 1988.

4 Barre-Sinoussi F et al: Isolation of a T-lymphotropic retrovirus from a patient at risk for acquired immune deficiency syndrome (AIDS). *Science* 220:868–871, 1983.

5 Clavel F et al: Isolation of a new human retrovirus from West African patients with AIDS. *Science* 233:343–346, 1986.

6 Poiesz BJ et al: Detection and isolation of type C retrovirus particles from fresh and cultured lymphocytes of a patient with cutaneous T-cell lymphoma. *Proc Natl Acad Sci USA* 77:7415–7419, 1980.

7 Uchiyama et al: Adult T-cell leukemia: Clinical and hematologic features of 16 cases. *Blood* 50:481–492, 1977.

8 Kalyanaraman VS et al: A new subtype of human T-cell leukemia virus (HTLV-II) associated with a T-cell variant of hairy cell leukemia. *Science* 218:571–573, 1982.

9 Ali M et al: No evidence of antibody to human foamy virus in widespread human populations. *AIDS Res Hum Retroviruses* 12:1473–1483, 1996.

10 Schweizer M et al: Markers of foamy virus infections in monkeys, apes, and accidentally infected humans: Appropriate testing fails to confirm suspected foamy virus prevalence in humans. *AIDS Res Hum Retroviruses* 11:161–170, 1995.

11 Griffiths DJ et al: A novel exogenous retrovirus sequence identified in humans. *J Virol* 71:2866–2872, 1997.

12 Rous P: A sarcoma of the fowl transmissible by an agent separable from the tumor cells. *J Exp Med* 13:397–411, 1911.

13 Ellermann V et al: Experimentelle leukeamie bei huhnern. *Zentralbl Bakteriol* 46:595–609, 1908.

14 Lai MM et al: Avian tumor virus RNA: A comparison of three sarcoma viruses and their transformation-defective derivatives by oligonucleotide fingerprinting and DNA-RNA hybridization. *Proc Natl Acad Sci USA* 70:2266–2270, 1973.

15 Stehelin D et al: DNA related to the transforming gene(s) of avian sarcoma viruses is present in normal avian DNA. *Nature* 260:170–173, 1976.

16 Vallee H et al: Sur la nature infectieuse de l'anemie do cheval. *C R Acad Sci* 139:331–333, 1904.

17 Sigurdsson B: Maedi, a slow progressive pneumonia of sheep: An epizootiological and pathological study. *Br Vet J* 110:255–270, 1954.

18 Narayan O et al: Biology and pathogenesis of lentiviruses. *J Gen Virol* 70:1617–1639, 1989.

19 Lignee M: Memoire et observations sur une maladie de sang, connue sous le nom d'anhemie hydrohemie cachexie aqueuse du cheval. *Rec Med Vet* 20:30, 1843.

20 Palsson PA: *Maedi and Visna in Sheep*. Amsterdam, North-Holland Publishing, 1976, pp. 17–43.

21 Van Der Maaten MJ et al: Isolation of a virus from cattle with persistent lymphocytosis. *J Natl Cancer Inst* 49:1649–1657, 1972.
22 Cork LC et al: Infectious leukoencephalomyelitis of young goats. *J Infect Dis* 129:134–141, 1974.
23 Crawford TB et al: Chronic arthritis in goats caused by a retrovirus. *Science* 207:997–999, 1980.
24 Clements JE et al: Biological characterization of the virus causing leukoencephalitis and arthritis in goats. *J Gen Virol* 50:423–427, 1980.
25 Narayan O et al: Biological characterization of the virus causing leukoencephalitis and arthritis in goats. *J Gen Virol* 50:69–79, 1980.
26 Gardner MB: The history of simian AIDS. *J Med Primatol* 25:148–157, 1996.
27 Pedersen NC et al: Isolation of a T-lymphotropic virus from domestic cats with an immunodeficiency-like syndrome. *Science* 235:790–793, 1987.
28 Kertayadnya G et al: Characteristics of a retrovirus associated with Jembrana disease in Bali cattle. *J Gen Virol* 74:1765–1778, 1993.
29 Baier M et al: Molecularly cloned simian immunodeficiency virus SIVagm3 is highly divergent from other SIV_{agm} isolates and is biologically active in vitro and in vivo. *J Virol* 63:5119–5123, 1989.
30 Gravell M et al: Infection of macaque monkeys with simian immunodeficiency virus from African green monkeys: Virulence and activation of latent infection. *J Med Primatol* 18:247–254, 1989.
31 Honjo S et al: Experimental infection of African green monkeys and cynomolgus monkeys with a SIVAGM strain isolated from a healthy African green monkey. *J Med Primatol* 19:9–20, 1990.
32 Johnson PR et al: Molecular clones of SIV_{sm} and SIV_{agm}: Experimental infection of macaques and African green monkeys. *J Med Primatol* 19:279–286, 1990.
33 Cichutek K et al: Lack of immune suppression in SIV-infected natural hosts. *AIDS* 7:S25–35, 1993.
34 Novembre FJ et al: SIV from stump-tailed macaques: Molecular characterization of a highly transmissible primate lentivirus. *Virology* 186:783–787, 1992.
35 Hunt RD et al: Transmission of naturally occurring lymphoma in macaque monkeys. *Proc Natl Acad Sci USA* 80:5085–5089, 1983.
36 Daniel MD et al: Isolation of T-cell tropic HTLV-III-like retrovirus from macaques. *Science* 228:1201–1204, 1985.
37 Khan AS et al: A highly divergent simian immunodeficiency virus (SIVstm) recovered from stored stump-tailed macaque tissues. *J Virol* 65:7061–7065, 1991.
38 Benveniste RE et al: Isolation of a lentivirus from a macaque with lymphoma: Comparison with HTLV-III/LAV and other lentiviruses. *J Virol* 60:483–490, 1986.
39 Joag SV et al: *Lentiviruses,* in *Fields Virology,* 3rd ed. Fields BN et al (eds). Philadelphia, Lippincott-Raven Publishers, 1996, pp. 1977–1996.
40 Perk K: Characteristics of ovine and caprine lentivirus infections. *Leukemia* 9:S98–100, 1995.
41 de la Concha-Bermejillo A et al: Ovine lentivirus infection: An animal model for pediatric HIV infection? *Arch Med Res* 26:345–354, 1995.
42 Gendelman HE et al: Tropism of sheep lentiviruses for monocytes: Susceptibility to infection and virus gene expression increase during maturation of monocytes to macrophages. *J Virol* 58:67–74, 1986.
43 Maury W: Monocyte maturation controls expression of equine infectious anemia virus. *J Virol* 68:6270–6279, 1994.
44 Narayan O et al: Activation of caprine arthritis-encephalitis virus expression during maturation of monocytes to macrophages. *Infec Immun* 41:67–73, 1983.
45 Sellon DC et al: Wild-type equine infectious anemia virus replicates in vivo predominantly in tissue macrophages, not in peripheral blood monocytes. *J Virol* 66:5906–5913, 1992.
46 Zink MC et al: Pathogenesis of visna/maedi and caprine arthritis-encephalitis: New leads on the mechanism of restricted virus replication and persistent inflammation. *Vet Immunol Immunopathol* 15:167–180, 1987.
47 Goerdt S et al: The mononuclear phagocyte-dendritic cell dichotomy: Myths, facts, and a revised concept. *Clin Exp Immunol* 105:1–9, 1996.
48 Xu H et al: Dendritic cells differentiated from human monocytes through a combination of IL-4, GM-CSF and IFN-gamma exhibit phenotype and function of blood dendritic cells. *Adv Exp Med Biol* 378:75–78, 1995.
49 Cameron PU et al: Preferential entry and productive infection of CD4 expressing lymphoid dendritic cells by macrophage-tropic HIV-1. *Adv Exp Med Biol* 378:429–433, 1995.
50 Cameron PU et al: The interaction of macrophage and non-macrophage tropic isolates of HIV-1 with thymic and tonsillar dendritic cells in vitro. *J Exp Med* 183:1851–1856, 1996.
51 Spira AI et al: Cellular targets of infection and route of viral dissemination after an intravaginal inoculation of simian immunodeficiency virus into rhesus macaques. *J Exp Med* 183:215–225, 1996.
52 Collman R: Human immunodeficiency virus type 1 tropism for human macrophages. *Pathobiology* 60:213–218, 1992.
53 Gendelman HE et al: Slow, persistent replication of lentiviruses: role of tissue macrophages and macrophage precursors in bone marrow. *Proc Natl Acad Sci USA* 82:7086–7090, 1985.
54 Meltzer MS et al: Role of mononuclear phagocytes in the pathogenesis of human immunodeficiency virus infection. *Annu Rev Immunol* 8:169–194, 1990.
55 Meltzer MS et al: Mononuclear phagocytes as targets, tissue reservoirs, and immunoregulatory cells in human immunodeficiency virus disease. *Curr Top Microbiol Immunol* 181:239–263, 1992.
56 Clements JE et al: Lentivirus infection of macrophages. *Immunol Series* 60:589–600, 1994.
57 Konno S et al: Pathology of equine infectious anemia. Proposed classification of pathological types of disease. *Cornell Vet* 60:393–449, 1970.
58 Sellon DC et al: Equine infectious anemia virus replication is upregulated during differentiation of blood monocytes from acutely infected horses. *J Virol* 70:590–594, 1996.
59 Sonza S et al: Human immunodeficiency virus type 1 replication is blocked prior to reverse transcription and integration in freshly isolated peripheral blood monocytes. *J Virol* 70:3863–3869, 1996.
60 Sierra MJ et al: Relationship between load of virus in alveolar macrophages from human immunodeficiency virus type 1-infected persons, production of cytokines, and clinical status. *J Infect Dis* 169:18–27, 1994.
61 Thieblemont N et al: Triggering of complement receptors CR1 (CD35) and CR3 (CD11b/CD18) induces nuclear translocation of NF-kappa B (p50/p65) in human monocytes and enhances viral replication in HIV-infected monocytic cells. *J Immunol* 155:4861–4867, 1995.
62 Levy RM et al: Central nervous system disorders in AIDS. *Immunol Ser* 44:371–401, 1989.
63 Georgsson G: Neuropathologic aspects of lentiviral infections. *Ann NY Acad Sci* 724:50–67, 1994.
64 Mankowski JL et al: Neurovirulent simian immunodeficiency virus replicates productively in endothelial cells of the central nervous system in vivo and in vitro. *J Virol* 68:8202–8208, 1994.
65 Clements JE et al: Molecular biology and pathogenesis of animal lentivirus infections. *Clin Microbiol Rev* 9:100–117, 1996.
66 Hurtrel M et al: Comparison of early and late feline immunodeficiency virus encephalopathies. *AIDS* 6:399–406, 1992.
67 Hurtrel B et al: Target cells during early SIV encephalopathy. *Res Virol* 144:41–46, 1993.
68 Anderson MG et al: Analysis of envelope changes acquired by SIVmac239 during neuroadaption in rhesus macaques. *Virology* 195:616–626, 1993.
69 Sharma DP et al: Derivation of neurotropic simian immunodeficiency virus from exclusively lymphocytetropic parental virus: Pathogenesis of infection in macaques. *J Virol* 66:3550–3556, 1992.
70 Hayman M et al: Neurotoxicity of peptide analogues of the transactivating protein tat from Maedi-Visna virus and human immunodeficiency virus. *Neuroscience* 53:1–6, 1993.

71 Giulian D et al: Study of receptor-mediated neurotoxins released by HIV-1-infected mononuclear phagocytes found in human brain. *J Neurosci* 16:3139–3153, 1996.
72 Barnhart HX et al: Natural history of human immunodeficiency virus disease in perinatally infected children: An analysis from the Pediatric Spectrum of Disease Project. *Pediatrics* 975:710–716, 1996.
73 Joshi VV et al: Pathologic pulmonary findings in children with the acquired immunodeficiency syndrome: A study of ten cases. *Hum Pathol* 16:241–246, 1985.
74 Mornex JF et al: Diffuse interstitial pneumopathies caused by lentivirus (HIV-1) in humans and animals. *Rev Malad Respir* 7:517–528, 1990.
75 DeMartini JC et al: Pathogenesis of lymphoid interstitial pneumonia in natural and experimental ovine lentivirus infection. *Clin Infect Dis* 17:S236–242, 1993.
76 Cordier G et al: Characterization of the lymphocytic alveolitis in visna-maedi virus-induced interstitial lung disease of sheep. *Clin Exp Immunol* 90:18–24, 1992.
77 Simon MA et al: Pathological features of SIV-induced disease and the association of macrophage infection with disease evolution. *AIDS Res Hum Retroviruses* 8:327–337, 1992.
78 Cordier G et al: In vivo activation of alveolar macrophages in ovine lentivirus infection. *Clin Immunol Immunopathol* 55:355–367, 1990.
79 Lujan L et al: Phenotypic analysis of cells in bronchoalveolar lavage fluid and peripheral blood of maedi visna-infected sheep. *Clin Exp Immunol* 91:272–276, 1993.
80 Lujan L et al: Ovine lentivirus (maedi-visna virus) protein expression in sheep alveolar macrophages. *Vet Pathol* 31:695–703, 1994.
81 Anderson AA et al: Quantitative analysis of immunohistological changes in the synovial membrane of sheep infected with Maedi-Visna virus. *Clin Immunol Immunopathol* 72:21–29, 1994.
82 Harkiss GD et al: Retroviral arthritis: Phenotypic analysis of cells in the synovial fluid of sheep with inflammatory synovitis associated with visna virus infection. *Clin Immunol Immunopathol* 60:106–117, 1991.
83 Swardson CJ et al: Effects of equine infectious anemia virus on hematopoietic progenitors in vitro. *Amer J Vet Res* 53:1176–1179, 1992.
84 McGuire TC et al: Immunopathogenesis of equine infectious anemia lentivirus disease. *Dev Biol Stand* 72:31–37, 1990.
85 Clabough DL et al: Immune-mediated thrombocytopenia in horses infected with equine infectious anemia virus. *J Virol* 65:6242–6251, 1991.
86 Fultz PN et al: Identification and biologic characterization of an acutely lethal variant of simian immunodeficiency virus from sooty mangabeys (SIV/SMM). *AIDS Res Hum Retroviruses* 5:397–409, 1989.
87 Fultz PN: SIVsmmPBj14: An atypical lentivirus. *Cur Top Microbiol Immunol* 188:65–76, 1994.
88 Israel ZR et al: Early pathogenesis of disease caused by SIVsmmPBj14 molecular clone 1.9 in macaques. *AIDS Res Hum Retroviruses* 9: 277–286, 1993.
89 Fultz PN et al: Unique lentivirus–host interactions: SIVsmmPBj14 infection of macaques. *Virus Res* 32:205–225, 1994.
90 Otsyula MG et al: Apparent lack of vertical transmission of simian immunodeficiency virus (SIV) in naturally infected African green monkeys, Cercopithecus aethiops. *Ann Trop Med Parasitol* 89:573–576, 1995.
91 Ruprecht RM et al: Animal models for perinatal transmission of pathogenic viruses. *Ann NY Acad Sci* 693:213–228, 1993.
92 Ochs HD et al: Intra-amniotic inoculation of pigtailed macaque (Macaca nemestrina) fetuses with SIV and HIV-1. *J Med Primatol* 22: 162–168, 1993.
93 Fazely F et al: Simian immunodeficiency virus infection via amniotic fluid: A model to study fetal immunopathogenesis and prophylaxis. *J Acq Immune Def Synd* 6:107–114, 1993.
94 Baba TW et al: Mucosal infection of neonatal rhesus monkeys with cell-free SIV. *AIDS Res Hum Retroviruses* 10:351–357, 1994.
95 Amedee AM et al: Genotypic selection of simian immunodeficiency virus in macaque infants infected transplacentally. *J Virol* 69:7982–7990, 1995.
96 Kennedy SS et al: The mammary gland as a target organ for infection with caprine arthritis-encephalitis virus. *J Comp Pathol* 95:609–617, 1985.
97 Schuitemaker H et al: Biological phenotype of human immunodeficiency virus type 1 clones at different stages of infection: Progression of disease is associated with a shift from monocytotropic to T-cell-tropic virus populations. *J Virol* 66:1354–1360, 1992.
98 Zhu T et al: Genotypic and phenotypic characterization of HIV-1 patients with primary infection. *Science* 261:1179–1181, 1993.
99 Royce RA et al: Sexual transmission of HIV. *NEJM* 336:1072–1078, 1997.
100 Rezikyan S et al: B-cell lymphomagenesis in SIV-immunosuppressed cynomolgus monkeys. *Int J Cancer* 61:574–579, 1995.
101 Colombini S et al: Detection of HHV-8-like DNA sequences in cynomolgus monkeys developing B-cell lymphomas. *AIDS Res Hum Retroviruses* 11:S75, 1995.
102 Miller CJ et al: The effect of contraceptives containing nonoxynol-9 on the genital transmission of simian immunodeficiency virus in rhesus macaques. *Fertil Steril* 57:1126–1128, 1992.
103 Miller CJ et al: Localization of SIV in the genital tract of chronically infected female rhesus macaques. *Am J Pathol* 141:655–660, 1992.
104 Miller CJ et al: Mechanism of genital transmission of SIV: A hypothesis based on transmission studies and the location of SIV in the genital tract of chronically infected female rhesus macaques. *J Med Primatol* 21:64–68, 1992.
105 Joag SV et al: Chimeric simian/human immunodeficiency virus that causes progressive loss of CD4+ T cells and AIDS in pig-tailed macaques. *J Virol* 70:3189–3197, 1996.
106 Allan JS et al: Infection of baboons with simian/human immunodeficiency viruses. *J Acq Immune Defic Syndr Hum Retrovirol* 9:429–441, 1995.
107 Uberla K et al: Animal model for the therapy of acquired immunodeficiency syndrome with reverse transcriptase inhibitors. *Proc Natl Acad Sci USA* 92:8210–8214, 1995.
108 Joag SV et al: Simian immunodeficiency virus SIVmac chimeric virus whose env gene was derived from SIV-encephalitic brain is macrophage-tropic but not neurovirulent. *J Virol* 69:1367–1369, 1995.
109 Stephens EB et al: Lymphocyte-tropic simian immunodeficiency virus causes persistent infection in the brains of rhesus monkeys. *Virology* 213:600–614, 1995.
110 Gibbs JS et al: Progression to AIDS in the absence of a gene for vpr or vpx. *J Virol* 69:2378–2383, 1995.
111 Dittmar MT et al: An in vitro assay for acute pathogenicity of immunodeficiency viruses. *Dev Biol Stand* 86:167–173, 1996.
112 Du Z et al: Identification of a *nef* allele that causes lymphocyte activation and acute disease in macaque monkeys. *Cell* 82:665–674, 1995.
113 Coffin JM: Retroviridae: The viruses and their replication, in *Fields Virology*, 3rd ed. Fields BN et al (eds). Philadelphia, Lippincott-Raven Publishers, 1996, pp. 1776–1848.
114 Dalgleish AG et al: The CD4 (T4) antigen is an essential component of the receptor for the AIDS retrovirus. *Nature* 312:763–767, 1984.
115 Bates P: Chemokine receptors and HIV-1: An attractive pair? *Cell* 86:1–3, 1996.
116 Gilboa E et al: A detailed model of reverse transcription and tests of crucial aspects. *Cell* 18:93–100, 1979.
117 Shank PR et al: Mapping unintegrated avian sarcoma virus DNA: Termini of linear DNA bear 300 nucleotides present once or twice in two species of circular DNA. *Cell* 15:1383–1395, 1978.
118 Hsu TW et al: Analysis of unintegrated avian RNA tumor virus double-stranded DNA intermediates. *J Virol* 28:810–818, 1978.
119 Grandgenett DP et al: A 32,000-dalton nucleic acid-binding protein from avian retravirus cores possesses DNA endonuclease activity. *Virology* 89:119–132, 1978.
120 Brown PO et al: Retroviral integration: Structure of the initial covalent product and its precursor, and a role for the viral IN protein. *Proc Natl Acad Sci USA* 86:2525–2529, 1989.

121 Brown PO: Integration of retroviral DNA. *Curr Top Microbiol Immunol* 157:19–48, 1990.
122 Gaynor RB: Regulation of HIV-1 gene expression by the transactivator protein Tat. *Curr Top Microbiol Immunol* 193:51–77, 1995.
123 Kingsman SM et al: The regulation of human immunodeficiency virus type-1 gene expression. *Eur J Biochem* 240:491–507, 1996.
124 Swanstrom R et al: *Retroviral Gene Expression: Synthesis, Assembly, and Processing of Viral Proteins.* Varmus HE et al (eds). Cold Spring Harbor, NY, Cold Spring Harbor Laboratory Press, 1997, chapter 7.
125 Sova P et al: Efficiency of viral DNA synthesis during infection of permissive and nonpermissive cells with vif-negative human immunodeficiency virus type 1. *J Virol* 67:6322–6326, 1993.
126 von Schwedler U et al: Vif is crucial for human immunodeficiency virus type 1 proviral DNA synthesis in infected cells. *J Virol* 67:4945–4955, 1993.
127 Rogel ME et al: The human immunodeficiency virus type 1 vpr gene prevents cell proliferation during chronic infection. *J Virol* 69:882–888, 1995.
128 Jowett JB et al: The human immunodeficiency virus type 1 vpr gene arrests infected T cells in the G2 + M phase of the cell cycle. *J Virol* 69:6304–6313, 1995.
129 Heinzinger NK et al: The Vpr protein of human immunodeficiency virus type 1 influences nuclear localization of viral nucleic acids in nondividing host cells. *Proc Natl Acad Sci USA* 91:7311–7315, 1994.
130 Strebel K et al: A novel gene of HIV-1, vpu, and its 16-kilodalton product. *Science* 241:1221–1223, 1988.
131 Terwilliger EF et al: Functional role of human immunodeficiency virus type 1 vpu. *Proc Natl Acad Sci USA* 86:5163–5167, 1989.
132 Willey RL et al: Human immunodeficiency virus type 1 Vpu protein induces rapid degradation of CD4. *J Virol* 66:7193–7200, 1992.
133 Sodroski J et al: Location of the trans-activating region on the genome of human T-cell lymphotropic virus type III. *Science* 229:74–77, 1985.
134 Arya SK et al: Trans-activator gene of human T-lymphotropic virus type III (HTLV-III). *Science* 229:69–73, 1985.
135 Felber BK et al: rev Protein of human immunodeficiency virus type 1 affects the stability and transport of the viral mRNA. *Proc Natl Acad Sci USA* 86:1495–1499, 1989.
136 Malim MH et al: The HIV-1 rev trans-activator acts through a structured target sequence to activate nuclear export of unspliced viral mRNA. *Nature* 338:254–257, 1989.
137 Aiken C et al: Nef stimulates human immunodeficiency virus type 1 proviral DNA synthesis. *J Virol* 69:5048–5056, 1995.
138 Garcia JV et al: Serine phosphorylation-independent downregulation of cell-surface CD4 by nef. *Nature* 350:508–511, 1991.
139 Guy B et al: HIV F/3′ orf encodes a phosphorylated GTP-binding protein resembling an oncogene product. *Nature* 330:266–269, 1987.
140 Miller MD et al: Expression of the human immunodeficiency virus type 1 (HIV-1) nef gene during HIV-1 production increases progeny particle infectivity independently of gp160 or viral entry. *J Virol* 69:579–584, 1995.
141 Schwartz O et al: Human immunodeficiency virus type 1 Nef increases the efficiency of reverse transcription in the infected cell. *J Virol* 69:4053–4059, 1995.
142 Roe T et al: Integration of murine leukemia virus DNA depends on mitosis. *EMBO Journal* 12:2099–2108, 1993.
143 Wei X et al: Viral dynamics in human immunodeficiency virus type 1 infection. *Nature* 373:117–122, 1995.
144 Ho DD et al: Rapid turnover of plasma virions and CD4 lymphocytes in HIV-1 infection. *Nature* 373:123–126, 1995.
145 Mansky LM et al: Lower in vivo mutation rate of human immunodeficiency virus type 1 than that predicted from the fidelity of purified reverse transcriptase. *J Virol* 69:5087–5094, 1995.
146 Pathak VK et al: Broad spectrum of in vivo forward mutations, hypermutations, and mutational hotspots in a retroviral shuttle vector after a single replication cycle: substitutions, frameshifts, and hypermutations. *Proc Natl Acad Sci USA* 87:6019–6023, 1990.
147 Coffin JM: HIV population dynamics in vivo: implications for genetic variation, pathogenesis, and therapy. *Science* 267:483–489, 1995.
148 Havlir DV et al: Nevirapine-resistant human immunodeficiency virus: Kinetics of replication and estimated prevalence in untreated patients. *J Virol* 70:7894–7899, 1996.
149 Richman DD et al: Nevirapine resistance mutations of human immunodeficiency virus type 1 selected during therapy. *J Virol* 68:1660–1666, 1994.
150 Kellam P et al: Zidovudine treatment results in the selection of human immunodeficiency virus type 1 variants whose genotypes confer increasing levels of drug resistance. *J Gen Virol* 75:341–351, 1994.
151 Molla A et al: Ordered accumulation of mutations in HIV protease confers resistance to ritonavir. *Nat Med* 2:760–766, 1996.
152 Simmonds P et al: Discontinuous sequence change of human immunodeficiency virus (HIV) type 1 *env* sequences in plasma viral and lymphocyte-associated proviral populations in vivo: Implications for models of HIV pathogenesis. *J Virol* 65:6266–6276, 1991.
153 Hu W-S et al: Role of reverse transcriptase in retroviral recombination, in *Reverse Transcriptase,* Skalka AM et al (eds). Cold Spring Harbor, NY, Cold Spring Harbor Laboratory Press, 1993, pp. 251–274.
154 Gu Z et al: Possible involvement of cell fusion and viral recombination in generation of human immunodeficiency virus variants that display dual resistance to AZT and 3TC. *J Gen Virol* 76:2601–2605, 1995.
155 Kellam P et al: Retroviral recombination can lead to linkage of reverse transcriptase mutations that confer increased zidovudine resistance. *J Virol* 69:669–674, 1995.
156 Moutouh L et al: Recombination leads to the rapid emergence of HIV-1 dually resistant mutants under selective drug pressure. *Proc Natl Acad Sci USA* 93:6106–6111, 1996.
157 Perelson AS et al: HIV-1 dynamics in vivo: Virion clearance rate, infected cell life-span, and viral generation time. *Science* 271:1582–1586, 1996.
158 Mellors JW et al: Prognosis in HIV-1 infection predicted by the quantity of virus in plasma. *Science* 272:1167–1170, 1996.
159 Choe H et al: The beta-chemokine receptors CCR3 and CCR5 facilitate infection by primary HIV-1 isolates. *Cell* 85:1135–1148, 1996.
160 Deng H et al: Identification of a major co-receptor for primary isolates of HIV-1. *Nature* 381:661–666, 1996.
161 Doranz BJ et al: A dual-tropic primary HIV-1 isolate that uses fusin and the beta-chemokine receptors CKR-5, CKR-3, and CKR-2b as fusion cofactors. *Cell* 85:1149–1158, 1996.
162 Dragic T et al: HIV-1 entry into CD4+ cells is mediated by the chemokine receptor CC-CKR-5. *Nature* 381:667–673, 1996.
163 Simmons G et al: Primary, syncytium-inducing human immunodeficiency virus type 1 isolates are dual-tropic and most can use either Lestr or CCR5 as coreceptors for virus entry. *J Virol* 70:8355–8360, 1996.
164 Asjo B et al: Replicative properties of human immunodeficiency virus from patients with varying severity of HIV infection. *Lancet* ii:660–662, 1986.
165 Feng Y et al: HIV-1 entry cofactor: Functional cDNA cloning of a seven-transmembrane, G protein-coupled receptor. *Science* 272:872–877, 1996.
166 Koot M et al: HIV-1 biological phenotype in long-term infected individuals evaluated with an MT-2 cocultivation assay. *AIDS* 6:49–54, 1992.
167 Koot M et al: Prognostic value of HIV-1 syncytium-inducing phenotype for rate of CD4+ cell depletion and progression to AIDS. *Ann Int Med* 118:681–688, 1993.
168 Tersmette M et al: Evidence for a role of virulent human immunodeficiency virus (HIV) variants in the pathogenesis of acquired immunodeficiency syndrome: Studies on sequential HIV isolates. *J Virol* 63:2118–2125, 1989.
169 Chesebro B et al: Identification of human immunodeficiency virus envelope gene sequences influencing viral entry into CD4-positive

HeLa cells, T-leukemia cells, and macrophages. *J Virol* 65:5782–5789, 1991.

170 De Jong J-J et al: Minimal requirements for the human immunodeficiency virus type 1 V3 domain to support the syncytium-inducing phenotype: analysis by single amino acid substitution. *J Virol* 66: 6777–6780, 1992.

171 Hwang SS et al: Identification of the envelope V3 loop as the primary determinant of cell tropism in HIV-1. *Science* 253:71–74, 1991.

172 Shioda T et al: Small amino acid changes in the V3 hypervariable region of gp120 can affect the T-cell-line and macrophage tropism of human immunodeficiency virus type 1. *Proc Natl Acad Sci USA* 89: 9434–9438, 1992.

173 Westervelt P et al: Identification of a determinant within the human immunodeficiency virus 1 surface envelope glycoprotein critical for productive infection of primary monocytes. *Proc Natl Acad Sci USA* 88:3097–3101, 1991.

174 Mariani R et al: High frequency of defective nef alleles in a long-term survivor with nonprogressive human immunodeficiency virus type 1 infection. *J Virol* 70:7752–7764, 1996.

175 Kirchhoff F et al: Absence of intact nef sequences in a long-term survivor with nonprogressive HIV-1 infection. *NEJM* 332:228–232, 1995.

176 Deacon NJ et al: Genomic structure of an attenuated quasi species of HIV-1 from a blood transfusion donor and recipients. *Science* 270: 988–991, 1995.

177 Kestler HW et al: Importance of the *nef* gene for maintenance of high virus loads and for development of AIDS. *Cell* 65:651–662, 1991.

178 Markovitz DM: Infection with the human immunodeficiency virus type 2. *Ann Int Med* 118:211–218, 1993.

179 Yamamoto JK et al: Experimental vaccine protection against homologous and heterologous strains of feline immunodeficiency virus. *J Virol* 67:601–605, 1993.

180 Issel CJ et al: Efficacy of inactivated whole-virus and subunit vaccines in preventing infection and disease caused by equine infectious anemia virus. *J Virol* 66:3398–3408, 1992.

181 Gudnadottir M: Experiments with inactivated visna-maedi vaccine. *Ann NY Acad Sci* 724:140–147, 1994.

182 Russo P et al: Caprine arthritis-encephalitis: Trial of an adjuvant vaccine preparation. I. Clinical and virological study. *Comp Immunol Microbiol Infect Dis* 16:131–136, 1993.

183 Vitu C et al: Caprine arthritis-encephalitis: Trial of an adjuvant vaccine preparation. II. Study of the antibody response. *Comp Immunol Microbiol Infect Dis* 16:137–144, 1993.

184 Cheevers WP et al: Caprine arthritis-encephalitis lentivirus (CAEV) challenge of goats immunized with recombinant vaccinia virus expressing CAEV surface and transmembrane envelope glycoproteins. *Vet Immunol Immunopathol* 42:237–251, 1994.

185 Daniel MD et al: Protective effects of a live attenuated SIV vaccine with a deletion in the nef gene. *Science* 258:1938–1941, 1992.

186 Baba TW et al: Pathogenicity of live, attenuated SIV after mucosal infection of neonatal macaques. *Science* 267:1820–1825, 1995.

187 Gao F et al: Human infection by genetically diverse SIVSM-related HIV-2 in west Africa. *Nature* 358:495–499, 1992.

188 Myers G et al: *Human Retroviruses and AIDS 1993*. Los Alamos, NM, Los Alamos National Laboratory, Theoretical Biology and Biophysics, 1993.

189 Louwagie J et al: Phylogenetic analysis of *gag* genes from 70 international HIV-1 isolates provides evidence for multiple genotypes. *AIDS* 7:769–780, 1993.

190 Ou CY et al: Independent introduction of two major HIV-1 genotypes into distinct high-risk populations in Thailand. *Lancet* 341: 1171–1174, 1993.

191 Ou C et al: Wide distribution of two subtypes of HIV-1 in Thailand. *AIDS Res Hum Retroviruses* 8:1471–1472, 1992.

192 McCutchan FE et al: Genetic variants of HIV-1 in Thailand. *AIDS Res Hum Retroviruses* 8:1887–1895, 1992.

193 Soto RL et al: HIV-1 Langerhans' cell tropism associated with heterosexual transmission of HIV. *Science* 271:1291–1293, 1996.

194 Kalish ML et al: The evolving molecular epidemiology of HIV-1 envelope subtypes in injecting drug users in Bangkok, Thailand: Implications for HIV vaccine trials. *AIDS* 9:851–857, 1995.

195 Gao F et al: The heterosexual human immunodeficiency virus type 1 epidemic in Thailand is caused by an intersubtype (A/E) recombinant of African origin. *J Virol* 70:7013–7029, 1996.

196 Robertson DL et al: Recombination in HIV-1. *Nature* 374:124–126, 1995.

197 Cornelissen M et al: Human immunodeficiency virus type 1 subtypes defined by env show high frequency of recombinant gag genes. The UNAIDS Network for HIV Isolation and Characterization. *J Virol* 70:8209–8212, 1996.

198 Huet T et al: Genetic organization of a chimpanzee lentivirus related to HIV-1. *Nature* 345:356–359, 1990.

199 Vanden Haesevelde M et al: Genomic cloning and complete sequence analysis of a highly divergent African human immunodeficiency virus isolate. *J Virol* 68:1586–1596, 1994.

200 Vanden Haesevelde MM et al: Sequence analysis of a highly divergent HIV-1-related lentivirus isolated from a wild captured chimpanzee. *Virology* 221:346–350, 1996.

201 Peeters M et al: Isolation and characterization of a new chimpanzee lentivirus (simian immunodeficiency virus isolate cpz-ant) from a wild-captured chimpanzee. *AIDS* 6:447–451, 1992.

202 Doolittle RF et al: *Retrovirus Phylogeny and Evolution*. New York, Springer-Verlag, 1990.

203 Swanstrom R et al: The aspartic proteinase of HIV-1. *Semin Virol* 1: 175–186, 1990.

Chapter 17

Immunology of human immunodeficiency virus

Scott Koenig
Anthony S. Fauci

Over the past two decades, considerable strides have been made in delineating the immunopathogenesis of the acquired immunodeficiency syndrome (AIDS).[1,2] While gaps persist in our complete understanding, a unified picture has begun to emerge to account for many of the aspects of immune abnormalities and viral persistence in infected individuals. Many of the key discoveries in the immunology of human immunodeficiency virus (HIV) disease have been facilitated by progress in related areas of virology, including antiviral therapeutics, the characterization of molecular diversity, and methods of viral quantitation. Likewise, progress in the immunology of HIV and AIDS has fostered fundamental and therapeutic advances in allied fields of infectious diseases and cancer.

The initial studies in the early 1980s that defined the syndrome, and those reported subsequently, documented immune defects in patients with AIDS as well as in patients with early clinical stages of disease.[3–5] These immune abnormalities provided a rational basis for the opportunistic infections first observed in these patients. They included the depletion of circulating CD4+ T lymphocytes, hypergammaglobulinemia and polyclonal B-cell activation, impaired induction of specific immune responses in vivo, and depression of T-cell, monocyte, and natural killer (NK) cell function.[5–7] With the isolation of HIV type 1[8–11] and a related virus, HIV type 2,[12,13] a large number of studies followed in the middle and late 1980s concerned with the tropism of HIV for particular cell types, identification of CD4 as the primary receptor of HIV,[14–16] and the functional abnormalities induced by HIV in normal lymphocytes and monocytes in vitro and HIV-infected subjects in vivo. Viral replication was observed in sites other than the peripheral blood, including the brain, lungs, and small bowel. At this time, the contribution of cytokines and monokines in augmenting or inhibiting HIV replication through autocrine- and paracrine-dependent mechanisms was first documented.[17,18] The importance of cytokines to immunopathogenesis continues to unfold. Recent observations have linked enhanced viral replication in patients infected with other pathogens to the elaboration of cytokines, and analogues of a family of chemokines have been added as potential antiviral agents.

Other efforts have been focused on identifying the natural and experimentally induced immune responses to HIV-1.[19–25] It was hoped that such studies would help to identify surrogates of protection and provide insights for prophylactic vaccine development and other immune-based therapies. These investigations have been concerned with the magnitude and quality of specific responses at different clinical stages and the heterogeneity of responses to different viral components. Many of these findings provided the rationale for therapies currently being explored in clinical trials. Key observations concerned with immune-dependent selection of viral variants evolved from some of these studies.[26,27]

In the early 1990s, a more systematic examination of HIV replication within lymphoid tissues was conducted to define the pathophysiologic consequences of infection in these regions.[28–30] These studies provided objective evidence for a continuum of destruction of various structural elements within the lymph node, spleen, and thymus and its intimate association with viral replication. It diminished the enthusiasm for autoimmune-based theories of T-cell depletion that were favored at that time and highlighted the imperative of therapeutic interventions to control viral replication in different tissue compartments.[31] Despite these observations, the primary mechanisms of CD4+ T-cell loss have not been elucidated fully. The majority of cells are presumed to be eliminated through direct viral infection. In addition, apoptosis or programmed cell death is thought to be responsible for loss of both CD4+ and CD8+ cells; however, other mechanisms of depletion have been proposed, including immune-mediated lysis, syncytia formation, and cellular necrosis.[32–34]

A greater appreciation for the biologic heterogeneity of HIV isolates occurred in the early 1990s, including differences in cell tropism, rates of replication, and cytopathicity.[35–39] Some viral isolates were found to be T-cell tropic (especially those passaged through T-cell lines), others exclusively monocytotropic, and a third group primarily monocytotropic but also able to infect primary, nontransformed T cells. Viral transmission to newly infected adult subjects and neonates was found to occur primarily with non-syncytial-inducing monocytotropic variants. Isolates that replicated rapidly and were more cytopathic and T-cell tropic often were isolated in later stages of disease, although exceptions were noted. Many of these properties were dictated by small sequence differences in envelope structure. Major shifts in viral populations in individuals were found to be influenced by processes of recurrent immune selection, especially early in the clinical course, and possibly by viral recombination. Since individuals with rapid progression often showed less viral diversity and impaired specific anti-HIV activity, this provided support to the concept of immune-dependent selection.[40]

The recognition of the immune selection of viral variants ultimately led to a reevaluation of natural and induced immunity and a greater appreciation of the resistance of primary isolates to immune regulation. This was highlighted by the inability of soluble CD4 to inhibit the replication of primary isolates as potently as the laboratory-passaged T-cell-tropic isolates.[41] Furthermore, antibody responses to subunit envelope vaccines, which were successful in inducing protective responses in animal model systems challenged with laboratory isolates, were uniformly ineffective in neutralizing primary viral isolates.[42] Significant efforts continue to address this formidable problem, including an exhaustive examination of native structure of the envelope protein.

As new antiretroviral agents became available and drug-induced mutations conferring resistance to these agents were identified rapidly, the primary tenets of viral replication were soon redefined. Initially, it was believed that after primary infection, viral replication entered a long latent phase sometimes interrupted by bursts of viral replication. Accelerated viral replication was thought to precede the development of AIDS. Currently, it is believed that viral replication and turnover of infected T cells are rapid and continuous.[43–46] The hematopoietic system replaces depleted T cells as the immune response attempts to limit viral replication. This mechanism is best appreciated during primary infection, which may present clinically as a mononucleosis-like syndrome. CD4+ T cells show a precipitous drop and are then partially restored within weeks when anti-HIV-specific immune responses are induced. Different clinical sequelae can follow. A minority of subjects (about 10 percent) progress to AIDS within 2 to 3 years after this primary infection; these individuals have been classified as rapid progressors. The majority of individuals develop AIDS typically within 10 years. In these patients, CD4+ T-cell counts have been noted to decline more precipitously about

1 to 2 years prior to the development of AIDS. The reason for this change in CD4+ T-cell count is not known. In a minority of infected subjects (5 to 10 percent), CD4+ T-cell counts remain stable (often defined as >500 cells/mm^3) for over 10 years, and it is predicted that individuals in this category may not develop AIDS even after 20 years. Rare subjects at high risk of infection through repeated exposures to HIV have been found to be resistant to infection, and the mechanisms of protection are being explored.

Recent advances in the arenas of clinical and basic science provide a basis for renewed optimism for controlling HIV replication. First, the addition of protease inhibitors to the antiviral armamentarium, along with combinations of nucleoside analogues (i.e., zidovudine and 3TC among others) and nonnucleosides, has resulted in substantial reductions (up to several $\log_{10}$) in the plasma viral load of some patients, including those with advanced disease (<100 CD4 cells/mm^3). Reduction in viral load is directly associated with marked CD4+ T-cell increases in many subjects, confirming the resilience of the immune system; however, total immune reconstitution is unlikely to occur. Second, the characterization of two distinct variants of chemokine receptors[2,47] provided a structural explanation for the tropism of T-cell and monocytotropic variants. This may foster development of new immune-based interventions.

The objective of this chapter is to describe the immunopathogenic mechanisms of HIV disease, highlight the abnormalities of immune function induced by HIV, and characterize the mechanisms by which HIV is regulated by the immune system.

THE TROPISM OF HIV AND IDENTIFICATION OF ITS RECEPTORS

The first major advance in AIDS research was the ability to isolate HIV (called HTLV-III and LAV at that time) from cultures of peripheral blood mononuclear cells (PBMCs) and lymph nodes from patients stimulated with mitogens.[8,11] Lymphoblasts and human tumor cell lines that expressed the CD4 molecule were identified as the cellular populations that could support viral growth.[14,15,48] Rarely, non-CD4-bearing cells could be infected under unusual circumstances in vitro or through secondary receptors such as galactosyl ceramides.[49,50] The selectivity of HIV for CD4-bearing cells is the result of binding of the viral envelope to the CD4 molecule, which serves as the primary receptor for the virus. The importance of this molecule was suggested originally by the finding that antibodies to some but not all determinants of CD4 could block infection with HIV.[51] With the elucidation of the x-ray crystal structure of CD4, independent faces could be distinguished that interacted with the major histocompatibility class (MHC) II molecule and HIV.[52] Thus selective blocking activities of anti-CD4 monoclonal antibodies could be explained by their localization to distinct faces of the molecule.[53]

Human cell lines that normally do not express CD4 and cannot be infected with HIV can be rendered susceptible to virus infection by transfecting the gene for CD4 and inducing CD4 expression.[54] However, it soon became apparent that other cell surface receptors might need to be expressed concomitantly with CD4. This was suggested by the observation that expression of the human CD4 in a murine cell line did not generate a permissive cell line for HIV, even though this cell line could support HIV replication through transfection of an infectious DNA clone of HIV.[55] This was confirmed more recently by development of transgenic mice with knockouts of the murine CD4 molecule complemented by the human CD4 analogue.[56] These animals were resistant to infection with HIV. Many years passed before insights into this elusive molecule were obtained. Among the candidates described were LFA-1, ICAM-1, and CD26, which may have incremental effects in promoting HIV infection, although conflicting results related to their significance in pathogenesis were obtained by others.[57–61]

A breakthrough in this area occurred with the demonstration that the chemokine receptor CXCR-4, also called *fusin* and *LESTR,* a heterotrimeric G protein-coupled receptor, was the coreceptor for entry and infection with T-cell-tropic strains of HIV, but not monocytotropic or primary isolates of HIV.[62] This was illustrated when antibodies to this receptor blocked entry and infection of the T-cell isolates, but not monocytotropic strains. The natural ligand for this receptor is stromal-derived factor 1 (SDF-1).[63,64] The identification of CXCR-4 as the T-cell-tropic coreceptor was reported soon after the demonstration that a combination of beta-chemokines, namely, RANTES, MIP-1-α, and MIP-1-β, could block infection with monocytotropic but not T-cell-tropic strains.[65] These same cytokines prevented envelope-mediated fusion by the monocytotropic lines. This quickly led to identification of the common receptor for these three chemokines, CCR-5, as a coreceptor for primary monocytotropic strains, again by complementing its expression in human and nonhuman cell lines that were not permissive for HIV infection[66–70] (reviewed in refs. 2 and 47). An "experiment of nature" that supported these findings was the demonstration that several individuals appeared to be naturally resistant to HIV infection. They were homozygous for a 32-base-pair deletion in the CCR-5 gene that prevented surface expression of the truncated protein; their PBMCs could not be infected with monocytotropic strains yet were susceptible to T-cell-tropic isolates.[71] Even heterozygosity for this gene defect, observed in about 20 percent of western European Caucasians, might provide some degree of protection against disease progression, based on reduced HIV replication efficiency in PBMCs of heterozygotes.[71–74] Additional chemokine receptors were shown to participate in fusion-mediated events; CCR-3-expressing cell lines also were permissive for infection with a subset of strains, and infection was prevented by the addition of eotaxin, the ligand for this receptor.[67,69] This latter receptor may serve as the coreceptor for isolates that have a dual tropism for monocytes and T cells. It is likely that other as yet unidentified chemokine coreceptors exist for HIV entry. Furthermore, it will be of interest to determine if transgenic mice expressing the various human chemokine homologues become suitable animal models for HIV disease.

HIV binding to the CD4 molecule is mediated primarily through the C4 region of gp120, although other variable and conserved domains of the envelope contribute to viral binding and entry. The CDR2-like loop of the CD4 domain 1 is the major contact site for interaction with gp120.[75] The relative infectivity of HIV-1 for a given cell line is dictated in part by the density of CD4. Recent studies also have shown that the envelope protein, especially the third hypervariable region (V3), participates in the binding to CCR-5.[65] Binding of the chemokine coreceptor may be independent of the association of envelope with CD4, but the latter may enhance the secondary binding of the chemokine receptor through conformational changes within the envelope protein, creating a high-affinity receptor.[76,77]

T CELLS: CHANGES OBSERVED IN VITRO AND IN VIVO

Infection of cells with HIV is accompanied by the loss of CD4 molecules from the cell surface; however, this can be variable depending on the vigor of viral replication. This is consistent with the persistence of CD4 on infected cells isolated from patients. Loss of CD4 has been attributed to expression of the regulatory protein nef.[78–80] Other surface molecules such as CD25 have been reported to be decreased in infected cells in vitro, but this is variable depending on the experimental conditions. Vpu also has been associated with maintaining CD4-gp160 complexes within the endoplasmic reticulum and enhancing CD4 degradation, possibly through a ubiquitin-dependent pathway, contributing to decreased surface expression.[81]

Transient modulation of CD4 from the surface of infected cells observed with the binding of HIV occurs without associated phosphorylation or endocytosis of CD4, which can be seen following activation with antigen or phorbol esters. In one experimental system, deletion of the cytoplasmic tail of CD4, necessary for phorbol ester-induced endocytosis, did not impede infection.[82] Thus viral entry is dependent on membrane fusion without endocytosis of CD4.

QUANTITATIVE AND PHENOTYPIC CHANGES IN CIRCULATING LYMPHOCYTES

Important changes are observed in both CD4+ and CD8+ cells of patients during their clinical course. The severity of CD4+ lymphocyte depletion correlates somewhat with clinical disorders in seropositive individuals, although measures of viral burden with phenotype are better predictors for clinical outcome.[5,83–87] Initial depression and recovery of CD4+ T cell counts observed in the majority of seropositive subjects is generally followed by a clinically latent phase characterized by a gradual and somewhat predictable CD4+ T cell loss over many years. There may be an abrupt acceleration of CD4 T cell decline within 1 to 2 years before the onset of AIDS, which frequently appears within 10 years and after CD4+ T cell counts decline below 200 cells/mm^3. Associated with overall decreases in CD4+ T cells and increases in CD8+ T cells before terminal stages of AIDS, patients show increased proportions of cells with activation markers and a decrease in cells bearing naive phenotypes.[88] For example, the proportion of cells that express CD45 Ro, DR+ phenotype increases over time, while the complementary phenotype (i.e., CD45 Ra, DR−) is decreased.[88,89] Since these changes are observed both in CD4+ and CD8+ cells, it is unlikely that HIV infection is directly causing the changes. More likely, when vigorous immune responses against HIV are induced and alterations in normal levels of cytokines occur, the phenotypic profiles of these populations are altered. Other observed changes include increases in the proportion of CD62L hi-bearing cells, another activation marker in both CD4 and CD8 cells (J. Margolick, personal communication), decreases in CD25 expression on CD4 cells, and increases in CD8 cells coexpressing CD38.[89–93] Variable changes in other adhesion molecules such as CD11 and CD18 have been reported.[89,94]

MECHANISMS OF CELL DEPLETION

HIV is cytopathic for CD4-bearing cells in vitro, although susceptibility may vary among cell lines. In vitro cytopathic effects may be manifested by the formation of syncytia among infected and uninfected cells.[32,95–97] These are fragile, multinucleated forms that erupt and release viral and cellular contents. Evidence for some syncytia formation in vivo has been derived from rhesus monkeys acutely infected with simian immunodeficiency virus (SIV) and in some tissues of infected humans, particularly within lymph nodes and the central nervous system (CNS). In the case of the latter, giant cell formation occurs primarily among macrophage and microglial cell types. Death of solitary infected cells can occur. Several mechanisms have been proposed for these observations. First, binding of HIV envelope to a cell, especially when cross-linked with agents such as antibody, can induce programmed cell death or apoptosis.[33,98] This appears to be dependent on Fas expression.[99,100] However, studies of infected lymph nodes from patients and animals experimentally infected with SIV demonstrate that most cells that undergo apoptosis are not infected with HIV or SIV.[101] This is consistent with the observation that both CD4+ and CD8+ cells seem to undergo apoptosis; the latter cell type is not normally susceptible to infection with HIV. Second, HIV envelope binding to internal and external membranes may cause disruption and cellular necrosis. However, this mechanism has been difficult to demonstrate in vivo. CD4+ T cells in contact with those expressing HIV-1 envelope have been observed to accumulate proteins involved in the regulation of cell cycling, including cyclin B and cdk1 kinase, suggesting arrest of proliferation at the G_2 phase of the cell cycle. These cells were observed to balloon and disappear with cyclin B synthesis.[102]

The binding of envelope to CD4 causes envelope shedding from virions. Since free gp120 is then available to bind to other uninfected CD4+ cells, this has been suggested as a potential source for CD4+ cell depletion by antibody-dependent or cell-mediated mechanisms.[103] The binding and cross-linking of envelope protein on uninfected CD4+ cells could promote apoptosis as described above,[104] possibly through induction of surface expression of Fas.[105] Again, firm evidence for these envelope-dependent cytopathic mechanisms operating in vivo is lacking.

Since the generation of immune responses to HIV following a primary infection is associated with marked reductions in plasma viremia, it must be presumed that elimination of infected CD4+ T cells contributes to cellular depletion. Since both neutralizing antibodies and class I restricted CTL can be detected in patients even during the late stages of HIV disease, these mechanisms may promote cell depletion in late-stage disease along with programmed cell death. The destruction of dendritic cells and other antigen-presenting cells by similar cytotoxic mechanisms may compromise immune system function. In summary, several mechanisms probably contribute to lymphoid cell depletion, including direct virus cytopathicity with envelope-dependent membrane disruption, antibody- and cell-mediated destruction of infected cells, and programmed cell death of activated but uninfected cells (Table 17–1).

SIGNALING DEFECTS IN T CELLS

Prior to the marked CD4+ T-cell depletion in HIV disease, T-cell functional responses are impaired, as manifested by depressed proliferative responses to antigens and impaired interleukin 2 (IL-2) production.[106] These defects occur in CD4+ T cells and

Table 17-1. Potential Mechanisms of the Functional and Quantitative Depletion of CD4+ T Lymphocytes

Direct HIV-mediated cytopathic effects (single-cell killing)
HIV-mediated formation of syncytia
Virus-specific immune responses
HIV-specific cytotoxic T lymphocytes
Antibody-dependent cellular cytotoxicity
Natural killer cells
Autoimmune mechanisms
Anergy caused by inappropriate cell signaling through gp120-CD4 interaction
Superantigen-mediated perturbation of T-cell subgroups
Programmed cell death (apoptosis)

SOURCE: Pantaleo G, Graziosi C, Fauci AS: The immunopathogenesis of human immunodeficiency virus infection. *N Engl J Med* 328:327–335, 1993.

CD8+ T cells from HIV-infected patients in the absence of productive viral replication. Efforts have been directed at determining if aberrant signaling occurs through stimulation of the T-cell receptor complex and CD4 and CD28 costimulatory pathways by examining cells derived from patients and normal lymphocytes cocultivated with envelope-derived proteins. Engagement of CD4 by gp120 appears to uncouple early events in signaling through the T-cell receptor, as manifested by impaired calcium mobilization, dissociation of p56lck from CD4,[107,108] and lack of induction of zeta-chain tyrosine phosphorylation.[109] Defects in p21ras-dependent pathways also have been observed using similar model systems.[110] These aberrations in signaling can occur in the absence of T-cell receptor costimulation.[111]

Cells from HIV-infected subjects, early in their clinical course, showed decreased levels of p56lck and increased levels of p59fyn in response to anti-CD3 stimulation, which correlated with their defects in proliferation. In this case, additional signaling through CD28 did not correct the abnormal tyrosine phosphorylation pattern in these cells, although proliferation was increased.[112] Others have observed that many of the major protein tyrosine kinases in cells from HIV-infected subjects are reduced, including p59fyn, p56lck, ZAP-70, and the zeta chain of the T-cell receptor, independent of the patient's clinical stage. Interestingly, cells from HIV-infected long-term nonprogressors had normal levels of these kinases. Furthermore, addition of a reducing agent, dithithreitol, reversed the kinase abnormalities, suggesting a possible mechanism and intervention for functional defects in T cells.[113] Likewise, abnormal CD45 phosphatase activity, which was reduced in cells from infected patients, could be restored by treatment with the antioxidants *N*-acetyl-L-cysteine and 2-mercaptoethanol.[112] Taken together, these studies demonstrate major defects in the critical signaling pathway for T-cell activation both in vitro and in vivo due in part to gp120 engagement of CD4.

Table 17-2. HIV Infection and Cytokines

	In vivo/Ex vivo	In Vitro	
Cytokine	Expression/ Production	Expression/ Production	Effect on HIV Replication
TNF-α/-β	↑	↑	↑
TGF-β	↑	?	⇅
IL-1	↑	↑	↑
IL-1ra	?	?	↓
IL-2	↓	↓	⇅
IL-3	↓	?	↑
IL-4	⇅	?	⇅
IL-6	↑	↑	↑
IL-7	?	?	↑
IL-8	↑	⇅	?
IL-10	⇅	?	⇅
IL-12	↓	↓	?
IL-13	?	?	↓
GM-CSF	?	↑	↑
M-CSF	?	↓	↑
IFN-α	↓(↑*)	↓	↓
IFN-β	?	?	↓
IFN-γ	⇅	↓	⇅

*Increased levels of "acid-labile IFN-α" are present in HIV-infected individuals.

SOURCE: Poli G, Fauci AS: Role of cytokines in the pathogenesis of human immunodeficiency virus infection, in *Human Cytokines: Their Role in Disease and Therapy*, BB Aggarwal, RK Puri (eds). Cambridge, MA, Blackwell Scientific, 1995.

ROLE OF CYTOKINES IN IMMUNOPATHOGENESIS

Viral propagation both in vitro and in vivo is influenced by the endogenous production or exogenous addition of cytokines[18] (Table 17–2). Activation of CD4+ PBMCs in vitro with antigen, mitogen, or phorbol esters is associated with release of certain cytokines and enhanced viral replication. Blockade of expression of some cytokines or prevention of their binding to target cells with antibodies or soluble receptors can prevent this viral replication. The sources for elevated levels of these cytokines in patients include cells infected with HIV and other opportunistic pathogens, the specific and nonspecific immune responses induced to HIV and these pathogens, noninfectious activation of cells by virus or viral products, and increased production of acute-phase reactants. It is difficult to extrapolate many of the in vitro findings to observations found in patients due to a variation in effects observed with different experimental conditions. These include the state of activation of cells, the source of donor cells, the mixtures of cell types in culture, the pleiotropic effects of cytokines, the variability in cytokine receptor expression, the multiplicity of infection of the virus used in culture, and the phenotype of viruses examined. However, there appears to be some conformity in the effects of certain of the cytokines examined in vitro, which might be correlated with clinical observations.

Interferon-α and interferon-β produce consistent reductions in viral replication in vitro. The former drug is approved as adjunctive therapy in AIDS patients with Kaposi's sarcoma,[114] while both have been approved for non-HIV-related indications. The antiviral effects do not appear to be virus-specific and are related to a common mechanism of induction of Janus (JAK) and STAT proteins. Clinical trials showed modest objective benefits and antiviral effects; however, this was associated with a tendency to greater toxicities and reduced benefits in patients with low CD4+ T cell counts.[115–117]

Tumor necrosis factor alpha (TNF-α) consistently induces virus replication in cells infected in vitro or in cells derived from infected patients.[118] Blockade of endogenous TNF production with anti-TNF or sTNF receptors following activation prevents the upregulation of virus production in T cells and macrophages.[119,120] The molecular basis of viral enhancement is related to the ability of TNF-α to activate NF-κB, a cellular transcription factor that can bind within the long terminal repeat sequences of HIV and enhance viral transcription.[121] Elevated plasma and tissue levels of TNF are observed also in HIV-infected subjects and are particularly elevated in subjects with coexisting opportunistic infections. However, attempts to reduce TNF effects in vivo either with pentoxifylline, thalidomide, or specific antibodies have not proven to reduce viral loads in early clinical trials.[122,123] Surface expression of TNF-α has been implicated in the polyclonal activation of B cells.[124]

Addition of interleukin 2 (IL-2) uniformly induces viral replication in vitro in association with activation of CD4+ T cells. During the induction of a normal immune response, IL-2 must be produced by CD4+ T cells; thus it is probable that as long as immune function is preserved in these patients, endogenous IL-2 secretion and cellular activation are associated with enhanced viral replication. Experimentally, this has been reproduced in patients by vaccination, which results in bursts of viral replication in vivo and enhanced viral replication in cells derived from these patients.[125,126] Other cytokines also may be involved in this process. When IL-2 is administered as a bolus or by continuous intravenous infusions, increased plasma viremia is observed, but these effects are transient and can be blocked with antiviral agents. This untoward effect is balanced by a significant polyclonal expansion of CD4+ T cells in patients following repeated intermittent administration.[127] Furthermore, the activation of CD8+ T cells by IL-2 may promote secretion of antiviral cytokines.

IL-6 is a potent regulator and enhancer of HIV replication in vitro;[128] furthermore, there is substantial evidence of its central role in B-cell abnormalities. Enhanced IL-6 and IL-6 mRNA production has been observed in PBMC and cells derived from lymph nodes and is conjectured to contribute to polyclonal B-cell activation and the increased incidence of B-cell lymphomas in HIV-infected subjects.[129,130] A small clinical trial with an anti-IL-6 monoclonal antibody was associated with reduction of acute-phase reactants and hypergammaglobulinemia.[131]

In most systems, the immunosuppressive cytokine IL-10 appears to reduce virus replication in vitro in activated macrophages and T cells.[132] The basis for the viral inhibition could be secondary to inhibition of secretion of other cytokines (e.g., TNF and IL-6)[133] and through impaired NF-κB/Rel A induction.[134] Because of the accessory cell function of macrophages, failure to induce coreceptors such as CD80 might interfere with T-cell activation and as a result inhibit T-cell activation and viral production. Preliminary studies of exogenous administration of IL-10 in HIV-infected subjects have resulted in transient decreases in plasma viremia (D. Weissman and A. S. Fauci, unpublished observations).

These antiviral effects of IL-10 superficially appear to be discordant with the proposed contribution of this TH2 cytokine (and others) in T-cell depletion and clinical progression by promoting apoptosis and inhibiting TH1 cytokine expression.[135–137] In accordance with its pleiotropic nature, IL-10 could promote salutary antiviral properties but inhibit favorable cell-mediated responses. In some studies, IL-10 production by PBMC from HIV-infected subjects appears to be increased compared with uninfected individuals, and some in vitro functional defects were improved by the addition of anti-IL-10 or cytokines associated with or promoting TH1 responses (e.g., IL-2, IL-12).[138–140] Others have found increases in IL-10 in PBMCs only in response to polyclonal activators but not constitutively.[141] On the other hand, IL-10 mRNA (among other cytokines) has been found to be increased in lymph nodes in subjects at all stages of disease.[142] While there is general agreement that cytokine dysregulation is implicated in the functional deterioration of infected patients, the evidence has not been consistent that global increases in TH2 cytokines and decreases in TH1 cytokines are temporally linked or uniformly observed in clinical progression of HIV infection. Differences in levels of particular cytokine mRNAs or protein can depend on the cell population or tissue compartment examined, the viral load or concomitant pathogens prevailing, and the clinical stage of disease. Finally, it is clear that in addition to the HIV-specific immune response, endogenous cytokines play a major role in the control of HIV replication. In this regard, the net level of HIV replication reflects a balance between HIV-inducing and HIV-suppressing cytokines. Perturbations of this balance can have profound effects on virus production.[2]

IMMUNE DEFECTS IN B CELLS

B-cell function and humoral immunity are markedly abnormal in HIV-infected subjects and patients with AIDS. These defects transcend the deficiencies in T-cell helper activities and may be a consequence of alterations in cytokine homeostasis. AIDS patients characteristically develop polyclonal B-cell activation manifested by hypergammaglobulinemia, spontaneous B-cell proliferation, and increased spontaneous secretion of immunoglobulin in vitro. Serum levels of IgG, IgA, and IgD typically are elevated.[143–146] Levels of secretory IgA are also increased.[147] In adults, IgM hypergammaglobulinemia is observed, while either hypogammaglobulinemia or hypergammaglobulinemia can be found in pediatric AIDS patients.[148,149] Changes in immunoglobulins can be seen in mucosal secretions, where the proportion of IgG to IgA is comparable in intestinal fluids in infected subjects, while increased ratios of IgA to IgG are found normally.[150] In HIV-infected children, IgE responses were found to be elevated, and poor clinical outcomes were associated with persistent elevations.[151]

In contrast to the increased spontaneous activation noted in B cells from AIDS patients, antigen-specific and nonspecific B-cell responses are impaired.[143] In vitro proliferative responses to antigens and mitogens are decreased, as is pokeweed mitogen (PWM)-induced immunoglobulin synthesis.[146] While in vivo responses of AIDS patients to protein and polysaccharide antigens are impaired,[143,152] the majority of HIV-infected subjects can be immunized with antigens, including HIV envelope proteins, to generate de novo immune responses.[153] Pathogen-specific antibody can be preserved in AIDS patients, even for some opportunistic pathogens such as cytomegalovirus (CMV), although functional responses such as neutralizing antibody may be diminished.[154] The consequences of impaired antibody responses are most notable for HIV-infected infants and children who have not been vaccinated previously or exposed to the spectrum of common viral and bacterial pathogens. Due to the absence of memory responses, serious bacterial infections can occur; prophylaxis with antibiotics can decrease the incidence of these infections. Supplemental immune globulin infusions can decrease morbidity and mortality in children who do not receive antibiotic prophylaxis.[155–157] Adults do not appear to derive similar benefits, presumably due to preformed antibodies to the common pathogens found in the unscreened immune globulin preparations.[158] Hyperimmune globulin preparations may provide additional benefits against certain pathogens such as respiratory syncytial virus in nonimmune HIV-infected children.[159]

The molecular basis of the hyperactivity of the B-cell compartment may be derived from a TNF-dependent mechanism. Among T cells infected with HIV in vitro, a small subset composed of blasts with membrane-associated TNF-α were able to induce polyclonal immunoglobulin production in vitro, which was blocked by antibodies to TNF or its receptor.[160] Similarly, T cells from infected individuals could induce the noncognate, contact-dependent production of immunoglobulin from B cells. The maintenance of this hyperactivity could be propagated by the B-cell growth-enhancing properties of IL-6, which is produced in increased amounts in HIV-infected subjects.[161] Endogenously produced IL-6 could sustain B-cell hyperactivity in an autocrine or paracrine fashion. In support of this concept, the treatment of a small number of lymphoma patients with a monoclonal antibody to IL-6 resulted in a reduction in acute-phase reactants, a normalization of hypoalbuminemia, and a reduction in serum and in vitro induced IgG and IgA levels.[131] While IL-6 production is felt to facilitate development of B-cell lymphoma, other factors contribute to B-cell transformation. Epstein-Barr virus (EBV) transcripts or proteins are observed in about 40 to 60 percent of lymphomas among HIV-infected individuals, especially those of monoclonal lineage.[162] Changes in the phenotypes and composition of the circulating B-cell population have been reported in HIV infection. Decreases in B cells expressing complement receptors (CR1 and CR2) have been observed, which may be caused by increased complement activation and immune complexes routinely found in HIV-infected subjects.[163,164] This could contribute to the sustained B-cell activation. Shifts in B-cell populations, including the proportion of CD5+ B cells have been reported.[165]

HIV or its envelope may directly affect B-cell responses. Despite the apparent inability of HIV to directly infect normal, untransformed B cells, the effects of viral proteins on B-cell activation and function may account for some of the observed in vivo changes. Purified virions and synthetic peptides derived from the envelope were observed to induce polyclonal activation.[166,167] It has been shown that gp120 will bind to certain variable heavy-chain frameworks (i.e., VH3), which alters the utilization of this immunoglobulin subfamily.[168] Specific sequences in VH3 have been identified that mediate binding to gp120 and may promote selective B-cell depletion.[169,170] B cells expressing VH3 in the germinal centers of HIV-infected subjects were depleted as compared with other VH subfamilies, while a normal distribution was observed in the peripheral blood or mantle zones of these nodes.[171] Elimination of the activated B cells within the germinal cells is believed to be due to programmed cell death.[172]

IMMUNE DEFECTS IN MONOCYTES AND MACROPHAGES

Monocytes and macrophages are infected with HIV in vivo[173–176] and in vitro[177–179] and contribute to the pathogenesis of HIV infection. This cell lineage can be infected directly through the binding of virus to CD4 and chemokine receptors and indirectly through Fc and complement receptors.[180–182] Infection of macrophages most often occurs with primary viral isolates with non-syncytial-inducing phenotypes and is dependent in large part on primary envelope sequences. The tropism of viral isolates for macrophage infection may be due to binding to particular chemokine receptors, but complementary chemokine receptor expression alone may not ensure infection with a T-cell-dependent isolate. Infected monocytes can be isolated from the circulation and along with dendritic cells, may promote dissemination of virus to different tissue compartments. Sites within the body in which macrophages are a major infected population are the brain (along with microglia), the bone marrow, lungs, and gastrointestinal (GI) tract. Macrophage infection may be responsible for the pathogenesis of encephalopathy and enteropathy.[173,183]

Although many monocyte activities appear to be preserved in AIDS patients, a number of functional abnormalities have been reported, including defective chemotaxis,[184,185] killing of certain microorganisms,[186] and antigen presentation in some but not all studies.[187] Abnormal function may be associated with high levels of circulating immune complexes.[188] In vitro infection of macrophages from uninfected individuals with HIV can induce functional abnormalities.[189] Given the relatively low proportion of circulating monocytes and tissue macrophages that are infected, it is unlikely that any of the defects observed are solely due to HIV infection of this cell type. Some of the defects observed in monocyte function may reflect deficient activation by T cells, since supplementing cultures with interferon-γ can reconstitute certain functional defects.[190,191] In addition, differences in composition of monocyte subpopulations in patients with progressive disease may contribute to functional abnormalities. For example, monocytes with a CD14-low, CD16-high phenotype may account for as many as 40 percent of circulating monocytes in AIDS patients.[192]

Chemotaxis is the monocyte function most frequently noted to be impaired in HIV-infected patients.[185] This defect is not specific to HIV infection, since many chronically ill patients with viral and malignant disorders have depressed chemotactic responses. Other activities that appear to be relatively preserved in monocytes derived from HIV-infected subjects include phagocytosis,[193] antibody-dependent cellular cytotoxicity (ADCC),[185] tumoricidal activity,[194] and microbicidal activity against toxoplasma, chlamydia, aspergillus, and candida.[190,193]

Inconsistent defects in antigen presentation have been reported from HIV-infected subjects.[195] Recall antigen responses are generally preserved, even in the cases of cocultures of syngeneic cells from twins discordant for HIV infection, but slight impairment of alloantigen-induced stimulation has been observed.[196] Others have found selective impairment of antigen presentation to T-cell clones in some, but not all HIV-infected subjects.[197]

In contrast to cells derived from infected patients, the in vitro infection of normal monocytes reduced anticandidal responses and ADCC activity.[189] Impaired anticryptococcal activity was found in peripheral blood monocytes but not alveolar macrophages infected in vitro with HIV, suggesting potential differences among macrophages of different tissue origin. Others have found that despite in vitro infection, phagocytic activity of macrophages is preserved.[198] One report suggested that HIV infection of macrophages contributed to T-cell apoptosis independent of the infection of T cells.[199]

In general, macrophages derived from AIDS patients[188] and those infected in vitro, including those of alveolar origin, demonstrate evidence of cellular activation.[200] Increases in inflammatory cytokines such as TNF-α, IL-1, IL-6, and IL-8, increased MHC class II expression, and superoxide anion production are frequent findings.[201,202] Increases in cytokine expression may be selective, since a reduction in production of hematopoetic cytokines (i.e., CSFs) by in vitro infected macrophages has been reported.[203]

Infection of cells of the monocytic lineage with HIV is intimately associated with the pathogenesis of neuropsychiatric abnormalities in AIDS. Infection of the CNS, observed in about 60 percent of AIDS patients, can be clinically silent or progress to meningoencephalitis and dementia. Histologic changes include neuronal loss and gliosis. Neurotoxins and products from infected and activated macrophages are believed to be responsible at least in part for pathologic changes in the CNS. Based on observations in the CNS of individuals with dementia and in in vitro model systems, gp120 and cytokines released from infected macrophages and microglia are thought to induce neuronal cell damage.[204] Mechanisms of toxicity include impaired uptake of excitatory amino acids and excess glutamate,[205–207] activation of adhesins in astrocytes,[208] and increased production of nitric oxide, arachadonic acid metabolites, platelet-activating factor, and the *N*-methyl-d-aspartate (NMDA) agonist cysteine.[209]

IMMUNE DEFECTS IN NATURAL KILLER CELLS

The natural killer (NK) cell population is a heterogeneous circulating subset of large granular lymphocytes that is mainly composed of cells expressing Fc receptor γ-III (CD16), believed to participate in immunosurveillance against tumors and virally infected cells. Functional defects in NK cell activity were observed in patients with advanced disease, but in vitro responses could be restored by supplementation with IL-2, Con A, and TPA.[7,210] Of interest are NK cell abnormalities in children who developed *Pneumocystis* pneumonia but who had normal CD4+ T-cell counts.[211] These findings are consistent with the reduced levels of NK cell-mediated lysis of targets expressing HIV antigens observed using cells from infected subjects. Depressed cytotoxicity was found to be independent of serum reactivity and was more impaired in AIDS patients.[212]

A recent retrospective analysis showed significant reductions in the major circulating CD16+ subpopulation of NK cells coexpressing CD56 in HIV-infected subjects without AIDS; expansion of CD16+, CD56− cells rarely found in HIV-uninfected individuals also was observed.[213] The intensity of CD16 expression was diminished in both subpopulations and may contribute to impaired function.

THE ROLE OF DENDRITIC CELLS AND FOLLICULAR DENDRITIC CELLS IN PATHOGENESIS

There has been a marked evolution in understanding of the contribution of dendritic cells to the pathogenesis of HIV infection. This is a heterogeneous population composed of circulating and tissue elements.[214] The circulating dendritic cells are derived from the bone marrow[215] and traffic within the blood, secondary lymphoid organs, and skin.[214,216] The dendritic cell within the skin is known as the *Langerhans cell*.[217] Other cell types include the lymphoid interdigitating cells, the circulating immature dendritic cell, and veiled cells within the afferent lymphatic system.[218] Cell surface molecules expressed by these dendritic cells include CD1a; CD83; the activation antigens CD40, CD80, CD86, and HLA-DR; Fc receptors CD32 and CD64; and a 55-kDa actin-bundling protein.[219–221] The primary function of these cells is to capture, process, and present antigens to T cells, particularly in the paracortex of lymph nodes; they are more efficient than other antigen presenting cells (APCs) such as macrophages. In fact, a subset of dendritic cells may be derived from monocytes.[222] The activation and maintenance of B-cell function are associated with another cell type, the follicular dendritic cell (FDC), which is possibly of stromal origin.[223]

Primary HIV infection at mucosal sites or in the skin probably involves the capture of virions by and/or infection of dendritic cells within the epithelium and migration of the infected dendritic cells to draining lymph nodes, where infection is established.[224] This progression of events was demonstrated in a model of vaginal infection with SIV.[225] Dendritic cells were found to be productively infected in vitro with monocytotropic isolates in some studies,[226–231] although this observation is not shared universally.[232] Productive infection of dendritic cells with HIV seems to be limited to those with a mature and activated phenotype.[233] The disparity in the results concerned with in vitro infection of dendritic cells could be due to the purity of the populations examined and culture conditions. Alternatively, viral isolates from particular geographic regions may infect dendritic cells more efficiently.[234] The ability to infect dendritic cells may depend on CD80 and possibly CD40 expression.[235–237] The absence of SP1, a transcription factor found in T cells, was thought to explain the failure of dendritic cells to be productively infected in one study.[238] Based on in vitro studies, dendritic cells pulsed with HIV can infect unactivated T cells efficiently and cause a disseminated, productive infection that is enhanced by the presence of activating cytokines such as IL-2 and IL-4 or specific antigen.[239–244] Productively infected dendritic cells have been identified in vivo, although few cells appear to be infected;[224,245,246] multinucleated cells with dendritic phenotypes have been recovered from tonsils and adenoids from asymptomatic individuals.[247]

Functional impairment in antigen presentation has been reported in dendritic cells derived from HIV-infected individuals,[248,249] although they were quite efficient in inducing HIV antigen-specific responses in vitro in the absence of exogenous antigen.[248] On the other hand, Langerhans cells from HIV-infected twins were competent in antigen presentation.[138] Given the limited number of dendritic cells productively infected with HIV, it is unlikely that antigen-presenting function is severely impaired during the clinical course of HIV disease.

With regard to FDCs, productive infection of T cells and macrophages is associated with the release of approximately 10^{10} virions daily;[250–252] many of these virions are captured by FDCs within germinal centers of lymph nodes, spleen, and the GI tract.[28,29,253,254] The majority of HIV associated with FDCs in vivo appears to be surface bound and complexed with antibody and complement. While debate persists about the infectability of FDCs by HIV,[255] in an SIV model of infection, FDCs appeared to lack spliced mRNA transcripts and therefore appeared not to be infected.[256] Thus the viral reservoir associated in complexes with FDCs may be impervious to the normal immune mechanisms generated to destroy infected cells. The resilience of this captured virus is highlighted by the compelling observation that complexes of HIV and neutralizing antibodies are still infectious when presented by FDCs.[257] The evolution of clinical disease and AIDS is associated with destruction of the FDCs[28,29,253] (Fig. 17–1). The mechanism inducing this marked distortion in lymphoid architecture is unclear, although in one SIV study the degeneration of germinal centers seemed to require CD8+ T-cell infiltration.[258]

IMMUNE RESPONSE TO HIV

There are many components of the immune system that respond to infection with HIV. Many of these responses have been associated with inhibition of viral replication. This is based on in vitro and ex vivo studies of the naturally induced responses detected in subjects from the various clinical stages of HIV infection.[19–25] Evaluation of the HIV-specific responses during primary HIV infection has been particularly enlightening, since the sequelae of long-term immunosuppression and infections with opportunistic infections did not cloud these analyses.

In addition to salutory immune responses, mechanisms have been identified in which specific immunity paradoxically enhances viral replication.[259–261] This could contribute to the failure of the immune system to regulate HIV replication effectively over the lifetime of an infected individual. Insufficient localization of specific immune responses at the sites of primary and persistent infection may lessen the positive impact of seemingly potent systemic immune responses. Protective immunity against mucosal infections may be more challenging due to the relative paucity of cellular infiltrates and the requisite for secretory immunity in these compartments.

Successful protective responses against HIV are believed to include the generation of envelope-specific antibodies with neutralizing activity and HIV-specific cytotoxic T cells to multiple HIV proteins. However, the participation of components of the natural or non-antigen-specific immune system, which previously were believed to be unessential in ameliorating HIV replication, is thought to be more significant.[262,263] This includes the secretion of cytokines with antiviral properties, especially by activated CD8+ cells, irrespective of their antigenic specificity.[263]

Primary infection at mucosal sites is initiated by the introduction of cell-free and cell-associated virions that are sequestered by Langerhans cells at epithelial surfaces. It is unclear whether sufficient virion production occurs at this time to promote any specific immune responses. Furthermore, some responses, such as the induction of CTL, are not usually observed at mucosal epithelial surfaces, even though CTL responses have been observed recently in vaginal epithelium following SIV infection.[264] Most likely, the focus of infection is transferred to draining lymph nodes and the peripheral circulation. The seeding of secondary sites with viral propagation in macrophages and T cells and virion transfer to sites of germinal cell development produce sufficient antigen to initiate specific immune responses in both T- and B-cell-dependent areas of lymph nodes, tonsils, and spleen.[45] On average, weeks to months may elapse from time of viral exposure until detectable systemic immune responses are found. However, due to issues in sampling human subjects, local immune responses could have occurred much earlier and were missed. In some individuals, such as commercial sex workers, where multiple exposures occur to HIV at mucosal sites, induction of cytotoxic immune responses may be generated more effectively and may

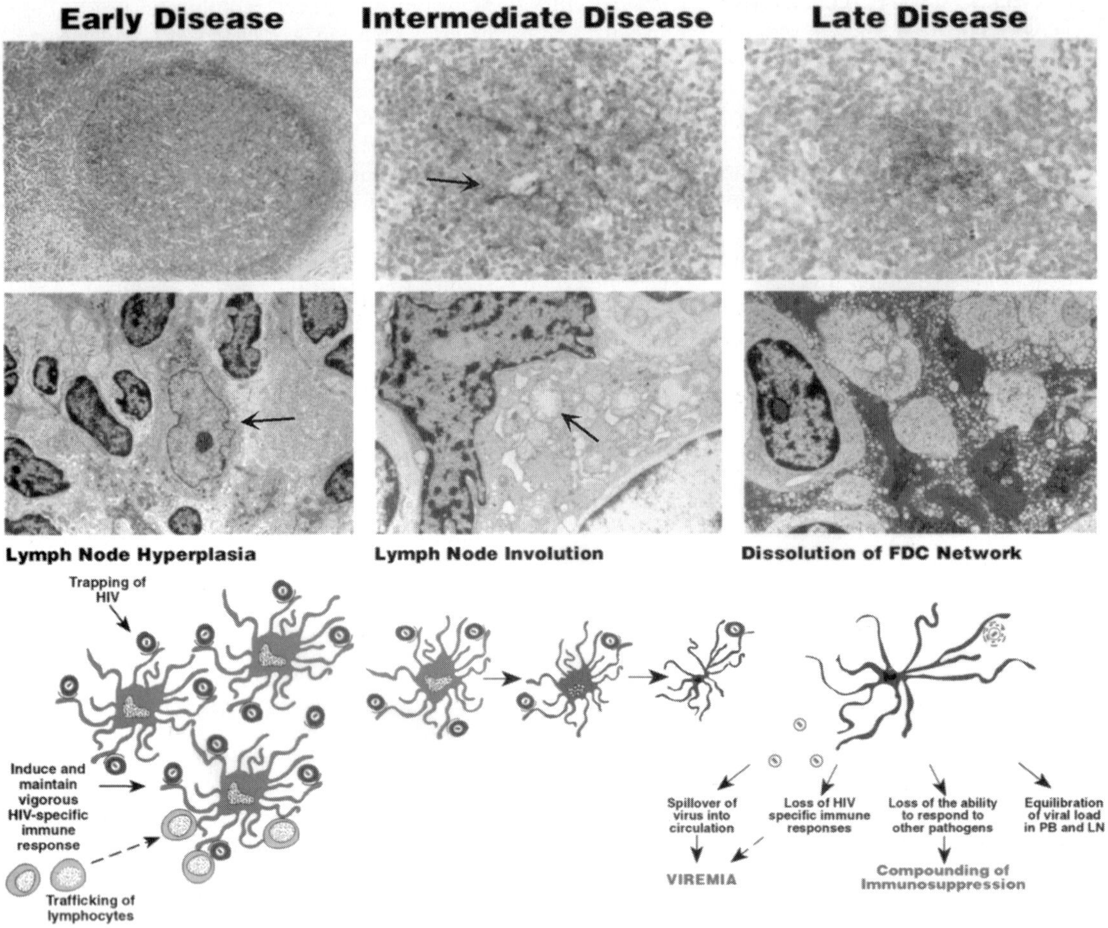

Fig 17–1 Lymph node germinal centers during various stages of HIV disease. During early disease an intact follicular dendritic cell (FDC) network (staining pink with a CD21 monoclonal antibody) is seen within the germinal center (*upper panel*). At this point individual FDCs appear healthy by electron microscopy (*arrow, middle panel*). During this period HIV particles are trapped by the processes of the FDC and initiate a vigorous humoral immune response by the germinal center B cells. CD4+ T cells migrate into the area and are exposed to virus (*lower panel*). During intermediate stage disease FDCs begin to degenerate, as indicated by clumping of the fine dendritic network (clumped red staining by antibody to CD21, *upper panel*) and by swollen organelles on electron microscopy (*arrow, middle panel*). At this point the efficiency of the FDC in trapping virions is diminished (*lower panel*). During advanced-stage disease the FDC network is virtually destroyed, with minimal staining by antibody to CD21 (*upper panel*) and necrotic-appearing, amorphous cells by electron microscopy (dark-staining material, *middle panel*). At this point, the destroyed FDCs are incapable of trapping virus, which now is readily detectable in blood. The loss of FDC function contributes to the profound immunosuppression of advanced-stage disease (*lower panel*). *(From Fauci AS: Multifactorial nature of human immunodeficiency virus disease. Science 262:1011, 1993.)*

contribute to the protection observed in this group at high risk of infection.[265]

CTL RESPONSES

CTL responses have been detected in a subset of individuals during primary HIV infection, coincidental with a decrease in plasma viremia and prior to significant neutralizing antibody responses.[266] The qualitative nature of the CTL response could predicate the ultimate clinical course. T-cell subsets (both CD4+ and CD8+ T cells) can be divided into families based on the variable (V) region of the beta chain of the T-cell receptor. There are 24 Vβ families within the T-cell receptor repertoire. In examining the diversity of the CD8+ CTL response during primary infection, it was observed that some individuals had a marked expansion of an individual Vβ family, while others had more marginal expansions of multiple Vβ families.[267] Those individuals with restricted CD8+ T-cell expansions appeared to be at greater risk for disease progression.[268] The basis of such a clinical outcome is unclear at present but may involve the rapid deletion of the expanded, high-affinity, HIV-specific CTL clones as well as the selection of viral variants because of the restricted nature of the CTL response. In contrast, in patients who generate a broad spectrum of responsiveness with respect to both epitope and protein targets and the diversity of the T-cell repertoire, the CTL response may be best able to handle the mixture of viral variants or quasi-species that evolve in any infected individual.[269] The initial observation that CTL can contribute to immune selection was suggested by the progressive changes in sequences within epitopes in particular individuals over time with subsequent changes in CTL responses.[270,271] It was then observed that adoptive transfer of a single expanded autologous CTL clone directed to a conserved epitope resulted in selection of viral variants with deletions and changes within the T-cell epitope.[272] More recently, CTL selection of new viral variants was observed in the setting of a primary infection with HIV[273] and later in the course of infection.[274] Yet the dominance of a given viral species may not correlate with the frequency of a particular CTL response.[275]

The inadequacy of the CTL response to eliminate viral persistence could be attributed to several mechanisms. The first, alluded to above, suggests the constant requirement for generating primary CTL responses to new specificities due to immune-based selection. Since control of viral replication is incomplete in most subjects, it would seem that a point would be reached when primary HIV-specific CTL could no longer be generated as CD4+ T cells decline and other immune functions are compromised.[276] In addition, there is a marked shift in the composition of the CD8+ T-cell population following acute infection, with expansion of total CD8+ T cells and CD8+, CD28− T cells in particular.[277,278] Induction and expansion of CTLs in the latter subpopulation may be less efficient due to the absence of a vital CD28-CD80 costimulatory pathway.[279,280] Persistence of these activated CTLs, especially those coexpressing CD38, could be subject to signals inducing apoptosis. Second, there is some experimental evidence that viral variants actually can inhibit CTL effector function against wild-type viruses.[281,282] Infected cells may be less susceptible to lysis as a consequence of nef-dependent downregulation of MHC class I expression, required for the presentation of processed antigen.[283] Finally, the expansion of certain CD8+, CD57+ cells has been associated with the production of factors that inhibit cytotoxic function;[284,285] cells with similar activity are observed in patients undergoing bone marrow transplantation.

While it seems logical that individuals who maintain relatively normal CD4+ T-cell counts for prolonged periods might have the most vigorous specific immune responses, including CTL, this has not been consistently observed. In fact, in one study, those HIV-infected individuals with normal CD4+ T-cell counts among long-term survivors consistently had lower CTL precursors, while the most vigorous CTL responses were observed in individuals with modestly reduced counts (300 to 700 CD4+ T cells/mm^3) and increased viral loads.[286] Others have found that subjects with the lowest recoverable virus among a small number of patients examined for CTL activity tended to generate the most diverse CTL responses.[287] As would be expected, patients with advanced HIV disease have reduced or absent HIV-specific CTL activity. However, progression to AIDS can develop in the presence of significant CTL activity.[272] These studies imply that clinical outcomes cannot be predicted solely on the presence of a particular CTL response.

NONCYTOLYTIC REGULATION OF HIV BY CD8+ T CELLS

In addition to the destruction of HIV-infected cells by CD4+ and CD8+ MHC-restricted CTLs, activated CD8+ T cells added to cultures of infected PBMCs from HIV-infected patients were found to inhibit HIV replication.[288,289] This inhibition occurred independent of the donor source of the CD8+ T cells, suggesting that the effect was not MHC-restricted. HIV-infected CD4+ T cells, either derived from HIV-infected patients or seronegative donor cells acutely infected with HIV in vitro, could be inhibited by activated CD8+ T cells from both HIV-infected and uninfected subjects, although the magnitude of the effect varied greatly among studies. The disparity in observed suppressive activity may reflect quantitative differences in viral load, multiple sites of activity for regulating viral replication, or qualitative or quantitative differences in CD8+ T-cell factors produced by infected and uninfected subjects.

The inhibitory effect of the CD8+ T cells did not require direct contact with the CD4+ T cells, since activated CD8+ T cells separated by a membrane filter from HIV-infected cells could still inhibit HIV replication;[290] however, the magnitude of the effect was greater if the cells were in contact with each other. The induction of the anti-HIV effect in CD8+ T cells could be achieved with different stimulating agents including mitogens and antigen; inhibition could be observed with both mixed populations and specific clones, including HIV-specific and non-HIV-specific CTLs.[291] In fact, the in vivo transfer of both HIV-specific and non-HIV-specific CTL clones in a hu-PBL-SCID model of HIV infection could inhibit viral replication independent of MHC restriction.[262]

The factors mediating this inhibitory effect have not been entirely defined. CD8+ T cells produce a number of well-characterized cytokines that have HIV inhibitory properties in vitro.[18] However, antibodies that neutralize many of the activities of these cytokines do not diminish the full anti-HIV activity of the activated CD8+ T cells. Some of the discrepancy in defining the mediators may reflect secretion of a mixture of cytokines, some of which have inhibitory properties and others of which stimulate HIV replication.[292] Chemokines produced by CD8+ T cells, including MIP-1-α, MIP-1-β, and RANTES, also might contribute to the inhibition; however, it is expected that as yet to be defined cytokines are responsible for the inhibition.[293,294]

NEUTRALIZING ANTIBODIES

Neutralizing antibodies to HIV are thought to remove and/or inactivate free circulating infectious virus, resulting in the prevention of virus spread and propagation. Inactivation appears to be an irreversible process and can occur prior to fusion with permissive cells.[295,296] This is similar to other viral systems such as respiratory syncytial virus, where in vivo production or passive transfer of neutralizing antibodies directly correlates with protection against infection and fusion-dependent infection is impaired in vitro. It is generally believed, but unproven, that consistently high levels of neutralizing antibody with broad cross-reactivity would favor a better clinical course, as has been described in some HIV-infected patients who are long-term nonprogressors.[297] It is also thought that the presence of antibodies with broad neutralizing activity is a requirement for the prevention of primary infection, both at mucosal sites and in the circulation. However, experimental and clinical data are somewhat contradictory with respect to the potency of neutralizing antibodies in conferring protection against infection.

Natural history studies of primary HIV infection indicate the initial detection of neutralizing antibody responses following the downregulation of the initial burst of viremia and often after the detection of cell-mediated immune responses.[298] It is suggested that neutralizing activity matures over time and that the earliest detectable responses are directed against a limited spectrum of linear epitopes, which are viral-type specific.[299] After the initial CD4+ T-cell decline and decrease in initially high levels of plasma viremia, specificities of neutralizing antibodies appear to broaden. Responses seem to be directed against different conformational domains and exhibit properties of cross-neutralization against strains of a similar genotype or clade and even against distinct clades. Given these observations, it would seem that preformed neutralizing antibodies of appropriate specificity and titer could prevent or mitigate the course of infection. To this end, animal studies with subunit vaccine candidates have elicited protection that correlated with the development of neutralizing antibody responses in some cases.[300] It was observed, however, that many of these candidate subunit vaccines induced neutralizing responses of limited activity, due to their inability to neutralize primary (low-passaged and macrophage-tropic) isolates in vitro.[301,302] In one case, in vivo protection was achieved despite the failure to neutralize the primary isolate in vitro.[303] It was proposed that the resistance of primary isolates was a result of a relative increase in envelope glycoprotein density on primary isolates,[304] but this mechanism of resistance was subsequently shown not to be implicated.[305] Moreover, the situation is complicated by the ability of neutralizing antibodies to reduce the expression of some but not all variants in a given individual, leading to continual and progressive immune selection. Resistance to neutralization can occur by differences in single or multiple residues that can confer changes in the envelope conformation sufficiently to alter recognition by polyspecific neutralizing antibodies.[306,307] Furthermore, amino acid substitutions can change patterns of glycosylation and render isolates resistant to neutralization.[308] Apart from the selection process, with clinical progression, titers of neutralizing antibodies tend to wane. One hypothesis for the decline of neutralizing responses is the observed CTL-mediated lysis of B cells that produce neutralizing antibodies.[309]

Substantial efforts have been directed at defining neutralizing domains. Most of the functional responses are directed toward both linear and conformational epitopes on the envelope protein. Initial efforts were focused on defining sequences within the third variable domain (V3 loop or principal neutralizing domain) of gp120 responsible for inducing neutralizing responses. Both polyclonal antisera and monoclonal neutralizing antibodies to V3, experimentally induced or derived from infected individuals, were found to react with multiple regions of the V3 loop. X-ray crystallography of the V3 loop and a neutralizing monoclonal antibody have shown that the tip of the loop adopts a double-turn conformation.[310] While many of these anti-V3 antibodies were strain-specific, others appeared to have broader neutralizing activities, particularly those directed to the crown or tip and sometimes the base.[311–314] However, other domains within gp120 are as important as the V3 loop in inducing neutralizing activity. Among the more important regions are conformational sites that are responsible for binding CD4 (CD4bd), including C4 and domains within the V2 or V1-V2 interface. Neutralizing antibodies directed to regions within C1, C2, and C3 also have been identified.[315–318] Using a competitive binding assay, it appeared that neutralizing monoclonal antibodies to gp120 localized to one surface of the structure, whereas the nonneutralizing antibodies bound to a distinct, inaccessible region of the envelope complex.[319] Neutralizing antibodies that are directed to epitopes within V2, V3, and C4 appear to promote the dissociation of gp120 from gp41, mimicking the interactions of gp120 and its cellular receptor. However, antibodies to the CD4bd fail to induce this dissociation and therefore neutralize by a distinct process.[320] Broadly neutralizing antibodies that bind to linear sequences within gp41 also have been identified.[321–323] Similar regions may be important in inducing antibodies that prevent vertical transmission of HIV from mothers to newborns,[324] although studies differ in correlating the presence of functional antibody responses with prevention of transmission in humans and animal models.[325,326] Identification of unique neutralizing epitopes generated within the envelope after binding to CD4 has so far eluded full characterization. Recent studies have shown that neutralizing antibodies to gp120 also can impede the binding to chemokine receptors (e.g., CCR-5) without affecting interactions with CD4.[77,327]

Apart from the antigen specificity, constant region structure can influence neutralizing activity, since a switch from an IgG_1 to an IgG_3 antibody enhanced neutralization as a result of increased flexibility conferred by the elongated IgG_3 hinge region.[328] Furthermore, neutralizing activity does not appear to be class specific, since IgA responses possess antiviral activity.[329] Combinations of antibodies to different domains demonstrated synergistic neutralizing activities.[330,331]

Many neutralizing sera have limited or reduced potency against primary isolates. Since it was found that the native conformation of HIV envelope on the virion is oligomeric rather than monomeric in structure, it was thought that the limitations of functional responses was due to the failure to recognize native envelope conformations.[332] Neutralizing activity of a series of monoclonal antibodies correlated with binding to oligomeric forms of gp120 and was dependent primarily on its rate of association.[333] Immunization of animals with oligomeric forms tends to induce antibody responses more restricted to that conformation, while monomeric subunit proteins induce responses primarily to nonconformational domains.[334,335] However, such strategies have not yet yielded more potent neutralizing responses.

In addition to their ability to inhibit viral replication in vitro, passively transferred neutralizing antibodies have demonstrated some ability to prevent primary infection in experimental models of HIV or SIV infection. In certain experimental conditions, antibodies directed to cellular products such as MHC class I can contribute to neutralizing activity, since many of these cellular proteins become incorporated within the viral envelope.[336] Inhibition in the latter case occurs subsequent to virion binding.[337] However, due to the large numbers of virions and rapid virus turnover during acute infections, it is unlikely that neutralizing monoclonal antibodies administered passively could be effective therapeutically, and significant quantities would be required even in prophylactic settings. The binding of neutralizing antibodies to virions may not guarantee a favorable outcome. A large reservoir of extracellular HIV is sequestered on follicular dendritic cells complexed to antibody.[28,29,253,254,338] It was presumed that most complexed antibody was nonneutralizing; however, complexes of HIV and neutralizing antibodies are still infectious when they are trapped on follicular dendritic cells.[257] This raises doubt that antibody-dependent immunotherapeutic strategies can control viral replication.[339] Other concerns include the ability of antibody-complexed virions to bypass CD4-dependent pathways of infection and to utilize Fc or complement receptors and promote infection of normally nonpermissive cell types.[182,261,340] Furthermore, neutralizing antibodies do not affect cell-to-cell transmission even among T cells.[341]

ANTIBODY-DEPENDENT CELLULAR CYTOTOXICITY

Antibody-dependent cellular cytotoxicity (ADCC) is an immune mechanism by which cytolytic cells armed with antibody through their Fc receptors can be triggered to destroy any membrane-expressed or -associated protein recognized by the binding domains of the antibody. The major cell type mediating this response is the NK cell, which may induce lysis both through perforin and Fas-dependent pathways, although other cells bearing Fc receptors, including macrophages and granulocytes, can participate in ADCC responses. Since mice with knockouts of the gene coding for perforin have impaired viral clearance in vivo and reduced NK-dependent lytic responses in vitro, one might presume that ADCC activity also would be impaired in vivo and in vitro, although this has not been examined.[342–344] Similar impairment of NK-mediated responses in vitro has been observed with disruption of the gene that encodes the Fas ligand.[343,344] Effector cell activity, including ADCC, is lost in mice deficient in expression of the Fc gamma chain, a component of the low-affinity IgG receptor.[345] It would be of interest to know if such animals have impaired viral clearance as well.

It is unclear if ADCC responses contribute significantly to the regulation of HIV replication in vivo. In a murine model of AIDS (MAIDS), viral expression was enhanced in animals with knockouts of the perforin gene that would affect both CD8+ T-cell and NK-cell function, and presumably ADCC activity as well.[346] Sera from individuals newly infected with HIV often contain antibodies that can mediate ADCC responses.[347] This activity was detected prior to neutralization activity; because both ADCC activity and CTL responses initially appeared to be generated at similar times and coincidental with reductions of plasma viremia, it was thought that ADCC activity could contribute to controlling viral replication during a primary infection.[348,349] ADCC activity against HIV-infected targets is reduced in neonates compared with adults, and impairment of this response might contribute to the vertical transmission of HIV from infected mothers.[350] However, comparable ADCC activity is detected in seropositive mothers of both infected and noninfected neonates, suggesting that ADCC cannot prevent viral transmission effectively.[351,352] On the other hand, the clinical course of infected infants seems better in those with significant ADCC activity.[353] It is unclear if this is attributable to ADCC activity or merely due to better overall immune function in these patients. Similarly, in infected adults, ADCC activity declines with clinical progression,[354] although progression can be observed in some patients with stable ADCC serum activity.[355] This includes both the loss of antibodies mediating ADCC and effector cell function, which can be lost independent of each other in particular patients.[212,356]

ADCC activity is directed primarily against cells expressing or binding HIV envelope or protein fragments. Activity can be demonstrated with sera derived from vaccinated or infected patients or by using specific monoclonal antibodies directed against gp120 or gp41.[357–360] Sera obtained from HIV-2-infected subjects also can mediate ADCC activity; in most cases, activity is viral-specific, although some sera can demonstrate ADCC reactivities against both HIV-1- and HIV-2-infected targets, presumably due to the recognition of shared epitopes.[361,362] Sera from HIV-2-infected subjects and monkeys infected with SIV appear to share common reactivities in ADCC assays.[363] ADCC activity was demonstrated with cells derived from patients without adding sera to the in vitro assay; lysis was blocked by CD16+ cell depletion and with antibody directed to IgG, suggesting that the NK cells are primed with antibody to function in vivo.[364]

SUMMARY

Remarkable advances have been made in the past few years in the delineation of the immunopathogenic mechanisms of HIV disease. The natural course of infection from viral exposure and primary infection to advanced disease (AIDS) has been clearly described along with the structural and functional consequences on the immune system (Fig. 17–2). In addition to infection of T cells and macrophages, the importance of bone marrow-derived dendritic cells and FDCs as carriers and conduits of infection has been realized. The consequences of persistent activation of the various

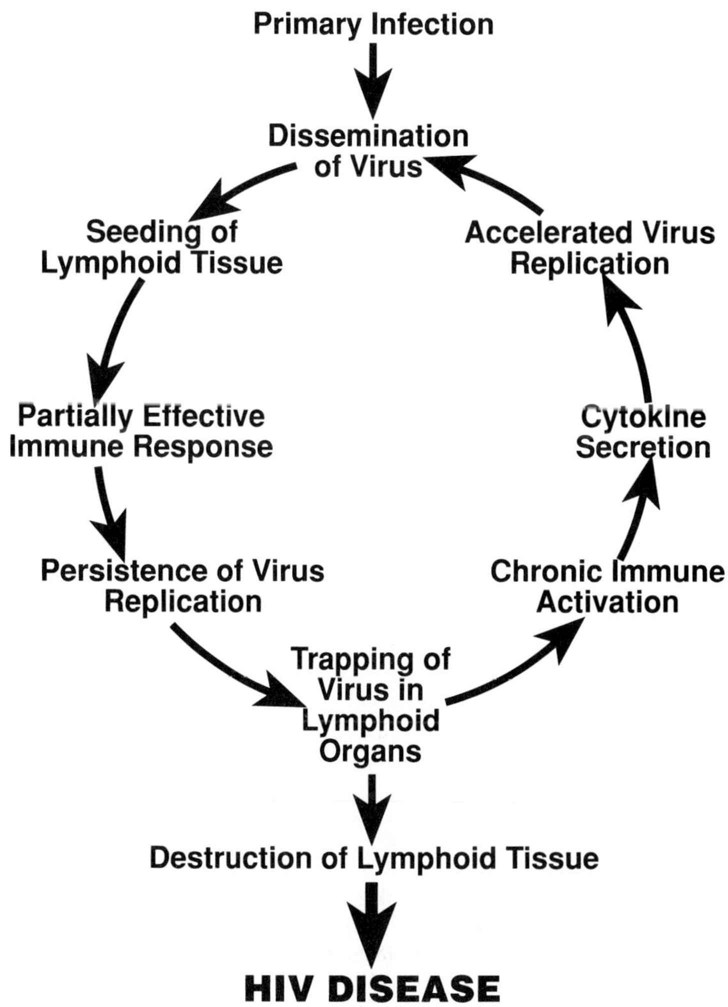

Fig. 17–2 The vicious cycle of HIV pathogenesis. *(From Pantaleo G, Fauci AS: New concepts in the immunopathogenesis of HIV infection. Annu Rev Immunol 13:487–512, 1995.)*

components of the immune system in patients with progressive disease and the sequelae of dysregulated cytokine production in promoting viral replication have been firmly established. Mechanisms responsible for T-cell depletion due to infection and viral proteins have been characterized. Newly defined coreceptors for HIV in addition to CD4 have created opportunities for novel therapeutic interventions. Finally, the elements of the immune system that inhibit viral replication continue to be deciphered, and the contributions of both the cellular and humoral responses in the selection of viral variants are better understood.

References

1 Fauci AS: Multifactorial nature of human immunodeficiency virus disease: Implications for therapy. *Science* 262:1011, 1993.
2 Fauci AS: Host factors and the pathogenesis of HIV-induced disease. *Nature* 384:529, 1996.
3 Masur H et al: An outbreak of community-acquired *Pneumocystis carinii* pneumonia: Initial manifestation of cellular immune dysfunction. *N Engl J Med* 305:1431, 1981.
4 Siegel FP et al: Severe acquired immunodeficiency in male homosexuals, manifested by chronic perianal ulcerative herpes simplex lesions. *N Engl J Med* 305:1439, 1981.
5 Lane HC et al: Correlation between immunologic function and clinical subpopulations of patients with the acquired immune deficiency syndrome. *Am J Med* 78:417, 1985.
6 Rook AH et al: Deficient, HLA-restricted, cytomegalovirus-specific cytotoxic T cells and natural killer cells in patients with the acquired immunodeficiency syndrome. *J Infect Dis* 152:627, 1985.
7 Rook AH et al: Interleukin-2 enhances the depressed natural killer and cytomegalovirus-specific cytotoxic activities of lymphocytes from patients with the acquired immune deficiency syndrome. *J Clin Invest* 72:398, 1983.
8 Barre-Sinoussi F: Isolation of a T lymphotropic retrovirus from a patient at risk for acquired immune deficiency syndrome (AIDS). *Science* 220:868, 1983.
9 Gallo R et al: Frequent detection and isolation of cytopathic retrovirus (HTLV-III) from patients with AIDS and at risk for AIDS. *Science* 224:500, 1984.
10 Levy JA et al: Isolation of lymphocytopathic retroviruses from San Francisco patients with AIDS. *Science* 225:840, 1984.
11 Popovic M et al: Detection, isolation, and continuous production of cytopathic retroviruses (HTLV-III) from patients with AIDS and pre-AIDS. *Science* 224:497, 1984.
12 Clavel F et al: Human immunodeficiency virus type 2 infection associated with AIDS in West Africa. *N Engl J Med* 316:1180, 1997.
13 Clavel F et al: Molecular cloning and polymorphism of the human immunodeficiency virus type 2. *Nature* 324:691, 1986.
14 Dalgleish AG et al: The CD4 (T4) antigen is an essential component of the receptor for the AIDS retrovirus. *Nature* 312:763, 1984.
15 Klatzmann D et al: T-lymphocyte T4 molecule behaves as the receptor for human retrovirus LAV. *Nature* 312:767, 1984.
16 McDougal JS et al: Binding of HTLV-III/LAV to T4+ T cells by a complex of the 110-kDa viral protein and the T4 molecule. *Science* 231:382, 1985.
17 Folks TM et al: Cytokine-induced expression of HIV-1 in a chronically infected promonocyte cell line. *Science* 238:800, 1987.
18 Poli G, Fauci AS: in *Human Cytokines: Their Role in Disease and Therapy, Role of cytokines in the pathogenesis of human immunodeficiency virus infection.* BB Aggarwal, RK Puri (eds). Cambridge, MA, Blackwell Scientific, 1995, p 421.
19 Walker BD et al: HIV-specific cytotoxic T lymphocytes in seropositive individuals. *Nature* 328:345, 1987.
20 Koenig S et al: Group specific, major histocompatibility complex class I restricted cytotoxic responses to human immunodeficiency virus-1 envelope proteins by cloned peripheral blood T cells from an HIV-infected individual. *Proc Natl Acad Sci USA* 85:8638, 1988.
21 Haynes BF et al: Toward an understanding of the correlates of protective immunity to HIV infection. *Science* 271:324, 1996.
22 Graham BS et al: Augmentation of human immunodeficiency virus type 1 neutralizing antibody by priming with gp160 in vaccinia-naive adults. The NIAID AIDS Vaccine Clinical Trials Network. *J Infect Dis* 167:533, 1993.
23 Putney SD et al: HTLV-III/LAV-neutralizing antibodies to an *E. coli*-produced fragment of the virus envelope. *Science* 234:1392, 1986.
24 Matthews TJ et al: Restricted neutralization of divergent human T-lymphotropic virus type III isolates by antibodies to the major envelope glycoprotein. *Proc Natl Acad Sci USA* 83:9709, 1986.
25 Palker TJ et al: Type-specific neutralization of the human immunodeficiency virus with antibodies to env-encoded synthetic peptides. *Proc Natl Acad Sci USA* 85:1932, 1988.
26 Goudsmit J: Genomic diversity and antigenic variation of HIV-1: Links between pathogenesis, epidemiology and vaccine development. *FASEB J* 5:2427, 1991.
27 McKeating JA et al: Characterization of HIV-1 neutralization escape mutants. *AIDS* 3:777, 1989.
28 Pantaleo G et al: HIV infection is active and progressive in lymphoid tissue during the clinically latent stage of disease. *Nature* 362:355, 1993.
29 Haase AT et al: Quantitative image analysis of HIV-1 infection in lymphoid tissue. *Science* 274:985, 1996.
30 Kourtis AP et al: Early progression of disease in HIV-infected infants with thymus dysfunction. *N Engl J Med* 335:1431, 1996.
31 Golding H et al: Identification of homologous regions in human immunodeficiency virus I gp41 and human MHC class II beta I domain I. Monoclonal antibodies against the gp41-derived peptide and patients' sera react with native HLA class II antigens, suggesting a role for autoimmunity in the pathogenesis of acquired immune deficiency syndrome. *J Exp Med* 167:914, 1988.
32 Lifson JD et al: AIDS retrovirus induced cytopathology: Giant cell formation and involvement of CD4 antigen. *Science* 232:1123, 1986.
33 Ameisen JC et al: Cell dysfunction an depletion in AIDS: The programmed cell death hypothesis. *Immunol Today* 12:102, 1991.
34 Ameisen JC et al: From AIDS to parasite infection: Pathogen-mediated subversion of programmed cell death as a mechanism for immune dysregulation. *Immunol Rev* 142:9, 1994.
35 Tersmette M et al: Evidence for a role of virulent human immunodeficiency virus (HIV) variants in the pathogenesis of acquired immunodeficiency syndrome: Studies on sequential HIV isolates. *J Virol* 63:2118, 1989.
36 Schwartz S et al: Rapidly and slowly replicating human immunodeficiency virus type 1 isolates can be distinguished according to target-cell tropism in T cell and monocyte cell lines. *Proc Natl Acad Sci USA* 86:7200, 1989.
37 Fenyo EM et al: Replicative capacity, cytopathic effect and cell tropism of HIV. *AIDS* 3:S5, 1989.
38 Hwang SS et al: Identification of the envelope V3 loop as the primary determinant of cell tropism in HIV-1. *Science* 253:71, 1991.
39 Shioda T et al: Macrophage and T cell-line tropisms of HIV-1 are determined by specific regions of the envelope gp120 gene. *Nature* 349:167, 1991.
40 Wolinsky SM et al: Adaptive evolution of human immunodeficiency virus-type 1 during the natural course of infection. *Science* 272:537, 1996.
41 Daar ES et al: High concentrations of recombinant soluble CD4 are required to neutralize primary human immunodeficiency virus type 1 isolates. *Proc Natl Acad Sci USA* 87:6574, 1990.
42 Mascola JR et al: Immunization with envelope subunit vaccine products elicits neutralizing antibodies against laboratory-adapted but not primary isolates of human immunodeficiency virus type 1. NIAID AIDS Vaccine Evaluation Group. *J Infect Dis* 173:340, 1996.
43 Perelson AS et al: HIV-1 dynamics in vivo viron clearance rate, infected cell lifespan, and viral generation time. *Science* 271:1582, 1996.

44 Ho DD et al: Rapid turnover of plasma virions and CD4 lymphocytes in HIV-1 infection. *Nature* 373:123, 1995.

45 Fauci AS: Multifactorial nature of human immunodeficiency virus disease: Implications for therapy. *Science* 262:1011, 1993.

46 Pantaleo G et al: New concepts in the immunopathogenesis of human immunodeficiency virus infection. *N Engl J Med* 328:327, 1993.

47 D'Souza MP et al: Chemokines and HIV-1 second receptors: Confluence of two fields generates optimism in AIDS research. *Nat Med* 2: 1293, 1996.

48 Klatzmann D et al: Selective tropism of lymphadenopathy associated virus (LAV) for helper-inducer T lymphocytes. *Science* 225:59, 1984.

49 Bhat S et al: Galactosyl ceramide or a derivative is an essential component of the neural receptor for human immunodeficiency virus type 1 envelope glycoprotein gp120. *Proc Natl Acad Sci USA* 88:7131, 1991.

50 Harouse JM et al: Inhibition of entry of HIV-1 in neural cell lines by antibodies against galacytosyl ceramide. *Science* 253:320, 1991.

51 Sattentau QJ et al: Epitopes of the CD4 antigen and HIV infection. *Science* 234:1120, 1986.

52 Brady RL, Barclay AN: in *The CD4 Molecule: Roles in T Lymphocytes and in HIV Disease, The Structure of CD4.* DR Littman (ed). New York, Springer-Verlag, 1996.

53 Lamarre D et al: The MHC-binding and gp120-binding functions of CD4 are separable. *Science* 245:743, 1989.

54 Maddon PJ et al: The T4 gene encodes the AIDS virus receptor and is expressed in the immune system and the brain. *Cell* 47:333, 1986.

55 Weiner DB et al: Human genes other than CD4 facilitate HIV-1 infection of murine cells. *Pathobiology* 59:361, 1991.

56 Lores P et al: Expression of human CD4 in transgenic mice does not confer sensitivity to human immunodeficiency virus infection. *AIDS Res Hum Retroviruses* 8:2063, 1992.

57 Pantaleo G et al: Human immunodeficiency virus (HIV) infection in CD4+ T lymphocytes genetically deficient in LFA-1: LFA-1 is required for HIV-mediated cell fusion but not for viral transmission. *J Exp Med* 173:511, 1991.

58 Jacotot E et al: HIV envelope glycoprotein-induced cell killing by apoptosis is enhanced with increased expression of CD26 in CD4+ T cells. *Virology* 223:318, 1996.

59 Lazaro I et al: Factors involved in entry of the human immunodeficiency virus type 1 into permissive cells: Lack of evidence of a role for CD26. *J Virol* 68:6535, 1994.

60 Oravecz T et al: CD26 expression correlates with entry, replication and cytopathicity of monocytotropic HIV-1 strains in a T-cell line. *Nat Med* 1:881, 1995.

61 Watkins BA et al: Expression of CD26 does not correlate with the replication of macrophage-tropic strains of HIV-1 in T-cell lines. *Virology* 224:276, 1996.

62 Feng Y et al: HIV-1 entry cofactor: Functional cDNA cloning of a seven-transmembrane, G protein-coupled receptor. *Science* 272:872, 1996.

63 Oberlin E et al: The CXC chemokine SDF-1 is the ligand for LESTR/fusin and prevents infection by T-cell-line-adapted HIV-1. *Nature* 382:833, 1996.

64 Bleul CC et al: The lymphocyte chemoattractant SDF-1 is a ligand for LESTR/fusin and blocks HIV-1 entry. *Nature* 382:829, 1996.

65 Cocchi F et al: The V3 domain of the HIV-1 gp120 envelope glycoprotein is critical for chemokine-mediated blockade of infection. *Nat Med* 2:1244, 1996.

66 Alkhatib G et al: CC CKR5: A RANTES, MIP-1 alpha, MIP-1 beta receptor as a fusion cofactor for macrophage-tropic HIV-1. *Science* 272:1955, 1996.

67 Choe H et al: The beta-chemokine receptors CCR3 and CCR5 facilitate infection by primary HIV-1 isolates. *Cell* 85:1135, 1996.

68 Deng H et al: Identification of a major co-receptor for many isolates of HIV-1. *Nature* 381:661, 1996.

69 Doranz BJ et al: A dual-tropic primary HIV-1 isolate that uses fusin and the beta-chemokine receptors CKR-5, CKR-3, and CKR-2b as fusion cofactors. *Cell* 85:1149, 1996.

70 Dragic T et al: HIV-1 entry into CD4+ cells is mediated by the chemokine receptor CC-CKR-5. *Nature* 381:667, 1996.

71 Liu R et al: Homozygous defect in HIV-1 coreceptor accounts for resistance of some multiply-exposed individuals to HIV-1 infection. *Cell* 86:367, 1996.

72 Dean M et al: Genetic restriction of HIV-1 infection and progression to AIDS by a deletion allele of the CKR5 structural gene. Hemophilia Growth and Development Study. Multicenter AIDS Cohort Study, Multicenter Hemophilia Cohort Study, San Francisco City Cohort, ALIVE Study. *Science* 273:1856, 1996.

73 Huang Y et al: The role of mutant CCR5 allele in HIV-1 transmission and disease progression. *Nat Med* 2:1240, 1996.

74 Samson M et al: Resistance to HIV-1 infection in caucasian individuals bearing mutant alleles of the CCR-5 chemokine receptor gene. *Nature* 382:722, 1996.

75 James W, Weiss RA, Simon JHM: in *The CD4 Molecule: Roles in T Lymphocytes and in HIV Disease, The Receptor for HIV: Dissection of CD4 and Studies on Putative Accessory Factors.* DR Littman (ed). New York, Springer-Verlag, 1996.

76 Trkola A et al: CD4-dependent, antibody-sensitive interactions between HIV-1 and its co-receptor CCR-5. *Nature* 384:184, 1996.

77 Wu L et al: CD4-induced interaction of primary HIV-1 gp120 glycoproteins with the chemokine receptor CCR-5. *Nature* 384:179, 1996.

78 Aiken C et al: Nef induces CD4 endocytosis: Requirement for a critical dileucine motif in the membrane-proximal CD4 cytoplasmic domain. *Cell* 76:853, 1994.

79 Brady HJ et al: CD4 cell surface downregulation in HIV-1 nef transgenic mice is a consequence of intracellular sequestration. *EMBO J* 12:4923, 1993.

80 Chen BK et al: CD4 down-modulation during infection of human T cells with human immunodeficiency virus type 1 involves independent activities of vpu, env, and nef. *J Virol* 70:6044, 1996.

81 Vincent MJ et al: The human immunodeficiency virus type 1 vpu protein: a potential regulator of proteolysis and protein transport in the mammalian secretory pathway. *Virology* 213:639, 1995.

82 Hoxie JA et al: Alterations in T4 (CD4) protein and mRNA synthesis in cells infected with HIV. *Science* 234:1123, 1986.

83 Mittelman A et al: Analysis of T cell subsets in different clinical subgroups of patients with the acquired immune deficiency syndrome. *Am J Med* 78:951, 1985.

84 Polk BF et al: Predictors of the acquired immunodeficiency syndrome developing in a cohort of seropositive homosexual men. *N Engl J Med* 316:61, 1987.

85 Goedert JJ et al: Effect of T4 count and cofactors on the incidence of AIDS in homosexual men infected with human immunodeficiency virus. *JAMA* 257:331, 1987.

86 Wong MT et al: Patterns of virus burden and T cell phenotype are established early and are correlated with the rate of disease progression in human immunodeficiency virus type 1-infected persons. *J Infect Dis* 173:877, 1996.

87 Mellors JW et al: Prognosis in HIV-1 infection predicted by the quantity of virus in plasma (see comments). *Science* 272:1167, 1996.

88 Mahalingam M et al: Abnormalities of CD45 isoform expression in HIV infection. *Clin Immunol Immunopathol* 81:210, 1996.

89 Benito JM et al: Quantitative alterations of the functionally distinct subsets of CD4 and CD8 T lymphocytes in asymptomatic HIV infection: Changes in the expression of CD45RO, CD45RA, CD11b, CD38, HLA-DR, and CD25 antigens. *J Acquir Immune Defic Syndr Hum Retrovirol* 14:128, 1997.

90 Mahalingam M et al: T cell activation and disease severity in HIV infection. *Clin Exp Immunol* 93:337, 1993.

91 Zola H et al: Patients with HIV infection have a reduced proportion of lymphocytes expressing the IL-2 receptor p55 chain (TAC, CD25). *Clin Immunol Immunopathol* 59:16, 1991.

92 Mocroft A et al: CD8+, CD38+ lymphocyte percent: A useful immunological marker for monitoring HIV-1 infected patients. *J Acquir Immune Defic Syndr Hum Retrovirol* 14:158, 1997.

93 Bofill M et al: Increased numbers of primed activated CD8+CD38+CD45RO T cells predict the decline of CD4 T cells in HIV-1 infected patients. *AIDS* 10:827, 1996.

94 Palmer S et al: Increased CD11/CD18 expression of the peripheral blood leucocytes of patients with HIV disease: Relationship to disease severity. *Clin Exp Immunol* 93:344, 1993.

95 Sodrowski JA et al: Role of the HTLV-III/LAV envelope in syncytium formation and cytopathicity. *Nature* 322:470, 1986.

96 Lifson JD et al: Induction of CD4-dependent cell fusion by the HTLV-III/LAV envelope glycoprotein. *Nature* 323:725, 1986.

97 Yoffe B et al: Fusion as a mediator of cytolysis in mixtures of uninfected CD4+ lymphocytes and cells infected by human immunodeficiency virus. *Proc Natl Acad Sci USA* 84:1429, 1987.

98 Foster S et al: gp120 induced programmed cell death in recently activated T cells without subsequent ligation of the T cell receptor. *Eur J Immunol* 25:1778, 1995.

99 Oyaizu N et al: Inhibition of CD4 cross-linking induced lymphocytes apopotosis by vesnarinone as a novel immunomodulating agent: Vesnarinone inhibits Fas expression and apoptosis by blocking cytokine secretion. *Blood* 87:2361, 1996.

100 Katsikis PD et al: Fas antigen stimulation induces marked apoptosis of T lymphocytes in human immunodeficiency virus infected individuals. *J Exp Med* 181:2029, 1995.

101 Finkel TH et al: Apoptosis occurs predominantly in bystander cells and not in productively infected cells of HIV- and SIV-infected lymph nodes. *Nat Med* 1:129, 1995.

102 Kolesnitchenko V et al: Human immunodeficiency virus 1 envelope-initiated G_2-phase programmed cell death. *Proc Natl Acad Sci USA* 92:11889, 1995.

103 Miskovsky EP et al: Studies of the mechanism of cytolysis by HIV-1 specific CD4+ human CTL clones induced by candidate AIDS vaccines. *J Immunol* 153:2787, 1994.

104 Wang ZQ et al: Deletion of T lymphocytes in human CD4 transgenic mice induced by HIV-gp120 and gp120-specific antibodies from AIDS patients. *Eur J Immunol* 24:1553, 1994.

105 Desbarats J et al: Fas CD95 expression and death-mediating function are induced by CD4 cross-linking on CD4+ T cells. *Proc Natl Acad Sci USA* 93:11014, 1996.

106 Lane HC et al: Qualitative analysis of immune function in patients with the acquired immunodeficiency syndrome. *N Engl J Med* 313: 79, 1985.

107 Hubert P et al: HIV-1 glycoprotein gp120 disrupts CD4− p56lck/CD3-T cell receptor interactions and inhibits CD3 signaling. *Eur J Immunol* 25:1417, 1995.

108 Kanner SB et al: HIV-1 down regulates CD4 costimulation of TCR/CD3 directed tyrosine phophorylation through CD4/p56lck dissociation. *J Immunol* 154:2996, 1995.

109 Goldman F et al: gp120 ligation of CD4 induces p56lck activation and TCR desensitization independent of TCR tyrosine phosphorylation. *J Immunol* 153:2905, 1994.

110 Jabado N et al: CD4 ligands inhibit the formation of multifunctional transduction complexes involved in T cell activation. *J Immunol* 158: 94, 1997.

111 Tian H et al: HIV envelope-directed signaling aberrancies and cell death of CD4+ T cells in the absence of TCR co-stimulation. *Int Immunol* 8:65, 1996.

112 Cayota A et al: CD4+ lymphocytes from HIV-infected patients display impaired CD45 associated tyrosine phosphatase activity which is enhanced by anti-oxidants. *Clin Exp Immunol* 104:11, 1996.

113 Stefanov I et al: HIV infection induced posttranslational modification of T cell signaling molecules associated with disease progression. *J Clin Invest* 98:1290, 1996.

114 Krown SE: Interferon and other biologic agents for the treatment of Kaposi's sarcoma. *Hematol Oncol Clin North Am* 5:311, 1991.

115 Lane HC et al: Anti-retroviral effects of interferon-alpha in AIDS-associated Kaposi's sarcoma. *Lancet* 2:1218, 1988.

116 Lane HC et al: Interferon-alpha in patients with asymptomatic human immunodeficiency virus (HIV) infection: A randomized, placebo-controlled trial. *Ann Intern Med* 112:805, 1990.

117 Lane HC: Interferons in HIV and related diseases. *AIDS* 8Suppl 3: S19–23, 1994.

118 Poli G et al: Tumor necrosis factor alpha functions in an autocrine manner in the induction of human immunodeficiency virus expression. *Proc Natl Acad Sci USA* 87:782, 1990.

119 Howard OM et al: Soluble tumor necrosis factor receptor: Inhibition of human immunodeficiency virus activation. *Proc Natl Acad Sci USA* 90:2335, 1993.

120 Butera ST et al: Regulation of HIV-1 expression by cytokine networks in a CD4+ model of chronic infection. *J Immunol* 150:625, 1993.

121 Duh E et al: Tumor necrosis factor alpha activates human immunodeficiency virus type 1 through induction of nuclear factor binding to the NF-kappa B sites in the long terminal repeat. *Proc Natl Acad Sci USA* 86:5974, 1989.

122 Walker RE et al: Inhibition of immunoreactive tumor necrosis factor-alpha by a chimeric antibody in patients infected with human immunodeficiency virus type 1. *J Infect Dis* 174:63, 1996.

123 Klausner JD et al: The effect of thalidomide on the pathogenesis of human immunodeficiency virus type 1 and *M. tuberculosis* infection. *J Acquir Immune Defic Syndr Hum Retrovirol* 11:247, 1996.

124 Macchia D et al: Membrane tumour necrosis factor-alpha is involved in the polyclonal B-cell activation induced by HIV-infected human T cells. *Nature* 363:464, 1993.

125 O'Brien WA et al: Human immunodeficiency virus-type 1 replication can be increased in peripheral blood of seropositive after influenza vaccination. *Blood* 86:1081, 1995.

126 Stanley SK et al: Effect of immunization with a common recall antigen on plasma viremia and in vitro virus isolation in HIV-1 infected individuals. *N Engl J Med* 334:1222, 1996.

127 Kovac JA et al: Controlled trial of interleukin-2 infusions in patients infected with the human immunodeficiency virus. *N Engl J Med* 335: 1350, 1996.

128 Poli G et al: Interleukin 6 induces human immunodeficiency virus expression in infected monocytic cells alone and in synergy with tumor necrosis factor alpha by transcriptional and post-transcriptional mechanisms. *J Exp Med* 172:151, 1990.

129 Emilie D et al: Administration of an anti-interleukin-6 monoclonal antibody to patients with acquired immunodeficiency syndrome and lymphoma: Effect on lymphoma growth and on B clinical symptoms. *Blood* 84:2472, 1994.

130 Emilie D et al: Interleukin-6 production in high-grade B lymphomas: Correlation with the presence of malignant immunoblasts in acquired immunodeficiency syndrome and in human immunodeficiency virus-seronegative patients. *Blood* 80:498, 1992.

131 Marfaing-Koka A et al: In vivo role of IL-6 on the viral load and on immunological abnormalities of HIV-infected patients. *J Acquir Immune Defic Syndr Hum Retrovirol* 11:59, 1996.

132 Montaner LJ et al: Interleukin-10 inhibits initial reverse transcription of human immunodeficiency virus type 1 and mediates a virostatic latent state in primary blood derived human macrophages in vitro. *J Gen Virol* 75:3393, 1994.

133 Weissman D et al: Interleukin 10 blocks HIV replication in macrophages by inhibiting the autocrine loop of tumor necrosis factor alpha and interleukin 6 induction of virus. *AIDS Res Human Retroviruses* 10:1099, 1994.

134 Romano MF et al: IL-10 inhibits nuclear factor-kappa B/Rel nuclear activity in CD3-stimulated human peripheral T lymphocytes. *J Immunol* 156:2119, 1996.

135 Clerci M et al: Type 1/type 2 cytokine modulation of T cell programmed cell death as a model for human immunodeficiency virus pathogenesis. *Proc Natl Acad Sci USA* 91:11811, 1994.

136 Shearer GM et al: Cytokines in immune regulation/pathogenesis in HIV infection. *Ciba Found Symp* 195:142, 1995.

137 Meyaard L et al: Changes in cytokine secretion patterns of CD4+ T cell clones in human immunodeficiency virus infection. *Blood* 84: 4262, 1994.

138 Blauvelt A et al: Modulation of T cell responses to recall antigens presented by Langerhans cells in HIV discordant identical twins by anti-interleukin (IL)-10 antibodies and IL-12. *J Clin Invest* 97:1550, 1996.

139 Clerici M et al: Role of interleukin-10 in T helper cell dysfunction in asymptomatic individuals infected with the human immunodeficiency virus. *J Clin Invest* 93:768, 1994.

140 Paganin C et al: Priming for high interferon-gamma production induced by interleukin-12 in both CD4+ and CD8+ T cell clones from HIV-infected patients. *J Clin Invest* 96:1677, 1995.

141 Chehimi J et al: Differential production of interleukin 10 during human immunodeficiency virus infection. *AIDS Res Hum Retroviruses* 12:1149, 1996.

142 Graziosi C et al: Lack of evidence for the dichotomy of TH1 and TH2 predominance in HIV infected individuals. *Science* 265:248, 1994.

143 Lane HC et al: Abnormalities of B-cell activation and immunoregulation in patients with the acquired immunodeficiency syndrome. *N Engl J Med* 309:453, 1983.

144 Chess Q et al: Serum immunoglobulin elevations in the acquired immunodeficiency syndrome (AIDS): IgG, IgA, IgM, and IgD. *Diagn Immunol* 2:184, 1984.

145 Papadopoulos NM et al: The presence of immunoglobulin D in endocrine disorders and diseases of immunoregulation, including the acquired immunodeficiency syndrome. *Clin Immunol Immunopathol* 32:248, 1984.

146 Anderson KC et al: Isolation and functional analysis of human B cell populations. *J Immunol* 134:820, 1985.

147 Vincent C et al: Secretory immunoglobulins in serum from human immunodeficiency virus (HIV)-infected patients. *J Clin Immunol* 12:381, 1992.

148 Pahwa SG et al: Defective B-lymphocyte function in homosexual men in relation to the acquired immunodeficiency syndrome. *Ann Intern Med* 101:757, 1984.

149 Pahwa R et al: Prematurity, hypogammaglobulinemia, and neuropathology with human immunodeficiency virus (HIV) infection. *Proc Natl Acad Sci USA* 84:3826, 1987.

150 Janoff EN et al: Intestinal mucosal immunoglobulins during human immunodeficiency virus type 1 infection. *J Infect Dis* 170:299, 1994.

151 Vigano A et al: Elevation of IgE in HIV-infected children and its correlation with the progression of disease. *J Allergy Clin Immunol* 95:627, 1995.

152 Carson PJ et al: Antibody class and subclass responses to pneumococcal polysaccharides following immunization of human immunodeficiency virus infected patients. *J Infect Dis* 172:340, 1995.

153 Redfield RR et al: A phase I evaluation of the safety and immunogenicity of vaccination with recombinant gp160 in patients with early human immunodeficiency virus infection. Military Medical Consortium for Applied Retroviral Research. *N Engl J Med* 324:1677, 1991.

154 Boppana SB et al: Virus specific antibody responses to human cytomegalovirus (HCMV) in HIV-1 infected individuals with HCMV retinitis. *J Infect Dis* 171:182, 1995.

155 Mofenson LM et al: Crossover of placebo patients to intravenous immunoglobulin confirms efficacy for prophylaxis of bacterial infections and reduction of hospitalizations in human immunodeficiency virus-infected children. The National Institute of Child Health and Human Development Intravenous Immunoglobulin Clinical Trial Study Group. *Pediatr Infect Dis J* 13:477, 1994.

156 Mofenson LM et al: Prophylactic intravenous immunoglobulin in HIV-infected children with CD4+ counts of 0.20 x 10^9/L or more: Effect on viral, opportunistic, and bacterial infections. The National Institute of Child Health and Human Development Intravenous Immunoglobulin Clinical Trial Study Group. *JAMA* 268:483, 1992.

157 Crow ME: Intravenous immune globulin for prevention of bacterial infections in pediatric AIDS patients. *Am J Health Syst Pharm* 52: 803, 1995.

158 Jablonowki H et al: The use of intravenous immunoglobulins in symptomatic HIV infection: Results of a randomized study. *Clin Invest* 72:220, 1994.

159 The Prevent Group: Reduction of respiratory syncytial virus hospitalization among premature infants and infants with brochopulmonary dysplasia using respiratory syncytial virus immune globulin prophylaxis. *Pediatrics* 99:93, 1997.

160 Macchia D et al: Membrane tumour necrosis factor-alpha is involved in the polyclonal B-cell activation induced by HIV-infected human T cells. *Nature* 363:464, 1993.

161 Boue F et al: HIV induced IL-6 production by human B lymphocytes: Role of IL-4. *J Immunol* 148:3761, 1992.

162 Shibata D et al: Epstein-Barr virus-associated non-Hodgkin's lymphoma in patients infected with the human immunodeficiency virus. *Blood* 81:2102, 1993.

163 Scott ME et al: In vivo decrease in the expression of complement receptor 2 on B cells in HIV infection. *AIDS* 7:37, 1993.

164 Munson LG et al: Decreased levels of complement receptor 1 (CD35) on B lymphocytes in persons with HIV infection. *Clin Immunol Immunopathol* 75:20, 1995.

165 Indraccolo S et al: B cell activation and human immunodeficiency virus infection. *J Clin Immunol* 13:381, 1993.

166 Schnittman SM et al: Direct polyclonal activation of human B lymphocytes by the acquired immune deficiency syndrome virus. *Science* 233:1084, 1986.

167 Nair MPN et al: Immunoregulatory activities of human immunodeficiency virus (HIV) protein: Effect of HIV recombinant and synthetic peptides on immunoglobulin synthesis and proliferative responses by normal lymphocytes. *Proc Natl Acad Sci USA* 85:6498, 1988.

168 Berberian L et al: A VH clonal deficit in human immunodeficiency virus-positive individuals reflects a B-cell maturational arrest. *Blood* 78:175, 1991.

169 Berberian L et al: Immunoglobulin VH3 gene products: Natural ligands for HIV gp120. *Science* 261:1588, 1993.

170 David D et al: Selective variations in vivo of VH3 and VH1 gene family expression in peripheral B cell IgM, IgD and IgG during HIV infection. *Eur J Immunol* 25:1524, 1995.

171 Berberian L et al: Effects of HIV infection on VH3 (D12 idiotope) B cells in vivo. *J Acquir Immune Defic Syndr* 7:641, 1994.

172 Muro-Cacho CA et al: Analysis of apoptosis in lymph nodes of HIV-infected persons: Intensity of apoptosis correlates with the general state of activation of the lymphoid tissue and not with stage of disease or viral burden. *J Immunol* 154:5555, 1995.

173 Koenig S et al: Detection of AIDS virus in macrophages in brain tissue from AIDS patients with encephalopathy. *Science* 233:1089, 1986.

174 Wiley CA et al: Cellular localization of human immunodeficiency virus infection within the brains of acquired immune deficiency syndrome patients. *Proc Natl Acad Sci USA* 83:7089, 1986.

175 Stoler MH et al: Human T cell lymphotropic virus type III infection of the central nervous sytem. *JAMA* 256:2360, 1986.

176 Vazeux R et al: AIDS subacute encephalitis: Identification of HIV-infected cells. *Am J Pathol* 126:403, 1987.

177 Ho DD et al: Infection of monocyte/macrophages by human T lymphotropic virus type III. *J Clin Invest* 77:1712, 1986.

178 Nicholson JKA et al: In vitro infection of human monocytes with human T-lymphotropic virus type III/lymphoadenopathy-associated virus (HTLV-III/LAV). *J Immunol* 137:323, 1986.

179 Gartner S et al: The role of mononuclear phagocytes in HTLV-III/LAV infection. *Science* 233:215, 1986.

180 Takeda A et al: Two receptors are required for antibody-dependent enhancement of human immunodeficiency virus type 1 infection: CD4 and Fc gamma R. *J Virol* 64:5605, 1990.

181 Laurence J et al: Human immunodeficiency virus infection of monocytes: Relationship to Fc-gamma receptors and antibody-dependent viral enhancement. *Immunology* 70:338, 1990.

182 Homsy J et al: The Fc and not CD4 receptor mediates antibody enhancement of HIV infection in human cells. *Science* 244:1357, 1989.

183 Heise C et al: Primary acute simian immunodeficiency virus infection of intestinal lymphoid tissue is associated with gastrointestinal dysfunction. *J Infect Dis* 169:1116, 1994.

184 Smith PD et al: Monocyte function in the acquired immune deficiency syndrome. *J Clin Invest* 74:2121, 1984.

185 Poli G et al: Monocyte function in intravenous drug abusers with lymphadenopathy syndrome and in patients with acquired immunodeficiency syndrome: Selective impairment of chemotaxis. *Clin Exp Immunol* 62:136, 1985.

186 Chaturvedi S et al: Macrophages from human immunodeficiency virus-positive persons are defective inhost defense against *Histoplasma capsulatum*. *J Infect Dis* 171:320, 1995.

187 Clerici M et al: Accessory cell function in asymptomatic human immunodeficiency virus infected patients. *Clin Immunol Immunopathol* 54:168, 1990.

188 Trial J et al: Phenotypic and functional changes in peripheral blood monocytes during progression of human immunodeficiency virus infection. Effects of soluble immune complexes, cytokines, subcellular particulates from apoptotic cells, and HIV-1-encoded proteins on monocytes phagocytic function, oxidative burst, transendothelial migration, and cell surface phenotype. *J Clin Invest* 95:1690, 1995.

189 Baldwin GC et al: Human immunodeficiency virus causes mononuclear phagocyte dysfunction. *Proc Natl Acad Sci USA* 87:3933, 1990.

190 Murray HW et al: Impaired production of lymphokines and immune γ-interferon in the acquired immunodeficiency syndrome. *N Engl J Med* 310:883, 1984.

191 Murray HW et al: In vitro and in vivo activation of human mononuclear phagocytes by interferon-gamma: Studies with normal and AIDS monocytes. *J Immunol* 138:2457, 1987.

192 Thieblemont N et al: CD14lowCD16high: A cytokine-producing monocyte subset which expands during human immunodeficiency virus infection. *Eur J Immunol* 25:3418, 1995.

193 Washburn RG et al: Phagocytic and fungicidal activity of monocytes from patients with acquired immunodeficiency syndrome. *J Infect Dis* 151:565, 1985.

194 Kleinerman ES et al: Activation of monocyte-mediated tumoricidal activity in patients with acquired immunodeficiency syndrome. *J Clin Oncol* 3:1005, 1985.

195 Clerici M et al: Multiple patterns of alloantigens presenting/stimulating cell dysfunction in patients with AIDS. *J Immunol* 146:2207, 1991.

196 Blauvelt A et al: Functional studies of epidermal Langerhans cells and blood monocytes in HIV infected persons. *J Immunol* 154:3506, 1995.

197 Fidler SJ et al: An early antigen-presenting cell defect in HIV-1-infected patients correlates with CD4 dependency in human T-cell clones. *Immunology* 89:46, 1996.

198 Nottet HS et al: Phagocytic function of monocyte-derived macrophages is not affected by human immunodeficiency virus type 1 infection. *J Infect Dis* 168:84, 1997.

199 Badley AD et al: Macrophage-dependent apoptosis of CD4+ T lymphocytes from HIV-infected individuals is mediated by FasL and tumor necrosis factor. *J Exp Med* 185:55, 1997.

200 Millar AB et al: Production of tumor necrosis factor-alpha by blood and lung mononuclear phagocytes from patients with human immunodeficiency virus related lung disease. *Am J Respir Cell Mol Biol* 5:144, 1991.

201 Enk C et al: Interleukin 1 activity in the acquired immunodeficiency syndrome. *Scand J Immunol* 23:491, 1986.

202 Buhl R et al: Activation of alveolar macrophages in asymptomatic HIV infected individuals. *J Immunol* 150:1019, 1993.

203 Esser R et al: Secretory repertoire of HIV-infected human monocytes/macrophages. *Pathobiology* 59:219, 1991.

204 Giulian D et al: The envelope glycoprotein of human immunodeficiency virus type 1 stimulates release of neurotoxins from monocytes. *Proc Natl Acad Sci USA* 90:2769, 1993.

205 Dreyer EB et al: The cost protein gp120 of HIV-1 inhibits astrocyte uptake of excitatory amino acids via macrophage arachidonic acid. *Eur J Neurosci* 7:2502, 1995.

206 Fine SM et al: Tumor necrosis factor alpha inhibits glutamate uptake by primary human astrocytes: Implications for pathogenesis of HIV-1 dementia. *J Biol Chem* 271:15303, 1996.

207 Bukrinsky MI et al: Regulation of nitric oxide synthase activity in human immunodeficiency virus type 1 (HIV-1) infected monocytes: Implications for HIV associated neurological disease. *J Exp Med* 181: 735, 1995.

208 Shrikant P et al: HIV glycoprotein 120 enhances intercellular adhesion molecule 1 gene expression in glial cells: Involvement of Janus kinase/signal C signaling pathways. *J Immunol* 156:1307, 1996.

209 Lipton SA et al: Update on current models of HIV-related neuronal injury: Platelet-activating factor, arachidonic acid and nitric oxide. *Adv Neuroimmunol* 4:181, 1994.

210 Rook AH et al: Interleukin 2 enhances the natural killer cell activity of acquired immunodeficiency syndrome patients through a gamma-interferon-independent mechanism. *J Immunol* 134:1503, 1985.

211 Bonagura VR et al: Dysfunction of natural killer cells in human immunodeficiency virus infected children with or without *Pneumocystis carinii* pneumonia. *J Pediatr* 121:195, 1992.

212 Tyler DS et al: Alterations in antibody dependent cellular cytotoxicity during the course of HIV-1 infection: Humoral and cellular defects. *J Immunol* 144:3375, 1990.

213 Hu PF et al: Natural killer cell immunodeficiency in HIV disease is manifest by profoundly decreased numbers of CD16+CD56+ cells and expansion of a population of CD16dimCD56- cells with low lytic activity. *J Acquir Immune Defic Syndr Hum Retrovirol* 10:331–40, 1995.

214 Steinman R et al: Maturation and migration of cutaneous dendritic cells. *J Invest Dermatol* 105:2S, 1995.

215 Reid CD et al: Interactions of tumor necrosis factor with granulocyte-macrophage colony-stimulating factor and other cytokines in the regulation of dendritic cell growth in vitro from early biopotent CD34+ progenitors in human bone marrow. *J Immunol* 49:2681, 1992.

216 Steinman RM et al: The dendritic cell system and its role in immunogenicity. *Annu Rev Immunol* 9:271, 1991.

217 Katz SI et al: Epidermal Langerhans cells are derived from cells originating in bone marrow. *Nature* 282:324, 1979.

218 O'Doherty U et al: Human blood contains two subsets of dendritic cells, one immunologically mature and the other immature. *Immunology* 82:487, 1994.

219 Ocklind G et al: Expression of CD54, CD58, CD14, and HLA-DR on macrophages and macrophage-derived accessory cells and their accessory capacity. *Immunol Lett* 31:253, 1992.

220 Zhou LJ et al: Human blood dendritic cells selectively express CD83, a member of the immunoglobulin superfamily. *J Immunol* 154:3821, 1995.

221 Mosialos G et al: Circulating human dendritic cells differentially express high levels of a 55-kDa actin-bundling protein. *Am J Pathol* 148:593, 1996.

222 Peters JH et al: Signals required for differentiating dendritic cells from human monocytes in vitro. *Adv Exp Med Biol* 329:275, 1993.

223 Liu YL et al: Follicular dendritic cells and germinal centers. *Int Rev Cytol* 166:139, 1996.

224 Armstrong GA et al: Follicular dendritic cells and virus-like particles in AIDS-related lymphadenopathy. *Lancet* 2:230, 1984.

225 Spira AI et al: Cellular targets of infection and route of viral dissemination after an intravaginal inoculation of simian immunodeficiency virus into rhesus macaques. *J Exp Med* 183:215, 1996.

226 Langhoff E et al: Replication of human immunodeficiency virus type 1 in primary dendritic cell cultures. *Proc Natl Acad Sci USA* 88:7998, 1991.

227 Beaulieu S et al: In vitro characterization of purified human thymic dendritic cells infected with human immunodeficiency virus type 1. *Virology* 222:214, 1996.

228 Cameron PU et al: The interaction of macrophage and non-macrophage tropic isolates of HIV-1 with thymic and tonsillar dendritic cells in vitro. *J Exp Med* 183:1851, 1996.

229 Ludewig B et al: Replication pattern of human imunodeficiency virus type 1 in mature Langerhans cells. *J Gen Virol* 76:1317, 1995.

230 Tsunetsugu-Yokota Y et al: Monocyte derived cultured dendritic cells are susceptible to human immunodeficiency virus infection and transmit virus to resting T cells in the process of nominal antigen presentation. *J Virol* 69:4544, 1995.

231 Patterson S et al: CD4 expression on dendritic cells and their infection by human immunodeficiency virus. *J Gen Virol* 76:1155, 1995.

232 Cameron PU et al: During HIV-1 infection most blood dendritic cells are not productively infected and can induce allogeneic CD4+ T cells clonal expansion. *Clin Exp Immunol* 88:226, 1992.

233 Weissman D et al: Three populations of cells with dendritic morphology exist in peripheral blood, only one of which is infectable with human immunodeficiency virus type 1. *Proc Natl Acad Sci USA* 92: 826, 1995.
234 Soto-Ramirez LE et al: HIV-1 Langerhans' cell tropism associated with heterosexual transmission of HIV. *Science* 271:1291, 1996.
235 Weissman D et al: Both a precursor and a mature population of dendritic cells can bind HIV. However, only the mature populations that expresses CD80 can pass infection to unstimulated CD4+ T cells. *J Immunol* 155:4111, 1995.
236 Pinchuk LM et al: The role of CD40 and CD80 accessory cell molecules in dendritic cell-dependent HIV-1 infection. *Immunity* 1:317, 1994.
237 Fagnoni FF et al: Role of B70/B7–2 in CD4+ T cell immune responses induced by dendritic cells. *Immunology* 85:467, 1995.
238 Granelli-Piperno A et al: Coexpression of NF-kappa B/Ral and Sp1 transcription factors in human immunodeficiency virus 1-induced, dendritic cell-T cell syncytia. *Proc Natl Acad Sci USA* 92:10944, 1995.
239 Pope M et al: Conjugates of dendritic cells and memory T lymphocytes from skin faciltate productive infection with HIV-1. *Cell* 78: 389, 1994.
240 Pinchuk LM et al: Cell-cell interactions regulate dendritic cell-dependent HIV-1 production in CD4+ T lymphocytes. *Adv Exp Med Biol* 378:461, 1995.
241 Pope M et al: Low levels of HIV-1 infection in cutaneous dendritic cells promote extensive viral replication upon binding to memory CD4+ T cells. *J Exp Med* 182:2045, 1995.
242 Weissman D et al: Cytokine regulation of HIV replication induced by dendritic cell-CD4-positive T cell interactions. *AIDS Res Human Retrovirus* 12:759, 1996.
243 Weissman D et al: The efficiency of acute infection of CD4+ T cells is markedly enhanced in the setting of antigen-specific immune activation. *J Exp Med* 183:687, 1996.
244 Ayehunie S et al: Acutely infected Langerhans cells are more efficiency than T cells in disseminating HIV type 1 to activated T cells following a short cell-cell contact. *AIDS Res Hum Retroviruses* 11:877, 1995.
245 Mcllroy D et al: Infection frequency of dendritic cells and CD4+ T lymphocytes in spleens of human immunodeficiency virus positive patients. *J Virol* 69:4737, 1995.
246 Hsia FJ et al: Low prevalence of HIV-1 proviral DNA in peripheral blood monocytes and dendritic cells from HIV-1 infected individuals. *AIDS* 9:398, 1995.
247 Frankel SS et al: Replication of HIV-1 in dendritic cell-derived syncytia at the mucosal surface of the adenoid. *Science* 272:115, 1996.
248 Roberts M et al: Dendritic cells from HIV-1 infected individuals show reduced capacity to stimulate autologous T cell proliferation. *Immunol Lett* 43:39, 1994.
249 Macatonia SE et al: Dendritic cell infection, depletion and dysfunction in HIV-infected individuals. *Immunology* 71:38, 1990.
250 Ho DD et al: Rapid turnover of plasma virions and CD4 lymphocytes in HIV-1 infection. *Nature* 373:123, 1995.
251 Perelson AS et al: HIV-1 dynamics in vivo: virion clearance rate, infected cell life-span, and viral generation time. *Science* 271:1582, 1996.
252 Wei X et al: Viral dynamics in human immunodeficiency virus type 1 infection. *Nature* 373:117, 1996.
253 Pantaleo G et al: Lymphoid organs function as major reservoirs for human immunodeficiency virus. *Proc Natl Acad Sci USA* 88:9838, 1991.
254 Fox CH et al: Lymphoid germinal centers are reservoirs of human immunodeficiency virus type 1 RNA (published erratum appears in *J Infect Dis* 165:1161, 1992). *J Infect Dis* 164:1051, 1991.
255 Tsunoda R et al: Follicular dendritic cells in vitro are not susceptible to infection by HIV-1. *AIDS* 10:595, 1996.
256 Reinhart TA et al: A new approach to investigating the relationship between productive infection and cytopathicity in vivo. *Nat Med* 3: 218, 1997.
257 Health SL et al: Follicular dendritic cells and human immunodeficiency virus infectivity. *Nature* 377:740, 1995.
258 Rosenberg YJ et al: Immunological and virological changes associated with decline in CD4/CD8 ratios in lymphoid organs of SIV-infected macaques. *AIDS Res Hum Retroviruses* 10:863, 1994.
259 June RA et al: Complement and antibody mediate enhancement of HIV infection by increasing virus binding and provirus formation. *AIDS* 5:269, 1991.
260 Robinson WE Jr et al: Antibody-dependent enhancement of human immunodeficiency virus type 1 (HIV-1) infection in vitro by serum from HIV-1-infected and passively immunized chimpanzees. *Proc Natl Acad Sci USA* 86:4710, 1989.
261 Takeda A et al: Antibody-enhanced infection by HIV-1 via Fc receptor-mediated entry. *Science* 242:580, 1988.
262 van Kuyk R et al: Clones human CD8+ cytotoxic T lymphocytes protect human-PBL-SCID mice HIV-1 infection by an HLA-unrestricted mechanism. *J Immunol* 153:4826, 1994.
263 Toso JF et al: Oligoclonal CD8 lymphocytes from persons with asymptomatic human immunodeficiency virus (HIV) type 1 infection inhibit HIV-1 replication. *J Infect Dis* 172:964, 1995.
264 Lohman BL et al: Antiviral cytotoxic T lymphocytes in vaginal mucosa of simian immunodeficiency virus infected rhesus macaques. *J Immunol* 155:5855, 1995.
265 Rowland-Jones S et al: HIV specific cytotoxic T cells in HIV exposed but uninfected Gambian women. *Nat Med* 1:59, 1995.
266 Koup RA et al: Temporal association of cellular immune responses with the initial control of viremia in primary human immunodeficiency virus type 1 syndrome. *J Virol* 68:4650, 1994.
267 Pantaleo G et al: Major expansion of CD8+ T cells with a predominant V beta usage during the primary immune response to HIV. *Nature* 370:463, 1994.
268 Pantaleo GP et al: The qualitative nature of the primary immune response to HIV infection is a prognosticator of disease progression independent of the initial level of plasma viremia. *Proc Natl Acad Sci USA* 94:254, 1997.
269 Rinaldo CR Jr et al: High levels of anti-HIV-1 memory cytotoxic T lymphocyte activity and low viral load are associated with lack of disease in HIV-1 infected long-term nonprogressors. *J Virol* 69:5838, 1995.
270 Haas G et al: Dynamics of viral variants in HIV-1 nef and specific cytotoxic T lymphocytes in vivo. *J Immunol* 157:4212, 1996.
271 Couillin I et al: Impaired CTL recognition due to genetic variations in the main immunogenic region of the HIV-1 nef protein. *J Exp Med* 180:1129, 1994.
272 Koenig S et al: Transfer of HIV-1 specific cytotoxic T lymphocytes to an AIDS patient leads to selection for mutant HIV variants and subsequent disease progression. *Nat Med* 1:304, 1995.
273 Borrow P et al: Antiviral pressure exerted by HIV-1-specific cytotoxic T lymphocytes (CTLs) during primary infection demonstrated by rapid selection of CTL escape virus. *Nat Med* 3:205, 1997.
274 Goulder PJR et al: Late escape from an immunodominant cytotoxic T-lymphocyte response associated with progression to AIDS. *Nat Med* 3:212, 1997.
275 Kalams SA et al: T cell receptor usage and fine specificity of human immunodeficiency virus 1 specific cytotoxic T lymphocyte clones: Analysis of quasispecies recognition reveals a dominant response directed against a minor in vivo variant. *J Exp Med* 183:1669, 1996.
276 McAdam S et al: Immunogenic HIV variant peptides that bind to HLA-B8 can fail to stimulate cytotoxic T lymphocyte responses. *J Immunol* 155:2729, 1995.
277 Caruso A et al: Expression of CD28 on CD8+ and CD4+ lymphocytes during HIV infection. *Scand J Immunol* 40:485, 1994.
278 Choremi-Papadopoulou H et al: Downregulation of CD28 surface antigen on CD4+ and CD8+ T lymphocytes during HIV-1 infection. *J Acquir Immune Defic Syndr* 7:245, 1994.
279 Fiorentino S et al: Predominant involvement of CD8+CD28− lymphocytes in human immunodeficiency virus-specific cytotoxic activity. *J Virol* 70:2022, 1996.

280 Borthwick NJ et al: Lymphocyte activation in HIV-1 infection: Functional defects of CD28− T cells. *AIDS* 8:431, 1994.
281 Meier UC et al: Cytotoxic T lymphocyte lysis inhibited by viable HIV mutants. *Science* 270:1360, 1995.
282 Klenerman P et al: The effects of natural altered peptide ligands on the whole blood cytotoxic T lymphocyte response to human immunodeficiency virus. *Eur J Immunol* 25:1927, 1995.
283 Schwartz O et al: Endocytosis of major histocompatibility complex class I molecules is induced by the HIV-1 nef protein. *Nat Med* 2: 338, 1996.
284 Sadat-Sowti B et al: An inhibitor of cytotoxic functions produced by CD8+CD57+ T lymphocytes from patients suffering from AIDS and immunosuppressed bone marrow recipients. *Eur J Immunol* 24:2882, 1994.
285 Legac E et al: CD4+CD7−CD57+ T cells: A new T lymphocyte subset expanded during human immunodeficiency virus infection. *Blood* 79:1746, 1992.
286 Ferbas J et al: Virus burden in long-term survivors of human immunodeficiency virus (HIV) infection is a determinant of anti-HIV CD8+ lymphocyte activity. *J Infect Dis* 172:329, 1995.
287 Harrer T et al: Cytotoxic T lymphocytes in asymptomatic long-term nonprogressing HIV-1 infection: Breadth and specificity of the response and relation to in vivo viral quasispecies in a person with prolonged infection and low viral load. *J Immunol* 156:2616, 1996.
288 Walker CM et al: CD8+ lymphocytes can control HIV infection in vitro by suppressing virus replication. *Science* 234:1563, 1986.
289 Walker CM et al: Inhibition of human immunodeficiency virus replication in acutely infected CD4+ cells by CD8+ cells involves a noncytotoxic mechanisms. *J Virol* 65:5921, 1991.
290 Walker CM et al: A diffusible lymphokine produced by CD8+ T lymphocytes suppresses HIV replication. *Immunology* 66:628, 1989.
291 Toso JF et al: Oligoclonal CD8 lymphocytes from persons with asymptomatic human immunodeficiency virus (HIV type 1) infection inhibit HIV-1 replication. *J Infect Dis* 172:964, 1995.
292 Kinter A et al: HIV replication in CD4+ T cells of HIV infected individuals is regulated by a balance between the viral suppressive effects of endogenous beta-chemokines and the viral inductive effects of other endogenous cytokines. *Proc Natl Acad Sci USA* 93:14076, 1996.
293 Baier M et al: HIV suppression by interleukin-16. *Nature* 378:563, 1995.
294 Moriuchi H et al: CD8+ T cell derived soluble factor(s) but not beta-chemokines RANTES, MIP-1alpha, and MIP-1beta, suppress HIV-1 replication in monocyte/macrophages. *Proc Natl Acad Sci USA* 93: 15341, 1996.
295 McDougal JS et al: Mechanisms of human immunodeficiency virus type 1 (HIV-1) neutralization: Irreversible inactivation of infectivity by anti-HIV-1 antibody. *J Virol* 70:5236, 1996.
296 Schutten M et al: Human antibodies that neutralize primary human immunodeficiency virus type 1 in vitro do not provide protection in an in vivo model. *J Gen Virol* 77:1667, 1996.
297 Montefiori DC et al: Neutralizing and infection-enhancing antibody responses to human immunodeficiency virus type 1 in long-term nonprogressors. *J Infect Dis* 173:60, 1996.
298 Pellegrin I et al: Kinetics of appearance of neutralizing antibodies in 12 patients with primary or recent HIV-1 infection and relationship with plasma and cellular viral loads. *J Acquir Immune Defic Syndr Hum Retrovirol* 11:438, 1996.
299 Moore JP et al: Development of the anti-gp120 antibody response during seroconversion to human immunodeficiency virus type 1. *J Virol* 68:5142, 1994.
300 Bruck C et al: HIV-1 envelope-elicited neutralizing antibody titres correlate with protection and virus load in chimpanzees. *Vaccine* 12: 1141, 1994.
301 Mascola JR et al: Immunization with envelope subunit vaccine products elicits neutralizing antibodies against laboratory-adapted but not primary isolates of human immunodeficiency virus type 1. *J Infect Dis* 173:340, 1996.
302 Keefer MC et al: Studies of high doses of a human immunodeficiency virus type 1 recombinant glycoprotein 160 candidate vaccine in HIV type 1 seronegative humans. *AIDS Res Hum Retroviruses* 10:1713, 1994.
303 Berman PW et al: Protection of MN-rgp120-immunized chimpanzees from heterologous infection with a primary isolate of human immunodeficiency virus type 1. *J Infect Dis* 173:52, 1996.
304 Klasse PJ et al: Quantitative model of antibody and soluable CD4 mediated neutralization of primary isolates and T cell line adapted strains of human immunodeficiency virus type 1. *J Virol* 70:3668, 1996.
305 Karlsson GB et al: Increased envelope spike density and stability are not required for the neutralization resistance of primary human immunodeficiency viruses. *J Virol* 70:6136, 1996.
306 Watkins BA et al: Resistance of human immunodeficiency virus type 1 to neutralization by natural antisera occurs through single amino acid substitutions that cause changes in antibody binding at multiple sites. *J Virol* 70:8431, 1996.
307 Yoshiyama H et al: Characterization of mutants of human immunodeficiency virus type 1 that have escaped neutralization by a monoclonal antibody to the gp120 V2 loop. *J Virol* 68:974, 1994.
308 Willey RL et al: Differential glycosylation, virion incorporation, and sensitivity to neutralizing antibodies of human immunodeficiency virus type 1 envelope produced from infected primary T lymphocyte and macrophage cultures. *J Virol* 70:6431, 1996.
309 Planz O et al: Specific cytotoxic T cells eliminate cells producing neutralizing antibodies. *Nature* 382:726, 1996.
310 Ghiara JB et al: Crystal structure of the prinicipal neutralization site of HIV-1. *Science* 264:82, 1994.
311 Burton DR et al: Efficient neutralization of primary isolates of HIV-1 by a recombinant human monoclonal antibody. *Science* 266:1024, 1994.
312 D'Souza MP et al: Evaluation of monoclonal antibodies to HIV-1 envelope by neutralization and binding assays: An international collaboration. *AIDS* 8:169, 1994.
313 Gaudin MC et al: Effective ex vivo neutralization of human immunodeficiency virus type 1 in plasma by recombinant immunoglobulin molecules. *J Virol* 70:2586, 1996.
314 Conley AJ et al: Neutralization of primary human immunodeficiency virus type 1 isolates by the broadly reactive anti-V3 monoclonal antibody, 447–52D. *J Virol* 68:6994, 1994.
315 McKnight A et al: Location, exposure, and conservation of neutralizing and nonneutralizing epitopes on human immunodeficiency virus type 2 SU glycoprotein. *J Virol* 70:4598, 1996.
316 Trkola A et al: Human monoclonal antibody 2G12 defines a distinctive neutralization epitope on the gp120 glycoprotein of human immunodeficiency virus type 1. *J Virol* 70:1100, 1996.
317 Shotton C et al: Identification and characterization of monoclonal antibodies specific for polymorphic antigenic determinants within the V2 region of the human immunodeficiency virus type 1 envelope glycoprotein. *J Virol* 69:22, 1995.
318 Gorny MK et al: Human anti-V2 monoclonal antibody that neutralizes primary but not laboratry isolates of human immunodeficiency virus type 1. *J Virol* 68:8312, 1994.
319 Moore JP et al: Antibody cross-competition analysis of the human immunodeficiency virus type 1 gp120 exterior envelope glycoprotein. *J Virol* 70:1863, 1996.
320 Poignard P et al: Neutralizing antibodies to human immunodeficiency virus type 1 gp120 induce envelope glycoprotein subunit dissociation. *J Exp Med* 183:473, 1996.
321 Muster Y et al: Cross-neutralizing activity against divergent human immunodeficiency virus type 1 isolates induced by the gp41 sequence. *J Virol* 68:4031, 1994.
322 Conley AJ et al: Neutralization of divergent human immunodeficiency virus type 1 variants and primary isolates by IAM-41-2F5 and anti-gp41 human monoclonal antibody. *Proc Natl Acad Sci USA* 91: 3348, 1994.
323 Purtscher M et al: A broadly neutralizing human monoclonal antibody against gp41 of human immunodeficiency virus type 1. *AIDS Res Hum Retroviruses* 10:1651, 1994.

324 Ugen KE et al: Vertical transmission of human immunodeficiency virus type 1: Seroreactivity by maternal antibodies to the carboxy region of the gp41 envelope glycoprotein. *J Infect Dis* 175:63, 1997.
325 Bal AK et al: Syncytium-inhibiting and neutralizing activity in maternal sera fail to prevent vertical transmission of human immunodeficiency virus type 1. *Pediatr Infect Dis J* 15:315, 1996.
326 Van Rompay KK et al: Vaccination of pregnant macaques protects newborns against mucosal simian immunodeficiency virus infection. *J Infect Dis* 173:1327, 1996.
327 Trkola A et al: Cross-clade neuralization of primary isolates of human immunodeficiency virus type 1 by human monoclonal antibodies and tetrameric CD4- IgG. *J Virol* 69:6609, 1995.
328 Cavacini LA et al: Influence of heavy chain constant regions on antigen binding and HIV-1 neutralization by a human monoclonal antibody. *J Immunol* 155:3638, 1995.
329 Burnett PR et al: Serum IgA mediated neutralization of HIV type 1. *J Immunol* 152:4642, 1994.
330 Laal S et al: Synergistic neutralization of human immunodeficiency virus type 1 by combinations of human monoclonal antibodies. *J Virol* 68:4001, 1994.
331 Vijh-Warrier S et al: Synergistic neutralization of human immunodeficiency virus type 1 by a chimpanzee monoclonal antibody against the V2 domain of gp120 in combination with monoclonal antibodies against the V3 loop and the CD4 binding site. *J Virol* 70:4466, 1996.
332 Moore JP et al: Primary isolates of human immunodeficiency virus type 1 are relatively resistant to neutralization by monoclonal antibodies to gp120 and their neutralization is not predicted by studies with monomeric gp120. *J Virol* 69:101, 1995.
333 Sattentau QJ et al: Human immunodeficiency virus type 1 neutralization is determined by epitope exposure on the gp120 oligomer. *J Exp Med* 182:185, 1995.
334 Broder CC et al: Antigenic implications of human immunodeficiency virus type 1 envelope quaternary structure: Oligomer-specific and sensitive monoclonal antibodies. *Proc Natl Acad Sci USA* 91:11699, 1994.
335 Van Cott TC et al: Lack of induction of antibodies specific for conserved, discontinuous epitopes of HIV-1 envelope glycoprotein by candidate AIDS vaccines. *J Immunol* 155:4100, 1995.
336 de Santis C et al: Role of HLA class I in HIV type 1-induced syncytium formation. *AIDS Res Hum Retroviruses* 12:1031, 1996.
337 Briant L et al: Inhibition of human immunodeficiency virus type 1 production in infected peripheral blood mononuclear cells by human leukocyte antigen class I specific antibodies: Evidence for a novel antiviral mechanism. *J Virol* 70:5213, 1996.
338 Fox CH et al: Lymphoid germinal centers are reservoirs of human immunodeficiency virus type 1 RNA. *J Infect Dis* 164:1051, 1991.
339 Heath SL et al: Follicular dendritic cells in human immunodeficiency virus infectivity. *Nature* 377:740, 1995.
340 Trischmann H et al: Lymphocytotropic strains of HIV type 1 when complexed with enhancing antibodies can infect macrophages via Fc gamma III, independently of CD4. *AIDS Res Hum Retroviruses* 11:343, 1995.
341 Pantaleo G et al: Effect of anti-V3 antibodies on cell-free and cell-to-cell human immunodeficiency virus transmission. *Eur J Immunol* 25:226, 1995.
342 Walsh CM et al: Immune function in mice lacking in the perforin gene. *Proc Natl Acad Sci USA* 91:10854, 1994.
343 Lowin B et al: Cytolytic T cell cytotoxicity is mediated through perforin and Fas lytic pathways. *Nature* 370:650, 1994.
344 Lowin B et al: A null mutation in the perforin gene impairs cytolytic T lymphocyte- and natural killer cell-mediated cytotoxicity. *Proc Natl Acad Sci USA* 91:11571, 1994.
345 Takai T et al: Multiple loss of effector cell functions in FcR gamma-deficient mice. *Int Rev Immunol* 13:369, 1996.
346 Tang Y et al: Control of immunodeficiency and lymphoproliferation in mouse AIDS: Studies of mice deficient in CD8+ T cells or perforin. *J Virol* 71:1808, 1997.
347 Connick E et al: HIV-specific cellular and humoral immune responses in primary HIV infection. *AIDS Res Hum Retroviruses* 12:1129, 1996.
348 Sawyer LA et al: Possible beneficial effects of neutralizing antibodies and antibody-dependent, cell-mediated cytotoxicity in human immunodeficiency virus infection. *AIDS Res Hum Retroviruses* 6:341, 1990.
349 Koup RA et al: Broadly reactive antibody-dependent cellular cytotoxic response to HIV-1 envelope glycoproteins precedes broad neutralizing response in human infection. *Viral Immunol* 4:215, 1991.
350 Merrill JD et al: Characterization of natural killer and antibody-dependent cellular cytotoxicity of preterm infants against human immunodeficiency virus-infected cells. *Pediatr Res* 40:498, 1996.
351 Jenkins M et al: Association between anti-human immunodeficiency virus type 1 (HIV-1) antibody-dependent cellular cytotoxicity antibody titers at birth and vertical transmission of HIV-1. *J Infect Dis* 170:308, 1994.
352 Broliden K et al: Antibody-dependent cellular cytotoxicity and neutralizing activity in sera of HIV-1 infected mothers and their children. *Clin Exp Immunol* 93:56, 1993.
353 Ljunggren K et al: IgG subclass response to HIV in relation to antibody-dependent cellular cytotoxicity at different clinical stages. *Clin Exp Immunol* 73:343, 1988.
354 Baum LL et al: HIV-1 gp120-specific antibody-dependent cell-mediated cytotoxicity correlates with rate of disease progression. *J Immunol* 157:2168, 1996.
355 Ojo-Amaize EA et al: Antibodies to human immunodeficiency virus in human sera induce cell-mediated lysis of human immunodeficiency virus-infected cells. *J Immunol* 139:2263, 1987.
356 Ahmad A et al: Evidence for a defect of antibody-dependent cellular cytotoxic (ADCC) effector function and anti-HIV gp120/41-specific ADCC-mediating antibody titers in HIV-infected individuals. *J Acquir Immune Defic Syndr* 7:428, 1997.
357 Tyler DS et al: Alterations in antibody-dependent cellular cytotoxicity during the course of HIV-1 infection: Humoral and cellular defects. *J Immunol* 144:3375, 1990.
358 Koup RA et al: Antibody-dependent cell-mediated cytotoxicity directed by a human monoclonal antibody reactive with gp120 of HIV-1. *AIDS* 5:1309, 1991.
359 Koup RA et al: Antigenic specificity of antibody-dependent cell-mediated cytotoxicity directed against human immunodeficiency virus in antibody-positive sera. *J Virol* 63:584, 1989.
360 Forthal DN et al: Functional activities of 20 human immunodeficiency virus type 1 (HIV-1) specific human monoclonal antibodies. *AIDS Res Hum Retroviruses* 11:1095, 1995.
361 Bjorling E et al: Hyperimmune antisera against synthetic peptides representing the glycoprotein of human immunodeficiency virus type 2 can mediate neutralization and antibody-dependent cytotoxic activity. *Proc Natl Acad Sci USA* 88:6082, 1991.
362 Norley SG et al: Demonstration of cross-reactive antibodies able to elicit lysis of both HIV-1 and HIV-2 infected cells. *J Immunol* 145:1700, 1990.
363 VonGegerfelt A et al: Specificity of antibody-dependent cellular cytotoxicity in sera from human immunodeficiency virus type 2-infected individuals. *AIDS Res Human Retroviruses* 9:883, 1993.
364 Tanneau F et al: Primary cytotoxicity against the envelope glycoprotein of human immunodeficiency virus-1: Evidence for antibody-dependent cellular cytotoxicity in vivo. *J Infect Dis* 162:837, 1990.

Chapter 18

Epidemiology, natural history, and pathogenesis of HIV infection

John Ambroziak
Jay A. Levy

The recognition of the human immunodeficiency virus (HIV) as a new infectious agent followed a striking rise in the presentation of patients, predominantly homosexual males, with Kaposi's sarcoma and *Pneumocystis carinii* pneumonia in the early 1980s. Epidemiological studies suggested a viral agent as the cause of the underlying immunosuppression, and HIV was soon isolated and linked to the acquired immunodeficiency syndrome (AIDS).[1–3]

These initial discoveries have spawned an intense worldwide effort to combat the spread and effects of HIV infection. Yet after more than a decade of research there is still much unknown about the precise mechanisms by which HIV causes disease and AIDS. HIV infection remains incurable, but recently treatable, as measured by length of survival. Research discoveries continue to reveal new avenues of investigation and lead to reevaluation of theories on the pathogenesis of AIDS and potentially effective therapies. The purpose of this chapter is to review what is currently understood about the epidemiology, natural history, and pathogenesis of HIV infection.

EPIDEMIOLOGY AND MECHANISMS OF HIV TRANSMISSION

The cumulative total of HIV infections worldwide rose to an estimated 20 million by late 1996 and is expected to double in the next six years.[4] The rate of increase in new AIDS cases varies statistically by gender and race, and analysis of the predominant means of transmission within these groups is important for developing methods to combat viral spread. Mathematical models have been used to predict current levels and extent of infection in the United States. HIV infection rates remain fairly constant among women and minorities, while the rate for white males is declining markedly.[5] It is estimated that 900,000 people in the United States are infected with HIV and over 500,000 individuals have died from AIDS. In the United States, AIDS is the leading cause of death of men between the ages of 25 and 40.[5]

The three principal means of HIV transmission are by blood or blood products, sexual contact, and passage from mother to child. The transmission of HIV was initially associated with sexual contact, blood transfusions, and intravenous drug use,[6] and epidemiological studies suggested an infectious agent in blood and genital fluids. With the recognition of maternal-child transmission,[7] infection *in utero* or via the vaginal canal were recognized as possible routes for the transmission of HIV. Transmission correlates with high levels of infectious virus in these different body fluids and the nature and duration of contact with these fluids.

BLOOD-BORNE TRANSMISSION

Molecular techniques have allowed quantitation of virus in the blood and have established a correlation between viral burden, disease stage, and CD4+ cell count.[8] Viremia is highest during the initial acute infection (up to 1 million particles/ml), then drops dramatically during the asymptomatic stage and rises steadily throughout progression to disease. Levels of more than 2 million virions/ml can be detected.[8] Analysis of viral burden is complicated by the estimation that the majority, perhaps as much as a 100,000-fold excess, of viral particles are defective.[8,9] Between 1 in 1000 and 1 in 10,000 PBMCs are believed to be infected in healthy HIV-seropositive individuals.[10,11] In AIDS patients this number can rise to around 1 in 10 PBMCs.[12] Asymptomatic individuals have on the order of five million PBMCs per milliliter of blood. Thus, a healthy seropositive individual would possess approximately 5000 infected cells/ml and 100 infectious viral particles/ml. With the ability to produce thousands of viral particles per day, the virally infected cells constitute the substantial source of infectious virus in the blood.[11]

In the early 1980s HIV infection was recognized primarily in homosexual men and in hemophiliacs and blood transfusion recipients. HIV in blood, and in blood products such as Factor VIII, infected thousands of hemophiliacs before the presence of the virus was recognized in these preparations. Solvent/detergent and heat treatment of blood products, along with improved donor screening techniques, have virtually eliminated the risk of receiving contaminated blood products.[13] Blood, containing infected cells and particles, transfused from an infected person is an extremely efficient means of transmission. Yet the risk of transmission is a consequence of the interdependent factors of disease stage, viral load, and perhaps the phenotype of the predominant host virus strain.[11]

HIV infection of intravenous drug users (IVDUs) represents another route of HIV transmission. Shared needles are the responsible vehicle, and risk of infection rises with the incidence of needle sharing and the viral load of the needle sharers.[14] Infection as a result of accidental needle sticks is not a major source of infection, as most sticks do not transfer appreciable amounts of blood. Infection results most often with deep wounds. Again, the viral load of the sample is the key factor in transmission incidence. Hepatitis B virus can be present at levels of 100 million to one billion particles per milliliter of blood.[15] Therefore, transmission of this agent by needle injury is much more common than similar transmission of HIV.

SEXUAL TRANSMISSION

The transmission of HIV virus among homosexual men was the focus of early epidemiological studies, but heterosexual transmission is the most important means of HIV spread worldwide today. A high prevalence of HIV infection has been observed in sex workers in parts of Africa and Southeast Asia, and this source is playing a key role in the spread of HIV.[16,17] In comparison, infections due to shared needles and contaminated blood products represent a small minority of new HIV infections worldwide.

The presence of virus in genital fluid is a major factor in transmission by sexual means. Seminal and vaginal cells, as well as fluids, can contain infectious virus. Infected cells would again be expected to be the major source of HIV. Higher levels of infected cells are also expected to coincide with the high viremia associated with acute infection and advanced disease. In fact, a progressive disease state in infective male partners has been shown to correspond with increased risk of transmission.[18,19] However, the number of infected cells in semen is highly variable, and studies fail to demonstrate a correlation between viral levels in the semen and clinical state.[20] There are also technical problems in assaying viral levels in genital fluids.

Studies have shown that the presence of other sexually transmitted diseases (STDs), such as gonorrhea, chlamydia, or syphilis, enhances the transmission of HIV.[21,22] One study has indicated that the transmission rate of HIV was substantially decreased in a population as a result of improved treatment for STDs.[23] Sexually transmitted diseases with their associated increase of inflammatory cells, often in the presence of ulcerative conditions, probably lead to increased numbers of virus-infected cells in the body fluids. In the presence of STDs, HIV can be present in as many as 1 in 20 cells in seminal fluid.[24]

In males, the virus is believed to be released from the prostate and secretory glands in addition to the testes.[25] In females, secretory glands can be a source of virus, as can infected cells in menstrual blood.[26] Early epidemiological studies indicated that for infection to occur, the virus required a point of entry such as irritated rectal mucosa or the ulcers associated with STDs. It is now known that healthy cells of the rectal mucosa and cervical epithelium can be directly infected.[27,28,29] The insertive partner, while at lower risk, can also be infected. This transmission probably occurs through cells in the urethra or foreskin. Lack of circumcision is a factor that increases the risk of HIV infection severalfold.[21,30]

TRANSMISSION OF HIV BY OTHER BODY FLUIDS

Since the risk of HIV transmission correlates with viral levels in body fluids, it is fortunate that other body fluids besides blood and genital fluids do not contain large quantities of infectious virus. Virus is occasionally detectable in saliva samples at low levels.[31,32] Urine and tears also contain low or undetectable levels of infectious virus, and infectious virus is undetectable in sweat or feces.[26] Breast milk can be a significant source of virus,[33] as discussed in the next section. Cerebrospinal fluid also contains high levels of virus but does not normally pose a transmission risk.[34]

MATERNAL-CHILD TRANSMISSION

Studies have shown that the rate of transmission from infected mothers to their newborns ranges from 13 to 35 percent.[35–37] About half of these cases appear due to infection *in utero*, while half are due to infection during birth. In support of in utero infection, virus has been found in cord blood, amniotic fluid, and placental tissue.[38,39] In support of peripartum transmission, twin studies have shown that the newborn delivered first has a significantly higher risk of infection, most likely because of having first contact with HIV-containing fluids in the vaginal canal.[40] Other evidence for infection at birth is the finding of virus in the newborn after one to three months, but not in the cord blood.[41,42]

While breast milk has been shown to contain high levels of virus that may be a source of transmission, this fluid also contains antiviral components.[33,43] Nevertheless, breast feeding by HIV-infected mothers is discouraged in countries where nutrition and the beneficial effects of colostrum are not needed for infant survival. The likelihood of transmission is increased for isolates that are either resistant to maternal neutralizing antibodies or actually enhanced by these antibodies.[44] The anti-HIV drug AZT has been shown to be useful in preventing HIV transmission to newborns and supports the prevention of transmission through control of viremia.[45,46]

The high level of viremia associated with acute HIV infection poses the most significant risk of virus transfer, both at delivery and through breast feeding. Yet the advanced disease state with its high virus load also carries a strong risk.[36]

NATURAL HISTORY

CLINICAL MANIFESTATIONS

Like other viral infections in humans, acute infection with HIV is often associated with specific clinical manifestations.[47,48] Within one to three weeks of contact with the virus, about one-half of patients report an acute mononucleosis-like illness. The symptoms include headache, muscle ache, sore throat, fever, and swollen lymph nodes. Also reported is an erythematous rash on the trunk and extremities that can distinguish HIV infection from other acute infections and is thus of particular clinical importance in early diagnosis. Infected individuals can also present with esophageal and anal canal ulcers, central nervous system disorders, and gastrointestinal problems, particularly diarrhea. Most of these symptoms subside within several weeks, but lymphadenopathy and malaise can persist for several months. This period of acute infection is associated with high levels of viremia and a great potential for transmission of the virus.

VIRAL KINETICS

HIV can be passed within the host by free virus or cell-to-cell transfer, and the number of human cell types infected or showing sensitivity to HIV infection is large (Table 18-1). CD4+ lymphocytes produce the highest levels of virus. Substantial replication of some viral isolates in macrophages can also take place. Other cell types vary in the amount of virus released, as measured in cell culture; some, such as dendritic cells, may produce low levels or maintain virus bound to the cell surface. The attached virus can be passed to circulating CD4+ cells.[26] It is known that cell-to-cell transfer is much more efficient for virus transmission than free virus or *de novo* infection.[49]

Viral infection involves the interaction of HIV with a cell sur-

Table 18-1. Human Cells Susceptible to HIV*

Brain	*Bowel*
Capillary endothelial cells	Columnar and goblet cells
Astrocytes	Enterochromaffin cells
Macrophages (microglia)	Colon carcinoma cells
Oligodendrocytes	*Other*
Choroid plexus	Myocardium
Ganglia cells	Renal tubular cells
Neuroblastoma cells	Synovial membrane
Glioma cell lines	Hepatocytes
Neurons (?)	Hepatic sinusoid endothelium
Skin	Hepatic carcinoma cells
Langerhans cells	Kupffer cells
Fibroblasts	Dental pulp fibroblasts
Hematopoietic	Pulmonary fibroblasts
T lymphocytes	Fetal adrenal cells
B lymphocytes	Adrenal carcinoma cells
Macrophages	Retina
NK cells	Cervix-derived epithelial cells
Megakaryocytes	Cervix (epithelium?)
Eosinophils	Prostate
Dendritic cells	Testes
Promyelocytes	Osteosarcoma cells
Stem cells	Rhabdomyosarcoma cells
Thymocytes	Fetal chorionic villi
Thymic epithelium	Trophoblast cells
Follicular dendritic cells	
Bone marrow endothelial cells	

* Susceptibility to HIV was determined by *in vitro* or *in vivo* studies.

face receptor, predominantly CD4, and subsequent fusion of the viral membrane with the cell membrane. Then entry of the viral core into the cytoplasm takes place. Through the mechanism of three viral enzymes (reverse transcriptase, integrase, and protease) the virus undergoes its replication cycle. First there is a duplication of the viral RNA into a double-stranded complementary DNA (cDNA) copy, using reverse transcriptase; then, integration of the viral cDNA into the cellular chromosome, using integrase. Next, production of messenger and viral RNA takes place, with translation into viral proteins. The processing of the transcribed polypeptides by protease leads to formation of an infectious particle that buds at the cell surface.

Recent results indicate that the virus interacts with additional receptors on the cell surface besides CD4.[50] These coreceptors are among a group of chemokine receptors. One coreceptor, CXCR-4, formerly called fusin/LESTR, appears to be expressed on the surface of many cells and is used principally by syncytium-inducing (SI) T-cell line tropic viruses.[51] The other coreceptor, CCR-5, the receptor for β-chemokines, is used primarily by nonsyncytium-inducing (NSI), often macrophage-tropic, viruses.[52–54] The discovery of this coreceptor was encouraged by the finding that β-chemokines can block HIV entry into cells.[55] Recent studies suggest that resistance to HIV infection, and perhaps delay in progression to disease, occurs in individuals whose CD4+ cells are either homozygous or heterozygous for a variant of the CCR-5 gene that has a 32-base-pair deletion.[56–58] In cells with this variant gene, the receptor is not expressed on the cell surface. These new observations are suggesting approaches for novel therapeutic modalities to prevent infection or spread of HIV in the host.

Some reports have indicated that the symptomatic phase associated with HIV infection represents a dynamic period of viral replication and cell infection and death.[59,60] Virus levels in the peripheral blood can reach one million particles/ml. These studies suggest that the viral replication cycle *in vivo* takes on the order of two days. These results imply that several hundred cycles of virus replication occur per year and several thousand cycles over the course of the average infection.[61,62] This level of replication distinguishes HIV from many other infectious human agents. If replication is uncontrolled after acute infection, the dynamics of this replicative pattern could be responsible for the eventual immune destruction observed in AIDS. The kinetics of virus replication in asymptomatic individuals remain to be elucidated.

Other biologic studies have shown that one infected cell produces up to 1000 virus particles in culture.[49,63] The majority of these may be defective and noninfectious.[9] Thus, a relatively small number of infected cells appear to be responsible for maintaining high viral loads. This observation emphasizes the importance of the already infected cell as the source of virus in HIV infection and thus as a target for antiviral therapies. Control of this source of HIV would be more effective than preventing only *de novo* virus infection in the host.[64] Persistently infected cells can serve as reservoirs for continual reseeding of virus in the host. Moreover, the viruses produced by these cells can have detrimental effects on normal cells through induction of apoptosis or cytotoxic T-cell responses against noninfected cells coated by viral proteins.[64]

STAGES OF HIV INFECTION

The pathogenesis of HIV infection can be considered as progressing through three stages (reviewed in Ref. 26). During the initial acute infection, or early stage, many CD4+ T cells and some macrophages are infected, and HIV replication produces high viremia levels that can approach 5000 infectious particles per milliliter of plasma. During this time, before an immune response can be mounted by the host, lymphoid tissues and other cells in the body become infected. As many as 250 billion cells could be infected in this early period, as measured by *in situ* PCR procedures.[65] CD4+ T cells decrease in numbers initially and CD8+ cells increase, then both return to near basal levels. This return to near normal levels occurs following the appearance first of antiviral cellular immune responses and later of antibodies to the virus. Viremia also decreases sharply concomitant with these immune responses, but a small number of infected cells continue to replicate virus. This continued replication of HIV, unless controlled by the immune system, leads to the eventual emergence of genetically divergent isolates that may escape antiviral immune responses.

Several months after primary infection the second, or asymptomatic, stage begins; this stage can last from one year to over a decade. During this period CD4+ cells, having returned to normal levels, often begin a slow decline in numbers. The virus is somewhat controlled during this stage, presumably by CD8+ cell antiviral activities (see below), and the length of this stage seems determined by the host's cellular immune response.[66] Eventually, in most infected people, a reduced CD4+ level mirrors an increase in viral load that plays a role in progression to the final, or symptomatic, stage. CD4+ loss and the appearance of a pathogenic virus strain are linked temporally, but their order is not conclusively known.

In general, viruses released by cells in an infected individual appear as populations of genetic variants of one dominant virus. These "quasispecies" can have distinct biologic differences, such as the ability to cause syncytium formation in culture, to be resistant to drugs, or to replicate with varying kinetics.[26] In this chapter we refer to recovered uncloned viruses as isolates because they represent the dominant virus present and most likely the one determining the extent of pathogenesis. The term "strain" will be used when the virus has been isolated and characterized in the laboratory.

CD4+ loss over time could be responsible for the reduction in CD8+ cell antiviral immune responses.[67] CD8+ cell function depends on adequate amounts of IL-2, produced by CD4+ cells. Possibly the declining CD8+ cell activity allows increased replication of a pathogenic HIV isolate, or a new and more pathogenic isolate leads to the final reduction of CD4+ numbers. Measurements of CD8+ cell responses, virus production, and CD4+ cell counts favor the former hypothesis.[66]

LONG-TERM SURVIVAL

Normally, progression to the symptomatic stage occurs after 5 to 8 years of infection. However, there are cases of a rapid decline in clinical state after infection, particularly with infection by pathogenic strains.[68] The longest time from infection to onset of symptoms has not been established, but some individuals have had documented infection for at least 18 years (Ref. 69 and unpublished observation). Certain characteristics are common to these long-term survivors (LTS). They have a low viral load, as determined by measurements of infected cells and free virus in peripheral blood. The viral isolates from these individuals are relatively noncytopathic and may grow to low levels in the blood. Antibodies to the autologous virus do not enhance infection. Furthermore, the CD8+ cell antiviral responses in these long-term survivors remain strong, in contrast to the decreased activity seen in most infected people progressing to disease.[70,71] This CD8+ antiviral response suppresses virus replication in CD4+ cells without killing the infected cell. The anti-HIV activity can be quantified by assaying virus replication in the presence of different ratios of CD8+ and CD4+ cells.[72] The reasons for the maintenance of this antiviral response by LTS or for its eventual loss and associated progression to disease are not yet understood. Recent studies have emphasized the importance of CD4+ cell Th-1 cytokines, particularly IL-2, in maintaining CD8+ cell activity.[67]

Long-term survival has also been associated with isolates possessing defective viral genomes, particularly with severe mutations in the *nef* gene. The *nef* accessory gene is required for progression to disease in SIV-infected macaques.[73] In one cohort of seven LTS infected from a common source, deletions in several regions of *nef* were detected.[74] However, other reports have revealed that only a few LTS possess defective *nef* sequences (Refs. 75 and 76 and unpublished observation). Defects have also been reported in other accessory genes of viruses from LTS.[77,78] In general, however, while mutant viral genomes can reveal sequences necessary for viral pathogenesis, they alone are not the cause of long-term survival in the majority of infected subjects. Instead, particular features of the subjects' immune systems, such as a strong CD8+ cell antiviral response, are likely responsible for a long asymptomatic course.

PATHOGENESIS OF HIV INFECTION

HEMATOPOEITIC SYSTEM

The pathogenic effects of HIV are often observed histologically in the lymphoid tissues and mirrored by a decrease in the function of the immune system. Even before a reduction in the number of CD4+ T cells is detectable, functional irregularities are apparent in a number of immune cells. The possible causes of these HIV-associated immune disorders are numerous.

Changes in the numbers of cell subsets can be demonstrated by flow cytometric techniques. For example, a decrease in CD4+ counts and an increase in CD8+ number are commonly seen in people infected with HIV. Specific subsets within the CD8+ fraction have also been shown to increase or decrease in relation to each other.[79,80] With progression to AIDS, activated cells (CD38+) increase in number[81] and memory cell (CD 26+) levels decrease.[82] Absolute and relative CD4+ and CD8+ T-cell counts have proven extremely valuable as correlates of clinical state and disease progression. They are less useful as markers of antiviral therapy.

HIV infection causes functional abnormalities in a variety of cell types. The abnormal activation of B cells leads to dysregulation and hypergammaglobulinemia. These features are particularly apparent in infected children.[7] B-cell dysfunction also plays a role in lymphadenopathy.[83] Macrophages show minor functional changes but are not often infected by HIV *in vivo*.[84,85] The function of NK cells is decreased. This finding could reflect direct infection of these cells[86] or a decrease in IL-12, which mediates their function.[87] Whether these effects are due to general responses to viral infection or specific effects of HIV infection remains to be determined.

In addition to reducing their numbers, HIV infection results in severe functional deficiencies in CD4+ helper T cells. As noted above, decreased CD4+ counts represent the first immune derangement associated with HIV infection,[88,89] and measurement of CD4+ levels remains a key diagnostic tool. Whether CD4+ cell reduction results from direct cell infection and destruction, secondary effects of immunologic dysfunction, or both is not yet certain. A decrease in CD4+ cell function is apparent before the decrease in numbers is detected.[90,91] Three functional abnormalities of CD4+ cells are observed sequentially: loss of response to recall antigens, followed by reduced proliferation to alloantigens and finally, by reduced proliferation to lectins (for example, PHA). CD4+ cells from AIDS patients show reductions in all three functions, while cells from healthy HIV-infected individuals exhibit normal responses.[90,92]

There are several possible reasons for the CD4+ cell abnormalities. Latent viral infection, in the absence of cell destruction, could alter membrane integrity and cytokine production. HIV may also infect CD4+ precursors or stromal cells in the thymus[93] and inhibit production of new cells. Deficiencies in CD4+ cell number or function may be due to production or accumulation of viral proteins, since the envelope proteins have been shown to decrease the mitogenic responses of lymphocytes and can be cytotoxic.[94,95] Some researchers report that HIV preferentially infects CD4+ memory T cells, leading to T-cell dysfunction.[96]

Another cause of loss in CD4+ cell function concerns the normal functional role of the CD4 molecule in signal transduction. When a natural ligand binds the CD4 molecule, a protein kinase cascade is initiated that results in protein phosphorylation and phenotypic changes. Extensive binding of the CD4 molecule by HIV, as well as subsequent CD4 downregulation, could hinder these normal processes. Some investigators believe that the loss of CD4+ cells, both infected and uninfected, is caused by the induction of apoptosis.[97] Finally, a number of cytokines are known to exert effects on HIV replication and CD4+ cell function. Their complex interplay is being extensively studied (see Chapter 17 for details).

While the effects of HIV on cells of the peripheral blood are significant, its effects on lymphoid tissue are also dramatic. Lymphoid organs play a key role in antiviral responses and appear to be the principal reservoir and site of replication of HIV.[65,98] After the high viremia associated with primary infection, immune activation causes proliferation of germinal centers and follicular dendritic cells (FDCs). FDCs are responsible for antigen presentation to B cells in the germinal centers and continually present HIV viral particles in the form of immune complexes. FDCs are eventually destroyed, probably through direct infection, cytotoxic T-cell activity, and general cytokine effects on the lymph node. A recent report has suggested that FDCs may in fact cause the spread of HIV in lymphoid tissue.[99] Normally, antibody-bound antigen associated with FDCs is noninfectious. Recent evidence suggests that this FDC-bound HIV could be capable of infecting CD4+ cells by being transformed from a neutralized to an infectious form by the FDCs.[99] These observations need further confirmation.

This process within the lymph node could be an especially efficient method of viral spread, since large numbers of CD4+ cells migrate through germinal centers, where they interact with B cells. As a result of HIV infection, lymph nodes exhibit follicular hyperplasia and an increase in secondary germinal centers filled with activated B cells. Throughout the course of the disease, the lymph node loses its normal architecture concomitant with a decrease in CD4+ cell counts and an increased viral load, reflecting an overall inability to control viral replication. In the final stage of the disease, the lymph node is atrophied with loss of normal architecture.

CENTRAL NERVOUS SYSTEM

Both adult and pediatric AIDS cases are characterized by a high level of central nervous system disorders attributed to the effects of HIV infection. Other lentiviruses are associated with brain disorders of sheep and goats (see Chapter 16). Visna virus can directly infect glial cells, astrocytes, and microglial cells.[100] In studies with human brain tissues, HIV has been found to infect macrophages and microglial cells.[101,102] Other cell types have also been found susceptible to the virus, for example, astrocytes and oligodendrocytes.[103,104] Moreover, HIV has been isolated from the cerebrospinal fluid of AIDS patients with neurologic symptoms such as meningitis and dementia, as well as from asymptomatic patients.[103,105]

The method of virus entry into the CNS is not understood. Initial brain infection requires the virus to cross the blood-brain barrier. This process could be accomplished by viral infection of brain capillary endothelial cells[106] and subsequent transfer to astrocytes.[107] Within the central nervous system, the virus could subsequently undergo mutational changes that would allow for spread to other cell types within the CNS and the development of disease. Viral isolates from the CNS show differences, both in biologic properties and in their envelope sequences, from the associated peripheral blood isolates.[108,109]

Another means for viral entry into the brain has been identified. Studies in animals have shown that limited numbers of T cells and peripheral macrophages can circulate through the CNS and could thus infect neural cells directly.[110] HIV has also been detected in developing fetal CNS tissue, indicating *in utero* CNS infection.[111] Furthermore, animal studies have suggested an increased susceptibility of the newborn brain to HIV replication, compared to the adult brain.[112]

Regardless of the mode of entry into the CNS, HIV causes debilitating pathologies. The spectrum of neurologic disorders includes HIV-associated dementia complex, sensory neuropathy, vacuolar myelopathy, and secondary conditions such as cytomegaloviral meningitis and cryptococcal meningitis. The mechanisms underlying HIV-associated neuropathology are not well understood but may include direct cell death from viral replication, viral protein toxicity, or disruption of normal cytokine levels (reviewed in Ref. 26). Consequent disruption of membrane integrity would have severe effects on neuronal cell function. Another possibility is that an increase in the number of macrophages in the CNS as a result of progression to disease, with consequent increased secretion of cytokines or toxic cellular products, could play an important role in neurologic pathologies.[113]

GASTROINTESTINAL SYSTEM

Gastrointestinal disorders are common during primary HIV infection and normally subside during the asymptomatic stage. Symptoms that later return with progression to disease include diarrhea, chronic malabsorption, and wasting. In Africa these common components of advanced disease are known as "slim disease."[114] They are sometimes caused by opportunistic parasitic infections (*Cryptosporidium* or *Microsporidium*), against which antimicrobials are usually ineffective. Yet symptoms occur in the absence of any detectable pathogens in about one-third of patients.[115] In these cases, HIV may be the proximate cause of disease.[27]

HIV can be detected in the bowel mucosa of symptomatic as well as asymptomatic patients.[27,116] It infects columnar epithelial cells, enterochromaffin cells responsible for normal bowel function, and macrophages in the lamina propria.[27,117] The lamina propria is considered to be the largest lymphoid organ in the human body, and the subsequent infection and destruction of CD4+ cells in this organ may play an important part in the pathogenesis of HIV disease in the bowel.[118] Again, similar to observations in the brain, specific bowel-tropic isolates have been described that have evolved separately from peripheral blood isolates.[116] The infected bowel can exhibit chronic inflammation and pathology, yet the pathogenesis of these conditions is not understood. Infection of macrophages and T cells could disrupt normal mucosal cytokine production. An increase in production of some cytokines, such as IL-6, can have detrimental effects on the bowel.[119,120] Increased cytokine release could lead to perturbation of membrane integrity and consequently to a disruption of water reabsorption function, leading to diarrhea. In addition, this compromise of normal GI function could allow for opportunistic infections that cause further bowel problems.

CONCLUSIONS

Early epidemiological studies linking AIDS to blood and genital fluids were essential to the identification of HIV. The routes of transmission defined in the early years of AIDS remain the same: blood, intimate sexual contact, and maternal-child transmission. Recognition of the modes of HIV transmission presented targets for intervention in the spread of HIV. Currently, the best hope for eventually controlling AIDS mortality worldwide lies in preventing new infections. Antiviral therapy may help reduce maternal-child transmission, but sexual transmission of HIV, as with other STDs, has proven to be difficult to control due to various social and biological factors. This problem, combined with the great length of time during which asymptomatic individuals can transmit the virus to others, has contributed to the extensive spread of HIV. Until effective clinical therapies or a vaccine are available, education must remain a primary means of prevention. Education and the availability of contraceptives have already measurably reduced the birth rate, and presumably the HIV transmission rate as well, in at least one African country.

While the study of HIV has revealed much about lentivirus pathogenesis, this viral infection remains basically resistant to treatment. Most therapies have focused primarily on the reduction of free virus as the target. Recent findings concerning viral load and kinetics and CD4+ cell turnover highlight the reflection of viral load on new rounds of CD4+ infection. Whether or not blocking replication of free virus will stabilize CD4+ cell numbers and prevent progression to disease is the key question (see Chapter 74). The large number of cells already infected in the host must be appreciated.

The early years of HIV research focused on elucidating the function of HIV gene products. The Tat protein has been the focus of several potential antiviral drugs. While much is understood about the structure and function of HIV gene products (see Chapter 16), their intra- and extracellular activities warrant further study. New extracellular roles have been discovered recently for Nef and Vpr, in addition to Tat. Vpr disrupts progression of the cell cycle and may allow for increased virus replication and production.[121] Nef has been shown to bind cellular factors and to have both positive and negative effects on T-cell activation, depending on its intracellular localization.[122] A more complete understanding of these and additional roles for the accessory proteins may reveal avenues for novel antiviral drug development.

More research needs to emphasize the virus-infected cell and its interactions with the human immune system. The virus-infected cell, as the major source of virus and new infection, is the underlying culprit in driving virus replication and deserves more attention as a therapeutic target.[64] In this regard, cell-mediated immune responses are crucial in maintaining the immunological control of HIV characterizing the asymptomatic state. Specifically, the CD8+ cell antiviral activity, initially present in infected individuals but found to decrease with progression to disease,[70,80] must be maintained. Another factor related to progression to disease concerns the shift from the production of type-1 to type-2 cytokines.[123] This shift can lead to a reduction in cell-mediated immune responses and subsequent advancement to disease.[67] Such findings have led to proposals for cytokine immunotherapy.[124,125]

Much remains unknown about potential beneficial host responses against HIV. The complicated relationship between cellular viral load, free viral load, viral kinetics, host-mediated immune responses and eventual progression to disease requires further study. Understanding the role of the genetic background of the host in preventing development of AIDS might also lead to new antiviral treatments. HIV continues to increase our understanding of host-virus interactions, and every new piece of information assists in the novel formulation, as well as reevaluation, of potential clinical therapies.

References

1 Barre-Sinoussi F et al: Isolation of a T-lymphotropic retrovirus from a patient at risk for acquired immune deficiency syndrome (AIDS). *Science* 220:868–871, 1983.
2 Gallo RC et al: Frequent detection and isolation of cytopathic retroviruses (HTLV-III) from patients with AIDS and at risk for AIDS. *Science* 224:500–503, 1984.
3 Levy JA et al: Isolation of lymphocytopathic retroviruses from San Francisco patients with AIDS. *Science* 225:840–842, 1984.
4 Mann J, Tarantola D (eds): *AIDS in the World.* Oxford University Press, 1996.
5 Rosenberg PS: Scope of the AIDS epidemic in the United States. *Science* 270:1372–1375, 1995.
6 Jaffe HW et al: Acquired immune deficiency syndrome in the United States: the first 1,000 cases. *J Infect Dis* 148:339–345, 1983.
7 Ammann A, Levy JA: Laboratory investigation of pediatric acquired immunodeficiency syndrome. *Clin Immunol Immunopathol* 40:122–127, 1986.
8 Piatak M et al: High levels of HIV-1 in plasma during all stages of infection determined by competitive PCR. *Science* 259:1749–1754, 1993.
9 Layne SP et al: Blocking of human immunodeficiency virus infection depends on cell density and viral stock age. *J Virol* 65:3293–3300, 1991.
10 Ho DD et al: Quantitation of human immunodeficiency virus type 1 in the blood of infected persons. *N Engl J Med* 321:1621–1625,1989.
11 Levy JA: The transmission of HIV and factors influencing progression to disease. *Am J Med* 95, 86–100, 1993.
12 Schnittman SM et al: Increasing viral burden in CD4+ T cells from patients with human immunodeficiency virus (HIV) infection reflects rapidly progressive immunosuppression and clinical disease. *Ann Intern Med* 113:438–443, 1990.
13 Petersen LR et al: Current estimates of the infectious window period and risk of HIV infections from seronegative blood donations. Fifth National Forum on AIDS, Hepatitis, and Other Blood-Borne Diseases, 1992, abstr P13, p 37.
14 Des Jarlais DC et al: International epidemiology of HIV and AIDS among injecting drug users. *AIDS* 6:1053–1068, 1992.
15 Ulrich PP et al: Enzymatic amplification of hepatitis B virus DNA in serum compared with infectivity testing in chimpanzees. *J Infect Dis* 160:1–8, 1989.
16 Willerford DM et al: Human immunodeficiency virus infection among high-risk seronegative prostitutes in Nairobi. *J Infect Dis* 167, 1414–1417, 1993.
17 Siraprapasiri T et al: Risk factors for HIV among prostitutes in Chiangmai, Thailand. *AIDS* 5, 579–582, 1991.
18 Osmond D et al: Time of exposure and risk of HIV infection in homosexual partners of men with AIDS. *Am J Pub Health* 78:944–948, 1988.
19 Saracco A et al: Man-to-woman sexual transmission of HIV: longitudinal study of 343 steady partners of infected men. *J AIDS* 6:497–502, 1993.
20 Krieger JN et al: Recovery of human immunodeficiency virus type 1 from semen: Minimal impact of stage of infection and current antiviral chemotherapy. *J Infect Dis* 163:386–388, 1991.
21 Cameron DW et al: Female to male transmission of human immunodeficiency virus type 1: risk factors for seroconversion in men. *Lancet* 2:403–407, 1989.
22 Hunter DJ, Maggwa BN: Sexual behavior, sexually transmitted diseases, male circumcision, and risk of HIV infection among women in Nairobi, Kenya. *AIDS* 8:93–99, 1994.
23 Grosskurth H et al: Impact of improved treatment of sexually transmitted diseases on HIV infection in rural Tanzania: randomised controlled trial. *Lancet* 346:530–536, 1995.
24 Levy JA: The transmission of AIDS: the case of the infected cell. *J Am Med Assoc* 259:3037–3038, 1988.
25 da Silva M et al: Detection of HIV-related protein in testes and prostates of patients with AIDS. *Am J Clin Path* 93:196–201, 1989.
26 Levy JA: HIV and the Pathogenesis of AIDS. Washington, DC, ASM Press, 1994.
27 Nelson JA et al: Human immunodeficiency virus detected in bowel epithelium from patients with gastrointestinal symptoms. *Lancet* 1: 259–262, 1988.
28 Phillips DM: The role of cell-to-cell transmission in HIV infection. *AIDS* 8:719–731, 1994.
29 Pomerantz RJ et al: Human immunodeficiency virus (HIV) infection of the uterine cervix. *Ann Int Med* 108:321–327, 1988.
30 Seed J et al: Male circumcision, sexually transmitted disease, and risk of HIV. *J AIDS Hum Retrovirol* 8:83–90, 1995.
31 Groopman JE et al: HTLV-III in saliva of people with AIDS-related complex and healthy homosexual men at risk for AIDS. *Science* 226: 447–449, 1984.
32 Levy JA, Greenspan D: HIV in saliva. *Lancet* 2:1248, 1988.
33 Van de Perre P et al: Postnatal transmission of human immunodeficiency virus type 1 from mother to infant. *N Engl J Med* 325:593–598, 1991.
34 Levy JA et al: Isolation of AIDS-associated retroviruses from cerebrospinal fluid and brain of patients with neurological symptoms. *Lancet* 2:586–588, 1985.
35 Newell ML et al: Risk factors for mother-to-child transmission of HIV-1. *Lancet* 339:1007–1012, 1992.
36 Rossi P: Maternal factors involved in mother-to-child transmission of HIV-1. Report of a Consensus Workshop, Siena, Italy, January 1992. *J AIDS* 5:1019–1029, 1992.
37 Scarlatti G et al: Polymerase chain reaction, virus isolation, and antigen assay in HIV-1-antibody-positive mothers and their children. *AIDS* 5:1173–1178, 1991.
38 Chandwani S et al: Pathology and human immunodeficiency virus expression in placentas of seropositive women. *J Infect Dis* 163: 1134–1138, 1991.
39 Mundy DC et al: Human immunodeficiency virus isolated from amniotic fluid. *Lancet* 2:459–460, 1987.
40 Goedert JJ et al: High risk of HIV-1 infection for first-born twins. *Lancet* 338:1471–1475, 1991.
41 Ehrnst A et al: HIV in pregnant women and their offspring: Evidence for late transmission. *Lancet* 338:203–207, 1991.
42 De Rossi A et al: Vertical transmission of human immunodeficiency virus type 1 (HIV-1): Lack of detectable virus in peripheral blood cells of infected children at birth. *AIDS* 6:1117–1120, 1992.
43 Newburg DS et al: A human milk factor inhibits binding of human immunodeficiency virus to the CD4 receptor. *Pediatr Res* 31:22–28, 1992.
44 Kliks SC et al: Features of HIV-1 that could influence maternal-child transmission. *J Am Med Assoc* 272:467–474, 1994.
45 Centers for Disease Control: Zidovudine for the prevention of HIV transmission from mother to infant. *MMWR* 43:285–287, 1994.
46 Connor M, Mofenson LM. Zidovudine for the reduction of perinatal human immunodeficiency virus transmission: pediatric AIDS Clinical Trials Group Protocol 076—results and treatment recommendations. *Pediatr Infect Dis J* 14:536–541, 1995.
47 Cooper DA et al: Acute AIDS retrovirus infection: definition of a clinical illness associated with seroconversion. *Lancet* 1:537–540, 1985.
48 Tindall B, Cooper DA: Primary HIV infection: host responses and intervention strategies. *AIDS* 5:1–14, 1991.

49 Dimitrov DS et al: Quantitation of human immunodeficiency virus type 1 infection kinetics. *J Virol* 67:2182–2190, 1993.
50 Levy JA: Infection by human immunodeficiency virus-CD4 is not enough. *N Engl J Med* 335:1528–1530, 1996.
51 Feng Y et al: HIV-1 entry cofactor: functional cDNA cloning of a seven-transmembrane, G protein-coupled receptor. *Science* 27:872–877, 1996.
52 Alkhatib G et al: CC-CKR-5: a RANTES, MIP-1α, MIP-1β receptor as a fusion cofactor for macrophage-tropic HIV-1. *Science* 272: 1955–1958, 1996.
53 Dragic T et al: HIV-1 entry into CD4+ cells is mediated by the chemokine receptor CC-CKR-5. *Nature* 381:667–673, 1996.
54 Deng HK et al: Identification of a major co-receptor for primary isolates of HIV-1. *Nature* 381:661–666, 1996.
55 Cocchi F et al: Identification of RANTES, MIP-1alpha, and MIP-1beta as the major HIV-suppressive factors produced by CD8+ T cells. *Science* 270:1811–1815, 1995.
56 Samson M et al: Resistance to HIV-1 infection in caucausian individuals bearing mutant alleles of the CCR-5 chemokine receptor gene. *Nature* 382:722–725, 1996.
57 Liu R et al: Homozygous defect in HIV-1 coreceptor accounts for resistance for some multiply-exposed individuals to HIV-1 infection. *Cell* 86:367–377, 1996.
58 Dean M et al: Genetic restriction of HIV-1 infection and progression to AIDS by a deletion allele of the CKR5 structural gene. *Science* 273: 1856–1861, 1996.
59 Ho DD et al: Rapid turnover of plasma virions and CD4 lymphocytes in HIV-1 infection. *Nature* 373:123–125, 1995.
60 Wei X et al: Viral dynamics in human immunodeficiency virus type 1 infection. *Nature* 373:117–122, 1995.
61 Perelson AS et al: HIV-1 dynamics in vivo: virion clearance rate, infected cell life-span, and viral generation time. *Science* 271:1582–1586, 1996.
62 Coffin JM: HIV population dynamics in vivo: implications for genetic variation, pathogenesis, and therapy. *Science* 267:483–489, 1995.
63 Levy JA et al: Plasma viral load, CD4+ cell counts, and HIV-1 production by cells. *Science* 271:670–671, 1996.
64 Levy JA: HIV research: a need to focus on the right target. *Lancet* 345:1619–1621, 1995.
65 Embretson J et al: Massive covert infection of helper T lymphocytes and macrophages by HIV during the incubation period of AIDS. *Nature* 362:359–362, 1993.
66 Levy JA: HIV pathogenesis and long-term survival. *AIDS* 7:1401–1410, 1993.
67 Barker E et al: Effects of TH1 and TH2 cytokines on CD8+ cell response against human immunodeficiency virus: implications for long-term survival. *Proc Natl Acad Sci USA* 92:11135–11139, 1995.
68 Kuritzkes DR et al: Rapid CD4+ decline after sexual transmission of a zidovudine-resistant syncytium-inducing isolate of HIV-1. *AIDS* 8: 1017–1019, 1994.
69 Buchbinder SP et al: Long-term HIV-1 infection without immunologic progression. *AIDS* 8:1123–1128, 1994.
70 Mackewicz CE et al: CD8+ cell anti-HIV activity correlates with the clinical state of the infected individual. *J Clin Invest* 87:1462–1466, 1991.
71 Mackewicz C, Levy JA: CD8+ cell anti-HIV activity: Nonlytic suppression of virus replication. *AIDS Res Hum Retrovirol* 8:1039–1050, 1992.
72 Walker CM et al: CD8+ T cells from HIV-1-infected individuals inhibit acute infection by human and primate immunodeficiency viruses. *Cell Immunol* 137:420–428, 1991.
73 Kestler HW et al: Importance of the *nef* gene for maintenance of high virus loads and for development of AIDS. *Cell* 65:651–662, 1991.
74 Deacon NJ et al: Genomic structure of an attenuated quasi species of HIV-1 from a blood transfusion donor and recipients. *Science* 270: 988–991, 1995.
75 Kirchhoff F et al: Brief report: absence of intact *nef* sequences in a long-term survivor with nonprogressive HIV-1 infection. *N Engl J Med* 332:228–232, 1995.
76 Michael NL et al: Functional characterization of human immunodeficiency virus type 1 *nef* genes in patients with divergent rates of disease progression. *J Virol* 69:6758–6769, 1995.
77 Iversen AKN et al: Persistence of attenuated *rev* genes in a human immunodeficiency virus type 1-infected asymptomatic individual. *J Virol* 69:5743–5753, 1995.
78 Michael NL et al: Defective accessory genes in a human immunodeficiency virus type 1-infected long-term survivor lacking recoverable virus. *J Virol* 69:4228–4236, 1995.
79 Choremi-Papadopoulou H et al: Downregulation of CD28 surface antigen on CD4+ and CD8+ T lymphocytes during HIV-1 infection. *J AIDS* 7:245–253, 1994.
80 Landay AL et al: An activated CD8+ T cell phenotype correlates with anti-HIV activity and asymptomatic clinical status. *Clin Immunol Immunopathol* 69:106–116, 1993.
81 Giorgi JV et al: Elevated levels of CD38+ CD8+ T cells in HIV infection add to the prognostic value of low CD4+ T cell levels: results of 6 years of follow-up. *J AIDS* 6:904–912, 1993.
82 Vanham G et al: Decreased expression of the memory marker CD26 on both CD4+ and CD8+ lymphocytes of HIV-infected subjects. *J AIDS* 6:749–757, 1993.
83 Jacobson DL et al: The evolution of lymphadenopathy and hypergammaglobulinemia are evidence for early and sustained polyclonal B lymphocyte activation during human immunodeficiency virus infection. *J Infec Dis* 163:240–246, 1991.
84 Ennen J et al: Decreased accessory cell function of macrophages after infection with human immunodeficiency virus type 1 *in vitro*. *Eur J Immunol* 20:2451–2456, 1990.
85 Patterson BK et al: Detection of HIV-1 DNA and messenger RNA in individual cells by PCR-driven *in situ* hybridization and flow cytometry. *Science* 260:976–979, 1993.
86 Fontana L et al: Deficiency of natural killer activity, but not of natural killer binding, in patients with lymphadenopathy syndrome positive for antibodies to HTLV-III. *Immunobiol* 17:425–435, 1986.
87 Chehimi J et al: *In vitro* infection of natural killer cells with different human immunodeficiency virus type 1 isolates. *J Virol* 65:1812–1822, 1991.
88 Gottlieb MD et al: *Pneumocystis carinii* pneumonia and mucosal candidiasis in previously healthy homosexual men. *N Engl J Med* 305: 1425–1431, 1981.
89 Mildvan D et al: Opportunistic infections and immune deficiency in homosexual men. *Ann Intern Med* 96:700–704, 1982.
90 Clerici M et al: Detection of three distinct patterns of T helper cell dysfunction in asymptomatic, human immunodeficiency virus-positive patients. Independence of CD4+ cell numbers and clinical staging. *J Clin Invest* 84:1892–1899, 1989.
91 Miedema F et al: Immunological abnormalities in human immunodeficiency virus (HIV)-infected asymptomatic homosexual men. *J Clin Invest* 82:1908–1914, 1988.
92 Shearer GM, Clerici M: Early T-helper cell defects in HIV infection. *AIDS* 5:245–253, 1991.
93 Bonyhadi ML et al: HIV induces thymus depletion in vivo. *Nature* 363:728–736, 1993.
94 Garry RF: Potential mechanisms for the cytopathic properties of HIV. *AIDS* 3:683–694, 1989.
95 Diamond DC et al: Inhibition of CD4+ T cell function by the HIV envelope protein, gp120. *J Immunol* 141:3715–3717, 1988.
96 Schnittman SM et al: Preferential infection of CD4+ memory T cells by human immunodeficiency virus type 1: Evidence for a role in the selective T-cell functional defects observed in infected individuals. *Proc Natl Acad Sci USA* 87:6058–6062, 1990.
97 Ameisen JC: Programmed cell death (apoptosis) and cell survival regulation: relevance to AIDS and cancer. *AIDS* 8:1197–1213, 1994.
98 Pantaleo G et al: HIV infection is active and progressive in lymphoid tissue during the clinically latent stage of disease. *Nature* 362: 355–358, 1993.
99 Heath SL et al: Follicular dendritic cells and human immunodeficiency virus infectivity. *Nature* 377:740–744, 1995.

100 Haase AT: Pathogenesis of lentivirus infections. *Nature* 322:130–136, 1986.

101 Tornatore C et al: Persistent human immunodeficiency virus type 1 infection in human fetal glial cells reactivated by T cell factor(s) or by the cytokines tumor necrosis factor alpha and interleukin-1 beta. *J Virol* 65:6094–6100, 1991.

102 Sharpless NE et al: Human immunodeficiency virus type 1 tropism for brain microglial cells is determined by a region of the *env* glycoprotein that also controls macrophage tropism. *J Virol* 66:2588–2593, 1992.

103 Cheng-Mayer C, Levy JA: Distinct biologic and serologic properties of HIV isolates from the brain. *Ann Neurol* 23:S58-S61, 1988.

104 Albright A et al: HIV-1 infection of cultured human adult oligodendrocytes. *Virol* 217:211–219, 1996.

105 Hollander H, Levy JA: Neurologic abnormalities and recovery of human immunodeficiency virus from cerebrospinal fluid. *Ann Intern Med* 106:692–695, 1987.

106 Moses et al: Human immunodeficiency virus infection of human brain capillary endothelial cells occurs via a CD4/galactosyl ceramide-independent mechanism. *Proc Natl Acad Sci USA* 90:10474–10478, 1993.

107 Levy JA: Pathogenesis of human immunodeficiency virus infection. *Microbiol Rev* 57:183–289, 1993.

108 Epstein LG et al: HIV-1 V3 domain variation in brain and spleen of children with AIDS: tissue-specific evolution within host-determined quasispecies. *Virol* 180:583–590, 1991.

109 Cheng-Mayer C et al: Isolates of human immunodeficiency virus type 1 from the brain may constitute a special group of the AIDS virus. *Proc Natl Acad Sci USA* 80:8575–8579, 1989.

110 Hickey WF et al: T-lymphocyte entry into the central nervous system. *J Neurosci Res* 28:254–260, 1991.

111 Lyman WD et al: Viral culture of HIV in neonates. *N Engl J Med* 328:814–815, 1993.

112 Buzy JM et al: HIV-1 in the developing CNS: developmental differences in gene expression. *Virol* 210:361–371, 1995.

113 Tyor WR et al: Unifying hypothesis for the pathogenesis of HIV-associated dementia complex, vacuolar myelopathy, and sensory neuropathy. *J AIDS Hum Retrovirol* 9:379–388, 1995.

114 Serwadda D et al: Slim disease: A new disease in Uganda and its association with HTLV-III infection. *Lancet* 2:849–852, 1985.

115 Antony MA et al: Infectious diarrhea in patients with AIDS. *Dig Dis Sci* 33:1141–1146, 1988.

116 Barnett S et al: Characterization of human immunodeficiency virus type 1 strains recovered from the bowel of infected individuals. *Virol* 182:802–809, 1991.

117 Levy JA et al: Detection of HIV in enterochromaffin cells in the rectal mucosa of an AIDS patient. *Am J Gastro* 84:787–789, 1989.

118 Kotler DP et al: Enteropathy associated with the acquired immunodeficiency syndrome. *Ann Intern Med* 101:421–428, 1984.

119 Birx DL et al: Association of interleukin-6 in the pathogenesis of acutely fatal SIVsmm/PBj-14 in pigtailed macaques. *AIDS Res Hum Retrovirol* 9:1123–1129, 1993.

120 Steffen M et al: Differences in cytokine secretion by intestinal mononuclear cells, peripheral blood monocytes, and alveolar macrophages from HIV-infected patients. *Clin Exp Immunol* 91:30–36, 1993.

121 Rogel ME et al: The human immunodeficiency virus type 1 *vpr* gene prevents cell proliferation during chronic infection. *J Virol* 69:882–888, 1995.

122 Baur AS et al: HIV-1 Nef leads to inhibition or activation of T cells depending on its intracellular localization. *Immunity* 1:373–384, 1994.

123 Clerici M et al: Changes in interleukin-2 and interleukin-4 production in asymptomatic, human immunodeficiency virus-seropositive individuals. *J Clin Invest* 91:759–765, 1993.

124 Clerici M, Shearer GM: The Th1-Th2 hypothesis of HIV infection: new insights. *Immunol Today* 15:575–581, 1994.

125 Kovacs JA et al: Increases in CD4 T lymphocytes with intermittent courses of interleukin-2 in patients with human immunodeficiency virus infection. *N Engl J Med* 332:567–575, 1995.

Chapter 19

Human T-cell lymphotropic virus and HTLV infection

Farley R. Cleghorn
William A. Blattner

Human T-cell lymphotropic virus type I (HTLV-I) was first isolated in 1979 from an African-American patient with cutaneous T-cell leukemia[1] and represented the culmination of a long search for human retroviruses. HTLV-I subsequently was associated etiologically with adult T-cell leukemia/lymphoma (ATL), a clinicopathologic entity first described in 1977 in Japan.[2] Other HTLV-I-associated diseases include a chronic neurologic disease called *tropical spastic paraparesis/HTLV-I-associated myelopathy* (TSP/HAM),[3] a chronic skin condition of children called *infective dermatitis*,[4] and a variety of inflammatory syndromes thought to result from immune perturbation. A second member of the human onco-retrovirus family, HTLV-II, was described in 1982[5] but is not unequivocally associated with any human disease.[6] HTLV-I and HTLV-II appear to be relatively ancient exogenous viruses of humans, are relatively poorly infectious, and environmental cofactors may amplify their spread and help maintain their low endemicity in certain populations.[7]

BIOLOGY

HTLV-I and HTLV-II are single-stranded RNA viruses that replicate through cDNA, a proviral intermediate, via reverse transcriptase, a viral enzyme.[8] This strategy seems to be central to the ability of retroviruses to induce lifelong infection and diseases of long latency (see Chap. 16). Although the precise mechanism for entering cells is not yet elucidated, cellular targets for HTLV-I infection include several types of T cells but primarily the CD4-positive lymphocyte, whereas HTLV-II preferentially infects CD8 cells.[9] This difference in cell tropism may account for the differences in clinical outcome of infection between these viruses. Infection is permanent, but only a small minority of cases will experience a clinical outcome as a result.

Known functional and regulatory genes located in the HTLV-I provirus include *gag* (group-specific antigen), *pol* (polymerase/integrase), and *env* (envelope) and a Px region that includes the *tax* (transcription activator) and *rex* (regulator of expression) regulatory genes. These genes encode for peptides with specific molecular weights that are expressed from infected cells. Host antibody responses to these peptides form the basis for serologic testing for these retroviruses.[10]

Available serologic assays employ a combination of whole virus and recombinant peptides to detect virus infection but until relatively recently could not reliably distinguish between HTLV-I and HTLV-II infection.[11] Screening assays include enzyme-linked immunoabsorbent assay (ELISA) formats using a variety of viral antigens, and the Western immunoblot is the standard confirmatory test.[12] Recent Western blot technology utilizes recombinant synthetic peptides both to confirm positivity and to attempt to distinguish virus type[13] (Fig. 19-1). The polymerase chain reaction technique (PCR) has proven useful in epidemiologic studies for precisely confirming virus type and more recently for quantifying viral load.[14] PCR also has been useful for confirming that infection in the absence of antibody is extremely rare.[15]

Phylogenetic analyses of HTLV-I sequences from around the world have shown that this virus is genetically very highly conserved when compared with the other group of human retroviruses, the lentiviruses HIV-1 and HIV-2.[16] The closest relative of the HTLV family of viruses is found in some old world primate species but not in those from the Americas.[17]

WORLDWIDE EPIDEMIOLOGY OF HTLV-I

HTLV-I is distributed at low endemicity worldwide but has unique macro- and microepidemiologic features. Virus prevalence varies significantly by geographic region, racial and/or ethnic group, and risk-group subpopulation.[18] Geographic clustering is evident in that adjacent national populations may have markedly different prevalence rates. Microgeographic clustering is also observed within endemic regions, with adjacent regions, villages, houses, and families having disparate prevalence rates.

Asia. Geographic clustering of HTLV-I was first documented in southern Japan (Kyushu, Shikoku, and Okinawa),[19] where population prevalence levels of up to 30 percent have been recorded, but infection also was seen in villages in Honshu and in Hokkaido among the aboriginal Ainu.[20] Based on *gag* and *env* sequencing, the virus prototype from Japan is termed *cosmopolitan* because it is found in other parts of the world, including Africa and the Caribbean, but very rarely in the rest of Asia. HTLV-I seems to be largely absent in mainland China, Taiwan, Korea, and Vietnam.[18] Melanesia, however, has an unexpectedly high seroprevalence rate, particularly in Papua New Guinea,[21] where a rate of 14 percent has been recorded in certain population groups. High rates are also noted in Australian aborigines and in some areas of the Solomon Islands but not in Polynesia,[22] and these Melanesian and Micronesian isolates display the greatest sequence diversity of all HTLV subtypes, implying that they diverted with these populations many thousands of years earlier.

Caribbean Basin. This is a well-studied endemic focus of HTLV-I infection. Soon after the description of ATL in Japan, it was observed that similar cases occurred among Caribbean migrants to the United States and the United Kingdom.[23] Serosurveys have since documented significant rates of positivity in Jamaica, Trinidad and Tobago, the French Antilles, Barbados, St. Lucia, Haiti, and the Dominican Republic.[24–27] Adjacent areas of South America, including Venezuela, Guyana, and Surinam, and some areas of Central America, including Panama and Honduras, harbor significant foci of seropositivity.[28,29] Infection seems to correlate with African-derived new world populations, fueling the speculation that HTLV-I was brought to the new world via the slave trade. In Trinidad, where the population is equally divided between Afro-Caribbeans and persons of Indo-Asian descent, and despite these two groups sharing a common environment for over 100 years, HTLV-I positivity is confined almost exclusively to persons of African descent.[25,30] These data support the concept of an African origin of the virus in the region. In Jamaica, a population survey provided no evidence of microgeographic clustering such as that reported in Japan.[31] A strong determinant of seropositivity seems to be socioeconomic group and may reflect host factors that serve to maintain low endemicity. Level of sexual exposure is also important, and men and women attending sexually transmitted disease (STD) clinics have markedly elevated rates of seropositivity in both Jamaica and Trinidad.[32,33] Among blood donors, usually healthy young adults, rates are generally lower than in other population groups.[34]

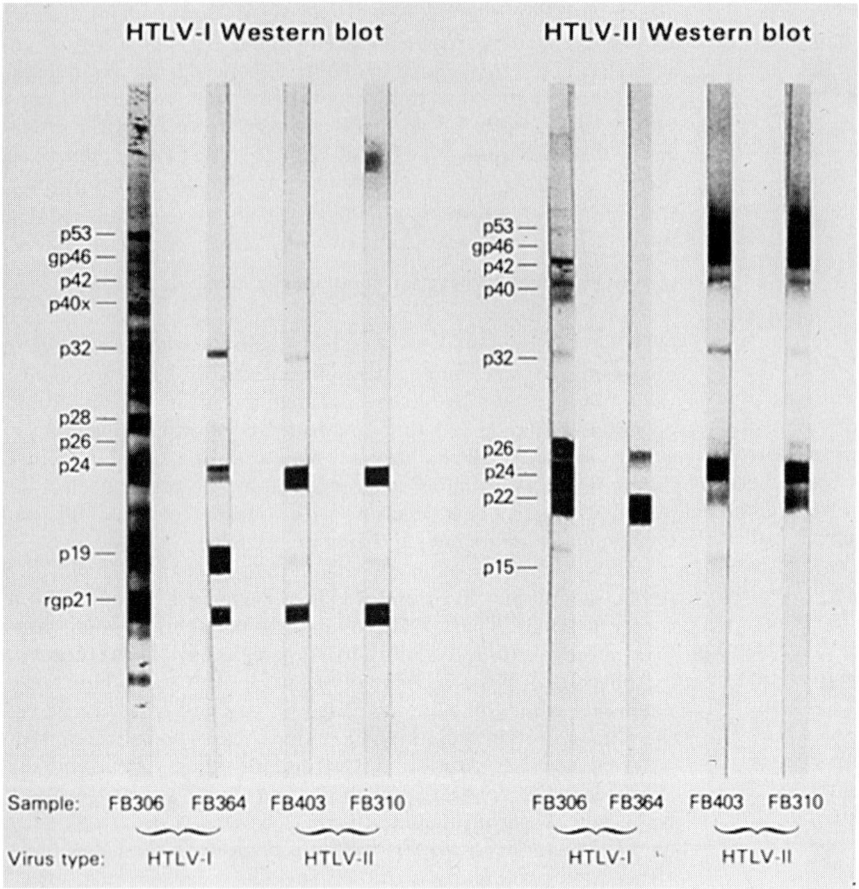

Fig. 19-1. Pattern of Western blot reactivity in HTLV-I and HTLV-II infections.

South and Central America. Endemic foci of HTLV-I have been observed in South and Central America, but the distribution of HTLV-I infection is markedly varied and detection is confounded by the coincidence of HTLV-II infection in many of the same regions. Along the Pacific Coast of Colombia, in an area with an unusually high rate of HTLV-I-associated neurologic disease, very high rates of HTLV-I seropositivity have been reported among persons largely of African descent.[35] Altitude is also a significant correlate of HTLV-I seropositivity in Colombia. Controlling for race, HTLV-I rates are higher in persons residing at low altitude; controlling for altitude, rates are higher in persons of African compared with Mestizo background. Other areas in South America with documented foci of HTLV-I include Brazil, Peru, and Chile.[36] The majority of seropositives are persons of African descent, except in Brazil, but some isolated Amerindian groups usually linked to endemic HTLV-II infection have been found to harbor HTLV-I. One study of Amerindians residing in southern coastal Chile identified foci of HTLV-I, and the authors speculated on the possibility of a trans-Pacific route of passage, where the virus might have been brought from those areas of Japan or Asia where HTLV-I is endemic.[37]

North America. HTLV-I infection has been documented in African-Americans, in certain Alaskan population groups, and in migrants from endemic areas. Blood donors in the United States have rates of HTLV-I/II infection of 0.43 per 1000, with approximately half the positives carrying HTLV-II.[38] Among HTLV-I-positive cases, the demographic profile of the positive donor includes direct or indirect links to known viral endemic areas.[39] Various population surveys including military populations show a similar pattern, with persons of ancestry in a viral endemic region having elevated rates of seropositivity.[40] Infection acquired early in life in a viral-endemic area can be carried to a nonendemic area and even passaged to the next generation. Examples of such migrant groups include persons born in Okinawa who migrated to Hawaii and individuals from the Caribbean who came to the United States.[41] Another source of seropositivity of persons residing in the United States is persons who have experienced sexual exposures as part of travel in viral-endemic areas or through marriage to a seropositive person from a viral-endemic area.[42]

Africa. Numerous countries, including Ivory Coast, Ghana, Nigeria, Zaire, Kenya, Tanzania, and South Africa, have elevated rates of HTLV-I seropositivity, but significant artifacts resulting from false-positive results on screening and confirmatory assays have made it difficult to precisely quantify rates.[43–45] Population-based surveys in Africa have not been specifically designed to fully characterize the patterns of HTLV-I occurrence, so detailed epidemiologic profiles have not been developed. In Zaire, an area of microgeographic clustering of HTLV-I was detected in the northern equatorial region by surveying HTLV-I among female prostitutes from different provinces residing in the capitol, Kinshasa.[46] Reports suggest that HTLV-I-associated neurologic disease is common in this area,[47] which is now also the epicenter for the Zairean HIV-1 epidemic.

Europe, the Middle East, and the Asian Subcontinent. In Europe, most infected individuals are migrants from more endemic areas.[18] In the Middle East, a focus of HTLV-I has been detected among Iranian Jews from northeastern Iran but residing now in Israel and New York.[48] Studies in Iran demonstrate a focus of viral endemicity among persons residing in the Mashad region.[49] The high frequency of intermarriage among the Mashad people could have amplified and sustained HTLV-I in this isolated population. Surveys in southern India are largely negative for HTLV-I despite the occurrence in the area of a neurologic disease very similar to TSP/HAM with occasionally demonstrable virus infection.[50] The Seychelles in the Indian Ocean also appear to be endemic for HTLV-I, probably again reflecting migration of peoples of African descent.[51]

DEMOGRAPHIC FEATURES AND EPIDEMIC BEHAVIOR OF HTLV-I

There is a consistent age-dependent increase in HTLV-I seroprevalence in practically all geographic areas studied. For example, the age-related HTLV-I prevalence patterns in Jamaica and Okinawa share similar features, although the overall prevalence of infection in Okinawa is higher than in Jamaica (Fig. 19-2). Characteristically, the rise in both male and female rates begins in adolescence, but prevalence levels off in males around age 40, while it continues to rise in females.[24,52] This may be explained by the reactivation of immunologically silent infections over time, continued exposure throughout life primarily via sexual exposure but with more efficient male-to-female transmission, and a cohort effect where declining rates of infection in younger birth cohorts give the appearance of rising rates in older birth cohorts.[53]

There is considerable evidence to document that new infections are taking place, in particular among sexually active populations such as attendees of STD clinics.[54] For example, the rates of seroconversion in STD clinics in Jamaica and Trinidad could potentially account for the age-dependent pattern and the female-to-male rate differential. In Japan, there is evidence to support a cohort effect due to a decline in infection rates in younger birth cohorts contributing to the apparent age-dependent rise.[55] Possible explanations for this declining rate include changes in standard of living leading to improved nutrition, changes in breast-feeding patterns, elimination of environmental cofactors that facilitate transmission, and declines in other sexually transmitted diseases that amplify transmission. Among migrants from Japan to Hawaii, HTLV-I rates were highest in those born in Okinawa, lower in first-generation Hawaiian born, and lowest in the grandchildren of migrants.[56] The likely factors explaining this pattern of declining prevalence include changes in environmental cofactors for transmission and improvement in socioeconomic status. Nevertheless, there is evidence in Japan of both more common male-to-female and less common female-to-male transmission in older HTLV-I-discordant couples, which may explain the continued rise in female prevalence after that in males plateaus.[57]

Table 19-1. Modes of Transmission of HTLV-I

Mode of transmission	Cofactor	Importance
Sexual		
Male to female	Inflammatory STD	++
	Elevated antibody titer	+
	Multiple sex partners	++
Female to male	Ulcerative STD	+
Male to male	Multiple sex partners	++
Parenteral		
Blood transfusion	Cellular components	++++
	Immunosuppressive therapy	++
Injection drug use	Sharing of "works"	+++
Mother-to-infant		
Transplacental	None known	
Breast feeding	Duration of breastfeeding	+++
	Maternal antibody titer	++

MODES OF HTLV-I TRANSMISSION

Table 19-1 lists the routes, modes, and cofactors associated with HTLV-I transmission, with a score of relative efficacy.

SEXUAL TRANSMISSION

Sexual transmission of HTLV-I occurs among married couples and sexually active population groups such as commercial sex workers and homosexual/bisexual men. Male-to-female, female-to-male, and male-to-male transmission has been documented. Cross-sectional surveys of heterosexual couples show an excess of couples concordant for HTLV-I infection; among discordant couples, the female partner is more likely than the male to be positive, except among younger couples, where the low prevalence in hus-

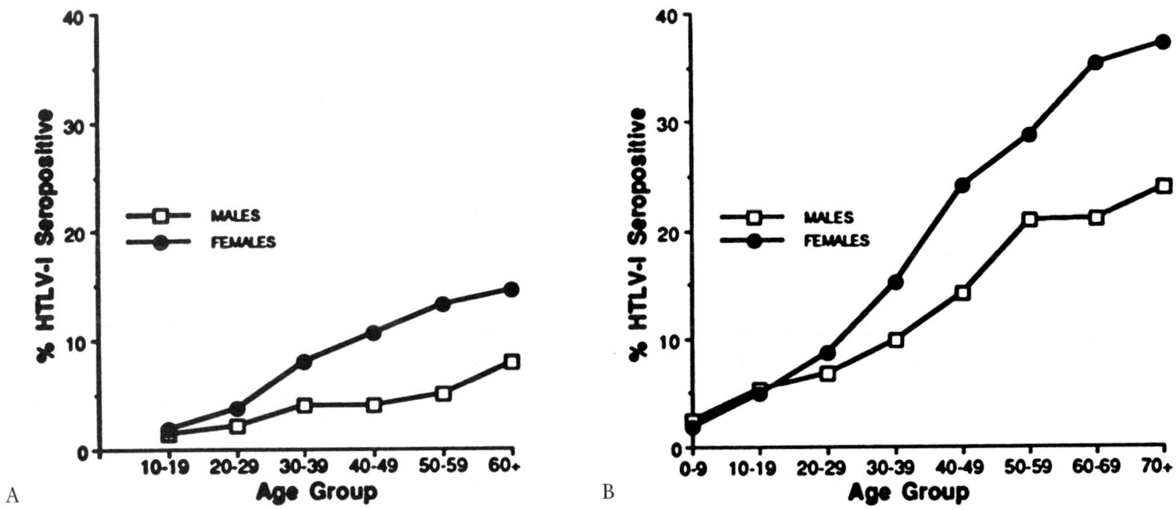

Fig. 19-2. Prevalence of HTLV-I antibodies by age in (*A*) Jamaica and (*B*) Japan.

bands approaches that in wives.[18] The difference in HTLV-I prevalence between men and women probably reflects the low efficiency of female-to-male transmission, which requires long-standing sexual exposure, except in the presence of cofactors that interrupt normal mucosal barriers.

Even in the absence of obvious cofactors, female-to-male transmission does occur, as seen in a group of Marine Corps veterans married to seropositive Okinawan women[42] and in a community-based cohort study conducted in the prefecture of Miyazaki, southwestern Japan, in which over 100 discordant married couples have been followed.[57] Seroconversions have been documented in both husbands and wives, with transmission taking place up to the seventh decade. Of 33 seronegative wives married to carrier husbands, 9 (27.3 percent) converted to antibody-positive status, whereas 4 (6.7 percent) of 60 initially seronegative husbands of carrier wives seroconverted. Based on these data, the incidence rate of male-to-female transmission (4.9 per 100 person-years) is 4.2 times higher than that of female-to-male transmission (1.2 per 100 person-years), with the 95 percent confidence interval around this estimate of relative risk being 1.3 to 13.5. In contrast, among 359 concordantly negative couples from the same community, the seroincidence was 0.048 per 100 person-years for females and zero for males over the same period.[58] The late seroconversion of a discordant partner with a long-standing sexual relationship may be explained in part by increases in virus titer, a marker of virus load that may occur as the couple ages. This relationship has been more directly documented using quantitative PCR; the presence of anti-*tax* antibody is also associated with heightened transmission in this setting.[59]

Markers of enhanced sexual activity are linked to HTLV-I transmission. A cross-sectional study conducted in 1989 in Fukuoka Prefecture, Japan, documented a significantly higher HTLV-I prevalence of 5.1 percent in female prostitutes, 5.7 percent in female STD patients, and 2.8 percent in male STD patients when compared with age- and sex-matched blood donor controls.[54] Among those with STDs, female patients with syphilis and gonorrhea and male patients with nongonococcal urethritis had a significantly higher HTLV-I prevalence than controls. Among attenders of an STD clinic in Jamaica, seropositivity in females but not males was associated with a large number of sexual partners.[32] In a group of homosexual men in Trinidad, a higher number of lifetime partners and longer duration of sexual activity were associated with HTLV-I seropositivity.[60] The coincidence of other STDs involving an ulcerative genital lesion appears to amplify the risk of horizontal HTLV-I transmission. In the Jamaican study, current diagnosis of syphilis, among other factors, was associated with HTLV-I positivity in the STD clinic population.[61] A study of Haitian women infected with HTLV-I ($n = 45$) and HIV-1 ($n = 95$) found a significantly higher coincidence of antibodies to herpes simplex virus type 2 (HSV-2) in both groups, consistent with the notion that recurrent disruptions of the mucous membranes caused by HSV-2 infections facilitate transmission of both viruses.[62]

Studies in Latin America have documented the role of sexual transmission of HTLV-I in commercial sex workers. In Peru, 467 prostitutes from the capital, Lima, had an overall prevalence of 21.8 percent compared with 3.1 percent overall among 510 antenatal clinic patients.[63] The estimate of annual HTLV-I incidence in this prostitute population over a 3-year period was 1.6 percent.[64] Further study of 400 sex workers in Lima showed that the prevalence of HTLV-I increased almost linearly with the duration of prostitution, reaching 16 percent in those with over 6 years' experience. In a multivariate analysis, duration of prostitution, lack of consistent condom use, and past infection with *Chlamydia trachomatis* were independent risk factors for HTLV-I infection.[65] In Paraguay, HTLV-I prevalence was 2.2 percent in 178 city prostitutes and 3.4 percent among 117 gay/bisexual men.[66] However, in Chile, where the population prevalence appears to be much lower, serologic testing of 502 prostitutes from Santiago revealed a 0.8 percent prevalence, similar to other population-based groups.[67] Additional evidence is available from other parts of the world to support enhanced HTLV-I transmission in population groups with greater sexual exposure.[68,69]

PARENTERAL TRANSMISSION

Transfusion involving the cellular components of blood is associated with transmission of HTLV-I; approximately 50 percent of recipients of 1 unit of HTLV-I-positive blood seroconvert.[70] Transfusion of plasma or cryoprecipitate is not associated with transmission, and whole blood or packed cells are less likely to be infectious if stored for prolonged periods (greater than 1 week), presumably because of the loss of white blood cell viability.[71] Elevated antibody titer (a surrogate for virus load) is not associated with increased risk for transmission.[72] Recipients on immunosuppressive drugs such as corticosteroids are more susceptible to infection, possibly due to a blunting of the immune response to HTLV-I in the recipient. Blood bank screening was implemented in the United States following reports of HTLV-associated myelopathy in transfusion recipients. U.S. donors with a positive Western blot have a 50 percent HTLV-I and a 50 percent HTLV-II distribution; risk factors for seropositivity include intravenous drug abuse, birthplace in a viral-endemic area, and sexual contact with a person with this profile.[73,74] Japanese studies clearly demonstrate that blood donor screening effectively prevents transfusion transmission.[75] Intravenous drug use is also a significant method for the spread of HTLV-I, but most transmission associated with intravenous drug use involves HTLV-II.[76]

MOTHER-INFANT TRANSMISSION

Mother-to-child transmission may account for up to 15 percent of all cumulative infections.[77] HTLV-I has been detected in breast milk and transmitted via breast milk in nonhuman primate and rabbit animal models.[78] Intervention trials done in Japan, where bottle feeding is widespread, showed that breast feeding accounts for most perinatal transmission.[79] Bottle-fed infants experienced a 1 to 2 percent seroconversion rate, whereas breast-fed infants experienced a 20 percent seroconversion rate. In Jamaica a similar rate of transmission also was seen.[80] Serial Western blots of seroconverting infants of HTLV-I-positive mothers show a pattern in which maternal antibodies are present in the first few months, but all bands usually disappear at about 6 months of age and new bands subsequently appear in association with native infection. For some infants, breast feeding had ceased several months prior to seroconversion, but latent HTLV-I viral infection was not detected by PCR of peripheral blood. Viral load measured by maternal antibody titer and viral antigen level on short-term culture is a significant predictor of transmission; presence of antibody to the tax antigen is also associated with transmission. Elevated HTLV-I transmission was reported in association with high-titer antibodies to certain envelope epitopes; this suggests that enhancing antibodies might contribute to transmission.[81] Approximately 2 to 5 percent of lifetime HTLV-I infections are linked to maternal-to-child transmission, and this early life infection may disproportionately contribute to the subsequent risk for adult T-cell leukemia.[82]

HTLV-I DISEASE ASSOCIATIONS

Since the first description of the link between adult T-cell leukemia/lymphoma (ATL) and HTLV-I, the list of possible associations has expanded greatly (Table 19-2). HTLV-I-associated diseases may be categorized as those resulting from direct integration of the virus in the transformed cell: the ATL model, and those where an indirect immunologic mechanism is postulated, the TSP/HAM model.

ADULT T-CELL LEUKEMIA/LYMPHOMA (ATL)

This clinical entity was first reported in Japan with a spectrum of clinical signs and symptoms including peripheral blood involvement by characteristic polylobated mononuclear cells called *flower* cells, hypercalcemia, lytic bone lesions, and cutaneous, nodal, and extranodal involvement with lymphoma exhibiting considerable pleomorphism.[2,83] HTLV-I originally was isolated in the United States from an African-American male patient presenting with features of classic ATL but originally diagnosed as having an aggressive variant of mycosis fungoides.[1] It now seems clear that in HTLV-I-endemic populations, skin involvement in ATL can mimic mycoses fungoides at early presentation, with a classic histopathologic picture including Pautrier microabscesses, but cases usually transform to prototypic ATL later in their clinical course.

Subsequent studies in Japan and the Caribbean and among migrants from these areas unequivocally linked HTLV-I to ATL.[23,84] Such evidence includes the concordance of geographic distribution of HTLV-I infection and ATL cases. ATL cases have been reported in Africa, North and South America, the Caribbean region, the Middle East, Taiwan, and Japan and in Australian aborigines.[85,86] ATL occurs with equal frequency in men and women despite the disproportionate occurrence of HTLV-I infection in women.[87–90] There is evidence that this gender-specific discordance between ATL incidence and HTLV-I prevalence could be explained by the fact that prenatal or perinatal exposure might carry the greatest risk for ATL occurrence.[88] For unexplained reasons, the peak incidence of ATL is in the fifties in Japan and a decade younger in the West Indies.[89] In persons under the age of 50, HTLV-I is the chief cause of lymphoma in viral-endemic areas.[90] The attributable risk of HTLV-I as a cause of leukemia/lymphoma is highest in the forties to fifties and thereafter declines. In Jamaica and Trinidad, over 70 percent of all lymphoid malignancies are attributable to HTLV-I exposure.[82,90] In some instances ATL occurs in the pediatric age group, with patients as young as 5 and 6 years of age reported, but these instances are extremely rare.[91]

The lifetime risk of developing ATL among healthy carriers is approximately 1 to 5 percent, but this figure might underestimate the attack rate for those infected early in life. In comprehensive studies conducted over an 8-year period in Jamaica and Trinidad, all cases of non-Hodgkin's lymphoma (NHL) in the population were ascertained and blood collected for HTLV-I determination. The world age-standardized NHL incidence rate in Jamaica was 1.9 ± 0.2 per 100,000 person-years and in Trinidad was 2.9 ± 0.4 per 100,000 person-years. Overall, the incidence of NHL increased with age and was higher in males than in females. In the HTLV-I-infected population, NHL incidence was inversely related to age, and age-specific rates were higher in males than in females. However, NHL incidence in those estimated to have acquired HTLV-I infection in childhood showed no sex difference, and 1 in 1300 such carriers (95 percent confidence interval 1 in 1100 to 1 in 1600) per annum were estimated to be at such risk (Fig. 19-3). For T-cell NHL, as proxy for adult T-cell lymphoma/leukemia (ATL), incidence was highest in those who were infected with HTLV-I early in life (perinatally or via breast milk), with a high sustained risk from early adulthood in both sexes. Thus, while overall NHL incidence rates reveal that HTLV-I endemicity does not impose an exaggerated lymphoma burden on these populations, the risk for lymphoma among carriers who acquire infection early in life is dramatic and is consistent with the hypothesis that virus exposure early in life is critical for lymphomagenesis.[82]

Table 19-2. HTLV-Associated Diseases

Age	Clinical entity	Strength of association
Children	Infective dermatitis	++++
	Persistent lymphadenopathy	+
	Infant death	?
Adults	Adult T-cell leukemia/lymphoma	++++
	Myelopathy	++++
	Infective dermatitis	++
	Uveitis	+++
	Arthritis	++
	Infiltrative pneumonitis	++
	Invasive cervical cancer	+
	Small cell carcinoma of lung	?

ATL subtypes

Four major categories of ATL have been characterized: acute or prototypical type, lymphoma type, chronic type, and smoldering type.[83] A feature of the natural history of this disease is for the more benign types to evolve into the more aggressive types. Acute ATL is an aggressive mature T-cell lymphoma with frequent leukemic involvement (80 percent of cases) with characteristic pleomorphic polylobulated cells, hypercalcemia (50 percent of cases), and cutaneous involvement (40 percent of cases ranging from maculo-papular rashes to tumorous lesions). Organ and extranodal involvement is common. Lymphoma-type ATL shares many features with acute ATL, but it is distinguishable by the absence of peripheral leukemic involvement. Chronic ATL presents as T-cell chronic lymphocytic leukemia, and a substantial proportion of patients have cutaneous involvement; nodal or extranodal in-

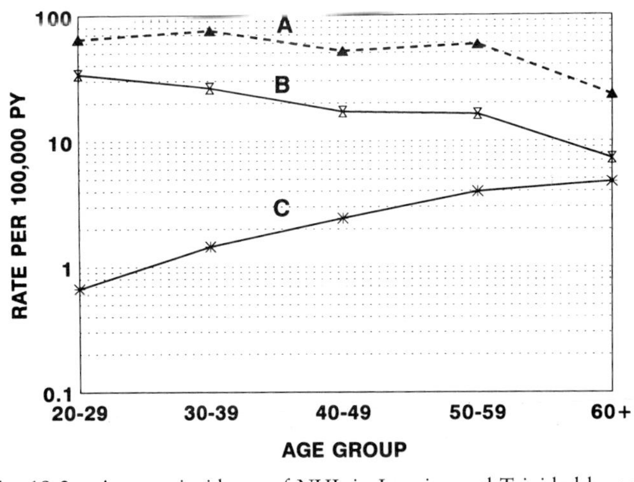

Fig. 19-3. Average incidence of NHL in Jamaica and Trinidad by age. Line A: T-cell NHL incidence in HTLV-I carriers infected during childhood. Line B: T-cell NHL incidence in total HTLV-I infected population. Line C: Overall NHL incidence in HTLV-I uninfected population.

volvement is rare, and hypercalcemia is absent. Smoldering ATL resembles mycosis fungoides/Sézary syndrome, with cutaneous involvement presenting as erythema or as infiltrative plaques or tumors, and Pautrier's microabscesses may be observed. The distribution of subtypes appears to vary by geography.[92]

In the vast majority of cases, HTLV-I antibodies are present in ATL patients; when studied, the HTLV-I virus is monoclonally integrated in the individual, but integration sites vary markedly between individuals.[93] In some cases of ATL, HTLV-I antibody is absent; in rare cases, defective virus is integrated in the tumor, with viral genes critical for transformation, notably *tax,* detectable by molecular techniques.[94]

The prognosis of patients with acute ATL and lymphoma-type ATL is poor; most die within 6 months of diagnosis.[95] Death usually results from rapid growth of tumor cells, hypercalcemia, bacterial sepsis, opportunistic infections such as *Pneumocystis carinii* pneumonia, and other infectious complications seen in patients with lymphoma-associated immunodeficiency. In Jamaica and Trinidad, a major cause of death is bacterial sepsis.[88] ATL has proven refractory to most conventional and experimental chemotherapeutic regimens. Anti-interleukin 2-receptor antibody linked with various toxins shows some promise in preliminary trials, as do combinations of antiretrovirals and interferon.[96] Recent evidence suggests that a promising approach to therapy lies in multiple-agent approaches combining antiretrovirals such as azidothymidine with cytokines such as gamma interferon.[97]

NEUROLOGIC AND OTHER DISEASES

A neurologic syndrome called *tropical spastic paraparesis/HTLV-I-associated myelopathy* (TSP/HAM) is etiologically linked to HTLV-I.[3] The syndrome results from demyelination of the long motor neurons of the spinal cord causing a variety of symptoms, sometimes acutely, including stiff gait, spasticity, lower extremity weakness, back pain, urinary incontinence and impotence, and rarely, ataxia. Lesions of the central nervous system are detected in some cases. Transfusion transmission of HTLV-I has been associated with dramatic examples of acutely progressive neurologic symptoms; in Japan, blood transfusion is a significant risk factor for TSP/HAM.[98] It is estimated that disease incidence is approximately half that of ATL.[99] Females are approximately two times more likely to develop TSP/HAM; in Jamaican cases, sexual transmission is a documented risk factor.[100] The majority of adult cases occur in the 30- to 50-year age group, but pediatric cases as young as 3 years of age do occur. These patterns suggest that the latency period for TSP/HAM is shorter than for ATL and that both early-life and adult exposure cause disease. Increased susceptibility to disease is observed in some patients with certain HLA profiles; carriers with this pattern have a heightened in vitro proliferative profile compared with controls. This suggests that an abnormal response to viral infection may predispose to this syndrome.[101] These data are consistent with the hypothesis of an indirect mechanism of pathogenesis whereby HTLV-I induces an autoimmune process through molecular mimicry between a viral and cellular antigen and/or through indirect cytopathic effects of infiltrating virus-negative CD8 cells in the central nervous system milieu.[102] The finding that the oligoclonal immunoglobulin bands in the cerebrospinal fluid of TSP/HAM patients react to HTLV-I antigens supports this hypothesis.[103] Viral antibody titers in TSP/HAM patients are markedly elevated, indicating the central role of the virus and loss of immunologic control in disease pathogenesis.[104] There is appreciable response to treatment with corticosteroids in some usually rapidly progressive cases in Japan, favoring an autoimmune etiology.

Most of the other conditions listed in Table 19-2 associated with HTLV-I also appear to involve an autoimmune/inflammatory pathogenesis. These include polymyositis of skeletal muscle,[105] large joint polyarthropathy among elderly patients,[106] infiltrative pneumonitis,[107] and uveitis.[108] In viral-endemic areas, 30 to 40 percent of idiopathic uveitis may be caused by the virus.[109] Other evidence for an immunologic abnormality includes parasitic infestations such as *Strongyloides stercoralis* that are refractory to treatment[110] and skin test anergy.[111] Depressed hemoglobin and lymphopenia have been reported in healthy HTLV-I carriers.[112] Infective dermatitis is an HTLV-I-associated syndrome in children; it also appears to involve HTLV-I-associated immunodeficiency that is manifested by refractory generalized eczema and saprophytic staphylococcal and streptococcal bacterial infections. In most cases, onset occurs in early life with persistence into adulthood[113]; some cases go on to develop ATL and TSP/HAM.[114]

IMPACT OF HTLV-I INFECTION ON OTHER INFECTIOUS DISEASES

HTLV-I infection may cause subclinical and clinical immunosuppressive effects that mediate increased susceptibility to certain bacterial and parasitic diseases, including *S. stercoralis*[110] and *Mycobacterium tuberculosis.*[115] In Japan, AIDS-like illnesses have been reported in some HTLV-I carriers.[116] Coinfection with HTLV-I and HIV-1 has been thought to result in acceleration of clinical immunosuppression and shortened survival in cross-sectional studies.[117] However, published data are all cross sectional and therefore subject to problems of interpretation. Thus HTLV-I infection in these patients may have been a marker of greater sexual exposure through common modes of transmission, or HTLV-I may have facilitated HIV-1 transmission in some way.[118] Prospective studies are lacking, largely because of the difficulty in finding prospective cohorts with known dates of infection, although there is additional evidence for clinical effects of coinfection, mainly with HTLV-II, in intravenous drug users in the United States.[119] Conversely, more recent studies of concomitant HTLV-I and HIV-1 infection demonstrate significant effects on the interpretation of immunophenotyping test results.[120] Coinfection alters the relationship between CD4 cell count and HIV disease stage, and such patients may have CD4 levels far above that normally associated with their degree of immune suppression, since these CD4 cells do not appear to mediate normal function.[121]

CONTROL OF HTLV-I INFECTIONS

PREVENTION

Guidelines are available from the Centers for Disease Control and Prevention for counseling of HTLV-positive persons. These recommendations include measures to limit sexual and maternal-infant transmission of the virus. For seropositive mothers, it is recommended that breast feeding be limited to the first 3 to 6 months of life. Condoms should be used to prevent viral transmission during sexual intercourse. While the efficacy of condoms for the prevention of HTLV-I and HTLV-II infection has not been proven, extension from studies of HIV-1 suggests that sexual transmission will be eliminated if condoms are used properly and consistently. The routine screening of blood donations for HTLV antibodies is now standard practice in the United States and Japan. If a unit is identified as positive, it is recommended that the blood be discarded.

TREATMENT

Diseases caused by HTLV-I infection are difficult to treat and consequently have a poor prognosis. ATL has proven refractory to most conventional and/or experimental chemotherapeutic regimens. Most patients with prototypical ATL die within 6 months of diagnosis, despite multiple-agent chemotherapy. Experimental approaches using monoclonal antibodies to the interleukin 2 receptor linked with cell toxins selectively targeted to the leukemic cells show some promise for the treatment of ATL. Preliminary analysis of phase I/II clinical trials using a combination of antiretrovirals and/or interferon have demonstrated remission in a small number of cases.

In inflammatory HTLV-I-associated diseases such as HAM/TSP and uveitis, treatment with corticosteroids benefits some patients, particularly those with rapidly progressive disease. Treatment of patients suffering from HAM/TSP with danazol, an androgenic steroid, has resulted in improvement in urinary and fecal incontinence but not in the underlying neurologic deficit. There are preliminary reports of clinical successes using high-dose vitamin C in these patients.

EPIDEMIOLOGY AND DISEASE ASSOCIATIONS OF HTLV-II

Much less is known about HTLV-II largely because until recently it was very difficult to distinguish this virus from HTLV-I by conventional serologic techniques. However, in investigations of collections of sera dating back to the 1960s, virtually every injection drug user population tested in the United States has shown evidence of HTLV-II infection. Prevalence rates range from 10 to 15 percent and higher. Amerindians residing in North, Central, and South America have varying rates of positivity for HTLV-II. Pockets of relatively high prevalence are encountered among the Seminoles in south Florida and the Pueblo and Navajo in New Mexico but not among various tribal groups in Alaska. In Central America, the Guaymi Indians, residing in northeastern Panama near the Costa Rican border, have high seroprevalence rates, but this is not the case for the Guaymi living in southwest Panama. There is also a characteristic age-dependent increase in the seroprevalence of HTLV-II antibodies. The most recent data from studies of endemic populations of Amerindians show age-related seroprevalence patterns similar to those of HTLV-I but without gender differences at any age. Unusually high rates of seropositivity in older groups of injecting drug abusers in the United States have been linked to the sharing of injection equipment, increasing the possibility of a "cohort effect" resulting from the use of different injection techniques. There is no evidence of a virus-positive/antibody-negative state.

Sexual transmission of HTLV-II has been difficult to study because of the high frequency of injection drug use among the study populations. In virtually every study of female prostitutes, injection drug use was the major risk factor for seropositivity. However, continuing studies of isolated Amerindians with no history of injecting drugs should shed further light on the epidemiology of this virus. In fact, a recent study of the Guaymi Indians in Panama has provided evidence for sexual transmission of HTLV-II consistent with patterns observed in cross-sectional studies of HTLV-I. However, the factors associated with transmission are not clearly defined.

The disease associations of HTLV-II also remain to be defined, but there are suggestive case reports of degenerative neurologic, hematologic, and infectious diseases. These are currently under investigation in a number of cohorts.

References

1 Poiesz BJ et al: Detection and isolation of type C retrovirus particles from fresh and cultured lymphocytes of a patient with cutaneous T-cell lymphoma. *Proc Natl Acad Sci USA* 77:7415–7419, 1980.

2 Takatsuki K et al: Adult T cell leukemia in Japan, in *Topics in Hematology,* S Seno et al (eds). Amsterdam, Excerpta Medica, 1976, pp 73–78.

3 Ijichi S Osame M: Human T-lymphotropic virus type I (HTLV-I)-associated myelopathy/tropical spastic paraparesis (HAM/TSP): Recent perspectives. *Intern Med* 34:713–721, 1995.

4 LaGrenade L et al: Infective dermatitis of Jamaican children: A marker for HTLV-I infection. *Lancet* 336:1345–1346, 1990.

5 Kalyanaraman VS et al: A new subtype of human T-cell leukemia virus (HTLV-II) associated with a T-cell variant of hairy cell leukemia. *Science* 218:571–573, 1982.

6 Rosenblatt JD et al: Relationship between human T-cell leukemia virus-II and atypical hairy cell leukemia: Serologic study of hairy cell leukemia patients. *Leukemia* 1:397–401, 1987.

7 Blattner WA: HTLV-I and HTLV-II, in *Cecil's Textbook of Medicine.* Baltimore, Williams & Wilkins, 1994.

8 Varmus H: Retroviruses. *Science* 240:1427–1435, 1988.

9 Igichi S et al: In vivo cellular tropism of human T-cell leukemia virus type II (HTLV II). *J Exp Med* 176:293–296, 1992.

10 Wong-Staal F, Gallo RC: Human T-lymphotropic retroviruses. *Nature* 317:395–403, 1985.

11 Cossen C et al: Comparison of six commercial human T-cell lymphotropic virus type I (HTLV-I) enzyme immunoassay kits for detection of antibody to HTLV-I and -II. *J Clin Microbiol* 30:724–725, 1993.

12 Lillehoj EP et al: Development and evaluation of a human T-cell leukemia virus type-I serologic confirmatory assay incorporating a recombinant envelope polypeptide. *J Clin Microbiol* 28:2653–2658, 1990.

13 Blomberg J et al: Type- and group-specific continuous antigenic determinants of HTLV: Use of synthetic peptides for serotyping of HTLV-I and -II infection. *J Acquir Immune Defic Syndr* 5:294–302, 1992.

14 Heneine W et al: Sensitive and specific polymerase chain reaction assays for diagnosis of human T-cell lymphotropic virus type I (HTLV-I) and HTLV-II infections in HTLV-I/II-seropositive individuals. *J Clin Microbiol* 30:1605–1607, 1992.

15 Pate EJ et al: Lack of viral latency of human T-lymphotropic virus type-I (HTLV-I). *N Engl J Med* 325:284, 1991.

16 Sherman MP et al: Evolutionary insights on the origin of human T-cell lymphoma/leukemia virus type I (HTLV-I) derived from sequence analysis of a new HTLV-I variant from Papua New Guinea. *J Virol* 66:2556–2563, 1992.

17 Homma T et al: Lymphoma in macaques: Association with virus of the human T-lymphotropic family. *Science* 225:716–718, 1984.

18 Blattner W: Retroviruses, in *Viral Infections of Humans: Epidemiology and Control,* AS Evans (ed). New York, Plenum Medical, 1989, pp 545–592.

19 Kajiyama W et al: Sero-epidemiologic study of antibody to adult T-cell leukemia virus in Okinawa, Japan. *Am J Epidemiol* 123:41–47, 1986.

20 Hinuma Y: Sero-epidemiology of adult T-cell leukemia virus (HTLV-I/ATLV): Origin of virus carriers in Japan. *AIDS Res* 2(suppl 1):S17-S22, 1986.

21 Yanagihara R et al: Human T lymphotropic virus type I infection in Papua New Guinea: High prevalence among the Hagahai confirmed by Western blot analysis. *J Infect Dis* 162:649–654, 1990.

22 Yanagihara R et al: Human T-lymphotropic virus type I infection in the Solomon Islands. *Am J Trop Med Hyg* 44:122–130, 1991.

23 Blattner W et al: The human type-C retrovirus, HTLV, in blacks from the Caribbean region, and relationship to adult T-cell leukemia/lymphoma. *Int J Cancer* 30:257–264, 1982.

24 Murphy EL et al: Human T-lymphotropic virus type I (HTLV-I) seroprevalence in Jamaica: I. Demographic determinants. *Am J Epidemiol* 133:1114–1124, 1991.

25 Blattner W et al: A study of HTLV-I and its associated risk factors in Trinidad and Tobago. *J Acquir Immune Defic Syndr* 3:1102–1108, 1990.

26 Riedel DA et al: A historical study of human T lymphotropic virus type I transmission in Barbados. *J Infect Dis* 159:603–609, 1989.

27 Bartholomew C et al: Racial and other characteristics of human T cell leukemia/lymphoma (HTLV-I) and AIDS (HTLV-III) in Trinidad. *Br Med J* 290:1243–1246, 1985.

28 Merino F et al: Natural antibodies to human T-cell leukemia/lymphoma virus in healthy Venezuelan populations. *Int J Cancer* 34: 501–506, 1984.

29 Reeves WC et al: Sero-epidemiology of human T-cell lymphotropic virus type-I in the Republic of Panama. *Am J Trop Med Hyg* 42:374–379, 1990.

30 Miller GJ et al: Ethnic composition, age and sex, together with location and standard of housing as determinants of HTLV-I infection in an urban Trinidian community. *Int J Cancer* 38:801–808, 1986.

31 Maloney EM et al: Human T-lymphotropic virus type I (HTLV-I) seroprevalence in Jamaica: II. Geographic and ecologic determinants. *Am J Epidemiol* 133:1125–1134, 1991.

32 Murphy EL et al: Sexual transmission of human T-lymphotropic virus type I (HTLV-I). *Ann Intern Med* 111:555–560, 1989.

33 Cleghorn FR et al: HIV-1 prevalence and risk factors among STD clinic attenders in Trinidad. *AIDS* 9:387–395, 1995.

34 Manns A et al: A prospective study of transmission by transfusion of HTLV-I and risk factors associated with seroconversion. *Int J Cancer* 51:886–891, 1992.

35 Maloney EM et al: A survey of the human T-cell lymphotropic virus type I (HTLV-I) in southwestern Colombia. *Int J Cancer* 44:419–423, 1989.

36 Cortes E et al: HIV-1, HIV-2, and HTLV-I infection in high-risk groups in Brazil. *N Engl J Med* 320:953–958, 1990.

37 Cartier L et al: Southernmost carriers of HTLV-I/II in the world. *Jpn J Cancer Res* 84:1–3, 1993.

38 Williams AE et al: Seroprevalence and epidemiological correlates of HTLV-I infection in U.S. blood donors. *Science* 240:643–646, 1988.

39 Lee HH et al: Relative prevalence and risk factors of HTLV-I and HTLV-II infection in U.S. blood donors. *Lancet* 337:1435–1439, 1991.

40 Blayney DW et al: The human T-cell leukemia/lymphoma virus (HTLV) in the southeastern United States. *JAMA* 250:1048–1052, 1983.

41 Blattner W et al: Modes of transmission and evidence for viral latency from studies of HTLV-I in Japanese migrant populations in Hawaii. *Proc Natl Acad Sci USA* 83:4895–4898, 1986.

42 Brodine SK et al: HTLV-I among U.S. marines stationed in a hyperendemic area: Evidence for female-to-male sexual transmission. *J Acquir Immune Defic Syndr* 5:158–162, 1992.

43 Delaporte E et al: Epidemiology of HTLV-I in Gabon (Western Equatorial Africa). *Int J Cancer* 42:687–689, 1988.

44 Lillo F et al: Detection of HTLV-I and not HTLV-II infection in Guinea Bissau (West Africa). *J Acquir Immune Defic Syndr* 4:541–542, 1991.

45 Madeleine MM et al: HTLV-I and HTLV-II worldwide distribution: Re-analysis of 4832 immunoblot results. *Int J Cancer* 54:255–260, 1993.

46 Wiktor SZ et al: Human T-cell lymphotropic virus type I (HTLV-I) among female prostitutes in Kinshasa, Zaire. *J Infect Dis* 161:1073–1077, 1990.

47 Kayembe K et al: A cluster of HTLV-I associated tropical spastic paraparesis in Equateur (Zaire): Ethnic and familial distribution. *J Neurol Neurosurg Psychiatry* 53:4-10, 1990.

48 Meytes D et al: Serological and molecular survey for HTLV-I infection in a high-risk Middle Eastern group. *Lancet* 336:1533–1535, 1990.

49 Nerurkar VR et al: Human T-cell lymphotropic virus type I in Iranian-born Mashhadi Jews: Genetic and phylogenetic evidence for common source of infection. *J Med Virol* 45:361–366, 1995.

50 Richardson JH et al: HTLV-I and neurological disease in south India. *Lancet* 1:1079–1080, 1989.

51 Lavanchy D et al: High seroprevalence of HTLV-I in the Seychelles. *Lancet* 337:248–249, 1991.

52 Hinuma Y: Sero-epidemiology of adult T-cell leukemia virus (HTLV-I/ATLV): Origin of virus carriers in Japan. *AIDS Res* 2(suppl 1):S17-S22, 1986.

53 Morofuji-Hirata M et al: Prevalence of antibody to human T-cell lymphotropic virus type I in Okinawa, Japan, after an interval of 9 years. *Am J Epidemiol* 137:43–48, 1993.

54 Nakashima K et al: Sexual transmission of HTLV-I among female prostitutes and patients with sexually transmitted diseases in Fukuoka, Kyushu, Japan. *Am J Epidemiol* 141:305–311, 1995.

55 Ueda K et al: Cohort effect on HTLV-I seroprevalence in Southern Japan. *Lancet* 2:979, 1989.

56 Ho GY et al: Declining seroprevalence and transmission of HTLV-I in Japanese families who immigrated to Hawaii. *Am J Epidemiol* 134: 981–987, 1991.

57 Stuver SO et al. Heterosexual transmission of human T-cell leukemia virus type I among married couples in southwestern Japan: An initial report from the Miyazaki Cohort Study. *J Infect Dis* 167:57–65, 1993.

58 Stuver SO, Mueller N: Re: Sexual transmission of HTLV-I among female prostitutes in Fukuoka, Japan (letter). *Am J Epidemiol* 142: 1247–1248, 1995.

59 Chen YMA et al: Sexual transmission of human T-cell leukemia virus type I associated with the presence of anti-tax antibody. *Proc Natl Acad Sci USA* 88:1182–1186, 1991.

60 Bartholomew C et al: Transmission of HTLV-I and HIV among homosexual men in Trinidad. *JAMA* 257:2604–2608, 1987.

61 Figueroa JP et al: Risk factors for HTLV-I among heterosexual STD clinic attenders. *J AIDS* 9:81–88, 1995.

62 Boulos R et al: HSV-II, syphilis and HBV infection in Haitian women with HIV-1 and HTLV-I infections. *J Infect Dis* 166:418–420, 1992.

63 Wignall FS et al: Sexual transmission of human T-lymphotropic virus type I in Peruvian prostitutes. *J Med Virol* 38:44–48, 1992.

64 Hyams KC et al: Three-year incidence study of retroviral and viral hepatitis transmission in a Peruvian prostitute population. *J AIDS* 6: 1353–1357, 1993.

65 Gotuzzo E et al: HTLV-I infection among female sex workers in Peru. *J Infect Dis* 169:754–759, 1994.

66 Zoulek G et al: A sero-epidemiological survey of antibodies to HTLV-I/II in selected population groups in Paraguay. *Scand J Infect Dis* 24: 397–398, 1992.

67 Suarez M et al: Prevalence of HTLV-I antibodies and possible risk factors in Chilean prostitutes. *Rev Med Chile* 121:614–617, 1993.

68 Brabin L et al: Patterns of migration indicate sexual transmission of HTLV-I infection in non-pregnant women in Papua New Guinea. *Int J Cancer* 44:59–62, 1989.

69 Van Doornum GJJ et al: Prevalence of human T-cell lymphotropic virus antibody among heterosexuals living in Amsterdam, Netherlands. *J Med Virol* 32:183–188, 1990.

70 Okochi K et al: A retrospective study on transmission of adult T cell leukemia virus by blood transfusion: Seroconversion in recipients. *Vox Sang* 46:245–253, 1984.

71 Manns A et al: Detection of early human T-cell lymphotropic virus type I antibody patterns during seroconversion among transfusion recipients. *Blood* 77:896–905, 1991.

72 Williams AE et al: Seroprevalence and epidemiological correlates of HTLV-I infection in U.S. blood donors. *Science* 240:643–646, 1988.

73 Lee HH et al: Relative prevalence and risk factors of HTLV-I and HTLV-II infection in US blood donors. *Lancet* 337:1435–1439, 1991.

74 Sullivan MT et al: Human T-lymphotropic virus (HTLV) types I and II infection in sexual contacts and family members of blood donors

who are seropositive for HTLV type I or II. *Transfusion* 33:585–590, 1993.

75 Kamihira S et al: Transmission of human T-cell lymphotropic virus type I by blood transfusion before and after mass screening of sera from seropositive donors. *Vox Sang* 52:43–44, 1987.

76 Briggs NC et al: Seroprevalence of HTLV-II infection with or without HIV-1 coinfection, among U.S. intravenous drug users. *J Infect Dis* 172:51–58, 1995.

77 Hino S et al: Mother-to-child transmission of human T-cell leukemia virus type-I. *Jpn J Cancer Res* 76:474–480, 1985.

78 Kinoshita K et al: Oral infection of a common marmoset with human T-cell leukemia virus type-I (HTLV-I) by inoculating fresh human milk of HTLV-I carrier mothers. *Jpn J Cancer Res* 76:1147–1153, 1985.

79 Ando Y et al: Transmission of adult T-cell leukemia retrovirus (HTLV-I) from mother to child: Comparison of bottle- with breast-fed babies. *Jpn J Cancer Res* 78:322–324, 1987.

80 Hirata M et al: The effects of breastfeeding and presence of antibody to p40tax protein of human T cell lymphotropic virus type-I on mother to child transmission. *Int J Epidemiol* 21:989–994, 1992.

81 Wiktor SZ et al: Mother-to-child transmission of human T-cell lymphotropic virus type-I (HTLV-I) in Jamaica: Association with antibodies to envelope glycoprotein (GP46) epitopes. *J Acquir Immune Defic Syndr* 6:1162–1167, 1993.

82 Cleghorn FR et al: Effect of HTLV-I infection on NHL incidence. *J Natl Cancer Inst* 87:1009–1014, 1995.

83 Shimoyama M: Diagnostic criteria and classification of clinical subtypes of adult T-cell leukaemia-lymphoma. *Br J Haematol* 79:428–437, 1991.

84 Gibbs WN et al: Non-Hodgkin's lymphoma in Jamaica and its relation to adult T-cell/lymphoma. *Ann Intern Med* 106:361–368, 1987.

85 Levine PH: Refining the case definition for ATL. *Int J Cancer* 59: 491–493.

86 Blattner W: Epidemiology of HTLV-I and associated diseases, in *Human Retrovirology: HTLV,* WA Blattner (ed). New York, Raven Press, 1990, pp 251–265.

87 Tajima K, Tominaga S: Epidemiology of adult T-cell leukemia/lymphoma in Japan. *Curr Top Microbiol Immunol* 115:53–66, 1985.

88 Murphy EL et al: Modelling the risk of adult T-cell leukemia/lymphoma in persons infected with human T-lymphotropic virus type I. *Int J Cancer* 43:250–252, 1989.

89 Gibbs WN et al: Non-Hodgkin's lymphoma in Jamaica and its relation to adult T-cell/lymphoma. *Ann Intern Med* 106:361–368, 1987.

90 Manns A et al: Age-associated HTLV-I risk in the development of non-Hodgkin's lymphoma. *Lancet* 342:1447–1450, 1993.

91 De Oliveira MS et al: Adult T-cell leukaemia/lymphoma in Brazil and its relation to HTLV-I. *Lancet* 336:987–990, 1990.

92 Broder S et al: T-cell lymphoproliferative syndrome associated with human T-cell leukemia/lymphoma virus. *Ann Intern Med* 100:543–557, 1984.

93 Yoshida M et al: Monoclonal integration of human T-cell leukemia provirus in all primary tumors of adult T-cell leukemia suggests causative role of human T-cell leukemia virus in the disease. *Proc Natl Acad Sci USA* 81:2534–2537, 1984.

94 Korber B et al: Polymerase chain reaction analysis of defective human T-cell leukemia virus type I proviral genomes in leukemic cells of patients with adult T-cell leukemia. *J Virol* 65:5471–5476, 1991.

95 Yamaguchi K et al: Pathogenesis of adult T-cell leukemia from clinical pathologic features, in *Human Retrovirology: HTLV,* WA Blattner (ed). New York, Raven Press, 1990, pp 163–171.

96 Waldmann TA: Adult T-cell leukemia: Prospects for immunotherapy, in *The Human Retroviruses,* RC Gallo, G Jay (eds). San Diego, Academic Press, 1991, pp 319–334.

97 Gill PS et al: Treatment of adult T-cell leukemia-lymphoma with a combination of interferon alpha and zidovudine. *N Engl J Med* 332: 1744–1748, 1995.

98 Osame M et al: Blood transfusion and HTLV-I associated myelopathy. *Lancet* 2:104–105, 1986.

99 Kaplan JE et al: The risk of development of HTLV-I-associated myelopathy/tropical spastic paraparesis among persons infected with HTLV-I. *J Acquir Immune Defic Syndr* 3:1096–1101, 1990.

100 Kramer A et al: Risk factors and cofactors for HAM/TSP in Jamaica. *Am J Epidemiol* 142:1212–1220, 1995.

101 Jacobson S et al: Immunological findings in neurological diseases associated with antibodies to HTLV-I: Activated lymphocytes in tropical spastic paraparesis. *Ann Neurol* 23(suppl):S196-S200, 1988.

102 LaGrenade L et al: HLA DRB1*DQB1* phenotype in HTLV-I-associated familial infective dermatitis may predict the development of HTLV-I-associated myelopathy/tropical spastic paraparesis. *Am J Med Genet* 61:37–41, 1996.

103 Jacobson S et al: HTLV-I-specific cytotic T lymphocytes in the cerebrospinal fluid of patients with HTLV-I-associated neurological disease. *Ann Neurol* 32:651–657, 1992.

104 Osame M et al: Chronic progressive myelopathy associated with elevated antibodies to human T-lymphotropic virus type I and adult T-cell leukemialike cells. *Ann Neurol* 21:117–122, 1987.

105 Morgan OS et al: HTLV-I and polymyositis in Jamaica. *Lancet* 2: 1184–1187, 1989.

106 Nishioka K et al: Chronic inflammatory arthropathy associated with HTLV-I. *Lancet* 1:441, 1989.

107 Sugimoto M et al: Bronchoalveolar T-lymphocytosis in HTLV-1-associated myelopathy. *Chest* 95:708, 1989.

108 Mochizuki M et al: HTLV-I uveitis: A distinct clinical entity caused by HTLV-I. *Jpn J Cancer Res* 83:236–239, 1992.

109 Mochizuki M: HTLV-I-associated uveitis. *Int Ophthalmol Clin* 35: 107–120, 1995.

110 Nakada K et al: High incidence of HTLV antibody in carriers of *Strongyloides stercoralis. Lancet* 1:633, 1984.

111 Tachibana N et al: Suppression of tuberculin skin reaction in healthy HTLV-I carriers from Japan. *Int J Cancer* 42:829–831, 1988.

112 Ho GYF et al: Markers of health status in an HTLV-I-positive cohort. *Am J Epidemiol* 136:1349–1357, 1992.

113 LaGrenade L et al: Infective dermatitis of Jamaican children: A marker for HTLV-I infection. *Lancet* 336:1345–1347, 1990.

114 LaGrenade L et al. TSP occurring in HTLV-I-associated infective dermatitis: Report of 2 cases. *West Ind Med J* 44:34–35, 1995.

115 Matsuzaki T et al: Diseases among men living in HTLV-I endemic areas in Japan. *Intern Med* 32:623–628, 1993.

116 Miyoshi I et al: ATLV in Japanese patients with AIDS. *Lancet* 2:275, 1983.

117 Bartholomew C et al: Progression to AIDS in homosexual men coinfected with HIV and HTLV-I in Trinidad. *Lancet* 2:1469–1470, 1987.

118 Cleghorn FR, Blattner WA: Editorial: Does human T-cell lymphotropic virus type I and human immunodeficiency virus type 1 coinfection accelerate acquired immunodeficiency syndrome? The jury is still out. *Arch Intern Med* 152:1372–1373, 1992.

119 Gotuzzo E et al: The impact of HTLV-I/II infection on the prognosis of sexually acquired cases of AIDS. *Arch Intern Med* 152:1429–1432, 1991.

120 Schecter M et al: Coinfection with human T-cell lymphotropic virus type I and HIV in Brazil. *JAMA* 271:353–357, 1994.

121 Volberding PA: Editorial: HIV, HTLV-I and CD4+ lymphocytes: Trouble in the relationship. *JAMA* 271:392–393, 1994.

Section 3
Herpesviruses, Human Papillomavirus, Hepatitis B Virus, Molluscum Contagiosum

Chapter 20
Biology of herpesviruses

Peter E. Pertel
Patricia G. Spear

Approximately 100 herpesviruses have been identified, with at least eight infecting humans.[1,2] All human herpesviruses are well adapted to their natural host, being endemic in all human populations studied and carried by a significant fraction of persons in each population. The human herpesviruses include herpes simplex viruses types 1 and 2 (HSV-1 and HSV-2), varicella-zoster virus (VZV), Epstein-Barr virus (EBV), cytomegalovirus (CMV), human herpesvirus 6 (HHV-6), human herpesvirus 7 (HHV-7), and the recently discovered human herpesvirus 8 (HHV-8) or Kaposi's sarcoma–associated herpesvirus. Disease caused by human herpesviruses tends to be relatively mild and self-limited in immunocompetent persons, although severe and quite unusual disease can be seen with immunosuppression.

A few key characteristics differentiate the herpesviruses from other viruses.[3,4] These include (1) a double-stranded linear DNA genome ranging in size from 125,000 to 250,000 base pairs, (2) an icosahedral capsid approximately 125 nm in diameter consisting of 162 capsomers, (3) an amorphous layer of viral proteins called the *tegument,* and (4) a lipid bilayer envelope containing viral glycoproteins. In addition to these structural elements that define members of the Herpesviridae family, all herpesviruses share biologic traits. These include expression of a large number of viral enzymes, assembly of the nucleocapsid in the cell nucleus, destruction of the cell during productive infection, and ability to establish latent infections in an infected host.

The pathology and epidemiology of herpesvirus infections depend not only on viral replication and associated cytotoxicity but also on the capacity of herpesviruses to establish latent infections. The term *productive infection* will be used here to describe, at the cell level, an infection in which the invading virus replicates to yield progeny virus and the cell is killed. *Latent infection* or *latency* means that the genome of the invading virus is stably maintained by the cell with only limited expression of viral genes, no production of progeny virus, and no evident virus-induced cytotoxicity. Latent infections can be converted to productive infections by factors and stimuli that have not yet been clearly defined. This conversion results in activation of virus replication, possibly at levels sufficient to cause clinical symptoms. Recurrence of disease due to periodic or sporadic activation of viral replication is an important feature of the pathology caused by HSV and, to a lesser extent, VZV. In addition, asymptomatic shedding of herpesviruses may play a significant role in transmission from person to person.[5–7]

TAXONOMY AND GENOMIC ORGANIZATION

The family Herpesviridae is further divided into three subfamilies based on biologic differences.[2,3] The alpha herpesviruses are neurotropic viruses that replicate relatively rapidly and infect a wide range of cells in cell culture. Examples include HSV-1, HSV-2, and VZV. The beta herpesviruses replicate slowly and are restricted in the types of cells productively infected in cell culture. Cells infected by beta herpesviruses often become enlarged. Examples include CMV, HHV-6, and HHV-7. The gamma herpesviruses are lymphotropic viruses that also replicate relatively slowly and are restricted in the types of cells productively infected. Examples include EBV and HHV-8. Some gamma herpesviruses are cofactors in malignancies. Except for the close relationship between HSV-1 and HSV-2, each of the human herpesviruses appears to be more closely related to biologically similar animal herpesviruses than to each other. This classification scheme based on biologic differences is for the most part concordant with evolutionary inferences that can be drawn from nucleotide sequence analysis.[2] In this chapter, HSV, EBV, and CMV will be discussed as the prototypes of their respective subfamilies.

The genomes of the various herpesviruses are clearly evolutionarily related but differ in size, in organization of unique and repeated sequences, and in gene content and order.[2,8–12] Although each virus encodes unique genes, a large fraction of the genes of herpesviruses are conserved among members of the family. These homologous genes are arranged in several colinear blocks (Fig. 20–1). The blocks are themselves arranged in the same order and orientation for members of any one subfamily of herpesviruses and in different orders and orientations for viruses from different subfamilies. Genes specific for a virus or subfamily tend to be at the genomic termini or in clusters between the blocks of homologous genes. Certain key regulatory proteins and genes expressed in latency tend to be different for members of the different subfamilies.[8]

It was recognized in the 1960s that there are two distinct serotypes of HSV, type 1 and type 2.[15,16] It also was noted that HSV-1 strains usually were isolated from labial, facial, and ocular lesions and from brain lesions in encephalitis, whereas HSV-2 strains usually were isolated from genital lesions and from newborn infants who became infected during delivery through an infected birth canal.[17] These distinctions, however, are not absolute. HSV-2 strains have been isolated at relatively high frequencies from sites more commonly associated with HSV-1 strains, and vice versa. Differences in HSV-1 and HSV-2 are subtle, and it is difficult to define HSV-1–specific and HSV-2–specific aspects of pathogenicity in human disease. It has been noted, however, that HSV-2 is more likely to cause recurrent disease at genital sites than at oral sites, whereas the converse is true for HSV-1.[18] One way to account for these differences is to postulate that HSV-1 and HSV-2 evolved from a common ancestor after establishment of this ancestor in separate ecologic niches defined by anatomic site and source of virus for inoculation.[19] If genital infections usually resulted from inoculation with virus shed from genital tissues and facial infections with virus shed from facial tissues, then conditions could be optimal for emergence of the two serotypes with subtle differences in properties dictated by differences in requirements for optimal maintenance within and transmission from the two anatomic sites.

Two EBV types, 1 and 2, also have been identified, although EBV-1 and EBV-2 are much more closely related to each other than are HSV-1 and HSV-2.[20] The most significant differences are in genes that have roles in growth transformation (EBNAs). Consistent with these observations, the ability of EBV-2 isolates to transform B cells in vitro is attenuated.[21]

Available information indicates that a single genetic map suffices for HSV-1 and HSV-2, although some homologous open

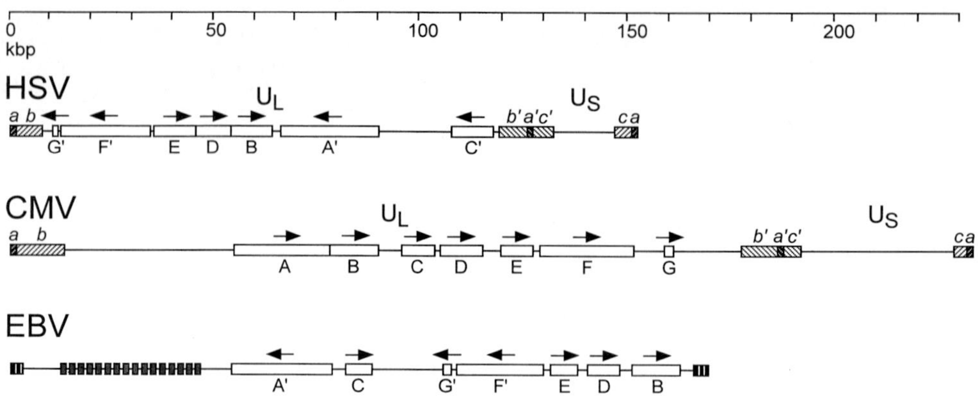

Fig. 20-1. The genomes of three representative alpha, beta, and gamma herpesviruses (HSV, CMV, and EBV) showing the positions of repeated sequences and of conserved gene blocks. The scale of these maps is in thousands of base pairs (kbp). The hatched boxes on the CMV and HSV maps represent repeated sequences present in two copies with inverted orientations. These repeated sequences divide the CMV and HSV genomes into unique long (U_L) and unique short (U_S) segments. The small shaded boxes on the EBV genome represent multiple repeated sequences all in the same orientation. The open boxes and letter designations represent conserved blocks of genes. The arrows denote the orientation of the blocks relative to CMV. These maps were adapted from Mocarski[14] and are based largely on the nucleotide sequence analyses of Kouzarides et al.,[9] McGeoch et al.,[12] and Baer et al.[13]

reading frames or noncoding regions may differ in length due to insertions or deletions of genetic information. This high degree of homology is consistent with the tremendous overlap in disease caused by HSV-1 and HSV-2. The order of homologous genes on the HSV and VZV genomes is for the most part colinear.[10,12] In addition, a few genes are found in one genome and not the other. On the other hand, comparison of the HSV genome with the EBV or CMV genome reveals only small blocks of colinear homologous genes, due in part to differences in gene order.[9,11,12] Divergence of the herpesviruses has been accompanied by rearrangements of the genomes (such as inversions and translocations), as well as by divergence of individual genes and distinctive additions or deletions of genetic information.

Inferences regarding the biology of new herpesviruses often can be drawn from what is known about closely related viruses. DNA sequence analysis of the HHV-8 genome initially revealed that this virus should be classified as a member of the *Rhadinovirus* genus of the gamma herpesvirus subfamily.[22] Herpesvirus saimiri (HVS) is the best characterized primate member of this genus.[23] Subsequent studies showed that HHV-8 infects B lymphocytes,[24] as does EBV, and that HHV-8 encodes proteins homologous to HVS proteins that could have a role in malignant transformation.[25] Further research into HHV-8 pathogenesis will no doubt be guided in part by previous and ongoing work on EBV and HVS.

MOLECULAR EPIDEMIOLOGY

Human herpesvirus infections are endemic. Transmission of virus usually requires intimate contact between persons. Often, the transmitting person is an asymptomatic shedder of infectious virus.[5–7] Sexual contact is a significant mode of transmission for several herpesviruses, including HSV and CMV,[26,27] but is not the only means by which virus can be passed from person to person. The detection of HHV-8 DNA in semen is consistent with sexual transmission of this virus.[28,29]

Strains of herpesviruses exhibit genetic variation. In theory, the biology of herpesviruses favors the generation and maintenance of a certain amount of genetic diversity, consistent with maintenance of function, among the viruses circulating within a human population at any given time. Every infected person is a long-term carrier of virus and may produce and shed virus periodically or continuously over a period of years in the face of pressures applied by protective immune responses. It is not surprising, therefore, that restriction endonuclease polymorphisms are easily detectable among epidemiologically unrelated strains of herpesviruses.[30] Use of as few as four or five endonucleases that cut the genome at 10 to 20 sites each is usually sufficient to differentiate between two HSV strains, of the same or different serotype, isolated from any two persons who are unacquainted. Conversely, virus isolates obtained sequentially from a single person or from known contacts exhibit no easily detectable restriction endonuclease polymorphisms. This has made it possible to trace the sources of infections occurring in clusters, such as in nosocomial outbreaks.[31,32] Similarly, restriction endonuclease polymorphism analyses have been used to show that persons latently infected with CMV or HSV can be superinfected with other strains.[33–35]

MOLECULAR BIOLOGY OF VIRAL REPLICATION AND LATENCY

Herpesvirus genomes encode approximately 100 or more proteins. Although a relatively large percentage of viral genes may not be essential for viral propagation in cell culture, all are most likely required for efficient viral function during naturally occurring infections. Many of these genes encode proteins that permit each herpesvirus to establish and maintain long-term infections in their natural hosts in ways that are biologically distinct for each virus.

Despite the fact that HSV infections outside the laboratory are, for the most part, limited to humans, the virus has an extremely broad host range. Many animal species can be experimentally infected with HSV, and many types and species of cultured cells will support HSV replication. On the other hand, the other human herpesviruses have a much more limited host range, are fastidious about the cell types in which they will replicate, and are often much more difficult to propagate in cell culture. Consequently, the molecular details of viral replication are much better understood for HSV than for the other human herpesviruses.

Herpesvirus infection is initiated by attachment of the virus to a susceptible cell. Viral glycoproteins in the virion envelope bind to components of the cell surface in a cascade of interactions that culminates in penetration of the nucleocapsid into the cell cytoplasm. After penetration, the nucleocapsid is transported to the cell nucleus. In productively infected cells, herpesvirus gene expression proceeds in a well-coordinated cascade.[36,37] Expression of the immediate-early (α) regulatory genes is necessary for the subsequent transcriptional activation and expression of the delayed-early (β) and late (γ) genes of the lytic cascade required for viral replication. In latently infected cells, the immediate-early (and delayed-early and late genes) ordinarily will not be expressed. The factors that determine whether immediate-early genes will not be expressed, permitting the establishment of latency, or will be expressed, initiating the cascade of viral gene expression required for viral replication, have not been defined for any herpesvirus. Viral DNA replication and nucleocapsid assembly are in the cell nucleus. Subsequent envelopment occurs by budding of the nucleocapsid through the inner nuclear membrane prior to release from the cell.

VIRAL ENTRY

The observation that HSV infects a wide range of cells implies that the virus uses highly conserved cellular molecules to effect entry or can use different molecules depending on the type of cell infected. The limited range of cells infected by EBV is in part due to the limited expression of the cellular molecule, CD21, that serves as a receptor for virus binding to cells.[38,39] In contrast, although the range of cultured cells that support CMV replication is also restricted, this is not always due to an inability of virus to enter cells but rather to a block in subsequent viral gene expression.[36,40]

For HSV, about a dozen virus-encoded glycoproteins have been identified in the virion envelope, although only five have been implicated in the process of viral entry.[41] Electron microscopy of virions labeled with gold-tagged antibodies (Fig. 20-2) has permitted the demonstration that three of these glycoproteins (gB, gC, and gD) constitute three morphologically distinct spikes projecting from the virion envelope.[42] Initial binding of HSV to cells is mediated by attachment to heparan sulfate. Heparan sulfate, which is closely related in structure to soluble heparin, is a major glycosaminoglycan moiety of ubiquitous cell surface proteoglycans. Both gB (UL27) and gC (UL44) are heparin-binding proteins, and either glycoprotein, acting independently, can mediate the initial adsorption of virus to cells. Glycoprotein C, however, probably makes the first contact with the cell surface. Penetration of HSV also may involve interaction with cell surface heparan sulfate. Initial binding of HSV to heparan sulfate may function to concentrate virus on the cell surface and thus facilitate subsequent interactions with other cellular receptors.

Penetration of HSV occurs by fusion of the virion envelope with the cellular plasma membrane.[41] Endocytosis of the virion is not required for viral entry. At least four viral glycoproteins, gB, gD (US6), gH (UL22), and gL (UL1), and possibly the tegument protein UL25 are required for penetration. Transfected cells that express gD are resistant to HSV infection due to a block in penetration but not adsorption. This latter observation suggests that cell-associated gD may somehow compete for a cell surface component required for interaction with virion-associated gD during penetration. Recently, a cell surface protein capable of mediating HSV entry into normally resistant cells was identified.[43] This protein, designated *herpesvirus entry mediator* (HVEM), is a member of the tumor necrosis factor/nerve growth factor (TNF/NGF) receptor family and has a key role in HSV infection of T cells. Interestingly, cell-associated gD can interfere with HSV entry via HVEM (Warner MS, Montgomery RI, Spear PG, unpublished data). Other cell surface proteins that can mediate HSV entry into other cell types have been identified recently and are under study.[43a,43b]

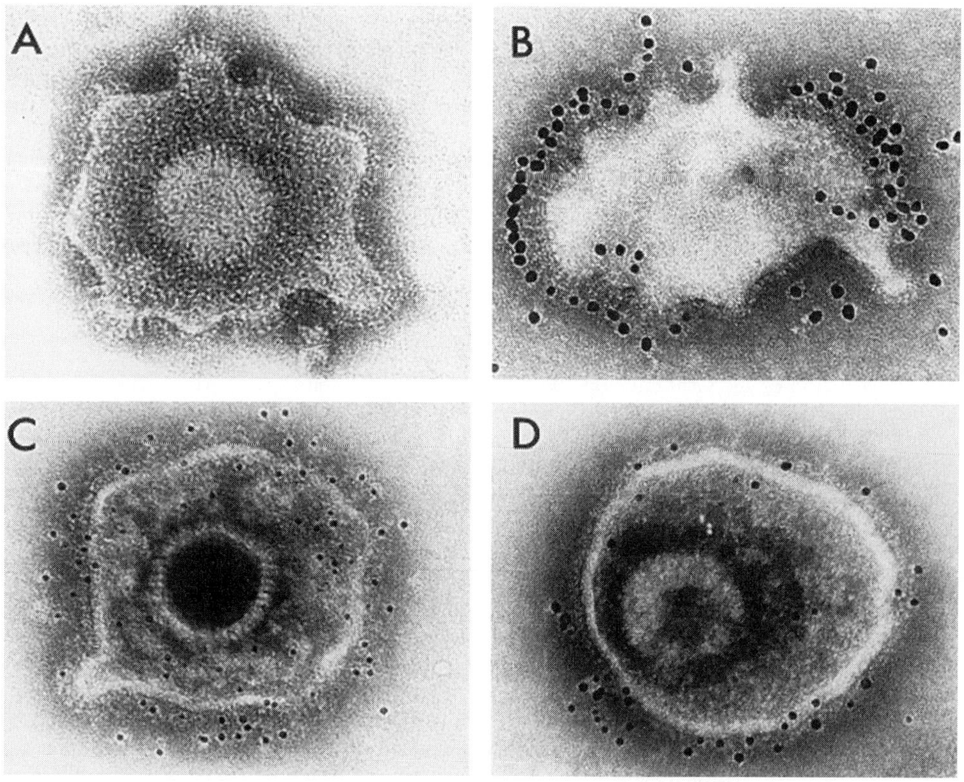

Fig. 20-2. Electron micrographs of negatively stained HSV showing different kinds of spikes projecting from the virion envelope. The most prominent spikes are composed of gB, as shown by the decoration of these spikes with gold-labeled anti-gB (*b*). Similarly, long, slender structures, difficult to resolve, are gC (*c*), and some of the short, fuzzlike structures are gD (*d*). No antibody was added in panel *a*. Similar figures were published by Stannard et al.[42] (*Courtesy of L. M. Stannard.*)

Initial attachment of EBV to B lymphocytes is mediated by interaction of viral gp350/220 with CD21, a receptor for the complement component C3d.[44] The ability of EBV to infect B cells correlates with the expression of CD21. It was thought originally that CD21 expression was limited to B cells. However, CD21 has been detected on nasopharyngeal carcinoma cells and also may be expressed on normal epithelial cells. In addition, T lymphocytes can express low levels of CD21. Thus CD21 also may mediate attachment of EBV to other cell types, including epithelial cells and T cells. Subsequent penetration of EBV is also thought to be mediated in part by gp350/220. The interaction of gp350/220 with CD21 results in the cross-linking of CD21. Subsequent patching and capping of CD21 and surface immunoglobulin are associated with the endocytosis of virus into smooth vesicles. In the vesicle, the EBV envelope presumably fuses with the vesicle membrane, resulting in release of the nucleocapsid into the cell cytoplasm. In addition to endocytosis, direct fusion of the EBV envelope with the cell membrane has been described with lymphoblastoid cell lines and may represent the primary route of EBV entry into epithelial cells. Fusion may be in part mediated by a viral oligomer containing gp85 and gp25, homologues of HSV gH and gL, along with a third glycoprotein, gp42/38, that has no known HSV homologue. A monoclonal antibody specific for an epitope on gp42/38 can block viral entry into B cells but not epithelial cells, indicating that molecular interactions required for entry with the two cell types are different. The interaction of EBV with other cell surface proteins specific to B cells or epithelial cells may be required because expression of CD21 is not sufficient for entry. Interestingly, gp110, the homologue of HSV gB, may be essential for viral assembly and egress whereas HSV-1 gB is not.[45]

As with HSV, initial attachment of CMV is mediated by binding of viral glycoproteins to cell surface heparan sulfate.[44,46] Glycoprotein complex II (gC-II) is the predominant component of the viral envelope that has heparin-binding activity. This complex, which is not homologous to HSV gC, is composed of two groups of distinct glycoproteins that are linked by disulfide bonds. CMV gB (UL55) also has heparin-binding activity but does not appear to mediate initial attachment. Instead, CMV gB appears to be involved in viral penetration, although a role for CMV gB in mediating attachment has not been excluded.

In addition to heparan sulfate, other cellular proteins have been implicated as receptors or coreceptors for CMV entry.[44,46] These include (1) class I human leukocyte antigen (HLA) molecules, (2) a fibroblast membrane protein, (3) a protein approximately 30 to 34 kDa in size, and (4) an aminopeptidase (CD13). Interaction of CMV with class I HLA heavy chains is dependent on initial binding of beta$_2$-microglobulin to virus. It has been suggested that this binding is followed by cross-linking of the class I heavy chains by virion-associated beta$_2$-microglobulin and subsequent endocytosis. However, more recent evidence suggests that entry of CMV occurs by fusion of the viral envelope with the cell plasma membrane and not by endocytosis. Thus the interaction of CMV with cellular HLA heavy chains may lead to noninfectious entry into cells. The fibroblast membrane protein is 92.5 kDa in size and was identified by an anti-idiotypic antibody directed against a CMV gH (UL75)–specific neutralizing monoclonal antibody. This 92.5-kDa protein is thought to be a possible receptor for CMV gH, which appears to have a role in viral penetration but not viral binding. The 30- to 34-kDa cellular protein has been identified in a variety of cell types by studying the ability of CMV to bind to cellular proteins. This protein appears to be annexin II. Because annexins are involved in cell-cell fusion, roles in viral penetration and viral-induced cell fusion are implied. CD13 appears to mediate CMV binding to monocytes and macrophages. It remains to be determined which cell surface proteins can mediate infectious entry of CMV.

INTRACELLULAR SYNTHESIS OF VIRAL COMPONENTS

Once the nucleocapsid enters the cytoplasm of the cell, it is transported to the vicinity of a nuclear pore, and the genome is delivered to the nucleus.[14,20,47] Transportation of the nucleocapsid to the nucleus is most likely mediated by specific interactions of the nucleocapsid with the cellular cytoskeleton. Parental viral DNA circularizes on entry into the nucleus. There the viral genes are transcribed by cellular RNA polymerase II under control of viral regulatory components, some of which are virion components. In productive infection, the immediate-early or α genes, which encode mostly regulatory proteins, are transcribed first. For HSV, optimal transcription of the α genes requires the activity of a viral regulatory protein called *α trans-inducing factor* (αTIF) or VP16. This viral regulatory protein is a virion constituent localized between the capsid and envelope and is delivered to the cell along with the viral genome. Homologous genes have been identified in EBV (BPLF-1) and in CMV (pp71).

Once the α genes have been transcribed and the α proteins translated, one or more of these proteins enables the transcription of the delayed-early or β genes.[14,20,47] The β genes encode enzymes and other proteins required for viral DNA replication. Most herpesviruses encode enzymes that can phosphorylate nucleosides and therefore also can activate nucleoside analogue inhibitors of viral DNA replication. In addition, all herpesviruses encode a DNA polymerase, which is responsible for genomic replication during lytic infection and is the target of nucleoside analogue inhibitors. For HSV, these enzymes are thymidine kinase (UL23) and DNA polymerase (UL30). Following α and β gene expression and DNA replication, the late or γ genes are expressed. The γ genes encode most of the virion structural proteins and glycoproteins.

Herpesviruses and certain other DNA viruses have provided excellent experimental systems for the study of eukaryotic gene expression and its regulation, in part because these viruses use the cell machinery for transcription of viral DNA to RNA and subsequent transcript processing to yield functional mRNAs.[14,20,47] The virus superimposes on this cell machinery its own regulatory factors that aid in targeting cell transcription factors to virus-specific nucleotide sequences. Interestingly, HSV differs from other DNA viruses and from eukaryotic cells in that most HSV genes expressed during productive infection are free of introns (intervening sequences that are removed from RNA transcripts by splicing to yield the functional mRNAs). In productively infected cells, RNA splicing is inhibited by the HSV protein ICP27 (UL54). One can speculate that expression of ICP27 homologues and evolution toward intron-free genes facilitate the expression of viral genes in preference to cell genes during a productive infection. In contrast, herpesvirus genes expressed in latently infected cells are usually spliced.

After synthesis of herpesvirus proteins in the cytoplasm, most of the proteins are transported to the nucleus, where they serve as regulatory factors, enzymes involved in DNA replication, or structural components of the nucleocapsid.[14,20,47] Viral glycoproteins are made on membrane-bound ribosomes and become distributed to all the membranes of the cell except the mitochondrial membranes. Synthesis of viral glycoproteins is similar to synthesis of cellular glycosylated proteins.

ASSEMBLY AND EGRESS OF VIRIONS

Herpesvirus nucleocapsids are assembled in the cell nucleus.[48] The nucleocapsids then acquire an envelope by budding through patches of the inner nuclear membrane that have been modified to contain viral glycoproteins. Virions can be observed in the perinuclear space and in cytoplasmic vesicles. Subsequent events involved in egress are not clearly understood.[4] The enveloped particles released into the perinuclear space may then be transported out of the cell by membrane-bound vesicles and the Golgi apparatus. Processing of viral glycoproteins may occur along the way. Alternatively, the enveloped virions in the perinuclear space may lose their envelopes by fusing with a cytoplasmic membrane. The nucleocapsids would then be reenveloped by budding through another cytoplasmic membrane. Whichever pathway of envelopement proves to be correct, the final stage of virion egress from the infected cell requires fusion of a transport vesicle with the cell plasma membrane.

FATE OF THE CELL THAT PRODUCES VIRUS

Herpesviruses kill the cells in which they replicate, at least in cell culture. For HSV, a viral gene product, virion host shutoff (VHS) protein (UL41), introduced into the cell along with the nucleocapsid causes degradation of preexisting cytoplasmic mRNAs such that cell protein synthesis is immediately inhibited. Other viral factors produced after infection inhibit or alter various host functions, including DNA replication and RNA processing.[49] In contrast, CMV initially stimulates host cell DNA, RNA, and protein synthesis, and effective CMV replication is dependent on this stimulation.[14] Later in the replicative cycle, host macromolecule synthesis is inhibited.

A hallmark of alpha herpesvirus infections in vivo is the presence of polykaryocytes.[50] Herpesvirus-induced cell-cell fusion may function as an alternative method for spreading virus from cell to cell and could facilitate evasion of host immune responses.

LATENCY

The ability of herpesviruses to persist for the life of their natural hosts depends in large part on their ability to establish latent infections. Latency occurs when the viral genome is stably maintained in the cell nucleus with expression of only a limited subset of viral genes. The latently infected cell is not killed by the virus, and viral gene products expressed actually may stimulate cell division. Virions or infectious virus cannot be recovered from latently infected tissue immediately after its removal from an experimental animal or human cadaver. However, activation of latent virus to the replicating state, yielding infectious virus, often can be achieved by in vitro cultivation of the explanted latently infected tissue.

Only limited information is available about the state and expression of herpesvirus genomes during latency. These data are principally for HSV in neurons and for EBV in B lymphocytes. In both cases the target cell is ordinarily in a nondividing state. EBV can induce the proliferation of latently infected B cells, causing cell division even in the absence of antigenic stimulation. HSV is not known to induce the proliferation of latently infected cells. This apparent difference may be related to the normal clearance of B cells and the need for EBV to maintain a reservoir of infected cells. Thus the observed differences in viral gene expression during latency noted for EBV and HSV may in part reflect the need for EBV to regulate cell proliferation.

The site of latency for HSV is sensory ganglia of nerves innervating the site of initial infection.[51] Infection of the sensory neurons occurs during initial HSV infection when the nerve endings are exposed to the virus. Virus is subsequently transported up the axons to the cell bodies. The HSV genomes present in ganglia of latently infected animals and humans are probably episomal and circular, in contrast to virion-associated genomes, which are linear.

Although gene expression by HSV is apparently not required during a latent infection, analyses of latently infected animal and human cells reveal the presence of transcripts from one specific region of the viral genome[51] (Fig. 20-3). These latency-associated transcripts (LATs) are transcribed from the DNA strand opposite that encoding one of the immediate-early proteins ICP0 or IE110. A relatively large transcript gives rise to a stable intron, from which two different spliced forms are derived. Open reading frames contained within these transcripts may be expressed.

The expression of LATs is not abolutely essential for the establishment of latency or for the reactivation of latent virus in animal models, and LATs can be detected during productive infections.[51] However, the significance of LATs in latency is suggested by observations that LAT expression is a good marker for the latent state induced by wild-type virus and that LAT-negative mutants may be somewhat impaired in their ability to reactivate from latency.

Subsequent reactivation of latent HSV can result after exposure to a variety of stimuli.[51] The mechanism by which virus is reactivated is unknown. Virus is subsequently transported down the axon to the site of initial infection or nearby. The frequency and clinical severity of reactivation depend on several factors, including immunocompetence of the infected host and severity of the initial infection. Presumably, the larger number of peripheral cells infected during a severe initial outbreak will result in a larger number of infected sensory neurons. Interestingly, HSV-1 reactivates more readily from trigeminal and cervical sensory ganglia, whereas HSV-2 reactivates more readily from sacral ganglia.[18,54] This correlates with the tendency for HSV-1 to cause recurrent orolabial disease and for HSV-2 to cause recurrent genital disease. The reasons for this are not known but may be secondary to differences in the cell or viral proteins needed for lytic growth in each cell type.

EBV establishes latent infections in B lymphocytes.[20] In latently infected B cells, the viral genome usually consists of a closed circular episome that is not integrated into the cellular DNA, although exceptions have been reported. Expression of two viral genes, a protein required for viral episome replication (EBNA-1) and a membrane protein that blocks signaling via the B-cell receptor (LMP-2), may represent the baseline state of latency in quiescent cells in vivo.[55,56] Based on the types of cells examined and the environmental conditions, the number of other viral genes expressed in a latent infection may vary.

At least 11 viral proteins expressed during latency have been defined in cultures of lymphoblastoid cells immortalized by EBV.[20] These include Epstein-Barr nuclear antigens (EBNAs) and viral latent membrane proteins (LMPs). Maintenance and controlled

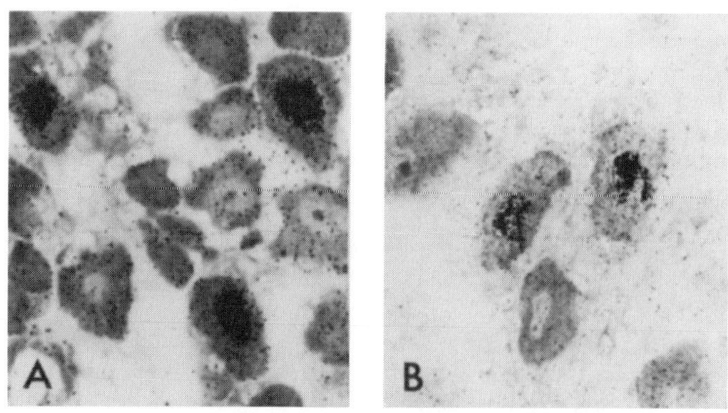

Fig. 20-3. Detection of HSV-1 LAT in neurons of peripheral ganglia by in situ hybridization and autoradiography. The black autoradiographic grains are localized over nuclei of some of the neurons in mouse tissue (*a*) and human tissue (*b*) taken from latently infected subjects. Experimental details are given in publications by Stevens et al.[52,53] (*Courtesy of J. G. Stevens.*)

replication of the EBV episome require EBNA-1. This protein interacts with the origin of DNA replication for latent EBV (ori-p) and may be involved in the partitioning of EBV episomes to the progeny of dividing cells by interacting with chromosomal proteins. The protein LMP-2 inhibits the switch from latent to lytic EBV infection by influencing transmembrane signal transduction via interaction with protein tyrosine kinases.

The proteins EBNA-2, EBNA-3A, EBNA-3C, EBNA-LP, and LMP-1 all appear to have roles in growth transformation of B lymphocytes.[20] These proteins appear to function by interacting with cell signaling pathways. For example, LMP-1 interacts with human proteins (TRAFs) that are involved in tumor necrosis factor receptor family signaling,[57] whereas EBNA-2 transactivates, in addition to other viral and cellular gene products, the protein tyrosine kinase c-fgr. This kinase is a member of the *src* oncogene family and may be involved in the regulation of B-cell growth. Expression of all these viral proteins in vivo, however, usually will induce cytotoxic responses by natural killer cells and T cells.

Two additional EBV products that may have a role in latency include small nonpolyadenylated Epstein-Barr–encoded RNAs (EBERs), which are expressed in both lytic and latent infections,[20] and the protein BHRF-1, which is an EBV homologue to the human oncogene *Bcl*-2. The function of EBERs is not known, whereas BHRF-1 can protect B cells from apoptosis and can delay the terminal differentiation of epithelial cells. However, neither EBERs nor BHRF-1 is required for B-cell transformation in vitro. The possibility exists that these EBV products are not dispensible in vivo, where mediators of immunity can influence the process.

Epidemiologic studies first implicated leukocytes as a possible site of CMV latency. CMV can be transmitted by blood transfusions, and the risk of infection can be decreased substantially by using leukocyte-depleted blood.[58–60] CMV DNA has been detected in monocytes, lymphocytes, and polymorphonuclear cells.[14] CMV infection of myeloid precursers and of monocytes is often restricted in that only immediate-early gene products are expressed. Differentiation of monocytes into macrophages can result in productive infection. In addition, replication of CMV in monocytes and macrophages does not necessarily result in the release of virus. This appears to be due to disaggregation of the microtubule network. Disruption of the microtubule network also may allow virus to avoid intracellular degradation and detection by the immune system. Recently, latency-associated transcripts were detected in CMV-infected granulocyte-macrophage progenitor cells.[61,62] These transcripts are derived from both strands of the CMV genome at the site encoding the immediate-early proteins IE1 and IE2. One unspliced and two spliced transcripts have been detected, and their expression appears to correlate with latent infections. These transcripts may function to downregulate expression of IE1 and IE2.

CMV immediate-early antigens without any evidence of productive viral infection have been detected in many cell types, including endothelial and epithelial cells. Latent CMV infection of endothelial cells is especially intriguing because of the possibility that virus can be transmitted to monocytes and macrophages migrating across the vessel wall. Transmission of CMV between endothelial cells and monocytes and macrophages has been described.[63]

At present, little is known about the molecular biology of HHV-8 latency, although HHV-8 may latently infect B cells.[24] HHV-8 homologues to cellular G protein–coupled receptor proteins and to cellular cyclins have been identified and were shown recently to be expressed in Kaposi's sarcoma (KS) tissue and in AIDS-related body cavity–based lymphomas.[25] Cellular G protein–coupled receptor proteins and cyclins function in regulation of cell proliferation, differentiation, and gene expression. CMV also encodes G protein–coupled receptor homologues, and these genes are transcribed during infection.[64,65] In addition, CMV infection induces cell cyclins along with two tumor suppressor proteins, p53 and the retinoblastoma gene product.[66]

TRANSFORMATION OF INFECTED CELLS

Most, if not all, DNA viruses encode proteins that can stimulate certain cell activities. For example, papillomaviruses and EBV induce the proliferation of latently infected cells, overriding normal controls on cell division. The epidermal hyperplasias or warts induced by papillomaviruses and the lymphoproliferation caused by EBV are usually benign proliferations unless immune responses are inadequate or unless secondary factors contribute to the viral-induced transformation to cause malignant transformation of the infected cells.

Normally, expression of additional EBV genes, including those which induce sustained proliferation of B cells in the absence of antigenic stimulation, will induce cytotoxic responses by natural killer cells and T cells. These responses account for the lymphoproliferation seen in infectious mononucleosis and control the virus-induced B-cell proliferation in the vast majority of immunocompetent persons. In persons with congenital or acquired immunodeficiencies, virus-induced B-cell proliferation may occur relatively unchecked and can result in polyclonal or monoclonal lymphomas. Monoclonality probably results from mutations during EBV-induced cell proliferation that confer a selective advantage to the mutated cell. EBV also has been implicated as a causal factor in Burkitt's lymphoma, Hodgkin's lymphoma, lymphoproliferative syndromes, and nasopharyngeal carcinoma, along with the hyperproliferative disorder oral hairy leukoplakia in persons with AIDS.

The role of HHV-8 in malignant transformation has not been established. Based on its close relationship to other gamma herpesviruses that are associated with malignancies, such as EBV and HVS, it seems likely that HHV-8 has a causal role in some malignancies. HHV-8 DNA has been detected in KS lesions and AIDS-related body cavity–based lymphomas.[1,67] Polymerase chain reaction (PCR) in situ hybridization has been used to identify HHV-8 DNA sequences in both endothelial and spindle cells found in KS lesions.[68] Also, initial seroepidemiologic studies show a correlation between antibodies to HHV-8–associated proteins and the development of KS.[69] Although HHV-8 DNA sequences are not routinely detected in established KS cell cultures, one study reported that HHV-8 could be isolated from a KS cell line and propagated in cell culture.[70]

CMV also has been associated with several malignancies, including prostatic carcinoma, cervical carcinoma, adenocarcinoma, and KS.[14] However, the evidence to support a causal role for CMV in these malignancies is confounded by the high prevalence of CMV in the general population and by the ability of CMV to infect a wide range of cells in vivo. Thus, although CMV is capable of modifying cell metabolism and can cause cell transformation in cell culture, there is no definitive evidence that CMV is the cause of any malignancy.

There is also no evidence that HSV is causally associated with any human malignancy. Early suspicions that HSV might be an etiologic agent of cervical carcinoma were based mostly on seroepidemiologic studies.[71] These suspicions have been lessened, if not laid to rest, by recent findings that papillomavirus DNA, not HSV DNA, can be detected regularly in cervical carcinomas. Also, there is no evidence that HSV induces the proliferation of latently infected cells. Although it has not been ruled out that HSV could be a cofactor in the causation of cervical carcinoma and other tumors, evidence for or against such a role would be difficult to obtain. Experimental models of HSV transformation have not yielded clues as to reliable viral markers in cells putatively transformed by HSV. The introduction of certain fragments of the HSV genome into cells in vitro has been associated with malignant transformation of the cells.[72] In contrast to cells transformed by other DNA viruses, however, it has not been possible to demonstrate that the transformed phenotype required retention of any of the viral DNA or expression of any particular HSV protein.

PATHOGENESIS

Human herpesvirus infections are highly prevalent, and the diseases they cause tend to be relatively mild and self-limited. The importance of cell-mediated immunity in controlling herpesvirus replication and limiting reactivation of latent virus in vivo is underscored by the increase in frequency and severity of disease in persons with suppressed cell-mediated immunity. Examples of diseases caused by HSV, EBV, and CMV are listed below. These different viruses share a number of common pathogenetic mechanisms, although they cause very different diseases. VZV causes chickenpox and shingles. HHV-6 and HHV-7 both cause roseola infantum. In addition, HHV-6 can cause hepatitis and pneumonitis. No clinical syndrome associated with a primary HHV-8 infection has yet been identified.

HSV PATHOGENESIS

HSV can cause gingivostomatitis, herpes labialis, keratoconjunctivitis, cutaneous herpes, genital herpes, encephalitis, meningitis, and neonatal herpes. The nature and severity of disease depend on several factors, including site of virus inoculation, age and immune status of the host, and undoubtedly genetic variation in virus strains or infected persons. Immune responses to viral antigens can, in some instances, cause as much or more damage in affected tissues as the cytopathology associated with viral replication. This kind of immunopathology appears to be important in cases of herpetic keratitis,[73] where there is deep stromal damage, but probably does not figure as importantly in other kinds of herpetic lesions or disseminated disease.

Infection with HSV is initiated by contact of virus with mucosa or abraded skin.[74] Replication of HSV in cells of the epidermis and dermis follows, resulting in cellular destruction and inflammation. Clinically, vesicles on an inflammatory base are noted.[75] Microscopically, multinucleated giant cells, focal cellular necrosis, and ballooning of infected cells are noted. During an initial infection, HSV can spread via the lymphatics to regional lymph nodes. Further spread of virus is limited by both humoral and cell-mediated immune mechanisms. It is during an initial infection that virus gains access to sensory neurons, allowing establishment of latent infection. In animal models, HSV can be detected in sensory nerve ganglia within 2 days of infection. Limited viral replication follows in neural tissue, allowing virus to migrate back down axons to sites near the inoculation site. This phenomenon, along with contiguous spread of virus in the cells of the epidermis and dermis, may explain the large surface area affected during a primary HSV infection. Ultimately, the host immune response in immunocompetent persons will control viral replication and allow healing of lesions.

Reactivation and replication of latent HSV can be induced by multiple stimuli, including ultraviolet light, immunosuppression, fever, pneumococcal pneumonia, and trauma to the latently infected neuron. The severity of symptoms associated with reactivation can vary substantially and may be related to the amount of replicating virus, the virulence of the HSV strain, and the integrity of the host immune system.[74] Virus reactivation and replication occur periodically in asymptomatic persons. Virus can be detected even in the absence of symptoms and signs of disease.[76–78]

Because HSV rarely causes severe or disseminated disease in adults, except when cell-mediated immunity is compromised, it seems likely that cell-mediated immune mechanisms are most important for preventing the spread of infection and controlling viral replication. However, humoral immune mechanisms also appear to play important roles in controlling infection. HSV glycoproteins expressed on the surface of the viral envelope or infected cells are targets for neutralizing antibodies and antibody-dependent cell-mediated cytotoxicity, respectively.[79–81] In addition, monoclonal antibodies against viral glycoproteins have been shown to protect against neurologic disease and to prevent the establishment of latency in animal models.[79,80,82] The role of these antibodies in human infections is not clear, but the quantity of neutralizing and antibody-dependent cell-mediated cytotoxic antibodies does correlate inversely with disseminated disease in newborns.[83–85] Interestingly, high titers of antibodies correlate with high frequency and severity of recurrent disease in adults.[54,86,87] The reason is not clear, but the high titers of antibodies appear to reflect a more severe primary infection. More severe primary infections correlate with an increase in frequency and severity of recurrent disease[87] and, therefore, with repeated antigenic stimuli.

Cell-mediated immunity directed against HSV-infected cells involves natural killer cells, activated T cells, and macrophages.[88–93] Both major histocompatibility complex (MHC) class I and class II restricted T cells have direct cytotoxic effects against HSV-infected cells.[88,89] Cytokines released by lymphocytes may have direct antiviral activity or may act to regulate other components of the host immune response. Whether the immune responses that control localized disease are the same as those which prevent disseminated disease is not known. Qualitative or quantitative differences in the responses may exist. In addition, differences in immune responses among infected persons may at least in part account for observed differences in clinical disease that are typically noted. Because neurons do not express MHC class I or II antigens, T cells may not be able to recognize HSV-infected neurons.[94] In cells that express class I MHC, presentation of antigenic peptides to MHC class I restricted T cells is inhibited by a viral protein, ICP47.[95–97] ICP47 blocks peptide translocation to the cell compartment where class I molecules are assembled.

In attempts to identify HSV antigens that can induce protective immunity in experimental animal systems, attention has been focused mostly on the virion envelope glycoproteins. However, for many viruses, including CMV and HSV, cytotoxic T cells can recognize and kill cells that express viral proteins not normally displayed on the cell surface.[98,99] The reason is that T cells recognize principally the peptide fragments of antigen produced by catabolic processes and presented on cell surfaces in association with MHC molecules. It is therefore difficult to predict which antigens are most important in inducing protective cell-mediated immune responses. Possibly many of the approximately 100 proteins encoded by HSV contribute to the induction of protective immunity, making it difficult to identify a few key immunogens.

Some of the viral glycoproteins expressed by HSV not only may induce immune responses but also may modulate immune effector mechanisms.[100] In addition to its heparin-binding activity and role in viral adsorption, HSV gC binds to the C3 fragments C3b and iC3b and is responsible for the expression of complement receptors on infected cell surfaces. Virions expressing gC appear to be somewhat protected against complement-mediated neutralization. In addition, HSV-1 gC can protect infected cells from complement-dependent lysis. Moreover, interaction of HSV-1 gC, but not HSV-2 gC, with C3b can accelerate decay of this pivotal component of the complement cascade. In infected cells, gE (US8) alone or gE-gI (US7) heterodimers can bind to the Fc region of immunoglobulin G (IgG), accounting for the expression of Fc receptors on the surface of HSV-infected cells. Binding of nonspecific IgG by virions can interfere with antibody-mediated and complement-dependent neutralization. In addition, IgG bound to cell surface Fc receptors protects HSV-infected cells against complement-dependent and cell-mediated immune lysis. The signficance of these observations in persons infected with HSV remains unknown.

Despite the ability of HSV to infect many cell types, HSV disease is often localized to the body surface at the site of inoculation and to the sensory ganglia of nerves communicating with this site. Undoubtedly, an effective immune reponse is responsible in part for limiting the spread of infection. The possibility exists, however, that there are nonimmunologic barriers to the spread of infection in the normal adult. For example, certain cell types in fully differentiated tissues may not be able to support HSV replication, due either to inaccessibility or lack of required cell surface receptors or to lack of other factors needed for biosynthesis of viral components. Clearly, expression of cell surface heparan sulfate and perhaps precise patterns of sulfation are required for efficient binding of virus to cells. Recent studies demonstrate that specific cell surface proteins serve as coreceptors for HSV entry into specific cell types. A newly discovered member of the TNF/NGF receptor family designated HVEM mediates entry into human T cells.[43] Other cell surface receptors mediate HSV entry into other cell types.

HSV-1 can cause sporadic cases of encephalitis. It has been proposed that virus may spread via neurons from peripheral ganglia to the brain.[101–104] The frequency at which HSV-1 enters the brain is not known, but HSV DNA has been detected in human brain tissue in the absence of encephalitis.[105–108] It is not unreasonable to assume that different strains of HSV-1 will differ in neurovirulence. However, attempting to assess which viral genes mediate neurovirulence has been problematic. Many HSV genes, including thymidine kinase, have been implicated in neurovirulence. In animal models, mutations within or deletions of these genes will attenuate neurovirulence. Recently, deletion of a gene designated γ_1 34.5 (ICP34.5) was shown to ablate neurovirulence in mice.[109] It appears that γ_1 34.5 enables HSV-1 to replicate in central nervous system tissue but is not essential for replication in many cell types in vitro. Mutant virus that does not express γ_1 34.5 can still establish and reactivate from a latent infection, although both events occur less efficiently than with wild-type virus.[110–112] Unfortunately, convincing correlation with clinical disease in humans is not yet available.

EBV PATHOGENESIS

Diseases caused by EBV include mononucleosis, hepatitis, encephalitis, and lymphoproliferative syndromes. EBV initially infects epithelial cells in the oropharynx.[113] The B cells in adjacent lymphoid tissue are then infected, and virus disseminates throughout the lymphoreticular system. Clinical symptoms and signs typically are not seen in young children but are seen in adolescents and adults. Symptoms and signs of infection may in large part result from the inflammatory response directed against EBV.

The humoral immune response to an EBV infection consists of specific antibodies directed against viral antigens and heterophile antibodies. Heterophile antibodies probably result from polyclonal stimulation of immunoglobulin synthesis in EBV-infected B cells and consist mostly of immunoglobulin M (IgM) molecules, some of which can bind to animal red blood cell antigens.[114] The presence of these antibodies will cause the agglutination or hemolysis of these red blood cells. Heterophile antibodies are detected in approximately 90 percent of persons with infectious mononucleosis due to EBV, and their presence can be used to confirm the diagnosis.[115] Antibodies directed against platelets, neutrophils, nuclear antigens, and ampicillin have all been reported.[116] These antibodies may have a role in mediating some of the complications of infectious mononucleosis, such as the rash that develops in over 70 percent of infectious mononucleosis patients treated with ampicillin.

Early in an EBV infection a mononuclear lymphocytosis consisting mostly of natural killer and T cells specific for EBV is noted.[113] Cytotoxic T cells can suppress growth and activation of EBV-infected B cells in vitro and most likely also in vivo. The importance of cytotoxic T cells in controlling EBV replication in vivo is suggested by the abnormally high levels of EBV-infected B cells in persons with diseases associated with suppressed cell-mediated immunity, such as persons with AIDS and persons receiving immunosuppressive medications. The cytotoxic T cells are directed against epitopes on LMP-1, LMP-2, and several EBNAs, but not EBNA-1. This is consistent with the expression of EBV proteins known to be required for B-cell immortalization and proliferation. Early in infectious mononucleosis the predominant latently infected B cell is probably similar to the proliferating B cell described in vitro in terms of the number of EBV proteins expressed. However, the developing T-cell response destroys these cells but is unable to eliminate cells in the proposed baseline state of latency.

EBV can modulate the immune response generated in infected persons. EBV encodes a protein that can degrade C3b and iC3b.[117] In addition, cell-mediated immune responses may be attenuated by one of several different mechanisms. First, EBV encodes a gene, BCRF-1, that is homologous to interleukin-10.[118] Interleukin-10 inhibits cytokine synthesis by MHC class II restricted T cells.[119] BCRF-1 has been shown to inhibit interferon-γ synthesis by T cells and natural killer cells.[120] Interferon-γ can inhibit proliferation of EBV-infected B cells.[121] Second, EBV can downregulate expression of MHC class I antigens, resulting in decreased cell lysis by cytotoxic T cells.[122]

Ultimately, the immune response generated in immunocompetent persons controls viral replication, and the number of infected B cells circulating in the body drops about 100- to 10,000-fold.[113] This drop correlates with the development of EBV-specific cytotoxic T cells. These cytotoxic T cells persist for the lifetime of the infected host, probably because of the continued presence of latently infected B cells that periodically reactivate or express additional proteins that can be recognized by the immune system. Also, EBV can be isolated from the oropharynx for 12 to 18 months after the resolution of clinical disease and then intermittently in both immunocompetent and immunosuppressed persons.[7]

Many of the symptoms and signs of infectious mononucleosis, including pharyngitis, fever, lymphadenopathy, and splenomegaly, may in part be a direct consequence of the host immune response.[113] Pharyngitis most likely results from lytic virus replication in epithelial cells along with the resulting inflammation. The systemic symptoms, including fever, malaise, and headaches, may result from the immune response directed against the infected B cells. Treatment of infectious mononucleosis with high doses of acyclovir stops viral replication in infected cells but does little to attenuate clinical symptoms.[123–125] Corticosteroids, however, do have a significant effect on decreasing the symptoms and signs associated with mononucleosis but are used only in selected situations.[126,127]

CMV PATHOGENESIS

CMV can cause mononucleosis, hepatitis, chorioretinitis, pneumonitis, colitis, and congenital cytomegalic inclusion disease. Infection with CMV usually is initiated by contact of virus with cells of the oropharynx or the genital tract or by transfusion of contaminated blood.[128] CMV infections are typically subclinical. The most common clinical manifestation is a self-limited mononucleosis, although disease can be quite severe and life-threatening in immunosuppressed persons.

Clinical disease most likely results from viral cytolysis and the host's inflammatory response.[128] However, additional pathology may result from abortively infected cells. The hallmark of CMV disease on histology is the cytomegalic inclusion-bearing cell.

Neutralizing antibodies directed against CMV can decrease the efficiency of viral transmission and can attenuate clinical disease.[128] Antibodies directed against gB and gH can neutralize CMV infectivity in vitro. However, cell-mediated immunity appears to be much more important in controlling CMV replication. The incidence of severe CMV disease is markedly increased in persons with suppressed cell-mediated immunity, and the risk of CMV disease correlates with the degree of immunosuppression.[129–131] Cell-mediated immunity against CMV involves activated T cells, natural killer cells, and macrophages. The cytotoxic T-cell response can be both MHC class I and class II restricted. Transfer of CD8+ cytotoxic T-cell clones to immunodeficient bone marrow transplant recipients may be able to restore protective immunity.[132] The immunosuppressive agents used to prevent graft rejection by transplant recipients can have profound and specific effects on either CMV latency or replication.[133–136]

CMV infection itself is immunosuppressive. Normal monocyte, T-cell, and natural killer cell function can all be inhibited.[137–139] The mechanism is not fully understood. However, cellular G protein–coupled receptor gene homologues encoded by CMV are transcribed in infected cells.[64,65,140] Also, CMV infection of monocytes or lymphocytes reduces interleukin-1 and interleukin-2 production and responsiveness.[137] Thus signal transduction in CMV-infected cells may be significantly altered and possibly account for the decreased immune function noted.

CMV has been suspected of contributing to the progressive immunosuppression noted in persons infected with the human immunodeficiency virus (HIV). The immediate-early gene region of CMV can transactivate the HIV promoter, and bidirectional enhancement of virus replication in cells infected with both CMV and HIV can occur.[141,142] However, the clinical significance of these observations is not clear.

CMV also encodes proteins that may modulate immune effector mechanisms. CMV-infected cells express Fc receptors.[143] As with HSV, nonspecific binding of IgG may reduce antibody-mediated neutralization and cellular cytotoxicity. CMV expresses proteins that are antigenically related to HSV gE and have Fc binding activity.[144,145] Induction of Fc receptor expression by CMV can allow HIV to infect fibroblasts.[146] The ability of CMV to bind beta$_2$-microglobulin (the light chain of the MHC class I antigen) may protect virus from neutralizing antibodies.[147,148] In addition, CMV encodes a protein homologous to the MHC class I heavy chain (UL18).[149] This homologue can associate with beta$_2$-microglobulin and was thought initially to sequester beta$_2$-microglobulin and prevent effective surface expression of the MHC class I antigen.[150] However, although MHC class I antigen expression is reduced in CMV-infected cells, UL18 does not appear to mediate this reduction.[151]

ANTIVIRAL AGENTS

Most of the drugs now in use for therapy of herpesvirus infections are nucleoside analogues or other agents that interfere with viral DNA replication. One of these medications is acyclovir.[152] Acyclovir is highly selective against cells infected with HSV or other herpesviruses that encode thymidine kinases.[153–155] This selectivity is based on properties of two of the viral enzymes involved in DNA replication. First, acyclovir is initially phosphorylated to the monophosphate form by a viral-encoded thymidine kinase (TK) but not by cellular kinases.[152,156] Subsequent phosphorylation to the active triphosphate form is by cellular kinases. Second, viral DNA polymerase is more sensitive to inhibition by phosphorylated acyclovir than are cell DNA polymerases.[152,157,158] Unfortunately, mutations in either of these viral enzymes can render virus resistant to acyclovir. For the most part, clinically significant disease caused by resistant viral mutants is limited to immunosuppressed patients. Most acyclovir-resistant isolates are deficient in TK production, although missense mutations in the viral TK or in the viral DNA polymerase gene also can confer resistance.[159] Although resistant HSV isolates can be selected for after prolonged therapy with acyclovir, reactivated virus causing subsequent recurrences often retains susceptibility to the medication.[160,161] Valacyclovir is a prodrug of acyclovir that has increased oral bioavailability and is rapidly metabolized to acyclovir.[162]

Acyclovir is less effective against CMV, apparently because CMV does not encode a TK. Ganciclovir is more effective against CMV than acyclovir. Although generation of ganciclovir monophosphate requires HSV TK in HSV-infected cells,[163] initial phosphorylation in CMV-infected cells is by a CMV protein kinase, phosphotransferase (UL97).[164,165] Resistance to ganciclovir can result from mutations in this protein kinase.[164–166]

Newer nucleoside analogues include penciclovir and famciclovir. Penciclovir, like acyclovir, also requires initial phosphorylation by viral TK.[167] Although penciclovir inhibits viral DNA polymerase less effectively than acyclovir, high intracellular levels of the phosphorylated drug and its longer intracellular half-life result in viral inhibition similar to that achieved with acyclovir.[168,169] Famciclovir is itself inactive, but it is converted to penciclovir following absorption through the intestinal wall.[170] Ganciclovir, penciclovir, or famciclovir cannot be used to treat TK-deficient strains of HSV. In contrast, strains resistant to acyclovir because of mutations in the HSV DNA polymerase may still be sensitive to one or more of these medications.[171] However, because most resistant strains are deficient in TK production, foscarnet therapy should be considered for clinically significant disease caused by acyclovir-resistant HSV and VZV isolates.[172] Foscarnet is a pyrophosphate analogue that noncompetitively inhibits the viral DNA polymerase.[173–175] Isolates of HSV, CMV, and VZV that are resistant to foscarnet because of mutations in the viral DNA polymerase have been described.[176–180] Because foscarnet requires intravenous administration, topical application of trifluridine may be considered in select patients.[181] Both cellular and viral-encoded TK can initiate phosphorylation of trifluridine.[182] As a result, trifluridine is too toxic to be used systemically but can be used topically to treat TK-deficient strains of herpesviruses.

Vidarabine is an analogue of adenosine that is highly effective at inhibiting HSV and VZV replication.[183] The mechanism by which vidarabine inhibits viral replication is not known. Although vidarabine inhibits viral DNA synthesis, it is not an absolute chain terminator.[184] Vidarabine can be used to treat TK-deficient viral strains, but foscarnet is more efficacious and is currently recommended.[172] Specific therapies are discussed in greater detail in Chap. 21.

As more is learned about the molecular interactions essential for herpesvirus replication and for the establishment of latency, attention is likely to be focused on developing new drugs or agents that can block interactions specifically required by the virus. Known inhibitory agents, even if not therapeutically useful, can provide structural information needed to design clinically acceptable drugs with antiviral activity. For example, analogues of heparin might bind selectively to HSV and block its adsorption to cells without possessing all the other pharmacologic activities of heparin. Preliminary results indicate that topical derivatives of heparin may be useful for preventing genital HSV infections.[185] Similarly, finding compounds that can block the interaction between HSV and entry mediators such as HVEM may lead to the development of medications that can prevent initial HSV infections.

Clues about essential and potentially inhibitable molecular interactions also come from findings that cells expressing certain HSV gene products are resistant to infection by or replication of HSV. As mentioned earlier, cells expressing HSV gD are resistant to HSV entry.[186,187] In addition, viral gene expression is aborted in cells expressing a mutant form of the HSV regulatory protein VP16.[188] In both instances, it is likely that the viral protein expressed by the infected cell saturates sites on cell components required for interaction with the infecting virus. When the cell components have been identified and the nature of the virus-cell interactions defined, it may be possible to design drugs that can block the required interactions without toxicity to uninfected cells.

VACCINES

Currently available vaccines prevent or attenuate clinical disease but do not necessarily prevent infection. The goal in vaccination has been to induce immunity that is equivalent to that induced during recovery from natural disease and which often confers long-lasting protection against another episode of the disease. Vaccine development poses greater challenges in the case of herpesviruses because recovery from natural disease is not associated with elimination of virus and does not always protect against another episode of disease.

Live-attenuated, killed, and recombinant subunit herpesvirus vaccines have all been studied. Whole-virus vaccines have the advantage of exposing the immune system to all viral antigens. Live-attenuated vaccines have tended to produce longer-lasting immunity than killed preparations. However, live-attenuated herpesvirus vaccines may be capable of establishing latent infections. The subsequent risks are not clear, and there is concern that vaccine recipients who subsequently become immunosuppressed may develop disease caused by reactivated virus. Two avirulent HSV strains have been shown to generate lethal recombinants in mice.[189] Thus recombination between an attenuated vaccine strain and a superinfecting wild-type strain could occur. Because several herpesviruses have been associated with malignancies in humans, the long-term safety of any live-attenuated vaccine needs careful study. The establishment of a latent infection is not a concern with subunit vaccines. However, effective subunit vaccines require knowledge as to which viral proteins are the best immunogens for protective immunity.

Live-attenuated VZV vaccines are effective at decreasing the incidence of chickenpox.[190–197] The attenuated strains in the vaccines can induce latent infections.[198,199] Although long-term follow-up is relatively limited, the rate at which zoster develops in vaccine recipients appears to be no greater and may even be lower than the incidence after natural infection.[200–202] Vaccination with a live-attenuated CMV strain has significantly reduced the incidence of severe CMV disease in previously uninfected renal transplant recipients.[203–205] No clinical benefit, however, was noted in patients seropositive for CMV before vaccination. As of yet, there is no evidence that the attenuated CMV vaccine strain can establish a latent infection.[205,206] Preliminary results indicate that a recombinant CMV gB subunit vaccine is well tolerated and induces significant increases in antibody titers.[207]

In addition to preventing initial disease, another goal of vaccination may be to bolster the natural immunity of persons already infected and therefore prevent recurrent disease. For HSV, several different recombinant subunit vaccines have been tested successfully in animal models.[208–211] In persons seronegative for HSV-2, immunization with a subunit vaccine containing both HSV-2 gB and gD has resulted in humoral and cellular immune responses equivalent to or greater than those typically seen with natural infections.[212] In another study of persons with recurrent genital herpes, recipients of a HSV-2 gD subunit vaccine had fewer and less severe recurrences than placebo recipients.[213] The vaccine recipients in this study had higher titers of neutralizing antibodies. The feasibility of nucleic acid vaccines has been demonstrated in other systems.[214,215] Recently, a nucleic acid vaccine encoding HSV-2 gB was shown to be immunogenic and to protect mice from HSV-2 disease.[216]

SUMMARY

Despite the remarkable diversity of the human herpesviruses with respect to the diseases they cause, latent infection and subsequent reactivation of viral replication are key aspects of the biology and pathology of them all. The prevalence and epidemiology of herpesvirus-induced diseases are determined in large part by the fact that latently infected persons experience periodic reactivation and production of transmissible virus, whether or not clinical symptoms accompany the virus production. The management of immunocompromised patients is complicated by the facts that most of us carry one or more latent herpesviruses and that reactivation of these viruses can be devastating in the absence of normal immune responses. In immunocompetent persons, however, it is principally HSV, and to a lesser extent VZV, that causes recurrent disease through reactivation of latent virus. This kind of disease poses difficult but interesting challenges for prevention and treatment.

ACKNOWLEDGMENTS

We thank Drs. John Phair, Richard Longnecker, and Stephen Miller for critical reviews of this chapter.

References

1 Chang Y, Cesarman E, Pessin MS, et al: Identification of herpesvirus-like DNA sequences in AIDS-associated Kaposi's sarcoma. *Science* 266:1865–1869, 1994.

2 Roizman B, Baines J: The diversity and unity of Herpesviridae. *Comp Immunol Microbiol Infect Dis* 14:63–70, 1991.

3 Roizman B, Carmichael LE, Deinhardt F, et al: Herpesviridae: Definition, provisional nomenclature and taxonomy. *Intervirology* 16: 201–217, 1981.

4 Steven AC, Spear PG: Herpesvirus Capsid Assembly and Envelopment, in Structural Biology of Viruses, W Chiu, R Burnett, R Garcea (eds). New York, Oxford University Press, 1997.

5 Collier AC, Meyers JD, Corey L, et al: Cytomegalovirus infection in homosexual men: Relationship to sexual practices, antibody to human immunodeficiency virus, and cell-mediated immunity. *Am J Med* 82:593–601, 1987.

6 Bryson Y, Dillon M, Bernstein DI, et al: Risk of acquisition of genital herpes simplex virus type 2 in sex partners of persons with genital herpes: A prospective couple study. *J Infect Dis* 167:942–946, 1993.

7 Miller G, Niederman JC, Andrews L-L: Prolonged oropharyngeal excretion of Epstein-Barr virus after infectious mononucleosis. *N Engl J Med* 288:229–232, 1973.

8 Gompels UA, Nicholas J, Lawrence G, et al: The DNA sequence of human herpesvirus-6: Structure, coding content, and genome evolution. Virology 209:29–51, 1995.

9 Kouzarides T, Bankier AT, Satchwell SC, et al: Large-scale rearrangement of homologous regions in the genomes of HCMV and EBV. *Virology* 157:397–413, 1987.

10 Davison AJ, McGeoch DJ: Evolutionary comparisons of the S segments in the genomes of herpes simplex virus type 1 and varicella zoster virus. *J Gen Virol* 67:597–611, 1986.

11 Davison AJ, Taylor P: Genetic relations between varicella-zoster virus and Epstein-Barr virus. *J Gen Virol* 68:1067–1079, 1987.

12 McGeoch DJ, Dalrymple MA, Davison AJ, et al: The complete DNA sequence of the long unique region in the genome of herpes simplex virus type 1. J Gen Virol 69:1531–1574, 1988.

13 Baer R, Bankier AT, Biggin MD, et al: DNA sequence and expression of the B95–8 Epstein-Barr virus genome. Nature 310:207–211, 1984.

14 Mocarski ES: Cytomegalovirus and Their Replication, in *Virology,* vol 2, 3d ed, BN Fields, DM Knipe, PM Howley (eds). Philadelphia, Lippincott-Raven, 1996, pp 2447–2492.

15 Plummer G: Serological comparison of the herpes viruses. *Br J Exp Pathol* 45:135–141, 1964.

16 Schneweis KE: Serologische Untersuchungen zur Typendifferenzierung des Herpesvirus hominis. *Z Immunitatsforsch Exp Ther* 124: 24–48, 1962.

17 Nahmias AJ, Dowdle WR: Antigenic and biologic differences in herpesvirus hominis. *Progr Med Virol* 10:110–159, 1968.

18 Lafferty WE, Coombs RW, Benedetti J, et al: Recurrences after oral and genital herpes simplex virus infection: Influence of site of infection and viral type. *N Engl J Med* 316:1444–1449, 1987.

19 Gentry GA, Lowe M, Alford G, Nevins R: Sequence analyses of herpesviral enzymes suggest an ancient origin for human sexual behavior. *Proc Natl Acad Sci USA* 85:2658–2661, 1988.

20 Kieff E: Epstein-Barr Virus and Its Replication, in *Virology,* vol 2, 3d ed, BN Fields, DM Knipe, PM Howley (eds). Philadelphia, Lippincott-Raven, 1996, pp 2343–2396.

21 Rickinson AB, Young LS, Rowe M: Influence of the Epstein-Barr virus nuclear antigen EBNA 2 on the growth phenotype of virus-transformed B cells. *J Virol* 61:1310–1317, 1987.

22 Moore PS, Gao SJ, Dominguez G, et al: Primary characterization of a herpesvirus agent associated with Kaposi's sarcoma. *J Virol* 70: 549–558, 1996.

23 Fleckenstein B, Desrosiers RC: Herpesvirus saimiri and Herpesvirus ateles, in *The Herpesviruses,* vol 1, B Roizman (ed). New York, Plenum Press, 1982, pp 253–332.

24 Ambroziak JA, Blackbourn DJ, Herndier BG, et al: Herpes-like sequences in HIV-infected and uninfected Kaposi's sarcoma patients. *Science* 268:582–583, 1995.

25 Cesarman E, Nador RG, Bai F, et al: Kaposi's sarcoma-associated herpesvirus contains G protein–coupled receptor and cyclin D homologues which are expressed in Kaposi's sarcoma and malignant lymphoma. *J Virol* 70:8218–8223, 1996.

26 Josey WE, Nahmias AJ, Naib ZM: The epidemiology of type 2 (genital) herpes simplex virus infection. *Obstet Gynecol Surv* 27:295–302, 1972.

27 Chretien JH, McGinniss G, Muller A: Veneral causes of cytomegalovirus mononucleosis. *JAMA* 238:1644–1645, 1977.

28 Lin J-C, Lin S-C, Mar E-C, et al: Is Kaposi's sarcoma–associated herpesvirus detectable in semen of HIV-infected homosexual men? *Lancet* 346:1601–1602, 1995.

29 Monini P, De Lellis L, Fabris M, et al: Kaposi's sarcoma–associated herpesvirus DNA sequences in prostate tissue and human semen. *N Engl J Med* 334:1168–1172, 1996.

30 Hayward GS, Frenkel N, Roizman B: Anatomy of herpes simplex virus DNA: Strain differences and heterogeneity in the locations of restriction endonuclease cleavage sites. *Proc Natl Acad Sci USA* 72: 1768–1772, 1975.

31 Buchman TG, Roizman B, Adams G, Stover BH: Restriction endonuclease fingerprinting of herpes simplex virus DNA: A novel epidemiological tool applied to a nosocomial outbreak. *J Infect Dis* 138: 488–498, 1978.

32 Hammer SM, Buchman TG, D'Angelo LJ, et al: Temporal cluster of herpes simplex encephalitis: Investigation by restriction endonuclease cleavage of viral DNA. *J Infect Dis* 141:436–440, 1980.

33 Buchman TG, Roizman B, Nahmias AJ: Demonstration of exogenous genital reinfection with herpes simplex virus type 2 by restriction endonuclease fingerprinting of viral DNA. *J Infect Dis* 140:295–304, 1979.

34 Spector SA, Hirata KK, Neuman TR: Identification of multiple cytomegalovirus strains in homosexual men with acquired immunodeficiency syndrome. *J Infect Dis* 150:953–956, 1984.

35 Drew WL, Sweet ES, Miner RC, Mocarski ES: Multiple infections by cytomegalovirus in patients with acquired immunodeficiency syndrome: Documentation by Southern blot hybridization. *J Infect Dis* 150:952–953, 1984.

36 Stinski MF: Sequence of protein synthesis in cells infected by human cytomegalovirus: Early and late virus-induced polypeptides. *J Virol* 26:686–701, 1978.

37 Honess RW, Roizman B: Regulation of herpesvirus macromolecular synthesis: I. Cascade regulation of the synthesis of three groups of viral proteins. *J Virol* 14:8–19, 1974.

38 Jondal M, Klein G, Oldstone MBA, et al: Surface markers on human B and T lymphocytes: VIII. Association between complement and Epstein-Barr virus receptors on human lymphoid cells. *Scand J Immunol* 5:401–410, 1976.

39 Ahearn JM, Harward SD, Hickey JC, Fearon DT: Epstein-Barr virus (EBV) infection of murine L cells expressing recombinant human EBV/C3d receptor. *Proc Natl Acad Sci USA* 85:9307–9311, 1988.

40 DeMarchi JM: Nature of the block in the expression of some early virus genes in cells abortively infected with human cytomegalovirus. *Virology* 129:287–297, 1983.

41 Spear PG: Entry of alpha herpesviruses into cells. *Semin Virol* 4:167–180, 1993.

42 Stannard LM, Fuller AO, Spear PG: Herpes simplex virus glycoprotein associated with different morphological entities projecting from the virion envelope. *J Gen Virol* 68:715–725, 1987.

43 Montgomery RI, Warner MS, Lum BJ, Spear PG: Herpes simplex virus-1 entry into cells mediated by a novel member of the TNF/NGF receptor family. *Cell* 87:427–436, 1996.

43a Warner MS, Geraghty RJ, Martinez WM, et al: A cell surface protein with herpesvirus entry activity (Hve B) confers susceptibility to infection by mutants of herpes simplex virus type 1, herpes simplex virus type 2, and pseudorabies virus. *Virology* 246:179–189, 1998.

43b Geraghty RJ, Krummeracher L, Cohen GH, Eisenberg RJ, Spear PG. Alphaherpesvirus entry mediated by poliovirus receptor related protein 1 and poliovirus receptor. *Science* 280:1618–1620, 1998.

44 Cooper NR: Early Events in Human Herpesvirus Infection of Cells, in *Cellular Receptors for Animal Viruses,* E Wimmer (ed). Plainview, NY, Cold Spring Harbor Laboratory Press, 1994, pp 365–388.

45 Herrold RE, Marchini A, Fruehling S, Longnecker R: Glycoprotein 110, the Epstein-Barr virus homologue of herpes simplex virus glycoprotein B, is essential for Epstein-Barr virus replication in vivo. *J Virol* 70:2049–2054, 1996.

46 Compton T: Towards a definition of the HCMV entry pathway. *Scand J Infect Dis* S99:30–32, 1995.

47 Roizman B, Sears AE: Herpes Simplex Viruses and Their Replication, in *Field's Virology,* vol 2, 3d ed, BN Fields, DM Knipe, PM Howley (eds). Philadelphia, Lippincott-Raven, 1996, pp 2231–2295.

48 Morgan C, Ellison SA, Rose HM, Moore DH: Structure and development of viruses as observed in the electron microscope. *J Exp Med* 100:195–202, 1954.

49 Fenwick ML, Walker MJ: Suppression of the synthesis of cellular macromolecules by herpes simplex virus. *J Gen Virol* 41:37–51, 1978.

50 Spear PG: Membrane Fusion Induced by Herpes Simplex Virus, in *Viral Fusion Mechanisms,* J Bentz (ed). Boca Raton, FL, CRC Press, 1993, pp 201–232.

51 Fraser NW, Valyi-Nagy T: Viral, neuronal and immune factors which may influence herpes simplex virus (HSV) latency and reactivation. *Microb Pathog* 15:83–91, 1993.

52 Stevens JG, Haarr L, Porter DD, et al: Prominence of the herpes simplex virus latency-associated transcript in trigeminal ganglia from seropositive humans. *J Infect Dis* 158:117–123, 1988.

53 Stevens JG, Wagner EK, Devi-Rao GB, et al: RNA complementary to a herpesvirus alpha gene mRNA is prominent in latently infected neurons. *Science* 235:1056–1059, 1987.

54 Reeves WC, Corey L, Adams HG, et al: Risk of recurrence after first episodes of genital herpes Relation to HSV type and antibody response. *N Engl J Med* 305:315–319, 1981.

55 Qu L, Rowe DT: Epstein-Barr virus latent gene expression in uncultured peripheral blood lymphocytes. *J Virol* 66:3715–3724, 1992.

56 Tierney RJ, Steven N, Young LS, Rickinson AB: Epstein-Barr virus latency in blood mononuclear cells: Analysis of viral gene transcription during primary infection and in the carrier state. *J Virol* 68: 7374–7385, 1994.

57 Mosialos G, Birkenbach M, Yalamanchili R, et al: The Epstein-Barr virus transforming protein LMP1 engages signaling proteins for the tumor necrosis factor receptor family. *Cell* 80:389–399, 1995.

58 Tolpin MD, Stewart JA, Warren D, et al: Transfusion transmission of cytomegalovirus confirmed by restriction endonuclease analysis. *J Pediatr* 107:953–956, 1985.

59 Lang DJ, Ebert PA, Rodgers BM, et al: Reduction of postperfusion cytomegalovirus-infections following the use of leukocyte depleted blood. *Transfusion* 17:391–395, 1977.

60 Kane RC, Rousseau WE, Noble GR, et al: Cytomegalovirus infection in a volunteer blood donor population. *Infect Immun* 11:719–723, 1975.

61 Kondo K, Kaneshima H, Mocarski ES: Human cytomegalovirus latent infection of granulocyte-macrophage progenitors. *Proc Natl Acad Sci USA* 91:11879–11883, 1994.

62 Kondo K, Mocarski ES: Cytomegalovirus latency and latency-specific transcription in hematopoietic progenitors. *Scand J Infect Dis Suppl* 99:63–67, 1995.

63 Waldman WJ, Knight DA, Huang EH, Sedmak DD: Bidirectional transmission of infectious cytomegalovirus between monocytes and vascular endothelial cells: An in vitro model. *J Infect Dis* 171:263–272, 1995.

64 Welch AR, McGregor LM, Gibson W: Cytomegalovirus homologues of cellular G protein-coupled receptor genes are transcribed. *J Virol* 65:3915–3918, 1991.

65 Chee MS, Satchwell SC, Preddie E, et al: Human cytomegalovirus encodes three G protein–coupled receptor homologues. *Nature* 344: 774–777, 1990.

66 Jault FM, Jault JM, Ruchti F, et al: Cytomegalovirus infection induces high levels of cyclins, phosphorylated Rb, and p53, leading to cell cycle arrest. *J Virol* 69:6697–6704, 1995.

67 Cesarman E, Chang Y, Moore PS, et al: Kaposi's sarcoma–associated herpesvirus-like DNA sequences in AIDS-related body-cavity-based lymphomas. *N Engl J Med* 332:1186–1191, 1995.

68 Boshoff C, Schulz TF, Kennedy MM, et al: Kaposi's sarcoma–associated herpesvirus infects endothelial and spindle cells. *Nature Med* 1:1274–1278, 1995.

69 Gao S-J, Kingsley L, Hoover DR, et al: Seroconversion to antibodies against Kaposi's sarcoma–associated herpesvirus-related latent nuclear antigens before the development of Kaposi's sarcoma. *N Engl J Med* 335:233–241, 1996.

70 Foreman KE, Friborg J, Kong W-P, et al: Propagation of a human herpesvirus from AIDS-associated Kaposi's sarcoma. *N Engl J Med* 336:163–171, 1997.

71 Rawls WE: Herpes Simplex Viruses and Their Roles in Human Cancer, in *The Herpesviruses,* vol 3, B Roizman (ed). New York, Plenum Press, 1985, pp 241–255.

72 Galloway DA, McDougall JK: The oncogenic potential of herpes simplex viruses: Evidence for a "hit-and-run" mechanism. *Nature* 302: 21–24, 1983.

73 Metcalf JF, Kaufman HE: Herpetic stromal keratitis: Evidence for cell-mediated immunopathogenesis. *Am J Ophthalmol* 82:827–834, 1976.

74 Corey L, Spear PG: Infections with herpes simplex viruses. *N Engl J Med* 314:686–691, 1986.

75 Whitley RJ: Herpes Simplex Virus, in *Field's Virology,* vol 2, 3d ed, BN Fields, DM Knipe, PM Howley (eds). Philadelphia, Lippincott-Raven, 1996, pp 2297–2342.

76 Douglas JM Jr, Davis LG, Remington ML, et al: A double-blind, placebo-controlled trial of the effect of chronically administered oral acyclovir on sperm production in men with frequently recurrent genital herpes. *J Infect Dis* 157:588–593, 1988.

77 Spruance SL: Pathogenesis of herpes simplex labialis: Excretion of virus in the oral cavity. *J Clin Microbiol* 19:675–679, 1984.

78 Rattray MC, Corey L, Reeves WC, et al: Recurrent genital herpes among women: Symptomatic versus asymptomatic viral shedding. *Br J Vener Dis* 54:262–265, 1978.

79 Eisenberg RJ, Cerini CP, Heilman CJ, et al: Synthetic glycoprotein D–related peptides protect mice against herpes simplex virus challenge. *J Virol* 56:1014–1017, 1985.

80 Balachandran N, Bacchetti S, Rawls WE: Protection against lethal challenge of BALB/c mice by passive transfer of monoclonal antibodies to five glycoproteins of herpes simplex virus type 2. *Infect Immun* 37:1132–1137, 1982.

81 Norrild B, Shore SL, Cromeans TL, Nahmias AJ: Participation of three major glycoprotein antigens of herpes simplex virus type 1 early in the infectious cycle as determined by antibody-dependent cell-mediated cytotoxicity. *Infect Immun* 28:38–44, 1980.

82 Dix RD, Pereira L, Baringer JR: Use of monoclonal antibody directed against herpes simplex virus glycoproteins to protect mice against acute virus-induced neurological disease. *Infect Immun* 34:192–199, 1981.

83 Prober CG, Sullender WM, Yasukawa LL, et al: Low risk of herpes simplex virus infections in neonates exposed to the virus at the time of vaginal delivery to mothers with recurrent genital herpes simplex virus infections. *N Engl J Med* 316:240–244, 1987.

84 Sullender WM, Miller JL, Yasukawa LL, et al: Humoral and cell-mediated immunity in neonates with herpes simplex virus infection. *J Infect Dis* 155:28–37, 1987.

85 Kohl S, Frazier JP, Pickering LK, Loo LS: Normal function of neonatal polymorphonuclear leukocytes in antibody-dependent cellular-cytotoxicity to herpes simplex virus-infected cells. *J Pediatr* 98:783–785, 1981.

86 Pass RF, Whitley RJ, Whelchel JD, et al: Identification of patients with increased risk of infection with herpes simplex virus after renal transplantation. *J Infect Dis* 140:487–492, 1979.

87 Zweerink HJ, Corey L: Virus-specific antibodies in sera from patients with genital herpes simplex virus infection. *Infect Immun* 37:413–421, 1982.

88 Yasukawa M, Zarling JM: Human cytotoxic T cell clones directed against herpes simplex virus-infected cells: I. Lysis restricted by HLA class II MB and DR antigens. *J Immunol* 133:422–427, 1984.

89 Yasukawa M, Shiroguchi T, Kobayashi Y: HLA-restricted T lymphocyte-mediated cytotoxicity against herpes simplex virus-infected cells in humans. *Infect Immun* 40:190–197, 1983.

90 Yasukawa M, Zarling JM: Autologous herpes simplex virus-infected cells are lysed by human natural killer cells. *J Immunol* 131:2011–2016, 1983.

91 Lopez C, Kirkpatrick D, Read SE, et al: Correlation between low natural killing of fibroblasts infected with herpes simplex virus type 1 and susceptibility to herpesvirus infections. *J Infect Dis* 147:1030–1035, 1983.

92 Ching C, Lopez C: Natural killing of herpes simplex virus type 1–infected target cells: Normal human responses and influence of antiviral antibody. *Infect Immun* 26:49–56, 1979.

93 Wagner H, Feldmann M, Boyle W, Schrader JW: Cell-mediated immune response in vitro: 3. The requirement for macrophages in cytotoxic reactions against cell-bound and subcellular alloantigens. *J Exp Med* 136:331–343, 1972.

94 Zinkernagel RM, Doherty PC: Immunological surveillance against altered self components by sensitised T lymphocytes in lymphocytic choriomeningitis. *Nature* 251:547–548, 1974.

95 Hill A, Jugovic P, York I, et al: Herpes simplex virus turns off the TAP to evade host immunity. *Nature* 375:411–415, 1995.

96 Fruh K, Ahn K, Djaballah H, et al: A viral inhibitor of peptide transporters for antigen presentation. *Nature* 375:415–418, 1995.

97 York IA, Roop C, Andrews DW, et al: A cytosolic herpes simplex virus protein inhibits antigen presentation to CD8+ T lymphocytes. *Cell* 77:525--535, 1994.

98 Martin S, Courtney RJ, Fowler G, Rouse BT: Herpes simplex virus type 1-specific cytotoxic T lymphocytes recognize virus nonstructural proteins. *J Virol* 62:2265–2273, 1988.

99 Reddehase MJ, Koszinowski UH: Significance of herpesvirus immediate early gene expression in cellular immunity to cytomegalovirus infection. *Nature* 312:369–371, 1984.

100 Dubin G, Fishman NO, Eisenberg RJ, et al: The role of herpes simplex virus glycoproteins in immune evasion. *Curr Top Microbiol Immunol* 179:111–120, 1992.

101 Stroop WG, Schaefer DC: Production of encephalitis restricted to the temporal lobes by experimental reactivation of herpes simplex virus. *J Infect Dis* 153:721–731, 1986.

102 Barnett EM, Jacobsen G, Evans G, et al: Herpes simplex encephalitis in the temporal cortex and limbic system after trigeminal nerve inoculation. *J Infect Dis* 169:782–786, 1994.

103 Davis LE, Johnson RT: An explanation for the localization of herpes simplex encephalitis? *Ann Neurol* 5:2–5, 1979.

104 Johnson RT: The pathogenesis of herpes virus encephalitis: I. Virus pathways to the nervous system of suckling mice demonstrated by fluorescent antibody staining. *J Exp Med* 119:343–356, 1964.

105 Fraser NW, Lawrence WC, Wroblewska Z, et al: Herpes simplex type 1 DNA in human brain tissue. *Proc Natl Acad Sci USA* 78:6461–6465, 1981.

106 Baringer JR, Pisani P: Herpes simplex virus genomes in human nervous system tissue analyzed by polymerase chain reaction. *Ann Neurol* 36:823–829, 1994.

107 Jamieson GA, Maitland NJ, Wilcock GK, et al: Latent herpes simplex virus type 1 in normal and Alzheimer's disease brains. *J Med Virol* 33:224–227, 1991.

108 Sequiera LW, Jennings LC, Carrasco LH, et al: Detection of herpes-simplex viral genome in brain tissue. *Lancet* 2:609–612, 1979.

109 Chou J, Kern ER, Whitley RJ, Roizman B: Mapping of herpes simplex virus-1 neurovirulence to gamma-1 34.5, a gene nonessential for growth in culture. *Science* 250:1262–1266, 1990.

110 Perng GC, Ghiasi H, Slanina SM, et al: High-dose ocular infection with a herpes simplex virus type 1 ICP34.5 deletion mutant produces no corneal disease or neurovirulence yet results in wild-type levels of spontaneous reactivation. *J Virol* 70:2883–2893, 1996.

111 Perng GC, Thompson RL, Sawtell NM, et al: An avirulent ICP34.5 deletion mutant of herpes simplex virus type 1 is capable of in vivo spontaneous reactivation. *J Virol* 69:3033–3041, 1995.

112 Robertson LM, MacLean AR, Brown SM: Peripheral replication and latency reactivation kinetics of the non-neurovirulent herpes simplex virus type 1 variant 1716. *J Gen Virol* 73:967–970, 1992.

113 Rickinson AB, Kieff E: Epstein-Barr Virus, in *Field's Virology*, vol 2, 3d ed, BN Fields, DM Knipe, PM Howley (eds). Philadelphia, Lippincott-Raven, 1996, pp 2397–2446.

114 Henle G, Henle W: The Virus as the Etiologic Agent of Infectious Mononucleosis, in *The Epstein-Barr Virus*, MA Epstein, BG Achong (eds). New York, Springer-Verlag, 1979, pp 297–320.

115 Evans AS, Niederman JC, Cenabre LC, et al: A prospective evaluation of heterophile and Epstein-Barr virus-specific IgM antibody tests in clinical and subclinical infectious mononucleosis: Specificity and sensitivity of the tests and persistence of antibody. *J Infect Dis* 132:546–554, 1975.

116 Schooley RT: Epstein-Barr Virus (Infectious Mononucleosis), in *Principles and Practice of Infectious Diseases*, 4th ed, GL Mandell, JE Bennett, R Dolin (eds). New York, Churchill-Livingstone, 1995, pp 1364–1377.

117 Mold C, Bradt BM, Nemerow GR, Cooper NR: Epstein-Barr virus regulates activation and processing of the third component of complement. *J Exp Med* 168:949–969, 1988.

118 Hsu DH, de Waal Malefyt R, Fiorentino DF, et al: Expression of interleukin-10 activity by Epstein-Barr virus protein BCRF1. *Science* 250:830–832, 1990.

119 Fiorentino DF, Zlotnik A, Vieira P, et al: IL-10 acts on the antigen-presenting cell to inhibit cytokine production by Th1 cells. *J Immunol* 146:3444–3451, 1991.

120 Vieira P, de Waal-Malefyt R, Dang MN, et al: Isolation and expression of human cytokine synthesis inhibitory factor cDNA clones: homology to Epstein-Barr virus open reading frame BCRFI. *Proc Natl Acad Sci USA* 88:1172–1176, 1991.

121 Gosselin J, Menezes J, Mercier G, et al: Differential interleukin-2 and interferon-gamma production by human lymphocyte cultures exceptionally resistant to Epstein-Barr virus immortalization. *Cell Immunol* 122:440–449, 1989.

122 Masucci MG, Torsteindottir S, Colombani J, et al: Down-regulation of class I HLA antigens and of the Epstein-Barr virus-encoded latent membrane protein in Burkitt lymphoma lines. *Proc Natl Acad Sci USA* 84:4567–4571, 1987.

123 van der Horst C, Joncas J, Ahronheim G, et al: Lack of effect of peroral acyclovir for the treatment of acute infectious mononucleosis. *J Infect Dis* 164:788–792, 1991.

124 Ernberg I, Andersson J: Acyclovir efficiently inhibits oropharyngeal excretion of Epstein-Barr virus in patients with acute infectious mononucleosis. *J Gen Virol* 67:2267–2272, 1986.

125 Andersson J, Britton S, Ernberg I, et al: Effect of acyclovir on infectious mononucleosis: A double-blind, placebo-controlled study. *J Infect Dis* 153:283–290, 1986.

126 Bender CE: The value of corticosteroids in the treatment of infectious mononucleosis. *JAMA* 199:529–531, 1967.

127 Schumacher HR, Jacobson WA, Bemiller CR: Treatment of infectious mononucleosis. *Ann Intern Med* 58:217–228, 1963.

128 Britt WJ, Alford CA: Cytomegalovirus, in *Field's Virology*, vol 2, 3d ed, BN Fields, DM Knipe, PM Howley (eds). Philadelphia, Lippincott-Raven, 1996 pp. 2493–2523.

129 Pertel P, Hirschtick R, Phair J, et al: Risk of developing cytomegalovirus retinitis in persons infected with the human immunodeficiency virus. *J Acquir Immune Defic Syndr* 5:1069–1074, 1992.

130 Sirianni MC, Volpi A, Soddu S, et al: Immune response to cytomegalovirus in patients with acquired-immunodeficiency syndrome related complex (ARC) and AIDS. *Eur J Epidemiol* 3:439–441, 1987.

131 Quinnan GV Jr, Burns WH, Kirmani N, et al: HLA-restricted cytotoxic T lymphocytes are an early immune response and important defense mechanism in cytomegalovirus infections. *Rev Infect Dis* 6: 156–163, 1984.

132 Riddell SR, Watanabe KS, Goodrich JM, et al: Restoration of viral immunity in immunodeficient humans by the adoptive transfer of T cell clones. *Science* 257:238–241, 1992.

133 Weir MR, Irwin BC, Maters AW, et al: Incidence of cytomegalovirus disease in cyclosporine-treated renal transplant recipients based on donor/recipient pretransplant immunity. *Transplantation* 43:187–193, 1987.

134 Pass RF, Reynolds DW, Whelchel JD, et al: Impaired lymphocyte transformation response to cytomegalovirus and phytohemagglutinin in recipients of renal transplants: Association with antithymocyte globulin. *J Infect Dis* 143:259–265, 1981.

135 Cheeseman SH, Rubin RH, Stewart JA, et al: Controlled clinical trial of prophylactic human-leukocyte interferon in renal transplantation: Effects on cytomegalovirus and herpes simplex virus infections. *N Engl J Med* 300:1345–1349, 1979.

136 Dowling JN, Saslow AR, Armstrong JA, Ho M: Cytomegalovirus infection in patients receiving immunosuppressive therapy for rheumatologic disorders. *J Infect Dis* 133:399–408, 1976.

137 Kapasi K, Rice GP: Cytomegalovirus infection of peripheral blood mononuclear cells: Effects on interleukin-1 and -2 production and responsiveness. *J Virol* 62:3603–3607, 1988.

138 Schrier RD, Rice GP, Oldstone MB: Suppression of natural killer cell activity and T cell proliferation by fresh isolates of human cytomegalovirus. *J Infect Dis* 153:1084–1091, 1986.

139 Carney WP, Hirsch MS: Mechanisms of immunosuppression in cytomegalovirus mononucleosis II. Virus-monocyte interactions. *J Infect Dis* 144:47–54, 1981.

140 AbuBakar S, Boldogh I, Albrecht T: Human cytomegalovirus stimulates arachidonic acid metabolism through pathways that are affected by inhibitors of phospholipase A2 and protein kinase C. *Biochem Biophys Res Commun* 166:953–959, 1990.

141 Skolnik PR, Kosloff BR, Hirsch MS: Bidirectional interactions between human immunodeficiency virus type 1 and cytomegalovirus. *J Infect Dis* 157:508–514, 1988.

142 Davis MG, Kenney SC, Kamine J, et al: Immediate-early gene region of human cytomegalovirus trans-activates the promoter of human immunodeficiency virus. *Proc Natl Acad Sci USA* 84:8642–8646, 1987.

143 Banks TA, Rouse BT: Herpesviruses: Immune escape artists? *Clin Infect Dis* 14:933–941, 1992.

144 Xu-Bin, Murayama T, Ishida K, Furukawa T: Characterization of IgG Fc receptors induced by human cytomegalovirus. *J Gen Virol* 70: 893–900, 1989.

145 Balachandran N, Oba DE, Hutt-Fletcher LM: Antigenic cross-reactions among herpes simplex virus types 1 and 2, Epstein-Barr virus, and cytomegalovirus. *J Virol* 61:1125–1135, 1987.

146 McKeating JA, Griffiths PD, Weiss RA: HIV susceptibility conferred to human fibroblasts by cytomegalovirus-induced Fc receptor. *Nature* 343:659–661, 1990.

147 Grundy JE, McKeating JA, Griffiths PD: Cytomegalovirus strain AD169 binds beta 2 microglobulin in vitro after release from cells. *J Gen Virol* 68:777–784, 1987.

148 McKeating JA, Griffiths PD, Grundy JE: Cytomegalovirus in urine specimens has host $beta_2$ microglobulin bound to the viral envelope: A mechanism of evading the host immune response? *J Gen Virol* 68: 785–792, 1987.

149 Beck S, Barrell BG: Human cytomegalovirus encodes a glycoprotein homologous to MHC class-I antigens. *Nature* 331:269–272, 1988.

150 Browne H, Smith G, Beck S, Minson T: A complex between the MHC class I homologue encoded by human cytomegalovirus and b2 microglobulin. *Nature* 347:770–772, 1990.

151 Browne H, Churcher M, Minson T: Construction and characterization of a human cytomegalovirus mutant with the UL18 (class I homologue) gene deleted. *J Virol* 66:6784–6787, 1992.

152 Elion GB, Furman PA, Fyfe JA, et al: Selectivity of action of an antiherpetic agent, 9-(2-hydroxyethoxymethyl) guanine. *Proc Natl Acad Sci USA* 74:5716–5720, 1977.

153 Datta AK, Colby BM, Shaw JE, Pagano JS: Acyclovir inhibition of Epstein-Barr virus replication. *Proc Natl Acad Sci USA* 77:5163–5166, 1980.

154 Crumpacker CS, Schnipper LE, Zaia JA, Levin MJ: Growth inhibition by acycloguanosine of herpesviruses isolated from human infections. *Antimicrob Agents Chemother* 15:642–645, 1979.

155 Collins P, Bauer DJ: The activity in vitro against herpes virus of 9-(2-hydroxyethoxymethyl)guanine (acycloguanosine), a new antiviral agent. *J Antimicrob Chemother* 5:431–436, 1979.

156 Fyfe JA, Keller PM, Furman PA, et al: Thymidine kinase from herpes simplex virus phosphorylates the new antiviral compound, 9-(2-hydroxyethoxymethyl)guanine. *J Biol Chem* 253:8721–8727, 1978.

157 Derse D, Cheng YC, Furman PA, et al: Inhibition of purified human and herpes simplex virus-induced DNA polymerases by 9-(2-hydroxyethoxymethyl)guanine triphosphate: Effects on primer-template function. *J Biol Chem* 256:11447–11451, 1981.

158 Furman PA, St Clair, Fyfe JA, et al: Inhibition of herpes simplex virus-induced DNA polymerase activity and viral DNA replication by 9-(2-hydroxyethoxymethyl)guanine and its triphosphate. *J Virol* 32: 72–77, 1979.

159 Field AK, Biron KK: "The end of innocence" revisited: Resistance of herpesviruses to antiviral drugs. *Clin Microb Rev* 7:1–13, 1994.

160 Straus SE, Takiff HE, Seidlin M, et al: Suppression of frequently recurring genital herpes: A placebo-controlled double-blind trial of oral acyclovir. *N Engl J Med* 310:1545–1550, 1984.

161 McLaren C, Corey L, Dekket C, Barry DW: In vitro sensitivity to acyclovir in genital herpes simplex viruses from acyclovir-treated patients. *J Infect Dis* 148:868–875, 1983.

162 Weller S, Blum MR, Doucette M, et al: Pharmacokinetics of the acyclovir pro-drug valaciclovir after escalating single- and multiple-dose administration to normal volunteers. *Clin Pharmacol Ther* 54:595–605, 1993.

163 Ashton WT, Karkas JD, Field AK, Tolman RL: Activation by thymidine kinase and potent antiherpetic activity of 2′- nor 2′-deoxyguanosine (2′NDG). *Biochem Biophys Res Commun* 108:1716–1721, 1982.

164 Sullivan V, Talarico CL, Stanat SC, et al: A protein kinase homologue controls phosphorylation of ganciclovir in human cytomegalovirus-infected cells. *Nature* 358:162–164, 1992.

165 Littler E, Stuart AD, Chee MS: Human cytomegalovirus UL97 open reading frame encodes a protein that phosphorylates the antiviral nucleoside analogue ganciclovir. *Nature* 358:160–162, 1992.

166 Biron KK, Fyfe JA, Stanat SC, et al: A human cytomegalovirus mutant resistant to the nucleoside analogue 9-([2-hydroxy-1-(hydroxymethyl)ethoxy]methyl)guanine (BW B759U) induces reduced levels of BW B759U triphosphate. *Proc Natl Acad Sci USA* 83:8769–8773, 1986.

167 Larsson A, Stenberg K, Ericson AC, et al: Mode of action, toxicity, pharmacokinetics, and efficacy of some new antiherpesvirus guanosine analogues related to buciclovir. *Antimicrob Agents Chemother* 30:598--605, 1986.

168 Earnshaw DL, Bacon TH, Darlison SJ, et al: Mode of antiviral action of penciclovir in MRC-5 cells infected with herpes simplex virus type 1 (HSV-1), HSV-2, and varicella-zoster virus. *Antimicrob Agents Chemother* 36:2747–2757, 1992.

169 Hodge RA, Perkins RM: Mode of action of 9-(4-hydroxy-3-hydroxymethylbut-1-yl)guanine (BRL 39123) against herpes simplex virus in MRC-5 cells. *Antimicrob Agents Chemother* 33:223–229, 1989.

170 Vere Hodge RA, Sutton D, Boyd MR, et al: Selection of an oral prodrug (BRL 42810; famciclovir) for the antiherpesvirus agent BRL 39123 [9-(4-hydroxy-3-hydroxymethylbut-l-yl)guanine;penciclovir]. *Antimicrob Agents Chemother* 33:1765–1773, 1989.

171 Boyd MR, Bacon TH, Sutton D, Cole M: Antiherpesvirus activity of 9-(4-hydroxy-3-hydroxy-methylbut-1-yl)guanine (BRL 39123) in cell culture. *Antimicrob Agents Chemother* 31:1238–1242, 1987.

172 Balfour HH Jr, Benson C, Braun J, et al: Management of acyclovir-resistant herpes simplex and varicella-zoster virus infections. *J Acquir Immune Defic Syndr* 7:254–260, 1994.

173 Eriksson B, Oberg B, Wahren B: Pyrophosphate analogues as inhibitors of DNA polymerases of cytomegalovirus, herpes simplex virus and cellular origin. *Biochim Biophys Acta* 696:115–123, 1982.

174 Datta AK, Hood RE: Mechanism of inhibition of Epstein-Barr virus replication by phosphonoformic acid. *Virology* 114:52–59, 1981.

175 Helgstrand E, Eriksson B, Johansson NG, et al: Trisodium phosphonoformate, a new antiviral compound. *Science* 201:819–821, 1978.

176 Fillet AM, Visse B, Caumes E, et al: Foscarnet-resistant multidermatomal zoster in a patient with AIDS. *Clin Infect Dis* 21:1348–1349, 1995.

177 Eriksson B, Oberg B: Characteristics of herpesvirus mutants resistant to phosphonoformate and phosphonoacetate. *Antimicrob Agents Chemother* 15:758–762, 1979.

178 Baldanti F, Sarasini A, Silini E, et al: Four dually resistant human cytomegalovirus strains from AIDS patients: Single mutations in UL97 and UL54 open reading frames are responsible for ganciclovir- and foscarnet-specific resistance, respectively. *Scand J Infect Dis Suppl* 99:103–104, 1995.

179 Baldanti F, Underwood MR, Stanat SC, et al: Single amino acid changes in the DNA polymerase confer foscarnet resistance and slow-growth phenotype, while mutations in the UL97-encoded phosphotransferase confer ganciclovir resistance in three double-resistant human cytomegalovirus strains recovered from patients with AIDS. *J Virol* 70:1390–1395, 1996.

180 Derse D, Bastow KF, Cheng Y: Characterization of the DNA polymerases induced by a group of herpes simplex virus type I variants selected for growth in the presence of phosphonoformic acid. *J Biol Chem* 257:10251–10260, 1982.

181 Kessler HA, Hurwitz S, Farthing C, et al: Pilot study of topical trifluridine for the treatment of acyclovir-resistant mucocutaneous herpes simplex disease in patients with AIDS (ACTG 172). *J Acquir Immun Defic Syndr Hum Retrovirol* 12:147–152, 1996.
182 Heidelberger C: On the molecular mechanism of the antiviral activity of trifluorothymidine. *Ann NY Acad Sci* 255:317–325, 1975.
183 Gephart JF, Lerner AM: Comparison of the effects of arabinosyladenine, arabinosylhypoxanthine, and arabinosyladenine 5'-monophosphate against herpes simplex virus, varicella-zoster virus, and cytomegalovirus with their effects on cellular deoxyribonucleic acid synthesis. *Antimicrob Agents Chemother* 19:170–178, 1981.
184 Pelling JC, Drach JC, Shipman C Jr: Internucleotide incorporation of arabinosyladenine into herpes simplex virus and mammalian cell DNA. *Virology* 109:323–335, 1981.
185 Herold BC, Siston AM, Bremer J, Kirkpatrick R, Wilbanks G, Fuged P, Peto C, Cooper M: Sulfated carbohydrate compounds prevent microbial adherence by sexually transmitted disease pathogens. *Antimicrob Agents Chemother* 41:2776–2780, 1997.
186 Campadelli-Fiume G, Arsenakis M, Farabegoli F, Roizman B: Entry of herpes simplex virus 1 in BJ cells that constitutively express viral glycoprotein D is by endocytosis and results in degradation of the virus. *J Virol* 62:159–167, 1988.
187 Johnson RM, Spear PG: Herpes simplex virus glycoprotein D mediates interference with herpes simplex virus infection. *J Virol* 63:819–827, 1989.
188 Friedman AD, Triezenberg SJ, McKnight SL: Expression of a truncated viral trans-activator selectively impedes lytic infection by its cognate virus. *Nature* 335:452–454, 1988.
189 Javier RT, Sedarati F, Stevens JG: Two avirulent herpes simplex viruses generate lethal recombinants in vivo. *Science* 234:746–748, 1986.
190 Gershon AA, Steinberg SP: Live attenuated varicella vaccine: Protection in healthy adults compared with leukemic children. National Institute of Allergy and Infectious Diseases Varicella Vaccine Collaborative Study Group. *J Infect Dis* 161:661–666, 1990.
191 Gershon AA, Steinberg SP, Gelb L, et al: Live attenuated varicella vaccine: Efficacy for children with leukemia in remission. *JAMA* 252: 355–362, 1984.
192 White CJ, Kuter BJ, Hildebrand CS, et al: Varicella vaccine (VARIVAX) in healthy children and adolescents: Results from clinical trials, 1987 to 1989. *Pediatrics* 87:604–610, 1991.
193 Gershon AA, Steinberg SP: Persistence of immunity to varicella in children with leukemia immunized with live attenuated varicella vaccine. *N Engl J Med* 320:892–897, 1989.
194 Asano Y, Nagai T, Miyata T, et al: Long-term protective immunity of recipients of the OKA strain of live varicella vaccine. *Pediatrics* 75:667–671, 1985.
195 Brunell PA, Shehab Z, Geiser C, Waugh JE: Administration of live varicella vaccine to children wtih leukaemia. *Lancet* 2:1069–1073, 1982.
196 Asano Y, Albrecht P, Vujcic LK, et al: Five-year follow-up study of recipients of live varicella vaccine using enhanced neutralization and fluorescent antibody membrane antigen assays. *Pediatrics* 72:291–294, 1983.
197 Asano Y, Nakayama H, Yazaki T, et al: Protection against varicella in family contacts by immediate inoculation with live varicella vaccine. *Pediatrics* 59:3–7, 1977.
198 Gelb LD, Dohner DE, Gershon AA, et al: Molecular epidemiology of live, attenuated varicella virus vaccine in children with leukemia and in normal adults. J Infect Dis 155:633–640, 1987.
199 Williams DL, Gershon AA, Gelb LD, et al: Herpes zoster following varicella vaccine in a child with acute lymphocytic leukemia. *J Pediatr* 106:259–261, 1985.
200 Hardy I, Gershon AA, Steinberg SP, LaRussa P: The incidence of zoster after immunization with live attenuated varicella vaccine. A study in children with leukemia. *N Engl J Med* 325:1545–1550, 1991.
201 Lawrence R, Gershon AA, Holzman R, Steinberg SP: The risk of zoster after varicella vaccination in children with leukemia. *N Engl J Med* 318:543–548, 1988.
202 Brunell PA, Taylor-Wiedeman J, Geiser CF, et al: Risk of herpes zoster in children with leukemia: Varicella vaccine compared with history of chickenpox. *Pediatrics* 77:53–56, 1986.
203 Plotkin SA, Starr SE, Friedman HM, et al: Effect of Towne live virus vaccine on cytomegalovirus disease after renal transplant: A controlled trial. *Ann Intern Med* 114:525–531, 1991.
204 Plotkin SA, Higgins R, Kurtz JB, et al: Multicenter trial of Towne strain attenuated virus vaccine in seronegative renal transplant recipients. *Transplantation* 58:1176–1178, 1994.
205 Balfour HH, Welo PK, Sachs GW: Cytomegalovirus vaccine trial in 400 renal transplant candidates. *Transplant Proc* 17:81–83, 1985.
206 Plotkin SA, Huang ES: Cytomegalovirus vaccine virus (Towne strain) does not induce latency. *J Infect Dis* 152:395–397, 1985.
207 Pass RF, Duliege A-M, Boppana SB, et al: Immunogenicity of a recombinant CMV gB vaccine (abstract). *Pediatr Res* 37:185A, 1995.
208 Stanberry LR, Myers MG, Stephanopoulos DE, Burke RL: Preinfection prophylaxis with herpes simplex virus glycoprotein immunogens: factors influencing efficacy. *J Gen Virol* 70:3177–3185, 1989.
209 Berman PW, Vogt PE, Gregory T, et al: Efficacy of recombinant glycoprotein D subunit vaccines on the development of primary, recurrent, and latent genital infections with herpes simplex virus type 2 in guinea pigs. *J Infect Dis* 157:897–902, 1988.
210 Stanberry LR, Burke R, Myers MG: Herpes simplex virus glycoprotein treatment of recurrent genital herpes. *J Infect Dis* 157:156–163, 1988.
211 Stanberry LR, Bernstein DI, Burke RL, et al: Vaccination with recombinant herpes simplex virus glycoproteins: Protection against initial and recurrent genital herpes. *J Infect Dis* 155:914–920, 1987.
212 Langenberg AG, Burke RL, Adair SF, et al: A recombinant glycoprotein vaccine for herpes simplex virus type 2: Safety and immunogenicity. *Ann Intern Med* 122:889–898, 1995.
213 Straus SE, Corey L, Burke RL, et al: Placebo-controlled trial of vaccination with recombinant glycoprotein D of herpes simplex virus type 2 for immunotherapy of genital herpes. *Lancet* 343:1460–1463, 1994.
214 Ulmer JB, Donnelly JJ, Parker SE, et al: Heterologous protection against influenza by injection of DNA encoding a viral protein. *Science* 259:1745–1749, 1993.
215 Wolff JA, Malone RW, Williams P, et al: Direct gene transfer into mouse muscle in vivo. *Science* 247:1465–1468, 1990.
216 Kriesel JD, Spruance SL, Daynes RA, Araneo BA: Nucleic acid vaccine encoding gD2 protects mice from herpes simplex virus type 2 disease. *J Infect Dis* 173:536–541, 1996.

Chapter 21
Genital herpes

Lawrence Corey
Anna Wald

Genital herpes simplex virus (HSV) infection is a disease of major public health importance, having markedly increased in prevalence throughout the world during the last two decades. The morbidity of the illness, its high recurrence rates, and its complications, such as aseptic meningitis and neonatal transmission, have made this disease of great concern to patients and health care providers. Multiple interactions between HSV and HIV, both on epidemiologic and clinical levels, have further emphasized the importance of this infection.

HISTORY

The word herpes (from the Greek, "to creep") has been used in medicine for at least 25 centuries. Cold sores (herpes febrilis) were described by the Roman physician Herodotus in 100 AD.[1] Genital herpes was first described by the French physician John Astruc in 1736, and the first English translation appeared in his treatise on venereal disease in 1754.[2] The disease also appeared to be well recognized by nineteenth century venereologists. In 1893 Unna diagnosed genital herpes in 9.1 percent of 846 prostitutes visiting his infirmary.[3] In 1886 Diday and Doyon published the monograph *Les Herpes genitaux,* in which they observed that genital herpes often appeared after a venereal infection such as syphilis, chancroid, or gonorrhea. They also described cases of recurrent genital herpes.[4]

Fluid from oral-labial infection was shown to be infectious to other humans in the late nineteenth century. The disease was successfully transferred to rabbits in the early twentieth century, and HSV was grown in vitro in 1925.[5–7] In 1921 Lipshultz inoculated material from genital herpetic lesions into the skin of humans, eliciting clinical infection within 48 to 72 hours in six persons and within 24 days in one case. In other experiments, he observed that rabbits developed corneal infection more readily with strains originating from genital sites than oral-labial sites. Although he surmised that there were epidemiologic and clinical differences between oral and genital herpes, most workers felt that the viruses of genital and labial herpes were identical.[8] In the early 1960s, Schneeweiss in Germany and Dowdle and Nahmias in the United States reported that HSV could be divided by neutralization tests into two antigenic types, and that there was an association between the antigenic type and the site of viral recovery.[9–12] These observations led to the benchmark studies of genital herpes in the late 1960s.

EPIDEMIOLOGY

SEROEPIDEMIOLOGY OF HSV INFECTION

Accurate evaluation of the seroprevalence to HSV-1 and HSV-2 has been markedly enhanced by the development of type specific serologic assays. These assays allow the detection of HSV-2 in the presence of HSV-1 antibodies and vice versa.[13,14] Most of these assays utilize purified type specific proteins such as glycoprotein gG1, and glycoprotein gG2, which are antigenically distinct between the two subtypes. The gG1 and gG2 assays are quite good in evaluating persons with longstanding HSV infections.[15] Another assay using an immunoblot format that identifies several type specific antibodies, for example, gG2 and ICP-35 complex, has also been developed.[14] It is the most sensitive assay for detecting recent HSV seroconversion. The Western blot assay has a sensitivity greater than 98 percent and a specificity greater than 98 percent for distinguishing HSV-1 specific and HSV-2 specific antibodies. Assays that utilize prototype viral antigens are inaccurate and should not be utilized for clinical diagnosis or seroepidemiologic studies.[16,17]

Prevalence of antibody to HSV increases with age and correlates with socioeconomic status.[12,18–22] Serosurveys of western populations in the post-World War II era found that 80 to 100 percent of middle-aged adults of lower socioeconomic status possessed antibodies to HSV, as compared to 30 to 50 percent of adults of higher socioeconomic groups.[23–25] In the United States in the 1970s, HSV-1 antibodies were detected in about 50 percent of high and 80 percent of lower socioeconomic class persons by age 30.[25] In Western Europe the prevalence of HSV-1 infection in young adults appears 10 to 20 percent higher than in the United States.[26] In STD clinics in the United States about 60 percent of attendees have HSV-1 antibodies.

Antibodies to HSV-2 are not routinely detected in sera until puberty, and antibody prevalence rates correlate with past sexual activity. Antibody prevalence rates of HSV-2 are higher in African-American than white populations.[15,27,28] Symptomatic infection appears relatively more commonly in whites.[29] Recent evidence suggests prior HSV-1 antibody increases the frequency of subclinical HSV-2 infection.[30] This observation and differential health care behavior may explain the differences in prevalence of symptomatic genital herpes in different racial groups. In the United States, seroprevalence of HSV-2 has been evaluated in two nationwide surveys.[15,31] As these studies employ a variety of techniques to test a random and representative sample of adults, they represent the most reliable estimates of HSV-2 in the general population. These studies showed that the HSV-2 seroprevalence has increased from 16.4 to 21.7 percent of adults in the United States. The cumulative lifetime incidence of HSV-2 reaches 25 percent in white women, 20 percent in white men, 80 percent in African-American women and 60 percent in African-American men (Fig. 21-1).

Other serologic studies conducted in more select populations support the high prevalence of HSV-2 infection worldwide (Table 21-1). The HSV-2 seroprevalence appears lower in Europe, including Great Britain and Australia. Few serologic studies of HSV-2 in the general population of developing countries have been conducted, but among STD clinic attendees the prevalence is very high, suggesting endemic levels of HSV-2 infection.

The frequency of HSV-2 antibody is higher among persons recruited from STD clinics and among homosexual men. Consistently among studies, the presence of HSV-2 antibody is closely related to the lifetime number of sexual partners, age of sexual debut and a history of other STDs. As such, it can serve as a serologic marker for sexual behavior in different populations.

Incidence rates for HSV infections are difficult to estimate as most infections are subclinical. A 15-year study of 839 adolescent women in Sweden showed that 50 percent of the cohort had acquired HSV-1 and 22 percent acquired HSV-2 by the end of the study.[45] In a study of women attending the Seattle STD Clinic, the annual rate of acquisition was 3 percent.

PREVALENCE OF GENITAL HSV INFECTIONS

The reported prevalence of genital herpes depends upon the demographic and clinical characteristics of the patient population

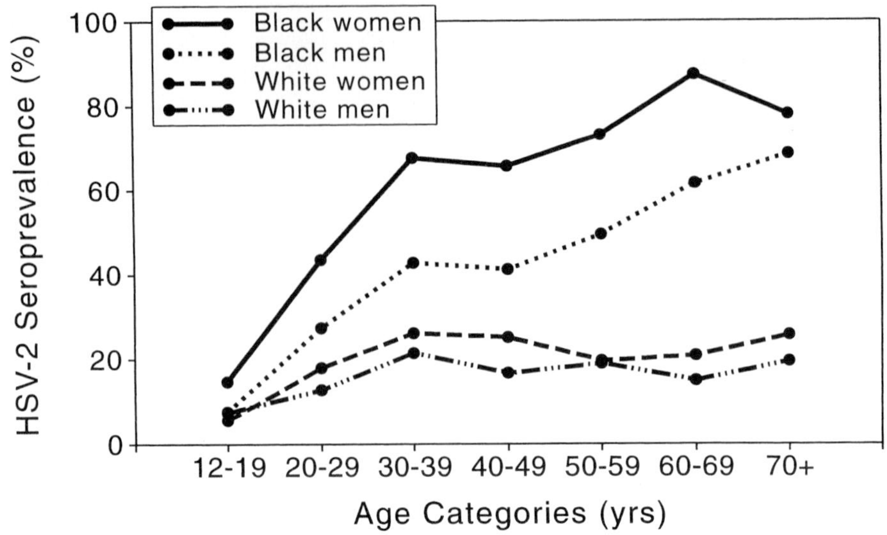

Fig. 21-1. Seroprevalence of HSV-2 in the United States, according to gender and race. *(Adapted from DT Fleming et al.*[31]*)*

studied and whether clinical and/or laboratory techniques are used for diagnoses. Seroepidemiologic studies have shown a wide disparity between antibody prevalence and clinical infections, indicating that many persons acquire subclinical infection (Table 21-1).[12,46] Reasons for lack of recognition of the infection include mild disease in most affected persons, attenuation of symptoms in those with prior HSV-1 infection, location of lesions in difficult to examine areas, for example, the perianal region, and differential access to health care and health care behavior in various populations. As such, there are great differences in the prevalence of HSV-1 and HSV-2 infection versus the frequency of symptomatic genital and oral-labial herpes seen by medical practitioners. HSV has been isolated from 0.3 to 5.4 percent of males and 1.6 to 10 percent of females attending STD clinics.[47–49] In non-STD clinic patient populations, HSV has been isolated from the genital tract in from 0.25 to 5.0 percent of patients. Many of these patients are asymptomatic.[30,50,52] In STD clinics seeing a high proportion of non-Caucasians, genital herpes is reported only ⅛ to 1/12 as frequently as *Neisseria gonorrhoeae* infection.[53] Student health centers seeing middle- and upper-class young adults, in whom the prevalence of gonococcal infection is very low, report that genital HSV infections are seven to 10 times more common than gonorrhea.[54] Similarly, in developing countries HSV-2 often has been an infrequent cause of genital symptoms. However, with the use of sensitive laboratory methods such as PCR, HSV has been shown to be a frequent and often predominant cause of genital ulcers.[55,56]

The prevalence of genital herpes has increased markedly between the early 1960s and 1990s. In Britain, reports of patients with genital herpes in STD clinics increased six-fold between 1972 and 1994.[41] Initial visits to physicians in the United States for first episode genital HSV increased tenfold, from 16,986 in 1970 to 160,000 in 1995 per 100,000 patient visits.[34,57] Concomitant with this increase in genital HSV has been an increase in neonatal HSV in the United States. In King County, Washington, the incidence of neonatal HSV has risen from 2.6 cases per 100,000 live births in the years 1966 to 1969 to 4.8 in 1970 to 1973, 7.4 in 1974 to 1977, 11.9 in 1978 to 1981, 15.7 in 1982 to 1985, 12.0 in 1986 to 1989, 11.7 in 1990 to 1993, and 11.4 in the years 1994 to 1995 (Fig. 21-2).[58] The concomitant rise in reported neonatal HSV infection seen throughout the United States and the results of serologic surveys discussed above suggest that in many population groups there has been a marked increase in HSV-2 infections during this time period.[19,58]

SEXUAL TRANSMISSION OF HSV

The frequency of transmission of HSV-2 is influenced by gender, past HSV-1 infection, and frequency of sexual activity with a person with known infection. Transmission of HSV between sexual partners has been addressed most often in prospective studies of serologically discordant couples, that is, in couples in whom one partner has and one does not have HSV-2. Longitudinal studies of such couples have shown that the transmission rate approximates 12 percent per year.[59,60] Several studies have described couples in which HSV-2 has not been transmitted despite frequent sexual activity. Whether this is owing to genetic or acquired resistance is unclear. Women and HSV seronegative persons have higher rates of acquisition than men and HSV-1 seropositive persons. In one study the attack rate among seronegative women approached 30 percent per year.[59] This increased risk for acquisition among women compared to men is evident in the 5 to 10 percent higher seroprevalence of HSV-2 antibodies among women than men. The reasons probably include anatomic differences that lead to greater mucosal surface area exposed in the genital area of women compared to men, a higher frequency of recurrences among men, and possibly a lower perception of discomfort in men with active lesions than in women.[61,62] This latter feature may lead to increased sexual activity when lesions are present and hence higher transmission rates. Sexual contact with persons with undiagnosed genital herpes may lead to higher transmission rates. In a study of 66 source partners who were interviewed and examined, one-third had a history of recurrent genital herpes, one-third had a clinical history of recurrent genital lesions consistent with herpes, and one-third denied a history of such lesions.[63] Median time of the relationship before transmission occurred was 3 months and the median number of sexual encounters was 24, suggesting that HSV is transmitted rather easily. The discrepancy in the ease of transmission noted in this study versus those of stable couples suggests that diagnosis of genital herpes in the potential source partner and awareness of both partners as to the existence of a transmissible STD may help reduce the risk of transmission. In both types of studies and in case reports, most episodes of transmission occur during episodes of subclinical shedding (discussed in the following). In prospective studies of HSV acquisition, 70 percent of newly acquired cases of genital HSV-2 develop genitourinary complaints around the time of acquisition, albeit many times these are mild and atypical for HSV disease.[59] The disease pattern in the person who acquired the disease does not reflect the

Table 21-1. The HSV-2 Seroprevalence in Selected Populations

Study setting	Number of persons tested	Percent with HSV-2 infection	Percent with history of genital herpes, among persons seropositive for HSV-2
General population			
United States population survey, 1990*[31]			
Men	6407	17.8	9.3
Women	6687	25.6	9.1
Family practice, Seattle WA[27]			
Men	351	13	26
Women	610	29	26
Family planning clinic, (women) Pittsburgh, PA[32]	4527	21.6	12.6
University students, South Carolina[33]	1093	4.3	0
San Francisco neighborhood survey, CA[28]			
Men	601	25	19
Women	611	41	13
Women's Clinic, Albuquerque, NM[34]	587	31	11.1
Lesbians, Seattle, WA (J. Marrazzo, personal communication)	133	13	41
Other Countries			
Blood Donors, London, UK[35]	1325	7.6	19
Pregnant women, Sao Paulo, Brazil[36]	655	39	8.2
Household survey of women, Costa Rica[37]	766	39.4	1.1
Pregnant women, Sydney, Australia[38]	229	14.5	0
Pregnant women, Stockholm, Sweden[39]	1000	33	NA
Military recruits, Italy[40]	1169	0.01	NA
Health care personnel, Italy[40]	411	4.8	NA
Homosexual men, Italy[40]	397	55	10
High risk settings			
STD clinic, Seattle WA, USA[30]	776	43	22
High risk homosexual men, Seattle, USA	572	26	51
STD clinic, Australia			42‡
Men	80	35	
Women	27	55	
STD clinic, London, UK[41]			
Men	294	17.3	39.2
Women	347	24.5	30.1
STD clinic, Sydney, Australia, heterosexual men[42]	300	65	24
STD clinic, Goteborg, Sweden[43]			
Men	1143	14	30
Women	475	26	30
STD clinic, heterosexuals, Italy†[44]	783	35	14
STD clinic, homosexuals, Italy[44]	158	69	14
Prostitutes, Senegal	272	80	NA
STD clinic, Lima, Peru	395	83	NA
Nairobi prostitutes, Kenya	115	61	NA
Prostitutes, HIV+ Kinshasa, Zaire	181	95	NA
Prostitutes, HIV− Kinshasa, Zaire	187	75	NA

* From National Health and Nutrition Examination Survey, III.
† No difference in HSV-2 seroprevalence in men and women.
‡ Separate percentage for each gender not available.
NA, not available.

disease pattern of the source partner. Fifty-eight percent of patients with newly acquired genital herpes presented within 5 days of last sexual contact and 95 percent within 14 days of sexual intercourse, confirming the short incubation period noted in experimental human and animal studies.[8,64]

PATHOGENESIS OF INFECTION

Transmission of HSV infections most frequently occurs through close contact with a person who is shedding (excreting) virus at a peripheral site, mucosal surface, in genital or oral secretions. Since HSV is readily inactivated at room temperature and by drying, aerosol and fomitic spread are unusual means of transmission.[65–68] Infection occurs via inoculation of virus onto susceptible mucosal surfaces (e.g., the oropharynx, cervix, conjunctivae) or through small cracks in the skin. HSV infection is associated with focal necrosis and ballooning degeneration of cells, production of mononucleated giant cells, and eosinophilic intranuclear inclusions (Cowdry type A bodies).[69] The initial cellular response is predominantly polymorphonuclear, followed by lymphocytic response. When viral replication is restricted, lesions reepithelialize.

Concomitant with initial infection, HSV ascends peripheral sensory nerves and enters sensory or autonomic nerve root ganglia where latency is established (see Chap. 20).[68–71] Using cocultiva-

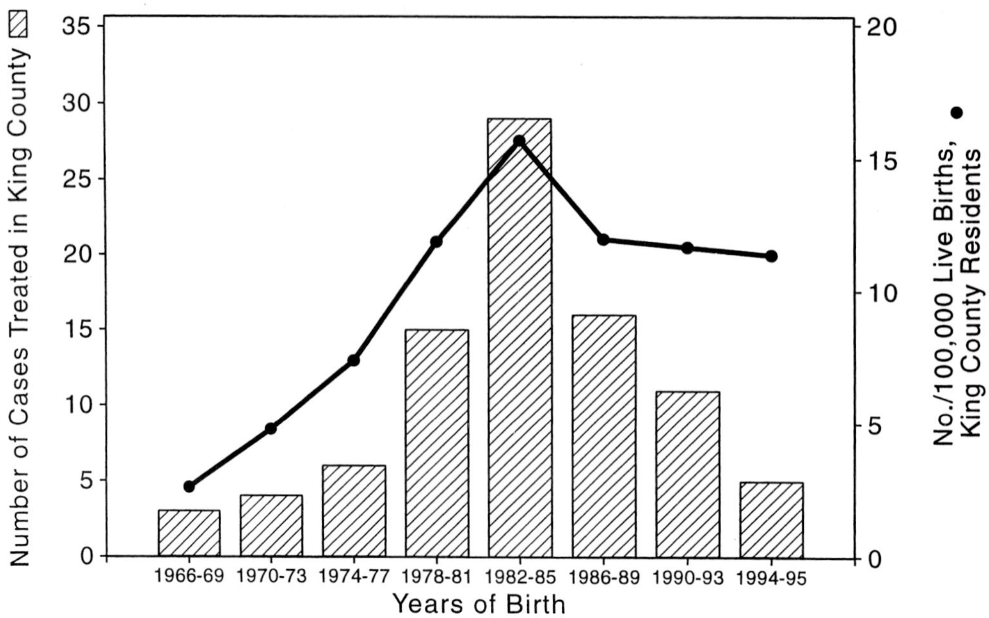

Fig. 21-2. Incidence of neonatal HSV infection in King County, Washington, 1966 to 1995.

tion techniques HSV-2, and rarely HSV-1, have been isolated from sacral nerve root ganglia.[70] The biological mechanism by which latency is established and the nature of the virus–cell interaction that results in latency are incompletely understood (see Chap. 20). Latency can be established after both symptomatic and asymptomatic initial infection. Available evidence suggests that all HSV seropositive persons have latent virus in nerve ganglia. As discussed in the following, it appears nearly all HSV-2 seropositive persons intermittently reactivate infection with HSV shedding occurring for a limited time period on mucosal surfaces. Recrudescences of disease may be clinically symptomatic or asymptomatic. Reinfection with different strains of virus has also been demonstrated; however, this appears to be a very infrequent event and recurrences are almost always caused by reactivation of the initial strain of virus from latently infected ganglia.[72,73]

The molecular mechanisms by which HSV intermittently reactivates are unknown. This issue is discussed in Chapter 20. The factors that influence the frequency of that reactivation also are largely unknown. In experimental systems many HSV genes influence neuroinvasion and spread. When the region containing the latency associated transcripts of HSV-2 is inserted into an HSV-1 virus, increasing reactivation in sacral nerve root ganglia has occurred, indicating that viral factors influence reactivation.[74]

Host factors also appear operative in influencing reactivation. Immunocompromised patients have both more frequent and more severe reactivations. Both HSV-1 and HSV-2 encode for proteins that are directed at subverting host T-cell responses. One protein in particular, ICP-47 (infected cell protein no. 47), interacts with the transporter activity protein (TAP) to prevent the interaction between HSV specific peptides to HLA class I molecules. This downregulates certain HSV-1 peptides with HLA Class I antigen on the cell surface and subverts the host CD8+ CTL response to HSV.[75–77]

Biopsies of herpetic lesions have shown that initially the predominant infiltrating cell is the CD4+ lymphocyte.[78] Staining of such lesions shows the presence of activation markers on these CD4 bearing cells. These include IL-2 receptor, DR+, ICAM−1+ within 2 to 4 days; later, the lesions are infiltrated with CD8+ T cells. Recently, Koelle et al. demonstrated that clearance of HSV-2 from genital lesions is associated with the ability to detect cytolytic killing to HSV-2 in lesional T cells.[79] Most of this CTL activity appears to be in the CD8 fraction of T

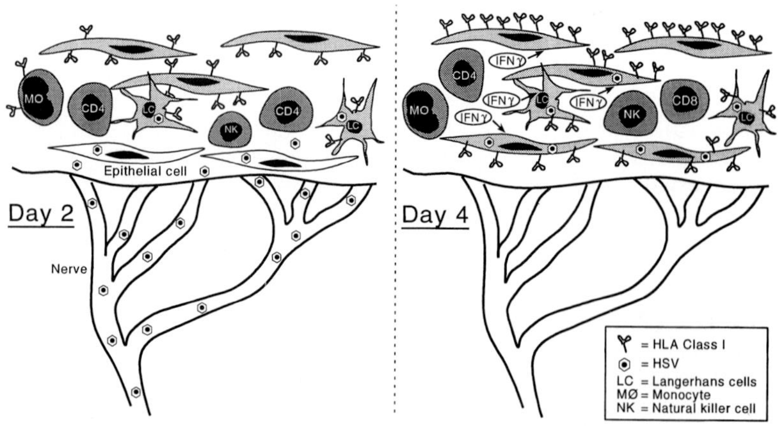

Fig. 21-3. Immunological Evolution of a Herpetic Lesion. Day 2 of clinical lesion maturation. HSV released from infected neurons has infected adjacent epithelial cells. With the expression of the immediate-early gene ICP47, TAP is inhibited, preventing the transport of peptides into the ER resulting in a decrease in the surface expression of HLA class 1/peptide complexes. CD4+ T cells and natural killer (NK) cells have migrated to the lesion. Antigen presenting cells (including monocytes and Langerhans cells) present HSV antigens to HSV-specific CD4+ T cells, stimulating the production of both type 1 and type 2 cytokines. Day 4–5 of clinical lesion maturation. IFN-g, produced by NK cells and activated HSV-specific CD4+ T cells, upregulates the expression of HLA class 1/peptide complexes on the surface of HSV-infected cells. HSV-specific CD8+ CTL precursors that migrate into the lesion are subsequently activated. Effector CTL (CD8 and CD4) lyse HSV-infected cells, preventing the spread of HSV to neighboring cells. (Courtesy of Drs. Posarad, Koelle, and Corey.)

lymphocytes. Figure 21-3 illustrates a schematic model of host responses to HSV reactivation. This includes early CD4+ infiltrating T cells which produce γIFN and other cytokines in response to HSV antigen. γIFN in particular upregulates cellular HLA class I expression that can then overcome the virus' ability to downregulate this response.[77] Infiltration of CD8+ T cells into the lesion then occurs and helps clear virus. This model recognizes the multifactorial aspects of host T-cell responses and helps explain why both deficits in CD4 and CD8+ HSV specific T cells are associated with more severe disease.

CLINICAL MANIFESTATIONS OF GENITAL HERPES

The severity and frequency of clinical manifestations and recurrence rate of genital herpes are influenced by viral and host factors such as viral type, prior immunity to autologous or heterologous virus, gender, and immune status of the host. The influence of other host factors such as age, race, site of inoculation, or genetic background on the acquisition of infection or expression of disease are poorly understood. Many HSV infections (both HSV-1 and HSV-2) are subclinical and the differences in persons with symptomatic versus clinically silent disease have not been defined. Moreover, identical strain of virus may have markedly different patterns of reactivation between persons. Even within an individual, poor correlations exist in the duration of consecutive episodes or in the interval between recurrences.

FIRST EPISODE OF GENITAL HERPES

The clinical manifestations of genital herpes differ greatly between first versus recurrent episode of HSV. First episodes of genital herpes often are associated with systemic symptoms, a prolonged duration of lesions and viral shedding, and involve multiple genital and extragenital sites.[82] Patients who are experiencing true primary infection (i.e., the first infection with either HSV-1 or HSV-2) have more severe illness than patients who have clinical or serological evidence of prior HSV-1 infection.[83–85] In most surveys, about 50 percent of persons who present with their first episode of symptomatic genital herpes have primary infection with either HSV-1 or HSV-2.[30] Most persons with nonprimary first episodes of genital HSV infection have serological evidence of past HSV-1 infection; acquisition of HSV-1 infection in persons with prior HSV-2 infection is rare.[86] About 25 percent of persons with their first clinical episode of symptomatic genital herpes already have serologic evidence of HSV-2 at presentation, indicative of past asymptomatic acquisition of HSV-2.[87] Thus, their initial clinical episode is their first recognized episode of past infection and does not indicate recent acquisition. Isolates recovered from sequential recurrences almost invariably have identical restriction enzyme patterns.

Genital HSV-1 infections have been reported with increasing frequency, and genital HSV-1 may account for the majority of persons presenting with primary genital herpes in several parts of the world.[88–92] Between 1 and 30 percent of true primary genital HSV are caused by HSV-1.[82,93] Most genital HSV-1 infections are primary infections, as genital HSV-1 recurs much less frequently than genital HSV-2 infections.[62,82,94,95]

Prior oral-labial HSV-1 infection appears to protect against the acquisition of genital HSV-1 disease.[86] However, genital HSV-1 disease does not protect completely against acquisition of genital HSV-2 infection, as sequential infections have been described.[96,97] Prior HSV-1 infection also ameliorates the severity of first episodes of genital herpes.[30,82] Persons with first episode nonprimary genital HSV-2 infection are less likely to have systemic symptoms and have a shorter duration of symptoms and signs than persons with primary genital herpes caused by either HSV-1 or HSV-2. However, prior HSV-1 infection does not appear to alter the subsequent rate of recurrences of genital HSV-2 disease.[62]

Primary genital herpes

Primary genital HSV-2 and primary genital HSV-1 infections are characterized by frequent and prolonged systemic and local symptoms (Fig. 21-4). Fever, headache, malaise, and myalgias are reported in nearly 40 percent of men and 70 percent of women with primary HSV-2 disease ($p < 0.05$). Systemic symptoms appear early in the course of the disease, usually reach a peak within the first 3 to 4 days after onset of lesions, and gradually recede over the subsequent 3 to 4 days.

Pain, itching, dysuria, vaginal or urethral discharge, and tender inguinal adenopathy are the predominant local symptoms of disease. The severity of local symptoms, duration of lesions, and viral shedding appear similar in patients with primary HSV-1 and primary HSV-2 disease. Painful lesions are reported in 95 percent of men (mean duration 10.9 days) and 99 percent of women (mean duration 12.2 days) with primary HSV infection. Dysuria, both external and internal, appears more frequently in women (83%) than in men (44%). The isolation of HSV from the urethra and urine of both men and women with primary genital herpes suggests that, in addition to external dysuria resulting from urine touching active genital HSV lesions, HSV urethritis and/or cystitis may account for the higher frequency and longer duration of dysuria in women.

Urethral discharge and dysuria are noted in about one-third of men with primary HSV-2 infection. HSV can be isolated from a urethral swab or from first-voided urine of these men. The urethral discharge is usually clear and mucoid, and the severity of dysuria is often out of proportion to the amount of urethral discharge elicited on genital exams. Gram stain of the urethral discharge usually reveals between five and 15 polymorphonuclear leukocytes per oil-immersion field. Occasionally a mononuclear cell response is seen.

The clinical symptoms of pain and irritation from lesions gradually increase over the first 6 to 7 days of illness, reach their maximum intensity between days 7 and 11 of disease, and gradually recede over the second week of illness. Tender inguinal adenopathy usually appears during the second and third week of disease and often is the last symptom to resolve. Inguinal and femoral lymph nodes generally are firm, nonfluctuant, and extremely tender to palpation. Suppurative lymphadenopathy is a very uncommon manifestation of genital herpes.

Clinical Signs and Duration of Viral Shedding in Primary Genital Herpes. In both men and women with primary genital HSV infection, widely spaced bilateral pustular or ulcerative le-

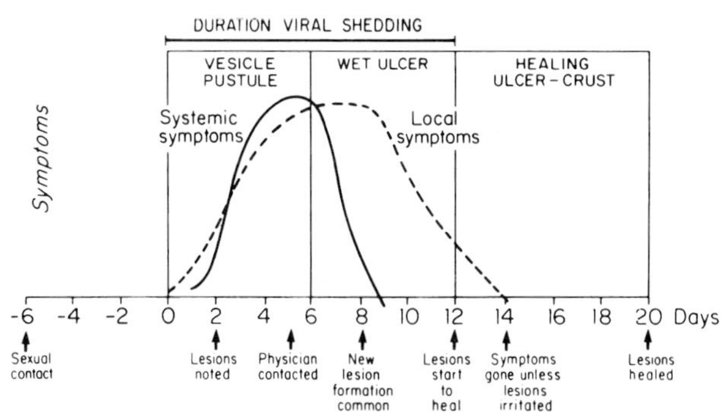

Fig. 21-4. Clinical course of primary genital herpes.

sions on the external genitalia are the most frequent presenting sign (plates 25 and 28). Lesions are characteristically described as starting as papules or vesicles that rapidly spread over the genital area. At the time of the first clinic visit, multiple small pustular lesions that coalesce into large areas of ulcerations are usually present. The size and shape of the ulcerative lesions vary greatly between patients. These ulcerative lesions persist from between 4 and 15 days until crusting and/or re-epithelialization occurs. In general, lesions in the penile and mons areas crust over before complete re-epithelialization ensues. Crusting does not occur on mucosal surfaces. Residual scarring from lesions is uncommon. New lesion formation (the development of new areas of vesiculation or ulceration during the course of infection) occurs in over 75 percent of patients with primary genital herpes. New lesions usually form between days 4 to 10 of disease. The median duration of viral shedding, as defined from onset of lesions to the last positive culture, is 12 days. The mean time from the onset of lesions to complete reepithelialization of all lesions appears slightly longer in women (19.5 days) than in men (16.5 days).

Frequency and Appearance of HSV Cervicitis in First Episodes of Genital Herpes. From 70 to 90 percent of women with first episode HSV-2 infection have HSV cervicitis.[82,90] This compares to a 15 to 20 percent isolation rate of HSV-2 from the cervix among women who present with recurrent external genital lesions.[82,98] Primary genital HSV cervicitis may be symptomatic (purulent or bloody vaginal discharge) or asymptomatic.[30,99] Areas of diffuse or focal friability and redness, extensive ulcerative lesions of the exocervix, or severe necrotic cervicitis (plate 14) may be seen. HSV infection of the cervix usually involves the squamous epithelium of the exocervix in contrast to the mucopurulent cervicitis of *C. trachomatis* and *N. gonorrhoeae* infection. Clinical differentiation may be difficult, although cervical ulceration and necrosis are highly correlated with HSV cervicitis.

Pharyngeal Infection. HSV of the pharynx is commonly seen in association with primary genital herpes and may be the presenting complaint in about 20 percent of patients with either primary HSV-1 or primary HSV-2 infections. Both HSV-1 and HSV-2 may cause pharyngitis and may be associated with oral-genital exposure to the source contact.[100,101] In children, autoinoculation of the genital area during the course of primary HSV-1 gingivostomatitis may be seen occasionally. HSV pharyngitis is seen much less frequently in patients with nonprimary first episode genital herpes or patients with recurrent genital herpes (1%). In the authors' experience, among persons with primary genital herpes who complained of sore throat during the acute episode of the disease, HSV was isolated from the pharynx in 70 percent. Viral cultures of the pharynx from 20 patients with primary HSV-2 who did not complain of sore throat did not yield HSV, which indicates that HSV pharyngitis is usually symptomatic. Clinical signs of HSV pharyngitis may vary from mild erythema to a diffuse ulcerative pharyngitis.[100–103] The inflammatory response to these large areas of ulceration may produce a whitish exudate; when wiped away the extensive ulceration may be visualized. In rare cases severe swelling of the posterior pharynx resulting in obstruction of the airway may occur.[104] Extension of the ulcerative posterior pharyngeal lesions into the anterior gingival area may occur. Most patients with HSV pharyngitis have tender cervical nodes, and constitutional symptoms, such as fever, malaise, myalgia, and headache, are common. Many are misdiagnosed as having streptococcal pharyngitis or infectious mononucleosis.

HSV-1 pharyngitis is common in teenagers and college students and is often caused by primary HSV-1 infection. The mode of transmission is kissing often during subclinical oral shedding. Reactivation of HSV in the pharynx rarely leads to symptomatic pharyngitis. Instead, recurrent oral-labial lesions or asymptomatic oral shedding are seen. Reactivation of HSV-2 in the trigeminal ganglia occurs much less frequently than reactivation of trigeminal nerve root latent HSV-1 infection.[101]

COMPLICATIONS OF GENITAL HERPES

The complications of genital herpes are related both to local extension and to spread of virus to extragenital sites. Central nervous system involvement and fungal superinfection are also frequently encountered. Complications of primary genital herpes occur more frequently in women than in men.

Central nervous system complications

Aseptic Meningitis. Central nervous system involvement may occur in several forms, including aseptic meningitis, transverse myelitis, or sacral radiculopathy.[105–107] In one series of patients with primary genital HSV-2 infection, stiff neck, headache, and photophobia on two consecutive examinations was reported in 36 percent of women and 13 percent of men ($p < 0.001$). Hospitalization was required for clinically overt aseptic meningitis in 6.4 percent of women and 1.6 percent of men with primary HSV-2 infections.[82] A study of primary genital herpes in the early 1900s reported a high frequency of CSF pleocytosis in patients without overt clinical evidence of meningeal irritation, suggesting that meningeal involvement may be a frequent occurrence with primary genital herpes.[108]

Both HSV-1 and HSV-2 have been isolated from CSF, although nuchal rigidity and isolation of HSV-2 are much more common.[109,110] HSV aseptic meningitis is more frequently associated with genital HSV-2 infection, whereas HSV encephalitis in older children or adults is usually associated with oral HSV-1 infection.[62,111–113] Fever, headache, vomiting, photophobia, and nuchal rigidity are the predominant symptoms of HSV aseptic meningitis. Meningeal symptoms usually start from 3 to 12 days after onset of genital lesions. Symptoms generally reach a maximum 2 to 4 days into the illness and gradually recede over 2 to 3 days. The CSF in HSV aseptic meningitis is usually clear, and the opening pressures may be elevated. White blood cell counts in CSF may range from 10 to over 1000 cells per cubic millimeter (mean 550). The pleocytosis is predominantly lymphocytic in adults, although early in the course of disease and in neonates a predominantly polymorphonuclear response may be seen. The CSF glucose in usually more than 50 percent of the blood glucose, although hypoglycorrhachia has been reported, and the CSF protein is slightly elevated.[114] HSV may be isolated from the CSF, although HSV DNA PCR assay is a more sensitive diagnostic test (see section on diagnosis). The differential diagnosis of HSV aseptic meningitis includes diseases that result in neurological involvement and genital ulcerations: sacral herpes zoster, Behcet's syndrome (plate 30), collagen vascular disease, inflammatory bowel disease, and porphyria.

Aseptic meningitis associated with genital herpes appears to be a benign, albeit uncomfortable, disease in immunocompetent persons. Signs and symptoms of encephalitis are unusual, and neurological sequelae are rare. Use of systemic antiviral chemotherapy of primary genital herpes decreases the subsequent development of aseptic meningitis.[115] Controlled trials of intravenous acyclovir for established HSV meningitis have not been conducted. However, we recommend that intravenous acyclovir 5 mg/kg q 8 hours be given for hospitalized symptomatic patients. Once symptoms are resolved, oral antiviral therapy, preferably with valaciclovir can be resumed. Oral antiviral agents should not, however, be utilized for patients with HSV-1 encephalitis.

Other Neurological Complications. Both autonomic nervous system dysfunction and transverse myelitis have been described in association with genital HSV infection.[106–108] Symptoms of autonomic nervous system dysfunction include hyperesthesia or anesthesia of the perineal, lower back, or sacral regions, and urinary retention and constipation. The last complication occurs more frequently among women and men with HSV proctitis.[116,117] Physical examination reveals a large bladder, decreased sacral sensation, and poor anal sphincter tone. In men, impotence and absent bulbocavernosus reflexes may occur. CSF pleocytosis may be present in some patients. Electromyography usually reveals slowed nerve conduction velocities and fibrillation potentials in the affected area, and urinary cystometric exam shows a large atonic bladder. Most cases gradually resolve over 4 to 8 weeks.[118–121]

Transverse myelitis occasionally occurs in association with primary genital HSV infection.[118,122,123] Decreased deep-tendon reflexes and muscle strength in the lower extremities, as well as the previously described autonomic nervous system signs and symptoms, are present. In one reported case, significant residual dysfunction was present years later.[122] Whether autonomic nervous system dysfunction results from viral invasion of the central nervous system or an unusual immunologic response to infection is unknown.

Extragenital lesions

The development of extragenital lesions during the course of infection is a common complication of first episode primary genital herpes and is seen more commonly in women than men. Extragenital lesions are most frequently located in the buttock, groin, or thigh area, although finger and eye can also be involved. Among patients with primary HSV-2, 9 percent develop extragenital lesions, most commonly on the buttocks.[124] Among patients with primary HSV-1, 25 percent develop extragenital lesions, most commonly in or around the mouth. Characteristically, the extragenital lesions developed after the onset of genital lesions, often during the second week of disease. The distribution of lesions on the extremities and/or areas near the genital lesions and their occurrence later in the course of disease suggest that the majority of extragenital lesions develop by autoinoculation of virus or by viral reactivation in another part of the affected dermatome rather than viremic spread.[125] However, the recent demonstration of HSV DNA in plasma of patients with primary HSV suggests that viremic spread may also be a factor in these lesions. Prior to universal use of gloves in health care settings, HSV-1 was commonly isolated from herpetic infections of the hand.[65] One recent survey of herpetic infections of the hand found HSV-2 much more common than HSV-1.[126]

Disseminated infection

Blood-borne dissemination evidenced by the appearance of multiple vesicles over widespread areas of the thorax and extremities occurs rarely in persons with primary mucocutaneous herpes.[127,128] Cutaneous dissemination usually occurs early in the disease and is often associated with aseptic meningitis, hepatitis, pneumonitis, or arthritis.[129,130] Other complications of primary genital HSV-2 infection include monarticular arthritis, hepatitis, thrombocytopenia, and myoglobinuria.[131–136] Pregnancy may predispose to severe visceral dissemination of primary genital HSV disease.[137–139] Severe mucocutaneous and occasionally visceral dissemination of disease may occur in patients with atopic eczema.[140–142] In immunosuppressed patients, especially those with impaired cellular immune responses, reactivation of genital HSV infection can be associated with viremic spread of virus to multiple organs.[143–147] These patients may develop interstitial pneumonia, hepatitis, and pneumonitis, similar to the manifestations of disseminated infection of the neonate. Disseminated visceral infections in the immunosuppressed and pregnant patient have high mortality and should be treated with systemic antiviral chemotherapy.

Local extension of disease

Both HSV-1 and HSV-2 have been shown to be rare causes of pelvic inflammatory disease.[148] Some patients with primary cervical HSV infection may manifest lower abdominal pain and adnexal uterine tenderness. Occasionally, this represents dual infection with other sexually transmitted pathogens such as *N. gonorrhoeae* and *C. trachomatis*. However, extension of HSV infection into the uterine cavity has been reported, as well as laparoscopic evidence of vesicular lesions on the fallopian tube from which HSV has been isolated.[148]

Superinfection

Bacterial superinfection of genital herpes in immunocompetent patients is uncommon. In rare cases, pelvic cellulitis presenting as an advancing erythema and swelling of the perineal area is encountered. In such patients systemic antimicrobial therapy should be administered.

Fungal vaginitis, however, is frequently encountered during the course of initial genital herpes. In one series, yeast vaginitis was reported in 14 percent of women with first episodes of genital disease.[82] In another study of women attending an STD clinic, concurrent yeast infection was reported significantly more frequently in women with genital herpes than those without.[30] Characteristically, vaginal fungal infection develops during the second week of disease and is associated with a change in character of the vaginal discharge, and re-emergence of local symptoms such as vulvar itching and irritation. Typical hyphal yeast forms can be demonstrated on potassium hydroxide examination of vaginal secretions. If symptomatic, appropriate treatment is recommended (see Chap. 45).

Summary of the clinical course of initial genital herpes

First episode genital HSV infection is a disease with both systemic and local manifestations. Over one-half of the patients with primary genital herpes suffer from constitutional complaints, and one-third complain of headache, stiff neck, and mild photophobia during the first week of disease.

Patients with serological evidence of prior HSV-1 infection are less apt to have systemic symptoms and have a lower rate of complications and a shorter duration of disease than persons with true primary genital herpes. Neutralizing antibody to herpes simplex virus has been shown to inactivate extracellular virus and interrupt the spread of HSV infection.[149] In addition, a cellular immune response to HSV antigens appears earlier in persons with nonprimary genital HSV than in persons with true primary infection.[98] It is likely that both of these immune mechanisms account for the clinical differences between primary and nonprimary first episodes of genital infection.

Untreated primary genital herpes is a disease of significant morbidity warranting prompt diagnosis and treatment. We recommend initiation of oral antiviral therapy of all persons with a presumptive clinical diagnosis of first episode genital herpes. Confirmation of the diagnosis via culture of virus from lesions or demonstration of viral antigen or DNA in the genitourinary tract should be sought. All patients with first episode genital herpes should be treated with oral antiviral drugs. Early use of therapy will reduce the frequency of systemic manifestations of disease and prevent local extension of lesions into the upper genital tract. Moreover, early use of oral antivirals prevents the frequent development of new lesions that occur during the latter part of an episode. In general, patients tend to note the resolution of headache, fever, and fatigue within 48 hours of initiating therapy with acyclovir, famciclovir, or valacyclovir. Lesions will continue to extend for the initial 48 hours of therapy, but the frequency of new lesions will decrease. Healing may take 7 to 10 days. We prefer to use at least 10 days of therapy with first episode infection, as reactivation of virus with a new crop of vesicles is quite common in the initial 30 days post healing of primary genital HSV-2. In our experience, early discontinuation of therapy tends to exacerbate this phenomenon. Besides initiation of therapy, definite diagnosis and subsequent counseling about the nearly universal likelihood of reactivation and the potential for transmission of infection are the most important messages the treating clinician must convey to the patient with first episode genital herpes. These latter issues are best discussed after symptoms and signs of disease abate at a later visit and are discussed more fully later in the chapter.

RECURRENT GENITAL HERPES: CLINICAL SIGNS AND SYMPTOMS

In contrast to first episodes of genital infection, the symptoms, signs, and anatomic sites of infection of recurrent genital herpes are localized to the genital region.[82,98,150] Local symptoms such as pain and itching are mild to moderate compared to initial genital infection, and the duration of the episode usually ranges from 6 to 12 days (Table 21-2). About 90 percent of persons with recurrent genital herpes develop prodromal symptoms in some episodes; the development of symptoms prior to appearance of lesions occurs in about 60 percent of the episodes.[151] Prodromal symptoms vary from a mild tingling sensation, occurring 0.5 to 48 h prior to the eruption, to shooting pains in the buttocks, legs, or hips 1 to 5 days prior to the episode. In many patients the symptoms of sacral neuralgia are the most bothersome part of the episode. In about 20 percent of episodes patients experience prodromal symptoms without subsequent lesions. Whether HSV is present on mucosal surfaces more frequently during these prodromal only episodes is unclear.

As with initial genital disease, symptoms of recurrent genital herpes tend to be more severe in women (see Table 21-2). In several studies, painful genital lesions are reported more frequently (60–90%) in women (mean duration 5.9 days), compared with men (30–70%, 3.9 days, respectively). In addition, pain is reported to be more frequent and more severe in women compared with men.[61] Dysuria is reported in 25 percent of women with recurrent disease. Most reported only external dysuria, and isolation of HSV from the urethra is uncommon in both sexes (3–9%).

Lesions of recurrent genital HSV are usually confined to one side, with an area of involvement approximately one-tenth that of primary genital infection (plate 25). Untreated, the average duration of viral shedding from the onset of lesions is about 4 days; and the mean time from the onset of lesions to crusting of lesions averages between 4 and 5 days for both men and women (see

Table 21-2. Selected Clinical Signs of Recurrent Genital Herpes in Patients Followed at the University of Washington Genital HSV clinic

	Men $n = 218$	Women $n = 144$
Percent experiencing prodromal symptoms	53	43
Percent with pain	67*	88
Mean duration pain, days (range)	3.9(1–14)†	5.9
Mean duration itching, days (range)	4.6(1–16)	5.2(1–15)
Percent with dysuria	9	27
Percent with tender lymph nodes	23	31
Mean duration tender nodes, days (range)	9.2(1–25)†	5.9(1–15)
Percent with bilateral lesions	15‡	4
Percent forming new lesions during episode	43‡	28
Mean number of lesions at onset of episode, days (range)	7.5(1–25)	4.8(1–15)
Mean time to crusting, days (range)	4.1(1–15)	4.7(2–13)
Mean time to healing, days (range)	10.6(5–25)	9.3(4–29)
Mean during viral shredding from lesions, days (range)	4.4(1–20)	4.1(2–14)

* $p < 0.01$ by chi square.
† $p < 0.01$ by student's t = test
‡ $p < 0.05$ by chi square.

Table 21-2). The mean time from onset of vesicles to complete reepithelialization of lesions is about 6 to 10 days. Considerable variability exists in the severity and duration of disease both among patients and in a patient between episodes. Some recurrences have only one to two lesions lasting 2 to 3 days, whereas others may be associated with 15 to 20 lesions lasting 12 to 16 days. Although symptoms of recurrent genital disease are more severe in women, objective signs of disease are relatively similar in the two sexes. Only about 15 to 30 percent of women who present with recurrent genital lesions experience concomitant cervical infection. When present, the duration of cervical viral shedding is short, occurs early in the episode and is often without visible cervical lesions, unless routine colposcopy is performed (see HSV cervicitis section that follows below).

"ATYPICAL" HSV REACTIVATION

Whereas the classical clinical findings of genital HSV are described above, recent studies have illustrated the diverse clinical spectrum of genital HSV infection. For example, in a recent survey of randomly selected women in an STD clinic, HSV was isolated from 33 percent of women with genital lesions that lacked the characteristic appearance of vulvar ulcers; many of these lesions were small linear ulcerations, thought to be caused by trauma or yeast vaginitis.[30] HSV was also isolated from cervical ulcerations, some of which could be seen only with colposcopy. HSV can often be identified from nonconcentric genital ulcers without an erythematous base (plates 26 and 29). Perhaps these findings illustrate that when an infection is as prevalent as HSV-2, varied clinical signs and symptoms are to be "expected." These observations indicate that all genital lesions, regardless of appearance should be evaluated for herpes. Laboratory diagnostic tests such as viral cultures, or detection of HSV antigen or DNA should be used in patients with lesions, and type specific serologic assays to identify those with past infection should be employed.

Recurrence rate of genital HSV infection

The major morbidity of recurrent genital herpes is its frequent reactivation rate. Nearly all HSV-2 seropositive persons reactivate HSV-2 in the genital region. Moreover, because of the extensive area innervated by the sacral nerve root ganglia, reactivation of HSV-2 is widespread over a large anatomic area.

A prospective study of 457 patients with documented first episode genital herpes infection has shown that 90 percent of patients with genital HSV-2 developed recurrences in the first 12 months of infection.[62] The median recurrence rate was 0.33 recurrences/month. Most patients experienced multiple clinical reactivations. After primary HSV-2 infection, 38 percent of patients had at least six recurrences and 20 percent had more than 10 recurrences in the first year of infection. Men had slightly more frequent recurrences than women, median five recurrences per year compared with four (Fig. 21-5). Also, patients whose primary infection lasted more than 34 days had more frequent recurrences than those who healed faster, median eight compared with 4.3 recurrences per year, respectively. This finding is supported by the guinea pig model in which the number of ganglia that express the HSV latency transcripts correlate with subsequent recurrences.[152] Patients with primary genital HSV-2 infection who have a more prolonged initial episode develop high titers of HSV-2 complement-independent neutralizing antibody in convalescent sera and are more likely to develop recurrences than those who do not develop anti-HSV neutralizing antibody.[86,153] Development of high titers of complement-independent neutralizing antibody in convalescent-phase sera after primary infection may reflect a high degree of antigenic exposure and/or a large number of latently infected cells in sacral nerve root ganglia. In the mouse model of mucocutaneous HSV infection, high levels of neutralizing antibody in convalescent sera have been associated with increased numbers of latently infected ganglionic cells.[154]

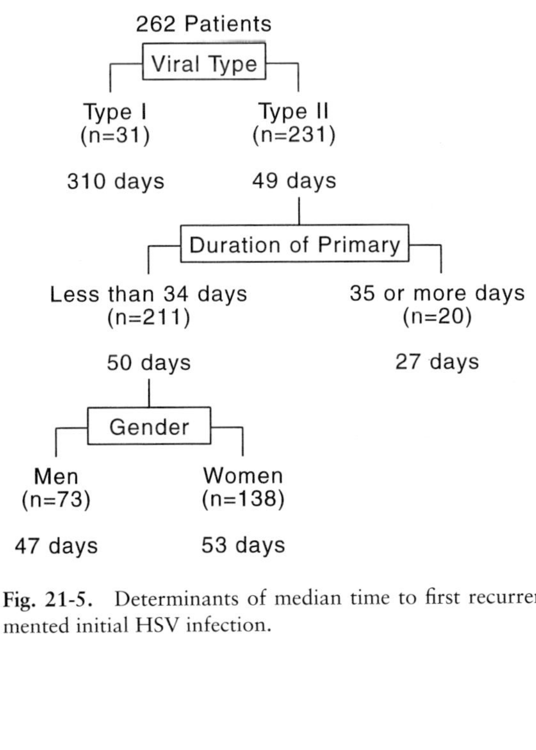

Fig. 21-5. Determinants of median time to first recurrence after documented initial HSV infection.

Recently, long term cohort studies indicate that the frequency of symptomatic recurrences gradually decrease over time of acquisition. Over the initial years of infection, the reported recurrence rate decreases by a median of one recurrence per year. As discussed below, almost all patients studied with recurrent symptomatic genital HSV also experience episodes of subclinical shedding. In general, these subclinical shedding episodes account for one-third to one-half of the total episodes of HSV reactivation as measured by viral isolation.

Reactivation, both symptomatic and subclinical, is less frequent with genital HSV-1 versus genital HSV-2 infection. Overall, 60 percent of patients with genital HSV-1 will recur clinically in the first year of follow up. However, rates of clinical reactivation average only 0.11 per month (1/year); and only 5 percent of persons with genital HSV-1 average more than four recurrences yearly, almost always in the first year of infection. In fact, frequent recurrences of genital herpes in persons with past genital HSV-1 suggest recent acquisition of genital HSV-2.

OTHER CLINICAL SYNDROMES ASSOCIATED WITH GENITAL HSV INFECTION

HSV cervicitis

HSV may involve the cervix alone, without involvement of the external genitalia. Cervical HSV infection may be asymptomatic or may present as a mucopurulent cervicitis (plate 14). In a recent survey of women attending an STD clinic, HSV was isolated from the cervix of 4 percent of randomly selected women attendees.[30] Of these women with HSV cervicitis, half had concomitant first episode genital lesions, 15 percent had evidence of recurrent genital lesions as well as HSV cervicitis infection; and 35 percent had only HSV cervicitis. Evidence of cervical lesions on routine speculum examination was present in 50 percent of these women, and an additional 15 percent of women had HSV lesions present on colposcopy. Overall, colposcopy detected 65 percent of women with HSV cervicitis. Papanicolaou smear revealed evidence of HSV cervicitis in 60 percent of women from whom HSV was isolated. Thus, even the most detailed clinical examination and cytologic testing will pick up only 65 to 70 percent of cervical HSV infection. Cervical HSV shedding is an occult site of reactivation of importance in transmission of HSV to infants and sexual partners.

Herpes simplex proctitis

HSV has been isolated from rectal mucosal and rectal biopsies in men and women with symptoms of rectal pain and discharge.[117,155–158] In the early 1980s among 100 consecutive homosexual men who presented to an STD clinic with symptoms of rectal discharge and pain, HSV was isolated from rectal swabs and/or rectal biopsies in 23 percent.[158] In men with nongonococcal proctitis, HSV was the most frequent pathogen isolated.

Unlike gonococcal proctitis, HSV proctitis is commonly associated with fever, systemic symptoms, severe rectal pain, discharge, tenesmus, and evidence of sacral autonomic nervous system dysfunction.[117,123,155–157,159,160–162] Patients usually present with acute onset of rectal pain, discharge, tenesmus, constipation, and bloody and/or mucoid rectal discharge. Fever, malaise, and myalgia are common, and urinary retention, dysesthesia of the perineal region, and impotence may be reported. External perianal lesions are seen in about one-half of the cases. Anoscopy and/or sigmoidoscopy generally reveal a diffuse, friable rectal mucosa, although occasionally discrete ulcerations of the rectal mucosa may be present (plates 73 and 74). In most cases the pathology is limited to the lower 10 cm of the rectum. Rectal biopsies of involved mucosa generally reveal diffuse ulcerations and lymphocytic infiltration. If multiple histological sections are performed, intranuclear inclusions may be demonstrated in rectal biopsies in about 40 percent of cases.[117] Both HSV-1 and HSV-2 have been isolated from patients with HSV proctitis.[117,157] Controlled clinical evaluation of the use of systemic acyclovir shows clinical benefit.[162] Most episodes of HSV proctitis are associated with the initial acquisition of HSV-1 or HSV-2. Although reactivation of infection in the perianal area is common and often subclinical in heterosexual and homosexual men and women, overt proctitis is uncommon with HSV-1 or HSV-2 reactivations.

Anorectal HSV infection may also be seen in women. Over three-quarters of anorectal HSV infections in women are asymptomatic, and there appears to be little association between anorectal HSV and anal intercourse (recent or past).[30] Reactivation of latent sacral ganglionic HSV infection may result in asymptomatic perianal shedding both among women and heterosexual men who deny anal intercourse.

Recurrent aseptic meningitis

Benign recurrent lymphocytic meningitis, or Mollaret's meningitis, is a syndrome characterized by recurrent episodes of aseptic meningitis lasting 3 to 7 days and resolving without neurologic sequelae.[163] The CSF shows protein elevation and predominantly mononuclear pleocytosis. Recent studies have demonstrated HSV DNA and the intrathecal persistence of HSV antibodies in the spinal fluid of patients with benign recurrent lymphocytic meningitis, indicating that HSV is the etiologic agent for many, if not most, cases of this disease.[164–167]

Recurrent episodes of aseptic meningitis following initial episodes of genital HSV-2 infection complicated by aseptic meningitis have been described.[168] In one series of 27 patients with HSV-2 meningitis associated with first-episode genital HSV-2, recurrent meningitis was noted in five patients, headache in association with genital recurrences in four, and possible recurrent meningitis in seven. Thus 16 (27%) patients appeared to have recurrent HSV reactivation in the CNS. Of interest, although HSV-2 was isolated from the CSF in most patients during the first episode disease, the virus was not isolated in any patients with recurrent meningitis. The inability to culture HSV from the CSF in recurrent episodes of aseptic meningitis has hindered the diagnosis until the advent of PCR assay and methods to detect HSV-specific intrathecal antibodies. Among 13 patients who met strict diagnostic criteria for benign recurrent lymphocytic meningitis, 11 had HSV DNA and HSV-specific antibodies recovered from the CSF, and the remaining two patients had intrathecal HSV-2 antibodies.[166] HSV-2 appears to be more frequently involved than HSV-1 and only a fraction of patients have a history of genital herpes.[166,167,169] Anecdotal reports and the authors' experience support the use of antiviral therapy to shorten or prevent the episodes.[169]

Genital ulcerations

HSV infection causes 40 to 60 percent of genital ulcerations in patients presenting to gynecologic practices or STD clinics in the United States.[170,171] The varied size, symptoms, and appearance of genital HSV lesions may make clinical diagnosis of genital ulcerations, especially single genital ulcerations difficult. HSV may be isolated from many lesions attributed by patients to trauma or irritation (plates 26 and 29). In addition, clinical differentiation of genital ulcerations caused by HSV, *Treponema pallidum,* and *Haemophilus ducreyi* is often uncertain (see Chap. 64). The sensitivity of a viral culture for detecting HSV in a lesion is only 50 percent, as the ulcer persists beyond the time virus is shed from the lesion. Thus, lack of isolation of HSV from a genital lesion does not rule out HSV as the etiologic agent. As almost all studied HSV-2 seropositive persons reactivate, the demonstration of HSV-2 seropositivity in a person with a recurrent genital ulceration strongly supports HSV-2 as the cause of the ulceration.

SUBCLINICAL REACTIVATION OF HSV

Subclinical or asymptomatic viral shedding is an important aspect of the clinical and epidemiologic understanding of genital herpes, as most episodes of sexual and vertical transmission appear to occur during such shedding.[59,172,173] HSV has been cultured from the lower genitourinary tract of women and men in the absence of genital ulcerations or other lesions. In women the anatomic sites of asymptomatic shedding include the cervix, vulva, anus, and urethra. In men asymptomatic shedding occurs from the penile skin, urethra, and anus. Transmission of genital herpes can occur by sexual contact with a person who is shedding HSV subclinically.[63,173–175]

Frequency of swabbing of the genital mucosa, the anatomic sites sampled and the technique to detect HSV correlate with the ability to detect subclinical shedding. In a study of 27 women who obtained daily samples from the cervix and the vulva, 9 percent of women who were sampled for less than 50 days had subclinical shedding compared with 83 percent of women who were sampled for a longer time.[176] Sampling the perianal region, in addition to the cervicovaginal and vulvar areas, increases the frequency of detection by one-third, and HSV DNA PCR assays detect HSV on mucosal surfaces two to three times as frequently as viral isolation.[177,178] Subclinical episodes of HSV reactivation share several characteristics with clinical episodes: (1) 25 percent of episodes last more than 1 day; (2) 17 percent of subclinical versus 22 percent of clinical episodes involve more than one anatomic site; (3) subclinical shedding is most likely to occur in temporal proximity to recurrences; and (4) women with frequent recurrences have frequent subclinical shedding.[177]

Development of PCR assays for HSV DNA has markedly broadened our understanding of the pathogenesis of subclinical HSV-2 infection. PCR is more sensitive for detecting HSV in genital lesions as well as on mucosal surfaces. Detailed evaluations have shown the specificity of the PCR assay. Figure 21-6 depicts the pattern and frequency of subclinical shedding in a man and a woman with genital HSV-2 infection. As shown in the diagram, shedding occurs in "clusters" of time, and subclinical shedding often occurs prior to episodes of genital lesions or culture positivity.

Subclinical HSV reactivation is highest in the 6 months after acquisition of infection. During this time period, HSV can be isolated from genital sites a mean of 6 percent of days by viral isolation and 20 to 35 percent of days by HSV PCR. Over the course of infection the frequency of HSV shedding decreases (Fig. 21-7). Persons with genital herpes for 5 to 10 years appear to have about half the subclinical shedding as women with disease of less than 2 years' duration. After 10 years the frequency of subclinical shedding appears to be about one-third of that within the early acquisition period. These estimates represent averages, as individual variability is great.

Great variability exists in the frequency of HSV shedding in the genital tract, whether measured by PCR or viral isolation. In the last several years, there has been increasing recognition of perianal reactivation of HSV, which relates to the overlapping dermatomal innervation of this area with the vulvar area in women and the

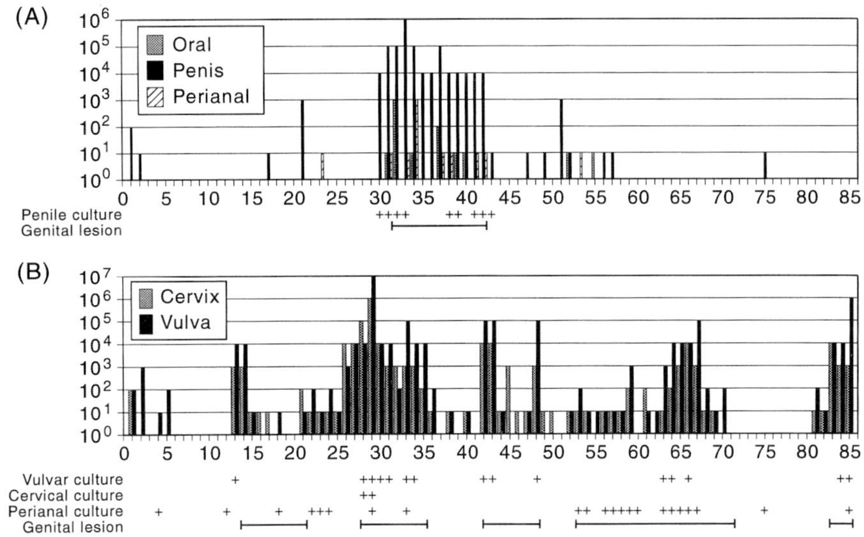

Fig. 21-6. Clinical and virologic shedding pattern as detected by viral culture and HSV DNA polymerase chain reaction in a man (A) and a woman (B). The man began obtaining daily viral cultures around day 30 after acquisition of genital HSV-2 infection. The woman was within 6-months of genital HSV-2 acquisition when she was enrolled into the study.

penile/scrotal area of men. During subclinical reactivation, HSV DNA can be detected by PCR in multiple anatomic areas. Studies in which the cervical, vulvar, and perianal sites are sampled show less difference in the frequency of HSV isolation and HSV DNA detection than studies in which only the cervical and/or vulvar sites are sampled.

Among men, the most common site of shedding is penile skin, followed by the perianal area. Shedding can also occur from the urethra and from the semen, especially close to the time of acquisition, and transmission of HSV via infected semen has been documented.[179] However, semen cultures rarely yield virus despite an early report of high rate of HSV isolation from seminal secretions in men undergoing vasectomy.[180,181] It is likely that the penile skin shedding is the most important source of transmission from men to women.

The existence of frequent subclinical shedding implies that the control of genital herpes will depend on more than prevention of sexual encounters during recurrences of lesions, as transmission can occur at times when no lesions are noted. Counselors of patients with genital herpes need to emphasize this potential for infectivity and provide appropriate strategies to decrease risk to patients' sexual partners.

THE PROBLEM OF UNRECOGNIZED RECURRENT GENITAL HERPES

Several recent studies have suggested that the vast majority of HSV-2 seropositive persons who deny having genital lesions are not truly asymptomatic, but have genital lesions that they do not recognize as being genital herpes. This observation has been demonstrated in three separate studies, in two different clinical set-

Fig. 21-7. Frequency of detection of HSV in 39 persons, according to time since acquisition of genital HSV-2 disease.

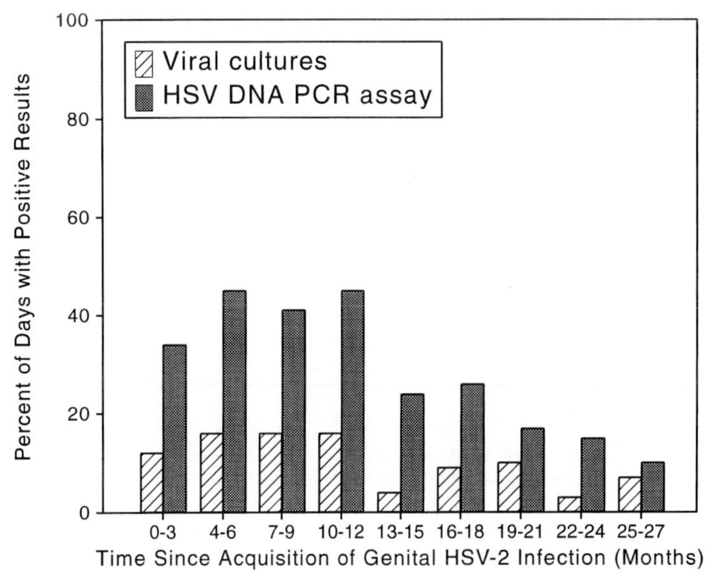

tings. The initial study was conducted by Langenberg et al. in a gynecology clinic in a public hospital.[182] In this study HSV-2 seropositive women unaware of genital herpes were instructed by a paramedical research assistant on the clinical signs and symptoms of genital disease. Pictures of genital HSV lesions were shown to them and the nature of HSV transmission and reactivation explained. The women were then asked to attend the clinic for any subsequent genitourinary complaints. Of 62 such women, 48 percent presented with recognizable genital lesions of HSV. Symptomatic genital herpes was the most common genitourinary complaint in this group of women during follow up. Previously, yeast vaginitis, nonspecific trauma associated with intercourse, and a variety of other explanations were given as the etiology of the ulcerations.

Similar findings were reported by Frenkel et al. in a group of pregnant women.[183] Most recently, Wald et al. have shown that in a general medicine clinic 57 percent of HSV-2 seropositive women, who initially denied genital lesions, were, after a counseling session, shown to be clinically symptomatic.[184] These data suggest that accurate serologic testing with an appropriate counseling session can effectively identify persons with symptomatic disease. As sexual contact with such persons is an important factor in HSV transmission, such an approach may be useful in containing the epidemic spread of this infection.

One of the critical questions in the area of subclinical genital HSV is whether the frequency of subclinical reactivation among persons denying genital lesions is higher, lower, or more varied than those with symptomatic infection. This question has been recently addressed by us in the following manner: 37 HSV-2 seropositive women without a history of genital herpes were enrolled in a study involving daily home cultures. Of these 37 women, all but six had HSV-2 reactivation during follow up. The frequency of subclinical reactivation was about 3 percent of days, similar to women with clinical disease. Unexpectedly, the duration of clinical recurrences tended to be shorter in those who previously denied genital lesions compared to women who recognized their herpetic lesions. These data help explain the unrecognized nature of these lesions. Yet, the major differences between HSV-2 seropositive persons who are aware of having genital herpes versus those not aware of having genital herpes is patient and provider education. Reactivation of HSV-2 is frequent in both populations.

GENITAL HERPES VIRUS INFECTION IN THE IMMUNOCOMPROMISED PATIENT

Although much of the literature on HSV infections in the immunosuppressed patient has concentrated on oral-labial disease, the increasing prevalence of genital herpes has resulted in an improved awareness of the consequences of genital herpes in this population. Immunocompromised patients have frequent and prolonged mucocutaneous HSV infections.[185–187] Over 70 percent of renal and bone marrow transplant recipients who have serologic evidence of past HSV infection reactivate latent HSV infection within the first month after transplantation.[188,189] Mucocutaneous HSV infections in the immunocompromised host may be associated with systemic complaints, prolonged local symptoms, and durations of viral shedding greater than 30 days.

Recurrent genital herpes in immunosuppressed patients often results in the development of large numbers of vesicles that coalesce into deep, often necrotic ulcerative lesions.[190] Dissemination of virus may occur. Ramsey et al. reported the isolation of HSV-2 from lung parenchyma of one of 15 adult bone marrow transplant recipients who developed herpes simplex virus pneumonitis.[191] The administration of prophylactic acyclovir prior to bone marrow transplantation has decreased the incidence of reactivated HSV disease.[192,193] Several studies have demonstrated the benefit of acyclovir in shortening the clinical and virologic course of mucocutaneous HSV infection in the immunocompromised patient.[194] In general most episodes of mucocutaneous herpes in the immunosuppressed should be treated with oral or intravenous antiviral agents.

HSV IN PATIENTS WITH HIV INFECTION

Both case-control and cohort studies have shown that prior HSV-2 infection is associated with acquisition of HIV.[195–201] Although the magnitude of the estimates of the relative risk for HIV seroconversion among persons with genital herpes has varied from 1.2 to 8.5, most studies that examined the association found a positive association with a relative risk of two to three, and no studies have found a negative association.[202] The elevated risk has been found in male to male, male to female, and female to male transmission. These studies have focused on the HSV status of the person acquiring HIV, as few studies of HIV transmitters have been done for methodological reasons. However, Cameron et al. found a 4.7 higher risk of HIV seroconversion among men who acquired a genital ulcer from a sex worker compared with men who did not.[203] Thus epidemiologic data support the role of genital herpes and other ulcerative STDs in fueling the HIV epidemic in developed and developing countries.

In the United States, the risk of HIV transmission attributable to genital ulcers may be especially great among heterosexuals who are currently the fastest growing segment of the HIV-infected population. The proportion of persons with AIDS who acquired HIV from heterosexual contact has increased from 3 percent between 1981 to 1987 to 10 percent between 1993 to 1995.[204] This increase is especially prominent among women, for whom heterosexual contact rivals injection drug use as the most frequent risk factor for HIV infections.[205] Epidemiologic studies conducted in this country suggest that HSV-2 infection doubles the risk of HIV acquisition in the heterosexual population, and those at risk for HIV are more likely to have HSV-2 infection than the general population.[198]

Laboratory studies have provided supportive evidence that HSV may be an important cofactor for HIV expression. The HSV regulatory proteins ICPO and ICP4 can upregulate the rate of HIV replication in vitro.[206] Herpetic lesions are associated with an influx of activated CD4-bearing lymphocytes, which may result in increased expression of HIV on mucosal surfaces.[207] In vivo, HSV-1 and HIV coinfection of epithelial cells results in a higher copy number of HSV virions.[208] Recently, Schacker et al. have detected HIV virions in nearly all genital herpes lesions in HSV and HIV infected persons, providing virologic confirmation of epidemiologic observations that HSV facilitates HIV transmission (T. Schacker, personal communication).

HSV infections are among the most common clinical presentations and manifestations of HIV infection. Almost all homosexual men with HIV infection possess antibodies to HSV: 80 to 90 percent with HSV-1 and 80 to 95 percent to HSV-2.[196,199] Of interest, in patients with both HSV-1 and HSV-2 antibodies, reactivation of genital lesions appears to be more frequent than of oral lesions.[101]

Although anecdotal observations suggest that patients with HIV have more frequent and prolonged episodes, with slower response to acyclovir, even in the absence of overt acyclovir resistance, few studies have examined the impact of HIV on the natural history of HSV infection. A small fraction of HIV and HSV infected patients will present with persistent chronic mucocutaneous ulcerations often involving large areas of perianal, scrotal, or penile skin.[209] Pain and lesions may be present for months and secondary candidal infections are extremely common. Among persons with high CD4 counts (>400), the frequency of disease or subclinical shedding has not been studied. In a recent study of 68 HIV and HSV-2 infected men who obtained daily viral cultures from the genital tract, HIV-related immunosuppression had only a modest effect on the rate and duration of clinical recurrences of genital herpes (T. Schacker, personal communication). However, the rate of subclinical shedding was significantly increased when compared with HIV negative controls, a mean 7.3 percent of days versus 1.1 percent of days without lesions on which a viral culture was obtained, respectively. The most common site of shedding was the perianal area. CD4 count below $200/m^3$ conferred an increased risk of subclinical shedding in the men with HIV infections. Similar observations were made in a cross-sectional study of HIV seropositive women: HSV was isolated in 13 percent of women with HIV infection compared with 3.6 percent of women without HIV infection.[210]

Most HSV infections in persons with HIV infection will respond to acyclovir, albeit slowly. Many of these patients benefit from chronic suppressive therapy. However, some patients who initially respond to acyclovir may develop thymidine-kinase deficient mutants for which standard antiviral therapy is ineffective (see the following).

GENITAL HSV INFECTIONS IN PREGNANCY

One of the major concerns to patients with genital herpes is the effect of disease on pregnancy and the neonate. Neonatal herpes is a disease of high mortality and morbidity (see Chap. 85).[211–213] Transmitting this STD to a newborn has devastating effects on the parents.

Both congenital and intrapartum transmission of HSV infection have been described.[214,215] When evaluating the pregnant woman with genital herpes, it should be remembered that the severity of the clinical disease, incidence of cervicitis, duration and titer of viral shedding, and potential of developing viremia differ between patients with first episode infections compared to those with recurrent infection. Relative risk of transmission to the neonate and management of disease vary accordingly.

EPIDEMIOLOGY OF HERPES IN PREGNANCY

The prevalence of genital HSV infection during pregnancy as well as the relative incidence of neonatal HSV infection is influenced by the socioeconomic status, age and past sexual activity of the patient population studied. In the United States serologic evidence of past HSV-2 infection is present in about 30 percent of middle-class women attending prenatal clinics; the percentage is 50 to 70 percent in nonwhite lower socioeconomic obstetrical populations. Despite this high serologic prevalence, clinical evidence of HSV is much less prevalent. In Seattle, where an obstetric population has a 30 percent prevalence of HSV-2, a past or current history of genital HSV is present in 8 percent of women.

Neonatal HSV infection is not a reportable disease in the United States. Estimates of the incidence of neonatal herpes have varied from 1 in 3000 to 1 in 20,000 live births.[212] The overall frequency of neonatal HSV infection in the United States has been estimated to be approximately 1 in 7500 live births, or about 700 cases yearly nationally. In many areas neonatal herpes has increased in frequency over the last decade. In King County, Washington, the rate is now 16 per 100,000 live births (see Fig. 21-2).[58]

Recent studies have shown that the highest risk for transmitting HSV in the perinatal period occurs during the acquisition of HSV at or near the time of labor. This helps explain the wide variability in frequency of neonatal herpes worldwide. Obstetrical populations with high HSV-2 prevalence have a low incidence of neonatal HSV infection. Populations with high risk of acquiring HSV in pregnancy have the highest neonatal HSV infection rates. Contraceptive and behavioral practices markedly influence the epidemiology of neonatal HSV infection. Scandinavia and the west coastal areas of the United States appear to have the highest neonatal HSV rates (about 1 in 3000 live births).

CLINICAL COURSE OF GENITAL HERPES IN PREGNANCY

Most of the clinical manifestations of recurrent genital herpes, including the frequency of subclinical vs. clinical infection and the duration of lesions, pain, and constitutional symptoms are similar in pregnant and nonpregnant women.[216,217] The frequency and severity of recurrences appear to increase over the course of pregnancy.[217] Visceral dissemination of HSV in pregnant women acquiring primary genital disease has been described, especially if infection is acquired in the third trimester.[137–139] Routine antiviral therapy for first episode HSV is not required in pregnancy but may be given for severe disease. Intravenous acyclovir should be initiated in pregnant women who have evidence of disseminated infection, especially hepatitis, pneumonitis, or coagulopathy.

EFFECTS OF HSV ON PREGNANCY OUTCOME

Studies in the 1960s in lower socioeconomic class populations suggested that genital HSV infection was associated with an increased frequency of spontaneous abortion and premature delivery.[218,219] These studies also suggested that primary HSV cervicitis had a higher risk of complications than other aspects of disease. Brown et al. accumulated 28 cases of women who acquired first episode genital HSV in pregnancy.[220] Pregnancy morbidity was only seen in the 15 women with clinical primary infection; that is, those with fever, constitutional symptoms, and severe lesions. Serologic and clinical evidence of nonprimary infection was not associated with pregnancy morbidity. Neonatal HSV and prematurity were most frequently seen in women who acquired primary genital infection during the third trimester.[220]

Several potential explanations may account for these differences in neonatal morbidity among women with primary versus recurrent genital HSV infection. With primary disease, both hematogenous spread of HSV as well as ascending chorioamnionitis may result in neonatal infection and disease.[221] Recurrent vulvar genital herpes is usually not associated with cervicitis. In fact, little evidence currently exists to suggest that women with recurrent genital herpes have increased rates of neonatal morbidity. Several clinical series and a recent population based study of women with recurrent genital HSV in pregnancy suggested no effect of clinical recurrent infection on neonatal outcome including birth weight and gestational age.[216,217,222]

TRANSMISSION OF HSV TO THE NEONATE

Almost all cases of neonatal herpes are perinatally acquired. The infant acquires infection at the time of delivery through contact with HSV.[211,212,223] In fact, a recent survey has shown that although HSV seroconversion occurs in about 3 percent of pregnancies, HSV acquisition is associated with little pregnancy morbidity, except when it occurs close to delivery.[224] Over 70 percent of infants with neonatal HSV infection are born to mothers who lack symptoms or signs of HSV lesions at delivery. Figure 21-8 depicts the frequency of subclinical HSV shedding at the time of labor and its relationship to neonatal HSV from studies conducted at the University of Washington. The risk of transmission of neonatal herpes to the infant from a woman with primary HSV infection is about 50 percent. HSV-2 infection from a woman with past HSV-1 and new HSV-2 infection is 20 percent and the risk of neonatal transmission in women with recurrent HSV-2 is less than 1 percent.[222,225–227]

These data suggest that HSV-2 specific antibodies protect from disease acquisition. The decreasing frequency of neonatal transmission from 50 percent in primary infection to 20 percent in those with past HSV-1 and newly acquired HSV-2 to less than 1 percent among those with recurrent HSV-2 strongly supports the protective role of maternal antibodies. These data support studies by Yeager et al. showing low levels of neutralizing antibodies in infants with severe neurologic HSV-2 infection.[228] Although titers of HSV shed from mucosal surfaces are higher in first versus recurrent episodes of infection, recent data suggest that many of the infants born to mothers with recurrent genital herpes have been exposed to high titers of HSV at delivery.

Factors determining whether an exposed infant becomes infected are not completely defined and include viral titer, local environmental and immune factors, use of fetal monitoring devices, cellular immune response of the neonate, and titer of maternal antibody in serum and/or amniotic fluid.[228,229]

MANAGEMENT OF PREGNANT WOMEN WITH GENITAL HERPES

The management of the pregnant women with genital HSV must be individualized and based on the clinical course of disease in the mother as well as the availability of virological and serologic methods of diagnosis. Although additional critical information is needed before optimal management of women with genital herpes can be recommended, some guidelines concerning the use of diagnostic virological tests and of cesarean section can be made.

The acquisition of primary disease in pregnancy carries the risk of potential transplacental transmission of virus to the neonate. In some women, primary infection will result in spontaneous abortion; albeit this appears to be relatively uncommon. One common question raised by patients with first episodes of genital herpes during pregnancy who do not abort is the use of amniocentesis to determine if intrauterine infection, and hence a congenitally infected child, is present. Recent evidence suggests that false-positive as well as false-negative information can occur from this procedure.[230] Uninfected infants have been delivered, despite the antepartum isolation of HSV from amniotic fluid. In addition, antiviral substances in amniotic fluid may make isolation of virus from the infant difficult. Thus, amniocentesis at present does not appear to be a reliable test for predicting the presence or absence of a congenitally infected infant. The vast majority of pregnant women with recurrent genital herpes deliver normal infants, and routine amniocentesis is not recommended in these women.

Criteria for laboratory screening and surveillance, as well as delivery procedures for women with recurrent genital HSV infections, are the most frequently encountered questions of obstetricians handling pregnant women with genital herpes. It is obvious that the high prevalence rate of HSV-2 infection in pregnancy (antibody prevalence 30–60% depending on the population studied) and the low incidence of neonatal disease (1:6000–1:20,000 live births) indicate that only a few infants are at risk of acquiring disease. Cesarean section is therefore not routinely warranted for all women with recurrent genital disease. As intrapartum transmission of infection accounts for the vast majority of cases, only those women who shed HSV at the time of delivery need be considered for abdominal delivery. Several studies have shown no correlation between recurrences or viral shedding prior to delivery, and the presence of viral shedding at term.[216,217,222] As such, weekly cytologic and virologic monitoring is no longer advocated.

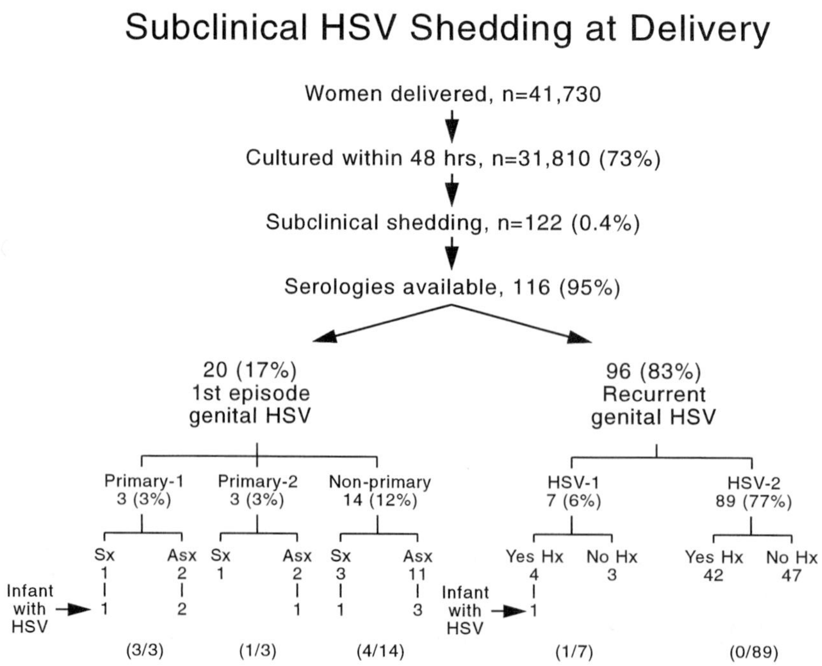

Fig. 21-8. Frequency of HSV isolation from cervix and vulva of women in labor in relation to the type of HSV infection and to transmission of infection to the neonate.

Unfortunately, a rapid and reliable diagnostic method to detect asymptomatic cervical viral shedding of HSV is not available. Although rapid assays such as ELISA, FA, and routine DNA hybridization methods have equal sensitivity to viral cultures from specimens from genital lesions, they have reduced sensitivity as compared to viral isolation for asymptomatic shedding. As shedding is a relatively uncommon event, these assays also have low positive predictive values for detecting genitourinary HSV infection at the time of delivery. In addition, tests that detect viral shedding lack specificity as most women with recurrent disease who shed virus at delivery do not transmit the infection.

The risk of transmitting neonatal HSV among women who are HSV seropositive is less than 2 percent. Patients with recurrent genital herpes should be encouraged to come to the delivery room early at the time of delivery. At this time, careful examination of the external genitalia and the cervix should be performed. In addition, a swab of the cervix and/or vulvar area for viral isolation should be performed. Women who have no clinical evidence of lesions should be delivered vaginally. The presence of active lesions of the cervix or external genitalia, that is, clinical evidence of herpes virus infection of the lower genital tract, are indications for abdominal delivery.[231] This policy will result in the exposure of some infants to episodes of cervical and/or vulvar shedding. Only a few infants exposed to maternal secretions containing HSV develop neonatal herpes.[227] Identifying such infants and communicating the HSV exposure to the attending pediatrician are necessary.[232,233] Currently, most experts advise obtaining viral cultures from the throat, nasopharynx, eyes, and rectum of these infants immediately and then at 5- to 10-day intervals. Any clinical evidence of lethargy, skin lesions, or other symptoms of neonatal HSV should be evaluated promptly. All infants from whom HSV is isolated after 24 hours of delivery should be treated with systemic antiviral chemotherapy.

Definitive studies on the relationship between the duration of ruptured membranes in women with clinically apparent lesions and transmission of HSV to the infant are lacking. Delivery of infants by cesarean section, even from women with intact membranes, will occasionally result in neonatal herpes.[232] Prolonged contact with infected secretions may increase the relative risk of acquisition of disease. Many authorities recommend that if membranes have been ruptured for over 4 to 6 hours, cesarean section should no longer be considered for protection against HSV transmission. However, studies of neonatal HSV infection in Seattle have shown that transmission can occur from exposure to only external genital lesions, that is, from women who are culture positive only on vulvar and not cervicovaginal swabs. Thus, for women with recurrent genital herpes who have active external genital lesions at the time of labor, we still recommend abdominal delivery, providing that no evidence of cervical involvement has been demonstrated by prior virological monitoring techniques and/or cervical cytological techniques.

Prevention of HSV acquisition in pregnancy

The key to prevention of neonatal HSV is the prevention of acquisition of genital HSV-1 or HSV-2 infection late in pregnancy. Several approaches are possible. In high incidence areas, such as the west coast of the United States and Scandinavia, a case can be made for serologic screening in the third trimester to identify women at risk. Risk exists in HSV seronegative women with an HSV-1 or HSV-2 seropositive partner or HSV-1 seropositive women with an HSV-2 seropositive partner. This requires the availability of accurate serologic assays for both the pregnant woman and her HSV-2 seropositive partner. Counseling to avoid sexual contact, including oral-genital contact, in late pregnancy is recommended. Greater appreciation of potential to acquire HSV-1 via oral-genital sex in late pregnancy is needed, as nearly 30 percent of neonatal HSV is caused by HSV-1.

Another approach is to serologically screen only women and to counsel about the risk of acquisition in the late third trimester. The disadvantage of this approach is that only about 20 percent of couples have discordant HSV serologies and are "at risk."[234] In low prevalence settings, where neonatal HSV is uncommon, the cost of serologic screening may outweigh the benefits.

Infants born by cesarean section to women prior to the rupture of membranes or by vaginal delivery to women with no evidence of recent HSV infection are at minimal risk of developing HSV infection and most hospitals do not recommend segregating the infant from the rest of the newborn nursery. If a more cautious approach is desired, the infant can be put into an Isolette to make hospital personnel aware of the necessity to use wound and skin precautions and proper hand washing techniques.

Infants born of women at risk of transmitting disease to the neonate (i.e., women with active lesions) should be placed in isolation.[235] Viral cultures, liver function studies, and CSF examinations should be obtained and the infant should be observed closely for the first month of life. Any symptoms of neonatal disease (e.g., poor feeding, fever, hypothermia, skin lesions, or central nervous system signs such as seizures) should be investigated expeditiously for evidence of neonatal HSV infection.[233,236] Management of contact between infant and mother should also be handled on an individual basis. In women who acquire primary genital herpes late in pregnancy, the high incidence of developing extragenital lesions and the potential of viremia suggest that separation between mother and infant is warranted until therapy has produced a clinical and virological response. As recurrent genital herpes is rarely associated with frequent dissemination of disease or the development of extragenital lesions in exposed extremities, protection of the infant from exposure to infected genital secretion is adequate. When handling the infant in the hospital, the mother should wear a gown and observe proper hand washing techniques. We allow rooming in with the mother once she has been taught protective measures and is cognizant of the importance of washing her hands between touching her genitalia and then touching the infant. Oral-labial herpes is a greater risk for postnatal acquisition of HSV infection by the newborn than genital herpes.[237] Thus, nursery personnel and other adults with external labial lesions caused by HSV should also be excluded from intimate contact with the newborn infant.[238]

Antivirals in pregnancy

Controversy exists regarding the use of antiviral therapy during pregnancy. Since the incidence of neonatal HSV-2 is low among women with recurrent genital herpes, the use of oral antivirals in late pregnancy to prevent neonatal HSV would not be cost effective; one would treat 99 to 100 women to prevent one case. However, the incidence of cesarean delivery is much higher, and studies are underway to evaluate if routine antiviral suppression is effective in reducing subclinical shedding of HSV and the frequency of abdominal delivery without increasing the risk to the infant via vaginal delivery. Until these studies are completed, no recommendations can be given.

DIAGNOSIS OF GENITAL HERPES

CLINICAL DIAGNOSIS

The differentiation between genital HSV infection and other infectious or noninfectious etiologies of genital ulceration may be difficult. If multiple grouped vesicles are present or if there is a history of prior lesions of similar size, duration, and character,

HSV infection is the most likely etiology of the ulceration. Lesions of genital herpes are usually painful when touched and this clinical sign may be useful in differentiating coalesced genital herpetic ulcers from other etiologies such as *T. pallidum*. It should, however, be remembered that occasionally both organisms may coexist in the same lesion.[239] A persistent, tender, large ulcerative lesion in a patient at risk of *T. pallidum* infection, especially one in whom nontender, rubbery bilateral inguinal adenopathy is present, should raise the suspicion that both pathogens may be present. Epidemiologic setting is helpful in determining the relative probability of genital herpes versus other infections. For example, in the United States most genital ulcerations in heterosexual persons will be caused by HSV. However, in other populations *H. ducreyi* and *T. pallidum* may be more prevalent.

Both primary and recurrent HSV infection are accompanied by tender lymphadenopathy. The inguinal nodes on palpation are usually mildly tender, nonfixed, and only slightly firm. Suppuration, commonly seen with *H. ducreyi* and/or lymphogranuloma venereum, is only rarely seen in genital HSV infection. Nontender, rubbery, firm lymph nodes are more commonly seen with *T. pallidum* infection. Because of the diversity of the signs and symptoms of HSV infections, laboratory confirmation of the etiology of genital ulcers should be sought in nearly all cases.[116]

Noninfectious causes of genital ulcerations, such as inflammatory bowel disease (Crohn's disease) or mucosal ulcerations associated with Behcet's syndrome, may also be confused with genital herpes. These noninfectious causes usually are associated with ulcers that persist for much longer periods of time than those associated with recurrent genital herpes. In addition, the lesions themselves appear larger and deeper than those typically seen in genital HSV infection. A history of persistent lesions waxing and waning with the symptoms of bowel disease is usually elicited in those who have genital ulcerations as mucocutaneous manifestation of Crohn's disease. Persistent oral lesions, conjunctivitis, and/or central nervous system disease may help differentiate Behcet's syndrome from recurrent genital herpes. The overlap between primary genital HSV infection with conjunctivitis and aseptic meningitis and Behcet's syndrome may, however, cause diagnostic confusion (plate 30). Persistent lack of laboratory evidence of HSV infection is often useful in establishing the clinical diagnosis of these noninfectious entities.

LABORATORY DIAGNOSIS

Laboratory confirmation of genital herpes should be performed on all persons in whom a definitive clinical diagnosis cannot be made. Knowledge of the diagnosis is useful in (1) explaining the potential infectivity during episodes of lesions; (2) identifying persons at risk for transmitting infection subclinically; (3) selecting women at future risk for transmitting the infection to the neonate; and (4) confirming the diagnosis in those in whom antiviral chemotherapy is prescribed. Viral isolation, HSV DNA detection by PCR, and HSV antigen detection by EIA or FA are all useful assays. The rapid appearance of HSV in tissue culture (1–4 days) makes viral isolation a very useful assay, especially if the isolate can be subtyped (HSV-1 vs HSV-2).

Demonstration of a rise in anti-HSV antibody titer in sera drawn early and after an episode of disease has limited utility. Serodiagnosis is useful for documenting first episode infections for clinical studies. Less than 10 percent of patients with recurrent episodes of disease experience a serological rise in antibody titer between acute and convalescent sera.[86]

The development of type specific serologic methods provides the opportunity to determine if a person is an asymptomatic HSV carrier. Such accurate, type specific assays will be marketed presently and will hopefully replace the currently available tests which do not differentiate reliably between antibodies to HSV-1 and HSV-2. As most HSV appears to be transmitted from persons who have undiagnosed disease or asymptomatic infection, more active identification of HSV-2 carriers should be initiated in high prevalence populations. Past infection with HSV-2 can be identified by the presence of specific HSV-2 antibodies in serum. It appears that nearly all persons with HSV-2 antibodies reactivate virus periodically and hence are potential transmitters of infection.

COUNSELING/PREVENTION

Because of its chronicity, for many persons the diagnosis of genital herpes brings with it significant long-term complications. Most patients diagnosed with genital herpes report feelings of depression and isolation and fear of rejection and discovery.[240,241] These feelings tend to subside, although not completely, with time. A survey of members of the American Social Health Association support groups showed that 50 percent of respondents experienced depression and feelings of rejection, even after many years of living with the disease.[241] The distress associated with the diagnosis of HSV is exacerbated by the frequent difficulties in obtaining an accurate diagnosis and the difficulties health care providers often have in dealing with the emotional and sexual issues that surround the diagnosis. During the acute illness, the patient is often too concerned with the physical illness and with having the diagnosis of an STD to comprehend the chronic nature of the infection and the caution that must be exercised to prevent the spread of the infection. Thus, the best strategy for counseling is to ask the patients to return after the primary illness resolves to deal with the long-term issues posed by having an incurable STD. At the first visit, palliation of symptoms is the most important objective. In addition to antiviral therapy, local measures such as sitz baths or drying the genital area with a hair dryer can decrease the discomfort of lesions.

Clinicians should emphasize the recurrent and highly variable natural history of herpes and explain the potential for transmission during subclinical shedding. However, it is also important to reassure the patients that they will be able to continue to have intimate relationships, despite the infection. Women are often concerned regarding the potential for having healthy children and need reassurance that the risk of transmission during delivery is minimal for women with recurrent genital herpes. Patients need to be encouraged to tell potential sexual partners of their infection, to abstain during recurrences, and to use condoms consistently at other times. It is useful to reinforce these issues over several visits and to see patients at their first recurrence to confirm their ability to recognize recurrences. Many patients are dismayed at their first recurrence because they realize that this infection will recur, whereas others are relieved that the symptoms are much milder than those during the primary episode. Most patients resent the lack of predictability of the disease as much as the discomfort. Attempts by patients to control the recurrences often include avoidance of certain foods, vitamin supplements and stress reduction. Scientific evaluation of the benefit of these methods is lacking and fraught with difficulties. Despite the common perception that stress causes recurrences, a prospective study suggested that stress follows recurrences.[242]

Strategies for the control of genital herpes have not been well defined. A combination of methods are likely to be needed to contain the current epidemic of genital herpes. For persons with recognized HSV infection, behavioral change is the most important tool for protection of sexual partners. Although we routinely advocate the use of condoms for prevention of HSV, their effectiveness has not been extensively evaluated. Given the wide anatomic distribution of HSV, the protection offered by a condom is most likely incomplete. While nonoxynol-9 has been shown protective in models of mice vaginitis, human data are lacking.[243] Antiviral therapy has been shown to effectively suppress subclinical shedding.[244] As such, chronic antiviral therapy may result in decrease of HSV transmission to sexual partners. Thus chronic suppression of viral reactivation may become one of the strategies for HSV control in selected settings. Given that most people with HSV-2 infection have mild symptoms and unrecognized disease, the public health impact of suppressive therapy in discordant couples is likely to be limited.

Since most persons with HSV-2 infection do not have a history of genital herpes, serologic testing to identify those who are infected may also play an important role in control of genital herpes. Behavioral change and, possibly, chronic antiviral therapy can then be used as methods for control of genital herpes among people identified on serologic testing as HSV-2 infected. The settings in which serologic screening may be useful have not been identified, but such a strategy may be fruitful among pregnant women and STD clinic attendees. Among pregnant women, it is crucial to identify those who are seronegative for HSV-2 but whose partners have HSV-2, as it is the acquisition of HSV during late pregnancy that is associated with the highest risk of infection of the fetus.[224]

THERAPY OF GENITAL HERPES

The therapy of genital herpes includes the following goals: (1) preventing infection (i.e., prophylactic therapy); (2) shortening the clinical course of disease, including the frequency of complications of primary infection such as aseptic meningitis and urinary retention; (3) preventing the development of latency and subsequent clinical recurrences after initial genital infection; (4) preventing subsequent recurrences of disease in those with established latency; (5) decreasing the transmission of disease; and (6) eradicating established latent infection. Despite major inroads in the therapy of genital herpes over the last 13 years, only some of these goals have been achieved by the available therapeutic interventions. Guidelines for evaluation of new therapies for genital herpes infections have been proposed.[245]

NUCLEOSIDE ANALOGS

Acyclovir

The mainstay of the therapy of genital HSV infection are formulations of nucleoside analogs, most often used in an oral form. Acyclovir (ACV) was the first effective antiviral developed and used for the therapy of genital herpes. ACV is an acyclic nucleoside analog that is a substrate for HSV-specified thymidine kinase.[246,247] Acyclovir is selectively phosphorylated by HSV-infected cells to ACV-monophosphate (ACV-MP). Cellular enzymes then phosphorylate ACV-MP to ACV-triphosphate, a competitive inhibitor of viral DNA polymerase.[248–250] ACV-TP is incorporated into the growing DNA chain of the virus and causes chain termination.

ACV has potent in vitro activity against both HSV-1 and HSV-2.[251] In animal models, topical or systemic ACV markedly reduces the severity of mucocutaneous HSV infections and, if administered within 96 hours after inoculation of virus, prevents ganglionic latency.[249] Numerous trials of ACV in primary and recurrent genital herpes have been conducted. In primary genital HSV infection, intravenous ACV (5 mg/kg q 8 h for 5 days), oral ACV 200 mg (5 times/day for 10–14 days) and topical ACV (5% in polyethylene glycol ointment) each reduce the duration of symptoms and viral shedding and speed healing.[94,95,115,252] Systemic therapy prevents new lesion formation. Because of the high incidence of urethral, cervical, and oral infections in first episode infections, oral acyclovir is preferable to topical. The clinical effect of acyclovir on first episode infection is considerable, reducing fever and constitutional symptoms within 48 hours of initiating therapy and rapidly relieving symptoms. As such, therapy should be initiated in all patients with presumptive first episode genital HSV who present with active lesions. The authors' personal recommendation is to initiate therapy with 400 mg tid per day (Table 21–3). Higher doses of acyclovir (800 mg 5×/day) do not offer additional benefit nor does the addition of topical to oral medication.[93] We initiate therapy with a presumptive clinical diagnosis. If an alternative diagnosis is made and cultures are negative, then therapy can be discontinued. Because the natural history of disease is for symptoms to progressively increase over the first week, early initiation of therapy is recommended even in patients who present with few lesions. Oral acyclovir is also effective in treatment of first episode of HSV proctitis in homosexual men.[162] Although treatment of first episode infection markedly shortens the course of first episode, it has no discernible effect on the long-term natural history of recurrences.[95,253] As such, all patients need to be counseled about the natural history, and high rate of recurrences, especially among those with HSV-2 infection, potential complications (including neonatal herpes), and risk of transmission to sexual partners.

Valacyclovir

A major limitation of acyclovir has been poor oral availability as only a small fraction—10 to 20 percent of the dose—is absorbed.[254] As such, an effort has been made to manufacture a compound that would result in higher blood levels of acyclovir. Valacyclovir, an ester of acyclovir, is rapidly and almost completely converted to acyclovir by hepatic enzymes and increases the bioavailability of acyclovir to 54 percent.[255] Therefore, an oral dose of 1000 mg valacyclovir results in blood levels of drug similar (area under the curve) to those of intravenous acyclovir.[256] Valacyclovir has been evaluated for the treatment of genital herpes in two studies.[257,258] In a double-blind, placebo controlled trial of 987 patients with recurrent genital herpes who initiated therapy at the first sign or symptom of a recurrence, valacyclovir was shown to provide significant reduction in the duration of the lesion and accompanying discomfort.[257] Time to complete resolution of signs and symptoms was decreased from a median of 5.9 days in placebo recipients to 4.0 days in valacyclovir recipients. Healing of lesions was faster in valacyclovir recipients (4.1 days) than placebo (6.0 days) as was resolution of viral shedding (2 days for valacyclovir and 4 days for placebo recipients). Of interest, the frequency of aborted episodes, defined as those that did not progress beyond prodrome or a macular/papular lesion, was significantly higher in the valacyclovir than the placebo group. Among patients receiving therapy with valacyclovir 500 mg bid, 31 percent had an aborted episode compared to 21 percent of placebo recipients. No differences were noted between the group that received valacyclovir 500 mg bid and 1000 mg bid, and therefore, the recommended dose is 500 mg bid for 5 days. Adverse effects were rare and did not occur at a different rate in placebo or valacyclovir recipients. As expected from experience with acyclovir, headache and nausea were the most frequent complaints. Another study of 739 patients with recurrent genital herpes that compared valacyclovir 500 mg bid with acyclovir 200 mg five times a day for 5 days did not find any significant differences between the two regimens.[258]

Valacyclovir 1000 mg bid has been compared to acyclovir

Table 21-3. Recommended Regimens of Antiviral Chemotherapy for Mucocutaneous HSV Infection

Indication	Drug	Dose	Duration	Comments
First episode genital herpes	Acyclovir Acyclovir Valacyclovir Famciclovir	200 mg po 5×/day 400 mg po 3×/day 500 mg–1000 mg po 2×/day 250 mg po 3×/day	10–14 days	Therapy has substantial benefit for all clinical and virologic aspects of the infection. Patients who have not healed after 2 weeks of therapy should be treated for additional 7 days.
First episode of herpes proctitis	Acyclovir	400 mg po 5×/day	10–14 days	
Recurrent genital herpes	Acyclovir Acyclovir Valacyclovir Famciclovir	400 mg po 3×/day 200 mg po 5×/day 500 mg po 2×/day 125 mg po 2×/day	5 days	Therapy shortens episode by 1–2 days. May be useful in patients with prolonged recurrences or significant distress during recurrences.
Suppressive therapy	Acyclovir Valacyclovir* Famciclovir	400 mg po 2×/day 500 mg po 1×/day 250 mg po 2×/day		Benefits of suppressive therapy are usually evident after 3–6 months of daily antiviral treatment. However, unless contraindications develop, it is preferable to continue therapy for at least 1 year
Aseptic meningitis	Acyclovir, intravenous	5 mg/kg q 8 h		After clinical improvement, oral administration of valacyclovir is recommended for a total of 10–14 days of treatment

* Patient with very frequent recurrences (≥10 per year) may benefit from valacyclovir 250 mg po bid.

200 mg five times a day for 10 days for therapy of first episode genital herpes.[259] No significant differences were noted between acyclovir and valacyclovir and both were well tolerated. The efficacy of valacyclovir has also been evaluated for suppression of herpes recurrences.[260] Valacyclovir 500 mg once daily was compared to placebo in 382 patients with a history of at least eight recurrences per year. The study continued until first recurrence or for 16 weeks. At that time, 69 percent of valacyclovir recipients were recurrence free, compared to 9.5 percent of placebo recipients. Studies comparing valacyclovir 500 mg once daily to other doses and to acyclovir for 1 year of suppression of recurrent genital herpes indicate that valacyclovir 500 mg po once daily is effective for patients with nine or fewer recurrences per year. However, in patients with more than 10 recurrences per year, valacyclovir 250 mg po bid or 1000 mg once daily is more effective.[261] Also in progress are studies to evaluate the use of valacyclovir for genital herpes in persons with HIV infection.

Valacyclovir 8 grams/day has been evaluated in clinical trials for the prevention of cytomegalovirus disease in immunocompromised patients. A syndrome of thrombotic microangiopathy has been described in about 3 percent of patients with HIV infection, bone marrow and renal transplant recipients who received this high dose of valacyclovir for a median of 53 days (range 8–100 days). The relationship between valacyclovir and this syndrome is uncertain at this time and no immunocompetent patient or patient receiving 3 grams or less of valacyclovir daily has developed thrombotic microangiopathy.[262] It appears that the prolonged administration of very high doses of the drug rather than immunocompromise per se may be associated with this syndrome.

Famciclovir

Famciclovir is a prodrug of penciclovir, a nucleoside analog that effectively inhibits replication of HSV-1 and HSV-2. Similar to acyclovir, penciclovir requires viral thymidine kinase for phosphorylation to monophosphate, and cross resistance with acyclovir is common.[263] Penciclovir triphosphate inhibits viral DNA synthesis with a similar in vitro activity to acyclovir.[264] The intracellular half-life of penciclovir appears longer than that of acyclovir (>10 hours). Oral famciclovir is 77 percent bioavailable.[265] The safety of famciclovir has been evaluated in several clinical trials, and the drug appears to be well-tolerated.[266] The most common reported adverse effects were nausea, headache, and diarrhea, occurring in similar proportion of famciclovir and placebo recipients. Although laboratory evaluation of famciclovir recipients did not indicate any deleterious effects, a lower dose is advised for patients with impaired creatinine clearance.

The efficacy of oral famciclovir for the treatment of recurrent genital herpes has been evaluated in a randomized, placebo-controlled study. In a patient-initiated trial of 467 subjects with recurrent genital herpes, famciclovir recipients compared to placebo recipients had significantly reduced healing time (median 3.8 days for famciclovir recipients vs 4.8 days for placebo recipients), viral shedding (1.7 vs 3.3 days), and duration of all symptoms (3.2 vs 3.7 days).[267] Famciclovir 125 mg twice daily was effective; higher doses did not confer additional benefit for immunocompetent patients with recurrent genital herpes.

In blinded studies comparing famciclovir with acyclovir 200 mg five times daily for the treatment of first episode genital herpes, the two drugs appeared comparable in their ability to effect viral shedding, lesion healing, and resolution of symptoms.[268] Preliminary analyses of studies also indicate that famciclovir is effective and well-tolerated when taken daily. In a study of 375 women with recurrent genital herpes who received famciclovir or placebo for 120 days, 78 percent of participants receiving famciclovir 250 mg bid remained recurrence-free compared to 42 percent of placebo recipients. Once-daily famciclovir in doses from 125 to 500 mg was substantially less effective.[269] In another study of 455 patients with recurrent genital herpes, the median time to first clinical recurrence was 11 months among patients receiving famciclovir 250 mg bid compared to 1.5 months for placebo recipients.[270] The median time to first virologically confirmed recurrence was greater than 1 year in famciclovir recipients versus 2.7 months in placebo recipients. It is not clear why a lower dose of famciclovir is effective for episodic treatment (125 mg bid) compared with suppressive treatment (250 mg bid). Famciclovir 500 mg bid has also been studied as suppressive therapy for genital herpes in HIV-infected persons.[271] In a crossover, double-blinded study of 48 patients who obtained daily cultures from the genital area, the relative risk of viral shedding was 0.15 (95% CI, 0.06–0.42) during famciclovir administration compared with placebo. In a paired analysis of 26 persons who completed both arms of the study, HSV-2 was isolated on 9.7 percent of days on placebo, compared to 1.3 percent of days on famciclovir, an 87 percent reduction. The number of days of lesions was also reduced from 13.7 percent of days on placebo to 4.4 percent on famciclovir. This study showed that daily oral antiviral therapy effectively reduces the frequency of recurrences as well as the frequency of clinical and subclinical viral shedding in immunocompromised HIV-infected patients.

Despite similar levels of inhibition of HSV replication in vitro by penciclovir and acyclovir, famciclovir and valacyclovir appear to have different effects in the murine model of HSV infection. During acute infection with HSV-1 in immunosuppressed mice, famciclovir was more effective than valacyclovir for healing of clinical signs and reducing the ability to isolate virus from skin and brain stem.[272] In addition, mice treated with famciclovir had better survival than mice treated with valacyclovir when therapy was initiated several days after inoculation.[273] Ganglia explanted from mice treated with famciclovir were less likely to yield infectious virus, or to reactivate virus, than ganglia from valacyclovir-treated mice. Thus it appears that therapy of early HSV infection with famciclovir in mice may ameliorate the natural history of the disease. The mechanism underlying this phenomenon is not understood at this time and the implications of these findings for therapy of humans are not clear. As people are usually treated several days after acquisition of the infection when ganglia have already become infected, administration of famciclovir at that time may not alter the natural history of the infection. Studies to further elucidate these observations are in progress.

Treatment of recurrent genital herpes

Oral ACV, famciclovir, and valaciclovir have all been shown to be of benefit in reducing the duration of recurrent attacks of genital herpes.[274,275] A series of studies have demonstrated that both physician and patient initiated therapy reduces the duration of lesions and shortens the time virus can be isolated from lesions. Patient-initiated therapy tends to offer greater benefit owing to earlier initiation of drug than physician-initiated therapy.[274] The recent studies of episodic therapy of genital herpes show that the clinical benefit of treatment of recurrences may be greater than previously appreciated, and should receive more attention in the treatment of genital herpes. This increased benefit may reflect both marginally better performance of the newer antiviral agents in comparison to acyclovir as well as a more carefully designed evaluation schedule during the clinical trials. Regardless of the agent chosen, therapy should be initiated by the patient at the first sign or symptom of a recurrence. Such management requires education of patients regarding the manifestations of genital herpes and provision of an appropriate supply of the antiviral drug for use at home. The currently recommended doses are shown in Table 21-3. Not all episodes or patients with recurrent HSV require antiviral therapy. In immunocompetent patients, episodes will self heal with supportive care. In persons with severe symptomatic episodes, episodic antiviral therapy is useful. Most immunosuppressed patients require therapy.

Topical antiviral therapy also has some benefit in recurrent genital HSV. Both the antiviral and the delivery base affect the outcome. In the United States a 5 percent topical acyclovir preparation in polyethylene glycol produced an antiviral effect but little clinical benefit.[94] In Europe where the preparation is a 5 percent acyclovir preparation in an aqueous cream, more consistent therapeutic benefit has been achieved.[276] No enhanced benefit is seen if both the oral and topical preparations are utilized simultaneously.[277]

Suppressive therapy

Recurrence rates of genital herpes vary in individuals over time. Most patients who seek medical attention for symptomatic genital HSV report from five to eight recurrences per year.

Several studies have shown that daily oral ACV therapy among patients with frequently recurring genital HSV (four to 12 episodes per year) is effective in preventing clinical recurrences of genital herpes.[278–282] Acyclovir in doses of 200 mg two to five times daily for up to 6 years will prevent recurrences in 65 to 85 percent of patients as long as therapy is continued. In a 5-year study of suppressive acyclovir, the mean number of breakthrough recurrences declined from 1.7 during the first year to 0.8 during the fifth year of suppression.[283] Suppressive therapy in persons with frequently recurring disease produces considerable relief of symptoms and can provide major medical and psychosocial benefit.[240] Isolates recovered from patients who have received long-term acyclovir therapy do not differ in their susceptibility from pretreatment isolates.[284]

The dose of oral ACV used for suppressive therapy of genital herpes has varied. Early studies suggested that 200 mg capsules taken two, three, four, or five times a day were of relatively similar efficacy.[278] For long term therapy, simple and convenient dosage regimens are required to achieve maximum compliance. Recent studies have shown that 400 mg bid or 200 mg four times daily are the best initial starting dosages in the immunocompetent patient.[281] The newer nucleoside analogues may provide more convenient dosing regimens but have not shown better efficacy than acyclovir 400 mg bid. More than 90 percent of persons with frequently recurring genital herpes who are immunocompetent have a significant reduction in the number of clinical recurrences on suppressive therapy. Even among those on suppressive therapy, breakthrough recurrence will, however, still occur. About 25 percent of persons on suppressive therapy will develop a breakthrough recurrence each 3-month period.[281] Thus, it is likely that most patients on chronic suppressive therapy will, at some time, develop a breakthrough. Compared with untreated recurrences, breakthrough recurrences are associated with milder symptoms, shorter duration of viral shedding, and shorter duration of lesions.[278,285]

A study of subclinical shedding in women with recently acquired genital herpes who received daily acyclovir 400 mg po bid showed that subclinical shedding was reduced 94 percent.[244] The women obtained daily viral cultures and the rate of subclinical shedding was reduced from 5.8 to 0.37 percent of days of cultures. Of interest, the clinical effect of acyclovir was less pronounced than the virologic effect as the frequency of lesions was reduced only 66 percent. However, these data suggest that chronic antiviral therapy may be effective in reducing the risk of HSV transmission to sexual partners. Since HSV DNA remains detectable on 8 percent of days of suppressive acyclovir therapy, further study of the ability of the antiviral drugs to interrupt transmission is required before such a recommendation can be made.

Because frequently recurring genital herpes may plague a patient for years, many patients desire to take oral ACV for prolonged periods. Preclinical animal studies of ACV showed no drug related carcinogenicity, effect on fertility, or abnormal fetal development.[286] Acyclovir has been shown to have mutagenic potential in two of 22 in vitro systems, but the implications of the results for long-term suppressive therapy are unknown. Chronic suppressive therapy taken at doses of 200 mg five times a day or 200 mg two times a day have had no effect on spermatic function in males.[287] Side effects of daily suppressive oral ACV were uncommon in a large multicenter trial and trials of smaller numbers of patients treated for up to 6 years.[283,284] Allergic reactions to acyclovir are rare and successful desensitization has been reported.[288]

One of the major issues facing the clinician with a patient with genital herpes is the use of intermittent versus chronic suppressive acyclovir therapy. A common criteria on which to base this decision is the number of outbreaks and the severity of the outbreaks. Patients with frequently recurring genital herpes who have considerable physical discomfort, emotional upset, and potential for transmission of infection to sexual partners are candidates for chronic suppressive therapy.[289] Studies indicate that it takes from 5 to 7 days of therapy before clinical effect can be seen.[278] Persons who have up to four genital recurrences per year are probably best managed with supportive care and acute intermittent oral therapy. Similarly, persons with more frequent recurrences who are minimally symptomatic may also be best served by supportive or intermittent therapy. The cost of chronic therapy ($1.50–2.50 per day) may affect this decision.

Clear gaps exist in our knowledge of the relative effectiveness of the three orally available agents for treatment of genital herpes. In addition, only acyclovir has been demonstrated to reduce subclinical viral shedding, although such data should also be forthcoming for the newer agents and are already available for famciclovir in HIV-infected persons. The main reason to demonstrate a reduction in subclinical viral shedding is to evaluate the usefulness of antiviral agents for interruption of sexual, and possibly perinatal, transmission of HSV. However, such studies have not been done and the degree of protection offered by such therapy is unknown. Lack of definitive data on the effect on viral shedding in pregnant women also precludes routine recommendation of acyclovir in that setting, despite promising preliminary data on the effect of antiviral treatment on the rate of abdominal deliveries in women with first episode HSV in pregnancy.[290]

Acyclovir in pregnancy

Although acyclovir is not teratogenic in animals, until studies better defining its role and safety in pregnancy are available, the routine use of oral acyclovir in pregnancy cannot be advocated. A pharmacokinetic evaluation of acyclovir in the third trimester of pregnancy showed that the disposition of acyclovir in pregnant women appears similar to that in other adults.[291] A potential concern is the development of obstructive uropathy in the newborns secondary to acyclovir crystals. However, no such abnormalities were observed in this study, or in a much larger number of infants with neonatal herpes treated with prolonged, high dose, intravenous acyclovir.[292]

Glaxo-Wellcome, in collaboration with the Centers for Disease Control, maintains a voluntary registry of women who received acyclovir and valacyclovir during pregnancy. The data are evaluated at six-month intervals. As of 1996, 636 women who received acyclovir in the first trimester were reported. Fifteen (2.3%) of the children had birth defects compared to a background rate of 3 percent. No consistent pattern of abnormalities has been noted. Although the number of women evaluated is insufficient to exclude a small increase in the rate of congenital abnormalities, the lack of a significant increase in the incidence of defects and of pattern to the abnormalities reported is reassuring. The safety and pharmacokinetics of valacyclovir and famciclovir in pregnancy have not been established.

Emergence of resistance

In vitro resistance to acyclovir can result from thymidine kinase (TK) deficient, TK altered, or DNA polymerase resistant strains of HSV. TK deficiency is the most common mechanism of resistance of HSV to acyclovir.[293–296] Animal studies have suggested that TK deficient mutants are less virulent and less able to establish neural latency.[297] However, some acyclovir resistant strains appear to make enough TK to establish ganglionic latency, and reactivate, especially in immunocompromised patients.[298] Disease caused by strains with DNA polymerase mutations has also been reported.[299] Acyclovir resistant strains of HSV have been recovered from patients who have never been treated with ACV.[294–296] About 3 percent of isolates obtained from immunocompetent patients demonstrate in vitro resistance to acyclovir. The frequency of in vitro resistance has not changed from the time prior to availability of acyclovir and does not appear increased among patients who received several years of daily suppressive acyclovir.[284] Furthermore, among women followed longitudinally with daily viral cultures, about 3 percent of isolates were acyclovir-resistant in vitro. The demonstration of acyclovir resistance in vitro in immunocompetent persons generally has not been associated with clinical failure of acyclovir therapy. An exception is a report of genital herpes with an HSV-2 strain characterized by an altered TK.[298,300] In this person, all isolates recovered from multiple recurrences had an altered TK and acyclovir did not offer clinical benefit.

The vast majority of ACV resistant isolates have been from immunocompromised patients undergoing multiple courses of acyclovir for established infection.[250] However, the frequency of acyclovir-resistance in HIV infected patients appears low and the risk factors for the development of resistance have not been well-defined. Thus, continued surveillance of HSV strains associated with breakthrough recurrences and/or persistent mucocutaneous HSV is needed. At present, routine in vitro testing of HSV isolates for acyclovir sensitivity is not recommended. However, isolates from patients with persistent HSV infections unresponsive to acyclovir, especially those with advanced HIV disease, should have testing for ACV resistance. In this setting, in vitro resistance appears to correlate well with acyclovir failure.[301] Most acyclovir-resistant HSV infections require therapy with alternative agents. As famciclovir has a similar mechanism of action, most acyclovir resistant strains are also famciclovir resistant. Treatment with high-dose continuous infusion of acyclovir has also been reported as successful.[302]

THERAPY OF ACYCLOVIR RESISTANT HSV

Foscarnet

Foscarnet is a viral DNA polymerase inhibitor similar in structure to phosphonoacetic acid. In vitro it has potent antiviral activity and has been effective in speeding the healing of lesions in animal models.[303] It is an insoluble compound and can be effectively administered only intravenously or topically. One study demonstrated in men a reduction in time to healing with 0.3 percent foscarnet cream as compared to placebo.[304] However, a collaborative Canadian trial of foscarnet cream 0.3 percent in men and 1 percent in women, demonstrated little overall effect on reducing symptoms or lesions.[305]

Systemic toxicity during intravenous administration limits the use of foscarnet to patients who fail acyclovir therapy because of development of resistance. In this population, however, foscarnet has become the preferred agent. Foscarnet infusion healed 81 percent of 26 patients with acyclovir resistant HSV infection.[306] A comparative study of foscarnet 40 mg/kg IV Q8 hours and vidarabine 15 mg/kg q day showed that foscarnet therapy led to healing of all eight patients, whereas all patients assigned to vidarabine failed therapy.[307] Adverse reactions are frequent but only rarely require discontinuation of therapy. The most common toxicities are renal insufficiency and metabolic disturbances, especially hypophosphatemia. Recurrences of HSV after foscarnet therapy can be either acyclovir-sensitive or acyclovir-resistant. HSV resistance to foscarnet has also been reported, usually in the setting of prolonged foscarnet therapy.[308] In that setting, the addition of acyclovir can be beneficial.

Cidofovir

Another nucleotide analog with good activity against herpes viruses is cidofovir, an acyclic nucleoside phosphonate. Unlike acyclovir, which requires phosphorylation by HSV-specified enzymes, cidofovir is phosphorylated only by cellular enzymes. Therefore, cidofovir is active against HSV strains with a deficient or altered thymidine kinase and, in fact, it appears more active against these isolates than against wild-type strains.[309] Topical and intravenous cidofovir has been used successfully to heal acyclovir-resistant lesions in patients with AIDS and after marrow transplant.[310,311] A recently completed randomized, double-blind, placebo-controlled trial of topical cidofovir gel 0.3 or 1.0 percent in 30 patients with AIDS who did not respond to acyclovir therapy showed that 10 of 20 cidofovir recipients healed by at least 50 percent compared with none of the placebo recipients. Most patients treated with topical cidofovir ceased viral shedding. No systemic reactions were noted; however, 23 percent of cidofovir recipients had mild or moderate local cutaneous adverse effects. A trial of topical cidofovir in healthy men with recurrent genital herpes showed decreased duration of lesions and viral shedding.[312] However, as long term toxicity studies of cidofovir showed tumors in animals, further development of the drug for immunocompetent persons has been slowed. Because of the potential for renal toxicity with intravenous administration, use of topical cidofovir is preferred for treatment of genital herpes. Availability of safer agents for therapy of herpes in healthy persons suggests that cidofovir will be an important therapeutic alternative only in the immunocompromised population.

Trifluridine

Trifluridine is a potent antiviral agent; toxicity precludes its systemic administration. However, trifluridine is frequently used for treatment of ophthalmic herpes infections. A series of 26 patients with AIDS and mucocutaneous herpes unresponsive to acyclovir demonstrated complete healing in seven patients and partial healing in 14 patients.[313] Anecdotal reports also suggest that the use of interferon-α may potentiate the antiviral effects of trifluridine.[314] These agents may be useful in some patients.

OTHER ANTIVIRALS

Several other therapies for genital HSV have been attempted with a variety of topical medications. Medications for which no therapeutic benefit can be demonstrated are listed in Table 21-4.

IMMUNOTHERAPY

The use of HSV antigens to boost host immune responses has been a longstanding area of HSV research. In animal models, administration of HSV vaccines with varying adjuvants has been associated with reduction in the frequency of reactivation. In people, a double-blind, placebo-controlled trial of a recombinant gD2 vaccine in alum was shown to reduce the recurrence rate of genital HSV by 25 percent.[279] In a follow-up study, a recombinant gD2 gB2 vaccine (10 μg) in MF-59 reduced the severity of the HSV recurrence after immunization but did not reduce recurrence rates.[315] These effects are clinically modest but demonstrate the principle that immunotherapy offers promise as therapy for genital herpes. Several new approaches to immunotherapy are under investigation. The ability to reduce disease severity for a prolonged time period is an attractive therapeutic alteration for many patients.

PROPHYLAXIS OF INFECTION

Currently, there is no proven completely effective means of prophylaxis of HSV. Barrier forms of contraception, especially condoms, may decrease transmission of disease.[37,59] However, transmission of disease may still occur despite the use of condoms when viral shedding occurs in areas of the genital tract not covered by a condom. Spermicides contain the topical surfactant nonoxynol 9, which inactivates HSV in vitro. Nonoxynol 9 has been shown to be ineffective in the treatment of established genital HSV infection.[85] No data are available, however, to determine if it would be effective in decreasing transmission of disease.

The high prevalence of asymptomatic and atypical HSV infection implies that development of an effective HSV vaccine is the best approach to the prevention of HSV. Prophylactic subunit protein vaccines have been tested and shown effective in a variety of animal models.[316] The effort has concentrated on glycoprotein D and B as the immune response to these glycoproteins appears to induce high levels of neutralizing antibodies. A trial of an HSV vaccine composed of a glycoprotein mixture elicited low levels of antibody titers and did not protect against infection.[317] A recombinant HSV-2 gD and gB vaccine in a novel MF-59 adjuvant emulsion induced humoral and cellular immunity comparable to that observed in natural infection.[318] However, in an efficacy trial of partners discordant for HSV-2 infection, the vaccine did not afford clinically useful protection from infection. Other vaccines under development include attenuated live vaccines, replication-defective viral mutants and live virus vectors expressing subunit protein.[152,316,319–321] Recently, a DNA vaccine encoding gD2 has

Table 21-4. Ineffective Therapies for Genital Herpes

Vidarabine	Povodine iodine	Isoprinosine
Idoxuridine	Topical surfactants	2-deoxy-D-glucose
Edoxuridine	Photodynamic dyes	BCG vaccine
Ether	Topical interferon α	Lysine
Chloroform	Transfer factor	Nonoxynol 9

shown some protection in animal models.[322,323] These products are currently in preclinical or early clinical stages of development.

SUMMARY

Genital HSV infection is a disease of major public health importance. In the last two decades genital herpes infection has increased in prevalence in many population groups, especially white, middle-class men and women between the ages of 15 and 35 years. First episode genital HSV infection is a disease of multiple anatomic sites, lasts 3 to 4 weeks, and has a high rate of complications. In contrast, episodes of recurrent genital disease are of much milder intensity and duration. The major morbidity of recurrent genital herpes is its frequency of recurrences, its chronicity, and its effects on the patient's personal relationships and sexuality. The transmission of disease to the neonate is a major concern. Studies over the last decade have demonstrated effectiveness of safe antiviral compounds in reducing many of the clinical manifestations of genital herpes. However, HSV-2 infection is still epidemic in most parts of the world. Greater attention to the diagnosis of the asymptomatic carrier and greater emphasis on the recognition of HSV as a cause of genital ulceration worldwide are needed. This is especially relevant with recent data showing that HSV-2 infection is a risk factor for acquisition and transmission of HIV. Further investigations on the mechanism of recurrence and risk factors associated with recurrence will hopefully provide the tools to better control this disease. In the meantime, knowledge of the natural history of the disease will aid the physician in providing the patient with the information necessary to understand this complex entity, attempt to decrease transmission to sexual partners and neonates through education, and explain the long-term complications of the illness. In this way the clinician may do much toward allowing the patient to cope with the psychological and physical components of this illness.

References

1 Wildy P: Herpes history and classification, in *The Herpes Viruses.* Kaplan AS (ed.) New York, Academic. 1973, pp. 1–25.

2 Astruc J: *De Morbis Venereis Libri Sex.* Paris, 1736.

3 Hutfield D: History of herpes genitalis. *Br J Vener Dis* 42:263, 1996.

4 Diday P et al: *Les Herpes Genitaux Paris, Masson et Cie,* 1886.

5 Baum O: Uber die Ubentragbarkeit des Herpes Simplex auf die kaninchen Hourhaut. *Derm Wochenshr* 70:105, 1920.

6 Cruter W: Das Herpes virus sein aetiologische und klinische Bedeutung. *Munich Med Wochenschr* 71:1058, 1924.

7 Parker F et al: Studies on filterable viruses: II. Cultivation of herpes virus. *Am J Pathol* 1:337, 1925.

8 Lipschutz B: Untersuchungen uber die Aetiologie der Krankheiten der Herpes gruppe (Herpes zoster, Herpes genitalis, Herpes febrillis). *Arch Dermatol Symp* (Berlin) 136:428, 1921.

9 Dowdle W et al: Association of antigenic type of Herpes virus hominis with site of viral recovery. *J Immunol* 99:974, 1967.

10 Nahmias A et al: Antigenic and biologic differences in Herpesvirus hominis. *Prog Med Virol* 10:110, 1968.

11 Nahmias A et al: Relation of pock size on chorioallantoic membrane to antigenic type of Herpesvirus hominis. *Proc Soc Exp Biol Med* 174:1022, 1968.

12 Nahmias A et al: Antibodies to herpesvirus hominis types 1 and 2 in humans: patients with genital infections. *Am J Epidemiol* 92:539, 1970.

13 Lee F et al: Detection of herpes simplex virus type 2 specific antibody with glycoprotein G. *J Clin Microbiol* 22:642–644, 1985.

14 Ashley R et al: Comparison of Western blot and gG-specific immunodot enzyme assay for detecting HSV-1 and HSV-2 antibodies in human sera. *J Clin Microbiol* 26:662–667, 1988.

15 Johnson R et al: A seroepidemiologic survey of the prevalence of herpes simplex virus type 2 infection in the United States. *N Engl J Med* 321:7–12, 1990.

16 Ashley R et al: Inability of enzyme immunoassays to discriminate between infections with herpes simplex virus type 1 and 2. *Ann Intern Med* 115:520–526, 1991.

17 Ashley R et al: Underestimation of HSV-2 seroprevalence in a high-risk population by microneutralization assay. *Sex Trans Dis* 20:230–235, 1993.

18 Rawls W et al: Measurement of antibodies to herpes virus types 1 and 2 in human sera. *J Immunol* 104:599, 1970.

19 Rawls W et al: Genital herpes in 2 social groups. *Am J Obstet Gynecol* 110:682, 1971.

20 Wentworth B et al: Seroepidemiology of infections due to members of the herpesvirus group. *Am J Epidemiol* 94:496, 1971.

21 Josey W et al: The epidemiology of type 2 (genital) herpes simplex virus infection. *Obstet Gynecol Suv* 27:295, 1972.

22 Nahmias A et al: Infection with herpes simplex virus 1 and 2. *N Engl J Med* 19:667, 1973.

23 Duenas A et al: Herpes virus type 2 in a prostitute population. *Am J Epidemiol* 98:483, 1972.

24 Porter D et al: Prevalence of antibodies to EB virus and other herpesviruses. *JAMA* 208:1675, 1979.

25 Guinan M et al: Genital herpes simplex virus infection. *Epidemiol Rev* 7:127–146, 1988.

26 Daling J et al: Sexual practices, sexually transmitted diseases, and the incidence of anal cancer. *N Engl J Med* 317:973–977, 1987.

27 Oliver L et al: Seroprevalence of herpes simplex virus infections in a family medicine clinic. *Arch Fam Med* 4:228–232, 1995.

28 Siegel D et al: Prevalence and correlates of herpes simplex infections: the population-based AIDS in multiethnic neighborhoods study. *JAMA* 268:1700–1708, 1992.

29 Corey L et al: Infections with herpes simplex viruses. *N Engl J Med* 314:686–691, 1986.

30 Koutsky L et al: Underdiagnosis of genital herpes by current clinical and viral-isolation procedures. *N Engl J Med* 326:1553–1539, 1992.

31 Fleming DT, et al: Herpes simplex virus type 2 in the United States, 1976 to 1994. *New Engl J Med* 337:1105–1111, 1997.

32 Breinig M et al: Epidemiology of genital herpes in Pittsburgh: serologic, sexual and racial correlates of apparent and inapparent herpes simplex infections. *J Infect Dis* 161:299–305, 1990.

33 Gibson J et al: A cross-sectional study of herpes simplex virus types 1 and 2 in college students: occurrence and determinants of infection. *J Infect Dis* 162:306–312, 1990.

34 Becker T et al: Genital herpes infections in private practice in the United States. *JAMA* 253:1601–1603, 1985.

35 Cowan F et al: Antibody to herpes simplex virus type 2 as serological marker of sexual lifestyle in populations. *BMJ* 309:1325–1329, 1994.

36 Weinberg A et al: Herpes simplex virus type 2 infection in pregnancy: asymptomatic viral excretion at delivery and seroepidemiologic survey of two socioeconomically distinct populations in Sao Paulo, Brazil. *Rev Inst Med Trop Sao Paulo* 35:285–290, 1993.

37 Oberle M et al: Herpes simplex virus type 2 antibodies: high prevalence in monogamous women in Costa Rica. *Am J Trop Med Hyg* 41:224–229, 1989.

38 Cunningham A et al: Herpes simplex virus type 2 antibody in patients attending antenatal or STD clinics. *Med J Aust* 158:525–528, 1993.

39 Forsgren M et al: Prevalence of antibodies to herpes simplex virus in pregnant women in Stockholm in 1969, 1983 and 1989: implications for STD epidemiology. *Int J STD AIDS* 5:113–116, 1994.

40 Pasquini P et al: Prevalence of herpes virus type 2 antibodies in selected population groups in Italy. *Eur J Clin Microbiol Inf Dis* 7:54–57, 1988.

41 Cowan F et al: Relationship between antibodies to herpes simplex virus (HSV) and symptoms of HSV infection. *J Infect Dis* 174:470–475, 1996.

42 Bassett I et al: Herpes simplex virus type 2 infection of heterosexual men attending a sexual health centre. *Med J Aust* 160:697–700, 1994.

43 Lowhagen G et al: Epidemiology of genital herpes infections in Sweden. *Acta Derm Venereol* (Stockh) 70:330–334, 1990.

44 Mele A et al: Genital herpes infection in outpatients attending a sexually transmitted disease clinic in Italy. *Eur J Epidemiol* 4:386–388, 1988.

45 Christenson B et al: A 15 year surveillance study of antibodies to herpes simplex virus types 1 and 2 in a cohort of young girls. *J Infect Dis* 25:147–154, 1992.

46 Stavraky K et al: Sexual and socioeconomic factors affecting the risk of past infections with herpes simplex virus type 2. *Am J Epidemiol* 118:109–121, 1983.

47 Jeansson S et al: Genital herpesvirus hominis infection: a veneral disease. *Lancet* 1:1064, 1970.

48 Wentworth B et al: Isolation of viruses, bacteria and other organisms from venereal disease clinic patients: methodology and problems associated with multiple isolations. *Health Lab Sci* 10:75, 1973.

49 Jeansson S et al: On the occurrence of genital herpes simplex virus infection. *Acta Derm Venereol* 54:479, 1974.

50 Rauh J et al: Genital surveillance among sexually active adolescent girls. *J Pediatr* 90:844, 1977.

51 Vesterinen E et al: Clinical and virological findings in patients with cytologically diagnosed gynecologic herpes simplex infection. *Acta Cytol* (Baltimore) 21:199, 1977.

52 Knox G et al: Comparative prevalence of subclinical cytomegalovirus and herpes simplex virus in the genital and urinary tracts of low-income urban women. *J Infect Dis* 140:419, 1979.

53 US Department of Health and Human Services: Public Health Service, Centers for Disease Control, Atlanta. *STD Fact Sheet,* 35th ed. 1981, pp. 5–12.

54 Sumaya C et al: Genital infections with herpes simplex virus in university student populations. *Sex Trans Dis* 7:16, 1980.

55 Kamya M et al: The high prevalence of genital herpes among patients with genital ulcer disease in Uganda. *Sex Trans Dis* 22:351–354, 1995.

56 Morse S et al: Comparison of clinical diagnosis and standard laboratory and molecular methods for the diagnosis of genital ulcer disease in Lesotho: association with human immunodeficiency virus infection. *J Infect Dis* 175:583–589, 1997.

57 Centers for Disease Control and Prevention: *Sexually Transmitted Disease Surveillance.* 1995.

58 Sullivan-Bolyai J et al: Neonatal herpes simplex virus infection in King County, Washington: increasing incidence and epidemiological correlates. *JAMA* 250:3059–3062, 1983.

59 Mertz G et al: Risk factors for the sexual transmission of genital herpes. *Ann Intern Med* 116:197–202, 1992.

60 Bryson Y et al: Risk of acquisition of genital herpes simplex virus type 2 in sex partners of persons with genital herpes: a prospective couple study. *J Infect Dis* 167:942–946, 1993.

61 Sacks S et al: Randomized, double-blind, placebo-controlled, clinic-initiated, Canadian multicenter trial of topical edoxudine 3.0% cream in the treatment of recurrent genital herpes. *J Infect Dis* 164: 665–672, 1991.

62 Benedetti J et al: Recurrence rates in genital herpes after symptomatic first-episode infection. *Ann Intern Med* 121:847–854, 1994.

63 Mertz G et al: Frequency of acquisition of first-episode genital infection with herpes simplex virus from symptomatic and asymptomatic source contacts. *Sex Trans Dis* 12:33–39, 1985.

64 Stanberry L et al: Genital herpes in guinea pigs: pathogenesis of the primary infection and description of recurrent disease. *J Infect Dis* 146:397–404, 1982.

65 Stern H et al: Herpetic whitlow, a form of cross-infection in hospitals. *Lancet* 2:871, 1959.

66 Selling B et al: An outbreak of herpes simplex among wrestlers (herpes gladiatorum). *N Engl J Med* 170:979, 1964.

67 Cesario T et al: Six years' experience with herpes simplex virus in a children's home. *Am J Epidemiol* 90:416, 1969.

68 Perl T et al: Transmission of herpes simplex virus type 1 infection in an intensive care unit. *Ann Int Med* 117:584–586, 1992.

69 Naib Z: Exfoliative cytology of viral cervico-vaginitis. *Acta Cytol* (Baltimore) 10:126, 1966.

70 Barringer J et al: Recovery of herpes simplex virus from human trigeminal ganglions. *N Engl J Med* 188:648, 1973.

71 Cook M et al: Pathogenesis of herpetic neuritis and ganglionitis in mice: evidence for intra-axonal transport of infections. *Infect Immunol* 7:272, 1973.

72 Barringer J: Recovery of herpes simplex virus from human sacral ganglions. *N Engl J Med* 291:828, 1974.

73 Warren K et al: Isolation of latent herpes simplex virus from the superior cervical and vagus ganglions of human beings. *N Engl J Med* 298:1068–1069, 1978.

74 Buchman T et al: Demonstration of exogenous genital reinfection with herpes simplex virus type 2 by restriction endonuclease fingerprinting of viral DNA. *J Infect Dis* 140:295–304, 1979.

75 Schmidt O et al: Exogenous reinfection is an uncommon occurrence in patients with symptomatic genital herpes. *J Infect Dis* 149:645–646, 1984.

76 Yoshikawa T et al: The characteristic site-specific reactivation phenotypes of HSV-1 and HSV-2 depend upon the latency-associated transcript region. *J Exp Med* 184:659–664, 1996.

77 Koelle D et al: Herpes simplex virus infection of cultured human fibroblasts and keratinocytes inhibits recognition by cloned CD8+ cytotoxic T lymphocytes. *J Clin Invest* 91:961–968, 1993.

78 York I et al: A cytosolic herpes simplex virus protein inhibits antigen presentation to CD8+ T lymphocytes. *Cell* 77:525–535, 1994.

79 Tigges M et al: Human herpes simplex virus (HSV)-specific CD8+ CTL clones recognize HSV-2 infected fibroblasts after treatment with IFN-gamma or when virion host shutoff functions are disabled. *J Immunol* 156:3901–3910, 1996.

80 Cunningham A et al: Evolution of recurrent herpes simplex lesions. An immunohistologic study. *J Clin Invest* 75:226–233, 1985.

81 Koelle D et al: Resolution of recurrent HSV-2 infection is temporally correlated with infiltration of cytotoxic lymphocytes. *21st International Herpesvirus Workshop,* DeKalb, Illinois, 1996.

82 Corey L et al: Clinical course of genital herpes simplex virus infections in men and women. *Ann Intern Med* 48:973, 1983.

83 Kaufman R et al: Clinical features of herpes genitalis. *Cancer Res* 33: 1446, 1973.

84 Adams H: Genital herpetic infection in men and women: clinical course and effect of topical application of adenine arabinoside. *J Infect Dis* 133:A151, 1976.

85 Vontver A et al: Clinical course and diagnosis of genital herpes simplex virus infection and evaluation of topical surfactant therapy. *Am J Obstet Gynecol* 133:548, 1979.

86 Reeves W et al: Risk of recurrence after first episodes of genital herpes: relation to HSV type and antibody response. *N Engl J Med* 305: 315, 1981.

87 Bernstein D et al: Serologic analysis of first episode nonprimary genital herpes simplex virus infection. *Amer J Med* 77:1055–1060, 1984.

88 Smith I et al: The incidence of herpesvirus hominis antibody in the population. *J Hyg* (Lond) 65:395, 1967.

89 Kalinyak J et al: Incidence and distribution of herpes simplex virus types 1 and 2 from genital lesions in college women. *J Med Virol* 1: 175, 1977.

90 Barton I et al: Association of HSV-1 with cervical infection. *Lancet* 2:1108, 1981.

91 Cheong W et al: Clinical and laboratory study of first episode genital herpes in Singapore. *Int J STD AIDS* 1:195–198, 1990.

92 Wooley P et al: Incidence of herpes simplex virus type-1 and type-2 from patients with primary (first attack) genital herpes in Sheffield. *Int J STD AIDS* 1:184–186, 1990.

93 Wald A et al: A randomized, double-blind, comparative trial comparing high and standard dose oral acyclovir for first-episode genital herpes infections. *Antimicrobiol Agents and Chemo* 38:174–176, 1994.

94 Corey L et al: Double blind placebo controlled trial of topical acy-

clovir in first and recurrent episodes of genital herpes simplex virus infection. *N Engl J Med* 106:1313, 1982.

95 Mertz G et al: Double-blind placebo-controlled trial of oral acyclovir in the first episode genital herpes simplex virus infection. *J Amer Med Assoc* 252:1147–1151, 1984.

96 Kit S et al: Sequential genital infections by herpes simplex viruses types 1 and 2: restriction nuclease analyses of viruses from recurrent infections. *Sex Trans Dis* 10:67–71, 1983.

97 Samarai A et al: Sequential genital infections with herpes simplex virus types 1 and 2. *Genito Med* 65:39–41, 1989.

98 Guinan M et al: Course of an untreated episode of recurrent genital herpes simplex infection in 27 women. *N Engl J Med* 304:759, 1981.

99 Josey W et al: Genital herpes simplex infection in the female. *Am J Obstet Gynecol* 96:493, 1966.

100 Embil J et al: Concurrent oral and genital infection with an identical strain of herpes simplex virus type 1. *Sex Trans Dis* 8:70–72, 1981.

101 Lafferty W et al: Recurrences after oral and genital herpes simplex virus infection: influence of anatomic site and viral type. *N Engl J Med* 316:1444–1449, 1987.

102 Evans A et al: Acute pharyngitis and tonsilitis in University of Wisconsin students. *JAMA* 190:699, 1964.

103 Glezen W et al: Acute respiratory disease of university students with special reference to the etiologic role of herpes virus hominis. *Am J Epidemiol* 101:111, 1975.

104 Tustin A et al: Life threatening pharyngitis caused by herpes simplex virus type 2. *Sex Trans Dis* 6:23, 1979.

105 Ross C et al: Herpes simplex meningoencephalitis. *Lancet* 2:682, 1961.

106 Klastersky J et al: Ascending myelitis in association with herpes simplex virus. *N Engl J Med* 187:182, 1972.

107 Caplan L et al: Urinary retention probably secondary to herpes genitalis. *N Engl J Med* 197:920, 1977.

108 Ravaut P et al: Les reactions nerveuses au cours de herpes genitaux. *Ann Derm Syph* (Paris) 5:481, 1904.

109 Olson L et al: Herpesvirus infections of the human central nervous system. *N Engl J Med* 272:1271, 1967.

110 Skoldenberg B et al: Herpes simplex virus 2 and acute aseptic meningitis. *Scand J Infect Dis* 7:227, 1975.

111 Craig C et al: Different patterns of neurologic involvement with herpes simplex virus types 1 and 2: isolation of herpes simplex virus from the buffy coat of two adults with meningitis. *J Infect Dis* 127: 365, 1973.

112 Morison R et al: Adult meningoencephalitis caused by herpesvirus hominis type 2. *Am J Med* 56:540, 1974.

113 Whitley R et al: Adenine arabinoside therapy of biopsy-proved herpes simplex encephalitis: National Institute of Allergy and Infectious Diseases Collaborative Antiviral Study. *N Engl J Med* 297:389–394, 1977.

114 Brenton D: Hypoglycorrhachia in herpes simplex type 2 meningitis. *Arch Neurol* 37:317, 1980.

115 Corey L et al: Intravenous acyclovir for the treatment of primary genital herpes. *Ann Int Med* 98:914, 1983.

116 Corey L et al: Genital herpes simplex virus infection: current concepts in diagnosis, therapy and prevention. *Ann Int Med* 98:973, 1983.

117 Goodell S et al: Herpes simplex virus: proctitis. *N Engl J Med* 309: 868, 1983.

118 Goldmeier D et al: Urinary retention and intestinal obstruction associated with anorectal herpes simplex virus infection. *Br Med J* 1: 425, 1975.

119 Oates J et al: Retention of urine in anogenital herpetic infection. *Lancet* 1:691, 1978.

120 Riehle R et al: Transient neuropathic bladder following herpes simplex genitalis. *J Urol* 122:263, 1979.

121 Jacome D et al: Herpes genitalis and neurogenic bladder and bowel. *J Urol* 124:752, 1980.

122 Shturman-Ellstein R et al: Myelitis associated with genital herpes in a child. *J Ped* 88:523, 1976.

123 Samarasinghe P et al: Herpetic proctitis and sacral radio-myelopathy: a hazard for homosexual men. *Br Med J* 2:365, 1979.

124 Benedetti J et al: Frequency and reactivation of nongenital lesions among patients with genital herpes simplex virus. *Amer J Med* 98: 237–242, 1995.

125 Crane L et al: Herpetic whitlow: a manifestation of primary infection with herpes simplex virus type 1 and 2. *J Infect Dis* 137:855, 1978.

126 Gill J et al: Herpes simplex virus infections of the hand. A profile of 79 cases. *Amer J Med* 84:89, 1988.

127 Kipping R et al: Generalized infection with herpes simplex. *Br Med J* 10:247, 1948.

128 Nahmias A: Disseminated herpes simplex virus infections. *N Engl J Med* 282:684, 1979.

129 Ruchman I et al: Recovery of herpes simplex virus from the blood of a patient with herpetic rhinitis. *J Lab Clin Med* 35:434, 1950.

130 Auch-Moedy J et al: Fatal disseminated herpes simplex virus infection in a healthy child. *Am J Dis Child* 135:45, 1981.

131 Friedman H et al: Acute monarticular arthritis caused by herpes simplex virus and cytomegalovirus. *Am J Med* 69:241, 1980.

132 Shelley W: Herpetic arthritis associated with disseminated herpes simplex virus and cytomegalovirus. *Am J Med* 69:241, 1980.

133 Flewett T et al: Acute hepatitis due to herpes simplex in an adult. *J Clin Pathol* 22:60, 1969.

134 Joseph T et al: Disseminated herpes with hepatoadrenal necrosis in an adult. *Am J Med* 56:735, 1974.

135 Whittaker J et al: Severe thrombocytopenia after generalized HSV-2 infection. *So Med J* 72:864, 1978.

136 Schlesinger J et al: Myoglobinuria associated with herpes group viral infections. *Arch Intern Med* 138:422, 1978.

137 Goyette R et al: Fulminant hepatitis during pregnancy. *Obstet Gynecol* 43:191, 1974.

138 Young E et al: Disseminated herpesvirus infection associated with primary genital herpes in pregnancy. *JAMA* 235:2731, 1976.

139 Koberman T et al: Maternal death secondary to disseminated herpesvirus hominis. *Am J Obstet Gyn* 137:742, 1980.

140 Wenner H: Complications of infantile eczema caused by virus of herpes simplex: (a) Description of the clinical characteristics of an unusual eruption and (b) identification of an associated filterable virus. *Am J Dis Child* 67:247, 1944.

141 Mailman C et al: Recurrent eczema herpeticum. *Arch Dermatol* 89: 815, 1964.

142 Wheeler Jr C et al: Eczema herpeticum, primary and recurrent. *Arch Dermatol* 93:162, 1966.

143 St Geme J et al: Impaired cellular resistance to herpes simplex virus in Wiskott-Aldrich syndrome. *N Engl J Med* 173:229, 1965.

144 Sutton A et al: Fatal disseminated herpesvirus hominis type 2 infection in an adult with associated thymic dysplasia. *Am J Med* 56:545, 1974.

145 Keane J et al: Herpesvirus hominis hepatitis and disseminated intravascular coagulation: occurrence in an adult with pemphigus vulgaris. *Arch Dermatol* 93:1312, 1976.

146 Linnemann C et al: Herpesvirus hominis type 2 meningo-encephalitis following renal transplantation. *Am J Med* 61:703, 1976.

147 Schneidman D et al: Chronic cutaneous herpes simplex. *JAMA* 241: 592, 1979.

148 Lehtinen M: Detection of herpes simplex virus in women with acute pelvic inflammatory disease. *J Infect Dis* 152:78–81, 1985.

149 Notkins A: Immune mechanisms by which the spread of viral infections is stopped. *Cell Immunol* 11:478, 1974.

150 Parker J et al: Herpes genitalis: clinical and virological studies. *Br J Vener Dis* 43:212, 1967.

151 Sacks S: Frequency and duration of patient-observed recurrent genital herpes simplex virus infection: characterization of the nonlesional prodrome. *J Infect Dis* 150:873–877, 1984.

152 Burke R et al: Detection and characterization of latent HSV RNA by in situ and northern blot hybridization in guinea pigs. *Virology* 181: 793–797, 1991.

153 Zweerink H et al: Virus specific antibodies for HSV-2 in sera from patients with genital herpes virus infection. *Inf Immunol* 37:413–421, 1982.

154 Klein R et al: Orofacial herpes simplex virus infection in hairless mice: latent virus in trigeminal ganglia after topical antiviral treatment. *Inf Immunol* 20:130, 1978.

155 Waugh M: Anorectal Herpesvirus hominis infection in men. *J Am Vener Dis Assoc* 3:68, 1976.

156 Levine J et al: Herpesvirus hominis (type 1) proctitis. *J Clin Gastroenterol* 1:225, 1979.

157 Goldmeier D: Proctitis and herpes simplex virus in homosexual men. *Br J Vener Dis* 56:111, 1980.

158 Quinn T et al: The etiology of anorectal infection in homosexual men. *Am J Med* 71:395, 1981.

159 Curry J et al: Proctitis associated with herpes virus hominis type 2 infection. *Can Med Assoc J* 119:485, 1978.

160 Goldmeier D: Herpetic proctitis and sacral radiculomyelopathy in homosexual men. *Br Med J* 2:549, 1979.

161 Jacobs S et al: Acute motor paralytic bladder in renal transplant patients with anogenital herpes infection. *J Urol* 123:426, 1980.

162 Rompalo A et al: Oral acyclovir for treatment of first-episode herpes simplex virus proctitis. *J Amer Med Assoc* 259:2879–2881, 1988.

163 Bruyn G et al: Mollaret's meningitis: differential diagnosis and diagnostic pitfalls. *Neurology* 12:745–753, 1962.

164 Yamamoto L et al: Herpes simplex virus type 1 DNA in cerebrospinal fluid of a patient with Mollaret's meningitis. *N Engl J Med* 325: 1082–1085, 1991.

165 Picard F et al: Mollaret's meningitis associated with herpes simplex type 2 infection. *Neurology* 43:1722–1727, 1993.

166 Tedder D et al: Herpes simplex virus infection as a cause of benign recurrent lymphocytic meningitis. *Ann Intern Med* 121:334–338, 1994.

167 Schlesinger Y et al: Herpes simplex virus type 2 meningitis in the absence of genital lesions: improved recognition with use of the polymerase chain reaction. *Clin Infect Dis* 20:842–848, 1995.

168 Bergstrom T et al: Primary and recurrent herpes simplex virus type 2-induced meningitis. *J Infect Dis* 162:322–330, 1990.

169 Cohen B et al: Herpes simplex type 2 in a patient with Mollaret's meningitis: demonstration by polymerase chain reaction. *Ann Neurol* 35:112–116, 1994.

170 Chapel T et al: Microbiological flora of penile ulcerations. *J Infect Dis* 137:50, 1978.

171 Kinghorn G et al: Pathogenic microbial flora of genital ulcers in Sheffield with particular reference to herpes simplex virus and Haemophilus ducreyi. *Br J Vener Dis* 58:377, 1982.

172 Brown Z et al: Neonatal herpes simplex virus infection in relation to asymptomatic maternal infection at the time of labor. *N Engl J Med* 324:1247–1252, 1991.

173 Rooney J et al: Acquisition of genital herpes from an asymptomatic sexual partner. *N Engl J Med* 314:1561, 1986.

174 Mertz G et al: Transmission of genital herpes in couples with one symptomatic and one asymptomatic partner: a prospective study. *J Infect Dis* 157:1169–1177, 1988.

175 Corey L: The current trend in genital herpes. Progress in prevention. *Sex Trans Dis* 21:S38–44, 1994.

176 Stenzel P et al: Herpes simplex in genital secretions. *Sex Trans Dis* 14:17–22, 1987.

177 Wald A et al: Virologic characteristics of subclinical and symptomatic genital herpes infections. *N Engl J Med* 333:770–775, 1995.

178 Wald A et al: Frequent genital HSV-2 shedding in immunocompetent women. *J Clin Invest* 99:1092–1097, 1997.

179 Moore D et al: Transmission of genital herpes by donor insemination. *JAMA* 261:3441, 1989.

180 Douglas J et al: A double-blind placebo-controlled trial of the effect of chronic oral acyclovir on sperm production in men with frequently recurrent genital herpes. *J Infect Dis* 157:588–593, 1988.

181 Centifano Y et al: Herpes virus type 2 in the male genitourinary tract. *Science* 318:1972, 1978.

182 Langenberg A et al: Development of clinically recognizable genital lesions among women previously identified as having "asymptomatic" HSV-2 infection. *Ann Intern Med* 110:882–887, 1989.

183 Frenkel L et al: Clinical reactivation of herpes simplex virus type 2 infection in seropositive pregnant women with no history of genital herpes. *Ann Intern Med* 118:414–418, 1993.

184 Wald A et al: Genital HSV-2 shedding in women with HSV-2 antibodies but without a history of genital herpes. *36th Interscience Conference on Antimicrobial Agents and Chemotherapy,* New Orleans, Louisiana, 1996.

185 Montgomerie J et al: Herpes simplex virus infection after renal transplantation. *Lancet* 2:867–871, 1969.

186 Wade J et al: Intravenous acyclovir to treat mucocutaneous herpes simplex virus infection after marrow transplantation: a double-blind trial. *Ann Intern Med* 96:265–269, 1982.

187 Whitley R et al: Infections caused by the herpes simplex virus in the immunocompromised host: natural history and topical acyclovir therapy. *J Infect Dis* 150:323–329, 1984.

188 Pass R et al: Identification of patients with increased risk of infection with herpes simplex virus after renal transplantation. *J Infect Dis* 140:487, 1979.

189 Meyers J et al: Infection with herpes simplex virus and cell-mediated immunity after marrow transplant. *J Infect Dis* 142:338, 1980.

190 Whitley R: Mucocutaneous herpes simplex virus infections in immunocompromised patients. *Am J Med* 73:236, 1982.

191 Ramsey P et al: Herpes simplex virus pneumonia: clinical presentation and pathogenesis. *Ann Intern Med* 97:813, 1982.

192 Saral R et al: Acyclovir prophylaxis of herpes-simplex-virus infections: a randomized double-blind controlled trial in bone-marrow-transplant recipients. *N Engl J Med* 305:63, 1981.

193 Gold D et al: Acyclovir prophylaxis of herpes simplex virus infection. *Antimicrobiol Agents Chemother* 31:361–367, 1987.

194 Straus S et al: Oral acyclovir to suppress recurring herpes simplex virus infection in immunodeficient patients. *Ann Int Med* 100:522, 1984.

195 Greenblatt R et al: Genital ulceration as a risk factor for human immunodeficiency virus infection. *AIDS* 2:47–50, 1988.

196 Stamm W et al: Association between genital ulcer disease and acquisition of HIV infection in homosexual men. *J Amer Med Assoc* 260: 1429–1433, 1988.

197 Boulos R et al: Herpes simplex virus type 2 infection, syphillis, and hepatitis B virus infection in Haitian women with human immunodeficiency virus type 1 and human T lymphotropic virus type 1 infections. *J Infect Dis* 166:418–420, 1992.

198 Hook E et al: Herpes simplex virus infection as a risk factor for human immunodeficiency virus infection in heterosexuals. *J Infect Dis* 165:251–255, 1992.

199 Holmberg S et al: Prior HSV type 2 infection as a risk factor for HIV infection. *J Amer Med Assoc* 259:1048–1051, 1988.

200 Keet I et al: Herpes simplex virus type 2 and other genital ulcerative infections as a risk factor for HIV-1 acquisition. *Genitourin Med* 66: 330–333, 1990.

201 Telzak E et al: HIV-1 seroconversion in patients with and without genital ulcer disease. *Ann Intern Med* 119:1181–1186, 1993.

202 Dickerson M et al: The causal role for genital ulcer disease as a risk factor for transmission of human immunodeficiency virus: an application of the Bradford Hill criteria. *Sex Trans Dis* 23:429–440, 1996.

203 Cameron DW et al: Female to male transmission of human immunodeficiency virus type 1: risk factors for seroconversion in men. *Lancet* 2:403–407, 1989.

204 Centers for Disease Control and Prevention: First 500,000 AIDS cases—United States, 1995. *MMWR* 44:81–84, 1995.

205 Centers for Disease Control and Prevention: Update: AIDS among women—United States. *MMWR* 44:81–84, 1994.

206 Albrecht M et al: The herpes simplex virus immediate-early protein, ICP4 is required to potentiate replication of human immunodeficiency virus in CD4+ lymphocytes. *J Virol* 63:1861–1868, 1989.

207 Koelle D et al: Direct recovery of herpes simplex virus (HSV)—specific T lymphocyte clones from recurrent genital HSV-2 lesions. *J Infect Dis* 169:956–961, 1994.

208 Kucera L et al: Human immunodeficiency virus type 1 (HIV-1) and herpes simplex virus type 2 (HSV-2) can coinfect and simultaneously replicate in the same human CD4+ cell: effect of coinfection on in-

fectious HSV-2 and HIV-1 replication. *AIDS Res Hum Retro* 6:641–647, 1990.

209 Siegel F et al: Acquired immunodeficiency in male homosexuals manifested by chronic perianal ulcerative herpes simplex lesions. *N Engl J Med* 305:1439–1444, 1988.

210 Augenbraun M et al: Increased genital shedding of herpes simplex virus type 2 in HIV-seropositive women. *Ann Intern Med* 123:845–847, 1995.

211 Nahmias A et al: Newborn infection with Herpesvirus hominis types 1 and 2. *J Pediatr* 75:1194, 1969.

212 Nahmias A et al: Infectious diseases of the fetus and newborn infant, in Remington JS, Klein JO (eds.) *Herpes Simplex.* Philadelphia, WB Saunders, 1983, pp. 636–678.

213 Stagno S et al: Herpes virus infections of pregnancy. Part II: Herpes simplex virus and varicella zoster infection. *N Engl J Med* 313:1327, 1985.

214 Florman A: Intrauterine infection with herpes simplex virus: resultant congenital malformations. *JAMA* 225:129, 1973.

215 Chalub E et al: Congenital herpes simplex type II infection with extensive hepatic calcification, bone lesions and cataracts: complete postmortem examination. *Dev Med Child Neurol* 19:527, 1977.

216 Vontver L et al: Recurrent genital herpes simplex virus infection in pregnancy: infant outcome and frequency as asymptomatic recurrences. *Am J Obstet Gynecol* 143:75, 1982.

217 Brown Z et al: Genital herpes in pregnancy: risk factors associated with recurrences and asymptomatic shedding. *Am J Obstet Gynecol* 153:24–30, 1985.

218 Naib Z et al: Association of maternal genital herpetic infection with spontaneous abortion. *Obstet Gynecol* 35:260, 1970.

219 Nahmias A et al: Perinatal risk associated with maternal genital herpes simplex virus infection. *Am J Obstet Gynecol* 110:825, 1971.

220 Brown Z et al: Effects on infants of first episode genital herpes during pregnancy. *N Engl J Med* 317:1247–1251, 1987.

221 Hain J et al: Ascending transcervical herpes simplex infection with intact fetal membranes. *Obstet Gynecol* 56:106, 1980.

222 Arvin A et al: Failure of antepartum maternal cultures to predict the infant's risk of exposure to herpes simplex virus at delivery. *N Engl J Med* 315:796–800, 1986.

223 Whitley R et al: The natural history of genital herpes simplex virus infection of mother and newborn. *Pediatrics* 66:489, 1980.

224 Brown Z et al: Acquisition of herpes simplex virus during pregnancy. *N Engl J Med* 337:509–515, 1997.

225 Tejani N et al: Subclinical herpes simplex genitalis infections in the perinatal period. *Am J Obstet Gynecol* 135:547, 1979.

226 Yeager A et al: Genital herpes simplex infections: effect of asymptomatic shedding and latency on management of infections in pregnant women and neonates. *J Invest Dermatol* 83:53s–56s, 1984.

227 Prober C et al: Low risk of herpes simplex virus infections in neonates exposed to the virus at the time of vaginal delivery to mothers with recurrent genital HSV infections. *N Engl J Med* 316:240–244, 1987.

228 Yeager A et al: Relationship of antibody to outcome in neonatal herpes simplex virus infections. *Infect Immunol* 29:532, 1980.

229 Parvey L et al: Neonatal herpes simplex virus infection introduced by fetal monitor scalp electrodes. *Pediatrics* 65:1140, 1980.

230 Zervoudakis I et al: Herpes simplex in the amniotic fluid of an unaffected fetus. *Obstet Gynecol* 55:16s, 1980.

231 Prober C et al: The management of pregnancies complicated by genital infections with herpes simplex virus. *Clin Infect Dis* 15:1031–1038, 1992.

232 Light I et al: Neonatal herpes simplex infection following delivery by cesarean section. *Obstet Gynecol* 44:496, 1974.

233 Whitley R et al: Changing presentation of herpes simplex virus infection in neonates. *J Infect Dis* 158:109–116, 1988.

234 Kulhanjian J et al: Identification of women at unsuspected risk of primary infection with herpes simplex virus type 2 during pregnancy. *N Engl J Med* 326:916–920, 1992.

235 Committee on Fetus and Newborn and Committee on Infectious Diseases: Perinatal herpes simplex virus infections. *Pediatrics* 66:147, 1980.

236 Sullivan-Bolyai J et al: Presentation of neonatal HSV infections: implications for a change in therapeutic strategy. *Ped Inf Dis* 5:309–314, 1986.

237 Light I: Postnatal acquisition of herpes simplex virus by the newborn infant: a review of the literature. *Pediatrics* 63:480, 1979.

238 Linnemann C et al: Transmission of herpes-simplex virus type 1 in a nursery for the newborn: identification of viral isolates by DNA "fingerprinting." *Lancet* 1:964, 1978.

239 Chapel T et al: Simultaneous infection with Treponema pallidum and herpes simplex virus. *Cutis* 24:191, 1979.

240 Carney O et al: The effect of suppressive oral acyclovir on the psychological morbidity associated with recurrent genital herpes. *Genitourin Med* 69:457–459, 1993.

241 Catotti D et al: Herpes revisited: still a cause of concern. *Sex Trans Dis* 20:77–80, 1993.

242 Rand K et al: Daily stress and recurrence of genital herpes simplex. *Arch Intern Med* 150:1889–1893, 1990.

243 Whaley K et al: Nonoxynol-9 protects mice against vaginal transmission of genital herpes infections. *J Infect Dis* 168:1009–1011, 1993.

244 Wald A et al: Suppression of subclinical shedding of herpes simplex virus type 2 with acyclovir. *Ann Intern Med* 124:8–15, 1996.

245 Corey L et al: Evaluation of new anti-infective drugs for the treatment of genital infections due to herpes simplex virus. *Clin Infect Dis* 15(s1):99–107, 1992.

246 Elion G et al: Selectivity of action of an antiherpetic agent, 9-(2-Hydroxyethoxymethyl) guanine. *Proc Natl Acad Sci USA* 74:5716, 1977.

247 Schaeffer H et al: 9-(2-Hydroxyethoxymethyl) guanine activity against viruses of herpes group. *Nature* 272:583, 1978.

248 Brigden D et al: The clinical pharmacology of acyclovir and its prodrug. *Scand J Infect Dis Suppl* 47:33, 1985.

249 Dorsky D et al: Acyclovir: drugs 5 years later. *Ann Intern Med* 207:859–874, 1987.

250 Erlich K et al: Acyclovir-resistant herpes simplex virus infections in patients with the acquired immunodeficiency syndrome. *N Engl J Med* 320:293–296, 1989.

251 Crumpacker C et al: Growth inhibition by acycloguanosine of herpes virus isolated from human infections. *Antimicrobiol Agents Chemother* 15:642, 1979.

252 Bryson Y et al: Treatment of first episodes of genital herpes simplex virus infections with oral acyclovir: a randomized double-blind controlled trial in normal subjects. *N Engl J Med* 308:916–920, 1983.

253 Corey L et al: Risk of recurrence after treatment of first episode genital herpes with intravenous acyclovir. *Sex Trans Dis* 12:215–218, 1985.

254 de-Miranda P et al: Pharmacokinetics of acyclovir after intravenous and oral administration. *J Antimicrobiol Chemo* 12 Suppl B:29–37, 1983.

255 Burnette T et al: Purification and characterization of a rat liver enzyme that hydrolyzes valaciclovir, the L-valyl ester prodrug of acyclovir. *J Biol Chem* 270:15827–15831, 1995.

256 Soul-Lawton J et al: Absolute bioavailability and metabolic disposition of valaciclovir, the L-Val ester of acyclovir, following oral administration to humans. *Antimicrobiol Agents and Chem* 36:2759–2764, 1995.

257 Spruance S et al: A large-scale, placebo-controlled, dose-ranging trial of peroral valacyclovir for episodic treatment of recurrent herpes genitalis. *Arch Int Med* 156:1729–1735, 1996.

258 Bodsworth N et al: Valaciclovir versus aciclovir in patient-initiated treatment of recurrent genital herpes: a randomised, double-blind clinical trial. *Genitourin Med* 73:110–116, 1997.

259 Fife K et al: Valaciclovir versus acyclovir in the treatment of first-episode genital herpes infection: results of an international, multicenter, double-blind randomized clinical trial. *Sex Trans Dis* 24:481–486, 1997.

260 Patel R et al: Valacyclovir for the suppression of recurrent genital HSV infection: a placebo controlled study of once-daily therapy. *Genitourin Medicine* 73:105–109, 1997.

261 Tyring S et al: Once daily valacyclovir for suppression of genital herpes—results from a large international study. *55th Annual Meeting American Academy of Dermatology,* San Francisco, California, 1997.

262 Chulay J et al: Long-term safety of valacyclovir for suppression of herpes simplex virus infections. *34th Annual Meeting of IDSA,* New Orleans, LA, USA, 1996.

263 Hodge R et al: The mode of action of penciclovir. *Antiviral Chem and Chemo* 4 S 1:13–24, 1993.

264 Weinberg A et al: In vitro activities of penciclovir and acyclovir against herpes simplex virus types 1 and 1. *Antimicrobiol Agents Chemo* 36:2037–2038, 1992.

265 Pue M et al: Pharmacokinetics of famciclovir in man. *Antiviral Chem and Chemo* 4(s1):47–55, 1993.

266 Saltzman R et al: Safety of famciclovir in patients with herpes zoster and genital herpes. *Antimicro Agents Chemo* 38:2454–2457, 1994.

267 Sacks S et al: Patient-initiated, twice-daily oral famciclovir for early recurrent genital herpes. A randomized, double-blind multicenter trial. *JAMA* 276:44–49, 1996.

268 Loveless M et al: Treatment of first episode genital herpes with famciclovir. *35th Interscience Conference on Antimicrobial Agents and Chemotherapy,* San Francisco, California, 1995.

269 Mertz G et al: Oral famciclovir for suppression of recurrent genital herpes simplex virus infection in women. *Arch Intern Med* 157:343–349, 1997.

270 Diaz-Mitoma F et al: Famcicovir suppression of recurrent genital herpes. *36th Interscience Conference on Antimicrobial Agents and Chemotherapy,* New Orleans, LA, 1996.

271 Schacker T et al: Famciclovir for the suppression of symptomatic and asymptomatic herpes simplex virus reactivation in HIV-infected persons. A double-blind, placebo-controlled trial. *Ann Intern Med* 128: 21–28, 1998.

272 Field H et al: Comparison of efficacies of famcyclovir and valaciclovir against herpes simplex virus type 1 in a murine immunosuppression model. *Antimicrobiol Agents Chemother* 39:1114–1119, 1995.

273 Thackray A et al: Differential effects of famciclovir and valacyclovir on the pathogenesis of herpes simplex virus in a murine infection model including reactivation from latency. *J Infect Dis* 173:291–299, 1996.

274 Reichman R et al: Treatment of recurrent genital herpes simplex infections with oral acyclovir: a controlled trial. *J Amer Med Assoc* 251:2103–2107, 1984.

275 Nilsen A et al: Efficacy of oral acyclovir in treatment of initial and recurrent genital herpes. *Lancet* ii:572, 1982.

276 Fiddian A et al: Topical acyclovir in the treatment of genital herpes: a comparison with systemic therapy. *J Antimicrob Chemother* 12 (Suppl. B):67–77, 1983.

277 Kinghorn G et al: Efficacy of combined treatment with oral and topical acyclovir in first episode genital herpes. *Genitourin Med* 62:186, 1986.

278 Douglas J et al: A double blind study of oral acyclovir for suppression of recurrences of genital herpes simplex virus infection. *N Engl J Med* 310:1551–1556, 1984.

279 Straus S et al: Suppressing of frequently recurring genital herpes: a placebo-controlled double blind trial of oral acyclovir. *N Engl J Med* 310:1545–1550, 1984.

280 Halsos A et al: Oral acyclovir suppression of recurrent genital herpes: a double-blind, placebo-controlled crossover study. *Acta Dermato Venerol* 65:59–63, 1985.

281 Mindel A et al: Dosage and safety of long term suppressive therapy for recurrent genital herpes. *Lancet* i:926–928, 1988.

282 Kaplowitz L et al: Prolonged continuous acyclovir treatment of normal adults with frequently recurring genital herpes simplex virus infection. The Acyclovir Study Group. *JAMA* 265:747–751, 1991.

283 Goldberg L et al: Long-term suppression of recurrent genital herpes with acyclovir. *Arch Dermatol* 129:582–587, 1993.

284 Fife K et al: Recurrence and resistance patterns of herpes simplex virus following cessation of >6 years of chronic suppression with acyclovir. *J Infect Dis* 169:1338–1341, 1994.

285 Mertz G et al: Long term acyclovir suppression of frequently recurring genital herpes simplex virus infection: a multi-center double blind trial. *J Am Med Assoc* 260:201–206, 1988.

286 Tucker W: Preclinical toxicology of acyclovir: an overview. *Amer J Med, Acyclovir Symp* 27–30, 1982.

287 Douglas J et al: A double-blind, placebo-controlled trial of the effect of chronic oral acyclovir on sperm production in men with frequently recurrent genital herpes. *J Infect Dis* 157:588, 1988.

288 Henry R et al: Successful oral acyclovir desensitization. *Ann Allergy* 70:386–388, 1993.

289 Gold D et al: Acyclovir prophylaxis for herpes simplex virus infection. *Antimicrobiol Agents Chemother* 31:361–367, 1987.

290 Scott L et al: Acyclovir suppression to prevent cesarean delivery after first-episode genital herpes. *Obstet Gynecol* 87:69–73, 1996.

291 Frenkel L et al: Pharmacokinetics of acyclovir in the term human pregnancy and neonate. *Amer J Obstet Gyn* 164:569–576, 1991.

292 Whitley R et al: Predictors of morbidity and mortality in neonates with herpes simplex infections. *N Engl J Med* 324:450–454, 1991.

293 Coen D et al: Two distinct loci confer resistance to acycloguanosine in herpes simplex virus type 1. *Proc Natl Acad Sci USA* 77:2265–2269, 1980.

294 McLaren C et al: In vitro sensitivity to acyclovir in genital herpes simplex viruses from acyclovir treated patients. *J Infect Dis* 148:868–875, 1983.

295 Barry D et al: Clinical and laboratory experience with acyclovir-resistant herpes viruses. *J Antimicrobiol Chemother* 18(Suppl B):75–84, 1986.

296 Nusinoff-Lehrman S et al: Recurrent genital herpes and suppressive oral acyclovir therapy: relationship between clinical outcome and in vitro drug sensitivity. *Ann Int Med* 204:686–690, 1986.

297 Field H et al: Pathogenicity in mice of strains of herpes simplex virus which are resistant to acyclovir in vitro and in vivo. *Antimicrobiol Agents Chemother* 17:209–216, 1980.

298 Sasadeusz J et al: Spontaneous reactivation of thymidine kinase-deficient, acyclovir-resistant type 2 herpes simplex virus: masked heterogeneity or reversion? *J Infect Dis* 174:476–482, 1996.

299 Sacks S et al: Progressive esophagitis from acyclovir-resistant herpes simplex. Clinical roles for DNA polymerase mutants and viral heterogeneity. *Ann Intern Med* 111:893–899, 1989.

300 Kost R et al: Brief report: Recurrent acyclovir-resistant genital herpes in an immunocompetent patient. *N Engl J Med* 329:1777–1782, 1993.

301 Safrin S et al: Correlation between response to acyclovir and foscarnet therapy and in vitro susceptibility result for isolates of herpes simplex virus from human immunodeficiency virus-infected patients. *Antimicrobiol Agents Chemother* 38:1246–1250, 1994.

302 Engel J et al: Treatment of resistant herpes simplex virus with continuous-infusion acyclovir. *JAMA* 263:1662–1664, 1990.

303 Alenius S et al: Therapeutic effects of foscarnet sodium and acyclovir on cutaneous infection due to herpes simplex virus type 1 in guinea pigs. *J Infect Dis* 145:569–573, 1982.

304 Wallin J et al: Topical treatment of recurrent genital herpes infection with foscarnate. *Scand J Infect Dis* 17:165–172, 1985.

305 Sacks S et al: Clinical course of recurrent genital herpes and treatment with foscarnet cream. *J Infect Dis* 155:178–186, 1987.

306 Safrin S et al: Foscarnet therapy for acyclovir-resistant mucocutaneous herpes simplex virus infection in 26 AIDS patients: preliminary data. *J Infect Dis* 161:1078–1084, 1990.

307 Safrin S et al: A controlled trial comparing foscarnet with vidarabine for acyclovir-resistant mucocutaneous herpes simplex in the acquired immunodeficiency syndrome. *N Engl J Med* 325:551–555, 1991.

308 Safrin S et al: Foscarnet-resistant herpes simplex virus infection in patients with AIDS. *J Infect Dis* 169:193–196, 1994.

309 Mendel D et al: Biochemical basis for increased susceptibility to cidofovir of herpes simplex viruses with altered or deficient thymidine kinase activity. *Antimicrobiol Agents Chemother* 39:2120–2122, 1995.

310 Lalezari J et al: Treatment with intravenous *(S)*-1[3-Hydroxy-2(Phosphonylmethoxy)propyl]-cytosine of acyclovir resistant mucocutane-

ous infection with herpes simplex virus in a patient with AIDS. *J Infect Dis* 170:570–572, 1994.

311 Snoeck R et al: Successful treatment of progressive mucocutaneous infection due to acyclovir- and foscarnet-resistant herpes simplex virus with *(S)*-1(3-Hydroxy-2-Phosphonylmethoxypropyl) cytosine (HPMPC). *Clin Infect Dis* 18:570–578, 1994.

312 Sacks S et al: A randomized, double-blind placebo-controlled pilot study of cidofovir topical gel for recurrent genital herpes. *International Society for Antiviral Research,* Fukushima, Japan, 1996.

313 Kessler H et al: Pilot study of topical trifluridine for the treatment of acyclovir-resistant mucocutaneous herpes simplex disease in patients with AIDS (ACTG 172). *J Acq Immune Def Synd Hum Retrovirol* 12:147–152, 1996.

314 Birch C et al: Clinical effects and in vitro studies of trifluorothymidine combined with interferon-alpha for treatment of drug-resistant and -sensitive herpes simplex virus infections. *J Infect Dis* 166:108–112, 1992.

315 Straus S et al: Immunotherapy of recurrent genital herpes with recombinant herpes simplex type 2 glycoproteins D and B: results of a placebo-controlled vaccine trial. *J Infect Dis* 176:1129–1134, 1997.

316 Burke R: Development of a herpes simplex virus subunit glycoprotein vaccine for prophylactic and therapeutic use. *Rev Infect Dis* 13: S906–911, 1991.

317 Mertz G et al: Herpes simplex virus type-2 glycoprotein-subunit vaccine: tolerance and humoral and cellular responses in humans. *J Infect Dis* 150:242–249, 1984.

318 Lagenberg A et al: A recombinant glycoprotein vaccine for herpes simplex type 2: safety and efficacy. *Ann Intern Med* 122:889–898, 1995.

319 Gallichan W et al: Mucosal immunity and protection with intranasal immunization with recombinant adenovirus expressing herpes simplex virus glycoprotein B. *J Infect Dis* 168:622–629, 1993.

320 Burke R: Current developments in herpes simplex virus vaccines. *Virology* 4:187–197, 1993.

321 Boursnell M et al: A genetically inactivated herpes simplex virus type 2 (HSV-2) vaccine provides effective protection against primary and recurrent HSV-2 disease. *J Infect Dis* 175:16–25, 1997.

322 Bourne N et al: DNA immunization against experimental herpes simplex virus infection. *J Infect Dis* 173:800–807, 1996.

323 Kriesel J et al: Nucleic acid vaccine encoding gD2 protects mice from herpes simplex virus type 2 disease. *J Infect Dis* 173:536–541, 1996.

Chapter 22

Cytomegalovirus

W. Lawrence Drew
Michael P. Bates

INTRODUCTION

Human cytomegalovirus (HCMV) is a member of the herpesvirus family. Its name results from its property of enlarging the cells that it infects. HCMV is a common human pathogen, infecting 0.5 to 15 percent of infants and approximately 50 percent of the adult population in developed countries. It is particularly prominent as a pathogen in immunocompromised patients.

HCMV has a 230-kb linear, double-stranded DNA genome that has a complex arrangement of inverted repeats and unique sequences that exist as four possible isomers and encode approximately 200 open reading frames. The nucleocapsid is surrounded by tegument and enveloped within a lipid bilayer that carries a number of virally encoded proteins. HCMV depends on the transcription and translation machinery of the host during growth in permissive cells. The expression of HCMV genes is temporally regulated and can be divided into immediate-early, early, and late phases. The immediate-early (IE) genes are transcribed in the absence of *de novo* viral protein synthesis. Their protein products play regulatory roles in determining the timing of early and late gene expression. Early proteins perform many functions, including viral DNA replication. Their synthesis depends on IE gene expression. Following DNA replication, late gene expression encodes proteins involved in the generation of progeny virus (Fig. 22-1).[1]

PATHOGENESIS

The pathogenesis of HCMV infection is a function of the complex interplay between the virus and the host in the course of the viral life cycle. The virus seeks to penetrate cells, evade host immunity, express its genes in a temporally regulated cascade, replicate its DNA, produce progeny virus, and spread to new cellular hosts. In response to changes in the host environment, HCMV may need to establish latency and reactivate at a later time when the conditions for replication are more favorable. During this series of interactions with the host, the virus may cause cellular damage resulting in disease. One major question in HCMV pathogenesis is whether cellular damage is caused directly by the viral lytic infection or indirectly by the immune response of the host. In some cases of HCMV disease, it seems clear that cellular damage results from a direct cytopathic effect. One such example is retinitis in severely immunocompromised AIDS patients, where blindness occurs as a result of a necrotizing infection by the virus.[2,3] The beneficial effects of ganciclovir therapy support this notion. In contrast, HCMV pneumonitis frequently manifests subtle histologic alterations in the face of life-threatening clinical symptomotology and extensive inflammation accompanied by mild viral replication, suggesting that immune-mediated injury is the primary pathologic mechanism.[4–6] In other instances, both direct and indirect forces seem to be at work.

Two major effectors of immune mediated injury stimulated by HCMV infection have been postulated. First, the upregulation and release of cytokines, such as tumor necrosis factor (TNF)-alpha, interferon (IFN)-gamma, and interleukin (IL)-2, leads to cellular cytotoxicity, either directly or by way of immune induction. Second, immune-mediated tissue injury may be effected by CD8+ cytotoxic T lymphocytes (CTL) directed against HCMV infected target cells.[4,7]

Another manifestation of the effect of HCMV on host immunity, perhaps leading to disordered immunity, is graft-versus-host disease (GVHD). HCMV has been associated with the development of chronic graft-versus-host disease in allogeneic bone marrow transplant recipients. The association of HCMV infection with GVHD and rejection may reflect an enhanced response to allogeneic stimulation mediated by increased MHC class II expression on the surface of infected cells.[8,9] Similarly, the increased expression of cellular adhesion molecules, such as ICAM-1, may encourage inappropriate inflammation.[10–12] Recently, HCMV has been shown to induce the development of autoantibodies specific to the human cell surface protein CD13, a proposed receptor for HCMV cellular entry. This observation may explain the relationship between HCMV and GVHD.[13] In the mouse system, murine CMV can exacerbate GVHD by inducing allospecific CD8+ CTL.[7]

HCMV is capable of cooperating with other viruses to cause disease. Patients who develop HCMV viremia following orthotopic liver transplantation for chronic hepatitis C virus (HCV) infection incur a significantly greater risk of severe recurrence of HCV. The mechanism is unknown, but the authors speculate that suppression of cell-mediated immunity by HCMV led to the recurrence.[14]

HIV-1 replication in human placental syncytiotrophoblast cells in vitro has been shown to be markedly increased by concomitant infection with HCMV. HCMV immediate early gene expression was necessary for this effect. HCMV infection in the same cells was converted from nonpermissive to permissive by prior infection with HIV-1. This conversion was dependent on HIV *tat* gene expression.[15] Most importantly, the US28 gene of HCMV encodes a β-chemokine receptor that is homologous to human CCR5 and CXCR4. US28 has been shown to facilitate infection of CD4+ human cell lines by both HIV-1 and HIV-2.[16,17] Although it is unclear whether HCMV acts as an accomplice of HIV in vivo to allow infection of CCR5-negative/CXCR4-negative cell types, these data raise questions about the role of this ubiquitous virus in HIV pathogenesis.

VIRAL GENE EXPRESSION AND HOST CELL INTERACTIONS

IE gene expression results in the production of two polypeptides that have been implicated in both positive and negative regulation of many viral and cellular genes (E2F-1/-2/-3,DNA polymerase-alpha).[18–21] The HCMV IE proteins upregulate the expression of NF-kB, a transcription factor that is critically important in the induction of the viral replication cycle through its association with the major immediate early promoter-enhancer (MIEP) of HCMV (see the following).[19] The *trans*-activation of NF-kB is accomplished through interactions between IE72 and chromatin, but there is no direct binding with DNA. Presumably, this function is mediated by binding to other proteins expressed in the nucleus.

The 72-kDa protein encoded by the immediate early (*ie*) 1 region functions as an autoregulatory trans-activator by binding to its own promoter. IE72 also functions in concert with the other major *ie* gene product of HCMV, IE86, to activate early gene expression. A deletion mutant of *ie* 1 is replication defective and has been proposed as a gene therapy vector.[22] The 86-kDa gene product of *ie* 2 is a major regulator of early gene activation and

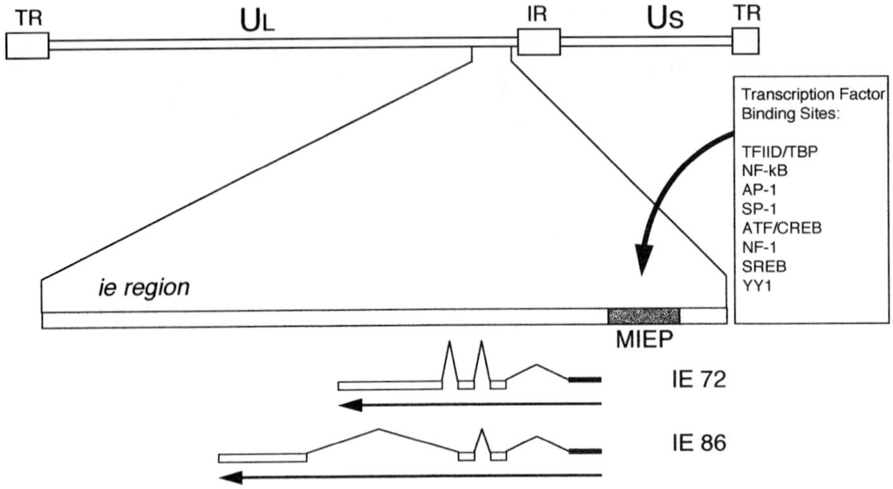

Fig. 22-1. The HCMV genome with the unique long (UL), unique short (Us), and flanking repeats (TR, IR) depicted. The immediate early region is enlarged and shows the location of the major immediate early promoter-enhancer (MIEP) and the exon/intron structure of the two major immediate early gene products, IE72 and IE86. The arrows indicate the direction of transcription/translation (adapted from Mocarski, ref 1).

exerts a repressive effect on the MIEP resulting in the shutoff of *ie* 1/*ie* 2 expression. IE86 has also been described as a promiscuous *trans*-activator of a host of cellular promoters. The mechanism by which IE86 accomplishes this is unclear, but the fact that there is no known consensus sequence for IE86 binding suggests that the *trans*-activation may be a result of protein–protein interactions between IE86 and host transcription factors. The DNA polymerase promoter of HCMV (UL54) is activated by binding of the cellular transcription factor SP-1, perhaps as a ternary complex in association with IE86 and the basal transcription apparatus. The production of SP-1 is itself upregulated by the IE proteins of HCMV.[23]

The TATA binding protein (TBP) and the tumor suppressor proteins p53 and the retinoblastoma protein (Rb) have all been shown to associate with IE86, suggesting that IE86 may be involved in the regulation of cell growth through interactions with proteins that influence the cell cycle. The HCMV IE proteins induce cell cycle arrest at G1/S and at G2/M by affecting the intracellular levels of cyclins, phosphorylated Rb, and p53(H13, H9). The location of the cell cycle block is dependent on the state of the cell at the time of infection. These interactions enable HCMV to manipulate the internal milieu of the cell to its advantage. When the cell cycle is blocked in G1, for example, the cell is ripe with the building blocks necessary for DNA synthesis, such as nucleotides and transcription factors.[24] This favors HCMV replication. Differential expression of the *ie* genes may influence the course of viral replication in different cell types and in response to extracellular signals received by the infected cell. The complex interplay between HCMV and its host is greatly influenced by the functions of these two IE proteins.[1,25]

Both of these IE genes are under the transcriptional control of a strong enhancer sequence, MIEP, that contains a large number of mammalian transcription factor binding sites (AP-1, SP-1, NF-kB, ATF/CREB, NF-1, SREB, TFIID/TBP). The MIEP can also be activated by binding of the HCMV tegument protein pp71, which is carried into the host cell as a component of the virion. Thus, transcriptional activation of these immediate early (*ie*) genes can proceed very early following viral entry, as transcription factors present in the host cell bind and activate the MIEP, independent of viral protein synthesis.[1] Negative regulation of the MIEP also occurs. Upstream of the MIEP, a sequence termed the modulator has been shown to bind cellular factors (YY1) leading to MIEP repression.[26] These regulatory elements provide an opportunity to modulate the infectious cycle of HCMV depending on the state of the host cell.[1,25]

Following DNA replication and the synthesis of late proteins in the nucleus, virion assembly occurs. Immature viral particles acquire tegument and envelope as they bud through the inner nuclear membrane. Final egress from the cell appears to occur in endosomes.[27]

CELLULAR TROPISM

HCMV has a broad range of target cells, although most cell types are nonpermissive for HCMV replication. The clinical manifestations of HCMV infection demonstrate the range of cell types that HCMV is capable of infecting. Meningoencephalitis, retinitis, enteritis, vasculitis, pneumonitis, myocarditis, lymphadenitis, hepatitis, adrenalitis, and pancreatitis resulting from HCMV infection have all been described.[28] When immunohistochemical techniques are applied to HCMV infected tissues, a variety of susceptible cells are identified, including smooth muscle cells, inflammatory cells, glial cells, neurons, hepatocytes, myocytes, and such ubiquitously distributed cells as endothelial cells, epithelial cells, and fibroblasts, which are the major targets of HCMV.[12,25] The presence of stromal cell types (e.g., fibroblasts) in virtually all tissues may explain the vast distribution of HCMV.

Tropism may be restricted by the presence of a specific receptor on a particular cell at a particular time. The wide range of cell types susceptible to infection with HCMV argues that the cellular receptor for HCMV is widely distributed or that there are many HCMV receptors.[29] Interstrain variation in envelope glycoprotein expression may also influence cellular tropism.[12]

HCMV successfully penetrates many cell types, but is able to replicate permissively in only a few. Cell type-specific expression of HCMV appears to be determined by the transcriptional activity of the MIEP.[30,31] Thus, cellular tropism is influenced to a greater degree by the restrictions placed on MIEP activity than by restricted entry into various cell types. A deletion mutant of murine cytomegalovirus that results in a block in IE gene expression exhibits altered cell and tissue tropism, lending credence to this model.[32]

VIRAL ENTRY

HCMV enters the cell in two stages: attachment and penetration. Adsorption to the plasma membrane is mediated initially by binding to heparan sulfate moieties on the plasma membrane surface. Penetration proceeds following specific binding to putative HCMV receptors. The plasma membrane and the envelope of

HCMV fuse, resulting in release of the nucleocapsid into the host cell cytoplasm.[29] By unknown mechanisms, the nucleocapsid and viral tegument proteins are transported to the nucleus, where HCMV gene expression commences. Following viral entry, cellular factors decide the outcome of HCMV infection.[25] If the MIEP is allowed to activate IE genes, the cascade of gene expression proceeds and productive, lytic infection ensues. If, on the other hand, there is a block to MIEP induction, infection is aborted or latency is established.

The HCMV envelope glycoproteins that participate in viral entry are gB, gH/gL, and gcII. Humoral immunity directed at gB has been detected in convalescent phase sera and has been shown to block viral entry, cell-to-cell transmission, and syncytia formation in HCMV infected cells.[33,34] Supporting data demonstrate a specific interaction between host cell surface receptor(s) and gB.[35]

Several host cell surface molecules have been identified as possible receptors for HCMV. The cellular aminopeptidase CD13 has been postulated as a receptor for HCMV, but the viral ligand is unknown.[29,34,36,37] A 34-kDa protein that may be annexin II is thought to bind gB specifically and participate in cell-to-cell spread.[29] Finally, a 92.5-kDa molecule present on the surface of human embryonic lung fibroblasts was identified as a putative receptor for HCMV gH.[38] Monoclonal antibodies directed at this receptor were able to block plasma membrane/HCMV envelope fusion in a specific and dose dependent manner. Following binding of this protein to HCMV gH, the 92.5-kDa putative receptor was phosphorylated and an increase in intracytoplasmic calcium was noted, suggesting a possible mechanism by which membrane fusion occurs.[34,39]

Certain cellular oncogenes and transcription factors such as c-fos, c-jun, c-myc, NF-kB, and SP-1 have been shown to be transcriptionally activated on membrane binding of inactivated viral particles. This effect is mediated by the binding of gB and gH to their cellular receptors.[40] It appears that HCMV makes use of cellular signal transduction pathways to modify the cellular environment in preparation for viral entry (Fig. 22-2).

IMMUNITY TO HCMV

The immune response to HCMV infection is heterogeneous, with contributions from the humoral and cell-mediated arms. Both CD4+ and CD8+ T-cell responses have been detected in seropositive patients, but the CD8+ CTL response appears to be the most important of these. Some investigators have postulated that HCMV-specific CD4+ Th cells are necessary for the generation of a specific CD8+ CTL response.[41] Deficiencies in CD8+ CMV-specific CTL responses have been implicated in the progression of disease.[42] The multiplicity of proteins that the virus has devoted to the avoidance of CTL recognition argues strongly that CTL are pivotal in the host defense against HCMV.[43]

gB, the major envelope glycoprotein of HCMV, has been identified as a target for CTL; but the major targets for CTL are the tegument proteins pp65 and pp150.[44–47] pp65 Makes up approximately 95 percent of the tegument. In one study, between 70 and 90 percent of all HCMV-specific CTL recognized pp65 specifically.[47]

Adoptive transfer of CD8+ CMV-specific CTLs has been successful in preventing HCMV infection in immunocompromised marrow transplant recipients.[42,44,45] In the murine system, viral load has been implicated as a determinant in the likelihood of reactivation from latency during immunosuppression.[48] Reddehase and colleagues demonstrated that they could decrease the viral DNA load in organs and reduce the rate of recurrence of productive infection by treating preemptively with CTL immunotherapy. They were not able to achieve complete clearance of viral DNA. They suggest that clinical trials of adoptive immunotherapy be continued.[49]

EVASION OF HOST IMMUNITY

MIEP inactivity in monocytes seems to allow HCMV to evade host immunity and achieve latent infection.[37] As we will discuss later, through latency HCMV is permitted to persist in the host for life. However, latency is not the only mechanism by which HCMV evades host immunity. In monocyte derived macrophages, HCMV infection has been shown to result in a disordered intracellular microtubule structure. Disruption of the Golgi apparatus occurs without accompanying cellular lysis. This disruption of intracellular transport pathways interferes with antigen presentation at the cell surface. In this way, HCMV avoids exposure to the immune system.[37,51]

Perhaps the most startling revelations regarding HCMV's ability to escape the host immune system come from the study of genes in the unique short region of the viral genome. Cytotoxic T cells (CTL) recognize virally encoded peptides in association with MHC class I molecules at the cell surface. HCMV interferes with

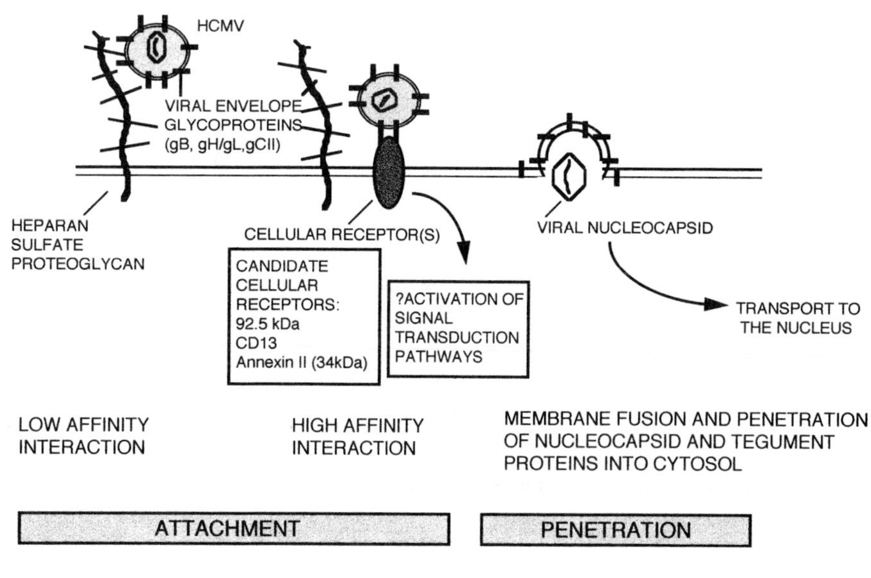

Fig. 22-2. Hypothetical model of viral entry (adapted from Compton, ref. 29).

this process at multiple steps. The viral glycoprotein encoded by US3 impairs the egress of MHC class I heavy chains from the endoplasmic reticulum (ER), thus preventing proper antigen presentation.[51] The products of the US2 and US11 genes trigger the rapid degradation of MHC class I molecules by translocating them out of the ER and into the cytosol where they are targeted to the proteasome for destruction.[43,52] The US6 gene product disturbs the intracellular loading of MHC class I molecules with peptide by interdicting the translocation function performed by TAP, the transporter associated with antigen processing.[53] These four glycoproteins allow HCMV to escape detection by host CTL (Fig. 22-3).

Cells that fail to express MHC class I molecules on their surface are targeted for destruction by natural killer (NK) cells. According to the "missing self" hypothesis, NK cells possess cell surface receptors for MHC class I molecules termed killer inhibitory receptors (KIRs). On binding of MHC class I molecules to KIRs, target cell lysis is inhibited. However, the absence or alteration of MHC class I molecules, as in the case of HCMV infected cells expressing US2, US3, US6, or US11 as discussed in the preceding, should leave the cell vulnerable to NK cell cytotoxicity. Recent data have shown that the UL18 gene of HCMV encodes an MHC class I homologue that binds to the leukocyte immunoglobulin-like receptor (LIR-1), a cellular glycoprotein expressed on monocytes and B cells, and related to KIR.[54] Furthermore, expression of the UL18 protein in an MHC class I-negative, NK-sensitive cell line protected the cells from lysis by NK cells.[55]

LATENCY

Fundamental to one's understanding of HCMV pathogenesis is the concept of latency. Defined, latency is the demonstration of the persistence of the viral genome in host cells without any evidence of viral replication or the production of infectious virus.[56] During the course of a typical HCMV infection in an immunocompetent person, the acute phase of the infection may be marked by a mononucleosis-like syndrome, or may be clinically silent. Subsequently, HCMV achieves latency and will remain as a lifelong persistent infection.

Mocarski's group has reported the existence of two latency-associated transcripts in bone marrow-derived granulocyte-macrophage precursors.[57,58] They have called these CMV latent transcripts (CLTs). These mRNAs are encoded by the *ie* 1/ *ie* 2 region and are unspliced. Importantly, these transcripts can only be detected in latently infected cells from seropositive healthy people and not at all in seronegative people. Thus, they serve as a marker of HCMV latency and may play a role in the establishment and maintenance of latency. These CLTs have also been identified in CD33+ progenitors of myeloid and dendritic cells.[59,60]

Recently, monocytes have been shown to be a site of HCMV latency. Nelson's group has demonstrated reactivation of HCMV following allogeneic stimulation from macrophages expressing dendritic cell markers.[56] Although HCMV gets into undifferentiated cells, such as monocytes and their progenitors, it is unable to replicate owing to MIEP repression. However, on differentiation to macrophages, the MIEP is activated, the *ie* genes are expressed, and productive infection proceeds. Undifferentiated cells provide an environment where the virus can persist in the latent state.[26,61–63]

Other investigators have confirmed the finding that HCMV latently infects bone marrow progenitor cells, and have suggested that CD34+ cells only reactivate HCMV following differentiation to macrophages.[63] These data dovetail with the clinical observation that HCMV infection is associated with graft failure in bone marrow transplant patients.[64–67]

Bone marrow progenitor cells of the granulocyte/monocyte lineage are not the only cells where HCMV resides in a latent state. HCMV DNA has been detected in human microvascular endothelial cells without any evidence of cytopathic effect, suggesting

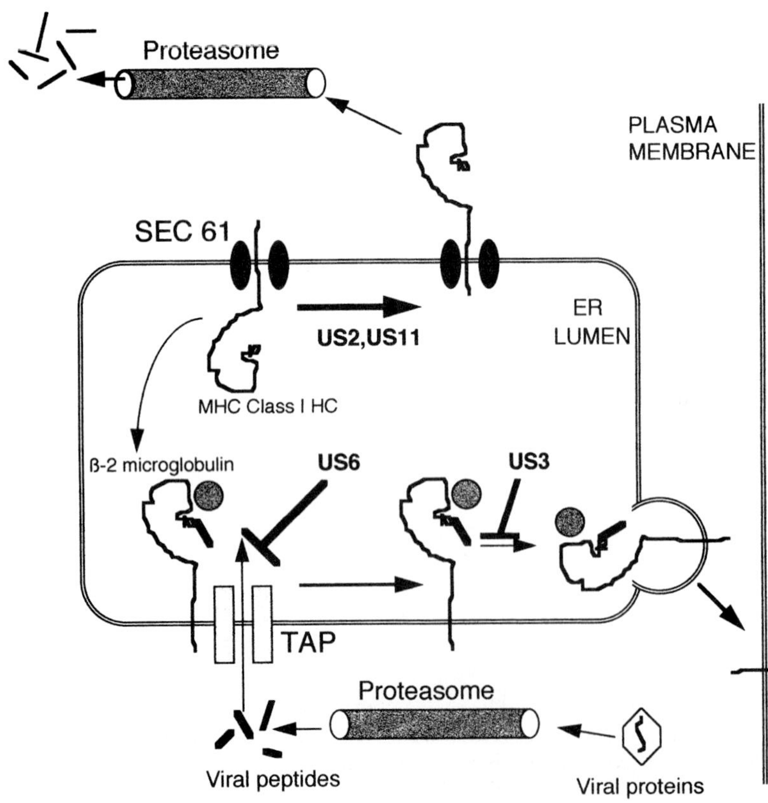

Fig. 22-3. MHC class I heavy chain is normally translocated into the ER lumen by the SEC 61 complex where it associates with β-2 microglobulin and is loaded with viral peptide that has been processed by the proteasome in the cytosol and transported into the ER by TAP, the transporter associated with antigen processing. Subsequently, the complex is transported out of the ER, through the Golgi, and presented at the plasma membrane for antigen recognition. The CMV proteins US2, US3, US6, and US11 interfere with this process at different steps, as indicated. US2 and US11 dislocate MHC Class I HC back into the cytosol where it is degraded by the proteasome. US6 blocks peptide loading of MHC Class I HC by inhibiting TAP-mediated transport of viral peptide into the ER. US3 blocks egress of the MHC/peptide complex from the ER lumen (adapted from ref. 43; Davis-Poynter NJ and Farrell HE, *Semin Virol* 8:369–376, 1998.)

latency. Murine CMV has recently been shown to reside latently in bone marrow, alveolar macrophages, T lymphocytes, and endothelial cells by in situ PCR.[68,69] Large-vessel endothelial cells and bone marrow stromal cells have also been shown to harbor latent HCMV.[37,63]

Reactivation from the latent state has classically been associated with immunosuppression, but the mechanism has remained a mystery. As noted in the preceding, we now know that allogeneic stimulation and exposure to a rich milieu of cytokines and growth factors results in the activation of signal transduction pathways, the generation of increased levels of intracellular transcription factors, and the promotion of differentiation in some cell types, such as monocytes. Agents that stimulate monocytes to differentiate; such as retinoic acid, phorbol esters, and certain cytokines and growth factors (IFN-gamma, TNF-alpha, IL-4, GMCSF) lift the block to IE gene expression and lead to reactivation of latent HCMV.[26,60] Elucidation of the molecular details of these processes will require further attention.

TRANSMISSION

The systemic nature of HCMV infection with multiorgan involvement suggests that the virus is efficiently spread throughout the body. One model implicates peripheral blood monocytes as vectors for HCMV spread. It had been known for some time that HCMV could be transmitted by blood transfusion and by allogeneic transplantation of organs.[28,70] It was also recognized that the likelihood of infection was decreased when blood was depleted of white cells prior to transfusion, implicating leukocytes as a vector for the spread of HCMV. The monocyte carries HCMV in the latent state. In response to chemokines and other mediators of inflammation, monocytes adhere to activated vascular endothelial cells expressing increased levels of adhesion molecules and migrate into tissues where they differentiate into macrophages. This leads to reactivation of HCMV from the latent state and facilitates local cytopathology and intercellular transmission. It has been shown that monocyte–endothelial cell interactions allow for bidirectional transmission of HCMV.[71] Since both monocytes and endothelial cells have been shown to be capable of harboring HCMV latently, this model would predict the existence of multiple sites of HCMV persistence.[7,12]

Another suspect implicated in the hematogenous spread of HCMV is the circulating endothelial cell. As a result of HCMV infection, these endothelial cells detach from the basement membrane and circulate until their inordinate size causes them to be trapped in small vessels, where they can transmit HCMV to microvascular endothelial cells and surrounding tissues.[12,37] It is notable that the endothelial cells lining small vessels and capillaries are the ones predominantly infected by HCMV.[72]

HCMV also spreads to adjacent cells via direct cell-to-cell contact. Productive replication in macrophages is accompanied by compartmentalization of HCMV into vacuoles that are frequently seen at cellular contact points. As such, the macrophage may play a role in cell to cell transmission of HCMV.[73] Pereira and colleagues have shown that the US9 gene of HCMV is required for cell-to-cell spread in polarized retinal epithelium.[74]

Epithelial cells are the most likely participant in interindividual transmission of HCMV. Secretions containing either free virions or cell-associated virus are capable of spreading HCMV.[72]

HCMV AND ATHEROSCLEROSIS

The conventional wisdom regarding HCMV reactivation and disease has been that it is limited to those individuals who are systemically immunosuppressed, such as is the case with AIDS patients and recipients of solid organ or bone marrow transplants. However, recent new data implicate HCMV as the cause of disease in selected immunocompetent individuals. There is mounting evidence that HCMV may play an etiologic role in the development of atherosclerosis and restenosis following angioplasty in patients with coronary artery disease. HCMV DNA has been found in the wall of atherosclerotic vessels and accelerated atherosclerosis has been correlated with HCMV seropositivity in heart transplant recipients.[75] Epstein and colleagues were able to show that HCMV was present in the smooth muscle cells of a high percentage of restenotic coronary arteries following angioplasty. They further demonstrated that levels of the tumor suppressor protein p53 were elevated in the lesions that were HCMV+, and that the *ie* 2 gene product IE86 was bound to p53. p53 is a transcription factor that functions as a tumor suppressor by inducing cell cycle arrest in response to DNA damage. The block in cell cycle progression and the activation of DNA repair mechanisms allow the cell to fix the damage before proceeding on to replication and cell division. Alternatively, the cell death program is activated. The induction of these processes by p53 provides protection from abnormal cellular proliferation. p53 mutants have been identified in many human cancers.[76] The authors proposed that the mechanical trauma of angioplasty led to the reactivation of latent HCMV within the vessel wall. The subsequent proliferation of smooth muscle cells occurred as a result of the antagonistic effects of IE86 on p53 function, resulting in coronary restenosis.[77] Furthermore, the p53 that was isolated in these cells was wild-type, not mutant. The implication was that IE86 somehow interfered with wild-type p53 function (Fig. 22-4).

This report sparked a flurry of papers, most in support of these findings. It was subsequently suggested that infection of endothelial cells with HCMV abolished the apoptotic response to serum starvation by sequestering p53 in the cytoplasm.[78] Several clinical studies of patients with atherosclerotic disease supported the hypothesis of a causal role for HCMV.[79,80] One group argued that IE 86 functioned as a transcriptional repressor that was recruited to the target genes of p53 by virtue of its physical interaction with p53.[81] Because IE86 may interfere with the p53 mediated effect on cell cycle control, Bonin and McDougal assessed the G1 checkpoint function of p53 in the presence of IE86. They confirmed IE86 binding to p53. However, they also demonstrated that the ability of p53 to elicit growth arrest in G1 in response to DNA damage was intact.[82] Other investigators noted that the increase in p53 was owing to stabilization of the protein. p53 appeared to be sequestered into discrete foci within the nucleus, possibly representing replication centers.[83]

Additional studies hypothesized that latently infected circulating monocytes are recruited to sites of vascular injury. HCMV infection has been shown to increase levels of IL-2, IFN-gamma, IL-6, TNF-alpha, and IL-1 in vascular cells. As a result of these increases in cytokine production, adhesion molecules, such as ICAM-1, VCAM-1, and ELAM-1, are upregulated and mediate the association of leukocytes with infected endothelial cells.[12] Inflammatory conditions of vascular tissue result in the further induction of cytokine and growth factors as well as stimulation of HCMV reactivation. Both processes are mediated by an increase in NF-kB.[84] NF-kB is a transcription factor that mediates cellular activation. Interestingly, there are multiple NF-kB binding sites in the MIEP of HCMV. By upregulating the expression of NF-kB, HCMV creates a situation that is conducive to productive viral infection, while providing for the activation of the MIEP. NF-kB provides a link between cellular activation and the induction of viral gene expression under the control of the MIEP.

HCMV is reactivated following interaction with endothelial cells and with oxidized low density lipoprotein (oxLDL).[62] In an

HL-60 cell line expressing the HCMV MIEP and a reporter gene, it has been shown that the combination of endothelial cells and oxLDL led to a sevenfold increase in MIEP activity. Moreover, it was shown that the binding of oxLDL to vascular smooth muscle cells, endothelial cells, fibroblasts, and macrophages led to an increase in NF-kB activity.[62] The same group showed that reactive oxygen intermediates generated in vascular smooth muscle cells in response to HCMV infection enhance MIEP activity and stimulate viral gene expression.[85] HCMV infected monocytes are also capable of transmitting the virus to endothelial cells and vascular smooth muscle cells in culture.[62]

Although the data are suggestive, a causal role for HCMV in coronary restenosis has not been proven. This special case of putative HCMV pathogenesis is important because the host is, as far as we know, immunologically normal. The implications for the participation of HCMV and other herpesviruses in the pathogenesis of vascular disease are enormous. Given the prevalence of coronary disease in Western society, the clinical ramifications are obvious.

The study of HCMV pathogenesis has been hampered by the strict species specificity of the virus and its narrow host cell range for productive infection. The lack of an animal model has also presented researchers with significant challenges in deciphering the pathogenetic mechanisms by which HCMV exerts its effects on the human host.[25] Most of what has been learned in vitro has resulted from the study of productive infection in cultured human fibroblasts. Data from the study of HCMV in a variety of cell systems are accumulating and are gradually providing a clearer view of HCMV infection in humans. The picture that is emerging reveals a virus that interacts with its host on many levels and in enormously complex and clever ways. Given that there is nothing known about the majority of the proteins that the genome of HCMV is predicted to encode, we are in the very early stages of our understanding of this remarkable virus.

EPIDEMIOLOGY

In the developed or industrialized nations, approximately one-half of the adult population is seronegative for HCMV antibody. This is in marked contrast to the prevalence in the underdeveloped countries of the world where more than 90 percent of the population is seropositive by the age of 2 years. The probable explanations for this are that in the underdeveloped countries the living conditions are more crowded, there is more close and repeated contact with infected urine, and more frequent breast feeding of

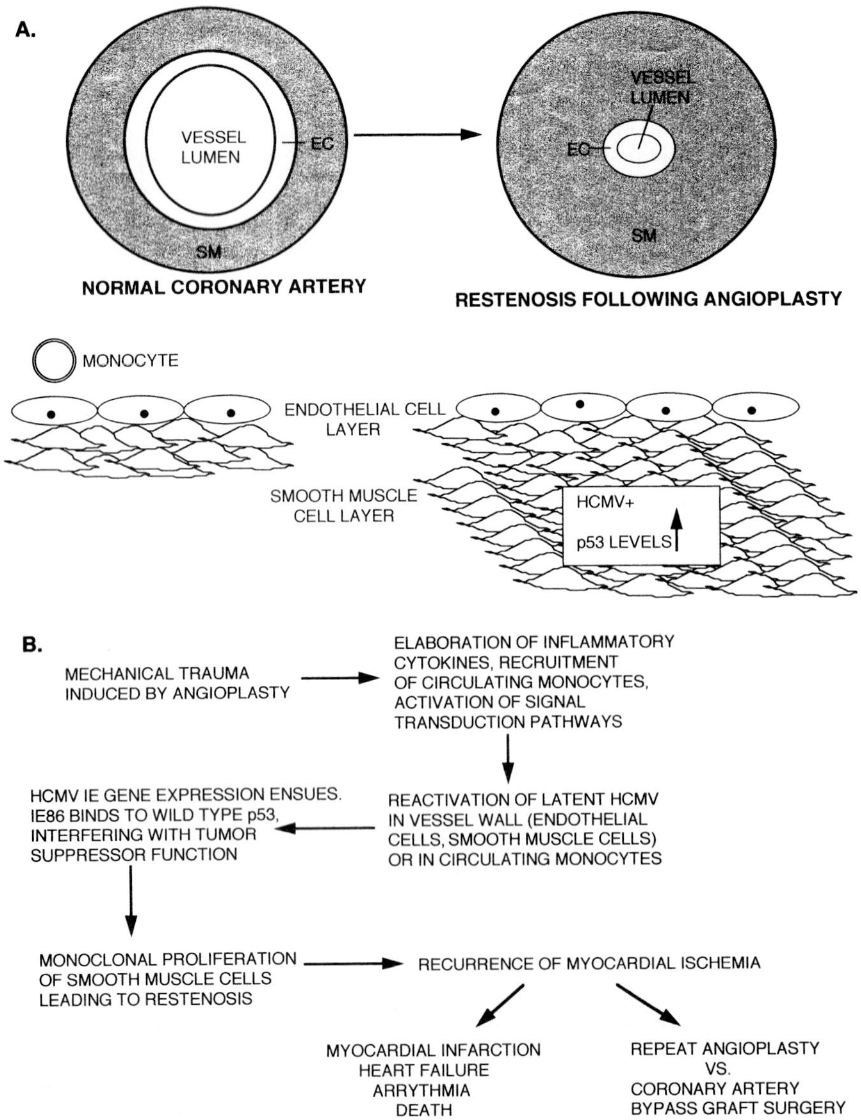

Fig. 22-4. Hypothetical model of the role of HCMV in the development of coronary restenosis following angioplasty. Panel A shows the effect of a monoclonal proliferation of smooth muscle cells within the vessel wall on the cross-sectional diameter of the lumen.

infants. In the developed countries, there is a large pool of uninfected adults who then acquire this virus at a slow rate, that is, approximately 1 to 2 percent seroconversions per year. It appears that these seroconversions result from close contact with virus-positive individuals. Such contact may be sexual with exchange of body fluids, including saliva, but other types of close contact may bring about transmission. For example, adults may be infected during maternal or paternal contact with a virus-positive child, or by blood transfusion or organ transplantation. In this chapter we will concentrate on evidence supporting the role of sexual transmission as an effective means of spreading the virus. In so doing we will consider the evidence in two different settings, heterosexual and homosexual.

HCMV AS A HETEROSEXUALLY TRANSMITTED INFECTION

In the United States only 10 to 15 percent of adolescents have antibodies to HCMV. However, during early adulthood the rate of seropositivity rapidly increases so that by age 35 approximately 50 percent show serologic evidence of past infection.[86] The evidence that many of these infections are sexually transmitted may be summarized as follows:

1. The virus does not spread readily among adults by ordinary, nonsexual, person-to-person contact, even during prolonged exposure to individuals known to be excreting the virus.[87–89] For example, among military recruits living in close contact with a recently infected index case, no seroconversions occurred. Also, among health care workers in close contact with actively infected patients, few, if any, seroconversions can be attributed to their professional activities.[89–91]
2. The prevalence of HCMV antibody more than doubles during the years of beginning sexual activity (age of 15 to 35 years).[86,92]
3. HCMV has been isolated from the cervix of 13 to 23 percent of women attending clinics for suspected venereal disease.[93,94] Knox et al. found that the prevalence of HCMV shedding in the genital tract of inner-city women with high rates of infection in adolescence decreased steadily with age, from a peak of 15 percent at 11 to 14 years of age to an undetectable level at age 31.[95] Most likely these results reflect the age at acquisition, that is, women acquiring the virus at age 30 would probably excrete the virus for the same duration as a newly infected adolescent.
4. Among seronegative women attending an STD clinic the rate of seroconversion is 10 to 12 percent per year versus 1 to 2 percent per year in the general population. Seroconverters had more sex partners and more new sex partners than nonseroconverters and were more likely to have gonorrhea, chlamydia, or pelvic inflammation.[96] At seroconversion *Chlamydia trachomatis* was isolated from the cervix in 14 versus 3 percent of nonseroconverters. Signs of upper genital tract infection were present in 8 percent of seroconverters versus 2 percent of nonseroconverters. All culture-positive seroconverters demonstrated cervical HCMV shedding and one-third were shedding from urine also.
5. HCMV has been isolated from semen; the prevalence of HCMV in semen among random donors for artificial insemination was 0.4 percent.[97,98]
6. Active HCMV infection (virus recovered from cervix and a positive HCMV IgM antibody titer) was described in the female sexual partner of a man whose semen had been virus positive during the preceding 5 months. In addition, Chretien et al. reported HCMV mononucleosis in two men after sexual contact with a woman whose cervix and urine were HCMV-positive.[99] Evidence of recent HCMV infection was also found in another female sexual contact of one of the two male patients, whereas roommates of these patients who were not their sexual partners had negative HCMV complement fixation (CF) antibody titers.
7. Cytomegalovirus proctitis has been reported in a woman who had "vigorous receptive anal intercourse for 4 consecutive days."[100] One week later she developed symptoms of proctitis and colonic biopsy revealed cellular inclusions characteristic of HCMV, whereas cultures were negative for herpes simplex and *Neisseria gonorrhea*. Serologic results were consistent with acute HCMV infection. She had both vaginal and anal intercourse with an additional three to four different men during the preceding 6 months, so the exact source of infection was not clear.

EVIDENCE OF REINFECTION WITH HCMV AMONG HETEROSEXUALS

Huang et al. were the first to show that reinfection may occur with different strains of HCMV.[101] Two different strains of HCMV were recovered from infants born of the same mother. Subsequently Chandler et al. studied cultures from the cervix, urine, and throat of eight women attending a sexually transmitted disease (STD) clinic.[102] Four of the eight women were infected with more than one strain of HCMV, two concurrently from different sites and two serially.

HCMV AS AN STD AMONG HOMOSEXUAL MEN

The initial documentation of high rates of HCMV infection in homosexual men resulted from prevalence studies performed at the San Francisco City Clinic in 1979.[103] Urinary excretion of HCMV was noted in 14 of 90 (7.4 percent) homosexual men but in none of 101 heterosexual men attending the same STD clinic ($p < 0.005$). Similarly, antibody to HCMV was detected in 130 of 139 (93.5 percent) homosexual men but in only 38 of 70 (54.3 percent) heterosexual men ($p < 0.005$).

In a subsequent prospective study of 237 homosexual men participating in the Western Study Group Hepatitis Vaccine Trial at the San Francisco City Clinic, a high prevalence of HCMV IgG serum antibody (206 of 237, 86.9 percent) was noted.[104] Of the 32 men lacking HCMV antibody on initial testing, 22 experienced seroconversion within 9 months of follow-up, for an attack rate of 71 percent during this time period. During a mean follow-up period of 14.3 months range, 2 to 20) 66 of the 206 initially seropositive men (32 percent) excreted HCMV from the urine on one or more occasions. Among 52 subjects from whom a sample of both semen and urine were obtained at single visit, the prevalence of HCMV excretion in semen (346 percent) was over four times greater than the prevalence of cytomegaloviruria (7.7 percent, $p = 0.001$, McNemar's test). Semen therefore appears to be nearly five times as likely to yield virus as urine when cell culture is used to detect the presence of HCMV. Clearly, the widespread occurrence of HCMV viruria and "virusemenia" in this population makes exposure to the virus all but inevitable and accounts for the extraordinarily high attack rate of HCMV infections among seronegative homosexual men. Among the men who were seropositive on initial testing, those who excreted HCMV during the study period were significantly younger (mean age, 26.6 years) than those who did not (mean age 32.7 years; $p < 0.01$). A Seattle study has reported that on a single visit, 36 percent of homosexual men were culture positive for HCMV, with virus most commonly recovered from semen. The estimated mean duration of semen positivity was 22 months versus 9 months for urine.[105]

In the San Francisco studies, questionnaires concerning demographic data, clinical histories, and sexual practices were completed by 78 homosexual men (54 of whom were initially seropositive and 24 of whom were initially seronegative, including 17 of the 22 seroconverters and seven of the nine who remained persistently seronegative). Information was obtained regarding the frequency of participation in the following sex practices: kissing, oral–anal contact (oral role), oral–anal (anal role), fellatio (oral role), fellatio (genital role), anal intercourse (active role), and anal intercourse (passive role).[104] Only passive anal intercourse correlated with the initial presence of anti-HCMV antibody or with seroconversion to this virus during the course of the study. Of 59 men who engaged in passive anal intercourse, HCMV antibody was present in 96.6 percent. In contrast, of the 19 men who did not engage in this practice, antibody was present in only 73.7 percent ($p < 0.01$). The latter figure does not differ significantly from the prevalence of HCMV antibody among heterosexual men attending a venereal disease clinic. These data suggest that exposure of the anorectal mucosa to HCMV-infected semen constitutes the major route of acquisition of HCMV infection by homosexual men.

REINFECTION WITH HCMV IN HOMOSEXUAL MEN

Data on the prevalence of HCMV IgM antibody suggest that homosexual men experience repeated episodes of HCMV infection. HCMV IgM antibody was detected on one or more occasions in the sera of more than 90 percent of the homosexual men and tended to appear, disappear, and reappear over time.[104] In contrast, IgM antibody to HCMV was detected in only 3.8 percent of 103 serum specimens randomly collected from volunteer male blood donors. HCMV IgM antibody was detected in a significantly ($p < 0.05$) higher proportion of serum samples from the 206 initially seropositive men (67 percent of 1136 samples) than in the postconversion samples obtained from the 22 seroconverters (53 percent of 86 samples). The higher prevalence of HCMV IgM antibody in long standing seropositive men than in recent seroconverters suggests that the former group is continually activating latent virus (see the following) or being reinfected with exogenous strains of the virus.

To determine whether more than one HCMV infection actually occurs in homosexual men, we analyzed multiple virus isolates from autopsy tissues of each of four AIDS patients by use of a restriction endonuclease polymorphism assay allowing comparison of the genetic relatedness of clinical isolates of HCMV.[106] This method had the distinct advantage of not requiring purification of virus or viral DNA and requires only relatively small numbers of infected cells from which total DNA is extracted. Each of the four patients we studied had at least two different strains of HCMV as determined by BamHI restriction site polymorphisms revealed by Southern blot analysis. Multiple HCMV infections in AIDS patients have been documented by Spector et al.[107] These results indicate that double infections with HCMV do occur in patients with AIDS but may represent terminal HCMV superinfections in patients already immunocompromised. Others have shown that reinfection with HCMV can occur in immunocompromised patients. For example, Chou showed that HCMV-seropositive renal transplant recipients can acquire HCMV infection from donor kidneys.[108]

To further investigate HCMV reinfection among homosexual men, we have investigated a cohort of homosexual men without AIDS for the excretion of more than one strain of HCMV. Isolates were obtained at intervals from urine or semen and compared for molecular relatedness by the Southern blot method described in the preceding. Among 17 men followed for an average of 7 months, eight excreted more than one strain. Two of these individuals were HIV antibody negative, indicating that more than one strain of HCMV can be acquired by homosexual men even in the absence of HIV infection. This should not be surprising given the high titer of virus in semen and the frequency of anal receptive intercourse among homosexual men. In effect, anal receptive intercourse may be equivalent to an intravenous injection of virus given the potential for multiple bleeding points in the traumatized anorectal mucosa.

In a recent report from Seattle, serial isolates from 11 homosexual men were available for restriction fragment analysis.[105] Five subjects were seronegative for HIV, and six were seropositive for HIV. Subsequently, two seronegative subjects developed antibody to HIV. Four of the 11 subjects shed more than one strain of HCMV. Three subjects, all HIV antibody positive, shed two different strains. Four different strains of HCMV were evident in the one HIV seronegative subject, two of which persisted over time. At the initial visit a single strain was isolated from semen; 15 months later, a different strain was isolated from his throat. A urine isolate, collected 17 months after his first visit, contained a mixture of the two previously isolated strains; throughout the genome, all bands present in both the previous isolates were seen. HCMV was isolated from both semen and urine 24 months after the initial visit. This study provides additional evidence that infection with multiple strains of HCMV is a relatively common occurrence among homosexual men with and without HIV infection and is not restricted to severely immunosuppressed individuals.

PREVENTION OF SEXUAL TRANSMISSION

VACCINE

An effective vaccine to prevent infection might be desirable for population groups at high risk for acquiring HCMV, for example, seronegative women contemplating pregnancy. A Towne strain live, attenuated vaccine has been under development and evaluation for many years.[109] In a clinical trial, seronegative women exposed to seropositive infants, were partially protected by this vaccine as compared to placebo recipients.[110] Furthermore, it has been shown to protect seronegative kidney transplant recipients from serious HCMV disease owing to receipt of a kidney from a seropositive donor.[111] Peptide-based vaccines or recombinant HCMV protein in a canary-pox vector are also being considered.[111–114] However, vaccine-induced immunity might be incomplete since, as discussed in the preceding, infection with "wild" HCMV may not prevent infection with additional strains of HCMV. It is possible that the multiple reinfections with wild virus strains observed in homosexual men may result from extraordinarily intense exposure of anorectal mucosa to high titer virus in semen, and that vaccines might be considerably more efficacious among heterosexuals experiencing penile–vaginal sexual contact with a limited number of partners.

CONDOMS

We performed a study to evaluate the potential of condoms to prevent HCMV transmission by semen.[115] Five different types of latex condoms were used. The strain of HCMV used was AD-169 at a median titer of 10, 4.5 ICID50 as determined by the Reed-Meunch titration. A 2-mL aliquot of the virus suspension was placed in a rinsed condom, which was then stretched over the shaft of a disposable plastic 35-cc syringe container. The condom was then sealed at its open end with tape. Two milliliters of Eagle's minimal essential medium (MEM) containing 10 percent fetal calf serum was then placed in a second rinsed condom. This second condom was placed over the HCMV containing condom, unrolled three-quarters of the way up the syringe shaft, and sealed with tape, to serve as a potential receptacle for any HCMV transmitted across the barrier provided by the first (inner) condom.

In the first part of the experiment three such test devices were assembled and incubated at 37°C for 15, 30, and 60 min, respectively. After incubation the solutions in the inner and outer condoms were cultured separately. Twelve repetitions of this procedure were completed using different types of condoms. HCMV was recovered in all cultures taken from inner condoms and from none of the outer condoms, indicating that no transmission occurred across the condom membranes.

The second set of experiments served as an attempt to more closely mirror in vivo condom use by simulating the trauma associated with sexual intercourse. Although imposing an external force on the condoms, the test device was thrust up and down 100 times in 5 minutes. The solutions from the inner and outer condoms were then cultured as in the preceding. Five repetitions of this procedure were completed, again using different types of condoms.

HCMV was recovered in all cultures taken from the inner condoms, except for one specimen, which was toxic in tissue culture. No virus was recovered from any of the outer condoms.

These results suggest that condoms might effectively block the sexual transmission of HCMV. Even after mimicking the trauma of sexual intercourse, no virus leaked from the inner condom.

CLINICAL SYNDROMES

CONGENITAL AND NEONATAL INFECTION

Approximately 10 percent of newborns congenitally infected with HCMV show clinical evidence of disease, such as microcephaly, intracerebral calcification, hepatosplenomegaly, and rash. From 6000 to 7000 infants may be born each year with unilateral or bilateral hearing loss and mental retardation resulting from congenital HCMV infection. Mothers of almost all infants with these stigmata had a primary infection during pregnancy.

Full-term and otherwise healthy infants who acquire HCMV during or shortly after birth (including perhaps transmission from breast milk) usually show no ill effects. However, premature infants may develop clinical findings, including hepatosplenomegaly, respiratory deterioration, rash, and fever. A peculiar gray pallor may also occur.

INFECTION IN ADULTS

Although most HCMV infections acquired in young adulthood are asymptomatic, patients may develop clinical illness resembling infectious mononucleosis caused by Epstein-Barr virus (EBV), but with minimal pharyngitis and lymphadenopathy. These patients develop atypical lymphocytosis similar to those with EBV infection, but have a negative heterophile antibody test.

POSTTRANSFUSION INFECTION

Transmission of HCMV by blood transfusion most often results in an asymptomatic infection; if symptoms are present, they typically resemble infectious mononucleosis as in the preceding. Fever, splenomegaly, atypical lymphocytosis (and mild hepatitis) usually begin 3 to 5 weeks after transfusion.

INFECTION IN IMMUNOCOMPROMISED PATIENTS

Several different HCMV syndromes occur in immunocompromised patients including retinitis, colitis, esophagitis, and central nervous system disease, for example, polyradiculopathy, encephalitis. These syndromes are especially common in AIDS patients. Pulmonary disease occurs in 20 to 40 percent of recipients of bone marrow transplants and appears as an interstitial pneumonia.

DIAGNOSIS

CYTOLOGY/HISTOLOGY

Microscopically, the hallmark of HCMV infection is the large (cytomegalic) 25- to 35-μ cell containing a large central, basophilic intranuclear inclusion. The inclusion is referred to as an "owl's eye" because it is separated from the nuclear membrane by a halo. These inclusions are clearly seen with Papanicolaou's or hematoxylin eosin stain. Clusters of small intracytoplasmic inclusions may also be seen in HCMV-infected cells and are best visualized with Wright's and Giemsa stains. Cytological and histologic observations are not sensitive measures of HCMV infection, but they are rather specific and more diagnostic of HCMV disease than isolation of virus in culture. However, histologic examination of a small piece of lung biopsy tissue obtained transbronchoscopically may be insensitive because of sampling error.

HCMV ANTIGEN AND DNA DETECTION

In an effort to provide a rapid diagnosis, monoclonal antibodies have been used to directly detect HCMV antigens in tissues, and was present in blood and bronchoalveolar lavage (BAL) specimens. Antigen detection in tissue is more sensitive than histologic examination for detecting HCMV infection, but whether or not cases in which no inclusions are revealed by histologic examination represent true instances of HCMV disease is less clear. Detection of antigenemia is more sensitive than detecting viremia by culture and offers the possibility of a quantitative assay. It has been increasingly used in bone marrow transplant recipients and AIDS patients.

Recent efforts have been directed at assaying HCMV DNA by hybrid capture or PCR. The former is now commercially available as a quantitative test. These assays are more sensitive than culture and at least comparable to antigenemia assays. Quantitative assays may be particularly useful for documenting HCMV disease and for monitoring therapy but are not commercially available as yet.

CULTURE

Culture has been regarded historically as the definitive method or gold standard for detecting HCMV infection. However HCMV grows only in diploid fibroblast cell cultures and may require at least 4 to 6 weeks because the characteristic CPE develops very slowly in specimens with very low titers of the virus. More rapid culture results may be achieved by culture amplification of a specimen. In this procedure specimens are inoculated by centrifuging them in a shell vial seeded with diploid fibroblast cells. Specimens are examined after 1 to 2 days of incubation by indirect immunofluorescence for either immediate early (IE) antigen or a combination of IE and early antigen (EA).

Interpretation of culture results for HCMV may be difficult, particularly in immunosuppressed patients. For example, HCMV may be present in saliva or urine in up to 60 to 90 percent of transplant recipients or patients with AIDS. Thus, recovery of virus from these sites does not prove that HCMV is the cause of a patient's pneumonia or fever. The diagnosis of HCMV disease is made on the basis of a combination of factors: (1) HCMV-positive cultures of tissue; (2) the presence in tissue of (a) pathognomonic cells with intranuclear inclusion bodies and (b) HCMV antigen or nucleic acid; and (3) the absence of other pathogenic organisms. Patients with HCMV-positive cultures of lung tissue or fluids and in which no other pathogens are identified with diagnostic bronchoscopy may have invasive HCMV pneumonia, but the diagnosis is more secure if tissue involvement is documented by the presence of inclusions, antigens, or viral nucleic acid within cells.

Recent studies of antigen and DNA based assays suggest that culture is no longer the gold standard and that these assays are more sensitive, while retaining the specificity of virus isolation.

SEROLOGY

Seroconversion is usually an excellent marker for primary HCMV infection, but IgG titer rises, even fourfold or greater, are not diagnostic of newly acquired infection. HCMV-specific IgM antibody develops during primary infection, but it may reappear during reactivation of latent HCMV. In homosexual men, IgM antibody is so prevalent that it is not useful as a positive diagnostic test. The high prevalence of IgM antibody in the sera of homosexual men is presumably a result of reactivation of HCMV, although repetitive exposure to differing strains of the virus may account for its presence in some individuals.

TREATMENT

GANCICLOVIR

Structure and mechanism of action

Ganciclovir (DHPG, Cytovene) is a nucleoside analog that differs from acyclovir (Zovirax) by a single carboxyl side chain. This structural change confers on the drug approximately 50 times more activity than acyclovir against HCMV. Acyclovir has low activity against HCMV, since it is not well phosphorylated in HCMV infected cells. This is owing to the absence of the gene for thymidine kinase (TK) in HCMV. Gancyclovir, however, is active against HCMV because it is phosphorylated by another viral-encoded enzyme (UL97) present in HCMV-infected cells. Then, cellular enzymes convert it to the active compound, ganciclovir triphosphate. Gancyclovir triphosphate acts to inhibit HCMV DNA polymerase.

Pharmacology and dosage

Both intravenous and oral ganciclovir are approved for treatment of HCMV retinitis. When administered by intravenous infusion over 1 hour in the usual dosage of 5 mg/kg, peak blood levels are approximately 6 to 15 mg/mL, and the serum half-life is 2.9 hours. The drug is given two times daily during initial induction (2 to 3 weeks) and maintenance therapy consists of 5 mg/kg once daily. Since the drug undergoes renal excretion, the dosage must be reduced with impaired renal function. Current oral therapy is 3 grams daily but higher doses may prove to be more effective.

Clinical use

Administration of ganciclovir is indicated for the treatment of acute HCMV infection, but other herpes viruses (specifically, herpes simplex virus (HSV)-1, HSV-2, and varicella zoster virus (VZV)) are also susceptible to the drug since enzymes induced by these viruses do phosphorylate the drug. Patients with severe HCMV infection frequently have illnesses caused by other herpes viruses, and a bonus of ganciclovir therapy may be an associated improvement of HSV and VZV infections. Gancyclovir is probably also active against Epstein-Barr virus.

Initial response in retinitis (improvement or stabilization in vision or ophthalmoscopic appearance) occurs in approximately 75 percent of treated patients. By comparison, the disease is relentlessly progressive in 90 percent of patients if left untreated. Visual-field defects present at the onset of therapy do not reverse, but a decrease in visual acuity caused by edema of the macula may improve with treatment. Maintenance therapy throughout the remaining life of the patient appears critical because the virus is only suppressed by ganciclovir and is not eliminated. Even with continued maintenance therapy, progression of HCMV retinitis usually occurs. This may result from poor drug compliance, low blood levels, impaired delivery of drug to retina, or viral resistance to the drug. Retinal detachment may occur as the necrotic retina scars and thins. Intravitreal injection has been used in certain special situations, such as in patients in whom neutropenia limited the systemic use of the drug. Sustained intravitreal release has been accomplished using a surgically implantable device, and this approach may gain acceptance but appears to require accompanying systemic treatment. Oral gancyclovir is not absorbed well but in sufficient dose may be nearly as effective as the intravenous form.

Colitis owing to HCMV may improve with ganciclovir therapy, although a recent study revealed that 14 days of ganciclovir therapy was only marginally more effective than administration of placebo. This study was confounded in part by the effects of antidiarrheal therapies that were used in both arms of the study.

Resistance

Erice et al. reported three patients whose clinical course suggested the emergence of resistance and whose HCMV isolates exhibited increases in the concentration of ganciclovir required to inhibit the virus in tissue culture over baseline determinations. A subsequent study in AIDS patients revealed that after three months of continuous ganciclovir therapy, approximately 10 percent of patients are excreting resistant strains of HCMV.[116] In virtually all these resistant isolates, there is a mutation in the pre encoding phosphorylating enzyme (ul97). These strains usually remain sensitive to foscarnet, which may be used as alternate therapy.

Toxicity

Approximately one-third of patients discontinue ganciclovir therapy owing to toxicity. The following organs are adversely affected.

Hematopoiesis. Sixteen percent of patients receiving the drug develop neutrophil counts of <500/mm. Neutropenia may occur early but often develops during later therapy. The leukopenia is usually reversible, but at least five patients are known to have had irreversible suppression. Many patients have low white blood counts before beginning therapy, so the contribution of ganciclovir to leukopenia may not be entirely clear. Moreover, the combination of ganciclovir with zidovudine may be especially toxic.

Ganciclovir dosage should be reduced when absolute neutrophil counts fall below 750/mm3 or discontinued when severe leukopenia occurs (absolute neutrophil counts <500/mm3). The drug may be resumed when neutrophil counts have risen to safe levels, preferably >750/mm3. Discontinuation of therapy is necessary in patients whose neutrophils do not increase during dosage reduction. Cytokines, such as granulocyte, colony-stimulating factor (G-CSF), are effective in reversing ganciclovir-induced neutropenia. Thrombocytopenia (platelet count <20,00/mm3) occurs in 9 percent of patients receiving the drug.

Other Organ Systems. Adverse effects on the central nervous system (CNS) occur in 17 percent of patients. Confusion is the most common symptom, occurring in 3 percent of patients, and 2 percent of patients experience convulsions, dizziness, headaches, or abnormal thinking. Overall, 15 percent of patients have gastrointestinal disturbances. Nausea is the most frequent complaint (5 percent), followed by vomiting (4 percent), abnormal liver function tests (3 percent), and diarrhea (2 percent).

FOSCARNET

Structure and mechanism of action

Foscarnet, also known as phosphonoformate, phosphonoformic acid, or PFA, is a pyrophosphate that inhibits the DNA polymerase of HCMV. Specifically, the drug blocks the pyrophosphate-binding site of the viral DNA polymerase, preventing cleavage of pyrophosphate from deoxyadenosine triphosphate. This action is relatively selective in that HCMV DNA polymerase is inhibited at concentrations less 1 percent of that required to inhibit cellular DNA polymerase. Unlike such nucleosides as acyclovir and ganciclovir, foscarnet does not require phosphorylation intracellularly to be an active inhibitor of viral DNA polymerases. This biochemical fact becomes especially important in regard to viral resistance, since the principal mode of viral resistance to nucleoside analogues is a mutation that eliminates phosphorylation of the drug in virus-infected cells. Since foscarnet does not require phosphorylation, it can be used to treat patients with ganciclovir-resistant HCMV. Resistance to foscarnet can develop due to mutations in DNA polymerase.

Pharmacology

Recommended initial therapy with foscarnet consists of 60 mg/kg intravenously every 8 hours or 90 mg/kg every 12 hours. A recent study of maintenance dosage indicated that 120 mg/kg/day was superior to 90 mg/kg/day.[117]

Cerebrospinal fluid (CSF) concentrations of foscarnet are approximately 40 percent of serum levels. Excretion is entirely renal without a hepatic component. Oral bioavailability is very low rendering this route impractical.

Clinical use

Palestine et al. reported a randomized control trial of foscarnet in the treatment of HCMV retinitis in AIDS patients.[118] Patients were assigned to receive either no therapy or immediate treatment with intravenous foscarnet. The mean time to progression of retinitis was 3 weeks in the control group versus 13 weeks in the treatment group, thereby proving that foscarnet is effective therapy. Also, an excellent antiviral effect was achieved in the treatment group (i.e., nine of 13 of the treated group had positive blood cultures for HCMV at entry, and all nine had cleared the blood by the end of the 3-week induction period).

In a more recent study foscarnet was compared with ganciclovir in the treatment of sight-threatening HCMV retinitis.[119] The two drugs were equivalently effective in treating retinitis. The mean time to progression of retinitis was approximately 56 days in both groups. The notable difference in the study was that the patients treated with foscarnet had a 4-month longer survival time than those receiving ganciclovir. The explanation for the difference in survival time is not clear but seems partly attributable to differences in the ability to take concurrent antiretroviral medications. Presumably, it was more difficult to continue a patient on concurrent zidovudine therapy while taking ganciclovir because of additive myelosuppression. Now that cytokines (e.g., granulocyte macrophage colony stimulating factor [GM-CSF] and G-CSF) and other antiretrovirals (lamivudines ddI, ddC, d4r) without extreme myelosuppressive toxicity are available, it should be possible for patients to continue receiving antiretroviral medications while taking ganciclovir.

There has not been a placebo-controlled study of foscarnet in the treatment of HCMV gastrointestinal disease but several comparisons with ganciclovir suggest that they are equivalent.[120]

Toxicity

Adverse effects include renal impairment, anemia, hypocalcemia (especially ionized calcium), hypomagnesemia, and hypophosphatemia. It is important to measure renal function frequently and adjust dosage accordingly to minimize toxicity. It also appears that daily infusion of 1 liter of saline may reduce nephrotoxicity during maintenance therapy.

CIDOFOVIR

In June 1996, Cidofovir, or HPMPC, was approved by the FDA for the treatment of HCMV retinitis. This drug is a departure from previous nucleoside analogues since it appears to the cell as a nucleotide. It has a phosphonate moiety attached to a cytosine analogue and does not require phosphorylation by virus induced enzyme. It is therefore active against the majority of ganciclovir-resistant viruses that have resistance mutations in the UL97 phosphorylating gene. The drug also has an extremely long half-life permitting it to be administered as infrequently as every 2 weeks during maintenance treatment.[121,122] Cidofovir is nephrotoxic, especially to the proximal renal tubule but this can apparently be diminished by prehydration and comcomitant probenecid therapy. Renal function and toxicity must be monitored carefully and and proteinuria or a rising creatinine are reasons for dosage reduction, interruption, or discontinuation. Despite its potential for toxicity, the drug is effective and convenient and it will find a niche in anti-HCMV therapy.

IMMUNE GLOBULIN

HCMV immune globulin prepared from a pool of high titered donors appears to provide added benefit when combined with ganciclovir for the treatment of HCMV pneumonia in bone marrow transplant recipients. Controlled trials of the therapy have not been reported. There have been conflicting reports regarding any additive benefits in the treatment of HCMV retinitis in AIDS patients but a randomized, blinded trial of immunoclonal antibody is planned.

References

1 Mocarski ES: Cytomegaloviruses and their replication, in *Fields virology*, 3rd ed. Fields B et al (eds). 1996, pp. 2447–2492, Lippincott-Raven, Philadelphia.
2 Miceli MV: Cytomegalovirus replication in cultured human retinal pigment epithelial cells. *Curr Eye Res* 8:835, 1989.
3 Heinemann MH: Characteristics of cytomegalovirus retinitis in patients with acquired immunodeficiency syndrome. *Am J Med* 92:12s, 1992.
4 Grundy JE et al: Is cytomegalovirus pneumonitis in transplant recipients an immunopathological condition? *Lancet ii*:996, 1987.
5 Shepp DH et al: Activity of 9-[2hydroxy-1-(hydroxymethyl) ethoxymethyl]guanine in the treatment of cytomegalovirus pneumonia. *Ann Intern Med* 103:368, 1985.
6 Zaia JA: The biology of human cytomegalovirus infection after bone marrow transplantation. *Int J Cell Cloning* 4(Suppl 1):S135, 1986.
7 Bruggeman CA et al: Pathogenicity: Animal models. *Scand J Inf Dis* 99(Suppl):S43, 1995.
8 Sedmak DD et al: The role of vascular endothelial cells in transplantation. *Arch Path Lab Med* 115:260, 1991.
9 Waldman WJ et al: Endothelial HLA class II induction mediated by allogeneic T cells activated by cytomegalovirus-infected cultured endothelial cells. *Transplant Proc* 25:1493, 1993.
10 Lautenschlager I et al: Induction of ICAM-1 on hepatocytes preceedes the lymphoid activation of acute liver allograft rejection and cytomegalovirus infection. *Transplant Proc* 25:1429, 1993.
11 Lautenschlager I et al: ICAM-1 on hepatocytes as a marker for immune activation of acute liver allograft rejection. *Transplantation* 56: 1495, 1993.
12 Sinzger C, Jahn G: Human cytomegalovirus cell tropism and pathogenesis. *Intervirology* 39:302, 1996.
13 Soderberg C et al: Cytomegalovirus-induced CD-13 specific autoimmunity: A possible cause of graft-versus-host disease. *Transplantation* 61:600, 1996.
14 Rosen HR et al: Cytomegalovirus viremia: Risk factor for allograft cirrhosis after liver transplantation for hepatitis C. *Transplantation* 64:721, 1997.
15 Toth FD et al: Interactions between human immunodeficiency virus type 1 and human cytomegalovirus in human term syncytiotrophoblast cells coinfected with both viruses. *J Virol* 69:2223, 1995.
16 Rucker J et al: Utilization of chemokine receptors, orphan receptors, and herpesvirus-encoded receptors by diverse human and simian immunodeficiency viruses. *J Virol* 71:8999, 1997.
17 Pleskoff O et al: Identification of a chemokine receptor encoded by human cytomegalovirus as a cofactor for HIV-1 entry. *Science* 276: 1874, 1997.
18 Sajovic S et al: Identification of a viral kinase that phosphorylates specific E2Fs and pocket proteins. *Mol Cell Biol* 17:6459, 1997.
19 Yurochko AD et al: Human cytomegalovirus upregulates NF-kB activity by transactivating the NF-kB p105/p50 and p65 promoters. *J Virol* 69:5391, 1995.
20 Hayhurst GP et al: CCAAT box-dependent activation of the TATA-less human DNA polymerase-alpha promoter by the human cytomegalovirus 72 kd major immediate-early protein. *J Virol* 69:182, 1995.
21 Poma EE et al: The human cytomegalovirus IE1-72 protein interacts with the cellular p107 protein and relieves p107 mediated transcriptional repression of an E2F-responsive promoter. *J Virol* 70:7867, 1996.
22 Mocarski ES et al: A deletion mutant in the human cytomegalovirus gene encoding IE1491aa is replication defective due to a failure in auto regulation. *Proc Natl Acad Sci USA* 93:11321, 1996.
23 Luu P, Flores O: Binding of SP-1 to the immediate-early protein-responsive element of the human cytomegalovirus DNA polymerase promoter. *J Virol* 71:6683, 1997.
24 Dittmer D, Mocarski ES: Human cytomegalovirus infection inhibits G1/S transition. *J Virol* 71:1629, 1997.
25 Plachter B et al: Cell types involved in replication and distribution of human cytomegalovirus. *Adv Virus Res* 46:195, 1996.
26 Sinclair J, Sissons P: Latent and persistent infections of monocytes and macrophages. *Intervirology* 39:293, 1996.
27 Tooze J et al: Progeny vaccinia and human cytomegalovirus particles utilize early endosomal cisternae for their envelopes. *Eur J Cell Biol* 60:163, 1993.
28 Ho M: Cytomegalovirus, in *Principles and practice of infectious diseases,* 4th ed. Mandell G et al (eds). 1995, Churchill Livingstone, New York.
29 Compton T: Towards a definition of the HCMV entry pathway. *Scand J Inf Dis Suppl* 99:20, 1995.
30 Baskar JF et al: The enhancer domain of the human cytomegalovirus major immediate-early promoter determines cell type-specific expression in transgenic mice. *J Virol* 70:3207, 1996.
31 Baskar JF et al: Developmental analysis of the cytomegalovirus enhancer in transgenic animals. *J Virol* 70:3215, 1996.
32 Cavanaugh VJ et al: Murine cytomegalovirus with a deletion of genes spanning *Hind*III-J and -I displays altered cell and tissue tropism. *J Virol* 70:1365, 1996.
33 Navarro D et al: Humoral immune response to functional regions of human cytomegalovirus glycoprotein B. *J Med Virol* 52:451, 1997.
34 Keay S, Baldwin B: Update on the 92.5 kDa putative HCMV fusion receptor. *Scand J Inf Dis Suppl* 99:32, 1995.
35 Boyle K, Compton T: Receptor-binding properties of a soluble form of human cytomegalovirus glycoprotein B. *J Virol* 72:1826, 1998.
36 Soderberg C et al: Definition of a subset of human peripheral blood mononuclear cells that are permissive to human cytomegalovirus infection. *J Virol* 67:3166, 1993.
37 Fish KN et al: Cytomegalovirus persistence in macrophages and endothelial cells. *Scand J Inf Dis Suppl* 99:34, 1995.
38 Baldwin B et al: Molecular cloning and expression of receptor peptides that block human cytomegalovirus/cell fusion. *Biochem Biophys Res Comm* 219:668, 1996.
39 Keay S, Baldwin B: Evidence for the role of cell protein phosphorylation in human cytomegalovirus/host cell fusion. *J Gen Virol* 77: 2597, 1996.
40 Yurochko AD et al: The human cytomegalovirus UL55 (gB) and UL 75 (gH) glycoprotein ligands initiate the rapid activation of SP-1 and NF-kB during infection. *J Virol* 71:5051, 1997.
41 Reusser P et al: Cytomegalovirus-specific T cell immunity in recipients of autologous peripheral blood stem cell or bone marrow transplants. *Blood* 89:3873, 1997.
42 Riddell SR: Pathogenesis of pneumonia in immunocompromised hosts. *Semin Respir Infect* 10:199, 1995.
43 Wiertz E et al: Sec61-mediated transfer of a membrane protein from the endoplasmic reticulum to the proteasome for destruction. *Nature* 384:432, 1996.
44 Riddell SR, Greenberg PD: Therapeutic reconstitution of human viral immunity by adoptive transfer of cytotoxic T cell clones. *Curr Top Microbiol Immunol* 189:9, 1994.
45 Riddell SR et al: Restoration of viral immunity in immunodeficient humans by the adoptive transfer of T cell clones. *Science* 257:238, 1992.
46 Walter EA et al: Reconstitution of cellular immunity against cytomegalovirus in recipients of allogeneic bone marrow by transfer of T cell clones from the donor. *N Engl J Med* 333:1038, 1995.
47 Wills MR et al: The human cytotoxic T Lymphocyte response to cytomegalovirus is dominated by structural protein pp65: frequency, specificity, and T cell receptor usage of pp65-specific CTL. *J Virol* 70:7569, 1996.
48 Reddehase MJ et al: The conditions of primary infection define the load of latent viral genome in organs and the risk of recurrent cytomegalovirus disease. *J Ex Med* 179:185, 1994.
49 Steffens H et al: Preemptive CD8 T cell immunotherapy of acute cytomegalovirus infection prevents lethal disease, limits the burden of latent viral genomes, and reduces the risk of viral recurrence. *J Virol* 72:1797, 1998.

50 Fish KN et al: A novel mechanism for persistence of human cytomegalovirus in macrophages. *J Virol* 70:1855, 1996.

51 Jones TR et al: Human cytomegalovirus US3 impairs transport and maturation of MHC class I heavy chains. *Proc Natl Acad Sci USA* 93:11327, 1996.

52 Wiertz E et al: The human Cytomegalovirus US11 gene product dislocates MHC class I heavy chains from the endoplasmic reticulum to the cytosol. *Cell* 84:769, 1996.

53 Kwangeog A et al: The ER-luminal domain of the HCMV glycoprotein US6 inhibits peptide translocation by TAP. *Immunity* 6:613, 1997.

54 Cosman D et al: A novel immunoglobulin superfamily receptor for cellular and viral MHC class I molecules. *Immunity* 7:273, 1997.

55 Reyburn HT et al: The class I MHC homologue of human cytomegalovirus inhibits attack by natural killer cells. *Nature* 386:514, 1997.

56 Soderberg-Naucler C et al: Reactivation of latent cytomegalovirus by allogeneic stimulation of blood cells from healthy donors. *Cell* 91: 119, 1997.

57 Kondo K et al: Human cytomegalovirus latent gene expression in granulocyte-macrophage progenitors in culture and in seropositive individuals. *Proc Natl Acad Sci USA* 93:11137, 1996.

58 Kondo K, Mocarski ES: Cytomegalovirus latency and latency-specific transcription in hematopoietic progenitors. *Scand J Inf Dis Suppl* 99: 63, 1995.

59 Kondo K et al: Human cytomegalovirus latent infection of granulocyte-macrophage progenitors. *Proc Natl Acad Sci USA* 91:11879, 1994.

60 Hahn G et al: Cytomegalovirus remains latent in a common precursor of dendritic and myeloid cells. *Proc Natl Acad Sci USA* 95:3937, 1998.

61 Sinclair JH, Sissons P: HCMV: Pathogenesis and models of latency. *Semin Virol* 5:249, 1994.

62 Guetta E et al: Monocytes harboring cytomegalovirus: Interactions with endothelial cells, smooth muscle cells, and oxidized low-density lipoprotein. *Circ Res* 81;8, 1997.

63 Zhuravskaya T et al: Spread of human cytomegalovirus after infection of human hematopoietic progenitor cells: Model of HCMV latency. *Blood* 90:2482, 1997.

64 Sing GK et al: Preferential suppression of myelopoiesis in normal human bine marrow cells after in vitro challenge with human cytomegalovirus. *Blood* 75:10090, 1965.

65 Simmons P et al: Mechanisms of cytomegalovirus-mediated myelosuppression: Perturbation of stromal cell function versus direct infection of myeloid precursors. *Proc Natl Acad Sci USA* 87:1386, 1990.

66 Winston DJ et al: Delay in platelet recovery after bone marrow transplantation: Impact of cytomegalovirus infection. *Am J Med* 106:128, 1984.

67 Verdonck LF et al: Cytomegalovirus infection causes delayed platelet recovery after bone marrow transplantation. *Blood* 78:844, 1991.

68 Koffron AJ et al: Cellular localization of latent murine cytomegalovirus. *J Virol* 72:95, 1998.

69 Koffron AJ et al: Direct evidence using in situ PCR that the endothelial cell and T lymphocyte harbor latent murine cytomegalovirus. *Scand J Inf Dis Suppl* 99:61, 1995.

70 Britt WJ, Alford CA: Cytomegalovirus, in *Fields virology,* 3rd ed. Fields B et al (eds). 1996, pp. 2493–2523, Lippincott-Raven, Philadelphia.

71 Waldman WJ et al: Bidirectional transmission of infectious cytomegalovirus between monocytes and vascular endothelial cells: An *in vitro* model. *J Inf Dis* 171:263, 1995.

72 Singzer C et al: Fibroblasts, epithelial cells, endothelial cells, and smooth muscle cells are major targets of human cytomegalovirus infection in lung and gastrointestinal tissues. *J Gen Virol* 76:741, 1995.

73 Fish KN et al: Growth kinetics of human cytomegalovirus are altered in monocyte-derived macrophages. *J Virol* 69:3737, 1995.

74 Maidji E et al: Accessory human cytomegalovirus glycoprotein US9 in the unique short component of the viral genome promotes cell to cell transmission of virus in polarized epithelial cells. *J Virol* 70:8402, 1996.

75 Epstein SE et al: The role of infection in restenosis and atherosclerosis: Focus on cytomegalovirus. *Lancet* 348:s13, 1996.

76 Levine A: p53, the cellular gatekeeper for growth and division. *Cell* 88:323, 1997.

77 Speir E et al: Potential role of human cytomegalovirus and p53 interaction in coronary restenosis. *Science* 265:391, 1994.

78 Kovacs A et al: Cytoplasmic sequestration of p53 in cytomegalovirus-infected human endothelial cells. *Am J Path* 149:1531, 1996.

79 Nieto FJ et al: Cohort study of cytomegalovirus infection as a risk factor for carotid intimal-medial thickening, a measure of subclinical atherosclerosis. *Circulation* 94:922, 1996.

80 Zhou YF et al: Association between prior cytomegalovirus infection and the risk of restenosis after coronary atherectomy. *N Engl J Med* 335:629, 1996.

81 Tsai H et al: Human cytomegalovirus immediate-early protein IE2 tethers a transcriptional repression domain to p53. *J Biol Chem* 271: 3534, 1996.

82 Bonin LR, McDougall JK: Human cytomegalovirus IE2 86-Kd protein binds p53 but does not abrogate G1 checkpoint function. *J Virol* 71:5861, 1997.

83 Fortunato EA et al: p53 and RPA are sequestered in viral replication centers in the nuclei of cells infected with human cytomegalovirus. *J Virol* 72:2033, 1998.

84 Vossen R et al: Cytomegalovirus infection and vessel wall pathology. *Intervirology* 39:213, 1996.

85 Speir E et al: Role of reactive oxygen intermediates in cytomegalovirus gene expression and in the response of human smooth muscle cells to viral infection. *Circ Res* 79:1143, 1996.

86 Wentworth BB, Alexander ER: Seroepidemiology of infections due to members of the herpesvirus group. *Am J Epidemiol* 94:496-507, 1971.

87 Wenzel RP et al: Cytomegalovirus infection: A seroepidemiologic study of recruit population. *Am J Epidemiol* 97:410–414, 1973.

88 Betts RF et al: Epidemiology of cytomegalovirus infection in end stage renal disease. *J Med Virol* 4:89–96, 1979.

89 Tolkoff-Rubin NE et al: Cytomegalovirus infection in dialysis patients and personnel. *Ann Intern Med* 89:625–628, 1978.

90 Dworsky ME et al: Occupational risk for primary cytomegalovirus infection among pediatric health-care workers. *N Engl J Med* 309: 950–953, 1983.

91 Gerberding JL et al: Risk of transmitting the human immunodeficiency virus, cytomegalovirus, and hepatitis B virus to health care workers exposed to patients with AIDS and AIDS-related conditions. *J Infect Dis* 156:1–8, 1987.

92 Stern H, Elek SD: The incidence of infection with cytomegalovirus in a normal population. A serological study in greater London. *J Hyg* (Camb) 63:79–87, 1985.

93 Jordan MC et al: Association of cervical cytomegalovirus with venereal disease. *N Engl J Med* 288:932–934, 1973.

94 Wentworth BB et al: Isolation of viruses, bacteria and other organisms from venereal disease clinic patients: Methodology and problems associated with multiple isolations. *Health Lab Sci* 10:75-81, 1973.

95 Knox GE et al: Comparative prevalence of subclinical and herpes simplex virus infections in the genital and urinary tracts of cytomegalovirus mononucleosis. *J Infect Dis* 170:419–422, 1979.

96 Coonrod D et al: Association between cytomegalovirus seroconversion and upper genital tract infection among women attending a sexually transmitted disease clinic: A prospective study. *J Infect Dis* 177: 1188–1193, 1998.

97 Lang DJ et al: Cytomegalovirus in semen: Persistence and demonstration in intracellular fluids. *N Engl J Med* 291:121–123, 1974.

98 Tjiam KH et al: Sexually communicable micro-organisms in human semen samples to be used for artificial insemination by donor. *Genitourin Med* 63:116–118, 1987.

99 Chretien JH et al: Venereal causes of cytomegalovirus mononucleosis. *JAMA* 238:1644–1645, 1977.

100 Rabinowitz M et al: Sexually transmitted cytomegalovirus proctitis in a woman. *Am J Gastroenterol* 83:885–887, 1988.

101 Huang E-S et al: Molecular epidemiology of cytomegalovirus infections in women and their infants. *N Engl J Med* 303:958–962, 1980.
102 Chandler SH et al: Isolation of multiple strains of cytomegalovirus from women attending a clinic for sexually transmitted diseases. *J Infect Dis* 155:655–660, 1987.
103 Drew WL et al: Prevalence of cytomegalovirus infections in homosexual men. *J Infect Dis* 143:188–192, 1981.
104 Mintz L et al: Cytomegalovirus infections in homosexual men: An epidemiological study. *Ann Intern Med* 99:326–329, 1983.
105 Collier AC et al: Identification of multiple strains of cytomegalovirus in homosexual men. *J Infect Dis* 159:123–126, 1989.
106 Drew WL et al: Multiple infections with CMV in AIDS patients: Documentation by Southern blot hybridization. *J Infect Dis* 150:952, 1984.
107 Spector SA et al: Detection of human cytomegalovirus in clinical specimens by DNA-DNA hybridization. *J Infect Dis* 150:121–126, 1984.
108 Chou S: Acquisition of donor strains of cytomegalovirus by renal transplant recipients. *N Engl J Med* 314:1418–1423, 1986.
109 Plotkin SA et al: Vaccines for varicella-zoster virus and cytomegalovirus: Recent progress. *Science* 265:1383–1385, 1994.
110 Adler SP et al: Immunity induced by primary human cytomegalovirus infection protects against secondary infection among women of childbearing age. *J Infect Dis* 171(1):26–32, 1995.
111 Plotkin SA et al: Multicenter trial of towne strain attenuated virus vaccine in seronegative renal transplant recipients. *Transplantation* 58(11):1176–1178, 1994.
112 Diamond DJ et al: Development of candidate HLAA*0201 restricted peptide-base vaccine against human cytomegalovirus infection. *Blood* 90:1751–1767, 1997.
113 Britt WJ: Vaccines against human cytomegalovirus: Time to test. *Trends Microbiol* 4:34–38, 1996.
114 Gonczol E et al: Preclinical evaluation of an ALVAC (canarypox): Human cytomegalovirus glycoprotein B vaccine candidate. *Vaccine* 13:1080–1085, 1995.
115 Katznelson S et al: Efficacy of the condom as a barrier to the transmission of cytomegalovirus. *J Infect Dis* 150:155–157, 1984.
116 Drew WL et al: Prevalence of resistance in patients receiving ganciclovir for serious cytomegalovirus infection. *J Infect Dis* 163:716–719, 1991.
117 Jacobson MA et al: Foscarnet therapy for ganciclovir-resistant cytomegalovirus retinitis in patients with AIDS. *J Infect Dis* 163:1348–1351, 1991.
118 Palestine AG et al: A randomized, controlled trial of foscarnet in the treatment of cytomegalovirus retinitis in patients with AIDS. *Ann Intern Med* 115:665–673, 1991.
119 Jabs DA: Studies of ocular complications of AIDS research group, in collaboration with the AIDS clinical trials group. Mortality in patients with the acquired immunodeficiency syndrome treated with either foscarnet or ganciclovir for cytomegalovirus retinitis. *N Engl J Med* 326:213–220, 1992.
120 Blanshard C et al: Treatment of AIDS-associated gastrointestinal cytomegalovirus infection with foscarnet and ganciclovir: A randomized comparison. *J Infect Dis* 172:622–628, 1995.
121 Lalezari JP et al: (S)-1-[3-hydroxy-2-(phosphonylmethoxy) propyl]cytosine (cidofovir): Results of a phase 1/11 study of a novel antiviral nucleotide analogue. *J Infect Dis* 171:788–796, 1995.
122 Lalezari JP et al: Intervenous cidofovir for peripheral cytomegalovirus retinitis in patients with AIDS. *Ann Intern Med* 126:257–263, 1997.

Chapter 23

Epstein-Barr virus infection

Karen S. Slobod
John W. Sixbey

DEFINITION

Herpesviruses are classified according to biologic characteristics into three subfamilies: the *alpha, beta,* and *gamma herpesviridae*[1] (see Chap. 20). The gamma herpesvirus subfamily, distinguished on the basis of establishing latent infection in lymphocytes, contains both the *Lymphocryptovirus* and *Rhadinovirus* genera defined by similarities in genome structure, gene organization, and relatedness of major viral proteins. These gamma herpesvirus genera include two members that infect humans and are implicated in oncogenesis. One of these, the Epstein-Barr virus (EBV, also called *human herpesvirus 4*) is the prototype *Lymphocryptovirus.* Kaposi's sarcoma herpesvirus (KSHV, or *human herpesvirus 8*) is a member of genus *Rhadinovirus.*[2] In this chapter we emphasize select aspects of EBV biology as they relate to sexual transmission and to clinical manifestations in the context of the general immunosuppression that accompanies human immunodeficiency virus (HIV) infections (for more general reviews, see Chap. 20 and refs. 3 and 4).

HISTORY

Denis Burkitt, a medical missionary to East Africa in the 1950s, first postulated an infectious agent as the cause for a common childhood tumor (Burkitt's lymphoma) based on the epidemiologic characteristics of this disease in equatorial Africa.[5] Using lymphoma samples provided by Burkitt, Tony Epstein and his student, Yvonne Barr, established the first permanent human lymphocytic cell lines[6] and by electron microscopy discovered a new herpesvirus with distinct antigenic and biologic characteristics.[7–9] Paramount among these was the ability of this virus to confer unlimited growth potential to B lymphocytes in vitro.[10,11] Seroepidemiologic studies by Werner and Gertrude Henle indicated that like other herpesviruses, EBV infection was widespread,[12,13] providing an apparent incongruity of ubiquitous asymptomatic carriage of this first candidate human tumor virus. Global distribution and high seroprevalence suggested that the virus might play a role in a very common disorder as well, and the fortuitous seroconversion of a technician in the Henle laboratory during the course of infectious mononucleosis led to the identification of EBV as the causal agent of this much studied lymphoproliferative syndrome.[14] Subsequent nucleic acid hybridization analyses have implicated EBV as an etiologic agent in nasopharyngeal carcinoma,[15,16] Hodgkin's disease,[17–19] unusual T-cell lymphomas,[20,21] and polyclonal B-lymphoproliferative disorders.[22,23] While historically much of EBV research has been focused on the oncogenicity of latent EBV proteins expressed in human tumors, a reexamination of events surrounding viral acquisition at mucosal sites draws attention to relatively new and unexplored areas of EBV biology: the pathologic contribution from EBV replication, reinfection, and genetic recombination.

EPIDEMIOLOGY

Antibody to EBV can be detected in 90 to 95 percent of the population by adulthood.[12] Primary exposure often occurs in the first years of life, with seroconversion evident before the age of 5 years in 50 percent of children studied in the United States and Great Britain.[24,25] In economically advantaged communities, primary infection may be delayed until adolescence or early adulthood,[26] at which time acquisition of virus produces the clinical syndrome acute infectious mononucleosis.

VIRAL SHEDDING AND TRANSMISSION

After initial exposure, EBV establishes a latent infection that persists for the life of the host. The lifelong virus carrier state is accompanied by asymptomatic viral shedding that provides a readily available source of infectious virus for person-to-person spread. Suspicion that infectious mononucleosis was related to an orally transmitted pathogen (hence the expression "kissing disease"[27]) was confirmed by the demonstration of cell-free virus in throat washings and saliva of infectious mononucleosis patients.[28,29] That intimate contact is required for transmission of virus was verified by epidemiologic studies wherein susceptible roommates of college students with acute infectious mononucleosis were shown to be at no greater risk for EBV seroconversion than the uninfected student population at large.[30,31] In young children, the route may be more indirect, associated with smaller virus inoculums and inapparent symptomatology. After recovery from acute infectious mononucleosis, EBV can be detected readily in the oropharynx for at least 18 months.[32] In healthy seropositive adults followed prospectively over 15 months, 90 percent shed EBV at some point, as detected by the standard lymphocyte transformation assay, with 25 percent shedding virus on every testing occasion.[33] Immunocompromised patients have still higher rates of viral shedding,[34] and increased levels of EBV excretion into oropharyngeal secretions are characteristic of individuals infected by HIV-1.[35,36]

Identification of EBV at oropharyngeal sites,[28,29,32] together with the experimental infection of mucosal epithelium derived from normal human cervix,[37] raised the possibility of broader mucosal involvement including the genital tract. In fact, infectious EBV can be recovered from genital mucosa of women with acute infectious mononucleosis, suggesting that virus is either conveyed from the oropharynx to distant mucosal sites by trafficking EBV-infected lymphocytes or that infection has been initiated by introduction of exogenous virus at that anatomic site. Transmissibility of genital virus is suggested by the successful isolation in the lymphocyte transformation assay of EBV from filtrates of cervical washings[38] as well as from vulvar ulcerative lesions.[39] Analogous to the persistent shedding of virus from oropharyngeal sites, EBV also can be recovered from the cervix of women without serologic evidence for recent EBV infection.[38] Indeed, the prevalence of EBV DNA in cervical samples from women attending sexually transmitted disease clinics ranges from 28 to 40 percent by polymerase chain reaction (PCR) analyses.[40–42] A possible etiologic role for EBV in subclinical genital lesions was indicated by a study of koilocytotic lesions of the vulva, since EBV DNA was detected in almost half of vulvar biopsies at sites of acetowhite lesions after application of 3 percent acetic acid.[43] In contrast, 11 percent of cell samples from normal vulvar mucosa contained EBV DNA.

In healthy, sexually active uncircumcised men, EBV DNA was detected by PCR in cells scraped from the coronal sulcus of the glans penis in 13 percent of study participants.[42] Forty-eight percent of EBV-seropositive men with urethral discharges secondary to gonococcal infection had EBV DNA detected in their genital tract secretions,[44] representing either lymphocyte-associated virus within the cellular inflammatory infiltrate or cell-free infectious virus. Although the transmissibility of cell-associated virus by the genital route remains to be determined, infection via transfer of latently infected cells can occur.[45] For example, the introduction of EBV-infected cells by blood transfusion[46–48] or tissue transplantation[49,50] causes both asymptomatic seroconversion and clinical disease.

Despite obvious epidemiologic implications of this mucosal distribution of EBV, no studies to date have directly addressed either oral-genital or sexual transmission of EBV, nor the possibility of acquiring classic infectious mononucleosis after genital tract infection. Indeed, the current understanding of events during primary EBV infection is remarkably limited and, given the expanding disease associations of the virus, requires careful reexamination. Although there have been few molecularly based epidemiologic studies of EBV infection, there now exist useful genotypic markers to facilitate such efforts.

EBV GENOTYPES AND COINFECTION

EBV isolates can be categorized broadly into two types now called *EBV-1* and *EBV-2* (formerly types A and B). Each is distinguished on the basis of polymorphisms in the genes that encode the EBV nuclear antigens (EBNAs), specifically EBNA2, 3A, 3B, and 3C.[51–53] EBNA2 differs more extensively between genotypes than the other EBNA proteins[52,53] and is primarily responsible for the biologic differences between type 1 and type 2. Specifically, type 1 strains transform primary B lymphocytes in vitro with greater efficiency than type 2 EBV, resulting in a cell growth phenotype readily maintained in culture.[54,55] Such polymorphisms in the EBNA genes generate immunologic responses that are both type-specific and cross-reactive. Although antibodies to EBNA2 and 3A are partially cross-reactive between types, the antibody responses to EBNA3B and 3C are largely type-specific.[56,57] Similarly, both type-specific and cross-reactive cytotoxic T-cell responses can be detected.[58–60]

Once thought to be restricted in its geographic distribution,[61] EBV-2 (like EBV-1) circulates widely in all human populations.[40,62,63] Coinfection with both EBV-1 and EBV-2 has been reported in from 9 to 27 percent of immunocompetent adults,[40,62] suggesting either the simultaneous acquisition of both types during primary infection or, more probably, reinfection on a second exposure. Although it has been long assumed that persistent carriage of EBV by a healthy host precludes second infections,[63] the independent acquisition of a second virus is suggested by a study of EBV genotypes in throat and genital washings of women at a sexually transmitted disease (STD) clinic.[40] Not only were coinfections more common in the STD study population, perhaps reflecting multiple exposures, but disparate EBV types were found in the oropharynx versus genital tract of a single participant. Such anatomic segregation of types is consistent with two separate introductions of virus into the same host. Unlike the case with herpes simplex 1 and 2, neither EBV genotype showed a predisposition toward one specific anatomic location.

Coinfection with type 1 and type 2 EBV is especially apparent in immunocompromised patients,[40,64–66] such as recipients of bone marrow or organ transplants and HIV-1-infected individuals. The increased load of endogenous virus that accompanies immune suppression[34] facilitates detection of the spectrum of resident virus in this clinic population. Moreover, immune impairment itself may render this group more susceptible to repeated infection from new viral exposures, whether in the form of administered blood products or multiple sexual partners.

In addition to the type 1 and type 2 classification of EBV, individual strains within the two major types can be distinguished based on size differences of EBNA proteins on immunoblots.[63,67] All EBNA-encoding genes contain repeat regions, the number of which vary between individual isolates. Such variability is also visible on DNA blots as restriction fragment length polymorphisms.[68] Strain-specific markers have been used to document spread of EBV infection between family members and from transplant donor to recipient.[68,69] Unlike with type differences, however, presence of multiple strains does not necessarily reflect repeated infection,[67] because intratypic diversity also may be generated within an individual by heterologous recombination between repeat sequences during replication of endogenous virus.

IMMUNOLOGY AND PATHOGENESIS

An elusive aspect of EBV biology is how a ubiquitous and persistent pathogen that normally achieves a natural rapport with its host may on occasion be highly pathogenic years after primary infection. New clinical settings characterized by enhanced viral exposure and immunosuppression, when viewed against the traditional EBV diseases Burkitt's lymphoma and nasopharyngeal carcinoma, are informative with regard to EBV pathophysiology.

MUCOSAL DETERMINANTS OF INFECTION

Consideration of EBV as a sexually transmitted agent highlights interactions between virus and cells at mucosal surfaces, where the major disease manifestations of the virus occur. In fact, it is only by viewing infection within the context of epithelial and lymphoid tissue interrelationships that a unified view of EBV pathogenesis emerges. For example, the anatomic distribution of EBV-positive Burkitt's lymphoma (salivary gland, breast of lactating women, gut, genitourinary tract) suggests a virus-initiated tumor affecting mucosa-associated lymphoid tissue (MALT).[70] Detection of viral DNA in breast milk[71] and at genital sites[38,44] further supports virus dissemination patterned after the physiologic circulation of mucosa-associated lymphocytes. Similarly, oropharyngeal epithelium is involved in the EBV-induced epithelial cell malignancy, nasopharyngeal carcinoma, as well as oral hairy leukoplakia of AIDS.[72]

A regular exchange of virus between epithelium and circulating lymphocytes first became evident in studies of primary EBV infection, where the detection of EBV DNA and RNA in desquamated epithelial cells from throat and cervical washings indicated epithelial cell foci of EBV replication.[38,73–75] Viral recombinants generated in oropharyngeal epithelium subsequently can be recovered in peripheral lymphocytes.[76] Despite the proclivity of EBV to remain latent in lymphocytes in vitro, virus transfer between cell types is almost certainly bidirectional, with viral reactivation occurring in circulating and intraepithelial B lymphocytes.[77,78] Mucosal seeding by trafficking, latently infected lymphocytes has been demonstrated convincingly in an organ transplant recipient who developed oropharyngeal shedding of virus strains acquired from transfused blood.[48] Moreover, cell-to-cell spread of virus in immune hosts also may be influenced by the presence of secretory antibody at mucosal surfaces. EBV-specific IgA facilitates uptake of EBV into epithelial cells via the polymeric immunoglobulin receptor while concurrently neutralizing infection of B lymphocytes by competing for the viral ligand of the B cell receptor.[79,80]

EPITHELIAL CELL-DERIVED RECOMBINANT EBV

Although lymphocyte culture has provided suitable models for study of EBV latency and virus-induced lymphoproliferation, systems permissive of EBV replication have not been available to address biologic issues raised by viral shedding at mucosal surfaces. EBV infection in acquired immune deficiency syndrome (AIDS) patients has been particularly instructive by providing the opportunity to observe replicative EBV infection in the epithelial setting.[72] Figure 23–1*a* shows a cross section through the epithelial lesion oral hairy leukoplakia, with abundant viral replication in the outer, more differentiated layers of epithelium. Analysis of this lesion has shown that markers of viral latency, characteristic of B-cell infection, are absent in this replicative infection of epithelium.[81–84]

An additional distinguishing attribute of this lesion is frequent coinfection with both type 1 and type 2 EBV,[65] along with the presence of defective EBV genomes[85–88] and intertypic recombinants.[76,89] Such genomic variability at mucosal sites may generate novel viral determinants capable of disturbing the usual virus-host balance in healthy carriers. For example, defective EBV genomes identified in hairy leukoplakia[86] have the potential of enhancing replication of standard latent EBV genomes,[90] thereby inducing the exuberant viral replication found in oral hairy leukoplakia. Other variants show loss of the EBNA2 gene critical for in vitro transformation of B lymphocytes,[65,85,87] which also may alter the usual course of EBV infection. Recent detection of type 1 and 2 recombinants[76,89,91] indicates not only coinfection of the human host but also superinfection of a single cell by two distinct and replicating virus types. Moreover, there is now unequivocal evidence that such epithelium-derived EBV mutants can disseminate via lymphocytes,[76] demonstrating not only their infectivity but also a role for epithelium in viral seeding of peripheral blood lymphocytes.

The larger issue is to what extent EBV biology in oral hairy leukoplakia reflects events in healthy virus carriers. EBV coinfection and recombination have been described in the general population,[40,62,76,85,91,92] and intertypic recombinants have been detected in peripheral blood lymphocytes.[91] In addition, nontransforming variants of EBV, capable of replication in the oropharynx, appear to be transmissible between healthy hosts.[85] Although the pathophysiologic significance of recombinant strains remains in question, defective nontransforming virus has been implicated in a rare form of chronic active EBV infection in an 8-year-old child.[92] Furthermore, defective EBV in the absence of prototypical virus has been found in sporadic Burkitt's lymphoma.[93]

CELL-MEDIATED IMMUNE CONTROL IN CHRONIC EBV CARRIERS

In vitro studies have indicated that the overall size of the EBV-infected B-cell pool is largely controlled by CD8+, HLA class I-restricted, EBV-specific cytotoxic T lymphocytes (CTLs). Impaired CTL responses in immunosuppressed patients, as seen in transplant recipients or HIV-1-infected individuals,[34,94] leads to an expansion of that pool and potentially fatal lymphoproliferative disease. The contribution of virus-specific CTLs in immune regulation of EBV-induced lymphoproliferation has been made clear by recent therapeutic interventions involving adoptive transfer of virus-specific T lymphocytes to restore immunity against EBV infection in bone marrow transplant recipients.[95–97]

Of the nine EBV proteins constitutively expressed during latent infection in cultured lymphoblastoid cell lines (see Chap. 20), only a subset (EBNA3A, 3B, and 3C) provides what appear to be dominant CTL targets (with some responses also seen to EBNA1, EBNA2, EBNA-LP, latent membrane protein 1 and 2 (or LMP1 and LMP2)).[98,99] Apart from deficient CTL activity, downregulation of latent gene expression in vivo also may facilitate the escape of infected cells from immune destruction. Three patterns of latent gene expression (latency I, II, and III) first observed in cultured cells[100] have parallels in EBV-associated tumors. In Burkitt's lymphoma (latency I), for example, only a single viral antigen is expressed, reducing tumor susceptibility to EBV-specific CTL surveillance.[101] By contrast, immunoblastic B-cell lymphomas (latency III) typical of immunocompromised patients express the full spectrum of EBV latent proteins and remain sensitive to CTL control if intact.

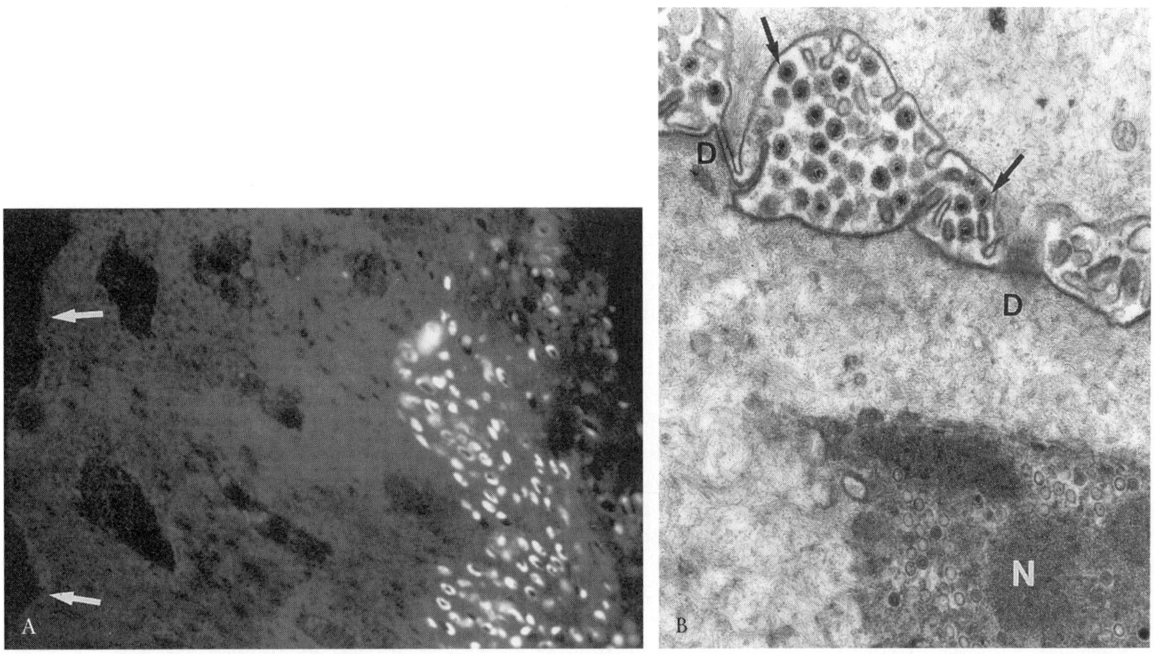

Fig. 23–1 EBV replication in oral hairy leukoplakia of AIDS. (*a*) A cross section of the mucosal lesion immunostained for EBV immediate-early antigen BZLF1 demonstrates replication in the upper layers of thickened epithelium. Arrows indicate the basal epithelial layer. (*b*) Electron micrograph of interepithelial space showing abundant mature EBV virions (*arrow*). Nucleus (*N*) contains immature virus particles (*D*, desmosomes).

CLINICAL MANIFESTATIONS

INFECTIOUS MONONUCLEOSIS

Primary EBV infection in infancy or early childhood is usually subclinical, but when delayed until the second decade of life, it manifests as infectious mononucleosis in up to 50 percent of patients. A self-limiting lymphoproliferative disease, the syndrome consists of fever, headache, pharyngitis, lymphadenopathy, and general malaise. Resolution of symptoms may take weeks to months, but primary infection is always followed by the establishment of a permanent viral carrier state.[45] Diagnostic features of acute infection include the appearance of heterophile antibodies and a prominent atypical lymphocytosis, reflecting the unusually strong T-cell response elicited by virally infected B cells. Predominantly CD8+,[102,103] the reactive T cells are comprised of both nonspecific and HLA-restricted EBV-specific cytotoxic T cells. The exaggerated nature of the T-cell response suggests that the syndrome is largely immunopathologic in nature. The greater frequency of symptomatic infection in adolescence may relate not to age but rather to a larger inoculum of transmitted virus and the ensuing T-cell reaction.[4]

AIDS-RELATED MANIFESTATIONS OF EBV INFECTION

HIV-related immunosuppression disrupts the usual homeostasis achieved between EBV and host, increasing the risk for both reactivation of latent EBV and acquisition of coinfecting strains. Reduced immune control results in elevated levels of EBV in the oropharynx as well as blood of HIV-infected patients,[35,36] similar to what has been described in transplant recipients.[34,96] There is some evidence to suggest that episodes of EBV reactivation may have clinical consequences. Most EBV malignancies in the population at large are preceded by antibody responses indicative of an enhanced level of viral activity[104–106]; deregulation of the virus-host balance may favor emergence of a malignant cell clone. Medical consequences of the high EBV burden in AIDS are reflected in unique pathology as well as in the increased frequency of otherwise rare EBV diseases.

Oral hairy leukoplakia

Oral hairy leukoplakia is a proliferative EBV-induced mucocutaneous epithelial cell disease and the first pathologic manifestation of replicative EBV infection,[72] making the lesion unique in EBV biology. It is seen in up to 25 percent of homosexual men with AIDS but has been reported as well in other immunocompromised patients and healthy individuals.[72,76] Clinically, the lesion is an asymptomatic, poorly demarcated keratotic area with a corrugated or "hairy" surface varying in size from a few millimeters to extensive lingual and oral mucosal involvement. Typically on the lateral borders of the tongue, the whitish, slightly raised lesion is often mistaken for thrush. Histopathologic features include a thickening of epithelium, with characteristic balloon cells resembling koilocytes, and a hyperkeratosis resulting in microscopic hairlike projections. An abundance of viral particles can be seen in the outer layers of epithelium (Fig. 23–1*b*), consistent with the notion that EBV replication is linked to terminal differentiation of cells.[37,74] Epithelial dysplasia is not a feature of these lesions, and malignant transformation of oral hairy leukoplakia has not been reported.

EBV-associated malignancies in AIDS

Non-Hodgkin's lymphoma, 60 times more common in AIDS patients than in the general population,[107] can be divided morphologically into Burkitt-like and immunoblastic lymphomas, both of which have a higher association with EBV (30 to 40 percent and 75 to 80 percent, respectively) in AIDS than in non-AIDS groups.[108,109] Tumors may carry either type 1 or type 2 virus,[110–112] reflecting the relative prevalence of each genotype within the HIV-infected population. Burkitt's lymphomas appear early in the course of AIDS, prior to profound immunosuppression, whereas immunoblastic lymphomas typically occur in late-stage AIDS when cellular immunity is compromised. The timing of immunoblastic lymphomas may be explained by their expression of latent viral proteins LMP1 and EBNA2 (type III pattern of EBV latency)[113] that in an immunocompetent host provide ample targets for EBV-specific cytotoxic T cells. Appearance of the malignancy coincidental with diminished immune surveillance suggests an opportunistic proliferation similar to posttransplant lymphoproliferative disease.

Hodgkin's lymphomas in the setting of AIDS contain EBV in 75 to 90 percent of the cases,[114,115] reflecting the unusually high frequency in the HIV-infected population of mixed-cellularity and lymphocyte-depletion subtypes[116] known to be most closely associated with EBV in the general population.[17,18] Although conclusive studies regarding an increased frequency of Hodgkin's disease in AIDS are lacking, disproportionate distribution of subtypes and unfavorable clinicopathologic features make the entity distinct to AIDS.[114,116]

Two malignancies that are not associated with EBV in the general population but which consistently contain the viral genome in patients with HIV-1 infection are leiomyosarcoma and primary central nervous system lymphoma (PCNSL). Leiomyosarcoma, a mesenchymal malignancy with smooth muscle differentiation, has been shown by in situ cytohybridization to contain EBV in affected muscle cells of both children and adults with HIV infection.[117,118] Similarly, AIDS-related PCNSL is uniformly EBV-positive.[119,120] The monoclonality of each malignant process, shown by size homogeneity of the fused terminal repeats of the EBV genome, indicates that infection of the malignant clone occurred prior to neoplastic expansion, providing a compelling argument for a contribution by EBV to the proliferative process. Again, both tumors occur at a much higher frequency in HIV-infected patients than in the population at large.

TREATMENT

The nucleoside analogue acyclovir is ineffective in the treatment of latent EBV infection characteristic of viral-induced lymphoproliferation but, as a potent inhibitor of EBV DNA polymerase, can inhibit EBV replication. Although capable of blocking viral shedding from the oropharynx in infectious mononucleosis patients, the drug does not reduce the load of latently infected B cells in the peripheral blood or affect the disease course. In contrast, acyclovir effectively reverses the lytic lesion of oral hairy leukoplakia, although cessation of treatment often results in a recurrence of lesions within 1 to 4 months.[121,122]

EBV-positive AIDS-related lymphomas often are refractory to conventional chemotherapy, with rare complete remissions and an absence of durable clinical responses, especially for PCNSL.[123,124] Adoptive immunotherapy, successfully pioneered for the immunoprophylaxis and therapy of posttransplant lymphoproliferative disease,[96,97] may be applicable to AIDS patients with EBV-associated tumors. Other strategies under consideration include pharmacologic modulation of EBV expression by azacytidine, an inhibitor of DNA methyltransferase, with the intent of converting a tumor with limited viral antigen expression to one with a latency III phenotype amenable to immune recognition and destruction.[125]

PREVENTION AND CONTROL

Largely because of the global significance of EBV-related malignancies, concerted efforts toward vaccine development are underway. One prototype subunit vaccine is based on the abundant viral envelope glycoprotein gp350 that binds the B-lymphocyte receptor and elicits neutralizing antibody against infectious virus.[126–128] Other strategies focus on the use of peptides derived from latent antigens to stimulate cytotoxic T cells central to the control of EBV-infected B lymphocytes.[98,99,129] With respect to precautions in clinical settings, physical isolation of patients with acute EBV infections is not required. However, individuals with a recent history of acute EBV infection should not be selected as blood or tissue donors when possible because of the enhanced viral load accompanying primary infection.

REFERENCES

1 Roizman B: Herpesviridae, in *Fields Virology*, 3d ed, BN Fields et al (eds). Philadelphia, Lippincott-Raven, 1996, chap 71, pp 2221–2230.

2 Moore PS et al: Primary characterization of a herpesvirus agent associated with Kaposi's sarcoma. *J Virol* 70:549, 1996.

3 Klein G: *Advances in Viral Oncology*, vol 8. New York, Raven Press, 1987, pp 103–259.

4 Rickinson AB, Kieff E: Epstein-Barr Virus, in *Fields Virology*, 3d ed, BN Fields et al (eds). Philadelphia, Lippincott-Raven, 1996, chap 75, pp 2397–2446.

5 Burkitt D: A children's cancer dependent on climatic factors. *Nature* 194:232, 1962.

6 Epstein MA, Barr YM: Cultivation in vitro of human lymphoblasts from Burkitt's malignant lymphoma. *Lancet* 1:252, 1964.

7 Epstein MA et al: Virus particles in cultured lymphoblasts from Burkitt's lymphoma. *Lancet* 1:702, 1964.

8 Epstein MA et al: Morphological and biological studies on a virus in cultured lymphoblasts from Burkitt's lymphoma. *J Exp Med* 121:761, 1965.

9 Henle G, Henle W: Immunofluorescence in cells derived from Burkitt's lymphoma. *J Bacteriol* 91:1248, 1966.

10 Pope JH et al: Transformation of foetal human leukocytes in vitro by filtrates of a human leukaemic cell line containing herpes-like virus. *Int J Cancer* 3:857, 1968.

11 Nilsson K et al: The establishment of lymphoblastoid cell lines from adult and from fetal human lymphoid tissue and its dependence on EBV. *Int J Cancer* 8:443, 1971.

12 Henle G et al: Antibodies to EB virus in Burkitt's lymphoma and control groups. *J Natl Cancer Inst* 43:1147, 1969.

13 Henle W, Henle G: Seroepidemiology of the Virus, in *The Epstein-Barr Virus*, MA Epstein, BG Achong (eds). Berlin, Springer-Verlag, 1979, pp 61–78.

14 Henle G et al: Relation of Burkitt tumor associated herpes-type virus to infectious mononucleosis. *Proc Natl Acad Sci USA* 59:94, 1968.

15 Zur Hausen H et al: EBV DNA in biopsies of Burkitt tumours and anaplastic carcinomas of the nasopharynx. *Nature* 228:1956, 1970.

16 Wolf H et al: EB viral genome in epithelial nasopharyngeal carcinoma cells. *Nature New Biol* 244:245, 1973.

17 Weiss LM et al: Epstein-Barr viral DNA in tissues of Hodgkin's disease. *Am J Pathol* 129:86, 1987.

18 Weiss LM et al: Detection of Epstein-Barr viral genomes in Reed-Sternberg cells of Hodgkin's disease. *N Engl J Med* 320:502, 1989.

19 Anagnostopoulos I et al: Demonstration of monoclonal EBV genomes in Hodgkin's disease and Ki-1-positive anaplastic large cell lymphoma by combined Southern blot and in situ hybridization. *Blood* 74:810, 1989.

20 Jones JF et al: T-cell lymphomas containing Epstein-Barr viral DNA in patients with chronic Epstein-Barr virus infections. *N Engl J Med* 318:733, 1988.

21 Harabuchi Y et al: Epstein-Barr virus in nasal T-cell lymphomas in patients with lethal mid-line granuloma. *Lancet* 1:128, 1990.

22 Hanto DW et al: Clinical spectrum of lymphoproliferative disorders in renal transplant recipients and evidence for the role of Epstein-Barr virus. *Cancer Res* 41:4253, 1981.

23 Craig FE et al: Posttransplant lymphoproliferative disorders. *Am J Clin Pathol* 99:265, 1993.

24 Porter DD et al: Prevalence of antibodies to EB virus and other herpesviruses. *JAMA* 208:1675, 1969.

25 Pereira MS et al: EB virus antibody at different ages. *Br Med J* 4:526, 1969.

26 Henle G, Henle W: Observations on childhood infections with the Epstein-Barr virus. *J Infect Dis* 121:303, 1970.

27 Hoagland RJ: The transmission of infectious mononucleosis. *Am J Med Sci* 229:262, 1955.

28 Chang RS, Golden HD: Transformation of human leukocytes by throat washings from infectious mononucleosis patients. *Nature* 234:359, 1971.

29 Gerber P et al: Oral excretion of Epstein-Barr virus by healthy subjects and patients with infectious mononucleosis. *Lancet* 2:988, 1972.

30 Sawyer RN et al: Prospective studies of a group of Yale University freshman: I. Occurrence of infectious mononucleosis. *J Infect Dis* 123:263, 1971.

31 Halle TJ et al: Infectious mononucleosis at the United States Military Academy: A prospective study of a single class over 4 years. *Yale J Biol Med* 47:182, 1974.

32 Miller G et al: Prolonged oropharyngeal excretion of Epstein-Barr virus after infectious mononucleosis. *N Engl J Med* 288:229, 1973.

33 Yao QY et al: A re-examination of the Epstein-Barr virus carrier state in healthy seropositive individuals. *Int J Cancer* 35:35, 1985.

34 Yao QY et al: In vitro analysis of Epstein-Barr virus:host balance in long-term renal allograft recipients. *Int J Cancer* 35:43, 1985.

35 Alsip GR et al: Increased Epstein-Barr virus DNA in oropharyngeal secretions from patients with AIDS, AIDS-related complex, or asymptomatic human immunodeficiency virus infections. *J Infect Dis* 157:1072, 1988.

36 Ferbas J et al: Frequent oropharyngeal shedding of Epstein-Barr virus in homosexual men during early HIV infection. *AIDS* 6:1273, 1992.

37 Sixbey JW et al: Replication of Epstein-Barr virus in human epithelial cells infected in vitro. *Nature* 306:480, 1983.

38 Sixbey JW et al: A second site for Epstein-Barr virus shedding: The uterine cervix. *Lancet* 1:1122, 1986.

39 Portnoy J et al: Recovery of Epstein-Barr virus from genital ulcers. *N Engl J Med* 311:966, 1984.

40 Sixbey JW et al: Detection of a second widespread strain of Epstein-Barr virus. *Lancet* 2:761, 1989.

41 Voog E et al: Prevalence of Epstein-Barr virus and human papillomavirus in cervical samples from women attending an STD clinic. *Int J STD AIDS* 6:208, 1995.

42 Naher H et al: Subclinical Epstein-Barr virus infection of both the male and female genital tract: Indication for sexual transmission. *J Invest Dermatol* 98:791, 1992.

43 Voog E et al: Demonstration of Epstein-Barr virus DNA in acetowhite lesions of the vulva. *Int J STD AIDS* 1:25, 1994.

44 Israele V et al: Excretion of Epstein-Barr virus from the genital tract of men. *J Infect Dis* 163:1341, 1991.

45 Henle G, Henle W: The Virus as Etiologic Agent of Infectious Mononucleosis, in *The Epstein-Barr Virus*, MA Epstein, BG Achong (eds). Berlin, Springer-Verlag, 1979, pp 297–320,

46 Gerber P et al: Association of EB-virus infection with the post-perfusion syndrome. *Lancet* 1:593, 1969.

47 Blacklow NR et al: Mononucleosis with heterophil antibodies and EB virus infection: Acquisition by an elderly patient in hospital. *Am J Med* 51:549, 1971.
48 Alfieri C et al: Epstein-Barr virus transmission from a blood donor to an organ transplant recipient with recovery of the same virus strain from the recipient's blood and oropharynx. *Blood* 87:812, 1996.
49 Gratama JW et al: Eradication of Epstein-Barr virus by allogeneic bone marrow transplantation: Implications for sites of viral latency. *Proc Natl Acad Sci USA* 85:8693, 1988.
50 Cen H et al: Epstein-Barr virus transmission via the donor organ in solid organ transplantation: Polymerase chain reaction and restriction fragment length polymorphism analysis of IR2, IR3, and IR4. *J Virol* 65:976, 1991.
51 Adldinger HK et al: A putative transforming gene of Jijoye virus differs from that of Epstein-Barr virus prototypes. *Virology* 141:221, 1985.
52 Dambaugh T et al: U2 region of Epstein-Barr virus DNA may encode Epstein-Barr virus nuclear antigen 2. *Proc Natl Acad Sci USA* 81: 7632, 1984.
53 Sample J et al: Epstein-Barr virus type 1 (EBV-1) and 2 (EBV-2) differ in their EBNA-3A, EBNA-3B, and EBNA-3C genes. *J Virol* 64:4084, 1990.
54 Rickinson AB et al: Influence of the Epstein-Barr virus nuclear antigen EBNA2 on the growth phenotype of virus-transformed B cells. *J Virol* 61:1310, 1987.
55 Cohen J et al: Epstein-Barr virus nuclear protein 2 is a key determinant of lymphocyte transformation. *Proc Natl Acad Sci USA* 86: 9558, 1989.
56 Rowe M et al: Distinction between Epstein-Barr virus type A (EBNA2) isolates extends to the EBNA3 family of nuclear proteins. *J Virol* 63:1031, 1989.
57 Sculley TB et al: Expression of Epstein-Barr virus nuclear antigens 3, 4, and 6 is altered in cell lines containing B type virus. *Virology* 171: 401, 1989.
58 Moss DJ et al: Cytotoxic T-cell clones discriminate between A- and B-type Epstein-Barr virus transformants. *Nature* 331:719, 1988.
59 Burrows SR et al: An Epstein-Barr virus-specific cytotoxic T cell epitope in EBNA 3. *J Exp Med* 171:345, 1990.
60 Burrows SR et al: An Epstein-Barr virus-specific cytotoxic T cell epitope present on A- and B-type transformants. *J Virol* 64:3974, 1990.
61 Zimber U et al: Geographic prevalence of two types of Epstein-Barr virus. *Virology* 154:56, 1986.
62 Apolloni A, Sculley TB: Detection of A-type and B-type Epstein-Barr virus in throat washings and lymphocytes. *Virology* 202:978, 1994.
63 Yao QY et al: The Epstein-Barr virus carrier state: Dominance of a single growth-transforming isolate in the blood and in the oropharynx of healthy virus carriers. *J Gen Virol* 72:1579, 1991.
64 Sculley TB et al: Coinfection with A- and B-type Epstein-Barr virus in human immunodeficiency virus-positive subjects. *J Infect Dis* 162: 643, 1990.
65 Walling DM et al: Coinfection with multiple strains of Epstein-Barr virus in human immunodeficiency virus-associated hairy leukoplakia. *Proc Natl Acad Sci USA* 89:6560, 1992.
66 Yao QY et al: Frequency of multiple Epstein-Barr virus infections in T-cell-immunocompromised individuals. *J Virol* 70:4884, 1996.
67 Gratama JW et al: Detection of multiple "Ebnotypes" in individual Epstein-Barr virus carriers following lymphocyte transformation by virus derived from peripheral blood and oropharynx. *J Gen Virol* 75: 85, 1994.
68 Katz BZ et al: Fragment length polymorphisms among independent isolates of Epstein-Barr virus from immunocompromised and normal hosts. *J Infect Dis* 157:299, 1988.
69 Gratma JW et al: EBNA size polymorphism can be used to trace Epstein-Barr virus spread within families. *J Virol* 64:4703, 1990.
70 Wright DH: Histogenesis of Burkitt's Lymphoma: A B-cell Tumor of Mucosa-Associated Lymphoid Tissue, in *Burkitt's Lymphoma: A Human Cancer Model*, GM Lenoir et al (eds). Lyons, International Agency for Research on Cancer, 1985, pp 37–45.
71 Junker AK et al: Epstein-Barr virus shedding in breast milk. *Am J Med Sci* 320:220, 1991.
72 Greenspan JS et al: Replication of Epstein-Barr virus within the epithelial cells of oral "hairy" leukoplakia, an AIDS-associated lesion. *N Engl J Med* 313:1564, 1985.
73 Wolf H et al: Persistence of Epstein-Barr virus in the parotid gland. *J Virol* 51:795, 1984.
74 Sixbey JW et al: Epstein-Barr virus replication in oropharyngeal epithelial cells. *N Engl J Med* 310:1225, 1984.
75 Lemon SM et al: Replication of EBV in epithelial cells during infectious mononucleosis. *Nature* 268:268, 1977.
76 Walling DM et al: Epstein-Barr virus coinfection and recombination in non-human immunodeficiency virus-associated oral hairy leukoplakia. *J Infect Dis* 171:1122, 1995.
77 Tao Q et al: Evidence for lytic infection by Epstein-Barr virus in mucosal lymphocytes instead of nasopharyngeal epithelial cells in normal individuals. *J Med Virol* 45:71, 1995.
78 Anagnostopoulos I et al: Morphology, immunophenotype, and distribution of latently and/or productively Epstein-Barr virus infected cells in acute infectious mononucleosis: Implications for the interindividual infection route of Epstein-Barr virus. *Blood* 85:744, 1995.
79 Sixbey JW, Yao QY: Immunoglobulin A-induced shift of Epstein-Barr virus tissue tropism. *Science* 255:1578, 1992.
80 Gan YJ et al: Epithelial cell polarization is a determinant of the infectious outcome of immunoglobulin A-mediated entry by Epstein Barr virus. *J Virol* 71:519, 1997.
81 Gilligan K et al: Epstein-Barr virus small nuclear RNAs are not expressed in permissively infected cells in AIDS-associated leukoplakia. *Proc Natl Acad Sci USA* 87:8790, 1990.
82 Thomas JA et al: Epstein-Barr virus gene expression and epithelial cell differentiation in oral hairy leukoplakia. *Am J Pathol* 139:1369, 1991.
83 Niedobitek G et al: Epstein-Barr virus infection in oral hairy leukoplakia: Virus replication in the absence of a detectable latent phase. *J Gen Virol* 72:3035, 1991.
84 Lau R et al: Epstein-Barr virus expression in oral hairy leukoplakia. *Virology* 195:463, 1993.
85 Sixbey JW et al: A transformation-incompetent, nuclear antigen 2-deleted Epstein-Barr virus associated with replicative infection. *J Infect Dis* 163:1008, 1991.
86 Patton DF et al: Defective viral DNA in Epstein-Barr virus-associated oral hairy leukoplakia. *J Virol* 64:397, 1990.
87 Walling DM et al: The Epstein-Barr virus EBNA2 gene in oral hairy leukoplakia: Strain variation, genetic recombination, and transcriptional expression. *J Virol* 68:7918, 1994.
88 Walling DM, Raab-Traub N: Epstein-Barr virus intrastrain recombination in oral hairy leukoplakia. *J Virol* 68:7909, 1994.
89 Yao QY et al: Isolation of intertypic recombinants of Epstein-Barr virus from T-cell-immunocompromised individuals. *J Virol* 70:4895, 1996.
90 Miller G et al: Epstein-Barr virus with heterogeneous DNA disrupts latency. *J Virol* 50:174, 1984.
91 Burrows JM et al: Identification of a naturally occurring recombinant Epstein-Barr virus isolate from New Guinea that encodes both type 1 and type 2 nuclear antigen sequences. *J Virol* 70:4829, 1996.
92 Alfieri C, Joncas JH: Biomolecular analysis of a defective nontransforming Epstein-Barr virus (EBV) from a patient with chronic active EBV. *J Virol* 61:3306, 1987.
93 Razzouk BI et al: Epstein-Barr virus DNA recombination and loss in sporadic Burkitt's lymphoma. *J Infect Dis* 173:529, 1996.
94 Birx DL et al: Defective regulation of Epstein-Barr virus infection in patients with acquired immunodeficiency syndrome (AIDS) or AIDS-related disorders. *N Engl J Med* 314:874, 1986.
95 Papadopoulos EB et al: Infusions of donor leukocytes to treat Epstein-Barr virus-associated lymphoproliferative disorders after allogeneic bone marrow transplantation. *N Engl J Med* 330:1185, 1994.
96 Rooney CM et al: Use of gene-modified virus-specific T lymphocytes to control Epstein-Barr virus-related lymphoproliferation. *Lancet* 345:9, 1995.

97 Heslop HE et al: Long-term restoration of immunity against Epstein-Barr virus infection by adoptive transfer of gene-modified virus-specific T lymphocytes. *Nature Med* 2:551, 1996.

98 Khanna R et al: Localisation of Epstein-Barr virus cytotoxic T cell epitopes using recombinant vaccinia: Implications for vaccine development. *J Exp Med* 176:169, 1992.

99 Murray RJ et al: Identification of target antigens for the human cytotoxic T cell response to Epstein-Barr virus (EBV): Implications for the immune control of EBV-positive malignancies. *J Exp Med* 176: 157, 1992.

100 Rowe M et al: Differences in B cell growth phenotype reflect novel patterns of Epstein-Barr virus latent gene expression in Burkitt's lymphoma cells. *EMBO J* 6:2743, 1987.

101 Rooney CM et al: Epstein-Barr virus-positive Burkitt's lymphoma cells not recognized by virus-specific T cell surveillance. *Nature* 317:629, 1985.

102 Sheldon PJ et al: Thymic origin of atypical lymphoid cells in infectious mononucleosis. *Lancet* 1:1153, 1973.

103 Reinherz EL et al: The cellular basis for viral induced immunodeficiency: Analysis by monoclonal antibodies. *J Immunol* 125:1269, 1980.

104 Henle G, Henle W: Epstein-Barr virus-specific IgA serum antibodies as an outstanding feature of nasopharyngeal carcinoma. *Int J Cancer* 17:1, 1976.

105 De The G et al: Epidemiological evidence for causal relationship between Epstein-Barr virus and Burkitt's lymphoma from Ugandan prospective study. *Nature* 274:756, 1978.

106 Mueller N et al: Hodgkin's disease and Epstein-Barr virus: Altered antibody patterns before diagnosis. *N Engl J Med* 320:689, 1989.

107 Beral V et al: AIDS-associated non-Hodgkin lymphoma. *Lancet* 337: 805, 1991.

108 Hamilton-Dutoit SJ et al. AIDS-related lymphoma: Histopathology, immunophenotype, and association with Epstein-Barr virus as demonstrated by in situ nucleic acid hybridization. *Am J Pathol* 138:149, 1991.

109 Subar M et al: Frequent *c-myc* oncogene activation and infrequent presence of Epstein-Barr virus genome in AIDS-associated lymphoma. *Blood* 72:667, 1988.

110 Boyle MJ et al: Subtypes of Epstein-Barr virus in human immunodeficiency virus-associated non-Hodgkin's lymphomas. *Blood* 78: 3004, 1991.

111 Gunthel CJ et al: Association of Epstein-Barr virus types 1 and 2 with acquired immunodeficiency syndrome-related primary central nervous system lymphomas. *Blood* 83:618, 1994.

112 Shibata D et al: Epstein-Barr virus-associated non-Hodgkin's lymphoma in patients infected with the human immunodeficiency virus. *Blood* 81:2102, 1994.

113 Hamilton-Dutoit SJ et al: Epstein-Barr virus-latent gene expression and tumour cell phenotype in acquired immunodeficiency syndrome-related non-Hodgkin's lymphomas: Correlation of lymphoma phenotype with three distinct patterns of viral latency. *Am J Pathol* 143:1072, 1993.

114 Tirelli U et al: Hodgkin's disease and human immunodeficiency virus infection: Clinicopathologic and virologic features of 114 patients from the Italian cooperative group on AIDS and tumors. *J Clin Oncol* 13:1758, 1995.

115 Herndier BG et al: High prevalence of Epstein-Barr virus in the Reed-Sternberg cells of HIV-associated Hodgkin's disease. *Am J Pathol* 142:1073, 1993.

116 Serraino D et al: Increased frequency of lymphocyte depletion and mixed cellularity subtypes of Hodgkin's disease in HIV-infected patients. *Eur J Cancer* 29A:1948, 1993.

117 McClain KL et al: Association of Epstein-Barr virus with leiomyosarcomas in children with AIDS. *N Engl J Med* 332:12, 1995.

118 Zetler PJ et al: Primary adrenal leiomyosarcoma in a man with acquired immunodeficiency syndrome (AIDS): Further evidence for an increase in smooth muscle tumors related to Epstein-Barr virus infections in AIDS. *Arch Pathol Lab Med* 119:1164, 1995.

119 MacMahon EME et al: Epstein-Barr virus in AIDS-related central nervous system lymphoma. *Lancet* 338:969, 1991.

120 Hamilton-Dutoit SJ et al: In situ demonstration of Epstein-Barr virus small RNAs (EBER1) in acquired immunodeficiency syndrome-related lymphomas: Correlation with tumour morphology and primary site. *Blood* 82:619, 1993.

121 Greenspan D et al: Efficacy of desciclovir in the treatment of Epstein-Barr virus infections in oral hairy leukoplakia. *J AIDS* 3:571, 1990.

122 Resnick L et al: Regression of oral hairy leukoplakia after orally administered acyclovir therapy. *JAMA* 259:384, 1988.

123 Kaplan LD et al: Clinical and virologic effects of recombinant human granulocyte-macrophage colony-stimulating factor in patients receiving chemotherapy for human immunodeficiency virus-associated non-Hodgkin's lymphoma: Results of a randomized trial. *J Clin Oncol* 9:929, 1991.

124 Levine AM: Acquired immunodeficiency syndrome-related lymphoma. *Blood* 80:8, 1992.

125 Robertson KD et al: Pharmacologic Activation of Expression of Immunodominant Viral Antigens: A New Strategy for the Treatment of Epstein-Barr Virus-Associated Malignancies, in *Mechanisms in B-Cell Neoplasia*, M Potter, F Melchers (eds). New York, Springer-Verlag, 1994, pp 145–154.

126 Pearson G et al: Relation between neutralization of Epstein-Barr virus and antibodies to cell-membrane antigens induced by the virus. *J Natl Cancer Inst* 45:989, 1970.

127 Tanner J et al: Soluble gp350/220 and deletion mutant glycoproteins block Epstein-Barr virus adsorption to lymphocytes. *J Virol* 62:4452, 1988.

128 Morgan AJ: Epstein-Barr virus vaccines. *Vaccine* 10:563, 1992.

129 Spring SB et al: Issues related to development of Epstein-Barr virus vaccines. *J Natl Cancer Inst* 88:1436, 1996.

Chapter 24

Biology of genital human papillomaviruses

Denise A. Galloway

GENERAL PROPERTIES AND CLASSIFICATION

Papillomaviruses are a group of small DNA viruses that primarily induce epithelial cell proliferation, or papillomas, in higher vertebrates. Infections are strictly genus- or species-specific, and there is considerable tropism among the viruses for particular anatomic sites. Viral particles are nonenveloped, have an icosahedral symmetry, and encapsidate a double-stranded circular genome of 7.9 kb that is associated with cellular histones.[1] To date, papillomaviruses have not been efficiently propagated in tissue culture, and therefore, little is known about the virus life cycle; much of what is known about the function of viral genes comes from studies using individual cloned genes in various cellular or in vitro assays. Unlike most other virus groups, types are not based on antigenic diversity, but rather on DNA homology (see the following). Nearly a hundred human papillomaviruses (HPVs) have been detected by PCR-based assays, and the genomes of approximately 75 types have been molecularly cloned and completely sequenced. The sequences are available through Genbank or the HPV sequence database WWW home page (http://hpv-web.lanl.gov/).

More than 30 HPV types infect the genital tract. The consequences of infection with genital HPVs varies, and at least some of the variation is type-specific, as discussed in detail elsewhere in this volume. The genital HPVs have been grouped into high- and low-risk types, based on the potential of the infected cells to progress to carcinoma.[2] For example, approximately 50 percent of invasive squamous cell cancers of the cervix (SCC) harbor the high-risk HPV 16, whereas only 1 of 932 SCCs collected worldwide contained the low-risk HPV 6; intermediate-risk types each contributed a small percent of the total HPV positivity.[3]

GENOME STRUCTURE AND FUNCTION

Sequence analysis of cloned viral genomes has shown that the genetic organization of all human and animal papillomaviruses is well conserved. The genomic map of HPV 16 is depicted in a linear form in Fig. 24-1. All eight open reading frames (ORFs) are located on one strand of DNA, and accordingly, transcription of viral genes has been shown to use only one strand as template.[4] The ORFs E6, E7, E1, E2, E4, E5 are designated as early, and L1 and L2 are late, based on the expression of only the early region in bovine papillomavirus-1 (BPV-1) transformed cells and expression of the late region in productively infected cells.[5,6] (E3 and E8 are not present in all genomes and have not been shown to code for viral proteins.) An approximately 850-bp segment between L1 and E6 is devoid of ORFs and has been variously designated as the noncoding region (NCR), upstream regulatory region (URR), or long control region (LCR). This region contains a number of *cis*-acting sequences necessary for viral DNA replication and the regulation of transcription.

Transcription of the viral genome is very complex with many alternatively, and multiply, spliced RNAs, mostly in low abundance (see Fig. 24-1).[4] Transcription initiates at several different promoters, although early and late genes seemingly share at least some of the same promoters. All of the early RNAs terminate at a polyadenylation site at nucleotide (nt) 4215, and the late RNAs use a poly-A site at nt 7321. Characterization of the mRNAs indicate that some genes, for example, E7 or E5, are translated only from bi- or poly-cistronic messages, although the low-risk viruses have an additional promoter for expression of E7.[7] An mRNA encoding L2 has not been unambiguously identified though the L2 protein has been readily detected.[5,8] Additionally, some ORFs are spliced together to encode fusion proteins (e.g., E1^E4), whereas other ORFs encode multiple products (e.g., E2, E2C, E2M, and possibly E6, E6*, E6**). Thus, although all genital HPVs encode 8 ORFs, the exact number of viral proteins that are expressed during infection is not known precisely.

Knowledge about the function of HPV gene products is incomplete because of the limited ability to study HPV infections in vitro. Table 24-1 summarizes information about the products encoded by the ORFs and their presumed functions and will be discussed in more detail in the following.

VIRION STRUCTURE

The three-dimensional structure of several papillomavirus virions has been determined by cryoelectron microscopy and image analysis as shown in Fig. 24-2.[9,10] Capsids are approximately 60 nm in diameter and are composed of 72 pentameric capsomers arranged on a skewed icosahedral lattice with a triangulation number of 7 dextro. The shell, made of L1 protein, is approximately 2 nm thick and appeared much smoother on the internal surface than the external surface with a fairly contiguous density. Capsomers extended radially 6 nm from the shell and appeared as five-pointed stars. Intercapsomer interactions were restricted to the shell. Twelve capsomers are pentavalent (contacting five neighboring capsomers), and 60 capsomers are hexavalent. The capsomers are composed of five subunits of L1 with an axial dimple of 3 nm. The location of the minor capsid protein, L2, was not apparent in the image reconstructions, although additional density in the dimples of the pentavalent capsomers suggests that L2 is located at the vertices. At a resolution of 3.5 nm, capsids generated by self-assembly of L1 are identical to authentic HPV virions, and no differences were observed when L2 was also present in the capsid.[11]

TAXONOMY AND PHYLOGENETIC RELATIONSHIP

The family *Papovaviridae* includes the genus *Papillomavirus* and the genus *Polyomavirus*, although recent studies indicate that the divergence in virion diameter, genome size, transcriptional organization, and other aspects of their biology merit the designation as subfamilies rather than genera. Papillomaviruses are widespread in higher vertebrates, including a plethora of human viruses with tropisms for cutaneous and mucosal epithelia. Originally HPV types were based on less than 50 percent homology as determined in liquid hybridization assays, but DNA sequence data revealed more extensive homology among types.[12] Based on criteria adopted by the Papillomavirus Nomenclature Committee, types are defined as having less than 90 percent homology of the aggregate E6, E7, and L1 ORF DNA sequences. A new type can only be assigned once the complete 7.9-kb genome has been cloned. HPV subtypes have between 2 and 10 percent sequence divergence, and variants of a type have less than 2 percent divergence. The extent of intratypic variability may differ among types. For instance, there is no evidence of subtypes of HPV 16, with sequence variation running around 1 percent. On the other hand,

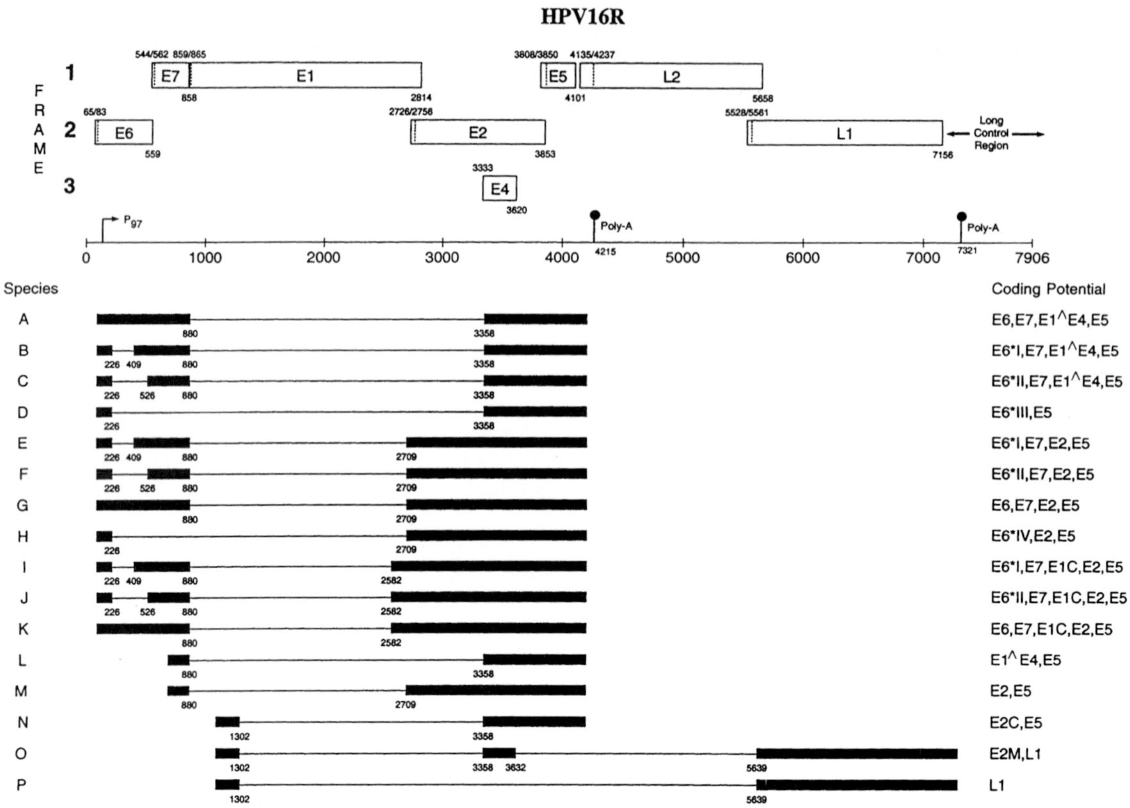

Fig. 24-1. Genome organization and RNA transcription pattern of HPV 16. The location of the HPV 16 ORFs in the correct reading frame is shown on top. The two numbers above the ORF correspond to the nucleotide (nt) start of the ORF followed by the nt start of the first ATG, using the revised sequence, HPV16R. Located below the genome are reported mRNA species; the solid bars are the exons and the thin lines are the introns. The numbers indicate the 5′ and 3′ boundaries of the introns. Contributed by C. Baker to the HPV database (http://hpv-web.lanl.gov/).

Table 24-1. Characterization of Proteins Encoded by HPV ORFs

ORF	Proteins	Approx. size	Functions	Refs.
E1	E1	68 kDa	Binds origin of replication; ATP-dependent helicase	(35,173–175)
	E1C	8 kDa	Unknown; encoded by several HPV mRNAs	
	E1N	23 kDa	Unknown; detected in BPV-1 transformants	(176)
E2	E2	48 kDa	Site-specific (ACCN$_6$GGT) transcription factor; heterodimerizes with E1 to facilitate replication initiation	(29,177–179)
	E2C	28 kDa	Lacks transactivation domain, may function to inhibit E2	(180)
E3		Unknown	Only present in BPVs	
E4	E1^E4	17 kDa and smaller processed forms	Very abundant protein; contains few codons of E1 fused to E4; interacts with cytokeratins	(31,181,182)
E5	E5	10 kDa	Promotes proliferation through growth factor signaling pathways (low-risk); transforming activity in vitro	(183–185)
E5b		Unknown	Only present in HPV 6, 11	
E6	E6	150 a.a.	Eliminates functional p53 (high-risk); alters transcription	(55,57,58)
	E6*, E6**	40–60 a.a.	Unknown, predicted in high-risk HPVs	(28)
E7	E7	100 a.a, migrates 20 kDa (high-risk)	Promotes proliferation by inactivating Rb and CKI function	(68,92,93,111)
E8	E8^E2	28 kDa	Only present in BPVs and HPV 6	
L1	L1	55 kDa	Major capsid protein, sufficient for self-assembly into capsid, neutralizing epitopes	(5,186,187)
L2	L2	50–60 kDa, migrates as 72 kDa	Minor capsid protein, function unknown	(5)

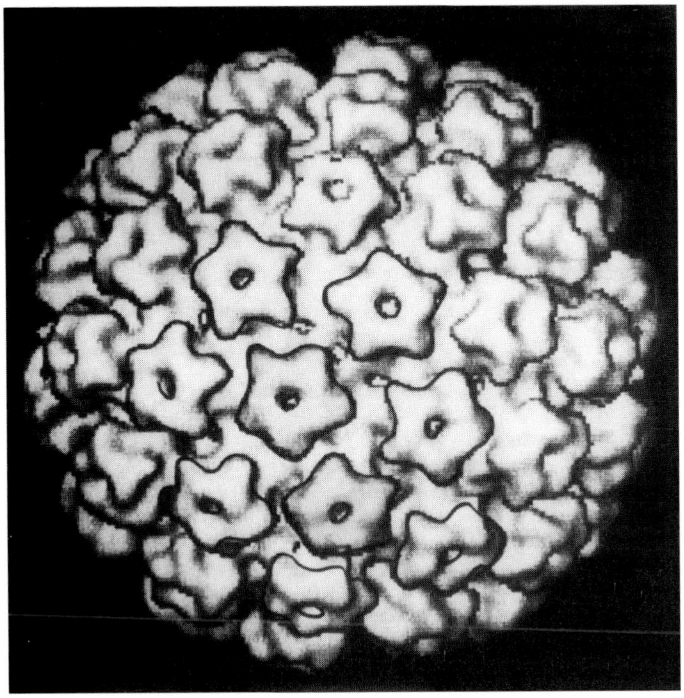

Fig. 24-2. Structure of the HPV virion. A three-dimensional reconstruction of cryoelectronmicrographs of a vaccinia virus-expressed HPV 1 capsid containing L1 and L2. Taken from Hagensee ME, Olson NH, Baker TS, et al. Three-dimensional structure of vaccinia virus-produced HPV-1 capsids. *J Virol* 1994;68:4503–4505.

a few subtypes of HPV 6 and HPV 45 have been found. Although HPV types clearly vary in their biological properties, it is largely unknown whether subtypes or variants have distinct biological behavior.

The genetic relationships among HPV types have been examined by the construction of phylogenetic trees based on various segments of the genome.[13] An example of a tree based on a partial L1 sequence that is frequently used in a PCR-based detection scheme with consensus primers is shown in Fig. 24-3.[14] The phylogenetic trees that were established based on the sequence of a segment of the consensus amplimer seemed to be highly related to trees based on more complete sequencing of the E6, E7, or L1 regions of the genome. This implies that the rate of evolution is constant throughout the genome. An important implication of the analysis is that HPV types with the same phylogenetic group have related biological behavior. Cutaneous versus mucosal types are in different branches, and cancer-related versus benign types are in separate groups. Importantly, novel sequences that are identified by PCR amplification of genital tract specimens were associated with disease in a way that could be predicted from their phylogenetic relationship to other mucosal papillomaviruses.[15]

VIRAL LIFE CYCLE

It has been difficult to study the life cycle of papillomaviruses because the full infectious life cycle has not been recapitulated in vitro. Viral infection or transfection of viral DNA into keratinocytes grown in monolayer cultures results in limited transcription and replication, without formation of infectious progeny, and a gradual loss of viral DNA.[16] Infectious virus has been produced in a xenograft system in which HPV 11 virus was used to infect fragments of tissue that were then implanted under the renal capsule of nude mice.[17] Characterization of viral transcripts produced in the xenografts has provided a great deal of information about

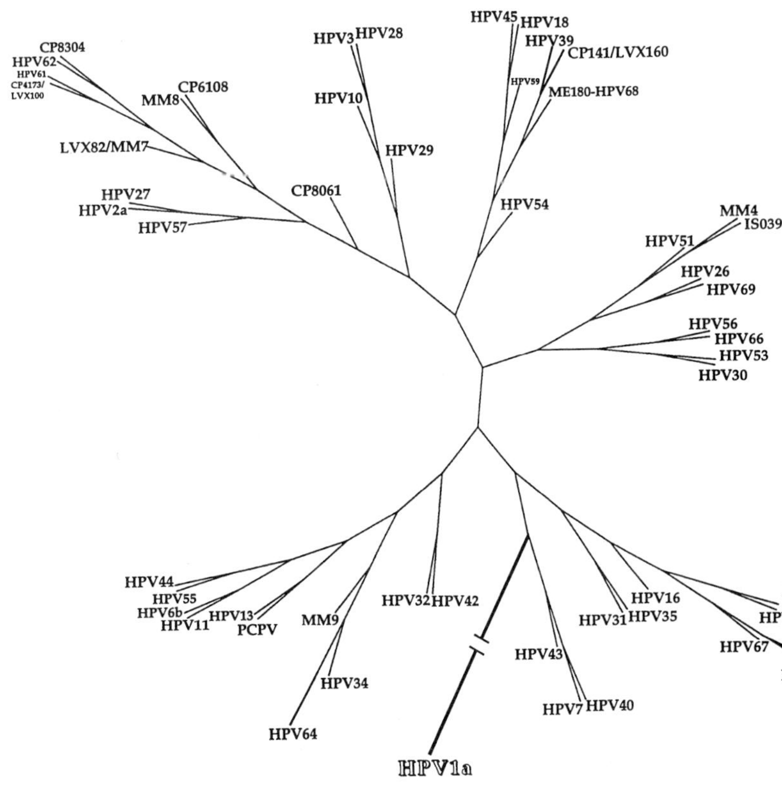

Fig. 24-3. Phylogenetic relatedness of genital HPVs. A phylogenetic tree based on maximum-likelihood evaluation of the My09/My11 consensus primer PCR fragment from the L1 gene. Taken from Bernard HU, Chan SY, Manos MM. Identification and assessment of known and novel human papillomaviruses by polymerase chain reaction, restriction digestion fingerprinting, nucleotide sequence, and phylogenetic algorithms. *J Infect Dis* 1994;170:1077–1085.

HPV 11 transcription.[18] Analyses of naturally occurring lesions have provided complementary results. Viral transcripts have been analyzed in cell lines harboring episomal HPV genomes, grown in monolayers or organotypic cultures.[19,20] On induction of complete keratinocyte differentiation, viral DNA replication, late gene expression, and formation of viral particles were observed, confirming the dependence of viral gene expression on the differentiated state of the host cell.[21,22] These in vitro observations are consistent with the restriction of vegetative HPV replication and formation of progeny to the most terminally differentiated layers of the epithelium. The recent techniques to introduce HPV genomes into keratinocytes followed by differentiation in organotypic cultures provide a means to do genetic analyses.[19]

ATTACHMENT, ENTRY, AND UNCOATING

Despite the exquisite species and cell type specificity of HPV infections, studies with labeled viral particles have shown that HPVs bind promiscuously to a wide range of cell types.[23,24] The inclusion of reporter DNA with the particles showed that entry also occurred in many cell types, indicating that the restriction of viral tropism is not owing to a cell type-specific receptor or coreceptor. Recently the $\alpha6$ integrin has been proposed as a candidate receptor based on the ability of VLPs to bind $\alpha6$ integrin, and for binding to be inhibited by anti-$\alpha6$ integrin antibodies and the $\alpha6$ integrin ligand, laminin.[25] The potential for $\alpha6$ integrin to serve as a receptor for papillomaviruses is consistent with its expression on basal epithelium; yet it is not clear how it can explain binding to many cell types. The L1 protein apparently mediates binding to the cell; VLPs containing L1 only can bind and can block binding of L1/L2 containing virions.[23] There is no information about the mechanism of entry into the cell, translocation to the nucleus, or uncoating of the viral genome.

TRANSCRIPTION OF VIRAL GENES

Transcription of HPV genes is tightly coordinated with the differentiated state of the cell, as evidenced by different RNA transcripts in different layers of the epithelium.[26,27] Expression of E1 and E2 is thought to occur in basal cells to maintain episomal replication of the HPV genome. Transcription of E6 and E7 is required to promote proliferation of parabasal cells, in order to provide the replication machinery for viral DNA replication. In the high-risk viruses E6 and E7 transcription is directed from a single promoter, p97 for HPV 16 and p105 for HPV 18, whereas the low-risk viruses use separate promoters for E6 and E7.[28,29] A basal level of transcription from the p97/p105 promoter is regulated by the keratinocyte-dependent enhancer in the NCR, and can be repressed by binding of E2 to its cognate recognition sequences located adjacent to the p97/p105 TATA boxes.[29,30] A viral transcript encoding the first few codons of E1 fused to the E4 ORF appears to be the major viral transcript in HPV-infected cells and specifies the viral protein designated E1^E4.[31] Regulation of the E1^E4 promoter is not well understood; however, this promoter appears to be used for transcription of the late gene products, L1 and L2, and both the capsid proteins and E1^E4 are only expressed in the most differentiated layers of the epithelium.[32] Late gene expression is also governed at the level of usage of the polyadenylation site, since late mRNAs do not terminate at the early poly A site at nt 4215 but continue to the site at nt 7321 (see Fig. 24-1).

VIRAL REPLICATION

It is widely believed that papillomaviruses have two modes of replication: stable replication of the episomal genome in basal cells, and runaway, or vegetative, replication in more differentiated cells to generate progeny virus. The initial stages of infection may involve limited amplification of the viral genome to maintain a stable but low copy number of viral genomes in basal cells. The origin of replication is located in the noncoding region and contains an AT-rich region, a region with dyad symmetry repeats to which E1 binds, and an adjacent E2 binding sequence.[33,34] E1 is the origin binding protein and has ATP-dependent helicase activity and interacts with the cellular polymerase–primase complex.[35,36] Although E2 is not absolutely required for replication in vitro, it strongly stimulates replication in vitro and is necessary for replication in vivo, presumably by recruiting other components to the preinitiation complex.[37,38] Apart from the origin-dependent initiation of replication, all other factors required for viral replication are encoded by the cell. It is unclear what regulates the switch from episomal to vegetative replication, except that it may depend on factors only found in terminally differentiating cells. One study with BPV-1 found that episomal replication occurred in proliferating cells, and extensive amplification of viral DNA only occurred in growth arrested cells.[39]

VIRUS ASSEMBLY AND RELEASE

There are no experimental models to study virus assembly or release. Viral particles have been observed in the nucleus of infected cells in the granular layer of the epithelium, where packaging of the genome likely occurs. There is no evidence that HPV infections are cytolytic; release of viral particles is a result of degeneration of desquamating cells.

ROLE OF HPVS IN CANCER

A role for human papillomaviruses (HPV) in the etiology of anogenital cancers has been firmly established based on a large number of molecular and epidemiologic studies. In a recent survey of approximately 1000 invasive cervical tumors obtained from 22 counties worldwide, 93 percent had HPV DNA detected by PCR, 50 percent of which was HPV 16.[3] No significant variation in positivity was found among countries, though the rates of cervical cancer varied markedly. Almost all studies using PCR are in agreement, finding over 75 percent of cervical cancers to contain HPV DNA.[40] The association of HPV with other genital tract tumors has been less well studied, and although the prevalence of HPV appears to be lower than in the cervix, consistent associations have been reported.[41] The epidemiologic and clinical relationship between preneoplastic lesions and HPV-containing anogenital cancers will be discussed elsewhere in this volume; this section will focus on the biological characteristics of high-risk HPVs that lead to the development of neoplasia.

E6 and E7 are the two viral genes that are invariably retained and expressed in tumors, and these two oncoproteins from the high-risk types, but not from low-risk types, are sufficient to immortalize cells in culture.[42–44] Immortalization studies have shown that E6 and E7 can independently extend the life span of cells in culture; however, efficient escape from crisis requires both E6 and E7 and also involves additional cellular changes.[45] Immortalized cell lines are not tumorigenic when assayed in nude mice, but tumorigenic derivatives could be established spontaneously with long-term culture or induced by carcinogen treatment.[46,47] Tumorigenicity is accompanied with additional cytogenetic changes. Taken together the current evidence suggests that the high-risk HPV E6 and E7 oncoproteins provide several critical functions for the development of neoplasia. First, E7 disrupts the signal that normally prevents a cell from entering S phase once the cell has left the basal layer. The increased number of proliferating cells increases the number of cells that are available as targets for additional genetic alterations, or "hits," that lead to neoplasia. Second, both E6 and E7 bypass damage-induced DNA checkpoints and other growth arrest signals. Inactivation of cell cycle checkpoints allows genetic instability, and the failure to eliminate cells that have undergone potentially deleterious changes contributes to the development of neoplasia. Third, E6 activates the expression of telomerase, allowing the continued proliferation of cells.[48] The development of invasive cancer, or tumorigenicity in animals, requires the activation of genes that favor penetration of the basement membrane, altered interactions with the matrix to permit growth in the stroma or other tissues, and new growth factor requirements. Additional cytogenetic changes accompany tumorigenicity. Inactivation of checkpoints allows the continued genetic instability that gives rise to the new genetic changes required for tumorigenicity; however, it is unclear whether the viral oncogenes directly promote expression of genes involved in invasion and metastasis.

Predictions about the role of HPV in neoplasia obtained from experimental studies are consistent with the natural history of cervical cancer. Among women who develop squamous intraepithelial lesions (SIL), the time from first detection of viral DNA to lesions is short, approximately 2 years, though factors like number of partners and infection with other STDs may influence the interval.[49] Even mildly dysplastic lesions show an increase in proliferation and polyploidization. These changes result as a direct consequence of expression of E6/E7. The median age of carcinoma in situ (CIS) in the United States is 29, indicating that approximately a decade has elapsed between the initial infection and severe dysplasia.[50,51] CIS lesions are characterized by their aneuploid DNA content and thus reflect the genetic instability that accompanies prolonged expression of E6/E7. The preneoplastic lesions can regress spontaneously. One principal explanation for their regression is likely to be an effective immune response, and generalized T-cell deficiency has been associated with increased dysplasia.[52] Other explanations may include the fact that some, perhaps most, alterations will be deleterious, resulting in cell death. The median age of invasive cervical cancer in the United States is 49, indicating that additional changes required for invasion and metastasis are acquired slowly over time.

FUNCTIONS OF E6 AND E7

The genital HPV E6 proteins are approximately 150 amino acids in length and contain four cys-x-x-cys motifs involved in binding zinc.[53,54] E6 proteins have activities that activate or repress various heterologous promoters.[55,56] HPV 16 E6 binds to p53 in concert with a cellular ubiquitin conjugating enzyme, E6AP, and targets p53 for degradation.[57,58] HPV 6 E6 has a greatly reduced ability to bind p53 in vitro, it does not target p53 for degradation in vitro, and the intracellular level of p53 in cells expressing 6E6 is unaffected.[57,59,60] Sedman et al. found that mutant p53 could cooperate with 16E7 to immortalize human keratinocytes, suggesting that the inactivation of p53 might be the sole function of E6 in immortalization; however, mutant p53 could not substitute for E6 in the transformation of rodent fibroblasts.[61] Using mutants of 16E6 that resulted in degradation of p53 but failed to immortalize human embryonic kidney cells in cooperation with 16E7, Nakagawa et al. concluded that degradation of p53 was necessary but not sufficient for E6-mediated immortalization.[62] HPV 16 E6 has been shown to bind other cellular proteins also, such as ERC-55, paxcillin, and hDLG, but the significance to the viral life cycle or to the induction of neoplasia is unknown at this time.[63–66]

The genital HPV E7 proteins are approximately 100 amino acids and contain two cys-x-x-cys repeats in the carboxy terminal half of the protein that bind zinc.[67] The amino terminal half of E7 shares two conserved regions of homology (CR1 and CR2) with the E1A oncoproteins of adenoviruses and with the SV40 T antigen. All of these oncoproteins bind to the retinoblastoma (Rb) tumor suppressor, p105Rb, and other Rb-related pocket proteins, such as p107 and p130, through a well defined motif, LxCxE present in CR2.[68,69] HPV 16 E7 binds Rb much more strongly both in vitro and in vivo than does HPV 6 E7, and transformation activity parallels Rb binding activity.[70,71] Interestingly, HPV 1 E7 has been shown to bind Rb with high affinity, though it failed to transform cells.[72] In that study, 1 E7 was not able to transactivate an E2F responsive promoter, suggesting that although 1 E7 bound Rb, it was not able to inactivate the tumor suppressor activity of Rb, that is, sequestering E2F transcription factor.[73] Several studies have shown that mutated 16E7 proteins that were unable to bind to Rb were transformation-deficient, although one study has shown that immortalization of keratinocytes might not involve Rb binding.[74–80] Although Rb binding was required for transformation, a number of mutated E7 constructs were fully competent to bind Rb yet were still transformation-deficient.[78,79] Residues in CR1 of E1A have been implicated in the release of E2F from Rb; however, the CR1 domain of HPV 16 E7 does not appear to disrupt the Rb–E2F interaction.[81–83] Alternatively, some other function of E7 in addition to Rb binding may be necessary for transformation. Mutations in the amino terminal region of both E1A and E7 also result in transformation-deficient oncoproteins. This region of E1A oncoprotein can bind to p300, a CREB-related transcription factor.[84,85] However, no p300 binding activity has been identified for E7. Furthermore, E1A constructs mutated in the p300 binding domain can complement E1A proteins mutated in the Rb binding domain, whereas HPV 16 E7 constructs mutated in the Rb binding domain could not complement E1A proteins mutated in the p300 binding domain.[86] Additionally, mutations affecting the zinc fingers found in the carboxy terminal end of E1A and E7 have both shown to be transformation-deficient.

DISRUPTION OF CELL CYCLE CONTROL

In normal epithelium, proliferation is restricted to a few cells in the basal layer; suprabasal cells exit the cell cycle and undergo terminal differentiation. Experimental studies have shown that high-risk E7 prevents quiescence resulting in proliferating cells throughout the epithelium.[87,88] Although the molecular mechanism that imposes a G1 arrest on epithelial cells as they leave the basal layer is not fully known, both Rb and the cyclin-dependent kinase (CDK) inhibitor (CKI) p21 have been implicated. p21 Associates with the G1 cyclin/CDK complexes, preventing the phosphorylation of Rb and other critical targets required for progression into S phase.[89] The E7 protein is capable of uncoupling proliferation and differentiation, allowing cellular and viral replication in cells expressing differentiation markers.[87,88,90] The mechanism likely involves both release of E2F and binding to $p21^{cip1}$.[91–93]

Large hyperchromatic nuclei characteristic of polyploid nuclei are observed in cells engineered experimentally to express E7 or E6/E7, as well as in HPV associated lesions. This observation suggests that that the viral oncoproteins can disrupt the S/M checkpoint that insures that S phase does not reinitiate without an intervening round of mitosis. Inactivation of p53 has been shown to disrupt the mitotic spindle checkpoint, and recent studies have suggested that p21 is required for S/M coordination, though the mechanism is not known.[94,95] Thus E7 bypasses control of epithelial cell proliferation, and both E6 and E7 may contribute to the development of polyploidy by disrupting the S/M checkpoint.

In response to DNA damage cells arrest in the G1 and G2 phases of the cell cycle, presumably to allow time to repair the

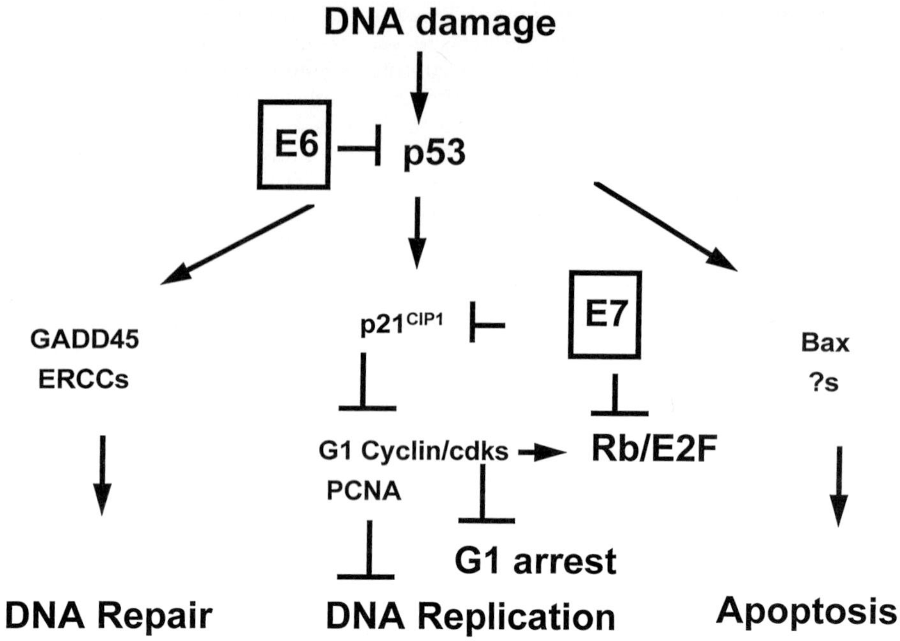

Fig. 24-4. Interaction of HPV oncogenes with DNA damage pathways. DNA damage induces cell cycle arrest and DNA repair or apoptosis. The HPV oncogenes interact with the pathway in various ways to bypass arrest and apoptosis.

damage before initiating DNA synthesis or mitosis.[96] Arrest in G1 is dependent upon the ability of a cell to induce p53, which results in the transactivation of a number of p53 responsive genes, the most critical of which appears to be p21^{cip1}.[97,98] By binding to cyclin/CDK complexes, p21 inhibits progression from G1 into S phase. Induction of p21 also inhibits PCNA-dependent DNA replication, though short-range DNA synthesis required for repair is not affected.[99,100] Other genes involved in DNA repair are also transactivated by p53. As an alternative to growth arrest, cells can undergo apoptosis in response to DNA damage. The decision as to which pathway to take is not completely understood but is influenced by cell type-specific factors, the presence or levels of p53, and conflicting signals for growth proliferation and growth arrest.[101] p53-Inducible genes such as Bax can promote apoptosis.

Both E6 and E7 are able to bypass DNA damage-induced interest; the pathways are distinct for the two viral oncogenes and are summarized below and in Fig. 24-4. Elimination of p53 by HPV 16 E6 leads to low levels of p21 and efficient bypass of the DNA damage-induced G1 checkpoint.[102,103] The use of mutated E6 proteins demonstrated that the ability to abrogate G1 arrest was completely correlated with E6-mediated degradation of p53.[60] The inability of HPV 6 E6 to bypass a DNA damage-induced growth arrest reinforces that 6E6 is not able to inactivate p53. HPV 16 E7, but not 6E7, bypasses a damage-induced G1 checkpoint independently of p53 through mechanisms that are not completely understood.[102,104,105] Inactivation of Rb by 16E7 obviates the requirement for cyclin D/CDK4 activity, and the subsequent release of E2F transcription factors from Rb activates the transcription of genes required for S phase, including cyclin E, which has been shown to be required for S phase entry.[106–109] Accordingly, cyclin E has been shown to be elevated in E7 expressing cells.[110] Inactivation of CKI-mediated growth arrest signals likely involves additional activities of E7 that include direct binding to CKIs.[92,93,111]

ADDITIONAL CELLULAR FACTORS

A great deal of interest has focused on the observation that integration of HPV sequences into the cellular genome frequently accompanies progression to malignancy.[112,113] Unlike retroviruses there is no specific viral integration site, but the frequent disruption of the early region has been postulated to provide a means to increase E6/E7 gene expression by either eliminating transcriptional repression by E2 or exchanging the viral 3′ end of the E6/E7 RNA that contains a RNA destabilizing element for a more stable 3′ end encoded by cellular sequences.[114,115] The chromosomal site into which HPV sequences integrate is nonspecific or at least occurs on many different chromosomes. Integration of HPV genomes has been reported to occur preferentially at fragile sites, perhaps because the chromatin structure provides easier access for recombination complexes.[116–118] Some studies have found integrated HPV sequences in proximity to cellular proto-oncogenes, but consistent activation of the oncogenes as a consequence of HPV integration has not been demonstrated.[116,117,119] Although integration of HPV sequences into the cellular genome is a frequent feature of invasive carcinomas, it is not obligatory as some HPV 16–positive tumors retain only episomal genomes.[120–122]

The identification of consistently observed chromosomal abnormalities in cervical carcinomas has been hampered by the difficulty of obtaining a sufficient number of metaphases for karyotypic analyses. Early studies found that cervical carcinomas were frequently aneuploid or tetraploid, and reported frequent alterations in chromosomes 1, 3, and 11.[123–125] Loss of heterozygosity has also been reported for 3p.[126] Comparative genome hybridization identified overrepresentation of 3q as a pivotal genetic change that marked the transition from severe dysplasia to invasive cancer.[127] A gain of 3q was observed in 1/13 severe dysplasias and in 9/10 invasive cervical cancers.

HPV-immortalized human epithelial cells are generally not tumorigenic, but long-term passage in culture can spontaneously give rise to tumorigenic derivatives, or they can be induced by treatment with carcinogens.[46,47] These experimentally derived tumor cell lines have been used to identify genes that may be responsible for the conversion to malignancy. Cytogenetic changes that accompany the progression to tumorigenicity were studied in a HPV 18–immortalized cell line, 18-11.[128] A striking but unstable aberration of chromosome 3 occurred very early after establishment of the cells in culture. Postcrisis, the length of the derivative three stabilized, but the long arm contained a complex rearrangement of other chromosomes. Concomitant with the development of tumorigenicity the ETS2 oncogene that maps to 21q22 was translocated to the derivative #3.[129] A similar translocation of ETS2 to 3qter was observed in the carcinogen-induced tumorigenic line. Importantly, cytogenetic analyses of cervical cancers have frequently reported changes in chromosome 3, suggesting that the model systems mimic authentic tumor development.[125]

IMMUNE RESPONSE TO HPV INFECTION

Because of the lack of authentic viral antigens and the difficulty in unambiguously identifying HPV-negative populations, it has been difficult to study the immune response to HPV infections. Additionally, HPV infections seemingly fail to produce a robust immune response, perhaps because of their restricted intraepithelial location. However, several lines of evidence suggest that papillomaviruses eventually generate effective immunity. The majority of HPV-associated lesions regress spontaneously, accompanied by lymphocyte infiltration of the lesions.[130] Conversely, immunosuppression is associated with reactivation of HPV. Infected individuals were shown to harbor the same HPV 16 variant over time, despite contact with new partners, yet they acquired new HPV types, suggesting that infection results in type-specific protection.[131] Studies in animals support the hypothesis that neutralizing antibodies protect in a type-specific manner against papillomavirus infection.

ANTIBODIES AND T CELLS

Many studies have shown that human sera have antibodies that react with HPV proteins.[132] The earliest studies used HPV virions extracted from tissues but did not take into account the heterogeneity of virus types. The next generation of antigen targets relied on bacterially expressed fusion proteins or synthetic peptides and used assays in which only antibodies that recognized linear epitopes would be detected. In most individuals these antibodies recognize capsid proteins, particularly L2, and the correlation with other parameters of infection was weak. Antibodies to other HPV proteins have been reported, but the results were more variable. Several groups have demonstrated that the prevalence of antibodies to the HPV 16 or 18 E7 protein is increased in cases with cervical cancer compared with age-matched controls.[133,134] However, only 25 to 50 percent of patients with HPV DNA-proven cancers have antibodies to E7 from the homologous HPV type, and these appear to develop as a consequence of prolonged exposure to the tumor rather than as a prognostic indicator of tumor development.

The newest generation of antigen targets are HPV capsids, or VLPs, of defined specificity that are obtained from recombinant vaccinia viruses or baculoviruses expressing L1 or L1 plus L2. Using capsids in an ELISA, it has been shown that infected individuals have "type-specific" (at least not broadly cross-reactive) antibodies to a conformational epitope(s) on the L1 protein and that these antibodies correlate strongly with a history of HPV-associated disease.[135–137] Experimentally infected animals generate similar antibodies that have been shown to be neutralizing.[138] Neutralization of human papillomaviruses has largely been restricted to assays measuring inhibition of HPV 11 production in xenografts, but those studies have found neutralizing antibodies in human sera.[139,140] Systems to assay neutralization of other types using pseudovirions are being developed.[141] It has been interesting to note that the tempo of development of serum anticapsid antibodies is very slow. Among women thought to be newly infected with HPV 16, the median time to seroconversion was approximately 1 year.[45] Viral titers were low, that is, a mean of 1:100. The duration of detectable antibodies has been more difficult to determine. In a cross-sectional study, HPV-1 antibodies were found to wane over 10 years; however, a recent longitudinal study in an STD clinic population suggested that antibodies to genital types routinely persist for decades (Grubert T, Shoultz D, Koutsky L, et al., in preparation).[135]

Although neutralizing antibodies may be useful in preventing infection, the cell-mediated immune response is likely to be important in controlling reactivation and regression of infections. Individuals with congenital T-cell deficiencies or who are immunosuppressed iatrogenically show increased evidence of HPV-associated disease.[52] HIV-positive men and women show increased levels of HPV DNA in the genital tract and an increased prevalence of dysplasia.[142,143] HPV infections elicit an inflammatory response at the lesion, but the cellular nature of the response and the viral antigen specificity remain to be better characterized.[130] Several studies have been able to demonstrate that HPV antigens introduced into mice can generate lymphoproliferative and cytotoxic responses.[52] Demonstrating T-cell responses in humans has been more difficult, perhaps because of problems in obtaining suitable cells and reagents, or because there are very small numbers of circulating HPV-specific precursors. Early studies looking at lymphoproliferative responses in vitro or delayed-type hypersensitivity suggested that T-cell responses were most abundant in people whose warts regressed spontaneously, while few responses were found in people with first episode warts or warts of long duration.[144] Low levels of lymphocyte proliferation to HPV antigens or peptides have been reported in normal women and in women attending colposcopy clinics.[145–147] In a more recent study, lymphoproliferative responses to E6 and E7 were associated with clearance of HPV infection and regression of lesions.[148] The detection of cytolytic T-cell (CTL) responses to HPV antigens has also been difficult, with many negative results.[149] Surprisingly, T-cell clones of defined specificity to the E4 protein of HPV 1 were the first to be established.[150] Recently, CTLs to the high-risk oncoproteins have been detected in the peripheral blood, draining lymph nodes and tumors of cervical cancer patients, whereas none were detected in healthy controls.[151]

Normal squamous cell epithelium of the cervix and epithelium from low-grade lesions do not express HLA class II molecules, indicating that the infected epithelial cell itself does not present antigen.[152] However, in a proportion of invasive cervical cancers, tumor cells have been shown to turn on the expression of class II DR molecules and to downregulate the expression of class I MHC at the cell surface accompanied by transcriptional downregulation of the transporter genes.[153–155] There is no evidence to indicate that this strategy to disrupt antigen presentation is mediated by a viral gene.

VACCINE POSSIBILITIES

A strong argument in favor of HPV vaccines is the encouraging results that have been achieved in animal papillomavirus models. Prophylactic vaccination with virus or recombinant capsid proteins has been shown to fully or partially protect against virus challenge or at least accelerate rejection. Several studies have suggested that immunogens that contain conformational epitopes found on the intact virus provide better protection than denatured immunogens. Dogs immunized with native, but not denatured, recombinant canine oral papillomavirus (COPV) L1 VLPs were fully protected from challenge.[156] Calves vaccinated with purified BPV 2 virus were fully protected from fibroma or fibropapillomavirus formation after challenge, whereas calves vaccinated with

BPV 2 L1 or L2 fusion proteins developed fibromas or fibropapillomas, respectively, that regressed rapidly postchallenge in comparison with unvaccinated calves.[157] Similar results were reported for another cutaneous bovine papillomavirus, BPV-1, and an L2 fusion protein from a mucosal virus, BPV 4, protected against challenge by BPV 4 via the palate.[158,159] Early studies showed that rabbits could be protected from papilloma formation by vaccination with cottontail rabbit papillomavirus (CRPV or Shope virus), and more recent studies have shown that either L1 or L2 CRPV-fusion proteins could confer immunity.[160–162] Interestingly, only the intact, nondenatured, full-length L1 fusion protein provided protection that was interpreted to indicate that conformational epitopes were likely to be important.[163] Many of these studies also concluded that the generation of a neutralizing antibody response was important in the success of a prophylactic vaccine. In the dog model, protection could be conferred by passive transfer of antibody.[156] Neutralizing antibodies (NA) are efficiently generated to intact viruses or capsids and frequently react with conformational epitopes on the L1 protein.[164] Weaker NA activity can be generated with L1 fusion proteins, and the success in generating NA and protective responses was related to the adjuvant that was used with the fusion proteins.[165] The relative contribution of L1 versus L2 in generating NA and in conferring protection has been controversial; it is unclear whether the different results are related to biological differences among the papillomaviruses or technical differences in the preparation or administration of the immunogens.

Both cutaneous and mucosal bovine papillomaviruses seem to be responsive to therapeutic vaccination. Both L2 and E7 fusion proteins (but not E2) have reduced the number, severity, and duration of lesions, and the partial protection conferred by some preparations of L1 resulted in an amelioration of the course of lesion formation and regression.[159,165,166] Animal models have also suggested the possibility of generating an antitumor response. When mice were inoculated with fibroblasts expressing HPV 16 E6 or E7, they could reject challenge by a melanoma cell line expressing the HPV oncogenes; the response was antigen, MHC, and CD8 restricted.[167,168] A peptide from HPV 16 E7 that was shown to bind to a specific MHC allele was found to protect mice from a syngeneic HPV 16 tumor in an MHC-restricted fashion.[169] Vaccinia virus recombinants expressing the BPV E5, E6, or E7 genes could retard the development of tumors resulting from challenge with a BPV-transformed cell line in syngeneic rats.[170] Extension of the latency period for tumor development versus abrogation or regression of tumor was speculated to be related to the dose of immunogen, the adjuvant used, or the immunization protocol.

Currently, a number of vaccine studies in humans have been initiated, though it is too early to assess the efficacy of the vaccines, or in most cases even the immunogenicity of the preparations.[171] The first trials have focused on immunotherapy for cervical cancer. Borysiewicz et al. vaccinated late-stage cancer patients with a vaccinia virus recombinant expressing modified E6 and E7 genes from HPV 16 and 18.[172] Apart from demonstrating that the vaccine was safe, they found that many of the patients had an impaired immune response to recall antigens; however, one patient demonstrated a clear CTL response to the HPV antigens. This approach as well as similar strategies using E7 protein or peptides are being examined both in cancer patients and in women with preneoplastic lesions.[171] Early trials aimed at prophylactic vaccines have begun using HPV capsids as immunogens.

Although the vaccination studies in animal models provide encouragement there are many questions that remain unanswered, some of which are unique to papillomaviruses, others of which are common for many vaccines. The lack of infectious virus that can be propagated either in tissue culture or in animals presents a serious problem for preclinical testing of HPV vaccines. The prophylactic vaccines used in animals did not address the efficacy of providing immunity in the genital tract or other mucosal sites, nor was the duration of immunity studied. However, epidemiologic data provide some support for the notion that protection against HPV infection in adolescence and in young adults might have a big impact in reducing the incidence of condyloma, dysplasia, and cervical cancer. Whether the generation of neutralizing antibody will be sufficient to achieve sterilizing immunity or whether cell-mediated immunity will also be required for prophylactic vaccines is not clear at this time. The experience with BPV vaccines also provides optimism for the feasibility of therapeutic vaccines, both in mediating regression of HPV infection and in antitumor activity. Yet it is unclear which component of the T-cell response should be targeted, and assays to measure the T-cell response are not well developed. Equally the animal experiments have looked at protection from tumor challenge rather than elimination of existing tumor. Despite these problems, vaccination to protect against HPV infection and to modulate the progression of HPV disease may well be a tractable problem.

References

1 Howley PM. Papillomavirinae: the viruses and their replication. In: Fields BN, Knipe DM, Howley PM, eds. *Fields virology*. 3rd ed. Philadelphia: Lippincott-Raven, 1996, pp. 2045–2076.

2 zurHausen H. Molecular pathogenesis of cancer of the cervix and its causation by specific human papillomavirus types. In: zurHausen H, ed. *Human pathogenic papillomaviruses*. Heidelberg: Springer Verlag, 1994, pp. 131–156.

3 Bosch FX et al. Prevalence of human papillomavirus in cervical cancer: a worldwide perspective. *J Natl Cancer Inst* 1995;87:796–802.

4 Baker CC. The genomes of the papillomaviruses. In: O'Brien SJ, ed. *Genetic maps: locus maps of complex genomes*. Cold Spring Harbor, NY: Cold Spring Harbor Laboratory Press, 1993, pp. 134 –146.

5 Heilman CA et al. Cloning of human papillomavirus genomic DNAs and analysis of homologous polynucleotide sequences. *J Virol* 1980; 36:395–407.

6 Lorincz AT et al. A new type of papillomavirus associated with cancer of the uterine cervix. *Virology* 1987;159:187–190.

7 Smotkin D et al. Oncogenic and nononcogenic human papillomaviruses generate the E7 mRNA by different mechanisms. *J Virol* 1989; 63:1441–1447.

8 Firzlaff JM et al. Detection of human papillomavirus capsid antigens in various squamous epithelial lesions using antibodies directed against the L1 and L2 open reading frames. *Virology* 1988;164:467–477.

9 Baker TS et al. Structures of bovine and human papillomaviruses—analysis by cryoelectron microscopy and three-dimensional image reconstruction. *Biophys J* 1991;60:1445–1456.

10 Belnap DM et al. Conserved features in papillomavirus and polyomavirus capsids. *J Mol Biol* 1996;259:249–263.

11 Hagensee ME et al. Three-dimensional structure of vaccinia virus-produced HPV-1 capsids. *J Virol* 1994;68:4503–4505.

12 Coggin J, zurHausen H. Workshop on papillomaviruses and cancer. *Cancer* Res 1979;39:545–546.

13 Myers G et al. *Human Papillomaviruses, 1996. A compilation and analysis of nucleic acid and amino acid sequences.* Los Alamos: Los Alamos National Laboratory, 1994.

14 Gravitt PE, Manos MM. Polymerase chain reaction-based methods for the detection of human papillomavirus DNA. In: Munoz M, Bosch FX, Shah KV, et al., eds. *The epidemiology of human papillomavirus and cervical cancer*. Lyon: IARC Scientific, 1992, pp. 121–133.

15 Bernard HU et al. Identification and assessment of known and novel human papillomaviruses by polymerase chain reaction, restriction di-

gestion fingerprinting, nucleotide sequence, and phylogenetic algorithms. *J Infect Dis* 1994;170:1077–1085.

16 Taichman LP, LaPorta RF. The expression of papillomaviruses in epithelial cells. In: Salzman NP, Howley PM, eds. *The Papovaviridae,* vol. 2: *The papillomaviruses.* New York: Plenum, 1986, pp. 109–139.

17 Kreider JW et al. Morphological transformation in vivo of human uterine cervix with papillomavirus from condylomata acuminata. *Nature* 1985;317:639–641.

18 Stoler MH et al. Infectious cycle of human papillomavirus type 11 in human foreskin xenografts in nude mice. *J Virol* 1990;64:3310–3318.

19 Frattini MG et al. In vitro synthesis of oncogenic human papillomaviruses requires episomal genomes for differentiation-dependent late expression. *Proc Natl Acad Sci USA* 1996;93:3062–3067.

20 Pray TR, Laimins LA. Differentiation-dependent expression of E1–E4 proteins in cell lines maintaining episomes of human papillomavirus type 31b. *Virology* 1995;206:679–685.

21 Meyers C et al. Biosynthesis of human papillomavirus from a continuous cell line upon epithelial differentiation. *Science* 1992;257:971–973.

22 Dollard SC et al. Production of human papillomavirus and modulation of the infectious program in epithelial raft cultures. *Genes Dev* 1992;6:1131–1142.

23 Roden RB et al. Interaction of papillomaviruses with the cell surface. *J Virol* 1994;68:7260–7266.

24 Muller M et al. Papillomavirus capsid binding and uptake by cells from different tissues and species. *J Virol* 1995;69:948–954.

25 Evander M et al. Identification of the alpha6 integrin as a candidate receptor for papillomaviruses. *J Virol* 1997;71:2449–2456.

26 Barksdale SK, Baker CC. Differentiation-specific expression from the bovine papillomavirus type 1P2443 and late promoters. *J Virol* 1993; 67:5605–5616.

27 Chow LT et al. Human papilloma virus gene expression. In: Steinberg BM, Brandsma JL, Taichman LB, eds. *Papillomaviruses.* Cold Spring Harbor, NY: Cold Spring Harbor Press, 1987, pp. 55 –72.

28 Smotkin D, Wettstein FO. Transcription of human papillomavirus type 16 early genes in a cervical cancer and a cancer-derived cell line and identification of the E7 protein. *Proc Natl Acad Sci USA* 1986; 83:4680–4684.

29 Thierry F, Yaniv M. The BPV1-E2 trans-acting protein can be either an activator or a repressor of the HPV 18 regulatory region. *EMBO J* 1987;6:3391–3397.

30 Romanczuk H et al. Mutational analysis of *cis* elements involved in E2 modulation of human papillomavirus type 16 P97 and type 18 P105 promoters. *J Virol* 1990;64:2849–2859.

31 Nasseri M et al. A human papillomavirus type 11 transcript encoding an E1^E4 protein. *Virology* 1987;159:433–439.

32 Doorbar J et al. Identification of the human papillomavirus-1a E4 gene products. *EMBO J* 1986;5:355–362.

33 Chiang C et al. Viral E1 and E2 proteins support replication of homologous and heterologous papillomavirus origins. *Proc Natl Acad Sci USA* 1992;89:5799–5803.

34 DelVecchio AM et al. Transient replication of human papillomavirus DNAs. *J Virol* 1992;66:5949–5958.

35 Seo Y et al. Bovine papilloma virus-encoded E1 protein contains multiple activities required for BPV DNA replication. *Proc Natl Acad Sci USA* 1993;90:702–706.

36 Yang L et al. The E1 protein of bovine papilloma virus 1 is an ATP-dependent DNA helicase. *Proc Natl Acad Sci USA* 1993;90:5086–5090.

37 Ustav M, Stenlund A. Transient replication of BPV-1 requires two viral polypeptides encoded by the E1 and E2 open reading frames. *EMBO J* 1991;10:449–457.

38 Yang L et al. Activation of BPV-1 replication in vitro by the transcription factor E2. *Science* 1991;353:628–632.

39 Burnett S et al. Loss of bovine papillomavirus DNA replication control in growth-arrested transformed cells. *J Virol* 1989;63:2215–2225.

40 Anonymous. *IARC Monographs on the evaluation of carcinogenic risks to humans.* Lyon: IARC, 1995.

41 Daling JR, Scherman KJ. Relationship between human papillomavirus infection and tumours of anogenital sites other than the cervix. In: Munoz N, Bosch FX, Shah KV, et al., eds. *The epidemiology of cervical cancer and human papillomavirus.* Lyon: IARC, 1992, pp. 223 –241.

42 Schwarz E et al. Structure and transcription of human papillomavirus sequences in cervical carcinoma cells. *Nature* 1985;314:111–114.

43 Hawley-Nelson P et al. HPV 16 E6 and E7 proteins cooperate to immortalize human foreskin keratinocytes. *EMBO J* 1989;8:3905–3910.

44 Münger K et al. The E6 and E7 genes of the human papillomavirus type 16 together are necessary and sufficient for transformation of primary human keratinocytes. *J Virol* 1989;63:4417–4421.

45 Carter JJ et al. The natural history of human papillomavirus type 16 capsid antibodies among a cohort of university women. *J Infect Dis* 1996;174:927–936.

46 Hurlin PJ et al. Progression of human papillomavirus type 18-immortalized human keratinocytes to a malignant phenotype. *Proc Natl Acad Sci USA* 1991;88:570–574.

47 Garrett LR et al. Interaction of HPV-18 and nitrosomethylurea in the induction of squamous cell carcinoma. *Carcinogenesis* 1993;14:329–332.

48 Klingelhutz AJ et al. Telomerase activation by the E6 gene product of human papillomavirus type 16. *Nature* 1996;380:79–82.

49 Shoultz DA et al. Epidemiology and modes of transmission. In: vonKrogh G, Gross G, eds. *Human papillomaviruses.* Boca Raton, FL: CRC Press, 1997, pp. 83–97.

50 Devesa S et al. Recent trends in cervix uteri cancer. *Cancer* 1989;64: 2184–2190.

51 Wiggins CL et al. *Cancer in western Washington state, Seattle,* 37th ed. Seattle: Fred Hutchinson Cancer Research Center, 1993.

52 Tindle RW, Frazer IH. Immune response to human papillomaviruses and the prospects for human papillomavirus-specific immunization. In: zurHausen H, ed. *Human pathogenic papillomaviruses.* Heidelberg: Springer Verlag, 1994, pp. 217–253.

53 Barbosa MS et al. Papillomavirus polypeptides E6 and E7 are zinc-binding proteins. *J Virol* 1989;63:1404–1407.

54 Grossman SR, Laimins LA. E6 protein of human papillomavirus type 18 binds zinc. *Oncogene* 1989;4:1089–1093.

55 Sedman SA et al. The full-length E6 protein of human papillomavirus type 16 has transforming and trans-activation activities and cooperates with E7 to immortalize keratinocytes in culture. *J Virol* 1991; 65:4860–4866.

56 Etscheid BG et al. The E6 protein of human papillomavirus type 16 functions as a transcriptional repressor in a mechanism independent of the tumor suppressor protein, p53. *Virology* 1994;205:583–585.

57 Werness BA et al. Association of human papillomavirus types 16 and 18 E6 proteins with p53. *Science* 1990;248:76–79.

58 Scheffner M et al. The HPV-16 E6 and E6-AP complex functions as a ubiquitin-protein ligase in the ubiquitination of p53. *Cell* 1993;75: 495–505.

59 Crook T et al. Degradation of p53 can be targeted by HPV E6 sequences distinct from those required for p53 binding and trans-activation. *Cell* 1991;67:547–556.

60 Foster SA et al. The ability of human papillomavirus E6 proteins to target p53 for degradation in vivo correlates with their ability to abrogate actinomycin D-induced growth arrest. *J Virol* 1994;68: 5698–5705.

61 Sedman SA et al. Mutant p53 can substitute for human papillomavirus type 16 E6 in immortalization of human keratinocytes but does not have E6-associated trans-activation or transforming activity. *J Virol* 1992;66:4201–4208.

62 Nakagawa S et al. Mutational analysis of human papillomavirus type 16 E6 protein: transforming function for human cells and degradation of p53 in vitro. *Virology* 1995;212:535–542.

63 Chen JJ et al. Interaction of papillomavirus E6 oncoproteins with a putative calcium binding protein. *Science* 1995;269:529–531.

64 Tong X, Howley PM. The bovine papillomavirus E6 oncoprotein interacts with paxillin and disrupts the actin cytoskeleton. *Proc Natl Acad Sci USA* 1997;94:4412–4417.
65 Lee SS et al. Binding of human virus oncoproteins to hDlg/SAP97, a mammalian homolog of the *Drosophilia* discs large tumor suppressor protein. *Proc Natl Acad Sci USA* 1997;94:6670–6675.
66 Kiyono T et al. Binding of high risk human papillomavirus E6 oncoproteins to the human homologue of the *Drosophilia* discs large tumor suppressor protein. *Proc Natl Acad Sci USA* 1997;94: 11612–11616.
67 Munger K et al. Interactions of HPV E6 and E7 with tumor suppressor gene products. *Cancer Surv* 1992;12:197–217.
68 Dyson N et al. The human papilloma virus-16 E7 oncoprotein is able to bind to the retinoblastoma gene product. *Science* 1989;243:934–937.
69 Davies R et al. Human papillomavirus type 16 E7 associates with a histone H1 kinase and with p107 through sequences necessary for transformation. *J Virol* 1993;67:2521–2528.
70 Munger K et al. Complex formation of the human papillomavirus E7 proteins with the retinoblastoma tumor suppressor gene product. *EMBO J* 1989;8:4099–4105.
71 Gage JR et al. The E7 proteins of the nononcogenic human papillomavirus type 6b (HPV-6b) and of the oncogenic HPV-16 differ in retinoblastoma protein binding and other properties. *J Virol* 1990; 64:723–730.
72 Schmitt A et al. Comparison of the properties of the E6 and E7 genes of low- and high-risk cutaneous papillomaviruses reveals strongly transforming and high Rb-binding activing for the E7 protein of the low-risk human papillomavirus type 1. *J Virol* 1994;68:7051–7059.
73 Chellappan SP et al. The E2F transcription factor is a cellular target for the RB protein. *Cell* 1991;65:1053–1061.
74 Storey A et al. Mutations of the human papillomavirus type 16 E7 gene that affect transformation, transactivation and phosphorylation by the E7 protein. *J Gen Virol* 1990;71:965–970.
75 Edmonds C, Vousden KH. A point mutational analysis of human papillomavirus type 16 E7 protein. *J Virol* 1989;63:2650–2656.
76 Heck DV et al. Efficiency of binding the retinoblastoma protein correlates with the transforming capacity of the E7 oncoproteins of the human papillomaviruses. *Proc Natl Acad Sci USA* 1992;89:4442–4446.
77 Watanabe S et al. Mutational analysis of human papillomavirus type 16 E7 functions. *J Virol* 1990;64:207–214.
78 Banks LM et al. Ability of the HPV16 E7 protein to bind RB and induce DNA synthesis is not sufficient for efficient transforming activity in NIH3T3 cells. *Oncogene* 1990;5:1383–1389.
79 Phelps WC et al. Structure-function analysis of the human papillomavirus type 16 E7 oncoprotein. *J Virol* 1992;66:2418–2427.
80 Jewers RJ et al. Regions of human papillomavirus type 16 E7 oncoprotein required for immortalization of human keratinocytes. *J Virol* 1992;66:1329–1335.
81 Ikeda MA, Nevins JR. Identification of distinct roles for separate E1A domains in disruption of E2F complexes. *Mol Cell Biol* 1993;13: 7029–7035.
82 Stirdivant SM et al. Human papillomavirus type 16 E7 protein inhibits DNA binding by the retinoblastoma gene product. *Mol Cell Biol* 1992;12:1905–1914.
83 Huang PS et al. Protein domains governing interactions between E2F, the retinoblastoma gene product, and human papillomavirus type 16 E7 protein. *Mol Cell Biol* 1993;13:953–960.
84 Egan C et al. Mapping of cellular protein-binding sites on the products of early-region 1A of human adenovirus type 5. *Mol Cell Biol* 1988;8:3955–3959.
85 Arany Z et al. E1A-associated p300 and CREB-associated CBP belong to a conserved family of coactivators. *Cell* 1994;77:799–800.
86 Davies RC, Vousden KH. Functional analysis of human papillomavirus type 16 E7 by complementation with adenovirus E1A mutants. *J Gen Virol* 1992;73:2135–2139.
87 Blanton RA et al. Expression of the HPV16 E7 gene generates proliferation in stratified squamous cell cultures which is independent of endogenous p53 levels. *Cell Growth Differ* 1992;3:791–802.
88 Halbert CL et al. The E6 and E7 genes of human papillomavirus type 6 have weak immortalizing activity in human epithelial cells. *J Virol* 1992;66:2125–2134.
89 El-Deiry WS et al. WAF1, a potential mediator of p53 tumor suppression. *Cell* 1993;75:817–825.
90 Cheng S et al. Differentiation-dependent up-regulation of the human papillomavirus E7 gene reactivates cellular DNA replication in suprabasal differentiated keratinocytes. *Genes Dev* 1995;9:2335–2349.
91 Demers GW et al. Abrogation of growth arrest signals by human papillomavirus type 16 E7 is mediated by sequences required for transformation. *J Virol* 1996;70:6862–6869.
92 Funk JO et al. Inhibition of CDK activity and PCNA-dependent DNA replication by p21 is blocked by interaction with the HPV-16 E7 oncoprotein. *Genes Dev* 1997;11:2090–2100.
93 Jones DL et al. The human papillomavirus E7 oncoprotein can uncouple cellular differentiation and proliferation in human keratinocytes by abrogating p21[Cip1]-mediated inhibition of cdk2. *Genes Dev* 1997;11:2101–2111.
94 Cross SM et al. A p53-dependent mouse spindle checkpoint. *Science* 1995;267:1353–1356.
95 Waldman T et al. Uncoupling of S phase and mitosis induced by anticancer agents in cells lacking p21 [see comments]. *Nature* 1996; 381:713–716.
96 Hartwell LH. Defects in a cell cycle checkpoint may be responsible for the genomic instability of cancer cells. *Cell* 1992;71:543–546.
97 Kuerbitz SJ et al. Wild-type p53 is a cell cycle checkpoint determinant following irradiation. *Proc Natl Acad Sci USA* 1992;89:7491–7495.
98 Brugarolas J et al. Radiation-induced cell cycle arrest compromised by P21 deficiency. *Nature* 1995;377:552–557.
99 Waga S et al. The p21 inhibitor of cyclin-dependent kinases controls DNA replication by interaction with PCNA. *Nature* 1994;369:574–578.
100 Luo Y et al. Cell-cycle inhibition by independent CDK and PCNA binding domains in p21[Cip1]. *Nature* 1995;375:159–161.
101 Bates S, Vousden KH. p53 in signaling checkpoint arrest or apoptosis. [Review] [68 refs]. *Curr Opin Genet Dev* 1996;6:12–18.
102 Demers GW et al. Growth arrest by induction of p53 in DNA damaged keratinocytes is bypassed by human papillomavirus 16 E7. *Proc Natl Acad Sci USA* 1994;91:4382–4386.
103 Kessis TD et al. Human papillomavirus 16 E6 expression disrupts the p53-mediated cellular response to DNA damage. *Proc Natl Acad Sci USA* 1993;90:3988–3992.
104 Slebos RJ et al. p53-dependent G1 arrest involves pRB-related proteins and is disrupted by the human papillomavirus 16 E7 oncoprotein. *Proc Natl Acad Sci USA* 1994;91:5320–5324.
105 Hickman ES et al. Cells expressing HPV16 E7 continue cell cycle progression following DNA damage induced p53 activation. *Oncogene* 1994;9:2177–2181.
106 Matsushime H et al. D-type cyclin-dependent kinase activity in mammalian cells. *Mol Cell Biol* 1994;14:2066–2076.
107 Ohtani K et al. Regulation of the cyclin E gene by transcription factor E2F1. *Proc Natl Acad Sci USA* 1995;92:12146–12150.
108 Geng Y et al. Regulation of cyclin E transcription by E2Fs and retinoblastoma protein. *Oncogene* 1996;12:1173–1180.
109 Ohtsubo M et al. Human cyclin E, a nuclear protein essential for the G1-to-S phase transition. *Mol Cell Biol* 1995;15:2612–2624.
110 Zerfass K et al P. Sequential activation of cyclin E and cyclin A gene expression by human papillomavirus type 16 E7 through sequences necessary for transformation. *J Virol* 1995;69:6389–6399.
111 Zerfass-Thome K et al. Inactivation of the cdk inhibitor p27KIP1 by the human papillomavirus type 16 E7 oncoprotein. *Oncogene* 1996; 13:2323–2330.
112 Schwarz E et al. DNA sequence and genome organization of genital human papillomavirus type 6b. *EMBO J* 1983;2:2341–2348.
113 Yee C et al. Presence and expression of human papillomavirus sequences in human cervical carcinoma cell lines. *Am J Pathol* 1985; 119:361–366.

114 Thierry F, Howley PM. Functional analysis of E2-mediated repression of the HPV18 P105 promoter. *New Biologist* 1991;3:90–100.

115 Jeon S, Lambert PF. Integration of human papillomavirus type 16 DNA into the human genome leads to increased stability of E6 and E7 mRNAs: implications for cervical carcinogenesis. *Proc Natl Acad Sci USA* 1995;92:1654–1658.

116 Popescu NC et al. Viral integration, fragile sites, and proto-oncogenes in human neoplasia. *Hum Genet* 1990;84:383–386.

117 Cannizzaro LA et al. Regional chromosome localization of human papillomavirus integration sites near fragile sites, oncogenes, and cancer chromosome breakpoints. *Cancer Gen Cytogen* 1988;33:93–98.

118 Smith PP et al. Viral integration and fragile sites in human papillomavirus-immortalized human keratinocyte cell lines. *Genes Chrom Cancer* 1992;5:150–157.

119 Durst M et al K. Papillomavirus sequences integrate near cellular oncogenes in some cervical carcinomas. *Proc Natl Acad Sci USA* 1987;84:1070–1074.

120 Cullen AP et al. Analysis of the physical state of different human papillomavirus DNAs in intraepithelial and invasive cervical neoplasm. *J Virol* 1991;65:606–612.

121 Cole JS III, Gruber J. Progress and prospects for human cancer vaccines. *J Natl Cancer Inst* 1992;84:18–23.

122 zur Hausen H. Viruses in human cancers. *Science* 1991;254:1167–1173.

123 Atkin NB, Baker MC. Chromosome 1 in 26 carcinomas of the cervix uteri. *Cancer* 1979;44:604–613.

124 Atkin NB, Baker MC. Nonrandom chromosome changes in carcinoma of the cervix uteri: II. Ten tumors in the triploid-tetraploid range. *Cancer Genet Cytogenet* 1984;13:189–207.

125 Mullokandov MR et al. Genomic alterations in cervical carcinoma: losses of chromosome heterozygosity and human papilloma virus tumor status. *Cancer Res* 1996;56:197–205.

126 Yokota J et al. Loss of heterozygosity on the short arm of chromosome 3 in carcinoma of the uterine cervix. *Cancer Res* 1989;49:3598–3601.

127 Heselmeyer K et al. Gain of chromosome 3q defines the transition from severe dysplasia to invasive carcinoma of the uterine cervix. *Proc Natl Acad Sci USA* 1996;93:479–484.

128 Smith PP et al. Cytogenetic analysis of eight human papillomavirus immortalized human keratinocyte cell lines. *Int J Cancer* 1989;44:1124–1131.

129 Montgomery KD et al. Genetic instability of chromosome 3 in HPV-immortalized and tumorigenic human keratinocytes. *Genes Chrom Cancer* 1995;14:97–105.

130 Coleman N et al. Immunological events in regressing genital warts. *Am J Clin Pathol* 1994;102:768–774.

131 Xi L et al. Analysis of human papillomavirus type 16 variants indicates establishment of persistent infection. *J Infect Dis* 1995;172:747–755.

132 Galloway DA. Serological assays for the detection of HPV antibodies. In: Munoz N, Bosch FX, Shah KV, et al., eds. *The epidemiology of cervical cancer and human papillomavirus*. Lyon: IARC, 1992, pp. 147–161.

133 Jochmus-Kudielka I et al. Seroreactivity against HPV 16 E4 and E7 proteins in renal transplant recipients and pregnant women. *J Invest Dermatol* 1992;98:389–390.

134 Mandelson MT et al. The association of human papillomavirus antibodies with cervical cancer risk. *Cancer Epidemiol Biomarkers Prev* 1992;1:281–286.

135 Carter JJ et al. Use of HPV1 capsids produced by recombinant vaccinia viruses in an ELISA to detect serum antibodies in people with foot warts. *Virology* 1994;199:284–291.

136 Carter JJ et al. HPV-1 capsids expressed in vitro detect human serum antibodies associated with foot warts. *Virology* 1993;195:456–462.

137 Kirnbauer R et al. A virus-like particle enzyme-linked immunosorbent assay detects serum antibodies in a majority of women infected with human papillomavirus type 16. *J Natl Cancer Inst* 1994;86:494–499.

138 Jochmus I et al. Major histocompatibility complex and human papillomavirus type 16 E7 expression in high-grade vulvar lesions. *Hum Pathol* 1993;24:519–524.

139 Christensen ND, Kreider JW. Antibody-mediated neutralization in vivo of infectious papillomaviruses. *J Virol* 1990;64:3151–3156.

140 Christensen ND et al. Detection of human serum antibodies that neutralize infectious human papillomavirus type 11 virions. *J Gen Virol* 1992;73:1261–1267.

141 Roden RB et al. In vitro generation and type-specific neutralization of a human papillomavirus type 16 virion pseudotype. *J Virol* 1996;70:5875–5883.

142 Palefsky JM et al. Anal intraepithelial neoplasia and anal papillomavirus infection among homosexual males with group IV HIV disease. *JAMA* 1990;263:2911–2916.

143 Kiviat NB et al. Association of anal dysplasia and human papillomavirus with immunosuppression and HIV infection among homosexual men. *AIDS* 1993;7:43–49.

144 Chardonnet Y et al. Cell-mediated immunity to human papillomavirus. *Clin Dermatol* 1985;3:156–164.

145 Strang G et al. Human T cell responses to human papillomavirus type 16 L1 and E6 synthetic peptides: identification of T cell determinants, HLA-DR restriction and virus type specificity. *J Gen Virol* 1990;71:423–431.

146 Cubie HA et al. Lymphoproliferative responses to fusion proteins of human papillomaviruses in patients with cervical intraepithelial neoplasia. *Epidemiol Infect* 1989;103:625–632.

147 Kadish AS et al. Cell-mediated immune responses to E7 peptides of human papillomavirus (HPV) type 16 are dependent on the HPV type infecting the cervix whereas serological reactivity is not type-specific. *J Gen Virol* 1994;75:2277–22784.

148 Kadish AS et al. Lymphoproliferative responses to human papillomavirus (HPV) type 16 proteins E6 and E7—outcome of HPV infection and associated neoplasia. *J Natl Cancer Inst* 1997;89:1285–1293.

149 Beverley PC et al. Strategies for studying mouse and human immune responses to human papillomavirus type 16. *Ciba Found Symp* 1994;187:78–96.

150 Steele JC et al. Production and characterization of human proliferative T-cell clones specific for human papillomavirus type 1 E4 protein. *J Virol* 1993;67:2799–2806.

151 Evans EM et al. Infiltration of cervical cancer tissue with human papillomavirus-specific cytotoxic T-lymphocytes. *Cancer Res* 1997;57:2943–2950.

152 Warhol MJ, Gee B. The expression of histocompatibility antigen HLA-DR in cervical squamous epithelium infected with human papilloma virus. *Mod Pathol* 1989;2:101–104.

153 Glew SS et al. HLA class II antigen expression in human papillomavirus-associated cervical cancer. *Cancer Res* 1992;52:4009–4016.

154 Conner ME, Stern PL. Loss of MHC Class-1 expression in cervical carcinomas. *Int J Cancer* 1990;46:1029–1034.

155 Cromme FV et al. Loss of transporter protein encoded by the TAP-1 gene is highly correlated with loss of HLA expression in cervical carcinomas. *J Exp Med* 1994;179:335–340.

156 Suzich JA et al. Systemic immunization with papillomavirus L1 protein completely prevents the development of viral mucosal papillomas. *Proc Natl Acad Sci USA* 1995;92:11553–11557.

157 Jarrett WFH et al. Studies on vaccination against papillomaviruses: a comparison of purified virus, tumour extract and transformed cells in prophylactic vaccination. *Vet Rec* 1990;126:449–452.

158 Pilacinski WP et al. Immunization against bovine papillomavirus infection. *Ciba Found Symp* 1986;120:136–156.

159 Campo MS et al. Prophylactic and therapeutic vaccination against a mucosal papillomavirus. *J Gen Virol* 1993;74:945–953.

160 Evans CA et al. Antiviral and antitumor immunologic mechanisms operative in the Shope papillomas-carcinoma system. *Cold Spring Harbor Symp Quant Biol* 1962;27:453–462.

161 Lin Y et al. Effective vaccination against papilloma development by immunization with L1 or L2 structural protein of cottontail rabbit papillomavirus. *Virology* 1992;187:612–619.

162 Christensen ND et al. The open reading frame L2 of cottontail rabbit papillomavirus contains antibody-inducing neutralizing epitopes. *Virology* 1991;181:572–579.
163 Lin Y et al. Cottontail rabbit papillomavirus L1 protein-based vaccines: protection is achieved only with a full-length, nondenatured product. *J Virol* 1993;67:4154–4162.
164 Christensen ND, Kreider JW. Neutralization of CRPV infectivity by monoclonal antibodies that identify conformational epitopes on intact virions. *Virus Res* 1991;21:169–179.
165 Jin XW et al. Bovine serological response to a recombinant BPV-1 major capsid protein vaccine. *Intervirology* 1990;31:345–354.
166 Jarrett WFH et al. Studies on vaccination against papillomaviruses: prophylactic and therapeutic vaccination with recombinant structural proteins. *Virology* 1991;184:33–42.
167 Chen L et al. Induction of cytotoxic T lymphocytes specific for a syngeneic tumor expressing the E6 oncoprotein of human papillomavirus type 16. *J Immunol* 1992;148:2617–2621.
168 Chen L et al. Human papillomavirus type 16 nucleoprotein E7 is a tumor rejection antigen. *Proc Natl Acad Sci USA* 1991;88:110–114.
169 Feltkamp MC et al. Vaccination with cytotoxic T lymphocyte epitopes-containing peptide protects against a tumor induced by human papillomavirus type 16-transformed cells. *Eur J Immunol* 1993;23: 224–229.
170 Menequzzi G et al. Vaccinia recombinants expressing early bovine papilloma virus (BPV1) proteins: retardation of BPV1 tumour development. *Vaccine* 1990;8:199–204.
171 McNeil C. HPV vaccine treatment trials proliferate, diversify [news]. *J Natl Cancer Inst* 1997;89:280–281.
172 Borysiewicz LK et al. A recombinant vaccinia virus encoding human papillomavirus types 16 and 18, E6 and E7 proteins as immunotherapy for cervical cancer [see comments]. *Lancet* 1996;347:1523–1527.
173 Thorner LK et al. DNA-binding domain of bovine papillomavirus type 1 E1 helicase: structural and functional aspects. *J Virol* 1993; 67:6000–6014.
174 Ustav M et al. Identification of the origin of replication of bovine papillomavirus and characterization of the viral origin recognition factor E1. *EMBO J* 1991;10:4321–4329.
175 Wilson VG, Ludes-Meyers J. A bovine papillomavirus E1-related protein binds specifically to bovine papillomavirus DNA. *J Virol* 1991; 65:5314–5322.
176 Thorner L et al. The product of the bovine papillomavirus type 1 modulator gene (M) is a phosphoprotein. *J Virol* 1988;62:2474–2482.
177 Androphy EJ et al. Bovine papillomavirus E2 transacting gene product binds to specific sites in papillomavirus DNA. *Nature* 1987;325: 70–73.
178 Hirochika H et al. Functional mapping of the human papillomavirus type 11 transcriptional enhancer and its interaction with the transacting E2 protein. *Genes Dev* 1988;2:54–67.
179 Mohr IJ et al. Targeting the E1 replication protein to the papillomavirus origin of replication by complex formation with the E2 transactivator. *Science* 1990;250:1694–1699.
180 Liu JS et al. The functions of human papillomavirus type 11 E1, E2, and E2C proteins in cell-free DNA replication. *J Biol Chem* 1995; 270:27283–27291.
181 Doorbar J et al. Specific interaction between HPV-16 E1^E4 and cytokeratins results in collapse of the epithelial cell intermediate filament network. *Nature* 1991;352:824–827.
182 Roberts S et al. Cutaneous and mucosal human papillomavirus E4 proteins form intermediate filament-like structures in epithelial cells. *Virology* 1993;197:176–187.
183 Conrad M et al. The E5 protein of HPV-6, but not HPV-16, associates efficiently with cellular growth factor receptors. *Virology* 1994; 200:796–800.
184 Gu Z, Matlashewski G. Effect of human papillomavirus type 16 oncogenes on MAP kinase activity. *J Virol* 1995;69:8051–8056.
185 Stoppler MC et al. The E5 gene of HPV-16 enhances keratinocyte immortalization by full-length DNA. *Virology* 1996;223:251–254.
186 Kirnbauer R et al. Papillomavirus L1 major capsid protein self-assembles into virus-like particles that are highly immunogenic. *Proc Natl Acad Sci USA* 1992;89:12180–12184.
187 Hagensee ME et al. Self-assembly of human papillomavirus type 1 capsids by expression of the L1 protein alone or by coexpression of the L1 and L2 capsid proteins. *J Virol* 1993;67:315–322.

Chapter 25
Genital human papillomavirus

Laura A. Koutsky
Nancy B. Kiviat

At least 35 of the over 100 different human papillomavirus (HPV) types primarily infect genital epithelium.[1,2,3] The great diversity of HPV types reflects the ability of this group of viruses to exploit the different microenvironments of the largest organ in humans—the skin. To some extent, the epithelial tropism of different HPV types corresponds to different clinical manifestations (Table 25-1). For example, HPV 2 and 4 are often detected in common warts of the hands,[4,5,6] while HPV 6 is the type that is most frequently detected in genital warts.[7,8,9] Although most external genital warts are positive for HPV 6 or 11 DNA, and most invasive squamous cell cancers of the genital tract and anus are positive for HPV 16, 18, 31, or 45 DNA,[10] squamous intraepithelial lesions (SILs) of the cervix, vagina, vulva, penis, and anus are associated with many different HPV types.[11]

DEFINITIONS

The majority of newly acquired genital HPV infections appear to be subclinical and asymptomatic. Clinically visible manifestations of HPV include warts that may be condylomatous, papular, flat, or keratotic in appearance. Subclinical infections may appear as flat "aceto-white" lesions that are visible with colposcopic magnification of epithelium that has been treated with a mild acetic acid (vinegar) solution, or as SILs that are diagnosed microscopically on the basis of characteristic cytologic and histologic features.[12] For some individuals, detection of HPV DNA in genital specimens is the only evidence of infection. Recent studies demonstrate that many adults without clinical, microscopic, or molecular evidence of HPV infection have serum antibodies to specific HPV types indicating past infection.[7,13,14,15,16,17,18] A number of years after initial infection, some individuals with HPV are at risk of developing squamous cell carcinomas.[19] HPV-related anal and genital tract neoplasms are addressed in Chapter 59. The main focus of this chapter is the clinical and epidemiologic features of external genital warts. Benign genital HPV infections that are asymptomatic and detected only by colposcopy, microscopy, or molecular hybridization assays will also be discussed.

HISTORY

Written descriptions of condylomatous warts of the genital tract and anus date as far back as the first century A.D. (see reviews by Oriel and Rosenbaum).[20,21] Within the first decade of this century, the viral etiology of both common skin warts and genital warts was demonstrated.[22] During the 1930s, work with the cottontail rabbit papillomavirus (CRPV) provided important clues as to the role of this family of viruses in the development of tumors.[23,24]

Although the cytologic manifestations now known to be characteristic of cervical HPV infection were first described in 1956,[25] it was not until the 1970s that these cellular changes were attributed to HPV infection.[26,27] Also during this decade, the genetic heterogeneity of HPVs was first demonstrated through use of molecular hybridization techniques.[28,29,30,31] Throughout the 1980s and 1990s, several epidemiologic and molecular studies provided firm evidence linking specific HPV types with the development of most genital tract and anal cancers.[10,19,31,32,33,34,35,36]

PATHOGENESIS

HPVs are epitheliotropic, and their replication depends on the presence of differentiating squamous epithelium.[37,38] Viral DNA, but not structural (capsid) protein, can be detected in the lower layers of the epithelium.[39] Capsid protein and infectious virus are found in the superficial differentiated cell layers. HPV infected epithelium characteristically has a hyperplastic prickle cell layer (acanthosis) with a stratum corneum consisting of only one or two layers of parakeratotic cells. The dermal papillae are elongated, and there is a sharp border with the dermis (Fig. 25-1). Koilocytes, which are mature squamous cells with a large, clear perinuclear zone, may be scattered throughout the outer cell layers. The nuclei of koilocytes may be enlarged and hyperchromatic, and double nuclei are often seen.[40] Ultrastructural studies show virus in some of the cell nuclei. Although koilocytes are thought to represent a specific cytopathic effect of HPV, koilocytotic features are often subtle, and other cellular changes may mimic koilocytic changes. Thus, detection of koilocytes is not a sensitive or reliable predictor of cervical HPV infection.[41]

PREVALENCE AND INCIDENCE

PREVALENCE

The point prevalence of genital HPV infection detected by polymerase chain reaction (PCR)-based methods among populations of women with cytologically normal Pap smears is summarized in Table 25-2. The HPV prevalence among cytologically normal women has ranged from 44.3[42] to 1.5 percent.[43] The weighted average of HPV prevalence among 12,595 cytologically normal women presented in the table is 16.2 percent (weight proportional to sample size). HPV16 appears to be the most common type among cytologically normal women, as well as the most common cancer-associated type.[44] A study that reported the lowest prevalence was conducted among women who had not experienced sexual intercourse,[43] and the one that reported highest prevalence was conducted among sexually active young women.[42] In general, sexually active younger women are more likely than older women to have HPV DNA detected in genital tract specimens.

Genital HPV infection is also common in men. A study in Croatia reported that 19.8% of 338 cervical scrapes from women and 26.6% of 79 urethral swabs from men were positive for HPV DNA by slot-bolt hybridization.[45] Among heterosexual men and women with multiple sex partners attending an STD clinic, 23% of 162 women had HPV DNA detected by a PCR-based method in specimens obtained from the oral cavity, cervix, labia minora, anus, or rectum, while 28% of 85 men had HPV DNA detected in specimens from the oral cavity, urethra, coronal sulcus, anus, or rectum.[46] In a study of HPV infection among 50 consecutive pairs of male and female sex partners attending an STD clinic, HPV DNA was detected by PCR in 72% of cervical or vulvovaginal specimens from women and 63% of penile, scrotal, or urethral specimens from men.[47] Among voluntary Finnish Army conscripts, HPV DNA was detected by PCR in 47 (16.5%) of 2850 penile shaft or urethra samples.[48] In a group of healthy men aged 18 to 23 years, HPV DNA was detected by PCR in urethra spec-

Table 25-1. Clinical Manifestations Associated with Different HPV Types*

Clinical manifestation	HPV types
Skin Lesions	
Plantar warts	1, 2, 4
Common warts	2, 4, 26, 27, 29, 57
Flat warts	3, 10, 28, 49
Butcher's warts	7
Benign EV lesions	2, 3, 10, 12, 15, 19, 36, 46, 47, 50
EV (benign or malignant)	5, 8, 9, 10, 14, 17, 20–25, 37
Nonwarty skin lesions	37, 38
Genital	
Condylomata acuminata	6, 11, 42–44, 54
Noncondylomatous lesions and/or CIN	6, 11, 16, 18, 30, 31, 33, 34, 35, 39, 40, 42, 43, 51, 52, 55, 56, 57–59, 61, 62, 64, 67–70
Carcinoma	16, 18, 31, 33, 35, 39, 45, 51, 52, 54, 56, 66, 68
Nongenital mucosal	
Mouth (focal epithelial hyperplasia)	13, 32
Laryngeal papilloma	6, 11, 30
Maxillary sinus papilloma	57
Carcinoma (head/neck/lung)	2, 6, 11, 16, 18, 30

* Adapted from de Villiers et al.[6]

imens from eight (12%) of 66 men with normal epithelium and from 10 (26%) of 39 men with aceto-white epithelium.[49] In case-control studies of the male role in the epidemiology of cervical cancer in Colombia and Spain, cell samples for detection of HPV DNA were collected from the distal urethra and the external surface of the glans and coronal sulcus of the penis. In Colombia, 26% of husbands of 210 cases and 19% of husbands of 262 controls were positive for HPV DNA by PCR,[50] whereas in Spain, 18% of husbands of 183 cases and 4% of husbands of 171 controls were positive for HPV DNA.[51]

Serologic assays for specific HPV types using conformationally correct antigen targets in the form of viruslike particles (VLPs) have only recently been developed. Seroprevalence studies using VLPs as antigen suggest that, among women without clinically evident HPV-related disease, 3% to 43% have antibodies to HPV 16, and 9% to 25% have antibodies to HPV 6 or 11.[7,13,15,16,17,18] The wide range of seroprevalence estimates may be due in part to differences in populations surveyed and to use of different assays, capsid antigen preparations, or cutpoints for distinguishing seropositives from seronegatives.

Current evidence suggests that over 50% of sexually active adults have been infected with one or more genital HPV types. The majority of these infections are subclinical, unrecognized, and benign (Fig. 25-2).

GEOGRAPHIC DISTRIBUTION

Recent studies on the evolution of papillomaviruses (Chapter 24) suggest that the known HPV types have existed in nearly identical molecular form since the beginning of the human species.[52] As shown in Table 25–2, the prevalence of genital HPV infection and the distribution of specific genital HPV types appears to be similar in different regions of the world. However, studies of invasive cervical cancers obtained from different regions of the world suggest that variants of HPV types may segregate according to geography. Based on DNA homology, HPV16 isolates have been

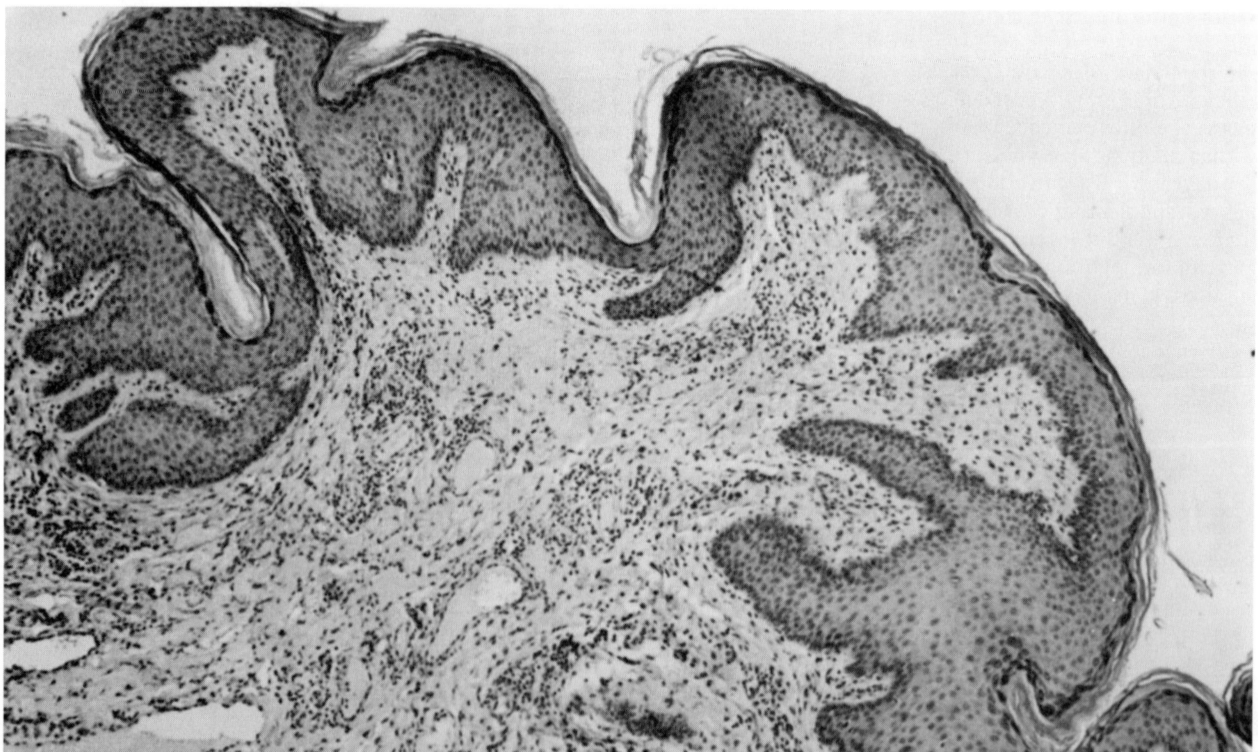

Fig. 25-1. Biopsy of condyloma acuminatum, showing acanthosis, elongated dermal papillae, and sharp border with dermis. H&E stain (*courtesy of E. Stolz.*)

Table 25-2. HPV DNA Detection Rates by PCR Amplification among Women with Cytologically Negative Pap Smears

Reference	Study population	No. of subjects	Sites tested	HPV types tested for	Age of subjects (range, mean or SD)	Percentage HPV positive	Percentage HP-16/18 positive
ter Meulen[180]	Gynecology clinic, Tanzania	[261]	Cervix	HPV-6,-11,-16,-18,-31,-33, -35,-39,-40,-45,-51, X	15–70; 30.9 years	[47.9]	[16.9]
Wheeler[42]	University Health Service, USA	357	Cervix	HPV-6,-11,-16,-18,-31,-33, -35,-39,-45,-51,-52,-54,-59, PAP 88, PAP 238A, W 13B	18–47; 23 years	44.3	8 (HPV-16)
Kjaer[104]	Random sample, Greenland	129[a]	Cervix	HPV-11,-16,-18,-33	20–39 years	43.4	35
Pao[181]	Clinic, Taiwan	102	Cervico-vaginal	HPV-6,-11,-16,-18,-33	NA	42.2	9.8
Lambropoulos[182]	Gynecology clinic, Greece	201	Cervix	HPV-16,-18, X	17–45 years	40.8[c]	7.5
Becker[183]	Gynecology clinics, USA	309	Cervix	HPV-6,-11,-16,-18,-31,-33, -35,-39,-45,-51,-52,-53,-54, -56,-58,-59, PAP 88, W 13B, PAP 238A	18–40; 26 years	40.1	11.7
Kjaer[104]	Random sample, Denmark	126[a]	Cervix	HPV-11,-16,-18,-33	20–39 years	38.9	44.4
Critchlow & Koutsky[78]	University, USA, sexually active	183	Cervix, vulvo-vaginal	HPV-6,-11,-16,-18,-31,-33, -35,-45, X	18–20 years	35	14
Bauer[63]	University Health Service, USA	442[b]	Cervix	HPV-6,-11,-16,-18,-31,-33, -35,-39,-45,-51,-52, W 13B, PAP 88, PAP 155, PAP 251, PAP 238B, X	Mean, 22.9 years; SD, 4.2	32.5[b]	NA
Seck[184]	Infectious Disease Service, Senegal	47[c]	Cervix	HPV-6,-11,-16,-18,-31,-33, -35, X	NA	24.5[c]	NA
Czeglédy[185]	Family planning clinic, Kenya	77	Cervix	HPV-6,-11,-16,-18,-31,-33	Mean, 25.8 years	19.5	10.4
Schiffman[186]	Health Maintenance Organization clinics, USA	453	Cervico-vaginal	HPV-6,-11,-16,-18,-26,-31, -33,-35,-39,-40,-42,-45,-51, -52,-53,-54,-55,-57,-59, PAP 38, PAP 155, PAP 238A, PAP 251, PAP 291, W 13B	Mean, 34 years	17.7	2.9
Engels[187]	STD clinic, Kenya	97	Cervix	HPV-6,-11,-16,-18,-31,-33, X	Mean, 28 years; SD, 9.7	16.5	NA
Melkert[188]	Screening, Netherlands	156	Cervix	HPV-6,-11,-16,-18,-31,-33, X	Mean, 15–34 years	14.1	3.8
Melkert[188]	Hospital, Netherlands	2320	Cervix	HPV-6,-11,-16,-18,-31,-33, X	Mean, 15–34 years	13.9	3.9
Muñoz[189]	Random sample, Colombia	98	Cervix	HPV-6,-11,-16,-18,-31,-33, -35, X	Mean, 47.5 years	13.3	11.2
van Doornum[190]	STD clinic, Netherlands, ≥5 partners 6 months before entry	108[d]	Cervix	HPV-6,-11,-16,-18,-33	Mean, 29 years	11.9[d]	10.2
Bosch[191]	Random sample, Colombia	181	Cervix	HPV-6,-11,-16,-18,-31,-33, -35, X	19–70; 39.2 years	10.5	3.3
Melkert[188]	Hospital, Netherlands	1826	Cervix	HPV-6,-11,-16,-18,-31,-33, X	35–55 years	6.6	1.5
Bosch[191]	Random sample, Spain	193	Cervix	HPV-6,-11,-16,-18,-31,-33, -35, X	18–68; 36.1 years	4.7	0.5
Muñoz[189]	Random sample, Spain	130	Cervix	HPV-6,-11,-16,-18,-31,-33, -35, X	Mean, 52.3 years	4.6	3.1
Melkert[188]	Screening, Netherlands	1555	Cervix	HPV-6,-11,-16,-18,-31,-33, X	35–55 years	4.2	0.9
Nishikawa[121]	Gynecology clinic, non-pregnant women, Japan	52	Cervix	HPV-16,-18,-33	18–73; 38.5 years	3.8 (HPV-16 only)	3.8 (HPV-16 only)
Engels[187]	Family planning clinic, Kenya	109	Cervix	HPV-6,-11,-16,-18,-31,-33, X	Mean, 28 years; SD, 9.7	3.7	NA
Critchlow & Koutsky[78]	University, USA, no reported coitus	56	Cervix, vulvo-vaginal	HPV-6,-11,-16,-18,-31,-33, -35,-45, X	18–20 years	3.6	0.0
Rylander[43]	Adolescent clinic, Sweden, no reported coitus	130	Cervix	HPV-6,-11,-16,-18,-31,-33, -39,-40,-45,-55,-56, X	10–25; 18 years	1.5 (HPV-6 only)	0.0
Fairley[192]	Clinic, Australia, no reported coitus	55	Vagina	HPV-6,-11,-16,-18,-31,-33, X	13–41; 18 years	0.0	0.0

NA, not available; SD, standard deviation; X, primers

[a]Each group includes three women with dysplasia.

[b]Excludes cases with cervical dysplasia and condylomatous atypia.

[c]Excludes cases with cervical dysplasia in HIV (human immunodeficiency virus)-negative cases.

[d]Excludes three cases with Pap IIIa smear.

[ ] estimated percentage.

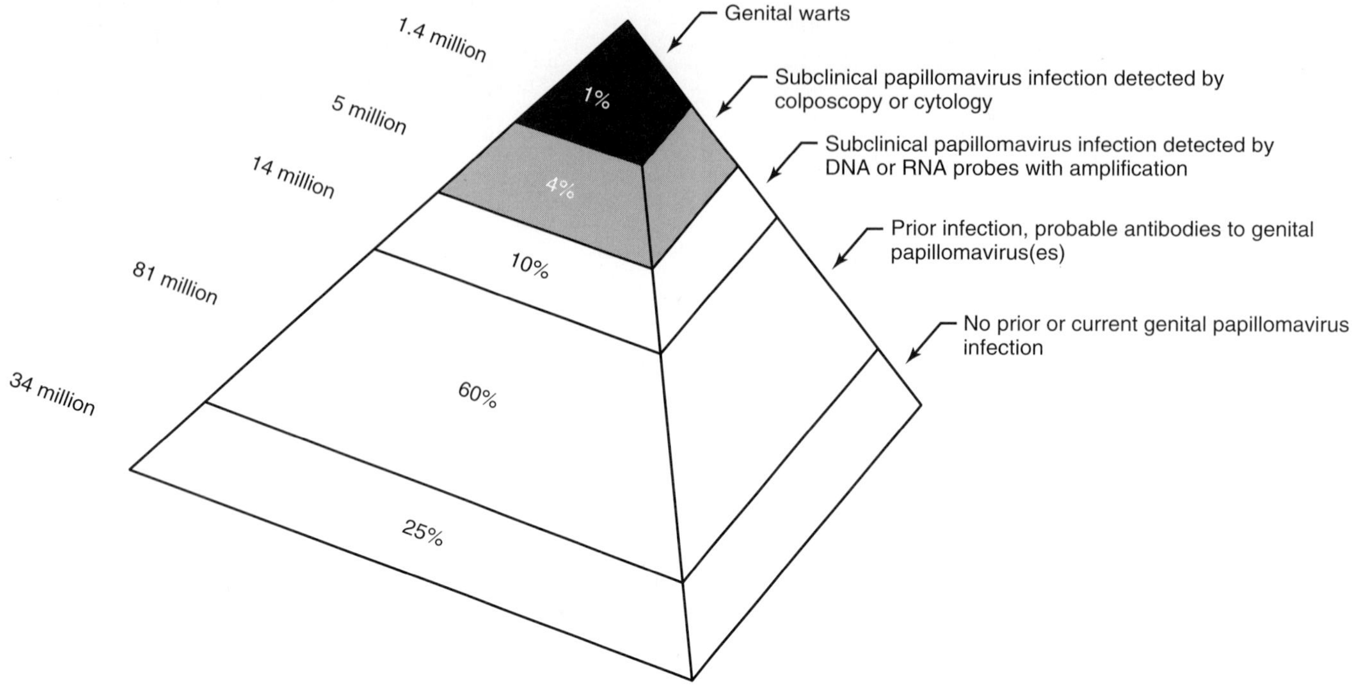

Fig. 25-2. Estimated prevalence of genital HPV infection among sexually active men and women 15–49 years of age in the United States.

classified into 5 major lineages, including Asian variants, American-Asian variants, European variants, African-1 variants, and African-2 variants.[53,54] Compared to the HPV16 prototype, non-European variants generally have greater nucleotide sequence divergence than European variants. Among European women with cervical cancer, European variants predominate, while African-1 and African-2 variants are more common in Africa.[55]

TIME TRENDS

In the United States, an eightfold increase in the age- and gender-adjusted incidence of genital warts was reported between the periods 1950–1954 and 1975–1978 (from 13 per 100,000 to 106 per 100,000).[56] During these years, rates of other STDs were increasing dramatically in Europe and North America and the population of sexually active young adults was also increasing.[57] The prevalence of genital warts reported by STD clinics in England and Wales nearly doubled from 1971 to 1979.[57] In the United States, a survey of physicians in private practice indicated a 4.5-fold increase in the number of first consultations for genital warts between 1966 and 1984.[58] This trend resembles that seen in England and Wales. Data on trends in the prevalence of genital HPV infection detected by molecular methods are not available. As with other STDs, it is possible that the prevalence of genital HPV infection in many countries has remained static or even decreased during the last 10 years (Chapter 4).

Few HPV incidence data are currently available. In one mass screening conducted between 1985 and 1986, focusing on a cohort of 22-year-old women in Kuopio, Finland, HPV infection was determined by cytological examination of Pap smears. The prevalence of HPV infection was about 3% among 1,289 women at the beginning of the study, and the annual incidence among 1,069 women followed for one year was estimated to be 7%.[59] A population-based study in Rochester, Minnesota reported an incidence of genital warts of 1.06 per 1,000 population in the late 1970s.[56] In Borås, Sweden, the incidence of genital warts was estimated to be 2.4 per 1,000 population in 1990.[60] In both the Rochester and the Borås studies, the incidence of genital warts was 30% to 40% higher in women than in men. Although these studies are population based, the reported incidence would be an underestimate, since the sensitivity of both cytological and clinical diagnoses of HPV infection is much lower than the sensitivity of diagnoses based on detection of HPV DNA. Unfortunately, population-based incidence data for HPV DNA detection have not been published.

In a cohort of STD clinic attendees with multiple sex partners, 110 women were followed over a period of 155.1 person-years with a total number of 411 visits, and 48 men were followed for a total of 65.4 person-years with 172 visits.[46] At entry to the study, 23 women and 15 men were positive for HPV by PCR, while during the follow up another 35 women and 14 men became HPV positive. In this small study of a unique population, the incidence of HPV infection was similar for men and women. It would be worthwhile to examine incidence rates in several other population samples.

TRANSMISSION

SEXUAL TRANSMISSION

Genital HPV infections are transmitted primarily through sexual contact. Sexual transmission of clinically evident HPV infection was noted in 1954, when Barrett et al.[61] reported on 24 women with genital warts who noticed the warts 4 to 6 weeks after their husbands had returned from the Far East. All husbands reported sexual contact with women while overseas, and all husbands had recently had penile warts. Oriel observed that 64% of 88 partners of individuals with genital warts developed warts, and newly developed warts were more infectious than older lesions.[20] Other data supporting the sexual transmission of HPV include the fact that HPV DNA is rarely found in genital tract specimens of women who have not had vaginal intercourse.[43,62] In addition, studies among young women show a positive trend between increasing numbers of sex partners and increasing prevalence of genital HPV infection.[42,62,63] In a recent study of 604 women attending a state university between 1992 and 1994, HPV DNA was detected by PCR in cervicovaginal lavage specimens of only 2 (3%) of 76 women who reported no prior vaginal intercourse, 9 (7%) of 137 women with one male sex partner, 79 (33%) of 243 women with two to four partners, and 78 (53%) of 148 women with five or more male partners.[62] The relationship between the increased prevalence of genital HPV infection and number of sex partners has been documented not only for women but also for men.[48]

These results suggest that among sexually active adults, risk of genital HPV infection with each new sex partner is high. Unlike certain bacterial STDs,[64] genital HPV does not appear to require core groups (small segments of the sexually active portion of the population with very high rates of partner change) to sustain high rates of infection in communities throughout the world.[65] To what extent the high prevalence of genital HPV infection can be attributed to a high rate of infectivity, a long duration of infectivity, or a combination of the two is currently not known.

Concordance of specific HPV types among sex partners has been demonstrated. Schneider et al.[66] examined sex partners of 156 women with genital HPV infection and found 87% of 61 men who were positive for HPV were infected with viral types identical to those detected in cervical specimens from their female partners. Baken et al.[47] showed that among a consecutive series of 45 couples presenting to an STD clinic, HPV type-specific concordance between partners was more common than predicted by chance ($p = .009$).

It is thought but not proven that moisture and abrasion of the epithelial surface enhance transmission of HPV. There are no data that conclusively address the question of whether condoms provide an effective barrier for HPV transmission.

NONSEXUAL TRANSMISSION

The transfer of HPV by fomites is important in the transmission of skin warts;[67] whether this occurs with genital HPV types is not known. Digital transmission may occur. HPV 16 DNA has been detected in finger lesions,[68] and molecular evidence of HPV 1, 2, and 4 (types that cause plantar and common skin warts) has been found in genital tract lesions.[69] Blood-borne transmission of HPV has not been reported.

Although rare, perinatal transmission does occur. As discussed in Chapter 80, a small minority of infants born to women with genital warts during pregnancy develop laryngeal papillomatosis,[70] and perinatal transmission appears to play a role in cases of condylomata developing within the first week of life.[71,72,73]

SUSCEPTIBILITY TO HPV INFECTION

Some papillomavirus-related lesions such as focal epithelial hyperplasia and the macular-papular warts seen in individuals with epidermodysplasia verruciformis appear to be influenced by genetic predisposition.[74] To date, no direct evidence is available regarding an association between HPV infection and HLA haplotypes. However, recent data demonstrate an association between certain HLA class II haplotypes and increased risk of cervical intraepithelial neoplasia and invasive cancer.[75,76] A study by Ellis et al.[77] found a significant association between HLA-B7 and an HPV16 variant with a particular change at one of the three potential cytotoxic T-lymphocyte (CTL) epitopes in the E6 region. They speculated that changes of this epitope might affect CTL responses and allow for escape from immune surveillance directed at prototype HPV 16 E6 in HLA-B7 individuals. This finding has not yet been confirmed by others.

Generally, an increased genital HPV prevalence has been observed among patients with immune-related disorders. Numerous studies have consistently demonstrated a high prevalence of HPV among HIV seropositive populations. Using PCR-based methods, HPV prevalence has ranged from 41 to 74% among HIV seropositive women and from 21 to 49% among HIV seronegative women.[78] The increased HPV prevalence in HIV seropositive men is similar to that seen among HIV seropositive women. A study conducted by Kiviat et al.[79] among men presenting to a community-based clinic for HIV serologic screening found that HIV seropositive men were 3.1 times (95% CI, 1.6–5.8) more likely to be positive for HPV DNA by PCR than HIV seronegative men and that HIV seropositive men more often had infection with multiple types as compared with seronegative men (44% versus 23%). Similar findings have been reported by others.[80,81,82,83] One interpretation for the increased prevalence among HIV seropositive individuals is that HIV-induced immunosuppression leads to reactivation of viruses which are otherwise undetectable.

Renal allograft recipients are at high risk of genital HPV infection. Halpert et al. found cytological evidence of HPV infection in 18 of 81 (22%) renal allograft recipients and in 2 of 81 (2.5%) hospitalized immunocompetent controls matched for age, race, and age at first coitus.[84] Recently, Ogunbiyi et al.[85] compared HPV16 prevalence detected by PCR among 133 renal allograft recipients and 145 controls. HPV16 DNA was detected in 47% and 12.4% of the allograft recipients and controls, respectively. Similar findings have been reported by others.[86] A study by Alloub et al.[87] reported a significantly higher prevalence of HPV 16 or 18 DNA in allograft recipients (27%) than in controls (6%), but the overall HPV prevalence and the prevalence of HPV 6 or 11 was similar for the two groups of patients.

RISK FACTORS

Although the morbidity rates for STDs such as syphilis, gonorrhea, and chlamydia are higher among single, divorced, and separated persons than among married persons, none of ten studies that examined marital status and HPV infection found a significant association.[42,88,89,90,91,92,93,94,95,96] Of nine studies that examined a relation between education level and HPV detection, only one found an increased rate of HPV DNA detection that was significantly associated with a lower level of education (only among Hispanic women).[97] A study by Bauer et al.[98] reported a similar, although not significant, trend.

As noted above, many recent studies have demonstrated a strong and consistent association between increasing number of sex partners and increasing likelihood of detecting HPV DNA in genital tract specimens. A study by Burk et al.[62] examined the relationship between HPV infection among women and the behavioral characteristics of their regular male partners. The lifetime number of partners of the woman's male partners and duration of her sexual relationship were positively associated with HPV detection among women.

Data on the association between smoking and HPV infection are inconclusive. Increased detection of genital HPV infection was found to be associated with current smoking,[94] past smoking,[99] and even the number of smokers in the household,[62] whereas a significantly lower HPV prevalence for former smokers than for women who had never smoked was reported in one study.[98] In another two studies,[90,100] smoking correlated with a high HPV prevalence in univariate analysis, but the association was diminished after adjusting for number of sex partners and other covariates. Most studies have failed to link smoking to HPV detection.[42,62,89,90,91,92,93,94,95,97,98,99,101,102,103,104]

Several lines of evidence suggest that HPV infection may be influenced by hormonal factors. Estrogen stimulation enhances expression of the HPV16 E6 and E7 genes in SiHa cervical carcinoma cells.[105] Oral contraceptive (OC) use has been associated with condylomata acuminata.[106] Anecdotal reports suggest that during pregnancy, when levels of estrogen and progesterone are high, condylomata acuminata increase in size in some women.[107] The relationship of OC use to HPV infection is difficult to ascertain, given the strong correlation between OC use and sexual activity. Although some studies report an association between use of hormonal contraceptives and detection of HPV DNA independent of correlated variables such as sexual activities,[100,108,109] most studies do not.[42,97,62,98,89,90,91,99,93,94] Use of OCs may represent a surrogate marker for sexual behavior that places a woman at high risk for genital HPV infection.

Some studies show a significantly higher HPV prevalence in pregnant women than in nonpregnant women[95,110,111,112] and a decreasing prevalence post partum.[111,112,113] In addition, an association between high levels of HPV DNA and pregnancy has been reported in one study,[111] and an association between increased risk of HPV infection and increasing number of pregnancies was reported in two other studies.[97,114] The increased HPV detection rate among pregnant women may result from hormonal effects, since estrogens and progestagens show a steady increase during pregnancy and decrease post delivery. Alternatively, slight immune tolerance or local physiologic change during pregnancy may be responsible for the increased detection rates. It should be noted, however, that most studies failed to find a significant association between increased HPV prevalence and pregnancy.[115,116,117,118,119,120,121,122,123] One methodologic difficulty in studies of the effect of pregnancy on HPV detection is lack of comparable controls.

NATURAL HISTORY

It is generally accepted that HPV infection may be detectable only transiently. In a follow-up study of 72 college women tested at weekly intervals over 10 weeks, the prevalence of HPV DNA by PCR was 36.1% at the entry visit and varied from 20.8% to 47.2% during any given week during the follow-up.[124] Of 42 HPV positive women, 12 were positive one or two times, 11 were positive four to seven times, and 19 were positive eight to ten times. Different or new HPV types were observed in 50% of the HPV positive individuals. The findings of transiently detected infection have been reported by others.[125,126,127,128] A study by Hildesheim et al. found that 26% of 393 cytologically normal women were HPV positive at enrollment and 26.2% at the time of their return visit over a median interval of 14.9 months.[129] Of 141 HPV positive women, 64 were positive at both visits and 77 at either visit. The number of women who had the same type of HPV between the enrollment and return visit was not reported. Another cohort study of 276 women showed prevalence of HPV decreasing from 21% to 8.3% between enrollment and return visit (mean interval of 2-years).[130] In two women only, the same HPV type persisted. Taken together, all studies suggest that in the majority of cases, HPV infection may be transient. Only a small subset of women had an infection that could be persistently detected over a 2-year interval. However, it is still not clear whether genital HPV infections are entirely eliminated by the host or merely become suppressed at a level below detection, possibly through immunological mechanisms.

Data concerning determinants associated with HPV persistence are scarce. HIV seropositive women are more likely to shed HPV persistently than those who are seronegative.[83,131] Hildesheim et al.[129] reported that HPV persistence was age and type related. Women over 29 years of age were more likely to be HPV DNA positive on two visits (65%) than those less than 25 years of age (32%), and persistence over two visits was higher among women infected with HPV types known to be cancer associated (45%) than those infected with other types (24%). A recent study by Brisson et al.[132] of 179 women 18 to 49 years of age with normal cytology showed the same association between persistence and cancer-associated HPV types found by Hildesheim et al. but the opposite relationship for age-related persistence. Factors such as longer duration of hormonal contraceptive use, increased viral load at initial visit, and history of penile condyloma in sex partners were associated with persistence in the Brisson et al. study.[132] Interpretation of the results from these studies is limited because (1) prevalent cases of HPV infection were used; (2) data were from only two time points in each study, and each used a different interval between the points; and (3) persistence was defined according to detectable HPV DNA rather than type concordance. However, these preliminary data do suggest the possibility of identifying determinants that influence the potential for per-

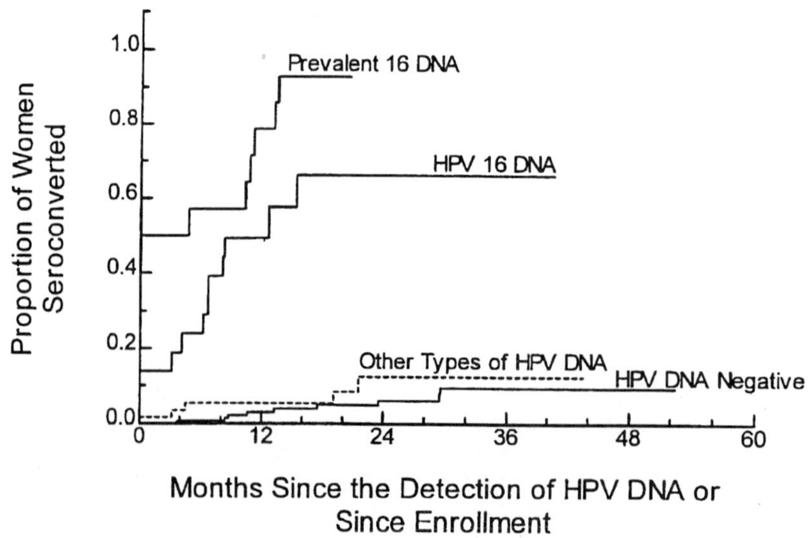

Fig. 25-3. Kaplan-Meier survival analysis using seroconversion as outcome. Lines represent proportion of women who seroconverted among women in whom HPV DNA was not detected (Neg = negative; n = 227), among women with incident HPV infections of types other than 16 (n = 64), among women with incident HPV 16 infections (n = 25), and among women with HPV 16 DNA detected at enrollment (n = 19). Women could contribute to more than one group if their HPV DNA status changed from HPV DNA negative to positive or from HPV DNA other-type positive to HPV 16 DNA positive during follow-up. (*Reprinted from Carter et al,[14] with permission.)*

sistence. Factors such as hormones, nutrition, cigarette smoking, pregnancies, and other genital tract infections may have important impacts on the course of HPV infection, but have not yet been studied sufficiently.

After infection by HPV 16, serum antibodies develop in most women but they appear to develop slowly. A recent study of women attending a public university[14] (Fig. 25-3) showed that, overall, 67% of women with incident HPV 16 infection and 94% of those with prevalent HPV 16 infection developed HPV 16 antibodies. In comparison, only 5% of women with incident genital HPV infection of other HPV types and 4% of those who were repeatedly negative for HPV DNA showed HPV 16 seroconversion. Importantly, among women with incident HPV 16 infection, the median time to seroconversion was 8.3 months.

Although simultaneous coinfection with different HPV types has been commonly observed, little is known about the role of cross-protective immunity between HPV types. It is unclear whether persons with certain types of HPVs are at increased or decreased risk for acquisition of other types as compared to those without, given the same exposures. It is currently unknown whether an initial infection with a specific HPV type confers immunity against reinfection with the same type of virus. Recently, a study by Xi et al.[133] characterized persistence of HPV 16 infection at the variant level. Seventy subjects who were repeatedly HPV 16 DNA positive two to eight times over an 8- to 32-month interval showed the same predominant variant at every visit. Sequencing of clones from a subset of specimens indicated that many women were infected by more than one variant but that only one major variant seemed to predominate over time, whereas minor variants appeared to be more transient. These results suggest that HPV 16 establishes a persistent infection in which a single variant predominates, while coinfection may result in minor populations of HPV 16 variants.

CLINICAL MANIFESTATIONS

Two clinical manifestations of genital HPV infection are important to diagnose: (1) genital warts that can be visualized without the aid of magnification, and (2) squamous intraepithelial lesions (SILs) of the cervix that are detected by routine cytologic screening of the cervical squamocolumnar junction. Although colposcopic examination and HPV DNA testing of genital tract epithelium would reveal SIL and HPV infection of the vagina, vulva, anus, or penis in a high proportion of sexually active adults, the clinical significance of SIL at sites other than the cervix (and perhaps the anus) is not clear. As discussed in Chapter 59, there is good support for the idea that high-grade cervical SIL represents an early stage in the development of invasive cervical cancer. In the anal canal, the dentate line corresponds to a squamocolumnar junction similar to that of the cervix. Individuals who engage in anoreceptive intercourse are at increased risk for high-grade SIL of the anus,[79,80,81,82,83] and by analogy to the cervix they may be at increased risk for invasive anal cancer. The clinical diagnosis and management of SIL and cancers of the genital tract is discussed in Chapter 59.

GENITAL WARTS

Individuals presenting with genital warts rarely report symptoms other than the appearance of new bumps or growths on their genitalia. Occasionally, patients will report itching, burning, pain, or bleeding. Some, perhaps most, individuals with genital warts never become aware of their presence. Women with external genital warts may report an abnormal vaginal discharge, which probably is due to a coexisting vaginal infection such as bacterial vaginosis and not HPV.[134]

Most genital warts occur on the penis, scrotum, urethral meatus, and perianal area in men and on the introitis, vulva, perineum, and perianal area in women. Less often, they may be found on the cervix and vaginal walls in women and the pubic area, upper thighs, or crural folds in both men and women.[135,136,137,138,139,140] Because genital warts frequently occur with more than one lesion on one genital site and with lesions on different genital sites, it is important to examine the entire genitalia. Speculum exam for vaginal and cervical warts is recommended for women with external genital warts. Colposcopy is indicated for women with cervical warts, anoscopy for men and women with recurrent perianal warts and a history of anoreceptive intercourse, and urethroscopy for men with warts at the distal urinary meatus and terminal hematuria or abnormal urinary stream. Use of mild (3% to 5%) acetic acid solutions to detect "subclinical" HPV infections of the external genitalia is not recommended because the predictive value and therapeutic benefit of this procedure has not been established.

Condyloma acuminatum appearing on the lips, tongue, or palate is a rare manifestation of infection by genital HPV types.[141,142] Some patients with oral condylomata will have concomitant genital or anal warts, and most give a history of oral sex. Transmission of HPV by orogenital contact is clearly possible.

The four morphologic types of genital warts are condylomata acuminata, which have a cauliflowerlike appearance (Fig. 25-4);

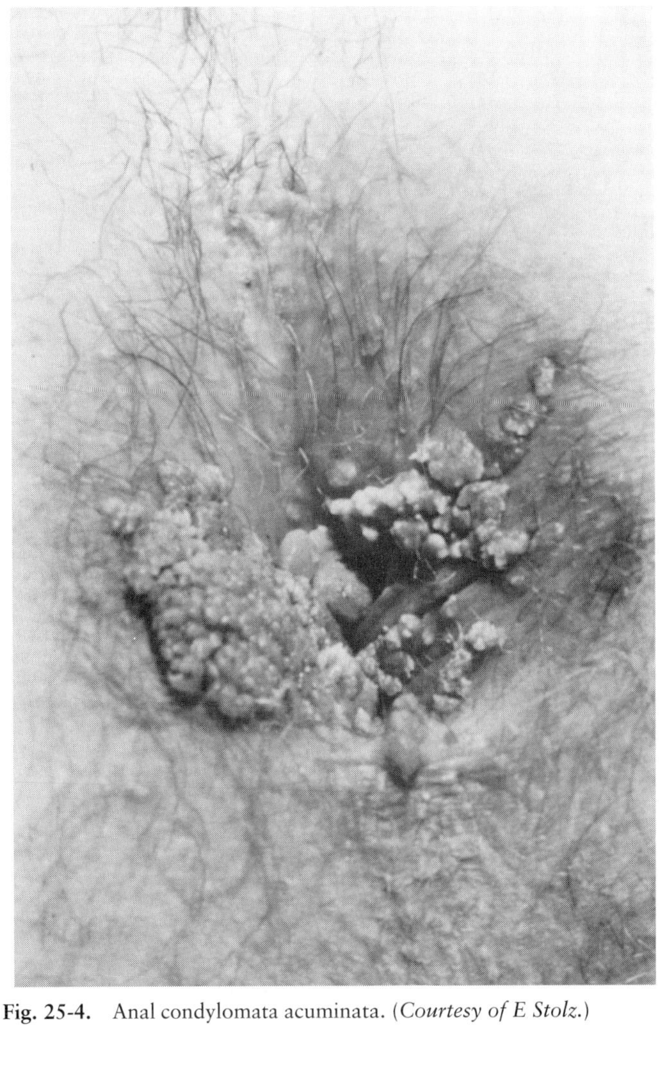

Fig. 25-4. Anal condylomata acuminata. (*Courtesy of E Stolz.*)

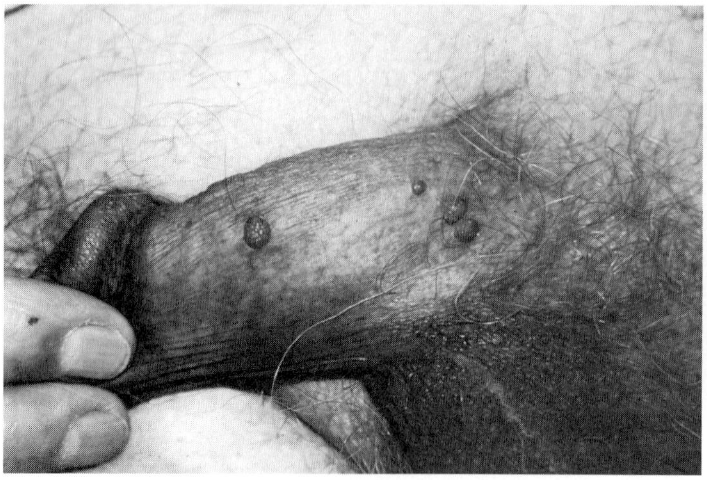

Fig. 25-5. Papular penile warts. (*Courtesy of KR Beutner.*)

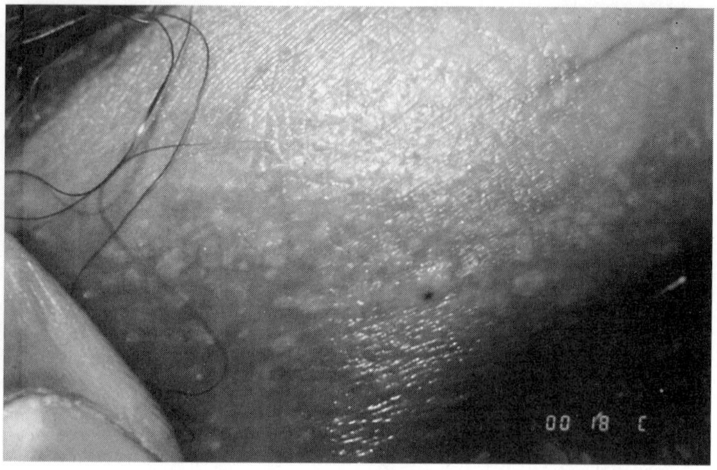

Fig. 25-7 Flat-topped macular warts. (*Courtesy of KR Beutner.*)

papular warts, which are flesh-colored, dome-shaped papules, usually 1–4 mm in diameter (Fig. 25-5); keratotic warts, which have a thick, crustlike layer and may resemble common skin warts or seborrheic keratosis (Fig. 25-6); and flat-topped papules, which appear macular to slightly raised (Fig. 25-7).[22,26,135,143,144,145,146,147] In general, condylomas are most frequently detected on moist, partially keratinized epithelium, papular and keratotic warts on fully keratinized epithelium, and flat papular warts on either partially or fully keratinized epithelium. Regardless of morphology and anatomic location, most genital warts are caused by HPV 6 and to a lesser extent HPV 11 and other HPV types.[8,9,63] A variant of dome-shaped and flat-topped papules, often referred to as "bowenoid papullosis," shows high-grade SIL on histology and is usually hyperpigmented and positive for HPV 16 DNA.[148]

Some individuals, particularly those with reduced cell-mediated immunity due to HIV, immunosuppressive therapy, Hodgkin's disease, or pregnancy develop very large genital warts. On rare occasions, these large warts become locally invasive, destructive but nonmetastasizing tumors that are called giant condylomas or Buschke-Lowenstein tumors.[149] These tumors are usually positive for HPV 6 DNA.

The differential diagnosis for genital warts includes papular anatomic structures such as skin tags (acrochordons), pearly penile papules, vestibular papillae, sebaceous (Tyson's) glands, melanocytic nevi, and acquired papular lesions including molluscum contagiosum, Crohn's disease, seborrheic keratosis, lichen planus, lichen nidus, and condyloma latum.[150,151,152,153,154,155,156]

Macular or flat lesions considered in the differential diagnosis of genital warts include psoriasis, seborrheic dermatitis, circinate balanitis of Reiter's syndrome, Bowen's disease, erythroplasia of Queyrat on the glans penis, and HPV-associated squamous cell cancers.[150,157,158] If the diagnosis of warts is questionable, a skin biopsy of the lesion may be performed.

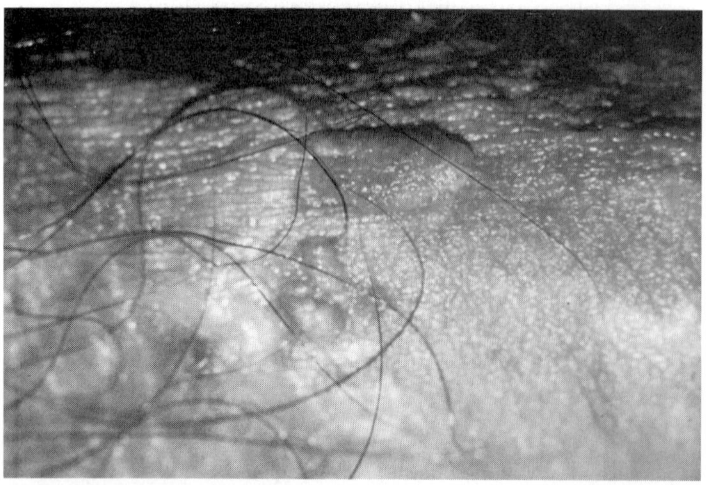

Fig. 25-6. Keratotic penile warts. (*Courtesy of KR Beutner.*)

MANAGEMENT

Although tests for HPV DNA detection and typing are commercially available, it is not clear how they should be used to manage patients with genital HPV infection. Such tests, however, may improve the management of women with mildly abnormal Pap smears (Chapter 59). As noted above, the prevalence of genital HPV infection is high among sexually active adults, multiple epithelial sites may be infected, and multiple HPV types may be present. Diagnosis and treatment of subclinical genital HPV infections in young adults would be a monumental undertaking, and with the exception of high-grade SIL, of unclear benefit but appreciable risk of scarring, hypo- or hyperpigmentation, and pain.[159,160,161] Although the clinical and morphologic manifestations of HPV infection are usually cleared with treatment, it is likely that virus persists in at least a few epithelial cells in many, if not most individuals. Treatment of genital warts is usually effective at inducing a wart-free state and may reduce the amount of infectious virus present. Treatment of cervical SIL, particularly high-grade SIL, reduces a woman's risk of invasive cervical cancer (Chapter 59).

In most settings, patients with genital warts are examined and treated for other STDs. Their current sex partners are also offered examination and treatment for macroscopically visible warts and other STDs. These visits provide an opportunity to counsel and educate. Counseling sessions involve educating patients about their diagnosis, treatment options, probability of recurrences, relationship of HPV infection to cancers, and infectivity. Most patients with genital warts are contagious to uninfected sex partners.[162] Treatment with clearance of warts probably reduces infectivity, but data addressing this issue are currently not available. Whether individuals with asymptomatic HPV infection are as contagious as patients with genital warts is unknown.

GENERAL PRINCIPLES OF TREATING GENITAL WARTS

Small warts of short duration (less than one year) respond better to therapy than large warts of long duration.[163] Although there are no data to show that treatment reduces the probability of transmission, it might. Without treatment, genital warts may disappear, stay the same, or grow larger in size or number.[164,165,166,167] Most genital warts are treated because they are aesthetically unpleasant. Clinical trials suggest clearance rates are similar for the more widely accepted treatment modalities. Clearance rates have ranged from 32% to 88% (from 32% to 79% for the same treatment evaluated in different studies).[168] Post-treatment recurrence rates are not well defined, because few subjects have been studied and follow-up protocols have not been standardized. For example, in some studies a recurrence is defined as a new wart at the same site detected within a six-month follow-up period, whereas in another study a recurrence is defined as new warts in the same anatomic area arising two to four months after initiation of therapy.

Choice of treatment is guided by patient preference, with consideration given to the patient's age and ability to comply with moderately complicated directions, to the location and number of warts, and to the clinician's training. Several treatment sessions are usually required to achieve a wart-free state. Thus, time spent counseling patients as to the high probability of recurrence during the first six months of therapy and the need for multiple treatment sessions is important. There is no need to use expensive and toxic therapies as first line therapy. Also, there are no data to support use of multiple rather than a single type of treatment on a single wart. Referral to a specialist is indicated for patients with extensive or refractory disease, cervical warts, or warts on the rectal mucosa.

Genital wart therapies are classified as patient-applied or provider-administered. Patient applied treatments include podofilox (Condylox™) solution and gel, and imiquimod (Aldara™) cream. To self-treat, patients must be able to identify and reach the warts and to follow the treatment application instructions. The provider-administered treatments include topical treatments—cryotherapy, podophyllin resin, trichloroacetic acid (TCA), or bichloroactetic acid (BCA); excisional treatments—curettage, electrosurgery, scissors excision, or laser vaporization; or injectable treatments—interferon or 5-fluorouracil/epinephrine gel implant.

Podofilox 0.5% solution or gel is an antimitotic agent purified from podophyllin resin. Unlike podophylin, podofilox has a stable shelf life, does not need to be washed off after application, and is less likely to cause systemic toxicity.[168,169,170] Treatment consists of twice-daily application by a cotton-tipped swab for three days followed by no treatment for four days for up to four weeks. Imiquimod 5% cream, which stimulates the production of interferon and other cytokines,[171,172] is applied to warts with fingers three times per week (every other night) for up to 16 weeks. The treatment area is washed with mild soap and water six to ten hours after application of imiquimod cream. For both of these patient-applied therapies the prescribing clinician provides the first application, instructing the patient in proper use. Imiquimod and podofilox have not been approved for treatment of perianal, rectal, urethral, vaginal, or cervical warts. Safety for use in pregnant patients has not been established for either agent.

Cryotherapy, which destroys the wart and a small area of surrounding tissue through freezing, is recommended for small warts that are not extensive. One to six freeze-thaw cycles per wart per treatment session may be required. Most patients will require one to two treatment sessions per week for an average of four to six weeks. A cryoprobe, modified Q-tip, or fine spray is used to apply liquid nitrogen to each wart. Cryotherapy may be painful, and a local anesthetic is recommended unless only one or two small warts are being treated. Safety and efficacy are highly dependent on clinician skills and training. Podophyllin resin, an antimitotic plant compound, is applied to warts as a 10% to 25% solution in ethanol or tincture of benzoin and allowed to dry. One to four hours after treatment, the compound is completely washed off. It is applied to the warts by a clinician using a cotton-tipped swab once to twice a week for up to six weeks. Applications are limited to 0.5 mL or 10 cm^2 per treatment session to decrease the potential for systemic effects such as bone marrow depression. Podophyllin is not used in pregnancy. Trichloroacetic or bichloroacetic acid in 80% to 90% solution may be used to treat small moist warts. The solution is applied by the clinician to each wart. Treatment may be repeated weekly for up to six weeks. Due to the low viscosity of these solutions and risk of local irritation, care must be taken to reduce contact of the solution with surrounding normal epithelium. Some clinicians recommend the application of sodium bicarbonate (baking soda) to the uninvolved surrounding epithelium to remove unreacted acid.

Warts may be removed by curettage, electrosurgery, excision by scissors or scalpel, or laser vaporization. Local anesthetic is applied before the excisional procedure is performed. Simple office surgery is often used for extensive or large warts and for treatment of warts during pregnancy. Electrosurgery is contraindicated for patients with cardiac pacemakers or for lesions proximal to the anal verge.

Other treatments, including intralesion injection of interferon and 5-fluorouracil/epinephrine gel implants, have been shown to be as effective as the modalities discussed above in clearing warts that are small in number and size. Side effect profiles and expense have limited the use of these alternative treatment modalities.[173,174,175]

All wart treatments may cause mild local irritation and infrequently cause serious pain or systemic effects. If complete wart clearance is not achieved within six weeks for provider-applied therapies or at the end of the manufacturer's specified treatment schedule for patient-applied therapies, use of a different treatment, performance of a skin biopsy, or referral to a specialist is recommended.

FOLLOW-UP

After warts have cleared and possible complications of therapy have resolved, there is no need for further follow up of immunocompetent patients. However, because genital wart recurrences are much more common in immunosuppressed patients, it may be helpful to provide these patients with repeated evaluations over an extended period of time. Annual cervical cytologic screening is recommended for women with or without genital warts, and the presence of genital warts per se is not an indication for cervical colposcopy.

PREVENTION

Genital HPV infections are so prevalent and so often asymptomatic that risk of infection with one or more HPV types appears to be high, even among individuals with relatively few sex partners. Currently, there are insufficient data on the efficacy of condoms in preventing HPV transmission. Abstinence or lifelong mutual monogamy undoubtedly reduces risk of infection, since virgins are rarely positive for genital types of HPV DNA.

Prophylactic vaccines for genital HPV infection are currently under development. Because the virus cannot be grown in tissue culture, attention has focused on subunit vaccines. A potential candidate for the subunit vaccine is a combination of the major (L1) and minor (L2) capsid proteins of HPV, which self-assemble into conformationally correct viruslike particles.[176] Although phase one vaccine trials are just beginning in humans, prophylactic vaccination for oral mucosal warts in beagles and fibroepithelial warts in rabbits and cattle has proven to be highly effective.[177,178,179] Potential impediments to genital HPV vaccine programs include the complexities of developing vaccines that will protect against the large number of HPV types that infect genital epithelium and the long interval between infection and development of the outcome of primary importance—cancer.

References

1 zur Hausen H: Roots and perspectives of contemporary papillomavirus research. *J Cancer Res Clin Oncol* 122:3, 1996.

2 Shamanin V et al: Specific types of human papillomavirus found in benign proliferations and carcinomas of the skin in immunosuppressed patients. *Cancer Res* 54:4610, 1994.

3 de Villiers EM: Human pathogenic papillomaviruses: an update, in *Curr Top Microbiol Immunol* 86:1, H zur Hausen (ed), 1994.

4 Chen SL et al: Characterization and analysis of human papillomaviruses of skin warts. *Arch Dermatol Res* 285:460, 1993.

5 de Villiers EM et al: Molecular cloning of viral DNA from human genital warts. *J Virol* 40:932, 1981.

6 de Villiers EM: Minireview. Heterogeneity of the human papillomavirus group. *J Virol* 63:4898, 1989.

7 Greer CE et al: Human papillomavirus (HPV) type distribution and serological response to HPV type 6 virus-like particles in patients with genital warts. *J Clin Microbiol* 33:2058, 1995.

8 Langenberg A et al: Dual infection with human papillomavirus in a population with overt genital condylomas. *J Am Acad Dermatol* 28: 434, 1993.

9 Sugase M et al: Human papillomavirus in exophytic condylomatous lesions on different female genital regions. *J Med Virol* 34:1, 1991.

10 Bosch FX et al and International Biological Study on Cervical Cancer (IBSCC) Study Group: Prevalence of human papillomavirus in cervical cancer: a worldwide perspective. *J Natl Cancer Inst* 87:796, 1995.

11 IARC Working Group: Studies of Cancer in Humans, in *IARC Monographs on the Evaluation of Carcinogenic Risks to Humans,* vol 64. Lyon, 1995, pp 142–163.

12 Wright TC et al: Precancerous Lesions of the Cervix, in *Blaustein's Pathology of the Female Genital Tract* 4th ed, R Kurman (ed). New York, Springer-Verlag, 1994, pp 229–277.

13 Carter JJ et al: Use of human papillomavirus type 6 capsids to detect antibodies in people with genital warts. *J Infect Dis* 172:11, 1995.

14 Carter JJ et al: The natural history of human papillomavirus type 16 capsid antibodies among a cohort of university women. *J Infect Dis* 36:174, 1996.

15 Heim K et al: Serum IgG, IgM, and IgA reactivity to human papillomavirus types 11 and 6 virus-like particles in different gynecologic patient groups. *J Infect Dis* 172:395, 1995.

16 Nonnenmacher B et al: Serologic response to human papillomavirus type 16 (HPV-16) virus-like particles in HPV-16 DNA-positive invasive cervical cancer and cervical intraepithelial neoplasia grade III patients and controls from Colombia. *J Infect Dis* 172:19, 1995.

17 Shah KV et al: Antibodies to human papillomairus 16 and subsequent in situ or invasive cancer of the cervix. *Cancer Epidemiol Biomarkers and Prev* 6:233, 1997.

18 Wideroff L et al: Evaluation of seroreactivity to human papillomavirus type 16 virus-like particles in an incident case-control study of cervical neoplasia. *J Infect Dis* 172:1425, 1995.

19 IARC Working Group: Studies of Cancer in Humans, in *IARC Monographs on the Evaluation of Carcinogenic Risks to Humans,* vol 64. Lyon, 1995, pp 87–231.

20 Oriel JD: Natural history of genital warts. *Br J Vener Dis* 47:1, 1971.

21 Rosenbaum J: *The Plague of Lust. Being a History of Venereal Disease in Classical Antiquity, and Including Detailed Investigations into the Cult of Venus and Phallic Worship, Brothels, etc.* Paris, C. Carrington, 1901.

22 Rowson KEK, Mahy BWJ: Human papova (wart) virus. *Bacteriol Rev* 31:110, 1967.

23 Rous P, Beard JW: Carcinomatous changes in virus-induced papillomas of the skin of the rabbit. *Proc Soc Exp Biol Med* 32:578, 1935.

24 Rous P, Kidd JG: The carcinogenic effect of papilloma virus on the tarred skin of rabbits. I. Description of the phenomenon. *J Exp Med* 67:399, 1938.

25 Koss LG, Durfee GR: Unusual patterns of squamous epithelium of the uterine cervix: cytologic and pathologic study of koilocytotic atypia. *Ann NY Acad Sci* 63:1245, 1956.

26 Meisels A, Fortin R: Condylomatous lesions of the cervix and vagina. I. Cytologic patterns. *Acta Cytol* 20:505, 1976.

27 Purola E, Savia E: Cytology of gynecologic condyloma acuminatum. *Acta Cytol* 21:26, 1977.

28 Gissmann L, zur Hausen H: Human papilloma viruses: physical mapping and genetic heterogeneity. *Proc Natl Acad Sci USA* 73:1310, 1976.

29 Gissmann L et al: Human papilloma viruses (HPV): characterization of four different isolates. *Virology* 76:569, 1977.

30 Orth G et al: Characterization of a new type of human papillomavirus that causes skin warts. *J Virol* 24:108, 1977.

31 Gissmann L, zur Hausen H: Partial characterization of viral DNA from human genital warts (condylomata acuminata). *Int J Cancer* 25:605, 1980.

32 IARC Working Group: Molecular Mechanisms of Carcinogenesis, in *IARC Monographs on the Evaluation of Carcinogenic Risks to Humans,* vol 64. Lyon, 1995, pp 233–260.

33 Phelps et al: The human papillomavirus type 16 E7 gene encodes transactivation and transformation functions similar to those of adenovirus E1A. *Cell* 53:539, 1988.

34 Matlashewski G et al: Human papillomavirus type 16 DNA cooperates with activated ras in transforming primary cells. *EMBO J* 6: 1741, 1987.

35 Dürst M et al: Molecular and cytogenic analysis of immortalized human primary keratinocytes obtained after transfection with human papillomavirus type 16 DNA. *Oncogene* 1:251, 1987a.

36 Kaur P, McDougall JK: Characterization of primary human kerati nocytes transformed by human papillomavirus type 18. *J Virol* 62: 1917, 1988.

37 Cripe TP et al: Transcriptional regulation of the human papillomavirus-16 E6-E7 promoter by a keratinocyte-dependent enhancer, and by viral E2 trans-activator and repressor gene products: implications for cervical carcinogenesis. *EMBO J* 6:3745, 1987.

38 Gloss B et al: The upstream regulatory region of the human papillomavirus-16 contains an E2 protein-independent enhancer which is specific for cervical carcinoma cells and regulated by glucocorticoid hormones. *EMBO J* 6:3735, 1987.

39 Blanton RA et al: Epithelial cells immortalized by human papillomaviruses have premalignant characteristics in organotypic culture. *Am J Pathol* 138:673, 1991.

40 Koss LG, Durfee GR: Cytological changes preceding the appearance of in situ carcinoma of the uterine cervix. *Cancer* 8:295, 1955.

41 Kiviat N et al: Prevalence of genital papillomavirus infection among women attending a college student health clinic or a sexually transmitted disease clinic. *J Infect Dis* 159:293, 1989.

42 Wheeler CM et al: Determinants of genital human papillomavirus infection among cytologically normal women attending the University of New Mexico. *Sex Transm Dis* 20:286, 1993.

43 Rylander E et al: The absence of vagina human papillomavirus 16 DNA in women who have not experienced sexual intercourse. *Obstet Gynecol* 83:735, 1994.

44 Schiffman MH: Recent progress in defining the epidemiology of human papillomavirus infection and cervical neoplasia. *J Natl Cancer Inst* 84:394, 1992.

45 Grce M et al: Increase of genital human papillomavirus infection among men and women in Croatia. *Anticancer Res* 16:1039, 1996.

46 van Doornum et al: Regional distribution and incidence of human papillomavirus infections among heterosexual men and women with multiple sexual partners: a prospective study. *Genitourin Med* 70: 240, 1994.

47 Baken LA et al: Genital human papillomavirus infection among male and female sex partners: prevalence and type specific concordance. *J Infect Dis* 171:429, 1995.

48 Hippelainen M: Prevalence and risk factors of genital human papillomavirus (HPV) infections in healthy males; a study on Finnish conscripts. *Sex Transm Dis* 20:321, 1993.

49 Kataoka A: Human papillomavirus infection of the male diagnosed by southern-blot hybridization and polymerase chain reaction: comparison between urethra samples and penile biopsy samples. *J Med Virol* 33:159, 1991.

50 Munoz N: Difficulty in elucidating the male role in cervical cancer in Colombia, a high risk area for the disease. *J Natl Cancer Inst* 88:106, 1996.

51 Bosch FX et al: Male sexual behavior and human papillomavirus DNA: key risk factors for cervical cancer in Spain. *J Natl Cancer Inst* 88:1060, 1996.

52 Ong CK et al: Evolution of human papillomavirus type 18: an ancient phylogenetic root in Africa and intratype diversity reflect coevolution with human ethnic groups. *J Virol* 67:6424, 1993.

53 Chan SY et al: Molecular variants of human papillomavirus type 16 from four continents suggest ancient pandemic spread of the virus and its co-evolution with humankind. *J Virol* 66:2057, 1992.

54 Yamada T: Human papillomavirus type 16 variant lineages in United States populations characterized by nucleotide sequence analysis of the E6, L2, and L1 coding segments. *J Virol* 69:7743, 1995.

55 Yamada T: Human papillomavirus type 16 sequence variation in cervical cancers: a worldwide perspective. *J Virol* 71:2463–2472, 1997.

56 Chuang TY: Condyloma acuminatum in Rochester, Minnesota, 1950–1978. *Arch Dermatol* 120:469, 1984.

57 Aral SO, Holmes KK: Epidemiology of Sexual Behavior and Sexually Transmitted Diseases, in *Sexually Transmitted Diseases,* 2nd ed, KK Holmes et al (eds). New York, McGraw-Hill, 1990, pp 126–141.

58 Becker TM et al: Genital human papillomavirus infection: a growing concern. *Obstet Gynecol Clin N Am* 14:389, 1987.

59 Syrjanen K et al: Prevalence, incidence, and estimated life-time risk of cervical human papillomavirus infection in a nonselected Finnish female population. *Sex Transm Dis* 17:15, 1990.

60 Persson G et al: Symptomatic genital papillomavirus infection in a community. Incidence and clinical picture. *Acta Obstet Gynecol Scand* 75:287, 1996.

61 Barrett TJ et al: Genital warts—a venereal disease. *JAMA* 154:333, 1954.

62 Burk RD et al: Sexual behavior and partner characteristics are the predominant risk factors for genital human papillomavirus infection in young women. *J Infect Dis* 174:679, 1996.

63 Bauer HM et al: Genital human papillomavirus infection in female university students as determined by a PCR-based method. *JAMA* 265:472, 1991.

64 Brunham RC, Plummer FA: A general model of sexualy transmitted disease epidemiology and its implications for control. *Med Clin N Am* 74:1339, 1990.

65 Brunham RC, Plummer FA: A general model of STD epidemiology and its implications for control. *Med Clin N Am* 26:138, 1991.

66 Schneider A et al: Sub-clinical human papillomavirus infection in male sexual partners of female carriers. *J Urol* 140:1431, 1988.

67 Bunney MH: *Viral Warts: Their Biology and Treatment.* New York, Oxford University Press, 1982, p 10.

68 Rüdlinger R et al: HPV 35 positive bowenoid papulosis of the anogenital area and concurrent HPV-35 positive verruca with bowenoid dysplasia of the periungual area. *Arch Dermatol* 125:655, 1989b.

69 Krzyzek RA et al: Anogenital warts contain several distinct species of human papillomavirus. *J Virol* 36:236, 1980.

70 Sundararaj AS et al: Anal and laryngeal papillomata in an 8 month old child. *Int J STD AIDS* 2:213, 1991.

71 Tang CK et al: Congenital condylomata acuminata. *Am J Obstet Gynecol* 131:912, 1978.

72 Cohen BA et al: Anogenital warts in children: clinical and virologic evaluation for sexual abuse. *Arch Dermatol* 23:1575, 1990.

73 Obalek S et al: Childhood condyloma acuminatum: association with genital and cutaneous human papillomaviruses. *Pediatric Dermatology* 10:101, 1993.

74 zur Hausen H: Papillomavirus infection—a major cause of human cancers. *Biochem Biophys Acta* 1288:55, 1996.

75 Apple RJ et al: Comparison of human leukocyte antigen DR-DQ disease associations found with cervical dysplasia and invasive cervical carcinoma. *J Natl Cancer Inst* 87:427, 1995.

76 Apple RJ et al: HLA DR-DQ associations with cervical carcinoma show papillomavirus-type specificity. *Nat Genet* 6:157, 1994.

77 Ellis JRM: The association of an HPV16 oncogene variant with HLA-B7 has implications for vaccine design in cervical cancer. *Nature Med* 1:464, 1995.

78 Critchlow CW, Koutsky LA: Epidemiology of Human Papillomavirus Infection, in *Genital Warts: Human Papillomavirus Infection,* A Mindel (ed). London, Edward Arnold, 1995, pp 53–81.

79 Kiviat NB et al: Association of anal dysplasia and human papillomavirus with immunosuppression and HIV infection among homosexual man. *AIDS* 7:43, 1993.

80 Law CLH et al: Factors associated with clinical and sub-clinical anal human papillomavirus infection in homosexual men. *Genitourin Med,* 67:92, 1991.

81 Critchlow CW et al: Association of HIV and HPV infection among homosexual men presenting to a public health department HIV antibody screening clinic. *Arch Int Med* 152:1673, 1992.

82 Palefsky JM et al: Risk factors for anal human papillomavirus infection and anal cytologic abnormalities in HIV-positive and HIV-negative homosexual men. *J AIDS* 7:599, 1994.

83 Breese PL et al: Anal human papillomavirus infection among homosexual and biosexual men: prevalence of type-specific infection and association with human immunodeficiency virus. *Sex Transm Dis* 22: 7, 1995.

84 Halpert R et al: Human papillomavirus infection and low genital neoplasia in female renal allograft recipients. *Transplant Proc* 17:93, 1985.

85 Ogunbiyi OA et al: Prevalence of anal human papillomavirus infection and intraepithelial neoplasia in renal allograft recipients *Br J Surg* 81:365, 1994.

86 Fairley CK et al: Prevalence of HPV DNA in cervical specimens in women with renal transplants: a comparison with dialysis-dependent patients and patients with renal impairment. *Nephrol Dial Transplant* 9:416, 1994.

87 Alloub MI et al: Papillomavirus infection and cervical intraepithelial neoplasia in women with renal allografts. *Br Med J* 298:153, 1989.

88 Xu S et al: Clinical observation on vertical transmission of human papillomavirus. *Chung-Hua Fu Chan Ko Tsa Chih* 30:457, 1995.

89 Reed BD et al: Factors associated with human papillomavirus infection in women encountered in community-based offices. *Arch Fam Med* 2:1239, 1993.

90 Fairley CK et al: Human papillomavirus infection and its relationship to recent and distant sexual partners. *Obstet Gynecol* 84:755, 1994.

91 Karlsson R et al: Lifetime number of partners as the only independent risk factor for human papillomavirus infection: a population-based study. *Sex Transm Dis* 22:119, 1995.

92 Fisher M et al: Cervicovaginal human papillomavirus infection in suburban adolescents and young adults. *J Pediatr* 119:821, 1991.

93 Meekin GE: Prevalence of genital human papillomavirus infection in Wellington women. *Genitourin Med* 68:228, 1992.

94 Davidson M et al: The prevalence of cervical infection with human papillomaviruses and cervical dysplasia in Alaska Native women. *J Infect Dis* 169:792, 1994.

95 Villa LL, Franco EL: Epidemiologic correlates of cervical neoplasia and risk of human papillomavirus infection in asymptomatic women in Brazil. *J Natl Cancer Inst* 81:332, 1989.

96 Muckerman DR: Sub-clinical human papillomavirus infection in a high-risk population. *J Am Osteopath Assoc* 94:545, 1994.
97 Hildesheim A et al: Determinants of genital human papillomavirus infection in low-income women in Washington, D.C. *Sex Transm Dis* 20:279, 1993.
98 Bauer HM et al: Determinants of genital human papillomavirus infection in low-risk women in Portland, Oregon. *Sex Transm Dis* 20: 274, 1993.
99 Rohan T et al: PCR-detected genital papillomavirus infection: prevalence and association with risk factors for cervical cancer. *Int J Cancer* 49:856, 1991.
100 Ley C: Determinants of genital human papillomavirus infection in young women. *J Natl Cancer Inst* 83:997, 1991.
101 Venuti A et al: Determinants of human papillomavirus types 16 and 18 infections in the lower female genital tract in an Italian population. *Eur J Gynaec Oncol* 15:205, 1994.
102 Moscicki AB: Human papillomavirus infection in sexually active adolescent females: Prevalence and risk factors. *Pediatr Res* 28:507, 1990.
103 Marrero M: Detection of human papillomavirus by nonradioactive hybridization. *Diagn Microbiol Dis* 18:95, 1994.
104 Kjaer SK: Risk factors for cervical human papillomavirus and herpes simplex virus infections in Greenland and Denmark: a population based study. *Am J Epidemiol* 131:669, 1990.
105 Mitrani-Rosenbaum S: Oestrogen stimulates differential transcription of human papillomavirus type 16 in SiHa cervical carcinoma cells. *J Gen Virol* 70:2227, 1989.
106 Schneider A, Koutsky LA: Natural history and epidemiological features of genital HPV infection, in *Epidemiology of Cervical Cancer and Human Papillomavirus,* IARC Scientific Publ No 119, N Munoz et al (eds.). Lyon, IARC, 1992, pp 25–52.
107 Fife KH et al: Symptomatic and asymptomatic cervical infections with human papillomavirus during pregnancy. *J Infect Dis* 156:904, 1987.
108 Lorincz AT et al: Temporal associations of human papillomavirus infection with cervical cytologic abnormalities. *Am J Obstet Gynecol* 162:645, 1990.
109 Negrini BP et al: Oral contraceptive use, human papillomavirus infection, and risk of early cytological abnormalities of the cervix. *Cancer Res* 50:467, 1990.
110 Saito J et al: Detection of human papillomavirus DNA in the normal cervices of Japanese women by the dot-blot (Vipa Pap) method. *Asia Oceania J Obstet Gynecol* 18:283, 1992.
111 Czegledy J et al: Detection of human papillomavirus deoxyribonucleic acid by filter in situ hybridization during pregnancy. *J Med Virol* 28:250, 1989.
112 Schneider A et al: Increased prevalence of human papillomaviruses in the low genital tract of pregnant women. *Int J Cancer* 40:198, 1987.
113 Rando RF et al: Increased frequency of detection of human papillomavirus deoxyribonucleic acid in exfoliated cervical cells during pregnancy. *Am J Obstet Gynecol* 16:150, 1989.
114 Gopalkrishna V et al: Increased human papillomavirus infection with the increasing number of pregnancies in Indian women. *J Infect Dis* 171:254, 1995.
115 Basta A et al: Human papillomavirus virus (HPV) infections of the uterine cervix, vagina and vulva in women of childbearing age. *Ginekol Pol* 65:563, 1994.
116 Delvenne P et al: Detection of human papillomavirus DNA in biopsy-proven cervical squamous intraepithelial lesions in pregnant women. *J Reprod Med* 37:829, 1992.
117 de Roda-Husman AM et al: HPV prevalence in cytomorphologically normal cervical scrapes of pregnant women as determined by PCR; the age-related pattern. *J Med Virol* 46:97, 1995.
118 Freitag P et al: Prevalence of HPV infection and histologic correlations. *Ceska Gynecol* 61:150, 1996.
119 Kemp EA et al: Human papillomavirus prevalence in pregnancy. *Obstet Gynecol* 79:649, 1992.
120 Kuhler-Obbarius C et al: Polymerase chain reaction-assisted papillomavirus detection in cervicovaginal smears: stratification by clinical risk and cytology reports. *Virchows Arch* 425:157, 1994.
121 Nishikawa A et al: Relatively low prevalence of human papillomavirus 16, 18, and 33 DNA in the normal cervices of Japanese women shown by polymerase chain reaction. *Jpn J Cancer Res* 82:532, 1991.
122 Peng TC et al: Prevalence of human papillomavirus infections in term pregnancy. *Am J Perinatol* 7:189, 1990.
123 Soares VR et al: Human papillomavirus DNA in unselected pregnant and non-pregnant women. *Int J STD AIDS* 1:276, 1990.
124 Wheeler CM: Short-term fluctuations in the detection of cervical human papillomavirus DNA. *Obstet Gynecol* 88:261, 1996.
125 Schneider A et al: Repeated evaluation of human papillomavirus 16 status in cervical swabs of young women with a history of normal papanicolaou smears. *Obstet Gynecol* 79:683, 1992.
126 Reeves WC et al: Human papillomavirus infection and cervical cancer in Latin America. *N Engl J Med* 320:1437, 1989.
127 Rosenfeld WD et al: Follow up evaluation of cervical vaginal human papillomavirus infection in adolescents. *J Pediatr* 121:301, 1992.
128 Moscicki AB et al: Variability of human papillomavirus DNA testing in a longitudinal cohort of young women. *Obstet Gynecol* 82:578, 1993.
129 Hildesheim A et al: Persistence of type specific human papillomavirus infection among cytologically normal women. *J Infect Dis* 169:235, 1994.
130 Evander M et al: Human papillomavirus infection is transient in young women: a population-based cohort study. *J Infect Dis* 171: 1026, 1995.
131 Vernon SD et al: A longitudinal study of human papillomavirus DNA detection in human immunodeficiency virus type 1 seropositive and seronegative women. *J Infect Dis* 169:1108, 1994.
132 Brisson J et al: Determinants of persistent detection of human papillomavirus DNA in the uterine cervix. *J Infect Dis* 173:794, 1996.
133 Xi LF et al: Analysis of human papillomavirus type 16 variants indicates establishment of persistent infection. *J Infect Dis* 172:747, 1995.
134 Kinghorn GR: Genital warts: incidence of associated genital infections. *Br J Dermatol* 99:405, 1978.
135 Bonnez W et al: A randomized, double-blind, placebo-controlled trial of systemically administered interferon-α, -β, or γ in combination with cryotherapy for the treatment of condylomata acuminatum. *J Infect Dis* 167:824, 1993.
136 Condylomata International Collaborative Study Group: Randomized placebo-controlled double-blind combined therapy with laser surgery and systemic interferon-α2a in the treatment of anogenital condylomata acuminata. *J Infect Dis* 167:824, 1993.
137 Handley JM: Subcutaneous interferon alpha 2a combined with cryotherapy vs cryotherapy alone in the treatment of primary anogenital warts: a randomized observer blind placebo controlled study. *Genitourin Med* 67:297, 1991.
138 Bellina JH: The use of the carbon dioxide laser in the management of condyloma acuminatum with eight-year follow-up. *Am J Obstet Gynecol* 147:375, 1983.
139 Ferenczy A: Laser therapy of genital condylomata acuminata. *Obstetr Gynecol* 63:703, 1984.
140 Syed TA et al: Management of genital warts in women with human leukocyte interferon-alpha vs podophyllotoxin in cream: a placebo-controlled, double-blind, comparative study. *J Mol Med* 73:255, 1995.
141 Judson FN: Condyloma acuminatum of the oral cavity: a case report. *Sex Transm Dis* 8:218, 1981.
142 Lutzner MA et al: Different papillomaviruses as the causes of oral warts. *Arch Dermatol* 118:393, 1982.
143 von Krogh G, Wikstrom A: Efficacy of chemical and/or surgical therapy against condylomata acuminata: a retrospective evaluation. *Inter J STD AIDS* 2:333, 1991.
144 Wikstrom A: Clinical and serological manifestations of genital human papillomavirus infection. *Acta Derm Venereol Suppl* 193:10, 1995.

145 Happonen HP et al: Topical idoxuridine for treatment of genital warts in males. A double blind comparative study of 0.25% and 0.5% cream. *Genitourin Med* 66:254, 1990.
146 Condylomata International Collaborative Study Group: A comparison of interferon alpha-2a and podophyllin in the treatment of primary condylomata acuminata. *Genitourin Med* 67:394, 1991.
147 Meisels A, Fortin R: Condylomatous lesions of the cervix: II. Cytologic, colposcopic and histopathologic study. *ACTA Cytologica* 21: 379, 1977.
148 Broker TR: Structure and genetic expression of papillomaviruses. *Obstet Gynecol Clin N Am* 14:329, 1987.
149 Ananthakrishnan N et al: Loewenstein-Buschke tumour of penis—A carcinomimic. Report of 124 cases with review of the literature. *Br J Urol* 53:460, 1981.
150 Fitzpatrick JE, Gentry RH: Nonvenereal Diseases of Male Genitalia, in *Dermatology* 3rd ed, vol 1, SL Moschella, HJ Hurley (eds). Philadelphia, WB Saunders, 1992, pp 1013–1014.
151 Gonzalez E: Molluscum Contagiosum and Other Viruses, in *Dermatology* 3rd ed, vol 1, SL Moschella, HJ Hurley (eds). Philadelphia, WB Saunders, 1992, p 64.
152 Jakubovic HR, Ackerman AB: Structure and Function of Skin: development, morphology, and physiology, in *Dermatology,* third ed, vol 1, SL Moschella, HJ Hurley (eds). Philadelphia, WB Saunders, 1992, p 64.
153 Gibson LE, Perry HO: Papulosquamous Eruptions and Exfoliative Dermatitis, in *Dermatology,* third ed, vol 1, SL Moschella, HJ Hurley (eds). Philadelphia, WB Saunders, 1992, pp 629–636.
154 Gibson LE, Perry HO: Papulosquamous Eruptions and Exfoliative dermatitis, in *Dermatology,* third ed, vol 1, SL Moschella, HJ Hurley (eds). Philadelphia, WB Saunders, 1992, pp 607–622.
155 Oriel JD: Sexually transmitted diseases in children: human papillomavirus infection. *Genitourin Med* 68:80, 1992.
156 Koh HK, Ghawan J: Tumors of the Skin, in *Dermatology,* third ed, vol 1, SL Moschella, HJ Hurley (eds). Philadelphia, WB Saunders, 1992, pp 1721–1808.
157 Webster SB: Nontreponemal Sexually Transmissible Diseases, in *Dermatology,* third ed, vol 1, SL Moschella, HJ Hurley (eds). Philadelphia, WB Saunders, 1992, pp 987–1007.
158 Koh HK, Ghawan J: Tumors of the Skin, in *Dermatology* third ed, vol 1, SL Moschella, HJ Hurley (eds). Philadelphia, WB Saunders, 1992, pp 1735–1737.
159 Beutner KR et al: Patient-applied podofilox for treatment of genital warts. *Lancet* 1:831, 1989.
160 Reid R: Genital condulomas, intraepithelial neoplasia, and vulvodynia. *Obstetr Gynecol Clin N Am* 23:917, 1996.
161 Duus BR: Refractory condylomata acuminata: a controlled clinical trial of carbon dioxide laser versus conventional surgical treatment. *Genitourin Med* 61:59, 1985.
162 Barrett TJ: Genital warts—a venereal disease. *JAMA* 154:333, 1954.
163 McCance DJ: Natural history of genital warts. *Br J Vener Dis* 47:1, 1971.
164 Monsonego J et al: Randomized double-blind trial of recombinant interferon-beta for condyloma acuminatum. *Genitourin Med* 72:111, 1996.
165 Kirby PK et al: Tolerance and efficacy of recombinant human interferon gamma in the treatment of refractory genital warts. *Am J Med* 85:183, 1988.
166 Eron LJ et al: Interferon therapy for condylomata acuminata. *N Engl J Med* 315:1059, 1986.
167 Condylomata International Collaborative Study Group: Recurrent condylomata acuminata treated with recombinant interferon alpha-2a. *JAMA* 265:2684, 1991.
168 Stone KM: Human papillomavirus infection and genital warts: update on epidemiology and treatment. *Clin Infect Dis* 20(Suppl 1):S91, 1995.
169 Beutner KR, von Krogh G: Current status of podophyllotoxin for the treatment of genital warts. *Semin Dermatol* 9:148, 1990.
170 Mazurkiewicz W, Jablonska S: Clinical efficacy of Condyline (0.5% pokophyllotoxin) solution and cream versus podophyllin in the treatment of external condulomata acuminata. *J Dermatol Treat* 1:123, 1990.
171 Kinghorn GR et al: An open, comparative, study of the efficacy of 0.5% podophyllotoxin lotion and 25% podophyllotoxin solution in the treatment of condylomata acuminata in males and females. *Int J STD AIDS* 4:194, 1993.
172 Wade TR, Ackerman AB: The effects of resin of podophyllin on condylomata acuminata. *Am J Dermatopathol* 6:109, 1984.
173 Swinehart JM et al: Relationship of genital wart burden to therapeutic response to fluorouracil/epinephrine injectable gel. *Int J STD AIDS* 1997;8:639–42.
174 Swinehart JM et al: Intralesional fluorouracil/epinephrine injectable gel for treatment of condylomata acuminata: a phase III clinical study. *Archiv Dermatol,* 1997;133:67–73.
175 Beutner KR, Ferenczy A: Therapeutic approaches to genital warts. *Am J Med* 102(5A):28.
176 Kirnbaurer R et al: Efficient self-assembly of human papillomavirus type 16 L1 and L1-L2 into virus-like particles. *J Virol* 67:6929, 1993.
177 Suzich JA et al: Systemic immunization with papillomavirus L1 protein completely prevents the development of viral mucosal papillomas. *Proc Natl Acad Sci USA* 92:11553, 1995.
178 Christensen ND et al: Immunization with viruslike particles induces long-term protection of rabbits against challenge with cottontail rabbit papillomavirus. *J Virol* 1996;70:960–965.
179 Kirnbauer R et al: Virus-like particles of bovine papillomavirus type 4 in prophylactic and therapeutic immunization. *Virology* 219:37, 1996.
180 ter Meulen J et al: Human papillomavirus (HPV) infection, HIV infection and cervical cancer in Tanzania, East Africa. *Int J Cancer* 51: 515, 1992.
181 Pao CC et al: Detection of human papillomaviruses in cervicovaginal cells using polymerase chain reaction. *J Infect Dis* 161:113, 1990.
182 Lambropoulos AF et al: Detection of human papillomavirus using the polymerase chain reaction and typing for HPV 16 and 18 in the cervical smears of Greek women. *J Med Virol* 43:228, 1994.
183 Becker TM. Sexually transmitted diseases and other risk factors for cervical dysplasia among southwestern Hispanic and non-Hispanic white women. *JAMA* 271:1181, 1994.
184 Seck AC et al: Cervical intraepithelial neoplasia and human papillomavirus infection among Senegalese women seropositive for HIV-1 or HIV-2 or seronegative for HIV. *Int J STD AIDS* 5:189, 1994.
185 Czeglédy J et al: High-risk human papillomavirus types in cytologically normal cervical scrapes from Kenya. *Med Microbiol Immunol (Berl)* 180:321, 1992a.
186 Schiffman MH et al: Epidemiologic evidence showing that human papillomavirus infection causes most cervical intraepithelial neoplasia. *J Natl Cancer Inst* 85:958, 1993.
187 Engels H et al: Cervical cancer screening and detection of genital HPV infection and chlamydial infection by PCR in different groups of Kenyan women. *Ann Soc Belg Med Trop* 72:53, 1992.
188 Melkert PWJ et al: Prevalence of HPV in cytomorphologically normal cervical smears, as determined by the polymerase chain reaction, is age-dependent. *Int J Cancer* 53:919, 1993.
189 Muñoz N et al: The causal link between human papillomavirus and invasive cervical cancer: a population-based case-control study in Colombia and Spain. *Int J Cancer* 52:743, 1992.
190 van Doornum GJ: Prevalence of human papillomavirus infections among heterosexual men and women with multiple sexual partners. *J Med Virol* 37:13, 1992.
191 Bosch FX et al: Human papillomavirus and cervical intraepithelial neoplasia grade III/carcinoma in situ: a case-control study in Spain and Colombia. *Cancer Epidemiol Biomarkers Prev* 2:415, 1993.
192 Fairley CK et al: The absence of genital human papillomavirus DNA in virginal women. *Int J STD AIDS* 3:414, 1992.

Chapter 26
Viral hepatitis

Stanley M. Lemon
Miriam J. Alter

HISTORY AND DEFINITIONS

Although viral hepatitis is unquestionably an ancient disease, it is only in recent years that an appreciation has emerged of the diversity of infectious agents capable of causing the clinical syndrome of acute hepatitis. The era of modern hepatitis virology began with the discovery of Australia antigen by Blumberg and associates in 1965 and the subsequent association of this antigen with hepatitis B.[1,2] Knowledge in this area has since continued to expand rapidly, and at least five distinctly different human viruses (classified as hepatitis A through E) are now generally recognized to be causative agents of acute and/or chronic viral hepatitis (Table 26-1).

Hepatitis A virus (HAV), hepatitis B virus (HBV), hepatitis C virus (HCV), hepatitis D virus (formerly hepatitis delta virus, HDV), and hepatitis E virus (HEV) all share a remarkable tropism for the liver despite profound differences in their physical structure, pathobiology, and epidemiology. Each of these viruses is a cause of clinically overt acute hepatitis associated with frank jaundice. The severity of the liver disease which frequently accompanies acute infection with these viruses generally distinguishes them from cytomegalovirus and Epstein-Barr virus, which typically cause much milder liver dysfunction during primary infections. Within the United States, almost all cases of acute hepatitis are caused by infection with HAV (49%), HBV (34%), or HCV (15%) (Sentinel Counties Study, Centers for Disease Control and Prevention). These acute hepatitis virus infections cannot be distinguished from each other without serologic testing. Acute hepatitis represents a considerable disease burden within the United States, with more than 45,000 cases reported each year. These represent only a fraction of all cases, however, because it is estimated that only 1 out of every 5–10 cases may be reported to public health authorities. Fulminant hepatic failure and death occur in a very small proportion of patients with acute hepatitis A or B, but these clinical endpoints are rarely associated with acute HCV infection in the United States.[3,4]

The major burden of disease due to hepatitis virus infections stems from the chronic liver damage that occurs in individuals who develop persistent infections. The proportion of persons who become persistently infected is highly dependent on the infecting virus. Persistent infections are extremely rare with HAV. On the other hand, up to 85% of persons infected with HCV fail to clear the virus, and most eventually develop chemical and histologic evidence of chronic liver disease.[5] HBV has an intermediate tendency to establish persistence, with the risk of persistent infection highly dependent upon the age and immunologic competence of the individual.

It is appropriate to focus attention on the hepatitis viruses in a textbook concerned with sexually transmitted diseases. Although these are systemic infections that are also commonly transmitted by other means, sexual activity may profoundly influence the risks for acquisition of both HAV and HBV infections. To some extent, sexual behavior may also determine the risk of infection with HCV and HDV. Individuals with a history of multiple sex partners and those who have had other sexually transmitted diseases are at increased risk for infection with HBV and, to a lesser extent, HAV and HCV. Vaccines have been available for the prevention of hepatitis B (and with it hepatitis D) for the past decade and a half and have more recently become available for hepatitis A.[6] These vaccines provide a means of prevention unavailable for other sexually transmitted diseases, and their use should be highly encouraged in populations at risk for hepatitis infections. This chapter will discuss the epidemiology and pathobiology of the hepatitis viruses, and the use of hepatitis vaccines in populations at risk for STDs. Aspects of the management of patients with viral hepatitis are considered in Chapter 67.

HEPATITIS A

HEPATITIS A VIRUS

Physical characteristics and replication cycle

HAV is classified as the type species of the genus *Hepatovirus* of the family *Picornaviridae*. The virus is a small (27 nm), spherical, nonenveloped particle.[7] Its RNA genome is single stranded, positive sense, and approximately 7.5 kb in length.[8] The genome organization includes a 5′ nontranslated segment 734 bases in length,[9] a long open reading frame encoding a polyprotein of 2227 amino acids, and a short 3′ noncoding region which terminates in a 3′ poly(adenylic acid) tract (Fig. 26-1). A small genome-linked protein (VPg) is covalently attached to the 5′ end of virion RNA.[10] Genome-length cloned cDNA and RNA derived from it are infectious in cell cultures.[11]

Within the infected cell, virion RNA acts as messenger for synthesis of a large polyprotein, which is cotranslationally processed by the virus-specified $3C^{pro}$ proteinase into both structural and nonstructural proteins[12,13] (Fig. 26-1). Three capsid proteins (VP1, VP2, and VP3, ranging from 222 to 280 amino acid residues in length) have been demonstrated in purified virus preparations.[14] Virion RNA also serves as template for (-)-strand RNA synthesis, which acts in turn as template for synthesis of more (+)-strand genomic RNA. This newly synthesized (+)-strand RNA is either used for further rounds of replication or packaged within the capsid proteins for export from the hepatocyte across the apical canalicular membrane into the bile. As with other picornaviruses, replication occurs in the cytoplasm of the infected cell and RNA transcription proceeds asymmetrically, with an excess of (+)-strand molecules synthesized under direction of the virus-specified $3D^{pol}$ RNA-dependent RNA polymerase.

Alone among the human hepatitis viruses, HAV may be propagated in cell cultures with reasonable efficiency. However, in most in vitro systems, HAV does not produce a cytopathic effect; there is no shutdown in host cell protein synthesis such as occurs with poliovirus infection.[15,16] A variety of primate cell lines are permissive for HAV, but primary isolation of wild-type virus is difficult and frequently entails a period of several weeks (or longer) between inoculation of cell cultures and the first detection of viral antigen.[17,18] Thus, virus isolation is not a viable approach to diagnosis. Furthermore, virus yields from cell culture are relatively low. Nonetheless, the ability of this virus to be propagated in cell culture has made it possible to develop conventional formalin-inactivated vaccines (see below).

No significant antigenic differences have been found among strains collected from widely separated geographic regions.[19,20] Substantial evidence suggests that the critical antigen(s) of HAV are "assembled," or conformationally determined, structures rather than linear structures determined solely by the primary

Table 26-1. Human Hepatitis Viruses

Virus (infection)	Taxonomic classification[1]	Genome[2]	Viral envelope	Modes of transmission[3]	Persistent infection	Disease associations[4]
Hepatitis A Virus (Infectious hepatitis)	*Picornaviridae (Hepatovirus)*	L/ss RNA 7.5 kb	No	ET ST PT (rare)	Extraordinarily rare	AH, FH
Hepatitis B Virus ("Homologous serum hepatitis")	*Hepadnaviridae (Orthohepadnavirus)*	C/ds DNA 3.2 kb	Yes	HT ST NT PT	Common in infants and immunocompromised persons	AH, FH CH HCC
Hepatitis C Virus (Parenterally-transmitted NANB hepatitis)	*Flaviviridae (Hepacivirus)*	L/ss RNA 9.6 kb	Yes	PT ST (occasional) NT (occasional)	85% of all infected persons	AH CH HCC
Hepatitis D Virus (Hepatitis D, or delta hepatitis)	Unassigned *(Deltavirus)*	C/ss RNA 1.7 kb	Yes	PT ST (occasional)	Common if patient is an HBV carrier	AH, FH CH
Hepatitis E Virus (Enterically-transmitted NANB hepatitis)	Unassigned (Hepatitis E-like viruses)	L/ss RNA 7.2 kb	No	ET	Never	AH, FH

[1]Virus family (Genus)
[2]L = linear, C = circular; ss = single-stranded, ds = partially double-stranded; kb = kilobases.
[3]Documented modes of transmission: ET, enteric transmission; HT, horizontal transmission (see text); NT, perinatal transmission; PT, percutaneous transmission; ST, sexual transmission.
[4]AH = acute hepatitis, FH = fulminant hepatitis; CH = chronic hepatitis and cirrhosis; HCC = hepatocellular carcinoma

amino acid sequences of the capsid protein. Analysis of HAV using neutralizing murine monoclonal antibodies indicates the presence of an immunodominant antigenic site on the virus capsid that is involved in antibody-mediated neutralization. Genomic sequencing of viral escape mutants selected during growth of the virus in the presence of neutralizing monoclonal antibodies has shown that such resistance can be conferred by substitutions at amino acid residues within VP3 and VP1 which contribute to this site.[21] The conformational nature of the HAV antigen has prevented development of a vaccine based on expression of antigen from recombinant cDNA.

Pathobiology

Chimpanzees, several species of marmosets, and New World owl monkeys are susceptible to HAV and may be infected by either oral or percutaneous inoculation of virus.[22,23] Although disease in these primates is usually mild compared with symptomatic infections in adult humans, the course of the infection is otherwise very similar. Infection of the hepatocyte is central to the pathogenesis of hepatitis A. Studies with animal models have provided conflicting evidence for the replication of virus within the gastrointestinal epithelium, even though relatively large amounts of virus are present in feces 1–4 weeks after exposure.[24] However, the most recent data support replication of the virus within crypt cells of the small intestine.[25]

Fecal shedding of the virus reaches its maximum just prior to the onset of hepatocellular disease, at which point the individual is probably maximally infectious. HAV, presumably replicated predominantly within hepatocytes, is present in the bile and feces.[26] Viral antigen also has been detected within the cytoplasm of hepatocytes, as well as within germinal centers of the spleen and lymph nodes and in some primates along the glomerular basement membrane.[27] There is a extended viremia which persists for several weeks during the prodrome and early clinical phase of the illness; it roughly parallels the shedding of virus in the feces but is of much lower magnitude.[28] At the onset of hepatic inflammation in experimentally infected primates, the titer of infectious virus is greatest in liver, followed by feces and then serum. The situation is likely to be similar in infected humans. Viral antigen

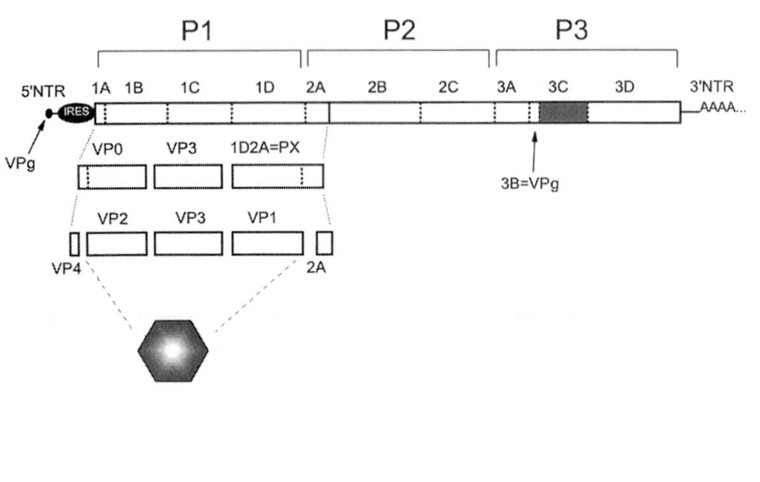

Fig. 26-1 Genomic organization of HAV. The 7.5 kb single-stranded (+)-sense RNA genome has a 5′ untranslated region (5′NTR) approximately 740 bases in length, followed by a long open reading frame (boxed region). The 5′ terminus of the RNA is covalently linked to a small viral protein (VPg). There is a short 3′ untranslated region, followed by a poly(adenylic acid) tail. Translation is under direction of an internal ribosome entry site (IRES) which is located within the 5′NTR. This leads to synthesis of a large polyprotein which is cotranslationally processed by a viral proteinase (3Cpro) into capsid precursor proteins, VP0, VP2, PX (representing the P1 segment of the polyprotein), and a series of proteins which are active in replication and which include the RNA polymerase 3Dpol (P2–3 segments). PX and VP0 undergo further cleavage to VP4 and VP1 following packaging of the viral RNA.

may be detected in the feces as late as two weeks after the onset of symptoms, but chronic fecal shedding of virus has not been observed.[29] Epidemiologic studies noting the disappearance of HAV from closed populations with the passage of time argue against the existence of such shedding.[30] However, relatively prolonged shedding of the virus has been reported in infected premature infants.[31]

The mechanisms responsible for hepatocellular damage are poorly characterized.[32] However, type A hepatitis appears to be due to an immunopathologic response to infection of the hepatocyte, rather than to a direct cytopathic effect of the virus. HLA-restricted, virus-specific, cytotoxic, CD8+ T cells have been recovered from the liver of persons with acute hepatitis A.[33–35] Virus-specific cytotoxic T cells have been shown to secrete γ-interferon, which likely stimulates the recruitment of additional, nonspecific inflammatory cells to the site of virus replication within the liver.[36]

Immunity

Antibody to the virus (anti-HAV) generally appears in the serum concurrent with the earliest evidence of hepatocellular disease (Fig. 26-2). This early antibody is comprised largely of IgM, although IgG may also be present shortly after the onset of symptoms.[37] IgG anti-HAV persists for life and confers protection against reinfection.[38] Re-exposure of seropositive individuals may lead to increases in anti-HAV titer but is not associated with liver disease.[39] Both fecal and serum IgA anti-HAV have been described,[40] but the role of secretory immunity in protection against HAV infection appears to be very limited.[41] Both NK cell and virus-specific, HLA-restricted cytotoxic T-cell activities have been described.[33,35,42] Along with the induction of interferon synthesis, such cellular effector mechanisms are likely to play an important role in clearing virus from the infected liver.

Transmission

With a few notable exceptions, the spread of HAV between individuals is always due to fecal-oral transmission. Virus transmission is facilitated by conditions which favor fecal-oral spread, including sexual practices involving oral-anal contact (see below). Saliva may contain very small amounts of infectious HAV.[43] The potential for household transmission and even common-source outbreaks is enhanced by the large amounts of virus present in feces and the extraordinary physical stability of the virus.[44] Virus is concentrated from contaminated coastal waters by filter-feeding shellfish; hepatitis A may result if such shellfish are ingested inadequately cooked or uncooked.

Percutaneous transmission of HAV has been documented with transfusion of blood and blood products, but such instances are relatively rare because the frequency of viremia (which only occurs during acute infection) is exceptionally low in blood donor populations. However, illicit injection-drug use has been shown to be an important risk factor for hepatitis A in some populations. Although it is not widely appreciated, it seems likely that HAV is often transmitted percutaneously among injection-drug users (IDUs) who share paraphernalia for the preparation and injection of drugs.[44] Viremia persists for several weeks during acute infection,[28,43] and the exceptional physical stability of the virus (which exceeds that of HBV or HCV) would favor such transmission. Epidemiologic data are consistent with the percutaneous transmission of HAV among IDUs. Within the United States, the reported frequency of hepatitis A among such individuals has remarkably paralleled that of hepatitis B and hepatitis C, peaking in the late 1980s and since declining substantially.

EPIDEMIOLOGY

Population studies

Overall, evidence suggests that hepatitis A has become less prevalent in developed nations during the past several decades, most likely as a result of continuing improvements in sanitation.[47] Because of this trend, the percentage of the adult population susceptible to the virus has undoubtedly increased and will probably continue to do so. The prevalence of antibody was only 15%–25% in American military populations sampled in the late 1970s and early 1980s (SM Lemon, unpublished data).

In the United States, the prevalence of anti-HAV is clearly related to age as well as to socioeconomic factors.[47] The age-related nature of antibody prevalence in some Western countries appears to be due largely to a cohort effect created by the decreasing incidence of HAV infection. In some developed countries the median age of infection has been shown to be increasing.[47] Significant international differences exist in the age-related prevalence of anti-HAV, however. In contrast to the United States and Northern Europe, infection still occurs during early childhood in many developing nations,[50] often at an age at which specific symptoms of hepatitis A are minimal or absent (see below). This situation may be changing, however, as sanitary conditions improve in these countries, leading to increased susceptibility to the virus among young adults. The potential impact of this effect is typified by an epidemic of hepatitis A in Shanghai which reportedly involved over 300,000 persons in early 1988.[51]

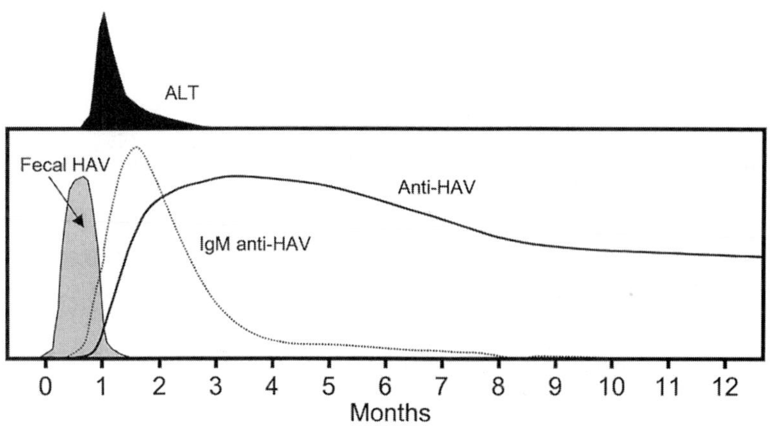

Fig. 26-2 Typical clinical and virologic course of hepatitis A virus infection. Temporal patterns are shown for the fecal excretion of HAV, the short-lived IgM specific anti-HAV response, and the long-lasting total anti-HAV response. At the top is shown the serum ALT pattern, which reflects the acute liver injury associated with this infection.

Endemic hepatitis A

The vast majority of HAV infections occur sporadically, presumably as a result of person-to-person spread of virus, and in many cases may not be recognized as hepatitis. In an ongoing study conducted in four "sentinel" counties within the United States by the Centers for Disease Control and Prevention (CDC), 49% of the cases of sporadic viral hepatitis were due to HAV. In these counties during 1983–1995, the average annual incidence of hepatitis A was 14.7 per 100,000 persons and ranged from 0.6 to 100.7 per 100,000 persons depending on the county and year (Beth P. Bell, personal communication[51a]). Preschool daycare facilities, especially those enrolling children under the age of two years, may play a significant role in the spread of HAV. In one study, up to 40% of all cases of hepatitis A within one American community were either related to attendance at a daycare center or exposure to a child enrolled in such a facility.[52] The majority of infected children under the age of 2 years do not become icteric and are not recognized as having hepatitis. Nevertheless, such children appear to efficiently shed virus, and transmission of virus from them is facilitated by their lack of toilet training. Subsequent infection of older siblings, parents, and baby-sitters (all of whom are more likely to develop classic signs of hepatitis) is therefore common.

Sexual transmission

Hepatitis A, like other predominantly enteric infections, may be transmitted during sexual activity. However, the importance of sexual behavior in determining the risk of HAV infection is likely to vary widely among different populations. Sexual transmission undoubtedly plays a greater role in the spread of HAV in industrialized nations which have good public health sanitation systems than in developing nations with inadequate sanitary and water systems where HAV is highly endemic. Sexual behavior can influence the prevalence of antibodies to HAV in developed countries, although this is not invariably the case. For example, a survey of Danish men who were reactive in various serologic tests for syphilis revealed a higher anti-HAV prevalence among homosexuals (36%) than among heterosexuals (20%).[53] Moreover, the prevalence of anti-HAV correlated with the number of episodes of syphilis in younger homosexual males. Yet another study involving STD patients suggested that the presence of anti-HAV was related to the number of lifetime sexual partners.[54]

In an early study from Seattle, 30% of 102 gay men recruited from an STD clinic in Seattle had anti-HAV antibodies, compared with only 12% of age- and socioeconomically matched heterosexual males.[55] The risk of previous infection was related to age, number of sex partners, and duration of homosexuality. In a more recent study from San Francisco, 28% of homosexual and bisexual men aged 17–22 years had serologic evidence of past infection.[55] Anti-HAV seropositivity was independently associated with Hispanic ethnicity, less than a high school education, and a history of ≥50 lifetime male sexual partners. Recent infection was documented in 3.3% of susceptible men. It was independently associated with insertive anal intercourse and the sharing of contaminated needles.[46] In contrast, in a study carried out in Madrid, Spain, a region where hepatitis A is moderately endemic, there were no differences in the prevalence of anti-HAV in homosexual and heterosexual men.[56] At an average age of 28–29 years, 43%–47% of these men were positive for anti-HAV antibodies.[56] However, a history of oral-anal contact was associated with anti-HAV seropositivity independent of sexual orientation.

In the Seattle study,[55] an annual infection rate of 22% was observed when seronegative gay men were followed prospectively. Men reporting frequent oral-anal exposure were found to be at significantly increased risk of becoming infected with HAV.[55] In retrospect, it is apparent that an epidemic of hepatitis A had occurred among gay men in Seattle at the time of this study. Most of the men who were studied had been homosexual for many years (mean = 12.4 years for those without anti-HAV). If the annual risk of acquiring hepatitis A were constant at 22%, the expected antibody prevalence would have been far greater than the observed 30%. Similar epidemics of hepatitis A have been described among urban gay men in Copenhagen, Amsterdam, Melbourne, London and other large, cosmopolitan Western cities in recent years.[57–62] Risk factors for the acquisition of hepatitis A in these studies have generally paralleled those determined in the Seattle outbreak. In a case-control study of a community-wide outbreak of hepatitis A in New York City, HAV infection was more prevalent in homosexual and bisexual men with >1 anonymous sex partner, a history of group sex, or participation in active oral-anal or digital-anal intercourse.[61]

In addition, a number of acute HAV infections were noted among gay men participating in the hepatitis B vaccine trial conducted in New York City during the mid-1970s.[61] One in five men was anti-HAV-positive at the start of this study, and an annual attack rate of about 4.5% was noted during the two years of follow-up. These cases were evenly distributed among the population at risk and did not appear to occur in identifiable groups or clusters.

Despite this evidence for sexual transmission of HAV, hepatitis A differs from most other sexually transmitted diseases in at least two important ways. First, infection with the virus produces solid immunity so that symptomatic reinfection never occurs.[38,62a] Second, the infected individual is infectious for a relatively brief period of time. There is no prolonged carrier state. Although there has been little effort to formally model the sexual transmission of HAV, these facts suggest that several conditions may be required to sustain sexual transmission of HAV within a population. These include: (1) a high degree of susceptibility among the population at risk, as defined by negative tests for anti-HAV, (2) sexual promiscuity, so that multiple partners may be exposed during the relatively brief period when virus is shed, and (3) sexual practices facilitating fecal-oral spread of virus. Epidemics of hepatitis A which have been observed among urban gay men have generally included all of these elements and further suggest that the introduction of virus into the sexually active population may be an additional requirement.[55,57,59–61] At times, the sexual transmission of HAV can figure prominently in determining community-wide rates of hepatitis A. In Melbourne during 1991, over 80% of all reported cases were in males, and over half of these males were known to be homosexual.[59]

CLINICAL MANIFESTATIONS OF HEPATITIS A

In the individual patient, acute illness due to hepatitis A virus is indistinguishable from that due to hepatitis B or hepatitis C.[1] The incubation period of hepatitis A is relatively short, averaging about 4 weeks (Fig. 26-2). Under the age of three years, fewer than 1 in 10 infected children develop symptoms of hepatitis, whereas most infected adults are symptomatic.[64] Symptoms are often abrupt in appearance, although there may be a prodromal period of low grade fever, malaise, headaches, and myalgias. Anorexia, nausea, and vomiting occur early in the illness, and diarrhea is not uncommon, especially among children.[1] The specific diagnosis of viral hepatitis, however, is often not suggested until the occurrence of dark urine or jaundice. Serum aminotransferase elevations are similar in magnitude to those seen in acute hepatitis B, although they generally do not persist as long. Most infected individuals will have normal aminotransferase levels by 6 weeks after the onset of symptoms, although 10%–20% of cases may have minor enzyme abnormalities persisting for up to 3 months and occasionally longer.

Other than a single case report,[65] chronic viral hepatitis has not been associated with HAV infection. However, it has been suggested that in rare instances HAV infection may trigger the onset of chronic autoimmune liver disease.[66] Although jaundice may occasionally be prolonged for several weeks or more ("cholestatic hepatitis"), it is not indicative of severe hepatocellular disease and uniformly resolves with time.[67] Occasional cases of "relapsing hepatitis A" have been noted. These patients have symptomatic and chemical evidence of recurrent hepatitis, usually occurring within several months of acute type A hepatitis.[67,68] The pathobiology of this condition is uncertain, but it always resolves without progression to chronic hepatitis. Hepatitis A accounts for less than 10% of all cases of fulminant hepatitis,[69] and the mortality in acute symptomatic hepatitis A is probably less than 0.1%–0.2%.

DIAGNOSIS OF HEPATITIS A

The diagnosis of hepatitis A rests entirely on serologic methods (Table 26-2). Anti-HAV is usually measured by solid-phase enzyme-linked immunosorbent assay (ELISA). Absence of anti-HAV is strong evidence against current infection with HAV. However, the detection of anti-HAV in a patient with hepatitis does not prove infection is recent or responsible for current symptoms. A specific serodiagnosis requires the demonstration of IgM anti-HAV, which is present in virtually all patients with acute hepatitis A (Fig. 26-2). IgM anti-HAV may be detected by sensitive antibody-capture immunoassays for as long as 6 months after the onset of symptoms.[70,71]

Prevention of Hepatitis A

Passive immunization. Immune globulin (IG), if administered within two weeks of exposure, is 80%–90% effective in protecting against illness associated with HAV infection.[72] Infection is also probably prevented if IG is given soon enough after exposure. IG confers immediate protection against hepatitis A, while hepatitis A vaccine does not produce protective levels of antibodies to HAV until 2–4 weeks after active immunization (see next section). Thus, IG continues to have an important role in the management of exposed persons.[73,74] Postexposure prophylaxis with IG (0.02 mL/kg intramuscularly) is recommended for household and sexual contacts of patients with hepatitis A.[74] Postexposure prophylaxis is generally not recommended in the setting of a common source outbreak, because such outbreaks are usually recognized only well into their course, when IG may no longer be effective in prevention of disease. Unfortunately, in recent years IG has become increasingly scarce due to the decision by one major manufacturer to exit the market.

Active immunization. Whole cell inactivated vaccines have largely replaced IG for preexposure prophylaxis of hepatitis A.[6] Hepatitis A vaccines contain formalin-inactivated viral particles that are produced in cell culture, purified, and adsorbed to aluminum hydroxide.[75,76] Immunization elicits serum neutralizing antibodies (anti-HAV) which protect against both infection and disease.[77]

At present, two similar vaccines are licensed in the United States: Havrix (SmithKline Beecham) and Vaqta (Merck). Both are produced from virus grown in infected human diploid fibroblasts. Each vaccine is available in adult and pediatric/adolescent formulations. Comparative clinical trials of these vaccines have not been reported, but they appear to be comparable with respect to their clinical performance. Reactogenicity is relatively low and similar to that reported with hepatitis B vaccines. The most common adverse events include soreness at the site of intramuscular injection, which occurs in 21%–56% of recipients. Fever has been reported in up to 4%.[78,79] Anaphylaxis, Guillain-Barré-Landry syndrome and more obscure neurologic syndromes have been reported rarely.[79] For adults over 17–18 years of age, both vaccines are given on a two-dose schedule, usually with 6–12 months intervening between doses. The package insert should be reviewed for specific details concerning administration.

Efficacy trials of hepatitis A vaccines have been limited to children, but it is reasonable to assume that similarly impressive results would be achieved in adults who develop comparable anti-HAV responses. In a randomized, placebo-controlled trial carried out among children aged 2–16 years in Monroe County, New York, a single 25 U dose of Vaqta provided complete protection against symptomatic hepatitis A during a seasonal outbreak of disease (95% confidence interval = 87%–100%).[80] The last case of hepatitis in an immunized child occurred 18 days after vaccine administration. Similar protection was observed in Thai children who had completed a primary immunization series with two 360 El. unit doses of Havrix (95% confidence interval = 74%–98%).[81] Immunization also has been shown to prevent asymptomatic infection.[82]

Hepatitis A vaccine is recommended for persons at increased risk of hepatitis A.[74] This includes homosexual men, IDUs, international travelers to hepatitis A endemic regions, and others. The decision to use vaccine in any risk group should reflect the perceived risk, the potential severity of infection, and the relatively high cost of the vaccine (about U.S. $50 per dose at retail).[6,73] However, there are few cost-benefit analyses available to help guide such decisions.

HEPATITIS B

HEPATITIS B VIRUS

Physical and chemical characteristics

HBV, an hepadnavirus, is one of a family of related DNA viruses infecting the livers of a variety of avian and mammalian species. The HBV virion (also known as the Dane particle) is a complex, double-shelled 42 nm spherical particle with an outer surface envelope surrounding a core structure containing a small DNA genome (Fig. 26-3). This genome is unique among human viruses in that it is a circular DNA molecule which is double-stranded for 50%–85% of its length, with a total genome length equivalent to double-stranded DNA of approximately 3200 base pairs[83,84]. The genomes of a number of HBV strains have been molecularly cloned and fully sequenced (Fig. 26-4). The partially double-stranded DNA consists of a long (-)-sense (i.e., antimessenger sense) strand and a shorter (+)-sense strand, which overlap at their 5′ ends[85]. Within the (+)-strand, there are four overlapping open reading frames utilizing all three translation frames (i.e., encoding different amino acids from the same nucleotide sequences). Given the small size of the genome, this parsimonious use of the genomic DNA provides for a relatively large amount of genetic information. There are no segments of the DNA that are not translated into protein. The four open reading frames encode a DNA polymerase/reverse transcriptase, the core protein (and the closely related precore protein, which is converted to the "e" protein by posttranslational processing), a family of three surface envelope proteins with common carboxy termini (see below), and the "X" protein. This latter protein has been described as having

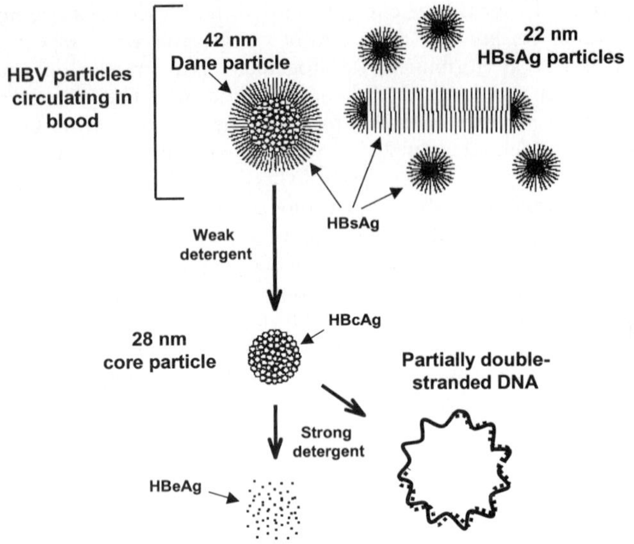

Fig. 26-3. Structure of HBV. A variety of HBV particles are present in the blood of an infected person. These include the 42-nm diameter infectious virion (Dane particle) and usually a much greater number of smaller, noninfectious, spherical or elongated HBsAg particles. Treatment of the Dane particle with weak detergent removes the surface envelope (HBsAg), leaving a smaller core particle (HBcAg). Stronger detergent treatment disrupts the core, releasing soluble HBeAg and the partially double-stranded DNA genome. (Modified from a figure courtesy of Dr. AJ Cann, Leicester University).

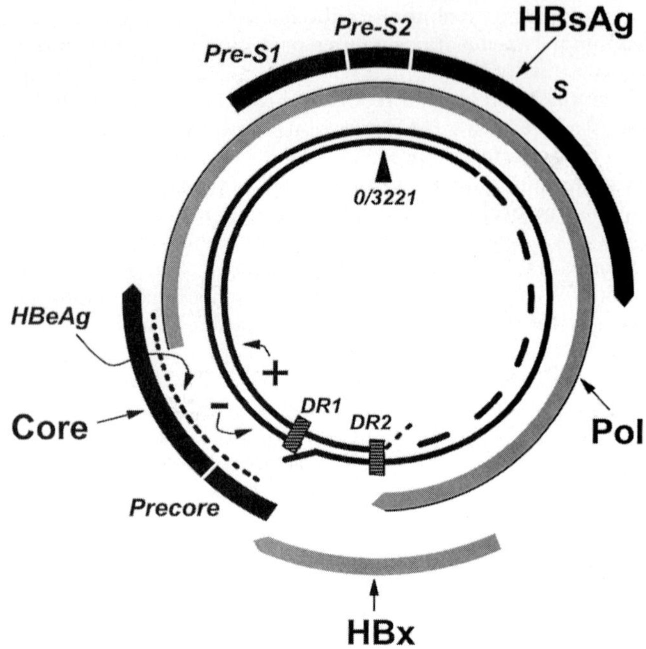

Fig. 26-4. Organization of the circular 3.2 kb HBV genome. At the center of the figure is a schematic depicting the complementary linear full-length (-)-strand and partial (+)-strand DNAs which are held in a relaxed circular conformation by the cohesive overlap formed by their 5′ ends. The solid lines represent DNA present within Dane particles, while the large dashed line represents the (+)-strand DNA segment that is synthesized following entry of the virus into the cell. Small boxes represent the two direct repeat elements (DR1 and DR2). The four overlapping open-reading frames are shown at the periphery: HBsAg (which encodes Pre-S1, Pre-S2, and the S envelope proteins), DNA polymerase/reverse transcriptase (pol), X, and Core (which encodes both HBcAg, and HBeAg).

numerous interactions with host cell proteins and is a nonspecific transactivator of host cell transcription.[86,87] However, its precise role in viral replication and the pathogenesis of hepatitis B disease remains obscure.

The DNA genome of HBV replicates via reverse transcription of an intermediate RNA molecule (the "pregenome"), directed by the viral DNA polymerase/reverse transcriptase.[85] The replication cycle of HBV thus resembles in gross detail that of the RNA-containing retroviruses, including the human immunodeficiency virus (HIV) (see Chap.00). Indeed, the genomic organizations of these viruses bear some superficial similarities (Fig. 26-5). The principal difference in their replication cycles is that in HBV it is the DNA

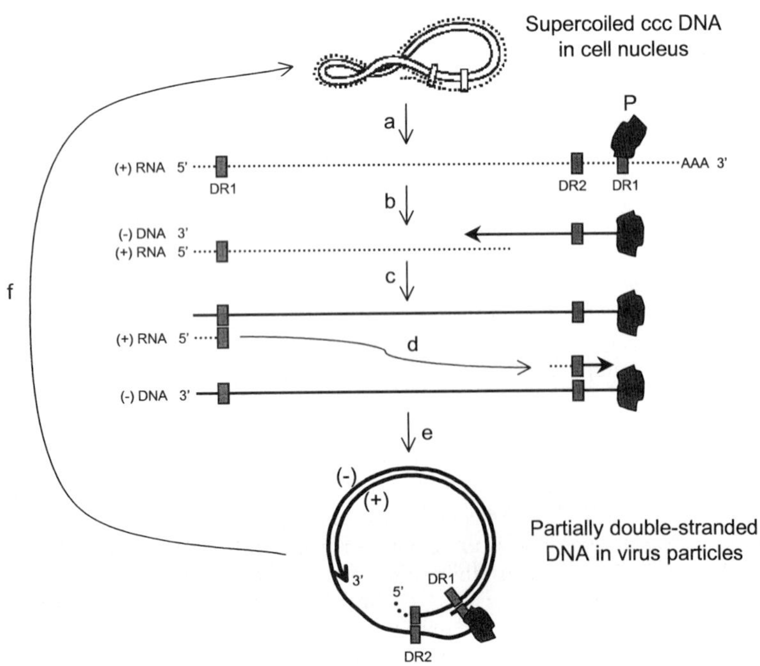

Fig. 26-5 Schematic depicting the HBV replication cycle. The transcriptionally active form of the viral DNA is the completely double-stranded, supercoiled cccDNA that is present within the nucleus of the cell (shown at top of the figure). (a) RNA transcription from cccDNA results in a greater-than-genome length (+)-strand RNA "pregenome" containing two copies of the DR1 direct repeat. (b) Protein-primed (P) reverse transcription with associated degradation of the pregenomic RNA template is carried out by the viral DNA polymerase/reverse transcriptase and leads to production of genome-length (-)-strand DNA (c). This occurs within immature core particles and is the step in replication that is blocked by lamivudine. Subsequent RNA-primed synthesis of the (-)-strand DNA (d) results in the partially double-stranded form of the genome found in mature virions (e). Completion of DNA synthesis, removal of the primer moieties, and repair of the DNA strands leads to new cccDNA following infection of a subsequent cell by mature virions (f). (Modified from a figure courtesy of Dr. AJ Cann, Leicester University).

form of the genome that is exported from the cell in virus particles, while in HIV and other retroviruses it is the RNA form. The clinical significance of the similarities in the replication cycles of HBV and HIV is reflected in their shared sensitivity to antiviral suppression by certain nucleoside analog inhibitors of reverse transcriptase, such as lamivudine.[88]

In addition to the genomic DNA, the core of the HBV particle contains the DNA polymerase/reverse transcriptase, which also has an associated RNase H activity. The DNA polymerase is active in situ within the core particle in the presence of appropriate deoxynucleoside triphosphates, using as a template the single-stranded region of the circular HBV genome.[89] The major core protein is a 21-kDa molecule with specific antigenic activity (hepatitis B core antigen, or HBcAg). HBcAg may be released from the intact virion by detergent treatment, which removes the surface envelope and leaves an intact 27 nm core particle. More vigorous disruption of the virus core results in the release of an antigenically distinct, soluble viral antigen (HBeAg, see Fig. 26-3).[90] HBeAg is closely related to the core protein, as it is the product of proteolytic processing of the precore molecule.[91] The DNA sequences unique to the precore region contain a signal sequence that directs the precore protein into a secretory pathway (see Fig. 26-4). During this process, both the amino terminal signal peptide and a carboxy terminal peptide are cleaved from the precore protein to generate HBeAg. Thus, although the soluble HBeAg and particulate HBcAg have completely distinct antigenic specificities, these molecules have identical amino acid sequences throughout much of their length. The immune responses to these closely related molecules are comprised of very different Th cell subsets.[92] It is possible that the function of HBeAg may be to modulate the cellular immune response to HBV in a manner that promotes viral persistence.

Hepatitis B variants with mutations within the precore region have been described.[89] These precore mutants are unable to express HBeAg due to the presence of a stop codon within the precore region (see Fig. 26-4). Such viruses retain the ability to replicate and express the core protein (HBcAg). They may appear in the course of chronic HBV infection, in association with an HBeAg to anti-HBe seroconversion (despite the continuing presence of HBV DNA), or they may be the cause of new infections (see below). In some situations, such mutant HBVs have been associated with clinically aggressive forms of liver disease.

The surface envelope surrounding the virus core is a complex structure containing as its major antigen a 24 kDa glycoprotein (hepatitis B surface antigen, or HBsAg, also called the S protein and previously known as "hepatitis associated antigen," or "Australia antigen"). An antigenic determinant common to all strains of hepatitis B ("a") is associated with HBsAg. In addition, two pairs of mutually exclusive allelic antigens ("y" and "d," "w" and "r") have been defined.[97] Of the four possible major subtype combinations, only three ("ayw," "adw," and "adr") have been found with any degree of frequency, and these occur in distinct, but possibly changing, geographic and demographic distributions. Also present in the Dane particle envelope are two related proteins, pre-S1 (42 kDa) and pre-S2 (36 kDa). The pre-S1, pre-S2, and S molecules all share the 226 amino acids of the S protein at their carboxy terminus: they are coterminal translation products of the open reading frame encoding the S-protein, but they represent products of translation from different AUG initiation codons and are derived from distinct mRNAs[83,84] (see Fig. 26-4). The roles of pre-S1 and pre-S2 in the biology of HBV remain controversial, although pre-S2 has been proposed to contain the virion receptor binding site. The inclusion of these antigens in future vaccines may result in improved immunogenicity (see below). HBsAg is usually produced in excess by infected hepatocytes, and incomplete 22 nm spherical or extended HBsAg particles greatly outnumber intact Dane particles in the blood of most BV carriers (Fig. 26-3). These particles, as well as the surface envelope of the Dane particle, also contain host cell derived materials, including human albumin.

Replication cycle of HBV

Attempts to propagate HBV in conventional cell cultures generally have not been successful. However, cells transfected with cloned HBV genomic DNA produce Dane particles which are detectable by electron microscopy and infectious for chimpanzees.[98,99] Such cells have been useful in dissecting the molecular steps in HBV replication and in assessing the response of HBV to candidate antiviral agents. However, no type of cultured cell is fully permissive for viral replication.

Early studies with the duck hepadnavirus (duck hepatitis B virus, or DHBV) and subsequent work with HBV led to the conclusion that replication of these DNA viruses proceeds via an RNA genomic intermediate.[85] This conclusion was based on the identification of immature intracellular core particles containing full-length RNA genomic intermediates and reverse transcriptase activity, and the observation that synthesis of (-)-strand viral DNA is not inhibited by actinomycin-D (which typically blocks DNA-directed but not RNA-directed DNA synthesis). Current concepts concerning the replication of HBV may be summarized briefly as follows (see Fig. 26-5).[83,84] After attachment and penetration of the hepatocyte, synthesis of the incomplete (+)-strand of the gapped virion DNA is accomplished, possibly under direction of a cellular enzyme(s). Ligation of the gapped DNA by cellular enzyme(s) results in a fully double-stranded circular DNA molecule (covalently closed circular DNA, or "cccDNA").

This supercoiled episomal DNA does not replicate by a DNA-dependent DNA synthesis mechanism and serves only a transcriptional role.[100] Nonetheless, its amplification and persistence in the cell is central to the replication cycle of the virus. The cccDNA serves in the nucleus as template for subgenomic (+)-strand RNA transcripts for the envelope proteins (S, pre-S1, and pre-S2), as well as a somewhat greater than full-length (+)-sense RNA genomic intermediate (the viral "pregenome"). There is only a single poly(adenylic acid) addition site located within the core gene, and all the messenger RNAs are therefore 3′ coterminal. The core protein and the DNA polymerase are translated from pregenomic RNA (the latter by a process of "leaky" ribosome scanning), while the X protein appears to be expressed from a unique transcript. The pregenomic RNA serves a dual role, however, as it is also encapsidated within immature cytoplasmic core particles along with the DNA polymerase (reverse transcriptase). Within these immature core particles, the long (-)-sense DNA strand is synthesized by reverse transcription of the pregenomic RNA, probably with concomitant degradation of the RNA directed by an associated RNase H activity. Subsequently, (+)-sense DNA is replicated from the full-length (-)-strand, but this process is prematurely interrupted by the completion of viral assembly and release of virus from the cell. The result is a partially double-stranded DNA molecule encapsidated within the Dane particle (see Fig. 26-5).

The mechanism by which the cellular pool of supercoiled cccDNA is expanded is uncertain. It has been suggested that amplification might be the result of intracellular nuclear reinfection with immature Dane particles;[100] alternatively, it might result from exogenous reinfection of the hepatocyte by additional virions. Either way, it is important to note that the maintenance of the cellular pool of supercoiled HBV DNA is not dependent upon the viral reverse transcriptase activity. The pool of supercoiled cccDNA is not reduced by treatment with reverse transcriptase inhibitors such as lamivudine, which otherwise may be very active in suppressing viral DNA synthesis and thus HBV replication. This feature of the replication cycle has very important implications for the response of infected individuals to antiviral therapies.

On a single cell level, antiviral nucleoside analogs such as lamivudine will suppress replication, but they will not eliminate the infection. Thus, such drugs may ultimately prove to be suppressive rather than curative, much as acyclovir is not curative for genital herpes infections. During viral replication, double-stranded HBV DNA may become integrated at a low frequency into host chromosomal DNA. However, this process is not obligatory for viral replication, as it is with conventional retroviruses, and appears to be a random event.

Pathobiology

Following exposure, virus presumably gains access to the liver via the blood stream. HBsAg is found within the cytoplasm of hepatocytes, whereas HBcAg is usually restricted to the hepatocyte nucleus. There is evidence that HBV may also replicate within certain mononuclear cells of the bone marrow or blood,[101] but the liver is the primary site of HBV replication. This tropism may result in part from the involvement of tissue-specific virus enhancer regions and promoters regulating HBV gene expression, the presence of virus-specific receptors on only certain cell types, or both. There is no evidence for replication of the virus at mucosal surfaces.

Acute hepatitis B

The majority of infections are self limited (Fig. 26-6, top panel). HBsAg may appear in the blood as early as six days after percutaneous exposure, although this interval is usually 1–2 months after mucosal exposure.[102] Shortly afterwards, circulating Dane particles, HBeAg, and DNA polymerase may be detected. This stage of detectable viremia is often brief. HBsAg synthesis is more abundant and typically more persistent, however, and it may be detected for up to five months or in some cases even longer.[102] The first humoral immune response to the virus, consisting of IgM antibody to HBcAg (IgM anti-HBc), develops shortly after the appearance of HBsAg.[103,104] Following the disappearance of circulating DNA polymerase and HBeAg, antibody to HBeAg (anti-HBe) may also be detected. Almost all (95%–99%) healthy adults who are infected with HBV will eventually clear HBsAg from the circulation, and most, but not all, will develop antibody to HBsAg (anti-HBs). There may, however, be a delay of weeks to months prior to the first appearance of anti-HBs, even after the disappearance of HBsAg. During this so-called "window period," anti-HBc and anti-HBe are the only serum markers of HBV infection. Symptoms of hepatitis usually develop after HBsAg has been circulating in the blood for 3–6 weeks and usually occur while HBsAg is still present (in approximately 90% of patients). Symptoms may develop during the "window period," however, or even after the appearance of anti-HBs.[103] The appearance of anti-HBs signals the resolution of the infection. This antibody is protective against reinfection[63] and represents responses against the S, pre-S1, and pre-S2 proteins. Anti-HBc and anti-HBs usually persist for years following infection.

Chronic hepatitis B

A small proportion (1%–5%) of infected adults are not able to resolve the infection and become chronic HBsAg carriers (Fig. 26-6, bottom panel). Such individuals frequently have little or no evidence of acute liver disease when initially infected. Development of the chronic carrier state is more frequently seen in individuals who are immunocompromised (those with underlying HIV infection).[105] Almost all infants who are infected neonatally become carriers. HBsAg may persist in the blood of these individuals for years in large and relatively constant amounts and may be associated with the presence of either HBeAg or anti-HBe.

Carriers who are positive for HBeAg usually have circulating Dane particles and detectable DNA polymerase activity;[106] such carriers should be considered to be especially infectious.[107,108] Chronic HBsAg carriers typically have very high titers of anti-HBc and usually do not have anti-HBs. Atypical individuals, however, may have both HBsAg and anti-HBs directed against a different

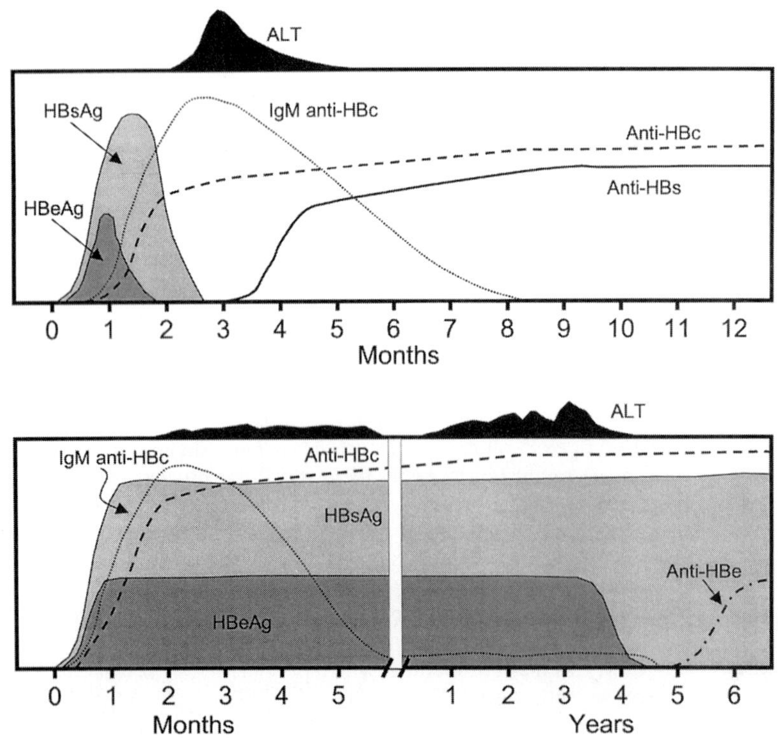

Fig. 26-6 Top: Typical virologic and serologic course of acute, self-limited HBV infection. Bottom: Typical virologic and serologic course in a patient with acute HBV infection in which the infection is not cleared and persistent HBV infection becomes established. Clinical evidence of hepatitis (e.g., ALT elevation) is often very limited during the acute stages of such infections. Late clinical complications include cirrhosis and hepatocellular carcinoma. Persistently infected patients with chronic hepatitis B can be distinguished from those with acute hepatitis B by the presence of high titer IgM antibody to HBcAg. The degree of virus replication during the chronic phase of the infection is reflected in the presence of serum HBeAg and serum HBV DNA (not shown). Patients with chronic HBV may undergo a late seroconversion event in which HBeAg and HBV DNA are lost and anti-HBe appears. This is associated with an improved prognosis and is the primary endpoint for antiviral therapy.

HBsAg subtype.[109] While most persistent HBsAg carriers are asymptomatic and do not have evidence of significant liver disease, a minority have elevated serum aminotransferases and varying degrees of inflammation and fibrosis on liver biopsy. The histologic lesion may progress in some cases to cirrhosis and liver failure. The hepatitis D virus (HDV) may play an important role in promoting severe liver disease in some patients with HBV infection (see below). The presence of HBeAg often correlates with significant liver disease, and seroconversion from HBeAg to anti-HBe in carriers with chronic hepatitis is frequently followed by resolution of liver function abnormalities [110] (Fig. 26-6, bottom panel). This is the desired endpoint in interferon treatment of chronic hepatitis B infection (along with clearance of HBV DNA, see Chap. 67) and has been shown to correlate with long-term survival.[111]

Because immunosuppressed patients are less likely to develop overt signs of hepatitis, and because replication of large quantities of virus occurs in many completely healthy carriers, it seems likely that the host immune response is intimately involved in the expression of liver disease. Much has been learned about this process in recent years from studies of transgenic mice expressing HBV proteins, as well as from infected humans. HBV-specific cytotoxic T cells have been shown to be directed against epitopes within both the core and surface proteins.[112–118] The local expression of gamma interferon (IFN-γ) and other cytokines by these virus-specific CD8+ cytotoxic effector cells may serve to recruit monocytes and other inflammatory cell types to the site of infection. These appear to contribute significantly to the inflammatory process, but they are less specifically directed than the CD8+ cells. Thus, hepatitis associated with HBV infection appears to be immunopathologically mediated rather than a direct result of virus-induced cytopathology. These cellular immune responses play a central role in resolution of the acute infection. CD8+ cells have been shown to be capable of inhibiting a posttranscriptional step in virus replication.[116] Individuals who fail to develop an acute immune response leading to hepatitis following acute infection with HBV are probably more likely to go on to become chronic carriers than those who do develop hepatitis. However, it is interesting to note that long-term persistence of the viral DNA has been documented by sensitive assays even in individuals who have appeared to resolve the infection and who have robust cytotoxic T cell responses.[119,120]

Liver cancer

There is a strong association between persistent HBV infection and primary carcinoma of the liver.[119,120] Infection with HBV usually precedes the development of hepatocellular carcinoma by years, although the tumor occasionally develops during childhood. Integrated HBV DNA is present within tumor tissue in some individuals, but this is not always the case, and there is no specific site at which the viral DNA is integrated into the host genome. Apparently random integration of viral DNA may disrupt normal control of cellular growth and differentiation in some cases.[119,120] However, it seems more likely that hepatocellular cancer usually develops as part of a multi-step process in which chronic inflammation, associated with hepatocellular regeneration and increased cellular proliferation, plays a prominent role. Free radicals produced as a product of the ongoing inflammatory response may cause damage to cellular DNA, ultimately contributing to the evolution of hepatocellular carcinoma. A similar mechanism of carcinogenesis may account for liver cancer in patients who are infected with HCV, which does not replicate through a DNA intermediate and which thus never integrates its genetic information into the host cell genome (see below). Mutations within tumor suppressor genes have been noted in many HBV-related hepatocellular carcinomas.[126–128] An additional factor that may contribute to the oncogenic potential of HBV is the promiscuous transcriptional transactivating activity of the HBx protein.[129,130]

The association of HBV with hepatocellular carcinoma is found worldwide, but hepatocellular carcinoma is a significant problem mainly in those countries where the HBsAg carrier rate is high and neonatal transmission of virus frequent. Not surprisingly, immunization with hepatitis B vaccine has been shown to reduce the risk of hepatocellular carcinoma.[131]

Immunity

Infection with HBV is marked by the development of antibodies directed against each of the individual viral antigens: anti-HBs, anti-HBc, and anti-HBe (Table 26-2; see Fig. 26-6). Of these, the antibody most clearly associated with protection is anti-HBs.[63] Protection afforded by anti-HBs extends to all HBV subtypes, although HBV variants with potential "escape" mutations in the S protein have been recognized in recent years.[132,133] Very recent evidence suggests that the evolution of such escape mutations may contribute to some vaccine breakthroughs in immunized infants who are born to HBV-carrier mothers. The presence of anti-HBe in the blood of a HBsAg carrier generally correlates with reduced infectivity,[108,134,135] but there is no evidence that anti-HBe by itself has any protective effect. Although anti-HBs account for the protection afforded by immunization, it is very likely that memory T cells also contribute to durable immunity in those who have recovered from hepatitis B.

Transmission

The transmission of HBV may be categorized into four general modes: percutaneous, sexual, perinatal, and "horizontal" (defined as occurring in the absence of recognized percutaneous, sexual, or perinatal exposure). Blood is the major source of virus for transmission, and it may contain a very high titer of virus. However, transfusion has become a very infrequent cause of hepatitis B over the past two decades due to the exclusion of paid donations from

Table 26-2. Common Diagnostic Markers of Hepatitis Virus Infections

Infection	Diagnostic marker	Significance of marker
HAV	Anti-HAV	Past or present infection, immunity to HAV
	IgM Anti-HAV	Recent acute infection with HAV
HBV	HBsAg	Current acute or chronic infection with HBV
	HBeAg	High titer HBV carrier, high infectivity
	HBV DNA	Current infection (quantitative measure of viremia)
	Anti-HBs	Immunity to HBV (vaccine or natural infection)
	Anti-HBc	Past or present infection with HBV
	IgM Anti-HBc	Recent acute infection with HBV
	Anti-HBe	Reduced viral replication (except with precore mutants)
HCV	Anti-HCV (ELISA)	Probable infection with HCV (~15% may have cleared infection)
	Anti-HCV (RIBA)	Recombinant immunoblot confirms screening ELISA
	HCV RNA	Definitive evidence of current infection (bDNA or RT-PCR assay)
HDV	Anti-HD	Active or recent infection with HDV

the donor pool and the introduction of sensitive methods for detecting HBsAg and anti-HBc in donor units. Hepatitis B remains relatively common among IDUs, but rates are down significantly over those of the late 1980s. This may reflect safer injection practices associated with AIDS education efforts and mirrors reductions in hepatitis A and hepatitis C among IDUs. Occupational exposures to blood remain a source of infection for health care workers, but this is relatively uncommon due to the requirement for immunization in the workplace and adherence to universal precautions.

Overall, HBV is most commonly transmitted by inapparent percutaneous or mucosal exposures. HBsAg has been found in the saliva, vaginal secretions, and semen of infected individuals, and the presence of Dane particles has been confirmed in saliva by electron microscopy.[136] HBV DNA can be detected by nucleic acid hybridization in both saliva and semen of many HBeAg-positive carriers.[137,138] Southern blot analyses have shown that the quantity of virus in saliva and semen is usually one thousandfold less than that present simultaneously in the blood but still may be as high as 10^6 genome copies per mL.[137] HBV carriers with high serum titers of virus are more likely to have virus detectable in these secretions by these relatively insensitive methods. Most of this virus appears to be extracellular. Its presence in saliva and semen presumably reflects leakage from the circulation, and not the replication of virus at oropharyngeal or genital sites. Although studies directly examining the infectivity of various body fluids are limited, virtually any body fluid or secretion from an HBeAg-positive HBV carrier should be considered to be infectious.

Transmission of HBV from HBsAg carriers to their household contacts is well documented.[139] In addition, multiple epidemiologic surveys suggest that "horizontal" transmission to young children is probably the most common means of transmission of this virus worldwide.[140] The exact mechanism by which this occurs is not known, however. Early experiments demonstrated that HBV-containing serum was infectious when given orally to susceptible individuals,[141] but the virus inoculum used in these studies included large amounts of exogenous protein which may have protected the virus from inactivation by mucosal enzymes, gastric acid, or bile. Attempts to transmit HBV to susceptible nonhuman primates by oral administration of infectious saliva were unsuccessful, even though saliva transmitted infection when inoculated percutaneously.[142,143] Such evidence suggests that the oropharynx is a relatively hostile portal of entry for HBV, but it is compatible with anecdotal reports that bites by infected individuals may transmit infection. It is probable that most "horizontal" transmission within families and among young children is due to inapparent percutaneous exposures to saliva or blood.[140] Such exposures may be relatively infrequent but are apt to occur repeatedly over an extended period of close contact with a persistently infected carrier.

Numerous studies indicate that sexual intercourse is associated with transmission of HBV. Studies on sexual transmission carried out among gay men during the 1970s pointed strongly to participation in rectal intercourse and exposure to large numbers of sexual partners as primary risk factors[144,145] (see below). In addition to more recent epidemiologic evidence supporting frequent sexual transmission of HBV among heterosexuals,[146,147] human semen has been shown to transmit infection when instilled into the vagina of susceptible gibbons.[142]

Finally, HBV is commonly transmitted from HBsAg carrier mothers to their infants at or near birth.[108,135] As infected infants usually become chronic carriers, often for life, perinatal transmission of virus contributes disproportionately to maintenance of the carrier pool in areas of high HBV endemicity. Perinatal transmission is also frequent following acute maternal HBV infection in the third trimester. The presence of maternal HBeAg is associated with an increased risk of transmission of virus to the newborn.[108,135] While intrauterine infection may occur, most infections are probably acquired at the time of birth. Transmission may be due to direct contamination of the infant's circulation with maternal blood at the time of delivery. The presence of HBsAg and anti-HBc in cord blood does not necessarily indicate that infection has occurred, however, as both may disappear with time. Cord blood IgM anti-HBc is not helpful in identifying infection in newborns. If the infant has no evidence of infection by the fourth month of life, he or she has a high probability of remaining free of infection subsequently (although late "breakthrough" infections occur in a small proportion of immunized infants). There is no epidemiologic evidence to incriminate breast feeding as a major factor in transmission of the virus. Immunization is very effective in preventing maternal-infant transmission of HBV (see below).

EPIDEMIOLOGY

Population studies

There are dramatic differences in the prevalence of HBV in various regions of the world.[108] In parts of Southeast Asia and sub-Saharan Africa, >90% of the population may have serologic evidence of past or current HBV infection, and 10%–20% of adults may be HBsAg-positive. In contrast, among a total of 2,163 New York City volunteer blood donors tested in the 1970s, only 7.2% had past exposure to HBV, and only 0.4% were HBsAg-positive.[148] Striking differences in HBsAg carrier rates have also been noted between ethnically disparate groups living within the same geographic area.[149] Within the United States, the seroprevalence generally increases with age and lower socioeconomic status and is higher among African Americans and Asian Americans.[144,148] Serologic studies indicate that health care workers are at increased risk of HBV infection unless they are immunized. Infection in this setting is largely acquired through inapparent means, but it correlates strongly with exposure to blood.[150]

Sexually transmitted hepatitis B among homosexual men

Sexual transmission of HBV was first suggested by the occurrence of acute hepatitis B among sexual contacts of HBsAg carriers.[151] An increased prevalence of HBsAg and anti-HBs was noted subsequently among prostitutes and individuals attending STD clinics.[144,152–154] Overall, however, the most striking serologic evidence relating HBV transmission to sexual practices was found among homosexual men prior to the AIDS epidemic and the subsequent educational campaigns promoting safe sex practices. Of over 600 New York City homosexual men who were solicited for study through recognized gay-oriented organizations and health clinics in the mid-1970s, 4.6% were found to be HBsAg carriers and 51.1% were found to have had past infection to the virus as evidenced by HBsAg or anti-HBs positivity.[144] These men were predominantly Caucasian, under 40 years of age, and highly educated. Female homosexuals were not at increased risk for infection, as only 6.3% had anti-HBs and none were carriers. Of the gay men evaluated in this study, 23% gave a past history of viral hepatitis, and in these individuals the total seroprevalence was 65%. There was a high degree of correlation between numbers of previous sex partners and serologic evidence of past HBV infection. Of those with fewer than 10 sex partners during the previous six months, only 30.9% had been infected with HBV, compared with 60.5% of those with more than 10 sex partners.[144] The highest rates for HBsAg (7.5%) were found among men reporting predominant or exclusive involvement in rectal intercourse, while those reporting oral-genital sex had significantly lower rates for both HBsAg (2.3%) and anti-HBs (39% vs. 51%). The duration of homosexuality was also related to past HBV infection and was more important than age at the time of screening. Injection drug use did not appear to be an important variable. A high prevalence of HBV infection has since been documented among gay men in many other studies.[145,148,152,155–157] Working from the estimate that approximately 4% of North American Caucasian men are exclusively homosexual, Dietzman et al.[155] estimated that approximately 27% of adult males with serologic evidence of HBV infection in 1977 had acquired it through a homosexual exposure.

Several factors account for the high risk of HBV infection among gay men that was noted in these early studies. One of the most important was the number of sexual partners. The typical homosexual male frequenting Denver's steam baths in the late 1970s had eight different male sexual contacts per month.[158] These contacts were largely anonymous and could total as many as 1000 over the lifetime of a gay man. In addition, the relatively high HBsAg carrier rate found among homosexual men in these studies meant that such anonymous sexual contacts often involved repeated exposure to HBsAg-positive partners. Schreeder et al.[145] estimated that the average openly homosexual male had 4.2 sexual contacts with HBsAg-positive men annually. However, these studies were conducted in the years immediately preceding licensure of the hepatitis B vaccine and the recognition of AIDS. Immunization coupled with the adoption of safer sex practices by many homosexual men appears to have altered the epidemiology of HBV in this high risk group. Although the overall incidence of hepatitis B increased within the United States from 1982 to 1988, the proportion of hepatitis B cases among men that were associated with homosexual activity fell from 30% to 12% in four sentinel counties studied by the CDC.[147] In contrast, the proportion attributed to heterosexual contact increased from 10% to 20% among men and from 22% to 34% among women during this same period. Nonetheless, in a study published as recently as 1995,[159] serologic evidence of previous HBV infection among homosexual men living in high risk, inner city neighborhoods of San Francisco was positively associated with numbers of lifetime sexual partners, as well as with nonwhite ethnicity and a history of injection drug use in a sexual partner. In sharp contrast to homosexual men, there are no data showing an increased risk of hepatitis B among gay women. This may be due in part to a lower number of sex partners among gay women. For example, in the years preceding the AIDS epidemic, Szmuness et al.[144] found that gay men in New York had a mean of 20 sex partners over a six month interval, compared with only 1.6 for gay women.

Receptive or insertive anal intercourse is a second important factor influencing the risk of acquisition of HBV among gay men.[144,145] Nonspecific proctitis may result from receptive anal intercourse, and breakdown of normal mucosal barriers may facilitate transmission of virus. In one study, over a quarter of homosexual men had experienced rectal bleeding during a four month period. This was related both to the number of sex partners and to participation in receptive anal intercourse.[145] In this same study, insertive oral-anal contact was also associated with HBV infection. In contrast, oral-genital or oral-oral contact between homosexual men had little apparent influence on the risk of becoming infected with HBV. These findings were confirmed in a more recent prospective study of homosexual men enrolled in the Multicenter AIDS Cohort Study.[157] In this study, 19.8% of initially seronegative men seroconverted to HBV during a 30-month period. Insertive anal intercourse was the major risk factor identified for HBV seroconversion, raising the possibility that transurethral exposure may be important in acquisition of the infection.[157] Based on a similar analysis of new HIV infections and a comparison of the prevalence of each virus, the investigators concluded that HBV is transmitted 8.6-fold more efficiently than HIV among homosexual men.[157]

These data suggest that traumatic sexual practices that lead to small breaks in the skin and mucosa play a prominent role in the transmission of HBV by facilitating exposure to virus in blood. In one survey, 1 out of 5 gay men reported rectal bleeding after intercourse and 9%–16% had fissures, cracks, or tears in the rectum or anal skin over a 12-month period.[160] In yet another study, 13 of 22 HBsAg-positive gay men were found to have rectal mucosal lesions, usually consisting of multiple, punctate bleeding points within 6 cm of the anal verge.[160] HBsAg was identified in swab specimens from such lesions, as well as in swabs taken from apparently normal rectal mucosa and anal sphincters. HBsAg was identified in feces from these men, a finding which may in part explain the risk of infection associated with insertive oral-anal contact and anal intercourse.

Another important factor in the transmission of HBV among homosexual men is that HBsAg-positive homosexual men are often HBeAg-positive. Approximately 65% of HBsAg-positive homosexual men are positive for HBeAg while anti-HBe may be detected in 25%.[162–164] In contrast, only about 10% of asymptomatic, HBsAg-positive blood donors are HBeAg-positive. This difference most likely reflects relatively recent acquisition of the infection by many homosexual men. The presence of HBeAg correlates with high replicative activity of the virus and is associated with an increased risk of heterosexual[139] and maternal-infant transmission of HBV.[108,135] Thus, its frequent presence in homosexual men implies a high risk of infectivity. The titer of HBeAg correlates directly with the amount of virus present in semen and saliva.[108,135] Cellular immunodeficiency due to HIV in dually infected persons may result in higher levels of HBV viremia and enhanced potential for transmission.[165–167]

Many HBsAg-positive homosexual men have at least chemical evidence of chronic liver disease. In the New York City study, 62% of male homosexual carriers had total serum alanine aminotransferase (ALT) levels of greater than 40 Karmen units, and 48% had levels greater than 60 Karmen units.[144] These rates are roughly twice those seen in other groups of asymptomatic carriers. Looked at in another way, Hentzer et al.[152] found elevated serum ALT levels in 9 out of 95 asymptomatic gay men. Eight of these individuals were HBsAg-positive. The implications of these findings for the long-term health of these carriers have not been studied carefully. However, studies in other populations indicate that such individuals are at risk for developing cirrhosis. Similarly, the risk of primary liver carcinoma among HBsAg-positive homosexuals is not well established. However, hepatocellular carcinoma has not emerged as a major problem in gay men with AIDS, and there is no evidence that this risk is increased by immunosuppression due to HIV infection.

Heterosexual transmission of HBV

Extensive evidence also supports the transmission of HBV by heterosexual contact. Sexual partners of HBsAg-positive carriers frequently have serologic evidence of HBV infection.[139,151] In one study, either HBsAg or anti-HBs was found in 27% of spouses of HBsAg carriers but only in 11% of spouses of noncarrier controls.[144] Although nonsexual, household contacts of HBsAg carriers may also have serologic evidence of past HBV infection,[139] the risk appears to be greater for sexual partners of index cases. The sexual partners of individuals with acute hepatitis B are clearly at increased risk of acquiring infection when compared with other members of the household. Mosley[168] reported that 18% of susceptible cohabiting spouses eventually became infected with HBV whereas other family members generally did not. Similarly, Koff et al.[169] found that 3 of 13 sexual partners, compared with 0 of 68 nonsexual domestic contacts, became infected with HBV in this setting. The risk of heterosexual transmission appears to be higher when the HBsAg-positive partner has detectable serum HBV DNA.[170] This is not surprising, since the amount of virus in saliva and semen is related to the magnitude of the viremia.[137] While it is likely that virus is transmitted by vaginal intercourse, it is difficult to assess the role of inapparent percutaneous or mucosal exposures resulting from the sharing of razors, toothbrushes, or other personal articles between partners. Available data do not support a major role for salivary exchange in the transmission of virus between sex partners.[171,172]

In one study, the prevalence of HBV infection among white heterosexuals attending a clinic for sexually transmitted diseases in Arizona, who were without other risk factors such as injection drug use, was related to numbers of previous sex partners.[146] Serum markers of HBV infection were present in 21% of those with 5 or more sex partners during the preceding four months, but in only 6% of those with fewer than 5 partners. A similar correlation existed for total numbers of lifetime sex partners, among both male and female clinic patients. In addition, a similar survey of heterosexual college students without other risk factors for HBV acquisition also demonstrated a positive correlation between numbers of previous sex partners and risk of HBV infection.[173] During the past 5 years, 40% to 50% of reported cases of acute hepatitis B in the United States were contracted through heterosexual exposure (Centers for Disease Control and Prevention, unpublished data).

Subsequent studies in a number of diverse populations, from San Francisco to Mwanza, Tanzania, have confirmed a strong association between higher numbers of recent or lifetime sexual partners and the risk of HBV infection among heterosexual persons.[159,174–177] Indeed, this association exists even among individuals with acute hepatitis B in Taiwan, a country with a very high overall prevalence of HBV infection.[174] In addition, an increased risk of HBV infection has been observed in heterosexual persons with a past history of STDs, particularly syphilis but also gonorrhea or herpes simplex virus type 2 seropositivity.[175–180] It is not clear whether this association is simply indicative of common risk factors for HBV and these other STDs, or whether it reflects an increased risk of transmission of HBV to persons who have active ulcerative genital lesions.

CLINICAL MANIFESTATIONS OF HBV INFECTION

Many adults infected with HBV probably have silent infections which result in permanent and solid immunity. Only one-third of seropositive homosexual men relate a past history of viral hepatitis.[144] However, in a placebo-controlled trial of an HBV vaccine conducted among homosexual men in New York City, 64% of infections in placebo recipients were associated with clinical evidence of disease.[63] The onset of illness is generally more insidious than in hepatitis A, and evidence of hepatocellular disease resolves more slowly. The incubation period is usually from 40 to 110 days, but it may be shortened by large inoculum or percutaneous exposures or prolonged by administration of partially protective immune globulin preparations.[102] A small proportion (1% or less) of icteric adults develop acute hepatic failure, and about three out of four of these unfortunate patients will die as a result of their infection in the absence of liver transplantation.[181] Fulminant disease may be more common following infection with precore mutants.[182] HBV is responsible for about half of all patients with fulminant hepatitis, although infection with HDV may be the immediate cause of severe disease in many of these patients (see below). As a rule, elderly patients tolerate acute hepatitis more poorly than younger individuals.

Approximately 15%–20% of patients develop a transient serum-sickness-like illness during the prodromal or early acute stage of hepatitis B.[183,184] This syndrome is characterized by an erythematous macular, maculopapular, or occasionally urticarial skin rash, polyarthralgias, and frequently frank arthritis. The arthritis may be migratory, is frequently symmetrical, and may involve both large joints of the extremities and the proximal interphalangeal joints of the hands. Synovial fluid findings are variable, but leukocyte counts as high as 90,000/mL^3 (often with a predominance of neutrophils) have been reported. Serum aminotransferases are usually elevated and may be the best clue to the proper diagnosis.

A striking feature of hepatitis B is the development of persistent infection. Out of 429 hospitalized patients with acute icteric hepatitis B, 43 became persistent carriers of HBsAg in one study.[185] Overall, however, the frequency with which acute infection leads to the chronic carrier state is undoubtedly much lower, as these hospitalized patients represented a selected population. Among normal adults, progression to the chronic carrier state (HBsAg-positive for >6 months) may occur in 1% or less. A long-term follow-up study of American soldiers who were infected by administration of contaminated yellow fever vaccine in 1941–1942 failed to identify a significant number of HBsAg carriers.[186] Up to a third of chronic HBsAg carriers develop histologic evidence of chronic hepatitis with fibrosis, while the remainder have a more benign disease characterized by minimal inflammatory changes on liver biopsy or no histologic changes at all.[186] While chronic hepatitis B may progress to cirrhosis and death, it more frequently remits spontaneously even in moderately advanced cases.[187] Although most persistent HBV infections are well tolerated by the host, a wide variety of immunopathological conditions are associated with persistent circulating HBsAg, including generalized necrotizing vasculitis (polyarteritis nodosa),[188–190] chronic membranous and membranoproliferative glomerulonephritis,[191] and essential mixed cryoglobulinemia.[192] The latter condition, however, is much more frequently associated with hepatitis C.[193,194]

DIAGNOSIS OF HBV [HEPATITIS B] INFECTION

The diagnosis of HBV infection is based on serology (see Table 26-2). Approximately 90% of patients with acute hepatitis B have detectable HBsAg when they first present for medical care.[103] This antigen may be detected by any of a variety of sensitive assay methods, most commonly enzyme-linked immunosorbent assay. Approximately 10% of patients with acute HBV infection are HBsAg-negative, however, and these cases are more difficult to document. In such patients, anti-HBc is uniformly present while anti-HBs may be found in some. Anti-HBs and anti-HBc generally are detected by solid-phase immunoassay, and both persist for many years after acute infection; their presence is not diagnostic of acute hepatitis B. In contrast, specific tests for IgM anti-HBc have proven very useful in the diagnosis of acute infection.[103] IgM anti-HBc may be detected by antibody-capture immunoassay in almost all cases of acute hepatitis B. This antibody marker generally persists after acute infection for 6–24 months. While many chronic HBsAg carriers have persistent IgM anti-HBc, the titer is usually substantially lower than that found in acute infection, and it is usually not detected in commercial assays (thus preserving IgM anti-HBc as a specific marker for acute infection). The IgM antibody is often 7S rather than 19S IgM in chronic carriers.[195] The presence of HBeAg in an HBsAg-positive individual suggests a high degree of infectivity.[107,108] Conversion of HBeAg to anti-

HBe in a patient with chronic hepatitis B generally signals a resolution of hepatocellular disease (see Fig. 26-6, bottom panel), and in some cases even heralds an end to the HBsAg carrier state.[110] Overall, however, the clinical value of HBeAg/anti-HBe testing is questionable.

PREVENTION

Hepatitis B vaccines are highly effective and provide protection against hepatitis B (and hepatitis D) by stimulating the production of neutralizing antibodies against HBV (anti-HBs).[6] Since homosexual men have historically had very high hepatitis B attack rates, early placebo-controlled clinical trials of these vaccines focused on this important risk group. Immunization was shown to reduce the incidence of hepatitis B among homosexual men by 90%–95%[63,160,196] and to similarly protect health care workers with frequent exposure to blood.[197] Protection became evident within weeks of the first 2 doses of vaccine in homosexual males, even though the incubation period of hepatitis B is often 6 weeks or longer. These results suggest some degree of postexposure protection. In general, protection correlates with anti-HBs titers >10 mIU/mL.[63,196] Immunization also prevents perinatal infection in infants born to HBsAg-positive mothers. For maximal benefit in this setting, vaccine should be administered within 12 hours of birth in combination with hepatitis B immune globulin.[198] Immunized infants appear to be protected against hepatitis B for at least 8 years.[199,200]

Symptomatic hepatitis B has almost never been observed in immunized persons who develop anti-HBs >10 mIU/mL, even though anti-HBs may fall to nondetectable levels in up to 50% of such persons within 5–10 years.[201] It is likely that continued protection against hepatitis B reflects the establishment of good immunologic memory by the vaccine. Some vaccine recipients may develop anti-HBc, which is indicative of HBV infection, but they almost always do so in the absence of disease.[160,201]

Subunit hepatitis B vaccines contain recombinant HBsAg produced in the yeast *Saccharomyces cerevisiae*. These have replaced earlier, chemically-inactivated, subviral particle vaccines that were produced from plasma collected from chronic HBsAg carriers (plasma-derived vaccine). Two recombinant vaccines, Recombivax HB (Merck) and Engerix-B (SmithKline Beecham) are licensed for use within the United States. Both contain purified HBsAg particles adsorbed on aluminum hydroxide and preserved with thimerosal.[202,203] In general, these vaccines are comparable to each other in terms of safety and efficacy. However, the vaccines are provided in several different formulations and dosage strengths, making it essential that the package insert be carefully examined for details concerning administration. Hepatitis B vaccines are very safe.[201,204] Adverse events are usually confined to mild injection site reactions (up to 22% of immunized persons), while fever and other systemic symptoms are only infrequently reported. There are anecdotal reports of Guillain-Barré-Landry syndrome in some recipients of hepatitis B vaccines, but it is not clear whether the vaccine played a causal role in such cases.[205] Anaphylaxis is a rare complication,[205] but it is important that epinephrine always be available for immediate use.

A usual immunization course includes 3 doses of the vaccine. The final booster dose should be given at least 4–6 months after the initial two-dose primary immunization series, as this enhances peak antibody levels and ensures more durable protection. All three doses can be administered on an accelerated, monthly, schedule in the hope of quickly stimulating immunity,[206,207] but this may reduce final anti-HBs titers and thus the duration of protection, and should be followed by a final booster dose at least 4–

Table 26-3. Persons for Whom Hepatitis B Vaccination Is Recommended

Preexposure
All infants
Adolescents 11–12 years old
Health-care and public safety workers at risk for blood or needle-stick exposures
Clients and staff of institutions for the developmentally disabled
Hemodialysis patients
Homosexually active men
Heterosexually active men and women (history of STD or multiple partners)
Users of illicit injectable drugs
Recipients of certain blood products
Household members and sexual partners of HBV carriers
Adoptees from countries with endemic HBV (and other children in household)
Children of immigrants and refugees from countries endemic for HBV
Inmates of long-term correctional facilities
International travelers to HBV-endemic areas
Postexposure
Infants born to HBV-positive mothers
Health-care workers with percutaneous or mucosal exposure to human blood
Sexual partners of persons with acute HBV infection

6 months later. Almost all healthy infants, children or young adults who receive a series of three intramuscular doses of a recombinant hepatitis B vaccine develop protective levels of anti-HBs.[202,203] Immunogenicity may be reduced in persons over 40 years of age or who are otherwise immunocompromised (including persons with asymptomatic HIV infection).[6] Immunocompromised patients should receive larger doses of vaccine in anticipation of a poor response.

Current recommendations for use of hepatitis B vaccines center on a four-fold hepatitis B reduction strategy (Table 26-3). This strategy includes (1) prevention of mother-to-infant transmission, (2) routine infant immunization, (3) routine adolescent immunization of 11–12 year olds, and (4) "catch-up" immunization of children, high risk adolescents, and adults who have not been previously immunized.[201] Individuals with a history of an STD and those with multiple sexual partners (>1 in the previous 6 months) should be offered vaccine. Most patients seen in STD clinics should be considered candidates for vaccination. Anti-HBs testing is not routinely recommended following immunization, and there are no recommendations for late booster doses of vaccine.

HEPATITIS D

CLINICAL VIROLOGY

Because HDV is a defective virus, its replication is absolutely dependent upon simultaneous HBV infection for essential helper functions. Thus, HDV infects only patients with active HBV infection. The HDV virion is a 35 nm particle found in the blood.[208,209] It has an outer envelope consisting of HBsAg and an amorphous core containing a viral protein, hepatitis delta antigen (HDAg), complexed with a small, circular single-stranded RNA molecule 1.7 kb in length.[210] This genomic RNA has a very high G+C content and extensive intramolecular complementarity, resulting in its assuming a rodlike, predominantly double-stranded secondary structure. Both genomic and antigenomic sense RNA is present in the liver of infected individuals. Replication of the viral RNA is thought to occur by a "rolling circle" mechanism under direction of a cellular polymerase, with nascent RNA molecules capable of autocatalytic cleavage and self-ligation. The HDV antigen is a highly basic phosphoprotein which forms oligomers and has RNA-binding activity.[211,212] It is encoded by the antigenomic sense RNA, making HDV a (-)-stranded RNA virus. The provision of HBsAg, encoded by the HBV genome, is the only helper function required for HDV replication.

HDV infection may occur as a coinfection with acute hepatitis B in an individual who was previously susceptible to HBV, or as a superinfection in an HBV carrier.[213] Either type of infection may result in severe hepatitis with fulminant disease and death.[214] Coinfections are often marked by a biphasic serum aminotransferase response, while superinfections may be associated with transient (at times permanent) suppression of HBV replication markers. Those who survive acute coinfections usually go on to complete recovery and are not at increased risk of becoming chronic HBV carriers. On the other hand, HBV carriers surviving HDV superinfections frequently become carriers of HDV with clinically aggressive chronic liver disease.[213] The diagnosis of HDV infection is generally dependent upon demonstration of antibody to HDAg (anti-HD) as this is the only widely available test (see Table 26-2). Acute HDV/HBV coinfections are distinguished from HDV superinfection of a chronic HBsAg carrier by measurement of IgM anti-HBc, which is present in the former and absent in the latter. Indeed, persons presenting with what appears to be acute type B hepatitis who lack this serum marker should be suspected of having HDV superinfection.

EPIDEMIOLOGY OF HDV

HDV is found in the blood of anti-HD positive HBsAg carriers, and the prevalence of anti-HD among American carriers is strongly associated with illicit injection drug use, hemophilia, or a history of multiple transfusions.[215,216] Geographic differences in the distribution of HDV are striking, however, and anti-HD is significantly more prevalent among HBsAg carriers from Middle Eastern and Mediterranean countries. Outbreaks of fulminant hepatitis D with high mortality rates have been reported among the indigenous populations of Venezuela and other South American countries, possibly representing widespread superinfection of HBsAg carriers.[217]

SEXUAL TRANSMISSION OF HDV

The extent to which HDV may be sexually transmitted remains unclear. HBsAg-positive homosexual men have a low prevalence of anti-HD compared with other carrier groups, particularly IDUs.[215,218–220] Accordingly, a smaller percentage of homosexual men presenting with acute HBsAg-positive hepatitis in Los Angeles were found to have anti-HD, compared with IDUs.[213] These men also had a lower overall mortality than IDUs with acute hepatitis B, reflecting their lower frequency of HDV infection. Nonetheless, HDV coinfection was found in 14% of homosexual men from Los Angeles with acute HBsAg-positive hepatitis,[213] many of whom denied a history of transfusions or injection drug use. Another survey found anti-HD antibodies in 9%– 15% of HBsAg-positive homosexual men living in Los Angeles and San Francisco but in only 0%–1% of HBsAg-positive homosexual men in Chicago and Pittsburgh.[218] In the West Coast groups, the presence of anti-HD was correlated with numbers of previous sex partners, as well as injection drug use. In contrast, of 60 homosexual men with acute hepatitis B who were identified through the Sentinel Counties Study of the CDC, none had concomitant HDV infection.[219] Thus, except for reports from the west coast of the United States,[213,218] HDV infection appears to be a relatively rare cause of hepatitis among homosexual men. A similar absence of HDV infection among homosexual men with HBV infection was observed in Sydney, Australia.[220] Fewer studies have focused on the potential for heterosexual transmission of HDV. However, a recent multivariate analysis of patients with acute hepatitis D in Italy, a country with a generally high prevalence of HDV infection among HBsAg carriers, identified a history of having had >2 sex partners in the preceding 6 months as a significant risk factor for acquisition of the disease.[220]

Although sexual transmission of HDV is uncommon, the severity of liver disease accompanying acute and chronic HDV infections makes the potential for such transmission a concern worthy of continuing attention. However, there is no specific means for prevention of HDV infection other than immunization with hepatitis B vaccine, which provides protection by preventing the helper virus infection required for HDV replication.

HEPATITIS C

INTRODUCTION

HCV was identified and shown to be the cause of almost all cases of non-B posttransfusion hepatitis in the late 1980s.[221,222] The virus establishes a persistent infection in the majority of infected persons, many of whom develop evidence of chronic inflammatory liver disease.[5] These chronically infected persons are at risk for cirrhosis and to a lesser extent hepatocellular carcinoma.[223,224] HCV infection accounts for 15% of acute viral hepatitis cases within the United States. However, it is by far the leading cause of chronic viral hepatitis and is present in over 40% of persons with chronic liver disease. The morbidity and mortality associated with HCV infection is due to its unique propensity to cause persistent infection in most persons, a feature that distinguishes this virus from other hepatitis viruses. The specific mechanisms underlying viral persistence are not known.

Although it has been controversial, the balance of evidence now favors the occasional sexual transmission of HCV. The risk of infection with HCV, like HBV, has been independently related to numbers of sexual partners in some STD clinic studies.[179,225] However, transmission of HCV is much more frequently associated with risks for percutaneous exposure such as sharing of paraphernalia for preparing and injecting drugs among illicit injection drug users. Although the risk of HCV infection has been shown to correlate with numbers of partners and/or specific sexual practices in some studies of homosexual men,[226,227] the risk of infection is overwhelmingly more closely tied to injection drug use.[226–229] Thus, sexual transmission of HCV appears to occur with a much lower efficiency than sexual transmission of HBV,[230,231] although the reasons underlying this difference are not well explained by any data.

HEPATITIS C VIRUS

HCV has recently been classified within the genus *Hepacivirus* of the family *Flaviviridae,* in part because of a distant phylogenetic relationship with yellow fever virus and other classical flaviviruses.[232,233] However, HCV has a number of unusual biological features that distinguish it from other flaviviruses. These include most notably the ability to establish persistent infections in the majority of infected persons.

Virus structure and replication

The single-stranded, (+)-strand RNA genome of HCV contains a single large open reading frame (Fig. 26-7).[232,233] This follows a relatively lengthy 5′ nontranslated region of approximately 342 bases, which contains an internal ribosome entry site (IRES) that directs the 5′ cap-independent initiation of viral translation.[234] The polyprotein encoded by the open reading frame undergoes posttranslational cleavages directed by both host cell and virus-encoded proteinases (see Fig. 26-7).[235–237] Signal sequences within the amino terminal third of the polyprotein direct its secretion into the endoplasmic reticulum (ER). Several cleavages directed by host cell signalase produce a series of structural proteins which include the nucleocapsid protein, two envelope glycoproteins, E1 and E2, and a small membrane-associated protein, p7 or NS2A. The nucleocapsid protein remains within the cytoplasm. E1 and E2 become heavily glycosylated within the ER and the Golgi, but details of the viral assembly and secretion process remain obscure.[238,239] E2 contains a highly variable domain near its amino terminus (HVR-1 domain), which is likely to form an immunogenic loop on the surface of the virion and which may interact with neutralizing antibodies.[240,241] As such, it might be quite analogous to the V3 loop of HIV-1.

At least 6 nonstructural proteins are derived from the remainder of the polyprotein (see Fig. 26-7). The functions of these proteins are only partly understood. They include NS2B (which with the adjacent NS3 sequence demonstrates cis-active metalloproteinase activity at the NS2B/NS3 cleavage site),[237,242] NS3 (a serine proteinase/NTPase/RNA helicase),[243,244] NS4A (serine proteinase accessory factor),[245] NS4B, NS5A, and NS5B (RNA-dependent RNA polymerase).[246] Efforts to develop effective antiviral inhibitors of HCV replication have driven extensive studies of these proteins, which have included high resolution X-ray crystallographic analysis of the NS3 proteinase domain complexed with its accessory factor, NS4A. Noncovalent association of NS4A with the NS3 proteinase domain is required to achieve full proteinase activity. The NS4A molecule forms extensive interactions with NS3, becoming an integral part of a b-barrel structure that flanks the proteinase active site. This complex is a prime target for development of new small molecule inhibitors of viral replication.

Negative-sense replicative intermediates of the viral RNA have been demonstrated in the liver and serum.[246] However, few details of the replication cycle of HCV are known because the virus undergoes only low-level replication in any cell culture system studied to date. Several B- and T-cell derived lymphoid cell lines may be permissive for HCV replication to a limited extent,[248,249] but the in vitro systems that are available for virus propagation are insufficient for biochemical characterization of the virus and its replication. Infectious molecular cDNA clones of the HCV genome have recently been developed.[250,251] The infectivity of RNA transcribed from these clones has been established by the demonstration of hepatitis associated with viremia in chimpanzees who were transfected in vivo by direct intrahepatic injection. These clones should benefit many aspects of HCV research, including the search for more fully permissive cell culture systems.

Genetic and antigenic heterogeneity

Different strains of HCV are classified as distinct "genotypes" based on the extent of nucleotide sequence divergence.[252] Genotype 1b strains appear to be more refractory to interferon therapy than non-1b strains, but there is no good evidence for other differences in the pathogenicity of various genotypes. The genetic distance between some genotypes is large enough to suggest that there are biologically significant serotypic differences as well. However, only low level homologous protection is evident when chimpanzees are challenged twice with the same strain of HCV.[253] The absence of a permissive cell culture system has precluded the development of specific virus neutralization assays and the formal determination of viral serotypes.

NATURAL HISTORY AND PATHOGENESIS OF HCV [HEPATITIS C] INFECTIONS

Current understanding of the natural history and pathogenesis of HCV must be considered incomplete, as many points remain in question. However, available data indicate that about 85% of all infections lead to virus persistence, and that this is often associated with evidence of chronic liver disease (Fig. 26-8). After many years, this process may culminate in cirrhosis and liver failure, or the development of hepatocellular carcinoma.

Acute hepatitis C

The primary cell type infected by the virus is the hepatocyte. However, there is some evidence for infection of lymphoid cells,[254] and it is possible that this plays an important role in pathogenesis.

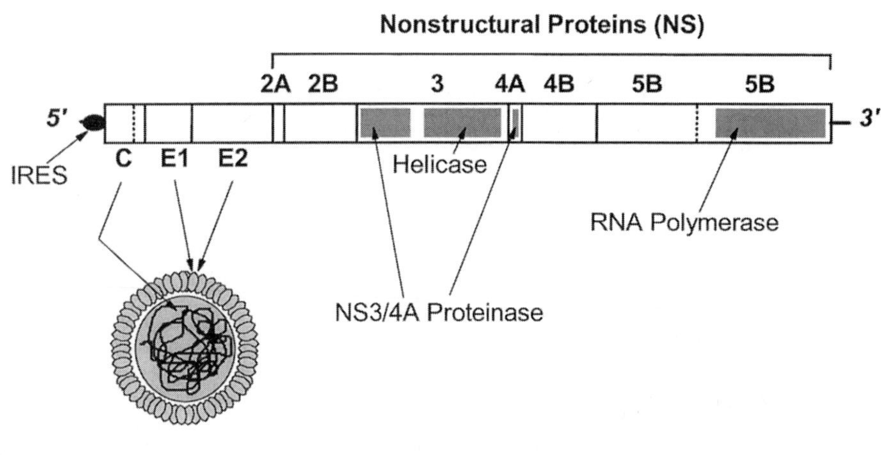

Fig. 26-7 Organization of the 9.6 kb (+)-strand RNA genome of HCV. As in HAV (Fig. 26-1), the translation of a large polyprotein is directed by an IRES located within the 5′ nontranslated RNA. This polyprotein is subsequently processed into the structural proteins, core (C), and the two envelope glycoproteins (E1 and E2) by cellular signalase following translocation of part of the polyprotein into the endoplasmic reticulum. Following a cis-active cleavage at NS2/NS3 directed by a metalloproteinase activity, the NS3 protease directs further processing of the polyprotein, resulting in additional nonstructural proteins that are involved in viral replication. The fully active protease is a complex of NS3 and NS4A. NS3 also contains an RNA helicase, while NS5B possesses RNA-dependent RNA polymerase activity. These HCV proteins are prime targets for development of future anti-viral drugs.

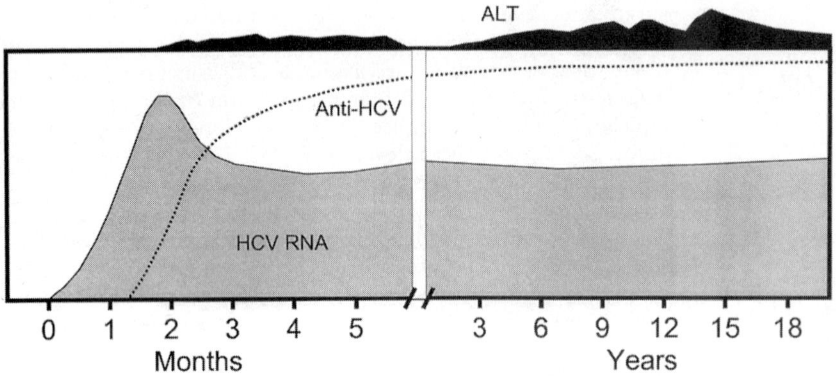

Fig. 26-8 Typical virologic and serologic course of persistent HCV infection. Acute infection is often marked by little clinical evidence of hepatitis, despite the presence of relatively high levels of viral RNA in the blood that are detected by RT-PCR or sensitive bDNA hybridization assays. Anti-HCV detected by ELISA assays reflects specific antibody responses to a number of the viral proteins. Viremia is generally constant, while serum ALT levels can fluctuate significantly. The latter correlate poorly with the extent of histologic abnormalities in the liver. Late clinical complications include cirrhosis and hepatocellular carcinoma.

Early studies in transfused individuals indicated that most HCV infections are associated with minimal symptoms and only rarely with identifiable jaundice. In contrast, patients presenting to physicians with acute hepatitis C are much more likely to be icteric.[5] They are thus likely to represent only a small fraction of all acute infections. Quantitatively, virus replication appears to be greatest shortly after infection with the magnitude of the viremia highest during this period (Fig. 26-8). Viremia subsequently declines with the appearance of antibody to viral proteins and T-cell mediated immunity to HCV, and in most persons it remains constant at a relatively fixed level for many years.[5] However, in a poorly defined minority of infected persons the infection may be self-limited and viral persistence may not be established. The clinical outcome of the acute HCV infection may be dependent upon the vigor of the cellular immune response to the infection.[256]

Chronic hepatitis C

Approximately two-thirds of persons who become infected with HCV go on to develop persistent or intermittent elevations in serum ALT levels.[5] At liver biopsy, these individuals may have intrahepatic inflammation and fibrosis, the extent of which is not well correlated with the magnitude of serum enzyme elevations. 15% to 30% of those with chronic hepatitis C will ultimately develop cirrhosis.[5,223,257,258] Cirrhosis may be present within as little as 60 months of the initial infection but is identified more often in persons who have been infected for decades. Even with histologically established cirrhosis, many patients will have no symptoms and will continue to lead normal lives. Nonetheless, in a poorly defined proportion of these patients the disease eventually progresses to the point where the patient becomes symptomatic with evidence of end-stage liver disease. Some patients, usually with well established cirrhosis, develop primary hepatocellular carcinoma.[224]

The major challenge to clinical investigators has been the discovery of specific markers that are predictive of progression of chronic hepatitis C to a clinically significant disease state. This remains an exceptionally difficult problem. There is no good correlation between biochemical markers and the extent of fibrosis or the presence or absence of cirrhosis. Indeed, many patients with advanced cirrhosis have no obvious biochemical abnormalities.[258] In addition, quantitative measurements of the viremia ("virus load") have not been proven to be useful in determining the extent of disease.[259] However, antibody-positive individuals who have normal ALT levels and who test persistently negative for viral RNA are at low risk for significant liver disease. About 15% of all anti-HCV positive individuals will fall into this category; these individuals may have successfully cleared the infection.

Many years of infection (>20–30) appear to be required in most cases for the clinical expression of end-stage cirrhosis or the development of hepatocellular carcinoma.[258] Many individuals with clinically advanced hepatitis C also have a history of excessive alcohol intake. It is suspected that excessive alcohol ingestion may act additively if not synergistically with HCV infection in promoting liver disease.[260–262] Mechanisms underlying the development of liver cancer in patients with HCV infection have not been established. However, it is likely that cancer occurs as a result of chronic, long-standing inflammation in the liver, as with hepatitis B-related cancers (see above).

Destruction of the liver cell is probably not caused by direct cytotoxic effects of HCV infection, but rather by immunopathological mechanisms. Liver injury most likely results from the direct action of virus-specific cytotoxic T-cells, as well as from secondary mediators of inflammation (such as gamma interferon) that are released as a result of the vigorous virus-specific T cell response.[260–262] Thus, T-cell mediated responses have two effects on the disease process. They may suppress virus replication and lower the magnitude of viremia. However, in the absence of eliminating the virus altogether, cytotoxic T-cell responses also stimulate significant inflammation within the liver and are likely to be the proximate cause of both ALT elevation and fibrosis.

The frequency with which HCV infection leads to clinically overt liver disease has yet to be well established. In a retrospective cohort study of transfused individuals carried out in the United States, overall mortality was not increased in persons who had been infected with HCV 18 years earlier.[258] Moreover, the risk of liver-specific mortality in infected individuals was only marginally increased over that of uninfected control subjects receiving equivalent numbers of transfusions. Although this study provides some level of comfort concerning this infection, this may be misleading. Most of the subjects were middle-aged or older at the time of transfusion and subsequent infection with HCV. The impact of HCV infection may be quite different in individuals who are infected in the second and third decades of life. Furthermore, when studied 18–20 years after their infection, as many as a third of these patients with transfusion-transmitted hepatitis C had elevated serum ALT activities indicative of chronic hepatitis. Moreover, among those patients from this group who underwent liver biopsy, approximately one-third had established cirrhosis.[266]

Consistent with this latter view, HCV is at present the leading cause of liver transplantation in the United States and an important cause overall of liver-related mortality. The CDC currently estimates that 8–10,000 persons die each year in the United States due to liver disease associated with HCV infection.[267] This is about one-third the number of AIDS-related deaths at present. Concerns have been raised that HCV-associated mortality may increase significantly over the next two decades, in view of the recognition that there are large numbers of asymptomatically infected persons who are at present in the third and fourth decades of life.[267] Most of these persons probably acquired their infection due to limited injection-drug use many years ago. Age-related seroprevalence data collected within the United States suggest that there has been a significant expansion of this pool of infected persons in recent decades.

Extrahepatic disease manifestations

Extrahepatic manifestations of HCV infection are relatively common and include most prominently glomerulonephritis and type II mixed cryoglobulinemia associated with vasculitis.[194,268,269] Such individuals have circulating immune complexes containing viral RNA. Other potentially associated clinical conditions include porphyria cutanea tarda, sicca syndrome, and a variety of autoimmune diseases.

DIAGNOSIS OF HVC [HEPATITIS C] INFECTION

Serologically, infection is marked by the presence of antibodies to several viral proteins: core, NS3, NS4, and NS5[270,271] (see Table 26-2). The presence of such antibodies may be detected by ELISA assays originally developed for screening of blood donations. When such tests are found to be positive, confirmatory assays (such as a recombinant immunoblot, or RIBA, assay) should be run to confirm the presence of antibodies to the virus. The demonstration of these antibodies signifies infection and not immunity. Positive reactions in new tests for antibodies to E2 also correlate with serum RNA positivity,[272] and thus are not likely to reflect immunity. RT-PCR detection of viral RNA in serum is useful for confirmation of serological results and for assessing the replicative activity of the virus.[273] Branched DNA hybridization assays are less sensitive but offer greater quantitative precision.[274,275] These assays are particularly useful for assessing the response to interferon therapy (see Chap. 67).

EPIDEMIOLOGY OF HEPATITIS C

Transmission of HCV occurs by both percutaneous and mucosal exposures. However, the overwhelming risk factor in almost all studies is a history of illicit injection drug use. Because active HCV infections are highly prevalent among IDUs, exposure to HCV occurs early in the career of an IDU who shares paraphernalia for the preparation and injection of drugs with others. Thus, HCV is one of the first infections contracted by most IDUs. In contrast to direct percutaneous transmission, the sexual transmission of this virus appears to be very inefficient. Sexual behavior is usually of secondary importance in determining the risk of HCV infection. However, there are a number of studies which relate sexual practices or numbers of sex partners to infection with HCV. Maternal-infant transmission of HCV also occurs at much lower rates than with HBV but is increased when the mother is infected with HIV.[276,277]

Sexual transmission of HCV

Three general types of studies have attempted to document the sexual transmission of HCV. These include cross-sectional studies of populations who are at a high risk of acquiring sexually transmitted diseases (such as homosexual men or prostitutes), studies of sexual partnerships in which one partner is known to be infected with HCV, and case-control studies of individuals who are infected with HCV. Each of these types of studies provides some support for the sexual transmission of HCV, but each also indicates that sexual transmission plays a limited role in determining the epidemiology of hepatitis C.

Osmond et al.[227] studied 735 homosexual or bisexual men in San Francisco. They found HCV antibodies in only 4.6% of these men, while 81% had one or more markers of HBV infection. When percutaneous exposures were controlled for, the risk of HCV infection was marginally greater in those with >50 sex partners/year, or >25 oral receptive or anal receptive partners. In contrast, HBV infection was much more strongly correlated with these risk factors.[227] In a similar study, 2.9% of 1058 homosexual men included in the Pittsburgh arm of the Multicenter AIDS Cohort Study were found to be anti-HCV positive.[226] Multivariate analysis found that injection drug use was the most important risk factor. However, seropositivity to HCV was significantly associated with a history of previous STD (syphilis, rectal gonorrhea) and anal receptive or insertive intercourse, but not with numbers of sexual partners.[226] These studies support a minor role for sexual transmission in determining the risk of HCV infection in homosexual men.

However, other studies have generated somewhat contradictory results. For example, Buchbinder et al.[229] studied 435 gay men attending a municipal STD clinic in San Francisco. Five percent of non-IDUs were seropositive for HCV, whereas 25% of homosexually active IDUs were anti-HCV positive. There was no independent association between HCV infection and any sexual risk factor on multivariate analysis.[229] Another study of homosexual men carried out in Sydney, Australia found 7.6% of homosexual men to be seropositive.[228] Using a case-control approach, the risk of HCV infection was found to be independent of sexual practices or numbers of sexual partners. In fact, men without HCV infection were significantly more likely to have engaged in unprotected insertive or receptive oral-anal intercourse. The only recognized risk factors for HCV infection in this study were injection drug use and infection with HIV-1.[228]

Taken in aggregate, these studies suggest that sexual behavior plays only a relatively minor role in determining the risk of HCV infection among homosexual men and that sexual transmission of the virus is relatively inefficient. Studies in prostitutes and other high risk heterosexual populations generally confirm this impression.

In separate studies carried out in Taipei, Taiwan and Fukuoka, Japan, HCV seroprevalence rates among female prostitutes ranged from 6% to 12%.[278,279] The presence of HCV infection correlated with the length of time in prostitution and a history of syphilis. However, similar correlations were lacking among female prostitutes who were studied in Somalia.[280] When non-IDU women attending an inner city STD clinic in Miami were studied, 4.4% were seropositive for HCV, compared with 22% for HBV and 7% for HIV.[225] Multivariate analysis indicated that HCV infection was more likely in women with >10 heterosexual partners in the preceding 5 years, those engaging in sexual practices more than once per week, and those with previous HBV or HIV infection.[225] A similar study carried out in Baltimore confirmed the association between numbers of sex partners (i.e., having had >1 sex partner in the previous month) and HCV infection among non-IDU patients attending an STD clinic.[179] In addition, this study found that the risk of infection was increased in men who reported a lack of condom use with sex during the month preceding their visit to the clinic.[179] In general, the risk of HCV infection is generally greater in STD clinic patients who are over 29–30 years of age.[179,231]

A number of studies have demonstrated that the rate of transmission of HCV within sexual partnerships is relatively low.[281–286] For example, Osmond et al.[282] documented HCV infection in only 2 of 31 exposed female partners of infected hemophilic men, compared with 0 of 81 partners of noninfected hemophilics. Similarly, Hallam et al.[283] found only 3 of 104 longstanding sexual partners of infected hemophilic patients to be seropositive for anti-HCV. Each of the infected partners had other risk factors for infection. In another study, Eyster et al.[284] found that female sexual partners of multitransfused men were approximately 8.5 times more likely to be infected with HIV than HCV if their partner was infected with either virus. In an STD clinic population, Thomas et al.[287] demonstrated that the non-IDU female sexual partners of HCV-positive men were 4 times more likely to be infected with HCV than the female partners of HCV-negative men. No association was found for the male sexual partners of HCV-positive women. Thus, these studies document a low risk of male to female transmission within stable sexual partnerships. Fewer data address the issue of female to male transmission, but there is no evidence that transmission is increased in this direction.

It is possible, but not well documented, that HIV infection might increase the low risk of transmission of HCV within a sexual partnership. In a study of non-IDUs at risk for sexually transmitted diseases, Lissen et al.[288] reported HCV infection to be about twice as prevalent in stable, heterosexual partners of HIV-infected persons (9.2%) as in the partners of those without HIV infection (4.1%). However, Eyster et al.[284] found that only 5 of 164 female sexual partners of multitransfused men who were infected with both HIV and HCV were seropositive for HCV.[284]

Although these results indicate a relatively low rate of transmission of HCV within stable heterosexual partnerships, it is important to note that cohabiting sexual partners are at a significantly increased risk of infection compared to other household contacts of HCV-infected persons.[289–291] This risk may be increased with older age and longer duration of marriage or sexual exposure.[289,291] Furthermore, in at least one study, the results of nucleotide sequence analysis of virus present in blood support the interspousal transmission of HCV.[289] Whether such infection occurs as a result of sexual intercourse or through other close, nonsexual contact remains uncertain.

Additional evidence for the occasional sexual transmission of HCV comes from a multivariate analysis of potential risk factors for HCV infection identified in a case-control study of blood donors in Sweden. HCV infection was independently correlated with injection drug use, blood transfusion, previous hospitalization, tattoos, and a history of previous STDs.[292] Among those non-IDU who did not have a history of blood transfusion, the prevalence of antibodies to herpes simplex virus type 2 was significantly increased in those infected with HCV compared to those without HCV infection. A case-control study of blood donors in the United States identified a history blood transfusion, injection drug use, intranasal cocaine use, and "sexual promiscuity" (defined as a history of STD, sex with a prostitute, and/or five or more partners per year) as significantly associated with HCV infection.[293]

All of these studies are consistent with the notions that HCV may be sexually transmitted occasionally and that sexual behavior may influence the risk of HCV infection. In addition, 15% of the reported cases of acute hepatitis C in the United States during the past 5 years appear to be contracted through sexual activity, of which two-thirds involved an anti-HCV positive sexual partner.[294] However, it is clear from these studies that the sexual transmission of HCV is significantly less efficient than sexual transmission of HBV or HIV and that risk factors for percutaneous transmission are overwhelmingly more important in determining the epidemiology of HCV.

PREVENTION AND PATIENT COUNSELING

Prevention

Efforts to develop a recombinant HCV vaccine based on envelope proteins expressed in eukaryotic cells have met with only limited success. Infection was prevented in immunized chimpanzees following challenge with a low-dose, homologous inoculum.[295] However, numerous technical difficulties hinder the development of vaccines, including the apparent lack of a robust protective immune response and the presence of substantial genetic and probably antigenic heterogeneity among different HCV isolates. It is very unlikely that a vaccine will become available in the near future. Similarly, passive immunotherapy with pooled immune globulin (IG) offers little promise of protection against HCV. Some early studies suggested that pooled immune globulin might protect against disease, although not infection.[296] However, protection was not observed in all studies. Moreover, IG preparations that are currently on the market are made from plasma pools from which donor units containing HCV antibodies have been excluded. Such preparations are less likely to be protective than the IG lots used in early studies of passive prophylaxis of non-A, non-B hepatitis. An experimental study in chimpanzees found that neither immune globulin manufactured from screened plasma nor immune globulin prepared from high-titered anti-HCV positive plasma administered 1 hour after exposure to HCV prevented infection or disease.[297]

Patient counseling

As indicated above, there is substantial evidence that HCV is only occasionally transmitted during sexual intercourse. Numerous partner studies demonstrate that the risk of transmission between individuals who are in a stable, monogamous relationship is quite low, although not completely absent. Thus, most experts do not routinely recommend the use of barrier prophylaxis by monogamous couples when one is found to be infected with HCV. Such a view is based in part on the absence of any data that condom usage would lower the already very low rates of transmission between sexual partners. On the other hand, many exposed individuals are relatively young, and there is clear evidence that HCV is a significant pathogen, albeit with a long clinical latent period. Furthermore, as detailed above, virus transmission has been documented between cohabiting sexual partners. Thus, recommendations for or against the use of condoms in this setting cannot be undertaken lightly or with any great degree of certainty. It is most important that the health care provider make available to the patient the appropriate information concerning the risk and potential consequences of HCV transmission during sex. The decision regarding the use of barrier prophylaxis must ultimately be made by the affected individuals.

NEW CANDIDATE "HEPATITIS" VIRUSES

Recently, a new candidate human hepatitis virus was identified. This virus (provisionally termed "GB virus C", or "hepatitis G virus") is often transmitted during blood transfusions and has been suggested to be the cause of liver disease in some patients who have acute or chronic hepatitis without evidence of infection with any of the 5 viruses listed in Table 26-1.[298,299] However, this putative association with liver disease is very doubtful given more recent studies.[300] GB virus C is a (+)-strand, enveloped RNA virus which, like HCV, has many features in common with the flaviviruses. At the genetic level, however, it shows many differences from HCV and cannot be considered to be simply an HCV variant. Viremia is quite common in healthy blood donors (1.7%).[299]

Much more work needs to be done to determine the specific disease associations (if any) of this virus. Thus far, there is no evidence for sexual transmission of this virus.

References

1 Blumberg BS et al: A "new" antigen in leukemia sera. *JAMA* 191: 541, 1965.

2 Prince AM: An antigen detected in the blood during the incubation period of serum hepatitis. *Proc Natl Acad Sci USA* 60:14, 1968.

3 Rakela J et al: Fulminant hepatitis: Mayo Clinic experience with 34 cases. *Mayo Clin Proc* 60:289, 1985.

4 Farci P et al: Hepatitis C virus-associated fulminant hepatic failure. *N Engl J Med* 335:631, 1996.

5 Alter MJ et al: The natural history of community-acquired hepatitis C in the United States. *N Engl J Med* 327:1899, 1992.

6 Lemon SM, Thomas DL: Vaccines to prevent viral hepatitis. *N Engl J Med* 336:196, 1997.

7 Feinstone SM et al: Detection by immune electron microscopy of a viruslike antigen associated with acute illness. *Science* 182:1026, 1973.

8 Cohen JI et al: Complete nucleotide sequence of wild-type hepatitis A virus: comparison with different strains of hepatitis A virus and other picornaviruses. *J Virol* 61:50, 1987.

9 Brown EA et al: The 5′ nontranslated region of hepatitis A virus: secondary structure and elements required for translation in vitro. *J Virol* 65:5828, 1991.

10 Weitz M et al: Detection of a genome-linked protein (VPg) of hepatitis A virus and its comparison with other picornaviral VPgs. *J Virol* 60:124, 1986.

11 Cohen JI et al: Hepatitis A virus cDNA and its RNA transcripts are infectious in cell culture. *J Virol* 61:3035, 1987.

12 Allaire M et al: Picornaviral 3C cysteine proteinases have a fold similar to chymotrypsin-like serine proteinases. *Nature* 369:72, 1994.

13 Schultheiss T et al: Cleavage specificity of purified recombinant hepatitis A virus 3C proteinase on natural substrates. *J Virol* 69:1727, 1995.

14 Lemon SM et al: Protease digestion of hepatitis A virus: disparate effects on capsid proteins, antigenicity, and infectivity. *J Virol* 65: 5636, 1991.

15 Glaser JB, Nadler JP: Hepatitis B virus in a cardiopulmonary resuscitation training course. Risk of transmission from a surface antigen-positive participant. *Arch Intern Med* 145:1653, 1985.

16 Gauss-Muller V, Deinhardt F: Effect of hepatitis A virus infection on cell metabolism in vitro. *Proc Soc Exper Biol Med* 175:10, 1984.

17 Daemer RJ et al: Propagation of human hepatitis A virus in African Green Monkey kidney cell culture: primary isolation and serial passage. *Infect Immun* 32:388, 1981.

18 Binn LN et al: Primary isolation and serial passage of hepatitis A virus strains in primate cell cultures. *J Clin Microbiol* 20:28, 1984.

19 Lemon SM, Binn LN: Antigenic relatedness of two strains of hepatitis A virus determined by cross-neutralization. *Infect Immun* 42:418, 1983.

20 Robertson BH et al: Genetic relatedness of hepatitis A virus strains recovered from different geographic regions. *J Gen Virol* 73:1365, 1992.

21 Ping L-H, Lemon SM: Antigenic structure of human hepatitis A virus defined by analysis of escape mutants selected against murine monoclonal antibodies. *J Virol* 66:2208, 1992.

22 Dienstag JL et al: Experimental infection of chimpanzees with hepatitis A virus. *J Infect Dis* 132:532, 1975.

23 LeDuc JW et al: Experimental infection of the New World owl monkey (*Aotus trivirgatus*) with hepatitis A virus. *Infect Immun* 40:766, 1983.

24 Dienstag JL et al: Faecal shedding of hepatitis-A antigen. *Lancet* i: 765, 1975.

25 Asher LVS et al: Pathogenesis of hepatitis A in orally inoculated owl monkeys (*Aotus trivergatus*). *J Med Virol* 47:260, 1995.

26 Schulman AN et al: Hepatitis A antigen particles in liver, bile, and stool of chimpanzees. *J Infect Dis* 134:80, 1976.

27 Mathiesen LR et al: Localization of hepatitis A antigen in marmoset organs during acute infection with hepatitis A virus. *J Infect Dis* 138: 369, 1978.

28 Lemon SM et al: In vivo replication and reversion to wild-type of a neutralization-resistant variant of hepatitis A virus. *J Infect Dis* 161: 7, 1990.

29 Coulepis AG et al: Detection of hepatitis A virus in the feces of patients with naturally acquired infections. *J Infect Dis* 141:151, 1980.

30 Skinhoj P et al: Hepatitis A in Greenland: importance of specific antibody testing in epidemiologic surveillance. *Am J Epidemiol* 105: 140, 1977.

31 Rosenblum LS et al: Hepatitis A outbreak in a neonatal intensive care unit: risk factors for transmission and evidence of prolonged viral excretion among preterm infants. *J Infect Dis* 164:476, 1991.

32 Alter MJ et al: The changing epidemiology of hepatitis B in the United States. Need for alternative vaccination strategies. *JAMA* 263:1218, 1990.

33 Vallbracht A et al: Cell-mediated cytotoxicity in hepatitis A virus infection. *Hepatology* 6:1308, 1986.

34 Vallbracht A et al: Liver-derived cytotoxic T cells in hepatitis A virus infection. *J Infect Dis* 160:209, 1989.

35 Fleischer B et al: Clonal analysis of infiltrating T lymphocytes in liver tissue in viral hepatitis A. *Immunology* 69:14, 1990.

36 Maier K et al: Human gamma interferon production by cytotoxic T lymphocytes sensitized during hepatitis A virus infection. *J Virol* 62: 3756, 1988.

37 Locarnini SA et al: The antibody response following hepatitis A infection. *Intervirology* 8:309, 1977.

38 Decker RH et al: Serologic studies of transmission of hepatitis A in humans. *J Infect Dis* 139:74, 1979.

39 Villarejos VM et al: Hepatitis A virus infection in households. *Am J Epidemiol* 115:577, 1982.

40 Yoshizawa H et al: Diagnosis of type A hepatitis by fecal IgA antibody against hepatitis A antigen. *Gastroenterology* 78:114, 1980.

41 Stapleton JT et al: The role of secretory immunity in hepatitis A virus infection. *J Infect Dis* 163:7, 1991.

42 Kurane I et al: Human lymphocyte responses to hepatitis A virus-infected cells: interferon production and lysis of infected cells. *J Immunol* 135:2140, 1985.

43 Cohen JI et al: Hepatitis A virus infection in a chimpanzee: duration of viremia and detection of virus in saliva and throat swabs. *J Infect Dis* 160:887, 1989.

44 Siegl G et al: Stability of hepatitis A virus. *Intervirology* 22:218, 1984.

45 Centers for Disease Control and Prevention: Hepatitis A among drug abusers. *MMWR* 37:297, 1988.

46 Katz MH et al: Seroprevalence of and risk factors for hepatitis A infection among young homosexual and bisexual men. *J Infect Dis* 175:1225, 1997.

47 Frosner GG et al: Decrease in incidence of hepatitis A infections in Germany. *Infection* 6:259, 1978.

48 Szmuness W et al: The prevalence of antibody to hepatitis A antigen in various parts of the world: a pilot study. *Am J Epidemiol* 106:392, 1977.

49 Szmuness W et al: Distribution of antibody to hepatitis A antigen in urban adult populations. *N Engl J Med* 295:755, 1976.

50 Burke DS et al: Age-specific prevalence of hepatitis A virus antibody in Thailand. *Am J Epidemiol* 113:245, 1981.

51 Halliday ML et al: An epidemic of hepatitis A attributable to the ingestion of raw clams in Shanghai, China. *J Infect Dis* 164:852, 1991.

51a Bell BP et al: The diverse patterns of hepatitis A epidemiology in the United States: implications for vaccination strategies. *J Infect Dis,* in press, 1998.

52 Hadler SC et al: Hepatitis A in day-care centers: a community-wide assessment. *N Engl J Med* 302:1222, 1980.

53 Kryger P et al: Increased risk of infection with hepatitis A and B viruses in men with a history of syphilis: relation to sexual contacts. *J Infect Dis* 145:23, 1982.
54 McFarlane ES et al: Antibodies to hepatitis A antigen in relation to the number of lifetime sexual partners in patients attending an STD clinic. *Br J Vener Dis* 57:58, 1981.
55 Corey L, Holmes KK: Sexual transmission of hepatitis A in homosexual men: incidence and mechanism. *N Engl J Med* 302:435, 1980.
56 Ballesteros J et al: Are homosexual males a risk group for hepatitis A infection in intermediate endemicity areas? *Epidemiol Infect* 117: 145, 1996.
57 Hoybye G et al: An epidemic of acute viral hepatitis in male homosexuals: etiology and clinical characteristics. *Scand J Infect Dis* 12: 241, 1980.
58 Centers for Disease Control and Prevention: Hepatitis A among homosexual men—United States, Canada, and Australia. *MMWR* 41: 155, 1992.
59 Stewart T, Crofts N: An outbreak of hepatitis A among homosexual men in Melbourne. *Med J Aust* 158:519, 1993.
60 Leentvaar-Kuijpers A et al: An outbreak of hepatitis A among homosexual men in Amsterdam, 1991–1993. *Int J Epidemiol* 24:18, 1995.
61 Henning KJ et al: A community-wide outbreak of hepatitis A: risk factors for infection among homosexual and bisexual men. *Am J Med* 99:132, 1995.
62 Sundkvist T et al: Outbreak of acute hepatitis A among homosexual men in East London. *Scand J Infect Dis* 29:211, 1997.
62a Lemon SM: Type A viral hepatitis: new developments in an old disease. *N Engl J Med* 313:1059, 1985.
63 Szmuness W et al: Hepatitis B vaccine: demonstration of efficacy in a controlled clinical trial in a high-risk population in the United States. *N Engl J Med* 303:833, 1980.
64 Lednar WM, Lemon SM et al: Frequency of illness associated with epidemic hepatitis A virus infections in adults. *Am J Epidemiol* 122: 226, 1985.
65 Inoue K et al: Chronic hepatitis A with persistent viral replication. *J Med Virol* 50:322, 1996.
66 Vento S et al: Identification of hepatitis A virus as a trigger for autoimmune chronic hepatitis type 1 in susceptible individuals. *Lancet* 337:1183, 1991.
67 Gordon SC et al: Prolonged intrahepatic cholestasis secondary to acute hepatitis A. *Ann Intern Med* 101:635, 1984.
68 Glikson M et al: Relapsing hepatitis A. Review of 14 cases and literature survey. *Medicine (Baltimore)* 71:14, 1992.
69 Rakela J et al: Hepatitis A virus infection in fulminant hepatitis and chronic active hepatitis. *Gastroenterology* 74:879, 1978.
70 Decker RH et al: Diagnosis of acute hepatitis A by HAVAB®-M, a direct radioimmunoassay for IgM anti-HAV. *Am J Clin Path* 76:140, 1981.
71 Lemon SM et al: Specific immunoglobulin M response to hepatitis A virus determined by solid-phase radioimmunoassay. *Infect Immun* 28:927, 1980.
72 Winokur PL, Stapleton JT: Immunoglobulin prophylaxis for hepatitis A. *Clin Infect Dis* 14:580, 1992.
73 Lemon SM, Shapiro CN: The value of immunization against hepatitis A. *Infect Agents Dis* 3:38, 1994.
74 Advisory Committee on Immunization Practices: Prevention of hepatitis A through active or passive immunization. *MMWR* no RR-15, 1996.
75 Andre FE et al: Inactivated candidate vaccines for hepatitis A. *Prog Med Virol* 37:72, 1990.
76 Lewis JA et al: Use of a live attenuated hepatitis A vaccine to prepare a highly purified, formalin-inactivated hepatitis A vaccine. in *Viral Hepatitis and Liver Disease,* FB Hollinger et al (eds). Baltimore, Williams and Wilkins, 1991, p 94.
77 Lemon SM et al: The early antibody response to hepatitis A vaccine. *J Infect Dis* (in press), 1997.
78 Clemens R et al: Clinical experience with an inactivated hepatitis A vaccine. *J Infect Dis* 171 (Suppl 1):S44-S49, 1995.
79 SmithKline Beecham Pharmaceuticals: Hepatitis A vaccine, inactivated. Package insert, Havrix. Philadelphia, PA, 1995.
80 Werzberger A et al: A controlled trial of a formalin-inactivated hepatitis A vaccine in healthy children. *N Engl J Med* 327:453, 1992.
81 Innis BL et al: Protection against hepatitis A by an inactivated vaccine. *JAMA* 271:1328, 1994.
82 Purcell RH et al: Inactivated hepatitis A vaccine: active and passive immunoprophylaxis in chimpanzees. *Vaccine* 10 (Suppl 1):S148-S151, 1992.
83 Ganem D, Varmus HE: The molecular biology of the hepatitis B viruses. *Ann Rev Biochem* 56:651, 1987.
84 Lau J, Wright T: Molecular virology and pathogenesis of hepatitis B. *Lancet* 342:1335, 1993.
85 Summers J, Mason WS: Replication of the genome of a hepatitis B-like virus by reverse transcription of an RNA intermediate. *Cell* 29: 403, 1982.
86 Lin Y et al: Hepatitis B virus X protein is a transcriptional modulator that communicates with transcription factor IIB and the RNA polymerase II subunit 5. *J Biol Chem* 272:7132, 1997.
87 Doria M et al: The hepatitis B virus HBx protein is a dual specificity cytoplasmic activator of Ras and nuclear activator of transcription factors. *EMBO J* 14:4747, 1995
88 Dienstag JL et al: A preliminary trial of lamivudine for chronic hepatitis B infection. *N Engl J Med* 333:1657, 1995.
89 Robinson WS: DNA and DNA polymerase in the core of the Dane particle of hepatitis B. *Am J Med Sci.* 270:151, 1975.
90 Takahashi K et al: Demonstration of hepatitis B e antigen in the core of Dane particles. *J Immunol* 122:275, 1979.
91 Ou J-H et al: Hepatitis B virus gene function: the precore region targets the core antigen to cellular membranes and causes the secretion of the e antigen. *Proc Natl Acad Sci USA* 83:1578, 1986.
92 Milich DR et al: The hepatitis B virus core and e antigens elicit different Th cell subsets: Antigen structure can affect Th cell phenotype. *J Virol* 71:2192, 1997.
93 Hasegawa K et al: Association of hepatitis B viral precore mutations with fulminant hepatitis B in Japan. *Virology* 185:460,1991.
94 Naoumov NV et al: Precore mutant hepatitis B virus infection and liver disease. *Gastroenterology* 102:538, 1992.
95 Bahn A et al: Selection of a precore mutant after vertical transmission of different hepatitis B virus variants is correlated with fulminant hepatitis in infants. *J Med Virol* 47:336, 1995.
96 Liang TJ et al: Hepatitis B virus precore mutation and fulminant hepatitis in the United States. A polymerase chain reaction-based assay for the detection of specific mutation. *J Clin Invest* 93:550, 1994.
97 Bancroft WH et al: Detection of additional antigenic determinants of hepatitis B antigen. *J Immunol* 109:842, 1972.
98 Sureau C et al: Production of hepatitis B virus by a differentiated human hepatoma cell line after transfection with cloned circular HBV DNA. *Cell* 47:37, 1986.
99 Acs G et al: Hepatitis B virus produced by transfected HepG2 cells causes hepatitis in chimpanzees. *Proc Natl Acad Sci USA* 84:4641, 1987.
100 Tuttleman JS et al: Formation of the pool of covalently closed circular viral DNA in hepadnavirus-infected cells. *Cell* 47:451, 1986.
101 Korba BE et al: Hepadnavirus infection of peripheral blood lymphocytes in vivo: woodchuck and chimpanzee models of viral hepatitis. *J Virol* 58:1, 1986.
102 Krugman S et al: Viral hepatitis, type B: studies on natural history and prevention re-examined. *N Engl J Med* 300:101, 1979.
103 Lemon SM et al: IgM antibody to hepatitis B core antigen as a diagnostic parameter of acute infection with hepatitis B virus. *J Infect Dis* 143:803, 1981.
104 Gerlich WH et al: Diagnosis of acute and inapparent hepatitis B virus infections by measurement of IgM antibody to hepatitis B core antigen. *J Infect Dis* 142:95, 1980.
105 Rustgi VK et al: Hepatitis B virus infection in the acquired immunodeficiency syndrome. *Ann Intern Med* 101:795, 1984.
106 Hindman SH et al: "e" antigen, Dane particles, and serum DNA polymerase activity in HB_sAg carriers. *Ann Intern Med* 85:458, 1976.

107 Alter HJ et al: Type B hepatitis: the infectivity of blood positive for e antigen and DNA polymerase after accidental needlestick exposure. *N Engl J Med* 295:909, 1976.
108 Okada K et al: e antigen and anti-e in the serum of asymptomatic carrier mothers as indicators of positive and negative transmission of hepatitis B virus to their infants. *N Engl J Med* 294:746, 1976.
109 Tabor E et al: Coincident hepatitis B surface antigen and antibodies of different subtypes in human serum. *J Immunol* 118:369, 1977.
110 Hoofnagle et al: Seroconversion from hepatitis B e antigen to antibody in chronic type B hepatitis. *Ann Intern Med* 94:744, 1981.
111 Niederau C et al: Long-term follow-up of HBeAg-positive patients treated with interferon alfa for chronic hepatitis B. *N Engl J Med* 334:1422, 1996.
112 Chisari FV et al: Functional properties of lymphocyte subpopulations in hepatitis B virus infection. I. Suppressor cell control of T lymphocyte responsiveness. *J Immunol* 126:38, 1981.
113 Chisari FV et al: Functional properties of lymphocyte subpopulations in hepatitis B virus infection. II. Cytotoxic effector cell killing of targets that naturally express hepatitis B surface antigen and liver-specific lipoprotein. *J Immunol* 126:45, 1981.
114 Ferrari C et al: Identification of immunodominant T cell epitopes of the hepatitis B virus nucleocapsid antigen. *J Clin Invest* 88:214, 1991.
115 Rehermann B et al: Differential cytotoxic T-lymphocyte responsiveness to the hepatitis B and C viruses in chronically infected patients. *J Virol* 70:7092, 1996.
116 Tsui LV et al: Posttranscriptional clearance of hepatitis B virus RNA by cytotoxic T lymphocyte-activated hepatocytes. *Proc Natl Acad Sci USA* 92:12398, 1995.
117 Tokino T et al: Chromosome deletions associated with hepatitis B virus integration. *Virology* 185:879, 1991.
118 Penna A et al: Hepatitis B virus (HBV)-specific cytotoxic T-cell (CTL) response in humans: Characterization of HLA class II-restricted CTLs that recognize endogenously synthesized HBV envelope antigens. *J Virol* 66:1193, 1992.
119 Penna A et al: Long-lasting memory T cell responses following self-limited acute hepatitis B. *J Clin Invest* 98:1185, 1996.
120 Rehermann B et al: The hepatitis B virus persists for decades after patients' recovery from acute viral hepatitis despite active maintenance of a cytotoxic T-lymphocyte response. *Nature Med* 2:1104, 1996.
121 Beasley RP et al: Hepatocellular carcinoma and hepatitis B virus: a prospective study of 22,707 men in Taiwan. *Lancet* ii:1129, 1981.
122 Ikegami H et al: An age-related change in susceptibility of rat brain to encephalomyocarditis virus infection. *Int J Exp Pathol* 78:101, 1997.
123 Rogler CE et al: Deletion in chromosome 11p associated with a hepatitis B integration site in hepatocellular carcinoma. *Science* 230:319, 1985.
124 Hino O et al: Hepatitis B virus integration site in hepatocellular carcinoma at chromosome 17;18 translocation. *Proc Natl Acad Sci USA* 83:8338, 1986.
125 Wang J et al: Hepatitis B virus integration in a cyclin A gene in a hepatocellular carcinoma. *Nature* 343:555, 1990.
126 Scorsone KA et al: *p53* Mutations cluster at codon 249 in hepatitis B virus-positive hepatocellular carcinomas from China. *Cancer Res* 52:1635, 1992.
127 Hsia CC et al: RB tumor suppressor gene expression in hepatocellular carcinomas from patients infected with the hepatitis B virus. *J Med Virol* 44:67, 1994.
128 Slagle BL: p53 mutations and hepatitis B virus: Cofactors in hepatocellular carcinoma. *Hepatology* 21:597, 1995.
129 Feitelson MA, Duan LX: Hepatitis B virus x antigen in the pathogenesis of chronic infections and the development of hepatocellular carcinoma. *Am J Pathol* 150:1141, 1997.
130 Kew MC: Increasing evidence that hepatitis B virus x gene protein and p53 protein may interact in the pathogenesis of hepatocellular carcinoma. *Hepatology* 25:1037, 1997.
131 Lee CL, Ko YC: Hepatitis B vaccination and hepatocellular carcinoma in Taiwan. *Pediatrics* 99:351, 1997.
132 Carmen WF et al: Vaccine-induced escape mutant of hepatitis B virus. *Lancet* 326:325, 1990.
133 Waters JA et al: Loss of the common "A" determinant of hepatitis B surface antigen by a vaccine-induced escape mutant. *J Clin Invest* 90: 2543, 1992.
134 Beasley RP et al: The e antigen and vertical transmission of hepatitis B surface antigen. *Am J Epidemiol* 105, 94, 1977.
135 Stevens CE et al: Vertical transmission of hepatitis B antigen in Taiwan. *N Engl J Med* 292:771, 1975.
136 Macaya G et al: Dane particles and associated DNA-polymerase activity in the saliva of chronic hepatitis B carriers. *J Med Virol* 4:291, 1979.
137 Jenison SA et al: Quantitative analysis of hepatitis B virus DNA in saliva and semen of chronically infected homosexual men. *J Infect Dis* 156:299, 1987.
138 Davison F et al: Detection of hepatitis B virus DNA in spermatozoa, urine, saliva, and leucocytes of chronic HBsAg carriers: a lack of relationship with serum markers of replication. *J Hepatol* 4:37, 1987.
139 Perrillo RP et al: Hepatitis B e antigen, DNA polymerase activity, and infection of household contacts with hepatitis B virus. *Gastroenterology* 76:1319, 1979.
140 Davis LG et al: Horizontal transmission of hepatitis B virus. *Lancet* i:889, 1989.
141 Krugman S et al: Infectious hepatitis: evidence for two distinctive clinical, epidemiological, and immunological types of infection. *JAMA* 200:365, 1967.
142 Scott RM et al: Experimental transmission of hepatitis B virus by semen and saliva. *J Infect Dis* 142:67, 1980.
143 Alter HJ, Purcell RH et al: Transmission of hepatitis B to chimpanzees by hepatitis B surface antigen-positive saliva and semen. *Infect Immun* 16:928, 1977.
144 Szmuness W et al: On the role of sexual behavior in the spread of hepatitis B infection. *Ann Intern Med* 83:489, 1975.
145 Schreeder MT et al: Hepatitis B in homosexual males: prevalence of HBV infection and factors related to its transmission. *J Infect Dis* 146:7, 1982.
146 Alter MJ et al: Hepatitis B virus transmission between heterosexuals. *JAMA* 256:1307, 1986.
147 Alter MJ et al: The changing epidemiology of hepatitis B in the United States. Need for alternative immunization strategies. *JAMA* 263: 1218, 1990.
148 Szmuness W: Large-scale efficacy trials of hepatitis B vaccines in the USA: baseline data and protocols. *J Med Virol* 4:327, 1979.
149 Gust ID et al: A seroepidemiologic study of infection with HAV and HBV in five Pacific islands. *Am J Epidemiol* 110:237, 1979.
150 Dienstag JL, Ryan DM: Occupational exposure to hepatitis B virus in hospital personnel: infection or immunization? *Am J Epidemiol* 115:26, 1982.
151 Hersh T et al: Nonparenteral transmission of viral hepatitis B (Australia antigen-associated hepatitis). *N Engl J Med* 285:1363, 1971.
152 Hentzer B et al: Viral hepatitis in a venereal clinic population. *Scand J Infect Dis* 12:245, 1980.
153 Frosner GG et al: Prevalence of hepatitis B antibody in prostitutes. *Am J Epidemiol* 102:241, 1975.
154 Orduna A et al: Infection by hepatitis B and C virus in non-intravenous drug using female prostitutes in Spain. *Eur J Epidemiol* 8:656, 1992.
155 Dietzman DE et al: Hepatitis B surface antigen (HB_sAg) and antibody to HB_sAg: prevalence in homosexual and heterosexual men. *JAMA* 238:2625, 1977.
156 Lim KS et al: Role of sexual and non-sexual practices in the transmission of hepatitis B. *Br J Vener Dis* 53:190, 1977.
157 Kingsley LA et al: Sexual transmission efficiency of hepatitis B virus and human immunodeficiency virus among homosexual men. *JAMA* 264:230, 1990.
158 Judson FN et al: Screening for gonorrhea and syphilis in the gay baths—Denver, Colorado. *Am J Public Health* 67:740, 1977.
159 Siegel D et al: Hepatitis B virus infection in high-risk inner-city neighborhoods in San Francisco. *Hepatology* 22:44, 1995.

160 Szmuness W et al: A controlled clinical trial of the efficacy of the hepatitis B vaccine (Heptavax B): a final report. *Hepatology* 1:377, 1981.
161 Reiner NE et al: Asymptomatic rectal mucosal lesions and hepatitis B surface antigen at sites of sexual contact in homosexual men with persistent hepatitis B virus infection. *Ann Intern Med* 96:170, 1982.
162 Murphy BL et al: Serological testing for hepatitis B in male homosexuals: special emphasis on hepatitis B e antigen and antibody by radioimmunoassay. *J Clin Microbiol* 11:301, 1980
163 Szmuness W et al: Prevalence of hepatitis B "e" antigen and its antibody in various HBsAg carrier populations. *Am J Epidemiol* 113: 113, 1981.
164 Tedder RS et al: Contrasting patterns and frequency of antibodies to the surface, core, and e antigens of hepatitis B virus in blood donors and in homosexual patients. *J Med Virol* 6:323, 1980.
165 Mai AL et al: The interaction of human immunodeficiency virus infection and hepatitis B virus infection in infected homosexual men. *J Clin Gastroenterol* 22:299, 1996.
166 Gilson RJC et al: Interactions between HIV and hepatitis B virus in homosexual men: effects on the natural history of infection. *AIDS* 11:597, 1997.
167 Bodsworth N et al: The effect of concurrent human immunodeficiency virus infection on chronic hepatitis B: a study of 150 homosexual men. *J Infect Dis* 160:577, 1989.
168 Mosley JW: The epidemiology of viral hepatitis: an overview. *Am J Med Sci* 270:253, 1975.
169 Koff RS et al: Contagiousness of acute hepatitis B: Secondary attack rates in household contacts. *Gastroenterology* 72:297, 1977.
170 Tassopoulos NC et al: Detection of hepatitis B virus DNA in asymptomatic hepatitis B surface antigen carriers: relation to sexual transmission. *Am J Epidemiol* 126:587, 1987.
171 Centers for Disease Control and Prevention: Lack of transmission of hepatitis B to humans after oral exposure to hepatitis B surface antigen-positive saliva. *MMWR* 27:247, 1978.
172 Glaser JB, Nadler JP: Hepatitis B virus in a cardiopulmonary resuscitation training course. Risk of transmission from a surface antigen-positive participant. *Arch Intern Med* 145:1653, 1985.
173 Lemon SM, Ping L-H: Antigenic structure of hepatitis A virus, in *Molecular Aspects of Picornavirus Infection and Detection*, B Semler, E Ehrenfeld (eds). Washington, American Society for Microbiology, 1998, p 193.
174 Hou M-C et al: Heterosexual transmission as the most common route of acute hepatitis B virus infection among adults in Taiwan—the importance of extending vaccination to susceptible adults. *J Infect Dis* 167:938, 1993.
175 Baddour LM et al: Risk factors for hepatitis B virus infection in black female attendees of a sexually transmitted disease clinic. *Sex Transm Dis* 15:174, 1988.
176 Rosenblum LS et al: Heterosexual transmission of hepatitis B virus in Belle Glade, Florida. Belle Glade Study Group. *J Infect Dis* 161: 407, 1990.
177 Corona R et al: Risk factors for hepatitis B virus infection among heterosexuals attending a sexually transmitted diseases clinic in Italy: role of genital ulcerative diseases. *J Med Virol* 48:262, 1996.
178 Jacobs B et al: Sexual transmission of hepatitis B in Mwanza, Tanzania. *Sex Transm Dis* 24:121, 1997.
179 Thomas DL et al: Hepatitis C, hepatitis B, and human immunodeficiency virus infections among non-intravenous drug-using patients attending clinics for sexually transmitted diseases. *J Infect Dis* 169: 990, 1994.
180 Kvinesdal BB et al: Risk factors for hepatitis B virus infection in heterosexuals attending a venereal disease clinic in Copenhagen. *Scand J Infect Dis* 25:171, 1993.
181 Mathiesen LR et al: Hepatitis type A, B, and non-A non-B in fulminant hepatitis. *Gut* 21:72, 1980.
182 Sterneck M et al: Hepatitis B virus genomes of patients with fulminant hepatitis do not share a specific mutation. *Hepatology* 24:300, 1996.
183 Sergent JS: Extrahepatic manifestations of hepatitis B infection. *Bull Rheum Dis* 33:1, 1983.
184 Duffy J et al: Polyarthritis, polyarteritis and hepatitis B. *Medicine* 55: 19, 1976.
185 Redeker AG: Viral hepatitis: clinical aspects. *Am J Med Sci* 270:9, 1975.
186 Seeff LB et al: A serologic follow-up of the 1942 epidemic of post-vaccination hepatitis in the United States Army. *N Engl J Med* 316: 965, 1987.
187 Lam KC et al: Deleterious effect of prednisolone in HBsAg-positive chronic active hepatitis. *N Engl J Med* 304:380, 1981.
188 Sergent JS et al: Vasculitis with hepatitis B antigenemia: long-term observations in nine patients. *Medicine* 55:1, 1976.
189 Guillevin L et al: Treatment of polyarteritis nodosa related to hepatitis B virus with short term steroid therapy associated with antiviral agents and plasma exchanges. A prospective trial in 33 patients. *J Rheumatol* 20:289, 1993.
190 Darras-Joly C et al: Regressing microaneurysms in 5 cases of hepatitis B virus related polyarteritis nodosa. *J Rheumatol* 22:876, 1995.
191 Conjeevaram HS et al: Long-term outcome of hepatitis B virus-related glomerulonephritis after therapy with interferon alfa. *Gastroenterology* 109:540, 1995.
192 Levo Y et al: Association between hepatitis B virus and essential mixed cryoglobulinemia. *N Engl J Med* 296:1501, 1977.
193 Misiani R et al: Hepatitis C virus infection in patients with essential mixed cryoglobulinemia. *Ann Intern Med* 117:573, 1992.
194 Agnello V et al: A role for hepatitis C virus infection in type II cryoglobulinemia. *N Engl J Med* 327:1490, 1992.
195 Sjogren MH et al: Clinical significance of low molecular weight (7–8S) immunoglobulin M antibody to hepatitis B core antigen in chronic hepatitis B virus infections. *Gastroenterology* 91:168, 1986.
196 Francis DP et al: The prevention of hepatitis B with vaccine: report of the Centers for Disease Control multi-center efficacy trial among homosexual men. *Ann Intern Med* 97:362, 1982.
197 Szmuness W et al: Hepatitis B vaccine in medical staff of hemodialysis units: efficacy and subtype cross-protection. *N Engl J Med* 307:1481, 1982.
198 Stevens CE et al: Yeast-recombinant hepatitis B vaccine: efficacy with hepatitis B immune globulin in prevention of perinatal hepatitis B virus transmission. *JAMA* 257:2612, 1987.
199 Marion SA et al: Long-term follow-up of hepatitis B vaccine in infants of carrier mothers. *Am J Epidemiol* 140:734, 1994.
200 Xu ZY et al: Long-term efficacy of active postexposure immunization of infants for prevention of hepatitis B virus infection. *J Infect Dis* 171:54, 1995.
201 Centers for Disease Control and Prevention: The hepatitis B virus: a comprehensive strategy for eliminating transmission in the United States through universal childhood vaccination. *MMWR* 40:1, 1991.
202 Merck and Company: Package insert, Recombivax HB. West Point, PA, Inc, 1995.
203 SmithKline Beecham Pharmaceuticals: Package insert, Engerix-B. Philadelphia, PA 1994.
204 Hadler SC, Margolis HS: Hepatitis B immunization: vaccine types, efficacy, and indications for immunization, in *Current Clinical Topics in Infectious Diseases*, JS Remington, MN Swartz. Boston, Blackwell Scientific Publications, 1992, p 282.
205 Stratton KR et al: Adverse events associated with childhood vaccines other than pertussis and rubella: summary of a report from the Institute of Medicine. *JAMA* 271:1602, 1994.
206 Jilg W et al: Vaccination against hepatitis B: comparison of three different vaccination schedules. *J Infect Dis* 160:766, 1989.
207 Hadler SC et al: Effect of timing of hepatitis B vaccine doses on response to vaccine in Yucpa Indians. *Vaccine* 7:106, 1989.
208 Rizzetto M et al: The hepatitis B virus-associated d antigen: isolation from liver, development of solid-phase radioimmunoassays for d antigen and anti-d and partial characterization of d antigen. *J Immunol* 125:318, 1980.
209 Rizzetto M et al: d agent: association of d antigen with hepatitis B

surface antigen and RNA in serum of d-infected chimpanzees. *Proc Natl Acad Sci USA* 77, 6124. 1980.

210 Wang K-S et al: Structure, sequence and expression of the hepatitis delta (d) viral genome. *Nature* 323:508, 1986.

211 Chang M-F et al: Human hepatitis delta antigen is a nuclear phosphoprotein with RNA-binding activity. *J Virol* 62:2403, 1988.

212 Wang J, Lemon SM: Hepatitis delta virus antigen forms dimers and multimeric complexes in vivo. *J Virol* 67:446, 1993.

213 De Cock KM et al: Delta hepatitis in the Los Angeles area: a report of 126 cases. *Ann Intern Med* 105:108, 1986.

214 De Cock KM et al: Hepatitis B virus DNA in fulminant hepatitis B. *Ann Intern Med* 105:546, 1986.

215 Rizzetto M et al: Epidemiology of HBV-associated delta agent: geographical distribution of anti-delta and prevalence in polytransfused HBsAg carriers. *Lancet* i:1215, 1980.

216 Rosenblum L et al: Sexual practices in the transmission of hepatitis B virus and prevalence of hepatitis delta virus infection in female prostitutes in the United States. *JAMA* 267:2477, 1992.

217 Hadler SC et al: Delta virus infection and severe hepatitis: an epidemic in the Yucpa Indians of Venezuela. *Ann Intern Med* 100:339, 1984.

218 Solomon RE et al: Human immunodeficiency virus and hepatitis delta virus in homosexual men: a study of four cohorts. *Ann Intern Med* 108:51, 1988.

219 Weisfuse IB et al: Delta hepatitis in homosexual men in the United States. *Hepatology* 9:872, 1989.

220 Bodsworth NJ et al: Hepatitis delta virus in homosexual men in Sydney. *Genitourin Med* 65:235, 1989.

221 Choo Q-L et al: Isolation of a cDNA clone derived from a blood-borne non-A, non-B viral hepatitis genome. *Science* 244:359, 1989.

222 Kuo G et al: An assay for circulating antibodies to a major etiologic virus of human non-A, non-B hepatitis. *Science* 244:362, 1989.

223 Jeffers LJ et al: Prevalence of antibodies to hepatitis C virus among patients with cryptogenic chronic hepatitis and cirrhosis. *Hepatology* 15:187, 1992.

224 Saito I et al: Hepatitis C virus infection is associated with the development of hepatocellular carcinoma. *Proc Natl Acad Sci USA* 87: 6547, 1991.

225 Daikos GL et al: Hepatitis C virus infection in a sexually active inner city population. The potential for heterosexual transmission. *Infection* 22:72, 1994.

226 Ndimbie OK et al: Hepatitis C virus infection in a male homosexual cohort: risk factor analysis. *Genitourin Med* 72:213, 1996.

227 Osmond DH et al: Comparison of risk factors for hepatitis C and hepatitis B virus infection in homosexual men. *J Infect Dis* 167:66, 1993.

228 Bodsworth NJ et al: Hepatitis C virus infection in a large cohort of homosexually active men: independent association with HIV-1 infection and injecting drug use but not sexual behaviour. *Genitourin Med* 72:118, 1996.

229 Buchbinder SP et al: Hepatitis C virus infection in sexually active homosexual men. *J Infect* 29:263, 1994.

230 Weinstock HS et al: Hepatitis C virus infection among patients attending a clinic for sexually transmitted diseases. *JAMA* 269:392, 1993.

231 Fiscus SA et al: Hepatitis C virus seroprevalence in clients of sexually transmitted disease clinics in North Carolina. *Sex Transm Dis* 21: 155, 1994.

232 Houghton M et al: Molecular biology of the hepatitis C viruses: Implications for diagnosis, development and control of viral disease. *Hepatology* 14:381, 1991.

233 Major ME, Feinstone SM: The molecular virology of hepatitis C. *Hepatology* 25:1527, 1997.

234 Lemon SM, Honda M: Internal ribosome entry sites within the RNA genomes of hepatitis C virus and other flaviviruses. *Semin Virol* (in press). 1997.

235 Hijikata M et al: Gene mapping of the putative structural region of the hepatitis C virus genome by in vitro processing analysis. *Proc Natl Acad Sci USA* 88:5547, 1991.

236 Hijikata M et al: Two distinct proteinase activities required for the processing of a putative nonstructural precursor protein of hepatitis C virus. *J Virol* 67:4665, 1993.

237 Reed KE et al: Hepatitis C virus-encoded NS2–3 protease: Cleavage-site mutagenesis and requirements for bimolecular cleavage. *J Virol* 69:127, 1995.

238 Dubuisson J et al: Formation and intracellular localization of hepatitis C virus envelope glycoprotein complexes expressed by recombinant vaccinia and Sindbis viruses. *J Virol* 68:6147, 1994.

239 Dubuisson J, Rice CM: Hepatitis C virus glycoprotein folding: disulfide bond formation and association with calnexin. *J Virol* 70:778, 1996.

240 Kato N et al: Humoral immune response to hypervariable region 1 of the putative envelope glycoprotein (gp70) of hepatitis C virus. *J Virol* 67:923, 1993.

241 Lesniewski RR et al: Hypervariable 5′-terminus of hepatitis C virus E2/NS1 encodes antigenically distinct variants. *J Med Virol* 40:150, 1993.

242 Pal-Ghosh R, Morrow CD: A poliovirus minireplicon containing an inactive 2A proteinase is expressed in vaccinia virus-infected cells. *J Virol* 67:4621, 1993.

243 Kim JL et al: Crystal structure of the hepatitis C virus NS3 protease domain complexed with a synthetic NS4A cofactor peptide. *Cell* 87: 343, 1996.

244 Yao NH et al: Structure of the hepatitis C virus RNA helicase domain. *Nature Struct Biol* 4:463, 1997.

245 Lin C et al: A central region in the hepatitis C virus NS4A protein allows formation of an active NS3-NS4A serine proteinase complex in vivo and in vitro. *J Virol* 69:4373, 1995.

246 Behrens SE et al: Identification and properties of the RNA-dependent RNA polymerase of hepatitis C virus. *EMBO J* 15:12, 1996.

247 Lanford RE et al: Lack of detection of negative-strand hepatitis C virus RNA in peripheral blood mononuclear cells and other extrahepatic tissues by the highly strand-specific rTth reverse transcriptase PCR. *J Virol* 69:8079, 1995.

248 Shimizu YK et al: Evidence for in vitro replication of hepatitis C virus genome in a human T-cell line. *Proc Natl Acad Sci USA* 89:5477, 1992.

249 Shimizu YK, Yoshikura H: Multicycle infection of hepatitis C virus in cell culture and inhibition by alpha and beta interferons. *J Virol* 68:8406, 1994.

250 Kolykhalov AA et al: Transmission of hepatitis C by intrahepatic inoculation with transcribed RNA. *Science* 277:570, 1997.

251 Yanagi M et al: Transcripts from a single full-length cDNA clone of hepatitis C virus are infectious when directly transfected into liver of a chimpanzee. *Proc Natl Acad Sci USA* 97:8738, 1997.

252 Simmonds P et al: A proposed system for the nomenclature of hepatitis C viral genotypes. *Hepatology* 19:1321, 1994.

253 Farci P et al: Lack of protective immunity against reinfection with hepatitis C virus. *Science* 258:135, 1992.

254 Lerat H et al: Specific detection of hepatitis C virus minus strand RNA in hematopoietic cells. *J Clin Invest* 97:845, 1996.

255 Feinstone SM et al: Transfusion-associated hepatitis not due to viral hepatitis type A or B. *N Engl J Med* 292:767, 1975.

256 Missale G et al: Different clinical behaviors of acute hepatitis C virus infection are associated with different vigor of the anti-viral cell-mediated immune response. *J Clin Invest* 98:706, 1996.

257 Kage M et al: Long-term evolution of fibrosis from chronic hepatitis to cirrhosis in patients with hepatitis C: Morphometric analysis of repeated biopsies. *Hepatology* 25:1028, 1997.

258 Seeff LB et al: Long-term mortality after transfusion-associated non-A, non-B hepatitis. *N Engl J Med* 327:1906, 1992.

259 Romeo R et al: Lack of association between type of hepatitis C virus, serum load, and severity of liver disease. *J Hepatol* 3:183, 1996.

260 Takase S et al: The alcohol-altered liver membrane antibody and hepatitis C virus infection in the progression of alcoholic liver disease. *Hepatology* 17:9, 1993.

261 Oshita M et al: Increased serum hepatitis C virus RNA levels among alcoholic patients with chronic hepatitis C. *Hepatology* 20:1115, 1994.

262 Alemy-Carreau M et al: Lack of interaction between hepatitis C virus and alcohol in the pathogenesis of cirrhosis. A statistical study. *J Hepatol* 25:627, 1996.
263 Koziel MJ et al: Intrahepatic cytotoxic T lymphocytes specific for hepatitis C virus in persons with chronic hepatitis. *J Immunol* 149: 3339, 1992.
264 Rehermann B et al: Quantitative analysis of the peripheral blood cytotoxic T lymphocyte response in patients with chronic hepatitis C virus infection. *J Clin Invest* 98:1432, 1996.
265 Koziel MJ et al: Hepatitis C virus (HCV)-specific cytotoxic T lymphocytes recognize epitopes in the core and envelope proteins of HCV. *J Virol* 67:7522, 1993.
266 Seeff LB: Natural history of hepatitis C. *Hepatology* 26:21S, 1997.
267 National Institutes of Health: NIH Consensus Development Conference Panel statement: management of hepatitis C. *Hepatology* 26 (Suppl 1):2S, 1997.
268 Johnson RJ et al: Membranoproliferative glomerulonephritis associated with hepatitis C virus infection. *N Engl J Med* 328:465, 1993.
269 Marcellin P et al: Cryoglobulinemia with vasculitis associated with hepatitis C virus infection. *Gastroenterology* 104:72, 1993.
270 Bresters D et al: Enhanced sensitivity of a second generation ELISA for antibody to hepatitis C virus. *Vox Sang* 62:213, 1992.
271 Silva AE et al: Diagnosis of chronic hepatitis C: Comparison of immunoassays and the polymerase chain reaction. *Am J Gastroenterol* 89:493, 1994.
272 Lesniewski R et al: Antibody to hepatitis C virus second envelope (HCV-E2) glycoprotein: A new marker of HCV infection closely associated with viremia. *J Med Virol* 45:415, 1995.
273 Garson JA: The polymerase chain reaction and hepatitis C virus diagnosis. *FEMS Microbiol Rev* 14:229, 1994.
274 Bresters D et al: Comparison of quantitative cDNA-PCR with the branched DNA hybridization assay for monitoring plasma hepatitis C virus RNA levels in haemophilia patients participating in a controlled interferon trial. *J Med Virol* 43:262, 1994.
275 Nomura H et al: Usefulness of HCV-RNA assays in efficacy evaluation of interferon treatment for chronic hepatitis C: Amplicor(TM) HCV assay and branched DNA probe assay. *J Infect* 34:249, 1997.
276 Reinus JF et al: Failure to detect vertical transmission of hepatitis C virus. *Ann Intern Med* 117:881, 1992.
277 Wejstål R et al: Mother-to-infant transmission of hepatitis C virus. *Ann Intern Med* 117:887, 1992.
278 Wu JC et al: Prevalence, infectivity, and risk factor analysis of hepatitis C virus infection in prostitutes. *J Med Virol* 39:312, 1993.
279 Nakashima K et al: Sexual transmisssion of hepatitis C virus among female prostitutes and patients with sexually transmitted diseases in Fukuoka, Kyushu, Japan. *Am J Epidemiol* 136:1132, 1992.
280 Watts DM et al: Low risk of sexual transmission of hepatitis C virus in Somalia. *Trans R Soc Trop Med Hyg* 88:55, 1994.
281 Everhart JE et al: Risk for non-A, non-B (type C) hepatitis through sexual or household contacts with chronic carriers. *Ann Intern Med* 112:544, 1990.
282 Osmond DH et al: Risk factors for hepatitis C virus seropositivity in heterosexual couples. *JAMA* 269:361, 1993.
283 Hallam NF et al: Low risk of sexual transmission of hepatitis C virus. *J Med Virol* 40:251, 1993.
284 Eyster ME et al: Heterosexual co-transmission of hepatitis C virus (HCV) and human immunodeficiency virus (HIV). *Ann Intern Med* 115:764, 1991.
285 Setoguchi Y et al: Analysis of nucleotide sequences of hepatitis C virus isolates from husband-wife pairs. *J Gastroenterol Hepatol* 9:468, 1994.
286 Gordon SC et al: Lack of evidence for heterosexual transmission of hepatitis C. *Am J Gastroenterol* 87:1849, 1992.
287 Thomas DL et al: Sexual transmission of hepatitis C virus among patients attending sexually transmitted diseases clinics in Baltimore—An analysis of 309 sex partnerships. *J Infect Dis* 171:768, 1995.
288 Lissen E et al: Hepatitis C virus infection among sexually promiscuous groups and the heterosexual partners of hepatitis C virus infected index cases. *Eur J Clin Microbiol Infect Dis* 12:827, 1993.
289 Kao JH et al: Intrafamilial transmission of hepatitis C virus: the important role of infections between spouses. *J Infect Dis* 166:900, 1992.
290 Diago M et al: Intrafamily transmission of hepatitis C virus: sexual and non- sexual contacts. *J Hepatol* 25:125, 1996.
291 García-Bengoechea M et al: Intrafamilial spread of hepatitis C virus infection. *Scand J Infect Dis* 26:15, 1994.
292 Shev S et al: Risk factor exposure among hepatitis C virus RNA positive Swedish blood donors—the role of parenteral and sexual transmission. *Scand J Infect Dis* 27:99, 1995.
293 Mannucci PM, Colombo M: Virucidal treatment of clotting factor concentrates. *Lancet* ii:782, 1988.
294 Alter MJ et al: Hepatitis C. *Infect Dis Clin North Am* 12:13, 1998.
295 Choo Q-L et al: Vaccination of chimpanzees against infection by the hepatitis C virus. *Proc Natl Acad Sci USA* 91:1294, 1994.
296 Knodell RG et al: Development of chronic liver disease after acute non-A, non-B post-transfusion hepatitis: role of [gamma]-globulin prophylaxis in its prevention. *Gastroenterology* 72:902, 1977.
297 Krawczynski K et al: Effect of immune globulin on the prevention of experimental hepatitis C virus infection. *J Infect Dis* 173:822, 1996.
298 Simons JN et al: Isolation of novel virus-like sequences associated with human hepatitis. *Nature Med* 1:564, 1995.
299 Linnen J et al: Molecular cloning and disease association of hepatitis G virus: a transfusion-transmissible agent. *Science* 271:505, 1996.
300 Alter MJ et al: Acute non-A-E hepatitis in the United States and the role of hepatitis G virus infection. *N Engl J Med* 336:741, 1997.

Chapter 27
Molluscum contagiosum

John Munroe Douglas, Jr.

DEFINITION AND HISTORY

Molluscum contagiosum is a benign papular condition of the skin which is often sexually transmitted in adults. It is caused by the molluscum contagiosum virus (MCV), a member of the poxvirus family. Its characteristic appearance was first described in 1817 by Bateman, who labeled the disorder "molluscum," a common term then for pedunculated lesions, and described it as "contagiosum" to signify its apparent transmissibility, which he felt was due to the "milky fluid" which could be expressed from the lesions.[1–3] In 1841, Henderson and Paterson each described in this fluid cellular elements with large intracytoplasmic inclusion bodies (subsequently termed Henderson-Paterson, or molluscum, bodies), which they felt were responsible for causation and transmission of the disease.[1–3] Subsequent reports of transmission of infection to humans by direct inoculation of lesion material supported an infectious etiology. The findings of tiny "elementary bodies" within the molluscum bodies by Lipschutz in 1911, and of disease transmission by a "filterable agent" by Juliusberg in 1905 and Wile and Kingery in 1919, suggested a viral agent.[1–3] In 1933 Goodpasture demonstrated a marked similarity between the cellular inclusions and elementary bodies of molluscum contagiosum, fowl pox, and vaccinia and concluded that these infectious agents all belonged to the same family of viruses.[3,4] Historically considered a minor clinical problem, over the past decade molluscum contagiosum has become a common and often severe condition in patients with HIV infection.[5–7]

BIOLOGY

Although never convincingly replicated in cultured cells, MCV has been purified from skin lesions and is considered to be a poxvirus on the basis of size, structure, chemical composition, and physical and genomic characteristics.[3,8,9,9a] Previously unclassified, MCV has recently been designated as a new poxvirus genus, molluscipoxvirus.[10] Ultrastructural studies of MCV reveal a particle much like vaccinia virus, with which it has been most extensively compared: brick-shaped, approximately 300 × 220 × 100 nm in volume, with a biconcave viral core enclosed by an inner membrane and an outer envelope.[3,9,11] The viral genome consists of a single molecule of linear double-stranded DNA 180–200 kilobases long; like the DNA of other poxviruses, it has terminal regions with intrastrand covalent links, inverted repeats, and blocks of tandem direct repetitions.[8,9] The genetic organization of MCV appears to be similar to that of vaccinia virus, and there is a high degree of homology, although not antigenic cross-reactivity, between their major envelope proteins.[9,9a,12]

Attempts at experimental cultivation of MCV have been frustrating and have limited the study of its life cycle. With one recent exception,[12a] infection has not been transmitted to laboratory animals, and even human transmission studies are only variably successful.[2,3,8] The virus cannot be grown in cell culture, a situation parallel to that of human papillomavirus (HPV), presumably because of the need for highly differentiated keratinocytes, which cannot be maintained in vitro. Virus derived from lesions will, however, cause functional changes in a variety of cell lines, inducing interferon production and induction of a characteristic cytopathic effect (CPE) with rounding of cells.[2,3,9,13] Ultrastructural studies indicate that virus particles penetrate the cell by phagocytosis, undergo envelope uncoating, and progress to the stage of free virus cores; however, the subsequent step, second-stage uncoating of the inner membrane to release viral DNA into the cytoplasm, fails to occur in cell culture, thus blocking completion of the replication cycle.[3,13]

The inability to propagate virus in cultured cells has also limited characterization of MCV subtypes. Recently, however, DNA restriction endonuclease techniques have identified two subtypes, MCV-1 and MCV-2, with evidence also of subtype variants and of a possible third subtype.[9,14–18] MCV-1 and MCV-2 are closely related in nucleotide sequence and genome organization; however their restriction maps differ substantially, in contrast to the restriction-site conservation seen with other poxviruses.[9] Furthermore, minor subtype variants have been described, which result from variations in length of terminal restriction fragments and from changes in restriction sites.[9,15,16]

EPIDEMIOLOGY

Characterization of the epidemiology of molluscum contagiosum has been limited by several factors. In most patients the lesions cause few problems and are self-limited.[1,2,19–22] Thus, it is likely that many infected patients do not seek medical attention, and there are few population-based data concerning those who do, since molluscum contagiosum is not a reportable disease. Furthermore, the inability to cultivate MCV in cell culture has restricted studies of virus transmission, asymptomatic infection, and seroprevalence and has forced epidemiologic studies to rely on detection of characteristic lesions by physical examination.[2]

MCV appears to be spread by both sexual and nonsexual routes of transmission, with transmission enhanced by warmth and humidity.[1–3,19–24] The suspicion that genital molluscum contagiosum is sexually transmitted is supported by indirect evidence, including lesion location, a frequent history of contact with multiple sexual partners and prostitutes, the history and presence of other STDs, the presence of genital lesions in sexual partners, and peak ages of occurrence (20 to 29 years) which are similar to those of other STDs.[2,19–21,25–28] There is no information about the efficiency of sexual transmission of MCV. The nonsexual form of the disease occurs primarily in children. It involves the face, trunk, and upper extremities and appears to be transmitted by direct contact with the skin of infected individuals and/or fomites.[1–3,22–24] Several studies have associated molluscum contagiosum with baths, swimming, or the use of gymnastic equipment and towels.[1–3,22,24]

Data on rates of genital molluscum contagiosum are limited. Summary data from the STD clinic system of the United Kingdom, published until 1986, documented a quadrupling of cases in England from the early 1970s through the mid 1980s, when approximately 3 cases per 100,000 population were reported.[25] This increase paralleled that for cases of genital herpes and warts, which were 7 and 25 times more common, respectively.[29] In the United States, a survey among private physicians from 1966 to 1983 demonstrated a similar trend, with an 11-fold increase in visits by adults for molluscum contagiosum.[26] Published data since the mid-1980s has largely focused on the increased rates of infection in patients with AIDS, 5 to 18 percent of whom are diagnosed with molluscum contagiosum.[30–33] Rates of nonsexual molluscum contagiosum are estimated from patients identified in dermatology clinics and in population-based surveys, mostly children with extragenital lesions.[1,2,22–24,34] While uncommon in North America and Europe, accounting for only 0.1 to 1.2 percent of patients attending dermatology clinics,[1,22] infection was noted during community surveys among villagers in Fiji and New Guinea in 4.5 percent and 7 percent of the population, respectively.[22,23] Most cases were in children, and in surveys restricted to children in Fiji, New Guinea, and Japan prevalence rates have ranged from 6 to 22 percent.[22–24]

Molecular epidemiologic studies indicate that MCV-1 occurs more commonly than MCV-2, although there is substantial geographic variability.[7,9,17,18] There is no association between subtype and anatomic site, as there is with HPV and with herpes simplex virus (HSV), or between subtype and lesion morphology. However, MCV-2 appears to occur more frequently in adults than in children, especially in those who are HIV-infected.[9,17] Although mixed infections with both MCV-1 and MCV-2 and with subtype variants have been described, they are uncommon, and studies of family members with molluscum contagiosum and of multiple lesions from the same patient usually reveal identical subtypes.[18] Seroepidemiologic studies of MCV are limited in number and difficult to compare because of varying techniques and lack of adequate controls.[2,3,23,35–37] Current assays do not distinguish between antibodies to MCV-1 and to MCV-2.[37]

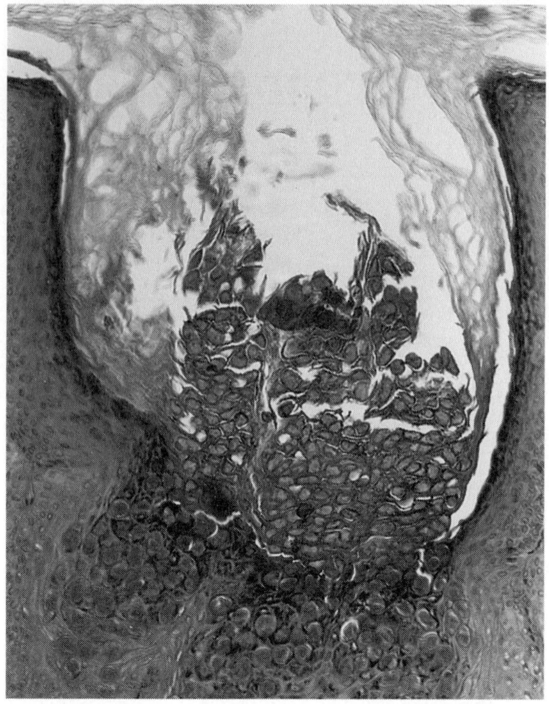

Fig. 27-1. Biopsy of a molluscum contagiosum lesion showing an area of epidermal hyperplasia surrounding a cystic lobule. Keratinocytes in the upper epidermis as well as those desquamated into the lobule, demonstrate large, round intracytoplasmic molluscum bodies. Hematoxylin and eosin stain. *(Courtesy of BA Werness.)*

PATHOGENESIS, PATHOLOGY, AND IMMUNOLOGY

MCV has the most limited range of tissue tropism of any poxvirus. Infection occurs only in the epidermis, and dissemination does not occur even in profoundly immunocompromised hosts, as it does in the case of vaccinia virus.[8,9] It is likely that a host factor produced by highly differentiated keratinocytes is required for productive viral replication, which also limits replication in cultured cells.[8] Transmission is a result of skin inoculation, probably following microscopic abrasions. Spread to "disseminated skin" sites probably occurs by external autoinoculation, with hematogenous or lymphatic spread unlikely.[6] Although some poxviruses can establish persistent infection in cell culture, there is no convincing evidence of persistence in vivo, and the issue of persistence has not been clarified for MCV.[8] While the high rate of infection in adults with AIDS raises the question of possible reactivation from subclinical infection in the setting of immunosuppression,[5,7] the predominantly nongenital distribution in these previously sexually active persons suggests that reinfection is more likely. The mechanism by which MCV stimulates basal cell proliferation and induces its benign tumors is under evaluation. A protein homologous to epidermal and α-transforming growth factors has been identified in vaccinia and other poxviruses.[8,9] Although an initial report suggesting the presence of a homologous gene in MCV[38] was not confirmed, the possibility of a different MCV growth factor remains a consideration.[6,9]

The pathologic changes induced by MCV infection are very characteristic[1–3,11] (Figure 27-1). Lesions consist of focal areas of hyperplastic epidermis surrounding cyst-shaped lobules which are filled with keratinized debris and degenerating molluscum bodies. In the basal layer, the nuclei and cytoplasm of the keratinocytes are enlarged; this is the only layer in which mitotic figures are seen. In the spindle layer, cells begin to display cytoplasmic vacuolization, enlargement, and then replacement by eosinophilic compartmentalized globules, the molluscum bodies, which are contained in well-defined sacs and which compress the nuclei to the cell periphery.[39] In the granular layer, the molluscum bodies become more homogeneous with loss of their internal structural markings and are finally desquamated into the cystic lobules.[1–3,11] Dermal changes are usually limited to stromal proliferation, although inflammation occurs in up to 20 percent of clinical lesions, with infiltration of the necrotic epithelium by lymphocytes, histiocytes, neutrophils, and occasionally multinucleated giant cells.[2,3,11,40]

The importance of host immunity in the control of MCV remains poorly characterized. In the epidermis, the inflammatory infiltrate is usually minimal: the superficial location of infection beyond the intact basement membrane and the sequestration of virions within the cytoplasmic sac are both thought to provide protection from immune recognition.[6,8,9,41] However, there are inflammatory cells in the dermis, and the epidermal inflammation which occurs commonly after trauma may result from disruption of these anatomic barriers, with a subsequent immune response which often precedes resolution of lesions.[6,9]Additionally, the greater prevalence of lesions in children than adults suggests the acquisition of host resistance with age.[22 23,34] Finally, the increase in rates and severity of infection in patients with AIDS indicates that intact cell-mediated immunity (CMI) is important in the control of MCV, as it is for vaccinia virus.[8] However, it is not clear whether a decrease in CD4 cells, Langerhans cells, or another component of CMI is responsible for more severe disease in AIDS patients.[5] The role of humoral immunity has not been defined, although the presence of low levels of antibody in most patients regardless of disease duration suggests that it must be minor.[2,35,36]

CLINICAL MANIFESTATIONS

The incubation period of molluscum contagiosum averages two to three months, with a range of one week to six months.[1,2] Most patients are asymptomatic, the diagnosis being made incidental to

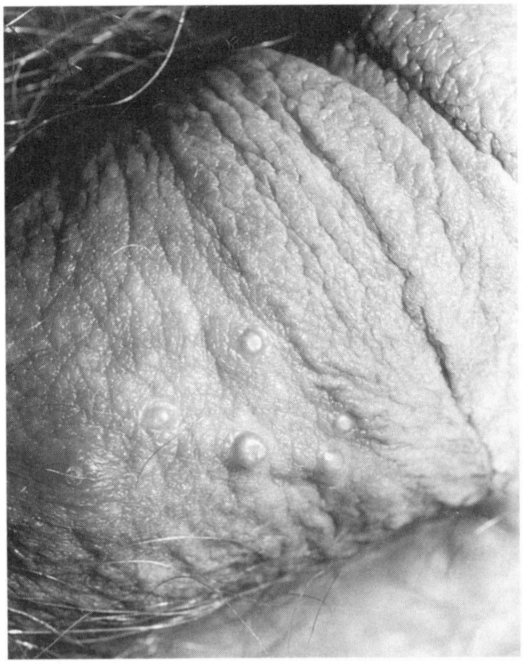

Fig. 27-2. Penile molluscum contagiosum lesions in an immunocompetent host, with typical dome shape and central umbilication. *(Courtesy of CAM Rietmeijer.)*

another problem. A minority of patients complain of itching or tenderness.[1,2,19–22] Lesions begin as tiny papules which grow over several weeks to a diameter of 3 to 5 mm, occasionally enlarging to 10 to 15 mm, producing the "giant molluscum."[1,2] The flesh-colored papules are smooth, firm, and dome-shaped, with a highly characteristic central umbilication from which caseous material can be expressed (Figure 27-2). In adults, lesions most often occur on the thighs, inguinal region, buttocks, and lower abdominal wall and less commonly on the external genitalia and perianal region, a pattern contrasting with the distribution of genital warts.[2,19–20] Children more typically develop lesions on the face, trunk, and upper extremities, often with a linear distribution suggesting autoinoculation by scratching; lesions on the palms, soles, and mucous membranes are rare.[1,2,19–20,22,24] Lesions are usually more widespread in children than in adults, and while adults with genital disease rarely develop extragenital lesions, 10 to 50 percent of infected children have lesions in the genital region.[22] The average duration of untreated disease is reported to be approximately two years, ranging from two weeks to four years; individual lesions usually resolve within two months.[20,22,23,42] Recurrences after clearance occur in 15 to 35 percent of patients;[22,42] whether these represent new infections or exacerbation of subclinical infections is unclear.

While normal hosts usually have 10 to 20 lesions, immunocompromised patients may develop hundreds of lesions.[5–7,19–22,43–44] Widespread involvement of eczematous areas has been described in patients with atopic dermatitis and attributed to skin disruption, use of topical steroids, and/or an underlying immunologic disorder.[43–44] Patients with frankly abnormal CMI are also at risk of developing extensive disease. Cases have been described in patients with sarcoidosis, epidermodysplasia verruciformis, lymphoma, and leukemia, and in those receiving immunosuppressive therapy,[2,6,7] although one review of molluscum contagiosum in children with cancer indicated that the prevalence was no higher than in normal hosts.[45] In contrast, patients with HIV infection clearly experience an increased rate of infection. First noted in the early years of the AIDS epidemic,[46–47] molluscum contagiosum in HIV-infected persons was recognized as a common problem by the late 1980s.[5–7,30–32] Both the prevalence and the severity of disease increase with advancing immunodeficiency,[5,30–33] with lesions occurring in up to one-third of patients with CD4 counts of 100 cells/mm or lower.[48] Rates of clinic visits for molluscum contagiosum are reported to be 38-fold higher for HIV-infected men than for uninfected men, and 140-fold higher for those with AIDS. These rate ratios are substantially greater than those for either HSV or condyloma.[33] The majority of lesions occur on the face and neck, especially in the beard area, where they are apparently spread by shaving; anogenital infection is relatively uncommon[5,48] (Figure 27-3). Outbreaks with extensive lesions are common, and giant molluscum lesions are noted in up to 10 percent of patients.[5]

The most frequent complication of infection, "molluscum dermatitis," appears 1 to 15 months after the onset of lesions in up to 10 percent of patients.[2,6,7,20,49] It consists of a sharply bordered eczematoid reaction 3 to 10 cm in diameter around an individual lesion, may involve only a portion of lesions, and usually disappears as the lesion resolves. Lesions of the eyelid may induce a unilateral conjunctivitis. The pattern is usually that of a chronic follicular or papillary conjunctivitis, but corneal changes with a punctuate epithelial keratitis similar to that of trachoma can also occur.[2,7] Other inflammatory conditions seen in association with molluscum contagiosum include folliculitis, sycosis barbae, erythema annular centrifugum, and pseudoleukemia cutis.[2,7] Although it has been suggested that molluscum contagiosum lesions, like genital warts, worsen during pregnancy, there is little information on this issue.[20,21] Infection does not appear to affect the outcome of pregnancy, and while lesions have been reported in a child as young as one week old, no documented case of maternal-fetal transmission has been reported.[21]

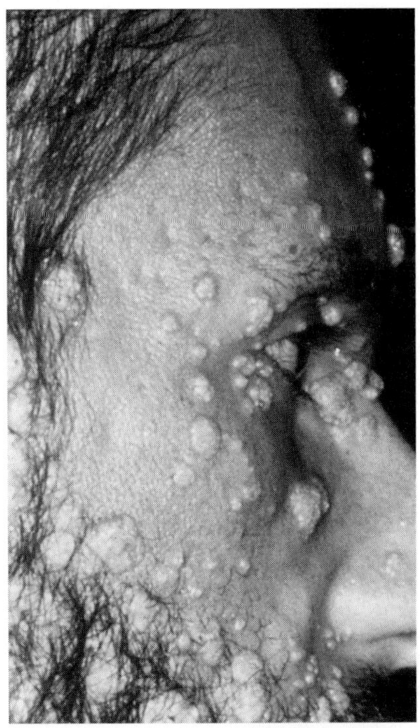

Fig. 27-3. Severe facial molluscum contagiosum in a man with AIDS, with extensive involvement of the skin of the periocular and beard areas. *(Courtesy of DL Cohn.)*

DIAGNOSIS

The clinical diagnosis is usually made easily on the basis of the characteristic, pearly, umbilicated papules with caseous centers found on the face, trunk, extremities, or genital region.[2,7,19] Lesions are most frequently misdiagnosed as common or genital warts or keratoacanthomas.[2,7,19] Other considerations in the differential diagnosis include syringomas, plane warts, lichen planus, epithelial and intradermal nevi, sebaceous adenomas, histiocytomas, seborrheic and atopic dermatitis, basal cell epitheliomas, and infection with HSV and varicella zoster virus. In patients with HIV infection, basal cell carcinoma and disseminated cryptococcosis are also considerations.[2,7,19,50] In atypical cases the diagnosis can be confirmed by demonstrating the pathognomonic enlarged epithelial cells with intracytoplasmic molluscum bodies on cytologic or histologic studies (see Figure 27-1).[2,7,19] Other diagnostic approaches include detection of MCV antigen by fluorescent antibody, of viral particles by electron microscopy, and of MCV DNA by dot blot and in situ hybridization assays.[2,51,52] Although not a diagnostic test, the CPE induced by MCV may be confused with that of HSV. Up to one-half of MCV lesions will induce CPE in cell culture,[53] and one laboratory reported that up to 10 percent of genital lesion specimens producing CPE were caused by MCV.[54]

Additional diagnostic concerns include screening for other STDs in those with genital lesions[19,28] and the possibility of an immunodeficiency, such as HIV infection, in those with widespread lesions. The issue of whether genital lesions in children should prompt a sexual abuse investigation is unresolved, although the presence of extragenital lesions suggests autoinoculation of the genital region, supporting a nonsexual route of transmission.[55]

TREATMENT AND PREVENTION

Treatment of molluscum contagiosum is generally simple and accomplished by eradicating lesions with mechanical destruction or techniques to induce local epidermal inflammation.[2,6,7] While therapy hastens resolution of individual lesions and may thereby reduce autoinoculation and transmission to others, the high frequency of recurrences and the benign and self-limited nature of the infection must be weighed against the pain and potential for scarring induced by destructive therapies, especially in children.[2,6,7] Few controlled treatment studies have been performed.

The simplest and most widely used methods are excisional curettage and expression of the lesion core by direct pressure. These procedures are often followed by cauterization of the lesion base with electrodessication or a chemical agent such as phenol, silver nitrate, trichloroacetic acid, or iodine.[2,6,7] Cryotherapy with liquid nitrogen is an alternative mode of direct destruction.[2,6,7] For tiny lesions which may be difficult to curette or express, topical application of irritating agents is recommended, although this often requires multiple treatments.[2,6,7] One of the few randomized controlled trials yet reported noted a cure rate of 95 percent with self-applied 0.5% podophyllotoxin cream versus 16 percent with placebo.[56] No therapy is very effective in immunocompromised patients because of the increased occurrence of new lesions.[5,7] In HIV-infected patients, intralesional alpha interferon results in shrinkage of most injected lesions but has no benefit on surrounding lesions;[57] likewise, daily administration of systemic interferon is ineffective.[58] Examination and treatment of sexual partners have been recommended,[2,7,19] but there are no data on the benefit of this practice for either prevention of reinfection or detection of new infections.

References

1 Low RC: Molluscum contagiosum. *Edinburgh Med J* 53:657, 1946.

2 Brown ST et al: Molluscum contagiosum. *Sex Transm Dis* 8:227, 1981.

3 Postlethwaite R: Molluscum contagiosum: a review. *Arch Environ Health* 21:432, 1970.

4 Goodpasture EW: Borreliotoses: Fowl-pox, molluscum contagiosum, variola-vaccinia. *Science* 77:119, 1933.

5 Schwartz JJ, Myskowski PL: Molluscum contagiosum in patients with human immunodeficiency virus infection. *J Am Acad Dermatol* 27:583, 1992.

6 Epstein WL: Molluscum contagiosum. *Seminars in Dermatology* 11: 184, 1992.

7 Gottlieb SL, Myskowski PL: Molluscum contagiosum. *Int J Dermatol* 33:453, 1994.

8 Buller RM, Palumbo GJ: Poxvirus pathogenesis. *Microbiol Rev* 55: 80, 1991.

9 Porter CD et al: Molluscum Contagiosum Virus, in *Molecular and Cell Biology of Sexually Transmitted Diseases,* D Wright, L Archard (eds). London, Chapman and Hall, 1992, pp 233–257.

9a Senkevich TG et al: Genome sequence of a human tumorigenic poxvirus: prediction of specific host response-evasion genes. *Science* 273: 813, 1996.

10 Esposito JJ: Family; poxvirus group; poxviridae in classification and nomenclature of viruses. Fifth Report. *Arch Virol* 2:91, 1992.

11 Reed RJ, Parkinson RP: The histogenesis of molluscum contagiosum. *Am J Surg Pathol* 1:161, 1977.

12 Blake NW et al: Characterization of a molluscum contagiosum virus homolog of the vaccinia virus p37k major envelope antigen. *J Virol* 65:3583, 1991.

12a Buller RM et al: Replication of molluscum contagiosum virus. *Virology* 213:655, 1995.

13 McFadden G et al: Biogenesis of pox-viruses: transitory expression of molluscum contagiosum early functions. *Virology* 94:297, 1979.

14 Darai G et al: Analysis of the genome of molluscum contagiosum virus by restriction endonuclease analysis and molecular cloning. *J Med Virol* 18:29, 1986.

15 Porter CD, Archard LC: Characterisation by restriction mapping of three subtypes of molluscum contagiosum virus. *J Med Virol* 38:1, 1992.

16 Bugert JJ, Darai G: Stability of molluscum contagiosum virus DNA among 184 patient isolates: evidence for variability of sequences in the terminal inverted repeats. *J Med Virol* 33:211, 1991.

17 Thompson CH et al: Clinical and molecular aspects of molluscum contagiosum infection in HIV-1 positive patients. *Int J STD AIDS* 3: 101, 1992.

18 Scholz J et al: Epidemiology of molluscum contagiosum using genetic analysis of the viral DNA. *J Med Virol* 27:87, 1989.

19 Cobbold RJC, MacDonald A: Molluscum contagiosum as a sexually transmitted disease. *Practitioner* 204:416, 1970.

20 Felman YM, Nikitas JA: Sexually transmitted molluscum contagiosum. *Dermatol Clinics* 1:103, 1983.

21 Wilkin JK: Molluscum contagiosum venereum in a women's outpatient clinic: a venereally transmitted disease. *Am J Obstet Gynecol* 128:531, 1977.

22 Postlethwaite R et al: Features of molluscum contagiosum in the north-east of Scotland and in Fijiian village settlements. *J Hyg* (Lond) 65:281, 1967.

23 Sturt RJ et al: Molluscum contagiosum in villages of the West Sepik district of New Guinea. *Med J Aust* 2:751, 1971.

24 Niizeki K et al: An epidemic study of molluscum contagiosum: relationship to swimming. *Dermatologica* 169:197, 1984.

25 Chief Medical Officer of the Department of Health and Social Security: Sexually transmitted diseases: extract from the annual report. *Genitourin Med* 61:204, 1985.

26 Becker TM et al: Trends in molluscum contagiosum in the United States, 1966–1983. *Sex Transm Dis* 13:18, 1986.

27 Oriel JD: The increase in molluscum contagiosum. *Br Med J* 294:74, 1987.
28 Radcliffe KW et al: Molluscum contagiosum: a neglected sentinel infection. *Int J STD AIDS* 2:416, 1991.
29 Public Health Laboratory Service Communicable Disease Surveillance Centre: Sexually transmitted disease in Britain: 1985–6. *Genitourin Med* 65:117, 1989.
30 Matis WL et al: Dermatologic findings associated with human immunodeficiency virus infection. *J Dermatol* 17:746, 1987.
31 Hira SK et al: Cutaneous manifestations of human immunodeficiency virus in Lusaka, Zambia. *J Am Acad Dermatol* 19:451, 1988.
32 Coldiron BM, Bergstrasser PR. Prevalence and clinical spectrum of skin disease in patients infected with human immunodeficiency virus. *Arch Dermatol* 125:357, 1989.
33 Coopman SA et al: Cutaneous disease and drug reactions in HIV infection. *New Engl J Med* 328:1670, 1993.
34 Murray MJ et al: Molluscum contagiosum and herpes simplex in Maasai pastoralists: refeeding activation of virus infection following famine? *Trans R Soc Trop Med Hyg* 74:371, 1980.
35 Epstein WL et al: Viral antigens in human epidermal tumors: localization of an antigen to molluscum contagiosum. *J Invest Dermatol* 40:51, 1963.
36 Shirodaria PV, Matthews RS: Observations on the antibody responses in molluscum contagiosum. *Br J Dermatol* 96:29, 1977.
37 Konya J, et al: Enzyme-linked immunosorbent assay for measurement of IgG antibody to molluscum contagiosum virus and investigation of the serological relationship of the molecular types. *J Virol Meth* 40:183, 1992.
38 Porter CD, Archard LC: Characterization and physical mapping of molluscum contagiosum virus DNA and location of a sequence capable of encoding a conserved domain of epidermal growth factor. *J Gen Virol* 68:673, 1987.
39 Shelley WB, Burmeister V: Demonstration of a unique viral structure: The molluscum viral colony sac. *Br J Dermatol* 115:557, 1986.
40 Henao M, Freeman RG: Inflammatory molluscum contagiosum. *Arch Dermatol* 90:479, 1964.
41 Viac J, Chardonnet Y: Imunocompetent cells and epithelial cell modifications in molluscum contagiosum. *J Cutan Pathol.* 17:202, 1990.
42 Hawley TG: The natural history of molluscum contagiosum in Fijiian children. *J Hyg* (Camb) 68:631, 1970.
43 Solomon LM, Telner P: Eruptive molluscum contagiosum in atopic dermatitis. *Can Med Assoc J* 95:978, 1966.
44 Pauly CR et al: Atopic dermatitis, impaired cellular immunity, and molluscum contagiosum. *Arch Dermatol* 114:391, 1978.
45 Hughes WT, Parham DM: Molluscum contagiosum in children with cancer or acquired immunodeficiency syndrome. *Pediatr Infect Dis J* 10:152, 1993.
46 Reichert CM et al: Autopsy pathology in the acquired immunodeficiency syndrome. *Am J Pathol* 112:357, 1982.
47 Redfield RR et al: Severe molluscum contagiosum infection in a patient with human T cell lymphotrophic (HTLV-III) disease. *J Am Acad Dermatol* 13:821, 1985.
48 Koopman RJ et al: Molluscum contagiosum: A marker for advanced HIV infection. *Br J Dermatol* 126:528, 1992.
49 Kipping HF: Molluscum dermatitis. *Arch Dermatol* 103:106, 1971.
50 Durden FM, Elewski B: Cutaneous involvement with *Cryptococcus neoformans* in AIDS. *J Am Acad Dermatol* 30:844, 1994.
51 Hurst JW et al: Direct detection of molluscum contagiosum virus in clinical specimens by dot blot hybridization. *J Clin Microbiol* 29: 1959, 1991.
52 Forghani B et al: Direct detection of molluscum contagiosum virus in clinical specimens by in situ hybridization using biotinylated probe. *Molec Cell Probes* 6:67, 1992.
53 Hovenden JL, Bushell TE: Molluscum contagiosum: possible culture misdiagnosis as herpes simplex. *Genitourin Med* 67:270, 1991.
54 Dennis J et al: Molluscum contagiosum, another sexually transmitted disease: its impact on the clinical virology laboratory. *J Infect Dis* 151:376, 1985.
55 Schactner L, Hankin D: Reply to, Is genital molluscum contagiosum a cutaneous manifestation of sexual abuse in children? *J Am Acad Dermatol* 14:848, 1986.
56 Syed TA et al: Topical 0.3% and 0.5% podophyllotoxin cream for self-treatment of molluscum contagiosum in males: A placebo-controlled, double-blind study. *Dermatol* 189:65, 1994.
57 Nelson MR et al: Intralesional interferon for the treatment of recalcitrant molluscum contagiosum in HIV antibody positive individuals: a preliminary report. *Int J STD AIDS* 6:351, 1995.
58 Tappero et al: Cutaneous manifestations of opportunistic infection in patients infected with human immunodeficiency virus. *Clin Microb Rev* 8:440, 1995.

CHAPTER 28

Biology of *Chlamydia trachomatis*

Julius Schachter

TAXONOMY

Chlamydia trachomatis, an important pathogen of humans, is one of four species within the genus *Chlamydia.*[1] Properties of the four species are shown in Table 28-1. *C. psittaci* is a common pathogen of avian species and domestic mammals but only involves humans as a zoonosis.[2] *C. pneumoniae* is a common respiratory pathogen of humans that has been implicated as a possible cause of coronary artery disease; it is thought to infect only humans.[3] *C. pecorum* is a pathogen of domestic animals.[4] Some *C. psittaci* strains are sexually transmitted in their natural hosts, and one—the guinea pig inclusion conjunctivitis (GPIC) agent—may offer a potentially useful animal model for the study of sexually transmitted chlamydial infections.[5,6]

Chlamydia psittaci, C. pneumoniae, and *C. pecorum* cannot be easily differentiated in the laboratory. DNA hybridization assays and the use of monoclonal antibodies are required to differentiate these three species, although use of electron microscopy may provide presumptive identification of *C. pneumoniae* because its elementary bodies (described below) may be pear-shaped rather than coccoid.

Chlamydia trachomatis is readily differentiated on the basis of two relatively simple laboratory tests (see Table 28-1). The simpler involves staining infected cells with iodine to determine whether the inclusions contain glycogen: *C. trachomatis* inclusions do, while inclusions of the other species do not. The second and less reliable test involves testing for susceptibility to sulfonamides: *C. trachomatis* strains are susceptible and other chlamydiae are usually resistant. Each of these species contains many different strains possessing a variety of serologic and biologic properties. Unfortunately, technical restrictions dictated by the chlamydial growth cycle have limited studies on the physiology of these organisms, and markers for more sophisticated attempts at speciation have therefore not been identified.

The need for better tools for speciation is particularly acute within *C. trachomatis.* This species contains four biovars that are probably different organisms.[1,7] The murine and swine biovars are not known to infect humans. The three serovars causing lymphogranuloma venereum (LGV) constitute a third biovar, the LGV biovar. The fourth biovar, the trachoma biovar, includes those strains causing the more common genital tract diseases (urethritis, cervicitis, salpingitis, infant diseases, etc.) and trachoma. DNA homology within the latter two *C. trachomatis* biovars is almost complete. The mouse biovar is less related to *C. trachomatis* (30–40% homology), but there is essentially no homology (less than 10%) between *C. trachomatis* and *C. psittaci.*

The trachoma and LGV biovars of *C. trachomatis* are related serologically but differ in the diseases they produce, in the type of cells they parasitize (in vivo and in vitro), in their experimental host range, and in a variety of other biological properties related to the infectious process (Table 28-2). The trachoma biovar has a very limited host spectrum in terms of susceptible cell types. In the natural host it appears to infect only squamocolumnar cells; its strains are not efficient in infecting macrophages. LGV strains are more invasive and appear to be more efficient at replication in macrophages. Neither biovar will grow in polymorphonuclear leukocytes.

The chlamydiae are distinguished from all other microorganisms on the basis of a unique growth cycle (Fig. 28-1).[1] This cycle involves an alternation between two highly specialized morphologic forms, one adapted to an intracellular and the other to an extraellular environment. Because of this cycle, chlamydiae have been placed in their own order and family (Chlamydiales, Chlamydiaceae). They are obligate intracellular parasites and cannot be cultured on artificial media. Chlamydiae are restricted to an intracellular life style because they lack the ability to synthesize high-energy compounds. Thus, they depend on the host cell to supply them with ATP and necessary nutrients. Moulder has called them "energy parasites."[8] They lack a system for electron transport, have no cytochromes, cannot synthesize ATP or GTP, and do not preferentially use glutamate.

The growth cycle initially involves attachment to and penetration of susceptible host cells.[9,10] The attachment process may involve specific receptor sites; presence of these sites could determine which cells are naturally susceptible. Attachment of *C. trachomatis* to susceptible host cells is apparently mediated by heparinsulfatelike molecules which act as a bridge between sites on the susceptible host cells and sites on the elementary body.[11] Attachment to the specific sites on the susceptible host cell apparently triggers receptor-mediated endocytosis. Once the chlamydiae penetrate the cell they remain within an endosome throughout the growth cycle, and they specifically inhibit phagolysosomal fusion. Heat-killed or antibody-treated chlamydiae are not ingested at an enhanced rate and fail to inhibit phagolysosomal fusion. These two properties, induced phagocytosis and prevention of phagolysosomal fusion, are probably the major virulence factors of this organism.

HISTORY

Human diseases caused by *Chlamydia trachomatis* have been recognized since antiquity.[12] Trachoma is described in Egyptian papyri. LGV was probably described by John Hunter in the eighteenth century. The genital tract infections, such as nongonococcal urethritis and neonatal ophthalmia caused by *C. trachomatis,* were not recognized until it was possible to categorize these conditions, following the identification of the gonococcus. With the introduction of ocular (Credé) prophylaxis with silver nitrate drops to prevent ophthalmia neonatorum and of cultural and smear methods of diagnosing gonococcal infections, it became apparent that conjunctivitis in infants and urethritis in adult males both had nongonococcal forms.

C. trachomatis was first visualized in 1907 by Halberstaedter and Prowazek in stained conjunctival scrapings taken from orangutans that had been inoculated with human trachomatous material. They quickly identified the typical intracytoplasmic inclusions, but initially they assumed that the organism was a protozoan. Shortly thereafter, similar inclusions were identified in human material from trachoma cases and then in conjunctival scrapings taken from infants with inclusion blennorrhea. Inclusions were then found in the genital tracts of mothers of the af-

Table 28-1. Usual Properties of *Chlamydia* spp.

Property	*C. trachomatis*	*C. psittaci*	*C. pneumoniae*	*C. pecorum*
Sulfonamide susceptibility	+	–	–	–
Iodine-staining inclusions	+	–	–	–
Natural host	Human	Birds, lower mammals	Human	Sheep, cattle, swine

fected infants and in the urethras of the fathers. In the first decade of this century the presence of these inclusions was associated with nongonococcal urethritis.[13]

C. trachomatis was first isolated from patients with lymphogranuloma venereum. In the 1930s the growth cycle of the LGV organism (as seen following intracerebral inoculation in mice and then in eggs) was noted to be similar to that found for the psittacosis organism, which had been isolated during the psittacosis pandemic of 1929–1930. The trachoma agent proved more difficult to recover, not being infective for mice. It was isolated by inoculation of embryonated hens'-egg yolk sacs by T'ang and associates in the 1950s.[14] These results were soon confirmed by a number of research teams in different parts of the world. In retrospect, it is likely that a previous isolation claim by Macchiavello was probably valid, but it was not confirmed and the isolate was lost. The first isolate of *Chlamydia* (other than LGV agents) from the genital tract was made in 1959 by Jones, Collier, and Smith, who recovered *C. trachomatis* from the cervix of the mother of an infant with ophthalmia neonatorum.[15] In 1964 chlamydiae were first recovered from the urethras of men epidemiologically associated with conjunctivitis cases.[16,17]

For a number of years there were very few groups actively pursuing the study of chlamydial genital tract infections. One of the reasons for this lack of interest was the lack of a technology which lent itself to screening large numbers of specimens. All of the early isolation studies (from 1960 to 1965) were performed using yolk-sac isolation procedures and thus were not clinically relevant, because they could take up to six weeks to provide definitive answers. Dunlop and his colleagues at the Institute of Ophthalmology in London were the pioneering group that provided much of the impetus for continued research on chlamydial genital tract infections. In a series of studies they found that a number of anatomic sites of the genitourinary system could be infected with *Chlamydia* and showed that approximately one-third of men with nongonococcal urethritis were carrying the organism in their urethras.[18–20]

A major technical breakthrough by Gordon and his colleagues in developing a tissue culture isolation procedure for *C. trachomatis* made it possible to: (1) screen large numbers of specimens, and (2) obtain the result of an isolation attempt in 48 to 72 hours, which made the diagnosis clinically useful.[21] Again, English workers were in the forefront of applying this test, and a number of research groups in England independently published studies finding that one-third to one-half of men with nongonococcal urethritis had chlamydial infections.[22–25] The clinical syndromes associated with these infections rapidly expanded.[26] These syndromes are listed in Table 28-3 and discussed in Chapters 29, 30, and 83.

EPIDEMIOLOGY

SEXUALLY TRANSMITTED CHLAMYDIAL INFECTIONS

There appear to be two major modes of transmission of *C. trachomatis*. LGV, wherever it is found, appears to be always sexually transmitted. In industrialized western society virtually all *C. trachomatis* infections are sexually transmitted. Men who acquire infection with non-LGV *C. trachomatis* strains usually develop

Table 28-2. Properties of the LGV and Trachoma Biovars of *C. trachomatis*

Properties	LGV	Trachoma
I. Sulfonamide susceptibility	+	+
II. Iodine-staining inclusions	+	+
III. Host spectrum		
A. Natural host: humans	+	+
1. Mucosal surfaces	–	+
2. Lymphoid	+	–
B. Produce follicular conjunctivitis in subhuman primates	–	+
C. Lethal to mice (intracerebral)	+	–
IV. Growth in cell culture		
A. Form plaques	+	–
B. Marked enhancement by centrifugation	–	+
C. Infectivity enhanced by treating cells with DEAE	–	+
D. Infectivity reduced by treating cells with neuraminidase	–	+
E. Infectivity blocked by saturating cell surface with heat-killed homologous organism	–	+

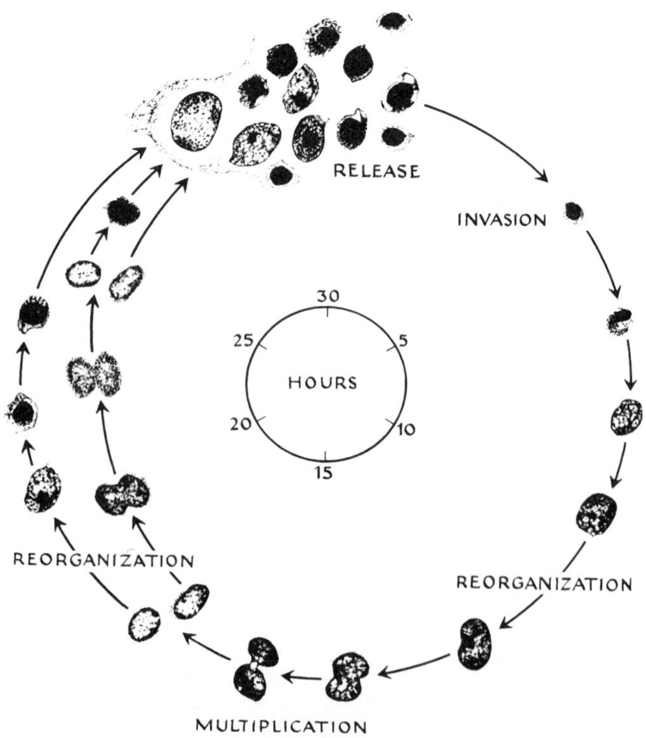

Fig. 28-1. Growth cycle of the chlamydiae. (*From JW Moulder.*[7])

Table 28-3. Human Diseases Caused by Chlamydiae

Species	Serovar*	Disease
C. psittaci	Many unidentified serotypes	Psittacosis
C. pneumoniae	TWAR	Respiratory disease
C. trachomatis	L1, L2, L3	Lymphogranuloma venereum
C. trachomatis	A, B, Ba, C	Hyperendemic blinding trachoma
C. trachomatis	B, D, E, F, G, H, I, J, K	Inclusion conjunctivitis (adult and newborn), non-gonococcal urethritis, cervicitis, salpingitis, proctitis, epididymitis, pneumonia of newborns

* Predominant, but not exclusive association of serovar with disease.
Adapted from J Schachter.[26]

nongonococcal urethritis one to three weeks postinfection. Because chlamydiae are obligate intracellular parasites and can only survive by a replicative cycle that results in death of the infected host cells, they must be considered to be pathogens at all times and are not part of the normal flora of the male or female genital tract. They do not always produce clinically apparent infections, however. For specific discussions of the epidemiology of these sexually transmitted infections see Chapters 29 and 30.

If infective genital tract discharges are inoculated into the eye either during sexual activity or by hand to eye contact, conjunctivitis may develop.[12,26,27] The disease caused by the trachoma biovar is called inclusion conjunctivitis, reflecting the diagnostic cytologic findings. In adults it is an acute follicular conjunctivitis which tends to follow a self-limited course. Keratitis and micropannus are common. Occasionally the disease persists beyond a few months and clinical features consistent with the diagnosis of trachoma may develop. Visual debility is rare. However, the regular appearance of corneal involvement (with the exception of Herbert's peripheral pits) similar to that found in classical trachoma, has led some workers to suggest that chlamydial infection of the eye represents a spectrum—from mild, self-limited, acute, follicular conjunctivitis to chronic trachoma. The clinical picture is determined by the immunologic status of the host: previous exposure and hypersensitivity result in more severe disease, and reinfections or complicating bacterial infections interfere with spontaneous healing.[12,26,27]

Infants exposed to *Chlamydia* by passage through the infected birth canal may also acquire the infection and can develop a number of diseases, including conjunctivitis and pneumonia (see Chapter 83). At least 60 to 70 percent of exposed infants acquire chlamydial infection.[28] Thus, both horizontal and vertical transmission of *C. trachomatis* occur in industrialized society. Neither *C. pneumoniae* nor *C. psittaci* is sexually transmitted in humans.

ENDEMIC TRACHOMA

Child-to-child transmission is the most common method of chlamydial transmission in trachoma endemic areas.[12,26,27,29] In many developing countries trachoma is endemic, and in some it is hyper- or holoendemic. Several hundred million people are known to be afflicted with trachoma, and millions have been blinded. In holoendemic areas children acquire the infection very early, either from persistently infected adults in their families or from exposure to other infected children. In some communities, all are infected by two years of age. Poor hygiene and unsanitary conditions contribute to the spread of the organism. Flies act as mechanical vectors in spreading infective ocular discharges. The disease begins as an acute mucopurulent conjunctivitis (often complicated by secondary bacterial infections) that becomes a chronic follicular keratoconjunctivitis, sometimes accompanied by a significant pannus (corneal neovascularization) formation.

In hyperendemic areas, active disease usually wanes when the children are 6 to 10 years old. Most of the children will be left with minor sequelae when the disease becomes inactive, and there will be no effect on vision. Some children with moderate to severe trachoma will develop badly scarred conjunctivae as a result of the necrosis of follicles. This scarring in the upper tarsal plate of the conjunctiva may with time result in distortion of the upper eyelid. The inturned upper lid margin causes the eyelashes to abrade and ultimately break down the corneal epithelium. It may take 25 or 30 years for this process to fully evolve, as the scars contract with age. The blindness seen in adults over 40 years of age usually reflect early childhood trachoma. In a hyperendemic area age-specific blindness rates at age 60 may be 20 percent or more.[30]

SERVOAR DISTRIBUTION

There are few studies aimed at determining the distribution of serovars in a community. There appear to be no biological markers associated with the different serovars that would tend to make such typing relevant from either a clinical or a public health viewpoint. In trachoma endemic areas there are usually only one or two serovars recovered in a community.[27,31] Most infections within a household appear to be of the same serovar.

The genital serovars (see Table 28-3) are not evenly distributed. L2 appears be the most common of the LGV serovars, and the D and E serovars are the most commonly recovered trachoma biovars.[32] The A and C serovars have never been recovered from the genital tract, but the B serovar, which is commonly associated with endemic trachoma, has also been shown to cause genital tract infection. Specific monoclonal antibodies are available which can distinguish among the different serovars, but until this identification becomes more meaningful it will remain a research procedure.

Finer typing of *C. trachomatis* strains has been possible by genotyping the major outer membrane protein (MOMP) gene.[33,34] This appears to be the most variable of the genes that have been studied to date. It has four variable domains that may reflect specific antigenic sites that are under selective immunologic pressures.[35] Use of a combination of monoclonal antibodies together with genotyping has verified that there are 18 major serovars of *C. trachomatis,* but because of nucleotide (usually coding amino acid) changes within serovars, multiple genovars can be detected. To date, the study of these genovars has had limited application. Efforts to associate specific genovars and serovars with more invasive disease or with more inflammatory changes are underway.

BIOLOGY

DEVELOPMENTAL CYCLE

It is the developmental cycle of chlamydiae that sets them apart from all other bacteria. There are some differences in inclusion morphology within the chlamydiae, but all species appear to have essentially identical developmental cycles. The cycle may be divided into several steps: (1) initial attachment of the infectious particle, or elementary body, to the host cell; (2) entry into the cell; (3) morphologic change to the reticulate particle, with intracellular growth and replication; (4) morphologic change of reticulate particles to elementary bodies; and finally (5) release of the infectious particles.

The elementary body (EB), is relatively resistant to the extracellular environment but is not metabolically active. This particle changes to a metabolically active and dividing form called the reticulate body (RB, or initial body) at some time within the first 6 to 8 hours after entering the host cell. This reorganization process is poorly understood. EBs are approximately 350 nm in diameter and have an electron-dense center; RBs are approximately 1 μm in diameter and do not appear to be electron dense.

After reaching the reticulate body stage, chlamydiae synthesize their own macromolecules—RNA, DNA, and protein—using the host-cell pool of precursors.[36] Glycogen accumulates within the inclusions of *C. trachomatis*, reaching levels detectable by iodine stain at approximately 30 to 48 hours postinfection.[37] The RBs divide by binary fission from approximately 8 hours to approximately 18–24 hours postentry. This is the stage of greatest metabolic activity, when the organisms are most sensitive to inhibitors of cell-wall synthesis and inhibitors of bacterial metabolic activity. At approximately 18 to 24 hours postentry, some of the RBs reorganize into the smaller infectious EBs. RBs are approximately 1 um in diameter and do not appear to be electron dense; the EBs are approximately 350 nm in diameter and have an electrondense center. Beyond 18 to 24 hours, the numbers of EBs increase and this form appears to predominate, although both EBs and RBs are found in the inclusion.

The entire cycle takes place within the phagosome, which obviously undergoes a large increase in size. There is considerable transport of molecules across the phagosome membrane during the cycle as metabolites and ATP enter the inclusion and ADP is excreted. As the EBs multiply there is active traffic of lipids from the Golgi apparatus into the inclusion.[37] At some time between 48 and 72 hours the cell ruptures, releasing the infectious elementary bodies. Phagolysosomal fusion does not occur until the death of the cell is imminent. This inhibition has been attributed to a chlamydial surface antigen because antibody-treated EBs do not inhibit phagolysosomal fusion.

The RBs are not stable outside the host cell. Thus, as part of their unique growth cycle, the chlamydiae appear to have evolved two morphologic entities—the compact, stable EB, which successfully persists in the extracellular environment and is responsible for cell-to-cell and host-to-host transmission, and the highly labile RB, which represents the metabolically active and vegetative form that is noninfective and does not survive outside the host cell.

The elementary body is toxic. If the host cell ingests many particles (on the order of 100 EBs) it may die with no resultant progeny.[38] Also, large concentrations of *Chlamydia* inoculated intravenously into mice will kill the animals; this "toxic death" appears to be a result of damage to the vascular endothelium. Chlamydiae do not produce an extracellular toxin.

Attachment

The attachment of *C. psittaci* and the LGV biovar of *C. trachomatis* to cells is highly efficient, as is penetration. Saturation of cultured host cell's surface is not observed.[39] Heating these organisms prevents attachment, and the host cells have a trypsin-sensitive attachment site that is quickly regenerated.[40] In contrast, the trachoma biovar attaches inefficiently, saturation can be demonstrated, and heating the organism does not inhibit attachment, nor does trypsinization of host cells keep them from attaching.[39,41] The trachoma biovar may have a more specialized attachment site than the LGV biovar; this may explain its more limited host range.

The initial contact of the chlamydial EB with the susceptible host cell may involve a specific receptor-ligand interaction, but no such structures have been clearly identified. Attachment appears to be mediated by heparin-sulfate-like molecules which act as a bridge between a specific receptor on the chlamydial particle and another on the susceptible host cell.[11] It is likely that this attachment process initiates a receptor-mediated endocytosis.

For some strains, attachment may be charge-dependent. DEAE-dextran pretreatment of cells leads to marked enhancement of attachment and entry of the trachoma biovar, but not of *C. psittaci* or the LGV biovar.[39] Treatment with negatively charged molecules such as heparin can inhibit chlamydial infectivity and elute EBs from the surface of host cells. The attachment of *Chlamydia* to host cells and inhibition of phagolysosomal fusion are inhibited by specific antibody, by mild heat treatment (56°C for 30 minutes) or trypsinization.[40,42] However, surface proteolysis of L2 EBs did not impair infectivity, although the major outer membrane protein (MOMP) was dramatically cleaved and largely removed from the surface.[43] Polyclonal antibody to MOMP neutralized infectivity, but did not inhibit attachment or penetration.[44] Similarly, monoclonal antibody to a species-specific *C. trachomatis* MOMP antigen can neutralize infectivity but not reduce attachment to susceptible cells.[45] Monoclonal and polyclonal antibodies to many different chlamydial antigenic sites (usually specific for variable domains of MOMP, but also including some to heat shock and other proteins) have been found to neutralize infectivity in vitro. The function of antibodies to these sites in naturally occurring infections is uncertain.

Cell entry

Once attached, the EB is rapidly internalized by the host cell. If a mixture of EBs and *E. coli* or yeast are presented to susceptible host cells, the chlamydiae will be preferentially ingested.[40] Many of the cells that the chlamydiae infect are not considered phagocytes. Moulder has stressed the differentiation of host cells into professional and nonprofessional phagocytes and that chlamydiae induce phagocytosis by the nonprofessional phagocytes.[46] The mechanism of chlamydial uptake is controversial.

Ultrastructural studies on the entry of chlamydiae into susceptible cells suggest that they enter through clathrin-coated pits. This suggests that chlamydial entry is via a pathway similar to receptor-mediated endocytosis.[47] However, inhibitors of receptor-mediated endocytosis such as monodansylcadaverine or amantadine did not inhibit LGV biovar uptake in HeLa cells.[48]

Intracellular growth

The chlamydial particle enters the cell within an endosome and stays within that endosome through its entire life cycle. But phagolysosomal fusion does not take place.[10] The inhibitor appears to be a surface protein antigen and is found on cell walls isolated from EBs.[49] The inhibitory signal is not present on the RB surface, as after RBs are ingested there is fusion.[50] Inhibition is specific to the chlamydial phagosome, as fusion can take place in other phagosomes in the same cell.[51]

Approximately 8 hours after entry into the cell, the EB (diameter approximately 350 nm) has changed into a RB, which has a diameter of approximately 800 to 1000 nm. The rigid structure of the EB is lost, and the RB is more permeable than the EB, allowing it to take up ATP and required nutrients. The inclusion and the RB act essentially as a reverse mitochondrion, with ATP and other nutrients entering the inclusion from the host cell.[52] The sequential synthesis of selected outer membrane proteins appears to reflect their putative function within the elementary body. Structural rigidity of the organism is maintained by disulfide bonds within the major outer membrane protein, which represents 60% of the outer membrane's weight.[53] The other cysteine-rich proteins of approximately 60 kDa and 15 kDa are synthesized relatively late in the cycle.[54]

The RBs divide by binary fission for approximately 20 to 24 hours. After that time, some of the RBs become EBs by a condensation process which is not clearly understood. Other RBs continue to divide. After replication of the RBs there is budding and blebbing of the outer membrane. Intermediate forms are also seen (see Fig. 28-1). The mature inclusion contains hundreds, even thousands, of elementary bodies. The entire cytoplasm of the cell may be displaced by the inclusion. Throughout the infectious cycle there is an inhibition of phagolysosomal fusion, and only at the very end is lysomal enzyme activity noted.[55]

MORPHOLOGY AND COMPOSITION

The chlamydiae are structurally complex microorganisms which possess cell walls and membranes quite analogous in structure to the cell walls of gram-negative bacteria[56] (Fig. 28-2). However, the cell walls of chlamydiae do not contain significant quantities of muramic acid. It is likely that the chlamydial cell wall is unique among bacterial species and probably represents a specialized structure compatible with the requirements of the chlamydial growth cycle. Traces of muramic acid have been found, but in quantities inadequate to maintain structural integrity by a peptidoglycan layer.[57]

The chlamydial cell wall consists of subunits approximately 20 nm in diameter arranged in a regular geometric pattern (Fig. 28-3).[58] The outer membrane of *Chlamydia* contains a MOMP which is approximately 30% of the weight of the organism and approximately 60% of the weight of the outer membrane.[59] The size of this protein varies by serovar, with a molecular weight range of 38–43 kDa.[60] It appears to be the major structural protein and functions in maintaining the structural integrity of the cell wall.[59] It is a cysteine-rich protein which is linked by disulfide bonds to itself and to two other proteins, of approximately 15 and 60 kDa, to maintain structural rigidity.[61,62]

Although this statement is probably too simplistic, it is likely that the major structural changes that occur when the EB changes to an RB represent a reduction of the disulfide links within the EB outer membrane. RB outer membrane structure is in some respects similar to that of the EB, although with less disulfide bridging between MOMP and the other cysteine-rich proteins.[53,61] In the beginning of the growth cycle MOMP is reduced to the monomeric form, and it is found in the outer membrane throughout the chlamydial life cycle, whereas the other chlamydial proteins are synthesized later in the cycle.[53,54,61] It is likely that the synthesis of these other proteins is regulated so that they appear at the time the EBs will form and are oxidized into the complex that is important for structural rigidity of the EB. Enzyme-mediated oxidation-reduction reactions are probably important in the differentiation of particle types.

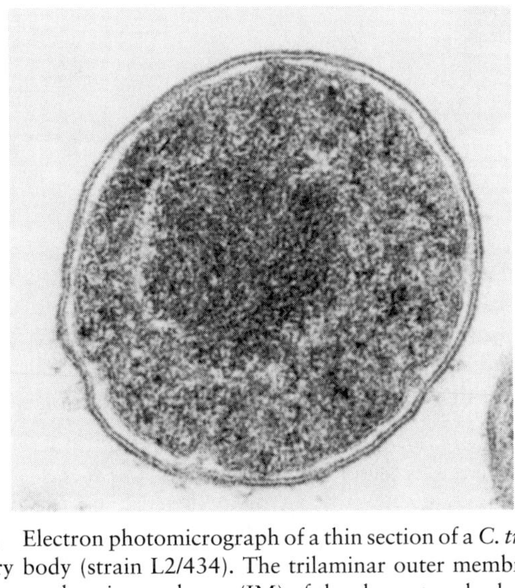

Fig. 28-2. Electron photomicrograph of a thin section of a *C. trachomatis* elementary body (strain L2/434). The trilaminar outer membrane (OM) and inner cytoplasmic membrane (IM) of the elementary body are shown at 118,000× magnification. (*From HD Caldwell.*[59])

Supporting the concept that the EB-RB transformation is partly dependent on reduction of disulfide bonds is the observation that reduced and alkylated MOMP functions as a porin.[63] EBs in the presence of dithiothreitol showed increased glutamine oxidation, reduced infectivity, decreased osmotic stability, and staining characteristics of the RB.[64] This would be consistent with a structural change that is also important in the developmental cycle, as the outer membrane would be permeable to the nutrients required for RB metabolism. MOMP is apparently a transmembrane protein, with surface antigenic components responsible at least in part for serovar, serogroup, and species-specific reactivity.[65,66] The common group antigen, an LPS, may be released from the particles by treatment with detergents such as deoxycholate.[67]

The chemical composition of the organism appears to be approximately 35% protein and 40–50% lipid. Both RNA and DNA are found, although reticulate particles, being metabolically active, have more RNA. Chlamydia do not appear to be able to utilize thymidine,[68] and there is no detectable thymidine kinase.[69] It is likely that requirements for DNA synthesis are met through a uridine and thymidylic synthetase pathway. The host cell's thymidine kinase may play a role.

Electron micrographs have shown the regular arrangement of spikelike protuberances, which occur in only a limited area of the elementary body (Fig. 28-4).[70] The function of these projections is not known, but from their arrangement it is likely that they are involved in attachment and possibly in transfer of molecules into or out of the EB particle.

Chlamydia appear to contain a number of penicillin-binding proteins.[71] The lack of muramic acid and peptidoglycan does not seem to jibe with the effects of penicillins. If one assumes that the ultimate effect of penicillin is the inhibition of cross-linking between tetrapeptide side chains of peptidoglycan, it would be reasonable to assume that chlamydiae have similar cross-linked tetrapeptides. These must link up with something other than peptidoglycan. Cycloserine, an inhibitor of tetrapeptide synthesis, is active against *Chlamydia* and its effect can be reversed by d-alanine, suggesting that such linkage occurs.[72]

GROWTH AND CULTURE

Because chlamydiae are obligatory intracellular parasites, it is necessary to supply a living host cell to support their growth. Tissue culture isolation procedures have made chlamydial isolation clinically relevant. The organism can be recovered from patients in 48 to 72 hours, a time period consistent with other bacteriologic procedures. A number of cell lines have been used as host cells, and a variety of treatments, physical or chemical, have been employed to increase the susceptibility of these cells to chlamydial infection.[12,73]

Modification of the host cells' charge by pretreatment of the monolayers with DEAE-dextran will enhance attachment by non-LGV *C. trachomatis* strains.[74] The single most important step in enhancing infection is centrifugation of the inoculum onto the tissue culture monolayer.[21,75] With the exception of LGV strains, the

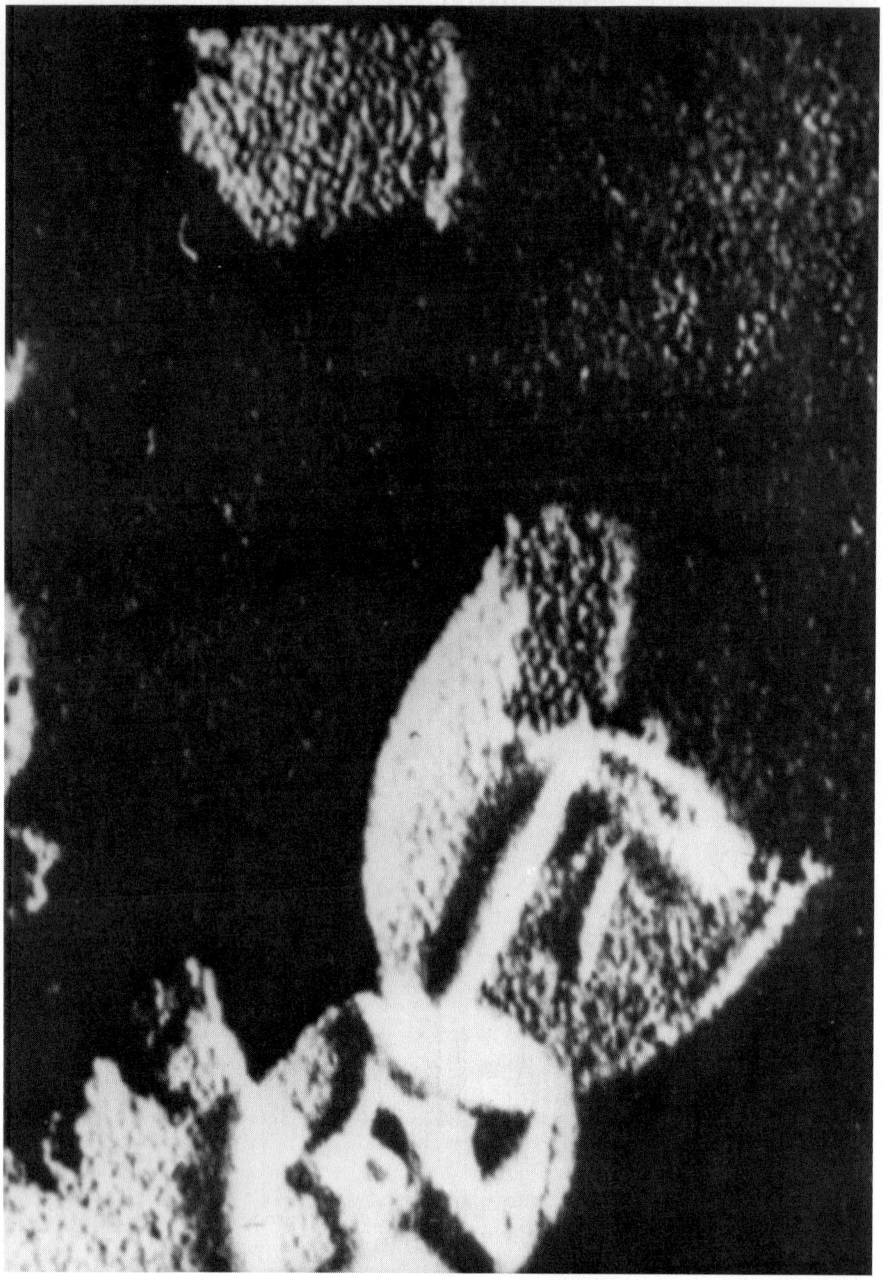

Fig. 28-3. Fine structure of cell wall of meningopneumonitis organism. Shadowed preparation showing regular geometric arrangement of subunits approximately 20 nm in diameter. Approximately 75,000× magnification. (*From A Matsumoto and GP Manire.*[56])

C. trachomatis strains are not efficient at attaching to and infecting cells in vitro. Indeed, a convenient method of differentiating LGV from the trachoma biovar strains is to measure the enhancement of infectivity achieved with centrifugation, for it is minimal with the LGV strains and $>10^2$ for the non-LGV strains. The centrifugal forces used (about 2500 g) are probably inadequate to sediment the chlamydial particles, and the effects may be on the cultured cell membranes.

The growth of chlamydiae within the cell requires that the cell receive its essential nutrients. If the cell is starved, or if depletion experiments are performed with essential amino acids, some nutrients can be found to be growth limiting for chlamydiae, although often this reflects the requirements of the host cell more than those of the chlamydiae. The growth of *Chlamydia* in cell culture can be regulated by the amino acid concentration in the medium. Deprivation of the essential amino acids can render productive chlamydial infections to a nonproductive state. Addition of the required amino acids will then trigger growth of the chlamydiae.[77]

The most commonly used procedure involves treatment of host cells with cycloheximide before or after centrifugation of the inoculum.[76] (See Chapter 53 for a detailed discussion of these methods.) Synthetic abilities of the host cell are stopped by the action of cycloheximide, and under these conditions, *C. psittaci* required isoleusine, valine, and phenylalanine.[78] *C. trachomatis* appears to require histidine, while *C. psittaci* does not.[79] Different *C. trachomatis* serovars can show different nutritional requirements.[79] Cysteine is needed for the production of the cysteine-rich proteins that are important in EB rigidity. Cysteine deprivation will, in fact, prevent the final differentiation of EBs from RBs, but replication during the RB phase appears to be almost normal.[80] The sensitivity of *Chlamydia* to amino acid concentrations may have impor-

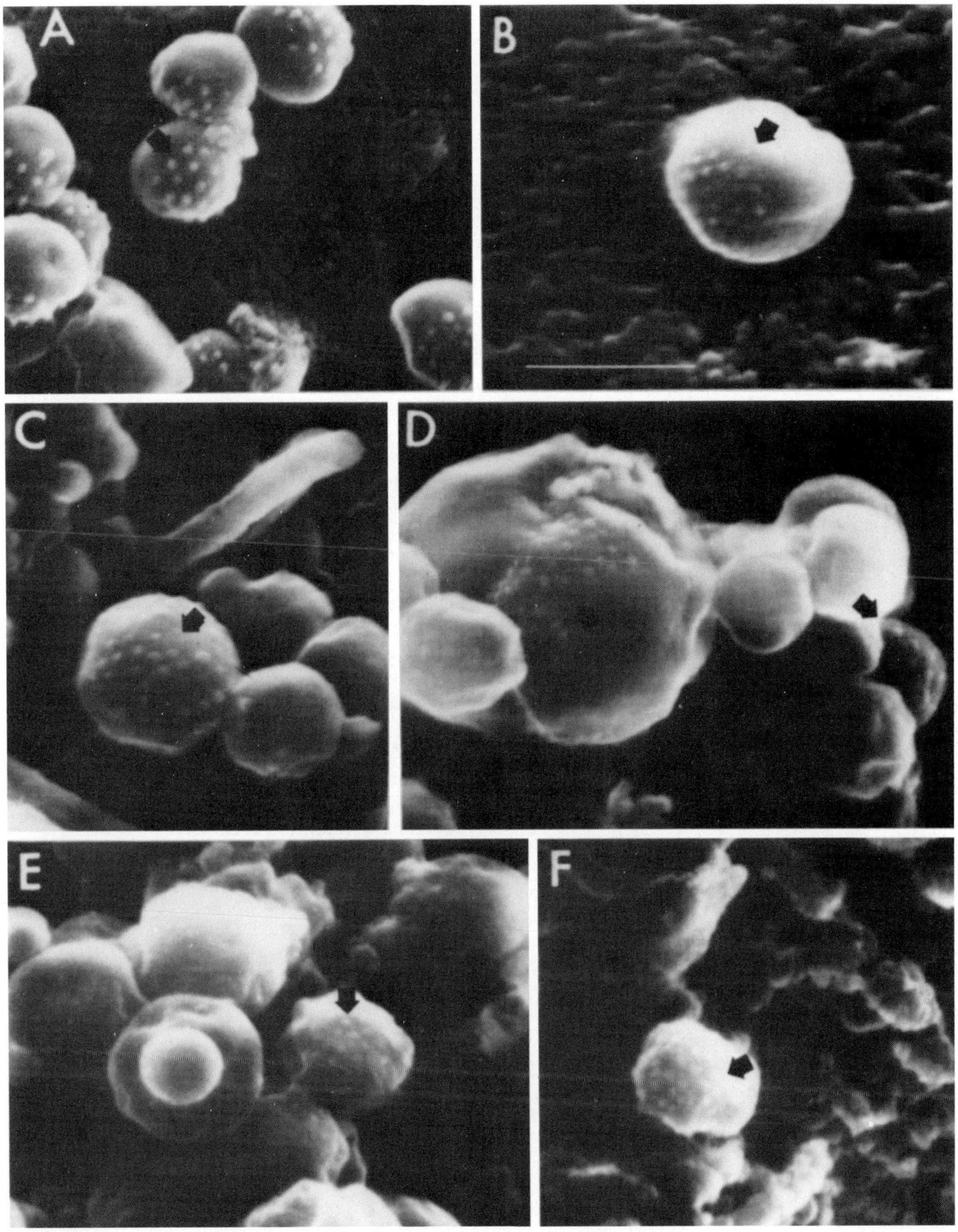

Fig. 28-4. Scanning electron micrograph of two strains of *C. psittaci* and four strains of *C. trachomatis* settled onto L cells (a) *C. psittaci* (6BC) (b) *C. psittaci* (feline pneumonitis) (c) *C. trachomatis* (mouse pneumonitis) (d) *C. trachomatis* (440L) (e) *C. trachomatis* (G17) (f) *C. trachomatis* (UW57). Arrows point to prominent arrays of projections. The bar in (b) represents 0.5 μm at 50,000× magnification. (*From WM Gregory et al.*[70])

tant biological implications. The action of gamma interferon in reducing chlamydial replication and infectivity may be a direct result of reduced tryptophan levels in *Chlamydia*-infected cells.[81]

RBs can use amino acids derived from either the host-cell nutrient pool or from degradation of host protein. L cells and *C. psittaci* require L-isoleucine, as neither synthesizes it. If L-isoleucine is added to an infected L-cell population carried in minimal medium, both *Chlamydia* and the L cells will replicate.[78] Inhibition of L-cell metabolism in a deficient medium will allow chlamydiae to grow; they are obviously using small amounts of the amino acid released by degradation of host protein.

RBs harvested at 20 hours, but not EBs purified from *C. psittaci* and *C. trachomatis* infected cells, can support ATP-dependent and antibiotic-susceptible synthesis of proteins. MOMP and 12.5 and 60 kDa cysteine-rich protein are produced at a lesser rate than is found in infected cells.[82] Chlamydiae are capable of incorporating carbon from glucose-6-phosphate, pyruvate, and isoleucine into a trichloroacetic acid insoluble fraction. This activity was shown using a mixture of EBs and RBs and is ATP-dependent.[83] Chlamydial inclusions and RBs function, in a sense, as reverse mitochondria, with ATP entering and ADP being excreted.[52]

Cyclic AMP inhibits chlamydial growth, and the action has been shown to be on the RB-to-EB transformation.[84] RBs appear to have a receptor protein for cyclic AMP.[85] Hormone levels may affect chlamydial growth and metabolism. Estradiol enhances the growth of *C. psittaci* and *C. trachomatis* in HeLa cells.[86,87]

GENETICS

Technical considerations have prevented extensive genetic analysis of *Chlamydia*. Difficulties in developing a genetic system and lack of suitable markers have restricted studies. Thus, little is known concerning the biological aspects of chlamydial genetics. The DNA of *C. trachomatis* strains have a G plus C content of approximately 44–45%.[88] At $6 - 8.5 = 10^5$ base pairs, chlamydiae have one of the smallest bacterial genomes (approximately one-half the size of neisserial or rickettsial DNA).[89] DNA homology within chlamydial species is virtually complete, but surprisingly (in view of their similarities), there is no interspecies homology. Restriction endonuclease analysis may provide the basis for molecular fingerprinting some chlamydial strains.[90] MOMP genotyping is likely to be more useful for molecular epidemiology studies.[33,34]

Relatively few *C. psittaci* strains have been analyzed for DNA homology or for the presence of plasmids. Some do contain plasmids different from the common cryptic plasmid of *C. trachomatis*. All *C. trachomatis* serovars contain a 4.4 MDa plasmid.[91] It is present as a multimeric form. Restriction endonuclease cleavage patterns of the plasmid differed for the single LGV strain compared to the other *C. trachomatis* strains tested. Functions of the plasmid genes are not known, although some of the gene products are expressed during *C. trachomatis* infection in cell culture. The gene products appear relatively late in the developmental cycle, during the multiplication of RBs and condensation from RB to EB.[90] Polypeptides encoded by these plasmids have been synthesized in an in vitro transcription translation system, and the polypeptides were not immunoreactive with antiserum prepared against chlamydiae,[92] but antiserum from infected individuals will recognize some of the plasmid gene products.[93] The sequence of the 16S RNA genes of *C. psittaci* and *C. trachomatis* has been determined, and there is only a 5% difference between the two species.[94] The sequence is similar to that of other eubacteria.

Chlamydial LPS has been successfully cloned into *E. coli* and is expressed in the outer membrane.[95] The MOMP genes of the various serovars have been cloned and sequenced. Because of MOMP's important structural and antigenic role, studies of the gene responsible for its synthesis have been of particular interest. The amino acid sequence of MOMP is now known for all serovars.[96,97] The L1 serovar MOMP is 371 amino acids long, the B and L2 MOMPs are 372 amino acids long, and the C MOMP is 375 amino acids long. The molecular weights fall between 39.5 and 40.5 kDa. MOMP genes actually encode for a 22-amino-acid leader signal peptide at the N-terminal region. There are five conserved and four variable domains within the genes, and two of the variable sequences encode for hydrophilic segments. The most variable segments are approximately 11 amino acids long and occur one each in the amino-terminal half and the carboxyl-terminal half of the MOMP. It is likely that these sites are responsible for subgroup- or serovar-specific antigenic reactivity.

PATHOGENESIS

The pathogenesis of any of the infections with *C. trachomatis* has not been elucidated. It is clear that lymphogranuloma venereum is a systemic infection involving lymphoid tissues. In vitro studies have shown the organisms are capable of replicating within macrophages.[98] To date all information suggests that non-LGV *C. trachomatis* strains have a very limited host range in vivo. They appear to be almost exclusively parasites of squamocolumnar-columnar epithelial cells. Because they are obligate intracellular parasites and kill host cells at the end stages of their growth cycle, these chlamydial strains must cause some cell damage where they persist. There is no in vivo evidence for latency in the sense of persistence of nonreplicating chlamydiae.

The disease process and clinical manifestations of chlamydial infections probably represent the combined effects of tissue damage from chlamydial replication and inflammatory responses to chlamydiae and the necrotic material from destroyed host cells. There is an abundant immune response to chlamydial infection (in terms of circulating antibodies or cell-mediated responses) and there is now evidence that chlamydial diseases result in part from hypersensitivity or are diseases of immunopathology.[12,27,99,100] The putative sensitizing antigen has been identified as belonging to the HSP60 class of heat shock proteins.[101] It may be synthesized by chlamydiae in cells where replication of the organism has been actively suppressed by the action of gamma interferon, and thus ongoing sensitization may occur.

There must be some sort of protective immune response to the organisms, because chlamydial infections tend to follow a fairly self-limited acute course, resolving into a low grade persistent infection which may last for years. These infections may be activated by a variety of stimuli, of which steroids represent one class. Other reactivating agents are not yet known but must exist, as spontaneous exacerbations occur.[102]

LGV is a truly lymphoproliferative disease, and the other chlamydiae appear to be capable of causing a more localized lymphoproliferative response, in the sense that they can induce follicle formation in the mucous membranes. Although such a response is most well known for the conjunctiva (trachoma and inclusion conjunctivitis), follicular cervicitis and probably follicular urethritis (cobblestone appearance of Waelsch urethritis) are recognized entities. Follicles induced by *C. trachomatis* are true lymphoid follicles with germinal centers.

Trachoma has long been considered a disease in which reinfection is important.[27] It has been speculated that hypersensitivity to chlamydial antigens in vaccine trials explains the deleterious outcome observed after inadequate vaccination and the more severe disease seen after heterotypic infection.[12,27] Resistance to reinfection appears to be predominantly serovar specific. In nonhuman primates, repeated (weekly) conjunctival instillation of *C. trachomatis* results in a disease with many of the manifestations of trachoma, including conjunctival scarring.[103] Similarly, in an experimental salpingitis model, it was found that severe salpingitis in nonhuman primates was also in part dependent on previous exposure to chlamydiae.[100] A common pathologic end point of chlamydial infection is scarring of the affected mucous membranes. This is what ultimately leads to blindness in trachoma and to infertility and ectopic pregnancy after acute salpingitis.

In the guinea-pig inclusion-conjunctivitis (GPIC) model, a triton-soluble extract of EBs induced an ocular hypersensitivity reaction when dropped onto the conjunctiva of previously infected animals, but it did not cause the same reaction in naive animals.[99] The reactive material appears to be genus specific, as similar results were obtained when the same extract was dropped onto the eyes of nonhuman primates that had been infected with the trachoma agent.[104]

The current prevalent theory is that much of the chlamydial disease is due to delayed hypersensitivity reactions to specific *Chlamydia* heat-shock proteins (HSP).[101] These HSPs are similar to the heat-shock proteins of other organisms.[105] HSP60 contains antigenic sites that are specific to chlamydiae, but it also has sites that are shared with mycobacteria and *Escherichia coli* and even with humans. Thus, the possibilities that part of chlamydial disease may be due to autoimmune reactions or that other infections could sensitize a person to worse disease following exposure to chlamydiae have also been considered. It is clear that low-level infections can produce relatively high quantities of HSP60 and that women who suffer from tubal-factor infertility and ectopic pregnancy often have high levels of antibody to *Chlamydia* HSP60.[105,106] It should be stressed that these are still theories and that direct proof from either human or animal studies has not been generated.

There are no satisfactory animal models for genital *C. trachomatis* infection. Nonhuman primates are susceptible to ocular and genital infections with the trachoma biovar. Much has been learned about the pathogenesis and immunity in ocular infections. Data suggesting that prior exposure is important in the poor outcome after oviduct infection have also been obtained in this model.[100] However, because of expense and difficulty of obtaining a large number of nonhuman primates, attempts have been made to develop models in smaller animals. The genital tract of female mice that have been treated with progesterone can be infected, and ascending infections can result in salpingitis and infertility.[107] Some workers have attempted to exploit naturally occurring chlamydial infection in smaller animals. The *C. psittaci* guinea pig inclusion conjunctivitis agent and the mouse pneumonitis biovar of *C. trachomatis* are both capable of infecting genital tracts of their natural host.[5,6,108] They are sexually transmitted and can cause tubal-factor infertility as a result of ascending infection in the female genital tract.[109–111]

DIAGNOSIS

The diagnosis of chlamydial diseases is discussed in Chapter 53.

ANTIMICROBIAL SUSCEPTIBILITY

There is no universally accepted protocol for testing the antibiotic susceptibility of *C. trachomatis*. A number of different procedures have been used, and the data presented in Table 28-4 present the range of results obtained for inhibitory levels in tissue culture systems. The simplest procedures involve infection of cell culture with a standard inoculum followed by addition of an antibiotic-containing medium. After an appropriate incubation period inclusion counts are performed, and the concentration of antibiotic resulting in 50% or 100% reduction in inclusion count is accepted as the minimum inhibitory concentration (MIC). This procedure tends to overestimate the activity of the drugs tested. A more rigorous test involves blind passage of inclusion-negative monolayers, in an effort to assure that the drugs in question actually killed the *Chlamydia*. In this test, the minimum concentration where no inclusions are detected on passage is considered to be the minimal cidal level.[112]

The most rigorous test of antimicrobial activity involves attempts to sterilize established infections in cell culture systems. In this test, the tissue culture monolayers are infected with *C. trachomatis* for approximately 48 hours, and then different drug levels are added to the infected cell culture systems. After a subsequent 24-hour incubation period, the cell cultures are washed and passed to determine whether the chlamydiae have been eradicated. This procedure is likely to underestimate the effective levels of drugs, since the antibiotics are added after the time they would be most active. (That time is during active replication or metabolism, which peaks at less than 48 hours.) In addition, the technique suffers from technical objections concerning potential carry-over of drugs into the second passage. This possibility is particularly present with those antimicrobials that are lipid soluble or that would have high intracellular penetration, as simple washing would not remove the drug from the monolayers and subsequent inoculum for the second passage.

Table 28-4. Minimum Inhibitory Concentration (MIC) of Antimicrobial Agents for *C. trachomatis*

Drug	MIC (μg/mL or U/mL)
Rifampin	0.005 – 0.25
Tetracyclines	0.03 – 1
Azithromycin	0.03 – 1
Erythromycin	0.1 – 1
Ofloxacin	0.5 – 1
Ampicillin	0.5 – 10
Penicillin	1 – 10
Sulfamethoxazole	0.5 – 4
Clindamycin	2 – 16
Spectinomycin	32 – 100
Gentamicin	500
Vancomycin	1,000

Citation adopted from previous edition.

Chlamydia trachomatis is susceptible to sulfonamides.[1] The organisms produce their own folic acid, and the enzymes in this synthetic pathway are susceptible to the action of the sulfonamides and to trimethoprim. Sulfonamides have been clinically effective in trachoma and lymphogranuloma venereum, but they are not used in treating most genital tract infections with *Chlamydia* because these drugs are not active against other organisms producing similar diseases.[26]

Azithromycin is currently considered the drug of choice for treating chlamydial infection.[113] Aside from excellent in vitro activity, this drug demonstrates prolonged bioavailability, which permits single-dose administration, and it accumulates within cells. Single-dose therapy with azithromycin has been shown to be as effective as a week-long course of doxycycline in treating chlamydial infection, but likely results in much better compliance, especially in nonstudy situations. The drug is similar to erythromycin in in vitro assays with MIC <1.0 mg/mL.[114]

Tetracyclines and erythromycin were formerly considered the drugs of choice in managing chlamydial genital tract infections. The organisms are highly susceptible in vitro and in vivo to the action of these antibiotics,[26,112] and resistance to these drugs has never been shown to occur naturally. Although there are documented treatment failures where chlamydiae have been isolated from patients following treatment, the recovered agents have been found to be wholly susceptible to the antibiotics. There is a suggestion that there may be some relative resistance to erythromycin and tetracycline, but there are no data to suggest that this has reached clinically relevant levels.[115,116] Rifampin, which is highly active in vitro, has not been widely used to treat human chlamydial infections. Resistance to this drug can be readily developed by passage in the laboratory in the presence of low concentrations of the antibiotic.[117]

Aminoglycosides are not active against *Chlamydia*, and this has led to their widespread use in controlling bacterial contamination in clinical specimens being tested for the presence of *Chlamydia*. Common antifungal drugs such as amphotericin-B and nystatin are also inactive against *Chlamydia*, as are the nitroimidazoles used to treat *Trichomonas* infections.

Penicillins are active against *Chlamydia* in vitro, but they are generally not clinically useful. By analogy from animal studies it has been calculated that levels on the order of 20 to 30 million units of penicillin per day would be required for antichlamydial activity in vivo. Cephalosporins are not active. Chlamydiae do have a cell wall similar to that of other bacteria, and its synthesis can be inhibited by penicillins, but only in the early phases of the growth cycle. Addition of penicillins to infected cells in vitro cannot be expected to show marked activity after 16 to 20 hours of infection, as at that stage active cell-wall synthesis is minimal. It is likely that one of the cell-wall inhibitors will ultimately be found to be clinically active against chlamydiae. There are now several studies that show a week of amoxicillin at 500 mg three times daily is effective in treating chlamydial infection in pregnant women. Many quinolones are active against chlamydia in vitro, but only ofloxacin has been clinically useful to date.

IMMUNOLOGY

There is little knowledge concerning the structure and chemistry of chlamydial antigens.[107] The biological role of antibodies or cell-mediated immunity (CMI) resulting from exposure to chlamydial antigens in either enhancing or protecting against disease or infection is also not yet clear. Much of the difficulty in studying chlamydial antigens is due to technical problems in obtaining adequate quantities of organisms for the physicochemical fractionation procedures that are commonly used to study antigenic structure. Thus, these organisms are ideal candidates for study by modern techniques of molecular biology and genetics. What is clear is that the chlamydiae are highly complex organisms which contain antigens of genus, species, subspecies, and serovar specificity.[118]

The most easily detected antigen is the chlamydial group antigen, shared by all members of the genus. This antigen is responsible for the complement-fixing reactions that have been commonly used to diagnose psittacosis or lymphogranuloma venereum. The group antigen is heat stable and periodate sensitive, and it can be extracted from infected tissues with ether or with detergents such as sodium lauryl sulfate or sodium deoxycholate. The reactive moiety was found to be a keto-deoxyoctanoic acid. Other, apparently protein, group antigens have been identified but have not been characterized. The major genus-specific antigen has been identified as the LPS.[119]

Chlamydial EBs and RBs contain an LPS antigenically similar to that of some gram-negative bacteria (*Acinetobacter calcoaceticus* and Re mutants of *Salmonella typhimurium*). Chlamydial LPS demonstrates a positive limulus lysate test. It is structurally similar to the lipid A and KDO core of LPS from rough (Re) mutants of *Salmonella typhimurium*.[120] Its chemical composition is also similar to that of *Salmonella typhimurium* LPS, but it appears to contain a unique constituent, 3-hydroxydocosanoic acid.[121] Chlamydial LPS has two antigen sites. One is identical to that of *Acinetobacter calcoaceticus* and *Salmonella typhimurium*, and the other is *Chlamydia* specific.[122] *Acinetobacter* LPS can be used as the CF antigen for antichlamydial antibodies, but not all sera that are positive against the chlamydial antigen will react to the *Acinetobacter* LPS.[120]

The antigens responsible for delayed hypersensitivity tests, such as the Frei test, which has been used in diagnosing lymphogranuloma venereum, have not been studied using modern techniques. The major antigen here is probably the LPS common group antigen because it is heat stable and sensitive to periodate. *C. psittaci* strains have been used successfully to prepare Frei antigens. There also appear to be specific antigens involved in delayed hypersensitivity responses, as more specific antigenic preparations can be prepared by acid extraction from the crude group antigen.

Species-specific antigens appear to be shared by all members of a chlamydial species. They have been demonstrated by indirect hemagglutination, immunodiffusion with sonicated organisms, and crossed immunoelectrophoresis with solubilized organisms. MOMP has an important species-specific antigen.[65,66] Another species-specific antigen, common to *C. trachomatis*, has been purified to homogeneity by immunoabsorption with monospecific antibody.[123] It is pronase and heat sensitive and of large molecular weight (1.55×10^5 Da). Antibody to this antigen is found in convalescent human sera from patients with lymphogranuloma venereum and those with high levels of antibody following other *C. trachomatis* infections.

The subspecies- or serovar-specific antigens are common only to selected strains within chlamydial species. These antigens have been the basis for a variety of serologic tests used for the classification of *C. trachomatis* isolates. They appear to be associated with the mortality observed following intravenous inoculation of mice with large quantities of viable chlamydiae. This death is termed a "toxic death" because it cannot be accounted for by multiplication of the organism; deaths occur within 24 hours, before a single cycle of replication can occur. The "toxic" affect of chlamydiae can be prevented by preincubation of the inoculum with hyperimmune serum. This "toxin"-neutralization is strain-specific and was first used to classify a variety of *C. psittaci* isolates.[124] A similar approach was used with *C. trachomatis* isolates, and it was found that immunization of mice could prevent lethality from homotypic toxic challenge. A mouse toxicity prevention test (MTPT) was developed which yielded a number of specific *C. trachomatis* serovars.[125,126] These serovars are identical to those shown by the microimmunofluorescence test (micro-IF).[127] The responsible antigens appear to be on the MOMP molecule.

To date, 18 serovars of *C. trachomatis* have been identified. A, B, and C serovars are usually associated with hyperendemic blinding trachoma in developing countries; D through K have been associated with oculogenital disease in industrialized societies; and L1, L2, and L3 are LGV serotypes. These serovars fall into two broad complexes (B and C) by micro-IF. Each complex shows extensive cross reaction within the complex but little reaction with the other complex. Serovar-specific monoclonal antibodies are now available for typing purposes.

The major outer-membrane protein appears to contain antigens of serovar, serogroup, and species specificity.[65,66,128] Minor genus-specific reactivity has also been shown. MOMP and the 60–62 kDa and 12–15kDa proteins may be copurified by sarkosyl extraction of EBs. The 60–62 kDa proteins are important immunogens and are often found as a doublet.[129] It is now clear that one of these is a cysteine-rich structural protein, while the other is a loosely bound HSP60. While MOMP appears to be the immunodominant antigen, there may be a more selective response to 60–62 kDa proteins. The latter proteins are surface exposed and have species-specific antigens. In contrast, the 15 kDa proteins are not on the EB surface. They contain antigens of species and biovar specificity.[130] Monoclonal antibodies directed against MOMP have been shown to be capable of neutralizing infectivity in cell culture and are protective against toxic effects seen in mice after intravenous inoculation of live EBs. They can also neutralize infectivity for ocular infection in subhuman primates.[131] Monoclonal antibodies against nonsurface subspecies, species-specific epitopes, or the LPS neither protected mice nor neutralized infectivity for the eye. The neutralization reactions usually appear to be serovar or serogroup specific.[132]

The outer membrane of *Chlamydia* is a particularly interesting structure because in the EB it represents a target for immune attack. There have been a number of functions identified with putative protective antigens in the outer membrane. These functions, including specific attachment, enhanced phagocytosis, and phagolysosomal fusion inhibition, are all neutralized by specific antibody. Although a number of protein antigens have been identified, and MOMP and other proteins induce neutralizing antibody, no virulence antigen has been specifically identified.

CONTROL OF CHLAMYDIAL INFECTION BY THE HOST

In the majority of chlamydial infections only a relatively small proportion of cells at affected sites are found to be infected. Because each inclusion releases hundreds of viable EBs and relatively few nearby cells are infected, there must be control mechanisms that limit infectivity. The mechanisms are not clear, although T-cell functions seem important. Lymphokines have been shown to have an inhibitory effect on chlamydiae.[133] *Chlamydia trachomatis* is sensitive to alpha, beta, and gamma interferons.[134] The last of these appears to be most active. The lymphokine which inhibits *Chlamydia* in human macrophages and in mice has been identified as gamma interferon.[135,136] The interferon appears to delay the developmental cycle so that the RBs persist for a longer period of time.[137,138] This may result in persistent inapparent infection and may also play a role in immunopathogenesis. The mode of action appears to be the same as in other systems and involves depletion of tryptophan, making tryptophan unavailable to the chlamydiae.[81] The effect is reversible by addition of exogenous tryptophan.

It is likely that mechanisms such as the apparent effect of gamma interferon represent control of infection rather than protection against new infection. They may be involved in clearance. It is possible that neutralizing antibody plays a role, but even the mechanism by which neutralizing antibody would act is not known. Antibody against MOMP has been shown to neutralize infectivity, but surprisingly, it did not interfere with chlamydial attachment, ingestion, or inhibition of phagolysosomal fusion.[44]

IMMUNITY

Immunity induced by chlamydial infection is not well understood. It is clear that single infections will not result in solid immunity to reinfection. Multiple infections, homo- or heterotypic, are common. Unfortunately, the natural infection is not readily quantifiable in terms of inoculum size, and thus relative degrees of immunity may exist which are overcome with a sufficiently large challenge. Some immunity probably develops following initial or serial infection. In screening studies, younger women are found to have higher cervical infection rates than older women, who often have higher antibody levels. This speculation is also consistent with the observation that many isolate-negative individuals attending STD clinics have IgM antibody to the organism.[139] This antibody could result from recent exposure and rapid resolution of the infection or its ablation by an immune response.

The only human chlamydial infection which has been subjected to extensive vaccine studies is trachoma. Unfortunately, these studies were performed without a sophisticated knowledge of the chlamydial immune response. These results have been summarized elsewhere.[12,27] The results from field studies on vaccine trials and infection of human volunteers and subhuman primates indicate that there is a short-lived relative immunity to reinfection with homotypic challenge. Heterotypic infection may result in more severe disease, as may also occur following vaccination with a poor (that is, nonprotective) immunogen.

Data from ocular infection with *C. psittaci* in guinea pigs and *C. trachomatis* in subhuman primates suggest an important role for antibody in host defense.[140–142] Antibody is capable of neutralizing chlamydial infectivity in cell culture. There are many possible modes of action. Antibody can inhibit attachment of the organism to the surface of a nonprofessional phagocyte, or result in failure to inhibit phagolysosomal fusion, or prevent a morphologic shift of the EBs and RBs by cross-linking surface proteins. Antibody may opsonize. Antibody that blocks attachment of *C. psittaci* to L cells enhances attachment to macrophages.[143]

There are now many in vitro studies showing that immunization with purified, synthesized, or recombinant peptides can induce neutralizing antibodies. Synthetic vaccines have been developed, sometimes by artificially juxtaposing synthesized conjugates of T-helper sites with selected B-cell sites predicted to result in neutralizing antibody and finding that such antibodies are indeed generated. In some instances, these immunizing peptides have been linked by genetic manipulation and expressed in *E. coli*. One interesting approach was incorporation of such peptides into a polio vaccine vector.[144] While it has been relatively easy to induce neutralizing antibodies as assayed in vitro, these approaches are aimed at inducing neutralizing antibody while not sensitizing the host to deleterious outcome on subsequent exposure to *Chlamydia* through exposure to heat-shock proteins. The vaccines have so far failed to protect animals from subsequent challenge.

Chlamydia do not appear to survive well in polymorphonuclear leukocytes (PMN).[145] It is possible that antibody-enhanced phagocytosis plays an important role in clearance of infection and in resistance to reinfection. Chlamydia are rapidly internalized by human PMNs, and the majority are rendered noninfectious within one hour. Most of the EBs are found in PMN phagosomes where lysosomal fusion has occurred.[146] The mechanism of killing by PMNs is not known, but it is likely that oxygen-dependent and oxygen-independent mechanisms are involved. Killing is still seen in the presence of inhibitors such as azide or cyanide.[145] Both species of chlamydiae act as polyclonal stimulators of B-lymphocytes.[147] Stimulation can be effected in mice that are LPS nonresponders, suggesting that something other than the genus-specific antigen is responsible.

Leukocytes clearly play an important role in resistance to infection and in clearance of primary infection. T-cell deficient mice do not produce significant levels of antichlamydial antibody.[148] Lymphocyte transformation in vitro and delayed hypersensitivity reactions are also T-cell dependent. They can be found in heterozygous mice and in mice who received thymus transplants but are not observed in the nude athymic mouse.[149,150]

Williams and colleagues have exploited the athymic mouse model of respiratory infection with the mouse pneumonitis biovar of *C. trachomatis* to dissect the immune response.[148,150–152] Results of these studies have suggested a defense role for both antibody and CMI responses. Both CD4+ and CD8+ T cells have protective roles in animal models.[153] The predominant accumulating evidence suggests that Th1-type cell responses involving CD4+ T-helper cells are likely to play an important role in protective immunity.[154,155] However, the actual mechanism of immunity is unclear, and the demonstration that cytotoxic CD8+ T lymphocytes are capable of lysing chlamydia-infected cells suggests that these cells too could play a role.[156]

VACCINE AND VIRULENCE FACTORS

Because the responsible surface antigens would be likely vaccine candidates, efforts to identify the factors responsible for attachment, enhanced uptake, and inhibition of phagolysosomal fusion will continue to be stressed. All evidence to date suggests that MOMP must be an extremely important antigen in some of these activities. Inhibition of these virulence determinants appears to be serovar specific. The only antigenic sites of that specificity that have been clearly identified are on MOMP. A likely alternative approach to vaccine development will be to use information obtained from sequence analysis of the MOMP genes to synthesize peptides reflecting the variable (presumed serovar specific) sites on the protein.[96] Because these variable sequences are fairly short—approximately eleven amino acids long—their synthesis should be relatively easy. Incorporation of the synthetic peptides into appropriate carriers could allow development of experimental vaccines and tools for identifying virulence factors.

The importance of T cells in immunity appears to be a recurring theme. Both humoral and CMI responses are T-cell dependent. Identification of specific T-cell recognition sites on the EB surface (or on MOMP) may be crucial to understanding chlamydial immunity, particularly because they may not be the antigenic epitopes.

A real problem with vaccine development will be generating immune responses that appear to be better than those that occur after natural infection. While much progress is being made on the microbiologic front, particularly in cloning the MOMP genes and identifying the potential antigenic sites, it is clear that considerable input from immunologists will be required to generate optimal methods for antigen presentation to enhance mucous-membrane immunity. Even if protective immune responses can be induced by a vaccine, the ultimate success of such a vaccine will depend, in part, on the antigenic stability of the organism. There is evidence of a high degree of immunologic variation within the variable regions of MOMP, which is at the moment the likeliest antigen candidate for use in a vaccine. Identification of high rates of DNA polymorphism in the MOMP gene among prostitutes in Nairobi suggest the possibility of immune selection and evasion, which may present further problems for would-be developers of a vaccine.[157]

References

1 Moulder JW: Order Chlamydiales and family Chlamydiaceae, in *Manual of Systematic Bacteriology*, vol 1, NR Krieg (ed). Baltimore, Williams and Wilkins, 1984, p 729.

2 Meyer KF: The host spectrum of psittacosis-lymphogranuloma venereum (PL) agents. *Am J Ophthalmol* 63:1225, 1967.

3 Grayston JT et al: Evidence that *Chlamydia pneumoniae* causes pneumonia and bronchitis. *J Infect Dis* 168:1231, 1993.

4 Fukushi H, Hirai K: *Chlamydia pecorum*—the fourth species of genus *Chlamydia*. *Microbiol Immunol* 37:516, 1993.

5 Murray ES: Guinea pig inclusion conjunctivitis virus. I. Isolation and identification as a member of the psittacosis-lymphogranuloma-trachoma group. *J Infect Dis* 114:1, 1964.

6 Mount DT et al: Experimental genital infection of male guinea pigs with the agent of guinea pig inclusion conjunctivitis and transmission to females. *Infect Immun* 8:925, 1973.

7 Storz J et al: Advances in Detection and Differentiation of Chlamydiae from Animals, in *Chlamydial Infections: Proceedings of the 8th International Symposium on Human Chlamydial Infections,* J Orfila et al (eds). Bologna, Italy, Societa Editrice Escuapio, 1994, pp 563–573.

8 Moulder JW: Intracellular parasitism: life in an extreme environment. *J Infect Dis* 130:300, 1974.

9 Byrne GI: Requirements of ingestion of *Chlamydia psittaci* by mouse fibroblasts (L cells). *Infect Immun* 14:645, 1976.

10 Friis RR: Interaction of L cells and *Chlamydia psittaci:* entry of the parasite and host responses to its development. *J Bacteriol* 110:706, 1972.

11 Zhang JP, Stephens RS: Mechanism of *C. trachomatis* attachment to eukaryotic host cells. *Cell* 69:861, 1992.

12 Schachter J, Dawson CR: *Human Chlamydial Infections*. Littleton, MA, PSG, 1978.

13 Lindner K: Gonoblennorrhoe, einschlussblennorrhoe und trachoma. *Albrecht von Graefes Arch Ophthalmol* 78:380, 1911.

14 T'ang FF et al: Trachoma virus in chick embryo. *Natl Med J China* 43:81, 1957.

15 Jones BR et al: Isolation of virus from inclusion blennorrhoea. *Lancet* 1:902, 1959.

16 Jones BR: Ocular syndromes of TRIC virus infection and their possible genital significance. *Br J Vener Dis* 40:3, 1964.

17 Rose L, Schachter J: Genitourinary aspects of inclusion conjunctivitis. *Invest Ophthalmol* 3:680, 1964.

18 Dunlop EM et al: Relation of TRIC agent to "non-specific genital infection". *Br J Vener Dis* 42:77, 1966.

19 Dunlop EM et al: Infection by TRIC agent and other members of the Bedsonia group; with a note on Reiter's disease. 3. Genital infection and disease of the eye. *Trans Ophthalmol Soc UK* 86:321, 1966.

20 Dunlop EMC et al: Genital infection in association with TRIC virus infection of the eye. III. Clinical and other findings. Preliminary report. *Br J Vener Dis* 40:33, 1964.

21 Gordon FB, Quan AL: Isolation of the trachoma agent in cell culture. *Proc Soc Exp Biol Med* 118:354, 1965.

22 Darougar S et al: Chlamydial infection. Advances in the diagnostic isolation of *Chlamydia*, including TRIC agent from the eye, genital tract, and rectum. *Br J Vener Dis* 48:416, 1972.

23 Oriel JD et al: Infection with *Chlamydia* group A in men with urethritis due to *Neisseria gonorrhoeae*. *J Infect Dis* 131:376, 1975.

24 Richmond SJ et al: Chlamydial infection. Role of *Chlamydia* subgroup A in non-gonococcal and post-gonococcal urethritis. *Br J Vener Dis* 48:437, 1972.

25 Dunlop EMC et al: Isolation of *Chlamydia* from the urethra of a woman. *Br Med J* 2:386, 1972.

26 Schachter J: Chlamydial infections (in 3 parts). *N Engl J Med* 298: 428, 490, 540, 1978.

27 Grayston JT, Wang S: New knowledge of chlamydiae and the diseases they cause. *J Infect Dis* 132:87, 1975.

28 Schachter J et al: Prospective study of perinatal transmission of *Chlamydia trachomatis*. *JAMA* 255:3374, 1986.

29 Jones BR: The prevention of blindness from trachoma. *Trans Ophthalmol Soc UK* 95:16, 1975.

30 Schachter J, Dawson CR: The epidemiology of trachoma predicts more blindness in the future. *Scand J Infect Dis* Suppl 69:55, 1990.

31 Treharne JD: The community epidemiology of trachoma. *Rev Infect Dis* 7:760, 1985.

32 Kuo CC et al: Immunotypes of *Chlamydia trachomatis* isolates in Seattle, Washington. *Infect Immun* 41:865, 1983.

33 Dean D et al: Comparison of the major outer membrane protein variant sequence regions of B/Ba isolates: a molecular epidemiologic approach to *Chlamydia trachomatis* infections. *J Infect Dis* 166:383, 1992.

34 Lampe MF et al: Nucleotide sequence of the variable domains within the major outer membrane protein gene from serovariants of *Chlamydia trachomatis*. *Infect Immun* 61:213, 1993.

35 Stephens RS et al: High-resolution mapping of serovar-specific and common antigenic determinants of the major outer membrane protein of *Chlamydia trachomatis*. *J Exp Med* 167:817, 1988.

36 Moulder JW: The relation of the psittacosis group (Chlamydiae) to bacteria and viruses. *Annu Rev Microbiol* 20:107, 1966.

37 Weiss E: Comparative metabolism of rickettsiae and other host dependent bacteria. *Zentralbl Bakteriol [Orig]* 206:292, 1968.

38 Kellogg KR, et al: Toxicity of low and moderate multiplicities of *Chlamydia psittaci* for mouse fibroblasts (L cells). *Infect Immun* 18: 531, 1977.

39 Kuo CC et al: Effect of polycations, polyanions, and neuraminidase on the infectivity of trachoma-inclusion conjunctivitis and lymphogranuloma venereum organisms' HeLa cells: sialic acid residues as

possible receptors for trachoma-inclusion conjunction. *Infect Immun* 8:74, 1973.

40 Byrne GI, Moulder JW: Parasite-specified phagocytosis of *Chlamydia psittaci* and *Chlamydia trachomatis* by L and HeLa cells. *Infect Immun* 19:598, 1978.

41 Lee CK: Interaction between a trachoma strain of *Chlamydia trachomatis* and mouse fibroblasts (McCoy cells) in the absence of centrifugation. *Infect Immun* 31:584, 1981.

42 Hatch TP et al: Attachment of *Chlamydia psittaci* to formaldehyde-fixed and unfixed L cells. *J Gen Microbiol* 125:273, 1981.

43 Hackstadt T, Caldwell HD: Effect of proteolytic cleavage of surface-exposed proteins on infectivity of *Chlamydia trachomatis*. *Infect Immun* 48:546, 1985.

44 Caldwell HD, Perry LJ: Neutralization of *Chlamydia trachomatis* infectivity with antibodies to the major outer membrane protein. *Infect Immun* 38:745, 1982.

45 Peeling R et al: In vitro neutralization of *Chlamydia trachomatis* with monoclonal antibody to an epitope on the major outer membrane protein. *Infect Immun* 46:484, 1984.

46 Moulder JW: Comparative biology of intracellular parasitism. *Microbiol Rev* 49:298, 1985.

47 Hodinka RL, Wyrick PB: Ultrastructural study of mode of entry of *Chlamydia psittaci* into L-929 cells. *Infect Immun* 54:855, 1986.

48 Ward ME, Murray A: Control mechanisms governing the infectivity of *Chlamydia trachomatis* for HeLa cells: mechanisms of endocytosis. *J Gen Microbiol* 130:1765, 1984.

49 Eissenberg LG et al: *Chlamydia psittaci* elementary body envelopes: ingestion and inhibition of phagolysosome fusion. *Infect Immun* 40:741, 1983.

50 Brownridge E, Wyrick PB: Interaction of *Chlamydia psittaci* reticulate bodies with mouse peritoneal macrophages. *Infect Immun* 24:697, 1979.

51 Eissenberg LG, Wyrick PB: Inhibition of phagolysosome fusion is localized to *Chlamydia psittaci*-laden vacuoles. *Infect Immun* 32:889, 1981.

52 Hatch TP et al: Adenine nucleotide and lysine transport in *Chlamydia psittaci*. *J Bacteriol* 150:662, 1982.

53 Newhall WJ: Biosynthesis and disulfide cross-linking of outer membrane components during the growth cycle of *Chlamydia trachomatis*. *Infect Immun* 55:162, 1987.

54 Hatch TP et al: Synthesis of disulfide-bonded outer membrane proteins during the developmental cycle of *Chlamydia psittaci* and *Chlamydia trachomatis*. *J Bacteriol* 165:379, 1986.

55 Doughri AM et al: Mode of entry and release of chlamydiae in infections of intestinal epithelial cells. *J Infect Dis* 126:652, 1972.

56 Matsumoto A, Manire GP: Electron microscopic observations on the fine structure of cell walls of *Chlamydia psittaci*. *J Bacteriol* 104:1332, 1970.

57 Garrett AJ et al: A search for the bacterial mucopeptide component, muramic acid, in Chlamydia. *J Gen Microbiol* 80:315, 1974.

58 Matsumoto A, Manire GP: Electron microscopic observations on the effects of penicillin on the morphology of *Chlamydia psittaci*. *J Bacteriol* 101:278, 1970.

59 Caldwell HD et al: Purification and partial characterization of the major outer membrane protein of *Chlamydia trachomatis*. *Infect Immun* 31:1161, 1981.

60 Salari SH, Ward ME: Polypeptide composition of *Chlamydia trachomatis*. *J Gen Microbiol* 123:197, 1981.

61 Hatch TP et al: Structural and polypeptide differences between envelopes of infective and reproductive life cycle forms of *Chlamydia* spp. *J Bacteriol* 157:13, 1984.

62 Newhall WJ, Jones RB: Disulfide-linked oligomers of the major outer membrane protein of chlamydiae. *J Bacteriol* 154:998, 1983.

63 Bavoil P et al: Role of disulfide bonding in outer membrane structure and permeability in Chlamydia trachomatis. *Infect Immun* 44:479, 1984.

64 Hackstadt T et al: Disulfide-mediated interactions of the chlamydial major outer membrane protein: role in the differentiation of chlamydiae? *J Bacteriol* 161:25, 1985.

65 Caldwell HD, Schachter J: Antigenic analysis of the major outer membrane protein of Chlamydia spp. *Infect Immun* 35:1024, 1982.

66 Stephens RS et al: Monoclonal antibodies to *Chlamydia trachomatis*: antibody specificities and antigen characterization. *J Immunol* 128:1083, 1982.

67 Jenkin HM et al: Species-specific antigens from the cell walls of the agents of meningopneumonitis and feline pneumonitis. *J Immunol* 86:123, 1961.

68 Pelc SR, Crocker TT: Differences in utilization of labelled precursors for the synthesis of deoxyribonucleic acid in cell nuclei and psittacosis virus. *Biochem J* 78:1, 1961.

69 Lin HS: Inhibition of thymidine kinase activity and deoxyribonucleic acid synthesis in L cells infected with the meningopneumonitis agent. *J Bacteriol* 96:2054, 1968.

70 Gregory WW et al: Arrays of hemispheric surface projections on *Chlamydia psittaci* and *Chlamydia trachomatis* observed by scanning electron microscopy. *J Bacteriol* 138:241, 1979.

71 Barbour AG et al: *Chlamydia trachomatis* has penicillin-binding proteins but not detectable muramic acid. *J Bacteriol* 151:420, 1982.

72 Moulder JW et al: Inhibition of the growth of agents of the psittacosis group by D-cycloserine and its specific reversal by D-alanine. *J Bacteriol* 85:707, 1963.

73 Stamm WE: Diagnosis of *Chlamydia trachomatis* genitourinary infections. *Ann Intern Med* 108:710, 1988.

74 Kuo C et al: Primary isolation of TRIC organisms in HeLa 229 cells treated with DEAE-dextran. *J Infect Dis* 125:665, 1972.

75 Weiss E, Dressler HR: Centrifugation of rickettsiae and viruses onto cells and its effect on infection. *Proc Soc Exp Biol Med* 103:691, 1960.

76 Ripa KT, Mardh PA: Cultivation of *Chlamydia trachomatis* in cycloheximide-treated McCoy cells. *J Clin Microbiol* 6:328, 1977.

77 Bader JP, Morgan HR: Latent viral infections of cells in culture. VI. Role of amino acids, glucose, and glutamine in psittacosis virus propagation in L cells. *J Exp Med* 106:617, 1958.

78 Hatch TP: Competition between *Chlamydia psittaci* and L cells for host isoleucine pools: a limiting factor in chlamydial multiplication. *Infect Immun* 12:211, 1975.

79 Allan I, Pearce JH: Amino acid requirements of strains of *Chlamydia trachomatis* and *C. psittaci* growing in McCoy cells: relationship with clinical syndrome and host origin. *J Gen Microbiol* 129(Pt 7):2001, 1983.

80 Stirling P et al: Interference with transformation of chlamydiae from productive to infective body forms by deprivation of cysteine. *FEMS Microbiol Lett* 19:133, 1983.

81 Byrne GI et al: Introduction of tryptophan catabolism is the mechanism for gamma-interferon-mediated inhibition of intracellular *Chlamydia psittaci* replication. *Infect Immun* 53:347, 1986.

82 Hatch TP et al: Synthesis of protein in host-free reticulate bodies of *Chlamydia psittaci* and *Chlamydia trachomatis*. *J Bacteriol* 162:938, 1985.

83 Weiss E, Wilson NN: Role of exogenous adenosine triphosphate in catabolic and synthetic activities of *Chlamydia psittaci*. *J Bacteriol* 97:719, 1969.

84 Ward ME, Salari H: Control mechanisms governing the infectivity of *Chlamydia trachomatis* for HeLa cells: modulation by cyclic nucleotides, prostaglandins, and calcium. *J Gen Microbiol* 128(Pt 3):639, 1982.

85 Kaul R, Wenman WM: Cyclic AMP inhibits developmental regulation of *Chlamydia trachomatis*. *J Bacteriol* 168:722, 1986.

86 Bose SK, Goswami PC: Enhancement of adherence and growth of *Chlamydia trachomatis* by estrogen treatment of HeLa cells. *Infect Immun* 53:646, 1986.

87 Moses EB et al: Enhancement of growth of the chlamydial agent of guinea pig inclusion conjunctivitis in HeLa cells by estradiol. *Curr Microbiol* 11:265, 1984.

88 Kingsbury DT, Weiss E: Lack of deoxyribonucleic acid homology between species of the genus *Chlamydia*. *J Bacteriol* 96:1421, 1968.

89 Kingsbury DT: Estimate of the genome size of various microorganisms. *J Bacteriol* 98:1400, 1969.

90 Peterson EM, de la Maza LM: Characterization of *Chlamydia* DNA by restriction endonuclease cleavage. *Infect Immun* 41:604, 1983.
91 Palmer L, Falkow S: A common plasmid of *Chlamydia trachomatis*. *Plasmid* 16:52, 1986.
92 Joseph T et al: Molecular characterization of *Chlamydia trachomatis* and *Chlamydia psittaci* plasmids. *Infect Immun* 51:699, 1986.
93 Comanducci et al: Humoral immune response to plasmid protein pgp3 in patients with *Chlamydia trachomatis* infection. *Infect Immun* 62:5491, 1994.
94 Weisburg WG et al: Eubacterial origin of chlamydiae. *J Bacteriol* 167: 570, 1986.
95 Nano FE, Caldwell HD: Expression of the chlamydial genus-specific lipopolysaccharide epitope in *Escherichia coli*. *Science* 228:742, 1985.
96 Stephens RS et al: Diversity of *Chlamydia trachomatis* major outer membrane protein genes. *J Bacteriol* 169:3879, 1987.
97 Pickett MA et al: Complete nucleotide sequence of the major outer membrane protein gene from *Chlamydia trachomatis* serovar L1. *FEMS Microbiol Lett* 1987:185, 1987.
98 Kuo CC: Cultures of *Chlamydia trachomatis* in mouse peritoneal macrophages: factors affecting organism growth. *Infect Immun* 20: 439, 1978.
99 Watkins NG et al: Ocular delayed hypersensitivity: a pathogenetic mechanism of chlamydial-conjunctivitis in guinea pigs. *Proc Natl Acad Sci USA* 83:7480, 1986.
100 Patton DL et al: Distal tubal obstruction induced by repeated *Chlamydia trachomatis* salpingeal infections in pig-tailed macaques. *J Infect Dis* 155:1292, 1987.
101 Morrison RP et al: Chlamydial disease pathogenesis. The 57-kD chlamydial hypersensitivity antigen is a stress response protein. *J Exp Med* 170:1271, 1989.
102 Beatty WL et al: Morphologic and antigenic characterization of interferon gamma-mediated persistent *Chlamydia trachomatis* infection in vitro. *Proc Natl Acad Sci USA* 90:3998, 1993.
103 Taylor HR et al: An animal model of trachoma II. The importance of repeated reinfection. *Invest Ophthalmol Vis Sci* 23:507, 1982.
104 Taylor HR et al: Pathogenesis of trachoma: the stimulus for inflammation. *J Immunol* 138:3023, 1987.
105 Wagar EA et al: Differential human serologic response to two 60,000 molecular weight *Chlamydia trachomatis* antigens. *J Infect Dis* 162: 922, 1990.
106 Toye B et al: Association between antibody to the chlamydial heat-shock protein and tubal infertility. *J Infect Dis* 168:1236, 1993.
107 Tuffrey M et al: Infertility in mice infected genitally with a human strain of *Chlamydia trachomatis*. *J Reprod Fertil* 78:251, 1986.
108 Barron AL et al: Immune response in mice infected in the genital tract with mouse pneumonitis agent (*Chlamydia trachomatis* biovar). *Infect Immun* 44:82, 1984.
109 Schachter J et al: Hydrosalpinx As a Consequence of Chlamydial Salpingitis in the Guinea Pig, in *Chlamydial Infections: Proceedings of the 5th International Symposium on Human Chlamydial Infections*, PA Mardh et al (eds). New York, Elsevier, 1982, p 454.
110 Swenson CE et al: *Chlamydia trachomatis*-induced salpingitis in mice. *J Infect Dis* 148:1101, 1983.
111 Swenson CE, Schachter J: Infertility as a consequence of chlamydial infection of the upper genital tract in female mice. *Sex Transm Dis* 11:64, 1984.
112 Ridgway GL et al: A method for testing the antibiotic susceptibility of *Chlamydia trachomatis* in a cell culture system. *J Antimicrob Chemother* 2:71, 1976.
113 Martin DH et al: A controlled trial of a single dose of azithromycin for the treatment of chlamydial urethritis and cervicitis. The Azithromycin for Chlamydial Infections Study Group. *N Engl J Med* 327: 921, 1992.
114 Agacfidan A et al: In vitro activity of azithromycin (CP-62,993) against *Chlamydia trachomatis* and *Chlamydia pneumoniae*. *Antimicrob Agents Chemother* 37:1746, 1993.
115 Mourad A et al: Relative resistance to erythromycin in *Chlamydia trachomatis*. *Antimicrob Agents Chemother* 18:696, 1980.
116 Jones RB et al: Partial characterization of *Chlamydia trachomatis* isolates resistant to multiple antibiotics. *J Infect Dis* 162:1309, 1990.
117 Schachter J: Rifampin in chlamydial infections. *Rev Infect Dis* 5(Suppl 3):S562, 1983.
118 Schachter J, Caldwell H: Chlamydiae. *Annu Rev Microbiol* 34:285, 1980.
119 Nurminen M et al: The genus-specific antigen of *Chlamydia*: resemblance to the lipopolysaccharide of enteric bacteria. *Science* 220: 1279, 1983.
120 Nurminen M et al: Immunologically related ketodeoxyoctonate-containing structures in *Chlamydia trachomatis*, Re mutants of *Salmonella* species, and *Acinetobacter calcoaceticus* var. *anitratus*. *Infect Immun* 44:609, 1984.
121 Nurminen M et al: Chemical characterization of *Chlamydia trachomatis* lipopolysaccharide. *Infect Immun* 48:573, 1985.
122 Brade L et al: Antigenic properties of *Chlamydia trachomatis* lipopolysaccharide. *Infect Immun* 48:569, 1985.
123 Caldwell HD et al: Antigen analysis of chlamydiae by two dimensional immunoelectrophoresis. II. A trachoma-LGV specific antigen. *J Immunol* 115:969, 1975.
124 Manire GP, Meyer KF: The toxins of the psittacosis-lymphogranuloma group of agents. III. Differentiation of strains by the toxin neutralization test. *J Infect Dis* 86:241, 1950.
125 Bell SD et al: Immunization of mice against toxic doses of homologous elementary bodies of trachoma. *Science* 130:626, 1959.
126 Alexander ER et al: Further classification of TRIC agents from ocular trachoma and other sources of the mouse toxicity prevention test. *Am J Ophthalmol* 63:1469, 1967.
127 Wang SP, Grayston JT: Immunologic relationship between genital TRIC, lymphogranuloma venereum, and related organisms in a new microtiter indirect immunofluorescence test. *Am J Ophthalmol* 70: 367, 1970.
128 Batteiger BE et al: Antigenic analysis of the major outer membrane protein of *Chlamydia trachomatis* with murine monoclonal antibodies. *Infect Immun* 53:530, 1986.
129 Newhall WJ et al: Analysis of the human serological response to proteins of *Chlamydia trachomatis*. *Infect Immun* 38:1181, 1982.
130 Zhang YX et al: The low-molecular-mass, cysteine-rich outer membrane protein of *Chlamydia trachomatis* possesses both biovar- and species-specific epitopes. *Infect Immun* 55:2570, 1987.
131 Zhang YX et al: Protective monoclonal antibodies recognize epitopes located on the major outer membrane protein of *Chlamydia trachomatis*. *J Immunol* 138:575, 1987.
132 Lucero ME, Kuo CC: Neutralization of *Chlamydia trachomatis* cell culture infection by serovar-specific monoclonal antibodies. *Infect Immun* 50:595, 1985.
133 Byrne GI, Faubion CL: Lymphokine-mediated microbistatic mechanisms restrict *Chlamydia psittaci* growth in macrophages. *J Immunol* 128:469, 1982.
134 Czarniecki CW et al: Interferon-Induced Inhibition of *Chlamydia trachomatis*: Dissociation from Other Biological Activities of Interferons, in *Interferons as Cell Growth Inhibitors and Antitumor Factors: Proceedings of a Schering Corporation-UCLA Symposium*, RM Friedman et al (eds). New York, Liss, 1986, pp 467–480.
135 Rothermel CD et al: Gamma-interferon is the factor in lymphokine that activates human macrophages to inhibit intracellular *Chlamydia psittaci* replication. *J Immunol* 131:2542, 1983.
136 Byrne GI, Kreuger DA: Lymphokine-mediated inhibition of *Chlamydia* replication in mouse fibroblasts is neutralized by anti-gamma interferon immunoglobulin. *Infect Immun* 42:1152, 1983.
137 Rothermel CD et al: Chlamydia trachomatis-induced production of interleukin-1 by human monocytes. *Infect Immun* 57:2705, 1989.
138 Shemer Y, Sarov I: Inhibition of growth of *Chlamydia trachomatis* by human gamma interferon. *Infect Immun* 48:592, 1985.
139 Philip RN et al: Fluorescent antibody responses to chlamydial infection in patients with lymphogranuloma venereum and urethritis. *J Immunol* 112:2126, 1974.
140 Ahmad A et al: Resistance to reinfection with a chlamydial agent (guinea pig inclusion conjunctivitis agent). *Invest Ophthalmol Vis Sci* 16:549, 1977.

141 Barenfanger J, MacDonald AB: The role of immunoglobulin in the neutralization of trachoma infectivity. *J Immunol* 113:1607, 1974.

142 Rank RG, Barron AL: Humoral immune response in acquired immunity to chlamydial genital infection of female guinea pigs. *Infect Immun* 39:463, 1983.

143 Gardner M: Differences Between the Interaction of *Chlamydia psittaci* (6BC) with Professional (Mouse Macrophages) and Nonprofessional (Mouse Fibroblasts) Phagocytes, in *Abstracts of the Annual Meeting of the American Society for Microbiology*. Washington DC, American Society for Microbiology, 1977, abstr D6.

144 Murdin AD et al: A poliovirus hybrid expressing a neutralization epitope from the major outer membrane protein of *Chlamydia trachomatis* is highly immunogenic. *Infect Immun* 61:4406, 1993.

145 Yong EC et al: Toxic effect of human polymorphonuclear leukocytes on *Chlamydia trachomatis*. *Infect Immun* 37:422, 1982.

146 Yong EC et al: Degradation of *Chlamydia trachomatis* in human polymorphonuclear leukocytes: an ultrastructural study of peroxidase-positive phagolysosomes. *Infect Immun* 53:427, 1986.

147 Levitt D et al: Both species of chlamydia and two biovars of *Chlamydia trachomatis* stimulate mouse B lymphocytes. *J Immunol* 136: 4249, 1986.

148 Williams DM et al: The role of antibody in host defense against the agent of mouse pneumonitis. *J Infect Dis* 145:200, 1982.

149 Rank RG et al: Chronic chlamydial genital infection in congenitally athymic nude mice. *Infect Immun* 48:847, 1985.

150 Williams DM et al: Cellular immunity to the mouse pneumonitis agent. *J Infect Dis* 149:630, 1984.

151 Williams DM et al: Primary murine *Chlamydia trachomatis* pneumonia in B-cell-deficient mice. *Infect Immun* 55:2387, 1987.

152 Williams DM et al: Role of natural killer cells in infection with the mouse pneumonitis agent (murine *Chlamydia trachomatis*). *Infect Immun* 55:223, 1987.

153 Igietseme JU et al: Role for CD8+ T cells in antichlamydial immunity defined by *Chlamydia*-specific T-lymphocyte clones. *Infect Immun* 62:5195, 1994.

154 Cain TK, Rank RG: Local Th1-like responses are induced by intravaginal infection of mice with the mouse pneumonitis biovar of *Chlamydia trachomatis*. *Infect Immun* 63:1784, 1995.

155 Su H, Caldwell HD: CD4+ T cells play a significant role in adoptive immunity to *Chlamydia trachomatis* infection of the mouse genital tract. *Infect Immun* 63:3302, 1995.

156 Beatty PR, Stephens RS: CD8+ T lymphocyte-mediated lysis of *Chlamydia*-infected L cells using an endogenous antigen pathway. *J Immunol* 153:4588, 1994.

157 Brunham RC et al: The epidemiology of *Chlamydia trachomatis* within a sexually transmitted diseases core group. *J Infect Dis* 173: 950, 1996.

Chapter 29

Chlamydia trachomatis infections of the adult

Walter E. Stamm

Since the early 1970s, *Chlamydia trachomatis* has been recognized as a genital pathogen responsible for an increasing variety of clinical syndromes, many closely resembling infections caused by *Neisseria gonorrhoeae* (Table 29-1). Because many practitioners have lacked access to facilities for laboratory testing for chlamydia, these infections often have been diagnosed and treated without benefit of microbiological confirmation. Newer, noncultural diagnostic tests have in part now addressed this problem, making specific diagnosis much more widely available. However, diagnostic tests are still not available to many clinicians in industrialized countries and to most providers in developing countries. Unfortunately, many chlamydial infections, particularly in women, are difficult to diagnose clinically and elude detection because they produce few or no symptoms and because the symptoms and signs they do produce are nonspecific. The high prevalence of these infections in many parts of the world thus in large part has resulted from inadequate laboratory facilities for their detection and eventual treatment, coupled with the nonspecific and minimal signs and symptoms chlamydial infections produce, the lack of familiarity clinicians have with these infections, and the lack of resources directed toward the development of programs for screening of high-risk patients, contact tracing, and treatment of infected partners.

EPIDEMIOLOGY

Chlamydial infections of the genital tract have a worldwide distribution, and are prevalent in both industrialized countries and in the developing world. The World Health Organization (WHO) estimates that 89 million new cases of genital chlamydial infections occurred worldwide in 1995.[1] In the United States, 4 to 5 million cases of chlamydial infection occur annually at an estimated cost of $2.4 billion dollars.[2] Since chlamydial infections first became a reportable disease in the United States in 1986, the number of reported cases in both men and women have increased each year to current rates of 290/100,000 women and 52/100,000 men (Fig. 29-1).[2] The greater number of reported cases in women than men reflects current screening practices, which focus mainly on women. In 1995, 477,638 cases were reported, making *C. trachomatis* the most common reportable disease in the United States.[3] In selected countries and in parts of the United States where intensive chlamydia control programs have been instituted, dramatic reductions in prevalence have been observed. In Sweden, for example, the number of cases of *C. trachomatis* infection was reduced by more than 50 percent over a 7-year period, falling from 38,200 in 1987 to 13,600 in 1994.[4] Similar declines have been seen in the Pacific Northwest and in Wisconsin after the institution of control programs (see the following).

Chlamydial infections of the genital tract are primarily caused by serovars D, E, F, G, H, I, J, and K.[5] A remarkably similar distribution of serovars has been observed worldwide, with the D, E, and F serovars being most prevalent and C class serovars less prevalent.[6] Infections caused by the former serovars are also associated with higher inclusion counts and with young age.[7] Among rectal infections in homosexual men, the D and G serovars are particularly prevalent for reasons as yet unexplained.[8] Several studies have suggested that the F and G serovars may produce less symptomatic and/or less inflammatory infections than strains of other serovars.[9,10] Paradoxically, variant F serotype strains have been seen more often in women with upper genital tract infection.[11]

Using molecular analyses of the chlamydial MOMP, it has become increasingly evident that polymorphism within the MOMP gene is common among isolates from patients who are highly sexually active and frequently exposed to chlamydial infection.[12] Allelic polymorphism thus may produce antigenic variation that provides the organism with the ability to evade the immune response. Less antigenic variation in MOMP has been observed in strains isolated from less sexually active populations.[13]

INFECTIONS IN MEN

The prevalence of chlamydial urethral infection has been assessed in populations of men attending general medical clinics, STD clinics, adolescent medicine clinics, and student health centers and ranges from 3 to 5 percent of asymptomatic men seen in general medical settings to 15 to 20 percent of all men seen in STD clinics.[5,14–17] Among military personnel, Podgore et al. found an 11 percent prevalence of asymptomatic urethral chlamydial infection compared with a 2 percent prevalence of urethral gonococcal infection.[18] Rates of chlamydial urethral infection of 13 to 15 percent also have been reported among sexually active boys attending adolescent medicine clinics.[19,20] Among men, the prevalence and site of mucosal infection as judged by positive culture appear to be strongly correlated with both age and sexual preference. Of 1221 patients screened for urethral infection in an STD clinic, 5 percent of homosexual men and 14 percent of heterosexual men had positive urethral cultures for *C. trachomatis*, and in both groups prevalence decreased in each 5-year period from age 19 to age 39 (Fig. 29-2). This striking age-related prevalence has been demonstrated repeatedly in both men and women. In other studies, both nongonococcal urethritis (NGU) and postgonococcal urethritis (PGU) were caused by *C. trachomatis* less frequently in homosexual men than in heterosexual men.[21] The prevalence of chlamydial infection generally has been higher in nonwhites than whites. In one screening study, 19 percent of nonwhite and 9 percent of white heterosexual males had urethral chlamydial infection.[17] Evidence of chlamydial infection has been infrequent in sexually inexperienced populations of men.

Chlamydial infection is a cause of acute proctitis in homosexual men who practice receptive rectal intercourse without condom protection.[22–24] Thus, both urethral and rectal chlamydial infections contributed to the high prevalence of serum antibody to *C. trachomatis* in homosexual men in the pre-AIDS era.

Pharyngeal infection with *C. trachomatis* has been demonstrated in 3 to 6 percent of men and women attending STD clinics and correlates with a history of recent orogenital contact.[25] Most such infections are asymptomatic. Among adolescents attending a teen clinic, only 1 percent were culture-positive for *C. trachomatis* in the pharynx.[26] Earlier serologic studies suggesting an etiologic role for *C. trachomatis* in nonstreptococcal community-acquired pharyngitis have not been supported by more recent attempts to isolate *C. trachomatis* from patients with pharyngitis.[27–29] The earlier serologic studies most likely were measuring antibodies against *Chlamydia pneumoniae*.

The overall incidence of *C. trachomatis* infection in men has not been well defined, since in most countries these infections are not officially reported, are not microbiologically confirmed, and

Table 29-1. Clinical Parallels Between Genital Infections Caused by *N. gonorrhoeae* and *C. trachomatis*

	Resulting clinical syndrome	
Site of infection	*N. gonorrhoeae*	*C. trachomatis*
Men		
Urethra	Urethritis	NGU, PGU
Epididymis	Epididymitis	Epididymitis
Rectum	Proctitis	Proctitis
Conjunctiva	Conjunctivitis	Conjunctivitis
Systemic	Disseminated gonococcal infection	Reiter's syndrome
Women		
Urethra	Acute urethral syndrome	Acute urethral syndrome
Bartholin's gland	Bartholinitis	Bartholinitis
Cervix	Cervicitis	Cervicitis, cervical metaplasia
Fallopian tube	Salpingitis	Salpingitis
Conjunctiva	Conjunctivitis	Conjunctivitis
Liver capsule	Perihepatitis	Perihepatitis
Systemic	Disseminated gonococcal infection	Reactive arthritis

often may be asymptomatic, thus escaping detection. In the United States, the number of reported cases of chlamydial infection in men is thought to be artifactually low because of the infrequent use of chlamydia diagnostic tests in men (see Fig. 29-1).

The transmissibility of genital chlamydial infections from females to males has not been extensively studied. In one study, male partners of women who had either chlamydial or gonococcal cervicitis were found to be infected with these agents 28 and 81 percent of the time, respectively.[30] Male partners of women with dual infections also were infected more often with gonorrhea than with chlamydia (77 and 28%, respectively).[30] Although this study suggests that *N. gonorrhoeae* is more transmissible than *C. trachomatis*, the differing lengths of incubation period of these two agents and differing efficiency of isolation from the urethra could explain the results. A more recent study by Quinn and colleagues utilized PCR rather than a culture to estimate rates of transmission, and demonstrated that although 42 percent of male partners of infected women were urethral culture-positive, 68 percent were PCR positive.[31] The genotypes of the chlamydial strains were identical in both partners as well. This study suggests that transmission

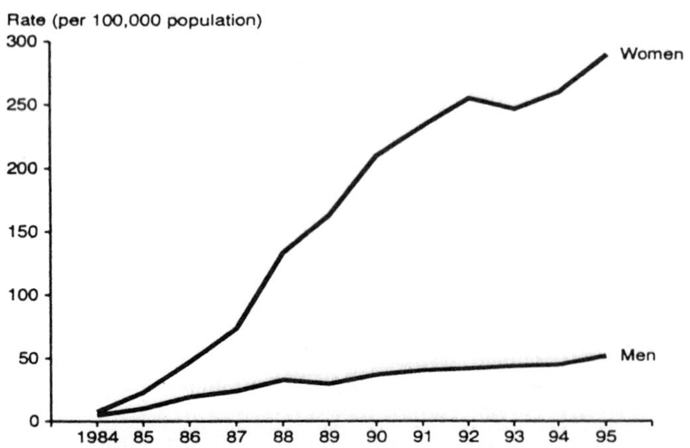

Fig. 29-1. Reported cases of *C. trachomatis* infections in the United States by year and gender.

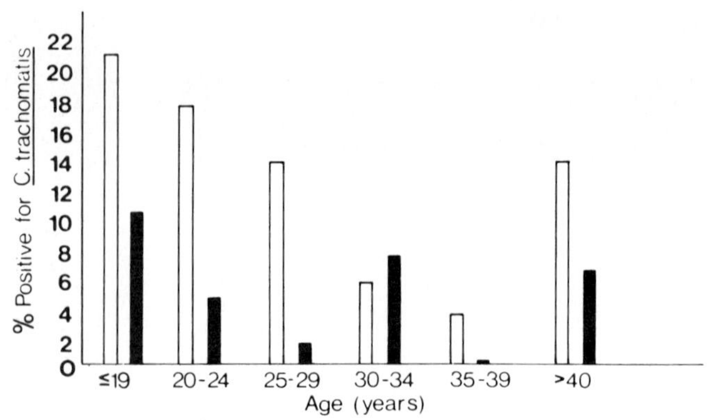

Fig. 29-2. Prevalence of *C. trachomatis* urethral infection by age in men attending an STD clinic. *Open bars* = heterosexual men; *solid bars* = homosexual or bisexual men.

from men to women and from women to men may be equally efficient.

INFECTIONS IN WOMEN

The prevalence of chlamydial infection has been studied in pregnant women, in women attending gynecology or family planning clinics, in women attending STD clinics, in college students, and in women attending general medicine or family practice clinics. Prevalence of infection in these studies has ranged widely from 3 to 5 percent in asymptomatic women to over 20 percent in women seen in STD clinics.[31–53] During pregnancy, 5 to 7 percent of women generally have been culture-positive, although a 21 percent prevalence in a population of inner city black women and a 26 percent prevalence among pregnant Navaho women have been reported.[46–48] Demographic factors associated with an increased risk of chlamydial isolation in at least several studies include young age, nonwhite race, single marital status, use of oral contraceptives, and measures of sexual activity such as a new partner or multiple sexual partners.[31,35,44,45] The proportion of sexually active women with positive cervical cultures for *C. trachomatis* has been highest for women aged 15 to 21 and declines strikingly thereafter, whereas the prevalence of serum antibody to *C. trachomatis* increases with age until about 30, when it plateaus at approximately 50 percent (Fig. 29-3). Sexually inexperienced populations rarely exhibit chlamydial cervical infections. In a study evaluating a 50 percent sample of all sexually active Alaskan Inuit

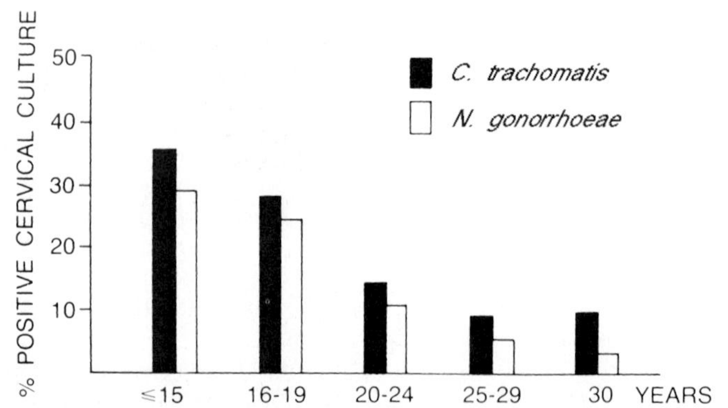

Fig. 29-3. Prevalence of *C. trachomatis* and *N. gonorrhoeae* cervical infection by age in women attending an STD clinic. *Open bars* = *N. gon-*

women living in remote villages, 114 (23%) of 493 had cervical infection with *C. trachomatis*.[53] It has been demonstrated repeatedly that in sexually active populations in which little diagnostic testing and/or specific treatment is being used, the prevalence of infection may thus reach surprisingly high levels. This reflects the asymptomatic nature of chlamydial infection and the ability of the infection, when untreated, to persist for months or years.

The incidence of *C. trachomatis* genital infection has been even less well defined in women than men. Because the infection produces no specific symptoms, is rarely confirmed microbiologically, and is often not reported, few reliable incidence data are yet available. The increasing number of reported cases in the United States among women in recent years undoubtedly reflects increased use of diagnostic testing and more frequent screening of high risk women (see Fig. 29-1).

Transmissibility of chlamydia also has been poorly defined in women. A comparative study of partners of men with either chlamydial or gonococcal urethritis found that these women were infected 45 and 80 percent of the time, respectively.[30] Among female partners of men with both infections, 45 percent had chlamydial infection and 64 percent had gonorrhea. Quinn and colleagues found that 57 percent of female partners of infected men were infected as judged by culture but 70 percent were positive as judged by PCR.[31]

NATURAL HISTORY OF CHLAMYDIAL INFECTION

Several studies in the United States indicate that approximately 5 percent of neonates acquire chlamydial infection perinatally, yet antibody prevalence in later childhood before onset of sexual activity may exceed 20 percent.[54] The acquisition of infection during childhood has not yet been well documented, but could occur from infected siblings (in whom infection acquired perinatally may persist for more than 1 year) or from parents or other adults via sexual abuse.[55] Childhood upper respiratory, eye, or middle ear infections with *C. trachomatis* might explain this rise in antibody prevalence between the neonatal period and adolescence, as could chlamydial genital infections acquired by children as a result of sexual abuse (see Chap. 72). Alternatively, crossreacting antibody to *Chlamydia pneumoniae* strains producing upper respiratory infections during childhood could account for some or all of this apparent increase in the seroprevalence to *C. trachomatis* (see Chap. 15).

In adolescence, the incidence of culture-positive symptomatic genital chlamydial infections rises sharply, as does antibody prevalence. Asymptomatic infection also occurs commonly, and long-lived but unrecognized urethral, rectal, and cervical infections undoubtedly occur. Unrecognized, asymptomatic, or minimally symptomatic infections of the upper genital tract also occur and have been termed "silent salpingitis." Both rectal and urethral infections contribute to the high antibody prevalence found in homosexual men.

Much remains to be learned about the natural history of genital infections owing to *C. trachomatis*, but on the basis of the knowledge of the natural history of trachoma and of limited studies of untreated men, nonpregnant women, and children, subacute and chronic asymptomatic infection of genital mucosal surfaces undoubtedly occurs.[32,56,57] The reported occurrence of chlamydial respiratory infection during immunosuppression suggests that impaired immunity may be followed by re-emergence of symptomatic infection from a chronic latent focus.[58,59] Recrudescence of ocular trachoma years after leaving an endemic area also has been shown to occur during topical cortisone therapy.[60] It is not certain yet whether pregnancy, also a state associated with depressed cell-mediated immunity, may be associated with reactivation of genital chlamydial infection. Current evidence indicates that chlamydial infection has not been a clinically evident problem in AIDS patients.[61] Similarly, the interactions between ocular trachoma, lymphogranuloma venereum (LGV), and non-LGV genital and perinatal infection have not been extensively studied in parts of the world where all of these strains are present in the same populations.[62] It is not known, for example, whether the epidemiology or clinical manifestations of genital chlamydial infections are altered in LGV or trachoma endemic areas.[62] Recent studies have called attention to the relatively high rate of recurrent infection with *C. trachomatis* in young, sexually active populations. In some studies, up to 20 to 30 percent of women have had evidence of recurrent infection within 6 months of an initial infection.[63,64] Recurrent infections may be with the same or a different serovar or genotype.[63] Mixed infections with two or more strains are evident in 3 to 8 percent of more highly sexually active populations.[65]

CLINICAL MANIFESTATIONS

Genital infections caused by *C. trachomatis* closely parallel those owing to *N. gonorrhoeae* in terms of clinical manifestations (see Table 29-1). Both organisms preferentially infect columnar or transitional epithelium of the urethra, with extension to the epididymis; the endocervix, with extension to the endometrium, salpinx, and peritoneum; and the rectum. Both organisms can produce extensive subepithelial inflammation, epithelial ulceration, and scarring. Rarely, both organisms can produce systemic manifestations. In general, infections caused by *C. trachomatis* tend to be less abrupt in onset and are more often characterized by no symptoms or by milder symptoms than is the case for gonococcal infections.

INFECTIONS IN MEN

Urethritis

Although Koch's postulates have not been specifically fulfilled, persuasive evidence suggests that *C. trachomatis* causes 35 to 50 percent of NGU in heterosexual men. In the 1970s and 1980s, the frequency of chlamydial isolation in men with recent onset of NGU was remarkably consistent from study to study, despite differences in patient population and methodology.[66–77] However, recent studies suggest that the proportion of NGU cases attributable to chlamydia may be declining in regions where chlamydia control programs have been in place.[78] When female partners of *C. trachomatis*-positive and *C. trachomatis*-negative men with NGU were examined, 60 to 75 percent of the former and 0 to 10 percent of the latter had chlamydial cervicitis, evidence that is consistent with sexual transmission of *C. trachomatis* having resulted in NGU.[72–75] Immunotyping (or, more recently, genotyping) of isolates from both partners has shown concordance of immunotypes or genotypes in most couples.[31] Serum IgM antichlamydial antibody is found frequently in chlamydia culture-positive men with NGU but rarely in culture-negative men with NGU.[74] Finally, placebo-controlled treatment trials of men with NGU or therapeutic trials utilizing drugs such as spectinomycin, which have little effect on chlamydia, indicate that most men given placebo or ineffective therapy for *C. trachomatis* remain culture-positive and symptomatic until effective treatment is given.[75–77] Elimination of chlamydia thus coincides with resolution of symptoms. Although *C. trachomatis* has not been experimentally inoculated into the human urethra, baboons and chimpanzees develop chlamydial urethritis accompanied by serologic evidence of infection after urethral inoculation.[79]

Clinically, chlamydia-positive and chlamydia-negative NGU

cannot be differentiated on the basis of signs or symptoms.[76] Both usually present after a 7- to 21-day incubation period with dysuria and mild to moderate whitish or clear urethral discharge. Examination reveals no abnormalities other than the discharge in most cases; associated adenopathy, focal urethral tenderness, and meatal or penile lesions should suggest herpetic urethritis. Neither abnormal prostatic examinations nor prostatic inflammation have been convincingly linked to chlamydial urethritis.

C. trachomatis urethral infection is more often asymptomatic than gonococcal urethral infection, and when symptoms occur, they are milder with chlamydial urethritis.[17,80] However, most men with asymptomatic chlamydial urethral infection exhibit ongoing inflammation as defined by persistent urethral leukocytosis [>−4 polymorphonuclear leukocytes (PMNS) per × 1000 field] on Gram stains of urethral secretions or persistent pyuria in a first-void urine. Leukocyte esterase testing also can be used to identify patients with asymptomatic chlamydial urethritis.[81,82]

Postgonococcal urethritis occurring in heterosexual men, like NGU, frequently results from infection with *C. trachomatis.*[83] These patients probably acquire gonorrhea and chlamydial infection simultaneously but, because of the longer incubation period of *C. trachomatis,* develop a biphasic illness if their original gonorrhea is treated with an agent that does not eradicate chlamydia. It is possible that acute gonococcal infection causes reactivation of a latent chlamydial infection but there is little evidence to support this premise. Coinfection with these two agents occurs in from 15 to 35 percent of heterosexual men with gonorrhea but rarely in homosexual men. In areas where chlamydial control programs have been in place, the frequency of chlamydial coinfection among men with gonorrhea has declined to 5 to 10 percent. Of men infected with both chlamydia and *N. gonorrhoeae* who are treated with penicillin, ampicillin, gentamicin, or spectinomycin, 80 percent or more develop symptomatic PGU, or urethral leukocytosis without symptoms.[66,68,83]

Epididymitis

Berger and coworkers have shown that *C. trachomatis* causes most cases of what was previously termed idiopathic epididymitis in young, heterosexually active males.[84,85] In these and subsequent studies, chlamydial and gonococcal epididymitis usually was associated with urethritis caused by *C. trachomatis* and/or *N. gonorrhoeae* in patients who were less than 35 years of age and sexually active, whereas patients with epididymitis who were older than 35 years generally had Gram-negative bacterial infections and a history of urologic disease or instrumentation (see Chap. 53). Currently, about 70 percent of acute epididymitis in young sexually active men appears to be attributable to chlamydial infection (see Chap. 53). Clinically, chlamydial epididymitis presents as unilateral scrotal pain, swelling, tenderness, and fever in a young male who often has associated chlamydial urethritis (NGU). The urethritis, however, may often be asymptomatic and evident only as urethral inflammation on Gram stain. Men with chlamydial epididymitis improve rapidly with tetracycline treatment, supporting the causal role of *C. trachomatis.*[85]

Chlamydia trachomatis also produces mild epididymitis in monkeys after introduction of the organism into the vas deferens.[86] Antibody production, stimulation of cell-mediated immunity to chlamydial antigens, histologic findings, and subsequent recovery of *C. trachomatis* from the monkey's urethra support the causative role of *C. trachomatis* in this model.[86,87] However, the epididymitis is mild, organisms have not been recovered from the epididymis, and the effects of repeated inoculation have not been studied. Thus, animal experiments have not yet elucidated the pathogenesis of chlamydial epididymitis.

Prostatitis

Despite continued study, the role of *C. trachomatis* in causing nonbacterial prostatitis remains controversial (see Chap. 54). Mardh and coworkers reported that only 13 percent of patients with nonbacterial prostatitis had antibodies to *C. trachomatis* in serum or in expressed prostatic secretions, and none had positive cultures from expressed prostatic secretions.[88] They speculated that negative cultures could have resulted from the antichlamydial effects of spermine and zinc in prostatic secretions.[89] Nilsson reported recovery of *C. trachomatis* from the expressed prostatic secretions of 26 men with acute NGU, all of whom were considered to have cytologic evidence of prostatitis.[90] Bruce and colleagues also reported frequent isolation of chlamydia from urine, prostatic fluid, and prostatic expressate of men with nonbacterial prostatitis.[91] However, these studies have not convincingly demonstrated the presence of chlamydia in the prostate itself, and the definition of prostatitis used is disputed. Poletti and colleagues performed transrectal biopsies of the prostate in 30 men with known positive urethral cultures for *C. trachomatis* and a diagnosis of nonbacterial prostatitis based on prostatic tenderness or swelling on digital palpation; the organism was recovered from 10 of 30 prostatic specimens.[92] These studies require confirmation, and taken together are inconclusive regarding the role of *C. trachomatis* in nonbacterial prostatitis. Further studies should utilize a careful case definition (including cell counts in expressed prostatic secretions), conventional histologic studies, immunohistochemical study of biopsied tissue, serologic studies, sensitive molecular techniques to assess the presence of chlamydia (i.e., PCR and in situ DNA hypridization) in the prostate, and evaluation of response to therapy.

Proctitis

The chronic, indolent form of LGV that results from secondary spread of *C. trachomatis* of the LGV immunotypes from the genitalia to the rectum, usually in women, is discussed in Chapter 17. *C. trachomatis* of non-LGV immunotypes also has been isolated from the rectal mucosa of infants, heterosexual women, and homosexual men.[5,6] The clinical manifestations of rectal infection in infants and adult women have not been studied extensively. Those seen in homosexual men are described elsewhere in this volume.

Prospective evaluation of homosexual men indicates that *C. trachomatis* of either the genital immunotypes D to K or LGV immunotypes can produce proctitis.[22–25] The LGV immunotypes usually produce a primary ulcerative proctitis and a histopathologic picture of giant cell formation and granulomas similar to that seen in acute Crohn's disease. Non-LGV immunotypes produce milder infections, ranging from asymptomatic infection to symptomatic proctitis resembling gonococcal proctitis with rectal pain and bleeding, mucous discharge, and diarrhea. Most *C. trachomatis*-infected patients have abnormal numbers of PMNs in their rectal Gram stain, and on sigmoidoscopy, those with symptoms exhibit friable rectal mucosa and often mucopus. In the pre-AIDS era, *C. trachomatis* appeared to be responsible for up to 15 percent of proctitis cases seen in homosexual males, and treatment with tetracycline promptly cured these patients.[93]

Reiter's Syndrome

Both Reiter's syndrome (urethritis, conjunctivitis, arthritis, and characteristic mucocutaneous lesions) and reactive tenosynovitis or arthritis without the other components of Reiter's syndrome have been related to genital infection with *C. trachomatis.* Studies of untreated men with characteristic Reiter's syndrome using the microimmunofluorescent (micro-IF) antibody assay indicate that preceding or concurrent infection with *C. trachomatis* is present in more than 80 percent of cases (see Chap. 61).[94–96] Many men with Reiter's syndrome also exhibit marked lymphocyte stimulation by chlamydial antigens in in vitro blastogenesis assays.[95] Fluorescein-conjugated monoclonal antibodies have been used to demonstrate what appear to be *C. trachomatis* elementary bodies in the joint fluid and synovial biopsies of patients with Reiter's syndrome, suggesting dissemination of chlamydial antigen beyond the mucosal site of entry in such patients.[97] However, viable chlamydial cannot be recovered from the joint fluid or synovium of these patients and demonstration of chlamydial DNA in the joint fluid/synovium has been reported by some groups but not by others.[98–100] Recently, cloned T cells from the synovium of patients with Reiter's syndrome have been demonstrated to recognize the chlamydial 57-kDa HSP and the chlamydial 18-kDa histone-like protein.[101]

Like postenteric (salmonella, shigella, yersinia) arthritides, sacroiliitis, and spondylitis, Reiter's syndrome occurs with increased frequency in patients with the HLA-B27 haplotype.[102–104] The Class 1 HLA-B27 haplotype appears to confer a tenfold increased risk of developing Reiter's syndrome, and 60 to 70 percent of persons with the syndrome are HLA-B27 positive.[102–104] However, among a large series of HLA-B27-positive men with chlamydial urethritis but with no other manifestations of Reiter's syndrome, none went on to develop Reiter's syndrome after onset of therapy with a tetracycline.[104]

INFECTIONS IN WOMEN

Cervicitis

Although many women with chlamydia isolated from the cervix have no signs or symptoms of infection, at least a third generally have local signs of infection on examination.[105,106] Most commonly found are mucopurulent discharge (37% of women) and hypertrophic ectopy (19%). Hypertrophic ectopy refers to an area of ectopy that is edematous, congested, and bleeds easily (see Chap. 46). Cervical follicles can sometimes be visualized colposcopically in women with chlamydial infection of the cervix, but this finding has been uncommon in our experience and that of others.[41] Paavonen et al. reported that colposcopic features of immature squamous metaplasia of the zone of ectopy are associated with chlamydial infection.[106] The number of PMN leukocytes in cervical mucus is correlated with chlamydial infection of the cervix. Brunham et al. reported that > 10 PMN leukocytes per × 1000 field was best correlated, although this criterion has been extensively debated.[107] Attention to careful collection of the specimen, and to selective counting of PMNs in cervical mucus, rather than in areas containing vaginal epithelial cells, is important. Based on clinical experience and cumulative studies published to date, a cutoff of > 30 PMN leukocytes per × 1000 field in Gram-stained smears of cervical mucus appears best correlated with chlamydial (or gonococcal) cervicitis. There appears to be a wide range of normal leukocyte values in women without cervical infection, likely owing to the influence of the menstrual cycle, contraceptive practices, sexual activity, and other infections. Women who exhibit signs of chlamydial cervicitis (mucopurulent discharge, hypertrophic ectopy) yield greater numbers of chlamydial inclusion-forming units on primary isolation in tissue culture than women who have chlamydial infection without cervicitis.[108] Whether infections associated with cervicitis have been more recently acquired has not been established, but may be the case.

The prevalence of *C. trachomatis* infection is greater in women with ectopy than in those without ectopy.[109] Ectopy may predispose women to chlamydial infection by exposing a greater number of susceptible columnar epithelial cells, making infection more likely on exposure. Alternatively, ectopy may increase the shedding of *C. trachomatis* from the cervix, or *C. trachomatis* infection of the cervix may cause ectopy. Cervical ectopy is normally present in 60 to 80 percent of sexually active adolescents and then declines in prevalence in the third and fourth decades. This may help explain the high prevalence of cervical chlamydial infections in adolescents. Oral contraceptives also have been associated with an increased risk of cervical *C. trachomatis* infection, probably because their use promotes ectopy; the increased risk appears limited to oral contraceptive users with ectopy.[35,105]

Clinical recognition of chlamydial cervicitis depends on a high index of suspicion and a careful cervical examination. There are no genital symptoms that are specifically correlated with chlamydial cervical infection. As discussed previously, findings on examination suggestive of chlamydial infection include easily induced endocervical bleeding, mucopurulent endocervical discharge, and edema within an area of ectopy. The differential diagnosis of mucopurulent discharge from the endocervical canal in a young, sexually active woman includes gonococcal endocervicitis, salpingitis, endometritis, IUD-induced inflammation, or other causes (see Chap. 46). Gram stain of appropriately collected mucopurulent endocervical discharge from patients with chlamydial endocervicitis also usually shows greater than 30 PMN leukocytes per × 1000 field, absence of gonococci, and only occasional other bacteria. Similarly, the observation of purulent (yellow or green) colored cervical discharge on a cervical swab collected from such patients (a positive "swab test"; see Chap. 46) correlates with the presence of chlamydial and/or gonococcal infection.[107] Unfortunately, the majority of women with chlamydial infection cannot be distinguished from uninfected women either by clinical examination or by these simple tests and thus require the use of specific diagnostic testing.

Nearly all women with endocervical chlamydial infection have or develop antibodies to *C. trachomatis* in serum as assessed by the micro-IF assay. Only 20 to 30 percent exhibit IgM antibody at the time of diagnosis, however, suggesting that many newly diagnosed cervical infections in women are not recent but long-lived. Local cervical antibody has been reported in only 30 to 50 percent of cases, but in our experience over 70 percent of culture-positive women have local antibody.[109] Sequential culturing of untreated women has demonstrated that chlamydial infection of the cervix may persist for weeks or months without development of symptoms, or may spontaneously resolve.[32,42]

The relation of chlamydial cervical infection to cytologic atypia, including reactive and metaplastic atypia and dysplasia, is discussed in Chap. 48. The cervical Pap smear frequently shows a characteristic pattern of inflammation in chlamydial infection, which can alert the cytopathologist and clinician to the need for further tests for chlamydia. The Pap smear itself, however, cannot be used as a sensitive or specific indicator of chlamydial infection of the cervix.

Urethritis

Screening studies in STD clinics suggest that of women cultured for *C. trachomatis* at both the cervix and urethra, approximately 50 percent of positive women yield chlamydia from both sites and 25 percent from either site alone.[35,37,72] Paavonen reported that women who had *C. trachomatis* in their cervix and urethra were more likely to complain of dysuria than women with cervical infection alone. Isolated urethral infection, without cervical infection, appears to increase in prevalence with age.[37] Case reports have previously suggested that symptoms of dysuria and frequency occur in women with chlamydial urethritis, pyuria, and no bacteriuria or other urinary pathogens, and a prospective evaluation of young women with the acute urethral syndrome (dysuria and frequency without bacteriuria of $<10^5$ conventional uropathogens per mL of urine) has implicated chlamydia as an important cause of dysuria in young, sexually active women.[36,110] Of 16 women with sterile pyuria, 10 had cultural and/or serologic evidence of infection with *C. trachomatis,* compared with less than 10 percent of women from the same population who lacked urinary symptoms or who had coliform cystitis.[36] Women with chlamydial infection who were given placebo remained culture-positive and symptomatic until given active antimicrobial therapy, whereas those given doxycycline improved rapidly.[111]

Although urethral symptoms may develop in some women with chlamydial infection, the majority of female STD clinic patients with urethral chlamydial infection do not have dysuria or frequency. Even in women with chlamydial urethritis causing the acute urethral syndrome, signs of urethritis (urethral discharge, meatal redness, or swelling) are infrequent.[36] However, the presence of mucopurulent cervicitis in a woman with dysuria and frequency should suggest the diagnosis. *C. trachomatis* urethritis should be suspected in young, sexually active women with dysuria, frequency, and pyuria, especially if they have had a new sex partner within the last month or a sex partner with NGU. Other correlates of chlamydial urethral syndrome include duration of dysuria of more than 7 to 10 days, lack of hematuria, and lack of suprapubic tenderness. An abnormal urethral Gram stain showing >10 PMNs per oil immersion field in women with dysuria but without coliform bacteriuria supports the diagnosis of chlamydial urethritis but is also found in women with gonococcal or trichomonal infection of the urethra.

Bartholinitis

Like gonococci, *C. trachomatis* may produce an exudative infection of Bartholin's ducts. Davies et al. studied 30 women who had clinical evidence of bartholinitis, and isolated *N. gonorrhoeae* and *C. trachomatis* from the ductal exudate of 24 and 9 women, respectively.[112] Of the nine chlamydia-positive women, seven had concurrent gonorrhea, but two were sex partners of men with NGU and had no evidence of gonococcal infection. Purulent infections of Bartholin's ducts may thus be owing to chlamydial infection, either alone or with concurrent gonococcal infection.

Endometritis

Histologic evidence of endometritis, often with immunohistologic and/or cultural evidence of *C. trachomatis,* is present in nearly one-half of patients with chlamydial mucopurulent cervicitis and can be demonstrated in nearly all patients with chlamydial salpingitis. The presence of endometritis in patients with chlamydial cervicitis also correlates with a history of abnormal vaginal bleeding (see Chaps. 50 and 64).

It is now clear that *C. trachomatis* infection is associated with endometritis.[113–119] Mardh and coworkers first described two women from whom *C. trachomatis* was recovered by uterine aspiration, despite negative cervical cultures.[113] Both women exhibited signs of salpingitis and had serologic evidence of chlamydial infection. Concomitant endometritis probably explains the menorrhagia and metrorrhagia often seen in women with salpingitis. These studies, like previous evidence gathered in monkeys infected with *C. trachomatis,* indicate that chlamydia cervicitis probably spreads through the endometrial cavity to reach the fallopian tubes.[116] Subsequent studies have shown that chlamydial endometritis is characterized by infiltration of the endometrial stroma by plasma cells, and infiltration of the endometrial superficial epithelium by PMN leukocytes. Besides nonpuerperal endometritis, Wager and coworkers have shown an association of intrapartum fever and late postpartum endometritis with untreated antenatal *C. trachomatis* infection.[120] Others have confirmed this association (see Chap. 64).

Salpingitis

The proportion of acute salpingitis cases owing to *C. trachomatis* varies geographically and with the population studied. In Sweden, Mardh and colleagues found that 19 of 53 women with salpingitis had chlamydial infections of the cervix and that of those with cervical infection who had laparoscopy, six of seven grew *C. trachomatis* in a culture from the fallopian tube.[121] These authors found that 80 percent of 60 consecutive women with acute salpingitis had antibodies to *C. trachomatis,* with 37 percent exhibiting serologic evidence of acute chlamydial infection. Other serologic studies of women with salpingitis also suggest a prominent etiologic role of chlamydia.[122–124] Studies in Seattle in women with laparoscopically confirmed salpingitis and histologically confirmed endometritis indicate that 80 to 90 percent have proven chlamydial or gonococcal infection, usually confirmed in the upper genital tract, with the proportion having either chlamydial or gonococcal infection being approximately equal.[117,122] An interesting treatment study by Rees and colleagues further supports the role of chlamydia in salpingitis.[125] Among 343 women randomly treated for gonorrhea with either penicillin or tetracycline, a significantly greater proportion of those who received penicillin went on to develop salpingitis; persistence of cervical *C. trachomatis was* associated with many but not all cases of salpingitis. As discussed in Chapters 49 and 50, and elsewhere, many cases of chlamydial salpingitis are associated with mild or absent symptoms or signs, despite progressive tubal scarring, resulting in pregnancy or infertility.[126–130] Such studies have given rise to the term "silent salpingitis" attributable to chlamydia. Studies in animal models (see Chaps. 49 and 50) also demonstrate the causative role of chlamydia in salpingitis and in the production of tubal scarring and infertility.[131,132]

Perihepatitis (Fitz-Hugh-Curtis Syndrome)

Since its original description by Fitz-Hugh and Curtis, perihepatitis occurring after or with salpingitis has been considered a complication of gonococcal infection. However, studies in the last 15 years suggest that chlamydial infection is in fact more commonly associated with perihepatitis than is *N. gonorrhoeae* (see Chap. 51), probably accounting for the majority of cases.[133–135] Perihepatitis should be suspected in young, sexually active women who develop right-upper-quadrant pain, fever, nausea, or vomiting. Evidence of salpingitis may or may not be present on examination. A recent study has demonstrated that perihepatitis is strongly associated with extensive tubal scarring, adhesions, and inflammation observed at laparoscopy, as well as with high titers of antibody to the 57-kDa chlamydial heat shock protein.[136]

OTHER CHLAMYDIAL INFECTIONS IN ADULTS

Since *C. trachomatis* causes a distinctive pneumonia syndrome in neonates (see Chap. 66), several studies have assessed the etiologic role of chlamydia in adults with pneumonia. Case reports and small studies suggest that *C. trachomatis* is an occasional cause of pneumonitis in immunocompromised adults.[137,138] Tack and coworkers isolated *C. trachomatis* from the lower respiratory secretions of five immunosuppressed patients with pneumonia and from one patient with acute bronchitis.[137] *C. trachomatis* was also isolated from the eye and nasopharynx and from bronchial brushings in three of these patients. However, none of these six patients developed serologic evidence of *C. trachomatis* infection, and all had concomitant cytomegalovirus infection. On the other hand, Meyers and coworkers demonstrated sustained IgM and IgG antibody rises to *C. trachomatis* in three patients who developed interstitial pneumonia after marrow transplantation, but lung tissue examined by culture and fluorescent antibody techniques from these patients and from 63 other transplant patients with idiopathic pneumonia provided no evidence of chlamydial infection.[138] More recently, histologic or cultural evidence of *C. trachomatis* infection could not be demonstrated in 48 lung biopsies from AIDS patients with pneumonia.[61] Komaroff and coworkers reported serologic evidence of recent chlamydial infections in 4 out of 19 adults with community-acquired pneumonia not owing to other common bacterial or viral pathogens.[139] However, in retrospect these likely represented antibodies to *C. pneumoniae* rather than to *C. trachomatis*. At this point, there is no evidence to suggest that *C. trachomatis* causes community-acquired pneumonia or other respiratory infections in adults.

Chlamydia trachomatis may on occasion produce culture-negative endocarditis and serologic studies in one patient suggested that meningoencephalitis resulted from chlamydial infection.[140–142] Other uncommon infections in adults, including peritonitis and postmenopausal vaginitis, have been attributed to chlamydia.[143,144]

DIAGNOSIS

Chapter 74 discusses in detail the cytologic, cultural, antigen-detection, DNA hybridization, nucleic acid amplification, and serologic methods for diagnosis of *C. trachomatis* infections. Aspects relevant to deciding whom to test, what test to use, the collection of specimens, and the interpretation of results in adult patients are presented here.

Being an intracellular pathogen, *C. trachomatis* requires a cell culture system for propagation in the laboratory. Thus, cell culture has been the gold standard test for the detection of *C. trachomatis* for years.[6] However, its stringent requirements both in terms of technical expertise and specimen transport make cell culture impractical in settings in which neither a cold chain nor a cell culture system can be maintained. Further, a carefully collected sample of columnar epithelial cells from the cervix or urethra is necessary and specimens composed purely of polymorphonuclear cells or mucopurulent discharge are not adequate.[6] For culture, specimens may be collected with a cotton-tipped swab (those with wooden sticks should not be used as they are inhibitory to chlamydia). For endocervical specimens, a cytobrush may result in an increase in the sensitivity of culture as more cells are collected.[6] Specimens must be placed in specific transport media and refrigerated until they are inoculated within 24 hours onto cell culture plates.

Owing to the inadequacies, cost, and technical difficulties of cell culture, the development of nonculture tests has been a major research priority over the last 15 years. As a result, many nonculture diagnostic tests for *C. trachomatis* are now commercially available.[6,145] The first of these tests used antigen detection, generally of chlamydia lipopolysaccharide (LPS) or MOMP, as a means of detecting chlamydial elementary bodies in genital specimens. The most widely used of these assays are the DFA and enzyme immunoassay (EIA) tests. In general, when obtained from the cervix, these tests detect between 60 and 85 percent of infections relative to culture.[146,147] The DFA, when done by an experienced technician, has a sensitivity of 80 to 85 percent, but overall sensitivity depends both on the experience of the person performing the test and on collection of an adequate specimen.[147,148] Sensitivity of the EIAs generally are in the range of 60 to 80 percent compared with culture, and vary by assay (see Table 29-1).[145–147,149] Although the DFA test is highly specific (>99 percent), the EIA requires a confirmatory assay with a blocking antibody or with DFA to eliminate false positive results. Results of antigen detection tests can usually be obtained within 1 to 2 days. Several simplified rapid antigen detection tests that can be done on-site and provide immediate results while the patient is in the clinic are also available. Unfortunately, the performance of these tests has been disappointing; most have yielded unacceptably low sensitivities relative to culture and their use is discouraged until performance can be improved.[147,150]

The first commercially available diagnostic test to use nucleic acid hybridization was GenProbe, which detects but does not amplify chlamydial nucleic acid and has performance characteristics on endocervical and urethral specimens comparable to that of DFA and the best EIAs.[6] The advantage of all of the nonculture tests outlined in the preceding in comparison with culture is their ease of use in settings where transport or maintenance of specimens at colder temperatures is problematic or where cell culture is not available, and because their low cost. However, the hope that they might be useful as a noninvasive means of diagnosing chlamydial infection by testing urine has not been realized. The sensitivities of these assays when applied to urine have been unacceptably low, often in the 40 to 50 percent range as compared with culture.[151]

The most exciting recent development in chlamydial diagnostic testing has been that of automated methods for the detection of amplified *C. trachomatis* DNA or RNA. The two most widely used methods are LCR and PCR, both of which can be used for cervical, urethral, and urine specimens from males and females. The specificity of these tests has consistently been above 99 percent.[6,147] Another methodology, transcription-mediated amplification (TMA), amplifies chlamydial ribosomal RNA, and appears to have performance characteristics similar to LCR and PCR.[152] LCR and PCR target nucleotide sequences on the plasmid of *C. trachomatis*, which is present in multiple copies within each elementary body. The TMA assay targets a ribosomal RNA sequence. The lower limit of detection of these tests is in the range of 1 to 10 elementary bodies (as compared to 10,000 elementary bodies for EIA).

In order to define the performance of these newer amplification tests, a new gold standard other than cell culture generally has been utilized; this requires reevaluation of specimens that are negative by culture and positive by an amplification test. Confirmation is first attempted using DFA on the cytospin of the culture transport medium. If this is negative, then PCR or LCR is repeated using a probe directed against a different nucleotide target sequence, namely a chromosomal MOMP gene sequence. An alternative approach now that three amplification assays are available would be to confirm one amplification assay with a second similar assay. Using this expanded gold standard, LCR when applied to first-catch urine (FCU; the first 10–30 mL of stream) has a sensitivity of approximately 90 to 96 percent for the detection of chlamydial urethritis in males, and 69 to 96 percent for chlamydial urethritis and/or cervicitis in females.[153–157] Sensitivity of LCR performed on endocervical specimens has ranged from 81 to 100 percent.[155,158,159] Compared with the performance of cell culture, LCR generally detects 15 to 40 percent more infected persons, with a concomitant increase in estimated prevalence of 4 to 5 percent. On balance, these studies indicate that LCR performed on endocervical specimens is consistently more sensitive than culture, and that its performance on FCU is sensitive enough to provide a means of noninvasive testing for the diagnosis of chlamydial infection of the urethra and the cervix in women.

The performance of PCR in the diagnosis of chlamydial infection has also been evaluated relative to the expanded gold standard described in the preceding. Among males, its sensitivity when performed on FCU has generally been 87 to 100 percent.[160–164] The test has detected up to approximately 40 percent more infections than urethral culture in some studies.[162] In at least one study, however, PCR performed on male urine specimens was significantly less sensitive than LCR, possibly owing to PCR-specific inhibitors present in fresh urine.[153] Among females, PCR performed on FCU has demonstrated a sensitivity of 82 to 93 percent.[162,165] Unexpectedly, performance of PCR on endocervical specimens has been variable, with sensitivities ranging from 60 to 92 percent.[162–165] The presence of inhibitors in endocervical mucous is thought to be responsible for this variability in PCR sensitivity; in one study effecting a reduction of sensitivity of 15 percent.[165] The effect of inhibitors on the routine performance of LCR and PCR on endocervical specimens and perhaps on urine specimens, requires further study. In addition to the use of first-void urine, the newer amplification tests may make it possible to use other novel specimens for the diagnosis of *C. trachomatis* infection. In women, self-collected swabs of the vaginal introitus, or self-collected tampons, offer unique approaches that may be useful in screening programs.

SEROLOGIC TECHNIQUES

Serologic tests have not been widely used for the diagnosis of chlamydial genital tract infections other than LGV. Several major problems have precluded their use. First, the baseline prevalence of antibody in populations of sexually active persons who are at risk of *C. trachomatis* infection is high, often ranging from 45 to 65 percent of persons tested. The high prevalence of seropositivity in culture-negative, asymptomatic patients presumably reflects either previous infection or persisting, chronic asymptomatic infection not easily detected with current culture techniques. Second, the lack of an abrupt onset of symptoms in many chlamydia infected patients means that patients often are seen during periods when IgM antibody or rising or falling titers of IgG antibody cannot be demonstrated, and hence these serologic parameters of recently acquired infection often are absent. This particularly applies to women. Onset of symptoms is more abrupt in men with NGU, and seroconversion or IgM antibody can be documented in most men. Third, superficial genital tract infection (urethritis, cervicitis) generally produces micro-IF antibody titers in the range of 1:8 to 1:256, but rarely higher. Of men with NGU who were initially seronegative but later developed IgG antibody to chlamydia, 60 percent developed titers between 1:8 and 1:32, whereas 40 percent were between 1:64 and 1:256. In women, higher antibody titers (>1:256) have more often been seen in women with salpingitis and even higher titers (often >1:1024) in women with perihepatitis. Finally, crossreacting antibody rises owing to *Chlamydia pneumoniae* may obfuscate serodiagnosis. These issues are discussed in more detail elsewhere in this volume.

WHEN TO USE DIAGNOSTIC TESTING

All women suspected of having *C. trachomatis* genital infections on the basis of symptoms, signs, or exposure history, including women with suspected mucopurulent cervicitis, endometritis, pelvic inflammatory disease, acute urethritis, or acute proctitis, as well as women whose male partners have gonorrhea or NGU, should have specific diagnostic testing. As described in the preceding, the diagnosis of many of these conditions is difficult to establish on clinical grounds alone, and the presence of a positive chlamydial test thus is of great value in confirming the suspected diagnosis. Although women in these categories should be empirically treated with antibiotics while test results are pending, the specific confirmation of *C. trachomatis* infection clarifies the diagnosis, improves the patient's understanding of her illness, probably enhances compliance with therapy, and facilitates management of sexual partners. Although "syndromic treatment" of women with chlamydia-associated syndromes (i.e., empiric treatment without testing) is an acceptable strategy where costs prohibit laboratory testing, the benefits attributable to testing argue for its use where affordable.

Second, unrecognized *C. trachomatis* infections should be identified by appropriate screening of asymptomatic women in high-risk groups. Universal screening of all women attending STD clinics or other clinics (e.g., family planning clinics, juvenile detention centers, and abortion clinics) where the prevalence of infection exceeds 10 to 12 percent appears to be an effective and cost-efficient strategy.[166–169] In other clinical settings where the overall prevalence of chlamydial infection is less than five to six percent, selective screening may be a more effective strategy. In this circumstance, physicians should screen women who have specific risk factors associated with chlamydial infections including adolescent age range, a new sexual partner, multiple sexual partners, racial/ethnic backgrounds found to be at high risk in the local setting, and signs of cervicitis.[147,168] Strong consideration should be given to screening all unmarried pregnant women and all pregnant women with one or more of these risk characteristics, especially adolescents.

In men, given both the relative paucity of serious complications that arise from *C. trachomatis* infections and the considerably greater proportion of infections that can be accurately diagnosed on clinical grounds alone, both specific diagnostic testing and screening for *C. trachomatis* infections should be given a lower priority than in women. Thus, when resources limit the numbers of tests that can be done (e.g., in public health clinics), the tests available should be used primarily for diagnosis and screening in women. However, knowledge of the etiologic role of *C. trachomatis* in NGU has prognostic implications (>90% cure rate for patients positive for *C. trachomatis* compared with 50% for those who are negative) and fosters the need for more aggressive identification and treatment of female partners. Specific diagnostic testing thus provides a number of benefits, even though infected men with symptoms or signs of urethritis should be treated empirically before the test results are known.

Up to one-third of heterosexual men with *C. trachomatis* urethral infection attending STD clinics lack symptoms of urethritis.[17] Further, asymptomatic chlamydial urethritis is surprisingly prevalent (five to seven percent) among young men in inner city high schools.[170,171] Screening of young men for asymptomatic *C. trachomatis* infection has been difficult because of the absence of a noninvasive and patient-acceptable diagnostic technique and because of the infrequency with which young men come into contact with health care facilities. The availability of chlamydia testing on first void urine using LCR or PCR now makes screening of large numbers of young men possible in settings such as high schools or other clinics. Asymptomatic partners of women with mucopurulent cervicitis, pelvic inflammatory disease, or asymptomatic chlamydial infection should also be screened and then given empirical therapy. The use of empirical therapy without specific testing foregoes an opportunity to identify still other sexual contacts who should be evaluated and treated and thus fosters continuation

Table 29-2. Diagnosis of *C. trachomatis* Infections in Men*

Associated findings	Clinical criteria	Laboratory criteria: Presumptive	Laboratory criteria: Diagnostic
NGU	Dysuria, urethral discharge	Urethral GS with 5 or more PMN/high-power (×1000) field; pyuria on FVU	Positive culture or nonculture test (urethra or FVU)
Acute epididymitis	Fever, epididymal or testicular pain, evidence of NGU, epididymal tenderness or mass	As for NGU	As for NGU; positive test on epididymal aspirate
Acute proctitis (non-LGV strain)	Rectal pain, discharge, bleeding; abnormal anoscopy (mucopurulent discharge, pain, spontaneous or induced bleeding)	Rectal GS with 1 or more PMN/high-power (×1000) field	Positive culture or direct FA (rectal)
Acute proctocolitis (LGV strain)	Severe rectal pain, discharge, hematochezia; markedly abnormal anoscopy (as above) with lesions extending into colon; fever lymphadenopathy	Rectal GS with 1 or more PMN/high-power (×1000) field	Positive culture or direct FA (rectal); complement fixation antibody titer

* GS = Gram stain; PMN = polymorphonuclear leukocytes; NGU = nongonococcal urethritis; FA = fluorescent antibody; FVU = first-void urine; LGV = lymphogranuloma venereum. Reproduced with permission from the *Annals of Internal Medicine*.

of the epidemic and reinfection of the patient. In homosexual men with suspected proctitis, *C. trachomatis* testing should be done to confirm the suspected diagnosis. Tables 29-2 and 29-3 summarize diagnostic criteria for various *C. trachomatis* infections in men and women, respectively.

THERAPY

Although in vitro susceptibility testing for *C. trachomatis* has not been rigorously standardized, studies to date have found little strain-to-strain variation in minimum inhibitory concentrations of individual antimicrobials against chlamydia.[6] The most active drugs against *C. trachomatis* in tissue culture are rifampin and the tetracyclines, followed by macrolides, sulfonamides, some fluoroquinolones, and clindamycin.[6] Unlike gonococci, there has been no apparent emergence of antimicrobial resistance.

The majority of clinical evidence regarding the effectiveness of various antimicrobials against *C. trachomatis* has been accumulated in men with NGU (Table 29-4). Two general principles have emerged from these studies: penicillin, ampicillin, cephalosporins, and spectinomycin in single-dose regimens given for treatment of gonorrhea usually do not eradicate concomitant chlamydial infection, and seven or more days of treatment with tetracyclines or macrolides eradicates *C. trachomatis* from nearly all men, at least as determined by short-term follow up.[172–182] However, chlamydial infection recurs three to six weeks after treatment in five to ten percent of these men and cannot be clearly designated as reinfection or relapse. Most such recurrences are of the same immunotype as the original infecting strain, and nearly all cause recurrent clinical evidence of urethritis. In addition, despite apparent elimination of *C. trachomatis,* 10 to 15 percent of men develop persisting or relapsing symptoms, perhaps owing to simultaneous infection with another agent.

In men with NGU, trials using either placebos or agents such as spectinomycin, which are ineffective against *C. trachomatis*, have clearly established the greater effectiveness of specific antimicrobial treatment in eliminating both signs and symptoms of infection and in eradicating chlamydia. Clinical trials indicate that tetracycline hydrochloride, doxycycline, minocycline, triple tetracycline, erythromycin, and trimethoprim-sulfamethoxazole all achieve comparable clinical cure rates of approximately 85 to 95 percent in men with chlamydial NGU (see Chap. 52). Of the newer fluoroquinolones, ofloxacin also has reported cure rates in this range, whereas ciprofloxacin has been associated with more frequent failures and should not be used for the treatment of NGU.[183–185] Although relatively ineffective against *C. trachomatis* in vitro and when administered as a single dose, amoxicillin, when

Table 29-3. Diagnosis of *C. trachomatis* Infections in Women*

Associated findings	Clinical criteria	Laboratory criteria: Presumptive	Laboratory criteria: Diagnostic
Mucopurulent cervicitis	Mucopurulent cervical discharge, cervical ectopy and edema, spontaneous or easily induced cervical bleeding	Cervical GS with greater than 30 PMN/high-power (×1000) field in nonmenstruating women	Positive culture or nonculture test (cervix, FVU)
Acute urethral syndrome	Dysuria-frequency syndrome in young sexually active women; recent new sexual partner; often more than 7 days of symptoms	Pyuria, no bacteriuria	Positive culture or nonculture test (cervix or urethra or FVU)
PID	Lower abdominal pain; adnexal tenderness on pelvic exam; evidence of MPC often present	As for MPC; cervical GS positive for gonorrhea; endometritis on endometrial biopsy	Positive culture or nonculture test (cervix, FVU, endometrium, tubal)
Perihepatitis	Right upper quadrant pain, nausea, vomiting, fever; young sexually active women; evidence of PID	As for MPC and PID	High-titer IgM or IgG antibody to *C. trachomatis*

* GS = Gram stain; PMN = polymorphonuclear leukocytes; PID = pelvic inflammatory disease; MPC = mucopurulent cervicitis. Reproduced with permission from the *Annals of Internal Medicine*.

Table 29-4. Summary of Selected Studies Evaluating Oral Antimicrobial Treatment of *C. trachomatis* Urethritis in Men

Regimen	Efficacy*	Reference
Minocycline, 200 mg stat., then 100 mg q 12 h for 6 days	11/12 (92%)	175
Tetracycline, 500 mg qid for 7 days	35/35 (100%)	76
Erythromycin stearate, 500 mg q 12 h for 2 weeks	30/31 (97%)	176
Doxycycline, 200 mg for 2 days, then 100 mg for 12 days	50/52 (96%)	177
Deteclo, qd for 7 days	11/12 (92%)	173
Deteclo, qd for 21 days	16/16 (100%)	
Minocycline, 200 mg stat., then 100 mg bid for 6 days	39/40 (98%)	178
Rifampin, 600 mg qd for 6 days	52/53 (98%)	
Erythromycin stearate, 500 mg q 12 h for 15 days	27/30 (90%)	180
Lymecycline, 300 mg q 12 h for 10 days	21/24 (88%)	
Lymecycline, 300 mg q 12 h for 20 days	18/21 (86%)	
Pivampicillin, 750 mg tid for 7 days	19/22 (86%)	172
Doxycycline, 200 mg for 1 day, then 100 mg for 6 days	56/57 (98%)	194
Trimethoprim-sulfamethoxazole, 160 and 800 mg bid, respectively, for 10 days	18/20 (90%)	
Erythromycin, 500 mg bid for 10 days	18/23 (78%)	
Trimethoprim-sulfadiazine, 160 and 500 mg, respectively, in 1 tablet bid for 14 days	18/19 (95%)	75
Tetracycline, 250 mg qid for 7 days	21/24 (88%)	181
Tetracycline, 500 mg qid for 7 days	33/36 (92%)	
Rosaramicin, 250 mg qid for 7 days	38/42 (90%)	
Amoxicillin, 750 mg tid for 10 days	6/6 (100%)	179
Ciprofloxacin, 750 mg bid for 7 days	11/20 (55%)	185
Ciprofloxacin, 1000 mg bid for 7 days	13/18 (72%)	185
Doxycycline, 100 mg bid for 7 days	15/16 (94%)	189
Minocycline, 100 mg Qd for 7 days	19/19 (100%)	189
Doxycycline, 100 mg bid for 7 days	23/23 (100%)	78
Azithromycin, 1.0 g single dose	27/30 (90%)	78
Doxycycline, 100 mg bid for 7 days	29/29 (100%)	187
Azithromycin, 1.0 g single dose	34/34 (100%)	187

* Studies cited here performed chlamydia cultures before, just after, and 2 to 3 weeks following completion of treatment; efficacy, as expressed in this table, equals the number of patients with negative chlamydia cultures on visit 2 or 3 divided by the number of patients returning for follow-up visits 2 and 3. Eradication of chlamydia was usually, but not always, associated with clinical resolution of signs and symptoms.

given as 750 mg PO tid for 10 days, apparently eliminated chlamydia from 6 men with NGU followed for 24 to 48 days.[179] Pivampicillin in high dosage gave similar results.[172] Although symptoms usually subsided as cultures became negative in these studies, the possibility cannot be excluded that latent chlamydial infection persisted after amoxicillin or pivampicillin treatment.

Azithromycin, with a half-life of 5 to 7 days, excellent intracellular and tissue penetration, and in vitro activity against *C. trachomatis* in the 0.25 μg/mL range is an important new agent for treatment of chlamydial infection.[186] It is the first drug to offer the advantage of single-dose therapy, an approach that is particularly attractive in potentially less compliant patients, such as adolescents or those with few or no symptoms.[186–189] However, individuals treated with azithromycin should still abstain from sex for seven days after receiving therapy; earlier resumption of sexual activity with use of single-dose therapy is a concern, and could theoretically result in transmission of an unresolved infection to sex partners. Whereas the procurement cost of azithromycin is considerably higher than that of doxycycline ($9–15 vs. $1–2), cost-effectiveness analyses support the hypothesis that the compliance assured with single-dose therapy may make it a more cost-effective therapy.[190,191] Wherever possible, directly observed single-dose therapy should be used, maximizing compliance. The recommended length of therapy for NGU using tetracycline or doxycycline has ranged from 7 to 21 days. However, in 2 studies in which 7 days of therapy were compared with 21 days of therapy with tetracycline or minocycline, no difference was found.[174,175] Thus, there is as yet no evidence that prolongation of tetracycline therapy beyond one week is necessary, provided that sex partners can be treated concurrently.

Fewer studies have assessed the effectiveness of antimicrobial treatment of uncomplicated cervical or urethral chlamydial infection in women (Table 29-5). Those data available suggest that tetracycline, 500 mg qid for 7 days, successfully eliminates *C. trachomatis* from the cervix through at least 3 weeks of follow up.[182,192–197] Erythromycin, when given as 500 mg PO qid for 7 to 14 days, is also effective as is ofloxacin, 200 mg PO bid. A small double-blind, placebo-controlled trial indicates that doxycycline, 100 mg PO bid for 10 days, successfully eliminated *C. trachomatis* from the cervix and urethra of women with the acute urethral syndrome.[111]

Azithromycin given as a 1-gram single dose was shown to be comparable to 7 days of doxycycline therapy for treatment of uncomplicated chlamydial infection of the cervix.[187] The advantages of single dose directly observed therapy argue for its use in young women with uncomplicated cervical infection. Treatment options in pregnancy remain somewhat limited as neither doxycycline nor ofloxacin can be used. Erythromycin given as a 2-gram daily dose achieves a cure in 84 to 94 percent of treated women, but up to half of women develop significant gastrointestinal side effects and cannot complete the course of therapy.[198–200] A 1-gram daily dose for 7 days is better tolerated but less efficacious. The efficacy of azithromycin in pregnancy has not been studied extensively. In one small study, azithromycin effected cure of chlamydial infection in 11 of 15 pregnant women.[201] Although the risk of adverse fetal effects with azithromycin is thought to be low, con-

Table 29-5. Summary of Selected Studies Evaluating Antimicrobial Treatment of *C. trachomatis* Cervicitis in Women

Regimen	Efficacy*	Reference
Deteclo, 300 mg bid for 7 days	20/20 (100%)	192
Oxytetracycline, 250 mg qid for 14 days	49/50 (98%)	176
Oxytetracycline, 250 mg qid for 21 days	145/161 (90%)	182
Erythromycin, 500 mg bid for 15 days	13/17 (76%)	180
Lymecycline, 300 mg bid for 10 days	18/20 (90%)	
Lymecycline, 300 mg bid for 20 days	14/14 (100%)	
Trimethoprim-sulfadiazine, 160 and 500 mg, respectively, in 1 tablet bid for 14 days	15/15 (100%)	75
Doxycycline, 100 mg bid for 10 days	15/15 (100%)	
Doxycycline, 200 mg stat., then 100 mg bid for 9 days	55/58 (95%)	194
Erythromycin, 500 mg bid for 10 days	36/39 (92%)	
Trimethoprim-sulfamethoxazole, 160 and 800 mg, respectively, in 1 tablet for 10 days	37/40 (93%)	
Tetracycline, 500 mg qid for 7 days	21/22 (95%)	196
Erythromycin, 250 mg qid for 7 days	12/12 (100%)	
Sulfisoxazole, 500 mg qid for 10 days	8/8 (100%)	
Ciprofloxacin, 500 mg bid for 7 days	30/35 (86%)	193
Pivampicillin, 700 mg bid for 7 days	26/26 (100%)	195
Doxycycline, 100 mg bid for 7 days	17/17 (100%)	189
Minocycline, 100 mg qD for 7 days	16/16 (100%)	189
Ofloxacin, 300 mg bid for 7 days	26/28 (93%)	184
Doxycycline, 100 mg bid for 7 days	22/22 (100%)	184
Doxycycline, 100 mg bid for 7 days	72/73 (99%)	187
Azithromycin, 1.0 g single dose	78/78 (100%)	187

cerns have been raised regarding the adequacy of a single 1-gram dose in pregnancy, particularly since the volume of distribution of the drug is markedly elevated, its breakdown in the liver is accelerated, and absorption may not be assured. Consequently, routine therapy with single-dose azithromycin during pregnancy requires further study before it can be recommended routinely. Other options include amoxicillin, which has a cure rate approximately equal to that of erythromycin and less frequent gastrointestinal intolerance.[100,199,202] However, because the efficacies of these regimens in the pregnant patient may be low, a test of cure should be performed two weeks after the completion of therapy using culture or antigen detection, or at three weeks using an amplification test.

Treatment of other chlamydia-related syndromes is discussed in individual chapters on salpingitis, epidymitis, and so forth.

PREVENTION

Since many chlamydial infections are asymptomatic, it has become clear that effective control must involve periodic testing of individuals at risk. As the cost of extensive screening may be prohibitive, various approaches to defining target populations at increased risk of infection have been evaluated. One strategy has been to designate patients attending specific high prevalence clinic populations for universal testing. Such clinics would include STD, juvenile detention, and some family planning clinics. This approach, however, fails to account for the majority of asymptomatic infections, since attendees at high prevalence clinics often do so because of symptoms or suspicion of infection. Consequently, selective screening criteria have been developed for use in various clinical settings.[204–208] Among females, young age (generally, <21 years) is a critical risk factor for chlamydial infection in almost all of these studies. Other risk factors include the presence of mucopurulent cervicitis; multiple, new, or symptomatic male sex partners and lack of barrier contraceptive use. These findings have given rise to criteria for selective screening of women. In some settings, screening based solely on young age (generally, <25 years) may be equally as sensitive as criteria that incorporate behavioral and clinical measures.[209,210]

The effectiveness of selective screening in reducing the prevalence of chlamydial infection in women has been demonstrated in several studies. In the Pacific Northwest, where extensive screening began in family planning clinics in 1988 and in STD clinics in 1993, prevalence declined from 10 to 12 percent in the late 1980s and 4 to 5 percent in 1995.[2] Similar trends have occurred in association with screening programs elsewhere.[211,212] Additionally, evidence that screening can effect a reduction in upper genital tract disease recently has been published. In a study in Seattle, women in a large health maintenance organization who satisfied selective screening criteria for chlamydial infection were randomized to one of two arms: an intervention arm in which women were tested for chlamydial cervical infection, and a control arm characterized by standard care.[213] Subjects in the intervention (screening) arm experienced a marked reduction in the 1-year incidence of symptomatic PID as assessed by clinical record review and patient report of symptoms compatible with PID (odds ratio, 0.44; 95 percent confidence interval, 0.20, 0.90). This finding was especially notable given that chlamydia prevalence in the study population was low (3.5 percent), and that chlamydia screening programs were already ongoing in the area.

The practical implementation of screening programs in settings with low to moderate chlamydia prevalence requires that the prevalence at which selective screening becomes cost-effective relative to universal screening must be defined. Toward this end, a number of investigators have undertaken cost-effectiveness analyses. Most of these analyses have concluded that universal screening is preferred in settings with chlamydia prevalence above three to seven percent.[166–168,203] Depending on the criteria used, selective screening is likely to be more cost-effective when prevalence falls below these numbers.

Among asymptomatic males, risk factors for chlamydial infection have been less extensively explored and effectiveness of screening programs targeting males is not known. One approach has been to screen males for the presence of polymorphonuclear leukocytes with the leukocyte esterase (LE) test on urine in order to identify asymptomatic infected males. Such males are then tested specifically for chlamydial infection, or treated empirically. Most of the studies examining this issue have used culture to define chlamydial infection, and have found the sensitivity of the LE test in predicting chlamydial urethritis to be 41 to 85 percent among asymptomatic males, with specificities of 75 to 95 percent.[169–171] Most authors have thus concluded that the LE test is insufficiently sensitive to provide a reliable means of deciding which asymptomatic males should be further evaluated or treated for chlamydial infection. In one study that used LCR to define chlamydial infection, the sensitivity of LE in predicting infection in asymptomatic males was 59 percent and the negative predictive value 98 percent.[81] Further study based on populations universally screened with amplified DNA tests is necessary to more clearly define the optimal role of LE in reducing the cost, but maintaining the performance of, a comprehensive strategy employing urine-based testing. However, in settings where the cost of specific diagnostic tests such as LCR and PCR prohibits their routine implementation, use of the inexpensive LE test may be cost-effective, particularly if it is combined with simple risk assessment to detect a higher pretest probability of disease.

References

1 World Health Organization: Sexually transmitted diseases. Press release WHO/64; 25 August 1995.
2 Centers for Disease Control: *Chlamydia trachomatis* genital infections—United States, 1995. *MMWR* 46:193–198, 1997.
3 Centers for Disease Control: The leading nationally notifiable infectious diseases—United States, 1995. *MMWR* 45:883–884, 1996.
4 Mardh PA: Is Europe ready for STD screening? *Genitourin Med* 73: 96–98, 1997.
5 Schachter J: Chlamydial infections. *N Engl J Med* 298:428, 1978.
6 Schachter J et al: Chlamydia, in *Manual of Medical Microbiology*, 6th ed., Murray PR et al. (eds). 1995, pp. 669–677.
7 Workowski KA et al: Association of genital infection with specific *Chlamydia trachomatis* serovars and race. *J Infect Dis* 166:1445–1449, 1992.
8 Barnes RC et al: Comparison of *Chlamydia trachomatis* serovars causing rectal and cervical infections. *J Infect Dis* 156:953–958, 1987.
9 Batteiger BE et al: Correlation of infecting serovar and local inflammation in genital chlamydial infection. *J Infect Dis* 160:332–336, 1989.
10 Workowski KA et al: Clinical manifestations of genital infection due to *Chlamydia trachomatis* in women: Differences related to serovar. *Clin Infect Dis* 19:756–760, 1994.
11 Dean DE et al: Major outer membrane protein variants of *Chlamydia trachomatis* are associated with severe upper genital tract infections and histopathology. *J Infect Dis* 172:1013–1020, 1995.
12 Brunham RC et al: *Chlamydia trachomatis* from individuals in a sexually transmitted core group exhibit frequent sequence variation in the MOMP (omp1) gene. *J Clin Invest* 94:458–463, 1994.
13 Lampe MF et al: Sequence conservation in the major outer membrane protein gene among *Chlamydia trachomatis* strains isolated from the upper and lower urogenital tract. *J Infect Dis* 172:589–592, 1995.
14 Schachter J et al: Are chlamydial infections the most prevalent venereal disease? *JAMA* 231:1252, 1975.
15 Thelin I et al: Contact tracing in patients with genital chlamydial infection. *Br J Vener Dis* 56:259, 1980.
16 McMillan A et al: Chlamydial infection in homosexual men: Frequency of isolation of *Chlamydia trachomatis* from the urethra, anorectum, and pharynx. *Br J Vener Dis* 57:47, 1981.
17 Stamm WE et al: *Chlamydia trachomatis* urethral infections in men. Prevalence, risk factors, and clinical manifestations. *Ann Intern Med* 100:47, 1984.
18 Podgore JK et al: Asymptomatic urethral infections due to *Chlamydia trachomatis* in male military personnel. *J Infect Dis* 146:828, 1982.
19 Sadof MD et al: Dipstick leukocyte esterase activity in first-catch urine specimens. A useful screening test for detecting sexually transmitted diseases in the adolescent male. *JAMA* 2S8:1932, 1987.
20 Adger H et al: Screening for *Chlamydia trachomatis and Neisseria gonorrhoeae* in adolescent males: Value of first catch urine examination. *Lancet* 2:944, 1984.
21 Bowie WR et al: Etiologies of postgonococcal urethritis in homosexual and heterosexual men: Roles of *Chlamydia trachomatis* and *Ureaplasma urealyticum*. *Sex Transm Dis* 5:151, 1978.
22 Stamm WE et al: *Chlamydia trachomatis* proctitis, in *Chlamydial Infections*, PA Mardh et al. (eds). Amsterdam, Elsevier, 1982, pp. 111–115.
23 Goldmeier D et al: Isolation of *Chlamydia trachomatis* from the throat and rectum of homosexual men. *Br J Vener Dis* S3:184, 1977.
24 Quinn TC et al: *Chlamydia trachomatis* proctitis. *N Engl J Med* 305: 195, 1981.
25 Jones RB et al: *Chlamydia trachomatis* in the pharynx and rectum of heterosexual patients at risk for genital infection. *Ann Intern Med* 102:757, 1985.
26 Weinstein LS et al: Low prevalence of *Chlamydia trachomatis* in the oropharynx of adolescents. *Pediatr Infect Dis* 5:660, 1986.
27 Komaroff AL et al: Serological evidence of chlamydial and mycoplasmal pharyngitis in adults. *Science* 221:927, 1983.
28 Gerber MA et al: Role of *Chlamydia trachomatis* in acute pharyngitis in young adults. *J Clin Microbiol* 20:993, 1984.
29 Husseltein et al: Frequency of *Chlamydia trachomatis* as a cause of pharyngitis. *J Clin Microbiol* 22:858, 1984.
30 Lycke E et al: The risk of transmission of genital *Chlamydia trachomatis* infection is less than that of genital *Neisseria gonorrhoeae* infection. *Sex Transm Dis* 7:6, 1980.
31 Quinn TC et al: Epidemiologic and microbiologic correlates of *Chlamydia trachomatis* infection in sexual partnerships. *JAMA* 276: 1737–1742, 1996.
32 McCormack WM et al: Fifteen month follow-up study of women infected with *Chlamydia trachomatis*. *N Engl J Med* 300:123, 1979.
33 Oriel JD et al: Chlamydial infections of the cervix. *Br J Vener Dis* 50:11, 1974.
34 Hilton AL et al: Chlamydia A in the female genital tract. *Br J Vener Dis* 50:1, 1974.
35 Brunham R et al: Epidemiological and clinical correlates of *C. trachomatis* and *N. gonorrhoeae* infection among women attending an STD clinic. *Clin Res* 29:47A, 1981.
36 Stamm WE et al: Causes of the acute urethral syndrome in women. *N Engl J Med* 303:409, 1980.
37 Paavonen J et al: Genital chlamydial infections in patients attending a gynecological outpatient clinic. *Br J Vener Dis* 54:2S7, 1978.
38 Ripa KT et al: *Chlamydia trachomatis* cervicitis in gynecologic outpatients. *Obstet Gynecol* 52:698, 1978.
39 Schachter J et al: Chlamydiae as agents of sexually transmitted diseases. *Bull WHO* 54:245, 1976.
40 Persson K et al: Prevalence of nine different microorganisms in the female genital tract. *Br J Vener Dis* S5:429, 1979.
41 Oriel JD et al: Infection of the uterine cervix with *Chlamydia trachomatis*. *J Infect Dis* 137:443, 1978.
42 Johannisson G et al: Genital *C. trachomatis* infection in women. *Obstet Gynecol* 56:671, 1980.
43 Robertson P et al: Failure to identify venereal disease in lesbian population. *Sex Transm Dis* 8:75, 1981.
44 Saltz GR et al: *Chlamydia trachomatis* cervical infections in female adolescents. *J Pediatr* 98:981, 1981.
45 Bowie WR et al: Prevalence of *C. trachomatis* and *N. gonorrhoeae* in two populations of women. *Can Med Assoc J* 124:1477, 1981.
46 Harrison HR et al: *Chlamydia trachomatis* infection in pregnancy: Epidemiology and outcomes, abstracted (no S16). Read at the Twenty-first Interscience Conference on Antimicrobial Agents and Chemotherapy. Washington, DC, American Society for Microbiology, 1981.

47 Hammerschlag MR et al: Prospective study of maternal and infantile infection with *Chlamydia trachomatis*. *Pediatrics* 64:142, 1979.

48 Martin DH et al: Prematurity and perinatal mortality in pregnancies complicated by maternal *Chlamydia trachomatis* infection. *JAMA* 247:1585, 1982.

49 Martin DH et al: High prevalence of chlamydial infections in inner city obstetrical population, abstracted (no 515). Read at the Twenty-first Interscience Conference on Antimicrobial Agents and Chemotherapy. Washington, DC, American Society for Microbiology, 1981.

50 Chandler JW et al: Ophthalmia neonatorum associated with maternal chlamydial infections. *Trans Am Acad Ophthalmol Otolaryngol* 83: 302, 1977.

51 Frommell GT et al: Chlamydial infection of mothers and their infants. *J Pediatr* 95:28, 1979.

52 Harrison HR et al: Cervical *Chlamydia trachomatis* and mycoplasmal infections in pregnancy. Epidemiology and outcomes. *JAMA* 250:1721, 1983.

53 Toomey KE et al: Unrecognized high prevalence of *Chlamydia trachomatis* cervical infection in an isolated Alaskan population. *JAMA* 258:53, 1987.

54 Black SB et al: Serologic evidence of chlamydial infection in children. *J Pediatr* 98:6S, 1981.

55 Hammerschlag MR: Diagnosis of chlamydial infection in the pediatric population. *Immunol Invest* 26:151–156, 1997.

56 Stamm WE et al: Asymptomatic *Chlamydia trachomatis* urethritis. *Sex Transm Dis* 13:163, 1986.

57 Bell TA et al: Chronic *Chlamydia trachomatis* infections in infants. *JAMA* 267:400–402, 1992.

58 Tack KJ et al: Isolation of *Chlamydia trachomatis* from the lower respiratory tract of adults. *Lancet* 1:116, 1980.

59 Ito il et al: Pneumonia due to *Chlamydia trachomatis* in an immunocompromised adult. *N Engl J Med* 307:95, 1982.

60 Ormsby HL et al: Topical therapy in inclusion conjunctivitis. *Annu J Ophthalmol* 35:1811, 1952.

61 Moncada JV et al: Prevalence of *Chlamydia trachomatis* lung infection in patients with acquired immune deficiency syndrome. *J Clin Microbiol* 23:986, 1986.

62 Ballard RC et al: The epidemiology of chlamydial infections of the eye and genital tract in South Africa. Third International Meeting on Sexually Transmitted Diseases, Antwerp, Belgium, 1980.

63 Stamm WE et al: Repeated genital infections with *C. trachomatis*; prevalence and risk factors, in *Chlamydial Infections,* Oriel D et al. (eds). Cambridge, England, Cambridge University Press, 1986, pp. 499–503.

64 Blythe MJ et al: Recurrent genitourinary chlamydial infections in sexually active female adolescents. *J Pediatr* 121:487–493, 1992.

65 Barnes RC et al: Detection of multiple serovars of *Chlamydia trachomatis* in genital infections. *J Infect Dis* 152:985–989, 1985

66 Holmes KK et al: Etiology of nongonococcal urethritis. *N Engl J Med* 292:1199, 1975.

67 Oriel JD et al: Chlamydial infection: Isolation of *Chlainvdia* from patients with non-specific genital infection. *Br Vener Dis* 48:429, 1972.

68 Richmond S et al: Chlamydial infection: Role of *Chlamydia* subgroup A in non-gonococcal and post-gonococcal urethritis. *Br J Vener Dis* 48:437, 1972.

69 Dunlop EMC et al: Chlamydia and non-specific urethritis. *Br J Vener Dis* 2:575, 1972.

70 Alani MD et al: Isolation of *Chlamydia trachomatis* from the male urethra. *Br J Vener Dis* 53:88, 1977.

71 Terho P: *Chlamydia trachomatis* in NGU. *Br J Vener Dis* 54:251, 1978.

72 Paavonen J: *Chlamydia trachomatis*-induced urethritis in female partners of men with nongonococcal urethritis. *Sex Transm Dis* 6: 69, 1979.

73 Lassus A et al: Erythromycin and lymecycline treatment of chlamydia-positive and chlamydia-negative NGU: A partner controlled study. *Acta Derm Venereol (Stockh)* 59:278, 1979.

74 Bowie WR et al: Etiology of nongonococcal urethritis: Evidence of *Chlamydia trachomatis* and *Ureaplasma urealyticum*. *J Clin Invest* 59:735, 1977.

75 Paavonen J et al: Treatment of NGU with trimethoprim-sulpha-diazine and with placebo: A double-blind partner-controlled study. *Br J Vener Dis* 56:101, 1980.

76 Handsfield HH et al: Differences in the therapeutic response of chlamydia-positive and chlamydia-negative forms of nongonococcal urethritis. *J Am Vener Dis Assoc* 2:5, 1976.

77 Prentice MJ et al: NGU: A placebo controlled trial of minocycline in conjunction with laboratory investigations. *Br J Vener Dis* 52:269, 1976.

78 Stamm WE et al: Azithromycin for empirical treatment of the nongonococcal urethritis syndrome in men. A randomized double-blind study. *JAMA* 274:545–549, 1995.

79 Taylor-Robinson D et al: Microbiological, serological and histopathological features of experimental *Chlamydia trachomatis* urethritis in chimpanzees. *Br J Vener Dis* 57:36, 1981.

80 Schwartz SL et al: Persistent urethral leucocytosis and asymptomatic chlamydial urethritis. *J Infect Dis* 140:614, 1979.

81 Marrazzo JM et al: Implementation and findings of a community-based chlamydia screening program using urine ligase chain reaction. 1996 National STD Prevention Conference, December 9–12, Tampa, FL, 1996.

82 Schafer MA et al: Evaluation of urine based screening strategies to detect *Chlamydia trachomatis* among sexually active asymptomatic young males. *JAMA* 270:2065–2070, 1993.

83 Oriel JD et al: Infection with *Chlamydia* group A in men with urethritis due to *Neisseria gonorrhoeae*. *J Infect Dis* 131:376, 1975.

84 Berger RE et al: *Chlamydia trachomatis* as a cause of acute "idiopathic" epididymitis. *N Engl J Med* 298:301, 1978.

85 Berger RE et al: Etiology, manifestations, and therapy of acute epididymitis: Prospective study of 50 cases. *J Urol* 121:750, 1979.

86 Moller BR et al: Experimental epididymitis and urethritis in grivet monkeys provoked by *Chlamydia trachomatis*. *Fertil Steril* 34:275, 1980.

87 Berger RE et al: Epididymitis induced in *Macaca nemestrina with Chlamydia trachomatis* (personal communication).

88 Mardh PA et al: Role in *Chlamydia trachomatis* in non-acute prostatitis. *Br J Vener Dis* 54:330, 1978.

89 Mardh PA et al: Inhibiting effect on the formation of chlamydial inclusions in McCoy cells by seminal fluid and some of its components. *Invest Urol* 17:510, 1980.

90 Nilsson S et al: Isolation of *Chlamydia trachomatis* from the urethra and from prostatic fluid in men with signs and symptoms of acute urethritis, in Studies on *C. trachomatis* as a cause of lower urogenital tract infections. *Thesis Acta Dermatovener* Suppl 93, 1981.

91 Bruce AW et al: The role of chlamydiae in genitourinary disease. *J Urol* 126:625, 1981.

92 Poletti F et al. Isolation of *Chlamydia trachomatis* from the prostatic cells in patients affected by nonacute abacterial prostatitis. *J Urol* 134:691, 1985.

93 Rompalo AM et al: Potential value of rectal-screening cultures for *Chlamydia trachomatis* in homosexual men. *J Infect Dis* 153:888, 1986.

94 Kousa M et al: Frequent association of chlamydial infection with Reiter's syndrome. *Sex Transm Dis* 5:57, 1978.

95 Martin DH et al: Urethral chlamydial infections in men with Reiter's syndrome, in *Chlamydial Infections,* Mardh PA et al. (eds). Amsterdam, Elsevier, 1982, pp. 107–111.

96 Bowie WR: personal communication, 1981.

97 Keat A et al: *Chlamydia trachomatis* and reactive arthritis—the missing link. *Lancet* 1:72–74, 1987.

98 Wordsworth BP et al: Chlamydial DNA is absent from the joints of patients with sexually acquired reactive arthritis. *Br J Rheumatol* 29: 208–210, 1990.

99 Poole E et al: A search for *Chlamydia trachomatis* in synovial fluids from patients with reactive arthritis using PCR and antigen detection methods. *Br J Rheumatol* 31:31–34, 1992.

100 Taylor-Robinson D et al: Detection of *Chlamydia trachomatis* DNA in joints or reactive arthritis patients by PCR. *Lancet* 340:81–82, 1992.

101 Hill-Gaston JS et al: Identification of 2 *Chlamydia trachomatis* antigens recognized by synovial fluid T cells from patients with chlamydia-induced arthritis. *J Rheumatol* 23:130–136, 1996.

102 Keat AC et al: *Chlamydia trachomatis* and reactive arthritis: The missing link. *Lancet* 1:72, 1987.

103 Brewerton DA et al: Reiter's disease and HLA 27. *Lancet* 2:996, 1973.

104 Keat AC et al: Role of *Chlamydia trachomatis* and HLA-B27 in sexually acquired reactive arthritis. *Br Med J* 1:605, 1978.

105 Harrison HR et al: Cervical *Chlamydia trachomatis* infection in university women: Relationship to history, contraception, ectopy and cervicitis. *Am J Obstet Gynecol* 153:244, 1985.

106 Paavonen J et al: Colposcopic manifestations of cervical and vaginal infections. *Obstet Gynecol Surv* 43:373, 1988.

107 Brunham RC et al: Mucopurulent cervicitis—the ignored counterpart in women of urethritis in men. *N Engl J Med* 311:1, 1984.

108 Hobson D et al: Quantitative aspects of chlamydial infection of the cervix. *Br J Vener Dis* 56:156, 1980.

109 Richmond SJ et al: Antibodies to *Chlamydia trachomatis* in cervicovaginal secretions. *Sex Transm Dis* 7:11, 1980.

110 Wallin JE et al: Urethritis in women attending an STD clinic. *Br J Vener Dis* 57:50, 1981.

111 Stamm WE et al: Treatment of the acute urethral syndrome. *N Engl J Med* 304:956, 1981.

112 Davies JA et al: Isolation of *Chlamydia trachomatis* from Bartholin's ducts. *Br J Vener Dis* 54:409, 1978.

113 Mardh PA et al: Endometritis caused by *Chlamydia trachomatis. Br J Vener Dis* 57:191, 1981.

114 Gump DW et al: Endometritis related to *Chlamydia trachomatis* infection. *Ann Intern Med* 95:61, 1981.

115 Hamark B et al: Bacteriological cultures from the endometrial cavity in patients with acute salpingitis. *Acta Obstet Gynecol Scand* (Suppl)93:55, 1981.

116 Moller BR et al: Salpingitis og endometritis forirsaget af *Chlamydia trachoniatis. Ugeskr Laeger* 172:3319, 1980.

117 Wasserheit JN et al: Microbial causes of proven pelvic inflammatory disease and efficacy of clindamycin and tobramycin. *Ann Intern Med* 104:187, 1986.

118 Sweet RL et al: Failure of beta-lactam antibiotics to eradicate *Chlamydia trachomatis* in the endometrium despite apparent clinical cure of acute salpingitis. *JAMA* 250:2641, 1983.

119 Paavonen J et al: Prevalence and manifestations of endometritis among women with cervicitis. *Am J Obstet Gynecol* 152:280, 1985.

120 Wager GP et al: Puerperal infectious morbidity: Relationship to route of delivery and to antepartum *Chlamydia trachomatis* infection. *Am J Obstet Gynecol* 138:1028, 1980.

121 Mardh PA et al: *Chlamydia trachomatis* infection in patients with acute salpingitis. *N Engl J Med* 296:1377, 1977.

122 Eschenbach DA et al: Polymicrobial etiology of acute pelvic inflammatory disease. *N Engl J Med* 293:166, 1975.

123 Treharne JD et al: Antibodies to *Chlamydia trachomatis* in acute salpingitis. *Br J Vener Dis* 55:26, 1979.

124 Simmons PD et al: Antichlamydial antibodies in pelvic inflammatory disease. *Br J Vener Dis* 55:419, 1979.

125 Rees E: The treatment of pelvic inflammatory disease. *Am J Obstet Gynecol* 138:1041, 1980.

126 Mardh PA: Ascending chlamydial infection in the female tract, in *Chlamydial Infections.* Oriel D et al. (eds). London, Cambridge University Press, 1986, pp. 173–185.

127 Svensson L et al: Differences in some clinical and laboratory parameters in acute salpingitis related to culture and clinical findings. *Am J Obstet Gynecol* 138:1017, 1980.

128 Bowie WR et al: Acute pelvic inflammatory disease in outpatients. *Ann Intern Med* 95:685, 1981.

129 Osser S et al: Epidemiologic and serodiagnostic aspects of chlamydial salpingitis. *Obstet Gynecol* 59:206, 1982.

130 Brunham RC et al: Etiology and outcome of acute pelvic inflammatory disease. *J Infect Dis* 158:510, 1988.

131 Moller BR et al: Experimental pelvic inflammatory disease provoked by *Chlamydia trachomatis* and *Mycoplasma hominis* in grivet monkeys. *Am J Obstet Gynecol* 138:990, 1980.

132 Patton D et al: *Chlamydia trachomatis* salpingitis in the pig-tailed macaque, in *Chlamydial Infections,* Mardh PA et al. (eds). Amsterdam, Elsevier, 1982, pp. 399–405.

133 Muller-Schoop JW et al: *Chlamydia trachomatis* as a possible cause of peritonitis and perihepatitis in young women. *Br J Vener Dis* 1: 1022, 1978.

134 Wolner-Hanssen P et al: Periheparitis in chlamydial salpingitis. *Lancet* 1:901, 1980.

135 Dalaker K et al: *Chlamydia trachomatis* as a cause of perihepatitis associated with pelvic inflammatory disease. *Br J Vener Dis* 57:41, 1977.

136 Eckert LO et al: Prevalence and correlates of antibody to chlamydial heat shock protein in women attending sexually transmitted disease clinics and women with confirmed pelvic inflammatory disease. *J Infect Dis* 175:1453–1468, 1997.

137 Tack Kj et al: Isolation of *Chlamydia trachomatis* from the lower respiratory tract of adults. *Lancet* i:116, 1980.

138 Meyers JD et al: *Chlamydia trachomatis* infection as a cause of pneumonia after human marrow transplantation. *Transplantation* 36: 130, 1983.

139 Komaroff AL et al: *Chlamydia trachomatis* infection in adults with community-acquired pneumonia. *JAMA* 245:1319, 1981.

140 Schachter J: Human *Chlamydia psittaci* infection in chlamydial infections, in *Proceedings of the Sixth International Symposium on Human Chlamydial Infections,* Oriel D et al. (eds). London, Cambridge University Press, 1986.

141 vander Bel-Kahn JM et al: *Chlamydia trachomatis* endocarditis. *Am Heart J* 95:627, 1978.

142 Myhre EB et al: *Chlamydia trachomatis* infections in a patient with meningoencephalitis. *N Engl J Med* 304:910, 1981.

143 Lannigan R et al: *Chlamydia trachomatis* peritonitis and ascites following appendectomy. *Can Med Assoc J* 123:295, 1980.

144 Goldmeier D et al: Chlamydial vulvovaginitis in a post menopausal woman. *Lancet* 2:476, 1981.

145 Stamm WE: Laboratory diagnosis of chlamydial infection, in *Chlamydial Infections Proceedings of the 7th International Symposium on Human Chlamydial Infections*, Bowie WR et al. (eds). Cambridge, England, Cambridge University Press, pp. 459–470, 1990.

146 Black CM: Current methods of laboratory diagnosis of *Chlamydia trachomatis* infections. *Clin Microbiol Rev* 10:160–184, 1997.

147 Marrazzo JM et al: New approaches to the diagnosis, treatment, and prevention of chlamydial infections. *Curr Topics Infect Dis*, in press.

148 Stamm WE et al: Diagnosis of *Chlamydia trachomatis* infection by direct immunofluorescence staining of genital secretions—a multicenter trial. *Ann Int Med* 101:683–641, 1984.

149 Clark A et al: Multicenter evaluation of the AntigEnz chlamydia enzyme immunoassay for diagnosis of *Chlamydia trachomatis* genital infection. *J Clin Microbiol* 30:2762–2764, 1992.

150 Kluytmans JA et al: Evaluation of Clearview and Magic Lite tests, polymerase chain reaction, and cell culture for detection of *Chlamydia trachomatis* in urogenital specimens. *J Clin Microbiol* 31: 3204–3210, 1994.

151 Schwebke JR et al: Use of a urine enzyme immunoassay as a diagnostic tool for *Chlamydia trachomatis* urethritis in men. *J Clin Microbiol* 29:2446–2449, 1991.

152 Carpenter Weet al: A transcriptionally amplified DNA probe assay with ligatable probes and immunochmical detection. *Clin Chem* 39: 1934–1938, 1993.

153 Stary A et al: Comparison of DNA amplification methods for the detection of *Chlamydia trachomatis* in first-void urine from asymptomatic military recruits. *Sex Transm Dis* 23:97–102, 1996.

154 Chernesky MA et al: Diagnosis of *Chlamydia trachomatis* infection in men and women be testing first-void urine by ligase chain reaction. *J Clin Microbiol* 32:2682–2685, 1994.

155 Ridgway GL et al: Comparison of the ligase chain reaction with cell culture for the diagnosis of *Chlamydia trachomatis* infection in women. *J Clin Pathol* 49:116–119, 1996.

156 Schachter J et al: Noninvasive tests for diagnosis of *Chlamydia trachomatis* infection: Application of ligase chain reaction to first-catch urine specimens of women. *J Infect Dis* 172:1411–1414, 1995.
157 Lee H et al: Diagnosis of *Chlamydia trachomatis* genitourinary infection in women by ligase chain reaction assay of urine. *Lancet* 345: 213–216, 1995.
158 Rumpianesi F et al: Detection of *Chlamydia trachomatis* by a ligase chain reaction amplification method. *Sex Transm Dis* 23:177–180, 1996.
159 Schachter J et al: Ligase chain reaction to detect *Chlamydia trachomatis* by a ligase chain reaction amplification method. *Sex Transm Dis* 23:177–180, 1996.
160 Mahony J et al: Confirmatory polymerase chain reaction testing for *Chlamydia trachomatis* in first-void urine from asymptomatic and symptomatic men. *J Clin Microbiol* 30:2241–2245, 1992.
161 Bauwens JE et al: Diagnosis of *Chlamydia trachomatis* urethritis in men by polymerase chain reaction assay of first-catch urine. *J Clin Microbiol* 31:3013–3016, 1993.
162 Quinn TC et al: Diagnosis by AMPLICOR PCR of CT in urine samples from women and men attending sexually transmitted disease clinics. *J Clin Microbiol* 34:1401–1406, 1996.
163 Toye B et al: Diagnosis of *Chlamydia trachomatis* infections in asymptomatic men and women by PCR assay. *J Clin Microbiol* 34: 1395–1400, 1996.
164 Bianchi A et al: An evaluation of the polymerase chain reaction (Amplicor) *Chlamydia trachomatis* in male urine and female urogenital specimens. *Sex Transm Dis* 21:196–200, 1994.
165 Pasternack R et al: Detection of CT infections in women by Amplicor PCR: comparison of diagnostic performance with urine and cervical specimens. *J Clin Microbiol* 34:995–998, 1996.
166 Trachtenberg AI et al: A cost-based decision analysis for Chlamydia screening in California family planning clinics. *Obstet Gynecol* 71: 101–108, 1988.
167 Genc M et al: A cost-effectiveness analysis of screening and treatment for *Chlamydia trachomatis* infection in asymptomatic women. *Ann Intern Med* 124:1–7, 1996.
168 Sellors JW et al: Effectiveness and efficiency of selective vs. universal screening for Chlamydial infection in sexually active young women. *Arch Intern Med* 152:1837–1844, 1992.
169 Genc M et al: An economic evaluation of screening for *Chlamydia trachomatis* in adolescent males. *JAMA* 270:2057–2064, 1993.
170 Sadof MD et al: Dipstick leukocyte esterase activity in first-catch urine specimens: A useful screening test for detecting sexually transmitted diseases in the adolescent male. *JAMA* 258:1932–1934, 1987.
171 Shafer MA et al: Evaulation of urine-based screening strategies to detect *Chlamydia trachomatis* among sexually active asymptomatic young males. *JAMA* 270:2065–2070, 1993.
172 Johannison G et al: Susceptibility of *Chlamydia trachomatis to* antibiotics in vitro and in vivo. *Sex Transm Dis* 6:50, 1979.
173 Thambar IV et al: Double-blind comparison of two regimens in the treatment of NGU. *Br J Vener Dis* 55:284, 1979.
174 Bowie WR et al: Therapy for nongonococcal urethritis: Double-blind randomized comparison of two doses and two durations of minocycline. *Ann Intern Med* 95:306, 1981.
175 Prentice M et al: Non-specific urethritis: A placebo-controlled trial of minocycline in conjunction with laboratory investigations. *Br J Vener Dis* 52:269, 1976.
176 Oriel JD et al: Comparison of erythromycin stearate and oxytetracycline in the treatment of non-gonococcal urethritis. *Scott Med J* 22: 375, 1977.
177 Perroud HM et al: L'hyclate de doxycycline dans le traitment des uretrites non-gonocciques. *Schweiz Med Wochenschr* 108:412, 1978.
178 Coufalik ED et al: Treatment of nongonococcal urethritis with rifampicin as a means of defining the role of *Ureaplasma urealyticum*. *Br J Vener Dis* 55:36, 1979.
179 Bowie WR et al: Eradication of *Chlamydia trachomatis* from the urethras of men with NGU by treatment with amoxiciilin. *Sex Transm Dis* 8:79, 1981.
180 Lassus A et al: Erythromycin and lymecycline treatment in chlamydia-positive and chlamydia-negative nongonococcal urethritis: A partner-controlled study. *Acta Derm Venereol (Stockh)* 59:278, 1979.
181 Stamm WE et al: Comparison of rosaramicin and tetracycline for the treatment of NGU, in *Current Chemotherapy and Infectious Diseases,* Nelson JD et al. (eds). Washington, DC, American Society for Microbiology, 1980, vol 1, pp 269–270.
182 Rees E et al: Chlamydia in relation to cervical infection and pelvic inflammatory disease, in *Nongonococcal Urethritis and Related Infections,* Hobson D et al. (eds). Washington, DC, American Society for Microbiology, 1977, pp 67–77.
183 Arya O et al: Evaluation of ciprofloxacin 500 mg twice daily for one week in treating uncomplicated gonococcal, chlamydial and nonspecific urethritis in men. *Genitourin Med* 62:170, 1986.
184 Hooton TM et al: Ofloxacin versus Doxycycline for Treatment of Cervical Infection with *Chlamydia trachomatis*. *Antimicrob Agents Chemother* 36:1144–1146, 1992.
185 Hooton TM et al: Ciprofloxacin compared with doxycycline for nongonococcal urethritis: Ineffectiveness against *Chlamydia trachomatis* due to relapsing infection. *JAMA* 264(11):1418–1421, 1990.
186 Stamm WE: Azithromycin in the treatment of uncomplicated genital chlamydial infections. *Am J Med* 3A:195–225, 1991.
187 Martin DH et al: A controlled trial of a single dose of azithromycin for the treatment of chlamydial urethritis and cervicitis. *N Engl J Med* 327:921–925, 1992.
188 Lister PJ et al: Comparison of azithromycin and doxycycline in the treatment of non-gonococcal urethritis in men. *J Antimicrob Chemother* 31:185–192, 1993.
189 Romanowski B et al. Minocycline compared with doxycyline in the treatment of nongonococcal urethritis and mucopurulent cervicitis. *Ann Intern Med* 119:16–22, 1993.
190 Magid D et al: Doxycycline compared with azithromycin for treating women with genital *Chlamydia trachomatis* infections: An incremental cost-effectiveness analysis. *Ann Intern Med* 124:389–399, 1996.
191 Haddix AC et al: The cost-effectiveness of azithromycin for *Chlamydia trachomatis* infections in women. *Sex Transm Dis* 22:274–280, 1995.
192 Waugh MA et al: Triple tetracycline (Detecio) in the treatment of chlamydial infection of the female genital tract. *Br J Venear Dis* 53: 96, 1977.
193 Ahmen-Jushuf IH et al: Ciprofloxacin treatment of chlamydial infection of the urogential tract in women. *Genitourin Med* 64:14, 1988.
194 Johannison G: Studies on *Chlamydia trachomatis* as a cause of lower urogenital tract infection. *Acta Derm Venereol* 93:(suppl)29, 1981.
195 Cramers M et al: Pivampicillin compared wtih erythromycin for treating women with genital *Chlamydia trachomatis* infection. *Genitourin Med* 64:247, 1988.
196 Bowie WR: Seven to ten day antimicrobial regimens for *Chlamydia trachomatis* cervical infection. *Clin Res* 28:43A, 1980.
197 Hunter J et al: Response to treatment of chlamydial infection of uterine cervix. *Lancet* 2:848, 1979.
198 Alary M et al: Randomized comparison of amoxicillin and erythromycin in treatment of genital chlamydial infection in pregnancy. *Lancet* 344:1461–1465, 1994.
199 Silverman NS et al: A randomized prospective trial comparing amoxicillin and erythromycin for the treatment of *Chlamydia trachomatis* in pregnancy. *Am J Obstet Gynecol* 170:829–832, 1994.
200 Magat AH et al: Double-blind randomized study comparing amoxicillin and erythromycin for the treatment of *Chlamydia trachomatis* in pregnancy. *Obstet Gynecol* 81:745–749, 1993.
201 Bush MR et al: Azithromycin and erythromycin in the treatment of cervical chlamydial infection during pregnancy. *Obstet Gynecol* 84: 61–63, 1994.
202 Turrentine MA et al: Amoxicillin or erythromycin for the treatment of antenatal chlamydial infection: A meta-analysis. *Obstet Gynecol* 86:1021–1025, 1995.
203 Marrazzo JM et al: Performance and cost-effectiveness of selective screening for chlamydial infection in women: Implications for a national screening strategy. *Sex Transm Dis* 24:131–141, 1997.

204 Addiss DG et al: *Chlamydia trachomatis* infection in women attending urban midwestern family planning and community health clinics: Risk factors, selective screening, and evaluation of non-culture techniques. *Sex Transm Dis* 17(3):138–146, 1990.

205 Kent GP et al: Screening for *Chlamydia trachomatis* infection in a sexually transmitted disease clinic: Comparison of diagnostic tests with clinical and historical risk factors. *Sex Transm Dis* 15:51–57, 1988.

206 Magder LS et al: Factors related to genital *Chlamydia trachomatis* and its diagnosis by culture in a sexually transmitted disease clinic. *Am J Epidemiol* 128:298–308, 1988.

207 Stergachis A et al: Selective screening for *Chlamydia trachomatis* infection in a primary care population of women. *Am J. Epidemiol* 138: 143–153, 1993.

208 Weinstock HS et al: *Chlamydia trachomatis* infection in women: a need for universal screening in high prevalence populations? *Am J Epidemiol* 135(1):41–47, 1992.

209 Hillis SD et al: Targeting screening for chlamydial infections in women: Is young age enough? Abstracts of the Eleventh Meeting of the International Society for STD Research, New Orleans, LA, 27–30, August 1995.

210 Marrazzo JM et al: Selective screening criteria for chlamydial infection in women: a comparison of CDC screening recommendations with age and risk-based criteria. *Fam Plann Perspect* 29:158–162, 1997.

211 Addiss DG et al: Decreased prevalence of *Chlamydia trachomatis* infection associated with a selective screening program in family planning clinics in Wisconsin. *Sex Transm Dis* 20(1):28–35, 1993.

212 Katz BP et al: Declining prevalence of chlamydial infection among adolescent girls. *Sex Transm Dis* 23:226–229, 1996.

213 Scholes D et al: Prevention of pelvic inflammatory disease by screening for cervical chlamydial infection. *N Engl J Med* 334:1362–1366, 1996.

Chapter 30
Lymphogranuloma venereum

Peter L. Perine
Walter E. Stamm

Lymphogranuloma venereum (LGV) is one of the sexually transmitted diseases caused by *Chlamydia trachomatis*. A sporadic disease in North America, Europe, and Oceania, LGV is highly prevalent in parts of Africa, Asia, and South America. It is also known variously as *tropical* or *climatic bubo*,[1] *strumous bubo*,[2] *poradenitis inguinalis*,[3] *Durand-Nicolas-Favre disease*,[3,4] *lymphogranuloma inguinale*, and the *fourth, fifth*, or *sixth venereal disease*.[5] LGV is preferred because it is less easily confused with granuloma inguinale.

LGV is a chronic disease that has a variety of acute and late manifestations. Three stages of infection, more or less analogous to those of venereal syphilis, are recognized.[6] The primary lesion of LGV is a small, nonpainful genital papule that may ulcerate rapidly. The secondary stage is characterized by acute lymphadenitis with bubo formation (the inguinal syndrome) and/or acute hemorrhagic proctitis following rectal intercourse (the anogenitorectal syndrome) together with fever and other symptoms caused by systemic spread of infection. The vast majority of patients recover from LGV after the secondary stage without sequels, but in a few patients the persistence of *Chlamydia* in anogenital tissue incites a chronic inflammatory response and the development of genital ulcers, fistulas, rectal strictures, and genital elephantiasis. Antibiotic treatment during the secondary stage prevents these late complications, which otherwise may require surgical repair.

LGV is usually caused by one of three serovars of *C. trachomatis:* Ll, L2, and L3 (see Chap. 15). Other *C. trachomatis* strains occasionally have been isolated from infected tissue taken from patients who have symptoms compatible with genitoanorectal LGV.[7–9]

Throughout most of its history, LGV has been confused with other diseases, particularly with the lymphadenopathy of syphilis and genital herpes and the buboes of chancroid. Confusion was caused in part by the failure to recognize the common etiology of the different manifestations of LGV, which often were described as distinct clinical or pathologic entities. Durand, Nicolas, and Favre[4] established the disease as a clinical and pathologic entity in 1913, and Phylactos deduced a common etiology of climatic bubo and LGV in 1922,[10] but a major diagnostic advancement in the study of LGV was the development of a "specific" skin test by Frei in 1925.[11] This test established the etiology of LGV proctocolitis and rectal stricture.[12] In 1930, LGV *Chlamydia* were isolated from buboes by intracerebral inoculation of monkeys,[10] and LGV *Chlamydia* were grown in embryonated eggs in 1935.[13] The latter achievement made possible the commercial manufacture of large amounts of standardized antigen for Frei tests and serodiagnostic tests.

The first effective drugs for treatment of LGV were the sulfonamides, which were introduced in the late 1930s.[14] Although other drugs have since been developed for treatment of LGV[15] and serodiagnostic tests have been refined to give greater specificity, we still do not fully understand the pathogenesis of this disease.

A thorough review of the history of LGV is a study in itself and will not be undertaken here. The monograph on LGV published by Stannus in 1933[5] lists 933 references and, together with the excellent reviews published by Koteen in 1945[16] and Favre and Hellerstrom in 1954,[10] describes the historical background of the disease.

EPIDEMIOLOGY

LGV is a sporadic disease throughout North America, Europe, Australia, and most of Asia and South America. It is endemic in east[17] and west Africa,[18] India,[19] parts of Southeast Asia,[20] South America,[21] and the Caribbean.[22] Few countries require official notification of LGV cases, and the lack of standard diagnostic criteria renders reported cases somewhat suspect. Since 1950 no country in Europe has reported more than a few dozen cases of LGV annually,[21] and the average for the United States was 595 cases per year, with slight increases during the wars in Korea and Vietnam.[23] By contrast, one municipal clinic in Ethiopia reports several thousand cases of acute LGV annually.[17] Most of the reported LGV cases in nonendemic areas occur in sailors, soldiers, and travelers who acquire the infection while visiting or living in an endemic area.[20] Like other sexually transmitted diseases, LGV is more common in urban than in rural areas, among the sexually promiscuous, and among the lower socioeconomic classes.[22] Until recently, much of the reported epidemiology on LGV was based on cases diagnosed using clinical criteria or the results of serologic tests and/or Frei skin tests that were not specific for the disease. When such tests were used in large prevalence studies (e.g., in venereal disease clinics and municipal hospitals), a large segment of the population was found to have positive test results but no history or physical evidence of the disease. Many such studies conducted in the United States in the 1930s claimed that 20 to 40 percent of blacks and 2 to 5 percent of whites were or had at one time been infected with LGV.[10,16,24] Such studies probably demonstrated the high prevalence of other *C. trachomatis* infections in these highly selected patient populations rather than a true racial difference. Of interest are early reports from Africa and South America that stated that climatic bubo was uncommon in all but white expatriates.[25] Acute LGV occurs most frequently during the third decade, which corresponds to the age of peak sexual activity. Extragenital[10,16] and adolescent infections also have been reported,[10] and material from ruptured buboes and other infected tissue poses a risk to research and health care personnel.[26,27]

Acute LGV is reported much more frequently in men than in women, with the ratio often reaching 5:1 or greater.[28] This is because symptomatic infection is much less common in women, who usually are diagnosed during early infection only if they develop acute proctocolitis or, less commonly, inguinal buboes. Late complications such as hyperplasia, ulceration and hypertrophy of the genitalia (esthiomene), and rectal strictures are reported to be more frequent in women than in men.[16,24] Men who are recipients of anal intercourse also may present with acute proctocolitis rather than inguinal buboes[9] and may develop rectal strictures.[22]

The frequency of infection following exposure is unknown. LGV is probably not as contagious as gonorrhea. Primary herpetiform lesions, urethritis, cervicitis, proctocolitis, and chronic ulcerations are probably the most infectious forms of LGV. Although supporting evidence is limited, the endocervix is apparently the most common site of acute infection in women. The cervix may remain infected for periods of weeks or months, as has been demonstrated for other serovars of *C. trachomatis*.[29] Conjugal infections are said to be common. Congenital transmission does not occur, but infection may be acquired during passage through an infected birth canal.

PATHOGENESIS

Chlamydia cannot penetrate intact skin or mucous membrane; these organisms probably gain entry through minute lacerations and abrasions. Laboratory-acquired infections following inhalation of highly concentrated virulent cultures have been reported.[27]

LGV is predominantly a disease of lymphatic tissue.[31] The essential pathologic process is thrombolymphangitis and perilymphangitis with spread of the inflammatory process from infected lymph nodes into the surrounding tissue. The lymphangitis is marked by proliferation of endothelial cells lining the lymph vessels and the lymph channels in lymph nodes. Lymph nodes draining the site of primary infection rapidly enlarge and form small, discrete areas of necrosis surrounded by densely packed endothelial cells.[32] The necrotic areas attract polymorphonuclear leukocytes and enlarge to form characteristic triangular- or quadrangular-shaped "stellate abscesses." Inflammation mats the adjacent lymph nodes together by periadenitis, and as the inflammation progresses, abscesses coalesce and rupture, forming loculated abscesses, fistulas, or sinus tracts.

The inflammatory process lasts several weeks or months before subsiding. Healing takes place by fibrosis, which destroys the normal structure of lymph nodes and obstructs lymph vessels. The resulting chronic edema and sclerosing fibrosis cause induration and enlargement of the affected parts. Fibrosis also compromises the blood supply to the overlying skin or mucous membrane, and ulceration occurs. In the rectum this results in destruction and ulceration of the mucosa, transmural inflammation of the bowel wall, obstruction of lymphatic drainage, and formation of a fibrotic, inflammatory stricture. Numerous adhesions form that fix the lower part of the sigmoid and rectum to the wall of the pelvis and neighboring organs.[32,33]

Although the primary pathologic process in LGV may be localized to one or two groups of lymph nodes, the organisms spread systemically in the bloodstream and can enter the central nervous system.[34] Dissemination and local extension of disease are limited by host immunity. Delayed hypersensitivity (as evidenced by positive skin tests) and LGV-specific *Chlamydia* antibody can be demonstrated 1 to 2 weeks after infection.[35] Chlamydial cytoplasmic inclusions also can be demonstrated within tissue phagocytes early in the course of infection.[13] Host immunity ultimately limits chlamydial multiplication but may not eliminate these organisms from the body, and a state of latency ensues.[15] Viable *Chlamydia* have been isolated from late lesions as long as 20 years after initial infection.[36] Much of the tissue damage in LGV is probably caused by cell-mediated hypersensitivity to chlamydial antigens. Persistence of LGV in tissues or repeated infections by the same or related serovars of *C. trachomatis* may be important in developing systemic disease.[37] It is of interest that repeated subcutaneous or intravenous injections of Frei antigen were used to treat LGV in the 1930s with some success,[38] possibly by desensitizing the host to *Chlamydia*.

CLINICAL MANIFESTATIONS

PRIMARY LESION

The primary lesion of LGV may take one of four forms: a papule, an ulcer or erosion, a small herpetiform lesion, or nonspecific urethritis.[28] The most common is the nonindurated herpetiform ulcer that appears at the site of infection after an incubation period of 3 to 12 days or longer.[10,24,30,32] It may be asymptomatic and inconspicuous (although occasionally multiple and deeply erosive). It is found in 3 to 53 percent of patients,[39,40] heals rapidly, and leaves no scar.[28,32] The most common site of occurrence in men is the coronal sulcus, followed by the frenum, prepuce, penis, urethral glans, and scrotum.[10] In women it appears most commonly on the posterior vaginal wall, the fourchette, the posterior lip of the cervix, and the vulva.[6,10,39] If located intraurethrally, the ulcer or erosion may cause nonspecific urethritis with a thin, mucous purulent discharge.[16,20] Other uncommon types of primary lesions are balanitis,[30] nodular ulcerations,[10,16,32] and proctitis in both sexes, following rectal intercourse.

Primary LGV lesions in men may be associated with a lymphangitis of the dorsal penis and formation of a large, tender lymphangial nodule, or *bubonulus*.[10] Bubonuli may rupture and form draining sinuses and fistulas of the urethra as well as fibrotic, deforming scars at the base of the penis.[41] Lymphangitis is very often accompanied by local and regional edema, which may produce varying degrees of phimosis in men and genital swelling in women[30] (Table 30-1).

Cervicitis and urethritis are probably more common manifestations of primary LGV than reported statistics indicate.[30] The urethritis is usually asymptomatic and follows a mild couse. Cervicitis may extend locally and could conceivably cause perimetritis or salpingitis, which are known to occur in other genital chlamydial infections.[15,29]

INGUINAL SYNDROME

Inflammation and swelling of the inguinal lymph nodes are the most common manifestations of the secondary stage of LGV in men[20,24] and are the reason that most patients seek medical attention.[28] Other lymph nodes may be involved; the likelihood of such involvement depends on the location of the primary lesion (Table 30-2). The incubation period for this manifestation is 10 to 30 days, but it may be delayed for as long as 4 to 6 months after infection.[36,39] It is important to note that LGV also can occur as an acute symptomatic infection without apparent lymph node localization or tissue reaction at the point of infection.

The inguinal bubo is unilateral in two-thirds of cases[16,24] (Fig. 30-1). It begins as a firm, slightly painful mass that enlarges over 1 to 2 weeks. The inguinal bubo was described by William Wallace[42] in 1833:

> The skin becomes red; and is then found to be adherent to the surface of the tumour, over which it could be previously moved. The bubo then for the most part increases with rapidity; the pain becomes of a throbbing

Table 30-1. Lesions of Lymphogranuloma Venereum

Early	Late
Inguinal syndrome	
Primary genital lesion(s)	Genital elephantiasis
Genital ulcers	Genital ulcers
Inguinal buboes	
Bubonulus	
Anorectal syndrome	
Proctitis	Rectal stricture
	Lymphorrhoids
	Perirectal abscesses
	Anal fistula
Other	
Urethritis	
Cervicitis	Frozen pelvis
Salpingitis	Infertility
Parametritis	
Conjunctivitis	

Table 30-2. Site of Primary LGV Infection Determining Subsequent Lymphatic Involvement

Site of primary infection	Affected lymph nodes
Penis, anterior urethra	Superficial and deep inguinal
Posterior urethra	Deep iliac, perirectal
Vulva	Inguinal
Vagina, cervix	Deep iliac, perirectal, retrocrural, lumbosacral
Anus	Inguinal
Rectum	Perirectal, deep iliac

kind; some degree of fever sets in, marked by an acceleration of pulse, an increase of heat, loss of appetite, imperfect sleep, with a general feeling of indisposition.

The constitutional symptoms associated with inguinal buboes may be associated with systemic spread of *Chlamydia*. During this stage of infection, LGV organisms have been recovered from the blood and the cerebrospinal fluid of patients both with and without symptoms of meningoencephalitis and abnormal cerebrospinal fluid.[34,43,44] Other manifestations of systemic spread are hepatitis,[45,46] pneumonitis,[28] and possibly arthritis.[47] Erythema nodosum, erythema multiforme, and eyeground changes (papillary edema) are also reported.[16,30,44]

As the bubo enlarges, the male patient complains of severe pain in the groin. He may walk with a limp, bent at the waist in an attempt to limit pain. Within 1 to 2 weeks the bubo becomes fluctuant, and the skin overlying the bubo takes on a characteristically livid color ("blue balls") that predicts rupture of the bubo.[24]

Rupture through the skin usually relieves pain and fever.[16,44] Numerous sinus tracts are formed that drain thick, tenacious, yellowish pus for several days or weeks with little or no discomfort.[48] Healing takes place slowly, leaving callous and contracted scars in the inguinal region. The disappearance of the inguinal bubo usually marks the end of the disease in men, and the majority suffer no serious sequelae.[24,49] Bubonic relapse occurs in about 20 percent of untreated cases.[49]

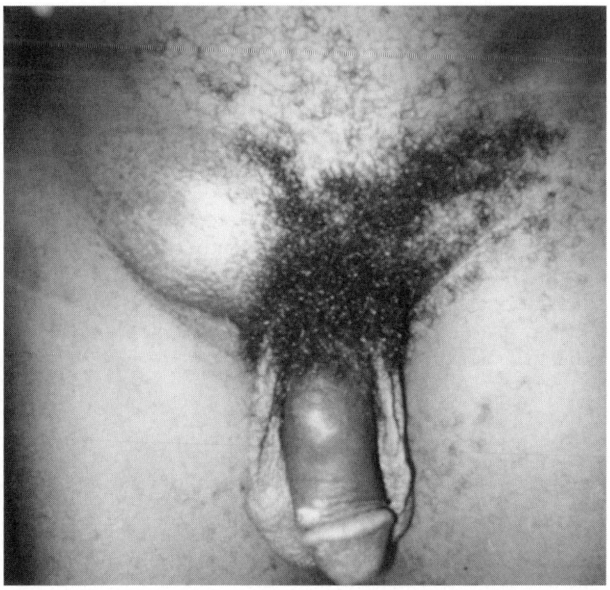

Fig. 30-1. Early inguinal syndrome of LGV showing superficial, primary preputial erosion, dorsal penile lymphangitis, and right inguinal bubo.

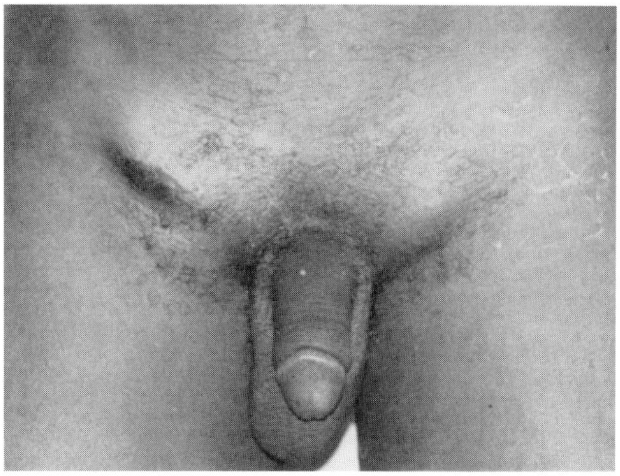

Fig. 30-2. Early inguinal syndrome of LGV showing a small vesicular primary lesion and bilateral inguinal lymphadenitis with cleavage of the enlarged right inguinal and femoral lymph nodes by the inguinal ligament, the characteristic "groove" sign.

Only about one-third of inguinal buboes become fluctuant and rupture; the others slowly involute and form firm, slowly resolving inguinal masses without undergoing suppuration.[16,24] In about 20 percent of cases the femoral lymph nodes are also affected and may be separated from the enlarged inguinal lymph nodes by Poupart's ligament; this process creates the "sign of the groove" that is said to be pathognomonic for LGV[28] (Fig. 30-2). Simultaneous involvement of the deep iliac lymph nodes occurs in about 75 percent of cases and may cause formation of a large pelvic mass that, fortunately, seldom suppurates.[30,44] Extragenital primary lesions produce lymphadenitis and bubo formation in the lymph nodes draining the lesions; these extragenital buboes do not differ symptomatically or pathologically from inguinal buboes.[16]

In large studies of LGV in women, only 20 to 30 percent present with the inguinal syndrome.[24,50] About one-third of female cases without proctitis, however, complain of lower abdominal and back pain, especially when supine.[44] This symptom is characteristic of involvement of the deep pelvic and lumbar lymph nodes and may be mistaken for acute appendicitis[28] or a tuboovarian abscess.[16,44] Numerous adhesions may form, fixing the pelvic organs together.[44]

Other infectious diseases causing inguinal lymphadenitis and bubo formation are plague, tularemia, and tuberculosis. More common causes of inguinal lymphadenitis without suppuration, which are frequently misdiagnosed as LGV, are genital herpes, syphilis, chancroid, and Hodgkin's disease.[30] Small lesions on the feet or lower extremities may cause significant inguinal adenopathy. In nonendemic areas, however, the syndrome is most frequently mistaken for an incarcerated inguinal hernia[51] or lymphoma.[52]

ANOGENITORECTAL SYNDROME

The subacute manifestations of this syndrome are proctocolitis and hyperplasia of intestinal and perirectal lymphatic tissue (lymphorrhoids). The chronic or late manifestations are perirectal abscesses, ischiorectal and rectovaginal fistulas, anal fistulas, and rectal stricture or stenosis.[22,30]

In men, the rectal mucosa can be inoculated directly with *Chlamydia* during receptive anal intercourse or by lymphatic spread from the male posterior urethra. In women, the rectal mucosa also

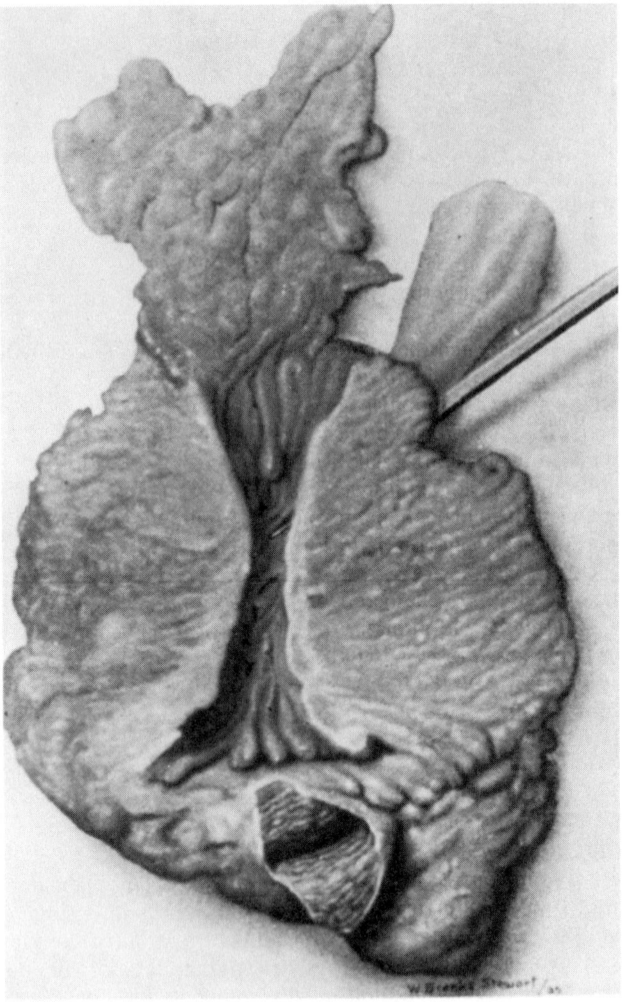

Fig. 30-3. Necropsy specimen of an LGV rectal stricture containing an ileosigmoidal fistula. *(From Lichtenstein.[60])*

can be inoculated directly with *Chlamydia* during anal intercourse, or it can be contaminated by migration of infectious vaginal secretions or by lymphatic spread from the cervix and posterior vaginal wall. The vast majority of patients with the anorectal syndrome are women or homosexual men.[50,53–57]

The early symptoms of rectal infection are anal pruritus and a mucous rectal discharge caused by local or diffuse edema of the anorectal mucosa. The mucosa becomes hyperemic and friable after a period of several weeks and bleeds easily when traumatized.[53,56,57] Multiple, discrete, superficial ulcerations with irregular borders appear on the mucosa and are gradually replaced by granulation tissue. A chronic inflammatory process invades the bowel wall, and noncaseous granulomas and crypt abscesses form.[53,56] With secondary bacterial infection of the rectal mucosa, the discharge becomes mucopurulent. If left untreated, the granulomatous process progressively involves all layers of the bowel wall. The muscle layers are replaced by fibrous tissue.[33,53] In women the rectovaginal septum may be eroded, and a rectovaginal fistula may be formed.[54] Contraction of the fibrous components of the granulation tissue over a period of months or years causes partial (stricture) or complete (stenosis) blockage of the rectum.[33,53,54]

Symptoms of proctocolitis include fever, rectal pain, and tenesmus.[16,22,54] The lower left quadrant of the abdomen is tender, and the pelvic colon may be palpably thickened. The rectal mucosa feels granular on digital examination, and movable, enlarged lymph nodes may be palpated immediately under the bowel wall.[54] There are no pathognomonic sigmoidoscopic findings. The inflammatory process may be localized to one segment of bowel or may occur at several different levels concurrently, but it is usually limited to that portion below the peritoneal reflection.[22,33,54]

Additional symptoms that occur with rectal stricture are varying degrees of constipation, passage of "pencil" stools, attacks of ileus with colic and abdominal distension, and weight loss.[24,30,53,58] The stricture usually forms 2 to 5 cm above the anocutaneous margin, where the perirectal lymphatic tissue is the richest.[22,54] It is usually annular or tubular in shape,[58] and its proximal margins are granular (Fig. 30-3). If the palpating finger can be introduced through the aperture of the nondistensible and rigid stricture, the mucous membrane above it has a normal consistency.[54] By contrast, the mucous membrane below the stricture generally shows ulcerative and granulomatous proctitis, which makes the digital examination very painful.[24] Although the stricture often is very narrow, complete bowel obstruction (rectal stenosis) is rare but may cause bowel perforation and peritonitis, which is the usual cause of death in LGV.[30,59]

The rectal mucosa below the stricture and the skin around the anus are frequent sites for formation of perirectal abscesses and anal fissures.[55,58] These also may occur as the only manifestation of chronic anogenitorectal LGV. Obstruction of the lymphatic and venous drainage of the lower rectum produces perianal outgrowths of lymphatic tissue that grossly resemble hemorrhoids but are called *lymphorrhoids*[60] or *perianal condylomas*.[58] Histologically, these anal tags are composed of dilated lymph vessels with perilymphatic inflammation.[16,24]

The clinical and histologic picture of early LGV proctocolitis is identical to that seen in inflammatory bowel disease,[61,62] and there has been considerable debate in the medical literature concerning a possible etiologic role for LGV in regional ileitis (Crohn's disease) and ulcerative colitis.[63] Schuller et al.[64] demonstrated specific LGV antibody in the sera of 38 of 55 patients with Crohn's disease, but subsequent studies showed no serologic evidence of *Chlamydia* infection in either Crohn's disease or ulcerative colitis.[65–67]

Several groups have isolated non-LGV *C. trachomatis* serovars from male homosexuals with proctocolitis.[9,56,57] The sigmoidoscopic and biopsy findings in these patients differ from those found in LGV infections; the inflammatory process is not as intense or as invasive as that caused by LGV serovars, and hypertrophic mucosal "follicles" predominate. Non-LGV proctocolitis may prove to be more common than that caused by LGV, but it is not known if non-LGV serovars will cause rectal stricture if left untreated.

The rectal stricture of LGV may resemble that caused by trauma, actinomycosis, tuberculosis, schistosomiasis, and malignancy.[22,30,58] It is most frequently mistaken for rectal cancer, and a biopsy should be taken to exclude this diagnosis. The incidence of rectal cancer in patients with LGV rectal stricture has ranged from 2 percent[68] to 5 percent.[69] In a study of 106 LGV patients who subsequently developed carcinoma, Rainey[69] proposed a causal relationship between LGV rectal stricture and the development of rectal cancer, hypothesizing that the chronic irritation of LGV predisposes the rectal stricture to malignant transformation.

ESTHIOMENE

Esthiomene (Greek, "eating away"), a primary infection affecting the lymphatics of the scrotum, penis, or vulva, may cause chronic progressive lymphangitis, chronic edema, and sclerosing fibrosis of the subcutaneous tissues of these structures.[24,50] This results in induration and enlargement of the affected parts and, ultimately, in ulceration. In the earliest stages the ulceration is superficial, but

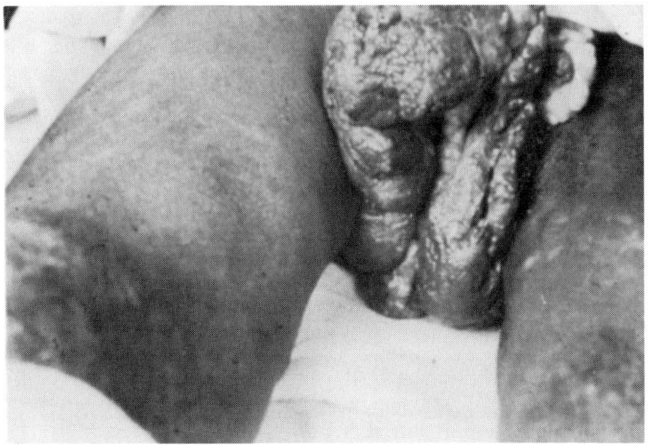

Fig. 30-4. Esthiomene of late lymphogranuloma venereum in a woman.

it gradually becomes more invasive and destructive. The vast majority of patients with esthiomene are women, and many authorities prefer to restrict the use of the term to this sex.

Chronic ulcerations are extremely painful. In women they are most common on the external surface of the labia majora, on the genitocrural folds, and on the lateral regions of the perineum[30] (Figs. 30-4 and 30-5). The edema may extend from the clitoris to the anus and interfere with normal function. Urethral and vaginal[16,24,50] stenoses and fistula formation have been reported.

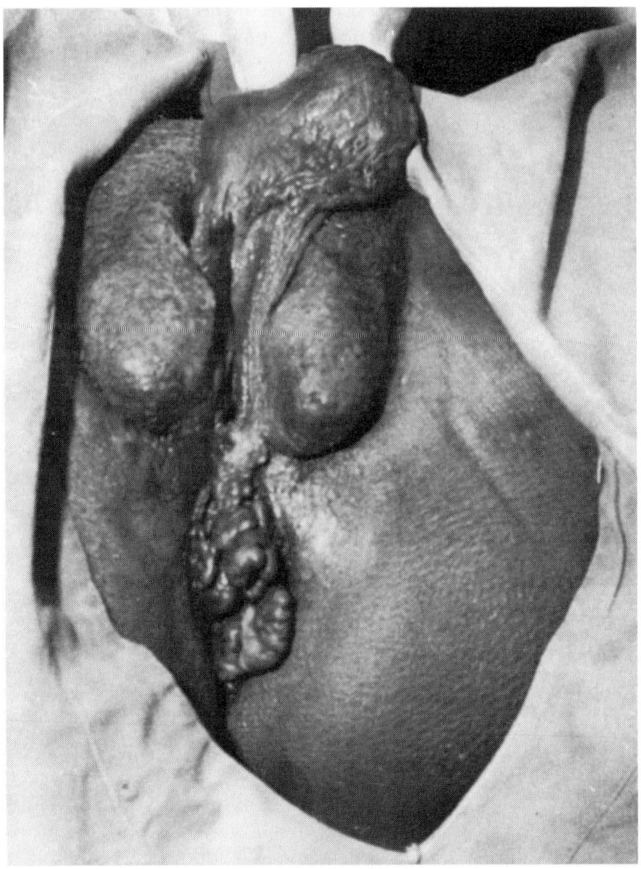

Fig. 30-5. Elephantiasis of the labia and clitoris in a woman with late lymphogranuloma venereum. *(Courtesy of M.I. Unit, Ibadan University, Nigeria.)*

OTHER MANIFESTATIONS

There is a tendency for women to develop papillary growths on the mucosa of the urethral meatus; these growths cause dysuria, frequency, and urinary incontinence with some perimeatal ulceration.[50] Penile, scrotal, or perineal sinuses may develop with or without urethral stenosis.[18,50] Coutts[30] refers to this symptom complex as the *urethrogenitoperineal syndrome.*

Penoscrotal elephantiasis appears from 1 to 20 years after infection.[30] It may affect only the prepuce, the prepuce and the penis, the scrotum alone, or all the male external genitalia. The genital tissue is indurated and often deformed. The scrotum may reach monstrous size, but this is unusual.[24] Other conditions such as filariasis and mycosis must be considered in the differential diagnosis.

Follicular conjunctivitis, often accompanied by lymphadenitis of the maxillary and posterior auricular nodes,[16] can occur at any stage of LGV. The conjunctiva is infected by autoinoculation of infectious genital discharge. This condition may be analogous to Parinaud's oculoglandular syndrome.[30]

Primary LGV lesions of the mouth and pharynx can occur as the result of fellatio or cunnilingus. This results in lymphadenitis of the submaxillary or cervical lymph nodes.[26] Cases of supraclavicular lymphadenitis with mediastinal lymphadenopathy and pericarditis also have been reported.[70,71] Coutts[47] has recovered LGV from the gallbladder wall (in cases of chronic cholecystitis) and from fibrous perihepatic (in cases of Fitz-Hugh-Curtis syndrome), abdominal, and pelvic adhesions.

Erythema nodosum and other skin manifestations occur in about 10 percent of LGV cases during the early stages of infection.[10] Their appearance may be precipitated by surgical manipulation of infected lymph nodes.[16] The malnutrition associated with rectal stricture was a frequent cause of pellagra in the preantibiotic era.[24]

DIAGNOSIS

Mild leukocytosis with an increase in monocytes and eosinophils frequently accompanies early bubonic and anogenitorectal LGV.[20,22,25] A more significant polymorphonuclear leukocytosis is found routinely in patients whose LGV buboes, abscesses, etc. are superinfected with pyogenic bacteria.[16] The only other clinical laboratory abnormality found with regularity is an elevated gammaglobulin concentration due to an increase of IgA, IgG, and IgM immunoglobulins.[17] Anticomplement activity is commonly associated with hypergammaglobulinemia.[72–74]

The diagnosis of LGV is usually based on (1) a positive Frei skin test, (2) a positive complement-fixation (CF) or other serologic test for LGV, (3) isolation of LGV *Chlamydia* from infected tissue and secretions in mice, embryonated eggs, or tissue culture, (4) histologic identification of *Chlamydia* in infected tissue, or (5) demonstration of *Chlamydia* by PCR in infected secretions or tissues. Although histopathologic changes in LGV are not unique, they are sufficiently distinct to differentiate LGV buboes, bubonuli, and rectal strictures from similar lesions caused by other sexually transmitted agents.[24,32,75]

FREI TEST

The original Frei test antigen utilized pus obtained from unruptured buboes, diluted in saline, and sterilized by heating.[11] Not only was the risk of bacterial or viral contamination of this antigen considerable, but it could easily be inactivated by overheating, and standardization of its potency was impossible.[76] Nevertheless, a positive test in a patient with clinical findings compatible with LGV generally indicated present or past infection. The successful culture of LGV in large amounts in the yolk sacs of chick embryos led to the commercial manufacture of a standardized skin test antigen (Lygranum) in 1940.[78] The test consisted of intradermal injections of 0.1 mL Lygranum into the skin of one forearm and a similar volume of control yolk sac material into the other forearm. The test was read at 48 hours, and a positive result was the development of a papule at least 6 × 6 mm in the principal diameter, provided that the papule produced by the control was 5 × 5 mm or smaller. The same antigen also was used in complement-fixation serodiagnostic tests for LGV[79] after Melczer and Sipos[80] demonstrated the complement-fixing property of LGV in 1937.

The Frei skin test usually becomes positive after the appearance of buboes 2 to 8 weeks after infection.[10,16,77] In the older literature it was said that the Frei test was positive in about 95 percent of patients with bubonic LGV and in about 90 percent of those with ulcerative genital elephantiasis.[6] The lack of sensitivity in the early stages of LGV is a distinct disadvantage.[46]

Since the Frei antigen is common to all *Chlamydia,* the specificity of a positive reaction has limited its diagnostic usefulness, particularly in the past two decades, when the prevalence of other chlamydial infections has risen considerably.[15] The Frei test tends to remain positive for several years and possibly for life despite treatment.[77,81] For these reasons, commercial manufacture of Frei antigen was discontinued in 1974.

COMPLEMENT-FIXATION SEROLOGIC TEST

The complement-fixation (CF) test is more sensitive and is positive earlier than the Frei test.[16,30,43] There is no correlation between the CF antibody titer and the intensity of the Frei reaction,[16,82] although in a given patient there is often close agreement between the two.[77] Like the Frei test, the CF test may result in cross-reactions in infections caused by other chlamydial infections, and the antibody may persist in high or low titer for many years.[77,83] In general, active LGV infections have CF titers of 1:64 or greater,[28,77,82–84] but high CF titers occasionally are found in asymptomatic patients and those with other chlamydial infections. Titers below 1:64 in a patient suspected of LGV on clinical grounds should be interpreted with caution.

Although a rise in CF titer of two or more dilutions may occur in early LGV,[82] most patients with documented LGV initially have high CF titers that show little difference between serum specimens obtained during acute infection and at 6 weeks into convalescence.[46,82] Variations in CF titer also can be caused by changes in both the concentration of test antigen and the test procedure.

NEUTRALIZING ANTIBODY

LGV-neutralizing antibody is measured by mixing test serum with virulent mouse brain emulsion[35]; if the test serum contains LGV antibody, the mixture will not produce meningoencephalitis when inoculated into the brains of mice.[16]

MICROIMMUNOFLUORESCENT (MICRO-IF) ANTIBODY TEST

The micro-IF test is considerably more sensitive and specific than the CF test[35,85,86]; although the micro-IF antibody reacts broadly with other *C. trachomatis* strains,[85] it is usually possible to demonstrate the antigenic type of the infecting strain by the pattern of reactivity.[9,17,35] In LGV, acute-phase serum usually contains very high titers of micro-IF antibody.[9,17,56] The major disadvantage of the micro-IF test is that it is used primarily in a few specialized research laboratories and is not routinely available.

OTHER SEROLOGIC TESTS

A radioisotope precipitation (RIP) test was used by Philip et al.[35] to detect LGV antibody. In this procedure, antiglobulin is used to precipitate otherwise nonsedimentable complexes of radiolabeled meningopneumonitis *Chlamydia* and *Chlamydia* antibody. The proportion of radioactivity removed from the system measures the amount of antibody present. The test is more sensitive than the micro-IF test, but unless specific LGV antigens are used, it suffers from the same lack of specificity as the CF test. It is also available in only a few specialized laboratories.

A trachoma LGV-specific antigen extracted from LGV *Chlamydia* grown in tissue culture has been used in a counterimmunoelectrophoresis test to detect antibodies in LGV patients.[87] It has about the same sensitivity and specificity as the micro-IF test.

Serovar-specific monoclonal chlamydial antibodies can be used to detect LGV in tissues or secretions. These antibodies have led to the commercial manufacture of test reagents and different test systems (e.g., enzyme-linked immunosorbent assay, or ELISA) that increase the availability of specific serodiagnostic tests for LGV.

ISOLATION OF LGV

Chlamydia can be isolated from infected tissue or secretions by inoculation of mouse brain, yolk sac, or tissue culture.[15,16,88] The recovery rate depends on the method used and the source of the inoculum. Bubo pus is the most practical clinical material to obtain and inoculate.[28] Wall et al.[82] compared the recovery rate from bubo biopsy or pus in mice and yolk sac; *Chlamydia* were cultured from 85 percent of patients, with a higher recovery rate in mice (98 percent) than in yolk sac (78 percent). Other studies report much lower recovery rates.[46,89]

For the past 15 years, HeLa-229[90] and McCoy[1] tissue-culture cell lines have been used to isolate LGV *Chlamydia.* The reported recovery rate from buboes, genital tissue, or rectal tissue ranges from 24 to 30 percent,[17,35,46] which is much lower than that reported for nongonococcal urethritis.[15,88]

CYTOLOGY

The elementary and inclusion bodies of *Chlamydia* can be visualized both outside and inside cells in secretions and infected tissues by using Giemsa's, iodine, and fluorescent antibody staining methods.[30,88,92] Cytology has not been very successful for the diagnosis of LGV,[32] often because of the frequent contamination of specimens by bacteria and other artifacts.

POLYMERASE CHAIN REACTION

Polymerase chain reaction (PCR) technology has been used recently to detect "signature" *C. trachomatis* nucleic acid specific for the organism in cases of urethritis, cervicitis, salpingitis, and other syndromes caused by this agent. The PCR utilizes complementary DNA primers to detect and amplify DNA sequences in the chlamydial cryptic plasmid or in the outer membrane protein (MOMP) of *C. trachomatis.*

For non-LGV infections, the PCR test provides additional sensitivity as compared with cell culture methods. A prospective study of an epidemic of LGV in the Bahamas in 1990[104] involving 47 consecutive patients with genital ulcers seen at an STD clinic in Nassau demonstrated the advantage of the PCR test for diagnosis of LGV in an area where other causes of genital ulcers and lymphadenopathy, including HIV, are common. Eight patients had LGV based on detection of *C. trachomatis* sequences consistent with the L2 serovar; 9 others had possible LGV, based on serum microimmunofluorescent *C. trachomatis* titers of 1:256 or greater. Inguinal lymphadenopathy or buboes were present in 15 of the 17 patients, meeting the laboratory criteria for definite or possible LGV, versus 7 of 30 not meeting laboratory criteria for diagnosis of LGV. The remaining 13 patients had laboratory criteria that confirmed genital herpes in 13 of the patients, chancroid in 6, and probable or possible genital herpes in 4.

OTHER DIAGNOSTIC PROCEDURES

Various radiologic procedures have been used in LGV. Lymphography demonstrates the extent of lymph node involvement but does not outline buboes or reveal specific changes.[93] Rectal strictures caused by LGV are said to be characteristic when seen on barium enema and quite different from cancer: The LGV stricture is elongated, in contradistinction to the stricture produced by cancer; it produces little alteration in the mucosal pattern of the bowel; and it has a tendency to form fistulas that tend to reenter the lumen of the rectum.[94,95]

TREATMENT

A number of different drugs have been used to treat LGV, but there is no singularly effective drug that will ensure bacteriologic cure. A major problem in evaluating a given drug is the relative lack of criteria by which efficacy can be measured.[96] The natural history of LGV is highly variable, and spontaneous remission is common.[44,49]

Sulfonamides were the first drugs to show efficacy in LGV by promoting reduction in the size of buboes, healing of fistulas, etc.[14,75,97] However, lesions were not sterilized despite many months of therapy,[14] and CF titers may show little or no change.[98] In experimentally infected mice, 20 percent remained infected with LGV despite the most extensive sulfonamide therapy.[97]

A number of different antibiotics have been used to treat LGV. Penicillin and streptomycin were the first to be used but were found ineffective, although penicillin has some activity against *Chlamydia* in vitro.[97] The next antibiotics used were the tetracyclines, which proved to be quite effective in the management of the primary and secondary stages of LGV.[49,83,99] Similar effectiveness was found with chloramphenicol,[96] erythromycin,[100] minocycline,[19] and rifampin.[101]

BUBONIC LGV

Greaves et al.[49] attempted the only comparative treatment study of bubonic LGV. The relative effectiveness of oral chlortetracycline, oxytetracycline, chloramphenicol, or sulfadiazine was compared with patients treated symptomatically with aspirin. The tetracyclines and chloramphenicol were given in a dosage of 500 mg qid for 14 days following a loading dose of 1 gm. Sulfadiazine was given in a dose of 2 gm initially, followed by 4 gm daily in divided doses for 10 to 28 days. The relative effectiveness of each drug was measured by the duration of inguinal adenopathy and the occurrence of bubonic relapse, sinus formation, or skin lesions after completion of therapy. Unfortunately, the average number of patients treated with each drug was 6.5, which limits the statistical validity of the results.

The duration of the bubo after treatment was the same in all the drug-treated groups and was not significantly shorter compared with the duration of the bubo in those given symptomatic therapy. Although specific chemotherapy had only a minimal effect in shortening the duration of the bubonic lesion (31 versus 69 days), there was a more frequent occurrence of complications among the symptomatically treated control group. There was a marked reduction in CF antibody titer in drug-treated patients, which suggests that the amount of LGV present in infected tissues was reduced, if not eliminated. Other workers have shown that lymph nodes that were proved to be infective before tetracycline were found to be negative after therapy.[102]

Minocycline, in a loading oral dose of 300 mg followed by 200 mg bid for 10 days, has been used with success to treat acute bubonic LGV and a limited number of cases of proctitis.[19] Only limited information is available on treatment of LGV with erythromycin.[100]

Although oral azithromycin in a 1-gm oral dose has been proven effective for treatment of chlamydial urethritis and cervicitis, its effectiveness in treating LGV is not known. While it may prove to be effective for single-dose treatment of LGV, such short-course therapy should not be used until further supporting evidence is available. The cost of this drug in single-dose therapy is likely to be prohibitive where the disease is highly prevalent.[92a]

Fever abates and patients usually experience prompt relief of bubo pain and tenderness and feel much improved 1 to 2 days after starting antibiotics.[17,20] The bubo seldom suppurates after therapy begins, but fluctuant buboes may require frequent needle-and-syringe aspiration to prevent rupture.[17]

ANOGENITORECTAL LGV

Banov[53] reported the immediate and long-term effects of chlortetracycline, oxytetracycline, chloramphenicol, and erythromycin in cases of rectal stricture. Criteria used to compare the different drugs were subjective, the patients were not randomly assigned treatments, and the dosage schedules were variable. With the exception of erythromycin (only three cases studied), all drugs were effective. Apparently these drugs reduced the inflammatory edema of the rectal stricture but had no effect on scar tissue. In contrast to bubonic LGV, antibiotics had no immediate effect on the titer of CF antibody. No case of anal or rectovaginal fistula was cured by drugs alone.

The response of proctocolitis to antibiotics is usually dramatic. Symptoms are completely relieved and the rectal mucosa heals within a few weeks after treatment.[22,56] Occasional tetracycline treatment failures in proctocolitis have been reported.[22,57]

The recommended antibiotic treatment for both bubonic and anogenitorectal LGV is tetracycline, 2 gm daily in divided doses for 2 to 4 weeks.[36] Dual infections with other sexually transmitted diseases are common in LGV patients,[16,22,30] and these should be treated appropriately.

SURGICAL TREATMENT

Surgical treatment of the acute inguinal syndrome should be limited to aspiration of fluctuant lymph nodes and occasional incision and drainage of abscesses.[22] Before the advent of sulfonamides, surgical extirpation of buboes was recommended,[22,25] although it was probably a prominent factor in the development of postoperative elephantiasis of the genitals by further blocking normal lymphatic drainage.[39] Under antibiotic coverage there is little risk that incision or aspiration of fluctuant buboes will lead to formation of sinuses.[20,51]

Spontaneous resolution of a fibrous LGV rectal stricture never occurs, but the inflammatory process and the diameter of the stricture may be improved dramatically by antibiotic treatment.[22,53] Dilatation of the stricture using elastic bougies under direct vision may be necessary but poses a significant risk of bowel perforation. It should be limited to soft, short strictures not extending above the peritoneal reflection and should be abandoned if the stricture splits easily or if bleeding occurs.[22]

A variety of different surgical procedures may be required for advanced rectal stricture. The indications for operation are bowel obstruction, persistent rectovaginal fistula, and gross destruction of the anal canal, anal sphincter, and perineum.[22] Plastic operations on the vulva, penis, and scrotum may be required for esthiomene and genital elephantiasis.[30] None of these procedures should be attempted without antibiotic treatment, and if possible, antibiotics should be given for several months before the decision to perform surgery is made.[103]

PREVENTION

Prevention of LGV in nonendemic areas is predicated on identification and treatment of sexual contacts of proved or suspected cases. These contacts should receive prophylactic antibiotic treatment if recently exposed to infection so as to prevent reinfection as well as to eliminate a potential reservoir. The increasing prevalence of anorectal LGV in male homosexuals in the United States should be kept in mind when a young male presents with symptoms of proctocolitis.

Control of LGV in endemic areas presents a formidable problem. Diagnostic and treatment facilities are very limited, and patients often do not seek medical attention until after late complications are well established. The only hope appears to be that with the passage of time the standards of living and hygiene in endemic areas will improve to the point where health education and medical care are readily available.

References

1 Godding CC: On non-venereal bubo. *Br Med J* 2:842, 1896.

2 Klotz HG: Uber die Entwickelung der sogenannten strumosen Bubonen und die indicationen fur die fruhzeitige Exstirpation derselben. *Berl Klin Wochenschr* 1:132, 1890.

3 Fiessinger N: Diagnostic des adenopathics chroniques. *J Des Pract* 39:162, 1925.

4 Durand M et al: Lymphogranulomatose inguinale subaigue d'origine génitale probable; peut-être venerienne. *Province Med (Paris)* 24:55, 1913.

5 Stannus HS: *A Sixth Venereal Disease.* London, Bailliere, Tindall and Cox, 1933.

6 Sokes JH et al: Lymphogranuloma venereum. *Am J Med Sci* 197:575, 1939.

7 Grayston JT, Wang SP: New knowledge of chlamydiae and the diseases they cause. *J Infect Dis* 132:87, 1975.

8 Schachter J, Meyer KF: Lymphogranuloma venereum: II. Characterization of some recently isolated strains. *J Bacteriol* 99:636, 1969.

9 Schachter J: Confirmatory serodiagnosis of lymphogranuloma venereum proctitis may yield false-positive results due to other chlamydial infections of the rectum. *Sex Transm Dis* 8:26, 1981.

10 Favre M, Hellerstrom S: The epidemiology, aetiology and prophylaxis of lymphogranuloma inguinal. *Acta Derm Venereol Suppl (Stockh)* 34:1, 1954.

11 Frei W: Eione neue Hautreaktion bei Lymphogranuloma inguinale. *Klin Wochenschr* 4:2148, 1925.

12 Frei W, Koppel A: Ulcus vulvae chronicum elephantiasticum (esthiomone) und sogennates Syphileme anorectal als Folgeerscheinungen der Lymphogranulomatosis inguinales. *Klin Wochenschr* 7:2331, 1928.

13 Miyagawa Y: Studies on the characteristics of *Miyagawanella* lymphogranulomatis. *Jpn J Exp Med* 26:157, 1956.

14 Jones H et al: Studies on lymphogranuloma venereum: III. The action of the sulfonamides on the agent of lymphohgranuloma venereum. *J Infect Dis* 76:55, 1945.

15 Schachter J: Chlamydial infections. *N Engl J Med* 298:428, 490, 540, 1978.

16 Koteen H: Lymphogranuloma venereum. *Medicine* 24:1, 1945.

17 Perine PL et al: Diagnosis and treatment of lymphogranuloma venereum in Ethiopia, in *Current Chemotherapy and Infections Diseases.* Washington, American Society for Microbiology, 1980, pp 1280–1282.

18 Osoba AO: Sero-epidemiological study of lymphogranuloma venereum in western Nigeria. *Afr J Med Sci* 6:125, 1977.

19 Sowmini CN et al: Minocycline in the treatment of lymphogranuloma venereum. *J Am Vener Dis Assoc* 2:19, 1976.

20 Abrams AJ: Lymphogranuloma venereum. *JAMA* 205:199, 1968.

21 Willcox RR: Importance of the so-called "other" sexually transmitted diseases. *Br J Vener Dis* 51:221, 1975.

22 Annamuthodo H: Rectal lymphogranuloma venereum in Jamaica. *Ann R Coll Surg Engl* 29:141, 1961.

23 Blount J: Personal communication, Venereal Disease Control Division, Centers for Disease Control and Prevention, Atlanta, Ga.

24 D'Aunoy R, von Haam E: Venereal lymphogranuloma. *Arch Pathol* 27:1032, 1939.

25 Butler CS: Climatic bubo. *US Nav Med Bull* 20:1, 1924.

26 Thorsteinsson SB et al: Lymphogranuloma venereum: A cause of cervical lymphadenopathy. *JAMA* 235:1882, 1976.

27 Harrop GA et al: New clinical conceptions of lymphogranuloma venereum. *Trans Assoc Am Physicians* 56:101, 1941.

28 Schachter J: Lymphogranuloma venereum and other nonocular *Chlamydia trachomatis* infections, in *Nongonococcal Urethritis and Related Infections,* D Hobson, KK Holmes (eds). Washington, American Society for Microbiology, 1977, pp 91–97.

29 Johannisson G et al: Genital *Chlamydia trachomatis* infection in women. *Obstet Gynecol* 56:671, 1980.

30 Coutts WE: Lymphogranuloma venereum: A general review. *Bull WHO* 2:545, 1950.

31 Schachter J, Osoba AO: Lymphogranuloma venereum. *Br Med Bull* 39:151, 1983.

32 Smith EB, Custer RP: The histopathology of lymphogranuloma venereum. *J Urol* 63:546, 1950.

33 Ault GW: Venereal disease of the anus and rectum. *Am J Syph* 21: 430, 1937.

34 Sabin AB, Aring CD: Meningoencephalitis in man caused by the virus of lymphogranuloma venereum. *JAMA* 120:1376, 1942.

35 Philip RN et al: Study of *Chlamydia* in patients with lymphogranuloma venereum and urethritis attending a venereal disease clinic. *Br J Vener Dis* 47:114, 1971.

36 Dan M et al: A case of lymphogranuloma venereum of 20 years duration: Isolation of *Chlamydia trachomatis* from perianal lesions. *Br J Vener Dis* 56:344, 1980.

37 Quinn TC et al: Experimental proctitis due to rectal infection with *Chlamydia trachomatis* in nonhuman primates. *J Infect Dis* 154:833, 1986.

38 Kornblith BA: Lymphogranuloma venereum: Treatment of 300 cases with special reference to the use of Frei antigen intravenously. *Am J Med Sci* 198:231, 1939.

39 Rothchild TPE, Higgins GA: Acute lymphogranuloma venereum: A short review with observations on the surgical implications and changing geographical distribution. *J Urol* 68:918, 1952.

40 Mehus A et al: Etiology of genital ulcers in Swaziland. *Sex Transm Dis* 10:33, 1983.

41 Hopsu-Havu VB, Sonck CE: Infiltrative, ulcerative, and fistular lesions of the penis due to lymphogranuloma venereum. *Br J Vener Dis* 49:193, 1973.

42 Wallace W: *A Treatise on the Venereal Diseases.* London, Burgess, Hill, 1833, p 348.
43 Beeson PB et al: Isolation of virus of lymphogranuloma venereum from blood and spinal fluid of a human being. *Proc Soc Exp Biol Med* 63:306, 1946.
44 von Haam EV, D'Aunoy R: Is lymphogranuloma inguinale a systemic disease? *Am J Trop Med Hyg* 16:527, 1936.
45 Bjerke JR, Hovding G Jr: Lymphogranuloma venereum with hepatic involvement. *Acta Derm Venerol (Stockh)* 57:90, 1977.
46 Schachter J et al: Lymphogranuloma venereum: I. Comparison of the Frei test, complement fixation test, and isolation of the agent. *J Infect Dis* 120:372, 1969.
47 Coutts WE: Contribution to the knowledge of lymphogranulomatosis venereum as a general disease. *J Trop Med Hyg* 39:13, 1936.
48 Prehn DT: Lymphogranuloma venereum and associated diseases. *Arch Dermatol Syphilol* 35:231, 1937.
49 Greaves AB et al: Chemotherapy in bubonic lymphogranuloma venereum. *Bull WHO* 16:277, 1957.
50 Torpin et al: Lymphogranuloma venereum in the female: A clinical study of ninety-six consecutive cases. Am *J Surg* 43:688, 1939.
51 Najafi JA et al: Surgical aspects of inguinal lymphogranuloma venereum. *Milit Med* 144:697, 1979.
52 Mauff AC et al: Problems in the diagnosis of lymphogranuloma venereum. S *Afr Med J* 63:55, 1983.
53 Banov L: Rectal stricture of lymphogranuloma venereum: Some observations from a five-year study of treatment with the broad spectrum antibiotics. *Am J Surg* 88:761, 1954.
54 Mathewson C Jr: Inflammatory strictures of the rectum associated with venereal lymphogranuloma. *JAMA* 110:709, 1938.
55 Greaves AB: The frequency of lymphogranuloma venereum in persons with perirectal abscesses, fistulae in ano, or both. *Bull WHO* 29:797, 1963.
56 Quinn TC et al: *Chlamydia trachomatis* proctitis. *N Engl J Med* 305: 195, 1981.
57 Levine JS et al: Chronic proctitis in male homosexuals due to lymphogranuloma venereum. *Gastroenterology* 79:563, 1980.
58 Saad EA et al: Ano-rectal-colonic lymphogranuloma venereum. *Gastroenterology* 97:89, 1962.
59 Jorgensen L: Lymphogranuloma venereum. *Acta Pathol Microbiol Scand* 47:113, 1959.
60 Lichtenstein LL: Rectal stricture: A clinical analysis of 58 cases with observations on 154 Frei-positive cases of lymphogranuloma inguinale. *Am J Surg* 31:111, 1936.
61 de la Monte SM et al: Follicular proctocolitis and neuromatous hyperplasia with lymphogranuloma venereum. *Hum Pathol* 16:1025, 1985.
62 Munday PE, Taylor-Robinson D: *Chlamydia* infection in proctitis and Crohn's disease. *Br Med Bull* 39:155, 1983.
63 Crohn BR et al: Regional ileitis, a pathologic and clinical entity. *JAMA* 99:1323, 1932.
64 Schuller JL et al: Antibodies against *Chlamydia* of lymphogranuloma venereum type in Crohn's disease. *Lancet* 1:19, 1979.
65 Swarbrick ET et al: *Chlamydia,* cytomegalovirus, and *Yersinia* in inflammatory bowel disease. *Lancet* 2:11, 1979.
66 Taylor-Robinson D et al: Low frequency of chlamydial antibodies in patients with Crohn's disease and ulcerative colitis. *Lancet 2:* 1162, 1979.
67 Mardh PA et al: Lack of evidence for an association between infection with *Chlamydia trachomatis* and Crohn's disease as indicated by micro-immunofluorescence antibody tests. *Acta Pathol Microbiol Scand [B]* 88:57, 1980.
68 Levin I et al: Lymphogranuloma venereum, rectal stricture and carcinoma. *Dis Colon Rectum* 7:129, 1964.
69 Rainey R: The association of lymphogranuloma inguinale and cancer. *Surgery* 35:221, 1954.
70 Sheldon WH et al: Lymphogranuloma venereum of supraclavicular lymph nodes with mediastinal lymphadenopathy and pericarditis. *Am J Med* 5:320, 1948.
71 Bernstein DI et al: Mediastinal and supraclavicular lymphadenitis and pneumonitis due to *Chlamydia trachomatis* serovars L1, L2, and L3. *N Engl J Med* 311:1543, 1984.
72 Lassus A et al: Auto-immune serum factors and IgA elevation in lymphogranuloma venereum. *Ann Clin Res* 2:51, 1970.
73 Sonck CE et al: Autoimmune serum factors in active and inactive lymphogranuloma venereum. *Br J Vener Dis* 49:67, 1973.
74 Williams RD, Gutman AB: Hyperproteinemia with reversal of the albumin: Globulin ratio in lymphogranuloma inguinale. *Proc Soc Exp Biol Med* 34:91, 1936.
75 Tucker HA: Inguinal lymphogranuloma venereum in the male. *Am J Syph Gon Vener Dis* 29:619, 1945.
76 Frei W: On the skin test in lymphogranuloma inguinale. *J Invest Dermatol* 1:367, 1938.
77 King AJ et al: Intradermal tests in the diagnosis of lymphogranuloma venereum. *Br J Vener Dis* 32:209, 1956.
78 Grace AW et al: A new material (Lygranum) for performance of the Frei test for lymphogranuloma venereum. *Proc Soc Exp Biol Med* 45: 259, 1940.
79 McKee CM et al: Complement fixation test in lymphogranuloma venereum. *Proc Soc Exp Biol Med* 44:410, 1940.
80 Melczer M, Sipos K: Komplementbindungsversuche bei lymphogranuloma inguinale. *Arch Dermatol Syphilol* 176:176, 1937.
81 Grace AW: Persistence of a positive Frei reaction after treatment of venereal lymphogranuloma with sulfonamide drugs. *Vener Dis Inform* 22:349, 1941.
82 Wall MJ et al: Studies on the complement fixation reaction in lymphogranuloma venereum. *Am J Syph Gon Vener Dis* 31:289, 1947.
83 Greaves AB, Taggart SR: Serology, Frei reaction, and epidemiology of lymphogranuloma venereum. *Am J Syph Gon Vener Dis* 37:273, 1953.
84 Goldberg J, Banov L Jr: Complement fixation titers in tertiary lymphogranuloma venereum. *Br J Vener Dis* 32:37, 1956.
85 Wang SP et al: A simplified method for immunological typing of trachoma-inclusion conjunctivitis-lymphogranuloma venereum organisms. *Infect Immun* 7:356, 1973.
86 Schachter J et al: Chlamydiae as agents of human and animal diseases. *Bull WHO* 49:443, 1973.
87 Caldwell HD, Kuo CC: Serologic diagnosis of lymphogranuloma venereum by counterimmunoelectrophoresis with a *Chlamydia trachomatis* protein antigen. *J Immunol* 118:442, 1977.
88 Paavonen I: Chlamydial infections: Microbiological, clinical and diagnostic aspects. *Med Biol* 57:152, 1979.
89 Shaffer MF et al: Use of the yolk sac of the developing chicken embryo in the isolation of the agent of lymphogranuloma venereum. *J Infect Dis* 75:109, 1944.
90 Kuo CC et al: Primary isolation of TRIC organisms in HeLa 229 cells treated with DEAE-dextran. *J Infect Dis* 125:665, 1972.
91 Gordon FB, Quan AL: Isolation of the trachoma agent in cell culture. *Proc Soc Exp Biol Med* 118:354, 1965.
92 Klotz SA et al: Hemorrhagic proctitis due to lymphogranuloma venereum serogroup L2. *N Engl J Med* 308:1563, 1983.
93 Osoba AO, Beetlestone CA: Lymphographic studies in acute lymphogranuloma venereum infection. *Br J Vener Dis* 52:399, 1976.
94 Annamunthodo H, Marryatt J: Barium studies in intestinal lymphogranuloma venereum. *Br J Radiol* 24:53, 1961.
95 Piersol GM et al: Lymphogranuloma venereum: A systemic disease. *Trans Assoc Am Physicians* 53:275, 1938.
96 Greenblatt RB: Antibiotics in treatment of lymphogranuloma venereum and granuloma inguinale. *Ann NY Acad Sci* 55:1082, 1952.
97 Rake G: Chemotherapy of lymphogranuloma venereum. *Am J Trop Med Hyg* 28:555, 1948.
98 Grace AW, Rake G: Complement fixation test for lymphogranuloma. *Arch Dermatol Syphilol* 48:619, 1943.
99 Wright LT et al: The treatment of lymphogranuloma venereum with Terramycin. *Antibiot Chemother* 1:193, 1951.
100 Banov L Jr, Goldberg J: Erythromycin treatment of lymphogranuloma venereum, in *Antibiotics Annual 1953–1954,* H Welch, F Mar-

tin-Ibanez (eds). New York, Medical Encyclopedia, 1953, pp 475–479.

101 Menke HE et al: Treatment of lymphogranuloma venereum with rifampicin. *Br J Vener Dis* 55:379, 1979.

102 Wright LT et al: Aueromycin: A new antibiotic with virucidal properties: 1. A preliminary report on successful treatment in twenty-five cases of lymphogranuloma venereum. *JAMA* 138:408, 1948.

103 Osoba AO: Medical treatment of late complications of lymphogranuloma venereum. *W Afr J Pharmacol Drug Res* 3:71, 1976.

104 Bauwens JE et al: Epidemic lymphogranuloma venereum during epidemics of crack cocaine use and HIV infection in the Bahamas. (in unpublished manuscript).

Chapter 31

Biology of *Neisseria gonorrhoeae*

P. Frederick Sparling

Neisseria gonorrhoeae (gonococci) is the etiologic agent of gonorrhea and its related clinical syndromes (urethritis, cervicitis, salpingitis, bacteremia, arthritis, and others). It is closely related to *N. meningitidis* (meningococci), the etiologic agent of one form of bacterial meningitis, and relatively closely to *N. lactamica,* an occasional human pathogen. The genus *Neisseria* includes a variety of other relatively or completely nonpathogenic organisms that are principally important because of their occasional diagnostic confusion with gonococci and meningococci.

This chapter is concerned principally with the microbiology, genetics, and pathogenicity of gonococci. Chapter 32 is concerned with the clinical syndromes caused by gonococci and their treatment. A discussion of diagnostic methods for gonococcal infections is found in Chap. 53 and 92.

HISTORY

Gonorrhea is one of the oldest known diseases of humans. There have been many reviews of the history of this disease, one of the best of which is the monograph by R.S. Morton.[1] Gonorrhea undoubtedly was known to the authors of the bible. The Book of Leviticus describes a person with urethral discharge. Proclamations that infected persons were to keep themselves from others for 7 days may indicate that they already knew the mean incubation period was 7 days. Biblical authors cautioned about transmission to social contacts and also about women copulating with afflicted men.

Hippocrates wrote extensively of gonorrhea in the fourth and fifth centuries BC. He called acute gonorrhea "strangury" and understood that it resulted from "the pleasures of Venus." The Roman physician Celsus was well aware of gonorrhea and its complications and was known to catheterize patients suffering from urethral stricture. In the second century Galen coined the word *gonorrhea*, by which he meant "flow of semen." Other early Greco-Roman physicians prescribed various treatments for gonorrhea, including sexual abstinence and the washing of the eyes of the newborn.

Knowledge of gonorrhea and other sexually transmitted diseases in Europe was scant until near the end of the Dark Ages. The term *clap*, which is still commonly used to refer to this disease, first appeared in print in 1378. The derivation of the word clap is unclear but possibly refers to the Les Clapier district of Paris in which prostitutes were housed in the Middle Ages. Other origins for the term clap are possible, but regardless it was clear in European writings of the late Middle Ages that the disease was associated with sexual intercourse.

After the arrival of syphilis in Europe in the late fifteenth century, considerable confusion existed regarding the relation between gonorrhea and syphilis. Great surgeons such as Ambroise Paré (sixteenth century) and John Hunter (eighteenth century) considered syphilis and gonorrhea to be different manifestations of a single disease. Hunter's conclusions were the result of a famous experiment in which he inoculated himself with material from a patient with gonorrhea; he acquired syphilis as a result. Distinction between these diseases was first clearly achieved by Philippe Ricord, but real understanding was only achieved after Neisser's description of *N. gonorrhoeae* in 1879 and Leistikow's and Löffler's cultivation of the organism in 1882.

The twentieth century brought new, safe, highly effective therapy for gonorrhea, replacing the sometimes horrific therapies used for centuries, including urethral astringents, soundings, and other mechanical devices. Sulfonamides were first introduced in 1936 and penicillin in 1943 for gonorrhea therapy. The second great development of this century concerns the revolution in our understanding of the pathogenic mechanisms of this fascinating organism, which started with the demonstration by Kellogg and his colleagues in 1963 that there are differences in virulence of gonococci with different colonial morphology.[2] These developments enable better understanding of how gonococci cause repeated infections in the same individual and may lead to development of an effective vaccine. (Boswell, Samuel Johnson's famous biographer, had at least 19 separate bouts of urethritis.)

EPIDEMIOLOGY

TRANSMISSION

Humans are the only natural host for gonococci. Gonococci survive only a short time outside the human body. Although gonococci can be cultured from a dried environment such as a toilet seat up to 24 h after being artificially inoculated in large numbers onto such a surface, there is virtually no evidence that natural transmission occurs from toilet seats or similar objects. Gonorrhea is a classic example of an infection spread by contact: Immediate physical contact with the mucosal surfaces of an infected person, usually a sexual partner, is required for transmission. (The single exception is the occasional epidemic among prepubescent females living together and sharing bath towels and similar objects.) Although meningococci can be spread by air droplet transmission over short distances, there is no evidence that gonorrhea is ever transmitted by such a mechanism.

STRAIN TYPING

For epidemiologic studies it is useful to differentiate one strain from another. Several techniques have been developed that can be used successfully for this purpose.

Auxotypes

A relatively cumbersome system for differentiating gonococcal strains based on their ability to grow on chemically defined media has been developed. This system was originally developed by B.W. Catlin and classifies strains as to whether they can grow without certain amino acids, purines or pyrimidines, or other specific nutrients.[3] A strain unable to grow on chemically defined media lacking proline is designated Pro^-, and a strain unable to grow without arginine is Arg^-. Naturally occurring gonococcal isolates exhibit remarkable diversity in their biosynthetic capacities, probably reflecting the biochemically rich environment of their human host, which provides the organisms with most of the compounds needed for growth. Genetic studies have shown that strains with a similar nutritional phenotype (e.g., Arg^-) may have multiple mutations in a single biochemical pathway.[4] The auxotyping system has been used successfully in a variety of epidemiologic studies.[5] Certain auxotypes are biologically and epidemiologically important. For instance, the Arg^- Hyx^- (hypoxanthine$^-$) Ura^- (uracil$^-$), or

AHU$^-$, auxotype typically is associated with multiple other properties, including resistance to killing by normal human serum; propensity for causing asymptomatic male urethral infection; increased likelihood for causing bacteremia, and others.[6] Because of the complexity of preparing the chemically defined media, and the short storage life of the media, the auxotyping technique is not widely used in clinical laboratories.

Serotyping

Investigators tried to develop a practical serotyping scheme for decades. The most useful and widely available technique for this purpose at present is based on monoclonal antibodies specific for various epitopes on outer membrane protein I (P.I, or Por).[7] Por occurs in two immunochemically distinct serogroups: PorA and PorB. By employing a set of monoclonal antibodies against PorA strains and another set against PorB strains, one can subdivide each of the serogroups into a wide variety of serovars (e.g., P.IA-6, P.IB-1), differing in their ability to react with certain members of the panel of monoclonal antibodies. Many dozens of specific serovars have been defined by these techniques.[5,7] By a combination of auxotyping and serotyping with anti-Por monoclonal antibodies, gonococci can be divided into over 70 different strains; the number may turn out to be much larger.

Antimicrobial susceptibilities

A third method to strain type gonococci is based on antimicrobial susceptibilities. This once was used widely and still may be employed as a useful adjunct to the auxotyping and serotyping schemes, but the ability of gonococci to transfer antibiotic resistance between strains seriously compromises the utility of this method for long-term epidemiologic studies.

Genotyping

Strain typing can be refined by determination of whether there are apparent significant differences in DNA sequences between strains. Although it is impractical to undertake full genomic sequencing, or even sequencing of one or a few specific genes, it is possible to use various tools of molecular biology to rapidly assess differences in DNA sequences. The first employed technique was restriction endonuclease digestion, with subsequent assessment of patterns of DNA bands separated on agarose gels.[8,9] Resolution of DNA bands may be difficult unless the technique employs enzymes that cut rare DNA sequences.[10] Another method is termed random-primed PCR, which uses short DNA primers that bind to multiple sites to generate a polymerase chain reaction–based ladder of DNA products, the sizes of which depend on the spacing of the homologous sequences scattered about the chromosome.[11] Reproducibility of this assay can be a problem. Perhaps most useful for epidemiologic purposes is a technique termed Opa typing, which uses *opa*-based PCR primers to generate DNA from each of the approximately 11 *opa* genes. These are then subjected to restriction enzyme digestion, and the resultant pattern of restriction fragment length polymorphisms (RFLP) is used to compare identities of strains.[12] Used in conjunction with other strain typing systems, genotyping offers additional and powerful resolving power.

BIOLOGY

MORPHOLOGY

Gonococci are gram-negative diplococci, nonmotile and non-spore-forming, which characteristically grow in pairs (diplococci) with adjacent sides flattened. In 1963 Kellogg showed that gonococci occur in multiple colony types when grown on a clear agar medium and viewed with obliquely transmitted light.[2] Small convex glistening type 1 and type 2 colonies were easily distinguished from the larger, flatter type 3 and type 4 colonies. The small colonies are now known to be piliated and are designated P^+; large colonies are nonpiliated (P^-) (Fig. 31-1). Colony types are variable, and although fresh isolates from patients usually are P^+, unselected transfer in vitro usually results in conversion to P^-.[2,13] Some P^- colonies are capable of subsequent reversion to P^+. Using human male prison volunteers as experimental subjects, Kellogg and his coworkers showed that after 69 in vitro passages, P^+ "type 1" colonies retained virulence but the P^- "type 4" colonies did

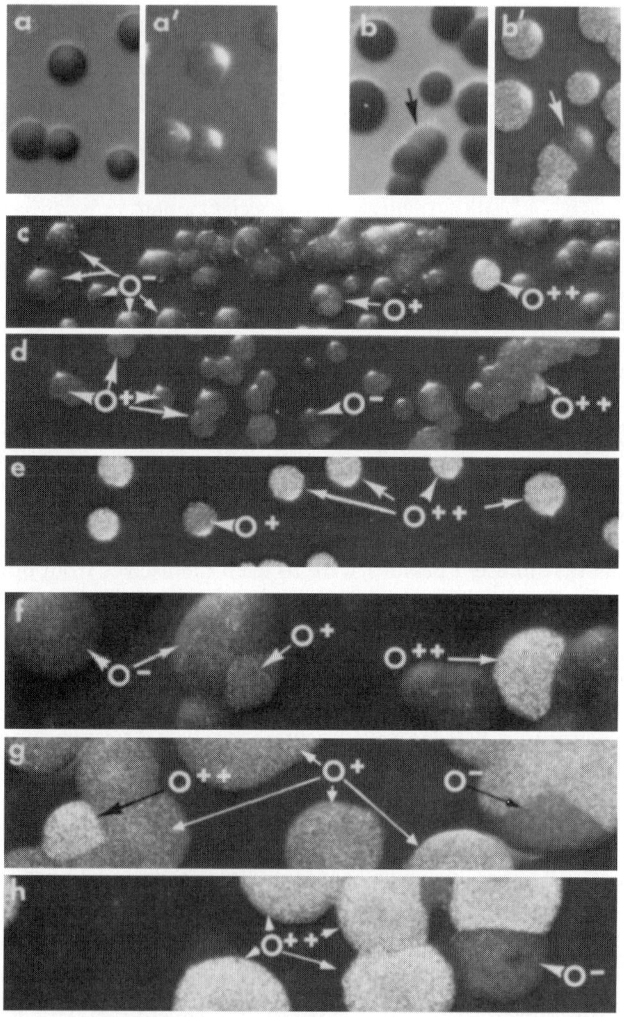

Fig. 31-1. Gonococcal colonial morphologies. A variety of sizes and forms are present in gonococci cultivated on clear medium, in vitro. Small colonies with darkly rimmed borders (a–e) contain heavily piliated organisms, whereas large colonies (f–h) are constituted of nonpiliated gonococci. Colonies of both piliated and nonpiliated organisms display variation in their color and opacity characteristics. Use of a diffusing substage reflector allows visualization of colony color (a and b) and is depicted here for very light (a) and very dark (b) colonies. Use of a polished substage mirror allows differentiation of colonial opacity variants (a′, b′, c–h). Transparent colony (O^-) populations are regularly "contaminated" by variants of intermediate (O^+) or marked (O^{2+}) colonial opacities (c). Similarly, O^- and O^{2+} colonies are found in O^+ preparations (d), and colonies of lesser opacity (O^- or O^+) appear in O^{2+} colony populations (e). These variants can also be found in otherwise homogeneous O^- (f), O^+ (g), and O^{2+} (h) populations of nonpiliated gonococcal colonies (courtesy of J. Swanson and L. Mayer).

not.[2] Recent studies have confirmed that P⁻ colonies have reduced ability to cause infection in male human volunteers (personal communication, J. Cannon and M.S. Cohen).

A second type of morphologically visible colonial variation concerns relative opacity of the colonies when viewed through a low-power microscope on clear media in appropriate lighting.[14,15] Opaque (Op) colonies are darker and more granular than transparent (Tr) colonies (see Fig. 31-1). The Op and Tr colony types undergo rapid reversible variations in vitro. The biochemical basis of the opaque-transparent colony variation is owing to variation in expression of a family of outer membrane proteins formerly designated protein II (P.II) but now designated Opa; Op colonies contain cells expressing Opa, whereas most transparent colonies contain cells that are not expressing Opa.[14–16]

Membrane structure

When gonococci are viewed in cross-section by transmission electron microscopy (TEM), they are seen to have a typical gram-negative outer membrane overlying a relatively thin peptidoglycan layer and cytoplasmic membrane. Meningococci contain a true polysaccharide capsule that is important to virulence, whereas gonococci lack such a structure. Frequently small blebs of outer membrane may be seen in TEM. Unlike *Escherichia coli* and many other enteric bacteria, gonococci are prone to release fragments of membrane into their surrounding environment; this may deliver toxic membrane components to distant sites and antigenic fragments that bind host antibodies.

PILI

The most important parts of the gonococcus from the pathogenic point of view concern surface molecules that are involved in attachment to, or invasion or injury of, the host or that serve as targets for host immune defenses. Among the best studied surface molecules are pili. Viewed by electron microscopy, pili are arranged in individual fibrils or fibrillar aggregates and cover virtually the entire outer cell surface of the organism (Fig. 31-2). Fibrillar pili actually are polymers composed of perhaps thousands of a subunit of about 18 kDa.[17] A great deal is now known about the structure of the pilin subunit, as assessed by x-ray crystallography.[18,19] Pili are known to increase adhesion to host tissues.[20]

ANTIGENIC AND PHASE VARIATION

Pili undergo two types of variations, at relatively high frequency: antigenic variation, in which strains shift the antigenic type of their pilus; and phase variation, in which strains switch between P^+ and P^- states. Immune sera raised in animals against a single purified pilus react relatively weakly with pili prepared from unrelated clinical isolates.[17] The pilus expressed by a single gonococcal strain is known to be able to undergo extensive antigenic variation, either during passage on agar plates, during growth in subcutaneous chambers implanted into experimental animals, or during natural infection of humans.[21–23] The complete structure of a number of pilin variants is well established.[23–26] There is a common N-terminal region and several variable domains in the midportion or carboxy terminus of the protein (Fig. 31-3). Several relatively invariant or common regions are scattered amid the variable domains, including two cysteines at amino acids 121 and 151 that form a disulfide bridge. The amino terminus is nearly identical in gonococci, meningococci, and several other organisms including *Bacteroides nodosus, Moraxella bovis,* and *Pseudomonas aeruginosa.*

MOLECULAR MECHANISMS

The mechanisms of pilus phase (P^+) ↔ (P^-) and antigenic (P^+_α) → (P^+_β) variation have been studied extensively by molecular biological techniques. There are one or sometimes two complete pilin genes on the chromosome.[25–30] The intact gene "expression site" contains an intact promoter region and ribosome binding site and encodes an unusual short 7 amino acid signal sequence and the 159 to 160 amino acids of the mature pilin subunit. There are six to eight "silent" regions scattered at various locales around the chromosome. Each silent locus contains various amounts of pilin sequences, but lacks a promoter region, and the 5′ end of the pilin structural gene. In some of these silent sites there are many different copies of incomplete pilin gene sequences arranged in a head-to-tail tandem repeat order, and many of these

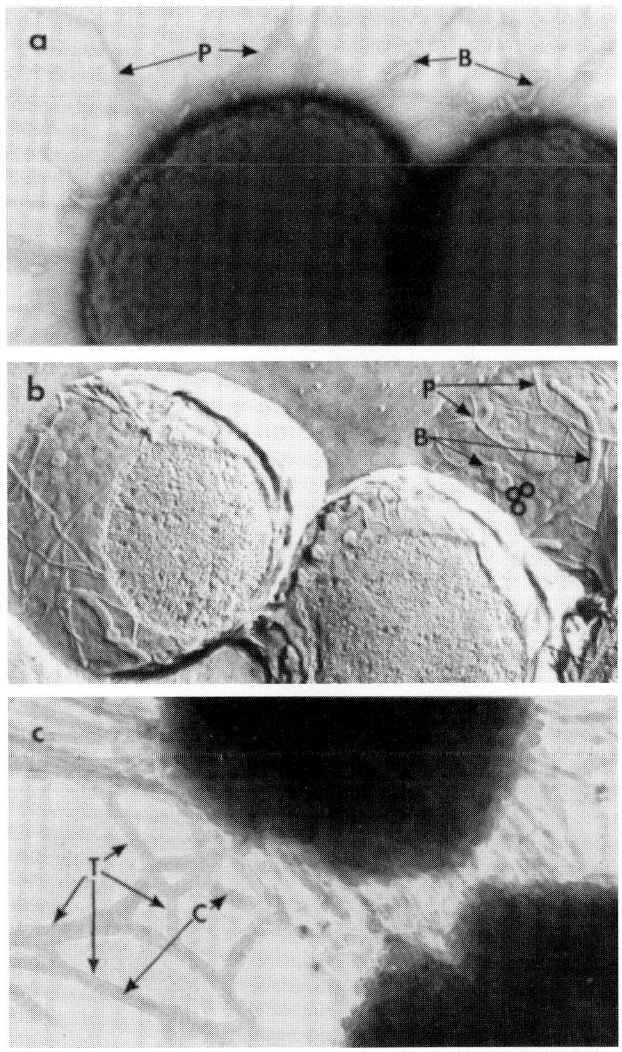

Fig. 31-2. Electron microscopic appearances of gonococcal surface constituents. Different methods of preparing gonococci for electron microscopic examination yield strikingly different views of these organisms' surface constituents. In negatively stained preparations (a), pili (P) appear as thin (approx 8-nm) structures that are clearly differentiated from evaginated *blebs* (B) of the outer membrane. These blebs occur as elongated, sausagelike forms or as small vesicles. The actual surfaces of gonococci have a rugose appearance that is poorly resolved in this micrograph. After freeze-fracture freeze-etching (b), both pili (P) and outer membrane blebs (B) are seen lying against the organisms' surfaces. The "pebbled" appearance of the gonococcal surface is punctuated by pits (examples encircled) (courtesy of J. Swanson and L. Mayer).

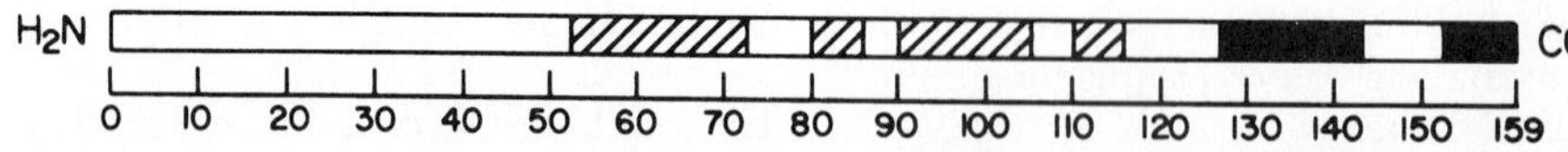

Fig. 31-3. Schematic diagram of variability of pilin structure as revealed by DNA sequencing of expressed *pil* genes in multiple clinical isolates of a single epidemic strain. In the semivariable regions (hatched), single amino acid substitutions were found. In the hypervariable regions (black), there frequently were insertions or deletions of one to several amino acids. White areas are constant regions. Results are typical of those found in vitro in three laboratory strains. Numbers refer to amino acid residues of mature pilins (from Sparling PF et al: *J Infect Dis* 153:196, 1986).

variant copies of pilin sequences are slightly different from each other. Nonreciprocal recombination events may move one of these silent variant copies of pilin sequence into the expression site, resulting in expression of an antigenically variant but fully functional pilus (antigenic variation). On occasion the variant copy of silent pilin DNA encodes a faulty peptide that when expressed results in a pilin that cannot be processed, assembled, secreted ("long pilin"), or anchored ("small" or secreted pilin) into a mature pilus, and the cell becomes P^- as a result.[28] Reversion back to a P^+ state in these instances occurs when a functional pilin sequence is moved from another variant silent copy into the expression site, replacing the faulty pilin sequences (phase variation) (Fig. 31-4).

Movements of pilin sequences between the silent and the expression sites are mediated by the homologous sequences that flank or are located at intervals within the pilin DNA at the silent and the expression sites and depend on a functional recombination system.[31] Occasionally a recombinational event results in deletion of the entirety of the 5′ and upstream regions of the structural gene in the expression site.[32] When this happens the organism becomes permanently nonpiliated since the necessary information to restore the pilus expression site is not contained within any of the silent copies.

Existence of three promoters for each pilin structural gene *(pilE)* suggests complex mechanisms for transcriptional control of pilus expression.[33] Indeed a *pilA pilB* sensor regulator system has been described that either induces or represses expression of *pilE*; it is not yet known which environmental factors affect the activity of this system.[34] Very recently an additional factor (integration host factor, or IHF) was described that also affects transcription of *pilE*.[35] Presumably these complex systems serve to provide fine control of the amount of expressed pili, although the biological advantage of such controls is unclear.

PORIN PROTEIN (POR)

When outer membranes are purified from gonococci and proteins are solubilized and examined by the technique of sodium dodecyl sulfate-polyacrylamide gel electrophoresis (SDS-PAGE), a number of proteins are visualized. Ordinarily the most prominent protein on such SDS-PAGE is a 34- to 36-kDa protein formerly designated P.I but now designated Por. Por is exposed on the surface of the outer membrane and in its native state in the membrane undoubtedly exists as a trimer.[36] In the outer membrane it is physically proximate to the lipo-oligosaccharide (LOS) and also to reduction modifiable protein (Rmp).[37,38] Por undoubtedly fulfills many functions for the gonococcus, including forming an anion-specific

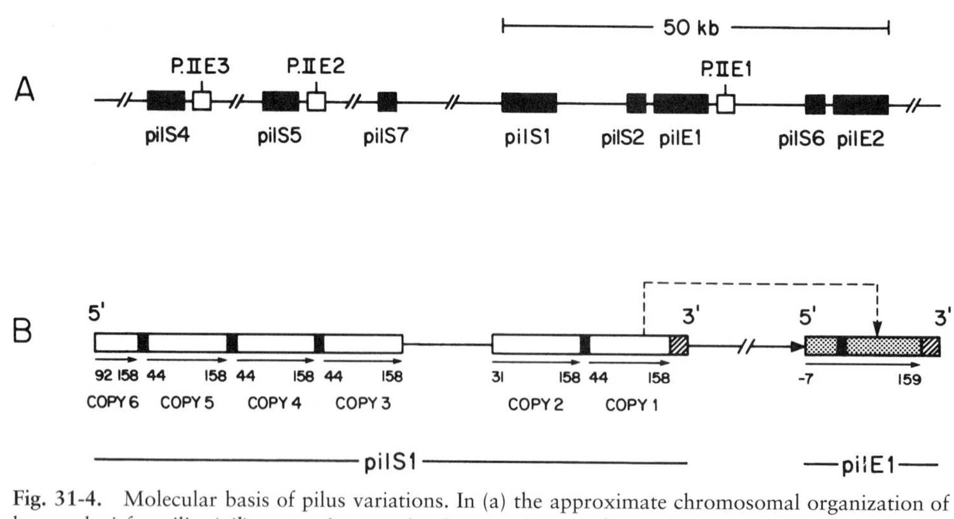

Fig. 31-4. Molecular basis of pilus variations. In (a) the approximate chromosomal organization of known loci for pilin *(pil)* or opacity proteins (*opa*, or P.II) is shown. In strain MS11 there are two complete ("expression") *pil* genes (*pil*E1, *pil*E2) and multiple incomplete ("silent") loci (e.g., *pil*S1) containing copies of the 3′ end of *pil* genes. In some instances, *opa* (P.II) genes are adjacent to *pil* loci (e.g., P.II E1), each encoding a complete Opa protein. In (b) is shown the organization of one silent locus (*pil*S1), which contains six slightly variant copies of the 3′ end of *pil* genes. Numbers below the bars indicate pilin amino acids encoded by the DNA. Solid bars or striped areas indicate constant regions in or around the *pil* genes; other constant DNA regions are omitted for simplicity. The dotted line and arrow refer to movement by recombination of DNA from one silent copy into an expression locus (*pil*E1), which is facilitated by homology between the constant regions. This may result in phase or antigenic variation, as described in the text (adapted principally from data of Haas R and Meyer TF, *Cell* 44:107, 1986).

channel through the lipid-rich outer membrane.[39,40] Por exists in two major chemically and immunologically distinct classes designated PorA and PorB. A given strain possesses either PorA or PorB but never both. As indicated in the preceding, monoclonal antibody serotyping schemes based on Por have been developed, and they have defined a number of antigenic variants of these two major families of porin protein.[7]

The primary structures of multiple Por proteins have been determined by DNA sequencing.[41,42] Their structure is similar to that of porin proteins in other gram-negative bacteria. Comparison of the sequence of PorA and PorB proteins reveals certain regions that are common to both proteins and others where there is considerable variation.[41–43] The regions of variability probably represent areas of antigenic diversity. The *porA* and *porB* genes are alleles of a single locus.[43]

OPACITY PROTEINS

The opacity-associated protein family designated Opa (formerly protein II, or P.II) comprises a family of closely related proteins involved in cell adhesion that share the property of heat modifiability.[14–16] These proteins vary in size from about 24 to about 28 kDa and when heated to 100°C take on a different conformation and exhibit a higher apparent molecular mass in SDS-PAGE. A given strain has the capacity to produce at least ten different variants of the Opa family, as judged by sizes and antigenic properties of the expressed Opa proteins.[44] A strain may express none of these or up to four or five different members of the Opa family simultaneously.[44] The Opa family undergoes both phase variations ($Opa^+ \leftrightarrow Opa^-$) and antigenic variation (OpaA → OpaB → OpaC → . . .), analogous to pilus variations.

Some Opa proteins promote adherence of cells in a colony and also promote adhesion of gonococci to epithelial cells.[45,46] Most Opa proteins result in increased colony opacity, whereas all Opa^- clones are transparent. The very high frequencies in variation of Opa proteins can easily be seen by examining colony morphologies under appropriate lighting; many colonies exhibit sectors varying in opacity, which reflects the variability in expression of Opa (see Fig. 31-1).

MECHANISMS OF OPA VARIATIONS

The genetic basis for phase and antigenic variation of the Opa family is now quite well understood and is different from that used to control the expression of pilus proteins. All *opa* genes from the gonococcal strains have been cloned and sequenced.[47–50] When Southern hybridizations are performed with the cloned *opa* gene, up to 12 *opa*-related restriction fragments of chromosomal DNA are visualized, indicating that there is a family of *opa* genes in the chromosome.[47–50] Each of the *opa* genes is a complete gene with its own promoter, and each is transcribed into RNA at all times.[48,49] Variation in expression of these genes is achieved by varying the number of an identical pentameric (CTCTT) repeat unit located immediately downstream from the ATG start codon, within the DNA that encodes the hydrophobic signal sequence, and upstream from the sequences coding for the mature structural protein.[48–50] When the number of these repeat units is evenly divisible by three (e.g., 9, 12, 15 . . .), the gene is translationally inframe and an Opa protein is expressed. Any other number of the pentameric repeat (e.g., 8, 10, 11, 13, 14 . . .) results in transcription of a gene that is translationally out-of-frame, and no Opa is expressed. The number of the pentameric repeat undergoes high-frequency variation, and this results in regulation of expression at the level of translation rather than the usual method for most genes of regulation at the level of transcription. Each *opa* gene contains two hypervariable domains, which may recombine with similar domains in other *opa* loci. Thus variable expression of *opa* genes results in antigenic variation, because of differences in structures encoded by different *opa* genes.

REDUCTION MODIFIABLE PROTEIN *(RMP)*

All pathogenic *Neisseria,* including all gonococci, contain an antigenically conserved Rmp protein (formerly designated Protein III, or P.III) of about 30 to 31 kDa that is characterized by its altered apparent molecular mass on SDS-PAGE under reducing conditions. The structural gene *rmp* was cloned and sequenced.[51] This protein is of interest in pathogenesis because many blocking antibodies that prevent serum bactericidal activity are directed against this antigen, as discussed in the following.

H.8 PROTEINS

A monoclonal antibody (MAb) designated H.8 reacts with a conserved antigen found on all gonococci and meningococci, and on *N. lactamica* and *N. cinerea,* but not on other nonpathogenic *Neisseria.*[52] In gonococci and meningococci there are at least two proteins containing an H.8 MAb-binding epitope. One is a lipoprotein containing five imperfect repeats of the peptide Ala-Ala-Glu-Ala-Pro (AAEAP) at the N-terminal region and an azurinlike sequence at the C-terminal region.[53,54] The azurins are copper-containing proteins that may be involved in electron transport. The function of the gonococcal azurinlike protein is not known. The second H.8 MAb-binding protein does not have azurin-related sequences and is made up primarily of 13 repeats of the AAEAP peptide. During convalescence from gonorrhea humans make antibodies against the H.8 proteins, but their roles pathogenesis are unknown.[55]

IRON- OR OXYGEN-REPRESSIBLE PROTEINS

Although all of the proteins discussed in the preceding with the possible exception of pili are expressed under all growth conditions, a variety of other proteins are expressed only under certain conditions, including iron starvation, anaerobic growth, or other limited-growth situations.[56–59] The iron-repressible proteins (Frps) include a 37-kDa protein and several in the approximate range of 65 to over 100 kDa.[56,57,60] The 37-kDa protein is designated ferric binding protein (Fbp) because it contains iron and is involved in iron transport.[61] Virtually all gonococci and meningococci express an antigenically conserved Fbp.[62] A 70-kDa protein designated FrpB on the outer membrane also is common to virtually all gonococci and meningococci.[63] Its function is unknown, although the predicted structure strongly suggests it is involved somehow in iron transport since it is a member of the TonB-box family, nearly all of which are receptors.[64] Many other iron-repressible proteins are now known to be receptors, either for transferrin (TF), lactoferrin (LF), or hemoglobin (Hb).[65–67] Each of these receptors binds its ligand (TF, LF, or Hb) with great specificity, and binding is required before iron is stripped from the ligand and transported into the cell. Each receptor is composed of a loosely surface-tethered lipoprotein and an integral membrane protein that appear to work together; their function in iron entry is dependent on transmission of energy to the outer membrane receptor by the inner membrane protein TonB.[68] Virtually all gonococci produce a functional TF and Hb receptor, although about half of gonococci do not produce a functional LF receptor.[66]

Presumably, these receptors are required to help scavenge available iron in vivo. Several additional proteins are expressed in considerable quantity during anaerobic growth.[58] Many of these growth-regulated proteins are expressed in vivo as evidenced by the ability of convalescent human sera to react with them in Western blots (unpublished data of W. McKenna and P.F. Sparling).

IGA$_1$ PROTEASES

All gonococci and meningococci but not other, nonpathogenic *Neisseria* produce a protease that recognizes both serum and secretory IgA$_1$ (but not IgA$_2$) as a substrate.[69] There are two genetically and biochemically distinct variants of the gonococcal IgA$_1$ protease, and there is a correlation between auxotype, Por serogroup, and the class of IgA$_1$ protease expressed by the strain.[70] Each of the IgA$_1$ proteases cleaves IgA$_1$ at the hinge region, resulting in release of Fab and Fc fragments.[69] Since secretory IgA is the principal arm of antibody-mediated defenses at mucosal surfaces, the *Neisseria* IgA$_1$ protease may be important in inactivation of mucosal immune defenses, but unfortunately no firm data are available to confirm this intuitively obvious conclusion. Surprisingly, loss of IgA$_1$ protease limits ability of gonococci to grow within epithelial cells, apparently because IgA$_1$ protease normally cleaves an intracellular protein (LAMP1) involved in phagosomal compartmentalization.[71] Loss of IgA$_1$ protease does not reduce infectivity of gonococci for human volunteers (personal communications, J. Cannon, M. Cohen, et al.).

One particularly interesting feature of the gonococcal IgA$_1$ protease was revealed by cloning and sequencing the entire structural gene for this protein.[72] The cell synthesizes a precursor protein of about 169 kDas that then is proteolytically cleaved twice to create a 45-kDa outer membrane protein and the mature 106-kDa IgA$_1$ protease molecule. The 45-kDa protein forms a channel through the membrane that allows export of the IgA$_1$ protease to the exterior.[72]

LIPO-OLIGOSACCHARIDE (LOS)

All gonococci express LOS on their cell surface, similar to the lipopolysaccharide (LPS) of other gram-negative bacteria. Gonococcal LOS contains a lipid A moiety and a core polysaccharide consisting of ketodeoxyoctanoic acid (KDO), heptose, glucose, galactose, and glucosamine and/or galactosamine.[73] The two-dimensional structure of gonococcal LOS is now well established.[74] Unlike other gram-negative bacteria, gonococci do not express a long polymeric sugar attached to this core, and thus the gonococcal LOS is considerably smaller than typical LPS of other bacteria. By both chemical and immunologic criteria there is intrastrain and interstrain variation in the nature of the core sugar antigens of LOS.[73,75,76] A single strain may make up to six variants of LOS, varying in apparent molecular mass from 3 to 7 kDas. Since the core sugars of LOS form antigens that are important in immune bactericidal reactions, phenotypic variation of these antigens may be pathogenically important.[77,78] Indeed, considerable evidence suggests that gonococci with "short" LOS are serum sensitive but able to invade eukaryotic cells, whereas gonococci with "long" LOS are serum resistant but noninvasive.[79–82] The biochemical and genetic mechanisms for phenotypic variation of gonococcal LOS has been elucidated; many genes involved in LOS core sugar assembly undergo high frequency phase variation by a mechanism similar to that involved in *opa* variations.[83] The terminal sugars on gonococcal LOS mimic the structure of certain human glycosphingolipids.[73]

Variation in LOS core sugar chain length has several important implications for pathogenesis. Gonococci vary in their ability to undergo sialylation of LOS (addition of host neuraminic acid to LOS by means of a bacterial sialyltransferase), because the site of sialylation is on a near-terminal LOS sugar that is variably expressed.[79,84] "Short" LOS is unable to be sialylated, whereas full-length LOS is readily sialylated.[80–82] Since sialylated gonococci are at least partially protected ("masked") from antibodies against both LOS and the closely neighboring Por molecule, they are more resistant to bactericidal attack.[85] On the other hand, "short" LOS gonococci, which are not sialylated and are serum-sensitive, are more able to invade certain epithelial cells.[79–82]

OTHER SURFACE STRUCTURES

Gonococcal peptidoglycan is similar to that of other gram-negative bacteria, containing a backbone of muramic acid and *N*-acetylglucosamine, but is rather unusual in the degree of its O-acetylation.[86] This may be relevant to the susceptibility of peptidoglycan fragments to biodegradation and to its inflammatory and other biological properties.[87]

Gonococci do not express a true polysaccharide capsule despite several early reports to the contrary. Gonococci do produce a surface polyphosphate, however, that may serve some of the functions of a polysaccharide capsule, including provision of a hydrophilic and negatively charged cell surface.[88] The role of the polyphosphate "pseudocapsule" in gonococcal biology and pathogenesis presently is unknown. Gonococci also bind charged polyanions to certain Opa proteins, which alters the surface charge of the cell and also the ability to be killed by normal human serum.[89] Gonococcal structures involved in pathogenesis are summarized in Table 31-1.

METABOLISM

Gonococci have complex growth requirements.[3] They utilize glucose, lactate, or pyruvate as sole sources of required carbon but cannot use other carbohydrates.[3] This forms the basis for the carbohydrate utilization tests used for decades to speciate neisserial organisms. When grown in media supplemented with serum, they exhibit different outer membrane proteins and altered attachment to human neutrophils.[90] The factor that seems to stimulate these phenotypic variations is lactate.[91] Human neutrophils release lactate as an end product of metabolism, with the result that gonococci growing in vivo might encounter lactate as a principal carbon source.[91] All gonococci (as well as other *Neisseria*) rapidly oxidize dimethyl- or tetramethyl-phenylenediamine, and this turns

Table 31-1. Some Gonococcal Structures Involved in Pathogenesis

Structure (abbreviation)	Function in infection
Por	(?) Insertion into host cell membranes
	Target for bactericidal, opsonic antibodies
Opa	Adherence
Rmp	Target for blocking antibodies
Pili	Adherence
	Resistance to neutrophils
Lipo-oligosaccharide	Tissue toxin
	Target for bactericidal, chemotactic antibodies
Peptidoglycan	Tissue toxin
Iron-repressible proteins	Iron uptake from transferrin, lactoferrin, hemoglobin
IgA$_1$ protease	(?) Escape from mucosal IgA$_1$

colonies pink and then black, forming the basis of the oxidase test.

Gonococci are capable of growth under anaerobic conditions if nitrite is provided as an electron acceptor.[92] Their growth is stimulated by 5% gaseous CO_2 or if additional bicarbonate is added to liquid or solid growth media. They produce abundant catalase, which undoubtedly helps to promote growth in the presence of otherwise toxic peroxides, but unlike most aerobes they do not produce appreciable amounts of superoxide dismutase. It has been postulated that they grow in vivo under relatively anaerobic conditions, although they ordinarily are grown in vitro under aerobic conditions.[58]

Gonococci have an absolute requirement for iron for growth. In humans the principal sources of iron for gonococci presumably are the serum glycoprotein transferrin and the mucosal glycoprotein lactoferrin. Gonococci possess an energy-requiring, iron-repressible system for scavenging iron from transferrin, lactoferrin, and hemoglobin; this is accomplished without evident synthesis of an iron-chelating siderophore.[57,65] Iron uptake from transferrin, lactoferrin, and hemoglobin is mediated by binding of the host protein to a specific gonococcal receptor.[65–67]

GROWTH

Gonococci do not tolerate drying and ordinarily must be plated onto appropriate media immediately on sampling patient secretions. As an alternative, gonococci may be put into one of several available transport media, in which they survive for up to 24 hours prior to being plated on definitive culture media. Growth is optimal at 35 to 37°C in a 5% CO_2 atmosphere, at a pH of about 6.5 to 7.5. When grown at relatively low pH (6.0–6.5), outer membrane composition is altered; below pH 6.0, no gonococci survive. (Vaginal secretions are quite acidic, but gonococci grow in the endocervix, where the pH is neutral.) Although certain nonpathogenic *Neisseria* grow at room temperature, gonococci do not grow well below 30°C, and they do not survive above 40°C.

A complex growth medium is required. Ordinarily this is in the form of either chocolate agar or similar complex agar containing inorganic iron and supplemental glucose, vitamins, and cofactors. Many less fastidious microorganisms also found in the same ecological niches (pharynx, cervix, and rectum) grow more readily than gonococci, and relatively selective media have been devised that utilize antibiotics to inhibit growth of nonpathogenic *Neisseria*. Vancomycin, colistin, and nystatin were widely used for this purpose, but some gonococci are quite sensitive to the concentrations of vancomycin used in the selective media. Other formulations now have been developed in which vancomycin is replaced with lincomycin or other antibiotics.

GENETIC SYSTEMS

There are two principal systems for performing genetic analysis of gonococci: transformation and conjugation. There are no known bacteriophages for gonococci (or meningococci), and a drug-resistance transposon system that functions well within the gonococcus has not been discovered. No presently available transposon is suitable for generalized chromosomal mutagenesis of the gonococcus. Seifert, So, and colleagues have developed a shuttle mutagenesis system that is extremely useful for genetic studies, in which a chloramphenicol acetyltransferase gene *cat* (or other antibiotic resistance genes) replaces β-lactamase (penicillinase) in a derivative of the transposon Tn3.[93] Other analogous shuttle mutagenesis systems have been developed.[94] The shuttle mutagenesis systems are excellent for creating mutations in a piece of cloned gonococcal DNA in *E. coli*, and for moving the cloned DNA containing the mutation back into the gonococcal chromosome by transformation, but these maneuvers require prior cloning of the gene of interest in an *E. coli* host.

TRANSFORMATION

Gonococci are quite unusual in their constitutive expression of competence for transformation by exogenous DNA. In competent gonococci, virtually every cell is competent at all stages of growth, quite unlike many other transformable species in which competence is restricted to certain phases of the growth cycle. However, only piliated (P^+) gonococci are competent for transformation.[95] The association between competence for transformation and expression of pili suggests that pili are involved directly in recognition or entry of transforming DNA. Mutations in *pil*E or in certain pilus-accessory genes dramatically reduce competence for transformation.[96]

Although most P^+ gonococci are highly competent, they only take up their own (homologous) DNA into the cell.[97,113] The structural basis for specificity in recognition of homologous DNA is uncertain. A 10-base pair sequence was described that seems to be responsible for selective entry.[99,100]

Because gonococci are piliated (competent) in vivo and are highly autolytic and release transforming DNA in a biologically active form, transformation may be used in nature to transfer genes between different gonococcal strains.[101] This might be important in transfer of chromosomal antibiotic resistance genes or pilin silent genes, among others. Indeed, Spratt has shown that gonococci probably are transformed in nature by DNA from other species, creating novel hybrid genes; this probably is important to evolution of the species, which exhibits a plastic, nonclonal structure.[102,103] A complete genomic map of the gonococcal chromosome will soon be available, when the entire DNA sequence of strain FA1090 is completed.

CONJUGATION

Many gonococci contain a 36-kb conjugal plasmid that efficiently mobilizes sexual transfer of certain other non–self-mobilizable plasmids such as the 4.5- or 7.2-kb penicillinase (Pc^r) plasmids.[104,105] The 36-kb conjugative plasmids also mobilize their own transfer with high efficiency, but they do not detectably mobilize chromosomal genes for transfer between gonococci.[106]

MUTAGENESIS

Although gonococci are highly variable in certain properties (particularly expression of pili, Opa, and LOS), they are relatively nonmutagenic. They are very susceptible to ultraviolet light but lack photoreactivation and error-prone repair systems and do not undergo ultraviolet mutagenesis under ordinary conditions.[107] The recombination systems of the gonococcus are not fully characterized yet. A gonococcal homologue of the *E. coli recA* gene has been cloned, and isogenic gonococci have been constructed lacking RecA function.[108] The gonococcal *recA* mutants show reduced frequencies of chromosomal transformation and of pilin antigenic variation.[31]

RESTRICTION AND MODIFICATION SYSTEMS

Gonococci are known to contain multiple restriction endonucleases and their corresponding methylases.[109] Transformation by plasmid DNA is markedly reduced when plasmids are introduced into gonococci across restriction barriers, but chromosomal transformation seems to be little influenced by restriction barriers.[110] Gonococci have DNA methylases for which there is no corresponding restriction endonuclease, which suggests that DNA methylation might be important to other biological functions including gene regulation.[109]

PLASMIDS

As indicated, many gonococci contain a 36-kb conjugal plasmid. Slightly larger derivatives of the 36-kb plasmid have been isolated that contain the tetracycline resistance (TC^r) *tet*M transposon.[111] A variety of gonococcal β-lactamase (penicillin-resistant, Pc^r) plasmids have been isolated and characterized. The two most frequent plasmids are either about 5.3 or 7.2 kb.[112] The Tc^r and Pc^r plasmids are discussed in the following under Antimicrobial Susceptibility.

Most gonococci also contain a 4.2-kb plasmid of unknown function *(cryptic plasmid)*. The DNA sequence of this plasmid has been determined.[113] Occasional gonococci can be isolated that do not contain the freely replicating (cytoplasmic) 4.2-kb cryptic plasmid, but they appear biologically normal.[114]

PATHOGENESIS

CLINICAL CORRELATIONS

Consideration of clinical manifestations of gonorrhea suggests many facets of the pathogenesis of the infection. Since gonococci persist in the male urethra despite hydrodynamic forces that would tend to wash the organisms from the mucosal surface, they must be able to adhere effectively to mucosal surfaces. Similarly, since gonococci survive in the urethra despite close attachment to large numbers of neutrophils, they must have mechanisms that help them to survive interactions with polymorphonuclear neutrophils. Since some gonococci are able to invade and persist in the bloodstream for many days at least, they must be able to evade killing by normal defense mechanisms of plasma, including antibodies, complement, and transferrin. Invasion of the bloodstream also implies that gonococci are able to invade mucosal barriers in order to gain access to the bloodstream. Repeated reinfections of the same patient by one strain strongly suggest that gonococci are able to change surface antigens frequently and/or are able to escape local immune mechanisms (Table 31-2).[115] The considerable tissue damage of fallopian tubes consequent to gonococcal salpingitis suggests that gonococci make at least one tissue toxin or that gonococci trigger an immune response that results in damage to host tissues. There is evidence to support many of these inferences.

Table 13-2. Mechanisms for Evasion of Host Defenses

Antigenic variation
Pili
Opa
Los
Blocking antibodies (serum-bactericidal resistance)
Rmp
Antibody cleavage
IgA_1, protease
Antigen release
Membrane blebs
Intracellular growth
(Facilitated by Por; certain Opas; short LOS)
Molecular mimicry (LOS)
Sialylation (serum-bactericidal resistance)

MODEL SYSTEMS

Studies of pathogenesis are complicated by the absence of a suitable animal model. A variety of animal models have been developed, each of which has certain utility, but no animal model faithfully reproduces the full spectrum of naturally acquired disease of humans. Considerable evidence about antigenic variation and interactions with neutrophils has been obtained from inoculation of subcutaneous chambers in guinea pigs or other animals. Cell cultures also provide means to study attachment and invasion. The best model system for many in vitro studies is organ culture of human tissues, particularly the fallopian tube system exploited successfully by McGee and colleagues.[116]

Investigators have recently utilized male human volunteers for critical studies of pathogenesis.[117] Evidence in human volunteers confirms high frequency of in vivo variation of pili and Opa; the role of pili (but not Opa) in initiation of mucosal infection (J.G. Cannon and M.S. Cohen, personal communication); and the apparent necessity of expression of a transferrin receptor, at least in a strain that does not express a functional lactoferrin receptor.[23,118,119] Expression of full-length LOS appears essential for maximal infectivity (J.G. Cannon, M.S. Cohen, personal communication). These studies in human volunteers are hopefully the prelude to efficient, rational, and safe tests of gonococcal vaccine candidates.

ADHERENCE

Two adherence ligands are well documented to be important: pili and Opa. Piliated gonococci adhere better to human columnar epithelial cells than to squamous cells and to human cells better than to nonhuman cells. Isolated pili adhere in vitro, and certain pilus antigenic variants exhibit selective ability to attach to particular cells under defined conditions in vitro.[20,120] Antibodies against pili decrease adherence of piliated gonococci to epithelial cells and red blood cells.[121–123] Similar evidence supports the role of Opa proteins in adherence: Gonococci expressing certain Opa proteins adhere better than Opa^- (transparent) gonococci to various cells, and a monoclonal antibody raised against one Opa protein inhibits adherence.[45,46,124] Antigenic variation of both pili and Opa may be biologically advantageous not only for escape from specific immune responses but also by providing specific adherence ligands for attaching to different niches in vivo. Recently, the cellular protein CD66 was identified as the host cell receptor for Opa.[125,126]

PILUS ADHESINS

Many studies have attempted to identify the portion of pilus protein involved in adhesion, and the cell receptor to which the pilus binds, without clear answers. Using conveniently available human red blood cells as a model cell, several laboratories showed that a cyanogen bromide cleavage fragment of pilin from amino acids 8 to 96 inhibits binding of whole pili, whereas other pilin fragments would not.[122] The thesis was advanced that a relatively invariant and immunorecessive pilus domain contains the ligand for cell binding.[122] Polyclonal sera raised against synthetic pilin peptides were studied for ability to block adherence of two unrelated P^+ gonococci to epithelial cells, and only sera against pilin peptides from amino acids 41 to 50 and 69 to 84 were effective.[127] These peptides are from relatively invariant regions of pilin.[128] However, many monoclonal antibodies that recognize specific or unique epitopes on pilin are more active in blocking adherence than monoclonal antibodies directed at common epitopes, which suggests that the pilin domain(s) involved in adherence actually are in variable region(s).[123] This is consistent with pilus vaccination studies of human volunteers, in whom protection extended only to the homologous isolate from which the pilus vaccine was prepared.[129]

In *E. coli* and other gram-negative bacteria, pili (or fimbriae) are associated with increased adherence, but the adhesin is not the pilin subunit but rather is a minor pilus-related protein.[130] Difficulties in identifying the gonococcal pilus adhesin might be owing to focusing research efforts entirely on pilin subunits. Gonococci contain several pilus-related proteins other than pilin.[131] At least one of these (PilC) has been proposed to be an adhesin independent of pili.[132] PilC is expressed on the outer membrane and undergoes high-frequency phase variation in its expression, like so many gonococcal cell surface molecules. Some evidence suggests PilC also may be located on the tip of the pilus and may be a tip-adhesion since antibodies against PilC decrease adherence.[133] PilC seems to play an important but still not fully defined role in gonococcal attachment.

Opa undoubtedly are important in infection since almost all isolates taken from patients are opaque or Opa expressing; the only exception is isolates taken from the female cervix near menses when most isolates are transparent.[134] Binding (adherence) to host cells is facilitated in an additive fashion by both Opa and Pili.[135] Once host cells have bound an Opa^+ Pil^+ gonococcus, they appear to undergo increased expression of an asialoglycoprotein cell-surface receptor for gonococcal LOS, thus presumably increasing the force and perhaps the frequency of attachment of other gonococci.[135]

INTERACTIONS WITH LEUKOCYTES

Gonococci were formerly referred to as *Neisseria intracellulare* because Gram-stain smears from human infections sometimes showed neutrophils covered with gonococci, which were assumed to be inside the cell. Pili are known to increase adherence of gonococci to human polymorphonuclear neutrophils, but they also increase resistance to phagocytosis and killing. In contrast to nonpiliated gonococci, which are readily ingested and killed by neutrophils, piliated gonococci attach well but are ingested relatively poorly.[136,137] Antipilus antibodies increase phagocytosis ("opsonization").[138,139] Thus pili increase epithelial cell adherence and decrease neutrophilic killing, and antipilus antibodies block epithelial adherence and increase phagocytic killing. Attachment to neutrophils is also increased by certain members of the Opa family.[140]

The majority of gonococci taken up by neutrophils are killed, but up to 2 percent of gonococci survive ingestion by neutrophils.[141] Work in Smith's laboratory has identified a 20-kDa gonococcal protein that seems to play an important role in resistance to intracellular killing by neutrophils.[142]

Neutrophils possess both oxidative and nonoxidative methods for killing intracellular bacteria. Oxidative killing depends on enzymes contained within the specific and nonspecific granules of neutrophils, whereas the nonoxidative mechanisms depend on a variety of cationic or basic lysosomal proteins. Gonococci are sensitive to damage by the oxidative products generated intracellularly during the neutrophilic respiratory burst but also are killed efficiently by neutrophils from patients with chronic granulomatous disease that lack the oxidative killing mechanism.[143] One neutrophilic protein involved in nonoxidative killing of gonococci is cathepsin G.[144] Gonococci containing certain alterations in penicillin-binding proteins show increased susceptibility to cathepsin G, which may explain the clinical observation that gonococci with low-level chromosomal resistance to penicillin are uncommonly isolated from the bloodstream.[144]

INVASION

Biopsies from patients with gonorrhea show gonococci partially imbedded within the cell surface (Fig. 31-5). Gonococci also can be seen within the epithelial cell, sometimes surrounded by cellular membranes. Shaw and Falkow employed a continuous culture of a human endometrial carcinoma cell to study variables affecting gonococcal invasion in vitro and found that invasion was increased when gonococci were grown in an iron-supplemented medium.[145] Other laboratories have confirmed this observation.[146] Studies with human fallopian tubes in organ culture have contributed significantly to understanding of the mechanisms of both adherence and invasion. Gonococci adhere selectively to mucus-secreting nonciliated cells of the fallopian tube and are gradually enfolded by pseudopods and engulfed by the host epithelial cell.[116] Gonococci appear to be able to multiply and divide intracellularly, although they do not invade laterally between cells.[116,147] Eventually some gonococci exit from the basal surface of the cell by a process termed exocytosis.[147] Once inside the epithelial cell, gonococci are immune to attack by antibody, complement, or neutrophils; their ability to survive to some degree inside epithelial cells suggests that they might be considered facultative intracellular parasites. As discussed in the preceding, invasion also is favored by expression of certain Opa proteins and by expression of "short" (nonsialylated) LOS.

IS POR A "TRIGGER" FOR INVASION?

The molecular mechanisms for invasion of epithelial cells are unknown. Several observations suggest that Por may play a role in invasion. Incubation of radiolabeled gonococcal membranes or whole bacteria with red blood cells results in transfer of the gonococcal porin from the bacterial cell surface into the red cell membrane.[148] No other protein is translocated into the red cell membrane. Using phospholipid bilayers or so-called black lipid membranes to quantitate rates of transfer of porin protein, Lynch et al. showed that gonococci containing PorA transfer Por into membranes more readily than gonococci containing PorB.[40] Since gonococci with PorA are more likely to cause disseminated disease than gonococci with PorB (see Chap. 32), these results are consistent with the hypothesis that translocation or spiking of host cells by Por may be an important step in invasion of the host cell. Possibly gonococci are bound closely to mucus-secreting nonciliated cells by adhesins such as pili or Opa, and after tight attachment might initiate penetration of the cell by spiking it with Por. These attractive ideas are still somewhat speculative, however. To date, it has not been demonstrated that gonococcal Por translocates into the surface membrane of epithelial cells, and it has not been shown that antibodies or peptides based on Por block gonococcal invasion. There is recent evidence, however, that porin channel activity is regulated during gonococcal growth in intact epithelial cells, and thus as of 1997 the Por invasion hypothesis is still alive.[149]

TISSUE DAMAGE

Gonococci produce a variety of extracellular products that might damage host cells including enzymes (phospholipase, peptidases,

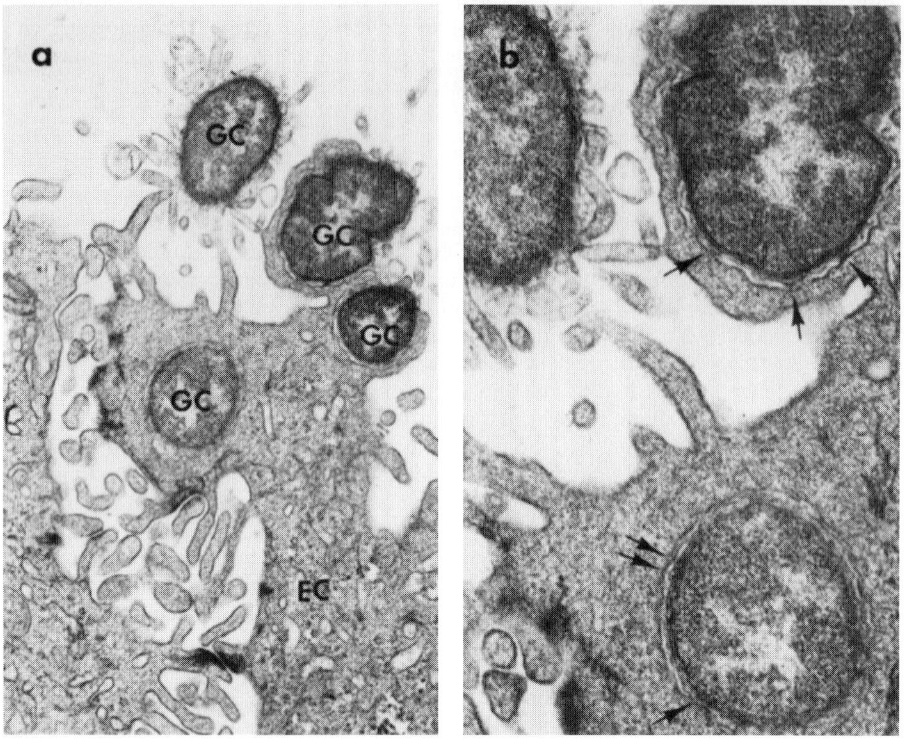

Fig. 31-5. Gonococcal–epithelial cell relation in cervical biopsies from a woman with acute gonorrhea. One of the exocervical epithelial cells (EC) seen in this electron micrograph (b is an enlarged portion of a) has closely adherent gonococci (GC). Some of the bacteria appear to be partially or completely endocytosed by the epithelial cells. Pili are not visible in this thin section and, in general, are usually difficult to visualize in thin-section preparations. Note the close apposition of gonococcal outer membrane and epithelial cell plasmalemma (arrows) and the apparent enfolding of the bacteria by the host's cervical cells (courtesy of D. Eschenbach and K. Holmes).

and others), but no true extracellular protein toxin has been identified. Tissue damage appears to be owing to two structural components of the cell surface: LOS and peptidoglycan.

Although gonococci do not attach to ciliated cells of fallopian tubes in organ culture, diminished beating of cilia is evident within hours after infection.[116] Electron micrographs demonstrate extrusion of ciliated cells, even though attached gonococci are only visible on adjacent nonciliated cells (Fig. 31-6). Similar effects are evident after purified gonococcal LOS is added to the fallopian tube model.[150] The toxic portion of LOS almost certainly is the lipid A portion, as would be expected.[150] Perhaps damage to ciliated cells results when membrane blebs containing lipid A are released from gonococci attached to nonciliated cells.

In addition to the unequivocal evidence that lipid A is a tissue toxin for gonococcal infections, there is also excellent evidence that fragments of the cell wall or peptidoglycan are capable of inducing damage in the human fallopian tube organ culture model.[151] Gonococcal peptidoglycan fragments also may be involved in the pathogenesis of inflammatory arthritis after bacteremic disease similar to the role of peptidoglycan fragments in a well-studied animal model of poststreptococcal arthritis.[152,153]

DISSEMINATION

SERUM RESISTANCE

The ability to resist the killing activity of antibodies and complement in normal human serum is closely related to the ability of gonococci to cause bacteremic illness with or without septic arthritis. A complex literature has evolved relating to the mechanisms of gonococcal resistance to serum antibodies and complement.

Most gonococci isolated from the bloodstream of patients are resistant to killing by serum from normal previously uninfected volunteers, whereas approximately two-thirds of isolates from mucosal infections are sensitive to killing by normal human serum.[6] Presumably the bactericidal activity of normal human serum for many gonococci results from previous exposure to common antigens shared by gonococci and other commensal bacteria. The nature of these common antigens and the bacteria on which they are carried are unknown.

Unstable serum resistance

Some gonococcal isolates are resistant to normal human serum on first isolation from mucosal surfaces but rapidly lose serum resistance on in vitro cultivation. This probably is owing to sialylation of full-length LOS in vivo, which results in phenotypic serum resistance. Nearly every isolate from patients with bacteremic disease exhibits stable serum resistance in vitro, which strongly suggests that unstable (phenotypically reversible) serum resistance is not biologically relevant to clinical gonococcal bacteremia.[6] The remainder of this discussion refers to stable (genotypic) serum resistance or serum sensitivity.

Immunochemistry

In normal human serum the principal bactericidal activity against serum-sensitive gonococci is found in the IgM fraction.[77,154] Bactericidal antibodies of the IgG class also occur in pooled human serum globulins or in convalescent sera. The antigens against which bactericidal complement-fixing antibodies are directed include LOS, although IgM and IgG bactericidal antibodies apparently recognize different epitopes on LOS.[77] Equal amounts of the complement "attack complex" are bound to the surface of both serum-sensitive and serum-resistant gonococci, suggesting that serum-resistant gonococci somehow are able to resist the otherwise lethal action of a fully formed complement attack complex.[155,156]

Blocking antibodies: role of Rmp

The interaction between serum antibodies, complement, and antigenic targets on LOS is complicated by the presence in many

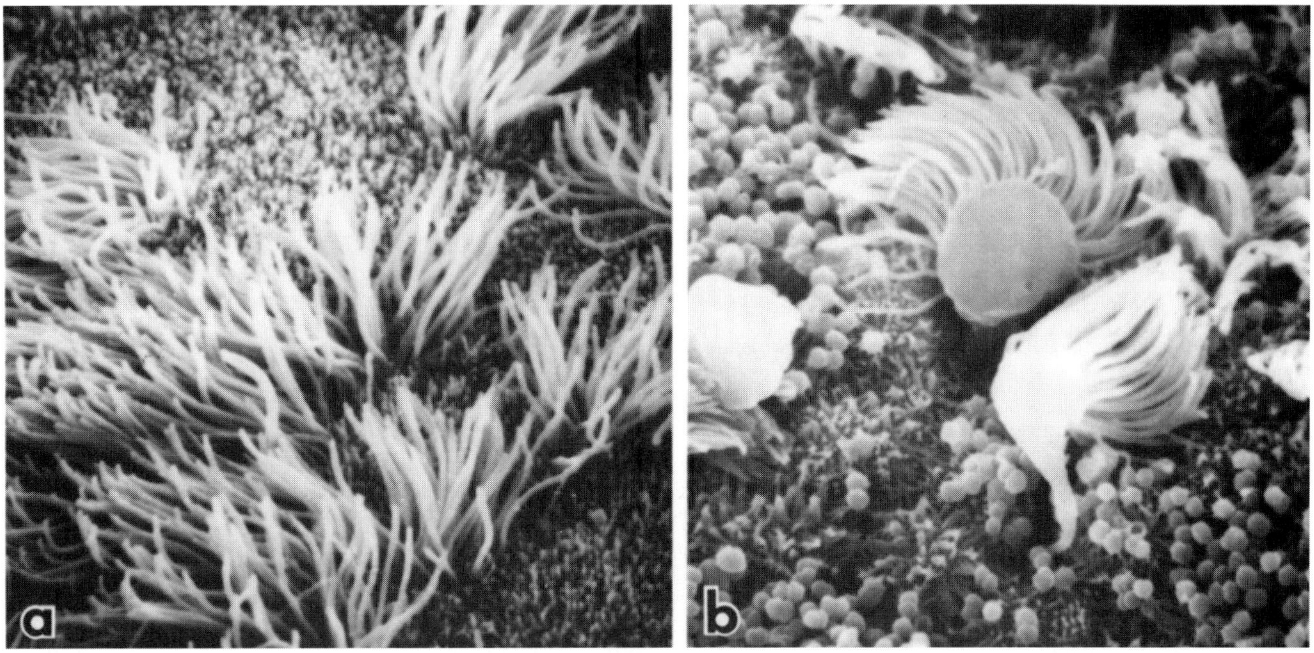

Fig. 31-6. Scanning electronic microscopy studies of normal, uninfected human fallopian tube mucosa showing (a) ciliated cells and nonciliated cells (the latter are covered with microvilli) and (b) human fallopian tube mucosa 20 hours after infection with a piliated clone of *N. gonorrhoeae*. In (b) note morphologically intact ciliated cells (far right and top), two sloughing ciliated cells (center), and gonococci attached almost exclusively to the microvilli of nonciliated cells but not attached to a sloughing ciliated cells. ×4000 magnification (from Z.A. McGee et al: *J Infect Dis* 143:413, 1981).

individuals of other non–complement-fixing IgG antibodies that recognize epitopes on Rmp. These *blocking antibodies* inhibit the ability of otherwise bactericidal IgM antibodies in normal human sera to effectively recognize their target on LOS.[154,157] The killing activity of sera frequently depends on the balance between non–complement-fixing blocking antibodies and complement-fixing bactericidal antibodies. Presumably the close physical proximity between Rmp and LOS accounts for the ability of anti-Rmp antibodies to block access of other antibodies to LOS. Recent evidence suggests that Rmp may be important not only for resistance to the bactericidal effects of human serum (and therefore for invasiveness), but also for successful transmission to the mucosal surfaces of sexual partners. Women with preexisting antibodies to Rmp were more likely to acquire infection from their infected partners than were other women who lacked antibodies to Rmp.[158] Presumably, antibodies to Rmp in genital secretions blocked otherwise protective antibodies in genital secretions.

In addition to the importance of Rmp to stable serum bactericidal resistance, the structure of Por probably also is important. Earlier work established several genetic loci that were important to serum resistance *(sac-1, sac-3)*, and each was very tightly linked to the *por* structural gene.[159] Subsequent genetic studies showed that creation of intragenic *por* hybrids, in which a crossover event occurred within *por*, markedly altered serum bactericidal resistance.[43] Thus the *sac* loci may well have represented alterations of Por, undetectable by the means available when those studies were conducted.

Chemotaxis

Serum resistance of gonococci also may relate to the pathobiological potential of infection at mucosal sites. Serum-resistant gonococci that cause bacteremia frequently cause asymptomatic relatively noninflammatory infections at the mucosal surface (see Chap. 32); this correlates with their relative inability to trigger a chemotactic response for neutrophils. In contrast, serum-sensitive isolates that rarely cause bacteremic disease but that frequently cause a marked inflammatory response at the mucosal surface elicit a much stronger chemotactic response in vitro.[160] Antibodies that elicit the C5a-dependent chemotactic response are directed against LOS antigens.[160] Since severe pelvic inflammatory disease is correlated with relatively high level sensitivity to serum killing in vitro, local tissue damage may reflect the ability of some gonococci to trigger a chemotactic response, resulting in increased local inflammation and tissue damage.[161]

DIAGNOSIS

Diagnostic procedures are discussed fully in Chap. 32, but the principles can be outlined briefly here.

The standard procedure for diagnosing symptomatic disease in men with urethritis is the Gram stain. In asymptomatic men or in women with genital infection, the Gram stain is less useful, however, and cultures are necessary. Cultures also are useful whenever one is considering the possibility of an antibiotic-resistant gonococcal strain. A variety of tests have been developed to detect gonococcal antigen in genital secretions. These include enzyme immunoassays with polyclonal sera against gonococcal antigens, monoclonal antibodies against gonococcal antigens, and a Limulus amoebocyte gelation test for lipid A: The enzyme immunoassays have achieved the most widespread use, but the gold standard still is culture. DNA–DNA hybridization has potential for rapid diagnosis of gonorrhea but is not practical yet. Polymerase chain reaction (PCR) and the variant termed ligase chain reaction (LCR) tests have been developed that offer great sensitivity, specificity, and convenience, since they can be used on urine samples. As of mid-1997, however, they are not widely available (see Chap. 92 for details).

Unfortunately, good diagnostic serologic tests have never been developed. Approximately one-half of infected persons develop antipilus antibodies in serum during convalescence, but the sensitivity of the test is not sufficiently high for its use in high-prevalence populations, and the specificity is too low to use as a screening test in low-prevalence populations. Serologic testing for diagnosing gonorrhea is still a problem for research.

A unique test that once had clinical promise uses competent piliated gonococci as a test system to detect gonococcal transforming DNA in patient secretions.[162] The principle of this test is that gonococci can be transformed only by their own DNA and that virtually every gonococcal infection leaves residual amounts of biologically active transforming DNA in the environment. It has not been widely utilized, however.

ANTIMICROBIAL SUSCEPTIBILITY

Gonococci are inherently quite sensitive to antimicrobial agents, compared with many other gram-negative bacteria. However, there has been a gradual selection for antibiotic-resistant mutants in clinical practice over the past several decades, and recently several different plasmids that mediate relatively high level antibiotic resistance have appeared. The consequence of these events has been to make penicillin and tetracycline therapy ineffective in most areas. Antibiotics such as spectinomycin, ciprofloxacin, and ceftriaxone are effective but more expensive than penicillin G and tetracycline. The epidemiologic trends in prevalence of antibiotic-resistant gonococci and proper treatment of antibiotic-susceptible and antibiotic-resistant gonococcal infections are discussed in Chap. 32. The biochemical and genetic basis for antibiotic resistance is discussed in this chapter.

PENICILLIN

Isolates obtained in the 1940s typically were inhibited by 0.01 μg/mL penicillin G or less. A gradual increase in prevalence and extent of resistance to penicillin occurred over the subsequent several decades; this was shown to be owing to the accumulation of several independent chromosomal mutations that affect cell surface structure. Three genetic loci resulting in low-level resistance to penicillin have been well studied, and results are reviewed elsewhere.[163] One of them *(penA)* results in alteration of penicillin-binding protein two (PBP2), decreasing the affinity of PBP2 for penicillin. The gene for altered gonococcal PBP2 was cloned and sequenced, with the interesting suggestion that it might be the result of gene transfer from another related species in nature, leading to a hybrid PBP2.[102] The other loci (*mtr* and *penB*) result in low-level resistance to many antibiotics in addition to penicillins. The *mtr* locus has been shown to encode an efflux-pump that reduces intracellular concentrations of antibiotics.[164] The *penB* locus appears to be indistinguishable from *por*, the structural gene for the major porin protein. Introduction of *penA*, *mtr*, and *penB* into a sensitive gonococcal strain results in an increase in the minimum inhibitory concentration (MIC) of penicillin G from 0.01 to about 1.0 μg/mL. There have been a number of reports of gonococci with chromosomally mediated resistance to penicillin in which the MIC for penicillin is 2 to 4 μg/mL.[115] The genetic and biochemical basis for increased resistance is unknown.

In 1976 a new type of gonococcal resistance to penicillin was first documented: The production of β-lactamase owing to the presence of plasmids that encoded production of a TEM-1 type of β-lactamase.[165] The first Pc^r (penicillinase-producing) gonococci contained either a 5.3- or a 7.2-kb plasmid. These two Pc^r plasmids are very closely related, and each carries approximately 40 percent of the common gram-negative μ-lactamase transposon Tn2.[166,167] Based on the molecular structure of the gonococcal and *Haemophilus ducreyi* Pc^r plasmids, there is strong suspicion that gonococci acquired the Pc^r plasmids from *H. ducreyi*.[168,169] The gonococcal Pc^r plasmids can be mobilized efficiently by the 36-kb gonococcal conjugal plasmid, helping to explain how Pc^r plasmids are spread to new gonococcal strains.[170]

TETRACYCLINE

Resistance to tetracycline (Tc) also has increased owing either to the additive effects of several chromosomal mutations or to acquisition of a tetracycline-resistance plasmid. Chromosomal loci mediating low-level resistance to tetracycline have been designated *mtr, penB,* and *tet*; two of these also are involved in low-level, non–β-lactamase-mediated penicillin resistance.[163] In aggregate these three loci result in an increase in the tetracycline MIC from about 0.25 to 2–4 μg/mL. Much higher levels of resistance (tetracycline MIC ≥ 64 μg/mL) are found in gonococci containing a 38-kb tetracycline-resistance (TC^r) plasmid, which is a derivative of the 36-kb conjugal plasmid. Hybridization studies show that the Tc^r plasmid contains *tetM,* which is carried on a transposon found in a variety of gram-positive and gram-negative microorganisms including many genital pathogens *(Gardnerella, Ureaplasma)*.[111] The Tc^r plasmids contain *tetM* in a position that does not inactivate conjugal function, and Tc^r gonococci can transfer this plasmid as well as Pc^r plasmids efficiently into other antibiotic-sensitive gonococci. The mechanism of resistance mediated by *tetM* involves production of a cytoplasmic protein that protects ribosomes from the action of tetracycline.

SPECTINOMYCIN

For many years there were only rare reports of gonococci exhibiting high-level resistance to spectinomycin (Spc), but in areas where this antibiotic has been used frequently because of the prevalence of Pc^r gonococci, Spc^r isolates are more common.[171] Single-step high-level resistance to Spc can be obtained relatively easily in the laboratory, and biochemical and genetic studies of Spc^r mutants and of naturally occurring Spc^r isolates show that they are virtually identical. The genetic locus *spc* maps within a cluster of chromosomal ribosomal genes and results in alteration of the ribosomal target on which Spc acts.[163]

OTHER ANTIBIOTICS

Streptomycin (Str) is not frequently used for therapy of gonorrhea at present, but many gonococci exhibit high-level resistance to Str. A locus for resistance to Str *(str)* maps near *spc,* and both are closely linked to those for resistance to tetracycline *(tet)*, rifampin *(rif)*, and others.[88]

Resistance to nalidixic acid and related DNA gyrase inhibitors is obtained easily in the laboratory with mutation frequencies of approximately 1×10^{-8}. In contrast, Spc^r mutants arise with a frequency of about 1×10^{-10} to 1×10^{-11}. Resistance to fluoroquinolones is increasing in certain regions, but is not yet a general problem.[172,173] Resistance to penicillins and tetracyclines is increasingly common in many parts of the world.[174,175]

HOST RESPONSE

Naturally acquired gonococcal infection results in serum antibodies against many gonococcal antigens including Pil, Por, Opa, Rmp, and LOS.[176,177] As would be expected, serum antibody responses are greater in patients who have bacteremia or salpingitis than in those who have uncomplicated mucosal infection. Studies of mucosal secretions demonstrate that uncomplicated genital infection often results in IgA and IgG antibodies against the homologous isolate.[178,179] The duration of the local mucosal antibody response after natural infection may be quite brief, however.[178] There also is a cellular immune response to natural gonococcal infection, although the cellular immunology of gonorrhea has been studied much less extensively than the humoral response.

VACCINES

The principal efforts to stimulate protective immunity to date have focused on use of P.I as an antigen. Intramuscular or subcutaneous inoculation with purified Pil results in both serum and mucosal antibodies that have antiadherence and opsonizing properties.[121,129,138] Limited in vitro studies of male volunteers vaccinated with a single antigenic type of pilus showed that there was partial protection against urethral challenge with the homologous strain.[180] Although the level of protection was modest, with only a 10- to 30-fold increase in the 50 percent infectious dose, this conceivably could result in clinically significant protection. Unfortunately challenge of vaccinated volunteers with a heterologous strain resulted in no protection (C.C. Brinton, presented at the International Pathogenic *Neisseria* Meeting, Montreal, 1982). A single antigenic type of pilus was used to vaccinate American military in a clinical trial, with the perhaps expected result that there was no protection against the diverse antigenic types of gonococci found in clinical practice.[129] It remains possible that a polyvalent pilus vaccine would be more effective or that a common pilin domain or pilus-related protein antigen will be discovered that is more broadly protective against mucosal and/or systemic gonococcal infection.

Other vaccines (including Por) are also under active investigation. The advantages of the recombinant Por vaccine include its ability to be purified from *E. coli* without contamination by other potentially confounding antigens such as the blocking antigen Rmp. Genital infection does not totally protect against reinfection by the same strain even within a few weeks of treatment, but partial protection against reinfection by the same Por serovar was demonstrated in a large study in Africa.[115,181] However, this result was not confirmed in another, differently designed study.[182]

Understanding of the pathogenesis of gonorrhea is now quite extensive. There is reason for some hope that this new information can be translated into protection against this common and sometimes serious infection. It remains for the future to determine whether this hope can be realized.

References

1 Morton RS (ed): *Gonorrhoea* [vol. 9 in the series Major Problems in Dermatology. A Rook (consulting ed)]. London, W.B. Saunders, 1977.

2 Kellogg DS et al: *Neisseria gonorrhoeae*: 1. Virulence genetically linked to clonal variation. *J Bacteriol* 85:1274, 1963.

3 Catlin BW: Nutritional profiles of *Neisseria gonorrhoea*, *Neisseria meningitidis*, and *Neisseria lactamica* in chemically defined media and the use of growth requirements for gonococcal typing. *J Infect Dis* 128:178, 1973.

4 Shinners EN et al: Arginine and pyrimidine biosynthetic defects in *Neisseria gonorrhoeae* strains isolated from patients. *J Bacteriol* 151: 295, 1982.

5 Hook EW III et al: Auxotype/serovar diversity and antimicrobial resistance of *Neisseria gonorrhoeae* in two mid-sized American cities. *Sex Transm Dis* 14:141, 1987.

6 Eisenstein BI et al: Penicillin sensitivity and serum resistance are independent attributes of strains of *Neisseria gonorrhoeae* causing disseminated gonococcal infection. *Infect Immunol* 15:834, 1977.

7 Knapp JS et al: Serological classification of *Neisseria gonorrhoeae* with use of monoclonal antibodies to gonococcal outer membrane protein 1. *J Infect Dis* 150:44, 1984.

8 Falk ES: Geneotypes and phenotypes of β lactamase producing strains of *Neisseria gonorrhoeae* from African countries. *Genitourin Med* 64:226–232, 1988.

9 Poh CL: Rapid in situ generation of DNA restriction endonuclease patterns for *Neisseria gonorrhoeae*. *J Clin Microbiol* 27:2784–2788, 1989.

10 Poh CL: Subtyping of *Neisseria gonorrhoeae* auxotype-serovar groups by pulsed-field gel electrophoresis. *J Med Microbiol* 38:366–370, 1993.

11 Camarena JJ: DNA amplification fingerprinting for subtyping *Neisseria gonorrhoeae* strains. *Sex Transm Dis* 22:128–136, 1995.

12 O'Rourke M et al: Opa-typing: A high-resolution tool for studying the epidemiology of gonorrhoea. *Mol Microbiol* 17:865–875, 1995.

13 Sparling PF et al: Colonial morphology of *Neisseria gonorrhoeae* isolated from males and females. *J Bacteriol* 93:513, 1967.

14 Walstad DL et al: Altered outer membrane protein in different colonial types of *Neisseria gonorrhoeae*. *J Bacteriol* 129:1623, 1977.

15 Swanson J: Studies on gonococcus infection: XIV. Cell wall protein differences among color/opacity colony variants of *Neisseria gonorrhoeae*. *Infect Immunol* 21:292, 1978.

16 Swanson J: Colony opacity and protein 11 compositions of gonococci. *Infect Immunol* 37: 359, 1982.

17 Buchanan TM: Antigenic heterogeneity of gonococcal pili. *J Exp Med* 151:1470, 1975.

18 Forest KT et al: Assembly and antigenicity of the *Neisseria gonorrhoeae* pilus mapped with antibodies. *Infect Immunol* 64:644–652, 1996.

19 Parge HE et al: Structure or the fibre-forming protein pilin at 2.6A resolution. *Nature* 378:32–38, 1995.

20 Buchanan TM: Attachment role of gonococcal pili: Optimum conditions and quantitation of adherence of isolated pili to human cells in vitro. *J Clin Invest* 61:931, 1978.

21 Lambden PR et al: The identification and isolation of novel pilus types produced by isogenic variants of *Neisseria gonorrhoeae* P9 following selection in vivo. *FEMS Microbiol Lett* 10:339, 1981.

22 Hagblom P et al: Intragenic recombination leads to pilus antigenic variation in *Neisseria gonorrhoeae*. *Nature* 315:156, 1985.

23 Seifert HS et al: Multiple gonococcal pilin antigenic variants are produced during experimental human infections. *J Clin Invest* 93:2744–2749, 1994.

24 Schoolnik GK et al: Gonococcal pili: Primary structure and receptor binding domain. *J Exp Med* 159:1351, 1984.

25 Meyer TF et al: Pilus expression in *Neisseria gonorrhoeae* involves chromosomal rearrangement. *Cell* 30:45, 1982.

26 Meyer TF et al: Pilus genes of *Neisseria gonorrhoeae*: Chromosomal organization and DNA sequence. *Proc Natl Acad Sci USA* 81:6110, 1984.

27 Nicolson IJ et al: Localization of antibody-binding sites by sequence analysis of cloned pilin genes from *Neisseria gonorrhoeae*. *J Gen Microbiol* 133:825, 1987.

28 Haas R et al: Release of soluble pilin antigen coupled with gene conversion in *Neisseria gonorrhoeae*. *Proc Natl Acad Sci USA* 84:9079–9083, 1987.

29 Segal E et al: Antigenic variation of gonococcal pilus involves assembly of separated silent gene segments. *Proc Natl Acad Sci USA* 83: 2177, 1986.

30 Swanson J et al: Gene conversion variations generate structurally distinct pilin polypeptides in *Neisseria gonorrhoeae*. *J Exp Med* 165: 1016, 1987.

31 Koomey M et al: Effects of *recA* mutations on pilus antigenic variation and phase transitions in *Neisseria gonorrhoeae*. *Genetics* 17:391, 1987.

32 Segal E et al: Role of chromosomal rearrangement in *N. gonorrhoeae* pilus phase variation. *Cell* 40:293, 1985.
33 Fyfe JAM et al: The *pilE* gene of *Neisseria gonorrhoeae* MS11 is transcribed from a σ^{70} promoter during growth in vitro. *J Bacteriol* 177:3781–3787, 1995.
34 Taha MK et al: Phosphorylation and functional analysis of PilA, a protein involved in the transcriptional regulation of the pilin gene in *Neisseria gonorrhoeae*. *Mol Microbiol* 15:667–677, 1995.
35 Hill SA et al: Integration host factor is a transcriptional cofactor of pilE in *Neisseria gonorrhoeae*. *Mol Microbiol* 23:649–656, 1997.
36 Blake MS et al: Purification and partial characterization of the major outer membrane protein of *Neisseria gonorrhoeae*. *Infect Immunol* 36:277, 1982.
37 Hitchcock PJ: Analyses of gonococcal lipopolysaccharide in whole cell lysates by sodium dodecyl sulfate-polyacrylamide gel electrophoresis: Stable association of lipopolysaccharide with the major outer membrane protein (Protein 1) of *Neisseria gonorrhoeae*. *Infect Immunol* 46:202, 1984.
38 Swanson J et al: Antigenicity of *Neisseria gonorrhoeae* outer membrane protein(s) Ill detected by immunoprecipitation and Western blot transfer with a monoclonal antibody. *Infect Immunol* 24(38): 668, 1982.
39 Young JD-E et al: Properties of the major outer membrane protein from *Neisseria gonorrhoeae* incorporated into model lipid membranes. *Proc Natl Acad Sci USA* 80:3831, 1983.
40 Lynch EC et al: Studies of porins: Spontaneously transferred from whole cells and reconstituted from purified proteins of *Neisseria gonorrhoeae* and *Neisseria meningitidis*. *Biophys J* 45:104, 1984.
41 Gotschlich EC et al: Porin protein of *Neisseria gonorrhoeae*: Cloning and gene structure. *Proc Natl Acad Sci USA* 84:8135, 1987.
42 Carbonetti NH et al: Molecular cloning and characterization of the structural gene for protein 1, the major outer membrane protein of *Neisseria gonorrhoeae*. *Proc Natl Acad Sci USA* 84:9084,1987.
43 Carbonetti NH et al: *Genetics* of protein I of *Neisseria gonorrhoeae*: construction of hybrid porins. *Proc Natl Acad Sci USA* 85:6841, 1988.
44 Black WJ et al: Characterization of *Neisseria gonorrhoeae* protein II phase variation by use of monoclonal antibodies. *Infect Immunol* 45: 453, 1984.
45 Sugasawara RJ et al: Inhibition of *Neisseria gonorrhoeae* attachment to HeLa cells with monoclonal antibody directed against a protein II. *Infect Immunol* 42:908, 1983.
46 Fischer SH et al: Gonococci possessing only certain P.II outer membrane proteins interact with human neutrophils. *Infect Immunol* 56: 1574, 1988.
47 Stern A et al: Opacity determinants of *Neisseria gonorrhoeae*: Gene expression and chromosomal linkage to the gonococcal pilus gene. *Cell* 37:447, 1984.
48 Stern A et al: Opacity genes in *Neisseria gonorrhoeae*: Control of phase and antigenic variation. *Cell* 47:61, 1986.
49 Stern A et al: Common mechanism controlling phase and antigenic variation in pathogenic *Neisseria*. *Mol Microbiol* 1:5, 1987.
50 Connell TD et al: Recombination among protein 11 genes of *Neisseria gonorrhoeae* generates new coding sequences and increases structural variability in the protein 11 family. *Mol Microbiol* 2:227, 1988.
51 Gotschlich EC et al: Cloning of the structural genes of three H8 antigens and of protein Ill of *Neisseria gonorrhoeae*. *J Exp Med* 164: 868, 1986.
52 Cannon JG et al: Monoclonal antibody that recognizes an outer membrane antigen common to the pathogenic *Neisseria* species but not to most nonpathogenic *Neisseria* species. *Infect Immunol* 43:994, 1984.
53 Gotschlich EC et al: Identification and gene structure of an azurin-like protein with a lipoprotein signal peptide in *Neisseria gonorrhoeae*. *FEMS Microbiol Lett* 43:253, 1987.
54 Kawula TH et al: Localization of a conserved epitope and an azurin-like domain in the H.8 protein of pathogenic *Neisseria*. *Mol Microbiol* 1:24 179, 1987.
55 Black JR et al: *Neisseria* antigen H.8 is immunogenic in patients with disseminated gonococcal and meningococcal infections. *J Infect Dis* 151:24, 650, 1985.
56 Norqvist A et al: The effect of iron starvation on the outer membrane protein composition of *Neisseria gonorrhoeae*. *FEMS Microbiol Lett* 4:71, 1978.
57 West SEH et al: Response of *Neisseria gonorrhoeae* to iron limitation: Alterations in expression of membrane proteins without apparent siderophore production. *Infect Immunol* 47:388, 1985.
58 Clark VL et al: Induction and repression of outer membrane proteins by anaerobic growth of *Neisseria gonorrhoeae*. *Infect Immunol* 55: 1359, 1987.
59 Keevil W et al: Physiology and virulence determinants of *Neisseria gonorrhoeae* grown in glucose, oxygen- or cystine-limited continuous culture. *J Gen Microbiol* 132:3289, 1986.
60 Mietzner TA et al: Identification of an iron-regulated 37,000-dalton protein in the cell envelope of *Neisseria gonorrhoeae*. *Infect Immunol* 45:410, 1984.
61 Mietzner TA et al: Purification and characterization of the major iron-regulated protein expressed by pathogenic *Neisseria*. *J Exp Med* 165:1041, 1987.
62 Mietzner TA et al: Distribution of an antigenically related iron-regulated protein among the *Neisseria* spp. *Infect Immunol* 51:60, 1986.
63 Black JR et al: Human immune response to iron-repressible outer membrane proteins of *Neisseria meningitidis*. *Infect Immunol* 54: 710, 1986.
64 Beucher M et al: Cloning, sequencing, and characterization of the gene encoding FrpB, a major iron-regulated, outer membrane protein of *Neisseria* gonorrhoeae. *J Bacteriol* 177:2041–2049, 1995.
65 Cornelissen C et al: Iron piracy: Acquisition of transferrin-bound iron by bacterial pathogens. *Mol Microbiol* 14:843–850, 1994.
66 Biswas GD et al: Characterization of *lbpA*, the structural gene for a lactoferrin receptor in *Neisseria gonorrhoeae*. *Infect Immunol* 63: 2958–2967, 1995.
67 Chen CJ et al: Identification and purification of a hemoglobin-binding outer membrane protein from *Neisseria gonorrhoeae*. *Infect Immunol* 64:5008–5014, 1996.
68 Braun V: Energy-coupled transport and signal transduction through the gram-negative outer membrane via TonB-ExbB-ExbD-dependent receptor proteins. *FEMS Microbiol Rev* 16:295–307, 1995.
69 Mulks MH et al: IgA protease production as a characteristic distinguishing pathogenic from harmless *Neisseriaceae*. *N Engl J Med* 299: 973, 1978.
70 Mulks MH et al: Immunoglobulin A, protease types of *Neisseria gonorrhoeae* and their relationship to auxotype and serovar. *Infect Immunol* 55:931, 1987.
71 Lin L et al: The *Neisseria* Type 2 Iga_1 protease cleaves LAMP1 and promotes survival of bacteria within epithelial cells. *Mol Microbiol* 24:1083–1094, 1997.
72 Pohlner J et al: Gene structure and extracellular secretion of *Neisseria gonorrhoeae* IgA protease. *Nature* 325:458, 1987.
73 Griffiss JM et al: Lipooligosaccharides: The principal glycolipids of the neisserial outer membrane. *Rev Infect Dis* 10:5287, 1988.
74 Gulati S et al: Immunogenicity of *Neisseria gonorrhoeae* lipooligosaccharide epitope 2C7, widely expressed in vivo with no immunochemical similarity to human glycosphingolipids. *J Infect Dis* 174: 1223–1237, 1996.
75 Demarco de Hormaeche R et al: Gonococcal variants selected by growth in vivo or in vitro have antigenically different LPS. *Microbial Pathogen* 4:289, 1988.
76 Apicella MA et al: Phenotypic variation in epitope expression of the *Neisseria gonorrhoeae* lipooligosaccharide. *Infect Immunol* 55:1755, 1987.
77 Apicella MA et al: Bactericidal antibody response of normal human serum to the lipooligosaccharide of *Neisseria gonorrhoeae*. *J Infect Dis* 153:520, 1986.
78 Griffiss JM et al: Physical heterogeneity of neisserial lipooligosaccharides reflects oligosaccharides that differ in apparent molecular

weight, chemical composition, and antigenic expression. *Infect Immunol* 55:1792, 1987.

79 Parsons NJ et al: Sialylation of lipopolysaccharide and loss of absorption of bacterial antibody during conversion of gonococci to serum resistance by cytidine 5′-monophospho-*N*-acetyl neuraminic acid. *Microbiol Pathogen* 7:63–72, 1989.

80 Smith H et al: Sialylation of *Neisseria* lipopolysaccharide: a major influence on pathogenecity. *Microbiol Pathogen* 19:365–377, 1995.

81 van Putten JPM: Phase variation of lipopolysaccharide directs interconversion of invasive and immunoresistant phenotypes of *Neisseria gonorrhoeae*. *EMBO J* 12:4043–4051, 1993.

82 van Putten JPM et al: Molecular mechanisms and implications for infection of lipopolysaccharide variation in *Neisseria*. *Mol Microbiol* 16:847–853, 1995.

83 Gotschlich EC: Genetic locus for the biosynthesis of the variable portion of *Neisseria gonorrhoeae* lipooligosaccharide. *J Exp Med* 180: 2181–2190, 1994.

84 Bramley J et al: A serum-sensitive, sialytransferase-deficient mutant of *Neisseria gonorrhoeae* defective in conversion to serum resistance by CMP-NANA or blood cell extracts. *Microbial Pathogen* 18:187–195, 1995.

85 Elkins C et al: Antibodies to N-terminal peptides of gonococcal porin are bacteridical when gonococcal lipolosaccharide is not sialylated. *Mol Microbiol* 5:2617–2628, 1992.

86 Rosenthal RS et al: Strain-related differences in lysozyme sensitivity and extent of O-acetylation of gonococcal peptidoglycan. *Infect Immunol* 37:826, 1982.

87 Melly MA et al: Ability of monomeric peptidoglycan fragments from *Neisseria gonorrhoeae* to damage human fallopian-tube mucosa. *J Infect Dis* 149:378, 1984.

88 Noegel A et al: Isolation of a high molecular weight polyphosphate from *Neisseria gonorrhoeae*. *J Exp Med* 157:2049, 1983.

89 Chen T et al: Heparin protects Opa⁺ *Neisseria gonorrhoeae* from the bactericidal action of normal human serum. *Infect Immunol* 63: 1790–1795, 1995.

90 Britigan B et al: Effect of growth in serum on uptake of *Neisseria gonorrhoeae* by human neutrophils. *J Infect Dis* 152:330, 1985.

91 Britigan BE et al: Phagocyte-derived lactate stimulates oxygen consumption by *Neisseria gonorrhoeae*. *J Clin Invest* 81: 318, 1988.

92 Knapp JS, Clark VL: Anaerobic growth of *Neisseria gonorrhoeae* coupled to nitrite reduction. *Infect Immunol* 46:176, 1984.

93 Seifert HS et al: Shuttle mutagenesis: A method of transposon mutagenesis for *Saccharomyces cerevisiae*. *Proc Natl Acad Sci USA* 83: 735–739, 1986.

94 Kahrs AF et al: Generalized transposon shuttle mutagenesis in *Neisseria gonorrhoeae*: A method for isolating epithelial Cell invasion-defective mutants. *Mol Microbiol* 12:819–831, 1994.

95 Biswas GD et al: Factors affecting genetic transformation of *Neisseria gonorrhoeae*. *J Bacteriol* 129:983, 1977.

96 Rudel T et al: Role of pili and the phase-variable PilC protein in natural competence for transformation of *Neisseria gonorrhoeae*. *Proc Natl Acad Sci USA* 92:7986–7990, 1995

97 Dougherty TJ et al: Specificity of DNA uptake in genetic transformation of gonococci. *Biochem Biophys Res Commun* 86:97, 1979.

98 Graves JF et al: Sequence-specific DNA uptake in transformation of *Neisseria gonorrhoeae*. *J Bacteriol* 152:1071, 1982.

99 Goodman SD et al: Identification and arrangement of the DNA sequence recognized in specific transformation of *Neisseria gonorrhoeae*. *Proc Natl Acad Sci USA* 85:6982, 1988.

100 Elkins C et al: Species-specific uptake of DNA by gonococci is mediated by a 10-base pair sequence. *J Bacteriol* 173:3911–3913, 1991.

101 Sarubbi FA et al: Transfer of antibiotic resistance in mixed cultures of *Neisseria gonorrhoeae*. *J Infect Dis* 130:660, 1974.

102 Spratt BG: Hybrid penicillin-binding proteins in penicillin-resistant strains of *Neisseria gonorrhoeae*. *Nature* 332:173–176, 1988.

103 Gibbs CP et al: Genome plasticity in *Neisseria gonorrhoeae*. *FEMS Microbiol Lett* 145:173–179, 1996.

104 Robert M et al: Conjugal transfer of R plasmids in *Neisseria gonorrhoeae*. *Nature* 266:630, 1977.

105 Eisenstein BI et al: Conjugal transfer of the gonococcal penicillinase plasmid. *Science* 195:998, 1977.

106 Biswas GD et al: High-frequency conjugal transfer of a gonococcal penicillinase plasmid. *J Bacteriol* 143:1318, 1980.

107 Campbell LA et al: Mutagenesis of *Neisseria gonorrhoeae*: Absence of error-prone repair. *J Bacteriol* 160:288, 1984.

108 Koomey JM et al: Cloning of the gene of *Neisseria gonorrhoeae* and construction of gonococcal *recA* mutants. *J Bacteriol* 169:790, 1987

109 Sullivan KM et al: Characterization of DNA restriction and modification activities in *Neisseria* species. *FEMS Microbiol Lett* 44:389, 1987.

110 Stein DC et al: Restriction of plasmid DNA during transformation but not conjugation in *Neisseria gonorrhoeae*. *Infect Immunol* 56: 112, 1988.

111 Morse SA et al: High-level tetracycline resistance in *Neisseria gonorrhoeae* is result of acquisition of streptococcal term determinant. *Antimicrob Agents Chemother* 30:664, 1986.

112 Perine PL et al: Evidence for two distinct types of penicillinase-producing *Neisseria gonorrhoeae*. *Lancet* 2:993, 1977.

113 Korch C et al: Cryptic plasmid of *Neisseria gonorrhoeae*: Complete nucleotide sequence and genetic organization. *J Bacteriol* 163:430, 1985.

114 Biswas GD et al: Construction of isogenic gonococcal strains varying in the presence of a 4.2-kb cryptic plasmid. *J Bacteriol* 167:685, 1986.

115 Faruki H et al: A community-based outbreak of infection with penicillin-resistant *Neisseria gonorrhoeae* not producing penicillinase (chromosomally mediated resistance). *N Engl J Med* 313:607, 1985.

116 McGee ZA et al: Pathogenic mechanisms of *Neisseria gonorrhoeae*: Observations on damage to human fallopian tubes in organ culture by gonococci of colony type I or type 4. *J Infect Dis* 143:413, 1981.

117 Cohen MS et al: Human experimentation with *Neisseria gonorrhoeae*: Rationale, methods, and implications for the biology of infection and vaccine development. *J Infect Dis* 169:532–537, 1994.

118 Jerse AE et al: Multiple gonococcal opacity proteins occurs during experimental urethral infection in the male. *J Exp Med* 179:911–920, 1994.

119 Cornelissen CN et al: Function and virulence studies of the gonococcal transferrin receptor. (Abstract). 10th International Pathogenic *Neisseria* Conference, Baltimore, MD. September 8–13, 1996, p. 552.

120 Lambden PR et al: Biological properties of two distinct pilus types produced by isogenic variants of *Neisseria gonorrhoeae* P9. *J Bacteriol* 141:393, 1980.

121 McChesney D et al: Genital antibody response to a parental gonococcal pilus vaccine. *Infect Immunol* 36:1006, 1982.

122 Schoolnik GK et al: A pilus peptide vaccine for the prevention of gonorrhea. *Prog Allerg* 33:314, 1983.

123 Virji M et al: The role of common and type-specific pilus antigenic domains in adhesion and virulence of gonococci for human epithelial cells. *J Gen Microbiol* 130:1089, 1984.

124 Bessen D et al: Interactions of gonococci with HeLa cells: Attachment, detachment, replication, penetration, and the role of protein 11. *Infect Immunol* 54:154, 1986.

125 Virji M et al: The N-domain of the human CD66a adhesion molecule is a target for Opa proteins of *Neisseria meningitidis* and *Neisseria gonorrhoeae*. *Mol Microbiol* 22:929–939, 1996.

126 Virji M et al: Carcinoembryonic antigens (CD66) on epithelial cells and neutrophils are receptors for Opa proteins of pathogenic *Neisseria*. *Mol Microbiol* 22:941–950, 1996.

127 Rothbard JB et al: Antibodies to peptides corresponding to a conserved sequence of gonococcal pilins block bacterial adhesion. *Proc Natl Acad Sci USA* 82:915, 1985.

128 Rothbard JB et al: Strain-specific and common epitopes of gonococcal pili. *J Exp Med* 160:208, 1984.

129 Boslego J et al: Efficacy trial of a parental gonococcal pilus vaccine in men. *Vaccine* 3:154–162, 1991.

130 Lindberg F et al: Gene products specifying adhesion of uropathogenic *Escherichia coli* are minor components of pili. *Proc Natl Acad Sci USA* 83:1891, 1986.

131 Muir LL et al: Proteins that appear to be associated with pili in *Neisseria gonorrhoeae. Infect Immunol* 56:1743, 1988.

132 Rudel T et al: Interaction of two variable proteins (PilE and PilC) required for pilus-mediated adherence of *Neisseria gonorrhoeae* to human epithelial cells. *Mol Microbiol* 6:3439–3450, 1992.

133 Rudel T et al: *Neisseria* PilC protein identified as type-4 pilus tip-located adhesin. *Nature* 373:357–359, 1995.

134 James JF et al: Color/opacity colonial variants of *Neisseria gonorrhoeae* and their relationship to the menstrual cycle, in *Immunobiology of Neisseria gonorrhoeae,* GF Brooks et al (eds). Washington, American Society for Microbiology, 1978, p. 338.

135 Porat N et al: *Neisseria gonorrhoeae* utilizes and enhances the biosynthesis of the asialoglycoprotein receptor expressed on the surface of the hepatic HepG2 cell line. *Infect Immunol* 63:1498–1506, 1995.

136 Densen P et al: Gonococcal interactions with polymorphonuclear neutrophils: Importance of the phagosome for bactericidal activity. *J Clin Invest* 62:1161, 1978.

137 Thongthai C et al: Studies in the virulence of *Neisseria gonorrhoeae*: Relation of colonial morphology and resistance to phagocytosis by polymorphonuclear leukocytes. *Infect Immunol* 7:373, 1973.

138 Siegel M et al: Gonococcal pili: Safety and immunogenicity in humans and antibody function in vitro. *J Infect Dis* 145: 300, 1982.

139 Virji M et al: Role of anti-pilus antibodies in host defense against gonococcal infection studied with monoclonal anti-pilus antibodies. *Infect Immunol* 49:621, 1985.

140 Swanson J et al: Studies on gonococcus infection: X. Pili and leukocyte association factor as mediators of interactions between gonococci and eukaryotic cells in vitro. *Infect Immunol* 24:1352, 1975.

141 Casey SG et al: *Neisseria gonorrhoeae* survive intraleukocytic oxygen-independent antimicrobial capacities of anaerobic and aerobic granulocytes in the presence of pyocin lethal for extracellular gonococci. *Infect Immunol* 52:384, 1986.

142 Parsons NJ et al: A determinant of resistance of *Neisseria gonorrhoeae* to killing by human phagocytes: An outer membrane lipoprotein of about 20 kDa with a high content of glutamic acid. *J Gen Microbiol* 132:3277, 1986.

143 Rest RF et al: Interactions of *Neisseria gonorrhoeae* with human neutrophils: Effect of serum and gonococcal opacity on phagocyte killing and cheiniluminescence. *Infect Immunol* 36:737, 1982.

144 Shafer W et al: Antigonococcal activity of human neutrophil cathepsin G. *Infect Immunol* 54:184, 1986.

145 Shaw JH et al: Model for invasion of human tissue culture cells by *Neisseria gonorrhoeae. Infect Immunol* 56:1625, 1988.

146 Heine RP et al: Tranferrin increases adherence of iron-deprived *Neisseria gonorrhoeae* to human endometrial cells. *Am J Obstet Gynecol* 174:659–666, 1996.

147 McGee ZA et al: Mechanisms of mucosal invasion by pathogenic *Neisseria. Rev Infect Dis* 5(suppl 4):5708, 1983.

148 Blake MS et al: Gonococcal membrane proteins: Speculation on their role in pathogenesis. *Prog Allerg* 33:298, 1983.

149 Rudel T et al: Modulation of neisserial Porin (PorB) by cytosolic ATP/GTP of target cells: Parallels between pathogen accomodation and mitochondrial endosymbiosis. *Cell* 85:391–402, 1996.

150 Gregg CR et al: Toxic activity of purified lipopolysaccharide of *Neisseria gonorrhoeae* for human fallopian tube mucosa. *J Infect Dis* 143: 532, 1981.

151 Melly MA et al: Ability of mononieric peptidoglycan fragments from *Neisseria gonorrhoeae* to damage human fallopian-tube mucosa. *J Infect Dis* 149:378, 1984.

152 Fleming TJ et al: Arthropathic properties of gonococcal peptidoglycan fragments: Implications for the pathogenesis of disseminated gonococcal disease. *Infect Immunol* 52:600, 1986.

153 Schwab JH et al: Association of experimental chronic arthritis with the persistence of group A streptococcal cell walls in the Irticular tissue. *J Bacteriol* 94:1728, 1967.

154 Rice PA et al: Characterization of serum resistance of *Neisseria gonorrhoeae* that disseminate: Roles of blocking antibody and gonococcal outer membrane proteins. *J Clin Invest* 70:157, 1982.

155 Harriman GR et al: Activation of complement by serum-resistant *Neisseria gonorrhoeae*: Assembly of the membrane attack complex without subsequent cell death. *J Exp Med* 156:1235, 1982.

156 Joiner KA et al: Studies on the mechanism of bacterial resistance to complement-mediated killing: IV. CSb-9 forms high molecular weight complexes with bacterial outer membrane constituents on serum-resistant but not on serum-sensitive *Neisseria gonorrhoeae. J Immunol* 131:1443, 1983.

157 Rice PA et al: Imnunoglobulin G antibodies directed against protein III block killing of serum-resistant *Neisseria gonorrhoeae* by immune serum. *J Exp Med* 164:1735, 1986.

158 Rice PA et al: Serum resistance of *Neisseria gonorrhoeae*. Does it thwart the inflammatory response and facilitate the transmission of infection? *Ann NY Acad Sci* 730:714, 1994.

159 Shafer WM et al: Identification of a the genetic site (sac-3) in *Neisseria gonorrhoeae* that affects sensitivity to normal human serum. *Infect Immunol* 35:764, 1982.

160 Densen P et al: Specificity of antibodies against *Neisseria gonorrhoeae* that stimulate neutrophil chemotaxis: Role of antibodies directed against lipooligosaccharides. *J Clin Invest* 80:78, 1987.

161 Rice PA et al: Natural serum bactericidal activity against *Neisseria gonorrhoeae* from disseminated, locally invasive, and uncomplicated disease. *J Immunol* 124:2105, 1980.

162 Jaffe HW et al: Diagnosis of gonorrhea using a genetic transformation test on mailed clinical specimens. *J Infect Dis* 146:275, 1982.

163 Cannon JG et al: The genetics of the gonococcus. *Ann Rev Microbiol* 38:111, 1984.

164 Shafer WM et al: Missense mutations that alter the DNA-binding domain of the MtrR protein occur frequently in rectal isolates of *Neisseria gonorrhoeae* that are resistant to faecal lipids. *Microbiology* 141:907–911, 1995.

165 Phillips L: P-Lactamase-producing penicillin-resistant gonococcus. *Lancet* 2:656, 1976.

166 Fayet O et al: P-Lactamase-specifying plasmids isolated from *Neisseria gonorrhoeae* have retained an intact right part of a Tn3-like transposon. *J Bacteriol* 149:136, 1982.

167 Chen S-T et al: Nucleotide sequence comparisons of plasmids pHDI31, pjbl, pFA3, and pFA7 and p-lactamase expression in *Escherichia coli, Haemophilus influenzae,* and *Neisseria gonorrhoeae. J Bacteriol* 169:3124, 1987.

168 Brunton J et al: Molecular nature of a plasmid specifying beta-lactamase production in *Haemophilus ducreyi. J Bacteriol* 148:788, 1981.

169 Anderson B et al: Common P-lactamase-specifying plasmid in *Haemophilus ducreyi* and *Neisseria gonorrhoeae. Antimicrob Agents Chemother* 25:296, 1984.

170 McNicol PJ et al: Transfer of plasmid-mediated ampicillin resistance from *Haemophilus* to *Neisseria gonorrhoeae* requires an intervening organism. *Sex Transm Dis* 13:145, 1986.

171 Boslego JW et al: Effect of spectinomycin use on the prevalence of spectinomycin-resistant and of penicillinase-producing *Neisseria gonorrhoeae. N Engl J Med* 317:272, 1987.

172 Kam KM et al: Quinolone-resistant *Neisseria gonorrhoeae* in Hong Kong. *Sex Transm Dis* 23:104–105, 1996.

173 Deguchi T et al: Quinolone-resistant *Neisseria gonorrhoeae:* Correlation of alterations in the Gyr A subunit of DNA gyrase and the ParC subunit of topoisomerase IV with antimicrobial susceptibility profiles. *Antimicrob Agents Chemother* 40:1020–1023, 1996.

174 Van Dyck E et al: Increasing resistance of *Neisseria gonorrhoeae* in west and central Africa. *Sex Transm Dis* 24:32–37, 1996.

175 Knapp JS et al: Molecular epidemiology in 1994, of *Neisseria gonorrhoeae* in Manila and Cebu City, Republic of the Philippines. *Sex Transm Dis* 24:2–7, 1996.

176 Lammel CJ et al: Antibody-antigen specificity in the immune response to infection with *Neisseria gonorrhoeae. J Infect Dis* 152:990, 1985.

177 Hook EW III et al: Analysis of the antigen specificity of the human serum immunoglobulin G immune response to complicated gonococcal infection. *Infect Immunol* 43:706, 1984.

178 McMillan A et al: Antibodies to *Neisseria gonorrhoeae*: A study of the urethral exudates of 232 men. *J Infect Dis* 140:89, 1979.

179 Tramont EC: Inhibition of adherence of *Neisseria gonorrhoeae* by human genital secretions. *J Clin Invest* 59:117, 1977.

180 Brinton CC Jr et al: The development of a neisserial pilus vaccine for gonorrhea and meningococcal meningitis, in *Seminars in Infectious Disease*, Weinstein L et al (eds). New York, Thieme Stratton, 1982, vol. 4, p. 140.

181 Plummer FA et al: Epidemiologic evidence for the development of serovar-specific immunity after gonococcal infection. *J Clin Invest* 83: 1472–1476, 1989.

182 Alcorn T et al: Absence of protective immunity from repeat infections by gonococci expressing the same Por protein. (Abstract). 10th International Pathogenic *Neisseria* Conference, Baltimore, MD. September 8–13, 1996, p. 9.

Chapter 32
Gonococcal infections in the adult

Edward W. Hook III
H. Hunter Handsfield

HISTORY

The major clinical manifestations of gonorrhea in men were described in ancient Chinese, Egyptian, Roman, and Greek literature as well as in the Old Testament.[1] The current term for the clinical syndrome referred to as gonorrhea (Greek, "flow of seed") is attributed to Galen (130 A.D.), who is said to have believed that the urethral exudate in males with gonorrhea was semen. However, there is little recorded evidence of awareness that urethral discharge in men was linked with morbidity for women until relatively recently. In 1879, *Neisseria gonorrhoeae* was demonstrated by Neisser in stained smears of urethral, vaginal, and conjunctival exudates,[2] making the gonococcus the second identified bacterial pathogen following the discovery of *Bacillus anthracis*. *N. gonorrhoeae* was first cultured in vitro by Leistikow in 1882, and effective antimicrobial therapy in the form of sulfonamides was first applied in the 1930s.[3] In 1962 the availability of Thayer-Martin medium[4] greatly facilitated the diagnosis of gonorrhea and may have contributed to subsequent increases in numbers of cases of gonorrhea reported in women. Since the mid-1960s, knowledge of the molecular basis of gonococcal–host interactions and of gonococcal epidemiology has increased to the point where there are few other microbial pathogens that are as well described.

N. gonorrhoeae initially infects noncornified epithelium, most often of the urogenital tract and secondarily of the rectum, oropharynx, and conjunctivae. It is transmitted almost exclusively by sexual contact or perinatally, and infection most often remains localized to initial sites of inoculation. Ascending genital infections (salpingitis, epididymitis) and bacteremia, however, are relatively common and account for most of the serious morbidity due to gonorrhea. These complications are most common in populations that lack ready access to effective diagnosis and therapy.

EPIDEMIOLOGY

INCIDENCE

Relatively few countries have reporting systems that permit accurate estimation of the true incidence of gonorrhea. Figure 32-1 shows the reported annual incidence of gonorrhea in the United States, Canada, and Sweden from 1955 through 1995.[5,6] Gonorrhea is rare in Canada and much of western Europe and remains relatively common in the United States as well as in much of the developing world. In the United States, recent changes in gonorrhea incidence reflect the influence of multiple, sometimes opposing trends for members of certain risk groups. At least part of the decline in gonorrhea in developed countries (including the United States) has been attributed to the impact of behavioral changes made to reduce risks of infection with human immunodeficiency virus (HIV). However, these changes have not occurred uniformly within the population. Although national data are not available, studies from several North American and European cities[7,8] suggest that gonorrhea rates in homosexual or bisexual men have declined precipitously, while rates in other groups have changed less. In addition, U.S. gonorrhea rates appear to have changed more for whites than for blacks and more among older age groups than in the young.

The incidence of gonorrhea varies with age (Fig. 32-2). Seventy-seven percent of reported cases in the United States in 1995 occurred in persons aged 15 to 29 years, with the highest rates occurring in the 15- to 19-year-old age group. The incidences in 15- to 19-year-old and 20- to 24-year-old women were 665 and 646 cases per 100,000 population, respectively. However, it is estimated that only about 50 percent of 15- to 19-year-old women in the United States were sexually experienced, compared with over 90 percent of the 20- to 24-year-old age group. Thus, despite similar overall rates, the reported incidence of gonorrhea was almost twice as high for sexually active adolescents as for sexually active women in the 20- to 24-year-old group.[5,9]

In the United States in 1995, reported cases of gonorrhea were more than 37-fold higher in African Americans than in whites, a difference only partly explained by greater attendance of nonwhites at public clinics, where reporting is more complete than in other health care settings.[5,10] Other demographic risk factors for gonorrhea include low socioeconomic status, early onset of sexual activity, unmarried marital status, and a history of past gonorrhea.[10,12] Studies in Seattle documented that about 25 percent of sexually active 16- to 18-year-old black females living in low-socioeconomic-level urban census tracts in 1986 to 1987 acquired gonorrhea each year.[11] Since the 1980s, illicit drug use and prostitution also have become increasingly associated with enhanced risk of gonorrhea, syphilis, and probably other sexually transmitted diseases (STDs) as well. In the past decade, male homosexuality has become less associated with gonorrhea because of changing sexual practices among many homosexual men as a consequence of concerns regarding AIDS. Despite this trend, the incidence of gonorrhea in men who have sex with men (MSM) may still be higher than in exclusively heterosexual persons.[13]

The incidence of gonorrhea in the United States is seasonal: The highest rates occur in late summer, whereas the lowest are in late winter and early spring, with nadirs tending to be about 20 percent lower than peaks.[10,14,15] The antimicrobial susceptibility of *N. gonorrhoeae* appears to fluctuate similarly.[15] The proportion of gonococcal isolates that are relatively resistant to penicillins and tetracyclines is slightly higher in late winter than in summer, possibly as a consequence of seasonal variation in antibiotic usage. Seasonal variations in sexual activity, access to health care, changing commitments in schedules of the young individuals at highest risk for gonorrhea, or other factors also may be involved in these seasonal fluctuations.

The efficiency of gonorrhea transmission depends on anatomic sites infected and exposed as well as the number of exposures. The risk of acquiring urethral infection for a man following a single episode of vaginal intercourse with an infected woman is estimated to be 20 percent, rising to an estimated 60 to 80 percent following four exposures.[16] The prevalence of infection in women named as secondary sexual contacts of men with gonococcal urethritis has been reported to be 50 to 90 percent,[16,17] but no published studies have carefully controlled for number of exposures. It is likely that the single-exposure transmission rate from male to female is higher than that from female to male, in part because of retention of the infected ejaculate within the vagina. The risk of transmission by other types of sexual contact is less well defined. Gonorrhea transmission through insertive or receptive rectal intercourse presumably is relatively efficient, and pharyngeal gonorrhea is readily acquired by fellatio.[18,19] Transmission of pharyngeal infection to other sites has been thought to be rare, but in a

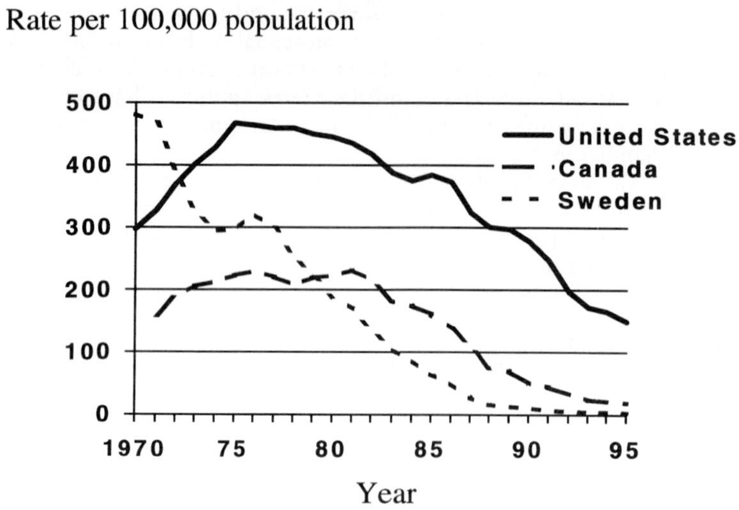

Fig. 32-1. Reported annual incidence of gonorrhea in the United States, Canada, and Sweden, 1955–1995.

recent study this route of exposure accounted for 26 percent of urethral gonorrhea in men who had sex with men (MSM).[13] It is possible that changing sexual practices among MSM in response to AIDS, specifically an increasing frequency of oral sex and decreased anal intercourse, have changed the population attributable risk of oral sex for urethral gonorrhea.

In women, use of hormonal contraception may increase the risk of acquiring gonorrhea,[20,21] and use of spermicides and/or the diaphragm clearly has a protective influence.[22,23] Transmission by fomites or through nonsexual contact is extremely rare but may account for rare cases of gonorrhea in infants.

Symptoms and the behavioral response to them also influence the transmission of gonorrhea. Previous reports that 80 percent of women with gonorrhea were asymptomatic were most often based on studies of women who were examined in screening surveys or who were referred to STD clinics because of sexual contact with infected men.[24] Symptomatic infected women who sought medical attention were thus often excluded from such surveys. However, as might be expected, more than 75 percent of women with gonorrhea attending acute care facilities such as hospital emergency rooms are symptomatic.[25] The true proportion of infected women who remain asymptomatic undoubtedly lies between these extremes. Appreciation of symptomatic infection in infected women is more difficult than in men because the clinical syndromes may be mistakenly attributed to other infectious processes, including urinary tract or vaginal infections.

Asymptomatically infected males and females contribute disproportionately to gonorrhea transmission, because symptomatic individuals are more likely to cease sexual activity and seek medical care. However, the presence of urogenital symptoms does not ensure that transmission will not occur. In a study of patients attending STD clinics in Baltimore, 38 percent of men and 46 percent of women presenting for symptom evaluation reported continued sexual activity after the onset of the symptoms that brought them to the clinic.[26] The reasons for continued sexual activity despite the presence of symptoms may include the relative lack of severity of symptoms early in the course of disease, denial, and for women, the nonspecificity of urogenital symptoms. The observation that many transmitters of gonorrhea (and other STDs) do not spontaneously cease sexual activity and seek care emphasizes the importance of taking active steps to bring the partners of infected persons to treatment.

Asymptomatic infections occur in men as well as women, and the percentage of infected men who are asymptomatic probably varies with duration of infection. In a cohort of 81 men who acquired urethral infection at a defined time, the mean time to development of symptoms was 3.4 days, and only 2 (2.5 percent) remained asymptomatic for 14 days[27] (Fig. 32-3). Although this study was performed in a geographic area where the strains of *N. gonorrhoeae* most likely to cause asymptomatic urethral infections were uncommon, the incidence of asymptomatic urethral gonococcal infection in the general population also has been es-

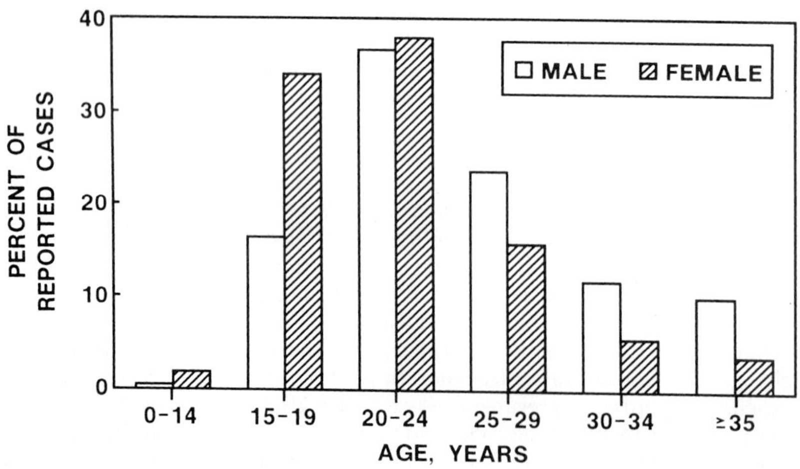

Fig. 32-2. Age and sex distribution of reported cases of gonorrhea in the United States, 1995.

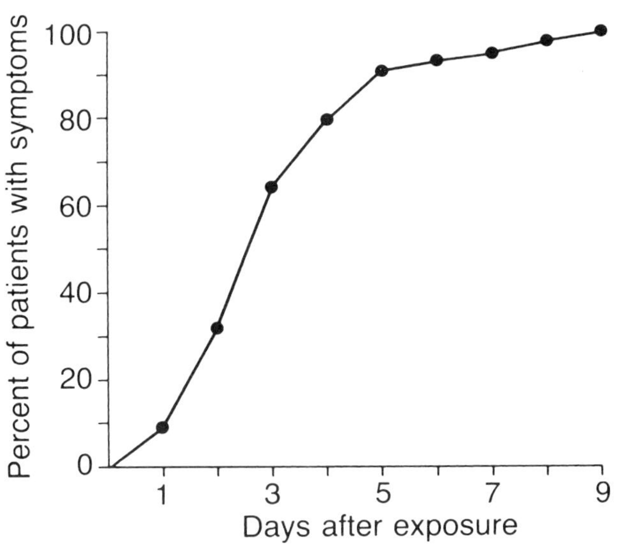

Fig. 32-3. Incubation period in 44 men with symptomatic gonococcal urethritis. (From Harrison et al.[27])

timated at approximately 1 to 3 percent.[28] The prevalence of asymptomatic infection may be much higher, approaching 5 percent in some studies, because untreated asymptomatic infections may persist for considerable periods.

PREVALENCE

The prevalence of gonorrhea within communities tends to be dynamic, fluctuating over time and influenced by a number of interactive factors. Mathematical models for gonorrhea within communities suggest that gonorrhea prevalence is sustained not only through continued transmission by asymptomatically infected patients but also by "core group" transmitters who are more likely than members of the general population to become infected and transmit gonorrhea to their sex partners.[29–31] Although members of the core group described in these mathematical models share a number of characteristics including geographic clustering (usually within inner cities) and low socioeconomic status, the core group is actually comprised of a number of heterogeneous subgroups. These include persons with repeated episodes of gonorrhea, those who fail to abstain from sex despite the presence of symptoms or knowledge of recent exposure, and patients who practice high-risk behaviors such as illegal drug use, prostitution, or prostitute patronage.[12,26,30] Finally, because the core group is defined primarily on behavioral grounds, membership in a core group is not a stable characteristic of an individual but may change over time. Several studies have provided empirical observations that support mathematical models of core-group transmission.[12,26,30]

While providing the focus for continued endemnicity of gonorrhea, core groups are not solely responsible for gonorrhea prevalence within communities. In terms of social behavior, disease prevalence is due to infections transmitted by both core-group and non-core-group members, the interaction between these two groups, and the movement of patients from one group to another. These factors fluctuate with changes in normative social behavior, disease-control efforts, and other epidemiologic factors. At present, gonorrhea prevention and control efforts are heavily invested in the concept of vigorous pursuit and treatment of infected core-group members and asymptomatically infected individuals. Because about 40 percent of asymptomatically infected men and many women who are asymptomatic indeed have clinical findings compatible with gonorrhea,[25,28] patient education designed to modify the behavior or response to mild symptoms also is an important albeit largely unexplored part of gonorrhea control. In addition, however, efforts to access the often-difficult-to-reach core-group transmitters are needed to assist in gonorrhea control. Mathematical models of core transmission theory suggest that because gonorrhea transmission is not 100 percent efficient, and because spontaneous cures occur, without hyperendemic transmission by core-group members, gonorrhea prevalence would decline, perhaps ultimately to zero.[29,31]

EPIDEMIOLOGIC CORRELATES OF GONOCOCCAL TYPES

A number of methods for gonococcal typing have been developed, as discussed in Chap. 31. Only auxotyping,[32] protein I–serotyping,[33] and the two used in combination have been used widely to study gonococcal epidemiology. Auxotyping classifies gonococci on the basis of stable nutritional requirements for a variety of amino acids and nucleosides, alone or in combination.[32] Examples of common auxotypes are strains that require arginine (Arg), proline (Pro), uracil (U), methionine (M), or arginine, hypoxanthine, and uracil (AHU) for growth. Gonococci requiring none of the substrates are termed *prototrophic* (Proto) or are referred to by some authors as *wild type.* Protein I–serotyping is based on the stable antigenic diversity of protein I, the protein present in largest quantity in the gonococcal outer membrane.[33] Protein I is divided into two mutually exclusive classes, protein IA and protein IB, each of which can be further subdivided into serovars in coagglutination assays using panels of protein IA– or protein IB–specific monoclonal antibody reagents. Each serovar is designated by its protein I type (IA or IB) and a numeral based on its coagglutination pattern (e.g., IA-4, IB-3). Using both auxotyping and serovar analysis, gonococci can be divided into a large number of auxotype/serovar (A/S) classes (e.g., AHU/IA-1, Pro/IB-3, Proto/IB-12), providing a highly discriminative tool for study of gonococcal epidemiology.[34]

Relatively large numbers (>50) of gonococcal A/S classes usually are present in most communities simultaneously,[34,35] and new strains can be detected over time. The distribution of isolates within A/S classes tends to be uneven, with a few A/S classes contributing disproportionately to the total number of isolates. These predominant A/S classes generally persist within communities for months or years. In most studies, many more A/S classes are detectable only intermittently or even only once during a sampling interval and then are not detected again. The factors that determine which A/S classes will become predominant and which will be seen only transiently may include biologic characteristics of the strain or the host. Alternatively, epidemiologic factors such as transmission by commercial sex workers or drug users and importation by travelers may be important.

By allowing individual strains of *N. gonorrhoeae* to be tracked, A/S classification has helped elucidate how gonococci are introduced and spread in communities. For example, during a 12-week study of consecutive patients with gonorrhea seen at a Seattle STD clinic,[34] 489 isolates were collected from 390 patients. These isolates could be divided into 57 different A/S classes. Some A/S classes were isolated only from heterosexual men and women (e.g., AHU/IA-1, AHU/IA-2), whereas others were isolated almost exclusively from homosexual or bisexual men (e.g., Arg/IB-2, Proto/IB-20). During the study, one strain (Proto/IB-3) was not detected until week 6 and over the next 2 weeks was isolated from 1 woman, 1 homosexual man, and 10 heterosexual men. During the next few weeks, isolates of this A/S class from heterosexual men continued to far outnumber those from women, and over the subsequent year, this strain became one of the predominant gonococcal A/S classes throughout the city. Interviews of the patients infected by the Proto/IB-3 strain early in the outbreak identified one infected female who acknowledged over 100 different sexual partners over the preceding 2 months, suggesting that she may have played an important role in the introduction and establishment of this gonococcal strain in the community. Thus the Proto/IB-3 strain may have become common in Seattle not because of specific biologic factors but because of its chance transmission to members of a core population by a high-frequency transmitter.

Some gonococcal strain types are associated with specific clinical manifestations of disease. In Seattle during the early 1970s, AHU/IA-1 and AHU/IA-2 strains caused more than 90 percent of asymptomatic urethral infections in men[36] and the majority of cases of disseminated gonococcal infections.[37] However, these A/S classes were less common in symptomatic men and in women with gonococcal salpingitis.[38] AHU/IA-1 and -2 strains grow more slowly than many other gonococci, are particularly susceptible to the penicillins and tetracyclines, and tend to be resistant to the complement-mediated bactericidal activity of normal human serum.[39] Since the 1970s, the prevalence of AHU/IA strains in Seattle has diminished markedly, as have the numbers of cases of disseminated gonococcal infection and asymptomatic urethral gonorrhea in men.[40] These changes occurred shortly after institution of contact tracing for gonorrhea and with routine treatment of asymptomatic male sexual partners of infected women. Thus it seems that AHU/IA strains may have accumulated in the population because of their ability to cause asymptomatic infection in men. When this selection pressure was reduced through partner notification and treatment of asymptomatic men, the prevalence declined.

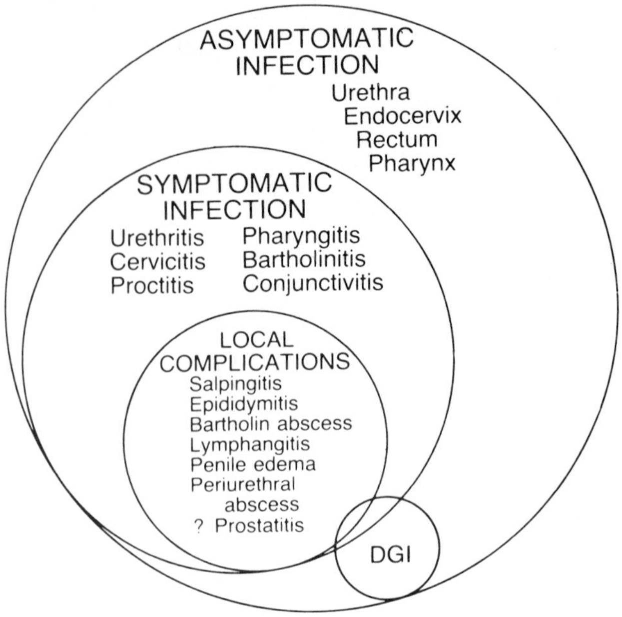

Fig. 32-4. Clinical spectrum of gonococcal infection (DGI, disseminated gonococcal infection).

PATHOLOGY

In adults, only mucous membranes lined by columnar or cuboidal, noncornified epithelial cells are susceptible to gonococcal infection. The initial event in gonococcal infection is the adherence of *N. gonorrhoeae* to mucosal cells in a process mediated by pili, Opa, and perhaps other surface proteins.[41,42] In fallopian tube organ culture models, the organism is then pinocytosed by the epithelial cells, which transport viable, sometimes dividing gonococci from the mucosal surface to subepithelial spaces.[43,44] Simultaneous with attachment of gonococci to nonciliated epithelial cells, gonococcal lipooligosaccharide (endotoxin) impairs ciliary motility and contributes to destruction of surrounding ciliary cells.[44] This process may promote further attachment of additional organisms. Progressive mucosal cell damage and submucosal invasion are accompanied by a vigorous polymorphonuclear leukocytic response, submucosal microabscess formation, and exudation of purulent material into the lumen of the infected organ. In untreated infections, polymorphonuclear leukocytes are gradually replaced by mononuclear cells, and abnormal round cell infiltration has been reported to persist for several weeks or months after gonococci can no longer be isolated.[43] The molecular mechanisms of gonococcal invasion and infection are more fully discussed in Chap. 31.

CLINICAL MANIFESTATIONS: UNCOMPLICATED GONOCOCCAL INFECTIONS

Despite the focus of many patients and even some clinicians on symptomatic local infections, clinical gonorrhea is manifested by a broad spectrum of clinical presentations including asymptomatic and symptomatic local infections, local complicated infections, and systemic dissemination. Figure 32-4 estimates the relative proportion of individuals with each of the major clinical syndromes and shows the interrelations between them in a simplified form.

URETHRAL INFECTION IN MEN

Acute anterior urethritis is the most common manifestation of gonococcal infection in men. The incubation period ranges from 1 to 14 days or even longer; however, the majority of men develop symptoms within 2 to 5 days, as was the case in 36 (82 percent) of 44 men with uncomplicated gonorrhea in one of the few studies in which the time of exposure could be clearly defined[27] (see Fig. 32-3). The predominant symptoms are urethral discharge or dysuria. Although initially scant and mucoid or mucopurulent in appearance, in most males the urethral exudate becomes frankly purulent and relatively profuse within 24 hours of onset[43] (Fig. 32-5). Dysuria usually begins after onset of discharge. Variable degrees of edema and erythema of the urethral meatus commonly accompany gonococcal urethritis. Approximately one-quarter of patients develop only a scant or minimally purulent exudate, grossly indistinguishable from that associated with nongonococcal urethritis,[45,46] and a minority never develop overt signs.[27,28] The severity of symptoms is partly determined by the infecting strain of *N. gonorrhoeae,* as discussed above. Without treatment, the usual course of gonococcal urethritis is spontaneous resolution over a period of several weeks, and before the development of effective antimicrobial therapy, 95 percent of untreated patients became asymptomatic within 6 months.[43] Subsequent asymptomatic carriage of *N. gonorrhoeae* may occur but probably is exceptional.

Complications of gonococcal urethritis include epididymitis (see Chap. 61); acute or chronic prostatitis (see Chap. 62); so-called posterior urethritis, which may be associated with stranguria and urinary urgency; seminal vesiculitis; and infections of Cowper's and Tyson's glands. These have been documented in-

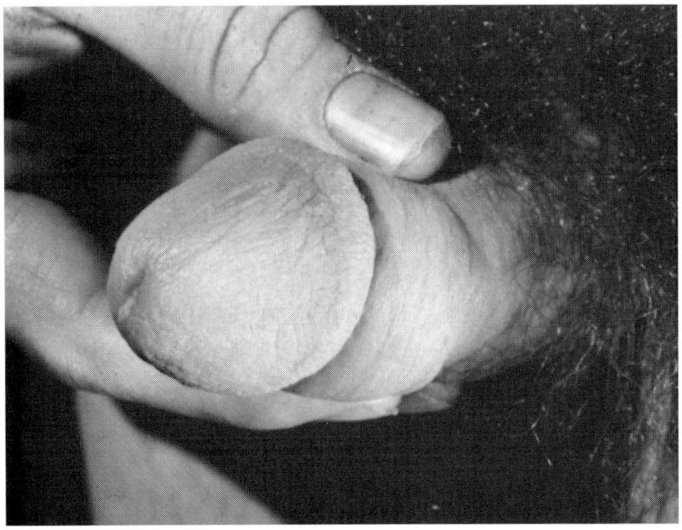

Fig. 32-5. Purulent urethral discharge and penile edema in a patient with gonococcal urethritis.

frequently using modern diagnostic techniques and are now rare in industrialized societies.

UROGENITAL INFECTION IN WOMEN

The endocervical canal is the primary site of urogenital gonococcal infection in women. Urethral colonization is present in 70 to 90 percent of infected women[47–49] but is uncommon in the absence of endocervical infection. However, after hysterectomy, the urethra is the usual site of infection.[50] Infection of the periurethral (Skene's) gland or Bartholin's gland ducts is also common but probably is rare in the absence of endocervical or urethral infection.

The incubation period for urogenital gonorrhea in women is less certain and probably more variable than in men, but most who develop local symptoms apparently do so within 10 days of infection.[51,52] The most common symptoms are those of most lower genital tract infections in women (see Chap. 57) and include increased vaginal discharge, dysuria, intermenstrual uterine bleeding, and menorrhagia, each of which may occur alone or in combination and may range in intensity from minimal to severe.[25,53] Although the physical examination may be normal, many infected women have cervical abnormalities that include purulent or mucopurulent cervical discharge, erythema and edema of the zone of ectopy, and mucosal bleeding that is easily induced by swabbing the endocervix.[53] Purulent exudate occasionally may be expressed from the urethra, periurethral glands, or the Bartholin's gland duct (Fig. 32-6). The clinical assessment of women for gonorrhea is often confounded, however, by the nonspecificity of these signs and symptoms and by the high prevalence of coexisting cervical or vaginal infections with *Chlamydia trachomatis, Trichomonas vaginalis, Candida albicans,* herpes simplex virus, and a variety of other organisms (see Chap. 57).

The manifestations of gonorrhea during pregnancy are not significantly different from those in nonpregnant women except that pelvic inflammatory disease is probably less common and pharyngeal infection appears to be more prevalent than in nonpregnant women.[54] Reported complications of genital gonorrhea in pregnancy include spontaneous abortion, premature rupture of fetal membranes, premature delivery, and acute chorioamnionitis (see Chap. 80), as well as ophthalmia neonatorum, pharyngeal infections, and other syndromes in the newborn (see Chap. 82).

RECTAL INFECTION

The rectal mucosa is infected in 35 to 50 percent of women with gonococcal cervicitis and is a frequent site of infection in homosexual men; it is the only site of infection in approximately 5 percent of women with gonorrhea and 40 percent of homosexually active men studied prior to recognition of the HIV epidemic.[47–49,55–59] In a study of men who had sex with other men (MSM) in 1993 and 1994, rectal infection was documented in 26 (25 percent) of 105 men infected at any anatomic site.[13] In women, rectal gonorrhea is usually asymptomatic, although some cases, especially in MSM, are associated with overt proctitis. Among MSM, rectal gonorrhea is due to direct inoculation through receptive rectal intercourse. In contrast, most rectal infections in women occur without acknowledged rectal sexual contact and are assumed to result from perineal contamination with infected cervical secretions. The prevalence of rectal infection in women is positively correlated with the duration of endocervical infection,[56] further supporting the thesis that infection is usually due to perineal contamination by cervicovaginal secretions. Rectal infection occurs rarely, if ever, in strictly heterosexual men.

The symptoms of rectal gonococcal infection range from min-

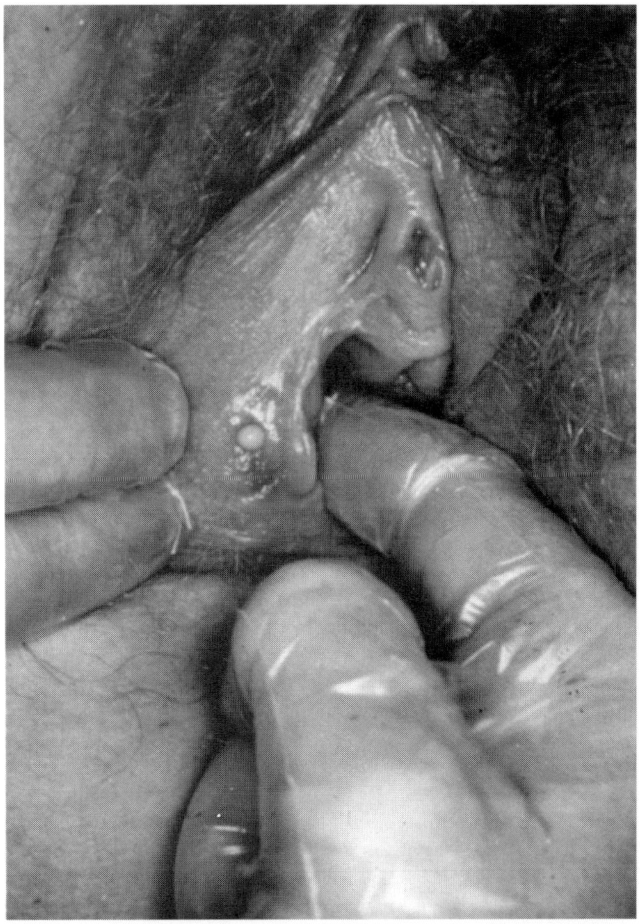

Fig. 32-6. Purulent exudate expressed from the Bartholin's gland duct of a woman with gonococcal Bartholin's gland abscess. *(From JA Davies et al:* Isolation of *Chlamydia trachomatis* from Bartholin's ducts. *Br J Vener Dis 54:409, 1978.)*

imal anal pruritus, painless mucopurulent discharge (often manifested only by a coating of stools with exudate), or scant rectal bleeding, to symptoms of overt proctitis, including severe rectal pain, tenesmus, and constipation.[56–58] External inspection of the anus only occasionally shows erythema and abnormal discharge, but anoscopy commonly reveals mucoid or purulent exudate (often localized to the anal crypts), erythema, edema, friability, or other inflammatory mucosal changes.[57] Several studies have suggested that fewer than 10 percent of rectal gonococcal infections in men and women are symptomatic, but many of these studies may have ignored or failed to elicit more subtle or ill-defined symptoms. Moreover, most studies have been affected by sample bias, failing to distinguish among patients being screened for gonorrhea, those attending spontaneously because of symptoms, and those responding to epidemiologic investigation of infected partners. One study[57] found that among MSM examined because they were sexual contacts of men with gonorrhea, 87 (57 percent) of 152 infected men had rectal symptoms, compared with 66 (41 percent) of 162 men from whom *N. gonorrhoeae* was not isolated ($p = 0.01$). However, infection with other pathogens was not investigated. A prospective study that controlled for the reason for the visit showed that while a history of recent exposure to a sexual partner with gonorrhea was common in asymptomatically infected patients, in patients attending the clinic for other reasons, *N. gonorrhoeae* was isolated from 31 (27 percent) of 114 symptomatic men but from only 6 (9 percent) of 64 asymptomatic men ($p < 0.01$).[58]

PHARYNGEAL INFECTION

Among patients with gonorrhea, pharyngeal infection occurs in 3 to 7 percent of heterosexual men, 10 to 20 percent of heterosexual women, and 10 to 25 percent of homosexually active men. In studies performed prior to the AIDS era, the pharynx was the sole site of infection in less than 5 percent of patients irrespective of gender or sexual orientation.[18,56,60–62] Among MSM, shifting prevalence of pharyngeal and rectal infection, as well as other published data, suggests that the frequency of fellatio has increased while the frequency of anal intercourse has declined in response to the HIV/AIDS epidemic. Gonococcal infection is transmitted to the pharynx by orogenital sexual contact and is more efficiently acquired by fellatio than by cunnilingus.[63]

Anecdotal reports suggest that gonococcal infection may cause acute pharyngitis or tonsillitis and occasionally is associated with fever or cervical lymphadenopathy, but over 90 percent of pharyngeal infections are asymptomatic.[18,60,61] Evaluation of pharyngeal symptoms is confounded, however, by the intriguing observation that among clients of STD clinics, sore throat and perhaps overt pharyngitis are correlated with a history of fellatio but not with isolation of *N. gonorrhoeae* or other sexually transmitted organisms.[18,63] Cunnilingus has not been associated with pharyngeal symptoms.

The clinical and epidemiologic significance of pharyngeal gonococcal infection may be greater than previously appreciated. The occasional occurrence of symptomatic pharyngitis and a possible increased risk of disseminated gonococcal infection in persons with pharyngeal gonorrhea[18] are countered by the usual absence of symptoms and a spontaneous cure rate that approaches 100 percent within 12 weeks of infection.[64,65] In addition, the transmission of pharyngeal gonorrhea to sex partners has been thought to be inefficient and relatively rare. However, in a recent study,[13] 17 (26 percent) of 66 MSM with urethral gonorrhea acknowledged insertive oral sex but not insertive anal sex in the preceding 2 months. In this study, insertive oral sex was independently associated with both urethral gonorrhea (odds ratio of 4.4, 95 percent confidence interval of 1.4, 9.4). Thus pharyngeal infections may now be an important source of urethral gonorrhea in MSM.

UNCOMPLICATED INFECTION OF OTHER SITES

Gonococcal conjunctivitis is rare in adults; it is most often seen in patients with concomitant anogenital gonorrhea, presumably due to autoinoculation.[66] Accidental conjunctival infection has been emphasized as a hazard for laboratory personnel working with *N. gonorrhoeae*.[67,68] An outbreak of 13 cases of gonococcal conjunctivitis was attributed to the cultural practice of ocular irrigation with urine.[69] Although usually described as a severe infection with a high risk of sequelae, mild or asymptomatic conjunctival gonorrhea infection occurs as well.

Primary cutaneous infection with *N. gonorrhoeae* has been reported[70–72] and usually presents as a localized ulcer of the genitals, perineum, proximal lower extremities, or finger. In many reports, simultaneous infection with other etiologic agents such as herpes simplex virus, *Haemophilus ducreyi*, and other pyogenic organisms was not excluded, and primary gonococcal infection could not be differentiated from secondary colonization of a preexisting lesion. Gonococcal infection of a congenitally patent median raphe duct of the penis is an uncommon but well-documented occurrence.[71] Such infections usually occur in patients with anogenital gonorrhea, but exceptions have been reported.[72]

DIFFERENTIAL DIAGNOSIS OF UNCOMPLICATED GONORRHEA

In males, gonococcal urethritis usually causes more florid signs and symptoms than nongonococcal urethritis and has a more abrupt onset, more prominent dysuria, and a urethral discharge that is more profuse and more purulent in appearance.[45,46] Additionally, the incubation period for gonorrhea usually is shorter than that of nongonococcal urethritis. Nonetheless, there is sufficient overlap in all these features that clinical differentiation is sometimes unreliable and must be corroborated by laboratory tests.[45] For the diagnosis of urogenital infection in women and for anorectal pharyngeal infection, clinical differentiation of gonococcal from other causes is even less reliable than for urethritis in men, and laboratory diagnosis is mandatory. Nonetheless, a careful history and use of clinical predictors of infection for directing presumptive therapy in populations at increased risk are appropriate and desirable because expeditious therapy is likely to reduce complications and reduce further transmission of infection. Differential diagnosis is discussed more completely in Chaps. 57, 58, 60, 61, and 62.

COMPLICATED GONOCOCCAL INFECTIONS

LOCAL COMPLICATIONS IN MEN

In men the most common local complication of gonococcal urethritis is epididymitis (see Chap. 61), a syndrome that occurred in up to 20 percent of infected patients prior to the availability of modern antimicrobial therapy.[43] At present, the most common causes of acute epididymitis in patients under age 35 are *C. trachomatis*, *N. gonorrhoeae*, or both organisms.[73] Patients with acute epididymitis tend to present with unilateral testicular pain and swelling, and most patients with gonococcal epididymitis have overt urethritis when they present.

Penile lymphangitis, sometimes associated with regional lymphadenitis, is an uncommon minor complication of gonococcal urethritis, as is penile edema ("bull-headed clap"), a syndrome that also may accompany nongonococcal urethritis or genital herpes.[74] The pathogenesis of penile edema is unclear; most such patients lack palpable cords or other clear signs of penile thrombophlebitis or lymphangitis. Postinflammatory urethral strictures were common complications of untreated gonorrhea in the preantibiotic era but are now rare.[43] Many such strictures, however, probably were related to repeated infection or were due to the caustic urethral irrigations used for treatment, and stricture is rare today if effective systemic antimicrobial therapy is instituted promptly. Periurethral abscesses also are rare.

LOCAL COMPLICATIONS IN WOMEN

Salpingitis

Acute salpingitis, or pelvic inflammatory disease, is the most common complication of gonorrhea in women, occurring in an estimated 10 to 20 percent of those with acute gonococcal infection.[75,76] Salpingitis is the most common of all complications of gonorrhea, as well as the most important in terms of public health impact, because of both its acute manifestations and its long-term sequelae (infertility, ectopic pregnancy, and chronic pelvic pain). Patients with gonococcal salpingitis usually present with various combinations of lower abdominal pain, dyspareunia, abnormal menses, intermenstrual bleeding, or other complaints compatible with intraabdominal infection.[77] On physical examination these patients usually are found to have lower abdominal, uterine, or adnexal tenderness, cervical motion pain, abnormal cervical discharge, and sometimes an adnexal mass or tuboovarian abscess.[77] Gram-stained smears of cervical secretions may show gram-negative intracellular diplococci. However, as in women with uncomplicated gonococcal cervicitis, the Gram stain is negative in 40 to 60 percent of women with gonococcal salpingitis. Other findings that may or may not be present include fever, leukocytosis, elevation of the erythrocyte sedimentation rate, and increased levels of C-reactive protein.[77] Women with gonococcal salpingitis often appear more acutely ill than women with nongonococcal salpingitis, are more often febrile (74 versus 22 percent), and are more likely to present during the first 3 days of symptoms (32 versus 15 percent).[77] Despite the apparently greater clinical severity of gonococcal salpingitis, laparoscopic studies show that the severity of tubal disease is similar in women with gonococcal or nongonococcal salpingitis.[77] The pathophysiology, differential diagnosis, and clinical spectrum of acute salpingitis are more fully discussed in Chap. 58.

Apart from salpingitis, Bartholin's gland abscess is the most common urogenital complication of gonorrhea in women. *N. gonorrhoeae* was isolated from the Bartholin's gland ducts of 52 (28 percent) of 183 women with urogenital gonorrhea, 10 of whom (6 percent) had enlargement and tenderness of the gland.[78] Other bacteria, including *C. trachomatis,* are responsible for many cases of bartholinitis, but tests for gonococcal infection are indicated for all women with this syndrome.

SYSTEMIC COMPLICATIONS: DISSEMINATED GONOCOCCAL INFECTION

Disseminated gonococcal infection (DGI), usually manifested by the acute arthritis-dermatitis syndrome, is the most common systemic complication of acute gonorrhea. The syndrome has been estimated to occur in 0.5 to 3 percent of patients with untreated mucosal gonorrhea, although the higher estimates were made in settings where the prevalence of gonococcal isolates likely to disseminate was high.[79–81] DGI results from gonococcal bacteremia and is most often manifested by acute arthritis, tenosynovitis, dermatitis, or a combination of these findings. Patients with these clinical manifestations are often stratified on the basis of culture results into proven, probable, and possible DGI.[82] Patients with positive cultures from blood, joint fluid, skin lesions, or otherwise sterile sources constitute less than 50 percent of DGI cases and are considered to have proven DGI.[79–82] In more than 80 percent of DGI patients, *N. gonorrhoeae* may be cultured from the primary mucosal site(s) of infection (anogenital or pharyngeal cultures) or from a sexual partner[79–82]; in the absence of positive blood or other sterile-site cultures, these patients are usually referred to as having probable DGI. Patients with an appropriate clinical syndrome and the expected response to therapy but with negative cultures for *N. gonorrhoeae* are referred to as having possible DGI. However, recognition of patients with DGI is sometimes delayed because of the wide variety of clinical findings associated with this syndrome and the mistaken assumption that patients with gonococcal bacteremia have genitourinary signs and symptoms, high fever, marked leukocytosis, or other signs of clinical toxicity.

The most common clinical manifestations of DGI are joint pain and skin lesions, leading some authors to utilize the term *arthritis-dermatitis syndrome.* Although the "classic" skin lesion of gonococcal dermatitis is a tender, necrotic pustule on an erythematous base, in many patients skin lesions also may evolve from or present as macules, papules, pustules, petechiae, bullae, or ecchymoses.[79–82] The skin lesions tend to be located on distal portions of the extremities and usually number fewer than 30.[80,82] Many patients with gonococcal dermatitis have arthralgia or tenosynovitis early in the disease, and frank arthritis with effusion tends to occur somewhat later. Approximately 30 to 40 percent of patients with DGI have overt arthritis.[79–82] Any joint may be involved, although DGI most often involves wrist, metacarpophalangeal, ankle, and knee joints. Synovial fluid cultures are rarely positive in patients with synovial fluid leukocyte counts of less than 20,000 per cubic millimeter, whereas cultures are often positive in patients with more than 40,000 white blood cells per cubic millimeter.[81,82] The manifestations of gonococcal arthritis and differentiation of this process from other acute arthritides are more fully discussed in Chap. 68.

Proving infection in patients with DGI is sometimes difficult. The bacteremia associated with DGI is not continuous, and positive blood cultures become less common as the duration of clinical signs and symptoms increases. Overall, only 20 to 30 percent of DGI patients have positive blood cultures.[79–82] In some areas, AHU/IA-1 and AHU/IA-2 strains of *N. gonorrhoeae* cause most cases of DGI; these strains also tend to be associated with asymptomatic urogenital infection, increased susceptibility to penicillin G, and resistance to the complement-mediated bactericidal activity of normal human serum.[80,81] Although most gonococci isolated from patients with DGI exhibit such "serum resistance," isolates from patients with suppurative arthritis are less resistant than those from patients who present with tenosynovitis or dermatitis.[81,83] These organisms also are more likely to be inhibited by the concentrations of vancomycin contained in selective media for gonococcal isolation from mucosal sites (e.g., modified Thayer-Martin medium) and by the sodium polyanethiosulfonate anticoagulant used in many blood culture media.[84–86] These problems may be overcome through use of alternative media; however, use of alternative media is relatively uncommon because of lack of knowledge of their availability. In addition, DGI is often not included in the differential diagnosis of acute, asymmetric arthritis or dermatitis in young, sexually active patients because of the erroneous expectation that patients with DGI are likely to have signs and symptoms of urogenital infection. Mucosal infection in patients with disseminated gonococcal infection often is asymptomatic. All these problems contribute to underdiagnosis.

Disseminated gonococcal infection is more common in women than in men.[79–82] In most cases, bacteremia probably begins 7 to 30 days after infection; in about half of women with DGI, the onset of symptoms occurs within 7 days following menstruation.[79–82] Several studies also have cited pregnancy and pharyngeal gonorrhea as risk factors for DGI.[18,79–82] Deficiency of complement either due to inherited complement deficiency or due to episodic complement deficiency in association with clinical flare-ups of other diseases such as lupus erythematosus may predispose individuals to gonococcal or meningococcal bacteremia.[80,81,87] Only a small percentage of patients with DGI, however, have complement deficiency syndromes, and routine screening of DGI patients for complement deficiency is probably not indicated. Such screening should be performed, however, in patients with second episodes of systemic gonococcal or meningococcal infection.[81,87]

The characteristic response to appropriate antimicrobial therapy has been utilized as evidence of DGI in patients from whom *N. gonorrhoeae* could not be isolated.[82] Over 90 percent of patients are subjectively improved within 48 hours of initiating therapy, and more than 90 percent of febrile patients become afebrile over the same period.[82] DGI due to PPNG[88] or gonococci with chromosomally mediated antibiotic resistance[89] has become apparent with failure to respond clinically to penicillin therapy; ceftriaxone or other antibiotics with proven activity against antibiotic-resistant gonococci should be used rather than penicillin for therapeutic trials in patients with suspected DGI.

Gonococcal endocarditis and meningitis

Gonococcal endocarditis is an uncommon complication of gonococcal bacteremia, occurring in an estimated 1 to 3 percent of patients with DGI.[79,80] Nonetheless, recognition of gonococcal endocarditis among patients with DGI is essential because of the possibility of rapidly progressive valvular damage with life-threatening consequences. The aortic valve appears to be infected most often in patients with gonococcal endocarditis, and in the pre-antibiotic era, most patients died of aortic valve incompetence and acute heart failure with 6 weeks.

Fewer than 25 cases of gonococcal meningitis have been reported. Case reports of this complication describe patients with typical presentations of acute bacterial meningitis, usually without typical findings of DGI.[90,91] *N. gonorrhoeae* is indistinguishable from *N. meningitidis* on Gram's stain of cerebrospinal fluid.

MENINGOCOCCAL INFECTIONS

Several reports have documented that infection or colonization with *N. meningitidis* may occur at all mucosal sites compatible with sexual transmission. Although rare in comparison with gonorrhea, meningococcal infections may mimic nearly all the clinical manifestations of gonorrhea. Pharyngeal colonization with *N. meningitidis* was documented in 17.2 percent of 2,224 patients attending an STD clinic from 1970 to 1972,[18] a rate comparable with that in the general population.[92] However, subgroups of patients attending STD clinics have been found to have differing rates of carriage. Among 398 STD clinic patients with gonorrhea, *N. meningitidis* was isolated from the oropharynges of 44 (52 percent) of 85 MSM, compared with 58 (19 percent) of 313 heterosexual men and women ($p < 0.0001$). In addition, *N. meningitidis* was isolated significantly less frequently from heterosexual African Americans than from heterosexual whites ($p < 0.0001$).[93] These prevalences parallel the relative frequencies with which these population groups acknowledge oral sex (MSM > heterosexual whites > heterosexual African Americans).[94] Other investigators reported a similar prevalence (42.5 percent) of pharyngeal meningococcal colonization in 815 homosexual men attending an STD clinic.[62]

Genital and anorectal colonization with meningococci also occurs. In studies conducted in STD clinics in the 1970s, the prevalence of urethral colonization with *N. meningitidis* was 0.2 to 0.4 percent in heterosexual men but was up to 1 percent in MSM.[95–97] In MSM, meningococci accounted for 15 (13 percent) of 114 urethral isolates of oxidase-positive, gram-negative diplococci, compared with 4 (1.1 percent) of such 368 urethral isolates from heterosexual men.[97] Similarly, 37 (21 percent) of 175 such isolates from the rectums of MSM were *N. meningitidis*.[97] In women, the prevalence of cervical, urethral, or rectal colonization with *N. meningitidis* was similar to that of urethral infection in heterosexual men.[92,95–97] However, in London, England, in the late 1980s, meningococci were isolated from only 11 (0.2 percent) of 5,571 urethral specimens in MSM, and only 4 percent of oxidase-positive, gram-negative diplococci were *N. meningitidis*.[98] In the same study, no meningococci were isolated from almost 25,000 urethral or cervical specimens from women or heterosexual men. Thus it is likely that the prevalence of anogenital meningococcal colonization varies geographically and over time. All suspicious anorectal or urethral isolates from homosexual men, as well as pharyngeal isolates from all patients, should be tested to distinguish *N. gonorrhoeae* from *N. meningitidis*.

The pathogenicity of anogenital meningococcal infection and the frequency with which it produces clinical disease are unclear, and no systematic studies have been performed to determine its mode of acquisition or the prevalence of infection in the sex partners of colonized patients. However, 50 to 80 percent of meningococcal isolates in this setting are serogroupable and hence presumably pathogenic; serogroups B, C, X, and Y account for most anogenital isolates.[62,93,95,96] Several case reports have linked meningococcal isolation to urethritis, epididymitis, vaginal discharge, acute salpingitis, and DGI-like syndromes.[40,92,95,96,98–101] Therapy has not been formally studied, but symptomatic rectal or genital meningococcal infections have been cured in small numbers of patients receiving treatment with regimens recommended by the Centers for Disease Control and Prevention for gonorrhea. Thus the preponderance of evidence suggests that genital meningococcal infection sometimes is sexually transmitted and, when detected, should be managed in the same manner as gonorrhea.

LABORATORY DIAGNOSIS

The laboratory diagnosis of gonococcal infections depends primarily on identification of *N. gonorrhoeae* at infected sites by microscopic examination of stained smears, by culture, or increasingly by immunochemical or genetic detection of the organism. Details of several techniques, and particularly culture, are included in Chap. 53.

IDENTIFICATION OF *NEISSERIA gonorrhoeae* IN SECRETIONS

Culture

Isolation of *N. gonorrhoeae* is the diagnostic standard for gonococcal infections. Currently available antibiotic-containing selective media (e.g., modified Thayer-Martin medium) have diagnostic sensitivities of 80 to 95 percent for promptly incubated specimens, depending in part on the anatomic site being cultured (Table 32-1). For urethral specimens from symptomatic men, cultures on selective and nonselective media are equally sensitive, because the concentration of gonococci in the urethra usually exceeds that of other flora. In contrast, selective media are preferred for culturing the endocervix, rectum, and pharynx, where other, less fastidious bacteria often outnumber *N. gonorrhoeae*.[85,86] The highest yield from all sites probably results when both selective and nonselective media are inoculated simultaneously with specimens obtained using separate swabs.[85,102,103] However, the incremental yield is small, and this procedure is probably not sufficiently cost-effective to be recommended for routine use.

For women, single cultures on most selective media detect 80 to 90 percent of cervical infections.[47,48,85,103] Although the urethra, Bartholin's gland ducts, and Skene's glands are commonly infected, they are rarely the sole site of infection in women with intact cervices and therefore are not usually cultured. In women who have undergone hysterectomies, however, urethral culture gives highest yield.[50] *N. gonorrhoeae* may be isolated from the anal canal of 35 to 50 percent of women with gonorrhea, and this is the sole site of infection in up to 5 percent.[47,48,55] Similarly, the pharynx is infected in about 5 to 20 percent of women with gonorrhea but is the sole site of infection in fewer than 5 percent.[18,47,48] The increased yield from sampling sites in addition to the cervix results in part from reduced sampling error. Thus the proportion of women found to have a positive culture from the anal canal or pharynx alone might be still lower if duplicate endocervical specimens were cultured routinely.[85,103] Accordingly, for women, cultures of the urethra, accessory gland ducts, anal canal, and pharynx should be considered optional, depending on symptoms, sites exposed, culture methods employed, and available resources.

The sites to be cultured in men also depend on sexual orientation and the anatomic sites exposed. For symptomatic heterosexual men, culture of urethral exudate alone is usually sufficient, but pharyngeal cultures may be useful for men with pharyngitis who practice cunnilingus or for men who have performed cunnilingus with a woman known to have gonorrhea.[18] Although screening of asymptomatic men for urethral gonorrhea has been recommended in the past, in many areas the prevalence of the AHU/IA strains that cause most asymptomatic infections has declined, and the yield of culture may be low enough to permit discontinuation of this practice. For example, at the Seattle-King County STD clinics in 1993 and 1994, *N. gonorrhoeae* was isolated with urethral cultures from only 6 (0.12 percent) of 5,179 men who had no symptoms of urethritis, no discharge on examination, and were not contacts of women with gonorrhea (authors' unpublished data). Similarly, only 34 (1 percent) of 3,271 men seen at a Birmingham, Alabama, STD clinic between January 1, 1994 and June 30, 1995 with positive cultures for *N. gonorrhoeae* were not treated at the time of their initial presentation to the clinic (authors' unpublished data). Among MSM, the rectum is infected almost as frequently as the urethra, although the actual yield depends on patients' specific sexual practices.[59,62,104] Isolated pharyngeal infection occurs in about 5 percent of infected homosexual men.[13,18,59,61,104] Although gonococcal urethritis is common, asymptomatic urethral infection is rare in this population.[59,62] Thus, in screening asymptomatic MSM for whom all three sites are potentially exposed, anorectal culture gives the highest yield, and pharyngeal cultures are desirable. However, these issues have not been thoroughly reexplored since the mid-1980s, when many urban homosexually active men made major changes in sexual behavior in response to the AIDS epidemic.

Table 32-1. Frequency of Isolation of *Neisseria gonorrhoeae* by Site from Patients with Uncomplicated Gonorrhea*

	N	Total positive number (%)	Only site positive, number (%)
Women†	162		
Endocervix		155 (96)	75 (46)
Anal canal		62 (38)	3 (2)
Pharynx		35 (22)	4 (3)
Heterosexual men	177		
Urethra		177 (100)	166 (94)
Pharynx		11 (6)	0
Homosexual men	355		
Urethra		205 (58)	146 (41)
Anal canal		177 (50)	109 (31)
Pharynx		62 (17)	18 (5)

* Analysis limited to patients for whom all indicated sites were cultured; single cultures on modified Thayer-Martin medium were used.

† Women who had undergone hysterectomy were excluded.

SOURCE: Data on women and heterosexual men are from Handsfield et al[59]; data on homosexual men are combined from Handsfield et al[59] and Tice and Rodriguez.[60]

Several reports have documented failure of vancomycin-containing selective culture media to support growth of vancomycin-sensitive gonococci.[84,105] The prevalence of such strains is highly variable but in the 1970s accounted for up to 30 percent of gonococcal isolates in some geographic areas.[84,86,105] The ability to culture these organisms also is inoculation-dependent, with greater inhibition occurring with smaller inocula.[84,86,105] Most vancomycin-sensitive strains belong to the AHU/IA or related A/S classes. Thus use of vancomycin-containing media in geographic areas where such strains are prevalent may selectively impair gonorrhea diagnosis and the yield of screening.

Stained smears

Gram's stain, methylene blue, acridine orange, and several other dyes have been used to prepare clinical material for microscopic examination for gonococci, but Gram's stain has been the most extensively studied. For examination of clinical material, a smear is considered positive for gonorrhea when gram-negative diplococci with typical morphology are identified within or closely associated with polymorphonuclear leukocytes (Fig. 32-7); it is considered equivocal if only extracellular organisms or morphologically atypical intracellular gram-negative diplococci are seen; and it is considered negative if no gram-negative diplococci are present. Nonpathogenic *Neisseriaceae* other than *N. meningitidis*, which are morphologically indistinguishable from *N. gonorrhoeae,* are generally not cell-associated. *Acinetobacter* species are bipolar-staining gram-negative bacilli that, contrary to earlier reports, are easily distinguished from *N. gonorrhoeae* by experienced microscopists. Table 32-2 shows the sensitivity and specificity of Gram-stained smears for various categories of genital and rectal infection relative to isolation of *N. gonorrhoeae.*

For evaluation of men with symptoms and signs of urethritis, the urethral smear is sufficiently sensitive and specific that culture may be considered optional for routine care.[106] This depends in part, however, on specimen collection technique and the experience of the microscopist. In addition, isolation of the organism is desirable to test for antimicrobial resistance. Accordingly, other than in settings where reliable surveillance for antibiotic-resistant gonococci is performed regularly, isolation of *N. gonorrhoeae* usually should be attempted. Although smears from the endocervix or rectum are less sensitive than those from the urethra, positive smears of properly collected specimens are highly specific when examined by experienced personnel, and they facilitate expeditious therapy of infected patients, especially when the index of suspicion is high.[75,106,107] For example, for women with mucopurulent cervicitis or salpingitis, an endocervical smear showing typical intracellular gram-negative diplococci supports the diagnosis of gonorrhea. On the other hand, smears have a low predictive value and are less cost-effective for screening asymptomatic women. Thus stained smears should be utilized as an adjunct to but not replacement for more specific tests. The sensitivity of anorectal smears for evaluation of patients with symptoms of proctitis is enhanced when the exudate is obtained by direct visualization using an anoscope rather than blindly,[108] even though anoscopy does not apparently improve the sensitivity of culture.[109] Smears are not commonly obtained from the urethra or accessory gland ducts of women but should be performed if abnormal exudate is expressed or the patient has had a hysterectomy. The Gram's stain smear has not been studied in pharyngeal gonococcal infection but is generally believed to be both insensitive and nonspecific; it is not recommended.

Table 32-2. Sensitivity and Specificity of Gram-Stained Smears for Detection of Genital or Anorectal Gonorrhea

Site and clinical setting	Sensitivity	Specificity*
Urethra		
Men with symptomatic urethritis	90–95	95–100
Men with asymptomatic urethral infection	50–70	95–100
Endocervix		
Uncomplicated gonorrhea	50–70	95–100
Pelvic inflammatory disease	60–70	95–100
Anorectum		
Blind swabs	40–60	95–100†
Anoscopically obtained specimens	70–80	95–100†

* Sensitivity = percent of patients with positive cultures who have positive gram-stained smears. Specificity = percent of patients with negative cultures whose gram-stained smears also are negative.

† The studies showing 95–100% specificity for anorectal smears did not report whether meningococcal infection was distinguished from gonorrhea. Until further data are available, a positive anorectal smear should be considered highly specific for either gonococcal or meningococcal infection.

SOURCE: Compiled from Handsfield et al,[28] Jacobs and Kraus,[45] Thin and Shaw,[48] Barlow and Phillips,[49] Wallin,[52] Rothenberg et al,[106] Wald,[107] William et al,[108] Deheragoda.[109]

Nonculture diagnostic techniques

In many clinical settings, specimens for detection of *N. gonorrhoeae* must be transported from collection sites to laboratories for testing, a process that may take several days and result in temperature variation or other circumstances that can jeopardize culture viability.[110] In recent years, reliable nonculture assays for gonorrhea detection have become available and are being utilized increasingly. In 1994 an estimated 20 million tests for gonorrhea diagnosis were performed in the United States, of which approx-

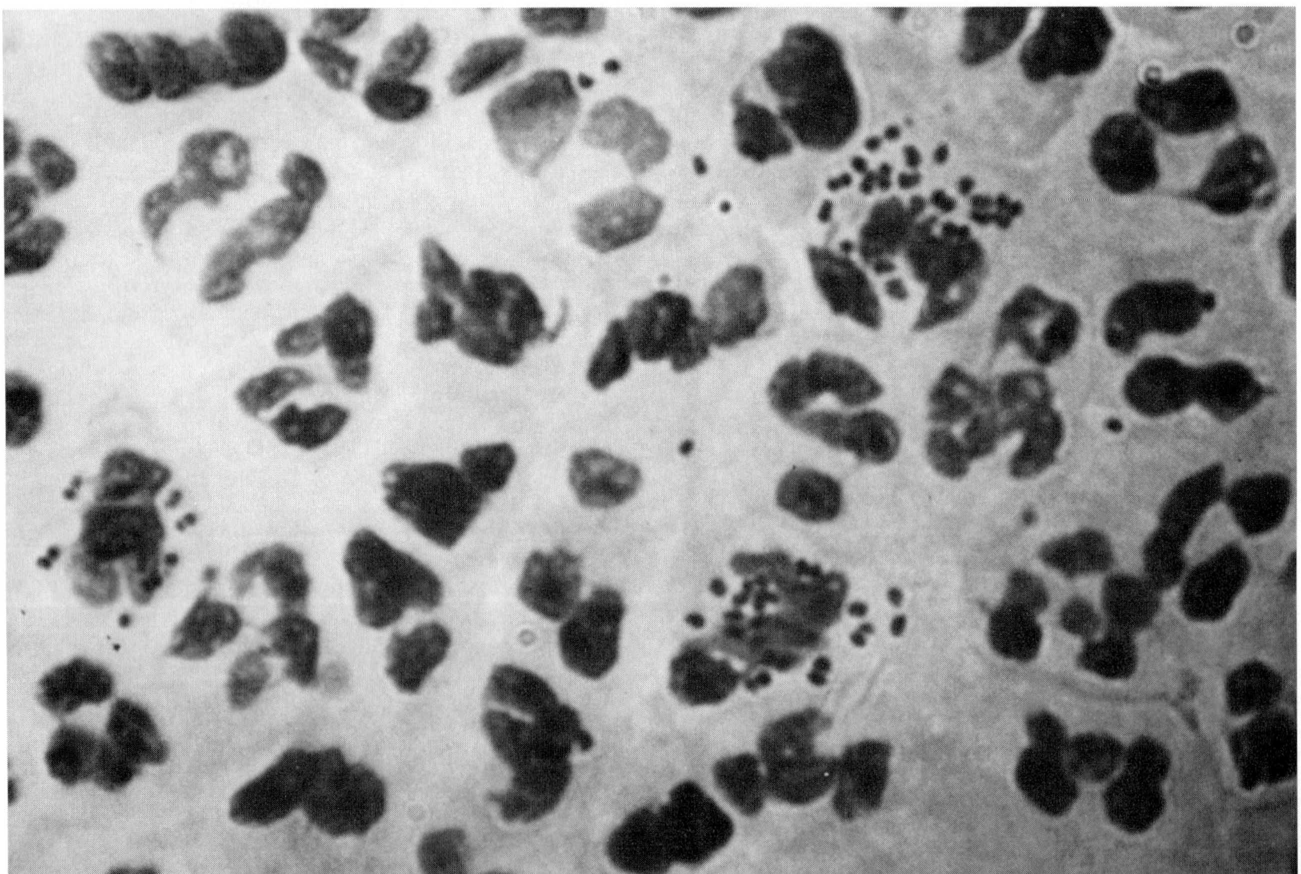

Fig. 32-7. Gram-stained smear showing polymorphonuclear leukocytes with intracellular gram-negative diplococci in urethral exudate from a man with gonococcal urethritis (× 1000).

imately 35 to 40 percent were nonculture tests (Susan DeLisle, Centers for Disease Control, personal communication). Given satisfactory performance of these tests, their continuing promotion by the manufacturers, and the fact that specimens collected for gonorrhea diagnosis with these tests also can be used frequently to test for *C. trachomatis*, their utilization is likely to continue to increase. At the same time, however, culture-based regional monitoring of gonococcal antimicrobial susceptibility is recommended to guide therapeutic choices.

Nonamplified DNA probe tests (e.g., Gen-Probe Pace 2) are the most widely utilized nonculture tests for gonorrhea diagnosis in the United States. This test, based on a single-stranded DNA probe designed to hybridize to *N. gonorrhoeae* rRNA, has been found to have sensitivities of 89 to 97 percent and specificity of 99 percent, has performed comparably to culture on selective media, and is often available for costs similar to culture.[111–113]

More recently, the first amplified nucleic–acid detection test for gonorrhea diagnosis, a ligase chain reaction (LCR) assay, has become available in the United States.[114,115] Assays based on polymerase chain reaction (PCR), transcription-mediated amplification (TMA), and other nucleic acid amplification technologies are also being developed. The LCR test has been found to be as sensitive as culture for detection of *N. gonorrhoeae* using swab specimens (sensitivity 95 to 98 percent)[114,115] but has the added advantage of being equally sensitive when first-void urine specimens are used,[115] allowing screening of men and women in settings where genital examinations are impractical. In addition, like the nonamplified tests mentioned above, a single specimen collected for LCR can be tested for both *N. gonorrhoeae* and *C. trachomatis*.

Fluorescein-conjugated antibodies have been employed to detect *N. gonorrhoeae,* but this method has not proved sufficiently sensitive or specific for routine use[118]; modifications using monoclonal antibodies remain under investigation. Immunologic or biochemical detection of gonococcal antigens or metabolic products, including surface proteins, endotoxin, and oxidase or other enzymes, also has been investigated but currently seems less promising than nucleic acid detection.

Collection of clinical specimens

Urethral exudate from men may be obtained by passage of a small swab or bacteriologic loop 2 to 4 cm into the urethra[28] or by collecting the first 15 to 30 mL of voided urine.[117,118] Although the latter method obviates the discomfort of passing a urethral swab or loop, collection and culture of urine are time-consuming, depend in part on the ability of the patient to provide a proper specimen, and require prompt processing for culture because the urine from some individuals is rapidly bactericidal for *N. gonorrhoeae.*[119] Similar specimen handling and transport have less effect on DNA amplification tests. For collection of endocervical specimens, the cervix should be cleansed of external exudate or vaginal secretions and a swab inserted 1 to 2 cm into the external os and rotated gently for up to 10 seconds.[120] When personal or logistic constraints preclude speculum examination, a vaginal specimen may be obtained by a clinician or the patient using a swab or a tampon.[121] With this technique, the sensitivity of LCR remains excellent, whereas there is a modest reduction in culture sensitivity and a marked reduction in the sensitivity of gram-stained smears.

None of the nucleic acid– or antigen-detection assays have been studied for clinical specimens from sites other than the urogenital tract. Only culture should be used to diagnose rectal or pharyngeal gonococcal infections. Anorectal specimens from patients without symptoms of proctitis may be obtained by blindly passing a swab 2 to 3 cm into the anal canal, using lateral pressure to avoid entering any fecal mass. If gross fecal contamination of the swab occurs, it should be discarded and another specimen obtained. For symptomatic patients, anorectal specimens should be obtained under direct vision using anoscopy, which increases the sensitivity of the smear.[108,109] Pharyngeal specimens are obtained by swabbing the posterior pharynx, including the tonsillar areas and faucial pillars.

SEROLOGIC DIAGNOSIS

Serologic tests have been developed to detect antibodies to *N. gonorrhoeae* or its components using complement fixation, immunoprecipitation, bacterial lysis, immunofluorescence, hemagglutination, latex agglutination, enzyme-linked immunoabsorbance, and other techniques.[122] Many of these methods have proved useful for studies of the immune response and pathogenesis of gonorrhea. However, most reported serodiagnostic tests have sensitivities of about 70 percent and specificities of about 80 percent for patients with uncomplicated gonorrhea and thus are not useful for screening, case finding, or diagnosis.[123,124]

THERAPY OF GONOCOCCAL INFECTIONS

ANTIMICROBIAL SUSCEPTIBILITY OF *N. gonorrhoeae* AND DEVELOPMENT OF RESISTANCE

While most gonococci remain susceptible to a variety of antimicrobial agents (e.g., penicillins, cephalosporins, tetracyclines, macrolides, quinolones, rifampin, and the aminoglycoside antibiotics), selection of strains with relative or absolute resistance is readily accomplished in the laboratory, and in vivo development of resistance continues to dictate changes in recommended therapy for gonorrhea. In general, this resistance is mediated through either the cumulative effect of sometimes multiple chromosomal mutations or by single-step acquisition of plasmids that encode for high-level resistance. Since many patients with gonorrhea are treated syndromically and formal agar dilution MIC determination for *N. gonorrhoeae* is time-consuming and not widely available, recommendations for gonorrhea therapy usually only consider regimens with efficacy of 95 percent or greater.[125] To accomplish this, both the United States and the World Health Organization utilize sentinel surveillance systems (see below) to monitor susceptibility and guide their gonorrhea treatment recommendations.

Prior to the mid-1930s, when sulfanilamide was introduced, gonorrhea therapy involved local genital irrigation with antiseptic solutions such as silver nitrate or potassium permangate.[3,43] By 1944, however, many gonococci had become sulfanilamide-resistant, and infection persisted in about one-third of patients treated with maximal doses. Fortunately, in 1943 the first reports of the near 100 percent utility of penicillin for gonorrhea therapy were published,[126] and by the end of World War II, as penicillin became available to the general public, it quickly became the therapy of choice. Since then, continuing development of antimicrobial resistance by *N. gonorrhoeae*[127,128] led to regular revisions of recommended gonorrhea therapy. From the 1950s until the mid-1970s, gradually increasing chromosomal penicillin resistance led to periodic increases in the amount of penicillin required for reliable therapy. Similar trends in MICs also were observed for macrolide and tetracycline antibiotics, the other two major antibiotics used at the time.[128] In 1976, however, strains of *N. gonorrhoeae* with high-level penicillin resistance due to plasmid-mediated beta-lactamase production were reported initially as having originated in West Africa and the Far East.[129] Thus, for the first time, through single-step plasmid acquisition, gonococci had become impervious to clinically useful doses of penicillin. About 10 years later, gonococci with high-level, plasmid-mediated resistance to tetracycline were first described,[130] further reducing the utility of the tetracycline family of drugs for gonorrhea treatment.

In addition to resistance to penicillin, tetracyclines, and erythromycin, in 1987, clinically significant chromosomally mediated resistance to spectinomycin, another drug recommended for gonorrhea therapy, was described in U.S. military personnel in Korea.[131] The data in that report provided empirical evidence of the effect of selective antimicrobial pressure on the development of antimicrobial resistance. In Korea, because of the high prevalence of PPNG, in 1981, spectinomycin had been adopted as the drug of choice for gonorrhea therapy. By 1983, however, reports of spectinomycin treatment failures were beginning to occur in patients with gonorrhea, and over the next 2 years, the prevalence of spectinomycin-resistant *N. gonorrhoeae* was noted to increase. The prevalence of PPNG declined from a peak of nearly 45 percent to approximately 13 percent during the period that spectinomycin was the drug of choice for gonorrhea therapy. These are among the best data to suggest that patterns of antimicrobial use for gonorrhea therapy within communities may contribute to development of antimicrobial resistance. Following recognition of the outbreak of spectinomycin-resistant gonococci in Korea, ceftriaxone became the drug of choice for treatment of gonorrhea in U.S. military personnel in that country.[131] Sporadic cases of spectinomycin-resistant gonorrhea have been reported elsewhere, but such strains remain rare in the United States, possibly related to relatively low utilization of this relatively expensive therapeutic agent.[132,133] In addition, the events that occurred in a relatively closed community represented by U.S. military personnel and a limited number of commercial sex workers may not apply elsewhere, and gonorrhea treatment regimens are not the sole determinants of resistance in *N. gonorrhoeae*. In Cleveland, Ohio, where fluoroquinolone antibiotics were not used for gonorrhea treatment in health department clinics, the prevalence of *N. gonorrhoeae* with decreased susceptibility to ciprofloxacin and other fluoroquinolones increased from 2 percent in 1991 to 16 percent in 1994.[134]

In 1986, as the problems of antimicrobial resistance in *N. gonorrhoeae* in the United States were becoming apparent, the CDC reinstituted sentinel surveillance of the antimicrobial susceptibility of *N. gonorrhoeae*.[135] In 1995, data from the systematic monthly testing of gonococcal isolates from 25 U.S. cities demonstrated that nearly 32 percent of isolates have one form or another of antimicrobial resistance.[136] The CDC sentinel surveillance system continues to document the substantial geographic diversity of antimicrobial-resistant *N. gonorrhoeae*.[135,136] Recently, this surveillance system has clearly identified an increasing proportion of isolates with decreased susceptibility to ciprofloxacin, one of the currently recommended treatments for gonorrhea.[136] These data confirm similar observations made in Seattle and Cleveland and suggest that, as has occurred in the Philippines and Far East, increasing fluoroquinolone resistance may soon limit the utility of this class of antibiotics for gonorrhea therapy as well.[137]

CHOICE OF TREATMENT REGIMENS FOR *N. gonorrhoeae*

The choice of antimicrobial agents for gonorrhea therapy is influenced by a variety of factors in addition to the antimicrobial activity of drugs for *N. gonorrhoeae*. Pharmacokinetic studies have demonstrated that serum levels of penicillin equal to or greater than three times the MIC of the infecting strain of *N. gonorrhoeae* for 8 hours are needed to reliably cure uncomplicated infection.[138] In general, single-dose, observed therapy is preferred for gonorrhea in order to overcome problems of patient compliance. In addition, the choice of antimicrobial agents for therapy is influenced by the probability that patients with acute gonococcal infection are coinfected or have been exposed recently to other STD agents. Among coinfecting agents for patients with gonorrhea in the United States, *C. trachomatis* is preeminent. Up to 10 to 20 percent of men and 20 to 30 percent of women with acute urogenital gonorrhea are coinfected with *C. trachomatis*.[10,46,76,139,140] In addition, substantial numbers of women with acute gonococcal infection have simultaneous *T. vaginalis* infections. For several decades it has been recommended widely that therapy for gonorrhea also be effective against incubating syphilis. However, more recent data suggest that incubating syphilis is relatively rare in gonorrhea patients in the United States and that the choice of treatment has no measurable effect on the frequency of syphilis.[138a] However, activity of selected agents against *Treponema pallidum* may remain an important consideration in some settings. In Africa and other areas where chancroid is prevalent, patients may have been exposed to *H. ducreyi* at the time of contraction of gonorrhea.

Since 1985, the treatment recommendations published by the CDC for the United States have recommended single-dose therapy with medications effective for eradication of *N. gonorrhoeae*, followed by therapy expected to eradicate *C. trachomatis* infections (currently either azithromycin or doxycycline). This approach has been shown to be effective for therapy of both infections.[139,140]

For over a decade, ceftriaxone, a third-generation cephalosporin, has been the most reliable single-dose regimen used for gonorrhea worldwide.[141] The dose of ceftriaxone currently recommended for therapy of uncomplicated gonorrhea by the CDC is a single intramuscular injection of 125 mg,[140,142] although in some settings 250 mg, the lowest unit dose commercially available, continues to be used. Either dose is highly effective for rectal and pharyngeal, as well as genital, gonorrhea.[143] Although a small percentage (<1 percent) of patients treated with ceftriaxone fail antimicrobial therapy, clinically significant ceftriaxone resistance has not been reported through 1995.[136,141] The major drawbacks of ceftriaxone therapy for gonorrhea are the requirement for parenteral administration and the potential (albeit low) for reactions of patients allergic to beta-lactam antibiotics. Cefixime, an orally absorbed cephalosporin with MICs for *N. gonorrhoeae* that are similar to ceftriaxone, provides a useful oral alternative to parenteral ceftriaxone and also was recommended by the CDC for gonorrhea in its *1993 STD Treatment Guidelines*.[140,141]

In 1984 a report was published describing the utility of norfloxacin, a new quinolone antibiotic, for treating antibiotic-resistant gonococcal infections.[144] Enthusiasm for gonorrhea therapy with earlier quinolones (nalidixic acid and rosoxacin) had been tempered by the tendency of gonococci to rapidly become resistant to the former and by the unacceptable neurotoxicity (primarily vestibular) of the latter.[145] Since that time, a number of other newer quinolones (ciprofloxacin, ofloxacin, enoxacin, fleroxicin, and others) have been evaluated as single-dose regimens with promising results.[141,145] On the other hand, reports of quinolone resistance among gonococcal isolates from the Philippines[146] and Southeast Asia, where some quinolone antibiotics are inexpensive and widely available, have raised important questions regarding the long-term utility of these otherwise relatively well tolerated, orally active antimicrobials for gonorrhea therapy. At present, most quinolones are no longer reliable in some Pacific and Asian countries, and as noted earlier, strains with low- and high-level resistance have been seen in several areas of the United States.[147] However, clinically important quinolone resistance remains uncommon in the United States, and the CDC continues to recommend use of either ciprofloxacin 500 mg or ofloxacin 400 mg as single-dose,[140] orally administered gonorrhea therapy in areas where decreased susceptibility to these agents is not a problem.

Each of the currently recommended treatment regimens has specific advantages and disadvantages that should be utilized to individualize therapy for gonorrhea. For example, single-dose oral regimens have potential benefits in terms of convenience and reduced risk for needle-stick exposures in health care workers. Quinolones are not recommended in pregnant women. For treatment of homosexual men with gonorrhea, the ceftriaxone regimen is preferred over other regimens. The strains of gonococci that occur in homosexual men are more likely to harbor the antibiotic resistance mutation (mtr),[148] which makes these organisms somewhat more resistant to antibiotics and thus results in higher treatment failure rates when alternate regimens are utilized. Similarly, while efficacious for anogenital gonorrhea, spectinomycin hydrochloride is not efficacious for treatment of pharyngeal gonorrhea[149] and is not recommended in homosexual men. Finally, particularly in settings such as public clinics where large numbers of patients are treated and funds are limited, cost considerations may lead to choice of one agent over another.

In addition to currently recommended regimens for treatment of uncomplicated gonorrhea, there are a substantial number of other antibiotics that have been demonstrated to be effective for gonorrhea therapy.[141,150] However, compared with the CDC-recommended ones, these drugs may not have any advantage over recommended regimens.[141]

FOLLOW-UP

Because all recommended regimens have cure rates that approach 100 percent, repeat cultures for test of cure are no longer recommended for all patients with gonorrhea.[140] Test-of-cure cultures should be used if an atypical regimen is used or medication compliance is uncertain.

MANAGEMENT OF SEX PARTNERS

Most authorities recommend treatment of all recent sex partners of patients with gonorrhea, prior to the availability of culture results, in order to prevent complications and curtail the transmission ("epidemiologic treatment").[149,151] The definition of *recent* depends on the clinical and epidemiologic settings; in most instances, all partners exposed within 2 weeks prior to the onset of symptoms or to diagnosis of the index case should be treated. For patients with asymptomatic gonococcal infection, however, extending contact tracing to 1 month may prove useful for prevention efforts.

PREVENTION

Properly used condoms provide a high degree of protection against acquisition and transmission of genital infection.[26,152] The diaphragm and cervical cap also may reduce transmission and acquisition of endocervical infection.[20,153,154] Topical spermicidal and bactericidal agents have been shown recently to clearly reduce the probability of infection by both *N. gonorrhoeae* and *C. trachomatis* in patients using these gels.[20,21,23] Urinating, washing, and douching after intercourse are assumed by many to be beneficial in prevention of gonorrhea, but controlled data are lacking. In addition, certain practices such as douching are now increasingly being associated with harmful outcomes. Prophylactic administration of antibiotics immediately or soon after sexual exposure clearly reduces the risk of infection.[27] However, this practice is likely to select and facilitate transmission of antibiotic-resistant strains of *N. gonorrhoeae*. In addition, except in very high-risk settings, routine antibiotic prophylaxis is unlikely to be cost-effective.

References

1 Rosebury T: *Microbes and Morals*. New York, Viking, 1971.

2 Kampmeier RH: Identification of the gonococcus by Albert Neisser. *Sex Transm Dis* 5:71, 1978.

3 Kampmeier RH: Introduction of sulfonamide therapy for gonorrhea. *Sex Transm Dis* 10:81, 1983.

4 Thayer JD, Martin JE: Selective medium for the cultivation of *N. gonorrhoeae* and *N. meningitidis*. *Public Health Rep* 79:49, 1964.

5 Division of STD Prevention. *Sexually Transmitted Diseases Surveillance, 1995*. Atlanta, U.S. Department of Health and Human Services, Public Health Service, Centers for Disease Control and Prevention, Sept. 1996.

6 Danielsson D, National Bacteriological Laboratory: Unpublished data, Orebro and Stockholm, Sweden, 1988.

7 Judson FN: Fear of AIDS and gonorrhea rates in homosexual men, letter. *Lancet* 2:159, 1983.

8 Handsfield HH: Decreasing incidence of gonorrhea in homosexually active men. *West J Med* 143:469, 1985.

9 Rice RJ et al: Gonorrhea in the United States 1975–1984: Is the giant only sleeping? *Sex Transm Dis* 14:83, 1987.

10 Barnes RC, Holmes KK: Epidemiology of gonorrhea: Current perspectives. *Epidemiol Rev* 6:1, 1984.

11 Rice RJ et al: Unpublished data.

12 Brooks GF et al: Repeated gonorrhea: An analysis of importance and risk factors. *J Infect Dis* 137:161, 1978.

13 Lafferty W et al: Sexually transmitted disease in men who have sex with men: Acquisition of gonorrhea and nongonococcal urethritis by fellatio and implications for STD/HIV prevention. *Sex Transm Dis* (*in press*).

14 Wright PA, Judson FN: Relative and seasonal incidences of the sexually transmitted diseases: A two-year statistical review. *Br J Vener Dis* 54:433, 1978.

15 Reynolds GH et al: The national gonorrhea therapy monitoring study: II. Trends and seasonality of antibiotic resistance of *Neisseria gonorrhoeae*. *Sex Transm Dis* 6(suppl):103, 1979.

16 Holmes KK et al: An estimate of the risk of men acquiring gonorrhea by sexual contact with infected females. *Am J Epidemiol* 91:170, 1970.

17 Hooper RR et al: Cohort study of venereal disease: 1. The risk of gonorrhea transmission from infected women to men. *Am J Epidemiol* 108:136, 1978.

18 Wiesner PJ et al: Clinical spectrum of pharyngeal gonococcal infections. *N Engl J Med* 288:181, 1973.

19 Tice RW, Rodriguez VL: Pharyngeal gonorrhea. *JAMA* 246:2717, 1981.

20 McCormack WM et al: Effect of menstrual cycle and method of contraception on recovery of *Neisseria gonorrhoeae*. *JAMA* 247:1292, 1982.

21 Louv WC et al: Oral contraceptive use and the risk of chlamydial and gonococcal infections. *Am J Obstet Gynecol* 160:396, 1989.

22 Cates W Jr et al: Sex and spermicides: Preventing unintended pregnancy and infection. *JAMA* 248:1636, 1982.

23 Louv WC et al: A clinical trial of nonoxynol-9 for preventing gonococcal and chlamydial infections. *J Infect Dis* 158:518, 1988.

24 Pedersen AHB, Bonin P: Screening females for asymptomatic gonorrhea infection. *Northwest Med* 70:255, 1971.

25 McCormack WM et al: Clinical spectrum of gonococcal infection in women. *Lancet* 2:1182, 1977.

26 Upchurch DM et al: Behavioral contributions to acquisition and transmission of *Neisseria gonorrhoeae*. *J Infect Dis* 161:938, 1989.

27 Harrison WO et al: A trial of minocycline given after exposure to prevent gonorrhea. *N Engl J Med* 300:1074, 1979.

28 Handsfield HH et al: Asymptomatic gonorrhea in men: Diagnosis, natural course, prevalence and significance. *N Engl J Med* 290:117, 1974.
29 Yorke JA et al: Dynamics and control of the transmission of gonorrhea. *Sex Transm Dis* 5:51, 1978.
30 Rothenberg RB: The geography of gonorrhea: Empirical demonstration of core group transmission. *Am J Epidemiol* 117:688, 1983.
31 May RM: The transmission and control of gonorrhea. *Nature* 291: 376, 1981.
32 Carifo K, Catlin BW: *Neisseria gonorrhoeae* auxotyping: Differentiation of clinical isolates based on growth responses on chemically defined media. *Appl Microbiol* 26:223, 1973.
33 Knapp JS et al: Serological classification of *Neisseria gonorrhoeae* with use of monoclonal antibodies to gonococcal outer membrane protein I. *J Infect Dis* 150:44, 1984.
34 Knapp JS et al: Epidemiology of gonorrhea: Distribution and temporal changes in *Neisseria gonorrhoeae* auxotype/serovar class. *Sex Transm Dis* 14:26, 1987.
35 Hook EW III et al: Determinants of emergence of antibiotic-resistant *Neisseria gonorrhoeae. J Infect Dis* 159:900, 1989.
36 Crawford G et al: Asymptomatic gonorrhea in men: Caused by gonococci with unique nutritional requirements. *Science* 196:1352, 1977.
37 Knapp JS, Holmes KK: Disseminated gonococcal infection caused by *Neisseria gonorrhoeae* with unique nutritional requirements. *J Infect Dis* 132:204, 1975.
38 Draper DL et al: Auxotypes and antibiotic susceptibilities of *Neisseria gonorrhoeae* from women with acute salpingitis: Comparison with gonococci causing uncomplicated genital tract infections in women. *Sex Transm Dis* 8:43, 1981.
39 Knapp JS et al: Phenotypic and epidemiologic correlates of auxotype in *Neisseria gonorrhoeae. J Infect Dis* 138:160, 1978.
40 Rompalo AM et al: The acute arthritis-dermatitis syndrome: The changing importance of *Neisseria gonorrhoeae* and *Neisseria meningitidis. Arch Intern Med* 147:281, 1987.
41 Pierce WA, Buchanan TM: Attachment role of gonococcal pili: Optimum conditions and quantitation of adherence of isolated pili to human cells in vitro. *J Clin Invest* 61:931, 1978.
42 King GL, Swanson J: Studies on gonococcus infection: XV. Identification of surface proteins of *Neisseria gonorrhoeae* correlated with leukocyte association. *Infect Immun* 21:575, 1978.
43 Pelouze PS: *Gonorrhea in the Male and Female.* Philadelphia, Saunders, 1941.
44 Gregg CR et al: Toxic activity of purified lipopolysaccharide of *Neisseria gonorrhoeae* for human fallopian tube mucosa. *J Infect Dis* 143: 432, 1981.
45 Jacobs NF, Kraus SJ: Gonococcal and nongonococcal urethritis in men: Clinical and laboratory differentiation. *Ann Intern Med* 82:7, 1975.
46 Handsfield HH: Gonorrhea and nongonococcal urethritis: Recent advances. *Med Clin North Am* 62:925, 1978.
47 Schmale JD et al: Observation on the culture diagnosis of gonorrhea in women. *JAMA* 210:312, 1969.
48 Thin RN, Shaw EJ: Diagnosis of gonorrhea in women. *Br J Vener Dis* 55:10, 1979.
49 Barlow D, Phillips I: Gonorrhea in women: Diagnostic, clinical, and laboratory aspects. *Lancet* 1:761, 1978.
50 Judson RN, Ruder MA: Effect of hysterectomy on genital infections. *Br J Vener Dis* 55:434, 1979.
51 Platt R et al: Risk of acquiring gonorrhea and prevalence of abnormal adnexal findings among women recently exposed to gonorrhea. *JAMA* 250:320, 1983.
52 Wallin J: Gonorrhea in 1972: A 1-year study of patients attending the VD unit in Uppsala. *Br J Vener Dis* 51:41, 1974.
53 Curran JW et al: Female gonorrhea: Its relation to abnormal uterine bleeding, urinary tract symptoms, and cervicitis. *Obstet Gynecol* 45: 195, 1975.
54 Corman LC et al: The high frequency of pharyngeal gonococcal infection in a prenatal clinic population. *JAMA* 230:568, 1974.
55 Klein EJ et al: Anorectal gonococcal infection. *Ann Intern Med* 86: 340, 1977.
56 Kinghorn GR, Rashid S: Prevalence of rectal and pharyngeal infection in women with gonorrhea in Sheffield. *Br J Vener Dis* 55:408, 1979.
57 Lebedeff DA, Hochman EB: Rectal gonorrhea in men: Diagnosis and treatment. *Ann Intern Med* 92:463, 1980.
58 Quinn TC et al: The polymicrobial origin of intestinal infections in homosexual men. *N Engl J Med* 309:576, 1983.
59 Handsfield HH et al: Correlation of auxotype and penicillin susceptibility of *Neisseria gonorrhoeae* with sexual preference and clinical manifestations of gonorrhea. *Sex Transm Dis* 7:1, 1980.
60 Tice AW, Rodriguez VL: Pharyngeal gonorrhea. *JAMA* 246:2717, 1981.
61 Bro-Jorgensen A, Jensen T: Gonococcal pharyngeal infections: Report of 110 cases. *Br J Vener Dis* 49:491, 1973.
62 Janda WM et al: Prevalence and site-pathogen studies of *Neisseria meningitidis* and *N. gonnorhoeae* in homosexual men. *JAMA* 244: 2060, 1980.
63 Sackel SG et al: Orogenital contact and the isolation of *Neisseria gonorrhoeae, Mycoplasma hominis,* and *Ureaplasma urealyticum* from the pharynx. *Sex Transm Dis* 6:64, 1979.
64 Wallin J, Siegel MS: Pharyngeal *Neisseria gonorrhoeae:* Colonizer or pathogen? *Br Med J* 1:1462, 1979.
65 Hutt DM, Judson FN: Epidemiology and treatment of oropharyngeal gonorrhea. *Ann Intern Med* 104:655, 1986.
66 Thatcher RW, Pettit TH: Gonorrheal conjunctivitis. *JAMA* 215: 1494, 1971.
67 Brians SC, Tight RR: Laboratory-acquired gonococcal conjunctivitis. *JAMA* 241:274, 1979.
68 Podgore JK, Holmes KK: Ocular gonococcal infection with little or no inflammatory response. *JAMA* 246:242, 1981.
69 Valenton MJ, Abendanio R: Gonorrheal conjunctivitis. *Can J Ophthalmol* 8:421, 1973.
70 Chapel T et al: The microbiological flora of penile ulcerations. *J Infect Dis* 137:50, 1978.
71 Robinson L, Alergant CD: Gonococcal infection of the penis. *Br J Vener Dis* 49:364, 1973.
72 Scott MJ Jr, Scott MJ Sr: Primary cutaneous *Neisseria gonorrhoeae* infections. *Arch Dermatol* 118:351, 1982.
73 Berger RE et al: Etiology, manifestations and therapy of acute epi didymitis: Prospective study of 50 cases. *J Urol* 121:750, 1979.
74 Wright RA, Judson FN: Penile venereal edema. *JAMA* 241:157, 1979.
75 Eschenbach DA et al: Polymicrobial etiology of acute pelvic inflammatory disease. *N Engl J Med* 293:166, 1975.
76 Holmes KK et al: Salpingitis: Overview of etiology and epidemiology. *Am J Obstet Gynecol* 138:893, 1980.
77 Svensson L et al: Differences in some clinical and laboratory parameters in acute salpingitis related to culture and serologic findings. *Am J Obstet Gynecol* 138:1017, 1980.
78 Rees E: Gonococcal bartholinitis. *Br J Vener Dis* 43:150, 1967.
79 Holmes KK et al: Disseminated gonococcal infection. *Ann Intern Med* 74:979, 1979.
80 Masi AT, Eisenstein BI: Disseminated gonococcal infection (DGI) and gonococcal arthritis (GCA): II. Clinical manifestations, diagnosis, complications, treatment and prevention. *Semin Arthritis Rheum* 10: 173, 1981.
81 O'Brien JA et al: Disseminated gonococcal infection: A prospective analysis of 49 patients and a review of pathophysiology and immune mechanisms. *Medicine* 2:395, 1983.
82 Handsfield HH et al: Treatment of the gonococcal arthritis-dermatitis syndrome. *Ann Intern Med* 84:661, 1976.
83 Rice PA, Goldenberg DL: Clinical manifestations of disseminated infection caused by *Neisseria gonorrhoeae* are linked to differences in bactericidal reactivity of infecting strains. *Ann Intern Med* 95:175, 1985.
84 Merrett S et al: *Neisseria gonorrhoeae* strains inhibited by vancomycin in selective media and correlation with auxotype. *J Clin Microbiol* 14:94, 1981.

85 Bonin P et al: Isolation of *Neisseria gonorrhoeae* on selective and nonselective media in a STD clinic. *J Clin Microbiol* 92:218, 1984.
86 Reichart CA et al: Comparison of GC-Lect and modified Thayer-Martin media for isolation of *Neisseria gonorrhoeae*. *J Clin Microbiol* 27:808, 1989.
87 Petersen BH et al: *Neisseria meningitidis* and *Neisseria gonorrhoeae* bacteremia associated with C6, C7, or C8 deficiency. *Ann Intern Med* 90:917, 1979.
88 Rinaldi RZ et al: Penicillin-resistant gonococcal arthritis: A report of four cases. *Ann Intern Med* 97:43, 1982.
89 Strader KW et al: Disseminated gonococcal infection caused by chromosomally mediated penicillin-resistant organisms. *Ann Intern Med* 104:365, 1986.
90 Sazeed ZA et al: Gonococcal meningitis: A review. *JAMA* 219:1730, 1972.
91 Rice RJ et al: Phenotypic characterization of *Neisseria gonorrhoeae* isolated from three cases of meningitis. *J Infect Dis* 153:362, 1986.
92 Apicella MA: *Neisseria meningitidis*, in *Principles and Practices of Infectious Diseases*, GL Mandell et al (eds). New York, Wiley, 1979, p 1640.
93 Handsfield HH et al: Unpublished data.
94 Laumann EO et al: *The Social Organization of Sexuality: Sexual Practices in the United States*. Chicago, University of Chicago Press, 1994.
95 Faur YC et al: Isolation of *N. meningitidis* from patients in a gonorrhea screening program: A four-year survey in New York City. *Am J Public Health* 71:53, 1981.
96 Judson FN et al: Anogenital infection with *Neisseria meningitidis in* homosexual men. *J Infect Dis* 137:458, 1978.
96a Winterscheid KK et al: Decreased susceptibility to penicillin G and Tet M plasmids in genital and ano-rectal isolates of *Neisseria menigitidis*. *Antimicrob Agents Chemother* 38:1661, 1994.
97 Carlson BL et al: Isolation of *Neisseria meningitidis* from anogenital specimens from homosexual men. *Sex Transm Dis* 7:71, 1980.
98 Maini M et al: Urethritis due to *Neisseria meningitidis* in London genitourinary medicine clinic population. *Int J STD AIDS* 3:423, 1992.
99 William DC et al: *Neisseria meningitidis:* Probable pathogen in two related cases of urethritis, epididymitis, and acute pelvic inflammatory disease. *JAMA* 242:1653, 1979.
100 Hagman M et al: *Neisseria meningitidis* in specimens from ureogenital sites: Is increased awareness necessary? *Sex Trans Dis* 18:228, 1991.
101 Conde-Glez CJ, Claderon E: Urogenital infection due to meningococcus in men and women. *Sex Transm Dis* 18:72, 1991.
102 Danielsson D, Johannisson G: Culture diagnosis of gonorrhea: A comparison of the yield with selective and non-selective gonococcal culture media inoculated in the clinic and after treatment of specimens. *Acta Derm Venereol (Stockh)* 53:75, 1973.
103 Judson FN, Werness BA: Combining cervical and anal-canal specimens for gonorrhea on a single culture plate. *J Clin Microbiol* 12: 216, 1980.
104 McMillan A, Young H: Gonorrhea in the homosexual man: Frequency of infection by culture site. *Sex Transm Dis* 5:146, 1978.
105 Windall JJ et al: Inhibitory effects of vancomycin on *Neisseria gonorrhoeae* in Thayer-Martin medium. *J Infect Dis* 142:775, 1980.
106 Rothenberg RB et al: Efficacy of selected diagnostic tests for sexually transmitted diseases. *JAMA* 235:49, 1976.
107 Wald ER: Diagnosis by Gram stain in the female adolescent. *Am J Dis Child* 131:1094, 1977.
108 William DC et al: The utility of anoscopy in the rapid diagnosis of symptomatic anorectal gonorrhea in men. *Sex Transm Dis* 8:16, 1981.
109 Deheragoda P: Diagnosis of rectal gonorrhea by blind anorectal swabs compared with direct vision swabs taken via a proctoscope. *Br J Vener Dis* 53:311, 1977.
110 Limberger RJ et al: Evaluation of culture and the Gen-Probe Pace 2 assay for detection of *Neisseria gonorrhoeae* and *Chlamydia trachomatis* in endocervical specimens transported to a state health laboratory. *J Clin Microbiol* 30:1662, 1992.
111 Panke ES et al: Comparison of Gen-Prove DNA probe test and culture for the detection of *N. gonorrhoeae* in endocervical specimens. *J Clin Microbiol* 29:883, 1991.
112 Granato PA, Franz MR: Evaluation of a prototype DNA probe test for the noncultural diagnosis of gonorrhea. *J Clin Microbiol* 17:632, 1989.
113 Hale YM et al: Evaluation of the Pace 2 *Neisseria gonorrhoeae* assay by three public health laboratories. *J Clin Microbiol* 31:451, 1993.
114 Ching S et al: Ligase chain reaction for detection of *Neisseria gonorrhoeae* in urogenital swabs. *J Clin Microbiol* 33:3111, 1995.
115 Smith KR et al: Evaluation of ligase chain reaction for use with urine for identification of *Neisseria gonorrhoeae* in females attending a sexually transmitted disease clinic. *J Clin Microbiol* 33:455, 1995.
116 Thin RNT et al: Direct and delayed methods of immunofluorescent diagnosis of gonorrhea in women. *Br J Vener Dis* 47:27, 1970.
117 Murray ES et al: New options for diagnosis and control of gonorrheal urethritis in males using uncentrifuged first voided urine (FVU) as a specimen for culture. *Am J Public Health* 69:596, 1979.
118 Luciano AA, Grubin L: Gonorrhea screening: Comparison of three techniques. *JAMA* 243:680, 1980.
119 McCutchan JA et al: Role of urinary solutes in natural immunity to gonorrhea. *Infect Immun* 15:149, 1977.
120 Ris HW, Dodge RW: Gonorrhea in adolescent girls in a closed population: Prevalence, diagnosis and treatment. *Am J Dis Child* 123: 185, 1972.
121 McCormack WM et al: Evaluation of the vaginal tampon as a means of obtaining cultures for *Neisseria gonorrhoeae*. *J Infect Dis* 128:129, 1973.
122 Sandstrom E, Danielsson D: A survey of gonococcal serology, in *Genital Infections and Their Complications*, D Danielsson et al (eds). Stockholm, Almqvist and Wiksell, 1975, p 253.
123 Holmes KK et al: Is serology useful in gonorrhea? A critical analysis of factors influencing serodiagnosis, in *Immunobiology of Neisseria gonorrhoeae*, GF Brooks et al (eds). Washington, American Society for Microbiology, 1978, p 370.
124 Dans PE et al: Gonococcal serology: How soon, how useful and how much? *J Infect Dis* 135:330, 1977.
125 Handsfield HH et al: Evaluation of new anti-infective drugs for the treatment of uncomplicated gonorrhea in adults and adolescents. *Clin Infect Dis* 15:(suppl 1):S123, 1992.
126 Mahoney JF et al: The use of penicillin sodium in the treatment of sulfonamide-resistant gonorrhea in men: A preliminary report. *Am J Gonorr Vener Dis* 27:525, 1943.
127 Martin JE et al: Comparative study of gonococcal susceptibility to penicillin in the United States, 1955–1969. *J Infect Dis* 122:459, 1970.
128 Sparling PF: Antibiotic resistance in the gonococcus, in *The Gonococcus*, RB Roberts (ed). New York, Wiley, 1978, p 111.
129 Phillips I: Beta-lactamase producing, penicillin-resistant gonococcus. *Lancet* 2:656, 1976.
130 Centers for Disease Control: Tetracycline-resistant *Neisseria gonorrhoeae*—Georgia, Pennsylvania, New Hampshire. *MMWR* 34: 563, 1985.
131 Boslego JW et al: Effect of spectinomycin use on the prevalence of spectinomycin-resistant and of penicillinase-producing *Neisseria gonorrhoeae*. *N Engl J Med* 317:272, 1987.
132 Ison CA et al: Spectinomycin-resistant gonococci. *Br Med J* 287: 1827, 1983.
133 Ashford WA et al: Spectinomycin-resistant penicillinase producing *Neisseria gonorrhoeae*. *Lancet* 2:1035, 1981.
134 Gordon SM et al: The emergence of *Neisseria gonorrhoeae* with decreased susceptibility to ciprofloxacin in Cleveland, Ohio: Epidemiology and risk factors. *Ann Intern Med* 125:465, 1996.
135 Centers for Disease Control: Sentinel surveillance system for antimicrobial resistance in clinical isolates of *Neisseria gonorrhoeae*. *MMWR* 36:585, 1987.

136 Fox KK et al. Antimicrobial resistance in *Neisseria gonorrhoeae* in the United States 1988–1994: The emergence of decreased susceptibility to fluoroquinolenes. *J Infect Dis* (*in press*).
137 Handsfield HH, Whittington WL: Antibiotic-resistant *Neisseria gonorrhoeae*: The calm before the storm? editorial. *Ann Intern Med* 125: 507, 1996.
138 Jaffe HW et al: Pharmacokinetic determinants of penicillin cure of gonococcal urethritis. *Antimicrob Agents Chemother* 15:587, 1979.
138a Peterman TA et al: Incubating syphilis in patients treated for gonorrhea: A comparison of treatment regimens. *J Infect Dis* 170:689, 1994.
139 Stamm WE et al: Effect of treatment regimens for *Neisseria gonorrhoeae* on simultaneous infections with *Chlamydia trachomatis*. *N Engl J Med* 310:545, 1984.
140 Centers for Disease Control: 1993 Sexually transmitted diseases guidelines. *MMWR* 42(RR-14):57, 1993.
141 Moran JS, Levine WC: Drugs of choice for the treatment of uncomplicated gonococcal infections. *Clin Infect Dis* 20(suppl 1):S47, 1995.
142 Handsfield HH, Hook EW III: Ceftriaxone for treatment of uncomplicated gonorrhea: Routine use of a single 125 mg dose in a sexually transmitted disease clinic. *Sex Transm Dis* 14:227, 1987.
143 Judson FN et al: Comparative study of ceftriaxone and spectinomycin for treatment of pharyngeal and anorectal gonorrhea. *JAMA* 253: 1417, 1985.
144 Crider SR et al: Treatment of penicillin-resistant *Neisseria gonorrhoeae* with oral norfloxacin. *N Engl J Med* 311:137, 1984.
145 Dallabetta GA, Hook EW III: Treatment of sexually transmitted diseases with quinolone antimicrobial agents, in *Quinolone Antimicrobial Agents,* JS Wolfson, DC Hooper (eds). Washington, American Society for Microbiology, 1989, p 125.
146 Joyce MP et al: In vitro sensitivity of *Neisseria gonorrhoeae* to quinolone antibiotics in the Republic of the Philippines, abstracted (no El 9), in *Abstracts of the Sixth International Pathogenic Neisseria Conference, Pine Mountain, Georgia,* 1988.
147 Centers for Disease Control: Fluoroquinolone resistance in *Neisseria gonorrhoeae*. *MMWR* 44:761, 1995.
148 Morse SA et al: Gonococcal strains from homosexual men have outer membranes with reduced permeability to hydrophobic molecules. *Infect Immun* 37:432, 1982.
149 Kraus SJ: Incidence and therapy of gonococcal pharyngitis. *Sex Transm Dis* 6(suppl):143, 1979.
150 Handsfield HH et al: Multicenter trial of single-dose azithromycin vs. ceftriaxone in the treatment of uncomplicated gonorrhea. *Sex Transm Dis* 21:107, 1994.
151 Hart G: Epidemiologic treatment for syphilis and gonorrhea. *Sex Transm Dis* 7:149, 1980.
152 Judson FN, Maltz AB: A rational basis for the epidemiologic treatment of gonorrhea in a clinic for sexually transmitted diseases. *Sex Transm Dis* 5:89, 1978.
153 Barlow D: The condom and gonorrhea. *Lancet* 2:811, 1977.
154 Stone KM et al: Personal protection against sexually transmitted diseases. *Am J Obstet Gynecol* 155:180, 1986.

Chapter 33

Biology of *Treponema pallidum*

Lola V. Stamm

CLASSIFICATION

Organisms of the genus *Treponema* are members of the order Spirochaetales, which contains two additional genera (*Borrelia* and *Leptospira*) of spiral-shaped pathogenic bacteria.[1] Treponemal species of public health significance include *Treponema pallidum* subspecies *pallidum* (agent of venereal syphilis), *T. pallidum* subspecies *pertenue* (agent of yaws), *T. pallidum* subspecies *endemicum* (agent of endemic syphilis), and *T. carateum* (agent of pinta). The *T. pallidum* subspecies are virtually identical based on their morphology, antigenic properties, and DNA homology. However, they exhibit differences in their geographic distribution, mode and severity of infection, and infectivity for different laboratory animals.[1] None of these spirochetes has been cultivated in vitro for sustained time periods.

Additional treponemal species are found in the human oral cavity, gastrointestinal tract, and genital tract.[1] In contrast to the *T. pallidum* subspecies, most of these spirochetes are cultivable and of limited pathogenic potential. However, *T. denticola,* an oral treponeme, is associated with periodontal disease.[2] Furthermore, a noncultivable pathogen-related oral spirochete (PROS) that is closely related antigenically to *T. pallidum* subspecies *pallidum* is associated with chronic periodontitis and acute necrotizing ulcerative gingivitis.[3] Data obtained from genomic DNA[4,5] and 16S rRNA[6] sequencing indicate that there is a closer relationship between *T. pallidum* subspecies *pallidum* and certain cultivable treponemes, such as *T. denticola,* than previously proposed based on DNA-DNA hybridization studies and percentage GC base composition.[7]

EPIDEMIOLOGY

T. pallidum subspecies *pallidum* was identified in 1905 by Schaudinn and Hoffman.[1] It is an obligate human parasite. There are no reservoirs for this organism in animals or the environment. Nearly all cases of venereal syphilis (hereafter referred to as syphilis) are acquired by direct sexual contact with lesions of an individual who has active primary or secondary syphilis. Transmission of syphilis occurs in approximately one-half of such contacts. Syphilis can be transmitted congenitally from an infected mother by transplacental passage of treponemes to the fetus. Less common modes of syphilis transmission include blood-borne (due to blood transfusion or sharing of needles), nonsexual personal contact, and accidental direct inoculation.

Syphilis is distributed worldwide but is particularly problematic in developing countries, where it is a leading cause of genital ulcer disease.[8] Historically, syphilis was distributed throughout the United States, but rates declined rapidly during the late 1940s after the introduction of penicillin therapy and broad-based public health programs. However, in the late 1980s and early 1990s, syphilis reemerged and has become focused in the urban and rural southern region of the United States and in large urban centers outside the South.[9,10] The demographics of syphilis also changed during this time period from a disease of white homosexual males to one that predominately affects heterosexual African-Americans.[9] The current distribution of syphilis by age shows that most cases are found in persons in their early 20s to early 30s.[9] This is in contrast to other bacterial sexually transmitted diseases that usually affect teens and young adults of less than 25 years of age.

STRUCTURE

T. pallidum subspecies *pallidum* is 6 to 20 μm in length with a diameter of 0.10 to 0.18 μm, which places it below the resolution of the light microscope.[1] The unstained organism can be visualized by dark-field or phase-contrast microscopy. Although *T. pallidum* subspecies *pallidum* stains poorly with aniline dyes, it can be stained by silver impregnation methods. Electron microscopy (EM) has proven useful for special clinical and investigational studies. *T. pallidum* subspecies *pallidum* has regular tight spirals with a coil wavelength of 1.1 μm and an amplitude of 0.2 to 0.3 μm. In contrast to some previous reports, this spirochete lacks a capsule.[11] Like gram-negative bacteria, *T. pallidum* subspecies *pallidum* has an outer membrane,[12–14] an inner (cytoplasmic) membrane, and a thin cell wall composed of peptidoglycan[15] (Fig. 33-1). However, unlike gram-negative bacteria, the *T. pallidum* subspecies *pallidum* outer membrane lacks lipopolysaccharide[16] and is more susceptible to disruption by routine physical manipulation of the organism (centrifugation, washing, in vitro incubation) and detergent treatment.[17–19] Additionally, two groups of investigators have shown by freeze-fracture EM that the *T. pallidum* subspecies *pallidum* outer membrane contains only rare integral membrane proteins, some of which are surface exposed.[20–22] These transmembrane proteins are referred to as treponemal rare outer membrane proteins (TROMPs) (Fig. 33-2). The relatively uniform size of the TROMP particles prompted initial speculation that they might represent only one species of protein.[20,21] However, it seems likely that *T. pallidum* subspecies *pallidum* must synthesize more than one species of TROMP in order to facilitate functions associated with survival and dissemination in the host. Interestingly, four to six putative TROMPs have been identified in *T. pallidum* subspecies *pallidum* outer membranes that were isolated by two different techniques.[13,14] One of these proteins (TROMP1) appears to have porin activity.[23] However, analysis of the *tromp1* gene indicates that it is part of a complex operon encoding a putative ATP-binding cassette (ABC) transport system.[5,23a]

T. pallidum subspecies *pallidum* is actively motile by virtue of flagella that are located in the periplasmic space.[24,25] The spiral shape of the organism and the unique location of the flagella enable this spirochete to retain motility in viscous fluids such as those found in the joint, eye, and extracellular matrix of the skin.[24] Three periplasmic flagella originate at each end of the treponemal cell and entwine the protoplasmic cylinder extending toward the cell center. The periplasmic flagella are composed of a hook-basal body complex and a flagellar filament made up of multiple proteins that are arranged into an outer sheath and a central core.[24,25] Genes encoding the protein subunits of the flagellar filament have been cloned and sequenced.[5,25] A large operon *(fla)* containing at least 17 genes encoding proteins associated with flagellar structure, assembly, and function has been identified recently.[4,26] The dedication of a significant portion of the *T. pallidum* subspecies *pallidum* genetic content to motility-related genes is in accordance with the important role that motility plays in invasion and dissemination.[5] *T. pallidum* subspecies *pallidum* also contains cytoplasmic filaments that are ribbonlike structures (7.0 to 7.5 nm wide) of unknown function that run the length of the organism.[5] An

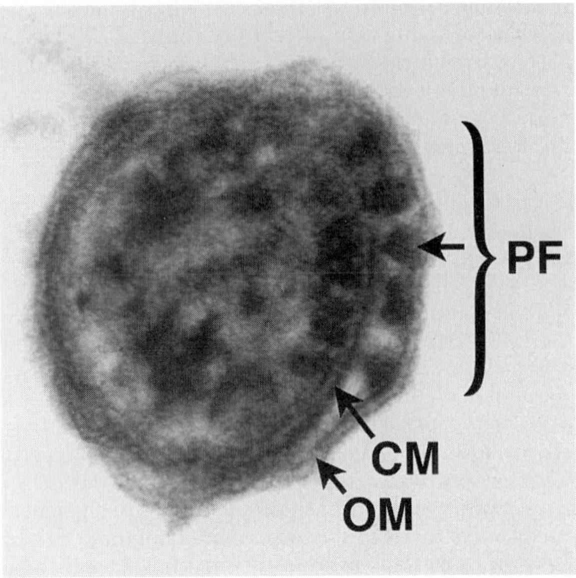

Fig. 33-1. Cross section of *T. pallidum* subspecies *pallidum* showing the outer membrane *(OM)*, periplasmic flagella *(PF)*, and cytoplasmic membrane *(CM)*. *(Courtesy of Steven J. Norris.)*

array of four to six cytoplasmic filaments lies just beneath the inner membrane and parallel to the periplasmic flagella.

CULTIVATION AND METABOLISM

T. pallidum subspecies *pallidum* remains one of the few pathogens of humans that has not been cultivated in vitro for extended time periods. For propagation, antigen preparation, and experimental studies, this spirochete is grown in rabbit testicles.[27] Limited growth of *T. pallidum* subspecies *pallidum* has been obtained in a tissue-culture monolayer of Sf1Ep cottontail rabbit epithelial cells under microaerobic conditions (1.5% O_2) at 34 to 35°C.[28,29] The generation time of 30 to 33 hours is similar to that estimated for organisms growing in vivo. *T. pallidum* subspecies *pallidum* is very sensitive to environmental conditions (temperature, O_2, pH) and to physical and chemical agents.

The small size of the single, circular chromosome (1000 kb) and the fastidious nature of *T. pallidum* subspecies *pallidum* suggest that this spirochete has metabolic limitations.[5,25] Due to its noncultivable nature and lack of genetic systems, knowledge of the metabolism of this bacterium is limited. Previous studies have shown that *T. pallidum* subspecies *pallidum* is capable of DNA, RNA, and protein synthesis.[30] Glucose is the major carbon and energy source, although pyruvate can be metabolized.[30] *T. pallidum* subspecies *pallidum* has an active glycolytic pathway but appears to lack a complete Krebs cycle.[30]

Much of what has been learned recently about the metabolism of *T. pallidum* subspecies *pallidum* has resulted from the cloning and expression of treponemal genes in *Escherichia coli.* For example, treponemal genes encoding the three enzymes necessary for proline biosynthesis have been identified.[31,32] An operon encoding homologues of proteins that facilitate high-affinity transport of glucose has been cloned and characterized.[33,34] The presence of treponemal genes encoding homologues of chemotaxis proteins (CheA, CheW, CheY) strongly suggests that *T. pallidum* subspecies *pallidum* has the ability to sense and respond to gradients of chemicals, such as nutrients, present in host tissues.[35] The results of a project to sequence the whole genome of *T. pallidum* subspecies *pallidum* will undoubtedly contribute useful information regarding the total metabolic capabilities of this spirochete and ultimately may provide clues to its in vitro cultivation.[5]

ANIMAL MODELS

Several animal models of *T. pallidum* subspecies *pallidum* infection have been investigated. With the exception of primates, infection of rabbits results in a pattern of infection and pathogenesis that is most similar to that of humans. The primary chancre, obtained following intradermal inoculation of rabbits with *T. pallidum* subspecies *pallidum,* closely resembles the lesion found in humans.[27] Additionally, treponemes disseminate and persist at other sites, despite the clearance of most organisms at the primary site. However, secondary lesions do not occur in older adult rabbits, and late manifestations have not been documented. Inbred hamsters[27,36] and guinea pigs[37] also have been used as animal models for syphilis. *T. pallidum* subspecies *pallidum* usually does not cause cutaneous lesions in these animal species, although systemic infection, lymphadenopathy, and humoral and cellular responses occur. However, since these animals are more susceptible

Fig. 33-2. Membrane architecture of *T. pallidum* subspecies *pallidum,* as demonstrated by freeze-fracture electron microscopy. The concave and convex outer membrane fracture *(OMF)* faces, corresponding to the outer and inner leaflets of the outer membrane, respectively, contain a very low concentration of intramembranous particles *(arrowheads)* that represent the TROMPs. In contrast, the convex inner membrane fracture *(IMF)* face, corresponding to the inner leaflet of the inner membrane, has a high concentration of intramembranous particles. *(Courtesy of Eldon M. Walker.)*

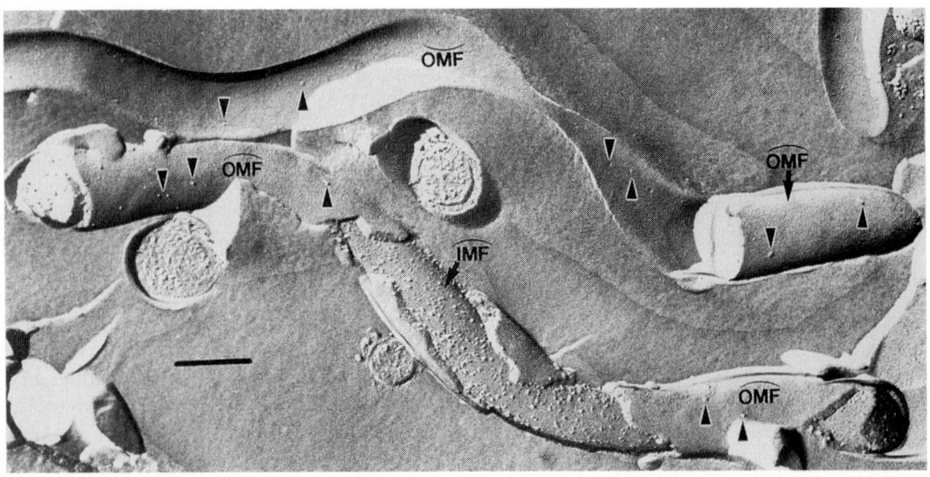

to infection with *T. pallidum* subspecies *endemicum* and *T. pallidum* subspecies *pertenue,* they have proven useful as models for endemic syphilis and yaws, respectively.[27,38]

PATHOGENESIS AND NATURAL COURSE OF UNTREATED SYPHILIS

PRIMARY STAGE

Syphilis is a chronic, systemic infection characterized by periods of active clinical disease that are interrupted by periods of latency. At this juncture, the factors involved in the pathogenesis of syphilis are incompletely understood. Following inoculation and penetration of mucosal surfaces or abraded skin, *T. pallidum* subspecies *pallidum* attaches to host cells and initiates multiplication. Treponemes are known to adhere to a variety of cell types,[39,40] putatively due to interaction with fibronectin[41–43] or other host cell receptors.[41] This initial attachment and multiplication are likely critical to the establishment of infection. Within a few hours, significant numbers of treponemes depart from the local site and are carried to the regional lymph nodes. The organisms disseminate to several organs and tissues via the circulation and exit through the tight junctions of vascular endothelial cells aided by their corkscrew motility.[44] The primary lesion develops at the site of inoculation 2 to 6 weeks after infection. The median incubation period (3 weeks) in humans suggests the introduction of an average inoculum of 500 to 1000 organisms.[45] The primary lesion begins as a painless indurated papule. The surface necroses to yield a hard-based, well-circumscribed, ulcerated lesion (chancre) that is teeming with infectious treponemes. Histopathologically, the chancre is characterized by an intense perivascular infiltration of plasma cells, lymphocytes (CD4+ and CD8+), and histiocytes with capillary endothelial proliferation, as well as eventual obliterative endarteritis.[45,46] *T. pallidum* subspecies *pallidum* is present in spaces between epithelial cells and within the invaginations or phagosomes of epithelial cells, fibroblasts, plasma cells, and the endothelial cells of small capillaries, within lymphatic channels, and in the regional lymph nodes. Lesion resolution and clearance of treponemes are largely attributed to cell-mediated immune mechanisms involving phagocytosis of treponemes by macrophages that have been activated by lymphokines released from antigen-specific sensitized T cells.[47] Van Voorhis et al.[47] recently have demonstrated that primary (and secondary) syphilitic lesions contain mRNA for interleukin 2 (IL-2), interferon-γ (IFN-γ), IL-12p40, and IL-10. These findings are consistent with a Th_1-predominant local cellular response that leads to macrophage activation resulting in clearance of treponemes. Additionally, in vitro data indicate that treponemal integral membrane lipoproteins activate monocytes-macrophages, B cells, and endothelial cells, suggesting that these molecules contribute to the immunopathogenesis of syphilis by mediating local inflammatory changes.[48–50] Clearance of treponemes is also enhanced by low levels of opsonic antibodies that serve to promote both ingestion and killing of organisms by macrophages.[51,52] Although the targets of opsonic antibodies have not been identified definitively, they appear to be pathogen-specific treponemal antigens.[53]

Despite the destruction of billions of treponemes by host immune responses, some organisms survive to cause chronic infection. Several mechanisms have been proposed for treponemal persistence: (1) an antigenically inert treponemal cell surface resulting from (a) a coat of host serum proteins[54] or (b) a paucity of outer membrane proteins,[20,21] (2) intracellular localization[55] or residence of treponemes within an immunoprotective niche,[56] (3) a subpopulation of treponemes resistant to phagocytosis,[57] and (4) premature downregulation of the local host immune response.[58] The mechanism with the most supportive data is that of the unique treponemal cell surface that appears to present few targets for the host immune response due to the paucity of the TROMPs.[20,21,59–61]

SECONDARY STAGE

Secondary syphilis represents the disseminated stage of disease that results from the multiplication and dissemination of treponemes throughout the body. *T. pallidum* subspecies *pallidum* is found in many different tissues despite the presence of high levels of antitreponemal antibodies.[62–64] The secondary stage occurs simultaneously with or up to 6 months after the healing of the primary lesion. It is characterized by a variety of manifestations that may include malaise, low-grade fever, headache, generalized lymphadenopathy, a generalized rash with lesions on the palms and soles, mucous patches in the oral cavity or genital tract, condylomata lata (wartlike lesions) in moist intertriginous regions, and alopecia. Deposition of immune complexes in the skin and kidneys may be involved in the dermal neutrophilic vascular reaction and glomerulonephritis that is seen at this stage.[65,66] The secondary stage lasts for several weeks or months and may relapse in approximately 25 percent of untreated patients. Pregnant women in the secondary stage of syphilis can infect the fetus in utero via transplacental passage of infectious treponemes.

LATENCY

Secondary lesions subside within a few weeks due to macrophage-mediated bacterial clearance and the treponemicidal activity of complement-dependent antibody, presumably directed against TROMPs.[59,61] While clinical symptoms are no longer apparent, serologic tests for detection of specific antibodies to *T. pallidum* subspecies *pallidum* remain positive, indicating that organisms are still present, particularly in the spleen and lymph nodes. This stage is termed latency. Early latent syphilis encompasses the first year of infection. Late latent syphilis, beginning 1 year after infection, is associated with relative immunity to relapse and increasing resistance to reinfection with the homologous treponemal strain. *T. pallidum* subspecies *pallidum* may still intermittently seed the bloodstream, since transfusion syphilis has been transmitted from patients with latent syphilis of many years' duration. Pregnant women with latent syphilis may infect the fetus in utero. However, the absence of exposed mucosal or genital lesions usually precludes venereal transmission. Latency can last for many years. Approximately two-thirds of untreated patients with latent syphilis will remain in this stage for the remainder of their lives. The occurrence of spontaneous cures is now doubtful.

TERTIARY STAGE

The tertiary or late stage of syphilis occurs in approximately one-third of untreated patients, presumably due to the waning of the host immune response. This stage may occur from months to many years after the initiation of latency. Treponemes invade the central nervous system (CNS), cardiovascular system, eyes, skin, and other internal organs, producing damage by virtue of their invasive properties and inflammation-provoking cellular components (lipoproteins) and by evoking the host delayed-type hypersensitivity response (DTH). Cardiovascular problems are usually due to local inflammation induced by the multiplication of treponemes within the wall of the aorta, which produces complications such as thoracic aortic aneurysm, aortitis, and/or aortic endocarditis. Neurosyphilis may be symptomatic or asymptomatic. The major clinical categories of symptomatic neurosyphilis are meningeal, meningovascular, and parenchymatous syphilis. The last category includes general paresis (destruction of brain parenchyma), tabes dorsalis (destruction of dorsal roots of the spinal column), or both (taboparesis). Gummas, destructive lesions that usually occur in skin, bones, or viscera, are likely to be the result of the DTH response to treponemal antigens. Gummas may occur singly or multiply and may vary in size from microscopic defects to large tumorlike masses. There are usually few treponemes present in these lesions. During the tertiary stage, transmission of syphilis by sexual contact does not occur; transmission of congenital syphilis rarely occurs.

SYPHILIS AND HUMAN IMMUNODEFICIENCY VIRUS (HIV)

There is a strong epidemiologic association between syphilis and HIV infection that represents more than concomitant transmission of sexually transmitted diseases.[67] Syphilis and other sexually transmitted diseases that produce genital lesions or evoke an inflammatory response are important risk factors for the acquisition and transmission of HIV.[68,69] Three features of the syphilitic chancre have been proposed to contribute to these processes: (1) the breach of the epithelial barrier creates a portal of entry (or exit) for HIV, (2) the influx of large numbers of macrophages and T cells provides an environment enriched with receptors for HIV, and (3) the production of cytokines by macrophages stimulated by treponemal lipoproteins may enhance HIV replication.[50]

Several studies have shown that clinical manifestations of syphilis may be altered in patients with concurrent HIV infection.[70,71] Although early CNS invasion is not more likely, such patients more often develop syphilitic meningitis, meningovasculitis, and ocular syphilis, even after therapy with intramuscular benzathine penicillin for early syphilis.[70] There is also a higher frequency of ulcerating secondary syphilis (often diagnosed in Europe as "malignant syphilis") that is characterized by rupialike ulcerating skin lesions and general symptoms such as severe fever and weakness.[67] The higher frequency of ulcerating secondary syphilis is hypothesized to be the consequence of immunodeficiency. The low mean CD4+ cell count found in this group of patients precludes the host's ability to clear treponemes from skin lesions or the CNS. While atypical serologic reactions have been observed in HIV-infected patients who have concurrent syphilis, the results of treponemal and nontreponemal serologic tests for syphilis are usually accurate for the majority of such patients.[70]

IMMUNITY AND VACCINATION

It is generally accepted that some degree of immunity to exogenous reinfection (so-called chancre immunity) eventually develops in humans who are infected with syphilis. This immunity is not complete, since it is incapable of eradicating the ongoing infection. In studies performed by Magnuson et al.[72] at Sing Sing Prison, male volunteers were inoculated intradermally with 10^5 virulent *T. pallidum* subspecies *pallidum* at a single site on the forearm. Control subjects with no prior history of syphilis developed dark-field-positive skin lesions at the inoculation site. Five subjects with previously untreated late latent syphilis did not develop skin lesions or show changes in serologic tests for syphilis (STS). In contrast, all 11 subjects with a previous history of early (primary or secondary) treated syphilis developed skin lesions and showed increased reactivity in STS. Among 26 subjects with previously treated latent syphilis, 10 developed skin lesions (1 dark-field-positive, 9 dark-field-negative) and showed increased reactivity in STS, 3 developed dark-field-negative skin lesions not associated with changes in STS, and 13 did not develop any skin lesions or changes in STS. The results of this study indicate that a long-term syphilis infection is required to produce immunity to exogenous reinfection and that immunity wanes some time following effective antimicrobial therapy.

Studies using the rabbit model of syphilis have confirmed the results observed with human subjects. Complete resistance to exogenous reinfection develops only after 3 to 6 months of prior infection.[27,36] Lewinski et al.[61] showed a positive correlation between immunity to exogenous reinfection and the presence of complement-dependent treponemicidal antibody in the sera of rabbits that were infected with *T. pallidum* subspecies *pallidum* for various time periods and then cured with penicillin prior to challenge. Their data suggest that the treponemicidal antibody measured by the "washed killing" assay is directed against the TROMPs and that the rarity of these proteins accounts for the slow mobilization of functional immune responses.

Both humoral and cell-mediated immune mechanisms play a role in the development of immunity to exogenous reinfection by *T. pallidum* subspecies *pallidum*. Previous studies have shown that passive transfer of serum or IgG from immune rabbits to naive recipient rabbits partially protects the latter animals when they are inoculated intradermally with *T. pallidum* subspecies *pallidum*.[73–77] Furthermore, serum or IgG from immune rabbits blocks attachment to and invasion of tissue-culture monolayer cells by treponemes,[39,40,44] promotes in vitro phagocytosis and killing of treponemes by macrophages,[51–53] and mediates complement-dependent treponemicidal activity.[59,61] Cellular immunity is of major importance in the healing of early lesions and the control of infection. Specifically sensitized T cells develop early in the course of infection. Clearance of treponemes is mediated by activated macrophages in conjunction with opsonic antibody.[8,53] Partial protection of rabbits from intradermal infection with *T. pallidum* subspecies *pallidum* has been achieved by transfer of lymphocytes from immune rabbits.[78]

The reemergence of syphilis in the United States and the recognition that syphilis is a risk factor for the acquisition and transmission of HIV infection have prompted renewed interest in a syphilis vaccine.[79] Miller[80] successfully immunized rabbits with unwashed cells of γ-irradiated *T. pallidum* subspecies *pallidum* (Nichols strain). The regimen required multiple immunizations over a course of 37 weeks using a total inoculum of 3.71×10^9 treponemes. Complete immunity to infection following intradermal challenge with the homologous strain persisted for 1 year. Due to the requirement for multiple doses of whole cells, this approach is impractical for immunization of humans. Recent efforts to develop a syphilis vaccine have focused on the use of recombinant-produced treponemal antigens.[25] Although most of these antigens were thought to be cell surface proteins, subsequent studies showed that they are subsurface and are unlikely to be primary targets of a host treponemicidal response.[60] While immunization with some of these proteins did alter the course of syphilis in the rabbit model, none elicited an immune response that conferred solid immunity to infection.[25]

Several investigators have hypothesized that an immune response to the TROMPs elicited by vaccination may prevent infection by *T. pallidum* subspecies *pallidum*.[53,60,61] Since the identities of the TROMPs remain in question, the functions of these proteins are unknown. Certain of the TROMPs likely mediate attachment to and invasion of host cells, acquisition of nutrients, and stabilization of cell structure. An immune response that would abrogate the ability of treponemes to accomplish requisite steps prior to early dissemination may prevent the establishment of infection. Data provided from the whole-genome sequencing project for *T. pallidum* subspecies *pallidum* should provide information regarding the identities and potential functions of the TROMPs.[5] Studies of the vaccinogenic potential of the TROMPs are contingent on obtaining greater quantities of these proteins via recombinant DNA technology. Until an effective vaccine can be developed, the prevention of syphilis will depend on the use of condoms and the detection and treatment of infected individuals.[45]

References

1 Smibert RM: Genus III: Treponema Schaudinn 1905, 1728[AL], in *Bergey's Manual of Systematic Bacteriology,* vol 1, Kreig NR, Holt JG (eds). Baltimore, Williams & Williams, 1984, pp 49–57.

2 Simonson LG et al: Quantitative relationship of *Treponema denticola* to severity of periodontal disease. *Infect Immun* 56:726, 1988.

3 Riviere GR et al: Identification of spirochetes related to *Treponema pallidum* in necrotizing ulcerative gingivitis and chronic periodontitis. *N Engl J Med* 325:539, 1991.

4 Limberger RJ et al: Organization, transcription and expression of the 5′ region of the *fla* operon of *Treponema phagedenis* and *Treponema pallidum. J Bacteriol* 178:4628, 1996.

5 Fraser CM et al: Complete genome sequence of *Treponema pallidum,* the syphilis spirochete. *Science* 281:375, 1998.

6 Paster BJ et al: Phylogenetic analysis of spirochetes. *J Bacteriol* 173: 6101, 1991.

7 Miao RM, Fieldsteel AH: Genetics of *Treponema:* Relationship between *Treponema pallidum* and five cultivable treponemes. *J Bacteriol* 133:101, 1978.

8 Lukehart SA: Immunology and pathogenesis of syphilis, in *Advances in Host Defense Mechanisms,* vol 8: *Sexually Transmitted Diseases,* Quinn TC, Gallin JI, Fauci AS (eds): New York, Raven Press, 1992, pp 141–163.

9 Nakashima AK et al: Epidemiology of syphilis in the United States, 1941–1993. *Sex Transm Dis* 23:16, 1996.

10 Thomas JC et al: Syphilis in the South: Rural rates surpass urban rates in North Carolina. *Am J Public Health* 85:1119, 1995.

11 Strugnell RA et al: *Treponema pallidum* does not synthesise in vitro a capsule containing glycosaminoglycans or proteoglycans. *Br J Vener Dis* 60:75, 1984.

12 Johnson RC, Ritzi DM, Livermore BP: Outer envelope of virulent *Treponema pallidum. Infect Immun* 8:294, 1973.

13 Blanco DR et al: Isolation of the outer membranes from *Treponema pallidum* and *Treponema vincentii. J Bacteriol* 176:6088, 1994.

14 Radolf JD et al: Characterization of outer membranes isolated from *Treponema pallidum,* the syphilis spirochete. *Infect Immun* 63:4244, 1995.

15 Radolf JD et al: Penicillin-binding proteins and peptidoglycan of *Treponema pallidum* subspecies *pallidum. Infect Immun* 56:1825, 1989.

16 Hardy PH Jr, Levin J: Lack of endotoxin in *Borrelia hispanica* and *Treponema pallidum. Proc Soc Exp Biol Med* 174:47, 1983.

17 Penn CW et al: The outer membrane of *Treponema pallidum:* Biological significance and biochemical properties. *J Gen Microbiol* 131: 2349, 1985.

18 Stamm LV et al: Changes in cell surface properties of *Treponema pallidum* that occur during in vitro incubation of freshly extracted organisms. *Infect Immun* 55:2255, 1987.

19 Cunningham TM et al: Selective release of the *Treponema pallidum* outer membrane and associated polypeptides with Triton X-114. *J Bacteriol* 170:5789, 1988.

20 Radolf JD et al: Outer membrane ultrastructure explains the limited antigenicity of virulent *Treponema pallidum. Proc Natl Acad Sci USA* 86:2051, 1989.

21 Walker EM et al: Demonstration of rare protein in the outer membrane of *Treponema pallidum* subspecies *pallidum* by freeze-fracture analysis. *J Bacteriol* 171:5005, 1989.

22 Bourell KW et al: *Treponema pallidum* rare outer membrane proteins: Analysis of mobility by freeze-fracture electron microscopy. *J Bacteriol* 176:1598, 1994.

23 Blanco DR et al: Porin activity and sequence analysis of a 31-kilodalton rare outer membrane protein (TROMP1). *J Bacteriol* 177: 3556, 1995.

23a Hardham JM et al: Identification and transcriptional analysis of a *Treponema pallidum* operon encoding a putative ABC transporter system, an iron-activated repressor protein homolog, and a glycolytic pathway enzyme homolog. *Gene* 197:47, 1997.

24 Charon NW et al: Spirochete chemotaxis, motility, and the structure of the spirochetal periplasmic flagella. *Res Microbiol* 143:597, 1992.

25 Norris SJ, *Treponema pallidum* Polypeptide Research Group: Polypeptides of *Treponema pallidum:* Progress toward understanding their structural, functional and immunologic roles. *Microbiol Rev* 57: 750, 1993.

26 Hardham JM et al: Identification and sequences of the *Treponema pallidum fliM′, fliY, fliP, fliQ, fliR,* and *flhB′* genes. *Gene* 166:57, 1995.

27 Turner TB, Hollander DH: *Biology of the Treponematoses.* Geneva, World Health Organization, 1957.

28 Fieldsteel AH et al: Cultivation of virulent *Treponema pallidum* in tissue culture. *Infect Immun* 32:908, 1981.

29 Cox DL: Culture of *Treponema pallidum. Methods Enzymol* 236: 390, 1994.

30 Cox CD: Metabolic activities, in *Pathogenesis and Immunology of Treponemal Infection,* Schell RF, Musher DM (eds). New York, Marcel Dekker, 1983, chap 4, pp 57–70.

31 Gherardini FC et al: Complementation of an *Escherichia coli proC* mutation by a gene cloned from *Treponema pallidum. J Bacteriol* 172:2996, 1990.

32 Stamm LV, Barnes NY: Nucleotide sequences of the *proA* and *proB* genes of *Treponema pallidum,* the syphilis agent. *DNA Sequence* 8: 63, 1997.

33 Stamm LV et al: Identification and sequences of the *Treponema pallidum mglA* and *mglC* genes. *DNA Sequence* 6:293, 1996.

34 Porcella SF et al: A *mgl*-like operon in *Treponema pallidum,* the syphilis spirochete. *Gene* 177:115, 1996.

35 Greene SG et al: Identification, sequences, and expression of *Treponema pallidum* chemotaxis genes. *DNA Sequence* 7:267, 1997.

36 Schell RF: Rabbit and hamster models of treponemal infection, in *Pathogenesis and Immunology of Treponemal Infection,* Schell RF, Musher DM (eds). New York, Marcel Dekker, 1983, chap 7, pp 121–135.

37 Wicher K, Wicher V: Experimental syphilis in the guinea pig. *Crit Rev Microbiol* 16:181, 1989.

38 Schell RF et al: LSH hamster model of syphilitic infection. *Infect Immun* 28:909, 1980.

39 Fitzgerald TJ et al: Characterization of the attachment of *Treponema pallidum* (Nichols strain) to cultured mammalian cells and the potential relationships of attachment to pathogenicity. *Infect Immun* 18:467, 1977.

40 Hayes NS et al: Parasitism by virulent *Treponema pallidum* of host cell surfaces. *Infect Immun* 17:174, 1977.

41 Fitzgerald TJ et al: Attachment of *Treponema pallidum* to fibronectin, laminin, collagen IV, and collagen I, and blockage of attachment by immune rabbit IgG. *Br J Venereal Dis* 60:357, 1984.

42 Baughn RE: Role of fibronectin in the pathogenesis of syphilis. *Rev Infect Dis* 9:S372, 1987.

43 Alderete JF et al: Identification of fibronectin as a receptor for bacterial cytoadherence. *Methods Enzymol* 236:318, 1994.

44 Thomas DD et al: *Treponema pallidum* invades intercellular junctions of endothelial cell monolayers. *Proc Natl Acad Sci USA* 85: 3608, 1988.

45 Lukehart SA, Holmes KK: Syphilis, in *Harrison's Principles of Inter-*

nal Medicine, 13th ed, Isselbacher KJ et al (eds). New York, McGraw-Hill, 1994, chap 133, pp 726–737.

46 Lukehart SA et al: Characterization of lymphocyte responsiveness in early experimental syphilis: II. Nature of cellular infiltration and *Treponema pallidum* distribution in testicular lesions. *J Immunol* 127:1361, 1980.

47 Van Voorhis WC et al: Primary and secondary syphilis lesions contain mRNA for Th1 cytokines. *J Infect Dis* 173:491, 1996.

48 Riley BS et al: Virulent *Treponema pallidum* activates human vascular endothelial cells. *J Infect Dis* 165:484, 1992.

49 Radolf JD et al: *Treponema pallidum* and *Borrelia burgdorferi* lipoproteins and synthetic lipopeptides activate monocytes/macrophages. *J Immunol* 154:2866, 1995.

50 Norgard MV et al: Activation of human monocytic cells by *Treponema pallidum* and *Borrelia burgdorferi* lipoproteins and synthetic lipopeptides proceeds via a pathway distinct from that of lipopolysaccharide but involves the transcriptional activator NF-kB. *Infect Immun* 64:3845, 1996.

51 Alder JD et al: Phagocytosis of opsonized *Treponema pallidum* subspecies *pallidum* proceeds slowly. *Infect Immun* 58:1167, 1990.

52 Baker-Zander SA, Lukehart SA: Macrophage-mediated killing of opsonized *Treponema pallidum. J Infect Dis* 165:69, 1992.

53 Shaffer JM et al: Opsonization of *Treponema pallidum* is mediated by immunogobulin G antibodies induced only by pathogenic treponemes. *Infect Immun* 61:781, 1993.

54 Alderete JF, Baseman JB: Surface-associated host proteins on virulent *Treponema pallidum. Infect Immun* 26:1048, 1979.

55 Sykes JA, Miller JN: Intracellular location of *Treponema pallidum* (Nichols strain) in the rabbit testis. *Infect Immun* 4:307, 1971.

56 Medici MA: The immunoprotective niche: A new pathogenic mechanism for syphilis, the systemic mycoses and other infectious diseases. *J Theor Biol* 36:617, 1972.

57 Lukehart SA et al: A subpopulation of *Treponema pallidum* is resistant to phagocytosis: Possible mechanisms of persistence. *J Infect Dis* 166:1449, 1992.

58 Fitzgerald TJ: The Th_1/Th_2-like switch in syphilitic infection: Is it detrimental? *Infect Immun* 60:3475, 1992.

59 Blanco DR et al: Complement activation limits the rate of in vitro treponemicidal activity and correlates with antibody-mediated aggregation of *Treponema pallidum* rare outer membrane protein. *J Immunol* 144:1914, 1990.

60 Radolf JD: Role of outer membrane architecture in immune evasion by *Treponema pallidum* and *Borrelia burgdorferi. Trends Microbiol* 2:307, 1994.

61 Lewinski MA et al: Treponemicidal antibody measured by the "washed-killing" assay correlates with immunity in experimental rabbit syphilis. *Sex Transm Dis* 22:31, 1995.

62 Hanff PA et al: Humoral immune response in human syphilis to polypeptides of *Treponema pallidum. J Immunol* 129:1287, 1982.

63 Baker-Zander SA et al: Antigens of *Treponema pallidum* recognized by IgG and IgM antibodies during syphilis in humans. *J Infect Dis* 151:264, 1985.

64 Stamm LV, Bassford PJ: Cellular and extracellular protein antigens of *Treponema pallidum* synthesized during in vitro incubation of freshly extracted organisms. *Infect Immun* 47:799, 1985.

65 Baughn RE et al: Characterization of the antigenic determinants host components in immune complexes from patients with secondary syphilis. *J Immunol* 136:1406, 1986.

66 Jorizzo JL et al: Role of circulating immune complexes in human secondary syphilis. *J Infect Dis* 153:1014, 1986.

67 Schöfer H et al: Active syphilis in HIV infection: A multicentre retrospective survey. *Genitourin Med* 72:176, 1996.

68 Quinn TC et al: The association of syphilis with risk of human immunodeficiency virus infection in patients attending sexually transmitted disease clinics. *Arch Intern Med* 150:1297, 1990.

69 Hutchinson CM et al: Characteristics of patients with syphilis attending Baltimore STD clinics: Multiple high-risk subgroups and interactions with human immunodeficiency virus infections. *Arch Intern Med* 151:511, 1991.

70 Marra CM: Syphilis and human immunodeficiency virus infection. *Semin Neurol* 12:43, 1992.

71 Flores JL: Syphilis: A tale of twisted treponemes. *West J Med* 163: 552, 1995.

72 Magnuson HJ et al: Inoculation syphilis in human volunteers. *Medicine* 35:33, 1956.

73 Turner TB et al: Effects of passive immunization on experimental syphilis in the rabbit. *Johns Hopkins Med J* 133:241, 1973.

74 Bishop NH, Miller JN: Humoral immunity in experimental syphilis: I. The demonstration of resistance conferred by passive immunization. *J Immunol* 117:191, 1976.

75 Weiser RS et al: Immunity to syphilis: Passive transfer in rabbits using serial doses of immune serum. *Infect Immun* 13:1402, 1976.

76 Titus RG, Weiser RS: Experimental syphilis in the rabbit: Passive transfer of immunity with immunoglobulin G from immune serum. *J Infect Dis* 140:904, 1979.

77 Blanco DR et al: Humoral immunity in experimental syphilis: The demonstration of IgG as a treponemicidal factor in immune rabbit serum. *J Immunol* 433:2693, 1984.

78 Schell RF et al: T-cell-mediated resistance, in *Pathogenesis and Immunology of Treponemal Infection,* Schell RF, Musher DM (eds). New York, Marcel Dekker, 1983, chap 17, pp 331–348.

79 Sparling PF et al: Vaccines for bacterial sexually transmitted infections: A realistic goal? *Proc Natl Acad Sci USA* 91:2456, 1994.

80 Miller JN: Immunity in experimental syphilis: VI. Successful vaccination of rabbits with *Treponema pallidum,* Nichols strain, attenuated by γ-irradiation. *J Immunol* 110:1206, 1973.

Chapter 34

Natural history of syphilis

P. Frederick Sparling

Know syphilis in all its manifestations and relations, and all other things clinical will be added unto you.

Sir William Osler, 1897

Syphilis is one of the most fascinating diseases of humans. Its remarkably variable and long-drawn-out course raises many unanswered questions about the nature of the host–parasite interaction. The disease has been of great historical importance not only for the practice of medicine but also because of its effect on many persons who played important roles in the history of the Western world. It was an extremely common infection only a few decades past, with prevalence in various autopsy series in the first half of the twentieth century of 5 to 10 percent.[1,2] In certain groups of low socioeconomic status studied in the prepenicillin era, syphilis affected 25 percent or more of the population.[3] Widespread use of antibiotics after World War II reduced the incidence of early syphilis to manageable proportions, and recognized new cases of late syphilis decreased. In the last decade, however, late syphilis (particularly neurosyphilis) has made a clinical comeback, perhaps reflecting the increase in early infectious syphilis and HIV that occurred in the late 1980s in many parts of the world. In this chapter, the origins of the disease are discussed briefly, and the course of the untreated and treated disease is analyzed.

ORIGINS

THE COLUMBIAN THEORY

Syphilis was epidemic in late fifteenth-century Europe, and the early stages apparently were often unusually severe by contemporary standards. The rapid spread and considerable effects of the disease throughout Europe in the last decade of the fifteenth century caused it to be termed the Great Pox, in contrast to another scourge, smallpox. The disease received its present name from the poem by Fracastoro in 1530 about the afflicted shepherd, Syphilis. The late complications of syphilis were recognized early and were frequently mentioned by many Elizabethan authors.

The late fifteenth-century European epidemic coincided with the return of Columbus from America in 1493, causing many to assume that the disease was acquired from natives in the West Indies and carried back to a nonimmune (and therefore particularly susceptible) population in Europe. Certainly, if this did occur, conditions were ripe for rapid transmission, because Europe was engaged in wars at that time, and the movement of the troops and their camp followers created a perfect vehicle for rapid spread of a sexually transmitted disease. On the other hand, there are biblical and ancient Chinese writings that are consistent with descriptions of late cutaneous syphilis, although other illnesses such as tuberculosis or leprosy could have caused similar descriptions to be written. An illness suggestive of syphilis apparently was not described in early American natives. These and other considerations led some to speculate that venereal syphilis did not arise suddenly in Europe after 1493 but may have been endemic already, only to become more widespread and severe as a consequence of the wars that coincided with the return of Columbus and his men.

THE ENVIRONMENTAL THEORY

Some scholars have suggested that venereal syphilis is merely a variant of other treponemal diseases that are common in other parts of the world. This idea, formerly championed by Hudson, was recently raised again in a slightly altered form by Hollander.[4,5] The notion is that *Treponema pallidum,* the causative agent of venereal syphilis, is really the same species as *T. pallidum* subspecies *pertenue,* the causative agent of yaws (a disabling cutaneous and osseous disease of the tropics); *T. pallidum* spp. *carateum,* the causative agent of pinta (a less destructive cutaneous disease found in certain parts of rural Central and South America); and *T. pallidum* spp. *bosnia,* the causative agent of nonvenereal syphilis (found in parts of the Near East and surrounding territory). According to this hypothesis, all treponematoses are merely variants of a single disease, the expression of which has been modified by environmental factors, especially temperature. Consistent with this idea is evidence by DNA–DNA hybridization of the close relationship between *T. pallidum* and *T. pallidum pertenue* and other studies that demonstrate their considerable antigenic similarities.[6,7] Although the various pathogenic treponemal species do exhibit some differences in host range in animals, this probably reflects relatively minor genetic variations.[8]

Current studies in several laboratories on the molecular genetics and immunology of *T. pallidum* may help to resolve questions of the relatedness of the pathogenic treponemes of humans, which is important to future considerations of programs for eradication of syphilis and other treponematoses.[9–11] It will remain for future historians to argue about the origins of syphilis; short of creation of an "Andromeda strain," it probably will never be possible to know for certain when and how any of the major infectious diseases arose.

THE COURSE OF UNTREATED SYPHILIS

The natural history of the disease, already quite well known in the nineteenth century, became even more clear after the discovery of *T. pallidum* by Schaudinn and Hoffmann in 1905 and after introduction of serological tests shortly thereafter.[12] In the following section an overview of the course of the disease is presented, followed by a more complete description of a few of the attempts at a definitive analysis of the natural course of the illness.

TRANSMISSION

The disease is usually acquired by sexual contact, with the obvious and important exception of congenital syphilis, where the infant acquires the infection by transplacental transmission of *T. pallidum.* Transmission by sexual contact requires exposure to moist mucosal or cutaneous lesions, and therefore a person ordinarily only is able to transmit syphilis during the first few years of infection, during the time of susceptibility to spontaneous mucocutaneous secondary relapses (see the following).

The rate of acquisition of syphilis from an infected sexual partner has been estimated at about 30 percent, based on a placebo-controlled study of the efficacy of various antibiotics in aborting syphilis in known contacts within the previous 30 days of patients with primary or secondary syphilis.[13] The ID_{50} of the rabbit-adapted Nichols strain of *T. pallidum* for human volunteers by intracutaneous inoculation was estimated to be 57 organisms, which was similar to the ID_{50} for rabbits; if the ID_{50} for humans of native or "street strains" of *T. pallidum* on mucosal surfaces is similar, exposure to a relatively few organisms suffices to initiate infection.[14]

Syphilis is a systemic disease shortly after its inception,[15] and women may transmit infection to their fetus in utero shortly after onset of infection.[15] Transmission to the fetus in utero has been documented as early as the ninth week of pregnancy.[16] Women remain potentially infectious for the fetus for many years, although the risk of infecting a fetus declines gradually during the course of untreated illness; after about 8 years there is little risk even in the untreated mother.

THE STAGES OF SYPHILIS

PRIMARY

The untreated illness typically results in a primary lesion, the chancre, 10 to 90 days (average 3 weeks) from exposure. The lesion is usually single but may be multiple, and although it is usually painless and associated with regional adenopathy, frequent exceptions occur. Primary lesions in nongenital sites may be particularly likely to have atypical appearance, especially in the anal area. Untreated, the primary lesion heals in a few weeks.

SECONDARY

Within a few weeks or months (or less commonly, coincident with the primary lesion) a variable systemic illness develops, characterized by low-grade fever, malaise, sore throat, headache, adenopathy, and cutaneous or mucosal rash. This secondary stage of illness may be accompanied by alopecia, and up to 10 percent of patients have mild hepatitis.[17] Rarely, a form of nephrotic syndrome develops.[18] Evolution of secondary lesions is a manifestation of widespread hematogenous and lymphatic dissemination of *T. pallidum,* as evidenced by the infectious transfer of disease to susceptible animals with blood, lymph nodes, liver biopsy, and cerebrospinal fluid.[15] A single sample of renal tissue was negative in an animal transfer test, consistent with other evidence that the pathogenesis of secondary syphilitic nephropathy involves deposition of immune complexes,[18] rather than infection of renal tissue by *T. pallidum.*[15,18]

There is interest in this possible role of depression of the cellular immune response in the observed waxing and waning of the lesions of early (primary and secondary) syphilis. Many investigators have observed depression of specific and nonspecific lymphocyte responses in vitro coincident with the lesions of early syphilis in humans and rabbits; the hypothesis that depression of cellular immune responses to *T. pallidum* antigens is in some way involved in recrudescence of active lesions in secondary syphilis is attractive but still unproved.[19–21] There is evidence for circulating immune complexes in early syphilis, which could be responsible for some of the clinical manifestations and perhaps contributes to the depression of cellular immune responses.[21] In this context, it is interesting to recall that old clinical and experimental observations established that there is temporary immunity to new infection during active early syphilis ("chancre immunity"), although individuals previously treated for early syphilis were susceptible to experimental infection.[14,22] The role of the immune responses in the pathogenesis of early syphilis and in resistance to infection is discussed elsewhere.[23–25]

LATENCY

By definition, persons with historical or serological evidence for syphilis but with no clinical manifestations have latent syphilis. This has been somewhat arbitrarily divided into early latency and late latency, on the basis of the time when untreated individuals are likely to have spontaneous mucocutaneous (infectious) relapses. In the Oslo study of untreated syphilis, secondary relapses occurred in 25 percent of patients, with most in the first year and a steadily decreasing incidence until 5 years had elapsed.[26] The U.S. Public Health Service therefore defines early (potentially infectious) latency as 1 year from onset of infection, whereas others prefer a longer interval before designating the infection as late latent. Since neurosyphilis may be asymptomatic or subtle, and cardiovascular syphilis also may be difficult to detect on physical examination, assignment of a diagnosis of latent syphilis requires both a careful physical examination and an examination of cerebrospinal fluid.

TERTIARY

The principal morbidity and mortality of syphilis in adults is owing to the variable occurrence of later manifestation illness in the skin, bones, central nervous system, or viscera, particularly the heart and great vessels.

Gumma

Late cutaneous and osseous manifestations formerly were very common, but have become exceedingly rare in present practice. These lesions (gummas) have characteristic gross and microscopic appearances. Because gummas usually responded dramatically and rapidly to specific therapy, they were classified as benign late syphilis, even though untreated they frequently led to destruction of soft tissues or bone. The pathogenesis of gummas was uncertain; spirochetes could be demonstrated in lesions, but limited experiments in previously infected humans suggested that gummas might have been the result of a hypersensitivity response to endogenous or exogenous *T. pallidum* antigen.[14,15] Lesions of late benign syphilis sometimes occurred for an extended period from as few as 2 to over 40 years from onset of infection. Gummas of critical organs (heart, brain, liver) could be fatal.

Cardiovascular

Involvement of the heart and aorta by *T. pallidum* occurred roughly 20 to 30 years following onset of infection. Spirochetes could be demonstrated in large numbers in the infected aorta at postmortem, but the critical effect was probably owing to a vasculitis of the vasa vasorum.[15] The most usual result was an aneurysm of the ascending aorta or other great vessels and aortic valve insufficiency and heart failure owing to dilatation of the aortic ring.

Neurological

Involvement of the central nervous system led to a number of different syndromes, occurring over an extended period from 1 or 2 years to more than 30 years from onset of infection. The pathogenesis of late central nervous system syphilis is not understood completely. In syphilitic meningitis, *T. pallidum* could be demonstrated easily in cerebrospinal fluid, and in general paresis (syphilitic meningoencephalitis) spirochetes were also easily demonstrable. The common denominator of these illnesses also may be a small-vessel vasculitis. In contrast, spirochetes could not be demonstrated in the spinal cord or other tissues in patients with tabes dorsalis, leading to the suggestion that loss of posterior column function in tabes dorsalis could have been the result of an immunologic attack on spinal cord tissue. Inability to create an animal model of neurosyphilis has greatly hindered further understanding of these devastating but interesting syndromes.

THE OSLO STUDY

Probably all of the important clinical manifestations of syphilis were recognized by physicians of the nineteenth century, prior to introduction by Wassermann in 1906 of the first serological test for syphilis. However, the fate of the individual untreated patient was uncertain, other than knowledge that some persons seemed to develop late destructive complications but others escaped unscathed. Our present understanding of this issue is based primarily on a large prospective study of patients conducted in Oslo from 1890 to 1910 by Professor Boeck, and followed up retrospectively by Bruusgaard and later by Gjestland et al.[26,27]

Boeck was concerned that therapy available in 1890 (principally mercurials) might be more toxic than the disease itself, and therefore instigated a study of the fate of selected patients with untreated early primary or secondary syphilis. Diagnosis was based strictly on clinical criteria, since neither dark-field microscopy nor serology was available for most of the initial phase of the study. Patients with lesions typical of early infectious syphilis were hospitalized until no longer infectious, but they were not treated. One-half of the males and three-fourths of the females were observed with lesions of secondary syphilis only. A total of 1978 different patients were entered into the study. Patients were hospitalized approximately 3 months, although a few remained in the hospital for 10 to 12 months, illustrating the long periods in which untreated patients were thought to be potentially infectious.

The most valuable data from the Oslo study came from a monumental follow-up and reappraisal conducted by Gjestland nearly 50 years after Boeck instigated the study. Follow-up information was obtained from 1949 to 1951 on over 80 percent of the 1404 patients in the original group who lived near Oslo, a remarkable figure considering the number of years that had passed. Only one-sixth had received any therapy (and of these, almost all received it late in the course), usually too little to be of any clinical importance. Several important findings emerged and are discussed in the following.

FREQUENCY OF SECONDARY RELAPSE

Prior to 1950, it was often stated that relapse of secondary syphilitis frequently was the result of inadequate therapy, which by interfering with the host immune response actually made it more likely that a patient would suffer later complications. Gjestland's observation that 23.6 percent of untreated patients suffered at least one secondary relapse clearly showed that waxing and waning was a normal part of the course of untreated syphilis. About one-fourth of patients with a relapse had more than one relapse. About 90 percent of secondary relapses occurred in the first year, and 94 percent within the first 2 years, but some occurred over 4 years later.

BENIGN LATE SYPHILIS (GUMMA)

This was the most frequent late (tertiary) manifestation, affecting 14.4 percent of males and 16.7 percent of females. The most frequently involved organs were skin (70 percent), bone (9.6 percent), and mucosa (10.3 percent). Only 10 percent of patients had gummas of more than a single type of tissue (e.g., bone and skin). Similar to secondary syphilis, gummas remitted only to recur later in the same or another site in about one-fourth of males and one-third of females, with up to seven discrete episodes. Gummas occurred anywhere from 1 to 46 years after onset of infection, usually within the first 15 years.

CARDIOVASCULAR SYPHILIS

No patients infected before age 15 developed late cardiovascular syphilis. Overall, 13.6 percent of males and 7.6 percent of females developed cardiovascular complications, usually within 30 to 40 years of onset. If persons under 15 were excluded, 14.9 percent of males and 8.0 percent of females developed cardiovascular syphilis. These figures, although frequently quoted in reviews of the Oslo study, are almost certainly an underestimate, since only a minority of the Oslo patients were autopsied, and the prevalence of cardiovascular syphilis was much higher in the autopsied group (Table 34-1). Since the clinical diagnosis of gumma was more obvious than that of other late forms of syphilis, it is possible that the incidence of gummas actually was not greater than that of cardiovascular or neurological syphilis.

NEUROSYPHILIS

Late syphilis of the nervous system developed in 9.4 percent of males and 5.0 percent of females. Curiously, although neurosyphilis did develop in persons infected before age 15, it did so rarely in persons infected after age 40 (0 of 28 males, 2 of 45 females). Onset from time of infection varied depending on the type of neurosyphilis; meningovascular disease typically occurred in the first 15 to 18 years of infection, whereas paresis occurred after 20 to 25 years and tabes after about 30 years. The frequency distribution of different types of neurosyphilis is shown in Table 34-2. Although recognized neurosyphilis was somewhat less common than either gumma or cardiovascular syphilis, it may have been the most important clinically by virtue of its occurrence at an earlier age than cardiovascular disease and its significant morbidity and mortality.

OTHER OBSERVATIONS

The probability of dying directly as a result of untreated syphilis in the Oslo study was 17.1 percent in males and 8 percent in

Table 34-1. Cardiovascular Syphilis in the Oslo Study of Untreated Syphilis: Comparison of Known Study Group with Autopsied Patients

	Percent in known study group	Percent in autopsied group
Uncomplicated aortitis		
Males	2.6	9.3
Females	2.9	11.2
Complicated aortitis (aortic insufficiency, aneurysms, coronary stenosis)		
Males	12.2	25.3
Females	5.1	10.4

Source: Gjestland.[26]

Table 34-2. Prevalence of Recognized Neurosyphilis in the Oslo Study of Untreated Syphilis

	Frequency	
Type	Males (n = 331)	Females (n = 622)
Diffuse meningovascular	3.6	1.7
General paresis	3.0	1.7
Tabes dorsalis	2.5	1.4
Gumma of brain	0.3	0.2
Total	9.4	5.0

Source: Gjestland.[26]

Table 34-3. Tertiary Syphilis in the Tuskegee Study

	Syphilitic study group	
Type	20-Year follow-up[31] (n = 159)	30-Year follow-up[32] (n = 90)
Benign late syphilis	6 (4%)	1 (1%)
Cardiovascular syphilis	10 (6%)	7* (8%)
Aneurysm	3	
Aortic insufficiency	5	
Aneurysm aortic insufficiency	2	
Neurological syphilis	7 (4%)	3* (3%)
Paresis	2	
Tabes	1	
Optic atrophy	2	
Tabes and optic atrophy	2	
Tabes, optic atrophy, aneurysm	1	
Total	23 (14%)	11 (12%)

* Specific types of illness not reported.

females after 40 years of infection. Syphilis was the second leading cause of death in males and fifth leading cause in females. (Tuberculosis was first in each group.) Life expectancy seemed to be reduced to an extent greater than could be attributed to the recognized specific late manifestations. Men fared less well than women, particularly regarding cardiovascular and neurosyphilis, where they ran a 2 to 1 risk compared to females of developing such complications. Overall, only 28 percent of patients developed recognized late complications; 72 percent survived to old age with no obvious ill effects. If autopsies had been performed more often, milder forms of late syphilis surely would have been discovered, so the often-quoted figure of 72 percent surviving without late complications certainly is too generous.

Despite flaws, particularly some uncertainty about the initial diagnosis in the absence of dark-field examination or serological tests for syphilis, nonrandomized selection of patients, absence of a suitably selected control group, insufficient autopsies (24 percent), and irregular performance of lumbar punctures, the Oslo study is highly valuable because of the large sample size, nearly total absence of treatment, excellent long-term follow-up, and entry of a reasonably homogeneous group of patients, each of whom was in the early stages of infectious syphilis.

THE TUSKEGEE STUDY

In 1932, a second study of the natural history of ostensibly untreated syphilis was undertaken by the U.S. Public Health Service in Macon County, Alabama, home of the Tuskegee Institute. This study, generally known as the Tuskegee study, has been harshly criticized on ethical grounds, because written informed consent was never obtained from the involved patients and because penicillin therapy was withheld after penicillin became widely available.[28,29] Indeed, the President of the United States recently officially apologized to the remaining survivors. It is commonly viewed as essentially racist because the study was limited to black males.[28,29] The rationale for the study apparently was the concept that the considerable toxicity of arsenicals, the principal antisyphilitic available at the time, might be worse than the disease, since the early results of the Oslo study indicated that the majority of untreated syphilitics suffered no late effects of the disease.[27] There was concern that the Oslo study was flawed by lack of proper controls and by insufficient rate of autopsies. There also was a question in the minds of many clinicians of the time about differences in the natural history of syphilis in different racial groups.

In 1932 a serological survey of men of Macon County, Alabama, revealed that about one-fourth had a positive test for syphilis. Those with infectious lesions of early syphilis were treated with arsenicals. A total of 412 other men who had a history of previous lesions of early syphilis but who no longer were considered infectious were enrolled in the study. Many of those received a short, subcurative course of arsenical therapy.[30] A matched group of 204 seronegative controls also was selected. The composition of these groups changed slightly with time; when some controls were later found to have acquired syphilis, they were switched to the syphilis group. All patients and controls received an entry physical exam, lumbar puncture, and chest films. An attempt was made to reexamine these men at periodic intervals, and to obtain as many autopsies as possible. Results of follow-up were excellent, since after 20 years only about 10 percent of patients were totally lost, and approximately two-thirds of patients who died had been autopsied.[30]

Results were published at intervals by different teams who conducted the periodic reviews.[30–33] Unfortunately, a comprehensive report never has been published. The principal finding was an increased mortality rate in the syphilitic group, estimated to be 20 percent loss of life expectancy at the 12-year follow-up and 17 percent at the 20-year follow-up.[31,33] Most of the excess mortality occurred in the first 20 years; little additional increment was noted in a report after 30 years.[32] As in the Oslo study, not all mortality could be directly attributed to specific lesions of late syphilis. Other significant differences between syphilitics and controls after 20 years included a higher frequency in the syphilitics of significant cardiac complaints and cardiac enlargement, a higher frequency of "arteriosclerosis," and a higher frequency of hypertension. After 30 years, remaining survivors had similar frequencies of hypertension, but a higher proportion of syphilitics had an abnormal electrocardiogram.[32]

Specific lesions of late syphilis were found in about 14 percent of syphilitics at the 20-year follow-up and in 12 percent of examined syphilitic survivors at the 30th year of the study.[31,32] The findings are summarized in Table 34-3. Cardiovascular syphilis was the most frequent finding; there was a roughly similar frequency of benign late syphilis (usually of bone) and of neurosyphilis. After 20 years of follow-up, cardiovascular or neurosyphilis was considered the primary cause of death in 30 percent of the infected men.[31]

THE ROAHN STUDY

A third large study of the natural course of syphilis was conducted by Paul Roahn, the results of which are available in a comprehensive monograph.[1] Unlike the Oslo or Tuskegee studies, this study was based entirely on a review of autopsy materials. Any study based on dead patients obviously has actual or potential bias toward poor outcomes, but the study nevertheless is of great value. A cross-sectional review was made of all autopsies conducted at Yale University School of Medicine from 1917 to 1941; among almost 4000 persons over age 20 at death, 9.7 percent had clinical, laboratory, or autopsy evidence of syphilis. (The hospital population was weighted toward lower socioeconomic groups, over 90% of whom were white.) About one-half of patients had received no therapy.

Overall, 51 percent of syphilitic patients had anatomic lesions attributable to syphilis at autopsy. Among untreated patients only, 39 percent had lesions attributable to syphilis. Among clinically diagnosed patients (diagnosis made during life), about 30 percent developed late anatomic lesions of syphilis (very similar to the Oslo study), and about 20 percent died because of syphilis. Most lesions were cardiovascular. Among 77 patients with untreated syphilis with late anatomic lesions at autopsy, 83 percent of lesions were cardiovascular, 7.6 percent were neurological, and 8.5 percent were gummas. Many patients had multiple lesions.

Patients with positive serological tests were more likely to have anatomic lesions and to have died because of them than those with negative serological tests, suggesting that persistence of positive VDRL-type tests was associated with disease activity. About one-fourth of patients with late lesions at autopsy had negative anticardiolipin serological tests before death, confirming once again the frequency of negative VDRL-type tests among patients with tertiary syphilis.

Syphilis was associated with reduced likelihood of living past 70 years of age. Part of the excess mortality may not have been due to morphologically recognized late complications.

In summary, the Rosahn study was similar in many respects to the other large studies (Oslo, Tuskegee). Each study demonstrated increased mortality due to syphilis and indicated that 15 to 40 percent of untreated patients develop recognizable late (tertiary) complications. The Tuskegee and Rosahn studies, which had the highest autopsy rates, showed the highest frequencies of cardiovascular syphilis. At least 60 percent of untreated patients did not develop late recognizable anatomic complications, and about 80 percent did not die primarily because of syphilis.

STUDIES IN THE ANTIBIOTIC ERA

No comprehensive study analogous to the studies cited in the preceding has been carried out in the past 30 years. There is clear evidence that penicillin treatment of acquired early syphilis almost always prevents late complications of the disease. There has been debate about the apparent persistence of *T. pallidum* in humans and animals after penicillin therapy, but there is little convincing evidence as to the importance of these observations.[15,34,35] Late clinically manifest neurosyphilis may be an exception; high-dose intravenous penicillin is probably indicated in an attempt to assuredly kill *T. pallidum* in the central nervous system of these patients.

Statistical studies published by the U.S. Public Health Service strongly suggest that intentional or unintentional antibiotic therapy of early syphilis is preventing some proportion of late syphilis.[36] There was a sharp decline in rates of reported early syphilis in the 1950s, followed by a threefold rise in the 1960s, which rates were maintained until the latter half of the 1980s, when a marked rise occurred in male homosexual and drug-using heterosexual populations. In contrast, there was only a minor secondary rise in reported early latent syphilis in the 1960s and 1970s, and a steady, continuous decline in late (tertiary) and late latent syphilis rates in the same interval (Table 34-4). Antibiotics apparently abort recognized late complications of syphilis.

Gumma and tabes dorsalis almost disappeared from the contemporary scene, although there are increasing reports of gummas of multiple organs in AIDS patients.[37] However, a survey of hospital records of patients with positive serologies in Denmark from the years 1961 to 1970 disclosed about equal numbers of patients with previously undiagnosed tabes, paresis, aortic insufficiency, and aortic aneurysm.[38] A variety of anecdotal experiences indicate that all of the classic forms of late syphilis of the central nervous system continue to turn up intermittently in large tertiary care hospitals, although diagnostic confusion is not at all uncommon in such patients.[39] Variant forms of neurosyphilis that are difficult to classify do occur, but they also occurred in the preantibiotic era.[39] Suggestions of the relatively common occurrence of subtle or highly atypical forms of neurosyphilis presenting primarily with seizures and peripheral neuropathies or pupillary abnormalities are difficult to evaluate, since a study that makes this claim is based to a considerable degree on positive fluorescent treponemal antibody-absorption (FTA-ABS) tests on cerebrospinal fluid.[40] This test is not standardized for this purpose, and its clinical meaning is suspect.

Table 34-4. Reported Rates of Syphilis in the United States of America, 1947–1977 (Representative Years)

	Case rates per 100,000		
	Primary secondary	Early latent	Late year late latent
1947	66.4	73.9	86.6
1952	6.9	24.0	69.1
1957	3.9	10.6	54.2
1962	11.5	10.7	43.3
1967	10.8	8.0	31.7
1972	11.8	10.1	21.0
1977	9.5	9.9	10.4

Source: Centers for Disease Control.[36]

There have been few recent studies to evaluate the prevalence of newly diagnosed cardiovascular syphilis. An interesting published in 1970 by Prewitt analyzed syphilitic patients seen at the Memphis-Shelby County (Tennessee) Venereal Disease Clinic for signs of aortic insufficiency.[41] All were over 35 years old and had a history of treatment for syphilis and/or a reactive FTA-ABS test. Of 317 patients examined, 26 (8 percent) had the murmur of aortic insufficiency, including 14 of 97 (14 percent) apparently untreated patients. The implication was that syphilitic aortic insufficiency may be much more common today than usually appreciated, at least in sexually transmitted disease clinics. One wonders whether the apparent long delay in onset of signs and symptoms, and the relatively mild form of the disease, was owing to partial or complete but inadvertent antibiotic therapy.

CONCLUSION

Syphilis is still common, particularly in certain sectors of the population. Late complications may be relatively less of a problem than in the preantibiotic era, but alertness to the possibility of late syphilis and awareness of the pleiotropic clinical manifestations of late syphilis are crucial if these forms of the disease are to be diagnosed and treated properly. The principal concern must be vigilance in finding, treating, and preventing early syphilis. Because all forms of syphilis, particularly certain types of late syphilis, are less common than in the glory days of syphilis as a clinical specialty, it is important to teach others and to remind ourselves of the multiple faces of the great actor, lues venerea.

Since syphilis is an independent risk factor for seropositivity to HIV, vigilance in diagnosis, therapy, and prevention of syphilis is now more important than ever.[42]

References

1 Roahn PD: Autopsy studies in syphilis. U.S. Public Health Service, Venereal Disease Division. *J Vener Dis Inf* 21(suppl):1947.

2 Symmers D: Anatomic lesions in late acquired syphilis: A study of 314 cases based on the analysis of 4,880 necropsies at Bellevue Hospital. *JAMA* 66:1457, 1916.

3 Olansky S et al: Untreated syphilis in the male Negro: Environmental factors in the Tuskegee study. *Public Health Rep* 69:691, 1954.

4 Hudson ER: Treponematoses and African slavery. *Br J Vener Dis* 40: 43, 1963.

5 Hollander DH: Treponematosis from pinta to venereal syphilis revisited: Hypothesis for temperature determination of disease patterns. *Sex Transm Dis* 8:34, 1981.

6 Fieldsteel AH: Genetics of Treponema, in *Pathogenesis and Immunology of Treponemal Infection,* RF Schell et al, (eds). New York, Marcel Dekker, 1983, p. 39.

7 Schell RF et al: Acquired resistance of hamsters to challenge with homologous and hieterologous virulent treponemes. *Infect Immunol* 37: 617, 1982.

8 Turner TB, Hollander DH: Biology of the treponematoses. *WHO Monogr Ser* 35:1, 1957.

9 Walfield AM et al: Expression of *Treponema pallidum* antigens in *Escherichia coli. Science* 216:522, 1982.

10 Stamm LV et al: Expression of *Treponema pallidum* antigens in *Escherichia coli* K-12. *Infect lmmunol* 36:1238, 1982.

11 Robertson SM et al: Murine monoclonal antibodies specific for virulent *Treponema pallidum* (Nichols). *Infect Immunol* 36:1076, 1982.

12 Schaudinn FR et al: Voridufiger Bericht uber das Vorkommen von Spirochaeten in syphilitischen Krakheitsproducten und bei Papillomen. *Arbeiten aus dem K Gesundheitsamte* 22:527, 1905.

13 Schroeter AL et al: Therapy for incubating syphilis: Effectiveness of gonorrhea treatment. *JAMA* 218:711, 1971.

14 Magnuson HJ et al: Inoculation syphilis in human volunteers. *Medicine* 35:33, 1956.

15 Turner TB et al: Infectivity tests in syphilis. *Br J Vener Dis* 45:183, 1969.

16 Harter CA et al: Fetal syphilis in the first trimester. *Am J Obstet Gynecol* 124:705, 1976.

17 Fehr J et al: Early syphilitic hepatitis. *Lancet* 2:896, 1975.

18 Gamble CN et al: lmmunopathogenesis of syphilitic glomerulonephritis: Elution of antitreponemal antibody from glomerular immune-complex deposits. *N Engl J Med* 292:449, 1975.

19 Levene GM et al: Reduced lymphocyte transformation due to a plasma factor in patients with active syphilis. *Lancet* 2:246, 1969.

20 Pavia CS et al: Selective in vitro response of thymus-derived lymphocytes from *Treponema pallidum*-infected rabbits. *Infect Immunol* 18: 603, 1977.

21 Baker-Zander SA et al: Serum regulation of in vitro lymphocyte responses in early experimental syphilis. *Infect Immunol* 37:568, 1982.

22 Chesney AM: Immunity in syphilis. *Medicine* 5:463, 1926.

23 Wicher K et al: Immunopathology of syphilis, in *Pathogenesis and Immunology of Treponemal Infection,* RF Schell et al (eds). New York, Marcel Dekker, 1983, p. 161.

24 Baughn RE: Immunoregulatory effects in experimental syphilis, in *Pathogenesis and Immunology of Treponemal Infection,* RF Schell et al (eds). New York, Marcel Dekker, 1983, p. 271.

25 Folds JD: Cell mediated immunity, in *Pathogenesis and Immunology of Treponemal Infection,* RF Schell et al (eds). New York, Marcel Dekker, 1983, p. 315.

26 Gjestland T: The Oslo study of untreated syphilis: An epidemiologic investigation of the natural course of syphilitic infection based on a restudy of the Boeck-Bruusgaard material. *Acta Derm Venereol* 35(Suppl [Stockh]34):I, 1955.

27 Bruusgaard E: Ober das schicksal der nicht specifisch behandelten leuktiker. *Arch Dermatol Syph* (Berlin) 157:309, 1929.

28 Brandt AM: Racism and research: The case of the Tuskegee syphilis study. *Hastings Cent Rep* December 1978, p 21.

29 Jones JH: *Bad Blood.* New York, Free Press, 1981.

30 Schuman SH et al: Untreated syphilis in the male Negro: Background and current status of patients in the Tuskegee study. *J Chronic Dis* 2: 543, 1955.

31 Olansky S et al: Untreated syphilis in the male Negro: X. Twenty years of clinical observation of untreated syphilitic and presumably non-syphilitic groups. *J Chronic Dis* 4:177, 1956.

32 Rockwell DH et al: The Tuskegee study of untreated syphilis. *Arch Intern Med* 114:792, 1964.

33 Heller JR Jr et al: Untreated syphilis in the male Negro: II. Mortality during 12 years of observation. *J Vener Dis Inform* 27:34, 1946.

34 Yobs AR et al: Do treponemes survive adequate treatment of late syphilis? *Arch Dermatol* 91:379, 1965.

35 Yobs AR et al: Further observations on the persistence of *Treponema pallidum* after treatment in rabbits and humans. *Br J Vener Dis* 44: 116, 1968.

36 Centers for Disease Control: Sexually Transmitted Disease Fact Sheet, ed 34. U.S. Department of Health, Education, and Welfare Publication 79-8195.

37 Kampmeier RH: Whatever has happened to locomotor ataxyl? (editorial). *J Am Vener Dis Assoc* 3:51, 1976.

38 Fischer A et al: Tertiary syphilis in Denmark 1961–1970: A description of 105 cases not previously diagnosed or specifically treated. *Acta Derm Venerol* (Stockh) 56:485, 1976.

39 Luxon L et al: Neurosyphilis today. *Lancet* 1:90, 1979.

40 Hooshmand H et al: Neurosyphilis: A study of 241 patients. *JAMA* 219:726, 1972.

41 Prewitt TA: Syphilitic aortic insufficiency: Its increased incidence in the elderly. *JAMA* 211:637, 1970.

42 Rabkin CS et al: Prevalence of antibody to HTLV-III/LAV in a population attending a sexually transmitted disease clinic. *Sex Transm Dis* 14:48, 1987.

Chapter 35

Early syphilis

Daniel M. Musher

EPIDEMIOLOGY

Reported syphilis peaked in the Western world in the years around World War II, but declined dramatically thereafter, coincident with the general availability of penicillin. In the United States, a significant resurgence of early syphilis occurred in the 1980s, owing to successive waves of disease, first in homosexual males and then in drug-abusing heterosexuals. The peak of this recent epidemic occurred in 1990, and since then there has been a steady decline in primary and secondary syphilis, as well as congenital syphilis. Between 1991 and 1995, total reported U.S. cases of primary and secondary syphilis declined from 43,500 to 16,787. Almost all states recorded decreases, with a few notable exceptions; incidence remained highest in the South and in African-Americans. Although the recent decline in early infectious syphilis has once again led some to speculate about the eradication of syphilis, it seems unlikely that this is possible in the near future.

PRIMARY SYPHILIS

Fourteen to 21 days after *T. pallidum* has been inoculated into a dermal site, a painless papule appears at the site of inoculation. Within a few days the papule grows to a size of 0.5 to 1.5 cm in diameter and ulcerates, producing the typical chancre of primary syphilis, a round or slightly elongated ulcer, 1 to 2 cm across, with an indurated margin (Fig. 35-1). The ulcer has a clear base, without an exudate being present. It is remarkable that genital ulcers of 1 to 2 cm in diameter are painless; this feature contributes importantly to the natural history of the infection, as will be shown in the following. Modest enlargement of inguinal lymph nodes, frequently bilaterally, is observed in the majority of patients who have genital lesions. Although solitary lesions are often thought to be typical, multiple lesions frequently occur.[1]

Because of their venereal origin, primary syphilitic chancres most frequently occur in the genital, perineal or anal area; however, any part of the body may be affected (Fig. 35-2). Most chancres are found on the penis of men, and on the labia, fourchette, or cervix of women. Therefore, syphilis is usually diagnosed in its primary stage in heterosexual men. In contrast, because the chancre is not visible in women and is also painless, syphilis is usually not diagnosed in women until the secondary stage. The same applies to chancres in the anus or rectum, which are particularly common in homosexual men. Although these lesions may cause pain on defecation or rectal bleeding, becoming confused with hemorrhoids or even a neoplasm, they often go unnoticed, as do those on the labia and cervix.[2] In the absence of treatment, syphilitic chancres heal spontaneously within 3 to 6 weeks. The mechanism for healing is obscure; some kind of local immunity is responsible, since secondary lesions regularly appear during or after the regression of the primary one.

DIFFERENTIAL DIAGNOSIS

As a general rule, syphilis should be considered as a possible cause of any ulcerating lesion of the genitalia or other erogenous zone. Differentiating a syphilitic chancre from chancroid, the soft chancre caused by *Haemophilus ducreyi,* may be impossible on clinical grounds, although a great degree of tenderness, a jagged border, a yellow exudate, or striking inguinal lymphadenopathy, especially if the overlying skin is thin and shiny, is suggestive of chancroid. A chancre that is smaller, but otherwise indistinguishable from that caused by syphilis, may be transiently present in lymphogranuloma venereum. Simple trauma to the penis, or a fixed drug eruption may cause lesions resembling a chancre. It is usually not a problem to distinguish lesions of herpes simplex virus infection from those of syphilis because herpes produces multiple small lesions on which a vesicle might be seen. However, coinfection by both organisms may occur, and secondary bacterial infection of a limited vesicular eruption may produce coalescent lesions that can be confused with syphilitic chancres.

LABORATORY DIAGNOSIS

The most specific and sensitive method for verifying the diagnosis of primary syphilis is the finding of treponemes with characteristic appearance by darkfield microscopic examination of fluid obtained from the surface of the chancre. This test result is nearly always positive if a good specimen is provided to an experienced observer, provided that there has been no prior therapy with antibiotics or application of ointments that render the reading difficult. If no exudate is present, abrading the chancre and adding a drop or two of saline yields an adequate specimen. False positive readings do not occur if trained observers are doing the study, even if the material has been obtained from oral lesions.

The darkfield examination is actually the only test that specifically establishes the diagnosis of primary syphilis. Antibody to cardiolipin, as measured by the RPR (rapid plasma reagin) test is present, often at a relatively low level ($\leq$1:16), in about 80% of patients at the time they come to medical attention for primary syphilis. Cardiolipin is a component of mammalian cells that is incorporated and, presumably, modified by *T. pallidum* so that the infected host generates antibody to it. Thus, in a manner of speaking, anticardiolipin antibody is an autoantibody; it is often called "nontreponemal antibody," terminology that is not advocated by the author of this chapter since the treponeme has certainly played a role in its evolution. In early syphilis, RPR reactivity reflects activity of disease. With treatment this reactivity is expected to disappear. The RPR is generally requested even when the darkfield examination is positive in order to provide a baseline for follow-up after therapy.

Tests that measure antibody to surface proteins of *T. pallidum* by a hemagglutination assay (TPHA or MHA-TP) are positive in about 90% of patients at the time they seek medical attention for a chancre. Thus, a negative result does not exclude the diagnosis. Once *T. pallidum* infection has caused the MHA-TP to be positive, this test remains positive for life. Thus, a positive result does not establish a diagnosis of primary syphilis in someone who has a lesion that might be syphilitic since antibody may be present as a result of some earlier infection. For these reasons, the search for treponemes by darkfield examination should be undertaken, even though it is time-consuming and requires trained personnel.

SECONDARY (DISSEMINATED) SYPHILIS

Lesions of secondary syphilis result from the hematogenous dissemination of treponemes during the evolution of the primary

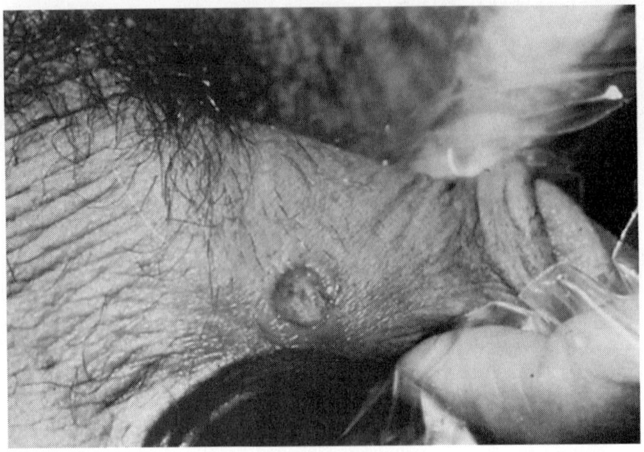

Fig. 35-1. Primary chancre of the shaft of the penis; typical clear-based lesion with indurated margin. *(Courtesy of E. Stolz.)*

syphilitic chancres, and the term "disseminated syphilis" might be more appropriate.[3] More than 3 weeks elapse between the deposition of *T. pallidum* in the dermis and emergence of these lesions; this delay in development, and the failure of the involved sites to develop into lesions that resemble primary chancres, reflect the development of some degree of humoral or cellular immunity. Lesions of secondary syphilis appear 4 to 10 weeks after the initial appearance of primary lesions and, therefore, in some patients there is an overlap, and a careful examination will disclose the primary chancre. Cases of "malignant" syphilis (lues maligna), in which disseminated lesions resemble primary chancres are exceedingly rare. Lues maligna resembles syphilis that occurs after intravenous injection of a large inoculum of *T. pallidum* into rabbits; since there has been no immune response during a primary stage of infection, widespread lesions resembling primary chancres appear. Host factors that permit this unusual clinical picture are unknown.

The initial finding in disseminated syphilis is said to be an evanescent macular rash that is usually overlooked by the patient and not observed by the physician. A few days later a symmetric papular eruption appears, involving the entire trunk and the extremities, including palms of the hands and soles of the feet. The papules are red or reddish brown, discrete, and usually 0.5 to 2 cm in diameter. They are generally scaly, although they may be smooth, follicular, or, rarely, pustular. Except for the involvement

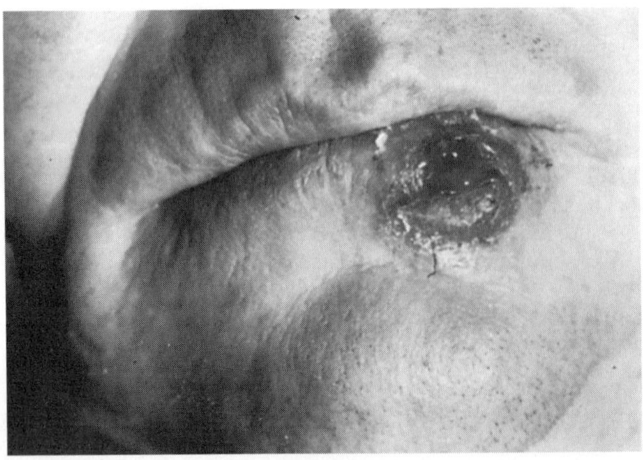

Fig. 35-2. Primary syphlitic chancre of the lip. *(Courtesy of E. Stolz.)*

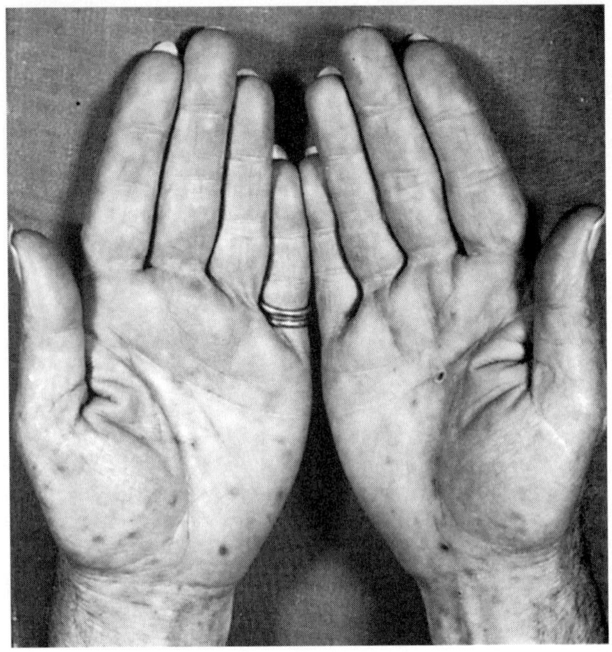

Fig. 35-3. Secondary syphilis: rash on palms.

of palms and soles (Figs. 35-3 and 35-4), syphilis may be difficult to distinguish from pityriasis rosea or psoriasis. Vesicles are said not to occur, although vesiculopustular lesions are seen on rare occasions and are common on the palms or soles. Circular (annular) lesions occur on the face of dark-skinned persons. Hypo- or hyperpigmentation may be seen. Alopecia (Fig. 35-5) occurs in some cases. Mucosal lesions, either small, superficial, ulcerated areas with grayish borders that resemble painless aphthous ulcers or larger gray plaques, also are common. Erosive gastritis has been documented in rare instances.

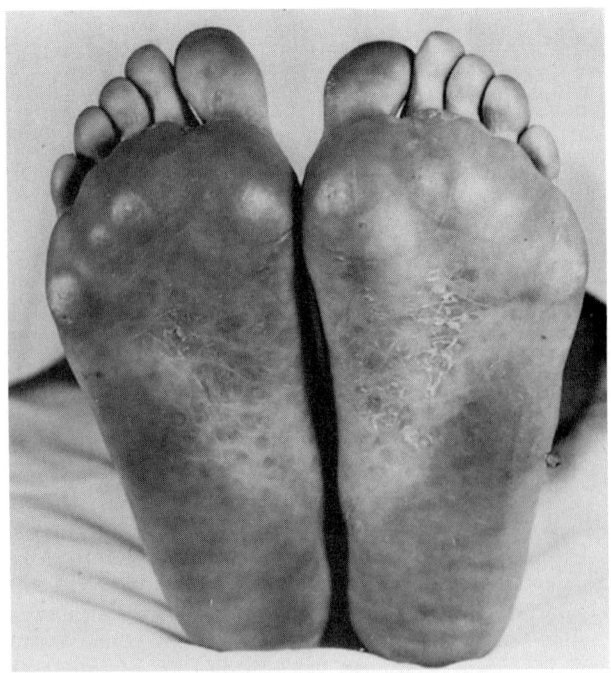

Fig. 35-4. Secondary syphilis: rash on soles of the feet.

Condyloma lata is a term used to describe large, raised, whitish or gray lesions found in warm, moist areas. These lesions were originally described as a manifestation of secondary syphilis, resulting from the effects of local skin breakdown in warm, moist areas; most frequently, the axilla and groin were involved. Today, it is far more common to observe condyloma in an area adjacent to a primary chancre, generally in the perineum or around the anus, resulting from direct spread of treponemes from the primary lesion. These lesions appear before or soon after the appearance of the generalized lesions of secondary syphilis. Thus, condyloma may represent an intermediate stage of infection, since they result from local extension from the chancre rather than from dissemination.

Secondary syphilis is a systemic disease, and interest in the dermatologic manifestations should not blind the physician to the presence of other symptoms, such as malaise, sore throat, headache, weight loss, low-grade fever, or muscle aches.[4] The presence of pruritus has received emphasis in the modern era, and it may be severe. Lymph node enlargement is present in the majority of patients. In one prospective study, 75% of infected persons had palpable inguinal nodes, and 38% had axillary, 28% posterior cervical, 18% femoral, and 17% epitrochlear nodes.[4] Periosteal inflammation was said to be clinically apparent in one-fourth of cases in the pretreatment era, with the skull, tibia, sternum, and ribs being involved most often. In a more recent study, technetium bone scan found lesions in a measurable proportion of cases, but these were asymptomatic; symptomatic bone involvement occurs only very rarely. Subclinical hepatitis can be detected by laboratory studies revealing elevated liver enzymes in about one-fifth of cases and is supported by histologic findings; occasionally, symptomatic hepatitis results.[5]

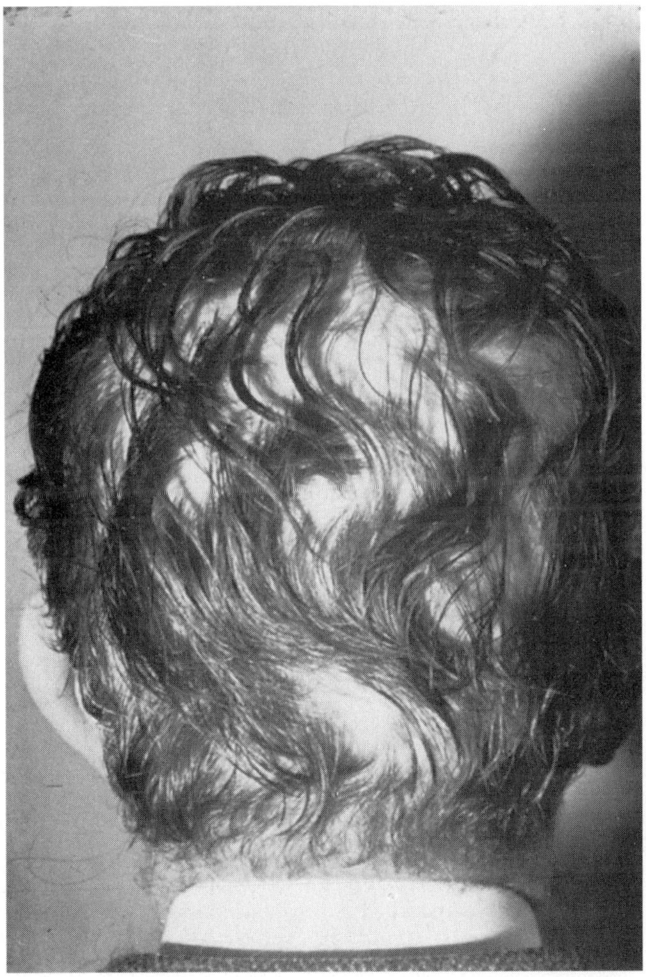

Fig. 35-5. Secondary syphilis: moth-eaten alopecia. *(Courtesy of E. Stolz.)*

Neurologic manifestations that appear in early syphilis have received increased attention in recent years, especially because of the relation with concurrent HIV infection, which is discussed in detail in the following. Prior to the occurrence of HIV infection, abnormalities in the cerebrospinal fluid (CSF)—including increased white blood cells, elevated protein, a positive Veneral Disease Research Laboratory (VDRL) test for anticardiolipin antibody, or the presence of viable *T. pallidum* organisms—were detected in up to 40% of cases of secondary syphilis in the absence of clinically apparent neurologic abnormalities.[6,7] However, no more than 1 to 2% of patients with secondary syphilis were found to have symptoms or signs of central nervous system involvement, including headache or meningismus.

Circulating immune complexes that contain treponemal outer membrane proteins and human fibronectin, antibody to these substances, and complement are uniformly present in secondary syphilis, and their deposition is thought to play a prominent role in the pathogenesis of syphilitic lesions.[8] When iritis, anterior uveitis, and glomerulonephritis or nephrotic syndrome occur in secondary syphilis, they are probably mediated entirely by deposition of complexes. Although syphilitic arthritis may be, in part, to such complexes, treponemes are also found in synovial fluid from affected joints, suggesting a dual pathogenesis that may not be unlike other bacterial arthritides.

DIFFERENTIAL DIAGNOSIS

The skin rash of secondary syphilis may be confused with pityriasis rosea, which it may closely resemble (although, of course, without a herald patch), psoriasis, especially if it is scaly, erythema multiforme or a drug eruption. Sometimes the diagnosis of nummular eczema is made, even by skilled observers. This author has even seen hot-tub folliculitis owing to *Pseudomonas* misidentified as secondary syphilis. Basically, unless lesions are present on the palms or soles, any cause of a generalized papular eruption may be confused with secondary syphilis. Finally, it may be difficult to diagnose syphilis in its secondary stage once the disease is considered; far more commonly, however, the physician has simply forgotten to entertain the diagnosis. For these reasons, serological tests for syphilis should probably be included in evaluations of sexually active adults who have a generalized skin eruption.

LABORATORY DIAGNOSIS

Treponemes can be found by darkfield examination of material obtained from skin lesions of secondary syphilis, but the skin needs to be abraded and saline applied by someone skilled in the technique; this test is usually not done. Serologic tests give far more distinctive results in secondary than in primary syphilis. Antibody to cardiolipin is always present, usually at a high dilution (RPR test reactive at ≥1:32). Rarely, a prozone phenomenon occurs, in which a blocking antibody obscures a positive reading in undiluted serum, but the positive reaction is readily apparent with dilutions. In doing the RPR test, most laboratories do not perform serum dilutions if the undiluted serum gives a negative result unless the physician specifically indicates that the diagnosis of syphilis is suspected clinically; therefore, in ordering an RPR in a case of suspected secondary syphilis, a request for dilutions should be specifically made. In secondary syphilis, the MHA-TP is always positive. Thus, a truly negative RPR or a negative MHA-TP in a patient with a disseminated rash that might be syphilitic actually excludes the diagnosis.

It is worth reiterating that the principal use of the MHA-TP is not to establish, but, rather, to exclude a diagnosis of syphilis after the primary stage, since a negative result is inconsistent with secondary, latent, or late syphilis.

LATENT SYPHILIS

The natural history of untreated secondary syphilis is marked by spontaneous resolution after a period of 3 to 12 weeks, leaving the patient entirely free of symptoms. This naturally attained asymptomatic state is called latency. In the pretreatment era, 25% of patients whose infection had become latent had a recrudescence of active, secondary syphilis.[9] Because these relapses usually occurred within 1 year of the onset of latency, this period was called early latency. Relapses after this time were very rare; therefore, after 1 year without recurrence of disease and before the onset of tertiary syphilis, untreated persons were said to have entered the late latent period. Patients with late latent syphilis are immune to reinfection with *T. pallidum*.[10]

DIAGNOSIS

At the present time, patients are diagnosed as having latent syphilis if they have a reactive RPR in the absence of any apparent signs of disease and the MHA-TP is positive. If a patient admits to having had a chancre or a skin rash for which he did not seek treatment and he now has a reactive RPR with a positive MHA-TP, the diagnosis of latent syphilis is apparent. However, this would be an unusual scenario. More often the serologic findings are present without any useful information in the medical history. From a public health point of view, such patients are regarded as if they have latent syphilis. It is worth noting, however, that such a diagnosis is problematic. On the one hand, these serologic abnormalities may have persisted after adequate treatment (the so-called serofast state) so that it may be difficult, especially in the absence of complete records or in a noncompliant patient, to be certain whether the patient has partially (inadequately) treated syphilis, latent syphilis, or adequately treated syphilis in which the serologic abnormalities persist. On the other hand, the positive serologic tests may indicate unrecognized active disease. Some patients may have an unrecognized chancre. Others may have had an unrecognized chancre that has healed and have not yet developed disseminated disease. Most ominously, the patient may have asymptomatic neurosyphilis, which can only be excluded by documenting a normal cerebrospinal fluid. This possibility is responsible for the recommendation that a spinal tap be done and the CSF be negative in order to establish the diagnosis of latency. Even though the majority of patients with reactive positive STS without signs of active syphilitic infection probably do not have true latent infection, only "presumptive latency" can be diagnosed in the absence of a documented normal CSF.

EARLY SYPHILIS AND HIV INFECTION

There is little to suggest that the dermatologic manifestations of syphilis are altered by HIV infection, nor has an increase in nondermatologic manifestations of secondary syphilis, such as hepatitis, arthritis, or osteitis, been specifically documented. This may not be surprising, since the lesions of secondary syphilis may be immunologically mediated, owing to deposition of circulating immune complexes.[11] Furthermore, minor abnormalities are likely to be overlooked in persons with advanced HIV infection because of the seriousness of their overall condition.

In contrast, concurrent HIV infection, whether before or after a diagnosis of AIDS has been made, appears to have a profound impact on neurologic involvement in syphilis.[12] As is discussed at length elsewhere in this volume, neurosyphilis has been seen more often and in younger patients in the past few years. Many cases have been described in the context of therapeutic failure with conventional doses of penicillin for primary or secondary syphilis. Numerous individual case reports and case series have documented the rapid progression of early syphilis to neurosyphilis, manifested as meningitis or cranial nerve defects (most commonly optic neuritis or deafness).[12–15] In the absence of treatment, these syndromes may progress to intracranial vasculitis and cerebrovascular accidents. The dubious term "quaternary neurosyphilis" has been revived to describe necrotizing encephalitis in an HIV-infected patient.[16] In many cases, the concurrent HIV infection has been documented for the first time only when neurologic complications appeared.

LABORATORY STUDIES

HIV-infected subjects tend to have positive STS with unusually high titers. Isolated case reports of secondary syphilis with a negative RPR result in an HIV-infected patient[17] may be the exceptions that prove the rule that the RPR is always reactive in secondary syphilis. The MHA-TP result is always positive in secondary infection.

TREATMENT OF SYPHILIS

Treatment schedules for syphilis are listed in standard textbooks as well as in brochures available from the Centers for Disease Control and Prevention and from state and city departments of public health. Especially with the advent of HIV infection, the subject is far more complicated than might have been imagined, and recommendations are being reformulated. Eventually, it may be best for physicians to evaluate each case individually, as is the custom for other diseases. It is worth noting that, even in the absence of HIV infection, some authorities have recommended higher doses of penicillin than were used in the past, although no tendency toward penicillin resistance has been found in *T. pallidum* and little or no evidence for better efficacy of higher doses has been provided.

PRIMARY OR SECONDARY SYPHILIS, NO HIV INFECTION

A single dose of 2.4 million units of benzathine penicillin appears to produce a clinical cure of primary or secondary syphilis. Persons who have been treated in this fashion are no longer contagious. Their lesions disappear, and late sequelae of tertiary syphilis do not occur. The RPR test returns to negative over 1 to 2 years in nearly all cases of treated primary infection, although some studies have recorded a serologic failure rate as high as 25%.[18,19] One poorly standardized study suggested that administering a second dose of benzathine penicillin causes the RPR test result to return to negative in every instance.[19] Clearly, some proportion of patients who are cured of their secondary syphilis retain low-grade VDRL reactivity throughout life (serofast state). These treatments may not produce a biologic cure; treponemes persist in lymph nodes, and probably the central nervous system of treated patients and experimental animals, a fact that becomes important in considering treatment of HIV-infected subjects.[20,21] The rarity of tertiary syphilis in the United States in the past three decades argues that, in practice, recommended doses of penicillin have been remarkably successful in curing syphilis.

In summary, in the absence of neurologic abnormalities and in subjects who do not have HIV infection it seems reasonable to treat persons who have primary or secondary syphilis with 2.4 million units of benzathine penicillin. Injection of 600,000 units procaine daily for 8 days yields equivalent efficacy. For patients who are unable to take penicillin, ceftriaxone (1 gm) intravenously every other day for 10 days (five doses) and erythromycin or tetracycline 500 mg, four times daily for 30 days are probably just as effective. Azithromycin has been used extensively in studies in Russia with good results, but additional studies are needed before a recommendation can be made.

LATENT SYPHILIS, NO HIV INFECTION

Latent syphilis presents a problem. As noted in the preceding, the diagnosis is based on a reactive RPR and MHA-TP tests in an asymptomatic subject. In the majority of instances in the United States today, this serologic result reflects previously treated rather than active infection. Nevertheless, the official recommendation that two treatments with benzathine penicillin, each of 2.4 million units, be given at weekly intervals unless neurosyphilis is also present, seems to be reasonable. Although many of these subjects may not require treatment, it is not possible to identify them, so all are treated as a public health measure.

A more complex problem arises from the CDC guidelines, which consider it "desirable" to perform a lumbar puncture in every patient with presumed latent syphilis in order to exclude asymptomatic neurosyphilis. It certainly is true that, in cases where suspicion of untreated or inadequately treated syphilis is high, this should be done. However, in many instances, other explanations for the reactive serology can be found. In such cases, an alternative approach is simply to treat with three doses of benzathine penicillin at weekly intervals, a therapeutic regimen that was standard for neurosyphilis in the 1960s and 1970s, and in which failures were documented very infrequently. Supporting this approach are the following considerations.

1. The vast majority of latent infections have been arrested or cured (i.e., no later appearance of tertiary syphilis) by two or three doses of benzathine penicillin, each of 2.4 million units.
2. For all the concern about treating proven neurosyphilis with benzathine penicillin because of low levels achieved in the CSF, there are very few well-documented case reports of therapeutic failure in the absence of HIV infection.
3. The CSF may be normal in some cases of neurosyphilis, so that lumbar puncture does not, with certainty, exclude the diagnosis. Some authorities have concluded that the likelihood of serious complications from lumbar puncture, as uncommon as they might be, still outweighs the potential benefits.[22]

In summary, then, it may be more practical to treat presumed latent syphilis with three doses of benzathine penicillin at weekly intervals and do no spinal tap unless neurological disease is present.

The response of latent syphilis to therapy is difficult to assess—since the patient is free of symptoms, the only possible response, barring the appearance of symptomatic tertiary syphilis, is a change in serologic test results. The RPR titer often remains unchanged (serofast state), or it may decline, but it usually does not return to negative. Rising titers suggest therapeutic failure (but see comments at end of this section on variability in titer results), in which case a CSF examination must be done and the patient must receive a more aggressive course of therapy.

TREATMENT OF PRIMARY AND SECONDARY SYPHILIS IN HIV-INFECTED PATIENTS

An early report suggested that HIV-infected patients with secondary syphilis respond only slowly to 2.4 million units of benzathine penicillin, both in terms of resolution of lesions and decline of RPR titer.[23] Two recent studies have suggested, however, that the response of early syphilis to therapy is not altered by HIV infection, and the CDC continues to recommend a single dose of 2.4 million units benzathine penicillin in this situation.[24,25]

What is, however, very impressive is the number of individual cases in which treatment of primary or secondary syphilis with benzathine penicillin is followed by rapid progression to neurosyphilis, a clinical finding that has been supported by documentation of persisting treponemes in the CSF of HIV-infected patients after treatment.[12,26–29] Those who continue to recommend a single dose of benzathine penicillin state that the percentage of all treated cases that fail is so small that they cannot recommend an increased penicillin dose for everyone. Some authorities, in contrast, believe that minimum therapy for primary or secondary infection without neurologic involvement in HIV-infected patients should be two doses each of 2.4 million units benzathine penicillin at weekly intervals and that three such doses would be preferable. However, there are no data to show that progression to neurosyphilis, the principal concern in this situation, is reduced by the more aggressive therapy. The same may be said for injection of 1.2 million units daily of procaine penicillin or of 1 g ceftriaxone on alternative days for 10 to 15 days. Erythromycin or tetracycline cannot be recommended because of failure to produce adequate levels in the CNS. If either is used in a case in which desensitization to penicillin cannot be achieved and ceftriaxone can not be given instead, both physician and patient should be fully aware of the need for close monitoring and the concern over failure to prevent neurologic disease.

TREATMENT OF LATENT SYPHILIS IN HIV INFECTION

Unlike the situation in non–HIV-infected persons, a measurable proportion (5–30%) of HIV infected persons with RPR ≥1:8 and no clinical signs of syphilis have abnormalities in the CSF that are consistent with neurosyphilis.[31] Accordingly, in such cases, lumbar puncture seems to be highly desirable. If negative, two or three doses of benzathine penicillin can be given. If positive, treatment should be given for neurosyphilis. If a lumbar puncture can not be done, many practitioners favor treatment with 20 million units of penicillin or 1 g ceftriaxone intravenously. It is not at all clear, however, that the rate of relapse to early neurosyphilis is any lower after this aggressive therapy than after daily administration of procaine penicillin or three doses of benzathine penicillin at weekly intervals.[30,31]

THERAPY OF THE PREGNANT PATIENT

A pregnant patient with primary or secondary syphilis should be treated with penicillin in the same dosages as in a nonpregnant patient. For any pregnant patient with primary or secondary syphilis who is allergic to penicillin, it seems reasonable to consider ceftriaxone, although series of cases showing efficacy have not been described. Erythromycin should not be used because it does not reliably cure an infected fetus.[32] Azithromycin may eventually prove to be more effective, but data have not been presented to date. Special care in followup is mandatory for both mother and child after treatment during pregnancy, since failure to prevent congenital syphilis by treating pregnant women with penicillin is well documented.[33]

JARISCH-HERXHEIMER REACTIONS

After treatment for primary or secondary syphilis, about one-third or two-thirds of patients, respectively, have a febrile reaction with chills, fever, arthralgias, headache, and transiently increased prominence of lesions. This is called a Jarisch-Herxheimer reaction and is owing to the release of treponemal constituents, presumably in an endotoxin-like reaction. The onset is within 4 to 6 hours after treatment, and it subsides within 24 hours. The symptoms may be impressive in their severity; in one small group of 35 cases in which temperatures were monitored by rectal probe, two patients had peak temperatures ≥103°F.[34] The Jarisch-Herxheimer reaction is not dependent on type or dose of antibiotic used, and should not be mistaken for a penicillin allergy. Jarisch-Herxheimer reactions are not an indication for discontinuance of treatment; most reactions can be managed by reassurance of the patient and aspirin or ibuprofen.

FOLLOW-UP

Serologic tests should be repeated at 6-month intervals in non–HIV-infected persons to document the return to a negative RPR. This is often overlooked in clinical practice. The argument is made that it always does return toward normal, and clinical failure is exceedingly unlikely. However: (1) documenting a return to negative does document the cure; (2) this also provides a baseline should the same patient later be found to have a reactive RPR (a common clinical occurrence); and (3) failure to respond, or especially a rising RPR, indicates the need for retreatment. It is important for the health provider to be aware of variability in testing kits and readers, such that a twofold difference is common and even four- and eightfold differences can be reported in the absence of any change. This explains why repeated tests to document a trend are recommended.

In those situations in which cure is not so certain—patients receiving therapy other than penicillin, infants treated in utero, and HIV-infected persons—follow-up must be especially rigorous. Serologic responses and, where indicated, clinical observations should be checked every 3 months for 1 to 2 years.

References

1. Chapel TA: The variability of syphilitic chancres. *Sex Transm Dis* 5: 68, 1978.
2. Drusin LM et al: Infectious syphilis mimicking neoplastic disease. *Arch Intern Med* 137:156, 1977.
3. Musher DM et al: Syphilis and yaws. In Schell RF et al (eds): *Pathogenesis and Immunology of Treponemal Infections*. New York, Marcel Dekker, 1983, pp. 101–120.
4. Chapel TA: The signs and symptoms of secondary syphilis. *Sex Transm Dis* 7:61, 1980.
5. Jozsa L et al: Hepatitis syphilitica: A clinico-pathological study of 25 cases. *Acta Hepatogastroenterol* 24:344, 1977.
6. Mills CH: Routine examination of cerebrospinal fluid in syphilis: Its value in regard to more accurate knowledge, prognosis and treatment. *Br Med J* 2:527, 1936.
7. Bauer TH et al: Spinal fluid examinations among patients with primary or secondary syphilis. *Am J Syph* 36:309, 1952.
8. Baughn RE et al: Characterization of the antigenic determinants and host components in immune complexes from patients with secondary syphilis. *J Immunol* 136:1406, 1986.
9. Clark EG et al: The Oslo study of the natural course of untreated syphilis: An epidemiologic investigation based on a re-study of the Boeck-Bruusgaard material. *Med Clin North Am* 48:613, 1964.
10. Magnuson HJ et al: Inoculation syphilis in human volunteers. *Medicine (Balt)* 35:33, 1956.
11. Jorizzo JL et al: Role of circulating immune complexes in human secondary syphilis. *J Infect Dis* 153:1014, 1986.
12. Musher DM et al: Effect of human immunodeficiency virus (HIV) infection on the course of syphilis and on the response to treatment. *Ann Intern Med* 113:872, 1990.
13. Johns DR et al: Alternation in the natural history of neurosyphilis by concurrent infection with the human immunodeficiency virus. *N Engl J Med* 316:1569, 1987.
14. Holtom PD et al: Prevalence of neurosyphilis in human immunodeficiency virus-infected patients with latent syphilis. *Am J Med* 93:9, 1992.
15. Katz DA et al: Neurosyphilis: A comparative study of the effects of infection with human immunodeficiency virus. *Arch Neurol* 50:243, 1993.
16. Morgello S et al: Quaternary neurosyphilis. *N Engl J Med* 319:1549, 1989.
17. Hicks CB et al: Seronegative secondary syphilis in a patient infected with the human immunodeficiency virus (HIV) with Kaposi sarcoma. *Ann Intern Med* 107:492, 1987.
18. Leslie N: Treatment of early infectious syphilis with benzathine penicillin G. In *Proceedings of World Forum on Syphilis and Other Treponematoses,* September 4–8, 1962, Washington, DC. Washington, DC, US Public Health Service, 1964, USPHS publication 997.
19. Fiumara NJ: Treatment of primary and secondary syphilis. Serological response. *JAMA* 243:2500, 1980.
20. Collart P et al: Significance of spinal organisms found, after treatment, in late human and experimental syphilis. *Br J Vener Dis* 40:81, 1964.
21. Yobs AR et al: Further observations on the persistence of *Treponema pallidum* after treatment in rabbits and humans. *Br J Vener Dis* 44: 116, 1968.
22. Wiesel J et al: Lumbar puncture in asymptomatic neurosyphilis. *Arch Intern Med* 145:465, 1985.
23. Frederick WR et al: Secondary syphilis and HIV infection (Abstr 1175). Abstracts of the 28th Interscience Conference. *Antimicrob Agents Chemother* 1988, p. 320.
24. Gourevitch MN et al: Effect of HIV infection on the serologic manifestations and response to treatment of syphilis in intravenous drug users. *Ann Intern Med* 118:350, 1993.
25. Hutchinson CM et al: Altered clinical presentations of early syphilis in patients with human immunodeficiency virus infection. *Ann Intern Med* 121:94, 1994.
26. Bayne LL et al: Acute syphilitic meningitis. Its occurrence after clinical and serologic cure of secondary syphilis with penicillin. G. *Arch Neurol* 43:137, 1986.
27. Jorgensen J et al: Neurosyphilis after treatment of latent syphilis with benzathine penicillin. *Genitourin Med* 62:129, 1986.
28. Berry CD et al: Neurologic relapse after benzathine penicillin therapy for secondary syphilis in a patient with HIV infection. *N Engl J Med* 316:1587, 1987.
29. Lukehart SA et al: Invasion of the central nervous system by Treponema pallidum: Implications for diagnosis and treatment. *Ann Intern Med* 109:855, 1988.
30. Dowell ME et al: Response of latent syphilis or neurosyphilis to ceftriaxone in persons infected with human immunodeficiency virus. *Am J Med* 93:481, 1992.

31. Malone JL et al: Syphilis and neurosyphilis in a human immunodeficiency virus type-1 seropositive population: Evidence for frequent serologic relapse after therapy. *Am J Med* 99:55, 1995.
32. El Tabbakh GH et al: Primary syphilis and nonimmune fetal hydrops in a penicillin-allergic woman. A case report. *J Reprod Med* 39:412, 1994.
33. McFarlin BL et al: Epidemic syphilis: Maternal factors associated with congenital infection. *Am J Obstet Gynecol* 170:535, 1994.
34. Young EJ et al: Studies on the pathogenesis of the Jarisch-Herxheimer reaction: Development of an animal mode and evidence against a role for classical endotoxins. *J Infect Dis* 146:606, 1982.

Chapter 36
Late syphilis

Morton N. Swartz
Bernadine P. Healy
Daniel M. Musher

Any discussion of late syphilis must begin with a brief recounting of the natural history of untreated infection in order to reorient the modern reader to what have become relatively uncommon manifestations of this common disease. (See Chap. 34 for a detailed discussion of this subject.) In the absence of treatment, primary syphilis is followed in almost every case by secondary syphilis which, in turn, is followed by latency. In the first year or two of latency a relapse to active (secondary) syphilis may recur in up to 25 percent of cases; this stage is called early latent syphilis. After 2 years, there are no relapses. Subjects are also immune to new primary infections. This stage is called late latent syphilis. There are no symptoms of disease, and the only signs of infection are the (usually) persistently elevated nonspecific serological tests (VDRL, RPR) and almost universally reactive specific treponemal tests (MHS-TP, TPHA, FTA-ABS). These tests are discussed in Chapter 35, Early Syphilis.

The outcome of late latent syphilis classifically is thought to follow the so-called "rule of thirds." In one-third of cases, the RPR becomes inactive, and there is no recurrence of disease; the only clue to infection ever having taken place is the persistence of antibody to outer membrane proteins of *Treponema pallidum*, manifest in the positive MHA-TP. In one-third of cases the RPR remains reactive, usually at a low level, and the MHA-TP is also positive, but there are no signs of disease. In the remaining one-third of patients, late syphilis occurs; about one-half of these patients have benign late syphilis, one-quarter have cardiovascular disease and one-quarter have neurologic disease. These proportions appear to be altered in the modern era, as discussed in the following. Characteristically, some degree of overlap occurs, so that some patients have two or, rarely, three forms of late syphilis.

The present chapter will review these three manifestations of late syphilis. We shall first discuss neurosyphilis that continues to be recognized in HIV-noninfected, but especially in HIV-infected persons. We will then go on to discuss cardiovascular and benign (gumma) syphilis that have become increasingly rare in the past two decades, although gummas are being reported more frequently in the last decade of the 20th century than in the previous 30 years.

NEUROSYPHILIS

The manifestations of central nervous system (CNS) syphilis, readily recognized by physicians practicing three or four decades ago, are unfamiliar to many physicians today as a result of the relative rarity of this condition. There were few recognized cases of neurosyphilis in the penicillin era, prior to and during the early years of the HIV epidemic, suggesting that recommended therapies for syphilis successfully prevented late complications. There has, however, been an increase in recent years in the incidence of acute syphilitic meningitis, an early form of neurosyphilis, associated with HIV infection and increasing recognition of a wide variety of later forms of neurosyphilis, including paresis, gummas, ophthalmic disease, and otologic complications. The clinical features and problems of treating neurosyphilis in HIV-infected persons are sufficiently distinctive that this subject will receive separate treatment at the end of this section.

The multitude of histopathologic reactions induced, anatomic sites involved, and clinical syndromes produced by neurosyphilis make classification complex. A helpful schema is that utilized by Merritt and colleagues in their classic monograph on neurosyphilis (Table 36-1).[1] Although this classification indicates the existence of distinctive individual forms of neurosyphilis, features of several of the entities commonly coexist, producing, for example, combinations of meningitis and vasculitis or tabes and paresis. This is not surprising when one considers that neurosyphilis fundamentally is a chronic meningitis capable of producing vascular and parenchymatous sequelae in the cerebrum and spinal cord. This scheme will be followed in the presentation of CNS syphilis in this chapter.

In the prepenicillin era, clinical neurosyphilis was an important element in the overall spectrum of syphilis, being found, for example, in 29 percent of 2263 cases seen at the Boston City Hospital.[1] The most common forms of nervous system involvement were asymptomatic neurosyphilis (31 percent) and tabes (30 percent) (Table 36-1). The incidence of paresis was probably underestimated since such patients were more likely to have been treated in psychiatric rather than general hospitals. In the antibiotic era, the successful treatment of early syphilis (and perhaps the unwitting treatment of latent syphilis when penicillin was administered for other infections) has made neurosyphilis an uncommon disorder in many parts of the world. In the United States, neurosyphilis declined as the cause of initial admissions to mental hospitals from a rate of 4.3 cases per 100,000 population in 1946 to 0.4 cases per 100,000 population in 1960. In Great Britain deaths from general paresis fell from an annual figure of about 600 in 1941 to 24 in 1968, this decrease reflecting both decreased incidence and increased efficacy of treatment.[2] In the United States, in 1976, the last year in which the Centers for Disease Control recorded separately the number of cases of neurosyphilis, there were 2903 reported cases of neurosyphilis out of a total of 71,761 reported cases of syphilis.[3]

The very early and frequent invasion of the meninges by *Treponema pallidum* during systemic dissemination of syphilitic infection is indicated by several lines of evidence. Abnormalities in the cerebrospinal fluid (CSF) have been noted in 13 percent of patients with untreated primary syphilis, 25 to 40 percent of patients with untreated secondary syphilis, and 14 percent of untreated patients with primary and secondary syphilis.[4–6] *Treponema pallidum* has been demonstrated, by animal inoculation, in the cerebrospinal fluid of 15 to 40 percent of patients with untreated primary and secondary syphilis even in the absence of other abnormalities.[1,7–9]

After the initial spirochetal invasion of the CNS during early syphilis, untreated infection may resolve spontaneously, persist as asymptomatic syphilitic meningitis, or progress to symptomatic acute syphilitic meningitis, a form that was uncommon in the preantibiotic era and was associated with inadequate therapy. Progression of early asymptomatic or symptomatic meningeal infection may lead to meningovascular syphilis (usually 5 to 12 years after primary infection) or the later forms of neurosyphilis such as tabes or paresis (usually 18 to 25 years). The progression often represents a continuum of changes rather than a series of

The authors acknowledge their indebtedness to Dr. Rudolph H. Kampmeier, noted scholar and teacher in the field of syphilis, whose chapter on benign neurosyphilis, from *Sexually Transmitted Diseases,* 2nd Ed., has been incorporated into the present chapter.

Table 36-1. Classification of Neurosyphilis[a]

Asymptomatic	31[b]
Early	
Late	
Meningeal	20
Acute syphilitic meningitis	6
Meningovascular	11[c]
Cerebral	
Spinal form	3
Parenchymatous	48
General paresis	12
Tabes dorsalis	30
Taboparesis (mixed)	3
Optic atrophy	3[d]
Gummatous	1
Cerebral form	
Spinal form	
Total	100

[a]After HH Merritt et al.[1]
[b]Distinction between early and late asymptomatic syphilis could not be made.
[c]"Deafness," comprising 1 percent of cases in HH Merritt et al., was included in this category.[1]
[d]"Optic neuritis," comprising 3 percent of cases in HH Merritt et al., was included in this category.[1]

discrete steps. It is unclear why some patients never develop neurosyphilis in the absence of treatment, whereas others do.

EARLY NEUROSYPHILIS: ASYMPTOMATIC

By definition, there are no clinical manifestations of asymptomatic neurosyphilis; this condition is, therefore, defined by the presence of abnormalities in the CSF in the absence of other findings of neurologic disease. The usual abnormalities include 10–100 WBC/mm^3 (nearly all of which are lymphocytes), a protein of 50–100 mg/dl and, in 90 percent of cases, a reactive nontreponemal antibody (VDRL) test in the CSF. Blood serology (RPR) is nearly always positive. Slight chronic meningitis and ependymitis (but no evidence of endarteritis or encephalitis) were observed at autopsy of an untreated patient with asymptomatic neurosyphilis who died of an intercurrent acute pneumococcal pneumonia.[1]

The likelihood of finding CSF abnormalities in persons with untreated syphilis increases until 12 to 18 months after initial infection, and the extent of the abnormalities is predictive of neurosyphilis.[10] Conversely, a completely normal CSF examination after 2 years of latent untreated syphilis affords reasonable assurance that neurosyphilis will not develop. Thus, because asymptomatic neurosyphilis tends, in the absence of therapy, to resolve or to progress, its frequency tends to decrease with the passage of time; one study reported that at 3, 10, and 20 years following onset, the frequency was 20, 12.9, and 6.3 percent, respectively, with a reciprocal increase in the incidence of symptomatic neurosyphilis.[11] Persistence of CSF abnormalities for more than 5 years after infection (called late asymptomatic syphilis), in the absence of treatment, was followed by the development of neurologic disease in up to 87 percent of patients.[4] It is clear from these considerations that, in some persons, asymptomatic neurosyphilis resolves spontaneously; in some it persists into advanced age, and some it progresses to neurosyphilis. Spontaneous resolution or persistence in the asymptomatic state does not imply protection against other forms of late syphilis.

EARLY NEUROSYPHILIS: SYMPTOMATIC

Even prior to the antibiotic era, acute syphilitic meningitis was relatively rare. In a 15-year (1920–1935) survey of records of three Boston hospitals, only 80 definite cases were found, appearing to account for 6 percent of all cases of neurosyphilis.[1] Syphilitic meningitis was recognized by Ehrlich when he was developing a regimen to treat syphilis at the beginning of the century and, for that reason, was called neurorecurrence. This syndrome is most common in young adults, in whom it generally appears after inadequate antimicrobial therapy for early syphilis, and it currently predominates in HIV-infected individuals (see the following).

ACUTE SYPHILITIC MENINGITIS

SYMPTOMS AND SIGNS. The incubation period in the majority of patients with syphilitic meningitis is less than 1 year. In about one-quarter of these patients, meningitis is the first clinical manifestation of syphilis. A small percentage of patients still have a secondary rash at the time of the meningitis.[12]

The clinical presentations of acute syphilitic meningitis may be divided into several patterns for convenience, but these categories overlap extensively. The principal neurologic manifestations include cranial nerve palsies (seen in 40 percent of cases) and signs of increased intracranial pressure. The involvement of multiple cranial nerves, particularly the third, sixth, seventh, and eighth, is consistent with an extensive basilar meningitis. Sensorineural deafness may occur in about 20 percent of patients, commonly in association with other cranial nerve palsies.[13] Deafness is often preceded by tinnitus and may develop rapidly, for example over 1 or 2 weeks. The hearing loss primarily involves higher frequencies; vestibular involvement is uncommon. Usually there are no other clinical findings to suggest syphilis and the CSF may be entirely normal. Thus, early acquired syphilis is a cause of potentially reversible, rapidly progressive, or sudden sensorineural deafness and must be considered in diagnosis, even in the absence of clinical findings of secondary syphilis or of overt lymphocytic meningitis.

Acute syphilitic hydrocephalus was seen in one-third of the cases of syphilitic meningitis reported by Merritt and Moore.[12] Symptoms usually develop 3 to 7 months after primary infection, but they can appear as many as 6 years later. The principal symptoms and signs are those of increased intracranial pressure; fever is only low-grade or may be absent.

Syphilitic meningitis with cerebral changes accounts for one-quarter of the cases of early neurosyphilis. The symptoms (seizures, aphasia, and hemiplegia) are a combination of those of increased intracranial pressure and those of focal cerebral involvement. Clinical findings usually include stiff neck, confusion or delirium, and papilledema. Occasionally, cranial nerve palsies are present and most commonly involve the third and sixth cranial nerves.

LABORATORY FINDINGS. In the extensive series reported by Merritt and Moore, the blood Wassermann reaction was positive in only 64 percent of patients.[12] However, this serologic test was less sensitive than more modern tests. The current serum RPR is positive in most cases of acute syphilitic meningitis. The CSF changes include elevated pressure, mononuclear pleocytosis of 10 to 200 cells per cubic millimeter (but occasionally as high as 1000 to 2000 cells per cubic millimeter), elevated protein concentration (up to 200 mg/dl), elevated globulin level, and a modest reduction in glucose in 45 percent of cases. The VDRL test on CSF is reactive in most, but not all cases. As has been noted, patients who present with isolated involvement of the eighth cranial nerve are likely to have a normal CSF with a nonreactive VDRL test.

Correlation between abnormal findings on auditory brainstem responses (suggesting occult brainstem involvement or cochlear nerve dysfunction) and CSF abnormalities was noted in one-quarter of patients with secondary or early latent syphilis, all of whom had normal neurological examinations.[14] Whether these preliminary findings indicate a subset of patients, who if untreated (or inadequately treated) would go on to develop sensorineural hearing loss associated with subsequent late syphilis, is not known.[15]

PATHOLOGIC CHANGES. The inflammatory process involves not only the meninges but also the ependyma (granular ependymitis). The meningeal infiltrate consists of lymphocytes and plasma cells located particularly in perivascular spaces. If the process becomes prolonged, fibroblastic organization ensues. Progressive inflammatory changes produce an endarteritis, which may result in thrombosis, vascular occlusion, and cerebral infarction. This process underlies the focal cerebral signs (aphasia, hemiplegia) and seizures that occur in some patients with acute syphilitic meningitis.

Acute syphilitic hydrocephalus develops as a result of obstruction, by organizing exudate, of CSF flow either from the posterior to middle cranial fossa (communicating hydrocephalus) or from the fourth ventricle (obstructive hydrocephalus). Cranial nerve abnormalities result from compression by basilar exudate and fibrous organization or, in the case of third nerve involvement, as a consequence of increased intracranial pressure.

DIAGNOSIS AND DIFFERENTIAL DIAGNOSIS. Diagnosis of acute syphilitic meningitis is based on the clinical picture of aseptic meningitis, lymphocytic response in the CSF (with or without mild hypoglycorrhachia), and reactive blood and CSF serology. A history of a recent chancre or secondary rash or the presence of generalized lymphadenopathy may suggest the diagnosis, but meningitis may be the first clinical manifestation of syphilitic infection.

Differential diagnosis includes the various causes of a lymphocytic meningitis, including enteroviruses, other spirochetes (*Leptospira* or *Borrelia* [Lyme disease]), mycobacteria, or fungi. Syphilis is likely to be accompanied by reactive serology, which does not, a priori, exclude any other diagnosis. Each of these other conditions is likely to have some unique epidemiologic, clinical and laboratory features pointing to the correct diagnosis. Acute syphilitic hydrocephalus may suggest the diagnosis of brain tumor, and the presence of low-grade fever and signs of increased intracranial pressure might raise the question of brain abscess; these conditions can be diagnosed by imaging techniques, either CT scan or magnetic resonance imaging (MRI).

The clinical features, particularly the distinctive skin lesion, and epidemiology of Lyme disease serve to distinguish it from secondary syphilis. When Lyme disease occurs in the absence of extrameningeal findings, the distinction between the two processes becomes more difficult. The sera and CSF of patients with the neurologic involvement of Lyme disease have been said to be nonreactive in nontreponemal tests.[16,17] However, the sera of 11 percent of patients with Lyme disease have been reported to show reactivity in the FTA-ABS test.[18] Furthermore, patients with syphilis show serologic reactivity with *Borrelia burgdorferi:* five of 18 patients with various stages (primary, secondary, latent, late) of syphilis had positive ELISA tests for Lyme disease, and 11 had positive IFA tests.[17] Utilizing the clinical and epidemiologic features of the two diseases as well as VDRL reactivity and *B. burgdorferi* antibody testing of serum and CSF, distinction between the meningeal syndromes of the two spirochetal diseases can be readily made.

MENINGOVASCULAR SYPHILIS

CEREBROVASCULAR SYPHILIS. Vascular neurosyphilis may involve any part of the central nervous system.[19] The common denominator is infarction secondary to syphilitic endarteritis. The process is almost invariably a meningovascular one, stemming from the chronic meningitis that underlies all forms of central nervous system syphilis. In the series of Merritt et al., 10 percent of patients had this form of neurosyphilis.[1] This disease usually occurs 5 to 12 years after initial syphilitic infection, which is earlier than the occurrence of paresis or tabes, and most patients are 30 to 50 years of age. Cerebrovascular neurosyphilis may occur concurrently with, or progress to general paresis or tabes and may be accompanied by Argyll Robertson pupils in the absence of these complications.

Symptoms and signs. The most common manifestations are hemiparesis or hemiplegia (83 percent of cases), aphasia (31 percent), and seizures (14 percent). Among 241 patients with neurosyphilis studied at the Medical College of Virginia, adult-onset seizure disorders were prominent in 24 percent; of those with seizures, 40 percent had cerebrovascular syphilis.[20] Twelve percent of patients have clinical evidence of more than one cerebral arterial occlusion. The most common involvement, by far, is the territory of the middle cerebral artery, but any other artery (anterior cerebral, posterior cerebral, basilar, posterior inferior cerebellar), on occasion may be occluded. The neurologic syndromes may be comparable to those caused by arteriosclerotic thrombotic lesions, but in neurosyphilis the site of thrombosis more often involves smaller branches, producing less extensive infarcts.

The onset of symptoms may be abrupt. However, about 50 percent of patients have premonitory symptoms of headache, dizziness, insomnia, memory loss, or mood disturbances lasting for weeks or months, probably consistent with diffuse arterial involvement. Psychiatric manifestations (personality and behavioral changes, slowing of mentation and speech) may be so prominent as to suggest the diagnosis of general paresis initially, until the onset of a stroke syndrome.[1,19]

Although distinctive occlusive cerebrovascular syndromes were features of cerebrovascular syphilis in the past when syphilis was more likely to run its course untreated or inadequately treated, nowadays the clinical picture may be atypical. An example[21] is that of a 64-year-old woman with a history of "drop attacks," suggesting vertebrobasilar artery disease, who was found to have positive blood and CSF serology and elevated CSF protein concentration (165 mg/dl) and cell count (40 cells per cubic millimeter). The attacks ceased after penicillin therapy.

Laboratory findings. Serum RPR is positive in meningovascular syphilis. The CSF changes are those usually seen in neurosyphilis, in keeping with a smoldering low-grade meningitis owing largely to occlusive vascular disease. The CSF VDRL test is positive in most, but not all cases. Angiographic changes include diffuse irregularity and "beading" of anterior and middle cerebral arteries and segmental dilatation of the pericallosal artery.[22] In contrast to the short, irregular sites of atherosclerotic disease, the areas of arterial narrowing in cerebrovascular syphilis tend to be longer and smoother. Vascular neurosyphilis, rather than atherosclerosis, is also suggested when angiographic changes occur in the supraclinoid portion of the internal carotid artery and the proximal portions of the anterior or middle cerebral arteries, in the absence of stenotic changes at the carotid bifurcation. Computed tomography (CT) shows low-density areas with variable degrees of contrast enhancement, consistent with multifocal infarctions. Magnetic resonance imaging shows focal regions of high signal intensity on T2-weighted sequences, compatible with foci of ischemia.[23]

Pathologic changes. The characteristic histologic changes of the arteritis of cerebrovascular neurosyphilis consist of infiltration by lymphocytes and plasma cells of the vasa vasorum, the adventitia and, ultimately, the media of large- and medium-sized arteries. Occlusion of the vasa vasorum results in destruction of the smooth muscle and elastic tissue of the media. Concentric proliferation of subintimal fibroblasts narrows the lumen progressively until it is occluded by thrombus formation. Infarction, subsequent scar formation, and cavitation (if the infarcted area is sizable) occur as in atherosclerotic cerebrovascular disease.

Diagnosis and differential diagnosis. The possibility of meningovascular syphilis should be considered when cerebrovascular accidents occur in a young adult, especially one who has none of the usual risk factors such as uncontrolled hypertension or findings suggestive of embolic cardiac disease. There may be a history of previously untreated or inadequately treated early syphilis. Since cerebrovascular syphilis is essentially always accompanied by some degree of meningitis, a lymphocytic pleocytosis in the CSF at the time of the thrombosis supports this diagnosis. A positive CSF serology is important in establishing the diagnosis. In the older age group, the problem is compounded by the greater likelihood of coexisting cerebral atherosclerosis, which may also be responsible for a stroke, even though the patient has meningeal (asymptomatic) neurosyphilis.

Differential diagnosis includes other causes of stroke syndromes such as hypertension (lacunar strokes), atherosclerotic vascular disease, cerebral emboli, or various types of cerebral vasculitis. Angiographic changes in cerebral vessels in systemic lupus erythematosus may be indistinguishable from those of syphilitic arteritis and those in polyarteritis nodosa may be somewhat similar.

MENINGOVASCULAR SYPHILIS OF THE SPINAL CORD. Meningovascular syphilis of the spinal cord consists principally of syphilitic meningomyelitis (the most common form) and spinal vascular syphilis (acute syphilitic transverse myelitis).[24] Spinal syphilis has always been rare, representing only about 3 percent of cases of neurosyphilis. It is almost always associated with cerebral involvement, but the disease of the cord may be preeminent. The basic underlying process is chronic spinal meningitis, which may result in parenchymatous degeneration of the cord directly or as a result of vascular thrombosis. Thus, the picture in some cases is predominantly that of chronic meningitis with cord damage (degeneration and atrophy of peripheral myelinated fibers); in other cases the picture is that of cord infarction or myelomalacia.[24]

Symptoms and signs. Syphilitic meningomyelitis usually occurs after a latent period of 20 to 25 years, at the same time as parenchymatous neurosyphilis might be expected. The onset is gradual. The earliest symptoms are weakness or paresthesias of the legs, progressing to paraparesis or paraplegia which is often asymmetric. Urinary and fecal incontinence and variable sensory disorders (pain and paresthesias) in the legs are prominent. On examination the legs are weak and spastic, and deep tendon reflexes are hyperactive; ankle clonus is present. Abdominal reflexes are absent, and extensor plantar responses can be elicited. The most frequent sensory abnormalities are loss of position and vibratory sense in the lower extremities, with a sensory level in about one-third of patients. The clinical picture may be more complex when meningomyelitis develops in the course of tabes or general paresis, or when spinal artery thrombosis supervenes, changing the spastic paraparesis to a flaccid paraplegia. Nowadays, the full-blown picture may not present itself, since antibiotic therapy can arrest progression of the process.

The classic manifestations of spinal vascular syphilis are those of a transection of the spinal cord, usually at a thoracic level, with abrupt onset of flaccid paraplegia, a sensory level on the trunk, and urinary retention. Most cases occur at about the same time after initial infection as does cerebrovascular syphilis. In some patients, transection of the cord is incomplete. After many years, in the absence of treatment, or as a result of antibiotic treatment that does not, of course, restore neurologic function, a "burned-out" state results, in which the neurologic findings persist but all laboratory evidence of active syphilitic infection disappears.

Laboratory findings. Blood serologic tests are regularly positive and CSF examination discloses the same abnormalities seen in other forms of syphilis (including a positive VDRL test), except in burned-out or old, treated cases.

Diagnosis and differential diagnosis. The diagnosis of syphilitic spinal thrombosis is made on the clinical picture of an abrupt flaccid paraplegia developing in a patient with consistent CSF abnormalities and reactive blood and CSF serologies. Other causes of a picture of acute transverse myelitis must be distinguished. Differential diagnosis of syphilitic meningomyelitis may include multiple sclerosis and subacute combined degeneration.

PARENCHYMATOUS NEUROSYPHILIS

GENERAL PARESIS. General paresis (also known as paretic neurosyphilis, dementia paralytica, and general paralysis of the insane) is a meningoencephalitis associated with direct invasion of the cerebrum by *T. pallidum*. The clinical illness is a chronic process that evolves over many years and declares itself in middle to late adult life. Untreated, the course is progressively downhill, terminating in death. This form of late syphilis develops 15 to 20 years after initial infection. Prior to World War II, patients with this disease made up 5 to 10 percent of all first admissions of psychotic patients to psychiatric hospitals.[25,26] Although this disease is now rare, it continues to account for about 10 percent of cases of neurosyphilis.[27]

Symptoms and signs. The clinical picture is that of a combination of psychiatric manifestations and neurologic findings that may mimic almost any type of psychiatric or neurological disorder. The illness is commonly insidious in onset but may occasionally become suddenly evident. The early features are usually of a psychiatric nature, and the course of illness is that of a dementing process. Early symptoms include gradual memory loss, impairment of intellectual function, and personality changes (Table 36-2). As the disease progresses, these symptoms are magnified and others appear, including defects in judgment, emotional lability, delusions, and inappropriate social or moral behavior. Grandiose delusions and megalomania, although dramatic manifestations traditionally considered classic features of general paresis, occur in only 10 to 20 percent of cases.[28] These delusions, often accompanied by hypomania, may take many forms, including those of great wealth or political power, extraordinary physical or intellectual prowess, or inappropriate social or political importance. Depression has been reported in some studies as the predominant presenting feature and the most common initial diagnosis in patients with paresis.[27]

Adult-onset seizures, noted in 15 to 20 percent of patients, may be the initial manifestation of paresis and may bring to medical attention a patient who has shown minimal or no evidence of mental aberrations.[28] In patients with paresis of apparently sudden clinical onset, the earliest indication of the disease may be a

Table 36-2. Symptoms of General Paresis[a]

Early	Late
Irritability	Defective judgment
Memory loss	Emotional lability (depression, agitation, euphoria)
Personality changes	Lack of insight
Impaired capacity to concentrate	Confusion and disorientation
Carelessness in appearance	Delusions of grandeur
Headache	Paranoia
Insomnia	Seizures

[a]After HH Merritt et al.[1]

seizure, transient ischemic attack, or apparent stroke with loss of consciousness (apoplectiform attacks), followed by hemiparesis, monoplegia, or aphasia. After such episodes, persisting confusion or psychotic behavior characteristic of paresis becomes apparent.

The most common neurologic findings in general paresis are pupillary abnormalities; flattening of the facial lines, tremors of the lips, tongue, facial muscles, and fingers; and impaired handwriting and speech (Table 36-3). The earliest speech disorder is faulty enunciation and slurring of consonants. Speech becomes progressively thicker, and the problem may be compounded by the development of dysnomia or global aphasia. Pupillary abnormalities are common in paresis and may be present in other forms of neurosyphilis. The pupils may be large, unequal, and sluggishly reactive to light and accommodation. Over the course of months, normal pupils may change to the Argyll Robertson type defined by the following characteristics: (1) the retina is sensitive (i.e., the eye is not blind); (2) the pupils are small and fixed, and do not react to strong light; (3) the pupils react normally to convergence-accommodation; (4) mydriatics (atropine) fail to dilate the pupils fully; and (5) the pupils do not dilate on painful stimuli. Argyll Robertson pupils are observed more frequently in tabes than in paresis.

As the untreated paretic process advances, apathy, hypotonia, unsteadiness, dementia, and physical deterioration become the major elements in the clinical picture. Frequent focal or generalized seizures accompany progressive deterioration and eventuate in a bedridden, paralyzed, incontinent state. The duration of untreated paresis ranges from a few months, in cases of sudden onset, to 4 or 5 years until death. Uncommonly, spontaneous but transitory remissions have occurred. The shorter the duration and the milder the symptoms at the institution of therapy, the better is the prognosis.

Communicating hydrocephalus has complicated a few cases of general paresis and, despite clearing of CSF abnormalities and improvement in hydrocephalus in some patients after treatment with large doses of penicillin, may account for either lack of clinical improvement or progressive deterioration.[29] The patients have had gait apraxia, akinetic mutism, incontinence, and pyramidal tract signs along with severe dementia. Isotope cisternograms have shown early ventricular entry of the radionuclide and absence of parasagittal radioactivity. CSF shunting has produced immediate improvement in several cases. Impairment of CSF absorption by chronic meningitis and meningeal fibrosis in general paresis appears to be the pathogenesis of this process. As noted in the preceding, the various forms of neurosyphilis do not necessarily exist as pure entities. Thus, in occasional patients with paresis, neurologic examination might reveal absent deep tendon reflexes in the lower extremities and loss of position and vibratory senses.

Laboratory findings. Nontreponemal serologic tests of blood and CSF are nearly uniformly positive in cases of paresis.[1,3,28,30,31] Other CSF findings are typical of those in neurosyphilis. The CSF may be normal in a patient whose neurosyphilis has been arrested by treatment, leaving persistent mental changes—a burned-out case as defined in the preceding. A positive serum VDRL often is a clue to presence of neurosyphilis.[32]

Specific antitreponemal antibody tests of CSF, such as FTA-ABS or MHA-TP, have been studied as a tool to diagnose neurosyphilis in the occasional case in which the CSF VDRL is nonreactive.[33–35] These tests are very sensitive, and they may be reactive as a result of diffusion of serum immunoglobulins into the CSF, or as a result of contamination of the CSF by a small amount of blood rather than because of local antibody synthesis in the CNS; for this reason, they should probably not be done.[36–38] Another approach is to examine intrathecal antibody synthesis using the CSF-IgG index, obtained by dividing the CSF to serum IgG ratio by the CSF to serum albumin ratio. A result >0.7 is indicative of IgG synthesis within the CNS, but this finding is consistent with a variety of infectious or inflammatory processes.[39,40] Specificity is provided by demonstrating that the antibody is produced intrathecally, as determined by an intrathecal *T. pallidum* antibody index >100,[41] defined as

$$\text{CSF-TPHA titer} \bigg/ \frac{\text{CSF albumin (mg/dl)} \times 10^3}{\text{serum albumin (mg/dl)}}$$

Better evidence for intrathecal antitreponemal antibody synthesis may be obtained if the serum:CSF ratio of TPHA is at least four times lower than the corresponding ratio for some other unrelated but ubiquitous antibody, such as adenovirus hemagglutinating antibody.[42] In a small number of patients with symptomatic neurosyphilis, CSF *T. pallidum*-specific IgM ELISA was found to have a sensitivity of 100 percent and a specificity of 98 percent.[43] However, CSF from patients with asymptomatic neurosyphilis was nonreactive. In another study, local synthesis of antitreponemal IgM antibodies within the CNS was found in 19 patients with untreated neurosyphilis by ratios of CSF IgM antibody levels to total CSF IgM in CSF that were 3- to 75-fold higher than corresponding serum levels.[44] The potential usefulness of the MHA-TP index has been confirmed, but tests for antitreponemal IgM antibodies in CSF rarely are performed. There is much interest in use of polymerase chain reaction test for *T. pallidum* as a means of diagnosing neurosyphilis, but the sensitivity and specificity are still unclear.[44a–d]

The use of CT scan in parenchymatous neurosyphilis may show extensive regions of decreased attenuation of the cerebral white matter, particularly in the frontal lobes and paraventricular areas of the parietal lobes, together with enlargement of cortical sulci and associated ventricular dilation, consistent with demyelinating disorders.[45] Cortical atrophy and multiple areas of hypodensity in both cerebellar hemispheres and in the brainstem, consistent with infarctions, may also be seen. Multiple nodular enhancing lesions

Table 36-3. Neurological Signs of General Paresis[a]

Sign	Percent
Common	
Pupillary abnormalities	57
Argyll Robertson pupils	26
Slurred speech	28
Expressionless facies	
Tremors (tongue, face, hands)	18
Impaired handwriting	
Reflex abnormalities	52
Uncommon	
Focal signs	2
Eye muscle palsies	
Optic atrophy	2
Extensor plantar responses	

[a]After Dewhurst[27] and Dawson-Butterworth.[28]

were observed at the base of the brain in one patient with meningovascular syphilis and cleared completely within 3 months after a 10-day course of intravenous penicillin.[46] Godt et al. found both enhancing lesions (gummas) and generalized cortical and subcortical atrophy in several patients with neurosyphilis.[47] Evidence of tertiary syphilis elsewhere, such as aortic aneurysm, may be used to support the diagnosis of neurosyphilis.

What should the physician conclude concerning an older adult with a history of prior treated early syphilis who years later has a reactive serum MHA-TP, atypical neurologic or psychiatric findings, and CSF abnormalities such as minimal pleocytosis and slightly elevated protein with a negative CSF VDRL? Is this a patient whose treponemal test reactivity merely represents prior infection and whose current neurologic syndrome has a nonsyphilitic etiology, or does he have active neurosyphilis in the absence of serum and CSF VDRL reactivity? The matter is controversial and opposing views have been stated.[32,47–49] Systematic application of some of the alternative approaches noted might help to resolve this difficult diagnostic dilemma.

Pathologic changes. Grossly, the brain in general paresis shows varying degrees of thickening of the meninges, consistent with chronic meningitis and fibrosis. Cerebral atrophy is prominent. The frontal pole and the tips of the temporal lobes are particularly involved. Demyelination of cerebral white matter is often present and usually correlates with the extent of cortical neuron loss.[50] A characteristic finding is that of granular ependymitis, formed of whorls of subependymal astrocytes. Microscopically, the changes consist of: (1) meningeal and perivascular infiltration with lymphocytes and plasma cells; (2) degeneration and loss of nerve cells; (3) proliferation of microglia and astrocytes; (4) iron deposition in vessel walls and in microglia; and (5) the presence of spirochetes in brain tissue.

Diagnosis and differential diagnosis. The diagnosis is based on the clinical picture, which is readily recognizable in its full-blown form but is more difficult to define when atypical or incomplete, together with characteristic spinal fluid abnormalities. Although the CSF is reputedly abnormal in all untreated cases of general paresis, the same changes may occur during the course of other types of neurosyphilis. Thus, the combination of preexisting CSF changes of asymptomatic syphilitic meningitis with a variety of organic brain syndromes may be misdiagnosed as general paresis. These syndromes include cerebral tumor, subdural hematoma, cerebral arteriosclerosis, Alzheimer's disease, multiple sclerosis, senile dementia, and chronic alcoholism. The findings on CT scan, the presence of pupillary changes, and a history of drug or alcohol abuse are helpful in correct diagnosis. Hallucinations are prominent in delirium tremens but are rare in general paresis. However, alcoholic deterioration and Korsakoff's psychosis may present a picture of memory loss, inappropriate behavior, mood swings, and poor judgment that is difficult to distinguish from paresis.

An adult-onset seizure disorder may be a manifestation of paresis or of an atypical form of neurosyphilis. Paresis can be excluded when CSF abnormalities are absent. When CSF changes of neurosyphilis are present, the question becomes one of whether the seizures represent epilepsy in a patient with asymptomatic neurosyphilis or whether they are the manifestations of syphilitic brain injury. The presence of focal neurologic findings in patients with neurosyphilis-induced seizures helps to resolve the question. The combination of seizures and focal findings may be found in both general paresis and meningovascular syphilis. Distinguishing between the two is probably not very important, since both are treated with penicillin.

TABES DORSALIS. In the prepenicillin era, tabes dorsalis accounted for about one-third of patients with neurosyphilis. Among several hundred patients with neurosyphilis treated in neurologic clinics in Poland from 1956 to 1965, tabes dorsalis was the most frequent diagnosis (44 percent), although in the majority, the process appeared to have "burned out," that is, there was an absence of CSF abnormalities, either spontaneously or as a result of the previous use of antibiotics to treat intercurrent infection.[51] In a study of late complications of syphilis involving about one-third of the population of Finland between 1963 and 1968, 66 cases of neurosyphilis were identified; of these, two-thirds involved tabes dorsalis.[52] In the 1960s, 30 cases of neurosyphilis (10 of tabes) were seen in one regional neurological center in England over a 3½ year period. Over the next 8½ years, only 16 cases, including four of tabes, were encountered.[53] These data support clinical observations in the United States that, in most developed countries, a patient with far-advanced tabes dorsalis is now a rarity. Some clinicians report seeing an increase in classical tabes in recent years (P.F. Sparling, personal communication).

Symptoms and signs. The onset of symptoms of tabes occurs in the majority of untreated patients in the fifth and sixth decades of life after an average latent period of 20 to 25 years. The early clinical features of tabes are lightning pains, paresthesias, diminished deep tendon reflexes (manifestations of posterior root and posterior column dysfunction), and poor pupillary responses to light. In more advanced stages of the disease, other symptoms and signs become prominent (Table 36-4). Lightning pains are sudden paroxysms of severe stabbing pains lasting for a few minutes at a time. These pains usually occur in the lower extremities but may be felt anywhere on the body. They may occur at long intervals or may persist in attacks lasting for several days at a time. Treatment with carbamazepine or related drugs may be effective.[54] Paresthesias are frequently felt on the legs or trunk. Hyperesthesia may be present in the areas involved by lightning pains; such areas may serve as trigger zones that precipitate bouts of pain when touched.

Visceral crises are related to lightning pains, tending to recur in attacks of marked severity that may mimic acute surgical emergencies. The most common form is a gastric crisis consisting of intense epigastric pain, nausea, and vomiting. Intestinal crises (ab-

Table 36-4. Symptoms and Signs of Tabes Dorsalis[a]

	Percent
Symptoms	
Lightning pains	75
Ataxia	42
Bladder disturbances	33
Paresthesias	24
Visceral crises	18
Visual loss (optic atrophy)	16
Rectal incontinence	14
Signs	
Pupillary abnormalities	94
Argyll Robertson pupils	48
Absent ankle jerks	94
Absent knee jerks	81
Romberg's sign	55
Impaired vibratory sense	52
Impaired position sense	45
Impaired touch and pain sense	13
Ocular palsies	10
Charcot's joints	7

[a]After HH Merritt et al.[1]

dominal pain and diarrhea), rectal crises (painful tenesmus), and laryngeal crises (pain in the larynx, hoarseness, stridor) are rare. In some patients, impotence and urinary retention or dribbling, resulting from an insensitive, hypotonic bladder, may be early symptoms of sacral root dysfunction.

Loss of vibration sense and inability to feel passive movement in joints are among the first detectable signs of this disease. Other sensory abnormalities include loss of deep pain perception and development of patchy areas of hypalgesia and hypesthesia over the trunk and extremities. Knee and ankle reflexes are almost always reduced or absent, whereas muscle strength is usually well preserved until the late stages. Plantar responses are flexor; the presence of Babinski's sign indicates the coexistence of meningovascular syphilis, general paresis, or some unrelated disorder of the CNS. Ataxia of gait is evident, and results of heel to-shin and finger-to-nose testing are abnormal. In addition to the broad-based, stamping gait, which becomes worse in the dark, abnormal findings include diminished vision owing to optic atrophy, Charcot's joint (unstable, painless, uninflamed, markedly enlarged joint with overproduction of bone owing to repeated trauma to this anesthetic structure, especially involving the knee), and mal perforans (a painless penetrating trophic ulcer on the plantar surface at the base of a toe). The spine (particularly the lumbar spine) may be the site of Charcot changes, characterized by dense irregular sclerosis, large parrot-beak osteophytes, scoliosis, and disk-space narrowing.[55] Although the lesion itself is painless, distressing pain may be produced by impingement of the hypertrophic bone or by a disk protruding on posterior nerve roots.[56]

Sluggish pupillary reactivity to light is an early finding in tabes; true Argyll Robertson pupil is a later feature of the disease. Involvement of cranial nerves (particularly the second, third, and sixth) is often overlooked in tabes. Primary optic atrophy appears as sharply defined, grayish white optic disks with conspicuous physiologic cupping, visible lamina cribrosa, and narrowed retinal arteries. If untreated, visual loss progresses to irreversible blindness over months to years. Ptosis and flabbiness of facial muscles probably contribute in a large measure to the so-called tabetic facies. Divergent strabismus may also result from third cranial nerve palsy. Oculomotor weakness is thought to be owing to an associated basilar meningitis, accounting for its occasional improvement after penicillin therapy. Eighth cranial nerve involvement (hearing loss with or without accompanying vestibular abnormalities) is not uncommon.

In the absence of treatment for syphilis, tabes appears 18 to 25 years after infection. The time from the onset of tabes to the development of ataxia may be 6 months to 25 years; the longer the duration of the pre-ataxic phase, the slower the subsequent course. In the prepenicillin era, far-advanced tabes was observed with complete incapacitation owing to joint deformity, loss of bladder control, blindness, ataxia, and deafness. Tabes may burn out with time, even in the absence of treatment. Lighting pains may persist even when early treatment has been successful; their presence, therefore, does not indicate continued syphilitic infection. Antibiotic treatment cannot reverse the extensive changes of advanced disease.

Laboratory findings. The laboratory findings in tabetic neurosyphilis are variable, depending on the stage of tabes, whether partial or full treatment has been administered in the past, and whether the process has spontaneously burned out. In the prepenicillin era, negative blood Wassermann reactions were reported in 12 to 42 percent of cases. In a 1972 study of seven patients with longstanding tabes, the blood Wassermann reaction was negative in six patients all of whom had been treated repeatedly but continued to have lightning pains and other manifestations of tabes.[54]

The CSF findings among 100 patients with tabes, including a large number of patients with old, arrested cases, were: (1) lymphocytic pleocytosis in 50 percent (practically all untreated cases); (2) elevated protein concentration (45 to 100 mg/dl) in 50 percent; and (3) reactive Wassermann test in 72 percent.[1]

Normal CSF can be found in the late stages of treated or burned out tabes in a patient who continues to have lightning pains and Charcot's joints; this finding reflects the irreversible damage already produced in the spinal cord and dorsal roots.

Diagnosis and differential diagnosis. A clinical diagnosis of tabes is most likely in a patient with lightning pains and ataxia who exhibits findings of absent deep tendon reflexes, Argyll Robertson pupils, and a positive Romberg sign. Early and atypical cases present greater problems in diagnosis, and only the results of serologic testing and spinal fluid examination may lead to the correct diagnosis. A mixed clinical picture of taboparesis may also be a source of diagnostic confusion.

Differential diagnosis includes a variety of neurologic disorders. Although knee and ankle jerks may be lost in meningovascular syphilis of the spinal cord, lightning pains and pupillary changes are not usually present; ultimately, hyperactive reflexes and extensor plantar responses develop. Adie's syndrome (absent deep tendon reflexes and myotonic pupil) can be distinguished from tabes by the fact that the pupil is not miotic. This syndrome also lacks the lightning pains and ataxia of tabes; serologic tests are negative and CSF examination is normal. Diabetic neuropathy may mimic tabes (diabetic pseudotabes) by producing sluggish pupillary reactivity, ptosis, pains, and ataxia and by absent deep tendon reflexes. However, in diabetic and other types of peripheral neuropathy, the pain is burning in character rather than shooting, as is typical of tabes, and the serologic findings are negative. Combined system disease is similar to tabes in producing ataxia and bladder disturbances, but lightning pains are not a feature. Extensor plantar responses are found in combined system disease but not in tabes.

OPTIC ATROPHY

Syphilitic optic atrophy, with the same ocular manifestations as occur in tabes dorsalis, may appear as an isolated manifestation of neurosyphilis.[57] The usual symptoms are those of progressive visual loss involving first one eye and then the other. As in cases of tabes, CSF abnormalities are usually present in the untreated patient. Optic atrophy may also result from prior syphilitic optic neuritis. The visual evoked response may make it possible to distinguish primary from postneuritic optic atrophy on the basis of a normal latency in the former.[58] Penicillin treatment can usually prevent further progression of visual loss.

GUMMAS OF THE NERVOUS SYSTEM

CEREBRAL GUMMAS. Intracerebral gummas are extremely rare; only one was encountered among 676 cases of neurosyphilis at the Boston City Hospital over a 15-year period in the prepenicillin era.[1] The features are those of a cerebral neoplasm, brain abscess, or tuberculoma. CSF findings are the same as in other forms of neurosyphilis but include increased CSF pressure. CT scan may reveal a low-density nonenhancing area, and angiography may show a hypervascular blush zone surrounding the focal area of gummatous necrosis.[59,60] The diagnosis may only be made when the patient is operated on for a suspected intracranial mass lesion. Curiously, the recent literature contains multiple anecdotal accounts of cerebral gummas, mostly in HIV infected persons.[60a–d]

GUMMA OF THE SPINAL CORD

Gumma of the spinal cord is fundamentally a granuloma of the meninges compressing the cord. The clinical picture is that of a cord tumor: root pains, spastic paraplegia, urinary and fecal incontinence, and loss of sensation below the lesion. The progression is subacute. The CSF findings consist of dynamic block, markedly elevated protein (over 350 mg/dl), and a positive nontreponemal serologic test.

CONGENITAL NEUROSYPHILIS

CLASSIFICATION AND CHRONOLOGY. The incidence of symptomatic congenital neurosyphilis has increased in recent years because of increased pregnancies in adolescents who do not seek prenatal care and increased exchange of sexual favors in return for illicit drugs. These issues are compounded by the prevalence of AIDS. The fetus acquires infection transplacentally from the mother, and this form of syphilis is essentially the only form that is not sexually transmitted. This subject is reviewed elsewhere and will not be discussed further in the present chapter.[61]

CURRENT "ATYPICAL" PRESENTATION OF NEUROSYPHILIS

During the past two decades, as the incidence of neurosyphilis has continued to decline, attention has been drawn to unusual patterns and atypical presentations of this disease.[20,21,62–66] One reason for this may simply be decreased familiarity among physicians with the full range of manifestations of neurosyphilis. It also is possible that the clinical features and the course of neurosyphilis have been modified by the use of inadequate doses of penicillin administered for the treatment of early or late syphilis or for the treatment of intercurrent illnesses during the latent stage of syphilis.

Hooshmand et al. claimed to have identified 241 cases in which neurosyphilis was diagnosed in one medical center between 1965 and 1970.[20] These investigators attempted to stress the importance of atypical presentative such as adult-onset seizures or mild symmetrical ptosis and a partial picture of tabes. Cerebrovascular accidents, confusional syndromes, and dementing illnesses (possible formes frustes of general paresis) were other presenting clinical manifestations. Since the cases described often did not have the full constellation of features characteristic of classical neurosyphilis (Argyll Robertson pupils, lightning pains, Charcot's joints), the diagnostic standards employed in this study are of paramount importance. They included one or another of the following sets of criteria: (1) positive blood FTA-ABS serology along with neurologic or ophthalmologic findings suggestive of neurosyphilis; (2) unexplained neurological illness with positive blood and CSF FTA-ABS tests and CSF showing more than five white blood cells per cubic millimeter; or (3) positive FTA-ABS results in blood and CSF in patients with progressive neurologic diseases in whom other etiologic considerations had been excluded. Only 49 percent of the patients had a reactive serum RPR and 56 percent had a reactive CSF VDRL. In almost 90 percent of the patients, the CSF cell counts were 10 or less per cubic millimeter, and in about 60 percent the protein level was in the normal range. Only 5 percent of patients had a clearcut clinical picture of paresis, although more than 50 percent had undergone earlier treatment for syphilis. Thus a substantial proportion of the patients in this series may not have had neurosyphilis at all, or they may have had sufficient prior treatment to alter the presentation. The use of a positive FTA-ABS on CSF to confirm the diagnosis in a sizable number of cases opens the conclusions of the study to question, since, as noted, this test gives false positive results. The same critique may be applied to other recent series of cases, purporting to show atypical manifestations of neurosyphilis in the modern era.[66]

A number of other case reports of rapid progression to neurosyphilis, atypical presentations of neurosyphilis and/or penicillin treatment failure that appeared in the 1970s appear, in retrospect, to represent cases of neurosyphilis in HIV-infected persons. This subject will be discussed in the following. With an incubation period of >10 years before the appearance of AIDS, HIV infection was certainly present in the population in the 1970s, although unrecognized until AIDS was first diagnosed in the early 1980s.

ANTIBIOTIC THERAPY

The introduction of penicillin in the 1940s strikingly simplified the therapy and improved the outcome of neurosyphilis. At first, repeated intramuscular injections of aqueous penicillin were administered every 3 to 4 hours for a total dosage of 2 to 3 million units over a period of 8 to 16 days.[12] By the early 1950s it was apparent that the administration of 6 to 10 million units of penicillin (as either procaine penicillin G or procaine penicillin in oil with aluminum monostearate) over a period of 18 to 21 days produced a good therapeutic response in over 90 percent of cases. In the occasional patient who did not respond, another course of penicillin at a higher dose was usually successful in arresting the infection. Return to normal function was not required as proof of efficacy. In one series of cases, spinal fluid findings indicated that the disease was arrested in each of 462 patients with various forms of neurosyphilis treated in this fashion.[67] In a multicenter study involving treatment of over 1000 patients with paresis, a total penicillin dosage of 6 million units was judged to be adequate.[68] Patients who required retreatment to arrest the infection had initially received less than 6 million units of penicillin.

As a result of these clinical field trials, for a period of two decades in the 1960s and 1970s treatment with 7.2 million units of benzathine penicillin G (2.4 million units intramuscularly weekly for three doses) was regarded as adequate for all forms of neurosyphilis. This conclusion was empirical, having been based on observations of clinical outcome.

The recommended dosages for the treatment of all forms of late syphilis were initially designed to maintain serum spirocheticidal levels of 0.031 unit or more per milliliter.[69] Understanding that 2.4 million units of benzathine penicillin produces serum levels ≤ 0.5 μg/ml, and that levels in CSF are probably no more than 2 percent of serum levels, it becomes clear that spirochetacidal levels are not achieved in the CSF of patients receiving this medication. Not surprisingly, therefore, penicillin was not detectable in the CSF of 12 of 13 patients who received especially high doses of benzathine penicillin G (3.6 million units per week for 4 weeks).[70] Even with administration of 600,000 units of aqueous procaine penicillin G intramuscularly daily, the peak CSF penicillin level 3 h after injection was less than 0.017 unit per milliliter.[70] Consistent with these observations is the reported isolation by rabbit inoculation of *T. pallidum* from the CSF of a patient who had been treated with 1.2 million units of benzathine penicillin G intramuscularly three times weekly for 3 weeks. It has been shown as well that treponemes may still be isolated from CSF after treatment.[9,71]

Other studies reinforced doubts raised about the adequacy of prior recommended doses of penicillin in the treatment of neurosyphilis. The long-term follow-up (average 17 years) of a group of 64 patients with general paresis treated with penicillin (3 to 30 million units, cumulative) indicated that 39 percent developed new neurological signs during that interval.[72] The new findings observed were major ones such as seizures, hemiparesis, paraplegia, tabes dorsalis, and their frequency was many times in excess of the prevalence rates for cerebrovascular disease or epilepsy in adults without syphilis but of comparable age. It is important to note, however, that some of these patients had not received recommended dosages of penicillin, and the progression of neurologic disease in older persons in the absence of CSF abnormalities is difficult to attribute to neurosyphilis. Hooshmand et al. reported 10 patients with tabes or meningovascular syphilis who continued to show clinical evidence of active neurosyphilis and continued CSF pleocytosis after what generally had been considered an adequate course of treatment (9 million units of penicillin G administered over 3 weeks).[20] Symptomatic improvement and clearing of the CSF pleocytosis followed intramuscular treatment with 1.2 million units of procaine penicillin G daily for a period of 3 weeks. In the same study, when 89 patients with neurosyphilis were followed up for at least 2 years after completion of a 3-week course of treatment with daily procaine penicillin G totaling ≥220 million units, five clinical failures were observed.[20] Four of these patients developed general paresis and one had an organic brain syndrome. CSF cell counts and protein values were normal in each case. Whether these "failures" represented further progression of the infection despite treatment or the consequences of already established structural changes is unclear from the report. Many of these patients had been treated with doses far in excess of generally recommended ones and still had progressive disease. It is certainly not clear that the outcome would have been better had even larger doses of penicillin been used to treat them.

During the 1970s, a few cases were reported in which benzathine or procaine penicillin in recommended dose failed to cure neurosyphilis. A careful reading of these case reports suggests that the failures represented early cases of neurosyphilis in HIV-infected persons.

As a result of these considerations, the World Health Organization and the Centers for Disease Control and Prevention no longer recommend benzathine penicillin to treat neurosyphilis. The most recent recommendations of the Centers for Disease Control[73] include the use of intravenous aqueous penicillin G 18 to 24 million units daily for 10 to 14 days or intramuscular procaine penicillin G 2.4 million units plus probenecid 500 mg by mouth four times daily for 10 to 14 days. This dosage of procaine penicillin is very painful. Some authorities recommend that the two higher dosage schedules be followed by benzathine penicillin because of the concept that duration of therapy may be as important as intensity (Table 36-5).

Table 36-5. Drug Regimens for Treatment of Neurosyphilis

1. Aqueous crystalline penicillin G: 18 to 24 million units intravenously daily (3 to 4 million units every 4 h) for 10–14 days followed by benzathine penicillin G 2.4 million units intramuscularly weekly for three doses
2. Aqueous procaine penicillin G: 2.4 million units daily intramuscularly plus probenecid 500 mg orally 4 times daily, both for 10–14 days, followed by benzathine penicillin G 2.4 million units intramuscularly weekly for three doses

Note:

1. Benzathine penicillin G: 2.4 million units by intramuscular injection each week for three doses is no longer recommended despite its apparent clinical efficacy over many years *(see text)*.
2. For patients who are allergic to penicillin, the official recommendation is that desensitization be undertaken, although some experts recommend a 3-week course of ceftriaxone, 1 gm daily, instead.

After Centers for Disease Control: MMWR 1997; 47:38.

FOLLOW-UP AND TREATMENT

Clinical (including CSF) examination should be done 3 months after antibiotic treatment of patients with neurosyphilis and then at 6 month intervals, until the CSF findings return to normal. Thereafter, reevaluation should be performed annually for several years. This is particularly important in patients who have been treated with alternative antibiotics, because limited data are available on the long-term efficacy of such therapeutic programs.

Normalization of CSF values may be taken as a reliable sign of antimicrobial efficacy of therapy. As noted, this response may be associated with a resolution of clinical findings or at least with a stabilization although, on occasion, clinical progression may occur. Such patients are often retreated, and with a more intensive regimen of penicillin when possible, despite the likelihood that there will be no further benefit.

In a minority of patients CSF abnormalities persist. Patients whose WBC count and protein do not decline after 6 months are often retreated, again with more intensive therapy when possible. Some patients simply maintain elevated WBC, protein and VDRL titers for several years despite multiple courses of therapy and although it may be difficult to argue against one or two courses of repeated therapy, it is unclear that any benefit results.[74]

A true failure of therapy may rarely occur, in which an initial normalization of CSF findings is followed by relapse; in such cases, repeat therapy needs to be given. If relapse has not occurred during a period of 2 years after therapy, the patient can generally be regarded as cured.

PROGNOSIS WITH TREATMENT

In the prepenicillin era, untreated or inadequately treated asymptomatic neurosyphilis progressed over a 5- to 18-year period to clinical neurosyphilis in 23 to 87 percent of cases; the percentage depended to some extent on the duration of the asymptomatic neurosyphilis when first diagnosed.[1,4] Although the optimal dosage, preparation, or duration of penicillin administration in the treatment of asymptomatic neurosyphilis was never established, penicillin clearly is effective therapy. Among 765 patients treated with varying dosages of penicillin (2.4 to more than 9 million units) for asymptomatic neurosyphilis, only one subsequently went on to develop symptomatic disease and was considered an unequivocal treatment failure.[75] Similarly, the results of penicillin therapy of acute syphilitic meningitis have been very good, with clearing of the CSF changes and lack of progression to parenchymatous neurosyphilis.

The immediate prognosis for a patient with cerebral arterial occlusion owing to meningovascular syphilis is usually better than that for a patient with a similar thrombosis on an atherosclerotic basis because of the younger age of the former and the greater likelihood that the arteries involved are smaller. Treatment, even in the prepenicillin days, was effective, and most patients had no further cerebrovascular accidents. Penicillin therapy has usually been effective in clearing the CSF changes and in preventing progressive clinical disease; obviously, it cannot reverse structural damage that has already occurred. The course of untreated general paresis is progressive, and the outcome is eventually fatal.

Early reports of results of penicillin treatment of paresis indicated a relatively low rate (6 to less than 20 percent) of failure of response in the CSF, of clinical progression, or of late complications.[76,77] Dissenting reports by Hooshmand et al. and Wilner and Brody have been discussed above. Among a group of 58 hospitalized patients with paresis treated with one or more courses of penicillin, 26 (45 percent) improved and were discharged from the hospital; this result indicates that this form of neurosyphilis is not hopeless, particularly when treatment is instituted as soon as clinical symptoms become evident, but response to therapy is by no means assured.[20,26,72]

The prognosis of tabes dorsalis is variable, and the disease can be compatible with long life. About 4 to 10 percent of untreated cases become spontaneously arrested at an early stage. In the prepenicillin era, treatment improved or arrested the clinical course in over 80 percent of cases. However, in view of the nature of the underlying pathology, disappearance of many of the clinical findings would not be expected. Similarly, many of the residual signs and symptoms may persist after penicillin therapy. The most satisfactory therapeutic results are achieved in early cases of tabes in which the CSF findings are markedly abnormal.

NEUROSYPHILIS IN HIV-INFECTED PERSONS

HIV infection has had a profound impact on the neurological manifestations of syphilis.[78,79] As has been pointed out above, during the 1960s and the early 1970s, newly diagnosed cases of proven neurosyphilis in the United States had become increasingly rare. As noted, this rarity was taken as evidence for efficacy of existing regimens used to treat early and latent syphilis. Beginning in the mid-1970s, an increasing number of case reports described patients with neurosyphilis that had a so-called atypical appearance. Although these reports antedated the formal recognition of AIDS, a perusal of individual case descriptions suggests that the persons affected were at high risk for, and, in retrospect, were likely to have had concurrent HIV infection. Because AIDS was first recognized in 1980, and the incubation period from the time of retroviral infection to the development of AIDS exceeds 12 years, HIV infection in the sexually active population was not rare in the 1970s.

With the description of AIDS and the subsequent development of serological tests to diagnose HIV infection, two important facts have become apparent: (1) neurosyphilis is a commonplace occurrence in HIV-infected patients even before the onset of AIDS; and (2) in this setting, the disease is not "atypical" but, in fact, presents with manifestations that are typical of early neurosyphilis as described (Table 36-6). It is important, therefore, to consider the effect of HIV infection on the natural history of syphilis and on the response to conventional treatment, after which the question of appropriate therapy will be discussed in depth.

ACUTE SYPHILITIC MENINGITIS. A review of the medical literature through 1989 revealed 42 cases in which neurosyphilis was thought to coexist with HIV infection (Table 36-6).[78] Five of the 42 patients had abnormal CSF, but were otherwise free of neurologic symptoms and were classified as asymptomatic; asymptomatic neurosyphilis is probably vastly more common in HIV-infected persons than suggested by this review, as shall be shown in the following. Acute syphilitic meningitis was present in 14 patients, as manifested by fever, headache, stiffness of the neck, and/or confusion. Five of these patients, and 15 others who lacked signs of meningitis, had cranial nerve abnormalities. Optic neuritis or neuroretinitis was most common, being diagnosed in 11 cases. Presenting symptoms included blurred vision and blindness; some patients had inflammatory cells in the vitreous or aqueous. Diffuse syphilitic neuroretinitis was also observed, this term being used to describe the presence of optic papillitis, retinal edema, vitreous inflammation and retinal vasculitis.[80] Six patients had involvement of the otic and vestibular branch of the eighth cranial nerve, presenting with deafness, sometimes quite sudden in onset (as described under early neurosyphilis), loss of balance or both. Others showed involvement of the third, fourth and sixth, the fifth, and the seventh cranial nerves, respectively, and several of those whose disease affected the second or eighth cranial nerve had some involvement of these other cranial nerves, as well. One patient had polyradiculopathy.

Table 36-6. Reported Cases of Neurosyphilis in HIV-infected Patients (as of 1990)[a]

Asymptomatic	5
Acute meningitis	25
Meningitis	9
Cranial nerve dysfunction	15
Polyradiculopathy	1
Meningovascular	11
General paresis	1

[a]After Musher et al.[78]

MENINGOVASCULAR SYPHILIS. Eleven of the 42 patients with coexisting HIV infection and syphilis had symptoms and signs of a cerebrovascular accident that varied depending on the location of the lesion and the presence or absence of infarction. Most had computerized axial tomography to confirm the presence of lesions, and two individuals had angiographic demonstration of multiple areas of narrowing, the typical beaded appearance of the cerebral arteries that is consistent with syphilitic vasculitis. In fact, two patients who originally presented with syphilitic meningitis but were not treated developed strokes owing to progression of untreated neurosyphilis. Finally, one patient had general paresis. All of the symptoms and signs are perfectly typical for meningovascular syphilis, as discussed in the preceding.

Some abnormality of the CSF was demonstrated in 38 of 39 cases in which a spinal tap was performed, and for any given parameter, 30 to 80 percent of CSF values were abnormal, consistent with early forms of neurosyphilis (Table 36-7). The CSF VDRL test, which provides the most specific diagnosis of neurosyphilis, was reactive in 79 percent of cases, emphasizing that CSF analysis does not provide a certain diagnosis, a worrisome situation but, as shown in the preceding, one that existed in the pre-AIDS era. Interpretation of abnormalities other than the CSF VDRL in patients with concurrent HIV infection is, admittedly, a problem, since the retroviral infection itself and the numerous other opportunistic infections associated with it may produce a variety of CSF changes.

Several studies of HIV-infected subjects have suggested that the prevalence of active neurosyphilis is between 1 and 2 percent. In the retrospective study by Katz and Berger, 1.5 percent of all patients attending a clinic for HIV-related disease were diagnosed as having neurosyphilis.[81] Finding neurosyphilis in a measurable percentage of any patient group in the United States in the 1980s was simply amazing. Holtom et al. screened 312 entrants to an AIDS clinic and found 71 with reactive RPR and MHA-TP tests.[82] Of these, 33 consented to have a lumbar puncture; three (10 percent) had reactive VDRL in the CSF. If the persons who underwent lumbar puncture were representative, the prevalence of neurosyphilis among entrants to an AIDS clinic would have exceeded 2 percent. Even if the prevalence was not this high (as was probably the case, since there was a bias toward doing a lumbar puncture in patients with more highly reactive serum RPR tests), it could not have been less than 1 percent (three of 312). Looking from a different point of view, Dowell et al. found that when 13 asymptomatic HIV-infected patients with serum RPR $\geq$1:4 submitted to a lumbar puncture, the CSF VDRL was reactive in seven (54 percent); five of these subjects had increased white blood cells in their CSF and six had elevated protein, as well.[83] Since clinics that provide care for HIV-infected patients find that 5 to 10 percent of all patients have serum RPR reactive at $\geq$1:4, these data are all consistent with a prevalence of asymptomatic neurosyphilis exceeding 2 percent in HIV-infected patients.[82,83]

Table 36-7. CSF Abnormalities in 42 Reported Cases of Coexisting Syphilis and HIV Infection[a]

	Cells	Protein (mg/dl)	Glucose (mg/dl)	VDRL(+)
Abnormality reported	29/34	28/34	11/32	31/39
Median abnormal values	173	125	37	1:4
Range of abnormal values	8–2000	46–1000	11–42	WR[b]–1:16

[a]After Musher et al.[78]
bWR = weakly reactive.
Note: A few, very rare examples of late syphilis are included to emphasize that no tissue or organ is immune to gummatous diseases and that there is therefore a need for the consideration of syphilis in differential diagnosis.

Several additional points need to be made about the relation between HIV infection and neurosyphilis. First, neurosyphilis occurs in persons whose HIV infection has not yet progressed to cause AIDS. Of 35 patients with concurrent neurosyphilis for whom the stage of HIV infection was reported, 17 had AIDS, four had AIDS-related complex and 14 had only serologic evidence of HIV infection.[78] In fact, the CD4 cell count may even exceed 500/mm^3 further supporting the notion that case reports of neurosyphilis from the 1970s may well have represented treponemal infection in HIV-infected persons. This observation serves as a reminder that, early in the course of HIV infection, subtle abnormalities in the host's immunologic capacity occur, increasing susceptibility to typical human pathogens such as *T. pallidum*, unlike the later course, in which a much greater degree of damage has been done to the immune system and infections owing to less pathogenic organisms predominate. Second, in 11 of 25 patients (44 percent) for whom data were available, the diagnosis of HIV infection was first made when the patient presented with neurosyphilis. Thus, neurosyphilis may be a sentinel infection in the recognition of HIV infection. Considering its rarity in the non-HIV infected population the diagnosis of neurosyphilis should strongly suggest the coexistence of HIV infection. Third, as was amply documented in several reported cases, the failure to treat asymptomatic neurosyphilis in HIV-infected persons may be followed by progression to symptomatic neurosyphilis, generally manifesting itself as a cerebrovascular accident. Recognition of the rapid progression to meningovascular syphilis in HIV infected persons was probably the first recognition of the coexistence of these diseases.[84] Finally, 16 of the 42 reported HIV-infected patients had previously been treated with penicillin for syphilis; five (31 percent) developed early neurosyphilis within 6 months of having received a recommended course of therapy, usually 2.4 million units of benzathine penicillin. Musher et al. have explained the association between early neurosyphilis and HIV infection by proposing that inadequate antimicrobial therapy for syphilis in an immunologically normal host may be analogous to adequate antibiotic therapy in an immunologically suppressed host.[78]

THERAPY OF NEUROSYPHILIS IN HIV-INFECTED PERSONS

It is best to state at the outset that there are, as yet, no reports of studies that give a scientific basis for treating neurosyphilis in HIV-infected persons. Just as the best regimen to treat primary or secondary syphilis in HIV-infected persons is not yet certain, the same is true of therapy for early neurosyphilis. A retrospective study observed patients for 6 to 24 months after treatment with 10 to 14 days of daily IV ceftriaxone.[83] The progression of syphilis in 33 of 43 (77 percent) patients, including six of seven who had documented neurosyphilis, appeared to be arrested. The remaining 10 patients (23 percent) either failed to respond to this therapy (one case) or had serologic evidence for reactivation of disease after an initial response (nine cases). The use of 1 versus 2 gm of ceftriaxone each day did not appear to have any impact on the outcome. Interestingly, in a small number of patients whose CSF was not examined and who received three doses of benzathine penicillin for what was presumed to be latent syphilis, the outcome was similar. This was consistent with the prediction that the rate of long-lasting responses might be no higher if intravenous penicillin were used since the basic problem is the immunologic status of the host, not antibiotic dosage.[78] A recent nonrandomized study of 11 patients treated with 18 to 24 million units of penicillin daily provided support for this hypothesis, showing that one patient relapsed and several others had no apparent response during a relatively short time of follow-up.[85,86]

ROUTINE CSF EXAMINATION IN HIV-INFECTED PERSONS WHO HAVE SEROLOGIC EVIDENCE FOR SYPHILIS

Should the CSF be examined in every patient who has early syphilis and concurrent HIV infection? This approach was taken routinely in the prepenicillin era in order to monitor therapy and to be certain that neurosyphilis did not develop. Opposing this approach is the argument that, in the past, CSF abnormalities including the presence of treponemes were found in up to 40 percent of patients with early syphilis, yet did not require an altered approach to penicillin therapy (see Chap. 35). It is also true, although perhaps it has been overstated, that CSF abnormalities may be present owing to the HIV infection itself, which would confound the situation. Finally, to do a lumbar puncture takes time and requires a suitable facility, a problem in some clinics that provide care to HIV-infected persons.

Favoring the routine use of lumbar puncture in HIV-infected persons who have latent syphilis of any duration (e.g., defined by a reactive serum RPR $\geq$1:4 without clinical signs of syphilis), is the observation that a substantial proportion may be found to have evidence of active neurosyphilis; for example, 10 to 30 percent may have a reactive CSF VDRL test.[82,83] Of all those infections that AIDS patients may develop, neurosyphilis may still be among the more readily treatable. Furthermore, as shown herein, repeated CSF analysis provides a means for following the results of treatment. Even this last point, however, may be overstated since repeated determinations of serum RPR may give equivalent insight into response or failure; lumbar puncture could then be reserved for those patients who have clinical or serological evidence for failure or for relapse. Data on the predictive value of routine or other serologic tests in this situation are not available at the present time.

Thus, at the time of this writing, we do not know whether CSF analysis should be performed routinely in every HIV-infected person who has a reactive VDRL. We think this study certainly should be done in patients who have symptoms or signs consistent with neurosyphilis, and in any stage of infection when a patient does not show an appropriate serologic response to therapy.

FOLLOW-UP CARE. It should be clear from these considerations that repeated, close evaluation is required for HIV-infected patients who have evidence of neurosyphilis. This is precisely what was done in the prepenicillin era, when less effective antimicrobial agents were used to treat syphilis in immunologically normal hosts. If, during the penicillin era but prior to the advent of HIV infection, individual practitioners thought they could afford to be somewhat cavalier in their serologic monitoring after treatment because the efficacy rate was so remarkably high, this is clearly not possible with HIV-infected persons. Recommendations to do followup serum and CSF studies at 3-month intervals should be followed. There is enough question about the efficacy of any recommended treatment and sufficient likelihood of a relapse even if initial therapy appears to be effective that a substantial sense of insecurity should characterize the approach of the treating physician to his or her patient.

CARDIOVASCULAR SYPHILIS

CLINICAL MANIFESTATIONS OF ACQUIRED CARDIOVASCULAR SYPHILIS

Since syphilis of the cardiovascular system becomes clinically manifest only in the tertiary stage of the disease, which is preceded by a latent period of 15 to 30 years, most patients are between 40 and 55 years of age; men are affected three times as often as women.

Cardiovascular syphilis in its tertiary phase may lead to aortic aneurysms, aortic insufficiency, coronary stenosis, and rarely myocarditis. Its clinical presentation is characterized by the functional disorder resulting from cardiac involvement and at times may be difficult to distinguish from other more common varieties of cardiac disease.[87]

Penicillin and other antibiotics appear to have nearly eliminated late cardiovascular syphilis, even in AIDS patients. It is unclear why this is so, since neurosyphilis and even gummas are no longer rare.

PATHOLOGY AND PATHOPHYSIOLOGY. The cardiovascular system is not clinically affected in the early stages of syphilis, but older studies showed it is involved morphologically in up to 80 percent of occurrences of the tertiary stage of the disease.[88] Clinical manifestations of cardiovascular syphilis occur in only about 10 percent of such occurrences, or less; the current literature contains only rare anecdotes of clinically evident cardiovascular syphilis. In the tertiary state, aortic, coronary ostial, valvular, and myocardial lesions of syphilis have been described, but aortitis is the most common lesion, accounting for the majority of clinical manifestations (Figs. 36-1 and 36-2).[89–91]

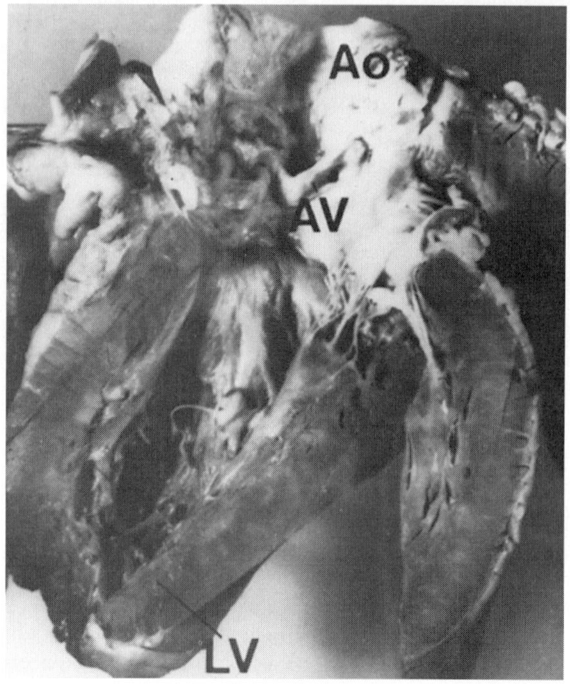

Fig. 36-2. Heart of a patient who died with syphilitic aortic insufficiency. The aortic valve leaflets are thickened and rolled. The proximal aorta (Ao) is involved by atherosclerotic plaques which demarcate the area of syphilitic aortitis. The left ventricle (LV) is hypertrophied and moderately dilated as a result of the long-standing aortic insufficiency.

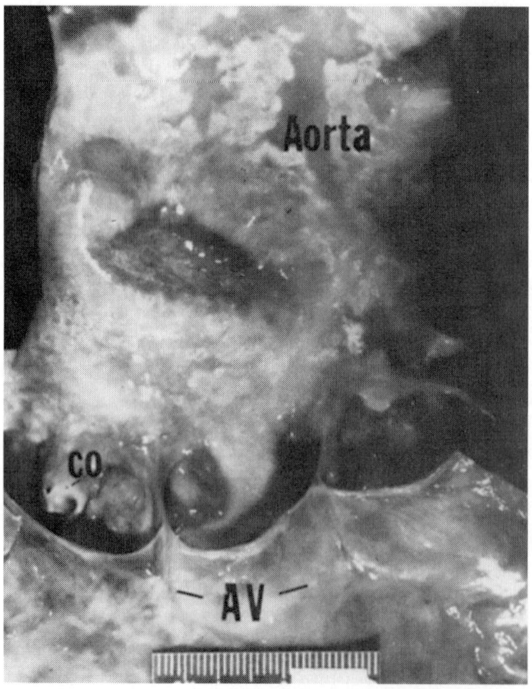

Fig. 36-1. Proximal aorta and aortic valve from a patient with syphilitic aortitis. The atherosclerotic process extensively involved the aortic root area and was less prominent in the distal aorta, which is the reverse of the atherosclerotic pattern ordinarily seen. The cusps of the aortic valve (AV) are thickened because of mild aortic insufficiency, and some intimal plaque is evident around the coronary ostia (CO), which may be critically narrowed in syphilis.

Treponema pallidum presumably spreads to the heart during the early stages of syphilis, possibly via the lymphatics, and the organisms lodge in the aortic wall, where they remain dormant for years. The spirochetes appear to have a predilection for the vasa vasorum of the aorta, particularly the proximal aorta, producing transmural inflammatory lesions resulting in endarteritis of these vessels. The proximal portions of the coronary arteries near the ostia sometimes are involved by the obliterative endarteritis. This inflammatory process, which is rich in perivascular lymphocytes and plasma cells, continues for years, long after evidence of early syphilis has passed. This suggests that the lesions of late cardiovascular syphilis have an immunologic basis, as has been proposed for other forms of tertiary syphilis.

Although the initial insult is primarily to the small nutrient vessels of the aorta, all three layers of aortic wall are affected by the process. Probably because of obliteration of the lumen of the vasa vasorum, the aortic media develops patchy necrosis with subsequent focal scarring. The medial destruction is also associated with the destruction of the important elastic tissue of the media, which sets the stage for subsequent aortic dilation and aneurysm formation. The adventitia, which contains the prominently inflamed vasa vasorum, undergoes fibrous thickening. The overlying aortic intima becomes diffusely diseased, with atherosclerotic changes involving virtually the entire intimal surface of the affected aorta. The extensive plaque formation has been described as "tree barking," and the calcification accompanying these complicated atherosclerotic plaques accounts for the eggshell calcifi-

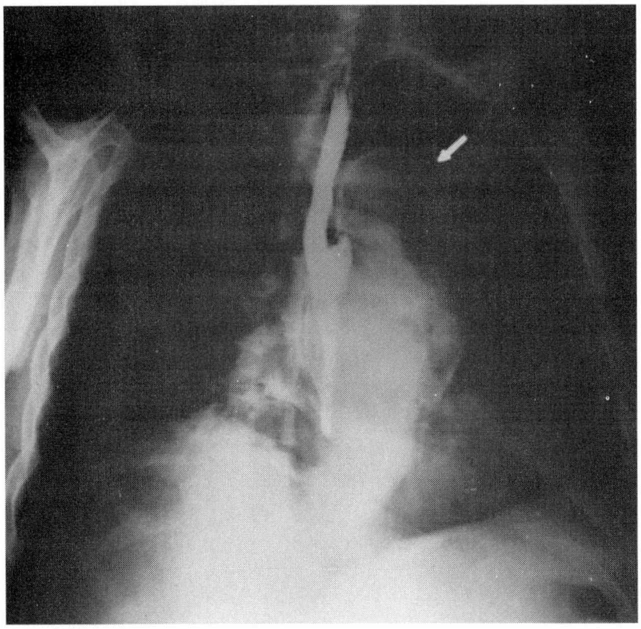

Fig. 36-3. Chest radiograph, after barium swallow, of a 56-year-old man with a history of incompletely treated syphilis. Marked calcification can be seen within the aneurysm of the ascending aorta *(arrow)*. (Courtesy BW Gayler.)

cation of the proximal aorta that is often evident radiographically (Fig. 36-3).

Rarely, syphilitic gummas (see the following) may infiltrate the aortic wall or myocardium culminating in a fibrous scar. Little is known of the clinical manifestations of gummas in the heart because of their rarity and the difficulty of clinical recognition, but is likely that the same complications of ventricular arrhythmias and the same valve dysfunctions that may occur in other granulomatous conditions affecting the heart, such as sarcoid, may also occur with syphilis.

AORTIC ANEURYSM

Syphilitic aneurysm, the most common manifestation of tertiary syphilis, virtually always involves the thoracic aorta, particularly the ascending aorta immediately at and above the sinuses of Valsalva. Over 60 percent of syphilitic aneurysms involve the ascending portion of the thoracic aorta and 25 percent involve the transverse arch.[92] Rarely, syphilitic aneurysms can occur, mainly in the innominate artery, where they may present with cerebral emboli.[92] These aneurysms are typically fusiform or saccular in type. Dissecting aneurysms do not occur, probably because of the medial scarring and wall thickening of the chronic inflammatory process.[89]

Characteristically, syphilitic aneurysms are present, asymptomatic, for may years before they are detected. Symptoms eventually develop because the aneurysm had encroached on surrounding structures or has ruptured. In some cases aneurysms erode through the chest wall and present as a chest wall mass. More typically the patient presents with persistent chest pain or with symptoms of a mass lesion compressing adjacent structures, such as hoarseness from recurrent laryngeal nerve pressure. A rare presentation may be with the superior vena cava syndrome, and in association with cough, dyspnea, dysphagia, and hemoptysis, may be misdiagnosed as lung cancer.[93] If aortic insufficiency is not present, there may be no detectable abnormalities on cardiac examination. The heart sounds have been described, however, as tambouric in quality, in part because of the dilated and noncompliant aorta. The chest radiograph may be normal or show a mediastinal mass with typical eggshell calcification outlining the aneurysm (see Fig. 36-3). This finding, however, may also be seen in severely atherosclerotic aortas or aortas from patients of advanced age and is not specific for syphilis. The precise definition of the aneurysm is achieved by aortic root angiography.

Management is largely dictated by symptoms. If a patient presents with evidence of an expanding aneurysm or with chest pain or symptoms of encroachment on adjacent tissue, surgical resection would be appropriate therapy.

CORONARY ARTERY DISEASE

The coronary arteries may be primarily involved in syphilis, but almost always only the ostia or the most proximal few millimeters of the coronary arteries are affected. The pathogeneis of the coronary arterial disease is an obliterative endarteritis. When the luetic process significantly narrows the coronary ostia, it may lead to ischemic heart disease, including angina pectoris or sudden death.[94] Probably because of the proximal nature of the coronary lesions, patients with syphilitic coronary disease typically die suddenly or develop chest pain rather than develop an acute occlusion of the left main coronary artery. Ordinarily, the acute coronary occlusion would involve such an extensive mass of left ventricular myocardium that the patient would not likely survive long enough to evolve a clinically apparent myocardial infarct. The diagnosis of syphilitic coronary disease should be considered in a patient who has been shown, by coronary angiography, to have isolated right or left main coronary ostial narrowing without atherosclerosis in the rest of the coronary tree and who has a history of syphilis or other signs of cardiovascular syphilis. At the present time, management of the symptomatic coronary ostial disease, particularly when the left coronary is involved, should be coronary artery bypass surgery; there is sufficient evidence now that patients with left main coronary narrowing have improved survival with surgery.[95]

AORTIC VALVE DISEASE

Pure aortic regurgitation without stenosis formerly was a common cardiovascular mainfestation of syphilis, occuring in roughly 30 percent of patients with tertiary syphilis of the cardiovascular system. The aortic regurgitation appears to be owing to aortic root dilation with stretching of the aortic valve, leading in many cases to widening of the aortic valve commissures, thickening of the aortic valve leaflets, and a variable amount of aortic valve incompetence.[89] Aortic insufficiency typically presents in patients who are 50 years of age or older. The degree of insufficiency may range from mild to severe and largely determines both the clinical course and its management.

Physical findings of luetic aortic insufficiency include diastolic blowing along the lower left sternal border, increased aortic second sound, and if the aortic insufficiency has been severe enough, a prominent left ventricle that is both hypertrophied and dilated. A tambourlike quality of the second heart sound has been commonly described in syphilitic aortic valve disease, probably owing to the aortic root dilation. If aortic stenosis also is present, the cause is highly unlikely to be syphilic.

The differential diagnosis of chronic pure aortic insufficiency (i.e., without a component of stenosis) includes healed infective endocarditis, congenitally malformed valves, Marfan's syndrome, ankylosing spondylitis, Reiter's syndrome, trauma with cusp dehiscence, or aging and aneurysm in a sinus of Valsalva. Cardiovascular syphilis can usually be distinguished from these other

Table 36-8. Causes of Aortic Regurgitation

	Syphilis	Ankylosing spondylitis	Marfan's syndrome	Rheumatic
Average age	50	45	30	45
Usual sex	Men	Men	Men	Men
Aortic regurgitation	+ + + +	+ + + +	+ + + +	+ + +
Mitral regurgitation	0	+	+ + +	+ + + +
Conduction disturbances	+	+ + + +	0	0
Aorta				
Adventitial scarring	+ + +	+ + +	0	0
Medial degeneration	+ + +	+ + +	+ + + +	0
Intimal proliferation	+ +	+ +	0	0
Limited to sinuses of Valsalva	0	+	0	0
Aortic cusp thickening	Focal	Diffuse	Focal	Diffuse
Anterior mitral leaflet thickening	0	+ +	+	+ + + +

conditions by findings including aortic root disease, a tricuspid aortic valve with normality of the other cardiac valves, and the absence of stigmata of metabolic and connective tissue diseases (Table 36-8).

Management of syphilitic aortic insufficiency is dictated by the symptoms and hemodynamic status of the patient. Congestive heart failure and chest pain are indications for valve replacement. Unfortunately, symptoms often develop at a time when the heart has already been hypertrophied and dilated, and despite valve replacement, a secondary valvular myocardiopathy remains. Technical aspects of surgery for syphilitic aortic insufficiency are generally no more difficult than for rheumatic valvular disease; the area of the sinuses of Valsalva and the most proximal aortic root tend to be scarred and thickened and therefore provide a good foundation for valve implantation. It should be stressed that the state of the aorta should be carefully assessed both before and after valve replacement. Progressive thoracic aortic dilatation can occur after aortic valve replacement for syphilitic aortic valve disease and may require surgical repair, as well.[95]

LATE BENIGN SYPHILIS

Late benign syphilis is a gummatous inflammatory process, proliferative or destructive, that involves structures generally not essential to the maintenance of life. The overwhelming majority of these manifestations occur in the skin and the bones, with a lesser frequency in the mucosae and certain of the viscera, muscles, and ocular structures. Resulting scar tissue may impair functions of the structures involved. In some ways, the classification is misleading, since gumma of the myocardium, brain, spinal cord, or trachea with stenosis may be anything but benign.[96]

INCIDENCE. A search of medical records at Vanderbilt University and Nashville General Hospitals disclosed only a single case in a 15-year period in the 1970s to 1980s. The recent literature (post-1990), however, contains multiple anecdotes of gummatous lesions of many organs (brain; bones; skin; others) mainly in HIV infected persons.[97–101] Thus, physicians still must be aware of this relatively rare form of syphilis. The most acceptable data concerning the frequency of late benign syphilis in an untreated population of syphilitic patients are those provided by the Boeck-Bruusgaard study. A critical review of this clinical material in 1955 showed that 15.8 percent of the 1147 patients in the study "sooner or later" developed late benign lesions of the skin, mucous membranes, or bones and joints. These manifestations occurred more frequently among women (17.3 percent) than men (13.7 percent). Among those observed to have late benign disease, 25 percent of the men and 34.7 percent of the women had from two to seven episodes of this manifestation.[102]

Table 36-9 shows the frequency with which late benign syphilis was encountered in the Vanderbilt syphilis clinic from 1925 to 1943. It must be emphasized that patients commonly had more than one tissue involved simultaneously. The decreased incidence of late disease with the passage of years (Fig. 36-4) was the result of intensive case finding followed by treatment of early and latent syphilis with arsenicals and after 1946, with penicillin.[103,104]

PATHOGENESIS. It is generally accepted that the gumma represents a maximal inflammatory (allergic) response to a few organisms. The demonstration of *Treponema pallidum* in this lesion is difficult; animal inoculation is rarely successful, silver stains usually are unrewarding; and instance of success with indirect immunofluorescence has been reported. From extensive experience in endemic syphilis, Grin of Yugoslavia proposed two explanations for gumma formation: (1) reactivation of treponemes in a sensitized patient with untreated or inadequately treated venereal or endemic syphilis; and (2) superinfection in a host already in an allergic state from a previous infection.[105] The best evidence in support of an allergic, or hypersensitivity, basis for the gumma was provided by Magnuson et al., who inoculated volunteers in Sing Sing Prison with the Nichols strain of *T. pallidum*. In the Sing Sing study, gummas developed only in persons with a history of previous syphilis. Among 26 inoculated prisoners who had been adequately treated earlier, 10 developed lesions (including one gumma) at the site of inoculation; of five who had been treated

Table 36-9. Distribution of Late Benign Lesions as to Site and Race, Vanderbilt, 1925–43

Site	Black	White
Skeletal (all types)	123	55
Skin	124	47
Upper respiratory tract (nose, throat, larynx)	50	19
Mucous membrane (mouth)	41	19
Eye (all types)	43	11
Visceral (liver, stomach, etc.)	23	14
Lower respiratory tract	2	2
Mediastinum	3	1
Lymph nodes	7	—
Genital tract (female)	4	—
Penis	3	2
Testes	3	1
Skeletal muscle	3	1
Totals	429	172

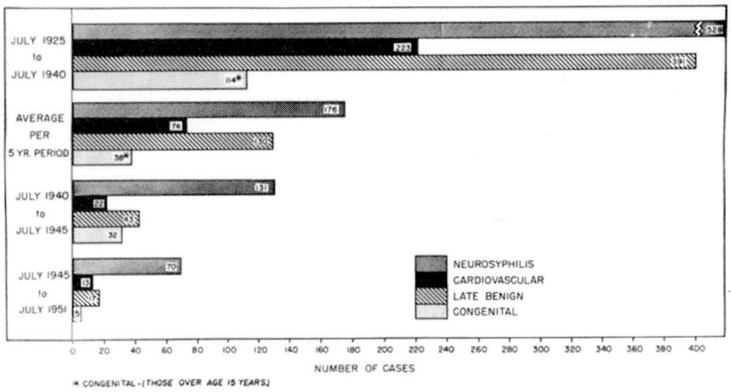

Fig. 36-4. The decrease in the incidence of late syphilis in the Vanderbilt University Hospital Syphilis Clinic. *Congenital = those over age 15. The experience of the first 15 years could not be broken down by 5-year periods; therefore, a 5-year average for this period is used for purposes of comparison. The figures marked by an asterisk represent the incidence of disease in which the diagnosis was made on ambulant clinic patients and does not include diagnoses made on ward patients. Unfortunately, figures subsequent to 1951 cannot be included; with the discontinuance of the syphilis clinic that year, the syphilitic patients were absorbed into the general medical and/or specialty clinics. Therefore, syphilitic disease was often not diagnosed and recorded. The diagnoses of syphilis that were made did not represent the critical diagnoses made in the syphilis clinic, which utilized history meetings and which included the consensus of three or four clinicians experienced in the disease. (From RH Kampmeier.[104])

adequately for congenital syphilis, one developed a gumma at the site of inoculation.[106] Magnuson et al. concluded that superinfection in a sensitized patient may explain gumma formation. However, Gjestland believed superinfection had a minor role in the Oslo patients who developed gummas.[107] That there may be other factors at times is suggested by the observations by members of the faculty at Vanderbilt University School of Medicine that osseous syphilis on occasion has followed local trauma in a person in a late latent stage.

PATHOLOGY. Syphilitic inflammation is generally relatively mild but chronic, and slow destruction of tissue leads to eventual fibrosis. The early inflammatory nodule has a granulomatous character closely resembling the lesion of tuberculosis. Grossly, gummas are nodules that may be found in any tissue or organ and may vary from microscopic size to many centimeters in diameter. The necrotic material in the larger nodules is of a gummy consistency, hence the term gumma. The histologic picture shows coagulative necrosis surrounded by lymphocytes and mononuclear cells; multinucleated giant cells appear only rarely. Ghosts of preexisting structures may be detected. The lesion is encapsulated by proliferating connective tissue with vascularized connective tissue extending outward from the necrotic area (Fig. 36-5). When the skin or mucous membrane is involved, an ulcer develops. Deep scarring accompanies the healing of gummas.

CLINICAL MANIFESTATIONS. It is well to recall Osler's words:

> Syphilis simulates every other disease. It is the only disease necessary to know. One then becomes an expert dermatologist, an expert laryngologist, an expert alienist, an expert oculist, an expert internist and an expert diagnostician.[108]

This aphorism may be put into other words as follows: The presence of any chronic inflammation, tumefaction or tumor, or destructive lesion of any tissue or organ of the body requires that syphilis be considered in the differential diagnosis.

SKIN

The late syphilid is considered first because of its frequency (see Table 36-9) and visualization as a prototype lesion involving tumefaction with or without softening (ulceration) and healing with scar formation. Two forms may appear: nodular or nodulo-ulcerative, and a solitary lesion.

NODULAR AND NODULO-ULCERATIVE LESIONS. Basically the nodular lesion is a deep indurated nodule that varies from pinhead to pea size and is brownish red in color. The multiple nodules are distributed usually in an arciform pattern with predilection for the face, the scapular and interscapular areas, and the extremities. They may remain for weeks or months and may heal without breaking down but still may show scarring. If nodular lesions break down to the nodulo-ulcerative form, they heal leaving an atrophic noncontractile scar (Figs. 36-6 to 36-8). If untreated, they will heal, but over time (up to years) new nodules appear at the margins of the previous site, advance in a serpiginous fashion and may eventually cover by scar an area as large as the whole back. Resolution of this syphilid is prompt under treatment. (A nonhealing area requires biopsy because of probable epithelioma.) A variant of this lesion on the palms or soles is a squamous or psoriasiform lesion without ulceration or scarring.

THE SOLITARY GUMMA. The solitary gumma is a subcutaneous process that involves the skin secondarily. It is more common on the thighs, buttocks, shoulders, forehead, and scalp. As it becomes necrotic, it has the characteristics of a "cold abscess," as in other granulomatous diseases. It may drain through one or more areas (Fig. 36-9).

SKELETON

Tertiary syphilis of bones is about as common as gumma of the skin (Figs. 36-10 and 36-11; see Table 36-9). Although the gumma

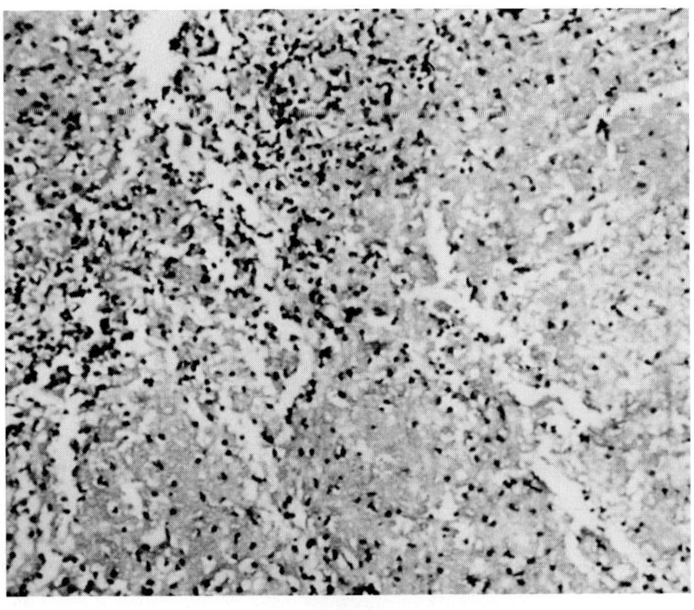

Fig. 36-5. Photomicrograph of a gummatous lesion in the testis of a 50-year-old black man. An ill-defined area of necrosis with architectural distortion is surrounded by scar and lymphocytic infiltrate. Giant cells are not detected in this lesion (H & E). (Courtesy of Dr. Robert Collins.)

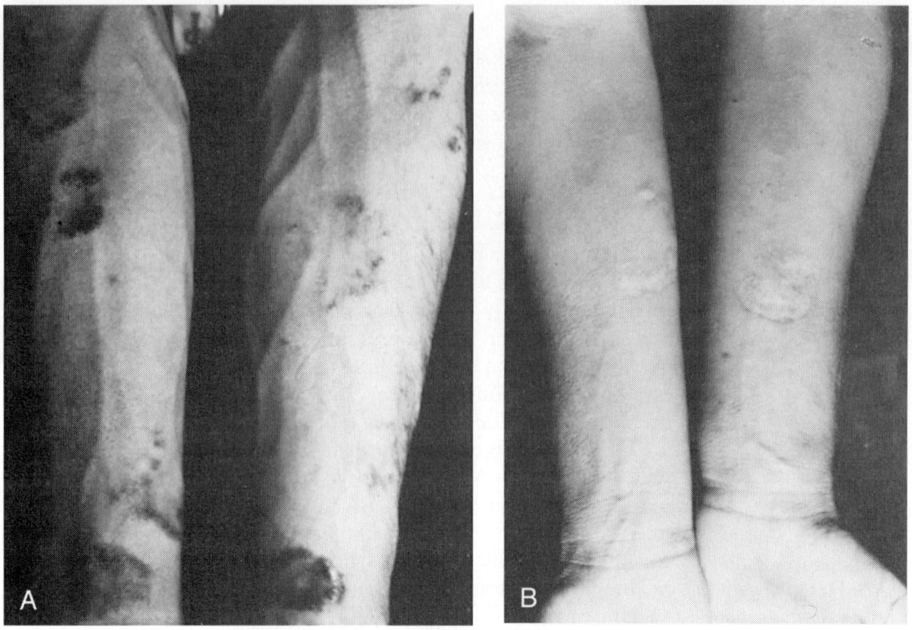

Fig. 36-6. (*a*) Nodular syphilid. (*b*) Characteristic residual scars from noduloulcerative syphilis. (From RH Kampmeier, *Essentials of Syphilology*, Philadelphia, Lippincott, 1943.)

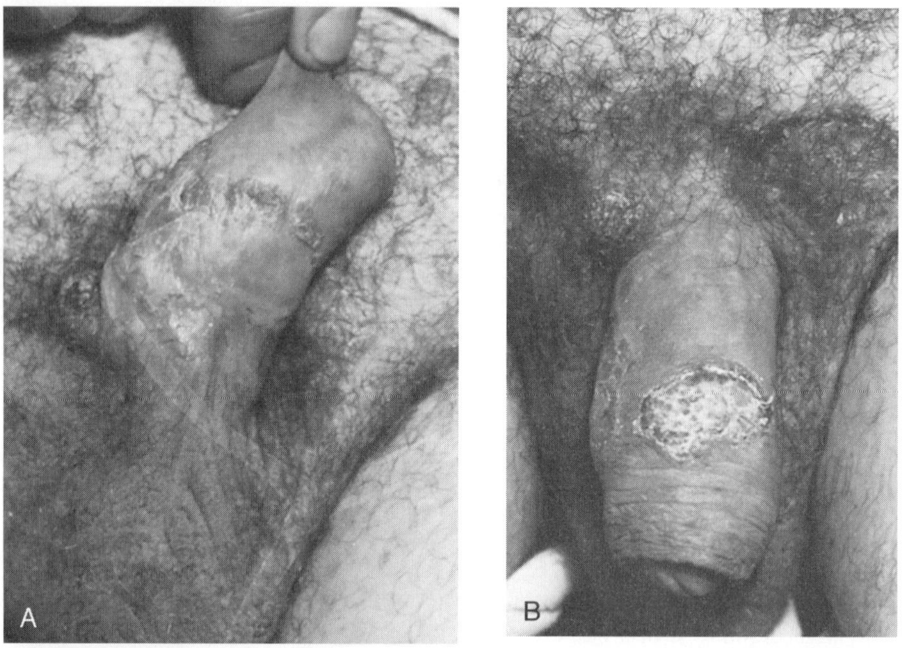

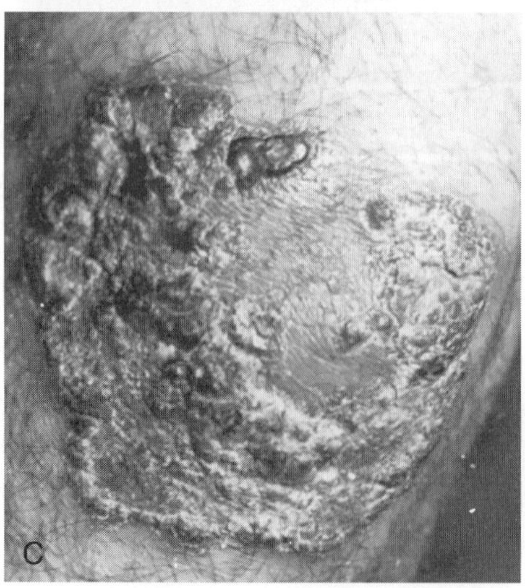

Fig. 36-7. (*a*) Nodular syphilid on inferior side of the penis. (*b*) Nodular syphilid of the pubic area and solitary gumma on dorsum of the penis. (*c*) Nodular syphilid of the knee. There were signs of aortic incompetency. (From RH Kampmeier, *Esentials of Syphilology*, Philadelphia, Lippincott, 1943.)

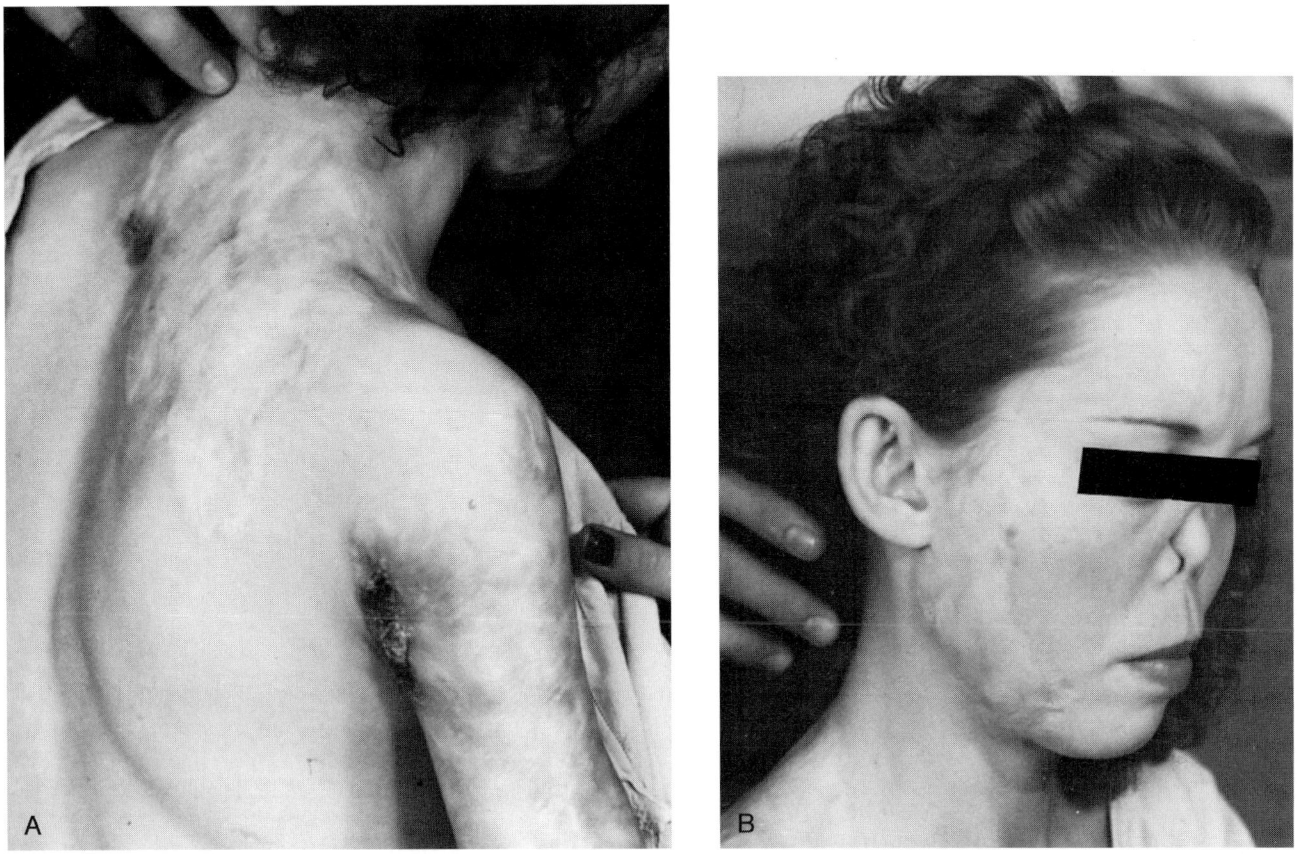

Fig. 36-8. (*a*) Atrophic scars on shoulder, arm, and (*b*) face following years of progressing noduloulcerative syphilids from congenital syphilis in a 14-year-old girl. An active area is visible at posterior axillary fold. Note the saddle-shaped nose. (From RH Kampmeier, *Physical Examination in Health and Disease,* Philadelphia, Davis, 1970.)

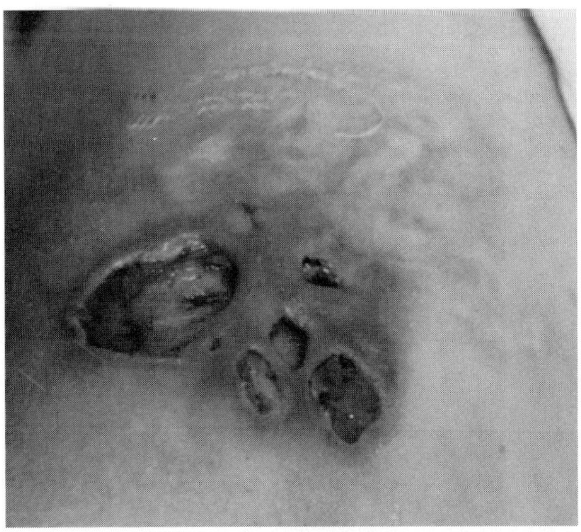

Fig. 36-9 Ulcerating solitary gumma of skin of 12 months' duration. Note scarring from spontaneous healing. Accompanying solitary ulcers on each shoulder and on the leg, 4 to 8 cm in diameter, began as pimples 7 months previously. (From RH Kampmeier, *Essentials of Syphilology,* Philadelphia, Lippincott, 1943.)

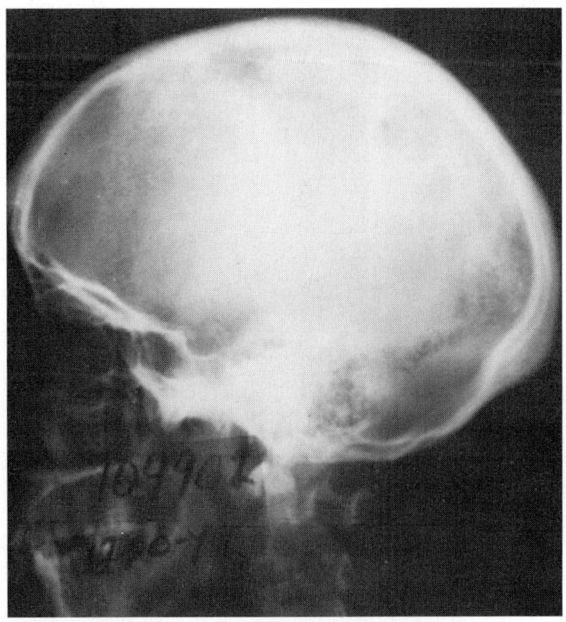

Fig. 36-10. Multiple areas of gummatous osteitis. (From RH Kampmeier.[103])

is a destructive process, it may be hidden by the osseous or periosteal reaction. A detailed radiologic study was made of 115 bones involved in 67 patients: tibia, 34; clavicle, 17; skull, 15; fibula, 15; humerus, five; rib, four; ulna, three; scapula, three; malar bone, two; mandible, two; and one each for facial bones, sternum, spine, radius, metacarpal, metatarsal, phalanx, patella, and ischium.[103] Although the basic lesion is the gumma, the radiographic manifestations were classified as follows:

Periostitis, periosteal thickening with increased density in laminated layers (27 bones).
Gummatous osteitis, destructive or osteomyelitic lesions, usually with periosteal or endosteal changes and sclerosis of the surrounding bone (72 bones).
Sclerosing osteitis, in which the increased density and periosteal change hide the gummatous lesion (16 bones).

The clinical characteristics include pain (especially nocturnal), tenderness, swelling, bony tumor, stiffness, and limited motion. Less common symptoms are heat, redness, and draining sinuses. Gumma of skeletal muscle is recognized by biopsy or by resolution of the tumor under therapy.

UPPER RESPIRATORY TRACT, MOUTH, AND TONGUE. Gummatous osteitis of the nasal bones, hard palate, and nasal septum, as well as perichondritis of the latter used to be relatively common (Figs. 36-12 and 36-13; see Table 36-9). Labial involvement may occur in the nodulo-ulcerative lesion of the face, as well as in a solitary gumma. Gumma of the tongue presents as a tumor (Fig. 36-14). Gumma of the soft palate leads to chronic ulceration, almost always with perforation. A history of chronic "sore throat" (actually difficulty in deglutition) lasting for weeks or months and the presence of an indolent ulcer are characteristic of tertiary involvement of the fauces and oropharynx. Deforming scars here provide the hallmark of such a process years before. Chronic hoarseness may result from tumefaction or ulceration and destruction of the epiglottis or laryngeal structures.

DIGESTIVE SYSTEM

The clinical picture of the rare gumma of the esophagus suggests carcinoma (Fig. 36-15).[110] Esophagoscopy may reveal an ulcer, tumor, or stricture. Gastric syphilis may mimic either a malignant or a benign gastric ulcer clinically and radiologically (Fig. 36-16).[111,112] Commonly, such patients have been operated on because of a mistaken diagnosis; others have required operation after antisyphilitic treatment resulted in obstructive scarring ("hourglass stomach").

Gumma of the liver is the most frequent type of gastro-intestinal tertiary syphilis. Some patients remain asymptomatic. However, there may be symptoms of low-grade fever, weight loss, and epigastric pain and tenderness. Splenomegaly often accompanies the disease. Healing of gumma of the liver leaves a characteristic scar and, if multiple, gross deformity of the liver (hepar lobatum).

MYOCARDIUM

Myocardial gummas, especially of the left ventricle and commonly asymptomatic, have been reported on occasion. Rarely, complete heart block has resulted from gummatous involvement of the atrioventricular bundle.[113]

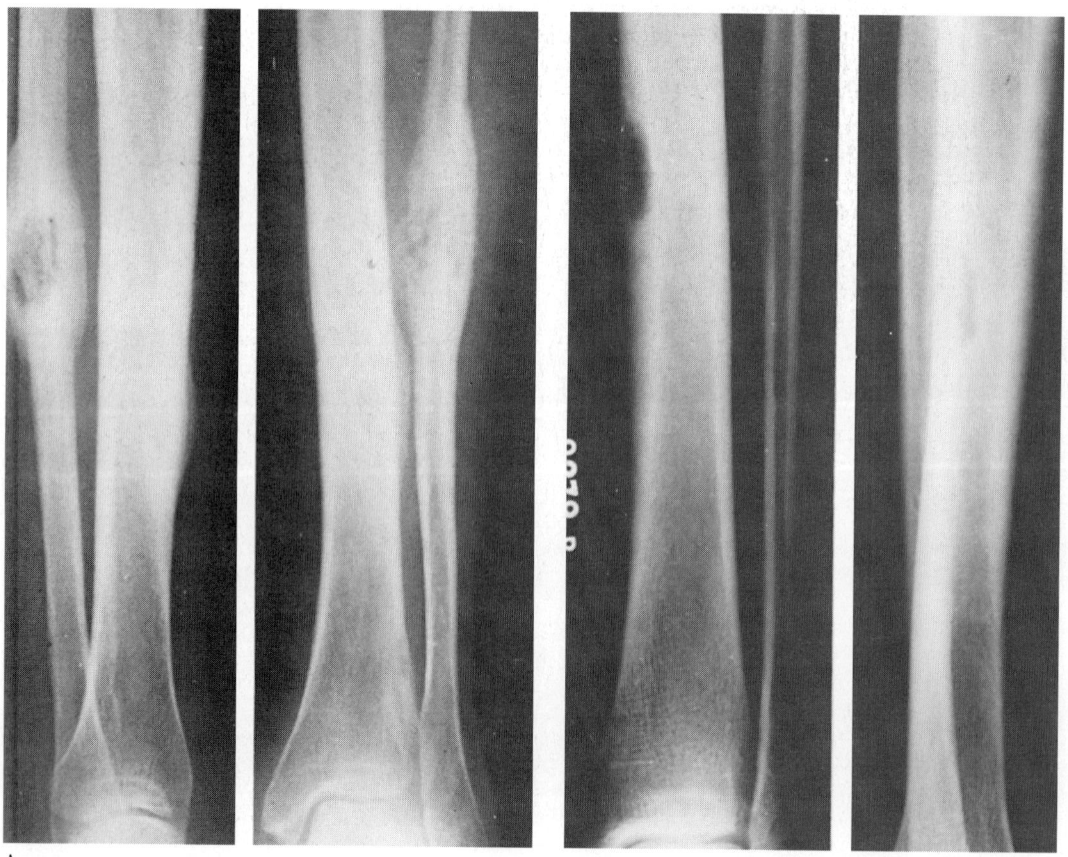

A B

Fig. 36-11. (*a*) Periostitis of tibia without destruction; gummatous destruction of fibula. (From RH Kampmeier, *Essentials of Syphilology,* Philadelphia, Lippincott, 1943.) (*b*) Destructive cystlike lesion (gumma) of cortex with periosteal elevation and thickening. (From ref 109)

Fig. 36-11 *(continued)* (*c*) Extensive, superficial destructive lesions in both tibias with almost complete absence of periosteal reaction; gummas with periosteal changes in the fibulas. (*d*) Sclerosing osteitis; the roentgenograph shows wavy outlines of dense sclerotic bone without destruction. (From ref 109)

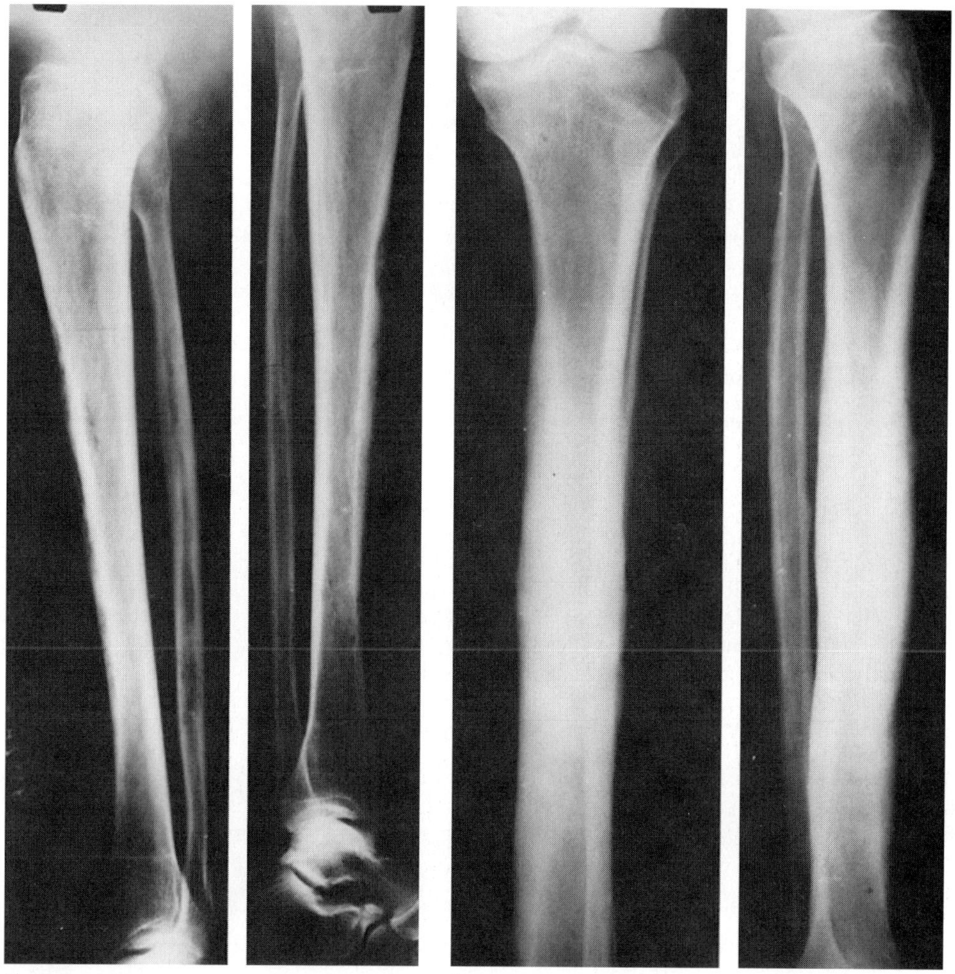

C D

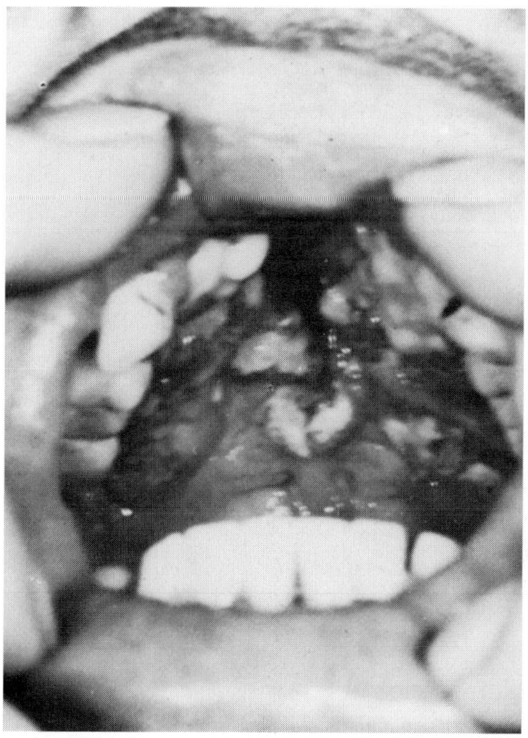

Fig. 36-12. Osteitis of hard palate with perforation. (From RH Kampmeier, *Physical Examination in Health and Disease,* Philadelphia, Davis, 1970.)

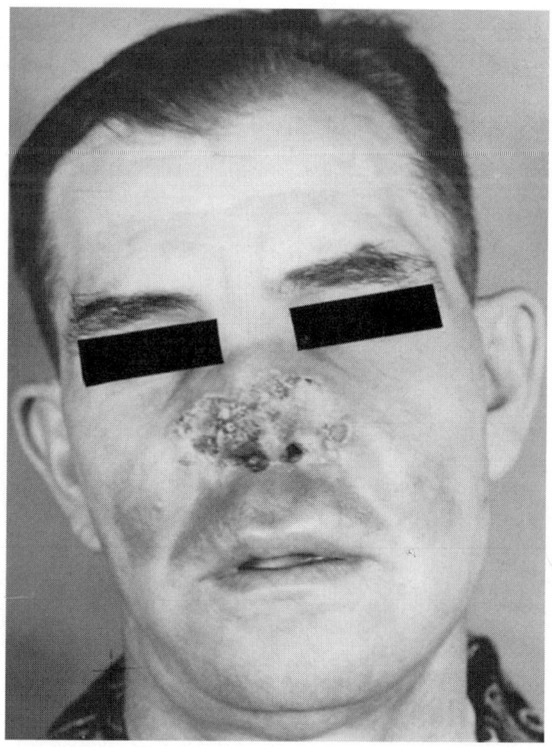

Fig. 36-13. Disease of the cartilagenous nasal septum.

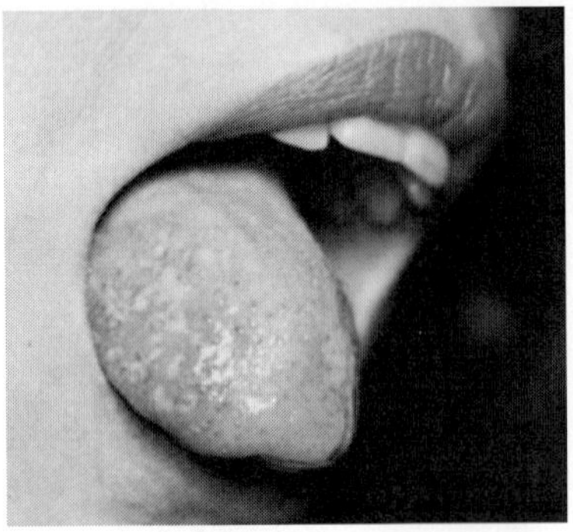

Fig. 36-14. Gumma of the tongue. (From RH Kampmeier, *Physical Examination in Health and Disease,* Philadelphia, Davis, 1970.)

DIAGNOSIS

To consider syphilis and include it in the differential diagnosis is one-half of the diagnosis. Gumma may involve virtually any organ (Fig. 36-17). Screening serologic tests are helpful because they are usually reactive, especially where there is extensive involvement of soft tissue (e.g., gumma of skin or liver). The serologic test results may be of high titer. The prozone phenomenon has been encountered in some cases, with serologic tests shown to be positive upon retesting in appropriate dilutions of serum. On the other hand a negative reaction may accompany a localized lesion, for example, as of bone.

TREATMENT

As shown in Fig. 36-4, late benign disease was approaching the vanishing point in the era before penicillin, and this trend was enhanced by the efficacy of penicillin therapy for early syphilis.[115–117] The evaluation of treatment in a rare disease is difficult, and there are no controlled studies of penicillin in any large series of patients. In 1948, after citing the first reported case of a syphilid treated with penicillin at the Mayo Clinic in 1944, Tucker reviewed the results of penicillin therapy in some detail in 34 patients with cutaneous lesions and in 16 with bone disease treated at the Johns Hopkins Hospital clinics.[115,116] Of the first 18 patients treated for a syphilid, two had relapses and were retreated. Sixteen patients who were followed for a mean of 911 days remained well after having received 1.7 million units of penicillin. Another 16 similar patients who received from 0.32 to 7.0 million units were well at the end of a mean of 364 days. The 16 patients who had syphilitic osteitis, osteomyelitis, and/or periostitis were treated with 0.6 to 7.0 million units of penicillin and were followed for a mean of 706 days. In one, although the bone lesion was under control, a syphilid developed 8 months later.

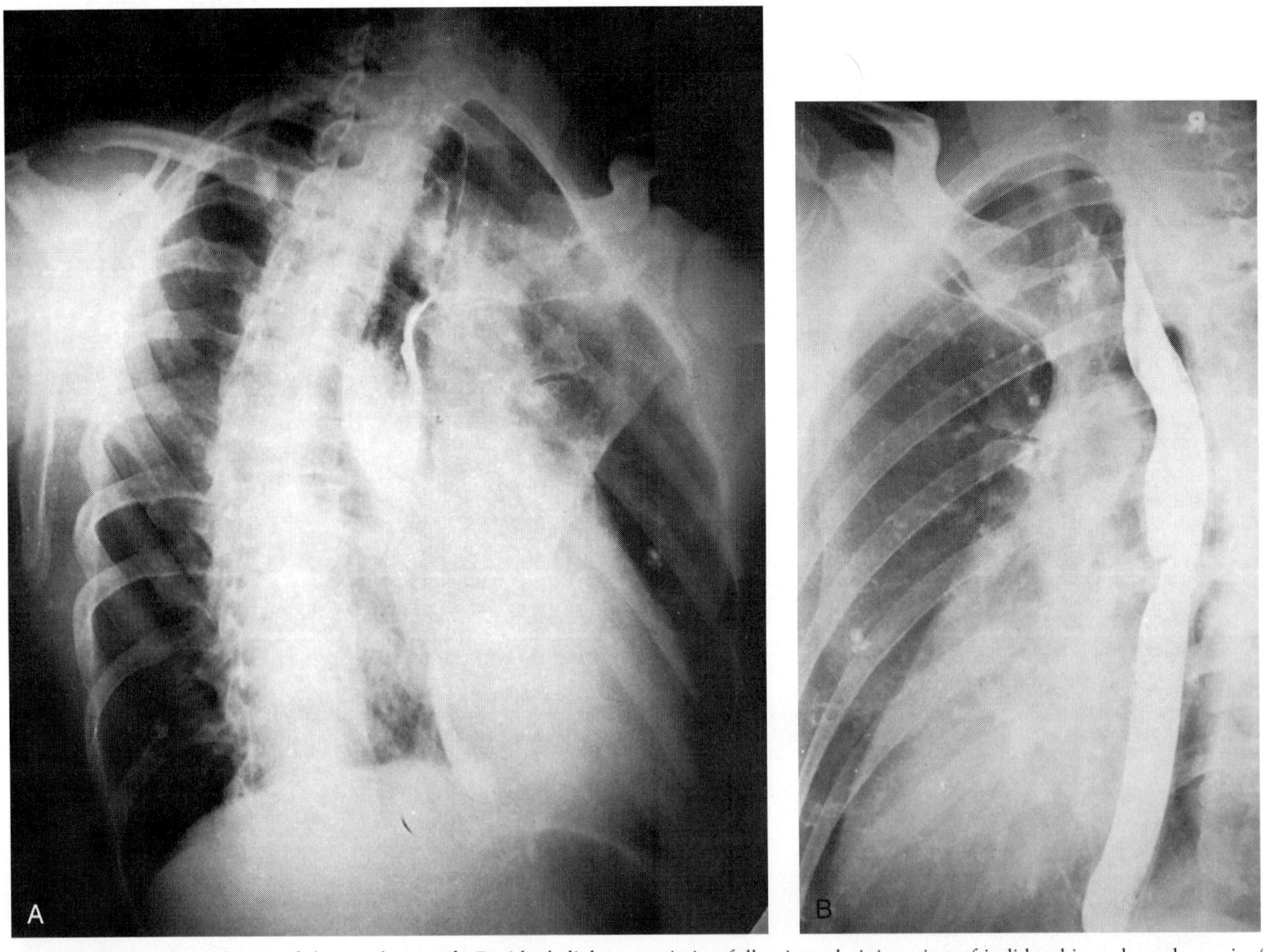

Fig. 36-15. (*a*) Obstructive lesion of the esophagus. (*b*) Residual slight constriction following administration of iodides, bismuth, and arsenic. (From RH Kampmeier and E Jones.)[110]

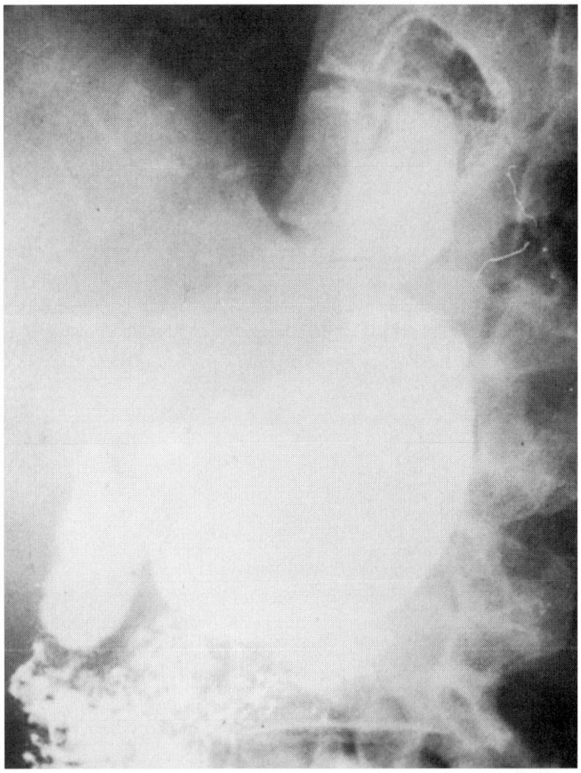

Fig. 36-16. Gummatous gastric ulcer. Radiological diagnosis of inoperable carcinoma. Resolution under bismuth and arsenic. (From RH Kampmeier, *Essentials of Syphilology,* Philadelphia, Lippincott, 1943.)

After Tucker had reviewed the experience at Johns Hopkins in the treatment of 34 patients with late benign syphilis, he concluded, "On the basis of reported data and an analysis of our own material, satisfactory results may be obtained in approximately 90% of such cases by the administration of a single course of penicillin alone." St. John, in his 1976 review of the literature on the treatment of late benign syphilis,[117] found no subsequent therapeutic trials and accepted Tucker's recommendation of treatment with "at least two million units of penicillin if not more." This conclusion still stands.

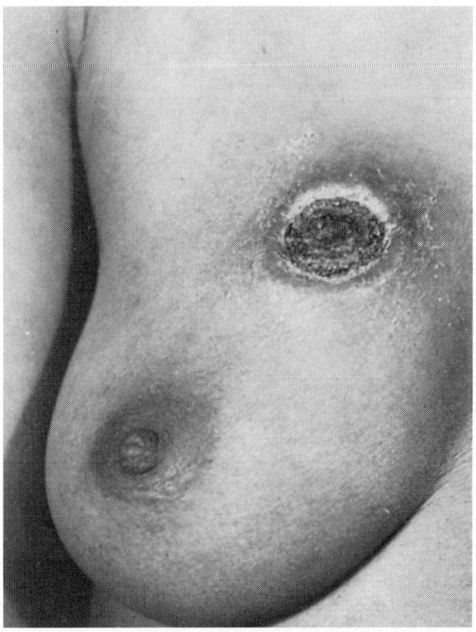

Fig. 36-17. Gumma of the breast. (From RH Kampmeier).[114]

References

1 Merritt HH et al: *Neurosyphilis.* New York, Oxford, 1946.
2 Martin JP: Conquest of general paresis. *Br Med J* 2:159, 1972.
3 Swartz MN: *Neurosyphilis,* in Holmes K et al. (eds). *Sexually Transmitted Diseases,* 2nd Ed. New York, McGraw-Hill, 1990.
4 Hahn RD et al: Asymptomatic neurosyphilis: A review of the literature. *Am J Syph Gon Vener Dis* 30:305, 1946.
5 Merritt HH: Early clinical and laboratory manifestations of syphilis of the central nervous system. *N Engl J Med* 223:446, 1940.
6 Dattner B: *The Management of Neurosyphilis.* New York, Grune & Stratton, 1944.
7 Chesney AM et al: Incidence of *Spirochaeta pallida* in cerebrospinal fluid during early stage of syphilis. *JAMA* 83:1725; 1924.
8 Stokes JH et al: *Modern Clinical Syphilology,* 3rd Ed. Philadelphia, Saunders, 1944, p. 8.
9 Lukehart SA et al: Invasion of the central nervous system by *Treponema pallidum:* implications for diagnosis and treatment. *Ann Intern Med* 109:855, 1988.
10 Moore JE et al: Asymptomatic neurosyphilis: VI. The prognosis of early and late neurosyphilis. *JAMA* 95:1637, 1930.
11 O'Leary PA et al: Cooperative clinical studies in the treatment of syphilis: Asymptomatic neurosyphilis. *Vener Dis Inf* 18:45, 1937.
12 Merritt HH et al: Acute syphilitic meningitis. *Medicine* 14:119, 1935.
13 Willcox RR et al: Nerve deafness in early syphilis. *Br J Vener Dis* 47: 401, 1971.
14 Löwhagen G-B et al: Central nervous system involvement in early syphilis. Part II. Correlation between auditory brainstem responses (ABR) and cerebrospinal fluid abnormalities. *Acta Derm Vernereol (Stockh)* 63:530, 1983.
15 Steckelberg JM et al: Otologic involvement in late syphilis. *Laryngoscope* 94:753, 1984.
16 Pachner AR et al: The triad of neurologic manifestations of Lyme disease: Meningitis, cranial neuritis, and radiculoneuritis. *Neurology* 35:47, 1985.
17 Russell H et al: Enzyme-linked immunosorbent assay and indirect immunofluorescence assay for Lyme disease. *J Infect Dis* 149:465, 1984.
18 Magnarelli LA et al: Cross-reactivity in serological tests for Lyme disease and other spirochetal infections. *J Infect Dis* 156:183, 1987.
19 Holmes MD et al: Clinical features of meningovascular syphilis. *Neurology* 34:553, 1984.
20 Hooshmand H et al: Neurosyphilis: A study of 241 patients. *JAMA* 219:726, 1972.
21 Joffe R et al: Changing clinical picture of neurosyphilis: Report of seven unusual cases. *Br Med J* 1:211, 1968.
22 Liebeskind A et al: Unusual segmental cerebrovascular changes. *Radiology* 106:119, 1973.
23 Holland BA et al: Meningovascular syphilis: CT and MR findings. *Radiology* 158:439. 1986.
24 Adams RA et al: Meningeal and vascular syphilis of the spinal cord. *Medicine* 23:181, 1944.
25 Catterall RD: Neurosyphilis. *Br J Hosp Med* 17:585, 1977.
26 Moore M et al: Role of syphilis of the nervous system in the production of mental disease. *JAMA* 107:1292, 1936.
27 Dewhurst K: The neurosyphilitic psychoses today: A survey of 91 cases. *Br J Psychiatry* 115:31, 1969.
28 Dawson-Butterworth K et al: Review of hospitalized cases of general paralysis of the insane. *Br J Vener Dis* 46:295, 1970.
29 Gimenez-Roldan S et al: Dementia paralytica: Deterioration from communicating hydrocephalus. *J Neurol Neurosurg Psychiatry* 42: 501, 1979.

30 Ch'ien L et al: Seronegative dementia paralytica: Report of a case. *J Neurol Neurosurg Psychiatry* 33:376, 1970.
31 Burke AW: Syphilis in a Jamaican psychiatric hospital: A review of 52 cases including 17 of neurosyphilis. *Br J Vener Dis* 48:249, 1972.
32 Musher DM et al: Evaluation and management of an asymptomatic patient with a positive VDRL reaction in, *Current Clinical Topics in Infectious Disease,* 9th ed. Remington JS et al (eds). New York, McGraw-Hill, 1988, p. 147.
33 Escobar MR et al: Fluorescent antibody tests for syphilis using cerebrospinal fluid: Clinical correlation in 150 cases. *Am J Clin Pathol* 53:886, 1970.
34 Mahony JDH et al: Evaluation of the CSF-FTA-ABS test in latent and tertiary treated syphilis. *Acta Derm Venereol (Stockh)* 52:71, 1972.
35 Jaffe HW et al: Tests for treponemal antibody in CSF. *Arch Intern Med* 138:252, 1978.
36 Madiedo G et al: False positive VDRL and FTA in cerebrospinal fluid. *JAMA* 244:688, 1980.
37 McGeeney T et al: Utility of the FTA-ABS test of CSF in the diagnosis of neurosyphilis. *Sex Transm Dis* 6:195, 1979.
38 Davis LE, Sperry S: The CSF-FTA test and the significance of blood contamination. *Arch Neurol* 6:68, 1979.
39 Vartdal F et al: Neurosyphilis: Intrathecal synthesis of oligoclonal antibodies to *Treponema pallidum. Ann Neurol* 11:35, 1981.
40 Pedersen NS et al: Specificity of immunoglobulins synthesized within the central nervous system in neurosyphilis. *Acta Pathol Microbiol Immunol* 90:97, 1982.
41 Prange HW et al: Relationship between neurological features and intrathecal synthesis of IgG antibodies to *Treponema pallidum* in untreated and treated human neurosyphilis. *J Neurol* 230:241, 1983.
42 Gschnait F et al: Cerebrospinal fluid immunoglobulins in neurosyphilis. *Br J Vener Dis* 57:238, 1981.
43 Lee JB et al: Detection of immunoglobulin M in cerebrospinal fluid from syphilis patients by enzyme-linked immunosorbent assay. *J Clin Microbiol* 24:736, 1986.
44 Müller F et al: Demonstration of locally synthesized immunoglobulin M antibodies to *Treponema pallidum* in the central nervous system of patients with untreated neurosyphilis. *J Neuroimmunol* 7:43, 1984/5.
44a Zoechling N et al: Molecular detection of *Treponema pallidum* in secondary and tertiary syphilis. *Br J Dermato* 136:683, 1997.
44b Tomberlin MG et al: Evaluation of neurosyphilis in human immunodeficiency virus-infected individuals. *Clin Inf Dis* 18:288, 1994.
44c Chung KY et al: Detection of *Treponema pallidum* by polymerase chain reaction in the cerebrospinal fluid of syphilis patients. *Yonsei Med J* 35:190, 1994.
44d Horowitz HW et al: Brief Report: Cerebral syphilitic gumma confirmed by the polymerase chain reaction in a man with human immunodeficiency virus infection. *N Engl J Med* 331:1488, 1994.
45 Ganti SR et al: Computed tomography of cerebral syphilis. *J Comput Assist Tomogr* 5:345, 1981.
46 Moskovitz BL et al: Meningovascular syphilis after "appropriate" treatment of primary syphilis. *Arch Intern Med* 142:139, 1982.
47 Godt P et al: The value of CT in cerebral syphilis. *Neuroradiology* 18:197, 1979.
48 Burke JN et al: Neurosyphilis in the antibiotic era. *Neurology* 35: 1368, 1985.
49 Jordan KG: Diagnostic criteria for neurosyphilis. *Neurology* 36: 1273, 1986.
50 Escobar A et al: *Neuro-Syphilis in Pathology of Central Nervous System,* Minkler J (ed). New York, McGraw-Hill, 1968, vol 3, p. 2448.
51 Towpik J et al: Changing patterns of late syphilis. *Br J Vener Dis* 46: 132, 1970.
52 Aho K et al: Late complications of syphilis: A comparative epidemiological and serological study of cardiovascular syphilis and various forms of neurosyphilis. *Acta Derm Venereol (Stockh)* 49:336, 1969.
53 Heathfield KWG: The decline of neurolues. *Practitioner* 217:753, 1976.
54 Ekbom K: Carbamazepine in the treatment of tabetic lightning pains. *Arch Neurol* 26:374, 1972.
55 McNeel DP et al: Charcot joint of the lumbar spine. *J Neurosurg* 30: 55, 1969.
56 Ramani PS et al: Cauda equina compression due to tabetic arthropathy of the spine. *J Neurol Neurosurg Psychiatry* 36:260, 1973.
57 Hahn RD: Tabes dorsalis with special reference to primary optic atrophy. *Br J Vener Dis* 33:139, 1957.
58 Kerty E et al: Visual evoked response in syphilitic optic atrophy. *Acta Ophthalmol* 64:553, 1986.
59 Kaplan JG et al: Luetic meningitis with gumma: Clinical, radiographic, and neuropathologic features. *Neurology* 31:464, 1981.
60 Tsai FY et al: Angiographic findings with an intracranial gumma. *Neuroradiology* 13:1, 1977.
60a Suarez JI et al: Cerebral syphilitic gumma in an HIV-negative patient presenting as prolonged focal motor status epilepticus. *New Engl J Med* 335:1159, 1996.
60b Inoue R et al: Cerebral gumma showing linear dural enhancement on magnetic resonance imaging—Case report. *Neurologia Medico-Chirurgica* 35:813, 1995.
60c Berger JR et al: Syphilitic cerebral gumma with HIV infection. *Neurology* 47:1282, 1992.
60d Tien RD et al: Neurosyphilis in HIV carriers: MR findings in six patients. *Am J Roentgenology* 158:1325, 1992.
61 Ingall D et al: Syphilis, in *Infectious Diseases of the Fetus and Newborn Infant,* 4th Ed. Remington JS et al (eds). Philadelphia, Saunders, 1993.
62 Koffman O: The changing pattern of neurosyphilis. *Can Med Assoc J* 74:807, 1956.
63 Lanigan-O'Keefe LM: Return to normal of Argyll-Robertson pupils after treatment. *Br Med J* 2:1191, 1977.
64 Modified neurosyphilis, editorial. *Br Med J* 2:647. 1978.
65 Jordan K et al: Bilateral oculomotor paralysis due to neurosyphilis. *Ann Neurol* 3:90, 1978.
66 Kolar OJ et al: Neurosyphilis. *Br J Vener Dis* 53:221, 1977.
67 Dattner B: Late results of penicillin therapy in neurosyphilis. *Trans Am Neurol Assoc* 77:127, 1952.
68 Hahn RD et al: The results of treatment in 1,086 general paralytics the majority of whom were followed for more than five years. *J Chronic Dis* 7:209, 1958.
69 Mohr JA et al: Neurosyphilis and penicillin levels in cerebrospinal fluid. *JAMA* 236:2208, 1976.
70 Yoder FW: Penicillin treatment of neurosyphilis: Are recommended dosages sufficient? *JAMA* 232:270, 1975.
71 Tramont EC: Persistence of *Treponema pallidum* following penicillin G therapy: Report of two cases. *JAMA* 236:2206, 1976.
72 Wilner E et al: Prognosis of general paresis after treatment. *Lancet* 2:1370, 1968.
73 Centers for Disease Control: 1997 STD treatment guidelines. *MMWR,* in press.
74 Dattner B et al: Criteria for the management of neurosyphilis. *Am J Med* 10:463, 1951.
75 Hahn RD et al: Penicillin treatment of asymptomatic central nervous system syphilis: I. Probability of progression to symptomatic neurosyphilis. *Arch Dermatol* 74:355, 1956.
76 Hahn RD et al: Penicillin treatment of general paresis (dementia paralytica). *Arch Neurol Psychiatry* 81:557, 1959.
77 Weickhardt G: Penicillin therapy in general paresis. *Am J Psychiatry* 105:63, 1948.
78 Musher DM et al: Effect of human immunodeficiency virus (HIV) infection on the course of syphilis and on the response to treatment. *Ann Intern Med* 113:872, 1990.
79 Musher DM: Syphilis, neurosyphilis, penicillin and AIDS. *J Infect Dis* 163:1201, 1991.
80 Folk JC et al: Syphilitic neuroretinitis. *Am J Ophthalmol* 95:480, 1983.
81 Katz DA et al: Neurosyphilis in acquired immunodeficiency syndrome. *Arch Neurol* 46:895, 1989.
82 Holtom PD et al: Prevalence of neurosyphilis in human immunodeficiency virus-infected patients with latent syphilis. *Am J Med* 93:9, 1992.

83 Dowell ME et al: Response of latent syphilis or neurosyphilis to ceftriaxone therapy in persons infected with human immunodeficiency virus. *Am J Med* 93:481, 1992.
84 Johns DR et al: Alteration in the natural history of neurosyphilis by concurrent infection with the human immunodeficiency virus. *N Engl J Med* 316:1569, 1987.
85 Gordon SM et al: The response of symptomatic neurosyphilis to high-dose intravenous penicillin G in patients with human immunodeficiency virus infection. *N Engl J Med* 331:1469, 1994.
86 Musher DM et al: Neurosyphilis in HIV-infected persons. *N Engl J Med* 331:1516, 1994.
87 Jackman JD, Radolf JD: Cardiovascular syphilis. *Am J Med* 87:425, 1989.
88 Webster B et al: Studies in cardiovascular syphilis: III. The natural history of syphilitic aortic insufficiency. *Am Heart J* 46:117, 1953.
89 Heggtveit HA: Syphilitic aortitis: A clinicopathologic autopsy study of 100 cases, 1950 to 1960. *Circulation* 29:346, 1964.
90 Roberts WC et al: Nonrheumatic valvular cardiac disease: A clinicopathologic survey of 27 different conditions causing valvular dysfunction. *Cardiovas Clin* 5:333, 1973.
91 Steel D: The roentgenological diagnosis of syphilitic aortitis: A review of forty proved cases. *Am Heart J* 6:59, 1930.
92 Tadavarthy SM et al: Syphilitic aneurysms of the innominate artery. *Radiology* 139:31, 1981.
93 Phillips PL et al: Syphilitic aortic aneurysm presenting with the superior vena cava syndrome. *Am J Med* 71:171, 1981.
94 Bulkley BH, Roberts WC: Atherosclerotic narrowing of the left main coronary artery: A necropsy analysis of 152 patients with fatal coronary heart disease and varying degrees of left main narrowing. *Circulation* 53:823, 1976.
95 Nancarrow PA, Higgins CB: Progressive thoracic aortic dilatation after valve replacement. *AJR* 142:669, 1984.
96 Kampmeier RH: Historical article: Clarification of the systemic manifestations of syphilis: especially in the tertiary stage. *Sex Trans Dis* 8:82, 1981.
97 Kearns G et al: Intraoral tertiary syphilis (gumma) in a human immunodeficiency virus-positive man: a case report. *J Oral & Maxillofacial Surg* 51:85, 1993.
98 Sule RR et al: Late cutaneous syphilis. *Cutis* 59:135, 1997.
99 Suarez JI et al: Cerebral syphilitic gumma in an HIV-negative patient presenting as prolonged focal motor status epilepticus. *N Engl J Med* 335:1159, 1996.
100 Kasmin F et al: Syphilitic gastritis in an HIV-infected individual. *Am J Gastroen* 87:1820, 1992.
101 Kastner RJ et al: Syphilitic osteitis in a patient with secondary syphilis and concurrent human immunodeficiency virus infection. *Clin Infect Dis* 18:250, 1994.
102 Clark EG, Danbolt N: The Oslo study of the natural course of untreated syphilis. *J Chronic Dis* 2:311, 1955.
103 Kampmeier RH: The late manifestations of syphilis: Skeletal, visceral and cardiovascular. *Med Clin North Am* 48:667, 1964.
104 Kampmeier RH: Comments on the present day management of syphilis. *South Med J* 46:226, 1953.
105 Grin EI: Epidemiology and Control of Endemic Syphilis: Report on a Mass Treatment Campaign in Bosnia. WHO Monography Series. Geneva, WHO, 1953.
106 Magnuson HJ et al: Inoculation syphilis in human volunteers. *Medicine* (Baltimore) 35:33, 1956.
107 Gjestland T: The Oslo study of untreated syphilis. *Acta Derm Venereol* (suppl) (Stockh) 35:34, 1955.
108 Bean RB, Bean WB: Sir William Osler Aphorisms from His Bedside Teachings and Writings. Springfield, IL, Charles C Thomas, 1961.
109 Francis HC, Kampmeier RH: The bone lesions in acquired tertiary syphilis. *South Med J* 36:556, 1943.
110 Kampmeier RH, Jones E: Esophageal obstruction due to gummata of esophagus and diaphragm. *Am J Med Sci* 201:539, 1941.
111 Harris S, Youmans JB: Syphilis of the stomach: A report of seven cases. *South Med J* 24:877, 1931.
112 Eusterman GB: Gastric syphilis: Observations based on 93 cases. *JAMA* 96:173, 1931.
113 Weinstein A et al: Complete heart block due to syphilis. *AMA Arch Intern Med* 100:90, 1957.
114 Kampmeier RH: Syphilis of the breast: Chancre and gumma. *Am Pract* 1:395, 1947.
115 Dexter DD, Tucker HA: Penicillin treatment of benign late gummatous syphilis: A report of twenty-one cases. *Am J Syph Gonor Vener Dis* 30:211, 1945.
116 Tucker HA: Penicillin in benign late and visceral syphilis. *Am J Med* 5:702, 1948.
117 St John RK: Treatment of late benign syphilis: Review of the literature. *J Am Vener Dis Assoc* 3(pt 2):146, 1976.

Chapter 37

Endemic treponematoses

André Meheus
Eugeni Tikhomirov

Treponemal infections include venereal syphilis and the endemic (nonvenereal) treponematoses (i.e., yaws, endemic syphilis, or bejel and pinta). The similarities between the clinical manifestations of the various treponemal diseases are remarkable. They all have initial lesions followed by more extensive secondary manifestations, and they all exhibit the phenomenon of latency. In general, virtually any lesion produced by the three endemic treponematoses also may be produced by venereal syphilis.[1]

The immune-response pattern in syphilis and the nonvenereal treponematoses is similar. This complicates the interpretation of reactive serologic tests for syphilis in patients who come from areas where endemic treponematoses are still common.

GLOBAL EPIDEMIOLOGY AND CONTROL

HISTORICAL CONTEXT

Since its creation in 1948, the World Health Organization (WHO) has made the fight against the endemic treponematoses a major priority. In close collaboration with UNICEF, in the period 1952–1964, the global endemic treponematoses control program (TCP) was launched, and it became a real success story: More than 50 million patients were treated with long-acting penicillin in 46 countries, reducing the overall disease prevalence by more than 95 percent. The control strategy subsequently was changed from a vertical program to one that was integrated into basic health services, and it was felt that this approach would cope with the remaining "last cases" in the community until eradication was achieved. Global eradication did not occur, however, and a number of transmission foci remained. By the end of the 1970s, resurgence of endemic treponematoses had occurred in many areas, and the World Health Assembly of the WHO alerted the international community.[2]

In the early 1980s, renewed control efforts were implemented in a number of countries (such as seven West African countries: Benin, Côte d'Ivoire, Ghana, Mali, Burkina Faso, Niger, and Togo). But again, the final blow to the endemic treponematoses was not given.

BARRIERS TO CONTROL AND ERADICATION

Barriers to sustaining control efforts up to eradication can be summarized as follows[3]:

There is a perception by health decision makers that these diseases are already fully under control.
The economic impact is not evident; children mainly are affected.
The diseases are not fatal.
Foci of diseases are mainly in remote, rural, poor populations (often ethnic minority groups).
Health services in areas affected are inadequate or absent; political commitment has not been translated in implementation of primary health care (PHC).
Single disease programs are not "fashionable."
The infections are not a threat to industrialized countries and to the leading classes in urban areas of the developing world.

The main motive for dealing with these diseases and working toward eradication is humanitarian, to protect children and communities from the crippling, invalidating, and disfiguring sequelae and, through endemic treponematoses control, to develop effective health services for remote and poor communities.

A comprehensive overview of the global epidemiology of the endemic treponematoses is available.[4] However, as reporting has become more and more incomplete, national and local statistics are increasingly unreliable. Articles in the scientific literature have become a major (fragmented) source of information.

ENDEMIC TREPONEMATOSES ESTIMATION IN 1996

The population actually at risk is estimated at 34 million (mainly infants, children, and to a lesser extent, adolescents and young adults).[5] They all live in the developing countries, with 21 million of them living in the so-called least developed countries (LDCs) (Fig. 37-1). The regions most affected are Africa and Southeast Asia, with some residual foci in Central and South America, the Middle East, and the Pacific Islands. The total number of cases (infectious, latent, and old cases) is estimated globally at 2.6 million, and infectious cases are estimated at 460,000, of which there are 400,000 cases in Africa. The prevalence of infectious cases is used for evaluating endemic treponematoses control programs. When infectious cases no longer appear in a geographic area, that area enters the consolidation phase of the control program. If serosurveillance indicates that transmission no longer occurs in the area, then the disease can be considered eradicated. The number of disabled persons due to endemic treponematoses is estimated at 260,000 globally.

YAWS

Yaws, also known as framboesia, pian, or buba, is caused by *Treponema pallidum* subspecies *pertenue (T. pertenue)*. Although *T. pertenue* has not been grown on artificial culture media, it has been grown successfully in rabbits and hamsters.

EPIDEMIOLOGY

Transmission of yaws occurs through direct contact with an infectious yaws lesion. It is usually contracted in infancy or childhood. Indirect transmission by flies *(Hippelates pallipes)* has been suggested. Congenital transmission does not occur. In sparsely dressed populations, transmission is obviously facilitated by close bodily contact when children are playing or sleeping together.

Yaws occurs primarily in the warm, humid, tropical areas of Africa, South Africa, South America, the Caribbean, Southeast Asia, and some Pacific Islands. Typically, yaws, like the other endemic treponematoses, is confined to populations with low standards of hygiene in remote areas with little or no health care; yaws is a disease found "at the end of the road."[6–8]

CLINICAL FEATURES

As in syphilis, the clinical manifestations of yaws are divided into early- (which includes primary and secondary lesions) and late-stage disease.[9]

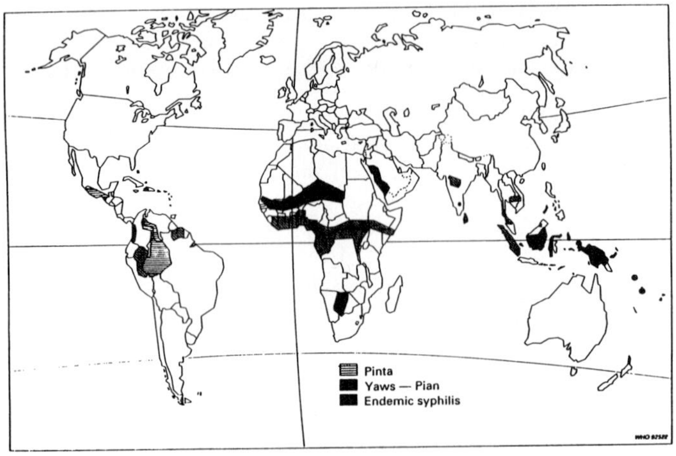

Fig. 37-1. Geographic distribution of the endemic treponematoses in the early 1990s.

Early-stage disease

Skin. An initial lesion develops at the point of entry of the treponeme (often the lower extremities) after an incubation period of 10 to 45 days or even longer. Systemic spread of the treponemes probably occurs during the incubation period. The initial lesion assumes a variety of appearances but usually progresses over a period of several weeks from a small papule to a proliferative papilloma, which exudes serum that is rich in treponemes and therefore highly infectious. The lesion may persist for 3 to 6 months and may ulcerate as a result of bacterial superinfection. The initial lesion heals spontaneously, often leaving a scar.

A first crop of secondary lesions may develop before the initial lesion has healed but may not appear for 1 to 2 years. Characteristic secondary lesions are the large, raised papillomas and papules from which exudation of highly infectious serum is a feature; in addition, a wide variety of lesions may appear on the skin and oral mucous membranes. Early lesions of the palms and soles include hyperkeratotic or squamous macular lesions, which may be combined with a papilloma. If such papillomas develop on the soles of the feet, walking becomes very painful, and the patient adopts a crablike gait (crab yaws). During the first 5 years of infection, there may be one or several relapses of early yaws lesions, separated by latent periods of variable duration. Each crop of secondary lesions may persist for more than 6 months; the lesions heal spontaneously and do not leave scars.

Change in climate may influence the number and distribution of early skin lesions. In the dry season, fewer lesions may be present, and they tend to be of the macular or papular type; papillomas tend to occur in the more humid body areas, such as the axillae and anal folds.

Bone. Many patients with yaws experience bone pain, which becomes worse at night and which may be accompanied by pathologic bone changes. Osteoperiostitis may involve the long bones and the bones of the hands and feet and presents as a polydactylitis of the fingers and goundou, a hypertrophic osteitis of the nasal process of the maxilla. The etiology of goundou and *sabre tibia* is still uncertain, but both conditions are commonly seen in yaws endemic areas.

Late-stage disease

Late active yaws lesions develop in about 10 percent of patients 5 to 10 years after the initial infection. Treponemes are microscopically scanty or absent in late lesions. Late lesions may involve the skin and subcutaneous tissues, including the skin of the palms and soles, the mucosae, and the bones and joints. In all these lesions, tissue destruction resulting in ulceration is common:

Gummas may involve the skin and the subcutaneous tissues or may be secondary to an underlying osteitis.
Hyperkeratosis of the soles and palms may result in atrophic skin and contractures of the fingers (ghoul hand).
Gangosa (rhinopharyngitis mutilans) is a destructive ulceration of the palate and nasal septum leading to collapse of the nose.
Juxtaarticular nodules are lumps of fibrous tissue that develop in the subcutis in the vicinity of joints, with a strong predilection for the sacrum, elbows, greater trochanter, capitulum fibulae, and malleolus externus.
The skin tends to react to trauma with pigmentary changes (hypopigmentation).

It is generally accepted that neurologic and cardiovascular complications and sequelae do not occur in yaws.

ENDEMIC SYPHILIS (BEJEL, DICHUCHWA)

Endemic syphilis is caused by *T. pallidum* subspecies *endemicum (T. endemicum)*. Transmission occurs via infectious lesions on the skin and mucous membranes, often through the use of common feeding utensils. Endemic syphilis is essentially a disease of hot, dry countries and used to be endemic in rural communities of the Middle East, Bosnia, Bulgaria, and Botswana, from where it is now practically eradicated. Major foci still exist in the Sahelian region of Africa, however.

CLINICAL FEATURES

Early-stage disease

Primary lesions are seldom seen. Patches on the mucous membranes, angular stomatitis, and papules and macules favoring the moist areas of the body are the most typical manifestations. Condylomata lata often occur and are comparable with those in yaws and venereal syphilis. Unlike venereal syphilis, however, the eruption may persist for many months or even years. In the early stage, a painful osteoperiostitis may occur, similar to the osteoperiostitis in yaws.[10]

Late-stage disease

Infections of skin, bones, and cartilage may lead to severe destruction, especially of the nose and palate (gangosa). On the skin, gummatous ulcers are characteristic. Periostitis with bone pain and gummas have been reported. Neurologic and cardiovascular involvement has not been reported, nor has congenital transmission.[10]

PINTA (CARATE, MAL DE PINTO)

Pinta is caused by *T. pallidum* subspecies *carateum (T. carateum)*. It is the most benign of the endemic treponematoses; the skin is the only organ affected. Transmission most probably occurs through direct skin contact; the disease is mainly transmitted in childhood. Pinta is now confined to native populations living in the remote rural areas of Central and South America (e.g., the Amazon basin).

CLINICAL FEATURES

Early-stage disease

After an incubation period of several weeks, initial lesions will appear in the form of an itchy erythematous papule, which may progress to an erythematosquamous plaque on the uncovered parts of the body accompanied by local lymphadenopathy. These lesions disappear spontaneously. In the secondary stage, widespread rashes or multiplication of papules develops. The lesions may persist for years and remain darkfield-positive for treponemes. Generalized lymphadenitis is common.

Late-stage disease

The late stage is characterized by pigmentary changes typical of pinta. At first, there are round, oval, or irregular patches of hyperpigmentation, ranging in color from red-purple to slate blue; later, achromic patches and skin atrophy develop. Pruritus is marked. These color changes are not necessarily synchronized, and patients may show the various stages simultaneously. A congenital form is not known.

TREATMENT OF THE ENDEMIC TREPONEMATOSES

The WHO recommends that patients and their contacts receive benzathine penicillin, 1.2 mU in a single intramuscular injection; children less than 10 years of age should be given half this dose.[1] Resistance to penicillin has not yet been demonstrated, but reports from areas as far apart as Papua New Guinea and Ecuador suggest reduced effectiveness of penicillin therapy in some yaws patients.[8,11] Distinction between relapse and reinfection has not been possible, but nevertheless, some health workers suggest doubling the recommended penicillin dosage.

Benzathine penicillin at the recommended dose will cure early lesions and prevent the development of destructive late lesions but often does not lead to seroreversal. Tetracycline, doxycycline, and erythromycin, at doses appropriate for syphilis, are alternatives in patients allergic to penicillin.

MAJOR ISSUES FOR RENEWED ACTION

Control strategies for the endemic treponematoses are well established and remain largely unchanged. Major issues to stimulate renewed action are[5]

1. A single, cheap, effective measure to stop transmission of these infections is available (single-dose injection of a long-acting penicillin); treponemes have not yet developed resistance to penicillin, but this could occur.
2. These infections are resurging and reemerging in large areas of the developing world, particularly in least developed countries.
3. Elimination and ultimately eradication globally are feasible.
4. Characteristics of at-risk populations are often poor, remote, end-of-the-road, ethnic minorities who are not covered at all or are underserved by health services.
5. Endemic treponematoses control can be used to establish or strengthen primary health care (PHC) and to dramatically increase confidence in and the use of health services. A high degree of community participation in control activities is assured nearly everywhere.
6. A high degree of decentralization of the health services with a true commitment to PHC is the best way to deal with these diseases.

A primary goal, therefore, should be a transfer of expertise on endemic treponematoses to the PHC networks and extension of their coverage, including outreach activities.[12]

References

1 Perine PL et al: *Handbook of Endemic Treponematoses.* Geneva, WHO, 1984.
2 World Health Organization: Control of Endemic Treponematoses. World Health Assembly Resolution WHA 31.58, 1978.
3 Hopkins DR: Control of yaws and other endemic treponematoses: Implementation of vertical and/or integrated programs. *Rev Infect Dis* 7(suppl 2):S338–342, 1985.
4 Meheus A, Antal GM: The endemic treponematoses: Not yet eradicated. *World Health Stat Q* 45:228–237, 1992.
5 World Health Organization: Informal Consultation on Endemic Treponematoses. Geneva, WHO/EMC/95.3, unpublished document.
6 Hervé V et al: Résurgence du pian en République Centrafricaine: Rôle de la population pymée comme réservoir de virus. *Bull Soc Pathol Exp* 85:342–346, 1996
7 Tharmaphornpilas P et al: Recurrence of yaws outbreak in Thailand, 1990. *Southeast Asian J Trop Med Public Health* 25:152–156, 1994.
8 Anselmi M et al: Yaws in Ecuador: Impact of control measures on the disease in the Province of Esmeraldas. *Genitourin Med* 71:343–346, 1995.
9 Engelkens HJH et al: Endemic treponematoses: I. Yaws. *Int J Dermatol* 30:71–83, 1991.
10 Engelkens HJH et al: Endemic treponematoses: II. Pinta and endemic syphilis. *Int J Dermatol* 30:231–238, 1991.
11 Backhouse JL et al: Failure of penicillin treatment of yaws on Karkar Island, Papua New Guinea: *Am J Trop Med Hyg* (submitted).
12 Meheus A: Integration of yaws control and primary health care. *Rev Infect Dis* 7(suppl 2):S284–288, 1985.

Chapter 38

Chancroid and *Haemophilus ducreyi*

Allan R. Ronald
William Albritton

DEFINITION

Chancroid is an acute ulcerative disease, usually of the genitals, often associated with inguinal adenitis or buboes, caused by infection with *Haemophilus ducreyi*, a gram-negative, facultative anaerobic bacillus that requires hemin (X factor) for growth.

HISTORY

Chancroid, or soft chancre (ulcus molle), was first differentiated from syphilis, or hard chancre, by Ricord and his pupil Bassereau in France in the 1850s.[1,2] At the University of Naples in 1889, Ducrey inoculated the skin of the forearm of three patients with purulent material from their own genital ulcer.[3] At weekly intervals he inoculated a new site with material from the most recent ulcer and was able to maintain serial ulcers through as many as 15 generations. He described the organism as a short, compact streptobacillary rod (1.5 × 0.5 μm) that is rounded at the ends and has an indentation at the sides. It was found both within and without neutrophils. He concluded that it was responsible for the soft chancre and further stated that others were incorrect in their attribution of a major role to the "common microorganisms of suppuration" in the pathogenicity of the ulcer or the bubo. Within 3 years this work was confirmed by Krefting, and Unna subsequently described the histology of the chancroidal ulcer and visualized the clumps and chains of gram-negative rods in the lesion.[4,5]

Sullivan in his review of chancroid in 1940 credited Lenglet in 1898 and Bezancon et al. in 1901 with the first successful cultures of *H. ducreyi*, although Himmel cited the successes of earlier investigators.[6,7] Teague and Deibert reported the isolation of *H. ducreyi* from up to 80 percent of patients with suspected clinical chancroid.[8] In subsequent studies they demonstrated that serum (rabbit or sheep), a red blood cell extract (rabbit), and casein digest or peptone were necessary to obtain good growth of *H. ducreyi* on agar media.[9] In 1946 Beeson confirmed that both serum and red cells were necessary to support the growth of the organism.[10]

In 1913 Ito carried out intradermal tests both with *H. ducreyi* from culture and with pus from a chancroidal bubo.[11] A papule, 8 mm or more in diameter, appearing between the third and seventh days, was interpreted as a positive test. In 1921 Reenstierna at the Pasteur Institute confirmed Ito's work.[12] The test became positive in over 90 percent of patients 2 or more weeks after the appearance of the genital ulcer. The value of the Ito-Reenstierna intradermal test was confirmed by Greenblatt and Sanderson, and an antigen was marketed for intradermal testing; it is no longer commercially available.[13]

Despite these substantial studies of chancroid, controversy as to its etiology persisted. In 1918 the British Medical Research Committee "found no sufficient evidence that what is clinically known as 'soft chancre' or 'soft sore' is a specific disease induced by a single species of microorganism."[14] Other historically relevant information can be found in the review of Sullivan in 1940, a series published as the "VDRL Chancroid Studies," and the reviews by Albritton, Morse, and Trees and Morse.[6,15–19]

EPIDEMIOLOGY

Genital ulcer disease (GUD) caused by *H. ducreyi* is endemic in many countries in the developing world. The World Health Organization (WHO) estimates that the annual incidence is about 7 million.[20] Outbreaks have been reported in a number of cities in industrialized countries, predominantly in the United States.[21–28] Chancroid is more prevalent in individuals from lower socioeconomic groups and has been common among military personnel.[22,29,30] Among American military during the Korean conflict, 32 percent of STDs were diagnosed as chancroid.[29] Uncircumcised men are about twice as susceptible to infection.[30] Among Australian troops during the Vietnamese conflict, 23 percent of men with chancroid were circumcised, compared with 60 percent of men with urethritis.[30] *H. ducreyi* is spread from person to person only by sexual contact with no proven role for fomites. It has not been described as being acquired from men having sex with men. Autoinoculation of fingers, conjunctiva, and other sites can occur.

During the past two decades, chancroid epidemics have been carefully studied in industrialized societies.[21–29] Prostitutes have been the usual reservoir of disease described in these epidemics. The exchange of sex for money or drugs, use of crack cocaine, and use of alcohol are major behavioral risk factors for chancroid.[23,28] The ratio of males to females with chancroid in most epidemics exceeds 10 to 1.

The annual incidence of chancroid decreased markedly in the United States between 1950 and 1978.[31] However, beginning in 1980, the annual number of reported cases rose dramatically to over 5000, even though underreporting was occurring.[32] By 1995, however, the number of reported cases had fallen below 1000, and large outbreaks were confined to endemic foci in New York City, New Orleans, and Jackson, Mississippi.[33] Recent evidence suggests that chancroid is now very rare in New Orleans. Ongoing vigilence is essential, as new disease outbreaks will occur as infected individuals travel to nonendemic areas and establish new foci of chancroid.

Genital ulcer disease caused by *H. ducreyi* is a major disease burden in many developing countries. In Malawi, over 50 percent of men presenting to an STD clinic have GUD.[34] In Nairobi, in an urban primary care clinic, 1 percent of adults visiting the clinic presented with GUD.[35] Among prostitutes in Nairobi, the prevalence of genital ulcers ranges from 5 to 25 percent, and *H. ducreyi* can be cultured from about half of the ulcers.[36] The risk of chancroid following coitus with a sexual partner with active genital ulcer disease was studied in Nairobi.[37] The source contacts of 10 men with chancroid were all women with genital ulcers. Among 29 secondary contacts of men with culture-proven chancroid, 17 women had ulcers.[37] It has been estimated that the probability of transmitting chancroid from an infected to an uninfected person during a single sexual exposure is 0.35.[38] The duration of infectivity in the absence of treatment for women is estimated to be 45 days. Although *H. ducreyi* can cause urethritis in men, the urethra is not a proven reservoir.[39] It is probable that individuals capable of transmitting the infection have ulcers. In women, ulcers are often subclinical, and sexual activity continues. Thus, commercial sex workers with ulcers are efficient reservoirs for dissemination of *H. ducreyi* to their clients.

In the absence of clinical cases of chancroid, the epidemiologic evidence supports the hypothesis that there is no subclinical reservoir of *H. ducreyi*. In a search for asymptomatic carriers among 213 commercial sex workers in the Gambia, only four were identified to be positive by polymerase chain reaction (PCR).[40] This is comparable to the rate of *H. ducreyi* carriage found earlier by culture technology.[37] Asymptomatic women with positive culture or PCR results for *H. ducreyi* may be incubating chancroid or may be transiently carrying the organism following recent sexual exposure. At present there is no evidence for an asymptomatic reservoir of infection among individuals without clinical findings of ulceration in the genital tract.

Epidemiologic studies of *H. ducreyi* require techniques to fingerprint strains and follow them within populations. Although a number of technologies have been used, ribotyping provides a high degree of discrimination with broad applicability. Brown and Ison, Sarafian et al., and Pilay et al. have found that ribotyping is reproducible and identifies approximately 17 specific types.[41–43] Although it has been used in outbreaks in the United States, the epidemiology of *H. ducreyi* in developing countries has not been studied with this technology.

BIOLOGY OF *H. DUCREYI*

TAXONOMY AND BIOCHEMISTRY

H. ducreyi is a gram-negative, facultative anaerobic bacillus that requires hemin (X factor) for growth, reduces nitrate to nitrite, and has a DNA guanosine-plus-cytosine content of 0.38 mole fraction.[17] The organism is small, nonmotile and non–spore-forming, and shows typical streptobacillary chaining on Gram stain. The ultrastructural characteristics of the *H. ducreyi* cell wall were described by Kilian and Theilade and Lwoff and Pirosky.[44,45] Hammond et al. demonstrated with the porphyrin test the absence of enzymatic activity in the hemin biosynthetic pathway.[46] *H. ducreyi* also lacks the ferrochelatase or heme synthetase that catalyzes the insertion of iron into the protoporphyrin nucleus.[46] These features, in addition to the guanosine-plus-cytosine content, are sufficient to include the organism among the hemin-requiring species of Pasteurellaceae. Although few unique biochemical characteristics are present, *H. ducreyi* can be differentiated from other hemin-requiring strains of *Haemophilus* by its lack of requirement for nicotinamide adenine dinucleotide (NAD, V factor); its failure to produce H_2S, catalase, or indole; and its production of alkaline phosphatase.[17–19] Nitrate reduction is characteristic of the genus, and all strains reported are oxidase-positive and catalase-negative. Otherwise in routine biochemical tests, most strains are inert other than a positive Voges-Proskauer reaction and weak acid production with glucose and arabinose. Although deficient in carbohydrate hydrolytic activity, *H. ducreyi* has a wide variety of peptide hydrolytic activities.[47] The Pasteur Institute strain CIP542 has been designated the type strain for the species. Biochemical characteristics of differential value are given in Table 38-1.

The taxonomy of *H. ducreyi* is uncertain. Transformation and DNA hybridization studies suggest that *H. ducreyi* is only distantly related to the true haemophili such as *H. influenzae*.[48,49] The sequencing studies of 16S rRNA confirms that *H. ducreyi* is a member of the Pasteurellaceae, and it has been assigned to cluster 4.[50,51] The lipo-oligosaccharide of *H. ducreyi* lacks repeating O-antigens, has a molecular mass of 3.5 to 6.0 kDa, and is similar to that of *N. gonorrhoeae* and *H. influenzae*.[52,53] The gal 1 epitope is present in paragloboside, a precursor of a major blood group antigen. This may enable *H. ducreyi* to evade host immune responses through antigenic mimicry.[52,53]

GROWTH AND NUTRITIONAL CHARACTERISTICS

H. ducreyi grows well on nutritionally enriched media. Chocolatized blood agar or hemoglobin agar with complex supplements such as IsoVitaleX (BBL) or CVA (Gibco) are satisfactory.[54] Growth is also possible on a more defined agar medium containing peptone, glucose, glutamine, and hemin, although some strains require cysteine and starch or albumin as well.[55] The requirement for albumin by some strains could explain the earlier findings of a nutritional requirement for serum.[10] Growth is best at 30 to 33°C in a water-saturated atmosphere, and some strains show improved growth with CO_2.[55] All isolates will grow anaerobically. Hemin requirements of *H. ducreyi* are higher than those of other hemin-requiring species, with most strains requiring 25 to 50 μg/mL for growth compared with 1 to 10 μg/mL for *H. haemoglobinophilus* or *H. influenzae*.[54] Dziuba et al. developed a liquid medium that contained a complex nitrogen source but was otherwise carefully defined.[55] Primary isolation growth conditions appear to be more pH-, moisture-, CO_2-, temperature-, and media-dependent than that required for working with laboratory-adapted strains.[55] Totten and Stamm described a clear broth and plate media and noted that the doubling time for *H. ducreyi* is about 3 hours, slower than many other bacteria and consistent with the 72-hour incubation time required to obtain visible colonies on solid media after primary isolation.[56] In this study they used catalase as a source of hemin.

H. ducreyi requires iron, lacks siderophores, and appears to obtain iron from intracellular sources by invading the cell or destroying it. Lee described four proteins that are upregulated by heme restriction.[57] Strum demonstrated that iron increases *H. ducreyi* virulence in a macaque primate model.[58] The iron could be provided in the injection fluid or by pretreating the monkey with

Table 38-1. Differential Biochemical and Nutritional Characteristics of *Haemophilus* spp. and Other Fastidious Gram-Negative Rods

	X factor required	V factor required	Lysine decarboxylase	Glucose, acid	Sucrose, acid	Lactose, acid	Catalase	Oxidase	Nitrate reductase	Alkaline phosphatase
H. ducreyi	+	–	–	V†	–	–	–	+	+	+
H. haemoglobinophilus	+	–	–	+	+	–	+	+	+	–
H. aphrophilus	–*	–	–	+	+	+	–	–	+	+
Actinobacillus actinomycetemcomitans	–	–	–	+	–	–	+	+	+	+
Eichenella corrodens	–	–	+	–	–	–	–	+	+	–
Cardibacterium hominis	–	–	–	+	+	–	–	+	–	–

* X factor is usually required on primary isolation but may not be needed after repeated passage. The porphyrin test, however, is positive.

† Variable.

injectible iron. A hemoglobin receptor has been characterized and is essential for uptake of iron from hemoglobin.[58a,58b]

IMMUNOLOGY, SEROLOGY, AND IMMUNOCHEMISTRY

Both cell- and humoral-mediated immunity occurs in response to infection with *H. ducreyi*. The cellular immune response has been characterized both with delayed hypersensitivity to *H. ducreyi* antigens and by the response in peripheral blood mononuclear cells to specific *H. ducreyi* antigens.[13,59] Of greater significance is the immunohistochemical studies in humans.[60,61] In both normal volunteers and in biopsies from chancroid lesions, a mononuclear infiltrate predominates and the infiltrate contains many CD4 and CD8 T lymphocytes and macrophages with a paucity of B-lymphocyte lineage.[60,62] The predominant response to *H. ducreyi* infection is a Th1 cell-mediated immune response.

The humoral immune response to *H. ducreyi* infection is being investigated.[63] Circulating IgG, IgM, and IgA are present in many patients with chancroid, and the specificity of the antibody response is enhanced by absorbing cross-reacting antibodies.[64] The lipo-oligosaccharide (LOS) appears to be a better antigen than outer membrane proteins, providing a reasonably sensitive and specific test using an adsorption immunoassay for seroepidemiologic studies.[64,65] Cross-reactivity with other bacterial species occurs, however, and the usefulness of serologic technologies for individual patients is less apparent.[65]

STRUCTURE

Several *H. ducreyi* antigens have been characterized. A major outer membrane protein with molecular weight of 40 kDa is present in all strains and is a member of the OmpA family of proteins.[66] An 18-kDa protein was also found in *H. ducreyi*, and it appears to be similar to the PAL protein in other *Haemophilus* species.[67]

Spinola et al. have identified pili on all strains of *H. ducreyi*.[68] These pili are very fine, tangled appendages, quite different from pili on other pathogens.[69] Purification has identified a pilin monomer that had a molecular mass of 24 kDa. The host cell receptor has not as yet been identified.

Several iron-regulated proteins have also been identified in *H. ducreyi* when grown under conditions in which access to iron and/or heme was limited.[57] These include the common (conserved) heme-regulated hemoglobin receptor.[58a,58b]

Cytotoxins and hemolysins have been characterized by several investigators.[69a–74a] Lagergard et al. observed cytotoxic activity against eukaryotic cells that could be neutralized with immune sera.[69a–70a] Palmer et al. and Totten et al. characterized hemolytic activity that is most apparent with horse erythrocytes.[73,74] Alfa et al. showed that the hemolytic and cytotoxic activity for human foreskin fibroblasts were caused by the same toxin, whereas other studies suggest that the cytotoxin and hemolysin are different proteins.[72] The precise roles of the cytotoxin and hemolysin in pathogenesis are unclear, but they may help to release hemoglobin from cells and may contribute to tissue damage and/or ulcer formation.

GENETICS

The *H. ducreyi* genome is being cloned. Electroporation technologies are able to transform *H. ducreyi* using the plasmid pLS88 as a shuttle vector, which has been sequenced in its entirety.[75–77] Isogenic mutants of *H. ducreyi* now can be constructed and the virulence properties of specific *H. ducreyi* mutants can be determined.

Strains of *H. ducreyi* can acquire 5.7- or 7.0-kDa ampicillin-resistance plasmids which contain the complete, functional Tn_2-like ampicillin-resistance transposon and are highly homologous with a 4.4-kDa *H. influenzae* plasmid, a 4.1-kDa *H. parainfluenzae* plasmid, and the 3.2- and 4.1-kDa plasmids from *Neisseria gonorrhoeae*.[78] Strains also have been shown to carry a plasmid identical to the gonococcal 3.2-mDa plasmid and a unique 2.6-mDa ROB-1 plasmid that confer resistance to penicillin.[79,80] Presumably the ampicillin transposon, although possibly of enteric origin, has been transposed into a group of related, small non–self-transmissible plasmids shared by several genera.[78] The ROB-1 plasmid is present in most strains of *H. ducreyi* from Thailand.[80] Nine plasmids have been characterized to date in *H. ducreyi*.[81] Their reassortment in various isolates can be used as a partial typing system.[26]

Self-transfer of antimicrobial-resistance plasmids and mobilization of non–self-transferable plasmids have been demonstrated in conjugative matings between *H. ducreyi* and other species.[82,83] The ability of *H. ducreyi* to accept and donate plasmids during conjugation suggests that widespread dissemination of antimicrobial-resistance determinants and other genes is possible in this species despite its limited genomic relatedness to other members of the genus *Haemophilus*.

VIRULENCE

Both in vitro and in vivo studies have been carried out to understand the virulence of *H. ducreyi*.[84–93] Attachment to human foreskin cell cultures, invasion of epithelial cell cultures, and cytopathic effect have all been used as markers for virulence.[93] Studies of pathogenesis and immune response have been done in the reduced temperature rabbit model, the primate model, a piglet model, and a human volunteer model.[88–91]

Protein exotoxins, which can be neutralized with immune serum, are presumably important determinants of virulence.[92] Earlier studies had shown that virulent strains of *H. ducreyi* are relatively resistant to phagocytosis and killing by human neutrophils and are resistant to complement-mediated killing by normal human sera.[94]

PATHOGENESIS

The pathogenesis of genital ulcers caused by *H. ducreyi* is being investigated in normal human volunteers and in animal models.[62,88–91] Trauma or abrasion is necessary for organisms to penetrate the epidermis. The inoculum size required for infection is greater than 10^4. In lesions, the organisms are present both within macrophages and neutrophils and also free in clumps in the interstitium.[62]

Histologic features have recently been characterized in two series of patients. The three discrete zones previously described in patients with chancroid do not seem to be as evident in these recent descriptions.[60–62,95] Naturally occurring human infections, human volunteer studies, and animal models all identify initial intraepidermidal lesions that consist of lymphocytes, macrophages, and granulocytes.[60–62,89–91] MHC class 2 HLA-Dr antigens are expressed by the inflammatory cells.[62] Vascular endothelial changes consisting of swelling, proliferation, and erythrocyte extravasation were noted.[60–62] The predominant Th1 response is consistent with the observation that patients with chancroid have increased levels of soluble IL-2 receptors in urine and serum.[96]

The lymphadenitis associated with genital ulcer disease is predominantly a pyogenic inflammatory response. The pathogenesis is unknown and the paucity of organisms in the bubo pus is also unexplained.

The role of the immune response in either susceptibility to chancroid or in its pathogenesis remains unexplored.

CLINICAL MANIFESTATIONS

The incubation period is usually between 4 and 7 days and is rarely less than 3 days or more than 10 days. No prodromal symptoms are recognized.

Males usually present with a complaint referrable directly to the ulcer or to inguinal tenderness. Depending on the site of the ulcer, women often present with less obvious symptoms, including pain on voiding, pain on defecation, rectal bleeding, dyspareunia, or vaginal discharge.[97] On occasion, patients of both sexes have been admitted with the diagnosis of acute nonreducible inguinal hernia.

The chancre begins as a tender papule surrounded by erythema. Over the course of 24 to 48 hours it becomes pustular, eroded, and ulcerated. Vesicles are not seen at any stage of the disease. The ulcer is usually quite painful in males, but it frequently is not noticed by females. The classical ulcer has ragged undermined edges, is sharply demarcated, and is without induration. The base of the ulcer is covered by a gray or yellow necrotic purulent exudate, and its friable granulomatous base often bleeds on scraping (Figs. 38-1 and 38-2). There is little inflammation of the surrounding skin. Several ulcers may merge to form giant ulcers (>2 cm) or serpiginous ulcers. Occasionally, lesions may remain pustular, the so-called dwarf chancroid, and resemble a folliculitis or pyogenic infection. One-half of men have a single ulcer, whereas in one study the mean number of discrete ulcers in women was 4.5.[97,98]

Most lesions in males are on either the external or internal surface of the prepuce, on the frenulum, or in the coronal sulcus (see Fig. 38-1). The glans, the meatus, and the shaft of the penis can also be involved. Edema of the prepuce is common. *H. ducreyi* can cause purulent urethritis and in an STD clinic in Nairobi, 1 to 2 percent of men who present with acute purulent urethritis are infected with *H. ducreyi*.[39]

In females the majority of lesions are at the entrance to the vagina and include lesions on the fourchette, labia, vestibule, and clitoris (see Fig. 38-2).[97,99] Longitudinal ulcers are often present at the posterior fourchette, and large periurethral ulcers are not uncommon. Vaginal wall ulcers can occur, usually by extension from the introitus, and are often painless. In a study of 34 women with chancroid, 5 had perianal ulcers and 3 had ulcerative lesions of the cervix.[97] Rectovaginal fistulas have been reported as a complication of chancroid. Extragenital lesions are less common but have been described on the breasts, fingers, and thighs, and within the mouth.

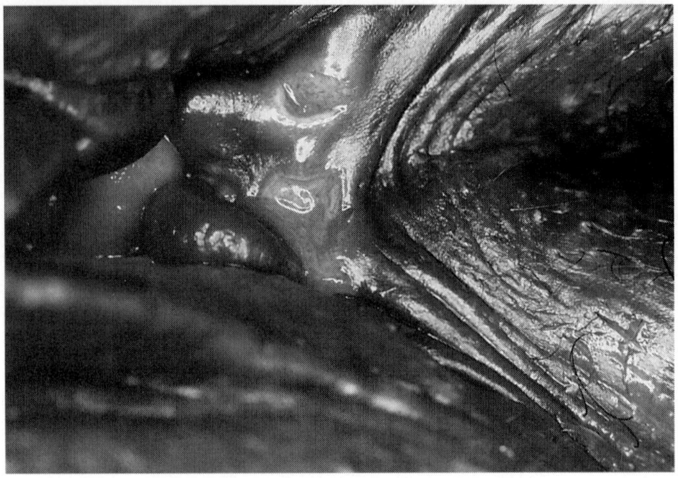

Fig. 38-2. Typical chancroidal ulcers in a female.

Chancroid may be confused with other GUD, including syphilis, genital herpes, and donovanosis.[35,98] The classic chancroid triad, which includes undermining of the ulcer edge, a purulent dirty gray base, and moderate to severe pain, are useful when present but less than half of men with chancroid have all three clinical findings. The differential diagnosis of genital ulcers is further discussed in Chap. 64.

Painful inguinal adenitis is a characteristic feature of chancroid and may be present in up to 40 percent of patients. The adenitis is unilateral in most patients, and erythema of the overlying skin is often present. Buboes can progress to become fluctuant with spontaneous rupture, and a large inguinal abscess can occur. Serpiginous spreading ulceration with destruction of both skin and soft tissue has been described (Fig. 38-3). Most patients with buboes greater than 5 cm in diameter on presentation either drain spontaneously or require drainage for resolution of symptoms. Bubo pus is usually thick, creamy, and viscous. Lymphadenitis and bubo formation are less common in females.[97]

Mild constitutional symptoms can accompany the illness. However, *H. ducreyi* has not been shown to cause systemic infection

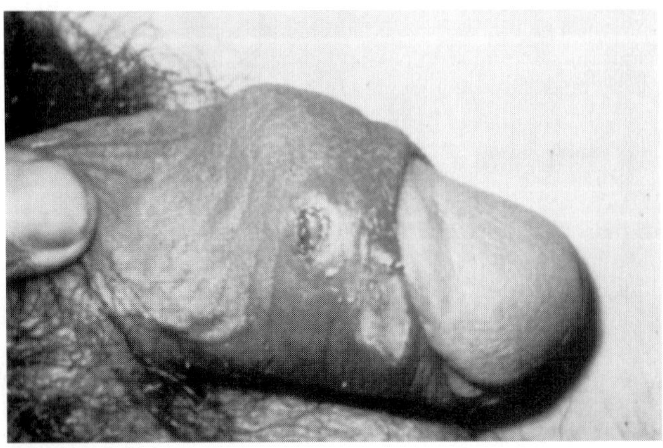

Fig. 38-1. Typical chancroidal ulcer in a male.

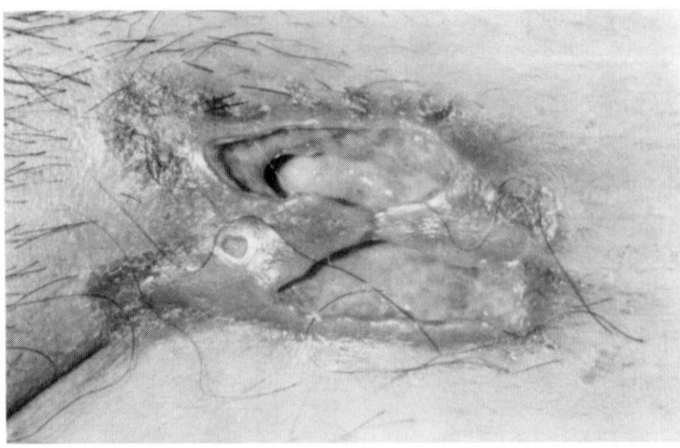

Fig. 38-3. Ruptured inguinal bubo in a patient with chancroid; extensive destruction of soft tissues and skin is evident.

or to spread to distant sites. Occasionally, superinfection with anaerobes including *Fusobacterium* spp. or *Bacteroides* spp. leads to gangrenous phagedenic ulceration and extensive destruction of genital tissue. Cicatrix formation with phimosis is a late complication of chancroid that may require circumcision.

H. ducreyi has not been noted to cause opportunistic infection or to become more invasive in immunocompromised hosts. It has not been reported to cause disease in infants born to women with active chancroid at delivery. However, acute conjunctivitis has been described.[100]

NATURAL HISTORY

Before the era of antimicrobial therapy, genital ulcer disease caused by *H. ducreyi* was a protracted illness with slow and often incomplete resolution. In one study, the mean duration of ulcer disease prior to hospitalization was 34 days, and for 479 men the average duration of hospitalization was 30 days.[101] Recurrence was common. In one study, following healing but on early return to prostitution, 26 percent of women were noted to have recurrent ulcers within 2 months and almost always at the site of the previous lesion.[99]

Occasionally, untreated genital ulcers and inguinal abscesses have been reported to persist for years.

LABORATORY DIAGNOSIS

The laboratory diagnosis of chancroid requires the identification of *H. ducreyi* from genital ulcer or bubo material and the exclusion of other diseases associated with similar clinical findings, especially ulcers caused by herpes simplex, syphilis, lymphogranuloma venereum, or granuloma inguinale.[17–19]

Either cotton or calcium alginate swabs are suitable for specimen collection. Swabs should be taken from the purulent ulcer base. The organism only survives 2 to 4 hours on a swab unless refrigerated at 4°C.[101] A thioglycolate hemin based transport media containing L-glutamine, bovine albumin fraction V, and vancomycin (3 mg/L) permits storage at 4°C for at least 24 hours and perhaps for as long as 7 days.[101] The numbers of *H. ducreyi* in ulcer exudates are substantial and probably are in the range of 10^7 to 10^9/mL of pus. On the other hand, organisms are rarely seen in bubo pus, and culture from the bubo is frequently sterile unless it has ruptured and an inguinal abscess is present. Ducrey made this observation in his classic paper in 1889.[3]

Direct examination of clinical material by a Gram's stain or electron microscopy can be misleading because of the polymicrobial flora of many genital ulcers.[18,103–105]

Primary isolation of *H. ducreyi* from genital lesions has been reported with varying success. Many field studies have used two primary isolation media to maintain culture sensitivity of at least 80 percent.[54,103,106–108] Gonococcal agar base with 1 percent bovine hemoglobin and 5 percent fetal calf serum or Meuller-Hinton agar base supplemented with 5 percent sterile horse blood are successfully used.[106] However, supplementation with 0.2 percent activated charcoal, 1 percent bovine hemoglobin, 1 percent CVA enrichment, and 3 mg/L of vancomycin is a single, relatively inexpensive media that appears to be able to replace other media for primary isolation of *H. ducreyi*.[109]

Small, nonmucoid, yellow-gray, semiopaque, or translucent colonies that can be pushed intact across the agar surface usually appear in 2 to 4 days but may appear as late as 7 days after inoculation. A water-saturated atmosphere containing 5 to 10% CO_2 and a reduced incubation temperature of 33°C are important for primary cultivation of *H. ducreyi*.[54,108]

Presumptive identification can be made by demonstrating short, gram-negative bacilli with occasional streptobacillary chaining from solid media and the inability of isolates to produce porphyrin from delta-aminolevulinic acid by the porphyrin test.[7,18,52] Confirmatory identification requires the demonstration of a hemin (X factor) requirement for growth and the absence of a requirement for NAD (V factor) on media otherwise nutritionally enriched and with the growth conditions previously described. The porphyrin test is the preferred method of demonstrating hemin requirement, and the oxidase test requires tetramethyl-*p*-phenylenediamine, as demonstrated by Nobre.[110]

The polymerase chain reaction (PCR) technology will shortly be commercially available for the diagnosis of *H. ducreyi* as well as for the other genital ulcer pathogens, HSV and *T. pallidum*.[111] Studies have compared PCR technology with culture, and PCR compares well with cultures with a sensitivity that exceeds 95 percent.[33,111–114] Initial technological problems have been resolved and this technology will become standard for definitive epidemiologic studies of genital ulcers.[113,114] During outbreaks of chancroid, early identification of *H. ducreyi* with initiation of appropriate treatment and control programs is critical.[33] PCR technology also permits sensitive and specific identification of *H. ducreyi* in laboratories remote from the outbreak.

Serologic diagnosis of chancroid has been useful in a number of seroepidemiologic studies using an enzyme-linked immunosorbent assay using either whole lysed *H. ducreyi* or lipoliposaccharide as the antigen source.[63–65] Serologic diagnosis of individual cases of chancroid has a sensitivity of between 60 and 80 percent, but it cannot differentiate between recent and remote infection.[65]

ANTIMICROBIAL SUSCEPTIBILITY

H. ducreyi were initially susceptible in vitro to tetracycline, streptomycin, chloramphenicol, sulfonamides, the penicillins, and trimethoprim. Recent studies from diverse regions have shown that clinically significant antimicrobial resistance has become common and has spread rapidly.[115–118] Plasmid-mediated antimicrobial resistance in *H. ducreyi* has been described for ampicillin, sulfonamides, chloramphenicol, tetracycline, streptomycin, and kanamycin.[17,18,79,80,118] Trimethoprim resistance mechanisms are not characterized. The macrolide antimicrobial agents (including erythromycin and azithromycin), the quinolones (including ciprofloxacin and fleroxacin), and the third-generation cephalospo-

Table 38-2. Antimicrobial Susceptibility of Clinical Isolates of *H. ducreyi*

	Range, mg/L	MIC_{50}, mg/L	MIC_{90}, mg/L
Sulfonamides*	0.25–128	64	128
Ampicillin*	0.03–128	16	128
Vancomycin	4–128	8	64
Tetracycline*	0.125–64	16	32
Trimethoprim	0.125–32	4	16
Kanamycin*	0.05–8	2	8
Chloramphenicol*	0.25–16	0.025	8
Rifampin	0.004–1	0.008	0.016
Erythromycin	0.0005–0.032	0.008	0.030
Ciprofloxacin	0.003–0.03	0.003	0.007
Ceftriaxone	0.001–0.004	0.002	0.002

* Antimicrobials currently associated with plasmid-mediated resistance in *H. ducreyi*.

SOURCE: After Hammond et al,[37] Sanson-Le Pors et al,[85] Slootmans et al,[86] Bilgeri et al,[87] Sturm,[88] and Bowmer et al.[108]

rins (including ceftriaxone, cefotaxime, and cefixime), all have very excellent in vitro activity against *H. ducreyi* (Table 38-2) with no proven resistance to date.

TREATMENT

Prior to the advent of antimicrobial agents, circumcision and saline soaks were standard therapy.[101] Sulfonamides were reported to be effective therapy for chancroid in 1938.[119] Five days of therapy were shown to be comparable to longer regimens and the average time to complete healing was less than 10 days. Prior to the emergence of β-lactamase producing strains of *H. ducreyi*, oral ampicillin was an effective regimen.[22]

During the 1970s, resistant strains of *H. ducreyi* emerged and treatment failures were common. During the Vietnam conflict, tetracycline and chloramphenicol were found to be ineffective regimens.[30] Clinical correlation with in vitro resistance was initially carried out in Nairobi in 1983.[120] Clinical failure could be anticipated if *H. ducreyi* were not eradicated from the ulcer within 72 hours of beginning therapy. Subsequent studies have shown that single-dose treatment with a variety of regimens is as effective as more prolonged therapy.[116,121–125] For several years trimethoprim–sulfonamide regimens were the drug of choice but resistance emerged initially in Thailand and subsequently in Kenya and Rwanda.[116,117,126,127] This resistance has spread widely and trimethoprim–sulfonamide combination should not be used unless there is no alternative.

Erythromycin is effective therapy for patients with chancroid.[38,123,128,130] No confirmed resistance has emerged and the organism remains very susceptible. A dose of 250 mg three times a day for 5 days is relatively inexpensive and effective.[129] The new macrolide, azithromycin, prescribed as a single oral dose of 1 g is also an effective, although much more expensive, regimen.[130,131]

The fluoroquinolones have been widely used for the treatment of chancroid and have given excellent results. A single dose of ciprofloxacin, 500 mg, cures over 95 percent of patients; fleroxacin, enoxacin, and presumably other fluoroquinolones are effective therapeutic agents for chancroid.[116,123–125]

Ceftriaxone, prescribed as a single intramuscular dose of 250 mg, has been an effective regimen.[131,132] However, a recent study found that 30 percent of patients concomitantly infected with HIV failed treatment.[133] This and other studies call into some question the efficacy of short-course or single-dose therapy in patients who have both HIV infection and chancroid. Further studies are needed to determine the effectiveness of regimens in patients concomitantly infected with HIV.[117]

A number of other regimens have been used successfully, including the oral combination of amoxicillin with clavulanic acid and intramuscular spectinomycin.[134,135]

Syndromic treatment is important for all patients with genital ulcers.[136] Both syphilis and chancroid should be treated with an appropriate algorithm at the point of first contact.

Relapse after complete healing occurs rarely and usually at the site of the original ulcer. Retreatment usually is successful. Reinfection occurs if the sexual partner is not treated, as there appears to be little or no immunity to *H. ducreyi* infection. All sexual partners of patients with clinical chancroid should be treated with the regimen used to successfully treat the index patient.

Aspiration of buboes has been the most effective management strategy and incision and drainage has been discouraged because of concerns that sinus formation would occur. However, in the modern era of effective antibacterial agents, incision and drainage is appropriate treatment and usually will be more effective.[137]

EPIDEMIOLOGIC ASSOCIATION WITH HUMAN IMMUNODEFICIENCY VIRUS-1

Chancroid has been established as an important risk factor for heterosexual spread of HIV.[137] In the initial studies, among 115 men presenting with genital ulcers, 63 percent of the HIV-1 seropositive men reported a prior episode of genital ulcers compared with 31 percent of HIV-1 seronegative men.[139] In a seroincidence study, of 429 initially HIV-negative men presenting with sexually transmitted infection acquired from a prostitute cohort where over 80 percent of the women were HIV-infected, acquisition of HIV was strongly correlated with both genital ulcer disease and the presence of a foreskin.[140] These independent risk factors increased the risk of seroconversion from less than 2 percent among 118 circumcised men with urethritis to 6 percent among 93 circumcised men who acquired genital ulcers to 29 percent in 55 uncircumcised men who presented with genital ulcers following sexual contact with an HIV-infected woman.[140]

Among female sex workers who had a very high seroincidence of HIV, 60 percent of seroconverting women experienced one or more episodes of genital ulcers prior to conversion compared to 45 percent of HIV seronegative women.[141] The risk increased with the number of ulcer episodes in a dose–response relationship.

Additional studies have confirmed the role of genital ulcers as portals of entry for HIV, and the association between genital ulcers and HIV-1 infection has been reported as well from elsewhere.[27,142,143] The risk appears to not only be present for HIV-1 but also for HIV-2.[144]

The biologic basis for enhanced HIV transmission in patients with chancroid is now apparent. *H. ducreyi* infection recruits CD4 lymphocytes and macrophages to genital surfaces, which cells are the principal early targets for HIV infection. In patients concomitantly infected with both HIV and *H. ducreyi*, the ulcer environment with activation of CD4 lymphocytes provides an ideal opportunity for latent HIV infection to become productive with excretion of virus into the ulcer exudate.[60] Studies have shown virus in ulcer secretions.[145,146] As a result of these biologic effects, the genital lesion becomes both a portal of entry and exit for retroviruses.

An intervention to control STDs including GUD has been successful in reducing HIV transmission.[147] Further studies to determine the effectiveness of various strategies to control GUD are underway.

PREVENTION AND CONTROL

The augmentation of the HIV epidemic by *H. ducreyi* has made chancroid control an urgent priority in all countries. Chancroid survives in populations in which many men are having sex with a few women and in which at least a significant minority of men are uncircumcised. In Western countries, chancroid control has been effective through widespread treatment of prostitutes with ulcers and prostitutes named as sexual contacts of men with ulcers.[21,148] However, most women do not seek treatment despite numerous ulcers and most commercial sex workers continue to be sexually active.[149] As a result, programs to trace and treat contacts are essential. In addition, effective syndromic treatment of genital ulcers at the point of first contact of the individual with the health care system and the widespread use of condoms by the clients of commercial sex workers has dramatically reduced the incidence of chancroid in Thailand and probably other countries.[149,150] Eradication of *H. ducreyi* from populations is an achievable goal. Although a vaccine may have a role, effective STD control programs should be able to achieve major reductions in the global incidence of chancroid.

References

1 Kampmeier RH: The recognition of *Haemophilus ducreyi* as the cause of soft chancre. *Sex Transm Dis* 9:212–213, 1982.
2 Bassereau PI: *Trait de Affections de la Peau Symptomatiques de la Syphilis*. Paris, J.B. Balliere, 1852.
3 Ducrey A: Experimentelle untersuchungen uber den ansteckungsstoff des weichen schankers und uber die bubonen. *Monatshr Prakt Dermatol* 9:387, 1889.
4 Krefting R: Ueber die fur ulcus molle specifische mikrobe. *Arch Dermatol Syphilis Erganzungshefte* 24:14, 1892.
5 Unna PG: Der streptobacillus des weichen schankers. *Monatshr Prakt Dermatol* 14:485, 1892.
6 Sullivan M: Chancroid. *Am J Syph* 24:482–521, 1940.
7 Himmel J: Contribution a l'etude de l'immunite des animaux vis-a-vis du bacille du chancre mou. *Ann Inst Pasteur* 15:928, 1901.
8 Teague O et al: The value of the cultural method in the diagnosis of chancroid. *J Urol* 4:543, 1920.
9 Teague O et al: Some observations on thc bacillus of unna-ducrey. *J Med Res* 43:61, 1922.
10 Beeson PB: Studies on chancroid: IV. The Ducreyi bacillus: Growth requirements and inhibition by antibiotic agents. *Proc Soc Exp Biol Med* 61:81, 1946.
11 Ito T: Klinische und bacteriologische studien iber ulcus molle and ducreysche streptobazillen. *Arch Dematol Syph* 116:341, 1913.
12 Reenstierna J: Chancre mou experimental chez le singe et la lapin. *Acta Dermatol Venereol* 2:1, 1921.
13 Greenblatt RB et al: The intradermal chancroid bacillary antigen test as an aid in the differential diagnosis of the venereal bubo. *Am J Surg* 41:384, 1938.
14 Pijper C: The bacillus Unna-Ducrey: A page from the history of bacteriology. *Med J S Afr* 16:89–91, 1920.
15 Deacon WE et al: VDRL chancroid studies: 1. A simplified procedure for the isolation and identification of *Haemophilus ducreyi*. *J Invest Dermatol* 26:399, 1956.
16 Kaplan W et al: VDRL chancroid studies: III. Use of Ducrey skin test vaccines on rabbits. *J Invest Dermatol* 26:415, 1956.
17 Albritton WL: Biology of *Haemophilus ducreyi*. *Microbiol Rev* 53: 377–389, 1989.
18 Morse SA: Chancroid and *Haemophilus ducreyi*. *Clin Microbiol Rev* 2:137–157, 1989.
19 Trees DL et al: Chancroid and *Haemophilus ducreyi*: An update. *Clin Microbiol Rev* 8:357–375, 1995.
20 World Health Organization Press Release: WHO/64. Sexually transmitted diseases three hundred and thirty-three million new, curable cases in 1995. Geneva, World Health Organization, 1995.
21 Blackmore CA et al: An outbreak of chancroid in Orange County, California: Descriptive epidemiology and disease-control measures. *J Infect Dis* 151:840, 1985.
22 Hammond GW et al: Clinical, epidemiological, laboratory and therapeutic features of an urban outbreak of chancroid in North America. *Rev Infect Dis* 2:867–879, 1980.
23 Dicarlo RP et al: Chancroid epidemiology in New Orleans men. *J Infect Dis* 172:446–452, 1995.
24 Jones C et al: Chancroid: Results from an outbreak in Houston, Texas. *S Med J* 83:1384–1389, 1990.
25 McCarley M et al: Chancroid: Clinical variants and other findings, 1986–1987. *J Amer Acad Dermatol* 19:330–337, 1988.
26 Flood JM et al: Multistrain outbreak of chancroid in San Francisco, 1989–1991. *J Infect Dis* 167:1106–1111, 1993.
27 Telzak EE et al: HIV-1 seroconversion in patients with and without genital ulcer disease. *Ann Intern Med* 119:1181–1186, 1993.
28 Chirgwin K et al: HIV infection, genital ulcer disease, and crack cocaine use among patients attending a clinic for sexually transmitted diseases. *Amer J Public Health* 81:1576–1579, 1991.
29 Asin J: Chancroid: A report of 1402 cases. *Am J Syph Gon Vener Dis* 36:483, 1952.
30 Hart G: Venereal disease in a war environment: Incidence and management. *Med J Aust* 1:808, 1975.
31 Schmid TP et al: Chancroid in the United States, reestablishment of an old disease. *JAMA* 258:3265, 1987.
32 Schulte JM et al: Chancroid in the United States. 1981–1990: Evidence for underreporting of cases. *MMWR* 41(no.SS-3):57–61, 1992.
33 Morse SA et al: Chancroid detected by polymerase chain reaction: Jackson, Mississippi, 1994–1995. *MMWR* 44:567–574, 1995.
34 Behets FMT et al: Sexually transmitted diseases and human immunodeficiency virus control in Malawi: A field study of genital ulcer disease. *J Infect Dis* 171:451–455, 1995.
35 Ndinya-Achola JO et al: Presumptive specific clinical diagnosis of genital ulcer disease (GUD) in a primary health care setting in Nairobi. *Int J AIDS STD* 7:201–205, 1996.
36 D'Costa LJ et al: Prostitutes are a major reservoir of sexually transmitted diseases in Nairobi, Kenya. *Sex Transm Dis* 12:64, 1985.
37 Plummer FA et al: Epidemiology of chancroid and *Haemophilus ducreyi* in Nairobi. *Lancet* 2:1293, 1983.
38 Brunham RC et al: Epidemiology of sexually transmitted diseases in developing countries. pp 61–80 in Research issues in human behavior and STD in the AIDS Era (ed.) Wasserheit J, S Aral and KK Holmes. *Amer Soc Microbiol* Washington DC, 1991.
39 Kunimoto DY et al: Urethral infection with *Haemophilus ducreyi* in men. *Sex Transm Dis* 15:37–39, 1988.
40 Hawkes S et al: Asymptomatic carriage of *Haemophilus ducreyi* confirmed by the polymerase chain reaction. *Genitourin Med* 71:224–227, 1995.
41 Brown TJ et al: Non-radioactive ribotyping of *Haemophilus ducreyi* using a digoxigenin labelled cDNA probe. *Epidemiol Infect* 110:289–295, 1993.
42 Sarafian SK et al: Molecular characterization of *Haemophilus ducreyi* by ribosomal DNA fingerprinting. *J Clin Microbiol* 29:1949–1954, 1991.
43 Pillay A et al: Ribosomal DNA typing of *Haemophilus ducreyi* strains: Proposal for a novel typing system. *J Clin Microbiol* 34:10, 1996.
44 Kilian M et al: Cell wall ultrastructure of strains of *Haemophilus ducreyi* and *Haemophilus piscium*. *Int J Systemat Bacteriol* 25:351, 1975.
45 Lwoff A et al: Determination du facteur de croissance pour *Haemophilus ducreyi*. *CR Seances Soc Biol* (Paris) 124:1169, 1937.
46 Hammond GW et al: Determination of the hemin requirement of *Haemophilus ducreyi*. Evaluation of the porphyrin test and media used in the satellite growth test. *J Clin Microbiol* 7:243, 1978.
47 Sturm AW et al: Enzymic activity of *Haemophilus ducreyi*. *J Med Microbiol* 18:181, 1984.
48 Albritton WL et al: Relatedness within the family *Pasteurellaceae* as determined by genetic transformation. *Int J Syst Bacteriol* 36:103–106, 1986.
49 DeLey JW et al: Inter- and intrafamilial similarities of rRNA cistrons of the *Pasteurellaceae*. *Int J Syst Bacteriol* 40:126–137, 1990.
50 Dewhirst FE et al: Phylogeny of 54 representative strains of species in the family *Pasteurellaceae* as determined by comparison of 16S rRNA sequences. *J Bacteriol* 174:2002–2013, 1992.
51 Rossau R et al: The development of specific rRNA-derived oligonucleotide probes for *Haemophilus ducreyi*, the causative agent of chancroid. *J Gen Microbiol* 137:277–285, 1991.
52 Melaugh W et al: Partial characterization of the major lipooligosaccharide from a strain of *Haemophilus ducreyi*, the causative agent of chancroid, a genital ulcer disease. *J Biol Chem* 267:13434–13439, 1992.
53 Melaugh W et al: Structure of the major lipooligosaccharide of *Haemophilus ducreyi* strain 35000 and evidence for additional glycoforms. *Biochemistry* 33:13070–13078, 1994.
54 Hammond W et al: Comparison of specimen collection and laboratory techniques for isolation of *Haemophilus ducreyi*. *J Clin Microbiol* 7:39, 1978.

55 Dziuba M et al: A study of the nutritional requirements of a selected *Haemophilus ducreyi* strain by impedance and conventional methods. *Curr Microbiol* 27:109–113, 1993.

56 Totten PA et al: Clear broth and plate media for culture of *Haemophilus ducreyi*. *J Clin Microbiol* 32:2019–2023, 1994.

57 Lee BC: Iron sources for *Haemophilus ducreyi*. *J Med Microbiol* 34: 317–322, 1991.

58 Sturm AW: Iron and virulence of *Haemophilus ducreyi* in a primate model. *Sex Transm Dis* 24:64–68, 1997.

58a Elkins C: Identification and purification of a conserved heme-regulated hemoglobin-binding outer membrane protein from *Haemophilus ducreyi*. *Infect Immunol* 63:1241–1245, 1995.

58b Elkins C et al: Characterization of the HgbA locus of *Haemophilus ducreyi*. *Infect Immunol* 63:2194–2200, 1995.

59 VanLaer L et al: In vitro stimulation of peripheral blood mononuclear cells (PBMC) for HIV- and HIV+ chancroid patients by *Haemophilus ducreyi* antigens. *Clin Exp Immunol* 102:243–250, 1995.

60 King R et al: An immunohistochemical analysis of naturally occurring chancroid. *J Infect Dis* 174:427–430, 1996.

61 Magro CM et al: A morphological study of penile chancroid lesions in human immunodeficiency virus (HIV)-positive and -negative African men with a hypothesis concerning the role of chancroid in HIV transmission. *Hum Pathol* 27:1066–1070, 1996.

62 Spinola SM et al: *Haemophilus ducreyi* elicits a cutaneous infiltrate of CD4 cells during experimental human infection. *J Infect Dis* 173: 394–402, 1996.

63 Desjardins M et al: Standardization of an enzyme immunoassay for human antibody to *Haemophilus ducreyi*. *J Clin Microbiol* 30:2019–2024, 1992.

64 Roggen EL et al: Enzyme immunoassays (EIAs) for the detection of anti-*Haemophilus ducreyi* serum IgA, IgG, and IgM antibodies. *Sex Transm Dis* 21:36–42, 1994.

65 Alfa MJ et al: Humoral immune response of humans to lipooligosaccharide and outer membrane proteins of *Haemophilus ducreyi*. *J Infect Dis* 167:1206–1210, 1993.

66 Spinola SM et al: The major outer membrane protein of *Haemophilus ducreyi* is a member of the OmpA family of proteins. *Infect Immunol* 61:1346–1351, 1993.

67 Spinola SM et al: The conserved 18,000-molecular-weight outer membrane protein of *Haemophilus ducreyi* has homology to PAL. *Infect Immunol* 64:1950–1955, 1996.

68 Spinola SM et al: Characterization of pili expressed by *Haemophilus ducreyi*. *Microbiol Pathogen* 9:417–426, 1990.

69 Brentjiens RJ et al: Fine tangled pili expressed by *Haemophilus ducreyi* are a novel class of pili. *J Bacteriol* 178:808–816, 1996.

69a Purven M et al: *Haemophilus ducreyi*, a cytotoxin-producing bacterium. *Infect Immunol* 60:1156–1162, 1992.

70 Lagergard T et al: Evidence of *Haemophilus ducreyi* adherence to and cytotoxin destruction of human epithelial cells. *Microbiol Pathogen* 14:417–431, 1993.

70a Lagergard T et al: Neutralizing antibodies to *Haemophilus ducreyi* cytotoxin. *Infect Immunol* 61:1589–1592, 1993.

71 Alfa MJ: Cytopathic effect of *Haemophilus ducreyi* for human foreskin cell culture. *J Med Microbiol* 37:43–50, 1992.

72 Alfa MJ et al: *Haemophilus ducreyi* hemolysin acts as a contact cytotoxin and damages human foreskin fibroblasts in cell culture. *Infect Immunol* 64:2349–2352, 1996.

73 Palmer KL et al: Identification of a hemolytic activity elaborated by *Haemophilus ducreyi*. *Infect Immunol* 62:3041–3043, 1994.

74 Totten PA et al: Characterization of the hemolytic activity of *Haemophilus ducreyi*. *Infect Immunol* 63:4409–4416, 1995.

74a Palmer KL et al: Cloning and characterization of the genes encoding haemolysin of *Haemophilus ducreyi*. *Mol Microbiol* 18:821–830, 1995.

75 Leong MG et al: Transformation of two reference strains of *Haemophilus ducreyi* to ampicillin resistance by electroporation. *Med Microbiol Lett* 1:338–346, 1992.

76 Hansen EJ et al: Use of electroporation to construct isogenic mutants of *Haemophilus ducreyi*. *Infect Immunol* 44:196–198, 1984.

77 Dixon LG et al: An analysis of the complete nucleotide sequence of the *Haemophilus ducreyi* broad-host-range plasmid pLS88. Plasmid 32:228–232, 1994.

78 Brunton J et al: Molecular epidemiology of beta-lactamase-specifying plasmids of *Haemophilus ducreyi*. *Antimicrobiol Agents Chemother* 21:857–863, 1982.

79 Anderson B et al: Common beta-lactams plasmid in *Haemophilus ducreyi* and *Neisseria gonorrhoeae*. *Antimicrobiol Agents Chemother* 25:296–297, 1984.

80 Maclean IW et al: Identification of a ROB-1 beta-lactamase in *Haemophilus ducreyi*. *Antimicrobiol Agents Chemother* 36:467–469, 1992.

81 McNicol PJ et al: The plasmids of *Haemophilus ducreyi*. *J Antimicrobiol Chemother* 14:561, 1984.

82 McNicol PJ et al: Characterization of a *Haemophilus ducreyi* mobilizing plasmid. *J Bacteriol* 165:657, 1986.

83 Deneer HG et al: Mobilization of nonconjugative antibiotic resistant plasmids in *Haemophilus ducreyi*. *J Bacteriol* 149:726–732, 1982.

84 Alfa MJ et al: *Haemophilus ducreyi* adheres but does not invade cultured human foreskin cells. *Infect Immunol* 61:1735–1742, 1993.

85 Lammel CJ et al: In vitro model of *Haemophilus ducreyi* adherence to and entry into eukaryotic cells of genital origin. *J Infect Dis* 167: 642–650, 1993.

86 Totten PA et al: *Haemophilus ducreyi* attaches to and invades human epithelial cells in vitro. *Infect Immunol* 62:5632–5640, 1994.

87 Brentjens RJ et al: *Haemophilus ducreyi* adheres to human keratinocytes. *Microbiol Pathogen* 16:243–247, 1994.

88 Purcell BK et al: A temperature-dependent rabbit model for production of dermal lesion by *Haemophilus ducreyi*. *J Infect Dis* 164:359, 1991.

89 Totten PA et al: A primate model for chancroid. *J Infect Dis* 169: 1284–1290, 1994.

90 Hobbs MM et al: Swine model of *Haemophilus ducreyi* infection. *Infect Immunol* 63:3094–3100, 1995.

91 Spinola SM et al: Experimental human infection with *Haemophilus ducreyi*. *J Infect Dis* 169:1146–1150, 1994.

92 Lagergard T et al: Neutralizing antibodies to *Haemophilus ducreyi* cytotoxin. *Infect Immunol* 61:1589–1592, 1993.

93 Alfa MJ et al: Use of tissue culture and animal models to identify virulence-associated traits of *Haemophilus ducreyi*. *Infect Immunol* 63:1754–1761, 1995.

94 Odumeru JA et al: Role of lipopolysaccharide and complement in susceptibility of *Haemophilus ducreyi* to human serum. *Infect Immunol* 50:495–499, 1985.

95 Freinkel AL: Histological aspects of sexually transmitted genital lesions. *Histopathology* 11:819–831, 1987.

96 Abeck D et al: Soluble interleukin-2 receptors in serum and urine of patients with chancroid and their response to therapy. *Int J STD AIDS* 1:282–284, 1990.

97 Plummer FA et al: Clinical and microbiologic studies of genital ulcers in Kenyan women. *Sex Trans Dis* 12:193, 1985.

98 Dangar Y et al: Accuracy of clinical diagnosis of genital ulcer disease. *Sex Transm Dis* 17:184–189, 1990.

99 Lao DG et al: Chancroid in women in Manila. *Am J Syph* 31:277, 1947.

100 Gregory JE et al: Conjunctivitis due to *Haemophilus ducreyi* infection. *Br J Vener Dis* 56:414, 1980.

101 Rauschkolb JE: Circumcision in treatment of chancroidal lesions of male genitalia. *Arch Dermatol Syph* 39:319, 1939.

102 Dangar Y et al: Transport media for *Haemophilus ducreyi*. *Sex Transm Dis* 20:5–9, 1993.

103 Borchardt KA et al: Simplified laboratory technique for diagnosis of chancroid. *Arch Dermatol* 102:190, 1970.

104 Marsch WC et al: Ultrastructural detection of *Haemophilus ducreyi* in biopsies of chancroid. *Arch Dermatol Res* 263:153, 1978.

105 Chapel T et al: The microbiological flora of penile ulcerations. *J Infect Dis* 137:50, 1978.

106 Dylewski J et al: Laboratory diagnosis of *Haemophilus ducreyi*: Sensitivity of culture media. *Diagn Microbiol Infect Dis* 4:241–245, 1986.

107 Sottnek FO et al: Isolation and identification of *Haemophilus ducreyi* in a clinical study. *J Clin Microbiol* 12:170, 1980.
108 Schmid GP et al: Enhanced recovery of *Haemophilus ducreyi* from clinical specimens by incubation at 33 versus 35°C. *J Clin Microbiol* 33:3257–3259, 1995.
109 Lockett AE et al: Serum-free media for the isolation of *Haemophilus ducreyi*. *Lancet* 338:326, 1991.
110 Nobre GN: Identification of *Haemophilus ducreyi* in the clinical laboratory. *J Med Microbiol* 15:243, 1982.
111 Orle KA et al: Simultaneous PCR detection of *Haemophilus ducreyi*, *Treponema pallidum*, and Herpes simplex virus Types 1 and 2 from genital ulcers. *J Clin Microbiol* 34:49–54, 1996.
112 Dangor Y et al: Antimicrobial susceptibility of *Haemophilus ducreyi*. *Antimicrob Agents Chemother* 34:1303–1307, 1990.
113 Chui L et al: Development of the polymerase chain reaction assay for the detection of *Haemophilus ducreyi*. *J Clin Microbiol* 31:659–664, 1993.
114 Johnson SR et al: Alterations in sample preparation increase sensitivity of PCR assay for diagnosis of chancroid. *J Clin Micribiol* 33: 1036–1038, 1995.
115 Knapp JS et al: In vitro susceptibilities of isolates of *Haemophilus ducreyi* from Thailand and the United States to currently recommended and newer agents for treatment of chancroid. *Antimicrobiol Agents Chemother* 27:1552–1555, 1993.
116 Plourde PJ et al: A randomized double-blind study of the efficacy of fleroxacin versus trimethoprim-sulfamethoxazole in men with culture-proven chancroid. *J Infect Dis* 165:949–952, 1992.
117 Bogaerts J et al: Failure of treatment for chancroid in Rwanda is not related to human immunodeficiency virus infection: In vitro resistance of *Haemophilus ducreyi* to trimethoprim-sulfamethoxazole. *Clin Infect Dis* 10:924–930, 1995.
118 Albritton WL et al: Plasmid-mediated sulfonamide resistance in *Haemophilus ducreyi*. *Antimicrobiol Agents Chemother* 21:159, 1982.
119 Hanschell HM: Sulfanilamide in the treatment of chancroid. *Lancet* 1:886, 1938.
120 Fast MW et al: Antimicrobial therapy of chancroid: An evaluation of five treatment regimens correlated with in vitro sensitivity. *Sex Transm Dis* 10:1, 1983.
121 Dylewski J et al: Trimethoprim-sulfamethoxazole in the treatment of chancroid: comparison of two single-dose treatment regimens with a five-day regimen. *J Antimicrobiol Chemother* 16:103–109, 1985.
122 Plummer F et al: Single-dose therapy of chancroid with trimethoprim-sulfamethoxazole. *N Engl J Med* 309:67–71, 1983.
123 Ballard RC et al: Treating chancroid: Summary of studies in southern Africa. *Genitourin Med* 65:54–57, 1989.
124 Naamara W et al: Treatment of chancroid with ciprofloxacin: a prospective, randomized clinical trial. *Am J Med* 82(Suppl.4A):317–320, 1987.
125 Bodhidatta LT et al: Evaluation of 500- and 100-mg doses of ciprofloxacin for the treatment of chancroid. *Antimicrobiol Agents Chemother* 32:723–725, 1988.
126 Taylor DN et al: Comparative study of ceftriaxone and trimethoprim-sulfamethoxazole for the treatment of chancroid in Thailand. *J Infect Dis* 152:1002–1006, 1985.
127 Van Dyck E et al: Emergence of *Haemophilus ducreyi* resistance to trimethoprim-sulfamethoxazole in Rwanda. *Antimicrobiol Agents Chemother* 38:1647–1648, 1994.
128 Plummer FA et al: Antimicrobial therapy of chancroid: Effectiveness of erythromycin. *J Infect Dis* 148:726, 1983.
129 Kimani J et al: Low dose erythromycin regimen for the treatment of chancroid. *E Afr Med J* 72:645–648, 1995.
130 Tyndall MW et al: Single dose azithromycin for the treatment of chancroid: A randomized comparison with erythromycin. *Sex Transm Dis* 21:231–234, 1994.
131 Martin DH et al: Comparison of azithromycin and ceftriaxone for the treatment of chancroid. *Clin Infect Dis* 21:409–414, 1995.
132 Bowmer MI et al: Single-dose ceftriaxone for chancroid. *Antimicrobiol Agents Chemother* 31:67, 1987.
133 Tyndall M et al: Ceftriaxone no longer predictably cures chancroid in Kenya. *J Infect Dis* 167:317–321, 1993.
134 Ndinya-Achola JO et al: Augmentin in the treatment of chancroid: Three day oral course. *Genitourin Med* 62:202, 1986.
135 Guzman M et al: Treatment of chancroid with a single dose of spectinomycin. *Sex Transm Dis* 19:291–294, 1992.
136 Bogaerts J et al: Simple algorithms for the management of genital ulcers: Evaluation in a primary health care centre in Kigali, Rwanda. *Bull World Health Org* 73:761–767, 1995.
137 Ernest AA et al: Incision and drainage versus aspiration of fluctuant buboes in the emergency department during an epidemic of chancroid. *Sex Transm Dis* 22:217, 1995.
138 Hayes RJ et al: The cofactor effect of genital ulcers on the per-exposure risk of HIV transmission in sub-Saharan Africa. *J Trop Med Hyg* 98:1–8, 1995.
139 Simonson JN et al: Human immunodeficiency virus infection among men with sexually transmitted diseases. *N Engl J Med* 319:274–278, 1988.
140 Cameron DW et al: Female to male transmission of human immunodeficiency virus type 1: Risk factors for seroconversion in men. *Lancet* ii:403–407, 1989.
141 Plummer FA et al: Cofactors in male-to-female sexual transmission of human immunodeficiency virus type 1. *J Infect Dis* 163:233–239, 1991.
142 Plourde PJ et al: Human immunodeficiency virus type 1 seroconversion in women with genital ulcers. *J Infect Dis* 170:313–317, 1994.
143 Figueroa JP et al: Rising HIV-1 prevalence among sexually transmitted disease clinic attenders in Jamaica: Traumatic sex and genital ulcers as risk factors. *J Acquir Immune Defic Syndr* 7:310–316, 1994.
144 Pepin J et al: HIV-2 infection among prostitutes working in the Gambia: Association with serological evidence of genital ulcer diseases and with generalized lymphadenopathy. *AIDS* 5:69, 1991.
145 Plummer FA et al: Detection of human immunodeficiency virus type-1 (HIV-1) in genital ulcer exudates of HIV-1 infected men by culture and gene amplification. *J Infect Dis* 161:810–811, 1990.
146 Kreiss JK et al: Isolation of human immunodeficiency virus from genital ulcers in Nairobi prostitutes. *J Infect Dis* 160:380, 1989.
147 Grosskurth H et al: Impact of improved treatment of sexually transmitted diseases on HIV infection in rural Tanzania: Randomized control trial. *Lancet* 346:530–536, 1995.
148 Jessamine PG et al: Rapid control of a chancroid outbreak: implications for Canada. *Can Med Assoc J* 142:1081, 1990.
149 Cameron WD et al: Condom use prevents genital ulcers in women working as prostitutes. Influence of human immunodeficiency virus infection. *Sex Transm Dis* 18:188–191, 1991.
150 Nelson KE et al: Changes in sexual behavior and a decline in HIV infection among young men in Thailand. *N Engl J Med* 335:297–303, 1996.

Chapter 39
Donovanosis

Nigel O'Farrell

HISTORY

Donovanosis is a chronic, progressive, mildly contagious bacterial infection that usually involves the genital region. The causative organism is a gram-negative bacillus, *Calymmatobacterium granulomatis*. The condition has been known under numerous terminologies, such as serpiginous ulceration of the groin, lupoid form of groin ulceration, ulcerating granuloma of the pudenda, granuloma genitoinguinale, granuloma venereum genitoinguinale, infective granuloma, granuloma inguinale tropicum, chronic venereal sores, and ulcerating sclerosing granuloma, but it is known more commonly as granuloma inguinale and granuloma venereum.[1] In the past, there has been considerable confusion between granuloma inguinale and lymphogranuloma venereum. Marmell and Santora[2] recognized this and recommended *donovanosis* as the most suitable name. Most authorities are gradually coming to accept this view.

The first description of donovanosis is attributed to McLeod, Professor of Surgery at the Medical College of Calcutta, in 1882.[3] He reported cases of serpiginous ulceration and formation of an imperfect cicatrix involving the scrotal and penile tissues in men and long-standing elephantiasis of the clitoris and labia in a woman. Subsequent cases were reported from British Guinea[4] and the United Kingdom.[5]

The causative organism was first described in 1905 by Donovan working in Madras.[6] He identified the characteristic Donovan bodies measuring 1.5 × 0.7 μm in macrophages and epithelial cells of the stratum malpighii. Difficulties in culturing the organism led to considerable debate about the causative agent. Aragao and Vianna[7] claimed to have cultured a pleomorphic bacterium from ulcer lesions and identified it as *C. granulomatis*.

Cornwall and Peck[8] cultured an organism that, when injected into rabbits, produced granulomatous lesions simulating donovanosis at the site of injection. Experimental transmission of the organism from one individual to another was reported by McIntosh in 1926.[9] DeMonbreun and Goodpasture[10] grew gram-negative bacilli of the *Aerogenes* group from ulcers and feces of patients with donovanosis in a filtrate of chick membrane in both the capsulated and noncapsulated forms. Greenblatt et al.[11] accomplished transmission of the disease into human volunteers by introducing material from a pseudobubo but were unable to grow the organism on the chorioallantois of chick embryos.[12]

Attempts at culture remained unconvincing until 1943 when Anderson[13] reported the isolation of the causative organism on the yolk sac of chick embryos and proposed a new genus, *Donovania*, and species, *granulomatis*.[14] Subsequent efforts to develop an artificial medium for the culture of *D. granulomatis* met with only limited success. Some growth was achieved using beef heart infusion agar and normal chick embryo yolk sacs with subsequent transfer to tryptose beef heart infusion broth and modified Levinthal's stock broth.[15] It would now seem that earlier claims of successful cultures may have been due to contamination. Positive skin reactions were demonstrated in human subjects with donovanosis after injection of bacterial antigen prepared from infected yolk sacs.[16]

A link between *C. granulomatis* and *Klebsiella* species was suggested on the evidence of antigenic cross-reactivity.[17] Goldberg[18] characterized the organism further and showed that two factors were necessary for growth: (1) a low oxidation-reduction potential, which could be satisfied by the use of a thioglycolate medium, and (2) a factor or factors in eggs, which could be substituted by the enzymatic digests of bovine albumin or soya meal.

Despite these developments, progress in donovanosis research was slow. After 1962,[19] there were no reports of successful culture until recently in Durban, where the bacteria were grown in a monocyte coculture system from biopsy specimens after pretreatment with amikacin: Multiplication of the bacteria was demonstrated, and extracellular dividing organisms were observed.[20]

PATHOGENESIS AND BIOLOGY

The first manifestation of donovanosis is usually a small, firm nodule in the genital region in skin that has been subjected to a degree of trauma. Most established infections are associated with poor standards of personal genital hygiene. Goldzieher and Peck[21] were the first to identify Donovan bodies in histologic sections of tissue in 1926 and described a large, swollen mononuclear cell containing the specific organisms. Pund and Greenblatt,[22] using Delafield's hematoxylin and eosin and Dieterle silver-impregnation staining methods, also described a large mononuclear cell 25 to 90 μm in diameter with intracytoplasmic cysts filled with deeply stained bodies that they regarded as pathognomonic of donovanosis. These cysts eventually rupture and release the infective organisms. Sehgal et al.[23] described gram-negative intra- and extracellular Donovan bodies with different morphologic features—coccoid, coccobacillary, and bacillary.

Electron microscopic studies have shown organisms with typical gram-negative morphology and a large capsule but no flagella. Filiform or vesicular protrusions may be seen on a corrugated cell wall.[24,25]

EPIDEMIOLOGY

In the preantibiotic era donovanosis was prevalent in many diverse geographic locations. Rajam and Rangiah[1] stated that the disease was distributed in both hemispheres and endemic in southern China; the East Indies; northern Australia; some countries of Central, South, and North America; and the West Indies. In the United States, Greenblatt[26] estimated a population prevalence of 5,000 to 10,000 cases in 1947. Nowadays significant numbers are found in only a few developing countries, although sporadic cases may occur in developed countries. A small epidemic of 20 cases was reported in 1984 in the United States.[27]

The main foci of donovanosis are in Papua New Guinea[28]; southern Africa, particularly the Durban-KwaZulu-Natal region[29] but also eastern Transvaal[30] and Zimbabwe[31]; northeast Brazil[32]; French Guyana[33]; and aboriginal communities in Australia.[34] Papua New Guinea seems to be the worst affected region; in 1980 donovanosis accounted for 46 percent of genital ulcers in women with genital ulcer disease.[35] The largest epidemic recorded was in Dutch South New Guinea between 1922 and 1952, when 10,000 cases were reported from a population of 15,000.[36] In Durban the numbers of donovanosis cases recorded in the annual reports of the medical officer of health have risen steadily from 312 in 1988 to 2,385 in 1995.[37] In a microbiologic study of genital ulcer disease among sexually transmitted disease (STD) clinic attenders in Durban, donovanosis was diagnosed in 11 percent of men[38] and 16 percent of women.[39] However, the true nature of the epidemic in Durban is still unclear: Diagnoses subsequent to 1988 were made on clinical grounds by a variety of staff and without laboratory confirmation. Elsewhere in Africa sporadic cases of donovanosis have been reported in recent times from Botswana,[40] the Central African Republic,[41] Gabon,[42] and Zambia.[43]

It has been questioned as to whether donovanosis is an STD because of the low incidence of the disease, the differences in the racial and sex distributions, uncertainty about the incubation period, infrequency of cases of conjugal infection, and the occurrence of primary extragenital lesions.[44] The condition undoubtedly has several unusual epidemiologic features that warrant close scrutiny.

The majority of cases are in the 20- to 40-year age group, i.e., the most sexually active. Most case series have recorded a preponderance of males, although in some studies with limited numbers of cases, such as in Zambia,[43] western Australia,[45] and eastern Transvaal, South Africa,[46] more women than men have been reported. Rajam and Rangiah[1] recorded 1,350 men and 562 women in their large series, and similar male-to-female ratios have been reported in Zimbabwe[31] and southeast India.[47] Higher male-to-female ratios of more than 6:1 have been reported from Papua New Guinea[28] and India.[48] In Durban, HLA studies showed an association between donovanosis and HLA-B57 and a trend toward resistance to disease with HLA-A23.[49]

The incubation period is uncertain. Sehgal and Prasad[50] found the average incubation period to be 17 days, but a range of 1 to 360 days has been reported.[51] Experimental production of typical donovanosis lesions was induced in humans 50 days after inoculation.[11]

Among sexual partners of index cases, wide variations in the rates of infection have been reported. In Papua New Guinea[28] and the United States[52] the coinfection rate was 1 to 2 percent, whereas in India rates of up to 50 percent were reported among marital partners examined.[47,53] A more recent study of 255 cases in India in which eight couples were examined found conjugal involvement in one pair only.[54] In many cases the disease is mild, particularly in men,[1] and examination of all regular sexual partners is recommended.

Transmission via fecal contamination of abraded skin was suggested as a possible mode of transmission by Goldberg.[19] Although he isolated the causative organism from feces, there are no subsequent reports to support this hypothesis. Cases in children have been attributed to sitting on the laps of infected adults.[55] Disseminated donovanosis has been reported in a neonate born to a mother with a large granulomatous lesion of the vulva who incurred a third-degree tear during delivery.[56]

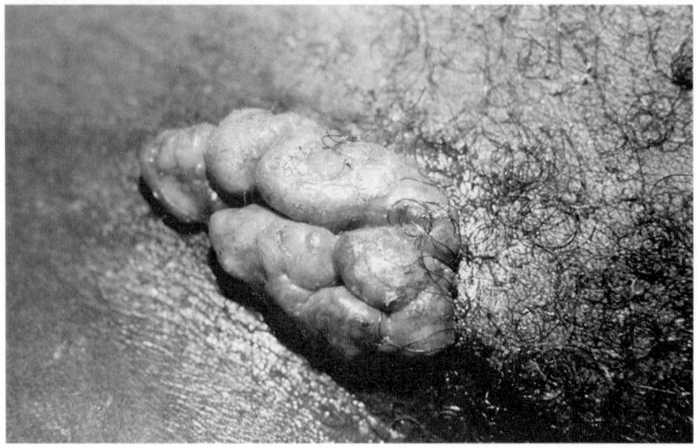

Fig. 39-2. Hypertrophic verruciform form of donovanosis in inguinal region.

CLINICAL MANIFESTATIONS

The first sign of infection is usually a firm papule or subcutaneous nodule that later ulcerates. Four types of donovanosis are described classically: (1) ulcerogranulomatous—the most common variant—nontender, fleshy, exuberant, single or multiple, beefy-red ulcers that bleed readily when touched (Fig. 39-1), (2) hypertrophic or verrucous type, an ulcer or growth with a raised, irregular edge, sometimes completely dry with a walnut like appearance (Fig. 39-2), (3) necrotic, usually a deep, foul-smelling ulcer causing tissue destruction (Fig. 39-3), and (4) sclerotic or cicatricial, characterized by extensive formation of fibrous and scar tissue.

The genitals are affected in 90 percent of cases and the inguinal region (Fig. 39-4) in 10 percent. The usual sites of infection are, in men, the prepuce, coronal sulcus (Fig. 39-5), frenum, and glans penis and, in women, the labia minora and fourchette (Fig. 39-6). A preponderance of cases has long been recognized in uncircumcised men.[57] Lesions of the cervix may mimic cervical carcinoma. Extragenital lesions occur in 6 percent of cases.[1,58] Sites of infection include the lip, gums, cheek, palate, pharynx, neck, nose, larynx, and chest. Extragenital lesions are usually associated with primary genital disease. On the rare occasions when primary extragenital lesions are diagnosed, the possibility of rhinoscleroma also should be considered.

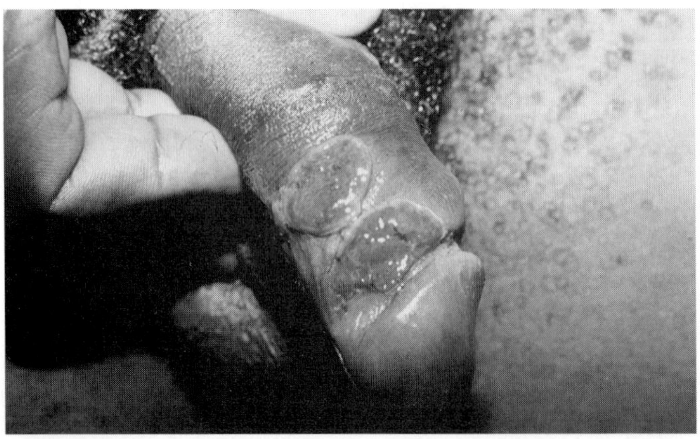

Fig. 39-1. Typical subpreputial ulcerogranulomatcus donovanosis lesions.

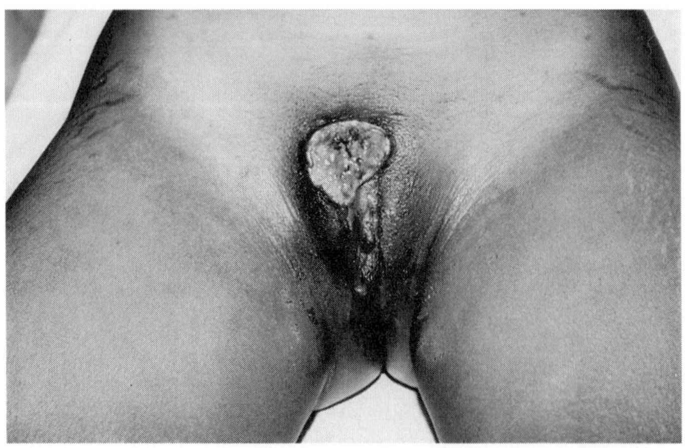

Fig. 39-3. Deep necrotic donovanosis ulcer causing tissue destruction.

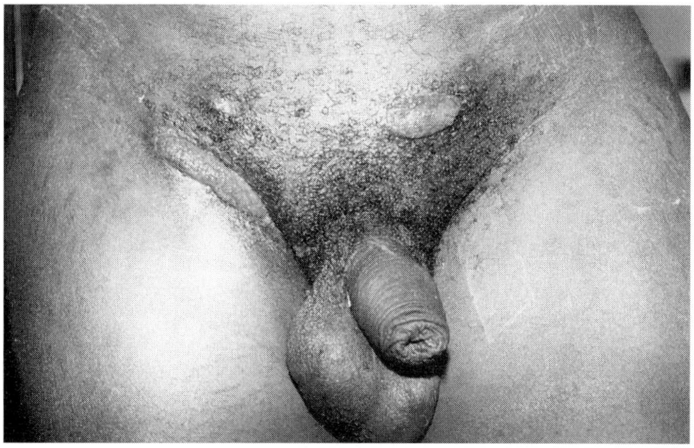

Fig. 39-4. Inguinal lesions of donovanosis.

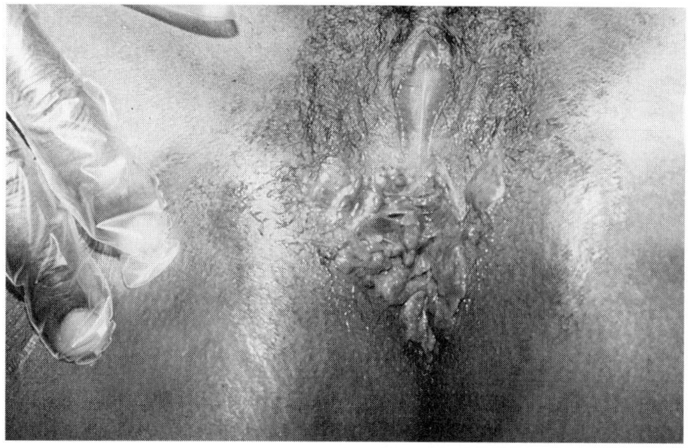

Fig. 39-6. Confluent donovanosis lesions at fourchette.

Lymphadenitis is an uncommon finding.[59] Disseminated donovanosis is rare; secondary spread to liver and bone may occur and is usually associated with pregnancy and cervical lesions. Donovanosis has a more aggressive course during pregnancy.[57,60,61] Polyarthritis and osteomyelitis are rare complications.[62]

DIAGNOSIS

Ulcerogranulomatous donovanosis lesions have a characteristic appearance and should be distinguished readily from the other classic STD causes of genital ulcer disease.[63] However, primary syphilitic chancres, secondary syphilis (condylomata lata), chancroid, and large herpetic ulcers can all be mistaken for donovanosis. Amebiasis and carcinoma of the penis also should be considered if tissue destruction or necrosis is present.

Tissue smears remain the mainstay method of diagnosis. Confirmatory specimens usually can be obtained as long as an adequate smear is prepared and antibiotic treatment has not been started. Most centers with experience with donovanosis have developed their own methods for maximizing the diagnostic yield from clinical specimens. Greenblatt and Barfield[64] advocated obtaining crush biopsy samples from the edges of lesions and stressed the importance of obtaining clean specimens for the preparation of tissue smears. Rajam and Rangiah[1] obtained material by means of a curette, forceps, the sharp end of a broken slide, or the edge of a safety razor blade and crushed the specimen between two slides and stained by the Leischmann or Giemsa methods. Rapid results have been achieved using material obtained with a chalazion spoon.[65] Other stains used include Delafield's hematoxylin and eosin,[22] Wright's,[66] and pinacyanole.[67] A 100 percent success rate was claimed using a slow-Giemsa (overnight) technique.[68] More recently, a modified Giemsa stain (RapiDiff) has yielded rapid results in a busy clinic environment[69] (Fig. 39-7). Donovan bodies also have been identified in Papanicolaou smears.[70]

Biopsy and histologic examination may be required for lesions that are small, dry, sclerotic, or necrotic. Giemsa or silver stains are the most effective methods for visualizing the organisms in tissue sections. The characteristic histologic picture shows chronic inflammation with infiltration of plasma cells and polymorphonuclear leukocytes[21]; the dermis shows a dense cellular infiltrate with large numbers of plasma or Pund cells. Ulceration and acanthosis with focal collections of polymorphonuclear leukocytes are found in the epidermis; elongation of rete ridges occurs in association with the hypertrophic variant.[23]

No serologic tests are currently in generalized use. Complement-fixation tests were developed and found to be quite sensitive.[15,16] An indirect immunofluorescent technique developed recently had a high sensitivity for established lesions but was not deemed suitable for early donovanosis ulcers. This test could be of use as an epidemiologic tool in population studies, however.[71]

Recently, the organism has been characterized further by the

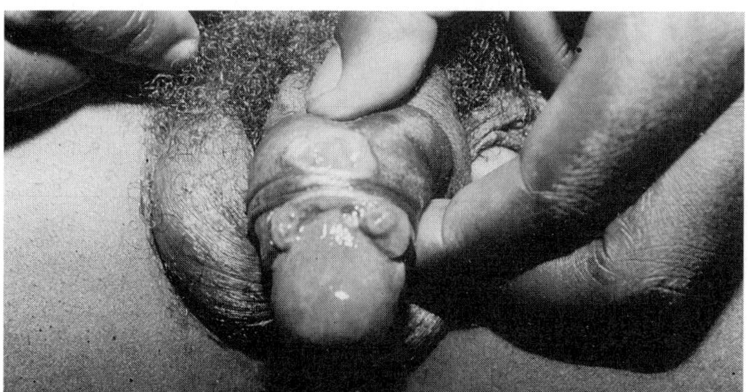

Fig. 39-5. Multiple ulcerogranulomatous penile lesions of donovanosis.

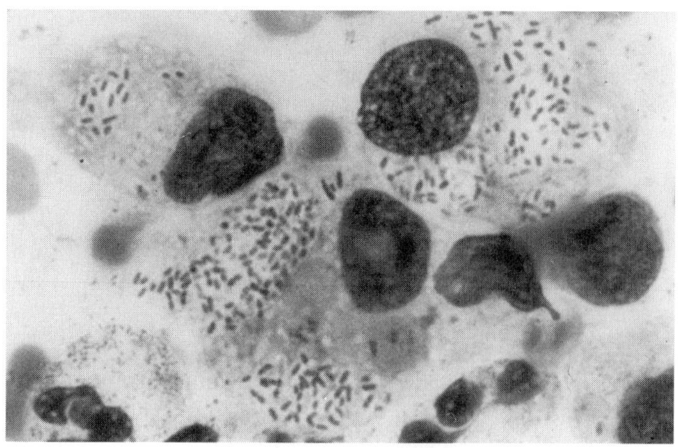

Fig. 39-7. Tissue smear stained by rapid Giemsa (RapiDiff) technique showing numerous Donovan bodies in monocytes.

development of molecular-based tests. A novel *Klebsiella*-like sequence amplified from DNA has been identified from genital donovanosis lesions using polymerase chain reaction (PCR) primers targeting the *phoE* gene; the sequence of PCR products was closely related to the *phoE* gene segments amplified from *K. pneumoniae*, *K. rhinoscleromatis,* and *K. ozaenae* cultures.[72] Other molecular work characterizing donovanosis using primers directed to the 16S rRNA gene has shown that amplified fragments restricted with EcoR1 and BamH1 produced three distinct bands; sequence analysis showed a homology of 90 percent for infected monocytes and biopsy specimens.[73] The development of a donovanosis-specific PCR undoubtedly would be an important step in further defining the taxonomy of the causative organism.

TREATMENT AND MANAGEMENT

Donovanosis is one of the few bacterial infections that could be treated in the preantibiotic era. Antimony compounds were used successfully for primary infections but had limited efficacy for recurrences or reinfections.

The first antibiotic shown to be effective for donovanosis was streptomycin in 1947.[74] Nowadays, various therapeutic treatments are used and probably reflect local availability of different drugs. Streptomycin has been used extensively in India and is effective for large lesions, although daily injections are required.[75] Chloramphenicol is used in Papua New Guinea,[76] cotrimoxazole in India[77] and South Africa,[78] and thiamphenicol in Brazil.[79] Healing is usually achieved with tetracycline, although resistance is reported.[80] Norfloxacin,[81] ciprofloxacin,[82] and high-dose ceftriaxone[83] are also effective. Erythromycin is recommended during pregnancy. Encouraging results have been shown with azithromycin; a course of 500 mg daily for 1 week cured extensive lesions involving the genitalia and groin in one man over a 5-month period.[84] Previously, most physicians have given long courses of antibiotics to patients with extensive lesions and advised that treatment be continued until healing was complete.[85] In view of the protracted course of the disease in many patients, azithromycin therapy is likely to be the most cost-effective way to manage extensive ulcers in the future.

COMPLICATIONS

Rajam and Rangiah[1] found carcinoma, either as a complication of or a sequel to long-standing donovanosis, to be a rare occurrence, seen in 0.25 percent of 2,000 cases. Positive reactivity with *D. granulomatis* antigens was found in 9 of 62 cases of carcinoma of the penis in Jamaica, but this work was not developed further.[86]

Nowadays the most frequent complication is pseudoelephantiasis (Fig. 39-8), which is more common in women and found in up to 5 percent of cases.[87] Surgical intervention may be indicated for advanced intractable lesions.[88] Stenosis of the urethra, vagina, or anus may occur in the sclerotic variant of donovanosis.[1]

The differential diagnosis between donovanosis and squamous cell carcinoma of the penis may be difficult. A therapeutic trial of antibiotic therapy always should be given, even if donovanosis is only a remote possibility.

Donovanosis ulcers may be coinfected with other sexually transmitted infections, particularly syphilis.[35,38] Such cases justify management by the syndromic approach with treatment for both conditions. However, it is important that these patients be followed, even when managed by primary health care workers, until complete healing is achieved. The presence of donovanosis ulcers does not preclude sexual intercourse,[89] and the risks of reinfection should be stressed at the initial consultation.

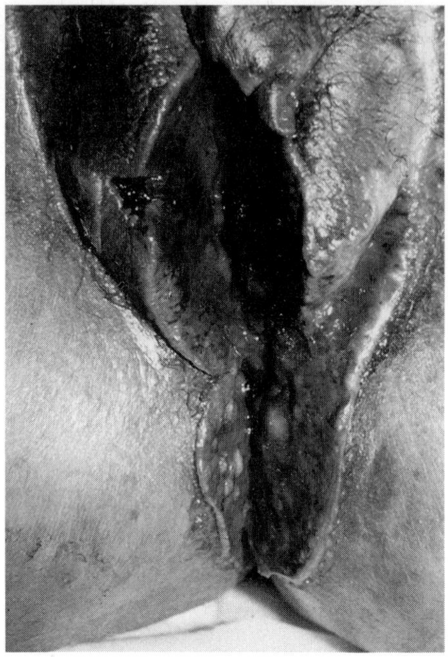

Fig. 39-8. Extensive vulval donovanosis with lymphedema and esthiomene.

DONOVANOSIS AND HIV INFECTION

The classic STDs, and genital ulcer diseases in particular, are significant risk factors for HIV in developing countries. In Durban, in a population where HIV infection had been introduced only recently, the proportion of men with donovanosis and HIV infection increased significantly as the duration of lesions increased, thereby suggesting that HIV was acquired via sexual intercourse in the presence of ulcers.[90]

The treatment of donovanosis may need to be modified in HIV-infected patients with significant immunosuppression. In India, HIV-positive patients with donovanosis had a high failure rate to first-line antibiotic therapy.[91] In Brazil, two AIDS patients with donovanosis failed to respond to conventional treatment with combinations of cotrimoxazole, tetracycline, and thiamphenicol.[92] Interestingly, two HIV-positive patients with oropharyngeal infections with *K. rhinoscleromatis*, an organism very similar to *C. granulomatis*, required prolonged courses of antibiotics before clinical cure.[93] However, among HIV-positive pregnant women without significant documented immunosuppression, the clinical presentation and response to treatment in donovanosis appeared to be unaltered by HIV.[94] Further clarification of the role of oral azithromycin in the management of donovanosis in HIV-positive patients is awaited.

PREVENTION AND CONTROL

Donovanosis is one of the most easily recognizable causes of genital ulcer disease clinically in endemic areas.[63] Because it is limited to a few specific geographic locations, global eradication is a realistic objective[95] that is justified if the high proportion of HIV transmissions attributable to genital ulcers is taken into consideration.[96] Such a program would need to appreciate the diverse nature of the communities affected and include careful appraisal of local customs and beliefs. Although communities in the donovanosis-endemic countries of Papua New Guinea, India, South Africa, Brazil, and Australia differ markedly, they all have similarities that may be relevant to donovanosis control: Most individuals with donovanosis in these communities are subject to social deprivation, low socioeconomic status, and poor standards of personal genital hygiene.

Commercial sex workers are one group that should be targeted. In India,[1] the United States,[27] and Papua New Guinea,[28] prostitutes have been identified as source contacts of index cases and usually have clinically detectable lesions. In Papua New Guinea, local sexual practices and beliefs may play a significant role in the spread of donovanosis: It is not unknown for many men to have sexual intercourse with a single woman during festival occasions[97]; furthermore, some men believe that impurities in their blood cause donovanosis ulcers and resort to self-mutilation in an attempt to "release" the cause of the problem.[98] It also should be noted that Papua New Guinea now has the highest reported per capita prevalence of HIV in the Pacific region.[99]

Since the overall prevalence of donovanosis in most endemic areas is low, mass surveys to identify cases or mass treatment campaigns are probably not justified. However, mass treatment of cases identified in house-to-house visits in Goilala, Papua New Guinea, was successful in controlling a localized epidemic in the 1950s.[55] This strategy merits further consideration as an HIV prevention measure in that country.

Poor understanding has in the past led patients with severe donovanosis to become shunned like lepers.[1] Many sufferers express profound feelings of shame, guilt, and embarrassment. Some have resorted to suicide. Greenblatt[26] has painted an emotive picture of the disease—"poorly understood and poorly handled, the disease becomes so loathsome that few clinics and fewer physicians are willing to treat those afflicted with it." Even now, extreme rejection is not unusual.[100]

In many developing countries, donovanosis patients are seen at STD clinics after attending primary health care centers where various treatment approaches have failed. Patients with donovanosis may need prolonged courses of antibiotics and require careful explanation and reassurance about a condition that they may have had for a long time. Where possible, this is probably best accomplished in STD clinics, where staff who have chosen to work with STD patients are well equipped to deal with such issues and can give patients individual attention with a sympathetic and nonjudgmental approach.[101] By contrast, patients with offensive genital ulcers seen in the primary health care setting are often perceived with disgust, disdain, or derision. Clearly, there is a need to educate health care workers about donovanosis in endemic areas and to raise community awareness of the importance of genital ulcer disease as a proven risk factor for HIV transmission.[102] Expanded access to drugs such as azithromycin would be a major step foward and contribute significantly to limiting compliance problems with therapies currently available.

References

1 Rajam RV, Rangiah PN: *Donovanosis (Granuloma Inguinale, Granuloma Venereum)*. Geneva, World Health Organization, WHO Monograph Series No 24, 1954, pp 1–72.

2 Marmell M, Santora E: Donovanosis: Granuloma inguinale. *Am J Syph* 34:83–90, 1950.

3 McLeod K: Precis of operations performed in the wards of the first surgeon, Medical College Hospital, during the year 1881. *Ind Med Gaz* 17:113–123, 1882.

4 Conyers JH, Daniels CW: The lupoid form of the so-called "groin ulceration" of this colony. *Br Guinea Med Annu* 8:13–29, 1896.

5 Galloway J: Ulcerating granuloma of the pudenda. *Br J Dermatol* 6: 133–150, 1897.

6 Donovan C: Medical cases from Madras General Hospital. *Ind Med Gaz* 40:411–414, 1905.

7 Aragao HD, Vianna G: Pesquizas sobre o granuloma venereo. *Mem Inst Oswaldo Cruz* 5:211–238,1913.

8 Cornwall LH, Peck SM: Etiology of granuloma inguinale. *Arch Dermatol Syph* 12:613–628, 1925.

9 McIntosh JA: The etiology of granuloma inguinale. *JAMA* 87:996–1002, 1926.

10 DeMonbreun WA, Goodpasture EW: Further studies on the etiology of granuloma inguinale. *Am J Trop Med* 13:447–468, 1933.

11 Greenblatt RB et al: Experimental and clinical granuloma inguinale. *JAMA* 113:1109–1116, 1939.

12 Dienst RB et al: Cultural studies on the "Donovan bodies" of granuloma inguinale. *J Infect Dis* 62:112–114, 1938.

13 Anderson K: The cultivation from granuloma inguinale of a microorganism having the characteristics of Donovan bodies in the yolk sac of chick embroyos. *Science* 97:560–561, 1943.

14 Anderson K et al: An etiologic consideration of *Donovania granulomatis* cultivated from granuloma inguinale (three cases) in embryonic yolk. *J Exp Med* 81:25–39, 1945.

15 Dunham W, Rake G: Cultural and serologic studies on granuloma inguinale. *Am J Syph* 32:145–149, 1948.

16 Anderson K et al: Immunologic relationship of *Donovania granulomatis* to granuloma inguinale. *J Exp Med* 81:41–50, 1945.

17 Rake G: The antigenic relationships of *Donovania granulomatis* (Anderson) and the significance of this organism in granuloma inguinale. *Am J Syph Gon Vener Dis* 32:150–158, 1948.

18 Goldberg J: Studies on granuloma inguinale: IV. Growth requirements of *Donovania granulomatis* and its relationship to the natural habitat of the organism. *Br J Vener Dis* 35:266–268, 1959.

19 Goldberg J: Studies on granuloma inguinale: V. Isolation of a bacterium resembling *Donovania granulomatis* from the faeces of a patient with granuloma inguinale. *Br J Vener Dis* 38:99–102, 1962.

20 Kharsany AB et al: Culture of *Calymmatobacterium granulomatis*. *Clin Infect Dis* 22:391, 1996.

21 Goldzieher M, Peck SM: Das venerische granulom. *Virchows Arch [A]* 259:795–814, 1926.

22 Pund ER, Greenblatt RB: Specific histology of granuloma inguinale. *Arch Pathol* 23:224–229, 1937.

23 Sehgal VN et al: The histopathology of donovanosis. *Br J Vener Dis* 60:45–48, 1984.

24 Kuberski T et al: Ultrastructure of *Calymmatobacterium granulomatis* in lesions of granuloma inguinale. *J Infect Dis* 142:744–749, 1980.

25 Chandra M et al: An ultrastructural study of donovanosis. *Ind J Med Res* 90:158–164, 1989.

26 Greenblatt RB: Socioeconomic aspects of granuloma inguinale. *J Vener Dis Inform* 28:181–183, 1947.

27 Rosen T et al: Granuloma inguinale. *J Am Acad Dermatol* 11:433–437, 1984.

28 Maddocks I et al: Donovanosis in Papua New Guinea. *Br J Vener Dis* 52:190–196, 1976.

29 O'Farrell N: Trends in reported cases of donovanosis in Durban, South Africa. *Genitourin Med* 68:366–369, 1992.

30 Wistrand R, Wegeroff F: Granuloma inguinale in the Eastern Transvaal. *S Afr Med J* 67:13–15, 1985.

31 Latif AS et al: The treatment of donovanosis (granuloma inguinale). *Sex Transm Dis* 15:27–29, 1988.

32 Jardim ML: Donovanose: Proposta de classificacao clinica. *An Bras Dermatol Sifilogr* 62:169–172, 1987.

33 Crenn Y et al: Les ulcerations genitales en Guyanne Francaise. *Med Trop* 48:15–18, 1988.

34 Mein J et al: Surveillance of donovanosis in the Northern Territory. *Venereology* 8:16–19, 1995.

35 Vacca A, MacMillan LL: Anogenital lesions in women in Papua New Guinea. *PNG Med J* 23:70–73, 1980.

36 Vogel LC, Richens J: Donovanosis in Dutch South New Guinea: History, evolution of the epidemic and control. *PNG Med J* 32:203–218, 1989.

37 O'Farrell N, Hoosen AA: Sexually transmitted diseases in South Africa: Epidemic donovanosis in Durban? *Genitourin Med* 73:76, 1997.

38 O'Farrell N et al: Genital ulcer disease in men in Durban, South Africa. *Genitourin Med* 67:327–330, 1991.
39 O'Farrell N et al: Genital ulcer disease in women in Durban, South Africa. *Genitourin Med* 67:322–326, 1991.
40 Veen J: Granuloma inguinale in Botswana. *Trop Geogr Med* 31:309–310, 1979.
41 Lala B et al: Efficacite d'un traitment univoque utilisant benzathine-penicilline et sulphamethoxazole-trimethoprime dans la cure des lesions ulceratives genitales en Centafique. *Med Afr Noire* 29:1–4, 1982.
42 Perret JL et al: Quel terrain pour la donovanose? *Med Trop* 51:359–361, 1991.
43 Bhagwandeen BS, Naik KG: Granuloma venereum (granuloma inguinale) in Zambia. *E Afr Med J* 54:637–642, 1977.
44 Goldberg J: Studies on granuloma inguinale: VII. Some epidemiological considerations of the disease. *Br J Vener Dis* 40:140–145, 1964.
45 Mitchell KM et al: Donovanosis in Western Australia. *Genitourin Med* 62:191–195, 1986.
46 Freinkel AL: Granuloma inguinale (donovanosis). *S Afr J STD* 4:43–47, 1984.
47 Lal S, Nicholas C: Epidemiological and clinical features in 165 cases of granuloma inguinale. *Br J Vener Dis* 46:461–463, 1970.
48 Sehgal VN, Jain MK: Pattern of epidemics of donovanosis in the "nonendemic" region. *Int J Dermatol* 27:396–399, 1988.
49 O'Farrell N, Hammond M: HLA antigens in donovanosis (granuloma inguinale). *Genitourin Med* 67:400–402, 1991.
50 Sehgal VN, Prasad AL: Donovanosis: Current concepts. *Int J Dermatol* 25:8–16, 1986.
51 Ramachander M et al: A study of donovanosis at Guntur. *Ind J Dermatol Venereol* 33:237–241, 1967.
52 Packer H, Goldberg J: Studies of the antigenic relationship of *D. granulomatis* in members of the tribe Escherichiae. *Am J Syph* 34:342–350, 1950.
53 Bedi BM et al: Clinico-epidemiological studies on 189 cases of donovanosis. *Ind J Dermatol Venereol* 41:1–3, 1975.
54 Sayal SK et al: A study of 255 cases of granuloma inguinale. *Ind J Dermatol* 32:91–97, 1987.
55 Zigas V: A donovanosis project in Goilala (1951–1954). *PNG Med J* 14:148–149, 1971.
56 Scott CW et al: Neonatal granuloma venereum. *Am J Dis Child* 85: 308–315, 1952.
57 Nair VG, Pandalai NG: Granuloma genitoinguinale. *Ind Med Gaz* 69:361–375, 1934.
58 Greenblatt RB et al: Extragenital granuloma inguinale. *Arch Dermatol Syph* 38:358–362, 1938.
59 Freinkel AL: Granuloma inguinale of cervical lymph nodes simulating tuberculous lymphadenitis: Two case reports and review of published reports. *Genitourin Med* 64:339–343, 1988.
60 Wilson LA: Pregnancy and labor complicated by granuloma inguinale. *JAMA* 95:1093–1095, 1930.
61 O'Farrell N: Donovanosis (granuloma inguinale) in pregnancy. *Int J STD AIDS* 2:447–448, 1991.
62 Lyford J et al: Polyarticular arthritis and osteomyelitis due to granuloma inguinale. *Am J Syph* 28:588–610, 1944.
63 O'Farrell N et al: Genital ulcer disease: Accuracy of clinical diagnosis and strategies to improve control in Durban, South Africa. *Genitourin Med* 70:7–11, 1994.
64 Greenblatt RB, Barfield WE: Newer methods in the diagnosis and treatment of granuloma inguinale. *Br J Vener Dis* 28:123–128, 1952.
65 Gollow M et al: Rapid diagnosis of granuloma inguinale. *Med J Aust* 144:502–503, 1986.
66 Cannefax GR: The technique of the tissue spread method for demonstrating Donovan bodies. *J Vener Dis Inform* 29:201 -204, 1948.
67 Greenblatt RB et al: A simple stain for Donovan bodies for the diagnosis of granuloma inguinale. *Am J Syph* 35:291–293, 1951.
68 Sehgal VN, Jain MK: Tissue section Donovan bodies: Identification through slow-Giemsa (overnight) technique. *Dermatologica* 174: 228–231, 1987.
69 O'Farrell N et al: A rapid staining technique for the diagnosis of granuloma inguinale (donovanosis). *Genitourin Med* 66:200–201, 1990.
70 de Boer AL et al: Cytologic identification of Donovan bodies in granuloma inguinale. *Acta Cytol* 28:126–128, 1984.
71 Freinkel AL et al: A serological test for granuloma inguinale. *Genitourin Med* 68:269–272, 1992.
72 Bastian I, Bowden FJ: Amplification of *Klebsiella*-like sequences from biopsy samples from patients with donovanosis. *Clin Infect Dis* 23: 1328–1330, 1996.
73 Kharsany AB et al: *Calymmatobacterium granulomatis:* In-Vitro Culture and Molecular Characterisation. Presented at the Fifth Joint Congress of the Sexually Transmitted Diseases and Infectious Diseases Societies of South Africa, Durban, South Africa, May 1995.
74 Barton RL et al: Granuloma inguinale treated with streptomycin. *Arch Dermatol Syph* 56:1–6, 1947.
75 Lal S: Continued efficacy of streptomycin in the treatment of granuloma inguinale. *Br J Vener Dis* 47:454–455, 1971.
76 Richens J: The diagnosis and treatment of donovanosis (granuloma inguinale). *Genitourin Med* 67:441–452, 1991.
77 Lal S, Garg BR: Further evidence of the efficacy of cotrimoxazole in granuloma venereum. *Br J Vener Dis* 56:412–413, 1980.
78 O'Farrell N: Clinicoepidemiological study of donovanosis in Durban, South Africa. *Genitourin Med* 69:108–111, 1993.
79 Jardim ML, Melo Z: Tratamento da donovaose com o tiafenicol. *An Bras Dermatol Sifilogr* 65:93–94, 1990.
80 Pariser RJ: Tetracycline-resistant granuloma inguinale. *Arch Dermatol* 113:988, 1977.
81 Ramanan C et al: Treatment of donovanosis with norfloxacin. *Int J Dermatol* 29:298–299, 1990.
82 Ahmed BA, Tang A: Successful treatment of donovanosis with ciprofloxacin. *Genitourin Med* 72:73–74, 1996.
83 Merianos A et al: Ceftriaxone in the treatment of chronic donovanosis in central Australia. *Genitourin Med* 70:84–89, 1994.
84 Bowden FJ et al: Pilot study of azithromycin in the treatment of genital donovanosis. *Genitourin Med* 72:17–19, 1995.
85 Hart G: Donovanosis in Australia. *Venereology* 8:15, 1995.
86 Goldberg J, Annamunthodo H: Studies on granuloma inguinale: VIII. Serological reactivity of sera from patients with carcinoma of penis when tested with *Donovania* antigens. *Br J Vener Dis* 42:205–209, 1966.
87 Sehgal VN et al: Pseudoelephantiasis induced by donovanosis. *Genitourin Med* 63:54–56, 1987.
88 Parkash S, Radhakrishna K: Problematic ulcerative lesions in sexually transmitted diseases: Surgical management. *Sex Transm Dis* 13:127–133, 1986.
89 O'Farrell N et al: Sexual behavior in Zulu men and women with genital ulcer disease. *Genitourin Med* 68:245–248, 1992.
90 O'Farrell N et al: Risk factors for HIV-1 in heterosexual attenders at a sexually transmitted diseases clinic in Durban. *S Afr Med J* 80:17–20, 1991.
91 Maniar JK, Desai V: Genital ulcer diseases and HIV status correlation in Bombay, India. Presented at the Eighth International Conference on AIDS, Abstract 3513, Amsterdam, 1992.
92 Jardim ML et al: Donovanose em pacientes portadores de AIDS: Relato de dois casos. *An Bras Dermatol Sifilogr* 65:175–177, 1990.
93 Paul C et al: Infection due to *Klebsiella rhinoscleromatis* in two patients infected with human immunodeficiency virus. *Clin Infect Dis* 16:441–442, 1993.
94 Hoosen AA et al: Granuloma inguinale in association with pregnancy and HIV infection. *Int J Gynaecol Obstet* 53:133–138, 1996.
95 O'Farrell N: Global eradication of donovanosis: An opportunity for limiting the spread of HIV-1 infection. *Genitourin Med* 71:27–31, 1995.
96 Hayes RJ et al: The cofactor effect of genital ulcers on the per-exposure risk of HIV transmission in sub-Saharan Africa. *J Trop Med Hyg* 98:1–8, 1995.
97 Jenkins C: Culture and sexuality: Papua New Guinea and the rest of the world. *Venereology* 6:55, 1993.

98 Jenkins C: Sex and society in Papua and New Guinea. Presented at the Ninth International Conference on AIDS, Abstract WS-D25–4, Berlin, 1993.

99 Purvis A: The global epidemic. *Time,* December 30, 1996–Jan 7 1997, pp 46–48.

100 Mein J et al: Donovanosis: sequelae of severe disease and successful azithromycin treatment. *Int J STD AIDS* 7:448–451, 1996.

101 O'Farrell N: Factors Contributing to the Rapid Increase in Heterosexual Transmission of HIV in Durban, South Africa: Donovanosis and Other Genital Ulcerative and Sexually Transmitted Diseases. M.D. thesis, University of Birmingham, England, 1995.

102 Dickerson MC et al: The causal role for genital ulcer disease as a risk factor for transmission of human immunodefiency virus. *Sex Transm Dis* 23:429–441, 1996.

Chapter 40

Genital mycoplasmas

David Taylor-Robinson
Jonathan G. Ainsworth
William M. McCormack

Organisms in the class Mollicutes ("soft skin") have devolved from ancestral anaerobic bacteria (clostridia) by gene deletion. Of the eight genera within the class, five, namely *Mycoplasma, Ureaplasma, Acholeplasma, Anaeroplasma,* and *Asteroleplasma,* comprise more than 120 species. Of these species, most belong to the genus *Mycoplasma.* The term "mollicutes" is sometimes used trivially to describe any of the organisms in the class, irrespective of genus or species, as is the term "mycoplasmas," which is used in this chapter. However, the term "ureaplasmas" is often used to refer to organisms within the genus *Ureaplasma.* Of the 16 mycoplasmas that have been detected in the human species, six appear to have the genitourinary tract as their primary site of colonization, as shown in Table 40-1. Because of orogenital contact, some of these are found occasionally in the oropharynx and, conversely, some of those mycoplasmas that have the oropharynx as their primary site of colonization are found in the genital tract.

Mycoplasma hominis and *Ureaplasma urealyticum* organisms (called originally T strains or T mycoplasmas and, trivially, ureaplasmas) are those isolated most frequently from the human genitourinary tract. Of species detected more recently, *Mycoplasma genitalium* requires polymerase chain reaction (PCR) technology for sensitive detection and has been found in men with nongonococcal urethritis. The current concepts of the role of these mycoplasmas, and others where appropriate, in human disease, particularly genital-tract disease, are the subject of this chapter. In addition, data concerning the possible role of mycoplasmas in AIDS are assessed. For further considerations of the biology and immunology of mycoplasmas, the reader is referred to several other reviews.[1–9]

EPIDEMIOLOGY

COLONIZATION OF INFANTS AND CHILDREN

Infants become colonized with genital mycoplasmas during passage through the birth canal; infants who are delivered by cesarean section are colonized less often than those delivered vaginally.[10–11] Ureaplasmas have been isolated from the genitalia of up to one-third of infant girls, and *M. hominis* from a smaller proportion.[10,12,13] These genital mycoplasmas are isolated even less frequently from the genitourinary tract of infant boys.[13] Mycoplasmas, mainly ureaplasmas, have also been isolated from the nose and throat of infants of both sexes.[10] Infant colonization figures vary from one population and from one study to another, depending upon the proportion of pregnant women who are colonized.

Neonatal colonization tends not to persist, particularly in boys, the proportion of infants who are colonized decreasing quite rapidly as they get older. Thus, genital mycoplasmas are seldom recovered from urine or genital-tract specimens from prepubertal boys, but 5 to 22 percent of prepubertal girls have been found to be colonized with ureaplasmas and 8 to 17 percent with *M. hominis.*[14–18] In sexually abused children, figures of as much as 48 and 34 percent, respectively, have been recorded.[18,19]

COLONIZATION OF ADULTS

After puberty, colonization occurs primarily as a result of sexual contact.[16,20–23] Sexually mature individuals without a history of sexual contact are colonized infrequently with genital mycoplasmas. Colonization increases in relation to the number of different sexual partners and the proportion of women colonized is greater than the proportion of men, which suggests that women are more susceptible to colonization with these organisms. In addition, the proportion of both men and women colonized with ureaplasmas is greater than the proportion colonized with *M. hominis.*

Genital mycoplasmas have been isolated more often from black than from white men and from black than from white women.[12,22,24–28] The latter was the case in a study that was carefully controlled for sexual experience.[29] Socioeconomic factors may be associated with the racial differences noted in colonization rates and in one study would seemed to have influenced the rates,[27] but the fundamental reason for the differences is unknown.

It is clear that some genital mycoplasmas can be isolated with considerable frequency from the genitourinary tract of men and women. It is against this background that studies of the role of these microorganisms in human disease must be viewed.

CLINICAL MANIFESTATIONS AND SEQUELAE

ROLE OF GENITAL MYCOPLASMAS IN DISEASES OF THE GENITOURINARY TRACT OF MEN

Nongonococcal urethritis

It is well established that *Chlamydia trachomatis* causes up to 50 percent of cases of nongonococcal urethritis, although sometimes less.[30] In assessing the role of mycoplasmas there are two prerequisites. First, *C. trachomatis* must be sought; second, the groups of men must be of comparable sexual experience because sexual experience is a major determinant of colonization.[20] Mycoplasmas were first associated with nongonococcal urethritis more than 40 years ago, but their role in this condition has been contentious. The results of studies based on cultural isolation do not indicate that *M. hominis* is likely to be a cause of nongonococcal urethritis.[2,31] The clinical response to various antimicrobial agents has also not supported the association of this mycoplasma with nongonococcal urethritis.[2,32,33]

In the case of ureaplasmas, in six studies[31,34–38] these organisms have been isolated significantly more often from patients with chlamydia-negative, nongonococcal urethritis than from patients who were chlamydia-positive or from control groups of men, or from both. In contrast, other workers have not found this to be the case.[39–41] If ureaplasmas are involved in the pathogenic process, it would be reasonable to find them in larger numbers than if they had only a commensal role and several investigators have reported quantitative data to support this hypothesis.[31,34,37,38] Persistent large numbers of ureaplasmas were noted in the urethra of a hypogammaglobulinemic man with recurrent urethritis.[42] Repeated antibiotic treatments correlated with symptomatic and microbiological cure.

An approach to understanding the role of ureaplasmas in nongonococcal urethritis is to treat patients with antibiotics that differentiate between these organisms and *C. trachomatis.* In one study, men were treated with aminocyclitols, which are active against ureaplasmas but not against chlamydiae, or with sulfisoxazole, which is active against chlamydiae but not against

Table 40–1 Primary Sites of Colonization, and Metabolism, of Mycoplasmas of Human Origin

Species	First Report of Isolation	Primary Site of Colonization		Metabolism of Glucose	Metabolism of Arginine
		Oropharynx	Urogenital Tract		
M. hominis	1937	No	Yes	−	+
M. fermentans	1952	Yes (?)	No (?)	+	+
M. salivarium	1953	Yes	No	−	+
*U. urealyticum**	1954	No	Yes	−	−
M. primatum	1955	No (?)	Yes	−	+
M. pneumoniae	1962	Yes	No	+	−
A. laidlawii	1964	Yes	No	+	−
M. orale	1964	Yes	No	−	+
M. buccale	1965	Yes	No	−	+
M. pirum	1968	?	?	+	+
M. faucium	1969	Yes	No	−	+
M. lipophilum	1974	Yes	No	−	+
M. genitalium	1981	No	Yes	+	−
A. oculi	1987	?	?	+	−
M. spermatophilum	1991	No	Yes	−	+
M. penetrans	1991	No	Yes	+	+

*Metabolizes urea.

ureaplasmas.[43] The clinical results suggested that both chlamydiae and ureaplasmas could cause urethritis. In another study, men who had nongonococcal urethritis were treated with rifampicin, which is active against chlamydiae but not against ureaplasmas.[33] The proportion of patients cured clinically was much smaller than that of another group who were given minocycline that is active against both kinds of microorganism. Of course, the extent to which the existence of *M. genitalium* in some of the patients in these studies, not appreciated at the time they were undertaken, may have affected the results and jeopardized the conclusions is unknown.

Serologic studies of the role of ureaplasmas in nongonococcal urethritis have been disappointing. The most informative study was one in which an enzyme immunoassay was used.[44] An ureaplasmal antibody response was demonstrated in 12 (67%) of 18 patients with nongonococcal urethritis. Ten (83%) of 12 had IgM antibody increases consistent with acute infection. On the other hand, of 40 ureaplasma-negative subjects, only four (10%) and three (7.5%) were IgG and IgM seropositive, respectively.

Perhaps the most convincing evidence linking ureaplasmas to nongonococcal urethritis comes from studies in which investigators inoculated themselves intraurethrally with ureaplasmal strains that had been isolated from patients who had nongonococcal urethritis. In a study in the United Kingdom, both subjects developed urethritis and a transient metabolism-inhibition antibody response.[45] In addition, ureaplasmas have been shown to cause urethritis in volunteer experiments in Germany and, more recently, in Japan.[30] In the latter study, the investigator subjected himself to four separate inoculations. The first resulted in colonization and a marked inflammatory response. The latter diminished with successive inoculations, so that by the fourth there was colonization but little inflammation. These observations are an indication of how ureaplasmas might be pathogenic yet be found in men who do not have urethritis.

Serovar 4 of *U. urealyticum* was associated with nongonococcal urethritis in one epidemiological study,[46] but, overall, the data reported so far do not suggest that specific serovars are regularly associated with specific clinical syndromes. Evaluation of the two biovars of *U. urealyticum* in nongonococcal urethritis might be revealing.

In summary, the data are supportive of ureaplasmas causing a few cases of nongonococcal urethritis, although it is unclear what proportion of the cases from which they can be recovered is actually due to ureaplasmas. The recovery of ureaplasmas from the urethra of a man who has nongonococcal urethritis does not necessarily mean that they are the cause of his disease.

M. genitalium was isolated originally from the urethras of two of 13 men with nongonococcal urethritis and subsequently its inoculation intraurethrally into male chimpanzees resulted in the development of urethritis in most of them, together with a late antibody response.[1,47,48] This suggests that late responses in humans could easily be missed unless widely separated paired sera are tested. Further attempts to repeat the original successful isolation by the use of culture failed. Several investigators tried to develop DNA probes, but this approach was superseded by the superior sensitivity of the PCR assay.[49,50] The availability of this assay provided the opportunity to evaluate or reevaluate the status of *M. genitalium* with respect to various clinical conditions, including nongonococcal urethritis. In several studies this mycoplasma has been detected more frequently, often significantly, in the urethra of men with nongonococcal urethritis than in men without this condition, the organisms being present often independently of *C. trachomatis*.[41,47,51–58] Furthermore, antibodies to *M. genitalium* have been detected by an enzyme immunoassay more often in the sera of men who are positive by PCR for *M. genitalium* than in the sera of those who are PCR negative (D. Taylor-Robinson and S.C. Lo, unpublished observation). Recently, strains of *M. genitalium* from men with nongonococcal urethritis have been isolated in mycoplasmal medium by using cell cultures as an intermediate.[59] In contrast to ureaplasmas, this mycoplasma appears to be quite strongly associated with acute nongonococcal urethritis. It has also been detected in the urethra of 12 to 20 percent of men with persistent or recurrent disease following an acute attack.[30,53] In one study (P Horner et al., unpublished data) men were followed up for 3 months and the detection of *M. genitalium* during this period was associated with chronic nongonococcal urethritis. Indeed, any person who was *M. genitalium*-positive during follow-up had chronic nongonococcal urethritis.

Prostatitis

Mårdh and Colleen recovered *M. hominis* from 10 percent of 79 patients with chronic prostatitis and from none of 20 normal age-matched controls.[60] Likewise, Peeters and associates isolated this mycoplasma from 10 (12%) of 85 men who had prostatitis of unknown origin and from two (4%) of 51 healthy men ($p = 0.26$).[61] Ureaplasmas were isolated from 40 (47%) of the patients and from 13 (26%) of the healthy men ($p = 0.02$). Hofstetter et al. studied men with what was described as urethroprostatitis.[62] Mycoplasmas, mainly ureaplasmas, were also isolated significantly more often and in greater numbers from patients with disease than from normal men who served as controls. Later, Brunner and colleagues associated ureaplasmas with prostatitis in 82 (13%) of 597 patients who had the disease, and Weidner and coworkers implicated these organisms in 46 (11%) of 412 men who had urethroprostatitis.[63,64] In contrast to these studies in which isolation has been successful, it is of interest that this has not been so in all. Thus, Meares, and Vinje et al. failed to recover ureaplasmas from men with chronic nonbacterial prostatitis.[65,66] Furthermore, two important issues are raised by these various studies. First, the accuracy of the diagnosis. It appears that chronic prostatitis has not always been truly chronic but sometimes "acute on chronic" or "acute urethritis on chronic prostatitis." Second, whether the organisms that have been detected have been derived entirely from the prostate or are "contaminants" that have come partly, or totally, from the urethra is unclear. With these aspects in mind, biopsies taken under transrectal ultrasound control from the prostates of 50 men with chronic prostatitis, defined by the Stamey technique, were found to contain chronic inflammatory cells but no microorganisms.[67] Most recently, *M. genitalium* was found by the use of PCR technology in 4 percent of prostatic biopsies from men with chronic idiopathic prostatitis.[68] It seems that a role for the genital mycoplasmas in the truly chronic condition can be no more than minimal.

Epididymitis

Most cases of epididymitis in heterosexual men less than 35 years of age are due to *N. gonorrhoeae* or *C. trachomatis*, whereas in older men and homosexuals, Gram-negative bacilli are usually responsible.[69–71] The recovery of *M. hominis* from an epididymal aspirate has been recorded once.[72] Furthermore, although ureaplasmas may be recovered from urethral specimens from some men who have epididymitis, recovery from percutaneous aspirates of the inflamed epididymis has also been recorded only once, in this instance in association with a greater than fourfold serologic antibody response.[73,74] The role of genital mycoplasmas seems to be meagre, but obviously they should not be discounted completely as a cause. Whether *M. genitalium* might be involved has not been determined.

Reiter's disease

Sexually acquired reactive arthritis (SARA) and the less common Reiter's disease, in which conjunctivitis also develops, occurs in men who have or have recently had nongonococcal urethritis, and less often in women. The disease is seen most often in those who are genetically predisposed, that is, who have the HLA-B27 histocompatibility antigen. When exposed to infectious and, possibly, other stimuli, these individuals develop the disease. There is considerable evidence that *C. trachomatis* is capable of initiating this pathophysiologic process, based principally on the detection of chlamydial elementary bodies and chlamydial DNA in joint material from some patients with SARA.[75,76] HLA-B27-positive men who have chlamydia-negative, nongonococcal urethritis are just as likely to develop arthritis as men who are chlamydia-positive.[77] This suggests that agents associated with nongonococcal urethritis other than *C. trachomatis* may play a role in SARA and Reiter's disease, but the role, if any, of *M. hominis*, ureaplasmas or *M. genitalium* in SARA or Reiter's disease is unclear. Serologic studies have been of limited utility,[2,78] and evidence for the involvement of ureaplasmas, not entirely convincing, is based on a specific response of synovial mononuclear cells to ureaplasmal antigens.[79,80] Attempts to isolate mycoplasmas from diseased joints have not been fruitful. *M. genitalium* has been detected in the joint of a patient with SARA by means of a PCR assay[81] and the results of seeking ureaplasmas by such technology are awaited.

ROLE OF GENITAL MYCOPLASMAS IN DISEASES OF THE GENITAL TRACT OF WOMEN

Bartholin's gland abscess

Genital mycoplasmas have been isolated from Bartholin's gland abscesses, but often they had ruptured or been opened surgically before specimen collection, so that it is not clear to what extent the results represent "contamination" of the abscesses by mycoplasmas present in the vagina.[2] This problem was overcome by Lee et al. who obtained percutaneous aspirates from 34 intact Bartholin's gland abscesses.[82] Eight abscesses contained Gram-negative bacilli and four contained *N. gonorrhoeae*. Twelve abscesses contained one or more vaginal microorganisms, including anaerobes and facultative organisms. Although genital mycoplasmas were isolated from vaginal specimens from most of the patients, *M. hominis* was isolated from only one, together with other vaginal organisms, and ureaplasmas from none of the aspirates. Thus, it would appear that genital mycoplasmas are not an important cause of Bartholin's gland abscesses. Whether they might have any role in less severe disease (Bartholinitis) has not been determined.

Bacterial vaginosis

Vaginal specimens from women who have bacterial vaginosis are positive for *M. hominis* more often, and contain larger numbers of the organisms, than specimens from women who do not have vaginosis.[23,83,84] Although mycoplasmas are resistant in vitro to metronidazole, this drug is often effective in treating bacterial vaginosis and at the same time eliminating *M. hominis* from many of the subjects.[85] This suggests that *M. hominis* proliferates in the milieu created by the other microorganisms and when the latter are eliminated, so too is *M. hominis*. Thus, although *M. hominis* could conceivably play a role in bacterial vaginosis as a primary pathogen, it is more likely to behave symbiotically with the other bacteria that are an integral part of this condition. The role played by ureaplasmas in bacterial vaginosis is even less well-defined. They have been associated with the condition less consistently than *M. hominis*, but they do occur a little more frequently and in larger numbers in women with bacterial vaginosis than they do in those without the disease.[84,86]

Preliminary evidence (Keane et al., unpublished data) suggests that *M. genitalium*, unlike *M. hominis*, behaves independently of bacterial vaginosis and has no role in the condition.

Pelvic inflammatory disease

Pelvic inflammatory disease is an ascending infection in which organisms present in the vagina and cervix invade the endometrium, fallopian tubes, and surrounding structures. *C. trachomatis* and *N. gonorrhoeae* are the organisms that are isolated most frequently from patients with pelvic inflammatory disease.[87–91] A mixture of aerobic and anaerobic bacteria has been implicated as a cause of this condition by some investigators.[92–95] It is against this background that the role of the genital mycoplasmas is considered.

In several studies, *M. hominis* was recovered more frequently from vaginal and cervical specimens taken from women who had pelvic inflammatory disease than from normal women.[88,92,95,96] However, *M. hominis* is often recovered from the lower genital tract of women who have bacterial vaginosis (see the preceding) and, as the aforementioned studies linking *M. hominis* to pelvic inflammatory disease did not include an assessment of bacterial vaginosis, the data are difficult to interpret. In any case, relating the microbial flora of the lower tract to changes in the upper tract is difficult and studies based on laparoscopy are much more relevant. In this regard, the study that first drew attention more than any other to the possibility that genital mycoplasmas might have a role in pelvic inflammatory disease was conducted by Mårdh and Westrom.[97] *M. hominis* was isolated from the tubes of four (8%) of 50 women with salpingitis, but not from those of women without salpingitis. More recently, in a study in which laparoscopy and endometrial biopsy were undertaken on 36 women with suspected pelvic inflammatory disease, *C. trachomatis* or *N. gonorrhoeae* was identified in 11 of 14 women with both salpingitis and endometritis, in two of nine with salpingitis or endometritis, and in none of 13 patients who had neither condition ($p < 0.0001$), but *M. hominis* organisms were not isolated from any of the patients.[90] On the other hand, in another laparoscopy study, *M. hominis* was isolated directly from the fallopian tubes of 11 percent of women with salpingitis but from only 3 percent of those without disease (Stacey, Munday, and Taylor-Robinson, unpublished data). However, the fact that it is rare to dissociate *M. hominis* from BV in the lower genital tract is a cautionary reminder to those who are ready to accept this mycoplasma in its own right as an unequivocal cause of pelvic inflammatory disease.

In several studies, antibody to *M. hominis* and fourfold rises in the titer of antibody to *M. hominis* were found more often among women who had pelvic inflammatory disease than among controls.[92,95,98] In several such studies the antibody titer rises were associated with the isolation of *M. hominis* from the lower genital tract or from the inflamed fallopian tubes.[99–101] In one study, an increased level of IgM antibody was found in 34 percent of patients with acute salpingitis and was associated with the isolation of *M. hominis* and with the presence of indirect hemagglutinating antibody to the mycoplasma.[102] The fact that there were high coinfection rates with other microorganisms[103] has led to the suggestion that epithelial damage caused by them allows contact between *M. hominis* and the immune system and thus an antibody elevation.[104] Damage to fallopian tube epithelium has also been studied in organ cultures. *N. gonorrhoeae* produced profound damage to the epithelium.[105] In contrast, *M. hominis* multiplied and persisted but did not cause damage.[106] However, scanning electron microscope examination showed that the organisms induced pathologic changes in the form of ciliary swelling.[107] This may be due to the effect of ammonia produced by mycoplasmal metabolism. Studies in intact animals may be more relevant than studies in organ cultures. Female grivet monkeys infected with *M. hominis* developed a self-limited acute salpingitis and parametritis.[108] Further studies in grivet monkeys have shown that ascending *M. hominis* infection of the genital tract must be preceded by mechanical injury to the epithelial barrier and that subsequent spread occurs via blood and lymph vessels rather than by the canalicular route.[109]

Ureaplasmas have been studied less extensively but they have been isolated directly from the fallopian tubes of patients with pelvic inflammatory disease, as well as from pelvic fluid obtained by culdocentesis from such patients.[87,97,110–112] However, their occurrence at both sites is rare and is usually in association with other known pathogens. In addition, the fact that most serological tests and inoculation studies in subhuman primates and in fallopian tube organ cultures have proved negative does not support a causal role for ureaplasmas.[106,113]

M. genitalium has been implicated in pelvic inflammatory disease. Twelve (39%) of 31 women with pelvic inflammatory disease who had not been infected with *N. gonorrhoeae* and had no antibody to *C. trachomatis* or *M. hominis* had a fourfold or greater rise in the titer of antibody to *M. genitalium* as measured by microimmunofluorescence.[114] However, some investigators have not found this to be the case.[115] Others have shown that approximately one-quarter of infertile women have antibody to *M. genitalium,* although there is no correlation with abnormal hysterosalpingograms as there is when antibody to *C. trachomatis* is associated with infertility.[116] *M. genitalium* adheres to human fallopian tube epithelial cells in culture[117] and has also been shown to cause lower genital tract inflammation as well as salpingitis in marmosets, grivet monkeys and baboons;[118] this finding suggests that the organism might do likewise in women.

In summary, there is some evidence to suggest that *M. hominis* may be a cause of pelvic inflammatory disease, but very little evidence that ureaplasmas have a similar role. The possibility that *M. hominis* plays a role only within the context of bacterial vaginosis needs to be addressed. *M. genitalium* is not involved in bacterial vaginosis and there is preliminary evidence to indicate that it could be an aetiological agent of pelvic inflammatory disease.

Postpartum and postabortal fever

Endometritis is the most common cause of postpartum fever, whether in the first 24 to 48 hours, or later. It occurs more often after cesarean section than after vaginal delivery, infections developing after vaginal delivery also tending to be less severe and often remitting spontaneously.

A relation between genital mycoplasmas and fever is least likely to be determined if it is based on vaginal colonization, unless the number of subjects studied is very large. In a study of over 300 women who were delivered consecutively at Boston City Hospital, no association was seen between *M. hominis* and postpartum fever.[119] However, Harrison et al. evaluated 1365 pregnant women and reported that *M. hominis* organisms, but not ureaplasmas, were associated with fever and/or endometritis after vaginal delivery (relative risk 7.3).[120] Furthermore, Berman et al. studied more than 1200 Navajo women and found that those undergoing cesarean section had a higher rate of postpartum endometritis if *M. hominis* was present on predelivery endocervical culture.[121] The association between vaginal colonization and postpartum fever is likely to be seen best when there is prolonged labor and prolonged rupture of the membranes.[122]

Employing protected transcervical catheters, Eschenbach et al. found that *Gardnerella vaginalis* was the most common endometrial isolate in early febrile postpartum women, but that nearly 20 percent had ureaplasmas as a sole isolate.[123] From three of 18 such patients, ureaplasmas were also isolated from the blood. Jones and Tobin avoided the vagina and cervix by examining the amniotic surface of placentas obtained at cesarean section; they found that patients whose placental cultures proved positive for *M. hominis* or ureaplasmas were more likely to be febrile after delivery than those who had negative cultures.[124] Williams and associates also avoided the vagina and cervix by taking intraoperative transabdominal specimens from 77 women undergoing cesarean sections.[125] Ureaplasmas were isolated from the lower uterine-segment of 6 (42%) of 15 women with endometritis compared to 4 (10%) of 40 uninfected controls. *M. hominis* was not isolated. There was a high degree of coisolation of virulent bacteria with the ureaplasmas, suggesting that the latter might play a symbiotic role in the pathogenesis of endometritis following cesarean section or could possibly just be a marker of the disease.

Seeking genital mycoplasmas in the blood is perhaps the best way of establishing a relationship between the organisms and fever. Genital mycoplasmas as well as other vaginal microorganisms can be found transiently in the bloodstream following vaginal delivery, but this transient invasion has not been associated with postpartum fever.[126] As detailed elsewhere, there have been many reports describing individual patients with postpartum fever, from the blood of whom *M. hominis* was isolated a day or more after delivery.[2,127] An antibody response was seen in nearly all cases.[119,128] In one study, *M. hominis* was isolated from the blood of nine of 125 febrile postpartum women, compared to none of 60 afebrile postpartum subjects ($p < 0.005$).[129] Very rarely, *M. hominis* spreads, even in an immunocompetent postpartum woman, to an extragenital site such as the brain and causes a major problem.[130] In addition, the association of *M. hominis* with febrile abortions is undoubted. Thus, in one study *M. hominis* was isolated from the blood of four of 51 women who had febrile abortions but from none of 53 women who had afebrile abortions. Antibody responses to *M. hominis* were detected in 50 percent of the women who had febrile abortions but in only two (14%) of 14 women who had afebrile abortions.

The role of *M. genitalium,* if any, in postpartum and postabortal fever has not been assessed.

In summary, it seems that *M. hominis* organisms are capable of causing postpartum and postabortal fever, and there is some but less evidence for ureaplasmas causing postpartum fever. This assumes that these organisms have been recovered from the blood and other sites in pure culture, at least in a proportion of cases. Otherwise, it is possible that genital mycoplasmas, particularly *M. hominis,* might be no more than a marker for bacterial vaginosis and not have a role in their own right.

ROLE OF GENITAL MYCOPLASMAS IN DISORDERS OF THE URINARY TRACT

Urinary calculi

When ureaplasmas were inoculated directly into the bladder or renal pelvis of rats, magnesium ammonium phosphate (struvite) calculi developed in the bladders of male, but not female, animals.[132] Since treating the animals with an inhibitor of urease (flurofamide) prevented stone formation, the production of calculi was presumably related to the urease activity of the ureaplasmas.[133] By virtue of such activity, ureaplasmas have also been shown to induce crystallization of struvite and calcium phosphates in urine in vitro.[134] Furthermore, ureaplasmas have been found more frequently in the urine and in the stones of patients with infection stones than they have in such specimens from patients with metabolic stones.[134] Although these findings suggest that ureaplasmas may have a role in the development of infection stones, they are likely to be implicated less often than other urease-positive bacteria.

Pyelonephritis and urinary tract infection

M. hominis does not appear to play a role in acute cystitis, similar isolation rates having been recorded for symptomatic women and controls, and the organism was not found in suprapubic aspirates.[135,136] However, ureaplasmas were cultured from four of 15 suprapubic aspirates taken from women with an acute urethral syndrome of unclear etiology.[137] In another study, ureaplasmas were recovered from suprapubic aspirates of urine from one-fifth of patients with urinary tract infections; in one-third they were the sole isolate.[138] However, there is as yet insufficient evidence to incriminate ureaplasmas as a cause of lower urinary tract infection in women.

Thomsen isolated *M. hominis* from the upper urinary tract of three women and ureaplasmas from the renal pelvis of two women who were in a group of 40 patients with chronic pyelonephritis.[139] In contrast, *M. hominis* was not isolated from the upper urinary tract of 40 patients with noninfectious urinary tract diseases. Only one of the three patients who harbored *M. hominis* had associated bacteriuria, but all three patients had an acute exacerbation of pyelonephritis; two of them developed antibody to *M. hominis*. In another study, *M. hominis* was isolated from the upper urinary tract of seven of 80 patients with acute pyelonephritis, in pure culture from four of them.[140] Antibodies to *M. hominis,* measured by indirect hemagglutination, were found in serum and in urine from some of these patients.[141] Ureaplasmas were isolated from the upper urinary tract of five patients, but the isolation rate was not statistically different from that for the control group.[140] In dogs, ureaplasmas have multiplied and survived for at least three weeks after being introduced into experimentally obstructed upper urinary tracts, causing severe interstitial nephritis accompanied by an antibody response.[142] However, there is no evidence that ureaplasmas cause this disease in humans and there is insufficient evidence to indicate that they cause acute pyelonephritis. In contrast, *M. hominis* appears to cause a small proportion of cases.

ROLE OF GENITAL MYCOPLASMAS IN DISORDERS OF REPRODUCTION

Involuntary infertility

A variety of mechanisms whereby mycoplasmas could conceivably reduce fertility in men and women has been proposed at one time or another, and they have been reviewed in detail elsewhere.[143] Ureaplasmas have been reported to decrease sperm motility and number and have been associated with an abnormal appearance of spermatozoa.[144–149] Elimination of ureaplasmas has been correlated with improvement in sperm motility, quantity, and appearance.[150–152] However, considering ureaplasmas alone has been a drawback in many studies since it may be that the elimination of other bacteria is the real reason for the beneficial effect. Furthermore, it should be noted that of 33 men who had ureaplasmas in semen, none had ureaplasmas isolated from the vas deferens, supporting the concept that sperm have first contact with ureaplasmas at the time of ejaculation.[153] The same conclusion was drawn from studying ureaplasmas in the genitourinary tract of bulls.[154]

Ureaplasmas have been isolated more often from genital specimens from infertile than from fertile couples by some investigators but not by others.[143,155–160] In several studies, ureaplasmas were recovered more often from endometrial specimens from infertile women that from fertile women.[161–163] However, the role of other organisms has rarely been considered, nor the possibility that ureaplasmas might be involved in only a small segment of infertility. In this regard, Cassell and colleagues found ureaplasmas twice as commonly in a subpopulation of women whose infertility was associated with a "male factor" than in other women.[28]

Treating infertile couples with antibiotics is clearly one way of defining the role of microorganisms in infertility. However, the results have been contradictory. As reviewed elsewhere, conception rates ranging from 23 to 84 percent have been recorded among ureaplasma-colonized infertile couples who were treated with tetracyclines.[2] Busolo et al. reported that conception had occurred in 5 (26%) of 19 doxycycline-treated patients in whom ureaplasmas in a concentration of 10^5 or more were eradicated; there were no conceptions among 29 couples in whom ureaplasmas persisted after treatment with doxycycline.[152] In another study, ureaplasmas were eradicated from 129 infertile couples; the 3-year conception rate was 60 percent compared to only 5 percent for 32 infertile couples in whom ureaplasmas could not be eliminated ($p < 0.001$).[164] In contrast, although others were able to eradicate ureaplasmas from 91 percent of infertile couples, the subsequent pregnancy rates were the same whether or not eradication had occurred.[156] Furthermore, in another study, after 1 year the conception rate among untreated ureaplasma-positive infertile women was 28 percent, similar to that among untreated ureaplasma-negative women (27%).[160] It is obvious that double-blind, placebo-controlled antibiotic studies of couples with unexplained infertility are likely to provide the best information. In this regard, Harrison et al. gave couples who had primary infertility of unknown cause either doxycycline or a placebo.[165] Although a 28-day course of the antibiotic eradicated *M. hominis* and ureaplasmas, the rate of conception (17%) was no greater in those given the antibiotic than in those given the placebo. The results of three other studies also failed to show an association between administration of tetracycline to ureaplasma-colonized couples and conception.[163,166,167] Thus, although ureaplasmas may be associated with altered sperm motility, there is no convincing evidence to implicate them as an important cause of infertility.

Habitual spontaneous abortion and stillbirth

In one study, ureaplasmas were found more often in endocervical specimens from women with a history of spontaneous abortion, especially recurrent spontaneous abortion, than from a control group of women,[168] but most investigators have not been able to relate lower genital tract colonization with ureaplasmas to fetal loss, although the possibility that a smaller subgroup was at higher risk could not be excluded.[2,120,169–171] Ureaplasmas have also been isolated more frequently from spontaneously aborted fetuses, stillborns, or premature infants than from induced abortions or normal full-term infants and the ability to isolate has not been entirely owing to superficial contamination; the organisms have been isolated from the lungs and from the brain, heart, and viscera.[2,172–177] Others have found a significant association between chorioamnionitis and mycoplasmal infection, the association being seen even when the duration of the rupture of the membranes was taken into account in the analyses.[176–184] Such membrane inflammation might be important in bringing about the poor outcome of pregnancy. Furthermore, there are serologic data to support the concept that ureaplasmal infections occur more commonly in women who have poor pregnancy outcomes than in those who have normal pregnancies.[185] Unfortunately, none of these observations answers the major question of whether abortion of the fetus occurs because mycoplasmas invade it and cause its death or whether they invade after the fetus dies for some other reason. Furthermore, the question of an etiological association is difficult to resolve, particularly as the role of other microorganisms has been ignored in most studies. This is of critical importance in view of the fact that ureaplasmas are to some extent part of the complex bacterial flora that comprises bacterial vaginosis and that this condition has been associated significantly with preterm labor and stillbirth.[186] In one study, however, bacterial vaginosis was excluded and women who were infected only with ureaplasmas were analyzed.[187] The T960 biovar was dominant in patients who had had a miscarriage and in those who delivered preterm. Nevertheless, the role of ureaplasmas is difficult to interpret because it is necessary to assume that a situation comprising a single microorganism truly exists and, furthermore, the outcome of pregnancy in those without ureaplasmas was not revealed.

There are reports of successful pregnancies occurring after antibiotic treatment of women who were colonized by ureaplasmas and who had had frequent abortions previously.[161,188,189] However, to postulate on the basis of this that mycoplasmal infection is a cause of reproductive failure seems inadvisable as specimens were not examined for other microorganisms and the treatment trials were largely uncontrolled or the numbers of persons studied were too few.[190]

Low birth weight

An observation in the early 1960s indicated that rates of low-birth-weight deliveries were unexpectedly low in pregnant women who had received tetracycline. Administration of tetracycline was not associated with any measurable demographic variable, and the possibility that the genital mycoplasmas might have been involved was mooted.[191,192] This notion was supported by finding that the rates of isolation of genital mycoplasmas from the nose and throat of newborn infants were roughly inversely proportional to birth weight[10] and that the occurrence of *M. hominis* and ureaplasmas in cervical specimens taken from women at their first antenatal visit was related to the low birth weight of their infants.[12] Other workers[176,181,183] agreed and the results of serological[193] and therapeutic[194] studies also supported the association of ureaplasmas with low birth weight. In the latter study,[194] women given erythromycin for 6 weeks during the third trimester had babies of a significantly greater mean birth weight (3331 g) than did those given a placebo (3187 g) ($p < 0.05$). However, not all investigators have been able to associate ureaplasmas with low birth weight.[195–197] Indeed, the true association is obscured by the fact that ureaplasmas constitute one of the components of the flora of bacterial vaginosis and that the latter has been associated with low birth weight.[198] This may account for any association that has been made between *M. hominis* and low birth weight.[199–200] Thus, the role of *M. hominis* is uncertain and whether ureaplasmas, and in particular the T960 biovar, have a role alone, as has been suggested,[187] or whether they play a part along with a variety of other microorganisms is still an issue.

ROLE OF MYCOPLASMAS IN IMMUNODEFICIENCY STATES

Patients with primary antibody deficiency disorders, agamma- and hypogammaglobulinemia, are particularly susceptible to mycoplasmal infections and there are reports of several different species being involved in sinusitis, pneumonia, cystitis, cellulitis, and osteomyelitis.[201] Furthermore, a small proportion of individuals with hypogammaglobulinemia develop suppurative arthritis in which mycoplasmas and particularly ureaplasmas, the latter often emanating from the genitourinary tract, are responsible for at least one-third of the joint infections.[201,202] In some of the cases involving ureaplasmas, more than one anatomical site may be affected; for example, arthritis has been associated with subcutaneous abscesses, persistent urethritis, and chronic urethrocystitis and cystitis.[203] In some patients, the arthritis responds to antibiotic therapy, whereas in others, the disease persists and so do the organisms in the joints for many months, despite antibiotic and antiinflammatory treatment, and γ-globulin replacement. All of the observations mentioned are based on the isolation of ureaplasmas by culture techniques. The development of the PCR for

U. urealyticum may prove useful in detecting nonviable ureaplasmas in joints and other sites.[204]

M. hominis causes infections in adults which do not involve the genitourinary tract, particularly if there is immunodeficiency. The sites implicated have been vascular, wounds, the central nervous system, joints, and the respiratory tract. Septicemia by *M. hominis* may occur in patients on immunosuppressive therapy and after organ transplantation, and sternal wound infections by this mycoplasma in heart or lung transplant patients appear particularly common.[205] Furthermore, polyarthritis with isolation of both *M. hominis* and ureaplasmas has been seen in a kidney allograft patient on an immunosuppressive regimen.[206] Indeed, 32 (48%) of 67 cases of extragenital *M. hominis* infection have been associated with immunosuppression or hypogammaglobulinemia.[207] Clearly, suppressed cell-mediated immunity or antibody deficiency, or both, play their part.

Association of mycoplasmas with HIV infection and AIDS

Early Observations. In the late 1980s, investigators in the United States, while searching for viruses in Kaposi's sarcoma (KS), extracted DNA from KS tissue and claimed to have transfected cell cultures, isolating a virus-like infectious agent.[208] Subsequent to this report of its existence in patients with AIDS, the virus-like agent was detected in a few patients with an acute fatal respiratory disease,[209] and, in addition, it was found to be lethal for silvered leaf monkeys.[210] Its electron microscopical appearance suggested that it might be a mycoplasma, but its intracellular location was contrary to the dogma of the time, namely that mycoplasmas do not invade epithelial cells. However, evidence that accrued subsequently showed that some mycoplasmas do enter such cells and that mycoplasmal generation of toxic oxygenated products may permit easier access by damaging the host cell membrane.[211,212] Irrespective of this, the virus-like infectious agent was cultured, found to be a mycoplasma, and termed *Mycoplasma incognitus*.[213] The use of several techniques confirmed its presence in the tissues and organs of patients with AIDS,[214] but it was later identified as *Mycoplasma fermentans*,[215] known to be of human origin. Before this, *M. fermentans* had been isolated rarely from the genitourinary tract, but more frequently from cell cultures as a contaminant, and was of unknown pathogeniticity. Nevertheless, despite another group subsequently detecting *M. fermentans* histochemically in various organs of only one of 42 autopsied subjects with AIDS,[216] the original observations gave rise to the notion that mycoplasmas, and *M. fermentans* in particular, might have importance in the pathogenesis of AIDS.

Observations In Vitro: Immune System Interaction. French and then Japanese workers noted that tetracyclines or a fluoroquinolone inhibited the cytopathic effect induced by HIV-1 or HIV-2 in lymphoblastoid leukemic (CEM) cells without suppressing virus growth.[217,218] This suggested that an antibiotic-susceptible agent, most probably a mycoplasma, was an important contributor to the cytopathic effect considered to be induced by HIV. This notion has been supported by several other investigators who have reported that various mycoplasmas, some of genital origin, in cell cultures usually enhance HIV replication and are able to bring about cell death.[219–222] In addition, *M. fermentans* was shown to be capable of fusing with the membrane of lymphoblastoid leukemic CD4+ (Molt-3) cells and CD4− (12E1) cells and also peripheral blood lymphocytes that remained intact, but which, nevertheless, may have had their function altered.[223] In this regard, subtle chromosomal changes and transformation have been found in C3H cells only after multiple passages with *M. fermentans* or *M. penetrans;* such transformation that can lead to the production of tumors in mice has been prevented by antibiotic treatment.[224]

By stimulating lymphocyte proliferation and cytokine production, mycoplasmas could enhance the replication of HIV in vivo. Numerous mycoplasmas are immune cell activators. They are mitogenic in vitro for lymphocytes, induce B-cell differentiation and trigger secretion of cytokines including interleukin-1 (IL-1), IL-2, IL-4, IL-6, tumor necrosis factor-α (TNF-α), interferons and granulocyte macrophage-colony stimulating factor.[225] Membrane lipoproteins from *M. fermentans* and *M. penetrans* are potent immunogens, triggering cellular proliferation, secretion of cytokines and IgG and IgM secretion from human myelomonocytic cell lines and monocytes.[226–228] Nonprotein membrane components, that is high molecular-weight material of *M. fermentans* and a glycolipid fraction of *M. penetrans*, have also been shown to be involved in mycoplasma-induced immune activation.[229–231] Apart from such activation, as oxidative stress results in transactivation of HIV-LTR[232] and various mycoplasma species enhance HIV-LTR-dependent gene expression,[233] HIV replication could be due, at least in part, to the production of reactive oxygen intermediates following cell infection with mycoplasmas.[234–235]

Further Observations In Vivo, Relating Particularly to *Mycoplasma fermentans*. In attempts to recover HIV from peripheral blood lymphocytes, French investigators reported that they had isolated *M. fermentans* from a small proportion of cell cultures that had been cocultivated with such blood cells from AIDS patients;[236] although this could have been due to tissue cell mycoplasmal contamination, it was consistent with the original detection of *M. fermentans* in AIDS patients.[214] In addition, *M. pirum,* hitherto recovered only from cell cultures, was isolated in the same way.[236] Thus, its image as a contaminant in search of an animal host may have been broken, although, if this is true, the mucosal site of origin of *M. pirum,* whether genitourinary, respiratory or intestinal, is unknown.

Other investigators obviously became interested in the topic. Thus, Chirgwin et al. isolated *M. fermentans* from the urine of 14 (8%) of 180 HIV-positive patients, but not from that of any of 38 HIV-negative individuals.[237] However, the development of a PCR assay for this mycoplasma[238] enabled much easier detection than by culture. In this regard, Dawson et al. reported that whereas they had detected *M. fermentans* in only 3 (7%) of 43 urine samples from HIV-positive patients by culture, they had detected it in 10 (23%) of the same urine samples by using the PCR technique, but not in any urine samples from 50 HIV-negative patients serving as controls.[239] Using this molecular method, Hawkins et al. detected *M. fermentans* DNA in the blood of about 11 percent of HIV-positive patients.[240] This raised the question of whether HIV-negative subjects might also be mycoplasma-positive. In a study in which *M. fermentans* was sought in different anatomical sites of HIV-seropositive and HIV-seronegative subjects, it was found in the throat of 23 percent, the urine of 7 percent, and the peripheral blood lymphocytes of 10 percent of HIV-positive homosexual patients,[241] the latter result being similar to that of the study mentioned previously.[240] Overall, in terms of relative proportions, the findings were similar to those found by another independent group.[242] However, *M. fermentans* was also found in about the same proportion of similar specimens from HIV-negative subjects, who were mainly homosexual men but also heterosexual women.[241] Furthermore, there was no significant association between the occurrence of *M. fermentans* and disease severity in the HIV-positive subjects, nor an association between the mycoplasma and viral load.[241] Investigators in

France, some of whom had made the earliest observations,[236] reported much later that they had detected *M. fermentans* by a PCR assay in the peripheral blood mononuclear cells of 6 percent of 154-seropositive patients and in 11 percent of 90 HIV-seronegative subjects.[243]

The various findings are indicative of the widespread distribution of *M. fermentans*. Although in one study, this mycoplasma was not found in the urethra of men with NGU,[244] it has been detected in the urine and throat of 20 percent and 19 percent, respectively, of medical students, assumed to be HIV-negative[245] and in the saliva of 44 percent of another immunocompetent group.[246] Thus, contrary to previous belief, *M. fermentans* would seem to have the oropharynx as much as, if not more than, the genitourinary tract as a site of colonization. Clearly, from either site it may become blood-borne. The extent to which it is then transient, intermittent or persistent might be germane in progression to AIDS, since it might be assumed that persistence would be most likely to help in progression or, alternatively, that progression with increasing immunodeficiency could lead to persistence. Examination of peripheral blood leucocytes and biopsied tissues from HIV-positive individuals has shown that *M. fermentans* is detectable on numerous occasions over months or years in some of them, despite repeated antibiotic administration (J Ainsworth, D Taylor-Robinson, unpublished data). Others have found *M. fermentans* more intermittently.[247] Whether intermittent or persistent existence does, in fact, lead to more rapid progression to AIDS is difficult to ascertain. So far, there is no evidence that this is the case; determination of the existence of *M. fermentans* in peripheral blood leucocytes of "fast" and "slow" progressors (disease-free with >500 CD4 cells/mm^3) has not revealed a difference.[245]

Serological investigations have not provided any real insight into the role of *M. fermentans* in AIDS.[248–250] Furthermore, although results of preliminary studies with macaque monkeys are provocative in indicating the ability of *M. fermentans* to cause immunosuppression, this approach to the problem can only ever provide results that are suggestive rather than decisive.[251,252]

Although the in vivo observations are somewhat negative in supporting a role for *M. fermentans* in the development of AIDS, two aspects are of interest. First, in an immunohistochemical study of renal tissue taken at autopsy from 203 patients with AIDS, 20 had evidence of AIDS-associated nephropathy and *M. fermentans* was detected in all the 15 renal tissue samples available from these patients.[253] Renal tissue from patients dying with AIDS but without renal disease or dying without AIDS showed no *M. fermentans*-specific staining. A case report from another group also described this association.[254] Second, as mentioned before, *M. fermentans* colonizes the oropharynx and may be a respiratory pathogen. In support of this contention, is its association with respiratory distress in adults.[255] It has also been detected in broncho-alveolar lavage specimens from 21 (28%) of 78 HIV-positive patients with pneumonia, but in none of such specimens from 46 HIV-negative patients examined for other reasons.[245] The behaviour of *M. fermentans* as an opportunist, and possibly as a pathogen, in this situation is apparent.

Observations on *Mycoplasma penetrans*. *Mycoplasma penetrans* was isolated originally from the urine of 6 (5%) of 113 HIV-positive individuals, but from none of 98 HIV-negative, age-matched, healthy volunteers.[256] This mycoplasma, as well as *M. pirum,* belongs to the same phylogenetic family defined by *M. pneumoniae* and is characterized by a prominent terminal portion, by which it penetrates and enters epithelial cells.[212] In the first serological investigation, antibodies to *M. penetrans,* measured by an enzyme-linked immunosorbent assay, were found in 20 to 40 percent of HIV-positive individuals, but in only 0.3 to 1.0 percent of various HIV-negative individuals,[257] an observation supported, in general, subsequently.[247,258,259] Thus, on this basis, and in contrast to the failure of the serological approach to indicate an association of some of the other mycoplasmas with HIV-positivity, *M. penetrans* has been regarded as uniquely HIV-associated. Although this mycoplasma is a strong activator of peripheral blood mononuclear cells in vitro,[260] it has not been detected by PCR assays in association with such cells from HIV-positive or HIV-negative subjects.[243,245,247] Furthermore, despite its original isolation from urine of HIV-positive men,[256] subsequently it has been found rarely or not at all in urine or throat specimens from such individuals.[245,247] There is, therefore, a discrepancy between the general failure to detect *M. penetrans* and the prevalence of antibody to it. One explanation for this could be that in both homosexuals and heterosexuals it is resident normally in an anatomical site that is not usually sampled, namely, the intestinal tract. In homosexuals, it could spread to the urethra and other sites through sexual activity and so stimulate antibodies, particularly under the influence of immunosuppression caused by HIV. Detection of *M. penetrans* in rectal specimens from two of 20 HIV-negative homosexual men is consistent with this notion, but more data are required.[245]

The report of antibodies to *M. penetrans* occurring more frequently in the sera of HIV-positive patients with Kaposi's sarcoma than in those of such individuals without Kaposi's sarcoma[261] has not found general support.[247,258] In addition, *M. penetrans* was not detected by use of a PCR assay in broncho-alveolar lavage specimens from 14 patients who had AIDS and evidence of Kaposi's sarcoma in the lung.[245] Thus, although *M. penetrans* could be a co-factor, together with HHV8, in the development of Kaposi's sarcoma, there is no substantive evidence to indicate that this is the case.

In conclusion, the possible role of mycoplasmas in AIDS has been the subject of several reviews.[8,236,262–265] However, although the results of studies in vitro indicate the ways in which *M. fermentans* and other mycoplasmas could hasten the onset and progression of AIDS, as yet there are few indications from studies in vivo that this is a reality.

DIAGNOSIS

The following comments are concerned mainly with *M. hominis* and the ureaplasmas, but are pertinent to other mycoplasmas that have been mentioned.

COLLECTION OF SPECIMENS

In men, *M. hominis* and the ureaplasmas colonize the urethral mucosa and can be found under the foreskin of uncircumcised men. Whether *M. genitalium* and other mycoplasmas occur under the foreskin has not been determined. In one study, intraurethral specimens were somewhat more productive than meatal specimens (86 vs 76% sensitivity) for the recovery of ureaplasmas and all men who were colonized with ureaplasmas were identified by one of these two specimens.[266] Also, *M. hominis* was recovered most often from the urethra of circumcised men (79% sensitivity), whereas the coronal sulcus was more likely to be colonized in uncircumcised men (83% sensitivity). In routine practice, the detection of mycoplasmas and ureaplasmas in the male genitourinary tract may be accomplished by collecting and testing an urethral swab specimen and/or a first-pass urine specimen. The latter is likely to prove less sensitive unless the specimen is centrifuged and the cellular deposit is tested.[267] High vaginal and endocervical swab specimens are likely to be more satisfactory than urethral swab or urine specimens for detecting the organisms in women. Avoiding contact with antiseptics, analgesics or lubricants is important since some kill mycoplasmas.[268] Swabs from whatever site should be expressed immediately in mycoplasmal or other transport medium, not broken off into the medium, and should never be allowed to dry.

If maintenance of viability is important, media used for transportation may be: (a) growth medium *(vide infra),* with or without the substrates metabolized by mycoplasmas and ureaplasmas; (b) nutrient broth enriched with, for example, 10 to 20 percent horse serum; or (c) sucrose-phosphate transport medium, designated 2SP, containing 10 percent heat-inactivated (56°C for 30 min) fetal calf serum, without antibiotics. The latter is used primarily for the transport of chlamydiae, but mycoplasmas may be recovered from the medium too, obviating the need to insert two swabs into the urethra.[269] If viability is not important, for example when specimens are to be used for antigen or DNA detection, then they may be taken and transported in phosphate-buffered saline (pH 7.2). If transport medium is not available, the swab, tissue specimen or urine should be taken to the laboratory as rapidly as possible and kept cool if this takes several hours. Even with a suitable transport medium, samples should be kept at 4°C and ideally should reach the laboratory within 24 hours. If transportation cannot be undertaken within a few days (5 at a maximum), the medium containing the specimen should be frozen to −70°C or placed in liquid nitrogen and transported in the frozen state. Concern over speed of transportation is less if the specimens are to be examined by noncultural methods.

Specimens that are received frozen in the laboratory may be kept indefinitely at −70°C or in liquid nitrogen and examined after rapid thawing in a 37°C water bath. Specimens received unfrozen should be examined promptly, if possible, rather than being frozen, because some loss of viability is inevitable through the freezing process.[270] It is feasible but undesirable to keep specimens at 4°C for a week or longer but if testing is not possible within this time, they should be frozen as indicated, but not at −20°C.

DETECTION OF ORGANISMS

Culture

The isolation of many mycoplasmas has depended on a medium comprising beef-heart infusion broth, available commercially as PPLO broth, supplemented with 10 percent (v/v) fresh yeast extract, 25 percent (w/v), and 20 percent (v/v) horse serum.[271] However, other sera, such as fetal calf serum, may improve the growth potential, and media of quite different formulations have been used satisfactorily for the isolation of both mycoplasmas and ureaplasmas.[272] In particular, SP4 medium, developed originally to cultivate spiroplasmas, has improved the isolation of not only the more fastidious mycoplasmas,[273] but also those more easily isolated, such as *M. hominis*.[270] Pretesting medium components for their ability to support growth and maintaining rigorous quality control, using a fastidious isolate, are important features of successful isolation.

Inoculation of specimens into liquid medium, which is diluted serially, followed by subculture to liquid or agar media, provides the most sensitive method for isolation.[274] Ureaplasma colonies, in particular, often fail to develop after putting a specimen directly onto agar medium, whereas color changes occur in liquid medium. For the latter to happen, advantage is taken of the metabolic activity of the organisms. Thus, 1.8 ml of medium, supplemented with phenol red (0.002%) and urea (0.1%), contained in a screw-cap vial of 2.5 ml capacity, is inoculated with, for example, 0.2 ml of the specimen. Further serial tenfold dilutions are made as deemed necessary *(vide infra)*, but in at least two further vials, that is to at least a 10^{-3} dilution of the specimen. The screw caps are secured and the vials are incubated at 37°C. As ureaplasmas possess a urease that breaks down urea to ammonia, their growth results in the medium, set initially at pH 6.0, changing in color from yellow to pink. In addition, the specimen is diluted in medium containing arginine (0.1%) and, again, in medium containing glucose (0.1%). *M. hominis* metabolizes arginine to ammonia, and raises the pH of the medium, set initially at 7.0, so that the color also changes from yellow to pink. Glucose-fermenting mycoplasmas, such as *M. genitalium,* metabolize this substrate to lactic acid, reducing the pH of the medium, set initially at 7.5 to 7.8, to less than 7.0, and thus changing the color from pink to yellow. Ureaplasmas usually produce a change within 24 to 48 hours or less and rarely thereafter, *M. hominis* less rapidly, but usually well within a week, whereas *M. genitalium* may take months to produce a change, if it does at all.

Serial dilution of specimens, as described, is valuable for various reasons, most notably for diluting antibodies, antibiotics and other inhibitors that may be present in the original specimen so that they lose their capacity to inhibit, for reducing the number of contaminating bacteria, if present, and for providing an estimate of the number of organisms in the original specimen; thus, the highest dilution at which a color change is seen may be regarded as containing one color-changing unit (ccu), assuming that there is even distribution and little aggregation of organisms.[274] As an example, a change up to the 10^{-5} dilution suggests that the original specimen contained 10^5 ccu (or 10^5 organisms).

To confirm that a mycoplasma has been isolated, aliquots of medium (0.1 or 0.2 ml) taken from liquid cultures that are just changing color, are introduced into fresh broth medium and onto agar medium. On the latter, colonies of the genital mycoplasmas develop best in an atmosphere of 95 percent N_2 plus 5 percent CO_2. Those of *M. hominis* have the classical "fried egg" appearance and are up to 200 to 300 μm in diameter. Colonies of *M. genitalium* are often much smaller and many do not have the typical appearance. Ureaplasmas produce the smallest colonies, 10 to 30 μm in diameter, which usually do not have a "fried egg" morphology because they lack the peripheral surface growth. On agar medium containing urea, 0.05 M HEPES buffer and a sensitive indicator of ammonia, that is manganous sulphate or better still calcium chloride, ureaplasmas produce colonies that are slightly larger and dark brown so that they are easier to detect.[275,276]

Commercial kits designed for the isolation and identification of *M. hominis* and ureaplasmas are available. Specialist laboratories are likely to have media of superior quality than in these, but successful use of the kits has been reported and they may be of particular value where the need to detect these microorganisms arises infrequently.[277,278]

Cultured organisms require specific identification and certain nonspecific features that are determined routinely during the course of isolation may give a lead. Thus, a specimen from the genitourinary tract that produces an alkaline color change without turbidity in medium containing arginine is most likely to contain *M. hominis,* and one that produces a similar change in medium containing urea is almost certain to contain ureaplasmas. Such clues narrow the range of specific antisera required to make a definitive identification. Incorporation of such antisera in filter-paper discs on agar to inhibit colony development (agar growth inhibition)[279] is widely used, but more than one antiserum to a species may be required to identify various strains of that species. Furthermore, distinguishing between *M. genitalium* and *M. pneumoniae* may require several techniques, more than one antiserum and perhaps monoclonal antibodies allied to Western blotting.[280] Agar growth inhibition has also been used to identify ureaplasmal serovars, although the metabolism-inhibition and complement-dependent mycoplasmacidal tests have been employed more often.[281] Epiimmunofluorescence or immunoperoxidase techniques used to stain colonies are advantageous in enabling different ureaplasmal serovars or, indeed, mycoplasmal species to be distinguished in mixtures.[281]

Antigen or DNA detection

Noncultural procedures have a particular place in the detection of mycoplasmas that are difficult to isolate in primary culture, for example *M. fermentans,* or are almost impossible to do so, for example, *M. genitalium.* Antigen detection tests have shown a lack of sensitivity and this has also been an obstacle to the development and use of DNA probes. Admittedly, 30 percent of urethral specimens from homosexual men proved positive for *M. genitalium* when tested with a DNA probe,[52] but the general difficulty of attaining sufficient sensitivity has led to the straightforward DNA probes being abandoned and a move toward the use of the PCR technique. In this regard, DNA primers specific for human ureaplasmas, *M. genitalium,* and *M. fermentans,* among others, have been developed and the method has been of considerable value diagnostically.[49,50,204,238] However, isolation of organisms through culture remains a worthy goal since quantitative results are more difficult to achieve with the PCR technique and it does not permit an assessment of antibiotic sensitivity or other biological features.

Serology

Detection of organisms, together with an antibody response to them, is the ultimate in diagnosis. Detection of an antibody response alone carries less weight and even less if reliance is placed on the existence of antibody in a single serum sample. Many serological tests have been used to measure antibodies to mycoplasmas[7,274] of which the complement fixation test, because of lack of sensitivity and specificity, is unsuitable for detecting antibodies to the genital mycoplasmas. The indirect hemagglutination technique is more sensitive and specific and has been used to detect antibody responses to *M. hominis* and *M. genitalium* in women with salpingitis.[7,274] It is, however, rather complex and difficult to reproduce, and is not used widely. In contrast, the metabolism-inhibition test is of greater specificity and has been used to detect antibody responses in various clinical settings. It does, however, require special expertise, a feature not needed with enzyme immunoassays that are becoming more widely employed. Thus, by use of a cell lysate ureaplasmal antigen and commercially available alkaline phosphatase conjugates, ureaplasmal responses were detected in two-thirds of patients with nongonococcal urethritis.[44] Furthermore, a modified enzyme immunoassay was used to measure changes in the levels of *M. hominis* antibody classes occurring in women with acute salpingitis.[100] The antigen comprised a soluble cell fraction that masked the serological diversity of different strains and allowed a single representative strain to be used; application of a heavy chain-specific second antibody followed by conjugated antispecies antibodies increased the overall sensitivity. Most recently, an enzyme immunoassay based on lipid-associated membrane proteins (LAMPs) of *M. penetrans* has been used to measure antibody to this mycoplasma,[257] as mentioned before, and the same method has been applied to detecting antibody to *M. genitalium.* The indirect immunofluorescence test has gained in popularity and is rapid, reproducible and quite sensitive and specific for measuring antibody to *M. genitalium,* there being less crossreactivity with *M. pneumoniae* than seen with some other methods.[7,274,282] The test has been used to detect antibody responses to *M. genitalium* in men with nongonococcal urethritis and in women with salpingitis.[7,114,274] Responses may develop slowly and collection of a second 'convalescent phase' serum sample too early could result in failure to detect a rise in the titer of antibody.

MANAGEMENT

Since mycoplasmal diagnostic facilities are often not available to clinicians, management should depend upon recognizing those clinical conditions for which mycoplasmas might be, at least, partially responsible and providing therapy that will be adequate to bring about clinical resolution and, at the same time, eliminate mycoplasmas. The involvement of *M. hominis* in pelvic inflammatory disease is such that initial antibiotic treatment should cover this mycoplasma, as well as *N. gonorrhoeae, C. trachomatis,* and anaerobes; cefoxitin and doxycycline, or clindamycin and gentamicin are recommended combinations. Tetracyclines are active against many strains of *M. hominis* as well as against *C. trachomatis,* which is a more important cause of pelvic inflammatory disease, but with the emergence of tetracycline-resistant *M. hominis,*[283] clindamycin is an obvious acceptable alternative.

The same sort of reasoning applies to the treatment of fever following abortion and normal vaginal delivery, in both of which *M. hominis* may be involved. As *M. hominis* is resistant to erythromycin, but not clindamycin, treatment of fever in these situations with the latter antibiotic appears to be warranted.

The weight of accumulated evidence indicates that *C. trachomatis, M. genitalium,* and occasionally ureaplasmas are causes of nongonococcal urethritis. The usual treatment of nongonococcal urethritis with a tetracycline is effective against *C. trachomatis* and against most ureaplasma isolates and probably most isolates of *M. genitalium,* although, so far, few of the latter have been available for testing. Azithromycin is sometimes used to treat nongonococcal urethritis. It is active against a wide range of mycoplasmas including all the genital mycoplasmas, although the ureaplasmas are the least susceptible to it.[284] Furthermore, about 10 percent of ureaplasmas are resistant to tetracyclines,[37,284–287] with about 40 percent of tetracycline-resistant strains exhibiting cross-resistance to erythromycin.[286] This is owing to the presence of the tetM DNA sequence described previously as a cause of *M. hominis* resistance.[283,287] Patients with nongonococcal urethritis due to tetracycline-resistant organisms usually have no clinical response to the administration of a tetracycline. This pattern is different from that seen in most treatment failures in which the symptoms of urethritis resolve while the patient is receiving a tetracycline and then recur 1 or 2 weeks after cessation of therapy. Thus, patients with nongonococcal urethritis who show no response to treatment with a tetracycline should be examined if possible for resistant ureaplasmas and should be treated with an alternative antibiotic active against these organisms—erythromycin or a quinolone (sparfloxacin).[284] In addition, infection with *M. genitalium* may result in persistent or recurrent urethritis, resolution of which may require prolonged treatment (>1 month) with a tetracycline or a macrolide, this mycoplasma being susceptible to these antibiotics in the same way as *M. pneumoniae.*[284]

Current data suggest that the detection of *M. genitalium* should signify antibiotic treatment directed against it. The other genital mycoplasmas can be isolated from specimens taken from the genitourinary tract of approximately one-half of normal, sexually experienced adults. Thus, culture of genital specimens from adults with an idiopathic disorder will result in isolation of either *M. hominis* or ureaplasmas, or both, from about one-half of such patients. To consider the organisms a cause of the disorder on the basis of such a predictable microbiological finding is not warranted, and to routinely provide antimycoplasmal therapy in such instances is not defensible.

References

1 Taylor-Robinson D et al: Urogenital mycoplasma infections of man: A review with observations on a recently discovered mycoplasma. *Isr J Med Sci* 17:524, 1981.

2 Taylor-Robinson D et al: Mycoplasmas in human genitourinary infections, in *The Mycoplasmas,* Tully, JG et al (eds). New York, Academic, 1979, vol 3, chap X.

3 Current insights in mycoplasmology. *Yale J Biol Med* 56:357,695, 1983.

4 Biology and pathogenicity of mycoplasmas. *Isr J Med Sci* 20:750, 800, 866, 1984.

5 International symposium on *Mycoplasma hominis*—a human pathogen. *Sex Transm Dis* 10(4 suppl):226, 1983.

6 Ureaplasmas of humans. *Pediatr Infect Dis* 5(6 suppl):S292, 1986.

7 Taylor-Robinson D: Immunology of genital mycoplasmal infections, in *Immunology of Sexually Transmitted Diseases,* Wright DJM (ed). Dordrecht, Kluwer Acad Publ, 1988, 163.

8 Taylor-Robinson D: Genital mycoplasmas. *Curr Opinion Infect Dis* 8:16, 1995.

9 Taylor-Robinson D: Infections due to species of *Mycoplasma* and *Ureaplasma:* An update. *Clin Infect Dis* 23:671, 1996.

10 Klein JO et al: Colonization of newborn infants by mycoplasmas. *N Engl J Med* 280:1025, 1969.

11 Taylor-Robinson D et al: The occurrence of genital mycoplasmas in babies with and without respiratory distress. *Acta Pediatr Scand* 73: 383, 1984.

12 Braun P et al: Birth weight and genital mycoplasmas in pregnancy. *N Engl J Med* 284:167, 1971.

13 Foy HM et al: Acquisition of mycoplasmata and T-strains during infancy. *J Infect Dis* 121:579, 1970.

14 Lee Y-H et al: The genital mycoplasmas: Their role in disorders of reproduction and in pediatric infections. *Pediatr Clin North Am* 21: 457, 1974.

15 Foy H et al: Prevalence of *Mycoplasma hominis* and *Ureaplasma urealyticum* (T-strains) in urine of adolescents. *J Clin Microbiol* 2: 226, 1975.

16 Iwasaka T et al: Hormonal status and mycoplasma colonization in the female genital tract. *Obstet Gynecol* 68:263, 1986.

17 Hammerschlag MR et al: Microbiology of the vagina in children: Normal and potentially pathogenic organisms. *Pediatrics* 62:57, 1978.

18 Hammerschlag MR et al: Colonization of sexually abused children with genital mycoplasmas. *Sex Transm Dis* 14:23, 1987.

19 Coury DL et al: *Ureaplasma urealyticum* and *Mycoplasma hominis* colonization among sexually abused children. *Pediatr Infect Dis* 5(6 suppl):S351, 1986.

20 McCormack WM et al: Sexual experience and urethral colonization with genital mycoplasmas: a study in normal men. *Ann Intern Med* 78:696, 1973.

21 McCormack WM et al: Sexual activity and vaginal colonization with genital mycoplasmas. *JAMA* 221:1375, 1972.

22 Shafer MA et al: Microbiology of the lower genital tract in postmenarchal adolescent girls: Difference by sexual activity, contraception and presence of non-specific vaginitis. *J Pediatr* 107:974, 1985.

23 Hill GB et al: Bacteriology of the vagina. *Scand J Urol Nephrol* 86(suppl):23, 1984.

24 Lee Y-H et al: Reevaluation of the role of T-mycoplasmas in nongonococcal urethritis. *J Am Vener Dis Assoc* 3:25, 1976.

25 Cassell GH et al: Incidence of genital mycoplasmas in women at the time of diagnostic laparoscopy. *Yale J Med Biol* 56:557, 1983.

26 Harrison HR: Prospective studies of *Mycoplasma hominis* in pregnancy. *Sex Transm Dis* 10(4 suppl):311, 1983.

27 McCormack WM et al: Colonization with genital mycoplasmas in women. *Am J Epidemiol* 97:240, 1973.

28 Cassell GH et al: Microbiologic study of infertile women at the time of diagnostic laparoscopy. Association of ureaplasmas with a defined subpopulation. *N Engl J Med* 308:502, 1983.

29 McCormack WM et al: Vaginal colonization with *Mycoplasma hominis* and *Ureaplasma urealyticum. Sex Transm Dis* 13:67, 1986.

30 Taylor-Robinson D: The history of nongonococcal urethritis. *Sex Transm Dis* 23:86, 1996.

31 Brunner H et al: Quantitative studies on the role of *Ureaplasma urealyticum* in non-gonococcal urethritis and chronic prostatitis. *Yale J Med Biol* 56:545, 1983.

32 Taylor-Robinson D: The role of mycoplasmas in non-gonococcal urethritis: A review. *Yale J Med Biol* 56:537, 1983.

33 Coufalik ED et al: Treatment of nongonococcal urethritis with rifampicin as a means of defining the role of *Ureaplasma urealyticum. Br J Vener Dis* 55:36, 1979.

34 Bowie WR et al: Etiology of nongonococcal urethritis: Evidence for *Chlamydia trachomatis* and *Ureaplasma urealyticum. J Clin Invest* 59:735, 1977.

35 Wong JL et al: The etiology of nongonococcal urethritis in men attending a venereal disease clinic. *Sex Transm Dis* 4:4, 1977.

36 Prentice JM et al: Non-specific urethritis: A placebo-controlled trial of minocycline in conjunction with laboratory investigations. *Br J Vener Dis* 52:269, 1976.

37 Hawkins DA et al: Unsuccessful treatment of non-gonococcal urethritis with rosoxacin provides information on the aetiology of the disease. *Genitourin Med* 61:51, 1985.

38 Hunter JM et al: *Chlamydia trachomatis* and *Ureaplasma urealyticum* in men attending a sexually transmitted diseases clinic. *Br J Vener Dis* 57:130, 1981.

39 Holmes KK et al: Etiology of nongonococcal urethritis. *N Engl J Med* 292:1199, 1975.

40 Taylor-Robinson D et al: *Ureaplasma urealyticum* and *Mycoplasma hominis* in chlamydial and non-chlamydial nongonococcal urethritis. *Br J Vener Dis* 55:30, 1979.

41 Jensen JS et al: *Mycoplasma genitalium:* A cause of male urethritis? *Genitourin Med* 69:265, 1993.

42 Taylor-Robinson D et al: *Ureaplasma urealyticum* causing persistent urethritis in a patient with hypogammaglobulinaemia. *Genitourin Med* 61:404, 1985.

43 Bowie WR et al: Differential response of chlamydial and ureaplasma-associated urethritis to sulphafurazole (sulfisoxazole) and aminocyclitols. *Lancet* 2:1276, 1976.

44 Brown MB et al: Measurement of antibody to *Ureaplasma urealyticum* by an enzyme-linked immunosorbent assay and detection of antibody responses in patients with nongonococcal urethritis. *J Clin Microbiol* 17:288, 1983.

45 Taylor-Robinson D et al: Human intra-urethral inoculation of ureaplasmas. *Q J Med* 46:309, 1977.

46 Shepard MC et al: Serological typing of *Ureaplasma urealyticum* isolates from urethritis patients by an agar growth inhibition method. *J Clin Microbiol* 8:566, 1978.

47 Tully JG et al: A newly discovered mycoplasma in the human urogenital tract. *Lancet* 1:1288, 1981.

48 Tully JG et al: Urogenital challenge of primate species with *Mycoplasma genitalium* and characteristics of infection induced in chimpanzees. *J Infect Dis* 153:1046, 1986.

49 Palmer HM et al: Development and evaluation of the polymerase chain reaction to detect *Mycoplasma genitalium. FEMS Microbiol Letts* 77:199, 1991.

50 Jensen JS et al: Polymerase chain reaction for detection of *Mycoplasma genitalium* in clinical samples. *J Clin Microbiol* 29:46, 1991.

51 Taylor-Robinson D et al: Microbiological and serological study of non-gonococcal urethritis with special reference to *Mycoplasma genitalium. Genitourin Med* 61:319, 1985.

52 Hooton TM et al: Prevalence of *Mycoplasma genitalium* determined by DNA probe in men with urethritis. *Lancet* 1:266, 1988.

53 Taylor-Robinson D et al: Occurrence of *Mycoplasma genitalium* in different populations and its clinical significance. *Clin Infect Dis* 17(suppl 1):S66, 1993.

54 Horner PJ et al: Association of *Mycoplasma genitalium* with acute non-gonococcal urethritis. *Lancet* 342:582, 1993.

55 Deguchi T et al: *Mycoplasma genitalium* in non-gonococcal urethritis. *Int J STD AIDS* 6:144, 1995.
56 Janier M et al: Male urethritis with and without discharge: A clinical and microbiological study. *Sex Transm Dis* 22:244, 1995.
57 Charron A et al: *Mycoplasma genitalium* as etiological agent of male urethritis in Southwest France, in *Abstracts of the 11th meeting of the International Society for STD Research,* New Orleans, 203, 1995.
58 Lackey PC et al: The etiology of nongonococcal urethritis (abstract 238). *Clin Infect Dis* 21:759, 1995.
59 Jensen JS et al: Isolation of *Mycoplasma genitalium* strains from the male urethra. *J Clin Microbiol* 34:286, 1996.
60 Mårdh P-A et al: Search for uro-genital tract infections in patients with symptoms of prostatitis: Studies on aerobic and strictly anaerobic bacteria, mycoplasma, fungi, trichomonads and viruses. *Scand J Urol Nephrol* 9:8, 1975.
61 Peeters MF et al: Role of mycoplasmas in chronic prostatitis. *Yale J Med Biol* 56:551, 1983.
62 Hofstetter A: Mykoplasmeninfektionen des Urogenitaltraktes. *Hautarzt* 28:295, 1977.
63 Brunner H et al: Studies on the role of *Ureaplasma urealyticum* and *Mycoplasma hominis* in prostatitis. *J Infect Dis* 147:807, 1983.
64 Weidner W et al: Ureaplasmal infections of the male urogenital tract, in particular prostatitis, and semen quality. *Urol Int* 4:5, 1985.
65 Meares EM Jr: Bacterial prostatitis vs "prostatosis": A clinical and bacteriological study. *JAMA* 224:1372, 1973.
66 Vinje O et al: Laboratory findings in chronic prostatitis—with special reference to immunological and microbiological aspects. *Scand J Urol Nephrol* 17:291, 1983.
67 Doble A et al: A search for infectious agents in chronic abacterial prostatitis using ultrasound guided biopsy. *Br J Urol* 64:297, 1989.
68 Krieger JN et al: Prokaryotic DNA sequences in patients with chronic idiopathic prostatitis. *J Clin Microbiol* 34:3120, 1996.
69 Harnisch JP et al: Aetiology of acute epididymitis. *Lancet* 1:819, 1977.
70 Berger RE et al: *Chlamydia trachomatis* as a cause of acute "idiopathic" epididymitis. *N Engl J Med* 298:301, 1978.
71 Hawkins DA et al: Microbiological survey of acute epididymitis. *Genitourin Med* 62:342, 1986.
72 Furness G et al: The relationship of epididymitis to gonorrhea. *Invest Urol* 11:312, 1974.
73 Doble A et al: Acute epididymitis: a microbiological and ultrasonographic study. *Br J Urol* 63:90, 1989.
74 Jalil N et al: Infection of the epididymis by *Ureaplasma urealyticum. Genitourin Med* 64:367, 1988.
75 Keat A et al: *Chlamydia trachomatis* and reactive arthritis: The missing link. *Lancet* 1:72, 1987.
76 Taylor-Robinson D et al: Detection of *Chlamydia trachomatis* DNA in joints of reactive arthritis patients by polymerase chain reaction. *Lancet* 340:81, 1992.
77 Keat AC et al: Role of *Chlamydia trachomatis* and HLA-B27 in sexually acquired reactive arthritis. *Br Med J* 1:605, 1978.
78 Taylor-Robinson D et al: The association of *Mycoplasma hominis* with arthritis. *Sex Transm Dis* 10(4 suppl):341, 1983.
79 Ford DK et al: Cell-mediated immune responses of synovial mononuclear cells in Reiter's syndrome against ureaplasmal and chlamydial antigens. *J Rheum* 7:751, 1980.
80 Horowitz S et al: *Ureaplasma urealyticum* in Reiter's syndrome. *J Rheumatol* 21:877, 1994.
81 Taylor-Robinson D et al: *Mycoplasma genitalium* in the joints of two patients with arthritis. *Eur J Clin Microbiol Infect Dis* 13:1066, 1994.
82 Lee Y-H et al: Microbiological investigation of Bartholin's gland abscesses and cysts. *Am J Obstet Gynecol* 129:150, 1977.
83 Paavonen J et al: *Mycoplasma hominis* in nonspecific vaginitis. *Sex Transm Dis* 10(4 suppl):271, 1983.
84 Rosenstein et al: Bacterial vaginosis in pregnancy: Distribution of bacterial species in different gram-stain categories of the vaginal flora. *J Med Microbiol* 44:1, 1996.
85 Koutsky LA et al: Persistence of *Mycoplasma hominis* after therapy: Importance of tetracycline resistence and of coexisting vaginal flora. *Sex Transm Dis* 10(suppl):374, 1983.
86 Gravett MG et al: Possible role of *Ureaplasma urealyticum* in preterm rupture of the fetal membrane. *Pediatr Infect Dis* 5(6 suppl):S253, 1986.
87 Sweet RL: Colonization of the endometrium and fallopian tubes with *Ureaplasma urealyticum. Pediatr Infect Dis* 5(6 suppl):S244, 1986.
88 Kinghorn GR et al: Clinical and microbiological investigation of women with acute salpingitis and their consorts. *Br J Obstet Gynaecol* 93:869, 1986.
89 Mårdh P: Introductory address: clinical and microbial etiology of pelvic inflammatory disease. *Sex Transm Dis* 11(4 suppl):428, 1984.
90 Wasserheit JN et al: Microbial causes of proven pelvic inflammatory disease and efficacy of clindamycin and tobramycin. *Ann Intern Med* 104:187, 1986.
91 Møller BR: The role of mycoplasmas in the upper genital tract of women. *Sex Transm Dis* 10(4 suppl):281, 1983.
92 Eschenbach DA et al: Polymicrobial etiology of acute pelvic inflammatory disease. *N Engl J Med* 293:166, 1975.
93 Mårdh P-A et al: *Chlamydia trachomatis* infection in patients with acute salpingitis. *N Engl J Med* 296:1377, 1977.
94 Dodson MG et al: The polymicrobial etiology of acute pelvic inflammatory disease and treatment regimens. *Rev Infect Dis* 7(suppl 4): S696, 1985.
95 Mårdh P: Mycoplasmal PID: A review of natural and experimental infections. *Yale J Med Biol* 56:529, 1983.
96 Møller BR et al: Chlamydia, mycoplasmas, ureaplasmas and yeasts in the lower genital tract of females. Comparison between a group attending a venereal disease clinic and a control group. *Acta Obstet Gynecol Scand* 64:145, 1985.
97 Mårdh P-A et al: Tubal and cervical cultures in acute salpingitis with special reference to *Mycoplasma hominis* and T-strain mycoplasmas. *Br J Vener Dis* 46:179, 1970.
98 Mårdh P-A et al: Antibodies to *Mycoplasma hominis* in patients with genital infections and in healthy controls. *Br J Vener Dis* 46:390, 1970.
99 Møller BR et al: *Chlamydia trachomatis, Mycoplasma hominis* and *Neisseria gonorrhoeae* infection in patients with signs of pelvic inflammatory disease. *Sex Transm Dis* 8:198, 1981.
100 Miettinen A et al: Enzyme immunoassay for serum antibody to *Mycoplasma hominis* in women with acute pelvic inflammatory disease. *Sex Transm Dis* 10(4 suppl):289, 1983.
101 Stacey CM et al: A longitudinal study of pelvic inflammatory disease. *Br J Obstet Gynaecol* 99:994, 1992.
102 Mårdh P-A: Increased serum levels of IgM in acute salpingitis related to the occurrence of *Mycoplasma hominis. Acta Pathol Microbiol Scand (B)* 78:726, 1970.
103 Mårdh P-A et al: Endometritis caused by *Chlamydia trachomatis. Br J Vener Dis* 57:191, 1981.
104 Lind K et al: Importance of *Mycoplasma hominis* in acute salpingitis assessed by culture and serological tests. *Genitourin Med* 61:185, 1985.
105 McGee ZA et al: Pathogenic mechanisms of *Neisseria gonorrhoeae:* Observations on damage to human fallopian tubes in organ culture by gonococci of colony type 1 or type 4. *J Infect Dis* 143:413, 1981.
106 Taylor-Robinson D et al: Growth and effect of mycoplasmas in fallopian tube organ cultures. *Br J Vener Dis* 50:212, 1974.
107 Mårdh P-A et al: Studies on ciliated epithelia of the human genital tract: 1. Swelling of the cilia of fallopian tube epithelium in organ cultures infected with *Mycoplasma hominis. Br J Vener Dis* 52:52, 1976.
108 Møller BR et al: Experimental infection of the genital tract of female grivet monkeys by *Mycoplasma hominis. Infect Immunol* 20:248, 1978.
109 Møller BR et al: Experimental infection of the genital tract of female grivet monkeys by *Mycoplasma hominis:* Effects of different routes of infection. *Infect Immunol* 26:1123, 1979.

110 Sweet RL et al: Use of laparoscopy to determine the microbial etiology of acute salpingitis. *Am J Obstet Gynecol* 134:68, 1980.
111 Solomon F et al: Infections associated with genital mycoplasma. *Am J Obstet Gynecol* 116:785, 1973.
112 Braun P et al: Tuboovarian abscess with recovery of T-mycoplasma. *Am J Obstet Gynecol* 117:861, 1973.
113 Møller BR et al: Attempts to produce gynaecological disease in grivet monkeys with *Ureaplasma urealyticum. J Med Microbiol* 14:475, 1981.
114 Møller BR et al: Serological evidence implicating *Mycoplasma genitalium* in pelvic inflammatory disease. *Lancet* 1:1102, 1984.
115 Lind K et al: Significance of antibodies to *Mycoplasma genitalium* in salpingitis. *Eur J Clin Microbiol* 6:205, 1987.
116 Møller BR et al: Serologic evidence that chlamydia and mycoplasmas are involved in infertility of women. *J Reprod Fertil* 73:237, 1985.
117 Collier AM et al: Attachment of *Mycoplasma genitalium* to the ciliated epithelium of human fallopian tubes, in *Recent Advances in Mycoplasmology,* G Stanek et al (eds). Stuttgart, Gustav Fischer Verlag, 1990, p. 730.
118 Taylor-Robinson D et al: Animal models of *Mycoplasma genitalium* urogenital infection. *Isr J Med Sci* 23:561, 1987.
119 McCormack WM et al: Genital mycoplasmas in postpartum fever. *J Infect Dis* 127:193, 1973.
120 Harrison HR et al: Cervical *Chlamydia trachomatis* and mycoplasmal infections in pregnancy. Epidemiology and outcomes. *JAMA* 250:1721, 1983.
121 Berman SM et al: Low birth weight prematurity, and post-partum endometritis. Association with prenatal cervical *Mycoplasma hominis* and *Chlamydia trachomatis* infections. *JAMA* 257:1189, 1987.
122 Caspi E et al: Isolation of *Mycoplasma* from the placenta after cesarean section. *Obstet Gynecol* 48:682, 1976.
123 Eschenbach DA et al: Bacterial vaginosis during pregnancy: An association with prematurity and postpartum complications. *Scand J Urol Nephrol* 86(suppl):213, 1984.
124 Jones DM et al: Isolation of mycoplasmas and other organisms from the placenta after caesarean section. *J Med Microbiol* 2:347, 1969.
125 Williams CM et al: Clinical and microbiological risk evaluation for post-Cesarian section endometritis by multivariate discriminant analysis: Role of intraoperative mycoplasma, aerobes, and anaerobes. *Am J Obstet Gynecol* 156:967, 1987.
126 McCormack WM et al: Isolation of genital mycoplasmas from blood obtained shortly after vaginal delivery. *Lancet* 1:596, 1975.
127 Eschenbach DA: *Ureaplasma urealyticum* as a cause of post partum fever. *Pediatr Infect Dis* 5(6 suppl):S258, 1986.
128 Wallace JR Jr et al: Isolation of *Mycoplasma hominis* from blood cultures in patients with postpartum fever. *Obstet Gynecol* 51:181, 1978.
129 Lamey JR et al: Isolation of mycoplasmas and bacteria from the blood of postpartum women. *Am J Obstet Gynecol* 143:104, 1982.
130 Zheng X et al: Isolation of *Mycoplasma hominis* from a brain abscess. *J Clin Microbiol* 35:992, 1997.
131 Harwick HJ et al: *Mycoplasma hominis* and abortion. *J Infect Dis* 121:260, 1970.
132 Friedlander AM et al: Production of bladder stones by human T mycoplasmas. *Nature* 247:67, 1974.
133 Texier-Maugein J et al: *Ureaplasma urealyticum*-induced bladder stones in rats and their prevention by flurofamide and doxycycline. *Isr J Med Sci* 23:565, 1987.
134 Grenabo L et al: Urinary infection stones caused by *Ureaplasma urealyticum:* A review. *Scand J Infect Dis* 53(suppl):46, 1988.
135 Stamm WE et al: Etiologic role of *Mycoplasma hominis* and *Ureaplasma urealyticum* in women with the acute urethral syndrome. *Sex Transm Dis* 10(4 suppl):318, 1983.
136 Thomsen AC: Occurrence and pathogenicity of *Mycoplasma hominis* in the upper urinary tract: A review. *Sex Transm Dis* 10(4 suppl): 323, 1983.
137 Gilbert GL et al: Bacteriuria due to ureaplasmas and other fastidious organisms during pregnancy: Prevalence and significance. *Pediatr Infect Dis* 5(6 suppl):S239, 1986.
138 McDonald MI et al: *Ureaplasma urealyticum* in patients with acute symptoms of urinary tract infection. *J Urol* 128:517, 1982.
139 Thomsen AC: The occurrence of mycoplasmas in the urinary tract of patients with chronic pyelonephritis. *Acta Pathol Microbiol Scand (B)* 83:10, 1975.
140 Thomsen AC: Occurrence of mycoplasmas in urinary tracts of patients with acute pyelonephritis. *J Clin Microbiol* 8:84, 1978.
141 Thomsen AC: Mycoplasmas in human pyelonephritis: Demonstration of antibodies in serum and urine. *J Clin Microbiol* 8:197, 1978.
142 Krieger JN et al: Evidence for pathogenicity of *Ureaplasma urealyticum* for the upper urinary tract derived from animal models. *Pediatr Infect Dis* 5(suppl):319, 1986.
143 Styler M et al: Mollicutes (mycoplasma) in infertility. *Fertil Steril* 44: 1, 1985.
144 Naessens A et al: Recovery of microorganisms in semen and relationship to sperm sample. *Fertil Steril* 45:101, 1986.
145 Fowlkes DM et al: T-mycoplasmas and human infertility: Correlation of infection with alterations in seminal parameters. *Fertil Steril* 26: 1212, 1975.
146 Busolo F et al: Mycoplasmic localization patterns on spermatozoa of infertile men. *Fertil Steril* 42:412, 1984.
147 Toth A et al: Light microscopy as an aid in predicting ureaplasma infection in human semen. *Fertil Steril* 30:586, 1978.
148 Hofstetter A et al: Genitale Mykoplasmenstämme als Ursache der männlichen Infertilität. *Helv Chir Acta* 45:329, 1978.
149 Meseguer M et al: Changes in semen parameters by incubation with *Ureaplasma urealyticum* strains, in *Recent Advances in Mycoplasmology,* G Stanek et al (eds). Stuttgart, Gustav Fischer Verlag, 1990, 745.
150 Swenson CE et al: *Ureaplasma urealyticum* and human infertility: The effect of antibiotic therapy on semen quality. *Fertil Steril* 31:660, 1979.
151 Toth A et al: *Ureaplasma urealyticum* and infertility: The effect of different antibiotic regimens on the semen quality. *J Urol* 128:705, 1982.
152 Busolo F et al: Microbial flora in semen of asymptomatic infertile men. *Andrologia* 16:269, 1984.
153 Taylor-Robinson D: Evaluation of the role of *Ureaplasma urealyticum* in infertility. *Pediatr Infect Dis* 5(6 suppl):S262, 1986.
154 Taylor-Robinson D et al: The isolation of T-mycoplasmas from the urogenital tract of bulls. *J Med Microbiol* 2:527, 1969.
155 Gnarpe H et al: Mycoplasma and human reproductive failure: 1. The occurrence of different mycoplasmas in couples with reproductive failure. *Am J Obstet Gynecol* 114:727, 1972.
156 Upadhyaya M et al: The role of mycoplasmas in reproduction. *Fertil Steril* 39:814, 1983.
157 de Louvois J et al: Frequency of mycoplasma in fertile and infertile couples. *Lancet* 1:1073, 1974.
158 André D et al: Rôle des mycoplasmes dans la stérilité. Étude de 150 femmes stériles. *J Gynecol Obstet Biol Reprod (Paris)* 7:51, 1978.
159 Matthews CD et al: The frequency of genital mycoplasma infection in human fertility. *Fertil Steril* 26:988, 1975.
160 Nagata Y et al: Mycoplasma infection and infertility. *Fertil Steril* 31: 392, 1979.
161 Stray-Pedersen B et al: Uterine T-mycoplasma colonization in reproductive failure. *Am J Obstet Gynecol* 130:307, 1978.
162 Koren Z et al: Irrigation technique for detection of *Mycoplasma* intrauterine infection in infertile patients. *Obstet Gynecol* 52:588, 1978.
163 Stray-Pedersen B et al: Infertility and uterine colonization with *Ureaplasma urealyticum. Acta Obstet Gynecol Scand* 61:21, 1982.
164 Toth A et al: Subsequent pregnancies among 161 couples treated for *T-mycoplasma* genital tract infection. *N Engl J Med* 308:505, 1983.
165 Harrison RF et al: Doxycycline treatment and human infertility. *Lancet* 1:605, 1975.
166 Matthews CD et al: T-mycoplasma genital infection: The effect of doxycycline therapy on human unexplained infertility. *Fertil Steril* 30:98, 1978.

167 Idriss WM et al: On the etiologic role of *Ureaplasma urealyticum* (T-mycoplasma) infection in infertility. *Fertil Steril* 30:293, 1978.
168 Foulon W et al: Epidemiology and pathogenesis of *Ureaplasma urealyticum* in spontaneous abortion and early premature labor. *Pediatr Infect Dis* 5(6 suppl):S353, 1986.
169 Harrison HR: Cervical colonization with *Ureaplasma urealyticum* and pregnancy outcome: Prospective studies. *Pediatr Infect Dis* 5(6 suppl):S266, 1986.
170 Munday PE et al: Spontaneous abortion—an infectious etiology? *Br J Obstet Gynecol* 91:1177, 1984.
171 Thomsen AC et al: The infrequent occurrence of mycoplasmas in amniotic fluid from women with intact fetal membranes. *Acta Obstet Gynecol Scand* 63:425, 1984.
172 Kundsin RB et al: The role of mycoplasmas in human reproductive failure. *Ann NY Acad Sci* 174:794, 1970.
173 Robertson JA et al: Serotypes of *Ureaplasma urealyticum* in spontaneous abortion. *Pediatr Infect Dis* 5(6 suppl):S270, 1986.
174 Caspi E et al: Early abortion and *Mycoplasma* infection. *Isr J Med Sci* 8:122, 1972.
175 Sompolinsky D et al: Infections with mycoplasma and bacteria in induced midtrimester abortion and fetal loss. *Am J Obstet Gynecol* 121:610, 1975.
176 Kundsin RB et al: *Ureaplasma urealyticum* incriminated in perinatal morbidity and mortality. *Science* 213:474, 1981.
177 Tafari N et al: Mycoplasma T strains and perinatal death. *Lancet* 1: 108, 1976.
178 Shurin PA et al: Chorioamnionitis and colonization of the newborn infant with genital mycoplasmas. *N Engl J Med* 293:5, 1975.
179 Cassell GM et al: Isolation of *Mycoplasma hominis* and *Ureaplasma urealyticum* from amniotic fluid at 16–20 weeks of gestation: Potential effect on outcome of pregnancy. *Sex Transm Dis* 10(4 suppl): 294, 1983.
180 Quinn PA et al: Chorioamnionitis: Its association with pregnancy outcome and microbial infection. *Am J Obstet Gynecol* 156:379, 1987.
181 Kundsin RB et al: Association of *Ureaplasma urealyticum* in the placenta with perinatal morbidity and mortality. *N Engl J Med* 310:941, 1984.
182 Hillier SL et al: The association of *Ureaplasma urealyticum* with preterm birth, chorioamnionitis, post partum fever, intrapartum fever and bacterial vaginosis. *Pediatr Infect Dis* 5(6 suppl):S349, 1986.
183 Embree JE et al: Placental infection with *Mycoplasma hominis* and *Ureaplasma urealyticum:* Clinical correlation. *Obstet Gynecol* 56: 475, 1980.
184 Gibbs RS et al: *Mycoplasma hominis* and intrauterine infection in late pregnancy. *Sex Transm Dis* 10(4 suppl):303, 1983.
185 Quinn PA: Evidence of an immune response to *Ureaplasma urealyticum* in perinatal morbidity and mortality. *Pediatr Infect Dis* 5(6 suppl):S282, 1986.
186 Hay PE et al: Abnormal bacterial colonisation of the genital tract and subsequent preterm delivery and late miscarriage. *Br Med J* 308:295, 1994.
187 Abele-Horn M et al: Association of *Ureaplasma urealyticum* biovars with clinical outcome for neonates, obstetric patients, and gynecological patients with pelvic inflammatory disease. *J Clin Microbiol* 35:1199, 1997.
188 Driscoll SG et al: Infections and first trimester losses: Possible role of mycoplasmas. *Fertil Steril* 20:1017, 1969.
189 Kundsin RB: Mycoplasma in genitourinary tract infection and reproductive failure. *Prog Gynecol* 5:275, 1970.
190 Quinn PA et al: Evidence supporting the role of genital mycoplasma infections in habitual spontaneous abortions, in *Proceedings of the Third Meeting of the International Organization for Mycoplasmology*, Custer, SD, September 1980.
191 Elder HA et al: The natural history of asymptomatic bacteriuria during pregnancy: The effect of tetracycline on the clinical course and the outcome of pregnancy. *Am J Obstet Gynecol* 111:441, 1971.
192 Elder HA et al: Effect of tetracycline on outcome of pregnancy in non-bacteriuric patients. Presented at the Eighth Interscience Conference on Antimicrobial Agents and Chemotherapy, New York, October 21–23, 1968.
193 Kass EH et al: Genital mycoplasmas as a cause of excess premature delivery. *Trans Assoc Am Physicians* 94:261, 1981.
194 McCormack WM et al: Effect on birthweight of erythromycin treatment of pregnant women. *Obstet Gynecol* 69:202, 1987.
195 Foy HM et al: Isolation of *Mycoplasma hominis,* T-strains, and cytomegalovirus from the cervix of pregnant women. *Am J Obstet Gynecol* 106:635, 1970.
196 Ross JM et al: The effect of genital mycoplasmas on human fetal growth. *Br J Obstet Gynecol* 88:749, 1981.
197 Zlatnick FJ et al: Chorionic mycoplasmas and prematurity. *J Reprod Med* 31:1106, 1986.
198 Hillier SL et al for the Vaginal Infection and Prematurity Study Group: Association between bacterial vaginosis and preterm delivery of a low-birth-weight infant. *N Engl J Med* 333:1737, 1995.
199 di Musto JC et al: *Mycoplasma hominis* type I infection and pregnancy. *Obstet Gynecol* 41:33, 1973.
200 Romano N et al: Mycoplasmas in pregnant women and in newborn infants. *Boll 1st Sieroter Milan* 55:568, 1976.
201 Gelfand EW: Unique susceptibility of patients with antibody deficiency to mycoplasma infection. *Clin Infect Dis* 17(suppl):250, 1993.
202 Furr PM et al: Mycoplasmas and ureaplasmas in patients with hypogammaglobulinaemia and their role in arthritis: Microbiological observations over twenty years. *Ann Rheum Dis* 53:183, 1994.
203 Webster ADB et al: Chronic cystitis and urethritis associated with ureaplasmal and mycoplasmal infection in primary hypogammaglobulinaemia. *Br J Urol* 54:287, 1982.
204 Blanchard A et al: Detection of *Ureaplasma urealyticum* by polymerase chain reaction in the urogenital tract of adults, in amniotic fluid, and in the respiratory tract of newborns. *Clin Infect Dis* 17(suppl 1): 148, 1993.
205 Steffenson DO et al: Sternotomy infections with *Mycoplasma hominis. Ann Intern Med* 106:204, 1987.
206 Burdge DR et al: Septic arthritis due to dual infection with *Mycoplasma hominis* and *Ureaplasma urealyticum. J Rheumatol* 15:366, 1988.
207 Meyer RD et al: Extragenital *Mycoplasma hominis* infections in adults: Emphasis on immunosuppression. *Clin Infect Dis* 17(suppl 1):243, 1993.
208 Lo S-C et al: A novel virus-like infectious agent in patients with AIDS. *Am J Trop Med Hyg* 40:213, 1989.
209 Lo S-C et al: Association of the virus-like infectious agent originally reported in patients with AIDS with acute fatal disease in previously healthy non-AIDS patients. *Am J Trop Med Hyg* 41:364, 1989.
210 Lo S-C et al: Fatal infection of silvered leaf monkeys with a virus-like infectious agent (VLIA) derived from a patient with AIDS. *Am J Trop Med Hyg* 40:399, 1989.
211 Taylor-Robinson D et al: Intracellular location of mycoplasmas in cultured cells demonstrated by immunocytochemistry and electron microscopy. *Int J Exp Pathol* 72:705, 1991.
212 Baseman JB et al: Interplay between mycoplasmas and host target cells. *Microbiol Pathogenesis* 19:105, 1995.
213 Lo S-C et al: Virus-like infectious agent (VLIA) is a novel pathogenic mycoplasma: *Mycoplasma incognitus. Am J Trop Med Hyg* 41:586, 1989.
214 Lo S-C et al: Identification of *Mycoplasma incognitus* infection in patients with AIDS: an immunohistochemical, in situ hybridization and ultrastructural study. *Am J Trop Med Hyg* 41:601, 1989.
215 Saillard C et al: Genetic and serologic relatedness between *Mycoplasma fermentans* strains and a mycoplasma recently identified in tissues of AIDS and non-AIDS patients. *Res Virol* 141:385, 1990.
216 Miller-Catchpole R et al: The incidence and distribution of *Mycoplasma fermentans* (*incognitus* strain) in the Chicago AIDS autopsy series: An immunohistochemical study. *Mod Pathol* 4:481, 1991.
217 Lemaître M et al: Protective activity of tetracycline analogs against the cytopathic effect of the human immunodeficiency viruses in CEM cells. *Res Virol* 141:5, 1990.

218 Nozaki-Renard J et al: A fluoroquinolone (DR-3355) protects human lymphocyte cell lines from HIV-1 induced cytotoxicity. *AIDS* 4:1283, 1990.
219 Lo S-C et al: Enhancement of HIV-1 cytocidal effects in CD4+ lymphocytes by the AIDS-associated mycoplasma. *Science* 251:1074, 1991.
220 Chowdhury M et al: Mycoplasma can enhance HIV replication *in vitro:* a possible cofactor responsible for the progression of AIDS. *Biochem Biophys Res Commun* 170:1365, 1990.
221 Sasaki Y et al: Mycoplasmas stimulate replication of human immunodeficiency virus type 1 through selective activation of CD4+ T lymphocytes. *AIDS Res Hum Retrovirus* 9:775, 1993.
222 Chowdhury M et al: Mycoplasma stimulates HIV-1 expression from acutely- and dormantly-infected promonocyte/monoblastoid cell lines. *Arch Virol* 139:431, 1994.
223 Dimitrov DS et al: *Mycoplasma fermentans* (incognitus strain) cells are able to fuse with T lymphocytes. *Clin Infect Dis* 17(suppl 1):305, 1993.
224 Tsai S et al: Mycoplasmas and oncogenesis: persistent infection and multistage malignant transformation. *Proc Natl Acad Sci USA* 92: 10197, 1995.
225 McGarrity GJ et al: Mycoplasmas and tissue culture cells, in *Mycoplasmas: Molecular Biology and Pathogenesis,* J Maniloff et al (eds). Amer Soc Microbiol, Washington DC, 1992, 445.
226 Rawadi G et al: Effects of *Mycoplasma fermentans* on the myelomonocytic lineage. *J Immunol* 156:670, 1996.
227 Kostyal DA et al: A 48-kilodalton *Mycoplasma fermentans* membrane protein induces cytokine secretion by human monocytes. *Infect Immunol* 62:3793, 1994.
228 Rawadi G et al: Mycoplasma membrane lipoproteins induce proinflammatory cytokines by a mechanism distinct from that of lipopolysaccharide. *Infect Immunol* 64:637, 1996.
229 Muhlradt PF et al: MDHM, a macrophage-stimulatory product of *Mycoplasma fermentans,* leads to *in vitro* interleukin-1 (IL-1), IL-6, tumor necrosis factor, and prostaglandin production and is pyrogenic in rabbits. *Infect Immunol* 59:3969, 1991.
230 Muhlradt PF et al: Involvement of interleukin-1 (IL-1), IL-6, IL-2 and IL-4 in generation of cytolytic T cells from thymocytes stimulated by a *Mycoplasma fermentans*-derived product. *Infect Immunol* 59: 3962, 1991.
231 Muhlradt PF et al: Purification and partial biochemical characterization of a *Mycoplasma fermentans*-derived substance that activates macrophages to release nitric oxide, tumor necrosis factor, and interleukin-6. *Infect Immun* 62:3801, 1994.
232 Schreck R et al: Reactive oxygen intermediates as apparently widely used messengers in the activation of the NF-kB transcription factor and HIV-1. *EMBO J* 10:2247, 1991.
233 Nir-Paz R et al: Mycoplasmas regulate HIV-LTR-dependent gene expression. *FEMS Microbiol Lett* 128:63, 1995.
234 Tryon V et al: Pathogenic determinants and mechanisms, in *Mycoplasmas: Molecular Biology and Pathogenesis,* J Maniloff et al (eds). Amer Soc Microbiol, Washington DC, 1992, 457.
235 Chochola J et al: Release of hydrogen peroxide from human T cell lines and normal lymphocytes co-infected with HIV-1 and mycoplasmas. *Free Rad Res* 23:197, 1995.
236 Montagnier L et al: Mycoplasmas as cofactors in infection due to the human immunodeficiency virus. *Clin Infect Dis* 17(suppl 1):309, 1993.
237 Chirgwin KD et al: Identification of mycoplasmas in urine from persons infected with human immunodeficiency virus. *Clin Infect Dis* 17(suppl 1):264, 1993.
238 Wang RY-H et al: Selective detection of *Mycoplasma fermentans* by polymerase chain reaction and by using a nucleotide sequence within the insertion sequence-like element. *J Clin Microbiol* 30:245, 1992.
239 Dawson MS et al: Detection and isolation of *Mycoplasma fermentans* from urine of human immunodeficiency virus type-1-infected patients. *Arch Pathol Lab Med* 117:511, 1993.
240 Hawkins RE et al: Association of mycoplasma and human immunodeficiency virus infection: Detection of amplified *Mycoplasma fermentans* DNA in blood. *J Infect Dis* 165:581, 1992.
241 Katseni VL et al: *Mycoplasma fermentans* in individuals seropositive and seronegative for HIV-1. *Lancet* 341:271, 1993.
242 Bébéar C et al: Mycoplasmas in HIV-1 seropositive patients. *Lancet* 341:758, 1993.
243 Kovacic R et al: Search for the presence of six *Mycoplasma* species in peripheral blood mononuclear cells of subjects seropositive and seronegative for human immunodeficiency virus. *J Clin Microbiol* 34: 1808, 1996.
244 Deguchi T et al: Failure to detect *Mycoplasma fermentans, Mycoplasma penetrans* or *Mycoplasma pirum* in the urethra of patients with acute nongonococcal urethritis. *Eur J Clin Microbiol Inf Dis* 15: 169, 1996.
245 Ainsworth J et al: Further observations on mycoplasmas that have been associated with AIDS. *IOM Letts* 4:1, 1996 (abstract).
246 Chingbingyong MI et al: Detection of *Mycoplasma fermentans* in human saliva with a polymerase chain reaction-based assay. *Arch Oral Biol* 41:311, 1996.
247 de Barbeyrac B et al: Mycoplasmas in patients infected by HIV-1. *IOM Letts* 4:69, 1996 (abstract).
248 Hakkarainen K et al: Serological responses to mycoplasmas in HIV-infected and non-infected individuals. *AIDS* 6:1287, 1992.
249 Tully JG et al: Titers of antibody to *Mycoplasma* in sera of patients infected with human immunodeficiency virus. *Clin Infect Dis* 17(suppl 1):254, 1993.
250 Horowitz S et al: Antibodies to *Mycoplasma fermentans* in HIV-seropositive and sernonegative patients. *IOM Letts* 3:354, 1994.
251 Davidson MK et al: Effects of *Mycoplasma fermentans* infection in pigtailed macaques (*Macaca nemustrinus*). *IOM Letts* 4:2, 1996 (abstract).
252 Reyes L et al: In vivo effects of *Mycoplasma fermentans* infection on the hemolymphatic cell populations of pigtail macaques. *IOM Letts* 4:74: 1996 (abstract).
253 Bauer FA et al: *Mycoplasma fermentans* (*incognitus* strain) infection in the kidneys of patients with acquired immunodeficiency syndrome and associated nephropathy. *Hum Pathol* 22:63, 1991.
254 Ainsworth JG et al: *Mycoplasma fermentans* and HIV-associated nephropathy. *J Infect* 29:323, 1994.
255 Lo S-C et al: Adult respiratory distress syndrome with or without systemic disease associated with infections due to *Mycoplasma fermentans. Clin Infect Dis* 17(suppl 1):259, 1993.
256 Lo S-C et al: Newly discovered mycoplasma isolated from patients infected with HIV. *Lancet* 338:1415, 1991.
257 Wang RY-H et al: High frequency of antibodies to *Mycoplasma penetrans* in HIV-infected patients. *Lancet* 340:1312, 1992.
258 Grau O et al: Association of *Mycoplasma penetrans* with human immunodeficiency virus infection. *J Infect Dis* 172:672, 1995.
259 Grau O et al: Serum IgG antibodies specific to *Mycoplasma penetrans* Triton X-114-extracted antigen in homosexual men during the course of HIV infection. *IOM Letts* 4:72, 1996 (abstract).
260 Sasaki Y et al: In vitro influence of *Mycoplasma penetrans* on activation of peripheral T lymphocytes from healthy donors or human immunodeficiency virus-infected individuals. *Infect Immun* 63:4277, 1995.
261 Wang RY-H et al: *Mycoplasma penetrans* infection in male homosexuals with AIDS: high seroprevalence and association with Kaposi's sarcoma. *Clin Infect Dis* 17:724, 1993.
262 Lo S-C: Mycoplasmas and AIDS, in *Mycoplasmas: Molecular Biology and Pathogenesis,* J Maniloff et al (eds). Amer Soc Microbiol, Washington DC, 1992, 525.
263 Taylor-Robinson D et al: Are mycoplasmas involved in the pathogenesis of AIDS? *Hutième Colloque des Cent Gardes,* 1993, 11.
264 Blanchard A et al: AIDS-associated mycoplasmas. *Ann Rev Microbiol* 48:687, 1994.
265 Brenner C et al: Mycoplasmas and HIV infection: from epidemiology to their interaction with immune cells. *Frontiers in Bioscience* 1:42, 1996.
266 Tarr PI et al: Comparison of methods for the isolation of genital mycoplasmas from men. *J Infect Dis* 133:419, 1976.

267 Furr PM et al: Prevalence and significance of *Mycoplasma hominis* and *Ureaplasma urealyticum* in the urines of a non-venereal disease population. *Epidem Inf* 98:353, 1987.
268 Furr PM et al: The inhibitory effect of various antiseptics, analgesics and lubricants on mycoplasmas. *J Antimicrob Chemother* 8:115, 1981.
269 Smith TF et al: Recovery of chlamydia and genital mycoplasma transported in sucrose phosphate buffer and urease color test medium. *Health Lab Sci* 14:30, 1977.
270 Tully JG et al: Evaluation of culture media for the recovery of *Mycoplasma hominis* from the human urogenital tract. *Sex Transm Dis* 10(suppl):256, 1983.
271 Freundt EA: Culture media for classic mycoplasmas, in *Methods in Mycoplasmology,* Razin S et al. (eds). Academic Press, New York, 1983, 127.
272 Shepard MC: Culture media for ureaplasmas, in *Methods in Mycoplasmology,* Razin S et al. (eds). Academic Press, New York, 1983, 137.
273 Tully JG et al: Enhanced isolation of *Mycoplasma pneumoniae* from throat washings with a newly modified culture medium. *J Infect Dis* 139:478, 1979.
274 Taylor-Robinson D: Genital mycoplasma infections. *Clin Lab Med* 9:501, 1989.
275 Shepard MC et al: Differential agar medium (A7) for identification of *Ureaplasma urealyticum* (human T-mycoplasmas) in primary cultures of clinical material. *J Clin Microbiol* 3:613, 1976.
276 Shepard MC et al: Calcium chloride as an indicator for colonies of *Ureaplasma urealyticum. Pediatr Infect Dis* 5(suppl):349, 1986.
277 Renaudin H et al: Evaluation des systèmes *Mycoplasma* PLUS et SIR *Mycoplasma* pour la détéction quantitative et l'étude de la sensibilité aux antibiotiques des mycoplasma genitaux. *Pathol Biol* 38:431, 1990.
278 Clegg A et al: High rates of genital mycoplasma infection in the highlands of Papua New Guinea determined both by culture and by a commercial detection kit. *J Clin Microbiol* 35:197, 1997.
279 Clyde WA: Mycoplasma species identification based on growth inhibition by specific antisera. *J Immunol* 92:958, 1964.
280 Morrison-Plummer J et al: Molecular characterization of *Mycoplasma genitalium* species-specific and cross-reactive determinants: Identification of an immunodominant protein of *M. genitalium. Isr J Med Sci* 23:453, 1987.
281 Taylor-Robinson D: Serological identification of ureaplasmas from humans, in *Methods in Mycoplasmology,* S Razin et al (eds), Vol 1, Academic Press, New York, 1983, 57.
282 Furr PM et al: Microimmunofluorescence technique for detection of antibody to *Mycoplasma genitalium. J Clin Pathol* 37:1072, 1984.
283 Roberts MC et al: Tetracycline-resistant *Mycoplasma hominis* strains contain streptococcal tet M sequences. *Antimicrob Agents Chemother* 28:141, 1985.
284 Taylor-Robinson D et al: Antibiotic susceptibilities of mycoplasmas and treatment of mycoplasmal infections. *J Antimicrob Chemother* 40:622, 1997.
285 Evans RT et al: The incidence of tetracycline-resistant strains of *Ureaplasma urealyticum. J Antimicrob Chemother* 4:57, 1978.
286 Taylor-Robinson D et al: Clinical antibiotic resistance of *Ureaplasma urealyticum. Pediatr Infect Dis* 5(6 suppl):S335, 1986.
287 Roberts MC et al: Dissemination of the tetM tetracycline resistance determinant to *Ureaplasma urealyticum. Antimicrob Agents Chemother* 29:350, 1986.

Chapter 41

Enteric bacterial pathogens: *Shigella, Salmonella, Campylobacter*

C. M. Thorpe
Gerald T. Keusch

In recent years, the recognized spectrum of sexually transmitted diseases has been broadened considerably. Perhaps most notable among the "new" sexually transmitted disease organisms are those that cause enteritis or proctitis, especially in gay males (the "gay bowel syndrome"). The clinical aspects of these syndromes are discussed elsewhere in this volume; this chapter reviews the microbiology and epidemiology of the bacteria most commonly associated with sexually transmitted enteritis.

EPIDEMIOLOGY

From the time of Moses, in one of the earliest published epidemiological studies, it was recognized that to control diarrheal disease one must control the spread of feces in the environment.[1] The recognized circle of transmission from oral ingestion to anal excretion to oral ingestion of the organism has led some to categorize the enteric bacterial diseases as filth diseases, and the role of feces, fingers, flies, fomites, food, fluids, and more recently, various forms of fornication, is well known. However, it must be remembered that the epidemiology of the individual agents is as much a consequence of their specific biological properties as it is the result of environmental (or host) factors.

SHIGELLA

Shigella are highly host-adapted bacteria, named for the Japanese microbiologist, Kiyoshi Shiga, who first described the organism and proved its role in disease. *Shigella* are natural pathogens only of humans and certain species of higher primates, and as a consequence, one human infection is almost invariably traceable to another human, although the route may deviate through food, fluids, or other indirect paths.[2] Another feature of importance is the capacity of small inocula to cause symptomatic infection. Experimental infections of human volunteers with a few hundred to a few thousand viable organisms is easily accomplished.[3] Hence, the principal route of infection for *Shigella* is by person-to-person contact spread. Since convalescent or asymptomatic carriers may have 10^2 to 10^3 bacteria per gram of stool, and active cases excrete 10^5 to 10^8 *Shigella* per gram of stool, it is easy to see how anal–oral spread can readily occur among close contacts of cases or carriers.

First noted in 1974, homosexually transmitted shigellosis has since been documented in many large U.S. cities.[4–7] In contrast to trends in prevalence of *Shigella* species in the general U.S. population, where *S. sonnei* has increased over the past two decades to the point where over 80% of the isolates are this species,[2] *S. flexneri* has accounted for the majority of cases among homosexuals.[8] The magnitude of this association is reflected in a greater than fivefold increase in *S. flexneri* isolates in adult males over this time period, in comparison with no change or a decrease in women and children, respectively. In addition, the median age of the patient with *S. flexneri* increased from 5 to 26 years.[8] Although it cannot be proven that this increase is accounted for primarily by transmission among homosexuals, the evidence is consistent with this view.[9] Shigellosis is a colonic disease and the organism is able to invade this organ.[2,3] In orally acquired infection, colonic lesions are most prominent in the rectum and become progressively less severe as the ileocecal junction is approached, indicating a tropism for the most distal portion of the bowel.[10] Thus, it is possible that direct inoculation of *Shigella* during anal intercourse could result in infection of the susceptible rectal mucosa. Alternatively, the practices of either fellatio after anal intercourse, or anilingus, could also lead to transmission of an oral infectious inoculum. In San Francisco, where concern for HIV infection altered sexual practices among male homosexuals during the first decade of the AIDS epidemic, the incidence of shigellosis decreased by 30% among the target group in a study from the mid-1980s.[11] Recent studies to assess HIV risk behavior among various groups suggest that the widespread adoption of condom use, which occurred among gay men in the 1980s, is not being maintained in some gay or heterosexual populations.[12–15] The use of recreational drugs seems to play a role in reducing condom use among high-risk populations, especially inhalant nitrites and cocaine.[16] Increases in unsafe sex practices may result in another upsurge in sexual transmission of enteric diseases.

SALMONELLA

The genus *Salmonella* is named for Daniel Salmon, the head of the U.S. Department of Agriculture when the prototype organism, *Salmonella cholerasuis,* was isolated from swine with cholera-like diarrhea. Today, there are just two recognized species of *Salmonella, S. enterica* (composed of multiple subspecies and serovars distinguished by somatic and flagellar antigen serology) and *S. bongori* (which is of less clinical interest since this species contains nonhuman pathogens). Most human pathogenic *Salmonella* are included in one subspecies of *S. enterica,* also named *enterica.* Based on this taxonomy, the correct but awkward formal nomenclature for the most common *Salmonella* isolate in the United States is now *S. enterica* ssp *enterica* serovar *enteritidis.* For simplicity in this chapter we will use the italicized serovar designation as a surrogate for the proper name, referring in this example simply to *Salmonella enteritidis.* Approximately 50% of the isolates that cause infections in the United States are either *Salmonella typhimurium* or *Salmonella enteritidis,* and 10 serovars account for over 80% of all human isolates.

Infections caused by these organisms may be traced to another human host, but as these strains are not highly human host-adapted, food (especially poultry, eggs, milk, or water) is most often implicated, and their presentation is generally a food-borne gastroenteritis (often classified as food poisoning with fever). Common-source outbreaks have been documented for a number of vehicles, including dried and whole milk, milk chocolate, poultry, pork, shellfish, and powdered eggs.[17] The surface of hen's eggs and the interior of cracked eggs have been known to be an important source. However, grade A uncracked eggs can also be infected transovarially or via micropores in the shells after laying, may be persistently culture positive, and be the source of clinical infection.[18]

Although such vehicles account for most outbreaks, person-to-person spread occurs, particularly among male homosexuals. Like shigellosis, spread of *Salmonella* between male sexual partners is promoted by direct anal–oral sexual practices and fellatio after anal intercourse. The minimal infectious dose in normal adult volunteers is around 10^5 organisms; inoculum size is reduced by 100-fold or more if it is protected in food or other vehicles with buffering capacity. Influencing this are such host factors as gastric acidity, composition of the normal bacterial flora, and age of the host.[17] Because acid pH rapidly and significantly reduces viability of salmonellae, the intermediate infectious dose needed and the efficacy of the normal gastric acid barrier may protect most individuals from direct transmission of *Salmonella* gastroenteritis during sexual activity. However, hypochlorhydric subjects or post-gastrectomy patients are clearly at greater risk of *Salmonella* infections, by whatever route of transmission.

Salmonella typhi and other causes of enteric fever are highly host-adapted to humans, and here the epidemiological route is always traceable to another human, whether a case or a carrier. Many interesting, intricate, and ingenious routings, however, can be involved in transmitting the inoculum to a susceptible new human host, but usually food or water vehicles are the direct carrier of the infecting dose. Volunteer studies using the virulent Quailes strain have demonstrated that at least 10^5 organisms in bicarbonate buffer are required to produce disease under these conditions. Although most typhoid fever in the United States is acquired abroad, the similarity in transmission between typhoid and nontyphoidal salmonellosis suggests that sexual transmission is possible.

CAMPYLOBACTER

The classification of *Campylobacter* has evolved considerably since 1963 when the first human isolates of this curved vibrio-like Gram-negative rod were assigned to the genus *Campylobacter* (derived from the Greek *campylo*, "curved," and *bacter*, "rod").[19] *Campylobacter* can be conveniently divided into two major groups on the basis of catalase activity; human pathogens are found only among the catalase-positive species (Table 41-1). The human pathogens can be further divided according to temperature tolerance. The existence of thermophilic species, defined as the ability to grow at 42 but not 25°C, was first reported by King in 1957, who described a group of "related Vibrios" exhibiting this property.[20] Since then, the use of better selective media has permitted the isolation and identification of several new species among thermophilic *Campylobacters*, including the most common species causing human illness, the hippurate-positive *C. jejuni*.[21] Two hippurate-negative thermophilic strains also cause human infection, *C. coli* and *C. lari* (formerly called *C. laridis*), the latter distinguished in part because of its nalidixic acid and cephalothin resistance.[22] However, because nalidixic acid-resistant strains of *C. jejuni* and *C. coli* are being seen with increasing frequency, this test no longer clearly distinguishes these strains from *C. lari*.[23] The thermophilic strains *C. jejuni* and *C. coli* account for almost all clinical isolates in most series.[24] A "thermo-intolerant" species, *C. fetus*, which grows well at temperatures ranging from 25 to 37°C, and is a rare cause of septicemic human infection, causes chronic bacteremic infections in gay men or immunocompromised hosts.

Human infections typically result from ingestion of contaminated food or liquids. *C. jejuni* is rapidly killed by gastric acid, but can survive for weeks in chilled milk or water.[25] The most common sources of infection are unpasteurized milk, undercooked poultry, and contaminated water sources. In common source outbreaks, around 25% of those exposed generally develop clinical illness. This is interesting since, in experimental studies in humans, ingestion of as few as 80 organisms can transmit *C. jejuni*.[26]

A second group of bacteria resembling *C. jejuni* were isolated from patients with diarrhea, especially from male homosexuals.[27] Although they resembled typical *Campylobacter* in being catalase- and oxidase-positive, microaerophilic, motile, curved Gram-negative rods, they could be distinguished by a distinct colonial morphology, and differences in some biochemical reactions and in growth temperature requirements.[28] For this reason they were designated "Campylobacter-like organisms" (CLOs); however, some CLOs have now been sufficiently characterized to raise them to species status. In some clinical series, *C. cinaedi* (formerly CLO type 1) and *C. fennelliae* (formerly CLO type 2) are the most common isolate from patients with "gay bowel syndrome."[29] However, because they are cephalothin sensitive, these organisms are likely to be missed if cephalothin-containing *Campylobacter* selective media are used.[27,30] A third related species, *C. upsaliensis*, has been described as an important cause of diarrhea.[31] It may be missed by the laboratory because it does not grow at 42°C and is not isolated on *Campylobacter* selective media. When looked for, *C. upsaliensis* appears to be an important cause of diarrhea in HIV-infected patients.[32]

On the U.S. West coast, the isolation rates for *C. jejuni* among homosexual men with diarrhea have been in the range of 5 to 10%.[33,34] In one of these studies, a variety of enteric pathogens were also found in two-fifths of asymptomatic homosexual subjects.[34] Together with the frequent finding of nonpathogenic protozoa in these asymptomatic gay men, this suggests the intensity of their exposure to infected feces. Another study carried out on the U.S. East coast found asymptomatic carriage of enteric pathogens in 12% of a sample of gay men.[35] Men who were pathogen positive, however, were more likely to be HIV seropositive than men without a pathogen, again suggesting that there is a more intense exposure to fecal pathogens as well as HIV-infected fluids among men who do not practice safe sex. A less likely explanation is that people with HIV are more likely to be colonized with enteric path-

Table 41-1. Classification of the Genus *Campylobacter*: Selected Characteristics

	Drug sensitivity					Growth temperature	
Species	Nalidixic acid	Cephalothin	Hippurate	H_2S	Nitrate	25°C	42°C
C. fetus	R	S	−	−	+	+	−
C. jejuni	S*	R	+	−	+	−	+
C. coli	S*	R	−	−	+	−	+
C. lari	R	R	−	−	+	−	+
C. cinaedi	S	S	−	−	+	−	−
C. fennelliae	S	S	−	−	−	−	−
C. hyointestinalis	R	S	−	+	+	±	+

R = resistance; S = susceptible; * indicates that resistant strains are being identified, resulting in classification difficulties.

Table 41-2. Relative Severity of Infections Owing to the Genus *Shigella*: Clinical Manifestations

	Frequency of isolation in the United States	Dysentery	Diarrhea	Hemolytic uremic syndrome	Other intestinal
S. dysenteriae type 1	Nil*	++++	++	+	+
S. flexneri	20–30%	++	+++	±	+
S. boydii	Nil	++	+++	0	+
S. sonnei	70–80%	+	++++	0	+

* Isolation of *S. dysenteriae* type 1 in the United States is rare and associated with travel from an endemic area of the world.

ogens than the normal population because of their underlying immunocompromise.

CLINICAL MANIFESTATIONS

Clinical manifestations infections caused by *Shigella, Salmonella,* and *Campylobacter* overlap, although there are distinctive features that help the clinician make a presumptive diagnosis.

SHIGELLA

Shigella are the classic cause of bacillary dysentery, a clinical syndrome characterized by the frequent passage of small volumes of frankly bloody, mucoid stools, accompanied by abdominal cramps, tenesmus, and fever.[36] Most episodes of shigellosis actually begin with watery diarrhea, which may or may not progress to the dysentery syndrome, largely dependent on the species involved (Table 41-2). *Shigella dysenteriae* type 1 causes the most severe illness, often progressing so rapidly from diarrhea to dysentery that the watery diarrhea stage is not even noticed, whereas *S. sonnei* generally causes only a self-limited watery diarrhea. *S. flexneri,* the predominant isolate in the homosexual population, is more virulent than *S. sonnei*, causing a much greater inflammatory response more commonly associated with bloody diarrhea and dysentery. New manifestations are also being seen in these patients. For example, a case of cutaneous shigellosis has been reported in a 22-year-old male homosexual who presented with a tender penile furuncle from which a pure culture of *S. flexneri* was isolated.[37]

SALMONELLA

Salmonella cause four clinical types of infection: acute gastroenteritis, enteric (typhoid) fever, septicemia with or without focal systemic lesions, as well as the asymptomatic carrier state (Table 41-3).[38] Enteric fever has become uncommon in the United States as the number of human host reservoirs has diminished, owing in large part to improved sanitation and case detection. There are now only some 500 cases per year, the vast majority of which are now imported from endemic areas abroad. The number of cases of salmonella gastroenteritis, however, has increased greatly over the past decade, primarily because of increasing use of potentially contaminated processed foods, the marked increase in the prevalence of *S. enteriditis* in hens' eggs, and poor food-storage practices that favor the multiplication of microorganisms.

Clinical manifestations of salmonella gastroenteritis, include fever, chills, headache, nausea, vomiting, abdominal pain, and diarrhea, and usually begin 24 to 48 hours after the organism is ingested.[39] Sporadic cases are generally not investigated by means of cultures and therefore go undiagnosed; in contrast, large common-source outbreaks are usually well studied by the public health system. Bacteremia is often detected if blood cultures are obtained early in the infection, and in the immunocompetent host is transient unless the isolate is a particularly invasive serovar, such as *S. dublin*. In AIDS patients, however, any *Salmonella* serovar can potentially cause clinically severe and continuous bacteremic illness.

Salmonella diarrhea is generally watery, often containing mucus and only on occasion, blood as well. Microscopic examination of the stool usually reveals a few red blood cells and large numbers of leukocytes.[17] In the rare patient, typical dysenteric symptoms

Table 41-3. Clinical Manifestations of Different Salmonella Serovars by Serogroup: Clinical Syndrome

Serogroup	Serovar	Host range (preference)	Acute gastroenteritis	Enteric fever	Septicemia	Focal invasive infections
A	Paratyphi A	Narrow (humans)	0	++	++++*	+†
B	Paratyphi B	Narrow (humans)	0	++	++++*	+†
B	Typhimurium	Broad‡	+++	±	+	+
B	Cholerasuis	Narrow (swine)	0	0	++++	++
C	Paratyphi C	Narrow (humans)	0	++	++++*	+†
D	Dublin	Broad‡	++	0	+++	+++
D	Enteritidis	Broad‡	++++	0	0	0
D	Typhi	Narrow (humans)	0	++++	++++*	++†

* Bacteremia occurs as part of the enteric fever syndrome.
† Invasion of gallbladder and Peyer's patches occur as part of the enteric fever syndrome.
‡ Most gastroenteritis strains are typically nonhost-adapted with a broad range of host perference.

can occur, including frankly bloody stools, tenderness over the sigmoid colon, and tenesmus. As in shigellosis, endoscopic examination of patients with *Salmonella* dysentery reveals colonic mucosal edema, hyperemia, friability, and petechial hemorrhages. Histological studies of colonic biopsies from these patients show mucosal inflammation, crypt abscess, and focal epithelial necrosis.[40,41]

CAMPYLOBACTER

Campylobacter jejuni causes a spectrum of illness resembling shigellosis, from self-limiting watery diarrhea to febrile bloody diarrhea with abdominal pain.[21,42,43] Diarrhea is often preceded by a prodromal febrile period and is accompanied by nausea, malaise, headache, myalgia, backache, and abdominal pain. After a day or so, the pain becomes colicky and diarrhea begins. Although frank blood or mucus is not frequently observed, microscopic examination demonstrates the presence of erythrocytes in most patients along with many inflammatory cells, as in *Salmonella* diarrhea. The fever is often short-lived, and acute diarrhea usually subsides in 2 to 3 days. In around 10% of patients, the abdominal pain and tenderness persists, or recurrent fever or diarrhea occurs. In some patients the intensity of abdominal pain and tenderness, accompanied by bloody diarrhea, leukocytosis with a left shift, and an elevated erythrocyte sedimentation rate, leads to the diagnosis of an acute surgical abdomen. Although appendicitis may indeed be present at laparotomy, more often only diffuse bowel inflammation and mesenteric adenitis are found. Sigmoidoscopy will reveal erythema, edema, granularity, exudation, and focal contact bleeding of colonic mucosa. Histologic examination is consistent with acute colitis, and toxic dilatation has been reported in such patients.[44,45]

Clinical disease owing to CLOs is similar to *C. jejuni*, with diarrhea, abdominal cramps, bloody stool, and even tenesmus. Proctocolitis is evident by endoscopic examination and histological examination of tissue biopsies, associated with anal discharge, pain, and fever. Mucosal friabilitiy, ulcers, crypt abscesses, and inflammation of the lamina propria are all present, similar to other bacterial inflammatory bowel diseases. These organisms are systemically invasive in homosexual men, in whom they can be isolated from blood, associated with systemic symptoms including fever, chills, and arthralgias.[46] *C. hyointestinalis*, previously believed to be a pathogen restricted to swine, has also been isolated from a male homosexual with proctitis.[47] This organism is similar to *C. fetus*, except that it produces H_2S in triple sugar iron agar, is often pigmented, and does not grow well at 25°C. Identification can be confirmed by other, more complex, laboratory tests.

Systemic invasion

All three of these pathogens can cause clinically severe bacteremia and persistent enteric infection in the setting of the acquired immune deficiency syndrome (AIDS). Shigellemia, previously considered a rare event in shigellosis, has been seen with increased frequency over the past decade with both *S. flexneri* and *S. dysenteriae* in the setting of immunocompromise.[48,49] Salmonella and possibly *Campylobacter* infections tend to be more severe, recurrent, or persistent when they occur in the HIV-positive host, often associated with bacterial infection outside the bowel. Recurrent *Salmonella* septicemia is well-described in the HIV-infected host, and usually occurs relatively late in the course of the disease.[51] In recognition of this, recurrent *Salmonella* septicemia has become part of the CDC surveillance definition of AIDS-defining illnesses.[52] The incidence of *Salmonella* bacteremia in the HIV-infected population is estimated to be between 46 and 384 per 100,00 persons, which is 100- to 1000-fold above the general population incidence of approximately 0.3 per 100,000. Not all *Salmonella* species are associated with more severe disease, and *Salmonella typhi*, for example, does not appear to be more invasive in immunosuppressed HIV patients.

Campylobacter infections are more likely to occur in patients with AIDS, with an incidence of laboratory-confirmed infection among AIDS patients of 519 cases per 100,000 population per year, which is almost 40 times the rate in the general population.[53] It is not established whether *Campylobacter* infections are more likely to be invasive in the HIV-infected; however, there are reports of *C. fetus, C. cinaedi, C. fennelliae,* and *C. lari* bacteremia in the HIV-infected patient.[50]

GROWTH, PHYSIOLOGY, AND CULTURE

SHIGELLA

The genus *Shigella* belongs to the tribe Eschericheae in the family Enterobacteriaceae and is closely related to *Escherichia coli*. Unlike *E. coli*, however, they are nonmotile and do not ferment lactose, although *S. sonnei* is able to do so slowly. Surprisingly for the potent illness they cause, shigellae are not very hardy bacteria; they do not survive well in high atmospheric temperatures, are subject to desiccation, may be overgrown by the acid-producing fecal flora, and quickly and quietly die in acidic stools.

Routine isolation and identification of *Shigella* in feces involves the use of selective media for presumptive diagnosis, followed by biochemical and serological agglutination reactions to confirm identity. Selective media are employed in order to suppress the growth of components of the normal fecal flora that might otherwise overgrow the pathogen, and to detect lactose fermentation by means of a color reaction, allowing a simplified search for nonlactose fermenting colonies. A variety of media have been developed for this purpose, such as MacConkey's bile salt, xylose-lysine-deoxycholate (XLD), Hektoen enteric (HE), and tergitol-7-triphenyltetrazolium chloride (T7T) agars. The yield of positives is enhanced by using more than one selective medium and by preliminary enrichment incubation in broth inhibitory to nonpathogens, such as Hajna's Gram-negative (GN) broth before plating to selective agar. Stool samples that cannot be rapidly processed should be inoculated to a holding medium, such as buffered glycerol-saline transport medium.

Lactose-negative colonies are picked and screened for their ability to ferment glucose (*Shigella* are positive) and produce gas (nearly all *Shigella* are negative). Triple sugar iron (TSI) agar slants are frequently used for this purpose. Glucose fermentation in the anaerobic portion of the tube, the butt, produces acid that turns the pH indicator yellow, whereas the slant exposed to the air remains red (alkaline) because the organism cannot aerobically metabolize lactose or sucrose. This pattern is identical to that of *Salmonella*; however, because the medium also detects H_2S production as a black reaction product (ferrous sulfide), the typically H_2S-positive *Salmonella* stand out from the H_2S-negative *Shigella*. The presumptive diagnosis of *Shigella* is supported by the lack of motility and may be confirmed by agglutination reactions using antisera to the group antigens of *S. dysenteriae* (A), *S. flexneri* (B), *S. boydii* (C), or *S. sonnei* (D). Further biochemical and serological identification is unnecessary for routine purposes, but may be useful for outbreak investigations.

SALMONELLA

The genus *Salmonella* is classified in the tribe Salmonellaeae, in the family Enterobacteriaceae. Like *Shigella*, *Salmonella* ferment glucose but not lactose or sucrose, and they are facultatively anaerobic. Unlike the former, *Salmonella* are invariably motile and almost always H_2S-positive. The strategy to isolate *Salmonella* is similar to that adopted for *Shigella*, using selective media and screening for the lactose-negative phenotype. *Salmonella* grow well on minimally selective media (such as MacConkey's), moderately selective media (including XLD, HE, and SS), and even on highly selective media (such as bismuth sulfite). Therefore, the latter is the most effective selective medium for isolating *Salmonella*, including *S. typhi*. Tetrathionate and selenite-F broth enrichment media are also satisfactory for *Salmonella* but are inhibitory to many *Shigella*.

However, identification of *Salmonella* to the serovar level is not simple. *S. typhi* is one of the readily identified serovars because it gives a characteristic alkaline slant-acid butt TSI pattern with no gas produced and just a trace of H_2S. Confirmation is obtained by negative citrate and ornithine decarboxylase reactions, and by serology. All of the rest of the more than 2300 members of the species *S. enterica* are distinguished by a combination of biochemical reactions and serological tests for somatic (O), and flagellar (H) antigens. Individual *Salmonella* possess multiple O and H antigens that result in agglutination reactions with specific antisera. Of all the *Salmonella*, *S. typhi* and *S. paratyphi* C alone possess an important capsular or envelope antigen named Vi, and the detection of Vi restricts the possibilities to these two organisms. The problem for routine diagnosis is that few non-reference laboratories maintain the necessary diversity of typing sera. Instead, clinical laboratories commonly use serogrouping, which is based on agglutination reactions using polyvalent grouping sera containing antibody to the major O antigens in the serogroup. These serogroups are designated by capital letters, A, B, C, and so on. Knowing that a gastroenteritis isolate is group B suggests it is *S. typhimurium*, whereas a group D isolate would suggest *S. enteritidis*, because these two organisms are the most common isolates. Serovar identity depends on distinguishing the pattern of H antigens present; however, this is much more difficult. In addition to needing a large number of individual typing sera, the organisms must be grown in broth culture to increase motility and develop flagellar antigens; only then can the ability of specific anti-H antibodies to immobilize the isolate be determined.

Fortunately, 75 to 80% of infections are caused by only 10 serotypes, and procedures using a small number of individual and pooled typing sera can be tailored to these limited number of possibilities. Identification of rare isolates is of particular value for surveillance and epidemiological studies; however, the diseases they cause are generally indistinguishable on clinical grounds. Reference public health laboratories, including state public health laboratories and the Centers for Diseases Control are available to carry out these studies in the United States.

CAMPYLOBACTER

The genus is composed of highly motile, oxidase-positive, curved Gram-negative rods. These properties originally suggested their identity as a *Vibrio*; however, *Campylobacter* are microaerophilic and nonfermentative, have a distinctive DNA composition, grow optimally in 5 to 6% O_2, grow poorly in air or under anaerobic conditions, and require CO_2, which distinguishes them from *Vibrios*. Antibiotic selective media were originally instrumental for the isolation of *Campylobacter jejuni*, but this precludes the growth of CLO species, which are quite sensitive to cephalothin used in many *Campylobacter*-selective media. Improved isolation of *Campylobacter* species may be achieved by growth on membrane filters.[54] A wet mount of fresh stool may reveal the characteristic darting, corkscrew motility of the organism under phase contrast microscopy, but the validity of this rapid method clearly depends on the experience of the observer.

Once isolated, identification of different *Campylobacter* species in the clinical laboratory relies on a few simple procedures, including growth characteristics at 25, 37, and 42°C, hippurate hydrolysis, nitrate reduction, H_2S production, and susceptibility to nalidixic acid and cephalothin (see Table 41-1). Unfortunately, results may not be clearcut because the test results can be variable, in part related to consistency of performance; for example, steady incubator temperature for temperature tolerance tests or use of fresh reagents for H_2S production. Distinguishing *C. jejuni* and *C. coli* from *C. lari* may also be difficult as increasing numbers of nalidixic acid resistant *C. jejuni* and *C. coli* are being isolated.[55] Unusual or uncertain isolates, including CLOs and in particular *C. hyointestinalis*, generally need to be sent to a reference laboratory for confirmation. PCR amplification of 23S rDNA sequences has improved the potential to identify these isolates and in the future this methodology is likely to be employed in clinical studies.

STRATEGY FOR ISOLATION OF ENTERIC PATHOGENS

Screening all stool samples from patients with diarrhea for *Shigella, Salmonella,* and *Campylobacter* has not been shown to be cost-effective. In one study in a University Hospital laboratory, the cost per positive culture was over $250, and pathogens were isolated in less than 10% of the stools examined.[56] However, when stools were screened first for fecal leukocytes and only the positives were plated, the cost per positive was reduced to $30, and 75% of the samples yielded a pathogen. Addition of patient-selection criteria may improve this further. For example, male homosexuals who present with proctitis should have the stool cultured on media that permit islation of *Campylobacter cinaedi, C. fennelliae,* and *C. lari*.

PATHOGENESIS

All of these organisms share a basic virulence trait that influences the kind of disease they produce, the ability to penetrate intestinal epithelial cells and cause tissue pathology.[57] Although there has been much progress in understanding the invasion mechanism, the more it is studied the greater is the apparent complexity. Differences in the site of and response to invasion among the pathogens also indicates that there are major biological differences between them. Invasion properties are clearly related to the small infectious dose of these organisms for humans, which is a crucial factor in the direct sexual transmission of infection. Various types of enterotoxins have been described in the three organisms; however, their role in pathogenesis remains uncertain.

SHIGELLA

The major pathology in shigellosis is in the colon, and this infection should be considered to be an inflammatory colitis owing to microbial invasion of the intestinal mucosa resulting in mucosal edema, hemorrhage, infiltration by inflammatory cells, hyperplasia of the crypt epithelium, and mucus discharge from goblet cells. Damage, death, and sloughing of epithelial cells lead to an inflammatory exudate in the colonic lumen and the stool.[58] This process requires the organism to invade the epithelium; deletion of genes required for invasion blocks pathogenesis of the disease process and no clinical manifestations occur.

However, in order to reach the colon, the organism must survive the gastric acid barrier. Recent studies have demonstrated that *Shigella* acquire the capacity to resist the lethal effects of acid as they reach the stationary phase in the growth curve. A set of genes associated with the expression of phase-specific sigma factor (sigma s) has been identified that regulate this property and permit transfer of the acid-resistant phenotype to an acid-sensitive recipient organism.[59] Because stationary phase growth is reached as the organism is excreted from the infected host into the environment, the acquisition of acid resistance at this precise time may directly benefit the organism. For example, this property would better equip *Shigella* to survive transit across the gastric acid barrier following ingestion by a new host. This feature of the growth cycle may account, at least in part, for the known extremely low oral infectious dose for *Shigella* spp.

Once past the stomach, *Shigella* transit to the colon where they invade the mucosa by inducing intestinal mucosal cells to initiate phagocytosis through signals transmitted by a group of microbial surface proteins called invasion plasmid antigens, or Ipas.[60] Although invasion of the mucosa was previously thought to occur at the epithelial cell apical membrane, more recent studies using cultured human intestinal epithelial cells demonstrate that the organisms cannot breach the microvillus surface, although they are able to invade from the serosal (basal) surface. In vivo experimental infections suggest that the most likely site of the initial invasion is the specialized antigen processing M cell. Once the organism has reached the basal surface of the epithelial cells it can then directly invade the epithelial cells from the lamina propria. The basis for the specificity of *Shigella* for invasion of colonic cells is not understood.

Like phagocytosis by leukocytes, microbial invasion of epithelial cells occurs within a host membrane bound vesicle. Invasion is quickly followed by lysis of the vesicle, multiplication of the bacteria within the cytoplasm, and direct spread to adjacent cells. As cell-to-cell spread continues, cell death ensues, apparently owing to apoptosis initiated in the process, which leads to the macroscopic epithelial ulcerations that are the pathologic hallmark of *Shigella* infection. Cell invasion, lysis, and ulceration are generally confined to the terminal ileum and colon, and there is clear tropism for the more distal segments of the colon, and the intensity of infection is greatest in the rectum and distal colon.[61]

In all *Shigella* species, the ability to invade host cells is controlled by multiple virulence genes, both structural and regulatory, that are encoded on plasmids as well as the chromosome.[62] Host cell actin and plastin, a host protein that bundles actin filaments into parallel bundles, co-localize in protrusions from the infected host cell containing the organism that lead to invasion of adjacent cells. The presence of these host proteins provide a glimpse into the organism's ability to subvert host mechanisms in order to achieve microbial invasion.[63] It is noteworthy that this process of cell-to-cell spread occurs entirely within the intracellular milieu, without a need for the organism to exit the host cell to reach the next target.

It was formerly thought that the intense inflammatory response in shigellosis was in response to host epithelial cell death, and therefore a mechanism to protect the host. Recent studies have totally redefined the paradigm of inflammation in shigellosis, and now it appears that the inflammatory response not only occurs early but is required if infection is going to lead to clinical disease.[64] After initial invasion of the lamina propria, the bacteria encounter macrophages which, in the process of ingesting them, become activated to secrete IL-1 and other cytokines.[65] In fact, there is a broad inflammatory cytokine response in plasma, mucosa, and intestinal secretions, which persists for weeks and lasts well into convalescence.[66,67] This may provide an explanation of prolonged anorexia in shigellosis, which contributes to the prolonged negative nitrogen balances in this infection.[68] The cytokine response also results in the recruitment of leukocytes that invade the epithelial layer from the basal side. This is associated with a marked increase in microbial translocation in the opposite direction across the epithelial layer. If the inflammatory cascade is interrupted, either by blocking the action of IL-1 using IL-1 receptor antagonist, or by preventing the chemokinesis of leukocytes by blocking the neutrophil surface antigen, CD18, with specific antibody, the subsequent inflammatory reaction is inhibited, microbial invasion is reduced, and clinical manifestations are prevented in animal models.[64,69] Thus, it is clearly the inflammatory response itself which leads to the major bacterial invasion across the mucosa, subsequent mass invasion of the epithelial cells from the basal surface, and extension of mucosal lesions as cell-to-cell invasion continues.

Because *Shigella* are non-motile, movement within cells and between adjacent cells is mediated by a complex interaction with the host cell cytoskeleton. Once the organisms are released from the phagocytic vesicle by lysis, an ATPase activity called IcsA, one of the products of a set of genes involved in intracellular spread (hence, IcsA), is expressed in the polar region of multiplying organisms.[70] This spatial localization of IcsA is now known to be owing to the action of an outer membrane protease, SopA, which cleaves IcsA at other sites on the surface of the organism, but not at the pole of dividing organisms.[71] As a consequence, actin polymerization occurs only at the pole where IcsA is present. In turn, this results in a jet-like propulsive force, termed the "actin motor," which pushes the organism in the direction opposite to the site of continuing actin deposition.[60] This process has been visualized by the use of fluorescein-tagged phalloidin, a fungal product that binds specifically to polymerized F-actin, revealing a comet-like tail streaming behind the moving organism. The force generated is sufficient to drive the bacterium across the cell cytoplasm to the plasma membrane, where an interaction with the host's calcium-dependent cell adhesin, cadherin, is required for the organism, still covered by the membrane of the originally infected host cell, to protrude into the adjacent host cell.[72] When these overlying host membranes subsequently pinch off, and the double membrane vesicle lyses, the organism enters the cytoplasm of the newly invaded cell.

Protein toxins may also contribute to disease pathogenesis. The best known, Shiga toxin produced by *S. dysenteriae* type 1, an inhibitor of eukaryotic cell protein synthesis resulting in target cell death, is present in the stool of dysentery patients.[73] It is believed that the toxin translocates from the bowel lumen to the systemic circulation, where it targets microvascular endothelial cells in the intestine and the renal glomerulus.[74] Endothelial cell damage contributes to the development of bloody stools and is the essential lesion in pathogenesis of hemolytic-uremic syndrome, a thrombotic renal microangiopathy that occurs in as many as 5% of patients infected by *S. dysenteriae* type 1.[73] Shiga toxin also targets differentiated intestinal villus epithelial cells in vitro that express a neutral glycolipid toxin receptor, but not less differentiated crypt-like cells.[75] This targeting results in villus cell damage and a reduction in the normal sodium absorptive function of these cells without altering the chloride secretion by the crypt cells. The net effect is the retention of sodium and water in the bowel lumen, which may contribute to the initial watery diarrhea phase of this illness. However, other Shigella species do not produce Shiga toxin and other mechanisms must be invoked for the watery diarrhea they cause, for example, two newly described Shigella enterotoxins. The first, Shet1, is encoded by a chromosomal gene in *S. flexneri* 2a but is not present in other Shigella species or *S. flexneri* serotypes.[76] The other, Shet2, is encoded by a plasmid gene and is highly homologous to a previously described plasmid-encoded toxin produced by enteroinvasive (Shigella-like) *E. coli*.[77] Both of these toxins have weak enterotoxic activity in vitro, and although humans develop neutralizing antibody when infected by toxin positive strains, which indicates the production of the antigen during the illness, it is unclear whether they play any role in pathogenesis of the clinical illness.

SALMONELLA

Although the minimum oral infectious dose of gastroenteritis strains of *Salmonella* in normal adult volunteers is around 10^5 organisms when the inoculum is given in an isotonic salt solution containing bicarbonate buffer, the infectious dose in natural infections may be much lower because the inoculum is usually ingested with food, which acts as a strong buffer against stomach acid. Recent evidence suggests that gastric acid may be an environmental signal used by the microorganism to initiate synthesis of virulence factors, and low pH is now known to transcriptionally upregulate at least 40 *Salmonella* genes.[78] Such signals appear to be a common mechanism used by microbes to regulate virulence genes, which are unnecessary for the organism's survival and growth outside the host. Although the role of these acid-regulated proteins in pathogenesis is still unclear, the postulate is that organisms surviving the acidic environment of the stomach have enhanced virulence properties when they enter the small bowel. Once in the host intestinal tract, virulent *Salmonella* are able to resist the lethal effects of cryptins, cationic antimicrobial peptides secreted by Paneth cells of the small bowel that permeabilize the bacterial cell membrane.[79,80] The implication of this finding is that serovars that cannot resist cryptin action are avirulent because the host is able to dispatch the bacterium. Secretory immunoglobulin A may also play a role in preventing *Salmonella* invasion.[81]

In contrast to shigellosis, salmonellosis is characterized by the translocation of organisms across the intestinal wall without disruption of the mucosal permeability barrier. Thus, this example of "bacterial-mediated endocytosis" must be distinct from the process by which *Shigella* are taken up. Molecular studies of *Salmonella* invasion mechanisms have been done with just a few serovars, primarily using *S. typhimurium*.[82,83] As far as known, the invasion process in *S. typhimurium* is similar to both other nontyphoidal salmonellas and *S. typhi*. Critical to this process is an invasion locus on the *Salmonella* chromosome termed *inv*, comprised of at least 14 genes that regulate the assembly and disassembly of appendages on the bacterial cell surface.[82,83] Assembly of these bacterial appendages is followed by host–cell membrane ruffling, the visual consequence of cytoskeletal rearrangements mediated by protein phosphorylations induced by the host–pathogen interaction. Disassembly of the appendages is also required for microbial uptake and transcytosis to occur. *Salmonella* then transit through the epithelial cell within membrane-bound vacuoles from the brush border to the basal membrane without multiplication or apparently harming the cell which they have traversed. In these properties, *Salmonella* invasion clearly differs from that of *Shigella*.

Nontyphoidal serovars may be recovered from the blood stream early in infection, unlike *S. typhi*, which is rapidly sequestered in host macrophages and cleared from circulation.[38,39] *S. typhi* subsequently causes a persistent bacteremia, which initiates the febrile clinical illness. After the initial bacteremia, nontyphoidal *Salmonella* are cleared and killed by normal host defenses, except for a few particularly invasive serovars (*S. typhimurium, S. enteritidis, S. dublin,* and *S. cholerasuis*).[39] The latter serovars possess virulence plasmids that promote multiplication in extra-intestinal tissues.[84] These plasmids all contain a highly conserved 8-kb region of DNA encoding a locus called *spv*, for *Salmonella* plasmid virulence, including at least four structural genes, *spv*ABCD, and a positive regulator, *spv*R. Another gene on the virulence plasmid, *rck*, mediates resistance to complement by blocking assembly of the terminal membrane attack complex on the bacterial surface.

Serovars causing invasive disease, including typhoid fever, require the ability to survive and multiply intracellularly within macrophages. One microbial locus promoting *Salmonella* survival within macrophages is *phoP/phoQ*, which consists of two genes, *phoP* and *phoQ*, which serves as a sensor for environmental signals and a regulator for adaptive response genes.[85,86] It is the adaptive regulated response of PhoP/Q regulated *Salmonella* genes that results in bacterial resistance to macrophage microbicidal mechanisms.

Host factors are also involved in determining the intracellular survival of *Salmonella* within the macrophage. The first host genetic locus regulating the host response to *Salmonella* was described on chromosome 1 in mice and named *ity* for its role in immunity and susceptibility to *S. typhimurium*, which actually causes a typhoid-like intracellular disease in mice.[87] Loci with similar functions in murine models using leishmania (*lsh* locus) and the mycobacterial vaccine strain, BCG (*bcg* locus) were described by other workers but later found to be descriptions of the same genetic region, which came to be known as *ity/lsh/bcg*. With the discovery of the human homologue genes, the locus has been renamed Nramp, for natural resistance-associated macrophage protein.[88] Nramp is presently known to consist of a family of at least three genes encoding a macrophage-specific membrane transport protein.[89]

CAMPYLOBACTER

Our understanding of the pathogenic mechanisms of *Campylobacter* lags behind that of *Shigella* and *Salmonella*; however, this is the subject of active investigation. In experimental human infections, a *Shigella*-like inoculum of around a hundred organisms is sufficient to cause disease in some volunteers.[26] Such small infectious doses are a property associated with organisms that have inducible acid tolerance responses and are invasive. There are some studies on *Campylobacter* invasion determinants, but none are purified thus far.[90,91] In reality, neither invasion or acid resistance have been well studied in *Campylobacter* species.

C. jejuni produces an enterotoxin that bears a resemblance to cholera toxin. Most watery-diarrhea-producing clinical isolates produce this heat-labile enterotoxin.[25] Similarities to cholera toxin include molecular weight (60–70 kDa), binding to GM1 ganglioside, ability to elongate CHO cells in culture (a property associated with activation of adenylate cyclase and increased intracellular cyclic AMP), similar B subunits, fluid secretion (enterotoxin activity) in suitable animal intestinal models, and neutralization by both anti-cholera toxin and anti-*E. coli* heat labile enterotoxin antibody.[25,92] Purification of the *C. jejuni* enterotoxin has not yet been reported and studies with strains in which the toxin is genetically altered have yet to be done.

Cytotoxicity can also be demonstrated by some *C. jejuni* culture supernatants.[93,94] The pathogenic significance of this toxin is unclear, as isolates causing diarrhea in children and animal models do not generally produce cytotoxin in vitro.[24,95] In some studies, this toxin is neutralized by antibody to Shiga toxin; however, the gene for the latter has not been detected in *Campylobacter* strains.[96] Interestingly, *Campylobacter* have been isolated from patients with hemolytic–uremic syndrome, which is strongly associated with Shiga toxin-producing organisms.[97,98] An alternative explanation, aside from toxin production by *Campylobacter*, is that the cause of the *Campylobacter*-associated hemolytic–uremic syndrome was undetected coinfection with a Shiga toxin producing serotype of *E. coli*.

Studies have been undertaken to determine the role of flagella in the interaction of *C. jejuni* with epithelial cells. Early results have shown that flagella are not involved in adherence of *C. jejuni* to epithelial cells but that one of the products of the flagellin gene, *fla A*, is required for internalization of *C. jejuni* by epithelial cells in vitro.[99]

ANTIMICROBIAL SUSCEPTIBILITY

SHIGELLA

Treatment of *Shigella* with appropriate and effective antibiotics decreases symptoms and may interrupt person-to-person spread. Many studies have established that, for *Shigella*, appropriate means an antibiotic that results in effective concentrations of the drug in both the lumen and the mucosa itself. Nonabsorbable antibiotics have been proved inferior because they cannot act on the invasive bacterial population in the tissues. The question of what constitutes an appropriate antibiotic today is not so easily answered, as antibiotic resistance in *Shigella* isolates has become increasingly important, both in North America and abroad.[100,101] The progressive acquisition by *Shigella* species of resistance to common, inexpensive antimicrobials, such as trimethoprim-sulfamethoxazole and ampicillin has created a problem, especially in the developing world, where oral therapy for some strains, in particular *S. dysenteriae* type 1 and *S. flexneri*, is now feasible only with a new quinolone, such as ciprofloxacin.[102] The Food and Drug Administration in the United States still considers this class of drugs to be risky in adolescents and children under the age of 17, because when given in industrial doses to rodents they result in cartilage and bone damage. A number of studies have shown that this risk is negligible in humans given the usual short course of treatment for these infections, especially when the benefits are measured in relation to the risks.[103] Initial studes suggest that azithromycin may also be a useful alternative oral drug, but this will be expensive in the developing world.[104] In Asia, multidrug-resistant *Shigella* strains remain susceptible to oral pivmecillinam; however, this drug is not available in the United States. There is some controversy over the utility of oral cefixime; however, the parenteral third generation cephalosporin, ceftriaxone, has been shown to be effective given by the parenteral route.[105–107]

SALMONELLA

Uncomplicated *Salmonella* gastroenteritis is a self-limiting disease; antibiotics are not recommended because they do not alter the course of clinical illness, might contribute to development of complications such as *C. difficile* colitis, and are known to prolong the period of excretion of bacteria in the stool, possibly placing others at risk for disease.[39] Although it initially appeared that the quinolones might alter this view, recent studies with these drugs have only confirmed the original recommendations.[108] Therefore, most experts consider that antimicrobials are not indicated in *Salmonella* diarrhea unless there are specific reasons to treat, such as underlying immunosuppression owing to HIV, chronic renal failure, sickle cell disease, or another cause of asplenia, or a patient with severe bloody diarrhea or septicemic invasive disease in the very old and very young. In AIDS patients, there is a high relapse rate after treatment of *Salmonella* bacteremia, suggesting that an aggressive approach to treatment of AIDS patients with positive blood cultures is appropriate. This should include several initial weeks of parenteral therapy followed by oral therapy totalling 6 to 8 weeks. Even with aggressive therapy relapses occur and indefinite prophylaxis may need to be considered.[109]

CAMPYLOBACTER

Like *Salmonella*, antibiotic therapy for *Campylobacter* enteritis has not been clearly shown to be beneficial, and therefore should be reserved for patients with more severe abdominal symptoms at the time of presentation, or with evidence of invasive disease, underlying medical problems such as AIDS or cirrhosis, or for patients at the extremes of age. Both macrolides and quinolones have been used for treatment. Although erythromycin has been used for many years, resistance has remained low at less than 5% of isolates in most developed countries and less than 20% in the developing world. In contrast, the frequency of isolation of quinolone-resistant strains has risen dramatically in several European countries and in some places the prevalence is already above 30%.[110,111] It has been speculated that this increase is secondary to widespread veterinary use of these agents; however, quinolone-resistant strains also emerge rapidly during therapy of human infection.[112] In addition, a recent report from the United Kingdom links foreign travel with acquisition of ciprofloxacin-resistant *Campylobacter* enteritis.[113] A single point mutation in one of the *Campylobacter jejuni* chromosomal gyrase genes, *gyr A*, is the usual mechanism of resistance in most isolates.[114] It has been suggested that treatment of *Campylobacter* infections with quinolones should be reserved for seriously ill patients who are unable to take macrolide antibiotics.[24] However, it should be noted that development of resistance to therapy during treatment with the macrolide antibiotics also appears to be increasing in the setting of treatment of AIDS patients with persistent infection, including resistance to both erythromycin and clarithromycin, and presumably this would extend to azithromycin as well.[32,115,116]

IMMUNE RESPONSE AND VACCINE DEVELOPMENT

SHIGELLA

Naturally acquired immunity in shigellosis is serotype-specific, as shown by early field studies using streptomycin-dependent vaccine strains.[117] Adult volunteers challenged with either virulent *S. sonnei* or *S. flexneri* are also protected against rechallenge with the same strain (approximately 70% protective efficacy).[118,119] There is some evidence that circulating serum antilipopolysaccharide (anti-LPS) antibodies confer homologous protection.[120,121] This is presumed to be mediated by leakage of serum IgG across the mucosal surface to the lumen in sufficient amounts to block further interactions of the pathogen with the epithelium.[122] That mucosal immunity to diarrheal pathogens may be mediated in the lumen is well illustrated by the protective effects of breast feeding on disease severity among infants in the developing world, as well as the ability of passively transferred oral immunoglobulin to both prevent and limit disease.[124,125] However, the nature of specific protective immune responses at the lumenal surface of the intestinal mucosa, whether induced by active oral or systemic immunization or passive oral immunization, remains unknown. Immune responses to the *Shigella* outer membrane proteins involved in invasion have been described, but their role in protection is still undefined.[126]

Vaccines comprised of *Shigella*-specific O-polysaccharides conjugated to potent immunogens have been developed because they can stimulate high serum concentrations of anti-LPS, and have been shown to be safe and immunogenic in humans.[127–129] Preliminary data using one of these constructs, composed of *Shigella sonnei* O-specific polysaccharide bound to recombinant *Pseudomonas aeruginosa* exoprotein A appears to confer type-specific protection against *S. sonnei* after only one injection.[130] Because it has been hypothesized that mucosal immunity is the most effective way to achieve protection against shigellosis, and because it is now understood that many virulent and potentially protective antigens will only be expressed in vivo in living organisms, a wide variety of oral live attenuated *Shigella* or *Shigella-E. coli* hybrid vaccine constructs have been described in the past several decades.[131–134] An oral live-attenuated *Shigella flexneri* hybrid vaccine has been used in field trials, but its efficacy could not be assessed because of the low incidence of cases in the study population.[135]

SALMONELLA

Immunity to *Salmonella* is complex and, because most of the work has focused on immunity in typhoid fever, the relevance of the findings to non–typhoidal disease remains to be shown. This is true even though many of these studies have employed serovars other than *S. typhi*, such as *S. typhimurium* and *S. enteritidis* in mouse experiments. However, these organisms induce a typhoid-like disease in mice and they are not at all representative of *Salmonella* gastroenteritis. There has been some work toward the development of vaccines for animals; however, the goal for these vaccines is to eliminate colonization of the animal intestine, because this is a source of infection for humans, and not to induce protective immunity to clinical infections. These model vaccines are not, of necessity, useful in humans since the nature of the immunity required may be very different to induce an anticolonization compared to an antidisease immunity. It is necessary to rethink many issues in salmonellosis, since it is now known that a large number of *Salmonella* virulence genes are activated only in vivo, and therefore experiments using killed in vitro grown organisms to define the important virulence antigens to target will surely miss detection of critical determinants.[136] However, this discussion is beyond the scope of this chapter.

Both cell-mediated and humoral responses are stimulated by infection, but antibodies to bacterial antigens appear to be sufficient to protect against *Salmonella* gastroenteritis in some models.[137] Local gut secretory IgA responses are probably important in the control of intestinal infection. For example, infection of highly susceptible mouse strains orally challenged with *S. typhimurium* is prevented by subcutaneous implantation of hybridoma cells synthesizing monoclonal IgA against a carbohydrate epitope on *S. typhimurium*.[138] This is reminiscent of human typhoid in which systemic antibodies raised in response to parenteral killed vaccines prevent infection, presumably by killing organisms in the initial dissemination phase from the intestine and before they are sequestered within mononuclear phagocytes, whereas antibody developed later during the bacteremic clinical phase of disease have no impact on the process.

There have been significant advances in the development of new vaccines for *S. typhi*, but not much progress in vaccines for control of nontyphoidal infections.[139] The traditional heat-killed, phenol-extracted whole typhoid vaccine is still useful, providing around 65% protection for a limited period, but at the cost of fever and local reactions following injection. A live, attenuated oral vaccine, prepared in lyophilized form for resuspension at the time of immunization, is now licensed.[140] The vaccine strain is invasive for macrophages but defective in its capacity to make UDP-galactose epimerase, an enzyme necessary for synthesis of the O polysaccharides of *Salmonella* LPS, and as a result it cannot survive for more than a few replication cycles. This is owing to the buildup of excessive levels of toxic metabolites within the cell; however, prior to death, the vaccine strain produces and delivers immunizing antigens to the intestinal immune system. Efficacy is somewhat lower than the heat-killed vaccine but is much longer-lasting. There is some concern about using this, as with any live vaccine, in AIDS patients; however, no data are available about its safety. There is also a new purified Vi polysaccharide vaccine that is safe and nonreactive, as effective as the multiple oral dose regimen of the live vaccine, and results in protection lasting for at least several years.[141] This vaccine may be used in children as young as 2 years of age, and is suitable for use in the HIV-infected individual at risk of *S. typhi*, for example, because of planned travel to a typhoid endemic country. New, genetically engineered live typhoid vaccine strains are also being developed, not only for immunization against typhoid but also for use as live vectors into which extraneous genes can be cloned for oral delivery of protective antigens from unrelated species.[142] Vi-protein conjugates are at present being evaluated as immunogens for infants under 2 year old, especially in endemic areas where infantile typhoid is prevalent.[143]

Prevention of non–typhoidal *Salmonella* infection is difficult because of the widespread natural reservoirs for these organisms and the multiplicity of antigenic determinants of the many different serovars. Non–vaccine strategies include hygienic improvements in the management of food animals to reduce colonization, and the decreased use of animal feed antimicrobials that are used to treat human illness in order to delay the emergence of drug resistance. Safe food preparation and storage practices and quality control testing of known commonly contaminated foods should be helpful as well, but may be difficult to implement. Vaccines for immunization of poultry, bovines, and ovines to prevent colonization and fecal shedding of *Salmonella* in the feces are one possible technical fix. Some progress has been made toward development of such vaccines, using strains containing mutations in critical bacterial genes, such as the aromatic amino acid synthesis genes or adenylate cyclase and the cyclic-AMP receptor.[144,145] If both safe and effective, these vaccines could also prove effective for human use as well.

CAMPYLOBACTER

Both human and animal studies suggest that infection with *C. jejuni* protects against later re-exposures.[26,146] Human volunteers who developed diarrhea after oral *C. jejuni* challenge were protected from symptoms on rechallenge 1 month later with the same strain, although colonization of the gastrointestinal tract occurred and the challenge strain was excreted in the stool.[26] There is evidence that infected patients make an antibody response to the organism that might play a role in immunity. Serum IgG antibody to enterotoxin was demonstrated in convalescent serum obtained 1 month following infection of children with enterotoxigenic strains of *C. jejuni*.[147] Humoral defects may be responsible for the persistence and severity of *C. jejuni* infections in patients with HIV, especially deficiency in synthesis of specific IgA.[148,149] Secretory IgA specific for *C. jejuni* is present in breast milk and studies from Mexico suggest that breast milk with high titres of anti-*C. jejuni* IgA will protect children from *Campylobacter* diarrhea in the first 6 months of age.[150] This protective antibody was directed against *Campylobacter* flagellar proteins, suggesting the potential importance of these proteins in protection and as vaccine candidates.

There are no established vaccines for *Campylobacter*. Oral *Campylobacter jejuni* vaccines have been tested in both primate and chicken models, and have been shown to induce specific anti-*Campylobacter* IgG and IgA responses.[151,152] In mice, oral vaccination with a *Campylobacter* whole-cell heat inactivated strain has a 50% protective efficacy at 6 weeks on challenge with live vaccine strain in the group receiving the mucosal adjuvant, *E. coli* heat labile enterotoxin B subunit.[153] There is, as yet, no evidence that the 62 kDa *Campylobacter* flagellin protein has potential as a vaccine candidate, since the role of anti-flagellin antibodies in protection has yet to be firmly established.[154] Effort is now being given toward the identification and characterization of the major antigenic proteins of *C. jejuni* to improve antigen selection, guided in part by their recognition by sera from recently infected patients.[155]

References

1 Deuteronomy 23:12–13.

2 Keusch GT et al: Shigellosis, in *Bacterial Infections of Humans: Epidemiology and Control, 3rd Ed,* Evans AS et al (eds). New York, Plenum, 1997, in press.

3 Levine MM et al: Pathogenesis of Shigella dysenteriae 1 (Shiga) dysentery. *J Infect Dis* 127:261–270, 1973.

4 Dritz SK et al: Patterns of sexually transmitted enteric diseases in a city. *Lancet* 2:3–4, 1977.

5 Owen RL et al: Venereal aspects of gastroenterology. *West J Med* 130:236–2446, 1979.

6 Bader M et al: Venereal transmission of shigellosis in Seattle-King County. *Sex Transm Dis* 4:89–91, 1977.

7 Drusin LM et al: Shigellosis: Another sexually transmitted disease? *Br J Ven Dis* 52:348–350, 1976.

8 Tauxe RV: The persistence of *Shigella flexneri* in the United States: The increased role of the adult male. *Am J Public Health* 78:1432–1435, 1988.

9 Quinn TC: Clinical approach to intestinal infections in homosexual men. *Med Clin N Am* 70:611–634, 1986.

10 Speelman P et al: Distribution and spread of colonic lesions in shigellosis: A colonoscopic study. *J Infect Dis* 150:899–903, 1984.

11 Department of Public Health, City and County of San Francisco: Shigellosis in San Francisco, 1977–1985. *San Francisco Epidemiol Bull* 2:1–3, 1986.

12 Buchbinder SP et al: Feasibility of human immunodeficiency virus vaccine trials in homosexual men in the United States: Risk behavior, seroincidence, and willingness to participate. *J Infect Dis* 174:954–961, 1996.

13 Hickson FC et al: No aggregate change in homosexual HIV risk behavior among gay men attending the Gay Pride festivals, United Kingdom, 1993–1995. *AIDS* 10:771–774, 1996.

14 Williams DI et al: A case control study of HIV seroconversion in gay men, 1988–1993: What are the current risk factors? *Genitourin Med* 72:193–196, 1996.

15 Ostrow DG et al: A case-control study of human immunodeficiency virus type 1 seroconversion and risk-related behaviors in the Chicago MACS/CCC cohort, 1984–1992. *Am J Epidemiol* 142:875–883, 1995.

16 Crosby GM et al: Condom use among gay/bisexual male substance abusers using the timeline follow-back method. *Addict Behav* 21: 249–257, 1996.

17 Turnbull PC: Food poisoning with special reference to Salmonella: Its epidemiology, pathogenesis and control. *Clin Gastroenterol* 8: 663–714, 1979.

18 St. Louis ME et al: The emergence of grade A eggs as a major source of *Salmonella enteritidis* infections. *JAMA* 259:2103–2107, 1988.

19 Cebald M et al: Teneur en bases de l'adn et classifications des vibrions. *Ann Inst Pasteur* 105:897–910, 1963.

20 King EO: Human infections with *Vibrio* fetus and a closely related *vibrio*. *J Infect Dis* 101:119, 1957.

21 Blaser MJ et al: *Campylobacter enteritis* in the United States. *Ann Int Med* 98:360–365, 1983.

22 Tauxe RV et al: Illness associated with *Campylobacter laridis*, a newly recognized *Campylobacter* species. *J Clin Microbiol* 21:222–225, 1985.

23 Sanchez R et al: Evolution of susceptibilities of *Campylobacter* spp to quinolones and macrolides. *Antimicrob Agents Chemother* 38: 1879–1882, 1994.

24 LaMont JT: *Campylobacter* infections, in *Gastrointestinal Infections: Diagnosis and Management,* LaMont TJ (ed). New York, Marcel Dekker, 1997, pp. 247–263.

25 Walker RI et al: Pathophysiology of *Campylobacter enteritis. Microbiol Rev* 50:81–94, 1986.

26 Black RE et al: Experimental *Campylobacter jejuni* infection in humans. *J Infect Dis* 157:472–479, 1988.

27 Quinn TC et al: Infections with *Campylobacter jejuni* and *Campylobacter*-like organisms in homosexual men. *Ann Intern Med* 101: 187–192, 1984.

28 Fennell CL et al: Characterization of *Campylobacter*-like organisms isolated from homosexual men. *J Infect Dis* 149:58–66, 1985.

29 Totten PA et al: *Campylobacter cinaedi* (spp nov.) and *Campylobacter fenneliae* (spp nov.): Two new *Campylobacter* species associated with enteric disease in homosexual men. *J Infect Dis* 151:131–139, 1985.

30 Grayson ML et al: Gastroenteritis associated with *Campylobacter cinaedi. Med J Austr* 150:214–215, 1989.

31 Goossens H et al: Is *Campylobacter upsaliensis* an unrecognised cause of human diarrhoea? *Lancet* 335:584–586, 1990.

32 Snidjers F et al: Prevalence of *Campylobacter*-associated diarrhea among patients infected with human immunodeficiency virus. *Clin Infect Dis* 24:1107–1113, 1997.

33 Siegel D et al: Predictive value of stool examination in acute diarrhea. *Arch Pathol Lab Med* 111:715–718, 1987.

34 Quinn TC et al: The polymicrobial origin of intestinal infections in homosexual men. *N Engl J Med* 309:576–582, 1983.

35 Laughton BE et al: Prevalence of enteric pathogens in homosexual men with and without acquired immunodeficiency syndrome. *Gastroenterology* 94:984–993, 1988.

36 Keusch GT: *Shigella* infections. *Clin Gastroenterol* 8:645–662, 1979.

37 Stoll DM: Cutaneous *shigellosis*. *Arch Dermatol* 122:22, 1986.

38 Rubin RH et al: *Salmonellosis: Microbiologic, Pathologic, and Clinical Features.* New York, Stratton Intercontinental Medical Book Corp., 1977.

39 Acheson DWK et al: Intestinal infections with *Salmonella* and *Yersinia* species, in *Gastrointestinal Infections: Diagnosis and Management,* LaMont TJ (ed). New York, Marcel Dekker,1997, pp. 149–189.

40 Mandal BK et al: Colonic involvement in salmonellosis. *Lancet* 1: 884–888, 1976.

41 Schofield PF et al: Toxic dilatation of the colon in salmonella colitis and inflammatory bowel disease. *Br J Surg* 66:5–8, 1979.

42 Butzler JP et al: *Campylobacter* enteritis. *Clin Gastroenterol* 8:737–765, 1979.

43 Karmali MA et al: *Campylobacter* enteritis in children. *J Pediatr* 94: 527–533, 1979.

44 Lambert ME et al: *Campylobacter* colitis. *Br J Med* 1:857–859, 1979.

45 Pockros PI et al: Toxic megacolon complicating *Campylobacter* enterocolitis. *J Clin Gastroenterol* 3:318, 1986.

46 Quinn TC et al: New developments in infectious diarrhea. *Disease-A-Month* 32:174–244, 1986.

47 Fennell CL et al: Isolation of "*Campylobacter hyointestinalis*" from a human. *J Clin Microbiol* 24:146–148, 1986.

48 Baskin DH et al: *Shigella* bacteremia in patients with the acquired immune deficiency syndrome. *Am J Gastroenterol* 82:338, 1987.

49 Huebner J et al: *Shigellemia* in AIDS patients: Case report and review of the literature. *Infection* 21:122–124, 1993.

50 Angulo FJ et al: Bacterial enteric infections in persons infected with human immunodeficiency virus. *Clin Infect Dis* 21(Suppl 1):S84–S93, 1995.

51 Sperver SJ et al: *Salmonellosis* during infection with human immunodeficiency virus. *Rev Infect Dis* 9:925–934, 1987.

52 Council of State and Territorial Epidemiologists: AIDS Program, Center for Infectious Diseases. Revision of the CDC surveillance case definition for acquired immunodeficiency syndrome. *Morbid Mortal Wkly Rep* 36(Suppl 1):1S–15S, 1987.

53 Sorvillo FJ et al: Incidence of campylobacteriosis among patients with AIDS in Los Angeles County. *J Acquir Immune Defic Synd* 4:598–602, 1991.

54 Steele TW et al: The use of membrane filters applied directly to the surface of agar plates for the isolation of *Campylobacter jejuni* from feces. *Pathology* 16:263–265, 1984.

55 Gaunt PN et al: Ciprofloxacin resistant *Campylobacter* spp. in humans: An epidemiological and laboratory study. *J Antimicrob Chemother* 37:747–757, 1996.

56 Guerrant RL et al: Evaluation and diagnosis of acute infectious diarrhea. *Am J Med* 78 (Suppl 6):91–98, 1985.

57 Formal SB et al: Invasive enteric pathogens. *Rev Infect Dis* 5:S702–S707, 1983.

58 Islam MM et al: Pathology of *shigellosis* and its complications. *Histopathology* 24:65–71, 1994.

59 Waterman SR et al: Identification of sigma s-dependent genes associated with the stationary-phase acid-resistance phenotype of *Shigella flexneri*. *Mol Microbiol* 21:925–940, 1996.

60 Zychlinsky A et al: Molecular and cellular mechanisms of tissue invasion by *Shigella flexneri*. *Ann NY Acad Sci* 730:197–208, 1994.

61 Speelman P et al: Distribution and spread of colonic lesions in shigellosis: A colonoscopic study. *J Infect Dis* 150:899–903, 1984.

62 Menard R et al: Bacterial entry into epithelial cells: The paradigm of *Shigella*. *Trends Microbiol* 4:220–226, 1996.

63 Adam T et al: Cytoskeletal rearrangments and the functional role of T–plastin during entry of *Shigella flexneri* into HeLa cells. *J Cell Biol* 129:367–381, 1995.

64 Perdomo JJ et al: Polymorphonuclear leukocyte transmigration promotes invasion of colonic epithelial cell monolayer by *Shigella flexneri*. *J Clin Invest* 93:633–643, 1994.

65 Zychlinsky A et al: Interleukin 1 is released by murine macrophages during apoptosis induced by *Shigella flexneri*. *J Clin Invest* 94:1328–1332, 1994.

66 Raqib R et al: Cytokine secretion in acute shigellosis is correlated to disease activity and directed more to stool than plasma. *J Infect Dis* 171:376–384, 1995.

67 Raqib R et al: Persistence of local cytokine production in shigellosis in acute and convalescent stages. *Infect Immunol* 63:289–296, 1995.

68 Rahman MM et al: Decreased food intake in children with severe dysentery due to *Shigella dysenteriae* type 1 infection. *Eur J Clin Nutr* 46:833–838, 1992.

69 Sansonetti PJ et al: Role of interleukin-1 in the pathogenesis of experimental shigellosis. *J Clin Invest* 96:884–892, 1995.

70 Mounier J et al: Secretion of *Shigella flexneri Ipa* invasins on contact with epithelial cells and subsequent entry of the bacterium into cells are growth stage dependent. *Infect Immunol* 65:774–782, 1997.

71 Egile C et al: SopA, the outer membrane protease responsible for polar localization of IcsA in *Shigella flexneri*. *Molec Microbiol* 23: 1063–1073, 1997.

72 Sansonetti PJ et al: Cadherin expression is required for the spread of *Shigella flexneri* between epithelial cells. *Cell* 76:829–839, 1994.

73 Keusch GT et al: Thrombotic thrombocytopenic purpura associated with *Shiga* toxins. *Semin Hematol* 34:106–116, 1997.

74 Acheson DWK et al: Translocation of Shiga-like toxins across polarized intestinal cells in tissue culture. *Infect Immunol* 64:3294–3300, 1996.

75 Kandel G et al: Pathogenesis of *Shigella* diarrhea. XVI. Selective targeting of *Shiga* toxin to villus cells of rabbit jejunum explains the effect of the toxin on intestinal transport. *J Clin Invest* 84:1509–1517, 1989.

76 Fasano A et al: *Shigella enterotoxin* 1: An enterotoxin of *Shigella flexneri* 2a active in rabbit small intestine in vivo and in vitro. *J Clin Invest* 95:2853–2861, 1995.

77 Nataro JP et al: Identification and cloning of a novel plasmid-encoded enterotoxin of enteroinvasive *Escherichia coli* and *Shigella* strains. *Infect Immunol* 63:4721–4728, 1995.

78 Foster JW et al: Adaptive acidification tolerance response of *Salmonella typhimurium*. *J Bacteriol* 172:771–778, 1990.

79 Lehrer RI et al: Defensins, endogenous antibiotic peptides of animal cells. *Cell* 64:229–230, 1991.

80 Selsted ME et al: Enteric defensins: Antibiotic peptide components of intestinal host defense. *J Cell Biol* 118:929–936, 1992.

81 Michetti P et al: Monoclonal secretory immunoglobulin A protects mice against oral challenge with the invasive pathogen *Salmonella typhimurium*. *Infect Immunol* 60:1786–1792, 1992.

82 Finlay BB: Molecular and cellular mechanisms of *Salmonella* pathogenesis. *Curr Top Microbiol Immunol* 192:163–185, 1994.

83 Galan J et al: The molecular genetic basis of *Salmonella* entry into mammalian cells. *Biochem Soc Trans* 22:301–306, 1994.

84 Guiney DG et al: Plasmid mediated virulence genes in non–typhoid *Salmonella* serovars. *FEMS Microbiol Lett* 124:1–10, 1994.

85 Miller SI et al: A two component regulatory system (phoPphoQ) controls *Salmonella* typhimurium virulence. *Proc Natl Acad Sci USA* 86: 5054–5058, 1989.

86 Garcia Vescovi E et al: The role of the *PhoP/PhoQ* regulon in *Salmonella* virulence. *Res Microbiol* 145:473–480, 1994.

87 Zwilling BS et al: Macrophage resistance genes: *Bcg/Ity/Lsh*. *Immunol Series* 60:233–245, 1994.

88 Vidal S et al: The *Ity/Lsh/Bcg* locus: natural resistance to infection with intracellular parasites is abrogated by disruption of the *Nramp*1 gene. *J Exp Med* 182:655–666, 1995.

89 Cellier M et al: Human natural resistance-associated macrophage protein: cDNA cloning, chromosomal mapping, genomic organization, and tissue-specific expression. *J Exp Med* 180:1741–1752, 1994.

90 Konkel ME et al: Adhesion to and invasion of Hep–2 cells by *Campylobacter* spp. *Infect Immunol* 57:2984–2990, 1989.

91 Konkel ME et al: Invasion-related antigens of *Campylobacter jejuni*. *J Infect Dis* 162:888–895, 1990.

92 Klipstein FA et al: Immunologic relationship of the B subunits of *Campylobacter jejuni* and *Escherichia coli* heat-labile enterotoxins. *Infect Immunol* 48:629–633, 1985.

93 Yeen WD et al: Demonstration of a cytotoxin from *Campylobacter jejuni*. *J Clin Pathol* 36:1237–1240, 1983.

94 Klipstein FA et al: Pathogenic properties of *Campylobacter jejuni*: Assay and correlation with clinical manifestations. *Infect Immunol* 50:43–49, 1985.

95 Florin I et al: Production of enterotoxin and cytotoxin in *Campylobacter jejuni* strains isolated in Costa Rica. *J Med Microbiol* 37:22–29, 1992.

96 Moore MA et al: Production of a Shiga-like cytotoxin by *Campylobacter*. *Microbial Pathogen* 4:455–62, 1988.

97 Delans RJ et al: Hemolytic uremic syndrome after *Campylobacter* induced diarrhea in an adult. *Arch Int Med* 144:1074–1076, 1984.

98 Miles TA et al: Haemolytic–uraemic syndrome in the Hunter: Public health implications. *Aust NZ J Public Health* 20:457–462, 1996.

99 Grant CC et al: Role of flagella in adherence, internalization, and translocation of *Campylobacter jejuni* in nonpolarized and polarized epithelial cell cultures. *Infect Immunol* 61:1764–1771, 1993.

100 Tauxe RV et al: Antimicrobial resistance of *Shigella flexneri* in the USA: The importance of international travelers. *J Infect Dis* 162: 1107–1111, 1990.

101 Ashkenazi S et al: Recent trends in the epidemiology of *Shigella* infections. *Clin Infect Dis* 17:897–899, 1993.

102 Sack RB et al: Antimicrobial resistance in organisms causing diarrheal disease. *Clin Infect Dis* 24: 102–105, 1997.

103 Schaad UB: Role of the new quinolones in pediatric practice. *Pediatr Infec Dis J* 11:1043–1046, 1992.

104 Khan WA et al: Treatment of *shigellosis*. V. Comparison of azithromycin and ciprofloxacin. A double, blind, randomized, controlled trial. *Ann Int Med* 126:697–703, 1997.

105 Ashkenazi S et al: A randomized, double blind study comparing cefixime and trimethoprim-sulfamethoxazole in the treatment of childhood shigellosis. *J Pediatr* 123:817–821, 1993.

106 Salam MA et al: Treatment of shigellosis: IV. Cefixime is ineffective in shigellosis in adults. *Ann Intern* Med 123:505–508, 1995.

107 Varsano I et al: Comparative efficacy of ceftriaxone and ampicillin for treatment of severe shigellosis in children. *J Pediatr* 118:207–215, 1991.

108 Akalin HE: Quinolones in the treatment of acute bacterial diarrhoeal diseases. *Drugs* 45(Suppl 3):114–118, 1993.

109 Nelson MR et al: *Salmonella, Campylobacter,* and *Shigella* in HIV-seropositive patients. *AIDS* 6:1495–1598, 1992.

110 Reina Borrell N et al A: Emergence of resistance to erythromycin and fluoroquinolones in thermo-tolerant *Campylobacter* strains isolated from feces 1987–1991. *Eur J Clin Microbiol Infect Dis* 11:1163–1166, 1992.

111 Velazquez JB et al: Incidence and transmission of antibiotic resistance in *Campylobacter jejuni* and *Campylobacter coli. J Antimicrob Chemother* 35:173–178, 1995.

112 Gaunt PN et al: Ciprofloxacin resistant *Campylobacter* spp. in humans: An epidemiological and laboratory study. *J Antimicrob Chemother* 37:747–757, 1996.

113 Goodman LJ et al: Empiric antimicrobial therapy of domestically acquired acute diarrhea in urban adults. *Arch Int Med* 150:541–546, 1990.

114 Piddock LJ: Quinolone resistance and *Campylobacter* spp. *J Antimicrob Chemother* 36:891–898, 1995.

115 Perlman DM et al: Persistent *Campylobacter jejuni* infections in patients infected with human immunodeficiency virus (HIV). *Ann Int Med* 1988;108:540–546.

116 Funke G et al: Development of resistance to macrolide antibiotics in an AIDS patient treated with clarithromycin for *Campylobacter jejuni* diarrhea. *Eur J Clin Microbiol Infect Dis* 13:612–615, 1994 .

117 Mel DM et al: Live oral Shigella vaccine: Vaccination schedule and the effect of booster dose. *Acta Microbiol Acad Sci Hung* 21:109–114, 1974.

118 Herrington D et al: Studies in volunteers to evaluate candidate Shigella vaccines: Further experience with a bivalent Salmonella typhi–*Shigella sonnei* vaccine and protection conferred by disease. *Vaccine* 8:353–357, 1990.

119 Kotloff KL et al: A modified Shigella volunteer challenge model in which the inoculum is administered with bicarbonate buffer: Clinical experience and implications for Shigella infectivity. *Vaccine* 13: 1488–1494, 1995.

120 Cohen D et al: Serum antibodies to liposaccharide and natural immunity to shigellosis in an Israel military population. *J Infect Dis* 157: 1068–1071, 1988.

121 Cohen D et al: Prospective study of the association between serum antibodies to lipopolysaccharide O antigen and the attack rate of shigellosis. *J Clin Microbiol* 29:386–389, 1991.

122 Robbins JB et al: Hypothesis for vaccine development: serum IgG LPS antibodies confer protective immunity to non–typohoidal *Salmonellae* and *Shigellae. Clin Infect Dis* 15:346–361, 1992.

123 Clemens JD et al: Breast feeding as a determinant of severity in shigellosis. *Am J Epidemiol* 123:710–720, 1986.

124 Tacket CO et al: Efficacy of bovine milk immunoglobulin concentrate in preventing illness after *Shigella flexneri* challenge. *Am J Trop Med Hyg* 47:276–283, 1992.

125 Hayani KC et al: Concentration of milk secretory immunoglobulin A against Shigella virulence plasmid associated antigens as a predictor of symptom status in Shigella-infected breast fed infants. *J Pediatr* 121:852–856, 1992.

126 Oaks EV et al: Serum immune responses to Shigella protein antigens in Rhesus monkeys and humans infected with *Shigella* spp. *Infect Immunol* 53:57–63, 1986.

127 Chu CY et al: Preparation, characterization and immunogenicity of conjugates composed of the O-specific polysaccharide of *Shigella dysenteriae* type 1 (Shiga's bacillus) bound to tetanus toxoid. *Infect Immunol* 59:4450–4458, 1992.

128 Taylor DN et al: Synthesis, characterization and clinical evaluation of conjugate vaccines composed of the O-specific polysaccharide of *Shigella dysenteriae* type 1, *Shigella flexneri* type 2, *Shigella sonnei (Pleisiomonas shigelloides)* bound to bacterial toxoids. *Infect Immunol* 61:3678–3687, 1993.

129 Cohen D et al: Safety and immunogenicity of investigational Shigella conjugate vaccines in Israeli volunteers. *Infec Immunol* 64:4074–4077, 1996.

130 Cohen D et al: Double blind vaccine-controlled randomised efficacy trial of an investigational *Shigella sonnei* conjugate vaccine in young adults. *Lancet* 349:155–159, 1997.

131 Formal SB et al: Oral vaccination of monkeys with an invasive *Escherichia coli* K-12 hybrid expressing *Shigella flexneri* 2a somatic antigen. *Infect Immunol* 46:465–469, 1984.

132 Black RE et al: Prevention of shigellosis by a *Salmonella typhi–Shigella sonnei* bivalent vaccine. *J Infect Dis* 155:1260–1265, 1987.

133 Lindberg AA et al: Aromatic-dependent Shigella strains as oral live vaccines, in *New Generation Vaccines: Vaccines against Shigella, Part II,* Woodrow GC et al (eds). New York, Marcel Dekker, 1990, pp. 677–687.

134 Sansonetti PJ et al: Construction and evaluation of a double mutant of *Shigella flexneri* as a candidate for oral vaccination against shigellosis. *Vaccine* 7:443–450, 1989.

135 Cohen D et al: Safety and immunogenicity of the oral *E. coli K12-S flexneri* 2a vaccine *(EcSf2a–2)* among Israeli soldiers. *Vaccine* 1994; 12:1436–1442.

136 Heithoff DM et al: Bacterial infection as assessed by in vivo gene expression. *Proc Natl Acad Sci USA* 94:934–939, 1997.

137 Eisenstein TK et al: Immunity to Salmonella infections, in *Enteric Infections and Immunity*, Paradise LJ et al (eds). Plenum Press, New York, 1996, pp. 57–78.

138 Michetti P et al: Monoclonal secretory immunoglobulin A protects mice against oral challenge with the invasive pathogen *Salmonella typhimurium. Infect Immunol* 60:1786–1792, 1992.

139 Levine MM et al: Attenuated *Salmonella* as live oral vaccines against typhoid fever and as live vectors. *J Biotechnol* 44:193–196, 1996.

140 Kollaritsch H et al: Randomized, double-blind placebo-controlled trial to evaluate the safety and immunogenicity of combined *Salmonella typhi Ty21a* and *Vibrio cholerae CVD 103–HgR* live oral vaccines. *Infect Immunol* 64:1454–1457, 1996.

141 Klugman KP et al: Immunogenicity, efficacy and serological correlate of protection of *Salmonella typhi Vi* capsular polysaccharide vaccine three years after immunization. *Vaccine* 14:435–438, 1996.

142 Ivanoff B et al: Vaccination against typhoid fever: Present status. *Bull WHO* 72:957–971, 1994.

143 Kossaczka Z et al: Synthesis and immunological properties of Vi and di-O-acetyl pectin protein conjugates with adipic acid dihydrazide as the linker. *Infect Immunol* 65:2088–2093, 1997.

144 Harrison JA et al: Correlates of protection induced by live Aro– *S. Typhimurium* vaccines in the murine typhoid model. *Immunology* 90:618–625, 1997.

145 Curtiss III R et al: Nonrecombinant and recombinant avirulent Salmonella vaccines for poultry. *Vet Immunol Immunopathol* 54:365–372, 1996.

146 Russell REG et al: Experimental *Campylobacter jejuni* infection in *Macaca nemestrina. Infect Immunol* 57:1438–1444, 1989.

147 Ruiz-Palacios GM et al: Serum antibodies to heat-labile enterotoxin of *Campylobacter jejuni. J Infect Dis* 152:413–416, 1985.

148 Perlman DM et al: Persistent *Campylobacter jejuni* infections in patients infected with human immunodeficiency virus (HIV). *Ann Int Med* 108:540–546, 1988.

149 Darbas H et al: Chronic diarrhea caused by *Campylobacter jejuni* in a patient with AIDS. *Pathol Biol* 36:888–890, 1988.

150 Ruiz-Palacios GM et al: Protection of breast fed infants against *Campylobacter* diarrhea by antibodies in human milk. *J Pediatr* 116:707–713, 1990.

151 Baqar S et al: Safety and immunogenicity of a prototype oral whole-cell killed *Campylobacter* vaccine administered with a mucosal adjuvant in non–human primates. *Vaccine* 13:22–28, 1995.

152 Cawthraw S et al: Isotype, specificity and kinetics of systemic and mucosal antibodies to *Campylobacter jejuni* antigens, including flagellin, during experimental oral infections of chickens. *Avian Dis* 32: 341–349, 1994.

153 Baqar S et al: Immunogenicity and protective efficacy of a prototype *Campylobacter* killed whole-cell vaccine in mice. *Infect Immunol* 63:3731–3735, 1995.

154 Khoury CA et al: A genetic hybrid of the *Campylobacter jejuni* flaA gene a LT-B of *Escherichia coli* and assessment of the efficacy of the hybrid protein as an oral chicken vaccine. *Avian Dis* 39:812–820, 1995.

155 Pei ZH et al: Identification, purification, and characterization of major antigenic proteins of *Campylobacter jejuni*. *J Biol Chem* 266: 16363–16369, 1991.

Chapter 42
Bacterial vaginosis

Sharon Hillier
King K. Holmes

Our knowledge of leukorrhea is unsatisfactory and incomplete. The majority of physicians neither appreciate the gross aspects of the condition nor discover the locality from which discharges arise, practically none of us possesses an adequate knowledge of the bacteria involved, and most clinicians admit that their curative efforts yield poor results.

Arthur H. Curtis (1913)[1]

DEFINITION

Bacterial vaginosis (BV) is the most prevalent cause of vaginal symptoms among women of childbearing age. Many primary care physicians perceive BV as a trivial and ill-defined syndrome of uncertain etiology, as primarily an aesthetic problem. These perceptions may explain why clinicians still commonly prescribe ineffective treatments for BV.

Bacterial vaginosis (nonspecific vaginitis) produces symptoms of slightly increased quantities of malodorous vaginal discharge. Although past conventional practice allowed the diagnosis of bacterial vaginosis only after excluding other causes of vaginal discharge, such as trichomoniasis, vulvovaginal candidiasis, or cervicitis, these conditions can undoubtedly coexist with bacterial vaginosis. Physical examination and analysis of vaginal fluid reveal the following: a thin homogeneous, white, uniformly adherent vaginal discharge; elevation of the pH of vaginal fluid above 4.5; development of a fishy odor after mixing vaginal fluid with 10% (wt/vol) KOH; and "clue cells" on microscopic examination of vaginal fluid. Whereas Gram stain of normal vaginal fluid shows a predominance of lactobacilli, the Gram stain of vaginal fluid from a woman with bacterial vaginosis shows a decrease or absence of lactobacilli, and a predominance of Gram-variable coccobacilli consistent with *Gardnerella vaginalis* or *Bacteroides* species. Culture of vaginal fluid reveals mixed flora that typically includes genital mycoplasmas, *Gardnerella vaginalis,* and anaerobic bacteria such as peptostreptococci, *Prevotella* spp., and *Mobiluncus* spp. Biochemical analysis of vaginal fluid from women with bacterial vaginosis usually shows characteristic changes thought to be caused by bacterial metabolism. The vaginal fluid contains an altered pattern of organic acids (e.g., increased succinate, decreased lactate); and abnormal amounts of putrescine, cadaverine, and trimethylamine, which probably contribute to the malodor. The pathogenesis of bacterial vaginosis remains far from clear. With little or no inflammation of the vaginal epithelium per se, the syndrome apparently represents a disturbance of the vaginal microbial ecosystem rather than a true tissue or epithelial infectin. However, recent work has demonstrated an increased risk for prematurity and chorioamnionitis among pregnant women with BV, as well as an association of BV with increased risk of pelvic inflammatory disease and with pelvic infection following obstetrical or gynecological surgery.

HISTORY

Nearly a century ago, Doderlein described a nonmotile bacillus that he considered to be the normal flora of the vagina of pregnant women.[2] The Doderlein bacillus later became known as *Lactobacillus.* In 1899, Menge and Kronig reported isolation of both facultative and strictly anaerobic microorganisms, as well as the Doderlein bacillus, from the vagina of most women.[3] These early studies established that normal vaginal flora includes a mixture of microorganisms, with *Lactobacillus* spp. as the predominant species.

"Leukorrhea," or white discharge from the vagina, became the focus of much research in the first quarter of the century. Some thought that vaginal discharge resulted from infection of the uterus, and treated the condition by curettage of the endometrium. In 1913, Curtis demonstrated that the endometria of women with leukorrhea lacked a white discharge, thus suggesting a vaginal, not endometrial, origin. He confirmed that the vaginal flora of clinically normal married women consisted of Doderlein's bacilli, and that the greater the deviation of vaginal flora from the normal state, the greater the likelihood of vaginal discharge. Curtis linked vaginal discharge with high concentrations of black-pigmented anaerobes, curved anaerobic motile rods, and anaerobic cocci, and with Gram-variable diphtheroidal rods that probably represented *Gardnerella.* Curtis' 1913 paper established three central themes: (1) that the discharge arose from the vagina, and not the uterus; (2) that women having white discharge did not have large numbers of Doderlein bacilli; and (3) that the presence of anaerobic bacteria in the vagina, especially anaerobic rods, correlated with vaginal discharge.

Research on vaginal flora continued in the early 1920s when Schroder reported three different types of vaginal flora that corresponded to the "rheinheitgrad" (grade of cleanliness) of the vagina.[4] He considered the flora of the first group, dominated by acid-producing rods (Doderlein's bacillus), as least pathogenic. A second group had a mixed flora with Doderlein bacillus in the minority. The third group, designated as the most pathogenic type of flora, had mixed vaginal flora with no Doderlein bacillus.

Despite observations by Curtis and Schroder linking vaginal discharge with a shift in vaginal flora (from predominance of lactobacilli to predominance of anaerobes), other workers attempted to attribute the symptoms of nonspecific vaginitis to a single microorganism. In 1950, Weaver again reported a link between lack of lactobacilli, presence of anaerobes spp., and nonspecific vaginitis.[5] However, the lack of association of other aerobic and facultative bacteria with discharge led him to conclude that no particular organisms caused this syndrome. The recognition of the association of *Gardnerella vaginalis* with nonspecific vaginitis by Gardner and Dukes in 1955 (discussed in the following) provided the first clear evidence that *Gardnerella vaginalis* caused nonspecific vaginitis.[6] However, because they failed (erroneously) to find an association between anaerobic bacteria and bacterial vaginosis, workers over the next 25 years tended to ignore the potential role of microorganisms other than *Gardnerella vaginalis.*

Confusion surrounding the etiology of this syndrome has prompted use of various names to describe bacterial vaginosis. Prior to 1955, leukorrhea or nonspecific vaginitis were the terms most frequently used. Gardner and Dukes first applied the name *Haemophilus vaginalis* vaginitis to this syndrome in 1955, and today some clinicians use the term *Gardnerella vaginalis* vaginitis or vaginosis to describe this syndrome, whereas others have used the term anaerobic vaginosis.[7] We prefer the term bacterial vaginosis rather than anaerobic vaginosis, since BV is associated with vaginal overgrowth not only by anaerobic bacteria, but also by certain species of facultative bacteria and genital mycoplasmas.[8,9] Since vaginal inflammation is not a feature of this infection, the term "vaginosis" has replaced the more familiar term "vaginitis." The term "vaginal bacteriosis" has been proposed to indicate an increase in vaginal bacteria, but bacterial vaginosis is still the name most commonly used to identify this syndrome.[10]

EPIDEMIOLOGY

PREVALENCE OF BV AND ASSOCIATED MICROORGANISMS

Data on prevalence vary widely, because of differing diagnostic criteria, and differences in clinical populations sampled as well as actual differences between populations. In a recent large U.S. study, 13,747 pregnant women at 23 to 26 weeks' gestation underwent evaluation for BV by standardized vaginal Gram stain criteria.[11] Although 16.3 percent of the women had BV, the prevalence varied widely by ethnicity, from a low of 6.1 percent of Asians, to 8.8 percent of Caucasian women, 15.9 percent of Hispanics, and 22.7 percent of African-American women.[11] Other studies have found antenatal BV prevalences of 5 percent among asymptomatic Italian women, 12 percent in Helsinki, 21 percent in London, 14 percent in Japan, 16 percent in Thailand, and 17 percent in Jakarta.[12–16]

In family planning clinics, BV prevalence was 14 percent among young Swedish women.[17] In Morocco, a three-city study of women with vulvo-vaginal or lower abdominal complaints showed BV based on clinical criteria in 19 percent of those attending family planning clinics, and in 24 percent of those attending primary health care clinics.[18] In Lima, Peru, BV was detected in 25 percent of asymptomatic women seen in family planning clinics; and in 23 percent of asymptomatic women and 37 percent of women with symptoms of vaginal discharge seen in a gynecology clinic.[19]

Women attending sexually transmitted disease clinics have had relatively high BV prevalence; for example, 24 to 37 percent of women attending STD clinics in Uppsala, Sweden, Seattle, Washington, Halifax, Nova Scotia, and Antananarivo, Madagascar.[20–23] In Thailand, 33 percent of female sex workers had BV, compared to the 16 percent prevalence found among pregnant Thai women.[24] The highest prevalence of BV reported in a large population-based sample of women was 51 percent among 4718 rural Ugandan women.[25] On the other hand, BV was diagnosed in only 18 percent of women hospitalized with complications of AIDS.[26] These and other data, in aggregate, suggest BV is common in most populations; is more common in STD clinics than in family planning or antenatal clinics; is more common among women with symptoms of vaginal discharge than among those without symptoms; has been related to ethnicity for unknown reasons; and is especially common in rural sub-Saharan Africans.

Sexually active women have vaginal carriage *G. vaginalis* more often than sexually inexperienced women, but nonetheless 10 to 31 percent of sexually inexperienced adolescent girls have had positive vaginal cultures for *G. vaginalis*.[27–29] Although these studies demonstrated *G. vaginalis* in sexually inexperienced females, considerable evidence supports sexual transmission of this organism. Gardner and Pheifer et al. detected *G. vaginalis in* the urethras of 79 and 86 percent of the male sex partners of women with BV, but not in male controls.[6,30] Piot et al. developed a system for biotyping strains of *G. vaginalis*, and showed that isolates from the vaginas of women with BV and from the urethras of their sex partners usually belonged to identical biotypes when strains were isolated within the same 24 hour period from both partners ($p < 0.005$).[31] However, in a longitudinal study women with a new sexual partner were no more likely to acquire a different biotype of *G. vaginalis* than were women who did not report having a new sexual partner (81 percent vs. 65 percent, $p = 0.15$).[32]

Ison and Easmon recovered both *G. vaginalis* and anaerobes at concentrations of 10^3 to 10^7 organisms per ml of semen from 16 percent of men attending a subfertility clinic, but did not examine the vaginal flora of the female sex partners.[33] However, another group studied urethral, rectal, and oral flora of 23 male consorts of women with BV and recovered *G. vaginalis* from only two of the urethral samples, one rectal sample, and none of the throat specimens.[34] None of the throat or urethral cultures from any of the men yielded *Mobiluncus* spp., but one rectal specimen yielded *M. curtisii*.[34] Four (17 percent) of the urethral samples yielded *Bacteroides* spp. and 12 (52 percent) yielded peptostreptococci. These authors concluded no evidence supported sexual transmission of these bacteria.

RISK FACTORS FOR BV

The published literature on the epidemiology of BV also offers somewhat conflicting evidence for the role of sexual transmission. Among postpubertal females, those reporting no sexual experience have had significantly lower prevalence of BV than have those with sexual experience.[27] Some studies but not others found BV associated with younger sexual debut.[27,34–36]Among college women, Amsel et al. found BV in 0 of 18 virgins versus 69 (24 percent) of 293 sexually experienced women ($p < 0.03$).[27] One study but not others found a relationship with numbers of lifetime or recent sex partners.[17,34–37] Longitudinal (cohort) studies provide the best evidence. Three cohort studies found that women having exposure to a new sex partner or multiple sex partners had an increased incidence of BV.[38–40] The lack of clear benefit of partner treatment in preventing recurrence of BV provides some evidence against heterosexual transmission, although such evidence is inconclusive, since the impact of such treatment on carriage of BV pathogens among men has not been studied.

Studies of lesbian couples provide further evidence for sexual transmission of BV.[41] Among 101 lesbians seeking gynecologic care, 29 percent had BV, and pairs of monogamous lesbians had high concordance in having BV. The likelihood of a female partner having BV was nearly 20 times greater if her partner had BV.[41] The authors concluded that this concordance probably reflected sexual transmission of BV.

Other epidemiological factors may also be important. A recent cohort study of 182 women demonstrating acquisition of BV was associated not only with having a new sex partner, and (as discussed in the following) with lack of H_2O_2-producing lactobacilli (hazard ratio 4.0, $p < 0.001$) but also with douching for hygiene (HR 2.1, $p = 0.05$). Both Amsel et al. and Holst et al. found use of an intrauterine device more common among women with BV than among other women (18.8 vs. 5.4 percent, $p < 0.001$, and 35 vs. 16 percent, $p < 0.03$, respectively).[27,34] In a prospective study, Avonts et al. reported a twofold increased incidence of BV among IUD users compared to oral contraceptive users.[38] A recent prospective study of female sex workers in Peru also found IUD use associated with more than a twofold increased risk of acquiring BV (Sanchez J, Holmes KK, unpublished). However, smoking status, history of abnormal Pap smears, days of menstrual flow, days since last menstrual period, form of menstrual protection, age at menarche, and years since menarche have not been associated with BV.[27,34]

ETIOLOGY

GARDNERELLA VAGINALIS

Leopold first reported the isolation of a small nonmotile nonencapsulated pleomorphic Gram-negative rod from the genitourinary tract of women with cervicitis in 1953.[42] Two years later, Gardner and Dukes isolated this organism, which they named *Haemophilus vaginalis*, from 92 percent of 141 women with "bacterial vaginitis," from 20 percent of women with *Trichomonas vaginalis* infection, from 4 percent of women with clinical moniliasis, and from none of 78 controls.[6] In an attempt to fulfill Koch's postulates, Gardner inoculated 15 women not infected by *H. vaginalis* with material from the vaginas of infected patients, and reproduced the manifestations of this condition in 11 of 15 women. However, inoculation of pure *H. vaginalis* resulted in these manifestations in only one of 13 women, despite isolation of *H. vaginalis* from the vagina of all of these women one or more weeks after inoculation. Both Brewer and Heltai confirmed the association between nonspecific vaginitis and *H. vaginalis*, but unlike Gardner and Dukes, they also isolated other organisms and concluded that *H. vaginalis* was not the sole etiology of nonspecific vaginitis.[6,43,44]

Lack of consensus on the taxonomic status of *G. vaginalis* added to the uncertainty surrounding the microorganism. In 1963, Zinneman and Turner recommended the reclassification of the organism to the genus *Corynebacterium,* because under optimal growth conditions, it became Gram-positive and formed polar granules.[45] Electron microscopy studies by Reyn et al. showed that the organism's cell wall resembled that of a Gram-positive bacterium, whereas Criswell's electron microscopic studies of the same strain indicated that the organism was more probably Gram-negative.[46,47] In 1980, Greenwood and Pickett resolved the issue by proposing a new genus, *Gardnerella,* "to include catalase and oxidase-negative, Gram-negative to Gram-variable bacteria with laminated cell walls, which produce acetic acid as the major end product of fermentation."[48]

The body of literature over the past 30 years has substantiated the association of *Gardnerella vaginalis* with bacterial vaginosis. However, with use of more sensitive culture media *G. vaginalis* can be isolated, often in high concentrations, from women with no signs of vaginal infection.[49] Many now believe that *G. vaginalis* somehow interacts with anaerobic bacteria and genital mycoplasmas (discussed in the following) to cause bacterial vaginosis.

ANAEROBIC BACTERIA

Anaerobic rods and cocci were first isolated from the vagina in 1897 and were found associated with vaginal discharge by Curtis in the early part of this century.[1,3] From 1947 to 1958, three studies found an association of black-pigmented anaerobic Gram-negative rods (the former *Bacteroides melaninogenicus* group) and other anaerobic Gram-negative rods, with vaginitis, and a decrease in prevalence of vaginal lactobacilli among those with vaginal discharge.[5,50,51] In 1979, Goldacre reported finding Gram-negative anaerobic bacilli significantly more commonly among women with "troublesome vaginal discharge" than among normal women, and concluded that the association between genitourinary symptoms and anaerobes warranted further study.[52] In 1980, Spiegel analyzed the vaginal fluid from 53 women with bacterial vaginosis using quantitative anaerobic cultures and gas–liquid chromatography to detect the short-chain organic acid metabolites of the vaginal flora.[8] She isolated *Bacteroides* spp. (now *Prevotella* and *Prophyromonas*) from 76 percent, and *Peptococcus* (now called *Peptostreptococcus*) from 36 percent of the women with bacterial vaginosis, and recovered both types of anaerobes significantly less often from normal women. The recovery of anaerobic species correlated directly with a decrease in lactate and an increase in succinate and acetate in the vaginal fluid. Paavonen later confirmed the presence of succinate and other short chain fatty acids in vaginal fluid from women with BV.[53] After metronidazole therapy, the anaerobic Gram-negative rods and peptostreptococci disappeared from the vagina, and lactate again became the predominant organic acid in the vaginal fluid. Spiegel concluded that anaerobes interacted with *G. vaginalis* to cause bacterial vaginosis. Others have since confirmed the association between anaerobes and BV.[9,34,54,55]

In our experience the anaerobic Gram-negative rods most commonly associated with BV include *Prevotella bivia*, the black-pigmented species belonging to the genera *Prevotella* and *Porphyromonas, Bacteroides ureolyticus,* and *Fusobacterium nucleatum.*[9] Members of the *Bacteroides fragilis* group (*B. fragilis, B. ovatus, B. vulgatus, B. thetaiotaomicron*), although common in the intestinal tract, are less common in the vagina and not associated with BV.[9]

The vaginal flora of most women includes anaerobic Gram-positive cocci (primarily peptostreptococci) but *P. prevotii, P. tetradius,* and *P. anaerobius* are the species most frequently recovered from women with BV.[9]

Although research during the early 1980s implicated another anaerobic microorganism, *Mobiluncus,* in BV, Kronig actually first observed a curved anaerobic rod by Gram stain of uterine discharge in 1895, and Curtis first isolated such an organism from the uterine discharge of women with postpartum fever.[56,57] Prevot suggested the name "*Vibrio mulieris*" in 1940.[58] Most early microbiologic studies failed to detect this nutritionally fastidious and strictly anaerobic microorganism, but in 1980, Durieux and Dublanchet isolated and characterized 18 strains of succinate-producing anaerobic curved rods from women with vaginal discharge.[59] Several researchers noted the association of this organism either with abnormal vaginal discharge or with clinical features of bacterial vaginosis.[60–64] Spiegel detected this organism by direct Gram stain of the vaginal fluid from 31 (51 percent) of 62 women with BV and from none of 42 normal controls.[64] In 1984, Spiegel and Roberts proposed the genus name *Mobiluncus* for this motile rod. Two species were described: *M. curtisii* and *M. mulieris.*[65] One study employed DNA probe, culture, or Gram stain to demonstrate *Mobiluncus* spp. in 68 percent of women with BV and another employed fluorescent monoclonal antibodies to detect *Mobiluncus* spp. in 50 percent of 107 women with and 17 (6 percent) of 291 women without clinical signs of BV.[19,66] Holst has reported the highest isolation rate for *Mobiluncus* spp., recovering *Mobiluncus* from the vagina or rectum from 29 (85 percent) of 34 women with BV.[61] The isolation of *Mobiluncus* spp. from only the rectum of seven of these women suggests that the gut may serve as a reservoir for this organism. In the vagina, *Mobiluncus* always occurs together with other organisms associated with BV, and has also been associated with gonorrhea. *Mobiluncus* spp. have most frequently been recovered from African-American women, but are not associated with young age at first intercourse, lifetime number of sexual partners, or having a new partner in the past month.[68]

Schwebke et al. have reported phenotypic variants of *M. mulieris* and *M. curtisii.*[69] The phenotypically and antigenically distinct *M. curtissii* strains are more frequently recovered from women with normal vaginal flora than from those with BV.[69] Recent studies have demonstrated serum antibody to *M. curtisii* very commonly in sexually experienced women (75 percent) (including many who denied a history of BV), and rarely in pediatric patients (6 percent) or virgins (0 percent).[70] The authors concluded that humoral antibody to *M. curtisii* may provide a useful serological marker for BV, and that BV may commonly go unrecognized in sexually experienced women.

GENITAL MYCOPLASMAS

Hunter and Long noted the association of genital mycoplasmas with vaginitis in 1958, recovering pleuropneumonia-like organisms (PPLO) from 48 percent of 39 women with vaginitis and 14 percent of 48 controls ($p < 0.05$).[51] Women harboring PPLO, later recognized as mycoplasmas, more often harbored other "abnormal" vaginal flora including anaerobic Gram-negative rods and trichomonads. In 1970, Mendel reported isolation of mycoplasmas from nearly half of patients with trichomoniasis or *Gardnerella vaginalis*, but without any specific disease.[71] Taylor-Robinson and McCormack first suggested in 1980 that *Mycoplasma hominis* could have a role in nonspecific vaginitis, either in symbiosis with *Gardnerella vaginalis* and other organisms or as a sole pathogen.[72] Pheifer et al. supported this hypothesis, by recovering *M. hominis* from 63 percent of women with BV and 10 percent of normal controls.[30] In 1982, Paavonen et al. also reported the association of BV with *M. hominis* and *G. vaginalis* in vaginal fluid.[53]

OTHER MICROORGANISMS

Women with BV do not have increased rates of vaginal colonization by *Escherichia coli* or other Gram-negative facultative bacteria, group B streptococci, coagulase-negative staphylococci, diphtheroids, or most species of viridans streptococci; but have had significantly increased rates of vaginal carriage of two species of viridans group streptococci, *Streptococcus acidominimus* and *Streptococcus morbillorum*.[73] However, vaginal colonization by *Enterococcus* occurs more frequently among women with *Lactobacillus*-predominant vaginal flora than among women with BV.[9]

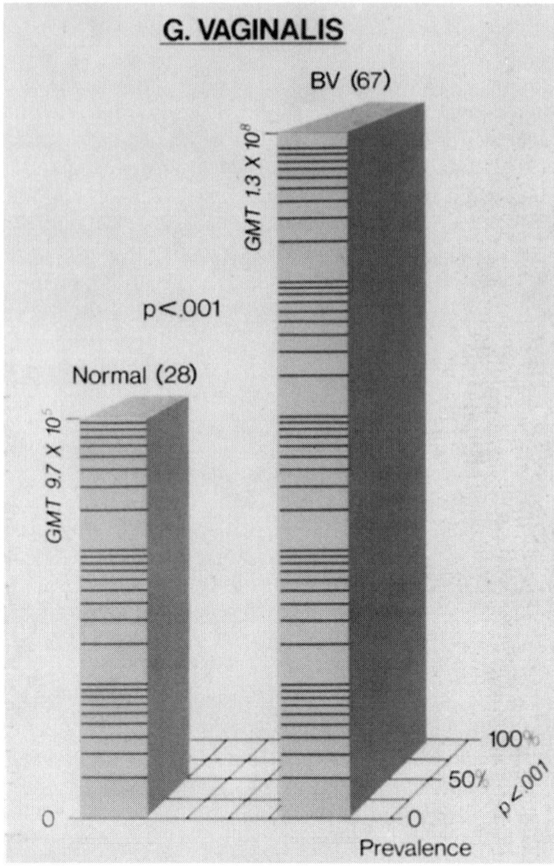

Fig. 42-2. The prevalence of *G. vaginalis* is nearly twice as high among women with bacterial vaginosis as among normal women. Among those colonized by *G. vaginalis*, the geometric mean concentration (GMT) of *G. vaginalis* for women with bacterial vaginosis is over 100 times higher than among normal women. (Courtesy of Eschenbach, DA, unpublished data.)

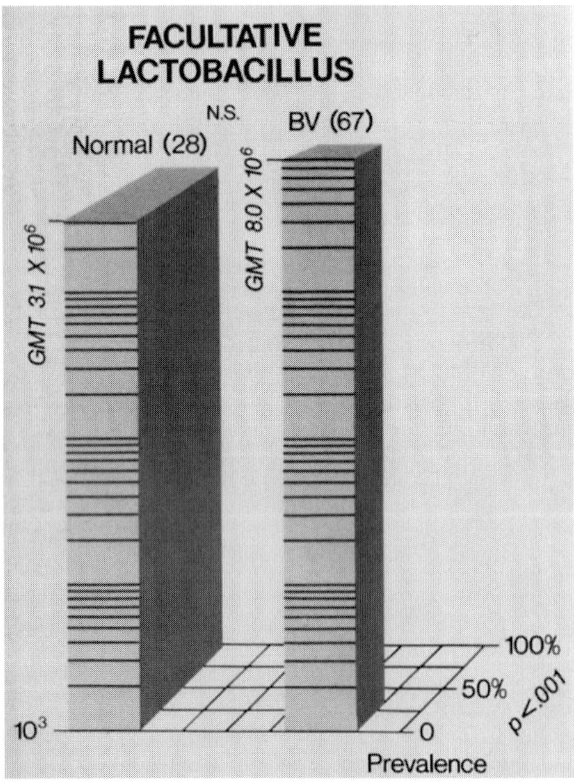

Fig. 42-1. Although the prevalence of lactobacilli is decreased among women with BV, the geometric mean concentration (GMT) of lactobacilli among those who are colonized is about the same for women with or without BV. (Courtesy of Eschenbach, DA, unpublished data.)

It is apparent that no single organism causes bacterial vaginosis. Our multivariate analysis found independent associations of BV with four categories of vaginal bacteria: *Mobiluncus* spp., anaerobic Gram-negative rods., *G. vaginalis*, and *M. hominis*.[74] The prevalence of each of these microorganisms is increased among women with BV. In addition, when present, these organisms are found at 100- to 1000-fold greater concentrations among women with BV than among normal women (Figs. 42-2 through 42-4) while lactobacilli are decreased among women with BV (Fig 42-1).

PATHOGENESIS

Bacterial vaginosis results from the replacement of the normal vaginal flora *(Lactobacillus)* with a mixed flora consisting of *Gardnerella vaginalis*, anaerobes, and *Mycoplasma hominis*. Thus, most studies of the pathogenesis of BV have focused on how the microbial ecosystem of the vagina becomes altered. In an effort to experimentally reproduce the signs and symptoms of bacterial vaginosis, Criswell et al. actually inoculated 29 normal pregnant women with 2 mL of suspension containing 2×10^{10} *G. vaginalis*. Seven (24 percent) of the 29 women developed clinical signs of infection over the 3 weeks postinoculation.[75] They did not assess whether anaerobic bacteria or genital mycoplasmas also appeared among those who acquired the clinical syndrome. In the grivet monkey model system, *Gardnerella vaginalis* or *Mobiluncus* sp. applied alone intravaginally did not cause signs of vaginitis.[76] However, inoculation of two monkeys with both *G. vaginalis* and *Mobiluncus* produced vaginal discharge in both monkeys after 5 days. These studies, together with epidemiologic data described in the preceding, are consistent with the notion that introduction of a particular set of organisms via sexual intercourse may initiate the change in vaginal flora characteristic of BV.

Lactobacillus spp. may help normal women to resist vaginal and cervical infection. Vaginal lactobacilli inhibit *G. vaginalis, Mobiluncus,* and *Bacteroides* species in vitro.[77] Some strains of *Lactobacillus* produce H_2O_2, and one case-control and four cross-sectional studies have demonstrated that H_2O_2-producing strains of lactobacilli more frequently colonize the vagina of normal women, compared to women with BV.[9,14,40,78–80] Further, during a prospective study, women colonized with H_2O_2-positive lactobacilli less often developed bacterial vaginosis than did those colonized with H_2O_2 negative lactobacilli.[40] The H_2O_2 produced by the vaginal lactobacilli may inhibit the growth of the anaerobic rod, *Gardnerella, Mobiluncus,* and *Mycoplasma* in the vagina either directly via the toxic activity of H_2O_2 or by reacting with a halide ion in the presence of cervical peroxidase as part of the H_2O_2-halide-peroxidase antibacterial system.[81] Chapter 14 presents more information on the role of lactobacilli in modulating vaginal flora.

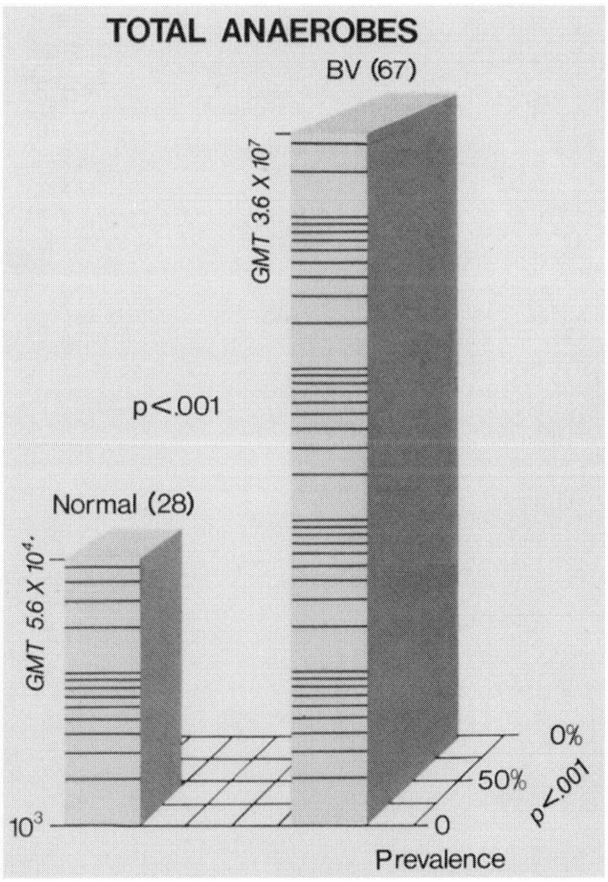

Fig. 42-3. We have isolated anaerobic bacteria from the vagina from approximately 60 percent of normal women and 100 percent of those with BV. Furthermore, the geometric mean concentration (GMT) of anaerobes was over 400 times higher among women with BV than among normal women from whom anaerobes were isolated. (Courtesy of Eschenbach, DA, unpublished data.)

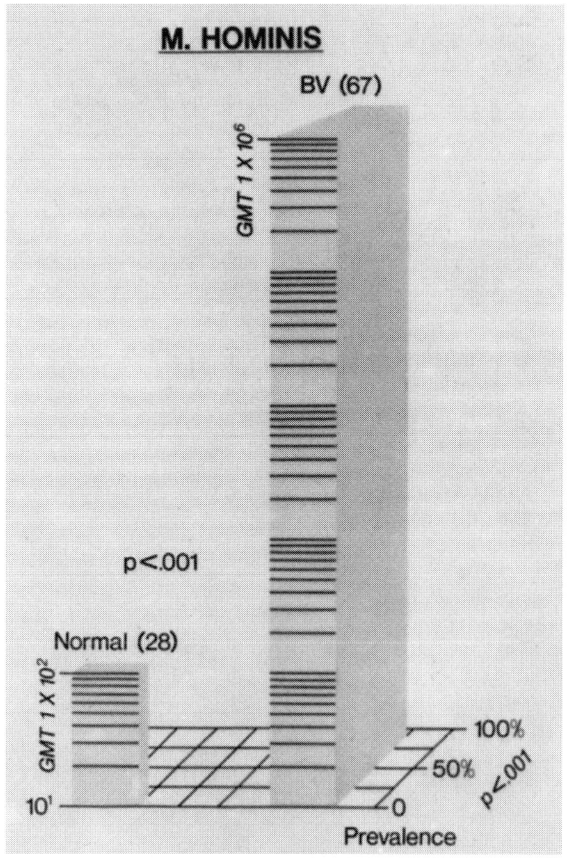

Fig. 42-4. We have isolated *Mycoplasma hominis* from 60 to 70 percent of women with BV and 20 percent of normal women. As with anaerobic bacteria and *Gardnerella vaginalis,* women with BV have geometric mean concentrations (GMT) several logs higher than normal women colonized by *M. hominis.* (Courtesy of Eschenbach, DA, unpublished data.)

So far, no host factor has been identified that increases susceptibility to BV. A possible exception is IUD use, but the mechanisms by which IUD use may increase the risk of BV are not understood.[38] The redox potential (Eh) of the vaginal epithelial surface is lower in women with BV than in normal women.[82] After the women with BV were treated with metronidazole, the redox potential of the vaginal epithelium returned to the normal range, a result suggesting that the low vaginal Eh was not a persistent underlying host factor.[82]

It is thought that amines produced by the microbial flora, perhaps by microbial decarboxylases, account for the characteristic abnormal fishy odor produced when vaginal fluid is mixed with 10 percent KOH. This so-called "whiff test" is thought to be owing to volatilization of aromatic amines, including putrescine, cadaverine, and trimethylamine at alkaline pH.[83,84] *Mobiluncus* is known to produce trimethylamine, but the other microbial sources of the amines are still unknown.[84] Recent data suggest that trimethylamine can be detected at relatively high concentrations in the vaginal fluid of bacterial vaginosis, with a median concentration of 5 mM.[85] The presence of trimethylamine in the vaginal fluid is thought to be largely responsible for symptoms of malodor experienced by women with BV.

The effects of altered patterns of organic acids are uncertain, although it has been shown that succinic acid produced by vaginal anaerobes inhibit the chemotactic response of white blood cells.[86] The vaginal fluid of women with BV has increased levels of endotoxin, sialidase, and the mucinase.[87–89] An increased host response to BV has been documented in the form of increased levels of interleukin-1α and prostaglandins in the cervical mucus of women with BV.[87,90] The effects of BV on the vaginal epithelium and on epithelial cell turnover have not yet been well studied. Nonetheless, the increased vaginal concentrations of anaerobic pathogens in BV may increase the risk of ascending upper genital tract infections, as discussed in the following.

CLINICAL MANIFESTATIONS

In a cross-sectional study of clinic patients, BV by Gram-stain criteria was significantly associated with symptoms of vaginal malodor (49 percent of patients with BV vs. 20 percent without BV) and vaginal discharge (50 percent of patients with BV vs. 37 percent without BV); and with signs of a nonviscous homogeneous, white, uniformly adherent vaginal discharge (69 percent women with BV vs. 3 percent without BV) (Table 42-1).[21] As noted in the preceding, the malodor is attributed to the abnormal

Table 42-1. Symptoms and Signs among 661 Randomly Selected Women Attending a Sexually Transmitted Disease Clinic*

	Bacterial Vaginosis (n = 311), %	No Bacterial Vaginosis (n = 350), %	Univariate		Multivariate†	
			Odds Ratio	P	Odds Ratio	P
Symptoms						
Chief complaint						
None	47	36	1.5	0.01	2.6	0.2
Abdominal pain	7	3	3.0	0.05	2.6	0.2
Vaginal bleeding	0.6	0.3	2.3	0.5	2.1	0.3
Vaginal discharge	17	7	2.9	<0.0001	2.6	0.01
Vulvar pruritus	8	18	0.4	<0.001	0.9	0.9
Other (dysuria, ulcers)	20	36	0.5		0.7	0.3
Odor	49	20	3.9	<0.001	3.4	<0.001
Increased discharge	50	37	1.7	0.001	1.3	0.005
Yellow discharge	24	17	1.6	0.01	1.2	0.08
Abdominal pain	45	35	1.5	0.01	1.2	0.4
Increased amount of menstrual bleeding	14	9	1.6	0.04	1.4	0.2
Prolonged menses	11	6	2.1	0.01	1.2	0.4
Intermenstrual bleeding	16	13	1.2	0.4	1.2	0.5
Signs						
Homogeneous discharge	69	3	77	<0.001	103	<0.001
Frothy discharge	2	0		0.007		
Increased discharge	9	4	2.3	0.02	1.5	0.001
Yellow vaginal dischargc	32	18	2.2	0.001	2.3	0.001
Ectopy (any)	51	52	1.0	0.8	1.1	0.8
Ectopy (≥50%)	7	8	0.8	0.4	1.2	0.8
Mucopus	28	21	1.5	0.03	1.2	0.4
Adnexal tenderness‡	28	21	1.5	0.03	1.2	0.4
Uterine tenderness	4	1	2.5	0.08	1.7	0.4
Cervical motion tenderness	3	0.6	4.6	0.04	2.8	0.2
Clinical diagnosis of PID	3	0		0.003		
Macroscopic warts	7	14	0.5	0.009	0.5	0.004
Amine-like odor of vaginal fluid in potassium hydroxide	43	1	88	<0.001	113	<0.001
pH ≥ 4.7	97	47	30	<0.001	23	<0.001
Mean pH + SD	5.0 ± 0.3	4.6 ± 0.3				
Microscopic result						
Any clue cells	81	6	69	M0.001	75	<0.001
Clue cells ≥ 20% of epithelial cells	78	5	72	<0.001	88	<0.001
Cervical Gram stain ≥ 30PMN/HPF	28	22	1.4	0.08	1.1	0.7
Vaginal wet mount ≥ 30 WBCs/HPF	40	34	1.3	0.2	1.4	0.1
Vaginal wet mount showing Predominance of lactobacilli	2	59	0.02	<0.001	0.02	<0.001

PID = pelvic inflammatory disease; PMNs = polymorphonuclear leukocytes; HPF = high power field; WBCs = white blood cells.

*Univariate and multivariate comparison of patients with and without gram stain criteria for bacterial vaginosis.

†Each sign was adjusted for age, race, parity, education, occupation, current smoking, age at first intercourse, lifetime sexual partners, *C. trachomatis, N. gonorrhoeae,* yeast, and herpes simplex virus in the analysis. Women with *Trichomonas vaginalis* were excluded from the analysis.

‡Adnexal tenderness scored as moderate to severe.

PID = pelvic inflammatory disease; PMNs = polymorphonuclear leukocytes; HPF = high power field; WBCs = white blood cells.

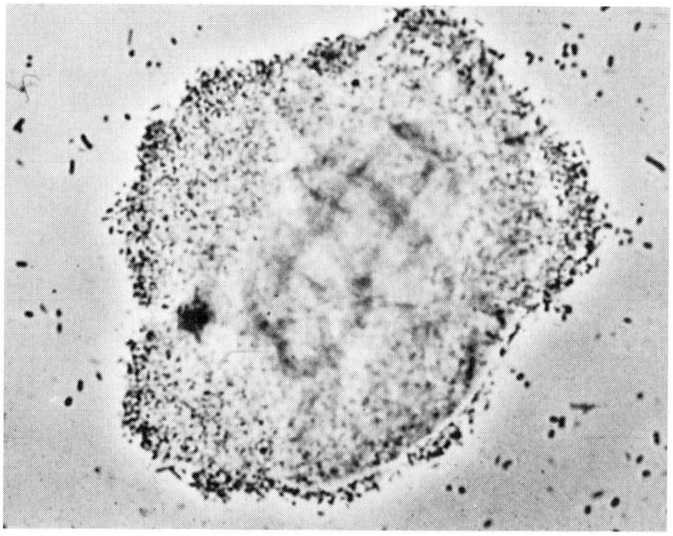

Fig. 42-5. Wet mount of vaginal fluid showing a typical clue cell from a woman with bacterial vaginosis. Note that the cell margins are obscured. (×1000 magnification.)

presence of amines, particularly trimethylamine. Of related interest is a syndrome of primary trimethylaminieria, a disorder of humans colloquially known as "fish-odor syndrome," owing to a recessively inherited defect in hepatic oxygenation of dietary trimethylamine.[91,92] Those affected can suffer from social isolation, depression, and attempted suicide—reminiscent of the psychosocial symptoms that can accompany BV. The discharge adheres uniformly to the vaginal walls, often visibly on the labia and fourchette before insertion of a vaginal speculum (color plate). Although one-third of women with BV describe their vaginal discharge as yellow, most studies have found no significant increase in the mean number of polymorphonuclear leukocytes in vaginal discharge in this syndrome. The observation by Rein et al. of an association of BV with a positive test for lactoferrin (a marker for PMN leukocytes) stands apart from other studies in this regard; in attempting to reconcile this finding with the generally accepted absence of pleocytosis, it was shown that BV-associated fluid was toxic for PMNs.[93] Another study confirmed that women having BV but no STD (gonorrhea, chlamydia, or trichomoniasis) had higher median vaginal fluid concentrations of lactoferrin compared to women without BV (531 vs. 29 ng/mL, $p = 0.04$).[94] In any case, the finding of PMNs in the wet mount should not exclude a diagnosis of BV.

Nearly all women with BV have a vaginal pH of ≥4.5 when measured with pH paper having an appropriate pH range, although this finding is by no means specific for BV. A fishy odor was noted when vaginal fluid was mixed with 10% KOH (the "whiff test") in 43 percent of those with BV versus 1 percent of those without BV. Microscopic evaluation of vaginal fluid at high power (400×) revealed clue cells in 81 percent of those with BV versus 6 percent of those without BV.[21] Clue cells are epithelial cells heavily coated with bacteria sufficient to obscure the cell borders (Fig. 42-5). The bacteria covering the clue cells include *Gardnerella vaginalis,* as well as anaerobes such as *Mobiluncus* (see color plates).

DIAGNOSIS

Self-diagnosis of vaginitis is usually incorrect. In a study of 552 women aged 16 or older, only 3 to 4 percent of women could accurately identify the symptoms associated with BV.[95] Many women believe vaginal malodor is owing to poor hygiene, or are embarrassed about the symptoms, and do not report this as a symptom to their health care provider. Thus, symptoms alone are not reliable for the diagnosis of bacterial vaginosis. Amsel et al. recommended basing the clinical diagnosis of bacterial vaginosis on the presence of at least three of the following four signs:[27] (1) characteristic homogeneous white adherent discharge; (2) vaginal fluid pH >4.5; (3) release of a fishy amine odor from vaginal fluid when mixed with 10 percent KOH; and (4) presence of clue cells (usually representing at least 20 percent of vaginal epithelial cells). These simple clinical tests are inexpensive and available in most office settings. We agree with the original observation of Gardner and Dukes that detection of clue cells is the most useful single procedure for diagnosis of BV, but demonstration of the other features serves to support the microscopic interpretation of presence of clue cells, and can support the diagnosis in resource-poor settings lacking microscopy. Evaluation of wet mounts of vaginal fluid is technically difficult and highly subject to interobserver variation. Therefore, determination of pH and amine odor can significantly enhance the accuracy of diagnosis of BV. In one recent study, the use of a visual test card for pH and trimethylamine (FemExam®, Litmus Concepts, Santa Clara, CA) was evaluated as a screening test for BV. Having both elevated vaginal pH and trimethylamine had a sensitivity of 86 percent (140/162) and specificity of 92 percent for detection of BV using this visual test card system.[85]

DISCHARGE

Douching, recent intercourse, menstruation, and concurrent infection all can alter the appearance of the discharge associated with BV. The white, nonfloccular discharge of BV adheres to the walls of the vagina, and is only slightly or moderately increased in amount over that normally seen. Absence of a discernable white homogeneous discharge should not rule out BV, if the other manifestations are present (Table 42-2).

VAGINAL FLUID PH

The vaginal fluid pH determination requires pH paper having appropriate range (pH 4.0 to 6.0). Commercially available pH paper suitable for this purpose includes colopHast (pH 4.0 to 7.0) (MCB Reagents, Gibbstown, NJ) pHydrion papers (pH 3.0 to 5.5) (Micro Essential Laboratory, Brooklyn, NY), or pH-fix (pH 3.6 to 6.1) (Gallard-Schlesinger Industries, Carleplace, NY). Vaginal pH is best determined by swabbing the lateral or posterior fornices of the vagina, and then placing the swab sample directly on the pH paper. Alternatively, the pH paper can be placed on vaginal fluid pooling in the speculum after removal from the vagina. The cervical mucus must be avoided since it has a higher pH (pH 7.0) than the vaginal fluid. Eschenbach et al. reported that none of 178

Table 42-2. Standardized Method for Scoring Gram-Stained Smears for Diagnosis of Bacterial Vaginosis

	Points Scored per Morphotype*				
Bacterial morphotype	None	1+†	2+†	3+†	4+†
Large Gram-positive rod	4	3	2	1	0
Small Gram-negative/variable rod	0	1	2	3	4
Curved negative/variable rod	0	1	1	2	2

*Score or 0 to 3 points, normal; 4 to 6, intermediate; 7 to 10, bacterial vaginosis.
†1+ <1/1000; 2+, 1-5/1000×; 3+, 6-30/1000×; 4+ >30/1000×.
Modified from Nugent RP et al. J Clin MIcrobiol 1991;29:297–301, by permission of the American Society for Microbiology.[103]

women with pH ≤4.4 had clue cells, whereas all of 257 women having ≥20 percent clue cells had vaginal pH ≥4.7.[21] Of these 257 women, 89 percent had a homogeneous discharge, an amine odor, or both. Vaginal fluid pH has the greatest sensitivity of the four clinical signs, but the lowest specificity.

ODOR

Vaginal malodor is the most common symptom of women with BV, and release of the "fishy" amine-odor from vaginal fluid after addition of 10 percent KOH greatly increases the detection of the malodor by the clinician. A drop of vaginal fluid should be placed on a glass slide and a drop of 10 percent KOH added, immediately releasing an amine odor as the pH of the mixture approaches the pKa of the amines (e.g., putrescine, cadaverine, histamine, trimethylamine), and amines that are no longer protonated become volatile. The odor then dissipates quickly. A coverslip placed over this preparation permits microscopic exam for the pseudohyphal forms associated with candidiasis. Although the KOH odor test was reportedly the most powerful single predictor for diagnosis of BV, this test may be the least sensitive of the four clinical tests for diagnosis of BV.[96] Eschenbach et al. reported a positive predictive value of only 76 percent for this test compared with Gram stain diagnosis of BV.[21] However, when an objective diamine test was used as a screening test for BV in 229 women, the detection of diamines was found to be 92 percent sensitive and 83 percent specific compared to identification of clue cells.[97] In another study of 164 women attending a genitourinary medicine clinic, the same colormetric diamine test had a 87 percent sensitivity and 98 percent specificity compared to Gram-stain criteria.[98] It is likely that the colorimetric tests for amines are more sensitive than the "whiff" test, which may explain the increased sensitivity of the chemical tests compared simply "sniffing" for amino odor.

WET MOUNT EXAM FOR CLUE CELLS

Clue cells are squamous vaginal epithelial cells covered with many vaginal bacteria, giving them a stippled or granular appearance. The borders are obscured or stipled owing to adherence of small rods or cocci, including *Gardnerella, Mobiluncus,* and other bacteria (see Fig. 42-5). Lactobacilli may also bind to exfollated vaginal epithelial cells, although seldom in high enough concentrations to mimic clue cells. We recommend that at least 20 percent of vaginal epithelial cells resemble clue cells to establish a diagnostic criterion for BV. However, when an experienced microscopist identifies only 1 to 20 percent of vaginal epithelial cells as clue cells, this is highly correlated with Gram-stain features of BV.[99]

A sample of vaginal fluid obtained with a swab and mixed on a glass slide with a drop of normal saline, is covered by a coverslip, and ten fields examined under high power (×400) for clue cells (and for detection of motile trichomonads). Clue cells represent the best single criterion for the diagnosis of BV.[21,100]

VAGINAL CULTURE

Cultures for *G. vaginalis* have little utility for the diagnosis of BV. *G. vaginalis* can be recovered from nearly all women with BV, but also from up to 58 percent of those without BV.[21] In one study, isolation of ≥3+ *G. vaginalis* by culture had a positive predictive value of only 49 percent with respect to composite clinical signs for the diagnosis of BV. Vaginal Gram stains had comparable sensitivity, but a much greater specificity and predictive value than vaginal cultures for *G. vaginalis.*[21] A positive vaginal culture for *G. vaginalis* in the absence of the clinical signs of BV does not warrant therapy. Likewise, *G. vaginalis* culture does not constitute "test of cure" since many women without clinical signs of BV have positive cultures for this organism following effective treatment.

GRAM-STAINED SMEARS OF VAGINAL FLUID

Dunkelberg first proposed the evaluation of vaginal Gram-stained smears for diagnosis of BV and Spiegel et al. later published specific guidelines.[101,102] A standardized 0- to 10-point scoring system

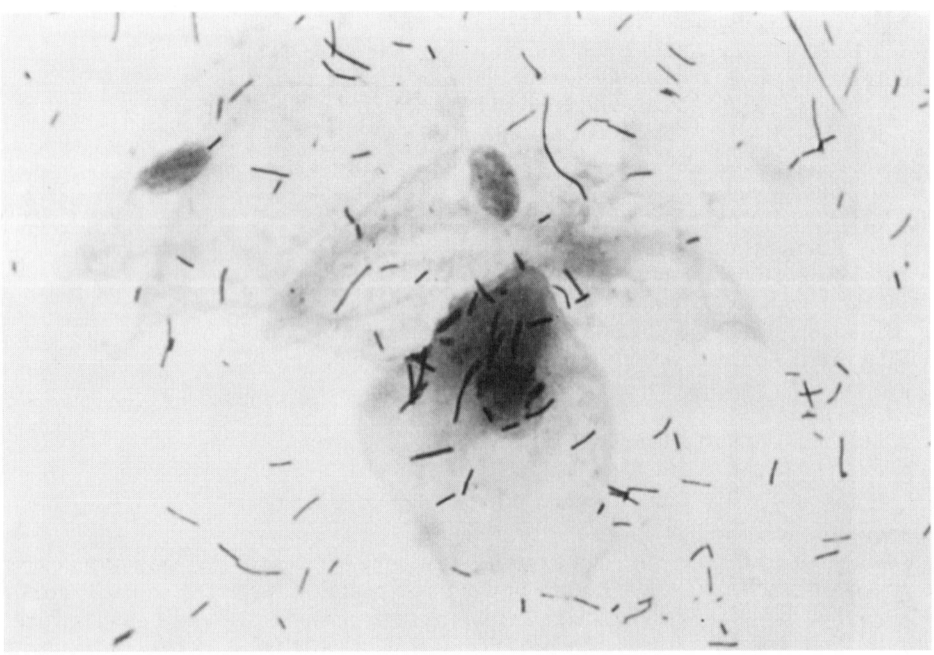

Fig. 42-6. Gram stain of normal vaginal fluid, showing gram-positive rods with blunt ends consistent with lactobacilli. (×1000 magnification.)

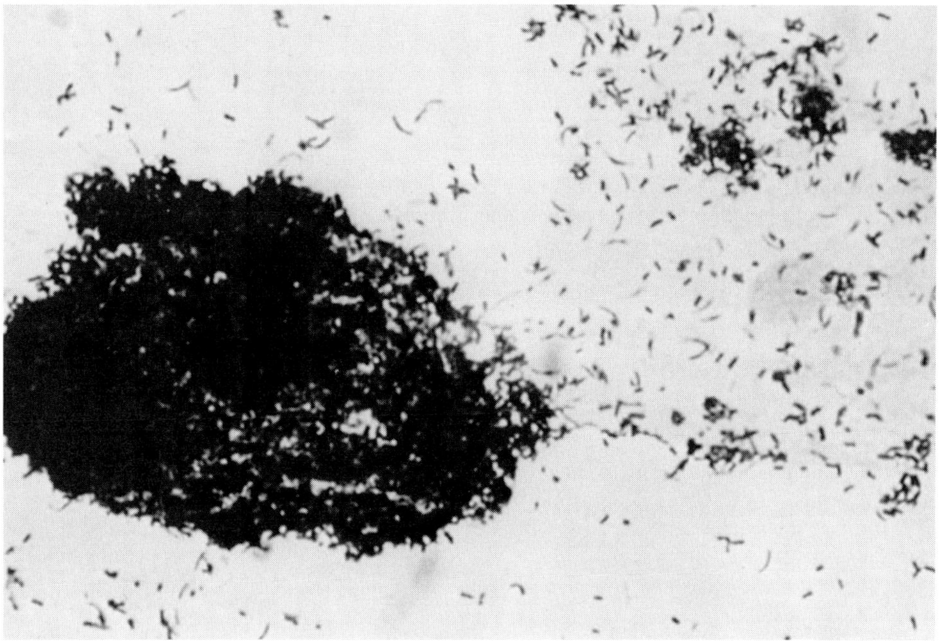

Fig. 42-7. Gram stain of vaginal fluid from a woman with bacterial vaginosis showing absence of lactobacilli and large numbers of Gram-negative or Gram-variable coccobacilli. Curved gram-variable rods are consistent with *Mobiluncus.* Note that epithelial cell on the left is a clue cell, whereas the epithelial cell to the right has clear margins. (×1000 magnification.)

for evaluation of Gram-stained vaginal smears was later developed based on three morphotypes: large Gram-positive rods (lactobacilli), small Gram-negative or variable rods (*Gardnerella* and anaerobic rods), and *Mobiluncus* (see Table 42-2).[103] This method, based on the shift in bacterial morphotypes from predominance of lactobacilli to predominance of *Gardnerella* and anaerobic bacterial morphotypes, including *Mobiluncus*, has had 89 percent sensitivity and 83 percent specificity for diagnosis of BV in comparison with clinical criteria,[104] and has had excellent inter-center reproducability (Figs. 42-6 and 42-7).[103,105] Two studies evaluating the Nugent Gram-stain criteria for diagnosis of bacterial vaginosis have reported sensitivities of 86 to 89 percent and specifies of 94 to 96 percent compared to the Amsel criteria.[99,106] In one of the studies, the Nugent and Spiegel methods were directly compared.[106] Evaluation of vaginal smears by the Nugent criteria yielded similar sensitivity (86 percent vs. 83 percent) and greater specificity (96 percent vs. 89 percent) compared to the Spiegel method. The vaginal smear for Gram-stain evaluation can be prepared at the same time that the wet mount is prepared by rolling (not streaking) the swab across the surface of a glass slide. After air drying, the slide can be stored for months or years prior to staining with no appreciable loss in quality. Self-obtained swabs have also been proven to be acceptable for preparation of Gram-stained vaginal smears.[107–108] The slide should be heat-fixed and stained as usual in the clinical lab. The advantages of Gram stain for diagnosis include interpretation by standardized objective criteria by a microbiologist, suitability for quick screening, and storage for batch reading or later confirmation if desired.

Oligonucleotide probes

A specific oligonucleotide probe test adjusted to detect only high concentrations ($>10^7$/mL vaginal fluid) of *G. vaginalis* was 95 percent sensitive and 79 percent specific for the diagnosis of BV in 113 women (Affirm VP III, Becton-Dickinson, Cockeysville, MD).[109] A commercially available 40-minute version of this test was 94 percent sensitive and 81 percent specific for the diagnosis of BV in an STD clinic population.[110] This test simultaneously detects *Candida* species as well as *Trichomonas vaginalis* and provides a laboratory-based option for detection of all three vaginal pathogens. The advantage of this system is that it is objective, detects mixed vaginal infections, and can be used in any setting approved for moderately complex laboratory tests.

DETECTION OF METABOLIC PRODUCTS

Several published methods for BV diagnosis involve detection of metabolic products of the microorganisms in the vaginal fluid of women with BV. Some of these tests have been modified for ambulatory clinic use, with commercial availability anticipated soon.

Determination of amines in vaginal fluid

As reported by Chen et al. and Brand and Galask, women with clinical signs of BV have diamines and polyamines in the vaginal fluid.[80,83] Chen found 87 percent sensitivity and 86 percent specificity for this test. As noted in the preceding, recently developed rapid card test for detection of trimethylamine combined with elevated pH in vaginal fluid (FemExam®, Litmus Concepts, Santa Clara, CA) had a sensitivity of 86 percent and a specificity of 92 percent for diagnosis of BV in a recent multicenter study of 606 women.[85] Others have reported that colorimetric detection of diamines provide 87 to 92 percent sensitivity for detection of BV.[97,98]

Proline aminopeptidase test

Some of the bacteria associated with BV (*G. vaginalis, Mobiluncus* spp.) produce proline aminopeptidase, whereas lactobacilli do not produce this enzyme. After incubation of vaginal fluid with enzyme substrate in a microtiter plate for 4 h at 35.5°C, rapid garnet green is added to produce a color reaction. A red or pink color indicates a positive test, whereas an orange or yellow color indicates a negative test. Among 500 consecutive women, Thomason reported 81 percent sensitivity and 96 percent specificity in comparison to clinical criteria for diagnosis of BV.[111] The advantages claimed for this test over gas chromatographic analysis of vaginal fluid included greater sensitivity and lower cost and time required. This test could be adapted for bedside use as a rapid colorimetric test. These rapid tests may prove useful for diagnosis of BV in offices lacking microscopy, and they have the potential advantage of objectivity and relative simplicity.

Succinate/lactate ratio

Many anaerobic Gram-negative rods produce succinate as a metabolic product, and lactobacilli produce lactate as a metabolic product. The ratio of succinate to lactate in vaginal fluid has been shown by gas–liquid chromolographic analysis to be increased in BV and has been used as a screening test for BV in clinical epidemiologic studies.[112]

TREATMENT

Gardner first described triple sulfa cream as a treatment for "*Haemophilus vaginalis* vaginitis" in 1955.[6] Subsequently, sulfa creams have been shown to have low efficacy and are inappropriate for treatment of BV. Over the past 15 years, numerous studies of various therapies for BV have repeatedly shown that only those antimicrobial compounds with broad activity against most anaerobic bacteria are highly effective for the treatment of this syndrome.

METRONIDAZOLE

Pheifer et al. first observed in 1978 that metronidazole used for vaginal trichomoniasis also cleared concurrent nonspecific vaginitis, and went on to demonstrate the efficacy of a 7-day metronidazole regimen for the latter condition.[30] Over the past 20 years, more than 50 articles have been published on the use of metronidazole for treatment of BV, giving consistent results.

Most of the carefully conducted clinical trials used the Amsel criteria for diagnosis of BV, and cure or improvement was usually defined as resolution of two or more of Amsel's criteria for diagnosis.[27] Outcome was generally assessed 1 week or 1 month after therapy. Several studies found that 10 to 15 percent of women who initially respond to therapy relapse by 1 month after treatment (Table 42-3).

Table 42-4. Side Effects Reported by Women Using Intravaginal Clindamycin or Oral Metronidazole in Double-Blind, Placebo-Controlled Direct Comparison Trials

Side Effects	Therapy: Intravaginal Clindamycin	Therapy: Oral Metronidazole
	n = 148	n = 129
Metallic taste	0%	3%
Gastrointestinal upset/nausea	3%	9%
Headaches	1%	2%
Vaginal irritation	3%	2%
Yeast vaginitis	12%	9%
Discontinued therapy owing to side effects	3%	5%

Adapted from references 119 and 120.

In a meta-analysis of metronidazole therapy treatment of BV, Lugo-Miro et al. reported initial cure in 87 percent of 280 women receiving oral metronidazole (400 to 500 mg) two to three times daily for 7 days, and an 86 percent response in 317 women receiving 5 days of oral therapy.[113] From this analysis of over 1200 women, there was a consistent finding that over 85 percent of women responded initially to metronidazole therapy. However, these authors reported that the 2-gm stat dose was equivalent to 7 days of oral therapy.

Our own analysis of six studies that compared the single 2-gm dose of metronidazole versus 800 to 1200 mg/day for 7 days and followed patients for at least 1 month after treatment shows that five of these six studies showed lower cure rates with the single dose (Table 42-4).[7,114] When results from the six studies are combined, a 2-gm single dose of metronidazole was significantly less effective than 7-day therapies (82 percent vs. 73 percent, p = 0.03) for treatment of BV.

Side effects of oral metronidazole include nausea, metallic taste, headaches and gastrointestinal distress. Swedberg et al. Reported unpleasant taste and nausea in half of their subjects, and decreased appetite or abdominal cramping in one-fourth.[118] Others have cited these side effects in only 15 percent of subjects (Table 42-4). Oral metronidazole also leads to a disulfiram-like reaction after alcohol consumption, which may decrease patient compliance.

To reduce systemic absorption of metronidazole and decrease side effects, intravaginal metronidazole therapies have been evaluated (Table 42-5). A 500-mg tablet of metronidazole used intra-

Table 42-3. Efficacy of Metronidazole for the Treatment of BV, with Outcome Evaluated 1 to 2 Weeks and >4 Weeks after Onset of Therapy*

Author	Ref	Cure 1 to 2 Weeks after Onset of Therapy† 2 g	Cure 1 to 2 Weeks after Onset of Therapy† 7 g	Cure >4 Weeks after Onset of Therapy 2 g	Cure >4 Weeks after Onset of Therapy 7 g
Blackwell et al.	7	16/20 (80%)	20/20 (100%)	10/20 (50%)	12/20 (60%)
Eschenbach et al.	114	27/33 (85%)	39/52 (93%)	24/25 (69%)	29/38 (82%)
Hovik et al.	115	—	—	18/20 (90%)	17/19 (89%)
Jerve et al.	116	—	—	70/83 (84%)	83/97 (87%)
Jones et al.	117	41/47 (87%)	30/33 (91%)	24/34 (71%)	22/28 (79%)
Swedberg et al.	118	39/46 (85%)	35/36 (97%)	20/34 (47%)	26/30 (87%)
Total et al.		124/148 (84%)	125/131 (95%) p‡ = 0.003	166/226 (73%)	191/232 (82%) p‡ = 0.03

*A comparison of 2 g single dose vs. 800–1200 mg daily dose for 7 days.

†In most studies, failure is defined by persistence or recurrence of three of four of the following: clue cells, amine odor, homogenous discharge, and elevated vaginal pH. For Swedberg, failure was defined by persistence or recurrence of clue cells.

‡Chi square test for comparison of efficacy of 2 vs. 7 g regimen.

Table 42-5. Efficacy of Intravaginal Clindamycin and Metronidazole for the Treatment of BV

Agent	Dosage	Frequency	Duration (Days)	No. Patients	Clinical Efficacy (%)*	Reference
Metronidazole	5 g 0.75%	bid	5	30	73	123
	5 g 0.75%	bid	5	49	71	124
	5 g 0.75%	bid	5	96	66	125
	500 mg	Once daily	7	19	74	121
	500 mg	Once daily	7	75	71	122
Clindamycin	5 g 2%	Once daily	7	16	94	129
	5 g 2%	bid	5	16	90	128
	5 g 2%	Once daily	7	66	77	130
	5 g 2%	Once daily	3	69	65	132
	5 g 2%	Once daily	3	23	82	131
	5 g 2%	Once daily	7	30	85	133
	5 g 2%	Once daily	7	53	87	134
	5 g 2%	Once daily	7	124	83	119
	5 g 2%	Once daily	7	25	61	120
	5 g 2%	Once daily	7	21	86	135

*Efficacy determined 1 month after therapy.

vaginally for seven days reportedly cured 14 (74 percent) of 19 women with BV, and 500-mg intravaginal pessaries cured 71 percent.[121,122] In the initial study of intravaginal 0.75 percent metronidazole gel used twice daily for 5 days, 26 (87 percent) of 30 women were free of BV 4 to 16 days after therapy; four (15 percent) of the women relapsed at the 1-month follow-up, giving a 73 percent cure rate at 1-month.[123] Livengood and his colleagues evaluated this same formulation of metronidazole gel in 49 women and reported cure rates of 78 percent and 71 percent at the first and second follow-up visits, respectively.[124] A comparison study of intravaginal metronidazole to triple sulfa cream showed higher efficacy of vaginal metronidazole.[125] Use of intravaginal metronidazole resulted in fewer side effects than were observed after use of oral metronidazole. None of the 53 subjects who used the metronidazole gel experienced nausea, headache, or complained of having a metallic taste during this placebo-controlled trial. A direct randomized comparison of metronidazole vaginal gel twice daily for 5 days versus oral metronidazole 500 mg twice daily for 7 days, showed that 5 weeks after therapy, BV was cured in 71 percent (29/41) of the intravaginal metronidazole group, 118 and in 71 percent (32/45) of the oral metronidazole group.[126] A once daily dosage of the 0.75 percent metronidazole gel, given over 5 days, has been approved for use in the United States, although published data on the efficacy of this regimen are not yet available.

In summary, metronidazole therapy used orally or intravaginally has been evaluated in hundreds of women with BV. These studies have consistently reported resolution of BV in 71 percent to 89 percent or more of women 1 month after therapy. In small trials, intravaginal therapies have had efficacy similar to that of oral metronidazole regimens with fewer side effects.

CLINDAMYCIN

Greaves et al. randomized 143 women to receive oral metronidazole, 500 mg bid, for 7 days or clindamycin 300 mg bid for 7 days.[127] The clinical efficacy at 1 week was 94 percent for the oral clindamycin group, compared to 96 percent for the oral metronidazole group. Overall, 16 percent of the clindamycin group and 22 percent of the metronidazole group reported adverse effects, none of which necessitated discontinuation of therapy. Oral clindamycin appeared as effective as metronidazole for treatment of BV, and was of particular interest for the treatment of pregnant women.

Intravaginal clindamycin for the treatment of BV has been evaluated in numerous studies.[119,120,128–136] Livingood et al. and Hillier et al. reported two dose-ranging studies of intravaginal clindamycin for BV.[128,129] In a placebo-controlled, double-blind, randomized trial, women received 5 gm of clindamycin cream at concentrations of 0.1 percent, 1.0 percent, or 2.0 percent to be used each night for 7 days. The authors concluded that 2.0 percent topical clindamycin was both clinically and microbiologically effective therapy for treatment of BV, whereas lower concentrations of clindamycin had lower clinical efficacy.

A placebo-controlled trial of 2 percent intravaginal clindamycin was then undertaken. At the first follow-up visit 50 (77 percent) of 66 women with BV given clindamycin and 17 (25 percent) of 69 women given placebo were free of BV.[130] At 1 month, 79 percent of clindamycin-treated patients remained free of BV. In a smaller, placebo-controlled trial of 3 days of intravaginal clindamycin therapy in women with BV, 22 of 23 responded initially and three additional patients developed recurrent BV at the second follow-up visit.[131]

Five double-blinded, placebo-controlled trials have been published comparing 7 days of intravaginal clindamycin cream (and twice daily oral placebo) to 7 days of oral metronidazole administered twice daily (and once daily placebo vaginal cream).[119,120,133–135] These studies were conducted in the United States, Germany, Switzerland, Austria, and Mexico. In all of these trials, intravaginal clindamycin vaginal cream was as efficacious as 7 days of oral metronidazole therapy for the treatment of BV after both 1 week and 1 month of follow-up (Fig. 42-8).

In two of these placebo-controlled, double-blind trials directly comparing intravaginal clindamycin to oral metronidazole, side-effects were also compared. These are summarized in Table 42-4.[119,120] Only 3 percent and 5 percent of women assigned to intravaginal clindamycin and oral metronidazole, respectively, discontinued treatment because of side effects. Metronidazole use was associated with a slightly increased incidence of gastrointestinal upset and nausea and metallic taste. Vaginal irritation was similar for both treatment groups. Yeast vaginitis occurred in a similar proportion of the two treatments groups. In summary, intravaginal therapies with metronidazole gel or clindamycin cream, as described in the preceding, are considered effective treatments for vaginal infections. Intravaginal therapies have been well tolerated. However, the costs of such therapies currently far exceed the cost of one-dose or 7 days of oral metronidazole.

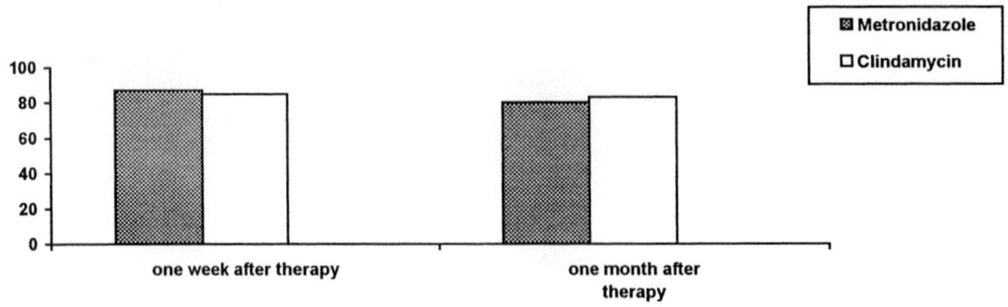

Fig. 42-8. Comparison of cure rates for bacterial vaginosis after 7 days of treatment with oral metronidazole or 2 percent intravaginal clindamycin cream. Results of five placebo-controlled, double-blind randomized trials, including nearly 500 women. (Data derived from references 119, 120, 133, 134, and 135.) At the first follow-up visits, 209 (85 percent) of 246 clindamycin-treated women and 213 (87 percent) of 245 metronidazole-treated were cured or improved. At the second follow-up visits, 195 (83 percent) of 235 clindamycin-treated women and 187 (80 percent) of 234 metronidazole-treated women were cured or improved.

In many developing country settings, especially in Latin America, topical intravaginal therapies with various mixtures of metronidazole, antifungal, antibacterial, antiseptic, and anti-inflammatory drugs are very commonly used for vaginal discharge.[137] We are not aware of any published data documenting the effectiveness of such peculiar preparations.

MICROBIOLOGICAL RESPONSE TO THERAPY WITH METRONIDAZOLE OR CLINDAMYCIN

Although metronidazole is active against Gram-negative anaerobes and *Mobiluncus mulieris,* it is less active against *G. vaginalis, Peptostreptococcus* spp., and *Mobiluncus curtisii,* and inactive against *M. hominis.*[138,139] *G. vaginalis* is more susceptible to the hydroxy metabolite of metronidazole than to the parent drug, but nonetheless, about 50 percent of women clinically cured after treatment with metronidazole remain colonized by *G. vaginalis. M. curtisii* is not susceptible to metronidazole in vitro, but is usually eradicated following metronidazole therapy. It is possible that inhibition or elimination of metronidazole-susceptible members of the vaginal flora in BV results in a decline in certain nonsusceptible members as well.

Clindamycin has activity against most of the microorganisms associated with BV, including *G. vaginalis* and *Mycoplasma hominis.* Figure 42-9 compares the microbiological response to therapy with intravaginal clindamycin or metronidazole during two separate clinical trials. Because a single laboratory performed the cultures, the results are combined.[123,129] The percentage with positive cultures for *G. vaginalis* decreased from 100 percent pretreatment to 79 percent post-therapy for the metronidazole-treated women, and to 19 percent for clindamycin-treated women. Clindamycin also had greater in vivo activity against *M. hominis* and anaerobic Gram-negative rods. Clindamycin, but not metronidazole, is active against lactobacilli. Therefore, it was not surprising that the prevalence of lactobacilli increased at the 1 week visit with metronidazole but not after therapy with clindamycin. However, paradoxically, by 1 month after treatment, the prevalence of vaginal lactobacilli in clindamycin-treated women was higher than in metronidazole-treated women. Vaginal colonization by *Escherichia coli* increased immediately after therapy with clindamycin, but returned to pretreatment rates 1 month after treatment. The activity of clindamycin against a broad spectrum of microbes including lactobacilli as well as *G. vaginalis*, anaerobes, and mycoplasmas probably led to an overgrowth of coliforms that was remarkably transient. Thus, although intravaginal clindamycin and metronidazole had considerably different microbiological effects, they produced similar clinical responses. Hill and Livengood reported similar findings with respect to clindamycin therapy.[140]

The types and number of lactobacilli found in the vaginal directly predict vaginal pH. Because of clindamycin activity against lactobacilli, the vaginal pH may stay elevated for 1 week after clindamycin treatment. For example, a vaginal pH of 4.5 or less was observed in 64 percent of metronidazole-treated women compared to 49 percent of clindamycin-treated women 1 week after therapy, despite similar clinical cure rates.[119] Oral metronidazole and vaginal clindamycin have produced similar long-term cure rates, although the long-term cure observed in these small studies suggests that the long-term recurrence rates approach 80 percent in the year after treatments.[141] Others have reported that true long-term recurrence over 5 to 9 years is 50percent but better data are needed.[142]

TREATMENT OF SEXUAL PARTNERS

Several placebo-controlled trials have demonstrated that treatment of the male partner(s) does not improve the clinical outcome of treatment of BV, or reduce recurrence.[118,136,143–146] For example, Moi and his colleaguesreported no differences in initial response of BV to therapy or in recurrence at 4 to 12 weeks after therapy for women whose partners were or were not treated with oral metronidazole.[144] In a double-blind, randomized trial, Vejtorp et al. observed no effect of treatment of the male partner on symptoms, clinical signs of BV, or isolation of *G. vaginalis* from the vagina 1 and 5 weeks after treatment of BV.[143] Similarly, Vutyavanich et al. reported that tinidazole treatment of male partners in Thailand had no effect on clinical response in the female, but was associated with a significant increase in side effects in the male partners who received tinidazole compared to placebo-treated men (22 percent vs. 7 percent, $p = 0.006$).[146] In a recent study in which women were treated for BV with clindamycin vaginal cream, and their male partners were randomly treated with oral clindamycin or placebo, recurrences of BV were unrelated to treatment of partners.[136]

Because all carefully controlled trials of male partners show no benefit of treatment of male partners, the U.S. Centers for Disease Control Guidelines for STD Treatment do not recommend routine treatment of male partners.[147] The discrepancy between data suggesting sexual acquisition of BV, and the lack of benefit of treating the male partner, remains puzzling. An explanation may await better understanding of the role of sexual exposure and of the male partner in transmission.

Fig. 42-9. Percent of vaginal cultures positive for various bacterial species before treatment, and at 1 week and 1 month posttreatment with intravaginal metronidazole or clindamycin.[123,129]

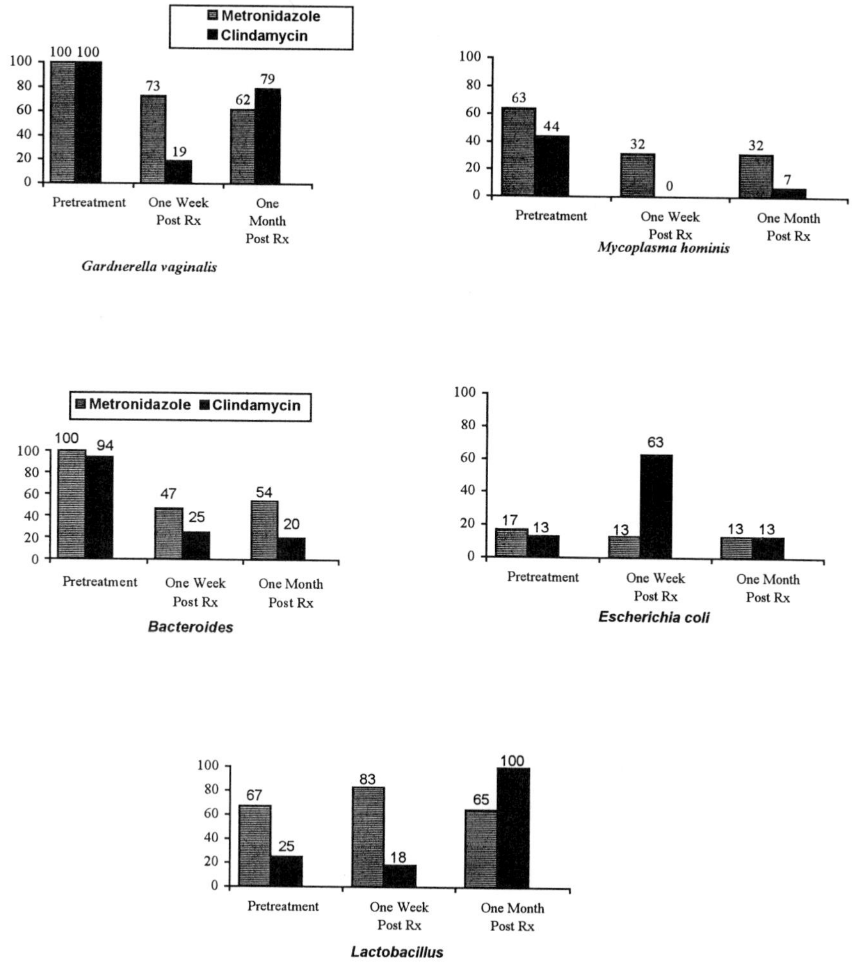

TREATMENT OF BV WITH OTHER ANTIMICROBIAL AGENTS

The relative efficacies of other antimicrobial therapies for treatment of BV are summarized in Table 42-6. Although sulfonamide creams have been used to treat BV for over 40 years, numerous studies document an unacceptably low efficacy for this product.

Tindazole has a reported efficacy of 43 to 95 percent, depending on the route of administration, dosage, and duration of therapy (see Table 42-6). Cephalosporins are generally less effective than metronidazole or clindamycin against BV, presumably because of their limited activity against anaerobic bacteria. Although ampicillin has been used as an alternative therapy for BV, especially in pregnancy, and has in vitro activity against *G. vaginalis*, ampicillin has given cure rates as low as 43 percent in studies with sufficiently long follow-ups. Lack of efficacy may be owing to production of beta lactamase by the anaerobic Gram-negative rods in the vagina of women with BV. Like clindamycin, ampicillin is

Table 42-6. Comparative Efficacy of Various Agents and Regimens Other than Metronidazole and Clindamycin for the Treatment of BV

	Regimen					
Agent	Route*	Dosage (mg)	Frequency	Duration (Days)	Clinical Efficacy (%)	Reference
Tinidazole	o	500	bid	5	95	148
	o	150	bid	7	43	149
	v	500	once daily	7	80	149
Cephadroxil	o	500	bid	7	64	150
Ampicillin	o	500	qid	7	43–48	151,152
Tetracycline	o	500	bid	7	50	153
Erythromycin	o	500	qid	7	23	154
Triple sulfonamide	v	500	bid	7	44–77	148,151
Ofloxacin	o	300	bid	7	28	155

*o = Oral; v = intravaginal.

also active against lactobacilli, and delays vaginal recolonization by lactobacilli.[152] The poor efficacy of ampicillin does not support its use for BV even during pregnancy.

Antimicrobial agents used for the treatment of chlamydial or gonococcal cervicitis, including tetracycline, erythromycin, and ofloxacin, have very limited activity against anaerobic bacteria. Furthermore, erythromycin has limited antibacterial potency at the acid pH of the vagina, even at the slightly less acid intravaginal pH characteristic of BV. These antimicrobial agents cure BV in only one-fourth to one-half of women, and are considered poor treatment choices.

ALTERNATIVE TREATMENTS FOR BV, INCLUDING RESTORATION OF NORMAL VAGINAL ECOLOGY

Because BV results from an ecological shift in the vaginal microflora, a number of researchers have evaluated therapies that either act as vaginal disinfectants or are aimed at restoring the vaginal ecosystem (Table 42-7). Chlorhexidine pessaries reportedly had 79 percent efficacy in 34 women with BV, but 48 percent had recurrence at 1 month posttreatment. Povidone-iodine inserted vaginally twice daily for 2 weeks was completely ineffective.[157] Studies reporting high success rates with povidone-iodine have usually had a very high incidence of spontaneous resolution of BV in the placebo group, suggesting potential problems with diagnosis, or in applying the data to populations in which the spontaneous resolution is low.

The efficacy of vaginal acidifiers in the form of gels, suppositories and acid-soaked tampons, has varied widely from 18 percent to 80 percent in several small studies. However, intermittent use over weeks is usually required. Vaginal acidifiers suppress, but do not kill, vaginal anaerobes, so may suppress without effecting a cure. Hydrogen peroxide douches have been advocated for BV treatment as an alternative to antimicrobial therapy, but data on this approach are limited.

Lactobacilli appear to be the primary microbiological deterrent to vaginal infection. However, lactobacilli found in yogurt do not bind vaginal epithelial cells to establish colonization of the vagina.[160] Therefore, therapies employing yogurt probably have little utility. Although Fredricsson et al. found that yogurt had only 7 percent efficacy for treatment of BV, another report claimed 88 percent efficacy for twice-daily douching with yogurt for 2 weeks.[160,161] Additional studies are required.

In a placebo-controlled trial of purified *Lactobacillus* spp. in suppositories, about half of the women receiving *Lactobacillus* improved during therapy, but only four of 29 women remained free of BV at the second follow-up visit.[162] Even though certain lactobacilli may play an important role in maintaining the normal vaginal flora, it remains to be determined whether the application of such lactobacilli is sufficient to restore the vaginal microflora. Another study evaluated the effectiveness of Gynoflor® (Medinova Ltd., Zurich, Switzerland), a tablet containing hydrogen peroxide producing *Lactobacillus acidophilus* in combination with 0.03 mg. of estriol.[163] Although preliminary results appear promising advocates of alternative or nature-based treatments for BV have not proven the efficacy of these therapies in large, well-controlled, randomized, double-blind trials.

BV IN PREGNANCY

BV during pregnancy has been linked to a significantly increased risk of preterm or low birthweight deliveries, intra-amnionic infection, histological chorioamnionitis, and postpartum endometritis. Is treatment necessary, or does BV resolve spontaneously during pregnancy? Two published studies have reported on the persistence of BV during pregnancy. The first study evaluated 762 pregnant women at 23 to 26 weeks' gestation and again at 31 to 36 weeks' gestation.[104] Women who used antibiotics during this interval were specifically excluded. In this study, 69 percent of women who had BV in the second trimester still had this syndrome in the third trimester. In a second study, bacterial vaginosis persisted in almost half of the women who had the condition initially and who went to term, that is, in 15 (47 percent) of 32, whereas the flora reverted to the intermediate stage in two women (6 percent) and to normal in 15 women (47 percent).[164] There was, however, a signficant association between bacterial vaginosis status at visit one and at visit three. Women who had the infection initially were more likely to have it at visit three than women who did not (15/32 versus 4/144, McNemar's test $x^2 = 0.05$). These data suggest that spontaneous clearance of BV does not occur in most pregnant women.

PRETERM LABOR, LOW BIRTH WEIGHT, AND PROM

In 1984, Minkoff et al. published a prospective study of perinatal morbidity in 233 women enrolled for prenatal care at 14 weeks' gestation and followed through delivery; women underwent vagi-

Table 42-7. Lack of Efficacy of Alternative Treatments for BV

Class	Type	Form and Use	No. of Women	Efficacy (%)	Follow-up (Days)	Reference
Disinfectant	Chlorhexidine 150 mg	Pessary	34	79	7	156
	Povidone-iodine	Pessary bid × 14 days	28	20	7	157
Acidifier	Lactic acid	Suppository	125	20	30	158
	Lactate pH 3.5, 5 g	Gel, daily × 7 days	31	77	7	159
	Lactate pH 3.8, 5 g	Gel, intermittent use × 6 weeks				
	Acetate	Gel	17	18	30	160
	5% Acetic acid	Tampon, bid × 7 days	32	38	30	161
Yogurt	Commercial pH < 4.5	Douche 10–15 mL bid × 14 days	32	88	30	161
	Commercial	Daily	14	7	30	160
Lactobacillus	Vivag; Pharmac-Vinci A/S, Denmark	Suppository bid × 6 days	28	43	1–4	162

Table 42-8. Studies Linking Bacterial Vaginosis with Preterm Birth and/or Low Birth Weight Delivery

Year	Author	Number of Women	Enrollment (Weeks)	OR (95% CI)	References
1986	Gravett	534	13–41	2.0 (1.1–3.5)	166
1986	Gravett	88	Delivery	3.8 (1.2–11.6)	167
1988	Martius	212	Delivery	2.3 (1.1–5.0)	74
1992	Kurki	790	8–17	6.9 (2.5–18.8)	168
1993	Riduan	490	16–20	2.0 (1.0–3.9)	169
1994	Holst	87	Delivery	2.1 (1.2–3.7)	170
1994	Hay	461	<16	5.5 (2.3–13.3)	171
1995	Meis	2929	28	1.8 (1.2–2.3)	172
1995	Hillier	10,397	23–26	1.4 (1.1–1.8)	173
1995	McGregor	559	<22	1.9 (1.2–3.0)	174

nal cultures for *Bacteroides* spp. and *M. hominis,* evaluation for BV (then called nonspecific vaginitis) based on clinical manifestations (vaginal pH >4.5, clue cells, amine odor), and cultures for *T. vaginalis,* yeast, herpes simplex virus, *C. trachomatis,* and facultative bacteria.[165] BV was diagnosed in 66 (30 percent) of 218 women. Subsquently, 35 (16 percent) patients developed preterm labor and received tocolysis; 50 percent of those who failed tocolysis had BV, compared to 29 percent of those whose labor stopped with tocolytic agents. In a stepwise logistic regression analysis of risk factors for perinatal morbidity, adjusting for maternal age, parity, previous premature delivery, abortion, and vaginal bacteria, isolation of *Bacteroides* spp. from the vagina was associated with preterm delivery (relative risk [RR] = 1.4, p <0.03), preterm premature rupture of membranes (PROM) (RR = 1.8, $p < 0.03$) and birth weight less than 2500 gm (RR = 1.8, $p < 0.04$). This study was the first to describe the association of vaginal anaerobic bacteria and of BV with perinatal complications. Several subsequent studies supported and extended these findings.

From 1984 through 1988, a series of studies linking BV to preterm delivery or low birth weight were published (Table 42-8).[74,166–174] One of these was a cross-sectional study of 534 consecutive pregnant women seen in a prenatal clinic at a mean gestational age of 32 weeks (range 13 to 41 weeks). BV was presumptively diagnosed by gas liquid chromatographic analysis of vaginal fluid demonstrating increased succinate: lactate ratios. In a multivariate analysis, BV was related to an increase in preterm labor (odds ratio [OR] = 2.0, $p < 0.5$), preterm PROM (OR = 2, $p < 0.05$), and delivery of a low birth weight infant (OR = 1.5, $p < 0.05$). In addition, BV was related to intrapartum fever (OR = 2.7, $p < 0.05$).[166] The increased levels of vaginal succinate relative to lactate in the vaginal fluid probably related to increased levels of anaerobic Gram-negative rods in the vagina.[8]

Two other studies have confirmed an association between obligately anaerobic Gram-negative rods (formerly *Bacteroides* spp.) and preterm delivery. Krohn et al. reported that vaginal colonization by *Prevotella bivia* (formerly *B. bivius*) or *B. fragilis* was associated with delivery before 34 weeks' gestation (RR = 2.0, $p < 0.05$); whereas vaginal colonization by *Lactobacillus* spp. was associated with a 40 percent decreased risk of preterm delivery (RR = 0.6, $p < 0.05$).[175] Similarly, a group of Australian investigators found vaginal colonization by *Bacteroides* spp. was associated with a 60 percent increased risk of delivery before 34 weeks' gestation.[176]

Over the next 4 years, four studies reported a link between BV, diagnosed by Gram-stained vaginal smear, and prematurity. In a case-control study of women in labor, women with BV had a two-fold increased risk of preterm delivery (OR = 2.3, $p < 0.05$); whereas vaginal lactobacilli had a sharply reduced risk of preterm delivery (OR = 0.2, $p < 0.05$).[74] In Finland, BV diagnosed at 8 to 17 weeks' gestation in 790 nulliparous women was associated with a increased risk of preterm labor ($p < 0.05$), preterm birth ($p < 0.01$) and preterm PROM ($p < 0.05$).[168] Among 783 pregnant women evaluated prenatally, BV by Gram-stained vaginal smear was associated with an increased incidence of preterm birth (OR 2.8, 95 percent CI 1.1, 7.4); and also with late miscarriages (OR 5.5, 95 percent CI 2.3, 13.3).[171] The two largest published studies evaluating the incidence and preterm birth among women with BV have been performed in the United States. Hillier et al. reported that women with Gram-stain evidence for BV plus vaginal pH > 4.5 at 23 to 26 weeks' gestation were 40 percent more likely to deliver an infant that was both preterm)<37 weeks') and low birthweight (<2500 gm).[173] Meis et al. similarly reported that BV diagnosed by Gram-stain at 28 weeks' gestation in a multicenter cohort was associated with a 80 percent increased incidence of delivery at <37 weeks' gestation (OR 1.8, 95 percent CI 1.2, 3.0),[172] whereas McGregor reported at 90 percent increased incidence of preterm birth in a cohort of women enrolled in Colorado.[174]

Thus, a series of studies in the United States, Scandinavia, and Australia that included women from different ethnic and socioeconomic groups have consistently reported an increased risk for preterm delivery or low birthweight among women colonized by BV-associated pathogens (anaerobic Gram-negative rods and *M. hominis*), and among those with clinical or Gram-stain evidence of BV; and some have noted a decrease in prematurity among those vaginally colonized by *Lactobacillus* spp.

CHORIOAMNIONITIS AND AMNIOTIC FLUID INFECTION

Several studies link BV with infection of the fetal placental membranes (chorioamnion) and amniotic fluid (Table 42-9), suggesting that ascension of vaginal microorganisms into the decidua, chorioamnion, or amniotic fluid, resulting in infection and inflammation at these sites, represents a probable mechanism by which BV can initiate labor and result in preterm delivery.

In a case-control study, BV diagnosed by Gram-stained vaginal smear was related to histological chorioamnionitis (OR = 2.6, $p = 0.05$) and to recovery of microorganisms from the chorioamnion (OR = 3.2, $p < 0.05$).[177] The possibility that the duration of membrane rupture or of premature labor caused the presence of bacteria or the inflammation of the chorioamnion was excluded

Table 42-9. Association of Bacterial Vaginosis with Placental and Amniotic Fluid Infection

Author, year	Outcome	Odds Ratio (95% CI)	References
Hillier et al., 1988	Chorioamnion infection	3.2 (1.1–6.6)	177
Hillier et al., 1988	Chorioamnionitis	2.6 (1.0–6.6)	177
Watts et al., 1990	Amnionitis	6.8 (3.2–14.6)	181
Silver et al., 1989	Intra-amniotic infection	2.6 (1.1–5.0)	180
Gravett et al., 1986	Amnionitis	2.1 (1.1–3.9)	167
Krohn et al., 1995	Intra-amniotic infection	1.5 (1.1–1.2)	182
Hillier et al., 1995	Amnionitis (intact membranes)	1.9 (1.1–3.3)	179

Table 42-10. Oral vs. Vaginal Clindamycin Treatment of Bacterial Vaginosis during Pregnancy: Effect on Outcome

			Preterm Birth		
Year	Author	Route	Clindamycin	Placebo	References
1994	McGregor	Vaginal	9/60 (15%)	5/69 (11%)	184
1995	Josoef	Vaginal	51/340 (15%)	46/341 (14%)	185
1995	McGregor	Oral	19/194 (10%)	31/165 (19%)*	174

*Women in the comparison group were untreated. (Relative risk 0.5, 95% confidence interval 0.3–0.9 treated compared to untreated women.)

in the analyses. *Fusobacterium* spp. and *Bacteroides* spp. both strongly associated with BV, were frequent isolates from the chorioamnion in a second study, and recovery of these two organisms from the placental membranes was associated with histological chorioamnionitis and preterm delivery.[178] Thus, BV has been directly linked with the isolation of BV-associated pathogens from the placenta and with histological chorioamnionitis, both of which have been related to preterm delivery.

Amniotic fluid infection results most commonly from invasion of lower genital tract bacteria through the placental membranes. The most frequent isolates recovered from the amniotic fluid of women with intact membranes are the microorganisms associated with BV, and women with BV are twice as likely to have invasion of the amniotic fluid as women with *Lactobacillus*-predominant vaginal flora.[179] A 2.6- to 2.7-fold increase in intra-amniotic infection among women with BV has been reported by Silver et al. and by Gravett.[167,180] Watts et al. reported a strong relationship of BV diagnosed at the time of C-section to clinically diagnosed amniotic fluid infection. Amniotic fluid infection occurred among 22 percent of women with a Gram stain diagnosis of BV compared to 4 percent of those with a *Lactobacillus*-predominant vaginal smear.[181] The largest study to evaluate the association between BV and amniotic fluid infection was by Krohn et al. prospective who reported women diagnosed as having BV in the second trimester of pregnancy were 50 percent more likely to develop a fever during labor compared to women having *Lactobacillus*-predominant flora.[182]

In summary, BV during pregnancy has consistently been related to chorioamnion infection, histological chorioamnionitis, and amniotic fluid infection. These three entities are strongly interrelated, and are associated with preterm delivery. Thus the key question of great current interest is whether prenatal treatment of BV can reduce perinatal morbidity, particularly preterm delivery.

TREATMENT OF BV DURING PREGNANCY FOR PREVENTION OF PRETERM BIRTH

Five published studies have evaluated treatment of BV in pregnancy as a means to prevent preterm birth. Because of the efficacy of clindamycin applied intravaginally for the treatment of BV, and early concerns with the potential teratogenicity of metronidazole in pregnancy, initial efforts to reduce preterm birth among women with BV focused on the use of intravaginal clindamycin (Table 42-10).[183–185] In a placebo-controlled trial involving 129 women, McGregor et al. found that the incidence of preterm birth actually was slightly higher among the women assigned to intravaginal clindamycin than among women assigned to placebo (15 percent vs. 11 percent).[184] In a larger study performed in Indonesia, Josoef et al. randomly assigned 681 women with BV to receive either clindamycin or placebo cream intravaginally, once daily for 7 days at a mean gestational age of 20 weeks.[185] Clindamycin-treated women had the same incidence of preterm birth as placebo-treated women (15 percent vs. 14 percent), with a trend toward a higher incidence of birth before 32 weeks' gestation and of low birthweight among the clindamycin-treated women.[185] These studies did not support use of clindamycin vaginal cream for prevenion of preterm birth among women with BV. It is not known whether the increase in vaginal *E. coli* colonization following use of clindamycin cream could be responsible for the trend toward an increased incidence of preterm birth among women using clindamycin cream.[129] Vaginal colonization by *E. coli* has been linked to an increased incidence of preterm and low birthweight delivery.[186]

Four published trials have evaluated oral regimens for treatment of BV during pregnancy. Oral clindamycin was evaluated in a prospective study that included only a historical control group. During the first phase of the study, when women with asymptomatic BV were not treated, 19 percent of 165 women with BV delivered preterm.[174] During the next phase of the study women were routinely screened and treated for BV with oral clindamycin 300 mg, bid for 7 days, and 10 percent of these women delivered preterm compared with 19 percent of these who remained untreated (RR = 0.5, 95 percent CI 0.3, 0.9).

Three randomized placebo-controlled trials have evaluated oral metronidazole, either alone or in combination with erythromycin, for prevention of preterm birth. Two studies were conducted among women who were considered at high risk of preterm birth because of a previous preterm delivery or low pregnancy weight.[187,188] In a study of 80 high-risk women with BV, 18 percent of those randomized to metronidazole versus 39 percent of those randomized to placebo delivered preterm ($p < 0.05$).[187] Hauth et al. evaluated oral metronidazole, 250 mg, tid for 7 days plus erythromycin 333 mg, tid for 14 days versus placebo in a population at high risk for preterm birth owing to previous preterm birth or having a prepregnancy weight of <50 kg (Table 42-11).[188] Among women with BV and a history of previous preterm delivery, the percent delivering preterm was 39 percent for those assigned to metronidazole plus erythromycin, versus 59 percent for those assigned to placebo (RR = 1.6 95 percent CI 1.1, 2.1).[188] However, a randomized trial of oral metronidazole in a low risk population of pregnant women failed to document a reduced in-

Table 42-11. Randomized Treatment Trials of Metronidazole vs. Placebo for Prevention of Preterm Delivery among Women with Bacterial Vaginosis

	Percent Preterm		
Author, Year	Treatment	Placebo	RR (95% CI)
Morales et al.[187]	8/44 (18%)	16/36 (39%)	0.3 (0.1–0.9)
Hauth et al.[188]*	54/172 (31%)	42/86 (49%)	0.5 (0.3–0.8)
McDonald et al.[189]	11/242 (4.5%)	15/238 (6.3%)	0.7 (0.3–1.7)

*Treatment group received erythromycin as well as metronidazole.
N Engl J Med 1995; 333:1732–1736.

Table 42-12. Postpartum Endometritis and Bacterial Vaginosis

		Postpartum Endometritis in Relation to Vaginal Flora		
Author	Ref	BV	Normal	OR (95% CI)
Watts et al.	181	23/75 (31%)*	28/350 (8%)	5.8 (3.0–10.9)†
Newton	194	21/76 (28%)‡	79/531 (15%)	2.2 (1.3–3.9)

*BV diagnosed by Gram stain

†Adjusted for maternal age, duration of labor, and duration of membrane rupture by multivariate analysis.

‡BV defined by presence of any two of the three in the amniotic fluid at the time of delivery: any anaerobes, *Gardnerella vaginalis,* or *Mycoplasma hominis.*

cidence of preterm among metronidazole-treated women, although the study lacked sufficient size to allow for statistical power to detect small decreases in incident preterm births.[189]

These studies suggest that treatment of pregnant women with BV who have previously had a preterm delivery may reduce the incidence of a subsequent preterm delivery. Large randomized trials are ongoing to evaluate whether routine screening for BV and treatment of all women with BV, including those who are asymptomatic and at low risk for preterm delivery can reduce the incidence of preterm birth in the latter group as well. The annual estimated cost for BV-associated complications in pregnancy are estimated at $500 million to $1 billion annually in the United States.[190] Estimated costs for screening the 4 million pregnant American women each year, and treating the 600,000 women found to have BV would be $5 to $17 million.[190] Assuming a prevention efficacy approaching that found in the previous randomized trials of metronidazole in pregnant women, these investments in screening and treatment would offer clear financial benefits.

The mechanisms by which BV causes prematurity and low birthweight are not completely understood. As discussed, BV-associated microorganisms ascend to cause infections of the decidua, placenta, or amniotic fluid. In addition, women with BV reportedly also have significantly elevated levels of endotoxin in vaginal fluid and others have suggested that the effects of endotoxin on activation of the prostaglandin system could provoke preterm labor.[191] Among 45 women having a termination of pregnancy in Sweden, the concentrations of prostaglandin E_2 and $F_{2\infty}$ were significantly higher in the cervical mucus of women with BV than among women without this syndrome. Thus, even in the absence of upper genital tract infection, other mechanisms BV-associated pathophysiologic factors might lead to preterm labor.[192]

OTHER COMPLICATIONS OF BV

POSTPARTUM ENDOMETRITIS

In a prospective study of risk factors for post-Cesarean endometritis in 462 women, those with BV diagnosed by Gram-strain had greatly increased risk of postpartum endometritis following Cesarean section compared to women with a *Lactobacillus*-dominant flora (OR 5.8, 95 percent CI 3.0, 10.9) after adjusting for possible confounding factors, including maternal age, length of labor, and duration of membrane rupture (Table 42-12).[181] Patients with BV also had increased rates of abdominal wound infection, and all of the documented wound infections were related to anaerobic bacteria. The endometrial aspirates from patients with BV who developed postpartum endometritis contained the microorganisms associated with BV.[181]

In a separate study, endometrial aspirates from 61 percent of patients with postpartum endometritis contained either the anaerobes associated with BV, *G. vaginalis*, or both. The anaerobes most frequently recovered included BV-associated *Bacteroides* spp., and *Peptostreptococcus* spp. *G. vaginalis* was the most common faculative Gram-negative rod isolated from both the endometrium and blood of patients with postpartum endometritis.[193]

The risk of postpartum endometritis remains high in patients with BV despite routine use of cephalosporin prophylaxis. Cephalosporin prophylaxis is presumably inadequate early because of the large number of bacteria contaminating the amniotic fluid of patients with BV or because the bacteria present are not highly susceptible to the cephalosporin used. The impact of antibiotic prophylaxis on patients with BV undergoing Cesarean section needs further study. Although women undergoing Cesarean section experience the highest risk for postpartum endometritis, and BV is a strong risk factor among patients who deliver by Cesarean section, BV also appears to increase the risk for postpartum endometritis among patients who deliver vaginally, specifically when amniotic fluid becomes contaminated with bacteria associated with BV during labor.[194] Invasion of anaerobes (most commonly *Prevotella bivia*), *G. vaginalis,* and *M. hominis* in the amniotic fluid resulted in a twofold increased risk of postpartum endometritis among patients delivered vaginally or by cesarean section (see Table 42-12).

VAGINAL CUFF CELLULITIS

Vaginal cuff cellulitis occurs when vaginal bacteria contaminate the operative field during a hysterectomy. Women with more virulent bacteria in the vaginal flora, present in the increased concentrations characteristic of BV, would be expected to have increased risk of vaginal cuff cellulitis following hysterectomy. In two separate studies, postabdominal hysterectomy cuff cellulitis occurred four times more commonly among patients with BV than patients with a normal *Lactobacillus*-dominant flora (Table 42-13). In one of the studies, *Trichomonas vaginalis* also was associated with a three-fold increase in cuff cellulitis; however, after adjusting for the BV, the relative risk of cuff cellulitis in those with *T. vaginalis* alone was not significantly increased.[195] A second study evaluated the association between clue cells and cuff cellulitis after abdominal hysterectomy and found a similar increased risk of infection among these with BV.[196]

Although selective treatment with antibiotics prior to surgery would be expected to reduce posthysterectomy infection related

Table 42-13. Cuff Cellulitis following Abdominal Hysterectomy: associated with Bacterial Vaginosis

		Vaginal Cuff Cellulitis in Relation to Vaginal Flora		
Author	Ref	BV	Normal	OR (95% CI)
Soper	195	11/32 (34%)	11/102 (11%)	4.3 (1.5–12.6)
Larsson	196	7/20 (35%)	4/50 (8%)	4.4 (1.4–13.3)

to BV, transient increases in other vaginal flora, including *E. coli* and enterococci, have been observed following certain types of therapy. Thus, the timing of the treatment of BV before the planned hysterectomy may be important. A controlled trial of BV treatment prior to hysterectomy is necessary to examine the possible reduction in postoperative infectious morbidity.

POSTABORTION PELVIC INFLAMMATORY DISEASE

Pelvic inflammatory disease (PID) is frequently caused by *Neisseria gonorrhoeae* and *C. trachomatis*. Many investigators have found PID following induced abortion related to *C. trachomatis*. Postabortal endometritis following induced first trimester abortion has also been related to BV. Postabortion PID occurred more commonly among patients with BV than among those with a *Lactobacillus*-dominant flora (OR = 2.4, 95 percent CI 1.1, 5.3).[197] *C. trachomatis* was also associated with postabortal PID (p = 0.06), but BV was more than twice as common as *C. trachomatis* infection, so that postabortion PID occurred in eight patients who had preoperative BV, two patients with preoperative *C. trachomatis* infection and 18 patients with neither. In a another study, 174 patients with BV underwent double-blind randomization to placebo or metronidazole prior to undergoing induced abortion.[198] Placebo-treated patients had higher rates of postabortal PID (OR = 30, 95 percent CI, 1, 11.8), suggesting that prior treatment of BV could significantly decrease infectious morbidity following termination of pregnancy.

PELVIC INFLAMMATORY DISEASE

The role of BV in spontaneous PID not associated with abortion or instrumentation of the uterus is less clear. Among randomly selected STD clinic patients, those with BV had adnexal tenderness significantly more often than patients with a *Lactobacillus*-dominant flora, suggesting that spontaneous PID occurring without instrumentation may also be related to BV.[21] In this study, the relationship between BV and adnexal tenderness persisted after adjusting by multifactorial analysis for infection with *N. gonorrhoeae* or *C. trachomatis*. Many of the bacteria recovered from the endometrium and fallopian tubes of patients with PID are those present in the vagina in high numbers among women with BV.[199] However, the proportion of women with BV who develop overt symptoms and signs of PID without instrumentation may be relatively low compared to the proportion of those infected with *N. gonorrhoeae* and *C. trachomatis*. Further, the interactions between *C. trachomatis, N. gonorrhoeae,* and facultative bacteria in producing PID is not known. Therefore, until recently it has seemed that treatment of asymptomatic nonpregnant women with BV to reduce PID could be viewed as optional, and of no proven benefit until further information is available. However, the risk of more subtle manifestations of endometritis attributable to BV may be greater than the risk of overt PID. A small amount of intermenstrual bleeding or increased bleeding with menses is a frequent occurrence in patients with endometritis and salpingitis. A randomized, double-blind trial was conducted among patients with BV who had these symptoms of abnormal bleeding. Abnormal bleeding resolved in all 11 patients treated with metronidazole and considered cured of BV versus only one (5 percent) of 11 placebo-treated patients not cured (p = 0.04).[200]

The foundation for our understanding of the connection between BV and upper-tract infections was laid in 1987, when Paavonen and colleagues published research showing that 29 percent of 31 patients who had histologic evidence of endometritis also had BV, whereas none of 14 controls without endometritis had BV.[201]

In 1995, Korn and colleagues published the findings of a case-control study in which they performed endometrial biopsies on 41 women who presented to an STD clinic complaining of vaginal discharge or pelvic pain.[202] All of the biopsies were examined for histopathologic evidence of plasma cell endometritis; and cultured for *N. gonorrhoeae, C. trachomatis, U. urealyticum, Mycoplasma hominis,* and facultative and anaerobic bacteria. None of the patients had culture or serologic evidence of *N. gonorrhoeae* or *C. trachomatis* infection.

Endometrial biopsies from the 22 women with BV were compared with those of the other 19 women, who were negative for BV on Gram-stain analysis of vaginal fluid. Ten (45 percent) of the 22 women with BV had plasma cell endometritis, compared with only one of the 19 women who served as controls. Microorganisms associated with BV were cultured from the endometria of nine of the 11 patients who had plasma cell endometritis, as well as from eight of the 30 patients who did not have that histologic diagnosis.[202]

In another study, endometrial biopsies were obtained on 178 consecutive women with suspected PID.[203] Endometrial specimens, as well as cervical swabs were tested for *N. gonorrhoeae* and *C. trachomatis*. Eighty-five of the patients also underwent laparoscopy to confirm a clinical diagnosis of salpingitis. Sixty-five percent, or 117, of the 178 patients had endometritis as confirmed by the presence of plasma cells and PMNs in the endometrial biopsy specimen. Among the patients with endometritis, 27 percent had *N. gonorrhoeae* present in the endometrium, whereas 13 percent had endometrial samples positive for *C. trachomatis*. Approximatley 50 percent of the patients with endometritis had anaerobic Gram-negative rods in their endometrial samples. A logistic regression analysis on the data showed that endometrial *N. gonorrhoeae* was associated with a 5.7 odds ratio for endometritis, as compared to odds ratio of 4.8 and 2.6 for endometrial *C. trachomatis* and anaerobic Gram-negative rods, respectively. The diagnosis of BV was associated with an endometritis odds ratio of only 1.1, suggesting that BV is not an independent risk factor in and of itself. However, when the anaerobic Gram-negative rods ascend and infect the endometrium, they are a cause of endometritis independent of STDs.

In a recent case-control study, 111 women with gonorrhea, chlamydia or BV, were compared to 24 women without any of these infections for plasma cell endometritis.[204] For the 5 percent of women with BV alone (those with coinfection by gonorrhea or chlamydia were excluded), plasma cell endometritis was detected in 42 percent, whereas endometritis was detected in only 13 percent of the controls (OR 6.4, 95 percent CI 1.7 to 35.0).[204] These studies suggest that women with BV may have clinically inapparent, or "silent" endometritis. However, whether BV-associated endometritis leads to salpingitis and infertility is the focus of ongoing studies.

BV AND HIV

As discussed in Chapter 14, there is growing body of evidence that suggests that the presence of BV, or absence of vaginal lactobacilli, may increase a woman's risk of acquiring HIV via heterosexual intercourse. Two cross-sectional studies have been published that report a twofold increased prevalence of HIV among Thai commercial sex workers and rural Ugandan women with BV compared to those women with *Lactobacillus*-predominant vaginal flora.[24,25]

A longitudinal study of pregnant and postnatal African women in Malawi found that women with BV were more likely to seroconvert to HIV than were women without clinical signs of BV.[205] HIV-seronegative pregnant women receiving prenatal care were followed during pregnancy and after delivery. All women were tested for HIV 6 months after delivery. BV was assessed by clinical signs (pH; clue cells; discharge; amine odor) during pregnancy and at least one postnatal visit. Among 1196 women enrolled, 27 seroconverted by the time of delivery and 97 seroconversions occured in the remaining women followed for a median of 2.5 years. BV during pregnancy was significantly associated with antenatal HIV seroconversion (OR 3.7, $p = 0.04$) as well as with postnatal HIV seroconversions (OR 3.5, 95 percent CI 1.5 to 8.3). In this population of women with a low prevalence of STDs, the attributable risk of BV for antenatal HIV seroconversion was 23 percent.[205] These data implicating BV as a risk factor for heterosexual acquisition of HIV also raise the question of whether a more aggressive approach to treatment of asymptomatic BV is warranted—especially in women at risk for heterosexual acquisition of HIV.

In other prospective studies, in the large study in the Rakai district of Uganda, HIV seroconversion also was significantly associated with BV (T. Quinn, personal communication); and in Mombasa, Kenya, absence of vaginal colonization by H_2O_2-producing lactobacilli was associated with HIV seroconversion among a cohort of female sex workers (Martin H, personal communication).

UNRESOLVED ISSUES IN PATIENT MANAGEMENT

HOW COMMON IS LATE RECURRENCE AND WHY DOES IT HAPPEN?

In 1955, Gardner noted that "before the advent of antibiotics and sulfonamides, the treatment of bacterial vaginitis was discouraging because eradication of the causative organism was difficult and recurrences were common."[6] Unfortunately, 35 years after Gardner made his initial observation, the treatment of BV can still be discouraging because of the high rate of recurrent infection. In studies, up to 70 percent of women develop recurrent BV within 3 months after therapy.[141] Others have reported that long-term recurrence rates are approximately 50 percent.[142] The reasons for recurrence are not understood. Four possible explanations include: (1) reinfection by a male partner colonized with BV-associated microorganisms; (2) recurrence due to the persistence of BV-associated microorganisms that were inhibited, but not killed, during therapy; (3) failure to reestablish the normal, and perhaps protective, *Lactobacillus*-predominant flora following therapy; and (4) persistence of another, yet-unidentified host factor in the patient making her susceptible to recurrence. Microbiologic studies have established that about half of women lack vaginal lactobacilli that produce H_2O_2 following therapy with clindamycin or metronidazole.[206] Some investigators have promoted the use of H_2O_2 douches for women with BV recurrences, but the utility of this approach is unproven.[207]

SHOULD MALE PARTNERS BE TREATED?

Although many women believe they have contracted BV from a male partner, no study to date has convincingly shown that treatment of the male partner decreases risk of recurrence. For this reason, we do not recommend routine treatment of the male partner at present, but do believe better data on this approach are needed. Randomized placebo-controlled trials of partner treatment, with long-term follow-up in monogamous couples, would be of interest; with better understanding of how men carry and transmit the organism responsible for BV necessary to guide such trials.

ARE OVER-THE-COUNTER PREPARATIONS OF LACTOBACILLI USEFUL?

A number of women have used over-the-counter lactobacilli products to attempt to reconstitute the vaginal flora. These include acidophilus milk, yogurt, or various *Lactobacillus*-containing capsules, and powders available from health food stores. Some of the earliest treatments for bacterial vaginosis involved attempts to restore the vaginal flora by application of *Lactobacillus* preparations.[208,209] Butler reported cure of 18 of 19 patients given from one to eight applications of pure culture of a human-derived strain of Doderlein bacillus at weekly intervals.[209] However, only 1 of 14 women were cured after applying yogurt intravaginally twice daily for 7 days.[160]

Bacteria found in an ecologic niche have uniquely adapted to that particular environment. However, the commercial strains of lactobacilli found in dairy products have adapted to the dairy food industry. Wood found that these commercial strains adhered to vaginal epithelial cells more poorly than human-derived strains of *Lactobacillus*.[210] Strains of lactobacilli that do not adhere well to vaginal epithelial cells may not successfully colonize the vagina. We have reported that 9 of 16 *Lactobacillus* preparations commercially available in the United States were contaminated with other bacteria, and five of 16 did not contain the H_2O_2-producing strains thought to be protective in the vagina.[211] It is unlikely that such products are of therapeutic value for the treatment or prevention of BV. Treatment of BV using H_2O_2-producing lactobacilli has been an unsuccessful therapeutic option, suggesting that recolonization of the vagina with exogenous lactobacilli will probably be of benefit as an adjunct to rather than as a replacement of, antimicrobial therapy.[162]

SHOULD WOMEN WITH SIGNS OF BV BE TREATED IF ASYMPTOMATIC?

In our experience, some women with BV are aware of a discharge or odor but discount it because it has been present for months or even years. Thus, many women who do not complain of symptoms acknowledge symptoms of odor or discharge on questioning. Furthermore, McGuire et al. interviewed women with signs but no symptoms of BV, and also women with symptoms but no signs of vaginal disease, and identified characteristic psychosexual profiles of each, suggesting psychological factors may influence perception of vulvo-vaginal symptoms.[212] Women with BV should be informed of their diagnosis, and treatment should be offered if requested. However, definitive recommendations for routine treatment of asymptomatic, nonpregnant women with BV await further studies defining risks of upper tract infection among women with BV and more information on the benefits treating BV to prevent HIV acquisition, as well as improved strategies to prevent late recurrence.

DOES BV CONTRIBUTE TO PID AMONG WOMEN UNDERGOING IUD INSERTION?

As noted earlier, three studies suggest IUD users are at increased risk for BV. A current deficiency in knowledge about BV concerns whether BV increases the risk of endometritis and salpingitis following IUD insertion. No prospective studies have yet examined this question, and no randomized controlled trials have examined whether BV treatment prior to IUD insertion reduces the risk of postinsertion infectious morbidity.

SHOULD HIV-INFECTED WOMEN WITH ASYMPTOMATIC BV RECEIVE BV TREATMENT?

Although there is no clear evidence that HIV infection increases the risk of BV or of complications of BV, one recent study in Kenya (Cohen C, Bukusi E, unpublished) suggests HIV infection may be particularly common in BV-associated PID. Whether or not HIV infection, and related immunosuppression, increase the risk of progression of BV to PID (as may be the case for chlamydial and gonococcal PID) remains to be determined, but it may be prudent to recommend treatment of asymptomatic BV in HIV-infected women. Essentially, more definitive guidelines on prevention of BV await better understanding of the risk factors, including host susceptibility factors for acquiring BV.

PREVENTION

Since the microbiologic and host risk factors for acquisition of BV are poorly understood, it is difficult to define useful approaches for the prevention of this condition. Since BV is associated with sexual activity, abstinence may represent the most effective (if least popular) means of prevention. Information on condom use and risk of BV is sketchy. One recent cohort study of female sex workers in Lima, Peru found no association of reported consistent condom use with decreased risk of acquiring BV (Sanchez J, Holmes KK, unpublished data). Since the role of sexual transmission in BV is not well defined, and concurrent treatment of male partners has not yet been shown to prevent recurrent BV, treatment of male sex partners cannot be recommended. Recolonization of the vagina with H_2O_2 lactobacilli may protect against infection by BV-associated organisms, but this has not yet been adequately evaluated. Similarly, treatment of BV has not yet been adequately evaluated as a method for preventing pregnancy and puerperal morbidity or postgynecological surgery morbidity. The role of IUD usage as a risk factor for BV requires further study, to confirm or refute the association, and assess the importance of IUD type to any relationships found. The role of genital hygienic practices in the male in protecting the female partner from BV warrants further study, as does the role of douching in increasing the risk among women.

References

1 Curtis AH: On the etiology and bacteriology of leucorrhoea. *Surg Gynecol Obstet* 18:229, 1914.

2 Doderlein A: *Das Scheidensekret und seine Bedeutung far das Puerperalfieber*. Leipzig: Durr, 1892.

3 Menge C, Kronig B: Bakteriologie des weiblichen Genitalkanales. *Monatschr Geburtsh* 9:703, 1899.

4 Schroder R: Zur pathogenese und Klinik des vaginalen Fluors. *Zentralb Gynakol* 38:1350, 1921.

5 Weaver JD et al: The bacterial flora found in nonspecific vaginitis vaginal discharge. *Am J Obstet Gynecol* 60:880, 1950.

6 Gardner HL, Dukes CD: *Haemophilus vaginalis* vaginitis. A newly defined specific infection previously classified "nonspecific vaginitis." *Am J Obstet Gynecol* 69:962, 1955.

7 Blackwell et al: Anaerobic vaginosis (nonspecific vaginitis): Clinical, microbiological and therapeutic findings. *Lancet* ii:1379, 1983.

8 Spiegel CA et al: Anaerobic bacteria in nonspecific vaginitis. *N Engl J Med* 303:601, 1980.

9 Hillier SL et al: The normal vaginal flora, H_2O_2-producing lactobacilli, and bacterial vaginosis in pregnant women. *Clin Infect Dis* 16(Suppl 4):S273, 1993.

10 Huth EJ: Bacterial vaginosis or vaginal bacteriosis? *Ann Int Med* 111: 553, 1989.

11 Goldenberg RL et al: Bacterial colonization of the vagina during pregnancy in four ethnic groups. *Am J Obstet Gynecol* 174:1618, 1996.

12 Cristiano L et al: Bacterial vaginosis: Prevalence in an Italian population of asymptomatic pregnant women and diagnostic aspects. *Eur J Epidemiol* 12:383–390, 1996.

13 Kurki T et al: Bacterial vaginosis in early pregnancy and pregnancy outcome. *Obstet Gynecol* 80:173, 1992.

14 Hay PE et al: A longitudinal study of bacterial vaginosis during pregnancy. *Brit J Obstet Gynecol* 101:1048, 1994.

15 Puapermpoonsiri S et al: Vaginal microflora associated with bacterial vaginosis in Japanese and Thai pregnant women. *Clin Infect Dis* 23: 748, 1996.

16 Riduan JM et al: Bacterial vaginosis and prematurity in Indonesia: association in early and late pregnancy. *Am J Obstet Gynecol* 169: 175, 193.

17 Nilsson U et al: Sexual behavior risk factors associated with bacterial vaginosis and *Chlamydia trachomatis* infection. *Sex Transm Dis* 24: 241–246, 1996.

18 Ryan CA et al: Reproductive tract infections in primary health care, family planning, dermatovenereology clinics: Implications for syndromic management in Arab Muslim women. *Sex Transm Infect* 74(Suppl 1):S95, 1998.

19 Sanchez SE et al: Rapid and inexpensive approaches to managing abnormal vaginal discharge or lower abdominal pain: An evaluation in women attending gynecology and family planning clinics in Peru. *Sex Transm Infect* 74(Suppl 1):S85, 1998.

20 Hallen A et al: Bacterial vaginosis in women attending STD clinic: Diagnostic criteria and prevalence of *Mobiluncus* spp. *Genitourin Med* 63: 386, 1987.

21 Eschenbach DA et al: Diagnosis and clinical manifestation of bacterial vaginosis. *Am J Obstet Gynecol* 158:819, 1988.

22 Hill LH et al: Nonspecific vaginitis and other genital infections in three clinic populations. *Sex Transm Dis* 10:114, 1983.

23 Harms G et al: Pattern of sexually transmitted diseases in a Malagasy population. *Sex Transm Dis* 21:315–320, 1994.

24 Cohen CR et al: Bacterial vaginosis and HIV seroprevalence among female commerical sex workers in Chiang Mai, Thailand. *AIDS* 9: 1093, 1995.

25 Sewankambo N et al: HIV-1 infection associated with abnormal vaginal flora morphology and bacterial vaginosis. *Lancet* 350:546, 1997.

26 Frankel RE et al: High prevalence of gynecologic disease among hospitalized women with human immunodeficiency virus infection. *Clin Infect Dis* 25:706–712, 1997.

27 Amsel R et al: Nonspecific vaginitis: Diagnostic criteria and microbial and epidemiologic associations. *Am J Med* 74:14, 1983.

28 Shafer MA et al: Microbiology of the lower genital tract in postmenarchal adolescent girls: Differences by sexual activity, contraception, and presence of nonspecific vaginitis. *J Pediatr* 107:974, 1985.

29 Bump RC et al: Sexually transmissable infections agents in sexually active and virginal asymptomatic adolescent girls. *Pediatrics* 77:488, 1986.

30 Pheifer TA et al: Nonspecific vaginitis. Role of *Haemophilus vaginalis* and treatment with metronidazole. *N Engl J Med* 298:1429, 1978.

31 Piot P et al: Biotypes of *Gardnerella vaginalis*. *J Clin Microbiol* 20: 677–679, 1984.

32 Briselden AM, Hillier SL: Longitudinal study of the biotypes of *Garnderella vaginalis*. *J Clin Microbiol* 28:2761–2764, 1990.

33 Ison CA, Easmon CSF: Carriage of *Gardnerella vaginalis* and anaerobes in semen. *Genitourin Med* 60:120, 1985.

34 Holst E et al: Bacterial vaginosis: Microbiological and clinical findings. *Eur J Clin Microbiol* 6:536, 1987.

35 Hillier SL et al: Association between bacterial vaginosis and preterm delivery of a low-birth-weight infant. *N Eng J Med* 333:1737, 1995.

36 Larsson PG et al: Is bacterial vaginosis a sexually transmitted disease? *Intern J STD AIDS* 2:362, 1993.

37 Evans BA et al: Risk profiles for genital infection in women. *Genitourin Med* 69:257, 1993.

38 Avonts D et al: Incidence of uncomplicated genital infections in women using oral contraception or an intrauterine device: A prospective study. *Sex Transm Dis* 17:23, 1990.

39 Barbone F et al: A follow-up study of methods of contracpetion, sexual activity, and rates of trichomoniasis, candidiasis and bacterial vaginosis. *Am J Obstet Gynecol* 163:510, 1990.

40 Hawes SE et al: Hydrogen peroxide-producing lactobacilli and acquisition of vaginal infections. *JID* 174:1058, 1996.

41 Berger BJ et al: Bacterial vaginosis in lesbians: a sexually transmitted disease. *Clin Infect Dis* 21:1402, 1995.

42 Leopold S: Heretofore undescribed organisms isolated from the genitourinary system. *US Armed Forces Med J* 4:263, 1953.

43 Brewer JL et al: *Haemophilus vaginalis* vaginitis. *Am J Obstet Gynecol* 74:834, 1957.

44 Heltai A, Taleghany P: Nonspecific vaginal infections: A critical evaluation of *Haemophilus vaginalis*. *Am J Obstet Gynecol* 77:144, 1959.

45 Zinneman K, Turner GC: The taxonomic position of *"Haemophilus vaginalis" (Corynebacterium vaginalis)*. *J Pathol Bacteriol* 85:213, 1963.

46 Reyn A et al: An electron microscope study of thin sections of *Haemophilus vaginalis* (Gardner and Dukes) and some possibly related species. *Can J Microbiol* 12:1125, 1966.

47 Criswell BS et al: *Haemophilus vaginalis* 594, a Gram-negative organism? *Can J Microbiol* 17:865, 1972.

48 Greenwood JR, Pickett MJ: Transfer of *Haemophilus vaginalis* Gardner and Dukes to a new genus, *Gardnerella: G. vaginalis* (and Dukes) comb. nov. *Int J Syst Bacteriol* 30:170, 1980.

49 Totten PA et al: Selective differential human blood bilayer media for isolation of *Gardnerella (Haemophilus) vaginalis*. *J Clin Microbiol* 15:141, 1982.

50 Hite KE et al: A study of the bacterial flora of the normal and pathologic vagina and uterus. *Am J Obstet Gynecol* 53:233, 1947.

51 Hunter CA, Long KR: A study of the microbiological flora of the vagina. *Am J Obstet Gynecol* 75:865, 1958.

52 Goldacre MJ et al: Vaginal microbial flora in normal young women *Br Med J* 1:1450, 1979.

53 Paavonen J et al: *Mycoplasma hominis* in nonspecific vaginitis. *Sex Transm Dis* 10:271, 1983.

54 Piot P et al: The vaginal microbial flora in nonspecific vaginitis. *Eur J Clin Microbiol* 1:301, 1982.

55 Fredricsson B et al: Gardnerella-associated vaginitis and anaerobic bacteria. *Gynecol Obstet Invest* 17:236, 1984.

56 Kronig I: Ober die Natur der Scheidenkeime, specieil aber das Vol kommen anaerober Streptokokken im Scheidensekret Schwangerel. *Zentralb Gynakol* 19:409, 1895.

57 Curtis AH: A motile curved anaerobic bacillus in uterine discharge. *J Infect Dis* 12:165, 1913.

58 Prevot AR: *Manuel de Classification et de Determination des Bacteries Anaerobics*. Paris, Masson et Cie, 1940.

59 Durieux R, Dublanchet A: Les "vibrions" anaerobies des leucorrhee. I. Technique d'isolemont et sensibilité aux antibiotiques. *Med Mal Infect* 10:109, 1980.

60 Hjelm E et al: Anerobic curved rods in vaginitis. *Lancet* ii:1353, 1981.

61 Holst E et al: Characteristics of anaerobic comma-shaped bacteria, recovered from the female genital tract. *Eur J Clin Microbial* 1:310, 1982.

62 Phillips I, Taylor E: Anaerobic curved rods in vaginitis. *Lancet* i:221, 1982.

63 Sprott MS et al: Characteristics of motile curved rods in vaginal secretions. *J Med Microbiol* 16:175, 1983.

64 Spiegel CA et al: Curved anaerobic bacteria in bacterial (nonspecific) vaginosis and their response to antimicrobial therapy. *J Infect Dis* 148:817, 1983.

65 Spiegel CA, Roberts MC: *Mobiluncus* gen nov, *Mobiluncus curtist*, subsp. curtisii sp. nov., *Mobiluncus curtisii* subsp. *holmesii* subsp. nov., and *Mobiluncus mulieris* sp. nov., curved rods from the human vagina. *Int J Syst Bacteriol* 34:177, 1984.

66 Roberts MC et al: Comparison of Gram stain, DNA probe, and culture for the identification of species of *Mobiluncus* in female genital specimens. *J Infect Dis* 152:74, 1985.

67 Thomason JL et al: Clinical and microbiological characterization of patients with nonspecific vaginosis associated with motile, curved anaerobic rods. *J Infect Dis* 149:801, 1984.

68 Hillier SL et al: Microbiological, epidemiological and clinical correlates of vaginal colonisation by *Mobiluncus* species. *Genitourin Med* 67:26, 1991.

69 Schwebke JR et al: Identification of two new antigenic subgroups within the genus *Mobiluncus*. *J Clin Microbiol* 29:2204, 1991.

70 Schwebke JR et al: Humoral antibody to *Mobiluncus curtissi*: A potential serological marker for bacterial vaginosis. *Clin Diag Labor Immun* 3:567, 1996.

71 Mendel EB et al: *Mycoplasma* species in the vagina and their relation to vaginitis. *Obstet Gynecol* 35:104, 1970.

72 Taylor-Robinson D, McCormack WM: The genital mycoplasmas. *N Engl J Med* 302:1003, 1980.

73 Rabe LK et al: Association of viridans group streptococci from pregnant women with bacterial vaginosis and upper genital tract infection. *J Clin Microbiol* 26:1156, 1988.

74 Martius J et al: Relationships of vaginal *Lactobacillus* species, cervical *Chlamydia trachomatis* and bacterial vaginosis to preterm birth. *Obstet Gynecol* 71:89, 1988.

75 Criswell BS et al: *Haemophilus vaginalis:* Vaginitis by inoculation from culture. *Obstet Gynecol* 33:195, 1969.

76 Mardh P-A et al: The grivet monkey as a model for study of vaginitis. Challenge with anaerobic curved rods and *Gardnerella vaginalis*, in *Bacterial Vaginosis*, P-A Mardh, D Taylor-Robinson (eds). Stockholm: Almqvist and Wiksell, 1984, p. 117.

77 Skarin A, Sylwan J: Vaginal lactobacilli inhibiting growth of *Gardnerella vaginalis, Mobiluncus* and other bacterial species cultured from vaginal content of women with bacterial vaginosis. *Acta Pathol Microbiol Immunot Scand.Sect B* 94:399, 1986.

78 Whittenbury R: Hydrogen peroxide formation and catalase activity in the lactic acid bacteria. *J Gen Microbiol* 35:13, 1964.

79 Eschenbach DA et al: Prevalence of hydrogen peroxide-producing lactobacillus species in normal women and women with bacterial vaginosis. *J Clin Microbiol* 27:251, 1989.

80 Hillier SL et al: The relationship of hydrogen peroxide-producing lactobacilli to bacterial vaginosis and genital microflora in pregnant women. *Obstet Gynecol* 79:369, 1992.

81 Klebanoff SJ et al: Control of the microbial flora of the vagina by H_2O_2-generating lactobacilli. *J Infect Dis* 164:94, 1991.

82 Holmes KK et al: Vaginal redox potential in bacterial vaginosis (nonspecific vaginitis). *J Infect Dis* 152:379, 1985.

83 Chen KCS et al: Amine content of vaginal fluid from untreated and treated patients with nonspecific vaginitis. *J Clin Invest* 63:828, 1979.

84 Brand JM, Galask RP: Trimethylamine: The substance mainly responsible for the fishy odor often associated with bacterial vaginosis. *Obstet Gynecol* 63:682, 1986.

85 Hillier SL et al: Improved reliability of diagnosis of bacterial vaginosis using an objective device for detection of elevated vaginal pH and trimethylamine. *Infect Dis Obstet Gynecol* 4:360, 1997.

86 Sturm, AW: Chemotaxis inhibition by *Gardnerella vaginalis* and succinate producing vaginal anaerobes: Composition of vaginal discharge associated with *G. vaginalis*. *Genitourin Med* 65:109, 1989.

87 Platz-Christensen JJ et al: Endotoxin and interleukin-1α in the cervical mucus and vaginal fluid of pregnant women with bacterial vaginosis. *Am J Obstet Gynecol* 169:1161, 1993.

88 Briselden AM et al: Sialidases (neuraminidases) in bacterial vaginosis and bacterial vaginosis-associated microflora. *J Clin Microbiol* 30: 663, 1992.

89 McGregor JA et al: Bacterial vaginosis is associated with prematurity and vaginal fluid mucinase and sialidase: Results of a controlled trial of topical clindamycin cream. *Am J Obstet Gynecol* 170:1048, 1994.
90 Platz-Christensen JJ et al: Increased prostaglandin concentrations in the cervical mucus of pregnant women with bacterial vaginosis. *Prostglandins* 43:133, 1992.
91 Dophin CT et al: Missense mutation in flavin-containing mono-oxygenase 3 gene, FM03, underlies fish-odour syndrome. *Nat Genet* 17:491–494, 1997.
92 Mitchell SC: The fish-odour syndrome. *Perspect Biol Med* 39:514–526, 1996.
93 Rein MF et al: Use of a lactoferrin assay in the differential diagnosis of female genitral tract infections and implications for the pathophysiology of bacterial vaginosis. *Sex Transm Dis* 23:517–521, 1996.
94 Heine PR et al: Vaginal fluid lactoferrin levels are elevated in women with lower reproductive tract infections. *Infect Dis Obstet Gynecol* 6:75, 1998.
95 Ferris DG et al: Women's use of over-the-counter antifungal medications for gynecologic symptoms. *J Family Prac* 42:595, 1996.
96 Bump RC et al: The prevalence, six-month persistence, and predictive values of laboratory indicators of bacterial vaginosis (nonspecific vaginitis) in asymptomatic women. *Am J Obstet Gynecol* 150:917, 1984.
97 O'Dowd TC et al: Evaluation of a rapid diagnostic test for bacterial vaginosis. *Brit J Obstet Gynecol* 103:336–370, 1996.
98 Sonnex C: The amine test: a simple, rapid, inexpensive method for diagnosing bacterial vaginosis. *Br J Obstet Gynecol* 102:160–161, 1995.
99 Schwebke JR et al: Validity of the vaginal Gram stain for the diagnosis of bacterial vaginosis. *Obstet Gynecol* 88:573–576, 1996.
100 Thomason JL et al: Statistical evaluation of diagnostic criteria for bacterial vaginosis. *Am J Obstet Gynecol* 162:155–160, 1990.
101 Dunkelberg WE: Diagnosis of *Haemophilus vaginalis* vaginitis by Gram-stained smears. *Am J Obstet Gynecol* 91:998, 1965.
102 Spiegel CA et al: Diagnosis of bacterial vaginosis by direct Gram stain of vaginal fluid. *J Clin Microbiol* 18:170, 1983.
103 Nugent RP et al: Reliability of diagnosing bacterial vaginosis is improved by a standardized method of Gram stain interpretation. *J Clin Microbiol* 29:297, 1991.
104 Hillier SL et al: Characteristics of three vaginal flora patterns assessed by Gram stain among pregnant women. *Am J Obstet Gynecol* 166: 938–944, 1992.
105 Joesoef MR et al: Reproducibility of a scoring system for Gram stain diagnosis of bacterial vaginosis. *J Clin Microbiol* 29:1730, 1991.
106 Thomason JL et al: Simplified Gram stain interpretive method for diagnosis of bacterial vagionsis. *Am J Obstet Gynecol* 167:16–19, 1992.
107 Morgan DJ et al: Comparison of Gram-stained smears prepared from blind vaginal swabs with those obtained at speculum examination for the assessment of vaginal flora. *Br J Obstet Gynecol* 103:1105–1108, 1996.
108 Schewbke JR et al: The use of sequential self-obtained smears for detecting changes in the vaginal flora. *Sex Transm Dis* 24:236–239, 1997.
109 Sheiness D, et al: High levels of *Gardnerella vaginalis* detected with an oligonucleotide probe combined with elevated pH as a diagnostic indicator of bacterial vaginosis. *J Clin Microbiol* 30:642, 1992.
110 Briselden AM , Hillier SL: Evaluation of Affirm VP microbial identification test for *Gardnerella vaginalis* and *Trichomonas vaginalis*. *J Clin Microbiol* 32:148, 1994.
111 Thomason JL et al: Proline aminopeptidase as a rapid diagnostic test to confirm bacterial vaginosis. *Obstet Gynecol* 71:607, 1988.
112 Gravett MG et al: Preterm labor asosciated with subclinical amniotic fluid infection and with bacterial vaginosis. *Obstet Gynecol* 67:229–237, 1986.
113 Lugo-Miro VI et al: Comparison of different metronidazole therapeutic regimens for bacterial vaginosis. A meta-analysis. *JAMA* 268: 92, 1992.
114 Eschenbach DA et al: A dose duration study of metronidazole for the treatment of nonspecific vaginosis. *Scand J Infect Dis Suppl* 40:73, 1983.
115 Hovik P: Nonspecific vaginitis in an outpatient clinic. *Scand J Infect Dis (Suppl)* 40:107, 1983.
116 Jerve F et al: Metronidazole in the treatment of nonspecific vaginitis (NSV). *Br J Vener Dis* 60:171, 1984.
117 Jones BM et al: *In vitro* and *in vivo* activity of metronidazole against *Gardnerella vaginalis, Bacteroides* spp. and *Mobiluncus* spp. in bacterial vaginosis. *J Antimicrob Chemother* 16:189, 1985.
118 Swedberg J et al: Comparison of single-dose vs. one-week course of metronidazole for symptomatic bacterial vaginosis. *JAMA* 254:1046, 1985.
119 Fischbach F et al: Efficacy of clindamycin vaginal cream versus oral metronidazole in the treatment of bacterial vaginosis. *Obstet Gynecol* 82:405, 1993.
120 Schmitt C et al: Bacterial vaginosis: treatment with clindamycin cream versus oral metronidazole. *Obstet Gynecol* 79:1020, 1993.
121 Bistoletti P et al: Comparison of oral and vaginal metronidazole therapy for nonspecific bacterial vaginosis. *Gynecol Obstet Invest* 21: 144, 1986.
122 Bro F: Metronidazole pessaries compared with placebo in the treatment of bacterial vaginosis. *Scand J Prim Health Care* 8:219, 1990.
123 Hillier SL et al: Efficacy of intravaginal 0.75% metronidazole gel for the treatment of bacterial vaginosis. *Obstet Gynecol* 81:963, 1993.
124 Livengood CH et al: Bacterial vaginosis: efficacy and safety of intravaginal mietronidazole treatment. *Am J Obstet Gynecol* 170:759, 1994.
125 Sobel JD et al: Comparative study of intravaginal metronidazole and triple sulfa therapy for bacterial vagiosis. *Infect Dis Obstet Gynecol* 4:66, 1996.
126 McGregor JA et al: Efficacy of Metrogel-vaginal– versus oral metronidazole for treatment of bacterial vaginosis: A randomized single-blind parallel comparison. *Eleventh Meeting International Society for STD Research*, New Orleans, Louisiana, Abstr. #003, 1995.
127 Greaves WL et al: Clindamycin versus metronidazole in the treatment of bacterial vaginosis. *Obstet Gynecol* 72:799, 1988.
128 Livengood CH et al: Bacterial vaginosis: Treatment with topical intravaginal clindamycin phosphate. *Obstet Gynecol* 76:118, 1990.
129 Hillier SL et al: Microbiologic efficacy of intravaginal clindamycin cream for the treatment of bacterial vaginosis. *Obstet Gynecol* 76: 407, 1990.
130 Stein GE et al: Placebo-controlled trial of intravaginal clindamycin 2% cream for the treatment of bacterial vaginosis. *Ann Pharmacother* 27:1343, 1993.
131 Dhar J et al: Treatment of bacterial vaginosis with a three day course of 2% clindamycin vaginal cream: A pilot study. *Genitourin Med* 70: 121, 1994.
132 Ahmed-Jushuf IH et al: The treatment of bacterial vaginosis with a 3 day course of 2% clindamycin cream: Results of a multicentre, double blind, placebo controlled trial. *Genitourin Med* 71:254–256, 1995.
133 Andres FJ et al: Clindamycin vaginal cream versus oral metronidazole in the treatment of bacterial vaginosis: A prospective, double-blind study. *South Med J* 85:1077, 1992.
134 Arrendondo JL et al: Clindamycin vaginal cream versus oral metronidazole in the treatment of bacterial vaginosis. *Arch AIDS STD* Res 6:183, 1992.
135 Higuera F et al: Bacterial vaginosis: A comparative, double-blind study of clindamycin vaginal cream versus oral metronidazole. *Curr Therap Res* 54:98–110, 1993.
136 Colli E et al: Treatment of male partners and recurrence of bacterial vaginosis: A randomised trial. *Genitourin Med* 73:267–270, 1997.
137 Garcia PJ et al: Syndromic management of sexually transmitted diseases in pharmacies: Evaluation and randomized intervention trial. *Sex Trans Infect* 74(Suppl 1):5, 1998.
138 Hill GB, Ayers OM: Antimicrobial susceptibilities of anaerobic bacteria isolated from female genital tract infections. *Antimicrob Agents Chemother* 27:324, 1985.

139 Koutsky LA et al: Persistence of *Mycoplasma hominis* after therapy: importance of tetracycline resistance and of co-existing vaginal flora. *Sex Trans Dis* 10:S374, 1983.

140 Hill GB, Livengood CH: Bacterial vaginosis-associated microflora and effects of topical intravaginal clindamycin. *Am J Obstet Gynecol* 171:1198, 1994.

141 Sobel JD et al: Long-term follow-up of patients with bacterial vaginosis treated with oral metronidazole and topical clindamycin. *J Infect Dis* 167:784–783, 1993.

142 Boris J et al: Six years observation after successful treatment of bacterial vaginosis. *Infect Dis Obstet Gynecol* 5:297–302, 1997.

143 Vejtorp M et al: Bacterial vaginosis: a double-blind randomized trial of the effect of treatment of the sexual partner. *B J Obstet Gynecol* 95:920, 1988.

144 Moi H et al: Should male consorts of women with bacterial vaginosis be treated? *Genitourin Med* 65:263, 1989.

145 Mengel MB et al: The effectiveness of single-dose metronidazole therapy for patients and their partners with bacterial vaginosis. *J Fam Prac* 28:163, 1989.

146 Vutyavanich T et al: A randomized double-blind trial of tinidazole treatment of the sexual partners of females with bacterial vaginosis. *Obstet Gynecol* 82:550, 1993.

147 Joesoef MR, Schmid GP: Bacterial vagnosis: Review of treatment options and potential clinical indications for therapy. *Clin Infect Dis* 20:S72, 1995.

148 Piot P et al: A placebo-controlled, double-blind comparison of tinidazole and triple sulfonamide cream for the treatment of nonspecific vaginitis. *Am J Obstet Gynecol* 147:85, 1983.

149 Heikkinen J, Vuoplala S: Anaerobic vaginosis: Treatment with tinidazole vaginal tablets. *Gynecol Obstet Invest* 28:98, 1989.

150 Qathne B et al: Cefadroxil as an alternative to metronidazole for the treatment of bacterial vaginosis. *Scand J Infect Dis* 21:585, 1989.

151 Malouf M et al: Treatment of *Haemophilus vaginalis vaginitis*. *Obstet Gynecol* 57:711, 1981.

152 Amsel R et al: Comparison of metronidazole, ampicillin, and amoxicillin for treatment of bacterial vaginosis (nonspecific vaginitis): Possible explanation for the greater efficacy of metronidazole, in *First United States Metronidazole Conference,* SM Finegold (ed). Biomedia Information Corp, New York, 1982.

153 Balsdon MJ et al: *Corynebacterium vaginals* and vaginitis: A controlled trial of treatment. *Lancet* i:501, 1980.

154 Durfee MA et al: Ineffectiveness of erythromycin for treatment of *Haemophilus vaginalis*-associated vaginitis. *Antimicrob Agents Chemother* 16:635, 1979.

155 Nayagam AT et al: Comparison of ofloxacin and metrondiazole for the treatment of bacterial vaginosis. *Int J STD AIDS* 3:204, 1992.

156 Ison Ca et al: Local treatment for bacterial vaginosis. *Br Med J Clin Res* 295:886, 1987.

157 Vander Meijden WJ et al: Treatment of clue-cell positive discharge with 200 povidone-iodine pessaries: A double-blind and placebo-controlled trial. *Eur J Obstet Gynecol* 24:299, 1987.

158 Boeke AJP et al: Effect of lactic acid suppositories compared with oral metronidazole and placebo in bacterial vaginosis: A randomized clinical trial. *Genitourin Med* 69:388, 1993.

159 Andersch B et al: Treatment of bacterial vaginosis with an acid cream: A comparison between the effect of lactate-gel and metronidazole. *Gynecol Obstet Invest* 21:9, 1986.

160 Fredriccson B et al: Ecological treatment of bacterial vaginosis. *Lancet* i:176, 1987.

161 Neri A et al: Bacterial vaginosis in pregnancy treated with yoghurt. *Acta Obstet Gynecol Scand* 72:17, 1993.

162 Hallen A et al: Treatment of bacterial vaginosis with lactobacilli. *Sex Transm Dis* 19:146, 1992.

163 Parent D et al: Therapy of bacterial vaginosis using exogenously-applied lactobacilli acidophili and a low dose of estroil. *Arzneim-Forsch/Drug Res* 46:68, 1996.

164 Hay PE et al: A longitudinal study of bacterial vaginosis during pregnancy. *Br J Obstet Gynecol* 101:1048, 1994.

165 Minkoff H et al: Risk factors for prematurity and premature rupture of membranes: A prospective study of the vaginal flora in pregnancy. *Am J Obstet Gynecol* 150:965, 1984.

166 Gravett MG et al: Independent association of bacterial vaginosis and *Chlamydia trachomatis* infection with adverse pregnancy outcome. *JAMA* 256:1899, 1986.

167 Gravett MG et al: Preterm labor associated with subclinical amniotic fluid infection and with bacterial vaginosis. *Obstet Gynecol* 67:229, 1986.

168 Kurki T et al: Bacterial vagionsis in early pregnancy and pregnancy outcome. *Obstet Gynecol* 80:173, 1992.

169 Riduan JM et al: Bacterial vaginosis and prematurity in Indonesia: Association in early and late pregnancy. *Am J Obstet Gynecol* 169: 175, 1993.

170 Holst E et al: Bacterial vaginosis and vaginal microorganisms in idiopathic premature labor and association with pregnancy outcome. *J Clin Microbiol* 32:176, 1994.

171 Hay PE et al: Abnormal bacterial colonization of the genital tract and subsquent preterm delivery and late miscarriage. *Br Med J* 308:295, 1994.

172 Meis PJ et al: The preterm prediction study: significance of vaginal infection. *Am J Obstet Gynecol* 173:1231, 1995.

173 Hillier SL et al: Association between bacterial vaginosis and preterm delivery of a low birth weight infant. *N Engl J Med* 333:1737, 1995.

174 McGregor JA et al: Prevention of premature birth by screening and treatment of common genital tract infections: results of a prospective controlled evaluation. *J Obstet Gynecol* 173:157, 1995.

175 Krohn MA et al: Vaginal Bacteroides species are associated with an increased rate of preterm delivery among among women in preterm labor. *J Infect Dis* 164:88, 1991.

176 McDonald HM et al: Vaginal infection and preterm labour. *Br J Obstet Gynecol* 98:427, 1991.

177 Hillier SL et al: Case control study of chorioamnionic infection and chorioamnionitis in prematurity. *N Engl J Med* 319:972, 1988.

178 Hillier SL et al: Microbial etiology and neonatal outcomes associated with chorioamnion infection. *Am J Obstet Gynecol* 165:955, 1991.

179 Hillier SL et al: The role of bacterial vaginosis and vaginal bacteria in amniotic fluid infection in women in preterm labor with intact fetal membranes. *Clin Infect Dis* 20 (Suppl 2):S276–278, 1995.

180 Silver HM et al: Evidence relating bacterial vaginosis to intraamniotic infections. *Am J Obstet Gynecol* 161:808, 1989.

181 Watts DH et al: Bacterial vaginosis as a risk factor for post-cesarean endometritis. *Obstet Gynecol* 75:52, 1990.

182 Krohn MA et al: The genital flora of women with intraamniontic infection. *JID* 171:1475, 1995.

183 Burtin P et al: Saftey of metronidazole in pregnancy: A meta analysis. *Am J Obstet Gynecol* 172:525, 1995.

184 McGregor JA et al: Bacterial vaginosis is associated with prematurity and vaginal fluid mucinase and silidase: Results of a controlled trial of topical clindamycin cream. *Am J Obstet Gynecol* 1048, 1991.

185 Joesoef MR et al: Intravaginal clindamycin treatment for bacterial vaginosis: Effects on preterm delivery and low birth weight. *Am J Obstet Gynecol* 175:1527, 1995.

186 Krohn MA et al: Vaginal colonization by *Escherichia coli* as a risk factor for very low birth weight delivery and other perinatal complications. *J Infect Dis* 175:606, 1997.

187 Morales WJ et al: Effect of metronidazole in patients with preterm birth in preceding pregnancy and bacterial vagionsis: A placebo-controlled, double-blind study. *Am J Obstet Gynecol* 171:345, 1994.

188 Hauth JC et al: Reduced incidence of preterm delivery with metronidazole and erythromycin in women with bacterial vaginosis. *N Engl J Med* 333:1732, 1995.

189 McDonald HM et al: Impact of metronidazole therapy on preterm birth in women with bacterial vaginosis flora (*Gardnerella vaginalis*): A randomised, placebo controlled trial. *Br J Obstet Gynecol* 104: 1391, 1997.

190 Oleen-Burkey MA, Hillier SL: Pregnancy complications associated with bacterial vaginosis and their estimated costs. *Infect Dis Obstet Gynecol* 3:149, 1995.

191 Sjoberg I, Hakansson S: Endotoxin in vaginal fluid of women with bacterial vaginosis. *Obstet Gynecol* 77:265, 1991.
192 Platz-Christensen JJ et al: Increased prostaglandin concentrations in the cervical mucus of pregnant women with bacterial vaginosis. *Prostaglandins* 43:133, 1992.
193 Watts H et al: Early postpartum endometritis: the role of bacteria, genital mycoplasmas and Chlamydia trachomatis. *Obstet Gynecol* 73:52, 1989.
194 Newton ER et al: A clinical and microbiologic analysis of risk factors for puerperal endometritis. *Obstet Gynecol* 75:402, 1990.
195 Soper DE et al: Bacterial vaginosis and trichomoniasis vaginitis are risk factors for cuff cellulitis after abdominal hysterectomy. *Am J Obstet Gynecol* 163:1016, 1990.
196 Larsson PG et al: Clue cells in predicting infections after abdominal hysterectomy. *Obstet Gynecol* 77:450, 1991.
197 Larsson PG et al: *C. mobiluncus* and clue cells as predictors of PID after first-trimester abortion. *Acta Obstet Gynecol Scand* 68:217, 1989.
198 Larrson PG et al: Incidence of pelvic inflammatory disease after first-trimester legal abortion in women with bacterial vaginosis after treatment with metronidazole: A double-blind, randomzied study. *Am J Obstet Gynecol* 166:100, 1992.
199 Soper DE et al: Observations concerning the microbial etiology of acute saplingitis. *Am J Obstet Gynecol* 170:1008, 1994.
200 Larsson PG et al: Treatment of bacterial vaginosis in women with vaginal bleeding complications or discharge and harboring. *Mobiluncus Gynecol Obstet Invest* 29:296, 1990.
201 Paavonen J et al: Microbiological and histopathological findings in acute pelvic inflammatory disease. *Br J Obstet Gynecol* 94:454–460, 1987.
202 Korn AP et al: Plasma cell endometritis in women with symptomatic bacterial vaginosis. *Obstet Gynecol* 85:387, 1995.
203 Hillier SL et al: Role of bacterial vaginosis-associated microorganisms in endometritis. *Am J Obstet Gynecol* 175:435, 1996.
204 Korn AP et al: Risk factors for plasma cell endometritis among women with cervical *Neisseria gonorrhoeae*, cervical *Chlamydia trachomatis*, or bacterial vaginosis. *Am J Obstet Gynecol* 178:987–990, 1998.
205 Taha TE et al: Bacterial vaginosis and distrubances of vaginal flora: Association with increased acquisition of HIV. *AIDS* 8,12:1699, 1998.
206 Agnew KJ, Hillier SL: The effect of treatment regimens for vaginitis and cervicitis on vaginal colonization by lactobacilli. *Sex Transm Dis* 22:269, 1995.
207 Winceslaus SJ, Calver G: Recurrent bacterial vaginosis: An old approach to a new problem. *I J STD AIDS* 7:284, 1996.
208 Mohler RW, Brown CP: Doderlein's bacillus in the treatment of vaginitis. *Am J Obstet Gynecol* 25:718, 1933.
209 Butler BC, Beakley JW: Bacterial flora in vaginitis. A study before and after treatment with pure cultures of Doderlein bacillus. *Am J Obstet Gynecol* 79:432, 1960.
210 Wood JR et al: *In vitro* and adherence *Lactobacillus* species to vaginal epithelial cells. *Am J Obstet Gynecol* 153:740, 1985.
211 Hughes VL, Hillier SL: Microbiologic characteristics of *Lactobacillus* products used for colonization of the vagina. *Obstet Gynecol* 75:244, 1990.
212 McGuire LS et al: Psychosexual functioning in symptomatic and asymptomatic women with and without signs of vaginitis. *Am J Obstet Gynecol* 137:600, 1980.

Chapter 43

Trichomonas vaginalis and Trichomoniasis

John N. Krieger
John F. Alderete

INTRODUCTION

Trichomonas vaginalis is a pathogenic protozoan commonly found in the human genitourinary tract of persons living in some areas. Transmitted primarily by sexual intercourse, this organism causes vaginitis in women and nongonococcal urethritis in men. *T. vaginalis* is also implicated in various other genitourinary syndromes. More than 200 million people worldwide are infected with this parasite annually.[1,2] Although accurate numbers are unknown, in 1975 it was estimated that *T. vaginalis* caused approximately 3 to 4 million infections per year in the United States alone and over 1.5 million cases in Great Britain.[3] However, the National Disease and Therapeutic Index, which provides estimates of initial visits for trichomonal vaginal infections seen by physicians in office practice, has shown a gradual decline from approximately 500,000 per year for the period 1970–1975 to approximately 200,000 or less per year for the period 1990–1995.[4]

Diagnosis and treatment of trichomoniasis are assuming a higher priority in STD control programs.[5] Documentation of infection with *T. vaginalis* indicates the need for counseling in behavioral changes to reduce the patient's risk for acquiring other STDs, including human immunodeficiency virus (HIV) infection. There is evidence that genital inflammation associated with vaginal trichomoniasis increases the transmission of HIV.[6,7] Epidemiological studies suggest that trichomoniasis is associated with a two- to fourfold increased rate of HIV transmission. Coinfection with *T. vaginalis* and HIV may result in epidemiological synergy with prolonged or augmented infectiousness of both infections.[7] Such epidemiological synergy may account for the explosive growth of the HIV pandemic in some populations. A strong association was also reported between maternal trichomoniasis and premature rupture of the membranes with concomitant preterm delivery.[8–11]

DEFINITION AND TAXONOMY OF THE PATHOGEN

Trichomonads are flagellated eukaryotic organisms belonging to the protozoan order Trichomonadida. There are more than 100 separate species. Most trichomonads are commensal organisms of the intestinal tract of mammals and birds. Of the three species found in humans, *T. vaginalis* is a parasite of the genitourinary tract, while *T. tenax* and *Pentatrichomonas hominis* are nonpathogenic trichomonads found in the oral cavity and large intestine, respectively.

T. vaginalis is a representative of one of the three most ancient eukaryotic lineages.[22] Although eukaryotic, *T. vaginalis* has properties similar to those of bacteria. The organism lacks mitochondria, 28S ribosomes, and regulated glycolysis. However, *T. vaginalis* has DNA sequences and peptides related to cell-division control molecules universal among yeasts and higher eukaryotes.[12]

HISTORY

In 1836 Donné described *T. vaginalis* in a preparation of fresh vaginal discharge. The protozoan was long regarded as a harmless inhabitant of the vagina.[14,16] This opinion was unchanged by Künstler's description of *T. vaginalis* in the female urinary tract in 1883 or by Marchand's description of *T. vaginalis* in the male urinary tract in 1884.[17–19] During the next 50 years many case reports were published, but clinicians were more interested in the diagnosis and treatment of syphilis and gonorrhea. By the 1950s the significant incidence of sexually transmitted diseases other than gonorrhea and syphilis had become apparent.[20] Investigators in the last 30 years have begun to view *T. vaginalis* as a potentially important sexually transmitted urogenital pathogen.[13,16,17,18]

BIOLOGY OF *TRICHOMONAS VAGINALIS*

Growth and multiplication of *T. vaginalis* are optimal in a moist milieu with temperature between 35°C and 37°C and pH between 4.9 and 7.5.[21] The organisms can be cultivated axenically in nutrient media designed to provide optimum Eh, pH, and antimicrobials to suppress other microorganisms.[15,22–24,26,28,33–36] The pH is a critical growth-limiting factor.

More robust, smaller organisms are observed at pH 5.5–5.8, whereas less motile, larger organisms are encountered at pH levels lower or higher than optimum. Recent clinical isolates readily attach to plastic and become ameboid in morphology. In batch cultures, parasites can have generation times of 4 to 6 hours but are capable of generation times greater than 150 hours.[37] The vaginal pH in trichomonal vaginitis is considered to fall within the range 5.5–6.0.[21,39] Clinical signs and symptoms are less prominent at lower pH levels. Winston suggested that smaller organisms are found in symptomatic women and larger, more rounded organisms are found in asymptomatic women, reflecting growth conditions within the vagina.[40] This suggestion perhaps indicates a need for better biological assays using purified parasite populations of defined morphology.

The influence of the normal vaginal flora and of local nonspecific environmental factors on the growth and pathogenicity of *T. vaginalis* requires further study. In most populations the great majority of women with trichomoniasis are infected simultaneously with other urogenital organisms with pathogenic potential, including *Ureaplasma urealyticum* and/or *Mycoplasma hominis* in over 90 percent, *Gardnerella vaginalis* in about 90 percent, *Neisseria gonorrhoeae* in approximately 30 percent, yeasts in approximately 20 percent, and *Chlamydia trachomatis* in approximately 15 percent.[1] *T. vaginalis* ingests and readily kills lactobacilli and other bacteria in vitro,[41–43] and thus it seems unlikely that trichomonads serve as "Trojan horse" vectors, which ingest other STD pathogens and carry them undamaged into a new human host.[42,43] The importance of coinfections remains unclear in the susceptibility of the host to trichomonal infection and in the clinical presentation of urogenital trichomoniasis. Given the recent findings that *T. vaginalis* degrades all classes of human immunoglobulins,[44] more attention should be given to the role of the numerous trichomonad proteinases that are found in the vagina[21,45–47] of predisposing patients with trichomoniasis to coinfection with other STD pathogens.[7]

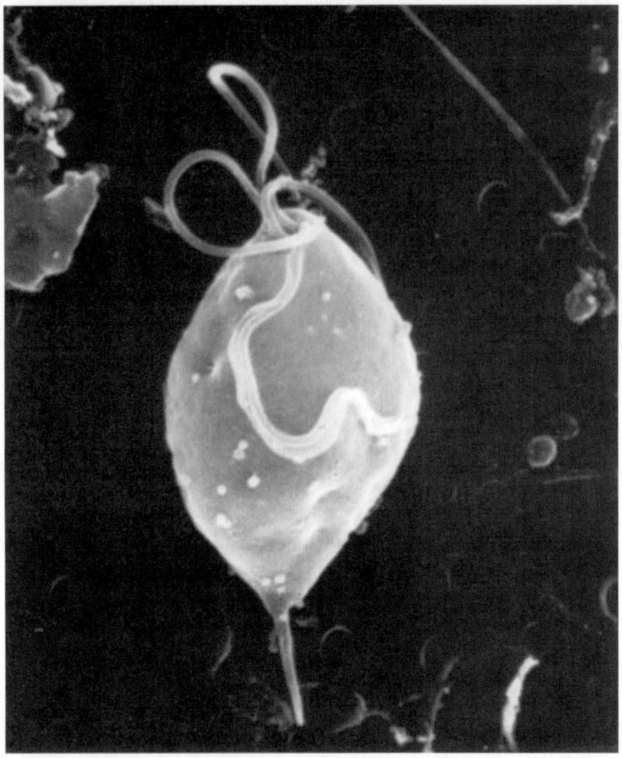

Fig. 43-1. Scanning electron micrograph of *Trichomonas vaginalis.* Three of the four anterior flagella (and the origin of the fourth), the undulating membrane with its trailing flagellum, and the axostyle protruding at the end of the body are clearly seen. ×6000 magnification. (*From A Warton, BM Honigberg, J Protozool 26:56, 1979.*)

The size and shape of *T. vaginalis* vary, depending on the vaginal microenvironment or on culture conditions. Typically, the organism has an oval or fusiform shape, with a mean length of 15 mm (the size of a leukocyte). Trichomonads demonstrate a characteristic erratic, twitching motility as they are propelled by four anterior flagella that originate in an anterior kinetosomal complex (Figure 43-1). A fifth flagellum is attached to the undulating membrane that originates from the kinetosomal complex and extends halfway down the organism. There is an anterior nucleus containing five chromosomes, a parabasal apparatus, a Golgi complex, and an axostyle that runs centrally through the cell to form a posterior tail, or "projection." Parallel to the axostyle and costa are three rows of large chromatic granules, which are believed to be hydrogenosomes because of their biochemical nature.[2,22,23] Reproduction is by mitotic division and longitudinal fission and occurs every 8 to 12 hours under optimal conditions. In contrast to most yeasts and vertebrate cells, *T. vaginalis* has a prolonged G2 period, comprising 50 to 58 percent of the cell population.[12] *T. vaginalis* is believed to exist only in trophozoite form, since a cyst form has never been described.

Cells of *T. vaginalis* are capable of phagocytosis. Vacuoles, particles, bacteria, viruses, and rarely, leukocytes and erythrocytes can be found within the cytoplasm. Specific association with erythrocytes (hemagglutination) results in hemolysis, and this association has been found to represent a nutrient acquisition mechanism for the parasite.[48,49] Particle recognition and phagocytosis appear to be mediated by both nonimmunological means and by specific immunological cell surface receptors similar to the Fc and complement receptors of polymorphonuclear leukocytes.[1] Older literature suggests that some treatment failures in patients with gonorrhea resulted from protection of viable gonococci within trichomonads. However, when *T. vaginalis* were mixed with suspensions of *N. gonorrhoeae*, *M. hominis*, or *C. trachomatis* in vitro, most gonococci were killed within 6 hours, and all mycoplasmas were killed within 3 hours.[42,43] Electron-microscopic studies revealed phagocytic uptake and destruction within the trichomonads. There was no evidence that *C. trachomatis* organisms persisted in mixed culture with *T. vaginalis*.[24]

T. vaginalis is an aerotolerant anaerobe. Growth is inhibited at high oxygen tensions due to deficiency of catalase,[14,16] but some multiplication can be observed in media equilibrated with air. This aerotolerance is attributed to the presence of active superoxide dismutase. Trichomonal energy metabolism appears unique, involving metabolism of pyruvate to lactate in the hydrogenosomes. These organelles contain pyruvate oxidizing enzymes (pyruvate-ferredoxin oxidoreductase) and hydrogenase that are linked by an electron transport protein of low redox potential. Although more information is required, this low-redox-potential protein appears to play a critical role in the action of antitrichomonal drugs. In common with most other parasitic protozoa, trichomonads are unable to synthesize purine ring structures or to interconvert purine nucleotides. However, washed cell suspensions can salvage the purine bases adenine and guanine and their nucleosides. Trichomonad nucleoside phosphorylase and nucleoside kinase activities appear to be responsible for conversion of the purine bases and nucleosides to nucleoside monophosphates.

Isoenzyme patterns (zymodemes) of *T. vaginalis* were evaluated in an attempt to characterize differences among isolates. The isoenzyme patterns of four enzymes (lactate dehydrogenase, malate dehydrogenase, hexokinase, and glucose phosphate isomerase) proved useful in classifying isolates into groups.[34] However, zymodeme patterns were not useful for distinguishing virulence potential or antimicrobial drug sensitivity.[34,35]

Numerous host macromolecules are known to coat the *T. vaginalis* cell surface.[25,26] These host-derived molecules are important to the survival of the parasite in vivo and contribute to the metabolism and pathogenicity of trichomoniasis, either through biological mimicry or through accumulation of nutrients from the host. These molecules include α1-antitrypsin,[28] α2-macroglobulin,[25] fibronectin,[25] lactoferrin and other iron-binding and iron-containing proteins,[29,30] lipoproteins,[26,27] and lipids.[26,27,49] Some evidence suggests that α1-antitrypsin, the major serine protease inhibitor in plasma, binds to specific receptors on the parasite cell surface, where it may protect the parasite from host-degrading enzymes.[28] Low-density lipoproteins derived from the host appear necessary for assembly of new parasite membranes.[26,27,49] Specific receptor-mediated acquisition of iron-binding proteins is important in the pathogenesis of trichomoniasis. Iron uptake, increased intracellular enzyme activity, and up-regulation of virulence genes[31,32] follow host lactoferrin binding by receptors on the parasites. [29,30] *T. vaginalis* also possesses hemolytic activity[33,49] that may be important for destruction of erythrocytes in menstrual blood, with release of iron, lipids, and fatty acids for parasite membrane biosynthesis.

A double-stranded RNA (dsRNA) virus, originally called "TVV," was described in *T. vaginalis*.[50] On electron microscopy this RNA was linear, 1.5 mm in length, and without hairpins or loops. Purification revealed icosahedral viruslike particles at densities ranging from 280 to 1,380 copies per cell.[50] A recent study suggested great divergence among the viruses from 16 *T. vaginalis* isolates.[51] Presence of the dsRNA was not correlated with metronidazole resistance.[53] The virus was found in 50 percent of 500 total clinical isolates examined. Interestingly, TVV-harboring *T. vaginalis* undergo phenotypic variation with respect to surface and cytoplasmic expression of a prominent immunogen, called "P270."[50,52] Virus-negative trichomonads also exhibit down-regulated expression of P270 mRNA, showing the influence of TVV on trichomonal gene and protein expression. More recently, the viral genome from the original isolate used to identify and purify the virus revealed a multisegmented nature with at least three segments, ranging in size from 4.3 to 4.8 kbp based on dsRNA size markers.[54] Furthermore, satellite dsRNAs were found in some virus-harboring trichomonal isolates.[55] The relationship of the virus to virulence and pathogenesis remains unknown.

EPIDEMIOLOGY, TRANSMISSION, AND RISK FACTORS

Data on the epidemiology of *T. vaginalis* are extensive and often conflicting.[14,16,20] The prevalence of trichomoniasis varies widely, depending on both the population studied and the diagnostic techniques.

TRANSMISSION

T. vaginalis is transmitted almost exclusively by sexual intercourse. In the past, however, there was active debate on the route for transmission.[14,56–61] Trichomonads survive for up to 45 minutes on toilet seats, washcloths, and clothing and in bath water.[61] Perinatal transmission occurs to about 5 percent of female children of infected mothers.[65,66] Such infections are usually self-limited, with progressive metabolism of maternal hormones.

The consensus view is that *T. vaginalis* is acquired by direct genital contact, as evidenced by (1) isolation of the organism from urogenital sites, (2) epidemiological data, and (3) human inoculation studies.[67] Thus, trichomoniasis is a urogenital infection. *T. vaginalis* is isolated most often from lower urogenital sites. In women these sites include the vagina, cervix, urethra, bladder, and Bartholin's and Skene's glands.[2,14,16,38,68,69] In men the organism has been isolated from the anterior urethra, external genitalia, prostate, epididymis, and semen.[5,16,20,70–73] The relative importance of different sites for transmission has not been defined. Thus, although nonvenereal transmission by contaminated fomites may explain reports of trichomoniasis in a few patients, such as sexually mature virgins, the data suggest that nonvenereal transmission of *T. vaginalis* is rare.[2,59,62–64]

The epidemiology of trichomoniasis is similar to that of other sexually transmitted diseases. The highest prevalence occurs during the years of peak sexual activity, in patients attending STD clinics, and in commercial sex workers.[20,67,112] Trichomoniasis is often associated with other STDs.[6,7] The high prevalence of *T. vaginalis* among sexual contacts of infected patients strongly supports the view that trichomoniasis is transmitted primarily by sexual contact (Table 43-1). In various studies *T. vaginalis* was isolated from 14 percent to 60 percent of male partners of infected women. Conversely, *T. vaginalis* was isolated from 67 percent to 100 percent of female partners of infected men.

Table 43-1. Epidemiological Data Suggesting that Trichomoniasis Is an STD*

Population, reference	Country, year	No. patients	Prevalence, %
Sexual contacts of men with trichomoniasis			
57	U.K., 1960	56	100
75	U.K., 1975	118	67
Sexual contacts of women with trichomoniasis			
76	U.K., 1960	30	60
77	U.K., 1963	207	45
56	U.S., 1959	31	42
78	Yugoslavia, 1959	364	39
75	U.K., 1957	24	33
17	Poland, 1961	50	30
79	U.S., 1965	94	28
80	U.K., 1978	37	22
81	Poland, 1969	641	20
82	U.K., 1980	21	14
83	U.S., 1993	147	22

* Updated from Krieger.[20,67]

Human inoculation studies also support the importance of sexual transmission and of the pathogenicity of the organism.[84] These investigations were done between 1940 and 1955, before the availability of effective therapy, and fulfilled Koch's postulates in both men and women. Intravaginal inoculation led to infection of up to 75 percent of women, regardless of the bacterial flora initially present (as definable at that time).[84] Findings characteristic of vaginal trichomoniasis occurred after a 5- to 28-day incubation period. Similar studies were conducted in men.[85] All five men injected with 4×10^6 *T. vaginalis* developed urethritis, and prostatitis occurred in two of them, a diagnosis based on microscopic examination of expressed prostatic secretions. Another man developed "moderately severe" urethral discharge containing trichomonads. The two remaining men experienced transient, mild urethral discharge. Although all five men developed urethritis within 24 hours of inoculation, trichomonads were demonstrated in urethral scrapings, urine, or prostatic fluid of only three men after 6 to 9 days. Trichomonads persisted for 13, 44, and 94 days, respectively, in these three men. None of five controls developed clinical manifestations following intraurethral inoculation with sterile medium.

EPIDEMIOLOGY IN WOMEN

Prevalence rates have ranged from 5 to 10 percent in women in the general population to as high as 50 to 60 percent in prison inmates and commercial sex workers (Tables 43-2, 43-3). Among women presenting with vaginal complaints, the prevalence of trichomoniasis has ranged from 18 to 50 percent. Women at high risk of acquiring other STDs[6] are often found to have coexistent trichomoniasis. For example, 30 to 50 percent of women with gonorrhea also have had *T. vaginalis* infection.[3,62,114]

An increased risk of trichomoniasis is described in individuals with multiple sex partners, poor personal hygiene, and low socioeconomic status.[10] One carefully controlled study of 13,816 pregnant women from six urban centers reported a prevalence rate of 12.6 percent.[9] Several investigations also have found a higher prevalence of trichomoniasis in blacks, multiparous women, women married at an early age, and during pregnancy.[1] Behavioral factors associated with an increased risk of *T. vaginalis* included greater numbers of sexual partners and 5 years or more of sexual activity. A history of gonorrhea has been associated with trichomoniasis, but women with a history of gonorrhea who used either barrier or oral contraception in the 6 months before becoming pregnant were less likely to be colonized.

EPIDEMIOLOGY IN MEN

Prevalence rates in different populations have ranged from 0 percent among asymptomatic men at low risk to 58 percent among adolescents at high risk for STDs (Table 43-4). Among randomly selected men attending an STD clinic, the prevalence of *T. vaginalis* was 6 percent in one recent study,[4,5] compared to rates of 1 to 19 percent among men with gonococcal urethritis.[20,67]

Among men infected with *T. vaginalis*, the strongest clinical association is with nongonococcal urethritis (Table 43-5), with prevalence rates ranging from 1 to 68 percent among men with NGU. Most studies suggest rates in the 5 to 15 percent range. Other urogenital syndromes associated with trichomoniasis in men have included prostatitis, urethral stricture, epididymitis, genital inflammations, "lower tract symptoms not responding to routine therapy," and infertility. Prevalence rates in these syn-

Table 43-2. *T. vaginalis* Prevalence in Various Female Populations*

Population, reference	Country, year	No. patients	Prevalence, %
Medical clinical patients			
13	Czechoslovakia, 1942	181	14
86	U.S., 1956	504	13
87	Pakistan, 1965	156	6
88	India, 1970	2,000	25
89	Poland, 1973	222,003	28
Obstetrics, gynecology, and family planning clinic patients			
13	Czechoslovakia, 1942	252	31
90	U.S., 1955	200	21
75	U.K., 1957	400	13
75	U.K., 1957	562	5
56	U.S., 1959	469	47
91	U.S., 1960	183	61
92	Poland, 1973	2,463	21
93	Philippines, 1986	87	5
94	South Africa, 1989	193	49
95	Belgium, 1989	248	2
9	U.S., 1991	13,816	13
96	Nigeria, 1991	500	32
Cancer survey patients			
90	U.S., 1955	300	13
56	U.S., 1959	1,848	18
97 normal	Sweden, 1969	13,000	7
preinvasive carcinoma	"	348	29
invasive carcinoma	"	47	30
98 normal	U.S., 1966	4,078	13
inflammation	"	166	47
neoplasia	"	46	28
99	Nigeria, 1991	2,224	3
100	India, 1994	63,265	5
Other populations			
Routine urine specimens 101	Japan, 1973	361	5
Admissions to medicine and surgery 40	England, 1974	441	8
Factory workers 102	Poland, 1990	1,918	13
University students 103	Nigeria, 1993	1,206	31

* Updated from Krieger.[70]

dromes have ranged from 4 to 100 percent in limited studies (Table 43-6).

Cross-sectional and longitudinal studies among men attending an STD clinic suggest that criteria for selection of men for evaluation of possible *T. vaginalis* infection should include the presence of nonchlamydial nongonococcal urethritis, recent sexual exposure to trichomoniasis, or a history of prior treatment for trichomoniasis or for nongonococcal urethritis.[5,71]

IMMUNOLOGY AND PATHOGENESIS

ANTIGENIC ANALYSIS OF THE PARASITE

Early characterization of the surface of *T. vaginalis* using traditional methods indicated considerable heterogeneity and strain differences among isolates.[14,16] Differential binding of fluorescein-conjugated plant lectins suggested significant variations in cell surface saccharides. A recent report indicated that the *T. vaginalis* cell structure has a lipophosphoglycan-like glycoconjugate.[145] The role of this complex in *T. vaginalis* lectinlike sugar reactions is unknown, as is its contribution to trichomonal virulence.

Early reports using polyclonal antisera in hemagglutination, gel immunodiffusion, and complement-fixation assays estimated the number of serotypes as between two and eight in Europe. Analysis by one- and two-dimensional electrophoresis showed a significant commonality (in contrast to heterogeneity) of trichomonal isolates based on total protein profiles.[146] Heterogeneity, as detected earlier among isolates, appeared to be due to a combination of factors. The presence or absence from the parasite surfaces of a repertoire of proteins, now known to be synthesized by all isolates, as well as different amounts of the synthesized proteins,[147–151] contributed to the variations described among isolates in the older literature. Immunofluorescence using patient sera and a monoclonal antibody against trichomonad surface immunogens revealed two prominent types of isolates.[149,152] Even more intriguing was the discovery that phenotypic variation for the surface (versus cytoplasmic) expression of immunogens varied with the presence of a double-stranded RNA virus.[50,52,153,154] The presence of virus-harboring and phenotypically varying trichomonads was confirmed in patients.[155]

The gene and protein of a representative immunogen associated with phenotypic variation, termed P270, have been shown to be organized with a repeated element.[157] This repeated element accounts for about 50 percent of the protein. One epitope was found within the repeat. All antibody to P270 in the sera of immunized animals and patients with trichomoniasis is directed against the repeated epitope. Thus, the remaining parts of the P270 are relatively immunorecessive, in contrast to the highly immunogenic epitope. The gene/protein structure was conserved in the laboratory strain cultivated in vitro for 10 years. Furthermore, P270 has been found in over 500 isolates from many geographic regions and retains the gene organization originally observed for the laboratory isolate.[157] Although a function for P270 is unknown, the

Table 43-3. *T. vaginalis* in Women at High Risk for Sexually Transmitted Diseases*

Population, reference	Country, year	No. patients	Prevalence, %
STD clinic patients			
104	U.K., 1954	600	46
75	U.K., 1957	400	21
61	U.K., 1960	126	40
17	Poland, 1961	152	41
105	U.K., 1965	1,424	32
80	U.K., 1978	508	8
106	U.S., 1978	255	88
62	U.S., 1980	400	33
182[a] Contacts of men with an STD	U.S., 1992	102	27
Attending for other reasons	"	177	15
108	Canada, 1990	247	7
62	U.S., 1980	400	32
109	India, 1995	215	16
110	France, 1988	392	3
111	Singapore, 1989	197	6
Commercial sex workers			
57	U.K., 1960	127	66
93	Philippines, 1986	1,284	39
112	Netherlands, 1986	60	16
112	U.S., 1986	300	4
113	Burkina Faso, 1990	127	17
(with gonorrhea) 114	Spain, 1991	89	40
Prisoners			
91	U.S., 1960	405	62
115	U.S., 1964	2,002	65
116	U.S., 1973	338	35
Victims of sexual assault			
117	U.K., 1992	110	6
118	U.S., 1990	204	15
119	U.K., 1990	124	12
Adolescents			
120	U.S., 1986	363	5
121	U.S., 1988	102	13
122	U.K., 1987	210	16
Women with vaginal complaints			
123	U.S., 1972	7,468	50
124	Sudan, 1988	403	18
125	India, 1989	150	20
126	U.S., 1989	157	33

* Updated from Krieger.[20]

highly stable nature of the molecule and gene suggest that it is essential.

The observations described above help explain the tremendous heterogeneity among *T. vaginalis* repeatedly noted in the literature. Investigators used monoclonal antibodies in indirect immunofluorescence assays, to describe significant variation. Such variation was also described among isolates from diverse geographical areas of North America.[158] The discovery of phenotypic variation, originally seen for P270[150] and other immunogens,[30,150] has also been noted for other properties, including hemolysis and hemagglutination,[33,48,49] adhesin synthesis and expression,[31,154] receptors for iron-binding and iron-containing proteins,[30] and sensitivity to complement lysis.[159] The possibility that expression of many trichomonad proteins and properties is under the control of environmental cues, such as iron, is under investigation.[30,31,159] A careful analysis of isolates, therefore requires attention to be given to the immunoreactives to specific trichomonad proteins when organisms are grown in a variety of experimental conditions.

HOST RESPONSE

Infection with *T. vaginalis* elicits cellular, humoral, and secretory immune responses. These responses do not protect the patient against repeated infection.[2,14] From a clinical standpoint, repeated infections are common. A history of prior treatment for trichomoniasis is a risk factor for current infection.[5]

Increased numbers of polymorphonuclear leukocytes represent the most obvious host response to infection with *T. vaginalis*. In some cases the inflammatory response is greater in patients who have high concentrations of organisms in their vaginal secretions.[160] A few reports indicate the ability of trichomonad molecules in extracts to chemoattract leukocytes.[161] Culture supernatants from live *T. vaginalis* organisms possess leukotriene B4, an eicosanoid neutrophil-activating factor.[162] Leukocytes have the potential to kill *T. vaginalis*, which are then fragmented and phagocytized by macrophages.[163] Macrophages may also be effector immune cells against trichomonads.[164]

COMPLEMENT

Component C3 of complement binds to acceptor sites on the *T. vaginalis* surface and leads to death of the parasite through activation of the alternative complement pathway.[159,166–169] It was also reported that sera of men infected with *T. vaginalis* possesses complement-fixing antibodies.[170] Nonetheless, persistent tricho-

Table 43-4. Prevalence of Trichomoniasis in Various Male Populations*

Population, reference	Country, year	No. patients	Prevalence, %
Gonococcal urethritis			
127	U.K., 1956	108	18
75	U.K., 1957	30	17
128	U.S., 1980 (unpublished)	141	10
17	Poland, 1961	96	4
85	U.K., 1953	285	1
129	Zimbabwe, 1987	218	1
130	Spain, 1987	1,370	2
131	South Africa, 1994	227	19
Asymptomatic men			
Civilian 75	U.K., 1957	22	0
Military 106	U.S., 1978	27	0
Prisoners			
132	Japan, 1969	191	4
132	Japan, 1969	1,303	3
17	Poland, 1961	34	0
82	U.K., 1980	227	0
University students			
103	Nigeria, 1993	840	16
Adolescents at high risk			
133	U.S., 1991	85	58
STD clinic			
76	U.K., 1960	50	8
Random men attending STD clinic			
5	U.S., 1992	300	6

* Includes patients with both gonococcal and nongonococcal urethritis.
SOURCE: Updated from Krieger.[20,67]

Table 43-5. Prevalence of Trichomoniasis in Men with Nongonococcal Urethritis*

Country, year	No. patients	Prevalence, %	Reference
Chile, 1959	2,482	68	134
U.K., 1956	75	41	127
U.K., 1960	179	2	19
U.S., 1975	118	1	135
U.S., 1992	121	17	5
Canada, 1960	324	11	18
U.K., 1957	326	15	75
U.K., 1960	2,300	6	57
U.K., 1965	1,646	6	105
U.K., 1953	310	6	58
France, 1954	288	12	136
France, 1991	225	2	137
Poland, 1961	128	11	17
Czechoslovakia, 1958	765	10	138
Zimbabwe, 1987	5,873	6	129
Japan, 1969	100	17	132

* Limited to men with nonchlamydial nongonococcal urethritis.
SOURCE: Updated from Krieger.[20,67]

monal infections in women are the hallmark of trichomoniasis, despite the presence of lytic complement during menstruation.[171] It has often been noted that symptoms of trichomoniasis are exacerbated shortly after menstruation,[3,20] the time at which high levels of complement are found in the vagina. Because active complement titers of menstrual blood vary among women,[171] patients with diminished levels of menstrual blood complement may have parasites that survive longer.

Multiple environmental factors may influence susceptibility to complement-mediated lysis.[159] Iron coupled with pH and generation time of the parasites is one example.[171–173] Active C3 removal may play a role in resistance to complement lysis; the mechanism of iron-induced resistance to lysis by complement appears to be induction of at least one membrane-associated cysteine proteinase that degrades C3. The pathogen may also shed bound C3 in the absence of proteinases. Cleavage of C3 by trichomonad proteinases results in the liberation of distinct peptides that may contribute to host pathology. Thus, variation in sensitivity of fresh isolates to complement-mediated lysis[170] may possibly be explained based on the iron status of the parasite and the differential induction of complement-degrading proteinases. Cultivation of *T. vaginalis* for evaluating complement resistance and other properties may be difficult, if the medium is deficient in factors and/or signals required for expression of such properties.

ANTIBODY RESPONSE

Trichomoniasis infection elicits humoral immune responses. Earlier studies demonstrated a serum antibody response among patients with trichomoniasis, by enzyme immunoassays and other techniques. Historically, sera and vaginal secretions from women were examined more often than sera and secretions from men. For example, of 23 infected women, 21 had IgG, 17 had IgM, and 6 had IgA antibodies against *T. vaginalis*.[181] Antibodies were shown to be directed against high-molecular-weight protein immunogens,[149] including P270, the phenotypically varying protein.[152,155] More recently, sera of patients were found to have IgG antibodies to the cysteine proteinases of *T. vaginalis*.[47,107] Data support the view that trichomonad cysteine proteinases are present in vivo, either through lysis of the parasite or through the parasite's secretion of these proteinases.[175,176] Immunoblot analysis using total trichomonad proteins probed with patient sera revealed complex banding patterns.[135] That individual patients had different patterns of reactivity has also been reported and is not surprising given the heterogeneity in expression of proteins and properties influenced by the environmental cues described above.

Table 43-6. Identification of *T. vaginalis* in Men with Urologic Conditions Other than Urethritis*

Syndrome	Country, year	No. patients	Prevalence, %	Reference
Prostatitis	U.S., 1980	26†	100	139
	Japan, 1966	70	28	140
	France, 1979	178	22	141
	Japan, 1960	946	9	142
Lower periotal tract symptoms not responding to "routine therapy"	U.S., 1972	46	71	143
Infertility	Japan, 1960	609	4	142

† All patients had "suspected" *T. vaginalis* urethritis or prostatitis.
* SOURCE: Krieger.[20,67]

Local antitrichomonal IgA, IgG, and IgM have been detected using numerous enzyme immunoassays. In one study, 76 percent of 29 women with acute trichomoniasis and 42 percent of women without current infection had specific IgA antibody.[177] The same assay detected no antibody in men with urogenital trichomoniasis.[80] Recent studies detected local (vaginal) antibody, mostly IgG, immunoreactive to a single surface protein and to numerous proteinases of *T. vaginalis*.[179,180] No IgG antibodies were detected by immunoprecipitation assays in the sera and vaginal washes from uninfected women.[107] The antibody responses in women during and after treatment are receiving attention.[178,179] The level of protection provided by the host antibody response remains undefined either for resolving current infection or for protecting against reinfection.

CLINICAL PRESENTATION AND LABORATORY MANIFESTATIONS

SITES OF INFECTION

T. vaginalis primarily infects vaginal epithelium and is less commonly isolated from the endocervix of infected women.[1,3] The urethra and Bartholin's and Skene's glands are other common sites of infection. Cultures of the urethra are positive in up to 90 percent of infected women. It is still unclear whether these areas harbor low numbers of trichomonads asymptomatically and are a source of reinfection or relapse due to alterations in vaginal microenvironment or other factors. Bladder infections due to *T. vaginalis* have also been reported, but actual differentiation from urethral infection has not been reliably demonstrated. Rare reports of extravaginal sites of *T. vaginalis* infection include isolation from the fallopian tubes of women with acute salpingitis, a perinephric abscess, and cerebrospinal fluid of a patient with meningitis.

In men, the urethra is the most common site for isolation. However, trichomonads have also been isolated from the external genitalia, epididymal aspirates, and prostate gland.[20,67] More recently, *T. vaginalis* was found in chronic perianal ulcerations in men.[182]

INFECTIONS IN WOMEN

The clinical manifestations of vaginal trichomonal infection vary from asymptomatic carriage to severe vaginitis. The presence or absence of symptoms has not been correlated with any specific host or parasite factor(s) and is likely to be complex. Patient symptomatology is multifactorial and clearly related to individual variations in perception. Host factors, which vary considerably during the course of the menstrual cycle, may influence the expression of certain trichomonad virulence factors. For example, iron regulates the expression of adhesins, receptors for iron-binding proteins, and complement resistance.[30–32,159] What role, if any, coexisting infections play in rendering the host more sensitive to trichomoniasis remains unknown. An inflammatory vaginal discharge may be present in many infected women who lack symptoms.[2,68]

The proportion of infected women who have symptoms ranges from 20 to 50 percent, depending on the population, selection criteria, and diagnostic methods.[2,4,20,182a] Indeed, some older studies suggested that the presence of *T. vaginalis* correlated poorly with symptoms and physical findings.[2,62] Unfortunately, these studies did not distinguish patients with cervicitis from those with vaginitis, and equally important, the existence of coinfections with other urogenital pathogens was not considered.

In most studies women with trichomonal vaginitis have had homogeneous vaginal discharge containing many polymorphonuclear leukocytes, which typically give the discharge a yellow-green color.[1] This appearance contrasts with the white floccular or clumped discharge of vulvovaginal candidiasis or the white to gray homogeneous discharge of bacterial vaginosis.[183] Abnormal vaginal bleeding, such as postcoital bleeding, may be due to cervicitis caused by *T. vaginalis* or by associated pathogens. Left untreated, vaginitis by *T. vaginalis* may develop into a chronic infection, characterized by intermittent symptoms or signs and less severe vulvovaginitis.[1,13]

Besides purulent vaginal discharge, the vulva may appear erythematous and edematous with evident excoriations. In many women the vagina and cervix also can appear erythematous and edematous. Small, punctate cervical hemorrhages with ulcerations, referred to as "colpitis macularis" or "strawberry cervix," can on occasion be found.[41] This finding is highly specific for trichomoniasis but is noted in only 2 to 5 percent of infected women on routine speculum examination.[16,20] With colposcopy, however, findings characteristic of "colpitis macularis" were present in 52 (44 percent) of 118 infected women and had high specificity for diagnosis of *T. vaginalis* infection.[68,160]

The signs and symptoms associated with vaginal trichomoniasis were evaluated in a carefully controlled study of 779 women attending an STD clinic.[68] *T. vaginalis* was detected by culture or wet-mount examination in 15 percent of this population. Statistical adjustments were made for coinfections and for demographic, behavioral, and other confounding variables. Trichomoniasis was significantly associated with symptoms of yellow vaginal discharge (odds ratio = 2.4) and vulvar itching (odds ratio = 3.0) and with signs of "colpitis macularis" (odds ratio = 241.0), purulent vaginal discharge (odds ratio = 8.0), vulvar erythema (odds ratio = 2.5), and vaginal erythema (odds ratio = 4.3). Vaginal fluid from women with "colpitis macularis" had a mean of 18 *T. vaginalis* organisms per 400× microscopic field, compared with a mean of 7 in women without "colpitis macularis" ($p < .003$).[160]

Abdominal pain, described in up to 12 percent of women,[16,62] may reflect severe vaginitis, regional lymphadenopathy, or conceivably endometritis or salpingitis due to *T. vaginalis* or another concurrent infection. Some studies suggest that *T. vaginalis* may be isolated more often from women with symptoms or signs of pelvic inflammatory disease than from control women.[184] *T. vaginalis* has been isolated from the pelvic organs and/or peritoneal fluid in a few women.[185] However, most authorities believe that presence of abdominal or adnexal tenderness suggests presence of other pathogens, particularly *N. gonorrhoeae* and *C. trachomatis*. Recent data suggest that *T. vaginalis* infection in women may also be associated with reproductive complications, including an increased risk of infection, post-cesarean infection, premature rupture of the membranes, and preterm birth.[8–11,186]

INFECTIONS IN MEN

T. vaginalis has been isolated from the urethras of 70 percent of men who have had recent sexual contact with infected women. However, 2 weeks after contact only 33 percent of the men were culture-positive.[77] This may be due to specific or nonspecific host immune factors that have antitrichomonal properties, such as the presence of zinc in prostatic fluid.[228,229] In epidemiological and clinical studies *T. vaginalis* has been associated with urethritis characterized by discharge, dysuria, and rarely, superficial penile ulcerations (see Tables 43-4 and 43-5).[20,67] In developed countries, *T. vaginalis* has been isolated from fewer than 15 percent of men with nongonococcal urethritis and usually from fewer than 5 percent of men without symptoms.[1] However, countries with a high prevalence of *T. vaginalis*, such as the eastern European and developing countries, have higher proportions of nongonococcal urethritis caused by this parasite.[20,67,70,187]

One well-controlled survey evaluated clinical manifestations of trichomoniasis among 447 men attending an STD clinic.[83] *T. vaginalis* was found in 33 (22 percent) of 147 sexual contacts of women with trichomoniasis and 17 (6 percent) of 300 randomly selected heterosexual men attending the same clinic. Men with trichomoniasis alone were more likely to complain of urethral discharge ($p < 0.01$), to have discharge on examination ($p < 0.03$), and to have inflammatory cells in urethral secretions ($p < 0.01$) than were men without *T. vaginalis*, *N. gonorrhoeae*, or *C. trachomatis* infection. *T. vaginalis* remained associated with nongonococcal nonchlamydial urethritis (odds ratio = 3.8) after adjustment for race, age, number of sex partners, exposure to a partner with trichomoniasis, and history of trichomoniasis, urethritis, or gonorrhea. A follow-up study documented spontaneous resolution in only 36 percent of untreated men, and one asymptomatic man had persistence of *T. vaginalis* throughout a 4-month period.[71] Nongonococcal nonchlamydial urethritis was documented in 12 (57 percent) of 21 men with *T. vaginalis* compared to only 2 (10 percent) after elimination of *T. vaginalis* as a result of treatment or spontaneous disappearance of the organism ($p < 0.001$) (Table 43-7). These findings suggest the following conclusions: (1) men with trichomoniasis often have symptoms of urethritis, (2) both spontaneous resolution of trichomoniasis and prolonged asymptomatic carriage occur in men with trichomoniasis, and (3) *T. vaginalis* is a treatable cause of urethritis among sexually active men.

Many studies describe prostate gland involvement in men with trichomoniasis, including the experimental studies described in the above discussion of transmission[85] as well as descriptive clinical studies (see Table 43-6). However, the importance of *T. vaginalis* in prostatitis remains unclear.[20] Identification of *T. vaginalis* in prostatic fluid was first reported by Drummond,[188] who identified the protozoa in prostatic secretions from four of five husbands of infected women. Other workers identified *T. vaginalis* in specimens obtained from 9 percent to 100 percent of patients with prostatitis.[19,140–143,189–191] Sylvestre et al. described prostatic involvement in 10 (29 percent) of 35 men with trichomonal urethritis.[18] Prevalence rates of up to 85 percent were reported for men who failed multiple courses of antimicrobials and for those who had long-standing symptoms.[85,106,190,192] Identification of *T. vaginalis* in prostate biopsies from symptomatic men, associated with inflammation, further supports a role for *T. vaginalis* in some cases of prostatitis.[72,191]

Less rigorous observations suggest that *T. vaginalis* may cause other genitourinary conditions, including balanoposthitis, other inflammations of the external genitalia, urethral stricture, epididymitis, and infertility. Inflammation of the glans penis (balanitis) and the foreskin (posthitis) were attributed to *T. vaginalis* infection by many investigators.[13,16,18,20,59,76,105] Balanitis was noted in 2 (11 percent) of 18 men with trichomoniasis reported by Watt and Jennison[76] and in 4 (4 percent) of 91 men reported by Wilson and Ackers.[82] Others suggest that both phimosis and "excessive length" of the prepuce increased the risk for trichomonal balanoposthitis.[18,139] *T. vaginalis* was the only pathogen isolated from chronic draining sinuses on the median raphe of the penis,[193–195] and the only pathogen identified as a cause of penile ulcers.[192,194]

Urethral strictures were noted in 5 (9 percent) of 56 men with trichomoniasis in Catterall's series.[57] Weston and Nicol found strictures in 11 (50 percent) of 22 men with persistent urethritis associated with *T. vaginalis*.[77] Urethral strictures were associated with long-standing and recurrent disease.[20,57,77,196] It is uncertain if preexisting urethral obstruction favored persistence of trichomonal urethritis or if trichomonal inflammation led to stricture formation. Congenital urethral abnormalities, such as hypospadias and meatal stenosis, were also suggested as risk factors for trichomoniasis.[59] Epididymitis caused by *T. vaginalis* was described by Liston and Lees in 1940.[197] There have been five more recent case descriptions.[73,198,199] None of the studies described in this paragraph and the last included control groups, and little consideration was given to other STD organisms, such as *C. trachomatis* or *N. gonorrhoeae*.

The high prevalence of *T. vaginalis* in some studies of infertile men, as well as adverse effects of *T. vaginalis* on sperm motility in vitro, led some workers to consider this parasite a cause of male infertility.[200–202] A recent study from India found *T. vaginalis* in 50 (4 percent) of 1,131 semen specimens.[202] Infected men were more likely to have abnormalities of sperm morphology and motility, along with abnormal seminal fluid viscosity and increased particulate debris, compared to the uninfected group. These abnormalities improved after treatment. However, *T. vaginalis* would appear to be an uncommon cause of infertility, since other studies have shown that *T. vaginalis* was highly prevalent in many populations of pregnant women. Finally, some observations suggest that *T. vaginalis* may be associated with both erectile dysfunction and premature ejaculation,[134,139] but there is no evidence for a causal relationship.

Table 43-7. Prevalence of Clinical Findings (Number, Percent) in 21 Men Before and After Resolution of *T. vaginalis* Infection*

Finding	*T. vaginalis** present	*T. vaginalis* absent	*p*
Symptomatic urethral discharge	13 (62)	3 (14)	<0.002
Urethral discharge on examination	12 (57)	5 (24)	0.03
≥5 PMN/hpf† of Gram stain	12 (57)	5 (24)	0.03
Urethritis†*	12 (57)	2 (10)	0.001
No. of PMN/hpf† of Gram stain (mean ± SD)	8 ± 7	2 ± 4	0.001

† Presence of at least polymorphonuclear leukocytes per 400× field of the gram-stained urethral smear.

* Urethritis was defined as presence of at least two of the following three criteria: symptomatic urethral discharge, presence of urethral discharge on physical examination, or presence of ≥5 PMN/hpf of the gram-stained urethral smear.

* SOURCE: Krieger.[67]

NEONATAL TRICHOMONAL INFECTION

Between 2 percent and 17 percent of female infants born to infected women have developed vaginal infections.[65] The neonatal vaginal epithelium resembles adult vaginal epithelium due to presence of maternal estrogens. Such mature epithelium is susceptible to *T. vaginalis* infection. Vaginal discharge may occur, but typical infections are asymptomatic. Metabolism of maternal estrogens occurs by 3 to 4 weeks of age, at which time the vaginal epithelium assumes a prepubescent state. At this time the epithelium may become relatively resistant to *T. vaginalis* infection and experience resolution of discharge.[2]

PATHOLOGY/HISTOPATHOLOGY

PATHOPHYSIOLOGY

Little is known regarding the pathogenesis of *T. vaginalis* infection. The absence of a satisfactory animal model and of genetic manipulation of trichomonads have hindered attempts to elucidate the pathogenetic mechanisms of *T. vaginalis*. A mouse subcutaneous abscess model[14,16,144] was found to correlate imperfectly with clinical findings in patients and, importantly, was inconsistent with the tropism of urogenital infection.[20,160,203] Intravaginal models have met with limited success.[204–206]

In vitro models have been developed to study the host-parasite interaction. The importance of contact-dependent extracellular killing of cells in monolayer culture has been established.[207,208] Kinetic analysis revealed that host-cell death was related to contact with *T. vaginalis*.[207] Filtrates of trichomonad cultures had no effect on cells in monolayer cultures.[207,208] That trichomonad microfilaments, but not microtubules, were important in the process of killing target cells was shown by the use of selective inhibitors. Hemolysis[49] also required direct contact between *T. vaginalis* and erythrocytes.[48,214] The ability to kill host cells likely promotes the survival of the parasite through nutrient acquisition. Erythrocytes, unlike epithelial cells,[27] provide essential cholesterol and fatty acids for trichomonal membranes,[48] an important consideration given the inability of *T. vaginalis* to synthesize lipids.[215,216] Both erythrocytes and epithelial cells may represent sources of iron.[29,30,48]

Interestingly, recognition and binding by trichomonads to host epithelial cells is mediated by at least four specific *T. vaginalis* surface proteins.[48,209] The adhesins identified using in vitro cell monolayers were also involved in the cytoadherence of *T. vaginalis* to vaginal epithelial cells.[209,210] Erythrocyte-binding ligands were distinct from those mediating epithelial-cell attachment by *T. vaginalis*.[48] The process of cytoadherence requires the continuous action of a trichomonad cysteine proteinase that is known to act upon the parasite surface, but not the host-cell surface, in an unknown fashion.[211] Recently, two specific surface cysteine proteinases of *T. vaginalis* were found to bind to host-cell surfaces, and amounts of these two proteinases correlated with cytoadherence and cytotoxicity.[212] Finally, molecular characterization of one of the adhesins revealed mimicry with malic enzyme.[32] Such mimicry of host molecules may provide a mechanism for evasion of host immune defenses by the parasite.

An ameboid morphology was observed for trichomonads adherent to vaginal epithelial cells but not epithelial cells in monolayer cultures.[212] The rate of signaling for transformation from the ellipsoid to ameboid form was related to the amount of adhesin on the parasite surface. A second signal received by adherent organisms led to induction of adhesin synthesis. These findings suggest that cytoadherence, which ultimately leads to cytotoxicity, is a dynamic, complex process involving a cascade of reactions.

Other studies have emphasized the importance of extracellular cytotoxins.[175,218] A factor from *T. vaginalis* culture filtrates that caused detachment and clumping of cultured cells has been identified.[175,190,220] Virulence of recent human isolates correlated with the level of β-hemolytic activity.[33]

These studies imply that *T. vaginalis* may possess a number of different virulence-associated characteristics. However, the relevance of these observations to the clinical presentation of disease in patients remains undefined. Continued investigations must define the aspects of the host-parasite relationship that promote growth and persistence of *T. vaginalis* in the vagina. Future work is also needed to clarify the sites of infection in the male, the mechanism(s) of cytotoxicity, and the immune evasion strategies of the parasite.

HISTOPATHOLOGY

T. vaginalis infection in women is commonly associated with increased blood vessel dilation in the surface epithelium and submucosa of the vagina and cervix. Blood vessel distention with local extravasation of blood (petechiae) produces the characteristic "strawberry cervix," or "colpitis macularis."[62,68] This sign is highly specific for trichomoniasis.

Mucopurulent cervicitis is also common among patients with trichomoniasis. *T. vaginalis* does not appear to be associated with any endocervical pathology on cervical biopsy,[222] but trichomoniasis does produce edema of the ectocervical squamous epithelium, desquamation, and an inflammatory exudate. Trichomonads have been shown to adhere to epithelial cells of the vagina and are also found in pooled vaginal fluid. Little direct evidence exists to show the parasites occur intracellularly. Cellular changes in the squamous epithelium that have been described with trichomoniasis include an increased number of parabasal cells, binucleation, nuclear enlargement, nuclear hyperchromasia, and perinuclear halos.

The cytological and histological changes described with *T. vaginalis* infection may be confused with koilocytotic atypia due to human papilloma virus infection and may sometimes mimic changes seen in mild dysplasia. However, no causal relationship has been established between cervical cancer and trichomonal vaginitis.[14,16,144] Studies that suggested such an association were based primarily on the high prevalence of *T. vaginalis* (10 to 30 percent) among patients with cervical cancer.[20] However, these studies did not control for other genital pathogens, such as human papilloma virus, that are now recognized as risk factors for cervical carcinoma. The consensus of expert opinion is that identification of *T. vaginalis* infection is a marker for other infections and behavorial risk factors that directly increase the risk of cervical dysplasia and carcinoma.[223–227]

Histopathological studies of urogenital trichomoniasis in men are limited. Men with trichomonal infections are more likely than uninfected men to show inflammation on gram-stained urethral smears.[5,83] The inflammatory process often resolves following treatment or spontaneous resolution of infection.[71] Prostate biopsy specimens from men with *T. vaginalis* infection show areas of inflammation surrounding *T. vaginalis* organisms.[72,191]

DIAGNOSIS

Diagnosis based solely on clinical signs and symptoms is unreliable, because the spectrum of infection is broad and other sexually transmitted pathogens cause similar signs and symptoms.[2,13,14,16,20,144] Diagnosis may prove particularly difficult in men, where infections are characterized by fewer organisms than infections in women.[5,16,20] High concentrations of zinc and other substances with antitrichomonal activity in prostatic secretions may help explain the lower concentrations of organisms in infected men.[5,222,229]

There is overlap between the clinical presentation of trichomoniasis and presentation of other infections: bacterial vaginosis and possibly other genital infections in women[1,239] and other types of nongonococcal urethritis in men.[20,230] Trichomonads in secretions can interfere with the Gram stain diagnosis or the proline aminopeptidase test for bacterial vaginosis.[231] Clue cells may not generally be found in women with trichomoniasis. One multicenter study of 7,918 pregnant women found that trichomoniasis was associated with reduced concentrations of vaginal lactobacilli. Women with trichomoniasis were more likely to have elevated vaginal pH, amine odor, milky discharge, or colonization by *Gardnerella vaginalis, Bacteroides* spp., or genital mycoplasmas than women with normal flora.[232]

LABORATORY DIAGNOSIS

Since the clinical manifestations of trichomoniasis vary and coexisting infections are common, diagnosis of *T. vaginalis* requires laboratory confirmation.

Direct microscopic examination

In clinical practice, diagnosis of trichomoniasis is most often based on examination of male urine or of a wet-mount preparation of vaginal discharge. In expert hands, this method has been found to be 50 to 70 percent sensitive in women but is less reliable in men.[5,20,69,233,234] Optimal diagnosis by wet mount depends on identification of motile protozoa.

Various staining methods include: Gram, Giemsa, Papanicolaou, periodic acid–Schiff, acridine orange, fluorescein, neutral red, and immunoperoxidase, among other techniques.[123,143,234–239] In spite of reports citing good results, staining methods are viewed as less accurate than direct examination by experienced microscopists.[20,62,240–242,242a]

Papanicolaou-stained smears can detect *T. vaginalis* in asymptomatic women during routine cytologic examinations.[1,4,69,242a] However, most reports comparing this method with wet mount and culture suggest a high percentage of false-positive and false-negative results[69,243] Further, the cytological features of inflammatory vaginal discharge associated with *T. vaginalis* and *C. trachomatis* may be similar.[126,244] One study of 290 asymptomatic women seen for routine gynecological examinations found that inflammation on the cervical Papanicolaou smear was more common among women with *T. vaginalis* and *C. trachomatis* infections, but the positive predictive value of inflammation was only 14 percent for trichomoniasis and 7 percent for chlamydial infection.[244] Confirmation using another method is recommended.[69] Use of monoclonal antibodies against *T. vaginalis* may improve the sensitivity and specificity of direct diagnosis in women.[69,155,245] Such methods have not been evaluated systematically in the male.

Culture

Culture techniques using a variety of liquid and semisolid media remain the "gold standard" for diagnosis of trichomoniasis.[69,75,233,240,246,247,249] Cultures are especially useful when relatively few organisms are present, for example, in women with chronic disease or in men.[5,36,62]

In research settings, obtaining multiple cultures or evaluating multiple sites has increased the rate of laboratory diagnosis. One study of 600 randomly selected women at high risk found that duplicate vaginal cultures using Feinberg-Whittington or modified Diamond culture medium resulted in a diagnosis of 82 and 78 cases, respectively, while the combination of the two cultures identified 88 infected women.[69] In comparison, wet-mount examination detected only 53 (60 percent) of the cases. Cytologic smears were interpreted as positive for *T. vaginalis* in 49 (56 percent) of the 88 culture-positive cases but also resulted in seven false-positive smears, and specimens from another 18 women with negative cultures were interpreted as "suspicious" for trichomoniasis. Similar studies of men found that evaluating multiple sites substantially increased the detection of *T. vaginalis*.[5,71]

The relative sensitivities of different culture media have not been determined adequately. One study evaluated six media, including all five media commercially available in the United States.[247] Sixty-five (17 percent) of 375 women had positive wet mounts, and all these positive results were confirmed by growth in at least one medium. Of 310 wet-mount-negative specimens, 37 (12 percent) grew *T. vaginalis*. Diamond and modified Diamond media detected 99 (97 percent) and 92 (90 percent) isolates compared with three formulations of Kupferberg medium that detected 77 (75 percent), 50 (49 percent), and 43 (42 percent) isolates, respectively. Lash medium also performed poorly. In vitro studies suggest that modified Diamond medium allows more prolific growth and is more suitable for detecting *T. vaginalis* than Kupferberg medium.[248]

Immunological and molecular methods

A variety of serologic techniques,[80,106,107,177,250] some with good sensitivity,[252] have been described to diagnose trichomoniasis. These assays have not proven specific for active infection or sensitive enough for diagnosis of individual infections.[2,20] Some studies found that serologic assays were less sensitive than culture or even wet-mount examination.[253] Alternative approaches have included antigen-detection immunoassays using monoclonal antibody[256] and nucleic acid–based tests.[257–260]

CLINICAL DIAGNOSIS IN WOMEN

Because the cause of vaginitis/vaginosis cannot be determined solely on the basis of symptoms or physical examination, laboratory methods are required.[39] While several studies showed that a purulent, yellow-green vaginal discharge is characteristic of trichomonal vaginitis,[62] discharge is absent in a varying percentage of cases. Thus, diagnosis of trichomoniasis depends on identification of *T. vaginalis* by wet mount, stains, cultures, or other methods described above.

Evaluation should begin with examination of vaginal fluid or discharge obtained during the speculum examination, using a cotton swab or wire loop.[2] The sample is mixed with one milliliter of body-temperature saline in a test tube, then examined using a microscope at low (100×) and medium (400×) power. Alternatively, one drop of saline may be placed on a microscope slide and the vaginal sample mixed directly in the saline on the slide. Using warmed saline or warming the slide is important for enhancing characteristic trichomonad motility. Optimally, the evaluation should use phase-contrast microscopy. With a standard microscope, the condenser should be racked down or the diaphragm closed to increase contrast. Diagnosis requires identification of motile trichomonads with characteristic motility, size, and morphology. Increased numbers of inflammatory cells, chiefly polymorphonuclear leukocytes, are also present in most cases of trichomonal vaginitis.

Culture is the method of choice for women at risk for trichomoniasis who have negative wet-mount examinations. As discussed above, cultures are far more sensitive and specific than other available diagnostic tests for identifying *T. vaginalis* in infected secretions,[36,62] particularly in women without symptoms or signs of vaginitis. For example, in one study of 177 inner-city women attending an STD clinic, 86 (49 percent) had positive cultures or wet mounts for *T. vaginalis*.[246] Culture was much more sensitive than the wet mount (98 percent versus 38 percent); symptoms were unreliable for diagnosis.

CLINICAL DIAGNOSIS IN MEN

Direct demonstration of *T. vaginalis* by microscopy is difficult in male genital or urine samples. Therefore, two strategies have been used for diagnosis/treatment in men: empirical therapy, based on epidemiological considerations, and culture. Conventional recommendations have focused on epidemiological treatment of sexual partners of infected women, without specific diagnosis.[261,262] Epidemiologic therapy is reasonable in situations where appropriate diagnostic facilities are unavailable. This approach will reduce subsequent transmission to uninfected women and limit the potential for reinfection of women following successful treatment. However, epidemiological therapy is limited by compliance with partner notification and tends to miss partners of asymptomatic women, since such women are less likely to be diagnosed.[5] A specific diagnosis of trichomoniasis in men could prompt identification of more infected males and enhance detection of additional infected women through partner notification.[5] Further, most infected men seen in an STD clinic setting did have symptoms.[83] Specific treatment is therefore of direct benefit to infected men.

Few studies have evaluated diagnosis of trichomoniasis in men. Although culture of *T. vaginalis* is ideal, the optimal site or specimen to culture in men is still debated.[16,20] Trichomonads can be recovered from varied sites, including the urethra, urine, external genitalia, epididymis, and prostate.[20,72] Saxena and Jenkins recently evaluated cultures of two sites in 85 high-risk men, using commercial medium.[133] Urine cultures were positive in 61 percent, and urethral cultures obtained after prostatic massage were positive in 39 percent. In another study of 447 men attending an STD clinic,[5] urethral and first-void urine cultures were positive in 80 percent and 68 percent, respectively, of the 50 cases that were positive at the external genital site alone. When combined, cultures of these two specimens detected 49 of the 50 cases.

Urethral swabs used to culture *N. gonorrhoeae* may also be used to culture *T. vaginalis*.[5] Combining a urethral swab specimen with a first-voided urine sediment might prove sensitive for evaluating possible *T. vaginalis* infection with a single culture, although this approach requires validation. In a natural history study, semen cultures proved valuable for documentation of infection in selected cases, including four instances when concomitant cultures of the external genitalia, urethra, and first-void urine sediment were all negative.[71]

ANTIMICROBIAL SUSCEPTIBILITY AND THERAPY

The treatment of trichomoniasis was revolutionized in 1958, when Cosar and Julou demonstrated the in vitro activity of metronidazole.[263] Metronidazole provided the first effective treatment for trichomoniasis and remains the mainstay for therapy despite development of a number of related drugs (tinidazole, ornidazole, nimorazole, tioconazole, etc.)[264–267]

ANTIMICROBIAL SUSCEPTIBILITY

T. vaginalis is susceptible to a limited number of antimicrobial agents.[268] Metronidazole and related drugs are highly effective. These 5′-nitroimidazoles are active largely against anaerobic or microaerophilic organisms. Ferredoxins, low-redox-potential proteins, play a major role in the energy metabolism of anaerobes but not that of aerobes. The 5′-nitroimidazoles require reduction of the nitro group to kill susceptible cells.[269] In *T. vaginalis* this reduction process is catalyzed by pyruvate-ferredoxin oxidoreductase. In essence, a short-lived reduction product, probably the protonated one-electron nitro radical anion, oxidizes susceptible DNA, causing strand breaks and subsequent cell death. The amount of damage depends on the base composition of the DNA. In general, nitroimidazoles damage DNA of a relatively high A+T content more readily than DNA with a low A+T content. *T. vaginalis*, *E. histolytica*, and clostridia have A+T contents that exceed 70 percent, and these organisms have low minimum lethal concentrations. Aerobic conditions interfere with the reduction process and diminish the trichomonacidal activity of 5′-nitroimidazoles.[270]

Most *T. vaginalis* isolates are highly susceptible to metronidazole and related 5′-nitroimidazole drugs. Minimal inhibitory concentrations are usually <1 μg/mL under anaerobic conditions.[270–272] Minimum trichomonacidal concentrations have ranged from 0.2 mg/mL to 16 μg/mL.[270–272] Effective concentrations measured under aerobic conditions are higher.[270,272,273] Large samples of isolates manifest a continuum of susceptibility. Treatment results generally correlate with in vitro susceptibility.[270,271]

Rare *T. vaginalis* isolates from patients who were not cured by metronidazole have in vitro resistance to high levels of the drug.[270,273–275] Metronidazole resistance can also be induced by prolonged exposure in vitro.[221,276] The mechanisms of resistance are not known. Testing for trichomonacidal concentrations of metronidazole under aerobic conditions enhances the difference between the minimum concentrations lethal to susceptible and to resistant organisms.[270,274,275] High aerobic values (>50 μg/mL) provide a good indication of clinically significant resistance, but these values are determined under conditions different from those prevailing with natural infection. Thus, in vitro susceptibility levels are unrealistically high and should not be regarded as representing blood levels needed to eliminate the infection.[274] Only large doses of metronidazole, at least 500 to 750 mg three times a day for 7 days, have been partially effective in the treatment of these cases. Successful treatment by combining topical and high-dose oral therapy was reported for some metronidazole-resistant infections.[277] High-dose intravenous metronidazole was used successfully to treat a patient who failed repeated oral therapy.[278]

In vitro activity by an antihelminthic benzimidazole, mebendazole, was observed,[268] but this compound has received limited clinical testing. In case reports, however, mebendazole proved unsuccessful for treatment of metronidazole-resistant infections.[279] Other compounds that have some activity against *T. vaginalis* in vitro or in animal models include nitropyrazole derivatives,[280] certain thiazides,[281] lipophilic tetracyclines,[282] and plant alkaloids.[283]

CURRENT TREATMENTS

Pharmacology

Peak serum levels following the oral administration of 500 mg of metronidazole are approximately 10 μg/mL. Peak serum levels following a single 2-g dose are about 40 μg/mL. The serum half-life is approximately 6 to 8 hours.[284] Pharmacokinetic problems are not responsible for treatment failures.[285] Metronidazole crosses the placenta readily. Other 5′-nitroimidazoles differ somewhat from metronidazole in their pharmacological behavior,[284] but none of these drugs offers any clear therapeutic advantages.[274,286]

Treatment recommendations

Because *T. vaginalis* often infects the urethra and periurethral glands, systemic chemotherapy is superior to topical treatment.[2] Therapy that treats only vaginal organisms may leave organisms at other sites, resulting in subsequent endogenous reinfection. Metronidazole is the treatment of choice for trichomoniasis in both women and men.

For women, the recommended regimen is metronidazole, 2 g by mouth, as a single oral dose.[261] This treatment is highly effective, with cure rates in the range of 82 to 88 percent.[144,270,287–289] Concomitant treatment of male sexual partners with a similar regimen is also recommended. Simultaneous therapy for sexual partners increases the cure rate to 95 percent or more with single-dose treatment.[144,287–289] Infected women and their sexual partners should be instructed to avoid intercourse until the patient and partner(s) are cured. An alternative regimen is metronidazole 500 mg twice daily for 7 days.[261] This regimen is recommended for patients who do not respond to single-dose therapy. A 2-g single oral dose once daily for 3 to 5 days, is recommended for patients who fail repeated treatment courses.

Relatively few studies have addressed treatment of trichomoniasis in men. A 7-day multidose metronidazole regimen proved highly effective in curing men.[105,129] The single-dose regimen has not been evaluated well. One report indicated a 43 percent failure rate with single-dose therapy.[129] Other investigators found that metronidazole, 2 g as a single oral dose, was highly effective in curing men.[71] HIV-positive individuals with trichomoniasis should receive the same treatment as persons who are HIV-seronegative.[261]

Adverse reactions and toxicity of metronidazole

Many patients taking metronidazole complain of a disagreeable or metallic taste. Nausea occurs in about 10 percent of patients taking a single 2-g dose.[144] Transient neutropenia with peripheral white blood cell counts of 100 to 1,400 were observed in 7.5 percent of patients treated with multiple doses of metronidazole.[290] Other patients experience a reaction similar to a disulfiram reaction, with nausea and flushing after ingesting ethanol. Therefore, patients should be cautioned to avoid alcohol while on treatment. Metronidazole may prolong the prothrombin time in patients taking warfarin,[291] presumably by competing for binding sites on serum proteins.

Animal data suggest that metronidazole may be both carcinogenic and mutagenic. After prolonged exposure to high doses of metronidazole, mice developed an excess of lung tumors,[292] but other species, such as hamsters, did not show a similar effect.[293] Metronidazole is mutagenic for certain bacteria that are good predictors of carcinogenic potential in animals.[263]

Human data suggest that metronidazole has limited carcinogenic or mutagenic potential. A cohort of 771 women followed for 15 to 25 years after treatment with metronidazole showed no significant increase of cancer morbidity and mortality over the expected rate.[294] These data confirm a shorter-term evaluation of the same cohort.[295] On balance, they suggest that the risk of short-term, low-dose metronidazole is extremely small. Based on these considerations, the Centers for Disease Control recommends that pregnant women with trichomoniasis may be treated after the first trimester with a single 2-g oral dose of metronidazole.[261]

OTHER THERAPIES

Immunization

A vaccine for active immunization against trichomoniasis (Solco Trichovac, Solco Co., Switzerland) is marketed in Europe. This vaccine consists of killed "aberrant lactobacilli" isolated from women with trichomoniasis.[296] The bacteria purportedly share numerous epitopes with *T. vaginalis*, such that antiserum generated against the bacteria was immunocross-reactive with the parasite surface. Using a variety of techniques, the immunocross-reactive nature was not confirmed.[297,298] Although some reports indicate a beneficial effect, the vaccine has not been evaluated in well-controlled, double-blind prospective studies. Based on the lack of adequate clinical trials and the absence of immunological evidence, the vaccine cannot be recommended.

Topical therapies

The wide variety of topical therapies proposed in earlier literature has fallen into disuse because these treatments have unacceptable failure rates. Topical therapy should be reserved for clinical situations in which systemic nitroimidazole therapy is contraindicated. Several newer agents may be considered in this unusual situation.

A metronidazole gel preparation is now approved for topical treatment of bacterial vaginosis.[261] This preparation has not been evaluated for treatment of trichomoniasis. However, earlier preparations of metronidazole had low efficacy compared to systemic therapy.

Clotrimazole, an imidazole antifungal, kills *T. vaginalis* after 48 hours of exposure to 100mg/mL in vitro.[299] This level of activity against protozoa was at least 50-fold lower than against fungi. One hundred milligrams applied intravaginally for 6 days was reported to cure 48 to 66 percent of patients, as determined by culture.[300] When cure was defined as relief of symptoms and elimination of the organism from the wet mount, the same course cured 61 to 81 percent of women.[263,301] Unpublished experience[2] suggests a cure rate of about 25 percent, perhaps equal to spontaneous resolution. However, this treatment may have a role in relieving symptoms in the first trimester of pregnancy, when metronidazole is not recommended.

Nonoxynol-9 has antitrichomonal activity and in a single case report proved effective topically against a *T. vaginalis* strain that exhibited high-grade resistance to metronidazole.[302] This patient had failed therapy with prolonged high-dose oral and intravaginal metronidazole and therapy with tinidazole. This case and published laboratory data suggest that intravaginal nonoxynol-9 deserves further study as a treatment for resistant trichomoniasis. However, trichomonal coinfection of the urethra, Skene's glands, and paraurethral glands would not likely be resolved by such therapy.

Povodone-iodine douches proved useful for treating metronidazole-resistant *T. vaginalis* in one study.[303] However, this therapy should be avoided in pregnancy because increased serum levels of iodine may suppress fetal thyroid development.[304] D-propranolol may prove useful as a topical spermacide and has antitrichomonal activity in vitro,[305] although this agent has not been evaluated in clinical trials. In contrast, topical lactobacillus treatment was unsuccessful for treatment of two patients with metronidazole-resistant *T. vaginalis* infections.[306]

PREVENTION AND CONTROL

Control of *T. vaginalis* infection can only be achieved through accurate diagnosis and treatment of infected individuals and of all recent sexual partners. Follow-up should optimally include both cultures and patient education to achieve compliance with therapy. Diagnosis of *T. vaginalis* indicates the need for appropriate evaluation and testing for other STDs and for counseling to change behaviors that increase the risk for STD acquisition.

References

1 Quinn TC, Krieger JN: Trichomoniasis, in *Tropical and Geographic Medicine*, 2nd ed, KS Warren, AAF Mahmoud (eds). New York, McGraw-Hill, 1990, p 358.

2 Rein MF, Muller M: *Trichomonas vaginalis* and Trichomoniasis, in *Sexually Transmitted Diseases*, 2nd ed. KK Holmes et al (eds). New York, McGraw-Hill, 1990, p 480.

3 Rein MF, Chapel TA: Trichomoniasis, candidiasis, and the minor venereal diseases. *Clin Obstet Gynecol* 18:73, 1975.

4 Centers for Disease Control and Prevention, Division of STD Prevention: *Sexually Transmitted Disease Surveillance, 1995*. Atlanta, U.S. Department of Health and Human Services, Public Health Service, September, 1996.

5 Krieger JN et al: Risk assessment and laboratory diagnosis of trichomoniasis in men. *J Infect Dis* 166:1362, 1992.

6 Laga M et al: The interrelationship of sexually transmitted diseases and HIV infection: Implications for the control of both epidemics in Africa. *AIDS* 5:555, 1991.

7 Wasserheit JN: Epidemiological synergy: Interrelationships between human immunodeficiency virus infection and other sexually transmitted diseases. *Sex Transm Dis* 19:61, 1992.

8 Read JS, Klebanoff MA: Sexual intercourse during pregnancy and preterm delivery: Effects of vaginal microorganisms: The Vaginal Infections and Prematurity Study Group. *Am J Obstet Gynecol* 168: 514, 1993.

9 Cotch MF et al: Demographic and behavioral predictors of *Trichomonas vaginalis* infection among pregnant women. *Obstet Gynecol* 78:1087, 1991.

10 Cotch MF: Carriage of *Trichomonas vaginalis* is associated with adverse pregnancy outcome: The Vaginal Infections and Prematurity Study Group. Interscience Conference on Antimicrobial Agents and Chemotherapy. American Society for Microbiology, Atlanta, 1990, abstr 681.

11 Minkoff H et al: Risk factors for prematurity and premature rupture of membranes: A prospective study of the vaginal flora in pregnancy. *Am J Gynecol* 150:965, 1984.

12 Riley DE et al: *Trichomonas vaginalis*: Dominant G2 period and G2 phase arrest in a representative of an early branching eukaryotic lineage. *J Eukaryot Microbiol* 41:408, 1993.

13 Jirovec O, Petru M: *Trichomonas vaginalis* and trichomoniasis. *Adv Parasitol* 6:117, 1968.

14 Honigberg BM: *Trichomonads Parasitic in Humans*. London, Springer-Verlag, 1989, p. 424.

15 Diamond LS: The establishment of various trichomonads of animals and man in axenic cultures. *J Parasitol* 43:488, 1957.

16 Honigberg BM: Trichomonads of Importance in Human Medicine, in *Parasitic Protozoa* , JP Kreier (ed). New York, Academic Press, 1978, vol 2, p 275.

17 Hoffmann B et al: Studies on trichomoniasis in males. *Br J Vener Dis* 37:172, 1961.

18 Sylvestre L et al: Urogenital trichomoniasis in the male: Review of the literature and report on treatment of 37 patients by a new nitroimidazole derivative (Flagyl). *Can Med Assoc* 83:1195, 1960.

19 Catterall RD: Diagnosis and treatment of trichomonal urethritis in men. *Br Med J* 2:113, 1960.

20 Krieger JN: Urologic aspects of trichomoniasis. *Invest Urol* 18:411, 1981.

21 Alderete JF et al: The vagina of women infected with *Trichomonas vaginalis* has numerous proteinases and antibody to trichomonad proteinases. *Genitourin Med* 67:469, 1991.

22 Muller M: Energy metabolism of ancestral eukaryotes: A hypothesis based on the biochemistry of amitochondriate parasitic protists. *Biosystems* 28:33, 1992.

23 Johnson PJ et al: Molecular analysis of the hydrogenosomal ferredoxin of the anaerobic protist *Trichomonas vaginalis*. *Proc Natl Acad Sci USA* 87:6097, 1990.

24 Street DA et al: Interaction between *Trichomonas vaginalis* and other pathogenic microorganisms of the human genital tract. *Br J Vener Dis* 60:31, 1980.

25 Peterson KM, Alderete JF: Host plasma proteins on the surface of pathogenic *Trichomonas vaginalis*. *Infect Immun* 37:755, 1982.

26 Peterson KM, Alderete JF: Selective acquisition of plasma proteins by *Trichomonas vaginalis* and human lipoproteins as a growth requirement for this species. *Molec Biochem Parasitol* 12:37, 1984.

27 Peterson K, Alderete JF: *Trichomonas vaginalis* is dependent on uptake and degradation of human low density lipoproteins. *J Exper Med* 160:1261, 1984.

28 Peterson K, Alderete JF: Acquisition of alpha 1-antitrypsin by a pathogenic strain of *Trichomonas vaginalis*. *Infect Immun* 40:640, 1983.

29 Peterson K, Alderete JF: Iron uptake and increased intracellular enzyme activity follow lactoferrin binding by *Trichomonas vaginalis* receptors. *J Exper Med* 160:398, 1984.

30 Lehker M, Alderete JF: Iron regulates growth of *Trichomonas vaginalis* and the expression of immunogenic proteins. *Molec Microbiol* 6:123, 1992.

31 Lehker M et al: The regulation by iron of the synthesis of adhesins and cytoadherence levels in the protozoan *Trichomonas vaginalis*. *J Exper Med* 174:311, 1991.

32 Alderete JF et al: Cloning and molecular characterization of two AP65 genes and adhesin proteins involved in *Trichomonas vaginalis* cytoadherence. *Molec Microbiol* 17:69, 1995.

33 Krieger JN et al: Beta-hemolytic activity of *Trichomonas vaginalis* correlates with virulence. *Infect Immun* 41:1291, 1983.

34 Proctor EM et al: Isoenzyme patterns of isolates of *Trichomonas vaginalis* from Vancouver. *Sex Transm Dis* 15:181, 1988.

35 Vohra H et al: Correlation of zymodeme patterns, virulence, and drug sensitivity of *Trichomonas vaginalis* isolates from women. *Indian J Med Res* 93:37, 1991.

36 Hess J: Review of current methods for the detection of *Trichomonas* in clinical material. *J Clin Pathol* 22:269, 1969.

37 Lehker M, Alderete JF: Properties of *Trichomonas vaginalis* grown under chemostat controlled growth conditions. *Genitourin Med* 66: 193, 1990.

38 Rein MF: *Trichomonas vaginalis,* in *Principles and Practice of Infectious Diseases*, 3rd ed. GL Mandell et al (eds). New York, Churchill-Livingstone, 1990, p 2115.

39 Spiegel CA: Vaginitis/vaginosis. *Clin Lab Med* 9:525, 1989.

40 Winston RM: The relation between size and pathogenicity of *Trichomonas vaginalis*. *J Obstet Gynaecol Br Commonw* 81:399, 1974.

41 Juliano C et al: In vitro phagocytic interaction between *Trichomonas vaginalis* isolates and bacteria. *Eur J Clin Microbiol Infect Dis* 10: 497, 1991.

42 Francioli P et al: Phagocytosis and killing of *Neisseria gonorrhoeae* by *Trichomonas vaginalis*. *J Infect Dis* 147:87, 1983.

43 Street DA et al: Interaction between *Trichomonas vaginalis* and other pathogenic micro-organisms of the human genital tract. *Br J Vener Dis* 60:31, 1984.

44 Provenzano D, Alderete JF: Analysis of human immunoglobulin-degrading cysteine proteinases of *Trichomonas vaginalis*. *Infect Immun* 63:3388–3395, 1995.

45 Coombs GH, North MJ: An analysis of the proteinases of *Trichomonas vaginalis* by polyacrylamide gel electrophoresis. *Parasitol* 86: 1, 1983.

46 Neale KA, Alderete JF: Analysis of the proteinases of representative *Trichomonas vaginalis* isolates. *Infect Immun* 58:157, 1990.

47 Bozner P et al: Proteinases of *Trichomonas vaginalis*: Antibody response in patients with urogenital trichomoniasis. *Parasitol* 105:387, 1992.

48 Lehker ML et al: Specific erythrocyte binding is an additional nutrient acquisition system for *Trichomonas vaginalis*. *J Exp Med* 171:2132, 1990.

49 Dailey DC et al: Characterization of *Trichomonas vaginalis* haemolysis. *Parasitol* 101:171, 1990.

50 Wang A et al: *Trichomonas vaginalis* phenotypic variation occurs only among trichomonads infected with the double-stranded RNA virus. *J Exp Med* 166:142, 1987.

51 Tai JH et al: The divergence of *Trichomonas vaginalis* virus RNAs among various isolates of *Trichomonas vaginalis*. *Exp Parasitol* 76: 278, 1993.

52 Khoshnan A, Alderete JF: *Trichomonas vaginalis* with a double-stranded RNA virus has upregulated levels of phenotypically variable immunogen mRNA. *J Virol* 68:4035, 1994.

53 Flegr J et al: The dsRNA of *Trichomonas vaginalis* is associated with virus-like particles and does not correlate with metronidazole resistance. *Folia Microbiol Praha* 32:345, 1987.

54 Khoshnan MA, Alderete JF: Multiple double-stranded RNA segments are associated with virus particles infecting *Trichomonas vaginalis*. *J Virol* 67:6950, 1993.

55 Khoshnan A et al: Unique double-stranded RNAs associated with the *Trichomonas vaginalis* virus are synthesized by viral RNA-dependent RNA polymerase. *J Virol* 68:7108, 1994.

56 Burch TA et al: Epidemiological studies on human trichomoniasis. *Am J Trop Med Hyg* 8:312, 1959.

57 Catterall RD, Nicol CS: Is trichomonal infestation a venereal disease? *Br Med J* 1:1177, 1960.

58 Lancely F: *Trichomonas vaginalis* infections in the male. *Br J Vener Dis* 29:213, 1953.

59 Trussell RE: *Trichomonas vaginalis and Trichomoniasis*. Springfield IL, Charles C. Thomas, 1947.

60 Wisdom AR, Dunlop EMC: Trichomoniasis: Study of its treatment in women: I. The disease and its treatment in women. *Br J Vener Dis* 41:90, 1965.

61 Willcox RR: Epidemiological aspects of human trichomoniasis. *Br J Vener Dis* 36:167, 1960.

62 Fouts AC, Kraus SJ: *Trichomonas vaginalis*: Reevaluation of its clinical presentation and laboratory diagnosis. *J Infect Dis* 141:137, 1980.

63 Rein MF, Holmes KK: Nonspecific Vaginitis, Vulvovaginal Candidiasis, and Trichomoniasis: Clinical Features, Diagnosis, and Management, in *Current Clinical Topics in Infectious Diseases*, JS Remington, MN Swartz (eds). New York, McGraw-Hill, 1983, p 281.

64 Short SL et al: Comparative rates of sexually transmitted diseases among heterosexual men, homosexual men, and heterosexual women. *Sex Transm Dis* 11:271, 1984.

65 al Salihi FL et al: Neonatal *Trichomonas vaginalis*: Report of three cases and review of the literature. *Pediatrics* 53:196, 1980.

66 Robinson SC, Halifax NS: Observations on vaginal trichomoniasis: I. In pregnancy. *Can Med Assoc J* 84:948, 1961.

67 Krieger JN: Trichomoniasis in men: Old issues and new data. *Sex Transm Dis* 22:83, 1995.

68 Wølner-Hanssen P et al: Clinical manifestations of vaginal trichomoniasis. *JAMA* 261:571, 1989.

69 Krieger JN et al: Diagnosis of trichomoniasis: Comparison of conventional wet-mount examination with cytologic studies, cultures, and monoclonal antibody staining of direct specimens. *JAMA* 259: 1223, 1988.

70 Kaneda Y et al: Effects of berberine, a plant alkaloid, on the growth of anaerobic protozoa in axenic culture. *Tokai J Exp Clin Med* 15: 417, 1990.

71 Krieger JN et al: Natural history of urogenital trichomoniasis in men. *J Urol* 149:1455, 1993.

72 Gardner J et al: *Trichomonas vaginalis* in the prostate gland. *Arch Pathol Lab Med* 110:430, 1986.

73 Fisher I, Morton RS: Epididymitis due to *Trichomonas vaginalis*. *Br J Vener Dis* 45:252, 1969.

74 Rajasekariah GR et al: A simple micropore system for experimental studies on trichomonad parasites. *J Parasitol* 75:997, 1989.

75 Whittington MJ: Epidemiology of infections with *Trichomonas vaginalis* in the light of improved diagnostic methods. *Br J Vener Dis* 33: 80, 1957.

76 Watt L, Jennison RF: Incidence of *Trichomonas vaginalis* in marital partners. *Br J Vener Dis* 36:163, 1960.

77 Weston TE, Nicol CS: Natural history of trichomonal infection in males. *Br J Vener Dis* 39:251, 1963.

78 Kostic P: Importance de l'étude de trichomonas chez l'homme. *Urologic Internationale* 9:171, 1959.

79 Scharpia HE: Studies on metronidazole (Flagyl) in the therapy of urogenital trichomoniasis in the male patient. *J Urol* 93:303, 1965.

80 Ackers JP et al: Absence of detectable local antibody in genitourinary tract secretions of male contacts of women infected with *Trichomonas vaginalis*. *Br J Vener Dis* 54:168, 1978.

81 Hofmann B, Malyszko E: Investigation of *Trichomonas vaginalis*: Incidence among inhabitants of Bialystok county using different laboratory methods. *Wiadomosci Parazytologi* 15:355, 1969.

82 Wilson A, Ackers JP: Urine cultures for the detection of *Trichomonas vaginalis* in men. *Br J Vener Dis* 56:46, 1980.

83 Krieger JN et al: Clinical manifestations of trichomoniasis in men. *Ann Intern Med* 118:844, 1993.

84 Hesseltine HC: Experimental human vaginal trichomoniasis. *J Infect Dis* 71:127, 1942.

85 Lancely F, McEntegart MG: *Trichomonas vaginalis* in the male: The experimental infections of a few volunteers. *Lancet* 1:668, 1953.

86 Feo LG: *Trichomonas vaginalis* infection in post-menopausal women. *Am J Obstet Gynecol* 72:1335, 1956.

87 Farooki MA, Sethi N: Genital trichomoniasis in 156 leukorrhoeic patients in Peshawar. *Medicus* 29:248, 1965.

88 Nagesha CN et al: Clinical and laboratory studies on vaginal trichomoniasis. *Am J Obstet Gynecol* 106:933, 1970.

89 Soszka S et al: Incidence of trichomoniasis in women from the Bialystok Province. *Wiadomosci Parazytologi* 19:275, 1973.

90 Kean BH: Urethral trichomoniasis in the female: A possible common denominator in recurrent *Trichomonas vaginalis* vaginitis and recurrent bacterial cystitis. *Am J Obstet Gynecol* 70:397, 1955.

91 Herbst S et al: Prevalence of *Trichomonas vaginalis* among female prison inmates and indigent prenatal patients in the Detroit area. *J Parasitol* 46:743, 1960.

92 Jusinska-Dubiel C et al: Vaginal trichomoniasis in women with gynecological diseases as seen in the material from the first obstetric and gynecologic clinic in Bialystok during the years 1969–1971. *Wiadomosci Parazytologi* 19:291, 1973.

93 Basaca-Sevilla V et al: Prevalence of *Trichomonas vaginalis* in some Filipino women. *S Asian J Trop Med Pub Hlth* 17:194, 1986.

94 O'Farrell N et al: Sexually transmitted pathogens in pregnant women in a rural South African community. *Genitourin Med* 65:276, 1989.

95 Avonts D et al: Sexually transmitted diseases and *Chlamydia trachomatis* in women consulting for contraception. *J R Coll Gen Pract* 39: 418, 1989.

96 Ogbonna CI et al: Studies on the incidence of *Trichomonas vaginalis* amongst pregnant women in Jos area of Plateau State, Nigeria. *Angew Parasitol* 32:198, 1991.

97 Bergreen O: Association of carcinoma of the uterine cervix and *Trichomonas vaginalis* infections: Frequency of *Trichomonas vaginalis* in preinvasive and invasive cervical carcinoma. *Am J Obstet Gynecol* 105:166, 1969.

98 Naguib SM et al: Epidemiologic study of trichomoniasis in normal women. *Obstet Gynecol* 27:607, 1966.

99 Konje JC et al: The prevalence of *Gardnerella vaginalis*, *Trichomonas vaginalis*, and *Candida albicans* in the cytology clinic at Ibadan, Nigeria. *Afr J Med Sci* 20:29, 1991.

100 Sardana S et al: Epidemiologic analysis of *Trichomonas vaginalis* infection in inflammatory smears. *Acta Cytol* 38:693, 1994.

101 Kawamura N: Studies on *Trichomonas vaginalis* in the urological field: VI. Clinical efficacy of various drugs. *Jpn J Urol* 64:281, 1973.

102 Grys E: Several years of observation of the incidence of *Trichomonas vaginalis* infections among female workers in a single industrial plant. *Wiadomosci Parazytologi* 36:201, 1990.

103 Anosike JC et al: Trichomoniasis amongst students of a higher institution in Nigeria. *Appl Parasitol* 34:19, 1993.

104 Mascall N: Some reflections on the *Trichomonas vaginalis*. *Br J Vener Dis* 30:156, 1954.

105 Wisdom AR, Dunlop EMC: Trichomoniasis: Study of the disease and its treatment: II. The disease and its treatment in men. *Br J Vener Dis* 41:93, 1965.

106 Kuberski T: Evaluation of the indirect technique for study of *Trichomonas vaginalis* infections, particularly in men. *Sex Transm Dis* 5: 97, 1978.

107 Alderete JF et al: Antibody in sera of patients infected with *Trichomonas vaginalis* is to trichomonad proteinases. *Genitourin Med* 67: 331, 1991.

108 Pereira LH et al: Cytomegalovirus infection among women attending a sexually transmitted disease clinic: Association with clinical symptoms and other sexually transmitted diseases. *Am J Epidemiol* 131: 683, 1990.

109 Iyer SV et al: Microbiological evaluation of female patients in STD clinics. *Indian J Med Res* 93:95, 1991.

110 Lefevre JC et al: Lower genital tract infections in women: Comparison of clinical and epidemiologic findings with microbiology. *Sex Transm Dis* 15:110, 1988.

111 Lim KB et al: Endocervical chlamydial infection in women attending a sexually transmitted disease clinic in Singapore. *Singapore Med J* 30:167, 1989.

112 Nayyar KC et al: Prevalence of genital pathogens among female prostitutes in New York City and in Rotterdam. *Sex Transm Dis* 13:105, 1986.

113 Damiba AE et al: Prevalence of gonorrhoea, syphilis, and trichomoniasis in prostitutes in Burkina Faso. *East Afr Med J* 67:473, 1990.
114 Vazquez F et al: Gonorrhea in women prostitutes: Clinical data and auxotypes, serovars, plasmid contents of PPNG, and susceptibility profiles. *Sex Transm Dis* 18:5, 1991.
115 Pereyra JA, Lansing JD: Urogenital trichomoniasis: Treatment with metronidazole in 20,002 incarcerated women. *Obstet Gynecol* 24: 499, 1964.
116 Ris HW, Dodge RW: Trichomoniasis and yeast vaginitis in institutionalized adolescent girls. *Am J Dis Child* 125:206, 1973.
117 Davies AG, Clay JC: Prevalence of sexually transmitted disease infection in women alleging rape. *Sex Transm Dis* 19:298, 1992.
118 Jenny C et al: Sexually transmitted diseases in victims of rape. *N Engl J Med* 322:713, 1990.
119 Estreich S et al: Sexually transmitted diseases in rape victims. *Genitourin Med* 66:433, 1990.
120 Shafer MA et al: Evaluation of fluorescein-conjugated monoclonal antibody test to detect *Chlamydia trachomatis* endocervical infections in adolescent girls. *J Pediatr* 108:779–783, 1986.
121 Oh MK et al: Sexually transmitted diseases and sexual behavior in urban adolescent females attending a family planning clinic. *J Adolesc Hlth Care* 9:67, 1988.
122 Mulcahy FM, Lacey CJ: Sexually transmitted infections in adolescent girls. *Genitourin Med* 63:119, 1987.
123 Perl G: Errors in the diagnosis of *Trichomonas vaginalis* infection. *Obstet Gynocol* 39:7, 1972.
124 Omer EF et al: Evaluation of the laboratory diagnosis of vaginal trichomoniasis in Khartoum. *J Trop Med Hyg* 91:292, 1988.
125 Poria VC et al: Study of candida and *Trichomonas vaginalis* in leucorrhoea. *J Indian Med Assoc* 87:184, 1989.
126 Bennett JR et al: The emergency department diagnosis of *Trichomonas* vaginitis. *Ann Emerg Med* 18:564, 1989.
127 Feo LG et al: *Trichomonas vaginalis* in urethritis of the male. *Br J Vener Dis* 32:233, 1956.
128 Butler WJ et al: Trichomoniasis: A male urethritis. In preparation.
129 Latif AS et al: Urethral trichomoniasis in men. *Sex Trans Dis* 14:9, 1987.
130 Hernanz JM et al: Urethritis caused by *Trichomonas vaginalis* in men: Epidemiology. *Medicina Cutanea Ibero-Latino-Americana* 15:213, 1987.
131 Pillay DG et al: Diagnosis of *Trichomonas vaginalis* in male urethritis. *Trop Geogr Med* 46:44, 1994.
132 Kawamura N: Studies on *Trichomonas vaginalis* in the urological field. Parts I-V. *Jpn J Urol* 60:15, 1969.
133 Saxena SB, Jenkins RR: Prevalence of *Trichomonas vaginalis* in men at high risk for sexually transmitted diseases. *Sex Transm Dis* 18: 138, 1991.
134 Coutts WE et al: Genitourinary complications of non-gonococcal urethritis and trichomoniasis in males. *Urol Int* 9:189, 1959.
135 Holmes KK et al: Etiology of nongonococcal urethritis. *N Engl J Med* 292:1199, 1975.
136 Durel P et al: Nongonococcal urethritis. *Br J Vener Dis* 30:69, 1954.
137 Lefevre JC et al: Clinical and microbiologic features of urethritis in men in Toulouse, France. *Sex Transm Dis* 18:76, 1991.
138 Jira J: Zur Kenntnis der männlichen Trichomoniase. *Zentralbl Bakteriol Parasitenkd Infektionskr Hyg (A)* 172:310, 1958.
139 Kuberski T: *Trichomonas vaginalis* associated with nongonococcal urethritis and prostatitis. *Sex Transm Dis* 7:135, 1980.
140 Kimura S: Studies on *Trichomonas vaginalis* in urological patients. *Jpn J Urol* 56:455, 1966.
141 Verges J: Les prostatites a trichomonas formes rondés (T.F.R.). *J Urol Nephrol* 85:357, 1979.
142 Ohmura K: Studies on the *T. vaginalis* infection in male genitourinary tracts. *Jpn J Parasitol* 9:510, 1960.
143 Summers JL, Ford ML: The Papanicolaou smear as a diagnostic tool in male trichomoniasis. *J Urol* 107:840, 1972.
144 Hager WD et al: Metronidazole for vaginal trichomoniasis: Seven day vs. single dose regimens. *JAMA* 244:846, 1980.
145 Singh BN: Lipophosphoglycan-like glycoconjugate of *Tritrichomonas foetus* and *Trichomonas foetus*. *Molec Biochem Parasitol* 57: 281, 1993.
146 Alderete JF: Antigenic analysis of several pathogenic strains of *Trichomonas vaginalis*. *Infect Immun* 39:1041, 1983.
147 Alderete JF et al: *Trichomonas vaginalis*: Electrophoretic analysis reveals heterogeneity among isolates due to high molecular weight trichomonad proteins. *Exper Parasitol* 61:244, 1986.
148 Alderete JF: Identification of immunogenic and antibody binding proteins on the membrane of pathogenic *Trichomonas vaginalis*. *Infect Immun* 40:84, 1983.
149 Alderete JF et al: Heterogeneity of *Trichomonas vaginalis* and discrimination among trichomonal isolates and subpopulations by sera of patients and experimentally infected mice. *Infect Immun* 49:463, 1985.
150 Alderete JF: *Trichomonas vaginalis* phenotypic variation may be coordinated for a repertoire of trichomonad surface immunogens. *Infect Immun* 55:1957, 1987.
151 Alderete JF, Neale KA: Relatedness of structures of a major immunogen in *Trichomonas vaginalis* isolates. *Infect Immun* 56:1849, 1989.
152 Alderete JF et al: Monoclonal antibody to a major surface immunogen differentiates isolates and subpopulations of *Trichomonas vaginalis*. *Infect Immun* 52:70, 1986.
153 Alderete JF et al: Phenotypic variation and diversity among *Trichomonas vaginalis* and correlation of phenotype with contact dependent host cell cytotoxicity. *Infect Immun* 53:285, 1986.
154 Alderete JF: Alternating phenotypic expression of two classes of *Trichomonas vaginalis* surface markers. *Rev Infect Dis* 10:S408, 1988.
155 Alderete JF et al: Phenotypes and protein-epitope phenotypic variation among fresh isolates of *Trichomonas vaginalis*. *Infect Immun* 55:1037, 1987.
156 Alderete JF, Kasmala L: Monoclonal antibody to a major glycoprotein immunogen mediates differential complement independent lysis of *Trichomonas vaginalis*. *Infect Immun* 53:697, 1986.
157 Dailey DC, Alderete JF: The phenotypically variable surface protein of *Trichomonas vaginalis* has a single, tandemly repeated immunodominant epitope. *Infect Immun* 59:2083, 1991.
158 Krieger JN et al: Geographic variation among *Trichomonas vaginalis*: Demonstration of antigenic heterogeneity using monoclonal antibodies and the indirect immunofluorescence technique. *J Infect Dis* 152: 979, 1985.
159 Alderete JF et al: Iron mediates *Trichomonas vaginalis* resistance to complement lysis. *Microb Pathol* 19:93–103, 1995.
160 Krieger JN et al: Characteristics of *Trichomonas vaginalis* isolates from women with and without colpitis macularis. *J Infect Dis* 161: 307, 1990.
161 Mason PR, Forman L: Polymorphonuclear cell chemotaxis to secretions of pathogenic and nonpathogenic *Trichomonas vaginalis*. *J Parasitol* 68:457, 1982.
162 Shaio MF et al: A novel neutrophil-activating factor released by *Trichomonas vaginalis*. *Infect Immun* 60:4475, 1992.
163 Rein MF et al: Trichomonacidal activity of human polymorphonuclear neutrophils: Killing by disruption and fragmentation. *J Infect Dis* 142:575, 1980.
164 Landolfo S et al: Natural cell-mediated cytotoxicity against *Trichomonas vaginalis* in the mouse: I. Tissue, strain, age distribution, and some characteristics of the effector cells. *Dev Comp Immunol* 4:11, 1980.
165 Martinotti MG et al: Role of cytoskeleton in natural cell-mediated cytotoxicity against *Trichomonas vaginalis*. *Microbiol* 5:389, 1982.
166 Gillin F, Sher H: Activation of the alternative complement pathway by *Trichomonas vaginalis*. *Infect Immun* 34:268, 1981.
167 Holbrook TW et al: *Trichomonas vaginalis*: alternative pathway activation of complement. *Trans R Soc Trop Med Hyg* 76:473, 1982.
168 Demes P et al: Fewer *Trichomonas vaginalis* organisms in vaginas of infected women during menstruation. *Genitourin Med* 64:22, 1988.
169 Demes P et al: Differential susceptibility of fresh *Trichomonas vaginalis* isolates to complement in menstrual blood and cervical mucus. *Genitourin Med* 64:176, 1988.

170 Jaakmees HP et al: Complement fixing antibodies in the blood sera of men infested with *Trichomonas vaginalis*. *Wiadomosci Parazytologi* 12:378, 1966.
171 Schumacher GFB et al: Immunoglobulins, proteinase inhibitors, albumin, and lysozyme in human cervical mucus. *Am J Obstet Gynecol* 129:629, 1977.
172 Cohen MS et al: Preliminary observation on lactoferrin secretion in human vaginal mucus: Variation during the menstrual cycle, evidence of hormonal regulation, and implications for infection with *Neisseria gonorrhoeae*. *Am J Obstet Gynecol* 157:1122, 1987.
173 Huggins GR, Preti G: Vaginal odors and secretions. *Clin Obstet Gynecol* 24:355, 1981.
174 Joiner KA: Complement evasion by bacteria and parasites. *Ann Rev Microbiol* 42:201, 1988.
175 Garber GE, Lemchuck-Favel LT: Characterization of extracellular protease of *Trichomonas vaginalis*. *Can J Microbiol* 35:903, 1989.
176 Lockwood BC et al: The release of hydrolases from *Trichomonas vaginalis* and *Tritrichomonas foetus*. *Molec Biochem Parasitol* 30: 135, 1988.
177 Ackers JP et al: Anti-trichomonal antibody in the vaginal secretions of women infected with *T. vaginalis*. *Br J Vener Dis* 51:319, 1975.
178 Sharma P et al: Anti-trichomonad IgA antibodies in trichomoniasis before and after treatment. *Folia Microbiol* 36:302, 1991.
179 Alderete JF et al: Vaginal antibody of patients with trichomoniasis is to a prominent surface immunogen of *Trichomonas vaginalis*. *Genitourin Med* 67:220, 1991.
180 Wos SM, Watt RM: Immunoglobulin subtypes of anti-*Trichomonas vaginalis* antibodies in patients with vaginal trichomoniasis. *J Clin Microbiol* 24:790, 1986.
181 Sayed FE, Bazex J: Chronic perianal ulcerations: Role of *Trichomonas vaginalis*? *Genitourin Med* 69:483, 1993.
182 Rein MF: Vulvovaginitis and Cervicitis, in *Principles and Practice of Infectious Diseases*, GL Mandell et al (eds). New York, John Wiley, 1985, p 729.
182a Pabst KM et al: Disease prevalence among women attending a sexually transmitted disease clinic varies with reason for visit. *Sex Transm Dis*19:88, 1992.
183 Hoosen AA et al: Sexually transmitted pathogens in acute pelvic inflammatory disease. *S Afr Med J* 76:251, 1989.
184 Hammond TL et al: Transvaginal-peritoneal migration of *Trichomonas vaginalis* as a cause of ascites: A report of two cases. *J Reprod Med* 35:179, 1990.
185 Heine P, McGregor JA: *Trichomonas vaginalis*: A reemerging pathogen. *Clin Obstet Gynecol* 36:137, 1993.
186 World Health Organization: Nongonococcal Urethritis and Other Sexually Transmitted Diseases. Geneva, WHO Technical and Reproductive Services, 1981.
187 Drummond AC: Trichomonas infestation of the prostate gland. *Am J Surg* 31:98, 1936.
188 Kawamura N: Trichomoniasis of the prostate. *Jpn J Clin Urol* 27: 335, 1973.
189 Gallai Z, Sylvestre L: The present status of urogenital trichomoniasis: A general review of the literature. *Appl Ther* 8:773, 1966.
190 Kurnatowska A et al: Rare cases of prostatitis caused by invasion of *Trichomonas vaginalis* with *Candida albicans*. *Wiadomosci Parazytologi* 36:229, 1990.
191 Fullilove REJ: *Trichomonas vaginalis* in men. *J Med Soc NJ* 80:94, 1983.
192 Soendjojo A, Pindha S: *Trichomonas vaginalis* infection of the median raphe of the penis. *Sex Transm Dis* 8:255, 1981.
193 Sowmini N et al: Infections of the median raphe of the penis: Report of three cases. *Br J Vener Dis* 49:469, 1972.
194 Pavithran K: Trichomonal abscess of the median raphe of the penis. *Int J Dermatol* 32:820, 1993.
195 Riba LW, Harrison RM: Strictures of the male urethra and *Trichomonas vaginalis*. *Surg Gynecol Obstet* 71:369, 1940.
196 Liston WG, Lees R: *Trichomonas vaginalis* infestation in male subjects. *Br J Vener Dis* 16:34, 1940.
197 Amar AD: Probable *Trichomonas vaginalis* epididymitis. *JAMA* 206: 417, 1967.
198 Krieger JN: Epididymitis, orchitis, and related conditions. *Sex Transm Dis* 11:173, 1984.
199 Bar CN, Fisch H: Infection and pyospermia in male infertility. *World J Urol* 11:76, 1993.
200 Tuttle JPJ et al: Interference of human spermatozoal motility by *Trichomonas vaginalis*. *J Urol* 118:1024, 1977.
201 Gopalkrishnan K et al: Semen characteristics of asymptomatic males affected by *Trichomonas vaginalis*. *J In Vitro Fert Embryo Transf* 7: 132b, 1990.
202 Assami K, Nakamura M: Experimental inoculation of bacteria-free *Trichomonas vaginalis* into human vaginae and its effect on the glycogen content of vaginal epithelia. *Am J Trop Med Hyg* 4:254, 1955.
203 McGrory T et al: The interaction of *Lactobacillus acidophilus* and *Trichomonas vaginalis* in vitro. *J Parasitol* 80:50, 1994.
204 McGrory T, Garber GE: Mouse intravaginal infection with *Trichomonas vaginalis* and role of *Lactobacillus acidophilus* in sustaining infection. *Infect Immun* 60:2375, 1992.
205 Street DA et al: Infection of female squirrel monkeys (*Saimiri sciureus*) with *Trichomonas vaginalis* as a model of trichomoniasis in women. *Br J Vener Dis* 59:249, 1984.
206 Krieger JN et al: Contact-dependent cytopathogenic mechanisms of *Trichomonas vaginalis*. *Infect Immun* 50:778, 1985.
207 Alderete JF, Pearlman E: Pathogenic *Trichomonas vaginalis* cytotoxicity to cell culture monolayers. *Br J Vener Dis* 60:99, 1984.
208 Arroyo R et al: Molecular basis of host epithelial cell recognition by *Trichomonas vaginalis*. *Molec Microbiol* 6:853, 1992.
209 Alderete JF et al: Specific parasitism by *Trichomonas vaginalis* of purified vaginal epithelial cells. *Infect Immun* 56:2558, 1988.
210 Arroyo R, Alderete JF: *Trichomonas vaginalis* surface proteinase activity is necessary for parasite adherence to epithelial cells. *Infect Immun* 57:2991, 1989.
211 Arroyo R, Alderete JF: Two *Trichomonas vaginalis* surface proteinases bind to host cells and are related to levels of cytoadherence and cytotoxicity. *Arch Med Res* 26:279–285, 1995.
212 Arroyo R et al: Signalling of *Trichomonas vaginalis* for amoeboid transformation and adhesion synthesis follows cytoadherence. *Molec Microbiol* 7:299, 1993.
213 Potamianos S et al: Lysis of erythrocytes by *Trichomonas vaginalis*. *Biosci Rep* 12:387, 1992.
214 Beach DH et al: Fatty acid and sterol metabolism of cultured *Trichomonas vaginalis* and *Tritrichomonas foetus*. *Molec Biochem Parasitol* 38:175, 1990.
215 Beach DH et al: Phospholipid metabolism of cultured *Trichomonas vaginalis* and *Tritrichomonas foetus*. *Molec Biochem Parasitol* 44: 97, 1991.
216 Garber GE et al: Isolation of a cell-detaching factor of *Trichomonas vaginalis*. *J Clin Microbiol* 27:1548, 1989.
217 Pindak FF et al: Contact-independent cytotoxicity of *Trichomonas vaginalis*. *Genitourin Med* 69:35, 1993.
218 Garber GE, Lemchuk-Favel LT: Characterization and purification of extracellular proteases of *Trichomonas vaginalis*. *Can J Microbiol* 35: 903, 1989.
219 Garber GE, Lemchuk-Favel LT: Association of production of cell-detaching factor with the clinical presentation of *Trichomonas vaginalis*. *J Clin Microbiol* 28:2415, 1990.
220 Tachezy J et al: Aerobic resistance of *Trichomonas vaginalis* to metronidazole induced in vitro. *Parasitology* 106:31, 1993.
221 Kiviat NB et al: Histopathology of endocervical infection caused by *Chlamydia trachomatis*, herpes simplex virus, *Trichomonas vaginalis*, and *Neisseria gonorrhoeae*. *Hum Pathol* 21:831, 1990.
222 Koss LG, Wolinska WH: *Trichomonas vaginalis* cervicitis and its relationship to cervical cancer. *Cancer* 12:1171, 1959.
223 Bertini B, Hornstein M: The epidemiology of trichomoniasis and the role of this infection in the development of carcinoma of the cervix. *Acta Cytol* 14:325, 1970.
224 Guijon FB et al: The association of sexually transmitted diseases with

cervical intraepithelial neoplasia: A case-control study. *Obstet Gynecol* 151:185, 1985.

225 Gram IT et al: *Trichomonas vaginalis* (TV) and human papillomavirus (HPV) infection and the incidence of cervical intraepithelial neoplasia (CIN) grade III. *Cancer Causes Control* 3:231, 1992.

226 Zhang ZF, Begg CB: Is *Trichomonas vaginalis* a cause of cervical neoplasia? Results from a combined analysis of 24 studies. *Intl J Epid* 23:682, 1994.

227 Krieger J, Rein M: Zinc-sensitivity of *Trichomonas vaginalis*: In vitro studies and clinical implications. *J Infect Dis* 146:341, 1982.

228 Krieger J, Rein M: Canine prostatic secretions kill *Trichomonas vaginalis*. *Infect Immun* 37:77, 1982.

229 Krieger J: Clinical Manifestations and Epidemiology of Urogenital Trichomoniasis in Me, in *Trichomonads Parasitic in Humans*, B Honigberg (ed). New York, Springer-Verlag 1989, p 235.

230 James JA et al: Is trichomoniasis often associated with bacterial vaginosis in pregnant adolescents? *Am J Obstet Gynecol* 166:859, 1992.

231 Hillier SL et al: Characteristics of three vaginal flora patterns assessed by Gram stain among pregnant women. Vaginal Infections and Prematurity Study Group. *Am J Obstet Gynecol* 166:938, 1992.

232 Rothenberg RB et al: Efficacy of selected diagnostic tests for sexually transmitted diseases. *JAMA* 235:49, 1976.

233 Fleury FJ: Diagnosis of *Trichomonas vaginalis* infection. *JAMA* 242: 2556, 1979.

234 Watt RM et al: Rapid assay for immunological detection of *Trichomonas vaginalis*. *J Clin Microbiol* 24:551, 1986.

235 Ridge AG: A rapid method for detection of *Trichomonas vaginalis*. *Med Lab Sci* 39:193, 1982.

236 Greenwood JR, Kirk-Hillaire K: Evaluation of acridine orange stain for detection of *Trichomonas vaginalis* in vaginal specimens. *Clin Micro* 14:199, 1981.

237 Martinez-Rodriguez HA et al: Adequate staining of *Trichomonas vaginalis* by McManus' periodic acid-Schiff stain. *Am J Clin Pathol* 59:741, 1973.

238 Bennett BD et al: Immunocytochemical identification of trichomonads. *Arch Pathol Lab Med* 104:247, 1980.

239 Nielsen R: *Trichomonas vaginalis*: II. Laboratory investigations in trichomoniasis. *Br J Vener Dis* 49:531, 1973.

240 Thomason JL et al: Comparison of four methods to detect *Trichomonas vaginalis*. *J Clin Microbiol* 26:1869, 1988.

241 Bickley LS et al: Comparison of direct fluorescent antibody, acridine orange, wet mount, and culture for detection of *Trichomonas vaginalis* in women attending a public sexually transmitted diseases clinic. *Sex Transm Dis* 16:127, 1989.

242 Weinberger MW, Harger JH: Accuracy of the Papanicolaou smear in the diagnosis of asymptomatic infection with *Trichomonas vaginalis*. *Obstet Gynecol* 82:425, 1993.

242a Spence MR et al: The clinical and laboratory diagnosis of *Trichomonas vaginalis* infection. *Sex Transm Dis* 7:168, 1980.

243 Bertolino JG et al: Inflammation on the cervical Papanicolaou smear: The predictive value for infection in asymptomatic women. *Fam Med* 24:447, 1992.

244 Chang TH et al: Monoclonal antibodies against *Trichomonas vaginalis*. *Hybridoma* 5:43, 1986.

245 Philip A et al: An agar culture technique to quantitate *Trichomonas vaginalis* from women. *J Infect Dis* 155:304, 1987.

246 Schmid GP et al: Evaluation of six media for the growth of *Trichomonas vaginalis* from vaginal secretions. *J Clin Microbiol* 27:1230, 1989.

247 Gelbart SM et al: Growth of *Trichomonas vaginalis* in commercial culture media. *J Clin Microbiol* 28:962, 1990.

248 Borchardt KA, Smith RF: An evaluation of an InPouchTM TV culture method for diagnosing *Trichomonas vaginalis* infection. *Genitourin Med* 67:149, 1991.

249 Mathews HM et al: Human serologic response to subcellular antigens of *Trichomonas vaginalis*. *J Parasitol* 73:601, 1987.

250 Matthews HM, Healy GR: Evaluation of two serological tests for *Trichomonas vaginalis* infection. *Clin Micro* 17:840, 1982.

251 Yule A et al: Detection of *Trichomonas vaginalis* antigen in women by enzyme immunoassay. *J Clin Pathol* 40:566, 1987.

252 Satapathy G et al: Trichomonal vaginitis: Evaluation of serological tests and identification of immunoreactive surface peptides. *Genitourin Med* 64:110, 1988.

253 Sibau L et al: Enzyme-linked immunosorbent assay for the diagnosis of trichomoniasis in women. *Sex Transm Dis* 14:216, 1987.

254 Sharma P et al: A comparison of wet mount, culture, and enzyme linked immunosorbent assay for the diagnosis of trichomoniasis in women. *Trop Geogr Med* 43:257, 1991.

255 Gombosova A, Valent M: Dot-immunobinding assay with monoclonal antibody for detection of *Trichomonas vaginalis* in clinical specimens. *Genitourin Med* 66:447, 1990.

256 Briselden AM, Hillier SL: Evaluation of affirm VP Microbial Identification Test for *Gardnerella vaginalis* and *Trichomonas vaginalis*. *J Clin Microbiol* 32:148, 1994.

257 Riley DE et al: Development of a polymerase chain reaction-based diagnosis of *Trichomonas vaginalis*. *J Clin Microbiol* 30:465, 1992.

258 Muresu R et al: A new method for identification of *Trichomonas vaginalis* by fluorescent DNA in situ hybridization. *J Clin Microbiol* 32:1018, 1994.

259 Rubino S et al: Molecular probe for identification of *Trichomonas vaginalis* DNA. *J Clin Microbiol* 29:702, 1991.

260 Centers for Disease Control: Sexually transmitted diseases treatment guidelines, 1993. *MMWR* 42(RR-14):1, 1993.

261 Lohmeyer H: Treatment of candidiasis and trichomoniasis of the female genital tract. *Postgrad Med J* 50:S78, 1974.

262 Goldman P: Metronidazole. *N Engl J Med* 303:1212, 1980.

263 Bhiraleus P et al: Rapid eradication of trichomonads by single-dosed nimorazole. *J Med Assoc Thai* 73:119, 1990.

264 Lossick JG: Treatment of *Trichomonas vaginalis* infections. *Rev Infect Dis* 4:801, 1982.

265 Lossick JG: Therapy of Urogenital Trichomoniasis, in *Trichomonads Parasitic in Humans*, BM Honigberg (ed). New York, Springer, 1989, p 326.

266 Donadio C: Tioconazole 2% cream in the treatment of *Trichomonas vaginalis* or mixed vaginal infections. *J Int Med Res* 14:50, 1986.

267 Sears SD, O'Hare J: In vitro susceptibility of *Trichomonas vaginalis* to 50 antimicrobial agents. *Antimicrob Agents Chemother* 32:144, 1988.

268 Edwards DI: Nitroimidazole drugs—action and resistance mechanisms: I. Mechanisms of action. *J Antimicrob Chemother* 31:9, 1993.

269 Muller M et al: In vitro susceptibility of *Trichomonas vaginalis* to metronidazole and treatment outcome in vaginal trichomoniasis. *Sex Transm Dis* 15:17, 1988.

270 Korner B, Jensen HK: Sensitivity of *Trichomonas vaginalis* to metronidazole, tinidazole, and nifurantel in vitro. *Br J Vener Dis* 52:404, 1976.

271 Meingassner JG et al: Studies on strain sensitivity of *Trichomonas vaginalis* to metronidazole. *Br J Vener Dis* 54:72, 1978.

272 Meingassner JG, Thurner J: Strain of *Trichomonas vaginalis* resistant to metronidazole and other 5′-nitroimidazoles. *Antimicrob Agents Chemother* 15:254, 1979.

273 Lossick JG et al: In vitro drug susceptibility and doses of metronidazole required for cure in cases of refractory vaginal trichomoniasis. *J Infect Dis* 153:948, 1986.

274 Krajden S et al: Persistent *Trichomonas vaginalis* infection due to a metronidazole-resistant strain. *Can Med Assoc J* 134:1373, 1986.

275 Kulda J et al: In vitro induced anaerobic resistance to metronidazole in *Trichomonas vaginalis*. *J Eukaryot Microbiol* 40:262, 1993.

276 Hamed KA, Studemeister AE: Successful response of metronidazole-resistant trichomonal vaginitis to tinidazole: A case report. *Sex Transm Dis* 19:339, 1992.

277 Dombrowski MP et al: Intravenous therapy of metronidazole-resistant *Trichomonas vaginalis*. *Obstet Gynecol* 69:524, 1987.

278 Pattman RS et al: Failure of mebendazole to cure trichomonal vaginitis resistant to metronidazole: Case reports. *Genitourin Med* 65: 274, 1989.

279 Escario JA et al: Antiparasitic activity of nine pyrazole derivatives against *Trichomonas vaginalis*, *Entamoeba invadens*, and *Plasmodium berghei*. *Ann Trop Med Parasitol* 82:257, 1988.
280 Herrero A et al: Synthesis and antiprotozoal properties of 1,2,6-thiadiazine 1,1-dioxide derivatives. *Archiv der Pharmazie Weinheim* 325: 509, 1992.
281 Katiyar SK, Edlind TD: Enhanced antiparasitic activity of lipophilic tetracyclines: Role of uptake. *Antimicrob Agents Chemother* 35: 2198, 1991.
282 Kaneda Y et al: In vitro effects of berberine sulphate on the growth and structure of *Entamoeba histolytica*, *Giardia lamblia*, and *Trichomonas vaginalis*. *Ann Trop Med Parasitol* 85:417, 1991.
283 Wood BA, Monro AM: Pharmacokinetics of tinidazole and metronidazole in women after single large oral dose. *Br J Vener Dis* 49: 475, 1975.
284 Robertson DH et al: Treatment failure in *Trichomonas vaginalis* infections in females: I. Concentrations of metronidazole in plasma and vaginal content during normal and high dosage. *J Antimicrob Chemother* 21:373, 1988.
285 Lossick JG: Treatment of sexually transmitted vaginosis/vaginitis. *Rev Infect Dis* 6(suppl):S665, 1990.
286 Underhill RA, Peck JE: Causes of therapeutic failure after treatment of trichomonal vaginitis with metronidazole: Comparison of single dose treatment with a standard regimen. *Br J Clin Pract* 28:134, 1974.
287 Dykers JR: Single dose metronidazole for trichomonal vaginitis. *N Engl J Med* 293:23, 1975.
288 Fleury FS: A single dose of two grams of metronidazole for *Trichomonas vaginalis*. *Am J Obstet Gynecol* 128:320, 1977.
289 Rodin P et al: Flagyl in the treatment of trichomoniasis. *Br J Vener Dis* 36:147, 1960.
290 Kazmier FJ: A significant interaction between metronidazole and warfarin. *Mayo Clin Proc* 51:782, 1976.
291 Rustia M, Shobik P: Induction of lung tumors and malignant lymphomas in mice by metronidazole. *J Natl Canc Inst* 48:421, 1972.
292 Federal Drug Administration: Metronidazole (Flagyl) box warning. FDA Drug Bull, April-May 1976.
293 Beard CM et al: Cancer after exposure to metronidazole. *Mayo Clin Proc* 63:147, 1988.
294 Beard CM et al: Lack of evidence for cancer due to use of metronidazole. *N Engl J Med* 301:519, 1979.
295 Pavic R, Stojkovic L: Vaccination with Solco Trichovac. Immunological aspects of a new approach for therapy and prophylaxis in women. *Gynakologische Rundschau* 23(suppl):7, 1983.
296 Gombosova A et al: Immunotherapeutic effect of the lactobacillus vaccine, Solco Trichovac, in trichomoniasis is not mediated by antibodies cross-reacting with *Trichomonas vaginalis*. *Genitourin Med* 62:107, 1986.
297 Alderete JF: Does lactobacillus vaccine for trichomoniasis, Solco Trichovac, induce antibody reactive with *Trichomonas vaginalis*? *Genitourin Med* 64:118, 1988.
298 Waitz JA et al: Chemotherapeutic evaluation of clotrimazole. *Appl Microbiol* 22:891, 1971.
299 Schnell JD: The incidence of vaginal candida and trichomoniasis infections and treatment of trichomonas vaginitis with clotrimazole. *Post Med J* 50:S79, 1974.
300 Legal HP: The treatment of trichomonas and candida vaginitis with clotrimazole vaginal tablets. *Post Med J* 50:S81, 1974.
301 Livengood CH, Lossick JG: Resolution of resistant vaginal trichomoniasis associated with the use of intravaginal nonoxynol-9. *Obstet Gynecol* 1991.
302 Wong CA et al: Povidone-iodine in the treatment of metronidazole-resistant *Trichomonas vaginalis*. *Aust NZ J Obstet Gynaecol* 30:169, 1990.
303 Vorherr H et al: Vaginal absorption of povodone-iodine. *JAMA* 244: 2628, 1980.
304 Farthing MJ et al: Effect of D-propranolol on growth and motility of flagellate protozoa. *J Antimicrob Chemother* 20:519, 1987.
305 van der Weiden R et al: Treatment failure in trichomoniasis and persistence of the parasite after *Lactobacillus* immunotherapy; two case reports. *Eur J Obstet Gynecol Reprod Biol* 34:171, 1990.

Chapter 44

Intestinal protozoa: *Giardia lamblia*, *Entamoeba histolytica*, *Cryptosporidium*, and new and emerging protozoal infections

Richard L. Guerrant
Cynthia L. Sears
Jonathan I. Ravdin

Enteric protozoan pathogens are increasingly recognized causes of diarrhea. This chapter reviews the biology of the major protozoan causes of diarrhea: *Giardia lamblia, Entamoeba histolytica,* and *Cryptosporidium.* These protozoa may sometimes be transmitted by sexual practices that enable fecal-oral spread; *Cryptosporidium* infections present particularly severe problems in patients with the acquired immunodeficiency syndrome (AIDS). Other intestinal protozoa that may also cause severe diarrhea in HIV-infected patients include *Cyclospora* and microsporidia, which are discussed at the end of the chapter.

GIARDIA LAMBLIA

HISTORY, EPIDEMIOLOGY, AND CLINICAL MANIFESTATIONS

History

Giardia lamblia was probably first discovered by the inventor of the microscope, Anton van Leeuwenhoek, when he examined his own diarrheal stool. In a letter to the Royal Society on November 4, 1681, he described "a number of animalcules approximately the size of a blood cell, with flattish bodies and several legs, moving much like a wood louse running up against a wall."[1] In 1859 Vilem D. F. Lambl described the parasite and called it *Cercomonas intestinalis.* However, since this organism was found in a number of asymptomatic individuals,[2] it was not considered to be a pathogen until it was repeatedly observed to be associated with diarrhea,[3–5] malabsorption,[6] and occasional tissue invasion.[7] Even the demonstration of experimental human infection in 36 percent of volunteers ingesting 10 to 25 *Giardia* cysts in water, and the presence of moderate to marked diarrheal symptoms in 60 percent of 15 infected individuals, left some question about the pathogenicity of this flagellated protozoan parasite.[8] There have since been numerous studies of the different strains of *Giardia,* its animal host-species specificities, its morphological and functional characteristics, its in vitro cultivation, and the possible mechanisms by which it may cause enteric disease. As with *Entamoeba histolytica,* the in vitro cultivation of *Giardia lamblia* has enabled the study of different strains at the molecular level.

Epidemiology

Several epidemiologic surveys have revealed that 2 to 9 percent of the population in many parts of the world excrete *Giardia lamblia* cysts.[9,10] Prevalence rates are higher in tropical areas and among travelers; exposed infants and children have the highest rates.[11,12] This skewed distribution of giardiasis toward children is in distinct contrast to amebiasis, where gain and loss of infections (with a median duration of 2 years) appears to be independent of age.[13] The geographic and age distribution, as well as increased frequencies of giardiasis in institutions where hygienic standards are difficult to maintain, indicate that spread occurs by the fecal-oral route.[3,14] The human volunteer studies by Rendtorff[8] suggest that ingestion of relatively small numbers of cysts in food or water or as a result of person-to-person contact results in infection. A foodborne outbreak was reported in which contamination of canned salmon apparently occurred after careful diaper changing of an infected infant.[15]

Waterborne giardiasis has been widely recognized in the last 15 years and is now the commonest reported parasitic infection in England and the United States.[16] Although first suggested by an outbreak of amebiasis and giardiasis in 1946 in a Tokyo apartment building where sewage-contaminated water was implicated (*Giardia* cysts were demonstrated in 80 percent of symptomatic individuals who did not have amebiasis),[4] attention was drawn to waterborne giardiasis by an outbreak in Aspen, Colorado in 1965, when 11 percent of skiers and 5 percent of residents were infected, and *Giardia* cysts were demonstrated in sewage that had contaminated the drinking water. A total of 23 additional outbreaks of giardiasis involving over 7,000 individuals in the United States subsequently implicated water which was inadequately sedimented and filtered, often despite bacteriologically adequate chemical disinfection.[16] These include a number of citywide outbreaks in Portland, Oregon; Aspen, Colorado; Rome, New York;[17] Camas, Washington; and Berlin, New Hampshire. In the Rome outbreak, cysts were found in city water which were shown to be infectious for beagle pups[17] (an experimental animal infection that had been described by Padchenko in the Russian literature in 1969). The greatest frequency of *Giardia lamblia* infections appeared to correlate with the season of greatest fecal contamination in a Colorado study.[18]

Studies of travelers from the United States and other countries to Leningrad and Moscow, summarized in a 1974 journal article,[19] noted impressive attack rates of giardiasis, ranging from 22 to 41 percent. In one of these studies the mean incubation period was 14 days, and 69 percent of those infected were symptomatic.

Besides humans, potential reservoirs include small animals such as beavers, which may be found contaminating even the remotest streams. As shown by Rendtorff in 1954,[20] *Giardia lamblia* cysts remain infectious for humans after holding in water for over 2 weeks. Furthermore, chemical disinfection of contaminated surface water is inadequate, especially when the water is cold, and appropriate flocculation, sedimentation, and filtration are necessary to remove infectious cysts. Cysts may also be killed by 2 to 5% phenol or Lysol. Transmission may also occur with contaminated, uncooked foods[15] or by person-to-person contact in families, nurseries, institutions, and day-care centers.[3,9,14] Fecal-oral and rectal-genital spread of *Giardia* have been implicated in homosexual men.[21,22,22a]

Clinical manifestations

In endemic areas the majority of *Giardia lamblia* infections are asymptomatic; however, a significant portion of residents and most previously uninfected travelers are symptomatic. The most characteristic symptoms include diarrhea of greater than 10 days' duration, cramping upper abdominal pain, bloating, flatulence, and weight loss.[17,19] Less commonly, nausea, vomiting, and fever may be seen.

Although the incubation period ranges from 1 to 8 weeks, symptoms often precede the first detectable fecal shedding of the parasites; the median prepatency period in one study (14 days) was 6 days longer than the median incubation period (8 days).[23] Thus, it may be necessary to examine upper small bowel aspirates or repeated fecal specimens to document a diagnosis of giardiasis. While the infection is usually self-limited,[8] symptoms may intermittently recur or persist for prolonged periods of up to months or even years.[24] The illness may last up to 6 or 7 weeks.[19]

Signs and symptoms of malabsorption, ranging from mild noninflammatory diarrhea, steatorrhea, or weight loss to a more severe celiac syndrome, especially in children,[6] are well documented, with malabsorption of D-xylose, fat, carotene, vitamin A, folate, and vitamin B_{12}.[5,25,26] Malabsorption may be especially severe in patients with achlorhydria,[25] immunodeficiency,[25,27] protein-calorie malnutrition,[28] or bacterial overgrowth[29] complicating their illnesses. In patients with hypogammaglobulinemia, giardiasis can be associated with mucosal inflammation, with villus flattening, and with lactase, maltase, or sucrase deficiency.[24,26,30] Likewise, giardiasis may mimic or accentuate the malabsorption seen in chronic pancreatitis.[31]

While giardia-induced diarrhea is usually noninflammatory, with only rare tissue invasion,[7] inflammatory proctitis and vaginitis have been reported.[32] For poorly understood reasons, patients with giardiasis may rarely develop eosinophilia, urticaria, or other symptoms, such as arthritis,[33] that are suggestive of an immune response to an antigen exposed during acute diarrhea. These symptoms respond to specific antigiardial therapy.[34]

STRUCTURE AND BIOLOGY OF THE ORGANISM

Named *"Giardia"* by Kunstier, who observed it in tadpole intestinal tracts in 1882, the genus was considered by Alexeieff and Dobell to be the same as the human flagellated protozoan. The genus and the disease are called *"Lamblia"* and lambliasis in eastern Europe; however, most authorities agree on the genus name *Giardia*. At least three species are recognized on the basis of morphology and host-species specificity.[35] Although species specificity is debated and size can be changed with host diet,[36] *Giardia lamblia* trophozoites usually measure 12 to 15μm long by 5 to 15μm wide and 1 to 4μm thick. Cysts are usually 8 to 12μm long by 7 to 10μm wide. Shaped like a horseshoe crab, with a rounded dorsal surface and concave ventral surface, the *Giardia lamblia* trophozoite has four pairs of flagella directed posteriorly from the lateral and ventral surfaces.

The trophozoite (Fig. 44-1) has a unique anterior ventral adhesive disk, to which are attached a clockwise spiral of microtubules and contractile elements. The disk has a posterior vent where beating ventral flagella appear to expel fluid that may help

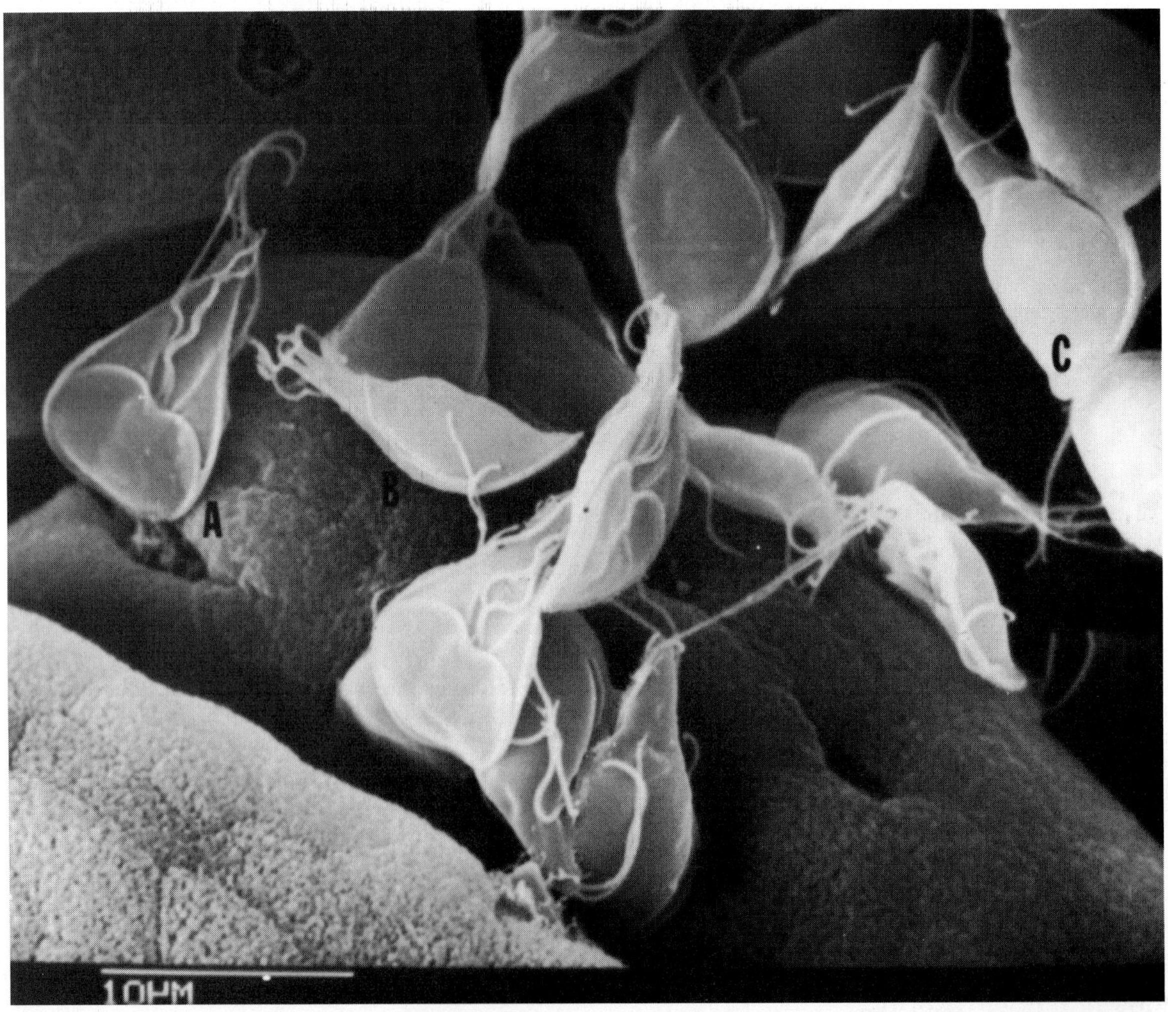

Fig. 44-1. Scanning electron micrograph of *Giardia lamblia* trophozoites from a jejunal biopsy of a patient with symptomatic giardiasis. (*A*) In the ventral view, flagella lead from the adhesive disk to the tapered posterior end. (*B*) In the lateral view, anterior flagella can be seen. (*C*) The dorsal view. (*Courtesy of R. L. Owen.*)

establish a mechanical suction for adherence of the parasite to mucosal or other surfaces.[38,39] Alternate suggestions for the disk's functions include contractile or grasping actions. The adhesive disk is divided into two lobes, the medial surfaces of which are the median groove. Two nuclei lie dorsal to the adhesive disk lobes, and the eight flagella appear to arise from basal bodies located anterior to the nuclei.

Endocytic or exocytic vacuoles that have been shown to concentrate ferritin or even bacteria are found adjacent to the disk and elsewhere.[40] There is evidence that *G. lamblia* have surface receptors for lectins such as wheat germ agglutinin and that these receptors can be blocked by specific carbohydrates.[41] In addition, a 56-kDa protease-activated *Giardia* lectin has been isolated by SDS-PAGE from a lipopolysaccharide (LPS)-sepharose column.[42]

The median body appears to be a tight packet of microtubules that lies between the posterior poles of the nuclei; it appears to be unique to *Giardia* species.[39] The median bodies of *G. lamblia* that infect humans, dogs, rabbits, and other mammals are characteristically claw-shaped and lie transversely across the trophozoite. *G. muris* trophozoites from rodents or birds have small, round central median bodies, and the long, narrow *G. agilia* trophozoites from amphibians have long, tear-shaped median bodies.[35–37]

As with *E. histolytica*, differences among *G. lamblia* strains as to isoenzyme patterns,[43] antigens and surface proteins,[44,45] and restriction endonuclease patterns[46] have been described. A double-stranded RNA virus has been described in the Portland I strain of *G. lamblia* that could infect another *G. lamblia* strain (WB).[47] Recent evidence on the antigenic variation of a cysteine-rich 170-kDa protein expressed on the surface of certain *G. lamblia* suggest frequent rearrangements at the gene locus as well as long tandem repeats in the DNA.[48,48a]

Trophozoites may encyst in response to a reduced pH, detachment, immunologic attack, or other hostile environments in vivo[39]; encystment has been accomplished in vitro using primary bile salts.[49] Apparently, after a single division in the cyst and a period of maturation, two daughter trophozoites can be induced to excyst in vitro by special conditions and reduced pH.[50]

GROWTH, PHYSIOLOGY, AND CULTURE

Although culture has not been successful with other *Giardia* strains, the human strain *G. duodenalis* (*G. lamblia*) has been grown in vitro, first symbiotically with *Candida guillermondii* and then axenically (without other bacteria or parasites) by Meyer.[51] In 1978, Bingham and Meyer successfully cultured trophozoites that were obtained in vitro from cysts shed by humans and monkeys.[50] As shown by Visvesvara, the conditions for culture of *G. lamblia* in vitro are similar to those for culture of *E. histolytica*. *G. lamblia* may be more oxygen tolerant, but both parasites require serum and cysteine.[52,53] Bile salts have been shown to support growth of *G. lamblia*.[53,54] giardia trophozoites can be preserved at low temperatures in glycerol or dimethyl sulfoxide.

The in vitro cultivation of giardia trophozoites has enabled definition of their growth curves, with doubling times of 7 to 40 hours noted by different investigators.[52,53] *G. lamblia* appear to facultatively metabolize glucose to ethanol acetate and carbon dioxide via a flavin-mediated electron-transport system rather than a cytochrome-mediated electron-transport system or a Krebs cycle.[55]

IMMUNOLOGY AND PATHOGENESIS

Immunology and host response

A substantial number of studies of humoral and cellular immune responses to *Giardia* infection reveal a complexity ranging from partial, protection to possible roles in pathogenesis. Evidence for acquired resistance includes the skewed age distribution toward children (in contrast to amebiasis)[13] the observation that long-term residents of endemic areas appear to have a lower infection rate than short-term residents,[56] and the tendency for individuals in endemic areas to be infected asymptomatically. In addition, prior infection appears to result in acquired resistance to *G. muris* infection in the mouse model.[57]

The nature of acquired resistance appears to be related in part to local antibody production. Although initial humoral responses to *G. lamblia* infection are predominantly IgM, there follows an IgA and IgG response[58] that correlates with the severity of the histologic jejunal lesion.[59] Although debated by others,[60] the findings of Zinneman suggested that patients with giardiasis had lower secretory IgA levels.[27] Of seven patients described by Hermans et al. who had type 2 IgA and IgM deficiency and nodular small bowel lymphoid hyperplasia, six had giardiasis that improved with therapy.[61] Ament et al. have shown that hypogammaglobulinemic patients who acquire giardiasis develop enteric symptoms and malabsorption.[62] However, the frequent occurrence of selective IgA deficiency without recognized problems with giardiasis suggests that other Ig classes or possibly still other factors are also involved in protection against symptomatic giardia infections.

Human serum kills *G. lamblia* trophozoites via activation of the classical complement pathway.[63] IgM-supported complement-dependent lysis of *G. lamblia* has been demonstrated. Anti-IgM treated mice develop heavy, prolonged infections (without any serum or local antibody responses) with *G. muris*.[65] Peyer's patch B cells show an early increase in surface IgM-bearing cells, followed by a switch to surface IgA-bearing cells with *G. muris* infection in mice.[66] The absence of severe disease with *G. lamblia* infections in AIDS patients (in contrast to cryptosporidial and mycobacterial infections, for example) militates against a major primary role for cellular immunity in preventing symptomatic giareliasis.

In the mouse model, transient protective immunity can be transferred by milk to suckling offspring, possibly at the cost of the nursing mother's effective intestinal immunity.[67] Whether this transient immunity is related to passive transfer of cellular or documented humoral immunity[68] or both remains to be determined. Murine and human biopsy studies have suggested roles for several types of cells in the pathogenesis and resistance in *G. lamblia* infection: microfolded epithelial (M) cells overlying Peyer's patches that have to do with processing giardia antigens, small lymphocytes that undergo intralumenal migration and directly attack the parasite, and intraepithelial large T lymphocytes or macrophages which are also involved.[37,39,69]

Evidence for a role for cell-mediated immunity in protection against *G. lamblia* infection again comes from the *G. muris* mouse model[70] in which athymic mice develop a prolonged *G. muris* infection.[71] Subsequent study has shown that the helper/inducer T lymphocytes (L3T4+), rather than the cytotoxic/suppressor (Ly-2+) subset, are responsible for clearance of murine *G. muris* infections.[72] Resistance to giardiasis may also be provided by toxic free fatty acids produced from breast milk by a bile-salt-stimulated lipase.[73,74]

The resistance to *G. lamblia* infection, however, is far from absolute. Normal human adults are usually susceptible to this widespread parasite; Rendtorff infected all 13 adults challenged with more than 100 cysts.[8] Despite the evidence for increased susceptibility when specific humoral or cellular responses are impaired or absent, the relative infrequency of giardiasis in most patients with IgA deficiency and the acquisition of incomplete resistance by athymic nude mice[70] show that resistance to *G. lamblia* infection is complex and may involve both local humoral and cellular immune responses.

The apparent increased frequency of giardiasis in patients with blood group A[75] may reflect less recognition of a parasite antigen similar to blood group A antigen,[76] or it may be related to other traits associated with blood group A, such as achlorhydria or differences in cell surface or mucus glycoproteins.

Pathogenesis

The initial stages in the pathogenesis of *G. lamblia* infection follow ingestion of a relatively small number of cysts (usually in water or by contact) and excystation of trophozoites in the upper small bowel, where multiplication apparently occurs. Larger inocula probably cause more severe infection.[8] Although gastric acidity may contribute to excystation,[50] several investigators have noted increased symptoms with giardiasis in hypochlorhydric or postgastrectomy patients.

There are several tantalizing hypotheses regarding the mechanism by which *G. lamblia* alters small bowel function or histology to cause disease. Some have suggested that the close adherence of many trophozoites mechanically impedes normal absorptive processes.[77] Holberton has shown evidence for a physical suction and some microvillus brush border damage under the ventral disk of giardia trophozoites that resulted in deformation of the gut cell cortex.[38] Imprints of the ventral disks have also been demonstrated in the microvillus brush border in the mouse model with *G. muris* infection.[78] However, this has not been shown in humans, nor do symptoms correlate with density or intensity of infection.[79] Instead, symptoms have been correlated with lymphocytic infiltration in the jejunal epithelium,[79] suggesting possible immunologic damage. Increased crypt cell production with lymphocytic infiltration has been noted in mice infected with *G. muris*.[80] Furthermore, Roberts-Thomson and Mitchell showed villus injury when T-lymphocytes were added to nude, athymic mice before infection with giardia protozoa.[71] Inflammatory responses with plasma cell infiltrates are also seen in segmentally damaged mucosa, especially in immunoglobulin deficiency states.[81]

Other researchers have described direct invasion of the mucosa by trophozoites in vivo.[82] Whether this tissue damage relates to cytotoxic or enterotoxic products of *G. lamblia* is unclear at present. Malabsorption and specific brush border enzyme deficiencies are well recognized in giardiasis.[26] These findings might be explained in part by increased epithelial cell turnover with increased villus-tip cell extrusion.[26,71] Others suggest that the parasite may compete with the host for nutrients.[77] Possible strain differences in pathogenicity based on differences in surface antigens, patterns of infection, and homologous immune responses have been suggested by studies in a gerbil model.

Finally, the interaction of *G. lamblia* with other microorganisms appears to be important in certain instances. Whether by host-tissue damage or by actual carriage of other microorganisms by giardia organisms,[40] severe malabsorption and steatorrhea with giardiasis has been associated with small bowel bacterial overgrowth.[20,28] Concentrations of 10^3 to 10^7 bacteria (mostly enteric coliforms) have been described with giardiasis and malabsorption or steatorrhea; in some instances the bacteria had to be eradicated before the symptoms resolved. Symptomatic responses to tetracycline without eradication of *G. lamblia* have also been noted.[85]

Bile salt deconjugation by bacterial overgrowth or by *Giardia* themselves has been postulated but has not been proved.[29] Smith and coworkers failed to confirm direct bile salt deconjugation by *G. lamblia*[86]; however, direct uptake of bile salts by the parasite may be significant and clearly enhances its growth.[87] Development of the in vitro culture techniques and the animal models of *Giardia muris* in mice offer considerable promise of improved understanding of the pathogenesis of giardiasis, as do recent studies in gerbils, rats, and mice.

DIAGNOSIS

Examination of fresh and concentrated stool specimens

The diagnosis of *G. lamblia* infection can often be made by examining fresh or concentrated fecal specimens in cases of diarrhea that persist beyond the prepatency period of 5 to 7 days. As summarized in Table 44-1, the prompt examination of a fresh diarrheal stool specimen may reveal the striking motile trophozoites of *G. lamblia* on an unstained direct wet-slide preparation or a specimen that has been trichrome-stained for cysts or trophozoites before or after concentration (Fig. 44-2).

The diagnosis of giardiasis is usually made by examining one to three stool specimens after concentration, using such methods as flotation in 33% zinc sulfate (after clarification by centrifugation in water) or formalin-ether sedimentation in approximately 10 mL of 10% formalin suspension with 3 mL ether. The concentrate is then stained with 1% potassium iodide saturated with iodine. While some report that three concentrated fecal specimens are adequate to diagnose the vast majority of cases, others have shown that as few as 34% of stool specimens from patients with the parasite in the upper small bowel were positive. Barium, kaolin products, oily laxatives, antibiotics, antacids, paregoric, enemas, and cotton swabs will greatly reduce the value of the microscopic examination.

A monoclonal antibody combination reagent for direct fluorescence detection of *Giardia* cysts and *Cryptosporidium* oocysts has proved useful in fecal microscopy.[87a] In addition, fecal antigen ELISAs (enzyme-linked immunosorbent assays) using polyclonal or monoclonal antibodies range in sensitivity and specificity from

Table 44-1. Diagnosis of *Giardia lamblia* Infection

Test	Sensitivity	Specificity
Microscopy		
Fresh fecal exam for motile trophozoites	Better with active diarrhea	Specific in experienced hands, but finding trophozoites does not prove disease causation
Stained, concentrated fecal exam		
Duodenal aspirate or string test	Approximately 34–98% May be more sensitive than stool exam early in illness and in children (83–86%)	
Jejunal biopsy/imprint	Approaches 100%	
Serologic tests:		
IFA using patient's cysts or trophozoites	89% of symptomatic patients	71–100%
Immunodiffusion (with sonicated cysts)	91%	Approaches 100%
IFA (with cultured trophozoites)	97% ≥ 1:16	85–100%
ELISA (with cultured trophozoites)	81%	88%

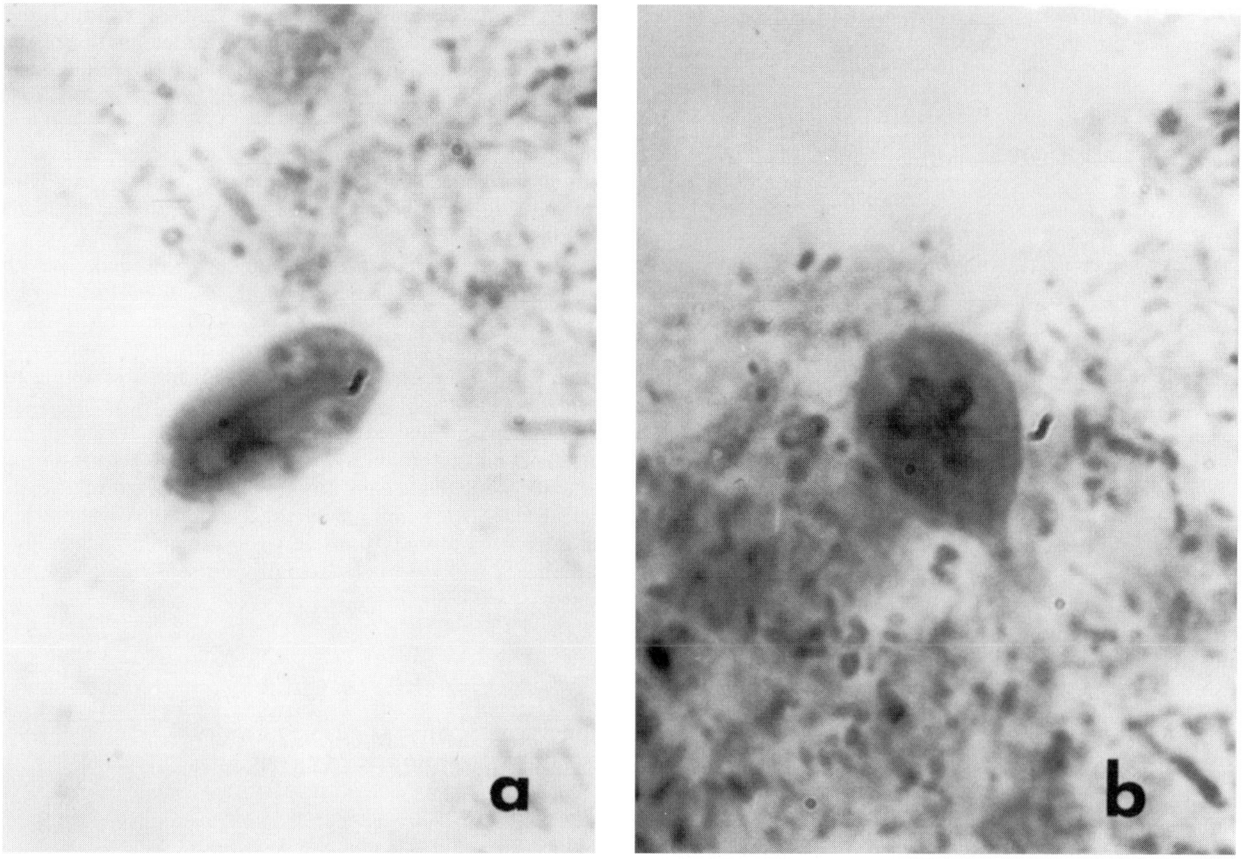

Fig. 44-2. *Giardia lamblia* (*a*) cyst and trophozoite (*b*) from fecal specimens of a patient with active giardiasis. Gomori-Wheatley trichrome stain, oil immersion ×640 magnification. (*Courtesy of G. R. Healy.*)

87 percent to 100 percent.[87b] Finally, DNA-based probes for *G. lamblia* are in development, but they are not yet widely useful.[89c]

Examination of small bowel contents or tissue

From studies in adult volunteers, several observers have reported an improved yield (although this is debated by some researchers) with examining duodenal aspirates or even small-bowel biopsies in patients whose fecal examinations are negative for *G. lamblia.*[88] When jejunal biopsy is performed, one should examine a Giemsa-stained sample of the "imprint" of the tissue, as well as the tissue itself, for the purple-stained trophozoites. Effective sampling of small bowel contents can also be accomplished, without intubation or biopsy, using the string test (Entero-Test, Hedeco, Palo Alto, California). This involves swallowing a gelatin capsule with one end of the 140-cm (or 90-cm for children) nylon line taped to the side of the mouth. Removing the string after 4 to 6 hours and examining the bile-stained mucus has been helpful in demonstrating *G. lamblia* trophozoites, particularly in young children and in adults early in their illness. When jejunal biopsy is performed, one should examine a Giemsa-stained sample of the "imprint" of the tissue as well as the tissue itself for the purple-stained trophozoites.

Serologic tests

Primarily because of limitations on antigen supply prior to in vitro cultivation of *Giardia,* little was known until recently about serologic responses to *G. lamblia* infections. In 1976 Ridley and Ridley, using an indirect fluorescent antibody (IFA) test and patient isolates of cysts and trophozoites as antigen, found that 32 of 36 cases (89 percent) of giardiasis with malabsorption gave positive results, whereas neither of two cases of giardiasis without malabsorption and none of 17 controls was positive. There was a crude correlation of severity of jejunal histopathology with antibody titer.[59] FA titers fell in 11 of 19 cases (58 percent) 1 month or longer after therapy. Of 34 patients with malabsorption (mostly after travel to tropical areas) but negative stool and biopsy studies for giardia trophozoites, 10 (29 percent) had significant IFA anti–*G. lamblia* titers, which suggests that available diagnostic tests by direct examination may miss clinically significant giardiasis. These investigators also noted that use of mature cysts gave less reproducible results.

Vinayak et al. used washed, concentrated, sonicated *Giardia* cysts from fecal specimens to develop an immunodiffusion test for giardiasis that was said to be 91 percent sensitive as well as negative in all 31 healthy or other-parasite-infected controls.[89] Visvesvara and colleagues have developed an IFA test using axenically cultured *G. lamblia* trophozoites as antigen.[90] They found antibody titers of 1:16 to 1:1024 among 29 of 30 patients with symptomatic giardiasis and 1:2 to 1:4 in 19 healthy controls. These positive titers could be absorbed with *G. lamblia* trophozoites in vitro. Fifteen patients with other parasitic infections for bacterial overgrowth syndromes had titers of ≤1:16. Smith et al. reported use of *G. lamblia* trophozoites cultivated in vitro in development of an ELISA that appeared to be specific and sensitive, with 81 percent of symptomatically infected patients developing antibody titer rises at 2 weeks to 15 months.[91] The sensitivity of an ELISA for detection of giardia antigen in feces has been

92 to 98 percent (probably more sensitive than fecal microscopy); the specificity is also high.[92–94]

GENETICS, ANTIMICROBIAL SUSCEPTIBILITY, AND THERAPY

Axenic cultivation of *G. lamblia* has enabled studies of the genetics of strain variation[46–48] as well as in vitro sensitivity testing to antiparasitic agents.[95] Because the natural history of giardiasis is usually self-limited but occasionally recurrent over long periods of time, studies of the clinical efficacy of antigiardial therapy are difficult at best. Table 44-2 summarizes the pertinent features of the drugs used to treat giardiasis. Quinacrine (Atabrine) 100 mg three times a day (t.i.d.) for 7 days, formerly the drug of choice in the United States, results in 80 to 100 percent cure rates,[9,25,96] but is no longer readily available.

Metronidazole (Flagyl) 250 to 750 mg t.i.d. for 10 days effects 70 to 95 percent cure rates, the cure rate varying with the dose.[25] Single daily doses of metronidazole of 1.6 to 2.0 g for 2 to 3 days also appear to be effective but may cause more gastrointestinal side effects. Other nitroimidazole derivatives, including tinidazole, nimorazole, and ornidazole (Ro 7-0207), have also been effective, with possibly fewer side effects when given for 1 to 7 days.[97]

Whether the mechanism of action of quinacrine is related to its relative distribution and then intercalation into DNA or to other membrane effects is currently unclear. The ability of nitroimidazoles to kill giardia protozoa may relate to inhibition of DNA synthesis, competition for reducing equivalents with electron-transport proteins, or other mechanisms that are not understood at present. As metronidazole is not officially approved in the United States for giardiasis and because of concern about its mutagenicity and carcinogenicity in some experimental animals, the potential risks should be weighed before this agent is used.

Furazolidone, which is available in liquid form for pediatric use, has also been suggested for treatment of giardiasis.[96] Tartrazine, which is in certain Latin American preparations of furazolidone, may be related to the serum sickness seen with this drug. Paromomycin has been used in pregnant patients with symptomatic giardiasis.[99]

Recent in vitro cultivation of *Giardia lamblia* has enabled studies of antigiardial activity of these agents.[95] Although the appropriate methods and standardized criteria remain to be determined, "4-day end point" killing of *Giardia* has been noted with 0.05 to 0.1 μg/mL quinacrine and with 0.05 to 6.4 μg/mL metronidazole.[35,51] Immobilization of the parasites by antigiardial agents in vitro has also been suggested.[100] Further definition of the in vitro inhibitory concentrations of these and other agents with axenically grown *Giardia* and amebas has recently become feasible and is under further study.

Epidemiologic control measures are needed, including improved hygienic and sanitary conditions as well as water treatment by means of flocculation, sedimentation, and filtration. In addition, recent developments in in vitro culture technique and animal models are now opening the potential for developing means to control giardiasis. The roles of external and in vivo environments, pH, mucus, specific parasite and intestinal surface receptors, gut motility, and interaction with bacterial or other flora in causing or controlling disease are among the current frontiers in giardiasis research. Despite tantalizing suggestions of a protective role for cellular or humoral immunity, it remains unclear at present whether a vaccine might actually worsen the disease process in giardiasis.

ENTAMOEBA HISTOLYTICA

HISTORY, EPIDEMIOLOGY, AND CLINICAL MANIFESTATIONS

History

For over a century, amebiasis has been recognized as an invasive enteric illness in humans. The clinical syndrome of amebiasis and effective therapy are well known. In recent years there has been a renewed interest in the pathogenesis of *Entamoeba histolytica* infections.

The early history of amebiasis has been reviewed extensively.[101] Although a British surgeon, Timothy Richard Lewis, first described amebas in human stool in 1869, Löesch is credited with the first description of amebic dysentery, in a patient from St. Petersburg, Russia, in 1875. Löesch also reproduced colitis in dogs by introducing the patient's stool orally or rectally. Koch first noted amebas in tissue specimens in 1887, and in 1893

Table 44-2. Agents Used in the Treatment of Giardiasis

Agent	Dosage	Cure rate	Side effects
Acridine derivative			
Quinacrine (Atabrine)	100 mg tid for 5–7 days	63–100%	Occasional: toxic psychosis; insomnia; headache; yellow sclerae, skin and urine; nausea; vomiting. Rare: exfoliative dermatitis. Contraindicated in patients with psoriasis.
	Pediatric: 6–8 mg/kg per day (or 2 mg/kg tid) for 5–7 days	84–93%	
*Nitroimidazoles**			
Metronidazole (Flagyl)	250 mg tid for 5–10 days	56–70%	Nausea, headache, metallic taste; occasional insomnia, diarrhea, vertigo, paresthesia, rash; rare mild disulfiramlike reaction with alcohol, ataxia, urethral burning, reversible neutropenia. (Single daily-dose metronidazole causes more gastrointestinal side effects; tinidazole reportedly causes fewer gastrointestinal side effects.)
	750 mg tid for 3–10 days	95%	
	1.6–2.0 g qd for 1–5 days	91%	
	Pediatric: 15–25 mg/kg per day (or 5 mg/kg tid) for 5–7 days	61–90%	
Tinidazole and others (nimorazole, ornidazole)	2 g PO for 1 dose	93–97%	
	125 mg bid for 7 days		
Nitrofurantoin			
Furazolidone (Furoxone)	100 mg tid for 7 days	72–92%	Occasional nausea, vomiting, headache; rare disulfiramlike reaction with alcohol, arthralgia, rash, urticaria, hemolysis, other blood dyscrasias.
	Pediatric: 1.5 mg/kg suspension qid for 7 days		

* Not approved in the United States for giardiasis.

Quincke and Roos first described amebic cysts. In 1903 Fritz Schaudinn named the parasite *Entamoeba histolytica* from its apparent capacity to destroy tissue. In 1912 Bernard Rogers found that emetine extracts from the ipecac root effectively cured amebic dysentery and liver abscesses. *E. histolytica* was definitively shown to be a human pathogen (as distinguished from the commensal *Entamoeba coli*) in human volunteer studies by Walker and Sellards in the Philippines in 1913.[102]

Epidemiology

Entamoeba species infect 10 percent of the world's population; although the vast majority of those infected are asymptomatic, invasive amebiasis is the third leading parasitic cause of death worldwide.[103] A distinct nonpathogenic species, *Entamoeba dispar*, has been identified by studies of isoenzyme patterns, genomic DNA, and ribosomal DNA.[104–106] *E. dispar*, morphologically indistinguishable from *E. histolytica*, does not invade the host or elicit a systemic immune response during transient intestinal infection. *E. dispar* infection is usually up to tenfold more prevalent than *E. histolytica* infection,[107] although foci of transmission of *E. histolytica* are often observed. Therefore, all invasive amebiasis syndromes result from *E. histolytica* infection. Although approximately 90 percent of *E. histolytica* intestinal infections are also asymptomatic, they typically induce a systemic antiamebic immune response.[108,109]

Epidemic outbreaks of amebiasis have been reported with food or water contamination from many areas.[4] However, endemic amebiasis as currently seen in the United States is acquired by the fecal-oral route, usually by person-to-person spread.[110] High-risk groups include mentally challenged institutionalized patients (with stool cyst excretion rates of up to 70 percent),[111] lower socioeconomic groups, recently immigrated Mexican-Americans in the southern United States,[111] and homosexual men (with cyst excretion rates in San Francisco and New York as high as 20 percent in the past).[112,115] However, the prevalence of *E. histolytica* infection in homosexual men has declined in the last decade; the decline has accompanied the alteration in sexual practices within this group.[114] Overall, the combined prevalence of *E. histolytica* and *E. dispar* in the United States is approximately 4 percent.[103] Travel to highly endemic areas such as Mexico, India, the Middle East, and South America also increases the risk of amebic infection.[115]

Sexual transmission of *E. histolytica* results in enteric infection with possible dissemination or in venereal infection in males and females. Sexually transmitted amebic colitis occurs primarily in sexually active homosexual men between 20 and 40 years of age, with analingus being a significant risk factor for acquisition of *G. lamblia and E. histolytica* infections. Penile and cervical amebiasis in conjugal partners is rare but reported.[116]

Clinical manifestations

Clinical syndromes with *E. histolytica* infection range from asymptomatic cyst excretion to acute rectocolitis, chronic nondysenteric intestinal disease (which can be confused with inflammatory bowel disease), typhloappendicitis, ameboma, or toxic megacolon. Extraintestinal amebiasis usually results from hepatic abscesses and may extend to pleuropulmonary disease, pericarditis, or peritonitis. Unusual extraintestinal manifestations include venereal genital lesions, cutaneous lesions, and brain abscess.

STRUCTURE OF THE ORGANISM

E. histolytica and *E. dispar* trophozoites range in size from 10 to 60 μm, with an average size of 25 μm. Trophozoites contain a single 3- to 5-μm nucleus with fine peripheral chromatin and a central nucleolus (Fig. 44-3). The cytoplasm consists of a clear ectoplasm and a granular endoplasm that contains numerous vacuoles (Fig. 44-4). Cysts of *E. histolytica* average 12 μm in diameter (range 5 to 20 μm), and depending on their maturity contain one to four nuclei that have the same morphology as trophozoite nuclei. Like other members of the order Amoebida, young *E. histolytica* cysts contain chromatoid bodies with smooth, rounded edges. Immature cysts may contain clumps of glycogen which stain with iodine.

Other members of the Entamoebidae family found in humans include *Entamoeba polecki, E. coli, E. gingivalis, Endolimax nana, Iodamoeba butschlii,* and *Dientamoeba fragilis*. *E. hartmanni* is recognized as a distinct species,[117] differing from *E. histolytica* in being smaller, having distinct antigenic differences, and being noninvasive.[117] Most experts agree that another nonpathogenic species of *Entamoeba* is the Laredo-like strain, which grows in culture at lower temperatures (25° to 30°C) and does not cause clinical disease.[118]

Extensive electron-microscopic studies of *E. histolytica* reveal no mitochondria; ribonucleoprotein exists in helical arrays in the cytoplasm.[119–121] Endoplasmic and ectoplasmic vesicles are bound by a 120-Å double-layered membrane, much like the outer limiting membrane.[120]

Amebas also contain a uroid area where vesicles are noted external to the cell membrane.[122] An external fuzzy glycocalyx measures 20 to 30 nm on bacteria-associated trophozoites from tissue and 5 nm on axenic amebas.[123] Actin and structures resembling microfilaments have been identified in amebic trophozoites,[124,125] and the actin gene has been cloned.[126] Microtubules have not been demonstrated. Apparent functions for microfilaments, but not for microtubules, have been described in studies of the cytopathogenic capacity of *E. histolytica*.[127–129]

The surface membrane of *E. histolytica* has been well characterized biochemically. Amebas are agglutinated by the lectin concanavalin A,[130] which may be a marker for degree of pathogenicity of different strains.[130,131] Using concanavalin A binding to stiffen the external surface membrane, Aley et al. isolated relatively pure membrane preparations of *E. histolytica*.[132] Petri et al. have isolated the galactose-inhibitable adherence lectin of *E. histolytica*.[133] Microfilament-dependent capping, or aggregation of receptors, for concanavalin A or fluorescent-tagged antiameba antibody has been shown on *E. histolytica*, and the capped membrane material has been characterized biochemically, but the capping capacity does not appear to correlate with virulence.[134,135] However, capping may help amebas avoid attack by host defenses.

GROWTH, PHYSIOLOGY, AND CULTURE

Life cycle

The life cycle of *E. histolytica* has been well characterized.[136,137] Cysts are the infective form of *E. histolytica* because they can survive outside the host for weeks to months in a moist environment. Infected individuals excrete up to 45 million cysts per day.[136] Ingestion of cysts from fecally contaminated sources is followed by excystation in either the small or the large bowel. The nuclei then divide to form eight nuclei (transient metacystic stage), cytoplasmic division occurs, and eight amebic trophozoites emerge.[102] The trophozoite population then resides in the large bowel, where tissue invasion may occur. *E. histolytica* cyst walls contain chitin, an oligosaccharide of *N*-acetyl-D-glucosamine, sialic acid, and other cyst-specific antigens.[138,139] Encystation is an active process: anaerobic glycolytic respiration and DNA synthesis occur.[130] The conditions that induce encystation, excystation,

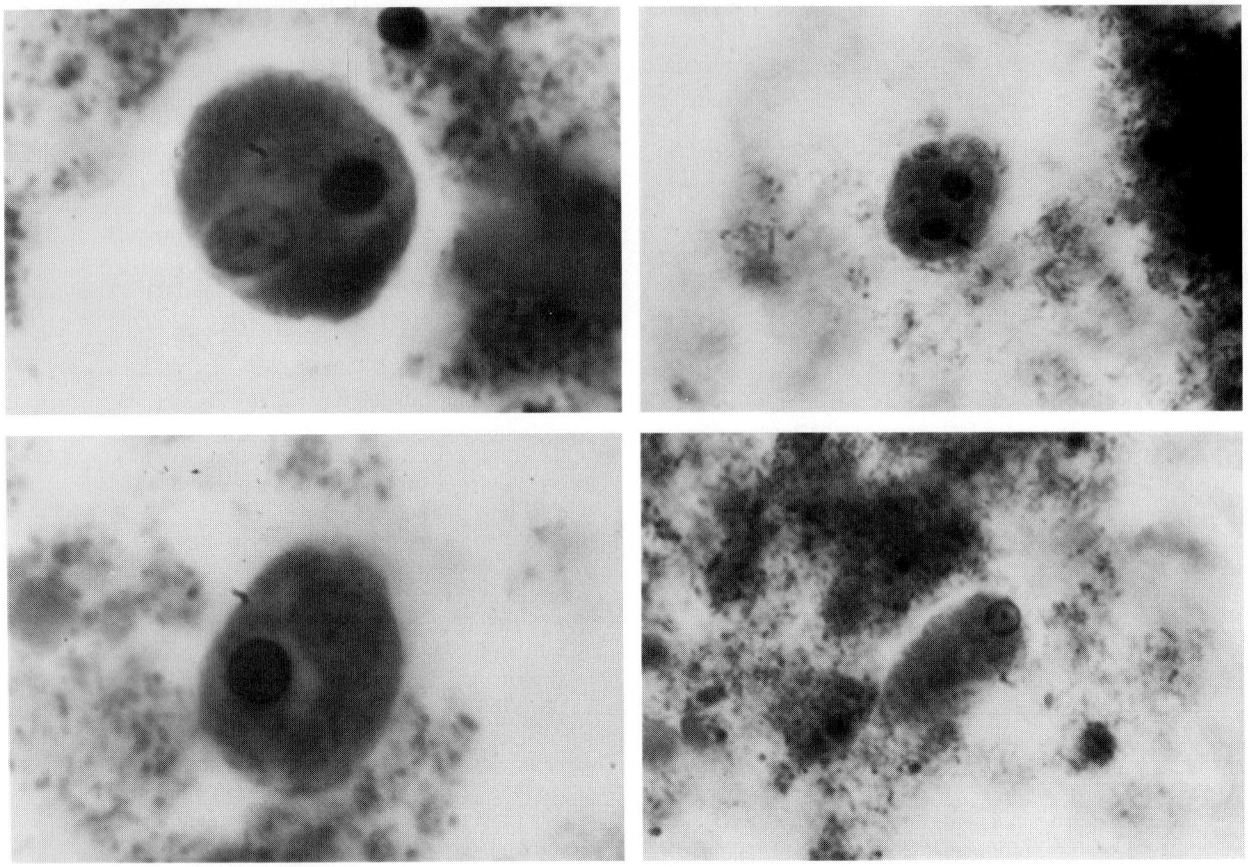

Fig. 44-3. *Entamoeba histolytica* trophozoites from fecal specimens of a patient with amebic colitis. Gomori-Wheatley trichrome stain, oil immersion. (*Right panel*) ×320 magnification. (*Left panel*) ×640 magnification. Note single nuclei with central, punctate karyosome, with delicate peripheral nuclear chromatin. The top two trophozoites also have an ingested red blood cell. (*Courtesy of G. R. Healy.*)

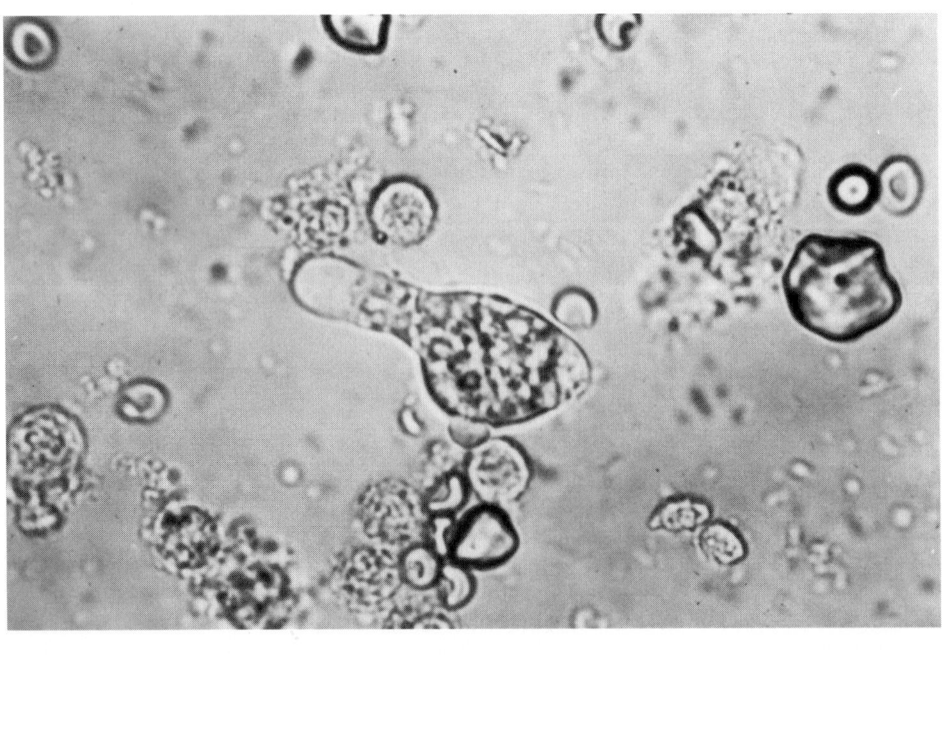

Fig. 44-4. *Entamoeba histolytica* trophozoites from a saline suspension of a vaginal specimen from a patient whose partner also had amebic colitis. A single typically motile trophozoite is seen.

and tissue invasion by amebas remain unclear and are the subject of current investigation.

Culture

Axenic cultivation of *E. histolytica* in medium without other organisms was first reported in 1961 by Diamond.[140] This was accomplished by microisolation of amebic cysts, which were then introduced into a monophasic medium seeded with crithidial trypanosomes. A liquid medium was reported in 1968, and the current medium in use (TYI-S-33: trypticase, yeast extract, iron, serum) was developed in 1978.[141] These culture techniques have made it possible to grow amebas in large numbers and to maintain cultures for prolonged periods. Clonal growth of *E. histolytica* in semisolid medium allows quantitative cultures for drug susceptibility testing and other laboratory studies.[142] Studies of axenic culture in vitro have clarified nutritional and other requirements for amebic growth. These include requirements for cysteine, riboflavin (B_2), vitamin B_{12}, iron, serum, optimal pH, and low oxygen tension.[141] Recently Clark has succeeded in establishing *E. dispar* in axenic culture.[143]

IMMUNOLOGY AND PATHOGENESIS

Immunology and host response

There is no evidence that intestinal colonization by *E. histolytica* elicits a protective host immune response.[144] However, extensive but anecdotal evidence indicates that cure of amebic colitis or liver abscess is followed by resistance to subsequent invasive amebiasis.[145,146] The mechanisms of immune defense against *E. histolytica* infection have not been fully characterized. Serum from both healthy controls and infected patients (with high antibody titers to *E. histolytica*) are amebicidal to trophozoites through activation of the alternate complement pathway.[147,148] However, trophozoites that cause invasive disease are resistant to complement-mediated lysis. Complement-resistant amebas can be selected in vitro by culture in normal human serum.[149,150] Serum antibodies and coproantibodies have been demonstrated to increase during invasive disease.[149,150]

A protective role for humoral immunity is suggested by the presence of antibody to the parasite's galactose-inhibitable adherence lectin.[151] Human immune sera can prevent amebic in vitro adherence,[151,152] despite the parasite's ability to aggregate and shed attached antibodies. The other *E. histolytica* antigens most frequently recognized by human immune sera have also been characterized,[153] which may be useful for development of diagnostic tests and vaccines. Lectin recombinant antigens (such as a 52-kDa fusion protein including the cysteine-rich LC3 section of the 170-kDa subunit),[154] as well as the entire 29-kDa surface antigen,[155] have recently been shown to conserve antigenicity.

Mucosal IgA immune responses have been studied in subjects cured of amebic liver abscess and colitis or with asymptomatic *E. histolytica* intestinal infections. Salivary sIgA to purified native galactose-inhibitable lectin has been found in subjects with amebic liver abscess[156] and colitis.[157] Fecal and salivary anti-LC3 sIgA responses occur in amebic colitis[158] and liver abscess; such patterns are absent or diminished in subjects with *E. dispar* infection.[158] Oral immunization of mice with the recombinant LC3 fusion protein and cholera holotoxin induced intestinal anti-LC3 IgA antibodies that inhibited amebic adherence in vitro.[159]

Cell-mediated immune (CMI) defense mechanisms appear to have a role in limiting invasive disease and possibly in resistance to recurrent invasion following pharmacologic cure.[144] Following invasive amebiasis, the CMI response consists of antigen-specific lymphocyte blastogenesis, with production of lymphokines (including gamma interferon) that activate monocyte-derived macrophages to kill *E. histolytica* trophozoites in vitro.[160–162] In addition, cured patients develop effective antigen-specific cytotoxic T-lymphocyte activity for *E. histolytica* trophozoites.[161] Purified native 260-kDa galactose-inhibitable lectin induced lymphocyte proliferation, gamma interferon production, and amebicidal activity in cultivated peripheral-blood mononuclear cells from subjects with serum antilectin IgG antibodies (indicating prior *E. histolytica* infection).[163] In addition, immunization of gerbils with native 260-kDa lectin induces a protective amebicidal cellular immune response.[164] However, in acute disease, CMI to *E. histolytica* is specifically depressed by a serum factor.[165] The high prevalence of *E. histolytica* intestinal infection in homosexual men with AIDS or certain other clinical manifestations of HIV infection without an increased incidence of invasive amebiasis[114] suggests that host resistance to the initial amebic invasion of the colonic mucosa does not involve CMI mechanisms.

Nonimmune host defenses may be most important in prevention of parasite attachment to and disruption of the colonic mucosa. In animal models, mucus trapping of *E. histolytica* trophozoites occurs,[166] and depletion of the colonic mucus blanket is always seen before parasite invasion.[167] *E. histolytica* elaborates a potent mucin secretagogue[168] that may contribute to depletion of the mucus layer. Chadee and coworkers demonstrated that purified rat and human colonic mucins, which are rich in galactose residues, are high-affinity receptors for the ameba's lectin, while mucin inhibits amebic adherence to and lysis of colonic epithelial cells in vitro.[169] Therefore, colonic mucin glycoproteins act as an important host defense by binding to the *E. histolytica* adherence lectin; however, this interaction may facilitate intestinal colonization by amebas and thus promote parasitism by *E. histolytica*.

Pathology

The pathology of human amebiasis provides clues to its pathogenesis. *E. histolytica* appears to exert a tissue lytic effect, for which the organism is named, whether in colon, liver, lung, or brain; this lytic effect leaves an amorphous, granular, eosinophilic material surrounding trophozoites in tissue[170] and can be studied in vitro. Consistent with the trophozoites' capacity to destroy leukocytes, inflammatory cells are found only at the periphery of amebic lesions and not adjacent to the trophozoites.[129,131,170,171]

The typical flask-shaped colonic ulcers are usually superficial, reaching only the muscularis mucosa level and separated by normal mucosa. Amebic trophozoites are seen in clusters in the periphery of necrotic areas. Light- and electron-microscopic studies have been alternatively interpreted as showing contact lysis of mucosal cells or diffuse mucosal damage prior to amebic invasion.[122,172] Current in vitro studies favor direct invasion and contact-dependent cytolysis by amebic trophozoites.

Liver pathology consists of the necrotic abscess and periportal fibrosis; however, the so-called abscess contains acellular, proteinaceous debris rather than white cells and is surrounded by a rim of amebic trophozoites.[170] Triangular areas of hepatic necrosis have been observed, possibly due to ischemia from amebic obstruction of portal vessels.[170] Periportal fibrosis alone, without trophozoites present, has been reported in patients with amebic colitis.[173] Whether this reflects past trophozoite invasion or host reaction to amebic antigens or toxins is currently unclear. "Amebic hepatitis" is a debated entity; liver function abnormalities commonly present with amebiasis are associated with periportal inflammation without demonstrable trophozoites.

Pathogenesis

The pathogenesis of invasive amebiasis can be divided into four steps: (1) colonization of the intestine with a virulent *E. histolytica* trophozoite, (2) disruption of mucosal barriers with adherence to colonic epithelial cells, (3) lysis of adherent epithelial cells and host inflammatory cells, and (4) resistance to host humoral and cellular defense mechanisms with deep tissue invasion. Recent in vitro studies have markedly increased our understanding of the biochemical and molecular mechanisms of the pathogenesis of invasive amebiasis.

Virulence

Current evidence indicates that there exist distinct pathogenic and nonpathogenic strains of *Entamoeba*. Sargeaunt and coworkers (reviewed in Ref. 158) demonstrated that starch gel electrophoresis of *E. histolytica* clinical isolates reveal patterns for the enzymes hexokinase, phosphoglucomutase, and glucosephosphate isomerase which are characteristic for invasive or noninvasive amebic infection at the time the sample was collected. The isoenzyme patterns are referred to as zymodemes. Sargeaunt[174] and others[175] proposed in 1986 that zymodeme studies reflect stable strain differences and that there was no need to treat individuals infected with *Entameoba histolytica* expressing a "nonpathogenic" zymodeme.

Many *Entamoeba* strains producing nonpathogenic zymodemes are now thought to be *E. dispar*. Epidemiologic studies of thousands of subjects confirm that *E. dispar* is not invasive, nor does it elicit a serum antibody response.[108,109] Tannich and coworkers were the first to demonstrate differences in genomic DNA between *E. histolytica* and *E. dispar*.[176] Recent studies by Clark and Diamond further characterized *E. dispar*.[106] Earlier studies indicating conversion of *E. dispar* to *E. histolytica* appear to be due to incomplete cloning of cultivated isolates.

In vivo experiments have drawn attention to the association of *E. histolytica* with bacteria (reviewed in Ref. 177). Associated bacteria facilitated early culture of *E. histolytica* in vitro, and Phillips et al. showed that bacteria were required for the establishment of invasive disease in germ-free guinea pigs infected with amebas grown with *Trypanosome cruzii*.[178] They interpreted the role of bacteria to be one of providing an environment which enables amebas to grow in the colon.[179] Wittner and Rosenbaum subsequently demonstrated that amebas required direct association with viable bacteria for virulence and that a soluble virulence factor could not be demonstrated.[180]

Recent axenic culture methods have allowed strains of amebas to retain virulence after prolonged periods (up to 9 years) of in vitro culture.[181] However, in vitro destruction of tissue-culture cells by axenic trophozoites is stimulated by parasite ingestion of viable bacteria.[182] Apparently these associated bacteria either accelerate the ameba's electron-transport system or increase its reducing capacity.[182] Viral particles have also been demonstrated in axenic amebas and can result in lysis of the amebas.[183] However, viral passage from amebic strains of higher virulence to less virulent strains does not consistently alter amebic virulence.[184]

Host nutritional factors appear to relate to the invasiveness of amebic infections. Weanling rats given protein-deficient diets are more susceptible to amebic infection; those already infected can eliminate the parasite when subsequently given high-protein diets.[184] High-carbohydrate, low-protein diets resulted in higher colonization but reduced tissue invasion compared with rats on a normal diet.[185] Faust and Read have noted an association of a poor nutritional state with more invasive amebic disease in humans.[186] Wanke and Butler reported a very high mortality for amebic colitis in malnourished patients in Bangladesh.[187] Although feeding of iron to experimental animals appears to increase the severity of experimental amebiasis, studies in humans do not reveal any correlation of invasive amebiasis with either serum iron or saturation of iron-binding proteins.[188] Finally, several investigators have noted an interesting association of ameba virulence with exposure of the parasite to cholesterol or with liver passage.[189,190] The increased virulence apparently persists for weeks after cholesterol exposure and is therefore not a temporary membrane or nutritional effect; it remains to be further elucidated.

Adherence mechanisms

E. histolytica trophozoites maintained in axenic culture must establish adherence in order to lyse target cells.[127,128] Ravdin and coworkers have demonstrated that in vitro adherence of *E. histolytica* trophozoites to Chinese hamster ovary (CHO) cells and human colonic mucins is exclusively mediated by the parasite's inhibitable surface lectin.[128,169,191] The galactose lectin also participates in amebic in vitro adherence to human leukocytes,[147,191] rat and human colonic mucosa and submucosa,[152] human erythrocytes,[128,192] Chang liver cells,[193] opsonized bacteria or bacteria with galactose-containing lipopolysaccharide,[194] and rat colonic epithelial cells.[169]

Ravdin and coworkers[195] produced monoclonal antibodies which inhibited amebic adherence to CHO cells. Utilizing the lectin's carbohydrate binding activity and lectin-specific monoclonal antibodies, Petri and coworkers isolated the *E. histolytica* adherence lectin.[196] Using ^{35}S-methionine, they metabolically labeled amebic proteins from a culture filtrate or detergent-solubilized amebas, which were then applied to an ASO affinity column. After washing, a peak of ^{35}S-methionine activity was eluted with galactose; with autoradiography, SDS-PAGE under reducing conditions demonstrated a 170-kDa metabolically labeled amebic protein (Fig. 44-5). Petri et al. confirmed that the purified amebic protein is the galactose-inhibitable lectin in three ways: (1) application of ^{35}S-methionine metabolically labeled amebic proteins to an adherence-inhibitory H8-5 antibody Affigel-10 column resulted in elution of the same protein; (2) on immunoblotting, the most adherence-inhibitory monoclonal antibody, F-14,[167] exclusively recognized the 170-kDa protein purified by ASO affinity chromatography; and (3) the lectin purified by H8-5 immunoaffinity chromatography bound to CHO cells in a galactose-specific manner and competitively inhibited adherence of viable amebas.

Subsequent studies determined that the galactose-inhibitable lectin consists of two subunits with masses of 170 kDa and 35 kDa.[197] The lectin has a mass of 260 kDa under nonreducing conditions. The 170-kDa subunit is highly antigenic and immunogenic. It contains the galactose-binding activity, as determined by recognition with adherence-inhibitory monoclonal antibodies and by the in vitro galactose-specific binding of an in vitro expressed PCR product based on 170-kDa subunit DNA.[198] The amebic genes encoding the 170-kDa subunit have been identified and sequenced,[199,200] as has the gene encoding the 35-kDa subunit.[201] The 35-kDa subunit is not antigenic and apparently exhibits fibronectin binding activity.[201] The 170-kDa subunit of the *E. histolytica* adherence lectin is the most prominent antigen immunoprecipitated by a pool of human immune sera (Fig. 44-6); immune sera from such diverse geographic regions as Mexico, India, the United States, South Africa, and Zaire all recognize this adherence protein on immunoblotting.[133,202,203]

A chitotriose-inhibitable lectin in *E. histolytica* homogenate which agglutinated erythrocytes was described by Kobiler and Mirelman.[204] In a high-ionic-strength buffer, amebic adherence to Henle cells was inhibitable by 40 percent with chitin.[205] The chitotriose-inhibitable lectin may have a role in encystation.[139] Arroyo and Orozco[206] produced monoclonal antibodies which inhibit parasite adherence and ingestion of fixed human erythrocytes by up to 60 percent and on immunoblotting recognized a 112-kDa *E. histolytica* surface protein. Carbohydrate specificity of this putative amebic adhesin is not described; apparently more than one amebic adhesin mediates adherence to erythrocytes.[135]

Cytolytic mechanisms

The pathology of invasive human amebiasis has a characteristic appearance: amebas are surrounded by amorphous granular debris, presumably due to tissue lysis.[170] Axenic *E. histolytica* trophozoites kill target cells only upon direct contact rather than via secreted cytotoxins.[127,128] Lectin-mediated adherence is required for lysis of target CHO cells, Chang liver cells, rat colonic epithelial cells, and human PMN or mononuclear cells.[128,188,191-193] Purified lectin is a cytotoxin which induces rapid reversible increases in target-cell $[Ca^{++}]_i$.[207] Amebic cytolytic activity is dependent on parasite microfilament function,[127,128] $[Ca^{++}]_i$,[207,208] Ca^{++}-dependent parasite phospholipase A (PLA) activity,[208,209] and maintenance of an acid pH in amebic endocytic vesicles.[210] Establishment of adherence by *E. histolytica* trophozoites is followed by a marked sustained elevation of target-cell $[Ca^{++}]_i$, , which contributes to but may not be totally sufficient for target-cell death.[207] Phorbol esters specifically augment amebic cytolytic activity.[211]

An 11-kDa *E. histolytica* ionophorelike *E. histolytica* protein induces lipid bilayers or vesicles of target cells to leak Na^+, K^+, and to a lesser extent Ca^{++}.[212–216] This protein, packaged in dense intracellular aggregates, can depolarize erythrocyte membranes.[214,215] The amebic ionophore apparently acts as a defense mechanism against ingested bacteria. Although it has been suggested, there is as yet no evidence that it directly participates in parasite cytolytic mechanisms. The gene encoding the ionophore has been sequenced.[216]

E. histolytica contains numerous proteolytic enzymes, including a cathepsin B protease,[217] an acidic protease,[218] a collagenase,[219] and a major neutral protease.[220] Proteases appear to be involved in dissolution of the extracellular matrix-anchoring cells and tissue structure.[220] *E. histolytica* enterotoxigenic activity[221,222] may induce a secretory diarrheal component.

In vivo models of amebic liver abscess[223,224] and in vitro studies[193] demonstrate that parasite adherence to and lysis of host polymorphonuclear leukocytes enhances tissue destruction by release of toxic neutrophil oxidative products. A further understanding of the biochemical and molecular basis for the pathogenicity of *E. histolytica* should aid in the development of a vaccine or pharmacologic strategies to combat this disease.

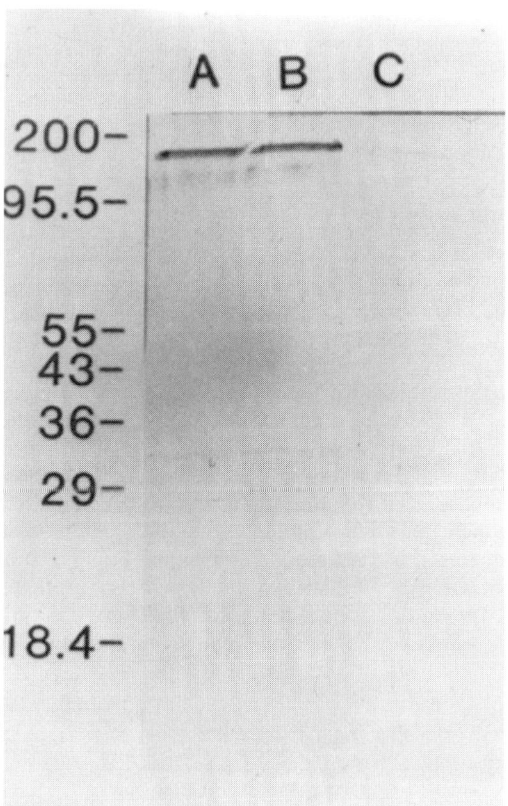

Fig. 44-5. Galactose inhibition of binding of the amebic adherence lectin to the asialoorosomucoid (ASOR) affinity column. Autoradiograph of SDS-PAGE of [^{35}S]methionine-labeled proteins eluted with galactose from an ASOR column to which conditioned medium (A), conditioned medium plus 0.5*M* dextrose (B), or conditioned medium plus 0.5*M* galactose (C) has been applied. The columns were extensively washed in 50 mM Tris, 200 mM NaCl, 10 mM $CaCl_2$, pH 7.35, and then eluted with 0.5*M* galactose in the above buffer. Galactose-eluted fractions were electrophoresed on 10% polyacrylamide gels and analyzed by autoradiography. (*From J Clin Invest 80:1238, 1987.*)

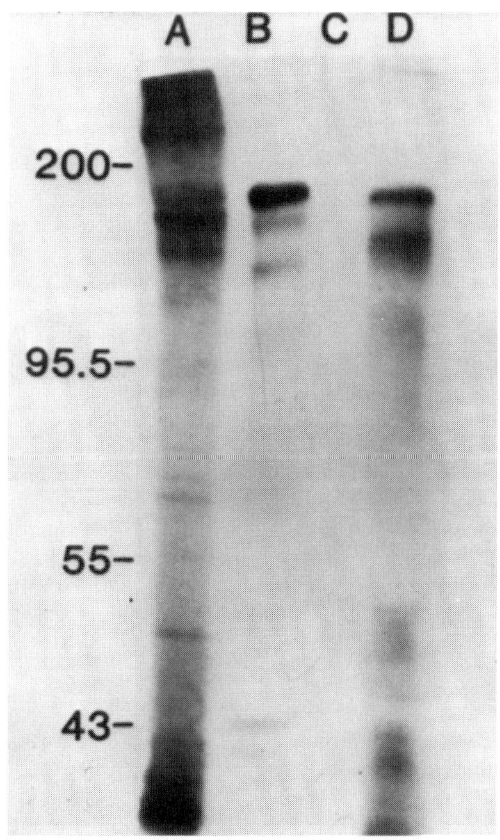

Fig. 44-6. Immunoprecipitation of [^{35}S]methionine metabolically labeled amebic protein with H8-5 and pooled human immune sera (PHIS). Autoradiograph of SDS-PAGE (10% acrylamide separating gel) of [^{35}S]methionine-labeled amebic proteins (A), immunoprecipitated with monoclonal antibody H8-5 (B), normal human serum (C), or PHIS (D). A 170-kilodalton metabolically labeled amebic protein was immunoprecipitated by lectin-specific H8-5 and PHIS and is the most intensively labeled antigen recognized by PHIS. (*From Infect Immun 55:2327, 1987.*)

DIAGNOSIS

Stool and proctoscopic examination

The key to laboratory diagnosis of colonic amebiasis is the stool examination. Three stool specimens or one purged specimen should be examined for maximum yield prior to use of barium, antacids, enemas, or antimicrobial or antiparasitic agents, which will interfere with the microscopic examination.[225,226] If fecal specimens cannot be examined immediately, they should be refrigerated or fixed. Trophozoites in stool will rapidly lyse at room temperature or at 37°C. A saline wet mount should first be examined to establish the presence of amebic trophozoites or cysts. Differentiation of *Entamoeba* species requires permanent stains (trichrome or iron-hematoxylin) following fixation in 10% formalin or polyvinyl alcohol to reveal characteristic nuclear morphology, as described above (see Figs. 44-3 and 44-4; Plate 67). The most common error in diagnosis is mistaking fecal leukocytes or macrophages for amebic trophozoites.[104] Of note, fecal leukocytes are usually pyknotic or absent in patients with amebic colitis, in contrast to patients with bacterial dysentery, possibly because of the direct toxic effect of amebas on leukocytes.[129,131,170]

The stool examination is positive in approximately 90 percent of patients with invasive amebic colitis[227]; however, if the stool examination is negative in a suspected case of amebic colitis, proctoscopy or colonoscopy is indicated.[228,229] The margin of a colonic ulcer should be scraped (not swabbed, as amebic trophozoites may adhere to cotton swabs) and appropriate stains made of the scraping material, which often shows the parasite. If tissue is obtained, a careful search for invading trophozoites should be made on routine hematoxylin and eosin (H&E)- and periodic acid–Schiff (PAS)-stained material.

In vitro cultivation

E. histolytica can be cultured from clinical specimens. Numerous culture media have been used, including liver extract (Cleveland and Collier), egg-infusion medium (Balamuth), and alcohol-egg extract of Nelson.[230] However, none is selective for *E. histolytica*. Both cysts and trophozoites can be cultured, a technique which can help differentiate *E. histolytica* from *E. coli, E. hartmanni*, and the Laredo strain of *E. histolytica*. Cleveland and Collier's medium can be made more selective by adding rice powder and antibiotics (penicillin and streptomycin).[118] Failure of the culture to grow at low temperatures excludes the Laredo-like strain, which grows well at 23°C.[118] These methods can be used to document amebiasis in patients. Zymodeme determination using starch gel electrophoresis of in vitro cultivates can be utilized to differentiate *E. dispar* from *E. histolytica*. However, this is a laborious technique that is available only in research laboratories.

Serology

Numerous techniques have been developed for study of the serologic response to *E. histolytica* infection (Table 44-3). All methods are highly specific; patients without exposure to *E. histolytica* are rarely positive. These tests are usually quite sensitive for detection of patients with amebic liver abscess or invasive colitis; *E. dispar* infection does not elicit a serum antiamebic antibody response, whereas asymptomatic *E. histolytica* infections do. Therefore, a negative serology is quite helpful in ruling out *E. histolytica* infection in an endemic area.[108,109] The indirect hemagglutination test (IHA) is the most widely used method at present in the United States.[149,231,232] The IHA uses antigen prepared from axenic cultures of *E. histolytica* (usually strain HK9). Serum is heat-inactivated and added in serial dilutions to sheep or human red blood cells sensitized with amebic antigens; hemagglutination is evaluated in comparison with known positive and negative controls.[233] IHA titers are usually elevated at the time of initial presentation with invasive amebiasis, often to titers of ≥1:1024,[231] and then fall to lower levels 2 to 11 years after therapy.[149,231,232]

When repeated exposure or persistent infection renders the IHA less useful,[232] the gel diffusion precipitin test, which remains positive for shorter periods following acute illness (6 months), may be helpful.[232] Serologic testing for amebiasis should be considered and may be quite helpful in differentiating inflammatory bowel disease from amebic colitis. Fewer than 2 percent of patients with inflammatory bowel disease and negative stool examinations for amebas have positive IHA titers.[231–233] Because of the widespread occurrence of amebiasis, patients in whom the diagnosis of inflammatory bowel disease is considered should have sera tested and stools examined for amebic infection, especially before steroid therapy is considered.

TREATMENT

At present, drug susceptibility of *E. histolytica* is based on clinical activity and nonquantitative observations. Quantitative, clonal growth of *E. histolytica* provides a method for drug evaluation that can be standardized for static and amebicidal activities.[234,235] Appropriate drug therapy of amebiasis must take into account drug distribution (absorption, penetration, excretion in the intestinal tract) and sites of amebicidal activity. For example, antibiotics are usually active only in colonic and not in hepatic disease. Drugs that are active in all tissues include metronidazole, tinidazole, dehydroemetine, and emetine hydrochloride.[227,236–238] Agents which may help eradicate gut luminal infection include diloxanide furoate, paromonycin, bismuth iodide, and diiodohydroxyquin.[228,238,239] Tetracycline and erythromycin have some activity in colonic disease and chloroquine may be active in hepatic disease.[227] Recommended drug regimens, including

Table 44-3. Systems in Use to Evaluate Serologic Response to Infection with *E. histolytica*

	Percent positive in			
Serologic test	Controls	Cyst passes	Rectocolitis	Liver abscess
Indirect hemagglutination	0–7	8–15	81–98	83–100
Indirect immunofluorescence			57	57
Countercurrent immunoelectrophoresis	0–1.7		87	95–100
Agar gel diffusion	0–18	1–52	55–95	80–100
Enzyme-linked immunosorbent assay (ELISA)		50		100
Complement fixation	0–16	28	85–90	83–100
Cellulose acetate membrane precipitation	0		100	
Immunoelectrophoresis			87	93
Latex agglutination	0		75	100
Thin layer immunoassay				79

dosages and possible adverse reactions, are outlined in Table 44-4.

PREVENTION AND BIOLOGICAL CONTROL

At present, prevention of amebiasis rests on interference with fecal-oral transmission by improved hygiene, sanitation, and water treatment; by abstaining from oral-anal-genital contact; and by proper isolation of index cases.[240] Numerous tantalizing but unexplored possibilities for biological control also exist. One approach would be to prevent commensal carriage in the human host; another, disregarding carriage, would be aimed at altering the parasite or host to avoid tissue invasion. Systemic and especially local intestinal immunity for alterations in microbial flora might well alter the parasite's carriage and shedding or its invasiveness. Recent isolation of the *E. histolytica* Gal/GalNAc adherence lectin and characterization of *E. histolytica* antigens further suggest the feasibility of vaccine development.

Certainly giardiasis and amebiasis rank among the widespread, often devastating human diseases for which the current renaissance of immunobiologic research holds great promise of many exciting developments. The groundwork that has been laid has already resulted in improved understanding of the biology of the giardia protozoa and amebas through in vitro culture and animal models. We now stand at the threshold of greatly improved understanding of the pathogenesis and, hopefully, eventual control of these two protozoan enteric parasitic infections.

CRYPTOSPORIDIUM

INTRODUCTION AND HISTORY

Organisms of the genus of *Cryptosporidium* are small (2 to 6 μm) coccidian protozoans that may inhabit the gastrointestinal, respiratory, and biliary tracts of a variety of animals including humans. In 1907, Tyzzer first described this parasite as a cause of asymptomatic infection in the gastric glands of the common laboratory mouse.[241] In 1955, Slavin reported the first case of symptomatic diarrheal disease in poultry due to *Cryptosporidium*.[242] The parasite was subsequently demonstrated to be a pathogen of many animals and to cause epidemics of diarrheal disease. However, the first instance of symptomatic human disease was recorded in 1976 in a young immunocompetent child.[243]

Human infection with *Cryptosporidium* was considered rare prior to 1982, the result of opportunistic infection with a pathogen outside its normal host range. With the recognition of AIDS in the early 1980s, an increasing number of cases of severe cryptosporidiosis were reported.[244] In 1983, an outbreak of symptomatic cryptosporidiosis among animal handlers stimulated clinical interest leading to the recognition of this parasite as an important diarrheal pathogen in the immunocompetent host.[245] Numerous waterborne and swimming pool outbreaks have since occurred, culminating in 1993 in the largest waterborne outbreak in U.S. history, involving over 400,000 people in Milwaukee. These outbreaks, along with studies in developing areas, have placed cryptosporidiosis among the leading causes of diarrhea worldwide.[246–250]

PATHOGENESIS

Historically, *Cryptosporidium* was assumed to be host-specific, similar to another coccidian parasite, *Eimeria*. Although the exact number of distinct species of *Cryptosporidium* is debated, recent studies indicate a limited number of valid species that can be distinguished by size, life-cycle characteristics, ability to transmit infection between animals (e.g., mammal to mammal vs. mammal to poultry), and chromosome pattern.[251–256] The primary mammalian species causing diarrheal disease is *Cryptosporidium parvum*.[252] A second species, infecting the stomach of mammals, is named *C. muris*.[241] Other apparent species include *C. baileyi* and *C. meleagridis* infecting poultry, as well as unnamed species infecting quail, guinea pigs, and possibly fish and reptiles.

Disease among animal hosts includes diarrhea in large mammals such as calves, piglets, lambs, foals, and goats; intestinal and respiratory disease in poultry; and asymptomatic carriage in most rodents. Persistent infection associated with diarrhea has been reported in nude (nu/nu) BALB/c mice infected at 6 days of age; when the mice were inoculated at 42 days of age, only asymptomatic infection developed.[257] These observations and the fact that AIDS patients manifest severe symptomatic disease suggest that T lymphocytes, particularly the T-helper subset, are important in recovery from infection and the development of protective immunity.[258] In general, young animals are more susceptible to infection, possibly because innate resistance develops or specific protective immunity is acquired as the animal matures. Experimentally, diarrheal disease develops in gnotobiotic animals monoinfected with *Cryptosporidium*, indicating that this parasite is a primary enteric pathogen.[259,260]

The life cycle of *Cryptosporidium* is similar to that of other coccidia (Fig. 44-7).[253,261] Infection is initiated when the host accidentally ingests oocysts. Although the infectious dose for many animal species is not clear, inoculation of 100 to 500 oocysts causes infection in 50 percent of Swiss-Webster mice.[262] A report of a researcher who acquired infection after a rabbit inoculated with *Cryptosporidium* coughed on him suggests that the infectious dose is also low in humans.[263] Indeed, studies in human volunteers demonstrate an estimated ID_{50} is 132 oocysts,[264] and some have estimated from mathematical modeling in the Milwaukee outbreak that the infectious dose may be as low as one oocyst for some individuals.[246,265]

The asexual cycle of *Cryptosporidium* is initiated when gastric acid and proteolytic enzymes in the upper small bowel cause the oocyst wall to dissolve at its single suture, resulting in a slitlike opening from which the four sporozoites can exit the oocyst.[266] The sporozoites are able to penetrate and parasitize the intestinal epithelial cells and potentially other epithelial surfaces contiguous to the gastrointestinal tract, such as respiratory or biliary tract epithelium. Within the host cells, sporozoites develop into trophozoites and subsequently into type I meronts. The type I meront releases six to eight merozoites capable of reinfecting the host epithelial cell. Some of these merozoites develop into type II meronts containing four merozoites. The merozoites released by type II meronts initiate the sexual cycle with the development of macrogamonts and microgamonts. Microgamonts are aflagellar but motile and fertilize macrogamonts, resulting in immature oocysts that develop within the intestinal epithelial cell. Oocysts released from the host epithelial cell are either thin- or thick-walled and immediately able to initiate infection (that is, fully sporulated). Thin-walled oocysts may excyst within the bowel, releasing sporozoites which reinfect the host epithelial cells. Thick-walled oocysts are excreted by the host and are known to be extremely hardy.

Thus, autoinfection of the host can occur due to either type I meronts or thin-walled oocysts. This may account for the ability of *Cryptosporidium* to cause sustained symptomatic infections in the immunocompromised host, potentially lasting for the life of the individual.[261]

In general, the pathogenesis of *Cryptosporidium* infections is poorly understood. In humans, detailed studies of intestinal histopathology and function are provided only by case reports of

Table 44-4. Treatment of *E. histolytic* Infections

Condition and drug	Dose and duration	Cure rate	Adverse reactions
Cyst passage			
Diloxanide furoate (obtain from CDC)	500 mg tid for 10 days	87–96%	Mild gastrointestinal upset (uncommon).
Diiodohydroxyquin (followed by tetracycline)	650 mg tid for 20 days	95%	Subacute optic neuropathy, dermatitis, diarrhea, headache. Avoid if hepatic disease or iodine intolerance present.
Paromomycin	300 mg/kg per day for 5–10 days	80–90%	Gastrointestinal upset.
Invasive colitis			
Metronidazole*	750 mg tid for 10 days 750 mg tid for 5 days† 2.4 g qd for 2–3 days† 50 mg/kg for 1 dose†	>90% >90% >90%	10–20% Gastrointestinal upset (less with divided dosage), disulfiram effect, bitter taste, seizures, possible carcinogenesis.
Tetracycline	250 mg qd for 14 days†	90%	Gastrointestinal upset, hepatotoxicity, fungal suprainfection, teeth discoloration.
Dehydroemetine	1–1.5 mg/kg per day IM for 5 days†	80–90%	25–50% Cardiotoxicity (tachycardia, hypotension, angina, electrocardiograph changes), neuromuscular (tremor, muscle tenderness, and weakness), gastrointestinal.
Liver abscess‡			
Metronidazole	750 mg tid for 5–10 days† or 2.4 g qd for 1–2 days†	99%	See above.
Dehydroemetine (followed by chloroquine)	1–1.5 mg/kg per day for 5 days† (600 mg qd for 2 days)	90% (60% Alone)	See above. Gastrointestinal upset, headache, pruritus.

* Alternate therapies to metronidazole with possibly less toxicity, but which are unavailable in the United States, include the following drugs: tinidazole, 50 mg/kg per day for 3 days (plus lumenal agent from the therapy for cyst passage), and tiberal, 15–30 mg/kg per day for 5 days (plus lumenal agent from the therapy for cyst passage).

† Plus lumenal agent from the therapy for cyst passage.

‡ Aspiration of abscess not necessary for cure, but in experienced hands it may decrease symptoms and recovery time. The only absolute indication is a lack of response or worsening while the patient is on medical therapy for 3–5 days.

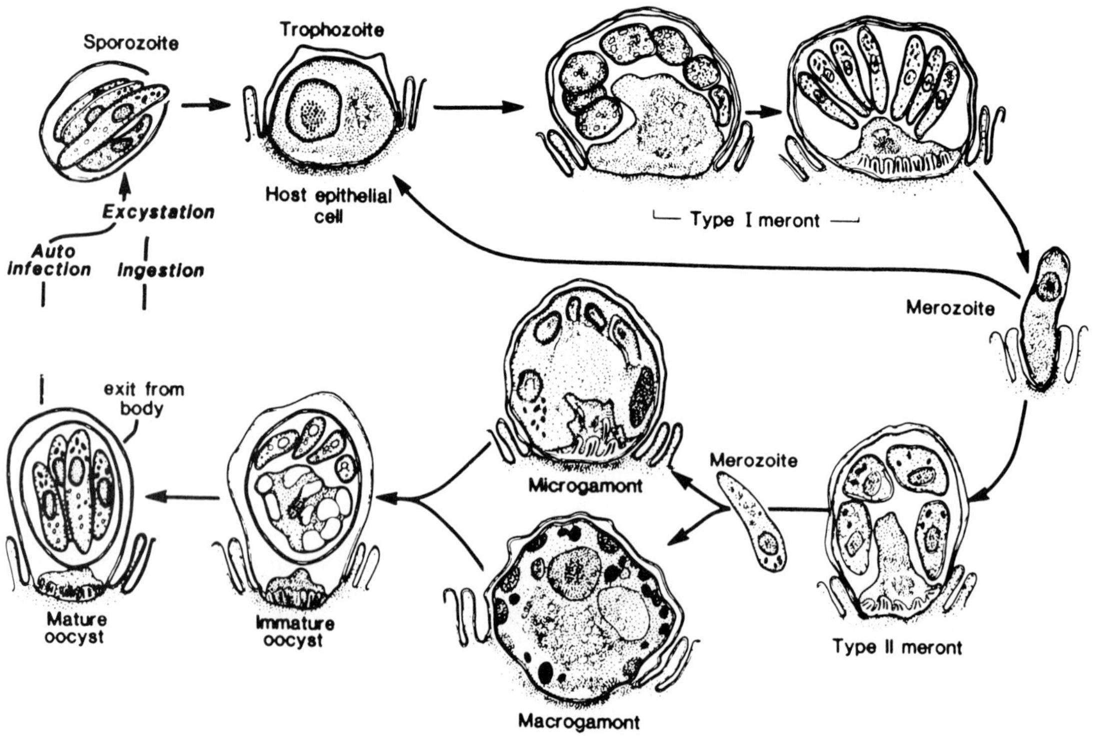

Fig. 44-7. Diagrammatic representation of the life cycle of *Cryptosporidium*. Sporozoites excyst from an oocyst and enter the microvillus of an epithelial cell, where they differentiate into trophozoites. Trophozoites undergo nuclear proliferation to form type I meronts. A merozoite leaves the type I meront to form either a type I or II meront. A merozoite leaves the type II meront to form microgamonts or a macrogamont. The microgamont fertilizes the macrogamont, which then develops into an oocyst. Oocysts sporulate in situ and either release sporozoites for autoinfection or pass from the body in the feces. (*From R Fayer, BLP Ungar, Microbiol Rev 50:458, 1986.*)

immunocompromised patients, primarily with the acquired immunodeficiency syndrome. Ultrastructural studies generally show that the intestinal mucosa are intact and the enterocytes well preserved.[268,269] Microvilli are displaced at the sites of parasite attachment to the enterocyte surface, and they may be elongated next to the parasite. In addition, "peaking" of the host-cell cytoplasm may occur at the point of attachment of the cryptosporidia.[267,268] In some infections, villous architecture by light microscopy is moderately to severely abnormal, revealing crypt elongation and villous atrophy.[270,271] However, significant diarrhea (≥1L/day) may occur with minimal histopathologic change in the gut.[269] The degree and cell content of the inflammatory infiltrate in the lamina propria of gut infected with *Cryptosporidium* in clinically affected patients has ranged from minimal[272] to substantial[269–271] and may include plasma cells, lymphocytes, macrophages, and/or polymorphonuclear leukocytes. One limitation of these human case reports is that it is often not clear how extensively the patients were evaluated for additional enteropathogens.

In animal studies the degree of pathologic abnormality has tended to correlate with the extent of infection and in some animals, including calves, lambs, and piglets, with the severity of clinical illness.[258,260,273,274] In rodents such as mice, rats, and guinea pigs, no obvious clinical illness occurs, and pathologic findings range from inapparent to moderate.[274,275] In studies of spontaneously infested guinea pigs, cryptosporidial organisms have been observed deep in the cytoplasm of M cells overlying Peyer's patches and associated with macrophages subjacent to the M cells. These observations suggest antigenic sampling by the intestinal immune system.[276]

The mechanisms by which *Cryptosporidium* causes diarrhea in either the immunocompetent or the immunocompromised host have not yet been elucidated. Both secretory (unaffected by fasting) and malabsorptive diarrhea have been reported in AIDS patients infected with *Cryptosporidium*.[269,277,278] D-xylose and vitamin B_{12} malabsorption, steatorrhea, and increased fecal alpha$_1$-antitrypsin clearance have been reported.[269,271,277,278] Radiographic studies have also showed results consistent with malabsorption, such as flocculation of the barium, mucosal thickening, and dilation in the small bowel.[279] Animal studies have confirmed lactase deficiency and xylose malabsorption in calves infected with *Cryptosporidium*.[258,273]

Detailed electron micrograph studies indicate that *Cryptosporidium* develops intracellularly in the host epithelial cell but is extracytoplasmic.[253,267] A striking electron-dense zone described as a "feeder organelle" forms at the interface between the parasite and the host cell.[253,267] It may be through this zone that the parasite receives nutrition and delivers products capable of stimulating intestinal secretion. The observation that voluminous, watery diarrhea may occur in the immunocompromised host might suggest production of an enterotoxin or neurohumoral products by the parasite. Experimental results to date are mixed.[280–282] Reports of enterotoxic effects do not distinguish the source of potential secretory products.[283,284] Indeed, Argenzio et al. suggest that the cytokines (such as tumor necrosis factor {TNF}) and macrophages seen in cryptosporidiosis may elicit prostaglandin-dependent secretion, possibly via secondary cells such as fibroblasts.[285,286] Studies in humans with cryptosporidiosis show villus tip damage and malabsorption.[287]

CLINICAL MANIFESTATIONS

Infection with *Cryptosporidium* has been documented in both immunocompetent and immunocompromised patient populations.[245,255,272,273,281,288,289] In immunocompetent hosts the majority of cases are sporadic and may involve either children or adults, in both the developed and developing world.[288] Infection has also been reported in animal handlers,[245,255] homosexual men,[271] travelers,[290,291] and contacts of infected individuals (for example, household contacts or hospital personnel).[255,289,292,293]

The clinical manifestations of cryptosporidiosis depend on the immune status of the host. In the immunocompetent host, infection results in a flulike, noninflammatory gastrointestinal illness characterized by malaise, anorexia, vomiting, abdominal pain and cramps, and sometimes fever. Blood and pus are not present in the stool and the fecal leukocyte examination is negative. Diarrhea lasts on average 6 to 14 days, although some patients will have a more prolonged illness, with diarrhea lasting a month or even, rarely, as long as 4 months.[272,289,294–296]

Diarrhea may occasionally be much more severe (for example, 17 liters of daily stool output) in immunocompromised hosts with defects in either humoral or cell-mediated immunity.[244,255,297] In these hosts, infection is frequently persistent and the resulting morbidity—for instance, in AIDS patients—may contribute to earlier mortality.[298] AIDS patients have been reported to develop extraintestinal infection involving the respiratory or biliary epithelium.[272,299–304] Although the contribution of respiratory cryptosporidiosis to clinical disease is unclear, individuals with biliary infection may present with the clinical picture of cholecystitis and may also be coinfected with cytomegalovirus.[272,304]

The incubation period of the infection is usually between 3 and 14 days.[255] Experimental data show that the parasite can complete its developmental cycle in 3 days.[261] Until recently, asymptomatic carriage of the oocysts in clinically unaffected populations has been thought to be infrequent. For instance, in three studies examining predominantly asymptomatic homosexual men attending sexually transmitted diseases clinics during the early 1980s, none of 375 individuals were found to have *Cryptosporidium* oocysts in their stools. In contrast, *Giardia lamblia* was found in 3.3 to 6.5 percent and *Entamoeba disbar* in 5.5 to 23.5 percent of the men.[305–307] In studies examining the prevalence of infection with *Cryptosporidium* in developed countries such as the United States, Australia, or Europe, rates of infection in situations other than outbreaks average 2.1 percent in symptomatic individuals (range = 0.26–22 percent).[249] Among controls, only 0.2 percent of stools were positive.[249,250] In contrast, infection rates have been highest in developing countries, with rates of 6.1 percent in individuals with symptoms (range 1.4–40.9 percent) and 1.5 percent in controls.[249,250,308–310] Persistent asymptomatic oocyst excretion may extend beyond clinical illness.[294,295,311–313] Oocyst excretion lasts an average of 7 days beyond illness but may, on occasion, extend for several weeks.[294,295]

Several potential modes of transmission for *Cryptosporidium* have been identified. Earlier studies documented the potential for animal-to-human spread, and *Cryptosporidium* is clearly a zoonotic infection.[245,255,272,288,297] Both domestic animals such as calves and companion animals such as puppies and kittens serve as potential sources of human infection. Increasing evidence indicates that person-to-person spread of this infection is important and is probably a major mode of transmission.[255,272,288,289,293] Since large numbers of *Cryptosporidium* oocysts can be present in feces and the infectious dose is quite small, it is very likely that fecal-oral contamination through sexual contact could play an important role in transmission.

Human-to-human transmission is particularly well illustrated by the reports of outbreaks of diarrhea associated with *Cryptosporidium* infection in day care centers,[295,314,315] and by reports of intrafamilial spread of infection in households showing that they are among the highest for any enteric pathogen.[247] In addition, waterborne outbreaks traced to surface water[316] or to sewage contamination of both chlorinated well water and fully treated municipal water have been reported.[246,317,318] *Cryptosporidium* oocysts have been identified in treated sewage effluents and surface waters, and several outbreaks have occurred with public swimming or wading pool exposure.[319,320] Unpasteurized apple cider has also been a source of *Cryptosporidium* infection.

Because the clinical syndrome associated with cryptosporidiosis is not unique, the differential diagnosis includes the extensive list of enteric pathogens which cause noninflammatory diarrhea. Rotaviruses and enterotoxigenic *Escherichia coli* are the leading causes of acute noninflammatory diarrhea worldwide, especially among young children; Norwalk-like viruses must also be considered. In immunocompromised individuals such as AIDS and bone marrow transplant patients, adenoviruses and coxsackieviruses may cause diarrhea.[321] The diagnosis of *Cryptosporidium* infection is especially important in patients with AIDS, as is the diagnosis of even more treatable causes of diarrhea in this setting. These causes include microsporidiosis and *Cyclospora* infection (described under "New and Emerging Protozoal Infections," below), as well as *Giardia lamblia*, *Strongyloides stercoralis*, and *Isospora belli,* all potential parasitic causes of noninflammatory diarrhea. Epidemiologic data such as travel history, food ingestion (for example, raw seafood), and recent antibiotic use may be helpful in prioritizing the diagnostic possibilities.[322] Cryptosporidiosis causes a substantial mortality (>30 percent) in HIV-infected patients with low CD4 counts, especially when the biliary tract is involved.[318,323]

DIAGNOSIS

The diagnosis of cryptosporidiosis is established by staining the stool with a modified acid-fast or immunofluorescence technique specific for the oocyst stage of *Cryptosporidium* and observing the characteristic oocyst morphology (Fig. 44-8). Examination of at least two fecal smears may be necessary for diagnosis,[294,324] and concentrating the stool may improve detection of the parasite, particularly in nonacute illness or in evaluation of contacts of infected individuals. Oocyst excretion may be intermittent; positive and negative smears from the same patient on the same day have been reported. In addition, a minority of the oocysts may not readily take up the acid-fast stain and may appear as empty holes in a fecal smear.[325] This variability in the staining characteristics of the oocysts does not hinder diagnosis in experienced hands.

A direct immunofluorescent antibody stain is sensitive and specific and may require less technician time.[324,326,327] Several enzyme-linked immunosorbent assay (ELISA) methods are available for detection of fecal cryptosporidial antigen; these are 83 to 95 percent sensitive in diarrheal specimens but may miss lighter infections or asymptomatic carriage.[324,328] ELISAs for detection of serum IgM and IgG antibodies to *Cryptosporidium* have been developed[329]; when both these tests were used, over 90 percent of the patients with cryptosporidiosis, including patients with AIDS, had detectable antibodies at the time of medical presentation. These ELISAs for detection of immunoglobulins should prove to be particularly helpful in epidemiologic studies of cryptosporidiosis.

PREVENTION OF INFECTION AND THERAPY

The primary therapy for all forms of diarrheal illness, including cryptosporidiosis, is fluid and electrolyte replacement. Rehydration may be oral or intravenous, depending on the clinical status and age of the patient. In studies to date, from 0 to 30 percent of immunocompetent patients have required hospital admission for intravenous rehydration during *Cryptosporidium* infections.[255,289,330–332] Although many drugs have been evaluated in animals or humans, no clearly effective pharmacologic therapy for cryptosporidiosis has emerged.[255,272,297,333–336] Paromomycin has shown modest benefit in a controlled study, but it fails to eradicate the parasite in immunocompromised patients.[337] Development of an effective specific therapy for cryptosporidiosis has been hindered by the lack of a simple model for testing of drug sensitivity. Although nonspecific antidiarrheal therapies such as kaolin plus pectin (Kaopectate), antimotility agents (loperamide, paregoric), or bismuth subsalicylate (Pepto-Bismol) may be helpful in controlling symptoms, their efficacy and safety in cryptosporidiosis have not been evaluated.

The thick-walled oocysts of *Cryptosporidium* are known to be very hardy and resistant to chlorine and numerous tested disinfectants. Only heat (boiling for 1 minute, at sea level), freezing,

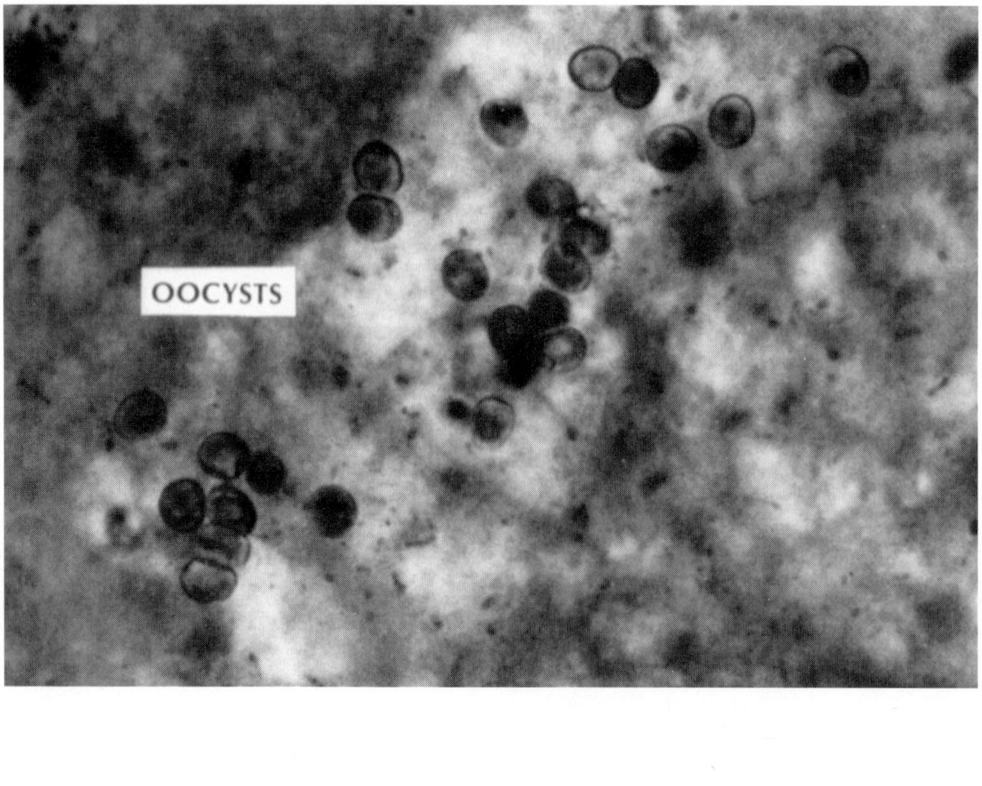

Fig. 44-8. *Cryptosporidium* oocysts stained with a modified acid-fast stain. Oocysts are approximately 4 to 6 μm in diameter.

and prolonged treatment (18 hours) with 10% formalin or 5% ammonia, have been shown experimentally to reduce the infectivity of the oocysts.[273,338,339] Therefore, careful hand washing and enteric precautions in the hospital setting are important to interrupt person-to-person spread of infection. Current USPHS/IDSA guidelines for prevention of opportunistic infections in HIV infected persons include avoidance of fecal exposure during sexual contact; careful hygiene, including hand washing in handling pets and avoidance of new pets under 6 months of age; precaution concerning exposure during travel; and possible boiling or filtering of drinking water.[339a] Future research to better understand the ecologic niches of this parasite will be important in the development of measures to control the spread of infection.

NEW AND EMERGING PROTOZOAL INFECTIONS

In addition to *G. lamblia, E. histolytica,* and *C. parvum,* additional intestinal protozoan infections are increasingly recognized. *Cyclospora cayetenensis* appears to be spread in contaminated water and is a potentially treatable cause of diarrhea in both normal hosts and in patients with AIDS.[340,341] Cyclospora infections are diagnosed with acid-fast stain of fecal specimens and are treated with sulfamethoxazole-trimethoprim.[342–346]

Microsporidial infections with *Enterocytozoon bienusi* or *Encephalitozoon* (formerly *Septata*) *intestinalis* are found predominantly in patients with AIDS and diarrhea and can be diagnosed with a special trichrome stain of fecal specimens.[347,348] However, their epidemiology and routes of transmission remain largely unknown. Importantly, these infections, especially *Encephalitozoon (Septata) intestinalis,* appear to respond to albendazole therapy.[349–351]

References

1 Leeuwenhoek AV: Letter no. 66 to the Royal Society, in *Tropical Medicine and Parasitology, Classic Investigations,* 1, BH Kean et al (eds). Ithaca, Cornell University Press. 1978, pp 4–5.

2 Monat HA, McKinney WL: Giardiasis: Question of pathogenicity. *US Naval Med Bull* 46:1204, 1946.

3 Ormiston G et al: Enteritis in a nursery home associated with *Giardia lamblia. Br Med J* 2:151, 1942.

4 Davis C, Ritdric LS: Clinical manifestations and treatment of epidemic amebiasis occurring in occupants of Mantetsu apartment building, Tokyo, Japan. *Am J Trop Med Hyg* 28:803, 1948.

5 Antia FP et al: Giardiasis in adults: Incidence, symptomatology and absorption studies. *Indian J Med Sci* 20:471, 1966.

6 Cortner JA: Giardiasis: A cause of celiac syndrome. *Am J Dis Child* 98:311, 1959.

7 Brandborg LL et al: Histological demonstration of mucosal invasion by *Giardia lamblia* in man. *Gastroenterology* 52:143, 1967.

8 Rendtorff R: The experimental transmission of human intestinal protozoan parasites: II. *Giardia lamblia* cysts given in capsules. *Am J Hyg* 59:209, 1954.

9 Petersen H: Giardiasis (lambliasis). *Scand J Gastroenterol* 7 (suppl 14):1, 1972.

10 Centers for Disease Control: Intestinal parasite surveillance; United States, 1976. *MMWR* 27:167, 1978.

11 Meuwissen JHE et al: Giardiasis. *Lancet* 2:32, 1977.

12 Court JM, Stanton C: The incidence of *Giardia lamblia* infestation of children in Victoria. *Med J Aust* 2:438, 1959.

13 Knight R: Epidemiology and transmission of giardiasis. *Trans R Soc Trop Med Hyg* 74:433, 1980.

14 Black RE et al: Giardiasis in day-care centers: Evidence of person-to-person transmission. *Pediatrics* 60:486, 1977.

15 Osterholm MT et al: An outbreak of food-borne giardiasis. *N Engl J Med* 304:24, 1981.

16 Craun GF: Waterborne giardiasis in the United States: A review. *Am J Public Health* 69:817, 1979.

17 Shaw PK et al: A communitywide outbreak of giardiasis with evidence of transmission by a municipal water supply. *Ann Intern Med* 87:426, 1977.

18 Wright RA et al: Giardiasis in Colorado: An epidemiologic study. *Am J Epidemiol* 105:330, 1977.

19 Brodsky RE et al: Giardiasis in American travelers to the Soviet Union. *J Infect Dis* 130:319, 1974.

20 Rendtorff RC, Holt CJ: The experimental transmission of human intestinal protozoan parasites: IV. Attempts to transmit *Entamoeba coli* and *Giardia lamblia* cysts by water. *Am J Hyg* 60:327, 1954.

21 Meyers JD et al: *Giardia lamblia* infection in homosexual men. *Br J Vener Dis* 53:54, 1977.

22 Schmerin MJ et al: Giardiasis: Association with homosexuality. *Ann Intern Med* 88:801, 1978.

22a Owen RL: Direct fecal-oral transmission of giardiasis, in *Giardia and giardiasis,* SL Erlandsen, EA Meyer (eds). New York, Plenum Press. 1984, pp 329–339.

23 Jokipii AMM, Jokipii L: Prepatency of giardiasis. *Lancet* 1:1095, 1977.

24 Cain GD et al: Malabsorption associated with *Giardia lamblia* infestation. *South Med J* 61:532, 1968.

25 Wolfe MS: Giardiasis. *JAMA* 233:1362, 1975.

26 Hartong WA et al: Giardiasis: Clinical spectrum and functional-structural abnormalities of the small intestinal mucosa. *Gastroenterology* 77:61, 1979.

27 Zinneman HH, Kaplan AP: The association of giardiasis with reduced intestinal secretory immunoglobulin. *Am J Dig Dis* 17:793, 1972.

28 Mayoral LG et al: Intestinal malabsorption and parasitic disease: The role of protein malnutrition. *Gastroenterology* 50:856, 1966.

29 Tandon BN et al: Mechanism of malabsorption of giardiasis: A study of bacterial flora and bile salt deconjugation in upper jejunum. *Gut* 18:176, 1977.

30 Tompkins AM et al: Bacterial colonization of jejunal mucosa in giardiasis. *Trans R Soc Trop Med Hyg* 72:32, 1978.

31 Sheehy TW, Holley P: *Giardia*-induced malabsorption in pancreatitis. *JAMA* 233:1373, 1975.

32 Kacker PP: A case of *Giardia lamblia* proctitis presenting in a VD clinic. *Br J Vener Dis* 49:318, 1973.

33 Goobar JP: Joint symptoms in giardiasis. *Lancet* 1:1010, 1977.

34 Harris RH, Mitchell JH: Chronic urticaria due to *Giardia lamblia. Arch Dermatol Syphilol* 59:587, 1949.

35 Meyer EA, Radulescu S: *Giardia* and giardiasis. *Adv Parasitol* 17.1, 1979.

36 Tsuchiya H: Changes in morphology of *Giardia canis* as affected by diet. *Proc Soc Exp Biol Med* 28:708, 1931.

37 Owen RL: The ultrastructural basis of *Giardia* function. *Trans R Soc Trop Med Hyg* 74:429, 1980.

38 Holberton DV: Attachment of *Giardia:* A hydrodynamic model. *J Exp Biol* 60:207, 1974.

39 Owen RL: The immune response in clinical and experimental giardiasis. *Trans R Soc Trop Med Hyg* 74:443, 1980.

40 Nemanic PC et al: Ultrastructural observations on giardiasis in a mouse model: II. Endosymbiosis and organelle distribution in *Giardia muris* and comparison with *Giardia lamblia. J Infect Dis* 140:222, 1979.

41 Hill DR et al: Lectin binding by *Giardia lamblia. Infect Immun* 34:733, 1981.

42 Lev B et al: Lectin activation in *Giardia lamblia* by host protease: A novel host-parasite interaction. *Science* 232:71, 1986.

43 Bertram MA et al: A comparison of isozymes of five axenic *Giardia* isolates. *J Parasitol* 69:793, 1983.

44 Smith PD et al: Antigenic analysis of *Giardia lamblia* from Afghanistan, Puerto Rico, Ecuador, and Oregon. *Infect Immun* 36:714, 1982.

45 Nash TE, Keister DB: Differences in excretory-secretory products and surface antigens among 19 isolates of *Giardia. J Infect Dis* 152:1166, 1985.

46 Nash TE et al: Restriction-endonuclease analysis of DNA from 15 *Giardia* isolates obtained from humans and animals. *J Infect Dis* 152: 62, 1985.

47 Wang AL, Wang CC: Discovery of a specific double-stranded RNA virus in *Giardia lamblia. Mol Biochem Parasitol* 21:269, 1986.

48 Adam RD et al: Antigenic variation of a cysteine-rich protein in *Giardia lamblia. J Exp Med* 167:109, 1988.

48a Nash T: Surface antigen variability and variation in *Giardia lamblia. Parasitol Today* 8:229–34, 1992.

49 Gillin FD et al: Encystation and expression of cyst antigens by *Giardia lamblia* in vitro. *Science* 135:1040, 1987.

50 Bingham AK, Meyer EA: *Giardia* excystation can be induced in vitro in acidic solutions. *Nature* 277:301, 1979.

51 Meyer EA: *Giardia lamblia:* Isolation and axenic cultivation. *Exp Parasitol* 39:101, 1976.

52 Visvesvara GS: Axenic growth of *Giardia lamblia* in Diamond's TPS-1 medium. *Trans R Soc Trop Med Hyg* 74:213, 1980.

53 Keister DB: Axenic culture of *Giardia lamblia* in TYI-S-33 medium supplemented with bile. *Trop Med Hyg* 487:77, 1983.

54 Gillin FD et al: Binary lipids support serum-free growth of *Giardia lamblia. Am Soc Microbiol* 641:53, 1986.

55 Lindmark DG: Energy metabolism of the anaerobic protozoon *Giardia lamblia. Mol Biochem Parasitol* 1:1, 1980.

56 Wright RA, Vernon TM: Epidemic giardiasis at a resort lodge. *Rocky Mountains Med J* 73:208, 1976.

57 Roberts-Thomson IC et al: Acquired resistance to infection in an animal model of giardiasis. *J Immunol* 117:2036, 1976.

58 Thompson A et al: Immunoglobulin-bearing cells in giardiasis. *J Clin Pathol* 30:292, 1977.

59 Ridley MJ, Ridley DS: Serum antibodies and jejunal histology in giardiasis associated with malabsorption. *J Clin Pathol* 29:30, 1976.

60 Jones EG, Brown WR: Serum and intestinal fluid immunoglobulins in patients with giardiasis. *Am I Dig Dis* 19:791, 1974.

61 Hermans PE et al: Dysgammaglobulinemia associated with nodular lymphoid hyperplasia of the small intestine. *Am J Med* 40:78, 1966.

62 Ament ME et al: Structure and function of the gastrointestinal tract in primary immunodeficiency syndromes: A study of 39 patients. *Medicine* 52:227, 1973.

63 Hill DR et al: Susceptibility of *Giardia lamblia* trophozoites to the lethal effect of human serum. *J Immunol* 2046:132, 1984.

64 Deguchi M et al: Mechanism of killing of *Giardia lamblia* trophozoites by complement. *J Clin Invest* 1296:79, 1987.

65 Snider DP et al: Chronic *Giardia muris* infection in anti-IgM-treated mice. *J Immunol* 4153:134, 1985.

66 Carlson JR et al: Response of Peyer's patch lymphocyte subsets to *Giardia muris* infection in BALB/c mice. *Cell Immunol* 51:97, 1986.

67 Stevens DP, Frank DM: Local immunity in murine giardiasis: Is milk protective at the expense of maternal gut? *Trans Assoc Am Physicians* 91:268, 1978.

68 Andrews JS Jr, Hewlett EL: Protection against infection with *Giardia muris* by milk containing antibody to *Giardia. J Infect Dis* 143:242, 1981.

69 Kraft SC: The intestinal immune response in giardiasis. *Gastroenterology* 76:877, 1979.

70 Stevens DP et al: Thymus dependency of host resistance to *Giardia muris* infection: Studies in nude mice. *J Immunol* 120:680, 1978.

71 Roberts-Thomson IC, Mitchell GF: Giardiasis in mice: I. Prolonged infections in certain mouse strains and hypothymic (nude) mice. *Gastroenterology* 75:42, 1978.

72 Heyworth MF et al: Clearance of *Giardia muris* infection requires helper inducer T lymphocytes. *J Exp Med* 1743:165, 1987.

73 Gillin FD, Reire, DS: Human milk kills parasitic intestinal protozoa. *Science* 221:1290, 1983.

74 Reiner DS et al: Human milk kills *Giardia lamblia* by generating toxic lipolytic products. *J Infect Dis* 825:154, 1986.

75 Zisman M: Blood-group A and giardiasis. *Lancet* 2:1285, 1977.

76 Ogilvie BM, Wilson, RI: Evasion of the immune response by parasites. *Br Med Bull* 32:177, 1976.

77 Barbieri D et al: Giardiasis in childhood: Absorption tests and biochemistry, histochemistry, light and electron microscopy of jejunal mucosa. *Arch Dis Child* 45:466, 1970.

78 Owen RL et al: Ultrastructural observations on giardiasis in a murine model: I. Intestinal distribution, attachment, and relationship to the immune system of *Giardia muris. Gastroenterology* 76:757, 1979.

79 Wright SG, Tomkins AM: Quantification of the lymphocytic infiltrate in jejunal epithelium in giardiasis. *Clin Exp Immunol* 29:408, 1977.

80 McDonald TT et al: Small intestinal epithelial cell kinetics and protozoal infection in mice. *Am Gastroenterol Assoc* 496:74, 1978.

81 Ament ME, Rubin CE: Relation of giardiasis to abnormal intestinal structure and function in gastrointestinal immunodeficiency syndromes. *Gastroenterology* 62:216, 1972.

82 Saha TK, Ghosh TK: Invasion of small intestinal mucosa by *Giardia lamblia* in man. *Gastroenterology* 72:402, 1977.

83 Blasevic M et al: *Giardia lamblia* infections in Mongolian gerbils: An animal model. *J Infect Dis* 222:147, 1983.

84 Aggawal A, Nash TE: Comparison of two antigenically distinct *Giardia lamblia* isolates in gerbils. *Am J Med Hyg* 325:36, 1987.

85 Leon-Barua R: The possible role of intestinal bacterial flora in the genesis of diarrhea and malabsorption associated with parasitosis. *Gastroenterology* 55:559, 1968.

86 Smith PD et al: In vitro studies on bile acid deconjugation and lipolysis inhibition by *Giardia lamblia. Dig Dis Sci* 700:26, 1981.

87 Forthing MJG et al: Effects of bile and bile salts on growth and membrane lipid uptake by *Giardia lamblia. Am Soc Clin Invest* 1727:76, 1985.

87a Garcia LS et al: Evaluation of a new monoclonal antibody combination reagent for direct fluorescence detection of *Giardia* cysts and *Cryptosporidium* oocysts in human fecal specimens. *J Clin Microbiol* 30:3255–57, 1992.

87b Addiss DG et al: Evaluation of a commercially available enzyme-linked immunosorbent assay for *Giardia lamblia* antigen in stool. *J Clin Microbiol* 29:1137–42, 1991.

87c Char S, Farthing MJG: DNA Probes for diagnosis of enteric infection. *Gut* 32:1–3, 1991.

88 Nash TE et al: Experimental human infections with *Giardia lamblia. J Infect Dis* 156:974, 1987.

89 Vinayak VK et al: Demonstration of antibodies in giardiasis using the immunodiffusion technique with *Giardia* cysts as antigen. *Ann Trop Med Parasitol* 72:581, 1978.

90 Visvesvara GS et al: An immunofluorescence test to detect serum antibodies to *Giardia lamblia. Ann Intern Med* 93:802, 1980.

91 Smith PD et al: IgG antibody to *Giardia lamblia* detected by enzyme-linked immunosorbent assay. *Gastroenterology* 80:1476, 1981.

92 Ungar BL et al: Enzyme-linked immunosorbent assay for the detection of *Giardia lamblia* in fecal specimens. *J Infect Dis* 90:149, 1984.

93 Green EL et al: Immunodiagnostic detection of *Giardia* antigen in feces by a rapid visual enzyme-linked immunosorbent assay. *Lancet* 691:2, 1985.

94 Nash TE et al: Usefulness of an enzyme-linked immunosorbent assay for detection of *Giardia* antigen in feces. *J Clin Microbiol* 1169:25, 1987.

95 Gillin FD, Diamond LS: Inhibition of clonal growth of *Giardia lamblia* and *Entamoeba histolytica* by metronidazole, quinacrine, and other antimicrobial agents. *J Antimicrob Chemother* 8:305, 1981.

96 Bassity S et al: The treatment of *Giardia lamblia* infection with mepacrine, metronidazole, and furazolidone. *J Trop Med Hyg* 73:15, 1970.

97 El-Masry NA et al: Treatment of giardiasis with tinidazole. *Am J Trop Med Hyg* 27:201, 1978.

98 Wolfe MS, Moede AL: Serum sickness with furazolidone. *Am J Trop Med Hyg* 27:762, 1978.

99 Davidson RA: Issues in clinical parasitology: The treatment of giardiasis. *Am J Gastroenterol* 79:256, 1984.

100 Jokipii L, Jokipii AMM: In vitro susceptibility of *Giardia lamblia* trophozoites to metronidazole and tinidazole. *J Infect Dis* 141:317, 1980.

101 Stitwell GG: Amebiasis: Its early history. *Gastroenterology* 28:606, 1955.
102 Walker EL, Sellards AW: Experimental entamoebic dysentery. *Philippine J Sci Trop Med* 8:253, 1913.
103 Walsh JA: Prevalence of *Entamoeba histolytica* infection, in *Amebiasis: Human Infection by Entamoeba histolytica*, JI Ravdin (ed). New York, Wiley, 1988, pp 93-105.
104 Sargeaunt PG et al: The differentiation of invasive and non-invasive *Entamoeba histolytica* by isoenzyme electrophoresis. *Trans R Soc Trop Med Hyg* 72:519–21, 1978.
105 Tannich E, Burchard GD: Differentiation of pathogenic from nonpathogenic *Entamoeba histolytica* by restriction fragment analysis of a single gene amplified in vitro. *J Clin Microbiol* 29:250–5, 1991.
106 Clark CG, Diamond LS: Ribosomal RNA genes of "pathogenic" *Entamoeba histolytica* are distinct. *Mol Biochem Parasitol* 49:297–302, 1991.
107 Gathiram V, Jackson TFHG: Frequency distribution of *Entamoeba histolytica* zymodemes in a rural South African population. *Lancet* 1:716–9, 1985.
108 Jackton TFHG et al: Seroepidemiological study of antibody responses to the zymodemes of *Entamoeba histolytica. Lancet* 1:716–9, 1985.
109 Ravdin JI et al: Association of serum anti-adherence, lectin antibodies with invasive amebiasis and asymptomatic pathogenic *Entamoeba histolytica* infection. *J Infect Dis* 162:768–72, 1990.
110 Krogstad DJ et al: Amebiasis: Epidemiologic studies in the United States, 1971–1974. *Ann Intern Med* 88:89, 1978.
111 Thompson JE et al: Amebic liver abscess: A therapeutic approach. *Rev Infect Dis* 7:171, 1985.
112 Markell EK et al: Intestinal protozoa in homosexual men of the San Francisco Bay area: Prevalence and correlates of infection. *Am Trop Med Hyg* 33:239, 1984.
113 Ortega HB et al: Enteric pathogenic protozoa in homosexual men from San Francisco. *Sex Transm Dis* 11:59, 1983.
114 Druckman DA, Quinn TC: *Entamoeba histolytica* infection in homosexual men, in *Amebiasis: Human Infection by Entamoeba histolytica,* JI Ravdin (ed). New York, Wiley, 1988, pp 563–575.
115 Pearson RD, Hewlett EL: Amebiasis in travelers, in *Amebiasis: Human Infection by Entamoeba histolytica*, JI Ravdin (ed). New York, Wiley, 1988, pp 556–562.
116 Thomas JA, Antonio AJ: Amebiasis of the penis. *Br J Urol* 48:269, 1976.
117 Goldman M et al: Antigenic analysis of *Entamoeba histolytica* by means of fluorescent antibody: II. *E. histolytica* and *E. hartmanni-hartmani. Exp Parasitol* 10:366, 1960.
118 Edelman MH, Spingarn CL: Cultivation of *Entamoeba histolytica* as a diagnostic procedure: A brief review. *Mt Sinai J Med (NY)* 43:27, 1976.
119 Miller JH et al: An electron microscopic study of *Entamoeba histolytica. J Parasitol* 47:S77, 1961.
120 El-Hashimi W, Pirtman F: Ultrastructure of *Entamoeba histolytica* trophozoites obtained from the colon and from *in vitro* cultures. *Am J Trop Med Hyg* 19:215, 1970.
121 Lushbaugh WB: Proteinase of *Entamoeba histolytica,* in *Amebiasis: Human Infection by Entamoeba histolytica,* JI Ravdin (ed). New York, Wiley, 1988, pp 219–231.
122 Pittman FE et al: Studies in human amebiasis: II. Light and electron-microscopic observations of colonic mucosa and exudate in acute amebic colitis. *Gastroenterology* 65:588, 1973.
123 Lushbaugh WB, Miller JH: Fine structural topochemistry of *Entamoeba histolytica* Schaudinn, 1903. *J Parasitol* 60:421, 1974.
124 Michel R, Schupp E: Cytoplasmic fibrils and their relation to ameboid movement of *Entamoeba histolytica,* in *Memorieas de la Conferencia Internacional Sobre Amibiasis,* B Sepulveda, LS Diamond (eds). Mexico City, Instituto Méxicano del Seguro Social, 1976, pp 300–310.
125 Meza I et al: Isolation and characterization of actin from *Entamoeba histolytica. J Biol Chem* 258:3936, 1983.
126 Edman E et al: Genomic and cDNA actin sequences from a virulent strain of *Entamoeba histolytica. Proc Natl Acad Sci USA* 84:3024, 1987.
127 Ravdin JI, et al: Cytopathogenic mechanisms of *Entamoeba histolytica. J Exp Med* 152:377, 1980.
128 Ravdin JI, Guerrant RL: The role of adherence in cytopathogenic mechanisms of *Entamoeba histolytica:* Study with mammalian tissue culture cells and human erythrocytes. *J Clin Invest* 68:1305, 1981.
129 Guerrant RL et al: The interaction between *Entamoeba histolytica* and human polymorphonuclear leukocytes. *J Infect Dis* 143:83, 1981.
130 Martinez-Palomo A et al: Selective agglutination of pathogenic strains of *Entamoeba histolytica* induced Con A. *Nature* 245:186, 1973.
131 Trissi D et al: Surface properties related to concanavalin A–induced agglutination. *J Exp Med* 145:652, 1977.
132 Aley SB et al: Plasma membrane of *Entamoeba histolytica. J Exp Med* 152:391, 1980.
133 Petri WA et al: Recognition of the galactose- or *N*-acetylgalactosamine-binding lectin of *Entamoeba histolytica* by human immune sera. *Infect Immun* 55:2327, 1987.
134 Calderon J, Avila EE: Antibody-induced caps in *Entamoeba histolytica:* Isolation and electrophoretic analysis. *J Infect Dis* 153:927, 1986.
135 Ravdin JI et al: Impedance measurements and cytotoxicity in the presence of bepridil, verapamil, and cytochalasin D. *Exp Parasitol* 60:63, 1985.
136 Barker DC, Swales LS: Characteristics of ribosomes during differentiation from trophozoite to cyst in axenic *Entamoeba* species. *Cell Differ* 1:297, 1972.
137 Neal RA: Phylogeny: The relationship of *Entamoeba histolytica* to morphologically similar amebae of the four-nucleate cyst group, in *Amebiasis: Human Infection by Entamoeba histolytica,* JI Ravdin (ed). New York, Wiley, 1988, pp 13–26.
138 Chayen A, Avron B: *Entamoeba histolytica,* antigens and amoebiasis, in *Parasite Antigens in Protection, Diagnosis and Escape. Current Topics in Microbiology and Immunology,* vol 120, M Parkhouse (ed). New York, Springer-Verlag, 1985.
139 Mirelman D, Avron B: Cyst formation in *Entamoeba,* in *Amebiasis: Human Infection by Entamoeba histolytica,* JI Ravdin (ed). New York, Wiley, 1988, pp 768–781.
140 Diamond LS: Axenic cultivation of *Entamoeba histolytica. Science* 134:336, 1961.
141 Diamond LS et al: A new medium for the axenic cultivation of *Entamoeba histolytica* and other *Entamoeba. Trans R Soc Trop Med* Hyg 72:431, 1978.
142 Gillin FD, Diamond LS: Clonal growth of *Entamoeba histolytica* and other species of *Entamoeba* in agar. *J Protozool* 25:539, 1978.
143 Clark CG: Axenic cultivation of *Entamoeba dispar* Brumpt 1925, *Entamoeba insolita* Geiman and Wichterman 1937, and *Entamoeba ranaram* Grassi 1879. *Eur J Microbiol* 42:590–593, 1995.
144 Salata RA, Ravdin JI: Review of the human immune mechanisms directed against *Entamoeba histolytica. Rev Infect Dis* 8:261, 1986.
145 DeLeon A: Prognostico tardio en el absceso hepatico amibiano. *Arch Invest Med (Mex)* 1(suppl 1):205, 1970.
146 Sepulveda B, Martinez-Palomo A: Immunology of amoebiasis by *Entamoeba histolytica,* in *Immunology of Parasitic Infections,* S Cohen, KS Warren (eds). Oxford, Blackwell Scientific Publications, 1982, p 170–191.
147 Ortiz-Ortiz L et al: Activation of the alternative pathway of complement by *Entamoeba histolytica. Clin Exp Immunol* 34:10, 1978.
148 Huldt G et al: Interactions between *Entamoeba histolytica* and complement. *Nature* 277:214, 1979.
149 Reed SL et al: Resistance to lysis by immune serum of pathogenic *Entamoeba histolytica. Trans R Soc Trop Med Hyg* 77:248, 1983.
150 Calderon J, Tovar R: Loss of susceptibility to complement lysis in *Entamoeba histolytica* HMI by treatment with human serum. *Immunology* 58:467, 1986.
151 Petri WA, Ravdin JI: Cytopathogenicity of *Entamoeba histolytica. Eur J Epidemiol* 3:123, 1987.
152 Petri WA et al: Recognition of the galactose- or *N*-acetyl-galactosamine-binding lectin of *Entamoeba histolytica* by human immune sera. *Infect Immun* 55:2327, 1987.

153 Joyce MP, Ravdin JI: Antigens of *Entamoeba histolytica* are recognized by immune sera from liver abscess patients. *Am J Trop Med Hyg* 38:74, 1988.
154 Soong CJG et al: A recombinant cysteine-rich section of the *Entamoeba histolytica* galactose-inhibitable adherence lectin is efficacious as a subunit vaccine in the gerbil model of ameobic liver abscess. *J Infect Dis* 171:645–651, 1995.
155 Soong CJG et al: Protection of gerbils from ameobic liver abscess by immunization with recombinant *Entamoeba histolytica* 29-kilodalton antigen. *Infect Immun* 63:472–477, 1995.
156 Kelsall BL, et al: Secretory immunoglobulin A antibodies to the galactose-inhibitable adherence protein in the saliva of patients with ameobic liver abscess. *Am J Trop Med Hyg* 51:454–459, 1994.
157 Carrero JC et al: Human secretory immunoglobulin A anti-*Entamoeba histolytica* antibodies inhibit adherence of ameoba to MDCK cells. *Infect Immun* 62:764–767, 1994.
158 Abou-el-Magd I et al: Humoral and mucosal IgA antibody response to a recombinant 52-kDa cysteine-rich portion of the *Entamoeba histolytica* galactose-inhibitable lectin correlates with detection of native 170-kDa lectin antigen in serum of patients with ameobic colitis. *J Infect Dis.* 174(1):157–162, 1996.
159 Beving DE et al: Oral immunization with a recombinant cysteine-rich section of the *Entamoeba histolytica* galactose-inhibitable lectin elicits an intestinal secretory IgA response that has *in vitro* adherence-inhibitory activity. *Infect Immun* 64:1473–1476, 1996.
160 Salata RA et al: Interaction of human leukocytes with *Entamoeba histolytica:* Killing of virulent amebae by the activated macrophage. *J Clin Invest* 76:491, 1985.
161 Salata RA et al: Patients treated for amebic liver abscess develop a cell mediated immune response effective in vitro against *Entamoeba histolytica*. *J Immunol* 136:2633, 1986.
162 Salata RA et al: The role of gamma interferon in the generation of human macrophages and T lymphocytes cytotoxic for *Entamoeba histolytica*. *Am J Trop Med Hyg* 37:72, 1987.
163 Schain DC et al: Human T lymphocyte proliferation, lymphokine production, and ameobicidal activity elicited by the *Entamoeba histolytica* galactose specific adherence protein. *Infect and Immun* 60: 2143–2146, 1992.
164 Schain DC et al: Development of amoebicidal cell-mediated immunity in gerbils (*Meriones unguiculatus*) immunized with the galactose-inhibitable adherence lectin of *Entamoeba histolytica*. *J Parasitol* 8: 563–568, 1995.
165 Salata RA et al: Immune sera suppress the antigen specific proliferative response in T lymphocytes from patients cured of amoebic liver abscess. The 34th Annual Meeting of the American Society of Tropical Medicine and Hygiene, Miami, Florida, November 5, 1985.
166 Leitch GJ et al: *Entamoeba histolytica* trophozoites in the lumen and mucus blanket of rat colons studied in vivo. *Infect Immun* 47:68, 1985.
167 Chadee K, Meerovitch E: *Entamoeba histolytica:* Early progressive pathology in the cecum of the gerbil *(Meriones unguiculatus)*. *Am J Trop Med Hyg* 34:283, 1985.
168 Chadee K et al: Mucin and nonmucin secretagogue activity of *Entamoeba histolytica* and cholera toxin in rat colon. *Gastroenterology* 100:986–997, 1991.
169 Chadee K et al: Rat and human colonic mucins bind to and inhibit the adherence lectin of *Entamoeba histolytica*. *J Clin Invest* 80:1245, 1987.
170 Brandt H, Perez-Tamyo R: The pathology of human amoebiasis. *Hum Pathol* 1:351, 1979.
171 Jarumilinta R, Kradolfer F: The toxic effect of *Entamoeba histolytica* on leukocytes. *Ann Trop Med Parasitol* 58:375, 1964.
172 Proctor EM, Gregory MA: The observation of a surface active lysosome in the trophozoites of *Entamoeba histolytica* from the lower colon. *Ann Trop Med Parasitol* 66:339, 1972.
173 Chanduri RN, Saba TK: Liver biopsy study in intestinal amoebiasis. *Calcutta Med J* 3:39, 1956.
174 Sargeaunt PG: Zymodemes of *Entamoeba histolytica,* in *Amoebiasis: Human Infection by Entamoeba histolytica,* JI Ravdin (ed). New York, Wiley, 1988, pp 370–387.
175 Allason-Jones E et al: *Entamoeba histolytica* as a commensal intestinal parasite in homosexual men. *N Engl J Med* 315:353, 1986.
176 Tannich E et al: Genomic DNA differences between pathogenic and nonpathogenic *Entamoeba histolytica*. *Proc Natl Acad Sci USA* 86: 5118–5122, 1989.
177 Mirelman D: Ameba-bacterial relationship in amebiasis, in *Amebiasis: Human Infection by Entamoeba histolytica,* JI Ravdin (ed). New York, Wiley, 1988, pp 351–369.
178 Phillips BP et al: Studies on the ameba-bacterial relationship in amebiasis: Comparative results of the intracecal inoculation of germ free, monocontaminated, and conventional guinea pigs with *Entamoeba histolytica*. *Am J Trop Med Hyg* 4:675, 1955.
179 Phillips BP et al: Studies on the ameba-bacterial relationship in amebiasis: II. Some concepts on the etiology of the disease. *Am J Trop Med Hyg* 7:392, 1958.
180 Wittner M, Rosenbaum RM: Role of bacteria in modifying virulence of *Entamoeba histolytica*. *Am J Trop Med Hyg* 19:755, 1970.
181 Diamond LS et al: A comparison of the virulence of nine strains of axenically cultivated *E. histolytica* in hamster liver. *Arch Invest Med (Mex)* 5 (suppl 2):423, 1974.
182 Bracha R, Mirelman D: Virulence of *Entamoeba histolytica* trophozoites: Effects of bacteria, microaerobic conditions, and metronidazole. *J Exp Med* 160:353, 1984.
183 Diamond LS et al: Viruses of *Entamoeba histolytica*: I. Identification of transmissible virus-like agents. *J Virol* 9:326, 1972.
184 Mattern CFF et al: Experimental amebiasis: IV. Amebal viruses and the virulence of *Entamoeba histolytica*. *Am J Trop Med Hyg* 28:653, 1979.
185 Ross GW, Knight R: Dietary factors affecting the pathogenicity of *Entamoeba histolytica* in rats. *Trans R Soc Trop Med Hyg* 6:560, 1973.
186 Faust EC, Read TR: Parasitologic surveys in Cali, Departmento del Valle, Columbia: V. Capacity of *Entamoeba histolytica* of human origin to utilize different types of starches in its metabolism. *Am J Trop Med Hyg* 8:293, 1959.
187 Wanke C, Butler T: Intestinal amebiasis in a hospital population in Bangladesh. The 25th Interscience Conference on Antimicrobial Agents and Chemotherapy, Minneapolis, Minnesota, 1985, paper 1566.
188 Diamond LS et al: *Entamoeba histolytica:* Iron and nutritional immunity. *Arch Invest Med (Mex)* 9 (suppl 1):329, 1978.
189 Lushbaugh WB et al: Effect of hamster liver passage on the virulence of axenically cultivated *Entamoeba histolytica*. *Am J Trop Med Hyg* 27:248, 1978.
190 Das SR, Ghoshal S: Restoration of virulence to rat of axenically grown *Entamoeba histolytica* by cholesterol and hamster liver passage. *Ann Trop Med Parasitol* 70:439, 1976.
191 Ravdin JI et al: The *N*-acetyl-D-galactosamine-inhibitable adherence lectin of *Entamoeba histolytica:* I. Partial purification and relation to amebic virulence in vitro. *J Infect Dis* 151:804, 1985.
192 Orozco ME et al: *Entamoeba histolytica:* Cytopathogenicity and lectin activity of avirulent mutants. *Exp Parasitol* 63:157, 1987.
193 Salata RA, Ravdin JI: The interaction of human neutrophils and *Entamoeba histolytica* increases cytopathogenicity for liver cell monolayers. *J Infect Dis* 154:19, 1986.
194 Bracha R, Mirelman D: Adherence and ingestion of *Escherichia coli* serotype 055 by trophozoites of *Entamoeba histolytica*. *Infect Immun* 40:882, 1983.
195 Ravdin JI et al: Production of mouse monoclonal antibodies which inhibit in vitro adherence of *Entamoeba histolytica* trophozoites. *Infect Immun* 53:1, 1986.
196 Petri WA et al: Isolation of the galactose-binding lectin which mediates the in vitro adherence of *Entamoeba histolytica*. *J Clin Invest* 80:1238, 1987.
197 Petri WA Jr. et al: Subunit structure of the glactose and *N*-acetyl-D-galactosamine-inhibitable adherence lectin of *Entamoeba histolytica*. *J Biol Chem* 264;3007–3012, 1989.
198 Kain KC, Ravdin JI: Galactose-specific adherence mechanisms of *Entamoeba histolytica,* a model for the study of enteric pathogens. *Methods Enzymol* 253:424–439, 1995.

199 Tannich B et al: Primary structure of the 170 kDa surface lectin of pathogenic *Entamoeba histolytica. Proc Natl Acad Sci* 88:1849–53, 1991.
200 Mann BJ et al: Sequence of a cysteine-rich galactose-specific lectin of *Entamoeba histolytica. Proc Natl Acad Sci* 88:3248–52, 1991.
201 McCoy JJ et al: Structural analysis of the light subunit of the *Entamoeba histolytica* galactose-specific lectin. *J Biol Chem* 24:223–31, 1993.
202 Petri WA et al: Antigenic stability and immunodominance of the Gal/GalNAc adherence lectins of *Entamoeba histolytica. Am J Med Sci* 297(3):163–165, 1989.
203 Ravdin JI et al: Correlation of clinical status and zymodeme analysis with serum Western blot recognition of *Entamoeba histolytica* antigens. The 36th Annual Meeting of the American Society of Tropical Medicine and Hygiene, Los Angeles, CA, December 1, 1987, abstr. 176.
204 Kobiler D, Mirelman D: Lectin activity in *Entamoeba histolytica* trophozoites. *Infect Immun* 29:221, 1980.
205 Kobiler D, Mirelman D: Adhesion of *Entamoeba histolytica* trophozoites to monolayers of human cells. *J Infect Dis* 144:539, 1981.
206 Arroyo R, Orozco E: Localización e Identificación de Adhemiba I, Una Proteína Que Participa en la Adhesión de *Entamoeba histolytica* a Eritrocitos Humanos y Celulas Epiteliales [abstract]. 10 Seminario Sobre Amibiasis, Mexico City, October 6–8, 1986.
207 Ravdin JI et al: The relationship of free intracellular calcium ions to the cytolytic activity of *Entamoeba histolytica. Infect Immun* 56: 1505, 1988.
208 Ravdin JI et al: Effect of calcium and phospholipase A antagonists on the cytopathogenicity of *Entamoeba histolytica. J Infect Dis* 152: 542, 1985.
209 Long-Krug SA et al: The phospholipase A enzymes of *Entamoeba histolytica:* Description and subcellular localization. *J Infect Dis* 152: 536, 1985.
210 Ravdin JI et al: Acid intracellular vesicles and the cytolysis of mammalian target cells by *Entamoeba histolytica* trophozoites. *J Protozool* 33:478, 1986.
211 Weikel CS et al: Phorbol esters specifically enhance the cytolytic activity of *Entamoeba histolytica. Infect Immun* 56:1485, 1988.
212 Lynch EC et al: An ion channel-forming protein produced by *Entamoeba histolytica. EMBOJ* 1:801, 1982.
213 Young JDE et al: Characterization of a membrane pore-forming protein from *Entamoeba histolytica. J Exp Med* 156:1677, 1982.
214 Rosenberg I, Gitler C: Subcellular fractionation of amoebapore and plasma membrane components of *Entamoeba histolytica* using self-generating percoll gradients. *Mol Biochem Parasitol* 14:231, 1985.
215 Young JDE, Cohn ZA: Molecular mechanisms of cytotoxicity mediated by *Entamoeba histolytica:* Characterization of a pore-forming protein (PFP). *J Cell Biochem* 29:299, 1985.
216 Leippe M et al: Primary and secondary structure of the pore-forming peptide of pathogenic *Entamoeba histolytica. EMBOJ* 11:3501–3506, 1992.
217 Lushbaugh WB et al: Purification of cathepsin B activity of *Entamoeba histolytica* toxin. *Exp Parasitol* 59:328, 1985.
218 Scholze H, Worries E: A weakly acidic protease has a powerful proteolytic activity in *Entamoeba histolytica. Mol Biochem Parasitol* 11: 293, 1984.
219 Mufioz MDL et al: The collagenase of *Entamoeba histolytica. J Exp Med* 155:42, 1982.
220 Keene WE et al: The major neutral proteinase of *Entamoeba histolytica. J Exp Med* 163:536, 1986.
221 McGowan K et al: *Entamoeba histolytica* causes intestinal secretion: Role of serotonin. *Science* 221:762, 1983.
222 Feingold C et al: Isolation, purification, and partial characterization of enterotoxin from extracts of *Entamoeba histolytica* trophozoites. *Infect Immun* 48:211, 1985.
223 Tsutsumi V et al: Cellular basis of experimental amebic liver abscess formation. *Am J Pathol* 117:81, 1984.
224 Chadee K, Meerovitch E: The pathogenesis of experimentally induced amebic liver abscess in the gerbil *(Meriones unguiculatus). Am J Pathol* 117:71, 1984.
225 Juniper K: Acute amebic colitis. *Am J Med* 33:377, 1962.
226 Ravdin JI, Guerrant RL: Current problems in diagnosis and treatment of amoebic infections, in *Current Clinical Topics in Infectious Diseases,* vol 7, JS Remington, MN Swartz (eds). New York, McGraw-Hill, 1986, pp 82–111.
227 Adams EB, MacLeod IN: Invasive amebiasis: I. Amebic dysentery and its complications. *Medicine* 56:315, 1977.
228 Ravdin JI: Intestinal disease caused by *Entamoeba histolytica,* in *Amebiasis: Human Infection by Entamoeba histolytica,* JI Ravdin (ed). New York, Wiley, 1988, pp 495–510.
229 Blumencranz H et al: The role of endoscopy in suspected amebiasis. *Am J Gastroenterology* 78:15, 1983.
230 Healy GR: Diagnostic techniques for stool samples, in *Amebiasis: Human Infection by Entamoeba histolytica,* JI Ravdin (ed). New York, Wiley, 1988, pp 635–649.
231 Healy GR: Serology, in *Amebiasis: Human Infection by Entamoeba histolytica,* JI Ravdin (ed). New York, Wiley, 1988, pp 650–663.
232 Patterson M et al: Serologic testing for amoebiasis. *Gastroenterology* 78:1185, 1980.
233 Kessel JF et al: Indirect hemagglutination and complement fixation tests in amebiasis. *Am J Trop Med Hyg* 14:540, 1965.
234 Cedeno JR, Krogstad DJ: Susceptibility testing of *Entamoeba histolytica. J Infect Dis* 148:1090, 1983.
235 Cedeno JR, Krogstad DJ: *In vitro* antiamebic drug activity, in *Amebiasis: Human Infection by Entamoeba histolytica,* JI Ravdin (ed). New York, Wiley, 1988, pp 723–733.
236 Powell SJ: Therapy of amebiasis. *Bull NY Acad Sci* 47:469, 1971.
237 Sunoto SH et al: Tiberal (Ro 7-0207-Roche) in the treatment of intestinal amoebiasis, Part II. *Paediatr Indones* 16:403, 1976.
238 Norris SM, Ravdin JI: The pharmacology of antiamebic drugs, in *Amebiasis: Human Infection by Entamoeba histolytica,* JI Ravdin (ed). New York, Wiley, 1988, pp 734–740.
239 Wolfe MS: Nondysenteric intestinal amebiasis: Treatment with diloxanide furoate. *JAMA* 224:1601, 1973.
240 Walsh JA: Transmission of *Entamoeba histolytica* infection, in *Amebiasis: Human Infection by Entamoeba histolytica,* JI Ravdin (ed). New York, Wiley, 1988, pp 106–119.
241 Tyzzer EE: A sporozoan found in the peptic glands of the common mouse. *Proc Soc Exp Biol* 5:12, 1907.
242 Slavin D: *Cryptosporidium meleagridis* (sp. nor.). *J Comp Pathol* 65: 262, 1955.
243 Nime FA et al: Acute enterocolitis in a human being infected with the protozoan *Cryptosporidium. Gastroenterology* 70:592, 1976.
244 Centers for Disease Control: Cryptosporidiosis: Assessment of chemotherapy of males with acquired immune deficiency syndrome (AIDS). *MMWR* 31:589, 1982.
245 Current WL et al: Human cryptosporidiosis in immunocompetent and immunodeficient persons. *N Engl J Med* 308:1252, 1983.
246 MacKenzie WR et al: A massive outbreak in Milwaukee of *Cryptosporidium* infection transmitted through the public water supply. *N Engl J Med* 331:161–167, 1994.
247 Newman RD et al: Household epidemiology *of Cryptosporidium parvum* infection. *Ann Intern Med* 120:500–505, 1994.
248 Fang G et al: Etiology and epidemiology of persistent diarrhea in northeastern Brazil: A hospital-based prospective case control study. *J Ped Gastro Nutr* 21:137–144, 1995.
249 Adal KA et al: *Cryptosporidium* and Related Species, in *Infections of the Gastrointestinal Tract,* MJ Blaser, PD Smith et al (eds). New York, Raven Press, 1107–1128, 1995.
250 Guerrant RL: An emerging highly infectious threat to our water supply. *Infect Agents Dis* 3(1):51–57, 1997.
251 Levine ND: Taxonomy and review of the coccidian genus *Cryptosporidium* (Protozoa, Apicomplexa). *J Protozool* 31:94, 1984.
252 Upton SJ, Current WL: The species of *Cryptosporidium* (Apicomplexa: Cryptosporidiidae) infecting mammals. *J Parasitol* 71:625, 1985.
253 Current WL, Reese NC: A comparison of endogenous development of three isolates of *Cryptosporidium* in suckling mice. *J Protozool* 33: 98, 1986.

254 Current WL et al: The life cycle of *Cryptosporidium baileyi* n sp (Apicomplexa, Cryptosporidiidae) infecting chickens. *J Protozool* 33: 289, 1986.
255 Fayer R, Ungar BLP: *Cryptosporidium* spp and cryptosporidiosis. *Microbiol Rev* 50:458, 1986.
256 Mead JR et al: *Cryptosporidium* isolate comparison using field inversion gel electrophoresis. *Am Soc Trop Med Hyg,* in press.
257 Heine J et al: Persistent *Cryptosporidium* infection in congenitally athymic (nude) mice. *Infect Immun* 43:856, 1984.
258 Moon HW et al: Intestinal cryptosporidiosis: Pathogenesis and immunity. *Microecol Therap* 15:103, 1985.
259 Tzipori S et al: Enterocolitis in pigs caused by *Cryptosporidium* sp purified from calf faeces. *Vet Parasitol* 11:121, 1982.
260 Heine J et al: Enteric lesions and diarrhea in gnotobiotic calves monoinfected with *Cryptosporidium* species. *J Infect Dis* 150:768, 1984.
261 Current WL, Haynes TB: Complete development of *Cryptosporidium* in cell culture. *Science* 224:603, 1984.
262 Ernest JA et al: Infection dynamics of *Cryptosporidium parvum* (Apicomplexa: Cryptosporidiidae) in neonatal mice (*Mus musculus*). *J Parasitol* 72:796, 1986.
263 Blagburn BL, Current WL: Accidental infection of a researcher with human *Cryptosporidium. J Infect Dis* 148:772, 1983.
264 DuPont HL et al: The infectivity *of Cryptosporidium parvum* in healthy volunteers. *N Engl J Med* 332:855–859, 1995.
265 Centers for Disease Control: Assessing the public health threat associated with waterborne cryptosporidiosis: Report of a workshop. *MMWR* 44:1–19, 1995.
266 Reduker DW et al: Ultrastructure of *Cryptosporidium parvum* oocysts and excysting sporozoites as revealed by high resolution scanning electron microscopy. *J Protozool* 32:708, 1985.
267 Vetterling JM et al: Ultrastructure of *Cryptosporidium wrairi* from the guinea pig. *J Protozool* 18:218, 1971.
268 Lefkowitch JH et al: Cryptosporidiosis of the human small intestine: A light and electron microscopic study. *Hum Pathol* 15:746, 1984.
269 Modigliani R et al: Diarrhoea and malabsorption in acquired immune deficiency syndrome: A study of four cases with special emphasis on opportunistic protozoan infestations. *Gut* 26:179, 1985.
270 Meisel JL et al: Overwhelming watery diarrhea associated with a *Cryptosporidium* in an immunosuppressed patient. *Gastroenterol* 70:1156, 1976.
271 Soave R et al: Cryptosporidiosis in homosexual men. *Ann Intern Med* 100:504, 1984.
272 Soave R, Armstrong D: *Cryptosporidium* and cryptosporidiosis. *Rev Infect Dis* 8:1012, 1986.
273 Tzipori S: Cryptosporidiosis in animals and humans. *Microbiol Rev,* 47:84, 1983.
274 Tzipori S et al: *Cryptosporidium:* Evidence for a single-species genus. *Infect Immun* 30:884, 1980.
275 Hampton JC, Rosario B: The attachment of protozoan parasites to intestinal epithelial cells of the mouse. *J Parasitol* 52:939, 1966.
276 Marcial MA, Madara JL: *Cryptosporidium:* Cellular localization, structural analysis of absorptive cell-parasite membrane-membrane interactions in guinea pigs, and suggestion of protozoan transport by M cells. *Gastroenterol* 90:583, 1986.
277 Koch KL et al: Cryptosporidiosis in a patient with hemophilia, common variable hypogammaglobulinemia, and the acquired immunodeficiency syndrome. *Ann Intern Med* 99:337, 1983.
278 Petras RE et al: Cryptosporidial enteritis in a homosexual male with an acquired immunodeficiency syndrome. *Cleve Clin Q* 50:41, 1983.
279 Berk RN et al: Cryptosporidiosis of the stomach and small intestine in patients with AIDS. *Am J Radiol* 143:549, 1984.
280 Garza DH et al: Enterotoxin-like activity in cultured cryptosporidia: Role in diarrhea. *Gastroenterology* 90:1424, 1986.
281 Casemore DP et al: *Cryptosporidium* species: A "new" human pathogen. *J Clin Pathol* 38:1321, 1985.
282 Guerrant RL et al: Parasitic causes of diarrhea: An overview, in *Pathophysiology of Secretory Diarrhea,* E Lebenthal, M Duffey (eds). Raven Press, Boston, 1990.
283 Guarino A et al: Human intestinal cryptosporidiosis: Secretory diarrhea and enterotoxic activity in Caco-2 cells. *J Infect Dis* 171:976–983, 1995.
284 Sears CL, Guerrant RL: Cryptosporidiosis: The complexity of intestinal pathophysiology. *Gastroenterol* 106:252–254, 1994.
285 Argenzio RA et al: Prostanoids inhibit intestinal NaCl absorption in experimental porcine cryptosporidiosis. *Gastroenterol* 104:440–447, 1993.
286 Argenzio RA et al: Glutamine stimulates prostaglandin-sensitive Na^+-H^+ exchange in experimental porcine cryptosporidiosis. *Gastroenterol* 106:1418–1428, 1994.
287 Goodgame RW et al: Intestinal function and injury in acquired immunodeficiency syndrome–related cryptosporidiosis. *Gastroenterol* 108:1075–1082, 1995.
288 Navin TR: Cryptosporidiosis in humans: Review of recent epidemiologic studies. *Eur J Epidemiol* 1:77, 1985.
289 Wolfson JS et al: Cryptosporidiosis in immunocompetent patients. *N Engl J Med* 312:1278, 1985.
290 Jokipii L et al: Cryptosporidiosis associated with traveling and giardiasis. *Gastroenterology* 89:838, 1985.
291 Soave R, Ma P: Cryptosporidiosis: Traveler's diarrhea in two families. *Arch Intern Med* 145:70, 1985.
292 Koch KL et al: Cryptosporidiosis in hospital personnel. *Ann Intern Med* 102:593, 1985.
293 Ribeiro CD, Plamer SR: Family outbreak of cryptosporidiosis. *Br Med J* 292:377, 1986.
294 Jokipii L, Jokipii AMM: Timing of symptoms and oocyst excretion in human cryptosporidiosis. *N Engl J Med* 3 15:1643, 1986.
295 Stehr-Green JK et al: Shedding of oocysts in immunocompetent individuals infected with *Cryptosporidium. Am J Trop Med Hyg* 36: 338, 1987.
296 Isaacs D et al: Cryptosporidiosis in immunocompetent children. *J Clin Pathol* 38:76, 1985.
297 Navin TR, Juranck DD: Cryptosporidiosis: Clinical, epidemiologic, and parasitologic review. *Rev Infect Dis* 6:313, 1984.
298 Navin TR, Hardy AM: Cryptosporidiosis in patients with AIDS. *J Infect Dis* 155:150, 1987.
299 Forgacs P et al: Intestinal and bronchial cryptosporidiosis in an immunodeficient homosexual man. *Ann Intern Med* 99:793, 1983.
300 Ma P et al: Respiratory cryptosporidiosis in the acquired immune deficiency syndrome. *JAMA* 252:1298, 1984.
301 Brady EM et al: Pulmonary cryptosporidiosis in acquired immune deficiency syndrome. *JAMA* 252:89, 1984.
302 Guarda LA et al: Human cryptosporidiosis in the acquired immune deficiency syndrome. *Arch Pathol Lab Med* 107:562, 1983.
303 Pitlik SD et al: Cryptosporidial cholecystitis. *N Engl J Med* 308:967, 1983.
304 Blumberg RS et al: Cytomegalovirus and *Cryptosporidium*-associated acalculous gangrenous cholecystitis. *Am J Med* 76:1118, 1984.
305 McMillan A, McNeillage GJC: Comparison of the sensitivity of microscopy and culture in the laboratory diagnosis of intestinal protozoal infection. *J Clin Pathol* 37:809, 1984.
306 Jokipii L et al: Frequency, multiplicity, and repertoire of intestinal protozoa in healthy homosexual men and in patients with gastrointestinal symptoms. *Ann Clin Res* 17:57, 1985.
307 Chaisson MA et al: A prevalence survey for *Cryptosporidium* and other parasites in healthy homosexual men in New York City. The 34th Annual Meeting of the American Society of Tropical Medicine and Hygiene, November, 1985, abstr 203.
308 Addy PAK, Aikins-Bekoe P: Cryptosporidiosis in diarrhoeal children in Kumasi, Ghana. *Lancet* 1:735, 1986.
309 Smith G, Ende J: Cryptosporidiosis among black children in hospital in South Africa. *J Infect Dis* 13:25, 1986.
310 Pape JW et al: Cryptosporidiosis in Haitian children. *Am J Trop Med Hyg* 36:333, 1987.
311 Hart CA et al: Gastroenteritis due to *Cryptosporidium:* A prospective survey in a children's hospital. *J Infect* 9:264, 1984.
312 Baxby D et al: Shedding of oocysts by immunocompetent individuals with cryptosporidiosis. *J Hyg Camb* 95:703, 1985.

313 Ratnam S et al: Occurrence of *Cryptosporidium* oocysts in fecal samples submitted for routine microbiological examination. *J Clin Microbiol* 22:402, 1985.
314 Centers for Disease Control: Cryptosporidiosis among children attending day care centers. *MMWR* 33:599, 1984.
315 Cordell RL, Addiss DG: Cryptosporidiosis in child care settings: A review of the literature and recommendations for prevention and control. *Pediatr Infect Dis J* 13:311–317, 1994.
316 Centers for Disease Control: Cryptosporidiosis—New Mexico, 1986. *MMWR* 36:561, 1987.
317 D'Antonio RG et al: A waterborne outbreak of cryptosporidiosis normal hosts. *Ann Intern Med* 103:886, 1985.
318 Goldstein ST et al: Cryptosporidiosis: An outbreak associated with drinking water despite state-of-the-art water treatment. *Ann Int Med* 124:459, 1996.
319 Musial CE et al: Detection of *Cryptosporidium* in water by using polypropylene cartridge filters. *Applied Environ Microbiol* 53:68, 1987.
320 Madore MS et al: Occurrence of *Cryptosporidium* oocysts in sewage effluents and select surface waters. *J Parasitol* 73:702, 1987.
321 Yolken RH et al: Infectious enteritis in bone-marrow transplant recipients. *N Engl J Med* 306:1009, 1982.
322 Symposium on Emerging Perspectives in Management and Prevention of Infectious Diseases: *Diarrheal Disease,* HC Neil (ed). *Am J Med* 78 (suppl 6B):63, 1985.
323 Vakil NB et al: Biliary cryptosporidiosis in HIV-infected people after the waterborne outbreak of cryptosporidiosis in Milwaukee. *N Engl J Med* 334:19–23, 1996.
324 Kehl KS et al: Comparison of four different methods for detection of *Cryptosporidium* species. *J Clin Microbiol* 33:416–418, 1995.
325 Weikel CS et al: Cryptosporidiosis in northeastern Brazil: Association with sporadic diarrhea. *J Infect Dis* 151:963, 1985.
326 Sterling CR, Arrowood MJ: Detection of *Cryptosporidium* sp. infections using a direct immunofluorescent assay. *Pediatr Infect Dis* 5: 139, 1986.
327 Garcia LS et al: Fluorescence detection of *Cryptosporidium* oocyst in human fecal specimens by using monoclonal antibodies. *J Clin Microbiol* 25:119, 1987.
328 Newman RD et al: Evaluation of an antigen capture enzyme-linked immunosorbent assay for detection of *Cryptosporidium* oocysts. *J Clin Microbiol* 31:2080–2084, 1993.
329 Ungar BLP et al: Enzyme immunoassay detection of immunoglobulin M and G antibodies to *Cryptosporidium* in immunocompetent and immunocompromised persons. *J Infect Dis* 153:570, 1986.
330 Holten-Andersen W et al: Prevalence of *Cryptosporidium* among patients with acute enteric infection. *J Infect Dis* 9:277, 1984.
331 Montessori GA, Bischoff L: Cryptosporidiosis: A cause of summer diarrhea in children. *Can Med Assoc J* 132:1285, 1985.
332 Marshall AR et al: Cryptosporidiosis in patients at a large teaching hospital. *J Clin Microbiol* 25: 172, 1987.
333 Weikel CS: Cryptosporidiosis: Diagnostic advances, treatment hurdles. *Hosp Ther* 13:109, 1988.
334 Centers for Disease Control: Update: Treatment of cryptosporidiosis in patients with acquired immunodeficiency syndrome (AIDS) *MMWR* 33:117,1984.
335 Portnoy D et al: Treatment of intestinal cryptosporidiosis with spiramycin. *Ann Intern Med* 101:202, 1984.
336 Collier AC et al: Cryptosporidiosis after marrow transplantation: Person-to-person transmission and treatment with spiramycin. *Ann Intern Med* 101:205, 1984.
337 White AC Jr et al: Paromomycin for cryptosporidiosis in AIDS: A prospective, double-blind trial. *J Infect Dis* 170:419–424, 1994.
338 Campbell I et al: Effect of disinfectants on survival of *Cryptosporidium* oocysts. *Vet Rec* 111:414, 1982.
339 Anderson BC: Moist heat inactivation of *Cryptosporidium* sp. *Am Public Health* 75:1433, 1985.
339a Kaplan JE et al and USPHS/IDSA Prevention of Opportunistic Infections Working Group: USPHS/IDSA guidelines for the prevention of opportunistic infections in persons infected with human immunodeficiency virus: an overview. *Clin Infect Dis* 21(supp 1):S12–S31,1995.
340 Huang et al: The first reported outbreak of diarrheal illness associated with *Cyclospora* in the United States. *Ann Intern Med* 123:409–414, 1995.
341 Wurtz R: *Cyclospora:* A newly identified intestinal pathogen of humans [Review]. *Clin Infect Dis* 18:620–623, 1994.
342 Connor BA et al: Pathologic changes in the small bowel in nine patients with diarrhea associated with a coccidia-like body. *Ann Intern Med* 119:377–382, 1993.
343 Hoge CW et al: Placebo-controlled trial of co-trimoxazole for cyclospora infections among travellers and foreign residents in Nepal *Lancet*, 345:691–693, 1995. [Erratum appears in *Lancet* 345(8956): 1060, Apr 22, 1995].
344 Ortega YR et al: *Cyclospora* sp.—a new protozoan pathogen of humans. *N Engl J Med* 328:1308–1312, 1993.
345 Pape JW et al: Cyclospora infection in adults infected with HIV: Clinical manifestations, treatment, and prophylaxis. *Ann lntern Med* l21: 654–657, 1994.
346 Shlim DR et al: An alga-like organism associated with an outbreak of prolonged diarrhea among foreigners in Nepal. *Am J Trop Med Hyg* 45:383–389, 1991.
347 Weber R et al: Improved light-microscopical detection of microsporidia spores in stool and duodenal aspirates. *N Engl J Med* 326:161–166, 1992.
348 Weber R et al: Detection of *Septata intestinalis* in stool specimens and coprodiagnostic monitoring of successful treatment with albendazole. *Clin Infect Dis* 19:342–345, 1994.
349 Molina JM et al: Disseminated microsporidiosis due to *Septata intestinalis* in patients with AIDS: Clinical features and response to albendazole therapy. *J Infect Dis* 171:245–249, 1995.
350 Blanshard C et al: Treatment of intestinal microsporidiosis with albendazole in patients with AIDS. *AIDS* 6:311–313, 1992.
351 Dieterich DT et al: Treatment with albendazole for intestinal disease due to *Enterocytozoon bieneusi* in patients with AIDS. *J Infect Dis* 169:178–183, 1994.

Chapter 45
Vulvovaginal candidiasis

Jack D. Sobel

EPIDEMIOLOGY

The earliest reports of vulvovaginal candidiasis (VVC) appear in the writings of Hippocrates and Galen. Frank is purported to have written the first clinical description in 1792.[1] A report by Wilkinson in 1894 is the earliest clinical description that also linked clinical manifestation with fungal etiology.[2]

Information on the incidence of VVC is incomplete, particularly since VVC is not a reportable entity. Furthermore, collecting data on VVC is hampered by inaccuracies of diagnosis of the condition. Data on incidence, where diagnostic data are based on definite clinical and mycological findings, are exceptional.[1] Moreover, most studies have been carried out in sexually transmitted disease (STD) clinics or in family planning or student health clinics, largely ignoring the private sector and older women. Most studies suggest a VVC prevalence of 5 to 15 percent, depending on the population studied.

Vulvovaginal candidiasis affects most females at least once during their lives, at an estimated rate of 70 to 75 percent,[3–5] of whom 40 to 50 percent will experience a recurrence.[5,6] A small subpopulation of probably fewer than 5 percent of all adult women has recurrent, often intractable episodes of VVC (Table 45-1). Diagnosis and therapy of VVC, together with lost productivity, result in an estimated cost of 1 billion dollars annually in the United States.[3] Statistical data in the United Kingdom derived from patients whose conditions were diagnosed at genitourinary medicine centers show a sharp increase in the annual incidence of VVC from 118 per 100,000 to 200 per 100,000 women during the last decade.[7] In the United States, candidiasis is currently the second most common cause of vaginal infections, with bacterial vaginosis (BV) the most common diagnostic entity.[8,9] The number of prescriptions written to treat yeast infections between 1980 and 1990 indicates that the incidence of VVC almost doubled during that time; approximately 13 million prescriptions were written in 1990.

Point-prevalence studies indicate that *Candida* species may be isolated from the lower genital tract of approximately 20 percent (occasional studies set the upper limit at 55 percent) of asymptomatic healthy women without abnormal vaginal discharge.[10–12] Among women with symptoms of vulvovaginitis, 29.8 percent had yeast isolated, confirming the diagnosis of VVC.[13] Most studies indicate that VVC is a frequent diagnosis among young women, affecting as many as 15 to 30 percent of symptomatic women visiting a clinician. Regrettably, the recent availability of over-the-counter antimycotics will further limit the ability to measure asymptomatic candida carriage and VVC in populations of women.

MICROBIOLOGY

Between 85 and 90 percent of yeast strains isolated from the vagina belong to the species *Candida albicans*. The remainder are non-*albicans* species, the commonest of which is *Candida glabrata (Torulopsis glabrata)*. Non-*albicans* species can also induce vaginitis, which is clinically indistinguishable from that caused by *C. albicans*; moreover, they are often more resistant to therapy.[12,14,15]

It has been claimed, but not proved, that the percentage of vaginal candida infections caused by non-*albicans* strains is rising dramatically.[16,17] The use of single-dose oral and topical regimens, together with the popularity of low-dosage azole maintenance regimens and the availability of over-the-counter antimycotics, have been blamed for the appearance of non-*albicans* species, given the lesser susceptibility of these species to azole agents. Nevertheless, two large multicenter studies failed to demonstrate any increase in the prevalence of VVC caused by non-*albicans* species.[18,19] It is of interest that anecdotal reports occasionally describe a natural high frequency of non-*albicans* VVC, often exceeding 50 percent.[20] After *C. albicans, C. glabrata* is by far the most frequent cause of acute and chronic vulvovaginitis. In the United States, diabetes mellitus has emerged as a major risk factor for *C. glabrata* vaginitis. Infrequent causes of fungal vaginitis include *C. parapsilosis* and *C. tropicalis*, although virtually every species of *Candida* has been associated with vaginitis.

Biotyping of *C. albicans* permitted early epidemiologic studies directed at identifying strains with specific tropism for the vagina.[21] Probably because of the limitations of biotyping methodology, no such tropism was identified. Similarly, no evidence emerged of vaginopathic strains of *C. albicans* demonstrating greater or lesser virulence that might explain why some women remain entirely asymptomatic despite being heavily colonized with *Candida* species, whereas other women develop severe symptomatic vaginitis. The concept of vaginopathogenicity, although somewhat simplistic, is not entirely without merit and may well be the result of switching phenotypic and virulence properties. DNA typing has provided a more reliable and reproducible method of answering these questions. Soll and coworkers, using computer assisted DNA-probe typing and including Southern blots, have presented data to support the concept of "vaginal tropism," in which selected organisms demonstrate adaptation to unique anatomic niches. [22] Such adaptation facilitates persistence and survival at certain anatomic sites, including the vagina.

Candida organisms are dimorphic, in that they may be found in humans in different phenotypic phases. In general, blastospores (blastoconidia) represent the phenotypic form responsible for transmission and spread, including the bloodstream phase, as well as the form associated with asymptomatic colonization of the vagina. In contrast, germinated yeast with production of mycelia most commonly (but not exclusively) constitute a tissue-invasive form usually identified in the presence of symptomatic disease.

CANDIDA VIRULENCE FACTORS

In order for species of *Candida* to colonize the vagina, they must first adhere to vaginal epithelial cells. *C. albicans* adheres in significantly higher numbers to such cells than do *C. tropicalis, C. krusei*, and *C. keyfer*.[23] This may explain the relative infrequency of the latter species causing vaginitis. All *C. albicans* strains appear to adhere equally well to both exfoliated vaginal and buccal epithelial cells. In contrast, there is considerable person-to-person variation in vaginal epithelial cell receptivity to candida organisms in adherence assays.[24] Nevertheless, such organisms do not show increased cell affinity for vaginal cells from women with VVC.[25] The significance of adherence in the pathogenesis of candidal vaginitis is suggested by the failure of a cerulean-resistant mutant of *C. albicans*, which adhered poorly, to induce vaginitis in an experimental murine model of candidiasis.[26] No epithelial cell receptor for *Candida* has yet been identified, and the yeast adhesin appears to reside with the surface mannoprotein.

Germination of candida cells enhances colonization[27] and facilitates tissue invasion. Using a mutant strain of *C. albicans* which failed to germinate at 37°C, Sobel and coworkers demonstrated

Table 45-1. Azole Therapy of Vaginal Candidiasis

Drug	Formulation	Dosage
Butoconazole (Femstat)	2% cream	5 gm × 3 days
Clotrimazole	1% cream	5 gm × 7–14 days
(Gynelotromin, Mycelex)	10% cream	5 gm single applic
	100-mg vaginal tab	1 tab × 7 days
	100-mg vaginal tab	2 tab × 3 days
	500-mg vaginal tab	1 tab once
Miconazole (Monistat)	2% cream	5 gm × 7 days
	100-mg vaginal supp	1 supp × 7 days
	200-mg vaginal supp	1 supp × 3 days
	1200-mg vaginal supp	1 supp once
Econazole	150-mg vaginal tab	1 tab × 3 days
Fenticonazole	2% cream	5 gm × 7 days
Tioconazole (Vagistat)	2% cream	5 gm × 3 days
	6.5% cream	5 gm single applic
Terconazole (Terazol)	0.4% cream	5 gm × 7 days
	0.8% cream	5 gm × 3 days
	80-mg vaginal supp	1 supp × 3 days
Fluconazole (Diflucan)	150-mg tab	single dose
Ketoconazole (Nizoral)	200-mg tab	2 tab × 5 days
Intraconazole (Sporonox)	100-mg tab	2 tab × 3 days

in vivo that nongerminating mutants were incapable of inducing experimental VVC.[27] The implications of this observation are that factors that enhance or facilitate germination might tend to promote symptomatic vaginitis, whereas measures that inhibit germination may prevent vaginitis in women who are asymptomatic carriers of yeast.[28]

Little is known regarding the role of candidal proteolytic enzymes, toxins, and phospholipase in determining the virulence of the organisms. A secreted aspartyl proteinase elaborated by pathogenic *Candida* species has been identified in vaginal secretions and is detected in women with symptomatic vaginitis but not in those with asymptomatic colonization.[29,30] These proteolytic enzymes, which have broad substrate specificity, destroy free and cell-bound proteins that impair fungal colonization and invasion. Levels of proteinase secretion by vaginal *C. albicans* isolates were greater in isolates obtained from symptomatic women than from asymptomatic carriers.[29] Several genes governing proteinase production have been cloned, and a strong correlation exists both in vitro and in experimental vaginitis between gene expression, aspartyl proteinase secretion, and ability to cause disease.[31] Mycotoxin—for example, gliotoxin—may act to inhibit phagocytic activity or suppress the local immune system. Gliotoxin has been found in vaginal secretions.[32]

High-frequency heritable switching occurs in colony morphology of most *Candida* species grown on amino acid–rich agar in vitro at 24°C.[33] The variant phenotypes represent, among other things, a varying capacity to form mycelia spontaneously and to express other virulence factors, such as drug resistance, adherence, and capacity to invade and survive in diverse body sites, as well as to cause disease. Although currently there is incomplete evidence that phenotypic switching occurs in vivo at 37°C, this is an attractive hypothesis to explain spontaneous in vivo transformation from asymptomatic colonization to symptomatic vaginitis. Fresh clinical vaginal isolates obtained from women with acute vaginitis have been found to be in a high-frequency mode of switching. These multiple phenotypes at a given site represent the same or related genetic strains.[34–36] Phenotypic transition occurs spontaneously but is facilitated by exogenous factors such as temperature and as yet unknown factors.

Overall adaptability of *C. albicans* to different microenvironments itself represents a factor of virulence. In one patient with recurrent VVC who was sampled extensively during three episodes of vaginitis, Soll observed colony phenotype switch with each recurrence of infection, even though DNA fingerprinting (genotype) of the infecting strain remained the same.[36] Vazquez et al., in a large longitudinal study of recurrent VVC, similarly reported an identical vaginal isolate genotype with each successive recurrence over several years, with only infrequent introduction of a new strain type of *C. albicans*.[37] Soll, using a sensitive DNA probe with great discriminatory ability, has recently shown that even though the same strain may persist long-term in the vagina, a certain degree of yeast genetic instability exists nevertheless, especially in the face of repeated courses of antifungal therapy.[38]

Recently, iron-binding by candida organisms has been shown to facilitate their virulence.[39] The ready availability of erythrocytes and hemoglobin in the vagina creates an ideal niche for yeast possessing erythrocyte-binding surface receptors.

PATHOGENESIS

Candida organisms gain access to the vaginal lumen and secretions predominantly from the adjacent perianal area.[40,41] VVC is seen predominantly in women of childbearing age, and in the majority of cases a precipitating factor is not identified to explain the transformation from asymptomatic carriage to symptomatic vaginitis. Two fundamental questions are critical in understanding the pathogenesis of VVC. The first relates to the mechanism whereby asymptomatic colonization of the vagina changes to symptomatic VVC. The second concerns the mechanism whereby some women suffer from repeated and chronic VVC.

Hurley and associates have fostered the view that *C. albicans* is never a commensal in the vagina, maintaining that clinicians can almost always detect vaginal pathology even in asymptomatic patients from whom such strains have been isolated.[5,6] Subsequent investigators, however, have not corroborated this view and have demonstrated that many women carry *C. albicans* in the vagina without symptoms or signs of vaginitis, usually with low concentration of yeast organisms.[10] These observations are compatible with the view that *C. albicans* may be either a commensal or a pathogen in the vagina and that changes in the host vaginal environment are usually necessary before the organism induces pathologic effects. The concept that *C. albicans* is never a commensal has been challenged as simplistic and excludes the possibility of the commensal organism inducing symptomatic infection due to spontaneous phenotype switching.[35]

PREDISPOSING FACTORS

Pregnancy

During pregnancy the vagina shows an increased susceptibility to infection by species of *Candida*, resulting in both a higher prevalence of vaginal colonization and as a higher rate of symptomatic vaginitis.[42] The rate of symptomatic vaginitis is maximally increased in the third trimester, and symptomatic recurrences are also more common during pregnancy.[15,42] It is generally thought that high levels of reproductive hormones, by providing a higher glycogen content in the vaginal tissue, provide an excellent carbon source for candida organisms.[43] A more complex mechanism seems likely, in that estrogen enhances adherence of yeast cells to the vaginal mucosa. A cytosol receptor, or binding system, for female reproductive hormones has been documented in *Candida albicans*.[44] Several investigators have demonstrated in vitro binding of female sex hormones to candida organisms as well as the capacity of certain hormones to enhance yeast mycelial formation and hence virulence.[44,45] Accordingly, it is postulated that the high levels of reproductive hormones encountered in pregnancy directly enhance yeast virulence. Not surprisingly, therefore, rates of cure of VVC are significantly lower during pregnancy.[1]

Contraceptives

Many small, poorly controlled studies have produced a plethora of conflicting conclusions. Several studies have shown increased vaginal colonization with species of *Candida* following high-estrogen-content oral contraceptive use.[1] Almost certainly, the same mechanism operative in pregnancy applies to the subjects of these studies. Some studies of women utilizing low-estrogen-content oral contraceptives have not found an increase in VVC.[46–49] Nevertheless, many investigators continue to identify oral contraceptives as predisposing to recurrent vulvovaginal candidiasis. Rahman and coworkers reported users of any contraceptive method more likely to harbor *Candida* organisms than nonusers.[50] Several studies found increased carriage of such yeasts in IUD users.[51,52] Peddie and coworkers[54] found an increased carriage in diaphragm and condom users, with or without use of spermicide. Barbone et al.,[49] as well as Hooton et al.,[55] reported an increased colonization associated with nonoxynol-9 use. Other risk factors may include the contraceptive sponge. Foxman, in an extensive study of risk factors in college students, identified no difference in risk between users of no birth control method and users of oral contraceptives, diaphragms, condoms, and spermicides.[48]

Diabetes mellitus

Vaginal colonization with *Candida* organisms is more frequent in diabetic women. Although uncontrolled diabetes predisposes to symptomatic vaginitis, most diabetics are not afflicted by such repeated infections.[1] It has become traditional to perform glucose tolerance tests in all women with recurrent VVC. The yield of these expensive studies is extremely low; testing, therefore, is not justified in premenopausal women. Occasionally women with recurrent VVC describe an association between "candy binges" and exacerbation of symptomatic vaginitis. However, for the most part dietary restrictions have no place in the routine management of yeast vaginitis.

Antibiotics

Onset of symptomatic VVC is frequently observed during courses of systemic antibiotics. Broad-spectrum antibiotics such as tetracycline, ampicillin, and oral cephalosporins are mainly responsible for exacerbation of symptoms. Not only is symptomatic vaginitis frequently precipitated, but vaginal colonization rates increase from approximately 10 percent to 30 percent.[56,57] Antibiotics, both systemic and topical agents, are thought to act by eliminating the protective vaginal bacterial flora.[57] The natural flora is thought to provide colonization resistance and also to prevent germination and thus superficial mucosal invasion. In particular, aerobic and anaerobic resident lactobacilli have been singled out as providing such a protective function. Auger and Joly found low numbers of lactobacilli in vaginal cultures obtained from women with symptomatic VVC.[59] Current concepts of a lactobacillus-yeast cell interaction include competition for nutrients as well as stearic interference by lactobacilli with receptor sites for *Candida* organisms on vaginal epithelial cells.[24] Other mechanisms include the elaboration of bacteriocins by lactobacilli which inhibit yeast proliferation and germination as well as a direct antibiotic-induced stimulatory effect on growth of *Candida* species.[59]

In spite of the evidence indicating a contributory role for antibiotics, most women who receive antibiotics do not develop symptomatic vaginitis. Moreover, the overwhelming majority of women with acute VVC have not been the recent recipient of antibiotics. It would appear that only a subpopulation of women, already colonized by potentially virulent species of *Candida*, are at risk of developing vaginitis following antimicrobial therapy.

Behavioral factors

The incidence of VVC increases dramatically in the second decade, corresponding to the onset of sexual activity. It peaks in the third and fourth decade, declining in females older than 40 years, until the permissive effect of hormone replacement therapy becomes apparent. Several studies have shown that sexual transmission of *Candida* organisms occurs during vaginal intercourse, although the role of nonsexual practices in introducing candida organisms into the lower genital tract has not been appraised.[41,60–63] Other studies have provided conflicting evidence as to the role, if any, of sexual behavior in causing symptomatic VVC.[3,48,49] The likelihood that sexual behavior may play a role in VVC is logical, but epidemiologic evidence is limited. Some authors suggest that recent sexual intercourse frequency is correlated with acute vaginitis,[48,63] and others have identified receptive orogenital sex.[64] In spite of anecdotal evidence, Foxman found no epidemiologic evidence incriminating female hygiene habits as risk factors for VVC.[48]

Miscellaneous

Among the putative factors that have contributed to the increased incidence of VVC in Western societies has been the use of tight, restricting, poorly ventilated clothing and nylon underclothing, resulting in increased local, perineal moisture and temperature.[1,65] The use of well-ventilated clothing and cotton underwear may be of value in preventing infection.[65] On the other hand, Foxman found no increased risk for VVC among wearers of tight clothing or noncotton underwear. [48] There is no evidence confirming that iron deficiency predisposes to infection.[66] Anecdotal evidence suggests that the use of commercial douches, perfumed toilet paper, chlorinated swimming pools, and feminine hygiene sprays contributes to symptomatic vaginitis. Chemical contact, local allergy, or hypersensitivity reactions may alter the vaginal milieu and permit the transformation from asymptomatic colonization to symptomatic vaginitis.

SOURCE OF INFECTION

Intestinal reservoir

Although the gastrointestinal tract may well be the initial source of colonization of the vagina by candida organisms, there is considerable controversy regarding the role of the intestinal tract as a source of reinfection in women with recurrent VVC.[67]

Species of *Candida* were recovered on rectal culture from 100 percent of women with recurrent VVC.[68] This observation has been the basis of the concept of a persistent intestinal reservoir. Reinoculation of the vagina occurs from the persistent rectal focus following apparent eradication of vaginal yeast by topical therapy. This hypothesis has been criticized, as several authors have found much lower concordance between rectal and vaginal cultures in patients with recurrent VVC.[41,42] The high rate of anorectal cultures in some studies likely reflects perineal and perianal contamination from the vaginal discharge. Moreover, VVC recurred frequently in women in the absence of simultaneously positive rectal cultures. Two controlled studies using oral nystatin treatment, which reduces intestinal yeast carriage, failed to prevent symptomatic recurrence of vaginal candidiasis.[69,70] Furthermore, some women had persistent intestinal yeast carriage and failed to develop vaginal colonization.

In spite of mounting skepticism, the possibility that persistent gastrointestinal tract carriage is a source of vaginal reinfection cannot be entirely dismissed, especially since the majority of *Candida* strains isolated from the rectum and the vagina are identical.[41,71] Women prone to recurrent VVC are not known to suffer from perianal or rectal candidiasis.

Sexual transmission

Penile colonization with candida organisms is present in approximately 20 percent of male partners of women with recurrent VVC (RVVC).[61,62] *Candida* organisms are most commonly found in uncircumcised, usually asymptomatic males in the vicinity of the coronal sulcus. Asymptomatic male genital colonization with species of *Candida* is four times more common in male sexual partners of infected women.[61] Infected partners usually carry identical strains.[41]

In spite of the aforementioned evidence indicating that sexual transmission does occur, the contribution of sexual transmission to the pathogenesis of infection remains unknown. From the prevalence of positive penile and urethral cultures, it appears that the role of sexual spread is limited. Hence, routine therapy of male partners, even those of women with RVVC, is unlikely to substantially reduce recurrence rates. Limited evidence is available that anogenital and particularly orogenital contact transmit infection.[64]

Relapse

After systemic and topical antibiotic therapy of VVC, negative vaginal candida cultures once more turn positive within 30 days in 20 to 25 percent of women, strongly supporting the hypothesis that vaginal relapse is responsible for RVVC.[1] Strains isolated before and after therapy are of the identical type in more than two-thirds of recurrences.[41] Symptomatic relief after clinically successful topical therapy of symptomatic vaginitis is accompanied by a drastic reduction in the number of viable yeast cells in the vagina. Small numbers of the microorganisms persist, however, within the vaginal lumen, generally in numbers too small to be detected by conventional vaginal cultures.[72] It is also conceivable that small numbers of *Candida* organisms might sojourn temporarily within superficial cervical or vaginal epithelial cells only to reemerge some weeks or months later.[73]

VAGINAL DEFENSE MECHANISMS

Humoral system

Patients with profound immunoglobulin deficiencies are not susceptible to vaginal yeast infections. Following acute VVC, systemic (IgM and IgG) and local (S-IgA) responses are elicited.[74,75] The protective role of vaginal antibodies is unknown. Patients with recurrent infection do not lack antibody.[76] Lower antibody titers have been described during active vaginal infections, which may reflect an adsorption effect. Recent studies by Polonelli and coworkers using an experimental animal model of vaginitis provide supportive evidence for a protective role of specific antibodies induced by immunization.[77] Elevated serum and vaginal IgE antibodies to *Candida* organisms were detected in some women with RVVC, even though the total IgE levels were normal.[78,79]

Phagocytic system

Although both polymorphonuclear leukocytes and monocytes play an important role in limiting systemic candidal infection and deep-tissue invasion,[80] these phagocytic cells are characteristically absent from vaginal fluid during VVC. Accordingly, these phagocytic cells are not thought to play a role in influencing mucosal colonization or even preventing superficial invasion of the vaginal epithelium by *Candida* organisms. In the rat model of experimental VVC, as in humans, histology of the vagina fails to demonstrate leukocytes in the vaginal fluid or stratified squamous epithelium. Polymorphonuclear cells can be seen concentrating within the underlying lamina propria but appear not to be presented with a chemotactic signal to induce migration into more superficial layers or vaginal fluid.

Cell-mediated immunity

Oral thrush, which correlates well with depressed cell-mediated immunity (CMI), is frequently seen in debilitated or immunosuppressed patients. This is particularly evident in patients with chronic mucocutaneous candidiasis or with AIDS. In this context *Candida* organisms are typically opportunistic pathogens. Accordingly, one might anticipate that lymphocytes similarly contribute to normal vaginal defense mechanisms, possibly preventing mucosal invasion by such organisms by the elaboration of cytokines such as gamma-interferon, which inhibits germ-tube formation.

The role of CMI is further emphasized by studies that investigated the role of impaired CMI in predisposing women to idiopathic RVVC. Virtually all adult women have positive cutaneous delayed hypersensitivity reactions, as well as in vitro lymphoblast proliferation response, to *Candida* antigens. Earlier studies reported cutaneous anergy and depressed lymphoblastic response to *Candida* antigens in women with RVVC.[80–84] The possibility of a subpopulation of suppressor lymphocytes or serum factors inducing suppression of local vaginal CMI was postulated.[83] In conflict with these observations, more recent studies using a variety of *Candida* antigens and measurement of cytokine elaboration demonstrated a normal systemic CMI response in this population.[85] They showed that the previously reported cutaneous anergy was transient only—the consequence and not the cause of RVVC—and that impaired systemic CMI was not involved in the pathogenesis of RVVC in these women. Several additional studies by Fidel et al., using the mouse vaginitis model, determined that systemic CMI has only a minor role in providing a normal defense function at the level of the vaginal mucosa.[86–88] These studies also demonstrated that local and systemic immunity to infection by *Candida* organisms could be induced by vaginal sensitization and that the immunity provided is partially protective in the vagina. Finally, they demonstrated a significant compartmentalization of the CMI system.[87,88]

The studies by Fidel et al. did not exclude the possibility of a local vaginal acquired defect in CMI predisposing to RVVC.[85–88] In this regard, Witkin et al. reported in vitro studies supporting an impaired CMI in women with RVVC.[89,90] They postulated that local elaboration of prostaglandin E2 by the patient's macrophages blocked local protective lymphocyte function, possibly by inhibiting interleukin-2 production.[91] According to this hypothesis, abnormal macrophage function could be the result either of local IgE antibodies to *C. albicans* in the vagina of women with RVVC or of inhibitory serum factors.[92] The exact protective mechanism of vaginal T lymphocytes has yet to be explained but appears to conform to a Th-1 profile.[87] Recent studies indicate unique subpopulations of vagina-specific lymphocytes.[140]

Vaginal flora

Probably the most important defense against both candidal colonization and symptomatic inflammation is the normal natural bacterial flora. Any newly arrived *Candida* organism, in order to survive and persist, must initially adhere to epithelial cells and then grow, proliferate, and germinate in order to colonize the vaginal mucosa successfully. Although microbial competition for nutrients has long been considered the most important source of competition, animal studies suggest that lactobacilli and *Candida* organisms frequently survive side by side.[93] The role of bacteriocins in inhibiting yeast growth and germination requires additional investigation.[59]

Miscellaneous defense mechanisms

Although not studied in the vagina, various natural secretions have been shown to possess considerable antifungal activity. Pollack et al. reported fungistatic and fungicidal activity against *C. albicans* of human parotid salivary histidine-rich polypeptides.[94]

MECHANISMS INVOLVED IN INVASION AND INFLAMMATORY RESPONSE

The mechanism whereby *Candida* organisms induce inflammation is not yet established. Yeast cells are capable of producing several extracellular proteases as well as phospholipase. The paucity of phagocytic cells in the inflammatory exudate possibly reflects the lack of chemotactic substances elaborated. Both blastoconidia and pseudohyphae are capable of destroying superficial cells by direct invasion.

During the symptomatic episode there is the conspicuous appearance of the germinated or filamentous forms of candida cells. Germinated organisms not only enhance colonization but represent the dominant invasive phase capable of penetrating intact epithelial cells and invading the vaginal epithelium, although only the very superficial layers are involved.[95] Although symptoms are not strictly related to the yeast load, VVC does tend to be associated with greater numbers of *Candida* organisms and with the germinated yeast phase.[95] Approximately 10^3 to 10^4 candida cells per milliliter of vaginal fluid may be recovered in both symptomatic and asymptomatic states.[1]

The clinical spectrum varies from an acute florid exudative form with thick white vaginal discharge and large numbers of germinated yeast cells, to the other extreme of absent or minimal discharge, fewer organisms, and yet severe pruritus. Based on this, it is suggested that more than one pathogenic mechanism may exist. In the presence of pruritus alone, hypersensitivity or immune mechanisms are likely to be involved.[96–98] Not infrequently, male partners of asymptomatic female carriers of *Candida* develop postcoital penile erythema and pruritus, which usually last several hours only.

CLINICAL MANIFESTATIONS

Acute pruritus and vaginal discharge are the usual presenting complaints, but neither symptom is specific to VVC, and neither is invariably associated with any obvious disease. The most frequent symptom is that of vulvar pruritus, which is present in virtually all symptomatic patients. Vaginal discharge is not invariably present and is frequently minimal. Although described as typically cottage-cheese-like in character, the discharge may vary from watery to homogeneously thick. Vaginal soreness, irritation, vulvar burning, dyspareunia, and external dysuria are commonly present. Odor, if present, is minimal and inoffensive. Examination frequently reveals erythema and swelling of the labia and vulva, often with discrete pustulopapular peripheral lesions. The cervix is normal, and vaginal epithelial erythema is present together with adherent whitish discharge. Characteristically, symptoms are exacerbated in the week preceding the onset of menstrual flow.

It is apparent that a clinical spectrum of VVC exists. In some patients a more exudative picture is apparent, with copious discharge and white plaques, satisfying the traditional description of vaginal thrush. At the other end of the spectrum are those patients with minimal discharge and severe erythema, particularly with extensive vulvar involvement which often extends into the inguinal and perianal regions. In general, a quantitative relationship exists between the classic signs and symptoms of VVC, notably pruritus and vulvitis, and the extent of genital yeast colonization. Several surveys indicate the unreliability of patient diagnosis.

Although *Candida* species occasionally cause extensive balanoposthitis in male partners of women with vaginal candidiasis, a more frequent event is a transient rash, erythema, and pruritus or a burning sensation of the penis which develops minutes or hours after unprotected intercourse. The symptoms are self-limiting and frequently disappear after showering. A history of postcoital penile rash was found in 20 percent of the partners of women with recurrent VVC (unpublished personal observation).

DIAGNOSIS AND TREATMENT

DIAGNOSIS

The lack of specificity of symptoms and signs precludes a diagnosis that is based on history and physical examination only. Neither clinical signs and symptoms alone nor culture confirmation of *Candida* should be regarded as a satisfactory basis for diagnosis.[99] Regrettably, both approaches are common in practice. In the Detroit Medical Center Candida Vaginitis Clinic, over 80 percent of physician-referred patients with a putative diagnosis of recalcitrant or recurrent VVC were found to have another cause of vaginitis and did not have VVC (personal observation). Bergman et al. emphasized that a patient's subjective symptoms are of no practical and consistent value in predicting VVC. The most specific symptom in genital candidiasis is pruritus without discharge, and even this criterion correctly predicted VVC in only 38 percent of patients.[100]

Most patients with symptomatic vaginitis may be readily diagnosed on the basis of microscopic examination of vaginal secretions (Fig. 45-1). Accordingly, a wet mount or saline preparation should routinely be done, not only to identify the presence of yeast cells and mycelia but also to exclude the presence of "clue cells" and motile trichomonads. A 10% potassium hydroxide (KOH) preparation is extremely valuable and even more sensitive in identifying germinated yeast (65 to 85 percent sensitivity). Large numbers of white cells are invariably absent in VVC and when present should suggest a mixed infection. Similarly, vaginal pH estimations reveal a normal pH (4.0 to 4.5) in VVC, and the finding of a vaginal pH in excess of 5.0 usually indicates bacterial vaginosis, trichomoniasis, or a mixed infection.

In spite of the value of direct microscopy, several studies have consistently revealed that up to 50 percent of patients with culture-positive symptomatic VVC (responding to antimycotic therapy) will have negative microscopy.[40] Thus, although routine cultures are unnecessary if the wet mount of KOH preparations shows yeast and mycelia, vaginal culture should be performed in the presence of negative microscopy if VVC is suspected on the

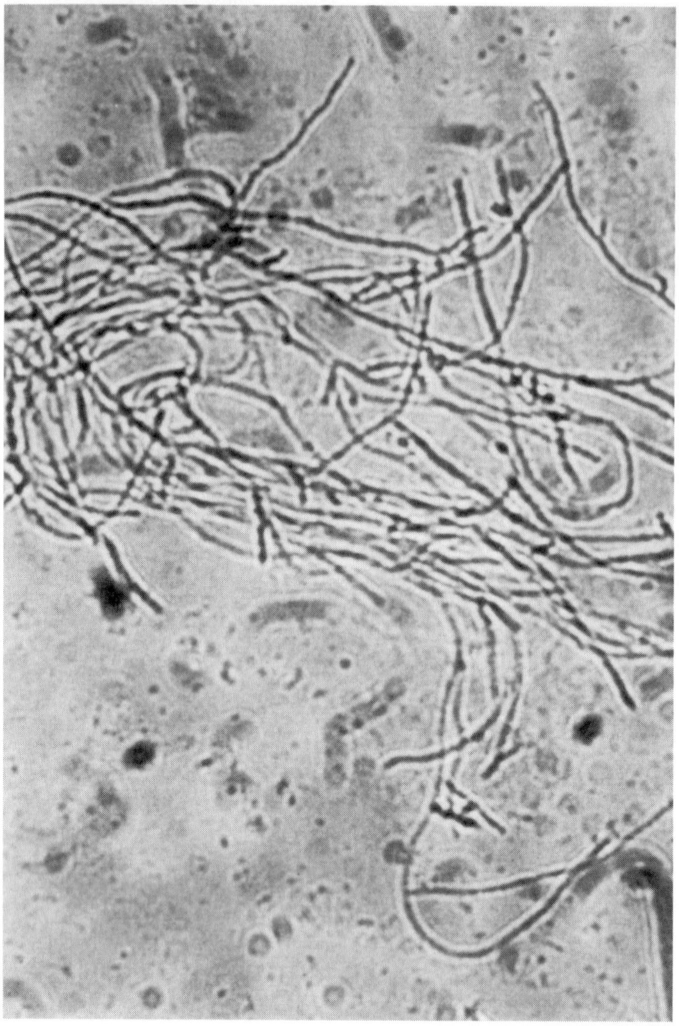

Fig. 45-1. Wet-mount examination of vaginal discharge from a woman with vulvovaginal candidiasis, showing mycelia. 1000 × magnification.

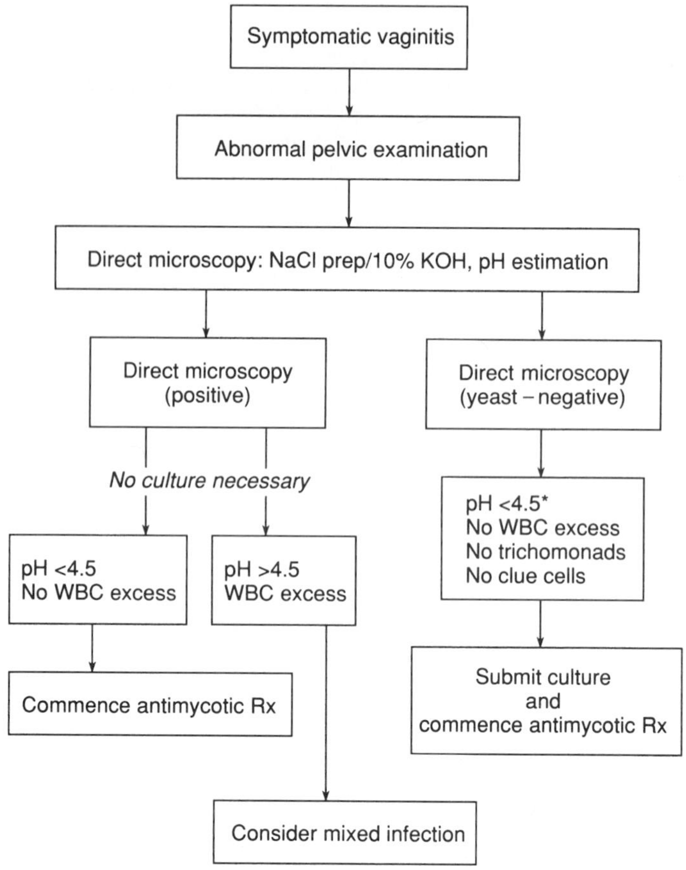

*Useful indication for Candida latex agglutination slide test.

Fig. 45-2. Algorithm for diagnosis and treatment of vulvovaginal candidasis.

basis of symptoms or signs (Fig. 45-2). Reliable clinical cultures can also be obtained using Nickerson's medium or semiquantitative "slide-stix" cultures. The PAP smear is unreliable as a diagnostic modality, being positive in only about 25 percent of patients with culture-positive symptomatic VVC.[101]

Although vaginal culture is the most sensitive method currently available for detecting candida cells, a positive culture does not necessarily indicate that the yeast is responsible for the vaginal symptoms.[102] Merson-Davies and coworkers[103] have shown that microscopy positive status usually correlates with relatively high yeast concentrations in vaginal secretions as confirmed by quantitative vaginal cultures. Their studies also suggested that in most women the yeast cell numbers correlate with severity of clinical signs and symptoms, and that commensal yeast vaginal carriage tends to be associated with lower numbers of vaginal yeast. Diagnosis of VVC requires a correlation of clinical findings, microscopic examination, and vaginal culture. Although some prefer to use a selective medium, there is no advantage in using Sabouraud agar, Nickerson's or Microstix-*Candida* media, or in adding antibiotics such as chloramphenicol to the isolation medium. There is no reliable serologic technique for the diagnosis of VVC.

Several commercial companies have reported success in achieving rapid and reliable diagnosis of candidal vaginitis, utilizing a latex agglutination slide technique employing polyclonal antibodies reactive with multiple species of *Candida* and directed against yeast mannan. One reported study revealed a sensitivity of 81 percent with a specificity of 98.5 percent.[102] Additional testing under clinical conditions, although confirming the reasonable sensitivity of the test, nevertheless found no advantage over standard microscopy.[104]

Most clinicians consider only trichomoniasis and bacterial vaginosis in the differential diagnosis of VVC. Given the profound differences in pH, PMN count, and Gram's stain appearance, these three common clinical infectious entities are easy to differentiate. More consideration is needed in the symptomatic patient in whom these three conditions have been excluded. The differential diagnosis of vulvovaginitis in the presence of normal pH, PMN count, and negative yeast cultures includes numerous noninfectious causes, including hypersensitivity, irritant and allergic vulvovaginitis, idiopathic focal vulvovestibulitis, cytolytic vaginosis, and physiologic leukorrhea.

TREATMENT

Acute vaginitis

A variety of highly effective topical azole agents are now available in a variety of formulations (Table 45-1).[105,106] No strong evidence exists that any one formulation results in superior cure rates, nor is there convincing evidence of the superiority of any specific azole over another azole in the treatment of VVC.[105,106] Overall cure rates for topical azole agents, defined as eradication of symptoms and mycologic-negative cultures, are of the order of 80 to 90 percent. Oral systemic azole agents achieve comparable or marginally higher therapeutic cure rates, and patients enjoy the convenience of oral administration, which eliminates local side effects and messiness. On the other hand, oral azoles suffer the drawback of potential systemic toxicity, which has limited the use of ketoconazole, although constituting a lesser consideration in prescribing intraconazole and fluconazole.

In spite of the wide therapeutic armamentarium available to practitioners, numerous management issues, some highly controversial, continue to permeate the clinical arena. None of the available agents or regimens fits all the desired properties of the ideal vaginal antifungal agent. None of them is fungicidal (that is, none achieves a greater than 99.9 percent killing of all *Candida* organism isolates within 24 h). Although capable of killing organisms, by strict definition azoles are fungistatic agents. This may be irrelevant when dealing with *C. albicans* strains, but in the presence of non-*albicans* species, including *C. tropicalis, C. parapsilosis,* and particularly *C. glabrata,* which are inherently less susceptible to all azoles, clinical failure is by no means infrequent.[107]

Several surveys have consistently shown that most women prefer the convenience of oral therapy.[108] Of the three oral azoles, ketoconazole, although the first effective systemic imidazole, is unlikely to gain widespread use in VVC due to a rare but serious hepatotoxicity.[109] Intraconazole 200 mg twice a day (single day) and fluconazole 150 mg (single-dose) are both highly effective triazoles, although neither achieves substantially higher cure rates than topical agents.[110–114] Oral agents cannot be expected to accomplish immediate local relief, hence severe local symptoms may necessitate adjunct topical treatment for the first 48 h.

Over the years, conventional use of vaginal antimycotics has been remarkably safe and free of untoward side effects. Certainly, no major morbidity or serious complications have been reported, although high-dose regimens of terconazole were associated with fever and flulike symptoms, which resulted in the withdrawal of this topical agent in high concentrations.[115] Mild to moderate vulvovaginal burning is an underestimated and not infrequent side effect of topical azoles. Accordingly, physicians should respect the preference of the patient when prescribing, both in relation to choice of route and the individual agent. Both intraconazole and fluconazole are extremely well tolerated, have good safety profiles, and are not comparable to ketoconazole with regard to risk of complications. Nevertheless, an untoward drug interaction was reported recently between intraconazole and astemizole or terfenadine (both commonly used antihistamines). Accordingly, the ideal antimycotic agent continues to elude us. Among the major shortcomings of the current agents is their relatively poor efficacy in vaginitis caused by non-*albicans* species of *Candida*, as well as the potential for *C. albicans* strains to become resistant to fluconazole (see later discussion of resistant yeast infections).

There has been a growing tendency to use shorter and shorter courses of both topical and oral agents.[105] Although justified on the basis of convenience and improved compliance, these new regimens have also been introduced to provide a marketing edge for one therapeutically equivalent agent over another. Testing the efficacy of short, often single-dose courses has not been subject to the same careful and thorough scrutiny as testing of the conventional 5-to 7-day regimens. Nevertheless, single-dose therapy by any route is effective in mild to moderate disease. Many of the single-dose drugs such as vaginal clotrimazole (500-mg suppository) and fluconazole (150-mg oral tablet) possess pharmacokinetic properties such that concentrations of the antimycotic persist in the vagina for up to 5 days following the single administration of these agents.[116,117] Hence, single-dose therapy may be more than "single-day" therapy. A recent study indicates that more severe vaginitis, particularly in women with recurrent VVC, should not be treated with single-dose therapy.[19]

Acute vaginitis in pregnancy

Management of VVC during pregnancy is more difficult, since clinical response tends to be slower and recurrences more frequent.[118–120] In general, most topical antifungal agents are effective, especially when prescribed for longer periods (1 to 2 weeks). Longer duration of therapy may be necessary to eradicate yeast infection. However, single-application high-dose topical therapy with clotrimazole has been shown to be effective in pregnancy and may be considered for the initial therapeutic attempt.[121] In the past nystatin was considered the drug of choice in the first trimester of pregnancy; however, all topical agents can be used throughout pregnancy. Oral azoles are contraindicated.

Management of recurrent vulvovaginal candidiasis (RVVC)

Prior to initiation of treatment, diagnosis must be confirmed by culture. Thousands of women carry the label of "RVVC" when their symptoms are in fact due to noninfectious etiologies such as allergic and hypersensitivity vulvitis. Following confirmation of VVC, every effort should be made to eliminate factors predisposing to VVC. However, in the majority of women no reversible or correctable causal factors are present.

Initial antimycotic therapy requires an induction course of either oral or vaginal antimycotic therapy, which must be continued daily until the patient is completely asymptomatic and a culture-negative status has been achieved. In RVVC, failure to initiate a maintenance regimen will result in a clinical relapse of VVC in 50 percent of patients within 3 months.[122] Maintenance-suppressive regimens include ketoconazole 100 mg daily and once-weekly regimens of either 500 mg clotrimazole suppositories or 100 mg fluconazole orally. All three maintenance regimens are effective in preventing breakthrough vaginitis.[123–125] The superior safety profile of fluconazole and clotrimazole have resulted in the latter two agents largely replacing ketoconazole suppressive prophylaxis. Whatever the maintenance regimen, cessation of therapy is accompanied by symptomatic relapse in half the women within a short time of stopping therapy.[122–125]

The role of treatment of male sexual partners was reviewed by Sobel, and no benefit was demonstrated in several large studies.[105] More recently, Fong evaluated systemic ketoconazole treatment of male partners and failed to reduce the recurrence rate in women with RVVC,[126] although Spinillo et al. did report decreased RVVC in women when attempts were made to eradicate *Candida* organisms in both partners.[127] Dennerstein reported a reduced rate of recurrence in RVVC in 15 patients during a 3-month period of depo-medroxyprogesterone acetate therapy.[128] In a small study using patients as their own controls, Hilton reported fewer episodes of VVC in women placed on oral yogurt.[129] Given the small numbers and lack of controls in this unblinded study, the role of yogurt in preventing *Candida* vaginitis remains unproved.

An alternative approach to long-term maintenance antifungal therapy is the use of hyposensitization with *Candida* antigen preparation. Two small studies achieved encouraging results.[98,130]

Resistant yeast infections

Vaginitis caused by azole-resistant strains of *C. albicans* is extremely rare, although fluconazole-resistant strains of *C. albicans* have recently been isolated from the oral cavity of males and females with AIDS.[131] It should be emphasized that azole-resistant strains of *C. albicans* are rarely the cause of RVVC. In contrast, RVVC is not infrequently due to non-*albicans* species, the majority of which show reduced susceptibility to all azoles. *C. glabrata (Torulopsis glabrata)* is particularly common, and approximately half the strains show reduced sensitivity to available azoles.[107,132] Boric acid 600 mg administered vaginally once daily in a gelatin capsule has been shown to be highly effective in this clinically resistant infection.[132,133] Therapy should be continued until cultures are negative (usually 10 to 14 days), and when a history suggests RVVC, a maintenance regimen of alternate day and then twice-weekly boric acid should be prescribed. Unfortunately, there is still little experience published on the efficacy of this maintenance regimen, and the long-term safety of intravaginal boric acid has not been confirmed.

The only alternative to vaginal boric acid in resistant infections is flucytosine cream. However, the latter agent is not available commercially and must be prepared by a pharmacist.[134] Flucytosine for vaginal use should be limited because of the potential for the acquisition of resistance.

VULVOVAGINAL CANDIDIASIS IN HIV-POSITIVE WOMEN

From the onset of the AIDS epidemic, both the prevalence and the significance of oral and esophageal candidiasis were recognized.[135] As the percentage and numbers of women with HIV grew in the 1980s, vaginal candidiasis was increasingly reported.[136,137]

The increased prevalence of oral candidiasis has been explained on the basis of the loss of oral mucosal CMI defense mechanisms, and the deficiency was thought also to apply to the vagina. Furthermore, given the enormous quantities of broad-spectrum antibiotics administered for prophylactic and therapeutic purposes to women with HIV, together with the women's progressive debilitation, one might similarly predict the frequent occurrence of symptomatic candida vaginitis, especially with severe immunodeficiency.

A 1987 report indicated that 24 HIV-infected women followed at the Walter Reed Army Medical Center had a history of unexplained chronic vaginal candidiasis for at least 1 year.[136] All the patients described had oral thrush and severe T-helper cell depletion and most were anergic. Within a 30-month follow-up, 80 percent of the patients developed other severe opportunistic infections. The authors emphasized that recurrent VVC was the presenting complaint, predating the recognition of oral thrush, and was frequently the only clinical indication of severe underlying immunodeficiency. HIV-associated RVVC was unique in having only temporary symptomatic improvement following use of intravaginal antifungal agents and in requiring constant therapy for control of symptoms. The authors concluded that HIV-positive women with RVVC are at serious risk for rapid progression to AIDS, as are males with recurrent oral thrush.[135] Rhoads et al. concluded that women with "chronic refractory" vaginal candidiasis should be tested for HIV[136] but did not define either word.

A subsequent report described candida vaginitis in 70 percent of an HIV-positive female cohort from Rhode Island.[137] In this study, VVC responded well to appropriate therapy but had a tendency to recur. The authors also reported increased severity and duration of episodes of VVC.[138] More than half the women with new onset of increased frequency or increased severity of candida vaginitis described their symptoms as originating 6 months to 3 years before the diagnosis of HIV infection had been considered. Over 90 percent of the women presenting with oral candidiasis had experienced new onset of increased frequency of vaginal candidiasis. The location and severity of candida infections in these HIV-positive women were closely related to degree of immunosuppression at the time the infection developed as measured by CD4 counts. Thirty percent of HIV-positive women with only vaginal candidiasis and no oral disease had CD4 counts identical to those of HIV-positive women without evidence of mucosal candidiasis. The authors concluded that mucosal infections by *Candida* organisms occur in a hierarchical pattern (first VVC, then oral, and finally esophageal candidiasis) in women with HIV infection, and that recurrent, often severe, vaginal candidiasis was common with little or no suppression of CD4 cells.[138]

A major limitation of the studies just discussed is the lack of information concerning diagnosis of candida vaginitis. Any epidemiologic information based on history only or on physical examination without KOH or culture confirmation is unreliable. A more definitive method of confirming the high prevalence of VVC in women with HIV should emerge from a prospective longitudinal cohort study of HIV-positive women compared to a matched cohort of HIV-negative women with similar risk factors. Such studies have only recently been initiated. In the absence of an HIV-negative control group, it is possible that the RVVC in HIV-positive women with high CD4 counts, as described by Imam et al.,[138] reflects background VVC prevalence in a sexually active group of women still possessing a sense of well-being. Moreover, if progressive loss in mucosal immunity accompanies the decline in CD4 cells, one would anticipate a further increase in frequency of RVVC accompanying advanced AIDS, but none of the published reports have described this occurrence. In contrast to the above studies, Duerr et al. observed that the rate of vaginal carriage of *Candida* organisms did not increase until the CD4 count dropped below 200 cells/μL.[139]

The issue of HIV testing in the presence of VVC remains controversial. Most women experiencing a single episode of VVC today are obviously not HIV-infected and clearly do not require testing. Even in the case of women with recurrent VVC, the issue is anything but clear, since most women with RVVC are HIV-negative. Only women with RVVC who have risk factors for HIV infection should be tested, but high-risk women should be tested anyway, regardless of the presence of candida vaginitis.

References

1 Odds FC: Candidosis of the genitalia, in *Candida and Candidosis*. A Review and Bibliography, 2nd ed. Bailliere Tindall, 1988, p 124.

2 Wilkinson JS: Some remarks upon the development of epiolyses with the description of new vegetable formation found in connection with the human uterus. *Lancet* 2: 448, 1894.

3 Reed BD: Risk factors for *Candida* vulvovaginitis. *Obstet Gynecol Surv* 47:551, 1992.

4 Berg AO et al: Establishing the cause of symptoms in women in a family practice. *JAMA* 251:6201, 1984.

5 Hurley R, De Louvois J: *Candida* vaginitis. *Postgrad Med J* 55:645, 1979.

6 Hurley R: Inveterate vaginal thrush. *Practitioner* 215:753, 1975.

7 Chief Medical Officer, Department of Health and Social Security: Annual Reports, 1976–1984 (England and Wales).

8 Centers for Disease Control: Nonreported sexually transmitted diseases. *MMWR* 38:61, 1979.

9 Fleury FJ: Adult vaginitis. *Clin Obstet Gynecol* 24:407, 1981.

10 Drake TE, Maibach HI: *Candida* and candidiasis: Culture conditions, epidemiology, and pathogenesis. *Postgrad Med J* 53:83, 1973.

11 Chow AW et al: Vaginal colonization with *Escherichia coli* in healthy women: Determination of relative risks by quantitative cultures and multivariate statistical analysis. *Am J Obstet Gynecol* 154:120, 1986.

12 Goldacre MJ et al: Vaginal microbial flora in normal young women. *Br Med J* 1:450, 1979.

13 McCormack WM Jr. et al: The incidence of genitourinary infections in a cohort of healthy women. *Sex Trans Dis* 21:66, 1994.
14 Sobel JD: Epidemiology and pathogenesis of recurrent vulvovaginal candidiasis. *Am J Obstet Gynecol* 152:926, 1985.
15 Morton RS, Rashid S: Candidal vaginitis: Natural history, predisposing factors, and prevention. *Proc R Soc Phid* 70(Suppl 4):3, 1977.
16 Cauwenbergh G: Vaginal candidiasis: Evolving trends in the incidence and treatment of non-*Candida albicans* infection. *Curr Probl Obstet Gynecol Fertil* 8:241, 1990.
17 Horowitz BJ et al: Evolving pathogens in vulvovaginal candidiasis: implications for patient care. *J Clin Pharmacol* 32:248, 1992.
18 Cotch MF et al: Vaginal Carriage of *Candida* spp in Pregnancy. Interscience Conference on Antimicrobial Agents and Chemotherapy, September 29, 1991, Chicago, Abstr 1251, p 307.
19 Sobel JD et al: Single oral dose fluconazole compared with conventional topical therapy of *Candida* vaginitis. *Am J Ob Gyn* 172:1263–1268, 1995.
20 Agatensi L et al: Vaginopathic and proteolytic species of *Candida* among outpatients attending a gynecological center. *J Clin Path* 44: 826, 1991.
21 O'Connor MI, Sobel JD: Epidemiology of recurrent vulvovaginal candidiasis: Identification and strain differentiation of *Candida albicans. J Infect Dis* 154:358, 1986.
22 Soll DR et al: Switching of *Candida albicans* during successive episodes of recurrent vaginitis. *J Clin Micro* 27:681, 1989.
23 King RD et al: Adherence of *Candida albicans* and other candida species to mucosal epithelial cells. *Infect Immun* 27:667, 1980.
24 Sobel JD et al: *Candida albicans* adherence to vaginal epithelial cells. *J Infect Dis* 143:76, 1981.
25 Trumbore DJ, Sobel JD: Recurrent vulvovaginal candidiasis: Vaginal epithelial cell susceptibility to *Candida albicans* adherence. *Obstet Gynecol* 67:810, 1986.
26 Lehner N et al: Pathogenesis of vaginal candidiasis: studies with a mutant which has reduced ability to adhere in vitro. *Sobaurudia* 24: 127, 1986.
27 Sobel JD et al: Critical role of germination in the pathogenesis of experimental candidal vaginitis. *Infect Immun* 44:576, 1984.
28 Sobel JD, Muller G: Ketoconazole prophylaxis in experimental vaginal candidiasis. *Antimicrob Agents Chemother* 25:281, 1984.
29 DeBernardis F: Evidence for a role for secreted aspartate proteinase of *Candida albicans* in vulvovaginal candidiasis. *J Infect Dis* 161: 1276, 1990.
30 DeBernardis F et al: Experimental pathogenicity and acid proteinase secretion of vaginal isolates of *Candida parapsilosis. J Med and Vet Mycol* 28:125, 1990.
31 DeBernardis F et al: Expression of *Candida albicans* SAP 1 and SAP 2 in experimental vaginitis. *Infect Immun* 63:1887, 1995.
32 Shah DT et al: In situ mycotoxin production by *Candida albicans* in women with vaginitis. *Gynecol Obstet Invest* 39:67, 1995.
33 Slutsky B et al: High frequency switching colony morphology in *Candida albicans. Science* 230:666, 1985.
34 Soll DR: High-frequency switching in *Candida albicans. Clin Microbiol Rev* 5:183, 1992.
35 Soll DR: High frequency switching in *Candida albicans* and its relations to vaginal candidiasis. *Am J Obstet Gynecol* 158:997, 1988.
36 Soll DR et al: Switching of *Candida albicans* during successive episodes of recurrent vaginitis. *J Clin Microbiol* 27:81, 1989.
37 Vazquez J et al: Karyotyping of *C. albicans* isolates obtained longitudinally in women with recurrent vulvovaginal candidiasis. *J Infect Dis* 170:1566, 1994.
38 Schroppel K et al: Evolution and replacement of *Candida albicans* strains during recurrent vaginitis demonstrated by DNA fingerprinting. *J Clin Microbiol* 32:2646, 1994.
39 Moors MA et al: A Novel Mechanism for Iron Acquisition by *Candida albicans*. Symposium on *Candida*, American Society of Microbiology. Baltimore MD, March 1993.
40 Bertholf ME, Stafford MJ: Colonization of *Candida albicans* in vagina, rectum, and mouth. *J Family Pract* 16:919, 1983.
41 O'Conner MI, Sobel JD: Epidemiology of recurrent vulvovaginal candidiasis: Identification and strain differentiation of *Candida albicans. J Infect Dis* 154:358, 1986.
42 Bland PB: Experimental vaginal and cutaneous moniliasis: Clinical and laboratory studies of certain monilias associated with vaginal, oral, and cutaneous thrush. *Arch Dermatol Syphil* 36:760, 1937.
43 McCourtie J, Douglas LG: Relationship between cell surface composition of *Candida albicans* and adherence to acrylic after-growth on different carbon sources. *Infect Immun* 32:1234, 1981.
44 Powell BL et al: Identification of a 173-estradiol-binding protein in *Candida albicans* and *Candida (Torulopsis) glabrata. Exp Mycology* 8:304, 1984.
45 Madani ND et al: *Candida albicans* estrogen-binding protein gene encodes an oxidoreductase that is inhibited by estradiol. *Proc Nat Acad Sci* 91:922, 1994.
46 Apisarnthanarax P et al: Oral contraceptives and candidiasis. *Cutis* 77, 1974.
47 Davidson F, Oates JK: The pill does not cause "thrush." *Br J Obstet Gynecol* 92:1265, 1985.
48 Foxman B: The epidemiology of vulvovaginal candidiasis: Risk factors. *Am J Public Health* 80:329, 1990.
49 Barbone F et al: A follow-up study of methods of contraception, sexual activity, and rates of trichomoniasis, candidiasis, and bacterial vaginosis. *Am J Obstet Gynecol* 163:510, 1990.
50 Rahman KM et al: General yeast infection in Bangladesh women using contraceptives. *Bangladesh Med Res Counc Bull* 10:65, 1984.
51 Parewijck W et al: Candidiasis in women fitted with an intrauterine contraceptive device. *Br J Obstet Gynecol* 95:408, 1988.
52 Spellacy WN et al: Vaginal yeast growth and contraceptive practices. *Obstet Gynecol* 38:343, 1971.
53 Davidson F: Yeasts and circumcision in the male. *Br J Vener Dis* 53: 121, 1977.
54 Peddie BA et al: Relationship between contraceptive method and vaginal flora. *Aust NZ J Obstet Gynecol* 24:217, 1984.
55 Hooton TM et al: Effects of recent sexual activity and use of the diaphragm on the vaginal microflora. *Clin Infect Dis* 19:274, 1994.
56 Caruso LJ: Vaginal moniliasis after tetracycline therapy. *Am J Obstet Gynecol* 90:374, 1964.
57 Oriel JD, Waterworth PM: Effect of minocycline and tetracycline on the vaginal yeast flora. *J Clin Pathol* 28:403, 1975.
58 Liljemark WF, Gibbons RJ: Suppression of *Candida albicans* by human oral streptococci in gnotobiotic mice. *Infect Immun* 8:846, 1973.
59 Auger P, Joly J: Microbial flora associated with *Candida albicans* vulvovaginitis. *Obstet Gynecol* 55:397, 1980.
60 Narayanan TK, Tao GR: Beta-indole-ethanol and beta-indolelactic acid production by *Candida* species: Their antibacterial and autoantibiotic action. *Antimicrob Agents Chemother* 9:375, 1976.
61 Rodin P, Kolator B: Carriage of yeasts on the penis. *Br Med J* 1:1123, 1976.
62 Thin RN et al: How often is genital yeast infection sexually transmitted? *Br Med J* 2:93, 1977.
63 Spinelli A et al: Recurrent vaginal candidiasis: Results of a cohort study of sexual transmission and intestinal reservoir. *J Reprod Med* 37:343, 1992.
64 Markos AR et al: Oral sex and recurrent vulvovaginal candidiasis. *Genitourin Med* 68:61, 1992.
65 Elegbe IA, Elegbe I: Quantitative relationships of *Candida albicans* infections and dressing patterns in Nigerian women. *Am J Public Health* 73:450, 1983.
66 Davidson F et al: Recurrent genital candidosis and iron metabolism. *Br J Vener Dis* 53:123, 1977.
67 De Sousa HM, Van Uden N: The mode of infection and infection in yeast vulvovaginitis. *Am J Obstet Gynecol* 80:1096, 1960.
68 Miles MR et al: Recurrent vaginal candidiasis: Importance of an intestinal reservoir. *JAMA* 238:1836, 1977.
69 Milne JD, Warnock DW: Effect of simultaneous oral and vaginal treatment on the rate of cure and relapse in vaginal candidosis. *Br J Vener Dis* 55:362, 1979.

70 Vellupillai S, Thin RN: Treatment of vulvovaginal yeast infection with nystatin. *Practitioner* 219:897, 1977.
71 Meinhof WL: Demonstration of typical features of individual *Candida albicans* strains as a means of studying sources of infection. *Chemotherapy* 28(Suppl 1):51–55, 1982.
72 Odds FC: Genital candidosis. *Clin Exp Dermatol* 7:345, 1982.
73 Garcia-Tamayo J et al: Human genital candidosis: Histochemistry, scanning, and transmission electron microscopy. *Acta Cytol* (Baltimore) 26:7, 1982.
74 Waldman RH et al: Immunoglobulin levels and antibody to *Candida albicans* in human cervicovaginal secretions. *Clin Exp Immunol* 10: 427, 1972.
75 Mathur S et al: Humoral immunity in vaginal candidiasis. *Infect Immun* 15:287, 1977.
76 Gough PM et al: IgA and IgG antibodies to *Candida albicans* in the genital tract secretions of women with or without vaginal candidosis. *Sabouraudia* 22:265, 1984.
77 Polonelli L et al: Idiotypic intravaginal vaccination to protect against candidal vaginitis by secretory, yeast killer toxin antiidiotypic antibodies. *J Immunol* 152:3175, 1994.
78 Mathur S et al: Immunoglobulin E anti-*Candida* antibodies and candidiasis. *Infect Immun* 18:257, 1977.
79 Witkin SS: IgE Antibodies to *Candida albicans* in Vaginal Fluids of Women with Recurrent Vaginitis. Meeting of the American Society of Microbiologists, Palm Springs, CA, 1987, Abstr 9, p 10.
80 Diamond RD et al: Damage to pseudohyphae of *Candida albicans* by neutrophils in the absence of serum in vitro. *J Clin Invest* 61:349, 1978.
81 Hobbs JR et al: Immunological aspects of candidal vaginitis. *Proc Res Soc Med* 70(Suppl 4):11, 1977.
82 Syverson RE et al: Cellular and humoral immune status in women with chronic *Candida* vaginitis. *Am J Obstet Gynecol* 123:624, 1979.
83 Witkin SS et al: Inhibition of *Candida albicans*–induced lymphocyte proliferation by lymphocytes and sera from women with recurrent vaginitis. *Am J Obstet Gynecol* 147:809, 1983.
84 Mathur S et al: Antiovarian and anti-lymphocyte antibodies in patients with chronic vaginal candidiasis. *J Reproduct Immunol* 2:247, 1980.
85 Fidel PL Jr. et al: Systemic cell mediated immune reactivity in women with recurrent vulvovaginal candidiasis. *J Infect Dis* 168:1458, 1993.
86 Fidel PL Jr. et al: Effects of preinduced *Candida*-specific systemic cell mediated immunity on experimental vaginal candidiasis. *Infect Immun* 62:1032, 1994.
87 Fidel PL Jr. et al: *Candida*-specific Th-1 responsiveness in mice with experimental vaginal candidiasis. *Infect Immun* 61:4202, 1993.
88 Fidel PL Jr. et al: Mice immunized by primary vaginal *C. albicans* infection develop acquired vaginal mucosal immunity. *Infect Immun* 63:547, 1994.
89 Witkin SS: Inhibition of *Candida* induced lymphocyte proliferation by antibody to *Candida albicans*. *Obstet Gynecol* 68:696, 1986.
90 Witkin SS et al: A macrophage defect in women with recurrent candida vaginitis and its reversal in vitro by prostaglandin inhibitors. *Am J Obstet Gynecol* 155:790, 1986.
91 Kalo-Klein A, Witkin SS: Prostaglandin E2 enhances and interferon gamma inhibits germ-tube formation in *Candida albicans*. *Infect Immun* 58:260, 1994.
92 Witkin SS: Immunologic factors influencing susceptibility to recurrent *Candida* vaginitis. *Clin Obstet Gynecol* 34:662, 1991.
93 Savage DC: Microbial interference between indigenous yeast and lactobacilli in the rodent stomach. *J Bacteriol* 98:1278, 1969.
94 Pollack JJ et al: Fungistatic and fungicidal activity of human parotid salivary histidine-rich polypeptides on *Candida albicans*. *Infect Immun* 44:702, 1984.
95 Sobel JD et al: Experimental chronic vaginal candidiasis in rats. *Sabouraudia* 23:199, 1985.
96 Kudelka NM: Allergy in chronic monilial vaginitis. *Ann Allergy* 29: 266, 1971.
97 Palacios HJ: Hypersensitivity as a cause of dermatologic and vaginal moniliasis resistant to topical therapy. *Ann Allergy* 37:110, 1976.
98 Rigg D et al: Recurrent allergic vulvovaginitis treatment with *Candida albicans* allergen immunotherapy. *Am J Obstet Gynecol* 162: 332, 1990.
99 Schaaf VM et al: The limited value of symptoms and signs in the diagnosis of vaginal infections. *Arch Intern Med* 150:1929, 1990.
100 Bergman JJ et al: Clinical comparison of microscopic and culture techniques in the diagnosis of Candida vaginitis. *J Family Pract* 18: 549, 1984.
101 Rosenberg M: Vaginal candidiasis: Its diagnosis and relation to urinary tract infection. *S Med J* 69:1347, 1976.
102 Evans EGV et al: Criteria for the diagnosis of vaginal candidosis: Evaluation of a new latex agglutination test. *Eur J Obstet Gynecol Reprod Biol* 22:365, 1986.
103 Merson-Davies LA et al: Quantification of *Candida albicans* morphology in vaginal smears. *Euro J Obstet Gynecol Reprod Biol* 42: 49, 1991.
104 Sobel JD et al: A new slide latex agglutination for the diagnosis of acute *Candida* vaginitis. *Am J Clin Pathol* 94:323, 1990.
105 Sobel JD: Therapeutic Considerations in Fungal Vaginitis, in *Chemotherapy of Fungal Diseases*, vol 14, Ryley JF (ed) Springer-Verlag, New York. 1990, p 365.
106 Reef S et al: Treatment options for vulvovaginal candidiasis: background paper for development of 1993 STD treatment recommendations. *Clin Infect Dis* 20:80, 1995.
107 Lynch ME, Sobel JD: Comparative in vitro activity of antimycotic against pathogenic vaginal yeast isolates. *J Med Vet Mycol* 32:267, 1994.
108 Tooley PJ: Patients and doctor preferences in the treatment of vaginal candidiasis. *Practitioner* 229:655, 1985.
109 Lewis JH et al: Hepatic injury associated with ketoconazole therapy: Analysis of 33 cases. *Gastroent* 86:503, 1984.
110 Silva-Cruz A et al: Itraconazole versus placebo in the management of vaginal candidiasis. *J Gynecol Obstet* 36:229, 1991.
111 Brammer KW: Treatment of vaginal candidiasis with a single oral dose of fluconazole. *Eur J Clin Microbiol Infect Dis* 7:364, 1988.
112 Kutzer E et al: A comparison of fluconazole and ketoconazole in the oral treatment of vaginal candidiasis: Report of a double-blind multicenter trial. *Eur J Obstet Gynecol Reprod Biol* 29:305, 1988.
113 Tobin MJ et al: Treatment of vaginal candidosis: A comparative study of the efficacy and acceptability of itraconazole and clotrimazole. *Genitourin Med* 68:36, 1992.
114 Osser S et al: Treatment of *Candida* vaginitis: A prospective randomized multicenter study comparing econazole with oral fluconazole. *Acta Obstet Gynecol Scand* 70:73, 1991.
115 Moebius UM: Influenza-like syndrome after terconazole. *Lancet* 2: 966, 1988.
116 Breuker G et al: Single-dose therapy of vaginal mycoses with clotrimazole vaginal cream 10%. *Mykosen* 29:427, 1986.
117 Ritter W: Pharmacokinetics fundamentals of vaginal treatment with clotrimazole. *Am J Obstet Gynecol* 152:945, 1985.
118 Lang WE et al: Nystatin vaginal tablets in treatment of candidal vulvovaginitis. *Obstet Gynecol* 8:364, 1956.
119 Wallenburg HCS, Wladimiroff JW: Recurrence of vaginal candidiasis during pregnancy: Comparison of miconazole and nystatin treatments. *Obstet Gynecol* 48:491, 1976.
120 McNellis D et al: Treatment of vulvovaginal candidiasis in pregnancy: A comparative study. *Obstet Gynecol* 50:674, 1977.
121 Lindeque BG, Van Niekerk WA: Treatment of vaginal candidiasis in pregnancy with a single clotrimazole 500 mg vaginal pessary. *S Am Med J* 65:123, 1984.
122 Sobel JD: Management of recurrent vulvovaginal candidiasis with intermittent ketoconazole prophylaxis. *Obstet Gynecol* 65:435, 1985.
123 Sobel JD: Recurrent vulvovaginal candidiasis: A prospective study of the efficacy of maintenance ketoconazole therapy. *N Engl J Med* 315: 1455, 1986.
124 Davison F, Mould RF: Recurrent genital candidosis in women and the effect of intermittent prophylactic treatment. *Br J Vener Dis* 54: 176, 1978.

125 Sobel JD: Fluconazole maintenance therapy in recurrent vulvovaginal candidiasis. *Int J Gynecol Obstet* 37:17, 1992.
126 Fong IW: The value of treating the sexual partners of women with recurrent vaginal candidiasis with ketoconazole. *Genitourin Med* 68: 174, 1992.
127 Spinillo A et al: Recurrent vaginal candidiasis: Results of a cohort study of sexual transmission and intestinal reservoir. *J Reprod Med* 37:343, 1992.
128 Dennerstein GJ: Depo-Provera in the treatment of recurrent vulvovaginal candidiasis. *J Reprod Med* 31:801, 1986.
129 Hilton E et al: Ingestion of yogurt containing *Lactobacillus acidophilus* as prophylaxis for candidal vaginitis. *Ann Int Med* 116:353, 1992.
130 Rosedale N, Braue K: Hyposensitization in the management of recurring vaginal candidiasis. *Ann Allergy* 43(4):250, 1979.
131 Ng TT, Denning DW: Fluconazole resistance in *Candida* in patients with AIDS: A therapeutic approach. *J Infect Dis* 26:117, 1993.
132 Redondo-Lopez V et al: *Torulopsis glabrata* vaginitis: Clinical aspects and susceptibility to antifungal agents. *Obstet Gynecol* 76:751, 1990.
133 Jovanovic R et al: Antifungal agents versus boric acid for treating chronic mycotic vulvovaginitis. *J Reprod Med* 36:593, 1991.
134 Horowitz B: Topical flucytosine therapy for chronic recurrent *Candida tropicalis* infections. *J Reprod Med* 31:821, 1986.
135 Klein RS et al: Oral candidiasis in high-risk patients as the initial manifestation of the acquired immunodeficiency syndrome. *N Engl J Med* 311:354, 1984.
136 Rhoads JL et al: Chronic vaginal candidiasis in women with human immunodeficiency virus infection. *JAMA* 257:3105, 1987.
137 Carpenter CCJ et al: Natural history of acquired immunodeficiency syndrome in women in Rhode Island. *Am J Med* 86:771, 1989.
138 Imam N et al: Hierarchical pattern of mucosal *Candida* infections in HIV-seropositive women. *Am J Med* 89:142, 1990.
139 Duerr A et al: Gynecologic Conditions in HIV-Infected Women in Brooklyn, New York. Eighth International Conference on AIDS/ Third STD World Congress, July 19–24, 1992, Amsterdam, Netherlands, Vol 2, Abstr PB 3051, B95.
140 Fidel PL Jr. et al: T lymphocytes in the murine vaginal mucosa are phenotypically distinct from those in the periphery. *Infect Immun* 64: 3793, 1996.

Chapter 46
Pubic lice

Stephan A. Billstein

The order Anaplura includes over 400 species of sucking lice, which are ectoparasites of mammals. Sucking lice are dorsoventrally compressed, wingless, and small, with retractable piercing-sucking mouthparts. One species is the cause of a common sexually transmitted disease: pubic lice, or "crabs."

Three species of lice infest human beings: *Phthirus pubis*, the crab louse; *Pediculus humanus humanus*, the body louse; and *Pediculus humanus capitis*, the head louse. This chapter focuses principally on pubic lice, but head and body lice will be considered briefly for purposes of comparison.

HISTORY

Lice have been constant companions of human beings since antiquity. Israeli scientists confirmed that the warriors in Bar Kochba's Jewish revolt against Rome 18 centuries ago were afflicted with lice. These lice were morphologically identical to *Pediculus capitis* (Anaplura: Pediculidae) that continue to afflict human populations today. The lice were discovered in the hair and clothes of archeological remains from caves in the Sudan desert.

LIFE CYCLE AND REPRODUCTION

Lice have five stages in their life cycle: egg (or nit), three nymphal stages, and the adult stage. All stages occur on the host. Sucking lice undergo a simple metamorphosis in which immature lice are morphologic miniatures of adults but have no reproductive ability.

The egg of the crab louse is smaller than the eggs of either the head or body louse, which measure approximately 0.8 mm long and 0.3 mm wide.[1] The nit is oval in shape and opalescent in color; it contains a cap (operculum) that comes off intact when the egg hatches (Fig. 46-1). An egg will hatch within 5 to 10 days after being incubated in the heat of the host's body. Interestingly, the young nymph emerges through the cap by sucking air into its body and expelling it from its anus until a cushion of compressed air is formed, which then pops the cap open and allows the nymph to escape.[2] Over a period of 8 to 9 days, the nymph produces three molts. The louse remains on the body and requires frequent blood meals after having hatched. When lice reach adulthood, mating occurs after approximately 10 hours and continues until the lice die. The female louse lays approximately four eggs per day.

In the case of the body louse, the egg case is attached to hair or clothing by a cementlike material secreted by the female louse. After hatching, the empty shell may stick to hair or clothing for some time. It is often difficult to remove by washing or shampooing or by vinegar or organic solvents. If all else fails, the empty egg cases eventually are moved away either by growth of the hair, by the use of a fine-tooth comb, or by cutting the hair.

Little is known about the actual life span of the adult louse. Under artificial conditions, lice have survived for about 1 month. Ambient temperature, humidity, and availability of human blood are thought to influence the life span of all types of human lice. Off the host, all stages of the louse can be expected to die within 30 days, regardless of temperature. Unfed adult head and body lice can survive for up to 10 days, whereas adult pubic lice rarely survive more than 24 hours off the host.[3] Lice leave the host voluntarily only when the host has died or becomes febrile or when there is close personal contact with another host.

The life of the louse is dependent on human blood. When ready to feed, the louse anchors its mouth to the skin, stabs an opening through the skin, pours saliva into the wound to prevent clotting, and pumps blood from the wound into its digestive system. During feeding, dark-red feces may be deposited on the skin.

The pubic louse has greatly enlarged middle and hind legs and claws; the abdomen is wider than it is long, giving it the appearance of a crab (Fig. 46-2). Pubic lice are about 1 mm in length. Adult head and body lice have a longer body (approximately 3 mm in females and 2 mm in males) and relatively shorter middle and hind legs (Fig. 46-3). The pubic louse has three parts: a head (with a pair of eyes), a thorax (with three pairs of legs), and a segregated abdomen. At the end of each leg, there is a hooklike claw and opposing thumb, which enable the louse to maintain its hold on hair (Fig. 46-4).

A difference between body and head lice and the pubic louse involves their grasping ability. The grasp of the pubic louse's claw matches the diameter of pubic and auxiliary hairs; hence pubic lice may be found not only in the pubic area (Fig. 46-5, see Color Plates) but also have been recovered from the axillae, beard areas of the face, eyelashes (Fig. 46-6), and eyebrows.[4,5] It is rare in these other areas and is probably mechanically moved to these areas via the fingers. The diameter of the head louse's grasp seems to be uniquely adapted to the diameter of the scalp hair. Therefore, it is very difficult to transplant head lice to other areas of the body.

Another difference between the species is that of egg laying. Adult female pubic lice and head lice glue their eggs to hairs, while the female body louse usually ovoposits on the fiber or in the seams of clothing.

The third difference is the rate of movement. Pubic lice seem to be the most sedentary. Nuttal and Payot[6] recorded pubic lice moving at a maximum of 10 cm in a day. Body lice can wander as much as 35 mm in a 2-hour period. Temperature, ambient humidity, and availability of a blood meal also influence the rate of movement. Lice do not like light and will move frantically to escape light.

EPIDEMIOLOGY AND TRANSMISSION

It is estimated by sales figures on pediculocides that more than 3 million cases of pediculosis are treated each year in the United States.[7] Most cases are due to head and pubic lice infestations. Infestation by body lice seems to be less common in this country. Infestations with pubic lice are more common in people of low socioeconomic status.[8] Epidemics of louse-borne relapsing fever and epidemic typhus are now rare, since the body louse is the only species implicated as their vector. Mass epidemics of these diseases have resulted when large populations have lived in unsanitary conditions as in times of famine, disaster, and war.

"Vagabond's disease" is a diagnosis made in persons who continually harbor these lice and whose skin becomes hardened and darkly pigmented as a result of frequent louse bites and patient response.

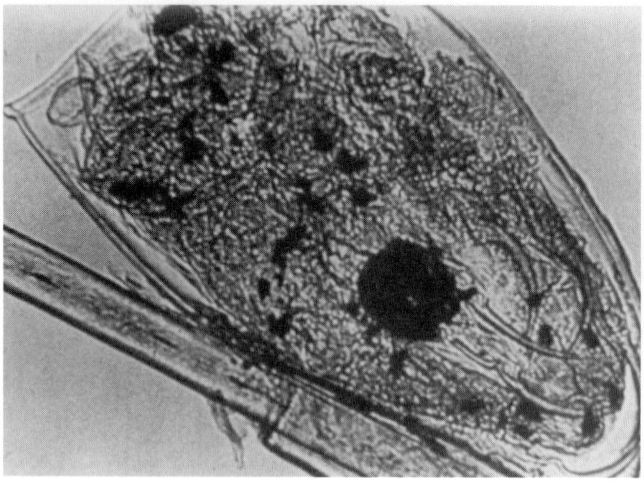

Fig. 46-1. Close-up micrograph of a louse nit (egg).

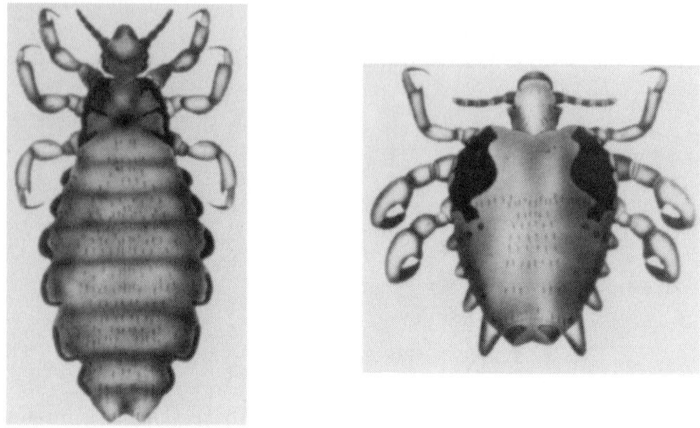

Fig. 46-3. Comparison of gross structure of *(left)* the head louse and *(right)* the pubic louse.

Phthirus pubis infestation is frequently associated with the presence of other sexually transmitted infections, and patients presenting with pubic lice should be examined for such infections.[9]

Human lice are transmitted from one person to another primarily by intimate contact. Although all types of human lice are relatively host-specific, crab lice occasionally have been reported to infest dogs. Both head and body lice are transmitted by sharing personal articles such as hairbrushes, combs, towels, or clothing. Pubic lice do not seem to spread as rapidly as other human lice when off the host. They have a shorter life span (24 hours compared with several days for other lice), and their movements are more lethargic. Sexual transmission is considered to be the most important means of pubic lice transmission. However, there are documented cases of transmission from toilet seats, beds, and egg-infested loose hairs dropped by infested persons on shared objects.

The population with the highest incidence of pubic lice is similar to that of gonorrhea and syphilis: single persons, ages 15 to 25 years. Prevalence of pubic lice infestation declines gradually to age 35 and is rare in persons older than age 35. Head lice are most common in children up to 6 years of age.

CLINICAL MANIFESTATIONS

Sensitivity to the effect of louse bites varies with the individual. When previously unexposed persons are bitten, there may either be no signs or symptoms or a slight sting with little or no itching or redness. At least 5 days must pass before allergic sensitization can occur. At that point, the main symptom is itching, which leads to scratching, erythema, irritation, and inflammation. An individual who has been bitten by a large number of lice over a short period of time may have mild fever, malaise, and increased irritability.

Ectoparasites produce a variety of immunologic responses in the host.[10] Apparently, many persons eventually develop some degree of immunity to the bite of the louse. Persons infested for a long time may even become oblivious to the lice on their bodies. The opposite also may occur. Excessive scratching may lead to superinfection. Characteristic small "blue spots" may appear in the skin as a result of the crab louse bites; these persist for several days. A tuboovarian inflammatory mass attributed to *Phthirus pubis* has been reported.

DIAGNOSIS

Diagnosis of lice infestation is made by (1) taking a careful history from the patient, (2) considering lice infestation as a possible or probable cause of the patient's signs and symptoms, and (3) careful examination of the patient. Both adult lice and their eggs (nits) are easily seen by the naked eye (see Figs. 46-5 and 46-6).

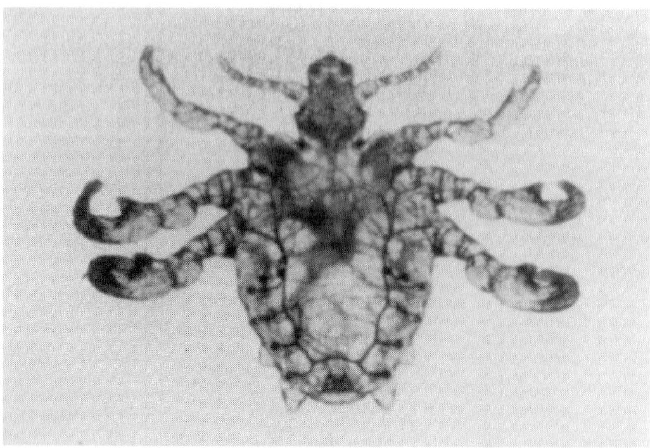

Fig. 46-2. Pubic louse after a recent blood meal. *(Courtesy of V. D. Newcomer.)*

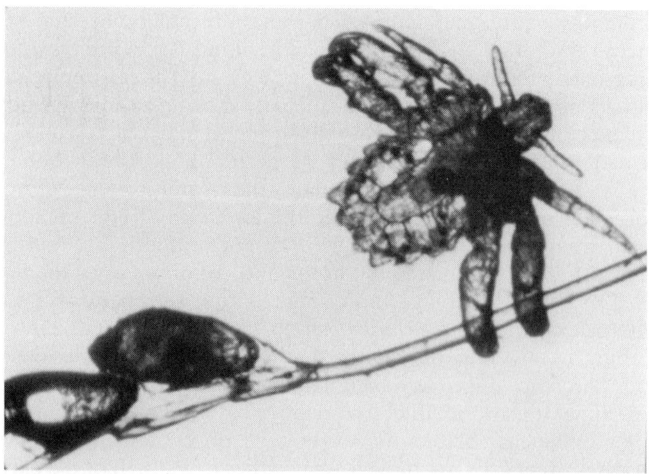

Fig. 46-4. Pubic louse and nits on a hair shaft. *(Courtesy of V. D. Newcomer.)*

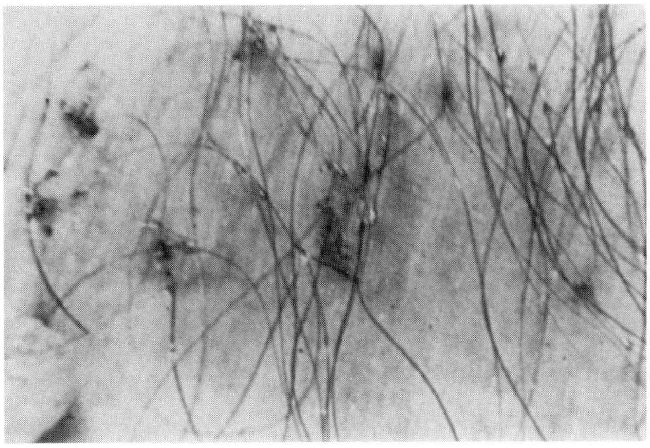

Fig. 46-5. Adult pubic lice and nits.

Head lice characteristically are found on the scalp surface with the nits attached to the hair. Since scalp hair grows at a rate of about 0.4 mm per day and nits of the head louse usually hatch within 9 days, most of the unhatched nits are within 5 mm of the scalp surface. Nits on scalp hair are usually cemented at an oblique angle, which helps to distinguish them from foreign material that slides up and down and frequently surrounds the hair.

Upon examination of the groin or pudendal area, pubic lice may be perceived as scabs over what first were thought to be "scratch papules." When taking a closer look, if nits appear on the hairs, the proper diagnosis becomes obvious. If the "crust" is removed and placed on a glass slide for microscopic examination, the crust often walks away before the cover glass is in place. When no adult lice are available, the demonstration of nits under the microscope also will confirm the diagnosis.

When one sees with the naked eye white flakes on the hair, other possible considerations are seborrheic dermatitis (dandruff flakes), hair casts, solidified globules of hair spray, and certain accretions on hair shafts.

MANAGEMENT

Treatment and disinfection regimens should be individualized. Ideally the regimen should employ a pediculocide that effectively will kill both the adults and the egg.[11] Also, examination of partners and other household contacts of the patient should be made so that both source and spread cases can be treated.

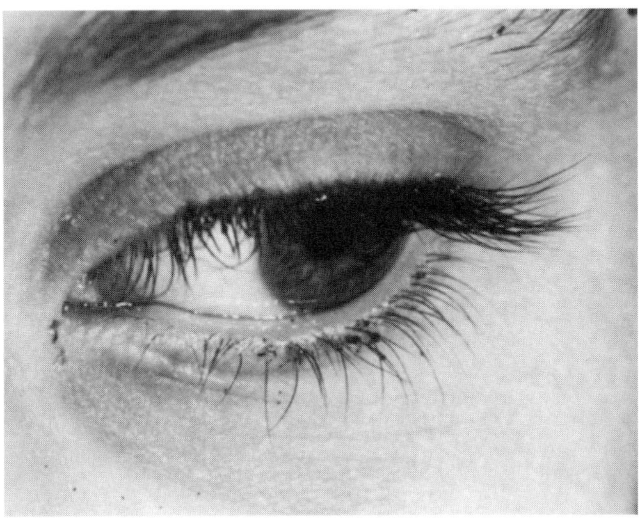

Fig. 46-6. Adult pubic lice and nits on eyelashes.

Both nonprescription and prescription medications are currently available. For these medications to be ovicidal, the pediculocide should remain in contact with the eggs for at least 1 hour. In my experience, the most effective nonprescription products contain pyrethrins and piperonyl butoxide.[12] Two products, Rid (liquid and shampoo) and Triple X (liquid and shampoo) contain 0.3% pyrethrins and 3.0% piperonyl butoxide. A single application of either of these compounds usually is effective on both adult lice and eggs. Recent studies[13,14] have indicated that a small percentage of patients will require reapplication 7 to 10 days after the first treatment. Rid has a fine-tooth comb in the package to help dislodge the dead nits on completion of treatment. The oldest marketed product in this group is A-200 Pyrinate (shampoo). It contains 0.165% pyrethrins and 2.0% piperonyl butoxide. This medication requires two applications 7 days apart, since the initial one is often not lethal for the nits. Other over-the-counter pediculocides currently available in the United States include Cuprex (0.31% tetrathdronaphthalene, 0.03% copper oleate) and Barc (0.18% pyrethrins, 2.2% piperonyl butoxide). They are allegedly less effective than the former drugs in treatment of lice infestations in a public health clinic setting.

Kwell, a 1% gamma benzene hexachloride preparation (lotion, shampoo, and cream), is the most commonly used prescription medication currently available. Scabene, marketed in late 1981, is the same formulation but is available only as a lotion. In the United States, gamma benzene hexachloride (lindane) also has been available at times as a commercial insecticide. In using the prescribed drug, the patient should be advised to divide the day into three 8-hour segments. A shower is taken before each of two applications. Each application must remain on the affected area for the 8-hour period, after which another shower is advised. After the third shower, no further application is required. Other prescription medications available include emulsions of benzyl benzoate 20% or greater, 10% sulfur ointment, and Eurax ointment (10% crotamiton). All three are effective but have disadvantages in that they require several daily applications and/or impart an unpleasant odor to and exuding from the patient.

The use of 1% gamma benzene hexachloride has several disadvantages. It can be absorbed percutaneously when applied to severely excoriated skin. Case reports have alluded to mild signs and symptoms of neurotoxicity when it has been ingested, applied too frequently, not washed off as directed, or used on massively excoriated skin. In one study,[15] 9 percent of a single dose was found in the urine in a badly excoriated patient in the 5 days following the treatment. No other studies, however, have shown blood, tissue, and urine levels.[16,17] Nonetheless, blood dyscrasias such as aplastic anemia and leukopenia have been described after use of lindane in agriculture and against ectoparasites in animals and humans, and lindane is reportedly cytotoxic in vitro for human hematopoietic progenitor cells.[18] Gamma benzene hexachloride use should be avoided in small children, pregnant women, and individuals with massive excoriations or multiple lesions over the scrotum.

Itching is an important feature of all lice infestations. The initial treatment with a pediculocide may be effective for killing both the adult lice and the eggs, but the itching may continue because of an allergic reaction and/or irritation. The possibility of posttreatment pruritus should be discussed with the patient; a mild topical antipruritic/anti-inflammatory cream or ointment may need to be prescribed. The patient should be reevaluated 4 to 7 days after initial treatment. Attention to these considerations is crucial, since it often prevents excessive pediculocide use and may prevent parasitophobia and feelings of "being unclean."

Additional prescription medications include 6% sulfur in petrolatum, which may be useful for infants who cannot tolerate other therapies; a 5% to 10% thiobendazole cream; DDT (currently not available in the United States; in addition, some strains are known to have been resistant to it); and malathion. Ovide Lotion, 0.5% malathion in 78% alcohol, was marketed in 1989 for the treatment of head lice. A previous preparation, Prioderm Lotion, marketed in 1983, is no longer available in the United States. Malathion is an organophosphate cholinesterase inhibitor. It is both pediculicidal and ovicidal. Sulfur atoms in malathion bond with sulfur groups on hair, giving a residual protective effect against reinfestation; this reaction takes a minimum of 6 hours and is maximal at 12 hours. Ovide Lotion is applied to dry hair until the scalp is moist, leaving it on for 8 to 12 hours (avoiding open flames or hair dryers) before rinsing. It has an unpleasant odor due to release of malodorous sulfhydryl compounds through hydrolysis. Also, until the alcohol dries, it is flammable.

A 1% primethrin creme rinse (Nix) is available as a prescription drug in the United States. Primethrin is a synthetic pyrethroid related chemically to the pyrethrins. It is photostable and thermostable and has a low mammalian toxic effect and a broad spectrum of insecticidal activity. Compared with pyrethrins, its marked stability in the presence of light is believed to give it residual activity. It has been shown to persist on the hair shaft for more than 10 days. Since complete ovicidal activity on initial contact is lacking, this residual property is believed to be the mechanism for overcoming this drawback. This prescription medication was introduced in the United States in 1986. The current package insert indication is for the treatment of head lice. Studies[13,14] have compared 1% primethrin marketed as a creme rinse with a shampoo (Kwell). Statistical significance was achieved in the studies on head lice showing a success rate of 97 to 99 percent eradication of the infestation using Nix versus a 43 to 85 percent success rate with the shampoo mixture. Another study[19] compared these two products for the treatment of pubic lice. This study showed, at 10 days after initial application, a 43 percent failure rate with primethrin and a 40 percent failure rate with the Kwell shampoo.

The current recommended administration of primethrin creme rinse is to apply it for 10 minutes after first thoroughly washing the infested area and then gently rinsing that area off. If signs and symptoms persist, another application may be warranted 7 to 10 days later.

All pediculocides interfere with the function of the louse nerve ganglion, leading to respiratory paralysis and death. An exception is the use of Vaseline on pubic lice attached to the eyelids or eyelashes; its action smothers lice by mechanical obstruction of the respiratory apparatus.

Chitin, an acetylated glycosamine polymer, is an important substance to insects. The substance that firmly binds the louse nit to hair has been shown to be chitinous in nature. Formic acid, a substance produced in large quantities by ant colonies, solubilizes chitin and assists in loosening or breaking the chitinous bond between nits and the hair. Gen-Derm Corporation (Northbrook, IL) has marketed an after-pediculocide nit removal system consisting of a cosmetically elegant creme rinse containing 8% formic acid that, when used with a specially toothed metal comb, greatly facilitates nit removal.

Ridding the patient's clothing and fomites of adult lice and nits is an important part of the treatment regimen. Laundering these items in hot water (125°F) or dry cleaning kills the adults, nymphs, or nits. Nonwashable items may be treated with any of a variety of pyrethrin-piperonyl butoxide-containing disinfectants (such as R and C spray, Li-Ban Spray, Black Flag, and Raid). It is important to inform the patient that these products should be used on inanimate or nonwashable items only.

CONTROL ASPECTS

In discussion of control of epidemic lice infestations with administrators of schools or institutions or control measures with and for an individual, the following set of guidelines can be recommended:

1. Document that lice are truly the cause of the problem.
2. Diagnose which louse species is involved.
3. Establish an effective therapeutic regimen, including
   a. Treatment of the individual with a pediculocide that kills adult lice and the nits.
   b. Environmental disinfection.
   c. Treatment of household and intimate contacts.
   d. Reassurance to the infested persons that they are not "unclean" and that they will get better.

Lice infestation may cause anxiety and embarrassment, but it is totally curable with no long-term effects.

References

1 Barnes AM, Keh B: The biology and control of lice on man. *Calif Vector Views* 6:7, 1959.
2 Slonka GF: Life cycle and biology of lice. *J School Health* 47:349, 1977.
3 Keh B, Poorbaugh JH: Understanding and treating infestations of lice on humans. *Calif Vector Views* 18:23, 1971.
4 Deschenes J et al: The ocular manifestations of sexually transmitted diseases. *Can J Ophthalmol* 25:177, 1990.
5 Skinner CJ et al: *Phthirus pubis* infestation of the eyelids: A marker for sexually transmitted diseases. *Int J STD AIDS* 6:451, 1995.
6 Nuttall GHF: Combating lousiness among soldiers and civilians. *Parasitology* 10:411, 1918.
7 Billstein SA, Mattaliano VJ Jr: The "nuisance" sexually transmitted diseases: Molluscum contagiosum, scabies, and crab lice. *Med Clin North Am* 74:1487, 1990.
8 Gillis D et al: Sociodemographic factors associated with *Pediculosis capitis* and *pubis* among young adults in the Israel Defense Forces. *Public Health Rev* 18:345, 1990–91.
9 Routh HB et al: Ectoparasites as sexually transmitted diseases. *Semin Dermatol* 13:243, 1994.
10 Allen JR: Host resistance to ectoparasites. *Rev Sci Tech* 13:1289, 1994.
11 Wierrani FW: *Phthirus pubis* as the cause of tubo-ovarian conglomerate tumor. Geburtshilfe-Frauenheilkd 53(10):721–722, 1993.
12 Billstein S, Laone P: Demographic study of head lice infestations in Sacramento County children. *Int J Dermatol* 18:301, 1979.
13 Brandenburg K et al: 1% Permethrin cream rinse vs 1% lindane shampoo in treating *Pediculus capitis*. *Am J Dis Child* 140:894, 1986.
14 Taplin D et al: Permethrin 1% creme rinse for the treatment of *Pediculus humanus* var *capitis* infestation. *Pediatr Dermatol* 3:344, 1986.
15 Juraneck D: Personal communication.
16 Rasmussen JE: The problem of lindane. *J Am Acad Dermatol* 5:507, 1981.
17 Shacter B: Treatment of scabies and pediculosis with lindane preparations: An evaluation. *J Am Acad Dermatol* 5:517, 1981.
18 Parent-Massin D et al: Lindane hematotoxicity confirmed by in vitro tests on human and rat progenitors. *Hum Exp Toxicol* 13:103, 1994.
19 Kalter DC et al: Treatment of *Pediculus pubis*. *Arch Dermatol* 123:1315, 1987.

Chapter 47

Scabies

Thomas A. E. Platts-Mills
Michael F. Rein

HISTORY

Scabies is one of the great epidemic diseases of humankind.[1,2] It is caused by the scabies mite or "itch mite" *Sarcoptes scabiei* (Fig. 47-1). Transmission of the mite occasionally can occur by touching an infected subject, but most commonly infection requires prolonged physical contact, i.e., sharing a bed or sexual contacts. The mite was first discovered by Bonomo in 1687, but this knowledge was not generally accepted until the details were worked out by Von Hebra in the nineteenth century. The pathophysiology of infection was most clearly demonstrated by Mellanby[3] in his elegant studies using conscientious objectors during World War II. Mellanby watched asymptomatic burrowing of the mites for 3 to 6 weeks, followed by the development of local and systemic pruritus and increased inflammation around the burrow. He also demonstrated that experimental reinfestation would produce itching within hours. These experiments provided very strong evidence that the patients had made an immune response. The timing of the response following reinfection and the associated itching implied that the mites had induced immediate hypersensitivity. Mellanby suggested that this immune response could be important in controlling infestation and that scratching was an effective method of dislodging the mites from the skin.

Adult scabies mites have a body structure and short legs that facilitate entry into the skin. Like all acarids, they have four pairs of legs and lay eggs. They are a member of the class that includes spiders, ticks, and chiggers, but they are most closely related to dust mites of the genus *Dermatophagoides*. The adult female is approximately 400 μm in length and is best seen with a hand lens. Mites can move rapidly on the skin (2 to 5 cm/min) when choosing a site to burrow. They penetrate down to the stratum granulosum and then extend their burrows by ½ in or less over the next month. Mite burrows concentrate on the hands and wrists, but they also can be found on axillary folds, breasts, the periumbilical area, and the penis. Arlian and Vyszenski-Moher[4] have demonstrated that scabies mites, especially the adult females, are selectively attracted to several lipids that are found in human skin. The lipids include odd-chain-length saturated (e.g., pentanoic and lauric) and unsaturated (e.g., oleic and linoleic) fatty acids as well as cholesterol and tripalmitin. The results suggest that lipids present on the skin of humans and other mammals may influence both the incidence of infection and also the distribution of mite burrows on the body. Once established in a burrow, the mites can lay eggs daily. The eggs are approximately 100 μm in length and can progress to the adult stage in about 10 days. The adult male is short-lived, but the females can live up to 6 weeks. Although the potential for multiplication is enormous, the average number of adult females on an infected normal host is less than 20. Adult mites deposit both eggs and fecal pellets in the burrows, and by analogy with dust mites, it is likely that digestive enzymes in the fecal pellets are important antigens for the immune response to scabies mites.[5,6]

IMMUNOLOGY AND PATHOGENESIS

Investigation of the immunopathology prior to 1980 demonstrated a cellular infiltrate and immunoglobulin deposits around lesions as well as circulating immune complexes. It also had been reported that the lesions contained IgE deposits. In 1980 Falk and Bolle[7] reported that patients with scabies had elevated total serum IgE and IgE antibodies to *Dermatophagoides pteronyssinus*. This result could have meant that scabies was common in atopic individuals or that infestation with *S. scabiei* produced an immune response including IgE antibodies that cross-react with dust mites. The latter view has been supported by studies showing extensive cross-reactivity between scabies mites and dust mites involving several different proteins.[8] Furthermore, in rabbits it has been demonstrated that immunization with *D. pteronyssinus* extract can protect the animals against infestation with scabies.[9]

Although it is now clearly established that the scabies mite induces IgE antibodies and immediate hypersensitivity, it is not certain that this response and the associated pruritus play a role in controlling infestation. The lesions around a mite burrow are infiltrated with inflammatory cells.[10,11] From experimental work with ticks, it is likely that the cellular immune response to scabies is comparable with cutaneous basophil hypersensitivity in experimental animals and that eosinophils and basophils could play a direct role in killing mites.[12] Although the immune response to scabies mites includes IgE antibodies, the relationship to atopy is not clear. Thus there are no reports that atopic individuals are significantly more likely to become infected. Equally, there is no clear evidence that becoming allergic to dust mites is protective against scabies in humans, as would be predicted from the results in rabbits.[9] The lesions are often eczematous or urticarial, in addition to the intense pruritus, all of these are in keeping with a pathogenesis related to immediate hypersensitivity.[13] Applying dust mite fecal antigens to the skin of patients with atopic dermatitis will induce a patch of eczema and a characteristic dermal infiltrate of eosinophils, basophils, and T cells.[14] A relation between atopic dermatitis and scabies has been reported. On the other hand, almost all adults with atopic dermatitis have high-titer IgE antibodies to dust mites that would be expected to cross-react with scabies mites and make serologic investigation difficult. In other cases of scabies, the lesions include urticaria or nodules as well as papular lesions. All of these could be related to a complex immune response including mast cells sensitized with IgE antibodies and a cellular response induced by cytokines released from Th2 cells and/or mast cells.

EPIDEMIOLOGY

Epidemics of scabies appear to cycle at approximately 10- to 30-year intervals.[1,2] The causes of epidemics are not clear, but poverty, sexual promiscuity, waning immunity, travel, and other factors may all contribute. Scabies can occur in any population but is reported to be less common among African Americans. The infestation appears to require prolonged contact for transmission and is thus more likely when partners spend the night together. Among young adults, sexual transmission is the most likely method of infection; however, tracing routes of infection is made difficult by the long, asymptomatic "incubation" periods. If multiple members of a family develop itching, the diagnosis is usually straightforward, and unlike most other venereal diseases, scabies can be transmitted by nonsexual contact within a family. Casual contact outside families is unlikely to transfer mites except from crusted scabies. For example, although scabies is frequent in school-age children, transmission in school is uncommon. Transmission to hospital staff is also rare, but some cases have been

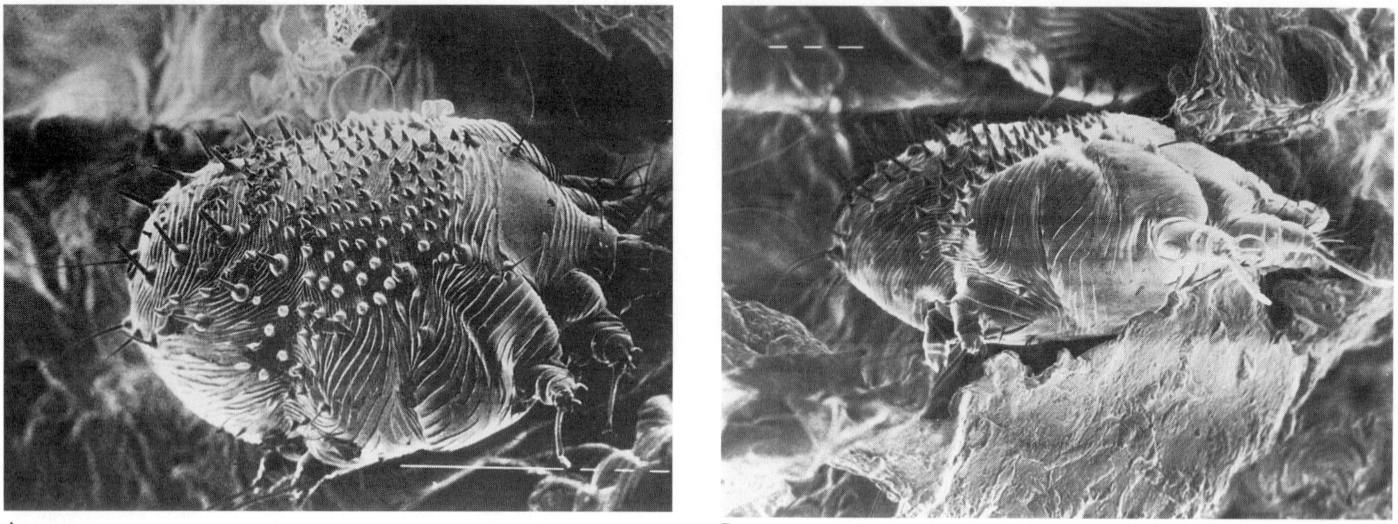

A B

Fig. 47-1 (*A,B*) Scanning electron micrographs of *Sarcoptes scabiei*. *(Courtesy of L. Arlian, Wayne State University.)*

reported. Crusted scabies can give rise to cases among hospital staff. When this happens, the infestation in these individuals is usually localized and not severe. However, occasional case reports have been made of severe scabies contacted from a patient with crusted scabies.[15] In another case where the scabies was lindane-resistant, 12 people were infected before the patient was cured with permethrin.[16] Fertile adult female mites generally transmit infection, and the heavier the infestation, the more likely transmission is to occur.

Transmission to humans from mange in animals can occur. In the dog, mange is caused by *S. scabiei* var. *canis*. This mite is very similar to the human scabies mite morphologically, but infection of humans is generally short-lived, lasting some 3 to 6 weeks (compared with the "seven-year itch" attributed to *S. scabiei* var. *homanis)*. The fact that infestation with mites derived from an animal does not give rise to typical burrows and is relatively short-lived may reflect differences in the mites. Thus they may be attracted by different fatty acids and may be more susceptible to killing by a basophilic or eosinophilic response in the skin. However, detailed studies of the killing of animal mites or the more severe variants of human scabies have not been carried out. Infection of several members of a family from a newly acquired animal can occur, but human-to-human transfer of the dog mite is thought to be rare. Thus animal-acquired scabies will only produce a few cases and does not usually require treatment of other members of the family.

CLINICAL MANIFESTATIONS

The most common manifestation of scabies is pruritic, papular, eczematous lesions on the sides of the fingers and in the interdigital webs (Figs. 47-2 and 47-3). The burrows are often diagnostic and sufficient to recommend specific treatment. Burrows also may be clearly visible on the wrists and elbows. By contrast, lesions elsewhere on the body are papular, nodular, crusted, or lichenified (see Plates 82 and 83). In all situations the lesions are inflamed and extremely pruritic; the pruritus initially may be restricted to the lesions but often becomes generalized. Diagnosis depends on thinking of scabies, demonstrating the mites by scraping or biopsy, and/or observing a response to specific therapy. Itching does not begin for 3 to 4 weeks after initial infestation, but reexposure may produce itching within hours.

SPECIAL FORMS OF SCABIES

Scabies can be difficult to diagnose both because of the wide range of skin lesions and because of atypical distribution. Some special

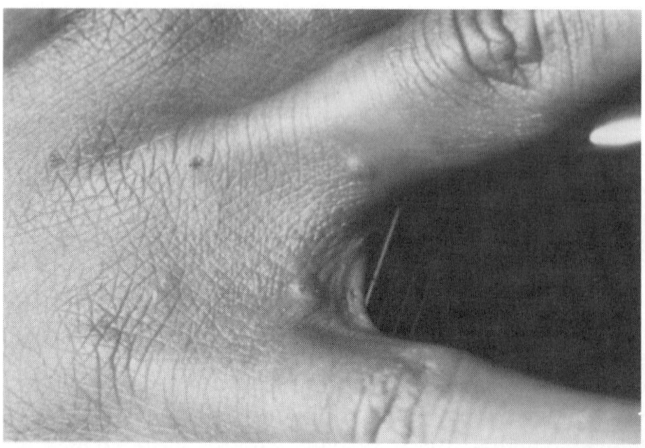

Fig. 47-2 Papules in the interdigital area, highly suggestive of scabies. *(Courtesy of E. Stolz.)*

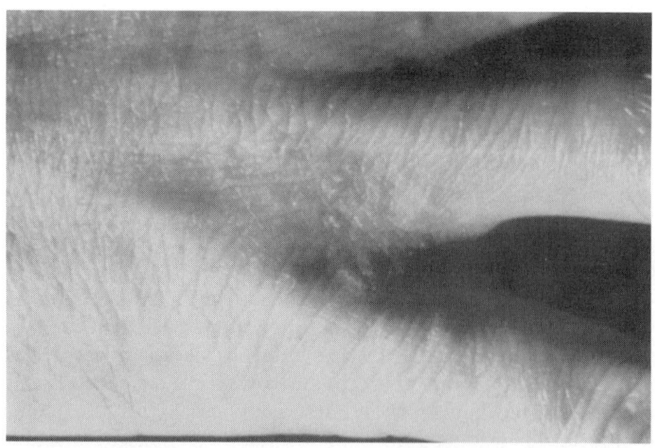

Fig. 47-3 Multiple scabietic burrows and papules are present on the finger webs. *(Courtesy of A. Hoke.)*

forms are worth describing, but scabies needs to be in the differential diagnosis of all pruritic skin diseases.

NODULAR SCABIES

Although unusual, nodular scabies is important to consider because the mildly pigmented, pruritic nodules can persist for months. Clinically, biopsy of the lesions may be necessary to exclude lymphomas of the skin. Diagnosis of scabies may become obvious from biopsy, but sometimes it will not. It is interesting that some cases of chronic atopic dermatitis develop similar nodules. In cases where the diagnosis is not clear from inspection, scrapes, or biopsy, it has to come from a history of scabies in a contact or a trial of specific treatment.

SCABIES INCOGNITO

Like all forms of inflammatory dermatitis, scabies responds to steroids either topically or systemically. In most cases this response is so poor that the diagnosis becomes obvious. However, in some cases steroid treatment may obscure the diagnosis, leading to a more chronic and widespread form that is easily confused with other generalized forms of eczema. These patients remain infectious, so they may come to light because of infection in other members of the family.

SCABIES IN INFANTS

In infants infection with scabies can give rise to failure to thrive or to generalized eczema. In young children widespread vesicles with an impetiginous appearance or secondary infection with *Staphylococcus aureus* is common.[17,18]

CRUSTED OR NORWEGIAN SCABIES

Crusted scabies is characterized by exuberant scaling lesions that are heavily infested with mites. The term *Norwegian scabies* refers to the country of original description of the syndrome and should be replaced by the more descriptive term *crusted scabies*.[19] The diagnosis is easily made once the possibility is considered. Unlike those with classic scabies, these patients can infect through casual contact. Whether this simply results from the large number of mites present or reflects a different strain of mites is not clear. However, most individuals who become infected because of contact with a case of crusted scabies develop typical scabies, suggesting that it is the host response that is abnormal. Detailed studies on the immunology of the response to crusted scabies have not been reported and would be interesting. The disease is seen commonly in patients who are physically or mentally disabled but also in patients with a defined immunologic defect or who are on immunosuppressive treatment. Therapy may require supportive treatment and antibiotics as well as repeated courses of specific treatment with acaricides.

SCABIES IN PATIENTS WITH HIV/AIDS

The immune response to *S. scabiei* is responsible for much of the symptomatology of the infestation as well as for its control. Thus it is hardly surprising that the clinical spectrum of scabies is different in patients with the acquired immunodeficiency syndrome (AIDS) than it is in those with normal immune systems. Although firm data are lacking, it is likely that a disproportionately large number of AIDS patients develop crusted scabies.[20–26] Although scabetic involvement of the face and scalp is relatively rare in normal adult hosts, AIDS patients often present with lesions in these areas. Likewise, the nails are involved with greater frequency than they are in normal hosts.[21,23] Unusual presentations of scabies in immunocompromised hosts may invite confusion with Darier-White disease (keratosis follicularis),[21,23] in which scaly papular lesions develop on the seborrheic areas of the body, including the trunk, face, scalp, and groin.[27] On the other end of the spectrum, patients may present with generalized pruritus and few lesions.[23] Scabies also should be considered in the differential diagnosis of AIDS patients with psoriasiform lesions, and some cases have been diagnosed initially as eczema.[24]

Pruritus is a hallmark of scabies in normal hosts, and even in patients with AIDS, pruritus may be quite marked. In other patients, however, perhaps as a consequence of a blunted immune response, pruritus may be markedly decreased, and this phenomenon seems to be associated with the conversion to crusted lesions.[21]

In AIDS patients as well as others, lesions of crusted scabies contain large numbers of mites, and the condition is highly contagious. Several cases of nosocomial transmission to other patients and to health care workers have been reported.[21] Transmission has occurred even in settings wherein the disease was quickly recognized and treated.[15] Crusted scabies results in a dramatic breakdown of integumentary defenses. When combined with the systemic immunodeficiencies of AIDS, it is hardly surprising that bacteremias have resulted. In addition to the usual bacterial pathogens associated with scabies, *S. aureus* and group A streptococci,[28] other streptococci, and gram-negative rods including *Enterobacter cloacae* and *Pseudomonas aeruginosa* have been recovered from the blood of septic AIDS patients with scabies. Although some authors have recommended prophylactic antibiotic treatment of scabetic AIDS patients,[24] it would seem that careful surveillance and a high level of suspicion are more appropriate in this group.

Treatment of crusted scabies in AIDS patients often requires prolonged application of scabecides. Weekly applications of lindane over 6 weeks have been successful in individual cases,[23,24,26] as have two or three applications at intervals of 48 to 72 hours.[23,27] Permethrin has been used in a smaller number of cases.[29] Concomitant use of a keratinolytic agent such as 6% salicylic acid is recommended.[23]

Difficulty is often encountered in treating crusted scabies in AIDS patients because of the high mite load and because of the difficulty in obtaining adequate penetration of topical scabecides through the crusts. Thus considerable interest has been generated in the oral treatment of scabies with ivermectin. Ivermectin is a derivative of one of the avermectins, a group of macrolide lactones with broad antiparasitic activity. It is widely used in the treatment of human oncocerciasis. In small series, the drug has been administered as a single oral dose of 200 μg/kg with excellent results, even in cases recalcitrant to topical therapy.[15,20,22] Multiple administrations of the same dose have been used in some patients as well.[30]

SCABIES AS A SEXUALLY TRANSMITTED DISEASE

That scabies is reliably transmitted during sexual intercourse is not questioned.[31] Although not all cases of adult scabies are so acquired, the disease is recognized as sexually transmitted.[31–33] As a consequence of this epidemiology, one can make certain clinical assumptions about the disease. First, because the sexually transmitted infections are diseases of lifestyle, individuals with one STD are at significantly higher risk of others to be infected. Thus patients diagnosed with scabies should be evaluated for other sexually transmitted diseases (e.g., chlamydial infection, HIV infection) that may be clinically silent but have greater eventual clinical significance.[31,32] Second, close household contacts and, particularly, sexual partners within the past month should be examined and treated if necessary.[32]

DIAGNOSIS

Typical scabies occurring within a family and presenting with burrows visible on the hands may be obvious by the time the patient has finished describing the symptoms. Furthermore, many atypical cases can be diagnosed because of an associated typical case that responds to specific treatment. In the isolated atypical case, the differential diagnosis includes many different pruritic dermatoses. Since the lesions of scabies can be eczematous, urticarial, or nodular, the list includes contact dermatitis, atopic dermatitis, infected atopic dermatitis, multiple insect bites, chiggers, dermatitis herpetiformis, papular urticaria, chronic urticaria, and mastocytosis.

TECHNIQUES FOR IDENTIFYING MITES IN LESIONS

Using a hand lens to examine burrows is standard practice. Burrows can be made more easily visible by allowing them to take up ink. After rubbing ink from a fountain pen on the area, the ink should be wiped off with alcohol, and ink in the burrows becomes visible[34] (see Color Plate).

Scraping of the skin with a no. 15 scalpel blade should be sufficiently vigorous to disrupt the top of burrows or papules.[35] The scrapings are transferred to a slide, covered with mineral or immersion oil and a coverslip, and examined for mites, eggs, and fecal pellets under a microscope (×20 or ×100) (Fig. 47-4). Samples also can be obtained from lesions using a needle or a curette.

Biopsy of atypical lesions may be helpful to identify mites or their eggs. However, it is important to remember that the typical adult case has only 12 live mites, so biopsies are only likely to be helpful if they are of the inflamed lesions. In general, punch biopsies are used, but an epidermal shave biopsy may be simpler and often can be carried out without local anesthetic on even a relatively uncooperative patient.[36]

THERAPY

The treatment of scabies is by topical application of acaricide; treatment generally requires only one to three applications depending on the agent used, but symptoms may persist for weeks. The cream should be applied to the trunk and limbs, and prescriptions should be for the required doses only. The major issues in treatment are efficacy, toxicity, and treatment of contacts or family members (Table 47-1).

CHOICE OF ACARICIDE AND TOXICITY

The treatment of choice is 5% permethrin cream; 30 gm is usually sufficient for an adult, and the cream should be removed after 12 hours (Table 47-2). Lindane cream 1%, crotamiton cream, and benzyl benzoate are also effective and may be important in some countries because they are cheaper than permethrin. However, in a range of studies over the last 10 years, permethrin has been consistently more effective than lindane.[37–39] Furthermore, 5% permethrin has been used successfully to treat cases that were resistant to lindane[39] or crotamiton.[40] These preparations are generally nontoxic when applied as directed.[41] However, lindane has significant toxicity when applied repeatedly or to children or old persons. Applying lindane immediately after a bath may predis-

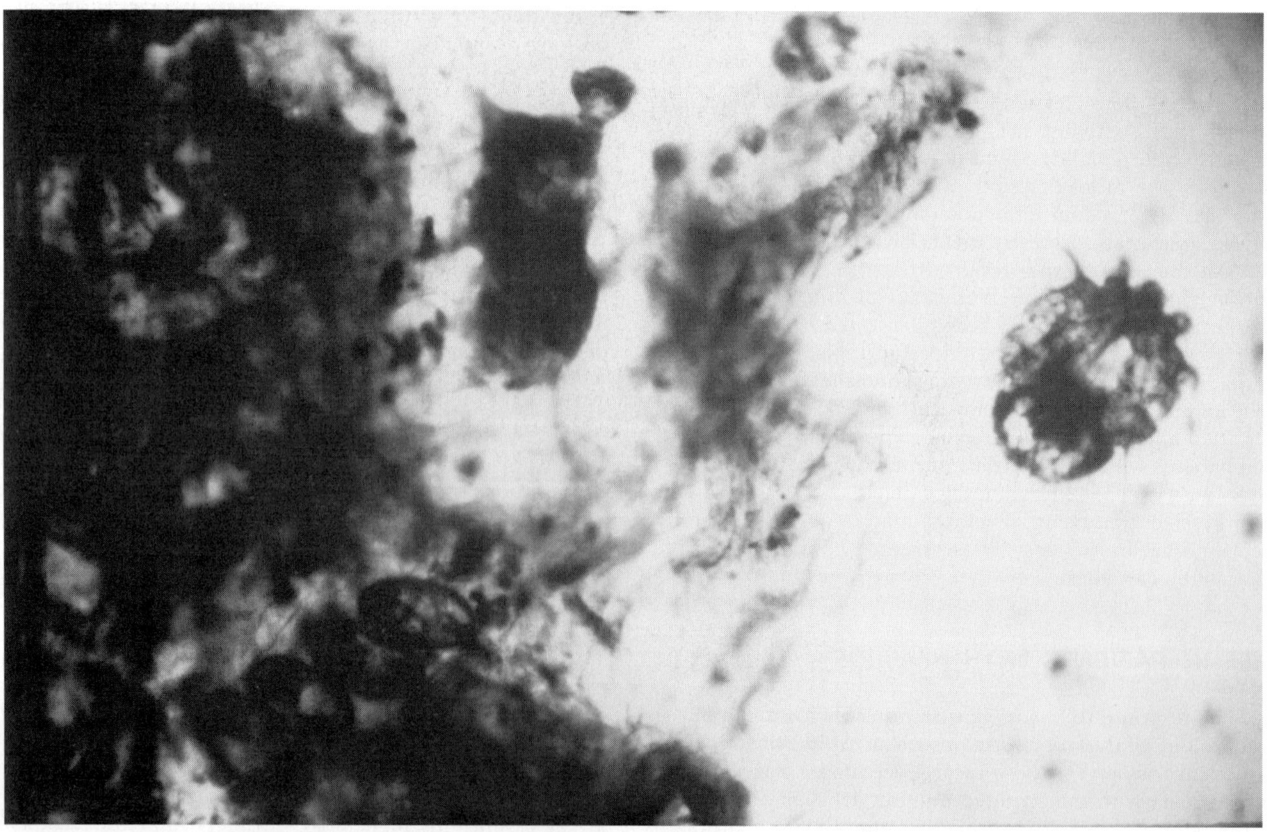

Fig. 47-4 Skin scrapings of unexcoriated papules fortuitously disclose adults, larva, eggs, and fecal pellets, any of which would be diagnostic.

Table 47-1. Pharmaceutical Agents Active against Scabies

Agent	Method of application	Trade name	Cure rates
Benzyl benzoate 25% solution	Topical	—	80–100%
Precipitated sulfur 6%	Topical	—	—
Crotamiton 10% cream (*N*-ethyl-*o*-crotonotoluidide)	Topical	Eurax	60%
Lindane 1% cream or lotion (gamma-benzene-hexachloride)	Topical	Kwell, Quellada, Scabend	65–86%
Permethrin 5%	Topical	Elimite	89–100%
Ivermectin (tested for treatment of animal infestation, mange)	Oral	—	>90%

pose to raising blood levels[42,43] and should be avoided. The main side effect is seizures, which were reported in 3 of 19 patients aged 65 to 93 years.[42] Seizures also have been reported in a 2-year-old child treated with lindane.[43]

TREATMENT OF CONTACTS

All symptomatic individuals should be treated and also sexual partners because they are likely to be infected. Most authorities recommend treating family members simultaneously, because the cure rate at 10 weeks is much higher. Treatment of family members and contacts may be the most important procedure to control spread of the disease. However, it is important to establish the diagnosis in the index case to prevent overtreatment.

TREATMENT OF THE ENVIRONMENT

Scabies mites can only live for a short time outside the body; however, the bedding and clothing should be cleaned. Scabies mites are killed by washing in hot water (130°F). It is not necessary to treat areas away from the bed (Table 47-3).

REPEATED TREATMENT AND ACAROPHOBIA

Occasional cases of crusted scabies or other atypical forms will require repeated courses of topical treatment or oral treatment. On the other hand, many patients try to repeat the treatment because of persistent symptoms. This carries a risk of sensitization and contact eczema that is then likely to be taken as further evidence of persistent scabies. Acarophobia is a well-recognized delusion. Affected patients believe they have something on or in their skin that may be specifically identified by them as scabies mites or other mites. These patients may create artifactual lesions or bite marks, and they will demand repeated courses of treatment. After carefully excluding the presence of parasites, one should manage these patients with reassurance, but some may require psychiatric help.

Table 47-2. Treatment of Scabies with 5% Permethrin Cream

- Massage cream in the skin from head to feet (30 gm is sufficient for an adult).
- Remove cream by washing after 12 hours.* Family and sexual partners should be treated simultaneously.
- Patients may experience burning of the skin and increased itching after application. In addition, patients should be warned that itching may persist for days or weeks after successful treatment.

*M Orkin and HI Maibach, *Semin Dermatol* 12:22, 1993.

Table 47-3. Diagnosis of Scabies

History and examination
- Burrows typically in finger webs examined with a hand lens
- Papular, crusted papules of eczematous lesions on hands, wrists, buttocks, breasts, penis, scrotum, and arms
- Local and generalized pruritus often worse at night
- Cluster of cases
- Specific response to acaricides

Diagnostic measures
- Ink test to identify burrows
- Skin scraping using a blade (no. 15) and transferring a slide to examine under a microscope
- Skin biopsy may be necessary to confirm diagnosis; microscopic examination can demonstrate mites, egg cases, and fecal pellets

OLDER TREATMENTS

Precipitated sulphur (5%) in petrolatum was used traditionally, but it is generally unacceptable (smell and straining) and unnecessary with the availability of permethrin. Similarly, crotamiton is no longer used because it is less effective than lindane or permethrin. Benzyl benzoate is important because it is effective and cheap, but it is no longer used in the United States.

GENERAL PRINCIPLES OF MANAGEMENT

Serious illness resulting from scabies is very rare except in infants and patients who develop crusted scabies. However, pruritus and infection of the lesions can create significant problems that require treatment. Given the presence of mite fecal pellets in the lesions, it is no surprise that itching persists for some period after killing of the mites. This requires antihistamines and reassurance. If itching remains severe, a short course of oral steroids is effective. In general, infection and crusting resolve once the mites are killed. However, both *S. aureus* and hemolytic streptococci may superinfect the lesions. If infection continues, systemic antibiotics may be required. The basic principle of treatment is to identify the mites and apply a topical acaricide in an adequate dose.

References

1 Orkin M, Maibach HI: Current concepts in parasitology: This scabies pandemic. *N Engl J Med* 298:496, 1978.
2 Orkin M: Resurgence of scabies. *JAMA* 217:593, 1971.
3 Mellanby K: *Scabies*. Oxford, England, Oxford University Press, 1943.
4 Arlian LG, Vyszenski-Moher DL: Response of *Sarcoptes scabiei* var. *canis* (Acari: Sarcoptidae) to lipids of mammalian skin. *J Med Entomol* 32:34–41, 1995.
5 Tovey ER et al: Mite faeces are a major source of house dust allergens. *Nature* 289:592–593, 1981.
6 Chua KY et al: Sequence analysis of cDNA coding for a major house dust mite allergens, Der p I. *J Exp Med* 167:175–182, 1988.
7 Falk ES, Bolle R: IgE antibodies to house dust mite in patients with scabies. *Br J Dermatol* 102:283, 1980.
8 Arlian LG et al: Cross-antigenicity between the scabies mite, *Sarcoptes scabiei*, and the house dust mite, *Dermatophagoides pteronyssinus*. *J Invest Dermatol* 96:349–354, 1991.
9 Arlian LG et al: Resistance and immune response in scabies-infested hosts immunized with *Dermatophagoides* mites. *Am J Trop Med Hyg* 52:539–545, 1995.
10 Frentz G et al: Immunofluorescence studies in scabies. *J Cutan Pathol* 4:191, 1977.
11 Hoering KK, Schroeter AL: Dermatoimmunopathology of scabies. *J Am Acad Dermatol* 3:237, 1980.

12 Michell EB, Askenase PW: Basophils in human disease. *Clin Rev Allergy* 1:127–128, 1983.
13 Falk ES, Bolle R: In vitro demonstration of specific immunological hypersensitivity to scabies mite. *Br J Dermatol* 103:367, 1980.
14 Mitchell EB et al: Cutaneous basophil hypersensitivity to inhalant allergens in atopic dermatitis patients: Elicitation of delayed responses containing basophils following local transfer of immune serum but not IgE antibody. *J Invest Dermatol* 83:290–295, 1984.
15 Corbett EL et al: Crusted ("Norwegian") scabies in a specialist HIV unit: Successful use of ivermectin and failure to prevent nosocomial transmission. *Genitourin Med* 72:115–117, 1996.
16 Meinking TL, Taplin D: Safety of permethrin vs lindane for the treatment of scabies. *Arch Dermatol* 132:959–962, 1996.
17 Hurwitz S: Scabies in babies. *Am J Dis Child* 126:226, 1973.
18 Burns BR et al: Neonatal scabies. *Am J Dis Child* 133:1031, 1979.
19 Parish LC: Scabies. *N Engl J Med* 332:611, 1994.
20 Aubin F, Humbert P: Ivermectin for crusted (Norwegian) scabies. *N Engl J Med* 332:612, 1995.
21 Orkin M: Scabies in AIDS. *Semin Dermatol* 12:9–14, 1993.
22 Meinking TL et al: The treatment of scabies with ivermectin. *N Engl J Med* 333:26–30, 1995.
23 Schlesinger I et al: Crusted (Norwegian) scabies in patients with AIDS: The range of clinical presentations. *South Med J* 87:352–356, 1994.
24 Skinner SM, De Villez RL: Sepsis associated with Norwegian scabies in patients with acquired immunodeficiency syndrome. *Cutis* 50:213–216, 1992.
25 Donabedian H, Khazan U: Norwegian scabies in a patient with AIDS. *Clin Infect Dis* 14:162–164, 1992.
26 Inserra DW, Bickley LK: Crusted scabies in acquired immunodeficiency syndrome. *Int J Dermatol* 29:287–289, 1990.
27 Baden HP: Darier-White disease (keratosis follicularis) and miscellaneous hyperkeratotic disorders, in *Dermatology in General Medicine*, 2d ed, TB Fitzpatrick et al (eds). New York, McGraw-Hill, 1979, pp 266–271.
28 Brook I: Microbiology of secondary bacterial infection in scabies lesions. *J Clin Microbiol* 33:39–40, 1995.
29 Waldmann BA: Crusted (Norwegian) scabies in an HIV-infected man. *Clin Cases Dermatol* 3:6–9, 1991.
30 Marty P et al: Efficacy of ivermectin in the treatment of an epidemic of sarcoptic scabies. *Ann Trop Med Parasitol* 88:453, 1994.
31 Schroeter A: Scabies: A venereal disease, in *Scabies and Pediculosis*, M Orkin et al (eds). Philadelphia, Lippincott, 1977, pp 56–59.
32 Centers for Disease Control and Prevention: 1993 sexually transmitted diseases treatment guidelines. *MMWR* 42(RR-14):95–97, 1993.
33 Brown S et al: Treatment of ectoparasitic infections: Reviews of the English-language literature, 1982–1992. *Clin Infect Dis* 20:S104–S109, 1995.
34 Woodley D, Sautat JH: The burrow ink test and the scabies mite. *J Am Acad Dermatol* 4:715, 1981.
35 Muller G et al: Scraping for human scabies: A better method for positive preparations. *Arch Dermatol* 107:70, 1973.
36 Martin WE, Wheeler CE Jr: Diagnosis of human scabies by epidermal shave biopsy. *J Am Acad Dermatol* 1:335, 1979.
37 Schultz MW et al: Comparative study of 5% permetrin cream and 1% lindane lotion for the treatment of scabies. *Arch Dermatol* 126:167–170, 1990.
38 Haustein UF, Hlawa B: Treatment of scabies with permethrin versus lindane and benzyl benzoate. *Acta Dermatol Venereol* 69:348–351, 1989.
39 Taplin D et al: Permethrin 5% dermal cream, a new treatment for scabies. *J Am Acad Dermatol* 15:995–1001, 1986.
40 Taplin D et al: Comparison of crotamiton 10% cream (Eurax) and permethrin 5% cream (Elimite) for the treatment of scabies in children. *Pediatr Dermatol* 7:67–73, 1990.
41 Drugs for sexually transmitted diseases. *Med Lett* 37:117–122, 1995.
42 Felman RH, Maibach HI: Percutaneous penetration of some pesticides and herbicides in man. *Toxicol Appl Pharmacol* 28:126, 1974.
43 Ginsberg CM et al: Absorbtion of lindane (gamma benzene hexachloride) in infants and children. *J Pediatr* 91:998, 1977.

PART VII STD CARE MANAGEMENT

Chapter 48
STD care management

King K. Holmes
Caroline A. Ryan

Medicine is a science of uncertainty and an art of probability

Sir William Osler

INTRODUCTION

Rapid advances in biomedical knowledge and technology provide clinicians with a continuously expanding armamentarium of diagnostic and therapeutic options. Biomedical and behavioral research also provide proven preventive interventions.[1–4] The public expects diagnostic certainty and effective medical care. Clinicians themselves grow increasingly dependent on advanced technology in diagnostic and therapeutic decision making. At the same time, resources for clinical care management become more constrained even in the best of circumstances, and new epidemiologic models call for greater outreach to resource-poor settings to achieve STD control.[5] Clinicians are increasingly forced to practice under conditions of great uncertainty. The desire to help and not to harm prompts the following questions: What is the true diagnosis? Which laboratory tests will help? What treatment will alleviate symptoms and cure infection? What evidence warrants treatment of sex partners? Which preventive interventions, if any, actually work?

The most appropriate answers to these questions depend on the clinical setting, the probability of various infections, the resources available, the expectations of patients, cultural constraints, and the overarching programmatic goals of the clinical service (e.g., primary patient care, public health STD clinic, family planning or prenatal clinic, etc.). Even in industrialized countries, recent crises in health care financing have made clinicians all too aware of the economic implications of their decision making. Diagnostic evaluation and disease treatment concern not only health benefits, but also economic costs.[6–11] A society lacking infinite resources to spend on health care can no longer focus only on the percentage of infections a new screening or treatment program detects, cures, or prevents; we now must examine the balance between costs and proven benefits.

This chapter examines the various approaches, both successful and unsuccessful, now used in the diagnosis and treatment of STDs in a variety of clinical settings and focuses on strategies clinicians can use to increase their effectiveness. We think (with due respect to William Osler) that medicine is a science of probability and an art of managing uncertainty.

DEFINITION AND GOALS OF STD CARE MANAGEMENT

STD care management requires managing care of both symptomatic and asymptomatic individuals. The major steps in effective STD care management include risk assessment and clinical evaluation; diagnostic or screening tests; diagnosis; treatment; and preventive or supportive measures, including risk reduction counseling, identification and treatment of partners, condom promotion, and efforts to ensure compliance with treatment and prevention measures.[12,13] The goals of STD care management are to cure or ameliorate the infection; prevent complications and sequelae of the infection, including complications related to pregnancy or family planning; prevent transmission of the infection to others; reduce HIV transmission; provide counseling on future risk reduction and, if necessary, on coping with chronic STD; and provide outreach for care management to exposed sex partners. In general, the earlier the diagnosis, treatment, and counseling, the greater the impact on preventing further transmission and complications.[1,14]

AN INTEGRATED APPROACH TO STD CARE MANAGEMENT

From inability to let alone; from too much zeal for the new and contempt for what is old; from putting knowledge before wisdom, and science before art and cleverness before common sense; from treating patients as cases; and from making the cure of the disease more grievous than the endurance of the same, Good Lord, deliver us.

Sir Robert Hutchinson

An integrated approach to STD care management begins with risk assessment (of sexual behaviors, specific exposures, and sociodemographic and other markers of high risk), history of reproductive health and past STDs, and clinical assessment (elicitation of specific symptoms and signs of STDs) (Fig. 48-1). Depending on available resources for testing, the results of these assessments may lead to confirmatory diagnostic tests (for symptomatic patients) or screening tests (for asymptomatic individuals judged to be at sufficiently high risk to warrant testing). In most settings, treatment of symptomatic patients is often started on a syndromic presumptive basis (i.e., it is selected to cover the most likely causes of the symptoms and signs); in industrialized countries treatment often begins while results of confirmatory tests are pending.[15] For certain syndromes, rapid tests may be used to narrow the spectrum of initial therapy (e.g., wet mount for women with vaginal discharge, Gram stain for men with urethral discharge and women with cervical mucopus, darkfield exam and rapid serologic test for syphilis for genital ulcer disease [GUD]).[16] After the institution of treatment, STD care management concludes with what has been termed "the four Cs": contact (sex partner) notification and treatment; condom promotion, where appropriate; counseling and education regarding reduction of future risk; and assurance of compliance with medication instructions (providing directly observed single dose therapy wherever possible).[13] A fifth "C" could be assurance of confidentiality. Although this outline specifically applies to care management for STDs, essentially the same steps apply to care management of most if not all diseases—with the preventive steps represented by the "4 Cs" differing for different diseases.

CLINICAL EVALUATION AND RISK ASSESSMENT

Patients may consult a clinician with a set of symptoms (manifestations of the disease perceived by the patient and either volun-

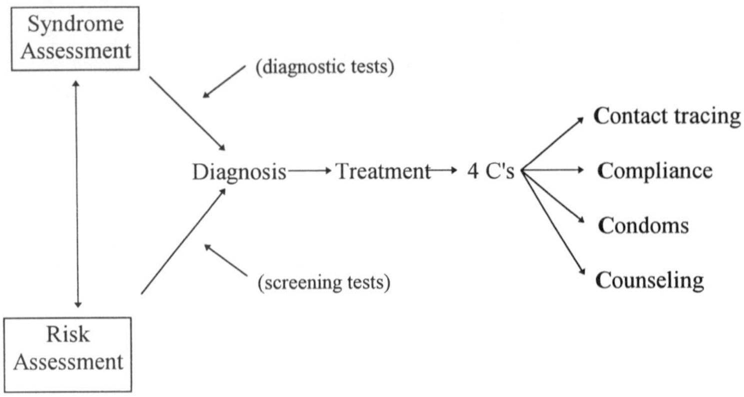

Fig. 48-1. Essential steps in STD care management.

teered or brought forth during the history taking), and signs (manifestations of the disease identified during the physical exam). Chapters 50 and 51 describe the approach to the physical examination of the male and female genitalia, as part of the clinical evaluation for STDs. Other individuals with sexually transmitted infections (STIs) may lack symptoms or fail to perceive symptoms that occur, or may perceive symptoms of infection but feel they are too trivial or too embarrassing to prompt them to seek care or to tell the clinician.[15,16]

Routine risk assessment can serve as a guide to selective clinical evaluation and selective laboratory testing for STDs in patients who do not report STD symptoms, and can also aid in the interpretation of any symptoms or signs that are presented.[17–22] Thus, clinical evaluation and risk assessment for STDs actually proceed concurrently; positive risk assessment prompts and guides the clinical evaluation for STDs, and conversely, clinical findings compatible with STDs should prompt risk assessment, since a positive STD risk assessment increases the probability that suspicious findings actually represent an STD. Chapter 49 reviews risk assessment for STD/HIV.

Clinicians will not know which patients need special clinical evaluation and testing for STDs and education and prevention counseling services unless they ask about risk. Surveys have shown that adolescents in particular will discuss their sexual behaviors and concerns, but usually will not bring up the subject unless asked.[23] A national survey showed that primary care physicians assessed sexual behavior for less than one-half of their patients.[24] Most communities urgently need collaboration between STD program and health education staff, clinicians, and other members of community-based organizations to develop risk assessment tools to help clinicians assess risk behavior, as well as counseling and educational materials to help in counseling high risk and STD-infected patients about how to recognize and reduce risk.

LABORATORY TESTING

Chapters 53, 71, 92, and 103 present different aspects of STD/HIV laboratory testing. Testing of symptomatic patients to establish the etiology of symptoms (diagnostic testing) is distinguished from testing of asymptomatic individuals brought to care as contacts of an infected person, or seeking care for reasons other than symptoms or signs of STDs (case finding tests) or testing of individuals identified through outreach to populations outside the clinic (screening). In this chapter, the term "screening" encompasses both case finding and screening, as defined in the preceding. Increasingly, risk assessment guides selective, cost effective allocation of resources for laboratory testing.[8,15,19,20]

Laboratory testing for specific causative infectious agents can provide the strongest evidence for infection and justification for treatment, and for preventive interventions including partner treatment. For *N. gonorrhoeae* and *H. ducreyi*, and to a some extent for viral pathogens, isolation of the pathogen also permits testing for sensitivity or resistance to antimicrobial agents. For syphilis, quantitative reagin antibody tests allow monitoring the response to therapy.[25] For cervicovaginal HPV infection, identification of oncogenic HPV types is under evaluation as a potential guide to prognosis and to the need for therapeutic intervention (see Chap. 25). Similarly, typing of genital HSV helps predict the likelihood of recurrence.[26] In addition, positive laboratory tests provide the most specific evidence of infection for surveillance purposes.

However, specific laboratory tests obviously are not available at some clinic sites, and even when tests are available, test results are often not available soon enough to guide therapy or partner management decisions during the initial patient visit. Further disadvantages of some laboratory tests include high cost and variable test performance. When intrinsic test characteristics or inadequate laboratory quality assurance lead to less than 100 percent sensitivity, treatment of symptomatic patients based only on positive test results rather than on syndromic diagnosis (see below) can lead to undertreatment. Even the diagnostic tests available for the more important STDs cannot be appropriately utilized where the test is too expensive or limited in availability.[27] Specimen collection procedures, such as pelvic examination for cervical samples, urethral swabbing, or veinpuncture for obtaining blood, may also present a disincentive for patients to seek testing or for providers to perform the test.[28] Less invasive sampling techniques, such as self-collected vulvovaginal swabs or urine for DNA amplification tests, or saliva collection for detection of antibody, helps to overcome these problems. Nonetheless, clinical, epidemiologic, technical, and resource considerations dictate the extent to which laboratory tests are useful in STD care management.

Even when resources permit rapid laboratory tests on specimens collected noninvasively, an additional practical concern is that rapid tests used to guide initial therapy of symptomatic patients often must be performed in an office or clinic without nearby laboratory support. This requires the clinician or office staff to do any tests needed to guide treatment of acute disease syndromes. For example the office or clinic-based laboratory analysis of a vaginal specimen is frequently performed to provide objective information regarding vaginal infections. A microscopic examination allows recognition of fungal hyphae indicative of vulvovaginal candidiasis, "clue cells" suggestive of bacterial vaginosis, and motile trichomonads indicative of trichomoniasis.[29] These microscopic tests for vaginal infection have been recently classified as "physician-performed microscopy" tests under the U.S. Clinical Laboratory Improvement Amendment of 1988, placing a new and greater diagnostic burden on U.S. clinicians in small offices choosing to maintain a laboratory.[30] Primary care clinicians have demonstrated high specificity but low sensitivity when identifying vaginal trichomoniasis and vulvovaginal candidiasis by microscopic techniques.[31] Correct microscopic diagnosis of bacterial vaginosis was even more difficult for clinicians. Clinicians were less accurate than a DNA probe test in diagnosing vaginal infections.[31] Thus, in general, a need remains for more reliable, but inexpensive and rapid clinic-based tests for the acute symptomatic STDs to guide prompt therapy.

Screening

Since many persons with sexually transmitted infection lack symptoms, screening is required to detect infection. Most studies of STDs are conducted in health care settings specifically intended for persons who do recognize symptoms; therefore, these studies usually overestimate the proportion of infected persons who are symptomatic. Conversely studies of STD screening in non–health care settings (such as in the community, jails, schools, or workplaces) or in health care settings for which STD treatment is not the primary function (such as antenatal or family planning clinics) suggest that the majority of persons with gonorrhea or chlamydia are asymptomatic. For example, among women seeking care for contraception or other gynecological reasons, 52 percent of those with gonorrhea and at least 70 percent of those with chlamydial infection showed neither symptoms nor signs of infection.[32,33] Four population-based studies of men found that 68 to 92 percent of those with gonorrhea reported no symptoms, and one reported that 92 percent of men with chlamydial infection reported no symptoms.[34–38] In a large community-based study in rural Uganda of individuals screened by urine LCR tests, 63 percent of men with gonorrhea and 92 percent of men with *C. trachomatis* infection reported no symptoms.[37] Neither the studies done in clinics serving symptomatic patients, nor the studies of prevalent STDs in largely asymptomatic populations, can give an accurate picture of the proportion of incident infections that actually cause inflammation or lesions, or the proportion of those with inflammation or lesions who perceive symptoms. For example, imagine an STD that caused severe symptoms in one-half of those infected, and that those with such symptoms immediately sought and obtained curative therapy. Investigators studying the symptomatic half would conclude that all had symptoms, whereas those studying the general population (from which the symptomatics had been quickly removed) would conclude that none had symptoms. The best approach to determining what proportion perceive symptoms and develop signs comes from studies of incident (new) infections in prospectively followed cohorts.

Nonetheless, the fact that many persons with an STI at any point in time, do not perceive symptoms has important implications for treatment of these STIs and for preventing complications and further transmission. Educating the public on STD symptom recognition, and providing access to treatment for symptomatic persons represent the essential first step in a prevention program, but no matter how much this enhances symptom recognition and access to health care, many cases of certain curable STDs will go unrecognized and untreated unless the persons are tested through other means. Other opportunities to identify and treat asymptomatically infected persons include screening in health care settings when persons present for other problems (such as in emergency rooms, family planning clinics, during routine or annual physical examinations, and during immunization visits for adolescents and adults) and screening in non–health care settings. Case findings can also be targeted through programs based on partner notification.

Establishing locally appropriate STD screening recommendations and policies should be priorities of STD control programs. For example, in the United States, various guidelines currently exist for screening for *C. trachomatis*, including the recommendation for screening all sexually active adolescent girls at least annually, or more frequently for those with new sex partners.[13] However, a study in San Diego, California, in 1995 showed that fewer than 50 percent of the primary care physicians caring for adolescents screened their sexually active adolescent female patients for chlamydial infection; screening of young men is far less common.[39] Sensitive and specific DNA amplification methods such as polymerase chain reaction, ligase chain reaction, and transcription-mediated amplification tests for detecting *N. gonorrhoeae* and *C. trachomatis* in urine should make screening more acceptable for both males and females.

DIFFERENT APPROACHES TO STD DIAGNOSIS

Health care providers have generally used either laboratory test-based etiologic diagnosis, or etiologic diagnosis based on clinical findings, for the etiologic diagnosis of many STDs in persons with symptoms and signs; and STD treatment guidelines in the past have largely focused on treatment of specific sexually transmitted infections, albeit sometimes with guidelines for management of a few syndromes as well (e.g., NGU, PID, epididymitis). However, in resource-poor settings, laboratory tests are not available, and because of low validity of etiologic diagnosis based on clinical findings, syndromic diagnosis has been increasing, leading to greater emphasis on guidelines for syndromic management of STDs.

Laboratory-based etiologic diagnosis

This involves identifying the organism causing symptoms, using microscopy or other laboratory tests. Even when testing is available, treatment is often initiated on the basis of syndromic diagnosis, while test results are pending.

Presumptive diagnosis of etiology based on clinical findings alone

This approach involves making a best guess as to the etiology of symptoms and signs, based on clinical experience. Even experienced STD service providers, however, often misdiagnose STDs when they rely only on their clinical experience in interpreting symptoms and signs. For example, numerous studies from Africa, the United States, and Jamaica have repeatedly demonstrated the inaccuracy of clinical impressions as to the etiology of genital ulceration.[40–48] In a South African study of 100 men and 100 women with genital ulcers; for example, clinicians correctly identified only about one-third of the cases of chancroid or syphilis in the men, about one-half of the cases in the women, and less than 10 percent of mixed infections.[45] Reasons cited for this low accuracy of clinical diagnosis include: (1) similarities in clinical appearance of various etiologies; (2) simultaneous infections with more than one organism; and (3) atypical appearance owing to longstanding disease, prior self-treatment with ineffective therapy, or concomitant HIV infection.[40–48]

Syndrome Diagnosis. In resource-poor settings the most practical approach is syndrome diagnosis, with or without risk assessment. This approach is less costly, and less technically demanding than laboratory-based or presumptive etiologic diagnosis based on clinical findings.[12] The World Health Organization (WHO) has recommended that national STD control programs in developing countries incorporate diagnostic and therapeutic flowcharts in their STD management guidelines.[12] The basis of the syndromic approach is the identification of a syndrome, that is, a set of easily elicited symptoms and easily recognized signs associated with a limited number of well-defined etiologies. The advantages of syndrome management include expedited care, treatment at the first visit, cost savings by not using expensive laboratory tests, and increased client satisfaction. Treatment at the first visit results in not losing the patient to follow-up before treatment is initiated, reducing further transmission and complications from untreated infections, and eliminating the need for a return visit for laboratory results. The use of flowcharts in STD management standardizes diagnosis, treatment, referral, and reporting, allowing for improved surveillance and program management. The significant limitations of the syndromic approach include the lack of utility for asymptomatic people with sexually transmitted infections; the relatively low sensitivity and specificity relative to laboratory testing for some infections; and the fact that many false positive diagnoses lead to unnecessary use of drugs, and to potential social problems attending a false positive diagnosis. Further, the quandary remains about when to attempt treatment of sex partners of individuals treated on the basis of syndromic diagnosis alone. In clinical settings where acquisition of infection by the patient from a steady sex partner (e.g., the husband) is likely—for example, in family planning clinics in many countries—reinfection of the patient would be very likely without treating the steady partner.

Design of flowcharts for syndromic diagnosis

As described in Chapter 100 and in a recent compilation of articles on syndromic management of STDs, a clinical flowchart, or algorithm, or decision tree, depicts a path of diagnostic reasoning.[50–61] The structure of a flowchart can be hierarchical or non-hierarchical.[50] In hierarchical algorithms, the presence of a single symptom is the limiting factor for entry, and one diagnosis excludes another. A non-hierarchical algorithm allows the consideration of several risk-markers, signs, or symptoms at once, and allows consideration of different diagnoses at the same time. To ensure efficient use for STD management, flowcharts should be adapted to the level of development of the health care system and the particular health care facilities for which they are intended. Culture specific perceptions about STDs, patterns of health seeking behavior, and expectations about health care to a large extent determine the usefulness of certain flowcharts.

Common STD Syndromes. The major STD syndromes include: dysuria and urethral discharge in men, testicular pain and swelling, genital ulceration, lower abdominal pain in women, and abnormal vaginal discharge. Several STD syndromes can be managed reasonably well using clinical flow charts for diagnosis. These include:

1. Genital ulcer syndrome, most commonly attributable to syphilis, genital herpes, or chancroid, less commonly to LGV or granuloma inguinale (donovanosis).
2. Urethral discharge syndrome in men, often attributable to gonorrhea and chlamydial infection, or to nongonococcal nonchlamydial urethritis. The latter has numerous potential etiologies, some still unproven or undefined yet often responsive to syndromic treatment.
3. The syndrome of testicular pain and swelling in heterosexually active men under the age of 35 most commonly reflects acute epididymitis due to the sexually transmitted pathogens *N. gonorrhoeae* or *C. trachomatis*. In heterosexual men over 35 years of age, particularly those with underlying genitourinary disease, coliform bacteria or *Pseudomonas* are more likely etiologies. Similarly, coliforms are the likely case of epididymitis in homosexual men who practice anal-insertive sex. No data suggest any modification in the current recommendations intended for heterosexual adolescents and young men to first exclude testicular torsion and trauma, and then treat with antimicrobials that cover *N. gonorrhoeae* and *C. trachomatis*.
4. Lower abdominal pain syndrome (pelvic inflammatory disease [PID]) caused by cervical pathogens *(N. gonorrhoeae, C. trachomatis)* and by less pathogenic vaginal bacteria (including vaginal anaerobes).
5. Mucopurulent cervicitis, caused by gonorrhea or chlamydial infection. Signs of yellow endocervical discharge, edema of the zone of cervical ectopy, and easily induced endocervical bleeding, with or without symptoms of abnormally yellow vaginal discharge, have been useful predictors of cervical infection in settings with high prevalence (prior probability) of gonococcal and chlamydial infection, particularly in women with positive risk assessment for cervical infection.[50–61] In such settings or patients, this syndrome remains potentially useful, supporting the diagnosis of PID and as a guide to syndromic management of cervical infection and/or to selective screening for cervical infection. However, in settings with low prevalence of gonococcal or chlamydial infection, MPC has a lower predictive value for such infections, useful as a criterion for selective diagnostic testing but not necessarily for treatment of these infections. The addition of risk assessment to identify women with risk factors *plus* signs of mucopurulent cervicitis or PID, has relatively low sensitivity, but relatively high specificity and positive predictive value for cervical infection.[50,54] However, critical factors in development and use of such algorithms include development of locally defined, culturally acceptable risk assessment algorithms; and the training, experience, and skill of the clinician in detecting manifestations of mucopururlent cervicitis or PID.[51,52]
6. Vaginal discharge syndrome in women, usually caused by bacterial vaginosis or trichomoniasis. The symptom of increased amount of vaginal discharge per se has not proven very useful for diagnosis either of cervical infection with *N. gonorrhoeae* or *C. trachomatis*, or of vulvovaginal candidiasis. In general, symptoms and signs of abnormal vaginal discharge have shown strong correlation with detection of bacterial vaginosis and trichomoniasis; and symptoms of vulvar pruritis and signs of vulvar inflammation have shown strong correlation with vulvovaginal candidiasis.[50,52,54,62] The true utility of algorithms dealing with vulvovaginal symptoms in many clinical settings lies in the management of vaginal infections. This seemingly trivial conclusion from several studies of syndromic management of vaginal discharge actually represents a potentially important practical advance in women's health care practice in developing countries. In contrast, a number of studies have found low utility of vulvovaginal symptoms for detecting cervical infection. Further, of the three major categories of abnormal vaginal discharge symptoms (abnormally increased amount, abnormal odor, or abnormally yellow color), only the latter (abnormally yellow color) has been consistently associated with cervical infection in studies published to date.[49,51,64] In developing countries classical hierarchical algorithms and risk score based algorithms for "vaginal discharge" have been tested and compared in a few countries and mainly in family planning or antenatal clinic attendees or female sex workers; unfortunately, few studies have been conducted in STD clinics or primary care or gynecology clinics that serve symptomatic women for whom the algorithms are intended.[50–61,63,64,66] One reason for the poor performance of algorithms for lower abdominal pain in detecting cervical gonococcal or chlamydial infection in most clinical settings has been the insensitivity and

the nonspecificity of the elicited symptom of low abdominal pain, except when coupled with signs of PID elicited by trained gynecologists.[51,52,54]

The term lower genital tract infection (LGTI) syndrome in women, as discussed in Chapter 57 has had a broader connotation, including abnormal in amount, color, or odor of vaginal discharge as well as vulvar and urethral symptoms. This definition encompasses disparate cervical vulvovaginal, and urinary infections with overlapping clinical manifestations. It is useful in calling attention to the need for further evaluation for such infections, and perhaps as an entry point to a flowchart that branches with different syndromes, but is not sufficiently specific to lead to treatment for cervical or vaginal infection.

In most developing countries, algorithms calling for treatment for gonococcal and chlamydial infection in men with urethral discharge and for treatment for syphilis and chancroid in men or women with genital ulcers have generally been found sensitive, specific, and preferable to presumptive etiologic diagnosis based on clinical findings.[40–47] However, in settings where genital herpes is common, chancroid uncommon, and serologic testing for syphilis feasible, other modified algorithms can defer antibiotics when herpetic vesicles are seen, withhold treatment for chancroid, and confirm syphilis serologically to guide partner notification. Even in these settings, for patients who may not return, or may expose others, initiating syphilis therapy at the first visit for genital ulcer is often best, even when a rapid syphilis serologic test is initially negative, since about one-third of patients with primary syphilis still have negative rapid plasma reagin or VDRL tests at the first clinic visit. Mathematical modeling suggests treatment and cure of primary syphilis would have a much greater impact on control of syphilis than would treatment of secondary or latent syphilis; therefore, prompt treatment of primary syphilis deserves high priority.

TREATMENT FOR STD, INCLUDING DIRECTLY OBSERVED THERAPY–SINGLE SESSION (DOTSS)

The diagnosis of a curable STD should lead to curative treatment. Curative antimicrobial therapy is available for all bacterial STDs, as well as for those caused by protozoa and ectoparasites.[12,13] In contrast, available drugs for viral STDs are suppressive but not curative; nonetheless, they can alleviate symptoms, prevent or delay complications, and in theory could reduce transmission from the patient who adheres to therapy without abandoning other protective measures. Significant barriers to curative treatment include patient failure to comply with a full course of medication, and failure of treatment providers to provide cheap and effective therapies for which compliance is easy. To address these problems, effective single-dose curative therapies have been developed for all of the major curable STDs (including early syphilis, chancroid, gonorrhea, trichomoniasis, chlamydial infections), together with guidelines promoting such therapies.

Development and promotion of STD treatment guidelines at national and local levels are particularly essential for the curable STDs. A recently published study showed that about half of the primary care physicians in the United States managing a patient with PID were unsure of or did not follow Center for Disease Control and Prevention (CDC) guidelines.[23] In much, if not most of the world, a large proportion of patients receive care from pharmacies or the informal medical sector, rather than from trained clinicians.[67] A recent study in Peru used standardized simulated patients presenting to pharmacies with one of four scripted scenarios for urethral discharge, vaginal discharge, genital ulcer, or PID. Over 80 percent of simulated patients were offered medication. However, effective, recommended medication was offered to as few as 0 and 1 percent of patients presenting PID or genital ulcer syndromes; and 4 percent of those presenting a vaginal discharge syndrome. Only 30 percent of those complaining of urethral discharge symptoms were offered recommended regimens active against both gonococcal and chlamydial infection.[68]

A further recent development in STD treatment involves monitoring therapy and assistant patients with chronic viral STD—especially HSV infection, HPV infection, HIV infection, and chronic hepatitis B or C, in self management. This was best illustrated to the public in the Broadway play *Rent,* when the actors all learned who had HIV infection when their pagers all beeped simultaneously to remind them to take their AZT. This approach increasingly involves case managers and systems designed to improve compliance, provide rapid access to nurses or pharmacists to address management of new symptoms, adverse effects, compliances, etc.

THE FOUR "CS"

The four "Cs," a term designed to encapsulate the preventive aspects of STD/HIV care management, refers to contact treatment or (partner notification, referral, and treatment); counseling on risk reduction; condom promotion; and efforts to facilitate compliance with treatment to prevent treatment failure as discussed above (see Chaps. 55 and 70). Although sound clinical reasons call for prevention in clinical practice, clinicians often fail to provide recommended clinical preventive services.[22,23,69] The current emphasis on short-term cost–benefit considerations in managed care programs in the United States (related to the short mean time that clients continue in any one managed care program) does not encourage preventive services. The inadequate reimbursement for preventive services, fragmentation of health care delivery, and insufficient time for clinicians to spend with patients to deliver the range of needed preventive services, exacerbate the problem. Recommendations for preventive services are issued regularly by government health agencies and their expert panels, by medical specialty organizations, voluntary associations, other professional and scientific organizations, and individual experts.[11,12] When these recommendations are inconsistent, as were recommendations from two medical specialty groups for preventing neonatal group B streptococcal infection, confusion may impede implementation of recommendations, until efforts to coordinate guidelines result in consensus.[70]

Skepticism about the effectiveness of education and counseling for STD/HIV prevention may dissuade some clinicians from offering such interventions. A half-hearted prevention effort might include patient education (e.g., simply telling people what to do, giving them an instructional pamphlet); mentioning male condoms; and with varying degrees of emphasis and success, advising patients to ask their contacts to come for treatment. Contact tracing and follow-up are often limited to certain categories of patients and partners and seldom thorough.[24] For example, gynecologists and family planning clinics provide little or no care to male partners of their female patients; female partners often shun those STD clinics that serve predominantly male patients; managed care programs generally provide no care to partners not enrolled in the same program as their patient; and student health services provide no care to nonstudents.[23,24] Urgent care clinics and emergency rooms provide little or no preventive care or follow-up. In developing countries where many if not most individuals seek care for STD-related symptoms from pharmacies or informal health care providers, counseling, partner notification, and condom promotion are very uncommon.[23] In the delivery of STD/HIV preventive services to adolescents by primary care physicians, higher levels of preventive service delivery were associated with female physician gender, specialization in obstetrics and gynecology, and more recent date of medical school graduation. Physicians practicing in health maintenance organizations reported providing significantly higher rates of preventive services to sexually active adolescents than did physicians in private practice.[24] In many settings, any contacts brought to treatment are regular partners, not the casual partners most likely to transmit infection. In summary, many clinicians emphasize the medical model almost exclusively, with little emphasis on effective behavioral preventive interventions.

Effective patient participation in prevention requires education, motivation, and counseling.[25] Although busy clinicians cannot fill all educational and counseling needs, they can start and guide the process. Patients with an STD can recognize their vulnerability to other STDs, including AIDS; an STD diagnosis presents a unique opportunity, or "teachable moment," where the messages of risk reduction counseling can have substantial potential for changing STD-related behaviors, particularly for adolescents and other high-risk groups.[26] Three studies have now demonstrated significant reduction in reported risk behavior and in subsequent incidence of one or more STDs through "client-centered" or "theory-based" individual or group counseling of patients in STD-clinic settings.[4,71,72] Jemmott et al. have recently demonstrated significantly greater reduction in risk behaviors reported by African-American adolescents by a safer-sex HIV-risk reduction intervention than by an abstinence-based intervention.[73] Thus, a new standard of STD care management should include the types of counseling shown to be effective—counseling that cannot be delivered in the 15-minute "slot" allocated for clinicians to see patients with STDs in many STD clinics or managed care settings, or in the even briefer and less confidential encounter typical of busy clinics in developing countries.

Similarly, clinicians in private practice, including those working in managed care, need to work with public health agencies to develop new strategies and techniques for community outreach for partner notification, and not rely solely on public sector staff to carry out this work.

POTENTIAL STEPS REQUIRED TO TREAT AND PREVENT STDS

Improving clinical care does not address the issues of subclinical and asymptomatic STIs, or poor treatment-seeking behavior by individuals with STD symptoms. Additional strategies needed include public education to promote awareness of STD symptoms and improve treatment-seeking behavior; access to treatment for symptomatic individuals; screening for asymptomatic infections; and treatment of partners of index cases. More comprehensive STD prevention strategies should address uninfected individuals through interventions at the individual- and population levels.[5]

Figure 48-2, modified from an analysis of TB prevention originally developed by M. Piot, highlights the potential steps for STD prevention, including steps up to and including STD care management.[74] The figure implies the focus of strategies needed to address different aspects of STD control; for example, prevention of exposure to or acquisition of an STD, screening and treating asymptomatic infection, education for improved symptom recognition, improving treatment seeking behavior and access to care, as well as improving STD care management per se. Each level, except for the third from the top on this diagram, represents an important point for public health or clinical intervention. Clinicians must recognize that STD care management focused only on diagnosis and treatment of patients seeking care for STD symptoms accomplishes little for the individual patient or for the population as a whole. This must be accompanied by partner notification, education of patients and public on STD symptom recognition, ensuring access to care for those who need it, screening for subclinical infection, and counseling on preventing exposure and preventing infection given exposure.[75]

It is essential to educate the population, especially youth, on the symptoms associated with STDs, while reinforcing an understanding that many STDs are often not symptomatic, especially in women. Health education programs for youth should nonetheless emphasize that once symptoms develop, further sexual contact should cease until appropriate care is obtained. Health seeking behavior is influenced by several factors apart from knowledge and awareness—particularly by access to effective, acceptable treatment. In developing countries, economic structural adjustment programs have affected uptake of services. A documented example of this occurred in Nairobi's large STD clinic where the introduction of fees led to a 60 percent reduction in attendance among men and a 35 percent reduction among women.[11]

EXAMPLES OF UNSUCCESSFUL APPROACHES TO ORGANIZING SYSTEMS FOR STD CARE MANAGEMENT

Although the failure of STD control throughout much of the world has resulted from inadequate resources and tools (e.g., lack of cheap, rapid effective diagnostic tests, and lack of trained personnel) equally important are lack of attention to each of the components of STD care management (see Fig. 48-1), and lack of intervention at each of the levels in the cascade (see Fig. 48-2). However, overlying these problems are a set of systematic, but correctable problems in the ways available resources are mobilized and organized to provide STD care management.

These systematic problems arise partly from attempting to im-

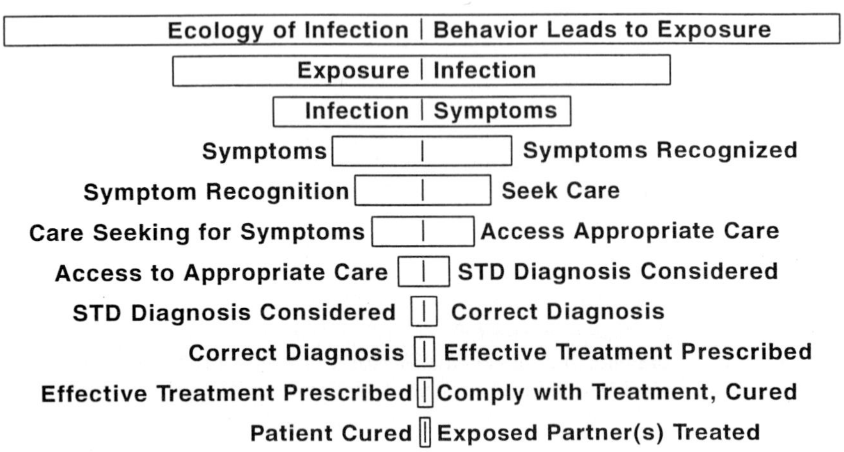

Fig. 48-2. Potential points for intervention through STD care management and other public health intervention, to reduce acquisition of STDs, and detected and treat asymptomatic and symptomatic infection that occur.

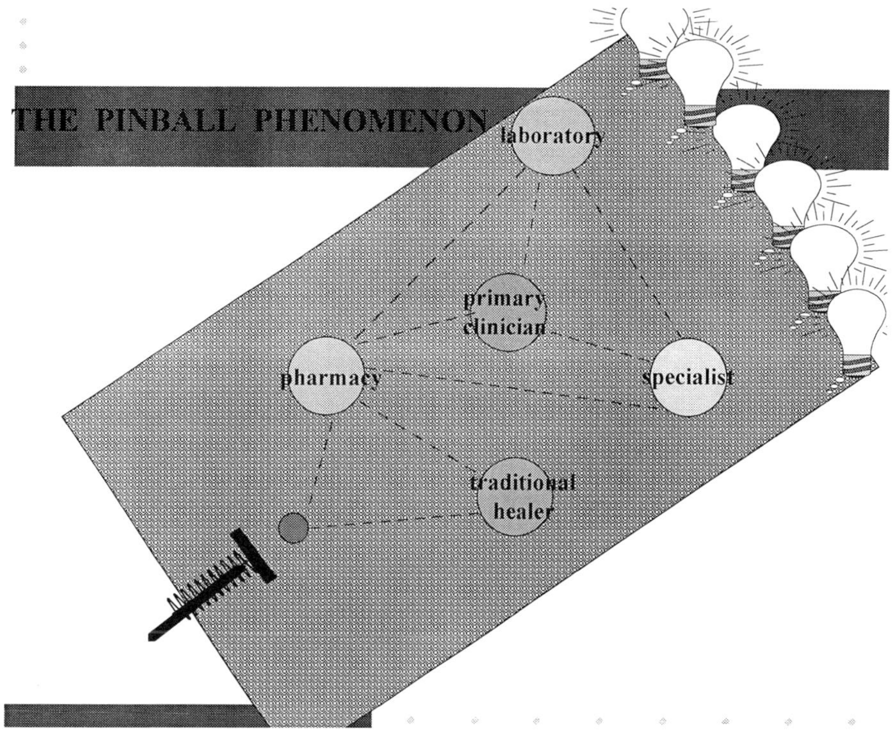

Fig. 48-3. The pinball approach to STD care management.

plement care management procedures not appropriate for the limited infrastructure and resources available; partly from attempting to reproduce systems used in industrialized countries, rather than adapting to local realities; and partly from constraints imposed by such realities. These problems are sufficiently common to be termed phenomena or syndromes indicative of a "sick" health care system.

THE "PINBALL" PHENOMENON

Figure 48-3 schematically depicts the path of many patients in their attempts to receive an STD diagnosis and treatment, particularly in developing countries where patients are required to visit several locations before being treated. Because of the stigmatization associated with STDs, and the inconvenience and costs associated with access to formal health facilities in either the public or the private health sectors, persons with STD-related symptoms often seek initial treatment in the informal sector. Drugs may be borrowed from other persons or purchased directly from licensed pharmacies, traditional medical practitioners, so-called "injectionists," or street-based drug peddlers. When the point of first encounter with the health care system for STD treatment is the informal health sector, over-the-counter purchase of ineffective types or doses of antibiotics is common, despite laws that regulate their distribution.[67,68] Treatment obtained from these sources is frequently expensive but inadequate or ineffective, patients do not receive the benefit of education or counseling or condom advice, and their sexual partners are not referred or treated.[53,54,68]

When this initial therapy is not successful, patients may eventually seek care in the formal health sector, where they may have to first visit a clinic for initial exam, then a laboratory for tests, then the clinic again to receive results of tests and prescription, then return to the pharmacy to buy the prescribed medication. Furthermore, the clinician may be reluctant to prescribe first-line, effective medication, preferring to initially try less effective but cheaper medications, reasoning that the patient will return if treatment fails; and then the cycle can be repeated. Successful navigation of this user-unfriendly system could be regarded as survival of the fittest. Few patients make all these visits, some never receive any treatment, and many never receive effective treatment. With most STDs, symptoms eventually resolve, but patients remain infectious, and at risk for late sequelae. Even in the formal health care sector, preventive services are minimal, owing to scarce resources, low prioritization of prevention in relation to curative treatment, inadequate provider training, and demands of patient flow and profit that often preclude prevention efforts.[52,56,57] Barriers to seeking care in the formal sector thus include the long waiting times; multiple return visits required to undergo laboratory testing, obtain test results, obtain prescriptions, fill prescriptions, return when treatment fails to relieve symptoms; and the cost of transportation, consultation, tests, and medications. All of this is aggravated by the social stigma of presenting with an STD in clinics where privacy and confidentiality are often lacking, and staff are often judgmental.[14] These social and financial barriers apply particularly to women, and improving their access to and use of STD services is a major challenge to STD control.[20,52]

THE "SUPPOSED-TO" SYNDROME

A corollary to the pinball phenomenon is the "supposed-to syndrome," best represented by antenatal screening for syphilis (Table 48-1). In this syndrome, the number of steps required to identify and treat pregnant women with syphilis foils the best of intentions of clinicians to prevent congenital syphilis. The alternative solution to these inconvenient systems of organization of services, as demonstrated by Temmerman et al., has been termed the "supermarket approach," or "one-stop shopping," in which patients undergo evaluation for all medical problems at one visit, receive an immediate syndromic diagnosis or rapid test (e.g., RPR test), and medication is provided with counseling at the first visit.[76]

Table 48-1. The "Supposed to" Syndrome for Antenatal Serologic Testing for Syphilis

Patient supposed to obtain antenatal care
Antenatal clinic supposed to stock supplies for venipuncture
Clinic supposed to obtain blood for syphilis serology
Clinic supposed to send blood to separate laboratory for testing
Laboratory supposed to have unexpired, good-quality serology reagents
Laboratory supposed to test blood
Laboratory supposed to return test results to antenatal clinic
Clinic supposed to record results of tests in patient record
Patient supposed to return for follow-up antenatal visit
Clinic supposed to stock benzathine penicillin G for treatment of seropositives
Clinic supposed to treat seropositives
Patient supposed to return for serologic test of cure

THE "BUNKER HILL" PHENOMENON

In this situation, the clinician is reluctant to treat the patient on the first or even the second visit, preferring to first have confirmation of a diagnosis by multiple laboratory tests. The approach resembles that of William Prescott on Bunker Hill on June 17, 1775 when, conserving his ammunition, he ordered his troops, "Don't one of you fire until you see the whites of their eyes" (Fig. 48-4). In an analogous way, the clinician treating a patient with a genital ulcer may state, "Don't treat for chancroid until you see three negative darkfield exams and two negative syphilis serologies." As with the pinball phenomenon in the preceding, the treatment finally offered is typically not first-line treatment, but less expensive and less effective treatment. Those who fail to respond clinically are expected to return again for a second attempt with the more effective but more expensive treatment. This was the approach and the reasoning taken by the U.S. Air Force at Clark Airbase in the Philippines for some time after the emergence of β-lactamase producing gonococci; it was considered cheaper to first use procaine penicillin for gonorrhea treatment, and reserve spectinomycin for the large proportion of airmen who failed initial treatment. This reasoning helps explain the continued use of ampicillin or tetracycline for treatment of gonorrhea in many developing countries through much of the 1980s and 1990s, even where most gonococci had become resistant to both drugs. This short-sighted approach increases the mean duration of infection and risks further transmission, failure of patients to return, and progression of disease; and the clinic also acquires a reputation for not giving prompt treatment. Reducing the duration of STDs among infected individuals is a time-honored method of preventing STDs in the population because reducing duration reduces the number of future partners exposed to infection. The impact of early detection and treatment on preventing STD transmission was illustrated by the trial of strengthened syndromic management of STD in Tanzania, demonstrating that early detection and treatment of common STD syndromes reduced the prevalence of active syphilis and of symptomatic urethritis in the general population.[77]

THE VENEREOLOGIST WHO CANNOT ADAPT TO A RESOURCE-POOR SETTING

The well-trained venereologist can adapt to make efficient, sensible use of the resources available in a resource-limited setting, thereby contributing to STD control. For example, in the Bahamas in the mid-1980s a major crack-cocaine epidemic led to related epidemics of GUDs and heterosexual HIV transmission. Implementation of syndromic treatment of genital ulcers in large numbers of patients (benzathine penicillin G plus a several-day course of erythromycin), together with highly effective notification and treatment of partners by the public health nursing service, brought the epidemic of GUDs under control.[78]

In contrast, in many other parts of the world, when confronted by overwhelming numbers of cases of STDs, which in turn fuel sexual transmission of HIV, specialists have often had a more schizophrenic professional existence, practicing dermatovenereol-

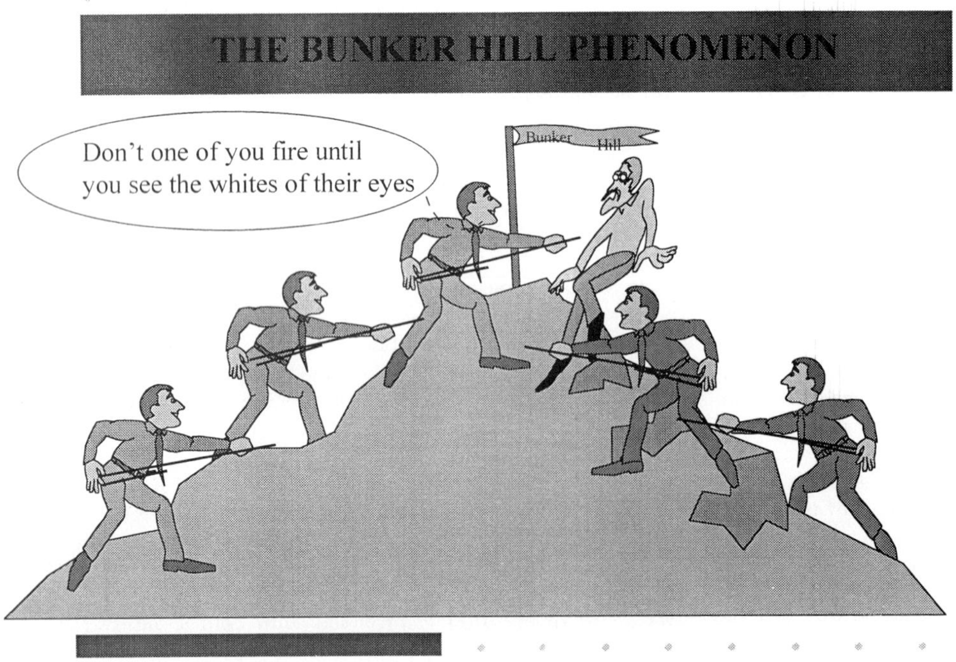

Fig. 48-4. The Bunker Hill approach to conserving ammunition, now malappropriated to STD care management, reserving treatment only to those with an absolutely proven STD infection.

Fig. 48-5. The venereologist who cannot adapt to a resource-limited setting. (A) high cost and low population coverage in the afternoon private office. (B) Poor quality and disincentive in the morning public clinic serving sex workers.

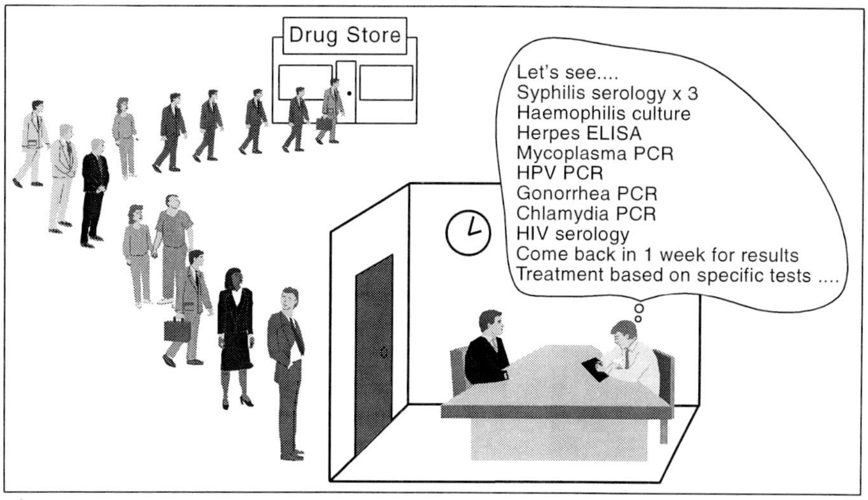
Drug Store
Let's see....
Syphilis serology x 3
Haemophilis culture
Herpes ELISA
Mycoplasma PCR
HPV PCR
Gonorrhea PCR
Chlamydia PCR
HIV serology
Come back in 1 week for results
Treatment based on specific tests ....

A

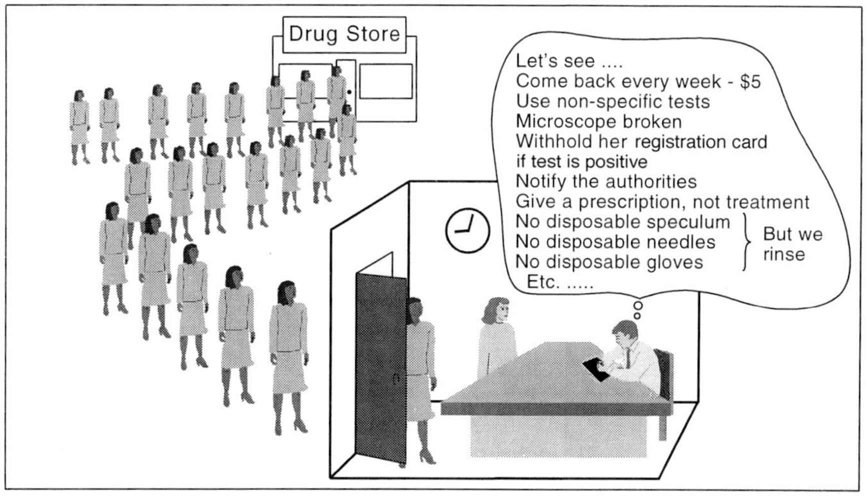

B

ogy just as they were trained in specialized centers in industrialized countries with patients able to afford the extensive evaluations offered at their afternoon private office, while using limited resources ineffectually in a hopeless effort to apply the same complex approach, but with inferior quality and disincentives, to the limited number of patients willing to confront the long waiting lines at their public clinic during the morning (Fig. 48-5). Those who choose not to wait at the public clinic and not to pay the high fees for all of the tests at the private office may initially seek care at a pharmacy or in the informal health sector. Sex workers threatened with loss of work if found infected at the public clinic often obtain prophylactic antimicrobials (perhaps from the pharmacy), before attending the public clinic for required screening exams.

Because of the relatively small proportion of all STDs that can be accommodated in either type of clinic, the contribution of the specialist to prevention and control of STDs in the population as a whole is modest at best. At worst, such practitioners can drain resources needed for efficient STD care management away into inefficient programs, thus actually impeding progress in STD control. In Russia in the 1990s, efforts to continue cost-intensive practices that may have been feasible when STDs were much less common and public health was funded to a greater degree, are no longer appropriate when the case load is now enormous.[79] Another example from the experiences of the authors, was provided by an initial proposal from STD specialists in one large country to expend one-third of the federal budget for STDs drugs on drugs for genital herpes, while not allocating any of the budget for doxycycline to treat chlamydia, because doxycycline was viewed as "too expensive." In the United States, a recent survey of public STD clinics found that a large proportion frequently often turned patients away (rather than expediting management when patient volume was high, so that all seeking care could be accommodated).[80] Thus, the problem of patient management that is inefficient and inadequate to accommodate demand when resources are scarce is not limited to developing countries. The problem becomes one of balancing the minimum level of acceptable services for the individual patient with the minimum level of services needed to interrupt transmission at the population level; and balancing adequate public sector efforts with adequate private sector efforts.

Instead, in resource-poor settings with overwhelming number of STDs, specialists need to refocus at least their public sector efforts at monitoring the etiology of STD syndromes and the antimicrobial susceptibility of STD pathogens, where possible; on increasing the numbers of clients served and improving access to efficient care in the public sector; and on training other primary care providers in syndromic management of the curable STD.

INTEGRATING STD CARE MANAGEMENT SERVICES INTO THE HEALTH CARE SYSTEM

The principal mission of national STD prevention programs is prevention of STD transmission and reduction of STD incidence. Related goals include reducing STD complications and costs, and reducing HIV transmission. Similarly, the principal missions of national AIDS control programs include preventing transmission of HIV and reducing the complications and costs of HIV infection. Surveillance and protecting the rights of individuals with HIV infection also are usually a priority. The clinical care management components of STD and AIDS programs have traditionally been organized vertically, and operated in separate facilities, such as STD clinics, and HIV/AIDS clinics, or in subspecialty dermatovenereology clinics, infectious diseases clinics, and gynecology or urology clinics, apart from other health care services. However, as the population affected by STD/HIV infection grows and becomes more diverse, as is currently happening in Eastern Europe, for example, and as is the case in many developing countries, there is an increasing emphasis on combining STD/HIV prevention and care management activities and integrating them into antenatal, family planning, and primary health care services.[14,20,52]

For example, in the United States, the vast majority of STD cases other than gonorrhea or syphilis are seen by individual private practitioners.[23] Among these practitioners, the largest percentages of total STD cases are seen by obstetricians and gynecologists, family practice physicians, and internists.[81] The specialists most likely to see large numbers of cases of STDs are OB/GYN, infectious disease, and emergency medicine.[81] By clinic type, the largest share of total STD cases are seen in family planning clinics, public STD clinics, and hospitals.[81] However, the types of institutions most likely to see large numbers of cases are military facilities, public STD clinics, and family planning clinics.[81]

In developing countries, within the formal health care sector, STD care is provided through an array of services and individuals, which include specialized STD clinics, general hospital outpatients, primary health care centers (PHCs), maternal and child

Table 48-2. Interrelationships Between Type of Health Care Delivery System, the Primary Goals of the System, the Relative Utility of Syndromic Diagnosis and Laboratory Testing (Diagnostic Testing and Screening), the STD of Greatest Potential Interest, and the Relationship Between Need and Availability of Resources for STD Care Management.

Comparison of STD delivery systems

Type of health care delivery system	Goal(s)	Utility of syndromic approach	Diagnostic testing	Screening	Prevalence of disease and importance in transmission/resources available for care
Family Planning Clinic	Protect reproductive health of client, couple and with respect to contraceptive use (i.e., prevent IUD-related infection, infertility)	—	+	+++ chlamydia gonorrhea	+−/+++
Antenatal Care Clinic	Prevent spontaneous abortion, complications of pregnancy, congenital and neonatal infections, puerperal morbidity and mortality	—	+	++++ syphilis gonorrhea chlamydia HIV trichomoniasis	+−/++++
Primary Health Care Clinic	Relief of symptoms	++++	++	++ chlamydia syphilis HIV per risk assessment	+/++++
STD Specialty Clinic	Prevent STD transmission, relief of symptoms, prevent HIV transmission/acquisition	++++	++	++++ syphilis HIV gonorrhea chlamydia per risk assessment	++++/+−
Female Sex Worker Clinic	Prevent STD transmission, prevent HIV transmission/acquisition	—	+	++++ syphilis HIV, BV gonorrhea chlamydia trichomoniasis	++++/+−
Adolescent/Teen Clinic	Prevent STD/HIV acquisition via education and counseling, relief of symptoms	++	+	++++ chlamydia	+++/−
Private Sector	Relief of symptoms	++++	++	++ chlamydia HIV	++/++++
Informal Sector	Relief of symptoms	++++	—	—	+++/++++

health facilities, family planning clinics, and clinicians in private practice.[14] Few of those providing care have specialist training.

In light of increasing efforts to integrate services, it is useful to recognize how the different approaches used for STD care management are related to the primary mission and goals pursued by each type of service. Rather than dwell on the shortcomings, limitations, or narrow perspective of each type of service, it seems more productive to recognize the different primary missions of that service, and improve on what each can contribute to STD care management and to STD/HIV prevention within the framework of its mission. Table 48-2 summarizes the relationship between a service's primary goals and the resulting emphasis on STD care management.

INTEGRATING STD SERVICES INTO BROADER REPRODUCTIVE HEALTH SERVICES

In some developing countries, women have less access than men to medical care. However, throughout the world, women access medical care through antenatal clinics and family planning clinics, which therefore offer unique opportunities for delivering STD care to women.

Family planning clinics

The International Conference on Population and Development held in Cairo in 1994 stressed that broadening the scope of family planning services could enhance their acceptability and effectiveness.[82] However, family planning clinics are less likely to reach adolescents, single sexually active women, including sex workers, and women who have completed their childbearing. STD rates found in women attending FP clinics reflect the rates among general population of low-risk women; with wide ranges in prevalence depending on the specific infection and on geographic region.[70–72] Since STD/HIV incidence and prevalence in urban areas generally considerably exceeds rates in rural areas, STD prevalence in rural family planning clinics is generally considerably lower than in urban clinics. The well-intended effort to implement syndromic management of STD in asymptomatic married women in rural family planning clinics—as opposed to STD care management of symptomatic women in urban primary care or gynecology clinics, or screening of sex workers—is reminiscent of the cartoon showing a man on his knees under a street lamp, a long distance away from his car, who explains, "I dropped my keys over there by my car where it is dark, but I'm looking for them here under the street lamp because I can see better."

The integration of STD/HIV with family planning services, although justified for a number of reasons, requires the program to integrate somewhat differing approaches and objectives.[83] Family planning clinics provide a commodity (contraceptives) to consumers, and tend to promote the methods most effective in preventing pregnancy, including long-acting contraceptive methods such as the IUD, sterilization, and injectable or implantable hormones, rather than reversible methods such as condoms that are less effective in preventing pregnancy, but that are effective in preventing STDs. STD services, on the other hand, follow the model common to the control of communicable disease. This model generally involves case identification, treatment, and follow-up of contacts and promotion of condoms. Reasons for integrating STD care management into family planning services include the need for women to know if they have an STD, or are at risk for STD/HIV and, ideally, to tailor contraceptive options and safer sex counseling to their needs. Family planners are particularly interested in ensuring safety of IUD insertion and of abortion; and therefore have particular interest in detecting and treating infection before performing these procedures. They are also concerned that women who begin contraception, especially those who then begin sexual activity, may acquire an STD that causes symptoms that could be erroneously attributed by the individual client, and eventually by all women, to the contraceptive method. This could lead to discontinuation of the contraceptive by the client, and eventually to decreased uptake of the method.

Promotion of dual contraceptive methods (e.g., hormonal plus barrier) is increasingly justified not only because certain clients, especially young single women, are not in stable or mutually monogamous relationships and are at high risk for both pregnancy and STD/HIV; but also because of data suggesting hormonal contraception not only increases risk of acquiring certain STDs, but also because hormonal contraceptives may increase shedding of HIV from cervical secretions from HIV-infected women, perhaps rendering them more infectious.[84]

The term reproductive tract infections (RTI), is increasingly used by women's health care workers to encompass cervical, uterine, and vaginal infections. Bacterial vaginosis in particular is referred to by some as an STD and by some as an RTI. In the family planning clinics–a setting where the diagnosis of STD is often not expected–the term RTI has the advantage of not provoking marital discord for management of diseases that do not currently warrant partner notification, such as BV or HPV infection; but also the disadvantage of potentially not emphasizing the need for partner treatment when this is essential (e.g., gonococcal or chlamydial infection).

Antenatal clinics

The primary mission of antenatal clinics is to maintain the health of the mother throughout pregnancy, ensuring uncomplicated pregnancy and a healthy newborn. Chapter 80 outlines the impact of STD on pregnancy and the newborn, and the importance of STD care management in pregnancy in preventing congenital infections and peripartum infections of the newborn, preterm rupture of membranes, amniotic fluid infection, and premature delivery, and puerperal infection of the mother. Antepartum screening for syphilis and neonatal ophthalmia prophylaxis rank among the most cost-effective of preventive health measures. On-site rapid serologic testing for syphilis in the antenatal clinic in developing countries can overcome the pitfalls of the "supposed-to syndrome," ensuring that infected women are detected and do receive treatment.[76] Antenatal detection of *C. trachomatis*, *N. gonorrhoeae*, bacterial vaginosis, trichomoniasis, group B streptococcal infection, hepatitis B virus, HTLV-1, and HIV all now represent potentially important steps that can lead to curative treatments, preventive treatments, vaccination, or avoidance of breastfeeding, to prevent the preceding complications. Because antenatal clinics serve women seeking obstetric care, rather than women with symptoms of STDs, syndromic diagnosis performs poorly in antenatal clinics, as in family planning clinics. Detection of these conditions requires laboratory testing, and simple, cheap, rapid tests are urgently needed to allow prompt detection and preventive interventions in antenatal clinics and family planning clinics.

INTEGRATING STD SERVICES INTO PRIMARY HEALTH CARE

Most countries attempt to provide most clinical services, including STD care, at the primary health care level. However, municipal STD clinics may serve large numbers of patients, especially men, and in developing countries, the informal health sector and pharmacies often represent the point of first encounter for STD care management. In industrialized countries, declining rates of STDs may warrant a stronger emphasis on STD care management in the public health sector, as STD control relies increasingly on outreach to marginalized unemployed populations not reached by managed care, and as the public sector must act effectively to contain outbreaks of imported STDs. This creates the paradoxical situation in which the relative importance of the public health infrastructure increases as the endemicity of STD declines. Nonetheless, primary care providers now diagnose the majority of STDs in the United States, and will likely assume an even greater role in STD prevention and control, because of the declining emphasis on provision of STD care management in some public health programs.[82] The primary goals of health care in the primary care setting tend to emphasize relief of symptoms, and preventing complications in individual patients served, rather than protecting the public health; services are very client-centered, directed toward the patient's perceived needs, and treatment is frequently based on syndromic management of the patient's symptoms. Advantages of STD care in the primary care setting include the ongoing relationships between the clinician and the individual, which can increase the likelihood of early STD detection and effective preventive interventions, such as regular clinician counseling. In addition, incorporating STD-related services into primary care may improve access to services, since primary care providers are much more numerous than public STD clinics, especially as public funding for public health programs decreases.[82] Because STD-related services provided in primary care clinics are not provided in isolation, but rather in the context of other medical problems, primary care clinics do not carry the stigma associated with STD clinics. Primary care providers can effectively coordinate the variety of health and social services available in the community and especially needed by those persons at highest risk for STDs and other infectious diseases, who often require multiple services.

As managed care organizations (MCOs) become the dominant providers of health care in the United States, many offer integrated delivery systems that can plan, organize, and deliver a continuum of health services to defined populations.[85] Public health agencies must develop the partnerships needed with various MCOs to deliver locally tailored, comprehensive STD care management and prevention services to an entire community. The MCOs usually also have the information services needed to monitor and evaluate these services.

Although development of STD care management services at the primary care level has the advantages of accessibility, lack of stigma, a full spectrum of services, and established provider–patient relationships, as noted in the preceding, disadvantages of service at the PHC level also are numerous. A recent study of adolescents enrolled in Massachusetts HMOs in 1992 found annual health care visits higher than the national average for adolescents (3.2 vs. 2.6, $p < 0.025$) but disclosed that fewer received Pap smears (18 percent vs. 41 percent, $p < 0.001$), and that the estimates of sexually active women tested for STD was lower (21 percent vs. 34 percent).[86] Further, among cases of congenital syphilis in Louisiana, those seen in a private health care plan were less often attributable to no or late prenatal care than those seen in a public system; but were more often attributable to no or inadequate prenatal screening or to failure to give treatment after a positive test.[87] In the United States, lack of confidentiality remains a problem for STD/HIV in MCOs, when diagnostic information or medications used are reported to insurers or to employers who purchase insurance. STD services at the PHC level tend to be less efficient and more rudimentary at the PHC level. Training in clinical evaluation and counseling may be lacking as well, especially in developing countries where the quality and effectiveness of services designed for STD care management at the PHC level, such as use of syndromic management flowcharts, require more extensive documentation.

COMMUNITY-BASED CLINICS

Community-based health providers such as urban community health centers, and school-based health clinics or other community-based clinics for teens and young adults, represent a particular type of primary health care which are potentially important sources of STD-related services because they serve patient populations with a high prevalence of STDs. Although many community-based health programs currently provide STD-related clinical services, most have not made STD control a priority despite its high prevalence in their patient population, and some lack expertise and essential technical resources in providing such services. Again, collaboration with local public health agencies or health care training institutions could improve the quality of services offered.

PUBLIC-SECTOR STD CLINICS FOR SEX WORKERS IN DEVELOPING COUNTRIES

Despite the ubiquitious presence of clinics for STD screening and prevention designed for sex workers in urban centers and port cities throughout the world, only limited attention has been given to the quality of care or efficacy of the STD care management provided in such clinics. Examples from industrialized countries and a few developing countries have demonstrated that rates of STDs can be lowered among the sex workers.[51,88–91] However, where sex workers are required to register with municipal authorities and attend clinics for regular periodic examinations, services generally are poor. Although the fees collected from the sex workers typically could pay for appropriate diagnostic testing, clinic personnel, and medications, these funds are seldom allocated to clinics' operation expenses. Neither male nor female condoms are provided in some clinics, the screening provided is noncomprehensive and of poor quality, and medications may not be provided free. The principal objective often appears to be preventing infected sex workers from working, rather than preventing and eliminating disease among the sex workers. Even where unregistered sex workers are likely to be arrested and put in jail, the common practice of revoking work permits when infection is found among registered sex workers provides a strong disincentive for sex workers to participate in the registration program (see Fig. 48-5). Indeed, there is an incentive to seek treatment elsewhere when symptoms of STD do occur, and to use prophylactic antibiotics and douche before routine screening exams to avoid detection of infection. The impact of such programs on reducing STD/HIV prevalence and incidence in sex workers is probably negligible in many developing countries. Indeed, when ineffective programs are in place, sex workers and clients may have a false sense of security from STDs, resulting in increased risk-taking behaviors.

PHARMACY-BASED STD CARE MANAGEMENT

As is the case for primary health care management, the goal of STD care management in pharmacies in developing countries is predominantly treatment and relief of symptoms presented by clients, together with sales of pharmaceutical products.[67] Pharmacy workers recognize STD syndromes in men better than STD syndromes in women as attributable to sexual transmission; conformance to published guidelines for STD treatment in pharmacies, even though partly learned from prescribing patterns of physicans, is very poor; and preventive practices are uncommon.[68] Because the reality is that many patients—especially men—receive STD treatment in pharmacies, especially in Latin America and Asia, there is an urgent need to upgrade the standards of care provided in pharmacies, and to promote STD/HIV prevention practices in these settings, while also improving recognition of STD syndromes, especially in women, and promoting referral to qualified clinicians of the more serious syndromes not well managed by pharmacists.[68,92]

CONCLUSION

The dynamic advances in medical technology and public expectations drive clinicians to use more and more services that are increasingly sophisticated and costly. This trend must be balanced by streamlined systems of care management that use common sense to apply available resources most efficiently in a patient-oriented manner. In addition, comprehensive systems must address each of the potential levels for intervention shown in Fig. 48-2. No longer should we use the old paradigm, simply asking what type of STD or RTI care management is required in various types of clinical settings to reduce the burden of STDs. Instead, we should ask what systems-wide sets of actions will solve the major reproductive health problems facing a population. For example, if it is still technically difficult to identify gonococcal and chlamydial infections in women in reproductive health clinics in resource-poor settings, but relatively easy to identify such infections in men, and if these men tend to obtain ineffective care in pharmacies, with no partner notification; then it may be important to improve the care management of urethritis in pharmacies to protect women from reproductive health consequences of gonococcal and chlamydial infection. For the women with undetected cervical infection, the old adage, "Your sex partner who develops urethritis is your best friend," underscores the major underutilized opportunity—partner notification—now available for detecting and treating these infections in developing countries. Similarly, to protect women in the general population from STDs, it may be more important to promote condom use by men engaging in commercial sex than to promote condom use by women seen in reproductive health clinics. Beginning with an understanding of the epidemiology and magnitude of the problems of AIDS and STDs, rather than only with the care to be provided clients of various clinics, will lead to the identification and undertaking of new and effective actions for reproductive health.

References

1 Grosskurth H et al: Impact of improved treatment of sexually transmitted diseases on HIV infection in rural Tanzania: Randomised controlled trial. *Lancet* 346:530, 1995.

2 Cohen MS et al: Reduction of concentration of HIV-1 in semen after treatment of urethritis: Implications for prevention of sexual transmission of HIV-1. *Lancet* 349:1868–1873, 1997.

3 Nelson KE et al: Changes in sexual behavior and a decline in HIV infection among young men in Thailand. *N Engl J Med* 335:297–303, 1996.

4 Kamb ML et al: HIV/STD prevention counseling for high-risk behaviors: Results from a multicenter, randomized controlled trial (Project RESPECT). *JAMA* 1998, in press.

5 Aral SO et al: Overview: Individual and population approaches to the epidemiology and prevention of sexually transmitted disease and human immunodeficiency virus infection. *J Infect Dis* 174 (Suppl 2): S127–123, 1996.

6 Hillis SD et al: New opportunities for chlamydia prevention: Applications of science to public health practice. *Sex Transm Dis* 22:197–202, 1995.

7 Washington AE, Katz P: Cost of and payment source for pelvic inflammatory disease: Trends and projections, 1983 through 2000. *JAMA* 266:2565–2569, 1991.

8 Scholes D et al: Prevention of pelvic inflammatory disease by screening for cervical chlamydial infection. *N Engl J Med* 334:1362–1366, 1996.

9 Begley CE et al: The incremental cost of screening, diagnosis, and treatment of gonorrhea and chlamydia in a family planning clinic. *Sex Transm Dis* 16:63–67, 1989.

10 Howell MR et al: Screening for *Chlamydia trachomatis* in asymptomatic women attending family planning clinics: A cost effectiveness analysis of three strategies. *Ann Intern Med* 128:277–284, 1998.

11 Moses S et al: Impact of user fees on attendance at a referral centre for sexually transmitted disease in Kenya. *Lancet* 340:463–466, 1992.

12 World Health Organization (WHO): Global Programme on AIDS, Management of Sexually Transmitted Diseases. Geneva, WHO, 1994. (WHO/GPA/TEM/94.1).

13 Centers for Disease Control and Prevention: 1998 Guidelines for treatment of sexually transmitted diseases. *MMWR* 47:1–111, 1998.

14 Adler MW: Sexually transmitted diseases control in developing countries. *Genitourin Med* 72:83–88, 1996.

15 Moses S et al: Health care-seeking behavior related to the transmission of sexually transmitted diseases in Kenya. *Am J Public Health* 84:1947–1951, 1994.

16 Ryan CA, Holmes KK: Editorial: How should clinical algorithms be used for syndromic management of cervical and vaginal infections. *Clin Inf Dis* 21:1456–1458, 1995.

17 Benjarattanaporn P et al: Men with sexually transmitted diseases in Bangkok: where to they go for treatment and why? *AIDS* 11(Suppl 1):S87–95, 1997.

18 Thomas T et al: Identifying cervical infection among pregnant women in Nairobi, Kenya: Limitations of risk assessment and symptom-based approaches. *Genitourin Med* 72:334–338, 1996.

19 Gertig DM et al: Risk factors for sexually transmitted diseases among women attending family planning clinics in Dar-es-Salaam, Tanzania. *Genitourin Med* 73(1):39–43, 1997.

20 Cates W Jr: A risk assessment tool for integrated reproductive health services. *Fam Plann Perspect* 29(1):41–43, 1997.

21 Mayaud P et al: Risk assessment and other screening options for gonorrhea and chlamydial infection in women attending rural Tanzanian antenatal care clinics. *Bull WHO* 73:621–630, 1995.

22 Gunn RA et al: Adolescent health care providers: Establishing a dialogue and assessing STD prevention practices. *Sex Transm Dis* 24: 90–93, 1997.

23 Moran JS et al: Survey of health care providers: Who sees patients needing STD services, and what services do they provide? *Sex Transm Dis* 22:67–69, 1995.

24 Maheux B et al: STD risk assessment and risk reduction counseling by recently trained family physicians. *Acad Med* 70(8):726–728, 1995.

25 Larsen SA et al: Syphilis, in *Laboratory methods for the diagnosis of sexually transmitted diseases.* Wentworth BB et al (eds). Washington, DC, American Public Health Association, 1991, pp. 1–52.

26 Corey L et al: Cellular immune response in genital herpes simplex virus infection. *N Engl J Med* 299:986–991, 1978.

27 Hitchcock PJ et al: Sexually transmitted diseases in the AIDS era: Development of STD diagnostics for resource-limited settings is a global priority. *Sex Transm Dis* 18:133–135, 1991.

28 Rietmeiier CA et al: Feasibility and yield of screening urine for *Chlamydia trachomatis* by polymerase chain reaction among high-risk male youth in field-based and other nonclinic settings. A new strategy for sexually transmitted disease control. *Sex Transm Dis* 24:429–435, 1997.

29 Easman CSF et al: Bacterial vaginosis: A diagnostic approach. *Genitourin Med* 68:134–138, 1992.

30 The Clinical Laboratory Improvement Amendments of 1988 (CLIA-88). *Fed Reg* 57(40), 1992.

31 Ferris DG et al: Office laboratory diagnosis of vaginitis. *J Fam Pract* 41(6):575–581, 1995.

32 Phillips RS et al: Gonorrhea in women seen for routine gynecologic care: Criteria for testing. *Am J Med* 85:177–182, 1988.

33 Schachter J et al: Screening for chlamydial infections in women attending family planning clinics: Evaluation of presumptive indicators for therapy. *West J Med* 1 38:375–379, 1983.

34 Handsfield HH et al: Asymptomatic gonorrhea in men: Diagnosis, natural course, prevalence, and significance. *N Engl J Med* 290:117–123, 1974.

35 Alexander-Rodriguez T, Vermund SH: Gonorrhea and syphilis in incarcerated urban adolescents: Prevalence and physical signs. *Pediatrics* 80:561–564, 1987.

36 Ellerbeck EF et al: Gonorrhea prevalence in Maryland state prisons. *Sex Transm Dis* 15:165–167, 1988.

37 Grosskurth H et al: Asymptomatic gonorrhea and chlamydial infection in rural Tanzanian men. *Br Med J* 312:277–280, 1996.

38 Quinn TC et al: Community-based screening for chlamydia and gonorrhea, by urine LCR in rural Uganda and the impact of mass antibiotic treatment, in *Chlamydial Infections. Proceedings of the Ninth International Symposium on Huna Chlamydial Infection.* Napa California, June 21–26, 1998, pp. 285–288.

39 Gunn RA et al: The changing paradigm of sexually transmitted disease control in the era of managed health care. *JAMA* 279(9):680–684, 1998.

40 Ndinya-Achola JO et al.: Presumptive specific clinical diagnosis of genital ulcer disease (GUD) in a primary health care setting in Nairobi. *Int J STD AIDS* 7:201–205, 1996.

41 Bogaerts J et al: Simple algorithms for the management of genital ulcers: Evaluation in a primary health care centre in Kigali, Rwanda. *Bull WHO* 73:761–767, 1995.

42 Plummer FA et al: Clinical and microbiologic studies of genital ulcers in Kenyan women. *Sex Transm Dis* 2:193–197, 1985.

43 O'Farrell N et al: Genital ulcer disease: accuracy of clinical diagnosis and strategies to improve control in Durban, South Africa. *Genitourin Med* 70:7–11, 1994.

44 DiCarlo RP, Martin DH: The clinical diagnosis of genital ulcer disease in men. *Clin Infect Dis* 25:292–298, 1997.

45 Dangor Y et al: Accuracy of clinical diagnosis of genital ulcer disease. *Sex Transm Dis* 17:184–189, 1990.

46 Morse SA et al: Comparison of clinical diagnosis and standard laboratory and molecular methods for the diagnosis of genital ulcer disease in Lesotho: Association with human immunodeficiency virus infection. *J Infect Dis* 175:583–589, 1997.

47 Behets F et al: Sexually transmitted diseases/human immunodeficiency virus control in Malawi: A field study of genital ulcer disease. *J Infect Dis* 171:451–455, 1995.

48 Braithwaite AR et al: Etiology of genital ulcer disease (GUD) in patients attending an STD clinic in Jamaica. International Congress of Sexually Transmitted Diseases, Seville, Spain, 19–22 October 1997 [Abstract no. P491].

49 Htun Y et al: A comparison of clinically-directed, disease-specific and syndromic protocols for the management of genital ulcer disease in Lesotho. *Sex Transm Infect* 74(Suppl 1):S23–S28, 1998.

50 Ryan CA et al: Risk assessment, symptoms and signs as predictors of vulvovaginal and cervical infections in urban U.S. STD clinic: Implications for use of STD algorithms. *Sex Transm Infect* 74(Suppl 1): S59–S76, 1998.

51 Wi T et al: Syndromic approach to detection of gonococcal and chlamydial infections among female sex workers in two Philippine cities. *Sex Transm Infect* 74(Suppl 1):S118–S123, 1998.

52 Ryan CA et al: Reproductive tract infections in primary health care, family planning, dermatovenereology clinics: Evaluation of syndromic management Morocco. *Sex Transm Infect* 74(Suppl 1):S95–S105, 1998.

53 Mayaud P et al: Validation of a WHO algorithm with risk assessment for vaginal discharge in Mwanza, Tanzania. *Sex Transm Infect* 74(Suppl 1):S77–S84, 1998.

54 Sánchez SE et al: Rapid and inexpensive approaches to managing abnormal vaginal discharge or lower abdominal pain: An evaluation in women attending gynecology and family planning clinics in Peru. *Sex Transm Infect* 74(Suppl 1):S85–S94, 1998.

55 Behets FM-T et al: Sexually transmitted disease are common in women attending Jamaican family planning clinics and appropriate detection tools are lacking. *Sex Transm Infect* 74(Suppl 1):S123–S127, 1998.

56 Bourgeois A et al: Prospective evaluation of a flowchart using a risk assessment for the diagnosis of STDs in primary healthcare centers in Libreville, Gabon. *Sex Transm Infect* 74(Suppl 1):S128–S131, 1998.

57 Kapiga SH et al: Evaluation of sexually transmitted diseases diagnostic algorithms among family planning clients in Dar es Salaam, Tanzania. *Sex Transm Infect* 74(Suppl 1):S132–S138, 1998.

58 Mayaud P et al: Risk scores to detect cervical infections in urban antenatal clinic attenders in Mwanza, Tanzania. *Sex Transm Infect* 74(Suppl 1):S139–S146, 1998.

59 Schneider H et al: Screening for sexually transmitted disease in rural South African women. *Sex Transm Infect* 74(Suppl 1):S123–S127, 1998.

60 Diallo MO et al: Evaluation of simple diagnostic algorithms for *Neisseria gonorrhoeae* and *Chlamydia trachomatis* cervical infections in female sex workers in Abidjan, Côte d'Ivoire. *Sex Transm Infect* 74(Suppl 1):S106–S111, 1998.

61 N'Doye I et al: Diagnosis of sexually transmitted infections in female prostitutes in Dakar, Senegal. *Sex Transm Infect* 74(Suppl 1):S112–S117, 1998.

62 Eckert LO et al: Vulvovaginal candidiasis: clinical manifestations, risk factors, and algorithm for case management. *OB/Gyn* 1998, in press.

63 Behets FM-T et al: Control of sexually transmitted disease in Haiti: Results and implications of a baseline study among pregnant women living in Cité Soleil shantytowns. *J Infect Dis* 172:764–771, 1995.

64 Behets FM-T et al: Management of vaginal discharge in women treated at a Jamaican sexually transmitted disease clinic: Use of diagnostic algorithms versus laboratory testing. *Clin Inf Dis* 21:1450–1455, 1995.

65 Brunham RC et al: Mucopurulent cervicitis—the ignored counterpart in women of urethritis in men. *N Engl J Med* 311:1–6, 1984.

66 Vuylsteke B et al: Clinical algorithms for the screening of women for gonococcal and chlamydial infection: Evaluation of pregnant women and prostitutes in Zaire. *Clin Infect Dis* 17:82–88, 1993.

66a Garnett GP, Aral SO, Hoyle DV, Cates Jr. W, Anderson RM: The natural history of Syphilis: Implications for the transmission dynamics and control of infection. *Sex Transm Dis,* 24:185–200, 1997.

67 Crabbé F et al: Prepackaged therapy for urethritis: The "MSTOP" experience in Cameroon. *Sex Transm Infect* 1998, in press.

68 Garcia PJ et al: Syndromic management of sexually transmitted disease in pharmacies: Evaluation and randomized intervention trial. *Sex Transm Infect* 74(Suppl 1):S153–S158, 1998.

69 Hessol NA et al: Management of pelvic inflammatory disease by primary care physicians. *Sex Transm Dis* 23:157–163, 1996.

70 Centers for Disease Control and Prevention: Decreasing incidence of perinatal Group B streptococcal disease—United States, 1993–1995. *MMWR* 46(21):473–477, 1997.

71 Shain RN et al: A controlled randomized trial of a risk-reduction intervention: Behaviors contributing to reduced infection rates at 12 months' follow-up. ISSTDR O 202, Seville, Spain, 19–22 October 1997.

72 The National Institute of Mental Health (NIMH) Multisite HIV Prevention Trial Group: The NIMH Multisite HIV Prevention Trial: Reducing HIV Sexual Risk Behavior. *Science* 280(5371):1889–1894, 1998.

73 Jemmott JB III et al: Abstinence and safer sex HIV risk-reduction intervention for African-American adolescents: A randomized controlled trial. *JAMA* 279:1529–1536, 1998.

74 Waller HT, Piot MA: The use of an epidemiological model for estimating the effectiveness of tuberculosis control measures. *Bull WHO* 41:75–93, 1969.

75 Fransen L et al: Health policies for controlling AIDS and STDs in developing countries. *Health Policy Planning* 6:148–156, 1991.
76 Temmerman M et al: STDs and pregnanacy, in *Control of sexually transmitted diseases: A handbook for the design and management of programs*. Dallabetta GA et al (eds). AIDSCAP/Family Health International, Arlington, VA, V–X11, 1996.
77 Mwijarubi E et al: Improved STD treatment significantly reduces prevalence of syphilis and symptomatic urethritis in rural Tanzania. Eleventh International Conference on AIDS, July 7–12, 1996. Vancouver [Abstract L.B.C.6062].
78 Gomez MP et al: Epidemic crack cocaine use, linked with epidemic genital ulcer diseases and heterosexual HIV infection in the Bahamas. Unpublished data.
79 Tikonova L et al: Epidemics of syphilis in the Russian Federation: Trends, origins, and priorities for control. *Lancet* 350:210–213, 1997.
80 Landry DJ, Forrest JD: Public health departments providing sexually transmitted disease services. *Fam Plann Perspect* 28(6):261–266, 1996.
81 Institute of Medicine: *The hidden epidemic: Confronting sexually transmitted diseases*. Washington, DC, National Academy Press, 1997, pp. 1–54.
82 Johnson BR: Implementing the Cairo agenda. *Lancet* 345(8954): 875–876, 1995.
83 Fox LJ et al: Improving reproductive health: Integrating STD and contraceptive services. *J Am Med Women's Assoc* 50(3–4):129–136, 1995.
84 Mostad SB et al: Hormonal contraception, vitamin A deficiency, and other risk factors for shedding of HIV-1 infected from the cervix and vagina. *Lancet* 350(9082):922–927, 1997.
85 Kitahata M et al: Care for persons with HIV infection in a managed care environment. *Am J Med* 104:511–515, 1998.
86 Thrall JS et al: Performance of Massachusetts HMOs in providing Pap smear and sexually transmitted disease screening to adolescent females. *J Adol Hlth* 22:184–189, 1998.
87 Berg DE, Toledo M, Kelso K, MacFarland L, Farley T: Changes in health care and the impact on congenital syphilis-Louisiana. 45th Annual Epidemic Intelligence Service (ETS) Conference, Atlanta, GA, April 22–26, 1996 [Abstract no. 10:35].
88 Stary A et al: Medical health care for Viennese prostitutes. *Sex Transm Dis* 18(3):159–165, 1991.
89 Laga M et al: Non-ulcerative sexually transmitted diseases as risk factors for HIV-1 transmission in women: Results from a cohort study. *AIDS* 7:95–102, 1993.
90 Holmes KK et al: Impact of gonorrhea control program, including selective mass treatment in female sex workers. *J Infect Dis* 174(Suppl 2): S230–239, 1996.
91 Ngugi EN et al: Focused peer-mediated education programs among female sex workers to reduce sexually transmitted disease and human immunodeficiency virus transmission in Kenya and Zimbabwe. *J Infect Dis* 174(Suppl 2):S240–247, 1996.
92 Tuladhar SM et al: The role of pharmacists in HIV/STD prevention: Evaluation of an STD syndromic management intervention in Nepal. *AIDS* 1998, in press.

Chapter 49

Individual-level risk assessment for STD/HIV infections

J. Randall Curtis
King K. Holmes

The medical and public health professions can play a central role in preventing STDs, including HIV infection, and in limiting the morbidity and mortality owing to STD/HIV infection by identifying individuals at risk for or with these infections as early as possible. Early identification allows the three-pronged approach to limiting morbidity and mortality in the high-risk individual: early detection and treatment of existing infection; risk-reduction counseling to prevent further transmission of infection; and instituting prophylactic measures for high-risk individuals not yet infected.[1–5] Although the literature on risk assessment and health overwhelmingly deals with environmental risk assessment, individual risk assessment is also a formal component of clinical patient care management in many areas of clinical medicine and social work. A few diverse examples include risk assessment for adverse pregnancy outcomes; prenatal genetic risk assessment prior to amniocentesis; ischemic heart disease; oral cancer prior to oral examination; childhood lead poisoning; psychiatric risk management; suicide risk in adolescents; and risk of child abuse as assessed by child protective agencies.[6–14]

Primary care, urgent care, and emergency department settings represent an underutilized but important setting for identifying individuals at moderate and high risk for HIV and STD infection, and often provide the first opportunity that health care professionals have to identify those with mild and sometimes protean symptoms of early infection. Specific categorical clinic settings that need to place particular emphasis on STD risk assessment include prenatal and family planning clinics and clinics serving sexually active adolescents. In 1993, a U.S. survey found that 32 percent of girls and 44 percent of boys in the ninth grade, and two-thirds of 12th graders were sexually experienced, and over one-half of the latter reported having had sex in the past 3 months.[15] Of the 20 percent of teenaged girls who become pregnant each year, approximately 80 percent have unintended pregnancies. Thus, risk assessment is needed for unintended pregnancy as well as for STDs, which are closely linked in teens. Other important settings for risk assessment include sexually transmitted disease clinics and HIV testing sites. These settings generally accomplish risk assessment as a part of their primary function.

There is also growing interest in methodologies for ecological or population-level risk assessment for disease in general and for STD/HIV infection in particular (see Chap. 88).[16,17] This chapter concerns individual-level risk assessment for STD and HIV infection, primarily in the clinical setting.

In STD/HIV care management, individual-level risk assessment has been most extensively evaluated, advocated, and used as a guide to selective screening for gonorrhea, chlamydial infection, and HIV infection.[18–30] STD/HIV risk assessment is now also widely used in initiating counseling on behavioral risk reduction, in use of prophylactic measures such as hepatitis B vaccine, and also (in conjunction with elicitation of symptoms and signs) for presumptive diagnosis of STDs, and for management of certain STD syndromes (see Chap. 26).[31] Table 49-1 summarizes the overall goals of risk assessment as an initial component of STD/HIV care management. Although a growing number of guidelines now address STD/HIV risk assessment, such guidelines often lack details on how to carry this out, and the literature still contains relatively few formal validations of the feasibility and utility of STD/HIV risk assessment in various settings.

GENERAL REQUIREMENTS FOR EFFECTIVE RISK ASSESSMENT AS A PUBLIC HEALTH STRATEGY

In general, risk assessment must have high sensitivity, specificity, and predictive value in discriminating between those at high and low risk. In addition, as noted in a World Health Organization Technical Report concerning antenatal care and risk ascertainment for preventing adverse pregnancy and maternal outcomes (but equally pertinent for STD/HIV risk assessment), effectiveness of risk assessment as a public strategy also requires meeting the following conditions.[32]

1. The whole population must be included in risk assessment screening.
2. Conditions screened for must include the important causes of mortality and mobidity.
3. Where increased risk is detected, appropriate referral or other action must be taken.
4. Adequate services must exist (e.g., at the referral level) to take such actions.
5. Those at risk must have access to such services.

It is also worth noting the obvious—that for a risk-based, selective intervention to be effective, those affected must have a risk profile different from those unaffected; and an intervention must exist that will alter favorably the natural history of the condition.

The WHO report cites the "inverse care law": Those at highest risk are least likely to have access to health care services.[32] A concern about risk assessment in the antenatal field has been that by focusing services on those at highest risk, attention will be diverted from developing needed services for all.[32] In the STD/HIV field, this concern must be countered by the epidemiologist's perspective that for these communicable diseases, intervention in those at highest risk, particularly those most likely to transmit infection, can benefit the entire population.[16]

DECISION ANALYSIS AND THE APPROPRIATE ROLE FOR RISK ASSESSMENT

RISK ASSESSMENT AS A COMPONENT OF SYNDROMIC MANAGEMENT OF STDS

In clinical decision analysis, identifying risk factors for STDs in patients with various sets of symptoms and signs increases the prior probability that a particular STI causes those signs and symptoms; this might lead to selective testing for that STI, to initiation of treatment while results of tests obtained are pending, or even to initiation of treatment without testing—especially if the prior probability of an STI becomes so high that confirmatory tests are not deemed cost effective. Figure 49-1 illustrates how risk assessment influences the potential for under-, over-, and correct diagnosis of an STI in a patient with a hypothetical STI-related syndrome, in a population where the prevalence of that STI is 10 percent, and the sensitivity and specificity of the symptoms and signs that make up the syndrome are 90 and 85 percent, respectively, for that STI. For a risk factor or combination of risk factors that carries an odds ratio for the STI of 10.0, the prevalence of

Table 49-1. Objectives of Risk Assessment in STD/HIV Care Management in Relationship to Patient Status

Patient status	Objectives of risk assessment
Symptomatic patient	Use risk assessment to determine the prior probability that a sexually transmitted infection causes the symptoms; guide testing and syndromic management
Asymptomatic patient, infection status unknown	Decision on whether or not to screen (cost-effective use of resources) or to use prevention or prophylaxis (e.g., postexposure antimicrobial prophylaxis or preventive treatment)
Known uninfected	Targeted counseling to decrease risky behavior to protect oneself; assess need for prophylaxis (e.g., HBV vaccination)
Known infected	Counsel to decrease risky behaviors: To protect others; To protect the patient against opportunistic infection, other sexually transmitted infections, and perhaps potential reinfection

STI among those with that risk factor would be 36 percent, and if treatment were offered, the probability of correct treatment of an STI, relative to the probability of overtreatment, is greatly increased among those who have both the syndrome and the risk factor.

Risk assessment is routinely used by clinicians as an adjunct to diagnosis and management of several STD syndromes, including unilateral intrascrotal pain and swelling (epididymitis); lower abdominal and pelvic pain in women (PID); vaginal discharge; proctitis; acute hepatitis; various STD-associated neurologic and rheumatologic syndromes; and the HIV-related clinical syndromes, including the primary infection syndrome, the generalized lymphadenopathy syndrome, various neurologic and hematologic syndromes, and other syndromes related to acquired immunodeficiency. Risk assessment is also potentially useful in managing mucopurulent endocervical discharge (see Table 57-5).

For some syndromes, simply age and sexual experience are sufficient to rule in or out the likelihood of an STI in the different diagnosis. For example, in evaluating testicular pain and swelling in an adolescent who is not be sexually active, the likely diagnoses are testicular torsion or trauma; in a sexually active young man the likely diagnoses are acute epididymitis owing to gonococcal or chlamydial infection; and in an older man in a mutually monogamous relationship the likely diagnoses are acute epididymitis caused by urinary pathogens. For other syndromes, more information on risky practices or partners is also useful. Risk assessment has been most extensively studied recently as an adjunct to syndromic management of vaginal discharge.[33–51]

It was hoped that risk assessment would be of sufficient aid in identifying women with cervical gonococcal or chlamydial infection, that those with vaginal discharge and positive risk assessment could be treated for cervical infection. Unfortunately, because abnormal vaginal discharge (especially increased amount or abnormal odor of the discharge) does not predict cervical infection, this approach was generally disappointing for identification of cervical infection; although risk factors for cervical infection usually can be identified, in most clinical settings even those with positive risk assessment have a prevalence of cervical infection too low to warrant routine treatment for it solely on the basis of positive risk assessment.

However, several findings of interest have emerged from these studies of women cited in the preceding.[52] (1) Risk factors now most widely used in North America for selection of women for screening for cervical infection (e.g., young age, single marital status, partner with recent symptoms of urethritis) were also predictive of cervical infection in many developing country settings; (2) locally defined risk factors, particularly perceived risk-taking behaviors of the male sexual partner (e.g., he is thought to have multiple sex partners, to have sex with prostitutes, to be bisexual, to use illegal drugs, or he travels and is frequently away from home) were also predictive of cervical infection, and in some settings where risk behaviors of females are much more proscribed than risk behaviors of males (e.g., Morocco) may be easier to include in a risk assessment interview than questions about the

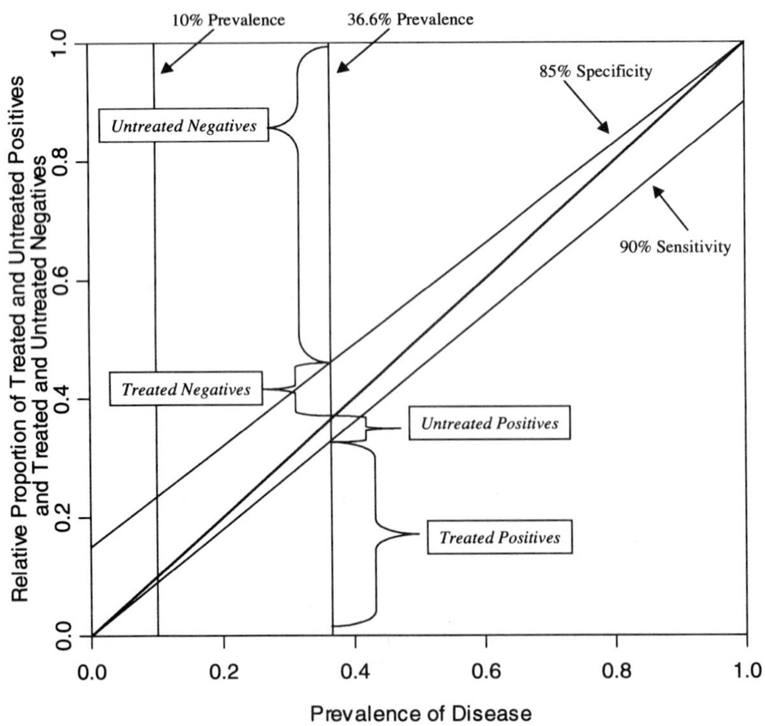

Fig. 49-1. The plot shows the impact of screening only those who are risk assessment (RA) positive in a population with 10 percent infection prevalence. In this example, the odds ratio for infection of RA positives against RA negatives was taken to be 10; this means that RA positives have a posterior probability of infection (i.e., prevalence) of 36.6 percent. The sensitivity and specificity of the diagnostic test was taken to be 90 and 85 percent, respectively. In this plot, the top line represents the stated specificity of 85 percent, the middle line the performance of a perfect test, and the bottom line represents the stated sensitivity of 90 percent. The left-hand vertical line in the plot represents the prevalence of infection in the entire population; the right-hand vertical line in the plot represents the prevalence of infection in the risk assessment-positive subset of the population. The division of the vertical, prevalence lines into four segments represents the performance of the diagnostic test. From top to bottom, the segments represents the relative proportion of patients in the following groups: untreated-negatives, treated-negatives, untreated-positives, or treated positives. The relative size of the four segments is determined by the prevalence of infection in the group tested, and the sensitivity and specificity of the diagnostic test. This plot is one way to examine the performance of a test across different levels of disease prevalence. Note that at 10 percent prevalence, the ratio of treated negatives/treated positives is 3/2; whereas at 36.6 percent prevalence, that ratio is 2/7. (Figure kindly provided by Barry N. Courtois.)

behavior of the woman herself; and (3) most importantly, when used as an adjunct to management of syndromes that actually predict cervical infection in women (e.g., mucopurulent cervicitis [MPC], lower abdominal pelvic pain and tenderness), then positive risk assessment did have positive predictive value sufficiently high to justify routine treatment of these syndromes for gonococcal or chlamydial infection in some settings (see Table 57-5).[37,39,40] The two caveats on the latter conclusion were that the signs of MPC and PID, if combined with risk assessment, were most predictive of cervical infection when the signs were demonstrated by more highly trained clinicians (e.g., gynecologists), especially in women seen in clinics that tend to serve symptomatic patients such as gynecology, STD, or primary care clinics, as opposed to family planning or antenatal clinics); and failure to identify risk factors for cervical infection does not necessarily have a sufficiently high negative predictive value to exclude cervical infection among women with signs of MPC or low abdominal or pelvic findings.[39,43]

Thus far, risk assessment has not been extensively evaluated as an adjunct to management of other STD syndromes, such as urethritis in men, urethral syndromes in women, genital ulcer disease, or most of the other syndromes listed in the preceding.

RISK ASSESSMENT AS A GUIDE TO SELECTIVE SCREENING FOR ASYMPTOMATIC INFECTION

In industrialized countries, the most extensive uses of STD/HIV risk assessment are probably to guide selective screening for chlamydial infections and HIV infection, and to a lesser extent, to guide selective screening for gonorrhea and syphilis. Age, gender, sexual behavior, recent symptoms of urethritis in a male partner, history of chlamydial infection, and recent history or presence of other STIs, all have been used (with or without signs of cervicitis) to guide selective testing for chlamydial infection.[20,27,28,53–57]

Beginning in 1972, the introduction of widespread screening of women for gonococcal infection, together with increased emphasis on treatment of partners exposed to gonorrhea, was associated with a reversal of trends in the incidence of reported gonorrhea in the United States. Screening of women was commonly selective, based on young age, female gender, nonmarried status, and race or ethnicity.[18,19] As the prevalence of gonorrhea has declined, the indications for cost-effective risk-based screening for gonorrhea have become less clear. Similarly, with primary and secondary syphilis essentially eliminated from 75 percent of U.S. counties, and with 1 percent of counties accounting for 50 percent of primary and secondary syphilis, the role of serologic screening for syphilis has greatly diminished, except during pregnancy to prevent congenital syphilis, and in geographic areas with continuing endemic transmission. However, a new emphasis on screening for gonorrhea and syphilis focuses less on individual risk assessment, and more on population characteristics, by screening in juvenile detention centers, jails, and prisons, where relatively high rates of these infections can still be found.[58–63] In addition, area of residence warrants increased emphasis as an indication for screening in view of the consistent link between census tract or region of the country and prevalence or incidence of these two infections.[19,64–68]

RISK ASSESSMENT IN HIV POST-EXPOSURE PREVENTION (PEP) OR STD PREVENTIVE TREATMENT

Prophylactic or preventive treatment (to prevent occurrence of infection or disease manifestations, respectively) are commonly provided to patients with known or suspected exposure to an STI. Administration of antiretroviral therapy following occupational exposure to HIV via needle stick or mucosal contamination is an example of the importance of risk assessment in guiding therapy. Recent recommendations from the CDC regarding PEP in the occupational setting use a combination of two risk assessments to guide therapy.[69] First, there is an assessment of the risk of exposure based on the source of the fluid and the volume and severity of the exposure. Second, there is a risk assessment of the HIV status of the source patient. The combination of these two risk are used to determine whether PEP is (1) not warranted; (2) to be considered as a basic regimen (two drugs); (3) to be recommended as a basic regimen (two drugs); or (4) to be recommended as an expanded regimen (three drugs).

Similarly, a form of risk assessment has occasionally been used for early postexposure prophylactic treatment of individuals potentially exposed to STDs, based on an assessment of the risk of infection in the sexual partner—for example, in the prophylactic treatment of men following sex with a prostitute.[70] More commonly, prophylactic or preventive treatment offered to individuals following known exposure to an STI, while test results from the exposed individual are pending (e.g., for *C. trachomatis* or *N. gonorrhoeae*); or even if initial screening test results are negative (e.g., for syphilis). In these cases, the risk assessment consists of defining whether the time of exposure of the individual to the person with a known STI fell within the period when that person was potentially infectious (e.g., within 2 weeks or less before recognition of symptoms of gonococcal urethritis); or was sufficiently recent that the exposed individual might still be in the incubation phase prior to seroconversion to a reactive serologic test for syphilis.

CHANGING ENVIRONMENT: THE EFFECT OF STD/HIV EPIDEMIOLOGY AND MANAGED CARE ON RISK ASSESSMENT

Efforts to modify sexual and drug use risk behaviors in order to decrease the transmission of HIV infection and other STDs has been effective in some selected populations, including older gay and bisexual men and some injection drug users.[71–73] Nonetheless, HIV seroprevalence continues to increase among other groups, particularly inner-city minorities, women, and young heterosexuals.[74] In addition, there is some evidence that moderate- or high-risk sexual behaviors more widespread in the general population than has been appreciated (see Chap. 4).[75–80] This changing epidemiology of HIV infection necessitates a broad approach to assessing risk behaviors. It is no longer adequate to concentrate HIV risk assessment solely on gay and bisexual men or injection drug users in some high-prevalence regions. Risk assessment should become a part of routine clinical care throughout the United States and in most parts of the world. As heterosexual transmission increases, risk assessment becomes increasingly difficult. Instead of simply assessing an individual's personal sexual and drug use history, it is important to assess the risk of the individual's sexual partners and social and sexual networks.

At the same time that HIV risk assessment is made more complicated by changing HIV epidemiology with increasing heterosexual transmission, the changing epidemiology of other STDs makes risk assessment for these infections more important. As the incidence of STDs is decreasing in many populations, it is returning to the "core risk groups," such as the inner-city poor. The individuals at risk are becoming harder to reach through public health efforts. Throughout the past decade, HIV and STDs are becoming increasingly more important among groups traditionally marginalized in our society. These groups, inner-city poor and minorities, and those with limited or no access to health care, are hardest to reach with prevention education. These groups are also likely to be mistrustful of efforts to identify risk behaviors by individuals or groups from outside their communities.

Although changing epidemiology makes risk assessment increasingly challenging, the changing patterns of health care delivery in the United States and elsewhere may provide opportunities that will facilitate systematic risk assessment. The increase in managed care and large systems of health care delivery offer the opportunity to define effective risk assessment practices in different communities and implement standardized and effective risk assessment strategies. For example, managed care organizations have the opportunity to identify risk assessment needs in their primary care base and implement standardized risk assessment instruments. These organizations represent systems that can be (1) evaluated, using performance measures to improve quality; (2) held accountable for process and outcomes; and (3) more easily targeted for incentives such as policies, coverage benefits, and so on. However, the incentives to not use resources in managed care settings could inhibit performance of risk assessment, testing, and counseling for STDs/HIV.

STD/HIV RISK ASSESSMENT IN CLINICAL SETTINGS: CURRENT RECOMMENDATIONS AND CURRENT PRACTICE

Many agencies and professional organizations have recommended that physicians routinely perform HIV and STD risk assessment and offer selected voluntary screening and counseling to those individuals with risk behaviors who are seen in clinical settings. Such organizations include the U.S. Preventive Services Task Force, the Centers for Disease Control and Prevention, the American Medical Association, the American College of Physicians, the Infectious Disease Society of America, the American Academy of Pediatrics, the American College of Obstetricians and Gynecologists, the American Academy of Family Physicians, the Canadian Planned Parenthood Association, and the Technical Guidance/Competence Working Group on Contraceptive Use convened by WHO and USAID.[29,30,81–93] Despite the proliferation of such recommendations, there is ample evidence that physicians do not routinely screen for sexual and drug-related risk behaviors among their patients. Clinicians attitudes toward clinical practice guidelines have been surveyed.[94] Several surveys of primary care physicians have found that less than half of physicians report that they regularly screen their patients for these risk behaviors.[95–99] A national survey reported in 1991 showed that fewer than 20 percent of physicians routinely obtain sexual histories and, even when their patients have symptoms classic for HIV infection, over 40 percent of these physicians do not ask about homosexual activities and over 60 percent do not ask about injection drug use.[99] The infrequent provision of preventive STD/HIV services to adolescents in a variety of health care settings is especially troubling.[100,101] In one survey, only 40 percent of providers reported screening all adolescents for sexual activity, for example.[100] Most data on the performance of primary care physicians in STD/HIV risk assessment and in STD/HIV-related risk behavior counseling has been limited to surveys of physicians. Physicians' self-reported practice of preventive health measures and counseling, however, overestimates actual practice patterns.[102,103] A recent study examined the actual practice of primary care physicians in screening for HIV risk behaviors through surveys of their patients and through a standardized patient examination. Most physicians did not routinely screen their patients for sexual or drug-related risk behaviors and even among standardized patients with classic presentations for HIV and STDs, risk assessment was highly variable.[104,105]

There are multiple reasons that physicians do not perform routine risk assessment. Physicians are under time constraints and have many routine health screening tasks to complete in a relatively brief encounter.[96,106] In addition, many physicians are uncomfortable taking a sexual history, particularly a history concerning homosexuality.[97,107–109] Regardless of the reasons, and despite widespread recommendations to the contrary, physician-initiated risk assessment is not being performed in most primary care settings.

BENEFITS OF RISK ASSESSMENT IN PREVENTION AND MANAGEMENT OF STDS/HIV AND THE COSTS OF MISSED OPPORTUNITIES

The benefits of appropriate risk assessment for HIV and STDs can be divided into two categories. First, the benefits to those with unidentified infection include preventing complications, limiting progression, and, where possible, curing infection. Second, the benefits to those who are at risk for infection but still uninfected include preventing acquisition of infection through risk reduction. In addition, in the reproductive health care setting, recommendations for STD risk assessment in the context of family planning and prenatal care cites the benefits to the client as helping to determine the following:[93]

1. What contraceptives, including dual method use, are best suited to the clients needs? For example, those at increased risk for STDs would be poor candidates for IUDs, but may be good candidates for barrier or dual methods.
2. What risk reduction counseling is needed?
3. Is testing or referral for STDs needed?
4. What diagnostic or treatment options are needed to decrease maternal and neonatal morbidity and mortality?

BENEFITS TO THOSE WITH UNIDENTIFIED HIV INFECTION

HIV risk assessment leading to selected voluntary HIV testing represents the first step in the provision of direct health benefits to individuals with undiagnosed HIV infection. Such health benefits include vaccinations, prophylactic therapies, and combination antiretroviral therapy that, together, can improve both the quantity and quality of life for these individuals. Recent improvements in combination antiretroviral therapy have made unprecedented strides in improving the survival and quality of life for persons with HIV infection.[110] With the improvements in the highly active antiretroviral therapy, it is being shown to be effective earlier in the course of HIV infection thereby increasing the importance of risk assessment to identify individuals early so that they can benefit from these therapies.[111] In addition, the myriad of prophylactic measures that can be instituted for primary prevention of opportunistic infections in persons with HIV infection makes it critically important that individuals with early HIV infection be identified and offered the appropriate prophylactic measures.[4,5] Many of these interventions, such as pneumococcal and other types of vaccinations and skin testing for identification of tuberculosis infection, will be most effective if performed as early as possible in HIV infection.

Another potential benefit of identifying individuals with HIV or STD infection is the possibility of notifying previous sexual partners of their risk for these infections. Partner notification is an underutilized public health measure. In one report, about 25 percent of HIV-positive gay and bisexual men reported that they did not intend to notify their sexual partners of their HIV status.[112] In a recent standardized patient study of primary care physicians, only 31 percent of physicians recommended partner notification to an HIV-positive individual presenting for primary care.[113] In a randomized controlled trial of partner notification, if individuals have full responsibility for notifying their partners, only 7 percent of the partners were notified. If, however, counselors were available to assist in partner notification, 50 percent of partners were successfully notified and, of the partners notified, 94 percent were unaware they had been exposed to HIV and 23 percent of those notified and tested were HIV-positive.[114] Voluntary partner notification programs have been found acceptable to HIV-positive individuals and have been successful at notifying individuals of their risk for HIV infection.[115–119] Despite the current inadequacy of recommending and producing partner notification, risk assessment and selected HIV and STD screening can lead to the identification of previous partners who would benefit from testing, early intervention, and risk-reduction counseling.

BENEFITS TO THOSE WITH OTHER UNIDENTIFIED STDS

The individual patient benefits of risk assessment and selective screening for chlamydial infection have been demonstrated by Scholes and colleagues, who showed more than a 50 percent reduction in the risk of PID among women randomly assigned to selective risk-based screening for *C. trachomatis* infection.[28] Similarly, risk assessment prior to IUD insertion to exclude those at risk of STDs is now the standard of care to prevent IUD-related PID.[120,121] For any of the curable STDs, risk-based screening followed by treatment can lead to secondary prevention of complications at the individual level and primary prevention of transmission at the population level.[17]

THE BENEFITS TO THOSE AT RISK BUT WITHOUT STD OR HIV INFECTION

The benefits of identifying HIV and STD risk to those without infection depend in large part on reducing risk behaviors in those with and without infection. There is evidence that risk assessment can play an important role in the prevention of further transmission of HIV and other STDs. For those with HIV infection, risk behavior screening and HIV testing can be the first step to behavioral interventions that can limit the transmission of HIV to those who are uninfected.[122] Such interventions have been successful in producing reported safer sexual behaviors among homosexual men and among heterosexual men and women.[123–125] Drug treatment, needle exchange programs, and primary care for drug users also decreased reported high-risk behavior among injection drug users.[123,126] Similarly, HIV-related behavioral risk reduction efforts, when added to the improving early diagnosis and treatment of curable STD, have undoubtedly contributed to the declining incidence of these other STDs.

For those individuals with HIV or STD risk behaviors who screen negative for infection, producing change in sexual risk behavior is more difficult. Some studies have shown that those testing negative for HIV are less likely to adhere to safer sex guidelines.[123,127] However, some HIV testing and counseling programs have reduced risky sexual behaviors in this group.[123,124,128,129] As discussed in Chapter 4, the NIMH multicenter trial and the CDC's Project Respect both achieved significant reduction in reported risk behaviors such as unprotected sex among individuals randomized to enhanced behavioral intervention; and the latter study also achieved a significant reduction in documented STD infection for a 6-month period.[130,131] HIV risk reduction may also be successful among HIV-negative injection drug users.[72,73,132]

THE COSTS OF MISSED OPPORTUNITIES FOR RISK ASSESSMENT

Studies examining the prevalence of unidentified HIV infection in urban and suburban emergency departments provide insight into the missed opportunities for risk assessment. Various estimates of seroprevalence over a period of several years ranged from 0.2 to 10.5 percent.[133–138] Two studies found that 70 percent of individuals with HIV infection were not recognized as having either HIV infection or HIV risk behaviors during the emergency department visit. Schoenbaum and Webber found that although HIV infection was recognized in 27 percent of men, it was recognized in only 13 percent of women.[134] Similarly, Lombardo and colleagues estimated that 60 percent of HIV-positive individuals admitted to a university hospital were not identified as having HIV infection.[139] The under-recognition of HIV infection in health care settings not only impacts on the care of individuals with HIV infection and eliminates the possibility of preventing HIV transmission through risk-reduction counseling, but it also potentially increases the risk of transmission of HIV infection to health care workers.[137]

There is considerable evidence of preventable morbidity and mortality occurring because individuals with undiagnosed HIV infection and other STDs are presenting for health care late in the course of their disease. Data from the HIV Costs and Services Utilization Study suggest that less than 45 percent of HIV-infected Americans were receiving medical care in 1996.[140] Hutchinson and colleagues found that 50 percent of clients with newly diagnosed HIV-infection at sexually transmitted disease clinics had fewer than 500 CD4 cells, and 12 percent had fewer than 200 CD4 cells.[141] These individuals would have benefited from earlier HIV testing and provision of primary care. Of patients diagnosed with *Pneumocystis carinii* pneumonia in 1991 at Johns Hopkins Medical Center, 33 percent were not previously known to be HIV-infected and 28 percent of individuals admitted to the hospital with previously unidentified HIV infection were admitted for preventable conditions.[142,143] The overall population-level costs of missed opportunities for STD/HIV risk assessment ultimately could exceed several billion dollars in direct medical costs in the United States—to the extent that risk assessment leads to selective early detection and treatment, to effective risk reduction counseling and education, and ultimately to the secondary prevention of complications and to primary prevention of transmission (see Chap. 99).[144] Widespread risk assessment for HIV (and STDs) and appropriate selected screening could potentially lead to the prevention of a substantial proportion of these illnesses.

METHODS FOR ASSESSING HIV AND STD RISK

TYPES OF RISK-BASED SCREENING FOR STDS/HIV

Screening for HIV infection or STDs can be implemented in a variety of different ways: Screening can be routine or selective, voluntary or mandatory, and confidential or anonymous. Screening is routine when HIV serology or STD screening cultures or serologies are offered to every individual regardless of risk profile. Selective screening involves testing following risk assessment; screening is recommended to those individuals for whom a certain level of risk is identified. Both routine and selected screening can be mandatory or voluntary and both can be anonymous or confidential. Each of these three facets of screening (who gets screened, whether it is voluntary, and whether it is anonymous) can be combined to make eight potential combinations. Most of the eight different approaches have important benefits and any one may be the method of choice in different settings. The role of mandatory screening involves complicated tradeoffs between the rights of the individual and the health of the public. The most common settings for mandatory screening involve incarceration and immigration, issues beyond the scope of this chapter that will not be discussed further.

Routine voluntary HIV or STD screening is indicated when the prevalence of infection exceeds a certain level, and when effective interventions are available. In this circumstance, the virtues of routine screening outweigh the potential harm of false positive tests because of the large number of infected individuals identified. In their seroprevalence study of sentinel hospitals in the United States, Janssen and colleagues recommended routine voluntary HIV screening for patients 15 to 54 years of age in hospitals with one or more patients with newly diagnosed AIDS per 100 discharges per year.[145] The cost-benefits of screening for STD infection depend on the cost of the various tests available, the prevalence of infection, and the costs of the specific STD and its complications and sequelae (see Chap. 29).

In the majority of health care settings throughout the world, however, routine testing for HIV infection or other STI is neither indicated nor feasible for a number of reasons. First, routine HIV testing may cause some high-risk individuals to avoid health care.[146,147] Second, in low-risk populations, a substantial proportion of those with positive screening tests would represent false positive tests. The costs, both financial and emotional, produced by a high proportion of false positive tests could be substantial. Individuals with false positive HIV serology may make unnecessary decisions to change careers, separate from sexual partners, remain childless, or have abortions.[146,148] Finally, routine testing in low-risk populations is unlikely to be a cost-effective approach to case finding.[149] Consequently, in many health care settings, selective voluntary screening based on risk assessment to identify individuals at increased risk for HIV or STD will remain the most effective method of targeting those individuals who should be offered HIV and STD screening. In addition, even in settings offering routine testing, risk assessment is still important in order to identify those who are uninfected with HIV or STDs but at high risk of acquiring infection.

STRATEGIES FOR CONDUCTING STD/HIV RISK ASSESSMENT

Ideally, STD/HIV risk assessment should be part of routine screening for all patients in most clinical settings. STD/HIV risk assessment could be accomplished in all patients if it were considered as part of a history and physical on a new patient and during an annual checkup for a patient in ongoing care. There are a number of additional circumstances under which STD/HIV risk assessment is especially important. For example, when a patient presents with the symptoms or signs of an STD- or HIV-related problem; when a patient is pregnant or wants to become pregnant; when a woman initiates contraceptive care; when a patient asks a question about an STD or HIV or about sex, and perhaps when men initiate phosphodiesterase-inhibiting drug therapy to restore potency.

Systematic methods to provide uniform HIV and STD risk assessment are an important component of identifying those at risk for infection. Systematic methods can include approaches targeting clients, clinicians, or clinics. Approaches targeting clients can include routine written screening instruments given to all new clients, computer-based screening programs designed to identify risk and educate, and written educational materials available to those interested. Approaches targeting clinicians include education in risk assessment methods, checklists or computer prompts to remind clinicians to assess risk, and the institutional expectation that risk assessment is a part of each new patient visit. System approaches can include all of the preceding methods when a clinic or health care system formalizes these methods. Also important are guidelines for clinicians, based on the strongest evidence (the best are from randomized controlled trials with comprehensive outcome measures), quality standards and performance indicators, health care contracting specifications, and so on.

Given the importance of risk assessment and the difficulties that clinicians have in routinely providing this screening, one solution is to develop a screening instrument that could be administered to all individuals seen in a health care setting. Such an instrument could be completed in a waiting room and used to signal physicians that follow-up questions and voluntary HIV or other STD testing may be indicated. Many clinicians have a medical history intake form to which HIV or other STD risk assessment questions could be added. In a survey of primary care physicians in California, 45 percent of physicians had a new patient intake questionnaire that contained some sexual history items. However, the vast majority of these questionnaires only inquired about sexual satisfaction and only 4 percent of physicians had intake forms that would identify persons at risk for HIV infection.[133]

Several sample HIV risk behavior questionnaires have been published, but none with the systematic input from the target population, and few have been formally validated.[152–154] The blood banking organizations have developed and tested questionnaires to identify potential blood donors at risk for HIV and other bloodborne infections.[152–154] However, these questionnaires have only been tested in a very specific population, persons presenting to donate blood. There have been several studies exploring the feasibility of HIV risk behavior screening among psychiatric inpatients.[155–157] These studies have shown that risk questionnaires can be successfully administered to this population, with a good correlation between questionnaire results and HIV seroprevalence.[155–157]

HIV risk behavior questionnaires have also been administered to college students.[79,158] Although HIV risk behaviors were found to be present in more than 20 percent of students, there has not been extensive work done validating these questionnaires. Kotloff and colleagues did find a high degree of internal consistency by using separate questions to assess the same risk behaviors and found reasonably high test-retest reliability for questions about sexual activities, drug use, and sexually transmitted diseases, suggesting these questions can reliably identify individuals at risk.[158]

An important question to address is whether a written HIV risk behavior questionnaire would be acceptable to patients and answered honestly in a health care setting. Written HIV risk questionnaires have been found highly acceptable to blood donors, psychiatric inpatients, and patients undergoing elective surgery.[154,155,159,160] Respondents may admit to “socially unacceptable” behaviors more often on a written questionnaire than in face-to-face interviews.[161] However, the acceptability of written, confidential (but nonanonymous) sexual and drug-related risk assessment to patients in most health care settings has not been formally tested, and this approach may be more problematic for low literacy populations, or those for whom English is a second language but for whom STD risk may be high.

Risk assessment in the individual clinician–patient encounter requires that clinicians ask culturally sensitive, understandable risk questions and provide an environment that allows patients to reveal potentially embarrassing or even illegal information. Table 49-2 shows one suggested approach to HIV or STD risk assessment involving some initial questions to be asked of all patients and follow-up questions when initial questions suggest that risk is present.[121] However, it is essential that questions be worded in a way that they are clear and unambiguous, and question 4 in Table 49-2, for example, "What can you tell me about your sexual life before this last year?," strikes some as provocative. There may be local or regional differences in language concerning sexual and drug use activity and it behooves clinicians to know these variations in language to maximize the effectiveness of their risk assessment.

FRAMING THE QUESTION IN RISK ASSESSMENT

In addition to using language, tone, and body language that suggests that the clinician will not be judgmental, it may also be helpful to use various "framing" tactics in risk assessment. One overall framing tactic is to tell patients that risk assessment for HIV and STD is an important part of health care delivery and that the clinician performs this type of risk assessment with all patients. For example, the American Social Health Association Personal Health History questionnaire begins by telling the patient, "In order to provide the best care for you today, and to understand your risk for certain infections, it is necessary for us to talk about your sexual practices."[162] The goal of this framing of risk assessment is to assure the patient that he or she was not singled out for risk assessment because of mannerisms, appearance, or race or ethnicity. Individual questions can also be framed to increase an individual's willingness to answer certain questions. For example, a clinician may say, "Many people have experimented with drugs such as cocaine or heroin" before asking an individual about past heroin use. This type of framing is not necessary in all circumstances, but may be helpful in some situations when a clinician believes that a patient may be reluctant to reveal risk behaviors.

Kassler and colleagues offer a series of additional framing statements giving "permission" to discuss taboo topics, and to introduce specific questions.[163] For example, "Many people are worried that they might be infected with the virus that causes AIDS; have you been concerned about that?" "Many women find it difficult to get their men to use condoms; has this been a problem for you?" "Many men have sex with other men. Have you ever had sex with another man?"

Respondents who do engage in sexual risk-taking and who also do perceive this as risky may nonetheless not report risk taking. Reasons for this at a clinical encounter may include fears that admitting risk could increase insurance rates, endanger employment, or lead to other discrimination, in addition to the usual concerns about embarrassment and loss of face. In an extensive review of this topic, Lee suggests use of an authorative source to justify sensitive questions.[164] Clinicians could not only offer the preceding framing statement, but could offer a more authoritative rationale, such as, "The American Medical Association now recommends asking patients about lifestyle and sexual behavior; to give you the best care I can, I need to ask you some questions so we can explore whether you are at risk for sexually transmitted infections."

Table 49-2. A Framework for Sexual History-Taking in the 1990s[121]

If you only have time to ask one question of each patient, a reasonable choice might be this: *What do you do to protect yourself from AIDS?* Responses can be used to examine STD risk in more detail, or reinforce safe behaviors.

If you have 2 to 5 minutes, you can ask these 10 questions to get a basic history (Ref 121 amplifies on the interpretation and follow-up of responses):

1. Have you had a sexual experience with another person in the past year?
2. (If yes), With how many different people in this year? One? Two or three? Four to 10? More than 10?
3. (If yes), In this year, have you had sex with men, women, or both?
4. What can you tell me about your sexual life before this last year?
5. Have you ever had a sexually transmitted disease of any kind?
6. Have you ever shared needles or infection equipment with another person for any reason?
7. Have you ever felt that a sex partner put you at risk for any reason?
8. What do you do to protect yourself from AIDS?
9. What do you do to protect yourself from unplanned pregnancy?
10. Is there anything else about your sexual lifestyle that I need to know to ensure good medical care?

TYPES OF INFORMATION RECOMMENDED BY EXISTING GUIDELINES FOR INCLUSION IN STD/HIV RISK ASSESSMENT

Many sets of practice guidelines, including the evidence-based and influential Guide to Clinical Preventive Services, recommend STD/HIV preventive interventions that depend on risk assessment. The lack of specificity, training, and validation of instruments for this purpose represents the "Achilles heel" of such recommendations.

The U.S. Title X 1982 guidelines (still under revision), which set standards of care for family planning services supported by federal funding, call for obtaining from males a history of sexual activity, STDs (including hepatitis B and HIV infection) and urological conditions; and from females, a comprehensive sexual history; partner history of intravenous drug use, multiple partners, history of STDs and HIV, bisexuality, STD history (including HBV and HIV); history of contraception usage; menstrual, obstetrical, and gynecologic history; Pap smear history (date of last Pap, any abnormal Pap smear, treatment for abnormal Pap smear); and history of in utero exposure to DES.

The CDC's *STD Clinical Practice Guidelines* advise obtaining a sexual history, a history of recent sexual activity, history of drug use, history of blood tests for syphilis and HIV infection, and history of hepatitis B vaccination.[165]

The *Guide to Clinical Preventive Services* from the U.S. Preventive Services Task Force, recommends that, "clinicians should assess risk factors for HIV infection by obtaining a careful sexual history and inquiry about injection drug use in all patients, and recommends preventive screening for infection with HIV "for all persons at unusual risk of infection."[29] This guide also recommends screening for asymptomatic *C. trachomatis* infection during pelvic examination for all sexually active female adolescents and for other women at high risk for chlamydial infection, based on history of prior STD, new or multiple sex partners, age under 25, inconsistent use of barrier contraceptives, cervical ectopy, being unmarried, and the local epidemiology of chlamydial infection. Routine screening for gonorrhea is recommended for asymptomatic women at high risk of gonorrhea, where high-risk groups include commercial sex workers (prostitutes), persons with a history of repeated episodes of gonorrhea, and young women (under age 25) with two or more sex partners in the past year, with actual risk depending on local epidemiology of gonorrhea. The guide does not recommend screening for genital herpes, but does suggest that clinicians consider asking all pregnant women at the first prenatal visit whether they or their sex partner(s) have had herpetic genital lesions. The guidelines do not address screening for trichomoniasis or bacterial vaginosis. Finally, the guide recommends advising all adolescent and adult patients about risk factors for STDs, and providing counseling about effective measurements to reduce risk.

> Assessment of risk should be based on a careful sexual and drug use history and consideration of the local epidemiology of STDs. Sexual history should include questions about number and nature of current and past sex partners (including same sex partners or partners who have injected drugs), any history of past STD infections, the use of condoms or other barrier protection, and particular high risk sexual practices such as anal intercourse.

Components of the preceding risk assessment were also included in recommendations for counseling to avoid unintended pregnancy or gynecologic cancers, and in selecting the interval at which women should receive cervical Pap smears.

A 1998 draft version of the *Specifications for STD Services* being prepared for the CDC to guide agencies in the purchase of medical insurance benefits suggests that the medical history include questions concerning: (1) a previous STD; (2) inconsistent or nonuse of condoms in a sexual relationship that is not mutually monogamous; (3) initiation of sexual activity in early adolescence; (4) intravenous drug use; (5) exchange of sex for money or drugs; (6) a new or multiple sex partners; and (7) partners with one or more risk factors.

Finally, the forthcoming Reproductive Health Services Guidelines, under preparation in the United States by the Centers for Disease Control, the Office of Population Affairs, and various professional groups, will contain evidence-based recommendations on an approach to risk assessment that integrates STD/HIV and family planning concerns.

SUMMARY OF SPECIFIC CATEGORIES OF INFORMATION NEEDED IN A COMPREHENSIVE STD/HIV RISK ASSESSMENT

DEMOGRAPHIC DATA

Key demographic data that may serve as potential markers for STD risk in some settings and are available on any clinical intake form include gender, area of residence, age, date of birth, and marital status. Educational level also may be helpful in some settings. All could be used to provide standard prompts to clinicians as to STD risk, and these alone could be sufficient in some settings to prompt screening or more comprehensive risk assessment for certain STDs.

SEXUAL HISTORY

The two main objectives of medical sexual history taking today are assessment of STD/HIV risk, and assessment of sexual function and dysfunction. The basic types of information sought include risk of exposure to STDs/HIV (whether or not the individual has ever had sex; and the number and "riskiness" of sex partners; types of sex practices and "riskiness" of these practices); and the risks of acquiring STDs if exposed (methods and consistency of methods used to prevent STDs).

CONTEXT OF RISK TAKING

A given sexual history may reflect high or low risk, depending on the ecological setting where sexual encounters occur (high or low STD prevalence); and the social context in which high-risk exposures occur (e.g., in drug-using situations) can provide the information needed to develop an individualized risk reduction plan.

STD HISTORY

The open-ended question, "Have you ever had a sexually transmitted disease of any kind?" identifies those who by definition have had high-risk exposure, and should lead to probing to identify specific infections that can be reacquired by reexposure within the originally infected sexual network, as well as those who can be chronic or recurrent or carry a risk of late sequelae. A formal checklist of the major STDs for self-administered questionnaires may elicit positive responses not elicited by the open-ended question.

PARTNER RISK BEHAVIORS

The question, "Have you ever felt that a sex partner put you at risk for any reason?" may uncover rape or abuse, as well as a history of a partner's high-risk behaviors (e.g., IDU, commercial sex, concurrent sex with others, multiple sex partners) or a history of an STD diagnosis or STD syndrome in a partner that should prompt STD screening. (Alternatively, asking, "Do you think your partner is at risk for STD or HIV infection?" removes any implied accusation that a partner is deliberately exposing the patient to STD or HIV.)

STD SYMPTOM REVIEW

The routine review of symptoms should include questions about dysuria; past or current genital sores or lesions; abnormal vaginal discharge (i.e., increased amount, abnormally yellow color, or abnormal odor); vulvar pruritis or burning; low abdominal or pelvic pain in the female; testicular pain or swelling; and skin rash. In general, such symptoms, when presented spontaneously or in response to an open-ended question as the chief complaint or reason for visit, have a higher predictive value for STDs than when elicited in response to a specific query or check-list.[37]

The Recommendations for Updating Selected Practices in Contraceptive Use (vol II), includes a section providing a rationale for various components of STD risk assessment in reproductive health programs.[93] The TG/CWG recommendations target developing countries, emphasize how specific risk factors differ from one country or population to another, and advise that reproductive health programs should try to establish what demographic characteristics, behavioral risk factors, and clinical symptoms and signs are associated with the various STDs seen in their own settings. The general categories of interest, and the rationale for their inclusion, are as follows.

YOUNG AGE

Young age (e.g., ≤20 vs. >20) is a risk factor in nearly all societies (especially true in females) both for physiologic reasons (cervical ectopy in the young female, less immunity), and behavioral reasons (more partners, rapid partner change, less condom use).[166–169]

PARTNERSHIP STATUS

Partnership status (single vs. married or living with regular partner) may or may not be a risk marker, depending on local customs. For example, in the United States, IUD use did not elevate risk of PID among women married or living with a partner.[120]

SEXUAL BEHAVIOR OF THE PATIENT OR PATIENT'S PARTNER(S)

A new partner or more than one partner within the past 2 or 3 months, and especially without consistent condom use, has been associated with increased risk of STDs and HIV in many studies.[123,170–172] Similarly, the patient's assessment that her or his partner has other sex partners is associated with increased STD risk (also, Alarcon, Johnson, and Holmes, unpublished data concerning risk of STDs and HIV among pregnant women in Peru).[173]

HISTORY OR SYMPTOMS OF STDS/RTIS IN THE PATIENT OR PARTNER

A history of STDs or PID or of syndromic treatment for a reproductive tract infection predicts increased risk of current STDs, particularly if the partner was not treated or the underlying risk behaviors persist.[25,53,173–175] Even with partner treatment, the persistence and rediffusion of an STD within wider sexual networks may not be adequately addressed. When the patient is aware that the partner has had recent symptoms of an STD, such as urethral discharge, genital sores, or pain when urinating, several studies document increased risk in the patient. Of course, the prevalence of STDs is also increased in association with several symptoms or signs of STDs in the patient her- or himself, particularly those symptoms presented as a chief complaint or a response to a general open-ended question such as, "Do you have any new symptoms that make you think you might have a genital infection?" and particularly those signs demonstrated by a well-trained and experienced clinicians who has had the opportunity for the educational feedback provided by reportedly comparing examination findings with laboratory test results.[37,48,49,176,177]

EXAMPLE OF COMPREHENSIVE STD/HIV RISK ASSESSMENT FORMAT: SELF-ADMINISTERED VERSUS FACE-TO-FACE INTERVIEW

Few clinical settings other than STD clinics—which already know their patients are at potential risk of STD/HIV—could allow the time needed for a clinician to carry out the preceding comprehensive risk assessment during a face-to-face interview. As discussed, self-administered questionnaires for STD/HIV risk assessment could be used to collect more comprehensive information, although more research is needed to assess the accuracy of this approach compared to face-to-face interviews for risk assessment in the clinical setting. Considerable experience suggests that computer-assisted interviews in clinical settings as well as in surveys can elicit more accurate information on sensitive topics than can face-to-face interviews.[178] Further, a self-administered patient intake form is commonly used in clinical settings for general medical risk assessment, and in the primary care setting, it is highly unlikely that a stand-alone STD/HIV risk assessment would be acceptable. Rather, an initial risk assessment not only should integrate STD and HIV risk assessment, but should be integrated into an overall risk assessment, that addresses risk for a variety of other medical and social problems.

Finally, self-administered risk assessment need not be limited to clinical settings, but could, for example, be included in a confidential setting in schools or even on computer websites directed toward young audiences—perhaps in a manner designed to encourage risk-takers to perceive the consequences of risk taking, and to motivate behavior change or further health care consultation. Obviously, all of these approaches are a high priority for future research and evaluation.

Whatever the method of administering questionnaires, important barriers to reporting sensitive risk behaviors exist. First, individuals who report high-risk sexual activities often do not perceive themselves at risk.[179–181] The magnitude of any STD/HIV risk perceived may be small relative to the hierarchy of other risks encountered by a poor, homeless urban adolescent, for example. Lack of education can impair perception of existing risk. Denial is a common defense mechanism when risk behaviors are unavoidable. Thus, specific questions about specific behaviors are essential in conjunction with questions about subjective perception of risk. Identification of gaps between perceived risk and actual risk highlights the need to change risk perception as one potential outcome of risk assessment. In this regard, it is important to distinguish perceived risk from perceived susceptibility.[182] Kowalewski and colleagues have critiqued current thinking on perceived risk and health behavior.[181]

The foregoing discussion illustrates the range of topics that could be addressed in an STD/HIV risk assessment; and some examples of how various agencies, professional groups, or experts suggest conducting STD/HIV risk assessment. Many of these recommendations have not yet been extensively evaluated in terms of feasibility or validity with respect to objective prediction of STD/HIV infection. Table 49-3 presents an example of a relatively comprehensive approach to individual-level STD/HIV risk assessment that has not yet been validated either for self-administered or face-to-face interviews. The table summarizes many of the key topics, offers ways they might be presented in a comprehensive face-to-face interview, and represents a point of departure for further work in this area. Although excessive for most clinical encounters, the more comprehensive approach may be appropriate for the patient who is positive for any of the risk factors elicited by the screening questions **or by the selected priority questions highlighted in bold type in the table.**

Table 49-3 does not include questions clinicians can use to identify the context of any risk-taking reported. Such questions can encourage further patient insight, and identify key avenues for counseling concerning skills, norms, misconceptions, and so on. For example, the clinician or counselor can ask, "Were there any avoidable circumstances that put you at that particular risk (e.g., not using a condom with a casual partner)? Is there anything you can think of that would make it hard for you to avoid taking that risk again?"

Table 49-3. A Comprehensive Approach to Individual-level STD/HIV Risk Assessment

DEMOGRAPHIC DATA:

Include date of birth, gender, race/ethnicity, residential zip code

FRAMING STATEMENT:

In order to provide the best care for you today, and to understand your risk for certain infections, it is necessary for us to talk about your sexual behavior.

SCREENING QUESTIONS:

1. Do you have any reason to think you might have an STD?

Yes ☐ No ☐

If so, what reason? ______

2. For all adolescents < 18 years old: Have you begun having any kind of sex yet?

Yes ☐ No ☐

STD HISTORY:

Have you ever had any sexually transmitted diseases or any genital infections?

Yes ☐ No ☐ If so, which ones? ______

Have you ever had:

Gonorrhea?	Yes ☐	No ☐
Chlamydia; NGU; urethritis; cervicitis or cervical infection?	Yes ☐	No ☐
PID (pelvic inflammatory disease, infection of the uterus)?	Yes ☐	No ☐
Syphilis?	Yes ☐	No ☐
Genital herpes?	Yes ☐	No ☐
Genital warts?	Yes ☐	No ☐
Trichomonas?	Yes ☐	No ☐
Bacterial vaginosis (nonspecific vaginitis)?	Yes ☐	No ☐

SEXUAL HISTORY

How old were you the first time you voluntarily had sexual intercourse? ______ years old

Have you had sex with men, women, or both? Men ☐ Women ☐ Both ☐

How many sex partners have you had in the past 3 months? ______

past 12 months? ______

in your lifetime? ______

How many days since the last time you had sex with your regular partner? ______ days

How many days since the last time you had sex with a "casual" (a nonregular) partner (e.g., a new partner who was not a regular sex partner)? ______ days

Did you use a condom the last time you had sex?

With your regular partner?	Yes ☐	No ☐
With a casual (nonregular) partner?	Yes ☐	No ☐

Do you always (consistently) use condoms to protect yourself from AIDS/STDs every time you have sex?

With your regular partner?	Yes ☐	No ☐
With other partners?	Yes ☐	No ☐
Have you ever used crack cocaine?	Yes ☐	No ☐
Have you ever exchanged sex for money or drugs?	Yes ☐	No ☐

ADDITIONAL HIV RISK ASSESSMENT

Have you ever injected yourself ("shot up") with drugs?	Yes ☐	No ☐
Have you ever had sex with anyone who had ever injected drugs?	Yes ☐	No ☐
Have you ever had sex with a gay or bisexual man?	Yes ☐	No ☐
Have you had a blood transfusion (since 1978)?	Yes ☐	No ☐

SEXUAL PRACTICES, LAST 2 MONTHS

(To guide examination and lab testing for patients assessed as being at risk for STD) *Now,* I'd like to ask what parts of your body have been exposed to an STD.

Male patient	**Partner's**		**Female patient**	**Partner's**	
Penis	Vagina	☐	Your vagina	Penis	☐
Anus	Penis	☐	Your anus	Penis	☐
Mouth	Penis/Vagina	☐	Your mouth	Penis/Vagina	☐

For MSM

Insertive anal sex past 12 months?	Yes ☐	No ☐
Receptive anal sex past 12 months?	Yes ☐	No ☐

Table 49-3. A Comprehensive Approach to Individual-level STD/HIV Risk Assessment *(Continued)*

STD SYMPTOM CHECKLIST:

Have you recently developed any of the following symptoms?

Male patient	
Discharge of pus (drip) from the penis	☐
Burning when you urinate?	☐
Genital lesion, sores, or rash?	☐
Rash on other parts of your body?	☐
Testicle pain or discomfort?	☐
Swollen lymph glands?	☐
Symptoms in your rectum (pain, mucous discharge, rectal bleeding)?	☐

Female patient	
Abnormal vaginal discharge (increased amount, abnormal odor, abnormal yellow color)?	☐
Itching or burning pain of your vulva or vagina?	☐
Burning when you urinate?	☐
Genital sores or lesions?	☐
Rash on other parts of your body?	☐
Low abdominal or pelvic pain or pain during sexual intercourse?	☐
Abnormal vaginal bleeding? (between your usual periods or after sex, for example?)	☐
Swollen lymph glands?	☐
Symptoms in your rectum (pain, mucous discharge, rectal bleeding)?	☐

PARTNER(S) CHARACTERISTICS

Do you think your partner is at risk for a STD/HIV?	Yes ☐	No ☐
Has your sex partner(s) done anything that may have put you at any risk?	Yes ☐	No ☐
Do you think your sex partner(s) has other sex partners besides you?	Yes ☐	No ☐
Do you think your sex partner exchanges sex for money or drugs?	Yes ☐	No ☐

Has your sex partner(s) had any sexually transmitted infection?

Ever?	Yes ☐	No ☐
Which one(s)? ____________		
Past 2 months?	Yes ☐	No ☐
Which one(s)? ____________		

Has your partner had any of the following?

Female patient	
Gonorrhea?	☐
Chlamydia or NGU?	☐
Syphilis	☐
Gential herpes?	☐
Genital warts?	☐
HIV infection or AIDS?	☐
Any genital symptoms, such as genital sores or discharge from the penis (urethritis)?	☐

Male patient	
Cervicitis?	☐
Any genital symptoms, such as genital sores or abnormal vaginal discharge?	☐
Any genital symptoms, such as sores or vaginal discharge?	☐

FUTURE RESEARCH AND TRAINING NEEDS

Future research needs include local definition of risk factors for STDs/HIV and evaluation of optional questions and methods (face-to-face interview, self-administered questionnaire, audio-computer–assisted questionnaire), for eliciting information about these risk factors in clinical settings, as well as in nonclinical settings. There is a need for particular emphasis on adolescents and young adults; for development of instruments for risk assessment that not only integrate STD and HIV risk assessment, but also integrate STD/HIV risk assessment with practical comprehensive social and medical risk assessment for clinical use. Finally the instruments and methods of administration should have demonstrated reliability and validity for predicting presence or absence of STD/HIV in a variety of clinical settings. Ideally, rational guidelines, such as the risk assessment component of the forthcoming USPHS Reproductive Health Guidelines, will provide a general model that can be widely used as a quality standard for purchasers, insurers, and providers of health care. There remains a clear need for improved performance of clinicians in assessing risk for STD/HIV infection. The approaches recommended by Boekeloo, Rabin, and colleagues provide examples of methods for educating clinicians.[183–185]

References

1 Cohen MS et al: A new deal in HIV prevention: Lessons from the global approach. *Ann Intern Med* 120:340–341, 1994.

2 Francis DP: Toward a comprehensive HIV prevention program for the CDC and the nation. *JAMA* 268(11):1444–1447, 1992.

3 Rhame FS, Maki DG: The case for wider use of testing for HIV infection. *NEJM* 320(19):1248–1254, 1989.

4 Kaplan K et al: Guidelines for prevention of opportunistic infection in HIV infected persons. *Clin Infect Dis* 21(suppl 1):S1–S141, 1995.

5 Kaplan JE et al (eds). USPHS/IDSA Prevention of Opportunistic Infections Working Group. Guidelines for prevention of opportunistic infection in HIV infected persons. *Clin Infect Dis* 25(suppl 3):S299–S335, 1997.

6 Adams MM et al: The pregnancy risk assessment monitoring system: design, questionnaire, data collection and response rates. PRAMS Working Group. *Paediatr Perinat Epidemiol* 5:333–346, 1991.

7 Carroll JC et al: Psychosocial risk factors during pregnancy. What do family physicians ask about? *Can Fam Phys* 40:1280–1289, 1994.

8 Bruce RA: Strategies for risk assessment of ischemic heart disease and total mortality. *Trans Assoc Life Insur Med Dir Am* 73:53–67, 1990.

9 Speight PM et al: The use of artificial intelligence to identify people at risk of oral cancer and precancer. *Br Dent J* 179:382–387, 1995.

10 Stefanak MA et al: Use of the Centers for Disease Control and Prevention childhood lead poisoning risk questionnaire to predict blood lead elevations in pregnant women. *Obstet Gynecol* 87:209–212, 1996.

11 Merrill JM et al: Why doctors have difficulty with sex histories. *South Med J* 83:613–617, 1990.

12 White GL Jr et al: Development of a tool to assess suicide risk factors in urban adolescents. *Adolescence* 25:655–666, 1990.

13 Fanshel D et al: Testing the measurement properties of risk assessment instruments in child protective services. *Child Abuse Negl* 18:1073–1084, 1994.

14 Wald MS, Woolverton M: Risk assessment: The emperor's new clothes? *Child Welfare* 69:483–511, 1990.
15 CDC Youth Risk Behavior Surveillance—United States, 1993. *Morb Mort Week Rep* 44(SS-1):1–56, 1995.
16 Rose G: Sick individuals—sick populations. *Int J Epidemiol* 14:32–38, 1985.
17 Aral SO et al: Overview: Individual and population approaches to the epidemiology and prevention of sexually transmitted diseases and human immunodeficiency virus infection. *J Infect Dis Supp* 174(S2): S127-S133, 1996.
18 Holmes KK: Screening and the detection of gonorrhea. *West J Med* 123:367–371, 1975.
19 Pederson AHB, Bonin P: Screening females for asymptomatic gonorrhea infection. *Northwest Med* 70:255–261, 1971.
20 Mertz KJ et al: Screening women for gonorrhea: Demographic screening criteria for general clinical use. *Am J Public Health* 87:1535–1538, 1997.
21 Marrazzo JM et al: Performance and cost-effectiveness of selective screening criteria for *Chlamydia trachomatis* infection in women. Implications for a national chlamydia control strategy. *Sex Transm Dis* 24:131–141, 1997.
22 Mosure DJ et al: Predictors of *Chlamydia trachomatis* infections among adolescents: A longitudinal analysis. *Am J Epidemiol* 144: 997–1003, 1996.
23 Howell MR et al: Screening for *Chlamydia trachomatis* in asymptomatic women attending family planning clinics: A cost-effectiveness analysis of three strategies. *Ann Intern Med* 128:277–284, 1998.
24 Hook EW III et al: Comparative behavioral epidemiology of gonococcal and chlamydial infections among patients attending a Baltimore STD clinic. *Am J Epidemiol* 136:662–672, 1992.
25 Addes DG et al: Decreased prevalence of *Chlamydia trachomatis* infection associated with a selective screening program in family planning clinics in Wisconsin. *Sex Transm Dis* 20:28–35, 1993.
26 Cohen DA et al: A school-based chlamydia control program using DNA amplification technology. *Pediatrics* 101:E1, 1998.
27 Centers for Disease Control and Prevention. Recommendations for the prevention and management of *Chlamydia trachomatis* infections, 1993. *Morb Mort Week Rep* 42(No. RR-12), 1993.
28 Scholes D et al: Prevention of pelvic inflammatory disease by screening for cervical chlamydial infection. *N Engl J Med* 334:1362–1366, 1996.
29 USPHS Prev. Services Task Force: *Guide to Clinical Prevention Services,* 2d Ed. Alexandria, Virginia, International Publishing, 1996.
30 Centers for Disease Control and Prevention: 1998 guidelines for treatment of sexually transmitted diseases. (Adaption printed March 1998) *Morb Mort Week Rep* 47(RR-1):1–116, 1998.
31 Mindel A et al (eds): Syndromic approach to STD management. *Sex Transm Infect* 74(suppl 1):S1-S178, 1998.
32 WHO (MSM) 92–4: Antenatal care and maternal health. How effective is it?
33 Dallabetta GA et al: Specificity of dysuria and discharge complaints and presence of urethritis in male patients attending an STD clinic in Malawi. *Sex Transm Infect* 74(suppl 1):S34-S37, 1998.
34 Moherdaui F et al: Validation of national algorithms for the diagnosis of sexually transmitted diseases in Brazil: Results from a multicenter study. *Sex Transm Infect* 74(suppl 1):S38-S43, 1998.
35 Alary M et al: Evaluation of clinical algorithms for the diagnosis of gonococcal and chlamydial infections among men with urethral discharge or dysuria and women with vaginal discharge in Benin. *Sex Transm Infect* 74(suppl 1):S44-S49, 1998.
36 Daly CC et al: Validation of the WHO diagnostic algorithm and development of an alternative scoring system for the management of women presenting with vaginal discharge in Malawi. *Sex Transm Infect* 74(suppl 1):S50-S58, 1998.
37 Ryan CA et al: Risk assessment, symptoms and signs as predictors of vulvovaginal and cervical infections in an urban U.S. STD clinic: IImplications for use of STD algorithms. *Sex Transm Infect* 74(suppl 1): S59-S76, 1998.
38 Mayaud P et al: Validation of a WHO algorithm with risk assessment for vaginal discharge in Mwanza, Tanzania. *Sex Transm Infect* 74(suppl 1):S77-S84, 1998.
39 Sánchez SE et al: Rapid and inexpensive approaches to managing abnormal vaginal discharge or lower abdominal pain: An evaluation in women attending gynecology and family planning clinics in Peru. *Sex Transm Infect* 74(suppl 1):S85-S94, 1998.
40 Ryan CA et al: Reproductive tract infections in primary health care, family planning, dermatovenereology clinics: Evaluation of syndromic management in Morocco. *Sex Transm Infect* 74(suppl 1):S95-S105, 1998.
41 Diallo MO et al: Evaluation of simple diagnostic algorithms for *Neisseria gonorrhoeae* and *Chlamydia trachomatis* cervical infections in female sex workers. *Sex Transm Infect* 74(suppl 1):S106-S111, 1998.
42 Ndoye I et al: Diagnosis of sexually transmitted infections in female prostitutes in Dakar, Senegal. *Sex Transm Infect* 74(suppl 1):S112-S117, 1998.
43 Wi T et al: Syndromic approach to detection of gonococcal and chlamydial infections among female sex workers in two Philippine cities. *Sex Transm Infect* 74(suppl 1):S118-S123, 1998.
44 Behets FM-T et al: Sexually transmitted disease are common in women attending Jamaican family planning clinics and appropriate detection tools are lacking. *Sex Transm Infect* 74(suppl 1):S123-S127, 1998.
45 Bourgeois A et al: Prospective evaluation of a flow chart using a risk assessment for the diagnosis of STDs in primary healthcare centers in Libreville, Gabon. *Sex Transm Infect* 74(suppl 1):S128-S131, 1998.
46 Kapiga SH et al: Evaluation of sexually transmitted diseases diagnostic algorithms among family planning clients in Dar es Salaam, Tanzania. *Sex Transm Infect* 74(suppl 1):S132-S138, 1998.
47 Mayaud Pet al: Risk scores to detect cervical infections in urban antenatal clinic attenders in Mwanza, Tanzania. *Sex Transm Infect* 74(suppl 1):S139-S146, 1998.
48 Mayaud P et al: Risk assessment and other screening options for gonorrhoea and chlamydial infections in women attending rural Tanzanian antenatal clinics. *Bull WHO* 73:621–30, 1995.
49 Behets FM et al: Management of vaginal discharge in women treated at a Jamaican sexually transmitted disease clinic: Use of diagnostic algorithms versus laboratory testing. *Clin Infect Dis* 21:1450–1455, 1995.
50 Thomas T et al: Identifying cervical infection among pregnant women in Nairobi, Kenya: Limitations of risk assessment and symptom-based approaches. *Genitourin Med* 72:334–338, 1996.
51 Gertig DM et al: Risk factors for sexually transmitted diseases among women attending family planning clinics in Dar-es-Salaam, Tanzania. *Genitourin Med* 73(1):39–43, 1997.
52 Dalabetta GA et al: Problems, solutions, and challenges in syndromic management of sexually transmitted diseases. *Sex Transm Infect* 74(suppl 1):S1-S11, 1998.
53 Handsfield HH et al: Criteria for selective screening for *Chlamydia trachomatis* infection in women attending family planning clinics. *JAMA* 255:1730–1734, 1986.
54 Sellors JW, Walter SD: A new visual indicator of chlamydial cervicitis?, in *Chlamydial Infections,* Stephens RS et al (eds). Proceedings of the Ninth International Symposium on Human Chlamydial Infection, San Francisco, CA, 1998, pp. 337–340.
55 Mosure DJ et al: Genital chlamydia infections in sexually active female adolescents: Do we really need to screen everyone? *J Adol Health* 20:6–13, 1997.
56 Stergachis A et al: Selective screening for *Chlamydia trachomatis* infection in a primary care population of women. *Am J Epidemiol* 138(3):143–153, 1993.
57 Johnson BA et al: Derivation and validation of a clinical diagnostic model for chlamydial cervical infection in university women. *JAMA* 264:3161–3165, 1990.
58 Bell TA et al: Sexually transmitted diseases in females in a juvenile detention center. *Sex Transm Dis* 12(3):140–144, 1985.

59 Shafer MA: Sexual behavior and sexually transmitted diseases among male adolescents in detention. (Editorial) *Sex Transm Dis* 21:181–182, 1994.
60 Oh MK et al: Sexual behavior and sexually transmitted diseases among male adolescents in detention. *Sex Transm Dis* 21:127–132, 1994.
61 Bickell NA et al: Human papillomavirus, gonorrhea, syphilis, and cervical dysplasia in jailed women. *Am J Public Health* 81:1318–20, 1991.
62 Holmes MD et al: Chlamydial cervical infection in jailed women. *Am J Public Health* 83(4):551–555, 1993.
63 Blank S et al: Incident syphilis among women admitted to a New York City women's correctional facility. Abstract presented at Twelfth Meeting of the International Society for STD Research. Seville, Spain, October 19–22, 1997 (Abstract no. P822).
64 Centers for Disease Control and Prevention: Assessment of sexually transmitted diseases services in city and county jails—United States, 1997. *Morb Mort Week Rep* 47:429–431, 1998.
65 Rothenberg RB: The geography of gonorrhea. *Am J Epidemiol* 117: 688–94, 1983.
66 Rothenberg RB, Potterat BA: Temporal and social aspects of gonorrhea transmission: the force of infectivity. *Sex Transm Dis* 2:88–92, 1988.
67 Rice RJ et al: Sociodemographic distribution of gonorrhea incidence: Implications for prevention and behavioral research. *Am J Public Health* 81:1252–1258, 1991.
68 Zenilman JM: New paradigms for sexually transmitted diseases surveillance and field studies. *Sex Transm Dis* 24:310–311, 1997.
69 Centers for Disease Control and Prevention: Public health service guidelines for the management of health-care worker exposures to HIV and recommendations for postexposure prophylaxis. *Morb Mort Week Rep* 47(No. RR-7), 1998.
70 Harrison WO et al: A trial of minocycline given after exposure to prevent gonorrhea. *N Engl J Med* 300:1074–1078, 1979.
71 Winkelstein W et al: The San Francisco men's health study: III. Reduction in human immunodeficiency virus transmission among homosexual/bisexual men, 1982–86. *Am J Public Health* 77:685–689, 1987.
72 van Ameijden EJC et al: Injecting risk behavior among drug users in Amsterdam, 1986 to 1992, and its relationship to AIDS prevention programs. *Am J Public Health* 84(2):275–281, 1994.
73 Moss AR, Vranizan K: Charting the epidemic: The case study of HIV screening of injecting drug users in San Francisco, 1985–1990. *Br J Addict* 87:467, 1992.
74 Centers for Disease Control and Prevention: Diagnosis and reporting of HIV and AIDS in states with integrated HIV and AIDS surveillance—United States, January 1994-June 1994. *Morb Mort Week Rep* 47(No. 15), 1998.
75 Campostrini S, McQueen DV: Sexual behavior and exposure to HIV infection: Estimates from a general-population risk index. *Am J Public Health* 83(8):1139–1143, 1993.
76 Leigh BC et al: The sexual behavior of US adults: Results from a national survey. *Am J Public Health* 83(10):1400–1408, 1993.
77 Stall R Catania J: AIDS risk behaviors among late middle-aged and elderly Americans. *Arch Intern Med* 154:57–63, 1994.
78 Avins AL et al: HIV infection and risk behaviors among heterosexuals in alcohol treatment programs. *JAMA* 271:515–518, 1994.
79 MacDonald NE et al: High-risk STD/HIV behavior among college students. *JAMA* 263:3155–3159, 1990.
80 Michael RT et al: Private sexual behavior, public opinion, and public health policy related to sexually transmitted diseases: A US-British comparison. *Am J Pub Health* 88:749–754, 1998.
81 Centers for Disease Control: Public Health Service guidelines for counseling and antibody testing to prevent HIV infection and AIDS. *Morb Mort Week Rep* 36:509–515, 1987.
82 Centers for Disease Control: Technical guidance on HIV counseling. *Morb Mort Week Rep* 42(RR-2):8–17, 1993.
83 American Medical Association: HIV blood test counseling. *Physician Guidelines*, 2d ed. Chicago, American Medical Association, 1993.
84 American Medical Association Guidelines for adolescent preventive services (GAPS): Recommendations and rationale. Chicago, American Medical Association, 1994.
85 American College of Physicans and Infectious Disease Society of America: Human immunodeficiency virus (HIV) infection. *Ann Intern Med* 120:310–319, 1994.
86 American Academy of Pediatrics, Committee on Adolescence: Sexually transmitted diseases. *Pediatrics* 94:568–572, 1994.
87 American Academy of Pediatrics: Condom availability for youth. *Pediatrics* 95:281–285, 1995.
88 American College of Obstetricians and Gynecologists: Human immunodeficiency virus infection. Technical Bulletin no. 169. Washington DC, American College of Obstetricians and Gynecologists, 1992.
89 American College of Obstetricians and Gynecologists: Condom availability for adolescents. Committee Opinion no. 154. Washington, DC, American College of Obstetricians and Gynecologists, 1995.
90 American Academy of Family Physicians: Age charts for periodic health examination. Kansas City, MO, American Academy of Family Physicians, 1994 (reprint no. 510).
91 Canadian Task Force on the Periodic Health Examination: Canadian guide to clinical preventive health care. Ottawa, Canada Communications Group, 1994, pp. 540–557.
92 Planned Parenthood Manual of Medical Standards and Guidelines, 1996.
93 Technical Guidance/Competence Working Group: Recommendations for updating selected practices in contraceptive use, Vol II. United States Agency for International Development (USAID), 1997.
94 Tunis SR et al: Internists' attitudes about clinical practice guidelines. *Ann Intern Med* 120:956–963, 1994.
95 Calabrese LH et al: Physicians' attitudes, beliefs, and practices regarding AIDS health care promotion. *Arch Int Med* 151:2257–2260, 1991.
96 Lewis CE, Montgomery K: The AIDS-related experiences and practices of primary care physicians in Los Angeles: 1984–89. *Am J Public Health* 80:1511–1513, 1990.
97 Lewis CE et al: The impact of a program to enhance the competencies of primary care physicians in caring for patients with AIDS. *J Gen Intern Med* 1(5):287–294, 1986.
98 Boekeloo BO et al: Frequency and thoroughness of STD/HIV risk assessment by physicians in a high-risk metropolitan area. *Am J Public Health* 81:1645–1648, 1991.
99 McCance KL et al: A survey of physicians' knowledge and application of AIDS prevention capabilities. *Am J Prev Med* 7(3):141–145, 1991.
100 Millstein Sget al: Delivery of STD/HIV preventive services to adolescents by primary care physicians. *J Adolesc Health* 19:249–257, 1996.
101 Blum RW et al: Don't ask, they won't tell: The quality of adolescent health screening in five practice settings. *Am J Public Health* 86: 1767–1772, 1996.
102 Hoppe RB et al: Residents' attitudes towards and skills in counseling: Using undetected standardized patients. *J Gen Intern Med* 5:415–420, 1990.
103 Woo B et al: Screening procedures in the asymptomatic adult: Comparison of physicians' recommendations, patients' desires published guidelines, and actual practice. *JAMA* 254:1480–1484, 1985.
104 Wenrich MD et al: Patient report of HIV risk screening by primary care physicians. *Am J Prev Med* 12:116–122, 1996.
105 Ramsey PG et al: History taking and preventive medicine skills among primary care physicians: An assessment using standardized patients. *Am J Med* 104:152–158, 1998.
106 Wechsler H et al: The physician's role in health promotion—a survey of primary care practitioners. *NEJM* 308:97–100, 1983.
107 Gemson DH et al: Acquired immunodeficiency syndrome prevention: Knowledge, attitudes, and practices of primary care physicians. *Arch Intern Med* 151:1102–1108, 1991.
108 Gerbert B et al: Primary care physicians and AIDS: Attitudinal and structural barriers to care. *JAMA* 266(20):2837–2842, 1991.

109 Hayward RA, Weissfeld JL: Coming to terms with the era of AIDS: Attitudes of physicians in US residency programs. *J Gen Intern Med* 8:10–18, 1993.

110 Palella FJ Jr: Declining morbidity and mortality among patients with advanced human immunodeficiency virus infection. *N Engl J Med* 338:853, 1998.

111 Fineberg MB et al: Report of the NIH Panel to define principles of therapy of HIV infection and Guidelines for the use of antiretroviral agents in HIV-infected adults and adolescents. *Ann Intern Med* 128: 1057–1100, 1998.

112 Kegeles SM et al: Intentions to communicate positive HIV-antibody status to sex partners. *JAMA* 259(2):216–217, 1988.

113 Curtis JR et al: Physicians' ability to provide initial primary care to an HIV-infected patient. *Arch Intern Med* 155(15):1613–1618, 1995.

114 Landis SE et al: Results of a randomized trial of partner notification in cases of HIV infection in North Carolina. *NEJM* 326(2):101–106, 1992.

115 Pavia AT et al: Partner notification for control of HIV: Results after 2 years of a statewide program in Utah. *Am J Public Health* 83(10): 1418–1424, 1993.

116 Giesecke J et al: Efficacy of partner notification for HIV infection. *Lancet* 338:1096–1100, 1991.

117 Rutherford GW et al: Partner notification and the control of human immunodeficiency virus infection: Two years of experience in San Francisco. *Sex Trans Dis* 18(2):107–110, 1991.

118 Wykoff RF et al: Notification of the sex and needle-sharing partners of individuals with human immunodeficiency virus in rural South Carolina: 30-month experience. *Sex Trans Dis* 18(4):217–222, 1991.

119 Cantor JC et al: Preparedness for practice: Young physicians' views of their professional education. *JAMA* 270(9);1035–1040, 1993.

120 Lee NC et al: The intrauterine device and pelvic inflammatory disease revisited: New results from the Women's Health Study. *Obstet Gynecol* 72:1–6, 1988.

121 Hatcher RA et al (eds): *Contraceptive Technology.* New York, Irvington Publishers, 1994.

122 Francis DP: Toward a comprehensive HIV prevention program for the CDC and the nation. *JAMA* 268(11):1444–1447, 1992.

123 Higgins DL et al: Evidence for the effects of HIV antibody counseling and testing on risk behaviors. *JAMA* 266(17):2419–2429, 1991.

124 Cleary PD et al: Behavior changes after notification of HIV infection. *Am J Public Health* 81(12):1586–1590, 1991.

125 Padian NS et al: Prevention of heterosexual transmission of human immunodeficiency virus through couple counseling. *J Acq Immune Def Syn* 6:1043–1048, 1993.

126 Watters JK et al: Syringe and needle exchange as HIV/AIDS prevention for injection drug users. *JAMA* 271:115–120, 1994.

127 Otten MW Jr et al: Changes in sexually transmitted disease rates after HIV testing and posttest counseling, Miami, 1988 to 1989. *Am J Public Health* 83(4):529–533, 1993.

128 Wenger NS et al: Reduction of high-risk sexual behavior among heterosexuals undergoing HIV antibody testing: A randomized clinical trial. *Am J Public Health* 81(12):1580–1585, 1991.

129 Kelly JA et al: Behavioral intervention to reduce AIDS risk activities. *J Consult Clin Psych* 57(1):60–67, 1989.

130 The NIMH Multisite HIV Prevention Trial: Reducing HIV sexual risk behavior. The National Institute of Mental Health (NIMH) Multisite HIV Prevention Trial Group. *Science* 280(5371):1889–1894, 1998.

131 Kamb ML et al: Efficacy of risk-reduction counseling to prevent human immunodeficiency virus and sexually transmitted diseases: a randomized controlled trial. Project RESPECT Study Group. *JAMA* 280: 1161–7, 1998.

132 Martin GS et al: Behavioural change in injecting drug users: Evaluation of an HIV/AIDS education programme. *AIDS Care* 2(3):275–279, 1990.

133 Lewis CE, Freeman HE: The sexual history-taking and counseling practices of primary care physicians. *West J Med* 147:165–167, 1987.

134 Schoenbaum EE, Webber MP: The underrecognition of HIV infection in women in an inner-city emergency room. *Am J Public Health* 83(3):363–368, 1993.

135 Marcus R et al: Risk of human immunodeficiency virus infection among emergency department workers. *Am J Med* 94:363–370, 1993.

136 Kelen GD et al: Unrecognized human immunodeficiency virus infection in emergency department patients. *NEJM* 318:1645–1650, 1988.

137 Kelen GD et al: Human immunodeficiency virus infection in emergency department patients. Epidemiology, clinical presentations, and risk to health care workers: The Johns Hopkins experience. *JAMA* 262(4):516–522, 1989.

138 Risi GF et al: Human immunodeficiency virus: Risk of exposure among health care workers at a southern urban hospital. *Southern Med J* 82(9):1079–1082, 1989.

139 Lombardo JM et al: Anonymous human immunodeficiency virus surveillance and clinically directed testing in a Newark, NJ, hospital. *Arch Intern Med* 151:965–968, 1991.

140 Bozzette S et al: Characteristics of HIV-infected patients receiving regular care in the US: Results from the HIV cost and services utilization study (HCSUS). 12th World AIDS Conference Geneva, June 28-July 3, 1998 [abstract no. 13229].

141 Hutchinson CM et al: CD4 lymphocyte concentrations in patients with newly identified HIV infection attending STD clinics. *JAMA* 266:253–256, 1991.

142 Gallant JE et al: The impact of prophylaxis on outcome and resource utilization in *Pneumocystic carinii* pneumonia. *Chest* 107(4):1018–1023, 1995.

143 Gallant JE et al: Prophylaxis for opportunistic infections in patients with HIV infection. *Ann Intern Med* 120(11):932–944, 1994.

144 Eng TR, Butler WT (eds): *The Hidden Epidemic: Confronting Sexually Transmitted Diseases.* Washington DC, Institute of Medicine, National Academy Press, 1997.

145 Janssen RS et al: HIV infection among patients in US acute care hospitals: Strategies for the counseling and testing of hospital patients. *NEJM* 327:448–452, 1992.

146 Lo B et al: Voluntary screening for human immunodeficiency virus (HIV) infection. *Ann Intern Med* 110:727–733, 1989.

147 Fehrs LJ et al: Trial of anonymous versus confidential human immunodeficiency virus testing. *Lancet* 2:379–382, 1988.

148 Meyer KB, Pauker SG: Screening for HIV: Can we afford the false positive rate? *NEJM* 317(4):238–241, 1987.

149 McCarthy BD et al: Who should be screened for HIV infection: A cost-effectiveness analysis. *Arch Intern Med* 153:1107–1116, 1993.

150 Soloway B, Hecht FM: Identifying patients at risk for HIV infection. *AIDS Clin Care* 2(10):85–88, 1990.

151 Antoniskis D et al: Importance of assessing risk behavior for AIDS: Why and how to obtain a relevant history. *Risk Assess* 83(5):138–152, 1988.

152 Kolins J, Silvergleid AJ: Creating a uniform donor medical history questionnaire. *Transfusion* 31:349–354, 1991.

153 Schneider DJ et al: Risk assessment for HIV infection: Validation study of a computer-assisted preliminary screen. *AIDS Educ Prevent* 3(3):215–229, 1991.

154 Locke SE et al: Computer-based interview for screening blood donors for risk of HIV transmission. *JAMA* 268:1301–1305, 1992.

155 Volavka J et al: Assessment of risk behaviors for HIV infection among psychiatric inpatients. *Hosp Commun Psych* 43(5):482–483, 1992.

156 Sacks MH et al: Self-reported HIV-related risk behaviors in acute psychiatric inpatients: A pilot study. *Hosp Commun Psych* 41(11): 1253–1261, 1990.

157 Carmen E, Brady SM: AIDS risk and prevention for the chronic mentally ill. *Hosp Commun Psych* 41(6):652–657, 1990.

158 Kotloff KL et al: A voluntary serosurvey and behavioral risk assessment for human immunodeficiency virus infection among college students. *Sex Trans Dis* 18(4):223–227, 1991.

159 Silvergleid AJ et al: Impact of explicit questions about high-risk activities on donor attitudes and donor deferral patterns: Results in two community blood centers. *Transfusion* 29(4):362–364, 1989.
160 Vipond MN et al: Questionnaire identification of surgical patients at risk of HIV infection. *J R Coll Surg Edinb* 35:305–307, 1990.
161 McEwan RT et al: Social survey in HIV/AIDS: Telling or writing? A comparison of interview and postal methods. *Health Educ Res* 7(2): 195–202, 1992.
162 American Social Health Association: *STD Counseling and Treatment Guide*. Research Triangle Park, NC, ASHA, Appendix B, 1995, pp. 243–246.
163 Kassler WJ et al: Sexually transmitted diseases, in *Health Promotion and Disease Prevention in Clinical Practice,* Woolf SH et al (eds): Baltimore, Williams & Wilkins, 1996, pp. 273–290.
164 Lee RM: *Doing Research on Sensitive Topics*. Thousand Oaks, CA, Sage, 1993.
165 *STD Clinical Practice Guidelines,* Atlanta, GA, Centers for Disease Control and Prevention, 1991.
166 Brabin L et al: Reproductive tract infections and abortion among adolescent girls in rural Nigeria. *Lancet* 345:300–304, 1995.
167 Duncan ME et al: First coitus before menarche and the risk of sexually transmitted disease. *Lancet* 335:338–340, 1990.
168 Duncan ME, et al: Teenage obstetric and gynecological problems in an African city. *Central Africa J Med* 40:234–244, 1994.
169 Critchlow CW et al: Determinants of cervical ectopia and of cervicitis: Age, oral contraception, specific cervical infection, smoking, and douching. *Am J Obstet Gynecol* 173(2):534–543, 1995.
170 Catania JA et al: Risk factors for HIV and other sexually transmitted diseases and prevention practices among US heterosexual adults: Changes from 1990 to 1992. *Am J Public Health* 85:1492–1499, 1995.
171 Lever J: Bringing the fundamentals of gender studies into safer-sex education. *Fam Plann Perspect* 27:172–174, 1995.
172 Aral SO et al: Sex partner recruitment as a risk factor for STD: Clustering of risk modes. *Sex Transm Dis* 18:10–17, 1991.
173 Faxelid E et al: Behaviour, knowledge and reactions concerning sexually transmitted diseases: Implications for partner notification in Lusaka. *East Afr Med J* 71:118–121, 1994.
174 Daly CC et al: Risk factors for gonorrhoea, syphilis and trichomonas infections among women attending family planning clinics in Nairobi, Kenya. *Genitourin Med* 70:155–161, 1994.
175 Sellors JW et al: Effectiveness and efficiency of selective vs. universal screening for chlamydial infection in sexually active young women. *Arch Intern Med* 152:1837–1844, 1992.
176 Germain M et al: Evaluation of a screening algorithm for the diagnosis of genital infections with *Neisseria gonorrhoeae* and *Chlamydia trachomatis* among female sex workers in Benin. *Sex Transm Dis* 24(2):109–115, 1997.
177 Gunn RA et al: Adolescent health care providers. *STD* 24:90–93, 1997.
178 Turner CF et al: Adolescent sexual behavior, drug use, and violence: Increased reporting with computer survey technology. *Science* 280: 867–873, 1998.
179 Molina LD, Basinait-Smith C: Revisiting the intersection between domestic abuse and HIV risk. *Am J Public Health* 88:1267–1268, 1998.
180 Moore JS et al: Interventions for sexually active, heterosexual women in the United States, in *Preventing AIDS: Theories and Methods of Behavioral Interventions,* DiClement RJ, Peterson JL (eds). New York, Plenum, 1994.
181 Kowalewski MR et al: Rethinking perceived risk and health behavior: A critical review of HIV prevention research. *Health Educ Behav* 24: 313–325, 1997.
182 Catania JA et al: Toward an understanding of risk behavior: An AIDS risk reduction model (ARRM). *Health Educ Q* 17:53–72,1990.
183 Rabin DL et al: Improving office-based physician's prevention practices for sexually transmitted diseases. *Ann Intern Med* 121:513–519, 1994.
184 Bowman MA et al: The effect of educational preparation on physician performance with a sexually transmitted disease-simulated patient. *Arch Intern Med* 152:1823–1828, 1992.
185 Rabin DL: Adapting an effective primary care provider STD/HIV prevention training programme. *AIDS Care* 10(suppl 1):S75-S82, 1998.

Chapter 50

Anatomy and physical examination of the female genital tract

Daniel O. Graney
Louis A. Vontver

INTRODUCTION

Any area of the body may be involved in sexually transmitted disease syndromes or in the differential diagnosis of these conditions. Clearly there is no single, optimal method for conducting the history and physical examination. The critical areas of interest are determined by the history, other physical findings, and conditions considered in the differential diagnosis. Many critical anatomical points may be important in some contexts but irrelevant in others. Thus, this chapter is an attempt to present succinctly one approach to "the routine examination." This approach is selective but is based on clinical experience in developing an efficient method for evaluating a large number of patients in a timely manner. Accurate physical examination of the female genital tract can also be used as an integral part of developing and using syndromic management plans for care of sexually transmitted diseases when laboratory support is either unavailable or prohibitively expensive.[1–3]

WHAT SHOULD BE INCLUDED IN THE ROUTINE EXAMINATION OF NONPREGNANT WOMEN FOR REPRODUCTIVE HEALTH CARE

Several guidelines have been developed for the physical examination of women for routine preventive care, family planning, and STDs. These include the U.S. Preventive Services Task Force *Guide to Clinical Preventive Services*; the two-volume *Recommendations for Updating Selected Practices in Contraceptive Use*, produced jointly by the World Health Organization, USAID, INTRAH (Program for International Training in Health, School of Medicine, University of North Carolina) and Pathfinder International, the *Guidelines for Adolescent Preventive Services*; the unpublished *Program Guidelines for Project Grants for Family Planning Services*, for recipients of so-called Title X funding in the United States; and the pending *Reproductive Health Guidelines* being coordinated in the United States by the Centers for Disease Control, the Office for Population Affairs, and certain professional societies.[4–6]

The U.S. Preventive Services Task Force recommends that screening examination of adult females include periodic screening for hypertension every 2 years (for women age 21 or older); measurement of height and weight, and assessment for obesity; and screening of sexually experienced women for cervical cancer by Papanicolaou smear every 3 years.[4] The Task Force found insufficient medical evidence to support routine clinical breast examination in women under 50 years of age. Neither did they find medical evidence to support routine thyroid examination. No medical evidence was found to support routine pelvic examination to screen for ovarian cancer, or to recommend for or against breast self-examination.

Until recently, recipients of federal Title X funding for family planning in the United States were not allowed to defer pelvic examination longer than 3 months for women receiving hormonal contraception. More recently, because of concerns that some women were avoiding contraception to avoid pelvic examination, some agencies have decided to "delink" provision of hormonal contraception from the pelvic examination. For example, Planned Parenthood of America informed its affiliates in 1998 that they could defer pelvic examination for 3 months, 6 months, 1 year, or even longer—in order to remove the requirement for pelvic examination as a possible disincentive to the use of hormonal contraception. Women electing other forms of contraception, such as tubal ligation, diaphragm, or IUDobviously would need a pelvic examination for evaluation of uterine anatomy or properly fitting a diaphragm. Some adolescent medicine specialists have been outspoken about the lack of evidence for benefit of routine pelvic examination for adolescents receiving hormonal contraceptives. There are few data on this issue, except for one nonrandomized study that found no adverse effect from delaying pelvic examination of adolescents seeking hormonal contraception for up to 6 months.[7]

It should be noted that such guidelines have so far arisen from the family planning field, not the STD/HIV field, and efforts are underway to develop interdisciplinary reproductive health guidelines, which should have considerable impact on what services are included in health care services purchased for women, funded through insurance programs, and provided by managed care organizations.

Clearly, for women found to be at high risk for STD, based on risk assessment—and for those with symptoms or signs suggestive of an STD, the minimal physical examination should include the following.

- Skin and hair (as indicated by symptoms or other findings)
- Throat and mouth (as indicated by symptoms)
- Inguinal examination for adenopathy
- External genitalia, including labia majora and minora, clitoris, introitus, perineum, anus, and perianal area
- Urethral meatus and Skene's glands
- Bartholin's glands
- Speculum examination, including vaginal walls and cervix (including Pap smear and tests for cervical and vaginal infection, as indicated)
- Bimanual examination (with rectovaginal examination, as indicated)

Further, even for asymptomatic women without risk factors for STDs, medical visits for reproductive health care may be the only source of medical care. For such women, a comprehensive initial physical examination, including pelvic examination, should be strongly encouraged, and the patient should be counseled on the desirability for such examination, and on any risks of deferring the examination, with documentation of counseling and referral in the patients' medical record.

General considerations in examination of the female genital tract

There are two major differences in the anatomy and the examination between male and female patients. First, in the female the genital tract is separate from the urinary tract. In the male we conduct a single genitourinary tract examination. The second major difference is that the critical reproductive organs in the female are located in the pelvis, and are therefore less accessible and less easily palpated.

In the female patient who presents to the STD clinic, few portions of the physical examination will yield as much information as the pelvic examination. Symptomatic pathology abounds and unsuspected pathology is found in a significant proportion of relatively asymptomatic women.

Rapport with the patient is always important in the physical examination but is especially critical in the female pelvic exam. Evidence of concern for a woman's problems at the initial interview will help provide needed rapport. The woman worried about sexually transmitted disease expects to have a pelvic examination and is understandably concerned about the findings. She will usually be very cooperative. A little effort on the part of the examiner in regard to her well-being and comfort during the pelvic examination will maintain that cooperation and enhance the diagnostic yield.

Some specific suggestions to establish and maintain rapport are as follows. Prior to the examination always wash your hands where the patient can see you. Unless you are checking for incontinence, have the patient void before the examination, as a full bladder is uncomfortable and inhibits the examination. Obtain urine for analysis, culture or ligase chain reaction as indicated.[8–11] Recognize that the dorsal lithotomy position is one of vulnerability. The patient's comfort may be improved by elevating the backrest, suggesting that the patient wear her shoes so that the stirrups do not cause discomfort, and providing a drape if desired but not draping if that is the desire of the patient. The speculum should be kept warm in a warming drawer or warmed with water just before the examination. All the equipment necessary for the examination should be present in the examination room, which should be private and quiet.

You should tell the patient what you are doing at each step. It will help the patient's anxiety if she is told of normal structures and normal findings during the examination. A mirror should be available to demonstrate specific findings to the patient, as the more involved the patient becomes in her own care the more apt she is to return for subsequent visits and necessary treatments. The pelvic examination is an opportunity to teach the patient about her anatomy and about the transmission of infectious disease.

The comfort of the examiner should not be overlooked. Equipment should be readily available, lighting should be good, and the examination table and stool should be at the right height. Most often, the standard examination proceeds according to an orderly sequence. This has two advantages. First, the sequence of the examination limits the opportunity for errors of omission in a busy clinical situation. Second, there is minimal need for the patient to move. During the examination any needed specimens should be obtained, and following the exam the findings should be recorded and correlated with the patient's history and complaints. The remainder of this chapter is organized to follow this suggested pattern of evaluation. The relevant considerations in routine examination of the female will be presented for each section of the physical examination, and critical anatomical principles will be considered for that area. We will present the examination and anatomical descriptions according to our own opinions, recognizing that some of these opinions are controversial and that other anatomists and clinicians may hold alternative, equally valid viewpoints.

THE EXTERNAL GENITALIA AND PERINEUM

PHYSICAL EXAMINATION

Ordinarily, the examination is initiated by having the patient sit on the examining table. If indicated, head and neck examination, inspection, palpation, percussion, and auscultation of the chest and examination of the breasts may be done in this position. Next, the patient is asked to lie supine. Skin, extremity, breast, cardiovascular, and abdominal examination may be conducted in this position, if indicated. Attention is then directed to the pelvic examination.

The examination begins with palpation of the inguinal nodes and inspection of the mons pubis and the external genitalia. The quantity and location of pubic hair is noted. The amount of pubic hair varies greatly in different racial groups. Normal hair growth for a southern European would imply hirsutism from androgen excess in an Asian woman. Nits on the shaft of the pubic hair are indicative of lice infestation. Freckles that move are probably lice.

The labia are separated and the vaginal introitus is inspected. Redness or erythema signifies an irritation that may be owing to infection with *Candida*, *Trichomonas vaginalis*, herpes simplex virus (HSV), or certain bacteria (e.g., toxic shock syndrome, streptococcal cellulitis). A uniformly adherent homogeneous white or gray discharge at the introitus is suggestive of bacterial vaginosis. Small tender fissures in the mucous membrane should arouse suspicion of genital herpes, as many genital HSV occurrences do not form classic ulcerations. Pigmented or nodular areas on the vulva may be owing to human papilloma virus infection or carcinoma in situ. Use of a magnifying glass or colposcope may help delineate small lesions that would be difficult to detect without magnification. Multifocal carcinoma in situ (i.e., involving more than one site on the cervix, vagina, and vulva) is being found more frequently in young women, and biopsies of suspicious areas of the vulva are important to rule out this disease. Pigmented areas may also be benign nevi or malignant melanomas (see Chap. 60). A suspicious area that is darkly pigmented with irregular borders should be removed by excisional biopsy for histologic inspection. The inspection for such lesions should include the frenulum and clitoris.

While the vulva are held apart, the woman should be asked to strain, cough, or otherwise perform a Valsalva maneuver. This will allow observation of any vaginal relaxation or stress incontinence. At this time the urethra with its associated periurethral (Skene's) glands should be palpated and milked by gentle finger pressure from above downward. If infection or a urethral diverticulum is present, a small amount of discharge may be evident at the urethral meatus or at the orifices of Skene's glands.

The greater vestibular glands (of Bartholin) are located at approximately 5 and 7 o'clock on the face of the posterior fourchette (Fig. 50-1). When these regions are explored with gentle pressure between the thumb and forefinger, the normal gland cannot be palpated and the region is not tender. However, an infected gland

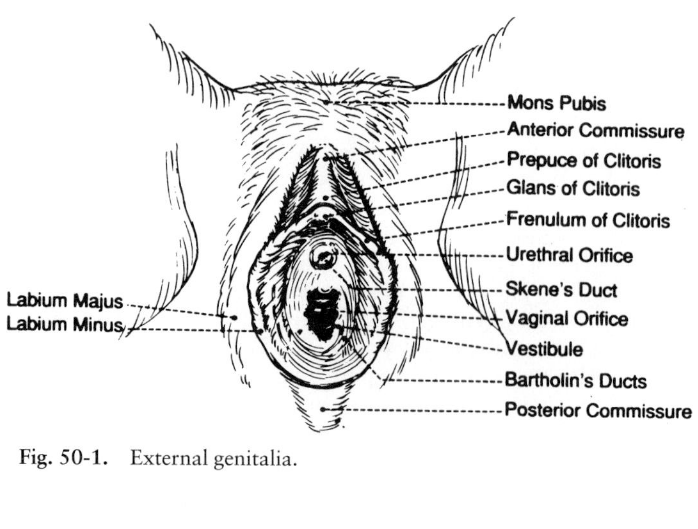

Fig. 50-1. External genitalia.

is extremely tender. Occasionally a small asymptomatic Bartholin's duct cyst can be seen as a convexity of the posterior fourchette and felt as a discrete cystic nodule in the position of the Bartholin's gland. If any palpable mass is discovered in this area in a perimenopausal or menopausal woman, it should be removed for histologic examination, as the incidence of carcinoma increases with age.

Anatomy of the perineum and external genitalia

The strict anatomical definition of the perineum is a diamond-shaped region bounded by the symphysis pubis anteriorly, coccyx posteriorly, and ischial tuberosities laterally. Projecting a line between the ischial tuberosities divides the diamond space into two triangles, the urogenital triangle anteriorly and the anal triangle posteriorly. Thus, both triangles share a common base with the apex of the urogenital triangle pointing anterosuperiorly and the anal triangle pointing posterosuperiorly. In lateral profile the floor of the perineum is shaped like a shallow V rather than appearing flat as implied by a two-dimensional drawing. The plane of the anal triangle is open and is filled only with fatty tissue. The plane of the urogenital triangle is closed or occupied by a thick triangular membrane, the urogenital diaphragm. The diaphragm closes the anterior floor of the perineum and defines the anterior wall of the ischiorectal fossa.

The region of the urogenital triangle contains two spaces, the superficial and deep perineal spaces (Figs. 50-2, 50-3, and 50-4). The superficial space can be imagined as a pair of spaces lying between the urogenital diaphragm and the skin of the labia majora. In fact, the two spaces are connected above the clitoris so that the space resembles an inverted U. It is bounded by the perineal fascia of the urogenital diaphragm that continues from the base of the diaphragm and reflects superiorly under the labial skin to join the membranous layer of superficial fascia of the abdomen above the symphysis pubis (see Figs. 50-2, 50-3, and 50-4). Because of these fascial attachments, a hematoma in the labia majora, that is, superficial pouch, expands superiorly into the abdominal wall but neither laterally to the thigh nor posteriorly to the ischiorectal fossa.

The contents of the superficial perineal pouch include the greater vestibular glands (Bartholin's), crura of the clitoris, bulbs of the vestibule, which are composed of elongated erectile tissue, and the overlying superficial perineal muscles.

The deep perineal space is a potential space within the urogenital diaphragm. It is formed by the superior and inferior fascia (perineal membrane) of the deep transverse perineal muscle that occupies the space. Together, the muscle and fascia form the urogenital diaphragm (see Figs. 50-3 and 50-4).

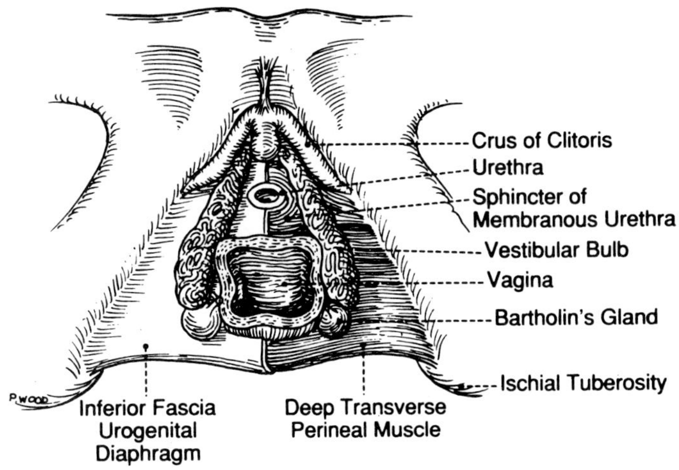

Fig. 50-3. Contents of the deep perineal pouch.

In the female, the contents of the deep perineal space include the deep transverse perineal muscle, and circular muscle fibers surrounding the urethra and vagina as these structures pierce the urogenital diaphragm.

Female Urethra. The female urethra measures 3 to 4 cm in length from the bladder neck to the meatus in the anterior vestibule of the vagina. Proximally the mucosa is composed of transitional epithelium gradually becoming stratified squamous as it courses distally. The lumen appears stellate in cross section because of extensive longitudinal folding of the mucosa. Beneath the mucosa is the lamina propria, rich in vascular and neural plexuses. The muscular coat, similar to other body tubes, is composed of a double layer of smooth muscle, with the inner fibers circularly arranged and the outer layer disposed longitudinally. As the urethra traverses the urogenital diaphragm, circularly arranged striated muscle fibers form an external sphincter of the urethra. These fibers are innervated by the internal pudendal nerve (somatic) in contrast to the internal urethral sphincter at the bladder neck, which is innervated by the pelvic splanchnic nerve (parasympathetic).

In essence, the entire length of the female urethra is paralleled by paraurethral glands that are tubuloalveolar outgrowths of the

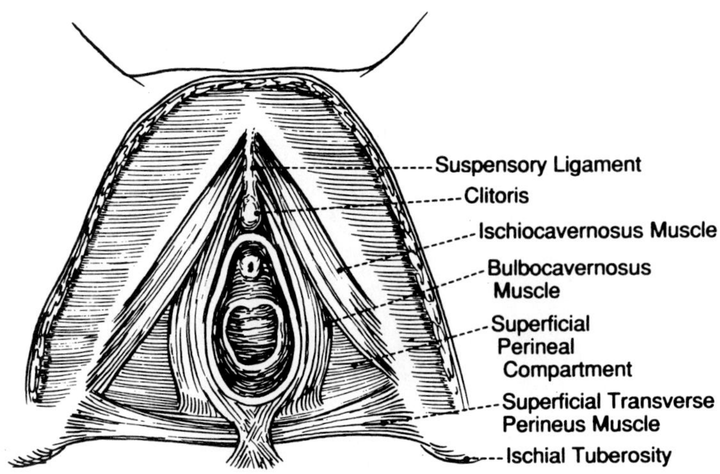

Fig. 50-2. Contents of the superficial perineal pouch.

mucosa. Located in the lamina propria, these glands have their openings on the posterior and posterolateral wall of the urethra (see Fig. 50-4). At the distal end of the urethra there are usually two larger glands, commonly identified as Skene's glands, whose ducts are visible on the posterior wall. Both Skene's glands and the paraurethral glands are vulnerable to infection.

More extensive review of female pelvic anatomy and histology may be found in recent texts.[14–16]

VAGINA, CERVIX, UTERUS, AND ADNEXAL STRUCTURES

Physical examination

Speculum Examination and Collection of Specimens for Microscopy and Culture. A warm speculum should be inserted into the vagina and opened to reveal the cervix. It should be inserted at an angle directed toward the hollow of the sacrum (Fig. 50-5). Care should be taken not to apply pressure against the urethra and anterior bony arch of the pubis. With the speculum in place, specimens may be obtained for pH determination and wet mount examination of vaginal fluid; vaginal fluid Gram stain and selected cultures, if indicated; and endocervical Gram stain and cultures and Pap smear. If there are no symptoms or signs of vaginal discharge or inflammation, no tests of vaginal fluid are usually done. If such symptoms or signs exist, a specimen of the vaginal discharge should be tested on pH paper to ascertain the vaginal pH, which is normally 4.5 or below. If the vaginal pH is above 4.5, it is suggestive of bacterial vaginosis or of trichomoniasis. Care should be taken to avoid mixing vaginal discharge with cervical mucus for determination of vaginal fluid pH, since cervical mucus has a pH of about 7.0. Vaginal discharge should also be mixed with saline for microscopic examination for motile trichomonads and clue cells; and with 10 percent potassium hydroxide for detection of a fishy, amine-like odor, characteristic of bacterial vaginosis, and for microscopic detection of fungal ele-

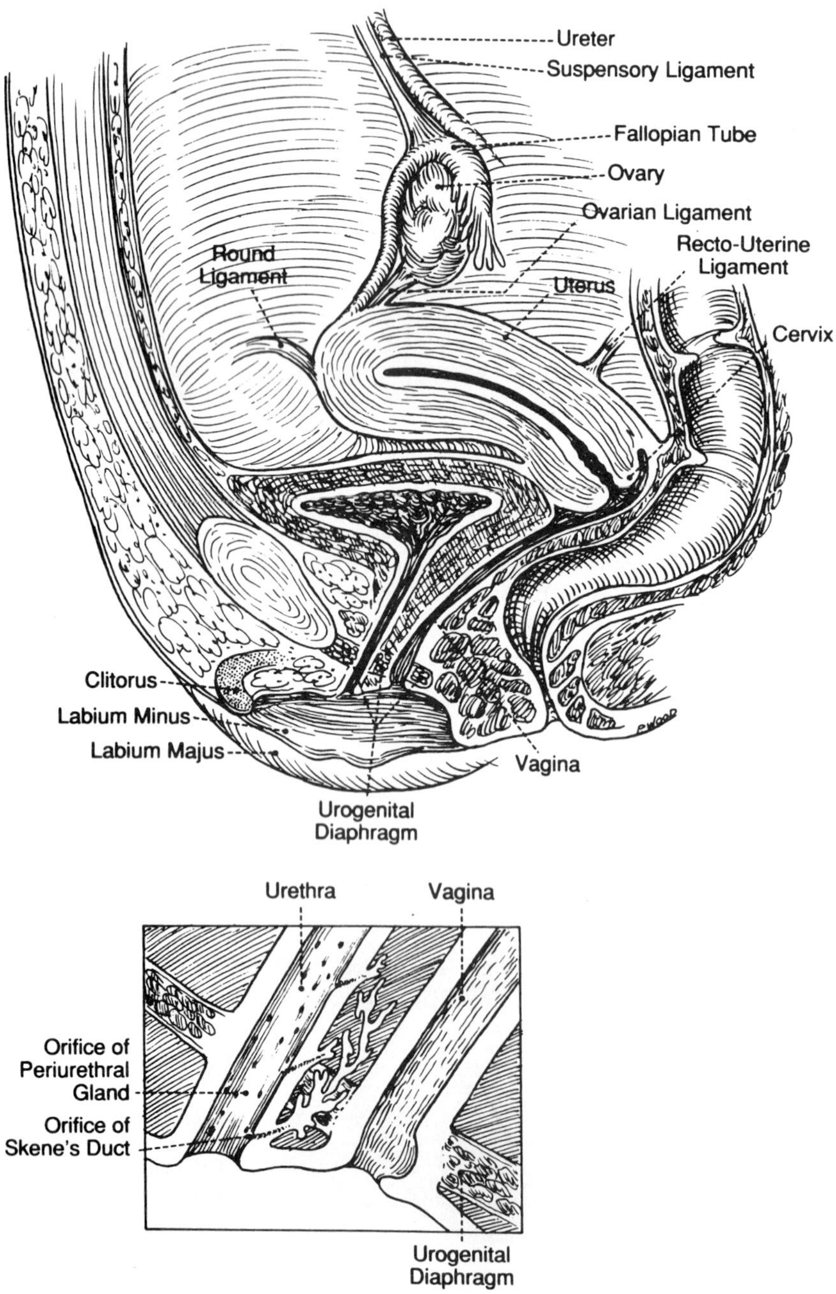

Fig. 50-4. Sagittal section of female pelvis. Inset shows magnification of urethra and urethral glands.

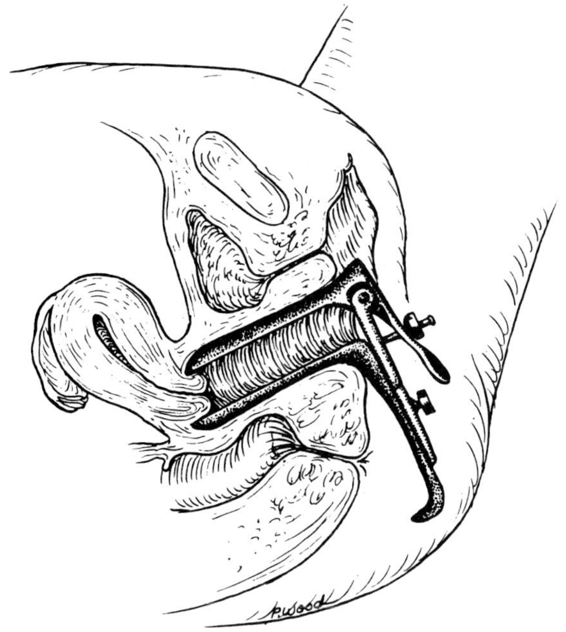

Fig. 50-5. Position of vaginal speculum.

ments (see Chap. 42). A Gram stain of a thinly smeared slide of vaginal discharge is useful for confirming the diagnosis of bacterial vaginosis. With rare exceptions (e.g., toxic shock syndrome), bacterial cultures of vaginal fluid are not useful. However, for detection of *Candida or Trichomonas vaginalis,* vaginal cultures are more sensitive than microscopic examination of vaginal fluid, especially in the absence of abnormal vaginal discharge.

For Pap smear, separate samples should be obtained from the ectocervix, including the transformation zone, using an Ayre's spatulum; and from the endocervix, using a cytobrush (see Chap. 48). We recommend annual cervical cytologic screening for sexually active women. Specimens for culture for gonorrhea and diagnosis of chlamydia by culture or antigen detection test can be taken from the endocervix. Ligase chain reaction assays of urine or urogenital swabs may also be used to detect gonorrhea and chlamydia.[8–11] A specimen of the endocervical mucus can also be obtained at this time, inspected for color (yellow color indicates increased numbers of PMN leukocytes), and used to prepare a Gram-stained smear for microscopic enumeration of PMN leukocytes in cervical mucus and for detection of gonococci. Nabothian cysts are a normal finding on the cervix (Fig. 50-6). They develop when squamous epithelium covers mucus-secreting columnar epithelium and the secretions cause a small cyst to form. These cysts rupture and reform throughout the reproductive years. While the speculum is still in place, colposcopy can be performed before and after applying dilute (3 percent) acetic acid or dilute lugol solution to the cervix. Colposcopy enables one to better visualize cervical, vaginal, and vulvar abnormalities such as dysplasia or infection with human papilloma virus, as well as cervical ulcers caused by HSV, or "strawberry cervix" caused by *T. vaginalis.* Colposcopy is clearly helpful to select lesions or areas for biopsy when evaluating a cervix after Pap smears have shown dysplasia. The role of colposcopy as an initial screening procedure is debated.

Bimanual Examination. After removal of the speculum, the first two fingers of the vaginal examining hand are lubricated and inserted into the vagina. The bladder should be compressed. This should cause no discomfort other than the sensation of needing to void. The cervix should be palpated and moved. Both it and the attached uterine body should be freely mobile without pain.

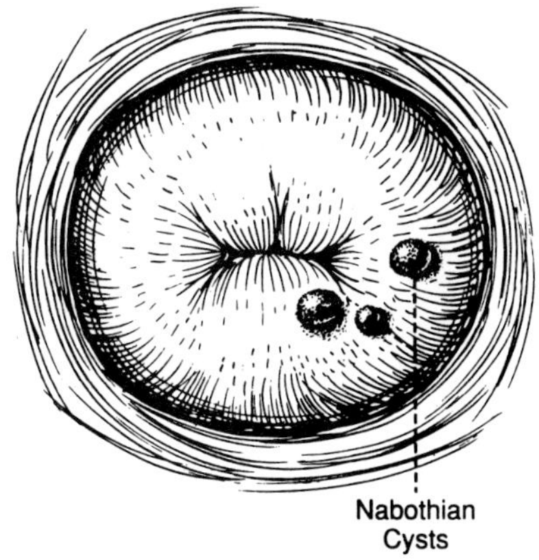

Fig. 50-6. Cervix, illustrating Nabothian cysts.

The body of the uterus is next located by providing suprapubic pressure with the abdominal hand to keep the uterus in the pelvic cavity. The two fingers of the examining vaginal hand should outline the uterus in its entirety. This is usually easy if the uterus is anterior. If it is in a mid or posterior retroflexed position, it will be more difficult to locate and may be best palpated on rectovaginal examination (Fig. 50-7). After noting the size, shape, position, mobility, consistency, and contour of the uterus, it is moved to the one side and the fingers of the examining hand are inserted into the right lateral vaginal fornix as far as possible (Fig. 50-8). The abdominal hand produces pressure on the right lower abdomen and the fingers of the vaginal hand are swept to the side to evaluate the adnexal structures consisting of the tube, ovary, round and cardinal ligaments, and the pelvic sidewall (Fig. 50-9). The same procedure is followed on the opposite side. (Some people prefer to change hands, using the left hand to examine the left side of the pelvis.) Only the ovaries should be palpable in the normal examination. Often they are not felt, especially if the patient is on birth control pills, which suppress the ovaries and decrease their size. A normal ovary in a menstruating nonsuppressed woman measures approximately $3 \times 3 \times 2$ cm. Any enlargement above 5 to 6 cm is an abnormal finding. Both pelvic sidewalls should be evaluated for enlargements of the lymph nodes. Ten-

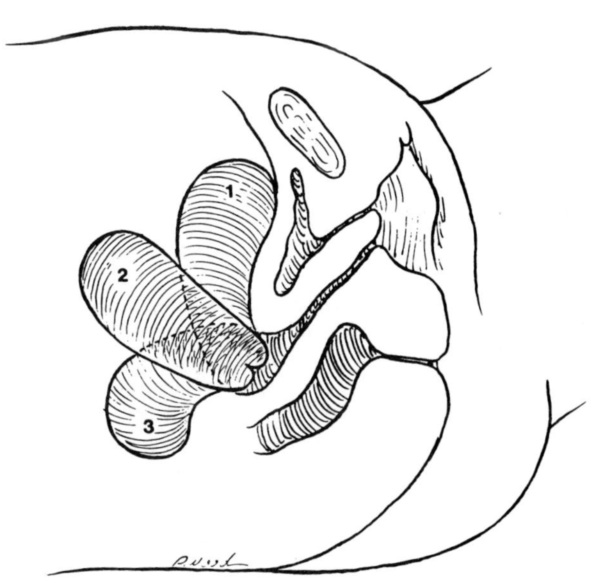

Fig. 50-7. Positions of the uterus: (1) anteverted, (2) midposition, and (3) retroflexed.

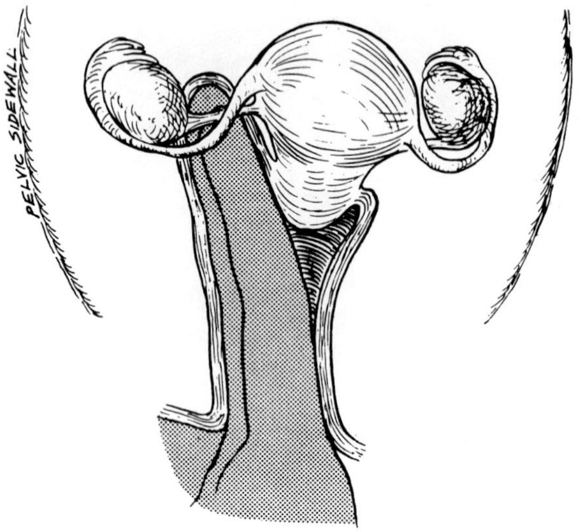

Fig. 50-8. Preparation for bimanual pelvic examination: placement of vaginal fingers (shaded).

derness of any of the pelvic structures is noted. The examination is concluded with a rectovaginal exam.

Rectovaginal Examination. After the patient is informed of the procedure, a well-lubricated middle finger is placed in the rectum and the index finger is simultaneously placed in the vaginal vault. The patient can often facilitate the rectal examination by relaxing the pelvic muscles during insertion of the fingers. The rectal finger carefully evaluates the entire rectal wall for nodularity or polygas. It is then placed against the cervix, which is felt through the rectal and vaginal wall. Pressure from the abdominal hand brings the uterus down so its entire posterior surface can be palpated with the rectal finger. This is the best method to examine the posterior wall of the uterus if it is in the mid- or posterior position in the pelvis. The uterosacral and cardinal ligaments can be put on tension by elevating the cervix and palpated for nodularity such as may be found with endometriosis. The posterolateral sidewalls of the pelvis should be swept with the rectal finger, and a stool specimen can be obtained if indicated for evaluation of occult bleeding. The American Cancer Society recommends annual testing for gastrointestinal bleeding beginning at age 50.

Throughout the pelvic examination a mental image of the pelvic organs should be formed, noting size, shape, consistency, mobility, contour, and tenderness. Practitioners often confirm or supplement their findings in physical examination with a transabdominal or transvaginal ultrasound. Ultrasound may be especially helpful in patients who are difficult to examine because of pain, fear, or obesity, and in patients who have physical findings of uncertain etiology. It is not as accurate as laparoscopy for the diagnosis of pelvic inflammatory disease. Ultrasound is specifically beneficial in evaluating suspected ectopic pregnancy and differentiating ovarian from uterine tumors, and can be used to evaluate other symptoms also.[15-17] All observations made should be accurately documented in the record. Correlation of the patient's complaints or historical data with the physical findings and the laboratory evaluation will often resolve the concerns of the patient and the questions of the examining physician.

Anatomy

Vagina. The vagina is a fibromuscular tube whose anterior and posterior walls are normally in contact with one another. A longitudinal ridge is present along the mucosal surface of both the anterior and posterior walls; from these ridges, secondary elevations called rugae extend laterally. The vaginal wall consists of three layers: (1) the mucous membrane, composed of stratified squamous nonkeratinized epithelium and an underlying lamina propria of connective tissue; (2) the muscular layer, composed of smooth muscle fibers disposed both longitudinally and circularly; and (3) the adventitia, a dense connective tissue that blends with the surrounding fascia.

There are no glands in the vaginal wall. During sexual stimulation the marked increase in fluid production in the vagina is believed to be caused by transudation across the vaginal wall.

The stratified squamous epithelium of the adult vagina is several layers thick. The basal layer is a single layer of cylindrical cells with oval nuclei. Above this area are several layers of polyhedral cells that appear to be connected together much like those of the stratum spinosum of the epidermis. Above these are several more layers of cells that are more flattened in appearance and accumulate glycogen in their cytoplasm, the significance of which is discussed in the following. They also exhibit keratohyalin granules intracellularly. This tendency toward keratinization, however, is not normally completed in the vaginal epithelium, and the surface cells always retain their nuclei.

The most superficial cells are desquamated into the vaginal lumen where their intracellular glycogen is converted into lactic acid, probably by the bacteria normally resident in the vagina. The resulting acidity is believed to be important in protecting the female reproductive system from infection by most pathogenic bacteria (see Chap. 13).

Estrogen stimulates the production of glycogen and maintains the thickness of the entire epithelium. Before puberty and after menopause, when estrogen levels are relatively low, the epithelium is thin and the pH is higher than in the reproductive years (neutral before puberty and 6.0 or higher after the menopause). The thinness of the epithelium and the relatively high pH of the vaginal milieu are among the factors that are thought to render females in these age groups more susceptible to vaginal infections.

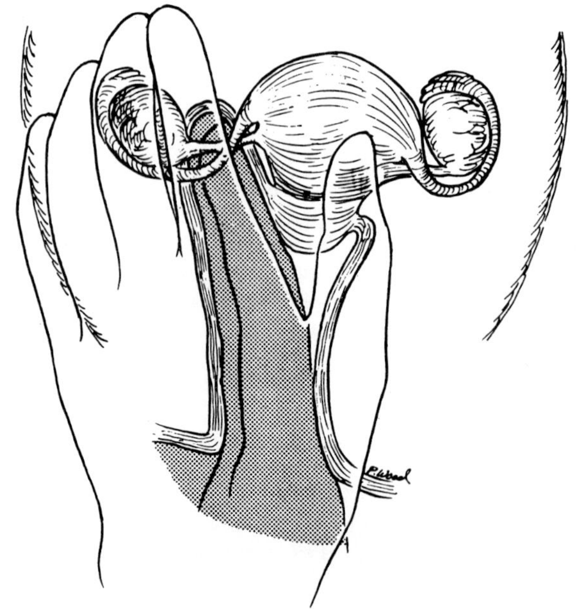

Fig. 50-9. Bimanual examination: comparing position of vaginal fingers (shaded) and abdominal hand.

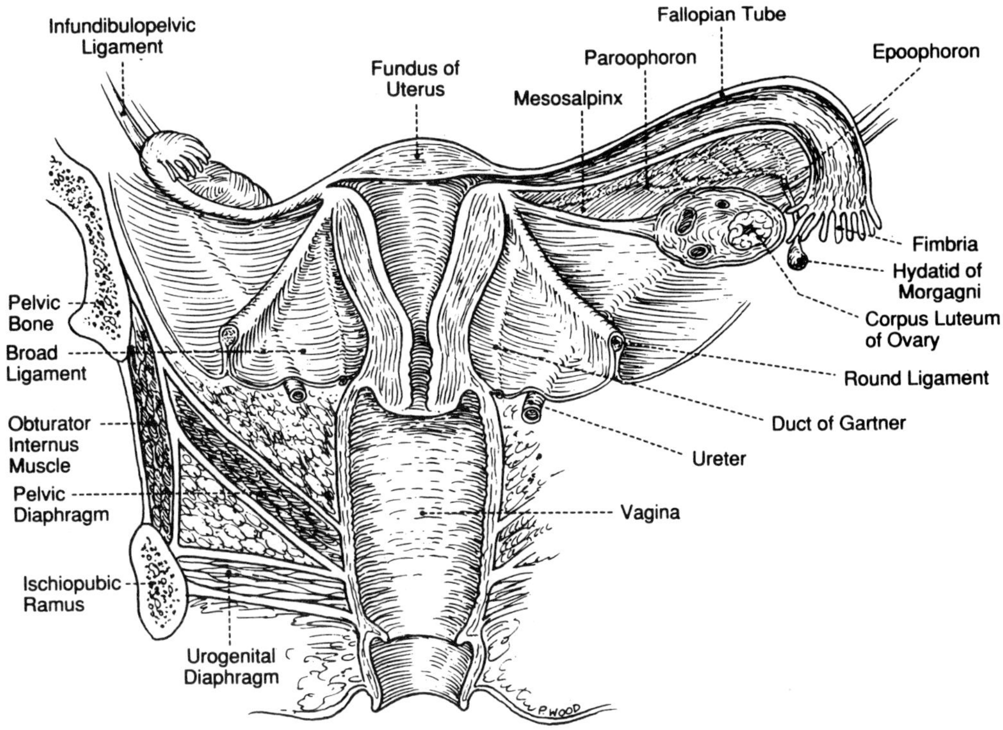

Fig. 50-10. Coronal section of pelvis illustrating broad ligament, endopelvic space, pelvic diaphragm, and urogenital diaphragm.

Uterus. The uterus has two major components: (1) the expanded upper two-thirds of the organ, the body of the uterus; and (2) the cylindrical lower one-third, the cervix (Figs. 50-10 and 50-11). The fundus is the rounded upper part of the body, superior to the points of entry of the uterine tubes. The isthmus is the short, slightly constricted zone between the body and the cervix.

The two main components of the uterus are rather different from one another in their structure and function.

Cervix. The cervix consists primarily of dense collagenous connective tissue. Only about 15 percent of its substance is smooth muscle. In the isthmus, the uterine lumen narrows down to form the internal os. Below this point the lumen widens slightly to form the cervical canal (or endocervical canal). Finally, a constricted opening, the external os, at the lower end of the cervix provides communication between the lumen of the cervix and that of the vagina.

Inside the cervix, the endocervical mucosa is arranged in a series of folds and ridges. A longitudinal ridge runs down the anterior wall and another down the posterior wall; from each of these, small folds (the *plicae palmatae)* run laterally. The resemblance of this arrangement to a tree trunk with upward-spreading branches has given rise to the term *arbor vitae uterina* to describe the endocervical mucosa.

The part of the cervix that projects into the vagina (the *portio vaginalis,* or ectocervix) is covered by stratified squamous, nonkeratinizing epithelium. Usually, in older women, this type of epithelium extends for a very short distance into the cervical canal,

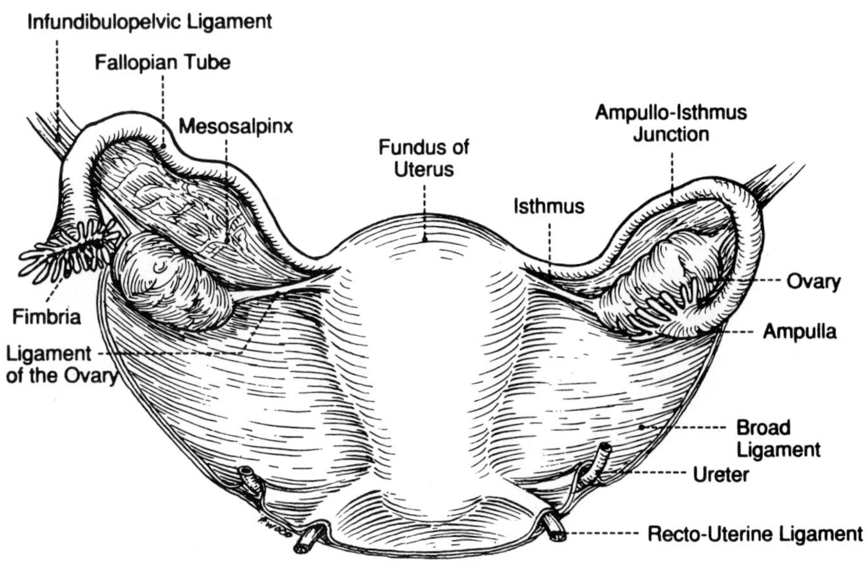

Fig. 50-11. Posterior view of broad ligament and female reproductive organs.

where it forms a rather abrupt junction with the simple columnar epithelium lining the rest of the canal. The site of the squamocolumnar junction varies, however. It may occur higher up in the cervical canal, or the columnar epithelium may actually extend out beyond the external os where it forms small patches known as physiologic eversion, or ectopy, on the vaginal surface of the cervix. Ectopy is usually present in adolescents, and decreases during the third and fourth decades of life. [see Fig. 50-6]

The mucosa contains large branched endocervical glands. In reality, they are not true glands but are merely deep grooves or clefts (sometimes called crypts) that serve to increase the surface area of the mucosa tremendously. The epithelium of both the mucosal surface and the "glands" is of the simple columnar type in which almost all the cells are mucus-secreting. A few ciliated cells are present. If the ducts of the glands become blocked, mucous secretion accumulates inside them to form small lumps just under the surface (see Fig. 50-6).

Unlike the mucous membrane of the body of the uterus, the endocervical mucosa does not slough off at menstruation. It does, however, respond to cyclic changes in the levels of the ovarian hormones, estrogen and progesterone. It secretes up to 60 mg of mucus a day throughout much of the cycle, but near the time of ovulation (midcycle), when estrogen secretion reaches a peak, the secretion rate increases tenfold and the abundant, clear mucus fills the cervical canal. It is less viscous than at other times during the cycle, and is easily penetrated by spermatozoa.

The production of progesterone by the corpus luteum after ovulation (or during pregnancy) changes the quantity and properties of mucus produced. It becomes more viscous, less abundant, and much less penetrable by spermatozoa. It acts as a plug to seal off the uterine cavity.

The Body of the Uterus. The wall of the body of the uterus is composed of three layers: (1) the endometrium, a glandular mucous membrane; (2) the myometrium or smooth muscle layer; and (3) the serosa.

ENDOMETRIUM

The function of the endometrium is to provide a suitable environment for the implantation and subsequent growth of the developing embryo. As such, it is a luxuriant mucosa with a large population of glycogen-secreting glands and a rich vascular network. However, if there is no developing embryo, most of the endometrium is sloughed off (causing the menstrual flow) and is regenerated again in the next menstrual cycle. This cyclic shedding and regeneration of the endometrium is under the control of the ovarian hormones, estrogen and progesterone. The rise and fall in ovarian hormone levels determine the rise and fall of the growth and shedding of the endometrium.

The endometrium varies from 0.5 mm to approximately 5 mm in thickness, depending on the stage of the menstrual cycle. It is at its greatest height a few days after ovulation, at about the time of expected implantation. It consists of a simple columnar epithelium and a highly cellular lamina propria (the endometrial stroma) in which there are large numbers of tubular uterine glands. The epithelium contains both ciliated and secretory cells.

The endometrium can be subdivided into a rather narrow, deeper layer next to the myometrium, the basalis, and a much thicker, more superficial layer, the functionalis. The latter receives its name because it is the portion that is shed during menstruation.

The arteries that supply the endometrium play an important role in the onset of menstruation. Circumferentially oriented arteries in the myometrium give off numerous branches toward the endometrium. As they enter this region, small basal arteries branch off to supply the basalis. The arteries then become highly contorted as they enter the functionalis and are known as coiled or spiral arteries. These arteries spasmodically contract late in the menstrual cycle that induces ischemia, necrosis, and eventually sloughing of the functionalis.

During the menstrual cycle, the endometrium passes through a number of phases. In the menstrual phase (approximately days 1 to 4 of a typical 28-day cycle) the functionalis is sloughed off; cellular debris and blood are discharged into the vagina. From day 5 until the time of ovulation (approximately day 14) the endometrium is in its proliferative phase. Epithelium in the persisting portions of uterine glands in the basalis grows out and covers the denuded surface. Estrogen from the growing follicles in the ovary promotes rapid proliferation of the epithelium, glands, and stroma. The endometrium may thicken by 2 to 3 mm at this time. Progesterone and estrogen from the corpus luteum stimulate the secretory phase (days 15 to 28), in which the epithelial cells begin to secrete. Accumulation of secretory products in the lumina of the glands, together with some edema of the stroma, causes the endometrium to increase further in height.

Late in the secretory phase, ovarian hormone levels drop and the changes that herald menstruation occur. Intermittent constrictions in the spiral arteries cause stasis of blood and ischemia of vessels and tissues in the area of supply. During the intervening periods of relaxation blood escapes from the weakened vessels, promoting menstrual hemorrhage.

MYOMETRIUM

The myometrium consists of bundles of smooth muscle fibers separated by strands of connective tissue. Four layers of smooth muscle have been distinguished, but their boundaries are poorly defined owing to overlap between adjacent layers. In the innermost and outermost layers, most of the muscle fibers are disposed longitudinally, whereas in the middle layers there are rather more circular fibers.

Estrogen is essential for the maintenance of normal size and function in myometrial smooth muscle cells.

SEROSA

The serosa is the peritoneal covering of the uterus; hence, only the pelvic portion of uterus has a serosa. The cervix has no serosa. The peritoneal reflections are discussed later in the chapter in the section on the broad ligament.

UTERINE TUBES

Fertilization and the earliest steps in development occur within the uterine tube. Therefore, these tubes must perform a number of tasks. As well as providing a suitable milieu for the gametes and transporting them to the site of fertilization in the midsection of the duct, they must also provide the nutritional support necessary for the embryo during segmentation and morula formation. In addition, transport mechanisms in the proximal portion of the oviduct must be such that the embryo arrives in the uterus at the appropriate time, both in terms of its own development and in terms of uterine receptivity.

GENERAL STRUCTURE

The uterine tubes lie in the upper margins of the broad ligament. Each is composed of four parts. Beginning at the distal end these are: (1) the infundibulum—the funnel-shaped end of the uterine tube that bears numerous delicate processes, the fimbriae, around the abdominal ostium; (2) the ampulla, or longest portion—it accounts for slightly more than half of the total length; (3) the isthmus—a narrow portion leading to the uterus; and (4) the intramural (or interstitial) portion—that part of the duct that extends through the wall of the uterus. At its end there is a minute ostium that connects the cavities of the uterus and uterine tube.

Three layers form the wall of the uterine tube: (1) the mucous membrane, characteristically composed of epithelium and lamina propria. The epithelium is of the simple columnar variety and contains two types of cells, ciliated and secretory. The lamina propria is loose connective tissue. (2) The muscular layer consists typically of two layers of smooth muscle, an inner circular and an outer longitudinal, but the boundary between the two is not distinct. In the intramural portion another longitudinal layer has been described, internal to the circular layer. (3) The serosa, which is typical of serosa elsewhere.

The mucous membrane and the muscular layer vary from one region of the duct to another. The structure and function of the various regions will now be discussed in more detail.

INFUNDIBULUM

When the oocyte leaves the ruptured follicle at ovulation, it is still surrounded by a mass of follicular cells that made up the bulk of the cumulus oophorus. The oocyte and its surrounding cells are now called the cumulus mass. The fimbriae of the infundibuium have the task of removing the cumulus mass from the site of follicular rupture on the ovary and transporting it into the ostium. Once contact is made, the cumulus mass begins to be transported over the fimbrial surface by ciliary action. The surface is richly ciliated and all the cilia beat toward the ostium. Since oocytes freed of cumulus cells are easily dislodged and are transported rather poorly, it is believed that the cumulus cells are essential for normal "pickup" and transport.

The epithelium of the fimbriae (and indeed, of the entire uterine tube) is sensitive to ovarian hormones. As estrogen concentration rises during the follicular phase of the cycle, the epithelium increases in height and reaches a maximum at midcycle. During the late luteal phase, cell height decreases. There is little evidence for deciliation and reciliation during the menstrual cycle in the human, but there is no doubt that withdrawal of estrogen will result in deciliation. The fimbriae of postmenopausal uterine tubes are largely devoid of cilia, whereas these from postmenopausal women who are on estrogen therapy are richly ciliated.

AMPULLA

The mucous membrane of the ampulla is thrown up into an elaborate system of longitudinal folds. Most of the lumen is thus reduced to a system of fine channels between the folds. Less than half of the epithelial cells are ciliated and they beat toward the isthmus (Fig. 50-12).

Fertilization occurs in the proximal portion of the ampulla. There are potentially two mechanisms for transporting the cumulus mass to this site: ciliary activity and smooth muscle contraction.

Although the role of the ciliated cells in the ampulla is fairly clear, the function of the secretory cells is less certain. Loss of cilia may be caused by infection leading to poor gamete transport with resultant infertility or ectopic pregnancy. Infection may also occlude the tube and persisting secretion may result in hydrosalpinx.

ISTHMUS

The elaborate mucosal folds of the ampulla give way rather abruptly to simpler, lower folds in the isthmus. Concomitant with a decrease in complexity of the mucosal folds is a marked increase in the thickness of the muscle layer. The ciliated cells of the mucosa beat toward the uterus.

The isthmus is perhaps the least understood portion of the uterine tube. It has the capacity of transporting spermatozoa distally toward the site of fertilization and later, conducting the developing embryo proximally. It is not known how the isthmus (or perhaps the intramural portion) controls the passage of cleaving eggs into the uterus.

INTRAMURAL PORTION

The lumen of the uterine tube becomes extremely narrow in the proximal isthmus and intramural portions. The mucosal folds are reduced to low ridges. The muscular layer, on the other hand, becomes thicker than in any other part of the tube. The large amount of muscle in this region might suggest that a sphincter exists that could close off the uterine tube and help to prevent the spread of infection. However, there are no reported observations documenting the existence of an anatomical sphincter.

BROAD LIGAMENT

The broad ligament represents a transverse double fold of peritoneum containing the uterus and the uterine adnexa (uterine tube and ligaments) as well as nerves, vessels, and lymphatics (see Figs. 50-4 and 50-5). Inferior to the sacral promontory the peritoneum covers the anterior surface of the sigmoid colon and dips to its lowest point overlying the posterior vaginal fornix. From this position it reflects superiorly over the fundus and body of the uterus and then anteriorly to cover the dome of the bladder. At the level of the pubic symphysis it reflects superiorly again onto the anterior abdominal wall. From either side of the body of the uterus the folded peritoneum is carried laterally to the wall of the pelvis, forming a transverse vertical partition, the broad ligament. This divides the inferior peritoneal cavity into an anterior vesicouterine (pouch of Douglas) and posterior rectouterine space.

SUSPENSORY LIGAMENT OF THE OVARY

The suspensory ligament (infundibulopelvic ligament) is an extension of the most superior and lateral part of the broad ligament. It is misnamed, as it provides no support for the ovary or uterus. In reality, it is merely a fold of peritoneum raised by the underlying ovarian vessels, nerves, and lymphatics as they course between the ovary and the retroperitoneum. It provides a potential route for the spread of infection from adnexal structures to the retroperitoneum and paraaortic nodes.

Ovary. The ovaries have two major functions: to nurture and release the female gametes, and to produce the female sex hormones, estrogen and progesterone. These functions entail considerable changes in ovarian structure, both cyclic changes during the reproductive years and long-term changes over the individual's lifetime.

The ovary is covered by a single layer of cells known as the germinal epithelium. This is actually a misnomer, since it does not give rise to germ cells, as was originally believed. The cells are cuboidal in the young individual but tend to become squamous with age. This epithelium is the source of most ovarian neoplasms. These masses may be detected on bimanual examination and can

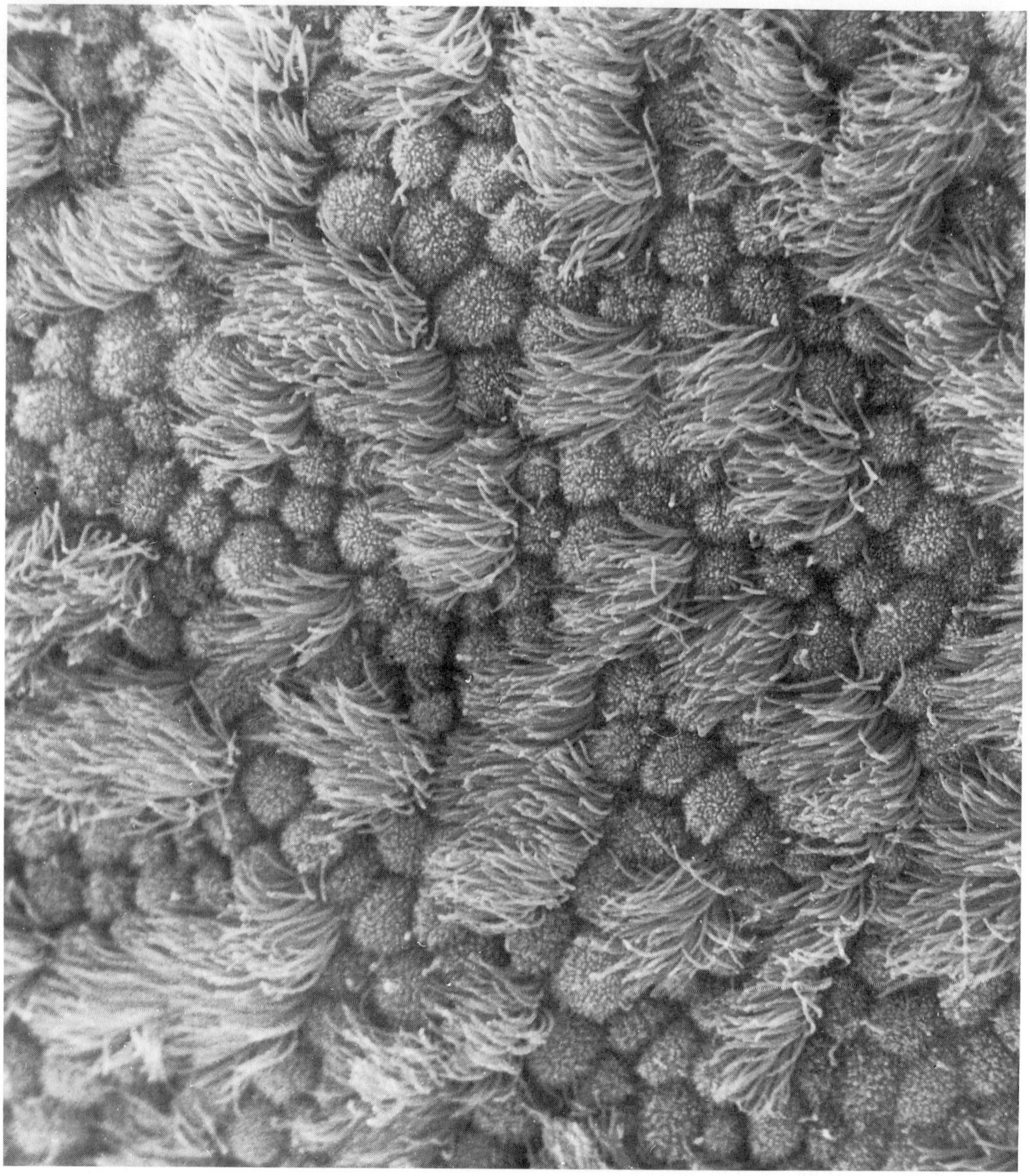

Fig. 50-12. Ampulla of the uterine tube from a 29-year-old woman in midcycle. Scanning electron micrograph illustrates distribution of ciliated and nonciliated cells. (Courtesy Dr. Penny Gaddum-Rosse.)

be confused with hydrosalpinx or more acute infectious processes, especially if the neoplasm undergoes torsion.

The substance of the ovary may be divided into an outer cortex and an inner medulla. The connective tissue stroma of the cortex contains many spindle-shaped cells that resemble fibroblasts and intercellular substance. In the outermost zone of the cortex, just under the epithelium, the ratio of intercellular material to cells is higher than elsewhere. The fibrous nature and relatively poor vascularity of this zone give it a whitish appearance that accounts for its name, the tunica albuginea. The stroma of the medulla is a loose connective tissue containing some smooth muscle cells, many elastic fibers, and large, tortuous blood vessels. The presence of elastic fibers and the convoluted nature of the blood vessels permit the ovary to adapt fairly readily to the large structural changes that occur in the organ during each menstrual cycle.

More extensive reviews of female pelvic anatomy and histology may be found in recent texts.[12–14]

BLOOD SUPPLY, LYMPHATIC DRAINAGE, AND INNERVATION OF THE PERINEUM AND EXTERNAL GENITALIA

Blood supply

The internal pudendal artery (Fig. 50-13) is an arterial trunk providing blood to all the perineal structures inferior to the pelvic diaphragm (see Figs. 50-10 and 50-14). It begins as a branch of the internal iliac artery located subperitoneally in the lateral pelvis. It exits the bony pelvis, crosses the sacrospinous ligament, and enters the ischiorectal fossa. At this point the artery along with the internal pudendal vein and nerve becomes enclosed by the obturator fascia forming the pudendal canal (of Alcock). As the artery enters the pudendal canal it gives off an inferior rectal artery that supplies the anorectal junction. The remaining portion of the internal pudendal artery reaches the base of the urogenital diaphragm and gives off a series of perineal branches. These supply the contents of both superficial and deep perineal spaces, including the vagina and urethra and clitoris.

The venous drainage of both perineal triangles parallels the arterial supply. There is also a rich submucosal venous plexus in the distal vagina. Distension of these submucosal veins can produce vaginal or vulvar varices. The inferior rectal veins join the internal pudendal vein just as it leaves the ischiorectal fossa at the lesser sciatic foramen. Both the rectal and vaginal submucosal plexuses penetrate the pelvic diaphragm to communicate with the endopelvic space. Here, vaginal veins may anastomose with uterine veins and inferior rectal veins with middle rectal veins.

Lymphatic drainage

As a general rule, lymphatic drainage follows the blood supply of a region. The lymphatic drainage of the perineum differs in this respect because there is a dual pathway. Deep lymphatics course upward following the pudendal veins, draining the deep parts of both urogenital and anal triangles. However, superficial lymphatics from the skin overlying the vulvar and anal areas course to the medial thigh where they communicate with superficial inguinal lymph nodes. Adenopathy of superficial inguinal nodes is well known in many vulvar and anal infections as well as in carcinoma of these regions.

Innervation

The motor and sensory innervation of the perineum is via fibers from sacral roots S2, S3, and S4 forming the pudendal nerve (Fig. 50-14). Originating from the sacral plexus in the presacral region, the pudendal nerve exits the pelvis via the greater sciatic notch, crosses the sacrospinous ligament, enters the pudendal canal, and accompanies the pudendal vessels. The branches of the internal pudendal nerve are the inferior rectal, perineal, and dorsal clitoral nerves, supplying these respective areas.

BLOOD SUPPLY, LYMPHATIC DRAINAGE, AND INNERVATION OF UTERUS AND VAGINA

Blood supply

The uterus and upper vagina lie within the endopelvic space, that is, between the pelvic peritoneum and the pelvic diaphragm. These

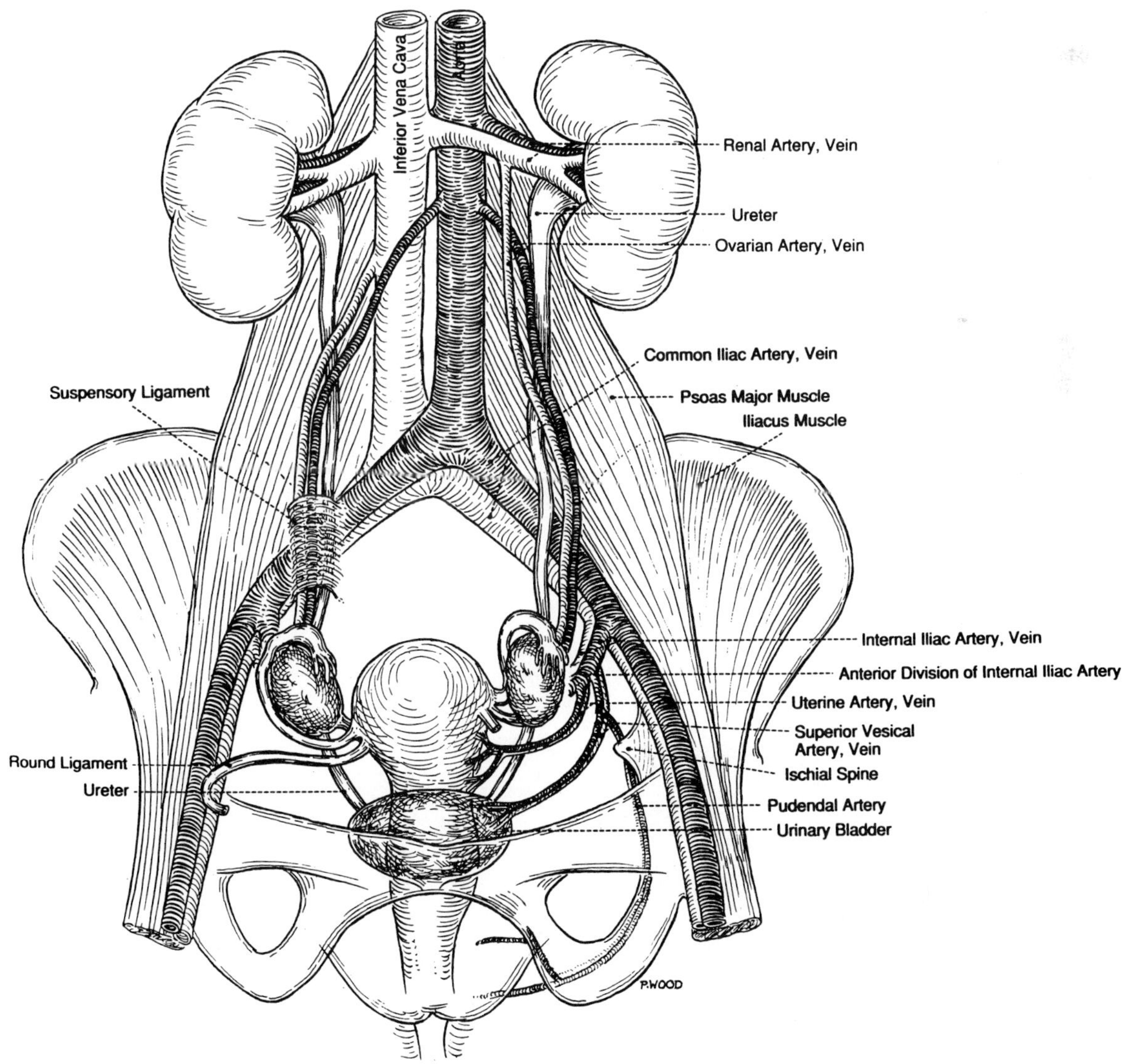

Fig. 50-13. Blood supply of female reproductive tract.

structures as well as the adjacent, rectum, bladder, and so on, are all supplied by a single arterial trunk, the internal iliac artery (see Fig. 50-13). It arises by division of the common iliac artery at the junction of the sacrum and the ilium. Descending in the laterial pelvis subperitoneally it gives off a series of visceral branches including rectal, uterine, and vesical. These course medially to enter the endopelvic space, at the base of the broad ligament. Before reaching the isthmus of the uterus the uterine artery crosses superior to the ureter, and gives branches to the vaginal fornix and cervix. Turning superiorly in the parametrial space of the broad ligament, a series of arterial branches is given to the body of the uterus until the artery anastomoses with the ovarian artery at the uterotubal junction.

The uterine vein is usually plexiform, coursing laterally in the base of the broad ligament before reaching the lateral pelvic wall. Here the plexus of veins forms a series of tributaries entering the internal iliac vein, which in turn empties into the inferior vena cava. Other veins in the endopelvic space include middle rectal veins draining the rectum.

The normal route of rectal venous flow is into the internal iliac vein. During pregnancy, the fetus may partially occlude the inferior vena cava when the woman is recumbent, increasing venous resistance and diminishing pelvic venous flow into the inferior vena cava. Because the middle rectal veins also communicate with the superior rectal branches of the inferior mesenteric vein, there is the potential that pelvic blood can ascend via the portal circulation. None of the pelvic veins contains valves, allowing blood to take the pathway of least resistance. Middle rectal veins also communicate with inferior rectal veins; these veins are tributaries of the internal pudendal vein that drains into the iliac veins before entering the inferior vena cava. Increased blood flow in these vessels, particularly in the last trimester of pregnancy, is a well-known cause of hemorrhoids.

Lymphatic drainage

A plexus of uterine lymphatics parallels the course of uterine veins, entering regional lymph nodes along the internal iliac artery. From these nodes lymph trunks ascend to paraaortic nodes in the retroperitoneum.

The endopelvic space is the primary pathway for both motor and sensory nerve fibers supplying the uterus (see Fig. 50-14). Sensory fibers from the uterine body descend in the parametrial space of the broad ligament to join other fibers from the cervix. These form a large plexus in the paracervical region termed the utero-vaginal plexus or Frankenhauser's ganglion. In the endopelvic space these fibers commingle with visceral afferents from other pelvic viscera, before entering the inferior hypogastric plexus. Ascending the sacral promontory the fibers join the superior hypogastric plexus and enter the sympathetic trunk via lumbar splanchnic nerves.

From sympathetic ganglia white rami communicans conduct fibers to the dorsal roots of spinal nerves T10 to T12.

The uterovaginal plexus also includes parasympathetic motor fibers from sacral roots that enter the endopelvic space directly, as well as sympathetic motor fibers that enter from the sympathetic trunk. Concentration of uterine sensory fibers in the uterovaginal plexus is the anatomical basis for a regional anesthetic procedure, paracervical block. It is accomplished by inserting the needle of a syringe into each lateral vaginal fornix and infiltrating the paracervical area with a local anesthetic. This will often provide adequate anesthesia for instrumentation of the cervix and uterus.

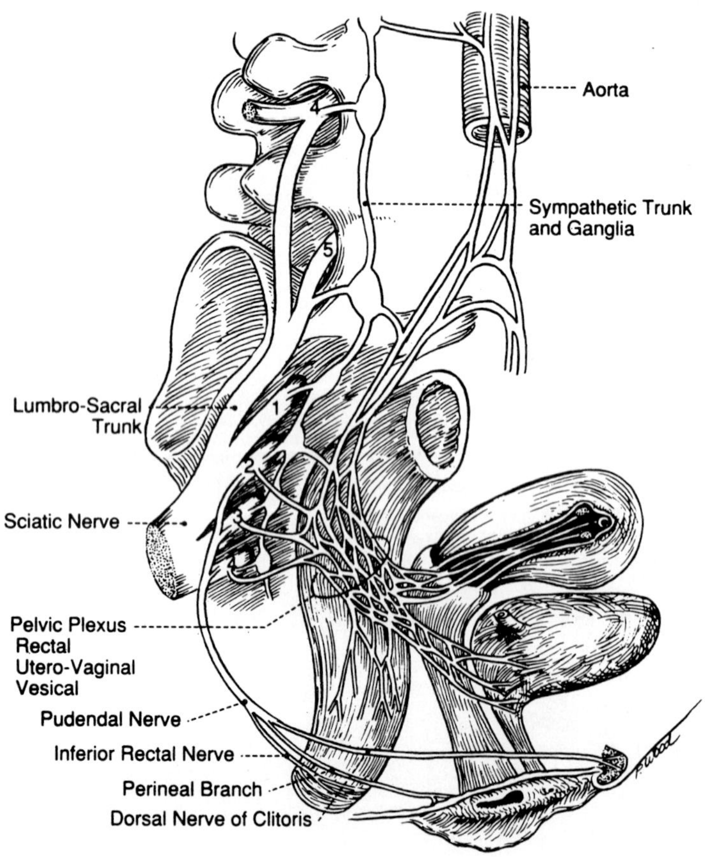

Fig. 50-14. Innervation of female reproductive tract.

BLOOD SUPPLY, LYMPHATIC DRAINAGE, AND INNERVATION OF THE OVARY AND UTERINE TUBE

Blood supply

The ovarian arteries arise as lateral branches from the abdominal aorta, descend in the retroperitoneal space, cross the ala of the sacrum, and enter the suspensory ligament of the ovary (see Fig. 50-13). As the ovarian artery enters the lateral edge of the broad ligament it courses medially between the two layers of the ligament, giving branches to the ovary and uterine tube.

The venous drainage of the structures in the superior part of the broad ligament is via the ovarian vein, which parallels the ovarian artery as the vein ascends in the retroperitoneal space. On the right side the ovarian vein is a tributary of the inferior vena cava, whereas on the left side it drains into the left renal vein.

Lymphatic drainage

Afferent lymphatics from the ovarian and uterine tube accompany ovarian vessels to paraaortic lymph nodes in the retroperitoneum. The fundus of the uterus is drained in part by this same route but also sends lymphatic vessels anteriorly paralleling the course of the round ligaments of the uterus. This bilateral course carries afferent lymphatics to inguinal lymph nodes on both sides of the pelvis.

Innervation

The suspensory ligament of the ovary is also the afferent neural pathway for the ovary and uterine tube (see Fig. 50-8). After reaching the retroperitoneum, these fibers join the superior hypogastric plexus, ascend briefly, and then enter a lumbar splanchnic to reach the sympathetic trunk. Ascending fibers leave the sympathetic trunk via rami communicantes to enter spinal sensory roots T10 to T12.

References

1 Ryan CA et al: Editorial: How should clinical algorithms be used for syndromic management of cervical and vaginal infections? *Clin Infect Dis* 21:1456–1458, 1995.

2 Ryan CA et al: Risk assessment, symptoms and signs as predictors of vulvovaginal and cervical infections in an urban US. STD clinic: implications for use of STD algorithms. *Sex Trans Infect* 74(Suppl 1): S59–S76, 1998.

3 Dalabetta G et al: Problems, solutions, and challenges in syndrome management of sexually transmitted diseases. *Sex Trans Infect* 74(Suppl 1):S1–S11, 1998.

4 US Preventive Services Task Force: Guide to clinical preventive services: Report of the US Preventive Services Task Force, 2nd ed. Baltimore, Williams & Wilkins, 1995.

5 The Technical Guidelines/Competence Working Group: Recommendations for Updating Selected Practices in Contraceptive Use. USAID & WHO, Vol. I, II, 1997.

6 Guidelines for Adolescent Preventive Services, Recommendations Monograph, 2nd ed. Chicago, Department of Adolescent Health, American Medical Association, 1995.

7 Armstrong KA et al: SMART START: An option for adolescents to delay pelvic examination and blood work in family planning clinics. *J Adolesc Hlth* 15:386–395, 1994.

8 Lee HH et al: Diagnosis of *Chlamydia trachomatis* genitourinary infection in women by ligase chain reaction assay of urine. *Lancet* 345: 213–236, 1995.

9 Schachter J et al: Noninvasive test for diagnosis of *Chlamydia trachomatis* infection: Application of ligase chain reaction to first-catch urine specimens in women. *J Infect Dis* 172:1411–1414, 1995.

10 Ching S et al: Ligase Chain reaction for detection of *Neisseria gonorrhoeae* in urogenital swabs. *J Clin Microbiol* 33(12):3111–3114, 1995.

11 Smith KR et al: Evaluation of ligase chain reaction for use with urine for identification of *Neisseria gonorrhoeae* in females attending a sexually transmitted disease clinic. *J Clin Microbiol* 33(2):455–457, 1995.

12 Fawcett DW: *A Textbook of Histology*, 12th ed. New York, Chapman & Hall, 1994.

13 Rosse C et al: *Hollinshead's Textbook of Anatomy*, 5th ed. Philadelphia, Lippincott, 1997.

14 Williams PL et al: *Gray's Anatomy*, 38th ed. London, Churchill Livingstone, 1995.

15 Schutter EM et al: Diagnostic value of pelvic examination, ultrasound, and serum CA 125 in postmenopausal women with a pelvic mass. An international multicenter study. *Cancer* 74(4):1398–1406, 1994.

16 Dodson MG: Use of transvaginal ultrasound in diagnosing the etiology of menometrorrhagia. *J Reprod Med* 39(5):362–372, 1994.

17 Goldstein SR: Early detection of pathologic pregnancy by transvaginal sonography. *J Clin Ultrasound* 18(4):262–273, 1990.

Chapter 51

Clinical anatomy, histology, and physical examination of the male genital tract

John N. Krieger
Daniel O. Graney

Any area of the body may be involved in sexually transmitted disease syndromes or in the differential diagnosis of these conditions. Clearly there is no single, optimal method for conducting the history and physical examination. The critical areas of interest are determined by the history, other physical findings, and conditions considered in the differential diagnosis. There are as many correct ways of eliciting historical data and physical findings as there are clinicians. Similarly, there are many critical anatomical points that may be important in some contexts yet irrelevant in others. Thus, this chapter reflects our bias and represents an attempt to succinctly present one approach to "the routine examination." Pertinent genitourinary tract anatomy and histology will be presented in the context of this examination. This approach is selective in the extreme, but it is based on our own clinical experience in developing an efficient method for evaluating a large number of patients in a timely manner.

Most often, the standard examination of a patient in our clinic proceeds according to an orderly sequence. The pertinent portions of the examination usually follow the outline in Table 51-1. Proceeding in this fashion has two advantages. First, there is an orderly sequence to the examination that limits the opportunity for errors of omission in a busy clinical situation. Second, there is a minimal need for the patient to move. Ordinarily, we initiate the examination by having the patient sit on the examining table. If necessary, head and neck examination and percussion and auscultation of the chest may be done in this position. Next, the patient is asked to lie supine. Cardiovascular examination may be conducted in this position, if indicated, and attention is directed to the abdominal examination. The patient is then asked to stand for examination of the groin and genitalia. Finally, the patient is asked to turn and bend over, placing his elbows on the examining table, for the rectal and prostate examination. In sum, there is minimal need for the patient to move from position to position if the examination is done in this order.

The remainder of this chapter is organized to follow this suggested pattern of evaluation. The relevant considerations in routine examination of the male are presented for each section of the physical examination; critical anatomical principles and histology are considered for that area. Throughout, we emphasize a practical approach and minimize use of Latin terms. This means that we present the anatomy according to our own opinions, recognizing that some of these opinions are controversial and that other anatomists or clinicians may hold alternative, equally valid, viewpoints.

There are two major differences in anatomy and examination between male and female patients. First, in the male we are talking about genitourinary tract examination. In the female there is a urinary tract and a separate genital tract. These two functions are combined in the male lower genitourinary tract, in which the urethra serves as a common conduit for the excretory functions of the urinary tract and for the reproductive functions of delivery of semen. The second major difference is that the critical reproductive organs in the male are all easily palpable. In contrast, the reproductive organs in the female are located in the pelvis and therefore may be examined less readily than the comparable structures in the male. The clinical implication is that examination of the male lower urinary tract and the entire male genital tract is readily accomplished and is straightforward in most patients.

EXAMINATION OF THE ABDOMEN AND GROIN

ABDOMEN

Complete details of the abdominal examination are beyond the scope of this chapter. However, brief mention is necessary of the pelvic organs, specifically the urinary bladder. This may be distended in patients with bladder outflow obstruction caused by an enlarged prostate or urethral stricture, and occasionally in patients with neurological dysfunction, as may occur with herpetic infections. The normal bladder is not palpable or percussible when it is empty or nearly empty because of its location in the pelvis. As the volume increases to approximately 125 to 150 mL, the dome of the bladder rises out of the pelvis into the lower abdomen and may project above the symphysis pubis. As it continues to fill, the bladder rises progressively toward the umbilicus. When the bladder contains 400 mL or more, it may be identifiable by observation as a bulge in the lower abdomen. Percussion over a distended bladder may cause the patient to experience a desire to void and may result in a change of the normal resonance of the lower abdomen on percussion to a dull note. The distended bladder may be palpated as a firm, round, and tender mass in the lower abdomen.

GROIN

The groin or inguinal region should be examined for the presence of adenopathy while the patient is lying supine on the examining table. The patient is then asked to stand and the inguinal area is again examined for the presence of hernia by direct palpation of the area and again by insertion of the index finger through the neck of the scrotum following the spermatic cord. Both examinations are done with the patient standing quietly and again while he is straining.

GENITALIA

PENIS

Examination

It is critical that the clinic staff instruct patients to refrain from voiding, if at all possible, prior to examination because signs of urethritis may not be apparent if the patient has recently voided. In fact, in symptomatic patients who do not have objective evidence of urethritis on examination or on the urethral smear, it is our practice to repeat the examination prior to the first urination of the day. Initially, attention is directed to examination of the skin. Use of a good light source and a hand lens is strongly recommended in evaluating possible lesions.

Attention is then directed to examination of the penis. In uncircumcised patients, the foreskin should be retracted to rule out phimosis with an obstructing small opening. This maneuver may reveal balanitis, condylomata, and occasionally, tumor, as the cause of a foul discharge. The glans and inner surface of the foreskin should be inspected to rule out presence of ulcers, vesicles,

Table 51-1. Routine STD Examination of the Male

General appearance
Skin
Abdominal examination
Groin
Hernia
Adenopathy
Genitalia
Penis
Prepuce
Urethral meatus
Shaft
Scrotum
Testes
Vasa
Epididymedes
Rectal examination
Sphincter tone
Fissure, hemorrhoids, or mass lesions
Prostate examination
Laboratory studies
Stool guaiac
Urethral smear
Urinalysis
Other

or warts. The location of the meatus is determined and the urethra is examined for presence of spontaneous discharge. If the location of the urethral meatus is abnormal, it can usually be found by following the midline along the undersurface of the penis. This is the most common location for an abnormal orifice and is termed *hypospadias.* Hypospadias is associated with a prepuce that does not completely encircle the glans but is incomplete on the lower surface. This is commonly termed a "hooded prepuce." Patients with more severe degrees of hypospadias, in which the urethral opening is located at the base of the penis or on the perineum, often have bifid, or split, scrotums. Rarely, the location of the urethral meatus may be on the upper surface of the phallus, a condition termed *epispadias.* In either hypospadias or epispadias, there is apt to be chordee, or an abnormal curvature of the phallus. Partial or complete duplication of the urethra may be noted. Commonly, patients with urethral duplications who present with urethritis have involvement of the accessory urethral meatus. The urethral meatus is examined by pinching the glans between the thumb and the forefinger at the 6 and 12 o'clock positions. This is important to exclude presence of meatal stenosis or intraurethral lesions, such as condylomata.

The shaft of the penis is palpated, looking for firm fibrosis plaques (characteristic of Peyronie's disease) and the urethra is palpated for evidence of induration. Induration is often secondary to infection, stricture (or scarring), or, rarely, tumor, abscess, or foreign body inserted by the patient. At this point, the urethra should be "milked" or stripped, beginning at the bulbous urethra (located at the perineal body, behind the scrotum in the midline) and proceeding to the meatus. This is necessary for evaluation for urethritis and may result in an expression of discharge at the meatus.

Anatomy

Major Divisions. There are two parts of the penis, the base, which is attached to the pubis, and the pendular portion. Underlying the penile skin there are three cavernous erectile bodies, the paired corpora cavernosa that are primarily concerned with erection, and the corpus spongiosum, which contains the urethra. These erectile bodies are separate structures at the base of the penis but become bound by fascia along the shaft of the penis (Fig. 51-1). The corpora cavernosa are cylindrical bodies in the shaft region but taper markedly at the base where they attach to the pubic ramus and perineal membrane. The corpus spongiosum has three parts; beginning at the perineum these are the bulb of the penis, the spongy portion, and the glans at the tip of the penis.

The base and proximal portion of the penile shaft are covered by thin muscles (see Fig. 51-1). The paired ischiocavernosus muscles overlie the crura and corpora cavernosa. Another pair of muscles, the buibospongiosus, overlies the corpus spongiosum.

Urethra and Glans. The urethra is named according to the part of the penis that it is traversing. Thus, in the penis the urethra is divided into bulbous, spongy, and glandular portions. The bulbous and spongy parts of the urethra are lined by a pseudostra-

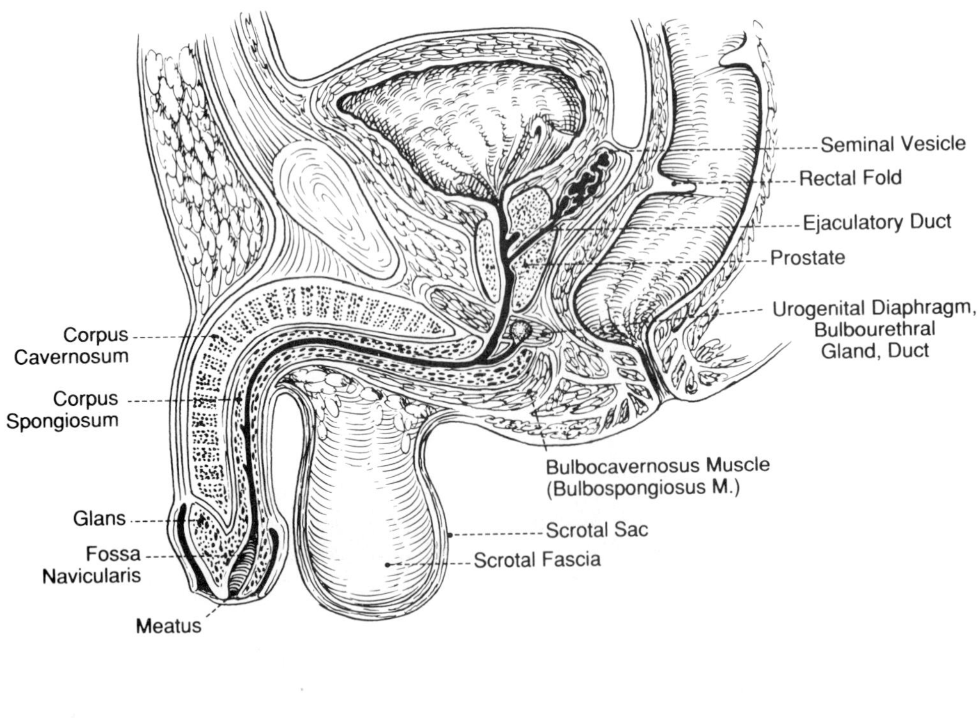

Fig. 51-1. Sagittal section of pelvis and male reproductive system.

tified columnar epithelium, except at the tip of the penis, termed *the fossa navicularis,* which is lined by stratified squamous epithelium. The epithelium contains small acini of mucous cells (glands of Littré) as well as mucosal and submucosal glands termed *urethral* or *periurethral glands* (Figs. 51-2, 51-3, and 51-4). These glands become infected and form abscesses.

On the superior surface of the corona of the glans penis, as well as on the undersurface near the frenulum, there are sebaceous glands, the glands of Tyson. These glands secrete a white cheesy type of material that with desquamating epithelial cells forms the smegma, a substance that accumulates between the prepuce and glans of uncircumcised men.

SCROTUM

Examination

Skin. The scrotum and its contents are examined next. Palpation of the scrotal skin may reveal small sebaceous cysts. These structures may be multiple and, on occasion, become quite large or develop infections. Malignant tumors of the scrotum are rare. In contrast, scrotal hemangiomas, bluish, vascular malformations, are common, and they may bleed spontaneously or following sexual activity. After the skin and subcutaneous tissues of the scrotum and perineum have been palpated, attention is directed to the intrascrotal contents.

Scrotal Compartments. The scrotum has two compartments that are divided in the midline. Each side is the mirror image of the other, and an identical examination is carried out for each scrotal compartment. The testis is the most anterior intrascrotal structure and must be examined carefully. The second most important structure in the scrotum is the epididymis, which lies immediately posterior to the testis.

Testis. Each testis should be palpated using two hands. Hard areas within the testicular parenchyma must be regarded as potentially malignant until proved otherwise. Testicular tumors are the most common genital urinary tract malignancy in men 20 to 40 years old. Transillumination of all scrotal masses should be routine. The patient is placed in a dark room and a strong light is applied to the back of the scrotum. Light is transmitted well through benign cystic structures, such as hydroceles or spermatoceles, but not through solid mass lesions, such as testicular tumors. Tumors may be nodular in consistency but are often smooth. The testis that has been replaced by tumor or damaged by a gumma is often insensitive to pressure, and the usual sick sensation produced by firm pressure on the testis is absent. The testis may be absent from the scrotum as a result of maidescent during development, a condition known as *cryptorchidism,* or as the result of abnormal mobility within the scrotal sac and inguinal ring, a condition known as *retractile testis.* An atrophic testis is small and flabby in consistency and may be hypersensitive. This may be congenital; following treatment of an undescended testes; the result of previous infection, such as mumps orchitis; or may follow torsion or previous surgery, such as hernia repair. Although sperm production may not occur in these organs, hormone production may continue. Very small (1.5 × 1 × 1 cm), abnormally firm testes in a young adult usually are attributable to Klinefelter's syndrome, a relatively common condition present in 0.2 percent of men and is

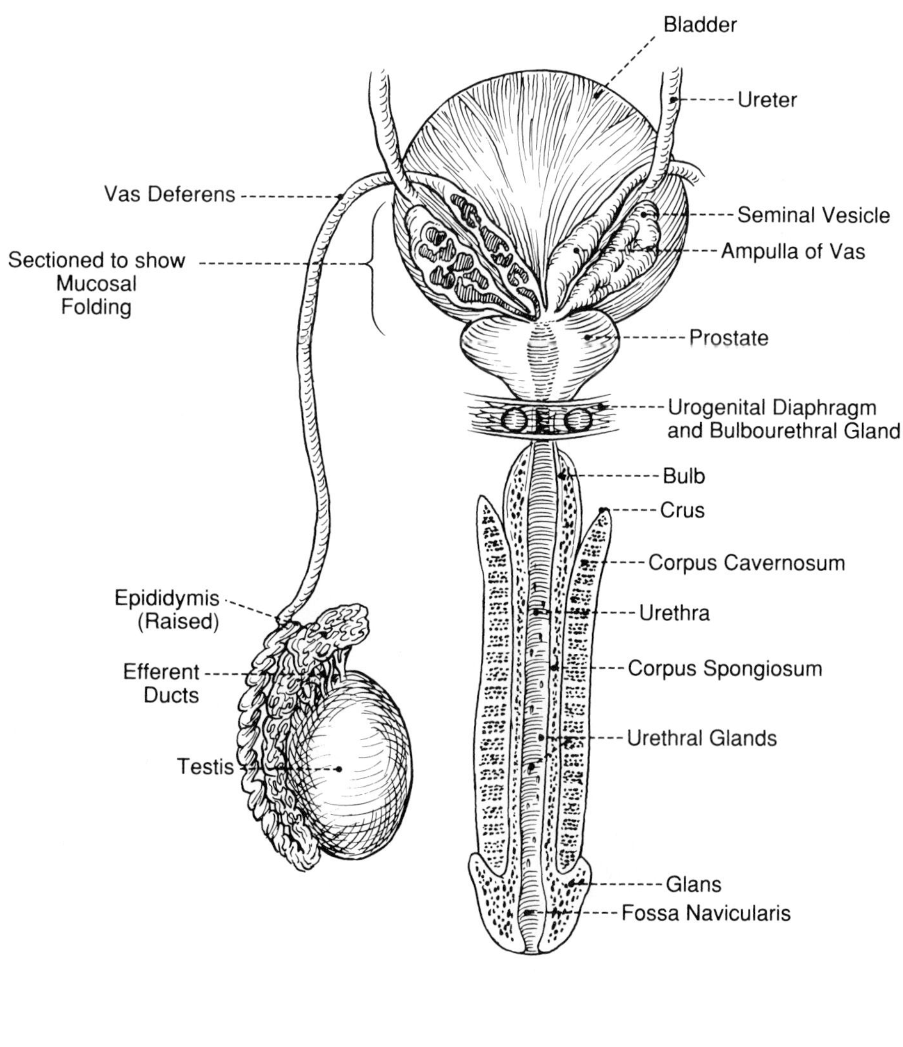

Fig. 51-2. Coronal section of male pelvis and urethra viewed posteriorly.

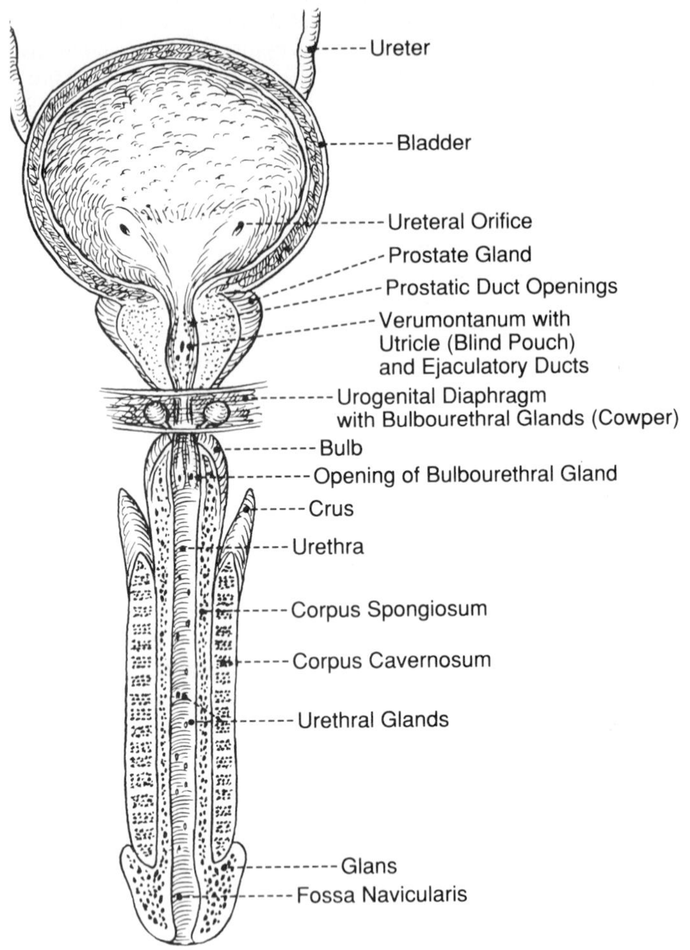

Fig. 51-3. Coronal section of male pelvis and urethra viewed anteriorly.

usually associated with infertility. Klinefelter's syndrome is associated with one Y and two X chromosomes. On occasion, the testis may twist within the scrotum, compromising its blood supply. This is termed *testicular torsion* and is one cause of acute scrotal pain and swelling.

Epididymis. The epididymis is a comma-shaped organ, that is usually applied closely to the posterior aspect of the testis. On occasion, however, the epididymis may be loosely applied to the testis. The epididymis should be carefully palpated for size, tenderness, and induration. Induration of the epididymis usually results from infection, as primary epididymal tumors are rare. It is often possible to feel the groove between the testis and the epididymis everywhere except superiorly, where the two structures are joined. During acute infections, the testis and epididymis are often indistinguishable, as both structures are involved in the inflammatory process. Tenderness is exquisite; swelling may be impressive and accompanied by an acute inflammatory hydrocele. In many men a small, ovoid mass, representing the appendix testis, a vestigial embryological structure, may be palpated near the groove between the upper pole of the testis and the epididymis. Occasionally, the appendix testis may twist, producing acute tenderness and swelling of the scrotum.

Spermatic Cord. The cord structures at the neck of the scrotum should be palpated between the thumb and index finger. The solid, rope-like vas is usually identified easily and may be followed to its junction with the tail of the epididymis. Other soft, stringy structures in the spermatic cord may be palpable but are usually not clearly defined. Swellings in the cord are usually cystic in nature (e.g., hydrocele or hernia) and are rarely solid (e.g., connective tissue tumor). Varicoceles represent collections of dilated veins, are usually present on the left side of the scrotum, are best demonstrated with the patient standing, and feel "like a bag of worms."

Anatomy

Testis. The testis fulfills two main functions: It produces sperm and it secretes male hormones. Production of sperm takes place in the seminiferous tubules, whereas the production of testoster-

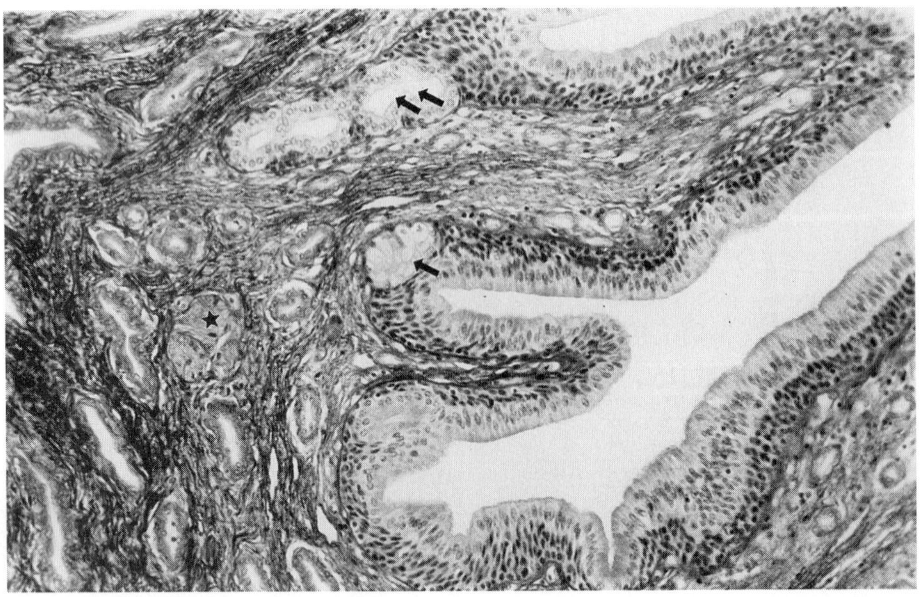

Fig. 51-4. Photomicrograph of the spongy portion of the penile urethra. Single arrow indicates intraepithelial gland of Littré. Double arrow indicates a crypt or lacuna formed by epithelial evagination. Star indicates periurethral submucosal glands. Human, iron hematoxylin aniline blue stain, ×135 in the original magnification.

one, the major male hormone, takes place in the tissue located between the tubules. Each testis contains approximately 400 to 600 seminiferous tubules. Individual tubules are up to 70 cm in length and are coiled along most of their length in order to be accommodated in a fascial compartment of the testis. These compartments are extensions of the outer fibrous capsule of the testis, the tunica albuginea. The seminiferous tubules join to form the rete testis, which is the connection to the excretory duct system.[1] The lining of the seminiferous tubules contains two main types of cells, the developing sperm cells and the Sertoli cells, which support and presumably "nurse" the sperm cells during their development process. Sperm are continuously produced in the testis from puberty to senility following an orderly sequence of events. In the testis this process takes about 64 days.[2–4] However, when they leave the testis, the sperm cells are immature and are unable to fertilize an egg.

Excretory Ducts. The excretory ducts transport sperm from the testis to the end of the male reproductive tract. The excretory ducts are composed of five elements, beginning from the testis: the efferent ducts, epididymis, vas, ejaculatory duct, and urethra.

EFFERENT DUCTS

There are approximately 12 efferent ducts, which are convoluted tubules connecting the rete testis to the epididymis. The epithelium lining the ductules contains both ciliated and nonciliated cells. Ciliary movement helps propel sperm toward the epididymis. On electron microscopy, the nonciliated cells are found to be lined by tall microvilli. Surrounding the epithelium are a thin basal lamina, lamina propria, and smooth muscle fibers oriented circularly.

EPIDIDYMIS

The epididymis receives the sperm and seminal fluid from each of the efferent ducts. The epididymis has three parts, the head, the body, and the tail. The initial segment of the epididymis is the head, which fuses with the efferent ductules. The epididymis continues inferiorly along the posterior surface of the testis as the body of the epididymis (see Fig. 51-2). At the inferior pole of the testis the epididymis thickens to form the tail.

Throughout its course the epididymis is lined by tall, thin columnar cells with nonmotile sterocilia (Fig. 51-5). In electron micrographs the sterocilia are found to be exceptionally long filamentous microvilli. In addition, the fine structure of these cells is typical of a cell that is both secretory (abundant rough endoplasmic reticulum and Golgi cisternae) and absorptive (epical vesicies and tubules).[5,6]

Within the epididymis, sperm undergo progressive maturation during their movement from the head to the tail. As sperm emerge from the testis they are infertile and relatively nonmotile. By the time they reach the tail of the epididymis, they are both motile and fertile.[7,8] The average time for sperm transit through the epididymis is 12 days.[9] The sperm and epididymal fluid together contribute about 10 percent of the ejaculate.

VAS

The vas is the continuation of the epididymal duct, with only slight modification of the epithelial surface but substantial thickening of the outer muscle coat. The thickness of the muscle coat produces the "whipcord" sensation when the vas is rolled between the thumb and forefinger during physical examination of the spermatic cord.

From the inferior pole of the testis, the vas ascends in the spermatic cord within the scrotum, until it reaches the superficial inguinal ring. After traversing the inguinal canal, the vas enters the preperitoneal space at the internal inguinal ring, where it courses inferiorly into the pelvis lying between the pelvic fascia and peritoneum. The terminal portion, or ampulla, of the vas is more dilated and fuses with the seminal vesicle to form the ejaculatory duct.

EJACULATORY DUCT

Traversing the substance of the posterior wall of the prostate, the ejaculatory duct opens into the prostatic urethra at the verumontanum, an oval-shaped mucosal excrescence.

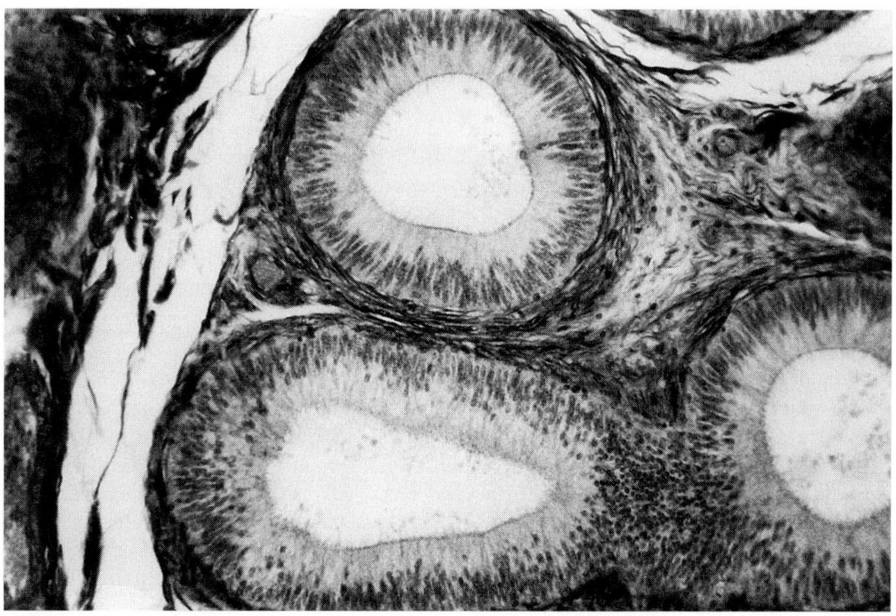

Fig. 51-5. Light micrograph of the ductus epididymis. Epithelium is composed of pseudostratified columnar cells with setereocilia. Human, Mallary azan stain, ×135 in the original magnification.

RECTUM AND PELVIC ORGANS

EXAMINATION

Inspection may reveal presence of external hemorrhoids, rectal fissures, or fistulas. Internal examination is then carried out by inserting a well-lubricated, gloved index finger into the anal canal. The sphincter tone is evaluated and the canal is examined for undue tenderness or induration. Presence of induration, rectal stenosis, or mass lesions may indicate the need for additional studies, such as anoscopy or procroscopy.

The prostate and seminal vesicles are palpated through the anterior rectal wall with the patient bent over the examining table. The normal prostate is about 4 cm in length and in width, about the size of the terminal segment of the thumb. The prostate is widest superiorly at the bladder neck. Two distinct "lobes" of the prostate are palpable, separated by a median sulcus, or indentation. Normally, the prostate gland is smooth, somewhat mobile, and nontender. The consistency is rubbery and resembles the tip of the nose.

One major problem in the prostate examination lies in differentiating firm areas. Differential diagnosis of a firm area in the prostate includes: cancer, calculi, infarction, granulomatous prostatitis, and nodular, benign hyperplasia. Even the most experienced examiner may have difficulty distinguishing among these possibilities on digital rectal examination.

Above the prostate it may be possible to feel soft, tubular seminal vesicles extending obliquely beneath the base of the bladder (see Fig. 51-2). Usually, clear presence of seminal vesicles on rectal examination indicates a pathological process. Most commonly, these patients have pelvic tumors such as prostate cancer or acute infectious processes.

Determination of the prostate specific antigen (PSA) level can prove helpful in evaluating patients with an abnormal prostate examination. Findings such as nodules, asymmetry, or loss of distinct sulci, suggest the possibility of prostate cancer. An elevated PSA provides further support for the possibility of cancer. Prostate biopsy is necessary for diagnosis. Elevation of the PSA and firm areas in the prostate may also occur following acute lower urogenital tract infections, such as prostatitis. In this setting reevaluation in several weeks may be appropriate.

Some authorities recommend annual PSA determination and rectal examination for all men over 50 years old.[1–3] These evaluations are also suggested for men over 40 if they have a family history of prostate cancer. Other investigators suggest that there is little evidence that routine PSA screening, with biopsies and aggressive treatment has improved the overall outcome for patients with prostate cancer. Lead-time and length-time biases may explain the results of many clinical series. Because aggressive diagnosis and treatment may be associated with considerable costs and morbidity, these authorities do not recommend routine screening.[4,5] Thus, the value of routine screening is debatable, but PSA testing is helpful for evaluating men with abnormal prostate glands on digital rectal examination.

ANATOMY

RECTUM

In the rectum, there are two to four permanent, semicircular transverse folds of the mucosa, which are termed rectal valves. They neither serve as valves nor support the feces, as suggested by some investigators. These valves are readily observed during endoscopy but may be lacerated during blind instrumentation of the rectum.

Microscopically, the mucosa of the rectum is composed of columnar absorptive cells, although goblet-type mucous cells are interspersed among the absorptive cells. Invaginations of the epithelial surface form straight, tubular colonic glands equivalent to the glands of Lieberkühn seen in the small intestine.

Rectoanal junction

The rectoanal junction is not a discrete point but a longitudinal mucosal fold extending superiorly from mucosa that is paler and flatter (Fig. 51-6). This gives the appearance of a horizontal band with teeth, hence the term *pectinate line* (Latin *pecten,* "comb"). The mucosal ridges forming the toothlike character of the line are termed *anal folds* or *columns* (of Morgagni). At the pectinate line between the base of the anal columns, the mucosa is redundant and outpockets to form the anal crypts. The epithelium of the anus, that is, distal to the pectinate line, is characterized by stratified squamous cells of the nonkeratinizing type.

Accessory sex glands

The male accessory sex glands include the seminal vesicles, prostate, and bulbourethral glands (Cowper's glands).

Seminal Vesicles. The seminal vesicles are paired, saccular glands with multiple foldings of their mucous membrane (Figs. 51-1 and 51-2). Embryologically they begin as tubular buds from the vas. Hence, the seminal vesicles join with the vas, forming a common ejaculatory duct.

The seminal vesicles are lined by multiple foldings of columnar epithelial cells (Fig. 51-7) with abundant Golgi, rough endoplasmic reticulum, and secretory granules in the apical cytoplasm. The mucosal folds of the seminal vesicles are supported by a moderate lamina propria, containing collagen and elastic fibers. There is also a substantial muscular coat, which is important in the emission of secretions.

The seminal vesicles secrete an alkaline, slightly yellowish viscid fluid which constitutes 60 to 70 percent of the ejaculate volume.[15] Fractionation by "split-ejaculate" techniques shows that the semen consists of a presperm prostatic fraction, a sperm-rich fraction, and a postsperm vesicular fraction.[16] Fructose and a variety of prostaglandins appear to be formed specifically by the seminal vesicle.[16,17,18] Fructose is the principal energy source for sperm motility, but the role of prostaglandins in male fertility is uncertain.

Prostate. The prostate gland is located between the bladder neck and the urogenital diaphragm (Figs. 51-1, 51-2, and 51-3). The prostate completely encircles the urethra.

Zones. The prostate gland is composed of three zones of tissue: a periurethral zone, surrounding the urethra; a wedge-shaped central zone, bounded by the ejaculatory duct, urethra, and base of the bladder; and a peripheral zone, composed of all remaining glandular tissue.[19,20]

The periurethral zone is composed of mucosal and submucosal glands penetrating the smooth muscle of the proximal urethra.[19,21,22] Benign hyperplasia originates in this region and may lead to obstruction of urinary outflow from the bladder.[19,23]

The central zone of the prostate is located between the urethra and ejaculatory duct. This area appears to be least susceptible to development of inflammatory, hyperplastic, or neoplastic disease.

The peripheral, or outer, zone is the portion of the prostate that is palpable on rectal examination.[20,24] It is lined by multiple

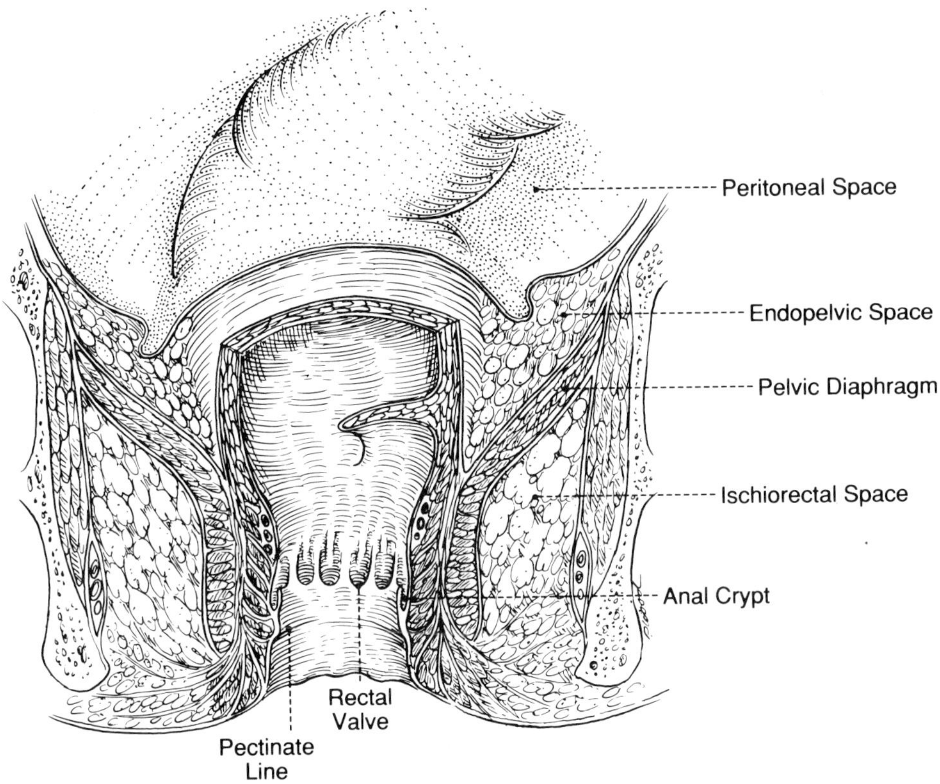

Fig. 51-6. Coronal section of male pelvis and rectoanal junction.

ducts (Fig. 51-8). The peripheral zone is also the region of the prostate that is most frequently involved in carcinoma and inflammation.[20]

Prostatic Secretions. The prostate contributes approximately 30 percent of the ejaculate volume, in the form of a thin, slightly opaque fluid.[15] The prostate gland appears to be important in protecting the male lower urogenital tract against infection, in providing enzymes for "liquefying" the semen after ejaculation, and in providing other components of the seminal fluid.[25] Normally the pH of prostatic fluid is around 7.[15] However, in men with well-documented bacterial prostatitis, the secretions alkalinize and may reach or exceed pH 8.[25] Zinc, magnesium, citric acid, and acid phosphatase in the ejaculate appear to originate in the prostatic secretions.[26–29]

Bulbourethral Glands (Cowper's Glands). These paired, pea-sized glands are located in the urogenital diaphragm (see Fig. 51-2). Their excretory ducts drain into the posterior urethra. The glands secrete a thin mucoid material during the excitatory stage

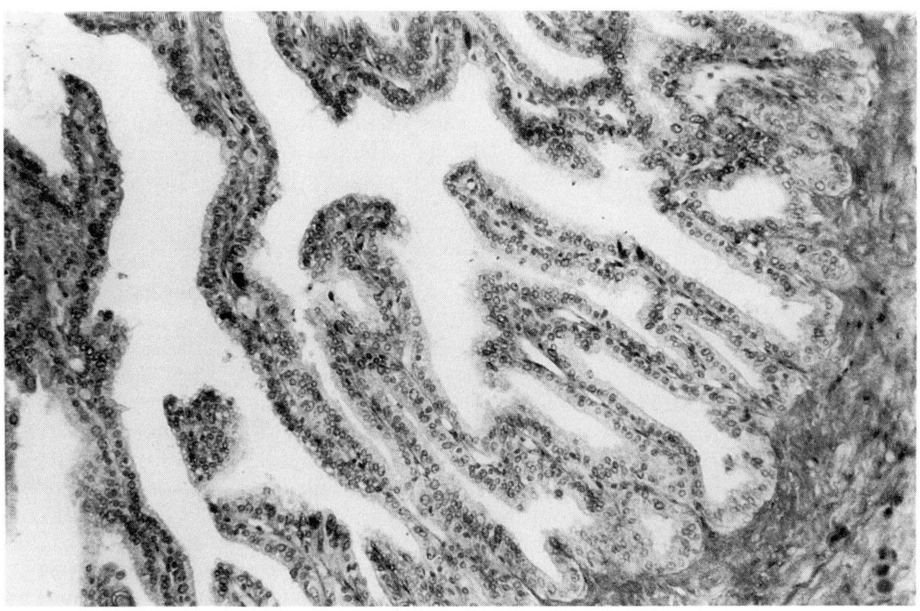

Fig. 51-7. Light micrograph of the seminal vesicle, illustrating multiple compound foldings of glands. Human, Mallory azan stain, ×135 in the original magnification.

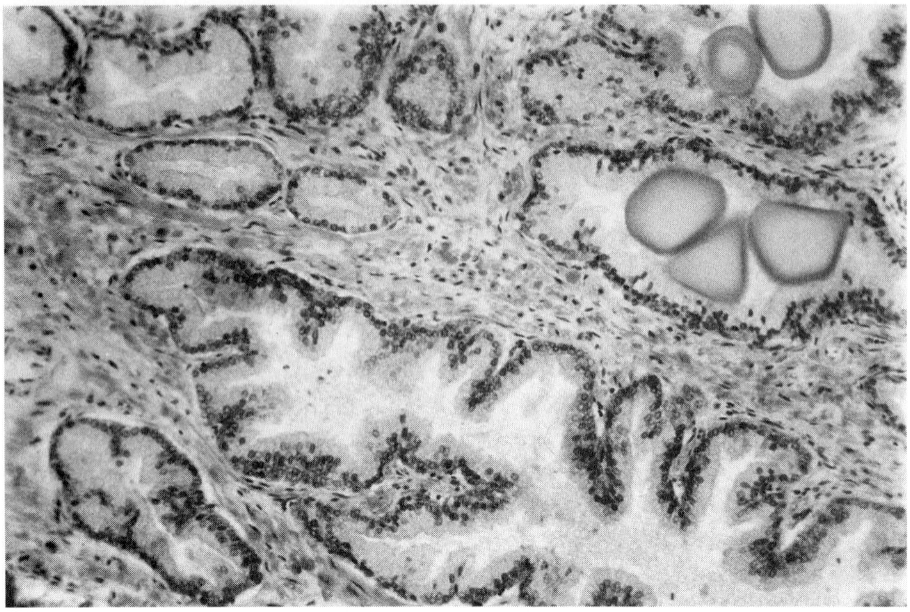

Fig. 51-8. Prostate gland of older man showing prostatic concretions and columnar epithelium. Human, H & E stain ×135 in the original magnification.

of sexual response, but the bulbourethral glands contribute only a minimal amount to the ejaculate. These glands are relatively immune to hyperplastic and neoplastic disease, although they can be involved in infections.[30]

BLOOD SUPPLY

ARTERIAL PATHWAYS (INTERNAL ILIAC ARTERY)

The pelvic organs in the male all receive their blood supply from the internal iliac artery. The internal iliac artery arises at the pelvic brim from the common iliac artery and immediately divides into an anterior and posterior division (Fig. 51-9).

Posterior division

The posterior division of the internal iliac artery provides small branches to the pelvic sidewall and has three branches that leave the pelvis, including the pudendal arteries.

The internal pudendal artery supplies the perineum (see Fig. 51-5). This includes all structures located in the ischiorectal fossa and superficial and deep pouches. As it leaves the pelvis via the greater sciatic notch, the pudendal artery gives off the inferior rectal artery and then enters the pudendal canal. The pudendal arteries have three areas of distribution: the anal canal, the perineum, and the phallus.

Anterior division

The anterior division of the internal iliac courses on the sidewall of the pelvis until it reaches the symphysis pubis, where it ascends the anterior abdominal wall. As it turns superiorly, the lumen of the vessel disappears and the vessel becomes a fibrous cord, the medial umbilical ligament. The internal iliac branches to form the middle rectal, superior, and inferior vesical arteries. The middle rectal artery supplies the rectum and has anastomosing branches with the superior rectal artery from the sigmoid. The superior vesicle artery supplies the fundus of the bladder, whereas the inferior vesicle artery supplies the bladder neck, seminal vesicle, vas deferens, and prostate. All these vessels anastomose with their members from the opposite side.

VENOUS AND LYMPHATIC PATHWAYS

Pelvic organs

Venous Drainage. The pelvic organs have abundant venous plexuses that give rise to larger veins that parallel the arterial pattern. These veins return blood from the pelvic organs to the internal iliac vein, which merges with the external iliac vessel to form the common iliac vein. This pathway joins the caval system of veins. Some blood in the perirectal region enters anastomotic channels in the mucosal plexus and ascends via the superior rectal vein to enter the portal drainage system.

Lymphatic Drainage. The lymphatic pathways from the pelvic organs follow the venous pattern. The first series of regional nodes are along the proximal parts of the internal iliac artery. From these nodes, lymphatic channels ascend to the aorta and the para-aortic lymphatic chain before entering the thoracic duct.

The sigmoid lymphatics follow the superior rectal veins to inferior mesenteric lymph nodes near the aorta.

Perineal structures

Venous Drainage. Most structures supplied by the pudendal artery are drained by veins that enter the internal pudendal vein. This vessel returns along a similar route to enter the internal iliac vein. There are two exceptions to this pattern: the anorectal region and the dorsum of the penis.

In the anorectal region blood may return via veins in the endopelvic space and eventually reach the vena cava through internal iliac tributaries or may continue superiorly to reach the superior rectal tributaries of the portal system. Increased venous pressure in this region, owing to increased venous resistance in either the portal system or the caval system, can result in anorectal hemorrhoids. The anorectal submucosal venous plexus is also a pathway for the spread of infection from the perianal and rectal areas to the endopelvic space.

The second nonpudendal venous pathway from the perineum is via the dorsal vein of the penis to the prostatic venous plexus at the neck of the bladder. These veins cross the urogenital diaphragm from the perineum to enter the endopelvic space. The prostatic veins are tributaries of the internal iliac system.

Lymphatic Drainage. The lymphatic drainage of the perineum differs from its venous drainage. In essence, all the skin and superficial structures of the perineum have lymphatics that course via the medial aspect of the thigh to the superficial inguinal nodes. Thus, anal and perianal ulcers caused by syphilis, chancroid, herpes simplex virus, or lymphogranuloma venereum cause inguinal lymphadenopathy. Channels from these nodes penetrate the fascia of the thigh at the saphenous opening to join the lymphatics from the leg. These lymphatic vessels course superiorly along the external iliac vein, then merge with paraaortic lymphatics.

An important exception is the lymphatic drainage of the testis, which does not follow the pattern described in the preceding. These lymphatics course superiorly in the spermatic cord, traverse the inguinal canal, and then ascend in the retroperitoneum with the testicular vein. In this manner the lymphatics reach the paraaortic lymph chain at the level of the renal vessels. This point is important clinically because metastases from testicular tumors do not cause inguinal adenopathy.

NERVE SUPPLY OF THE PERINEUM AND PELVIC ORGANS

The three neural components that must reach the perineal and pelvic structures are the somatic, parasympathetic, and sympathetic nerves.

Only the perineum is supplied by somatic fibers. These arise in spinal cord segments S-2, S-3, and S-4, and travel via the pudendal nerve to all the skin and structures of the anal and urogenital triangles (Fig. 51-10). The pudendal nerve leaves the pelvis along with the pudendal vessels, entering the pudendal canal after giving off the inferior rectal nerves. These supply the perineal skin, external anal sphincter, and the skin of the anal canal. The pudendal nerve then divides into a perineal branch, supplying the deep and superficial pouch structures, and the dorsal nerve of the penis, supplying the skin of the penis. Branches of the perineal division supply the urogenital diaphragm, superficial perineal muscle, and skin of the scrotum.

PARASYMPATHETIC NERVE SUPPLY

The parasympathetic innervation of the pelvic organs is also derived from spinal segments S-2, S-3, and S-4. However, these fibers originate from neurons in the intermediolateral gray rather than the ventral gray, which is the origin for fibers in the pudendal nerve. After these fibers leave the anterior sacral foramina, they join to form the pelvic splanchnic nerve (nervi erigentes), which contributes these fibers to the plexus surrounding the viscera. This is termed the pelvic plexus. These fibers traverse the plexus without synapsing and enter the walls of the pelvic organs, rectum, bladder, and prostate, where they synapse in intramural ganglia. Short postganglionic fibers are then relayed to the muscle fibers.

SYMPATHETIC NERVE SUPPLY

Sympathetic fibers to the pelvic viscera are believed to originate in the intermediolateral gray of the spinal segments T-12 to L-2.

After joining a spinal nerve, they enter a sympathetic ganglion for that segment but do not synapse in the ganglion. The fibers descend briefly in the sympathetic chain, then course medially to enter the superior hypogastric plexus anterior to the aorta. The preganglionic fibers descend in the plexus to the inferior hypogastric plexus, which divides around the lateral sides of the pelvic organs and becomes the pelvic plexus (rectal, vesical, or prostatic).

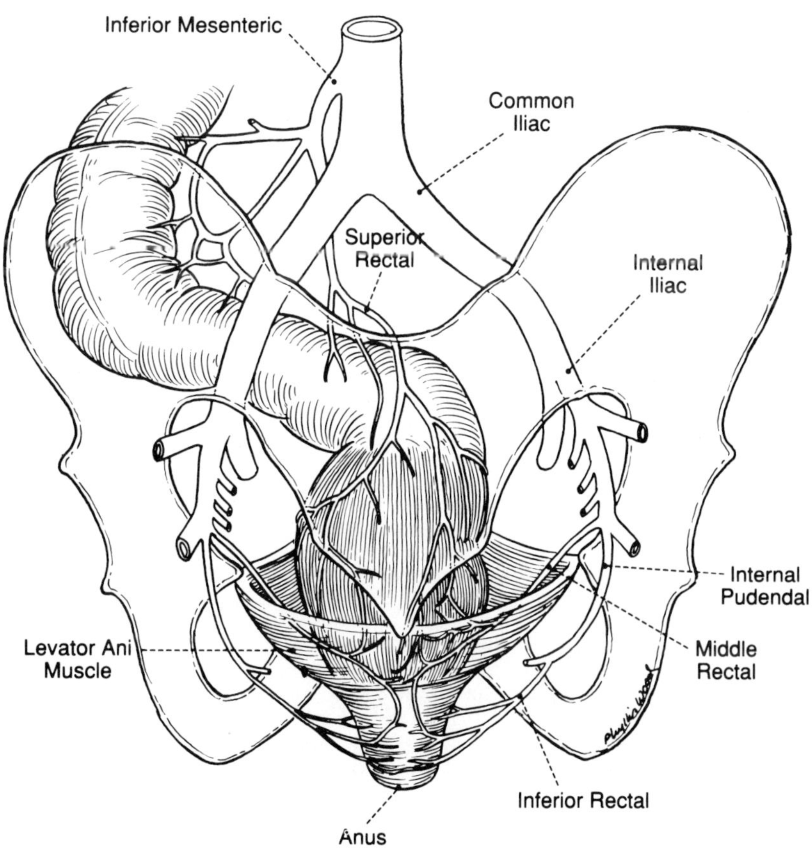

Fig. 51-9. Branches of the internal iliac artery and the distribution of the internal pudendal artery.

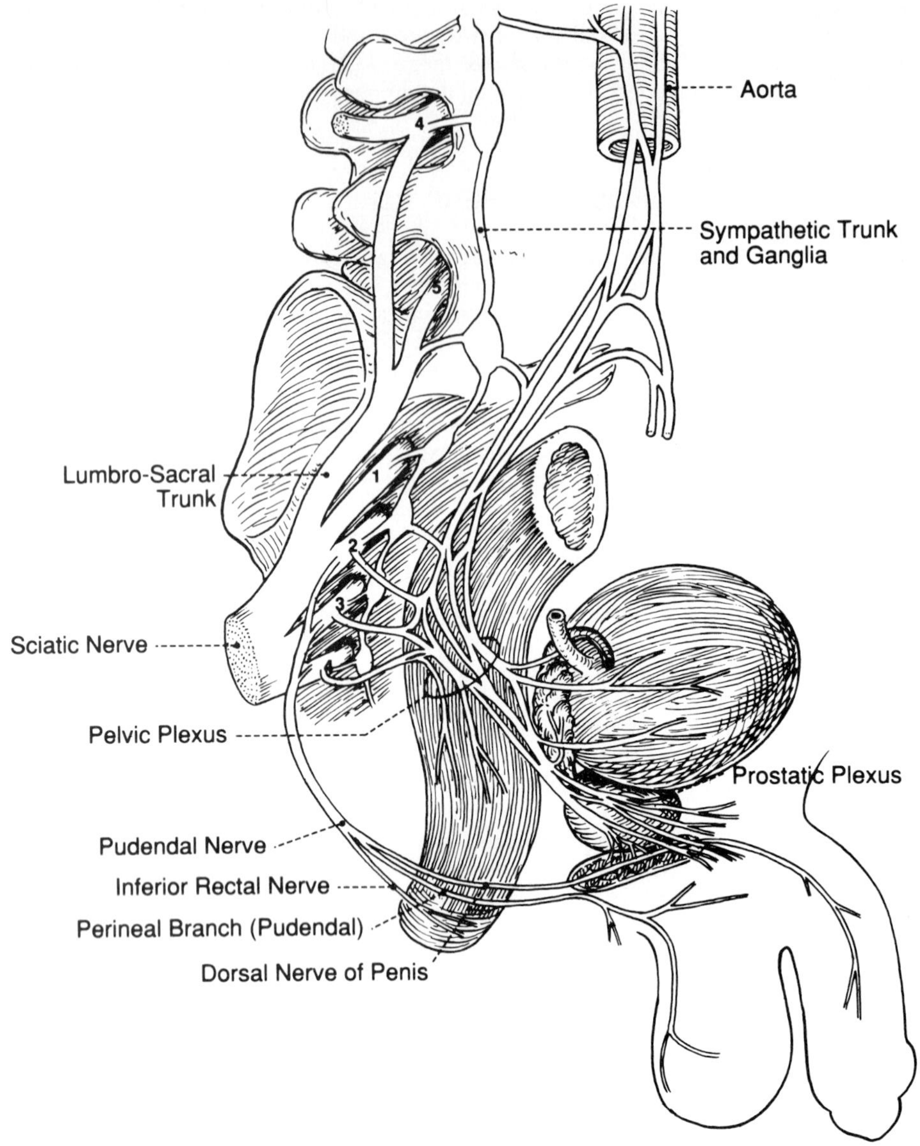

Fig. 51-10. Innervation of the pelvic viscera.

Synapses occur in the plexus or in the capsule of the organ innervated.

The pelvic plexus, therefore, is a mixture of parasympathetic and sympathetic fibers. In the region of the prostate, there is a group of fibers that course anteriorly at the upper edge of the urogenital diaphragm and supply the cavernous tissues of the penis (cavernous nerve). These fibers contain both parasympathetic and sympathetic components.

References

1 Roosen-Runge EC et al: The human rete testis. *Cell Tissue Res* 189: 409, 1978.
2 Roosen-Runge EC: The process of spermatogenesis in mammals. *Biol Rev* 37:343, 1962.
3 Clermont Y: Kinetics of spermatogenesis in mammals: seminiferous epithelium cycle and spermatogonial renewal. *Physiol Rev* 52:198, 1972.
4 Rowley MJ et al: Duration of transit of spermatozoa through the human male ductular system. *Fertil Steril* 21:390, 1970.
5 Holstein AF: Structure of the human epididymis, in ES Hafez (ed): *Human Semen and Fertility Regulation in Man.* St. Louis, Mosby, 1976, p. 23.
6 Hamilton DW: Structure and function of the epithelium lining the ductuli efferentes, ductus epididymis and ductus deferens in the rat, in *Handbook of Physiology,* sec 7: *Endrocrinology,* vol 5: *Male Reproductive System,* Hamilton DW et al (eds). Washington, American Physiological Society, 1975, p. 259.
7 Hinton BT: The epididymal microenvirornment. A site of attack for a male contraceptive? *Invest Urol* 18:1, 1980.
8 Hafez ES, Prasad MR: Functional aspects of the epididymis, in *Human Semen and Fertility Regulation in Men,* Hafez ESE (ed). St. Louis, Mosby, 1976, p. 31.
9 Hoffer A: The ultrastructure of the ductus deferens in man. *Biol Reprod* 14:425, 1976.
10 Chodak GW: Screening for prostate cancer. The debate continues. *JAMA* 272:813, 1994.
11 Epstein JI: Can insignificant prostate cancer be predicted preoperatively in men with stage T1 disease? *Semin Urol Oncol* 14:165, 1996.
12 Kuritzky L: PSA: to screen or not to screen. *Hosp Pract Off Ed* 31: 145, 1996.
13 Chodak GW: Screening for prostate cancer. *Eur Urol* 2:3, 1993.

14 Chodak GW: Urology. *JAMA* 271:1717, 1994.
15 Lundquist F: Aspects of the biochemistry of human semen. *Acta Physiol Scand* 19(Suppl)66, 1949.
16 Mann T: Biochemistry of semen, in *Handbook of Physiology,* sec 7: *Endocrinology,* vol 5, *Male Reproductive System,* Hamilton DW et al (eds). Washington, American Physiological Society, 1975, p. 461.
17 Eliasson R et al: Functions of male accessory genital organs, in *Human Semen and Fertility Regulation in Men,* Hafez ES (ed). St. Louis, Mosby, 1976, p. 44.
18 Polakoski KL et al: Biochemistry of human seminal plasma, in *Human Semen and Fertility Regulation in Men,* Hafez ES (ed). St. Louis, Mosby, 1976, p. 133.
19 McNeal JE: Regional morphology and pathology of the prostate. *Am J Clin Pathol* 49:347, 1968.
20 McNeal JE: The anatomic heterogeneity of the prostate. *Prog Clin Biol Res* 37:149, 1980.
21 Lowsley OS: Development of the human prostate with reference to the development of other structures at the neck of the bladder. *Am J Anat* 13:299, 1912.
22 LeDuc IE: The anatomy of the prostate and the pathology of early benign hypertrophy. *J Urol* 42:1217, 1939.
23 Franks LM: Benign nodular hyperplasia of prostate: review. *Ann Roy Coll Surg* 14:92, 1954.
24 Salander H et al: The histology of the dorsal, lateral and medial prostatic lobes in man. *Invest Urol* 18:479, 1981.
25 Fair AT et al: The pH of prostatic fluid: reappraisal and therapeutic implications. *J Urol* 120:695, 1978,
26 Eliasson R et al: Zinc in human seminal plasma. *Andrologie* 3:147, 1971.
27 Eliasson R et al: Magnesium in human seminal plasma. *Invest Urol* 9: 286, 1971.
28 Mann T: *The Biochemistry of Semen and of the Male Reproductive Tract.* New York, Wiley, 1964.
29 Huggins C: The prostatic secretion. *Harvey Lecture* 42:148, 1947.
30 Elbadawi A: Pathology of male accessory genital glands. II. Proliferative diseases and neoplasms, in Accessory Glands of the Male Reproductive Tract, Spring-Mills E et al (eds). Ann Arbor, Ann Arbor Science, 1979.

Chapter 52

Principles of treatment of sexually transmitted diseases

H. Hunter Handsfield

Most treatment decisions for STDs seem straightforward, made on the basis of the clinician's past experience and general knowledge, sometimes with reference to standardized guidelines such as those of the Centers for Disease Control and Prevention (CDC)[1] (See Appendix A) or the World Health Organization (WHO).[2] In reality, however, the basis for treatment decisions is complex. This chapter reviews the theoretical underpinnings of the antimicrobial therapy of sexually transmitted infections and discusses current controversies and dilemmas in the treatment of selected STDs.

APPROACHES TO TREATMENT

THERAPEUTIC GOALS

There are several goals of treatment for STDs (Table 52-1). From the perspective of the individual patient, the ultimate goal is *biological cure*, or eradication of the infecting organism from the host. For the bacterial STDs biological cure is closely linked to resolution of signs and symptoms and to the prevention of complications, but biological cure does not guarantee these outcomes. Biological cure is the norm for treatment of gonorrhea, chlamydial infection, trichomoniasis and chancroid and the intent, often difficult to document, for treatment of syphilis, but it remains elusive for the viral STDs. Whether or not biological cure is attainable or practical, the *amelioration of clinical manifestations* and the *prevention of sequelae* are always desired outcomes. For most patients these goals are achievable even for the incurable viral STDs such as genital herpes, genital warts, hepatitis B, and especially HIV infection. A fourth goal is *preventing transmission* of infection, which may be independent of biological cure. For example, benzathine penicillin treatment for syphilis may abort infectivity without curing the patient, and it is possible, albeit not yet known, that antiviral therapy may prevent transmission of genital herpes or HIV. It is still less certain whether current treatments can reduce the likelihood of transmission of human papillomavirus (HPV) to infected persons' sex partners. Finally, preventing transmission of infection by curative or suppressive therapy also contributes to the fifth goal of therapy, *community-based prevention*. In the paradigm represented by the reproductive rate of infection in the community ($R_0 = \beta cD$, Chapter 3), treatment shortens the mean duration of infection in the population (D) thereby reducing the reproductive rate (R_0). Thus, although biomedical approaches to diagnosis and treatment are often classified as secondary prevention (i.e., prevention of complications in the individual patient after infection has already occurred), early diagnosis and treatment also represent primary prevention at the population level.

TREATMENT STRATEGIES

The strategies for treating infected persons can be viewed as a continuum according to the timing of treatment after exposure or acquisition of infection and the specificity of the diagnosis (see Table 52-1). *Preexposure prophylaxis*, or true preventive therapy administered before or at the time of exposure, is a theoretically feasible but little-studied approach that has rarely been systematically employed as a prevention strategy, primarily among military personnel and commercial sex workers. *Postexposure prophylaxis* is treatment of an exposed person to prevent infection, clinical disease, and transmission to new sex partners. At a biological level, postexposure prophylaxis probably cures early infection rather than preventing it. Indeed, postexposure prophylaxis is most commonly used in the guise of "epidemiologic" treatment of exposed sex partners,[3] when in most cases the infection already is established rather than incubating. True postexposure prophylaxis, wherein exposed persons receive treatment within hours of exposure, has been shown to be effective in preventing chlamydial infection or gonorrhea[4] but has been rarely employed on a systematic basis. However, despite the rarity with which pre- or postexposure prophylaxis are employed as standardized STD prevention strategies, it seems likely that both are used, perhaps frequently, by some persons at risk or their health care providers.

Etiologic treatment, directed toward a specific pathogen, is the modern historical norm for most STDs in industrialized countries. Etiologic therapy usually but not invariably implies the use of a microbiologic test to identify the infecting pathogen. *Syndromic management*, of special interest in developing countries and other resource-poor settings, requires only determination of broad clinical manifestations together with risk assessment, followed by treatment of the main causes of the syndrome without attempting to identify the specific pathogen.[5] Examples include treating persons with cervicitis or urethritis for both gonorrhea and chlamydial infection; treating women with vaginal discharge (without cervicitis) for trichomoniasis and bacterial vaginosis; and treating persons with genital ulcer disease for both syphilis and chancroid. Some therapeutic strategies amount to a hybrid of etiologic and syndromic management, which might be termed "presumptive etiologic therapy," as when nongonococcal urethritis (NGU) is differentiated from gonorrhea and the patient is treated for presumptive chlamydial infection without attempting to identify *Chlamydia trachomatis*. Successful syndromic treatment requires knowledge of the etiologies of the syndromes treated and their local or regional epidemiology, as well as the susceptibility of the most common etiologic pathogens to locally available antimicrobial drugs. The benefit of syndromic management in population-based prevention may be more limited for STDs characterized by a high proportion of subclinical disease, such as chlamydial infection, than for those that usually cause overt clinical manifestations, such as chancroid. Similarly, syndromic treatment of gonorrhea reaches a greater proportion of infected men than women, and its success as a prevention strategy may require systematic presumptive therapy of all exposed partners, usually a daunting prospect. Syndromic management, including therapeutic recommendations for several syndromes, is addressed in chapters 48 and 102.

Mass treatment is the treatment of entire populations known to have substantial prevalences of infection, without attempting to diagnose infection in individuals. Mass treatment can be *universal*, if applied to all persons in a population, or it may be *selective*. Selective mass treatment is the treatment of population subgroups with high prevalences of infection or with marked behavioral risks, such as sex workers. Selective mass treatment may be repeated periodically if the target population remains at high risk.

There have been few studies of either selective or universal mass treatment in STD control.[6] Most dramatically, selective mass treatment was instrumental in almost eliminating yaws, pinta, and endemic syphilis in much of the developing world in the 1950s

Table 52-1. Therapeutic Goals and Treatment Strategies for Sexually Transmitted Diseases

Therapeutic goals
Biological cure
Amelioration of clinical manifestations
Prevention of sequelae
Prevention of transmission to partners, fetus, or newborn
Community-based prevention
Treatment strategies
Prophylactic treatment
Preexposure
Postexposure
Etiologic treatment
Syndromic management
Mass treatment
Universal
Selective

and 1960s. From 1950 through 1969, 50 million persons in 46 countries were treated with various forms of long-acting penicillin, and in some regions (e.g., Bosnia) one or more of these diseases were entirely eliminated.[7] Mass screening and selective mass treatment also may have contributed to the near-elimination of syphilis in China in the 1950s and 1960s,[8] and it helped curtail an outbreak of syphilis in sex workers and seasonal farm workers in California in the 1970s.[9] By contrast, in the Philippines a trial of selective mass treatment of female sex workers for gonorrhea resulted in only a modest, transient reduction in the prevalence of the infection in the treated women and had no significant effect on the rate of gonorrhea among U.S. military personnel, who accounted for most of their partners.[6] In Greenland, selective mass treatment in communities with high rates of gonorrhea resulted in only transient benefits in the least populated areas and no measurable benefit elsewhere, and the program was abandoned.[10] As a generalization, mass treatment appears to have been more effective in controlling syphilis and other treponemal infections than in controlling gonorrhea, probably due to differences in the two diseases' chronicity and incubation periods. The experience with gonorrhea suggests that this strategy is problematical in highly mobile populations with the potential for frequent reintroduction of infection.

As suggested by these examples, mass treatment usually has been directed toward a single STD or a few biologically similar infections. However, a current project in the Rakai district of Uganda is designed to assess the effect of periodic (approximately every 9 months) selective mass treatment in villages randomly selected for intervention compared with control villages.[11] In the intervention villages, all persons 15 to 49 years old are treated simultaneously for gonorrhea, chancroid, chlamydial infection, trichomoniasis, and bacterial vaginosis; this treatment is coupled with mass screening for syphilis and penicillin therapy for those found to be infected. The goals of this ambitious project are to assess the efficacy of selective mass treatment for STD on the incidence of HIV infection, the incidence and prevalence of the STDs themselves, and possible benefits on reproductive health. The trial is designed to test the hypothesis that STD control is effective in HIV prevention, not necessarily to demonstrate a widely applicable strategy.[11]

DIRECTLY OBSERVED TREATMENT, SINGLE SESSION

Directly observed treatment, single session (DOT-SS) has been a central theme of STD therapy since the beginning of the antimicrobial era; it anticipated by several decades the emergence of DOT-SS as a mainstay of tuberculosis therapy. Multiple-dose treatment for STDs initially was problematical, because only parenterally administered penicillin was available, most patients lacked health insurance, and many patients lacked convenient transportation to physicians' offices or public clinics. Moreover, many clinicians and public health authorities believed patients with STDs to be inherently unreliable and unlikely to comply with unsupervised, multiple-dose regimens. This belief probably remained common even after orally administered antibiotics became available and as transportation and access to health care improved. In actuality, persons with STDs may be no less likely to comply with therapy than others of similar education and socioeconomic level. However, therapeutic compliance is poor in most population groups, especially among persons without symptoms and those with trivial clinical manifestations. The need to curtail transmission adds a strong public health rationale for DOT-SS: whereas poor therapeutic compliance for most conditions has adverse effects only for the patient, for communicable diseases it affects the health of the patients' contacts and the community at large. Accordingly, DOT-SS remains a high priority for the curable bacterial STDs.

In both industrialized and developing countries, DOT-SS is the standard of care for patients with uncomplicated gonorrhea, early syphilis, and trichomoniasis, and it is increasingly so for chancroid, chlamydial infection, and NGU[1,2] (See Appendix A). Direct observation of treatment by the health care provider assures compliance and may be as important as using a single-dose regimen. When multiple-dose treatment must be used, the clinician should carefully counsel the patient about the necessity of compliance. When practical, even multiple-dose therapy for the curable bacterial STDs should be dispensed in the clinician's office, and ideally the clinician should observe the patient taking the first dose instead of giving a prescription to be filled elsewhere, especially when the patient must personally pay for the drug. In a study of women with acute pelvic inflammatory disease (PID) diagnosed in a hospital emergency department, 28% of patients interviewed after treatment acknowledged that they had not filled their prescriptions for doxycycline and only 31% completed the 10-day course of treatment.[12] More recently, 223 patients given a seven-day course of doxycycline for documented or presumptive chlamydial infection in two STD clinics were studied using a computerized system to monitor the timing and frequency with which their medication containers were opened. Even though the drug was given directly to patients in the clinic, 24% apparently took little or no doxycycline and only 25% took the drug as directed; 51% had intermediate levels of compliance.[13]

Single-dose regimens are not available—or, if available, are not optimally effective—for HPV infection, genital herpes, other viral STDs, or bacterial vaginosis, nor have available multiple-dose regimens been shown to cure the viral STDs or prevent their transmission. Accordingly, DOT-SS may be less important for viral than bacterial STDs. Treating late syphilis with recommended parenteral penicillin regimens requires administration by the clinician, except in special circumstances in which injections can be provided in nonclinical settings. But transmission to sex partners is not an issue in the management of patients with late syphilis, and self-administered oral therapy often is employed when penicillin is contraindicated.

MANAGEMENT OF SEX PARTNERS

TRADITIONAL PARTNER NOTIFICATION AND TREATMENT

For the curable bacterial STDs, it is traditionally recommended that patients' sex partners be personally examined, counseled, and treated. When practical, the partner should be managed by the provider or clinic that treats the index case, which is routine for public STD clinics in the United States and probably for many primary care clinics and practitioners. This approach also is increasingly being adopted by family planning clinics. Unfortunately, several structural factors often make it difficult for managed care organizations, clinicians in private practice, or specialized clinics to personally examine and treat their patients' sex partners. The partner may not belong to the same managed care plan as the patient, the partner of a university student or soldier may not be a student or belong to the military, or the partner may lack health insurance. Moreover, partner notification *per se* may not be reimbursed by insurance plans. It is sometimes asserted that gynecology practices or family planning clinics are not conducive to managing patients' male sex partners, although this should be amenable to clinician training and patient education.

In addition to these structural problems, concerns about confidentiality may lead the partner to seek a different provider, or the partner may be geographically remote. Moreover, physicians often view themselves as advocates for their patients, which may make them uncomfortable participating in partner notification, especially when the patient is reluctant to cooperate, even though failure to diagnose and treat partners amounts to suboptimal management of their own patients, who may be reinfected. Resistance to partner notification is currently strongest among some communities and individuals affected by HIV, who are concerned about stigma, discrimination, and confidentiality. For all these reasons, the public health sector has a responsibility to the community to facilitate partner management in the private sector. Public health agencies should work to persuade health maintenance organizations and managed care plans that the costs of partner notification and treatment are likely to be less than the costs of treating the reinfections and complications that otherwise will occur in the index patients.[14]

When any of these structural or other problems prevent personal examination by the clinic or physician who treated the index patient, the partner should be referred to specific provider or clinic known to be competent in STD management and sensitive to sexual health issues; it is probable that nonspecific advice to the patient like "make sure your partner gets checked" is often unheeded. Public health agencies have a responsibility to assure that clinical services are available to partners who cannot be treated by the index patient's provider, by providing care at public clinics or facilitating referral to alternate sources of care. Managed care plans should also fund out-of-plan treatment by public health agencies for enrollees who choose to seek STD care in the public sector.[14]

PATIENT-DELIVERED PARTNER THERAPY

An alternative to personal examination and treatment of the sex partner is to give the index patient drug for delivery to the partner, or a prescription in the partner's name. Experience in STD clinics in the United States suggests that referral of partners by either patients or trained counselors results in treatment of well under half the partners of persons with syphilis. Peterman et al. were able to locate and evaluate only 2,236 (19.8%) of 11,272 potentially exposed partners of persons with infectious syphilis,[15] and anecdotal reports from other public STD control programs suggest that the record is not substantially better for gonorrhea or chlamydial infection. Patient-delivered partner treatment is the historical norm for management of trichomoniasis in many settings, and anecdotal experience indicates that this strategy is commonly used in the management of other STDs. For example, 43 obstetrician-gynecologists who had treated at least one woman for chlamydial infection, gonorrhea, or PID in the preceding year were asked in an informal survey how frequently they had arranged for treatment of the sex partners without personal examination or referral. Only 6 (14%) had never done so, 19 (44%) did so rarely or occasionally, and 18 (42%) usually or always arranged for such treatment (Handsfield HH, unpublished data). A study in Sweden showed reinfection with *C. trachomatis* to be substantially less frequent in women given antibiotics to treat their partners than in those whose partners were referred for treatment.[16] However, the partner management strategies in that study were not randomly assigned and were employed sequentially over a few years, so that patient-delivered partner treatment may have been selectively employed among patients at inherently lower risk for reinfection, or the differing outcomes may partly reflect changing patterns of chlamydia epidemiology and transmission in the community.

Patient-delivered partner therapy has obvious disadvantages as well as potential benefits. It risks poor therapeutic compliance by the partner, virtually assures suboptimal understanding by the partner about the nature of the infection, misses an opportunity to screen the partner for other STDs and to bring still other partners to treatment, and may carry medicolegal risks in the event of an adverse drug reaction. Some patients may be unwilling or unable to deliver drug to some or all of their partners; persons at highest risk, such as teens or illicit drug users, may be the least effective in using this approach; and patients may be more successful in delivering treatment to their regular sex partners than to casual partners, although the latter may be most likely to continue to transmit infection. Controlled trials of patient-delivered therapy for chlamydial infection and gonorrhea are underway. Until the results are known, the standard approach should be to personally examine and treat the partners of patients with curable bacterial STDs. Nevertheless, patient-delivered treatment may be warranted for selected cases in which partner referral is unlikely to be effective or is unsuccessful. Only single-dose regimens with high safety profiles should be used in this manner.

CONCURRENT INFECTIONS

Many patients with STDs have concurrent infections, and treatment guidelines have often recommended therapy for undiagnosed STDs likely to coexist with the primary infection. Treatment of gonorrhea with regimens that would eradicate undiagnosed or incubating syphilis was once considered a high priority, based on the belief that both infections often were acquired simultaneously. However, a controlled study in Miami, Florida from 1985 to 1992, when gonorrhea was epidemic and syphilis resurgent, analyzed 98,441 cases of gonorrhea treated either with drugs active against *Treponema pallidum* (various regimens that included ceftriaxone, doxycycline, or erythromycin) or with spectinomycin, which is not effective against syphilis. New cases of primary syphilis within 6 weeks or secondary syphilis within 3 months following gonorrhea therapy were rare (2.1–5.6 cases per 10,000) and were not significantly different according to the treatment given.[17] Thus, in the United States (and probably in other industrialized countries) the activity of the selected antibiotic against *T. pallidum* and its efficacy against incubating syphilis are not important criteria in selecting routine therapy for patients with gonorrhea. It is unknown whether this conclusion is valid for developing countries or other settings with high rates of both gonorrhea and syphilis.

For the past two decades, recommendations for treatment of concurrent infections have been dominated by the high prevalence of chlamydial infection in patients with gonorrhea. In the 1970s and early 1980s, 10–20%of men and 20–40% of women with gonorrhea in industrialized countries were infected with *C. trachomatis*,[18] leading to recommendations of several authorities, such as CDC and WHO, that all patients with gonorrhea be treated with regimens effective against *C. trachomatis*[1,2] (See Appendix A). Treating only those patients with documented concurrent infection usually is impractical, because it is difficult to assure that the patient will return after the diagnosis is established, and excess clinic visits are costly. Moreover, financial constraints often preclude routine testing for *C. trachomatis* ,and the least expensive tests are insensitive. Thus, antichlamydial therapy is considered routine for all patients with gonorrhea, unless a sensitive assay for *C. trachomatis*, such as a DNA amplification test, is already known to be negative. Although some anecdotal reports suggest that the prevalence of chlamydial infection in persons with gonorrhea is declining in the United States, from 1993 through 1996 12–18%of heterosexual men and 25–35% of women with gonorrhea in King County, Washington, were also infected with *C. trachomatis*, rates comparable to those found in the 1970s and 1980s.[19] The prevalence of chlamydial infection in patients with gonorrhea also was stable in Columbus, Ohio from 1989 to 1992.[20] The impression that coinfection is less common than in past years may be due in part to the widespread use of relatively insensitive chlamydia tests, whereas both the early studies[18] and the recent King County data[19] were based on isolation of *C. trachomatis* by culture. Because the epidemiology of both gonorrhea and chlamydial infection is geographically variable and fluctuates over time, coinfection rates need to be repeatedly assessed in other areas of the United States and elsewhere.

Undoubtedly other combinations of simultaneous infection with treatable STDs are common, but few if any systematic studies are available. Infection with multiple pathogens, including herpes simplex virus (HSV), *Haemophilus ducreyi*, and *T. pallidum*, has been reported in patients with genital ulcer disease in the United States and in developing countries.[21] However, data are lacking on the prevalences of gonorrhea or chlamydial infection among patients with trichomoniasis, genital herpes, genital warts, syphilis, or chancroid. In the absence of definitive data, clinicians should test patients with any of these infections for locally prevalent curable STDs. In some instances, presumptive therapy based on local epidemiologic data may be indicated for selected patients, such as those who are unlikely to return for follow-up.

POST-TREATMENT TESTING

TEST OF CURE

Clinical follow-up and retesting to assess the response to therapy are common practices, especially in industrialized countries. Syphilis in particular requires clinical and serological follow-up, often for several months or years, in order to document cure[1,22] (See Appendix A). Clinical follow-up is generally recommended following treatment of chancroid, but prompt resolution of symptoms and signs are reliable indicators of cure, so that retesting for *H. ducreyi* rarely is indicated[1,23] (See Appendix A). Likewise, the clinical response of gonococcal or chlamydial urethritis in men usually is a reliable indicator of bacteriologic cure, although subclinical persistence after initial clinical improvement sometimes occurs[1,24,25] (See Appendix A). On the other hand, cervical, rectal or pharyngeal infections with *Neisseria gonorroeae* or *C. trachomatis* commonly are asymptomatic or have nonspecific manifestations, necessitating follow-up test of cure to assure eradication of the organism[1,25] (See Appendix A). But a test of cure rarely is practical in resource-poor settings and is relatively expensive, even in industrialized countries. Thus, an important decision in formulating treatment guidelines is the alternative between use of a highly effective but often costly treatment regimen to obviate the need for test of cure, versus the use of a less expensive and less effective regimen which requires retesting. For example, during the late 1970s and early 1980s, the U.S. Air Force continued to proclaim penicillin as the treatment of choice for gonorrhea despite high and rising rates of penicillin resistance, believing the cost of test of cure and persistent symptoms to be less than that of using a more expensive drug (spectinomycin) as routine therapy.[26] By contrast, in the early 1980s the percentage of β-lactamase-producing strains of *N. gonorrhoeae* in the United States rose above 5%, forcing a decision between continued use of the penicillins together with an increased investment in antimicrobial susceptibility testing and follow-up examinations for test of cure, at a cost of many millions of dollars in the public health sector; or switching to routine treatment with ceftriaxone, at an cost of a few million dollars more for medication in the public sector, but obviating the need for even more expensive susceptibility testing and routine test of cure. The latter alternative was chosen.

The currently recommended treatment regimens for gonorrhea and chlamydial infection are sufficiently reliable that routine test of cure clearly is not cost-effective. However, test of cure continues to be indicated when the treatment used has uncertain efficacy or if the potential consequences of persistent infection are especially severe (e.g., for all recommended antichlamydial regimens in pregnant women); when the susceptibility of *N. gonorrhoeae* to the antibiotic used is in doubt; or when therapeutic compliance cannot be reasonably assured[1] (See Appendix A). In developing countries, where test of cure is most problematic, it is especially important that highly effective DOT-SS be used wherever possible. For uncomplicated gonorrhea, retesting by culture normally is reliable 5–10 days after treatment is completed. However, it is generally recommended that test of cure for chlamydial infection be delayed until at least three weeks after completion of therapy, because of the possibility that *C. trachomatis* may be transiently suppressed but not eradicated.[27] Additionally, most testing is done with assays that detect chlamydial antigens or DNA that may persist for several days and occasionally as long as three weeks after viable organisms can no longer be isolated.[28,29]

RESCREENING

Delayed post-treatment testing, or rescreening, is designed primarily to detect reinfection rather than treatment failure. Studies in the 1960s and 1970s showed that *N. gonorrhoeae* was reisolated from approximately 10% of women treated for gonorrhea several weeks earlier, and most such infections were believed to result from reinfection. Accordingly, some authorities recommended routine rescreening of women with gonorrhea 1–2 months after treatment, and mathematical modeling suggested that rescreening women at high risk might contribute to control of gonorrhea. However, compliance was poor and the use-effectiveness and cost-effectiveness of rescreening were low,[30] and this strategy was largely ignored or was implemented transiently and then abandoned. More recent studies indicate that 10–20% of women treated for chlamydial infection have persistent or recurrent infection within the first year, with most cases detected within four months.[31,32] These results are consistent with the hypothesis that most reinfections are acquired from untreated sex partners or from reentry into high-risk partner networks. Epidemiologic studies and animal models suggest that reinfection with *C. trachomatis* carries an enhanced risk of PID and other serious outcomes,[31] making prevention or early detection of reinfection especially important. The development of diagnostic tests for *C. trachomatis* and *N. gonorrhoeae* that retain high sensitivity when performed on urine or self-obtained vaginal specimens,[33,34] obviating the requirement for a speculum examination and even the need to visit a clinical facility, may make rescreening more practical. In light of these developments, new studies of rescreening for gonorrhea and chlamydial infection are a high priority.

TREATMENT GUIDELINES

EVIDENCE-BASED GUIDELINES

CDC, WHO, professional societies, and several national, state, provincial, and local health departments promulgate and periodically update guidelines for the treatment of STDs[1,2,35] (See Appendix A). Historically, such guidelines were based on the consensus among members of expert committees, supported when possible by the results of controlled studies. More recently, notably in the development of CDC's 1993 and 1998 treatment guidelines for STDs[1,36] (See Appendix A) and in the guidelines developed by the U.S. Public Health Service and the Infectious Diseases Society of America for management of opportunistic infections in HIV-infected persons,[35] an "evidence-based" approach was employed. This method emphasizes a systematic review of the results of controlled trials and supplements those results with evaluations of the strength of the recommendations and the quality of the evidence behind them.[37] Unfortunately, important gaps exist in the quality of the evidence for most STD treatment recommendations, so that guidelines for many conditions continue to be based on incomplete data supplemented by expert opinion.

STANDARDS FOR EVALUATING EFFICACY OF STD TREATMENT

Most industrialized countries have regulatory agencies responsible for approving drugs for specific clinical indications, such as the U.S. Food and Drug Administration (FDA). In the early 1990s the Infectious Diseases Society of America made recommendations to the FDA concerning the data that should support approval of anti-infective drugs for treatment of the common STDs and offered guidelines for the conduct of clinical trials to document efficacy.[22–25,38–41] According to the guidelines for gonorrhea, chancroid, and uncomplicated chlamydial infection, microbiologic cure—i.e., eradication of the infecting pathogen—should be documented in $\geq$ 95 percent of patients in comparative, controlled trials. An intent-to-treat analysis should be used, wherein all patients assigned to a treatment regimen are analyzed regardless of later protocol violations, and the sample size should be sufficient to assure that the lower limit of the 95% confidence interval (CI) for the observed cure rate is $\geq$ 90 percent.[23–25] Except for chancroid, these goals should be achieved independently in women and men. These standards are independent of the antimicrobial susceptibility of *N. gonorrhoeae*, *C. trachomatis*, and *H. ducreyi* isolated from the study subjects, because individual treatment decisions typically must be made without knowledge of the susceptibility of the infecting strain. Similarly, because of geographic variability in the susceptibility of *N. gonorrhoeae* and *H. ducreyi*, studies designed to secure regulatory approval should be conducted at several geographically dispersed sites.[23,24] Qualitatively similar standards were recommended for approval of regimens for the treatment of genital herpes, syphilis, NGU, mucopurulent cervicitis, PID, bacterial vaginosis, trichomonal vaginitis, and yeast vulvovaginitis.[22,38–41] These recommendations were developed primarily to provide guidelines for regulatory approval, but they also are useful to assist clinicians and health planners in critically interpreting the strength of evidence presented in published reports.

EFFICACY VERSUS USE EFFECTIVENESS

Well-designed randomized controlled trials will define the *efficacy* of an antimicrobial drug, but often in highly selected populations that may not be representative of typical patients in most clinical settings. Such studies, if otherwise well designed and executed, may be said to have internal validity (i.e., the results are reliable in the population studied) but may not have external validity (i.e., applicability to patients in other settings).[42] Numerous factors affect the selection and enrollment of subjects in clinical trials, including decisions by patients to attend specific clinical facilities, the need for informed consent, the use of financial inducements, and the usual exclusion of patients with chronic medical conditions, alcoholism, substance abuse, and other factors that might adversely affect pharmacokinetics, other determinants of cure, or follow-up.[39] Thus, the *use effectiveness* of a regimen—its efficacy in typical infected persons in various settings—depends not only on the efficacy demonstrated in controlled studies, but on the proportion of the infected population reached with treatment, the presence of confounding clinical conditions, behavioral norms in the community, and the proportion of treated persons who comply with therapy. At a population level, the impact of treatment on transmission of the infection in the community also is influenced by various characteristics of those who receive treatment, such as whether they are frequent transmitters, members of an extensive network of sex partners, or the monogamous (e.g., marital) partners of high-frequency transmitters. Thus, clinicians and public health authorities need to critically assess the strength of evidence in clinical trials to determine whether or not it is valid to apply the (mostly favorable) results to their own patients.

PROBLEMS AND DILEMMAS IN TREATMENT OF SELECTED STDs

Dilemmas and controversies exist in the treatment of almost all STDs, usually because there are inadequate data to resolve differing opinions among the experts. Recommendations for management of specific STDs are presented in the chapters for those infections.

GONORRHEA

Pharmacokinetic considerations

In a classic analysis of studies designed to assess the efficacy of varying doses of penicillin against gonococcal urethritis, Jaffe et al correlated the cure rates with the treatment doses used, the resulting blood levels of penicillin, and the minimum inhibitory concentration (MIC) of penicillin for each patient's urethral isolate of *N. gonorrhoeae*.[43] With few exceptions, cure was assured when single-dose treatment produced plasma levels of penicillin that remained 3–4 times greater than the MIC of the infecting strain for at least 7 hours. Thus, the dose of penicillin selected for routine single-dose treatment should achieve this standard in relation to the maximum MIC of *N. gonorrhoeae* strains in the community. Unfortunately, soon after this study was published penicillin became untenable as routine therapy for gonorrhea in most of the world, owing to the spread of β-lactamase-producing gonococci. The validity of these guidelines is unknown for antibiotics other than penicillin and for gonococcal infection of anatomic sites other than the male urethra. While it seems likely that these standards may be valid for cephalosporins or other β-lactam antibiotics, their utility for the fluoroquinolones or other antibiotic classes is unknown.[24] The Jaffe study is now mainly of historical interest; its only practical purpose is perhaps to provide early guidance on the doses to be used in early clinical trials of new antibiotics.

Antimicrobial resistance

The potential for evolution and spread of *N. gonorrhoeae* strains with clinically significant antimicrobial resistance has been a concern since sulfonamides were first used to treat gonorrhea in the 1930s. However, the past decade has been one of relative stability in the susceptibility of *N. gonorrhoeae* in the United States and western Europe, where single-dose treatment with a newer cephalosporin (typically cefixime or ceftriaxone) or a fluoroquinolone (usually ciprofloxacin or ofloxacin) has retained nearly 100% efficacy for uncomplicated anogenital gonorrhea[1] (See Appendix A). However, the prevalence of gonococci with high-level fluoroquinolone resistance has been increasing for a decade in East Asia and some Pacific island countries.[44,45] For example, nearly half of all gonococci isolated from female sex workers in the Philippines in 1996 had ciprofloxacin MICs $\geq$ 4 mg/L (Whittington WL, Holmes KK, unpublished data), a level at which single-dose treatment probably would be ineffective. A similar trend also has been reported in India.[45a] Such strains were isolated only rarely in the United States through 1997,[45,45b] but eventual worldwide dissemination of gonococci with high-level fluoroquinolone resistance seems likely, as occurred with β-lactamase-producing gonococci from 1975 to 1985.[46] In addition, other gram-negative bacteria have acquired plasmids bearing genes that encode TEM-type β-lactamases active against the newer cephalosporins, so it seems there is a potential for the evolution of ceftriaxone-resistant *N. gonorrhoeae*. Simultaneous evolution and spread of both fluoroquinolone-resistant and cephalosporin-resistant gonococci might be disastrous, because few other practical single-dose options currently are available, so that research into new regimens and novel classes of antimicrobial agents for gonorrhea remains important.

CHLAMYDIAL INFECTION AND RELATED SYNDROMES

Single-dose versus multiple-dose therapy

The development of effective single-dose treatment for chlamydial infection with azithromycin was one of the most important advances in therapy of the bacterial STDs in the past two decades.[47] However, some controversy persists concerning the treatment regimen of choice, engendered by the cost of azithromycin, which varies from about $10.00 to $25.00 per gram in the United States, depending on the setting and formulation (powder versus capsules), whereas the standard seven-day course of doxycycline costs $.50 to $2.00. Mathematical modeling studies suggest that despite its high cost, DOT-SS with azithromycin is more cost-effective than giving doxycycline, even at relatively high rates of therapeutic compliance with multiple-dose therapy.[48,49] On the other hand, a recent study found no difference in the efficacy of azithromycin and doxycycline for treatment of cervical chlamydial infection, as measured by persistence of *C. trachomatis* 3–4 weeks after treatment; with either treatment, about 5% of patients had persistent or recurrent infection.[50] However, questions exist about that study's external validity. As for most clinical trials, limitations in interpreting the results arose from the research environment and the need for informed consent. Additionally, many women were enrolled only if their male sex partners consented to the women's participation as study subjects. This may have biased the study population in favor of women in committed partnerships, which in turn might be associated with enhanced compliance with multiple-dose treatment, but which would have no influence on compliance with DOT-SS.[51] It would be surprising if the use-effectiveness of DOT-SS with azithromycin and multiple-dose doxycycline in fact were equivalent to one another in most clinical settings, in view of the vagaries of therapeutic compliance. As cited above, both Brookoff[12] and Augenbraun et al.[13] found that about a quarter of patients prescribed or given doxycycline for known or presumed chlamydial infection failed to fill the prescription or took little or none of the drug.

A problem in interpreting the available studies is that the minimum dose of doxycycline or other tetracyclines required to eradicate *C. trachomatis* is unknown. Bowie and colleagues[52] reported that minocycline, which has pharmacokinetic characteristics and activity against *C. trachomatis* almost identical to those of doxycycline, was equally effective in regimens of 100 mg and 200 mg daily for 7 days. Cerin et al[29] found that all women with cervical or urethral chlamydial infection were negative by culture, direct immunofluorescence, and EIA within 6 days of starting an 8-day course of doxycycline in a dose of 200 mg initially then 100 mg daily. Stamm et al. showed that in persons with both gonorrhea and chlamydial infection, *C. trachomatis* was eradicated in 27 (93%) of 29 patients given 5 days treatment with tetracycline hydrochloride, 500 mg four times daily.[18] Unfortunately, few studies have followed patients for three weeks or longer in order to exclude transient suppression of the organism as the explanation for negative tests at earlier intervals. Hooton et al. showed that transient suppression occurs in some patients given ciprofloxacin for uncomplicated chlamydial infection,[27] and Brown et al. reported transient suppression of *N. gonorrhoeae* in patients treated with erythromycin.[53] In the absence of well-designed dose-ranging studies with several weeks' follow-up or direct comparative studies between doxycycline and azithromycin, it seems prudent to assume that treatment with doxycycline for less than 5 days (which occurred in up to half the patients treated by both Brookoff[12] and Augenbraun et al.[13]) is associated with a substantial risk of treatment failure.[51]

Another factor that contributes to uncertainty about DOT-SS versus multiple-dose therapy for chlamydial infection is the practical utility of cost-effectiveness considerations in driving therapeutic decisions. The clinic or agency treating the patient may experience no financial benefit from using a more expensive regimen, because the sequelae of chlamydial infection usually become apparent only after several months or years and often are treated by other providers or funded by other payment plans.[14] CDC recommends single-dose azithromycin and the 7-day doxycycline regimen as equal first-choice regimens for treatment of documented or presumed uncomplicated chlamydial infection and advises clinicians to use azithromycin whenever compliance with multiple-dose therapy is in doubt[1] (See Appendix A). Nevertheless, on balance it seems prudent to consider DOT-SS with azithromycin the routine first-line regimen except when the clinician is confident that the patient will comply with the doxycycline regimen, while recognizing that predicting compliance is difficult and often unreliable.[51] Certainly clinicians, health maintenance organizations, health care financing plans, and especially departments of public health should recognize their responsibilities to consider societal and long-range institutional costs in selecting regimens for routine use in STD therapy and to not make drug cost the sole criterion for selecting among the available treatment options.[14]

Treatment of pregnant women with chlamydial infection

The best treatment for pregnant women with chlamydial infection remains uncertain. Because the tetracyclines and fluoroquinolones are contraindicated in pregnancy, erythromycin (500 mg four times daily for 7 days) has been the historical recommendation for treatment, but this regimen is associated with a high rate of gastrointestinal intolerance and probably lower use effectiveness than either azithromycin or doxycycline. In the combined results of two studies, 20 (25%) of 80 women were unable to complete the erythromycin regimen.[54,55] In addition, pregnancy is associated with both an increased volume of distribution and accelerated metabolism of erythromycin, leading to reduced blood levels and a lower plasma half-life, potentially contributing to higher treatment failure rates. For these reasons CDC now recommends either erythromycin or a 10-day course of amoxicillin (500 mg three times daily) as co-equal regimen of choice for pregnant women with chlamydial infection[1] (See Appendix A). However, the treatment efficacy of the amoxicillin regimen varied from 98% in one study to 85% in two others;[54,56,57] for all three of these studies combined, 151 of 165 pregnant women were cured (90%, 95% CI 85.1–94.7%), suggesting that amoxicillin is less effective in pregnant women than either doxycycline or azithromycin in nonpregnant patients. The sulfonamides have been used but are less effective than other regimens and are contraindicated late in pregnancy. Azithromycin almost certainly is safe, but the only published study to date included only 15 pregnant women given single-dose azithromycin; although 14 apparently were cured, the enzyme immunoassay for *C. trachomatis*, an insensitive test, was used for test of cure.[55] More research is required before azithromycin can be recommended for routine treatment of pregnant women, but its use might be appropriate in patients who are unlikely to comply with multiple-dose therapy. A recent cost-effectiveness study advocated initial therapy with amoxicillin, followed by a test of cure and use of azithromycin in women with persistent infection.[58] In industrialized countries, test of cure with a sensitive assay such as culture or a DNA amplification test should be routine following treatment of all pregnant women for *C. trachomatis* infection.

Treatment of mucopurulent cervicitis

Nongonococcal mucopurulent cervicitis (MPC) has been described as the female counterpart to NGU in males.[59] Although antimicrobial therapy is effective in eradicating *C. trachomatis* in women with MPC, and eradication of chlamydial infection is associated with improvement in the signs of cervicitis,[60] few data exist on the response of nonchlamydial MPC to antimicrobial therapy. It is also unknown whether nonchlamydial, nongonococcal MPC leads to PID or other sequelae, or whether treatment modifies the risk of such outcomes. The central problem is that MPC remains an etiologic enigma; although many cases are due to *C. trachomatis* or *N. gonorrhoeae* and primary genital herpes often results in erosive cervicitis, in most cases the cause is unknown. CDC now recommends treating women with MPC only if chlamydial or gonococcal infection is documented or suspected on epidemiologic grounds, such as sexual exposure to a known case[1] (See Appendix A). Thus, MPC *per se* is not considered to warrant routine antimicrobial therapy, a recommendation that is likely to be controversial. There are no data on the efficacy of azithromycin against MPC, although DOT-SS with azithromycin is as effective as 7 days of doxycycline for treatment of men with nonchlamydial NGU.[61] Studies of the etiology, diagnosis, sequelae, and treatment of nonchlamydial, nongonococcal MPC are a high priority.

Recurrent nongonococcal urethritis

NGU, especially when not associated with *C. trachomatis* infection, often recurs in the absence of sexual reexposure or after intercourse only with a treated partner, and some men have repeated episodes over several months or years.[62] The syndrome is defined as the persistence or recurrence of urethritis within several weeks—there is no clear agreement on a more specific interval—in the absence of opportunities for reinfection, such as unprotected sex with new or untreated partners.[62] Aside from the associated psychological stress and inconvenience to patient and clinician alike, the importance of recurrent NGU is unknown; the syndrome has not been linked with epididymitis, infertility, urethral stricture, systemic complications, or morbidity in patients' sex partners. While some reports and clinicians' impressions have linked recurrent NGU with nonbacterial prostatitis, the two syndromes probably are distinct. The causes are unknown: *C. trachomatis* is rarely identified, only a small minority of cases may be due to *Trichomonas vaginalis*, infection with coliform bacteria or other uropathogen is uncommon, and most cases apparently are not caused by *Ureaplasma urealyticum* or other genital mycoplasmas.[62]

In view of these uncertainties, the choice of therapy is arbitrary. With the potential exception of treatment for possible trichomoniasis, no patient should be given anti-infective therapy, as often occurs, in the absence of objective evidence of urethral inflammation, such as mucopurulent discharge or urethral leukocytosis, or clear evidence of prostatitis. When NGU persists during therapy or first recurs within a few weeks of apparently successful treatment with doxycycline or a macrolide antibiotic, many experts first treat with metronidazole for possible trichomoniasis.[1] If signs persist or recur yet again, a common approach is to treat the patient with one of the standard NGU regimens—a 7-day course of erythromycin often is given if the previous episode was treated with doxycycline, and treatment with doxycycline for 7 days might be tried if azithromycin or erythromycin was used initially. Subsequent recurrences commonly are then treated with 3–4 week regimens of erythromycin,[62] doxycycline, or a fluoroquinolone. Some experts select these antibiotics because they achieve therapeutic levels in the prostate gland, although prostatitis has not been clearly documented as a component of the syndrome. On the other hand, many cases resolve spontaneously and antimicrobial therapy may not always be necessary. In a randomized comparison of 21 days of erythromycin versus placebo for persistent or recurrent NGU, resolution occurred within one month in 8 (24%) of 34 men given placebo compared with 13 (52%) of 25 men given erythromycin ($p = 0.03$).[62] With or without treatment, further recurrences remain common. Repeated treatment of the patients' sex partners probably is not indicated.

SYPHILIS

Antimicrobial susceptibility of *Treponema pallidum*

It is universally believed and repeatedly asserted that *T. pallidum* retains exquisite susceptibility to penicillin. Indeed, apart from a single isolate with high-level resistance to erythromycin,[63] *T. pallidum* has not been reported to have reduced susceptibility to an antibiotic to which it is generally sensitive. However, owing to inability to cultivate *T. pallidum*, standard in vitro methods cannot be used to measure antimicrobial susceptibility, and all the available indirect methods are too cumbersome to permit testing large numbers of isolates. Most testing of the antimicrobial susceptibility of *T. pallidum* was done early in the antibiotic era, and susceptibility results have been reported for only a handful of isolates in the past two decades. Moreover, antimicrobial susceptibility testing has not been reported for *T. pallidum* isolated from any patient following failure of penicillin therapy. Thus, while it is likely that penicillin resistance indeed is rare or nonexistent, the hypothesis that reduced susceptibility may contribute to persistent infection following treatment in fact has not been adequately tested. There is no known biological limitation on the ability of *T. pallidum* to develop penicillin resistance through either chromosomal mutation or acquisition of a resistance plasmid, and plasmid DNA has been identified in *T. pallidum*.[64] A high priority for clinical research is to attempt isolation of *T. pallidum* from patients with apparent treatment failure and subject the organism to antimicrobial susceptibility testing.

Treatment of neurosyphilis

The best penicillin regimen for treatment of neurosyphilis remains uncertain. Many of the largest studies were conducted in the first decade after penicillin became available and used formulations that are no longer are available; none met current standards of randomization, blinding, or statistical design; and the quality and duration of follow-up often were poor.[65,66] Nonetheless, those studies and the weight of clinical experience suggested that prolonged treatment with relatively low doses of penicillin is adequate to achieve clinical resolution, supporting the use of benzathine penicillin G. However, benzathine penicillin does not produce measurable levels of penicillin in cerebrospinal fluid (CSF).[67] Consistently achieving CSF penicillin levels that inhibit *T. pallidum* requires high doses of penicillin administered intravenously or intramuscular procaine penicillin (e.g., 2.4 million units daily) plus oral probenecid.[65,66] Nevertheless, one study showed that 37 (79%) of 47 patients with asymptomatic neurosyphilis responded to 2.4–2.5 million units of benzathine penicillin,[68] and the importance of achieving inhibitory penicillin levels in CSF remains uncertain.[65,66] Recommendations for high-dose therapy for neurosyphilis have been influenced by anecdotal reports of persistent *T. pallidum* in CSF or the development of overt neurosyphilis after treatment of early syphilis, especially in the presence of asymptomatic central nervous system involvement or immunodeficiency.[69–71] CDC now recommends treating patients with overt neurosyphilis or syphilitic uveitis for 10-14 days with high-dose penicillin intravenously or with procaine penicillin plus probenecid, but it acknowledges that some experts recommend following such therapy with 7.2 million units of benzathine penicillin.[1]

Treatment of syphilis in HIV-infected persons

Containment of treponemal infections probably depends largely on cellular immunity, and patients with impaired cellular immune function might be expected to require higher doses or more prolonged therapy with penicillin. Indeed, there have been several reports of syphilis complications in HIV-infected patients following standard therapy,[65,66,70,71] and such persons are at increased risk for treatment failure for tuberculosis and other infections dependent on cell-mediated immunity. A multicenter study has assessed the effect of supplementing standard benzathine penicillin G therapy with high-dose oral amoxicillin in the treatment of early syphilis, based on the hypothesis that enhanced levels of antibiotic in blood or CSF might improve the response to therapy, especially in patients with HIV infection.[72] Five hundred forty-one patients with primary, secondary, or early latent syphilis, of whom 101 were HIV-seropositive, were randomized to DOT-SS with 2.4 million units of benzathine penicillin or with the same regimen followed by amoxicillin, 2.0 g by mouth three times daily for 10 days. Serologically defined treatment failure was somewhat more common in HIV-infected than uninfected patients, especially in those with primary syphilis (adjusted odds ratio [OR] 7.6, 95% CI 1.3–44.2), and less common in those with secondary syphilis (OR 2.9, 95% CI 0.9–8.9) but the response was unrelated to the treatment regimen. Overall, serologically defined treatment failure occurred in 24% of patients at 3 months, 17% at 6 months, and 14% at 12 months following treatment. Only one clinically apparent treatment failure occurred, in an HIV-infected person who received routine therapy. *T. pallidum* was detected in CSF after treatment in 6 (46%) of 13 patients in whom it was found before treatment, but this finding was not apparently related to HIV status, treatment regimen, or the clinical or serological response to therapy.[72] While this study did not address the treatment of late syphilis or neurosyphilis, it suggests that the response to treatment of early infection usually is not affected by HIV, even when *T. pallidum* has penetrated the central nervous system. However, the study lacked statistical power to assure that the two regimens in fact are equally effective in HIV-infected and uninfected patients. Currently CDC recommends no modification of standard treatment in any patient with HIV infection, regardless of the stage of syphilis, but suggests longer and closer follow-up in those with HIV[1] (See Appendix A).

BACTERIAL VAGINOSIS

The most troublesome aspect of the management of bacterial vaginosis is the high recurrence rate. Although the efficacy of oral and topical metronidazole or clindamycin are 80% or more at one month following therapy, recurrence rates approach 80% within the year following therapy (Chapter 42). Recurrences have been associated with vaginal douching and with exposure to a new sexual partner. Treatment of patients' sex partners has not prevented recurrences and is not recommended.[1] Better measures for prevention of recurrence await better understanding of the transmission of BV, but counseling on avoidance of douching and on the apparent relationship with new partners may be warranted in women troubled by recurrent BV.

PELVIC INFLAMMATORY DISEASE

The dominant controversy in the treatment of PID revolves around the need for routine use of drugs active against anaerobic pathogens. While *C. trachomatis* and *N. gonorrhoeae* are the primary pathogens in most cases, *Bacteroides*, *Prevotella*, *Peptostreptococcus*, and other anaerobes are commonly isolated from infected fallopian tubes or the pelvic cul-de-sac, although contamination of the culture specimens cannot always be excluded.[73,74] In studies with brief follow-up periods, usually 3–6 weeks, clinical efficacy against acute PID has been documented for ofloxacin or other fluoroquinolone antibiotics with little or no activity against anaerobic bacteria, suggesting that the anaerobic component of infection resolves once *C. trachomatis* or *N. gonorrhoeae* is eradicated.[75] Some authorities consider such treatment to be adequate. However, it is possible that fallopian tube scarring may develop or persist despite clinical improvement, and few data are available on the frequency of infertility, ectopic pregnancy, chronic pelvic pain, or other sequelae in relation to the treatment regimen used.[73] Therefore, CDC and WHO recommend routinely including antibiotics with anaerobic activity such as metronidazole, clindamycin, cefotetan or cefoxitin in the regimens used to treat women with acute PID.[1,2] Doxycycline, once believed to have substantial activity against anaerobic bacteria, in fact is not active against most anaerobes isolated from women with PID.[76] Nevertheless, there is substantial clinical experience in apparently successful treatment of outpatients with a single dose of ceftriaxone followed by a 10-day course of doxycycline.[73]

GENITAL HERPES

The availability of valacyclovir and famciclovir as alternatives to orally administered acyclovir has expanded the options for treatment of patients with genital herpes. Although valacyclovir and famciclovir are promoted as requiring less frequent oral dosing than acyclovir, the pharmacokinetics of acyclovir in fact support its use 3 times daily rather than the 5 times daily schedule recommended by the manufacturer. Nonetheless, the improved bioavailability of the new drugs should reduce the frequency of suboptimal clinical responses, and the apparent efficacy of once daily dosing with valacyclovir for suppression of symptomatic outbreaks of recurrent herpes also is a useful advance. There are no apparent important advantages or disadvantages of valacyclovir compared with famciclovir; clinicians should select among them according to dosing convenience and price.

Suppressive therapy with acyclovir has been shown to markedly reduce the frequency of subclinical viral shedding and the viral titer when shedding occurs,[77] leading to speculation that treating chronically infected persons might reduce the risk of transmission to uninfected sex partners, in addition to the well-established benefit of suppressing symptomatic recurrences. However, treatment does not prevent all shedding, and small amounts of HSV can be found by culture or polymerase chain reaction in some patients while taking antiviral therapy.[78] Because the risk of transmission undoubtedly is influenced by inoculum size and certainly is related to the frequency of exposure, it is almost certain that suppressive antiviral therapy would reduce the risk of transmission, perhaps substantially. One clinician with experience in managing over 15,000 patients with genital herpes has never observed acquisition of infection by the partner of a patient receiving suppressive therapy with acyclovir or valacyclovir (M. Reitano, personal communication). However, it is possible that some persons taking suppressive therapy might become less cautious about avoiding exposure of partners, and it is virtually certain that expansion of routine treatment to large numbers of asymptomatically infected persons would be associated with substantial rates of poor therapeutic compliance, perhaps resulting in a paradoxical increase in transmission risk in the community. Until the results of controlled studies are available, antiviral therapy should not be used for the primary purpose of preventing transmission, and clinicians should assure that patients receiving suppressive therapy understand that transmission to uninfected partners may still occur.

Concerns have been raised that increasing use of antiherpetic chemotherapy might result in selection and spread of HSV strains with reduced susceptibility to acyclovir and related compounds. However, acyclovir-resistant HSV strains currently are rare in immunocompetent persons, and there is no evidence of rising prevalence during 15 years of increasingly widespread use of acyclovir. The first, preliminary, results from a national multicenter surveillance study documented acyclovir resistance in 3(0.6%, 95%CI 0.1–1.3%) of 504 isolates from patients with symptomatic genital herpes.[79] All three of the patients with resistant strains were also infected with HIV, and all had histories of repeated or continual therapy with antiherpetic drugs. Continued surveillance for antiviral resistance in HSV is a high priority.

The treatment of pregnant women with genital herpes is controversial because of theoretical concerns about harmful effects of acyclovir, valacyclovir, and famciclovir on the fetus. However, a registry of pregnant women given acyclovir, maintained jointly by the manufacturer and CDC, has not shown any apparent difference between the frequency or pattern of congenital anomalies and those in the general population.[80,81] CDC now suggests that use of acyclovir may be warranted for treatment of pregnant women with first-episode genital herpes.[1] It is less certain whether antiviral therapy is indicated to suppress clinical recurrences or asymptomatic shedding in pregnant women with genital herpes. Because clinically significant neonatal HSV infection is rare in children born to chronically infected women, it is unlikely that routine use of such treatment would measurably reduce the frequency of perinatal transmission. However, preliminary data suggest that by suppressing clinical outbreaks at term, antiviral therapy may prevent some cesarean sections and their attendant morbidity.[82] This issue requires continued study. The treatment of genital herpes is addressed comprehensively in Chapter 21.

HUMAN PAPILLOMAVIRUS INFECTION

Many questions surround the management of external genital warts and other HPV infections. Several treatments are available to ablate exophytic warts, but the very existence of multiple options reflects the inadequacy of all of them.[83] No practical treatment has been shown to eradicate HPV infection, nor has any therapy been shown to prevent recurrence of warts or transmission to sex partners. Perhaps more important, no proven treatment exists for subclinical infection with the high-risk HPV types associated with neoplasia, nor has any type of therapy been shown to modify the risk or natural course of dysplasia or cancer. Even if some form of chemotherapy eventually is shown to attenuate viral shedding, prevent transmission, or prevent HPV-related neoplasia, most infections are not accompanied by visible lesions (with or without magnification, application of acetic acid, or other methods), nor in many cases by identifiable histological abnormalities. Therefore, any therapy with significant population benefit would probably have to be systemically effective, and sensitive, low-cost tests to detect subclinical HPV infection also will be required. These facts underlie the current recommendations of CDC that routine screening currently need not include tests for HPV DNA or antigens on cytological specimens; that subclinical infection does not warrant attempts at ablative therapy in an attempt to eradicate HPV; that sexual partners of infected persons should be evaluated and treated only for overt, exophytic warts; and that despite the association of most cervical and anal dysplastic or neoplastic lesions with HPV, management of such lesions should not be influenced by the results of tests for the virus.[1] Of course, all these recommendations are subject to change as new knowledge becomes available in this rapidly evolving field. A national, multicenter randomized trial evaluating the utility of HPV DNA amplification tests in managing cervical cytologic abnormalities is currently underway in the United States. Other controversies regarding cervical cytology in screening and management of cervical cytologic abnormalities, and the markedly different approaches used in the United States, Canada, Europe, and elsewhere are addressed in Chapter 59.

References

1 Centers for Disease Control and Prevention: 1998 Guidelines for treatment of sexually transmitted diseases. *MMWR Morb Mortal Wkly Rep* 47(RR-1):1–116, 1998.

2 World Health Organization: Recommendations for the management of sexually transmitted diseases: report of the WHO Advisory Group

meeting on sexually transmitted diseases treatment. Global Program on AIDS and Sexually Transmitted Infections, WHO, Geneva, Switzerland, 1994.
3 Moore MB Jr et al: Epidemiologic treatment of contacts to infectious syphilis. *Public Health Rep* 78:966–970, 1963.
4 Harrison WO et al: A trial of minocycline given after exposure to prevent gonorrhea. *N Engl J Med* 300:1074–1077, 1979.
5 Vuylsteke B et al: Clinical flowcharts for the screening of women for gonococcal and chlamydial infection: evaluation of pregnant women and prostitutes in Zaire. *Clin Infect Dis* 17:82–88, 1993.
6 Holmes KK et al: Impact of a gonorrhea control program, including selective mass treatment, in female sex workers. *J Infect Dis* 174(Suppl 2):S230–239, 1996.
7 Grin EI, Guthe T: Evaluation of a previous mass campaign against endemic syphilis in Bosnia and Herzegovina. *Br J Vener Dis* 43:1–19, 1973
8 Cohen MS et al: Successful eradication of sexually transmitted diseases in the People's Republic of China: implications for the 21st century. *J Infect Dis* 174(Suppl 2):S223–229, 1996
9 Jaffe HW et al: Selective mass treatment in a venereal disease control program. *Am J Public Health* 69:1181–1182, 1979.
10 Evans AJ et al: Prolonged use of the Greenland method of treatment of gonorrhea. *Br J Vener Dis* 56:88–91, 1980.
11 Wawer MJ et al: Trends in HIV-1 prevalence may not reflect trends in incidence in mature epidemics: data from the Rakai population-based cohort, Uganda. *AIDS* 11:1023–1030, 1997.
12 Brookoff D: Compliance with doxycycline therapy for outpatient treatment of pelvic inflammatory disease. *South Med J* 87:1088–1091, 1994.
13 Augenbraun M et al: Compliance with doxycycline therapy in sexually transmitted diseases clinics. *Sex Transm Dis* 25:1–4, 1998.
14 Institute of Medicine: The Hidden Epidemic: Confronting Sexually Transmitted Diseases. Washington, National Academy Press, 1997.
15 Peterman TA et al: Partner notification for syphilis: a randomized, controlled trial of three approaches. *Sex Transm Dis* 24:511–518, 1997.
16 Ramstedt K et al: Contact tracing in the control of genital *Chlamydia trachomatis* infection. *Int J STD AIDS* 2:116–118, 1991.
17 Peterman TA et al: Incubating syphilis in patients treated for gonorrhea: a comparison of treatment regimens. *J Infect Dis* 170:689–692, 1994.
18 Stamm WE et al: Effect of treatment regimens for *Neisseria gonorrhoeae* on simultaneous infections with *Chlamydia trachomatis*. *N Engl J Med* 310:545–549, 1984.
19 Handsfield HH, Whittington WL: Stable prevalence of *Chlamydia trachomatis* infection in patients with gonorrhea. International Congress of Sexually Transmitted Diseases, Seville, Spain, 1997 (Abstr O157).
20 Mertz KJ et al: Trends in the prevalence of chlamydial infections: the impact of community-wide testing. *Sex Transm Dis* 24:169–175, 1997.
21 Morse SA et al: Comparison of clinical diagnosis and standard laboratory and molecular methods for the diagnosis of genital ulcer disease in Lesotho: association with human immunodeficiency virus infection. *J Infect Dis* 175:583–589, 1997.
22 Ronald AR et al: Evaluation of new anti-infective drugs for the treatment of syphilis. *Clin Infect Dis* 15(Suppl 1):S140-S147, 1992.
23 Ronald AR et al: Evaluation of new anti-infective drugs for the treatment of chancroid. *Clin Infect Dis* 15(Suppl 1):S108-S114, 1992.
24 Handsfield HH et al: Evaluation of new anti-infective drugs for the treatment of uncomplicated gonorrhea in adults and adolescents. *Clin Infect Dis* 15(Suppl 1):S123-S130, 1992.
25 Handsfield HH et al: Evaluation of new anti-infective drugs for the treatment of sexually transmitted chlamydial infections and related clinical syndromes. *Clin Infect Dis* 15(Suppl 1):S131-S139, 1992.
26 Berliner DS, No PU: Prevalence of penicillinase-producing *Neisseria gonorrhoeae* in Korea. *Av Space Envir Med* 57:1170–1175, 1986.
27 Hooton TM et al: Ciprofloxacin compared with doxycycline for nongonococcal urethritis: ineffectiveness against *Chlamydia trachomatis* due to relapsing infection. *JAMA* 264:1418–1421, 1990.
28 Workowski KA et al: Long-term eradication of *Chlamydia trachomatis* genital infection after antimicrobial therapy: evidence against persistent infection. *JAMA* 270:2071–2075, 1993.
29 Cerin Å et al: Chlamydia test monitoring during therapy. *Int J STD AIDS* 2:176–179, 1991.
30 Judson FN, Wolf FC: Rescreening for gonorrhea: an evaluation of compliance methods and results. *Am J Pub Health* 69:1178–1180, 1979.
31 Hillis SD et al: Recurrent chlamydial infections increase the risks of hospitalization for ectopic pregnancy and pelvic inflammatory disease. *Am J Obstet Gynecol* 176:103–107, 1997.
32 Kent CK et al: Factors associated with persistent and recurrent chlamydial infection in women. International Congress of Sexually Transmitted Diseases, Seville, Spain, 1997 (Abstr O232).
33 Lee HH et al: Diagnosis of *Chlamydia trachomatis* genitourinary infection in women by ligase chain reaction assay or urine. *Lancet* 345: 213–216, 1995.
34 Hook EW III et al: Diagnosis of *Neisseria gonorrhoeae* infections in women by using the ligase chain reaction on patient-obtained vaginal swabs. *J Clin Micro* 35:2129–2132, 1997.
35 Kaplan JE et al: USPHS/IDSA guidelines for the prevention of opportunistic infections in persons infected with human immunodeficiency virus: introduction. *Clin Infect Dis* 21(Suppl 1):S1-S11, 1995.
36 Levine WC et al: 1993 Sexually transmitted diseases treatment guidelines: introduction. *Clin Infect Dis* 20(Suppl 1):S1-S2, 1995.
37 Cook DJ et al: The relation between systematic reviews and practice guidelines. *Ann Intern Med* 127:210–216, 1997.
38 Hemsell DL et al: Evaluation of new anti-infective drugs for the treatment of acute pelvic inflammatory disease. *Clin Infect Dis* 15(Suppl 1):S53-S61, 1992.
39 Handsfield HH et al: Special issues in clinical trials of new anti-infective drugs for the treatment of sexually transmitted diseases. *Clin Infect Dis* 15(Suppl 1):S96-S98, 1992.
40 Corey L et al: Evaluation of new anti-infective drugs for the treatment of genital infections due to herpes simplex virus. *Clin Infect Dis* 15(Suppl 1):S99-S107, 1992.
41 McCutchan JA et al: Evaluation of new anti-infective drugs for the treatment of vaginal infections. *Clin Infect Dis* 15(Suppl 1):S115-S122, 1992.
42 Karras DJ: Statistical methodology II: reliability and validity assessment in study design, part B. *Acad Emerg Med* 4:144–147, 1997.
43 Jaffe HW et al: Pharmacokinetic determinants of penicillin cure of gonococcal urethritis. *Antimicrob Agents Chemother* 15:587–591, 1979.
44 Gordon SM et al: The emergence of *Neisseria gonorrhoeae* with decreased susceptibility to ciprofloxacin in Cleveland, Ohio: epidemiology and risk factors. *Ann Intern Med* 125:465–470, 1996.
45 Handsfield HH, Whittington WL: Antibiotic-resistant *Neisseria gonorrhoeae*: the calm before another storm? (Editorial). *Ann Intern Med* 125:507–509, 1996.
45a Ray K et al: Prevalence of antimicrobial resistance in *Neisseria gonorrhoeae* in New Delhi, India. 8th Interantional Congress on Infectious Diseases, Boston, Massachusetts, 1998 (Abstr 22.004).
45b Centers for Disease Control and Prevention: Fluoroquinolone-resistant *Neisseria gonorrhoeae*—San Diego, California, 1997. *MMWR Morb Mortal Wkly Rep* 47:405–408, 1998.
46 Handsfield HH et al: Epidemiology of penicillinase-producing *Neisseria gonorrhoeae* infections: analysis by auxotyping and serogrouping. *N Engl J Med* 306:950–954, 1982.
47 Martin DG et al: A controlled trial of a single-dose of azithromycin for the treatment of chlamydial urethritis and cervicitis. *N Engl J Med* 327:921–925, 1992.
48 Haddix AC et al: The cost-effectiveness of single-dose therapy for *Chlamydia trachomatis* infections in women. *Sex Transm Dis* 22: 274–280, 1995.
49 Magid D et al: Doxycycline compared with azithromycin for treating

women with genital *Chlamydia trachomatis* infections: an incremental cost-effectiveness analysis. *Ann Intern Med* 124:389–389, 1996.

50 Hillis SD et al: Doxycycline and azithromycin for prevention of chlamydial persistence or recurrence one month following treatment in women: a use-effectiveness study in public health settings. *Sex Transm Dis* 25:5–11, 1998.

51 Handsfield HH, Stamm WE. Treating chlamydial infection: compliance versus cost (Editorial). *Sex Transm Dis* 25:12–13, 1998.

52 Bowie WR et al: Therapy for nongonococcal urethritis: double-blind randomized comparison of two doses and two durations of minocycline. *Ann Intern Med* 95:306–311, 1981.

53 Brown ST et al: Comparison of erythromycin base and estolate in gonococcal urethritis. *JAMA* 238:1371–1373, 1977.

54 Magat AH et al: Double-blind randomized study comparing amoxicillin and erythromycin for the treatment of *Chlamydia trachomatis* in pregnancy. *Obstet Gynecol* 81:745–749, 1993.

55 Bush MR, Rosa C: Azithromycin and erythromycin in the treatment of cervical chlamydial infection during pregnancy. *Obstet Gynecol* 84:61–63, 1994.

56 Crombleholme WR et al: Amoxicillin therapy for *Chlamydia trachomatis* in pregnancy. *Obstet Gynecol* 76:896–897, 1990.

57 Silverman NS et al: A randomized, prospective trial comparing amoxicillin and erythromycin for the treatment of *Chlamydial trachomatis* in pregnancy. *Am J Obstet Gynecol* 170:829–832, 1994.

58 Heston WJ, Lenhart JG: A decision analysis to guide antibiotic selection for chlamydia infection during pregnancy. *Arch Fam Med* 6: 551–555, 1997.

59 Brunham RC et al: Mucopurulent cervicitis—the ignored counterpart in women of urethritis in men. *N Engl J Med* 311:1–6, 1984.

60 Brunham RC et al: Therapy of cervical chlamydial infection. *Ann Intern Med* 97:216–219, 1982.

61 Stamm WE et al: Azithromycin for empirical treatment of the nongonococcal urethritis syndrome in men: a randomized double-blind study. *JAMA* 274:545–549, 1995.

62 Hooton TM et al: Erythromycin for persistent or recurrent nongonococcal urethritis: a randomized, placebo-controlled trial. *Ann Intern Med* 113:21–26, 1990.

63 Stamm LV et al: In vitro assay to demonstrate high-level erythromycin resistance of a clinical isolate of *Treponema pallidum. Antimicrob Agents Chemother* 32:164–169, 1988.

64 Norgard MV, Miller JN. Plasmid DNA in *Treponema pallidum* (Nichols): potential for antibiotic resistance by syphilis bacteria. *Science* 213:553–555, 1981.

65 Rolfs RT: Treatment of syphilis, 1993. *Clin Infect Dis* 20(Suppl 1): S23-S28, 1995.

66 Hook EW III, Marra CM: Acquired syphilis in adults. *N Engl J Med* 326:1060–1069, 1992.

67 Ducas J, Robson HG: Cerebrospinal fluid penicillin levels during therapy for latent syphilis. *JAMA* 246:2583–2584, 1981.

68 Smith CA, et al. Benzathine penicillin G in the treatment of syphilis. *Bull WHO* 15:1087–1096, 1956.

69 Lukehart SA et al: Invasion of the central nervous system by *Treponema pallidum*:: implications for diagnosis and treatment. *Ann Intern Med* 109:855–862, 1988.

70 Musher DM, Baughn RE: Neurosyphilis in HIV-infected patients (Editorial). *N Engl J Med* 331:1516–1517, 1994.

71 Gordon SM et al: The response of symptomatic neurosyphilis to high-dose intravenous penicillin G in patients with human immunodeficiency virus infection. *N Engl J Med* 331:1469–1473, 1994.

72 Rolfs RT et al: A randomized trial of enhanced therapy for early syphilis in patients with and without human immunodeficiency virus infection. *N Engl J Med* 337:307–314, 1997.

73 Walker CK et al: Pelvic inflammatory disease: meta-analysis of antimicrobial regimen efficacy. *J Infect Dis* 168:969–978, 1993.

74 Soper DE: Pelvic inflammatory disease. *Infect Dis Clin North Am* 8: 821–840, 1994.

75 Soper De, et al: Microbial etiology of urban emergency department acute salpingitis: treatment with ofloxacin. *Am J Obstet Gynecol* 167:653–660, 1992.

76 Hasselquist MB, Hillier S: Susceptibility of upper-genital tract isolates from women with pelvic inflammatory disease to ampicillin, cefpodoxime, metronidazole, and doxycycline. *Sex Transm Dis* 18:146–149, 1991.

77 Wald A et al: Suppression of subclinical shedding of herpes simplex virus type 2 with acyclovir. *Ann Intern Med* 124:8–15, 1996.

78 Wald A et al: Frequent genital herpes simplex virus 2 shedding in immunocompetent women: effect of acyclovir treatment. *J Clin Invest* 99:1092–1097, 1997.

79 Reyes M et al: Acyclovir-resistant HSV: initial results from a national surveillance system. Thirty-fifth Annual Meeting, Infectious Diseases Society of America, San Francisco, 1997 (Abstr 55).

80 Andrews EB et al: Acyclovir in pregnancy registry: six years' experience. *Obstet Gynecol* 79:7–13, 1992.

81 Stone KM et al: Acyclovir pregnancy registry: an international registry to monitor birth outcomes following prenatal acyclovir exposure. Thirty-fifth Annual Meeting, Infectious Diseases Society of America, San Francisco, 1997 (Abstr 639).

82 Scott LL et al: Acyclovir suppression to prevent cesarean delivery after first-episode genital herpes. *Obstet Gynecol* 87:69–73, 1996.

83 Beutner KR: Therapeutic approaches to genital warts. *Am J Med* 102(Suppl 5A):28–37, 1997.

Chapter 53

Issues in the laboratory diagnosis of STDS

Stephen A. Morse
Consuelo M. Beck-Sagué
Per-Anders Mårdh

The saying "the chain is no stronger than its weakest link" applies to the laboratory diagnosis of sexually transmitted diseases (STDs). A number of factors may, depending on test technique and technology employed, influence the outcome of any diagnostic effort. These factors are: choice of sampling site (urethra, vagina, cervix, rectum, conjunctiva, nasopharynx, etc.); the sampling device (type, brand, and lot); sampling technique; composition of the transport medium; composition of the transport vial (different plastics may absorb organisms by differing degrees); physical storage and transport conditions; and contamination problems in the clinic and laboratory, particularly when using nucleic acid amplification techniques.

Other weak points in the diagnostic chain are failure of the clinician to provide appropriate information to the laboratory concerning patient history and recent antibiotic use, and a request for the wrong or inappropriate diagnostic test. Misinterpretation of the test result may occur due to a lack of knowledge by the clinician or misinformation at the laboratory level. Lack of communication between laboratory and clinic may interfere with proper diagnosis. Tests that are not appropriate for the population being tested, or failure to ensure confidentiality of persons tested for STDs, may render even accurate test results useless or harmful.

This chapter will discuss the concepts of sensitivity, specificity, positive and negative predictive values, evaluation of new diagnostic methods, and test applications. It will assist in determining which tests are appropriate for particular circumstances, and it will consider cost-benefit analysis of screening.

BARRIERS TO LABORATORY TESTING

Among the many difficulties in the management of STDs are that many of these infections are asymptomatic, that more than one may be present, and that many of them may present with very similar symptoms and signs. Thus, laboratory testing is often needed to establish if one or more of them have been acquired. Obtaining multiple specimens, such as urethral and cervical swabs, from both male and female patients (particularly children and adolescents) may be uncomfortable or traumatic for the patient. The need for such uncomfortable procedures may not be appreciated, especially by asymptomatic patients. The use of noninvasive specimens such as voided urine, or even a self-collected vaginal introitus specimen,[1,2,3] coupled with the use of highly sensitive techniques such as polymerase chain reaction (PCR) or ligase chain reaction (LCR) may address some of these concerns and may permit outreach for testing in settings where physical examination is not feasible, such as work sites, detention facilities, and schools.

Another obstacle to the proper management of STDs is the need for multiple laboratory tests to cover the range of possible agents that an individual may have acquired. Such testing is generally too expensive to be universally employed on a routine basis. In developing countries, limited resources and clinical/laboratory infrastructure often preclude any diagnostic testing. The development of rapid, inexpensive diagnostic tests that are still sensitive and specific is a top priority in the field of STDs.

ACCURACY OF DIAGNOSTIC TESTS

Laboratorians and clinicians must know how well a test performs clinically, especially if consideration is being given to replacing an existing test with a newer one, to adding a new test, or to eliminating an old test from the laboratory's menu. Clinical performance is comprised of two elements: (1) discrimination, or diagnostic accuracy; and, (2) decision, or efficacy.[4] Laboratory tests are employed to help answer questions about patient management. Clinical and laboratory data are usually integrated into a complex decision-making process based upon probabilities of disease, quality of the data available, effectiveness of various treatment/management alternatives, probability of outcomes, and value (and cost) of outcomes to the patient.[5] A single laboratory test result is often not the sole basis for a diagnosis or patient management decision, but it should provide diagnostic discrimination. Clinical accuracy, the most fundamental characteristic of the test itself as a classification device, measures the ability to discriminate between alternative states of health, that is, between diseased and nondiseased (Figure 53-1).

The usefulness of test data involves other factors or parameters that are properties of the circumstances of the clinical application rather than properties of the test system or device. These include the prior probability of disease (its prevalence), the possible outcomes and the relative values of those outcomes, the cost to the patient and others of incorrect information (false-positive and false-negative classifications), and the costs and benefits of various treatment options. Thus, in evaluating tests it is helpful to separate the discrimination of the tests per se from the interaction of this discrimination with external factors in the course of patient management (Table 53-1).[7,8]

The first step in evaluating a diagnostic test is to determine its technical performance. Does the test measure what it claims to measure? Is the test replicable? (Replicability, or precision, reflects the variance in a test result that occurs when the test is repeated on the same specimen.) The greater this variation, the less confidence one has in results based on a single test. However, a precise test is not necessarily a good test. A test may exhibit a high level of replicability yet be in error, that is, it may be unreliable. A test must exhibit agreement between the mean test result and the true biologic variable being measured in the sample. Evaluations of clinical tests should consider both the replicability and the reliability of the test.[7]

The four most commonly used measures of reliability of diagnostic test performance are sensitivity, specificity, predictive value, and likelihood ratio (Figure 53-2). These test characteristics concern the correct identification of subjects with and without the condition of interest and should be applicable to any diagnostic method. Perfect tests would give no false-negative or false-positive results; test sensitivity and specificity would be 100%. However, no test is perfect; some misclassification occurs with all testing.

SENSITIVITY (CLINICAL SENSITIVITY)

Sensitivity answers the question "Among patients who have the disease, what proportion or percentage will have a positive test?" It is the ratio of subjects with a positive test result to all infected subjects (true positive fraction). Test sensitivity is of maximum

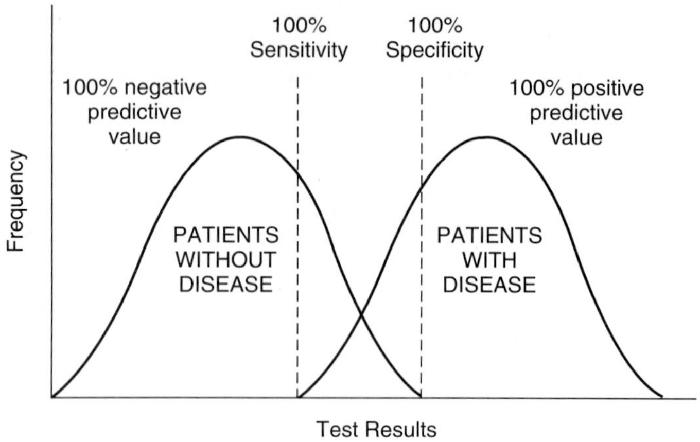

Fig. 53-1. Relationship of choice of cutoff value to selected test parameters for converting continuous valued test into dichotomous test result. (*From Albritton, 1996.*[6])

		REFERENCE STANDARD +	REFERENCE STANDARD −	
TEST	+	TRUE POSITIVE a	FALSE POSITIVE b	Predictive value (+) a/(a + b) Likelihood ratio (+) a(b + d)/b(a + c)
TEST	−	c FALSE NEGATIVE	d TRUE NEGATIVE	Predictive value (−) d/(c + d) Likelihood ratio (−) c(b + d)/d(a + c)
		Sensitivity a/(a + c)	Specificity d/(b + d)	Prevalence (a + c)/(a + b + c + d)

Figure 53-2. Binary table representation of important test parameters. (*From Albritton, 1996.*[6])

concern in patient populations having a high prevalence of disease, such as those seen in STD clinics. A high sensitivity suggests that the test is good for ruling out disease.[10] High sensitivity is also important when the treatment available is very cost-beneficial—treating pregnant women for early syphilis, for example—and when the consequences of false-negative tests are serious—for example, the consequences of false-negative tests for HIV in blood donors.

SPECIFICITY (CLINICAL SPECIFICITY)

Specificity answers the question "Among patients who do not have the disease, what proportion or percentage have a negative test?" It is the ratio of subjects with a negative test result to all uninfected subjects (true negative fraction). Test specificity is of maximum concern when testing patient populations having a low prevalence of disease, such as those seen in family planning clinics and most private practice settings. A high specificity suggests that the test is good for "ruling in" disease.[10] High specificity is also important when the consequences of a false-positive test are serious, as when the diagnosis itself, or the treatment, could have serious adverse effects. This consideration is generally important for STDs, because of the stigma associated with diagnosis of an STD.

Table 53-1. Evaluating and Applying the Results of Studies of Diagnostic Tests

Are the results of the study valid?
Primary guides:
- Was there an independent blind comparison with a reference ("gold") standard?
- Did the patient sample include an appropriate spectrum of patients to whom the diagnostic test will be applied in clinical practice?

Secondary guides:
- Did the results of the test being evaluated influence the decision to perform the reference standard?
- Were the methods for performing the test described in sufficient detail to permit replication?
- What were the results?
- Are likelihood ratios for the test results presented or data necessary for their calculation provided?

Will the test results help me in caring for my patients?
- Will the reproducibility of the test result and its interpretation be satisfactory in my setting?
- Are the results applicable to my patient?
- Will the results change my management?
- Will the patients be better off as a result of the test?

SOURCE: Adapted from Stephenson and Williams 1996.[9]

PREDICTIVE VALUE

In clinical practice, however, a clinician's question is: "If the patient has a positive test, how likely is he or she to have the disease?" (what is the predictive value of a positive test, or PVP?) or "If the patient has a negative test, how likely is he or she not to have the disease?" (what is the predictive value of a negative test, or PVN?). PVP and PVN are calculated from the arrangement shown in Figure 53-2. The PVP and PVN depend not only on the test sensitivity and specificity (stable properties of the test), but also on the prevalence of the disease in the population examined, which is (a+c)/N.[11] As prevalence of the disease decreases, the proportion of individuals with a positive test result who actually are infected falls, and the proportion of uninfected persons who are falsely identified as being infected rises (Table 53-2). In general, tests with high PVPs are desirable with conditions in which a false diagnosis can have profound consequences, either because therapeutic modalities are not benign or because of the psychosocial or medical implications associated with a particular diagnosis. By contrast, tests with high PVNs are desirable when it is essential not to miss any infections.[12]

Table 53-2. Effect of Decreasing Prevalence on Predictive Values of a Hypothetical Test with Sensitivity and Specificity of 95%

Actual Disease Prevalence (%)	Predictive Values Positive (%)	Predictive Values Negative (%)
1	16.1	99.9
2	27.9	99.9
5	50.0	99.7
10	67.9	99.4
20	82.6	98.7
50	95.0	95.0
75	98.3	83.7
100	100	

LIKELIHOOD RATIO

The likelihood ratio (LR, see Figure 53-2) allows clinicians to build on their clinical judgment, or estimated pretest probability. This is the estimated probability of a patient having a given disease, based on the known average prevalence of infection in the population or on history, physical examination, and other findings established before diagnostic testing.[5] The LR is calculated using the same figures used to calculate sensitivity and specificity; it is a ratio calculated by dividing the sensitivity (numerator) by 1 minus specificity (denominator). A positive LR expresses how much more likely a positive test is to occur in a patient with the disease in question than in a patient without the disease. A negative LR expresses how much more likely a negative test is to occur in a patient with the disease than in a patient without the disease; generally, a negative LR will be much less than 1. Using the nomogram provided in Figure 53-3, a straight line can be drawn from the pretest probability through the positive LR for a particular test to identify the post-test probability. Thus, the positive LR can be used to predict the probability of disease (given a positive test) in a particular patient (given the prior probability of infection).[5,8,13]

TEST EVALUATION

Understanding how diagnostic tests are evaluated helps in selecting tests for diagnostic or screening purposes. The evaluation of a new diagnostic test involves comparing its performance to the performance of methods in current use on an appropriate study population. Unless an appropriately broad spectrum of diseased and nondiseased persons is chosen for the study population, the

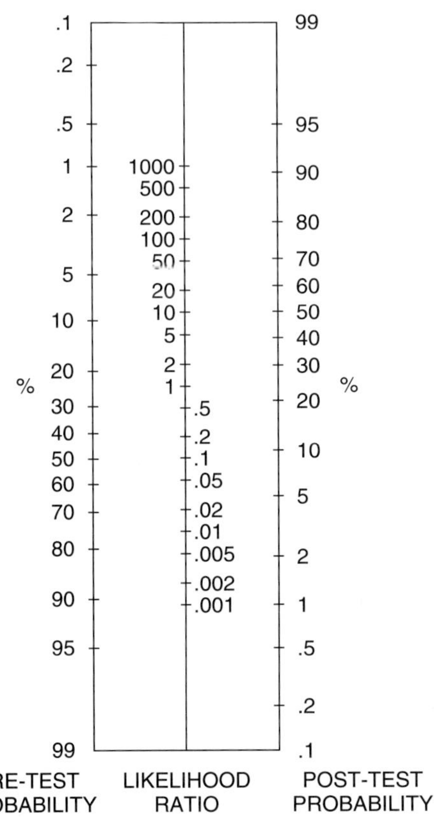

Figure 53-3. Nomogram for interpreting diagnostic test results. (*Adapted from Fagan, 1975.*[13])

diagnostic test may receive falsely high values for its "rule-in" and "rule-out" performances.[10] This failure to consider the heterogeneity of diseased and nondiseased populations in assessing test performance is termed *spectrum bias*.

Until recently, evaluation of a diagnostic test has begun with selection of a reference test (or "gold standard") for comparison; this standard is usually the most sensitive and specific of the established tests (see Figure 53-2). However, technologic advances in diagnostic test development, such as nucleic acid amplification tests for infections caused by *Chlamydia trachomatis*, illustrate the need for an "expanded gold standard."[14] For example, if cell culture is employed as the "gold standard," the sensitivity and specificity of the newer technology-based tests will depend on the performance of cell culture, which can vary greatly between laboratories.[15] Thus, the performance characteristics of tests may be distorted. A single reference test may not be suitable for all types of clinical specimens. Cell culture, which has been used as the "gold standard" for evaluating new diagnostic tests using urethral swab specimens from men and cervical and urethral swab specimens from women, has a sensitivity that is too low to be a suitable comparative method when used with urine specimens for the diagnosis of *C. trachomatis* infections.[16] Nucleic acid amplification and antigen-detection tests have been shown to be more suited to this purpose.[17–19] The concept of an "expanded gold standard" has, for most investigators, meant the use of at least two techniques based on different principles for comparing the performance of a new test.[20,21] This "expanded gold standard" is preferred when resolving disparate results by EIA[22] or PCR.[23]

For the purpose of DNA amplification test evaluations, investigators have developed various strategies to resolve discrepancies involving potential false-positive results.[5] If cell culture for *C. trachomatis* was one of the reference tests, analysis of discrepancies should (if possible) begin by reculturing the specimen and by using the direct fluorescent antibody (DFA) test on a cytospun preparation of the culture transport medium. If the discrepancy persists, the DNA amplification test is repeated;[24] a DNA amplification test using an alternate target has been recommended.[25] It has been argued that all test results, including false- and true-negative results, as well as discrepant positive results, should also be subjected to the same discrepant analysis.[26] However, due to the work load and costs involved, this has seldom been done. One caveat is that during reanalysis of true-negative results (see Figure 53-2), a positive result obtained with a test that is less sensitive than the test under evaluation will generally, if not almost always, be false positive.[27]

Classic diagnostic tests such as culture rely on the growth or nongrowth of a particular pathogen. Culture is seldom 100% sensitive, but when positive it is considered to be an indication of true infection. However, all culture-positive results should not be automatically accepted as true-positives, since the culture method may produce false-positive results. For example, cultivation of *C. trachomatis* in a microtiter plate tissue-culture system with multiple blind passages can result in cross-contamination between wells.[28]

Recent technologic advances in development of nonculture tests rely on the visual observation (e.g., DFA) or detection of component(s) of an organism (e.g., antigens, nucleic acid); these are continuously scaled tests. However, results are subjective and are interpreted in relation to a cutoff value or decision level established by the manufacturer (see Figure 53-1). All test scores at or beyond this cutoff value are considered positive; those below the cutoff value are considered negative. The cutoff value is set after establishing the clinical performance of the test. The performance data are described graphically, and the curve is referred to as a Relative Operating Characteristic or "ROC" plot (Figure 53-4).[4]

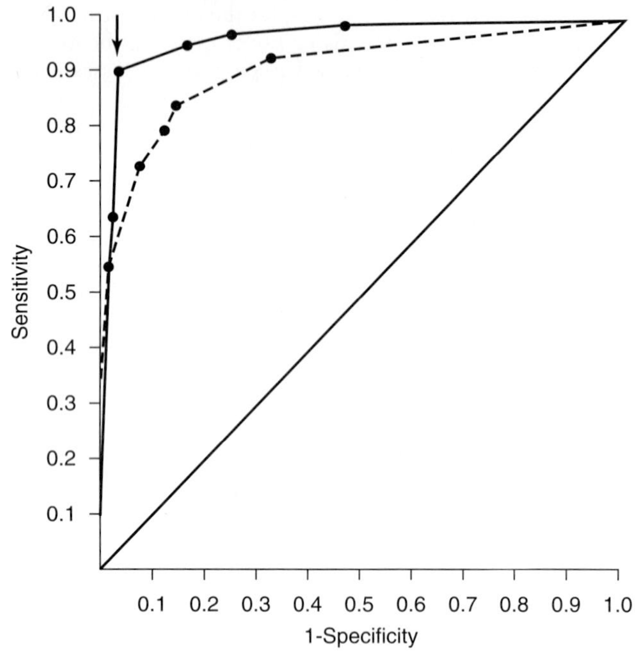

Figure 53-4. Relative operating characteristics (ROC) curves for two hypothetical assays using five different cutoff levels to define positivity. Each symbol represents the sensitivity and 1-specificity obtained at a different cut-off level, using known positive and negative specimens. Cut-off levels decrease as you move from left to right. The best cut-off level for Test 1 is indicated by the arrow; further increases in sensitivity occur at the expense of specificity. Sensitivity increases and specificity decreases as lower cut-off levels are used to define positive test results. The solid line indicates Test 1; the dashed line indicates Test 2. (*Adapted from Schwartz JS, 1988.*[29])

This plot represents the relationship between the true-positive fraction (sensitivity) and the false-positive fraction (1-specificity). Customarily, the true-positive fraction is plotted on the vertical axis and the false-positive fraction is plotted on the horizontal axis. Clinical accuracy, in terms of sensitivity and specificity, is displayed for the entire spectrum of decision levels (cutoff values). Selection of the test cutoff point should be based on the benefits of true-positive and true-negative results, the costs of false-positive and false-negative errors, and prevalence of the disease.[29]

Often a test is said to have a particular sensitivity and specificity. However, a test does not have a single sensitivity and specificity; rather, it has a continuum of sensitivities and specificities. By varying the cutoff (or decision level), any sensitivity from 0 to 100% can be obtained, and each one will have a corresponding specificity. For any test in which the distribution of results from the two categories of subjects (infected and not infected) overlaps, there will be inevitable trade-offs between sensitivity and specificity (see Figure 53-1). As the cutoff is varied, the sensitivity and specificity will move in opposite directions. The use of ROC curves is necessary in order to compare alternative diagnostic tests. For example, in Figure 53-4 the ROC curve for test 1 is farther up and to the left than that for test 2, indicating that test 1 is a better test because it has fewer false-positive results at any given level of test sensitivity. Using the ROC curve, a single-valued measure of accuracy can be calculated as the proportion of the area of the entire graph that lies beneath the curve. This value varies from 0.5 to 1.0. Thus, when the curve lies along the major diagonal, A = 0.5, no discrimination exists.

TEST APPLICATIONS

Clinical tests fall into several overlapping categories, depending on the situation in which they are used. The requirements for sensitivity and specificity are different for each category and may vary depending on the particular application.

SCREENING TESTS

Screening refers to the voluntary testing of a broad sector of the population that may be largely asymptomatic and is therefore important in the control of STDs. Screening can also be mandatory. For example, mandatory screening for syphilis currently is used on donated blood and in some states for persons seeking a marriage license. The actual disease prevalence of the population may be low. A positive result in a screening test does not always necessarily indicate the presence of the microorganism or a disease state; rather, it may prompt further testing. In contrast, a negative result implies that the patient does not have the disease or harbor the targeted microorganism. Therefore, high diagnostic sensitivity and very high negative predictive value are the most important performance characteristics of a screening test. These characteristics assume that false-positive results can be easily and inexpensively resolved and that the negative medical, psychological, and financial effects of false-positive results are acceptable.

CHOICE OF METHOD FOR SCREENING

The correct choice of a screening test involves a knowledge of the prevalence of the infectious disease one wants to study.[30] Thus, some screening methods may work well in high-prevalence populations but less well in low-prevalence populations. Differences in the prevalence of an STD may exist in different age, ethnic, or socioeconomic groups of persons in the same area. A difference in prevalence may even exist between different practitioners' offices. Within the same clinic, for instance, prevalence may differ among units seeing pregnant women, units for family planning, and gynecologic emergency rooms.

As stated earlier, the PVP and PVN of a test varies with disease prevalence. In a low-prevalence setting (1% prevalence), the PVP of a test with a sensitivity and specificity of 95% will only be 16%; however, in a high-prevalence population (20% prevalence) the same test will have a PVP of 83% (see Table 53-2). Conversely, the PVN of the same test will be 99.9% in the low-prevalence population and 98.7% in the high-prevalence population. This implies that there must be an exchange of information between the clinician and the diagnostic laboratory to assist in choosing the right technique for different test situations, and this exchange should include information regarding the prevalence of the disease in the population. With a low PVP, the chance that the answer given by the test is correct may not be higher than for an answer obtained by tossing a coin. Institution of screening programs for a treatable disease is associated with decreases in the prevalence of the disease.[31,32] Thus, the PVP of a test will decrease with duration of the screening program.

Screening tests are often used for populations with a low prevalence of infection. Therefore, most of the test results will be negative. In order to decrease the cost of screening, inexpensive nonspecific prescreening tests, such as the urine leukocyte esterase (ULE) test have been recommended for some screening situations. Identification of pyuria has been found useful for screening young men for urethritis.[33] Analysis of urine for pyuria was more useful than was the detection of leukocytes in stained urethral smears for predicting chlamydial infection in males.[34]

The ULE test has been shown to be a rapid and easy way to detect inflammatory changes in the urogenital tract.[35–38] The commercial test is a colorimetric assay in a dipstick format, which detects the presence of an esterase produced by polymorphonuclear leukocytes.[39] Thus, the ULE test can diagnose urethritis but cannot identify the specific cause of infection. Positive ULE test results occur with infections caused by a number of different microorganisms, including *C. trachomatis* and *N. gonorrhoeae*. The ULE test is recommended for prescreening adolescent males but not for prescreening women or males over 25 years of age, due to unsatisfactory performance.[40,41] The ULE test has been used in a screening algorithm to preselect urine samples from sexually active men for subsequent testing for *C. trachomatis*.[30,37,39]

The use of the ULE test as an approach to screening asymptomatic adolescent male populations appears feasible not only because of its acceptable sensitivity[21,33,42] but also because it is cheap, and therefore a cost-effective procedure.[30,43,44] Best results with ULE testing either alone or in combination with other tests are achieved only with the use of first void of the day urine specimens.

COST-EFFECTIVENESS, COST-BENEFIT RATIO, AND COST UTILITY

Cost-effectiveness of laboratory costs for STD refers to the cost per case of STD detected. *Cost-benefit ratio* refers to the costs of testing divided by the cost (either direct medical cost or direct plus indirect costs) of the disease prevented by testing. *Cost utility* refers to the cost of testing in relation to the quality of life preserved (for example, cost per disability-adjusted life-year saved, or DALY; or cost per quality-adjusted life-year preserved, or QALY). Most studies of the cost-benefit of laboratory testing consider only the benefit to the individual tested, not the impact on reduced transmission. Since STDs are communicable, such analyses underestimate the benefit to the population as a whole.

The low cost of the ULE test allows its use in mass screening programs for the detection of genital chlamydia infections.[45] ULE pre-screening can reduce the number of urine specimens to be tested by as much as 90% among men. The potential benefit of using urine specimens, as opposed to cervical or urethral specimens, for STD screening involves not only the costs for the laboratory tests but also reduced costs for scheduling patient examinations, facilities, and staff for collecting specimens by invasive sampling methods, and the lower costs of handling of specimens and test results, including notification and therapy of positive cases. The calculation of benefits of screening should also include the preventive costs of complications and sequelae. The cost saving, particularly in the long term, may be great, even taking into account short-term increases in costs due to the detection of positive cases requiring expenditure of additional health care resources.[44,46]

Even in very low-prevalence populations, screening for STDs having potentially devastating complications using inexpensive tests (for example, prenatal serologic screening for syphilis) will generally be cost-effective.[47,48] Conversely, even the use of expensive tests such as nucleic acid amplification tests may be cost-effective in high-prevalence populations.[46] Cost-effectiveness analyses have confirmed that screening for *C. trachomatis* infection using less sensitive antigen detection tests is cost-effective during routine gynecologic visits[49,50,51] and during pregnancy,[52] when prevalence of infection exceeds 6–8%, or even at lower prevalences.[53]

Screening asymptomatic adolescent males with urine-based tests for chlamydial infection was calculated to be cost-saving, primarily by reducing infection in female partners.[43] In general, men with STDs are more likely to be symptomatic than women and thus more likely to obtain treatment; in addition, the sequelae of most untreated bacterial STDs are not as devastating in men as in women. Therefore, unless the impact of preventing transmission of infection to women is taken into account, cost-benefit analyses would not favor screening asymptomatic men except in STD clinics and in very high-risk populations, such as those in drug-rehabilitation facilities, jails, and detention centers. However, it would be short-sighted to ignore the population-level benefits of screening and treating infected men for STD.

Multiple guidelines exist to help clinicians and laboratories determine for which populations screening for specific agents is appropriate (Table 53-3)[54–56] and, for a variety of agents, which populations should be screened (Table 53-4).[57] Such guidelines have become increasingly influential with purchasers and insurers of health care, with managed care organizations and individual clinical providers, and with the general population. These 1996 guidelines should be updated as new information accrues. For example, the strength of the recommendation for screening high-risk women for chlamydial infection is listed only as "B" (fair evidence to support the recommendation), but the recently published study by Scholes et al. showing that screening for chlamydia reduced PID incidence by over 50% should increase the strength of the recommendations to "A."[58] Further, guidelines from different professional medical associations differ considerably[57] (see Table 53-4). For example, the U.S. Public Health Service currently recommends voluntary HIV testing for all pregnant women.[59] The American Academy of Pediatrics recommends routine screening, with consent, of all pregnant women and HIV testing for all infants whose mother's HIV status is not known.[60] The U.S. Preventive Services Task Force (USPSTF) recommends routine HIV screening for women with certain behavioral risk factors; for the general pregnant population it recommends only that screening be available, offered, or discussed. The American Medical Association has proposed mandatory universal HIV testing of pregnant women.[56]

In selecting pathogens for which to screen, patients to screen, and tests to use in screening, it is vital to weigh issues such as availability of treatment options, risk of sequelae and complications among undetected cases, and most important, prevalence in the population, as well as the overall cost-benefit ratio of the patient management protocol. Some organizations have modified, for multiple reasons, the definition of those who should be screened more aggressively for STDs, using such formulas as "populations with high-risk sexual behaviors." This analysis has certain drawbacks.[56] First, some of the populations with the highest HIV or STD prevalence in both the developing and developed world report no high-risk behaviors and/or report consistent condom use.[59,61] Although most patients are very frank about their own and their partners' sexual behaviors to the best of their knowledge,[62] some may under-report their own sexual risk-taking

Table 53-3. WHO Recommendations for Where Genital Chlamydial Infections May Present in a Hypothetical District

STD clinics	Rheumatology clinics
Gynecologic clinics	Ophthalmology clinics
Urologic clinics	Family planning centers
Health centers	Maternity centers
Youth health centers	School health centers
Student health services	Drug addiction treatment centers

SOURCE: WHO, 1989;[54] Brabin, 1996[55] (revised).

Table 53-4. Recommended Screening Tests during the Periodic Health Examination for the Prevention of STDs

Age group (in years)	Interventions for general population	Strength of recommendation[a]	Interventions for high-prevalence/ High-risk populations	Strength of recommendation[a]
Birth–10			HIV testing (for infants of mothers at high risk for HIV)[b]	B
			RPR/VDRL (serological test for syphilis)	A
11–24	Screen with Papanicolaou (Pap) test (for females who are sexually active at present or in the past, at least every 3 years. If sexual activity may have started before age 21, begin Pap tests at age 18 or at first family planning visit/STD visit).	A	RPR/VDRL (serological test for syphilis)[c]	A
	Screen for chlamydia (for sexually active females <20 years old).	B	Screen for gonorrhea (for females)[d]	B
			HIV[e]	A
			Chlamydia (for females)[g]	B
25–64	Screen with Papanicolaou (Pap) test (for women who are or have been sexually active, at least every 3 years).	A	RPR/VDRL[c]	A
			Screen for gonorrhea (for females)[i]	B
			HIV[e]	A
			Chlamydia (for females)[j]	B
			Hepatitis B vaccine[k]	A
			Hepatitis A vaccine[l]	A
>64	Screen with Papanicolaou (Pap) test (for all women who have a cervix). Consider discontinuation of testing after age 65 years if previous regular screening showed consistently normal results.	B	Hepatitis A vaccine[m]	B
			HIV screen[e]	A
			Hepatitis B vaccine[k]	A
			RPR/VDRL[c]	A
Pregnant women	*During first visit:*		Screen for chlamydia (1st visit)[n]	B
	Screen for hepatitis B surface Antigen (HbsAg)	A	Gonorrhea (1st visit)[o]	B
	RPR/VDRL	A	HIV (1st visit)[p]	A
	Chlamydia (<25-year-olds)	B	HbsAg (3rd trimester)[q]	A
	Offer to screen for HIV (universal screening is recommended for states, counties, or cities with an increased prevalence of HIV infection among pregnant women. In low-prevalence areas the choice between universal and targeted screening may depend on other considerations).	A	RPR/VDRL (3rd trimester)[r]	A
			Bacterial vaginosis (2nd trimester)[s]	B
Detention centers, drug-rehabilitation centers, prisons			Screen for chlamydia	B
			Gonorrhea	B
			HIV, syphilis	

Source note and Footnotes continue on next page

behaviors, and some may be unaware of their partners' risk-behaviors. Clinicians often do not effectively elicit sexual histories, especially from asymptomatic patients.[63–65] Further, reporting of illegal drug use or prostitution could result in the patient's loss of parental rights and/or incarceration and these behaviors may be understated.[66,67]

Thus, it may prove impossible to monitor and evaluate clinician compliance with guidelines for screening "sexually active persons" or persons with "high-risk sexual behaviors," because it is difficult if not impossible to precisely define who these people are. There is probably no better surrogate for patient risk than the prevalence of infection in the clinical population in which the patient is sexually active (Table 53-5); and testing guidelines based on easily measured variables such as age, marital status, geographic location, and pregnancy are highly desirable.

Most screening tests require that the patient who tests positive return to the clinic for treatment of an often asymptomatic, poorly understood condition. In some settings, contacting the patient for treatment may be difficult. Pretest explanations of the implications of the diseases for which the patient is being screened, with reinforcement in the form of patient educational materials at a posttest counseling session, may be essential to increase the likelihood

SOURCE: U.S. Preventive Services Task Force. Guide to clinical preventive services, 2nd ed. Washington, DC: U.S. Department of Health and Human Services, 1996.

The following footnotes are quotations from the primary source:

[a]The letter "A" indicates that there is good evidence to support the recommendation that the condition be specifically considered in a period health examination, "B" indicates that there is fair evidence to support the recommendation that the condition be specifically considered in a period health examination. Because level of risk related to the patient's and/or his/her partner's behavior may be difficult or impossible to assess, and risk does not always reflect behaviors, clinicians should consider primarily local epidemiology, particularly prevalence of infection in the population being served, to determine whether interventions appropriate to the general or high prevalence populations should be used. Interventions for high risk are additional to those for general population.

[b]Infants born to high-risk mothers whose HIV status is unknown. Women at high risk include past or present injection drug users; persons who exchange sex for money or drugs and their sex partners; injection drug users, bisexual, or HIV-positive sex partners currently or in past; persons seeking treatment for STDs; blood transfusion during 1978–1985.

[c]Persons who exchange sex for money or drugs, and their sex partners with other STDs (including HIV); and sexual contacts of persons with active syphilis. Clinicians should also consider local epidemiology.

[d]Women who have two or more sex partners in the last year; a sex partner with multiple sexual contacts; exchanged sex for money or drugs; or a history of repeated episodes of gonorrhea. Clinicians should also consider local epidemiology.

[e]Men who had sex with men after 1975; past or present injection drug use; persons who exchange sex for money or drugs and their sex partners; injection-drug using, bisexual, or HIV-positive sex partner currently or in the past; blood transfusion during 1978–1985; persons seeking treatment for STDs. Clinicians should also consider local epidemiology.

[f]The ability of clinician counseling to influence this behavior is unproven.

[g]Sexually active women with multiple risk factors including history of STD; new or multiple sex partners; age under 25; nonuse or inconsistent use of barrier contraceptives; cervical ectopy. Clinicians should also consider local epidemiology of the disease in identifying other high-risk groups.

[h]Persons living in, traveling to, or working in areas where the disease is endemic and where periodic outbreaks occur (e.g., countries with high or intermediate endemicity; certain Alaska Native, Pacific Island, Native American, and religious communities); men who have sex with men; injection or street drug users. Vaccine may be considered for institutionalized persons and workers in these institutions, military personnel, and day care, hospital, and laboratory workers. Clinicians should also consider local epidemiology.

[i]Sexually active women including those with history of STD; new or multiple sex partners; age under 25; nonuse or inconsistent use of barrier contraceptives; cervical ectopy. Clinicians should also consider local epidemiology of the disease in identifying other high-risk groups.

[j]Sexually active women with multiple risk factors including history of STD; new or multiple sex partners; nonuse or inconsistent use of barrier contraceptives; cervical ectopy. Clinicians should also consider local epidemiology.

[k]Blood product recipients (including hemodialysis patients), persons with frequent occupational exposure to blood or blood products, men who have sex with men, injection drug users and their sex partners, persons with multiple recent sex partners, persons with other STDs (including HIV), travelers to countries with endemic hepatitis B.

[l]Persons living in, traveling to, or working in areas where the disease is endemic and where periodic outbreaks occur (e.g., countries with high or intermediate endemicity; certain Alaska Native, Pacific Island, Native American, and religious communities); men who have sex with men; injection or street drug users. Consider for institutionalized persons and workers in these institutions, military personnel, and day-care, hospital, and laboratory workers. Clinicians should also consider local epidemiology.

[m]Persons living in, traveling to, or working in areas where the disease is endemic and where periodic outbreaks occur (e.g., countries with high or intermediate endemicity; certain Alaska Native, Pacific Island, Native American, and religious communities); men who have sex with men; injection or street drug users. Consider for institutionalized persons and workers in these institutions, military personnel, and day-care, hospital, and laboratory workers. Clinicians should also consider local epidemiology.

[n]Women with history of STD or new or multiple sex partners. Clinicians should also consider local epidemiology. Chlamydia screen should be repeated in 3rd trimester if at continued risk.

[o]Women under age 25 with two or more sex partners in the last year, or whose sex partner has multiple sexual contacts; women who exchange sex for money or drugs; and women with history of repeated episodes of gonorrhea. Clinicians should also consider local epidemiology. Gonorrhea screen should be repeated in the 3rd trimester if at continued risk.

[p]In areas where universal screening is not performed due to low prevalence of HIV infection, pregnant women with the following individual risk factors should be screened: past or present injection drug use; women who exchange sex for money or drugs; injection drug-using, bisexual, or HIV-positive sex partner currently or in the past; blood transfusions during 1978–1985; persons seeking treatment for STDs.

[q]Women who are initially HBsAg negative who are at high risk due to injection drug use, suspected exposure to hepatitis B during pregnancy, multiple sex partners.

[r]Women who exchange sex for money or drugs, women with other STDs (including HIV), and sexual contacts of persons with active syphilis. Clinicians should also consider local epidemiology.

[s]Bacterial vaginosis may increase the risk of preterm birth, and, particularly among women with past history of preterm birth or pregravid weight <50 kg, treatment of bacterial vaginosis may reduce the risk of preterm birth.

of return for treatment of patients who are screened with other than rapid tests.

Diagnostic tests

Diagnostic tests are applied to persons suspected of having a particular infection. Diagnostic testing is usually a response to a patient's presentation with symptoms or signs of disease, to his or her identification as a sexual partner of a case of STD, or to some other indication of a particular infection. Therefore, the likelihood (prevalence) of disease among patients evaluated with diagnostic tests is expected to be high. Because the presence of the infectious agent can be important for treatment or prognosis, the specificity of a diagnostic test should be as high as possible without sacrificing sensitivity (refer to Figure 53-4 curves). Diagnostic tests have very high PVNs.

Algorithms for use in various clinical syndromes aid in the selection of diagnostic tests. In general, a variety of common syndromes and complications should prompt evaluation for sexually transmitted agents (See opening paragraphs to this book). However, clinical judgment must always be used to determine the need or indication for specific diagnostic tests. For example, sexually

Table 53-5. Prevalence of *C. trachomatis* and *N. gonorrhoeae* and Proportion with Both Infections in Different Populations of Women

C. trachomatis prevalance (%)	*N. gonorrhoeae* prevalence (%)	% *C. trachomatis* positive with *N. gonorrhoeae*	% *N. gonorrhoeae* positive with *C. trachomatis*	Reference
Family planning clinics				
20.7	7.4	–	–	Begley 1989[68]
9.8	<1.0	–	45.0	Schachter 1983[69]
10.5	0.7	–	47.4	Glenney 1988[70]
10.5	1.5	–	40.0	Winter 1990[71]
University students				
8.0	1.2	–	–	Harrison 1985[72]
Isolated Eskimo community				
23.0	6.0	15.0	57.0	Toomey 1987[73]
Adolescents				
23.0	10.0	–	–	Chacko 1984[74]
10.2	9.7	–	44.4	Golden 1984[75]
15.3	3.8	–	–	Shafer 1984[76]
12.0	8.0	–	–	Fraser 1981[77]
22.0	3.0	0.0	0.0	Saltz 1981[78]
19.0	6.0	–	–	Bump 1986[79]
14.5	0.0	0.0	0.0	Fisher 1987[80]
26.3	8.4	12.9	37.5	Jaffe 1986[81]
27.4	7.1	–	–	Smith 1988[82]
21.0	7.0	–	42.0	Eager 1985[83]
20.7	10.0	21.5	47.2	Beck-Sague 1998[84]
STD clinics				
13.0	–	15.0	–	Kent 1988[85]
21.5	20.7	–	37.5	Kinghorn 1981[86]
17.0	–	–	38.0	Magder 1988[87]
25.0	28.0	–	40.0	Persson 1979[88]
19.0	9.0	–	48.0	Richmond 1980[89]
31.0	20.0	–	63.0	Hilton 1974[90]
26.5	–	–	–	Woolfitt 1977[91]
15.7	13.8	–	–	Thelin 1980[92]
Prostitutes				
57.6	24.8	–	–	Bai 1995[93]
Prisoners				
27.0	8.0	7.0	–	Holmes 1993[94]

SOURCE: Brabin 1996[55] (revised).

active, nonpregnant adults with highly typical findings for genital herpes may not need HSV culture confirmation. Conversely, in a child presenting with genital vesicles or ulceration, where a diagnosis of genital herpes may have profound medicolegal implications, a culture-proven diagnosis is vital, as is ruling out other sexually transmitted diseases by definitive tests.[95]

Rapid tests

"Stat," "bed-side,", or "in-office" rapid tests, performed while the often symptomatic patient waits, provide a definitive diagnosis to guide therapy at the first point of contact and a strong impetus for compliance and partner referral (Table 53-6). Such tests, when positive, are extremely effective in prompting rapid, appropriate therapeutic action. Rapid tests are particularly important (1) when patients have symptoms or signs of acute infection and prompt treatment based on test results is needed, (2) when patients are not highly likely to return for results of tests and treatment, and (3) when the chain of events that lead to later diagnosis and treatment has many weak links (for example, syphilis serologic testing of pregnant women in many developing countries). However, the sensitivity of many rapid tests is suboptimal, and many are not definitive. Important exceptions are the Gram stain of urethral exudate for gonococcal urethritis in men and darkfield microscopy for lesion (primary and secondary) syphilis, which are definitive rapid tests;[96,97] and the rapid plasma reagin (RPR) test for syphilis. In the United States the Clinical Laboratory Improvement Act (CLIA) has set more rigorous standards for quality assurance in office-based laboratory testing, but this requirement now poses a major potential barrier to rapid testing for management of STD.

Confirmatory tests

Confirmatory tests are supplemental tests applied after obtaining a positive screening or diagnostic test result. An example of a confirmatory test is the fluorescent treponemal antibody absorption (FTA-ABS) test, which is used to confirm a positive RPR or veneral disease research laboratory (VDRL) test result. Confirmatory tests are also used to identify or otherwise characterize a microorganism (for example, *N. gonorrhoeae*) once it has been

Table 53-6. "Stat" (Bedside) Laboratory Tests for the Diagnosis of STDs

STD	Test
Syphilis	Rapid plasma reagin
	Darkfield microscopy
Gonorrhea	Gram stain of urethral exudate or smear (male)
	Gram stain of cervical exudate (female)
Chlamydia trachomatis	Endocervical swab for pus
	Leukocyte esterase test on first voided male urine
	Rapid ELISA tests
Bacterial vaginosis	Gram stain
	Wet mount for clue cells
	"Whiff test" for fish odor
	pH of vaginal fluid
	Rapid test card for amines and pH of vaginal fluid
Trichomoniasis	Wet mount for motile trichomonads
Genital herpes	Tzanck smear

cultured or presumptively identified. Specificity and positive predictive value are most important because these tests are applied in situations of high disease prevalence.

OTHER STRATEGIES FOR TEST USE

Case-finding

Case-finding occurs when a person presents for care for one reason and is tested for another disease for which that person is at increased risk. It also occurs when a person is identified as a sexual contact of an STD case and is then tested for that STD and others. In the case of STD testing, case-finding can occur in STD clinics when patients presenting with gonorrhea are also tested for syphilis and when sexual contacts of infected individuals are examined and tested.

Test-of-cure

A test-of-cure is not a separate clinical test category. The term has been used most often in regards to gonococcal and chlamydial infections and syphilis and refers to post-treatment testing to document effectiveness of therapy. Because highly effective treatments, often clinician-observed, exist for many STDs, response to treatment of these diseases does not need to be confirmed under most circumstances by a test-of-cure for compliant patients. Important exceptions to this general rule include syphilis, particularly during pregnancy, in congenital syphilis, and in late latent (tertiary "benign") neurologic and cardiovascular syphilis.[95] A fourfold or greater decline in titer of nontreponemal tests without subsequent rise in titer confirms response to therapy. Response of CSF abnormalities to treatment guides the management of neurosyphilis.

Persons treated with second- or third-line regimens should have a test-of-cure four to seven days after completion of therapy for gonococcal infections, or three weeks after treatment for chlamydial infections.[95] It is important to note that nucleic acid amplification tests such as PCR or LCR may detect *C. trachomatis* or *N. gonorrhoeae* nucleic acid remaining after completion of therapy and may yield false-positive results.[98]

In the case of cervical premalignant and malignant lesions associated with human papilloma virus, treatment often fails to entirely eradicate the original lesions, and recurrence is frequent. Therefore, close follow-up is an essential aspect of the management of these lesions.

Alternatives to diagnostic testing

Because of the high cost and infrastructure requirements of some of the most reliable tests, a syndromic approach is often espoused as an alternative to diagnostic testing in resource-poor settings; such settings may be found in both developing and industrialized countries.[99] According to this approach, common STD syndromes are managed with broad-spectrum antimicrobial treatments that are effective against most bacterial pathogens that cause the clinical syndrome. This approach is most effective for certain syndromes (such as urethritis in the male, pelvic inflammatory disease, and genital ulcer disease), but it has not been highly effective for cervical and vaginal infections, and of course it is not useful for screening for asymptomatic infection.

The syndromic approach has drawbacks. The clinical presentation of infection with one pathogen may mask the presence of another.[100] Persons presenting with one STD syndrome are at risk for other STDs that may be detected only by testing for other infections. Syndromic case management usually involves use of multiple antimicrobial agents, potentially promoting noncompliance and antimicrobial resistance. Finally, counseling and partner notification without a definitive diagnosis of an STD may be less effective. Nevertheless, implementation of the syndromic approach has been credited not only with the identification and treatment of thousands of cases of infections, but with marked reduction in HIV sexual transmission.[45]

Even with syndromic management, laboratory testing is essential to periodically reassess the appropriateness of the algorithms. As an etiologic agent is effectively treated, its prevalence in a population may decline, along with the relative proportion of cases of a syndrome it causes, necessitating changes in the recommended antimicrobial treatment. Periodic surveys of the etiologies of common syndromes will help ensure the continuing adequacy of the algorithm. Periodic culture surveys of antimicrobial susceptibilities are essential, since antimicrobial pressure inevitably results in the emergence of antimicrobial-resistant strains of some sexually transmitted pathogens.

Presumptive therapy is a more focused alternative, providing for treatment of commonly coexisting and more-difficult-to-diagnose infections in patients with a laboratory diagnosis of an STD. For example, since patients with gonorrhea are very frequently coinfected with *C. trachomatis* (see Table 53-5), it is recommended that treatments for proven gonorrhea include an agent effective against *C. trachomatis*, such as ceftriaxone and oral doxycycline or azithromycin, if *C. trachomatis* infection cannot be ruled out by specific testing.[95] Similarly, in populations with high chancroid prevalence it is recommended that proven syphilis be treated not only with benzathine penicillin G but also with a drug such as ceftriaxone that is curative for chancroid, if a definitive diagnosis cannot be made.

In many settings, syndromic treatment is inevitable. Even when diagnostic testing is performed, syndromic treatment (for example, for PID) is often desirable while test results are pending. Nonetheless, we recommend that wherever possible, a definitive laboratory diagnosis be made in patients with common STD syndromes such as genital ulcer disease or vaginal discharge.[95] The obvious advantages of a specific diagnosis include specific therapy (generally one agent); often, one clinician-observed dose; and more effective counseling and partner referral. A caveat is that insensitive tests, with intrinsically low negative predictive value or poor quality control, are a poor guide to specific therapy (as opposed to broader-spectrum therapy covering the major causes of a syndrome).

In many countries, the risk of HIV infection among patients diagnosed with some STDs, particularly syphilis and chancroid, is so high in most populations as to justify HIV counseling and screening in any patient with a confirmed diagnosis or reliable recent history of these diseases.[95,101] In other countries, diagnoses of other STDs may also warrant HIV counseling and screening in some populations.

IMPLICATIONS OF STD SCREENING AND DIAGNOSIS

In virtually all cases, the diagnosis of an STD has unique emotional and social implications. In certain groups of patients (such as children, or women in many settings), the diagnosis of an STD can trigger legal and social consequences having tremendous repercussions for the family and social networks. For these reasons, the decision to test and the choice of diagnostic test must be carefully assessed to ensure the maximum possible benefit. Only adolescents and adults who acknowledge consensual sexual activity should be screened or diagnosed with nonculture screening tests. In all cases where a potential legal use of test results or very negative social repercussions can reasonably be anticipated, definitive tests of very high specificity should be used.[95]

In children, physical examination findings which prompted the test, such as genital and/or anal or rectal lesions, tears, or other findings should be carefully documented, preferably photographically. For example, when diseases such as syphilis are suspected in these settings, darkfield microscopy and both nontreponemal and confirmatory treponemal tests should be used. The use of the fluorescent treponemal antibody stain of lesion material offers the opportunity to save the specimen for later review, which is not possible with darkfield microscopy.[102]

ERRONEOUS TEST RESULTS

Multiple reasons for false positive and false negative results exist. In many cases, a false positive, particularly with nonculture tests, results from the persistence of analyte after treatment. This is of particular importance in nucleic acid amplification tests.[103,104] Conversely, topical antimicrobial ointments and creams can render lesions such as primary syphilitic chancres negative by darkfield microscopy.[97] A wide variety of products to which patients have access and often resort can alter specimen quality, both in theory and in proven fact. Recent use of vaginal deodorants and spermicides can reduce the sensitivity of tests that depend on the organisms' viability; theoretically, douching may do the same. However, in well-controlled studies, reported frequent use of douches has not appeared to interfere with the sensitivity of nucleic acid probes or amplification tests and has, in fact, emerged as a risk factor for infection diagnosed by these methods.[84,105]

ANTIMICROBIAL SUSCEPTIBILITY

For some sexually transmitted agents, such as *T. pallidum* and *C. trachomatis*, where antimicrobial resistance is not yet a clinical issue, antimicrobial susceptibility testing is unnecessary. However, in the cases of *N. gonorrhoeae* and *H. ducreyi,* resistance to antimicrobials used routinely in treatment of gonorrhea and chancroid has been well documented, and geographical and temporal differences in antimicrobial susceptibilities have been observed.[106,107] Generation and revision of meaningful treatment guidelines depends on the periodic reassessment of emerging resistance, which should be done by antimicrobial susceptibility testing of a representative sample of viable organisms.[95] Sentinel events, such as decreased susceptibility to first- or second-line antimicrobials, require surveillance systems geared to early detection of emerging resistance.[106,107] In some U.S. facilities serving clients with STDs, antimicrobial susceptibility testing of patients with treatment failures constitutes an alternative strategy for identifying emerging resistance.[108]

However, just as it affects other issues relevant to the laboratory diagnosis of STDs, the current trend toward decreasing laboratory diagnosis may reduce the opportunities for early detection of emerging resistance.[108] The CDC-supported introduction of culture testing for gonorrhea in women in the early 1970s clearly led to increased awareness of and attention to gonococcal infection in women in the United States. Similarly, the introduction of tests for *C. trachomatis* infection into many patient settings has been credited with increased recognition of chlamydial disease.[31] Dramatic decreases in prevalence of chlamydial infection following the introduction of screening have been attributed to the treatment of large numbers of asymptomatic patients.[32] It is likely that any marked decreases in screening in the future, coupled with reduced diagnostic testing, would greatly compromise laboratory-based surveillance for sexually transmitted infections.[109] The strategy of repeated prevalence monitoring in sentinel sites and populations may become a more essential alternative for STD surveillance.

References

1 Wiesenfeld HC, et al: Self-Collection of Vaginal Introitus Specimens: A Novel Approach to *Chlamydia trachomatis* Testing in Women, in *Proceedings of the Eleventh Meeting of the International Society for STD Research,* abstr 40, 1995.

2 Lee HH et al: Diagnosis of *Chlamydia trachomatis* genitourinary infections in women by ligase chain reaction assay of urine. *Lancet* 345: 213, 1995.

3 Quinn TC: Nucleic Acid Amplification Assays for Sexually Transmitted Diseases, in *Nucleic Acid Amplification Technologies and Their Application to Disease Diagnosis*, HH Lee et al (eds). Natick, MA, Eaton, 1997, pp 201–232.

4 Swets JA: Measuring the accuracy of diagnostic systems. *Science* 240: 1285, 1988.

5 Grun L, Sheldon J: Does ligase chain reaction assay of urine in the diagnosis of *Chlamydia trachomatis* offer significant improvement over existing diagnostic tests?—a critical appraisal of the evidence. *Genitourin Med* 72:433, 1996.

6 Albritton WL et al: Human immunodeficiency virus testing for patient-based and population-based diagnosis. *J Infect Dis* 174 (suppl 2):S176, 1996.

7 Jaeschke R et al: User's guides to the medical literature. III. How to use an article about a diagnostic test. A. Are the results of the study valid? *JAMA* 271:389, 1994a.

8 Jaeschke R et al: User's guides to the medical literature. III. How to use an article about a diagnostic test. B. What are the results and will they help me in caring for my patients? *JAMA* 271:703, 1994.

9 Stephenson JM, Williams JG: Is rifabutin prophylaxis against *Mycobacterium avium* complex infection in HIV patients worthwhile? The net impact on patients suggest not. *Genitourin Med* 7:272, 1996.

10 Ransohoff DF, Feinstein AR: Problems of spectrum and bias in evaluating the efficacy of diagnostic tests. *N Engl J Med* 299:926, 1978.

11 Feinstein AR: *Clinical Biostatistics*. St. Louis MO, Mosby, 1977.

12 Washington JA: Evaluation of new in vitro diagnostic test procedures in clinical microbiology. *Infect Control Hosp Epidemiol* 10:77, 1989.

13 Fagan T: Nomogram for Bayes Theorem. *N Engl J Med* 293:257, 1975.

14 Schachter J et al: Nonculture tests for genital tract chlamydial infection. What does the package insert mean, and will it mean the same thing tomorrow? *Sex Transm Dis* 19:243, 1992.

15 Kluytmans JAJW et al: Evaluation of Clearview and Magic Lite tests, polymerase chain reaction, and cell culture for detection of *Chla-*

mydia trachomatis in urogenital specimens. *J Clin Microbiol* 31: 3204, 1993.

16 Smith TF, Weed LA: Comparison of urethral swabs, urine, and urinary sediment for the isolation of Chlamydia. *J Clin Microbiol* 2:134, 1976.

17 Stamm WE: Diagnosis of *Chlamydia trachomatis* genitourinary infection. *Ann Intern Med* 108:710, 1988.

18 Stary A et al: Screening for *Chlamydia trachomatis* in military personnel by urine testing. *Infection* 19:205, 1991.

19 Chernesky M et al: Detection of female *Chlamydia trachomatis* infection of the lower genital tract by testing first void urine in the ligase chain reaction. *Sex Transm Dis* 21(suppl):125, 1994.

20 Bassiri M et al: Ligase chain reaction for detection of *Chlamydia trachomatis* in urine of asymptomatic women. *J Clin Microbiol* 33: 898, 1994.

21 Domeika MA et al: Diagnosis of genital *Chlamydia trachomatis* infections in urine of asymptomatic males by polymerase chain reaction. *J Clin Microbiol* 32:2350, 1994.

22 Jang D et al: Effects of broadening the gold standard on the performance of chemiluminometric immunoassay to detect *Chlamydia trachomatis* antigens in centrifuged first void urine and urethral swab samples from men. *Sex Transm Dis* 19:315, 1992.

23 Scieux C et al: Evaluation of a chemiluminometric immunoassay for detection of *Chlamydia trachomatis* in the urine of male and female patients. *Eur J Clin Microbiol Infect Dis* 11:704, 1992.

24 Mahony JB et al: Chlamydia trachomatis confirmatory testing of PCR-positive genitourinary specimens using second set of plasmid primers. *Molec Cell Probes* 6:381, 1992.

25 Jachek G et al: Direct detection of *Chlamydia trachomatis* in urine specimens from symptomatic and asymptomatic men by using a rapid polymerase chain reaction assay. *J Clin Microbiol* 31:1209, 1993.

26 Hadgu A: The discrepancy in discrepant analysis. *Lancet* 348:592, 1996.

27 Schachter J et al: Letter. *Lancet* 348:1308, 1996.

28 Schachter J, Martin DH: Failure of multiple passages to increase chlamydial recovery. *J Clin Microbiol* 25:1851, 1987.

29 Schwartz JS et al: Human immunodeficiency virus test evaluation, performance, and use. Proposals to make good tests better. *JAMA* 259:2574, 1988.

30 Shafer MA et al: Evaluation of urine-based screening strategies to detect *Chlamydia trachomatis* among sexually active asymptomatic young males. *JAMA* 270:2065, 1993.

31 Centers for Disease Control and Prevention, Division of Sexually Transmitted Diseases Prevention: *Sexually Transmitted Disease Surveillance*, 1995. Atlanta, U.S. Department of Health and Human Services, Public Health Service, 1996.

32 Addiss DG et al: Decreased prevalence of *Chlamydia trachomatis* infection associated with a selective screening program in family planning clinics in Wisconsin. *Sex Transm Dis* 20:28, 1993.

33 Adger H et al: Screening for *Chlamydia trachomatis* and *Neisseria gonorrhoeae* in adolescent males: value of first-catch urine examination. *Lancet* 2:944, 1984.

34 Stamm W, Cole B: Asymptomatic *Chlamydia trachomatis* urethritis in men. *Sex Transm Dis* 13:163, 1986.

35 Sadof MD, et al: Dipstick leukocyte esterase activity in first-catch urine specimens. *JAMA* 258:1932, 1987.

36 Veeravahu M et al: Detection of leukocyte esterase in urine. A new screening test for nongonococcal urethritis compared to two microscopic methods. *Sex Transm Dis* 14:180, 1987.

37 O'Brien SF et al: Use of a leukocyte esterase dipstick in asymptomatic adolescent male detainees. *Am J Public Health* 78:1583, 1988.

38 Sellors JW et al: Screening urine with a leukocyte esterase strip and subsequent chlamydial testing of asymptomatic men attending primary care practitioners. *Sex Transm Dis* 20:152, 1993.

39 McNagny SE et al: Urinary leukocyte esterase test: a screening method for the detection of asymptomatic chlamydial and gonococcal infections in men. *J Infect Dis* 165:573, 1992.

40 Chow JM et al: Is urine leukocyte esterase a useful screening method to predict *Chlamydia trachomatis* infection in women? *J Clin Microbiol* 34:534, 1996.

41 Robinson AJ, Black CM. Screening for Sexually Transmitted Disease in the Male: In the Context of Pelvic Inflammatory Disease, in: *The Prevention of Pelvic Infection*, A Templeton (ed). London, RCOG Press, 1996, pp. 192–208.

42 Schwebke JR et al: Use of an enzyme immunoassay as a diagnostic tool for *Chlamydia trachomatis* urethritis in men. *J Clin Microbiol* 29:2446, 1991.

43 Genc M et al: An economic evaluation of screening for *Chlamydia trachomatis* in adolescent males. *JAMA* 270:2057, 1993.

44 Genc M et al: Cost-effectiveness of screening for *Chlamydia* using DNA amplification. *JAMA* 271:1741, 1994.

45 Grosskurth H et al: A community trial of improved treatment of sexually transmitted diseases in rural Tanzania: randomized controlled trial. *Lancet* 346:530, 1995.

46 Genc M, Mardh PA: A cost-effectiveness analysis of screening and treatment for *Chlamydia trachomatis* infection in asymptomatic women. *Ann Intern Med* 124:1, 1996.

47 Stray-Pedersen B: Economic evaluation of maternal screening to prevent congenital syphilis. *Sex Transm Dis* 10:167, 1983.

48 Williams K: Screening for syphilis in pregnancy: an assessment of the costs and benefits. *Community Med* 7:37, 1985.

49 Phillips RS et al: Use of a direct fluorescent antibody test for detecting *Chlamydia trachomatis* cervical infection in women seeking routine gynecologic care. *J Infect Dis* 156:575, 1987.

50 Nettleman MD, Jones RB: Cost-effectiveness of screening women at moderate risk for genital infections caused by *Chlamydia trachomatis*. *JAMA* 260:207, 1988.

51 Estany A et al: Early detection of genital chlamydial infection in women: an economic evaluation. *Sex Transm Dis* 16:21, 1989.

52 Nettleman M, Bell T: Cost-effectiveness of prenatal screening for *Chlamydia trachomatis*. *Am J Obstet Gynecol* 164:1289, 1991.

53 Handsfield HH et al: Criteria for selective screening for *Chlamydia trachomatis* infection in women attending family planning clinics. *JAMA* 255:1730, 1986.

54 World Health Organization: Guidelines for the Prevention of Genital Chlamydial Infections. Report on Two WHO Working Groups. *EUR/ICP/CDS* 199, Geneva, 1989.

55 Brabin L: Prevention of Pelvic Inflammatory Disease: Screening of High-Risk Groups, in *The Prevention of Pelvic Infection*, A Templeton (ed). London, RCOG Press, 1996, pp 160–80.

56 U.S. Prevention Services Task Force: *Guide to Clinical Preventive Services, 2nd ed.* Washington DC, U.S. Department of Health and Human Services, 1996.

57 Institute of Medicine: *The Hidden Epidemic: Confronting Sexually Transmitted Diseases*, TR Eng et al (eds). Washington DC, National Academy Press, 1997.

58 Scholes D et al: Prevention of pelvic inflammatory disease by screening for cervical chlamydial infection. *N Engl J Med* 334:1362, 1996.

59 Centers for Disease Control and Prevention: U.S. Public Health Service recommendations for human immunodeficiency virus counseling and voluntary testing for pregnant women. *MMWR* 55:1, 1995.

60 American Academy of Pediatrics: Provisional committee on pediatric AIDS 1995. *Pediatr* 95:303, 1995.

61 Tanfer K, et al: Condom use among US men, 1991. *Fam Plan Perspect* 25:61, 1993.

62 Briggs LP et al: The importance of social history for assessing sexually transmitted disease risk. *Sex Transm Dis* 22:348, 1995.

63 Padian NS et al: Reliability of sexual histories in heterosexual couples. *Sex Transm Dis* 22:169, 1995.

64 Maheux B et al: STD risk assessment and risk-reduction counseling by recently trained family physicians. *Academ Med* 70:726, 1995.

65 Blum RW et al: Don't ask, they won't tell: the quality of adolescent health screening in five practice settings. *Am J Public Health* 86:1767, 1997.

66 Birschfield M et al: Perinatal screening for illicit drugs: policies in hospitals in a large metropolitan area. *J Perinatol* 15:208, 1995.

67 Rhodes AM: Guardianship and the refusal of treatment. *Am J Maternal Child Nursing* 20:109, 1995.

68 Begley CE et al: The incremental cost of screening, diagnosis and treatment of gonorrhoea and chlamydia in a family planning clinic. *Sex Transm Dis* 16:63, 1989.
69 Schachter J et al: Screening for women attending family planning clinics. *West J Med* 138:375, 1983.
70 Glenney KF et al: The prevalence of positive test results for *Chlamydia trachomatis* by direct smear for fluorescent antibodies in a South Texas family planning population. *J Reprod Med* 33:457, 1988.
71 Winter L et al: Prevalence and epidemiologic correlates of *Chlamydia trachomatis* in rural and urban populations. *Sex Transm Dis* 17:30, 1990.
72 Harrison HR: Cervical *Chalmydia trachomatis* infection in university women: relationship to history, contraception, ectopy and cervicitis. *Am J Obstet Gynecol* 153:244, 1985.
73 Toomey KE et al: Unrecognized high prevalence of *Chlamydia trachomatis* cervical infection in an isolated Alaskan Eskimo population. *JAMA* 258:53, 1987.
74 Chacko MR, Lovchik J: *Chlamydia trachomatis* infection in sexually active adolescents: prevalence and risk factors. *Pediatrics* 73:836, 1984.
75 Golden N et al: Prevalence of *Chlamydia trachomatis* cervical infection in female adolescents. *Am J Dis Child* 138:562, 1984.
76 Shafer M et al: *Chlamydia trachomatis*: Important relationships to race, contraception, lower genital track infection, and Papanicolaou smear. *J Pediatr* 104:141, 1984.
77 Fraser JJ: Prevalence of cervical *Chlamydia trachomatis* and *Neisseria gonorrhoeae* in female adolescents. *Pediatrics* 71:333, 1983.
78 Saltz GR et al: *Chlamydia trachomatis* cervical infections in female adolescents. *J Pediatr* 98:981, 1981.
79 Bump RC et al: Sexually transmissible infectious agents in sexually active and virginal asymptomatic adolescent girls. *Pediatrics* 77:488, 1986.
80 Fisher M et al: *Chlamydia trachomatis* in suburban adolescents. *J Pediatr* 111:617, 1987.
81 Jaffe LR et al: *Chlamydia trachomatis* detection in adolescents. A comparison of direct specimen and tissue culture methods. *J Adolesc Health Care* 7:40, 1986.
82 Smith PB et al: Predominant sexually transmitted diseases among different age and sex groups of indigent sexually active adolescents attending a family planning clinic. *J Adolesc Health Care* 9:291, 1988.
83 Eager RM et al: Epidemiological and clinical factors of *Chlamydia trachomatis* in black, Hispanic, and white female adolescents. *West J Med* 143:37, 1985.
84 Beck-Sague CM et al: Detection of *Chlamydia trachomatis* cervical infection by urine tests among adolescents clinics. *J Adolesc Health* 22:197, 1998.
85 Kent GP et al: Screening for *Chlamydia trachomatis* infection in a sexually transmitted disease clinic: comparison of diagnostic tests with clinical and historical risk factors. *Sex Transm Dis* 15:51, 1988.
86 Kinghorn GR, Waugh MA: Oral contraceptive use and prevalence of infection with *Chlamydia trachomatis* in women. *Br J Vener Dis* 57: 187, 1981.
87 Madger LS et al: Factors related to genital *Chlamydia trachomatis* and its diagnosis by culture in a sexually transmitted disease clinic. *Am J Epidemiol* 128:298, 1988.
88 Persson K et al: Prevalence of nine different micro-organisms in the female genital tract. *Br J Vener Dis* 55:429, 1979.
89 Richmond SJ et al: Value and feasibility of screening women attending STD clinics for cervical chlamydial infections. *Br J Vener Dis* 56: 259, 1980.
90 Hilton AL et al: *Chlamydia* A in the female genital tract. *Br J Vener Dis* 50:1, 1974.
91 Woolfitt JMG, Watt L: Chlamydial infection of the urogenital tract in promiscuous and non-promiscuous women. *Br J Vener Dis* 53:93, 1977.
92 Thelin L et al: Contact tracing in patients with genital chlamydial infection. *Br J Vener Dis* 56:259, 1980.
93 Bai H et al: Prevalence of genital *Chlamydia trachomatis* infection in selected populations in China. *Sex Transm Dis* 22:383, 1995.
94 Holmes MD et al: *Chlamydia* cervical infection in jailed women. *Am J Public Health* 83:51, 1993.
95 Centers for Disease Control and Prevention: 1998 sexually transmitted diseases treatment guidelines. *MMWR* 47:1, 1998.
96 Ehret JM, Judson FN: Gonorrhea, in *Laboratory Methods for the Diagnosis of Sexually Transmitted Diseases*, BB Wentworth et al (eds). Washington DC, American Public Health Association, 1991, pp 53–94.
97 Creighton ET: Darkfield Microscopy for the Detection and Identification of *Treponema pallidum*, in *A Manual of Tests for Syphilis*, SA Larsen et al. (eds). Washington DC, American Public Health Association, 1990, pp 49–62.
98 Mardh PA, Domeika M: Prevention of Pelvic Inflammatory Disease by Reducing the Prevalence of Causative Agents by Screening Strategies, in *The Prevention of Pelvic Infection*, A Templeton (ed). London, RCOG Press, 1996, pp 154–157.
99 World Health Organization: *Management of patients with sexually transmitted diseases.* WHO Technical Report Series, 1991, p 810.
100 Morse SA et al: Comparison of clinical diagnosis, standard laboratory and molecular methods for the diagnosis of genital ulcer disease in Lesotho: association with HIV infection. *J Infect Dis* 175:583, 1997.
101 Jessamine PG, Brunham RC: Rapid control of a chancroid outbreak: implications for Canada. *Can Med Assoc J* 142:1081, 1990.
102 Hunter EF: Direct Fluorescent Antibody for *Treponema pallidum*, in *A Manual of Tests for Syphilis,* SA Larsen et al (eds). Washington DC, American Public Health Association, 1990, pp 63–69.
103 Ossewaarde JM et al: Efficacy of single dose azi thromycin versus doxycycline in the treatment of cervical infections caused by *Chlamydia trachomatis*. *Eur J Clin Microbiol Infect Dis* 11:693, 1992.
104 Vogels WH et al: *Chlamydia trachomatis* infection in a high-risk population. Comparison of polymerase chain reaction and cell culture for diagnosis and follow-up. *J Clin Microbiol* 31:1103, 1993.
105 Barbosa C et al: Recurrent *Chlamydia trachomatis* cervical infection in adolescent women. Thirty-Sixth Interscience Conference on Antimicrobial Agents and Chemotherapy, New Orleans, September 15–18, 1996, abstr K36.
106 Centers for Disease Control and Prevention: Decreased susceptibility of *Neisseria gonorrhoeae* to fluoroquinolones: Ohio and Hawaii, 1992–1994. *MMWR* 43:325, 1994.
107 Trees DL, Morse SA: Chancroid and *Haemophilus ducreyi*, an update. *Rev Clin Microbiol* 8:357, 1995.
108 Beck-Sague CM et al: Laboratory diagnosis of sexually transmitted diseases in facilities in the United States. *Sex Transm Dis* 23:342, 1996.
109 Schulte JM et al: Chancroid in the United States 1981–1990. Evidence for underreporting of cases. *MMWR* 41:57, 1992.

Chapter 54

Behavioral interventions for sexually transmitted disease prevention at the individual level

Martin Fishbein
Richard J. Wolitski
Lynda S. Doll

In order to prevent the spread of the acquired immune-deficiency syndrome (AIDS) and other sexually transmitted diseases (STDs), it is necessary to develop programs that can help individuals change their behavior. It is not who one is, but what one does, that largely determines whether or not an individual will be exposed to, or transmit, human immunodeficiency virus (HIV) and other STDs. Behavior also plays an important role in the treatment and management of HIV infection and other STDs. In this chapter we will consider the factors that influence behavior and point out their implications for developing effective behavior change interventions. Clearly, the more one understands the factors underlying the performance or nonperformance of any given behavior, the more likely it is that one can develop counseling strategies and interventions to reinforce or change that behavior successfully.

Unfortunately, many different behaviors can contribute to the spread of an STD. Consider, for example, May and Anderson's model[1] for the reproductive rate of an STD:

$$R_0 = \beta c D$$

where R_0 is the reproductive rate, β is the infectivity or transmissibility, c is the interaction rate between susceptibles and infectors, and D is a measure of duration of infectiousness.

Each of the parameters on the right-hand side of the equation can be influenced by behavior (Table 54-1). For example, transmissibility β can be lowered by increasing consistent and correct condom use or by delaying the onset of sexual activity (since younger females appear to be more susceptible than older females to acquiring an STD, if exposed). Transmissibility also can be reduced by vaccines, but people must participate in vaccine trials as vaccines are developed and must utilize vaccines once they are introduced. Decreasing the rate of new partner acquisition will reduce the sexual interaction rate c, and at least for bacterial STDs, duration of infectiousness D can be reduced through the detection and treatment of asymptomatic individuals or through early treatment of symptomatic clients. Thus increasing care-seeking behavior and/or participation in screening programs can affect the reproductive rate. Because STDs are important cofactors in the transmission of HIV infection, early detection and treatment of STDs also will influence HIV transmissibility β. Finally, D also can be influenced by patient adherence to medical treatment, as well as by adherence to or cooperation with partner notification.

Clearly, there are a number of different behaviors that, if changed or reinforced, could have an impact on the reproductive rate R_0 of HIV and other STDs. A critical question is whether it is necessary to consider each of these behaviors as a unique entity, or whether there are some more general principles that can guide our understanding of any behavior. Fortunately, even though every behavior is unique, theories of behavioral prediction and behavior change suggest that there are only a limited number of critical factors (or variables) underlying an individual's decision to perform or not perform a given behavior. Behavioral science theory and research also suggest that the most effective interventions will be those directed at a specific behavior. As will be seen below, every behavior has its own substantively unique determinants, and thus very different interventions are required to change different behaviors. Perhaps the most difficult part of developing any intervention is the identification of the behavior (or behaviors) that one wishes to change.

The selection of a behavior (or behaviors) to serve as the target of an STD/HIV risk-reduction intervention for a given individual, for example, should be based on sound epidemiologic evidence and a careful assessment of the client's sexual and drug-use history. Although many clinicians are reluctant to or feel uncomfortable about taking such histories, most clients (and particularly those coming in for STD screening or treatment or for an HIV test) view sexual and drug histories as a normal (and acceptable) part of a medical examination.[2–6] At the very least, these assessments should provide information about the number and types of partners (e.g., main or occasional), their HIV serostatus and risk, types of sex practiced, condom use, use of both injected and non-injected drugs, and for injecting drug users, information about the use of sterile syringes and disinfection of shared injection paraphernalia. It is only by taking such histories that one can identify the one or two behaviors that are putting the client at greatest risk for acquiring and transmitting HIV and other STDs. This behavior (or these behaviors) should serve as the target of an intervention.

All too often, however, interventions are directed at increasing the probability that one will reach a given goal (e.g., avoiding AIDS, staying healthy, losing weight) or at increasing the probability that one will engage in a category of behaviors (e.g., practicing safe sex, negotiating condom use, dieting) rather than at increasing the probability that one will engage in a specific behavior (e.g., always using a condom for vaginal sex with one's main partner, telling one's partner to always use a condom). The latter type of intervention is most likely to be successful in changing behavior.

The distinction between broad goals, behavioral categories, and specific behaviors is not always obvious. Among men, condom use is not a specific behavior but a behavioral category. That is, one does not just "use a condom." Instead, condoms are used for given sexual activities with specific partners, and the factors influencing the use of a condom for vaginal sex with one's main partner or spouse, for example, can be quite different from those underlying the use of condoms for vaginal sex with an occasional partner or the use of condoms for anal sex with one's main partner.[7–11] Further, while using a male condom is a behavior for men, it is a goal for women that may require influencing partner behavior. The substantive uniqueness of behavioral determinants can best be illustrated by briefly considering the four theories that have most strongly influenced health-related behavioral prevention research: the health belief model,[12–14] social cognitive theory,[15,16] the theory of reasoned action,[17–19] and the transtheoretical model of behavior change.[20–23]

Although other theories also could be considered (e.g., the theory of planned behavior,[24] the theory of self-regulation and self-control,[25] the theory of subjective culture and interpersonal relations,[26] the AIDS risk-reduction model,[27] and the information-motivation behavioral-skills model),[28] they have considerable overlap with the four we will describe below. Indeed, the latter two theories that apply specifically to HIV risk reduction were developed relatively recently and, to a certain extent, can best be seen as attempts to incorporate concepts from two or more of the

Table 54-1. Examples of Behaviors that Influence the Rate of Spread of Sexually Transmitted Diseases

Behaviors that reduce interaction between susceptibles and infectors
Delayed onset of sexual debut
Infrequent acquisition of new partners
Avoiding concurrent partnerships
Avoiding unprotected sex while symptomatic with an STD
Behaviors that reduce acquisition, if exposed
Using safer sex practices
Use of barrier prophylactic
Use of topical or systemic chemoprophlaxis agent
Use of vaccines
Delayed onset of sexual intercourse (young females most susceptible)
Obtaining early treatment for STD (to decrease HIV transmission)
Behaviors that reduce duration of infectivity
Early health care seeking if experiencing STD symptom
Undergoing routine STD screening
Adherence to therapy
Compliance with partner notification

existing general theories of behavior and behavior change (i.e., those which are not specific to any one health threat).

BEHAVIORAL THEORIES

THE HEALTH BELIEF MODEL (HBM)

According to the health belief model, the likelihood that someone will adopt (or continue to engage in) a health-protective behavior is primarily a function of two factors. First, the person must feel personally threatened by the disease. That is, he or she must feel personally susceptible to (or at risk for) a condition that is perceived to have serious negative consequences. Second, the person must believe that the benefits of taking the preventive action outweigh the perceived barriers to (and/or costs of) taking that action. Note that the costs and benefits of performing one behavior (e.g., always using a condom for vaginal sex with one's spouse) may be very different from those associated with performing another behavior (e.g., always using a condom for vaginal sex with an occasional partner). For example, while one might believe that always using a condom with one's spouse would lead to a loss of trust or would otherwise damage the relationship, this belief might not occur with respect to a new or occasional partner.

SOCIAL COGNITIVE THEORY (SCT)

Social cognitive theory also identifies two factors as primary determinants underlying the initiation and persistence of an adaptive behavior. First, the person must have self-efficacy with respect to the behavior. That is, the person must believe that she or he can (i.e., has the capability to) perform the behavior in question in the face of various circumstances or barriers that make it difficult to perform that behavior. Second, one must have some incentive to perform the behavior. More specifically, the expected positive outcomes of performing the behavior must outweigh the expected negative outcomes. Social cognitive theory has focused on three types of perceived (or expected) outcomes: physical outcomes (e.g., performing the behavior will protect me from HIV), social outcomes (e.g., performing the behavior will make my partner angry), and self-standards (e.g., performing the behavior will make me feel guilty).

THE THEORY OF REASONED ACTION (TRA)

According to the theory of reasoned action, performance or nonperformance of a given behavior is determined primarily by the strength of a person's intention to perform (or to not perform) that behavior, where *intention* is defined as the subjective likelihood that one will perform (or try to perform) the behavior in question. The intention to perform a given behavior is, in turn, viewed as a function of two basic factors: the person's attitude toward performing the behavior (i.e., one's overall positive or negative feeling about personally performing the behavior) and/or the person's subjective norm concerning the behavior (i.e., the person's perception that his or her important others think that he or she should or should not perform the behavior in question).

The theory of reasoned action also considers the determinants of attitudes and subjective norms. Attitudes are viewed as a function of behavioral beliefs (i.e., beliefs that performing the behavior will lead to certain outcomes) and their evaluative aspects (i.e., the evaluation of those outcomes); subjective norms are viewed as a function of normative beliefs (i.e., beliefs that a specific individual or group thinks one should or should not perform the behavior in question) and motivations to comply (i.e., the degree to which, in general, one wants or does not want to do what the referent thinks one should do). Generally speaking, the more one believes that performing the behavior will lead to positive outcomes and/or will prevent negative outcomes, the more favorable one's attitude will be toward performing the behavior. Similarly, the more one believes that specific referents (i.e., individuals or groups) think that one should (or should not) perform the behavior and the more one is motivated to comply with those referents, the stronger will be the perceived pressure (i.e., the subjective norm) to perform that behavior.

Based on these three theories, one can identify four factors that may influence an individual's intentions and behaviors: (1) the individual's perception that he or she is personally susceptible to acquiring a given disease or illness, (2) the individual's attitude toward performing the behavior, which is based on one's beliefs about the positive and negative consequences of performing that behavior, (3) perceived norms, which include the perception that those with whom the individual interacts most closely support the individual's attempt to change and that others in the community are also changing, and (4) self-efficacy, which involves the individual's perception that he or she can perform the behavior under a variety of difficult or challenging circumstances.

While there is considerable empirical evidence to support the role of attitude (or outcome expectancies), perceived norms, and self-efficacy as determinants of intention and behavior,[29–33] this is not always the case for perceived susceptibility (or perceived risk). Particularly with regard to HIV, there is growing evidence that perceived risk of exposure to HIV (or of getting AIDS) is, in most cases, unrelated to the likelihood that one will take preventive action.[34] In contrast, there does seem to be some evidence that perceived risk is related to seeking HIV testing[35,36] and, as will be seen below, to adherence to medical regimens. Nevertheless, it appears that although perceiving that one is at risk for AIDS may be a necessary first step in a behavior change process; whether one does or does not change depends primarily on attitudes, norms, or self-efficacy.[37]

The relative importance of these three factors as determinants of intention and behavior is expected to vary as a function of both the behavior and the population being considered. That is, while some behaviors are determined primarily by attitudinal considerations, others are determined primarily by norms or self-efficacy. Equally important, a given intention (or behavior) may be influenced primarily by attitudes in one population but be influenced primarily by norms or self-efficacy in another population.

For example, while sexually experienced U.S. male college students' intentions to always use condoms were found to be primarily under normative control, this same intention was found to be primarily under attitudinal control in a sample of sexually experienced male college students in Mexico City.[38]

In addition to considering attitudes, norms, and self-efficacy, it is also necessary to know the degree to which an individual is ready to adopt a new behavior. Behavior change is usually not a one-step, all-or-nothing process but often involves a series of steps that ultimately may lead to long-term maintenance of a new behavior. Clearly, different behavior change messages will be necessary for a person who has not even thought about adopting a health-protective behavior than for a person who is trying to adopt that behavior. The transtheoretical model of behavior change[20–22] directly addresses this issue.

THE TRANSTHEORETICAL MODEL OF BEHAVIOR CHANGE

According to this model, adoption of a new behavior involves five distinct stages of change (SOC). Many individuals who are performing risky behavior may have no intention to change that behavior or to adopt a given health-protective behavior (precontemplative stage). Any one of several events (e.g., perceiving that one is personally at risk for an illness) may then lead the individual to consider change and perhaps to form an intention to adopt the behavior immediately or at some time in the future (contemplative stage). This immediate intention is often accompanied by initial, perhaps exploratory attempts to adopt the behavior (preparation or ready-for-action stage). Then the new behavior is adopted (action stage), and ultimately, it becomes a routine part of one's life (maintenance stage). Movement through the stages is assumed to be sequential, although individuals may skip certain stages or relapse (at any stage) and then cycle back through the stages repeatedly before achieving long-term maintenance of the behavior.

In order to help people change their behavior, one should first determine where each person is on this continuum of behavior change and then develop interventions to help him or her move to subsequent, more advanced stages. Having discrete and immediate objectives for persons at risk of acquiring STDs or HIV infection allows one to more precisely target an intervention to the needs of individuals. For example, one can determine empirically which of the theoretical factors (e.g., norms, attitudes, or self-efficacy) one needs to focus on to move an individual from one stage to the next. Generally speaking, if a person has formed a strong intention (or made a strong commitment) to perform a given behavior, and if he or she has the skills and abilities necessary to perform that behavior, and if there are no environmental constraints to prevent behavioral performance, it is almost certain that the behavior will be performed.[37]

Thus, once risk assessment has been completed and a decision has been made to target a risky behavior, an important first step in developing any intervention is to assess the individual's intention to perform that behavior. Intention can be assessed easily by asking the client if he or she plans on starting (or continuing) to practice the risk-reducing behavior. For example, "Do you plan on using condoms every time you have sex with your boyfriend? How sure are you about this?" If the individual has already formed a strong intention to perform the behavior but has been unable to act on this intention, it is important to determine whether this is due to a lack of skills or to the presence of environmental constraints. Depending on which of these factors is operating, the intervention should be directed at either increasing the person's skills and abilities or removing or helping the individual overcome the environmental constraints.

If, on the other hand, the individual has not formed a strong intention to perform the behavior, then the intervention should be directed at increasing the individual's intention to perform the behavior. And, as indicated above, this will involve changing the person's attitude toward performing the behavior, his or her perceived normative pressure to perform the behavior, and/or his or her self-efficacy with respect to performing the behavior.

Thus it becomes necessary to rapidly assess the client's attitude toward, perceived norms concerning, and self-efficacy with respect to performing the behavior. For example, let us assume that the risk assessment indicated that a client was primarily at risk for acquiring or transmitting an STD (including HIV) because he did not consistently use condoms for vaginal sex with his occasional partners. And let us further assume that the client had no intention to consistently use condoms for vaginal sex with his occasional partners. Although there are standardized scaling procedures available for assessing attitudes, norms, and self-efficacy,[17,37] the following three questions will provide information to help guide an intervention:

Attitude: "Do you feel mostly positive or negative about always using condoms for vaginal sex with your occasional partners?"

Norms: "Would you say that most people who are important to you think you should or should not always use a condom when you have vaginal sex with your occasional partners?"

Self-efficacy: "Considering all the things that can get in the way or make it difficult to always use a condom, are you certain that you could always use a condom for vaginal sex with your occasional partners?"

If the client has a negative attitude toward using condoms, it is important to understand the client's beliefs about using a condom. That is, the client can be asked to describe what he thinks will happen if he always uses a condom for vaginal sex with his occasional partners. More specifically, the client can be asked to list the advantages and disadvantages (i.e., the "good" and "bad" things that will happen or the "outcomes") of always using a condom for vaginal sex with his occasional partners. The intervention can then be directed at decreasing beliefs that always using a condom for vaginal sex with occasional partners will lead to negative outcomes or at increasing beliefs that condom use will lead to positive outcomes.

If the client perceives that most important others are opposed to consistent condom use for vaginal sex with occasional partners, it is important to understand which important referents oppose or support such condom use. That is, the client can be asked to list specific others or groups who oppose his consistent condom use and to list specific others or groups who support his consistent condom use for vaginal sex with occasional partners. The intervention can then be directed at clarifying misperceptions or at pointing out others in the client's life who would support consistent condom use.

Finally, if the client indicates little self-efficacy with respect to condom use, it is important to understand the specific circumstances that are lowering the client's self-efficacy. Thus the client can be asked to list those things which make it difficult for him to consistently use condoms for vaginal sex with occasional partners (barriers) and to list those things which would make it easier for him to consistently use condoms (facilitators). The intervention can than be directed at helping the client overcome barriers or to find ways to facilitate condom use.

By understanding the client's behavioral, normative, and efficacy beliefs, it should be possible to tailor a theoretically appropriate intervention. Unfortunately, such theoretical considerations often are not taken into account in developing interventions. Consider, for example, counseling and testing for HIV infection.

HIV COUNSELING AND TESTING

HIV counseling and testing have been a major focus of federally supported HIV prevention efforts. Beginning in 1985, the U.S. government, in collaboration with state and local health departments, established a network of publicly funded HIV counseling and testing centers. The number of tests (and associated counseling sessions) provided at these centers has grown from 79,000 in 1985 to over 2.5 million in 1993. Initially, HIV counseling was directed toward providing information about the test itself and the meaning of positive and negative results. By 1987, the focus of counseling had shifted to emphasize prevention by encouraging risk-reducing behavior change. As Kamb et al.[39] point out however, this largely entailed informing clients about HIV transmission and then telling them how HIV infection could be avoided.[39] All too often this approach inundated clients with technical information about HIV and AIDS and used global prevention messages that were not tailored to a client's unique circumstances.[40] It should not be too surprising, then, to find out that initial reviews of studies evaluating HIV counseling and testing indicated little support for their efficacy or effectiveness in producing behavior change.[41,42] More recent reviews, including the one by Celum and Buchbinder in Chap. 70 of this book, also suggest that the evidence to date regarding the behavioral effects of HIV counseling and testing is, at best, mixed.[43]

At least three explanations may account in part for the mixed reviews of HIV counseling and testing: (1) the methods used to evaluate counseling and testing may be of concern,[42–44] (2) the actual practice of counseling (e.g., amount and quality of time spent) may vary from the ideal practice that would be expected to have an impact,[41] and (3) the model or approach to counseling may not be adequate to effect behavior change.

With regard to evaluation methods, concerns about the research methods utilized in some studies, including the lack of random assignment, failure to use control groups, and the array of outcome measures and time periods used, have raised questions about the comparison and interpretation of some studies.[42,43] A second set of methodologic concerns revolves around the complex problem of generalizing from evaluations of counseling and testing conducted as part of research studies to an assessment of the actual practice of counseling and testing in field settings.

Logistical issues such as the content and amount of time actually spent in counseling are also important to consider when evaluating counseling and testing activities. According to Kamb et al.[39] counseling for HIV prevention is "a process that engages the client in an interactive self-exploration of his or her behaviors in the context in which these behaviors take place, during which the counselor gives professional guidance, most often by helping the client arrive at a policy, plan of action, or behavior" (p. 100). Public Health Service (PHS) guidelines published in 1994 defined HIV counseling as a personalized and client-centered intervention designed to help initiate behavior change.[45] The guidelines also provided examples of elements to be included in counseling and testing services such as assessment of the client's risk, development of a risk-reduction plan, provision of support for initiating and maintaining behavior change, provision of referrals, and so on. In 1991, the Centers for Disease Control and Prevention (CDC) funded a qualitative case study and inventory of services provided by 43 publicly funded sites.[40] While not an evaluation, these case studies illustrate considerable discordance between counseling guidelines and actual practice. In general, investigators found counseling sessions to be factually correct and interactive. The extent and quality of individual risk assessments varied, however, and individualized risk-reduction plans were developed infrequently. Furthermore, average duration of posttest counseling was just 20 minutes for seropositive persons and 10 minutes for seronegative persons. The latter often consisted of general admonitions to reduce risk and seek testing again in the future.

While PHS guidelines[45] contain important instructions on objectives, techniques, and elements to be included in the counseling and testing process, it is not their goal to provide in-depth information regarding behavior-change models or theories. Yet, as we noted earlier, understanding and applying theory are critical to developing the relevant *counseling approach* for each client. Without the use of theory, these sessions may consist largely of information provision without adequate attention given to motivations for behavior change. Indeed, many counseling guidelines provide concrete step-by-step instructions on *what* to tell the client about risk behaviors and behavior change but fail to address important *psychosocial determinants* that facilitate or discourage individual behavior change.

There is now some clear and compelling evidence that theory-based, client-centered counseling (and testing) can be effective in reducing both risky behavior and incidence of STDs. The CDC, in collaboration with partners in five U.S. cities, conducted a randomized control trial (Project RESPECT)[39,46] to evaluate the efficacy of three interventions aimed at increasing correct and consistent condom use:

1. *Clinician education*: A brief, two-session health education intervention that was at that time similar to standard practice in many STD clinics. The first 5-minute educational message was given by the clinician who examined the participant during his or her initial clinic visit. The second was conducted when the client returned for HIV test results. During this second 5-minute session, the participant was informed about the limitations of the test, his or her personal HIV and STD risks were identified, and information about HIV transmission and prevention was provided.
2. *Prevention counseling*: A client-centered counseling intervention that was based on the health belief model and revised CDC guidelines for HIV counseling and testing.[45] Both sessions were conducted by HIV counselors who were skilled professionals who had undergone standardized training to give HIV test results and conduct counseling sessions. This intervention consisted of two 20-minute sessions that emphasized increasing the client's perception of risk, developing a personalized risk-reduction plan, identifying and discussing strategies for overcoming barriers to carrying out the plan, and support for behavior change. Information regarding the structure and content of the counseling sessions is available elsewhere.[39]
3. *Enhanced counseling*: A four-session, counselor-conducted client-centered counseling intervention based on the theories of behavior and behavior change described earlier in this chapter. More specifically, after receiving the same first session as that in prevention counseling, clients in this condition participated in three 1-hour sessions that emphasized changing client attitudes (session 2), building self-efficacy (session 3), and changing and reinforcing social norms (session 4). In addition, the client received skill training in both condom use and negotiating condom use, and at each of the first three sessions, an achievable behavioral goal was established. In the final session, a long-term, personalized risk-reduction plan was developed.

Clients attending five STD clinics (Baltimore, Denver, Long Beach, Newark, and San Francisco) were recruited for participation in the study. To be eligible, clients had to have come to the clinic for a diagnostic STD examination, engaged in vaginal sex in the past 30 days, be willing to have an HIV test, and be found to be HIV negative. In addition, men had to self-identify as heterosexual and report no sex with a man in the past 12 months. From August 1993 to June 1995, 5758 clients (3269 men and 2489 women) were enrolled and randomized (men and women separately) to one of the three counseling interventions described above or to a fourth "Hawthorne effect control" condition that was designed to evaluate the impact of repeated exposure to the study personnel, measurement instruments, and clinical assessments. All participants in the Hawthorne control group received the clinician education intervention, and all received an STD examination at baseline; about half were asked to complete a behavioral questionnaire at a 12-month follow up. In all but the Hawthorne control condition, behavioral questionnaires were administered at baseline, immediately after the intervention, and at 3, 6, 9, and 12 months. In addition, all clients (except for those in the Hawthorne control group) received a complete STD examination at baseline and at 6 and 12 months. Eighty-one percent completed all intervention sessions, but fewer completed enhanced counseling (72 percent) than either prevention counseling (86 percent) or clinician education (84 percent). Of all enrolled, follow-up was 70 percent at 3 and 6 months and 65 percent at 9 and 12 months.

Although data from the Hawthorne control group have not yet been analyzed, analyses of 6-month data, utilizing an intention-to-treat design (i.e., all respondents are included, whether or not they attended all intervention sessions), showed that all three interventions significantly increased condom use, with enhanced counseling leading to a significantly greater increase than either of the other two interventions. In addition, in comparison with clinician education, both prevention counseling and enhanced counseling led to significant decreases in incident STDs. Although not significant, those in enhanced counseling were less likely to acquire new STDs than those in prevention counseling.[46]

Whether these changes will be sustained at 12 months and whether secondary analyses considering only those who attended all counseling sessions will show even greater differences among the three interventions remains to be seen. It also will be important to evaluate the relative efficacy of the two counseling interventions in different subgroups. For example, it is important to determine whether the preceding results hold equally well for different ethnic groups, different age groups, or clients at different levels of risk. The answers to these and other questions will be important in deciding the implications for clinical practice. For example, different recommendations should be made if, compared with prevention counseling, enhanced counseling has a bigger impact on condom use and STD incidence for clients at higher risk. Although beyond the scope of this chapter, it should be clear that there are a number of issues involved in moving from a research trial to a clinical setting (e.g., subject payment, quality assurance, client retention). Nevertheless, these initial findings demonstrate that individually targeted, theory-based HIV counseling not only increases protective behavior (i.e., condom use) but also significantly reduces STD incidence.

ADHERENCE TO PROVIDER RECOMMENDATIONS

Individual behavior is important not only in the prevention of disease but also in its treatment. Patients' willingness and ability to adhere to the recommendations of their health care provider are essential components in the successful treatment of most health problems. It is widely acknowledged that from 30 to 60 percent of patients fail to take medication as prescribed.[47] This also has been shown to be the case for STD patients—only 63 percent of STD patients prescribed a 1-week course of tetracycline or erythromycin were adherent to treatment in one study.[48]

While the availability of directly observed single-dose treatments for gonorrhea, syphilis, and chlamydia has minimized the importance of patient adherence in the minds of some clinicians, adherence to provider recommendations nonetheless remains an important factor in the successful treatment of STDs. This is true for a number of reasons: (1) due to its increased cost, single-dose therapy may not always be available to all individuals, (2) single-dose therapies may be contraindicated for some patients, (3) single-dose therapies or vaccines are not available for all STDs (e.g., herpes, hepatitis A and B), and (4) patients are often required to adhere to recommendations to return for test-of-cure or other follow-up assessments. Furthermore, at least one author suggests that even adherence to single-dose therapies may not approach 100 percent if patients are required to fill their own prescription because of cost or other barriers.[49]

Regardless of a provider's belief regarding the relative importance of patient adherence in STD treatment, the role of adherence in the successful management of HIV infection cannot be overstated. Unwillingness to initiate or poor adherence to prophylactic drugs such as trimethoprim-sulfamethoxazole (TMP-SMX) may lead to potentially life-threatening opportunistic infections among patients with advanced HIV disease. In addition, inconsistent adherence to antiretroviral regimens, particularly protease inhibitors, may hasten the emergence of drug-resistant viral mutations. For example, periods of poor adherence or "drug holidays" from saquinavir have been associated directly with emergence of drug resistance.[50] Development of cross-resistant mutations may severely limit a given patient's treatment options and may lead to the transmission of HIV strains that are multidrug resistant if safer sex and injection practices are not followed.

Although some health care providers may assume that the serious outcomes associated with HIV disease would be sufficient to motivate consistent patient adherence to treatment, recent studies suggest otherwise. A review of clinical trial data suggests that from 5 to 21 percent of participants in some trials may not have taken antiretroviral medications as prescribed.[51] Not surprisingly, results from clinic-based studies suggest that adherence rates outside the clinical trial setting may be lower. Nonadherence rates for zidovudine (ZDV) monotherapy in published studies range from 12 percent[52] to 58 percent,[53] with results from other studies falling somewhere in between this range.[54–58]

At this time, only limited information is available regarding patient adherence to HIV treatments other than ZDV. Newly emerging data suggest that adherence also may be problematic for other agents as well. For example, in a small study of 40 patients receiving saquinavir monotherapy, the percentage of prescribed doses taken ranged from 69 to 98 percent.[50] Other studies indicate that there may be differences in the acceptance of and adherence to various antiretroviral and prophylactic regimens. A study of HIV-seropositive injecting drug users found that participants were somewhat more likely to accept treatment with ZDV compared with didanosine (DDI; 85 versus 74 percent).[59] Higher rates of acceptance were reported for initiation of PCP prophylaxis with TMP-SMX (94 percent). Similarly, this study and at least one other have observed better adherence rates for PCP prophylaxis than for antiretroviral regimens.[57,59] It is important to bear in mind, however, that these differences also may be influenced by factors such as prior experience with HIV treatment and the individual's disease stage (e.g., symptomatic versus asymptomatic).

The recognition that adherence presents a serious threat to the successful treatment of HIV and other STDs is only a first step toward addressing this problem. In order to improve patients' adherence to STD and HIV treatment, it is essential to understand the factors that contribute to poor adherence. More than 30 years of research has provided a wealth of information regarding the factors associated with adherence to treatment for a wide variety of health problems.[47,60] Across diseases and patient populations, five basic factors generally are associated with adherence: (1) characteristics of the disease or disorder (e.g., presence of symptoms, impact on cognitive abilities), (2) characteristics of the prescribed treatment regimen (e.g., frequency of administration, duration, side effects, cost), (3) patient characteristics (e.g., beliefs about treatment and disease outcomes, motivation, self-efficacy), (4) the relationship between the patient and the provider (e.g., rapport, communication, satisfaction with clinical interactions), and (5) the clinic or care setting (e.g., waiting time, convenience, reputation of clinic).[47]

While the ability of an individual health care provider to influence all these factors is limited, he or she can significantly improve patient adherence by addressing those factors which are amenable to change. In this section we will briefly illustrate how behavioral theory can assist providers in addressing one of these factors—patient characteristics.

PATIENT CHARACTERISTICS

Obviously, some patient characteristics, such as ethnicity, sex, and age, cannot be changed despite the best efforts of health care providers. While these types of demographic factors have been shown to be associated with adherence in some studies, they are not consistently associated with treatment adherence.[47] Attitudes, beliefs, and other perceptions of patients regarding their condition and its treatment, however, often are associated with adherence and *can* be influenced significantly by health care providers. In this section we will briefly discuss the four factors described earlier in this chapter as being primary determinants of health behavior.

Perceived susceptibility

In contrast to the finding that perceived susceptibility is unrelated to the likelihood that one will engage in any specific HIV risk-reduction behavior, perceived susceptibility, including the patient's beliefs that the diagnosis is accurate and that he or she is susceptible to a health threat and its recurrence, has been associated with adherence to provider recommendations in a number of studies.[61] With regard to treatment adherence, *perceived susceptibility* can best be viewed not only as the initial perception of risk of becoming ill but also, and perhaps more important, as the perception of increased morbidity and serious sequelae if treatment is not initiated, prematurely discontinued, or improperly followed.

Health care providers can easily assess a patient's perceived susceptibility by asking "What would happen to you if you stopped taking this medication?" In addition to questioning general susceptibility to disease, it is also important to inquire about the patient's perceived susceptibility when medications are not taken as prescribed. Questions such as "What do you think would happen if you stopped taking your pills for just a day or two?" and "What if you missed only one dose?" are useful in assessing perceived susceptibility. Information obtained by asking questions of this type can be used to address the patient's misperceptions regarding the consequences of not taking medications as prescribed.

Attitudes and beliefs

Patients' global assessment of the desirability of adhering to a specific treatment (i.e., their attitude regarding treatment) and their beliefs about the advantages and disadvantages associated with adhering to that treatment (which combine to form an individual's attitude) are often powerful factors influencing adherence. Messages given to patients about treatment efficacy should focus on the efficacy of the specific treatment regimen (e.g., two tablets, three times a day) rather than on just the general efficacy of the regimen (e.g., these tablets are very effective). Clearly, patients may believe that a particular drug is very effective but at the same time not believe that its effectiveness is significantly influenced by dosing instructions (e.g., take for 10 days, take with food). Patients may have different beliefs about (and perceive different barriers to) taking a given drug once a day than about taking it every 4 hours. Similarly, they may have different beliefs about the consequences of taking a given drug on an empty stomach than about taking that same drug with meals. Considerable research has been conducted regarding the role of beliefs (particularly beliefs regarding treatment efficacy) in adherence to provider recommendations. For example, patients who have negative beliefs regarding the efficacy of ZDV and the severity of its side effects are less likely to take the drug as prescribed,[53,55] whereas patients who strongly believe that ZDV prolongs life are more likely to be adherent.[56]

Assessment of patient attitudes and beliefs regarding treatment should focus on both the perceived benefits and drawbacks of the therapy. Simple questions such as "What do you see as the advantages and disadvantages of taking this drug as prescribed?" or "Do you have any concerns about taking this medication as prescribed?" can provide valuable insights into perceived negative outcomes associated with following a given treatment regimen. Providers should make sure to communicate their belief, even when treating routine conditions, that if the patient takes the medication as prescribed, it will be effective. With regard to side effects, it is important that patients are aware of side effects that may reasonably be encountered, their expected duration, and the steps that can be taken to cope with or alleviate their severity. In addition, patients should be made aware of the negative consequences of not adhering to the prescribed regimen or of discontinuing it prematurely.

Norms

Patients' perceptions of what others think they "should do" can influence their adherence. Patients who perceive more support from their family, friends, and important others with regard to initiating and maintaining therapy are more likely to be successful. A particularly important source of normative influence is the health care provider. For example, 74 percent of HIV-seropositive patients in one study indicated that encouragement by a health care provider was a reason for their initiation of ZDV therapy, whereas encouragement by family or friends was mentioned by 27 percent.[55] Care must be taken, however, not to inadvertently coerce patients into accepting a course of action that they do not feel comfortable with—the perception of undue *pressure* from a health care provider also can lead to poor adherence.[55] Perceived norms can be assessed by questions such as "Do you think that the people who are most important in your life think that you should take this medication as prescribed?" and "How supportive are they?" While changing perceptions of norms may be difficult, providers can try to encourage patients to elicit the support of others or can try to directly intervene with individuals accompanying the patient to a clinic visit to personally solicit their support. Health care providers also should communicate their own support for the patient's willingness to initiate and complete treatment.

Self-efficacy

Common sense tells us that individuals who do not believe that they will be able to overcome barriers to following their provider's instructions are likely to have poor adherence rates. While self-efficacy is a cognitive factor, it is influenced not only by the patient's self-perceived ability to perform a target behavior (e.g., taking pills on time) but also by the presence of real barriers to performing the behavior (e.g., work schedule, parenting responsibilities, dosing schedule, forgetfulness) that may interfere with adhering to a given treatment protocol. In some instances, working with the patient to develop practical strategies for overcoming these barriers may serve not only to increase self-efficacy but also to reduce the negative influence of barriers. Examples of these strategies include providing detailed written instructions regarding the treatment and follow-up plan, linking medication taking with daily activities (e.g., taking pills at meals or at bedtime), encouraging the use of pill boxes to organize daily or weekly supplies of medication, and promoting utilization of reminder systems including pill boxes or watches with alarms that alert the patient when it is time to take his or her medication. Barriers to adherence may be assessed by asking, "What would make it difficult for you to take this medication as prescribed?" Self-efficacy may be assessed by asking, "How confident are you that you can overcome these barriers and take this medication as prescribed?"

OTHER CONSIDERATIONS

It is important to recognize that emotional reactions to a diagnosis, preexisting psychological disorders, and cognitive impairment may significantly influence one's behavioral, normative, or efficacy beliefs and/or interfere with patients' decision-making processes and thereby influence treatment adherence. For example, depression, anxiety, and other psychiatric disorders have been associated with poorer adherence in a number of studies.[55,56,62,63]

It also should be kept in mind that past behavior is usually the best predictor of future behavior. While adherence varies with regard to the condition being treated and the characteristics of the treatment regimen, it is important to assess patients' prior adherence to other medications when initiating treatment. Furthermore, adherence within the first month of treatment has been found to predict adherence to therapy 1 and 7 years later.[64] This emphasizes the critical importance of early follow-up and intervention for patients who are prescribed treatment for chronic conditions, are undergoing ongoing prophylaxis, or are required to make lifestyle changes such as initiating and maintaining safer sex practices. While the first few months may be the most important, it is essential to remember that relapse can occur at any point in time. This emphasizes the importance of regular follow-up and ongoing reinforcement of adherent behavior, which can significantly improve long-term compliance.[65]

SUMMARY AND CONCLUSIONS

In this chapter we have tried to show how behavioral theory can serve as a framework for understanding, reinforcing, and changing health-related behavior. It is important to recognize that behaviors, even those which have been viewed as difficult (or impossible) to change (e.g., sexual and drug-using behaviors), can be changed and changed radically. It is also important to recognize that there are only a limited number of theoretical variables that influence and account for most of the variance in any given behavior. Generally speaking, once a person has formed a strong intention (or made a commitment) to perform a behavior, he or she is likely to perform that behavior given that the person has the necessary skills and there are no environmental constraints to prevent behavioral performance. If a person has not formed an intention to perform the behavior in question, this may be due to his or her attitude toward, perceived norms concerning, or self-efficacy with respect to performing the behavior in question. These variables are in turn determined by underlying beliefs about the perceived consequences of performing the behavior, the normative proscriptions of significant others, and perceived barriers to behavioral performance.

Since many behaviors can put a client at risk for acquiring or transmitting a given STD, a provider, through a risk assessment, should first identify the behavior or behaviors the client is engaging in that put the client at risk. Needless to say, good provider-patient communication is crucial for obtaining accurate risk assessments as well as other relevant information. The provider can then determine whether failure to engage in protective behavior is due to a lack of intention, a lack of skills, or the presence of environmental constraints. If failure is due to a lack of intention, the provider can rapidly assess the client's behavioral, normative, and efficacy beliefs. Discussion of these beliefs along with the establishment of a risk-reduction plan should help the client to change his or her behavior, thus reducing STD incidence.

With respect to adherence to provider recommendations concerning a treatment regimen, the provider should first clearly inform the client about the basis on which he or she has made the diagnosis (e.g., laboratory results, specific clinical symptoms). Second, the provider should elicit and listen to the patient's concerns regarding the diagnosis and treatment. In particular, the provider should obtain information about the client's beliefs about following the prescribed protocol, his or her perceptions of social support or opposition, and his or her beliefs about possible barriers to adherence. In addition, the provider should obtain information about prior adherence to other medical regimens as well as the client's intention to adhere to the medical protocol. The provider's response to these concerns should recognize the barriers faced by the patient, support information seeking (e.g., second opinion), and communicate the consequences of not initiating treatment, prematurely discontinuing treatment, or incorrectly following the treatment protocol. Following these recommendations should lead to an increase in client adherence.

In this chapter we have reviewed the evidence regarding the use of behavioral theory in motivating individual behavior change in two specific areas: HIV counseling and testing and adherence to STD/HIV treatment. It is important to note, however, that a growing scientific literature points to the usefulness of behavioral interventions in promoting and maintaining individual STD/HIV risk-related behavior change. For example, a number of HIV risk interventions using individual counseling models, skills training approaches, and small group activities for a wide range of at-risk populations have been developed, evaluated, and found to be effective.[66,67] The success of these approaches has been recognized and endorsed in an external scientific review sponsored by the National Institutes of Health.[68] The evidence regarding the success of behavioral interventions is now clear and points to the paramount need for clinics and individual health care providers to integrate these approaches into their daily patient care activities.

References

1 May RM, Anderson RM: Transmission dynamics and HIV infection. *Nature* 326:137–142, 1987.

2 Centers for Disease Control and Prevention: HIV prevention practices of primary-care physicians—United States, 1992. *MMWR* 42:988–992, 1994.

3 Croft CA, Asmussen L: A developmental approach to sexuality education: Implications for medical practice. *J Adolesc Health* 14:109–114, 1993.

4 Gemson DH et al: Acquired immunodeficiency syndrome prevention: Knowledge, attitudes, and practices of primary care physicians. *Arch Intern Med* 151:1102–1108, 1991.
5 Gerbert B et al: Are patients talking to their physicians about AIDS. *Am J Public Health* 80:467–468, 1990.
6 Lewis CE et al: Continuing medical education for AIDS: An organizational response. *AIDS Educ Prev* 5:263–271, 1993.
7 Corby NH et al: Using the theory of planned behavior to predict condom use among male and female injecting drug users. *J Appl Social Psychol* 26:52–75, 1996.
8 Jamner MS et al: Using the theory of planned behavior to predict intention to use condoms among female sex workers. *Psychol Health* (*in press*).
9 Montano DE, Kasprzyk D: Differential condom use by type of sex, type of partner, risk group, gender, and ethnicity. Poster presented at the VIIIth International Conference on AIDS, Amsterdam, the Netherlands, July 1992.
10 Kasprzyk D, Montano DE: Theory based identification of precursors to condom use. Poster presented at the IXth International Conference on AIDS, Berlin, Germany, June 1993.
11 Misovich SJ et al: Close relationships and elevated HIV risk behavior: Evidence and possible underlying psychological processes. *Gen Psychol Rev* (*in press*).
12 Becker MH: The health belief model and personal health behavior. *Health Educ Monogr* 2:324–508, 1974.
13 Becker MH: AIDS and behavior change. *Public Health Rev* 16:1–11, 1988.
14 Rosenstock IM: The health belief model and preventive health behavior. *Health Educ Monogr* 2:354–386, 1974.
15 Bandura A: *Social Foundations of Thought and Action: A Social Cognitive Theory.* Englewood Cliffs, NJ, Prentice-Hall, 1986.
16 Bandura A: Social cognitive theory and exercise of control over HIV infection, in *Preventing AIDS: Theories and Methods of Behavioral Interventions*, RJ DiClemente, JL Peterson (eds). New York, Plenum Press, 1994, pp 25–59.
17 Ajzen I, Fishbein M: *Understanding Attitudes and Predicting Social Behavior.* Englewood Cliffs, NJ, Prentice-Hall, 1980.
18 Fishbein M, Ajzen I: *Belief, Attitude, Intention and Behavior: An Introduction to Theory and Research.* Boston, Addison-Wesley, 1975.
19 Fishbein M et al: Using information to change sexually transmitted disease-related behaviors: An analysis based on the theory of reasoned action, in *Research Issues in Human Behavior and Sexually Transmitted Diseases in the AIDS Era*, J Wasserheit et al (eds). Washington, American Society for Microbiology, 1991, pp 243–257.
20 Prochaska JO, DiClemente CC: Stages and processes of self-change in smoking: Toward an integrative model of change. *J Consult Clin Psychol* 51:390–395, 1983.
21 Prochaska JO, DiClemente CC: Toward a comprehensive model of change, in *Treating Addictive Behaviors*, W Miller, N Healther (eds). New York, Plenum Press, 1986, pp 3–27.
22 Prochaska JO et al: In search of how people change: Applications to addictive behaviors. *Am Psychol* 47:1102–1114, 1992.
23 Prochaska JO et al: The transtheoretical model of change and HIV prevention: A review. *Health Educ Q* 21:471–486, 1994.
24 Ajzen I: From intentions to actions: A theory of planned behavior, in *Action Control: From Cognition to Behavior*, J Kuhl, J Beckman (eds). New York, Springer-Verlag, 1984, pp 11–38.
25 Kanfer FH: Self-regulation: Research, issues, and speculations, in *Behavior Modification in Clinical Psychology*, C Neuringir, JL Michael (eds). New York, Appleton-Century-Crofts, 1970, pp 178–220.
26 Triandis HC: *The Analysis of Subjective Culture.* New York, Wiley, 1972.
27 Catania JA et al: Toward an understanding of risk behavior: An AIDS risk reduction model (AARM). *Health Educ Q* 17:53–72, 1990.
28 Fisher JD, Fisher WA: Changing AIDS-risk behavior. *Psychol Bull* 111: 455–474, 1992.
29 Holden G: The relationship of self-efficacy appraisals to subsequent health related outcomes: A meta-analysis. *Soc Work Health Care* 16: 53–93, 1991.
30 Kraus SJ: Attitudes and the prediction of behavior: A meta-analysis of the empirical literature. *Person Soc Psychol Bull* 21:58–75, 1995.
31 Sheppard BH et al: The theory of reasoned action: A meta-analysis of past research with recommendations for modifications and future research. *J Consum Res* 15:325–343, 1988.
32 Strecher VJ et al: The role of self-efficacy in achieving health behavior change. *Health Educ Q* 13:73–92, 1986.
33 van den Putte B: 20 years of the theory of reasoned action of Fishbein and Ajzen: A meta-analysis. Unpublished manuscript, University of Amsterdam, the Netherlands, 1991.
34 Gerrard M et al: Relation between perceived vulnerability to HIV and precautionary sexual behavior. *Psychol Bull* 119:390–409, 1996.
35 Fichtner RR et al: Influence of perceived and assessed risk on STD clinic clients' acceptance of HIV testing, return for test results, and HIV serostatus. *Psychol Health Med* 1:83–98, 1996.
36 Irwin KL et al: The acceptability of voluntary HIV antibody testing in the United States—A decade of lessons learned. *AIDS* 10:1707–1717, 1996.
37 Fishbein M et al: *Factors Influencing Behavior and Behavior Change: Final Report.* Rockville, Md, National Institute of Mental Health, 1992.
38 Fishbein M: AIDS and behavior change: An analysis based on the theory of reasoned action. *Int J Psychol* 24:37–56, 1990.
39 Kamb ML et al: Project RESPECT Study Group: Quality assurance of HIV prevention counseling in a multi-center randomized controlled trial. *Public Health Reps* 111(suppl 1):99–107, 1996.
40 Macro International, Inc: *Assessment of CDC-Funded Counseling, Testing, Referral, and Partner Notification (CTPRN) Services for Prevention of HIV Transmission,* 1992. Atlanta, GA: Macro International, Inc.
41 Doll LS, Kennedy MB: HIV counseling and testing: What is it and how well does it work? in *AIDS Testing: A Comprehensive Guide to Technical, Medical, Social, Legal, and Management Issues*, G Schochetman, JR George (eds). New York, Springer-Verlag, 1994, pp 301–319.
42 Higgins DL et al: Evidence for the effects of HIV antibody testing on risk behaviors. *JAMA* 266:2419–2429, 1991.
43 Wolitski RJ et al: The effects of HIV counseling and testings on risk-related practices and help-seeking behavior. *AIDS Educ Prevent* 9(Suppl B):52–67, 1997.
44 Oakley A et al: Behavioral interventions for HIV/AIDS prevention. *AIDS* 9:479–486, 1995.
45 Centers for Disease Control and Prevention: *HIV Counseling, Testing, and Referral Standards and Guidelines.* Atlanta, CDC, 1994.
46 Kamb ML et al: Project RESPECT Study Group: A multi-center, randomized, controlled trial evaluating HIV prevention counseling (Project RESPECT): Preliminary results. Poster presented at the the XIth International Conference on AIDS, Vancouver, British Columbia, July 1996.
47 Meichenbaum D, Turk DC: *Facilitating Treatment Adherence: A Practitioner's Guidebook.* New York, Plenum Press, 1987.
48 Katz BP et al: Compliance with antibiotic therapy for *Chlamydia trachomatis* and *Neisseria gonorrhoeae. Sex Transm Dis* 19:351–354, 1992.
49 Bowie WR: Antibiotics and sexually transmitted diseases. *Infect Dis Clin North Am* 8:841–857, 1994.
50 Schapiro JM, et al: Causes of long term efficacy and/or drug failure in protease inhibitor monotherapy. Paper presented at the XIth International Conference on AIDS, Vancouver, British Columbia, July 1996.
51 Besch CL: Compliance in clinical trials (editorial). *AIDS* 9:1–10, 1995.
52 Samuels JE et al: Zidovudine therapy in an inner city population. *J Acquir Immune Defic Syndr* 3:877–883, 1990.
53 Muma RD et al: Zidovudine adherence among individuals with HIV infection. *AIDS Care* 7:439–447, 1995.
54 Broers B et al: A cohort study of drug users' compliance with zidovudine treatment. *Arch Intern Med* 154:1121–1127, 1994.
55 Nannis ED et al: Perceptions of AZT: Implications for adherence to medical regimens. *J Appl Biobehav Res* 1:39–54, 1993.
56 Samet JH et al: Compliance with zidovudine therapy in patients infected with human immunodeficiency virus, type 1: A cross-sectional study in a municipal hospital clinic. *Am J Med* 92:495–502, 1992.

57 Singh N et al: Determinants of compliance with antiretroviral therapy in patients with human immunodeficiency virus: Prospective assessment with implications for enhancing compliance. *AIDS Care* 8:261–269, 1996.

58 Wall TL et al: Adherence to zidovudine (AZT) among HIV-infected methadone patients: A pilot study of supervised therapy and dispensing compared to usual care. *Drug Alcohol Depend* 37:261–269, 1995.

59 Demas PA: Personal communication, February 1996.

60 Haynes RB et al: *Compliance in Health Care.* Baltimore, Johns Hopkins University Press, 1979.

61 Becker MH, Maiman LA: Sociobehavioral determinants of compliance with health and medical care recommendations. *Med Care* 13:10–24, 1975.

62 Chesney MA, Folkman S: Psychological impact of HIV disease and implications for intervention. *Psychiatr Clin North Am* 17:163–182, 1994.

63 Demas PA et al: HIV treatment adherence and psychosocial factors among injecting drug users. Paper presented at Society of Behavioral Medicine, San Diego, Calif, March 1995.

64 Dunbar J: Predictors of patient adherence: Patient characteristics, in *The Handbook of Health Behavior Change.* New York, Springer, 1990, p 348.

65 Bond CA, Monson R: Sustained improvement in drug documentation, compliance, and disease control: A four-year analysis of an ambulatory care model. *Arch Intern Med* 144:1159–62, 1984.

66 Choi KH, Coates TJ: Prevention of HIV infection (editorial). *AIDS* 8: 1371–1389, 1994.

67 Kalichman SC et al: Prevention of sexually transmitted HIV infection: A meta-analytic review of the behavioral outcome literature. *Ann Behav Med* 18:6–15, 1996.

68 National Institutes of Health: *Interventions to Prevent HIV Risk Behaviors.* Consensus development conference statement, Bethesda, Md, National Institutes of Health, 1997.

Chapter 55

Partner notification for sexually transmitted diseases and HIV infection

Richard B. Rothenberg
John J. Potterat

The epidemiologic investigation of persons exposed to infectious conditions has deep roots in public health practice. Although the time and place of origin are uncertain, such investigation has been a part of sexually transmitted disease (STD) control since the early nineteenth century.[1] In 1917, Osler[2] championed the development of a comprehensive educational and treatment campaign that included the use of social workers in venereal disease (VD) clinics. Although he did not specifically invoke the concept of tracing infectious contacts, he made an eloquent plea for the revision of attitudes and practices with regard to venereal diseases. In 1926, public health officials in New Jersey claimed to have the only continuous statewide program to detect "foci of venereal infection."[3] They stated:

> Under this plan the physicians ask their patients recently infected with gonorrhea or syphilis to tell the name and address of the person who infected them, if they know these facts. This information is transmitted by the physician on his case report to the State department of health. If the person named is a professional prostitute the information is passed on, without giving the name of the physician or his patient, to the police official having jurisdiction. If the person named is a child, a man or a woman who is apparently a clandestine prostitute, the information is transmitted to the health officer concerned [p. 335].

This quotation encapsulates both the epidemiologic process and its embedded social perceptions. In 1933, Munson[4] reported on the value of tracing clusters of venereal infections in rural upstate New York. Of special interest in his report—discussed later in this chapter—are several full-fledged sociograms (diagrams showing the interrelationships among groups of people) that antedate the coinage of that term.[5]

In 1937, U.S. Surgeon General Parran proposed that epidemiologic investigation of syphilis cases be part of a comprehensive national control strategy that also included screening, case reporting, public support for clinical treatment, and public education.[6,7] The recommendation languished until after World War II. In part because of the success of American military efforts at venereal disease follow-up in England and elsewhere during the war,[7,8] Dr. Parran's program was adopted at the National Communicable Disease Center (established in 1946),[9] and the epidemiologic investigation of persons with syphilis became a cornerstone of the program.

THE NAME OF THE PROCESS

Through much of its history, this process was known as *contact tracing*—identifying the sexual partners of infected persons, locating those partners, and ensuring their medical evaluation. In the 1980s, soon after the recognition of AIDS, and perhaps in response to the distant echoes quoted earlier, the name was changed by near universal consent to *partner notification.*[10–14] The term was meant to encompass two separate approaches:[14] *patient referral* (also called *self-referral),* the process whereby patients themselves are encouraged to notify partners at risk, and *provider referral,* wherein health care workers assist in notifying at-risk partners. The latter, in this formulation,[14] is viewed as the equivalent of contact tracing. The definitional distinctions are useful, but none of the terms captures an important feature of this epidemiologic activity—a process of investigation and discovery that may have important implications for understanding disease transmission and control.[1,15–19] Whatever the term of the moment, it is important to retain the dual nature of the activity: direct service to persons at risk and a basic source of epidemiologic information that can focus disease control efforts.[1]

DISTAL EFFORTS

Despite the central position of contact tracing in the early decades of the VD control program in the United States, surprisingly little published information is available on its deployment, its descriptive results, its use-effectiveness in bringing exposed persons to evaluation and treatment, and its impact on disease transmission. The vast majority of such information is in the form of programmatic data generated by federal, state, and local STD workers (Centers for Disease Control and Prevention, Division of Sexually Transmitted Disease Prevention, unpublished data). Such program narratives, a part of the reporting process required for federal funding, usually addressed the degree to which antecedent program activity met preestablished (and often arbitrary) federal guidelines. Their value in evaluating the process itself may thus be somewhat limited. Actual published reports during the period from the 1950s to the 1980s may suffer similarly from reporting bias. The vast majority were laudatory, reporting positive findings and stressing the importance of this technique for disease control.

The fundamental approach to the contact interview was established explicitly at the inception of the program in the United States[20] and was implicit in the activities of "American public health nurses" (p. 1)[21] working with American soldiers and airmen in England during World War II and in the Tyneside scheme, a system for seeking contacts that had been inaugurated in 1943.[22] These approaches presaged all the systems that have been used subsequently and which differ only in detail; techniques have been modified, however, to fit current conditions.[23] In brief, a conversation is held with an infected person during which the interviewer attempts to establish rapport, provide information to the patient about the disease and its treatment, discuss the manner in which the disease is transmitted, and elicit names and identifying information on all persons with whom the patient has had sexual contact within a defined period. An administrative system for recording contact information and for keeping track of follow-up was an integral part of the process. During this early period, most of the interviewees were men, and referral was usually by the provider, not the patient. Basic measures of effectiveness and productivity were quickly established: contact index (contacts elicited per interview), epidemiologic index (number of infected contacts per case), brought to treatment index (newly infected contacts not previously treated per case), and lesion-to-lesion index (number of early syphilis cases with infectious lesions per case).[24] Although alternate terms have been used to describe these measures, the basic approach of evaluating program results using measures of central tendency (e.g., mean indices) rather than distributions became a fixed feature of these efforts. In this initial report,[24] the authors note that the contact index varied by 10-fold in two areas during the same 6-month interval (from 0.43 contacts per case (area unidentified) to 4.97 contacts per case).[25]

Subsequent reports from Great Britain[8,26–42] and the United

States[25,43–63] provided further detail and explication but did not furnish a systematic overview of process or outcome measures of effectiveness. Such a systematic overview might be expected to provide a standard for some of the indices cited earlier, consensus concerning the time frames in which interviewing takes places, the establishment of a relationship between the amount and intensity of contact tracing and disease morbidity, and some overall measures of impact on disease transmission. With the exception of some attempts to link contact tracing to incidence, these were not forthcoming. Most of the reports adopt an idiosyncratic approach that, although frequently informative, does not permit an orderly overview of the field. For example, it is hard to establish a standard for the number of contacts that "should" be elicited per case. In the American literature, the average reported contact index (from those studies which either reported it or from which it could be calculated[24,25,44,45,47–49,51,55–57,62,63]) was 1.75 (range 0.43–4.96), and the epidemiologic index (contacts newly brought to treatment per case interviewed) was 0.36 (range 0.02-0.67). Reports from outside the United States had lower indices: 0.82 (range 0.08–1.56) and 0.20 (range 0.06-0.45), respectively.[8,26,27,29–31,34,35,40] Without information on patient selection, interviewing techniques, intensity of field follow-up, and perhaps most important, the underlying distribution of sex contacts in the general population and in the subpopulation at risk, these numbers are hard to interpret. Only a few of the studies provide information on the timeliness of contact follow-up,[41,47–49] and only several make an overt effort to relate specific local contact tracing efforts to the occurrence of disease.[34,47] In Alabama, investigators noted a peak in reported syphilis cases in 1965 and a marked decline in the two subsequent years, during which they initiated a program of intense interviewing and case investigation (referred to as a "blitz," presumably in reference to the German *Blitzkrieg).*[47] As they put it, ". . . Today more than ever before, exploitation is being performed on all infectious syphilis cases in Alabama" (p. 1365). A temporal approach to data presentation was not taken, but it appeared that the decline in secular trend preceded full implementation of the program, whose initial impact should have caused some increase in reported cases.

Several groups of investigators have sought to link contact tracing directly to changes in incidence. Researchers at Whitechapel Clinic in London noted that gonorrhea had declined by 20 percent during the decade of the 1960s compared with a 33 percent increase in England and Wales during the same period.[34] They pointed to the increased efficacy of case finding by interviewing infected men and a decreasing male-to-female ratio. The direct relationship between these activities and the changing morbidity pattern is hard to define, however, particularly in the absence of information on the proportion of their catchment population reached. In a similar study at Sheffield, a 35 percent decline in reported gonorrhea was noted between 1977 and 1982 compared with an 11 percent decline overall in England during the same period.[64] The authors felt that a number of factors pointed to the influence of contact tracing on the decline: Virtually 100 percent of cases were interviewed, the male-to-female ratio in Sheffield fell from 1.26 to 1.10, the proportion of gonorrhea cases that was discovered as a result of contact tracing efforts rose from 0.62 to 0.93, and they noted a decline in complications affecting women and children in Sheffield. In a later report, however, it was noted that the changing incidence could not be correlated directly with measures of efficiency of contact tracing.[65]

A contemporaneous report from Colorado Springs, however, gave further credence to these findings.[66] In comparing the period 1977–1979 to the period 1980–1982, the authors reported a 13 percent decline in gonorrhea in Colorado Springs, a 7 percent decline in the rest of Colorado, and a 3 percent decline in the United States. They noted a greatly improved contact tracing effort during the second interval compared with the first, owing in large measure to a successful partnership with military preventive medicine units in the area. In the second interval, about 93 percent of cases were interviewed, with an overall contact index of 1.9. Compared with the first interval, there was a marked decline in the male-to-female ratio among military personnel (from 12 to 4.7), a near doubling of the number of persons found through contact tracing, and more than double the proportion of gonorrhea cases discovered by this process in the second interval. The authors reported no substantial change in programmatic activity between the two intervals other than intensification of contact tracing and were able to effect this intensification without additional resources. Although cause and effect are not inextricably linked by such observations, the use of epidemiologic surrogates—a high proportion of cases affected by the process, declining incidence and sequelae of disease, an increasing proportion of cases found through intervention, a changing ratio of men to women, and a constancy of other activity—paints an optimistic picture for the potential impact of this process.

THE AIDS INTERREGNUM

With the advent of AIDS in the late 1970s and early 1980s, interest in contact tracing for other STDs dropped off noticeably. Several features of the new illness conspired to make contact tracing unacceptable: particular epidemiologic characteristics such as a high case-fatality proportion, a long incubation period, and no apparent treatment; sensitive societal circumstances with considerable opportunity for adverse social outcomes for those affected; and some of the social baggage associated with contact tracing.[3,47] Nonetheless, a burgeoning interest in the dynamics of disease transmission, coupled with biostatistical techniques for modeling transmission, served to underline some of the importance of information on contacts.

With roots in "classic epidemic theory," disease dynamics had been explored by Yorke and colleagues,[67] who used a model of interacting "compartments" to describe the transmission of gonorrhea. Their thinking led to the concept that small groups of sexual active persons, definable by stable demographic, geographic, and behavioral characteristics (so-called core groups),[68] are responsible for maintaining the endemicity of gonorrhea. A series of empirical studies demonstrated the existence of such groups by using a combination of data from disease reporting and from routinely acquired information about contacts.[19,69–73]

The epidemic of human immunodeficiency virus (HIV) was an impetus to further development of theories of disease transmission dynamics. Investigators developed and refined the use of compartments to explore potential scenarios for the spread of HIV[74–80] and for the potential effect of interventions.[81] Although these models are powerful tools for simulating the environment in which transmission takes place, they do not lend themselves readily to prediction[82] and were limited by the inadequacy of epidemiologic data for parameter estimation.[75] Such parameters—frequency of partner change, probability of transmission per sexual contact, duration of incubation period, and mixing patterns—are estimable in principle from contact tracing information.

For example, such information has been used to define the degree of assortative or disassortative mixing for gonorrhea.[83] In the examples examined, the investigators noted that mixing was assorative (like with like), with moderate to high rates of sexual contact within areas reporting the majority of cases of gonorrhea. The authors noted that there are problems related to the use of contact tracing data for identifying patterns of sexual mixing, but that ". . . these [problems] do not detract from the importance of acquiring better information, since the nature of these mixing patterns determines to a large extent the pattern of infection within a community and the appropriate policies to adopt for control of infection and disease" (p. 191). In a study that was similar in design but differed in some of its mathematical approaches, investigators used contact tracing data to estimate the preference matrix for women in choosing male partners.[84] They concluded that a proportional mixing model is not an adequate description of sexual partner choice and that models based on such assumptions may be awry. In similar work, some of these same investigators used contact tracing data to show that random-mixing models will probably overestimate the spread and final size of an epidemic,[85] again throwing into doubt the results of some models that were based on assumptions of random mixing. Rather than discrediting such models, however, the use of contact tracing data provides refinement and enhanced credibility. The same authors have explored the use of contact tracing data to estimate transmission probabilities.[17] From a large series of contact interviews, they described characteristics of the population and isolated 130 initially HIV-discordant same-sex and different-sex couples. Overall, they estimated the probability of transmission to be 0.44 for homosexual couples and 0.22 for heterosexual couples.

PROXIMAL EFFORTS

Despite this increased awareness of the value of contact tracing information in understanding transmission, there was considerable, often impassioned foment during the 1980s and early 1990s about the value, efficacy, cost-effectiveness, and ethics of contact tracing, whose name changed at about this time, as noted, to *partner notification*. A considerable body of opinion, both for[86–100] and against[101–107] was marshaled, primarily directed at the use of partner notification in HIV control. In summary, detractors felt that the technique had little proven value for relatively high cost, that the long, asymptomatic incubation made partner identification difficult, and that the failure to relate partner notification to a reduction in disease transmission is a serious drawback.[14] Proponents suggest that targeted HIV prevention is preferable to a generalized, nonspecific approach,[108] that a focused approach for interviewing is affordable, manageable, and can reach those at highest risk effectively, that the use of prophylaxis for *Pneumocystis carinii* pneumonia[109] and other conditions[110] and of antiretroviral therapy for maintenance of asymptomatic infection[111,112] and reduction of maternal-infant transmission[113,114] have contributed to the acceptability of early case finding to those at risk,[115,116] and that partner notification helps provide necessary medical care and support services to people with HIV.[117]

The critical subset of this debate, however, has concerned the potential for loss of confidentiality, violation of civil liberties, the possibility of discrimination, and the unwanted result that persons at risk might not seek medical care.[86,88,107,118–125] The fundamental tension is between the "two faces" of partner notification: the duty to warn endangered persons of risk and eliciting voluntary cooperation of patients in seeking persons known to them who may be at risk.[121] As these authors put it, ". . . Confusion between the two approaches has led many to mischaracterize processes that are fundamentally voluntary as mandatory, and processes that respect confidentiality as invasive of privacy" (p. 1158). In a thoughtful, lengthy discussion, they consider the legal genesis of these issues and conclude that those placed at risk have a moral right to know of it, and in that context, ". . . [n]either the principle of confidentiality nor the value attached to professional autonomy is an absolute" (p. 1163). They also make it clear that "contact tracing" does not pose these same ethical dilemmas, since it requires neither disclosure without the patient's consent nor loss of confidentiality. When these issues are considered at the level of a single case,[122,123] however, the complexity of such decisions and the need to avoid blanket legal requirements that constrain local judgment become manifest. An example of such complexity, perhaps not often considered, is the harm that may befall the original patient (particularly if a woman) if her identity becomes known to her partner(s).[124] In addition, the extent to which public health agencies and the law may go in restricting the behavior of those who are infected[120,121] is a complicated issue that is in some measure dependent on local circumstances and mores.

In any event, the vigorous debate over the ethics of partner notification and the establishment of acceptability, particularly to those most affected, have led to a rejuvenation of interest in studying the process. Since 1990, several dozen investigations have examined the techniques for interviewing and case investigation, the "yield" from such activity, the costs associated with the process, and in several instances, the influence on local secular trends. A number of these studies have been cast in an experimental mode: a comparison of a partner notification technique with some default condition. The results have a curiously atavistic quality[16,106,117,126–144] [Table 55-1 (HIV), Table 55-2 (gonorrhea and chlamydia), and Table 55-3 (syphilis)]. Contact indices have a familiar ring: For HIV, the average contact index in these studies was 2.45 (range 0.73–5.31) (see Table 55–1); for gonorrhea and chlamydia, 1.14 (range 0.79–1.57) (see Table 55–2); and for syphilis, 3.73 (range 1.81–6.25 for four observations) (see Table 55–3). As in the past, syphilis case finding appeared to have been more vigorous than that for gonorrhea (although it is uncertain, as it was in the past, to what extent this observation represents differences in the underlying distribution of sexual contacts). It important to note, however, that most publications from earlier years, and particularly those from programs in the United States, only reported identified, located partners. In the current studies, a number of investigators have rediscovered the fact that more people are named than can be identified.[106,143] Case finding for HIV appears to fall between the other two in its "yield," although, once again, there is little information on the underlying sexual activity of those at risk for HIV.

Another correspondence with the past is a similarity in the proportion of contacts infected and the epidemiologic index (infected contacts per case). For both syphilis and gonorrhea/chlamydia, about three contacts had to be located and examined to find another infected person. Results for HIV are lower, partly because of a greater reluctance on the part of patients to be tested. Finally, an important evocation of past studies is the difficulty of relating partner notification activity to underlying transmission and to changes in secular trend. The reported investigations are small, for the most part, and do not encompass a clearly defined group. Several of the studies do report an estimate of cost-effectiveness, either in the form of total costs ($62,500 per year[126]) or as cost per positive partner identified ($2203 per HIV-seropositive partner,[133] $1625 per HIV-seropositive partner,[128] and $1627 per syphilis case identified[143]). The only available comparison with the past (a different time, a different fiscal structure) was a cost of between $6.16 and $13.60 for a new case of gonorrhea brought to treatment.[51] These results are difficult to interpret. The cost per discovered case, though measured in dollars, is actually a relative metric used for comparison and should not be confused with real dollars. In addition, its method of calculation differs among the studies (certainly, there is little connection with similar metrics that are now 23 years old). But perhaps more important, although the cost-effectiveness measure is theoretically interpretable as a comparison among studies, it provides little general sense of how much such an activity should cost, nor whether the activity is expensive. A more comprehensive analysis demonstrated that the CDC's overall program of counseling, testing, referral, and partner notification was cost-beneficial, even using conservative as-

Table 55-1. Results of Selected Studies of Partner Notification for HIV Infection, 1990–1995

Study	Site	Number enrolled	Number interviewed	Partners named (CI)*	Partners located	Positives/tested (%)	Comment
Pavia, 1993[127]	Utah	308	244	890 (3.65)	489	193/433 (45) EI† = 0.79	Statewide experience Total cost = $62,500
Vernon, 1993[128]	Colorado	—	2837	4773 (1.68)	485	272/2550 (11) EI = 0.10	Statewide experience, 1986–1992
Spencer, 1993[129]	Colorado	231	226	239 (1.06)	188	17/80 (21) EI = 0.08	1988 results; cost per seropositive person identified = $1625
Hoffman, 1995[130]	Colorado	263	188	142 (0.76)	73	4/26 (15) EI = 0.02	Anonymous testing site
Hoffman, 1995[130]	Colorado	316	213	215 (1.01)	122	16/50 (32) EI = 0.08	Confidential testing site
Pattman, 1993[131]	Newcastle upon Tyne	89	89	80 (0.90)	80	25/80 (31) EI = 0.28	Tyneside scheme revisited
Landis, 1992[132]	No. Carolina	534	39	157 (4.03)	78	9/36 (25) EI = 0.23	Provider referral
Landis, 1992[132]	N. Carolina	534	35	153 (4.37)	10	5/25 (20) EI = 0.14	Patient referral (some partners not notified by patients were later located by the provider.)
CDC, 1994[133]	Pennsylvania	1	5+	124 (na)	124	44/121 (36) EI = na	A large network stemming from 1 person who named 4 others; 124 persons ultimately identified
Wycoff, 1991[118]	S. Carolina	119	91	485 (5.31)	290	41/280 (15)	Retesting yielded 8 more positives; decline in CI during study, possibly due to intervention
Rutherford, 1991[114]	San Francisco	145	51	135 (2.65)	59	7/34 (21) EI = 0.14	Total cost = $15,120; cost per sero-positive partner = $2203
Giesecke, 1991[16]	Göteberg	403	365	546 (1.55)	390	143/350 (41) EI = 0.39	53/143 positives were new; also see Giesecke, 1992

*CI = Contact Index, the number of partners elicited per infected person interviewed.
†EI = Epidemiologic Index, the number of infected partners per person interviewed.

sumptions.[145] The methods used did not permit individual examination of the program's components.

This overall, somewhat pessimistic view of the available data on partner notification is supported by an extensive survey and metaanalysis.[146–148] These investigators reviewed available studies of partner notification, recontacted original authors when possible, and attempted to evaluate these studies using standards of evidence. They confirmed, as noted here, that few conclusions could be drawn from the available data and felt that a more rigorous approach, particularly to the evaluation of components of the process, was needed to form practice guidelines based on observation and experimental trials.

Perhaps the difficulties, both past and present, stem from uncertainty as to how to measure the value and effectiveness of partner notification. As alluded to, investigators have attempted to examine "yield" (contact index, epidemiologic index, proportion of examined partners infected, rapidity of examination) without a standard against which to compare such parameters and without underlying information about the distribution of sexual activity in the population at risk. Alternatively, researchers have looked to cost-effectiveness, which also suffers, as noted, from a lack of clear standards or goals. The extent to which persons at risk accept the procedure and the degree to which the community accepts it are often considered but are clearly ancillary to the epidemio-

Table 55-2. Results of Selected Studies of Partner Notification for Gonorrhea (GC) and Chlamydial Infection (Ct), 1990–1995

Study	Site	Number enrolled	Number interviewed	Partners named (CI)*	Partners located	Positives/tested (%)	Comment
Ruden, 1993[135]	Stockholm	857	671	826 (1.23)	736	345/736 (47) EI = 0.37	GC; 161 new infections
Katz, 1992[136]	Indianapolis, IN	—	12,732	13,845 (1.09)	11,350	4035/11350 (36) EI = 0.32	Syph, GC, Ct; index = 1.09 if those with no contacts not counted
Kamwendo, 1993[117]	Orebro, Sweden	349	196	—	200	64/200 (33) EI = 0.33	GC, Ct; provides detail on joint infection as a function of PN
Ranstedt, 1991[138]	Göteberg, Sweden	425,	425	537 (1.26)	477	—	CT; initial screening study
Langille, 1992[139]	Nova Scotia	52	47	37 (0.79)	25	—	Ct; no detail on infection
Patel, 1994[140]	London	254	254	328 (1.29)	271	—	Ocular Ct; no detail on infection
Oh, 1995[141]	Birmingham	—	265	198 (0.75)	129	—	GC, Ct; adolescents; patient referral preferred
Andrus, 1990[107]	Portland, OR	164	164	258 (1.57)	189	—	Stresses high proportion of contacts that could not be found

*CI = Contact Index, the number of partners elicited per infected person interviewed.
†EI = Epidemiologic Index, the number of infected partners per person interviewed.

Table 55-3. Results of Selected Studies of Partner Notification for Syphilis, 1990–1995

Study	Site	Number enrolled	Number interviewed	Partners named (CI)*	Partners located	Positives/tested (%)	Comment
Gunn, 1995[142]	San Diego, CA	725	696	2091 (4.20)	1045	282/1045 (27) EI = 0.41	Also identified 473 high-risk associates; stressed difficulties in finding partners
Andrus, 1990[107]	Portland, OR	148	146	913 (6.25)	184	—	Stressed named contacts who could not be found; see Table 55-2
Romanowski, 1991[143]	Alberta, Canada	1089	1089	1969† (1.81)	—	249/1089 (13) EI = 0.23	131/826 men and 118/263 women dx'ed as a result of PN
Engelau, 1995[144]	Montgomery Co, Alabama	800	373	984 contacts (2.64) 1446 associates	679 1153	113/679; EI = 0.30 41/1153 (4)	Cost per case = $1627 compared to $771 in nonstudy period
CDC, 1991[145]	Philadelphia, PA	1					Network of 26 infected persons generated by single infectee; subsequent targeted screening yielded 100/372 positives (42 infectious syphilis).

*CI = Contact Index, the number of partners elicited per infected person interviewed.
†EI = Epidemiologic Index, the number of infected partners per person interviewed.

logic process. Finally, several studies have successfully related partner notification activity to declining incidence, but their success is clearly tied to the intensity of the intervention. For most partner notification reports, the usually small and undefined nature of the group exposed to the intervention is a substantial barrier to defining a connection between this disease control activity and the secular trend.

IN THE CONTEXT OF SOCIAL NETWORKS

Some reconceptualization of partner notification may be necessary to supply a context for its evaluation. One promising avenue for further development is the connection of this process to the larger field of social network analysis. Since the initial description of statistical and graphic methods for describing interactions among persons within a social group in the 1930s,[149] considerable knowledge about such interactions has accrued, and a sizable methodology has evolved.[150] Although proceeding in different channels, there have been some striking resemblances between the materials and methods of social network analysis and the techniques used for collection and analysis of partner notification data for STDs.[151] As noted earlier, Munson[4] in New York State drew classic sociograms to describe the interaction of persons with venereal disease. Since the 1970s, the federal STD control program has encouraged the use of the "lot system," an administrative technique for placing all sexually connected persons together and treating them as a subgroup.[151] In the early 1980s, investigators stressed the importance of evaluating the entire social milieu—and not just sexual contacts—in assessing children with gonorrhea.[152] Perhaps a milestone in the rapprochement between the two fields occurred with the publication of a sociogram describing the connections among 44 men from New York City and San Francisco who were afflicted with a then ill-defined serious illness that affected their immune system.[153] Shortly thereafter, Klovdahl[154] used the same data for more formal social network analysis, describing temporal and spatial relationships within the group.

Since these early efforts, a number of investigational teams have pursued the larger social context in which transmission of HIV and STDs takes place. Studies of injecting drug users in inner-city areas,[155,156] in small metropolitan areas,[157–160] and in rural communities[161–163] have all demonstrated the importance of social context for determining the potential for disease transmission. For example, the presence of persons who serve as bridges between groups has proved to be predictive of transmission from one bounded network to another.[164] Further, structural characteristics of networks and the central or noncentral position of infected persons within them may serve as either a barrier or facilitator of transmission.[158,159] Finally, in an area of low transmission, the changing character of a network over time serves as a marker for the decreasing likelihood of transmission.[165] In this example, the investigators were able to demonstrate a "thinning" out of network connections involving needle-sharing over a 3-year period of observations.

Taken together, these early observations have promise for defining a new context in which partner notification may be evaluated. The demonstration that network characteristics have an influence on the likelihood of transmission, that these characteristics change over time, and that risks can best be assessed in the social context in which they take place all underscore a changing view of the process of case interview and contact follow-up.[162] In addition, the social network approach provides more direct connection with theoretical modeling of disease transmission[166–168] and with a larger view of the interaction of groups for disease transmission.[169] Because evaluation in real time is difficult, since observational data do not prove cause-and-effect relationships, and because the virtual reality of modeling is always arguable, social networks may provide an important alternative and may enhance the use of more standard evaluative tools such as yield and cost-effectiveness.

The valuation of partner notification does not depend solely on its evaluation, however. The two faces of partner notification have their cognates in the dual nature of the process. By fulfilling the duty to warn, partner notification serves the interest of the person at risk. By seeking contacts in a confidential, humane way, it delivers data for understanding the dynamics of disease transmission and for establishing tools for disease control. Seen in its broader social context, partner notification appears to have intrinsic value. Without such context, cycles of enthusiasm and rejection are likely to continue.

References

1 Ramstedt K: An epidemiologic approach to sexually transmitted diseases: With special reference to contact tracing and screening. *Acta Derm Venereol (Stockh)* 157(suppl):S1-S45, 1991.

2 Osler W: Annual oration: The campaign against syphilis. *Lancet* 4891:792, 1917.

3 Casselman AJ, Patterson RS: Special articles: Difficulties encountered in venereal follow-up. *J Vener Dis Inform* 7:335–337, 1926.
4 Munson WL: Epidemiology of syphilis and gonorrhea. *Am J Public Health* 23:797–808, 1933.
5 Moreno JL: *Who Shall Survive? Foundations of Sociometry, Group Pyschotherapy, and Sociodrama.* Washington, Nervous and Mental Diseases Publishing Company, 1934.
6 Parran T: *Shadow on the Land.* New York, Reynal and Hitchcock, 1937.
7 Cutler JC, Arnold RC: Venereal disease control by health departments in the past: Lessons for the present. *Am J Public Health* 78: 372–376, 1988.
8 Wigfield AS: 27 years of uninterrupted contact tracing: The "Tyneside scheme." *Br J Vener Dis* 48:37–50, 1972.
9 Etheridge EW: *Sentinel for Health: A History of the Centers for Disease Control.* Berkeley and Los Angeles, California, University of California Press, 1992.
10 Centers for Disease Control and Prevention: Partner notification for preventing human immunodeficiency virus (HIV) infection—Colorado, Idaho, South Carolina, Virginia. *MMWR* 37:393, 401–396, 302, 1988.
11 Anonymous editor: *Guide to Public Health Practice: HIV Partner Notification Strategies.* Association of State and Territorial Health Officials NA, U.S. Conference of Local Health Officers, 1988.
12 Anonymous editor: *Consensus Statement from Consultation on Partner Notification for Preventing HIV Transmission.* Geneva, World Health Organization, Global Programme on AIDS and Programme of STD, 1989.
13 World Health Organization: Consensus statements on HIV transmission. *Lancet* 1:1396, 1989.
14 Toomey KE, Cates W: Partner notification for the prevention of HIV infection. *AIDS* 3(suppl 1):S57-S62, 1989.
15 Rothenberg RB, Potterat JJ: Strategies for Management of Sex Partners, in *Sexually Transmitted Diseases,* 2d ed, Holmes KK et al (eds). New York, McGraw-Hill, 1990.
16 Giesecke J et al: Efficacy of partner notification for HIV infection. *Lancet* 91:1096–1100, 1991.
17 Giesecke J et al: Partner notification as a tool for research in HIV epidemiology: Behavior change, transmission risk and incidence trends. *AIDS* 92:101–107, 1992.
18 Potterat JJ et al: Gonorrhea as a social disease. *Sex Transm Dis* 12: 25–32, 1985.
19 Rothenberg RB, Potterat JJ: Temporal and social aspects of gonorrhea transmission: The force of infectivity. *Sex Transm Dis* 15:88–95, 1988.
20 Ennes H, Bennett TB: The contact-education interview: Its functions, principles, and techniques in venereal disease contact investigation. *Am J Syphil Vener Dis* 29:647, 1945.
21 The venereal disease contact, editorial. *Br J Vener Dis* 21:1, 1945.
22 Johns HM: The social background of venereal disease: A report on an experiment in contact tracing and an investigation into social conditions. Tyneside experimental scheme in venereal disease control. *Br J Vener Dis* 21:26–34, 1945.
23 Potterat JJ et al: Partner notification: Operational considerations. *Int J STD AIDS* 2:411–415, 1991.
24 Ishkrant AP, Kahn HA: Statistical indices used in the evaluation of syphilis contact investigation. *J Vener Dis Inform* 29:13–19, 1948.
25 Ensley EJ et al: The 100-day experiment in contact investigation in Arkansas. *J Vener Dis Inform* 29:13–19, 1948.
26 Haworth MC: Tracing the contacts of male patients with acute gonorrhoea. *Br J Vener Dis* 30:36–37, 1954.
27 Dunlop EMC: Epidemiology of gonorrhea certain aspects of control of the disease in women with particular reference to contact tracing. *Br J Vener Dis* 39:109–112, 1963.
28 Burgess JA: A contact-tracing procedure. *Br J Vener Dis* 39:113–115, 1963.
29 Lamb AM: New methods of contact tracing in infectious venereal diseases. *Br J Vener Dis* 42:276–279, 1966.
30 Willcox RR et al: Contact investigation of male West Indian patients with gonorrhoea. *Br J Vener Dis* 42:167–170, 1966.
31 Muspratt B, Ponting LI: Improved methods of contact tracing. *Br J Vener Dis* 43:204–209, 1967.
32 Capinski TZ, Urbanczyk J: Value of re-interviewing in contact tracing. *Br J Vener Dis* 46:138–141, 1970.
33 Morton RS: Male:female ratios in the V.D. clinics of England and Wales. *Br J Vener Dis* 46:103–105, 1970.
34 Dunlop EM et al: Improved tracing of contacts of heterosexual men with gonorrhoea: Relationship of altered female to male ratios. *Br J Vener Dis* 47:192–195, 1971.
35 Bierre TH: Venereal disease: Case and contact finding. *N Z Med J* 77:380–384, 1973.
36 Willcox RR: International contact tracing in venereal disease. *WHO Chron* 27:418–422, 1973.
37 Contact tracing, editorial. *Br Med J* 3(92):75–76, 1974.
38 Rubin SG: Influence of contact tracing on sex ratios in gonorrhoea. *Public Health* 90:21–23, 1975.
39 Satin A: A record system for contact tracing. *Br J Vener Dis* 53:84–87, 1977.
40 Satin A, Mills A: Measuring the outcome of contact tracing. *Br J Vener Dis* 54:187–191, 1977.
41 Mills A, Satin A: Measuring the outcome of contact 2: The responsibilities of the health worker and the outcome of contact investigations. *Br J Vener Dis* 54:192–198, 1978.
42 Thin RN: Health advisers (contact tracers) in sexually transmitted disease. *Br J Vener Dis* 84:269–272, 1984.
43 Buchwald J et al: The venereal disease contact interview. *Public Health Rep* 75:1000–1006, 1960.
44 Hookings CE, Graves LM: Speed zone epidemiology: A preliminary report on benzathine penicillin G for gonorrhea in women. *Public Health Rep* 71:1142–1143, 1956.
45 Fiumaara NJ et al: An outbreak of gonorrhea in Massachusetts. *Am J Public Health* 49:924–936, 1959.
46 Glass LH: An analysis of some characteristics of males with gonorrhoea. *Br J Vener Dis* 43:128–132, 1967.
47 Smith WHY, Hill JJ: Domestic eradication of syphilis in Alabama. *J Med Assoc Ala* 37:1363–1369, 1968.
48 Pedersen AHB, Harrah WD: Follow-up of male and female contacts of patients with gonorrhea. *Public Health Rep* 85:997–1000, 1970.
49 Marino AF et al: Gonorrhea epidemiology: Is it worthwhile? *Am J Public Health* 62:713–714, 1972.
50 Jacobs CF et al: "Blitz" proves effective public health tool. *J SC Med Assoc* 123:416–418, 1971.
51 Blount JH: A new approach for gonorrhea epidemiology. *Am J Public Health* 62:710–713, 1972.
52 Brown WJ, Blount JH: The effectiveness of the epidemiological approach to syphilis control. *J Reprod Med* 11:123–124, 1973.
53 McCormack WM et al: Evaluation of two methods of following women who have been treated because of exposure to gonorrhea. *Am J Public Health* 64:714–716, 1974.
54 Hinman AR: Evaluation of gonorrhea control efforts. *J Am Vener Dis Assoc* 2(2):9–12, 1975.
55 Lee SS: Gonorrhea control measures: A study in New Hanover County, N.C. *Public Health Rep* 69(10):998–1007, 1954.
56 Gilstrap LC et al: Gonorrhea screening in male consorts of women with pelvic infection. *JAMA* 238(9):965–966, 1977.
57 Potterat JJ, Rothenberg RB: The case-finding effectiveness of a self-referral system for gonorrhea: A preliminary report. *Am J Public Health* 67(2):174–176, 1977.
58 Henderson RH: Control of sexually transmitted diseases in the United States: A federal perspective. *Br J Vener Dis* 53:211–215, 1977.
59 Judson FN, Wolf FC: Tracing and treating contacts of gonorrhea patients in a clinic for sexually transmitted disease. *Public Health Rep* 93:460–463, 1978.
60 Felman YM, Nikitas JA: Epidemiologic approach to control of sexually transmitted disease. *NY State J Med* 79:745–746, 1979.

61 Volkin LB et al: Epidemiologic follow-up study of patients with gonococcal pelvic inflammatory disease. *Sex Transm Dis* 6(4):267–269, 1979.

62 Potterat JJ et al: Gonococcal pelvic inflammatory disease: Case-finding observations. *Am J Obstet Gynecol* 138:1101–1104, 1980.

63 Merino HI, Richards JB: An innovative program of venereal disease case-finding, treatment and education for a population of gay men. *Sex Transm Dis* 4(2):50–52, 1977.

64 Talbot MD, Kinghorn GR: Epidemiology and control of gonorrhoea in Sheffield. *Genitourin Med* 61:230–233, 1985.

65 Talbot MD: Relation between incidence of gonorrhoea in Sheffield and efficiency of contact tracing: A paradox? *Genitourin Med* 62: 377–379, 1986.

66 Woodhouse DE et al: A civilian-military partnership to reduce the incidence gonorrhea. *Public Health Rep* 100:61–65, 1985.

67 Yorke JA et al: Dynamics and control of the transmission of gonorrhea. *Sex Transm Dis* 5:51–56, 1978.

68 Thomas JC et al: The development and use of the concept of a sexually transmitted disease core. *J Infect Dis* 174(suppl 2):S134, 1996.

69 Arya OP et al: Epidemiology and treatment of gonorrhoea caused by penicillinase-producing strains in Liverpool. *Br J Vener Dis* 54:28–35, 1978.

70 Arya OP et al. Epidemiology of penicillinase-producing *Neisseria gonorrhoeae* in Liverpool from 1977 to 1982. *J Infect* 8:70–83, 1984.

71 Alvarez-Dardet C et al: Urban clusters of sexually transmitted diseases in the city of Seville, Spain. *Sex Transm Dis* 12(3):166–168, 1985.

72 Zenilman JM et al: Penicillinase-producing *Neisseria gonorrhoeae* in Dade County, Florida: Evidence of core group transmitters and the impact of illicit antibiotics. *Sex Transm Dis* 15:45–50, 1988.

73 Hamers FF et al: Syphilis and gonorrhea in Miami: Similar clustering, different trends. *Am J Public Health* 85:1104–1108, 1995.

74 May RM, Anderson RM: Transmission dynamics of HIV infection. *Nature* 326:137–142, 1987.

75 May RM, Anderson RM: The transmission dynamics of human immunodeficiency virus (HIV). *Trans R Soc Lond [B]* 321:565–607, 1988.

76 Anderson RM, May RM: Epidemiologic parameters of HIV transmission. *Nature* 333:514–518, 1988.

77 Hyman JM, Stanley EZ: Using mathematical models to understand the AIDS epidemics. *Math Biosci* 90:415–473, 1988.

78 Blower SM et al: Drugs, sex and HIV: A mathematical model for New York City. *Philos Trans R Soc Lond* 321:171–187, 1991.

79 Blower S, Medley G: Epidemiology, HIV and drugs: Mathematical models and data. *Br J Addic* 87:371–379, 1992.

80 Jacquez JA et al: Modeling and analyzing HIV transmission: The effect of contact patterns. *Math Biosci* 92:119–199, 1988.

81 Blower SM, McLean AR: Prophylactic vaccines, risk behavior change, and the probability of eradicating HIV in San Francisco. *Science* 265:1451–1454, 1994.

82 Gail MH, Brookmeyer R: Methods for projecting the course of the AIDS epidemic. *J Natl Cancer Inst* 80:900–911, 1988.

83 Garnett GP, Anderson RM: Contact tracing and the estimation of sexual mixing patterns: The epidemiology of gonococcal infections. *Sex Transm Dis* 93:181, 1993.

84 Granath F et al: Estimation of a preference matrix for women's choice of male sexual partner according to rate of partner change, using partner notification data. *Math Biosci* 107:341–348, 1991.

85 Ramstedt K et al: Choice of sexual partner according to rate of partner change and social class of the partners. *Int J STD AIDS* 91:428, 1991.

86 Adler MW, Johnson AM: Contact tracing for HIV infection. *Br Med J* 296:1420–1421, 1988.

87 Echenberg DE: A new strategy to prevent the spread of AIDS among heterosexuals. *JAMA* 254:2129–2130, 1985.

88 Wykoff RF: Preventing the spread of AIDS. *JAMA* 255(13):1706–1707, 1986.

89 Gostin L, Curran WJ: AIDS screening: Confidentiality and the duty to warn. *Am J Public Health* 77:361–365, 1987.

90 Kegeles SM et al: Intention to communicate positive HIV antibody status to sex partners. *JAMA* 259:216–217, 1988.

91 Potterat JJ et al: Partner notification in the control of human immunodeficiency virus infection. *Am J Public Health* 89:874–876, 1989.

92 Zonana H: Warning third parties at risk of AIDS: APA's policy is a reasonable approach. *Hosp Commun Psychiatry* 40:162–164, 1989.

93 Judson FN: What do we really know about AIDS control? *Am J Public Health* 79:878–883, 1989.

94 Wein M: Duty to warn. *JAMA* 261:1355–1340, 1989.

95 Nissenbaum GD, Newark JD: A physician's duty to disclose that his patient has AIDS. *N Engl J Med* 86:123–125, 1989.

96 Isaacman SH, Closen ML: Notifying contacts of HIV infected patients: Strategies to use until health agencies assume responsibility. *Postgrad Med J* 85:42–44, 53–55, 59, 1989.

97 Lo B et al: Voluntary screening for human immunodeficiency virus (HIV) infection: Weighing the benefits and harms. *Ann Intern Med* 110:727–733, 1989.

98 Dimas JT, Richland JH: Partner notification and HIV infection: Misconceptions and recommendations. *AIDS Public Policy J* 4:206–211, 1989.

99 Jones JL et al: Partner acceptability of health department notification of HIV exposure. *JAMA* 264:1284–1286, 1990.

100 Taylor AF et al: Heterosexual and perinatal transmission of human immunodeficiency virus in a low prevalence community. *West J Med* 148:171–175, 1988.

101 Gostin L, Curran WJ: The limits of compulsion in controlling AIDS. *Hastings Cent Rep* 24–29, 1986.

102 Ohi G et al: Notification of HIV carriers: Possible effect on uptake of AIDS testing. *Lancet* 2:947–949, 1988.

103 Osbom JE: Sounding Board—AIDS: Politics and science. *N Engl J Med* 318(7):444–447, 1988.

104 Archer VE: Psychological defenses and control of AIDS. *Am J Public Health* 79(7):876–878, 1989.

105 Perry S: Warning third parties at risk of AIDS: APA's policy is a barrier to treatment. *Hosp Commun Psychiatry* 40:158–161, 1989.

106 Andrus JK et al: Partner notification: Can it control epidemic syphilis? *Ann Intern Med* 112:539–543, 1990.

107 Brandt AM: Sexually transmitted disease: Shadow on the land, revisited. *Ann Intern Med* 112:481–483, 1990.

108 DesJarlais DC et al: Targeted HIV-prevention programs. *N Engl J Med* 331:1451–1453, 1994.

109 Centers for Disease Control and Prevention: Guidelines for prophylaxis against pneumocystis carinii pneumonia for persons infected with human immunodeficiency virus. *MMWR* 38(suppl 5):S1-S9, 1989.

110 Gallant JE et al: Prophylaxis for opportunistic infections in patients with HIV infection. *Ann Intern Med* 120:932–944, 1994.

111 Volberding PV et al: Zidovudine in asymptomatic human immunodeficiency virus infection: A controlled trial in persons with fewer than 300 CD4-positive cells per cubic millimeter. *N Engl J Med* 322: 941–949, 1990.

112 Fischl MA et al: The safety and efficacy of zidovudine in the treatment of subjects with mildly symptomatic human immunodeficiency virus type 1 (HIV) infection. *Ann Intern Med* 112:727–737, 1990.

113 Connor EM et al: Reduction of maternal-infant transmission of human immunodeficiency virus type I with zidovudine treatment. *N Engl J Med* 331:1173–1180, 1994.

114 Peckham C, Gill D: Mother-to-child transmission of the human immunodeficiency virus. *N Engl J Med* 333:298–302, 1995.

115 Hilts PJ: Major changes for health system seen in wake of the AIDS finding: All those at risk are urged to take virus test. *New York Times* 1989.

116 Lambert B: In shift, gay men's health crisis endorses testing for AIDS virus. *New York Times* 1989.

117 Wycoff RF et al: Notification of the sex and needle-sharing partners of individuals with human immunodeficiency virus in rural South Carolina: 30-month experience. *Sex Transm Dis* 4:217–222, 1991.

118 Cates W et al: Partner notification and confidentiality of the index patient: Its role in preventing HIV. *Sex Transm Dis* 17:113–114, 1990.
119 Toomey KE: HIV infection: The dilemma of patient confidentiality. *Am Fam Phys* 40:955–959, 1990.
120 Bayer R, Toomey KE: Health law and ethics: HIV prevention and the two faces of partner notification. *Am J Public Health* 82:1158–1164, 1992.
121 Bayer R, Fairchfld-Carrino A: Health Law and Ethics: AIDS and the limits of control. Public health orders, quarantine, and recalcitrant behavior. *Am J Public Health* 83:1471–1476, 1993.
122 Smith ML, Martin KP: Confidentiality in the age of AIDS: A case study in clinical ethics. *J Clin Ethics* 4:236–241, 1993.
123 O'Brien RC: The legal dilemma of partner notification during the HIV epidemic. *J Clin Ethics* 4:245–252, 1993.
124 North RL, Rothenberg KH: Partner notification and the threat of domestic violence against women with HIV infection. *N Engl J Med* 329:1194–1196, 1993.
125 Woodhouse DE et al: *Ethical and Legal Issues in Social Network Research: The Real and the Ideal.* Washington, Social Networks, Drug Abuse and HIV Transmission NIDA Research Monograph 151, National Institutes of Health, 1995.
126 Pavia AT et al: Risk 1: Partner notification for control of HIV: Results after 2 years of a statewide program in Utah. *Am J Public Health* 93: 1418–1424, 1993.
127 Vemon TM et al: Colorado's HIV partner notification program. *Am J Public Health* 83(4):598, 1993.
128 Spencer NE et al: Partner notification for human immunodeficiency virus infection in Colorado: Results across index case groups and costs. *Int J STD AIDS* 4:26–32, 1993.
129 Hoffman RE et al: Comparison of partner notification at anonymous and confidential HIV test sites in Colorado. *J Acquir Immune Defic Syndr Hum Retrovirol* 8:406–410, 1995.
130 Pattman RS, Gould EM: Partner notification for HIV infection in the United Kingdom: A look back on seven years experience in Newcastle upon Tyne. *Genitourin Med* 93:94–97, 1993.
131 Landis SE et al: Results of a randomized trial of partner notification in cases of HIV infection in North Carolina. *N Engl J Med* 326(2): 101–106, 1992.
132 Anonymous: Notification of syringe-sharing and sex partners of HIV-infected persons, Pennsylvania, 1993–1994. *MMWR* 44(11):202–204, 1994.
133 Rutherford GW et al: Partner notification and the control of human immunodeficiency virus infection: Two years of experience in San Francisco. *Sex Transm Dis* 18(2):107–110, 1991.
134 Ruden AK et al: Endemic versus non-endemic gonorrhoea in Stockholm: Results of contact tracing. *Int J STD AIDS* 4:284–292, 1993.
135 Katz BP et al: Evaluation of field follow-up in a sexually transmitted disease clinic for patients at risk for infection with *Neisseria gonorrheoae* and *Chlamydia trachomatis*. *Sex Transm Dis* 19(2):99–104, 1992.
136 Kamwendo F et al: Gonorrhea, genital chlamydial infection, and nonspecific urethritis in male partners of women hospitalized and treated for acute pelvic inflammatory disease. *Sex Transm Dis* 20(3):143–146, 1993.
137 Ramstedt K et al: Contact tracing in the control of genital *Chlamydia trachomatis* infection. *Int J STD AIDS* 2:116–118, 1991.
138 Langifle DB, Shovelier J: Partner notification and patient education for cases of *Chlamydia trachomatis* infection in a rural Nova Scotia Health Unit. *Can J Public Health* 83(5):358–361, 1992.
139 Patel HC et al. Chlamydial ocular infection: Efficacy of partner notification by patient referral. *Int J STD AIDS* 5:244–247, 1994.
140 Oh MK et al: Sexual contact tracing outcome in adolescent chlamydial and gonococcal cervicitis cases. *J Adolesc Health* 1995.
141 Gunn RA et al: Syphilis in San Diego County 1983–1992: Crack cocaine, prostitution, and the limitations of partner notification. *Sex Transm Dis* 22(1):60–66, 1995.
142 Romanowski B et al: Epidemiology of an outbreak of infectious syphilis in Alberta. *Int J STD AIDS* 2:424–427, 1991.
143 Engelgau MM et al: Control of epidemic early syphilis: The results of an intervention campaign using social networks. *Sex Transm Dis* 22(4):203–209, 1995.
144 Centers for Disease Control: Alternative case-finding methods in a crack-related syphilis epidemic, Philadelphia. *MMWR* 40(5):77–80, 1991.
145 Holtgrave DR et al: Human immunodeficiency virus counseling, testing, referral, and partner notification services. *Arch Intern Med* 153: 1225–1230, 1993.
146 Oxman AD et al: Partner notification for sexually transmitted diseases: An overview of the evidence. *Can J Public Health* 85(suppl 1): S41-S47, 1994.
147 Rasooly I et al: A survey of public health partner notification for sexually transmitted disease in Canada. *Can J Public Health* 85(suppl 1):S48-S52, 1994.
148 Millson ME et al: Partner notification for sexually transmitted disease: Proposed practice guidelines. *Can J Public Health* 85(suppl 1): S53-S55, 1994.
149 Moreno JL, Jennings HH: Statistics of social configurations. *Sociometry* 1:342–374, 1938.
150 Wasserman S, Faust K: *Social Network Analysis: Methods and Applications*. Melbourne, Australia, Cambridge University Press, 1994.
151 Rothenberg RB, Narramore J: Commentary: The relevance of social network concepts to STD control. *Sex Transm Dis* 23:24, 1996.
152 Alexander WJ et al: Infections in sexual contacts and associates of children with gonorrhea. *Sex Transm Dis* 11(3):156–158, 1984.
153 Auerbach DM et al: Cluster of cases of the acquired immune deficiency syndrome: Patients linked by sexual contact. *Am J Med* 76: 487–492, 1984.
154 Klovdahl AS: Social networks and the spread of infectious diseases: The AIDS example. *Soc Sci Med* 21(11):1203–1216, 1985.
155 Neaigus A et al: The relevance of drug injectors' social networks and risk networks for understanding and preventing HIV infection. *Soc Sci Med* 38:67–78, 1994.
156 Neaigus A et al: *Using Dyadic Data for a Network Analysis of HIV Infection and Risk Behaviors Among Injecting Drug Users.* Washington, Social Networks, Drug Abuse and HIV Transmission NIDA Research Monograph 151, National Institutes of Health, 1995.
157 Rothenberg RB et al: *Social Networks in Disease Transmission: The Colorado Springs Study.* Washington, Social Networks, Drug Abuse and HIV Transmission NIDA Research Monograph 151, National Institutes of Health, 1995.
158 Woodhouse DE et al: Mapping a social network of heterosexuals at high risk for human immunodeficiency virus infection. *AIDS* 8:1331–1336, 1994.
159 Rothenberg RB et al: Epidemiologic correlates in the Colorado Springs study of social networks. *Social Networks* 17:273, 1995.
160 Rothenberg RB et al: Personal risk taking and the spread of disease: beyond core groups. *J Infect Dis* 174(suppl 2):S144, 1996.
161 Trotter RT et al: Network structure and proxy network measures of HIV, drug and incarceration risks for active drug users. *Connections* 18:89–104, 1995.
162 Trotter RT et al: Drug abuse and HIV prevention research: Expanding paradigms and network contributions to risk reduction. *Connections* 18(l):29–45, 1995.
163 Trotter TR et al: *Social Networks, Drug Abuse and HIV Transmission.* Washington, NIDA Research Monograph 151, National Institutes of Health, 1995.
164 Trotter RT, Baldwin SA: *Social Networks as a Predictive Map for HIV Transmission.* American Public Health Association Meeting, San Diego, CA, 1995.
165 Rothenberg RB et al: The statibility of networks over time, abstracted. *Am Public Health Assoc J* 1995.
166 Gupta S et al: Networks of sexual contacts: Implications for the pattern of spread of HIV. *AIDS* 3:807–817, 1989.
167 Morris M: Epidemiology and social networks: Modeling structured diffusion. *Sociol Methods Res* 22:99–126, 1993.
168 Morris M: Data Driven Network Models for the Spread of Infectious Disease, in *Epidemic Models: Their Structure and Relation to Data.* Cambridge, England, Cambridge University Press, 1994.
169 Wallace R: Traveling waves of HIV infection on a low dimensional socio-geographic network. *Soc Sci Med* 32:847–852, 1991.

CHAPTER 56

Support groups for people with HIV, HPV, and HSV infections

Judith B. Greenberg
Peggy Clarke

SOCIAL SUPPORT AND HIV/STD

There has been a growing trend in the United States toward delivery of mental health services through nonprofessionals. In a comprehensive review of social support theory and research, Vaux notes that several themes have contributed to this movement—too few providers to address the amount of psychological distress; the fact that many distressed people prefer to obtain support from relatives, friends, or traditional community caregivers; and the cultural gap between clients and mental health providers. It is generally agreed that social support can have a positive effect on well-being through a number of modes of support, including "emotional, advice/guidance, feedback, practical, financial/material and socializing."[1]

Because natural support groups such as family and friends may reject infected persons or may be unable to provide useful advice or information, a continuum of complementary social support programs delivered outside the traditional mental health community has evolved to address the care and prevention needs of persons with human immunodeficiency virus (HIV), human papillomavirus (HPV), or genital herpes simplex virus (HSV) infections. These programs range from individual counseling by peers to buddy systems, support groups with a high level of member involvement, and community level interventions including local and national telephone hotlines. In this chapter we focus on the support group, a mutual self-help group that provides emotional support and information about disease and treatment, as well as practical help in dealing with these chronic sexually transmitted diseases (STDs). In contrast to psychotherapy groups with psychiatrists or psychologists delivering a specific therapeutic intervention, formats of self-help group meetings vary and may include sharing of personal experiences, group discussions, and role-playing on a variety of topics pertinent to infected persons.

Support groups are found throughout the United States as well as in other countries. The database used by the National AIDS Hotline of the American Social Health Association (ASHA) lists 1,941 support groups for HIV-seropositive individuals in the United States and its territories. Such groups can be found in most large cities, sponsored by both community agencies and national groups such as ASHA.[2] To accommodate the varied support needs created by a widespread epidemic, numerous specialized HIV groups have evolved. Examples from Los Angeles and from the New York area include groups serving a number of special populations: people with addictive behaviors, heterosexual men and women, teens and people in their early twenties, women only, HIV-negative partners of infected individuals, Spanish-speaking individuals, Asian and Pacific Islanders, and people with hemophilia. Groups for the uninfected appear to constitute an emerging trend. These groups offer support in adopting and maintaining healthful behaviors and coping with the stress of a continuing epidemic. They include the Boston HIV-Negative Support Group for gay men, as well as groups to help youths reduce or eliminate behaviors that put them at risk, such as groups offered by the Gay Men's Health Crisis in New York.

With respect to HSV and HPV, ASHA has a network of approximately 110 local support groups throughout the United States and Canada. Groups have also been established in Australia and Mexico. These groups allow participants with these conditions to share experiences, knowledge, and support in a caring environment. The groups vary in size, but they average 10 to 20 in attendance at any one meeting, and larger groups sometimes split into smaller clusters for discussion. Genital herpes groups are typically made up of approximately 60 percent females and 40 percent males. The age range is usually 30 to 50 with a few people in their twenties, and members are typically educated, white, middle-class, and heterosexual. Each year an estimated 1,500 individuals in the United States participate in ASHA's support services for people with HPV or HSV. Efforts are being made to reach other populations.

In this chapter we describe the unique care and prevention functions of support groups, factors that affect the delivery of support group services, and scientific evidence for the role such groups can play in risk reduction. We conclude with a discussion of the benefits and challenges of support groups for HIV/STD and recommendations for future research and service delivery.

THE UNIQUE CARE AND PREVENTION FUNCTIONS OF SUPPORT GROUPS FOR HIV AND STD

Extensive observations in over 100 HIV support groups, responses from ASHA's hotlines, and surveys and verbal feedback from ASHA's group facilitators suggest that support groups perform a number of unique functions for their clients. They provide members with *an opportunity for sharing practical "experiential knowledge"* about everyday activities pertinent to their infections, knowledge that professionals often do not have.[3] For example, HIV group members may identify the most discreet pharmacies for purchasing AZT or other drugs that identify their purchasers as infected, or they may provide the names of the health professionals most sensitive to client issues. In an HPV group, members may discuss whether to have their genital warts removed. In genital herpes groups, members may discuss techniques for explaining the risks of asymptomatic shedding to prospective sexual partners.

Groups also provide *a place for resolving "ethical dilemmas"* for infected persons. A typical dilemma for those with herpes is whether one should ever have sexual relations without telling one's prospective partner about the infection.[4] Especially important from a public health standpoint, groups offer an optimal forum to effect the key components of promoting AIDS and STD risk-reduction identified by Fisher and Fisher: *education, motivation, and behavioral skills*, especially the social skills for practicing safer sexual behaviors such as condom negotiation.[5] Group members often discuss the issue of disclosing one's infection to a sex partner, and they may provide examples of why this is important and how to do it.

The group setting offers *opportunity for emotional release*, a place to talk about troublesome things that cannot be shared in public. For example, an HIV-seropositive mother who has not told her children may share her distress over cutting herself and refusing their assistance to clean up her wound. By providing a setting in which one can hear of others' experiences and anxieties and help others by listening and conveying understanding, groups provide *emotional support to rebuild self-image* and to counter depression and other negative feelings that often accompany chronic infections.

Groups provide an *opportunity to meet others* with whom one can build an independent support system apart from the group. Similarly, groups can provide a place for those with sexual infections to meet others who are infected for possible *intimate relationships*. While this aspect of groups is not typically addressed in the public health literature, it is apparent when one observes groups. Members express appreciation for the opportunity to meet others with whom disclosure and the possibility of spreading their infections are not issues. It is important that group members' views on dating within the group be allowed to surface in the group discussion and that guidelines for such behavior be made explicit.

Groups provide a *forum for a broad array of disease management strategies*. These range from techniques for stress management in herpes groups to nutrition guidance for HIV-seropositive groups. They also can facilitate needed referrals to professionals (for example, to drug treatment or to a physician) by destigmatizing treatment and explaining its benefits.[6] Finally, the ongoing nature of many support groups provides *opportunity for sustained support and intervention,* of special importance to those with HIV infection.

FACTORS THAT AFFECT THE DELIVERY OF SUPPORT GROUP SERVICES

GROUP STRUCTURE

A number of structural factors have the potential for impacting support group activity (Table 56-1). The degree of openness to new members, the duration of the group, and its format for delivery of activities all contribute to what actually happens with a particular support group. Attendance at open, continuing groups is likely to vary. In a six-month period, 79 new members of an ongoing, open HIV support group attended an average of 7 sessions, with a range of 1 to 22 sessions. Thirty-eight percent attended only one or two sessions.[7] Currently, ASHA's Groups for HSV and HPV are all open groups.

A qualitative study of 27 HIV positive gay men who had attended 26 different support groups in the Atlanta area (an average of three each) found that groups that promote a feeling of well-being for these men were small (8 to 12 members), closed groups. This study also recommended tailoring groups to an individual's need. It suggested that time-limited groups that focus on information about the infection and about resources may be the most suitable for individuals in the crisis stage of learning their serostatus, while continuing groups may be preferable for those who have accepted their diagnosis and are living with HIV.[8] These continuing groups might include a focus on wellness, sexuality, and the disease process.

Table 56-1. Group Structure and Its Effect on Support Group Services

Structural factor	Potential effects
Degree of Openness	
open to new members	Modeling of adjustment by seasoned members Ensures group's continuity Drop-in support
closed to a cadre of continuing members	Increased confidentiality Focus on evolving issues v. crisis of diagnosis
Duration	
time-limited	Focus on information and resources
continuing	Focus on members' continuing issues
Format	
member-directed rap	Less facilitator time needed Addresses personal issues Dynamics can get out of control Inaccurate information
facilitator-directed planned activities	Greater behavioral improvement in clients

Groups also vary over a continuum of format from spontaneous discussion to highly structured. Many support groups use a "rap" format wherein members initiate discussion of topics of interest to them and there is no formal agenda. Other groups may have predetermined topics for discussion. And moving to the very structured end of the continuum, some groups have a written agenda that is addressed at each meeting. For example, the Twelve Step model of Alcoholics Anonymous has been adapted for HIV support groups. Kendall's study of HIV support groups indicated that gay men preferred moderately structured groups whose members participate in a variety of activities, from role playing to group meditation, to unstructured open groups where discussions can deteriorate.[8] In support of this preference, a recent meta-analysis of group psychotherapy suggests that therapist-directed groups which focus on specific topics produce greater improvement in clients than less highly structured groups where discussion is more interactive.[9] Under ASHA's HSV and HPV model, all support groups must have an educational component, otherwise members might pass along inaccurate information. Moreover, dispelling false notions about the diseases helps with psychological adjustment. To facilitate the education process, ASHA groups can vary their formats, and facilitators encourage speakers on an occasional basis. All group leaders are provided a support group kit which includes suggestions for varying format and structure, in order to accommodate the changing needs of the group and to guarantee the educational objective (see "Support Group Resources" at the end of this chapter). Each group is required to have a medical advisor, who also may make presentations.

CHARACTERISTICS OF FACILITATORS

Support groups can be peer-facilitated by a member of the group, who is not necessarily a professional, or they can be directed by professional facilitators with formal training in group dynamics and behavioral change, who may or may not be infected. There are few scientific data to guide the selection of support group facilitators, although meta-analyses from the field of psychotherapy suggest that the outcome of individual counseling is not improved by either years of experience or by professional training in psychotherapy.[10] What appears to make the therapeutic relationship successful and contributes significantly to outcome of therapy are qualities and skills such as the ability to establish a positive bond with the client, and being perceived as "warm," "trustworthy," "nonjudgmental," and "empathetic".[11] These would also seem to be important qualities for support group facilitators, especially if members are to be recruited and retained.

Race/ethnicity and gender of facilitators are also factors to consider. Although reports are limited with respect to the effects of the facilitator's race on group processes when group members are of a different race, Sattler's review suggests that qualities of therapists such as competence, sensitivity, and warmth rather than race are associated with success or failure in group therapy.[12] However, since studies have focused on African American clients who were willing to participate with white therapists, they do not tell us whether the race of the group facilitator has an effect on recruitment. The sex of facilitators also has received limited attention. Existing research[13] and focus-group findings from a three-site women's-group intervention currently funded by the Centers for Disease Control (CDC)[14] suggest that the facilitator's sex can alter group participation or behavior.

A quality important to facilitation of support groups, whether peer or professional, is a commitment to the value of up-to-date knowledge, including technical information and services related to the particular infection as well as other referral resources that may be useful for the group. In some groups members may be quite knowledgeable about these topics. If they are not, it is important to see that this information is available either through a professional facilitator or through guest speakers.

Our own observations suggest that the ability to manage group dynamics is also important to a positive group experience. While some professionals may be well trained in running productive groups, it should not be assumed that all are. Group skills include setting and enforcing norms, such as not permitting members to monopolize the discussion or to use the group to obtain one-on-one crisis counseling. In particular, the facilitator needs to involve members in mutual assistance rather than take personal responsibility for addressing individual needs. It also is critical for public health that facilitators be committed to an agenda that includes both care and prevention for the group and that they be able to bring this agenda into the group, in which emotional support is generally the overriding concern. Existing research suggests that HIV groups often focus on mental health and substance issues and ignore or pay minimal attention to sexual risk prevention activities.[15,16] Similar analyses of HPV or HSV groups are not available.

NEEDS OF GROUP MEMBERS

A key to support-group success is meeting people's needs, and these may vary over time and with disease progression or type of infection. For example, newly diagnosed individuals may have very different needs from individuals who have known of their infections for a period of time. In the former case, group members may need help in accepting the fact that they are infected, as well as state-of-the-art information on the course of disease and treatment. In the latter case, individuals may need more assistance with continuing management of their health and behaviors. Thus, just as the infection phases of HIV affect individual counseling issues,[17] *stage and type of infection* is important to determining the activities of HIV groups. A study of seronegative and seropositive gay men, the latter with and without symptoms, indicated that seropositive men with symptoms scored highest on measures of death anxiety and were most likely to use formal help from medical or mental health professionals regarding death concerns.[18] A second study comparing asymptomatic and symptomatic persons found community support groups were most effective for those who were symptomatic for HIV infection, with respect to reducing the uncertainty and hopelessness.[19] Our experience suggests, however, that safer sex needs to be addressed at all levels of infection.

Needs may also vary with respect to members' social class, gender, and drug use. In HIV groups, better educated and more affluent group members may be more knowledgeable about the disease but less knowledgeable about financial assistance and Medicaid. When drug use is common in the group, especially use of injection drugs, time needs to be spent on safer drug behaviors and drug treatment issues, whereas these topics may be less relevant for group members who do not use drugs. Gender is also a mediating variable. Especially with respect to HIV issues, infected women have very different concerns than men, such as how to provide child care over the course of their infection and after their death.

RECRUITMENT

An aspect of groups that is often overlooked is how the group is promoted to prospective members. Getting a group off the ground may take considerable time and may involve a number of recruitment strategies. It is critically important to inform health care providers working with STD/HIV about related support group services so that they can refer their clients. However, for potential members who do not use health care services or who do not want to admit to health care providers that they are infected, information on groups can be sent to mass communication media such as newspapers, hotlines, and radio stations or to community outreach agencies. In particular, recruiting members of disadvantaged populations may be difficult. Having facilitators who are in close contact with potential members—individuals who work in settings such as outreach programs, drug treatment, HIV counseling and testing, or community clinics—may be helpful both for gaining access to clients and for establishing the level of trust necessary for participation. Interview feedback from group members indicates that common barriers to attendance include illness, in the case of HIV groups; drug relapse; a group setting that is considered unsafe; confidentiality concerns; scheduling conflicts with work, school, or other obligations; lack of transportation; and lack of child care.

SPONSORSHIP OF GROUPS

Sponsorship of groups also affects their functioning, including the potential for recruiting new members. Commercial or professional sponsorship of groups can provide credibility, resources, and organizing assistance. For example, national organizations such as ASHA offer free materials and technical assistance in starting and running HSV and HPV groups. Linkages with organizations such as Planned Parenthood or other local women's clinics that see infected individuals on a regular basis can strengthen the recruitment process. However, these clinics may attract picketers and the news media, which may cause concerns about confidentiality and in some cases about safety. Dr. Joel Fischer, Executive Director of SupportWorks, a regional clearinghouse for support groups, agrees that professional affiliation has benefits but offers the following caveat: "If decision-making power in the group lies with the members who share the problem being addressed, professional assistance can be useful. However, when the professionals take over the leadership of the group, it can interfere with members' learning how to advocate for themselves and furthers the myth that people with a problem cannot take care of or fend for themselves without professional assistance."[20]

HIV IN RURAL COMMUNITIES

The number of persons with AIDS living in rural areas has significantly increased between 1985 and 1992.[21] This includes seropositive individuals who relocate to rural areas, as well as those who have been living with infection in these communities. However, conversations with rural professionals illustrate that living in a rural community poses a number of constraints on group services for their clients. Because many rural clients go to metropolitan areas for diagnosis and treatment, and thereby may be included in a city's health statistics, moneys are not generally available for intervention and support in their areas of residence. HIV-seropositive individuals in rural areas are typically fewer in number and more isolated geographically than city residents, with transportation constraints for attendance at meetings that may be held 50 miles away.

Confidentiality may be more of a problem in those rural communities where tolerance for alternative lifestyles involving drug use or homosexuality is not very high. Picketing of group meetings, with possible violence toward members, is a concern. Therefore, the locations and the nature of groups are kept closely guarded, and those interested in attending are often screened before being told how to gain access to them. Also, because infected individuals may move in distinct and separate cultural circles (such as circles of gay men or of injecting drug users), a rural community that has only a few infected individuals may find it difficult to sustain a group of any size. Some rural groups, however, report success in sustaining groups with very diverse membership. One of these, Absolutely Positive +, Inc. in Georgia, initially recruited members through local free newspapers and grew from a beginning group of 5 individuals to 58 registered members within 11 months. Another agency, the Schoharie County AIDS Consortium in New York State addresses the issue of group size by including the families, children, and caretakers of people with AIDS.

Depending on available resources, rural communities may want to explore delivery of support through electronic methods such as telephone groups. Such groups can address the barriers of residing far from services, inability to attend meetings because of physical disability, concerns about physical appearance, anonymity concerns, or fear of joining a group. This alternative way of connecting with other infected people offers the opportunity to avail oneself of support through the community of one's choice, whether it be recovering drug users in the inner city or a group of professional men in the gay community.

One study of a 14-session group telephone intervention for safer sexual behaviors suggests that this method is promising. The intervention featured a toll-free number to join group sessions. Seventy percent of the men who began the group attended at least 10 of the 14 sessions. Compared with a control group of men assigned to a waiting list, treatment participants were significantly more likely to report protected anal or oral sex and significantly less likely to report any unprotected anal sex after treatment. Treated subjects significantly increased the proportion of anal sex acts that were protected, and this outcome was maintained through the 12-month follow-up assessment.[22] On the basis of a pilot study of a telephone group for three HIV-seropositive men in rural North Carolina, researchers suggest that three to four members seem to be the maximum number of participants that can effectively engage in a telephone group, as visual cues are not available to the practitioner or to the members.[23] The HIV/AIDS Project Development and Evaluation Unit of the School of Social Work at the University of Washington in Seattle is currently implementing pilot telephone support groups in rural areas of Washington for seropositive gay or bisexual men, heterosexual men, and women. Groups will be time-limited, and recruitment is moving beyond provider referrals to extensive use of the media.

HIGH-TECH SUPPORT GROUPS

There are other high-tech possibilities for support groups, including computerized support models on the Internet. These groups range from open forums with no facilitator, where individuals can call in with a question such as "I'm on these medications and having these symptoms, where do I turn now?" to one-on-one "chats" that can be set up as electronic mail. A study of 26 persons with AIDS randomly assigned to a home-care computer network suggests that computers not only served as a feasible system for delivering home-care nursing support but could also function as a medium for group participation.[24] The project nurse answered questions and facilitated group problem solving through an unrestricted bulletin board for any member to use and through answers to anonymous questions that all could read and retain. People with AIDS used the system at all hours of the day and night.

There also are new computer on-line services which will offer the opportunity to gain access to small numbers of individuals for more meaningful and supportive discussions that could include a facilitator. Although something may be lost in not having face-to-face contact, the Internet perhaps replaces our practice of letter writing for information and emotional support. With free public access to computer networks, the cost of participating in such groups should be no more than the cost of purchasing a household appliance such as a television set.

SUPPORT GROUPS IN OTHER COUNTRIES

The World Health Organization reports that HIV support groups are found in communities in Africa, Great Britain, Brazil, Thailand, and Australia. Information on these groups is best obtained directly through the specific country, as there is no international registry. A study of a support group organization for women, the Dimba of Senegal, suggests that support groups in developing areas such as this part of Africa may be quite different from those in more educated and affluent environments.[25] The Dimba groups address much broader objectives than support for STD patients, such as treatment for STDs, care for infant illnesses, and help with harvesting. Moreover, this organization serves as an activist political force for women, constituting a powerful counterforce to male dominance. Similarly, the existing tradition of mutual aid and support networks among women in sub-Saharan Africa could be an important resource for behavior change related to HIV/STD prevention in both men and women if recognized by health policy makers.[26]

Herpes support groups are found in other countries as well. There are at least 10 groups in Canada, representing most of the provinces. Canada has been slower than the United States to establish such support groups—Americans appear to be more oriented towards support and self-help. Seven of the Canadian groups were established in 1994 owing to special funding received by ASHA. Australia has one support group affiliated with ASHA. It is handled through the Sydney Sexual Health Centre, a part of the government's health system. In 1995, a group was established in Mexico City.

HIV SUPPORT GROUPS AND HIV RISK REDUCTION

A number of studies document the effectiveness of support groups for HIV-seropositive persons in helping them to cope with their illness (see, for example., Refs. 8, 27, and 28). Although several studies have linked lower levels of social support to high-risk sexual activity,[29,30] published studies of support groups and their effect on behavioral change related to transmission of infection are rare. Problems in conducting such research with existing groups include agencies' concerns about clients' feelings and confidentiality if research is imposed on an existing group; difficulty in obtaining control subjects, as most service organizations do not want to deny or delay access to their services, especially for HIV-positive clients; variable content that requires observation and recording of actual group activities; and high attrition rates, which can mean a long-term commitment for researchers if they are to secure enough subjects who have attended the group for more than one or two sessions.

A 1993 study of AIDS-related peer support groups in New York State described variations in support group services and assessed the effect of participation.[31] Researchers conducted semi-structured interviews with members of supervisory staff at six sponsoring agencies, observed groups, and debriefed facilitators about group sessions they did not observe themselves. The second phase of the study included structured surveys of 266 group participants in 22 peer groups run by six agencies. These groups had minimal structure, with group members allowed to set the course of discussion. Key findings from this extensive study include that "behavioral change related to preventing the infection of others was seldom a topic of group discussion." Neither peer education nor peer support groups showed significant effects on change in drug use or sexual behaviors; however, there was low prevalence of these risk behaviors at baseline.

In a more detailed look at one continuing group for HIV-positive, addicted people, Greenberg et al. combined group observations with interview responses of 100 study participants.[7] All participants were African American, and the group included gay men and heterosexual men and women. Two facilitators, a man and woman trained in both addiction and HIV issues, served as moderators. A sociologist observed 104 meetings of the open "rap" group before and during the year of the study, and members completed behavioral assessments at the beginning of group participation and approximately six months later . The objective in this study was twofold: to profile the topics covered by this group, especially those related to prevention, and to assess participant-reported risk behavior to see whether reductions occurred in those who attended the group most frequently.

To examine the content of group discussion, researchers defined a speaking turn as beginning when the topic was first introduced and ending when the speaker concluded or shifted to another topic. The number of turns per topic was aggregated to weight the content of discussion. Group members spent the most time on drug abstinence issues such as identifying and avoiding situations that trigger drug use (22 percent of group time). Other key areas of discussion were health issues (such as the latest treatment regimens and concerns about troublesome symptoms) and maintaining a positive attitude. Compared with other topics, sexual behaviors received considerably less attention (8 percent of group time). Discussion of sexual issues focused on how to inform a sex partner of one's serostatus, with members contributing their personal experience with disclosure. Sexual issues of particular relevance to women (such as sex during menstruation) and to gay men (such as risks from anal sex) were never discussed. There were no planned exercises that promoted modeling of safer sex behaviors such as how to use condoms correctly or how to insist upon their use. This failure to discuss sex issues may reflect both the public's persistent difficulty in talking about sex[32] and the failure of many medical professionals to talk about sexual issues with their clients.[33,34]

Frequency of group attendance was associated with maintenance of safe behavior already in existence at baseline or with positive change in only those behaviors that were most frequently discussed (see Table 56-2). Group attendance was unrelated to condom use, to reporting a high-risk partner (defined as a prostitute, injecting drug user, or stranger), or to number of sex partners.

Table 56-2. Association Between Group Attendance, Drug Treatment and Risk Behaviors

Behaviors	Residential Drug Treatment	Attending at ≥4 Group Meetings
Reduced frequency of drug use	2.218 (0.869-5.661)	3.072 (1.206-7.827)*
Increased months drug free	3.222 (1.259-8.243)*	2.608 (1.005-6.762)*
Reduced sex while high	6.186 (1.817-21.06)**	3.436 (1.093-10.80)*
Disclosed to all partners	1.832 (0.748-4.485)	2.533 (1.010-6.354)*

* $p < .05$ ** $i < .01$

Mutually adjusted odds ratios for association of risk reduction behaviors to (1) completion of residential treatment and (2) frequency of group attendance (with 95% confidence intervals), from multivariate models including demographics.

This study suggests the importance of the role of facilitator if support groups for drug users are to affect sexual behavior. Facilitators need to direct discussion towards safer sex practices and drug issues and to include skill-building for safer sex practices in the group's agenda, including skills for dealing with nonsexual intimacy and relationships. Providing classes or consultants to train facilitators and using guest speakers to address crucial issues may increase the effectiveness of this readily available intervention. Because infected individuals are primarily coming to groups for support, it appears critical to combine time for sharing of their common issues and problems with prevention activities. In addition, studies of intervention groups created for research purposes (for example, see References 35–37) suggest that groups that change behavior are typically time-limited, closed groups whose members tend to be homogeneous with respect to socioeconomic status, risky behavior such as drug injection or men having sex with men, and ethnicity.

CHALLENGES AND CONCLUDING COMMENTS

Support groups can offer a cost-effective expansion of both mental and public health services for promoting wellness in persons infected with HIV, HPV, or HSV. To the extent that support groups provide care and support for their clients, they perform an important mental health function. To the extent that they provide assistance with prevention of new infections in others, they also provide an important public health function. Moreover, groups can address multiple other health issues, including TB and drug issues. On the other hand, groups do not work for everyone. Some individuals have personal resources and prefer to address their concerns independently of a group. For example, ASHA's support groups for HPV and HSV have not worked well in the midwestern part of the United States, where a strong philosophy of independence appears to operate and geographic barriers may preclude attendance. And some people who encounter others who are very upset about an infection may begin to see their problems as worse than before they attended a group.[38]

Support groups offer a number of challenges to health professionals and communities. One challenge is prevention. While support groups may offer a prime opportunity to address prevention, many groups focus on emotional and resource support and ignore the spread of the virus. This seems to occur for three reasons: one, the members come with the idea of getting support, not a lecture on safer sex; two, facilitators are often unskilled in and uncomfortable with the areas of sexuality and behavioral change; and three, when facilitators do focus on prevention, they may target drug use to the exclusion of safer sex, especially in HIV support groups for drug-addicted individuals. Researchers should explore the feasibility of strategies for addressing this imbalance, such as training sessions for group facilitators. They should consider what even a short session might offer—for example, training about the special problems of STDs for HIV positive persons or an update on community speakers who could periodically address groups on such topics as prevention and safer sex role-playing. The incidental teaching model is one method that may be effective for support group settings.[39] Using this model, facilitators would identify and use "teachable moments" that occur in the natural discussion by members to interject brief intervention activities.

A second challenge is that of getting support for people in rural settings. Recruitment strategies used by one successful nonmetropolitan group include obtaining referrals from metropolitan agencies who see rural clients for testing and treatment, and placing ads in free newspapers with wide circulation. High-tech solutions may hold one possible answer, and research is needed on both feasibility and cost-effectiveness.

Maintaining confidentiality is another challenge. This has been a big problem in groups, since members may know one another outside the group setting and inadvertently let information slip. Fear of this happening may keep people from using support groups. Professionals need to devise strategies for group facilitators to minimize this issue, especially in large, open groups. One group employs a system of written contracts which are signed by members as part of their commitment to the group.

The maturing AIDS epidemic presents a special challenge for gay men's support groups because their needs have changed over the years, moving from "how to reduce risks with a condom" to more complex psychosocial issues. Interviews with 45 HIV-negative gay men illustrate recurring themes of grief and loss, shame (for failing to be "perfectly safe," for being a survivor when so many others have perished), and uncertainty about having the will and ability to be safe, not just for a year but probably for a lifetime.[40] There is also the issue of whether there can ever be a choice not to use condoms. A model of negotiated safety for gay male couples has been developed by the Victoria AIDS Council/Gay Men's Health Centre of Australia and may be appropriate for discussion in support group settings.[41] This model consists of a series of communication steps which proactively address critical issues such as unsafe sex outside the relationship. Other research suggests that a couple's approach to safer sex can be an important alternative to both individual and community approaches. This couple approach, which could include a shift in research emphasis towards an understanding of the process of negotiation, suggests that negotiated safety between regular partners with concordant serostatuses should not be equated with relapse.[42]

Another challenge for providers is the issue of how to identify those who need more intensive therapy than groups can offer. A major contribution to group research could be made by studies that predict which clients will derive greater benefit from support group participation and which clients need referral to other interventions.

Finally, groups typically do not address the broader social constraints such as economic conditions or discrimination that may impel individuals into high-risk behavior or depression. However, Wallerstein's discussion of Friere's empowerment model[43] suggests that using the group context to examine social roots of members' personal problems and to develop personal and social action plans could take support groups to the next step in health promotion.

SUPPORT GROUP RESOURCES

American Social Health Association (ASHA)
P.O. Box 13827
Research Triangle Park, NC 27709-9904
919-361-8400
Publishes *The Help Kit: A Guide to Organizing and Maintaining a Help Group* (1991). For a copy, call 919-361-8486 or write the Herpes Resource Center Coordinator at the address above. The following hotlines operated by ASHA provide current listings of support group resources:

National AIDS Hotline
(7 days/week, 24 hours/day)
1-800-342-AIDS

National Herpes Hotline
(Monday–Friday, 9 a.m.–7 p.m. ET)
919-361-8488

National STD Hotline
(Monday–Friday, 8 a.m.–11 p.m. ET)
1-800-227-8922

CDC National AIDS Clearinghouse
Rockville, MD
1-800-458-5231
A national toll-free reference service that includes referrals to local and national organizations. Provides national directories for community-based organizations providing HIV/AIDS services and hotlines (by state) and HIV/AIDS information services, including electronic bulletin boards.

AMERICAN SELF-HELP CLEARINGHOUSE
Northwest Covenant Medical Center
25 Pocono Road
Denville, NJ 07834-2995
201-625-7101
Provides directory of self-help group resources, including a listing of Self-Help Clearinghouses around the country and some HIV/STD agencies. Also, a free two-page handout on starting a self-help group.

THE UNITED STATES CONFERENCE OF MAYORS
1620 "Eye" Street, NW
Washington, DC 20006
202-293-7330
Publishes *The National Directory: Local AIDS Services,* a listing of resources including support groups throughout the country.

HIV-NEGATIVE SUPPORT NETWORK
P.O. Box 126
Boston, MA 02117-0126
Maintains a list of support services for HIV-negative gay and bisexual men in the United States.

ABSOLUTELY POSITIVE +, INC.
10800 Alpharetta Highway
Suite 200-M1
Roswell, GA 30076
Provides information on developing group support for rural individuals who are HIV-seropositive.

AHRTAG (Appropriate Health Resources and Technologies Action Group)
Farringdon Point
29–35 Farringdon Road
London EC1M 3JB, UK
Publishes a newsletter, *Aids Action*, which is free to readers in developing countries and includes support group information. Readers in developing countries can also order *Women and HIV/AIDS: An International Resource Book* at a reduced price by contacting: Pandora Press, HarperCollins UK, 77–85 Fulham Palace Rd. London W6, UK.

References

1 Vaux A: *Social Support: Theory, Research, and Intervention.* New York, Prager, 1988, pp 230, 296.
2 U.S. Conference of Mayors: *The National Directory: Local AIDS Services.* Washington DC, 1994.
3 Borkman T: Experiential knowledge: a new concept for the analysis of self-help groups. *Social Service Rev* 50:445–456, 1976.

4 Drob S, Bernard HS: Time-limited group treatment of genital herpes patients. *Internat J Group Psychother* 36:141, 1986.
5 Fisher JD, Fisher WA: Changing AIDS-risk behavior. *Psychol Bull* 111(3):455–474, 1992.
6 Madara, EJ: Self-help support groups: tapping into a growing empowerment movement. *Wellness Managem* 9:8–9, 1993.
7 Greenberg J et al: A community support group for HIV-seropositive drug users: is attendance associated with reductions in risk behaviour? *AIDS Care* 8:529–540, 1996.
8 Kendall, J: Promoting wellness in HIV-support groups. *J AIDS Nursing and AIDS Care* 3:28–38, 1992.
9 Burlingame GM et al: Group Psychotherapy Efficacy: A Meta-Analytic Perspective. Paper presented at the 103rd Annual Meeting of the American Psychological Association, New York, 1995.
10 Jacobson N: The overselling of therapy. *Fam Therapy Networker* 19: 40–47, 1995.
11 Miller S et al: No more bells and whistles. *Fam Therapy Networker* 19:53–63, 1995.
12 Sattler, JM: The Effects of Therapist-Client Racial Similarity, in *Effective Psychotherapy: A Handbook of Research,* AS Gurman, AM Razin (eds). New York, Pergamon Press, 1977, pp 284, 253.
13 Spitz HI, Spitz S: Clinical Considerations in Group Psychotherapy with Cocaine Abusers, in *Group Psychodynamics,* DA Halperin (ed). Chicago, Year Book Medical Publishers, 1989, p 166.
14 Gonzales V: The Use Of Formative Research to Develop Small Group Interventions. Paper presented at the 123rd Annual Meeting of the American Public Health Association, San Diego, 1995.
15 Hedge B, Glover LF: Group intervention with HIV seropositive patients and their partners. *AIDS Care* 2:147–154, 1990.
16 Green G: Social support and HIV [Editorial review]. *AIDS Care* 5:87–104, 1993.
17 Doll LS, Dillon BA: Counseling Persons Seropositive for Human Immundeficiency Virus Infection and Their Families, in *AIDS: Etiology, Diagnosis, Treatment, and Prevention,* VT Devita et al (eds). Philadelphia, Lippincott-Raven, 1997, pp 533–539.
18 Ramsey, P: The Effect of Community Support Groups on Psychosocial Adjustment, Uncertainty, and Hopelessness in Persons Infected with the Human Immunodeficiency Virus. Dissertation, University of Virginia School of Nursing, Charlottesville, 1990.
19 Catania, JA et al.: Coping with death anxiety: help-seeking and social support among gay men with various HIV diagnoses. *AIDS* 6:999–1005, 1992.
20 Fischer, J: Personal communication, July 17, 1995.
21 Buehler JW et al.: The migration of persons with AIDS: data from 12 states, 1985 to 1992. *Am J Public Health* 85:1552–1555, 1995.
22 Roffman RA: Telephone Group Counseling in Reducing Barriers to AIDS Prevention. Paper presented at Third Science Symposium on HIV Prevention Research: Current Status and Future Directions, Flagstaff AZ, August 1995.
23 Rounds KA et al: Linking people with aids in rural communities: the telephone group. *Social Work* 36:13–18, 1991.
24 Brennan PF, Ripich S: Use of a home-care computer network by persons with AIDS. *Internat J Technol Assessm in Health Care* 10:258–272, 1994.
25 Niang CI: The Dimba of Senegal: a support group for women. *Reproduct Health Matters* no 4:39–45, 1994.
26 Ulin PR: African women and AIDS: negotiating behavioral change. *Social Sci Med* 34:63–73, 1992.
27 DiPasquale JA: The psychological effects of support groups on individuals infected by the AIDS virus. *Cancer Nursing* 13:278–285, 1990.
28 Ribble D: Psychological support groups for people with HIV infection and AIDS. *Holist Nursing Pract* 3:52–62.
29 Folkman S et al: Stress, coping, and high-risk sexual behavior. *Health Psychol* 11:218–222, 1992.
30 Kelly JA et al: Outcome of cognitive-behavioral and support group brief therapies for depressed, HIV-infected persons *Am J Psychiatry* 150:1679–1686, 1993.
31 Messeri P et al: Peer Groups for HIV Risk Reduction and Social Support: Description of HIV Peer Group Activities and Assessment of Outcomes. Report prepared for the New York State Department of Health, AIDS Institute, March 9, 1994.
32 American Social Health Association: *Finding the Words: How to Communicate about Sexual Health.* Research Triangle Park, NC, 1994.
33 Ende J et al: The sexual history in general medicine practice. *Archives Intern Med* 144:558–561, 1984.
34 Centers for Disease Control: HIV prevention practices of primary-care physicians—United States, 1992. *MMWR* 42:988–992, 1994.
35 Kelly JA et al: The effects of HIV/AIDS intervention groups for high-risk women in urban clinics. *Am J Public Health* 84:1918–1922, 1994.
36 Hobfoll SE et al: Reducing inner-city women's AIDS risk activities: a study of single, pregnant women. *Health Psychol* 13:397–403, 1994.
37 Rotheram-Borus et al: Reducing HIV sexual risk behaviors among runaway adolescents. *JAMA* 266:1237–1241, 1991.
38 Manne S: Coping and adjustment to genital herpes: the effects of time and social support. *J Behav Med* 9:163–177, 1986.
39 Hart BM, Risley TR: *How to Use Incidental Teaching for Elaborating Language.* Lawrence KS, H and H Enterprises, 1982.
40 Johnston WI: *HIV-Negative: How the Uninfected Are Affected by AIDS.* New York, Plenum Press, 1995.
41 Davies PM et al: Science, Gay Men, and AIDS: New Directions for Research. Paper presented at the International AIDS Conference, abstrWS-DO7–6, (vol 9, p 110), Berlin, 1993.
42 Kippax S: Sustaining safe sex: a longitudinal study of a sample of homosexual men. *AIDS* 7:257–263, 1993.
43 Wallerstein N: Powerlessness, empowerment, and health: implications for health promotion programs. *Am J Health Promotion* 6:197–205, 1991.

Chapter 57

Lower genital tract infection syndromes in women

King K. Holmes
Walter E. Stamm

Differences in male and female anatomy and reproductive physiology account for the greater risk of complications of certain STDs in women and also for the greater difficulty in differential diagnosis of urogenital infections in women. In fact, the difficulty in diagnosing sexually transmitted urogenital infections in women undoubtedly results in delay of proper therapy, which further contributes to the higher risk of complications in women and to the further spread of infection in the community.

In heterosexual men, gonococcal and chlamydial infections appear limited to the anterior urethra in most cases, although the frequency of extension of infection to the posterior urethra and genital adnexae has not been well studied. Symptoms and signs of urethral discharge readily recognizable by both the patient and the clinician have come to represent the most monotonous aspect of venereology; knowledge of variations on this theme is limited.

On the other hand, in women several STD pathogens, including *Neisseria gonorrhoeae, Chlamydia trachomatis,* and herpes simplex virus (HSV), have predilection for infection of the urethra, cervix, and rectum simultaneously, producing more variable symptom patterns, each with a wide range of differential diagnostic possibilities. Furthermore, infections at any one site can produce poorly localized symptoms easy to erroneously ascribe to involvement of a contiguous site. For example, infections of the bladder, urethra, or vulva can produce similar symptoms, such as dysuria or dyspareunia. Finally, lack of appreciation of the differing clinical signs of specific genital infections in women can often be attributed to inadequate inspection of the genitalia because of poor clinical skills, lack of speculums in many developing countries, or simple reluctance to perform the examination (Fig. 57-1). These factors account for the vague terms still used to describe some of the urogenital syndromes in women, such as "nonspecific genital infection" and "lower genital tract infection"—terms that pose a barrier both to understanding these syndromes and to accurate clinical diagnosis and therapy.

Improved detection of gonococcal and chlamydial infections in women represents one of the major thrusts in venereology during the past 25 years. Beginning in the 1970s, culture diagnosis of gonorrhea in women became widely available in industrialized countries; and during the past decade newer tests for chlamydial infection have also become increasingly available. However, in developing countries there is still almost total reliance on contact tracing to detect and reduce the "female reservoir" of these infections. Because of the expense and limited availability of facilities for specific detection of *N. gonorrhoeae* or *C. trachomatis* in developing countries, there has been an unwarranted sense of futility about the prospects for diagnosis of lower genital infections in women. Uncertainty about the usual etiologies of inflammatory conditions of the urinary tract, vulva, vagina, and cervix in women, the lack of consistent application of available laboratory testing where needed, and the failure to exclude coinfections when analyzing the clinical manifestations of any one particular infection add to the confusion and vagueness concerning classification of urogenital inflammation in women. Clinicians experience further difficulty in differentiating true inflammatory conditions from noninflammatory conditions, including functional, psychosomatic genitourinary complaints.

Although the etiology of certain genitourinary and anorectal inflammatory conditions in women is still not well understood, it is becoming increasingly possible to presumptively identify many common and potentially serious STDs in women on the basis of clinical observations of symptoms and signs, supplemented with selective use of relatively simple screening and confirmatory laboratory tests. More precise diagnosis of urogenital infection in women could make a major contribution to improved control of several important STDs in the community, and should lead to improved management strategies for genital infection in the individual patient. An etiologic classification of urogenital inflammatory and "pseudo-inflammatory" syndromes in women is presented in Table 57-1; also, each syndrome is further discussed in this chapter. Chapter 50 introduces an approach to the anatomy and physical examination of the female genital tract and provides useful background for this chapter. Chapters 42, 43, and 45 discuss the three most common nonviral vaginal infections (bacterial vaginosis, trichomoniasis, vulvovaginal candidiasis, respectively), which are therefore not covered in detail here.

CYSTITIS AND URETHRITIS

EPIDEMIOLOGY AND ETIOLOGY

In the United States, women with symptoms of lower urinary tract infection (UTI) account for an estimated 7 million office visits to physicians in office practice each year.[1] In a community-based study in England, symptoms of dysuria and frequent urination occurred in as many as 20 percent of women per year.[2] A recent prospective study of young women in Seattle initiating contraceptive use demonstrated an incidence of acute cystitis of 0.5 to 0.7 percent per year.[3] Thus, this infection is exceedingly common and its incidence probably underestimated by surveys dependent on office visits. Symptoms of dysuria or frequency in women can usually be attributed to acute bacterial cystitis, urethritis, or vulvitis.

The incidence of acute bacterial cystitis is highest in women 20 to 25 years of age, and this condition is a particularly common cause of urinary symptoms among sexually active young women. Recent studies have identified sexual intercourse, spermicide or diaphragm-spermicide use, a history of a prior UTI, and recent antimicrobial exposure as independent risk factors for acute cystitis.[3–5] Among 263 women presenting to the Seattle STD clinic with urinary symptoms alone, or with both urinary and vaginal symptoms, but without clear signs of vaginal infection, 69 (26%) had "significant" bacteriuria ($\geq 10^5$ organisms/mL of urine).[6] A separate study of female students at the University of Washington showed that the traditional criterion of $\geq 10^5$ uropathogens per mL of urine is insensitive for diagnosis of acute bacterial cystitis in women who present with dysuria and frequency.[7] This criterion was originally established in studies of women with acute pyelonephritis, and in surveys of asymptomatic women who have a low prevalence of bladder infection. However, among female students with symptoms of dysuria, specimens obtained by suprapubic aspiration or urethral catheterization usually confirmed the presence of bladder infection, even when urines contained lower concen-

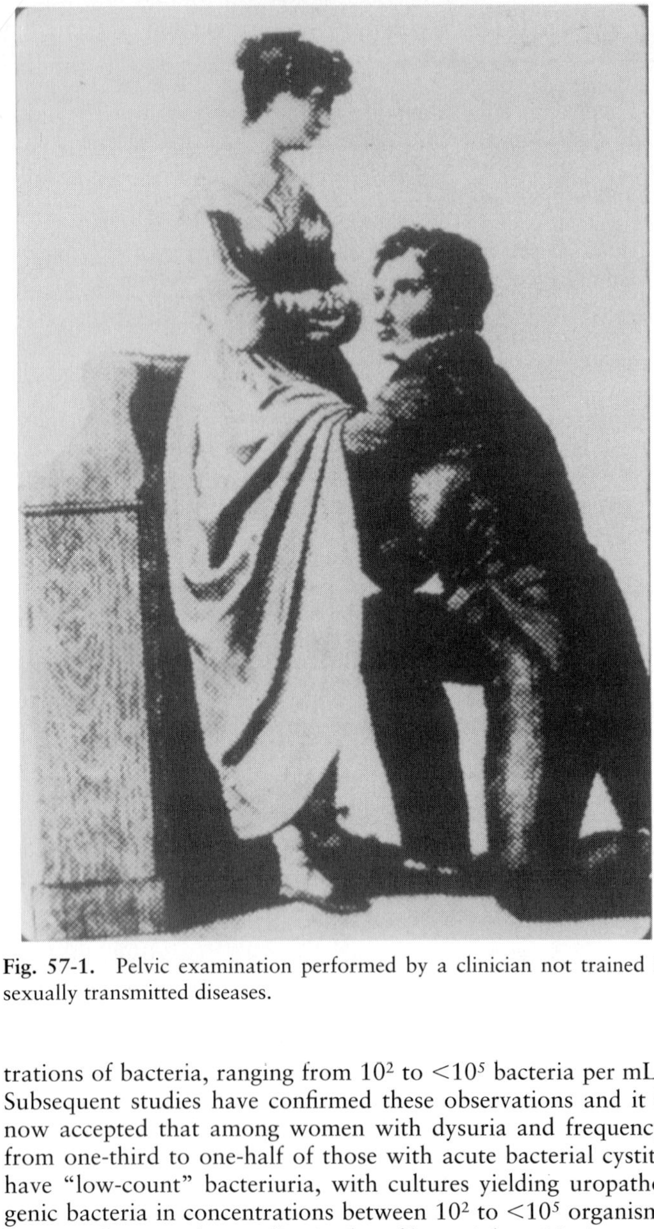

Fig. 57-1. Pelvic examination performed by a clinician not trained in sexually transmitted diseases.

trations of bacteria, ranging from 10^2 to $<10^5$ bacteria per mL.[7] Subsequent studies have confirmed these observations and it is now accepted that among women with dysuria and frequency, from one-third to one-half of those with acute bacterial cystitis have "low-count" bacteriuria, with cultures yielding uropathogenic bacteria in concentrations between 10^2 to $<10^5$ organisms per mL of urine. Almost all episodes of bacterial cystitis, irrespective of the urinary colony count, are accompanied by pyuria, and about 20 percent of patients have gross hematuria. The etiologic agents in women with acute uncomplicated cystitis are highly predictable, with *E. coli* causing 80 percent of cases. *S. saprophyticus* is the second most common pathogen, causing 5 to 15 percent of cases.[8] This organism has a seasonal variation in incidence (a summer/fall peak) and preferentially infects adolescents. Infections due to *E. coli* and *S. saprophyticus* cannot be distinguished clinically. *Proteus mirabilis, K. pneumoniae,* Enterobacter and enterococci collectively cause about 10 percent of cystitis cases.

The syndrome of dysuria and frequency in women whose urine does not contain $\geqq 10^2$ of the preceding uropathogens has been called the "urethral syndrome" or, in the presence of pyuria, the "dysuria-sterile pyuria syndrome."[9–11] In a 1980 study of female university students with the urethral syndrome who had sterile bladder urines, the etiology was found to be related to the presence or absence of pyuria. Infection with *C. trachomatis* was demonstrated in 10 of 16 women with pyuria but in only 1 of 16 women without pyuria ($p = 0.002$).[9] Pyuria was defined as more than eight leukocytes per mL of uncentrifuged midstream urine, approximately equivalent to 10 leukocytes per 400× microscopic field when 10 mL of urine have been centrifuged and the sediment resuspended in 1 mL of urine for microscopic examination under a coverslip. *N. gonorrhoeae* was not associated with the urethral syndrome in this population of university students.

However, in a 1970s study of indigent women attending a hospital emergency room, gonococcal infection was significantly correlated with dysuria, accounting for eight (61%) of 13 cases whose urine samples contained $<10^5$ uropathogens per mL.[12] Cultures for *C. trachomatis* were not obtained in that study. Thus, among young women with the urethral syndrome, and without bladder infection by uropathogens, the relative importance of gonococcal and chlamydial infection probably depends on the relative background incidence of these two infections in young women. HSV infections (especially primary infection), although not commonly found among women with the urethral syndrome, clearly can produce urethritis, dysuria, and pyuria in young sexually active women, and can be mistaken for bacterial cystitis if vulvar lesions are not prominent or carefully sought. Dysuria in women who do not have bacteriuria or urethral infection with STD pathogens is often attributable to vulvar inflammation caused by genital herpes or candida vulvovaginitis.[13–15] For example, Komaroff et al. reported that in young women, dysuria was attributable to vaginitis more often than to UTI because vaginitis was so much more common than UTI.[15]

DIAGNOSIS AND THERAPY

The characteristic features that help to differentiate the three major conditions that can result in dysuria in women are summarized

Table 57-1. Etiologic Classification of Lower Urogenital Inflammatory or "Pseudoinflammatory" Syndromes in Adult, Premenopausal Women

Syndrome	Usual microbial etiology	Other/idiopathic
Cystitis	Coliform bacteria *S. saprophyticus*	Interstitial cystitis
Urethritis	*N. gonorrhoeae* *C. trachomatis* HSV	
Vulvitis	HSV *C. albicans*	Vulvar papillomatosis Vulvar vestibulitis Essential vulvodynia Vulvar necrotizing fasciitis
Bartholinitis	*N. gonorrhoeae* *C. trachomatis* Facultative or anaerobic bacterial infection	
Vaginitis/ Vaginal discharge	*T. vaginalis* *C. albicans* *G. vaginalis,* mycoplasmas, and anaerobic bacteria	Desquamative inflammatory vaginitis Toxic shock syndrome Intravaginal use of detergents, chemicals, physical agents. Chronic tampon use, other retained foreign bodies Allergic vaginitis
Endocervicitis	*C. trachomatis* *N. gonorrhoeae* HSV	
Ectocervicitis	HSV *T. vaginalis* *C. albicans*	

in Table 57-2. The medical history, physical examination, and simple laboratory tests are all helpful in the differential diagnosis of dysuria. The optimal diagnostic approach to dysuria frequency varies, depending on the clinical setting and the likelihood of STD. Thus, in STD clinics, family planning clinics, teen clinics, or other settings where the prevalence of STDs is high, speculum exam is warranted to rule out STDs. In clinical settings or individual patients where the likelihood of an STD is low, the pelvic exam can be omitted. Urinalysis should be performed in all women with dysuria or frequency to detect pyuria. Microscopic examination of unspun urine using a hemocytometer or calibrated chamber is the most sensitive and specific test for the presence or absence of pyuria.[16] Alternatively, leukocytes can be counted after centrifugation of the urine followed by resuspension of the sediment in 1 mL of urine and enumeration of white cells in one to two drops of urine placed on a microscope slide under a coverslip. This method is slightly less accurate than the first method. Another simple test for pyuria involves the use of a "dipstick" to detect leukocyte esterase in urine. Although the sensitivity of the leukocyte esterase test appears lower than that of the chamber microscopy method for detection of pyuria, the simplicity and low cost of the test make it useful for screening women with dysuria in the clinic.[16] Among women with dysuria, pyuria usually is indicative of acute bacterial cystitis in women at low risk for STDs and may indicate either cystitis or urethritis in women at high risk for STDs. If pyuria is found microscopically or by leukocyte esterase test, the urine can also be examined microscopically for bacteriuria, either by (1) preparation of a Gram stain of a fresh, midstream, clean-catch, uncentrifuged urine specimen and examination with an oil immersion lens (the presence of one bacterial organism per field is correlated with quantitative isolation of $\geq 10^5$ bacteria per milliliter of urine); or (2) by examination of unstained, centrifuged urinary sediment of fresh urine under the high dry objective (detection of 100 organisms per field also correlates well with isolation of $\geq 10^5$ bacteria per milliliter of urine). These simple procedures should be readily available in any clinic. However, bacteria present in concentrations of $<10^5$ per mL of urine are not likely to be seen on Gram stain; hence this is not a sensitive test for bacteriuria. The use of urine cultures to confirm the diagnosis of acute cystitis, once universally recommended for all suspected cases, is now considered unnecessary for most women. In women with typical symptoms and signs of acute cystitis and a low risk of STDs, the uropathogens that would be identified by culture and their antimicrobial susceptibility profiles are highly predictable, obviating the need for culture (see Table 57-2). Cultures are most useful to confirm the diagnosis in cases of persistent or recurrent symptoms of UTI, when there are signs of pyelonephritis or other complications, or when there is a history of recent use of antimicrobials. If the patient has pyuria without bacteriuria and is considered to be at risk for STD, or has signs of mucopurulent endocervicitis, specimens from the endocervix and urethra should be tested for *N. gonorrhoeae* and *C. trachomatis*.

The diagnosis of urethritis owing to *C. trachomatis, N. gonorrhoeae,* or HSV rather than the diagnosis of bacterial cystitis is favored by a recent history of acquiring a new sex partner. Genital herpes is suggested by history of genital herpes, exposure to a partner with genital herpes, or the presence of genital lesions (which can also result in external dysuria). Symptoms or signs of abnormally yellow vaginal discharge, or pelvic pain or tenderness, or other signs of pelvic inflammatory diseases in the woman with internal dysuria suggest gonorrhea or chlamydial infection. Infection with *N. gonorrhoeae* or *C. trachomatis* is suggested by the presence of expressible urethral discharge (plate 4), inflammation of Skene's glands (plate 6), bartholinitis (plate 5), mucopurulent cervicitis (plates 15 and 16), or proctitis. Findings that favor cystitis rather than urethritis include a history of previous cystitis, history of onset of symptoms within 24 hours after sexual intercourse, prominent frequency or urgency as well as dysuria, and history of gross hematuria.[5,9] Cystitis is also suggested by a history of current spermicide or diaphragm use, which appear to increase the risk of cystitis in young women by altering the vaginal bacterial flora,[3,4] but which may be associated with decreased risk of cervical infection. Acute onset of severe dysuria leading to consultation within 4 days after onset favors a diagnosis of bacterial cystitis (or perhaps gonococcal urethritis), whereas a history of gradual onset of milder symptoms and long duration of symptoms before seeking therapy ($\geq$7 days) suggests chlamydial urethritis.[9] Suprapubic tenderness and microscopic hematuria are also highly suggestive of cystitis in the acutely dysuric patient.[9]

External dysuria (vulvar burning during urination) owing to vulvitis is produced most commonly by genital herpes or by vulvovaginal candidiasis.[14,15] Perhaps the less common conditions discussed in Chapters 64 and 65 can also produce this symptom. With trichomoniasis, no significant correlation was found with dysuria or frequency, after adjustment for coinfections.[17] The patient with external dysuria should be questioned about history of genital herpes or exposure to herpes, or about risk factors for vulvovaginal candidiasis, such as recent antibiotic use, or history of VVC.

Women with clinical findings suggestive of uncomplicated bacterial cystitis (or with microscopic evidence of pyuria and bacteriuria as well) should generally be treated with 3-day courses of

Table 57-2. Characteristic Features that Differentiate the Three Major Causes of Dysuria in Women

	Acute bacterial cystitis	Urethritis	Vulvitis
Predisposing factors	Previous cystitis Spermicide Onset of symptoms within 24 h after intercourse	New sex partner	History of genital herpes Partner with genital herpes Antibiotic use History of recurrent vulvovaginal candidiasis
Symptoms	Internal dysuria Duration of symptoms ≤4 days Frequency and urgency Gross hematuria	Internal dysuria Duration of symptoms often ≥7 days with chlamydial urethritis No hematuria	External dysuria Vaginal discharge (with herpes) Vulvar irritation, burning, pruritis, or lesions
Signs	Suprapubic tenderness	Mucopurulent cervicitis Vulvar lesions (with herpes)	Vulvar lesions Vulvitis Curdlike vaginal exudate
Laboratory	Pyuria Microscopic hematuria Rapid nitrite test Urine Gram stain Urine culture	Pyuria Urethral discharge or bartholinitis Endocervical exudate Cervical and urethral tests for *C. trachomatis* and *N. gonorrhoeae* Test lesion for HSV	No pyuria Test lesion for HSV Test vaginal discharge for *C. albicans*

.itimicrobial therapy.[18,19] If the temperature exceeds 38.3°C (101°F), symptoms have been present for longer than 1 week, or there is costovertebral angle pain or tenderness, the presence of pyelonephritis should be ruled out and longer treatment is needed.[19] Over 25 percent of coliform isolates from women with acute cystitis are currently resistant to sulfonamides, ampicillin, tetracyclines, and first-generation cephalosporins. These organisms, as well as *S. saprophyticus,* generally remain susceptible to sulfamethoxazole-trimethoprim, trimethoprim alone, nitrofurantoin, the fluoroquinolones, or amoxicillin-clavulanic acid. However, an increasing proportion (up to 10–15% in the United States) are now resistant to TMP/SMX, which may limit the effectiveness of this agent in those areas where resistance is frequent. Studies now suggest that 3 days of treatment with TMP, TMP/SMX, or a fluoroquinolone provides excellent results when treating acute cystitis.[18] Specific regimens include trimethoprim (100 mg PO q12h); TMP/SMX (160 plus 800 mg q12); ciprofloxacin (250 mg q12h); or ofloxacin (200 mg q12).[19] These 3-day regimens are more effective than single-dose therapy and as effective as 7 days of therapy. Further, both cost and rates of side effects are lower than those seen with 7 days of therapy. However, β-lactams and nitrofurantoin generally provide better cure rates with 7 days of therapy than with 3 days. Women suspected of having urethritis owing to chlamydia (because of pyuria without microscopic evidence of bacteriuria, together with other compatible clinical or epidemiological findings) should be treated with azithromycin (1.0 gm) or with a tetracycline regimen such as 100 mg doxycycline twice daily for 1 week while urine cultures are pending. The latter regimen was significantly more effective than placebo in curing symptoms of the urethral syndrome in women with pyuria and would also be adequate in many bladder infections caused by common uropathogens.[9] Male sex partners of women with suspected or confirmed gonococcal or chlamydial urethritis should be examined and tested to exclude urethral infection, or should be treated for exposure to these agents.

VULVOVAGINITIS AND VAGINAL DISCHARGE SYNDROMES

AGE-DEPENDENT DIFFERENCES IN VAGINAL ANATOMY, PHYSIOLOGY, AND FLORA

The normal anatomy, physiology, and microbial ecology of the vagina are age-dependent, and there are also obvious age-dependent differences in the source of vaginal infections (see Chap. 14).[20] These factors account for very different etiologies of vaginitis in neonates, infants and toddlers, prepubertal girls, and pre- and postmenopausal adults.

During the first month of life, the neonatal vagina, still under the influence of maternal estrogen, is lined by stratified squamous epithelium. From about 1 month of age until puberty, the vagina is lined by cuboidal cells, and the pH of vaginal fluid is normally about 7.0. After puberty, under the influence of estrogen, the vagina becomes lined by stratified squamous epithelium containing glycogen (Fig. 57-2). With growth of facultative H_2O_2-producing species of lactobacillus, such as *L. crispatus* and *L. jenseni* to concentrations of approximately 10^9/mL of vaginal fluid, lactic acid is produced from glycogen, and the pH falls to between 4.0 and 4.5 in normal adult women. The fall in pH, as well as the H_2O_2

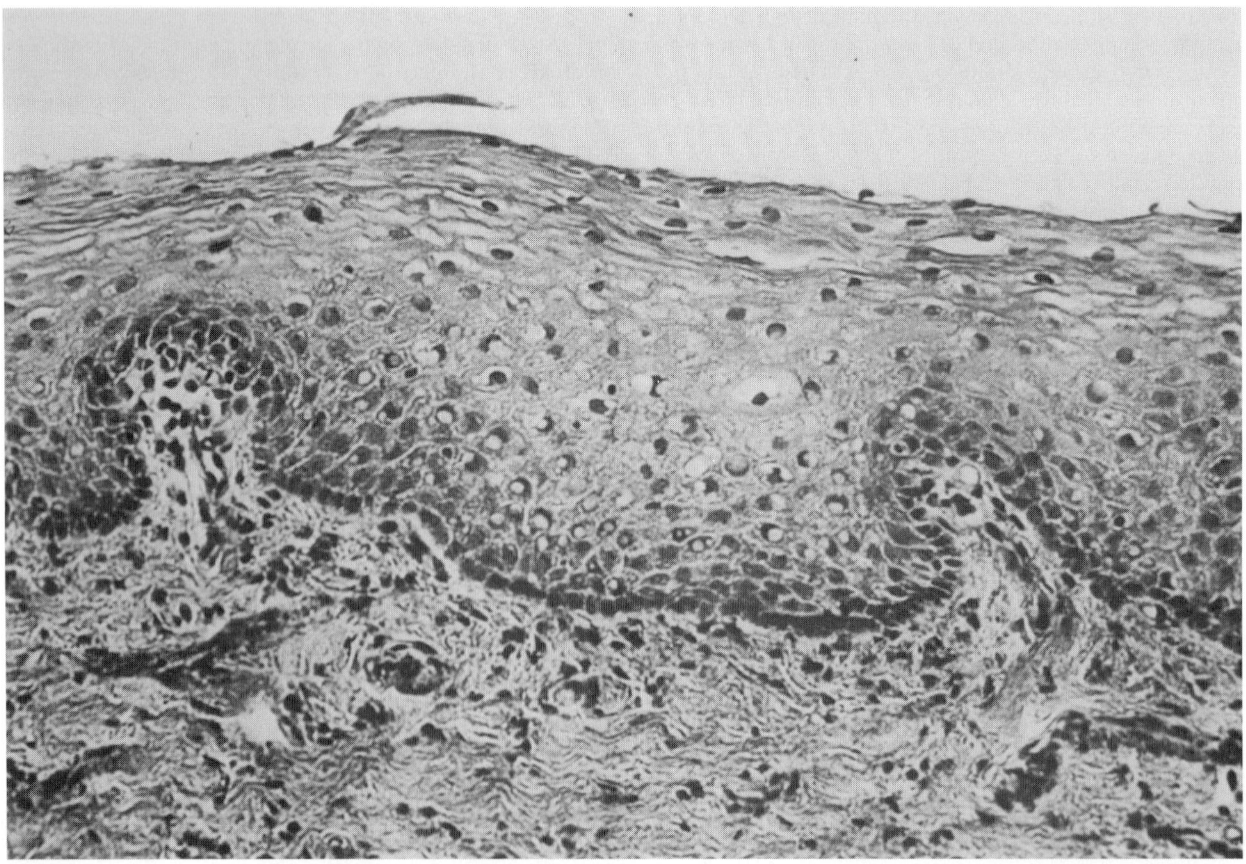

Fig. 57-2. Normal adult vaginal epithelium, showing the basal cell layer with overlying stratum spinosum. Note the absence of an overlying stratum corneum. The transit time for cells moving from the basal layer to the superficial surface of the vaginal epithelium has been estimated to be about 4 days, perhaps one-third that of normal epidermis.

production, are considered important in regulating the vaginal flora (see Chap. 14).[21,22] The oxidation-reduction potential (Eh) at the surface of the vaginal epithelium is approximately 0 ± 50 mV in the absence of bacterial vaginosis, but is much lower in bacterial vaginosis.[23]

The relative concentration of vaginal microbes has not been extensively characterized in neonates, infants, or prepubertal girls, but the facultative flora most often includes diphtheroids, *S. epidermidis*, γ-hemolytic streptococci, lactobacilli, and coliforms.[24,25] Coliforms are more common in the vagina before puberty (especially among toddlers still in diapers) than after puberty, whereas the reverse is true for lactobacilli, which dominate the vaginal flora of normal postpubertal women.

VAGINITIS IN PREMENARCHAL GIRLS

The neonatal vaginal squamous epithelium resists perinatally transmitted *N. gonorrhoeae* and *C. trachomatis* but is susceptible to perinatally transmitted vaginal candidiasis. Among older infants, the cuboidal vaginal epithelium is susceptible to *N. gonorrhoeae* and *C. trachomatis* but is resistant to candidiasis. Vaginal shedding of *C. trachomatis* does indeed sometimes appear after about 1 month of age in infants who were exposed perinatally but is not generally associated with overt signs of vaginitis in young infants. Vaginal infection by *N. gonorrhoeae* is rare among infants, and with few exceptions it is thought to represent postnatal acquisition.[26]

Among older premenarchal girls, the etiology of vaginal symptoms is correlated with puberty status and with the presence or absence of objective signs of abnormal vaginal discharge. For example, in a study of 54 premenarchal patients with suspected vaginitis and 52 age-matched controls, a microbial pathogen was isolated from the vagina from 14 of 26 with abnormal vaginal discharge, zero of 26 with suspected vaginitis who had no vaginal discharge, and zero of 52 control subjects (Table 57-3).[27] *N. gonorrhoeae* accounted for one-third of abnormal discharges in prepubertal girls, whereas *C. albicans* or "yeast" was isolated only from those premenarchal girls who were considered to be pubertal (Tanner stages II, III, or IV) on the basis of breast growth.

Streptococcus pyogenes (group A β-hemolytic streptococci) and *Shigella* sp. are also recognized as causes of purulent or bloody vaginal discharge in prepubertal girls.[28–31] Any species of *Shigella* may cause vaginitis in children, but *Shigella flexneri* has been most often implicated and represented a significantly higher proportion of isolates from the vagina than from all other sites in one retrospective study.[30] Shigella vaginitis is often chronic, causes a bloody vaginal discharge in about 50 percent of recognized cases, and is associated with diarrhea in only about one-quarter of cases. The predilection of shigella for prepubertal rather than adult vaginitis may be partly attributable to poor survival of this organism below a pH of 5.5.

The etiologic roles of group B *Haemophilus influenzae* and coagulase-positive staphylococci in prepubertal vaginitis are controversial. As indicated in Table 57-3, no specific bacterial pathogen is found in a large proportion of prepubertal girls with abnormal vaginal discharge. However, intravaginal foreign body and poor perineal hygiene are among the leading predisposing factors in young girls, among whom *Enterobius vermicularis* (pinworm) is an acknowledged cause of vulvovaginitis. Although *C. trachomatis* has not been implicated as a common cause of prepubertal vaginitis, this agent was isolated from the vagina from about one-quarter of girls with gonococcal vaginitis and appeared responsible for postgonococcal vaginitis following penicillin treatment in such cases.[32] The occurrence of *C. trachomatis* infection in prepubertal sexually abused girls has been documented in several studies (see Chap. 105).

VULVOVAGINAL SYNDROMES IN ADULT WOMEN

Vaginal infections in adult women rank among the most common problems in clinical medicine, being among the 25 most common reasons for consulting physicians in private office practice in the United States. The three most common types of vaginal infections in adult women are bacterial vaginosis, vulvovaginal candidiasis, and trichomoniasis (see Chaps. 42, 43, and 45).[33]

In the United States, the number of initial visits to private physicians' offices for trichomonal vaginitis declined slowly from an estimated 579,000 in 1966 to 190,000 in 1988, remaining fairly stable since then, with 175,000 visits in 1997 (see Fig. 4-17). However, initial visits for other conditions classified as "vaginitis" (presumably including bacterial vaginosis, not a true vaginitis, and vulvovaginal candidiasis) increased from an estimated 1,155,000 in 1966 to nearly 4.5 million per year during 1989, then declined to 3.1 million in 1997. (Genital herpes is discussed in Chapter 21 and vulvovaginal papilloma virus infections in Chapters 24 and 25.)

Other types of relatively well-characterized vaginitis syndromes in adults are attributable to microbial or chemical toxins or those associated with physical agents. The most serious and important to rule out is a destructive type of ulcerative vaginitis currently attributed to a toxin produced by *S. aureus* in women with toxic shock syndrome.[34,35] Vaginal ulceration and mixed infections have been associated with use of vaginal tampons, or other retained foreign bodies.[36,37] Cervical caps; detergent spermicides such as nonoxynol-9, or a vaginal antiseptic preparation containing policresulin (a condensation product of metacresol sulfonic acid and formaldehyde) can cause vaginitis and vaginal ulceration, as can various chemicals used in douching.[38–41] Vaginal inflam-

Table 57-3. Pathogens Isolated from Vaginal Cultures from 52 Premenarcheal Girls with Suspected Vaginitis and 52 Age-Matched Controls

	Prepubertal		Pubertal		
Pathogens isolated	Discharge present ($n = 12$)	Discharge absent ($n = 24$)	Discharge present ($n = 14$)	Discharge absent ($n = 2$)	Control subjects ($n = 52$)
Strep. pyogenes	0	0	1	0	0
N. gonorrhoeae	4	0	0	0	0
Shigella sonnei	1	0	0	0	0
C. albicans or "yeast"	0	0	8	0	0
*C. trachomatis**	0	0	0	0	0

*Specimens from 27 of 36 prepubertal girls with suspected vaginitis were cultured for *C. trachomatis*.
Source: Paradise et al.

ation also has been associated with use of various traditional vaginal preparations in some developing countries.[42–44]

In postmenopausal women, vaginal symptoms are very prevalent, and the usual forms of vaginal infection need to be considered and differentiated from vaginal atrophy.[45,46] The vaginal epithelium becomes thin with estrogen withdrawal, with decreased glycogen and increased pH. Lubrication occurs less often with sexual arousal, the introitus narrows, and the depth of the vagina decreases. These atrophic changes have been negatively correlated with frequency of intercourse and with circulating concentrations of gonadotrophins and androgens in postmenopausal women.[47] Treatment with intravaginal or systemic estrogen is effective. A possibly related syndrome, puerperal vaginal atrophy with dyspareunia, occurs postpartum in relation to the duration of breast-feeding, and is sometimes treated with topical estrogen.

A number of other perplexing, chronic vulvovaginal syndromes tend to involve women older than those most often affected by STD.[33,48] These include desquamative inflammatory vaginitis, a syndrome associated with purulent vaginal discharge, massive vaginal cell exfoliation with increased numbers of parabasal cells on vaginal smear, elevated vaginal pH, and Gram-positive cocci on Gram's stain of vaginal fluid; this syndrome usually responds to intravaginal 2 percent clindamycin cream.[49] Some experts view this syndrome as the most severe manifestation of what may represent a continuum of vaginitis caused by facultatative or aerobic microbial pathogens. Various other forms of irritant or allergic vulvovaginitis have also been described, including those caused by various intravaginal medications or personal hygiene products, latex condoms, and occasional instances in which vulvovaginitis seems to follow intercourse with a particular sex partner.[50] Vulvar vestibulitis and essential vulvodynia are other poorly understood vulvovaginal syndromes. Since the etiology of these syndromes remains unknown, treatment is empiric, and should be as conservative as possible. Vaginal aphthae, like oral and esophageal aphthae, have been described among women with HIV infection. Among women who present vulvovaginal symptoms with or without dyspareunia, but without objective physical evidence of vulvitis or vaginitis, psychological factors may sometimes be involved.[51]

DIFFERENTIAL DIAGNOSIS AND MANAGEMENT OF VAGINAL DISCHARGE

Symptoms or signs of abnormal vaginal discharge are usually attributable to vaginal infection. As shown in Table 57-4, in analyses adjusted for detection of cervical or vaginal infections, signs of increased profuse vaginal discharge among STD clinic patients were associated only with isolation of *T. vaginalis*; foul or fishy odor (after adding 10% KOH) was associated strongly with bacterial vaginosis and weakly with *T. vaginalis;* and yellow color of vaginal discharge was significantly associated with HSV, *T. vaginalis, N. gonorrhoeae,* and *C. trachomatis*.[13] The relationship of symptoms or signs of abnormal vaginal discharge to cervical infection has undergone reevaluation in recent years. Few recent studies have found statistically significant associations between symptoms of vaginal discharge and cervical infection; and where found, any associations could represent coincidental sexual acquisition of cervical infection together with trichomoniasis or bacterial vaginosis. Several studies have demonstrated no association of cervical infection with symptoms or signs of abnormally increased amount or abnormal odor of vaginal discharge.[13,52]

The initial assessment of the patient for vulvovaginal infection ideally should begin with an open-ended question about the reason for the clinic visit (i.e., the chief complaint), since a chief complaint of vaginal discharge is most predictive of vaginal infection. An alternative or intermediate step is a semistructured but non-leading question (e.g., "Do you have any abnormal genital symptoms?" or "Do you have any new symptoms that make you think you might have a vaginal infection or an STD?"). A nonspecific and leading question, such as "Do you have a vaginal discharge?" generates very nonspecific responses of low predictive value. More specific questions concerning abnormal vaginal discharge, as a follow-up to an initial open-ended question should probe the following three main types of abnormality and focus on recent changes in symptoms to further increase specificity of positive responses, such as, "Have you recently developed (1) an abnormal increase in the amount of vaginal discharge? (2) an abnormal and unpleasant odor of vaginal discharge? (3) an unusually yellow color of vaginal discharge?" Unfortunately, the terminology commonly used in clinical practice (i.e., "leukorrhea," or the equivalents in other languages) may have little utility.

Specific questions directed toward vulvar disease also should focus on the main types of vulvar abnormality and on recent changes in symptoms, such as: (1) "Have you recently developed abnormal itching or burning pain of the vulva (the opening of the vagina)? (2) any open sores or painful lesions? (3) any lumps or swellings?" Positive responses should lead to probing about past history of such symptoms, because of the recurrent nature of genital herpes or vulvovaginal candidiasis.

Vulvar and perineal inspection and speculum examination are indicated to establish the presence or absence of mucopurulent cervicitis, as well as signs of vulvovaginitis and also to identify other types of ectocervicitis (e.g., herpetic ulcerations), vulvovaginitis, vulvovaginal ulcers, and less common types of severe vulvovaginal pathology (see the following), and to identify specific microbial pathogens.

The amount, consistency, and location of the discharge within the vagina should be noted. A sample of discharge should then be removed with a swab from the vaginal wall, avoiding contamination with cervical mucus. The color of vaginal discharge should be noted in comparison with the white color of the swab. The pH should be determined directly by rolling the swab containing the specimen on appropriate pH indicator paper, which should show color variation with pH above and below 4.5. An additional specimen should be removed with a swab and mixed first with a drop of saline, then with a drop of 10 percent KOH, on a microscope slide. Any abnormal fishy (amine) odor released after mixing the specimen with KOH is noted, and separate coverslips are placed on both the saline and KOH wet mounts for microscopic examination to detect the presence and quantity of normal epithelial cells, clue cells, neutrophils, motile trichomonads, or fungal forms. The presence of any three of the four criteria described by Amsel et al. (homogeneous adherent white discharge, pH $\geq$ 4.5, clue cells and amine odor after mixing the discharge with 10% KOH) provides the usual basis for a clinical diagnosis of bacterial vaginosis.[53] A recently approved card test can be used by the clinician to screen for presence of elevated pH and trimethylamine.[54] Gram stain criteria or oligonucleotide probe testing are used on an increasing but still very limited basis (see Chap. 42).

Although the sensitivity and specificity of individual symptoms and signs as outlined above and in Table 57-5 are not high, in many patients, symptoms and signs combined with risk assessment and with pH and amine tests and microscopic wet mount findings correspond to a consistent pattern, and further studies are unnecessary. However, when symptoms or signs suggest a vaginal infection that cannot be confirmed by microscopic wet mount examination, further microbiological studies are indicated. Depending on the clinical findings, these further studies may include culture for *C. albicans,* culture for *T. vaginalis,* or Gram stain of vaginal fluid to differentiate between normal flora and the flora characteristic of bacterial vaginosis or other forms of vaginitis.[13,14] In women with prominent vaginal complaints but no

Table 57-4. Infections Associated with Signs of Vaginitis and Cervicitis on Physical Examination among 779 STD Clinic Patients

	Unadjusted			Adjusted		
	OR	(95%CI)*	*p*-value	OR	(95%CI)*,†	*p*-value
Speculum examination—yellow vaginal discharge§ (n = 69)						
GC	2.71	(1.73,4.24)	<.01	1.76	(1.06,2.92)	0.03
CT	2.79	(1.81,4.3)	<.01	3.06	(1.88,4.99)	<.01
GC or CT	2.85	(1.97,4.12)	<.01	2.79	(1.88,4.14)	<.01
TV	4.34	(2.8,6.72)	<.01	4.71	(2.84,7.79)	<.01
BV	1.76	(1.25,2.46)	<.01	1.30	(0.86,1.95)	0.21
TV or BV	1.94	(1.39,2.72)	<.01	1.84	(1.27,2.69)	<.01
CA	0.64	(0.42,0.96)	0.03	0.83	(0.65,1.06)	0.14
HSV	6.91	(3.1,15.4)	<.01	11.52	(5,26.56)	<.01
Speculum examination—profuse vaginal discharge (n = 56)						
GC	1.44	(0.7,2.96)	0.32	1.23	(0.57,2.67)	0.60
CT	1.11	(0.53,2.34)	0.78	1.33	(0.61,2.91)	0.47
GC or CT	1.05	(0.56,1.96)	0.89	1.14	(0.59,2.21)	0.70
TV	2.85	(1.54,5.25)	<.01	2.67	(1.31,5.32)	0.01
BV	1.72	(1,2.96)	0.05	1.49	(0.79,2.81)	0.22
TV or BV	1.94	(1.12,3.36)	0.02	2.18	(1.19,4.02)	0.01
CA	1.22	(0.67,2.24)	0.51	1.20	(0.85,1.69)	0.29
HSV	1.92	(0.64,5.72)	0.24	2.34	(0.76,7.17)	0.14
Speculum examination—foul/fish odor (n = 149)						
GC	1.58	(0.97,2.58)	0.07	0.79	(0.43,1.45)	0.45
CT	0.80	(0.47,1.37)	0.42	0.78	(0.4,1.52)	0.46
GC or CT	1.24	(0.82,1.87)	0.30	0.82	(0.5,1.34)	0.43
TV	5.63	(3.6,8.81)	<.01	3.35	(1.91,5.88)	<.01
BV	20.88	(12.31,35.44)	<.01	18.97	(10.61,33.93)	<.01
TV or BV	29.11	(15.41,55.01)	<.01	33.95	(16.76,68.77)	<.01
CA	0.57	(0.36,0.91)	0.02	1.02	(0.74,1.4)	0.90
HSV	0.91	(0.37,2.27)	0.84	1.47	(0.47,4.56)	0.51
Speculum examination—cervical mucopus (n = 182)						
GC	3.72	(2.37,5.83)	<.01	2.81	(1.69,4.66)	<.01
CT	5.64	(3.63,8.76)	<.01	5.14	(3.2,8.24)	<.01
GC or CT	4.94	(3.4,7.2)	<.01	5.10	(3.43,7.59)	<.01
TV	1.91	(1.23,2.97)	<.01	1.86	(1.1,3.15)	0.02
BV	1.05	(0.74,1.49)	0.77	0.83	(0.55,1.25)	0.37
TV or BV	1.18	(0.84,1.66)	0.34	0.94	(0.64,1.39)	0.76
CA	0.68	(0.45,1.03)	0.07	0.90	(0.71,1.14)	0.39
HSV	2.83	(1.37,5.86)	0.01	4.20	(1.95,9.04)	<.01
Speculum examination—cervical ectopy (n = 379)						
GC	1.33	(0.88,2)	0.18	1.33	(0.82,2.14)	0.24
CT	2.99	(1.95,4.58)	<.01	3.48	(2.16,5.59)	<.01
GC or CT	1.92	(1.37,2.68)	<.01	2.23	(1.57,3.17)	<.01
TV	0.68	(0.45,1.01)	0.06	0.67	(0.42,1.06)	0.09
BV	0.76	(0.56,1.02)	0.07	0.76	(0.54,1.06)	0.10
TV or BV	0.74	(0.55,0.98)	0.04	0.64	(0.47,0.88)	0.01
CA	1.01	(0.72,1.4)	0.97	1.02	(0.85,1.23)	0.83
HSV	1.22	(0.54,2.75)	0.64	1.51	(0.63,3.65)	0.36
Speculum examination—cervical bleeding on touch (n = 286)						
GC	1.41	(0.91,2.18)	0.13	1.02	(0.63,1.65)	0.94
CT	2.62	(1.7,4.04)	<.01	2.81	(1.77,4.45)	<.01
GC or CT	1.78	(1.25,2.53)	<.01	1.76	(1.22,2.54)	<.01
TV	1.32	(0.87,2.02)	0.19	1.53	(0.95,2.46)	0.08
BV	1.34	(0.98,1.82)	0.07	1.3	(0.91,1.84)	0.15
TV or BV	1.31	(0.96,1.77)	0.09	1.3	(0.93,1.81)	0.12
CA	0.81	(0.57,1.16)	0.26	0.91	(0.75,1.11)	0.37
HSV	3.07	(1.43,6.61)	<.01	3.66	(1.67,8.01)	<.01

*The odds ratios (OR) are in relation to those without stated sign.

†The adjusted confidence intervals are based on a logistic model that includes GC (*N. gonorrhoeae*), CT (*C. trachomatis*), TV (*T. vaginalis*), BV (bacterial vaginosis), CA (*Candida albicans*), and HSV. The adjusted confidence intervals for GC or CT and TV or BV are based on a logistic model that includes these each as single variables as well as CA and HSV.

§Color detected on white dacron swab.

Modified with permission from: Ryan CA, Courtois BN, Hawes SE, Stevens CE, Eschenbach DA, Holmes KK: Risk assessment, symptoms and signs as predictors of vulvovaginal and cervical infections in an urban U.S. STD clinic: Implications for use of STD algorithms. *Sex Transm Infect* 74(Suppl 1): S59–S76, 1998.

abnormal findings, all three of these additional microbiological tests may be indicated to differentiate vaginal infection from other causes of vaginal symptoms, including functional complaints.[98]

Usual treatments for vaginal infection are also summarized in Table 57-5. It is still common practice to prescribe metronidazole for bacterial vaginosis only for those who have complaints related to this condition. However, this perspective is changing because of the association of BV with PID, preterm delivery, and increased risk of HIV acquisition (see Chap. 42). Further studies of prenatal BV treatment are required to confirm the reported reduction in preterm delivery; until then, the need for routine screening for and treatment of BV in pregnancy is still debated.

Vulvar symptoms

Symptoms of vulvar pruritis or burning, of painful vulvar lesions, and of external dysuria, are most often associated with isolation of HSV or *C. albicans*. Primary genital herpes with cervicitis may also produce symptoms of increased or yellow vaginal discharge, whereas such symptoms do not typically seem to occur with vulvovaginal candidiasis (see Table 57-4).[13]

BARTHOLINITIS

Bartholin's gland infection can involve the main duct (which opens near the junction of the anterior ⅔ and posterior ⅓ of the labia majorum) as well as the minor ducts and glandular acini. Ductal inflammation and obstruction can lead to Bartholin's abscess or cysts, which can reach 1 to 8 cm in diameter. The etiology of bartholinitis commonly involves *N. gonorrhoeae*, or *C. trachomatis*; abscesses often contain enteric and vaginal gram negative rods and anaerobes.[55–58] The potential role of bacterial vaginosis as a risk factor for Bartholinitis (analogous to the role of BV or PID) remains undefined. Unusual etiologies include the respiratory pathogens *Streptococcus pneumoniae* and *Haemophilus* species.[59–61] Ductal exudate or aspirates from abscesses or cysts provide material for microbiologic diagnoses. The differential diagnosis of cysts includes benign tumors such as adenomas and hamartomas, as well as carcinoma—especially in post menopausal women. Treatment of Bartholinitis and Bartholin's abscess probably should cover gonococcal and chlamydial infection, as well as anaerobic bacteria—analogous to treatment of PID. Drainage of abscesses, and excision or marsupulization of cysts are commonly employed.

Table 57-5. Diagnostic Features and Management of Vaginal Infection in Premenopausal Adults

	Normal vaginal exam	Yeast vaginitis	Trichomonal vaginitis	Bacterial vaginosis (NSV)
Etiology	Uninfected; *Lactobacillus* predominant	*Candida albicans* and other yeasts	*Trichomonas vaginalis*	Associated with *G. vaginalis,* various anaerobic bacteria, and mycoplasma
Typical symptoms	None	Vulvar itching, burning, or irritation	Profuse purulent discharge	Malodorous, slightly increased discharge
Discharge:				
Amount	Variable; usually scant	Scant to moderate	Profuse	Moderate
Color*	Clear or white	White	Yellow	Usually white or gray
Consistency	Nonhomogeneous, floccular	Clumped; adherent plaques	Homogeneous	Homogeneous, low viscosity; uniformly coating vaginal walls
Inflammation of vulvar or vaginal epithelium	None	Erythema of vaginal epithelium, introitus; vulvar dermatitis common	Erythema of vaginal and vulvar epithelium; colpitis macularis	None
pH of vaginal fluid†	Usually ≤4.5	Usually ≤4.5	Often ≥5.0	Usually >4.5
Amine ("fishy") odor with 10% KOH	None	None	May be present	Present
Microscopy§	Normal epithelial cells; lactobacilli predominate	Leukocytes, epithelial cells; yeast, mycelia, or pseudomycelia in up to 80%	Leukocytes; motile trichomonads seen in 80 to 90% of symptomatic patients, less often in the absence of symptoms	Clue cells; few leukocytes; lactobacilli outnumbered by profuse mixed flora, nearly always including *G. vaginalis* plus anaerobic species, on Gram stain
Usual treatment	None	Miconazole, clotrimazole, or other imidazoles (see Chap. 45)	Metronidazole or tinidazole 2.0 g orally (single dose) Metronidazole 500 mg orally twice daily for 7 days	Metronidazole 500 mg orally twice daily for 7 days Intravaginal metronidazole gel or clindamycin cream
Usual management of sex partners	None	None; topical treatment if candidal dermatitis of penis is present	Examine for STD; treat with metronidazole, 2 gm p.o.	Examine for STD; no treatment if normal

*Color of discharge is determined by examining vaginal discharge against the white background of a swab.
†pH determination is not useful if blood is present
§To detect fungal elements, vaginal fluid is digested with 10% KOH prior to microscopic examination; to examine for other features, fluid is mixed (1 : 1) with physiologic saline. Gram's stain also is excellent for detecting yeasts and pseudomycelia and for distinguishing normal flora from the mixed flora seen in bacterial vaginosis, but is less sensitive than the saline preparation for detection of *T. vaginalis*.

CERVICITIS

Two types of cervicitis can be distinguished—*endocervicitis* (also known as *mucopurulent cervicitis*) and *ectocervicitis*. Causes of endocervicitis include *C. trachomatis, N. gonorrhoeae,* and herpes simplex virus. HSV infection can also be associated with ectocervicitis, and will be discussed separately in the following. The presence of cervical infection is not synonymous with the term "cervicitis," since not all infections are associated with demonstrable cervicitis, and vice versa. For example, a positive test for *C. trachomatis* in an endocervical specimen leads to a diagnosis of chlamydial infection of the cervix, not of necessarily to a diagnosis of chlamydial "cervicitis."

Mucopurulent cervicitis caused by *C. trachomatis* or *N. gonorrhoeae* must be differentiated from endo- and ecto-cervicitis caused by HSV, from ectocervicitis caused by *T. vaginalis,* from vaginitis, and from simple cervical ectopy without inflammation, a common condition (plate 13). Columnar epithelium lies in an exposed position on the ectocervix in the majority of adolescent girls at the onset of menarche. The prevalence of ectopy gradually declines through young adulthood.[62] The term ectropion, has also been used to describe the patulous parous cervix, which opens as the blades of a vaginal speculum are spread, to expose the endocervix. Ectopy or ectropion, when not associated with visible or microscopic evidence of mucopurulent exudate, or with colposcopic epithelial abnormalities, is a normal finding and requires no therapy. Recurrent genital herpes involving the cervix alone produces lesions of the endocervix and the ectocervical squamous epithelium. Ectocervicitis caused by trichomoniasis and vulvovaginal candidiasis are generally associated with vaginitis, as discussed below.

Endocervicitis

Urethritis in men represents the tip of the iceberg of infections caused by *C. trachomatis* and *N. gonorrhoeae*. Endocervicitis, together with subclinical urethral infections in both sexes, represents the portion of the iceberg that often goes unrecognized. The fact that urethritis in the male can result in detection and treatment of cervical infection led to the old adage in venereology: "The man who develops a discharge after sex with a woman could become that woman's best friend." At present, in most of the world, control of these infections unfortunately is based largely on the clinical diagnosis of urethritis in the male and on treatment of the female sex partners of men with urethritis. This is particularly so in developing countries, where specific laboratory tests for *N. gonorrhoeae* and *C. trachomatis* are rarely available. Because endocervicitis produces symptoms less often than male urethritis, and symptoms of endocervicitis that may occur (e.g., yellow vaginal discharge) are less distinctive than symptoms of urethritis, the careful assessment of clinical signs of mucopurulent cervicitis, and the appropriate use of laboratory tests for confirming MPC, as well as for screening for subclinical infection of the female, are of paramount importance in the control of gonococcal and chlamydial infections.

Infection of the cervix represents a reservoir for sexual or perinatal transmission of pathogenic microorganisms, and might lead to at least two possible types of complications in the female: (1) ascending intralumenal spread of pathogenic organisms from the cervix, producing endometritis and salpingitis; (2) ascending infection during pregnancy, resulting in chorioamnionitis, premature rupture of membranes, premature delivery, amniotic fluid infection, and puerperal infection.

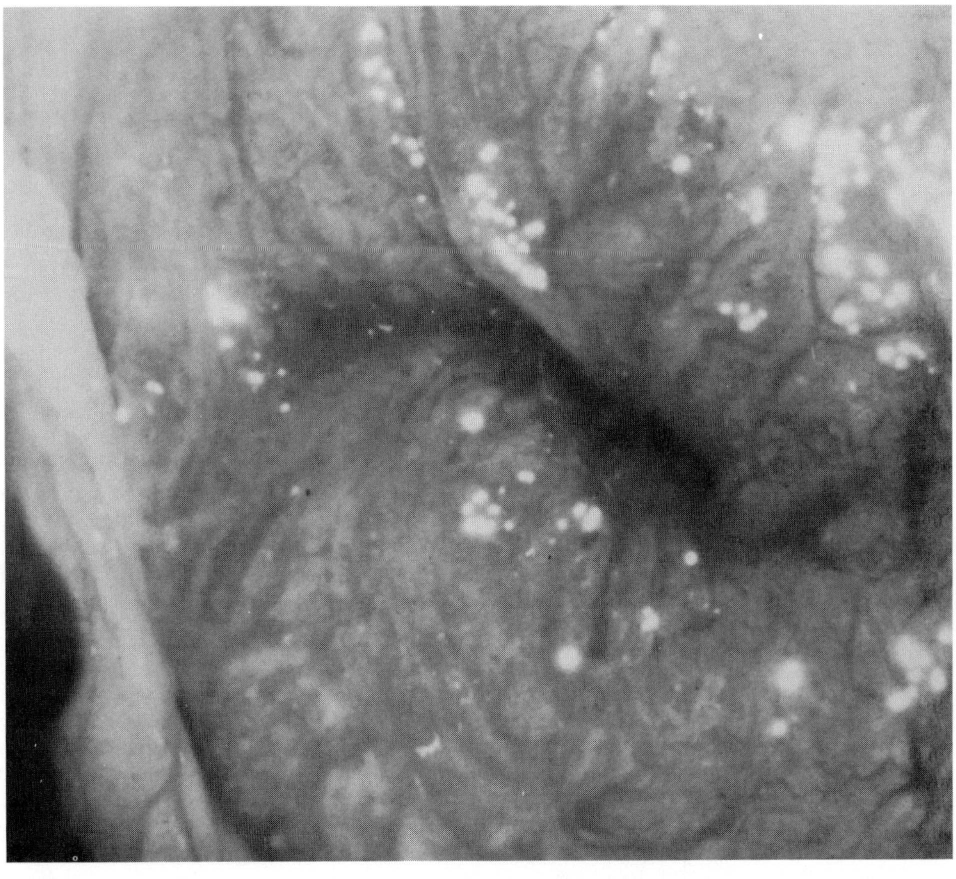

Fig. 57-3. Colpophotograph of the cervix infected with *C. trachomatis*, showing proliferation and dilation of subepithelial capillaries in the zone of ectopy.

The lack of widely recognized objective signs of cervical inflammation is illustrated by the confusing nomenclature for endocervicitis. Terms such as acute and chronic cervicitis, cervical erosion, cervical discontinuity, mucopurulent cervicitis, papillary cervicitis, follicular cervicitis, and hypertrophic cervicitis have all been used. This confusion results in part from the changes that occur in the cervix over the reproductive period and in part from difficulty in differentiating normal ectopic columnar epithelium from endocervicitis.[62–65] The latter differentiation is complicated by the fact that cervical ectopy (plate 13) appears correlated with detection of cervical infection by *C. trachomatis*.[62,66–68] Ectopy is present in the majority of younger teenage girls, and decreases steadily in prevalence with increasing age. Further, ectopy is significantly positively correlated with oral contraceptive use, and inversely correlated with smoking, independent of age.[62]

In this chapter, the term *mucopurulent endocervical discharge* (or *endocervical mucopus*) refers to yellow endocervical exudate or increased numbers of neutrophils in endocervical mucus as demonstrated by Gram's stain (see the following). The yellow color is thought to be caused by the presence of the "green enzyme" myeloperoxidase contained within polymorphonuclear neutrophils. *Mucopurulent endocervicitis* refers to the appearance of the inflamed endocervix on physical examination—optimally by colposcopy—with manifestations such as yellow endocervical discharge, edema and erythema of the zone of ectopy, and easily induced endocervical bleeding. *Endocervicitis* refers to histopathologic features of endocervical inflammation.

Definition and etiology of mucopurulent cervicitis

Rees et al. were particularly instrumental in initially establishing the relationship of *C. trachomatis* to mucopurulent cervicitis.[69] To further evaluate objective criteria for the clinical diagnosis of mucopurulent cervicitis, we studied 100 randomly selected women attending an STD clinic in Seattle for the correlation of selected cervical abnormalities with isolation of *C. trachomatis, N. gonorrhoeae,* and HSV.[70] The presence of yellow endocervical exudate, confirmed by the simple identification of yellow exudate on a white cotton-tipped swab specimen of endocervical secretions, correlated only with isolation of *C. trachomatis.* Mucopurulent secretions were present in 62 percent of women with cervical chlamydial infection and 12 percent of women with no cervical pathogen. Bleeding produced by collection of culture specimens from the endocervix, erythema (owing to increased vascularity), and edema of the zone of ectopy were also more common among women with *C. trachomatis* infection (Fig. 57-3). Examples of some of these findings are shown in color plates 15 and 16. Microscopic detection of increased numbers of neutrophils demonstrated by Gram stain within the faintly pink strands of endocervical mucus, collected after first removing ectocervical vaginal cells with a large swab, and examined as described in the following, was also correlated with isolation of *C. trachomatis* (Figs. 57-4 and 57-5).

In a subsequent study of a larger series of 779 women attending the Seattle STD clinic, when the prevalence of endocervical chlamydial and gonococcal infection by culture were 15 and 14 percent, respectively, we found that the presence of yellow mucopus collected from the endocervix and visualized on a white swab was independently correlated not only with isolation of *C. trachomatis*, but also with isolation of *N. gonorrhoeae* and of HSV from the endocervix, and with isolation of *T. vaginalis* from the vagina.[13] Figure 57-6 displays the proportion of all women with endocervical mucopus in that study found to have *N. gonorrhoeae, C. trachomatis*, HSV, or *T. vaginalis,* alone or in mixed infections; 38% had none of these pathogens (but in populations with lower prevalences of these pathogens (including the same Seattle Clinic today), smaller proportions of those with mucopus would have these infections). *N. gonorrhoeae* or *C. trachomatis* were isolated from 45 percent of those with endocervical mucopus and 14 percent of those without endocervical mucopus in this study. By multivariate analysis adjusting for other infections, chlamydial infection was also significantly associated with cervical ectopy and with cervical bleeding that was easily induced with a dacron swab (commonly mistermed cervical "friability" (see Table 57-4). Gonococcal and chlamydial infection, cervical HSV infection, and trichomoniasis all were also associated with signs of yellow vaginal discharge on speculum examination, but neither gonococcal nor chlamydial infection was associated with objective signs of profuse vaginal discharge.

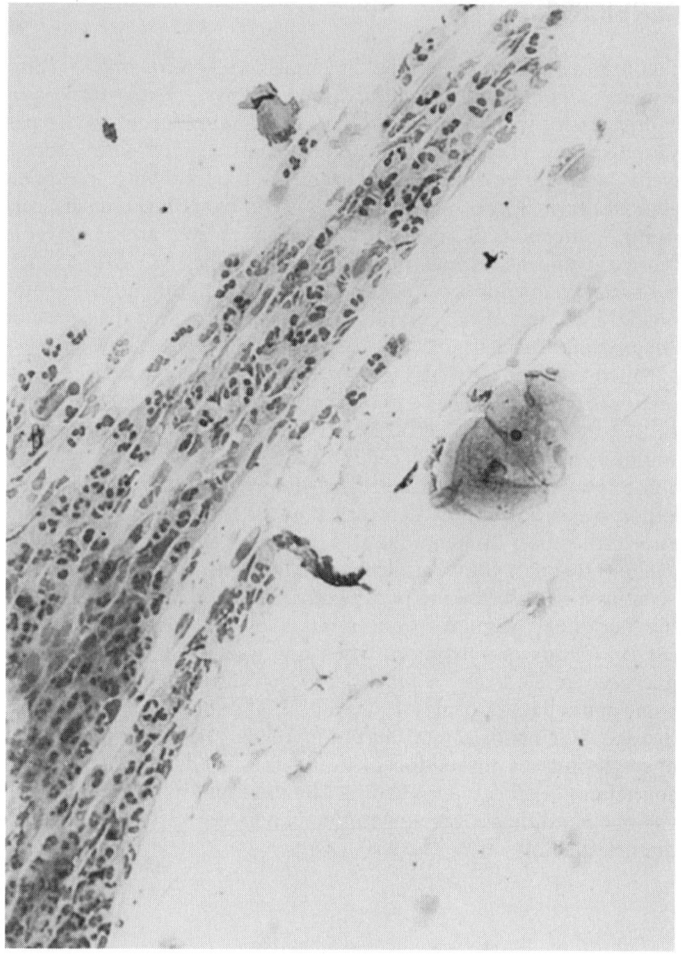

Fig. 57-4. Satisfactory smear of endocervical mucus from chlamydial mucopurulent cervicitis, showing many neutrophils in strands of mucus, with few contaminating vaginal squamous cells or bacteria.

Initial efforts to develop clinical algorithms for syndromic management of STDs were based on the premise that symptoms of vaginal discharge could identify women with increased risk of gonococcal and chlamydial infection, and that this could be the basis for improved control of these infections in the population. When this approach failed to identify women with increased prevalence of cervical infection, a modified approach was proposed by the World Health Organization, in which risk assessment was added to try to identify a subset of women with vaginal discharge who might have a higher prevalence of cervical infection, sufficient to warrant presumptive treatment for cervical infection. In general, although various locally derived strategies for risk assessment did help to identify those with increased prevalence, the positive predictive values for cervical infection were still too low to war-

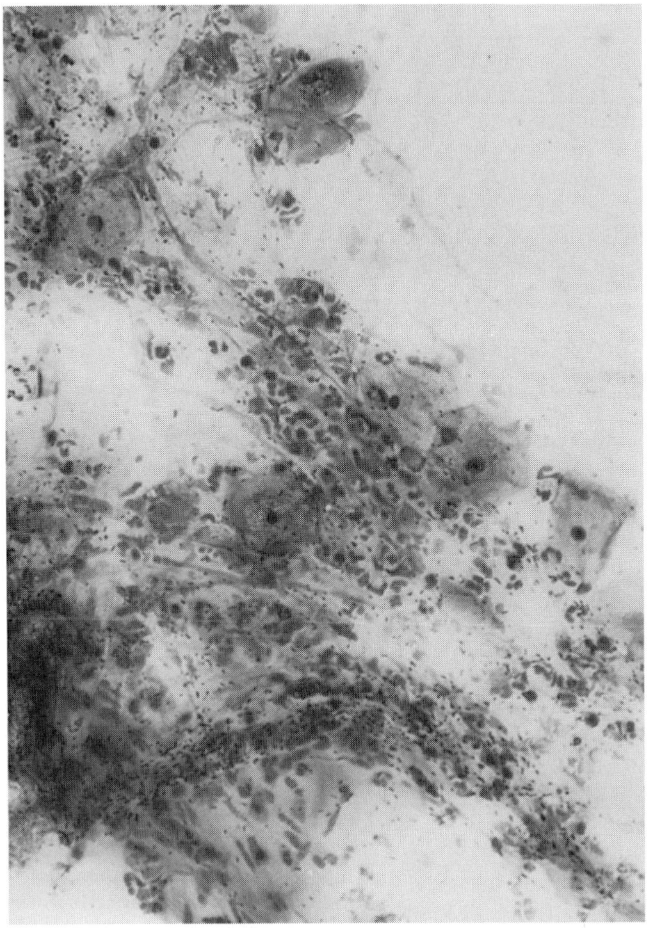

Fig. 57-5. Unsatisfactory smear of cervical mucus. Although moderate numbers of neutrophils are seen, the presence of many vaginal squamous cells and bacteria makes it difficult to tell whether the neutrophils originate in the cervix or the vagina.

rant routine treatment in most settings; the basic flaw was the lack of correlation of vaginal discharge symptoms with cervical infection.[71] The question then arises: If endocervical mucopus or other manifestations of cervicitis are the true clinical manifestations of cervical infection, would addition of risk assessment *after detection of mucopus,* help to further discriminate those with from those without cervical infection; and prove more useful for syndromic management algorithms in which speculum exam was performed? We are not aware of the evaluation of risk assessment for syndromic management of mucopurulent endocervical discharge, as opposed to syndromic management of vaginal discharge. Applying this more logical approach to the same data set of 779 women who had an overall prevalence of cervical gonococcal or chlamydial infection of 24 percent, the prevalence of cervical gonococcal or chlamydial infection was 57 percent among those with mucopus and positive risk assessment versus only 11 percent among those with no mucopus and negative risk assessment (Table 57-6). Such an approach might prove useful in various settings for deciding who to treat empirically and initiate presumptive partner treatment as well, who to test while deferring treatment, and who to offer neither treatment nor testing.

In various published studies, the recommended cutoff value indicative of MPC for the number of polymorphonuclear (PMN) leukocytes per 1000× microscopic field in endocervical mucus on Gram's stain for diagnoses of endocervical mucopus has been ≥10, ≥20, or ≥30. As shown in Table 57-7, in our study of 779 women, cutoff values of ≥10 neutrophils and ≥30 neutrophils per 1000× field in endocervical mucus both were significantly and independently associated with isolation of *N. gonorrhoeae, C. trachomatis*, and HSV, but only the lower value (≥10) was also associated with isolation of *T. vaginalis.*[13] With respect to detection of *N. gonorrhoeae* or *C. trachomatis*, the finding of ≥10 PMN/1000× field in cervical mucus had a sensitivity of 80.4 percent, a specificity of 48.3 percent, and a positive predictive value of 33 percent in this population, with its 24 percent prevalence of either infection. The finding of ≥30 PMN had a lower sensitivity of 46.6 percent, a higher specificity of 80.2 percent, and higher positive predictive value of 43 percent. Neither finding was as accurate as detection of yellow endocervical mucopus, which had a sensitivity of 52 percent, specificity of 82 percent, and positive predictive value of 48 percent.[13]

CHANGING PREVALENCE AND ETIOLOGY OF MUCOPURULENT ENDOCERVICAL DISCHARGE

During 1987, the diagnosis of nongonococcal urethritis was made in 30 percent of heterosexual men visiting the Seattle King County Department of Public Health STD Clinic at Harborview Medical Center with a new problem. In recent years, the proportion of new problem male visits associated with a diagnosis of urethritis has fallen, as has the proportion of urethritis cases associated with gonococcal or chlamydial infection. By 1997, the diagnosis of urethritis of any etiology was made in only 23 percent of new problem clinic visits by heterosexual men, with only 25 percent associated with gonococcal or chlamydial infection. By comparison, during 1987 the diagnosis of MPC was made by any of several clinicians in 18 percent of new problem visits by women, and in 1997, the diagnosis of MPC was again made in 18 percent of new problem visits by women. Gonococcal or chlamydial infection

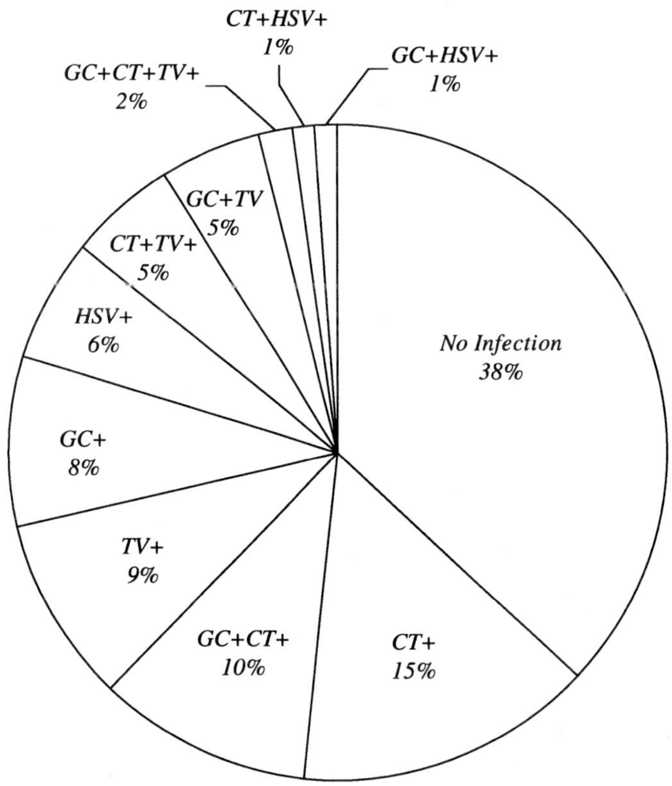

Fig. 57-6. Among 779 consecutive female STD clinic patients, 182 (23.4%) had signs of endocervical mucopus. This pie chart shows the percentage of those with endocervical mucopus no cervical infection, or cervical infection by *C. trachomatis* (CT), *N. gonorrhoeae* (GC), herpes simplex virus (HSV), or *T. vaginalis* (TV).

Table 57-6. Performance of Risk Assessment (RA) in Identifying Gonococcal and Chlamydial Infection among Women with and without Signs of Endocervical Mucopus

	Endocervical mucopus present		Endocervical mucopus absent	
	RA positive (n = 119)*	RA negative (n = 63)	RA positive (n = 314)	RA negative (n = 283)
% GC+	35	10	14	5
% CT+	37	27	12	7
% GC or CT+	57	21	23	11
Sensitivity**	78		70	
Specificity**	45		51	
Positive P.V.**	57		23	
Negative P.V.**	69		89	

*Risk assessment positive = partner with gonorrhea or chlamydia or 2 or more of the following: age <21, no use of barrier contraception, new partner in past 30 days, multiple partners in past 30 days.
**Sensitivity, specificity, and positive and negative predictive values for detection of GC and/or CT are presented separately for those with, and those without endocervical mucopus.

was found in 15.3 percent of those with MPC versus 4.8 percent of those without MPC during 1997 (odds ratio 3.6). These data suggest that in Seattle, as the prevalence of gonococcal and chlamydial infection has fallen, and as the experience of clinicians with diagnosis of mucopus has increased: the disparity between proportion of male patients diagnosed with urethritis and the proportion of women diagnosed with MPC by routine clinical examination has decreased; and even as the overall prevalence of gonococcal and chlamydial infection among all women and among women with MPC has fallen dramatically in the Seattle STD clinic over the past decade, the overall association between MPC and cervical infection remains high in this clinical setting.

CONSENSUS ON THE ASSOCIATION OF MUCOPURULENT CERVICITIS WITH CERVICAL GONOCOCCAL OR CHLAMYDIAL INFECTION

Several published studies on the prevalence of endocervical gonococcal and chlamydial infections, and on the prevalence of endocervical mucopus on speculum examination, are summarized in Table 57-8, in relation to the year and type of population studied.[13,70,72–88] Some but not all of these studies enrolled only women with symptoms, such as abnormal vaginal discharge or lower abdominal pain; many did not test for HSV or *T. vaginalis* infection. The prevalence of gonococcal or chlamydial endocervical infection ranged from as low as 2.7 percent in the US Region X family planning clinics in 1995 to 1996 to as high as 37 percent in female sex workers (FSW) in Cebu City, the Philippines.[84] The reported prevalence of endocervical mucopus observed by speculum ranged from 2.8 percent in Cebu FSW (perhaps representing insensitive screening for mucopus) to 50.7 percent (probably representing nonspecific detection of mucopus) in Moroccan family planning clinics enrolling women with symptoms of vaginal discharge or low abdominal pain.[52,84] This wide range reflects the importance (and difficulty) of training health care providers to accurately screen for this finding. Nonetheless, of the 19 studies cited, 16 found significant associations of endocervical mucopus (usually defined as a positive "swab test," meaning yellow color of endocervical discharge visualized on a white swab) with endocervical gonococcal or chlamydial infection (with OR ranging from 2.1–5.5); whereas the remaining three (all done in family planning or antenatal clinics) did find associations with increased numbers of PMN leukocytes in cervical mucus, or with induced endocervical bleeding. Sellors and Walter and Linder have also noted an association of endocervical infection with opaque (i.e., nontranslucent) cervical mucus, independent of yellow color of the mucus. Some studies also assessed and found associations with yellow vaginal discharge, or with increased numbers of leukocytes in vaginal smears.[13,78,81,89] This finding may be easier for clinicians to demonstrate in some settings than the demonstration of endocervical mucopus, but can reflect vaginal trichomoniasis as well. Many of these studies found no relationship of symptoms of vaginal discharge to presence or absence of endocervical gonococcal or chlamydial infection, as discussed earlier.

Although mucopurulent cervicitis has been significantly correlated with endocervical infection in most of these studies, the sensitivity, specificity, and predictive value have varied in different settings.[13,70,72–88,90–92] It is difficult to assess to what extent the variability is attributable to differences in patients, to differences in assessing mucopurulent cervicitis, or to differences in detection of infection. Our experience suggests that the correlation of isolation of *C. trachomatis* or *N. gonorrhoeae* from the cervix with detection of mucopurulent (yellow) endocervical discharge by an inexperienced clinician is initially low (in which case identification of increased numbers of neutrophils in cervical mucus by an experienced laboratory technician is more reliable); but with training and experience, the correlation improves.

The cause of mucopurulent cervicitis in the absence of proven gonococcal, chlamydial, or HSV infection or trichomoniasis remains uncertain. Various genital pathogens have been implicated, and it is likely that false negative tests for *C. trachomatis*, *N. gonorrhoeae*, or HSV account for some cases.[93] In addition, it seems possible that oral contraceptive use and cervical ectopy per se may be associated with endocervical inflammation.[93]

ECTOCERVICITIS

Routine colposcopic examination of female STD clinic patients has shown that cervical HSV infection is highly correlated with cervical ulcers or necrotic lesions (color plate 14), whereas trichomoniasis is correlated with colpitis macularis ("strawberry cervix"), and both *C. trachomatis* and cytomegalovirus infection of the cervix are correlated with colposcopic features of immature metaplasia.[94] Immature metaplasia was defined as faint acetowhite epithelium (white after application of acetic acid) with diffuse distal borders, occurring as finger-like projections within the transformation zone, at the central margin of a squamocolumnar junction advancing centrally into the zone of ectopy. In a further analysis, colpitis macularis (color plate 20) was identified without magnification in only two (2%) of 108 women with trichomoniasis but was seen by colposcopy in 49 (45%) of the 108 with trichomoniasis versus only six (1%) of 509 without trichomoniasis.[17] Cervical ulcerations or necrotic lesions were detected by colposcopy in 22 (65%) of 34 women with positive cervical cultures for HSV, and 11 (1.5%) of 745 with negative cultures for HSV.[95] *C. albicans*, like *T. vaginalis*, also can produce ectocervicitis, but both are associated with other manifestations of inflammation of the contiguous stratified squamous vaginal epithelium (plates 19 and 21).

Table 57-7. Percentage with Infection among 779 Randomly Selected Female STD Clinic Patients with and without Increased Concentrations of Polymorphonuclear (PMN) Leukocytes in Cervical Mucus or Vaginal Fluid*

	Percent infected with finding	Percent uninfected without finding	Unadjusted OR	Unadjusted (95% CI)†	Adjusted OR	Adjusted (95%CI)†,§
Cervical PMNs ≥ 10 (*n* = 457)						
GC	83.0%	54.8%	4.03	(2.38,6.81)	3.20	(1.82,5.63)
CT	79.5%	55.0%	3.17	(1.98,5.09)	2.82	(1.71,4.66)
GC or CT	80.4%	51.7%	3.84	(2.59,5.69)	3.73	(2.49,5.57)
TV	72.6%	56.2%	2.07	(1.34,3.2)	1.75	(1.07,2.86)
BV	61.3%	55.6%	1.27	(0.94,1.71)	1.04	(0.74,1.46)
TV or BV	63.5%	55.1%	1.42	(1.06,1.9)	1.24	(0.9,1.7)
CA	55.1%	60.2%	0.81	(0.58,1.13)	0.99	(0.83,1.2)
HSV	82.4%	57.2%	3.49	(1.44,8.5)	4.13	(1.67,10.23)
Cervical PMNSs ≥ 30 (*n* = 205)						
GC	44.3%	23.5%	2.60	(1.7,3.96)	2.23	(1.38,3.62)
CT	50.4%	22.1%	3.60	(2.4,5.4)	3.69	(2.37,5.74)
GC or CT	46.6%	19.8%	3.52	(2.48,5)	3.59	(2.48,5.18)
TV	33.3%	25.1%	1.49	(0.98,2.28)	1.17	(0.71,1.94)
BV	27.5%	24.8%	1.15	(0.83,1.61)	1.07	(0.73,1.58)
TV or BV	28.0%	25.1%	1.16	(0.84,1.6)	0.97	(0.68,1.39)
CA	18.7%	28.9%	0.57	(0.38,0.85)	0.82	(0.66,1.04)
HSV	47.1%	24.9%	2.68	(1.34,5.37)	3.67	(1.75,7.74)
Vaginal PMNs ≥ 10 (*n* = 491)						
GC	77.4%	61.2%	2.16	(1.34,3.5)	1.99	(1.17,3.39)
CT	79.5%	60.6%	2.52	(1.57,4.05)	2.41	(1.46,3.99)
GC or CT	76.2%	59.3%	2.19	(1.51,3.18)	2.45	(1.66,3.61)
TV	70.1%	62.2%	1.42	(0.93,2.17)	1.44	(0.88,2.34)
BV	63.8%	63.8%	1.00	(0.74,1.36)	1.03	(0.73,1.45)
TV or BV	63.2%	63.6%	0.99	(0.73,1.32)	1.03	(0.75,1.42)
CA	71.1%	61.1%	1.57	(1.1,2.25)	1.34	(1.1,1.63)
HSV	94.1%	61.2%	10.1	(2.47,41.7)	10.43	(2.51,43.39)
Vaginal PMNs ≥ 30 (*n* = 277)						
GC	50.0%	33.3%	2.00	(1.33,3.03)	2.13	(1.33,3.42)
CT	55.6%	32.0%	2.65	(1.78,3.96)	2.93	(1.89,4.53)
GC or CT	50.8%	30.7%	2.33	(1.67,3.26)	2.67	(1.87,3.810
TV	39.3%	34.9%	1.21	(0.81,1.81)	1.11	(0.7,1.78)
BV	36.6%	36.2%	1.02	(0.75,1.38)	1.06	(0.75,1.51)
TV or BV	35.9%	35.3%	1.02	(0.76,1.38)	1.02	(0.73,1.41)
CA	41.2%	33.8%	1.37	(0.98,1.92)	1.29	(1.07,1.56)
HSV	70.6%	33.6%	4.75	(2.23,10.09)	5.66	(2.54,12.62)

*Number of PMN leukocytes per 1000 × microscopic field.

†The odds ratios (OR) are in relation to the those without stated sign.

§The adjusted confidence intervals are based on a logistic model that includes GC, CT, TV, BV, CA, and HSV. The adjusted confidence intervals for GC or CT and TV or BV are based on a logistic model that includes these each as single variables as well as CA and HSV. Models will exclude BV, TV or TV/BV if finding is used as criteria for diagnosis.

Modified with permission from: Ryan CA, Courtois BN, Hawes SE, Stevens CE, Eschenbach DA, Holmes KK: Risk assessment, symptoms and signs as predictors of vulvovaginal and cervical infections in urban U.S. STD clinic: implications for use of STD algorithms. *Sex Transm Infect* 74(Suppl 1):S59–S76, 1998.

SPECIAL DIAGNOSTIC PROCEDURES FOR CERVICITIS

The presence of endocervicitis can be confirmed by a variety of supplementary diagnostic procedures, most of which should be available to clinicians specializing in treatment of genital infections of women. These include Gram's stain of endocervical mucus, cervical cytology, colposcopy, and cervical biopsy. The microbial etiology of endocervicitis can be presumptively established by Gram's stain of endocervical mucus and further substantiated by isolation of *C. trachomatis, N. gonorrhoeae,* or HSV, by detection of specific microbial antigens, or by detection of specific nucleic acid sequences from these pathogens.

Endocervical gram's stain

Just as sputum is difficult to evaluate microscopically when contaminated by oropharyngeal cells and flora, the endocervical mucus is difficult to evaluate microscopically when contaminated by vaginal cells and flora. The ectocervix is therefore generally wiped clean with a large swab before endocervical mucus is obtained for microscopy. Mucus is then obtained from the endocervical canal, rolled in a thin film over a slide, heat-fixed, and stained by Gram's stain. The slide is screened at low magnification (×100) to identify strands of cervical mucus containing PMN, as well as to evaluate the extent of contamination by vaginal squamous cells, and to select representative areas of cervical mucus for closer examination with the oil immersion lens. The number of polymorphonuclear (PMN) neutrophils per ×1000 field (oil immersion magnification) within strands of cervical mucus should then be counted in several representative fields. The presence of increased concentrations of PMN in mucus strands supports the diagnosis of cervicitis, unless heavy contamination by vaginal squamous cells (e.g., >100 squamous cells per slide) and by vaginal flora (e.g., >100 bacteria per ×1000 field overlying cervical mucus) suggest that the neutrophils may have originated in the vagina

Table 57-8. Prevalence of Endocervical Gonococcal and Chlamydial Infection (GC and CT) and of Mucopurulent Endocervical Discharge in Published Studies, and the Relationship of GC and/or CT to Various Manifestations of Cervicitis*

Author, year	Clinical setting	Percent with mucopus	Percent with GC ± CT	Findings associated with GC ± CT	Odds ratio*
Brunham 1982[70]	Seattle STD clinic	24	28.0	Mucopus	4.8
				≥10 PMN/1000 × field	8.0
Ryan 1984–1986[13]	Seattle STD clinic	23.4	24.0	Mucopus	5.1
				Induced bleeding	1.8
				Yellow vaginal discharge	2.8
				Ectopy	2.2
				≥30 PMN/1000 × field	3.6
Handsfield 1984[72]	Seattle family planning	14.2	9.7	Mucopus	3.0
				Induced bleeding	2.3
Thomas 1994[73]	Nairobi antenatal	7.3	10.8	Mucopus	2.6
				Induced bleeding	2.1
Mayaud 1992–1993[74]	Tanzania antenatal	4.5	8.4	Cervical discharge	2.7
				≥10 PMN/HPF	2.0
Behets[75]	Jamaica STD clinic	NA	34.0	Mucopus	2.1
				Induced bleeding	1.5
Mosure 1995–1996[76]	U.S. family planning Region VIIII	10.5†	3.7†	Mucopus	2.3
				Induced bleeding	2.1
	Region X	8.2†	2.7†	Mucopus	2.8
				Induced bleeding	2.5
Sellors 1989–1992[77]	Canada family planning, student and abortion clinics	—	6.3	Yellow mucopus	2.8
				Opaque cervical dis-	2.9
				charge	2.3
				Induced bleeding	
Alary 1993–1994[78]	Benin STD, antenatal clinics	14.3	7.8	Mucopus	2.8
				Pos. swab test	3.3
Daly 1994[79]	Malawi hospital outpatient clinic	19.5	19.5	Abnormal color of vaginal discharge	2.4
				Cervical motion tenderness	8.7
				Mucopus	2.7
				≥10 WBCs/HPF on vaginal wet mount	2.3
Sanchez 1996[80]	Peru gynecology and family planning clinics	27.7§	12.2	Profuse yellow vaginal discharge	4.1
				Induced bleeding	2.8
				≥10 PMN/HPF	2.3
Ryan 1995–1996[81]	Morocco primary care	35.9	10.1	Mucopus	2.1
				Yellow vaginal discharge	2.0
	Morocco family planning	50.7	5.4	Malodorous discharge	3.0
Diallo 1992–1993[82]	Côte d' Ivoire sex workers	20.2	35.0	Mucopus	4.8
				Induced bleeding	2.2
				Cx motion tenderness	1.6
				WBC ≥ 10/HPF	3.8
Ndoye 1990[83]	Senegal sex workers	11.8	24.9	Mucopus	2.6
				WBC ≥ 10/HPF in cervical fluid	3.5
				WBC ≥ 10/HPF in vaginal fluid	6.6
Wi 1994[84]	Philippines-sex workers				
	Manila	20.7	23.3	Mucopus	3.0
				≥20PMN/1000 × field	2.5
	Cebu City	2.8	37.0	≥20PMN/1000 × field	2.4
Behets 1995[88]	Jamaica family planning	4.3	14.1	None	—
Kapiga 1995[85]	Tanzania family planning	7.7	8.2	Induced bleeding	2.5
				Cx motion tenderness	2.4
Mayaud 1994[86]	Tanzania antenatal clinic	Not assessed	7.4	Yellow vaginal discharge	2.0
				≥20PMN/HPF	6.3
				≥5PMN/HPF	4.0

Table 57-8. Prevalence of Endocervical Gonococcal and Chlamydial Infection (GC and CT) and of Mucopurulent Endocervical Discharge in Published Studies, and the Relationship of GC and/or CT to Various Manifestations of Cervicitis* *(Continued)*

Author, year	Clinical setting	Percent with mucopus	Percent with GC ± CT	Findings associated with GC ± CT	Odds ratio*
Schneider 1994[87]	South Africa family planning clinic	22	14	Mucopus and/or induced bleeding	2.4

*Limited to statistically significantly elevated odds ratios
†Data for ages 20–24 only
§Mucopus defined as yellow or "brown" cervical mucus in this study.
Sources: See reference numbers throughout.

rather than in the endocervix. Common mistakes are to search areas of the smear other than cervical mucus strands to enumerate PMNs, or to enumerate mononuclear leukocytes rather than PMN. Contamination of the specimen with vaginal flora can also obfuscate the detection of gonococci in endocervical mucus by Gram's stain. As discussed elsewhere, detection of Gram-negative diplococci within neutrophils in properly collected endocervical mucus is highly specific, but gonococci can be identified by Gram's stain in only about 50 to 60 percent of women with cervical gonococcal infection.

Cytopathology

An estimated 50 million cervical Pap smears are performed by physicians in private office practices in the United States each year for detection of cervical neoplasia. Cervical cytological screening also can help identify women with cervicitis who require further microbiological studies.

The correlation of cervical intraepithelial neoplasia with human papilloma virus infection is described in Chapter 59. Cytological studies in STD clinic patients and in pregnant women have shown that *C. trachomatis* infection is significantly correlated with certain other epithelial cell changes and inflammatory cell patterns.[96] The epithelial cell changes include so-called reactive changes of metaplastic cells and endocervical cells. Inflammatory changes which are significantly correlated with *C. trachomatis* infection include the presence of transformed lymphocytes and of increased numbers of histiocytes and plasma cells, as well as increased numbers of neutrophils. Large, inclusion-containing vacuoles in endocervical and metaplastic cells also are correlated with *C. trachomatis* infection, but they are relatively nonspecific and are not present in the majority of women with chlamydial infection. Use of cytopathology to identify cervical inflammation in addition to cervical neoplasia, represents a potential but little used approach to control of cervical infections.

Colposcopy

Colposcopy has been increasingly used to evaluate women who have cervical cytological smears consistent with cervical intraepithelial neoplasia, and to obtain directed biopsies of colposcopically visible lesions. Colposcopy has potential utility for use in high-risk patients (e.g., in STD clinics) for screening examinations for cervical dysplasia, and for cervical infection.[94,97] Colposcopic features of papillomavirus infection and of dysplasia are described in Chapter 59. Colposcopic features of mucopurulent cervicitis are described in the preceding and are illustrated in plates 14, 15, 16, 19, and 20 and in Fig. 57-4. The sensitivity, specificity, and predictive value of colposcopy and cervicography as screening tests for dysplasia and cervical infection require further study in various clinical settings.

Histopathology

In patients with endocervicitis due to *C. trachomatis*, cervical biopsy may show intraepithelial inclusions, which are located in columnar or metaplastic cells. Such inclusions are best demonstrated by immunofluorescence or immunoperoxidase staining (Fig. 57-7). By electron microscopy with special stains, these can be shown to contain typical elementary and reticulate bodies of *C. trachomatis* (Figs. 57-8 and 57-9). Inflammation surrounds endocervical glands in a patchy distribution, and lymphoid follicles, containing germinal center cells (transformed lymphocytes) can be identified in about two-thirds of patients (Fig. 57-10). The majority of cervical biopsy specimens from patients with chlamydia-positive endocervicitis show superficial focal endocervical microulcerations, reactive endocervical cellular changes, stromal and epithelial cellular edema, dilatation and proliferation of subepithelial capillaries, and stromal inflammatory infiltration, predominantly by plasma cells.[98] These changes resemble those described in ocular trachoma.

There is surprisingly little recent information on the histopathology of cervical infection with *N. gonorrhoeae* or of initial and recurrent episodes of HSV cervicitis. We have observed that HSV infections differ from chlamydial and gonococcal infections in showing deep, necrotic ulceration with stromal infiltration predominantly by lymphocytes; whereas chlamydial cervicitis differs from gonococcal or HSV cervicitis in showing germinal centers and stromal infiltration predominantly by plasma cells.[98]

Confirmatory microbiological studies

To provide the best guide to therapy, patient counseling, and management of sex partners, a specific microbiological diagnosis is desirable in patients with cervicitis. This can be accomplished by isolation of *N. gonorrhoeae, C. trachomatis,* HSV, or *T. vaginalis;* by immunologic detection of microbial antigens; or increasingly by use of nucleic acid probes or DNA amplification/detection methods. A Gram stain of endocervical mucus is useful in patients with suspected endocervicitis, for detection of Gram-negative diplococci associated with neutrophils, as well as for quantitation of neutrophils. However, even if gonococci are identified by Gram stain, confirmatory test for *N. gonorrhoeae* is desirable, and culture testing has the advantage of allowing tests for beta-lactamase production, and antimicrobial sensitivity. The presence of cervical lesions suggestive of HSV infection warrants confirmatory testing for HSV (see Chap. 21). Viral isolation will permit differentiation of HSV-1 from HSV-2, which has prognostic importance, since HSV-1 is less likely than HSV-2 to cause recurrent genital herpes.

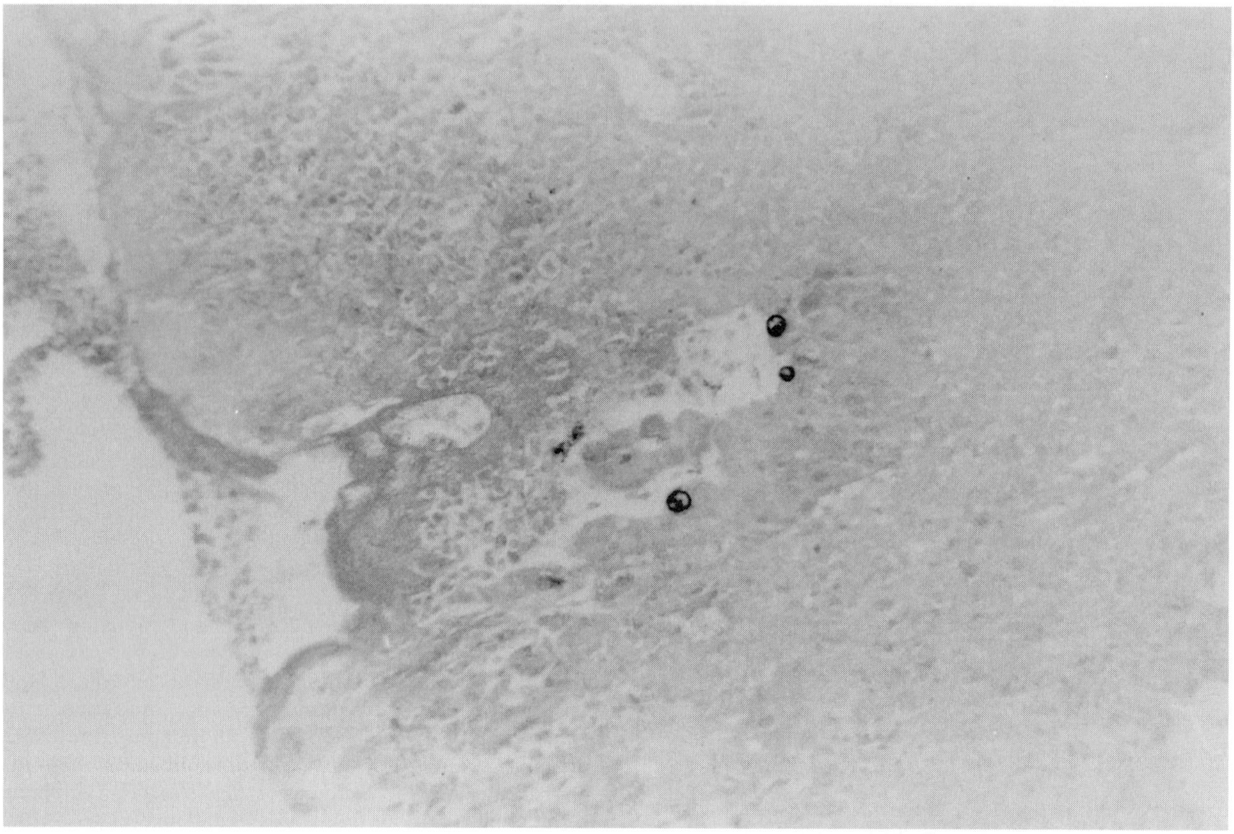

Fig. 57-7. Immunoperoxidase stain of a cervical biopsy specimen using monoclonal antibodies to *C. trachomatis* showing cervical intraepithelial chlamydial inclusions. (Courtesy of N. Kiviat.)

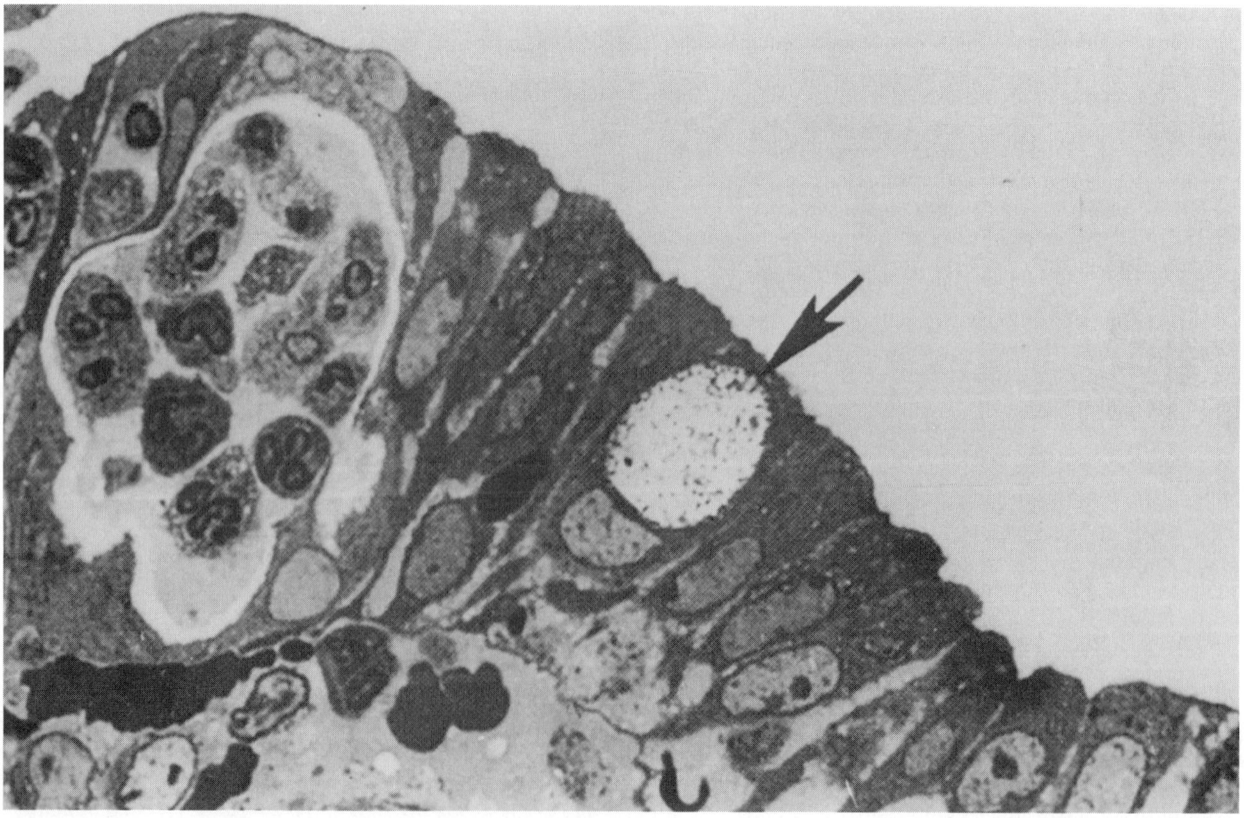

Fig. 57-8. Thin section of cervical biopsy showing a chlamydial inclusion in a columnar epithelial cell, compressing the nucleus to the base of the cell. Toluidine blue O stain, phase contrast, ×1000 magnification. (Courtesy of J Swanson.)

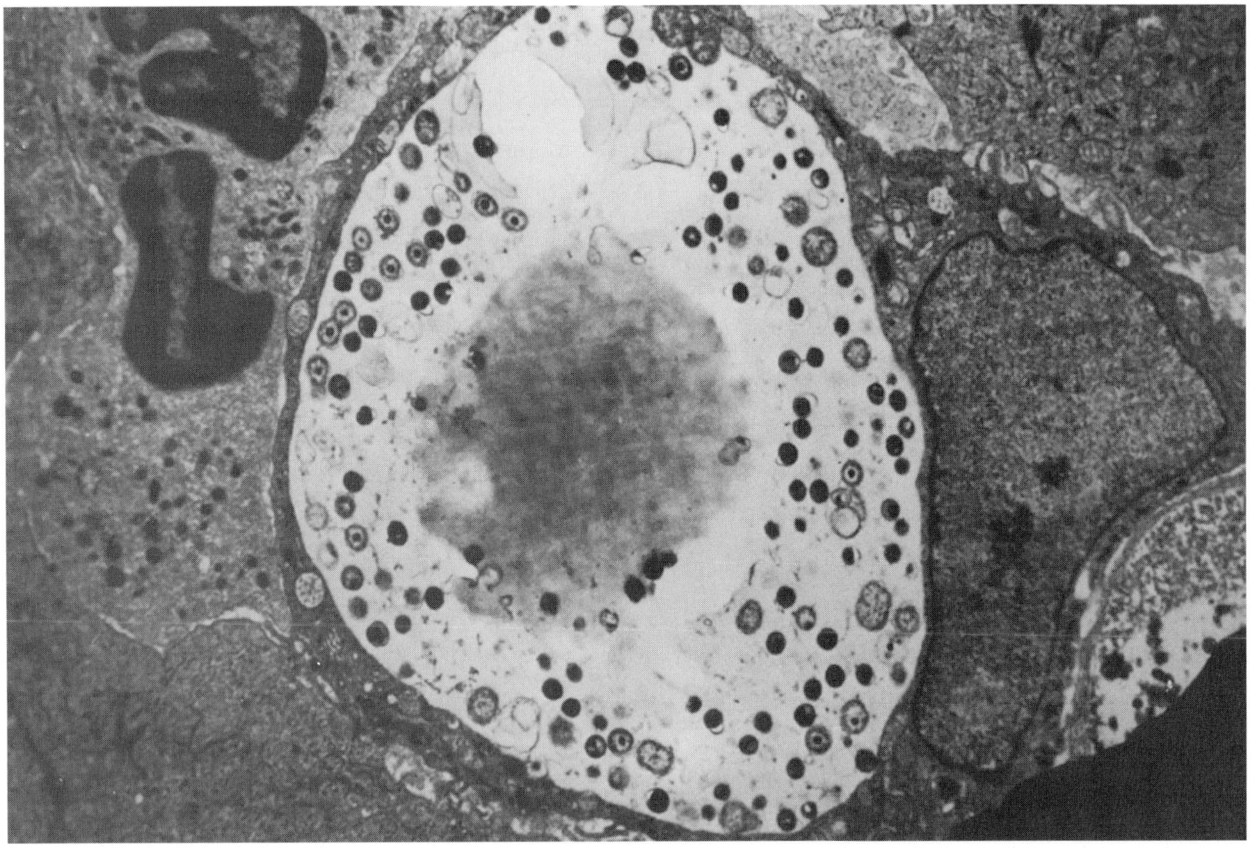

Fig. 57-9. Electron micrograph of a chlamydial inclusion in cervical biopsy tissue, showing compact elementary bodies, larger reticulate bodies, and intermediate forms that resemble bull's eyes. Uranyl acetate, lead citrate, ×12,000 magnification. (Courtesy of J. Swanson.)

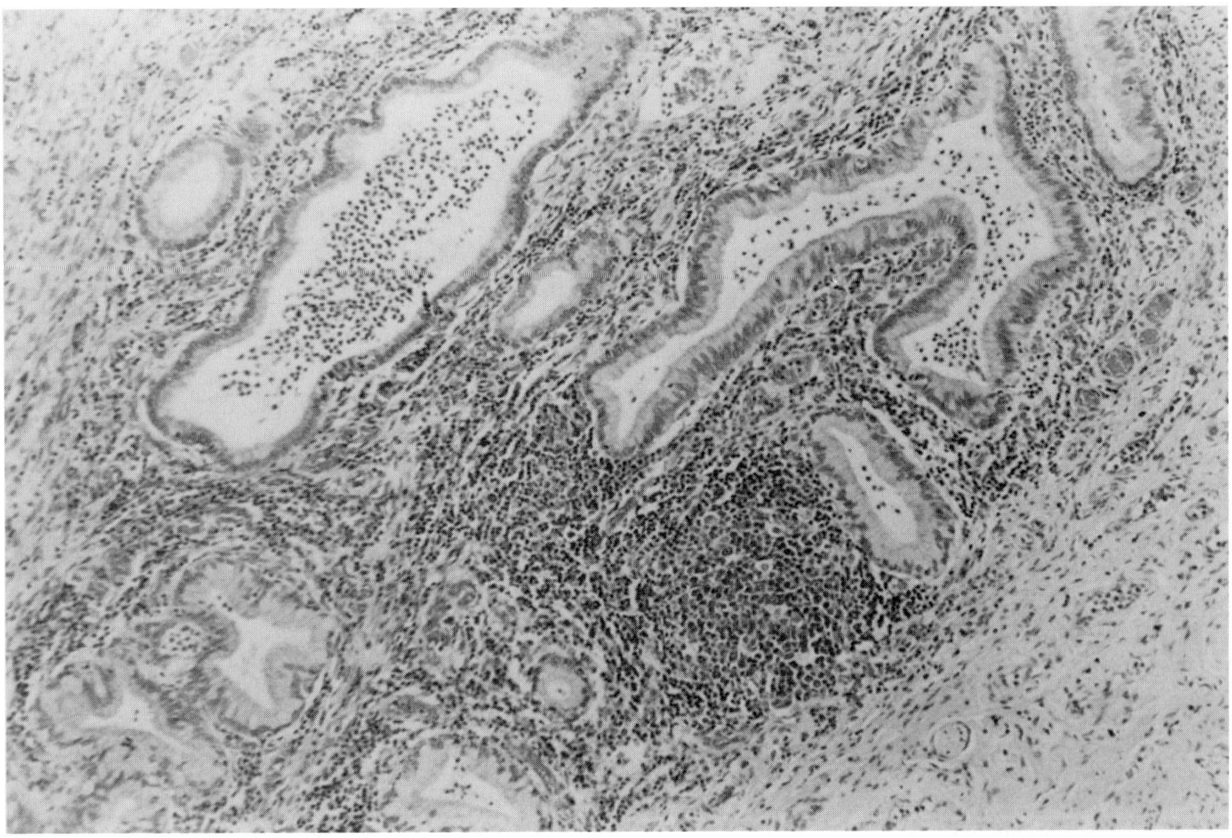

Fig. 57-10. Endocervical biopsy showing patchy periglandualr inflammation associated with chlamydial infection. Several gland lumena are filled with neutrophils, with intraepithelial infiltration by neutrophils, and are surrounded by mononuclear cells, predominantly plasma cells. A rounded germinal center containing transformed lymphocytes is present.

If colpitis macularis is seen, wet mount examination for motile trichomonads is usually positive.

TREATMENT FOR MUCOPURULENT CERVICITIS

The 1998 Centers for Disease Control guidelines for treatment of STD recommend "use of results of sensitive tests for *C. trachomatis* or *N. gonorrhoeae* (culture or nucleic acid amplification tests) to determine the need for treatment; but consideration of empiric treatment for a patient who has a suspected case of gonorrhea or chlamydial infection if the prevalences of these infections are high in the patient population, and the patient might be difficult to locate for treatment" after results of diagnostic tests become available.[99] A negative endocervical Gram stain for *N. gonorrhoeae* does not exclude gonorrhea. The guidelines also recommend that management of sex partners of women with MPC should be "appropriate for the identified or suspected STD," including examination and treatment for that STD; and further note that management of persistent MPC is unclear, since infection is not often found, and the need or benefit of further treatment is unproven.

However, among women with coexistent gonococcal and chlamydial infection of the cervix, persistence of *C. trachomatis* has been more common after single-dose ampicillin therapy than after therapy with trimethoprim-sulfamethoxazole; and persistence or development of cervicitis after therapy was correlated with persistence of *C. trachomatis.*[100] Treatment of women with gonococcal infection with 4.8 million units of procaine penicillin G plus probenecid was associated with a significantly higher rate of posttreatment cervicitis and pelvic inflammatory disease than was treatment with drugs effective against *C. trachomatis* (tetracycline or trimethoprim-sulfamethoxazole).[101] Treatment of cervical *C. trachomatis* infection with effective therapy for this pathogen (e.g., 500 mg of tetracycline hydrochloride four times daily for 7 days) has eliminated mucopurulent endocervical discharge in nearly all women within 3 weeks after completion of therapy.[102]

PREVENTION

When used correctly, the condom can probably be regarded as highly effective in preventing sexual transmission of pathogens that infect the columnar epithelium of the urethra and endocervix (e.g., *N. gonorrhoeae,* and *C. trachomatis*); moderately effective in reducing sexual transmission of pathogens that can infect the squamous epithelium of the vulva and penis (e.g., HSV, *Treponema pallidum, H. ducreyi*); and ineffective in reducing sexual transmission of pathogens that infect the cornified skin or the cutaneous appendages (e.g., *Sarcoptes scabiei, Phthirus pubis*) (see Chaps. 46 and 47). Other intravaginal barrier contraceptives, such as the diaphragm, might also be expected to reduce transmission of *N. gonorrhoeae* and *C. trachomatis,* especially when used with antimicrobial spermicides (see Chaps. 78 and 94).

OBSTETRIC, GYNECOLOGIC, AND SYSTEMIC COMPLICATIONS OF LOWER GENITAL TRACT INFECTIONS IN WOMEN

A high index of suspician for local complications or systemic disease is essential in evaluating women with symptoms or signs of lower genital tract infection.

The differential diagnosis of vulvovaginitis, or Bartholinitis includes potentially catastrophic diseases, including toxic shock syndrome (TSS) and necrotizing fasciitis of the vulva.[103–113] TSS associated with tampon use and menses is associated with temperature $>38.9°C$; systolic blood pressure <90 mmHg; rash with subsequent desquamation—especially on palms and soles; involvement of ≥ 3 of the following organ systems: GI, muscular, mucous membranes (vagina, conjunctiva, pharynx), renal, liver, blood (thrombocytopenia), or central nervous system; and negative tests for causes of similar illnesses (e.g., measles, leptospirosis, Rocky Mountain spotted fever).

Necrotizing fasciitis of the vulva arises from obstetrical or other trauma or episiotomy, vulvar abscess, or Bartholin's abscess, with predisposition for diabetic, alcoholic, or otherwise immunocompromised patients.[103–113] The process involves the superficial fascia and subcutaneous tissue (as opposed to necrotizing cellulitis, which occurs beneath deep fascia and involves muscle). Symptoms and signs often begin with tenderness, swelling, and erythema, progressing to an ecchymotic appearance with bullae and skin breakdown, eventually leading to anesthesia and loss of pain following destruction of superficial innervation. The etiology generally is either group A *Streptococcus pyogenes* or anaerobic plus/minus facultative anaerobic species that can produce gas in the tissue with foul odor. The histopathology includes polymorphonuclear infiltration, with necrosis of fat and superficial fascia, microabscesses and thrombi, and the presence of causative organisms visualized with special stains. Superantigens produced by β-hemolytic streptococci may contribute to local and systemic manifestations. Diagnosis is prompted by a high index of suspicion, and best confirmed by surgical exploration. Management is guided by the phrase, "Be bloody, bold, and resolute" with surgical debridement; together with prompt antimicrobial therapy that covers streptococci and staphylococci, Gram-negative pathogens, and anaerobes. In particular, clindamycin is commonly used, and some clinicians use hyperbaric oxygen or immunoglobulin therapy, although the benefits of these adjunctive approaches require further study.

Perhaps the most important aspect of the differential diagnosis of mucopurulent cervicitis is careful evaluation for complicating endometritis or salpingitis. As discussed in the following and in Chapter 50, endometritis, manifested by midline abdominal tenderness or menorrhagia, often with elevation of the erythrocyte sedimentation rate, C-reactive protein, or peripheral white count, and with characteristic histopathological evidence of endometritis, is often present among women with mucopurulent cervicitis. Among STD clinic patients with mucopurulent cervicitis studied at the University of Washington, at least 40 percent had histopathological evidence of plasma cell endometritis.[114] The classic study of Jacobsen and Westrom required the presence of purulent discharge in the vagina (leukocytes must outnumber other cell types) for the diagnosis of salpingitis.[115,116] It seems likely that such discharge is probably attributable to mucopurulent cervicitis in most if not all cases. Jacobsen and Westrom once stated they had never seen salpingitis laparoscopically in a patient who did not have a purulent vaginal discharge.[117] In contrast, U.S. gynecologists have not required the presence of mucopurulent cervicitis as a criterion for salpingitis, and in fact guidelines developed for diagnosis of salpingitis by a group of U.S. gynecologists and approved by the Obstetrics and Gynecology Infectious Disease Society did not include this criterion.[118]

Bacterial vaginosis may also predispose to endometritis and salpingitis caused by those pathogens characteristically found in the vagina in bacterial vaginosis.[119] Among the set of randomly selected Seattle STD clinic patients described in the preceding, bacterial vaginosis was significantly associated with a clinical diagnosis of PID; and even after adjusting for coinfections and other potential confounders, bacterial vaginosis was significantly associated with moderate to severe adnexal tenderness.[120] The role of MPC and the potential role of BV in predisposing to endometritis and salpingitis are illustrated in Fig. 57-11. Simultaneous mucopurulent cervicitis and bacterial vaginosis may be responsible for mixed tubal infections caused by the cervical pathogens *(N. gonorrhoeae, C. trachomatis),* together with the bacterial vaginosis-associated organisms. HIV infection with immunosuppression may increase the risk of PID, given cervical chlamydial or gonococcal infection or BV; and may increase the risk of tuboovarian abscess among women who develop PID. Evaluation of these and other possible models for the interrelationship between upper and lower genital tract infection could lead to clearer understanding of the pathogenesis of salpingitis. As discussed in Chapter 80, there is also a great deal of evidence for the importance of cervical and vaginal infection in causing complications of pregnancy, including chorioamnionitis and premature delivery; and evidence for a beneficial impact of detecting and treating such infections early in pregnancy. Increasing emphasis on proper management of these lower genital tract infections in pregnant women can be anticipated. Finally, there is ample evidence that mucopurulent endocervicitis, and endocervical gonococcal and chlamydial infections, are associated with increased risk of acquiring HIV infection, and with increased cervical shedding of HIV; growing evidence for an association of bacterial vaginosis with acquisition of HIV; and recent evidence that vulvovaginal candidiasis may be associated with increased risk of HIV.[121]

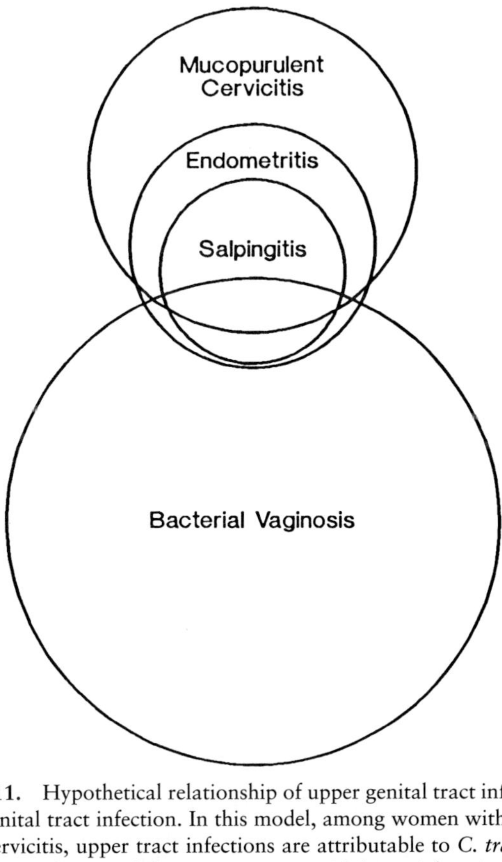

Fig. 57-11. Hypothetical relationship of upper genital tract infections to lower genital tract infection. In this model, among women with mucopurulent cervicitis, upper tract infections are attributable to *C. trachomatis* and *N. gonorrhoeae,* while among women with bacterial vaginosis, upper tract infections are attributable to bacterial vaginosis-associated vaginal organisms. Upper tract infections in women with both bacterial vaginosis and mucopurulent cervicitis may be owing to either or both sets of organisms. A second hypothesis advanced here is that salpingitis complicating mucopurulent cervicitis or bacterial vaginosis is associated with endometritis.

References

1 Schappert SM: Ambulatory care visits to physician offices, hospital outpatient departments, and emergency departments: United States, 1995, National Center for Health Statistics. *Vital Health Stat* 13(129), 1997.
2 Waters WE et al: Clinical significance Of dysuria in women. *Br Med J* 12:754, 1970.
3 Hooton TM et al: A prospective study of risk factors for symptomatic urinary tract infection in young women. *N Engl J Med* 335:468–474, 1996.
4 Fihn SD et al: Association between diaphragm use and urinary tract infection. *JAMA* 253:240, 1985.
5 Nicolle LE et al: The association of urinary tract infection with sexual intercourse. *J Infect Dis* 146:579, 1982.
6 Wong ES et al: Urinary tract infection among women attending a clinic for sexually transmitted diseases. *Sex Transm Dis* 11:18, 1984.
7 Stamm WE et al: Diagnosis of coliform infection in acutely dysuric women. *N Engl J Med* 307:463, 1982.
8 Latham RH et al: Urinary tract infections in young adult women caused by *Staphylococcus saprophyticus. JAMA* 250:3063, 1983.
9 Stamm WE et al: Causes of the acute urethral syndrome in women. *N Engl J Med* 303:409, 1980.
10 Panja SK: Urethral syndrome in women attending a clinic for sexually transmitted diseases. *Br J Vener Dis* 59:179, 1984.
11 Komaroff AL, Friedland G: The dysuria-sterile pyuria syndrome. *N Engl J Med* 3038:452, 1980.
12 Curran JW: Gonorrhea and the urethral syndrome. Sex *Transm Dis* 4:119, 1977.
13 Ryan CA et al: Risk assessment, symptoms and signs as predictors of vulvovaginal and cervical infections in urban U.S. STD clinic: Implications for use of STD algorithms. *Sex Transm Infect* 74(suppl 1): S59–S76, 1998.
14 Eckert LO et al: Vulvovaginal candidiasis: clinical manifestations, risk factors, and algorithm for case management. *OB/Gyn* 1998, in press.
15 Komaroff AL et al: Management strategies for urinary and vaginal infections. *Arch Intern Med* 138:1069, 1978.
16 Pfaller M et al: The usefulness of screening tests for pyuria in combination with culture in the diagnosis of urinary tract infection. *Diagn Microbiol Infect Dis* 6:207, 1987.
17 Wolner-Hanssen P et al: Clinical manifestations of vaginal trichomoniasis. *JAMA* 261:571, 1989.
18 Hooton TM et al: Randomized comparative trial and cost analysis of 3-day antimicrobial regimens for treatment of acute cystitis in women. *JAMA* 273:41–45, 1995.
19 Stamm WE, Hooton TM: Management of urinary tract infections in adults. *N Engl J Med* 329:1328–1334, 1993.
20 Cruickshank R, Shairnan A: The biology of the vagina in the human subject. II: The bacterial flora and secretion of the vagina at various age-periods, and their relation to glycogen in the vaginal epithelium. *J Obstet Gynaecol Br Emp* 41:208, 1934.
21 Eschenbach DA et al: Prevalence of hydrogen peroxide-producing *Lactobacillus* species in normal women and women with bacterial vaginosis. *J Clin Microbiol* 27:251, 1989.
22 Klebanoff SJ et al: Control of the microbial flora of the vagina by H_2O_2-generating lactobacilli. *J Infect Dis* 164:94–100, 1991.
23 Holmes KK et al: Vaginal redox potential in bacterial vaginosis (nonspecific vaginitis). *J Infect Dis* 152:379, 1985.
24 Hardy GC: Vaginal flora in children. *Am J Dis Child* 62:939, 1941.
25 Hammerschlag MR et al: Microbiology of the vagina in children: Normal and potentially pathogenic organisms. *Pediatrics* 62:57, 1978.
26 Gutman L, Holmes KK: Gonococcal infection, in *Infectious Diseases of the Fetus and Newborn Infant,* 3d ed, JS Remington, JO Klein (eds). Philadelphia, Saunders, 1989.
27 Paradise JE et al: Vulvovaginitis in premenarcheal girls: Clinical features and diagnostic evaluation. *Pediatrics* 70:193, 1982.

28 Heller RH et al: Vulvovaginitis in the premenarcheal child. *J Pediatr* 74:370, 1969.
29 Singleton AF: Vaginal discharge in children and adolescents. *Clin Pediatr (Phila)* 19:799, 1980.
30 Murphy TV, Nelson JD: Shigella vaginitis: Report of 28 patients and review of the literature. *Pediatrics* 63:511, 1979.
31 Schwartz RH et al: Vulvovaginitis in prepubertal girls: The importance of group A streptococcus. *South Med J* 75:446, 1982.
32 Rettig PJ, Nelson JD: Genital tract infection with *Chlamydia trachomatis* in prepubertal children. *J Pediatr* 99:206, 1981.
32 Centers for Disease Control: Nonreported sexually transmitted diseases. *Morb Mort Week Rep* 28:61, 1979.
33 Sobel JD. Vaginitis. *N Engl J Med* 337:1896–1903, 1997.
34 Larkin SM et al: Toxic shock syndrome: Clinical, laboratory, and pathologic findings in nine fatal cases. *Ann Intern Med* 96:858, 1982.
35 Paris AL et al: Pathologic findings in twelve fetal cases of toxic shock syndrome. *Ann Intern Med* 96:852, 1982.
36 Friedrich EG, Siegesmund KA: Tampon-associated vaginal ulcerations. *Obstet Gynecol* 55:149, 1980.
37 Barrett KF et al: Tampon-induced vaginal or cervical ulceration. *Am J Obstet Gynecol* 127:332, 1977.
38 Kreiss J et al: Efficacy of nonoxynol-9 contraceptive sponge use in preventing heterosexual acquisition of HIV in Nairobi prostitutes. *JAMA* 268:477–482, 1992.
39 Roddy RE et al: A dosing study of nonoxynol-9 and genital irritation. *Int J STD AIDS* 4:165–170, 1993.
40 Marquez-Monter H et al: Latrogenic vaginal membrane exfoliation. *Am J Obstet Gynecol* 110:1018–1020, 1971.
41 Kilmarx Phet al: Mucosal disruption due to use of a widely-distributed commercial vaginal product: Potential to facilitate HIV transmission. *AIDS* 12:767–773, 1998.
42 Brown RC et al: Vaginal inflammation in Africa (letter). *N Engl J Med* 327:572, 1992.
43 Irwin K et al: More on vaginal inflammation in Africa (letter). *N Engl J Med* 328:888–889, 1993.
44 Dallabetta GA et al: Traditional vaginal agents: use and association with HIV infection in Malawian women. *AIDS* 9:293–297, 1995.
45 Galask RP, Larsen B: Identifying and treating genital tract infections in postmenopausal women. *Geriatrics* 36:69, 1981.
46 Osborne NG et al: Genital bacteriology: A comparative study of premenopausal women with postmenopausal women. *Am J Obstet Gynecol* 135:195, 1979.
47 Leiblum S et al: Vaginal atrophy in the postmenopausal women. *JAMA* 249:2195, 1983.
48 Elsner P, Martins J (eds): *Vulvovaginitis*. New York, Dekker, 1993.
49 Sobel JD: Desquamative inflammatory vaginitis: A new subgroup of purulent vaginitis responsive to topical 2% clindamycin therapy. *Am J Obstet Gynecol* 171:1215–1220, 1994.
50 Elsner P, Maibach HL: Irritant and allergic contact dermatitis, in *Vulvovaginitis*, Elsner P, Martius J (eds). New York, Dekker, 1993, pp 61–82.
51 McGuire LS et al: Psychosexual functioning in symptomatic and asymptomatic women with and without signs of vaginitis. *Am J Obstet Gynecol* 137:600, 1980.
52 Ryan CA et al: Reproductive tract infections in primary health care, family planning, dermatovenereology clinics: Evaluation of syndromic management Morocco. *Sex Transm Infect* 74(suppl 1):S95–S105, 1998.
53 Amsel R et al: Nonspecific vaginitis: Diagnostic criteria and microbial and epidemiological associations. *Am J Med* 74:14, 1983.
54 Hillier SL et al: Improved reliability of diagnosis of bacterial vaginosis using an objective device for detection of elevated vaginal pH and trimethylamine (unpublished).
55 Rees E: Gonococcal bartholinitis. *J Vener Dis* 43(3):150–156, 1967.
56 Davies JA et al: solation of Chlamydia trachomatis from Bartholin's ducts. *J Vener Dis* 54(6):409–413, 1978.
57 Cheetham DR: Bartholin's cyst: Marsupialization or aspiration? *Am J Obstet Gynecol* 152(5): 569–570, 1985.
58 Lee YH et al: Microbiological investigation of Bartholin's gland abscesses and cysts. *Am J Obstet Gynecol* 129(2):150–153, 1977.
59 Westh H et al: Streptococcus pneumoniae infections of the female genital tract and in the newborn child. *Rev Infect Dis* 12(3):416–422, 1990.
60 Casin I et al: Biotypes, serotypes, and susceptibility to antibiotics of 60 Haemophilus influenzae strains from genitourinary tracts. *Genitourin Med* 64(3):185–188, 1988.
61 Christensen JJ et al: Haemophilus isolated from unusual anatomical sites. *Scand J Infect Dis* 22(4):437–444, 1990.
62 Critchlow CW et al: Determinants of cervical ectopia and of cervicitis: Age, oral contraception, specific cervical infection, smoking, and douching. *Am J Obstet Gynecol* 173(2):534–543, 1995.
63 Goldacre MJ et al: Epidemiology and clinical significance of cervical erosion in women attending a family planning clinic. *Br Med J* 11: 748, 1978.
64 Singer A: The uterine cervix from adolescence to the menopause. *J Obstet Gynaecol* 82:81, 1975.
65 Pixley E: Basic morphology of the prepubertal and youthful cervix: Topographic and histologic features. *J Reprod Med* 16:221; 1976.
66 Arya OP et al: Epidemiological and clinical correlates of chlamydial infection of the cervix. *J Vener Dis* 56:37, 1980.
67 Tait IA et al: Chlamydial infection of the cervix in contacts of men with nongonococcal urethritis. *J Vener Dis* 56:37, 1980.
68 Harrison HR et al: Cervical *Chlamydia trachomatis* infection in university women: Relationship to history, contraception, ectopy, and cervicitis. *Am J Obstet Gynecol* 153:244, 1985.
69 Rees E et al: Chlamydia in relation to cervical infection and pelvic inflammatory disease, in *Nongonococcal Urethritis and Related Infections,* Hobson D, Holmes KK (eds). Washington, American Society of Microbiology, 1977, p 67.
70 Brunham RC et al: Mucopurulent cervicitis: The ignored counterpart of urethritis in the male. N *Engl J Med* 311:1, 1984.
71 Dalabetta GA et al: Problems, solutions, and challenges in syndromic management of sexually transmitted diseases. *Sex Transm Dis* 74(suppl 1): S1–S11, 1998.
72 Handsfield HH et al: Criteria for selective screening for *Chlamydia trachomatis* infection on women attending family planning clinics. *JAMA* 255:1730, 1986.
73 Thomas T et al: Identifying cervical infections among pregnant women in Nairobi, Kenya: limitations of risk assessment and symptom-based approaches. *Genitourin Med* 72:334–338, 1996.
74 Mayaud P et al: Validation of a WHO algorithm with risk assessment for vaginal discharge in Mwanza, Tanzania. *Sex Transm Infect* 74(suppl 1):S77–S84, 1998.
75 Behets FM-T et al: Management of vaginal discharge in women treated at a Jamaican sexually transmitted disease clinic: Use of diagnostic algorithms versus laboratory testing. *Clin Inf Dis* 21:1450–1455, 1995.
76 Lefevre JC et al: Lower genital tract infections in women: Comparison of clinical and epidemiologic findings with microbiology. *Sex Transm Dis* 15:110–113, 1988.
77 Mosure DJ et al: A re-evaluation of selective screening criteria for women attending family planning clinics in the US, in *Chlamydial Infections*, Stephens RS et al (eds). San Francisco, International Chlamydia Symposium, 1998, pp 333–336.
78 Sellors JW, Walter SD: A new visual indicator of chlamydial cervicitis?, in *Chlamydial Infections,* Stephens RS et al (eds). San Francisco, Proceedings of the Ninth International Symposium on Human Chlamydial Infection, 1998, pp 337–340.
79 Alary M et al: Evaluation of clinical algorithms for the diagnosis of gonococcal and chlamydial infections among men with urethral discharge or dysuria and women with vaginal discharge in Benin. *Sex Transm Infect* 74(suppl 1):S44–S49, 1998.
80 Daly CC et al: Validation of the WHO diagnostic algorithm and development of an alternative scoring system for the management of women presenting with vaginal discharge in Malawi. *Sex Transm Infect* 74(suppl 1):S50–S58, 1998.

81 Sánchez SE et al: Rapid and inexpensive approaches to managing abnormal vaginal discharge or lower abdominal pain: An evaluation in women attending gynecology and family planning clinics in Peru. *Sex Transm Infect* 74(suppl 1):S85–S94, 1998.
82 Diallo MO et al: Evaluation of simple diagnostic algorithms for *Neisseria gonorrhoeae* and *Chlamydia trachomatis* cervical infections in female sex workers in Abidjan, Côte d'Ivoire. *Sex Transm Infect* 74(suppl 1):S106–S111, 1998.
83 N'Doye I et al: Diagnosis of sexually transmitted infections in female prostitutes in Dakar, Senegal. *Sex Transm Infect* 74(suppl 1):S112–S117, 1998.
84 Wi T et al: Syndromic approach to detection of gonococcal and chlamydial infections among female sex workers in two Philippine cities. *Sex Transm Infect* 74(suppl 1):S118–S123, 1998.
85 Kapiga SH et al: Evaluation of sexually transmitted diseases diagnostic algorithms among family planning clients in Dar es Salaam, Tanzania. *Sex Transm Infect* 74(suppl 1):S132–S138, 1998.
86 Mayaud P et al: Risk scores to detect cervical infections in urban antenatal clinic attenders in Mwanza, Tanzania. *Sex Transm Infect* 74(suppl 1):S139–S146, 1998.
87 Schneider H et al: Screening for sexually transmitted disease in rural South African women. *Sex Transm Infect* 74(suppl 1):S123–S127, 1998.
88 Behets FM-T et al: Sexually transmitted disease are common in women attending Jamaican family planning clinics and appropriate detection tools are lacking. *Sex Transm Infect* 74(suppl 1):S123–S127, 1998.
89 Linder LE et al: Clinical characteristics of women with chlamydial cervicitis. *J Reprod Med* 33:684–690, 1988.
90 Schafer M-A et al: *Chlamydia trachomatis:* Important relationships to race, contraception, lower genital tract infection, and Papanicolaou smear. *J Pediatr* 104:141, 1984.
91 Kent GP et al: Screening for *Chlamydia trachomatis* infection in a sexually transmitted disease clinic: Comparison of diagnostic tests with clinical and historical risk factors. *Sex Transm Dis* 15:51, 1988.
92 Swinker ML et al: Prevalence of *Chlamydia trachomatis* cervical infection in a college gynecology clinic: Relationship to other infections and clinical features. *Sex Transm Dis* 15:133, 1988.
93 Paavonen J et al: Etiology of cervical inflammation. *Am J Obstet Gynecol* 154:556, 1986.
94 Paavonen J et al: Colposcopic manifestations of cervical and vaginal infections. *Obstet Gynecol Survey* 43:373, 1988.
95 Koutsky LA et al: The frequency of unrecognized type 2 herpes simplex virus infection among women: Implications for the control of herpes. *Sex Transm Dis* 17:90–94, 1990.
96 Kiviat N et al: Cytologic manifestations of cervical and vaginal infections. I. Epithelial and cellular inflammatory changes. *JAMA* 253: 989, 1985.
97 Wilson JD: Value of colposcopy in genitourinary departments. *Genitourin Med* 64:100, 1988.
98 Kiviat N et al: Endometrial histopathology in patients with culture-proven upper genital tract infection and laparoscopically diagnosed acute salpingitis. *Am J Surg Pathol* 14:167–175, 1990.
99 Centers for Disease Control and Prevention: 1998 Guidelines for Treatment of Sexually Transmitted Disease. *Morb Mort Week Rep* 47:RR-1, 1997.
100 Brunham RC et al: Treatment of concomitant *Neisseria gonorrhoeae* and *Chlamydia trachomatis* infections in women: Comparison of trimethoprim-sulfamethoxazole with ampicillin-probenecid. *Rev Infect Dis* 4:91, 1983.
101 Stamm WE et al: Effect of *Neisseria gonorrhoeae* treatment regimens on simultaneous infection with *Chlamydia trachomatis. N Engl J Med* 310:545, 1984.
102 Brunham RC et al: Therapy of cervical chlamydial infection. *Ann Intern Med* 97:216, 1982.
103 Roberts DB, Hester LL Jr: Progressive synergistic bacterial gangrene arising from abscesses of the vulva and Batholin's gland duct. *Am J Obstet Gynecol* 114:285, 1972.
104 Golde S, Ledger WJ: Necrotizing fasciitis in postpartum patients. *Obstet Gynecol* 50:670, 1977.
105 Pruyn SC: Acute necrotizing fasciitis of the endopelvic fascia. *Obstet Gynecol* 52(suppl):S2–S4, 1978.
106 Addison WA et al: Necrotizing fasciitis of vulvar origin in diabetic patients. *Obstet Gynecol* 63:473–479, 1984.
107 Sutton GP et al: Group B streptococcal necrotizing fasciitis arising from an epistotomy. *Obstet Gynecol* 66:733–736, 1985.
108 Charles D, Larsen B: Streptococcal puerperal sepsis and obstetric infections. *Rev Infect Dis* 8:411–422, 1986.
109 Kruikshank SH, McLaughlin L; A de novo case of vulvar synergistic necrotizing fasciitis. *Obstet Gynecol* 69:516–518, 1987.
110 Roberts DB: Necrotizing fasciitis of the vulva. *Am J Obstet Gynecol* 157:568–571, 1987.
111 Hoffman MS, Turnquist D: Necrotizing fasciitis of the vulva during chemotherapy. *Obstet Gynecol* 74:483–484, 1989.
112 Frohlich EP, Schein M: Necrotizing fasciitis arising from Bartholin's abscess. *Isr J Med Sci* 25:644–647, 1989.
113 Stamenkovic I, Lew PD: Early recognition of potentially fatal necrotizing fasciitis. The use of frozen-section biopsy. *N Engl J Med* 310: 1689, 1984.
114 Paavonen J: Prevalence and manifestations of endometritis among women with cervicitis. *Am J Obstet Gynecol* 152:280, 1985.
115 Westrom L: Diagnosis, etiology and prognosis of acute salpingitis. Thesis. Student littatur, Lund, Sweden, 1976.
116 Westrom L: Incidence, prevalence and trends of acute pelvic inflammatory disease and its consequences in industrialized countries. *Am J Obstet Gynecol* 138:880, 1980.
117 Jacobsen L: Differential diagnosis of acute pelvic inflammatory disease. *Am J Obstet Gynecol* 138:1006, 1980.
118 Hager DW et al: Criteria for diagnosis and grading of salpingitis. *Obstet Gynecol* 61:113, 1983.
119 Hiller SL et al: Role of bacterial vaginosis-associated microorganisms in endometritis. *Am J Obs Gyn* 175:435–441, 1996.
120 Eschenbach DA et al: Diagnosis and clinical manifestations of bacterial vaginosis. *Am J Obstet Gynecol* 158:819, 1988.
123 Martin HL et al: Vaginal lactobacilli, microbial flora, and risk of HIV-1 and STD acquisition, (submitted).
122 Grosskurth H et al: Impact of improved treatment of sexually transmitted diseases on HIV infection in rural Tanzania: Randomised controlled trial. *Lancet* 346(8974):530–536, 1995.

Chapter 58

Pelvic inflammatory disease

Lars Weström
David Eschenbach

DEFINITION

Pelvic inflammatory disease (PID) comprises a spectrum of upper genital tract inflammatory disorders among women that includes any combination of endometritis, salpingitis, tubo-ovarian abscess, and pelvic peritonitis.[1] Use of the term *pelvic inflammatory disease* is restricted to infections of the upper genital tract caused by microorganisms that ascend from the cervix or vagina; the term excludes blood-born infections such as tuberculosis. Infections following delivery or induced abortion also are categorized separately as puerperal or postabortion infection.

Salpingitis, or infection of the fallopian tubes, is the most important feature of PID, and the terms *PID* and *salpingitis* are often used synonymously. In this chapter, we reserve the term *salpingitis* for women with visual confirmation of fallopian-tube infection. About two-thirds of women with a clinical diagnosis of PID in fact have salpingitis, while the remaining one-third have either other conditions or normal pelvic organs when laparoscopy is used to confirm a clinical diagnosis.[2] A small proportion of women with clinical PID have infection and inflammation of the endometrium and/or blood vessels and lymphatics adjacent to the uterus, but without visually recognized salpingitis.[3]

Women with salpingitis/PID present with a vast array of clinical manifestations that range from virtually none to severe. No symptom, clinical sign, or laboratory result or combination thereof is pathognomonic for PID. In most women with mild or uncharacteristic manifestations, the diagnosis of salpingitis is just not made. In fact, about two-thirds of cases of PID probably go unrecognized.[4] Attempts have been made to sharpen the diagnostic criteria for PID and to grade the severity of clinical manifestations,[5,6] but there are no accepted criteria or classification in the clinical diagnosis of salpingitis/PID. Chronic PID is an even more poorly defined entity that often designates patients with chronic pain or infertility caused by pelvic adhesions and other abnormalities from a prior episode of PID. Patients with chronic PID can have viable microorganisms sequestered in tissue or localized in walled-off tissue, but other patients have sterile areas of inflammation. Thus, the term *PID* has different meanings in various settings.

HISTORICAL REVIEW

In Ancient Greece, Aetius described drainage of pus through the vagina, indicating that early physicians not only diagnosed pelvic abscesses but also provided surgical treatment.[7] In the seventeenth and eighteenth centuries direct observations and dissection of human cadavers became acceptable, and in 1683 Mauriceau described inflammatory tumors of the uterine adnexa in puerperal infections.[8] In the 1700s, "adnexitis" was described in autopsy reports.

Noeggerath, in 1876, was the first physician who linked sexual transmission with infertility,[9] three years before Neisser identified the gonococcus. In the late nineteenth century, advances in bacteriology, pharmacology, anesthesiology, asepsis, and surgery opened the era of modern medicine. By the turn of the century, a number of important observations had been made with respect to PID; some immediately increased our understanding, but others were not fully understood until half a century later. Von Bumm established the sequence of cervical gonorrhea progressing to endometritis, salpingitis, and pelvic peritonitis in 1887.[10] Between 1892 and 1914, Wertheim, Schauta, Kelly, Martin, Schottmüller, and Barfuth isolated a variety of aerobic and anaerobic bacteria from the fallopian tubes and pelvic cavities of women with PID.[11]

In 1898, Nocard and Roux identified the causative organism of pleuropneumonia in cattle, later to be named *mycoplasmas*.[12] Kelling described the fundamentals of laparoscopy in 1902, and by 1910–12 Jacobaeus reported laparoscopy in humans.[13] In 1907, Halberstaedter and von Prowazek described inclusion conjunctivitis in experimental infections in primates,[14] and in 1910 Fritsch, Hofstätter, and Lindner[15] linked inclusion conjunctivitis with genital infection, later recognized as chlamydia. Successful attempts at conservative treatment of PID began in the 1920s[16] and were generally accepted by the 1930s. Sulfonamides were first used to treat PID in the 1930s.

In 1937, mycoplasmas were first isolated from the human genital tract.[17] By 1946, Falk demonstrated the ascending route of spread in PID,[18] and Ruddock in the United States and Palmaer in Paris pioneered modern laparoscopy.[13] *Chlamydia trachomatis* was identified by T'ang and co-workers in 1957,[19] and in 1959 the organism was isolated from the human genital tract.[20]

During the 1960s, laparoscopy was systematically used to provide an accurate diagnosis of salpingitis, and the vast array of clinical presentations became apparent.[2] Laparoscopy made possible accurate studies of the microbial etiology of salpingitis, and laparoscopy became the gold standard for diagnosis and research in PID. Mycoplasmas in 1970[21] and chlamydia in 1977[22,23] were isolated from the fallopian tubes of women with PID, and in 1975 the polymicrobial etiology of PID was described.[24] Echoing the theories of Noeggerath, Weström in 1975[25] quantitated the amount of infertility and ectopic pregnancy following salpingitis. During the 1980s and first half of the 1990s, our understanding of PID has further increased due to progress in microbiology, immunology, epidemiology, experimental animal models, and social and behavioral sciences.

MICROBIAL ETIOLOGY

Pelvic inflammatory disease is caused when microorganisms ascend from the vagina/cervix into the endometrium, fallopian tubes, and contiguous structures. Since a large number of species colonize the vagina and cervix, the microbial etiology of PID is best established by direct culture of upper genital tract tissue. Specimens potentially contaminated by vaginal/cervical flora include endometrium obtained by transcervical biopsy,[26,27] peritoneal fluid obtained by cul-de-sac puncture,[28] or abscess material from transvaginal drainage.[26] Direct uncontaminated specimens can be obtained from the pelvic cavity at laparoscopy or laparotomy.[21,26,29,30] Specimens from the cul-de-sac or peritoneal cavity may also contain microorganisms not present in infected tubes because of different competition between microorganisms at various sites.[30,31] Furthermore, comparisons among studies is difficult because of differences in the sample method (tissue biopsy, scraping, swabbing, aspiration), transport (media, time, temperature), laboratory identification techniques, and number of species sought.[26]

Isolates from the upper genital tract and abdominal cavity in PID are usually classified into sexually transmitted organisms (those never normally isolated from the genital tracts) and endogenous organisms (those often present in the lower genital tract), some of which may also be sexually transmitted.[31]

SEXUALLY TRANSMITTED ORGANISMS

Neisseria gonorrhoeae and *Chlamydia trachomatis* both cause PID, while the role of genital mycoplasmas remains unclear. Herpes simplex virus,[21,32] cytomegalovirus, and *Trichomonas vaginalis*[29,33] have been isolated from the pelvis, but systematic studies provide no convincing evidence that viral pathogens or protozoa cause PID.

Isolation of more than one sexually transmitted pathogen from the lower genital tract is common in acute PID. From one-fourth to three-fourths of young women with acute PID have *N. gonorrhoeae* and/or *C. trachomatis* isolated from the lower genital tract, although these bacteria are isolated less frequently from the upper genital tract of women with PID.[21,24,29,30,34,35] *Mycoplasma hominis*, *Ureaplasma urealyticum*, and *T. vaginalis* are also commonly present in the lower genital tract in PID.

N. gonorrhoeae

N. gonorrhoeae is the "classic" bacterial cause of PID. N. gonorrhoeae has been recovered from the cervix, endometrium,[31,36] fallopian tubes,[29,32,34,36] peritoneal fluid,[10,11,24,36] and serosal surface of the liver[37–39] in women with PID. The organism has not been isolated from normal fallopian tubes. Koch's postulates, establishing the organism as the causative agent of disease, have not been fulfilled because of difficulty of infecting animals with *N. gonorrhoeae*.[40] *N. gonorrhoeae* causes a cytotoxic effect,[41,42] and gonococcal endotoxin causes damage of tubal cilia in human organ culture experiments.[43]

Ten to 19 percent of women with *N. gonorrhoeae* in the cervix have clinical signs of acute PID.[44–46] Certain characteristics of gonococci appear related to a propensity to cause tubal infections rather than remain in the cervix, specific auxotypes and penicillin resistance,[47,48] the formation of transparent colonies on agar,[49,50] and certain serovars.[50,51] Women with *N. gonorrhoeae* and PID tend to have the onset of pain in the first part of the menstrual cycle, suggesting a rapid ascent of *N. gonorrhoeae* into the upper genital tract after loss of cervical mucus at menses.[52] In women with cervical *N. gonorrhoeae* and PID, the rate of recovery of gonococci from the upper genital tract is inversely related to the

Table 58-1. Rates of Isolation of *Chlamydia trachomatis* and *Neisseria gonorrhoeae* from the Cervix, and *N. gonorrhoeae* from Fallopian Tubes among Women with Acute Pelvic Inflammatory Disease.

Study	Number of patients	Cervical infection: *C. trachomatis*	Cervical infection: *N. gonorrhoeae*	Tubal/Abdominal infection: *C. trachomatis*	Tubal/Abdominal infection: *N. gonorrhoeae*
Henry-Suchet et al., France, 1980	17	6/16 (38%)	0/4	4 (24%)* 4/6†	1/4 (25%)* 0/4†
Møller et al., Denmark, 1981	166	37 (22%)	9 (5%)		
Mårdh et al., Sweden, 1981	60	23 (38%)	4 (7%)		
Gjønnaess et al., Norway, 1982	65	26/56 (46%)	5 (8%)	5/31 (16%) 4/5	0/65 0/5
Bevan et al., England, 1995	104	37 (36%)	14 (13%)	13 (13%) 13/37	3 (3%) 3/14
Mårdh et al., Sweden, 1977	53	19 (36%)	11 (17%)	6/20 (30%) 6/7	1/14 (7%) 1/2
Adler et al., England, 1982	78	4 (5%)	14 (18%)		
Ripa et al., Sweden, 1980	206	52/156 (33%)	39 (19%)		
Osser and Persson, Sweden, 1982	209	52/111 (47%)	41 (20%)		
Paavonen, Finland, 1979	106	27 (25%)	27 (25%)		
Paavonen et al., Finland, 1981	101	32 (32%)	25 (25%)		
Paavonen et al., Finland, 1980	228	69 (30%)	60 (26%)		
Eilard et al., Sweden, 1976	22	6 (27%)	7 (32%)	2 (9%) 1/6	1/22 (5%) 1/7
Bowie and Jones, Canada, 1981	43	22 (51%)	15 (35%)		
Livengood et al., United States, 1992	23	6 (26%)	9 (39%)	1 (4%) 1/6	6 (26%) 6/9
Eschenbach et al., United States, 1975	204	20/100 (20%)	90 (44%)	1/54 (2%)	7/54 (13%) 7/21
Sweet et al., United States, 1981	39	2 (5%)	18 (46%)	0/35 0/2	8/35 (23%) 8/18
Cunningham et al., United States, 1978	104	N.D.	56 (54%)		30/104 (29%) 30/56
Soper et al., United States, 1992	36	6 (17%)	25 (69%)	0 0/6	12 (37%) 12/25
Thompson et al., United States, 1980	30	3 (10%)	24 (80%)	3/30 (10%)	10/30 (33%) 10/24
Totals	1,904	449/1,528 (29%)	493/1,891 (26%)	35/372 (9%)* 29/75 (39%)†	79/491 (16%)* 78/185 (42%)†

* Isolation (%) of *C. trachomatis* and *N. gonorrhoeae* from the peritoneum of the total number of women studied.
† Isolation of *C. trachomatis* from the abdomen of those with *C. trachomatis* cultured from the cervix and isolation of *N. gonorrhoeae* from the abdomen of those with *N. gonorrhoeae* cultured from the cervix.
N.D. = Not Done

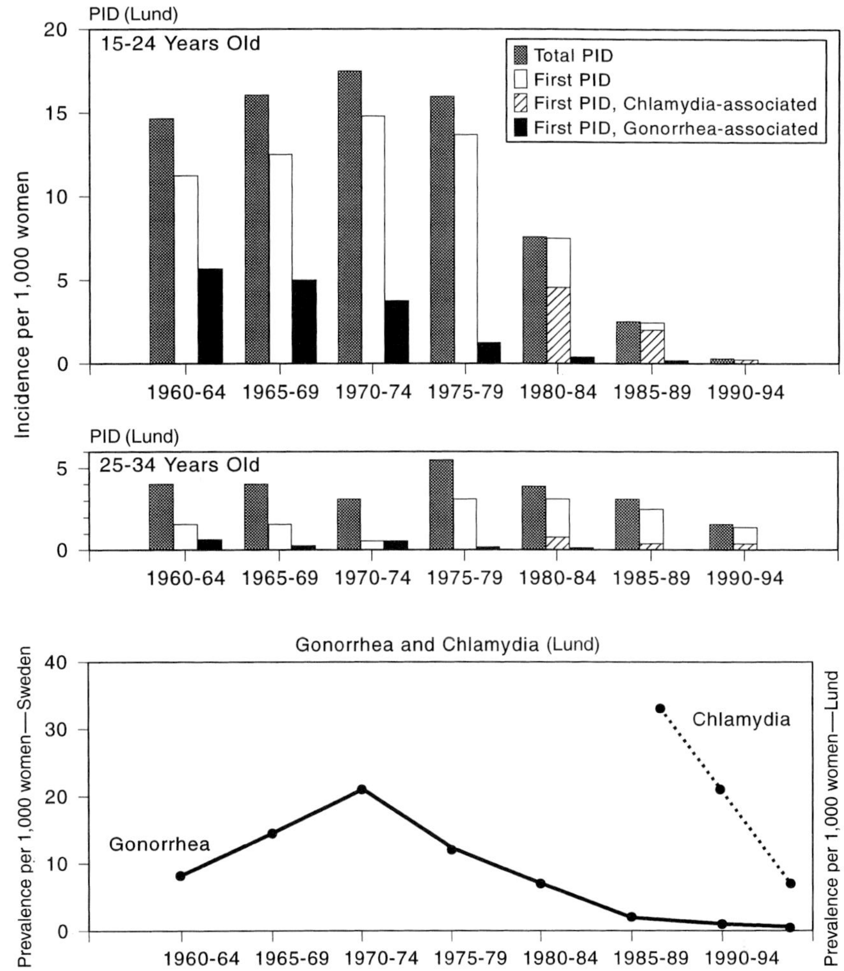

Fig. 58-1. Mean annual incidences of PID in women 15–24 and 25–34 years of age during five-year periods 1960–64 through 1990–94 in the city of Lund, Sweden, as well as the prevalences of gonorrhoea in Swedish women less than 25 years of age from 1960 to 1994 and of genital chlamydial infection in women in Lund from 1987 to 1994.

duration of pain,[29,53,54] possibly because *N. gonorrhoeae* causes severe symptoms that rapidly lead to a diagnosis, or because *N. gonorrhoeae* may gradually disappear from the fallopian tubes in the presence of inflammation, or both.

In Table 58–1 42 percent of 185 women with cervical *N. gonorrhoeae* and PID have had *N. gonorrhoeae* isolated from fallopian-tube or cul-de-sac specimens.[22–24,52,55–69] Many women with PID and *N. gonorrhoeae* also have *C. trachomatis* in the cervix, however, or they have other bacteria isolated from the fallopian tubes or peritoneum.[24] Thus, mixed infections are common with gonorrhea.

In populations with a high endemic rate of gonorrhea, a high proportion of PID is associated with gonorrhea. *N. gonorrhoeae* has been isolated from the lower genital tract in up to 70 to 80 percent of women with acute PID (see Table 58–1).[68,69] In regions with reliable statistics, the proportion of PID associated with gonorrhea increased in the 1960s, leveled, and then decreased in the 1980s, paralleling changes in the incidence of gonorrhea (Fig. 58–1).[45,46,70] In many U.S. populations, gonorrhea is currently found in 40 to 50 percent or more of patients with PID (Table 58–1); however, in populations without endemic gonorrhea, as Sweden, less than 5 percent of young women with PID have gonorrhea (Fig. 58–1).[46,70]

C. trachomatis

C. trachomatis is now established as an important etiological agent in acute and chronic PID. *C. trachomatis* has been isolated from the cervix, endometrium,[27,70–73] fallopian tubes,[22,23,60,73,74] and the liver capsule of women with PID.[75] Specific serum IgM and IgG antibody and titers increase significantly with primary PID associated with chlamydia.[24] In experimental infection of human fallopian-tube organ culture, *C. trachomatis* can be recovered for 5–7 days, and inclusions containing all forms of chlamydia are present in ciliated and nonciliated cells for 72 hours after inoculation.[76,77] Disruption of cell junctions and rupture of the cell occur with the release of elementary bodies.[77] Experimental chlamydial infection in primates produces salpingitis.[78,79] A single inoculation of *C. trachomatis* directly into the oviducts produces infection for several days, after which the organism is no longer recovered and inflammation subsides. The cellular response is complex and severe inflammation can result, however, particularly with repetitive *C. trachomatis* infection. Repeat infection contributes to development of a delayed hypersensitivity response, which appears important in chlamydial disease and its sequelae.[80]

In contrast to gonorrhea, and often despite severe tubal damage, chlamydial salpingitis may produce only mild clinical manifestations and can even be asymptomatic (see below). The age-distribution of women with chlamydia-associated PID parallels that of uncomplicated cervical chlamydia in the same population, with a peak incidence in sexually active teenagers. An estimated 10 percent of *C. trachomatis* cervical infections ascend to cause PID, although this proportion is less well established than with *N. gonorrhoeae*. In a population-based study, the mean annual incidence of infection per 1,000 sexually active teenagers was 97 for genital chlamydial infection and 14 for symptomatic PID associated with chlamydia; among women aged 25–29, the incidence was 46 for genital chlamydial infection and 3 for chlamydial PID.[81]

C. trachomatis was isolated from the cervix of 29 percent of the 1,528 women with PID in Table 1 (range 5–51 percent); in comparison, *N. gonorrhoeae* was isolated from the cervix of 26 percent of the 1,891 women (range 5–80 percent). Patients in studies with high rates of cervical *C. trachomatis* tended to have low rates of cervical *N. gonorrhoeae* and vice versa. About 20 to 30 percent of patients with *C. trachomatis* also have *N. gonorrhoeae*, however, and a similar percent with *N. gonorrhoeae* have *C. trachomatis*.[58,61–64,82] The combined results of most studies from Europe during the 1970s and 1980s indicated that *C. trachomatis* was isolated from 25 to 50 percent of women with PID while *N. gonorrhoeae* was found in 5 to 25 percent. American studies at the time showed higher rates of gonorrhea and lower rates of chlamydial infection than the European studies. A fourfold or greater change in IgG antibody titer to *C. trachomatis* was present in 25 percent of women with laparoscopically verified PID.[24,82]

In acute salpingitis, *C. trachomatis* has been isolated from the tubes/abdomen in 39 percent of those with cervical *C. trachomatis* infection, a percentage similar to that for recovery of N. gonorrhoeae from tubes of PID patients with gonorrhea (see Table 58-1). Recovery of *C. trachomatis* from tubes is apparently unaffected by the duration of symptoms, in contrast to the decreasing recovery of *N. gonorrhoeae* from tubes with increased duration of pain. As opposed to *N. gonorrhoeae, C. trachomatis*, has been isolated from the fallopian tubes of women with "chronic PID"[31,83–85] and occasionally from normal-appearing fallopian tubes.[85,86] *C. trachomatis* is uncommonly recovered from the cul-de-sac.[86,87]

Mycoplasmas and *Ureaplasmas*

Mycoplasma hominis has been isolated from the cervix, the endometrium,[88] and the fallopian tubes of women with laparoscopically verified salpingitis (Table 58-2).[21,24,57,69,89] The organism has not been isolated from normal fallopian tubes.[21,88] Direct inoculation of *M. hominis* into the oviducts of grivet monkeys provoked oviductal infection,[90,91] and a cytopathogenic effect was demonstrated after inoculation of human fallopian-tube organ culture with *M. hominis*.[92]

M. hominis is recovered frequently from the cervix[21,88,93–94] but infrequently (0–17 percent) from the upper genital tract of women with PID (see Table 58-2). Twenty to 40 percent of women with acute PID had significant change of antibody to *M. hominis* demonstrated by enzyme immunoassay (see Table 58-2).[94–6] In contrast to PID associated with *N. gonorrhoeae* and *C. trachomatis*, PID associated with *M. hominis* was evenly distributed in all age groups.[93]

On the other hand, *M. hominis* is frequently isolated from the lower genital tract of sexually active women,[21,97] and it is associated with bacterial vaginosis (BV) (see Chap. 42). Bacterial vaginosis has been implicated as a risk factor for PID. Thus, *M. hominis* may be either a risk marker or an independent risk factor in the pathogenesis of PID.

Mycoplasma genitalium has produced oviductal infections in marmosets, grivet monkeys, and baboons.[98,99] *M. genitalium* adheres to human fallopian-tube epithelial cells in organ cultures.[100] *M. genitalium* has been demonstrated by polymerase chain reaction (PCR) in cervical samples from 25 percent of women attending a Genito-Urinary-Medicine clinic.[101] A fourfold or greater increase in the serum antibody titers to *M. genitalium* was demonstrated in one-third of women with acute PID and no evidence of *N. gonorrhoeae*, *C. trachomatis*, or *M. hominis* infection.[102] These results were not subsequently confirmed, however, [103] and PCR studies for *M. genitalium* on tubal specimens of women with salpingitis could help further assess the role of *M. genitalium* in PID.

Ureaplasma urealyticum has been isolated from the fallopian tubes from 2 to 20 percent of women with PID (see Table 58-2), and a significant increase of serum metabolism-inhibiting antibody to *U. urealyticum* was documented in 20 percent of women with acute PID.[24] Attempts to produce tubal infection in monkeys with *U. urealyticum* have failed.[91] *U. urealyticum* is commonly found in the lower genital tract of sexually active women, and isolation rates are similar in healthy women and women with PID.[21,88,97,104] The role, if any, of *U. urealyticum* in PID appears minimal.

Table 58-2. Evidence of Genital Mycoplasma Infection among Women with Acute Salpingitis.

Study	Cervical isolation (%)	Tubal isolation (%)	Antibody titer change (%)
M. hominis			
Sweet et al., United States, 1979	73	4	
Eschenbach et al., United States, 1975	72	4	20
Mårdh and Weström, Sweden, 1970	62	8	
Thompson et al., United States, 1980	60	17	
Møller et al., Denmark, 1981	55		30
Mårdh et al., Sweden, 1981			40
Bevan et al., England, 1995	38	0	
U. urealyticum			
Eschenbach et al., United States, 1975	81	2	18
Mårdh and Weström, Sweden, 1970	56	4	
Sweet et al., United States, 1979	54	15	
Thompson et al., United States, 1980	33	20	
Henry-Suchet et al., France, 1980	24	17	
Sweet et al., United States, 1981		9	

Human immunodeficiency virus

There is no evidence that the human immunodeficiency virus (HIV) infection per se causes PID. Infection with HIV does influence the risk clinical manifestations of PID, however, as discussed below in the section Epidemiology and Risk Factors.

ENDOGENOUS AND MISCELLANEOUS ORGANISMS

Facultative and anaerobic bacteria are commonly isolated alone or together with *N. gonorrhoeae* or *C. trachomatis* from the endometrium, fallopian tubes, cul-de-sac, and/or abscesses of women with acute PID.[21,24,30,52,105–108] *Bacteroides* spp. (*disiens, fragilis, melaninogenicus*), *Prevotella bivius, Escherichia coli, Gardnerella vaginalis, Peptostreptococcus* spp. (*asaccharolyticus, anaerobius, magnus*), staphylococci, group B-D streptococci, *Actinomyces israeli, Campylobacter fetus*, clostridiae, and others have all been isolated from the upper genital tract of women with acute PID. Most of these bacteria are also found in normal vaginal flora, and several occur more often and in large concentrations among women with bacterial vaginosis (BV). Even respiratory pathogens such as *Haemophilus influenzae, Streptococcus pneumoniae*, and group A streptococci[24,30,31] are occasionally isolated from the tubes in salpingitis. Often more than one species from the vaginal flora are isolated from the patient, leading to the concept of "polymicrobial" PID.[24]

The microbial species associated with BV are frequently recovered from upper genital tract or cul-de-sac specimens of women with acute PID and deserve special mention.[109] Bacterial vaginosis has been associated with a clinical diagnosis of PID[110] and with histologic endometritis.[111] Among patients with a clinical diagnosis of PID, "BV-associated" bacteria were associated with histologic endometritis even when controlling for gonorrhea or chlamydia.[112] "BV-associated" bacteria have also been isolated from the upper genital tract of women with gonorrhea and PID in a polymicrobial infection.[24,105]

Isolation of "endogenous" bacteria from the upper genital tract appears more common in older women[29] and may be associated with severe suppurative disease,[24] IUD use,[113] recurrent PID,[52] and tuboovarian abscess.[24,33,105] Tuboovarian abscesses virtually always contain a mixture of facultative and anaerobic bacterial species.[114] In contrast, women with early mild salpingitis at laparoscopy generally have no anaerobic bacteria recovered from the upper genital tract.[31]

These observations could indicate a dynamic infectious process, evolving over time, in which a large proportion of cases of PID initially begin as an ascending gonococcal or chlamydial infection. If not treated, such infections might be followed days or weeks later by a "polymicrobial" stage and eventually by abscess formation. Alternatively, endogenous bacteria may ascend into the upper genital tract without a pre-existing cervical infection. At present, it is not fully known how or under what circumstances endogenous, predominantly vaginal, bacteria cause infection in an otherwise healthy fallopian tube, or if the tube needs to be "primed or compromised" by an earlier pathological process to enhance tissue invasion. Risk factors for ascending infection are discussed below.

PELVIC INFLAMMATORY DISEASE OF UNKNOWN ETIOLOGY

Although many different microbial species can be recovered from the upper genital tract in acute PID, no microorganisms are recovered in approximately 20 to 30percent of patients in recent studies. In one study, 30 (20 percent) of 151 women with laparoscopically verified acute salpingitis had no evidence of gonococcal, chlamydial, mycoplasmal, or other endogenous infection. In comparison with patients with PID of proven etiology, patients with unknown etiology were older (28 percent were > 30 years old), and more often they had a longer duration of pelvic pain (38 percent had > 3 days of pain), a normal erythrocyte sedimentation rate (ESR) (53 percent), and mild inflammatory changes at laparoscopy (53 percent).[115] Newer diagnostic techniques, such as PCR and antigen detection assays, may help study the etiology of infection in this group.

PATHOGENESIS

By definition, PID associated with sexually transmitted diseases (STDs) is caused by spread of microorganisms from the lower to the upper female genital tract.[1] The spread is canalicular, along mucosal surfaces from the vagina/cervix through the cervix to the endometrial cavity, the fallopian tubes, and into the abdominal cavity. The initial infection involves the mucosa and not the muscularis.[78] *N. gonorrhoeae* and *C. trachomatis* have been demonstrated by culture or antigen detection in epithelia of the cervix, endometrium, and fallopian tube in women with salpingitis.[73,116] Interruption of the fallopian tubes by cornual resection prevents STD-associated salpingitis.[18]

Some observations indicate that an intermittent ascent of microorganisms into the endometrial cavity and fallopian tubes might be a physiological phenomenon.[2,117] Spermatozoa, dyes, and particulate matter are transported from the vagina/cervix into the pelvic cavity.[118–120] With menses, the cervical mucus plug is lost, potentially allowing bacteria access to the endometrium. Endometrial blood is commonly present in the abdomen at menses in women undergoing peritoneal dialysis, potentially facilitating the movement of bacteria into and through the tube.[121] Observations in animal experiments also suggest that microorganisms may be transported through the genital tract without causing infection.[122] The fate of such ascended organisms would depend upon their viability, number, pathogenicity, and local defense mechanisms.

FACTORS INFLUENCING ASCENDING CANALICULAR SPREAD

Coitus-related factors

PID is rare in virgins,[123] and the frequency of sexual intercourse appears related to PID among monogamous women.[124] The role of spermatozoa in the active transport of microorganisms in PID is intriguing, but unknown. "Bacteriospermia" occurs, however, and spermatozoa with adherent microorganisms migrate through egg albumen and cervical secretion.[125,126] Spermatozoa with attached *C. trachomatis* have been identified in cul-de-sac fluid of women with salpingitis.[127] Experimental *C. trachomatis* infection in the cervix of pig-tailed macaques produced plasma-cell infiltrates in the tubes of mated but not of unmated animals, suggesting that mating was important to introduce chlamydia to the tubes.[128] On the other hand, symptoms of PID may begin weeks following sexual intercourse, and the use of condoms in women already infected with *N. gonorrhoeae* or *C. trachomatis* is not thought to be protective against PID.[124]

Iatrogenic procedures

Diagnostic and therapeutic procedures that disrupt the protective cervical barrier—such as dilatation and curettage, induced abortion, IUD-insertion, and hysterosalpingography—introduce bacteria into the endometrial cavity. In one series, these procedures preceded the onset of acute PID in 12 percent of women with PID.[2]

Sexual steroid hormones

A number of observations suggest that sexual steroid hormones might influence the pathogenesis of PID. The cervix provides a barrier against ascent of microorganisms into the endometrial cavity, and the production and characteristics of cervical mucus are highly influenced by sexual steroid hormones. During the estrogen phase of the menstrual cycle, cervical mucus is watery with glycoprotein molecules arranged in parallel rows, allowing penetration by spermatozoa.[129] In contrast, during the progesterone-dominated luteal phase, the water content of the secretion is low and glycoprotein molecules are arranged in an interlacing network that inhibits spermatozoa penetration.[129] By analogy, the likelihood of microorganism spread from the cervix to the endometrial cavity might be higher in follicular- than in luteal-phase mucus. In ovulating women, gonorrhea has been diagnosed more often in the follicular than in the luteal phase of the menstrual cycle,[130] and symptoms of STD-associated salpingitis more often start at menses or shortly after than in the luteal phase; this suggests that retrograde menstruation may play a role in the transport of bacteria into the fallopian tubes.[121,131,132]

Combination oral contraceptive pill (OCP) use is associated with protection against acute salpingitis.[133] The 36-month PID-related discontinuation rate was lower in women using levonorgestrel-medicated intrauterine devices (IUDs) (0.5) than among women using copper IUDs (2.0).[134] During a 2–3 year follow-up, PID was not found in ten high risk women with multiple partners on long-acting progesterone injections (Weström, unpubl.). *In vitro*, progesterone suppresses the growth of *N. gonorrhoeae*,[135] while 17-β-estradiol enhances the adherence and growth of *C. trachomatis* in a dose-dependent manner in human endometrial cells.[136] The addition of contraceptive progestins (and ethinyl estradiol) to cell cultures had no effect on the replication of *C. trachomatis*, however.[137]

In animal experiments, administration of estradiol to ovariectomized guinea pigs prolonged genital chlamydial infection and promoted upper genital tract infection.[138] In guinea pigs experimentally infected with the guinea-pig inclusion conjunctivitis (GPIC) agent, mestranol/norethynodrel enhanced the course of the infection and produced ascending infection not seen in untreated animals.[139] Progesterone alone given to the animals prevented acute endometritis.[140] On the other hand, the duration of experimental chlamydial infections in monkeys was not influenced by combined OCPs.[141]

The apparent protective effect of progestins against ascending infection may be explained by the production of luteal-type cervical mucus that inhibits bacterial penetration, and by the production of an inactive endometrium (which may inhibit bacterial attachment). Oral contraceptive pills appear to protect against PID in women infected with *C. trachomatis* but not in those with gonorrhea, however,[133] and these postulated effects of progesterone should protect against both infections. Thus, the mechanism of protection by sex steroid hormones remains unclear, but protection against overt *C. trachomatis* salpingitis raises the possibility that sex steroids down-regulate the immune response to *C. trachomatis*.

Miscellaneous factors

The ecological disturbance in the vaginal flora of women with BV includes a significant increase in the concentration of potentially pathogenic species (see Chap. 42), which may predispose to upper genital infection if the cervical barrier is breached. An increased risk of PID has been documented among women who douche.[142,143] Induced abortion also predisposes to PID,[144] presumably from the introduction of pathogenic cervical or vaginal bacteria into the endometrium.

The role of the IUD in the ascending spread of infection in the female genital tract has been controversial. A majority of epidemiological studies report higher incidences of PID in IUD-using women than in non-users. With IUD insertion, bacteria from the vagina/cervix are introduced into the endometrium along with the IUD.[145] Bacteria are also found to colonize the string and the main body of the IUD months to years after insertion.[146] Intrauterine devices also enhance cervical colonization by bacteria such as actinomyces,[147] predispose to bacterial vaginosis,[148] and cause impressions in the endometrium.[149] While all of these findings would be expected to enhance infection, the importance of one over another in the pathogenesis of PID remains uncertain (see below).

TUBAL INFLAMMATION

The presence of *N. gonorrhoeae* and *C. trachomatis* on genital mucosal surfaces starts a cascade of events involving humoral and cellulardefense mechanisms. These mechanisms can result in clearance of infection and/or provoke tissue damage. Because of the delicate anatomic constraints of fallopian-tube function in reproduction, tissue damage at this site can have important reproductive consequences. The fallopian-tubes events are discussed below.

Gonococcal strains that cause salpingitis differ from strains that cause disseminated gonococcal infection.[47–49] In a human fallopian-tube culture model, *N. gonorrhoeae* selectively adheres to and enters nonciliated cells, leaving ciliated cells uninfected. The ciliated cells soon undergo ciliostasis and sloughing, however.[41,42,150] Ciliary activity of tubes is significantly reduced within 24 hours when infected with gonococci and bathed in gonococcal supernatant, compared to uninfected controls.[43] This suggests that sloughing of ciliated cells and ciliostasis is mediated by a toxic cell-free product. The reduction in tubal ciliary activity also occurs from purified *N. gonorrhoeae* lipopolysaccharide[151] and from monomeric peptidoglycan fragments from *N. gonorrhoeae*.[152] Once inside nonciliated cells, gonococci are protected from immune-defense factors, traverse the cells, and eventually are released from the basal surfaces of the cells by exocytosis.[41,42]

In the natural disease, antibody binding to gonococcal lipooligosaccharide molecules and peptidoglycan in the fallopian tubes activates complement and initiates the prostaglandin cascade,[132] resulting in an intense acute inflammatory reaction that includes purulent secretion, edema, vasodilatation, and tissue destruction. Since rates of isolation of *N. gonorrhoeae* from the fallopian tubes in "gonorrhea-associated" salpingitis are inversely related to the duration of symptoms,[29,31,52] some investigators speculated that *N. gonorrhoeae* may soon succumb in the upper genital tract and other endogenous microorganisms may continue the tubal infection initiated by gonococci. Alternatively, gonococcal infection may produce more severe symptoms that lead women to seek health-care quickly; meanwhile, other pathogens produce more indolent symptoms, which result in delayed health-care seeking. The studies that led investigators to postulate the former hypothesis were performed before *C. trachomatis* was recognized to cause acute PID. Women with chlamydial PID generally have a clinically milder disease than women with gonococcal salpingitis[115] and tend to delay seeking medical care.[153]

Immunological defense mechanisms induced by a gonococcal infection appear to offer some defense against recurrent gonococcal salpingitis. Antibody against the principal outer-membrane protein of *N. gonorrhoeae* was associated with reduced risk of PID among women with recurrent gonococcal infection in a small study in the 1970s.[51] More recently, antibodies to gonococcal opacity proteins significantly reduced the risk of gonococcal salpingitis among prostitutes.[154]

C. trachomatis attaches to tubal epithelium and is engulfed by endocytosis in a membrane-lined vacuole.[76] *C. trachomatis* replicates within the cell, thereby protecting the organism from immune recognition. Infectious *C. trachomatis* elementary bodies are eventually released from the cytoplasmic inclusions into the lumen of the fallopian tube.[76] In human fallopian-tube organ culture, elementary bodies were observed to replicate with inclusion formation in both ciliated and nonciliated cells during a five-to-seven-day maintenance period of the cultures.[77] Similar findings were present in the oviducts of mice infected with murine–*C. trachomatis*.[155] Both cilia and ciliated cells were lost in chlamydial salpingitis in pig-tailed macaques.[78]

Chlamydial infections induce cytokines, including tumor necrosis factor (TNF), interferon (IFN), and interleukins (IL).[156–158] In PID, monocytes appear to produce increased amounts of IL-1 and IL-6 that in turn can induce scarring and tissue damage.[159] IFN-γ is present in cervical secretions of women with chlamydial cervicitis[160] and in the sera of women with acute PID.[161] IFN-γ may elicit further increase in monokine production, and it may induce expression of major histocompatibility complex (MHC) class II molecules on epithelial and endothelial cells and on macrophages. Expression of MHC II–bound exogenous antigens on epithelial cells activates an immune response directed against the expressing cells that in salpingitis could result in tubal cell destruction analogous to that demonstrated in ocular trachoma.[162]

Genital chlamydial infection also elicits a humoral immune response of local and serum IgA, IgM, and IgG antibodies. Serum IgG antibody to *C. trachomatis* was detected 6 years after chlamydia-associated PID.[163] Partial protection against re-infection with *C. trachomatis* has been demonstrated in animal experiments,[164–166] but this protective immunity appeared both short lived and serotype specific.[167] On the other hand, studies on CBA/nu mice[168] and B-cell deficient mice[169] indicate that cell-mediated immune mechanisms rather than antibody mechanisms play a dominant role in the resolution of chlamydial infection.

In experimental studies involving primates and mice, progressive tubal scarring occurs after repeated inoculations with *C. trachomatis*.[79,170] A single direct tubal inoculation with *C. trachomatis* in previously uninfected pig-tailed macaques produced self-limited infection with edema that spontaneously resolved, leaving no tubal scarring.[78] In contrast, tubal inoculation after either repeated cervical or tubal inoculations caused tubal occlusion and peritubal adhesions.[78,79] Analogous to clinical and experimental findings after repeated infection in ocular trachoma,[171,172] these findings suggest damage from immunologic responses to chlamydial antigens.[80] A cytokine response involving interferon gamma (INF-γ) and interleukins 2, 6, and 10 occurs with experimental fallopian tube infection.[173] While INF-γ can help destroy *C. trachomatis*, INF-γ also stimulates macrophages to intensify the inflammatory response. With acute infection, about 60 percent of the lymphocytes were CD8 cytotoxic lymphocytes; taken together with finding porforin, this suggests the presence of activated cytolytic T cells.[173] With repetitive inoculation of *C. trachomatis*, severe permanent tissue damage may result from immunopathogenic T cell responses.

Since CD4 T cell loss induced by HIV infection increases the risk of *C. trachomatis* salpingitis, it may be that CD8 T cells are relatively more important in immunopathology than are CD4 T cells. This is supported by the observation that chlamydial salpingitis in humans is associated with an increased number of individuals with HLA-A31.[174] HLA-A31 is a HLA class I molecule that presents cytoplasmically processed peptide antigen to CD8 cells.

CD4 T cells may also play a role in immunopathology, in part mediated by T cell delayed type hypersensitivity (DTH) responses. In experimental ocular trachoma, a DTH was reproduced by placing a 60 kilodalton (kD) chlamydial heat-shock protein (Chsp-60) on the conjunctiva of previously infected animals.[175] A human 60-kD heat shock protein (Hhsp-60) is present in humans, and both heat shock proteins share extensive amino-acid sequence homology.[176] A proliferative response by lymphocytes to conserved epitopes Chsp-60 and Hhsp-60 was demonstrated in 5 of 10 women with two or more episodes of PID, 1 of 9 with a single episode of PID, and 1 of 32 control women.[176] Pre-existing antibody to Chsp-60 was associated with a fivefold increased risk of developing chlamydial PID.[174] Antibody to Chsp-60 is also associated with severe tubal disease at acute infection,[177] and perihepatitis,[178] as well as with infertility[179] and tubal pregnancy.[180] These findings support the likelihood that *C. trachomatis* PID is, in part, an immune-mediated disease and that particularly severe inflammation can result from an immune response to Chsp-60.[80,181]

Antibody response to Chsp-60 appears to be in part genetically determined.[182] Several mechanisms could explain the role of Chsp-60 in the immunopathogenesis of chlamydial PID. First, antibody to Chsp-60 could reflect a shift in the immune response to a Th-2 dominant response and away from a protective cellular immune response. Second, immune complexes involving Chsp-60 antibody could stimulate excessive tissue inflammation. Third, because of the homology between Chsp-60 and human Hhsp-60, antibody to Chsp-60 could initiate an autoimmune response to self Hhsp-60, precipitating tissue injury.

Information from clinical and experimental studies suggests a profound difference in host-parasite interactions of tubal infections caused by *N. gonorrhoeae* compared to *C. trachomatis*. *N. gonorrhoeae* appears to induce an acute neutrophilic inflammatory response, while *C. trachomatis* often results in a more indolent, cell-mediated lymphocytic response, possibly a DTH response. In naturally occurring chlamydial salpingitis, however, neither a DTH nor human heat shock protein expression on tubal cells has been confirmed.

TUBOOVARIAN ABSCESS

Abscess formation is a late manifestation of PID. Neither *N. gonorrhoeae* nor *C. trachomatis* alone produce abscesses in animals or humans.[183] Instead, tuboovarian abscess (TOA) typically results from a mixture of facultative and anaerobic bacteria, where facultative bacteria dominate the early phase of infection and bacterial metabolic products produce an environment of low oxygen tension that favors the growth of anaerobic bacteria.[114,183] Anaerobic bacteria dominate the infection in tuboovarian and pelvic abscesses.[24,33,114]

TISSUE REPAIR

In the repair process, the replacement of dead tubal epithelial cells by ingrowing fibroblasts causes tubal scarring and eventual functional impairment of tubal function. Tubal deciliation,[78] intraluminal adhesions,[184] tubal occlusion, and peritubal adhesions occur after both natural infection in women[185] and experimental infections in animals.[183,186–188] These sequelae appear irreversible. These morphologic tubal changes can lead to infertility or tubal pregnancy (see below).

Tubal infection and scarring can be rapid; tubal infection and inflammation are initiated within hours for gonorrhea and within days for chlamydia, and tubal scarring begins within days of infection. In follow-up studies of women with STD-associated salpingitis, a delay in seeking care for more than 2 days after the onset of pain was associated with a threefold increase in infertility or ectopic pregnancy.[153] The infertility rate after chlamydial salpingitis in mice was inversely proportional to the time between inoculation and the start of tetracycline treatment.[187]

EPIDEMIOLOGY AND RISK FACTORS

We do not usually know accurately the incidence and prevalence of acute PID in a population, but considerable variation between populations clearly occurs. Patient surveys, outpatient visits, hospital discharge rates, retrospective self-reporting, and extrapolations from incidence figures of gonorrhea and chlamydia have all been used to study the epidemiology of PID. In most instances, however, PID is not a notifiable disease, and different methods were used to obtain information, including the use of ICD-codes, reporting agencies, and self-reporting. Furthermore, accurate clinical criteria do not exist for the diagnosis, and the diagnostic accuracy of standard clinical diagnosis assessed by laparoscopy is only about 65 percent.[2] In addition, about two-thirds of women with PID have so few or such mild symptoms that the diagnosis is not made. These latter cases are only identified if and when the late complications of tubal infection become evident. Thus, published figures on the epidemiology of PID are difficult to compare, and these data must be interpreted with caution. Trends in the incidence of PID over time are influenced by a number of factors, most importantly the prevalence of STDs in the population. Other factors that influence the rate of PID include demography (parous and/or married women have a lower incidence of PID than nulliparous, single, divorced, or widowed women[29]), economics, health-care characteristics of the population, sexual and "adolescent culture" attitudes, douching, smoking and drug habits, and contraceptive use.

REPORTED INCIDENCES AND TRENDS

In the United States, widely divergent figures on the estimated incidence of PID illustrate the difficulties with such estimates. During the 1980s, the annual estimated number of cases of PID varied from 857,000 cases (1980 data from the National Ambulatory Medical Care Survey, National Center for Health Statistics),[189] to 1,477,000 cases (based on average numbers of hospitalized cases in 1987–88 and outpatient cases in 1985–89)[190] to 2,000,000 cases (a 1984 community survey).[191] About 30 percent of cases of PID were hospitalized in the late 1980s.[192] In 1982, 14.2 percent, and in 1988, 10.8 percent of U.S. women 15–44 years of age reported that they had received treatment for PID.[193]

American data indicate a particularly high incidence of PID among young, nonwhite, single, or divorced women from urban areas.[189–93] Hospitalized cases of PID per 100,000 women peryear had decreased among African-American teenagers from 1,000 to 750, and had increased among white teenagers from 250 to 300 cases between 1972 and 1981.[194] Since 1980, the number of hospitalizations of women for acute PID peaked in 1992 at nearly 200,000; the number has fallen fairly steadily since then, to less than 90,000 in 1993 (Fig. 58–2).[195] The number of initial visits to physicians' offices for PID peaked in the mid-1980s at over 450,000 visits; the number has fallen sharply since 1993 to less than 250,000 in 1995 (Fig. 58–3).[195] In 1993, an estimated 313,000 women 15–44 years of age were diagnosed with PID in hospital emergency departments (National Ambulatory Medical Care Survey, National Center for Health Statistics),[196] and were not included in the visits to physicians' offices.

In England and Wales, hospital admissions for PID in women 15–44 years of age increased from 11,300 to 16,000 between 1975 and 1985. The incidence per 1,000 women increased from 1.3 to 1.8 in the 20-to-24-year age group and from 1.1 to 1.2 in the 25-to-29-year age group, but was virtually constant among teenagers and older women.[197]

In Sweden, hospital discharge rates for PID peaked in 1977 and have significantly decreased since.[70] The incidence of PID has been followed from 1960 in one region in Sweden, where one gynecological department cared for the female population, and about 90 percent of all cases were verified by laparoscopy. The total incidence of PID per 1,000 women 15–24 years of age increased to a peak of 17.5 in the mid-1970s and subsequently decreased to less than one in 1990–94 (Fig. 58–1).[198] Only minor changes in the incidence of PID occurred in the 30to 34-year age group over this time. The incidence of gonorrhea-associated PID per 1,000 women 15–24 years of age decreased from 6 in 1960–64 to none in 1990–94, paralleling a significant nationwide drop in gonorrhea rates after 1975. The incidence of chlamydia-associated PID per 1,000 women 15–24 years of age decreased from 6.3 in 1977 to less than one in 1994, in parallel with a local chlamydial-control program that markedly reduced chlamydial infection in women. Additionally, recurrent episodes of PID decreased from 21 percent of the total in 1960–64 to 4 percent in 1990–94, possibly from a lower risk of gonorrhea and chlamydia.[198] Thus,

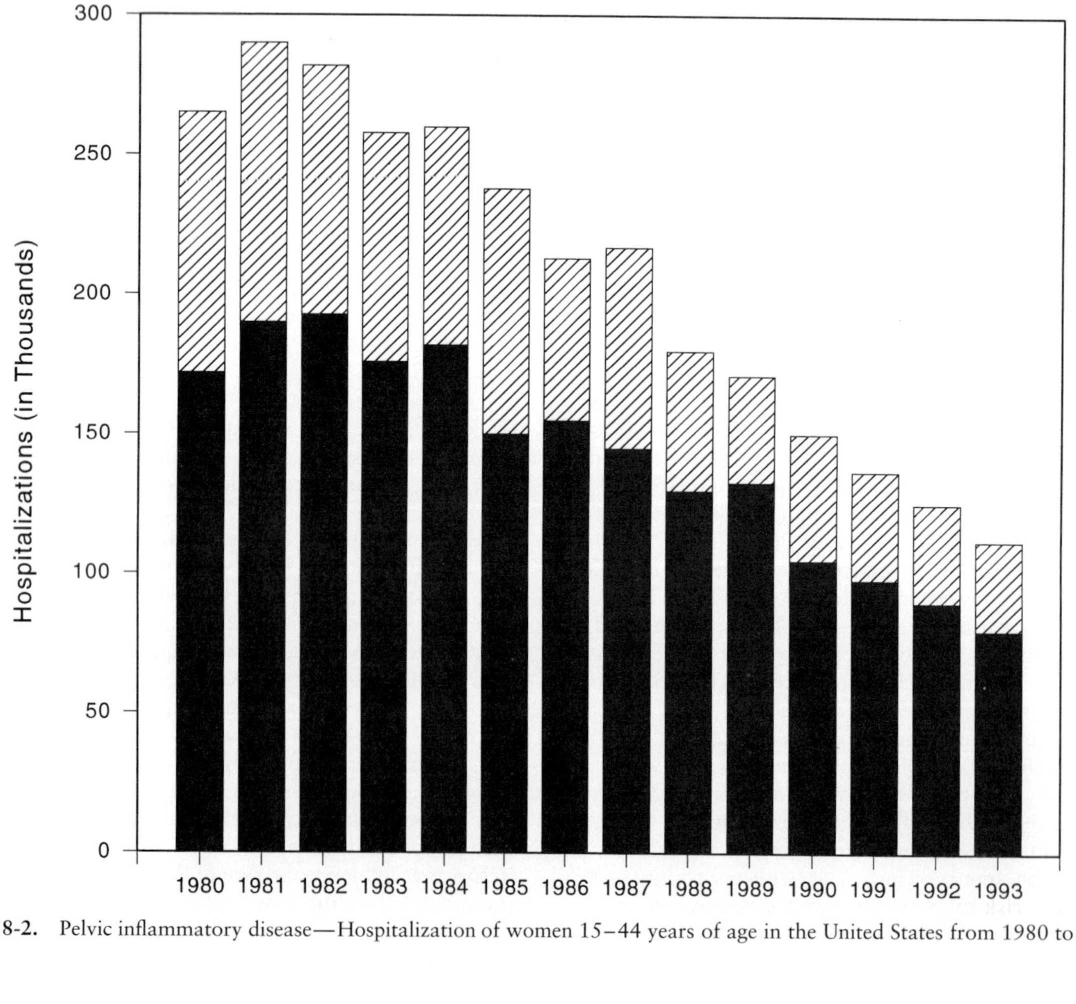

Fig. 58-2. Pelvic inflammatory disease—Hospitalization of women 15–44 years of age in the United States from 1980 to 1993.

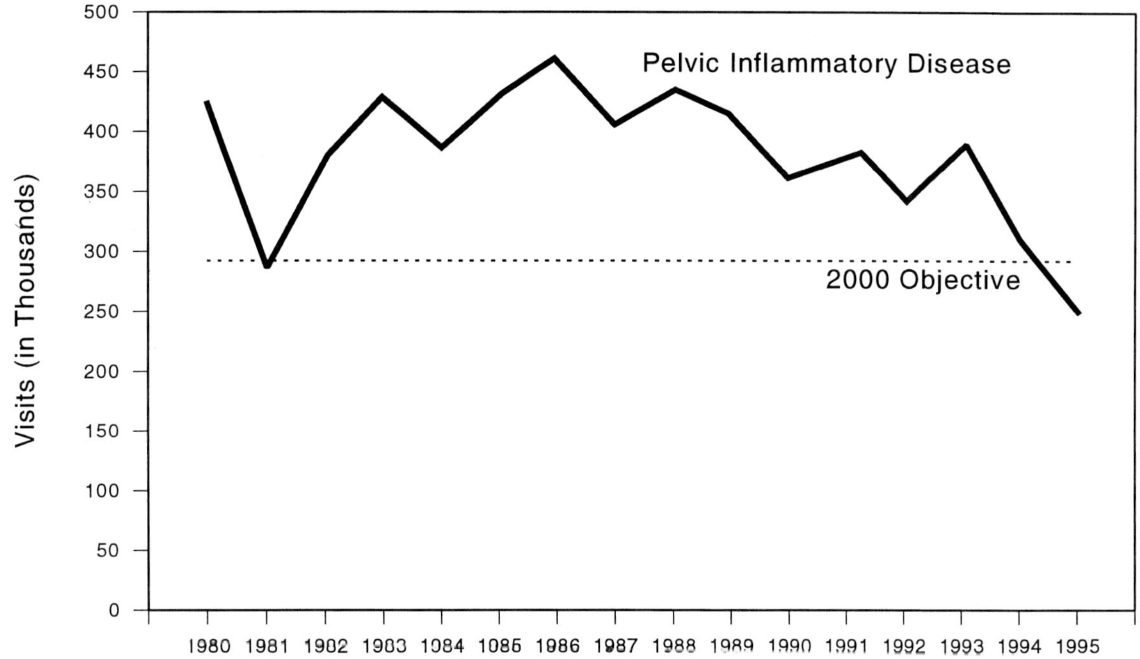

Fig. 58-3. Pelvic inflammatory disease—Initial visits to physicians' offices by women 15–44 years of age in the United States from 1980 to 1995, and the Healthy People Year 2000 Objective.

trends in STDs have a significant impact on the epidemiology of PID.

In developing countries, hospital admissions for PID provide a crude marker of PID as a public-health problem. It accounts for 17 to 40 percent of all gynecological admissions in the sub-Saharan region of Africa, 15 to 37 percent in Southeast Asia, and 3 to 10 percent in India.[199] The proportion of PID that is associated with STDs is not known, however, because postpartum and postabortal infections are also common.

As expected, tubal infertility is common in developing countries. Some sub-Saharan communities reported that up to 80 percent of infertility was associated with previous PID, and that 30–50 percent of reproductive age women are infertile.[200] Ectopic pregnancy was the most common surgical emergency in one center in Nairobi.[201] The ratio of ectopic to intrauterine pregnancy prior to 1980 was 1:88 in Benin and 1:91 in Kampala,[202] compared with 1:133 in Finland.[203] In summary, limited data indicate that PID and its consequences are common in most developing nations. Poverty, urbanization, lack of education, prostitution, and the low status of women constitute formidable challenges to controlling STDs and PID.

RISK MARKERS AND RISK FACTORS

Risk factors for PID that are possibly in the causal pathway after acquiring an STD include age, contraceptive use, coital frequency, douching, invasive diagnostic procedures, health-care behavior, and HIV infection. Knowledge of how risk factors cause PID could allow reduction of PID rates by education, counseling, or treatment.[124] By contrast, risk markers are variables associated with PID that in themselves do not cause the acquisition of organisms that cause PID, nor do they cause the ascent of organisms into the upper genital tract. Risk markers for PID include age, socioeconomic status, smoking, and drug and alcohol abuse. Age, smoking, and other risk markers for PID disappear in statistical models that adjust for gonorrhea and chlamydial infection. Risk markers and risk factors are interrelated and form a complex network.

Sexually transmitted diseases

Risk factors for the acquisition of STDs are discussed in Chap. 4. As discussed above, gonorrhea, chlamydial infection, and probably bacterial vaginosis represent the most important risk factors for PID based upon epidemiologic and etiologic studies.[46,194] A genital infection was diagnosed in about 50–65 percent of sexual partners of young women with PID, irrespective of the etiology of PID.[67,204] Declining rates of PID parallel control of gonorrhea and chlamydial infection in Sweden (see Fig. 58–1) and the United States. In Wisconsin, the institution of a chlamydial treatment program was followed by a drop in the rate of PID.[205] In Seattle, a randomized trial of screening high-risk women for chlamydial infection, and treating those found infected, demonstrated a 60-percent reduction in the rate of PID, in comparison with the control group of high-risk women assigned to receive usual care (which did not involve routine chlamydia screening).[206]

Age

Age is associated with PID, probably as a risk marker rather than a causal risk factor.[48,195] The risk of acquiring acute salpingitis is 1:8 for sexually active 15 year olds, and 1:16 for 16 year olds, compared to 1:80 for women 24 years of age.[207] The high number of sexual partners in younger women is associated with more frequent acquisition of STDs in this group. Women 20–24 years of age have the highest incidence of both STDs and PID, closely followed by teenagers.[207] After adjusting for sexual activity, however, sexually active teenage females have higher incidence of gonorrhea and chlamydia than any age group. The incidences of both STDs and PID decrease significantly with increasing age beyond the age of 24. Additionally, age is no longer associated with PID when gonorrhea and chlamydia are controlled, which further suggests that young age is related to PID through increased rates of these two STDs.[208] In high-risk women (e.g., commercial sex workers), increasing age is associated with increasing duration of prostitution and thus with increasing experience with prior gonococcal and chlamydial infections. The impact of history of infection on risk of PID should be viewed as a risk factor independent of the physiologic attributes of age per se.

Contraceptive use

The magnitude of the effect of contraception on PID is difficult to ascertain. Experimental studies of the influence of contraceptives on the pathogenesis of PID have been cited above. The use of different methods of contraception influences the risk of acquiring STDs, as well as the risk of progressing to PID. Some contraceptives, such as barrier methods, reduce the acquisition of STDs, while oral contraceptives may enhance the acquisition of chlamydial infection yet reduce the development of PID among those who have acquired chlamydial infection.[133] Use of IUDs has no known influence on STD acquisition, but it enhances the movement of bacteria from the cervix to the uterus/tubes. Behaviors that influence both contraceptive choice and PID could confound studies of the association of contraceptives with PID. Women using no contraception may tend to take sexual risks and pregnancy risks and have poor health-care utilization, which in concert can increase the rates of STDs, PID, and pregnancy. Contraceptives have not been randomly assigned to women to examine the influence of contraception per se on PID, so the influence of contraception on PID is generally assessed from case-control studies.

Barrier methods decrease the acquisition of STDs by providing a barrier between urethral exudate and contaminated semen and the cervix. Spermicidal agents offer a partial protection against STDs by a direct inhibitory effect on bacteria. Barrier and spermicidal use has been associated with modest reduction in PID.[124,209]

Overall, OCP use has generally been associated with a reduction of 40 to 60 percent in the rate of PID.[133] Among women with chlamydial infection, OCP use has been associated with a 70-percent reduction in risk of PID,[133] but OCPs do not appear to protect women with gonorrhea from PID.[133] The protective effect of OCPs on chlamydial PID, but not other forms of PID, raises the possibility that OCPs influence the immune response to chlamydia and thereby reduce inflammation in the fallopian tubes. This hypothesis is consistent with the finding that OCP users have had less severe damage of the fallopian tubes when PID is visualized laparoscopically, compared to IUD users or women who use no birth control.[210] Women in these studies used first- and second-generation combination OCPs with higher doses of steroids than most of the OCPs used today, however, and there is a complex interaction among OCP use, age, ectopy, and cervical infection.[211]

At least 20 controlled studies from the 1960s through the 1980s reported a two- to fourfold increased risk of PID or consequences of PID among users of IUDs compared to women using other or no contraceptives.[212,213] Women who use IUDs clearly have an increased risk of PID in the first 1–3 months following insertion of the device, probably related to the introduction of bacteria into the uterus with insertion.[214] After this immediate post-insertion period, the rate of PID decreases but remains above that of non-IUD users, based upon data from case-control studies of PID,[215] tubal infertility,[216,217] and ectopic pregnancy.[218] Later infections are probably related to the long-term colonization of the IUD and string surface demonstrated by bacteriologic and scanning electron microscope studies.[146,219] Uncontrolled prospective cohort studies of IUD users report low rates of PID, but since they lack non-IUD-using controls they cannot examine the sensitivity of detection of PID nor the impact of incomplete follow-up.[213] Thus, the prospective cohort data are not consistent with the controlled studies. Women who use IUDs appear to have more non-STD-associated PID than non-IUD users, as well as more PID associated with *N. gonorrhoeae* and *C. trachomatis*.[220,221] The rate of PID among IUD users can be reduced by screening for these two bacteria before insertion, and by recognizing early signs of infection such as abnormal vaginal discharge, vaginal bleeding, and mild abdominal pain. Progesterone-medicated IUDs may reduce the rate of PID compared to copper or non-medicated IUDs.[134]

The most recent studies of the association of prior IUD usage with tubal infertility and ectopic pregnancy are not subject to the bias of underdiagnosis or misdiagnosis of PID. Women using only copper IUDs have a threefold increased rate of tubal infertility after adjustment for variables associated with infertility,[222] and women using copper IUDs also have a threefold increased rate of ectopic pregnancy following IUD removal and after adjustment for variables associated with ectopic pregnancy.[218] The data on tubal infertility and ectopic pregnancy following IUD use are consistent with the increased rates of salpingitis noted in case-control studies of IUD users.

Douching and bacterial vaginosis

In the United States, douching is practiced more commonly among African Americans and is associated with low socioeconomic status. Women with PID report frequent douching more commonly than controls, even after adjustment for gonorrhea and chlamydial infection.[142] A recent confirmation of the link between douching and PID and a link between douching and ectopic pregnancy[223] raises the possibility that douching upsets the vaginal ecology or in some way enhances bacterial invasion of the uterus.

Among women undergoing induced, abortion those with bacterial vaginosis (BV) have a threefold increased rate of postabortion PID compared to those without BV. The increased rate of PID was reduced to baseline in a randomized treatment trial of BV.[144] Frequent intercourse has been implicated as a risk factor for PID.[124] The association between frequent intercourse and PID may be evident only in women with BV, however, (Wølner-Hanssen, unpubl.). Thus, BV, with its 20–1,000 fold increased concentration of a variety of bacteria in the lower genital tract, might interact with the frequency of intercourse in causing ascending infection.

Surgical procedures

Microorganisms are spread to the upper genital tract by surgical procedures—such as dilatation and curettage, hysterosalpingography, and IUD insertion—that breech the protective cervical barrier. Such procedures preceded the onset of PID in 12 percent of cases in one study.[2]

Smoking, alcohol, and illicit drug abuse

Cigarette smoking has been related to a twofold relative risk of PID.[124,224] A dose-response relationship was not observed, however,[224] and the relationship between smoking and PID is not consistent. The association between alcohol and illicit drug use, particularly cocaine, may occur because of an increased risk of PID from high STD rates in this population.[124]

Human immunodeficiency virus infection

Patients with HIV infection may have increased risk of PID, although several potential biases may distort the recognition and

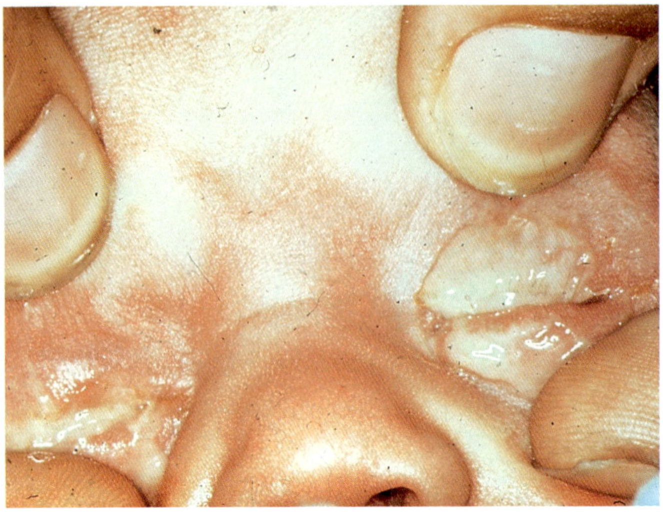

Plate 7. Neonatal gonococcal conjunctivitis. Note profuse purulent exudate.

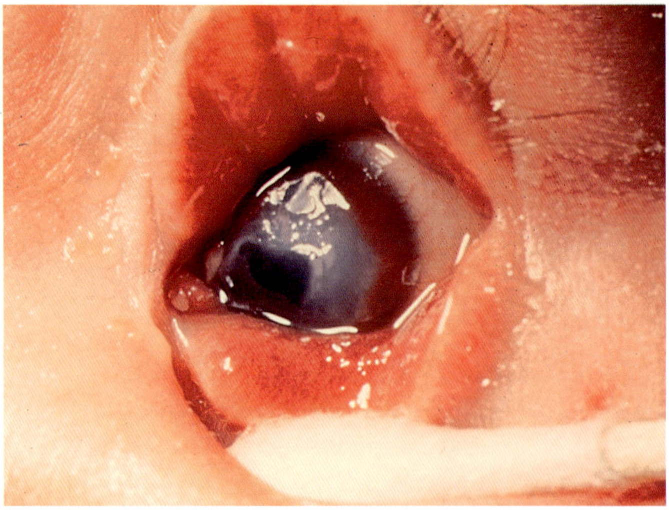

Plate 8. Neonatal conjunctivitis and keratitis. Both *Chlamydia trachomatis* and herpes simplex virus type 2 were isolated from the eye of this infant.

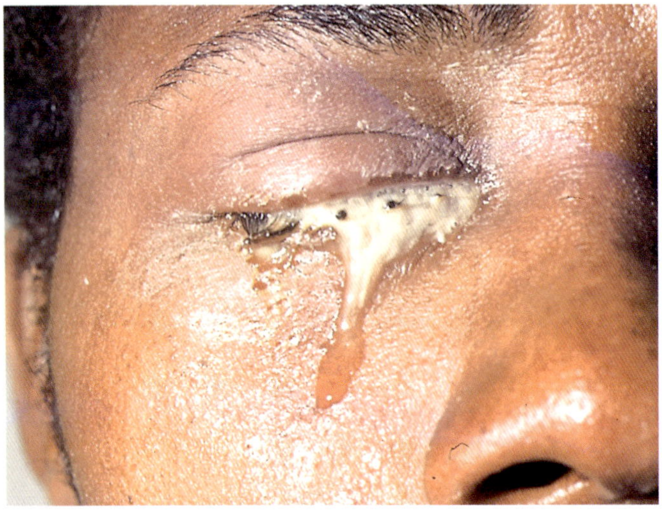

Plate 9. Acute gonococcal conjunctivitis in an adult.

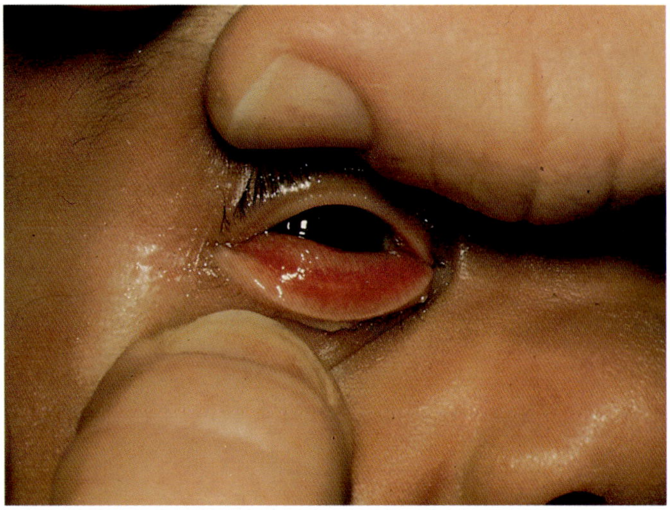

Plate 10. Acute recurrent chlamydial conjunctivitis in a two-month old infant. The follicular hyperplasia of the lower palpebral conjunctiva, seen in this recurrent infection, is usually not seen in the first episode of neonatal chlamydial conjunctivitis.

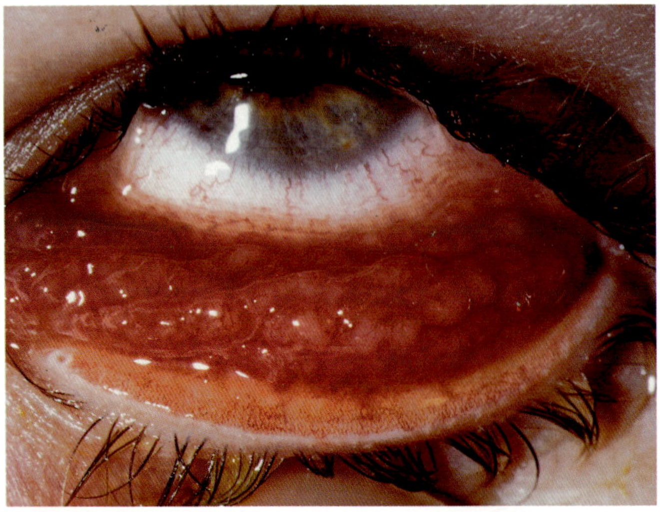

Plate 11. Paratrachoma in an adult, caused by a genital immunotype of *C. trachomatis*. Note the marked follicular appearance.

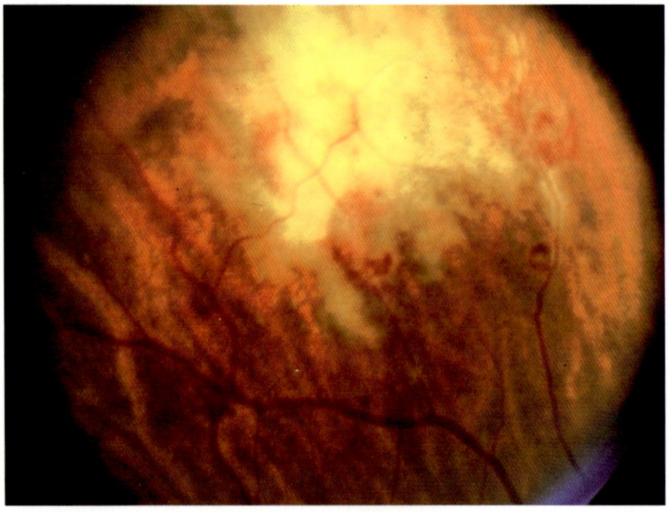

Plate 12. CMV chorioretinitis in a patient with AIDS.

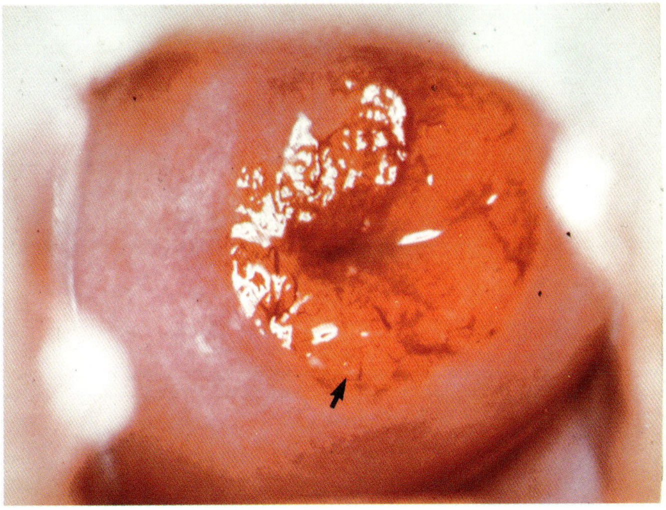

Plate 13. Cervical ectopy. Endocervical columnar epithelium is present in an ectopic position on the exocervix, giving a bright-red circumoral appearance. Note that the cervical mucus is clear, not purulent. However, also note the small vesicle (arrow) indicative of a very early primary HSV lesion, within the zone of ectopy.

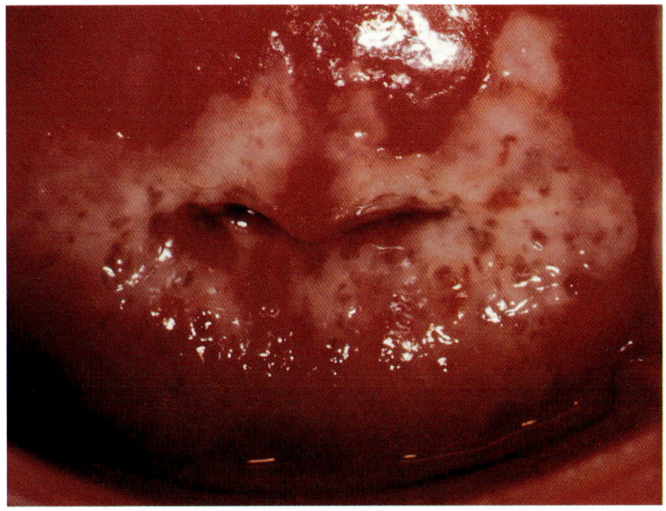

Plate 14. Severe primary HSV-2 cervicitis. HSV-2 produces both endocervicitis and ectocervicitis.

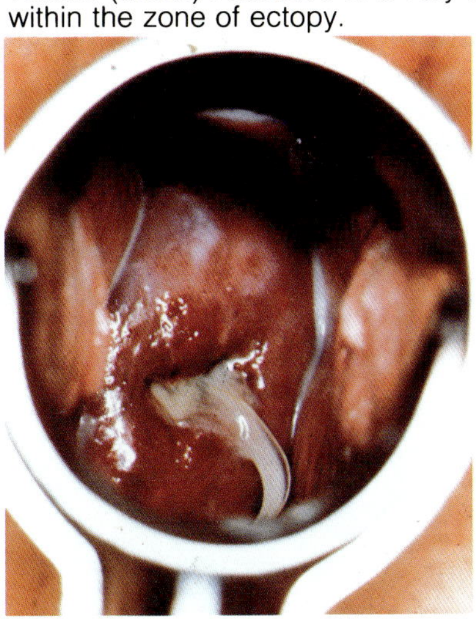

Plate 15. Mucopurulent cervicitis caused by *C. trachomatis*. Note pus mixed with mucus (indicating source from the endocervix); also note ectopy, edema, and bleeding.

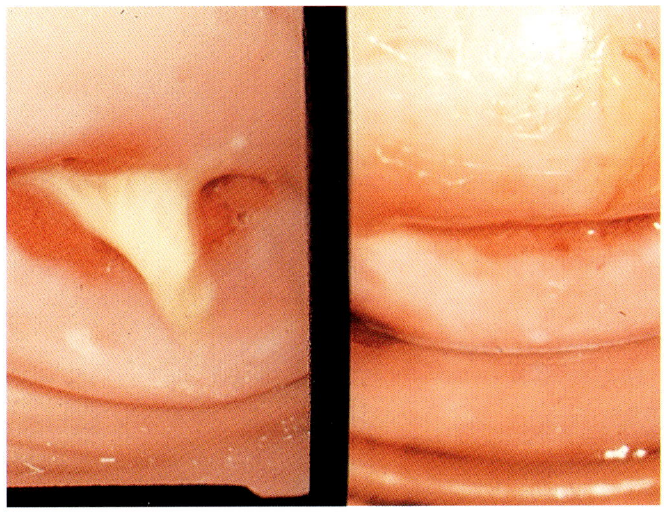

Plate 16. Mucopurulent cervicitis caused by *C. trachomatis*, before and after treatment with doxycycline.

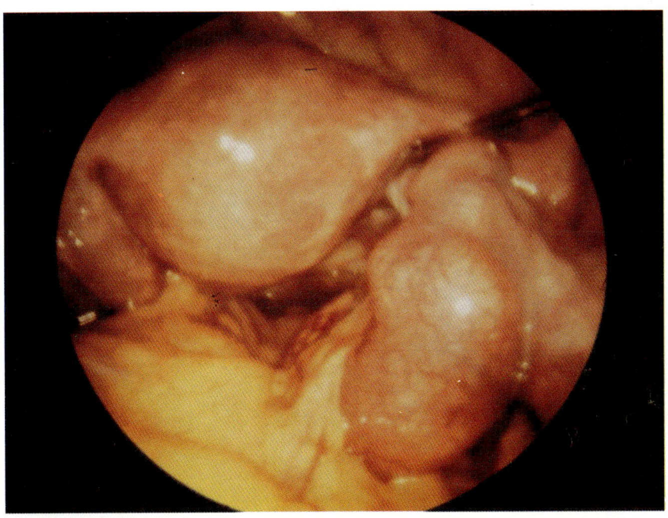

Plate 17. Proven chlamydial pyosalpinx. The right tube is swollen, tortuous, reddened, and filled with pus. The yellow omentum is adherent to the abdominal orifice of the tube.

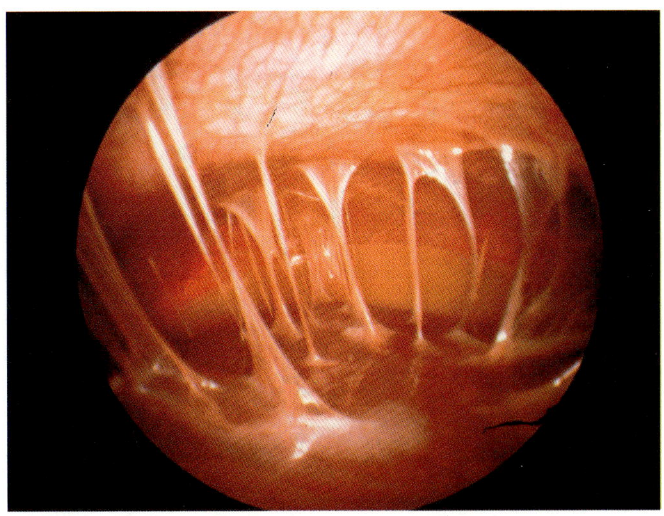

Plate 18. Laparoscopic view of perihepatic adhesions in a patient with Fitz-Hugh–Curtis syndrome of approximately six weeks duration.

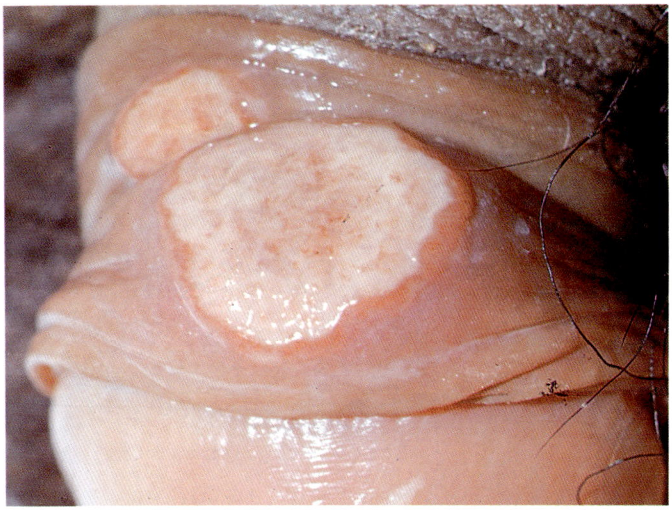

Plate 31. Chancroid ulcer involving the foreskin with "kissing" lesion of the penile shaft. Note serpiginous border of the ulcer, which is superficial and covered with a purulent exudate.

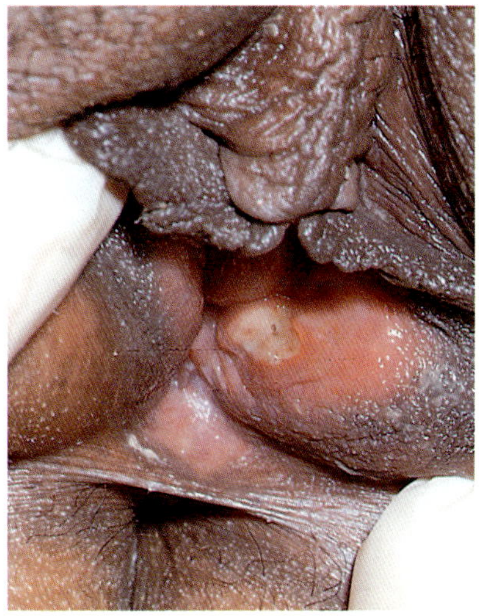

Plate 32. Chancroid ulcer of the fourchette in a female.

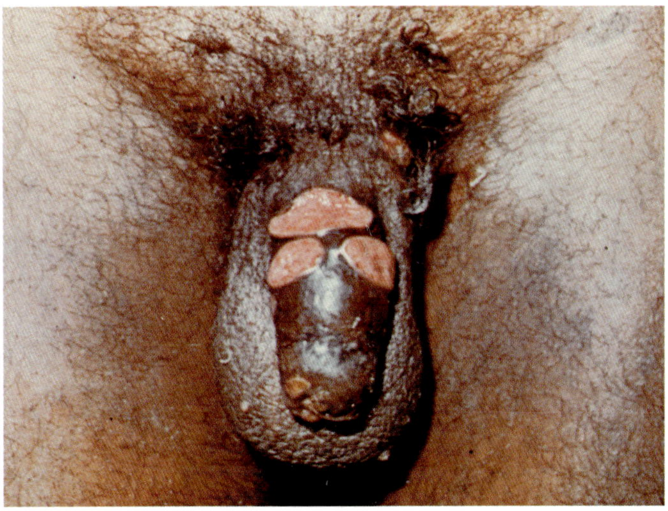

Plate 33. Diskoid form of donovanosis.

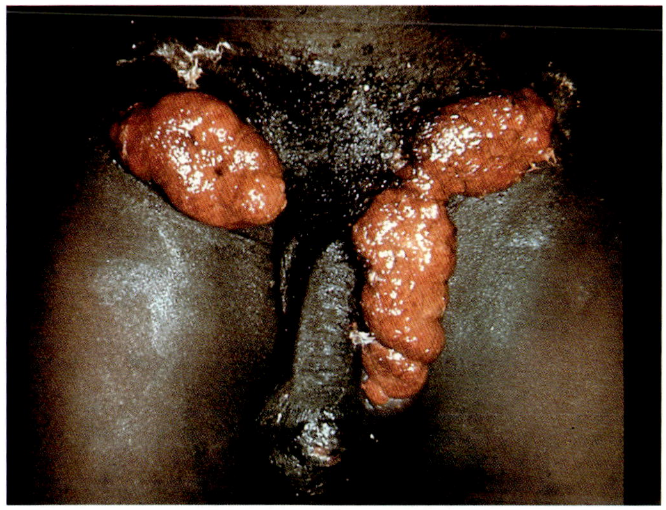

Plate 34. Donovanosis. Exuberant granulation tissue with lesions spreading from the penis and scrotum by continuity to one inguinal area, and also to the opposite inguinal area with an intervening skip area, producing pseudobuboes of both inguinal regions.

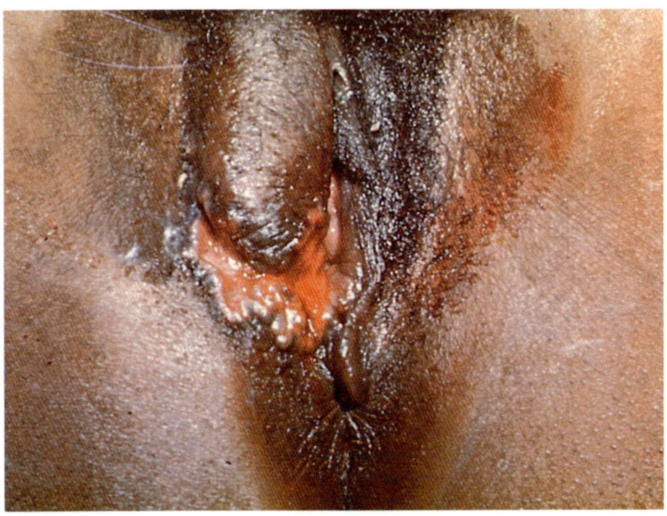

Plate 35. Donovanosis in the female with vulvar lymphedema.

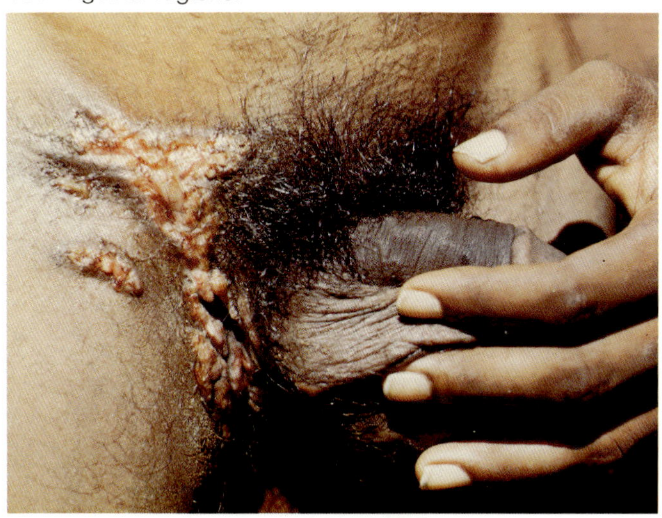

Plate 36. Verrucous form of donovanosis, with lesions spreading from the crural area to the inguinal area by continuity. Verrucous donovanosis is most often perianal.

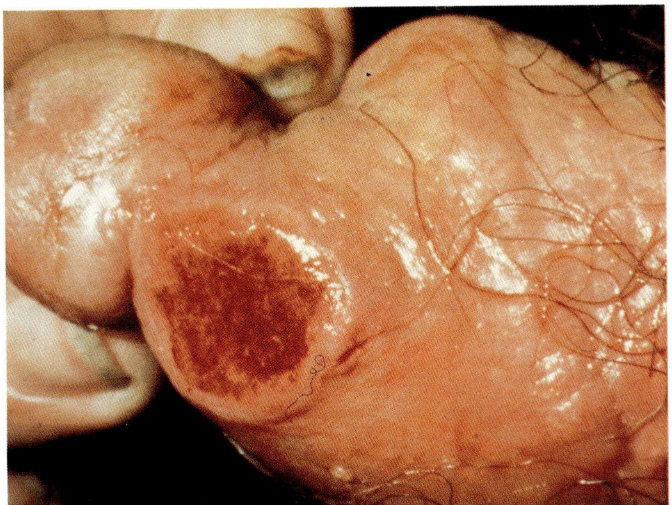

Plate 37. Primary syphilitic chancre of the penis. Note the rolled edges of the ulcer, the indurated button-like appearance, and the clean ulcer base.

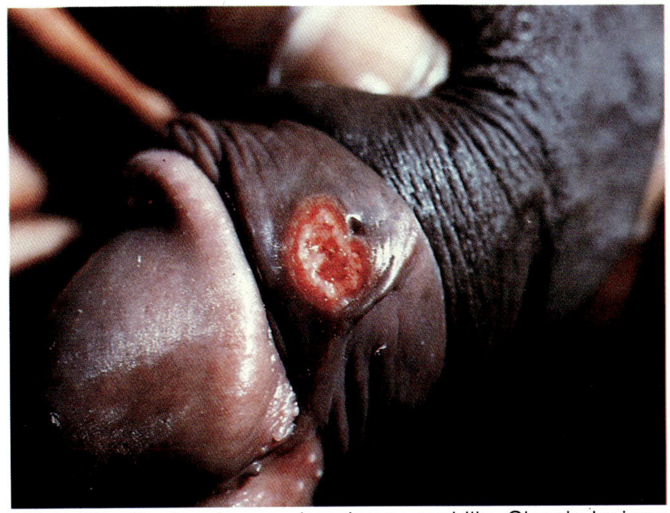

Plate 38. Penile chancre in primary syphilis. Classic lesions showing rolled indurated edges with clean ulcer base.

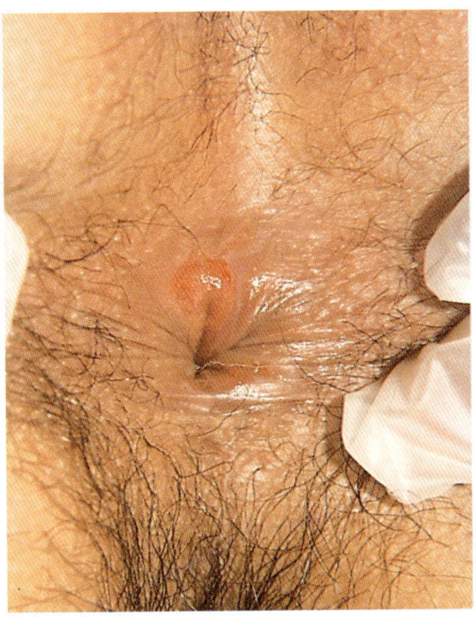

Plate 39. Primary perianal chancre in a homosexual man.

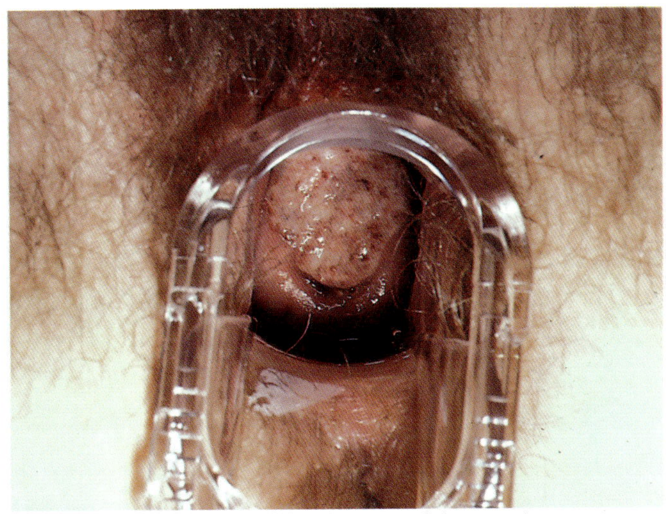

Plate 40. Primary syphilitic chancre of the cervix.

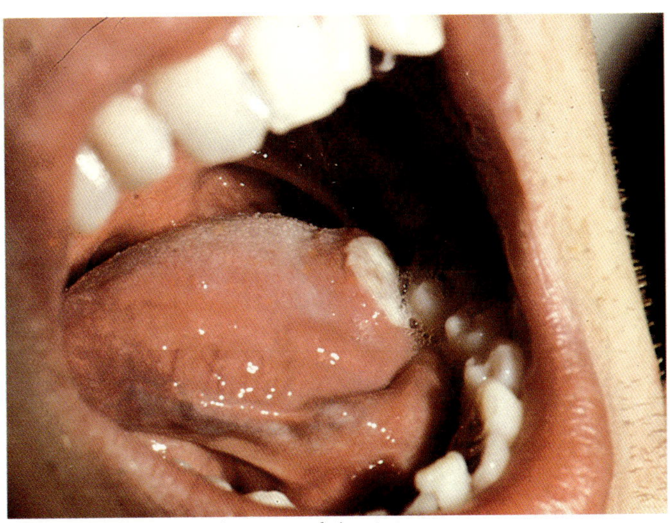

Plate 41. Primary chancre of the tongue.

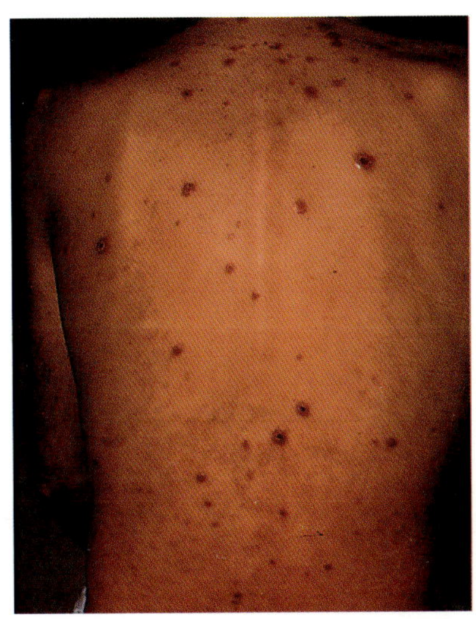

Plate 42. Pustular and macular lesions in secondary syphilis.

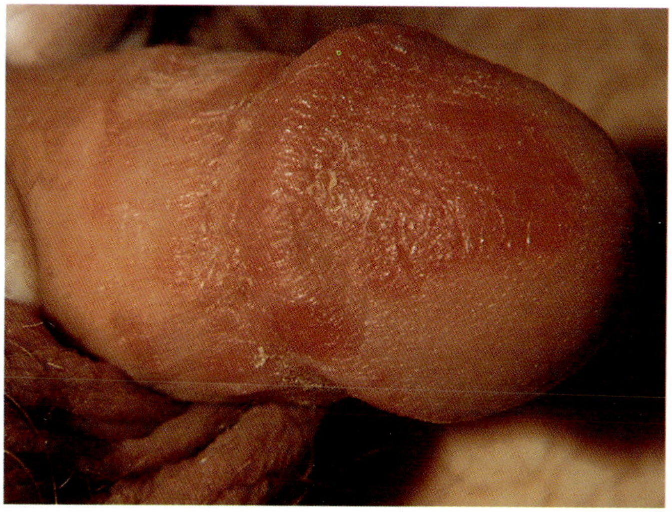

Plate 49. Seborrheic dermatitis of the glans and preputium of the penis. Red erythematous lesions, covered with yellowish-white scales. On the genitalia, seborrheic lesions are characteristically sharply defined.

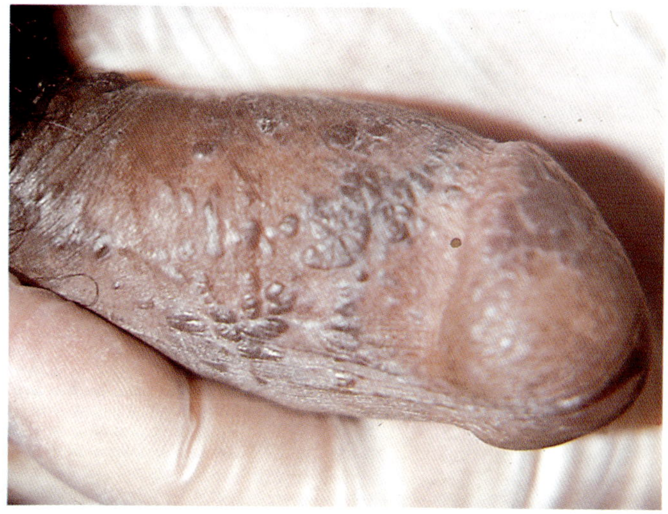

Plate 50. Lichen ruber planus of the penis. Brown, hyperpigmented papules on the penis. Reticulated white pattern on glans penis. Lichen ruber planus lesions may be flat, angular, and white linear striae (Wickham's striae) or atrophic variants can be seen.

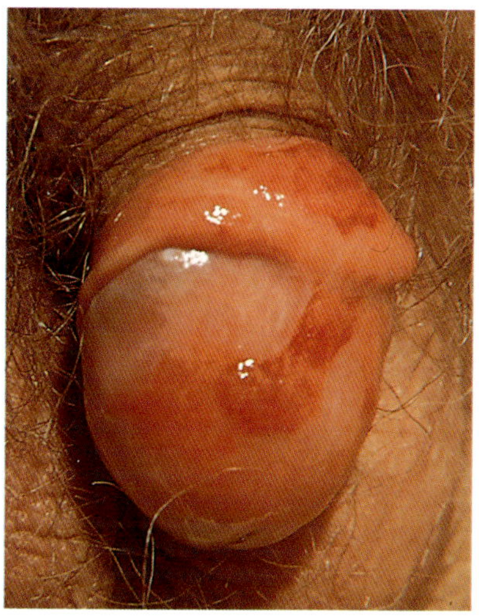

Plate 51. Plasmocellular balanitis. Patches of erythema with a shiny, smooth, and moist surface of glans and foreskin of the penis.

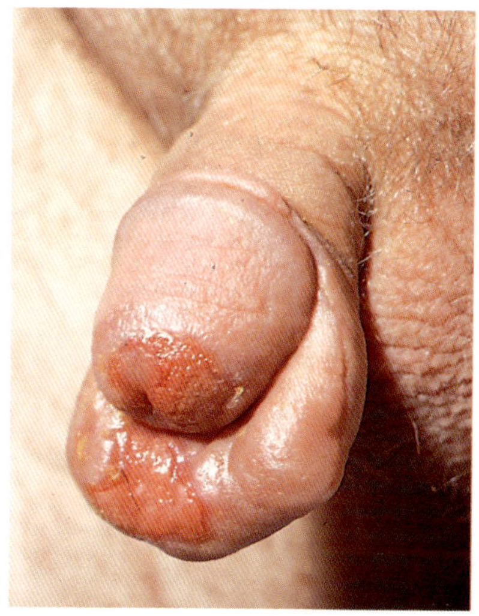

Plate 52. Erythroplasia of Queyrat. Red-colored, glazed, barely raised irregularly shaped plaques on glans and foreskin of the penis. These lesions also occur on the inner aspect of the vulva. Ulceration and crusting may occur.

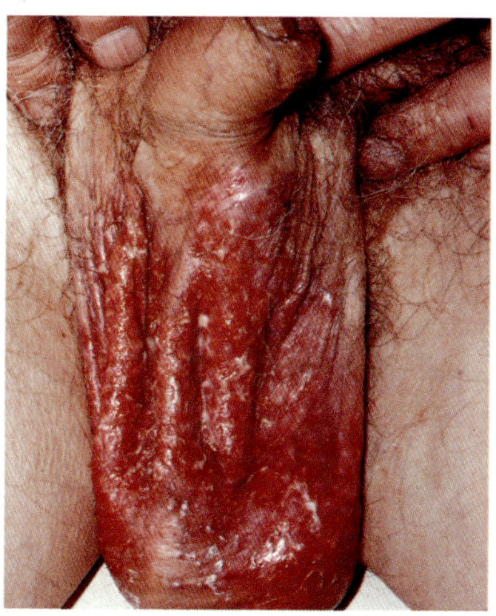

Plate 53. Scrotal candidiasis.

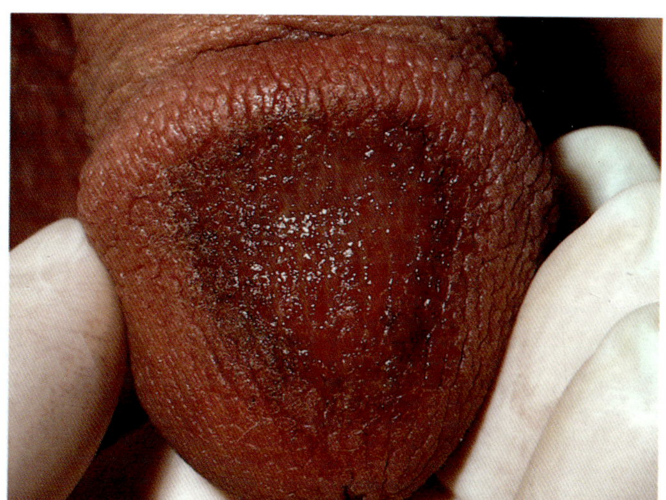

Plate 54. Fixed drug eruption of the glans penis due to tetracycline, showing an eroded surface and peripheral hyperpigmentation.

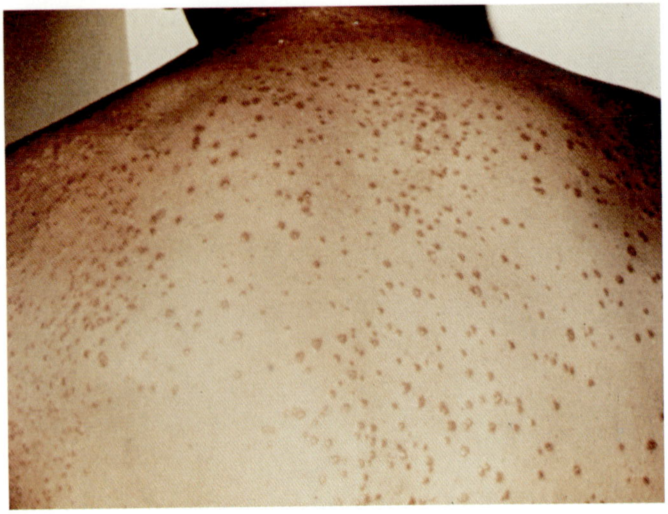

Plate 55. Droplike, or guttate, lesions of psoriasis. Such lesions are often seen with acute flares of the disease, often following streptococcal infection.

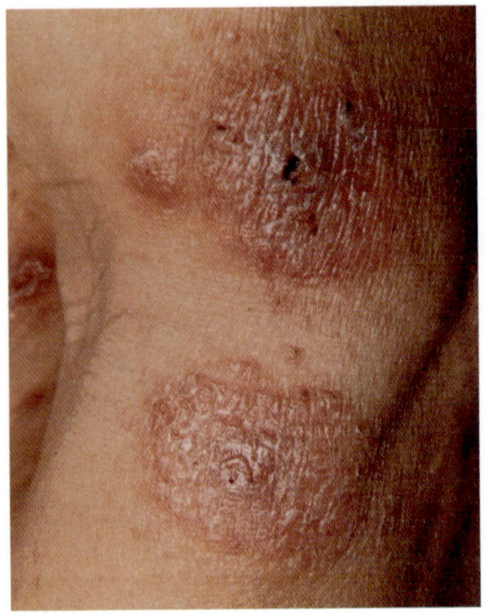

Plate 56. Morphologically these lesions look like psoriasis. In fact, they are psoriasiform lesions of secondary syphilis.

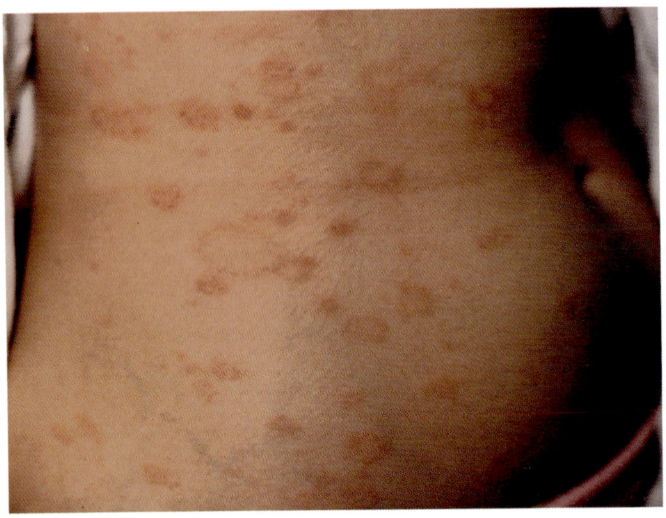

Plate 57. Characteristic lesions of pityriasis rosea.

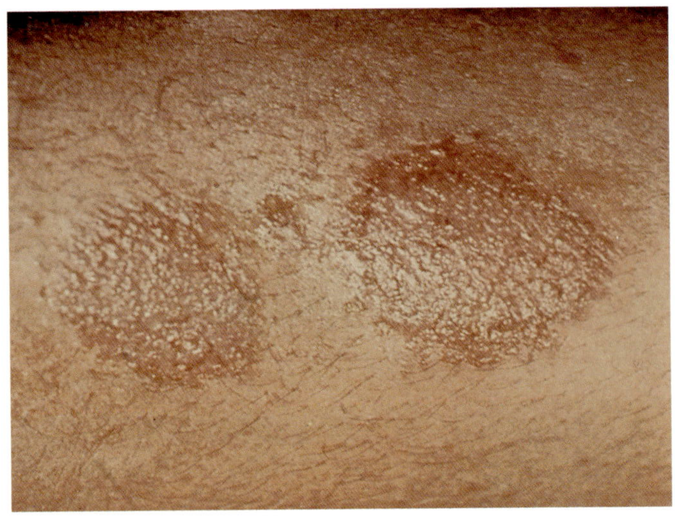

Plate 58. Scaling macules of nummular eczema.

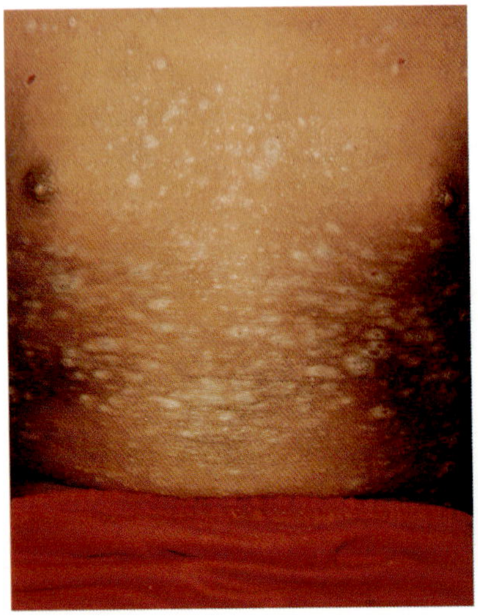

Plate 59. Lichen planus.

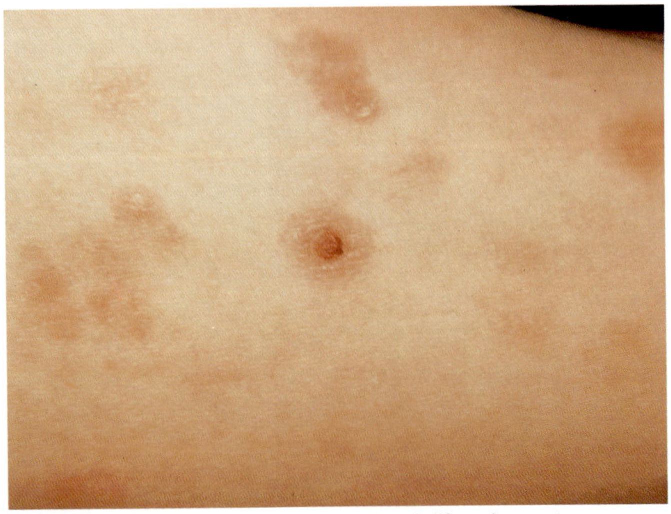

Plate 60. Pityriasis lichenoides et varioliformis acuta (PLEVA).

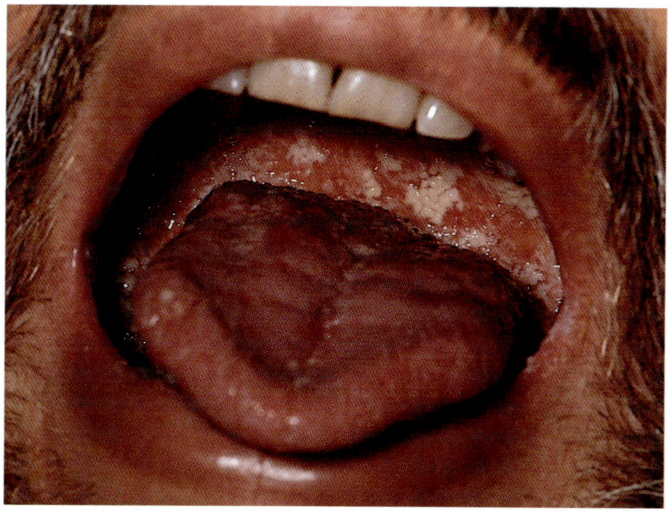

Plate 61. Oral thrush in a patient with HIV infection.

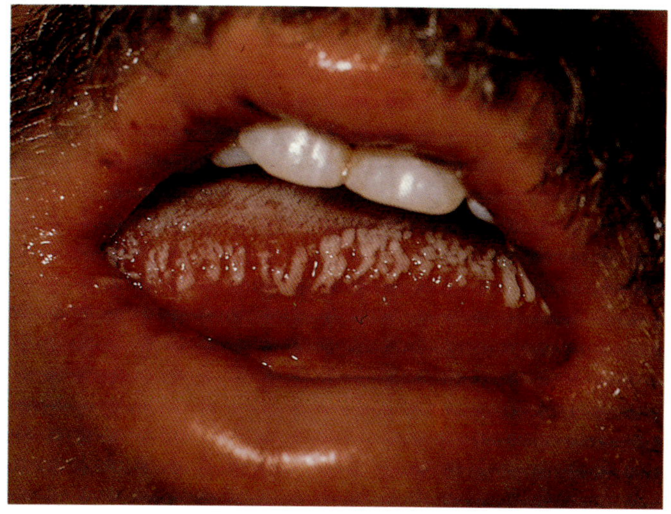

Plate 62. Oral hairy leukoplakia in a patient with HIV infection.

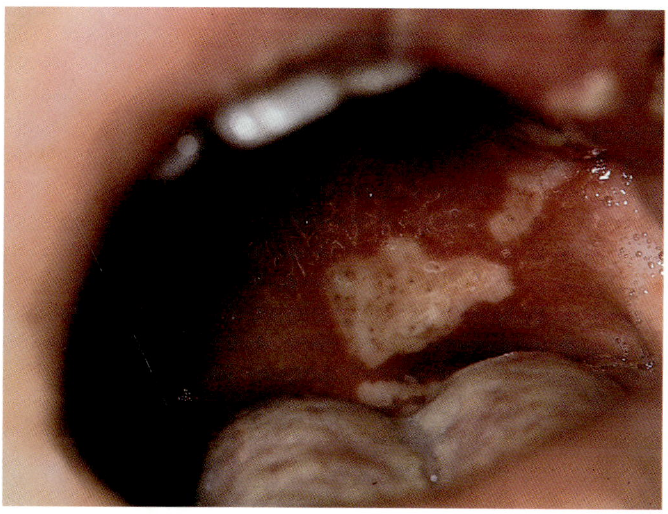

Plate 63. Oral herpes zoster (with cutaneous dissemination) in Group IVa HIV infection.

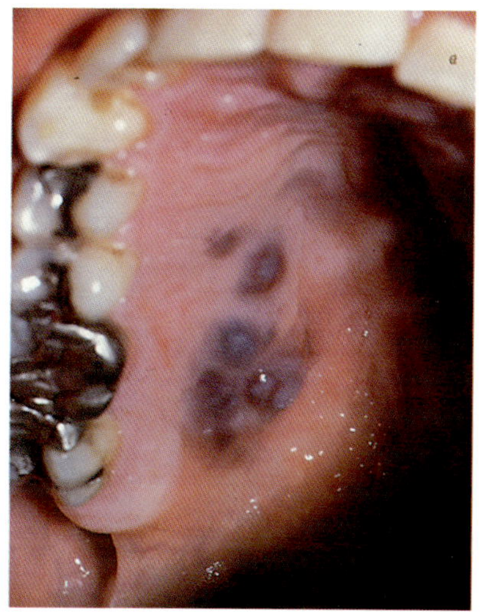

Plate 64. Kaposi's sarcoma in the palate as a manifestation of AIDS.

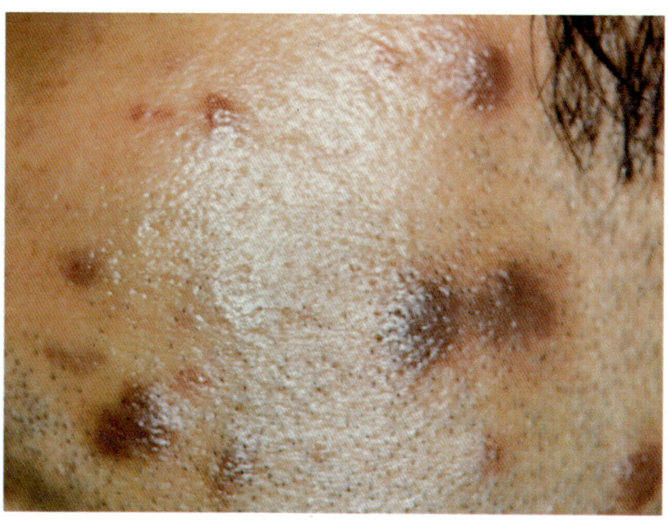

Plate 65. Kaposi's sarcoma on the face of a homosexually active man with AIDS.

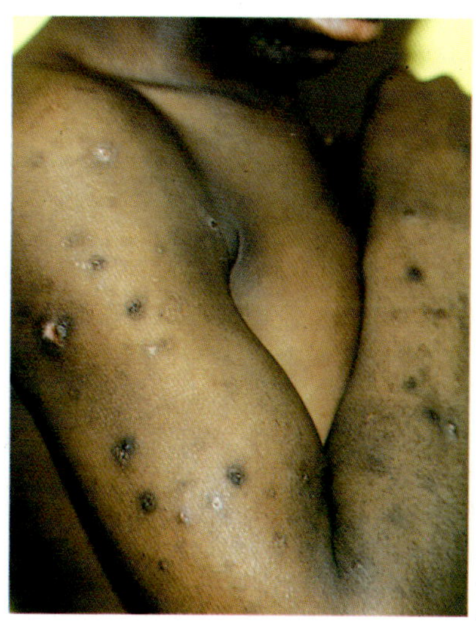

Plate 66. Pruritic excoriated rash on an African man with AIDS.

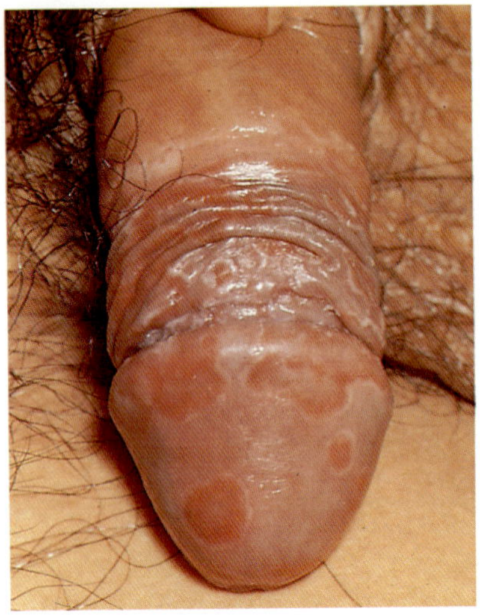

Plate 67. Circinate balanitis in Reiter's syndrome.

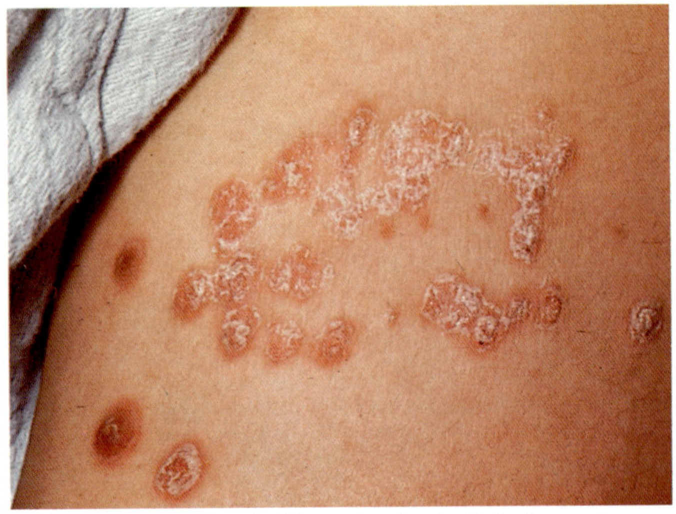

Plate 68. Keratodermia blenorrhagica in Reiter's syndrome.

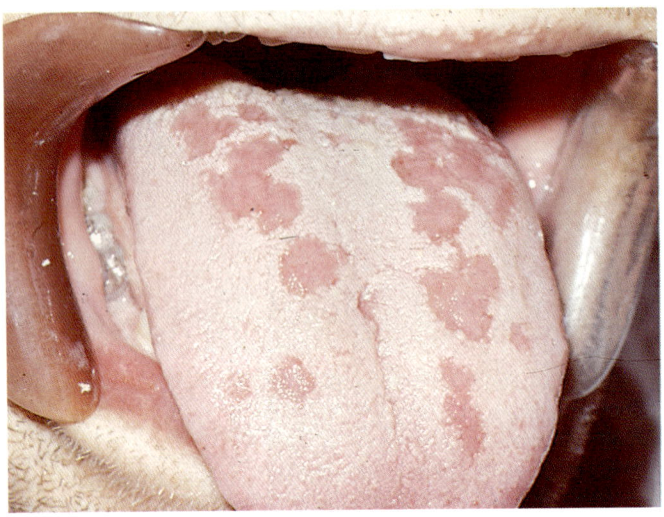

Plate 69. Superficial ulcerations of the tongue in Reiter's syndrome.

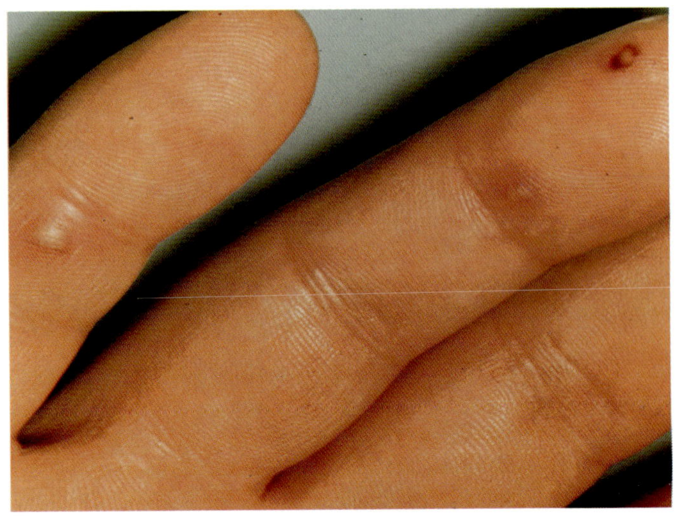

Plate 70. Typical distribution of skin lesions in disseminated gonococcal infection. Usually 5 to 20 such lesions are apparent on the extremities, generally sparing the face and trunk.

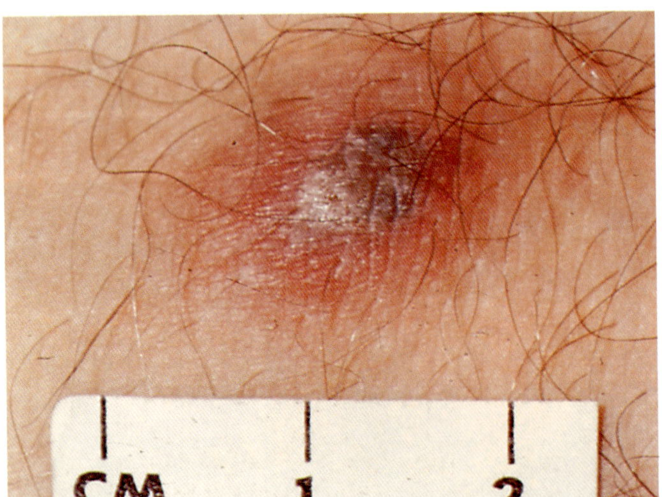

Plate 71. Hemorrhagic pustular lesion of disseminated gonococcal infection.

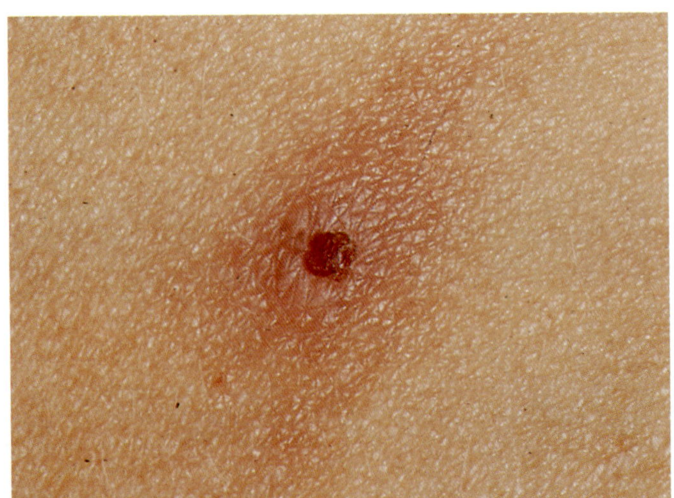

Plate 72. Crusted petechial lesion of disseminated gonococcal infection.

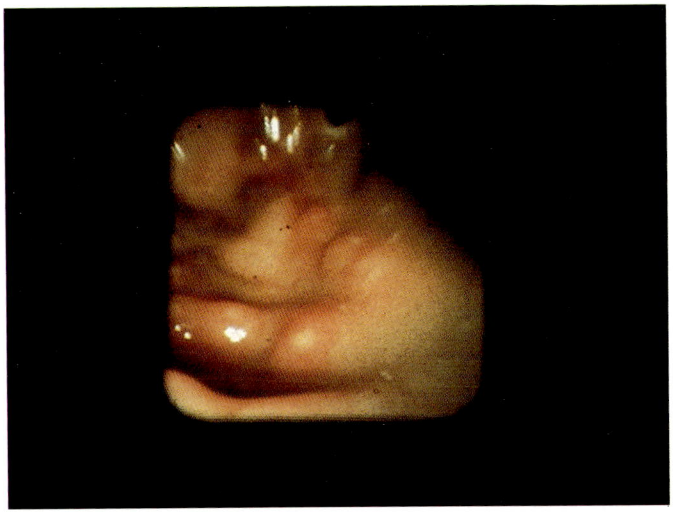

Plate 73. Short-bundle sigmoidoscopic view of the distal rectum in a patient with early primary anorectal herpes, showing intact vesiculopustules.

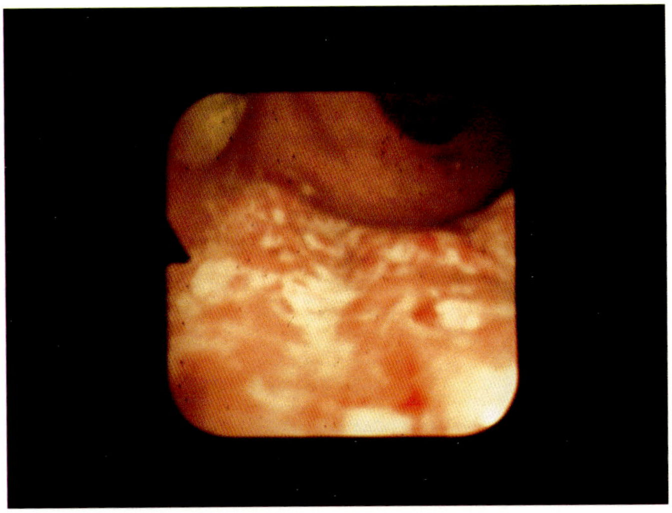

Plate 74. Short-bundle sigmoidoscopic view of primary anorectal herpes showing patchy bleeding and exudate extending up to 8 cm, with normal rectal mucosa above.

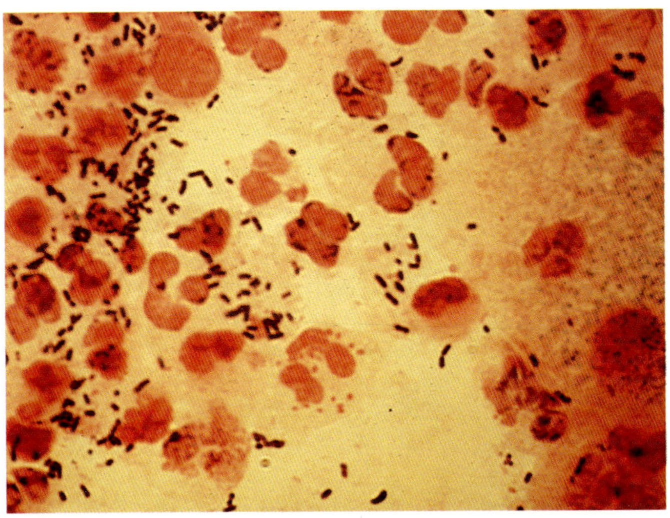

Plate 75. Gram-stained smear of exudate obtained at anoscopy showing one polymorphonuclear leukocyte containing gram-negative diplococci.

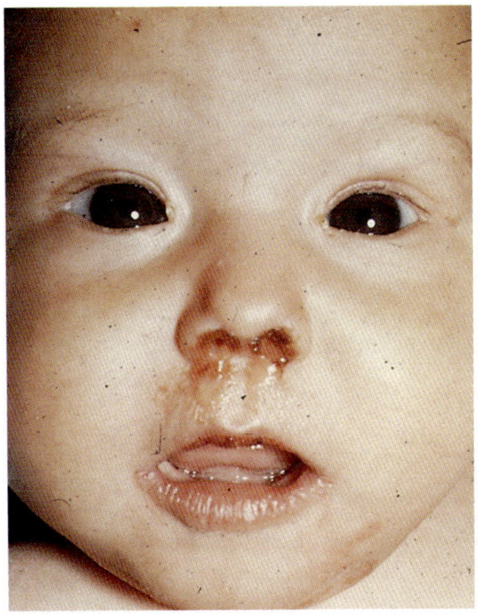

Plate 76. "Snuffles" associated with crusting and purulent nasal discharge in an infant with congenital syphilis.

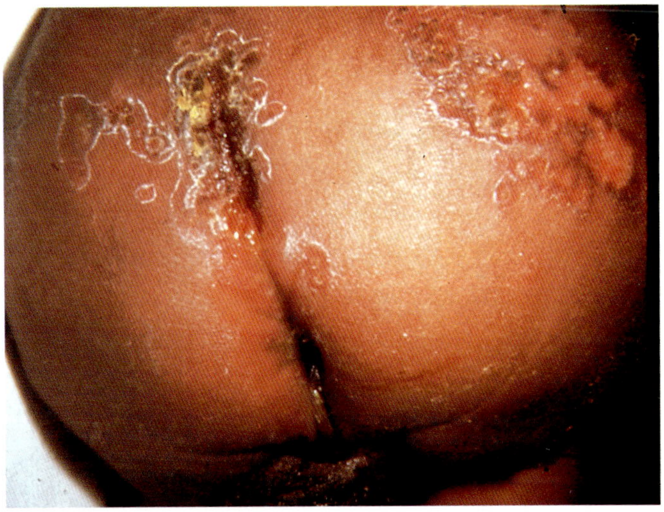

Plate 77. Neonatal HSV infection. Ulcers and crusted lesions on the buttocks.

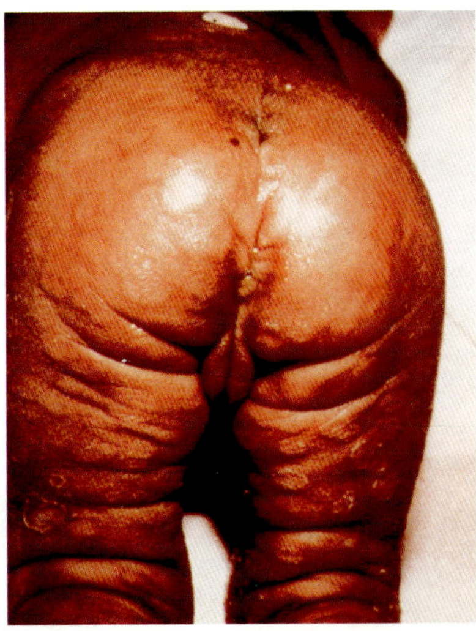

Plate 78. Congenital syphilis. Diffuse diskoid lesions associated with perianal lesions cover the entire body of this infant.

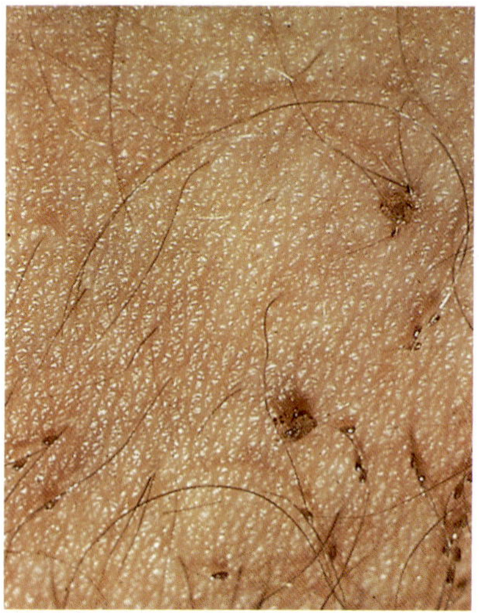

Plate 79. Heavy infestation with *Phthirus pubis,* showing nits (eggs) on pubic hair and adult crab lice holding onto pubic hairs.

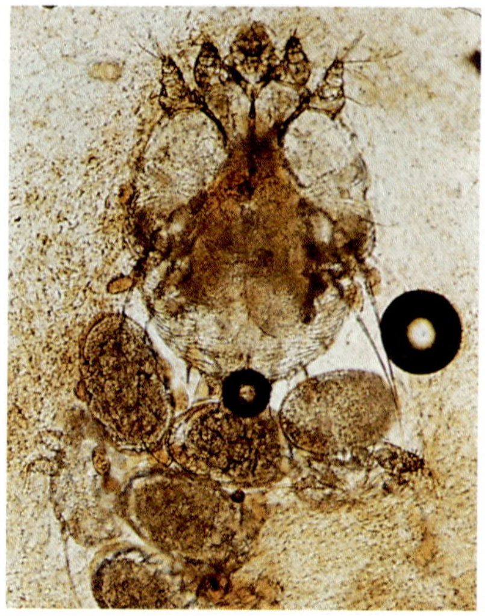

Plate 80. *Sarcoptes scabiei* mite with eggs in feces scraped from scabetic burrow.

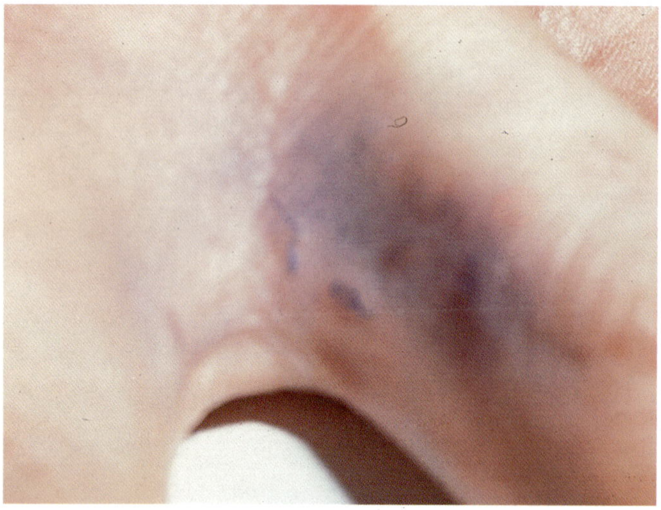

Plate 81. Intradermal burrow of scabies demonstrated by coating the skin with ink, then wiping away surface ink, leaving the intradermal burrow filled with ink.

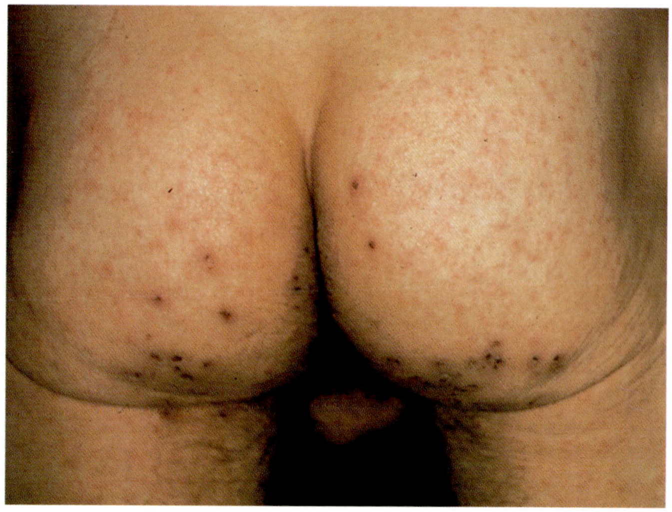

Plate 82. Grouped excoriations due to scabies on the lower buttocks, simulating dermatitis herpetiformis.

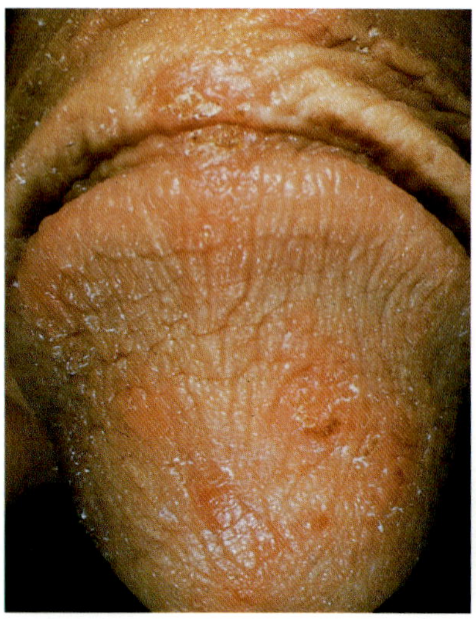

Plate 83. Scabies of the penis. Pyoderma of the penis is highly suggestive of scabies.

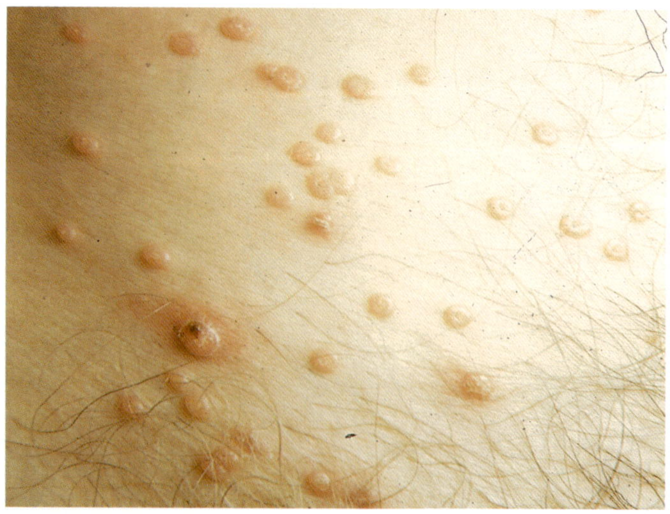

Plate 84. Molluscum contagiosum of the lower abdomen and suprapubic area in a patient with co-existing genital molluscum lesions. Note central umbilication and pale salmon color.

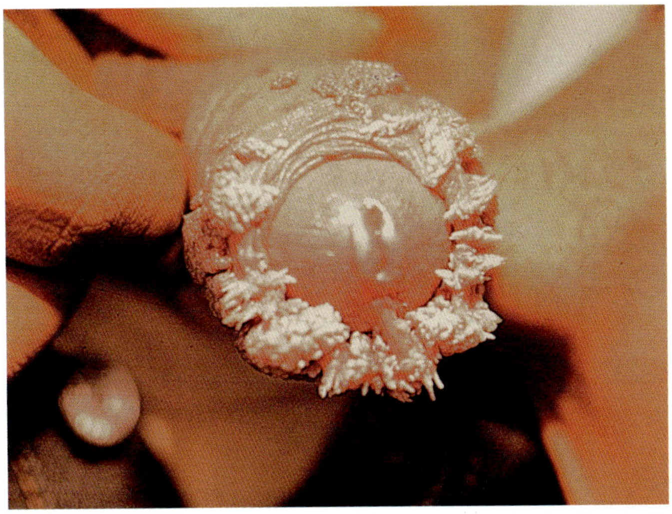

Plate 85. Extensive penile condylomata acuminata. Typically, exophytic visible condylomata of the external genitalia in the male and female are associated with HPV types 6 or 11.

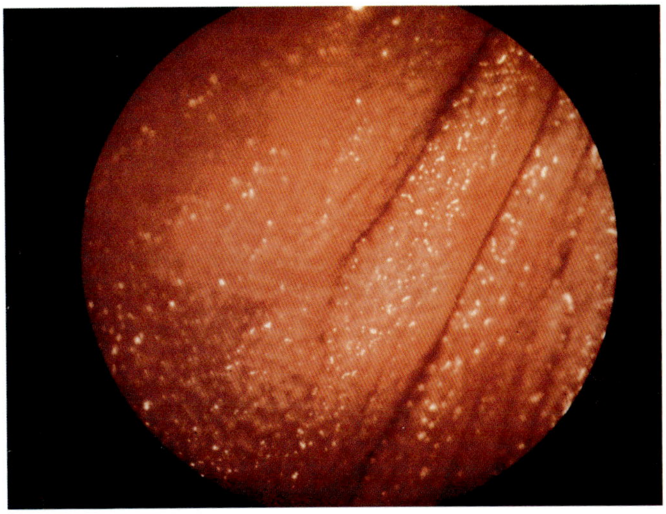

Plate 86. Vaginal asperities. Small somewhat-raised white dots diffusely scattered over the pink vaginal epithelium, following acetic acid treatment. Magnification 16×. It is suspected but not yet proven that these are associated with HPV infection of the vaginal epithelium.

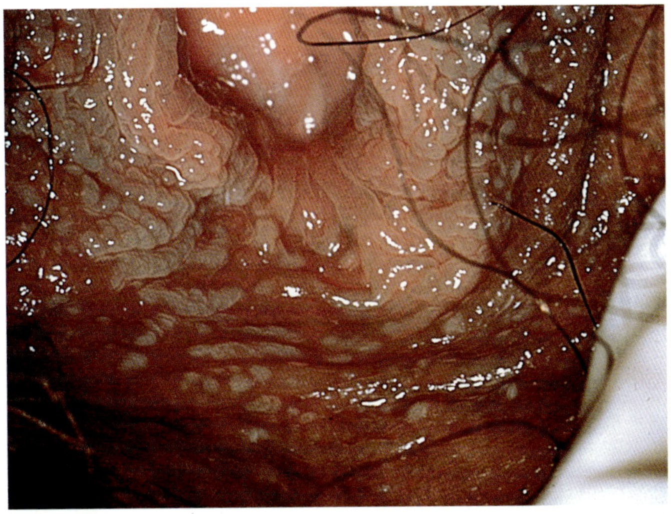

Plate 87. Appearance of "white epithelium" after application of acetic acid to the vulva. It is suspected that these lesions are associated with HPV infection.

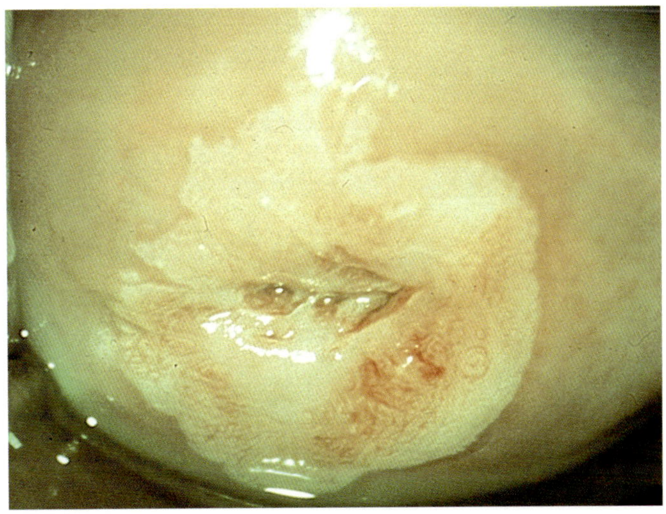

Plate 88. Appearance of "white epithelium" visualized with a colposcope through a green filter after application of acetic acid to the cervix. Opaque, white epithelium with sharp borders, as shown here, is associated with HPV infection.

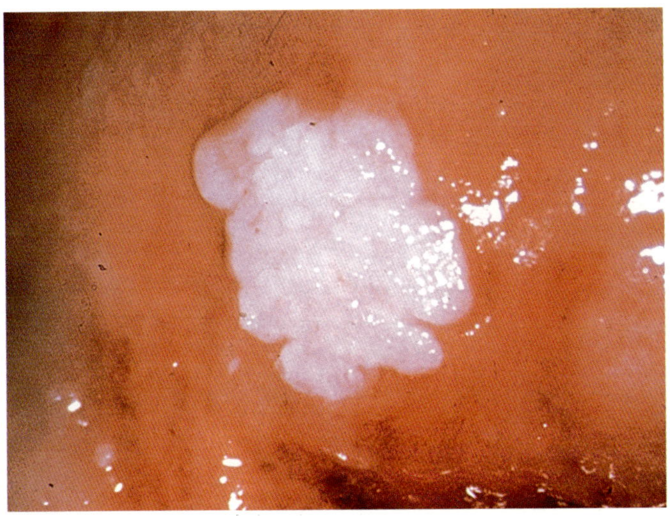

Plate 89. Cervical leukoplakia which is associated with dysplasia and cervical HPV infection.

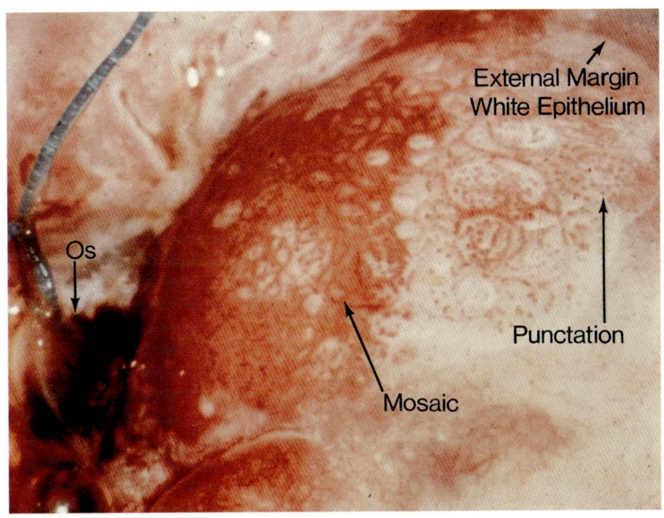

Plate 90. Severe dysplasia of the cervix as seen by colposcopy. This cervix displays features of punctation, mosaicism, and white epithelium.

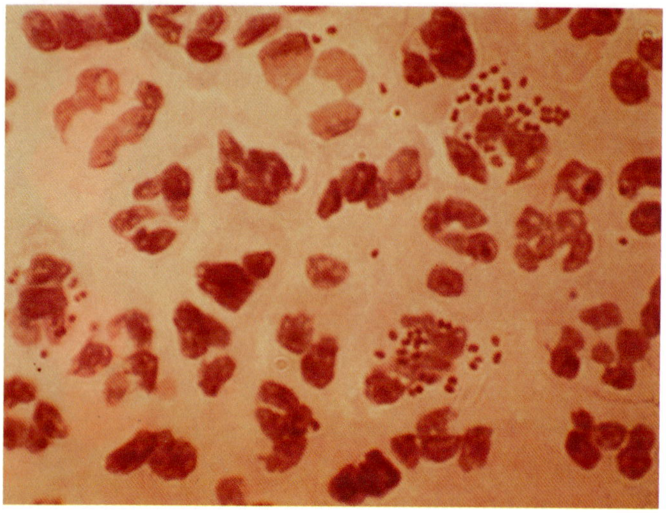

Plate 91. Gram stain of gonococcal urethritis, showing large number of Gram-negative intracellular diplococci.

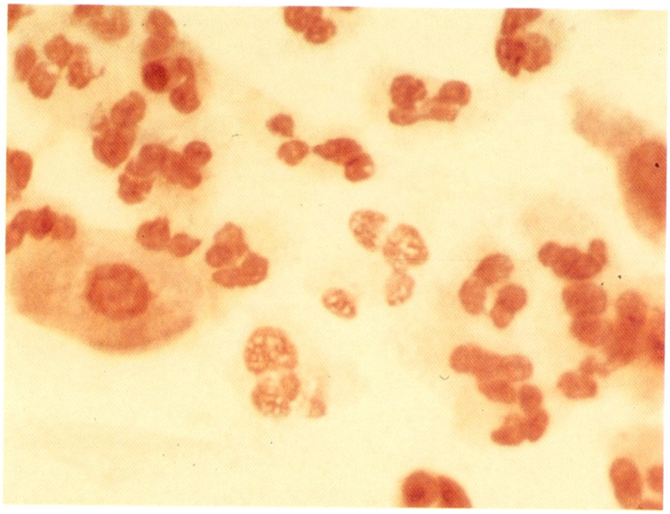

Plate 92. Smear from non-gonococcal urethritis. Note the presence of both polymorphonuclear leukocytes and occasional mononuclear leukocytes in the absence of Gram-negative diplococci.

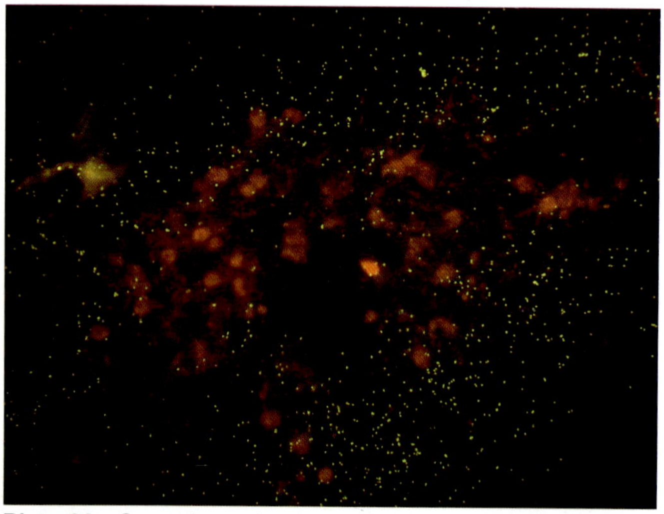

Plate 93. *C. trachomatic* elementary bodies visualized in endocervical exudate using fluorescein-conjugated species-specific monoclonal antibodies against *C. trachomatis*.

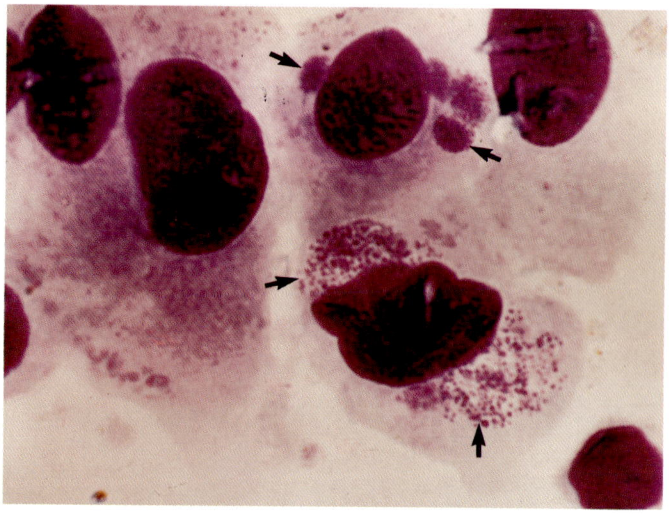

Plate 94. Giemsa-stained conjunctival scraping from neonatal inclusion conjunctivitis caused by *C. trachomatis* (arrows indicate chlamydial inclusions).

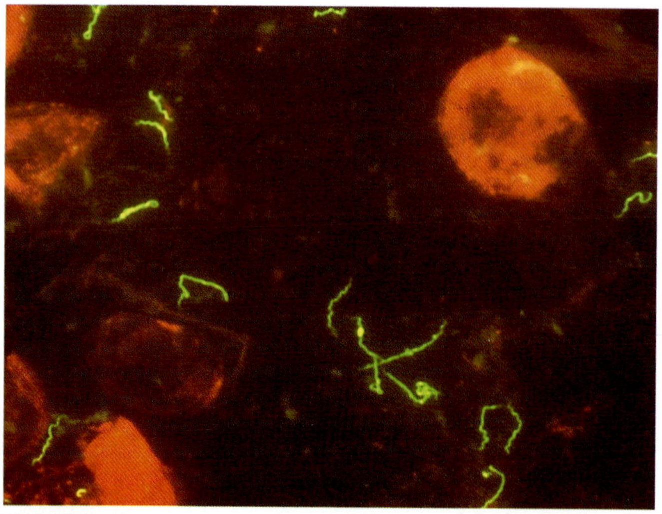

Plate 95. *Treponema pallidum* identified on direct smear from primary human chancre using species-specific fluoroscein-conjugated monoclonal antibody to *T. pallidum*.

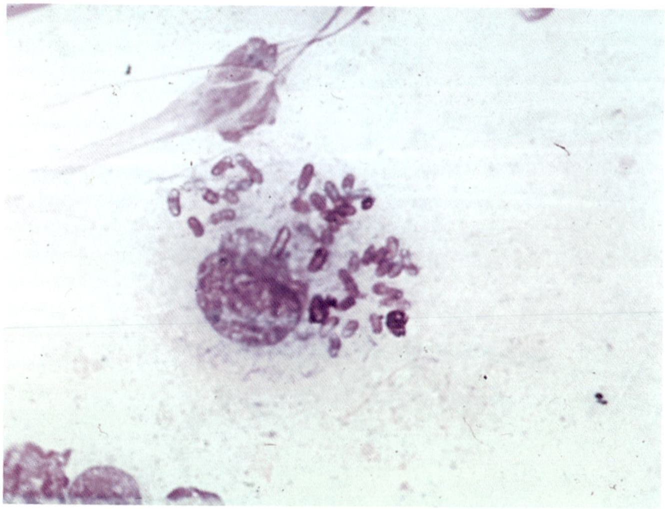

Plate 96. Impression smear from a punch biopsy obtained from the margin of a lesion of donovanosis and stained with Wright-Giemsa stain, showing typical donovan bodies.

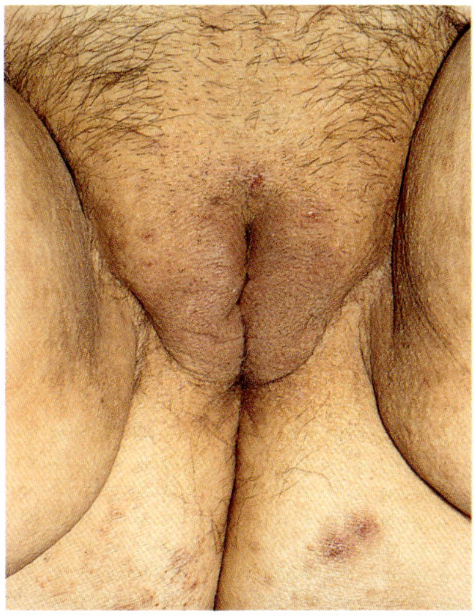

Plate 97. Neurodermatitis is produced by rubbing and scratching as seen here with thickening of the skin of the labia majora,excoriations, broken hairs,and erythema

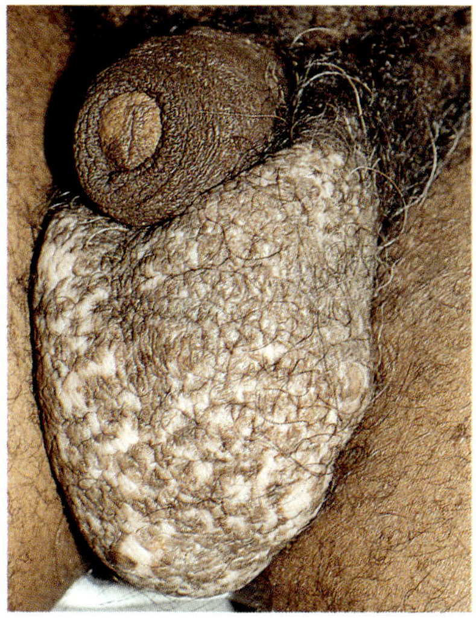

Plate 98. Remarkable thickening of the scrotum with white areas of postinflammatory hypopigmentation are typical of neurodermatitis in black skin.

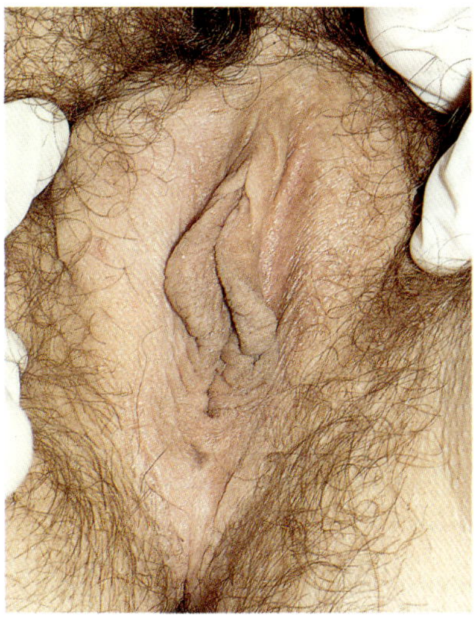

Plate 99. Excruciating pruritus was associated with the relatively subtle thickening of the right inner labium majus, manifested by slightly lighter color, mild thickening,and drier appearance than seen on the contralateral side.In addition, excoriations are visible, and fissures with scale suggestive of bacterial or yeast superinfection

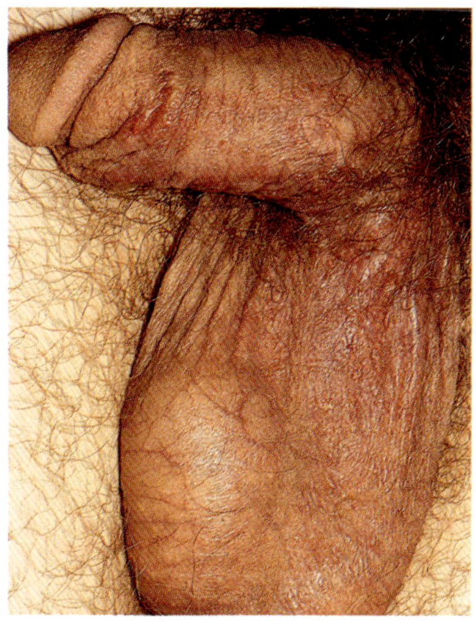

Plate 100. This red, scaling and crusted plaque of irritant contact dermatitis was produced by washing the area several times a day with a disinfectant intended for cleaning floors.

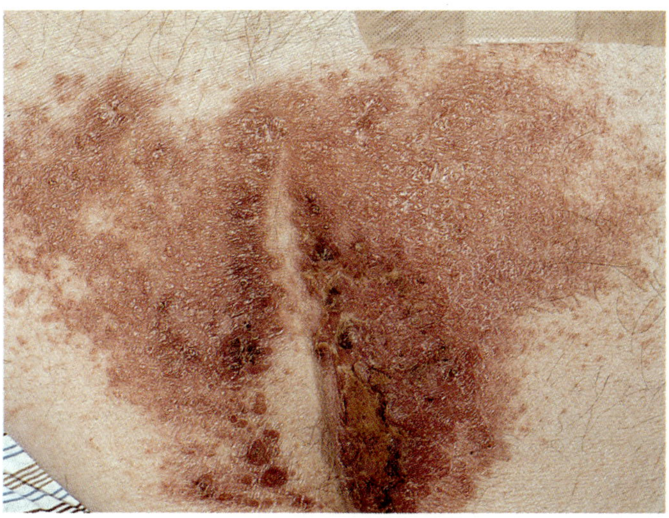

Plate 101. Erythema,exudation,and crusting is characteristic of allergic contact dermatitis in this patient who applied diphenhydramine (Benadryl) for itching. Positive results of patch testing,extreme pruritus,and time of onset are often more useful than morphology for differentiation from irritant contact dermatitis.

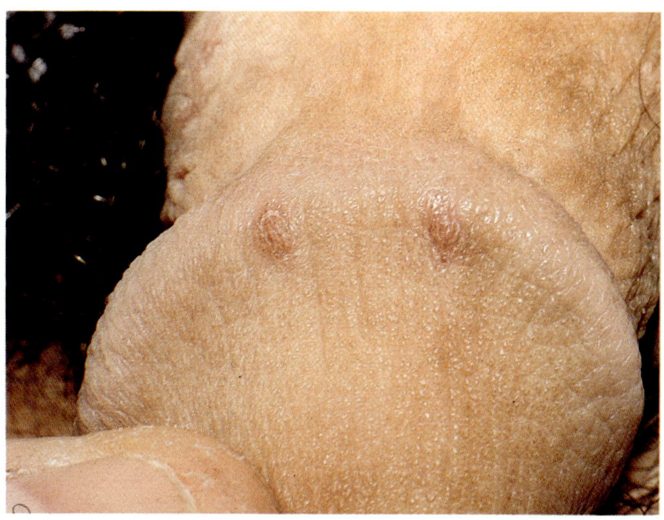

Plate 102. Two nondescript, red, scaling papules over the edge of the corona are characteristic of lichen planus but could also represent candida infection, psoriasis, or even scabies. An examination of other skin surfaces and the mouth may produce the diagnosis without a biopsy.

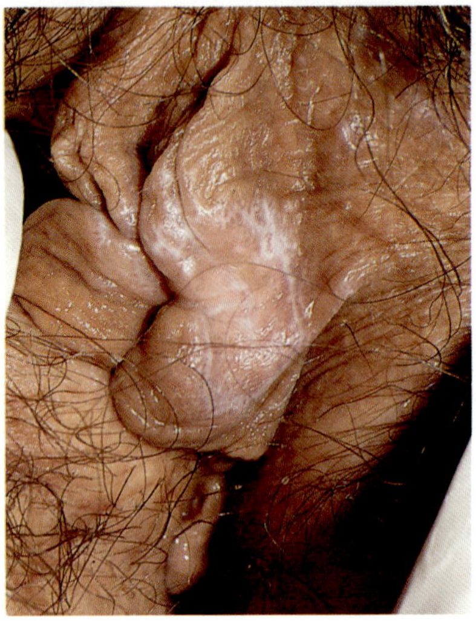

Plate 103. These white, branching striae are pathognomonic of lichen planus.

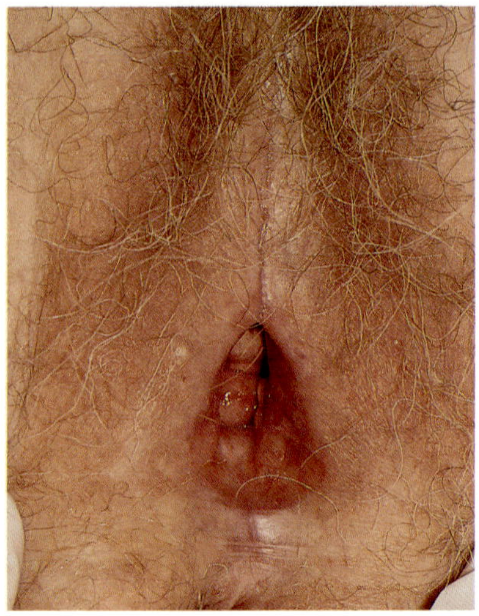

Plate 104. Endstage scarring with obliteration of the labia minora and clitoris, with remaining erosions of the vestibule (introitus) are characteristic of erosive lichen planus, but can be seen also with late lichen sclerosus, cicatricial pemphigoid, pemphigus vulgaris, or any other intensely inflammatory, chronic vulvar disease. The diagnosis requires the identification of specific lesions elsewhere or a characteristic biopsy.

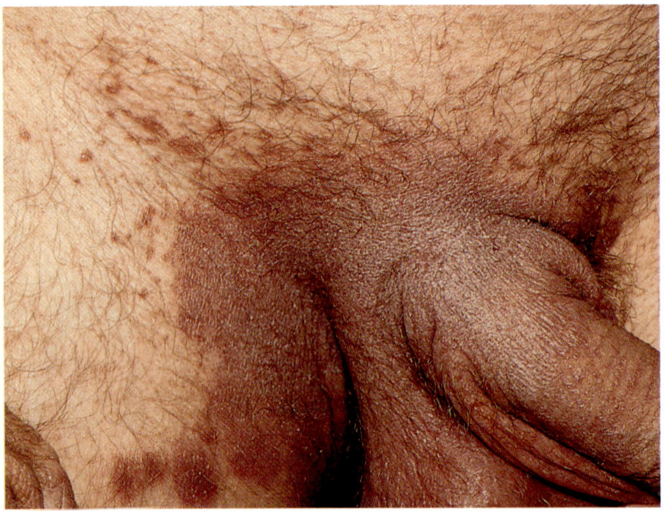

Plate 105. Psoriasis characterized by sharply demarcated, red, thickened plaques. Scale is present on the penis, although the classic heavy, silvery scale is often absent in the moist genital area.

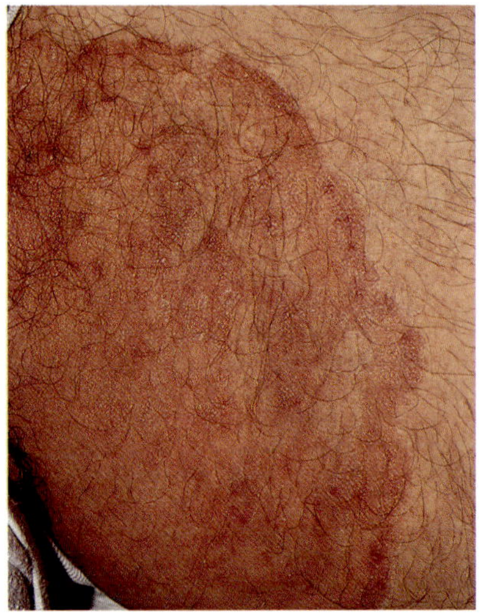

Plate 106. Red, scaling plaques with distinct margins and accentuation of disease at the borders are features of tinea cruris.

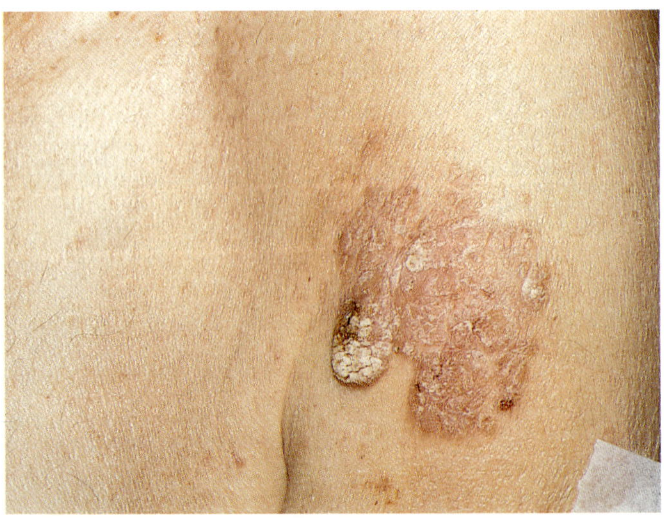

Plate 107. This sharply marginated, red, scaling, and hyperkeratotic plaque of Bowen's disease could easily be mistaken for psoriasis. However, the existence of a solitary plaque and a poor response to topical therapy should prompt a skin biopsy. Lesions may be more moist and less thickened, particularly on damp skin such as the modified mucous membranes and uncircumcised penis (erythroplasia of Queyrat).

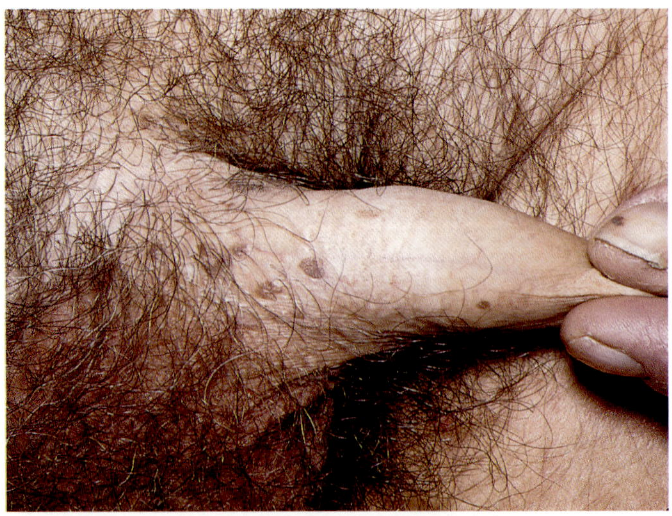

Plate 108. Bowenoid papulosis, a variant of squamous cell carcinoma in situ associated with human papillomavirus infection, resembles flat genital warts and may be pigmented, pink, or skin-colored.

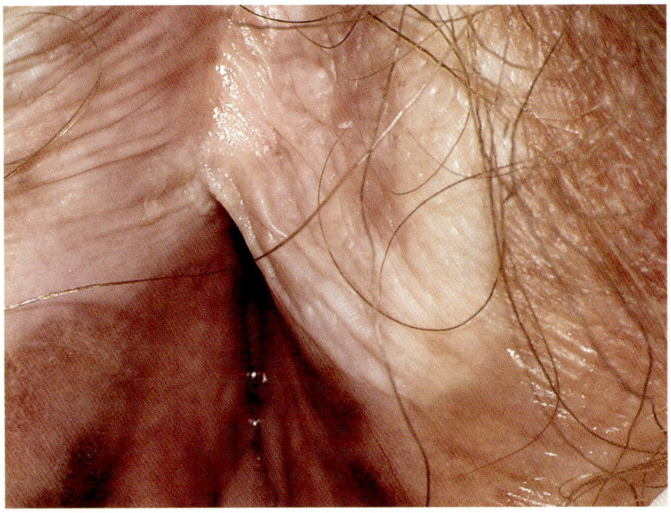

Plate 109. The wrinkling of this white plaque covering the modified mucous membranes of the anterior vulva is an extremely useful finding that differentiates lichen sclerosus from vitiligo, the white lesions of lichen planus, and postinflammatory hypopigmentation.

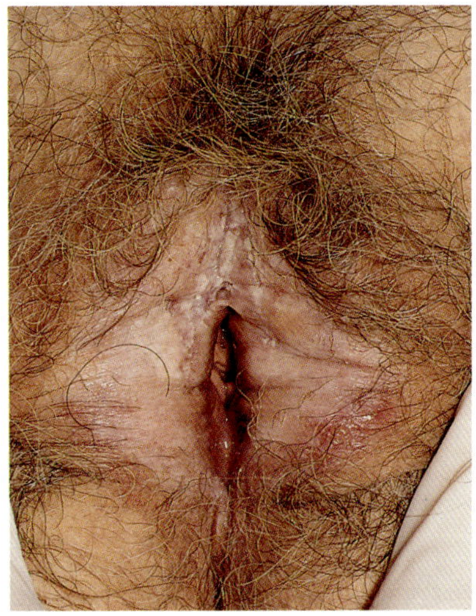

Plate 110. Late lichen sclerosus displays the characteristic hypopigmentation and fine wrinkling in association with loss of labia minora and clitoral hood to scarring.

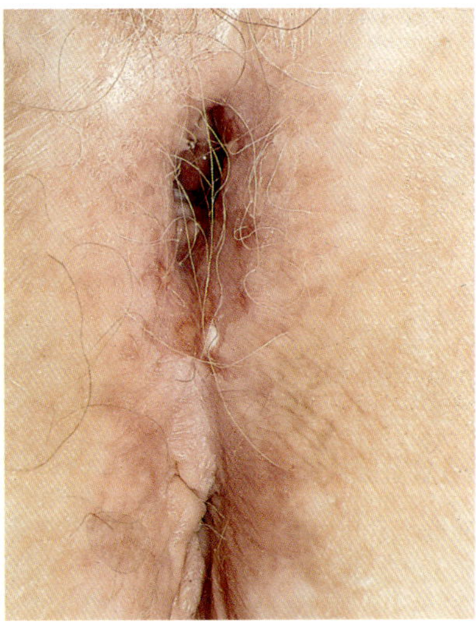

Plate 111. Kraurosis vulvae consists of severe scarring of the vulvae and narrowing of the introitus due to lichen sclerosus. The erosions at the introitus were firm on palpation and proved to be squamous cell carcinoma.

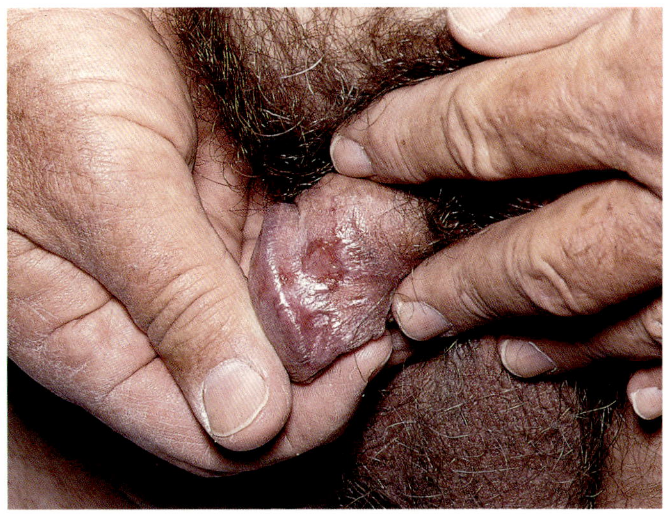

Plate 112. This nonspecific erosion due to a fixed drug eruption can be differentiated from ulcers caused by STD by its superficial nature and association with several other round, edematous plaques or blisters on keratinized skin, or oral lesions.

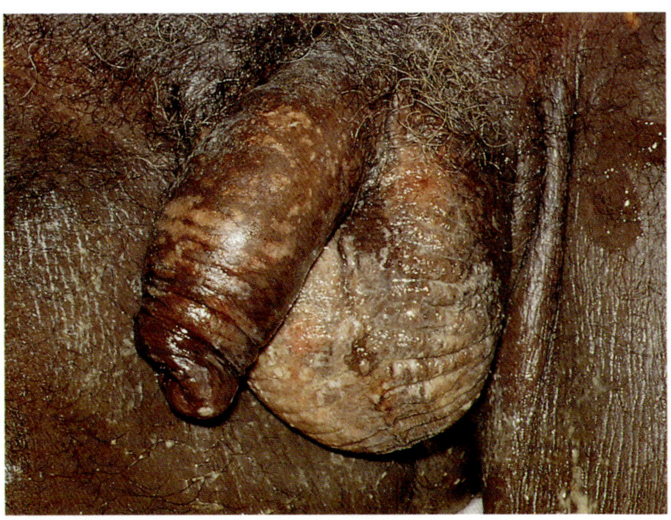

Plate 113. Intense inflammation with resulting necrosis and loss of the epidermis and exudation is characteristic of bullous erythema multiforme (Stevens-Johnson syndrome, toxic epidermal necrolysis).

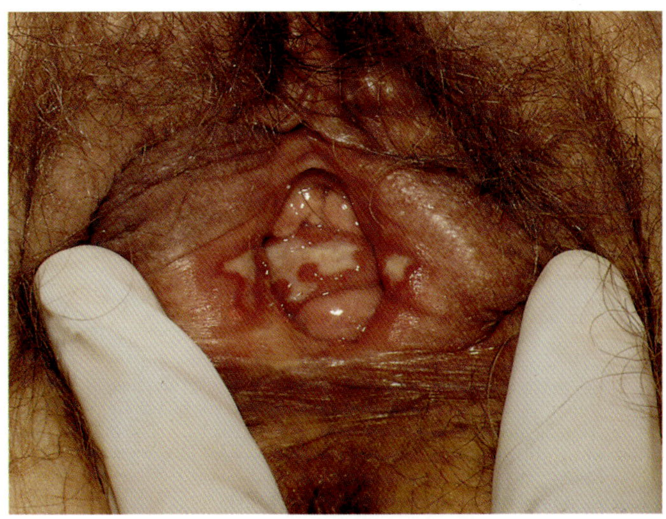

Plate 114. These aphthous ulcers show the characteristic larger size (as compared to oral lesions), peripheral red flare, and fibrin base. In the absence of a history of recurrence or oral aphthae, a biopsy may be required to rule out sexually transmitted causes.

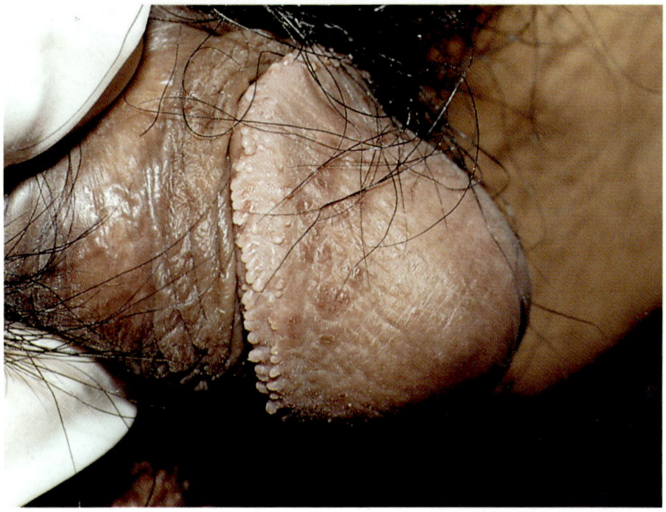

Plate 115. Pearly penile papules are differentiated from genital warts by their regular, monomorphous appearance in rows around the edge of the corona, and the dome-shaped rather than keratotic, acuminate tips to the papules.

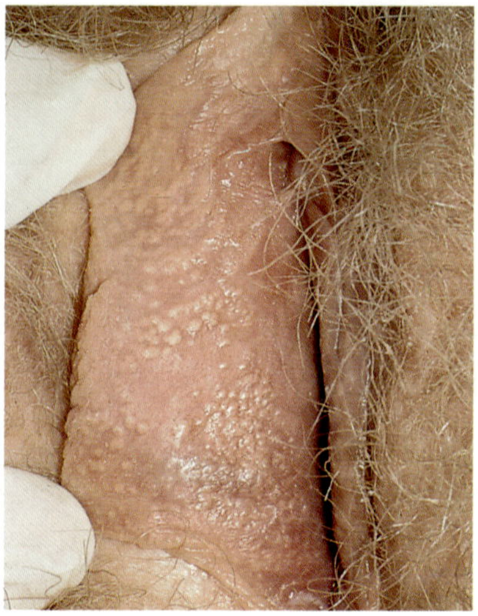

Plate 116. Fordyce spots represent enlarged sebaceous glands located primarily over the inner aspect of the labia minora although they can be seen elsewhere,including the penis.Individual papules are lobular and white, yellowish,or skin colored.

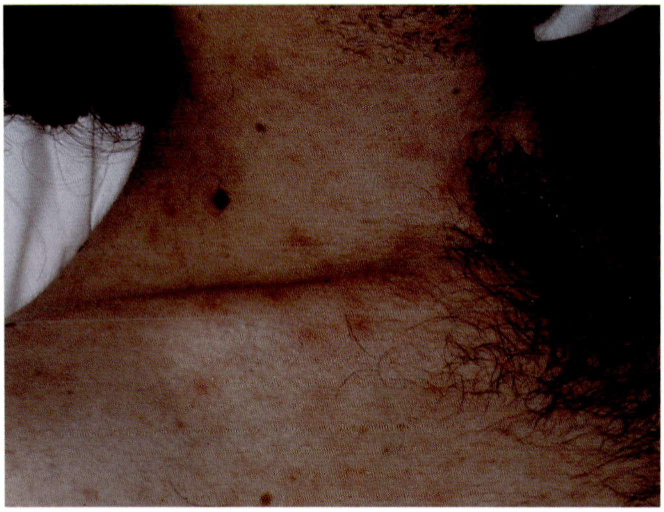

Plate 117. Erythematous macular and papular exanthem in acute HIV infection.*(Reproduced with permission from Handsfield HH. Atlas of Sexually Transmitted Diseases, McGraw-Hill, New York, 1992.)*

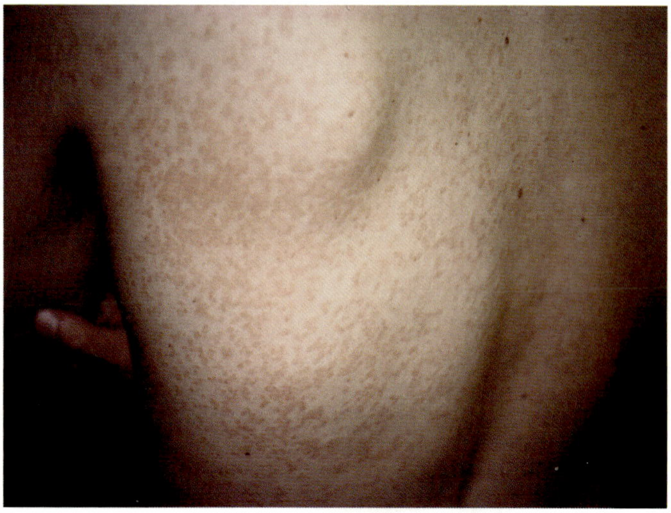

Plate 118. Generalized maculopapular rash due to drug hypersensitivity.

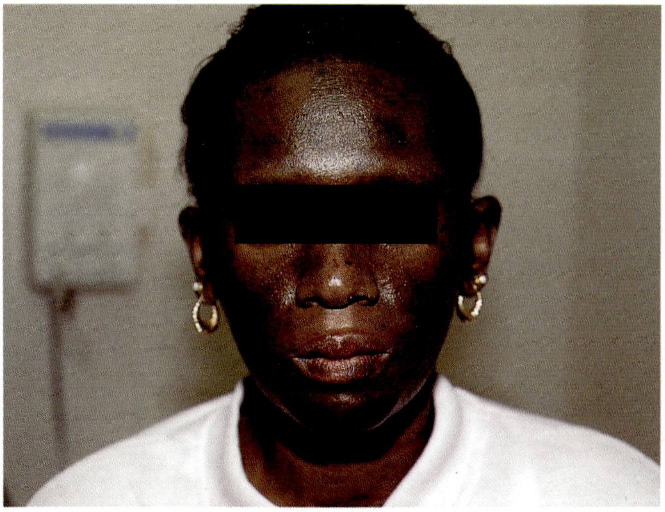

Plate 119. Hyperpigmentation associated with zidovudine (AZT) therapy.

incidence.[225] The seroprevalences of HIV were 15–17 percent among patients with PID compared to 2–3 percent among control women in two U.S. studies,[226,227] and they were elevated in patients with PID in Nairobi.[228] Infection with HIV may also influence the course and clinical manifestations of PID, particularly among patients with markedly suppressed immunity. pPatients with PID who were also HIV positive tended to have more abscesses[228,229] and more frequent surgical intervention[229,230] compared to HIV-seronegative women with PID. The Centers for Disease Control and Prevention (CDC) recommends early hospitalization and intravenous antibiotics for HIV-infected women with PID.[231]

CLINICAL MANIFESTATIONS

In response to the spread of microorganisms from the lower to the upper genital tract, and in some instances into the abdominal cavity, the host produces inflammatory mediators causing endometritis, salpingitis, peritonitis, or perihepatitis. Different etiologic agents (*N. gonorrhoeae, C. trachomatis*, etc.) tend to cause different clinical presentations, ranging from mild to severe (Fig. 58–4). Mild symptoms may not prompt patients to seek care and may allow physicians to miss the diagnosis. About two-thirds (range 30–75 percent) of infertile women with post-infection tubal obstruction report no history of prior PID,[4,232–235] indicating that subclinical infection accounts for the majority of PID and tubal infertility following PID. On the other hand, many patients who do receive a clinical diagnosis of PID have other conditions. The specificity of any one clinical and laboratory diagnostic procedure is low; up to one-third of women with pain and other clinical findings suggestive of PID in fact have other diseases or no disease.[29, 236–42] Thus, the clinical diagnosis of PID is incorrect about one-third of the time.

Subclinical disease (atypical PID, "silent" PID)

Historically, low abdominal or pelvic pain has been regarded as the symptom *sine qua non* to suspect acute PID.[2] As noted above, however, individuals with apparent subclinical infection identified in studies of post-infection stigmata of salpingitis—such as tubal occlusion, hydrosalpinx, infertility, and ectopic pregnancy—often give no past history of having had treatment for PID. On the other hand, in detailed focused interviews of infertile women with "no history of PID," medical visits for abdominal pain were reported by 60 percent of women with tubal occlusion, compared to 19 percent of those without tubal disease.[243] Thus, many who recall receiving no treatment for PID may nevertheless have experienced symptomatic PID, and may even have sought medical care.

Inflammation, or microorganisms, in the endometrium and fallopian tubes, and abnormal tubal ciliary function, can be found in women with no or few symptoms of PID. Histopathologic evidence of endometritis (≥10 plasma cells in any of six tissue sections) was found in 45 percent of women with mucopurulent cervicitis, including 65 percent of those with chlamydia-associated mucopurulent cervicitis.[27] Some of these patients had abnormal uterine bleeding or mild uterine tenderness, but no overt signs of salpingitis. Other studies have demonstrated *C. trachomatis* in the endometrium in 5 of 19 asymptomatic infertile women with serum antibody to chlamydia,[244] and in the fallopian tubes of 6 of 39 infertile women with no clinical or laparoscopic evidence of acute salpingitis.[245] Among asymptomatic women undergoing laparoscopic sterilization, plasma cells were present in the tubal mucosa of 47 percent of IUD users and 1 percent of those who have never used IUDs.[235]

Some evidence suggests C. *trachomatis* infection can persist without symptoms in fallopian tubes after treatment. In one study, *C. trachomatis* DNA and/or antigen was detected in fallopian tube biopsy specimens of 19 of 24 women undergoing surgery for post-infection tubal factor infertility (TFI).[83] Eight women had been treated for PID and six for chlamydial cervicitis. Such data requires confirmation.

Another study suggests that tubal pathology from prior PID appears unrelated to presence or absence of history of previous clinical symptoms. Among 59 women with TFI, abnormal ciliary-beat frequency in fallopian tube specimens, and structure measured by scanning and transmission electron microscopy, were identical in women with and without a history of overt PID.[246]

Thus, ascending infection can cause endometrial and tubal inflammation, resulting in tubal scarring, impaired tubal function, tubal occlusion, and infertility, even among those who report no prior treatment for PID. *C. trachomatis* is particularly implicated in subclinical PID, on the basis of (1) lack of prior history of PID among chlamydia-seropositive women with tubal damage[4,232]; (2) detection of chlamydial DNA or antigen among asymptomatic women with tubal infertility[83]; and (3) clinical manifestation of acute infection among those with symptomatic PID, as discussed below. These data further imply that the best method to prevent PID and its sequelae is the surveillance and control of lower genital tract infection, particularly chlamydial and gonococcal infections. Promotion of early symptom recognition and health-care seeking may also reduce the sequelae of PID.

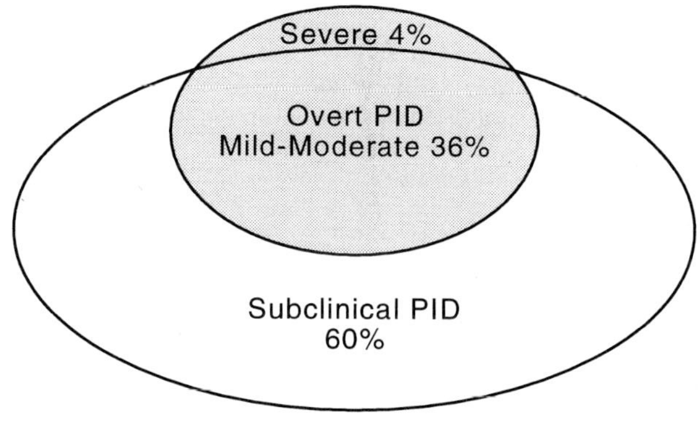

Fig. 58-4. Illustration of the probable proportions of clinical manifestations of PID.

Mild and moderately severe pelvic inflammatory disease

Most of the laparoscopically verified cases of overt PID have had mild to moderate symptoms and physical signs (see Fig. 58–4).[29] Up to 75 percent of women with mild or moderate PID are sexually active, are less than 25 years of age, and have gonococcal or chlamydial infection.[46,207,247]

In Table 58–3, the consecutive women routinely laparoscoped because of assumed PID all had low abdominal or pelvic pain for less than 3 weeks, cervical motion tenderness, and an increase of inflammatory cells in the cervical/vaginal secretion on microscopic wet mount.[2,29] Salpingitis was identified at laparoscopy in 65 percent of those with a clinical diagnosis of PID, but some of the remaining women without salpingitis had lower genital tract in-

Table 58-3. Percent Prevalence of Symptoms, Signs, and Laboratory Abnormalities among 807 Women Subjected to Laparoscopy because of Clinically Suspected Salpingitis. All Women had (as Inclusion Criteria) Abdominal Pain, Adnexal Tenderness, and Objective Evidence of Purulent Vaginal Discharge. (Refs 2, 29)

	Laparoscopic diagnosis			Laparoscopic diagnosis	
Symptoms	Salpingitis, % ($n = 623$)	No salpingitis*, % ($n = 184$)	Signs and laboratory abnormalities	Salpingitis, % ($n = 623$)	No salpingitis*, % ($n = 184$)
Abnormal discharge	55	56	Temperature > 38.0°C	41	20
Irregular bleeding	36	43	Palpable mass	49	25
Dysuria	19	20	ESR ≥ 15 mm/h	76	53
Vomiting	10	9	WBC > 10,000/ml blood†	59	33
Anorectal symptoms	7	3	Acute phase reactants‡	79	24
			Decreased isoamylases§	90	20

* Normal intraperitoneal findings; assumed to have lower genital tract infection or endometritis.
† WBC was determined in 186 cases of salpingitis and 54 controls with no salpingitis.
‡ Antichymotrypsin, orosomucoid, or acute-phase reactants including CRP, determined in 40 cases of salpingitis and 15 controls with no salpingitis.
§ Determined in peritoneal fluid in 57 cases of salpingitis and 20 controls without salpingitis.

fection.[2] The prevalence of selected symptoms in Table 58–3 was similar among women found to have salpingitis and those with no salpingitis, however, and no symptoms helped to distinguish the group with salpingitis.

Various combinations of symptoms and signs are also given in Table 58–4 for the proportions of 2,220 women in the Swedish study with and without salpingitis. A minimum of clinical and laboratory abnormalities (lower abdominal pain plus signs of a lower genital tract infection and cervical motion tenderness) was present in 16 percent of women with salpingitis. Sixty-one percent of women with salpingitis and 39 percent of those without salpingitis had these minimum abnormalities. The addition of an elevated ESR or temperature or an adnexal mass (especially two to three of these abnormalities) increased the possibility of salpingitis and decreased the possibility of no salpingitis. In fact, 84 percent of the women with salpingitis had the minimum criteria and at least one of the three additional abnormalities; however, so too did 36 percent of those with no salpingitis.

The general condition of the patient with mild or moderately severe PID is good. Pain associated with PID is usually subacute and slow in onset, bilateral, dull in character, and present in the lower abdomen or pelvis. Of women with PID who experienced pain within 7 days of the first menstrual day, 81 percent had gonococcal or chlamydial infection compared to 66 percent of those with premenstrual onset of pain.[131] A short period of pelvic pain (< 3 days) at time of presentation to the clinic was significantly correlated with gonorrhea-associated PID and with age > 30 years.[29] Women with chlamydia-associated PID more often reported a period of pain exceeding one week in duration (Table 58–5).[115] Deep dyspareunia is frequent in women with PID.[29]

A fever was reported by about one-half of women with gonorrhea-associated PID, but only by 22 percent of those with chlamydial PID (Table 58–5). Chills (reported by 12 percent of patients) have been strongly correlated with the isolation of *N. gonorrhoeae* and *Staphylococcus aureus* from the lower genital tract (Weström, personal communication). A palpable mass occurred slightly more often in women with gonorrhea than the other groups, and ESR > 30 mm/hr was associated with *C. trachomatis*. Irregular vaginal bleeding was also common and significantly associated with chlamydia-associated PID (Table 58–5).[115] The abnormal bleeding appears to be a manifestation of endometritis. Bleeding is often the only symptom (other than pelvic pain) of chlamydial PID.[243] One-fifth of women with PID reported dysuria,[2,29] reflecting the urethritis caused by gonorrhea and chlamydial infection. Nausea and vomiting are infrequent in mild to moderate PID and, if present, should provoke suspicion of a "surgical abdomen" such as appendicitis or a ruptured ectopic pregnancy.

Despite increased inflammatory cells in the cervical/vaginal discharge of all cases in the Swedish series, only slightly more than one-half of the patients with PID reported symptoms of increased or changed vaginal secretion (see Table 58–3).[29] Thus, symptoms of lower genital tract infection preceding PID go unnoticed or are not present.

Clinical symptoms and signs do not accurately predict the extent of tubal disease observed at laparoscopy.[248] Patients with tubal

Table 58-4. Correlation of Clinical and Laboratory Abnormalities with Laparoscopic Findings in 2,220 Cases, Given a Clinical Diagnosis of Acute Salpingitis. (Refs 2, 29)

	Laparoscopic diagnosis		
Clinical and laboratory abnormalities	Salpingitis, %	Normal or other, %	Percentage of women with salpingitis presenting the symptoms or signs
Low abdominal pain plus signs of an LGTI* plus cervical motion tenderness	61	39	16
As above plus one or more of the following: ESR ≥ 15 mm/h; temperature >38.0°C; palpable adnexal mass:			
+ one of the above abnormalities	78	22	28
+ two of the above abnormalities	90	10	39
+ all three abnormalities	96	4	17
		75	100

* LGTI = lower genital tract infection, as defined by the presence of inflammatory cells outnumbering other cellular elements on wet-mount examination of vaginal fluid.

Table 58-5. Prevalence of Clinical and Laboratory Abnormalities in Women with Laparoscopically Verified Acute Salpingitis Associated with Cervical Infection with *Neisseria gonorrhoeae, Chlamydia trachomatis,* or Neither Organism. (Ref 115)

Clinical or laboratory abnormality	Prevalence of clinical and laboratory abnormalities Gonorrhea, % (n = 19)	Chlamydia, % (n = 68)	Neither, % (n = 64)
Duration of pelvic pain:			
≤3 days	32	15	38
>10 days	21	41	27
Temperature >38.0°C	52	22	30
Palpable adnexal mass	52	25	20
ESR ≥ 30mm/hr	32	65	19
Irregular bleeding	25	40	30

occlusion or moderate-severe tubal adhesions are fairly equally distributed among patients with mild-moderate and those with severe clinical symptoms and signs.[25,234,249]

Severe pelvic inflammatory disease

Clinical manifestations of severe PID corresponds to classic textbook descriptions of PID, but severe manifestations account for only 5–10 percent of overt PID and even fewer of all PID cases. Severe PID has two general etiologic categories: (1) young patients with florid peritonitis, usually from gonorrhea; and (2) older patients with an abscess and no STD-associated disease.[2,29,247,249] In fact, severe PID was diagnosed in only about 3–4 percent of all patients with PID in Swedish and American studies.[29,247,249] This group represents only the tip of the iceberg of PID cases (see Fig. 58–4).

These patients can appear very ill. Patients with peritonitis usually have a short duration of symptoms (e.g., < 3 days), fever, chills, purulent vaginal discharge, nausea, vomiting, abdominal guarding, and other signs of diffuse peritonitis. The white blood count (WBC), erythrocyte sedimentation rate (ESR), and C-reactive protein (CRP) are usually elevated. Patients with an abscess have a more varied duration and severity of pain, but they are usually febrile with clinical or ultrasonographic evidence of an abscess.

Clinical manifestations of extragenital intra-abdominal spread of *N. gonorrhoeae* and *C. trachomatis*: periappendicitis and perihepatitis

Both *N. gonorrhoeae* and *C. trachomatis* may enter the abdominal cavity and cause inflammation of serosal surfaces.[250,251] Spread of gonococci from gonococcal salpingitis, causing periappendicitis, was described by Moritz in 1912,[252] and gonococcal perihepatitis was described in 1930 by Curtis[253] and in 1934 by Fitz-Hugh.[37]

Periappendicitis is serositis not involving the intestinal mucosa. Periappendicitis alone is found in 1 to 15 percent of appendices removed because of a preoperative diagnosis of acute appendicitis.[254] The majority (32/41) of patients with periappendicitis in one study were young women, and 8 of the 32 had "tubal abnormalities."[255] Periappendicitis must always be kept in mind; when an appendix is removed from a young woman, the appendix should be opened and the mucosal surface inspected. A normal-looking mucosal surface strongly suggests periappendicitis secondary to salpingitis. Of seven appendices removed from 112 women with bilateral salpingitis, all had histologically confirmed periappendicitis and all had chlamydial salpingitis. The appendix was adherent to the right fallopian tube in six of these women, indicating a direct spread of organisms from the infected tube to the appendiceal serosa, but *C. trachomatis* was not detected in the removed appendices.[256] On the other hand, an inflammatory mass involving both the appendix and the right tube with a normal left tube indicates primary appendicitis.[29]

Perihepatitis involves inflammation of the liver capsule and the adjacent peritoneum associated with PID. The liver parenchyma is normal.[37,251] In acute perihepatitis, filmy fibrinous deposits develop on the reddened liver capsule ("pepper-and-salt appearance") and avascular, initially soft, adhesions form between the liver capsule and the adjacent parietal peritoneum under the ribs (Fig. 58–5).[257,258] The adhesions eventually form dense "violin-string" adhesions between the liver capsule and the abdominal wall (Fig. 58–6), indicative of dense adhesions from prior perihepatitis.[258]

Although some women with laparoscopic perihepatitis report no local symptoms,[258] acute severe pleuritic right-upper-quadrant abdominal pain is a cardinal clinical sign of perihepatitis.[251,258] Its sudden dramatic onset mimics pleuritis or cholecystitis. Right-upper-abdominal tenderness, guarding, and slight liver enlargement on palpation are present. A friction rub is occasionally auscultated over the liver.[37]

In perihepatitis, the panel of conventional laboratory tests (ESR,WBC,CRP) usually are within the ranges seen in other cases of acute salpingitis.[178,258] Even liver-enzyme levels are most often normal,[178,257–59] but they may be slightly elevated in users of OCPs. A small amount of basal pleural fluid may be found on x-ray.[260] Ultrasonic examination of the gall bladder is normal in perihepatitis but should be performed to differentiate perihepatitis from gall-bladder disease.

Perihepatitis has been observed by laparoscopy in 5 to 15 percent of patients with acute salpingitis,[261,262] although a smaller proportion have clinical signs of perihepatitis.[257–62] Twenty-four of 38 women with laparoscopic signs of perihepatitis and salpin-

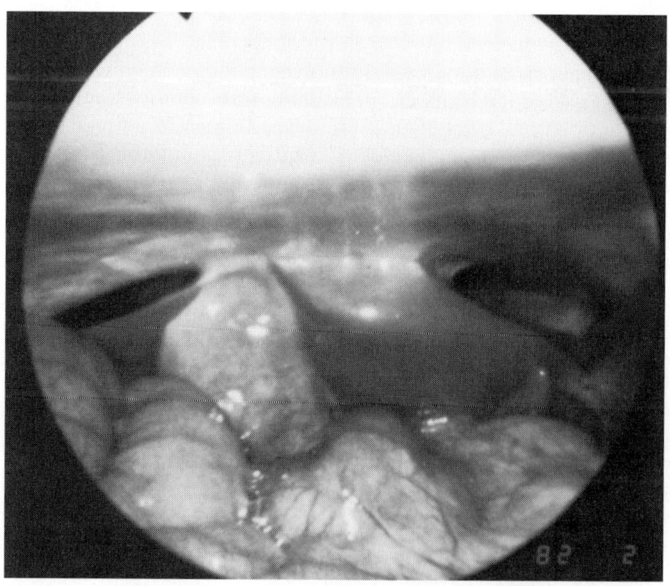

Fig. 58-5. Laproscopic view of an early stage Fitz-Hugh–Curtis syndrome with the liver surface closely adherent to the anterior abdominal wall.

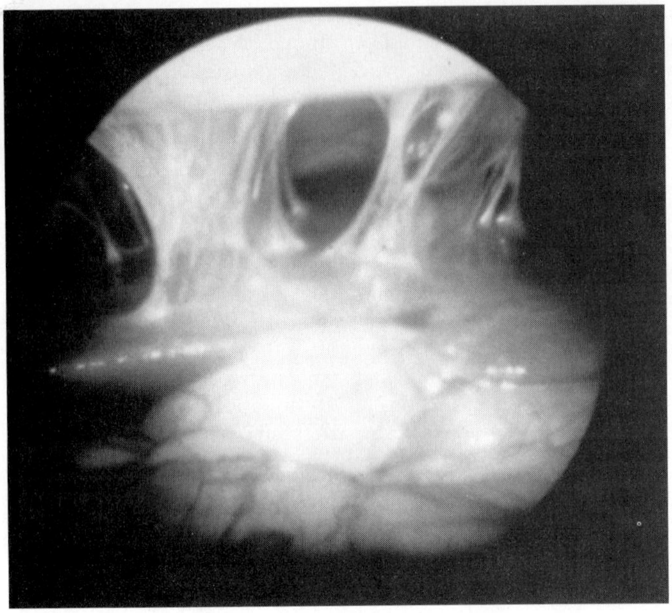

Fig. 58-6. Laproscopic view of a later stage Fitz-Hugh–Curtis syndrome demonstrating fibrous adhesions, including "violin string adhesions," between the liver surface and the anterior abdominal wall.

gitis had right-upper-quadrant abdominal pain.[261] Other conditions can cause upper-quadrant pain; laparoscopy can establish a definite diagnosis of acute perihepatitis.

Perihepatitis was initially associated with gonococcal PID,[37,253] but in most recent reports it has been associated with *C. trachomatis*.[251,258,259,262–64] *C. trachomatis* has been isolated from the liver capsule in women with perihepatitis.[258,264] An elevated serum antibody to *C. trachomatis* of ≥1:32 occurs in 70–75 percent of women with perihepatitis[251,259,262]; the geometrical mean titer of *C. trachomatis* antibody is higher among women with perihepatitis than among those with salpingitis alone.[259]

The pathogenesis of perihepatitis remains unclear. Fluid and particulate matter in the cul-de-sac rapidly move to the subdiaphragmatic spaces.[265] As suggested by the recovery of *N. gonorrhoeae* and *C. trachomatis* from the liver capsule in perihepatitis, microorganisms may move with this fluid-film. However, reports of perihepatitis in a man with gonorrhea,[266] in women with tubal ligation (Wøolner-Hanssen, personal communication), and after inoculation of *C. trachomatis* into the endometrial cavity of grivet monkeys with ligated oviducts[267] argue for an alternative hematogenous or lymphatic spread. An additional factor might involve a delayed hypersensitivity reaction to Chsp-60[178] or other chlamydial antigens, analogous to the proposed role of DTH in chlamydial salpingitis. In addition to the particularly high levels of antichlamydial serum antibody, noted above, women with perihepatitis are more likely to have serologic evidence of a prior infection with a heterologous chlamydial immunotype,[259] and less frequent use of OCPs,[241,258,260] which may reduce the cellular immune response.[268] Recently, antibody to Chsp-60 has been associated with laparoscopically verified perihepatitis.[178]

The clinical importance of perihepatitis lies in the differential diagnosis. Many women with perihepatitis do not report or lack symptoms from the concomitant genital infection Perihepatitis should always be considered in a young woman presenting with right-upper-quadrant abdominal pain or right sided pleuritic pain. Chest x-ray, ultrasonographic examination of the gall bladder, and gynecological examination, including tests for *N. gonorrhoeae* and *C. trachomatis*, can exclude other disease and reveal salpingitis and predisposing cervical infection.

DIAGNOSIS

As mentioned, no symptom or sign is pathognomonic of PID and, in fact, all symptoms have a low positive and negative predictive value for the diagnosis of PID.[2,29,237–41]

CLINICAL SIGNS

An increase in the inflammatory cells in the vagina has been a useful criterion because it is common in PID. This criterion is imprecise, lacks an accepted definition, and can reflect either cervical or vaginal inflammation, however. Mucopurulent cervicitis (MPC) is correlated with cervical infection[269,270] and therefore is a more logical clue to the presence of upper genital tract infection in women with pelvic pain. In populations at high risk for gonorrhea and chlamydia, MPC is common and has had relatively low positive predictive value of diagnosis of PID. In contrast, in a primary-care setting where cervical infection is less common, the clinical diagnosis of cervicitis among 95 women presenting with pelvic pain was 75 percent sensitive and 95 percent specific for the diagnosis of PID.[239] Since PID usually arises from lower genital tract infection, the absence of MPC or inflammatory cells carries a relatively high negative predictive value to exclude PID. In fact, none of the Swedish patients with laparoscopically documented PID presented with an entirely normal vaginal wet mount and clear cervical secretion.[2,29] In a recent report, a vaginal wet mount containing 3 or more WBC per high-powered field was more sensitive (87 percent) but less specific (38 percent) than the ESR, CRP, or periperul WBC among patients with signs of overt PID documented by endometrial biopsy or laparoscopy.[248]

In a meta-analysis of data from 14 studies on the diagnosis of PID, adnexal tenderness had a sensitivity of 95 percent but a low specificity of 74 percent; a palpable adnexal mass had a sensitivity of 48 percent and a specificity of 75 percent in predicting PID.[242] Other physical findings were even less predictive.

LABORATORY TESTS

Most laboratory tests used to diagnose PID are nonspecific. Furthermore, the sensitivity and specificity of laboratory tests have not been compared with laparoscopic diagnosis in most series. No laboratory test is either highly sensitive or specific for PID. However, a pregnancy test is required in all cases of suspected PID to exclude possible ectopic pregnancy, which represents a life-threatening complication of an early pregnancy.

Laboratory findings from Jacobson and Weström's study of Swedish women with PID are presented in Table 58–3.[2,29] An erythrocyte sedimentation rate (ESR) >15 mm/hr was present in 76 percent of patients with and in 53 percent of patients without laparoscopically verified PID. An elevated ESR has been significantly associated with laparoscopic staging of the inflammatory reactions (mild 60 percent, moderate 84 percent, and severe 89 percent),[29] and, in another data-set, with chlamydia-associated PID.[115]

Elevated levels of C-reactive protein (CRP) have had a sensitivity ranging from 70 percent to 93 percent, and a specificity ranging from 67 percent to 90 percent for PID.[236,271–73] The level of CRP also appears to reflect the severity of laparoscopically proven PID. The mean CRP was 47 mg/L (range 32–63) for mild tubal abnormalities, and 83 mg/L (range 65–103) for severe tubal disease.[272] An elevated CRP is a more sensitive and specific predictor of PID than an elevated ESR.[272] Furthermore, changes in CRP more accurately reflect the course of the infection and the effect of treatment than a change in ESR.

In the Jacobson-Weström study, the peripheral white blood cell count (WBC) exceeded 10,000 mm^3 in 59 percent of patients with laparoscopically verified PID and in 33 percent of patients with no PID.[2,29] The WBC was normal in 63 percent of patients with laparoscopically mild disease and in 20 percent of those with severe disease.[29] An elevated WBC was particularly associated with gonococcal PID in a Seattle study.[249]

Other serum markers have been examined in patients with PID, but they remain investigational. Antichymotrypsin levels were increased (> 140 percent of a reference pool) in 23 of 40 patients with PID and in none of 15 control women.[29,273] Ovarian cancer–associated tumor markers, both CA125 and tumor associated trypsin inhibitor (TATI) have been elevated in one-fourth to one-third of patients with proven PID.[230,274] Specific genital isoamylases (SGI) are produced in fallopian-tube epithelium and are present in peritoneal fluid.[275] The SGI level is high in peritoneal fluid of healthy women but is diminished or absent in tubal infections and pregnancy.[276] Ratios of the level of nonpancreatic isoamylases in peritoneal fluid and serum (P/S quotient) < 1.5 were found in 45 of 56 of patients with PID, in none of 22 women with lower genital tract infection, and in 1 of 18 control women.[276] This commercially available test is easy to perform, but it demands a cul-de-sac puncture. Larger studies are needed to confirm these results.

INVASIVE DIAGNOSTIC TECHNIQUES

Culdocentesis

Peritoneal fluid can be obtained by culdocentesis, which is easy to perform, especially with vaginal ultrasonography to guide the needle tip to available fluid.[275] Intrauterine pregnancy, a retroverted uterus, adynamic ileus, and fixed pelvic tumors contraindicate the procedure. A suspected abscess should not be punctured for a diagnosis. An increased WBC level in peritoneal fluid indicates intraabdominal inflammation. Combining two studies,[29,275] 21 out of 24 patients with proven PID and none of 36 control women had WBC counts > 3,100/mm in cul-de-sac fluid. Pure nonclotting blood in the aspirate indicates ongoing intraabdominal bleeding and usually is an indication for laparoscopy or laparotomy to exclude ectopic pregnancy or ruptured ovarian cyst.

Microbiological results on peritoneal fluid obtained by culdocentesis must be interpreted with caution because of potential contamination from vaginal organisms or unrecognized bowel puncture. Additionally, species recovered by culdocentesis in PID have often been different from those recovered from tubal specimens obtained simultaneously by laparoscopy.[30,31] *C. trachomatis* is rarely isolated from peritoneal fluid even in chlamydial salpingitis,[31] although detection of *C. trachomatis* antigen or DNA in peritoneal fluid has not been evaluated.

Endometrial biopsy

Endometrial biopsy specimens are easy to obtain under local anesthesia.[277] Histologic evidence of endometritis includes the polymorphonuclear leukocytes (PMNs) migrating through the endometrial epithelium and present within lumina of endometrial "glands," dense infiltration of the subepithelial stroma by plasma cells and lymphocytes, and germinal centers within the stroma.[36] Demonstration of histologic endometritis based upon detection both of plasma cells and of intraepithelial PMNs, had a sensitivity of 92 percent and a specificity of 87 percent with respect to detection of salpingitis by laparoscopy.[277] The distribution of endometrial inflammation may be patchy, and limited experience in other studies has given somewhat lower sensitivity and specificity.

Laparoscopy

Laparoscopy was introduced to study PID in the 1950s; after a series of publications during the 1960s through the 1980s,[2,23,237,238] laparoscopy became the gold standard to diagnose PID and to obtain specimens directly from the fallopian tubes. A review of laparoscopy in PID has been published recently.[234] Criteria used to define salpingitis observed through the laparoscope include tubal erythema, swelling, and exudate.[2] Laparoscopy is a valuable research tool to study the accuracy of the clinical diagnosis of PID; to correlate symptoms and signs with laparoscopy findings; and to study the microbiology, pathology, and prognosis. Laparoscopy is not practical for the majority of women with PID, however. Interpretation of laparoscopic findings are subjective and in need of interobserver and intraobserver reproducibility; in addition, the procedure has slight risks, is costly, and only rarely changes the management of PID. When fimbrial histopathologic criteria were used to diagnose tubal inflammation, laparoscopy had a sensitivity of only 50 percent and a specificity of 80 percent.[239] Histopathologic signs of fallopian-tube inflammation may be present in other conditions, however, and they have been reported in 65 percent of menstruating women without signs of salpingitis.[278]

Laparoscopy is valuable in selected circumstances; about 5 percent of women with clinically suspected PID have serious surgical conditions such as ectopic pregnancy, appendicitis, or a ruptured abscess that would be dangerous if left unrecognized.[2,29,30] Laparoscopy has been used increasingly to guide the percutaneous placement of catheters for drainage of abscesses or direct puncture of tuboovarian abscess.[279,280] Laparoscopy also benefits patients unresponsive to antibiotics where the only objective finding is pelvic tenderness. These patients do not usually have active infection, and laparoscopy identifies conditions such as painful adhesions from PID or other pelvic pathology such as endometriosis.

Ultrasonography

Ultrasound provides a noninvasive test to help diagnose and follow the course of severe PID. Findings in cases of severe PID include tuboovarian abscess, dilated fallopian tubes suggestive of pyosalpinx, excess fluid in the cul-de-sac, and enlarged polycystic ovaries.[281,282] These ultrasound findings were consistent with PID in 94 percent of patients with proven severe PID, in 80 percent of patients with moderate PID, and in 64 percent of patients with mild PID.[283] A vaginal probe has improved the efficacy of ultrasonographic diagnosis of PID; in one study, vaginal ultrasound—showing dilated tubes, thickening of the wall of the tube, or fluid within the tube—was 85-percent sensitive and 100-percent specific compared to plasma-cell endometritis among outpatients with pelvic pain.[284] Ultrasonography may be used to guide needles for the drainage of tuboovarian abscess in selected cases where the abscess is fixed to the vagina in the midline.[285,286]

Rapid technical development will probably give ultrasonography a significant role in the diagnosis of PID in the future, but at present the use of ultrasonography is limited because of the lack of sensitivity in patients with mild tubal abnormalities, who represent the majority of women with PID.

COMBINATIONS OF SYMPTOMS AND SIGNS IN THE DIAGNOSIS OF PELVIC INFLAMMATORY DISEASE

It is evident that individual symptoms and signs of PID have a low diagnostic accuracy. In two comprehensive surveys on the diagnosis of PID, in 1986[240] and in 1991,[242] a syndromic approach was used to evaluate the diagnosis of PID. In these analyses, increasing the number of positive indicators of PID increased the specificity but decreased the sensitivity, and a high sensitivity and good specificity were achieved only by integrating laparoscopy into the logistic models.[242] Nonetheless, in clinical practice, even in industrialized countries, a syndromic approach that is supplemented by simple laboratory tests for WBC and acute phase reactives and for pregnancy, plus cervical tests for gonorrhea and chlamydial infection, remain the usual practice (see Table 58–4).

In conclusion, the diagnosis of PID is difficult. In the absence of laparoscopy, the most obvious difficulty is to discriminate whether or not a genital infection has extended to the most important organ, the fallopian tubes, where infection potentially affects future reproduction. In the future, vaginal ultrasound and analyses of endometrial and/or cul-de-sac specimens seem to offer the best possibilities to diagnose PID without the use of laparoscopy.

DIFFERENTIAL DIAGNOSIS

Pelvic inflammatory disease is one of many diagnoses that must be considered in women with abdominal or pelvic pain. In the largest series of 814 consecutive women laparoscoped because of a clinical diagnosis of salpingitis, 12 percent had intraabdominal disorders other than PID.[2] The differential diagnosis of PID include other gynecological conditions and disorders of the gastrointestinal and urinary tract. Ectopic pregnancy and acute appendicitis are the most serious intraabdominal conditions to exclude. Despite the limitations of a direct microscopy of vaginal secretion, as mentioned above, a completely normal wet mount argues strongly against PID.[29]

GYNECOLOGICAL CONDITIONS OTHER THAN PELVIC INFLAMMATORY DISEASE

Ectopic pregnancy is the most common and important differential diagnosis in PID.[287,288] It is difficult to differentiate between an unruptured ectopic pregnancy and mild/moderate PID on clinical criteria alone. Thus, a pregnancy test should be done in all potentially fertile women with acute abdominal/pelvic pain. This test should detect at least 40 IU of chorionic gonadotropin per mL of urine or blood, and it should be performed even in women using contraception.

Other common gynecological diagnoses to consider include rupture, bleeding, or torsion of an ovarian cyst. In such instances, the pelvic pain is usually very acute in onset, unilateral, and severe. Laboratory tests are generally normal, and ultrasonography most often reveals a pelvic mass and/or fluid in the cul-de-sac. Pelvic endometriosis may mimic PID, but the history of pelvic pain is often of longer duration than in PID. The microbiologic tests will be normal, but the ESR may be elevated, and only laparoscopy will establish the diagnosis.

GASTROINTESTINAL DISEASES

Acute appendicitis is the most important differential diagnosis to exclude in this group. The clinical signs and laboratory test results overlap in appendicitis and PID, and up to 3 percent of women treated for PID have appendicitis.[2] A brief period of abdominal pain, pain originating in the central abdomen and moving to the right lower quadrant, nausea and vomiting, favoring a supine position, pallor, and abdominal guarding suggest appendicitis. If appendicitis cannot be excluded, laparoscopy should be performed and expectant management should not be considered.

Mesenteric lymphadenitis, regional ileitis, enteritis, and other manifestations of *inflammatory bowel disease* are other considerations in the differential diagnosis of PID. If appendicitis can be excluded, expectant management and use of appropriate laboratory tests will usually suffice. An explorative laparotomy is indicated in women with prostration and signs of diffuse peritonitis.

URINARY TRACT DISORDERS

Urinary tract infection and colic from renal or ureteral stones are unusual differential diagnostic problems in PID. Microscopy and culture of urine usually will reveal the diagnosis. About 20 percent of women with STD-associated PID have urinary symptoms.[2]

A stepwise algorithm for the differential diagnosis of PID includes the following: (1) A patient prostrate with signs of peritonitis needs hospitalization and/or an explorative laparoscopy/laparotomy. (2) A pregnancy test is needed; if positive, consider an ectopic pregnancy or other pregnancy complications. (3) If the pregnancy test is negative, and a wet mount or Gram stain of cervical/vaginal secretions is normal (i.e., shows no increase in PMNs or evidence of bacterial vaginosis [see Chap. 42]), consider ultrasonography to diagnose gynecological conditions other than PID, or a gastrointestinal/urinary disorder. (4) If the wet mount reveals WBCs, PID is probable but other intrapelvic conditions are not completely excluded; consider pelvic ultrasound and endometrial biopsy to increase the accuracy of diagnosis.

TREATMENT

Antimicrobial therapy is required to treat the infection present in PID. As previously noted, early antibiotic treatment in the first 3 days after the onset of symptoms reduced tubal infertility.[153] The choice of antimicrobial is necessarily empiric since therapy must begin before the microbial etiology is known. The ideal of providing antimicrobial therapy based upon the isolation, identification, and antimicrobial susceptibility of the offending pathogen is rarely achieved because collection and microbial testing of fallopian-tube specimens is neither practical nor desirable for the majority of cases, and test procedures are still not rapid enough to guide initiation of therapy. Therefore, the antimicrobial regimen must inhibit at least the most frequently expected microorganisms, including *N. gonorrhoeae, C. trachomatis,* and common aerobic and anaerobic isolates. At least two drugs are recommended by the CDC for the treatment of PID (Table 58–6).

Guidelines for the hospitalization of patients are available.[1] Hospitalization is necessary for patients with an unclear diagnosis, particularly if serious surgical disease cannot be excluded, or for patients who are seriously ill, who have abscesses, or who are unable to tolerate oral medication. It is also reasonable to hospitalize patients unlikely to be compliant taking antimicrobials. Less clear is the need for hospitalization of all patients with PID to provide the higher antimicrobial levels achieved with intravenous than with oral therapy alone. Randomized trial data are not yet available to compare either clinical or long-term outcome of inpatient versus outpatient therapy for PID. The recent trend toward office-based or home parenteral therapy for many infectious diseases[289] should be coupled with close gynecological follow-up if this course is followed instead of hospitalization.

Comprehensive assessment of efficacy of antimicrobial treatment of acute PID must include: (1) evaluation of the clinical response to acute infection; (2) elimination of *N. gonorrhoeae* and *C. trachomatis*, if present; (3) evaluation of subsequent relapse and/or recurrence rates; and (4) incidence of late sequelae, including infertility, ectopic pregnancy, and pelvic pain. No study to

Table 58-6. Inpatient and Outpatient PID Treatment Regimens

INPATIENT:
Regimen A
Cefoxitin 2 g IV every 6 hours, or cefotetan 2 g IV every 12 hours,
plus
Doxycycline 100 mg IV or orally every 12 hours
Regimen B
Clindamycin 900 mg IV every 8 hours,
plus
Gentamicin loading dose IV, or IM (2 mg/kg of body weight) followed by a maintenance dose (1.5 mg/kg) every 8 hours. The intravenous regimens should be continued for at least 48 hours after substantial clinical improvement, then followed by doxycycline 100 mg twice daily or clindamycin 450 mg 4 times daily (both orally) for a total of 14 days of therapy.
OUTPATIENT:
Regimen A
Cefoxitin 2 g IM plus probenecid, 1 g orally in a single dose concurrently, or ceftriaxone 250 mg IM or other parenteral third-generation cephalosporin (e.g., ceftizoxime or cefotaxime),
plus
Doxycycline 100 mg orally 2 times daily for 14 days.
Regimen B
Ofloxacin 400 mg orally 2 times daily for 14 days,
plus
Either clindamycin 450 mg orally 4 times a day, or metronidazole 500 mg orally 2 times daily for 14 days.

Table 58-7. First Pregnancies (Uterine and Ectopic) and Infertility (Tubal and Nontubal Factor Infertility) in 1,282 Patients and 448 Control Women Followed after Index Laparoscopy Related to Number of PID Episodes, Severity of Infection, and Age at Infection. (Refs 25, 198, 234)

		Pregnant		Infertile		
		Uterine*	Ectopic*	TFI†	Other	
PID episodes	*N*	*n*	*n*	*n*	*n*	RR‡
None	448	433	6	4	5	1.0
One (total)	1,015	852	61	79	23	6.3
Mild	320	300	9	4	7	(1.0)
Moderate	459	404	19	26	10	(2.4)
Severe	236	148	33	49	6	(8.5)
Age <25	783	676	34	60	13	(1.0)
Age 25–35	232	176	27	19	10	(1.8)
Two	198	124	24	46	4	16.2
≥Three	69	24	15	30	0	29.6
All PID	1,282	1,000	100	155	27	9.1

* First pregnancy after PID
† TFI = tubal factor infertility
‡ RR = Relative risk of post-infection tubal dysfunction (TFI/ectopic pregnancy)

date has evaluated all four outcome measurements, and the vast majority of studies have evaluated only the clinical response to infection. Factors that influence efficacy, besides the interval between symptoms and treatment, include the presence of *N. gonorrhoeae* (which improves the clinical outcome) and abscesses and prior PID (which worsen the clinical outcome).

A recent report summarizing the clinical cure rate of inpatient and outpatient regimens found clinical cure rates ranged from 60 to 100 percent.[290] Only 5 inpatient studies reported clinical cure rates less than 84 percent. Of these, one used metronidazole and penicillin, two used metronidazole and doxycycline, one used cefoxitin-doxycycline, and the other sulbactam-ampicillin-doxycycline. In a meta-analysis of 21 studies that met inclusion criteria, pooled cure rates were similar between the multiple-drug inpatient regimens of clindamycin-aminoglycosides (92 percent), cefoxitin-doxycycline (93 percent), cefotetan-doxycycline (94 percent) and ciprofloxacin (94 percent).[290] Thus, regimens A and B of Table 58–6 provide virtually identical clinical cure rates. Metronidazole-doxycycline had a pooled cure rate of only 75 percent. Single reports of multiple-drug inpatient regimens combining other cephalosporins (ceftizoxime, cefotaxime) or sulbactam ampicillin with doxycycline and ofloxacin alone also provided clinical cure rates of 88 to 100 percent.[290] Quinolones could also be combined with doxycycline and metronidazole for coverage.

Another review was conducted of 58 studies published between 1975 and 1990 involving 4,128 patients.[291] Clinical trials published between 1975 and 1979 reported an overall clinical cure rate of 86 percent, using regimens composed of penicillin and/or ampicillin, penicillin combined with an aminoglycoside, tetracycline and metronidazole, or tetracycline alone. None of these regimens would be acceptable today because they failed to provide comprehensive coverage for *C. trachomatis*, *N. gonorrhoeae,* and other anaerobic and facultative bacteria. In trials between 1980 and 1990, the clinical cure rate was 90.4 percent. Six antibiotic regimens (clindamycin-aztreonam, cefoxitin-doxycycline, ticarcillin-clavulanic acid, moxalactam alone, clindamycin-aminoglycoside and cefoxitin alone) provided clinical cure rates of 91 to 98 percent.[291] All of the regimens achieved over a 90-percent clinical response rate as reported in three or more papers, and all had significantly greater clinical response rates than penicillin combined with tetracycline, aminoglycosides, or metronidazole. Superior regimens judged on the highest clinical response rates, lowest toxicity, and adequate coverage of *C. trachomatis* included clindamycin-aztreonam and cefoxitin-doxycycline, where the clinical response rates were 98 percent and 95 percent, respectively.[291]

Currently no single intravenous drug provides coverage of both *N. gonorrhoeae* and *C. trachomatis*; two drugs are used to cover these two bacteria. As shown in Table 58–7, most facultative and anaerobic bacteria found in PID are effectively treated by the cephalosporins in regimen A, and by gentamicin and clindamycin in regimen B. Intravenous clindamycin provides adequate if not optimal *C. trachomatis* coverage.[292,293] Microbiologic cure rates were over 85 percent, with the exception of two studies—one of metronidazole-doxycycline-gentamicin (71 percent) and one of cefoxitin-doxycycline (85 percent).[290]

Outpatient regimens recommended by the CDC for the treatment of PID are also listed in Table 58–6. As with the intravenous regimens, they are designed to provide excellent *N. gonorrhoeae* and *C. trachomatis* inhibition and some aerobic and anaerobic coverage. Metronidazole could be added to improve coverage of anaerobic bacteria. In the meta-analysis report, only one outpatient regimen (cefoxitin-probenecid-doxycycline) was examined, and it had a pooled clinical cure rate of 95 percent.[290] Other outpatient regimens evaluated, including ofloxacin alone and sulbactam-ampicillin-doxycycline, had clinical cure rates of 95 to 100 percent.[290] A word of caution regarding outpatient therapy is necessary, however. Ofloxacin has inadequate activity to anaerobic pathogens, and it requires compliance with several days of therapy to cure *C. trachomatis* infection; the cephalosporin-doxycycline regimen has limited facultative and anaerobic bacteria coverage.[294] Furthermore, it is now apparent that the degree of tubal damage cannot be accurately assessed by the degree of laboratory or clinical findings,[249] and patients with severe tubal damage are often treated as outpatients. While intravenous therapy has not been shown to influence results, physicians must ensure that those treated as outpatients comply with treatment.

As expected, microbiologic cure rates of *N. gonorrhoeae* and *C. trachomatis* in the cervix are high with all regimens.[290] There are virtually no valid data on microbiologic cure rates at the fallopian-tube site following therapy, and endometrial specimens following therapy are potentially contaminated with vaginal/cervical bacteria. Thus, little has been established on the microbiologic cure of bacteria other than *N. gonorrhoeae* or *C. trachomatis*.

Also, few studies have followed patients for more than a few weeks to provide reliable data on relapse and recurrence of infection after therapy. Furthermore, with the one exception of the Swedish studies, infertility, ectopic pregnancy, and chronic pain have generally not been assessed after therapy.[185,295] Weström found that the subsequent infertility rate was 11–13 percent in patients treated with regimens such as penicillin-streptomycin, penicillin-chloramphenicol, ampicillin, and doxycycline.[296] The data suggested that most of the permanent damage occurred before antibiotic therapy was given, reinforcing the finding that the most important predictor of subsequent infertility is the degree of tubal damage when the infection was first observed.[25,296] However, more data are needed at least on tubal patency following therapy. While Weström found no influence of antibiotic regimens on tubal patency,[296] in one small study patients given doxycycline-metronidazole had a higher rate of tubal patency based upon hysterosalpingogram than those given penicillin-ampicillin-metronidazole.[297]

Women with an IUD should have it removed, usually after some interval of antibiotic therapy. All patients should be re-examined at 2 to 3, 7, and 21 days after the beginning of therapy to document a satisfactory clinical response and to obtain repeat cervical cultures. Patients with a slow response need more frequent examinations. All recent male sexual contacts of women with acute salpingitis, including those who are asymptomatic, should be examined, tested for gonococcal and chlamydial infection, and, if necessary, treated.

With the use of antibiotics that inhibit anaerobic bacteria, particularly *Bacteroides* sp., radical extirpative surgery during the acute phase of PID has decreased. Immediate surgical exploration is necessary to prevent septic shock in patients with a ruptured pelvic abscess, however. Early operative transvaginal drainage is the preferred method of treating a fluctuant pelvic abscess that becomes attached to the vagina in the midline of the cul-de-sac. More difficulty arises when an abscess that is not attached to the vagina requires transperitoneal drainage. Because even large masses do not always represent abscess formation, our current recommendation is that antibiotic therapy aimed particularly at anaerobes should be instituted and continued if the mass size declines. Surgical exploration can then be delayed unless a definite abscess is identified by the clinical course (the patient fails to improve clinically or the mass remains unchanged in size) or if an abscess is of substantial size (greater than 6 cm in diameter) as demonstrated by scans. With this approach, few patients require transabdominal drainage.

If surgical drainage is required, open laparoscopy is used to guide percutaneous placement of catheters into the large abscesses. Ultrasound-guided catheter drainage is also possible, but bowel injury from the catheter is probably more frequent than with laparoscopy. The catheter is used to drain pus and gently irrigate the abscess cavity. The catheter is left to drain for 24 to 48 hours or until drainage decreases and the patient's condition improves. Care must be taken to avoid bowel injury and to identify multiloculated abscesses. About 90 percent of large abscesses can be cured with percutaneous drainage[298,299] with the advantage of obviating extensive surgery. If abdominal exploration is necessary, the least-extensive surgery likely to be effective should be performed, particularly among women who wish to remain fertile. For women with a unilateral adnexal abscess or an abscess within loops of bowel, total abdominal hysterectomy and bilateral salpingo-oophorectomy represent surgical overkill. Simple drainage or even removal of a unilateral abscess without removal of the opposite tube and ovary and the uterus is usually successful when a patient receives an adequate antibiotic regimen that includes antibiotics to inhibit anaerobic species. This conservative approach is particularly mandatory for young women with a first episode of acute PID who may desire children in the future. Advances in microsurgery and *in vitro* fertilization are likely to continue in the future, and destructive surgery for acute infection is passé.

A limited number of patients with salpingitis suffer persistent abdominal pain without evidence of an abscess or adnexal pathology except for mild tenderness. If pain continues for several weeks, laparoscopy should be performed to rule out other pelvic pathology or pelvic adhesion, which can then by lysed. No discernible pelvic pathology is present in many instances, however. Thus, laparoscopy should be performed before repeated antibiotic courses are given to patients with persistent pelvic pain and with no objective evidence of salpingitis.

PROGNOSIS AND SEQUELAE

PROGNOSIS

The clinical course of acute PID may be protracted, but the vast majority of women have a complete clinical recovery, regardless of treatment.[296] In the industrialized countries, mortality from PID is unusual. In the United States, the mortality rate for PID was 0.29 per 100,000 female population 15–44 years of age in 1979.[300] The most common cause of death is rupture of an abscess with generalized peritonitis, a condition where mortality remains at 3–8 percent.[301,302]

SEQUELAE

Despite prompt diagnosis and treatment, sequelae are common. The most-feared complication of PID for women is an impaired ability to conceive. Tubal infertility is common following PID (Fig. 58-7)[25,198,303–306] Tubal and peritubal damage after PID results in not only infertility but also ectopic pregnancy, chronic pain, and gynecological morbidity. Antibiotic treatment has helped to reduce these complications. In comparable-size follow-up studies before (three studies of a total of 1,026 patients) and after (four studies of 954 patients) the use of antimicrobial therapy, the mean pregnancy rates in women attempting pregnancy after conservatively treated PID were 28 percent and 73 percent respectively.[185]

In the United States and Europe, it has been estimated that 10–15 percent of married and cohabiting couples fail to conceive after 1 year of unprotected sexual intercourse.[306] Among infertile couples, a global study showed a wide range from a few to over 50 percent of women had post-infection tubal occlusion with wide geographical variations.[306–308] In studies from industrialized countries, 10–15 percent of women in infertile couples have tubal abnormalities and/or pelvic adhesions.[309] The corresponding figure in African women was about 64 percent.[307]

As mentioned, many tubal infections severe enough to cause tubal infertility have no or mild symptoms. In 23 seroepidemiologic studies of IgG antibody to *C. trachomatis* among infertile women, a serum antibody titer of $\geq$ 1:8 was present in 68 percent of 1,466 women with, and 27 percent of 1,544 women without, tubal factor infertility (TFI).[234] IgG antibody was found in about 33 percent of 1,130 fertile controls. A titer of $\geq$ 1:32 was present in 75 percent of those with tubal infertility and 21 percent of those with other reasons for infertility.[234] In these studies, 30–60 percent of the infertile women reported no history of PID.

The most extensive prospective follow-up study on reproductive events after overt PID was conducted at the University of Lund in Sweden.[25,29,198,234,296,303,310] In brief review of these studies, 1,730 women underwent routine diagnostic laparoscopy because of a clinical suspicion of acute salpingitis during the 25 years from 1960 through 1984. Pelvic inflammatory disease was diagnosed in 1,282 and entirely normal conditions in 448. The latter women served as controls. Women who exposed themselves to pregnancy during the follow-up and either conceived or consulted because of infertility were compared to the controls. Details of the methods are given in reference 199 and the results are provided in Table 58–7.

Fertility

In this series, 96.7 percent of the controls and 78.0 percent of the patients with salpingitis had an intrauterine pregnancy after the index laparoscopy. Among those with intrauterine pregnancies, no difference was observed between patients and controls in the proportion resulting in normal term delivery, preterm delivery, stillbirth, and induced or spontaneous abortions.[25]

Infertility

Among the patients with salpingitis, 12.1 percent had post-infection TFI and 2.1 percent were infertile for other reasons (Table 58–6). The corresponding figures for the control women were 0.9 percent and 1.1 percent. An independent and significant factor in the rate of post-PID TFI was the number of PID episodes (Fig. 58–7*A*)[25,296] and the severity of the infection determined among women with only one PID episode (Fig. 58–7*B*).[25,296] In a report by this same group, mild tubal disease was observed significantly more often at laparoscopy among women who used OCPs than among women who did not use contraception or who used other methods.[311] With non-contraceptors as a reference group, tubal infertility after salpingitis was reduced by one third ($p < .01$) in women who used combined oral contraceptive pills at the time of the index laparoscopy, one-half in IUD users ($p < .05$), and not at all in users of barriers or other methods.[296] These results should be interpreted with caution because there was no information on the contraceptive method used after the PID episode. In an analysis of 443 women with STD-associated PID in this series, women who consulted after ≥ 3 days of abdominal pain had a 2.8 fold (95 percent confidence interval 1.3–6.1) increased risk of impaired fertility (tubal infertility or ectopic pregnancy) compared with those who consulted within 3 days.[153]

Among women with only one episode of PID, post-PID TFI did not correlate with the antibiotic treatment administered.[296] Studies on the influence of the microbial etiology of PID on post-PID fertility have given conflicting results. A more-favorable prognosis may occur after gonorrhea-associated PID than after non-gonococcal PID,[25] but no such difference was observed in other reports.[234,303,312,313] *C. trachomatis* associated PID has produced higher rates of infertility in other studies,[179,304] and recent re-analysis of the series from Lund also indicated a less-favorable fertility prognosis after chlamydia-associated PID than after PID without genital chlamydial infection. The odds ratio for TFI in chlamydia-associated PID versus non-chlamydial PID was 2.7 (95 percent CI 1.0–7.6) after adjustment for age, use of contraception, and gonorrhea-associated PID.[313] However, no difference was observed between women with chlamydia-associated PID and gonorrhea-associated PID in a subsequent report from that same group.[312]

Women less than 25 years of age have an overall better fertility prognosis after PID than older women (Figure 58–7C). There was no difference between the age groups in tubal infertility after PID, however; the difference was accounted for by a higher proportion of fertility from other causes and from ectopic pregnancy in older women, factors only partly related to PID (Fig. 58–7C).

In seroepidemiological studies of infertile and fertile women, attempts to correlate tubal infertility with serum antibody to *N. gonorrhoeae, C. trachomatis, M. hominis*, and *M. genitalium* have suggested a significant role of *N. gonorrhoeae*,[314–16] *C. trachomatis*,[232,312–17] and a possible role of *M. hominis*,[317,318] but no significant role of *M. genitalium* , in tubal infertility.[317]

In women with one episode of severely damaged tubes, fertility nonetheless remained in 62.7 percent (Table 58–7). Similarly, fertility was preserved in 63 percent in a series of women treated by colpotomy for pelvic abscess.[319] Thus, even in severely diseased tubes, fertility is preserved in over one-half of the cases, which argues against routine radical surgery in such women.

Ectopic pregnancy

In any population, the ratio of ectopic pregnancy (EP) to intrauterine pregnancy is related to the prevalence of fertile women exposed to pregnancy and the distribution of risk factors for EP. Accepted risk factors for EP besides salpingitis include increasing

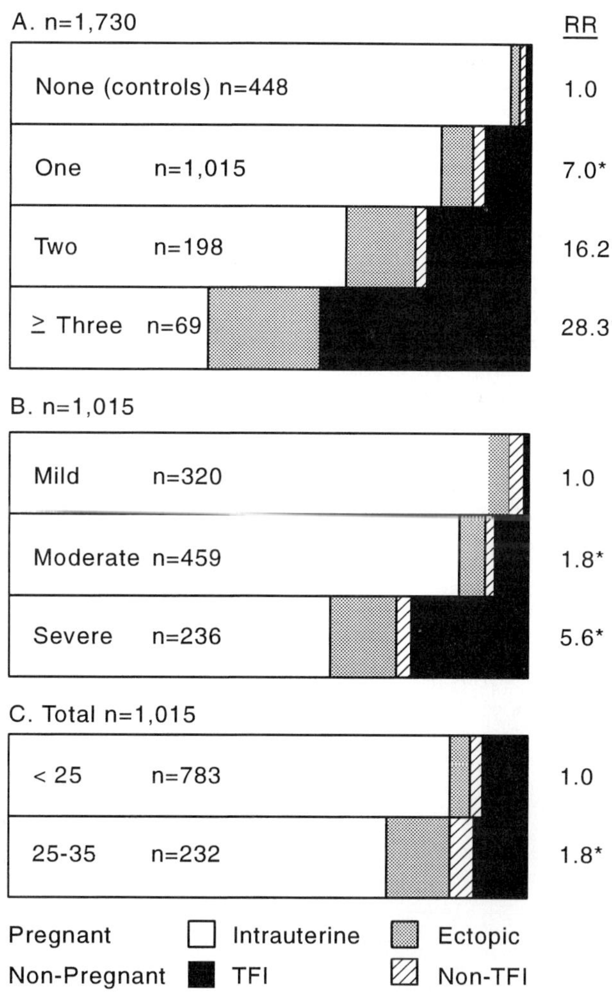

Fig. 58-7. Fertility and infertility after pelvic inflammatory diseases. *A*: Related to the number of PID episodes in one and the same woman; *B*: Related to laparoscopic severity of the inflammatory reactions in women with only one episode of PID; C: Related to the age of the patient at the time of her only episode of PID.

age, use of an IUD, postoperative tubal damage, and other tubal pathology.[203,320] Since 1970, significant increases have been observed in EP in the industrialized countries.[321–24] A 64-percent increase in annual hospital admissions for EP was observed in one study between 1970–74 and 1980–84.[323] In the United States, hospital admissions for ectopic pregnancy continued to increase until 1989, then began to fall (Fig. 58–8). The decline may reflect a growing trend toward outpatient management of ectopic pregnancy rather than a true decline in incidence, however; nearly one-half of all women with ectopic pregnancies in the United States are treated as outpatients.[324] Thus, the estimated number of ectopic pregnancies in the United States in 1992 was 108,800 (19.7 cases per 1,000 pregnancies), the highest level in more than two decades.[324] The epidemic increase in ectopic pregnancies has been explained by better diagnostic methods, increased use of IUDs, postponing the first pregnancy to an older age, and the epidemic of STDs. The impact of any individual factors has been difficult to evaluate, but in one report the increase in EP parallels an increase in STDs in the 1980s and the risk increases with the number of episodes of salpingitis.[325]

In the series from Lund, the first pregnancy after documented salpingitis was ectopic in 1.3 percent of the control women compared to 7.8 percent of patients who had had salpingitis. The ratio of EP:intrauterine pregnancy in all first pregnancies was 1:73 among the control women, and 1:15, 1:6, and 1:2.6 after one, two, and ≥ three episodes of salpingitis, respectively (Table 58–7; Fig. 58–7*A*). In women with only one episode of salpingitis, the corresponding figures were 1:36, 1:25, and 1:5.4 after mild, moderately severe, and severe PID, respectively (Table 58–7; Fig. 58–7*B*).

Age is consistently related to EP.[320,322] The ratio of EP:intrauterine pregnancy was 1:27.6 in patients with salpingitis less than 25 years of age and 1:8.4 in patients aged 25 to 35. Recent data indicate that women who have used an IUD in the past have an increased rate of EP.[218] In seven seroepidemiological case-control analyses, the mean prevalence of chlamydial serum antibody was 60 percent (range 32–71) in patients with EP and 24 percent (range 4–39) in control women.[234] Pelvic inflammatory disease has a "carry-over" effect for increased risk of EP even if the first pregnancy was intrauterine, such that an increased percentage of ectopic pregnancy was parallel to the severity of tubal damage (observed by laparoscopy) and the number of episodes of prior salpingitis.[325] If the first pregnancy was an ectopic, the risk for an EP in the following pregnancies was about 20 percent, regardless of prior PID history.[325]

Chronic pain

Abdominal or pelvic pain lasting longer than six months occurred in 16.7–18.1 percent of patients after one or more episodes of PID compared to only 1.7–5.0 percent in control women.[29,185,238,326] Chronic pain is related to the number of PID episodes, occurring in 11.8 percent with one episode, 30.0 percent with two episodes, and 66.7 percent after three or more episodes of PID.[326] In patients with chronic pain after PID, peritubal and periovarian adhesions at a second-look laparoscopy revealed that pain occurred in 9 percent with no visible adhesions and 91 percent in those with extensive adhesions.[326] Chronic pelvic pain correlated better with the extent of pelvic adhesions than to number of PID episodes.[326]

General gynecologic morbidity

A follow-up study of 1,200 women hospitalized for PID, compared to 10,507 control women, found that patients with PID had a 4.5 to 9.8 increased risk of hospitalization during the year follow-up period of 6.5–8.5 years for abdominal pain, "gynecologic" pain, endometriosis, hysterectomy, and ectopic pregnancy.[327] The rate of total gynecological operations (excluding laparoscopy for repeat PID) was 0.8 procedures per woman in 415 patients with PID compared to 0.1 per woman in 100 controls followed for 6 to 14 years.[25]

It is evident that serious long-term sequelae can result following PID. In fact, it has been estimated that one of four women with acute PID will suffer from one or more of the following: tubal infertility, ectopic pregnancy, chronic pelvic pain, or PID-related gynecological surgery. Apart from the economic and public-health consequences of PID and its sequelae,[196] the human suffering is unmeasurable in terms of a lowered quality of life and childlessness.

PREVENTION

Because treatment of PID has so far had only a limited impact upon sequelae of PID, prevention of PID is a higher priority. Prevention of PID would not only reduce the morbidity and costs from acute infection, but it would also potentially offer large cost savings of treating sequelae. Public-health efforts to control gonorrhea and chlamydia reduce the rate of PID. In fact, recent data indicate that control programs for chlamydia have a major

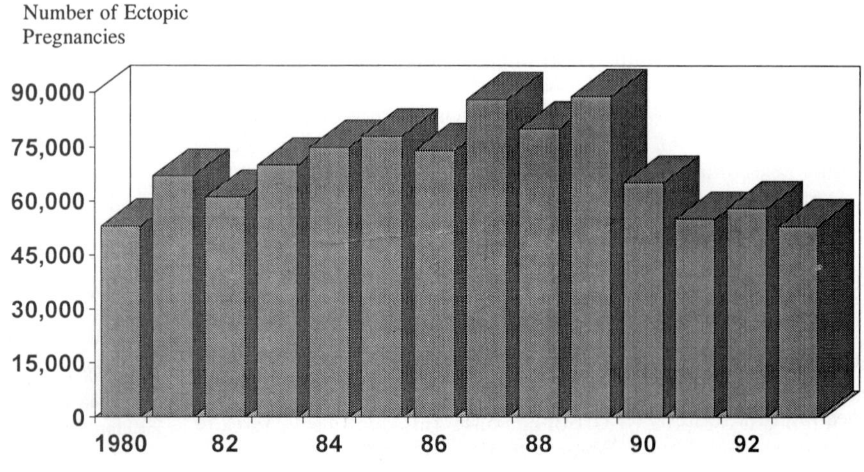

Fig. 58-8. Ectopic pregnancy—Hospitalization of women 15–44 years of age in the United States from 1980 to 1993.

impact on reducing PID rates.[205,206,328] A major justification for such infection-control programs is the reduction of PID and its sequelae.

While about one-half of women with acute PID have *C. trachomatis* identified by culture, new DNA amplification methods indicate that a cervical culture in some laboratories fails to detect about 30 percent of women with *C. trachomatis* actually present.[329] *C. trachomatis* is also particularly likely to produce mild symptoms[115] and thus chlamydia causes a disproportional amount of unrecognized PID.[241] Furthermore, tubal infertility may be more common following *C. trachomatis* than *N. gonorrhoeae* PID,[312] and the association between *C. trachomatis* and ectopic pregnancy is especially strong.[180,234] Thus, chlamydia-associated PID probably causes greater morbidity than currently estimated, simply from the proportion of all cases of PID associated with *C. trachomatis* by culture.

C. trachomatis infection is not controlled in most populations. While the United States has had a gonorrhea-control program in place for a quarter century, efforts to control chlamydia in the United States are just beginning and are at a very slow pace. Some barriers to *C. trachomatis* control relates to difficulties of identification. While *C. trachomatis* causes specific clinical manifestations in women such as cervicitis[269] and the urethral syndrome,[330] most *C. trachomatis* infections are asymptomatic or produce only nonspecific or mild symptoms,[331] resulting in a reservoir of *C. trachomatis* infection that is several times larger than the reservoir of *N. gonorrhoeae.1* Effective control programs require screening of asymptomatic men and women, and partner referral, rather than reliance only upon the identification and treatment of syndromes related to chlamydial infection.

Reduction in prevalence of *C. trachomatis* has followed widespread screening programs in Sweden,[332] and selective high-risk population screening in Wisconsin[205] and Region X of the United States.[205] In Wisconsin, selective screening begun in all family-planning clinics resulted in a 50-percent decline in prevalence in urban as well as nonurban clinics.[205] In Region X, the prevalence of *C. trachomatis* dropped after selective screening in family-planning clinics, and subsequently STD clinics, from 10.9 percent to 6.8 percent in two years,[328] with further declines to about 4% after six years. These programs were based upon use of relatively insensitive screening tests.

Ligase chain reaction (LCR) had excellent sensitivity (94 percent) and specificity (99 percent) for detecting chlamydia compared to an expanded gold standard defined as positive results from the Direct Fluorescent Antibody (DFA) and of an LCR assay performed with probes specific to the major outer-membrane protein gene. In the same patients, culture had a 65-percent sensitivity compared to the expanded gold standard.[333] Ligase chain reaction performed on urine samples of women appear more sensitive that a cervical culture. In a multicenter study of 1,937 women, LCR on first-voided urine samples was 94 percent sensitive and 99.9 percent specific, and the cervical culture was 65 percent sensitive and 100 percent specific in comparison to the expanded gold standard.[334] Similar results occurred in a larger study of 4,053 women.[329] Thus LCR on urine detected almost 30 percent more women than a cervical culture.

Thus, widespread clinic-based screening for chlamydial infection has reduced the prevalence of chlamydial infection at the population level—essentially shifting from prevalent infection to incident infection. A more recent report demonstrated that chlamydia screening also benefits the individual woman herself.[206] After criteria were established for selective screening of high-risk women enrolled in a managed health care plan, female enrollees meeting these criteria were randomly assigned to an intervention or a usual-care group. Women in the intervention group were invited to undergo cervical sampling for EIA and culture testing for chlamydial infection. Those who were postive for either test were treated. Women assigned to the usual-care group were not contacted or routinely screened for chlamydia. All participants were followed for 12 months, and the incidence of PID per 10,000 women-months was 8 in the intervention group versus 18 in the usual-care group (relative risk 0.44).[206] Thus, screening and treatment of a group at increased risk for chlamydia was feasible and reduced the rate of PID. Because the data suggest that a surprisingly high amount of *C. trachomatis* caused PID in this population, additional intervention studies are needed. It is apparent, however, that screening and treatment of asymptomatic women for *C. trachomatis* and *N. gonorrhoeae* reduce the prevalence of chlamydial infection at the population level, and they lower the risk of acute PID at the individual level and therefore urgently need widespread implementation.

References

1 Anonymous: Pelvic inflammatory disease, in 1993 Sexually Transmitted Diseases Treatment Guidelines. *MMWR,* 42:75, 1993.

2 Jacobson L, Weström L: Objectivized diagnosis of pelvic inflammatory disease. *Am J Obstet Gynecol ,* 105:1088, 1969.

3 Paavonen J, et al: Microbiological and histopathological findings in acute pelvic inflammatory disease. *Br J Obstet Gynaecol,* 94:454, 1987.

4 Sellors JW, et al: Tubal factor infertility: An association with prior chlamydial infection and asymptomatic salpingitis. *Fertil Steril,* 49: 451, 1988.

5 Monif GRG: Clinical staging of acute bacterial salpingitis and its therapeutic ramifications. *Am J Obstet Gynecol,* 43:489, 1982.

6 Hager WD, et al: Criteria for diagnosing and grading of salpingitis. *Obstet Gynecol,* 61:113, 1983.

7 Diepgen P: Die Frauenheilkunde der Alten Welt, in *Handbuch der Gynäkologie,* W Stoeckel (ed). Munich,, Verlag JF Bergman, 1937, vol XII. part 1, p 279.

8 Mauriceau F: *Traité des maladies des femmes grosses.* Dernière ed. Paris, 1683. (Cited in Viberg L. Acute Inflammatory Conditions of the Adnexa. *Acta Obstet Gynecol Scandinav,* 43:suppl 4, 1964).

9 Noeggerath E: Latent gonorrhea, especially with regard to its influence on fertility in women. *Trans Am Gynaecol Assoc,* 1:292, 1876.

10 Von Bumm E: Der Mikro-Organismus der gonorrhoischen Schleimhauterkrankungen Gonococcus Neisser.*Dtsch Med Wochenschr,* 11: 508, 1885

11 Diepgen P: Die Frauenheilkunde im Mittelalter und die Neuzeit bis zur Gegenwart, in *Handbuch der Gynäkologie,* W Stoeckel (ed). Munich, Verlag, JF Bergman, 1937, vol XII, part 2, p 367ff.

12 Nocard E, Roux ER: Le microbe de la péripneumonie. *Ann Inst Pasteur,* 12:240, 1898.

13 O. Wittman I: The history of peritoneoscopy, in *Peritoneoscopy,* I Wittman (ed.), Budapest, Akadémiai Kiadó (Hungarian Academy of Science), 1966, p 13.

14 Halberstaedter L, von Prowazek S: über Zelleneinschlüsse Parasitärer Natur beim Trachom. *Arbeiten aus dem Kaiserlichen Gesundheitsamte,* 26:44, 1907.

15 Fritsch HO, et al: Experimentelle Studien zur Trachomfrage. *Graefe's Archiv für Ophtalmologie,* 76:547, 1910.

16 Ahlström E: Die Behandlung nicht tuberkulöser Adnexentzündungen. *Acta Obstet Gynecol Scand,* 5:765, 1919.

17 Dienes L, Edsall G: Observations on the L-organism of Klineberger. *Proc Soc Exp Biol Med,* 36:740, 1937.

18 Falk HC: Interpretation of the pathogenesis of pelvic infections as determined by cornual resection. *Am J Obstet Gynecol ,* 52:66, 1946.

19 T'ang FF, et al: Studies on the etiology of trachoma with special reference to isolation of the virus in chick embryo. *Chin Med,* 75:429, 1957.

20 Jones BR, et al: Isolation of virus from inclusion blenorrhoeae. *Lancet* i;902, 1959.

21 Mårdh P-A, Weström L: Tubal and cervical cultures in acute salpingitis with special reference to *Mycoplasma hominis* and T-strain mycoplasmas. *Brit J Vener Dis,* 46:179, 1970.

22 Eilard T, et al: Isolation of chlamydia in acute salpingitis. *Scand J Infect Dis* (suppl), 9:82, 1976

23 Mårdh PA, et al: *Chlamydia trachomatis* infection in patients with acute salpingitis. *N Engl J Med* 296:1377, 1977.

24 Eschenbach DA, et al: Polymicrobial etiology of acute pelvic inflammatory disease. *N Engl J Med* 293:166, 1975.

25 Weström L: Effect of pelvic inflammatory disease on fertility. *Am J Obstet Gynecol* 121:707, 1975.

26 Mårdh PA, et al: Sampling, specimen handling, and isolation techniques in the diagnosis of chlamydial and other infections. *Sex Transm Dis,* 8:280, 1981.

27 Paavonen J, et al: Prevalence and manifestations of endometritis among women with cervicitis. *Am J Obstet Gynecol,* 152:280, 1985.

28 Douglas-Punktion. In *Atlas der gynekologischen Operationen,* O Kaser, et al (eds). Stuttgart, Georg Thieme Verlag, 1982, vol 2, p 15.

29 Weström L: *Diagnosis, aetiology, and prognosis of acute salpingitis* (Thesis) Lund, Sweden. Studentlitteratur, 1977.

30 Sweet RL et al: Microbiology and pathogenesis of acute salpingitis as determined by laparoscopy. What is the appropriate site to sample? *Am J Obstet Gynecol* 138:985, 1980.

31 Mårdh PA: An overview of infectious agents of salpingitis, their biology, and recent advances in methods of detection. *Am J Obstet Gynecol,* 138:933, 1980.

32 Paavonen J, et al: Endometritis and acute salpingitis associated with *Chlamydia trachomatis* and herpes simplex virus type 2. *Obstet Gynecol,* 65:288, 1985.

33 Heynemann T: Entzüüdungen der Adnexe, in *Biologie und Pathologie des Weibes,* L Seitz, A Amreich (eds). Berlin, Urban & Schwarzenberg, 1953, vol 5, p 19.

34 Møller BR, et al: Infection with *Chlamydia trachomatis, Mycoplasma hominis,* and *Neisseria gonorrhoeae* in patients with acute pelvic inflammatory disease. *Am Vener Dis Assocs,* 8:198, 1981.

35 Brihmer C, et al: Salpingitis: Aspects on diagnosis and etiology; a 4-year study from a Swedish hospital. *Eur J Obstet Gynecol Reprod Biol,* 3:211, 1987.

36 Kiviat NB, et al: Endometrial histopathology in patients with culture-proved upper genital tract infection and laparoscopically diagnosed acute salpingitis. *Am J Surg Pathol,* 14:167, 1990.

37 Fitz-Hugh T Jr: Acute gonococcic peritonitis of the right upper quadrant of women. *JAMA* 102;2094, 1934.

38 Stanley MM: Gonococcal peritonitis of the upper part of the abdomen in young women. *Arch Intern Med,* 78:1, 1946.

39 Mauro E: Le syndrome abdominal droit supérieur au cours des annexites gonococciques (syndrome de Fitz-Hugh) *Presse Med,* 46: 1919, 1938.

40 Arko RJ: An immunological model in laboratory animals for the study of *Neisseria gonorrhoeae. J Infect Dis,* 129(4):451, 1974.

41 Taylor-Robinson D, et al: Effect of *Neisseria gonorrhoeae* on human and rabbit oviducts. *Br J Vener Dis,* 50:279, 1974.

42 McGee ZA, et al: Pathogenic mechanism of *Neisseria gonorrhoeae*: Observations on damage to human fallopian tubes by gonococci of colony type 1 or 4. *J Infect Dis,* 143:413, 1981.

43 Mårdh PA, et al: Studies on ciliated epithelia of the human genital tract. III. Mucociliary wave activity of tissue organ culture of human fallopian tube challenged with *Neisseria gonorrhoeae* and endotoxin. *Br J Vener Dis,* 55:265, 1979.

44 Eschenbach DA: Acute pelvic inflammatory disease: Etiology, risk factors and pathogenesis. *Clin Obstet Gynecol,* 19:147, 1976.

45 Gisslén B, et al: Incidence, age distribution, and complications of gonorrhea in Sweden. *Bull World Health Organ,* 24:367, 1961.

46 Weström L: Incidence, prevalence, and trends of acute pelvic inflammatory disease and its consequences in industrialized countries. *Am J Obstet Gynecol,* 138:880, 1980.

47 Draper DL, et al: Auxotypes and antibiotic susceptibilities of *Neisseria gonorrhoeae* in women with acute salpingitis. *Sex Transm Dis,* 8:43, 1981.

48 Holmes KK, et al: Salpingitis: Overview of etiology and epidemiology. *Am J Obstet Gynecol,* 138:893, 1980.

49 Draper DL, et al: Comparison of virulence markers of peritoneal and fallopian tube isolates with endocervical *Neisseria gonorrhoeae* isolated from women with acute salpingitis. *Infect Immun,* 27:882, 1980.

50 Danielsson D, Sandström E: Serology of *Neisseria gonorrhoeae.* Demonstration with co-agglutination and immunoelectrophoresis of antigenic differences associated with color/opacity colonial variants. *Acta Path Microbiol Scandinav* (Section B), 88:39, 1980.

51 Buchanan TM, et al: Gonococcal salpingitis less likely to recur with *Neisseria gonorrhoeae* of the same principal outer membrane protein antigenic type. *Am J Obstet Gynecol,* 138:978, 1980.

52 Sweet RL, et al: Etiology of acute salpingitis: Influence of episode number and duration of symptoms. *Obstet Gynecol,* 58:62, 1981.

53 Curtis A. Bacteriology and pathology of fallopian tubes removed at operation. *Surg Gynecol Obstet,* 33:621, 1921.

54 Hundley JM, et al: Bacteriological studies in salpingitis with special reference to gonococcal viability. *Am J Obstet Gynecol,* 60:977, 1950.

55 Henry-Suchet J, et al: Microbiology of specimens obtained by laparoscopy from controls and from patients with pelvic inflammatory disease or infertility with tubal obstruction: Chlamydia trachomatis and ureaplasma urealyticum. *Am J Obstet Gynecol,* 138:1022, 1980.

56 Gjønnaess H, et al: Pelvic inflammatory disease: Etiologic studies with emphasis on chlamydial infection. *Obstet Gynecol,* 59:550, 1982.

57 Bevan CD, et al: Clinical, laparoscopic and microbiological findings in acute salpingitis: Report on United Kingdom cohort. *Br J Obstet Gynecol,* 102:407, 1995.

58 Mårdh P-A, et al: Antibodies to *Chlamydia trachomatis* and *Neisseria gonorrhoeae* in sera from patients with acute salpingitis. *Br J Vener Dis,* 57:125, 1981.

59 Adler MW, et al: Morbidity associated with pelvic inflammatory diseases. *Br J Vener Dis,* 58:151, 1982.

60 Ripa KT, et al: *Chlamydia trachomatis* infection in patients with laparoscopically verified acute salpingitis. *Am J Obstet Gynecol,* 138: 960, 1980.

61 Osser S, Persson K: Epidemiologic and serodiagnostic aspects of chlamydial salpingitis. *Obstet Gynecol,* 59:206, 1982.

62 Paavonen J: *Chlamydia trachomatis* in acute salpingitis. *Am J Obstet Gynecol,* 138:957, 1980.

63 Paavonen J, et al: *Chlamydia trachomatis* in acute salpingitis. *Br J Vener Dis,* 55:203, 1979.

64 Paavonen J, et al: Serologic evidence for the role of *Bacteroides fragilis* and *Enterobacteriaceae* in the pathogenesis of acute pelvic inflammatory disease. *Lancet* 1:293, 1981.

65 Bowie WR, Jones H: Acute pelvic inflammatory disease in outpatients and associates with *Chlamydia trachomatis* and *Neisseria gonorrhoeae. Ann Intern Med,* 95:685, 1981.

66 Livengood CH, et al: Pelvic inflammatory disease: Findings during inpatient treatment of clinically severe, laparoscopy-documented disease. *Am J Obstet Gynecol,* 166:519, 1992.

67 Cunningham FG, et al: The bacterial pathogenesis of acute pelvic inflammatory disease. *Obstet Gynecol,* 52;161, 1978.

68 Soper DE, et al: Microbial etiology of urban emergency department acute salpingitis: Treatment with ofloxacin. *Am J Obstet Gynecol,* 167;653, 1992.

69 Thompson SE, et al. The microbiology and therapy of acute pelvic inflammatory disease in hospitalized patients *Am J Obstet Gynecol,* 136:179, 1980.

70 Weström L. Decrease in the incidence of women treated in hospital for acute salpingitis in Sweden. *Genitourin Med,* 64:59, 1988.

71 Mårdh PA, et al: Endometritis caused by *Chlamydia trachomatis. Br J Vener Dis,* 27:191, 1981.

72 Jones RB, et al: Recovery of *Chlamydia trachomatis* from the endometrium of women at risk for chlamydial infection. *Am J Obstet Gynecol*, 155:35, 1986.
73 Kiviat NB, et al: Localization of *Chlamydia trachomatis* infection by direct immunofluorescence and culture in pelvic inflammatory disease. *Am J Obstet Gynecol*, 154:865, 1986.
74 Weström L, Mårdh PA: Chlamydial salpingitis. *Br Med Bull* 39:145, 1983.
75 Wølner-Hanssen P, et al: Isolation of *Chlamydia trachomatis* from the liver capsule in Fitz-Hugh Curtis syndrome. *N Engl J Med*, 306: 113, 1982.
76 Cooper MD, Jeffrey C: Scanning and transmission electron microscopy of bacterial attachment to mucosal surfaces with particular reference to human fallopian tube. *Scan Electron Microsc* Pr3;1183, 1985.
77 Cooper MD, et al: *Chlamydia trachomatis* infection of human fallopian tube organ cultures. *J Gen Microbiol*, 136:1109, 1990.
78 Patton DL: Immunopathology and histopathology of experimental chlamydial salpingitis. *Rev Infect Dis*, 7:746, 1982.
79 Patton DL, et al: The effects of *Chlamydia trachomatis* on the female reproductive tract of *Macaca nemestrina* after a single challenge following repeated cervical inoculations. *Obstet Gynecol*, 76:1271, 1990.
80 Morrison RP, et al: Immunology of *Chlamydia trachomatis* infections: immunoprotective and immunopathogenic responses. In: TC Quinn. *Advances in Host Defense Mechanisms. Vol. 8 Sex Transm Dis*. New York, Raven Press 1992:57.
81 Weström L: Chlamydial and gonococcal infection in a defined population of women. *Scand J Inf Dis*, 32(suppl):157S, 1982.
82 Treharne J, et al: Antibodies to *Chlamydia trachomatis* in acute salpingitis. *Br J Vener Dis*, 55:26, 1979.
83 Henry-Suchet J, et al: Microbiologic study of chronic inflammation associated with tubal factor sterility: Role of *Chlamydia trachomatis*. *Fertil Steril*, 47:274, 1987.
84 Patton DL, et al: Detection of *Chlamydia trachomatis* in fallopian tube tissue in women with postinfectious tubal infertility. *Am J Obstet Gynecol*, 171:95, 1994.
85 Shephard MK, Jones RB: Recovery of *Chlamydia trachomatis* from endometrial and fallopian tube biopsies in women with infertility of tubal origin. *Fertil Steril*, 52:232, 1989.
86 Stacey C, et al: *Chlamydia trachomatis* in the fallopian tubes of women without laparoscopic evidence of salpingitis. *Lancet*, 336: 960, 1990.
87 Sinei KA, et al: Isolation of *Chlamydia trachomatis* from fallopian tubes of healthy women undergoing tubal sterilization by minilaparotomy. *East Afr Med J*, 66:388, 1989.
88 Møller RB: The role of mycoplasmas in the upper genital tract of women. *Sex Transm Dis* 10(4 Suppl):5281–5284, 1983.
89 Sweet RL, et al: Use of laparoscopy to determine the microbiologic etiology of acute salpingitis. *Am J Obstet Gynecol*, 134:781, 1979.
90 Møller RB, et al: Experimental infection of the genital tract of female grivet monkeys by *Mycoplasma hominis*. *Infect Immun*, 20:248, 1978.
91 Møller BR, Freundt EA: Monkey animal model for study of mycoplasmal infections of the urogenital tract. In *Mycoplasma hominis, a human pathogen*. Mårdh P-A, Møller BR, McCormack WM (eds). *Sex Transm Dis* 10:359, 1983.
92 Mårdh PA, et al: Studies on ciliated epithelia of the human genital tract. I. Swelling of the cilia of fallopian tube organ cultures infected with *Mycoplasma hominis*. *Br J Vener Dis*, 52:52, 1976.
93 Miettinen A, et al: Epidemiologic and clinical characteristics of pelvic inflammatory disease associated with *Mycoplasma hominis, Chlamydia trachomatis* and *Neisseria gonorrhoeae*. *Sex Transm Dis*, 13: 24, 1986.
94 Lind K, et al: Importance of *Mycoplasma hominis* in acute salpingitis assessed by culture and serologic tests. *Genitourin Med*, 61:185, 1985.
95 Mårdh PA, Weström L: Antibodies to *Mycoplasma hominis* in patients with genital infections and healthy controls. *Br J Vener Dis*, 46:390, 1970.
96 Miettinen A, et al: Enzyme immunoassay for serum antibody to *Mycoplasma hominis* in women with acute PID. *Sex Transm Dis*, 10: 276, 1983.
97 McCormack WM, et al: Sexual activity and vaginal colonization with mycoplasmas. *JAMA*, 221:1375, 1972.
98 Taylor-Robinson D: The history of *Mycoplasma genitalium* in sexually transmitted diseases. *Genitourin Med*, 71:1, 1995.
99 Taylor-Robinson D, et al: Animal models of *Mycoplasma genitalium* urogenital infection. *Isr J Med Sci*, 23:561, 1987.
100 Collier AM, et al: Attachment of *Mycoplasma genitalium* to the Ciliated Epithelium of Human Fallopian Tube, in *Recent Advances in Mycoplasmology*. G Stanek et al (eds). Stuttgart, Gustav Fischer Verlag, 1990, p 730.
101 Palmer HM, et al: Detection of *Mycoplasma genitalium* in the genitourinary tract of women by the polymerase chain reaction. *Int J STD AIDS*, 2:261, 1991.
102 Møller BR, et al: Serological evidence implicating *Mycoplasma genitalium* in pelvic inflammatory disease. *Lancet*, 1:1102, 1984.
103 Lind K, Kristensen GB: Significance of antibodies to *Mycoplasma genitalium* in salpingitis. *Eur J Clin Microbiol*, 6:205, 1987.
104 Mårdh PA, Weström L: T-mycoplasmas in the genital tract of the female. *Acta Pathol Microbiol Scand* (Sec B), 78:367, 1970.
105 Soper DE, et al: Observations concerning the microbial etiology of acute salpingitis. *Am J Obstet Gynecol*, 170:1008, 1994.
106 Lip J, Burgoyne X: Cervical and peritoneal bacterial flora associated with salpingitis. *Obstet Gynecol*, 28:561, 1966.
107 Wasserheit JN, et al: Microbial causes of proven pelvic inflammatory disease and efficacy of clindamycin and tobramycin. *Ann Intern Med*, 104:187, 1986.
108 Berardi RS: Abdominal actinomycosis. *Surg Gynecol Obstet* 149; 257, 1979.
109 Weström L, Wølner-Hanssen P: Pathogenesis of pelvic inflammatory disease. *Genitourin Med*, 69:9, 1993.
110 Eschenbach DA, et al: Diagnosis and clinical features associated with bacterial vaginosis. *Am J Obstet Gynecol*, 158:819, 1988.
111 Korn AP, et al: Plasma cell endometritis in women with symptomatic bacterial vaginosis. *Obstet Gynecol*, 85:387, 1995.
112 Hillier SL, et al: Role of bacterial vaginosis-associated microorganisms in endometritis. *Am J Obstet Gynecol*, 175:435, 1996.
113 World Health Organization: Mechanisms of action, safety, and efficacy of intrauterine devices. *WHO Techn Rep Ser*, 75:35, 1987
114 Bieluch VM, Tally FP: Pathophysiology of abscess formation. *Clinics in Obstet Gynecol*, 10:93, 1983.
115 Svensson L, et al: Differences in some clinical and laboratory parameters in acute salpingitis related to culture and serological findings. *Am J Obstet Gynecol*, 138:1017, 1980.
116 Heinonen PK, et al: Anatomic sites of genital upper tract infection. *Obstet Gynecol*, 66:384, 1985.
117 Weisner D, et al: Bakteriologische Unersuchungen von Douglasflüssigkeit. *Geburtshilfe Frauenheilk*, 40:1118, 1980.
118 Amersbach R: Sterilität und Frigidität. *Münchener Medizinische Wochenschrift*, 77:225, 1930.
119 Egli G, Newton M: The transport of carbon particles in the human female reproductive tract. *Fertil Steril*, 12:151, 1961.
120 Keith LG, et al: New concepts on the causation of pelvic inflammatory disease. *Current Problems in Obstetrics, Gynecology and Fertility*, 9:3, 1986.
121 Halme J, et al: Retrograde menstruation in healthy women and in patients with endometriosis. *Obstet Gynecol*, 64:151, 1984.
122 Rank RG, Sanders MM: Ascending genital tract infection as a common consequence of vaginal inoculation with the guinea pig inclusion conjunctivitis agent in normal guinea pigs. In *Chlamydial Infection. Proceedings of the VIIth International Symposium on Human Chlamydial Infection*, WR Bowie et al (eds). Cambridge UK, Cambridge University Press, 1990, p 249.
123 Stemmer W. über die Ursachen von Eileiterentzündungen. *Zbl Gynäkol*, 63:1062, 1941.
124 Washington AE, et al: Assessing risk for pelvic inflammatory disease and its sequelae. *JAMA*, 266:2581, 1991.

125 Wølner-Hanssen P, Mårdh PA: In vitro tests of the adherence of *Chlamydia trachomatis* to human spermatozoa. *Fertil Steril*, 42:102, 1984.
126 Toth A, et al: Evidence of microbial transfer by spermatozoa. *Obstet Gynecol*, 59:556, 1982.
127 Friberg J, et al: *Chlamydia trachomatis* is attached to spermatozoa recovered from the peritoneal cavity of patients with salpingitis. *J Reprod Med*, 32:12120, 1987.
128 Patton DL, et al: The role of spermatozoa in the pathogenesis of *Chlamydia trachomatis* salpingitis in a primate model. *Sex Transm Dis*, 20:214, 1993.
129 Odeblad E: The functional structure of human cervical mucus. *Acta Obstet Gynecol Scand*, 47(suppl 1):57, 1968.
130 Koch ML, Baltimore MS: A study of cervical cultures taken in cases of acute gonorrhea with special reference to the phases of the menstrual cycle. *Am J Obstet Gynecol*, 54:861, 1947.
131 Sweet RL, et al: The occurrence of chlamydial and gonococcal salpingitis during the menstrual cycle. *JAMA*, 25:2062, 1986.
132 Rice PA, Schachter J: Pathogenesis of pelvic inflammatory disease. What are the questions? *JAMA*, 266:2587, 1991.
133 Wølner-Hanssen P, et al: Decreased risk of symptomatic chlamydial pelvic inflammatory disease associated with oral contraceptive use. *JAMA*, 263:54, 1990.
134 Luukkainen TJ, Allonen T: Protective effect of intrauterine release of levonorgestrel on pelvic infection; three years comparative experience of levonorgestrel-releasing intrauterine devices. *Obstet Gynecol*, 77: 261, 1991.
135 Morse SA, Fitzgerald TJ: Effect of progesterone on *Neisseria gonorrhoeae*. *Infect Immun*, 10:1370, 1974.
136 Maslow AS, et al: Estrogen enhances attachment of *Chlamydia trachomatis* to human endometrial cells in vitro. *Am J Obstet Gynecol*, 159:1006, 1988.
137 Kleinman D, et al: The effects of contraceptive hormones on the replication of *Chlamydia trachomatis* in human endometrial cells. *Contraception*, 35:533, 1987.
138 Pasley JN, et al: Effects of various doses of estradiol on chlamydial genital infection in ovariectomized guinea pigs. *Sex Transm Dis*, 12: 8, 1985.
139 Barron AL, et al: Chlamydial salpingitis in female guinea pigs receiving oral contraceptives. *Sex Transm Dis*, 15:169, 1988.
140 Pasley JN, et al: Absence of progesterone effects on chlamydial genital infection in guinea pigs. *Sex Transm Dis* 12:155, 1985.
141 Patton DL, et al: Oral contraceptives do not alter the course of experimentally induced chlamydial salpingitis in monkeys. *Sex Transm Dis*, 21:89, 1994.
142 Wølner-Hanssen P, et al: Association between vaginal douching and acute pelvic inflammatory disease. *JAMA*, 266:2587, 1990.
143 Scholes D, et al: Vaginal douching as a risk factor for acute pelvic inflammatory disease. *Obstet Gynecol*, 81:601, 1993.
144 Larsson PG, et al: Incidence of pelvic inflammatory disease after first-trimester legal abortion in women with bacterial vaginosis after treatment with metronidazole: A double blind randomized study. *Am J Obstet Gynecol*, 166:100, 1992.
145 Mishell DR, Moyer DL: Association of pelvic inflammatory disease with the intrauterine device. *Clin Obstet Gynecol*, 12:179, 1969.
146 Sparks H, et al: Bacteriological colonization of uterine cavity: Role of tailed intrauterine contraceptive device. *Br Med J*, 282:1189, 1981.
147 Valicenti JF, et al: Detection and prevalence of IUD-associated actinomyces colonization and related morbidity. A prospective study of 69,925 cervical smears. *JAMA*, 247:1149, 1982.
148 Holst E, et al: Bacterial vaginosis. Microbiology and clinical findings. *Eur J Clin Bact*, 6:536, 1987.
149 Moyer DC, Mishell DR: Reaction of human endometria to the intrauterine foreign body. *Am J Obstet Gynecol*, 111:66, 1971.
150 Carney FE Jr, Taylor-Robinson D: Growth and effect of *Neisseria gonorrhoeae* in organ cultures. *Br J Vener Dis*, 49:435, 1973.
151 Gregg CR, et al: Toxic activity of purified lipopolysaccharide of *Neisseria gonorrhoeae* for human fallopian tube mucosa. *J Infect Dis*, 143:432, 1981.
152 Melly MA, et al: Ability of monomeric peptidoglycan fragments from *Neisseria gonorrhoeae* to damage human fallopian-tube mucosa. *J Infect Dis*, 149:378, 1984.
153 Hillis SD, et al: Delayed care of pelvic inflammatory disease as a risk factor for impaired fertility. *Am J Obstet Gynecol*, 168:1503, 1993.
154 Plummer FA: Antibodies to opacity proteins (Opa) correlate with a reduced risk of gonococcal salpingitis. *J Clin Invest*, 93:1748, 1994.
155 Phillips DM, et al: Ultrastructure of *Chlamydia trachomatis* infection of the mouse oviduct. *J Ultrastruct Res*, 88:244, 1984.
156 Williams DM, et al: Tumor necrosis factor as a cytotoxin induced by murine *Chlamydia trachomatis* infection. *Infect Immun*, 57:1351, 1989.
157 Byrne GL, et al: Gamma interferon-mediated cytotoxicity related to murine *Chlamydia trachomatis* infection. *Infect Immun*, 56:2023, 1988.
158 Rothermel CD, et al: *Chlamydia trachomatis*-induced production of interleukin-1 by human monocytes. *Infect Immun*, 57:2705, 1989.
159 Witkin S, et al: Increased inducibility of inflammatory mediators from peripheral blood mononuclear cells in women with salpingitis. *Am J Obstet Gynecol*, 165:719, 1991.
160 Arno JN, et al: Interferon-gamma in endocervical secretions of women infected with *Chlamydia trachomatis*. *J Infect Dis*, 162:1385, 1990.
161 Grifo JA, et al: Interferon gamma in the diagnosis and pathogenesis of pelvic inflammatory disease. *Am J Obstet Gynecol*, 160:23, 1989.
162 Mabey DC, et al: Expression of MHC class II antigens by conjunctival epithelial cells in trachoma: Implications concerning the pathogenesis of blinding disease. *J Clin Ophthalmol*, 44:285, 1991.
163 Puolakkainen M, et al: Persistence of chlamydial antibodies after pelvic inflammatory disease. *J Clin Microbiol*, 23:924, 1986.
164 Rank RG, Batteiger BE: Protective role of serum antibody in immunology to chlamydial genital infection. *Infect Immun*, 57:299, 1989.
165 Wølner-Hanssen P, et al: Protective immunity in pig-tailed macaques after cervical infection with *Chlamydia trachomatis*. *Sex Transm Dis*, 18:21, 1991.
166 Johnson AP, et al: Immunity to reinfection of the genital tract of marmosets with *Chlamydia trachomatis*. *Br J Exp Pathol*, 62:606, 1981.
167 Grayston JT, et al: Trachoma vaccine studies in volunteer students of the National Defense Medical Center II. Response to challenge eye inoculation of egg-grown trachoma virus. *Chin Med J*, 8:312, 1961.
168 Tuffrey M, et al: Effect on *Chlamydia trachomatis* infection of the murine genital tract of adoptive transfer of congenic immune cells or specific antibody. *Br J Exp Pathol*, 66:427, 1985.
169 Ramsay KHG, et al: Resolution of chlamydial genital infection in B-cell deficient mice and immunity to reinfection. *Infect Immun*, 56: 1320, 1988.
170 Tuffrey M, et al: Severity of salpingitis in mice after primary and repeated inoculations with a human strain of *Chlamydia trachomatis*. *Exp Pathol*, 71:403, 1990.
171 Taylor HR, et al: Pathogenesis of trachoma: The stimulus for inflammation. *J Immun*, 138:3023, 1987.
172 Williams DM, Schachter J: Role of cell-mediated immunity in chlamydial infection: Implications for ocular immunity. *Rev Infect Dis*, 7:754, 1985.
173 Van Voorhis WC, Barrett LK, Cosgrove Sweeney C, et al: Analysis of lymphocyte phenotype and cytokine activity in the inflammatory infiltrates of the upper genital tract of female macaques infected with *Chlamydia trachomatis*. *J Infect Dis*, 174:647, 1996.
174 Kimani J, et al: Risk factors for *Chlamydia trachomatis* pelvic inflammatory disease among sex workers in Nairobi, Kenya. *J Infect Dis*, 173:1437, 1996.
175 Taylor HR, et al: Chlamydial heat shock proteins and trachoma. *Infect Immun*, 58:3061, 1990.
176 Witkin SS, et al: Proliferative response to conserved epitopes of the *Chlamydia trachomatis* heat-shock proteins by lymphocytes from women with salpingitis. *Am J Obstet Gynecol*, 171:455, 1994.

177 Eckert LO, et al: Prevalence and correlates of antibody to chlamydial heat shock protein in women attending sexually disease clinics and women with confirmed pelvic inflammatory disease. *J Infect Dis*, 175: 1453, 1997.
178 Money DM, et al: Antibodies to the chlamydial 60 kDa heat shock protein are associated with laparoscopically confirmed perihepatitis. *Am J Obstet Gynecol*, 176:870, 1997.
179 Toye B, et al: Association between antibody to the chlamydial heat shock protein and tubal infertility. *J Infect Dis*, 168:1236, 1993.
180 Brunham RC, et al: *Chlamydia trachomatis*-associated ectopic pregnancy: Serologic and histologic correlates. *J Infect Dis*, 165:1076, 1992.
181 Brunham RC, Peeling RW: *Chlamydia trachomatis* antigens: Role in immunity and pathogenesis. *Infectious Agents Disease*, 3:218, 1994.
182 Cerrone MC, et al: Cloning and sequence of the gene for heat shock protein 60 from *Chlamydia trachomatis* and immunologic reactivity of the protein. *Infect Immun*, 59:79, 1991.
183 Cox SM, et al: Role of *Neisseria gonorrhoeae* and *Chlamydia trachomatis* in intraabdominal abscess formation in the rat. *J Reprod Med* 36:202, 1991.
184 Nordenskjöld F, Ahlgren M: Laparoscopy in female infertility. *Acta Obstet Gynecol Scand*, 62:609, 1983.
185 Weström L: Long Term Consequences of PID. In *Genital Tract Infection in Women*, MJ Hare (ed). London, Churchill Livingstone, 1988, p 350.
186 Tuffrey, et al: Correlation with altered tubal morphology and function in mice with salpingitis induced by a human genital-tract isolate of *Chlamydia trachomatis*. *J Reprod Fertil*, 88:295, 1990.
187 Swensen CE, et al: The effect of tetracycline treatment on chlamydial salpingitis and subsequent infertility in the mouse. *Sex Transm Dis*, 13:40, 1986.
188 Patton DL, et al: Distal tubal obstruction induced by repeated *Chlamydia trachomatis* salpingeal infections in pig-tailed macaques. *J Infect Dis*, 155:1292, 1987.
189 Curran JW: Economic consequences of pelvic inflammatory disease in the United States. *Am J Obstet Gynecol*, 138:484, 1980.
190 Washington AE, Katz P: Cost of and payment source for pelvic inflammatory disease: Trends and projections, 1983 through 2000. *JAMA*, 266:2565, 1991.
191 Rolfs RT, et al: Epidemiology of pelvic inflammatory disease: Trends in hospitalizations and office visits 1979–1988. In: *Proceedings of the CDC and NIH Joint Meeting: Pelvic Inflammatory Disease: Prevention, Management, and Research in the 1990s*. Bethesda, MD, September 4–5, 1990.
192 *Division of STD/HIV Prevention Annual Report, 1989*. Atlanta, GA: Centers for Disease Control, 1989.
193 Aral SO, et al: Self-reported pelvic inflammatory disease in the United States. 1988. *JAMA* 266:2570, 1991.
194 Washington AE, et al. Pelvic inflammatory disease and its sequelae in adolescents. *J Adol Health Care*, 6:309, 1985.
195 Expert Committee on Pelvic Inflammatory Disease: Pelvic inflammatory disease: Research directions in the 1990s. *Sex Transm Dis*, 18:46, 1991.
196 Division of STD Prevention. Sexually Transmitted Disease Surveillance, 1995. U.S. Department of Health and Human Services, Atlanta,GA: Centers for Disease Control and Prevention, September, 1996.
197 Buchan H, Vessey M: Epidemiology and trends in hospital discharges for pelvic inflammatory disease in England 1975 to 1985. *Br J Obstet Gynaecol*, 96:1219, 1989.
198 Weström L, et al: Pelvic inflammatory disease and infertility. A cohort study of 1,844 women with laparoscopically verified disease and 657 control women with normal laproscopic findings. *Sex Transm Dis*, 19:185, 1992.
199 Kani J, Adler MW: Epidemiology of Pelvic Inflammatory Disease, in *Pelvic Inflammatory Disease*, GS Berger, L Weström (eds). New York, Raven Press, 1992, p 7.
200 Wasserheit JN: The significance and scope of reproductive tract infections among Third World women. *Int J Gynecol Obstet*, Suppl 3; 145S, 1989.
201 Carty MJ, et al: The role of gonococcus in acute pelvic inflammatory disease in Nairobi. *East Afr Med J*, 49:376, 1972.
202 Muir DG, Belsey MA: Pelvic inflammatory disease and its consequences in the developing world. *Am J Obstet Gynecol*, 138:913, 1980.
203 Mäkinen J: Ectopic pregnancy in Finland 1966–1986: *Annales Universitatis Turensis. Medica Odontologica*, 36:1, 1988.
204 Johansson E, et al: Gonorrhea, chlamydia, and urethritis in partners to women with acute salpingitis (in Swedish). *Läk Tidn*, 37:2974, 1988.
205 Addiss DG, et al: Decreased prevalence of *Chlamydia trachomatis* infection associated with a selective screening program in family planning clinics in Wisconsin. *Sex Transm Dis*, 20:24, 1992.
206 Scholes D, et al: Prevention of pelvic inflammatory disease by screening for cervical chlamydial infection. *N Engl J Med*, 334:1399, 1996.
207 World Health Organization: Pelvic inflammatory disease in Nongonococcal urethritis and other selected sexually transmitted diseases of public health importance. *WHO Techn Rep Ser*, 660:89, 1981.
208 Eschenbach D et al: Epidemiology of acute pelvic inflammatory disease. Abstract C03-088, *International Society for STD Research*, Banff, Canada, Oct 6–9, 1991.
209 Kelaghane J, et al: Barrier method contraceptives and pelvic inflammatory disease. *JAMA*, 248:184, 1982.
210 Wøolner-Hanssen P, et al: Laparoscopic findings and contraceptive use in women with signs and symptoms suggestive of acute salpingitis *Obstet Gynecol*, 66:233, 1985.
211 Critchlow CW, et al: Determinants of cervical ectopy and of cervicitis: Age, oral contraception, specific cervical infection, smoking and douching. *Am J Obstet Gynecol*, 173:534, 1995.
212 World Health Organization. Mechanisms of action, safety, and efficacy of intrauterine devices. *WHO Techn Rep Ser*, 75:35, 1987.
213 Kessel E: Pelvic inflammatory disease with intrauterine device use: A reassessment. *Fertil Steril*, 51:1, 1989.
214 Farley TMM, et al: Intrauterine devices and pelvic inflammatory disease: An international perspective. *Lancet*, 339:785, 1992.
215 Senanayake P, et al: Contraception and the etiology of pelvic inflammatory disease: New perspectives. *Am J Obstet Gynecol*, 138:852, 1980.
216 Cramer DW, et al: Tubal infertility and the intrauterine device *N Engl J Med*, 312:941, 1985.
217 Daling JR, et al: Primary tubal infertility in relation to the use of an intrauterine device. *N Engl J Med*, 312:937, 1985.
218 Basuki B, et al: Intrauterine device use and risk of tubal pregnancy: An Indonesian case-control study. *Int J Epidemiol*, 23:1000, 1994.
219 Marrie TJ, Costerton JW: A scanning and transmission electron microscopic study of the surfaces of intrauterine contraceptive devices. *Am J Obstet Gynecol*, 146:384, 1983.
220 Eschenbach DA, et al: Pathogenesis of acute pelvic inflammatory disease: Role of contraception and other risk factors. *Am J Obstet Gynecol*, 128:838, 1977.
221 Gump DW, et al: Evidence of prior pelvic inflammatory disease and its relationship to *C. trachomatis* antibody and intrauterine contraceptive device use in infertile women. *Am J Obstet Gynecol*, 146: 143, 1983.
222 Daling JR, et al: The intrauterine device and primary tubal infertility. *N Engl J Med*, 326:203, 1992.
223 Daling JR, et al: Vaginal douching and the risk of tubal pregnancy. *Epidemiol*, 2:40, 1991.
224 Marchbanks PA, et al: Cigarette smoking as a risk factor for pelvic inflammatory disease. *Am J Obstet Gynecol*, 162:639, 1990.
225 Irwin KI: Potential for bias in studies of the influence of human immunodeficiency virus infection on the recognition, incidence, clinical course, and microbiology of pelvic inflammatory disease. *Obstet Gynecol*, 84:463, 1994.
226 Safrin S, et al: Seroprevalence and epidemiologic correlates of human immunodeficiency virus infections in women with acute pelvic inflammatory disease. *Obstet Gynecol*, 75:666, 1990.
227 Sperling RS, et al: Seroprevalence of human immunodeficiency virus in women admitted to the hospital with pelvic inflammatory disease. *J Reprod Med*, 36:122, 1991.

228 Cohen C, et al: HIV and acute pelvic inflammatory disease: A laparoscopic study in Kenya (Abstr 113). *XI International Conference on AIDS*. Vancouver, Canada, July 1996.

229 Hoegsberg B, et al: Sexually transmitted diseases and human immunodeficiency virus infection among women with pelvic inflammatory disease. *Am J Obstet Gynecol*, 163:1135, 1990.

230 Korn AP, et al: Pelvic inflammatory disease in human immunodeficiency-virus infected women. *Obstet Gynecol*, 82:765, 1993.

231 Centers for Disease Control: Pelvic inflammatory disease: Guidelines for prevention and management. *MMWR*, 40:1, 1991.

232 Moore DE, et al: Increased frequency of serum antibodies to *Chlamydia trachomatis* in infertility due to distal tubal disease. *Lancet*, 2: 574, 1982.

233 Kane JL, et al: Evidence of chlamydial infection in infertile women with and without fallopian tube obstruction. *Fertil Steril*, 42:843, 1984.

234 Weström L: Consequences of Pelvic Inflammatory Disease, in *Pelvic Inflammatory Disease*, GS Berger, L Weström (eds). New York, Raven Press, 1992, p 101.

235 Smith MR, et al: Endosalpingitis: A frequent response to intrauterine contraception. *J Reprod Med*, 126:159, 1976.

236 Paavonen J, Weström L. Diagnosis of Pelvic inflammatory Disease, in *Pelvic Inflammatory Disease*, GS Berger, L Weström (eds). New York, Raven Press, 1992, p 49.

237 Jacobson L: Laparoscopy in the diagnosis of acute salpingitis. *Acta Obstet Gynecol Scand*, 43:160, 1964.

238 Falk V: Treatment of acute non-tuberculous salpingitis with antibiotics alone and in combination with glucocorticoids. *Acta Obstet Gynecol Scand*, 44(suppl 6):96, 1965.

239 Sellors J, et al: The accuracy of clinical findings and laparoscopy in pelvic inflammatory disease. *Am J Obstet Gynecol*, 164:113, 1991.

240 Hadgu A, et al: Predicting acute pelvic inflammatory disease: A multivariate analysis. *Am J Obstet Gynecol*, 155:954, 1986.

241 Wølner-Hanssen, et al: Laparoscopy in women with chlamydial infection and pelvic pain: A comparison of patients with and without salpingitis. *Obstet Gynecol*, 61:299, 1983.

242 Kahn JG, et al: Diagnosing pelvic inflammatory disease. A comprehensive analysis and considerations for developing a new model. *JAMA*, 266:2594, 1991.

243 Wølner-Hanssen P: Silent pelvic inflammatory disease: Is it overstated? *Obstet Gynecol*, 86:321, 1995.

244 Cleary RE, Jones RB: Recovery of *Chlamydia trachomatis* from the endometrium in infertile women with serum antichlamydial antibodies. *Fertil Steril*, 44:233, 1985.

245 Henry-Suchet J, et al: *Chlamydia trachomatis*associated with chronic inflammation in abdominal specimens from women selected for tuboplasty. *Fertil Steril*, 33:599, 1981.

246 Patton D, et al: A comparison of the fallopian tube's response to overt and silent salpingitis. *Obstet Gynecol*, 73:622, 1989.

247 World Health Organization: Pelvic inflammatory disease, in *Non-gonococcal urethritis and other selected sexually transmitted diseases of public health importance. WHO Techn Rep Series*, 660:89, 1981.

248 Perpert TF: Laboratory evaluation of acute upper genital tract infection. *Obstet Gynecol*, 87:730,1996.

249 Eschenbach DA, et al: Acute pelvic inflammatory disease: Association of clinical and laboratory findings with laparoscopic findings. *Obstet Gynecol*, 89:184, 1997.

250 Husebøo OS, et al: Acute perihepatitis. *Acta Chir Scand*, 145:483, 1979.

251 Wølner-Hanssen P, et al: Perihepatitis and chlamydial salpingitis. *Lancet*, 1:901, 1980.

252 Moritz E: Wurmvorsatzveranderungen nach Tubenentzündungen. *Zbl Geburtsh Gynäkol*, 70:404, 1912.

253 Curtis AH: A cause of adhesions in the right upper quadrant. *JAMA*, 94:1221, 1930.

254 Butler C: Surgical pathology of acute appendicitis. *Human Pathol*, 12:870, 1980.

255 Fink AS, et al: Periappendicitis is a significant clinical finding. *Am J Surg*, 159:564, 1990.

256 Mårdh PA, Wølner-Hanssen P: Periappendicitis in chlamydial salpingitis. *Surg Gynecol Obstet*, 160:304, 1985.

257 Litt IF, Cohen MI: Perihepatitis associated with salpingitis in adolescents. *JAMA*, 240:1253, 1978.

258 Wølner-Hanssen P. *Manifestations and Pathogenesis of Chlamydial Pelvic Inflammatory Disease*. Umeå, Sweden: Nyheternas Tryckeri AB, 1985.

259 Wang S-P, et al: *Chlamydia trachomatis* infection in Fitz-Hugh Curtis syndrome. *Am J Obstet Gynecol*, 13:1034, 1980.

260 Onsrud M, et al: Acute perihepatitis. *Acta Chir Scand*, 145:483, 1979.

261 Onsrud M: Perihepatitis in pelvic inflammatory disease. Association with intrauterine contraception. *Acta Obstet Gynecol Scand*, 59:69, 1980.

262 Paavonen J, et al: Association of infection with *Chlamydia trachomatis* with Fitz-Hugh Curtis syndrome. *J Infect Dis*, 144:176, 1981.

263 Müller-Schoop JW, et al: *Chlamydia trachomatis* as a possible cause of peritonitis and perihepatitis in young women. *Br Med J*, i:1022, 1978.

264 Henry-Suchet J, et al: Perihepatites (syndrome de Fitz-Hugh Curtis) infra-cliniques au cours de salpingites ou de sterilites tubaires. Cultures positives pour *Chlamydia trachomatis* dans les adherences perihepatiques. *Presse Med* 12:1725, 1983.

265 Schildt BE, Eisemann B: Peritoneal absorption of CR^{51}-tagged erythrocytes. Its influence by pneumoperitoneum and Fowler's position. *Acta Clin Scand*, 119:937, 1960.

266 Francis TI, Osoba AO: Gonococcal perihepatitis (Fitz-Hugh Curtis syndrome) in a male patient. *Br J Vener Dis*, 48:187, 1972.

267 Møller BR, Mårdh PA: Experimental salpingitis in grivet monkeys by *Chlamydia trachomatis*. *Acta Pathol Microbiol Scand* [B], 88:107, 1980.

268 Fitzgerald PN, et al: Depressed lymphocyte response to PHA in long-term users of oral contraceptives. *Lancet*, 1:15, 1973.

269 Brunham RC, et al: Mucopurulent cervicitis: The ignored counterpart in women of urethritis in men. *N Engl J Med*, 311:1, 1984.

270 Paavonen J, et al: Etiology of cervical inflammation. *Am J Obstet Gynecol*, 154:556, 1986.

271 Hemilä M, et al: Serum CRP in the diagnosis and treatment of pelvic inflammatory disease. *Arch Gynecol Obstet*, 241:177, 1987.

272 Lehtinen M, et al: Serum C-reactive protein determinations in acute pelvic inflammatory disease. *Am J Obstet Gynecol*, 154:158, 1986.

273 Jacobson L, et al: Plasma protein changes induced by acute inflammation of the fallopian tubes. *Acta Obstet Gynecol Scand*, 40:556, 1986.

274 Paavonen J, et al: Serum CA 125 levels in acute pelvic inflammatory disease. *Br J Obstet Gynaecol*, 96:574, 1989.

275 Skude G, et al: Isoamylases of genital tract tissue homogenates and peritoneal fluid. *Am J Obstet Gynecol*, 126:657, 1976.

276 Skude G, et al. Isoamylases in the Diagnosis of Acute Salpingitis, Iin *Progress in Clinical Enzymology*, DM Goldberg, et al (eds). New York, Masson, 1983, vol 2, p 277.

277 Paavonen J, et al: Comparison of endometrial biopsy and peritoneal fluid cytology with laparoscopy in the diagnosis of acute pelvic inflammatory disease. *Am J Obstet Gynecol*, 154:645, 1986.

278 Nassberg S, et al. Physiological salpingitis. *Am J Obstet Gynecol*, 67: 130, 1954.

279 Mecke H, et al: Pelviskopische Behandlung abszedierende Entzündungen im klienen Becken. *Geburtsh u Frauenheilk*, 48:479, 1988.

280 Reich H, et al: Laparoscopic treatment of tuboovarian and pelvic abscesses. *J Reprod Med*, 32:742, 1987.

281 Swayne LC, et al. Pelvic inflammatory disease. Sonographic-pathologic correlation. *Radiology*, 151:751, 1984.

282 Berland LL, et al: Ultrasound evaluation of pelvic inflammatory disease. *Radiol Clin North Amer*, 20:367, 1982.

283 Spirtos NJ, et al: Sonography in acute pelvic inflammatory disease. *J Reprod Med*, 27:312, 1982.

284 Cacciatore B, et al: Transvaginal sonographic findings in ambulatory patients with suspected pelvic inflammatory disease. *Obstet Gynecol*, 80:912, 1992.

285 Nelson AL, et al: Endovaginal ultrasonographically guided transvaginal drainage for treatment of pelvic abscesses. *Am J Obstet Gynecol*, 172:1926, 1995.

286 Aboulghar MA, et al: Ultrasonographically guided transvaginal aspiration of tuboovarian abscesses and pyosalpinges: An optional treatment for acute pelvic inflammatory disease. *Am J Obstet Gynecol*, 172:1501, 1995.

287 Jacobson L: Differential diagnosis of acute pelvic inflammatory disease. *Am J Obstet Gynecol*, 138:1006, 1980.

288 Weström L, Wølner-Hanssen P: Differential Diagnosis of Pelvic Inflammatory Disease, in *Pelvic Inflammatory Disease*, GS Berger, L Weström (eds). New York, Raven Press, 1992, p 79.

289 Tice AD: An office model of outpatient antibiotic therapy. *Rev Infect Dis*, 13(Suppl 2):S184, 1991.

290 Walker CK, et al: Pelvic inflammatory disease: Metaanalysis of antimicrobial regimen efficacy. *J Infect Dis*, 168:969, 1993.

291 Dodson, MG: Antibiotic regimens for treating acute pelvic inflammatory disease: An evaluation. *J Reprod Med*, 39:285, 1994.

292 Landers DV, et al. Combination antimicrobial therapy in the treatment of acute pelvic inflammatory disease. *Am J Obstet Gynecol*, 164:849, 1991.

293 Walters MD, Gibbs RS: A randomized comparison of gentamicin-clindamycin and cefoxitin-doxycycline in the treatment of acute pelvic inflammatory disease. *Obstet Gynecol*, 75:867, 1990.

294 Hasselquist MB, Hillier SL: Susceptibility of upper-genital tract isolates from women with pelvic inflammatory disease to ampicillin, cefpodoxime, metronidazole, and doxycycline. *Sex Transm Dis*, 18: 146, 1991.

295 Brunham RC: Therapy for acute pelvic inflammatory disease: a critique of recent clinical trials. *Am J Obstet Gynecol*, 148:235, 1984.

296 Weström L, et al: Infertility after acute salpingitis: Results of treatment with different antibiotics. *Curr Ther Res*, 26:752, 1979.

297 Paavonen J, et al: Factors predicting abnormal hysterosalpingographic findings in patients treated for acute pelvic inflammatory disease. *Int J Gynaecol Obstet*, 23:171, 1985.

298 Gerof SG, et al: Percutaneous catheter drainage of abdominal abscesses: A five year experience. *N Engl J Med*, 305:653, 1981.

299 Henry-Suchet J, et al: Laparoscopic treatment of tuboovarian abscesses. *J Reprod Med*, 29:579, 1984.

300 Grimes DA: Deaths due to STD. *JAMA*, 255:1727, 1986.

301 Pedowitz P, Bloomfield RD: Ruptured adnexal abscess with generalized peritonitis. *Am J Obstet Gynecol*, 88:721, 1964.

302 Rivlin ME, Hunt JA: Ruptured tubo-ovarian abscess: Is hysterectomy necessary? *Obstet Gynecol*, 50(suppl):518, 1977.

303 Weström L: Influence of sexually transmitted diseases on sterility and ectopic pregnancy. *Acta Eur Fertil*, 16:21, 1985.

304 Brunham RC, et al: Etiology and outcome of acute pelvic inflammatory disease. *J Infect Dis*, 158:510, 1988.

305 Cates W, et al: Sexually transmitted diseases, pelvic inflammatory disease, and infertility: An epidemiologic update. *Epidemiol Rev*, 12: 199, 1990.

306 Lenton EA, et al: Long-term follow-up of the apparently normal couple with complaint of infertility. *Fertil Steril* 28;913, 1977.

307 Cates W, et al: Worldwide patterns of infertility. Is Africa different? *Lancet*, 2:596, 1985.

308 World Health Organization: Infections, pregnancies, and infertility: Perspectives on prevention. *Fertil Steril*, 47:964, 1987.

309 Hull MG, et al: Population study of causes, treatment, and outcome of infertility. *Br Med J*, 291:1693, 1985.

310 Weström L: STD and infertility. *Sex Transm Dis*, 21 (suppl):32S, 1994.

311 Wøolner-Hanssen P: Oral contraceptive use modifies the manifestations of pelvic inflammatory disease. *Br J Obstet Gynaecol*, 93:619, 1986.

312 Svensson L, et al: Infertility after acute salpingitis—with special reference to *Chlamydia trachomatis* associated infections. *Fertil Steril*, 40:322, 1983.

313 Weström L: Consequences of genital chlamydial infections in women. *III European Chlamydial Meeting*. Vienna, September 11–14, 1996.

314 Mabey DC, et al. Tubal infertility in the Gambia, chlamydial and gonococcal serology in women with tubal obstruction compared with pregnant controls. *Bull WHO*, 63:1197, 1985.

315 Tjiam KH, et al: Prevalence of antibodies to *Chlamydia trachomatis, Neisseria gonorrhoeae,* and *Mycoplasma hominis* in infertile women. *Genitourin Med*, 61:175, 1985.

316 Robertson JN, et al: Chlamydial and gonococcal antibodies in sera of infertile women with tubal obstruction. *J Clin Pathol*, 40:377, 1987.

317 Møller RB, et al: Serological evidence that chlamydiae and mycoplasmas are involved in infertility in women. *J Reprod Fertil*, 73:237, 1985.

318 Gump DW, et al: Lack of evidence of association between genital mycoplasmas and infertility *N Engl J Med*, 310:937, 1984.

319 Rivlin ME: Clinical outcome following vaginal drainage of pelvic abscess. *Obstet Gynecol*, 61:680, 1983.

320 Thorburn J: Background factors of ectopic pregnancy II. Risk estimation by means of a logistic model. *Eur J Obstet Gynecol Reprod Biol*, 23:333, 1986.

321 Centers for Disease Control. Ectopic pregnancies—United States 1987. *MMWR*, 39:401, 1990.

322 Weström L, et al: Incidence, trends, and risks of ectopic pregnancy in a population of women. *Br Med J*, 82:15, 1981.

323 Krantz SG, et al: Time trends in risk factors and clinical outcome of ectopic pregnancy. *Fertil Steril*, 54:42, 1990.

324 Centers for Disease Control and Prevention: Ectopic pregnancy—United States, 1990–1992, *MMWR*, 44:46, 1995.

325 Joesoef R, et al: Recurrence of ectopic pregnancy: The role of salpingitis. *Am J Obstet Gynecol*, 165:46, 1991.

326 Weström L, Svensson L: Chronic pain after acute pelvic inflammatory disease, in P Belfort, et al (eds). *Advances in gynecology and obstetrics. Proc XIIth World Congr Gynecol Obstet, Rio de Janeiro*, Vol. 6, "General Gynecology." P Belford et al (eds). Casterton Hall, Lancashire, UK: 1988, p 265.

327 Buchan H, et al: Morbidity following pelvic inflammatory disease. *Br J Obstet Gynaecol*, 100:558, 1993.

328 Britten TF, et al: STDs and family planning clinics: A regional program for chlamydia control that works. *Am J Gynecol Health*, 6:24, 1992.

329 Schachter J, et al: Noninvasive test for diagnosis of *Chlamydia trachomatis* infection: Application of ligase chain reaction to first-catch urine specimens of women. *J Infect Dis*, 172:1411, 1995.

330 Stamm WE, et al: Causes of the acute urethral syndrome in women. *N Engl J Med*, 311:1, 1984.

331 Cates W Jr, Wasserheit JN: Gonorrhea, chlamydia, and pelvic inflammatory disease. *Curr Opin Infect Dis*, 3:10, 1990.

332 Herrmann B, et al; Genital *Chlamydia trachomatis* (Ct) infections in Uppsala County, Sweden 1985–1993: Has a changed STD legislation contributed to declining rates (Abstr 259)? *Eleventh Meeting of the International Society for STD Research*. New Orleans, LA, August 1995.

333 Burczak JD, et al: Application of LCR to the Detection of *Chlamydia trachomatis* in Urogenital Specimens from Men and Women, in *Chlamydial Infections,* J Orfila, et al, (eds). Bologna, Societa Editrice Escalopis 1944, pp 322–25, 1994.

334 Lee HH, et al: Diagnosis of *Chlamydia trachomatis* genitourinary infection in women by ligase chain reaction assay of urine. *Lancet* 345:213, 1995.

Chapter 59

Cervical neoplasia and other STD-related genital tract neoplasias

Nancy B. Kiviat
Laura A. Koutsky
Jorma Paavonen

PAST SUCCESSES AND CURRENT CHALLENGES FOR PREVENTION AND TREATMENT OF GENITAL TRACT NEOPLASIA

It is now well established that specific types of sexually transmitted human papillomaviruses (HPV) play a central role in the pathogenesis of most squamous cell cancers of the male and female genital tract. This makes HPV an STD with potentially life threatening consequences. In 1992 cervical cancer was the most common cause of STD-related death among U.S. women, with almost double the number of deaths attributed to invasive cervical cancer as to HIV (Fig. 59-1).[1] In 1994 it was estimated that the cost of treating cervical cancer and HPV exceeded $4.5 billion, more than any other single STD with the exception of HIV.[2] Forty years ago cervical cancer was considerably more common in the United States than it is today. Over the last 35 years there has been a 78% decrease in the incidence and mortality from invasive cervical cancer within the United States, primarily due to the establishment of cytology-based cervical cancer screening programs.[3–5] Cervical cancer control, based on the cytologic detection and eradication of preinvasive lesions, termed *intraepithelial lesions* or *cervical dysplasia,* is widespread in industrialized countries, but it is only rarely available in much of the developing world. Therefore, the global incidence of invasive cervical cancer has remained high. Currently, cervical cancer is the most common cause of cancer-related mortality among women in the developing world, and worldwide it is second only to breast cancer.[6,7] Of further concern is the fact that in many areas where the incidence of cervical cancer is already high, large numbers of women are now infected with HIV, raising the possibility that the incidence of cervical cancer may further increase. While the incidence of invasive cervical cancer has markedly decreased in the United States, the cost of cervical cancer control has dramatically increased over the last decade due to referral of many women with atypical squamous cells of undetermined significance (ASCUS) and cervical intraepithelial neoplasia Grade 1 (CIN 1) for colposcopy, biopsy, and often treatment. The challenge of the next decade will be to use our new understanding of the pathogenesis of cervical cancer to develop more cost-effective approaches for screening for CIN 2 and 3 and for management of women with ASCUS and CIN 1. To achieve this aim we will need to make significant changes in our approach to cervical cancer control. Recently developed highly sensitive and specific HPV assays and a variety of new technologies now available for collecting and automatically screening smears may prove useful in conjunction with traditional cytology (or conceivably might replace it).

This chapter reviews the successes and failures of our current approach to cervical cancer control and of our current histologic and cytologic classification systems. It summarizes recent trends in incidence of invasive cervical and other anogenital tract cancers (vagina, vulva, penis, and anus), discusses evidence that links genital and anal cancers with HPV, and offers practical guidelines for the prevention, diagnosis, and early treatment of precancerous lesions. We also present an overview of emerging technologies that will likely be applied to the diagnosis and management of these lesions in the future. In addition, we examine the changing epidemiology of cervical neoplasia in the setting of human immunodeficiency (HIV).

DEFINITIONS AND CLASSIFICATION OF LESIONS

INVASIVE SQUAMOUS CELL CANCER

A variety of different types of malignancies occur at all genital and anal sites, but the majority of tumors are of the squamous cell type (Table 59-1). As discussed below, all have been associated with HPV infection. Squamous cell lesions of the anal and genital tract which are felt to be neoplastic in nature are generally divided into (1) invasive cancer and (2) noninvasive lesions. The term *invasive* refers to tumors in which the malignant cells have penetrated the underlying basement membrane and have infiltrated into the stroma. Invasive squamous cancers are graded as well, moderately, or poorly differentiated. Grade 1, or well-differentiated carcinoma, most resembles normal squamous epithelium, with many keratinizing cells and keratin pearls present. Grade 2; or moderately differentiated cancer, shows less keratin formation, with greater nuclear polymorphism and more mitoses present. Grade 3, or poorly differentiated squamous cell cancer, is composed of cells with a high nuclear/cytoplasmic ratio and many mitotic figures, but no keratin formation.[8] Invasive cervical cancers are further classified as being either frankly invasive or microinvasive. The Society of Gynecologic Oncologists (SGO) guideline defines microinvasive cervical lesions as those in which the malignant cells have not penetrated more than 2 mm below the basement membrane and in which lymphatic or vascular invasion is absent. More recently it has been proposed that lesions in which the malignant cells have penetrated to a depth of 5 mm without vascular and/or lymphatic invasion, or lesions in which malignant cells penetrate to a depth of 3 mm but where vascular and/or lymphatic invasion is present, should be classified separately as *occult carcinoma.*[9] The term *microinvasive vulvar cancer* has also been introduced.

NONINVASIVE SQUAMOUS CELL EPITHELIAL LESIONS

Histologic classification and natural history of noninvasive squamous cell epithelial lesions of the cervix

The concept of precancerous lesions was first developed around the turn of the century, when it was noted that the normal cervical epithelium cells adjacent to invasive squamous carcinomas were often replaced by a full-thickness layer of cells morphologically identical to invasive tumor cells.[10,11] Such areas were termed *carcinoma in situ* (CIS). On the basis of retrospective studies of women with invasive squamous cell carcinoma in whom prior biopsies showed CIS,[12,13] as well as on the basis of prospective studies,[14] it became widely accepted that such lesions represented incipient cancers. In fact, the exact proportion of cases that would progress from CIS to invasive cervical carcinoma (ICC) if left untreated is still unknown. Estimates (based on eight studies) range

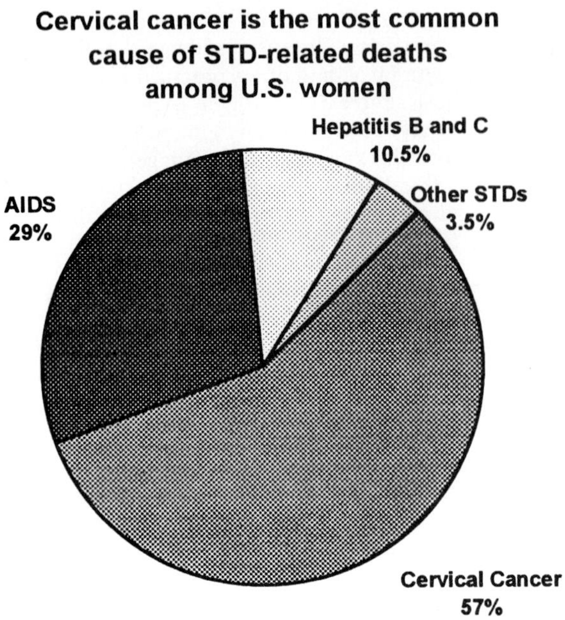

Fig. 59-1. Causes of STD-related deaths among U.S. women, 1973–1992. (*From Ebrahim SH et al*[1].)

from 0% to 71%, with a median of 34%.[14] Cervical cancer control today is based on cytologic detection and subsequent treatment of women harboring such lesions.

Other types of cervical lesions composed of less worrisome cells were subsequently described. The significance of these lesions was even less clear, but because the cells in these lesions shared some morphologic features of cells seen in CIS, it was proposed that these lesions (initially called *dysplasias* and later termed *cervical intraepithelial neoplasia*) represented the very earliest morphologic changes associated with cervical cancer. Despite the fact that little was known about the natural history of such lesions, several hierarchical systems for their classification were developed which supposedly reflected their potential biological behavior. In the most popular of these classification schemes, noninvasive cervical epithelial lesions were classified as mild, moderate, or severe dysplasia or CIS. Subsequently, natural history studies in which women with varying degrees of dysplasia were followed by cytology alone (as it was felt that biopsies might alter the natural history) were undertaken to clarify the nature of these lesions and to provide a basis for clinical management of women harboring such lesions. As summarized in Table 59-2, with the exception of the Richart and Barron study most investigators have reported extremely low rates of progression of mild dysplasia to CIS. Nevertheless, on the basis of the results of his natural history study, Richart concluded and popularized the idea that "dysplasia is simply an early cervical neoplasm and . . . although some spontaneous regressions do occur in the mild lesions, the vast majority of dysplasias ultimately evolve to carcinoma in situ and invasive carcinoma."[15] This view of dysplasia is inherent in the *cervical intraepithelial neoplasia* (CIN) classification scheme for cervical lesions proposed by Richart. This system advocates that mild, moderate, and severe dysplasia and CIS represent a morphologic and biologic continuum of progressive, consecutive stages in the development of invasive cancer. Lesions are classified as cervical intraepithelial grade lesion 1, cervical intraepithelial grade lesion 2, cervical intraepithelial grade lesion 3, or carcinoma in situ, according to the proportion of epithelium occupied by basaloid, undifferentiated cells (cells resembling the basal cell layer of the epithelium). CIN 1 lesions are conceptualized as having neoplastic, basaloid cells occupying the lower third of the epithelium, while in CIN 2 lesions basaloid cells occupy the lower third to two-thirds of the epithelium, and in CIN 3 the full thickness of the epithelium is occupied by undifferentiated basal type cells. The belief inherent in this system is that these are successive stages in development of invasive cancer and that most CIN 1, if left untreated, will progress to CIS. This view of the natural history of CIN 1 is dramatically different from that suggested by most natural history studies (see Table 59-2), which provide support for the view that mild dysplasia is generally a benign self-limited lesion with little malignant potential. The high rate of progression of CIN 1 detected in the Richart study most likely resulted from specific study entry criteria and the unique cytologic classification scheme employed. The fact that only women who had had three consecutive Pap smears showing mild dysplasia during the previous twelve months were eligible for enrollment in Richart's study biased the study population toward women with mild dysplasias that were unlikely to regress. Furthermore, the Okagaki cytologic classification used in the study by Richart and Barron differed markedly from that used today or from that used in the other studies shown in Table 59-2. Nevertheless, over the last 30 years the CIN classification system has been widely used for histologic classification of cervical pathology and has served as the basis for clinical management of women with cervical epithelial abnormalities. The view of the pathogenesis of cervical cancer inherent in the CIN classification system has led to aggressive treatment of all lesions classified as CIN. As discussed below, such an approach is increasingly being questioned in light of what we have learned about the role of HPV as a common self-limited STD and as the etiologic agent of most squamous cell genital tract neoplasia.

Table 59-1. Distribution (percent) of Genital and Anal Cancers by Histologic Type [Surveillance, Epidemiology, and End Results (SEER) Program, United States, 1973–1977]

	Cervix	Vagina	Vulva	Female anus	Male anus	Penis
Total N:	6549	353	876	394	230	370
Histologic types:*						
Carcinoma, NOS	11.0	7.2	3.8	3.3	2.2	3.5
Papillary carcinoma, NOS	0.4	2.2	3.1	0.3	0.9	5.4
Squamous cell carcinoma	75.6	67.0	74.4	49.2	44.3	85.4
Transitional cell carcinoma, NOS	0.1	0.7	0.1	30.2	22.2	0.5
Adenocarcinoma, NOS	7.2	6.1	1.3	10.4	22.2	—
Melanomas	—	3.6	6.4	1.9	—	1.6
Other tumors	5.7	13.2	10.9	4.7	8.2	3.6

* NOS = not otherwise specified.

Table 59-2. Development of Carcinoma in Situ among Women with Cytologic Evidence of Dysplasia: Summary of Four Studies

Principal author, year	Cytologic system*	Cytologic entry criterion	Cohort definition	Number in cohort	Months of follow-up	% progressing to ≥carcin in situ
Richart, 1969[11]	O[a]	3 dysplastic smears	Mild dysplasia	NS†	Projected progression at 60 months (life table analysis)	50
			Mod. dysplasia	NS		70
			Severe dysplasia	NS		95
			Any dysplasia			48
Patten, 1978[216]	P[b]	1 dysplastic smear	Mild dysplasia	3299	60 months	0.5
			Mod. dysplasia	661		2.4
			Severe dysplasia	125		10.4
Jordan, 1981[217]	WP[c]	2 negative smears	Mild dysplasia	708	60 months	1.1
			Mod. dysplasia	164		1.8
			Severe dysplasia	52		7.7
		3 dysplastic smears	Any dysplasia	65		19.0
Nasiell, 1983, 1986‡[219,229]	W[c]	1 dysplastic smear	Mild dysplasia	555	Projected progression at 60 months (life table analysis)	15.0
			Mod. dysplasia (no biopsy)	410		26.0
			Severe dysplasia (biopsy)	484		21.0

* Organization of cytologic classification scheme used to classify cytologic findings: O = Okagaki, P = Patten, W = World Health Organization.
† Numbers of subjects followed not specified.
‡ No difference in biopsied vs. nonbiopsied group for the mild dysplasia group.
[a] Okagaki T, et al: Diagnosis of anaplasia and carcinoma in situ by differential cell counts. *Acta Cytol* 6:343, 1962.
[b] Patten SF: Diagnostic cytology of the uterine cervix, in *Monographs in Clinical Cytology: Diagnostic Cytopathology of the Uterine Cervix*. New York, S Karger, 1978, p. 141.
[c] Charles EH, Savage EW: Cryosurgical treatment of cervical intraepithelial neoplasia. Obstet Gynecol Surv 35:539–548, 1980.

Histologic classification and natural history of noninvasive squamous cell epithelial lesions of the vagina, vulva, anus, and penis

The nomenclature for the precancerous states of vaginal, vulvar, anal, and penile squamous epithelium is similar to that of the cervix,[16] being termed vaginal intraepithelial neoplasia (VAIN 1, 2, 3), vulvar intraepithelial neoplasia (VIN 1, 2, 3), and intraepithelial neoplasia (AIN 1, 2, 3), and penile intraepithelial neoplasia (PIN 1, 2, 3). It is preferable to avoid using terms such as "Bowen's disease" or "Bowenoid papulosis." Although there appears to be a remarkable morphologic similarity between CIN and VIN, the risk for progression of VIN to invasive carcinoma is thought to be much lower than for CIN, with less than 10% progression among young women with normal immune systems.[17–21] Given this apparent low risk of progression, the management of patients with VIN should be as conservative as possible. Similarly, management of VAIN and PIN is conservative. Invasive vaginal carcinoma is rare, and less is known about the relationship between intraepithelial and invasive disease. VAIN is most often found in the upper third of the vagina, and the lesions are usually multifocal. In a recent study approximately one-half of the lesions were associated with concomitant cervical or vulvar intraepithelial neoplasia. Progression to invasive vaginal carcinoma occurred in two cases (9%), persistence of VAIN occurred in three (13%), and regression of VAIN occurred in 18 (78%).[22]

Classification of abnormal cervical epithelial cells detected by cytologic examination

The criteria Papanicolaou originally used over 50 years ago to make a cytologic diagnosis of invasive squamous cancer on vaginal aspirates are similar to those used today and include the presence of cells with characteristic nuclear and cytoplasmic changes in a background containing necrotic debris, old blood, and inflammation (termed a tumor diathesis).[23] Papanicolaou proposed that an increasing grade of dysplasia be assigned to abnormal but not clearly malignant cells as the nuclear to cytoplasmic ratio increased and as the nuclei increasingly resembled those of CIS. Abnormal individual cells were classified as showing superficial, intermediate, or "parabasal" cell dyskaryosis according to the normal cervical epithelial cell to which they bore the greatest resemblance.[24] Overall diagnoses were reported as one of five classes: class I, designated as the absence of atypical or abnormal cells; class II, atypical cells (reactive) but no malignant or premalignant cell changes; class III, atypical cells suggestive of but not diagnostic of malignancy; class IV, cells strongly suggestive of malignancy; and class V, changes consistent with malignancy.[25] The overall cytology slide diagnosis was based on the grade of the most abnormal cell present, regardless of the number of such cells present. Over time, pathologists have generally continued to classify individual abnormal cells in a manner similar to that proposed by Papanicolaou. The terminology has changed, with the designations of mild, moderate, and severe dysplasia replacing the original terms. A new classification scheme proposed by a 1988 National Cancer Institute Workshop on the Classification of Cervical and Vaginal Cytology and known as the Bethesda System has been introduced in an attempt to both standardize diagnoses and to improve inter- and intrapathologist reproducibility for the diagnosis of mild, moderate, and severe dysplasia.[194] This system, which has been widely adopted,[26] replaces the atypia-mild-moderate-severe dysplasia nomenclature. The term *atypical squamous cells of uncertain significance* (ASCUS) is used for cells felt to be abnormal but neither clearly reactive nor clearly dysplastic (Table 59-3). Moderate and severe dysplasias are regrouped into *high-grade squamous intraepithelial lesions* (HGSIL), with mild dysplasia and the changes suggestive of HPV (koilocytosis) grouped as *low-grade squamous intraepithelial lesions* (LGSIL). Although a corresponding revision of the histologic classification system has not formally occurred, the same "Bethesda" approach to classification of histologic lesions has been adapted by many pathologists.

Table 59-3. 1991 Bethesda System

Adequacy of the specimen
Satisfactory for evaluation
Satisfactory for evaluation but limited by . . . (specify reason)
Unsatisfactory for evaluation . . . (specify reason)
General categorization (optional)
Within normal limits
Benign cellular changes: see descriptive diagnosis
Epithelial cell abnormality: see descriptive diagnosis
Descriptive diagnoses
- *Benign cellular changes*
- Infection
  - *Trichomonas vaginalis*
  - Fungal organisms morphologically consistent with *Candida* spp
  - Predominance of coccobacilli consistent with shift in vaginal flora
  - Bacteria morphologically consistent with *Actinomyces* spp
  - Cellular changes associated with herpes simplex virus
  - Other[a]
- Reactive changes
  - Reactive cellular changes associated with:
  - Inflammation (includes typical repair)
  - Atrophy with inflammation ("atrophic vaginalis")
  - Radiation
  - Intrauterine contraceptive device (IUD)
  - Other[a]
- *Epithelial cell abnormalities*
- Squamous cell
  - Atypical squamous cells of undetermined significance: qualify[b]
  - Low-grade squamous intraepithelial lesion (LSIL) encompassing: HPV,[a] mild dysplasia/CIN 1
  - High-grade squamous intraepithelial lesion (HSIL) encompassing: moderate and severe dysplasia, CIS/CIN 2 and CIN 3
  - Squamous cell carcinoma
- Glandular cell
  - Endometrial cells, cytologically benign in a post-menopausal woman
  - Atypical glandular cells of undetermined significance: qualify[b]
  - Endocervical adenocarcinoma
  - Endometrial adenocarcinoma
  - Extrauterine adenocarcinoma
  - Adenocarcinoma, NOS
- *Other malignant neoplasms:* Specify
- *Hormonal evaluation* (applies to vaginal smears only)
  - Hormonal pattern compatible with age and history
  - Hormonal pattern incompatible with age and history: specify
  - Hormonal evaluation not possible due to: specify

[a] Cellular changes of human papillomavirus (HPV), previously termed *koilocytosis, koilocytotic atypia,* and *condylomatous atypia,* are included in the category of LSIL.
[b] Atypical squamous or glandular cells of undetermined significance should be qualified further, as to reactive or premalignant/malignant.
SOURCE: National Cancer Institute Workshop.[194]

Current controversies regarding cytologic and histologic classification of cervical epithelial pathology

It is well recognized that current schemes for histologic and cytologic classification of cervical, vulvar, and vaginal abnormalities have serious theoretical and practical shortcomings including poor intra- and interpathologist reproducibility and an inability to accurately predict risk of development of CIS and ICC. There have been several unsuccessful attempts to address poor interpathologist reproducibility for classification of specific grades of CIN. First the distinction between CIN 3 and CIS was abolished.[27–29] As noted above, the Bethesda cytologic classification system merges HPV related changes, i.e., koilocytosis and mild dysplasia (corresponding to a histologic diagnosis of CIN 1) into one category designated low-grade SIL and places moderate and severe dysplasia together into another category designated high-grade SIL.[30] These recommendations have generated a good deal of controversy, especially in regard to the lack of separation of HPV infection from mild dysplasia. This is despite the fact that with sensitive detection methods most mild dysplasia or CIN 1 is associated with HPV, and despite the low reproducibility for the morphologic distinction between koilocytosis and CIN 1. Another shortcoming of the current classification systems is that cytologic and histologic diagnoses do not very precisely assign risk of malignancy. In classifying lesions which have a high rate of regression as "neoplastic," the CIN terminology encourages aggressive treatment of women with such changes. The Bethesda System's use of the term squamous intraepithelial lesion as opposed to squamous intraepithelial neoplasia appears to be more appropriate terminology in light of the low malignant potential of most CIN 1 lesions. Furthermore, as we learn more about the clinical and microscopic manifestations of HPV infection and its role in the pathogenesis of cancer, it is no longer clear that CIN 1, 2, and 3 really do represent successive stages of one disease process. It now appears that CIN 1, CIN 2, and CIN 3 frequently are established concomitantly and early but differ with respect to when they are likely to be detected by cytology. CIN 3 may not always arise from slow progression from CIN 1, but may be a relatively common and early consequence of infection with high-risk types of HPV.[31] In summary, recent insights concerning the role of HPV in cervical cancer and in precancer lesions have thrown into doubt assumptions concerning the pathogenesis of cervical cancer inherent in our current histologic (and corresponding cytologic) classification systems.

INCIDENCE AND PREVALENCE

INVASIVE CERVICAL CANCER

International trends

Carcinoma of the uterine cervix is the second most common cancer in the world among women, and the most common cancer in many developing countries of Africa, South and Central America, Asia, and the Pacific, with crude incidence rates ranging from 4 cases per 100,000 in western Asia to 33 per 100,000 in the East Asian regions of Hong Kong, Korea, and Mongolia.[6] In 1980 it was estimated that there were 465,600 new cases of cervical cancer detected worldwide, making it the fifth most common cancer among both sexes, preceded only by cancers of the stomach, lung, breast, and colon or rectum. Fig. 59-2 shows the incidence of cervical and penile cancer estimated from data collected from tumor registries that were maintained in several countries in the years 1968–1971 and 1977–1982.[7,32] The incidence of cervical cancer declined in all of the areas shown except Recife, Brazil, whereas the incidence of penile cancer increased slightly in most areas between the two periods studied. There is a statistically significant positive correlation between the country-specific rates of cervical and penile carcinoma for these data.

U.S. trends

Data on the incidence, mortality, and survival rates of invasive cancer in the United States come from the Surveillance, Epidemiology, and End Results (SEER) Program, the part of the Surveil-

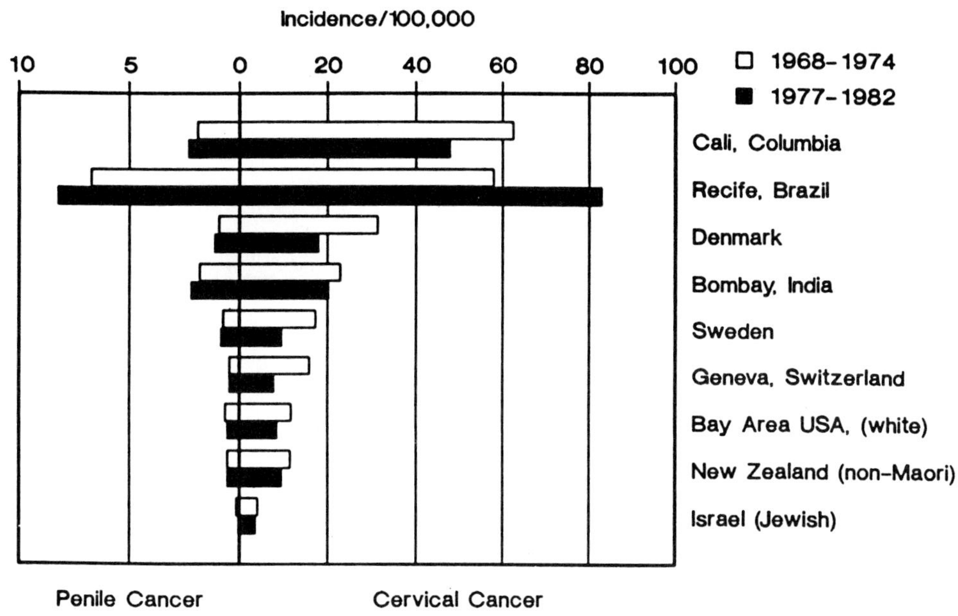

Fig. 59-2. Age-adjusted sex-specific incidence of invasive cancer of the cervix and penis in countries with established tumor registries during the years 1968–1974 and 1977–1982.

lance Program at the National Cancer Institute (NCI) that routinely collects cancer data from nine population-based cancer registries located throughout the United States. The National Center for Health Statistics (NCHS) provides cancer mortality data for the entire United States. The SEER data presented below are calculated for women only and are age-adjusted to the 1970 U.S. standard million.

From 1950 to 1991 the incidence of cervical cancer in the United States declined 76.6% among white women, with an estimated annual percent change of −3.3. From 1973 to 1992 mortality from cervical cancer declined by 43.0% among whites and 46.9% among blacks, with the estimated annual percent change in incidence of cervical cancer being −3.4 among black women, compared to −3.0 among whites. The 5-year relative survival among white women has increased from 59% (1950–1954) to 71.1% (1986–1991); among black women it has increased from 47% (1960–1963) to 56.2% (1986–1991).[5] The development and implementation of Pap smear screening for early detection of precancerous cervical lesions in the 1950s has generally been credited with a major portion of the dramatic decline in incidence and mortality.

Recently there has been a suggestion in countries such as England and Wales, where Pap smears have been used at less frequent intervals or where screening has focused on older women than in the United States, that the incidence and death rate for ICC may have increased among young women less than 35 years of age.[34–36] Similarly, in Canada, Australia, and New Zealand the incidence of ICC for younger women (40 years of age and younger) appears to have increased slightly during the 1970s.[37–40] Whether the slight increase in invasive cervical cancer incidence in American women (and particularly white women less than fifty years of age) noted for the 1986–1990 time interval is an indication of a true change or of statistical fluctuation is not yet known, but it might reflect an increase in oncogenic HPV infection among younger white women initiating sexual activity at earlier ages.[41] The changes in incidence of cancers of the cervix, vagina, vulva, penis, and anus since 1969 are shown in Table 59-4. While rates of cervical cancer have generally declined, the incidence of carcinomas at these other genital and anal sites has remained relatively low and steady over the past two decades, at least five times lower than the rates of cervical cancer, despite the fact that there is no routine screening for such lesions.[42,43] Thus, the combined incidence of cancers of the vagina, vulva, penis and anus equaled 26.3% of the incidence of cervical cancer in 1969–1971, increasing to 54% in 1986–1990.

In 1995 there were an estimated 15,800 new cases and 4,800 actual deaths from invasive cervical cancer in the United States. The U.S. mortality rate (1988–1992) for cervical cancer was 3.0 per 100,000, and for women diagnosed between 1983 and 1989, the 5-year relative survival rate was 66.8%. With an incidence of

Table 59-4. Age-Adjusted Genital and Anal Cancer Incidence for 1969–1971, 1973–1977, 1981–1985, and 1986–1990, All Races; SEER Programs, USA

	1969–1971 incidence per 100,000		1973–1977 incidence per 100,000		1981–1985 incidence per 100,000		1986–1990 incidence per 100,000	
	Females	Males	Females	Males	Females	Males	Females	Males
Cervix	16.7		12.4		8.0		8.7	
Vagina	0.6		0.7		0.7		0.6	
Vulva	1.8		1.6		1.5		1.7	
Penis		1.0		0.9		0.8		0.7
Anus	0.6	0.4	0.7	0.5	0.9	0.7	0.9	0.8

SOURCE: Krone MR et al.[48]

8.6 cases per 100,000 during 1988–1992, cancer of the cervix uteri was the third most common female genital tract malignancy, following cancers of the corpus uteri (20.9 per 100,00) and ovary (15.1 per 100,000). In comparison, the incidence of breast cancer among women was considerably higher (109.6 per 100,000). The incidence of cervical cancer declined during the 1973–92 period by 38.1% cancer of the corpus uteri declined by 27.6%, but the incidence of breast and ovarian cancer rose 25.3% and 4% respectively.[5]

Although carcinomas of the cervix, penis, vagina, vulva, and anus are morphologically similar and are felt to share a common sexually transmitted etiology,[27] the incidence of cervical cancer is from 5 to 50 times higher than most other squamous cell cancers of the genital tract. The exception is anal cancer among homosexual men. While anal cancer was rare among the general population even prior to the advent of HIV, the incidence of anal cancer among homosexual men at that time approached that of cervical cancer prior to Pap screening.[33] In 1980 Daling estimated the incidence of anal cancer among never-married men to be approximately 36/100,000.[33] Why cervical cancer and anal cancer in homosexual men are so much more common than the other HPV-related genital tract cancers is unclear. Interestingly, however, both of these types of cancer arise in areas where HPV commonly infects metaplastic epithelium. Metaplasia is the process by which much of the mucus-secreting columnar epithelium present on the portion of the ectocervix at birth is replaced by stratified squamous epithelium. As shown in Fig. 59-3, the surface epithelium of the endocervix and ectocervix undergoes dramatic changes (squamous metaplasia) throughout a woman's lifetime, presumably as a result of hormonal and physical influences as well as infection with various agents, including HPV. As this change occurs, the point at which the squamous epithelium abuts columnar epithelium (termed the squamocolumnar junction) progressively recedes up into the endocervical canal. The area of the cervix where the native mucus-secreting columnar epithelium has been replaced by squamous epithelium is termed the transformation zone, and it is within this area of metaplastic epithelium that most cervical pathology, including early cancer, occurs. A similar zone of active epithelial metaplasia is apparently present in the anal canal in the presence of HPV infection.

Age-specific rates

Among all races, the median age of diagnosis for carcinoma of the cervix is 48 years, about 20 years younger than the median age of diagnosis of carcinoma of the vagina (67 years), vulva (70 years), anus (females, 66 years; males, 63 years), and penis (66 years). As shown in Fig. 59-4, the incidence of all genital tract and anal cancers increases with age. The incidence of invasive cervical cancer increases with age, rising sharply to 15 per 100,000 between the ages of 20 and 35 years (premenopausal years), then fluctuating around 15–20 cases per 100,000 through the ninth decade of life. The age-specific incidence for other HPV-associated genital tract and anal cancers increases much more slowly and remains relatively low throughout life, except that of vulvar cancer, which increases sharply among women sixty years of age or older, up to about 20 cases per 100,000.

Ethnic comparisons

For all genital tract cancers except cancer of the vulva, the incidence is higher and five-year survival rate lower among African Americans than among whites. Overall in 1992, the incidence of carcinoma of the cervix was about 40% higher for black women than for white women (11 as compared to 7.8 per 100,000 for black and white women respectively). The disparity in cervical cancer incidence between white and black women is greatest among those over 50 years of age.

Mortality rates for HPV-related genital tract cancers have also remained considerably higher among African-Americans of all ages since the early 1970s. This may be related to the fact that while among whites, 51% of cervical tumors were localized at the time of diagnosis, among African Americans only 36% of tumors were detected without distinct spread or metastases at the time of diagnosis, with most cervical cancers (41%) already showing regional spread at diagnosis.[44] These racial differences in age and stage of cancer diagnosis may be related to varying access to and utilization of screening and treatment. However, the fact that survival is better for white women than for black women for each diagnostic stage of cancer suggests other factors are also of importance. Regardless of race, women among lower socioeconomic groups (lower income and education level), who until recently have had less access to Pap screening and gynecological services, have a higher risk of cervical cancer.[44,45]

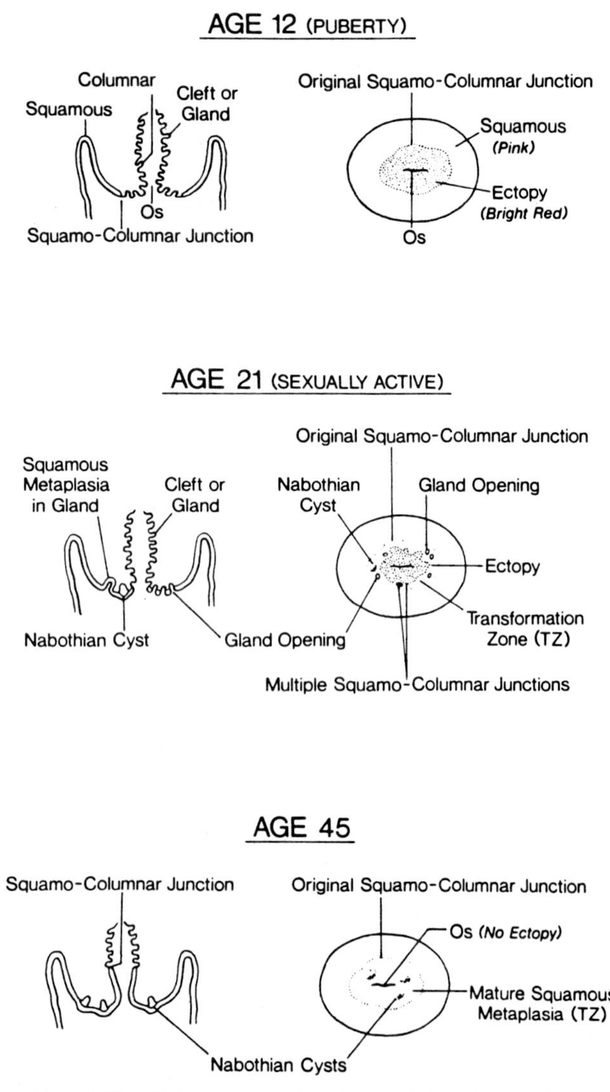

Fig. 59-3. These diagrams show the change in location of the squamo-columnar junction on the uterine cervix from menarche (12 years) through initiation of sexual activity (21 years) and menopause (45 years).

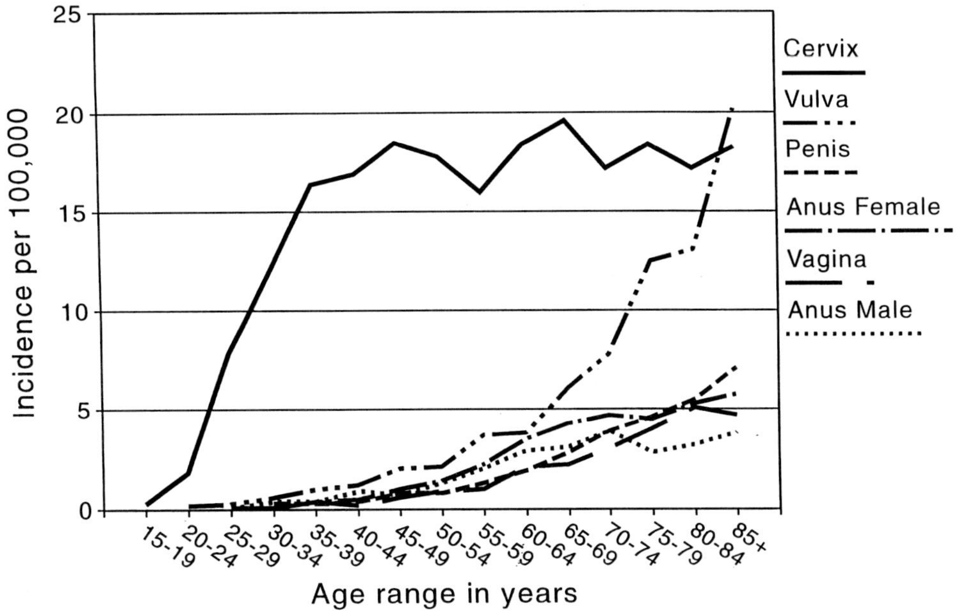

Fig. 59-4. Age- and sex-specific incidence of invasive cancers of the cervix, vulva, penis, anus, and vagina in the United States: Data from the SEER Program, 1986–1990. (*From Krone MR et al*[48].)

CERVICAL CARCINOMA IN SITU

Washington State's SEER Program has collected population-based data on the incidence of cervical carcinoma in situ (CIS) and invasive cervical cancer since the mid-1970s. As expected, the incidence of cervical carcinoma in situ is much higher than the incidence of invasive cervical cancer through the fourth decade of life. The age-adjusted rates of invasive cervical cancer and cervical carcinoma in situ were 7.9 and 62.4 per 100,000, respectively,[46] between 1987 and 1991 in the state of Washington. CIS has a younger age distribution, with incidence rates about thirty to over one hundred times higher than rates for invasive cervical cancer among adolescent and young adult females. The 1979–1981 and 1989–1991 incidence rates of histologically confirmed cases of CIS among women for the most populous county in Washington state, King County, are shown in Fig. 59-5. Interestingly, comparison of the age-specific incidence of CIS for 1979–1981 and 1989–1991 shows that there was a statistically significant increase in this diagnosis among young women 15 to 19 years of age between these two times. This increase is not likely to be completely related to changes in the classification of Pap smear findings which took place during this time. That the incidence of CIS might increase during this period is perhaps not surprising, given that current literature indicates an increase in sexual activity among young women in recent years.[47] This increased activity was accompanied by a marked increase in other STDs during and preceding this period.[48]

The true incidence of CIS for the youngest and older women is probably somewhat higher than is seen in Fig. 59-5, since the denominator in this figure includes women who, by virtue of never having had a Pap smear and/or of having had a hysterectomy, could not have had a diagnosis of cervical CIS. Using data from the Centers for Disease Control (CDC) Behavioral Risk Factor Survey[49] for Washington State, Fig. 59-6 presents the age specific CIS incidence rates for the 1989–1991 period adjusted for age-specific Pap smear and hysterectomy rates. Interestingly, for the years 1989 to 1991, the adjusted incidence rate for women 18 to 24 years of age (196 per 100,000) approximated the adjusted rate observed for women 25 to 34 years of age (212 per 100,000). This has important implications both for cervical cancer control strategies and, as discussed below, for modeling the relationship of HPV infection, CIN 1, CIS, and invasive cancer.

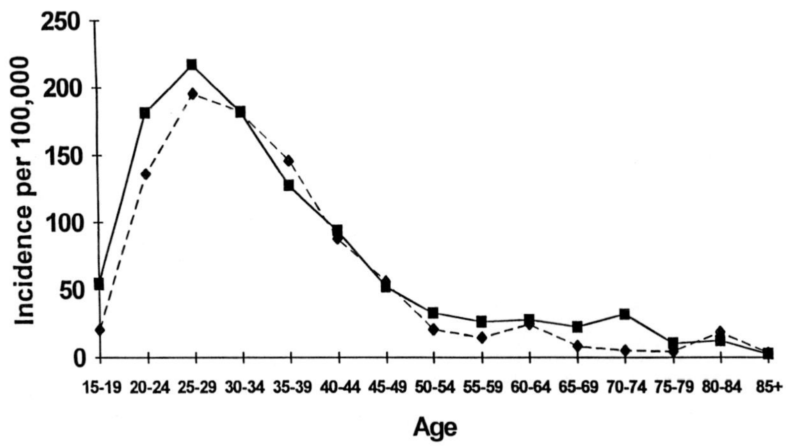

Fig. 59-5. Age-specific incidence of cervical carcinoma-in-situ, King County, Washington state. Solid line represents rates for 1989–1991; dashed line represents 1979–1981. (*From Krone MR et al*[48].)

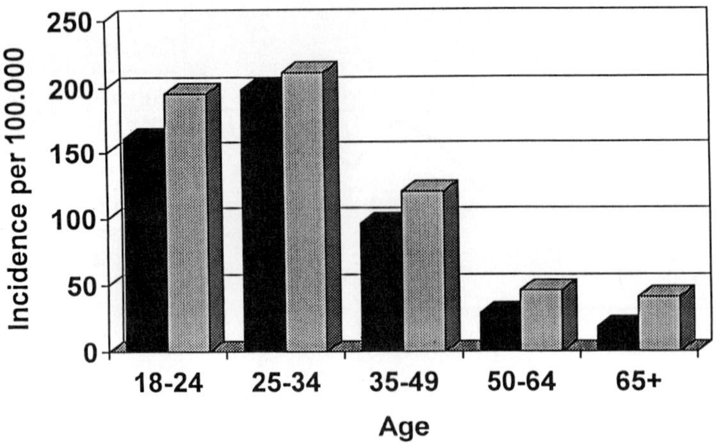

Fig. 59-6. Age-specific incidence of cervical carcinoma-in-situ, King County WA, 1989–1991. Solid bars represent unadjusted rates; shaded bars represent rates adjusted for Pap smear and hysterectomy. (*From Krone MR et al*[48].)

There are no good data on the prevalence of intraepithelial neoplasia or CIS of the vagina, vulva, anus, or penis in the general population, but it is thought that the prevalence of these lesions is much lower than for cervical neoplasia. VAIN 2–3 in the upper vagina usually represents a distal extension of CIN.[50,51,52] Since vaginal cancer is so uncommon until the seventh decade of life, screening for vaginal cancer has not received the same degree of emphasis as screening for cervical neoplasms; however, during the 1970s, concomitantly with the increasing interest in vulvar and vaginal HPV infections, the prevalence of VIN lesions reportedly increased.[18,52,53]

PREVALENCE OF CERVICAL INTRAEPITHELIAL NEOPLASIA (CIN)

Industrialized countries, including the United States, have had widespread Pap smear screening programs for over 25 years. However, interpretation and reporting of cytologic findings have never been well standardized, and even when pathologists use the same classification system it is difficult for their findings to be reproducible; thus, it is nearly impossible to compare results from different countries, laboratories, and time periods.[30] For example, during the early to mid-1980s, the prevalence of dysplasia in two similar STD clinics (Denver and Seattle) was 1.72% and 13.66%, respectively. The reported prevalence of cytologic changes consistent with CIN ranges from 0.43% to 24%, depending on the population studied and reporting system used, with most gynecology clinic populations reporting annual prevalences for CIN of about 2%[42,43] and with the highest prevalence reported for clinics serving sexually active females between the ages of 18 and 35 years. Hopefully, the recent adoption of the Bethesda classification system by many pathology laboratories will improve the interlaboratory correlation. As discussed below, standardization based on correlating the detection of HPV DNA with the detection of intraepithelial lesions may also prove useful.

ETIOLOGY

HISTORICAL OVERVIEW: EPIDEMIOLOGICAL DATA SUGGESTING THAT CERVICAL CANCER IS AN STD

The association between cervical cancer and sexual activity was noted as early as 1842, when Rigoni-Stern reported that cancer of the uterus (site unspecified) occurred less frequently among cloistered nuns than among married women.[54] Since this initial report, other studies have confirmed the association between various measures of sexual exposure and development of squamous cell neoplasms of the cervix,[55] anus,[56] and vulva.[57] Since 1950, at least three studies have documented a low incidence of mortality from cervical cancer among nuns.[58–60] In contrast, subsequent wives of husbands whose previous wife had cervical cancer have increased risk.[61] In most studies, total number of sex partners is strongly associated with risk of cervical neoplasia.[62,63] In 1981, Buckley et al. reported that among women reporting only one lifetime sex partner, those whose husbands reported six or more sex partners, appeared to have approximately a fourfold higher risk for cervical neoplasia than women whose husbands reported having had fewer than six partners.[64] Zunzunegui showed that among South American women residing in California, the total number of sex partners of the husband was highly associated with occurrence of ICC in the wife, whereas the woman's sex partner history was not.[65] Martinez, Graham, and Smith et al. have reported an increased occurrence of cervical cancer in partners of men with penile carcinoma.[66–68] Increased numbers of sex partners has also been associated with carcinoma of the anus.[56]

The epidemiologic evidence correlating sexual behavior with CIN and ICC as well as with cancers of the penis and anus[56,63,69,70] led to an extensive search for specific STD agents acting as carcinogens in genital and anal cancers. During the last 50 years attention has shifted from one organism to another about every ten years, from syphilis in the 1940s[71,72] to gonorrhea[73–76] and trichomoniasis.[77–81] Other pathogens implicated in one or more studies include mycoplasmas, *Gardnerella vaginalis,* cytomegalovirus,[82–88] and Epstein-Barr virus.[89–94] The relationship of other sexually transmitted bacterial, chlamydial,[95–100] protozoan, and fungal infections to genital tract neoplasia has also been evaluated, and although it is now clear that they are not independent causes of genital and anal cancers, their capacity to induce chronic inflammation or to produce mutagenic metabolites[101] may increase the risk of genital and/or anal carcinogenesis.

During the 1970s and early 1980s there was considerable interest in HSV 2 and cervical cancer.[63,102,103] The major problem in most seroepidemiologic studies linking cervical cancer to various STDs, including HSV, has been lack of careful matching of cases and controls for potential confounding factors, most importantly sexual behavior. With HSV 2 there was the additional difficulty in seroepidemiologic studies of discriminating between serum antibody responses to HSV 1 and HSV 2.[104–109] Recent epidemiologic and laboratory-based studies suggest that once HPV is taken into account, there is little evidence for an important role for HSV in the pathogenesis of cervical cancer.[110,111] However, a possible involvement in HSV 2 at some level in the causal pathway in some cases has not been ruled out.[112]

HPV TYPE AND GENITAL TRACT CANCERS

HPVs are classified into types, subtypes, or variants, based on DNA homology.[113–116] Clinical epidemiologic studies undertaken over the last 10 years have strongly supported the central role for specific types of HPV in the pathogenesis of squamous cell cancers of the genital tract. In addition, as discussed in Chapters 37 and 38, the molecular and biochemical evidence supporting a link between specific types of HPV and cancers of the genital tract and anus are quite strong. The genital HPVs are commonly referred to as high-risk or low-risk depending on their association with cancers. Oncogenic HPVs (i.e., high-risk HPVs) include 16, 18, 26, 31, 33, 35, 39, 45, 51, 54, 55, 58, 59, 64, and 68. The most common high-risk types include HPV types 16, 18, 45, and 56. HPV 6, 11, 42, 43, and 44 are considered to be low-risk, as they are almost never associated with invasive cancers.[117] Initially, due to differences in the populations studied, the type of material tested (fixed versus fresh, swabs versus biopsy), and most importantly, the variability of early methods of detecting HPV (with regards to sensitivity, specificity, and reproducibility), the early epidemiological studies of HPV and genital tract cancer showed a highly variable association between HPV and cancer. However, with the accurate PCR-based methodologies, numerous case control studies over the last decade have convincingly demonstrated that specific HPV types are the causal agent of most genital tract cancers. Using multiple probes for HPV, the prevalence of HPV DNA in invasive cervical squamous cell cancers has generally exceeded 75%,[118] with lower rates reported for adenocarcinomas and adenosquamous carcinomas. HPV 16 is the most frequent type of HPV detected in invasive squamous cell cancers of the cervix in most countries, with HPV 18 also frequent in adenocarcinomas.[118] Bosch et al. recently examined over 1000 cases of invasive cervical cancers from 22 countries from around the world for HPV DNA by PCR, using the L1 consensus primer and 26 type specific probes. Over 93% of cancers in this series were positive for HPV DNA (Table 59-5).[119] Cases were assayed for HPV DNA by PCR. No significant regional differences in the prevalence of specific types were noted. HPV DNA types 16, 45, and 18 were detected in 50%, 8%, and 14% of cases, respectively, with type 16 predominating in all countries except Indonesia and Algeria, where type 18 was more frequently detected. A number of case-control studies examining the association between specific HPV types and ICC have been performed, with most studies reporting relative risks for the association of HPV DNA and invasive cervical cancer ranging from about 10 to over 40 for the most recent PCR-based studies.[118,120] The HPV 16 link with cervical cancer does not appear to be a uniquely recent phenomenon, as Collins et al. showed that HPV 16 DNA could be detected from a similar proportion of cervical cancer specimens sampled in each decade beginning in 1932, the first year that stored specimens were available.[121]

Several cohort studies have examined the risk of development of CIN 2–3 in relationship to HPV type.[56] Lorincz et al. reported that 3 (15%) of 20 HPV positive women (tested by low-stringency Southern blot probed for 15 types of HPV), developed cervical or vaginal CIN, as compared to 9 (5%) of 195 who were HPV negative at study entry.[122] A high percentage of the women who developed CIN had a prior history of CIN. We enrolled and followed 241 randomly selected women presenting to an STD clinic who had no history of CIN and who were cytologically negative at study entry. Women were examined for the presence of HPV DNA (for HPV 6, 11, 31, 33, 35, 16, and 18 by Southern or dot blot hybridization), and for cytologic and colposcopic abnormalities, every four months for an average of 25 months until they developed biopsy-confirmed CIN 2–3 or ended follow-up, or until the study ended. Cumulative incidence of biopsy-confirmed CIN 2–3 at two years was 28% for those with HPV detected, as compared to 3% among those without HPV. CIN 2–3 developed in over 36% of those with either HPV 16 or 18 infection. Interestingly, almost all CIN 2–3 developed within the first two

Table 59-5. Prevalence of Individual HPV Types in Invasive Cervical Cancers by Geographical Region

HPV type	Region											
	Africa		Central and South America		Southeast Asia		Europe		North America		Total	
	No.	(%)	No.	(%)	No.	(%)	No.	(%)	No.	(%)	No.	(%)
HPV-16 and related												
HPV-16	79	(42.5)	255	(50.5)	42	(42.9)	56	(65.1)	33	(57.9)	465	(49.9)
HPV-31	5	(2.7)	35	(6.9)	1	(1.0)	5	(5.8)	3	(5.3)	49	(5.3)
HPV-33	5	(2.7)	18	(3.6)	2	(2.0)	1	(1.2)	0		26	(2.8)
HPV-35	4	(2.2)	10	(2.0)	1	(1.0)	1	(1.2)	0		16	(1.7)
HPV-52	4	(2.2)	16	(3.2)	2	(2.0)	3	(3.5)	0		25	(2.7)
HPV-58	5	(2.7)	11	(2.2)	2	(2.0)	1	(1.2)	0		19	(2.0)
HPV-18 and related												
HPV-18	33	(17.7)	48	(9.5)	31	(31.6)	7	(8.1)	9	(15.8)	128	(13.7)
HPV-39	0		13	(2.6)	1	(1.0)	0		0		14	(1.5)
HPV-45	23	(12.4)	37	(7.3)	8	(8.2)	2	(2.3)	8	(14.0)	78	(8.4)
HPV-59	0		14	(2.8)	1	(1.0)	0		0		15	(1.6)
HPV-68	4	(2.2)	2	(0.4)	1	(1.0)	3	(3.5)	1	(1.8)	11	(1.2)
Other												
HPV-6	0		1	(0.2)	0		0		0		1	(0.1)
HPV-11	0		1	(0.2)	0		0		0		1	(0.1)
HPV-56	6	(3.2)	3	(0.6)	3	(3.1)	2	(2.3)	2	(3.5)	16	(1.7)
Miscellaneous	5	(2.7)	16	(3.2)	4	(4.1)	1	(1.2)	0		26	(2.8)
Undetermined	2	(1.1)	8	(1.6)	0		1	(1.2)	1	(1.8)	12	(1.3)
HPV negatives	19	(10.2)	36	(7.1)	3	(3.1)	4	(4.7)	4	(7.0)	66	(7.1)
Total specimens	186		505		98		86		57		932	

SOURCE: Bosch FX et al.[119]

years of follow-up, with the majority developing within the first 6 months. We concluded that CIN 2–3 was an early and relatively common manifestation of HPV infection.[31]

HPV VARIANTS AND NEOPLASIA

Because only a minority of women infected with HPV-16 go on to develop cervical cancer, there is now considerable interest in the idea that different HPV-16 variants might have differing biological behaviors. The first HPV-16 to be cloned was from a cervical cancer removed from a German patient. This HPV is considered the HPV-16 prototype variant and is the variant commonly used in molecular studies of HPV. Comparison of the long control region (LCR) of the prototype HPV-16 genome to the LCR of HPV-16 variants identified in samples from approximately 700 women (most of whom had cancer), from various geographic regions throughout the world, shows the existence of multiple different HPV-16 variants which occur with variable frequency in all populations thus far examined.[123–126] A number of attempts have been made to classify these variants into groups, including assignment to one of five geographically based distinct phylogenetic branches[123,124] and comparison of the sequence of the sample HPV to that of the prototype HPV.[127] Yamada et al. examined invasive cervical cancers from 22 countries and found that 92% belonged to previously reported HPV 16 lineages, with 7.8% of cancers harboring HPV 16 variants with novel hybridization and or nucleotide changes. Most variants from European and North American samples were phylogenetically classified as European prototype (E), while samples from Africa were primarily classified as African.[128] It is possible that differences in certain amino acid sequences might have functional importance for biologic properties related to development of malignancy. Evidence for this has been provided by *in vitro* studies demonstrating that nucleotide alterations in the noncoding region of HPV-16 enhance promoter activity[127,129] or alter oncogenic potential in the presence of *ras* oncogene and hormone.[130] Clinical data suggesting that certain HPV variants may alter risk of clinical disease[129,131–134] include reports of an association between an HPV-16 variant with a base pair change at nucleotide 350 and persistence of detection of HPV DNA,[130] and existence of an HPV-18 subtype with apparently decreased oncogenic potential.[132] In addition, we have reported that HIV-seronegative women in Seattle infected with certain nonprototypelike (NPL) variants of HPV-16, as compared to prototypelike (PL) variants, were at greater risk of development of CIN 2–3 (Table 59-6).[127] It is possible that the oncogenic potential of HPV variants may vary in different populations if certain amino acid changes present in certain HPV-16 variants, in association with specific host HLA haplotypes, influence the host immune response to different HPV types or variants.[133] Presently, few data exist concerning the frequency of different HPV-16 variants in women with and without ICC and CIN 2–3. A recent study has evaluated HPV-16 variants in a large series of invasive cancers from around the world (N = 408), but it did not compare the prevalence of variants present in women with ICC to the prevalence of these variants in comparable women without ICC.[125] Hence, the risk for ICC associated with these variants in the geographical locations from which samples were obtained is unknown.

OTHER RISK FACTORS

Since only a subset of the many women infected with high risk types of HPV ever develop cervical cancer, there is a good deal of interest in identifying other factors (cofactors) that might act in conjunction with HPV to increase risk of development of cancer.

Measures of sexual behavior, hormone and contraceptive use, smoking, and diet

After adjusting for HPV, the association with cervical cancer with many of the traditional risk factors, such as number of sex partners, early age of first intercourse, parity, or other infectious agents, disappears or is greatly reduced. Likewise, while several case control studies during the 1980s linked current cigarette smoking with cancers of the cervix,[62,135–137] vulva,[57] anus,[56] and penis,[138] these studies did not adequately take into account confounding sexual exposures not measured by number of sex partners, or (most importantly) laboratory evidence of HPV infection. In more recent studies in which HPV was taken into account,[139,140] there was little support for smoking as a major risk factor for cervical cancer. Nonetheless, there is evidence that cervical mucus from cigarette smokers is more likely than mucus from nonsmokers to be mutagenic[141] and that cigarette smokers have a reduced Langerhans cell population in the cervix, suggesting the possibility of a local immunologic effect of smoking on cervical epithelium infected with HPV.[142] As regards oral contraceptives, conflicting results were obtained from earlier studies[143–148] where HPV was not assessed. At least two studies in which HPV was taken into account have found an association between oral contraceptive use and cervical cancer. Although these studies are not conclusive, there appears to be a slightly increased risk for cervical cancer associated with use, particularly long term use, of oral contraceptives.[148] Once the presence of HPV is taken into account, the role of other hormonal contraceptives[149–151] and of dietary factors is unclear.

Table 59-6. Risk for Biopsy-confirmed Cervical Intraepithelial Neoplasia (CIN) Grade 2-3 Associated with HPV16 Variants among University Students and among STD Clinic Patients

Cohorts	HPV 16 variant group*	No. (%) of CIN 2-3	No. of subjects	RR**	95% CI
University students	PL	4 (8.9)	45	1.0	
	NPL	5 (41.7)	12	6.5	1.6–27.2
STD clinic patients	PL	7 (12.3)	57	1.0	
	NPL	3 (33.3)	9	4.5	0.9–23.8

* PL = Prototypelike, NPL = nonprototypelike

** RR estimates adjusted for age (≤20, ≥21 years), lifetime number of sexual partners (≤5, ≥6 partners), HPV16 status at entry (positive, negative), ethnic group (white, nonwhite), and number of visits positive for HPV16 (1–3, ≥4 visits)

† 95% confidence interval

SOURCE: XI LF et al.[127]

Immunosuppression, including HIV infection

The importance of immune surveillance for prevention of HPV-associated neoplasia of both the skin and genital tract has been well documented.[152–154] For example, patients with a rare genetic defect of cell mediated immunity, epidermodysplasia verruciformis, have been particularly prone to developing multiple common skin warts, with up to one-third of these individuals going on to develop skin cancers at the site of such lesions.[155] Renal transplant patients also have increased risk for various manifestations of HPV infection, including genital warts and cervical neoplasia.[156,154] Patients with either iatrogenic or congenital immunosuppression have been 14 to 100 times more likely than those with a normal immune system to develop carcinoma in situ, the lesion most likely to progress to invasive disease.[157] Several investigators have also suggested, without adequate substantiation, that squamous cell cancers of the cervix in immunosuppressed women differ from those in nonimmunosuppressed women with respect to the types of HPV detected and to their natural history. For example, in immunosuppressed women squamous cell cancers are more often found with similar tumors at other genital sites and occur at a younger mean age, in comparison with such cancers in immunocompetent women.[157]

Women with HIV infection appear to be at increased risk for HPV and CIN. Odds ratios for the association between HIV and CIN have ranged from 1.0 to 14.7.[158–164] Detection of HPV, as well as the frequency of detecting CIN, increases with worsening immunosuppression.[164] Most of the studies of HIV and CIN report primarily on women with CIN 1, and CIN 2 with a minority of women in these studies having CIN 3/CIS. In immunocompetent women, CIN 1 has little malignant potential. If the effect of HIV is simply to increase expression of HPV, then the association between CIN and HIV does not constitute proof that HIV infection increases risk of invasive cervical cancer. Even though invasive cervical cancer has been added to the list of AIDS-defining illnesses, to date no population-based data from the United States or other countries support an association between HIV and invasive cervical cancer. Published data supporting such an association are currently limited to isolated case reports and small case series.[165–168] Indirect evidence supporting an association between HIV and invasive cervical cancer comes from reports and studies of invasive anal cancer in homosexually active, HIV-positive men. Recently, using a linkage between an AIDS database (Center for Disease Control HIV/AIDS Reporting System) and cancer registries from the same geographic locations, Melbye and colleagues[169] compared the number of expected cases of anal epidermoid cancer (based on general population rates) to the number of observed cases of epidermoid anal cancers, at and after the diagnosis of AIDS. By using this approach they found a significantly increased risk of anal cancer among patients with AIDS. However, when a similar approach was used to assess the association between cervical cancer and HIV infection there was only a small increase in the number of observed as compared to expected cases of invasive cervical cancer among women with AIDS. In addition, a study among 200 Kenyan women (mean age, 42 years) presenting with cervical cancer found an HIV seroprevalence of only 1.5%, an estimate that was comparable to the seroprevalence of 2% for the population from which the cases were detected.[170]

If HIV does increase the risk of cervical cancer in developing countries, our current inability to demonstrate an increased risk could reflect the fact that HIV infected women in these countries are dying of other opportunistic diseases before their cervical cancer develops or is detected. In the United States, where HIV infection has been introduced into the female population only relatively recently, and where most women have access to Pap screening and to diagnostic and treatment services for preinvasive lesions, it is perhaps not surprising that an association between HIV and invasive cervical cancer has not yet been detected.

Association between HLA haplotype and risk of HPV-related cancer

A number of recent studies have found associations between HLA class and HPV related neoplasia.[171–179] Apple et al. examined HLA class II haplotypes in relationship to both invasive cervical cancer and preinvasive lesions. DR-DQ haplotypes were associated with HPV-16-positive invasive cancers and CIS but not with mild or moderate dysplasia. Odunsi and colleagues reported that susceptibility for cancer and CIN was associated with DQB1*03, DQB1*04, and DRB1*11.[178] Specific HLA class-II alleles have also been associated with protection from cancer. Sastre reported on the possible protective effect of DR13,[179] and the DQA1-DQB1 haplotype was negatively associated with CIS but not with invasive cancer in the Apple study.[172]

INTEGRATING KNOWLEDGE OF THE BIOLOGY OF HPV INTO CLASSIFICATION OF CERVICAL PATHOLOGY

As the importance of HPV infection in development of benign and malignant cervical pathology has become clear, a number of attempts to update our current classification systems have taken HPV into account. For example, as it has become apparent that the morphologic changes classified as koilocytotic atypia and CIN 1 are most often associated with transient HPV infection, many pathologists have attempted to classify cervical lesions as either *condyloma* (regarded as being without malignant potential) or CIN (felt to be cancer precursors). Since it is now evident that specific types of HPV are associated with risk of cancer, it was proposed that morphology was associated with the type (high versus low risk type) of HPV that was present. However, while it is true that most CIN 3 lesions and a high percentage of CIN 2 lesions contain high-risk HPV types (primarily types 16 or 18), both high- and low-risk HPV types have been observed in low-grade lesions, with no recognizable difference in morphology.

Our current understanding of cancer and HPV has led to a fundamental rethinking of the relationship between CIN 1, CIN 2, CIN 3/CIS and ICC. Studies of the relationship between HPV infection and CIN show that detection of incident HPV DNA is followed within a relatively short period by development of CIN; and (as summarized above) cohort studies of initially cytologically negative subjects have suggested that high-grade intraepithelial neoplasia (CIN 3 and AIN 3) may be an early and quite common manifestation of HPV 16 infection. This raises questions as to the utility of a CIN 1 diagnosis as a marker for detection of women at risk for CIN 2–3. In our study summarized above, most CIN 2–3 was diagnosed within 6 months after detection of high-risk types of HPV.[31] Furthermore, detection of high risk types of HPV DNA was a better predictor of development of CIN 2–3 than was detection of CIN 1, and many of the women who developed CIN 2–3 never had evidence of a preceding CIN 1. Cuzick recently reported finding a high rate of biopsy proven CIN 2–3 among cytologically negative women who were without a previous history of CIN 1 and who had been referred for biopsy on the basis of a positive test for detection of high-risk types of HPV DNA.[180] It appears likely that at least some CIN 2–3 do not evolve from CIN 1, but are established de novo as CIN 2–3. The alternative dogma that CIN 3 lesions evolve slowly from preexisting CIN 1 has been supported by the observation that young women who develop CIN 1 appear more likely than those without CIN

1 to develop cervical cancer later in life.[181–183] On the other hand, numerous studies have documented that CIS does arise in women with previously negative smears. Such cases have been explained away as the result of sampling error, suboptimal Pap smears due to inflammation or blood, misinterpretation of cytologic findings, or rapid progression of LGSIL to HGSIL.[184,185] However, CIN 1 and CIN 3 may simply be distinct manifestations of infection with different types of HPV. These may have distinct natural histories, but these differences could be obscured if they are acquired concomitantly or sequentially.

That both lesions might be frequently seen in the same women would not be surprising, since both lesions are related to HPV and some women experience multiple HPV infections. Thus, just as CIN occurs more frequently in women with than without a history of vulvar warts, CIN 3 might be expected to occur more frequently among those with than without other manifestations of HPV infection. It is also possible that CIN 1 and CIN 2–3 are separate but concurrently established lesions which differ in their likelihood of detection by cytology, because of either their location or their growth characteristics. If this were the case, these lesions might be detected at different times. Support for this idea comes from studies which demonstrate that low-grade cervical dysplasia generally occurs distal to CIS.[186] Low-grade lesions may therefore be more accessible than high-grade lesions to sampling and colposcopic identification. Although CIN 2–3 lesions appear to be morphologically homogeneous, it is possible that they vary considerably in their malignant potential. Some lesions classified as consistent with CIN 2–3 may simply represent infection of metaplastic epithelium with specific types of HPV and spontaneously resolve, while others may persist and evolve into the true precursors of invasive cancers. These issues need further investigation, since determining whether CIN 1 lesions are simply markers of exposure to HPV (the etiologic agent of cervical cancer), or are truly cervical cancer precursor lesions, would influence our approach to cervical cancer control and allow us to devise appropriate clinical management of these lesions.

PRACTICAL ISSUES RELATED TO CERVICAL CANCER SCREENING

SENSITIVITY OF CYTOLOGIC SCREENING FOR DETECTION OF CIS

Our current approach of yearly cytologic screening with referral for colposcopy and biopsy, together with aggressive treatment of women with abnormal biopsies, has proved very effective for decreasing cervical cancer mortality. This despite the fact that identification of women with CIN 2–3 by detection of cytologic abnormalities appears only moderately sensitive and relatively nonspecific. False-negative smears have reportedly ranged from 1.1% to 62.5%.[187,188] In a recent study of women from a general screening population referred for colposcopy and biopsy on the basis of an abnormal cytologic smear or detection of HPV 16, 18, 31 or 33 DNA in cervical specimens, only 27 (33%) of 81 women who had CIN 2–3 on biopsy had HGSIL on Pap smear; 18 (22%) of the 81 had "borderline" changes (roughly the equivalent of ASCUS) or LGSIL on Pap smear, while 33 (41%) had a completely negative Pap smear and 3 smears were unsatisfactory.[180] Thus, the sensitivity and positive predictive value of any abnormal cytologic finding for biopsy confirmed CIN 2–3 were 56% and 35%, respectively. This low sensitivity for detection of CIN 2–3, along with the rising cost of traditional cytology-based cervical cancer control (due primarily to the increasing numbers of women with ASCUS and LGSIL being referred for further evaluation and testing), has raised interest in a number of new approaches to cervical cancer control. These include redesigning cytology-based screening strategies, in terms of screening interval and improving the sensitivity of cytology for detection of CIS, and instituting a more conservative (less aggressive) approach to the clinical management of ASCUS and CIN 1. New systems for preparation of monolayer slides and automated review systems for quality assurance (and potentially for primary screening) have become available over the last several years, and although it is not yet clear whether they are useful, it is likely that such technologies will become increasingly routine in cytology laboratories in the United States, in part because of the growing number of malpractice suits. Furthermore, given the importance of HPV in cancer, there has been growing interest in detection of HPV DNA as a basis for screening or for management of women with abnormal Pap smears.

SCREENING INTERVAL

In the United States, cervical cancer control involves yearly screening, commencing after the onset of sexual activity and continuing for life. Pap smears are performed every 3 years in Canada and every 5 years in Finland. Decreasing the screening interval to 1–3 years further decreases mortality only marginally. Thus, screening less frequently may be more cost-effective. In developing countries the invasive cervical cancer rate has reportedly decreased by 25% with a single screening between ages 40 and 50.[189]

COLLECTION OF SPECIMENS

Many studies have shown that false-negative cytologies frequently result from inadequate sampling in collection of specimens.[190,191] Past improvements to the sensitivity of cytology have been achieved by sampling the endocervical and ectocervical areas rather than the vaginal pool, as was the practice early in cytology,[187,192] and by using a wooden spatula rather than an aspirate.[187] More recently endocervical brushes have afforded better sampling of the squamocolumnar junction. The presence of endocervical cells on a smear increases the likelihood of detecting CIN.[193] For this reason some practitioners regard the presence of endocervical cells as an indication of smear adequacy. Other practitioners, however, claim that the presence of endocervical mucus alone is indicative of an adequate smear.[23] The Bethesda System defines an adequate transformation-zone sample in women of all ages as the presence of two clusters of endocervical or metaplastic squamous cells, with a cluster containing a minimum of 5 cells. Smears without endocervical or metaplastic groups are considered satisfactory for evaluation but limited by the absence of these cellular elements.[194] In addition to collection of endocervical samples, immediate (during the same examination) repeated sampling of the cervix can significantly increase the number of dysplastic cells present.[190]

NEW TECHNOLOGIES FOR PREPARATION AND REVIEW OF CYTOLOGIC SPECIMENS

Several systems have recently been developed for routine collection of exfoliated cervical cells in a liquid transport medium for preparation of monolayer slides for cervical cytology. Studies thus far show a sensitivity of monolayers for detection of cytologic abnormalities no lower than for conventional cytology, with an increase in detection of ASCUS and LGSIL reported in some studies.[195] At least one of these systems has received FDA approval for use in gynecologic cytology (ThinPrep, CYTYC Corporation). Advantages of this approach include the possibility (in most cases) of preparing multiple slides, and potentially the use of part of the liquid for additional assays for HPV or other STDs. Other advantages include elimination of fixation artifact and dense inflammation and blood, and increased visibility of cells.

Several automatic screeners have been developed and have recently received FDA approval in the United States for use in cytologic quality assurance programs (PapNet and Neopath). Potentially both systems could be adapted for primary screening and triage of slides that need attention, although they are not yet approved for such uses.

HPV DNA TESTING

The relatively low sensitivity and specificity of cytology for detection of CIS raise the question of the utility of HPV typing either in primary screening for CIN 2–3, or as an adjunctive test among women referred for abnormal cervical cytology. Cuzick and coworkers[180] reported on women screened by both cytology and HPV DNA testing. Women were referred for colposcopy and biopsy on the basis of either an abnormal cytologic smear or detection of HPV 16, 18, 31 or 33 DNA. The positive predictive value of detection of HPV for CIN 2–3 was 42%, similar to that of a cytologic diagnosis of HGSIL. Several large studies evaluating HPV DNA detection as an adjunctive or primary screening method are now underway. Detection of high-risk HPV DNA in a cervical specimen from women with ASCUS or LGSIL may help to classify patients as either high-risk or low-risk for the development and progression of cervical neoplasia.[196–201]

CYTOLOGY AT OTHER GENITAL TRACT SITES

Sampling of exfoliating cells has also been used for evaluation of other sites, including the vagina, vulva,[202] and anus.[203–207] Anal smears appear important in screening for anal cancer and precancer in homosexual men, a population known to be at high risk for this disease.

MANAGEMENT OF ABNORMAL CERVICAL CYTOLOGY

In recent years the cost and morbidity associated with the detection and treatment of ASCUS and low-grade cervical lesions has escalated, as the number of women reported as having minor smear abnormalities has strikingly increased.[208] A recent study suggests that since the widespread adaptation of the Bethesda System, (85% of laboratories in the United States used this classification system as of 1992), more women are being referred for further workup. It is unclear whether this results from the new classification scheme or from other factors.[26] This increase has occurred without a corresponding increase in HGSIL, perhaps suggesting a change in the diagnostic threshold for such lesions.[209] In any case, the cost-effectiveness (in terms of cancer prevention) of referring women with minor lesions for immediate colposcopy and biopsy has not been established. Given new insights into the role of HPV in cervical pathology, considerable controversy has arisen about the management of cervical cytologic findings of low-grade squamous intraepithelial lesions (LGSIL) or atypical squamous cells of unknown significance (ASCUS). Many experts now favor conservative, nonaggressive management, suggesting that such findings do not require immediate referral for colposcopy. In one study among 500 women who initially had an abnormal smear, 60% regressed after 7 years' median follow-up.[210] Two other large studies have assessed the feasibility of conservative management of CIN 1–2 (mild to moderate cervical dyskaryosis), and similarly found a low incidence of HGSIL (11–14%) during the rigorous cytologic follow-up ranging from 2 to 4.5 years.[211–213] However, the studies concluded that although cytologic surveillance is safe for initial management of mild to moderate cervical dyskaryosis, it may not be an efficient strategy for all women. In a study of 158 women with abnormal smears assigned to conservative management by Pap surveillance for 2 years, only 40 had not defaulted or had normal smears by the end of the 2 years. Among certain groups of women a policy of immediate referral to colposcopy may be the most cost effective strategy. Below, and in Figure 59-7, we summarize the interim guidelines drafted during a recent National Cancer Institute workshop for management of women with abnormal clinical cytology.

NATIONAL CANCER INSTITUTE INTERIM GUIDELINES FOR MANAGEMENT OF WOMEN WITH ABNORMAL CERVICAL CYTOLOGY[214]

ASCUS

Women with abnormal cytologic findings can be followed without colposcopy by repeat Pap smears every 4–6 months for 2 years until there have been 3 consecutive negative smears. If a second

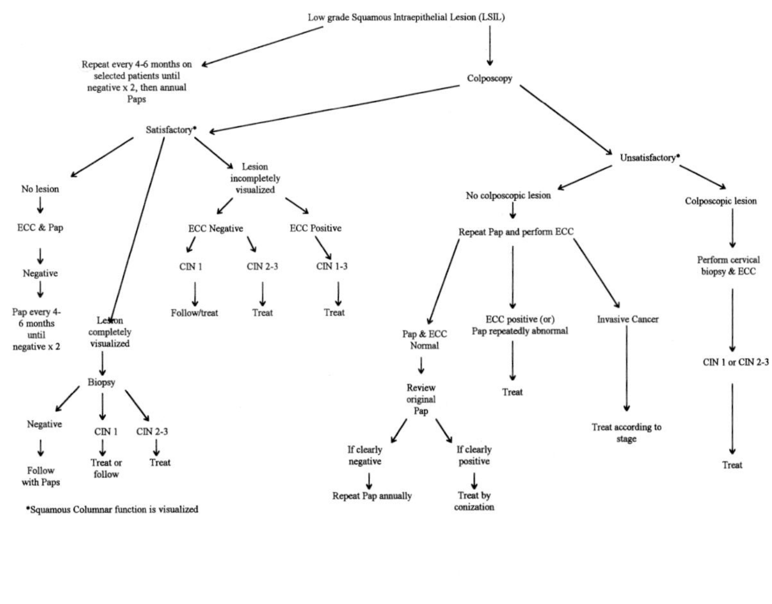

Fig. 59-7. Algorithm for managing Pap smear findings suggestive of a low-grade squamous intraepithelial lesion.

ASCUS report occurs in the 2-year period, the patient should be evaluated by colposcopy and colposcopically directed biopsy. If ASCUS is associated with severe inflammation and a specific diagnosis is established, the patient should be treated. Postmenopausal women with ASCUS should receive a course of topical estrogen therapy, and if the Pap smear is still abnormal after estrogen therapy colposcopy should be considered. For high-risk patients who have a history of abnormal Pap smears, or noncompliant patients likely to be lost to further long-term follow-up with ASCUS, immediate colposcopy should be considered.

Low-grade SIL (LGSIL)

Pap smears every 4–6 months for 2 years are adequate, assuming that the patients are reliable for follow-up. If reliable follow-up is not possible, colposcopy, biopsy, and (if appropriate) endocervical curettage is suggested. Those with persistent abnormalities should be referred for colposcopy and biopsy to obtain a tissue diagnosis. This involves a colposcopically directed loop electrosurgical excision procedure (LEEP) using a small-size loop, but not routine electroexcision of the whole transformation zone (T zone). Ablation of the T zone without histological confirmation is inappropriate. Following histological confirmation, the entire lesion and T zone can be excised (LEEP, CO2 laser) if the entire lesion is visualized and the limits of the T zone are seen (adequate colposcopy). If the entire lesion cannot be visualized (inadequate colposcopy), cervical conization (CO2 laser) should be considered.

High-grade SIL (HGSIL)

Patients with a cytological diagnosis of HGSIL should always be referred for colposcopy and directed biopsy, and if HGSIL is confirmed, nonpregnant patients should have excisional therapy aimed at removal of the entire lesion and T zone. Among pregnant patients, excisional therapy is preferred when there is suspicion of invasion. If histology confirms HGSIL without evidence of invasion, pregnant women are followed with repeat colposcopies, with treatment delayed to postdelivery.

Atypical endocervical glandular cells of undetermined significance (AEGUS)

Persistent findings of atypical glandular cells requires colposcopic examination and biopsy. Clinical management of women with a diagnosis of AEGUS varies depending on the clinical circumstances.

THE ROLE OF COLPOSCOPY IN CERVICAL CANCER CONTROL

During the last 50 years colposcopy has been used to evaluate women with atypical cervical cytology or with vaginal and vulvar intraepithelial neoplasia, to determine where to biopsy and to follow the evolution of lesions over time.[215,216] More recently, colposcopy has been used as a routine diagnostic test to detect specific cervicovaginal infections.[217] Colposcopic identification of epithelial pathology is possible because as cancers or intraepithelial lesions develop, the normal epithelium is replaced by a proliferating, crowded epithelium which is characterized by an altered optical density and an abnormal vasculature. With the cervix, the colposcopist first determines whether the colposcopic examination is adequate (i.e., whether the squamocolumnar junction and the whole lesion are visible). If the entire squamocolumnar junction cannot be seen (because a portion or all of the junction lies within the endocervical canal), the colposcopic examination is termed inadequate, or unsatisfactory. This situation occurs in approximately 15–20% of women, especially older women, and requires an endocervical curettage for diagnosis of any pathology present. Next, severity of the lesions is estimated and biopsies obtained from what appear to be the most serious lesions. Colposcopic criteria for diagnosis of different pathologic diagnoses are well established, and the reader is referred to a standard colposcopy textbook for a detailed discussion of this issue.[199,218] Generally, the size of the lesion, its appearance with and without the application of acetic acid, and its vascular pattern (best assessed with the use of a green filter) are used to classify changes. Concordance varies between colposcopic diagnoses and biopsies from 67% to 95%.[219–221] If a two-stage or greater discrepancy exists between colposcopically directed biopsies and cervical cytology, it is important to consider diagnostic or therapeutic conization by performing large-loop excision of the T zone (LLETZ). Although in the 1980s there was a great deal of enthusiasm for colposcopic detection of HPV infection, this approach is insensitive and nonspecific, and with the advent of commercially available HPV DNA assays it no longer seems logical. Colposcopy has also been used for aiding in evaluation of cervicitis and other cervical vaginal infections. A major problem with colposcopy is poor inter- and intraobserver reproducibility even among experienced colposcopists.[222] Although quality control is accepted as an integral part of the cytology laboratory's services, provision of similarly necessary safeguards for colposcopy are currently lacking.[223]

COLPOSCOPIC EXAMINATION OF THE PENIS AND ANUS

Colposcopic examination of the penis and anus has been used for evaluation of intraepithelial neoplasia at these locations.[224–226] Common manifestations of subclinical HPV infection in the male include sharply demarcated, slightly raised macules and papules with fine punctation. There have been reports that application of 5% acetic acid and colposcopy augment the detection and diagnosis of subclinical HPV infections and penile intraepithelial neoplasia (PIN). Detection of acetowhite epithelium, although useful for clinical examination, is not sufficiently specific and should not be used as a sole criterion for the diagnosis of HPV infection.[227]

CERVICOGRAPHY

Cervicography provides a 16× magnified colposcopic image of the cervix and a photograph taken with a 35-mm camera equipped with a special lens system and a light source. Since cervicograms can be obtained by a technician and sent off for an expert to read, it was hoped that this would provide a cost-effective approach to cervical cancer control in resource-poor settings.[228] In early studies[229,230] patients with atypical Pap smears were evaluated with repeat smear, cervicography, and colposcopy; cervicography appeared to have a sensitivity between that of a repeat smear and colposcopy for detection of CIN. However, among women not selected on the basis of abnormal cytologic smears, cervicography appears less specific than cytology for CIN. Unsatisfactory and defective cervicograms, especially in older women in whom the squamocolumnar junction is high up in the endocervical canal, have been a frequent problem, and cervicography has not been proven cost-beneficial.

TREATMENT OF GENITAL SQUAMOUS CELL NEOPLASIA

CERVICAL INTRAEPITHELIAL NEOPLASIA (CIN)

Once invasion has been ruled out by histologic examination of tissue and the extent of a lesion has been accurately established by colposcopy, the lesion can be destroyed by a variety of methods, including excision or ablation. Although treatment of CIN by various methods may be followed by recurrence of CIN, subsequent development of invasive cancer is quite rare.

Local biopsy excision

Local biopsy excision is appropriate for excision of a small, single focus of CIN 1 completely visualized by colposcopic examination, but it is not appropriate for multifocal disease or for lesions which extend into the endocervical canal.

Hysterectomy

Hysterectomy is an alternative treatment for CIS, if fertility is not important and when concomitant gynecologic indications for hysterectomy are present.

Cold-knife conization

Cold-knife conization has been widely employed as a definitive therapy for CIN in the past, but it has recently been replaced by simple outpatient procedures such as CO_2 laser conization, and most recently by loop electrosurgical excision procedure (LEEP). The recurrence rates after cold-knife conization are generally low if margins are negative; however, there is a relatively high complication rate, including postoperative hemorrhage, cervical stenosis and scarring, increased risk for subsequent preterm deliveries, and infertility.

Electrocautery

Although electrocautery was popular in the past, this approach is no longer recommended because of frequent complications and failure to eradicate lesions with deep crypt involvement.

Cryocautery

Introduced by Townsend and Ostergard[231] 25 years ago, cryocautery involves liquid nitrogen freezing of lesions. Treatment usually involves one or two 2–3 minute applications of a cold probe, which causes necrosis of the targeted area. Cryocautery is virtually painless and bloodless, and total reepithelialization is complete in 7 to 10 weeks. The value of cytology and colposcopy after treatment may be reduced as a result of scarring and of the fact that the squamocolumnar junction often recedes high up into the endocervical canal after squamous metaplasia during reepithelialization. Published failure rates (i.e., persistence of disease) after initial cryotherapy for CIN range from 8% for CIN 1 to 17% for CIN 3.[232–235] Failure is especially common among women with a positive endocervical curettage specimen (ECC), inadequate colposcopic examination, extensive lesions, or glandular involvement. Given the high rate of treatment failures, cryotherapy is no longer considered the treatment of choice for CIN lesions and is contraindicated in patients with CIN who have inadequate colposcopy, positive ECC, or extensive lesions.

CO_2 laser

Laser conization or vaporization treatment of CIN can be performed as an outpatient procedure and allows for precise tissue destruction under colposcopic guidance, minimal damage to surrounding tissue, low risk for postoperative hemorrhage, rapid healing with practically no scarring, and decreased risk for postoperative infections. A new squamocolumnar junction is formed at the external os and usually remains visible colposcopically, facilitating posttreatment cytologic and colposcopic evaluation. Concomitant multifocal intraepithelial lesions in the vagina or vulva can easily be treated simultaneously. Conization offers the advantage of a low failure rate (around 6%)[233,236,237] and the opportunity of histopathologic evaluation for degree of pathology and margins.

Large loop excision of the T zone (LLETZ)

Large loop excision of the T zone (LLETZ) is also called LEEP.[238–242] Prendiville et al.[238] use a fine wire loop diathermy for biopsy or excision of the whole T zone. This is a safe, effective, inexpensive, easily mastered outpatient procedure[243–246] which provides excellent quality tissue for histologic evaluation.[241] Reported recurrence rates have ranged from 5%, when lesions involved only one quadrant, to 26% when the lesions involved all four quadrants.[241] Morbidity of this procedure, as with laser or cold knife cone biopsies, is related to the volume, and probably the amount, of endocervical tissue excised. Potential problems include intra- and postoperative bleeding in 4–7% of women treated,[243–247] a figure well below the average complication rates reported with cold-knife conization or CO_2 laser conization,[248] and removal of excessive amounts of tissue which can result in an increased risk of preterm delivery and low birth weight.[249–251] Although there was initially a great deal of enthusiasm for a "see and treat" approach using the LLETZ, this approach has led to overtreatment of minor cytological abnormalities, with recent reports showing that 5–41% of "see and treat" LLETZ specimens are free of disease.[240,243,245,252]

Topical chemotherapy

Topical chemotherapy (bleomycin, 5-fluorouracil, beta-all-trans-retinoic acid, or interferons) has been used in the treatment of CIN with relatively poor success rates, due to its inability to eradicate CIN involving glandular crypts.

VAGINAL AND VULVAR INTRAEPITHELIAL NEOPLASIA

Although during the 1960s vulvectomy, and more recently skinning vulvectomy, were the standard treatments for vulvar carcinoma in situ (VIS), the high rate of spontaneous regression of VIN has prompted less aggressive treatment modalities. Excisional biopsy and CO_2 laser treatment have now largely replaced skinning vulvectomy in the treatment of VIN, including VIS. The CO_2 laser is useful because it is an efficient treatment of multifocal disease to a depth that allows for rapid healing with minimal scarring.[254]

PENILE AND ANAL INTRAEPITHELIAL NEOPLASIA

The spontaneous regression rate of subclinical (papular) penile papillomavirus infections, called penile intraepithelial neoplasia

(PIN) or Bowenoid papulosis, is not known; however, these lesions appear to have a low risk of progression. Lesions suggestive of PIN should be biopsied, and preferably treated with local ablation using CO_2 laser surgery or cryotherapy under colposcopic guidance. Perianal and anal condylomas are most difficult to treat; the anal area is very sensitive to pain, bleeding is a problem, and the lesions are easy to miss. Anal intraepithelial neoplasia (AIN) is extremely common among homosexual men, especially those with HIV infection.[205] In the absence of HIV infection, AIN 1 appears to have a natural history similar to that of CIN 1, with a low risk of progression (Kiviat, unpublished data). Perianal and intra-anal laser therapy is the most effective treatment for AIN.[255]

CERVICAL CARCINOMA

Treatment for early microinvasive carcinoma ranges from cervical conization to radical hysterectomy with pelvic node dissection and radiotherapy or chemotherapy. The overall recurrence rate is approximately 1%, regardless of the criteria used for case definition or the method of treatment. Hysterectomy with excision of the vaginal cuff is the current treatment of choice in cases with less than 3 mm invasion depth, without evidence of stromal or vascular involvement, and in which there is no confluence of tongues of invasive cells. Treatment of other forms of invasive cervical carcinoma (ICC) is based on the stage of disease defined by the International Federation of Gynaecology and Obstetrics (FIGO) classification.

VAGINAL AND VULVAR CARCINOMA

Treatment of vaginal cancer is more difficult because of anatomic considerations. Selection of treatment is based on the stage of the disease, the tumor volume, and location within the vagina. Most superficial lesions can be treated with vaginectomy. However, in general, surgical treatment can rarely be conservative because of the close proximity of the rectum and the bladder. Hence, ultraradical surgery with pelvic exenteration is often necessary. Cure rates are generally poor except in stage I disease. During the 1960s VAIN was treated by partial or total vaginectomy with or without radiation. Currently, less traumatic treatment modalities are used, including colposcopically directed excisional biopsies, cryotherapy, laser therapy, and topical 5-FU. Laser therapy has reported cure rates of 85–90%, whereas 5-FU has a high recurrence rate and can result in local toxicity, with frequent development of genital ulcerations.

PENILE AND ANAL CARCINOMA

Squamous cell carcinoma of the anus is usually treated by excision of the rectum and anus and formation of a permanent colostomy. Radiotherapy can in some cases be used for patients with tumors unsuitable for local excision. Anal cancer and its metastases in lymph nodes are particularly radiosensitive. Small tumors under 2 cm and carcinoma in situ arising at the anal margin can be excised locally. However, most anal cancers are not suitable for local excision.

Treatment of carcinoma of the penis includes excision of localized lesions, with margins of excision 2 cm proximal to the most proximal area of induration, when localized lesions are extensive. Radiotherapy is equally effective in the treatment of small localized lesions. With clinical and pathologic evidence of inguinal metastases, inguinal node dissection is carried out after treatment of the primary tumor. Definitive surgery is rarely possible in patients with inoperable nodal metastases or evidence of spread beyond the inguinal lymph nodes.

References

1 Ebrahim SH et al: Mortality related to sexually transmitted diseases in women, U.S., 1973–1992. Proceedings of the Eleventh Meeting of the International Society for STD Research, August 27–30, 1995, New Orleans LA.

2 Institute of Medicine, Committee on Prevention and Control of Sexually Transmitted Diseases, Division of Health Promotion and Disease Prevention: *The Hidden Epidemic: confronting sexually transmitted diseases,* TR Eng, WT Butler (eds). Washington, DC, National Academy Press, 1997.

3 Harlan LC et al: Cervical cancer screening: who is not screened and why? *Am J Public Health* 81:885–890, 1991.

4 National Cancer Institute, Division of Cancer Prevention and Control: *1987 Annual Cancer Statistics Review.* NIH Pub 88–2789, U.S. Department of Health and Human Services, Bethesda MD, 1988.

5 Kosary CL et al (eds): *SEER Cancer Statistics Review, 1973–1992: Tables and Graphs,* National Cancer Institute. NIH Pub 96-2789,— U.S. Department of Health and Human Services, Bethesda MD, 1995.

6 Parkin DM et al: Estimates of the worldwide frequency of sixteen major cancers in 1980. *Int J Cancer* 41:184, 1988.

7 Muir CS et al: *Cancer Incidence in Five Continents,* vol 5. Lyon, France, International Agency for Research on Cancer, Sci Pub 88, 1988.

8 Reagan JW, Fu YS: The uterine cervix, in *Principles and Practice of Surgical Pathology,* vol 2, SG Silverberg (ed.). New York, Wiley Medical Publications, 1983, p 1247.

9 Ferenczy A, Winkler B: Carcinoma and metastatic tumors of the cervix, in *Blaustien's Pathology of the Female Genital Tract,* 3rd ed, RS Kurman (ed). New York, Springer-Verlag, 1987, p 219.

10 Schauenstein W: Histologische Untersuchungen uber atypisches Plattenepithel an der Portio und an der Inneflache der Cervix uteri. *Archiv Fur Gynakologie* 85:576, 1908.

11 Schottlaender J, Dermauner F: *Zur Kenntnis des Uteruskarzinoms.* Berlin, Karger, 1912.

12 Lange P: Clinical and histological studies on cervical carcinoma. *Acta Pathol Microbiol Scand* 50(Suppl 143):13, 1960.

13 Jones HW Jr et al: Reexamination of biopsies taken prior to the development of invasive carcinoma of the cervix, in *Proceedings of the Third National Cancer Conference,* Philadelphia, Lippincott, 1956, p 678.

14 Spriggs AI et al: Progression and regression of cervical lesions. *J Clin Pathol* 33:517, 1980.

15 Richart RM, Barron BA: A follow-up study of patients with cervical dysplasia. *Am J Obstet Gynecol* 105:386–389, 1969.

16 Report of the International Society for the Study of Vulvar Disease Terminology Committee. Proceedings of the Eighth World Congress, Stockholm, Sweden. *J Reprod Med* 31:973, 1986.

17 Jeffcoate N: *Principles of Gynecology,* 5th ed. London, Butterworths, 1987.

18 Buscema J et al: Carcinoma in situ of the vulva. *Obstet Gynecol* 55: 225, 1980.

19 Jones RW et al: Carcinoma in situ of the vulva: A review of 31 treated and 5 untreated cases. *Obstet Gynecol* 68:4999, 1986.

20 Friedrich EG et al: Carcinoma in situ of the vulva: A continuing challenge. *Am J Obstet Gynecol* 136:830, 1980.

21 Crum CP et al: Human papillomavirus type 16 and early cervical neoplasia. *N Engl J Med* 310:880, 1984.

22 Aho M et al: *Natural history of vaginal intraepithelial neoplasia.* Cancer 68:195—197, 1991.

23 Koss LG: *Diagnostic Cytopathology,* 3rd ed. Philadelphia, JB Lippincott, 1979, p 337.

24 Papanicolaou GN: A survey of the actualities and potentialities of exfoliative cytology in cancer diagnosis. *Ann Med* 30:661, 1948.

25 Papanicolaou GN: *Atlas of Exfoliative Cytology.* Massachusetts, Commonwealth Fund by University Press, 1954.
26 Jones H: Impact of the Bethesda System. *Cancer* 76:1914–1918, 1995.
27 Cocker J et al: Consistency in the histological diagnosis of epithelial abnormalities of the cervix uteri. *J Clin Pathol* 21:67–70, 1968.
28 Siegler EE: Microdiagnosis of carcinoma in situ of the uterine cervix. A comparative study of pathologists' diagnoses. *Cancer* 9:463, 1956.
29 Kirkland JA: Atypical epithelial changes in the uterine cervix. *J Clin Pathol* 16:150, 1963.
30 Schiffman MH et al: Accuracy and interlaboratory reliability of human papillomavirus DNA testing by hybrid capture. *J Clin Microbiol* 33:545–550, 1995.
31 Koutsky L, et al: A cohort study of the risk of cervical intraepithelial neoplasia grade 2 or 3 in relation to papillomavirus infection. *N Engl J Med* 327:1272–1278.
32 Waterhouse J et al: *Cancer Incidence in Five Continents,* vol 3. Lyon, France, International Agency for Research on Cancer, Sci Pub 15, 1976.
33 Daling JR et al: Correlates of homosexual behavior and the incidence of anal cancer. *JAMA* 247:1988–90, 1982.
34 Draper GJ, et al: Changing patterns of cervical cancer rates. *Br Med J* 287:510, 1983.
35 McGregor JE: Mortality from carcinoma of cervix uteri in Britain. *Lancet* 2:774, 1978.
36 Cook GA, et al: Trends in cervical cancer and carcinoma in situ in Great Britain. *Br J Cancer* 50:367, 1984.
37 Armstrong B et al: Increasing mortality from cancer of the cervix in young Australian women. *Med J Aust* 1:460, 1981.
38 Bourne RG et al: Invasive carcinoma of the cervix in Queensland. *Med J Aust* 1:156, 1983.
39 Roberts AW et al: Invasive carcinoma of the cervix in young women. *Med J Aust* 2:333, 1985.
40 Green GH: Rising cervical cancer mortality in young New Zealand women. *NZ Med J* 89:89, 1979.
41 Holmes KK: Human ecology and behavior and sexually transmitted bacterial infections. *Proc Nat Acad Sci USA* 91:2448–2455, 1994.
42 British Co-operative Clinical Group: Cervical cytology screening in sexually transmitted diseases clinics in the United Kingdom. *Genitourin Med* 63:40, 1987.
43 Armstrong BK et al: *Cervical cytology in western Australia 1983. Reports to the Cancer Foundation of Western Australia.* NH and MRC Research Unit in Epidemiology and Preventative Medicine, University of Western Australia, 1984.
44 Miller BA et al (eds): *SEER Cancer Statistics Review: 1973–1990.* NIH Pub 93-2789, National Cancer Institute, Bethesda MD, 1993.
45 Devesa SS: Descriptive epidemiology of cancer of the uterine cervix. *Obstet Gynecol* 63:605–612, 1984.
46 Wiggins CL et al: *Cancer in Western Washington State 1974–1991.* Cancer Surveillance System, Fred Hutchinson Cancer Research Center, Seattle WA, 1993.
47 Roye CF: Abnormal cervical cytology in adolescents: A literature review. *J Adolesc Health* 13:643–650, 1992.
48 Krone MR et al: The epidemiology of cervical neoplasms, in *Intraepithelial Neoplasia of the Lower Genital Tract,* D Luesley et al (eds). New York, Churchill Livingstone, 1995, p. 49.
49 Centers for Disease Control and Prevention: Special focus: behavioral risk factor surveillance—United States, 1991. *MMWR Morb Mort Wkly Rep* 42:11–14, 1993.
50 Ferguson JH, Maclure JG: Intraepithelial carcinoma, dysplasia, and exfoliation of cancer cells in the vaginal mucosa. *Am J Obstet Gynecol* 87:326–336, 1963.
51 Timonen S et al: Dysplasia of the vaginal epithelium. *Gynecologica* 162:125–138, 1966.
52 Woodruff JD: Carcinoma in situ of the vagina. *Clin Obstet Gynecol* 24:485–501, 1981.
53 Campion MJ: Clinical manifestations and natural history of genital human papillomavirus infection. *Obstet Gynecol Clin North Am* 14: 363, 1987.
54 Rigoni-Stern D: Fatti statistici relativi alle malattie cancerose. *Gior Servire Progr Pathol Terup* 2:507, 1842.
55 Cramer DW: Uterine Cervix, in *Cancer Epidemiology and Prevention.,* D Schottenfeld, JF Fraumeni (eds). Philadelphia, WB Saunders, 1982, p 881.
56 Daling JR et al: Sexual practices, sexually transmitted diseases, and the incidence of anal cancer. *N Engl J Med* 317:973, 1987.
57 Newcomb PA et al: Incidence of vulvar carcinoma in relation to menstrual, reproductive, and medical factors. *J Natl Cancer Inst* 73:391, 1984.
58 Gagnon F: Contribution to the study of the etiology and prevention of cancer of the cervix of the uterus. *Am J Obstet Gynecol* 60:516, 1950.
59 Kinlen LJ et al: Meat and fat consumption and cancer mortality: a study of strict religious orders in Britain. *Lancet* 1:946, 1982.
60 Fraumeni JF et al: Cancer mortality among nuns: Role of marital status in etiology of neoplastic disease in women. *J Amer Cancer Inst* 42:455, 1969.
61 Kessler I: Venereal factors in human cervical cancer: evidence from marital clusters. *Cancer* 39:1912, 1977.
62 Harris RWC et al: Characteristics of women with dysplasia or carcinoma in situ of the cervix uteri. *Br J Cancer* 42:359, 1980.
63 Hulka BS: Risk factors for cervical cancer. *J Chron Dis* 35:3–11, 1982.
64 Buckley JD et al: Case-control study of the husbands of women with dysplasia or carcinoma of the cervix uteri. *Lancet* 2:1010–1015, 1981.
65 Zunzunegui MV et al: Male influences on cervical cancer risk. *Amer J Epidemiol* 123:302,1986.
66 Martinez I: Relationship of squamous cell carcinoma of the cervix uteri to squamous cell carcinoma of the penis among Puerto Rican women married to men with penile carcinoma. *Cancer* 24:777, 1969.
67 Graham S et al: Genital cancer in wives of penile cancer patients. *Cancer* 44:1870, 1979.
68 Smith PG et al: Mortality of wives of men dying with cancer of the penis. *Br J Cancer* 41:422–428, 1980.
69 Hall NEL et al: Penis, in *Cancer Epidemiology and Prevention.,* D Schottenfeld, JF Fraumeni (eds). Philadelphia, WB Saunders, 1982, p 958.
70 Schottenfeld D: Genetic and environmental factors in human carcinogenesis. *J Chronic Dis* 39:1021–30, 1986.
71 Kessler I: Etiological concepts in cervical carcinogenesis. *Gynecol Oncol* 12:S7, 1981.
72 Rojel J: The interrelation between uterine cancer and syphilis: a pathodemographic study. *Acta Pathol Microbiol Scand* 97:13, 1953.
73 Beral V: Cancer of the cervix: a sexually transmitted infection. *Lancet* 1:1037, 1974.
74 Lynge E et al: Cohort trends in incidence of cervical cancer in Denmark in relation to gonorrheal infection. *Acta Obstet Gynecol Scand* 64:291, 1985.
75 Starreveld AA et al: The latency period of carcinoma-in-situ of the cervix. *Obstet Gynecol* 62:348–352, 1983.
76 Furgyik S et al: Gonorrheal infection followed by an increased frequency of cervical carcinoma. *Acta Obstet Gynecol Scand* 59:521, 1980.
77 Papanicolaou GN et al: Vaginal cytology in trichomonas infestation. *Int Rec Med Gen Pract Clin* 168:551, 1955.
78 Thomas DB: An epidemiologic study of carcinoma in situ and squamous dysplasia of the uterine cervix. *Am J Epidemiol* 98:10, 1973.
79 Meisels A: Dysplasia and carcinoma of the uterine cervix. IV. A correlated cytologic and histologic study with special emphasis on vaginal microbiology. *Acta Cytol* 13:224, 1969.
80 Koss LG et al: Trichomonas vaginalis cervicitis and its relationship to cervical cancer. A histological study. *Cancer* 12:1171, 1959.
81 Patten SF Jr et al: An experimental study of the relationship between *Trichomonas vaginalis* and dysplasia in the uterine cervix. *Acta Cytol* 7:187, 1963.
82 Chandler SH et al: The epidemiology of cytomegaloviral infection in

women attending a sexually transmitted disease clinic. *J Infect Dis* 152:597, 1985.

83 Melnick JL et al: Association of cytomegalovirus (CMV) infection with cervical cancer: isolation of CMV from cell culture derived from cervical biopsy. *Intervirology* 10:115, 1978.

84 Pacsa A et al: Herpes virus antibodies and antigens in patients with cervical anaplasia and in controls. *J Natl Cancer Inst* 55:775, 1975.

85 Paavonen J et al: Genital *Chlamydia trachomatis* infection in patients with cervical atypia. *Obstet Gynecol* 54:289, 1979.

86 Hart H et al: Lack of association of cytomegalovirus antibody level with carcinoma of the uterine cervix. *Gynecol Obstet Invest* 14:300, 1982.

87 Albrecht T et al: Malignant transformation of hamster embryo fibroblasts following exposure to ultraviolet-irradiated human cytomegalovirus. *Virology* 55:53, 1973.

88 Nelson JA, et al: Transformation of NIH 3T3 cells with cloned fragments of human cytomegalovirus strain AD169. *J Virol* 43:83, 1982.

89 Brown ZA et al: Genital ulceration and infectious mononucleosis: report of a case. *Am J Obstet Gynecol* 127:673, 1977.

90 Lawee D, Shafir MS: Solitary penile ulcer associated with infectious mononucleosis. *Can Med Assoc J* 129:146–7, 1983.

91 Portnoy J et al: Recovery of Epstein-Barr virus for genital ulcers. *N Engl J Med* 311:966, 1984.

92 Sixbey JW et al: Replication of Epstein-Barr virus in human epithelial cells infected in vitro. *Nature* 306:480, 1983.

93 Sixbey JW et al: A second site for Epstein-Barr virus shedding: The uterine cervix. *Lancet* 2:1122, 1986a.

94 Sixbey JW et al: Human epithelial cell expression of an Epstein-Barr virus receptor. *Clin Res* 34:533A, 1986b.

95 Paavonen J et al: Cytologic findings in cervical chlamydial infection. *Med Biol* 58:174, 1980.

96 Paavonen J et al: Association of infection with Chlamydia trachomatis with Fitz-Hugh-Curtis syndrome. *J Infec Dis* 144:176, 1981.

97 Cevenini R et al: Cytological and histopathological abnormalities of the cervix in genital *Chlamydia trachomatis* infections. *Br J Vener Dis* 57:334, 1981.

98 Carr MC et al: *Chlamydia*, cervicitis, and abnormal Papanicolaou smears. *Obstet Gynecol* 23:27, 1979.

99 Schachter J et al: Chlamydia trachomatis and cervical neoplasia. *JAMA* 248:2134, 1982.

100 Paavonen J et al: Genital *Chlamydia trachomatis* infection in patients with cervical atypia. *Obstet Gynecol* 54:289, 1979.

101 Mackowiak PA: Microbial oncogenesis. *Amer J Med* 82:79, 1987.

102 Naib ZM et al: Genital herpetic infection. Association with cervical dysplasia and carcinoma. *Cancer* 23:940, 1969.

103 Vonka V et al: Prospective study on the relationship between cervical neoplasia and herpes simplex type 2 virus. I. Epidemiological characteristics. *Int J Cancer* 33:49, 1984.

104 Frenkel N et al: A DNA fragment of herpes simplex virus type 2 and its transcription in human cervical cancer tissue. *Proc Nat Acad Sci* 69:3784, 1972.

105 Galloway DA et al: The oncogenic potential of herpes simplex viruses: evidence for a "hit and run" mechanism. *Nature* 302:21, 1983.

106 Park M et al: Detection of herpes simplex virus type 2 DNA restriction fragments in human cervical carcinoma tissue. *EMBO Journal* 2:1029, 1983.

107 Prakash SS et al: Herpes virus type 2 and human papillomavirus type 16 in cervicitis, dysplasia and invasive cervical carcinoma. *Int J Cancer* 35:51, 1985.

108 McDougall JK et al: Cervical carcinoma: detection of herpes simplex virus RNA in cells undergoing neoplastic change. *Int J Cancer* 25:1–8, 1980.

109 McDougall JK et al: Herpes virus-specific RNA and protein in carcinoma of the uterine cervix. *Proc Natl Acad Sci USA* 79:3853, 1982.

110 Di Luca D et al: Simultaneous presence of herpes simple virus and human papillomavirus sequences in human genital tumors. *Int J Cancer* 40:763, 1987.

111 Macnab JC et al: Human papillomavirus in clinically and histologically normal tissue of patients with genital cancer. *N Engl J Med* 315: 1052–1058, 1986.

112 Zur Hausen H: Human genital cancer: synergism between two virus infections or synergism between a virus infection and initiative agents? *Lancet* 2:489, 1982.

113 Gissman L, Hausen HZ: Human papilloma virus DNA: physical mapping and genetic heterogeneity. *Proc Natl Acad Sci USA* 73: 1310–1313, 1976.

114 Gissman L et al: Human papilloma viruses (HPV): characterization of four different isolates. *Virology* 76:569–580, 1977.

115 Gissman L, zur Hausen H: Partial characterization of viral DNA from human genital warts (condylomata acuminata). *Int J Cancer* 25:605–609, 1980.

116 Orth G et al: Characterization of a new type of human papillomavirus that causes skin warts. *J Virol* 24:108–20, 1977.

117 Draper GJ et al: Changing patterns of cervical cancer rates. *Br Med J* 287:510, 1983.

118 International Agency for Research on Cancer Working Group: Studies Of Cancer In Humans, in *IARC Monographs on the Evaluation of Carcinogenic Risks to Humans,* vol 64. Lyon, France 1995, p 87.

119 Bosch FX et al: Prevalence of human papillomavirus in cervical cancer: a worldwide perspective. *J Natl Cancer Inst* 87:796–802, 1995.

120 Schiffman MH et al: Cervical cancer, in *Cancer Epidemiology and Prevention,* 2nd ed., D Schottenfeld, JF Fraumeni (eds). New York, Oxford University Press, 1996.

121 Collins JE et al: Detection of human papillomavirus DNA sequences by in situ DNA-DNA hybridization in cervical intraepithelial neoplasia and invasive carcinoma: a retrospective study. *J Clin Pathol* 41: 289, 1988.

122 Lorincz AT et al: Temporal associations of human papillomavirus infection with cervical cytologic abnormalities. *Am J Obstet Gynecol* 162:645–651, 1990.

123 Ho L et al: The genetic drift of human papillomavirus type 16 is a means of reconstructing prehistoric viral spread and the movement of ancient human populations. *J Virol* 67(11):6413–6423, 1993.

124 Chan SY et al: Molecular variants of human papillomavirus type 16 from four continents suggest ancient pandemic spread of the virus and its coevolution with humankind. *J Virol* 66:2057–2066, 1992.

125 Yamada T et al: Human papillomavirus type 16 variant lineages in United States populations characterized by nucleotide sequence analysis of the E6, L2, and L1 coding segments. *J Virol* 69:7743–7753, 1995.

126 Xi LF et al: Analysis of human papillomavirus type 16 variants indicates establishment of persistent infection. *J Infect Dis* 172:747–755, 1995.

127 Xi LF et al: Genomic variation of human papillomavirus type 16 and risk for high grade cervical intraepithelial neoplasia. *J Natl Cancer Inst* 89(11):796–802, 1997.

128 Yamada T et al: Human papillomavirus type 16 sequence variation in cervical cancers: a worldwide perspective. *J Virol.* 71:2463–2472, 1997.

129 May M et al: The E6/E7 promoter of extrachromosomal HPV-16 DNA in cervical cancers escapes from cellular repression by mutation of target sequences for YY1. *EMBO Journal* 13:1460–1466, 1994.

130 Mittal R et al: Multiple human papillomavirus type 16 glucocorticoid response elements functional for transformation, transient expression, and DNA protein interactions. *J Virol* 67:5656–9, 1993.

131 Londesborough P et al: Human papillomavirus (HPV) genotype as a predictor of persistence and development of high grade lesions in women with minor cervical abnormalities. *Int J Cancer* 69:364–368, 1996.

132 Hecht JL et al: Genetic characterization of the human papillomavirus (HPV) 18 E2 gene in clinical specimens suggests the presence of a subtype with decreased oncogenic potential. *Int J Cancer* 60:369–376, 1995.

133 Ellis JRM et al: The association of an HPV-16 oncogene variant with HLA-B7 has implications for vaccine design in cervical cancer. *Nature (Medicine)* 1:464–470, 1995.

134 Bavin PJ et al: Sequence microheterogeneity in the long control region of clinical isolates of human papillomavirus type 16. *J Med Virol* 39: 267–272, 1993.
135 Brinton LA et al: Cigarette smoking and invasive cervical cancer. *JAMA* 255:3265, 1986.
136 Clarke EA et al: Smoking as a risk factor in cancer of the cervix: additional evidence from a case-control study. *Am J Epidemiol* 115: 59–66, 1982.
137 La Vecchia C et al: Cigarette smoking and the risk of cervical neoplasia. *Amer J Epidemiol* 123:22, 1986.
138 Hellberg D et al: Penile cancer: Is there an epidemiologic role for smoking and sexual behavior: *Brit Med J* 295:1306, 1987.
139 Bosch FX et al: Risk factors for cervical cancer in Colombia and Spain. *Int J Cancer* 52:750–758, 1992.
140 Eluf-Neto et al: Human papillomavirus and invasive cancer in Brazil. *Br J Cancer* 69:114–119, 1994.
141 Holly EA et al: Mutagenic mucus in the cervix of smokers. *J Natl Cancer Inst* 76:983, 1986.
142 Barton SE et al: Effect of cigarette smoking on cervical epithelial immunity: a mechanism for neoplastic change? *Lancet* 2:652–654, 1988.
143 Celentano DD et al: The role of contraceptive use in cervical cancer: the Maryland cervical cancer case-control study. *Am J Epidemiol* 126:592–604, 1987.
144 Peters RK et al: Risk factors for invasive cervical cancer among Latinas and non-Latinas in Los Angeles County. *J Natl Cancer Inst* 77: 1063–1077, 1986b.
145 Vessey MP et al: Neoplasia of the cervix uteri and contraception: a possible adverse effect of the pill. *Lancet* 2:930–934, 1983a.
146 Vessey MP et al: Oral contraceptives and cervical cancer (Letter). *Lancet* 2:1358–1359, 1983b.
147 Andolsek L et al: Influence of oral contraceptives on the incidence of premalignant and malignant lesions of the cervix. *Contraception* 28: 505–519, 1983.
148 Beral et al: Oral contraceptive use and malignancies of the genital tract: results from The Royal College of General Practitioners' Oral Contraceptive Study. *Lancet* 2:1331–1335, 1988.
149 Thomas DB et al: Monthly injectable steroid contraceptives and cervical cancer. *Am J Epidemiol* 130:237–247, 1989.
150 Dabancens A et al: Intraepithelial cervical neoplasia in women using intrauterine devices and long-acting injectable progestogens as contraceptives. *Am J Obstet Gynecol* 119:052–1056, 1974.
151 Herrero R et al: Injectable contraceptives and risk of invasive cervical cancer: evidence of an association. *Int J Cancer* 46:5–7, 1990a.
152 Penn I et al: Cancers of the anogenital region in renal transplant recipients. *Cancer* 58:611–616, 1986.
153 Sillman FH et al: Anogenital papillomavirus infection and neoplasia in immunodeficient women. *Obstet Gynecol Clin North Am* 15:537–538, 1987.
154 Halpert R et al: Human papillomavirus and lower genital neoplasia in renal transplant patients. *Obstet Gynecol* 68:251–258, 1986.
155 Orth G: Epidermodysplasia verruciformis. A model for understanding the oncogenicity of human papillomaviruses. *CIBA Found Symp* 120:157–174, 1986.
156 Schneider V et al: Immunosuppression as a high-risk factor in the development of condyloma acuminatum and squamous neoplasia of the cervix. *Acta Cytol* 27:220–224, 1983.
157 Sillman F, Stanek A, Sedlis A et al: The relationship between human papillomavirus infection in renal transplant recipients. *Int J Dermatol* 30:785–789, 1984.
158 Schafer A et al: The increased frequency of cervical dysplasia-neoplasia in women infected with the human immunodeficiency virus is related to the degree of immunosuppression. *Am J Obstet Gynecol* 164: 593–599, 1991.
159 Schrager LK et al: Cervical and vaginal squamous cell abnormalities in women infected with human immunodeficiency virus. *J AIDS* 2: 570–575, 1989.
160 Vermund SH et al: High risk of human papillomavirus infection and cervical squamous intraepithelial lesions among women with symptomatic human immunodeficiency virus infection. *Am J Obstet Gynecol* 165:392–400, 1991.
161 Smith JR et al: Influence of HIV on lower genital tract neoplasia. *Antibiot Chemother* 43:150–155, 1991.
162 Laga M et al: Genital papillomavirus infection and cervical dysplasia—opportunistic complications of HIV infection. *Int J Cancer* 50: 45–48, 1992.
163 Kreiss JK et al: Human immunodeficiency virus, human papillomavirus, and cervical intraepithelial neoplasia in Nairobi prostitutes. *Sex Trans Dis* 19:54–59, 1992.
164 Smith JK et al: Is HIV infection associated with an increase in cervical neoplasia. *Br J Obstet Gynecol* 100:149–153, 1993.
165 Tirelli U et al: Malignant tumors other than lymphoma and Kaposi's sarcoma in association with HIV infection. *Cancer Detect Prevent* 12:267–272, 1988.
166 Maiman M et al: Human immunodeficiency virus infection and cervical neoplasia. *Gynecol Oncol* 38:377–382, 1990.
167 Rellihan MA et al: Rapidly progressing cervical cancer in a patient with human immunodeficiency virus infection. *Gynecol Oncol* 36: 435–438, 1990.
168 Schwartz LB et al: Rapidly progressive squamous cell carcinoma of the cervix coexisting with human immunodeficiency virus infection: clinical opinion. *Gynecol Oncol* 41:255–258, 1990.
169 Melbye M et al: High incidence of anal cancer among AIDS patients. *Lancet* 343:636–639, 1994.
170 Rogo KO, Kavoo-Linge: Human immunodeficiency virus seroprevalence among cervical cancer patients. *Gynecol Oncol* 37:87–92, 1990.
171 Apple RJ et al: Comparison of human leukocyte antigen DR-DQ disease associations found with cervical dysplasia and invasive cervical carcinoma. *J Natl Cancer Inst* 87:427–36, 1995.
172 Apple RJ et al: HLA DR-DQ associations with cervical carcinoma show papillomavirus-type specificity. *Nat Genet* 6:157–62, 1994.
173 Bartholomew JS, et al: Integration of high-risk human papillomavirus DNA is linked to the down-regulation of class I human leukocyte antigens by steroid hormones in cervical tumor cells. *Cancer Res* 57: 937–942, 1997.
174 Allen M et al: HLA DQ-DR haplotype and susceptibility to cervical carcinoma: indications of increased risk for development of cervical carcinoma in individuals infected with HPV 18. *Tissue Antigens* 48: 32–7, 1996.
175 Helland A et al: DQA1 and DQB1 genes in patients with squamous cell carcinoma of the cervix: relationship to human papillomavirus infection and prognosis. *Cancer Epidemiol Biomarkers Prev* 3:479–86, 1994.
176 Gregoire L et al: Association between HLA-DQB1 alleles and risk for cervical cancer in African-American women. *Int J Cancer* 57:504–7, 1994.
177 Coleman N et al: Analysis of HLA-DR expression on keratinocytes in cervical neoplasia. *Int J Cancer* 56:314–319, 1994.
178 Odunsi K et al: Susceptibility to human papillomavirus-associated cervical intra-epithelial neoplasia is determined by specific HLA DR-DQ alleles. *Int J Cancer* 67:595–602, 1996.
179 Sastre-Garau X et al: Decreased frequency of HLA-DRB1 13 alleles in Frenchwomen with HPV-positive carcinoma of the cervix. *Int J Cancer* 69:159–64, 1996.
180 Cuzick J et al: Human papillomavirus testing in cervical screening. *Lancet* 345:8964, 1995.
181 Brinton LA: *Epidemiology of cervical cancer—overview*. Lyon, France, International Agency for Research on Cancer, Sci Pub 119: 3–23, 1992.
182 Burghardt E: *Early Histological Diagnosis of Cervical Cancer*. Stuttgart, Germany, Thieme, 1973.
183 Stern E, Neely PM: Carcinoma and dysplasia of the cervix. A comparison of rates for new and returning populations. *Acta Cytol* 7: 357–361, 1963.
184 Sherman ME, Kelly D: High-grade squamous intraepithelial lesions and invasive carcinoma following the report of three negative Papanicolaou smears: screening failures or rapid progression. *Modern Pathol* 5:337–342, 1992.

185 Bamford PN et al: The natural history of cervical intraepithelial neoplasia as determined by cytology and colposcopic biopsy. *Acta Cytol* 27:48248–4, 1983.
186 Saito J et al: New human papillomavirus sequences in female genital tumors from Japanese patients. *Jpn J Cancer Res* 78:1081–7, 1987.
187 Richart RM, Vailant HW: Influence of cell collection techniques upon cytological diagnosis. *Cancer* 18:1474, 1965.
188 Rylander E: Negative smears in women developing invasive cancer. *Acta Obstet Gynecol Scand* 56:115, 1977.
189 Miller AF: Cervical Cancer Screening Programs: Management Guidelines. Geneva, WHO, 1992.
190 Sedlis A et al: Evaluation of two simultaneously obtained cervical smears: a comparison study. *Acta Cytol* 18:291, 1974.
191 Gay JD et al: False-negative results in cervical cytologic studies. *Acta Cytol* 29:1043, 1985.
192 Vooijs GP et al: Relationship between diagnoses of epithelial abnormalities and the composition of cervical smears. *Acta Cytol* 29:323, 1985.
193 Elias A et al: The significance of endocervical cells in the diagnosis of cervical epithelial changes. *Acta Cytol* 27:225, 1983.
194 National Cancer Institute Workshop: The revised Bethesda System for reporting cervical/vaginal cytologic diagnoses: report of the 1991 Bethesda Workshop. *JAMA* 267:1892, 1991.
195 Ferenczy A et al: Conventional cervical cytologic smears vs. ThinPrep smears. A paired comparison study on cervical cytology. *Acta Cytol* 40:1136–1142, 1996.
196 Lorincz AT et al: Human papillomavirus infection of the cervix: relative risk associations of 15 common anogenital types. *Obstet Gynecol* 79:328–337, 1992.
197 Cox JT et al: An evaluation of human papillomavirus testing as part of referral to colposcopy clinics. *Obstet Gynecol* 80:389–395, 1992.
198 Wright TC et al: Comparison of management algorithms for the evaluation of women with low-grade cytologic abnormalities. *Obstet Gynecol* 85:202–210, 1995.
199 Campion MJ et al: Progressive potential of mild cervical atypia: prospective cytological colposcopic, and virological study *Lancet* August 2:237–240, 1986.
200 Cuzick J et al: Human papillomavirus type 16 DNA in cervical smears as predictor of high-grade cervical cancer. *Lancet* 339:959–960, 1992.
201 Burger MPM, Hollema H, Pieters WJLM, Quint WGV: Predictive value of human papillomavirus type for histological diagnosis of women with cervical cytological abnormalities. *BMJ* 310:94–95, 1995.
202 Nauth H: Cytology of the exfoliative layer in normal and diseased vulvar skin. *Acta Cytol* 26:269, 1982.
203 Webb AJ: Cytologic diagnosis of anorectal and rectosigmoid lesions by a simple smear technique. *Acta Cytol* 23:524, 1979.
204 Medley Y: Anal smear test to diagnose occult anorectal infection with human papillomaviruses in men. *Br J Vener Dis* 60:205, 1984.
205 Kiviat NB et al: Association of anal dysplasia and human papillomavirus with immunosuppression and HIV infection among homosexual men. *AIDS* 7:43–49, 1993.
206 Critchlow CW et al: Association of human immunodeficiency virus and anal human papillomavirus infection among homosexual men. *Arch Intern Med* 152:1673–1676, 1992.
207 Palefsky JM et al: Anal intraepithelial neoplasia and anal papillomavirus infection among homosexual males with group IV HIV disease. *JAMA* 263:2911–2916, 1990.
208 Skegg DCG: Cervical screening blues. Lancet 345:1451–1452, 1995.
209 Raffle AE, Alden B, Mckenzie EFD: Detection rates for abnormal cervical smears: what are we screening for? *Lancet* 345:1469–1473, 1995.
210 Kirby AJ et al: Conservative treatment of mild/moderate cervical dyskaryosis: long-term outcome. *Lancet* 339:828–831, 1992.
211 Fletcher A, et al: Four and a half year follow up of women with dyskaryotic cervical smears. *BMJ* 301:641–664, 1990.
212 Robertson JJ et al: Risk of cervical cancer associated with mild dyskaryosis. *BMJ* 297:18–21, 1988.
213 Flannelly G et al: Management of women with mild and moderate cervical dyskaryosis. *BMJ* 308:1399–1403, 1994.
214 Kurman RJ et al: Interim guidelines for management of abnormal cervical cytology. *JAMA* 271:1866–1869, 1994.
215 Kolstad P et al: *Atlas of Colposcopy,* 2nd ed. Baltimore, University Park Press, 1977.
216 Coppleson M et al: *Colposcopy. A Scientific and Practical Approach to the Cervix and Vagina in Health and Disease,* 2nd ed. Springfield IL, Thomas, 1978.
217 Paavonen J et al: Significance of mild cervical cytologic atypia in a sexually transmitted disease clinic population. *Acta Cytol* 33:831–838, 1989.
218 Melamed MR et al: Nondiagnostic squamous atypia in cervico-vaginal cytology as a risk factor for early neoplasia. *Acta Cytol* 20:108, 1976.
219 Townsend DE et al: Abnormal Papanicolaou smears. Evaluation by colposcopy, biopsies, and endocervical curettage. *Am J Obstet Gynecol* 108:429–434, 1970.
220 Stafl A, Mattingly RF: Colposcopic diagnosis of cervical neoplasia. *Obstet Gynecol* 41:168–176, 1973.
221 McCord ML et al: Discrepancy of cervical cytology and colposcopic biopsy: is cervical conization necessary? *Obstet Gynecol* 77:715–719, 1991.
222 Sellors JW et al: Observer variability in the scoring of colpophotographs. *Obstet Gynecol* 76:1006–1008, 1990.
223 Benedet JL et al: A quality—control program for colposcopic practice. *Obstet Gynecol* 78:872–875, 1991.
224 Surawicz CM et al: Anal dysplasia in homosexual men; role of anoscopy and biopsy. *Gastroenterology* 105;658–666, 1993.
225 Kiviat NB et al: Association of anal dysplasia and human papillomavirus with immunosuppression and HIV infection among homosexual men. *AIDS* 7:43–49, 1993.
226 Palefsky JM et al: Risk factors for anal human papillomavirus and anal cytologic abnormalities in HIV positive and HIV negative homosexual men. *J Acquir Immun Defic Syndr* 7:599–606, 1994.
227 Mazzatenta C et al: Detection and typing of genital papillomaviruses in men with a single polymerase chain reaction and type-specific DNA probes. *J Am Acad Dermatol* 28:704–710, 1993.
228 Stafl A: Cervicography: a new method for cervical cancer detection. *Am J Obstet Gynecol* 139:815–825, 1981.
229 Spitzer M et al: Comparative utility of repeat Papanicolaou smears, cervicography, and colposcopy in the evaluation of atypical Papanicolaou smears. *Obstet Gynecol* 69:731–735, 1987.
230 Jones DE: Evaluation of the atypical Pap smear. *Am J Obstet Gynecol* 157:544–549, 1987.
231 Townsend DE et al: Cryocauterization for pre-invasive cervical neoplasia. *J Reprod Med* 6:171–176, 1971.
232 Charles EH, Savage EW: Cryosurgical treatment of cervical intraepithelial neoplasia. *Obstet Gynecol Surv* 35:539–548, 1980.
233 Stein DS et al: Laser vaporization in the treatment of cervical intraepithelial neoplasia. *J Reprod Med* 30:179–183, 1985.
234 Figge DC et al: Cryotherapy in the treatment of cervical intraepithelial neoplasia. *Obstet Gynecol* 62:353, 1983.
235 Richart RM et al: An analysis of "long-term" follow-up results in patients with cervical intraepithelial neoplasia treated by cryotherapy. *Am J Obstet Gynecol* 137:823–826, 1980.
236 Bellina JH et al: Carbon dioxide laser management of cervical intraepithelial neoplasia. *Am J Obstet Gynecol* 141:828–832, 1981.
237 Jordan JA et al: The treatment of cervical intraepithelial neoplasia by laser vaporization. *Br J Obstet Gynecol* 92:394, 1985.
238 Prendiville W et al: A low voltage diathermy loop for taking cervical biopsies: a qualitative comparison with punch biopsy forceps. *Br J Obstet Gynecol* 93:773–776, 1986.
239 Prendiville W et al: Large loop excision of the transformatin zone (LLETZ): a new method of management for women with cervical intra-epithelial neoplasia. *Br J Obstet Gynecol* 96:1054–1060, 1989.
240 Bigrigg MA et al: Colposcopic diagnosis and treatment of cervical dysplasia at a single clinic visit. *Lancet* 336:229–231, 1990.
241 Wright TC Jr et al: Treatment of cervical intraepithelial neoplasia

using the loop electrosurgical excision procedure. *Obstet Gynecol* 79: 173–178, 1992.

242 Prendiville W: Large loop excision of the transformation zone. *Clin Obstet Gynecol* 38:622–639, 1995.

243 Luesley DM et al: Loop diathermy excision of the cervical transformation zone in patients with abnormal cervical smears. *BMJ* 300: 1690–1693, 1990.

244 Bigrigg A et al: Efficacy and safety of large-loop excision of the transformation zone. *Lancet* 343:32–34, 1994.

245 Ferenczy A, et al: Loop electrosurgical excision procedure for squamous intraepithelial lesions of the cervix: advantages and potential pitfalls. *Obstet Gynecol* 87:332–337, 1996.

246 Large loop excision of the transformation zone (Editorial). *Lancet* 337:148–149, 1991.

247 Murdoch JB, et al: Histological incomplete excision of CIN after large loop excision of the transformation zone (LLETZ) merits careful follow up, not retreatment. *Br J Obstet Gynecol* 99:990–993, 1992.

248 Baggish MS: A comparison between laser excisional conization and laser vaporization for the treatment of cervical intraepithelial neoplasia. *Am J Obstet Gynecol* 155:39–44, 1986.

249 Forsmo S et al: Pregnancy outcome after laser surgery for cervical intraepithelial neoplasia. *Acta Obstet Gynecol Scand* 75:139–143, 1996.

250 Blomfield et al: Pregnancy outcome after large loop excision of the cervical transformation zone. *Am J Obstet Gynecol* 169:620–625, 1993.

251 Hagen B, Skjeldestad FE: The outcome of pregnancy after CO_2 laser conisation of the cervix. *Br J Obstet Gynecol* 100:717–720, 1993.

252 Alvarez RD et al: Prospective randomized trial of LLETZ versus laser ablation in patients with cervical intraepithelial neoplasia. *Gynecol Oncol* 52:175–179, 1994.

253 Kennedy AW et al: The role of the loop electrosurgical excision procedure in the diagnosis and management of early invasive cervical cancer. *Int J Gynecol Cancer* 5:117–120, 1995.

254 Reid R III: A new surgical technique for appendage-conserving ablation of refractory condylomas and vulvar intraepithelial neoplasia. *Am J Obstet Gynecol* 152:504–509, 1985.

255 Frisch M et al: Benign anal lesions and the risk of anal cancer. *N Engl J Med* 331:300–302, 1994.

Chapter 60
Urethritis in males

David H. Martin
William R. Bowie

DEFINITIONS

Urethritis, manifested by urethral discharge, dysuria, or itching at the end of the urethra, is the response of the urethra to inflammation of any etiology. The characteristic physical finding is urethral discharge, and the pathognomonic confirmatory laboratory finding is an increased number of polymorphonuclear leukocytes (PMNL) on Gram stain of a urethral smear or in the sediment of the first-voided urine. Urethritis is called gonococcal, or gonorrhea, when *Neisseria gonorrhoeae* is detected, and nongonococcal if *N. gonorrhoeae* cannot be detected. The term *nongonococcal urethritis* (NGU) is preferable to the term *nonspecific urethritis*, because NGU has specific causes and some of these have been elucidated. Of these, *Chlamydia trachomatis* and *Ureaplasma urealyticum* are the most frequent. NGU occurring soon after curative therapy for urethral gonorrhea is called *postgonococcal urethritis* (PGU).

HISTORY

In the 1800s, even prior to the discovery of *N. gonorrhoeae*, the existence of several types of urethritis was already suspected. By the 1880s, after the isolation of *N. gonorrhoeae* and the introduction of the Gram stain, differentiation of gonococcal from nongonococcal urethritis became possible. In the early 1900s, intracytoplasmic inclusions, which today are considered characteristic of chlamydiae, were seen in urethral smears of some men with urethritis. The development that had the greatest impact on clinical differentiation of gonococcal and nongonococcal urethritis, however, was the introduction of the sulfonamides and penicillins for treatment of urethritis. With penicillin in particular, gonococcal urethritis was curable, but NGU usually was not. Progress in therapy of NGU came with the introduction of tetracyclines and macrolides. Further insight into the etiology of NGU came with the discovery of *Ureaplasma urealyticum* in 1954[1] and the development of cell culture isolation techniques for *Chlamydia trachomatis* in 1965.[2]

ETIOLOGY

Organisms that are proved or are possible causes of sexually transmitted urethritis are listed in Table 60-1.

NEISSERIA GONORRHOEAE

The causal role of *N. gonorrhoeae* in male urethritis is well established. Several aspects that are important for management of gonococcal urethritis deserve reemphasis here. These include the frequency of asymptomatic infection, the increasing resistance of isolates of *N. gonorrhoeae* to traditional treatments, and the high frequency of concurrent *C. trachomatis* infection. Although most new cases of gonococcal urethritis are symptomatic, many studies have emphasized that gonococcal urethritis can be asymptomatic or minimally symptomatic.[3] As many as two-thirds or more of men in the community who are found to have urethral gonorrhea by routine screening or by contact-tracing have no symptoms at all, or they have such mild symptoms that they are able to ignore them. These are the men most likely to remain sexually active and to spread gonorrhea. For example, a population-based study of 5,867 men in rural Tanzania found that 27 percent had a positive urine leukoctye esterase dipstick test, and 2.5 percent reported a complaint of urethral discharge. Of those with a positive dipstick test or with symptoms, 158 had urethral gonorrhea (by Gram stain) or chlamydial infection (by antigen-detection immunoassay). Only 24 (15 percent) of those with either infection complained of symptoms or signs, and a further 30 (19 percent) had a discharge on examination, leaving 66 percent with neither symptoms nor signs.[4] Asymptomatic men in a U.S. study appeared especially likely to have the arginine-, hypoxanthine-, and uracil-requiring auxotrophs of *N. gonorrhoeae* that have often been associated with disseminated gonococcal infection.[5] Gradually increasing resistance of *N. gonorrhoeae* to penicillins resulted in the need for progressively higher doses of penicillin in conjunction with probenecid to obtain a cure. Penicillinase-producing *N. gonorrhoeae* strains appeared in 1976; they were initially most prevalent in Southeast Asia and Africa but have now spread worldwide. Chromosomally mediated resistance to penicillin has reached a level where even large doses of penicillin do not reliably eradicate the organism.[6] Additionally, high-level resistance to tetracycline is now well established in gonococci[7] throughout the world, and quinolone resistance has already become a widespread problem in Southeast Asia and the Philippines.[8,9]

CHLAMYDIA TRACHOMATIS

Since 1972, many studies have shown that *C. trachomatis* could be isolated from the urethras of 25 to 60 percent (usually 30 to 40 percent) of men who have NGU, 4 to 35 percent (usually 15 to 25 percent) of men with urethral gonorrhea, and 0 to 7 percent of men without obvious urethritis (Table 60-2). When asymptomatic men were screened to exclude pyuria, the rate of isolation was only 0 to 3 percent.[10] *C. trachomatis* has been less frequently isolated from homosexual men with NGU.[11,12] More recent studies suggest that *C. trachomatis* is a less frequent cause of NGU today.[13] These observations are consistent with the decrease in prevalence of *C. trachomatis* in the United States in general.[14–16]

Most patients with NGU seen in sexually transmitted disease (STD) clinics have existing antibody to *C. trachomatis* demonstrable in acute-phase sera by micro-immunofluorescence (micro-IF). It is unusual to document seroconversion or a fourfold increase in micro-IF antibody in such patients.[17] However, in a selected group of men who had relatively few sex partners and no previous history of urethritis, and who had had symptoms of NGU for less than 10 days, 9 of 10 who were culture-positive for *C. trachomatis* seroconverted.[10] IgM micro-IF antibody, a transiently detectable antibody that allows diagnosis of recent infection despite preexisting antibody, was detected in specimens from 16 of 20 men whose cultures were *C. trachomatis*–positive, com-

Table 60-1. Etiology of Sexually Transmitted Urethritis in Males

Gonococcal:
- *Neisseria gonorrhoeae**

Nongonococcal:
- *Chlamydia trachomatis,* 15–40%
- *Ureaplasma urealyticum,* 10–40%
- Neither, 20–40%
  - *Mycoplasma genitalium,* 15–25%
  - *Trichomonas vaginalis,* rare
  - Yeasts, rare
  - Herpes simplex virus, rare in the absence of obvious skin lesions
  - Adenoviruses, rare
  - *Haemophilus* sp., rare
  - Other bacterial ?
  - Other ???

* Rare cases of *Neisseria meningitidis* urethritis presenting like gonococcal urethritis have been reported (see text).

pared with 3 of 39 with NGU whose cultures were negative ($p >$ .0001).[10] These results suggested that recent acquisition of chlamydia, rather than reactivation of latent infection, was associated with urethritis in these men.

Postgonococcal urethritis (PGU) provides an opportunity for prospective assessment of the ability of *C. trachomatis* to produce urethritis. Gonorrhea has a shorter incubation period than chlamydial urethritis, so men with both infections can present with gonorrhea while the chlamydial urethritis is still incubating. When gonorrhea is treated with antimicrobials that do not eradicate *C. trachomatis*—such as single-dose penicillin, ampicillin, ceftriaxone, fluoroquinolones, or spectinomycin—PGU develops in most men who have concurrent *C. trachomatis* infections (see Table 60-2). The rate of development of PGU is much greater in patients infected with *C. trachomatis* than in men with gonorrhea without *C. trachomatis* infection. The rate of development of PGU is lower if an antimicrobial that is active against *C. trachomatis,* such as doxycycline, is used.

Selective eradication of *C. trachomatis* results in alleviation of urethritis in men infected with the organism.[10,18,19] Use of sulfonamides or rifampin, which are active against *C. trachomatis* but which overall have a poor record in the treatment of NGU, resulted in clinical responses in most men infected with *C. trachomatis,* but in a significantly smaller proportion of men without *C. trachomatis*.[10,18,19] However, a better response in *C. trachomatis*–positive NGU patients than in chlamydia-negative NGU is also observed with a broader-spectrum antimicrobial, tetracycline.[20] Persistence or recurrence of NGU within 6 weeks of initiation of a 7-day course of tetracycline, 2 gm per day, was seen in 17 percent of men whose cultures were *C. trachomatis*–positive, com-

Table 60-2. Recovery of *C. trachomatis* from Males with Nongonococcal Urethritis (NGU), Gonococcal Urethritis (GU), Postgonococcal Urethritis (PGU), and Symptomless Controls

Country	Investigator	Year	NGU*	GU*	PGU*	Controls	References
U.K.	Dunlop et al.	1972	44/99 (44)				108
U.K.	Oriel et al.	1972	49/135 (36)			0/31 (0)	22
U.K.	Richmond et al.	1972	40/103 (30)	32/99 (32)	17/21 (81)	5/92 (5)	109
U.K.	Oriel et al.	1975		15/44 (34)	11/23 (48)		110
U.K.	Oriel et al.	1975	33/133 (25)				111
U.S.A.	Schachter et al.	1975	27/76 (36)	2/18 (11)		0/57 (0)	112
U.S.A.	Smith et al.	1975	34/131 (26)				113
U.S.A.	Holmes et al.	1975	48/113 (42)	13/69 (19)	12/20 (60)	4/58 (7)	17
U.K.	Oriel et al.	1976	125/262 (48)	35/141 (25)		3/74 (4)	114
U.K.	Prentice et al.	1976	43/136 (32)				42
U.S.A.	Bowie et al.	1976	36/91 (40)				18
Sweden	Johannisson et al	1977	44/103 (43)		11/15 (73)		115
U.K.	Alani et al.	1977	116/385 (30)	13/118 (11)	9/59 (15)		23
U.K.	Vaughan-Jackson et al.	1977		30/95 (32)	26/49 (53)		41
U.S.A.	Bowie et al.	1977	23/69 (33)			1/39 (3)	10
U.S.A.	Segura et al.	1977	71/180 (39)				116
U.S.A.	Wong et al.	1977	21/67 (31)	4/99 (4)		3/85 (4)	62
Finland	Paavonen et al.	1978	39/75 (52)				24
Finland	Terho	1978	93/159 (58)			0/64 (0)	74
Finland	Terho	1978		38/133 (29)	30/50 (60)		117
Norway	Csango	1978	36/81 (44)				118
Sweden	Ripa et al.	1978	74/284 (26)	15/88 (17)			119
Switzerland	Perroud et al.	1978	124/238 (52)	32/139 (23)	15/19 (79)	1/40 (3)	120
U.S.A.	Bowie et al.	1978		23/121 (18)	10/26 (38)		40
U.S.A.	Bowie et al.	1978	78/211 (37)				11
U.S.A.	Smith et al.	1978		31/143 (22)			121
U.S.A.	Swartz et al.	1978	35/107 (33)	12/61 (20)		6/112 (5)	43
Finland	Lassus et al.	1979	75/181 (45)				25
U.K.	Coufalik et al.	1979	93/217 (43)				19
U.K.	Taylor-Robinson et al.	1979	263/726 (36)				122
Canada	Bowie et al.	1980	80/200 (40)				26
U.S.A.	Root et al.	1980	19/96 (20)				31
Denmark	Ibsen et al.	1988	82/188 (44)				102
France	Lefevre et al	1990	52/202 (26)	5/23 (22)			123
U.S.A.	Hooten et al.	1990	60/152 (39)				100
U.S.A.	Stamm et al.	1995	69/452 (15)				13

* Number of culture-positive/number examined (percent of culture-positive).

pared with 47 percent of those whose cultures were *C. trachomatis*–negative ($p = .01$). In a subsequent study with minocycline, persistent or recurrent NGU developed within 6 weeks of initiation of therapy in 17 percent of 78 *C. trachomatis*–positive men, compared with 35 percent of 133 men without *C. trachomatis* infection ($p > .005$).[11]

When the urethra of a nonhuman primate is infected experimentally,[21] discharge and pyuria are not usually detected. Urethral follicles develop, however, and urethral cultures may remain positive for *C. trachomatis* for as long as 3 months.

Etiology of *C. trachomatis*–negative NGU

Several types of data indicate that *C. trachomatis* is usually not the cause of urethritis when *C. trachomatis* is not isolated (assuming sensitive isolation procedures are used). If men had false-negative cultures, further culture attempts or nucleic acid–based tests might eventually demonstrate the organism. When initial urethral specimens are negative for *C. trachomatis,* however, they usually remain negative when the patients are followed without treatment.[20] Cervical cultures from female sex partners of men with *C. trachomatis*–negative NGU are likely to be *C. trachomatis*–negative.[17,22–25] In most cases of *C. trachomatis* culture–negative NGU, there is no serologic evidence of recent *C. trachomatis* infection.[10] *C. trachomatis*–negative NGU responds poorly to certain antimicrobials that are active against *C. trachomatis* such as the sulfonamides, rifampin, and the tetracyclines.[10,11,18,20,26]

Ureaplasma urealyticum**.** The most likely cause of many *C. trachomatis*–negative cases of NGU is *U. urealyticum.* Case-control studies of the association of *U. urealyticum* with NGU must account for the fact that urethral colonization is common in men without urethritis, and it is strongly correlated with the total number of female sex partners.[27] In general, *U. urealyticum* has been isolated more often from patients with NGU than from control groups when the control group was less sexually active than the NGU group, but not when the sexual activity of the two groups was comparable (reviewed by McCormack et al.[28]). Moreover, the serum antibody response to *U. urealyticum* in NGU has not been as impressive as the antibody response to *C. trachomatis.*[10]

Other evidence, however, is consistent with a pathogenic role for *U. urealyticum.* When men with relatively few sex partners and no previous episodes of urethritis were studied, the rate of isolation and the concentration of *U. urealyticum* in first-voided urine were significantly greater in men with *C. trachomatis*–negative NGU than in those with *C. trachomatis*–positive NGU or in a comparison group without urethritis.[10] In that study, the comparison group without urethritis had actually had more sex partners than the other groups.[10] Results in other studies are shown in Table 60-3. Although cases were not stratified by history of urethritis or number of sex partners in some studies, *U. urealyticum* was isolated more often from *C. trachomatis*–negative than from *C. trachomatis*–positive NGU patients in many of these studies. Data compiled from three Seattle studies[10,11,18] showed that *U. urealyticum* was isolated significantly more often from men with a first episode of urethritis than from those who had had previous episodes or from men without urethritis.

The results of selective eradication of *U. urealyticum* also support a pathogenic role in NGU. Sulfonamides and rifampin are active against *C. trachomatis,* whereas spectinomycin and streptomycin are active against *U. urealyticum,* but not against *C. trachomatis.* In men whose cultures were *C. trachomatis*–negative but *U. urealyticum*–positive, the urethritis responded poorly to sulfonamides and rifampin.[10,18,19] Urethritis responded well to streptomycin or spectinomycin when *U. urealyticum* was eradicated, but not when *U. urealyticum* persisted.[18] In another study, Shepard, using suboptimal doses of doxycycline to treat patients with NGU, showed that with the disappearance of *U. urealyticum,* symptoms disappeared; with the reappearance of *U. urealyticum,* symptoms recurred.[29] Cultures for *C. trachomatis* were not performed in this study, however. In yet another study, NGU persisted 6 to 12 days after onset of minocycline therapy significantly more often in men infected with tetracycline-resistant *U. urealyticum* than in those infected with tetracycline-sensitive *U. urealyticum,* and persistent NGU correlated with persistence of the tetracycline-resistant strains.[30] Root et al. also demonstrated that there was a strong correlation between the tetracycline resistance of *U. urealyticum* and the persistence of *U. urealyticum* after tetracycline treatment.[31]

Intraurethral inoculation of *U. urealyticum* has been performed in two men and several nonhuman primates. The first man developed dysuria and frequency of urination, associated with pyuria and positive cultures for *U. urealyticum.*[32] Symptoms and signs disappeared with eradication of the *U. urealyticum* by minocycline. The second man developed polymorphonuclear leukocyte (PMNL)–containing mucus threads in his urine, which persisted after minocycline treatment despite the eradication of *U. urealyticum.*[32] Intraurethral inoculation of *U. urealyticum* into nonhuman primates has resulted in colonization of the urethra for various periods of time, and it has been associated with increased numbers of PMNL in the endourethral smear in some animals.[33,34]

There are at least 14 serovars of *U. urealyticum*[35] of which perhaps only one or several produce urethritis. Shepard and Lunceford found serovar 4 in 52 percent of 122 isolates from men with NGU, compared with 25 percent of 125 isolates from asymptomatic, but not necessarily normal, men.[36] Other data indicated

Table 60-3. Recovery of *C. trachomatis* (C) and *U. urealyticum* (U) from Men with NGU

Country	Investigator	Year	C+U+	C+U−	C−U+	C−U−	Number	Reference
U.S.A.	Holmes et al.	1975	29 (26)*	19 (17)	41 (36)	24 (21)	113	17
U.K.	Prentice et al.	1976	9 (11)	16 (20)	38 (47)	18 (22)	81	42
U.S.A.	Bowie et al.	1976	21 (23)	15 (16)	42 (46)	13 (14)	91	18
U.S.A.	Bowie et al.	1977	11 (16)	15 (22)	35 (51)	8 (12)	69	10
U.S.A.	Wong et al.	1977	4 (13)	8 (27)	12 (40)	6 (20)	30	62
Finland	Paavonen et al.	1978	11 (15)	28 (37)	10 (13)	26 (35)	75	24
U.S.A.	Bowie et al.	1978	38 (18)	40 (19)	87 (41)	46 (22)	211	120
U.K.	Coufalik et al.	1979	58 (27)	35 (16)	70 (32)	54 (25)	217	19
U.K.	Taylor-Robinson et al.	1979	138 (19)	125 (17)	246 (34)	217 (30)	726	74
Canada	Bowie et al.	1980	22 (11)	58 (29)	73 (37)	47 (24)	200	26
U.S.A.	Root et al.	1980	8 (8)	11 (11)	50 (52)	27 (28)	96	31
Canada	Romanowski et al.	1993	32 (21)	14 (9)	48 (33)	55 (37)	149	92

* Number in subgroup (percent of total study).

that *U. urealyticum* serovar 4 was frequently associated with asymptomatic pyuria as well.[36] However, while some groups have also demonstrated an association of urethritis with serovar 4,[37] others have not.[38,39]

In contrast to the strong association between PGU and *C. trachomatis,* the association between PGU and *U. urealyticum* is weak. Among *C. trachomatis*–negative men with gonorrhea who received treatment with penicillins, which are not active against *U. urealyticum,* PGU developed in 11 (61 percent) of 18 who had *U. urealyticum,* compared with 5 (28 percent) of 18 without *U. urealyticum* infection ($p = .09$).[40] In two other studies involving cultures for *C. trachomatis and U. urealyticum, U. urealyticum* was not shown to be associated with PGU.[17,41]

The accumulated evidence cited above is consistent with a role for *U. urealyticum* as a urethral pathogen, but it does not prove that *U. urealyticum* is a cause of urethritis, it does not establish what proportion of urethritis cases can be attributed to this agent, and it does not resolve the question as to why colonization with *U. urealyticum* so often occurs without apparent urethritis. It is possible that only certain strains may produce urethritis, that urethritis occurs predominantly on first exposure to *U. urealyticum,* that only a proportion of men colonized by *U. urealyticum* are susceptible to development of urethritis, or that urethritis produced by *U. urealyticum* is frequently subclinical and self-limited.

Other causes of NGU

Even if both *C. trachomatis* and *U. urealyticum* are etiologic agents in NGU, neither organism can be isolated from 30 to 50 percent of heterosexual men with NGU (see Table 60–3). Moreover, this is true of the majority of homosexual men with NGU.[11]

The observation that *C. trachomatis*–negative, *U. urealyticum*–negative men responded least well to therapy with a tetracycline is consistent with a different etiology in these men. Of 46 such men, NGU persisted or recurred within 6 weeks after initiation of minocycline therapy in 24, or 52 percent.[11] All but 1 of these 24 men actually improved during minocycline therapy but subsequently had recurrent NGU soon after stopping therapy. This failure rate was significantly greater than that for men from whom *C. trachomatis* or *U. urealyticum* was initially isolated. Prentice et al. also found that men from whom neither organism was initially isolated showed good responses to treatment on short-term follow-up.[42] This initial response to therapy is consistent with but does not prove a bacterial or mycoplasmal etiology of *C. trachomatis*–negative, *U. urealyticum*–negative NGU.

Most other studies of the aerobic and anaerobic urethral flora have not yet revealed significant differences between *C. trachomatis*–positive and *C. trachomatis*–negative patients with NGU.[43,44] Early studies suggested a possible role for *Bacteroides ureolyticus,*[45,46] but more recent work has not demonstrated this organism more frequently among men with NGU than among normal men.[47] *Haemophilus influenzae* and *Haemophilus parainfluenzae* appear to cause urethritis infrequently.[48,49] Similarly, coliforms may cause a few cases of urethritis in homosexual men.[50] *N. meningitidis,* in particular, has been reported as a cause of urethritis relatively more often in areas such as western Europe, as the incidence of gonorrhea has dropped to very low levels. Today men with urethral smears positive for gram-negative diplococci in these countries may be relatively likely to have an infection caused by this organism, (*Staphylococcus saprophyticus*[44,54,55] and *Corynebacterium genitalium* type I[55,56]) in view of the rarity of *N. gonorrhoeae.*[51,52] Other organisms (*Haemophilus equigenitalis,* the agent of contagious equine metritis[53]), have been proposed as potential causes of NGU, but their role has so far been assessed only by one group or it has not been confirmed by other groups.

Mycoplasma genitalium was first implicated as a cause of NGU in 1981.[57] Further understanding of the role of this organism had to await the advent of modern DNA amplification technology, as this organism remains extremely difficult to isolate. Recent studies using the polymerase chain reaction assay have shown that *M. genitalium* is present in as many as 25 percent of men with NGU,[58,59] but it is present in only 6 percent of normal men.[60] These studies do not prove a causal relationship between this organism and NGU, but the consistency of the observations between centers is strongly supportive. So far *M. genitalium* has not been implicated as a cause of invasive or upper genital tract disease in either men or women, but further studies are needed.

Urethritis occurs in approximately 30 percent of men with primary genital herpes simplex virus (HSV) infection and in a much lower percentage of men with recurrent genital HSV infection.[61] Most, but not all, such patients have penile lesions. In comparative studies, however, HSV was not isolated at higher frequency from the urethra of men with NGU than from controls.[17,62] In one of these studies, HSV was isolated from 2 percent of 115 men with NGU, 6 percent of 53 men with gonorrhea, and 3 percent of 62 men without urethritis.[17] Cytomegalovirus was not isolated from the urethra from any of 60 men with NGU, 28 men with gonorrhea, or 20 men without urethritis.[17] Multiple other attempts to isolate viruses from men with NGU have been unrewarding, although adenoviruses have repeatedly been isolated from men with urethritis in Perth, Australia.[63]

Trichomonas vaginalis has been implicated in a surprisingly high proportion of NGU cases in the former Soviet Union, India, and Africa and in a few surveys done in South America. This has not been the experience in most European countries or in North America. It remains possible that there are regional differences in the role of *T. vaginalis* in NGU. Future studies of the etiology of NGU in countries that report high rates of documented *T. vaginalis* should employ simultaneous cultures for both *T. vaginalis* and *C. trachomatis.*

In four earlier North American studies, the proportion of cases of NGU in which *T. vaginalis* was detected was small.[17,44,62,64] In one of these, however, 9 (11 percent) of 85 men with NGU demonstrated seroconversion or increased indirect hemagglutination titers to *T. vaginalis* ($\geq 1:80$) in paired sera.[64] More recently, using cultures of both the urethra and a first-voided urine sample, Krieger et al. found that 18 percent of men with NGU in Seattle had trichomonas,[65] and that trichomoniasis was indeed associated with NGU.

In three studies of NGU,[17,44,62] yeasts were rarely detected. Therefore, although some men with candidal balanitis have symptoms of urethritis, *Candida* sp. are not a frequent cause of NGU.

Nonsexually transmitted causes of NGU

The proportion of cases of NGU that are not sexually transmitted has not been defined since *C. trachomatis* was recognized as a cause of NGU. Bacterial urethritis may occur in association with urinary tract infection, bacterial prostatitis, urethral stricture, phimosis, and secondary to catheterization or other instrumentation of the urethra. Urethritis is also described with congenital abnormalities, chemical irritation, and tumors. Allergic etiologies have been postulated, but the supporting evidence is very meager. Similarly, there is no proof as yet that repeated stripping of the penis, masturbation, use of caffeine and alcohol, too little or too much sexual activity, or eating of certain foods will result in urethritis. Stevens-Johnson syndrome may produce urethritis (see Plate 3).

EPIDEMIOLOGY

As discussed in Chap. 4, the incidence of NGU has surpassed that of gonococcal urethritis in men in the United States, England, and Wales. To some extent the relative increase in number of cases of NGU over the past 25 to 30 years was probably related in part to improved recognition of NGU[66] and in part to an increased incidence of infection with the major causes of NGU. In individual STD clinics during the 1970s the relative proportion of cases of urethritis that were nongonococcal varied from 19 to 78 percent,[67] and on college campuses more than 85 percent of urethritis was nongonococcal.[68]

For both gonorrhea and NGU, the peak age group affected is 20 to 24 years, followed by 15 to 19 years, and then 25 to 29 years. Some characteristics of men with gonorrhea and NGU differ, but not to the extent that the differences are diagnostic in individual cases. In a comparison between 113 men with NGU and 69 men with urethral gonorrhea, those with NGU were more often white, better educated, more likely to be students and less likely to be unemployed, members of a higher socioeconomic stratum, older at the age of first intercourse, and involved with fewer total sex partners.[17] Histories of previous gonorrhea were more frequent among men who had gonorrhea, while histories of NGU were more frequent among men with NGU.[17,69] There are no epidemiologic characteristics that will reliably separate *C. trachomatis*–positive and –negative NGU patients. Men with two or more previous episodes of NGU have a lower isolation rate of *C. trachomatis*[23] than those with one or no previous episode, but men with previous episodes of urethritis also have a lower isolation rate of *U. urealyticum*.[11]

INCUBATION PERIOD AND CLINICAL MANIFESTATIONS

COMPARISON BETWEEN GONORRHEA AND NGU

The symptoms and signs of gonococcal and nongonococcal urethritis differ quantitatively, but not qualitatively, so that in an individual case it is impossible to make an absolute distinction between the two on clinical grounds. Both may cause urethral discharge, dysuria, or urethral itching. Frequency, hematuria, and urgency are infrequent with either infection. In one study, 71 percent of 185 men with gonorrhea, but only 38 percent of 214 men with NGU, complained of both discharge and dysuria.[69] All but one man with urethral gonorrhea had urethral discharge, but 19 percent of men with NGU did not. Discharges are more profuse and usually purulent in men with gonorrhea but are generally scant and mucoid in men with NGU (see Plates 1 and 2). Especially with NGU, discharge may be detected only in the morning or noted as crusting at the meatus or as staining on underwear. Men with gonorrhea had a more abrupt onset and sought medical care sooner. More than three-fourths of the men who had gonorrhea, but less than one-half of those who had NGU, sought treatment within 4 days of onset of symptoms.[69] The usual incubation period is also shorter with gonorrhea. Gonorrhea usually develops 2 to 6 days after exposure, whereas NGU generally develops between 1 and 5 weeks after the likely time of acquisition of infection, with a peak at around 2 to 3 weeks. Longer incubation periods for both infections are seen, however, and a significant proportion of both groups of men remain asymptomatic.

In urethritis caused by HSV, dysuria is usually severe, the urethral discharge is scant relative to the severity of dysuria, and there may be localized urethral tenderness at the site of focal urethral ulceration. Regional lymphadenopathy and constitutional symptoms are common with primary HSV urethritis, probably even in the absence of penile lesions.

ASYMPTOMATIC URETHRAL INFECTION

The importance of asymptomatic urethral gonococcal and chlamydial infection cannot be overstressed. In the studies listed in Table 60-2, the rate of isolation of *C. trachomatis* was usually low in asymptomatic men seen in STD clinics. As noted above, however, high rates of asymptomatic infection have been documented. In three studies, *C. trachomatis* was isolated from 11 percent of asymptomatic soldiers, 11 percent of asymptomatic men attending an urban emergency department, and 7 percent of asymptomatic college students.[70–72] Just as with male partners of women with gonorrhea, male partners of chlamydia-infected women are at high risk of infection, and the infection is often asymptomatic. Among male contacts of infected women, Thelin et al. detected *N. gonorrhoeae* in 78 percent of male contacts of women with gonorrhea, and they detected *C. trachomatis* in 53 percent of male contacts of women with *C. trachomatis*.[73] Only 50 percent of the male partners infected with either organism were symptomatic.[73] The possibility of asymptomatic infection in the male partner should always be discussed with women who are being treated for proven or suspected chlamydial and gonococcal infections. Otherwise men who believe they cannot have an STD unless they have symptoms are not likely to seek therapy.

COMPARISON BETWEEN *C. TRACHOMATIS*–POSITIVE AND *C. TRACHOMATIS*–NEGATIVE NGU

In cases of NGU, a clinical distinction between a *C. trachomatis*–positive and a *C. trachomatis*–negative infection is not possible. Some investigators report that men whose *C. trachomatis* cultures are negative have more profuse and more purulent discharges,[10,17] but others have found the reverse.[23,74] In a study of men with and without NGU, *C. trachomatis* infection was associated with discharge but not dysuria, whereas *U. urealyticum* infection was associated with dysuria but not discharge.[62] However, in another study of symptomatic men with few or no PMNL on urethral smear, isolation of *U. urealyticum* did not correlate with symptoms of dysuria.[75] Given these discrepant results, clearly there are no clinical grounds for separating these two entities.

IMPORTANCE OF AN OPTIMAL EXAMINATION

When patients give a history of dysuria and/or urethral discharge but a discharge is not detected, the patient should be examined in the morning, after not voiding overnight, to enhance the likelihood of reaching a firm diagnosis.[76] In a study by Simmons in an STD clinic, 200 men with genitourinary symptoms in whom no firm diagnosis was made on the first visit were asked to return for reexamination in the morning prior to voiding. Among these men, 108 new infections were diagnosed; 5 had gonorrhea and 103 had NGU.[76]

Another study of symptomatic men with few or no PMNL on urethral smear also showed the value of repeat examination after a longer interval without voiding.[75] Furthermore, in that study, using pyuria as the criterion for urethritis, almost 80 percent of men with *C. trachomatis* had urethritis, whereas only one-third of symptomatic men without *C. trachomatis* had pyuria at the initial or on repeat visits.

OTHER MANIFESTATIONS OF URETHRITIS

Other manifestations of urethritis are unusual. A small proportion of patients with gonococcal or chlamydial urethritis will have conjunctivitis caused by *N. gonorrhoeae* or *C. trachomatis,* especially the latter, probably as a result of autoinoculation. Epididymitis develops infrequently today. Some patients with NGU present with Reiter's syndrome, or they develop it soon after their initial presentation. Inguinal lymphadenopathy is unusual, though it is occasionally seen in men with a severe inflammatory reaction to gonococcal urethritis. In the preantibiotic era it was said that prostatitis was a frequent complication of gonorrhea, but this is not the case today. In a study by Holmes et al.,[17] prostatic enlargement or tenderness was not significantly more common among patients with NGU (13 percent) than among those with gonorrhea or with no urethritis (4 percent). If present, it was always of minimal severity. Symptoms of hematuria, chills, fever, frequency, hesitancy, nocturia, urgency, perineal pain, scrotal masses, postvoid dribbling, or genital pain other than dysuria or urethral pain are not typical of urethritis; these suggest the presence of other genitourinary abnormalities such as classic urinary tract infection, acute prostatitis, a flare-up of chronic prostatitis, or acute epididymitis or orchitis.

DIAGNOSIS

The diagnosis of gonorrhea simply requires demonstration of *N. gonorrhoeae* by Gram stain, culture, or a reliable nonculture technique. In contrast, diagnosis of NGU requires not only exclusion of urethral infection with *N. gonorrhoeae* but also demonstration of the presence of urethritis based on the presence of an abnormal discharge and/or demonstration of PMNL in the urethral smear (Fig. 60-1, Table 60-4). Specific diagnostic tests for *C. trachomatis* are increasingly available (see Chaps. 28, 53, and 92), but there is no simple clinical or laboratory marker diagnostic of *C. trachomatis* or *U. urealyticum* infection. Rapid tests for the detection of *C. trachomatis* as a cause of urethritis thus far have proven to be insensitive (see Chaps. 53 and 92).

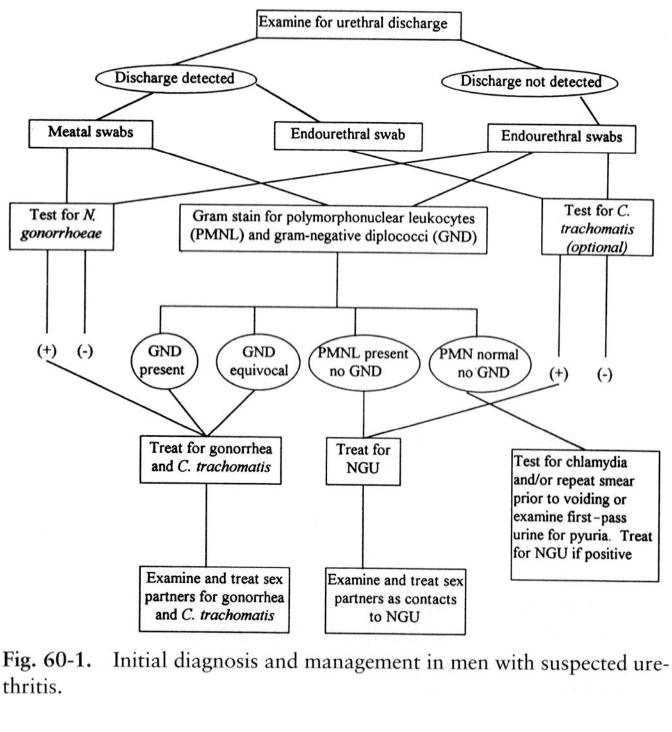

Fig. 60-1. Initial diagnosis and management in men with suspected urethritis.

CRITERIA FOR THE DIAGNOSIS OF URETHRITIS

For research purposes, the criteria used for diagnosis of urethritis have usually included presence of urethral discharge and of 20 or more PMNL in two or more of five random $\times 400$ microscopic fields of the sediment of the first 10 to 15 mL of urine collected when the patient has not voided for 4 h or longer.[10] These criteria are undoubtedly too restrictive. In a study of men with minimal or no discharge, there was a definite bimodal distribution of the numbers of PMNL in Gram-stained urethral specimens and in the first-voided urine; the presence of 15 or more PMNL in any of five random $\times 400$ microscopic fields of the sediment of the first-voided urine was correlated with a mean of more than four PMNL per field in five $\times 1000$ oil-immersion fields in Gram-stained specimens of urethral exudate, and either finding was regarded as abnormal.[77] Swartz et al. independently concluded that a mean of more than four PMNL per oil-immersion field on urethral smear correlated with urethritis.[43] In that study, there was more of a continuum from normal to abnormal.

Subsequent studies among symptomatic men with minimal or no urethral discharge show similarly strong correlations between the Gram stain and the first-voided urine sediment.[75] However, *C. trachomatis* was isolated from some men when neither the urethral Gram stain nor the first-voided urine sediment contained PMNL. In many other *C. trachomatis*–positive men, only the urine or the smear, but not both, showed increased PMNL. Isolation of *C. trachomatis* was more frequent from men with a urine positive for increased PMNL counts alone than from men with a positive smear alone. In another study, Root et al. noted that 7 of 18 *C. trachomatis*–positive men had five or fewer PMNL in "several representative fields" on urethral Gram stain.[31] Thus, use of smears or urines to provide objective evidence of urethritis is only a rough guide to the presence of urethral pathogens. Just as with gonorrhea, the inescapable conclusion is that a specific diagnostic test is necessary to exclude *C. trachomatis* infection in men with minimal or no evidence of urethritis.

Men who are symptomatic without objective evidence of urethritis (i.e., either discharge on examination or the presence of

Table 60-4. Management of Urethritis

1. Establish presence of urethritis
   a. Examine for urethral discharge
   b. Gram stain urethral discharge
   c. Reexamine if necessary in A.M. prior to voiding
2. Establish presence or absence of *N. gonorrhoeae*
   a. Gram stain
   b. Culture or nonculture test for *N. gonorrhoeae* if Gram stain is negative
3. Diagnostic test for *C. trachomatis*
4. If gonorrhea, treat with single-dose cefixime, 400 mg, or ciprofloxacin, 500 mg, or ofloxacin, 400 mg p.o.; or ceftriaxone, 125 mg IM, plus 7 days of doxycycline, 100 mg p.o. twice daily
5. If NGU, treat with 7 days of doxycycline, 100 mg p.o. twice daily, or azithromycin, 1 gm p.o. as a single dose
6. Evaluate and treat partner(s) appropriately—generally with same regimen used to treat the patient with urethritis, or guided by results of additional diagnostic tests.
7. Follow-up examinations (optional)
   a. 3–5 days after completing therapy with gonorrhea
   b. 2–4 weeks after completing therapy for NGU

PMNL in the stained urethral smear) should be reexamined in the morning without having voided overnight. The urethra should be stripped from the base to the meatus three or four times to detect urethral discharge. For Gram stain, any expressible urethral exudate can be obtained with a swab from the urethral meatus. When discharge is minimal or absent after an attempt to express discharge, a thin urethrogenital swab should be inserted 3 to 4 cm into the urethra. The patient should be warned that the procedure is moderately painful and that the next urination will also be painful. The swab is then rolled gently back and forth over a glass slide to cover an area of approximately 1 cm^2. The slide is then Gram-stained and scanned at a magnification of $\times 100$. Areas that have the largest numbers of PMNL are then examined under oil ($\times 1000$), and the number of PMNL in each of five such fields is recorded. While the PMNL are being enumerated, the slide should also be examined for gram-negative diplococci. For research purposes or for patients in whom the establishment of objective evidence of inflammatory urethritis is especially important (i.e., the male with recurrent urethritis), examination of a first-voided urine specimen is worthwhile. To detect PMNL in urine, the first 10 to 15 mL of urine voided should be collected and centrifuged at 400 *g* for 10 min. All but 0.5 mL of the supernatant is decanted, and the sediment is resuspended in the residual urine. Sufficient sediment is placed on a slide to cover an area of approximately 1 cm^2, and a coverslip is placed on the slide. The area under the coverslip is examined at a magnification of $\times 400$, and the number of PMNL in each of five randomly selected fields is enumerated.

LABORATORY DIFFERENTIATION BETWEEN GONORRHEA AND NGU

Although clinical suspicion that a patient with urethritis has either gonorrhea or NGU may be strong, the final distinction requires laboratory examination to determine if *N. gonorrhoeae* is present. The most rapid and least expensive procedure is microscopic examination of stained urethral exudate or material obtained with an endourethral swab. For experienced microscopists, the sensitivity, specificity, and positive predictive value of the finding of typical gram-negative diplococci inside the PMNL for the diagnosis of gonorrhea are close to 100 percent in men with urethritis (see Color Plate 91). A simple, one-step procedure using a stain such as methylene blue probably works equally well, though careful comparative studies have not been done. This procedure relies solely on morphologic characteristics, since color differences are not obtained with the single staining reagent. It should be noted, however, that in most clinical settings there is insufficient time to enumerate PMNL carefully in the urethral smear. Therefore, most clinicians accept the presence of any PMNL in smears from symptomatic men as adequate support for the diagnosis of NGU (see Color Plate 92). Thus, in a symptomatic case where the urethral smear contains increased numbers of PMNL, gonorrhea can be differentiated from NGU at the initial visit, and specific therapy can be given. Since the Gram stain misses up to 5 percent of gonococcal infections in men with urethritis under usual clinical circumstances, patients clinically diagnosed as having NGU on the basis of Gram stain should undergo further testing for *N. gonorrhoeae* if possible. Specific tests for the agents known to cause NGU will not influence therapeutic decisions at this point. When Gram-stained specimens are interpreted as being equivocal, with only extracellular typical or intracellular atypical gram-negative diplococci being detected, cultures for *N. gonorrhoeae* have been positive in 25 percent.[69] Such patients should be treated for gonorrhea (see Fig. 60-1), but cultures or DNA-based tests will establish the diagnosis definitively. Cultures are also necessary in cases that are positive by Gram stain when prior treatment has failed. The laboratory should be alerted that antibiotic resistance may be a problem, so that the organism can be referred to a laboratory able to perform susceptibility testing. Previously, it was frequently recommended to detect penicillin and tetracycline resistance. After treatment recommendations were changed to exclude the penicillins and tetracycline for treatment of gonorrhea, detection of resistance has become less of an issue; clinicians should know, however, that gonococci acquired in Asia are more likely to be resistant to the quinolones.[78] Additionally, in the United States a national surveillance system has been developed to provide consistent data on gonococcal resistance on a regular basis.

DETECTION OF *C. TRACHOMATIS* AND *U. UREALYTICUM*

Specific diagnosis of *C. trachomatis* urethritis requires culture or detection by one of the nonculture techniques (see Chaps. 29 and 92). While the diagnosis may be confirmed in some cases serologically, this approach is not practical.[10] Because *C. trachomatis* is an intracellular parasite of columnar epithelial cells, the preferable specimen is endourethral material rather than urethral exudate. In most circumstances, identification of *C. trachomatis* as the cause of NGU is not necessary, as an antibiotic therapy is the same for both chlamydia-positive and chlamydia-negative disease (see below). Furthermore, it is recommended that the partners of men with NGU be treated regardless of the etiology. As with the gonococcus, a specific diagnosis of *C. trachomatis* is useful for the purposes of surveillance, partner notification, and may be desired by some patients who wish to know the specific etiology of their disease.

DNA amplification techniques for identifying *C. trachomatis*[79,80] are more sensitive than culture for the detection of this organism. In fact, they are so sensitive that first-voided urine specimens may provide an adequate specimen.

Outside of research laboratories, cultures for *U. urealyticum* generally are not available. In men with obvious urethritis, the diagnostic yield of cultures for *U. urealyticum* from urethral swabs or first-voided urine is very similar. If urethritis is minimal or absent, an endourethral swab is preferable.[81] Because *U. urealyticum* is isolated from many men who have no urethritis,[27] however, isolation of this agent from a man with urethritis does not mean that it is causing the patient's symptoms. Hence, even if simple methods of detecting this organism were available, they would be of little practical use. Better correlations with disease are obtained when quantitative cultures in a liquid medium are performed, but such tests are obviously impractical in the usual clinical setting.

THERAPY

In many parts of the world, and in many smaller public-health and primary-care clinics, specific diagnostic tests for urethral pathogens are not available. Unfortunately, as noted previously, the clinical presentation is not adequately specific to differentiate between the causative organisms. In these circumstances, treatment should be based on the pathogens most likely to result in long-term sequelae, namely *N. gonorrhoeae* and *C. trachomatis*. While this approach seems intuitively correct, clinicians in the past frequently attempted to provide specific therapy based on their clinical impressions. In many cases, this resulted in inadequate treatment and continued chronic infection with one pathogen or the other. Recently, increased emphasis has been placed on "syndromic management" of STDs as an alternative to specific disease treatment, particularly in resource-poor settings (see Chaps. 48 and 102). In a recent study of syndromic management of all STD syndromes, this approach decreased rates of HIV transmission.[82]

In the case of male urethritis, syndromic management is relatively straight forward. Therapy for *N. gonorrhoeae* is best provided by single-dose oral therapy with certain oral cephalosporins or quinolones.[83] Among the oral cephalosporins, the best choice for gonorrhea is cefixime, 400 mg. The two recommended quinolones for this indication in the United States are ciprofloxacin, 500 mg, and ofloxacin, 400 mg. There are several other oral cephalosporins and quinolones that are also effective in single doses, but in the United States there is less experience with these drugs than with the recommended regimens. Ceftriaxone given as a single 125-mg intramuscular dose is also highly effective for gonococcal urethritis, but intramuscular administration is inconvenient and relatively expensive, since additional supplies and personnel time are required. Spectinomycin, 2 gm intramuscularly, remains very effective but has been largely supplanted by the quinolones for treating the patient allergic to the beta-lactam antibiotic class.

Tetracycline and doxycycline have been used most commonly as the antichlamydial component of dual-drug combinations for the syndromic management of male urethritis. Doxycycline is easier to comply with as it is administered as two daily 100-mg doses with food, if desired, in contrast to tetracycline, which must be taken as 500 mg four times daily on an empty stomach. Alternatives to doxycycline or tetracycline that could be included as part of dual-treatment regimens are erythromycin, four times daily for a week, and azithromycin, 1 gm orally as a single dose. There are few studies of dual-antibiotic therapy of urethritis, probably because there is little reason to doubt the efficacy of drugs already proven to be useful for treating *N. gonorrhoeae* and *C. trachomatis* infections individually. More data on tolerance would be helpful, though experience would suggest that significant increases in adverse events have not been a problem. The combination of cefixime, 400 mg orally, and azithromycin, 1 gm orally, given together for the treatment of gonococcal urethritis has been evaluated only in one small pilot study; a relatively high rate of gastrointestinal toxicity was noted (HH Handsfield, personal communication).

Two drugs currently are approved in the United States for the treatment of both *N. gonorrhoeae* and *C. trachomatis*. Ofloxacin, 400 mg followed by 300 mg bid to complete a seven-day course, is effective for both organisms, as is azithromycin, 2 gm as a single dose. However, the cost of these regimens is significantly higher than the cost of any of the recommended single-dose treatments for gonorrhea combined with fourteen doxycycline tablets. Furthermore, the single 2-gm dose of azithromycin frequently causes gastrointestinal side effects.[84]

It should be remembered that empiric dual-antibiotic therapy of urethritis in males requires that sex partners also be treated empirically for both organisms.

TREATMENT OF GONOCOCCAL URETHRITIS

Since the late 1980s STD treatment guidelines from the Centers for Disease Control and Prevention (CDC) have recommended dual-antibiotic therapy of men with gonococcal urethritis as discussed above for the syndromic management of urethritis. The primary rationale for this approach is that *C. trachomatis* is found in 15 to 40 percent of women with endocervical gonorrhea and 15 to 25 percent of men with gonococcal urethritis. Providing effective therapy for *C. trachomatis* in these patients eliminates the major cause of postgonococcal urethritis and also eliminates a number of potential male carriers of *C. trachomatis* who would otherwise disseminate the organism to future sex partners. The hypothesis that this approach benefits society as a whole by decreasing the population prevalence of *C. trachomatis* seems very reasonable, but it has never been tested specifically. Nonetheless, decreases in the prevalence of *C. trachomatis* in the United States over the past 10 years suggests that this policy may have had the desired effect, though it is not possible to separate the individual effects of a variety of public-health measures designed to control chlamydial infections that were also instituted during this time. Another potential benefit is that dual-antibiotic therapy with two drugs active against *N. gonorrhoeae* may slow the development of antibiotic resistance.

Arguments against dual therapy include increased cost and higher adverse event rates. Since the added cost of doxycycline is small and experience does not suggest substantial increases in toxicity rates, on balance the arguments favor dual-antibiotic therapy for gonococcal urethritis in males. In areas such as western Europe, where the incidence of both gonorrhea and chlamydial infections have decreased dramatically in the past decade, the argument for dual therapy becomes less compelling.

TREATMENT OF NGU

Results of treatment for NGU are not as good as for gonorrhea, even though almost every antimicrobial in clinical usage has been tried. In the 1950s tetracyclines, erythromycin, and a combination of sulfonamides and aminocylitols were recognized as being the most effective therapy. The basis for these observations has been clarified by subsequent research, because all three regimens are capable of eradicating *C. trachomatis*[10,18,20,85] and because tetracycline and erythromycin are also active against most strains of *U. urealyticum,* while spectinomycin eradicates *U. urealyticum* from the urethras of 60 to 70 percent of men.[10] Current recommendations for initial treatment of a previously untreated episode of NGU are to use doxycycline, 100 mg orally twice daily, or azithromycin 1 gm as a single dose.[13,83] A 1-gm powdered dose of azithromycin specifically formulated for treating STDs is available. The advantage of this dose form is that it is significantly cheaper than four 250-mg capsules. Alternative choices are 7 days of erythromycin base or stearate, 500 mg orally four times daily, or erythromycin ethylsuccinate, 800 mg orally four times daily, though the gastrointestinal tolerance of these regimens is poor. An empiric approach to this problem is to give half the recommended dose over a period of 2 weeks.

Anticipated response to 1 week of treatment with a tetracycline

In compliant patients who are not reexposed to new or untreated partners, all but approximately 5 percent of men will show definite and often total improvement by the end of treatment. Among men who initially respond and are followed for 4 to 6 weeks posttreatment, 30 to 35 percent will have recurrence or incomplete resolution of pyuria.[11] About one-half of these men will have symptoms of urethritis. Bowie et al. showed that the critical determinant of response was the etiology of the NGU rather than the amount of drug given or the duration of therapy.[11] Response to treatment was best in men infected with *C. trachomatis,* significantly worse in men infected with *U. urealyticum* alone, and significantly worse still in men from whom neither organism was initially isolated from urethral specimens. In contrast to these earlier results, more recent studies have not demonstrated any differences in clinical responses between men with and men without chlamydial infections.[13,86] In compliant patients, the high rates of recurrent or incomplete resolution of urethritis are not due to failure to eradicate *C. trachomatis.* A report of a "positive" posttreatment test for *C. trachomatis* should raise several considerations. With a nonculture test there is a considerable likelihood that the result is a false-positive. If it is felt to be a true-positive result, however, it is highly likely that the patient either did not take his medications or was reexposed to a new or untreated sexual partner. Tetracycline-resistant isolates of *C. trachomatis* have not yet been described. The situation is somewhat different with respect to *U. urealyticum,* where tetracycline resistance has been shown to account for a small proportion of treatment failures.[30]

Difficulties in assessment of treatment for NGU

Although many studies of treatment of NGU have been performed, an optimal drug, dosage, and duration of therapy has not been clearly established. Tetracycline regimens reported to be efficacious range from a single 300-mg dose of doxycycline to 21 days of tetracycline or minocycline. However, assessment of the reported efficacy of various antimicrobial regimens is often difficult because (1) until the mid-1970s most studies did not employ cultures for both *C. trachomatis* and *U. urealyticum,* (2) *C. trachomatis*–positive NGU may respond differently from *C. trachomatis*–negative NGU, (3) manifestations may spontaneously disappear in some cases even without specific therapy, (4) patients frequently remain sexually active so that relapse cannot be distinguished from reinfection, (5) patients frequently default, (6) the appropriate duration of follow-up assessment of results is debatable, (7) eradication of *C. trachomatis* and *U. urealyticum* does not ensure a lasting clinical cure, and (8) investigators have used different criteria to define a clinical cure. For example, most studies have used persistence of PMNL in either the first-voided urine specimen or in urethral secretions to define clinical treatment failures. The problem is that investigators have used different cell counts in their definitions, and the methods of counting and averaging cells also have varied considerably.

Duration of therapy

With short-term follow-up, tetracycline therapy has been consistently more effective than placebo.[20,42,87,88] A few investigators have concluded that longer courses of antimicrobial therapy are more effective than shorter courses.[87,89,90] Holmes et al. showed that a 7-day course of tetracycline was more effective than a 4-day course,[87] and in an unblinded study John showed that 21 days were better than 10 days, which in turn were better than 5 days.[89] Thambar et al. concluded that 3 weeks of triple tetracycline was better than 1 week of therapy, but patients on the longer regimen had a much shorter follow-up after cessation of therapy—a critical problem, as discussed below.[90] In contrast to these studies, others have not found a significant difference with longer courses of therapy.[11,88,91] Grimble and Amarasuriya did not show any marked differences between results with 4- to 10-day regimens of several different tetracyclines.[88] Helmy and Fowler had essentially identical results in a double-blind comparison between tetracycline, 500 mg four times daily for 7 days, and 250 mg four times daily for 14 days, and the results were also similar to those of unblinded treatment with 4- and 21-day regimens.[91] A double-blind comparison of two doses and two durations of minocycline has been performed in a study that included cultures for *C. trachomatis* and *U. urealyticum.*[11] Overall, persistent or recurrent NGU within 6 weeks of initiation of therapy was seen in 32 percent of men. Prolonging therapy from 7 to 21 days delayed, but did not diminish, the rate of recurrence, and the use of 100 mg daily gave results that were as good as those obtained with twice-daily treatment. A subsequent study showed that 250 mg of tetracycline four times daily for 7 days was as effective as 500 mg of tetracycline four times daily for 7 days in eradicating both *C. trachomatis* and *U. urealyticum* and in treating NGU.[26] More recently, it has been shown that minocycline, 100 mg nightly for 7 days, was equal to doxycycline, 100 mg twice daily for 7 days, for the treatment of NGU.[92] Whether regimens employing a tetracycline for less than 7 days would be effective for eradicating *C. trachomatis* and *U. urealyticum,* and for producing similar clinical responses in NGU, requires further study, but the weight of evidence argues strongly against treating for more than 7 days in the usual case.

Use of antimicrobials other than tetracyclines for NGU

Martin et al. clearly demonstrated the efficacy of azithromycin, 1 gm orally as a single dose, for uncomplicated chlamydial infections in women and men, including those with NGU.[93] Two small unblinded studies suggested that single-dose azithromycin would be effective also for chlamydia-negative NGU.[94,95] In a large randomized double-blind study of men with NGU regardless of etiology, Stamm et al. showed that the 1 gm dose of azithromycin was equivalent to doxycycline, 100 mg twice daily for 7 days.[13] In this study, both chlamydia-positive and -negative cases did equally well with azithromycin. Azithromycin is a proprietary drug and therefore costs more than even multiple doses of doxycycline, but the advantage with this drug is that directly observed therapy can be given, thereby guaranteeing compliance.

Less experience is available with other antimicrobials. Erythromycin stearate, 500 mg twice daily for 2 weeks, effectively eliminated *C. trachomatis*[84] and should also be active against *U. urealyticum.* Erythromycin stearate, 500 mg four times daily for 7 days (or equivalent doses of other forms of erythromycin), should also be effective. Erythromycin stearate, 250 mg four times daily for 7 days, resulted in failure to eradicate *C. trachomatis* from one-third of men with chlamydial urethritis.[75] Trimethoprim-sulfamethoxazole is active but not synergistic against *C. trachomatis*[96] and is not active against *U. urealyticum.* Several of the new quinolones, especially ciprofloxacin and ofloxacin, have in vitro activity against *C. trachomatis,* with quite variable activity against genital mycoplasmas.[97] Norfloxacin has no activity in vivo against *C. trachomatis.*[98] Clinically, ciprofloxacin has been associated with frequent treatment failures in men with chlamydia-positive NGU,[99,100] while ofloxacin, 200 to 300 mg twice daily for 7 days, has proven to be effective.[101,102]

Treatment of sex partners

As part of the management of urethritis, every attempt should be made to evaluate and treat the patient's sex partner(s). This procedure is widely accepted for partners of men with either gonorrhea or chlamydial infection, and it is equally appropriate for partners of men with NGU. Though it has not been clearly demonstrated that treatment of the partner diminishes the rate of recurrence of NGU in men, female partners need treatment for their own benefit. *C. trachomatis* is isolated from 30 to 60 percent of the female partners of men with gonococcal or nongonococcal urethritis[9,17,20,22,25,74] and has important sequelae in women (see Chaps. 29 and 58).[9] Furthermore, infected women (and men) constitute a major undiagnosed and untreated reservoir of *C. tracho-*

matis infection; ultimate control of *C. trachomatis* infection is unlikely to be achieved without reduction of this reservoir of infection. In general, the same regimens used to treat males with urethritis can be used to treat their female partners, though the tetracyclines should be avoided in pregnant women.

Management of recurrent or persistent NGU

Management of men with recurrent symptomatic NGU represents one of the most difficult problems in venereology. The median time for such recurrences is about 2 weeks after completing therapy.[11] Most men with recurrences of NGU are culture-negative for both *C. trachomatis* and *U. urealyticum*. However, some recurrences after intercourse with untreated partners are *C. trachomatis*–positive, particularly if the recurrent urethritis develops more than a few weeks after treatment. The initial step in management requires that the presence of urethritis again be documented by examining urethral secretions for the presence of PMNL to exclude patients with functional complaints or other disorders. This point cannot be overemphasized, because many men receive multiple courses of antibiotics for symptoms of recurrent urethritis even though they have no objective evidence of an ongoing inflammatory process. The patient should be questioned about compliance and unprotected sexual intercourse. When an exudate is present, it should be examined for *T. vaginalis* by culture, if available. Kreiger et al. recently pointed out that sensitivity is significantly enhanced by culturing both urethral secretions obtained by a swab and the sediment of a first-voided urine specimen.[65] Unfortunately, trichomonas culture is not a commonly available laboratory test and is likely to be less available in the future under managed care. In the absence of culture, trichomonas can be sought by mixing a drop of exudate with saline solution and looking for motile organisms. In persistent (as opposed to recurrent) NGU, the possibility of herpes simplex virus urethritis should be considered. Primary HSV urethritis typically lasts about 2 weeks. Urethral foreign bodies, periurethral fistula, and abscess should be excluded by palpation. Cultures or nonculture tests for *N. gonorrhoeae* and *C. trachomatis* should be repeated at least once. No firm guidelines for retreatment can be offered, since the cause of recurrent NGU is usually unknown. Since tetracycline-resistant *U. urealyticum* is a cause of persistent urethritis, however, treatment with a 1-week course of erythromycin, 500 mg four times daily, is reasonable if no other cause is detected at the time of examination. Such a regimen would also be expected to eradicate *C. trachomatis* should the patient have been reinfected with this organism. If both the male and his female partner have taken their initial course of therapy correctly, the partner usually is not re-treated unless the man is proven to have a chlamydial, gonococcal, or trichomonal infection as a cause of the recurrence. There is no established benefit to treating female partners if the male has only *U. urealyticum* or does not have any identifiable pathogen.

Most men will improve again on the second course of therapy, but approximately 30 percent will have further recurrences of symptoms. At this point, if the patient again can be demonstrated to have an inflammatory exudate, there are several considerations. If the second round of chlamydial and gonococcal cultures were negative, further studies for these organisms should not be done. Trichomoniasis remains a possibility, especially if nothing more than a wet prep examination of urethral secretions was done earlier, given the fact that this is an insensitive study.[65] Further attempts to document the presence of this organism should be pursued, including evaluation of the female partner. In the absence of sensitive cultures for *T. vaginalis,* an empiric trial of metronidazole, 2 gm as a single dose, would be reasonable at this point. If the patient again fails treatment and again Gram stain of urethral secretions shows PMNL, is there any value of further treatment? Hooton et al. suggested that a 3-week course of erythromycin, 500 mg four times daily, may be of benefit.[103] They found evidence of prostatic inflammation in many of these men, and it was this group that benefited most from treatment. Nonetheless, relapse rates were high. Men with inflammatory urethritis that persists after the above treatment approaches have been tried should be evaluated by a urologist who is experienced in dealing with such patients. The urologist should be made aware of the details of the patient's workup in order to avoid unnecessarily repeating expensive cultures and, more important, to avoid further empiric antibiotic trials. After urologic evaluation has ruled out anatomic problems (as it usually does[104]), whether or not chronic suppressive antibiotic therapy is justified is unknown. The best advice is not to treat further but to reassure the patient, using the counseling points listed below, and to follow. Many cases will resolve spontaneously over time.

The following issues should be discussed with the patient:

1. The likelihood of long-term sequelae such as infertility or cancer appears to be exceedingly low even in men who have recurrent urethritis after two therapeutic courses.
2. The risk of transmission of disease to partners is exceedingly low because these men do not have ongoing *C. trachomatis* infection, and other pathogens are usually not identified or are not important causes of sequelae in women.
3. Even if no treatment were given, symptoms would likely disappear over time in most of these men.
4. If the man has an ongoing monogamous sexual relationship (and which also holds true for the partner), there is no need for further treatment of the partner if both have received an initial course of therapy active against *C. trachomatis.*
5. Most of these recurrences will arise independent of resumption of sexual activity, and these recurrences do not mean that the partner has been "unfaithful."
6. Persistent or recurrent urethritis is not a presentation suggestive of AIDS.
7. Finally, as part of a general discussion with patients who have a sexually transmitted disease, men should be warned that one episode of urethritis does not provide immunity to subsequent episodes.

It should be noted that many patients complaining of persistent or recurrent symptoms of urethritis after treatment for a documented episode do not have any evidence of an inflammatory process, even after a careful search. In the authors' experience these are often well-educated men who are very health conscious, sometimes to the point of obsessiveness. Not infrequently this problem develops in a monogamous man who originally acquired a documented episode of urethritis following an illicit sexual encounter, suggesting that unresolved guilt feelings are contributing to the problem. Since most physicians simply represcribe antibiotics without attempting to document the presence or absence of an inflammatory process, the specialist often sees such patients after they have received many courses of a variety of drugs. These patients may benefit from a urological examination as much for reassurance as for anything else, though a urethral stricture may occasionally be discovered. The important point is that, rather than launching into a prolonged series of evaluations and empiric therapies as recommended above for the patient with documented inflammatory disease, counseling should be initiated early in the course for the patient with symptoms but without objective evidence of urethritis.

PROGNOSIS

Although frequent in the preantimicrobial era, local complications of urethral gonorrhea are now unusual in developed countries. Epididymitis occurs in 1 to 2 percent, seminal vesiculitis is rare, and prostatitis and prostatic abscess are almost never seen. Other unusual complications include abscess of Tyson's glands, penile edema secondary to dorsal lymphangitis or thrombophlebitis, inflammation of the urethral wall including periurethral abscesses and fistula, and regional lymphadenitis. Urethral strictures secondary to urethritis rarely occur now in the developed countries but remain significant problems in certain areas of the world. Other complications include inflammation of other sites concurrently infected—for example, the rectum—and disseminated gonococcal infection. NGU is generally a self-limited disease, and even without therapy the physical consequences to the individual are slight. One to 2 percent of both *C. trachomatis*–positive and *C. trachomatis*–negative men with NGU develop epididymitis, and another 1 to 2 percent develop conjunctivitis.[74] Urethritis is a manifestation of Reiter's syndrome, but it is unclear how frequently Reiter's syndrome develops as a consequence of NGU. Two studies indicate that the rate of development of Reiter's syndrome is not high in HLA-B27-positive men after initiation of therapy with a tetracycline for *C. trachomatis*–positive or *C. trachomatis*–negative NGU.[105,106] In one of the studies, however, men who were positive for *C. trachomatis* had more reactive arthritis than men who were chlamydia-negative.[105] Although approximately 20 percent of men with NGU have an increased number of PMNL in expressed prostatic secretions,[17] development of overt prostatitis is rare. In contrast to the infrequent physical consequences, the psychological impact of persistent urethritis or frequent recurrences of urethritis may be great. A thorough discussion of the issues mentioned above will usually greatly alleviate this distress.

PREVENTION

Preventive measures offered by health-care deliverers and health departments should include (1) the adequate recognition and treatment of patients with sexually transmitted diseases, (2) treatment of gonorrhea with regimens that will eradicate *C. trachomatis,* (3) improved contact-tracing to detect and treat partners exposed to either *N. gonorrhoeae* or *C. trachomatis* infection, and (4) increased availability of adequate diagnostic tests, especially for asymptomatic *C. trachomatis* infection. Urine-based diagnostic tests are now available. These tests are useful for screening hard-to-reach asymptomatic populations such as adolescents who are unlikely to attend a clinic for screening by one of the conventional tests. One hopes that the resources can be found to support the widespread application of this approach, which could lead eventually to control of chlamydial infections. Although much progress has been made in understanding the immunobiology of these infections, effective vaccines are not presently available.

A sexually active male can take several preventive measures. He can choose his partner carefully, avoid multiple partners, use a condom, or take prophylactic antimicrobials. There is no way that one can determine by intuition that a prospective new partner is free of genital pathogens. Proper use of a condom diminishes acquisition and transmission of many sexually transmitted diseases. Prophylactic antimicrobials are partially efficacious for prevention of urethritis (for example, 200 mg of minocycline or doxycycline soon after intercourse),[107] but use of prophylactic antimicrobials for relatively benign and easily treated infections cannot be justified.

References

1 Shepard MC: The recovery of pleuropneumonia-like organisms from Negro men with and without nongonococcal urethritis. *Am J Syph Gonorrhea Vener Dis* 38:113, 1954.

2 Gordon FB, Quan AL: Isolation of the trachoma agent in cell culture. *Proc Soc Exp Biol Med* 118:354, 1965.

3 Handsfield HH et al: Asymptomatic gonorrhea in men: diagnosis, natural course, prevalence, and significance. *N Engl J Med* 290:117, 1974.

4 Grosskurth H, et al. Asymptomatic gonorrhea and chlamydial infection in rural Tanzanian men. *BMJ* 312:277, 1996.

5 Crawford et al: Asymptomatic gonorrhea in men: Caused by gonococci with unique nutritional requirements. *Science* 196:1352, 1977.

6 Rice RJ et al: Chromosomally mediated resistance in *Neisseria gonorrhoeae* in the United States: Results of surveillance and reporting, 1983–84. *J Infect Dis* 153:340, 1986.

7 Knapp JS et al: Frequency and distribution in the United States of strains of *Neisseria gonorrhoeae* with plasmid-mediated, high level resistance to tetracycline. *J Infect Dis* 155:819, 1987.

8 Tapsall JW et al: Quinolone-resistant *Neisseria gonorrhoeae* isolated in Sydney, Australia, 1991 to 1995. *Sex Trans Dis* 23:425, 1996.

9 Anonymous: Resistance to gonococci isolated in the WHO Western Pacific Region to various antimicrobials used in the treatment of gonorrhea, 1 January–31 December 1994. *Communicable Diseases Intelligence* 19:495, 1995.

10 Bowie WR et al: Etiology of nongonococcal urethritis. Evidence for *Chlamydia trachomatis* and *Ureaplasma urealyticum. J Clin Invest* 59:735, 1977.

11 Bowie WR et al: Therapy for nongonococcal urethritis: Double-blind randomized comparison of two doses and two durations of minocycline therapy for nongonococcal urethritis. *Ann Intern Med* 95: 306, 1981.

12 Rodriguez-Pichardo A et al: Sexually transmitted diseases in homosexual males in Seville, Spain. *Genitourin Med* 67:335, 1991.

13 Stamm WE et al: Azithromycin for empirical treatment of nongonococcal urethritis syndrome in men: A randomized double-blind study. *JAMA* 274:545, 1995.

14 Jones RB: Treatment of *Chlamydia trachomatis* infections of the urogenital tract, in *Chlamydia Infections: Proceedings of the Seventh International Symposium on Human Chlamydial Infections,* WR Bowie, HD Caldwell, RP Jones (eds). Cambridge, UK, Cambridge University Press, 1990, pp. 490–518.

15 Britton TF et al: STDs and family planning: A regional program for chlamydia control that works. *Am J Gynecol Health* 6:24, 1992.

16 Patrick DM, Bowie WR: The epidemiology of *Chlamydia trachomatis* infection in British Columbia, in *Chlamydial Infections. Proceedings of the Eighth International Symposium on Human Chlamydial Infections,* J Orfila, GI Byrne, MA Chernesky, et al (eds). Bologna, Italy, Societa Editrice Escalapio, 1996.

17 Holmes KK et al: Etiology of nongonococcal urethritis. *N Engl J Med* 292:1199, 1975.

18 Bowie WR et al: Differential response to chlamydial and ureaplasma-associated urethritis to sulfafurazole (sulfisoxazole) and aminocyclitols. *Lancet* 2:1276, 1976.

19 Coufalik ED et al: Treatment of nongonococcal urethritis with rifampicin as a means of defining the role of *Ureaplasma urealyticum. Br J Vener Dis* 55:36, 1979.

20 Handsfield HH et al: Differences in the therapeutic response of chlamydia-positive and chlamydia-negative forms of nongonococcal urethritis. *J Am Vener Dis Assoc* 2:5, 1976.

21 DiGiacomo RF et al: Chlamydial infections of the male baboon urethra. *Br J Vener Dis* 51:310, 1975.

22 Oriel JD et al: Chlamydial infection: Isolation of chlamydia from

patients with non-specific genital infection. *Br J Vener Dis* 48:429, 1972.

23 Alani MD et al: Isolation of *Chlamydia trachomatis* from the male urethra. *Br J Vener Dis* 53:88, 1977.

24 Paavonen J et al: Examination of men with nongonococcal urethritis and their sexual partners for *Chlamydia trachomatis* and *Ureaplasma urealyticum*. *Sex Transm Dis* 5:93, 1978.

25 Lassus A et al: Erythromycin and lymecycline treatment in *Chlamydia*-positive and *Chlamydia*-negative nongonococcal urethritis—A partner-controlled study. *Acta Derm Venereol (Stockh)* 59:278, 1979.

26 Bowie WR et al: Tetracycline in nongonococcal urethritis. Comparison of 2 g and 1 g daily for 7 days. *Br J Vener Dis* 56:332, 1980.

27 McCormack WM et al: Sexual experience and urethral colonization with genital mycoplasmas: A study in normal men. *Ann Intern Med* 78:696, 1973.

28 McCormack WM et al: The genital mycoplasmas. *N Engl J Med* 288: 78, 1973.

29 Shepard MC: Quantitative relationship of *Ureaplasma urealyticum* to the clinical course of nongonococcal urethritis in the human male. *Colloq INSERM* 33:375, 1974.

30 Stimson JB et al: Tetracycline-resistant *Ureaplasma urealyticum*: A cause of persistent nongonococcal urethritis. *Ann Intern Med* 94:192, 1981.

31 Root TE et al: Nongonococcal urethritis: A survey of clinical and laboratory features. *Sex Transm Dis* 7:59, 1980.

32 Taylor-Robinson D et al: Human intraurethral inoculation of ureaplasmas. *Q J Med* 46:309, 1977.

33 Bowie WR et al: Genital inoculation of male *Macaca fascicularis* with *Neisseria gonorrhoeae* and *Ureaplasma urealyticum*. *Br J Vener Dis* 54:235, 1978.

34 Taylor-Robinson D et al: Urethral infection of chimpanzees by *Ureaplasma urealyticum*. *J Med Microbiol* 11:197, 1978.

35 Robertson JA, Stemke GW: Expanded serotyping scheme for *Ureaplasma urealyticum* strains isolated from humans. *J Clin Microbiol* 15:873, 1982.

36 Shepard MC, Lunceford CD: Serologic typing of *Ureaplasma urealyticum* isolates from urethritis patients by an agar growth inhibition method. *J Clin Microbiol* 8:566, 1978.

37 Cracea E et al: Serotypes of *Ureaplasma urealyticum* isolated from patients with nongonococcal urethritis and gonorrhea and from asymptomatic urethral carriers. *Sex Transm Dis* 12:219, 1985.

38 Black PT: Modifications of the growth inhibition test and its application to human T-mycoplasmas. *Appl Microbiol* 25:523, 1973.

39 Stemke GW, Robertson JA: Problems associated with serotyping strains of *Ureaplasma urealyticum*. *Diagn Microbiol Infect Dis* 3:311, 1985.

40 Bowie WR et al: Etiologies of postgonococcal urethritis in homosexual and heterosexual men: Roles of *Chlamydia trachomatis* and *Ureaplasma urealyticum*. *Sex Transm Dis* 5:151, 1978.

41 Vaughan-Jackson JD et al: Urethritis due to *Chlamydia trachomatis*. *Br J Vener Dis* 53:180, 1977.

42 Prentice MJ et al: Non-specific urethritis: A placebo-controlled trial of minocycline in conjunction with laboratory investigations. *Br J Vener Dis* 52:269, 1976.

43 Swartz SL et al: Diagnosis and etiology of nongonococcal urethritis. *J Infect Dis* 138:445, 1978.

44 Bowie WR et al: Bacteriology of the urethra in normal men and men with nongonococcal urethritis. *J Clin Microbiol* 6:482, 1977.

45 Fontaine EA et al: Anaerobes in men with urethritis. *Br J Vener Dis* 58:321, 1982.

46 Fontaine EA et al: Characteristics of a gram-negative anaerobe isolated from men with nongonococcal urethritis. *J Med Microbiol* 17: 129, 1984.

47 Woolley PD et al: Significance of *Bacteroides ureolyticus* in the lower genital tract. *International Journal of AIDS & STD* 3:107, 1992.

48 Sturm AW: *Hemophilus influenzae* and *Hemophilus parainfluenzae* in nongonococcal urethritis. *J Infect Dis* 153:165, 1986.

49 Facinelli B et al: *Haemophilus parainfluenzae* causing sexually transmitted urethritis: Report of a case and evidence for β-lactamase plasmid mobilizable to *Escherichia coli* by an Inc-W plasmid. *Sex Trans Dis* 18:166, 1991.

50 Barnes RC et al: Urinary tract infection in sexually active homosexual men. *Lancet* 1:171, 1986.

51 Hagman M et al: *Neisseria meningitidis* in specimens from urogenital sites: Is increased awareness necessary? *Sex Trans Dis* 18:228, 1991.

52 Conde-Glez CJ, Calderon E: Urogenital infection due to meningococcus in men and women. *Sex Transm Dis* 18:72, 1991.

53 Taylor CED et al: Serological response of patients with nongonococcal urethritis to causative organism of contagious endometritis. *Lancet* 1:700, 1979.

54 Hovelius B et al: *Staphylococcus saprophyticus* in the aetiology of nongonococcal urethritis. *Br J Vener Dis* 55:369, 1979.

55 Stamm WE, Holmes KK: Personal communication.

56 Furness G et al: *Corynebacterium genitalium* (non-specific urethritis *Corynebacterium*): Biologic reactions differentiating commensals of the urogenital tract from the pathogens responsible for urethritis. *Invest Urol* 15:23, 1977.

57 Tully JG et al: A newly discovered mycoplasma in the human urogenital tract. *Lancet* 1:1288, 1981.

58 Jensen JS et al: *Mycoplasma genitalium*, a cause of male urethritis. *Genitourin Med* 69:265, 1993.

59 Janier M et al: Male urethritis with and without discharge: a clinical and microbiological study. *Sex Trans Dis* 22:244, 1995.

60 Horner PJ et al: Association of *Mycoplasma genitalium* with acute non-gonococcal urethritis. *Lancet* 342:582, 1993.

61 Corey L et al: Genital herpes simplex virus infection: Clinical manifestations, course, and complications. *Ann Intern Med* 98:958, 1983.

62 Wong JL et al: The etiology of nongonococcal urethritis in men attending a venereal disease clinic. *Sex Transm Dis* 4:4, 1977.

63 Harnett GB et al: Association of gential adenovirus infection with urethritis in men. *Med J Aust* 141:337, 1984.

64 Kuberski T: *Trichomonas vaginalis* associated with nongonococcal urethritis and prostatitis. *Sex Transm Dis* 7:135, 1980.

65 Krieger JN et al: Risk assessment and laboratory diagnosis of trichomoniasis in men. *J Infect Dis* 166:1362, 1992.

66 McCutchan JA: Epidemiology of venereal urethritis: Comparison of gonorrhea and nongonococcal urethritis. *Rev Infect Dis* 6:669, 1984.

67 Wiesner PJ: Selected aspects of the epidemiology of nongonococcal urethritis, in *Nongonococcal Urethritis and Related Oculogenital Infections,* D Hobson, KK Holmes (eds). Washington, D.C., The American Society for Microbiology, 1977, p. 9.

68 McChesney JA et al: Acute urethritis in male college students. *JAMA* 226:37, 1973.

69 Jacobs NF, Kraus SJ: Gonococcal and nongonococcal urethritis in men. Clinical and laboratory differentiation. *Ann Intern Med* 82:7, 1975.

70 Podgore JK et al: Asymptomatic urethral infections due to *Chlamydia trachomatis* in male U.S. military personnel. *J Infect Dis* 146:828, 1982.

71 Karam GH et al: Asymptomatic *Chlamydia trachomatis* infections among sexually active men. *J Infect Dis* 154:900, 1986.

72 Kaplan JE et al: *Chlamydia trachomatis* infection in a male college student population. *J Am Coll Health* 37:159, 1989.

73 Thelin I et al: Contact-tracing in patients with genital chlamydial infection. *Br J Vener Dis* 56:259, 1980.

74 Terho P: *Chlamydia trachomatis* in non-specific urethritis. *Br J Vener Dis* 54:251, 1978.

75 Bowie WR: Treatment of chlamydial infections, in *Chlamydial Infections*, P Mardh et al (eds). New York, Elsevier, 1982, p. 231.

76 Simmons PD: Evaluation of the early morning smear investigation. *Br J Vener Dis* 54:128, 1978.

77 Bowie WR: Comparison of gram stain and first voided urine sediment in the diagnosis of urethritis. *Sex Transm Dis* 5:39, 1978.

78 Centers for Disease Control: 1985 Sexually Transmitted Diseases Guidelines. *MMWR* 38: 1989.

79 Bobo L et al: Diagnosis of *Chlamydia trachomatis* cervical infection by detection of amplified DNA with an enzyme immunoassay. *J Clin Microbiol* 28:1968, 1990.

80 Ostergaard L et al: Use of polymerase chain reaction for detection of *Chlamydia trachomatis*. *J Clin Microbiol* 28:1254, 1990.

81 Tarr PI et al: Comparison of methods for the isolation of genital mycoplasmas from men. *J Infect Dis* 133:419, 1976.

82 Grosskurth H et al: Impact of improved treatment of sexually transmitted disease on HIV infection in rural Tanzania: randomized controlled trial. *Lancet* 346:530, 1995.

83 Centers for Disease Control and Prevention: 1993 Sexually Transmitted Diseases Guidelines. *MMWR* 42:56, 1993.

84 Handsfield HH et al: Multicenter trial of single-dose azithromycin versus cetriaxone in the treatment of uncomplicated gonorrhea. *Sex Transm Dis* 21:107, 1994.

85 Oriel JD et al: Comparison of erythromycin stearate and oxytetracycline in the treatment of nongonococcal urethritis: Their efficacy against *Chlamydia trachomatis*. *Scott Med J* 22:375, 1977.

86 Hay PE et al: A reappraisal of chlamydial and non-chlamydial acute non-gonococcal urethritis. *Intern J STD & AIDS* 3:191, 1992.

87 Holmes KK et al: Studies of venereal diseases: III. Double-blind comparison of tetracycline hydrochloride and placebo in treatment of nongonococcal urethritis. *JAMA* 202:474, 1967.

88 Grimble AS, Amarasuriya KL: Nonspecific urethritis and the tetracyclines. *Br J Vener Dis* 51:198, 1975.

89 John J: Efficacy of prolonged regimens of oxytetracycline in the treatment of nongonococcal urethritis. *Br J Vener Dis* 47:266, 1971.

90 Thambar IV et al: Double-blind comparison of two regimens in the treatment of nongonococcal urethritis: Seven-day versus 21-day course of triple tetracycline (Deteclo). *Br J Vener Dis* 55:284, 1979.

91 Helmy N, Fowler W: Intensive and prolonged tetracycline therapy in non-specific urethritis. *Br J Vener Dis* 51:336, 1975.

92 Romanowski B et al: Minocycline compared with doxycycline in the treatment of nongonococcal urethritis and mucopurulent cervicitis. *Ann Intern Med* 119:16, 1993.

93 Martin DH et al: A controlled trial of a single dose of azithromycin for the treatment of chlamydia urethritis and cervicitis. *N Engl J Med* 327:921, 1992.

94 Stamm WE: Azithromycin in the treatment of uncomplicated genital chamydial infections. *Am J Med* 91:19S, 1991.

95 Lauharanta J et al: Single-dose oral azithromycin versus seven-day doxycycline in the treatment of non-gonococcal urethritis in males. *J Antimicrob Chemother* 31:177, 1993.

96 Johannisson G et al: Susceptibility of *Chlamydia trachomatis* to antibiotics in vitro and in vivo. *Sex Transm Dis* 6:50, 1979.

97 Wolfson JS, Hooper DC: The fluoroquinolones: Structure, mechanisms of action and resistance, and spectrum of activity in vitro. *Antimicrob Agents Chemother* 28:581, 1985.

98 Bowie WR et al: Failure of norfloxacin to eradicate *Chlamydia trachomatis* in nongonococcal urethritis. *Antimicrob Agents Chemother* 30:594, 1986.

99 Arya OP et al: Evaluation of ciprofloxacin 500 mg twice daily for one week in treating uncomplicated gonococcal, chlamydial, and nonspecific urethritis in men. *Genitourin Med* 62:170, 1986.

100 Hooten TM et al: Ciprofloxacin compared with doxycycline for nongonococcal urethritis: Ineffectiveness against *Chlamydia trachomatis* due to relapsing infection. *JAMA* 264:1418, 1990.

101 Mobabgab WJ et al: Randomized comparison of ofloxacin and doxycycline for chlamydia and ureaplasma urethritis and cervicitis. *Chemotherapy* 36:70, 1990.

102 Ibsen HHW et al: Treatment of nongonococcal urethritis: Comparison of ofloxacin and erythromycin. *Sex Transm Dis* 16:32, 1989.

103 Hooten TM et al: Erythromycin for persistent or recurrent nongonococcal urethritis: A randomized, placebo-controlled trial. *Ann Intern Med* 113:21, 1990.

104 Krieger J et al: Evaluation of chronic urethritis: Defining the role for endoscopic procedures. *Arch Intern Med* 148:703, 1988.

105 Keat A et al: Role of *Chlamydia trachomatis* and HLA-B27 in sexually acquired reactive arthritis. *Br Med J* 1:605, 1978.

106 Bowie WR et al: Unpublished observation.

107 Harrison WO et al: A trial of minocycline given after exposure to prevent gonorrhea. *N Engl J Med* 300:1074, 1979.

108 Dunlop EMC et al: Chlamydial infection: Incidence in "nonspecific" urethritis. *Br J Vener Dis* 48:425, 1972.

109 Richmond SJ et al: Chlamydial infection: Role of chlamydia subgroup A in nongonococcal and postgonococcal urethritis. *Br J Vener Dis* 48:437, 1972.

110 Oriel JD et al: Infection with chlamydia group A in men with urethritis due to *Neisseria gonorrhoeae*. *J Infect Dis* 131:376, 1975.

111 Oriel JD et al: Minocycline in the treatment of nongonococcal urethritis: Its effect on *Chlamydia trachomatis*. *J Am Vener Dis Assoc* 2:17, 1975.

112 Schachter J et al: Are chlamydial infections the most prevalent venereal diseases? *JAMA* 231:1252, 1975.

113 Smith TF et al: Isolation of chlamydia from patients with urethritis. *Mayo Clin Proc* 50:105, 1975.

114 Oriel JD et al: Chlamydial infection of the male urethra. *Br J Vener Dis* 52:46, 1976.

115 Johannisson G et al: *Chlamydia trachomatis* infection and venereal disease. *Acta Derm Venereal (Stockh)* 57:455, 1977.

116 Segura JW et al: Chlamydia and non-specific urethritis. *J Urol* 117: 720, 1977.

117 Terho P: *Chlamydia trachomatis* in gonococcal and postgonococcal urethritis. *Br J Vener Dis* 54:326, 1978.

118 Csango PA: *Chlamydia trachomatis* from men with nonogonococcal urethritis: Simplified procedure for cultivation and isolation in replicating McCoy cell culture. *Acta Pathol Microbiol Scand Sect B* 86: 257, 1978.

119 Ripa KT et al: *Chlamydia trachomatis* urethritis in men attending a venereal disease clinic: A culture and therapeutic study. *Acta Derm Venereol (Stockh)* 48:175, 1978.

120 Perroud HM, Miedyzbrodzka K: Chlamydial infection of the urethra in men. *B J Vener Dis* 54:45, 1978.

121 Smith TF et al: A comparison of genital infections caused by *Chlamydia trachomatis* and by *Neisseria gonorrhoeae*. *Am Soc Clin Pathol* 70:333, 1978.

122 Taylor-Robinson D et al: *Ureaplasma urealyticum* and *Mycoplasma hominis* in chlamydial and non-chlamydial non-gonococcal urethritis. *Br J Vener Dis* 55:30, 1979.

123 Lefevre J et al: Clinical and microbiological features of urethritis in men in Toulouse, France. *Sex Transm Dis* 18:76, 1991.

Chapter 61
Acute epididymitis

Richard E. Berger

DEFINITION AND HISTORY

The epididymis and vas deferens are derived from the wolffian system and mesonephric duct. The epididymis is a sausage-shaped structure positioned on the posterior aspect of the testicle. It consists of a single, delicate convoluted tubule 12 to 15 feet in length. The epithelium of the epididymis possesses stereocilia, which have no directional movement. The epididymis has been divided into six sections based on histological characteristics, which probably represent different functional capacities. Fluid and particulate matter are both secreted and absorbed by the epididymis. During passage through the epididymis sperm achieve motility and the potential to fertilize an ovum.

Inflammation of the epididymis causes pain and swelling, which is almost always unilateral and usually relatively acute in onset. Monteggro in 1804 was probably the first to describe the gross pathology of epididymitis and differentiate it from orchitis. Despres in 1879 suggested that epididymitis was due to the retention of semen related to the pain of urethritis. Subsequently, specific infectious forms, such as tuberculous and gonococcal epididymitis, have been well-recognized. With the advent of specific diagnostic criteria and effective antimicrobial therapy for gonorrhea and tuberculosis in the 1940s and 1950s, an increasing proportion of cases seen during the 1960s and 1970s were regarded as "idiopathic," often attributed to "straining" or reflux of sterile urine into the epididymis. However, recent studies have established the infectious etiology of most cases of epididymitis and the importance of sexually transmitted urethritis as a precursor of epididymitis.

Epididymitis is common, and it carries much morbidity in terms of suffering and loss of time from work. Because of epididymitis an estimated 634,000 patients sought treatment by American physicians in 1977.[1] In 1981 the National Institutes of Health estimated 500,000 cases of acute epididymitis to occur per year.[2] Researchers have reported that the incidence of epididymitis may range from one to four per 1,000 men per year.[3,4] In Great Britain, from 1963 to 1964, 13,600 claims were made for workman's compensation for epididymoorchitis.[5] In 1984, Baumgarten reported that 82 percent of men with work-related epididymitis returned to work after an average of 6 days.[6] However, 18 percent had prolonged symptoms or required surgical therapy. Epididymitis was reported in 1963 to account for more days lost from service than any other disease in the military, with over 20 percent of urologic admissions being caused by epididymoorchitis.[7–9]

With improved understanding of the etiology of epididymitis, the diagnosis and management of this condition is becoming more rational, leading to decreased morbidity and possibly to prevention of recurrences. Epididymitis may occur as a complication of urethral infection with *Neisseria gonorrhoeae* or *Chlamydia trachomatis,* or of genitourinary infection with enteric Gram-negative rods *Pseudomonas aeruginosa.* It may also occasionally occur as a complication of systemic infection with various pathogens, including *Mycobacterium tuberculosis, brucella* spp., *Streptococcus pneumoniae, Neisseria meningitidis, Treponema pallidum,* and various fungi. The proper management of these patients requires that an accurate etiologic diagnosis be established. The agent responsible must be identified, along with contributing factors that might lead to recurrences. In the case of epididymitis caused by *N. gonorrhoeae* or *C. trachomatis,* this would most certainly include treatment of the patient's sexual partners. In the case of epididymitis secondary to coliform urinary tract infection, primary genitourinary disease must be sought out and, if possible, treated. The term nonspecific epididymitis, which has been used in the past to denote patients who have epididymitis associated with nonspecific urethritis or with no obvious infection, should generally be avoided. Only those cases for which no etiologic agent can be determined after a careful search for known pathogens should be referred to as "idiopathic" (Table 61-1).

EPIDEMIOLOGY AND ETIOLOGY

EPIDIDYMITIS ASSOCIATED WITH BACTERIURIA

In prepubertal children, epididymitis is frequently associated with coliform or pseudomonas infection of the genitourinary tract (Table 61-2).[10,11] These children often have predisposing structural or neurologic abnormalities. Gierup et al. found that ten of 22 children who had epididymitis confirmed by surgical exploration had significant bacteriuria (e.g., $>10^5$ *E. coli*/ml of urine).[10] Prepubertal children had bacteriuria more often than postpubertal children. Pyuria with negative urine cultures occurred more often in older children. Cultures for *C. trachomatis* or *N. gonorrhoeae* were not performed, but these agents could be important among older boys who are sexually active. In a retrospective study, Gislason et al. found that approximately two-thirds of boys with epididymitis were postpubertal, 29 percent had pyuria, but only 12.5 percent had urine cultures that yielded conventional pathogens.[12] In adolescents with epididymitis, the age and sexual activity should be ascertained, as sexually transmitted pathogens may be important in such patients.

In postpubertal males less than 35 years of age, epididymitis is usually not attributable to coliforms, and the presence of *Ps. aeruginosa* is unusual. In various series, from 0 to 35 percent of sexually mature young men with epididymitis have had infection with coliform bacteria or *Ps. aeruginosa.*[1,9,13,14] This low prevalence may be partially owing to the low prevalence in this age group of structural disease predisposing an individual to urinary tract infections. Most males with congenital anomalies of the urinary tract have been discovered and treated surgically at an earlier age, whereas acquired structural or functional disorders of the male urinary tract, such as benign prostatic hypertrophy, develop later in life.[1] As shown in Table 61-3, six of 51 men less than 35 years of age in our series had coliform infection and one had infection with *Haemophilus influenzae.* All of those seven were homosexual men infected with Gram-negative rods, who regularly practiced anal-insertive intercourse.[15] No pathogen was identified in the two additional homosexual men in this series, but all nine homosexual men had many neutrophiles per 400 × microscopic field on Gram stain of midstream urine. Drach has previously noted that a history of anal intercourse was associated with chronic bacterial prostatitis.[16] Barnes et al. found that bacteriuria was more common among homosexual men than among heterosexual men in a venereal disease clinic population.[17] Of those with bacteriuria, 61 percent had urethral discharge, presumably owing to *E. coli* urethritis. Thus, we hypothesize that the occurrence of *E. coli* epididymitis in homosexual men may be owing to more frequent exposure of the urethra to pathogenic enteric bacteria during anal intercourse. Although Stamey et al. showed in 1971 that enteric pathogens isolated from the urine of women with urinary tract infections could be isolated from the

Table 61-1. Classification of Acute Epididymitis

Epididymitis due to infectious agents
- Associated with urethritis
- Associated with bacteriuria
- Associated with systemic infections

Epididymitis due to noninfectious causes
- Associated with trauma
- Associated with drugs (amiodarone)

urethra of their male sexual partners, coliform epididymitis appears to be uncommon in young heterosexual men.[18]

In contrast, among men over 35 years of age with epididymitis, up to 80 percent have coliform or *Ps. aeruginosa* urinary tract infection.[19] The high proportion of cases of epididymitis caused by coliform infections in older men may be owing to the decreasing incidence of sexually transmitted disease and an increased incidence of acquired genitourinary abnormalities. These patients may have a history of prostatic calculi, recent urinary instrumentation, neurogenic bladder, benign prostatic hypertrophy, or chronic bacterial prostatitis. We found only one of 17 patients over 35 years of age with epididymitis to have a sexually transmitted infection, whereas 12 of the 17 had coliform or pseudomonas infection (Table 61-3). Almost one-half of the patients over 35 years of age had pre-existing genitourinary pathology.

In military populations, epididymitis secondary to coliform bladder infections is unusual.[9,13,14,20,21] This may be owing to the predominantly young age and absence of underlying urinary abnormalities in military populations. Mittemeyer found underlying urinary abnormalities in only 3.4 percent of 610 patients with epididymitis.[14] In Mittemeyer's study, 70.1 percent were between the ages of 20 and 39; and in Shapiro's study, 75 percent of the patients were between 18 and 32.[13,14]

EPIDIDYMITIS ASSOCIATED WITH URETHRITIS

Epididymitis caused by *N. gonorrhoeae* or *C. trachomatis* is rare in prepubertal children, but in postpubertal children, these organisms must be suspected. No study to date of postpubertal children with epididymitis has assessed the sexual history, or has utilized appropriate cultures for sexually transmitted organisms as well as for conventional uropathogens.

Sexually transmitted organisms are the most common cause of epididymitis in heterosexual men under the age of 35 (Table 61-4).[1,16] In the preantibiotic era, Pelouze reported that epididymitis

Table 61-2. Microbial Etiology and Predisposing Factors in Acute Epididymitis

Prepubertal children
- Usual etiology: Coliforms, *Ps. aeruginosa*
- Usual etiology: Hematogenous spread from primary infected site
- Predisposing factors: Underlying genitourinary pathology

Men under 35
- Usual etiology: *C. trachomatis, N. gonorrhoeae*
- Unusual etiology: Coliform or *Ps. aeruginosa, Mycobacterium tuberculosis*
- Predisposing factors: Sexually transmitted urethritis

Men over 35
- Usual etiology: Coliforms or *Ps. aeruginosa*
- Unusual etiology: *N. gonorrhoeae, C. trachomatis, M. tuberculosis*
- Predisposing factors: Underlying structural pathology or chronic bacterial prostatitis

Table 61-3. Etiology of Acute Epididymitis in 68 Consecutive Men

Etiology	Heterosexual men >35 years old (*n* = 17)	Heterosexual men <35 years old (*n* = 42)	Homosexual men <35 years old (*n* = 9)
Coliform, *Ps. aeruginosa*	12	0	6
N. gonorrhoeae	0	9	0
C. trachomatis	1	18	0
N. gonorrhoeae plus *C. trachomatis*	0	1	0
H. influenzae	0	0	1
Trauma	0	2	0
Tuberculosis	1	0	0
Idiopathic	3	12	2

SOURCE: Berger RE, refs. 1, 15, 19.

occurred in 10 to 30 percent of cases of gonorrheal urethritis.[22] More recently, Watson found that 16 percent of patients with epididymitis in a young military population had gonorrhea, although only 50 percent of those with gonorrhea had urethral discharge.[23]

In our series of acute epididymitis, 28 of 42 men (67%) under 35 years of age had epididymitis secondary to *N. gonorrhoeae* or *C. trachomatis*. *N. gonorrhoeae* alone was isolated from the urethra from nine, *C. trachomatis* infection alone was found in 18, and both agents were recovered from one patient (Table 61-3). *C. trachomatis* was isolated as the sole pathogen from the epididymis in five of six men with *C. trachomatis* infection who underwent epididymal aspiration.

Characteristically, patients with epididymitis caused by *N. gonorrhoeae* or *C. trachomatis* are young and sexually active; they may have multiple sexual partners. Symptoms of urethritis may or may not be present. Nonetheless, even in patients who deny symptoms of urethritis, a urethral discharge may be expressible; a Gram-stained smear of an endourethral swab specimen may reveal ≥5 polymorphonuclear leukocytes per 1000 × field; or urinalysis may reveal pyuria. Underlying urinary tract abnormalities usually are not found.

In our series, 13 of 19 men with *C. trachomatis* epididymitis were referred from venereal disease clinics.[1,15,19] Therefore, this could represent a biased population and could overestimate the proportion of cases actually associated with *C. trachomatis*. However, other studies have confirmed our findings.[24,25] Among men with acute epididymitis, *C. trachomatis* infection was found by Melekos and Asbach in nine (53%) of 17 men less than age 40; by Colleen and Mårdh in 14 (33%) of 42 men less than age 35; and by Mulcahy et al. in 65 percent of men less than age 35.[24–26] Hawkins et al. and Lee found that men presenting with epididymitis often had nonspecific urethritis even in the absence of positive tests for *Chlamydia trachomatis* or *N. gonnorhoeae*.[27,28] These cases could be attributed to urethritis owing to other less common causes, or to the inability to isolate organisms such as *C. trachomatis*. Eley et al. found that they could increase detection of *C. trachomatis* in acute epididymitis by employing polymerase chain reaction (PCR) testing.[29] Future use of PCR testing for *C. trachomatis, N. gonorrhoeae*, and other urethral pathogens may allow more accurate determination of the role of the various organisms in epididymitis.

The argument has long been popular that epididymitis in young men is caused by the reflux of sterile urine down the vas deferens during straining, producing sterile inflammation. The popularity of this theory may be partly owing to the previous inability to

Table 61-4. Etiology of Acute Epididymitis

Study	Total No. men	Age <35; No./total (%)			Age >35; No./total (%)		
		GC	Ct	*E. coli*	GC	Ct	*E. coli*
Berger et al. (1978)	23		11/13 (3)			8/10 (80)	
Scheibel et al. (1983)	52	1/31 (3)	13/31 (42)			6/13 (46)	
Kristensen et al. (1984)	16	4/16 (25)	14/16 (88)				
Hawkins et al. (1986)	40		13/27 (48)		2/13 (15)	3/13 (23)	
Hawkins et al. (1986)	40	2/27 (7)	13/27 (48)	0/27	3/13 (23)	2/13 (15)	3/13 (23)
Berger et al. (1987)	51	9/51 (28)	19/51 (37)	6/51 (12)*			
Grant et al. (1987)	54	2/42 (5)	29/40 (73)	3/42 (7)		3/12 (25)	8/12 (67)
Melekos et al. (1987)	31		10/17 (59)	4/17 (24)		3/14 (21)	7/14 (50)
Mulcahy et al. (1987)	40	4/40 (10)	13/40 (33)	0			6/11 (55)
De Jong et al. (1988)	25	1/13 (8)	11/13 (85)	1/13 (8)		1/12 (8)	10/12 (83)
Kojima et al. (1988)	45	3/30 (10)	21/30 (70)			10/15 (67)	
Pearson et al. (1988)	27	1/27 (4)	7/29 (24)	0			
Doble (1989)	24†	1/24 (4)	10/24 (42)				
Hoosen et al. (1993)‡	144	76/134 (57)	46/134 (34)	4/134 (3)	1/10 (10)	2/10 (20)	3/10 (30)

* Six of nine homosexual men had coliform infection; one other had infection with *Haemophilus influenzae*. None of 42 heterosexual men had coliform infections.
† All less than 45 years old.
‡ Cut-off between younger and older men was age 40 years.
gc = gonorrhea; ct = *Chlamydia trachomatis* infection

recover a pathogenic organism from these patients. However, Shapiro noted only two of 52 patients had a history of straining prior to the onset of epididymitis.[13] Similarly, Mittemeyer noted such a history in only 6.6 percent of his population.[14] We studied two patients who had a history of strenuous lifting just before onset of epididymitis, and *C. trachomatis* was isolated from both of these patients.[19] Cathcart reported that 12 of 14 cases of epididymitis with a history of "strain" also had urethral discharge.[30] Although reflux of infected urine into the vas deferens may well be important in the production of epididymitis, reflux of sterile urine has not been shown to play an important role in causing epididymitis.

MISCELLANEOUS CAUSES OF EPIDIDYMITIS

Epididymitis may occur in systemic tuberculosis. In Mittemeyer's military series, 0.8 percent of patients had epididymitis owing to tuberculosis.[14] Halker reported that 75 percent of patients with renal tuberculosis had an episode of epididymitis.[31] Ross found the age of patients with tuberculous epididymitis to be between 20 and 40 years.[32] Medlar reported that no case of tuberculous epididymitis occurred without renal, prostate, or seminal vesicle involvement.[33] Sixty-four percent of patients with tuberculous epididymitis had bilateral involvement, in contrast with epididymitis caused by coliforms, *N. gonorrhoeae*, or *C. trachomatis*, which is nearly always unilateral. The presence of sterile pyuria in these men may cause confusion with other causes of sterile pyuria, such as nonspecific urethritis.[34] The incidence of tuberculous epididymitis may be increasing as this infection becomes more common in HIV infected men.[35]

Numerous other organisms that have been reported to cause epididymitis probably spread by a hematogenous route. These organisms include *Strep. pneumoniae, brucella* spp., *N. meningitidis, T. pallidum,* Nocardia spp., and numerous other bacteria.[36–41] *Haemophilis influenzue* type B has been isolated from the epididymis of children with acute epididymitis as well as in a homosexual man with epididymitis.[15,42,43] Salmonella epididymitis has also been reported in children with enteric salmonella infection.[44] Epididymitis may occur as a manifestation of disseminated fungal infections, such as histoplasmosis, coccidioidomycosis, blastomycosis, and cryptococcosis.[45,46] Candidal epidididymitis has also been reported.[47] Cytomegalovirus epididymitis has been reported in a patient with immunodeficiency syndrome.[45]

A new cause of epididymitis was reported by Gasparich et al., who reported a syndrome of epididymitis in 6 of 56 men taking the antiarrhythmic drug amiodarone.[3] Epididymal biopsy showed lymphocytic infiltration and fibrosis. Amiodarone levels in the epididymis were found to be 400 times higher than therapeutic blood levels in one patient. Reduction of the dosage of amiodarone resulted in resolution of epididymitis.

CLINICAL MANIFESTATIONS AND ETIOLOGIC DIAGNOSIS

The history of men with bacteriuria often suggests urinary tract infections. Frequency, urgency, and dysuria are common. There may be a history of symptoms suggestive of urinary tract obstruction, such as hesitancy or slow urinary stream, indicating conditions such as stricture and benign prostatic hypertrophy, predisposing to urinary tract infection. Men with epididymitis secondary to sexually transmitted pathogens often have a history of urethral discharge or dysuria. They usually have a history of recent sexual exposure. The patient with epididymitis secondary to tuberculosis will often have a prior history of pulmonary tuberculosis or a history of exposure.

Of 92 men in the military service with epididymitis, one-third had a sudden onset, and two-thirds a gradual onset.[21] A history of lifting or straining on onset of pain is probably not significant in determining the etiology of the epididymitis or in its differentiation from other intrascrotal conditions. In addition to severe scrotal pain, the patient may also complain of inguinal pain.[19] In severe cases, with the cord acutely swollen, flank pain may result from obstruction of the ureter as it crosses over the spermatic cord.[22] A history suggestive of urinary infection may or may not be present.[21,49] We found that only one of ten patients with coliform infections, and only six of 14 patients with *C. trachomatis* infection, had dysuria.[1]

On examination, the scrotum on the involved side may be red

and edematous. The degree of erythema may be greater in patients with coliform and gonococcal epididymitis than with *C. trachomatis* epididymitis. However, massive erythema and edema may occur even with *C. trachomatis* if left untreated. The testicle tends to ride in the normal position in the scrotum. The tail of the epididymis, which connects with the vas deferens, near the lower pole of the testes, is swollen first, and later swelling spreads to the head of the epididymis, near the upper pole of the testes. The groove between the epididymis and the testicle should be examined, as this will help to show whether the maximum swelling is in the testicle or the epididymis. The spermatic cord may be swollen and tender. If the patient has not recently voided, a urethral discharge may be present, but asymptomatic urethral infection without discharge is not uncommon. Watson found that 50 percent of the cases owing to *N. gonorrhoeae* did not have urethral discharge.[23] If no spontaneous discharge is noted, the urethra should be stripped and again examined. Digital rectal exam may reveal abnormalities suggestive of prostatitis in some cases.[13,20]

Gram stain of the urethral swab specimen will usually indicate the presence of urethritis and establish with a high degree of certainty whether its etiology is gonococcal or nongonococcal. In our series, the presence or absence of intracellular Gram-negative diplococci on Gram stain or urethral smear correlated in all cases with the results of culture for *N. gonorrhoeae*.[1] Nonetheless, urethral specimens should be tested for *N. gonorrhoeae* and *C. trachomatis* in all cases. Alternatively, tests of first-voided urine for *N. gonorrhoeae* and *C. trachomatis* using ligase chain reaction or polymerase chain reaction techniques, may also prove useful, though more experience with these tests is needed in men with epididymitis. First-voided and midstream urine specimens should next be examined for bacteria and white cells. Comparison of the urinary sediments in the first voided urine and midstream urine may reveal whether pyuria is coming from the urethra or the bladder. Gram stain of uncentrifuged midstream urine can be used to presumptively establish the diagnosis of bacteriuria in cases of epididymitis secondary to coliform or pseudomonas infections. The presence of greater than one Gram-negative rod per oil immersion field on Gram stain of one drop of unspun midstream urine is correlated with the presence of greater than 10^5 coliforms or pseudomonas spp. per milliliter of urine. Quantitative midstream urine culture should nonetheless be obtained in all cases of acute epididymitis. In our series, two-thirds of the cases of epididymitis not owing to Gram-negative rods or *N. gonorrhoeae* in men under 35 years of age were secondary to *Chlamydia trachomatis*.[1]

In certain difficult cases, the etiologic diagnosis of epididymitis may be aided by the use of epididymal aspiration cultures.[50] These cultures may be useful in patients with (1) indwelling urethral catheters; (2) failure to respond to initial antimicrobial therapy; (3) epididymitis found on surgical exploration for torsion of the testicle; and (4) recurrent epididymitis in which the etiologic agent is uncertain. If the patient had received prior antimicrobial therapy and the urine is sterile, the organism responsible for epididymitis may still be obtainable from aspirate cultures. Patients with indwelling urethral catheters often have multiple organisms in the urine, and therapy may be best selected on the basis of the organism(s) found on epididymal aspiration.

DIFFERENTIAL DIAGNOSIS OF ACUTE EPIDIDYMITIS

An algorithm for differential diagnosis and management of the patient with pain in the scrotal sac is presented in Fig. 61-1.[51] Acute epididymitis always must be differentiated from torsion of the testicle. In infants and prepubertal children, torsion of the testicle is much more common than acute epididymitis, and any acute swelling of the scrotum must be presumed to be torsion of the testicle unless proved otherwise. Quinto found that only 12 of 158 pediatric patients with scrotal swelling had epididymitis.[52] Children with epididymitis often have pyuria, whereas children with torsion generally do not have pyuria.

Boys with an acute scrotal condition should lead to immediate surgical exploration to perform detorsion and orchidopexy. Cases of suspected epididymitis in adolescents or young adults should be confirmed by Doppler and radionuclide scanning, since the incidence of torsion is also higher in this age group.

In consecutive cases of acute testicular swelling, Devillar noted that 11 of 13 patients under age 20 had torsion of the testicle.[53] In contrast, of all patients from 20 to 30 years old, only 10 percent had torsion of the testicle. Of 29 patients with acute epididymitis, only eight were under age 20. Barker also found that epididymitis was much more likely to be found in patients over 18 years of age than in patients less than 18 years of age, presumably because of increasing sexual activity and decreasing incidence of torsion with age.[54] As sexual mores have changed, however, and the age at first intercourse has decreased, the incidence of epididymitis has increased in patients less than 18 years of age.

A history of previous scrotal pain is more common in torsion of the testicle than in epididymitis, presumably owing to previous

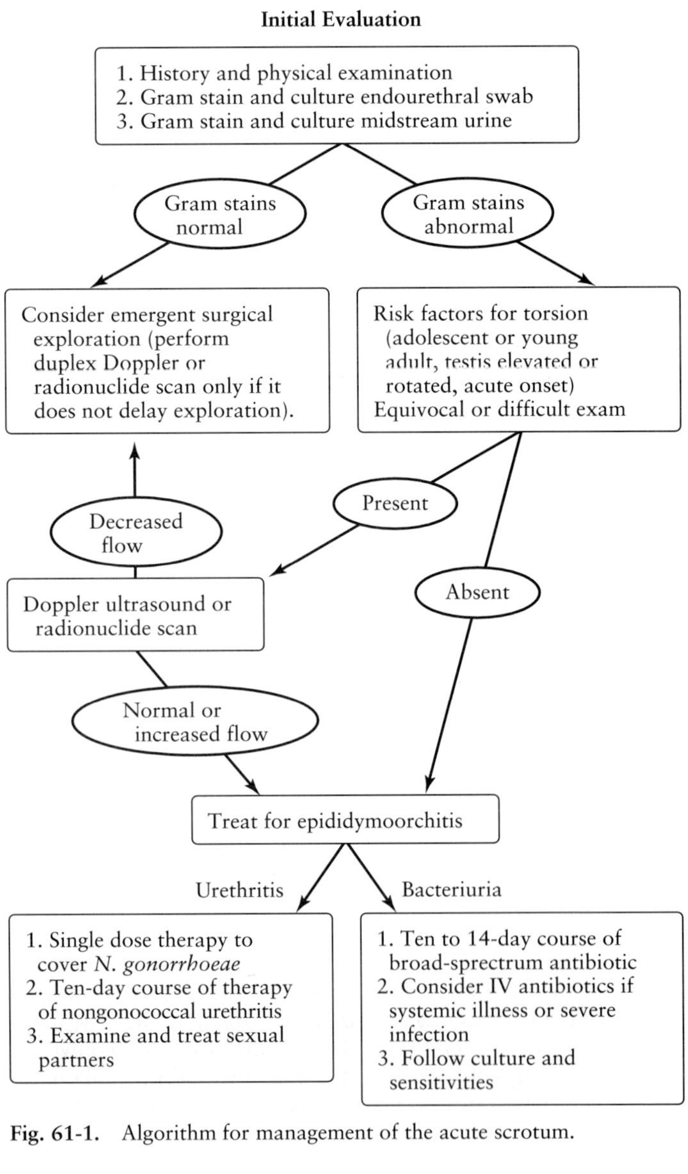

Fig. 61-1. Algorithm for management of the acute scrotum.

intermittent torsion. History of trauma to the testicle or of extreme exertion at the onset of pain may occur with either epididymitis or torsion of the testicle. Unless physical examination is performed early in the course of the acute scrotum, the physical examination in torsion and epididymitis may be very similar. Devillar noticed swelling of the testes in 28 percent of patients with epididymitis and in 77 percent of cases of torsion.[53] On the other hand, swelling of the epididymis alone occurred in 59 percent of cases of epididymitis and in 15 percent of torsion. In torsion of the testicle, sometimes examination of the opposite testicle will reveal that the epididymis is anterior. This indicates that the congenital abnormality that allows torsion of the testicle may also be present on the opposite side and is a clue to the diagnosis of torsion. In torsion also, the testicle is often high into the scrotum, whereas in epididymitis this is not usually the case. In epididymitis, the cord in the inguinal canal may be quite tender, whereas in torsion tenderness is generally limited to the scrotal contents.

Examination of the urine and urethral smear is a very helpful procedure in differentiating epididymitis from torsion of the testicle as discussed above. Barker and Raper noted that 31 of 32 patients with epididymitis had bacteriuria or pus cells in the urine, whereas none of 38 patients with torsion had bacteriuria or pyuria.[54] In Doolittle's series, eight of 11 patients with epididymitis had pyuria, whereas none of 19 with torsion had pyuria.[55] Evaluation should include examination of first-voided urine, which would yield a concentration of white cells higher than that observed in midstream urine in patients with urethritis. In Madsen's series, 49 of 50 patients with acute epididymitis had expressed prostatic secretions that were loaded with white blood cells.[56] Although Madsen did not examine urethral smears routinely, the finding of clear evidence of urethritis on smear would eliminate the need for performing rigorous rectal examination in most cases. Some authors consider a rigorous rectal exam in patients with epididymitis to be contraindicated because of the risk of exacerbating the symptoms or because of a possible risk of causing bacteremia in men with coliform or *Ps. aeruginosa* infection. Madsen reported no such exacerbations and neither did we in our series. However, we avoided prostatic massage on older patients with suspected coliform or *Ps. aeruginosa* infection.[1]

The Doppler stethoscope is a useful tool in the differential diagnosis of torsion and epididymitis.[57] It shows increased blood flow to the acutely inflamed epididymis and decreased blood flow to a testicle that has undergone torsion, cutting off its blood supply. The opposite testicle is used as a control. Care must be performed in interpreting Doppler ultrasound examinations, as hyperemia surrounding a necrotic testicle may produce a false positive signal for epididymitis. Compression of the spermatic cord at the external ring will cause the Doppler pulse to disappear if blood flow is coming from the testicle, but not if it is coming from scrotal vessels. Similarly, a hydrocele surrounding an inflamed epididymis may produce a falsely decreased signal. The use of radionuclide testicular scanning is also based on a finding of increased blood flow in epididymitis (Fig. 61-2). In Holder's series, 22 of 22 patients with acute epididymitis had increased blood flow and were correctly diagnosed.[58] Abu-Sleiman et al. found that a correct diagnosis could be made in 86 percent of cases.[59] False positives were noted in hydroceles and false negatives in late torsions and patients with retracted scroti.[60,61] Testicular tumor may also produce increased flow on testicular scan, resembling epididymitis.[62]

Color-coded duplex Doppler ultrasonography has recently proven valuable in the differential diagnosis of epididymitis and torsion. This method uses visual color coding of flow velocities in blood vessels superimposed on the gray scale ultrasonography. Increases or decreases in blood flow can be determined.[63,64] Wilbert et al. found that color coded Doppler ultrasonography had a sensitivity of 82 percent and a specificity of 100 percent for torsion.[65] For epididymitis the sensitivity was 70 percent and specificity was 88 percent. Falsely negative scans in torsion were generally owing to partial torsion with some residual blood flow in the testicle and epididymis. Magnetic resonance imaging has also been found to be accurate in the differential diagnosis of epididymitis and torsion in a small series.[66]

In all cases, unless the examiner can unequivocally rule out torsion of the testicle, scrotal exploration should be undertaken. After 4 hours of torsion, there is a significant risk of irreversible testicular infarction. A "wait and see" attitude is never justified. We have encountered one patient who had simultaneous epididymitis and testicular torsion.

Another common and potentially disastrous mistake in diagnosis of acute epididymitis is to overlook a testicular carcinoma (Fig. 61-3). The ages at which epididymitis and testicular tumors occur are similar, the peak ages of testicular tumors being between 18 and 32. Approximately one-quarter of patients with testicular tumors present with testicular pain. Therefore, although the presentation of a painless testicular mass almost always indicates a testicular tumor, the presence of pain does not rule out a tumor. In the early stages of epididymitis, swelling is limited to the epididymis, and differentiation from testicular tumor usually is not difficult. However, as epididymitis progresses and the testicle becomes more involved, the limits of inflammation are not easily defined. Furthermore, a testicular tumor may invade the epididymis and thus, on physical exam, mimic exactly the findings of acute epididymitis. Reactive hydrocele formation may further limit the usefulness of physical examination. In testicular tumors, the urine and urethral smear should show no evidence of inflammation. Failure of improvement in the size of swelling or pain in any young man being treated for epididymitis should lead to the suspicion that an incorrect diagnosis has been made. Scrotal exploration through an inguinal incision should be considered to

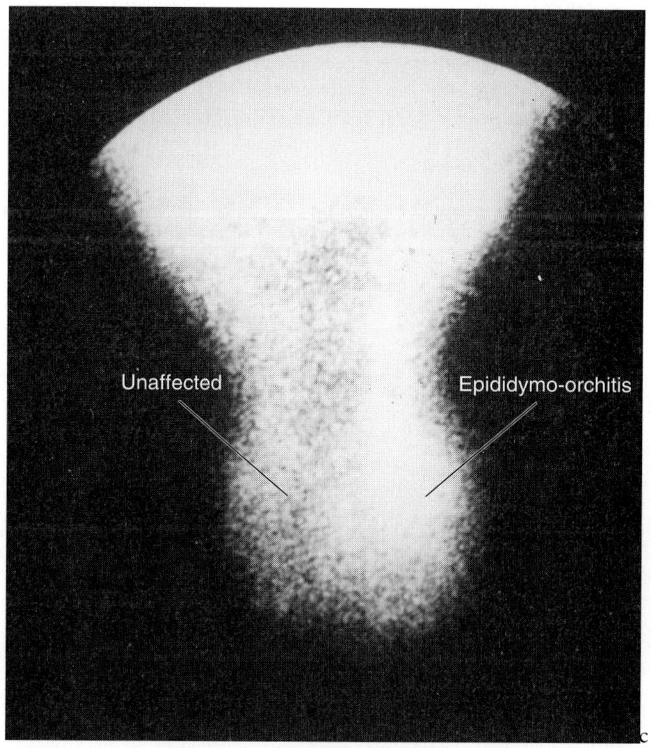

Fig. 61-2. Technetium radionuclide scan of patient with typical acute unilateral epididymoorchitis, showing increased uptake of Tc^{99} on the affected side, with normal uptake on the unaffected side.

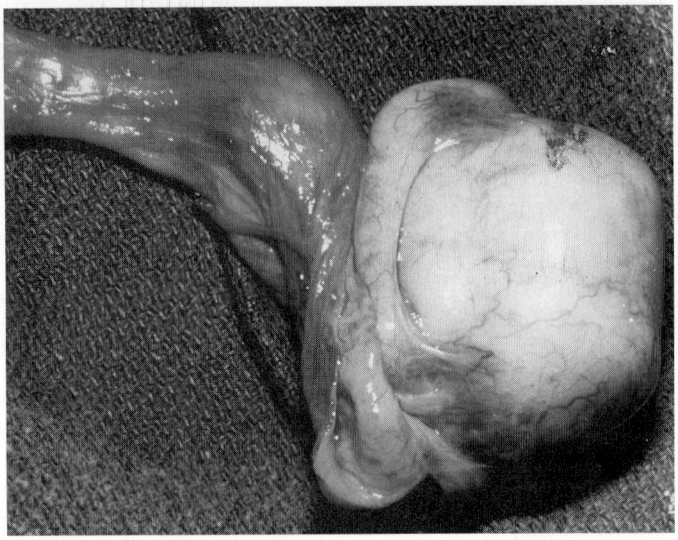

Fig. 61-3. Testicular seminoma that was misdiagnosed as epididymitis by three urologists. Cancer is sausage-shaped and elevated epididymis.

rule out carcinoma of the testicle. Transscrotal open or needle biopsy should never be performed when carcinoma of the testicle is suspected for fear of spreading tumor cells in the scrotal contents. Examination by ultrasound may be of value to confirm or deny the normalcy of the underlying testicular architecture.

Other common intrascrotal conditions that may present difficulties in diagnosis are presented in Table 61-5. Spermatocele and hydrocele are easily differentiated by transillumination. The scrotal varicosities of a varicocele disappear on assuming the supine position. A hernia protruding into the scrotum may sometimes present difficulties in diagnosis. However, this may be reducible as the patient lies down. Hernias are not transilluminable, and bowel sounds may occasionally be heard in the hernia contents. Other less common causes of confusion are testicular vasculitis from polyarteritis nodosa or other autoimmune disorders.[67,68] Epididymitis may occur after intravesical BCG (bacillus calmette-gerrin) instillation for treatment of carcinoma of the bladder.[69] Henoch-Schönlein purpura may present with bleeding into the epididymis. Men taking high doses of Amiodarone have been found to develop sterile epididymitis. The urine shows no pyuria, and there is no urethral discharge. Amiodarone has been found to be concentrated in the epididymis to over 400 times serum levels. The epididymitis is usually bilateral; however, it may be unilateral.[3]

COMPLICATIONS OF ACUTE EPIDIDYMITIS

SURGICAL COMPLICATIONS

Since the use of antibiotics, the incidence of surgical complications from epididymitis has decreased. From 1951 to 1955, Gartman used few antibiotics and had a 30 percent incidence of surgical complications.[20] From 1955 to 1959, he used antibiotics much more frequently, and had an 8 percent incidence of surgical complications. He noted an overall 10.2 percent complication rate in idiopathic epididymitis, and a 16.2 percent rate when a definite pathogen was found in the urine or urethra.

The most serious local complications of epididymitis are abscess formation and infarction of the testicle (Fig. 61-4). Both of these complications are clinically suggested by the failure of the patient to improve with appropriate bed rest and antibiotic therapy. Testicular infarction probably results from thrombosis of the spermatic vessels secondary to severe inflammation (Fig. 61-5).[19,70,71] Gangrene of the testicle may take place while the epididymis remains viable (Fig. 61-4). Costas suggested that the swollen spermatic cord may become compressed at the external ring and lead to vascular compromise of the testicle.[72] In Gartman's series, three of 310 cases resulted in gangrene of the testicle.[20] Abscess may be suggested by a "cold" area in the middle of a "hot" area on radionuclide scan. See et al. found that serial gray scale ultrasonography revealing progressive inhomogeneity was highly correlated with the development of abscess and the need for orchiectomy.[73] In Mittemeyer's series, 19 of 610 patients developed abscess formation that required surgical drainage.[14] Treatment requires surgical drainage and probably orchiectomy. In Gartman's series, 22 out of 310 patients developed hydroceles; however, only 11 of

Table 61-5. Common Differential Diagnosis of Acute Epididymitis in Adult Men

	Usual age	Pain	Onset	Past history of pain	Spermatic cord tenderness	Scrotal tenderness	Transillumination	Decrease in swelling on lying down	Fever	Location of swelling	Urethritis, pyuria, bacteriuria	Activity on testicular scan	Blood flow on Doppler ultrasonic
Epididymitis	Any	Mild–severe	Gradual to sudden	Infrequent	Frequent	Severe	No	No	Frequent	Posterior to testes	Yes	↑	↑
Torsion of testes	<30	Severe	Sudden	Frequent	Infrequent	Severe	No	No	Infrequent	Testes*	No	↓	↓
Testes tumor	18–32	None–mild	Gradual	Infrequent	No	None–mild	No	No	No	Testes	No	Normal or ↓	Normal
Hydrocele	Any	None–mild	Gradual	Infrequent	No	None	Yes	No	No	Entire hemiscrotum	No	Normal	Normal or ↓
Spermatocele	Any	None–mild	Gradual	Infrequent	No	None	Yes	No	No	Above testes†	No	Normal	Normal
Varicocele	Any	None–mild	Gradual	Infrequent	No	None	No	Yes‡	No	"Bag of worms"	No	Normal	Normal§
Hernia	Any	None–moderate	Gradual	Frequent	Frequent	None–mild	No	Yes¶	No	Above testes	No	Normal	Normal

* In torsion of testicle, epididymis of normal testicle may be anterior.
† Spermatocele may feel like "third testicle."
‡ Varicocele should disappear on lying down.
§ May get increased venous flow.
¶ Hernia may be reducible on lying down.

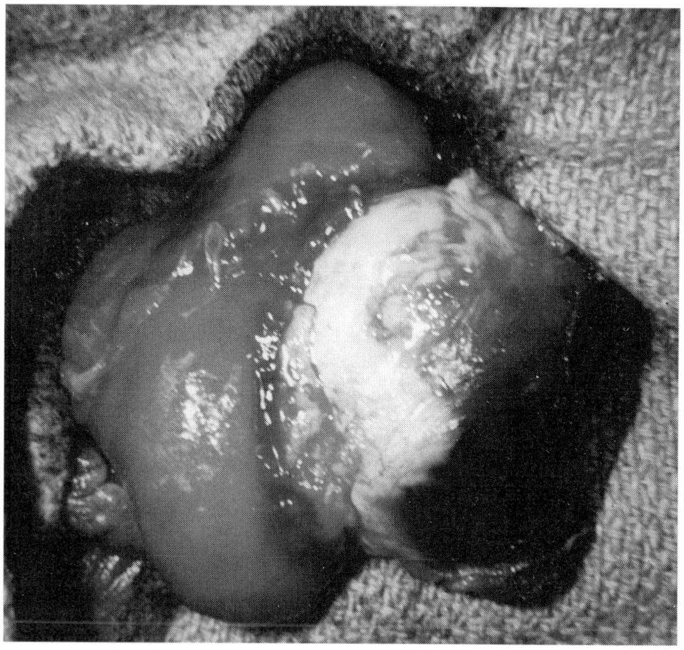

Fig. 61-4. Infarcted testis with infected epididymis in man with *Escherichia coli* epididymitis.

these failed to resolve after treatment of epididymitis and required surgical repair.[20]

Recurrence of epididymitis usually reflects lack of adequate treatment, failure to identify factors predisposing to reinfection, or inadequate suppression of a source of chronic infection. We have found an unusually high rate of complications in homosexual men with coliform epididymitis. Of six such men, one developed a testicular abscess, one developed contralateral epididymitis, and two relapsed after initial treatment.

Chronic epididymitis with chronic pain after the initial episode developed in 15 percent of Mittemeyer's cases.[14] It is not clear whether this is related to persistence of bacteria in the epididymis or whether it is owing to scarring or other factors. Chronic epididymitis is generally considered idiopathic and is notoriously unresponsive to antimicrobial therapy.

INFERTILITY

Another complication of acute epididymitis, although poorly documented, is decreased fertility. Patients with bilateral epididymitis and bilateral occlusion of the vas deferens or epididymis have virtually no potential for fertility. In some parts of sub-Saharan Africa where urethritis often goes untreated, epididymitis is a leading cause of male infertility.[74] Campbell noted that 40 percent of patients with bilateral epididymitis secondary to gonorrhea were sterile.[75] Pelouze reported involuntary infertility among 10.5 percent of men with only a history of gonococcal urethritis, 23 percent of men with history of unilateral epididymitis (Fig. 61-6), and 42 percent of men with history of bilateral epididymitis.[22] Gartman reported that among 18 azoospermic men with normal testes biopsies and patent vas deferens, only four had histories of bilateral epididymitis, but all were found to have fine scars that transected the epididymal tubules.[20] Gerris et al. found elevated chlamydia antibody titers in *tunica vaginalis* fluid in men with oligoasthenospermia, suggesting previous undetected chlamydia infection.[76] These data suggest that patients may have a subclinical form of epididymitis that may lead to asymptomatic scarring and decreased fertility. This intriguing observation may be analogous to the observation that among infertile women who have bilateral tubal obstruction (many of whom have serological evidence of past *C. trachomatis* infection), only about half have a past history of salpingitis (see Chapter 63). Since sperm transit through the epididymis is necessary for development of normal sperm function, it is possible that acute inflammation and damage to the epididymis could ultimately lead to decreased fertility even in the absence of occlusion of the epididymal tubules. Epididymal obstruction may be spontaneously reversible in some patients. Pelouze reported one patient who had a return of sperm and fertility after 5 years of apparent epididymal occlusion following gonococcal epididymitis.[22] The inflammation in acute epididymitis is not limited to the epididymis but also involves the testicle. Wolin found on testes biopsy during acute epididymitis that 20 of 28 patients had decreased spermatogenesis, and 9 of 28 had testicular

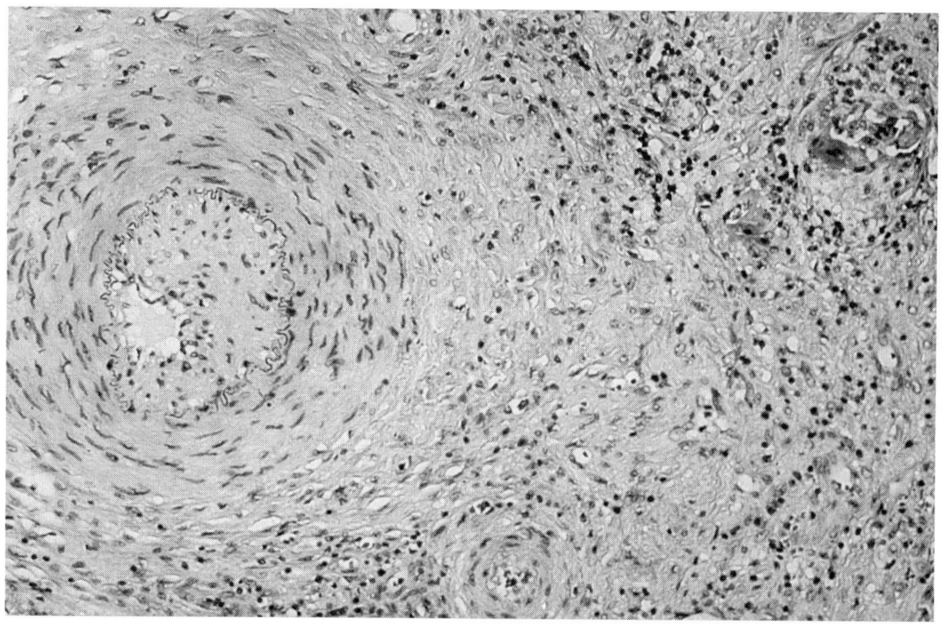

Fig. 61-5. Thrombosed artery in spermatic cord of man with *Escherichia coli* epididymitis.

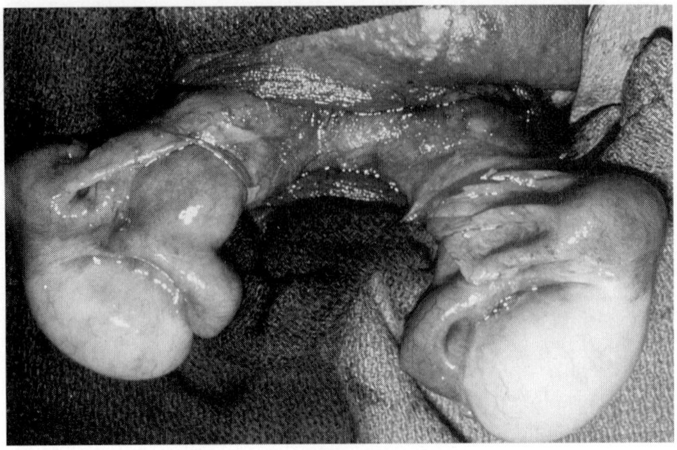

Fig. 61-6. Bilateral epididymitis in young man with *C. trachomatis* infection

inflammation.[9] Nilsson did aspiration biopsies on testicles in acute epididymitis and found that 16 of 22 showed inflammatory cells.[77] Follow-up biopsy of these testicles after 2 to 3 years showed that five of nine had reduced or absent spermatogenesis. Bietz found nonspecific toxic changes in the opposite testis 150 to 280 days following the onset of epididymitis.[78] Osegbe found thickened basement membranes, decreased spermatogenesis, and fibrosis in the contralateral testicle of men with clinical unilateral epididymitis.[79] Both Tozzo and we have found low sperm counts in a high proportion of patients with acute epididymitis.[1,80] Ludwig followed 46 patients with unilateral epididymitis from 8 days to 1 year.[81] He found initially that two-thirds had oligoesthenospermia. However, only 20 percent had long-term fertility disturbance as reflected in semen analysis, and only one had persisting sperm agglutinins after 1 year. In other unilateral conditions of the testicles, such as cryptorchidism and torsion of the testicle, decreased fertility has been demonstrated.[82,83] Whether unilateral testicular involvement in acute epididymitis can decrease fertility potential has not been definitively evaluated. Bandhauer found that nine of 48 men with acute unilateral epididymitis developed sperm agglutinins.[84] Ingerslev et al. found that 27 percent of men who had epididymitis developed serum antisperm agglutinating antibodies.[85] Heidenreich et al. and Ingerslev et al. found that antibodies often appeared in the early period after acute epididymitis; however, later the incidence of antibody titers usually decreased to nonsignificant levels.[85,86] Greskovich et al. found experimentally that early antibiotic therapy suppressed the antibody response, perhaps through a direct immunosuppressive effect, or through decreased antigenic load of killed sperm secondary to eradication of infection.[87] We have found that men without a history of clinical epididymitis, but with serological evidence of past exposure to *C. trachomatis*, have a significantly greater chance (50%) of having sperm autoantibody than do men without evidence of such exposure (16%).[88] In summary, bilateral epididymitis can lead to bilateral epididymal occlusion, a zoospermia, and infertility. Whether unilateral epididymitis, subclinical epididymitis, or epididymitis without occlusion, result in infertility remains unproven.

PATHOLOGY OF ACUTE EPIDIDYMITIS

The clinical manifestations of inflammation in acute epididymitis usually begin in the tail of the epididymis and spread to involve the rest of the epididymis and the testicle proper. Pelouze noted in 98 percent of cases of epididymitis, the clinical course suggested that the epididymis was inflamed before the vas became inflamed.[22] Early in the course of the disease, the epididymal ducts become distended with polymorphonuclear and mononuclear leukocytes that may actively phagocytize sperm.[89] The epithelium of the epididymis may be destroyed, and small abscesses form in the connective tissue, which is intensely hyperemic. In the stroma, lymphocytes may outnumber the polymorphonuclear leukocytes. Microabscesses may be present after 48 hours.[89] Later on, the columnar epithelium of the epididymis may become squamoid in appearance and plasma cells more frequent. Cronquist reported seven cases of epididymitis in which sperm penetrated the epithelium and basement lamina of the epididymis with a marked inflammatory reaction.[90] In biopsies in acute epididymitis, Wolin noted that 13 of 24 patients had epididymal tubular destruction with microabscesses and a predominance of polymorphonuclear leukocytes.[9] However, in the remaining 11 cases, there was predominantly lymphocytic infiltration with no tubular involvement. Perivascular mononuclear cell infiltration was prominent in some of these cases. We have also noted mononuclear cell infiltrate in the epididymis of men with chlamydial infection proven by fluorescent monoclonal antibody.[91] The interstitium is often infiltrated with neutrophils, small lymphocytes, plasma cells, and transformed lymphocytes. Neutrophils are often seen in the epididymal tubules and migrating through the epithelium.[91] As noted in the preceding, Wolin and Nilsson et al. described testicular inflammation.[9,77] The latter reported that Sertoli's cells were vacuolated, with cloudy cytoplasm. Furthermore, the organism responsible for epididymitis was isolated from the testicle in four patients. After 2 to 7 months, repeat biopsies showed decreased inflammation with an increased proportion of lymphocytes, macrophages, and plasma cells. After 2 to 3 years, there was atrophy, which was proportional to the degree of initial inflammation.

In summary, available data suggest that most cases of acute epididymitis begin in the tail of the epididymis, with an acute intralumenal exudate, tubular epithelial damage, and subjacent microabscesses. However, some cases show predominantly mononuclear and perivascular infiltration. Testicular involvement occurs and may lead to testicular atrophy. Unfortunately, these previous pathological studies have not employed comprehensive microbiological studies of etiology.

EXPERIMENTAL PATHOLOGY

Møller and coworkers has reported a primate model of *C. trachomatis* epididymitis in grivet monkeys.[92] Injection of *C. trachomatis* down the vas deferens produced a marked infiltration with polymorphonuclear leukocytes and lymphocytes through all layers of the spermatic cord. In the epididymis, the ducts were also filled with exudate containing mostly leukocytes and polymorphonuclear leukocytes. They were able to isolate *C. trachomatis* from the vas deferens but were unable to isolate it from the epididymis. We have used *Macaca nemistrina* as a primate model for chlamydial epididymitis, and after inoculation of *C. trachomatis* through the vas deferens, obtained mainly a mononuclear perivascular inflammation in the area of the epididymis.[93] Other models for acute and chronic epididymitis have been developed in mice and rats.[94–96] Lucchetta et al. have developed a model for epididymitis caused by *E. coli* in the rat, and we have developed a similar model in the rabbit.[97,98] Both models show a marked decrease in spermatogenesis following epididymitis. In a rat model See et al. found that the concentration of the antibiotic amdinocillin was actually increased in the infected testicle over the noninfected side.[98] Likewise, in a rat model Tartaglione et al. found increased concentrations of antibiotics on the infected side for sulfamethoxazole, tobramycin, doxycycline, and ampicillin.[99] Trimethoprim had similar levels in infected and noninfected sides. Doxycycline had the best tissue penetration of any antibiotic. Vieler et al. compared efficacy of treatment with cefotaxime, doxycycline, and ofloxacin in rats with experimental *E.* coli epididymitis.[100] Ofloxacin was the most efficacious at decreasing the number of organisms and histologic changes. Doxycycline was more effective than cefotaxime. Nielsen found that antibiotic therapy had no effect after abscess formation had taken place in a rat model.[101]

ROUTE OF SPREADS OF INFECTION

The route of spread of infection to the epididymis has been a subject of much debate. Much of the controversy was spawned originally by the idea that "idiopathic" epididymitis was caused by "sterile" inflammation from urine refluxing down the vas deferens while straining with a full bladder. This theory had implications both for workman's compensation from results of injuries sustained while working, and for the military, where prevention of epididymitis and loss of time from service was of great importance. Currently, most cases of epididymitis are thought to be infectious in origin. Therefore, the route of spread to the epididymis may be more of academic interest, since the spread of naturally occurring infection from the urethra, bladder, or prostate does not carry the same legal implications as reflux of sterile urine caused by strenuous work.

Experimentally, infective epididymitis has been produced by inoculation and intralumenal spread.[92] On numerous occasions, it has been demonstrated that urine from the bladder can reflux into the ejaculatory ducts and into the vas deferens in patients undergoing prostatectomy or in those with serious urinary pathology. Thind et al. have shown high voiding pressures and sphincter dysinergia in many patients who have had acute epididymitis.[102,103] On the other hand, Kohler was unable to produce reflux of radiographic contrast down the vas in patients recovering from acute epididymitis.[104] Similarly, Herwig was unable to demonstrate retrograde urination down the vas in patients with sterile urine.[105] Pelouze pointed out that the ejaculatory ducts contain no circular muscles, and for a peristaltic wave to carry urine in a retrograde fashion down the vas deferens, the seminal vesicle would have to first fill with urine and then contract and force the urine down into the epididymis.[22] Inflammation of the seminal vesicle during acute epididymitis has been demonstrated by gal lium scan and ultrasound.[106,107] We have noted grossly purulent semen in men who have epididymitis with minimal urethritis and no symptoms or signs attributable to prostatitis or seminal vesiculitis. Since the seminal vesicle is subject to the same intra-abdominal pressures as the bladder, perhaps straining could force infected seminal vesicle contents down the vas and into the epididymis. Reflux of urine therefore would not be necessary to explain the sudden onset of epididymitis with straining in these patients. In men with prostate obstruction, Kendall found positive vas cultures in only 15 percent of patients with positive urinary cultures without a catheter, but in 36 percent of infected patients who had a urethral catheter in place.[108] Orandi performed preprostatectomy vas cultures and found that 32 of 67 patients with positive urine cultures also had positive vas cultures.[109] He found none of 74 patients with negative urine cultures to have positive vas cultures. Reeves ligated only one vas deferens in 505 preprostatectomy cases.[110] He found a higher rate of epididymitis on the nonligated side. Perhaps a catheter or similar irritation from infection of the verumontanum may allow reflux of infected urine from the bladder down the vas deferens or lead to seminal vesiculitis with infection subsequently spreading to the epididymis.

Other theories have been proposed to explain how infection gets to the epididymis. Spread of organisms by continuity of surface down the vas has been questioned. Wesson suggested that organisms could spread to the vas by means of lymphatics.[111] He noted the frequent swelling of the spermatic cord in patients with epididymitis. Since the epididymis drains to hypogastric and iliac nodes and the prostate and seminal vesicles drain to the same area, spread by the way of lymphatic drainage was postulated. The lack of involvement of the testicle in some cases was attributed to the different lymphatic drainage of the two organs. Rolnick suggested that the spread could advance along the sheath of the vas, since this sheath is a continuation of the sheath of the prostate and seminal vesicles.[112] Infection that extended out of the prostate or seminal vesicles could thus travel along the sheath of the vas to the tail of the epididymis. Some infections, such as tuberculous, pneumococcal, fungal, and other infections, might well spread to the epididymis by a hematogenous route. However, this route is probably unusual for coliform or sexually transmitted organisms, since most often the offending organism can be found within the urethra or bladder.

TREATMENT

Symptomatic treatment of the patient with epididymitis is always indicated. Scrotal elevation provides for maximum lymphatic and venous drainage. The patient should be placed at bed rest with the scrotum elevated on a towel between his legs. The use of constricting scrotal supports while the patient is supine often only holds the scrotal contents between the patient's legs in a dependent position. If the patient is standing, gravity prevents proper drainage of the tissues and may increase swelling. The patient should remain at bed rest until the scrotal contents are nontender. If the pain should return after ambulation, the patient should again return to bed rest and scrotal elevation.

In view of the microbial etiology of the vast majority of cases of epididymitis, antibiotics should never be withheld in this condition. Nilsson has provided evidence that antibiotic treatment is superior to placebo in patients with coliform epididymitis, as well as in patients without coliforms.[113] Appropriate antibiotics can be chosen on the basis of culture and Gram stain of the urine and urethra, as outlined in Fig. 61-1. In patients with bacteriuria, initiation of broad spectrum parenteral antimicrobial therapy (e.g., tobramycin) is recommended. However, if ambulatory therapy is used for afebrile patients with mildly or moderately severe epididymitis, trimethoprim-sulfamethoxazole or a quinolone antibiotic provides activity against most enterobacteria. The organism recovered from the urine is also responsible for epididymitis and therapy can be modified on the basis of susceptibility tests on the isolate from urine.[1,55] In patients with indwelling urethral catheters who may have multiple organisms isolated from the urine and in patients who have been started on antibiotics who may have sterile urine, the use of epididymal aspiration cultures may identify the causal pathogen and provide needed antimicrobial sensitivity information.[50] Antibiotic treatment may need to be prolonged in some cases. We have isolated pathogenic organisms from the epididymis and testicular tissue for as long as 2 weeks after the beginning of appropriate antimicrobial therapy.

In patients with epididymitis associated with urethritis, cultures should initially be taken for both *N. gonorrhoeae* and *C. trachomatis.* Chlamydiae can be isolated from the urethra from approximately 20 percent of patients with gonorrhea, and theoretically could cause epididymitis even when *N. gonorrhoeae.* Patients with urethritis and acute epididymitis should therefore preferably be treated with a regimen active against β-lactamase positive strains of *N. gonorrhoeae* (e.g., ceftriaxone 250 mg intramuscularly), followed by 10 days of oral doxycycline (100 mg twice daily for 10 days) or by tetracycline hydroxychloride (500 mg orally four times daily for 10 days) to adequately cover chlamydial infection. Alternatively, ofloxacin 300 mg orally two times a day for 10 days is effective for both gonococcal and chlamydial infection, and active against most coliforms, and can also be used.[114]

Drainage of testicular abscesses or orchiectomy is seldom necessary in patients who receive early therapy with bed rest, scrotal elevation, and appropriate antimicrobials. Vordermark et al. found that, in patients who do not respond to antibiotics within 4 hours, epididymectomy hastened convalescence.[115–117] However, this has not been subjected to controlled study; in our experience, many patients require 48 to 72 hours to show improvement, but then do well. Epididymectomy may be indicated in an older group of patients after unsuccessful conservative treatment. Prophylactic vasectomy of the contralateral testicle has also been advocated during such procedures.[118]

Several nonantimicrobial treatments have been proposed for epididymitis. Smith found that patients with epididymitis had dramatic relief of pain after one or two injections of the spermatic cord with procaine hydrochloride. He noted that the relief of pain was not only immediate but lasted well beyond the period of local relief.[119] Kamat et al. reported on three groups of patients.[120] One group received antibiotics only, one group was treated with antibiotics plus oxyphenbutazone, and one group was treated with antibiotics plus infiltration of the spermatic cord with xylocaine hydrochloride. He found that patients treated with antibiotics plus oxyphenbutazone or antibiotics plus spermatic cord infiltration had quicker recovery than patients on antibiotics alone. His study was not blinded, however, and he did not report bacteriologic results. McClellan found antibiotic treatment to be better than symptomatic treatment alone.[121] He reported that the addition of paraenzyme or varidase also decreased the amount of swelling and percentage with residual chronic epididymitis. Lapides found that 35 of 47 patients with acute epididymitis were relieved by oxyphenbutazone alone.[122] He found decreased pain in these patients but no decrease in the amount of erythema or swelling. In a multicenter placebo study, Moore et al. found that prednisone had no value as adjuvant to antibiotic therapy in the treatment of epididymitis.[123] Thus, some clinicians believe that anesthetic infiltration of the spermatic cord and the use of oxyphenbutazone in addition to antibiotics may increase the comfort of a patient. However, it is not clear whether these forms of treatment provide better symptomatlc relief than the use of analgesics with antibiotics. The effect of such adjuvant therapy on the long-term sequelae of epididymitis is uncertain.

In patients in whom the etiologic agent is a sexually transmitted pathogen, treatment of epididymitis is not complete without treatment of the sexual partner(s). This, hopefully, will prevent recurrences in the patient as well as prevent disease in the partner. In a study by Berger et al., two of eight female partners of men with epididymitis were found to have chlamydia infection.[1] Robinson et al. found that 14 of 16 female consorts of men with chlamydial epididymitis had active cervical chlamydial infection.[1,124]

In the treatment of a patient with acute epididymitis, the decision must be made as to whether to pursue radiologic or endoscopic evidence for intrinsic genitourinary disease. Svend-Hansen found in patients under the age of 50 that only six of 43 men had abnormal excretory urograms; all six with abnormal findings had symptoms suggestive of urologic disease.[125] He concluded that in patients less than 50 years old, epididymitis in itself is not an indication for radiographic evaluation. This may well reflect the small proportion of cases of epididymitis that are owing to underlying urinary tract infection with coliforms or *Ps. aeruginosa* in younger men and thus the lower prevalence of genitourinary abnormalities. Similarly, we found no patient under the age of 35 years to have concurrent genitourinary pathology, whereas seven of 12 patients over the age of 35 with coliform infection had underlying pathology.[1] Kaver et al. also found that only patients over age 50 had urographic abnormalities.[126] All abnormalities were secondary to lower tract outflow obstruction. Certainly the presence of urethritis owing to *N. gonorrhoeae* or *C. trachomatis* does not suggest that the patient has an underlying genitourinary problem. On the other hand, the presence of a coliform urinary infection in a male always requires investigation. Patients with epididymitis owing to coliform or *Ps. aeruginosa* infection should also be evaluated after completion of antimicrobial therapy with four glass urine cultures for chronic bacterial prostatitis (see Chapter 53), as this may be a predisposing factor to recurrent epididymitis.

References

1 Berger RE et al: Etiology, manifestations and therapy of acute epididymitis: prospective study of 50 cases. *J Urol* 121:750–754, 1979.
2 U.S. Public Health Service, Sexually Transmitted Diseases, 1980, in Status Report, NIAID Study Group. Washington, DC: Government Printing Office, 1981, pp. 81–85.
3 Gasparich JP et al: Amiodarone-associated epididymitis: drug-related epididymitis in the absence of infection. *J Urol* 133:971–972, 1985.
4 Drotman DP: Epidemiology and treatment of epididymitis. *Rev Infect Dis* 4:S788–792, 1982.
5 Hanley HG: Non-specific epididymitis. *Br J Surg* 53:873–874, 1966.
6 Baumgarten H: Epididymitis in the workplace. *J Fla Med Assoc* 71: 21–22, 1984.
7 Bormel P: Current concepts of the etiology and treatment of epididymitis. *Med Bull US Army, Europe* 20:332, 1963.
8 Heap G: Acute epididymitis attributable to chlamydial infection—preliminary report. *Med J Aust* 1:718–719, 1975.
9 Wolin LH: On the etiology of epididymitis. *J Urol* 105:531–533, 1971.
10 Gierup J et al: Acute non-specific epididymitis in boys. A survey based on 48 consecutive cases. *Scand J Urol Nephrol* 9:5–7, 1975.
11 Megalli M et al: Reflux of urine into ejaculatory ducts as a cause of recurring epididymitis in children. *J Urol* 108:978–979, 1972.
12 Gislason T et al: Acute epididymitis in boys: a 5-year retrospective study. *J Urol* 124:533–534, 1980.
13 Shapiro SR et al: Acute epididymitis in Vietnam: review of 52 cases. *Milit Med* 138:643–645, 1973.
14 Mittemeyer BT et al: Epididymitis: a review of 610 cases. *J Urol* 95: 390–392, 1966.
15 Berger RE et al: Etiology and manifestations of epididymitis in young men: correlations with sexual orientation. *J Infect Dis* 155:1341–1343, 1987.
16 Drach GW: Sexuality and prostatitis: A hypothesis. *J Am Vener Dis Assoc* 3:87, 1976.
17 Barnes RC et al: Urinary tract infections in sexually active homosexual men. *Lancet* i:71, 1986.
18 Stamey TA et al: Recurrent urinary infections in adult women. The role of introital enterobacteria. *Cal Med* 115:1, 1971.
19 Berger RE et al: *Chlamydia trachomatis* as a cause of acute "idiopathic" epididymitis. *N Engl J Med* 298:301–304, 1978.
20 Gartman E: Epididymitis: A reappraisal. *Am J Surg* 101:736, 1961.
21 Ross WM et al: Nonspecific epididymitis in the military service. *US Armed Forces Med J* 8:841, 1957.
22 Pelouze PS: Epididymitis, in Pelouze PS (ed): *Gonorrhea in the Male and Female,* Philadelphia, WB Saunders, 1941, p. 240.
23 Watson RA: Gonorrhea and acute epididymitis. *Milit Med* 144:785–787, 1979.
24 Mulcahy FM et al: Prevalence of chlamydial infection in acute epididymo-orchitis. *Genitourin Med* 63:16–18, 1987.
25 Melekos MD et al: Epididymitis: aspects concerning etiology and treatment. *J Urol* 138:83–86, 1987.
26 Colleen S et al: Complicated infections of the male genital tract with emphasis on *Chlamydia trachomatis* as an etiological agent. *Scand J Infect Dis Suppl* 32:93–99, 1982.

27 Hawkins DA et al: Microbiological survey of acute epididymitis. *Genitourin Med* 62:342–344, 1986.

28 Lee CT et al: Epidemiology of acute epididymo-orchitis in Singapore. *Ann Acad Med Singapore* 18:320–323, 1989.

29 Eley A et al: Detection of *Chlamydia trachomatis* by the polymerase chain reaction in young patients with acute epididymitis. *Eur J Clin Microbiol Infect Dis* 11:620–623, 1992.

30 Cathcart CW: Epididymitis from muscular strain followed by tuberculosis of epididymis. *Edinburg Med J* 26:152, 1921.

31 Halker E: *Treatment of Renal Tuberculosis with Chemotherapeutics.* Nyt Nordisk Forlag, 1956.

32 Ross JC et al: Tuberculosis epididymitis: A review of 170 patients. *Br J Surg* 48:663, 1961.

33 Medlar EM et al: Post-mortem compared with clinical diagnosis of genitourinary tuberculosis in adult males. *J Urol* 61:1078, 1949.

34 Heaton ND et al: Tuberculous epididymo-orchitis: clinical and ultrasound observations. *Br J Urol* 64:305–309, 1989.

35 Wolf JS Jr et al: Tuberculous epididymo-orchitis: diagnosis by fine needle aspiration. *J Urol* 145:836–838, 1991.

36 McDonald JH et al: Acute pneumococcal epididymitis. *Ill Med J* 95: 304, 1949.

37 Mitchell CJ et al: Letter: Acute brucellosis presenting as epididymo-orchitis. *Br Med J* 2:557–558, 1974.

38 Khan MS et al: Epididymo-orchitis and brucellosis. *Br J Urol* 63:87–89, 1989.

39 Ibrahim AI et al: Genito-urinary complications of brucellosis. *Br J Urol* 61:294–298, 1988.

40 Davis WH et al: Meningitis presenting as epididymitis. *So Med J* 65, 1972.

41 Wheeler JJ et al: Nocardia epididymo-orchitis in an immunosuppressed patient. *J Urol* 136:1314–1315, 1986.

42 Lin YC et al: Acute scrotum due to *Haemophilus influenzae* type b. *J Pediatr Surg* 23:183–184, 1988.

43 Weber TR: *Hemophilus influenzae* epididymo-orchitis. *J Urol* 133, 1985.

44 Hakim A et al: Salmonella epididymo-orchitis in infancy and childhood. *Clin Pediatr (Phila)* 31:120–122, 1992.

45 James CL et al: Cryptococcal epididymo-orchitis complicating steroid therapy for relapsing polychondritis. *Pathology* 23:256–258, 1991.

46 Short KL et al: The use of ketoconazole to treat systemic blastomycosis presenting as acute epididymitis. *J Urol* 129:382–384, 1983.

47 Docimo SG et al: Candida epididymitis: newly recognized opportunistic epididymal infection. *Urology* 41:280–282, 1993.

48 Randazzo RF et al: Cytomegaloviral epididymitis in a patient with the acquired immune deficiency syndrome. *J Urol* 136:1095–1097, 1986.

49 Furness G et al: Epididymitis after the luminal spread of NSU corynebacteria and gram negative bacteria from the fossa navicularis. *Invest Urol* 11:486–488, 1974.

50 Berger RE et al: The clinical use of epididymal aspiration cultures in the management of selected patients with acute epididymitis. *J Urol* 124:60–61, 1980.

51 Shapiro R et al: Epididymo-orchitis. *Current Therapy of Infectious Disease,* Schlossberg D (ed). Mosby, St. Louis, 178–181, 1996.

52 Quinto O: Swelling of scrotum in infants and children and nonspecific epididymitis. *Acta Chir Scand* 110:417, 1956.

53 Devillar RG et al: Early exploratory in acute testicular conditions. *J Urol* 108:887–888, 1972.

54 Barker K et al: Torsion of the testis. *Br J Urol* 36:35, 1964.

55 Doolittle KH et al: Epididymitis in the prepuberal boy. *J Urol* 96: 364–366, 1966.

56 Madsen PO: Acute epididymitis vs. torsion of spermatic in military service. *J Urol* 83:169, 1960.

57 Perri AJ et al: The Doppler stethoscope and the diagnosis of the acute scrotum. *J Urol* 116:598, 1976.

58 Holder LE et al: Testicular radionuclide angiography and static imaging: Anatomy, scintigraphic interpretation, and clinical indications. *Radiology* 125:739, 1977.

59 Abu-Sleiman R et al: Scrotal scanning: present value and limits of interpretation. *Urology* 13:326–330, 1979.

60 Palestro CJ et al: Hydrocele and epididymitis mimicking testicular torsion on scrotal scintigraphy. *Clin Nucl Med* 18:910–911, 1993.

61 van Ahlen H et al: Static and dynamic radionuclide imaging in the diagnosis of the acute scrotum. *Urol Int* 47:20–24, 1991.

62 Hankins AJ: Testicular torsion and epididymitis demonstrated by radionuclide angiograms and static imaging. *J Natl Med Assoc* 71:981–983, 1979.

63 Fitzgerald SW et al: Color Doppler sonography in the evaluation of the adult acute scrotum [see comments]. *J Ultrasound Med* 11:543–548, 1992.

64 Middleton WD et al: Acute scrotal disorders: prospective comparison of color Doppler US and testicular scintigraphy. *Radiology* 177:177–181, 1990.

65 Wilbert DM et al: Evaluation of the acute scrotum by color-coded Doppler ultrasonography. *J Urol* 149:1475–1477, 1993.

66 Trambert M et al: Subacute scrotal pain: evaluation of torsion versus epididymitis with MR imaging. *Radiology* 175:53–56, 1990.

67 Shurbaji MS et al: Testicular vasculitis: implications for systemic disease. *Hum Pathol* 19:186–189, 1988.

68 Wright LF et al: Systemic necrotizing vasculitis presenting as epididymitis. *J Urol* 136, 1986.

69 O'Connell H et al: Delayed epididymitis following intravesical bacillus Calmette-Guerin administration. *Aust NZ J Surg* 63:70–72, 1993.

70 Rencken RK et al: Venous infarction of the testis—a cause of non-response to conservative therapy in epididymo-orchitis. A case report. *S Afr Med J* 78:337–338, 1990.

71 Eisner DJ et al: Bilateral testicular infarction caused by epididymitis. *Ajr Am J Roentgenol* 157:517–519, 1991.

72 Costas S et al: Incision of the external inguinal ring in acute epididymitis. *Br J Urol* 45:555–558, 1973.

73 See WA et al: Scrotal ultrasonography: a predictor of complicated epididymitis requiring orchiectomy. *J Urol* 139:55–56, 1988.

74 Arya OP et al: Correlates of venereal disease and fertility in rural Uganda. Presented at the Medical Society for the Study of Venereal Diseases, Malta, April 1975.

75 Campbell MF: Surgical pathology of epididymitis. *Ann Surg* 88:98, 1928.

76 Gerris J et al: A possible role of *Chlamydia trachomatis* as a causative agent in epydimal infertility. *Acta Eur Fertil* 16:179–182, 1985.

77 Nilsson S et al: Changes in the testis parenchyma caused by acute nonspecific epididymitis. *Fertil Steril* 19:748–757, 1968.

78 Bietz O: Fertilitatsuntersuchungen bei der unspezifischen Epididymitis. *Hautarzt* 10:134, 1959.

79 Osegbe DN: Testicular function after unilateral bacterial epididymo-orchitis. *Eur Urol* 19:204–208, 1991.

80 Tozzo PJ: Semen analysis in unilateral epididymitis. *NY State J Med* 68:2769–2770, 1968.

81 Ludwig VG et al: Epididymitis und fertilität: Behandlungsergebnisse bei akuter anspezifischer epididymitis. *Fortschr Med* 5:397, 1977.

82 Lipschultz LI et al: Testicular function after orchidopexy for unilateral undescended testicle. *N Engl J Med* 295:15, 1976.

83 Gartsch G et al: Testicular torsion: Late results with special regard to fertility and endocrine function. *J Urol* 124:375, 1980.

84 Bandhauer K et al: Spermagglutinins in diseases of epididymis. Presented at the 5th World Congress Fertil Steril, 1966, p. 781.

85 Ingerslev HJ et al: A prospective study of antisperm antibody development in acute epididymitis. *J Urol* 136:162–164, 1986.

86 Heidenreich A et al: Risk factors for antisperm antibodies in infertile men. *Am J Reprod Immunol* 31:69–76, 1994.

87 Greskovich F et al: Effect of early antibiotic treatment on the formation of sperm antibodies in experimentally induced epididymitis. *Arch Androl* 30:183–191, 1993.

88 Close CE et al: The relationship of infection with *Chlamydia trachomatis* to the parameters of male infertility and sperm autoimmunity. *Fertil Steril* 48:880, 1987.

89 Cunningham JH et al: The operative treatment and pathology of acute epididymitis. *J Urol* 7:139, 1920.
90 Cronquist S: Spermatic invasion of the epididymis. *Acta Pathol Microbiol Scand* 26:786, 1949.
91 Kiviat MD et al: *Chlamydia trachomatis* epididymitis diagnosed by fluorescent monoclonal antibody. *Urology* 30:395–397, 1987.
92 Møller BR et al: Experimental epididymitis and urethritis in grivet monkeys provoked by *Chlamydia trachomatis. Fertil Steril* 34:275, 1980.
93 Berger RE: Epididymitis after the experimental inoculation of the nonhuman primate with *Chlamydia trachomatis*, unpublished data.
94 Kuzan FB et al: A proposed mouse model for acute epididymitis provoked by genital serovar E, *Chlamydia trachomatis. Biol Reprod* 40: 165–172, 1989.
95 Jantos C et al: Experimental chlamydial epididymitis. *Urol Int* 44: 279–283, 1989.
96 Jantos CB et al: Experimental epididymitis due to *Chlamydia trachomatis* in rats. *Infect Immunol* 60:2324–2328, 1992.
97 Lucchetta R et al: Acute experimental *E. coli* epididymitis in the rat and its consequences on spermatogenesis. *Urol Res* 11:117–120, 1983.
98 Hackett RA et al: Experimental *Escherichia coli* epididymitis in rabbits. *Urology* 32:236–2340, 1988.
98a See WA et al: Bacterial epidedymitis in the rat: a model for assessing the impact of acute inflammation and epididymal antibiotic penetration. *J Urol* 144:780–784, 1990.
99 Tartaglione TA et al: Antimicrobial tissue penetration in a rat model of *E. coli* epididymitis. *J Urol* 146:1413–1417, 1991.
100 Vieler E et al: Comparative efficacies of ofloxacin, cefotaxime, and doxycycline for treatment of experimental epididymitis due to *Escherichia coli* in rats. *Antimicrob Agents Chemother* 37:846–850, 1993.
101 Nielsen OS: An experimental study of the treatment of bacterial epididymitis. *Scand J Urol Nephrol Suppl* 104:115–117, 1987.
102 Thind P et al: Assessment of voiding dysfunction in men with acute epididymitis. *Urol Int* 48:320–322, 1992.
103 Thind P et al: Is micturition disorder a pathogenic factor in acute epididymitis? An evaluation of simultaneous bladder pressure and urine flow in men with previous acute epididymitis. *J Urol* 143:323–325, 1990.
104 Kohler FP: An inquiry into the etiology of acute epididymitis. *J Urol* 87:918, 1962.
105 Herwig KR et al: Response of acute epididymitis to oxyphenbutazone. *J Urol* 106:890–891, 1971.
106 Krishnan R et al: Study of the seminal vesicles in acute epididymitis. *Br J Urol* 67:632–637, 1991.
107 Kiviat MD: Unpublished data.
108 Kendall AR: Rationale of prophylactic vasectomy. *J Urol* 89:712, 1963.
109 Orandi A et al: Vas culture, epididymitis and post-prostatectomy fever. *J Urol* 96:367–369, 1966.
110 Reeves JF et al: Prevention of epididymitis after prostatectomy by prophylactic antibiotics and partial vasectomy. *J Urol* 92:528, 1964.
111 Wesson MB: Epididymitis: importance of determining etiology. *J Urol* 85:960, 1961.
112 Rolnick HC: Infections along the sheath of the vas deferens. *J Urol* 85:960, 1925.
113 Nilsson T et al: Acute epididymitis: Investigation, etiology and treatment with doxycycline, in *Sexually Transmitted Disease (Symposium Proceedings),* Los Angeles, Science & Medicine Publishing, 1979, p. 38.
114 Centers for Disease Control and Prevention: 1998 Sexually transmitted diseases. Treatment guidelines. MMWR 1998 42 (No. RR-14).
115 Vordermark JS et al: Role of surgery in management of acute bacterial epididymitis. *Urology* 35:283–287, 1990.
116 Vordermark JS: Acute epididymitis: experience with 123 cases. *Milit Med* 150:27–30, 1985.
117 Vordermark JS et al: Testicular necrosis: a preventable complication of epididymitis. *J Urol* 128:1322–1324, 1982.
118 Hoppner W et al: Surgical treatment of acute epididymitis and its underlying diseases. *Eur Urol* 22:218–221, 1992.
119 Smith DR: Treatment of epididymitis by infiltration of spermatic cord with procaine hydrochloride. *J Urol* 46:74, 1941.
120 Kamat MH et al: Epididymitis. Response to different modalities of treatment. *J Med Soc NJ* 67:227–229, 1970.
121 McClellan DS et al: Effect of varidase on acute non-specific epididymitis. *J Urol* 84:6733, 1960.
122 Lapides J et al: Oxyphenbutazone therapy for mumps orchitis, acute epididymitis and osteitis pubis. *J Urol* 98:528–530, 1967.
123 Moore CA et al: Prednisone in the treatment of acute epididymitis: a cooperative study. *J Urol* 106:578–580, 1971.
124 Robinson AJ et al: Acute epididymitis: why patient and consort must be investigated. *Br J Urol* 66:642–645, 1990.
125 Svend-Hansen H et al: The value of routine intravenous urography in acute epididymitis. *Int Urol Nephrol* 9:245–248, 1977.
126 Kaver I et al: Epididymo-orchitis: a retrospective study of 121 patients. *J Fam Pract* 30:548–552, 1990.

Chapter 62
Prostatitis syndromes

John N. Krieger

HISTORY

Prostate disease, stones, obstruction, and infection were well known in antiquity. The Ebers Papyrus refers to prostatitis, urethritis, urinary retention, incontinence, and cystitis.[1] Bladder stones, often a consequence of prostatic or urethral obstruction, were found in Egyptian mummies. The ancient Egyptians used reeds, copper and silver tubes, and rolled palm leaves to treat urinary retention, which may have been due to stones, prostatic obstruction, or probably both. Practitioners who used these instruments the most became known as lithologists, the first specialists in medicine.

The Hindu Vedas contain procedures—which may be 4,000–5,000 years old—for relief of obstruction caused by prostatic disease and bladder stones. The Vedas also describe cannulas of wood and metal. Uroscopy, or examination of the urine, was a highly developed art before the time of Hippocrates (460–377 B.C.), who paid much attention to this examination. Herophilus of Chalcedonia, a well-known lithotomist, is credited with what is probably the earliest gross description of the prostate in his anatomic texts. Rufus of Ephesus described the "parastatus glandulus" (meaning "standing before"), a likely origin of the term *prostate*. Aristotle used the term *varicose parastatae* for what may well have been seminal vesicles.

At the beginning of the Christian era, Celsus (25 B.C. to A.D. 50) described catheterization and urethrotomy: "Circumstances sometimes render it necessary to draw off the urine by an operation; as in retention, or when the urethra has become collapsed from old age, or when a calculus or grumous blood has produced internal obstruction; . . . even a moderate degree of inflammation often prevents natural micturition. Now this operation is necessary not only in males, but sometimes in females, also. Hence, copper catheters are made for this purpose. . . . The practitioner should keep by him three for men, and two for females. . . . They ought to be somewhat curved."

By 1500, cystostomy, generally perineal, was in widespread use for removal of stones. On occasion this approach would also treat prostatic obstruction because it was necessary to remove portions of the prostate to obtain access to the stone.[1] Thus, the first prostatic surgery was probably unintentional and through a perineal incision.

DEFINITION, EPIDEMIOLOGY, AND OVERVIEW

"Prostatitis" is the diagnosis given to a large group of men who present with a variety of complaints referable to the lower urogenital tract and perineum.[2–5] By one estimate 50 percent of men experience symptoms of prostatitis at some time in their lives.[2] Data from the National Health Center for Health Statistics indicate that there were 76 office visits per 1,000 men per year for genitourinary tract problems, with prostatitis accounting for approximately 25 percent of these visits.

Many men remain symptomatic for prolonged periods. Patients frequently relate the onset of their condition to sexual activity, commonly to an episode of acute urethritis.[6] Antimicrobial treatment often results in transient relief of symptoms. Based on these observations, standard practice is to prescribe multiple courses of antibacterial therapy in the frequently vain hope that patients will experience lasting relief.[2,7,8] In our report of 75 men with chronic prostatitis, the average patient had received 10 weeks of unsuccessful antimicrobial treatment during the 3 months before evaluation.[9]

Clinical characterization of patients with prostatitis syndromes has not been carefully correlated with the pathologic classification of prostatitis.[2,8] Pathologic studies have not included sufficient clinical or microbiologic data. On the other hand, clinical studies rarely have found pathologic specimens to be helpful, probably reflecting the focal nature of the inflammatory response in patients with prostatitis.[10–12]

From a clinical standpoint, it is critical to distinguish men with lower-urinary-tract complaints associated with bacteriuria from the larger number of patients without bacteriuria.[8] Careful lower-urinary-tract localization studies classify most patients into four diagnostic groups: acute bacterial prostatitis, chronic bacterial prostatitis, nonbacterial prostatitis, and prostatodynia.[2,13] Considerable progress has been made in understanding the pathophysiology and in developing rational approaches for treatment of patients with acute and chronic bacterial prostatitis. Unfortunately, few reliable data are available on the etiology of nonbacterial prostatitis or prostatodynia. Thus, current therapy is unsatisfactory for most patients with prostatitis syndromes. Occasional men develop granulomatous prostatitis, a characteristic histologic reaction of the prostate to a variety of insults. Treatment of granulomatous prostatitis depends on accurate etiologic diagnosis.

PATHOGENESIS AND IMMUNE RESPONSE

Prostatic infection can occur despite the wide variety of defenses of the male lower urogenital tract against infection. These defenses include nonspecific mechanisms, such as mechanical factors and antimicrobial secretions, as well as the specific humoral and cellular limbs of the immune system.

NONSPECIFIC DEFENSES

Most infections of the urogenital ducts and accessory sex organs are caused by organisms that ascend through the urethra.[2] Thus, mechanical factors including urethral length, micturition, and ejaculation should provide some protection against infection, although the relative importance of such defenses is unclear. The oblique courses taken by some prostatic ducts and by the ejaculatory ducts have also been proposed as mechanical defense mechanisms.

Prostatic secretions contain several substances active against a wide spectrum of microorganisms.[2,14] A zinc-containing polypeptide, known as the prostatic antibacterial factor, is the most important antimicrobial substance secreted by the prostate. The prostate has higher concentrations of zinc than any other organ, and prostatic secretions of normal men contain high zinc levels.[15–19] The bactericidal activity of prostatic secretions against a wide range of gram-negative and gram-positive organisms is a direct function of zinc concentration. Zinc also inhibits other genital pathogens including herpes viruses,[20,21] *Candida albicans*,[22,23] *Trichomonas vaginalis*,[7,24,25] and *Chlamydia trachomatis*.[26] Men with well-documented chronic bacterial prostatitis have significantly lower levels of zinc in their prostatic fluid than controls,[16,17] but their serum zinc levels are within normal limits.[17] It is unclear whether the reduction of concentrations of zinc in the prostatic secretions of men with bacterial prostatitis precedes development of prostatic infection or reflects secretory dysfunction resulting from such infections.[18] Oral zinc supplements did not increase the concentration of zinc in prostatic secretions of men with bacterial prostatitis.[17]

The prostate gland secretes a number of other substances with antibacterial activity. Spermine and spermidine, which are responsible for the characteristic seminal aroma, have been studied in most detail.[19,27] These compounds possess activity primarily against gram-positive bacteria and appear to be of secondary significance in protecting the male lower genitourinary tract against infection.[19,28]

HUMORAL IMMUNITY

Many investigators have studied the serologic responses of men with bacterial prostatitis. Sera from men with acute bacterial prostatitis contain specific agglutinating antibodies against the infecting bacterial strains.[29–31] Titers remain elevated during persistent bacterial infection of the prostate, and changes in antibody titers reflect the response to antimicrobial therapy in some patients.[29,30] Controls had low titers of antibodies against gram-negative organisms of their own fecal flora, and similar low titers are present in men whose urethras are colonized by *Escherichia coli.* Serologic studies of men with bacterial prostatitis have had two significant technical limitations: First, most studies have employed an assay that does not distinguish specific immunoglobulin classes, and second, some patients with well-documented bacterial prostatitis have low titers of agglutinating antibodies.[2,29]

Local immunoglobulin production by the prostate appears to be an important defense of the lower urogenital tract against infection. Prostatic secretions from men with bacterial prostatitis contain high concentrations of immunoglobulin.[32–34] Several studies have demonstrated an antigen-specific antibody coating of bacteria isolated from patients with prostatitis.[35,36] An indirect solid-phase radioimmunoassay was used to measure the local immunologic response in a limited number of patients with well-documented bacterial prostatitis.[37–40] The antigen-specific antibody response in prostatic secretions (predominantly secretory IgA) was significantly greater than the serologic response.[37,39,40] The antigen-specific IgA response in prostatic secretions persisted longer than the prostatic IgG antigen-specific antibody or the serum antigen-specific responses.[38] Patients with nonbacterial prostatitis had a modest nonspecific increase in local class-specific immunoglobulins, whereas normal controls, with no history of urologic disease, had even lower levels of local prostatic antibodies.[40,41]

Men with prior episodes of *E. coli* bacteriuria, but with no bacteriologic evidence of prostatitis, had similar increases in antigen-specific antibody levels in their prostatic secretions.[40,41] These data suggest that bacteriuria in men may be associated with subclinical colonization of the prostate.[40–42] Comparable increases in local immunoglobulins were not detected in men with *Staphylococcus epidermidis* apparently localized to their prostates.[40]

CELLULAR IMMUNITY

Presence of leukocytes characterizes many inflammatory conditions of the male lower urinary tract, including cystitis, urethritis, and prostatitis syndromes.[13,43–47] Among men with prostatitis, patients with acute disease have a predominance of mononuclear cells in prostatic secretions, while patients with chronic disease have few cells of the monocyte-macrophage series.[48] One longitudinal study of prostatic secretions from 106 patients with prostatitis found that inflammation resolved in most patients with acute bacterial prostatitis and was episodic in patients with chronic bacterial or abacterial prostatitis.[49] The observation of phagocytosis of abnormal sperm by leukocytes in infertile men with pyospermia suggests one functional role of leukocytes in inflammatory conditions of the male lower urogenital tract.[50,51] Apart from these isolated findings, there are few data on the role of cellular host defenses in the male lower urinary tract.

Pathology

Prostatitis is usually a focal process with areas of acute or chronic inflammatory cells in close apposition to areas with normal architecture. Histologic findings compatible with prostatitis occur commonly in adult males. In an autopsy series, McNeal found evidence of prostatitis in 40 of 91 adult prostates.[10] Two cases involved the periurethral zone only, 24 cases involved the peripheral zone only, and 14 cases involved both zones. These data suggest that prostatitis usually arises as a focal inflammation in the peripheral zone and spills over into the periurethral zone in severe cases. Kohnen and Drach found some inflammation in 98 percent of 162 surgically resected hyperplastic prostates.[52] Both histologic and bacteriologic evidence of prostatitis may occur without endoscopic signs of inflammation.[11] Blacklock suggests that these findings may be explained by differences in the drainage patterns of prostatic ducts.[11] The peripheral prostatic ducts tend to drain at right angles to the ejaculatory ducts and, therefore, are vulnerable to infection by organisms ascending through the urethra. In contrast, ducts draining the periurethral zone tend to parallel the ejaculatory ducts and are more resistant to infection by organisms in the urethra.

As noted above, clinical, pathologic, and microbiologic data have seldom been carefully correlated in studies of prostatitis,[10,52] but clinical studies have seldom found pathologic specimens helpful, perhaps reflecting the focal nature of inflammation in patients with prostatitis.[10,12] In one recent study, 60 men with "chronic abacterial prostatitis" had transrectal prostatic ultrasound with transperineal biopsy of abnormal areas. Histologic examination revealed chronic inflammation, predominantly of low grade, in 53 (88 percent) of 60 patients.[53] No uropathogens were cultured. The same investigators found intraprostatic-antibody deposition in men with chronic abacterial prostatitis but not in controls, possibly suggesting an earlier infection. Although the authors describe sonographic findings characteristic of "prostatitis,"[54] extensive clinical experience indicates that such findings lack specificity.[55,56] It is difficult, or impossible, to distinguish prostatitis sonographically from other pathologic processes in the prostate. Other critical issues with these data include patient selection and limited attempts to correlate inflammatory cells in expressed prostatic secretions with inflammation in prostatic parenchyma or with microbiologic findings.

Laboratory assessment of etiology

The critical clinical issue is to distinguish patients with lower-urinary-tract complaints associated with bacteriuria, that is, patients who may have bacterial prostatitis, from the larger number of patients without bacteriuria.[2,18] Systematic studies have shown that approximately 10 percent of men with the clinical diagnosis of "prostatitis" have bacterial prostatitis.[9] Further classification of patients with prostatitis is based on careful bacteriologic assessment of the lower urinary tract using the technique of Meares and Stamey.[57] This method is based on cultures of specimens that are sequentially obtained during micturition (Table 62-1).

Attention to several technical points assures useful and reliable

Table 62-1. Procedure for Localization of Infection in the Lower Urinary Tract by Use of Segmented Urine Cultures

Specimen	Abbreviation	Description
Voided bladder 1	VB_1	Initial 5–10 mL of urinary stream
Voided bladder 2	VB_2	Midstream specimen
Expressed prostatic secretions	EPS	Secretions expressed from prostate by digital massage after midstream specimen
Voided bladder 3	VB_3	First 5–10 mL of urinary stream immediately after prostate massage

NOTE. Terminology is from Drach et al.[3]

information.[2,3,8,13] Quantitative bacteriologic methods and rapid transport to the laboratory are critical. The midstream urine should be found sterile during the localization procedure. The prepuce of uncircumcised men should be retracted, the glans cleansed, and the detergent rinsed because small amounts may falsely reduce bacterial counts. It is important to collect the initial few drops of the first-void urine (VB_1) specimen, since the bacterial concentrations may be significantly lower in the next few milliliters of urine. Finally, it may be necessary to repeat the localization procedure for men with inconclusive findings.

Unequivocal diagnosis of bacterial prostatitis requires that the colony count in the postmassage (VB_3) specimen exceed the count in the first-void (VB_1) specimen by at least 10-fold.[2,8,13,57] Many men with chronic bacterial prostatitis harbor only small numbers of bacteria in their prostates, however. Direct culture of the prostatic secretions is useful in this situation.[2,57,58] Often the colony counts in the expressed prostatic secretion (EPS) specimens are 1 or 2 logs higher than comparable counts in the VB_3 specimen. This difference reflects dilution of the small volume of prostatic secretions by urine in the VB_3 sample. A prominent characteristic of bacterial prostatitis is that the organism present in the VB_3 or in the EPS in significantly greater numbers than in the VB_1 may be isolated on multiple occasions and is identical to the organism causing episodes of bacteriuria.[57,58]

Isolation of gram-positive organisms, such as staphylococci and diphtheroids, which appear to "localize" to the prostate, is a major source of confusion to clinicians and in the literature.[2,18,59,60] In most cases such patients have neither a history nor bacteriologic documentation of bladder infection with these organisms.[2,13,18] Technical problems, such as failure to collect the initial portion of the VB_1 or having some of the detergent used to cleanse the glans fall into the collection bottle for the VB_1, account for part of the problem.[2] Furthermore, the VB_1 is the control for the VB_3. The EPS is useful in borderline cases only. Relying on the EPS may introduce some artifacts since prostatic fluid may acquire organisms during transit through the urethra, especially if the EPS drops "hang" at the fossa navicularis.

Microscopic evaluation of the EPS is useful to identify inflammation.[2,3,18] Presence of leukocytes and "oval fat bodies" (large lipid-laden macrophages) is characteristic of the prostatic inflammatory response. Various criteria have been used by researchers to define an abnormal number of leukocytes.[2,43,61] Most investigators agree that >20 leukocytes per high-power field represents significant inflammation. Most recent reports use a criterion of ≥10 leukocytes per high-power field.[3,18,43,62] There appears to be little value in counting the number of leukocytes in the EPS of men with objective evidence of urethral inflammation, especially among men at risk for sexually transmitted diseases.[8] Thus, we examine a urethral smear for inflammation before proceeding with a lower-urinary-tract localization study.[9,13]

Under certain circumstances, lower-urinary-tract localization studies may be misleading.[4] False impressions concerning excessive concentrations of leukocytes in the prostatic expressate occur in urethral disorders (such as urethritis, strictures, condylomata, or diverticula) or in men with noninfectious conditions of the prostate (such as uninfected prostatic calculi) or after ejaculation.[63] Isolated analysis or culture of the ejaculate without concomitant study of urethral and bladder specimens may be more misleading than isolated examination of prostatic secretions.[4] Semen contains fluids from several accessory glands besides the prostatic fluid. Furthermore, cytologic examination of semen is complicated by the difficulty of distinguishing immature sperm from leukocytes. Thus, diagnosis of prostatitis should not be based solely on seminal fluid analysis.[2,4]

Differential diagnosis

Lower-urinary-tract localization studies facilitate classification of most men with prostatitis syndromes into four diagnostic groups: acute bacterial prostatitis, chronic bacterial prostatitis, nonbacterial prostatitis, and prostatodynia (Table 62-2).[3,4,8,64]

Bacterial prostatitis is a common diagnosis in clinical practice

Table 62-2. Classification of Prostatitis Syndromes Based on Documentation of Bacteriuria and Segmented Urine Cultures

Syndrome	Bacteriuria*	Infection localized to prostate†	Inflammatory response in EPS^	Abnormal prostate on rectal exams§	Systemic illness¥
Acute bacterial prostatitis	+	+	+	+	+
Chronic bacterial prostatitis	+	+	+	–	+/–
Nonbacterial prostatitis	–	–	+	–	–
Prostatodynia	–	–	–	–	–

* Documented with identical organism shown to localize to a prostatic focus when the midstream urine culture is negative.

† Refer to text for diagnostic criteria.

^ Expressed prostatic secretions (EPS) containing ≥10 white blood cells per high-power (× 400) microscopic field when patient has no objective evidence of urethritis.

§ Abnormal findings include exquisite tenderness and swelling that may be associated with signs of lower-urinary-tract obstruction.

¥ Systemic findings frequently include signs of bacteremia. Signs of sepsis are common in patients with acute bacterial prostatitis. Patients with chronic bacterial prostatitis may become septic during acute symptomatic episodes of bladder bacteriuria.

and is a frequent indication for antimicrobial therapy. However, well-documented bacterial infections of the prostate, whether acute or chronic, are uncommon.[13,41] The great majority of patients with a diagnosis of "prostatitis" are adult men with perineal, lower-back, or lower-abdominal pain; urinary discomfort; or ejaculatory complaints.[9] Most have no history of bacteriuria, and there is little objective evidence of bacterial infection of the prostate. Thus, most patients with "prostatitis" may be classified in the groups of nonbacterial prostatitis or prostatodynia, conditions about which there are few firm data for rational therapeutic decisions.

CLINICAL MANIFESTATIONS, TREATMENT, AND COMPLICATIONS

ACUTE BACTERIAL PROSTATITIS

Clinical presentation

Acute bacterial prostatitis is seldom a subtle or difficult diagnosis.[2,18,58] Characteristic symptoms are those associated with lower-urinary-tract infection, such as increased urinary frequency, urgency, and dysuria. Patients also may complain of bladder outflow obstruction due to acute edema of the prostate. Signs of systemic toxicity are common and may include fever, malaise, and myalgias. The patient may suffer from high temperature, lower abdominal or suprapubic discomfort due to bladder infection, or urinary retention. The rectal examination is frequently impressive, with an exquisitely tender, tense, "hot" prostate on palpation. Urinalysis is abnormal with pyuria, and cultures will be positive for gram-negative facultative or aerobic rods or *Streptococcus faecalis.* Systemic leukocytosis is common, with increased numbers of segmented cells. Bacteremia may be present spontaneously or may result from overly vigorous rectal examinations.

Treatment

Antimicrobial therapy often results in dramatic improvement of signs and symptoms of acute bacterial prostatitis. Many drugs that do not penetrate into the prostate under normal conditions have proved effective for treating acute bacterial prostatitis.[2,18] Thus, drugs appropriate for treatment of bacteremia caused by enterobacteria, pseudomonads, or enterococci should be started after specimens have been obtained for urine and blood cultures. For men who require hospitalization, conventional therapy is the combination of an aminoglycoside plus a beta-lactam drug.[4,8] However, the fluoroquinolones or third-generation cephalosporins are attractive alternatives for monotherapy[65] of prostatitis known to be caused by Enterobacteriaceae spp. For men with less severe infections, a conventional choice has been the combination of trimethoprim and sulfamethoxazole,[2,18] although resistance of uropathogens to this combination is becoming more common. Beta-lactam drugs and the new fluoroquinolones are also useful as oral therapy for patients with acute bacterial prostatitis who do not require hospitalization. Previous urine culture and antimicrobial-sensitivity patterns may alert the clinician to the possibility of recurrence with antimicrobial-resistant microorganisms. Similarly, history of genitourinary instrumentation increases the probability of finding resistant nosocomial pathogens, such as *Pseudomonas* or *Enterobacter* species.

Patients with acute urinary retention require bladder drainage. In this situation, placement of a suprapubic cystostomy tube, either using a percutaneous trocar apparatus or by open surgery, is preferred. An indwelling transurethral catheter would pass through and obstruct drainage of the acutely infected prostate, increasing the risk for bacteremia and prostatic abscess.[2,8] General measures, including hydration, analgesics, and bed rest, are also indicated.[2,8,18,58]

Complications

A few patients with acute bacterial prostatitis experience complications.[2,7,65] Chronic bacterial prostatitis occasionally follows an episode of acute bacterial prostatitis. Men with chronic bacterial prostatitis often remain asymptomatic between acute episodes of bacteriuria. Prostatic abscess is a rare complication among patients who receive appropriate antimicrobial therapy for acute bacterial prostatitis.[7,8,65–67] The classic presentation of prostatic abscess is a fluctuant area in the prostate that is felt during rectal examination,[66,68,69] but many patients present with more subtle findings. Transrectal ultrasound and computerized tomography are especially valuable for diagnosis of prostatic abscess in men with such subtle findings.[70–73] Treatment includes drainage of the abscess, using a perineal, percutaneous, or transurethral approach, together with appropriate antimicrobial therapy.[72,73] In most situations, the transurethral approach is optimal.

Granulomatous prostatitis may develop during resolution of an episode of acute bacterial prostatitis.[2,74] Usually the patient is asymptomatic but has a hard area noted during rectal examination that arouses the suspicion of carcinoma. Areas of prostatic infarction may also complicate acute bacterial prostatitis. Such areas usually present as firm portions of the prostate, and their chief importance lies in the differential diagnosis of carcinoma.

Summary

Acute bacterial prostatitis is characterized by the abrupt onset of symptoms and dramatic findings on physical examination. Laboratory findings include bacteria in the midstream urine. Most patients respond readily to treatment, and the disease is self-limited in most cases.

CHRONIC BACTERIAL PROSTATITIS

Clinical presentation

Chronic bacterial prostatitis is an important cause of bacterial persistence in the male lower urinary tract.[2,18,58] Patients characteristically experience recurrent episodes of bacteriuria caused by the same bacterial species.[2,13] In fact, the most common cause of relapsing urinary tract infections in men is the persistence of small numbers of bacteria in the prostate.[2] Patients are often asymptomatic between episodes of bladder bacteriuria, and the prostate gland is usually normal on either rectal or endoscopic evaluation. Thus, careful lower-urinary-tract localization studies are critical for diagnosis of chronic bacterial prostatitis.[57] Diagnosis based solely on symptoms, numbers of leukocytes in EPS or semen, or prostate biopsy is inadequate.

Men with chronic bacterial prostatitis occasionally present with signs of a systemic illness. Small numbers of bacteria in the prostate do not cause systemic illness; however, with acute exacerbations, bladder bacteriuria and secondary sepsis may result from the prostatic focus of infection. This is especially true among older men, who may have the combination of prostatic obstruction and infection.

Gram-negative rods, including enterobacteria and pseudomonads, are by far the most important pathogens in chronic bacterial prostatitis.[12,13,18,58] Gram-positive cocci, such as *Streptococcus faecalis* or *Staphylococcus saprophyticus,* may cause a few cases.[18,75] Reports implicating many other organisms in the etiology of chronic bacterial prostatitis are difficult to evaluate because of methodological problems with case definitions, lack of documentation of bacteriuria caused by the alleged pathogen, or lack of immunological response by the prostate.[4,8,76,77]

Chronic bacterial prostatitis is associated with secretory dysfunction of the prostate gland.[18] Alterations include increased pH of prostatic secretions, changes in the ratio of lactic dehydrogenase (LDH) isozymes, and increased concentration of immunoglobulins. Other changes include decreases in specific gravity of prostatic secretions, prostatic antibacterial factor, cation concentrations (zinc, magnesium, and calcium), citric acid, spermine, cholesterol, acid phosphatase, and lysozyme. These findings suggest that bacterial prostatitis is associated with a generalized secretory dysfunction of the prostate gland.

Men with chronic bacterial prostatitis characteristically have episodes of symptomatic bladder bacteriuria caused by the same organism; these episodes are separated by asymptomatic intervals of varying length.[2,18] Lower-urinary-tract localization studies during episodes of bladder bacteriuria are worthless[2,57]; patients must be evaluated when their midstream urine is sterile. Occasionally it has been necessary to eradicate organisms present in the bladder urine and urethra with drugs, such as penicillin G or nitrofurantoin, to obtain diagnostic localization studies.[2]

Medical therapy

Medical management is effective in curing or suppressing bacterial prostatitis.[2,4,65] Effective antimicrobial therapy for localized bacterial infections depends upon achieving sufficient levels of an appropriate drug at the infected site. Unfortunately, many drugs penetrate prostatic parenchyma poorly.[78,79] Other antimicrobials that achieve good tissue levels, such as erythromycin, have an inappropriate spectrum for the pathogens in prostatitis.[2]

Trimethoprim-sulfamethoxazole has been the "gold standard" for treating chronic bacterial prostatitis.[4,65] Trimethoprim has two useful characteristics: It achieves adequate levels in prostatic parenchyma, and it is effective against most of the common bacterial pathogens.[2,80] Available studies have usually employed the combination of trimethoprim and sulfamethoxazole for men with well-documented chronic bacterial prostatitis. Long-term therapy with trimethoprim (80 mg) plus sulfamethoxazole (400 mg) taken orally twice daily for 4 to 16 weeks was superior to shorter treatment courses.[81,82] Follow-up studies showed that such long courses result in symptomatic and bacteriologic cure in approximately one-third of patients, symptomatic improvement during therapy in approximately another one-third (who relapse after stopping treatment), and no improvement in the remaining patients.[18,81–84] Single-agent treatment using trimethoprim alone has been studied less well. In theory, trimethoprim alone should produce comparable results to combination therapy, since sulfamethoxazole diffuses poorly into the prostatic parenchyma.[2,77]

During the past decade considerable success has been reported using several of the new fluoroquinolones to treat chronic bacterial prostatitis. In contrast to the beta-lactams, concentrations of many fluoroquinolones in prostatic fluid, in prostatic tissue, and in seminal fluid are relatively high compared to plasma levels.[85–89] Good results have been reported for men with chronic bacterial prostatitis, including some patients who failed therapy with trimethoprim-sulfamethoxazole.[85–89] Promising agents include norfloxacin, ciprofloxacin, ofloxacin, and enoxacin.[86–91] Available studies are difficult to compare, however, because investigators used varying diagnostic criteria and because there was a considerable range in duration of treatment and follow-up. Because relapse rate is the critical issue for evaluating treatment of prostatitis, patients cannot be considered cured without long-term follow-up. Further investigations, especially controlled studies, are needed to determine the role of the newer quinolones in treatment of chronic bacterial prostatitis.

Many other orally administered antimicrobials have been used to treat patients with chronic bacterial prostatitis. Most reports are hampered by imprecise case definitions, lack of sufficient microbiologic documentation or follow-up, or an abundance of patients "infected" with organisms generally considered urethral contaminants. Although it is difficult to draw definitive conclusions, the indanyl ester of carbenicillin,[92,93] doxycycline,[94] rosamicin,[95] erythromycin plus urinary alkalization with bicarbonate,[96,97] or drug combinations employing rifampicin plus trimethoprim[98] have been found useful for selected patients. Some investigators report success using aminoglycosides, administered parenterally[2] or by local injection into the prostate[99,100] for men with prostatitis who failed oral therapy.

In studies published through 1984, bacteria isolated from men with chronic bacterial prostatitis were generally antimicrobial-sensitive strains, even after multiple symptomatic episodes and prolonged courses of therapy.[2,8,18] Although bacterial resistance has seldom been a problem in chronic bacterial prostatitis, an infected prostate may become the focus of a persistent infection with recurrent bouts of bacteriuria and a risk for bloodstream infection. Although often identified in the prostates of asymptomatic men,[56,101] some studies suggest that calculi occur more often among men with chronic prostatitis. Infection of prostatic stones may serve as a persistent focus for bacteria that is difficult to eradicate with antimicrobial agents.[4,90,102–105] Other reasons offered for the difficulty in curing chronic bacterial prostatitis include difficulties in achieving high levels of drug in areas of infection within the prostate, changes in the pH of the prostatic fluid associated with infection that influence the diffusion of drugs into the prostate,[106–108] and the presence of biofilms[109,110] that protect bacteria from antimicrobial agents.

Men with chronic bacterial prostatitis who are not cured by antimicrobial therapy may be rendered asymptomatic by long-term suppressive treatment using low-dosage antimicrobial agents.[2,18] Since most patients are asymptomatic between episodes of bacteriuria, the goal of suppressive therapy is to prevent symptomatic episodes, despite persistence of bacteria in the prostate. Very low doses of agents are remarkably effective in preventing episodes of symptomatic bladder bacteriuria among men with chronic bacterial prostatitis. Drugs that have been used effectively include penicillin G, tetracycline, nitrofurantoin, naladixic acid, cephalexin, or trimethoprim-sulfamethoxazole.

The data presented above form the basis for a rational approach to antimicrobial therapy for men with chronic bacterial prostatitis. It is important to document a prostatic source of organisms causing bacteriuria by careful lower-urinary-tract cultures. If these cultures indicate chronic bacterial prostatitis, then a prolonged course of therapy—using an antimicrobial to which the organism is sensitive and that achieves good levels in the prostate—should be employed in an effort to cure the infection. During and after such therapy, lower-urinary-tract studies should be repeated to evaluate the therapeutic response. A second course of treatment using a drug with a different mechanism of action may be indicated for men with a persistent focus of prostatic infection. Men who are not cured may be treated with long-term, low-dose, suppressive medication to prevent colonization of the bladder and urethra with organisms from the prostate.

Surgical therapy

Surgery has a limited role in the treatment of patients with chronic bacterial prostatitis. Although complete surgical removal of the prostate by radical prostatectomy or cystoprostatectomy will cure bacterial prostatitis,[2] such surgery is a major undertaking that is associated with a significant incidence of complications. Thus, radical surgery is best reserved for patients with localized prostate cancer. For the rare men who have both carcinoma of the prostate and chronic bacterial prostatitis, radical prostatectomy may cure both conditions.

Subtotal prostatectomy (transurethral, retropubic, suprapubic, or visual laser ablation) is the most common procedure for treating benign prostate disorders. These procedures remove periurethral adenomatous tissue, leaving the surgical capsule of the prostate. The observation that most bacteria appear to be located in the peripheral prostatic tissue may explain why subtotal prostatectomy cures only about one-third of patients with well-documented chronic bacterial prostatitis.[2,18,111] Therefore, transurethral or open surgical procedures for removal of prostatic adenomas are best reserved for patients who have symptoms of lower-urinary-tract obstruction that persist after sterilization of the midstream urine.

Occasional studies report higher cure rates using transurethral resection to remove infected prostatic calculi and periurethral adenoma in men with chronic prostatitis.[112–114] "Radical" transurethral resection is necessary to remove all infected stones because the peripheral zone of the prostate contains the greatest foci of infection and stones.[11,105] The populations in most reports were defined poorly, and bacteriologic evaluation and follow-up were often inadequate to document the conclusion that 70 to 100 percent of patients were "cured."

Rare patients with chronic bacterial prostatitis associated with other obstructive lesions, such as urethral stricture disease, may benefit from surgery combined with antimicrobial therapy. Before recommending surgery it is essential to document the functional significance of such lesions by appropriate urodynamic and radiographic studies when the patient is not bacteriuric.

"NONBACTERIAL" PROSTATITIS

Clinical presentation

Men with "nonbacterial" prostatitis have both symptoms and inflammation of their prostatic secretions, but these patients have no history of bacteriuria and lack evidence of a bacterial infection localized to the prostate (see Table 62-2).[3] They complain of various perineal and pelvic symptoms.[9] Vague pain and discomfort is common and may be perineal, penile, urethral, suprapubic, infrapubic, scrotal, or inguinal in location. The discomfort may be described as either continuous or spasmodic and is described commonly as a "dull ache." Occasional patients complain of increased urinary frequency or dysuria or of pain on ejaculation. Systemic symptoms and signs are absent. Genital examination is usually unremarkable, and the prostate is normal on rectal examination.

Etiology

The etiology of nonbacterial prostatitis is unclear. Many workers have examined microbiologic, urodynamic, and psychological aspects. However, no study has been completely satisfactory with careful definition of the disease, adequate microbiologic evaluation, and psychological assessment. The evidence for various causes of nonbacterial prostatitis is summarized below. Although many of the agents are classified as bacteria, the standard classification of prostatitis syndromes considers these agents as potential causes of the nonbacterial prostatitis syndrome.

Chlamydia trachomatis. Mårdh and Colleen[115] obtained urethral specimens for culture of *Neisseria gonorrhoeae, Trichomonas vaginalis, Ureaplasma urealyticum, Mycoplasma hominis, Candida albicans,* anaerobic bacteria, and some viruses from 78 men with "nonacute prostatitis" and from 20 normal men. There were no significant differences between the cases and the controls. One-third of the men with chronic prostatitis had antibodies to *C. trachomatis,* compared with 3 percent of controls. Tetracycline treatment was superior to placebo in eliminating symptoms. In follow-up studies employing cultures and serology, however, these workers could not implicate *C. trachomatis* as the cause of idiopathic "prostatitis."[116–119] The authors concluded that chlamydiae were not important agents in "chronic prostatitis." Similarly, we could not culture *C. trachomatis* from the urethras of men with nonbacterial prostatitis or prostatodynia,[120] nor did we find an association of serologic or local immune responses to *C. trachomatis* with these syndromes. Doble and associates evaluated 60 men with the diagnosis of "chronic abacterial prostatitis" using transrectal prostatic ultrasound with transperineal biopsy of abnormal areas.[121] Chlamydiae were not cultured from the prostatic tissue of any patient, nor were they detected by immunofluorescence, and no subject had serum antibody titers against *C. trachomatis.*

In contrast, Bruce et al. examined early-morning urine, prostatic fluid, or semen from 70 men with "subacute or chronic prostatitis."[122] Of these men, 39 (56 percent) were infected with *C. trachomatis.* The microbiologic methods used in this study have been criticized, as has the finding of positive chlamydial cultures in 9 (17 percent) of 54 controls undergoing elective vasectomy.[123] In a follow-up study, Bruce and Reid evaluated 55 men with "prostatitis," including 31 "believed to have chlamydial prostatitis."[124] Only 6 cases met strict criteria for chlamydial prostatitis based on identification of the organisms by culture or immunofluorescence techniques. Japanese investigators identified *C. trachomatis* in the urethras of 20 percent of men with prostatitis.[125] Other investigators have reached similar conclusions.[126–128]

In support of a potential etiologic role, Poletti and associates isolated *C. trachomatis* from prostate cells obtained by transrectal aspiration biopsy of men with "nonacute abacterial prostatitis."[129] Abdelatif et al. evaluated transurethral prostate specimens with histologic evidence of chronic abacterial prostatitis using in situ hybridization.[130] Intracellular chlamydiae were detected in 7 (30 percent) of 23 cases. Shurbaji and associates also identified *C. trachomatis* in paraffin-embedded sections from 5 (31 percent) of 16 men with histologic evidence of prostatitis but in none of 19 cases of prostatic hyperplasia without significant inflammation.[131] Kobayashi and associates found peroxidase anti-peroxidase staining for chlamydiae in prostate biopsy tissue following therapy.[132] These studies suggest that chlamydiae may invade the prostate, that chlamydial antigen or DNA may persist in the prostate after treatment, and that presence of such antigen might be related to prostatitis.

Important criticisms of previous studies include absent or inappropriate controls, the fact that urethral specimens may not reflect prostatic infection, and problems with inhibition of cultures for *C. trachomatis* and other microorganisms by prostate tissue and secretions. Another reservation is that direct methods (such as microscopy, immunofluorescence, or in situ hybridization) may be insensitive for identification of defective organisms or organisms present in small numbers. Recent demonstration of chlamydial DNA and RNA by polymerase chain reaction (PCR) in culture-negative cases of trachoma (a chronic eye disease caused by *C. trachomatis*) has suggested that "live chlamydiae may remain at a site of infection and produce inflammation beyond the time at which microbial techniques are able to detect them."[133] Similar events may occur in chronic prostatitis. Another problem is that biopsy studies sampled abnormal areas only. Thus, the precise role of *C. trachomatis* in nonbacterial prostatitis deserves further study.

Ureaplasma urealyticum. In a study of over 700 patients, Weidner et al. found that high concentrations of *U. urealyticum* (>10^3/mL) in prostatic fluid, semen, or urine obtained after prostatic massage were associated with clinical signs and symptoms of "prostatitis."[134] A recent study identified "significant" concentrations of *ureaplasma* organisms in 18 (13 percent) of 143 men with prostatitis.[135] Treatment with either ofloxacin or minocycline resulted in clearance of the organisms in all cases and resolution of symptoms in 10 patients (71 percent). Isaacs and associates isolated *U. urealyticum* at concentrations >10^3/mL, without other organisms, from prostatic secretions of 11 (8 percent) of 131 men with chronic nonbacterial prostatitis, suggesting an etiologic role.[136] Other investigators, however, have been unable to implicate the genital mycoplasmas in nonbacterial prostatitis.[111,115] Additional studies of other, carefully defined patient populations employing immunologic and genetic probe techniques, and a comprehensive search for other potentially relevant pathogens, would be useful to further assess the purported role of *U. urealyticum* in prostatitis syndromes.

Trichomonas vaginalis. This has been proposed as causing varied urological conditions. Studies outlined in Chap. 57 suggest that *T. vaginalis* is indeed pathogenic in the male lower genitourinary tract, causing nongonococcal nonchlamydial urethritis and persistent infection. We isolated *T. vaginalis* and *C. trachomatis* with comparable frequencies from the urethras of men with chronic prostatitis syndromes.[9] *T. vaginalis* has been identified in urinary sediment, prostatic secretions, and prostatic parenchyma. In some studies the prevalence of trichomoniasis has exceeded 85 percent among men with symptoms of prostatitis that persisted despite antibacterial therapy.[137,138] These findings support previous reports of an association between *T. vaginalis* and prostatitis.[137–142] Some suggest that the highest prevalence is in men with long-term symptoms and in those who have not responded to standard antibacterial therapy.[138] Nonetheless, the precise role of *T. vaginalis* as a cause of nonbacterial prostatitis remains undefined. Assuming the organism does play a role in prostatitis, specific diagnosis would be necessary because treatment of trichomoniasis requires antimicrobials seldom prescribed for urogenital infections in men.

Other Organisms. Many other organisms are regarded as potential causes of chronic prostatitis and urethritis syndromes, including viruses, fungi, and anaerobic and gram-positive bacteria. In two Scandinavian studies, men with "chronic nonbacterial" prostatitis had prostate biopsies that were cultured for aerobic bacteria, anaerobic bacteria, and viruses.[143,144] Neither study demonstrated an etiologic role for such pathogens.

Of the proposed microbial causes of nonbacterial prostatitis the rate of gram-positive aerobic bacteria is the most controversial. Although their significance in this condition has been debated for more than 20 years, until recently the consensus was that these organisms are rarely, if ever, causative.[8,13,18,145] Nickel and Costerton revived this debate by localizing coagulase-negative staphylococci to the prostates of three men with "chronic prostatitis" that was refractory to antimicrobial treatment.[110] The bacteria were isolated in culture from prostate biopsies. Electron microscopy demonstrated "sparse and focal microcolonies adherent to the prostatic ductal walls," suggesting sequestration of resistant staphylococci within intraprostatic biofilms. In contrast, other investigators found that such organisms disappeared without treatment in all cases.[146]

In the preantibiotic era, *Neisseria gonorrhoeae* was a recognized cause of prostatitis and the most common cause of prostatic abscess.[147] However, gonococcal prostatitis has seldom been reported in the postantibiotic era. Two studies demonstrated antibody against *N. gonorrhoeae* in prostatic fluid of men whose cultures were negative.[118,148] In contrast other studies seldom identified *N. gonorrhoeae* as a cause of prostatitis.[4,13,120]

Controlled studies have shown no significant differences in anaerobic bacteriology between cases and controls,[146] but they employed outdated bacteriological methods. Of viruses that may be cultured from genitourinary sites, herpes viruses types 1 and 2[149–151] and cytomegalovirus[152–154] are the most likely causes of prostatitis, based on anecdotal reports.

Noninfectious causes

Some workers have proposed that nonbacterial prostatitis is not an infectious disease.[2,155–157] Prostaglandins,[2] autoimmunity,[158,159] psychological abnormalities,[160,161] neuromuscular dysfunction of the bladder neck[7,162–164] or urogenital diaphragm,[157] and allergy to environmental agents[165,166] have all been suggested as etiologic factors. For example, Mathur et al. found that 18 of 25 men with "prostatitis" had cytotoxic antisperm antibodies at significantly higher titers than normal patients.[158] None of these studies used carefully defined patient populations or comprehensive, simultaneous microbiologic methods.

Differential diagnosis and treatment

The differential diagnosis of nonbacterial prostatitis includes two important conditions, interstitial cystitis and carcinoma in situ of the bladder.[2,167] These disorders may present with irritative symptoms of the lower urinary tract that may mimic nonbacterial prostatitis. Thus, for selected patients it may be reasonable to obtain urine specimens for cytology and to perform careful endoscopic examination under anesthesia (in which the bladder is evaluated after overdistension), as well as to procure appropriate bladder specimens for biopsy.

Therapy is unsatisfactory for most men with nonbacterial prostatitis. Antimicrobial drugs are considered the first-line treatment.[4,9] Patients with recognized uropathogens respond to specific therapy, but few men receive an accurate diagnosis because diagnosis of fastidious organisms proves difficult in most clinical settings. For men without evidence of infection by recognized pathogens, antimicrobial treatment often results in temporary resolution. Symptoms frequently return following treatment, however. Most patients receive repeated courses of antimicrobials. Patients and their physicians often became frustrated following multiple courses of unsuccessful empirical therapy. The next section describes other diagnostic procedures and treatments that are commonly prescribed for men with nonbacterial prostatitis as well as those men with prostatodynia.

Summary

Nonbacterial prostatitis is defined by presence of inflammation among men with symptoms referable to the prostate but who do not meet the criteria for bacterial prostatitis. A wide variety of infectious and noninfectious causes have been implicated in the literature, but the etiology of this condition has not been clearly defined. Men with recognized uropathogens respond to specific treatment, but therapy is empirical and ineffective for many patients.

PROSTATODYNIA

Clinical presentation

Prostatodynia is characterized by pelvic, perineal, ejaculatory, and urinary complaints similar to those of patients with nonbacterial prostatitis. Systemic complaints are absent, and physical examination is usually unremarkable. In contrast to men with nonbacterial prostatitis, patients with prostatodynia have normal-appearing prostatic secretions with no evidence of inflammation (Table 62-2).[8,9,13]

Etiology and treatment

The etiology of prostatodynia remains unclear. Most studies combined patients with nonbacterial prostatitis and prostatodynia under a variety of terms, such as "prostatosis,"[61,157] or "abacterial prostatitis."[121,130,168] Thus, earlier comments on the lack of conclusive evidence of an infectious etiology for nonbacterial prostatitis apply also to prostatodynia. Many noninfectious factors have been proposed as the etiology of prostatodynia,[159] e.g., neuromuscular dysfunction of the bladder neck or urethra,[99,155,169,170] stress,[171] and other psychological factors.[161]

The literature implies that the causes of nonbacterial prostatitis and prostatodynia differ. Infectious, immunologic, or other structural causes were believed more important among men with nonbacterial prostatitis, while psychological factors were thought to be more important among men with prostatodynia.[2,4,171] To date, little objective evidence supports this conclusion. There are few differences in clinical presentation or historical risk factors for nonbacterial prostatitis and prostatodynia.[9] Furthermore, some studies suggest that the concentrations of inflammatory cells in prostatic secretions vary over time[49,62] or with sexual activity.[63] Thus, the distinction between nonbacterial prostatitis and prostatodynia may be less clear than appreciated by earlier investigators.

Current therapy is unsatisfactory for nonbacterial prostatitis. Recommended treatments include prostate massage, anti-inflammatory drugs, anticholinergic drugs, muscle relaxants, transurethral resection of the prostate, sitz baths, diathermy, exercises, physiotherapy, and psychotherapy.[2,18,112,113,157] Some clinicians recommend increased frequency of ejaculation to relieve "congestion," while others recommend abstinence from ejaculation, alcohol, coffee, tea, spicy foods, and so forth. There is little objective evidence that any of these treatments affects the natural history of either nonbacterial prostatitis or prostatodynia.

The best rationale for non-antimicrobial therapy involves use of alpha-adrenergic blockade to treat the neuromuscular dysfunction that some workers describe with nonbacterial prostatitis and prostatodynia.[7,162,163] Complaints of urinary hesitancy, poor or intermittent stream, or ejaculatory dysfunction may be manifestations of functional neuromuscular abnormalities. Small clinical series suggest that patients benefit from treatment with alpha-blocking agents such as phenoxybenzamine,[2] phentolamine,[7] or terazosin.[172] Documentation of neuromuscular abnormalities before therapy with appropriate urodynamic studies is prudent. There are several important reservations about treating neuromuscular abnormalities in patients with lower-urinary-tract symptoms. No study has included a substantial number of carefully defined patients with comprehensive microbiologic assessment. In addition, lower-urinary-tract infections and cystitis, for example, are commonly associated with abnormal urodynamic studies, and without appropriate cultures it may be impossible to distinguish such infections from overt neurological disorders.

Psychological factors may be important in the etiology and pathogenesis of nonbacterial prostatitis and prostatodynia. For example, Rosenbloom noted that men with "chronic prostatitis" frequently present with sexual dysfunction.[160] Smart found that patients with an abnormal personality inventory who had surgery for "chronic prostatitis" benefited only 20 percent of the time, compared to a 60 percent success rate for men who had a normal personality inventory.[112,113] Nilsson et al. conducted detailed psychiatric interviews and psychological testing in men with "chronic prostatitis" and found paranoid projection and severe anxiety associated with the absence of objective pathology.[161] Patients with abnormal psychological tests responded less well to antimicrobial treatment than did patients with normal tests. Two recent studies compared psychological findings in men with chronic prostatitis to men with chronic low-back pain[173] and men undergoing vasectomy[174]; depression and decreased interpersonal relationships were associated with chronic prostatitis. One major problem with these studies is that they could not distinguish between psychological factors as a cause of chronic prostatitis and psychological consequences of a chronic condition that did not respond to repeated courses of therapy.[173]

Patients routinely undergo a wide variety of invasive diagnostic procedures, such as cystoscopy, transrectal ultrasonography, excretory urography, and other imaging tests, urodynamic studies, and biopsies.[96,155,163] The recent literature contains many reports of surgical procedures to treat men with chronic prostatitis and related syndromes. These procedures include: transurethral and "subtotal resection" of the prostate,[96,112,113,175] balloon dilation of the prostate,[176] hyperthermia,[168,177–179] endourethral electrostimulation and laser radiation,[180,181] and even radical prostatectomy.[182,183] None of these small series has included adequate control groups or sufficient microbiologic and clinical data. Although such procedures might be effective in certain highly selected cases, our experience includes many men who failed operative therapy.

Summary

There is little or no objective evidence that men with prostatodynia benefit from antimicrobial therapy. It is possible that treatment with multiple courses of therapy may reinforce the patient's perception that he has a chronic debilitating disease, a factor that may lead him to wander from one physician to another in a vain search for effective therapy. Many other empirical treatments have been proposed but little objective data support routine use of any of these measures. Thus, there is a major need for carefully conducted studies to define the causes and optimal treatment for men with nonbacterial prostatitis and prostatodynia.

GRANULOMATOUS PROSTATITIS

Most men with prostatitis syndromes may be classified in one of the four categories described above. However, unusual patients have granulomatous prostatitis, a fifth category. Diagnosis is important because specific therapy may be necessary to resolve the infectious causes of granulomatous prostatitis.

Granulomatous prostatitis is a characteristic reaction of the prostate to a variety of insults. Patients may present with findings on rectal examination suggesting prostate cancer.[184] Others present with systemic symptoms or with lower-urinary-tract obstruction due to prostatic enlargement. Biopsy or examination of tissue removed at surgery is often necessary for diagnosis. Thus, granulomatous prostatitis is a histologic diagnosis not associated with a discrete clinical syndrome.

Histology

On gross examination the prostate appears indurated, and on rectal examination it is frequently nodular. The histologic pattern is that of a granulomatous reaction with lipid-laden histiocytes, plasma cells, and scattered giant cells. A prominent eosinophilic infiltrate is apparent in some cases. Recent reports suggest that the histologic findings range from a localized appearance resembling rheumatoid nodules often associated with a history of previous transurethral resection, to a more diffuse appearance, associated with systemic illness or idiopathic etiology.[185,186] Specific stains or cultures may be necessary to make an etiologic diagnosis.

Etiology

Granulomatous prostatitis is arbitrarily classified as "specific" when associated with particular granulomatous infections or as "nonspecific" in other cases. Recognized causes of nonspecific granulomatous prostatitis include acute bacterial prostatitis, prostatic surgery, and disorders associated with vasculitis.

Nonspecific granulomatous prostatitis

In many cases granulomatous prostatitis follows an episode of acute bacterial prostatitis or previous prostatic surgery.[2,74] Nonspecific granulomatous prostatitis occurs in two forms: a non-eosinophilic variety and an eosinophilic variety. Although neither variety is seen frequently in clinical practice (the eosinophilic variety is especially rare), both types are important clinically because they may be confused with prostatic carcinoma.

Some authors suggest that granulomatous prostatitis represents a tissue response of the foreign body type to extravasated prostatic fluid.[74] Acute signs and symptoms of bladder outlet obstruction associated with an enlarged, firm prostate that feels malignant characterize the clinical presentation. Fever and irritative-voiding symptoms may occur.

Eosinophilic granulomatous prostatitis, associated with fibrinoid necrosis and generalized vasculitis, may present as a serious systemic illness.[165] Because it occurs almost exclusively in patients with allergies, especially asthmatics, this entity is also known as "allergic granuloma of the prostate."[145] Granulomatous prostatitis has also been associated with other rheumatoid disorders, particularly Wegener's granulomatosis.[187–190]

Specific granulomatous prostatitis

There are a number of specific infectious causes of granulomatous reaction by the prostate. Tuberculous prostatitis is usually secondary to tuberculosis elsewhere in the genital tract.[191,192] Most patients have no symptoms referable to prostatic infection. On biopsy the granulomas frequently contain typical Langhans' giant cells and may be associated with caseous necrosis. Such infections are caused most often by *Mycobacterium tuberculosis* but have also been reported with atypical mycobacteria.[193,194]

With many of the deep mycoses, mycotic prostatitis may be secondary to systemic involvement.[195,196] Most such reported cases have been associated with blastomycosis,[195,197] coccidioidomycosis,[198–200] and cryptococcosis.[201,202] Histoplasmosis and paracoccidioidomycosis also occasionally involve the prostate.[195,203] A few cases of prostatitis due to candidiasis or aspergillosis have also been described.[204–206] Usually, mycotic prostatitis is part of a systemic hematogenous dissemination. This process may involve any fungal organism occurring in the genitourinary tract. Mycotic involvement of the prostate is probably more common than is generally appreciated, since such involvement is frequently asymptomatic and the prostate is often not specifically evaluated in autopsy protocols.[195]

Other unusual infectious causes of granulomatous prostatitis include actinomycosis, candidiasis, and syphilis (F. Mantz, personal communication).[207] Cases of granulomatous prostatitis have also been associated with brucellosis[208] and can be sequelae of sacral herpes zoster.[209] Granulomatous prostatitis may also complicate BCG therapy for bladder cancer.[210] Recent reports suggest that acquired immunodeficiency syndrome (AIDS) and human immunodeficiency virus (HIV) infection may be associated with an increased risk for granulomatous prostatitis,[211] and that the etiology may include pathogens such as the intracellular *Mycobacterium avium* complex.[212]

Diagnosis and treatment

Granulomatous prostatitis is perhaps most important in the differential diagnosis of an indurated, firm, or nodular prostate. Frequently the rectal examination of such patients raises the suspicion of prostatic carcinoma. Other causes of a nodular prostate include prostatic infarction, nodular benign prostatic hypertrophy, or a prostatic calculus. Biopsy of the prostate may be necessary for diagnosis. Use of appropriate stains and cultures to detect specific etiologic agents is important in cases where granulomatous prostatitis is a consideration.

Treatment of patients with granulomatous prostatitis generally involves appropriate and specific treatment of the primary disease. A few patients have symptoms directly referable to the granulomatous reaction in the prostate. Such men usually complain of obstructive voiding symptoms. In most cases the symptoms resolve with systemic therapy. Patients with urinary retention may be managed initially by percutaneous placement of a suprapubic cystostomy tube. Prostatectomy may be necessary if symptoms persist after an appropriate course of antimicrobial therapy.

CONCLUSION

Efforts to identify pathogens have been successful in small groups of men, such as those with bacterial or granulomatous prostatitis.[2,18,213] Although numerous studies have increased our understanding of chronic bacterial prostatitis,[2,18,40,76,107,214] this information has benefited only a small proportion of cases.

Accurate diagnosis is important to indicate specific therapy for men with active infections. Bacterial or granulomatous prostatitis may present with systemic symptoms and represent a source of organisms that can cause repeated episodes of bacteriuria of systemic infection. Such men respond well to specific treatment.

Diagnosis may also indicate the need to avoid inappropriate therapy for men who have no evidence of infection or anatomic or structural problems. We have algorithms and antimicrobial strategies for bacterial and granulomatous prostatitis. In contrast, there are few guidelines for managing the larger number of men who suffer long-term morbidity from other prostatitis syndromes. Some of these men may have infections with infectious agents and will respond to specific therapy. Chronic prostatitis syndromes may represent the most common indication for antimicrobial therapy in urology, but many men derive little benefit from such treatment. It is also important to limit other investigations and treatments to men with a reasonable chance to benefit from such treatment.

The psychological consequences are major. In our clinic over 50 percent of men with chronic prostatitis syndromes met criteria for depressive illness.[9,173] Other investigators also found that psychological abnormalities are common.[160,161] Depression, infection, and structural abnormalities may coexist in men with chronic prostatitis.[9] This observation supports the idea that depression may represent the response of some men to repeated courses of ineffective treatment. Appropriate medical treatment may limit these adverse psychological responses. It is possible that psychological abnormalities may be primary in other cases. Therefore it may be essential to refer these men for psychological assessment and intervention; this may be more appropriate and helpful than repeated courses of antimicrobial therapy for patients with prostatodynia without clear evidence of prostatic inflammation. Our data document reduced sexual activity, often related to concern about transmitting a "serious infection." Idiopathic lower-urinary-tract syndromes account for major morbidity in addition to costs of medications, urological procedures, and time away from work.

In summary, common, poorly understood prostatitis syndromes cause considerable morbidity in men. Specific therapy results in cure or improvement for men with infectious causes of prostatitis. Unfortunately, treatment is frequently empirical and often unsatisfactory because we have limited understanding of the causes and pathophysiology of these neglected disease syndromes.

References

1 Herman JR: *Urology: A View through the Retrospectoscope.* New York, Harper and Row, p. 192, 1973.
2 Stamey TA: *Pathogenesis and Treatment of Urinary Tract Infections.* Baltimore: Williams and Wilkins, 1980.
3 Drach GW et al: Classification of benign disease associated with prostatic pain: Prostatitis or prostatodynia? *J Urol* 120:266, 1978.
4 Lipsky BA: Urinary tract infections in men. *Ann Intern Med* 110:138, 1989.
5 Meares EM Jr: Prostatitis and related disorders, in *Campbell's Urology*, 6th ed. PC Walsh, AB Retik, TA Stamey, J Vaughan (eds). Philadelphia, W.B. Saunders, vol. 1, 1992, p. 807.
6 Bowie W: Urethritis in males, in *Sexually Transmitted Diseases*, 2d ed, K Holmes, P-A Mardh, P Sparling, P Weisner, W Cates, S Lemon, W. Stamm (eds). New York, McGraw-Hill, 1990, p. 627.
7 Kaneko S et al: Bladder neck dysfunction: The effect of the alpha-adrenergic blocking agent phentolamine on bladder neck dysfunction and a fluorescent histochemical study of bladder neck smooth muscle. *Invest Urol* 18:212, 1980.
8 Krieger JN: Prostatitis syndromes: Pathophysiology, differential diagnosis and treatment. *Sex Transm Dis* 11:100, 1984.
9 Krieger J, Egan K: Comprehensive evaluation and treatment of 75 men referred to chronic prostatitis clinic. *Urology* 38:11, 1991.
10 McNeal JE: Regional morphology and pathology of the prostate. *Am J Clin Pathol* 49:347, 1968.
11 Blacklock NJ: Anatomical factors in prostatitis. *Br J Urol* 46:47, 1974.
12 Schmidt JD, Patterson MC: Needle biopsy study of chronic prostatitis. *J Urol* 96:519, 1966.
13 Krieger J, McGonagle L: Diagnostic considerations and interpretation of microbiological findings for evaluation of chronic prostatitis. *J Clin Microbiol* 27:240, 1980.
14 Stamey TA et al: Antibacterial nature of prostatic fluid. *Nature* 218: 444, 1968.
15 Marmar JL et al: Values for zinc in whole semen, fractions of split ejaculate and expressed prostatic fluid. *Urology* 16:478, 1980.
16 Marmar JL et al: Semen zinc levels in infertile and postvasectomy patients and patients with prostatitis. *Fertil Steril* 26:1057, 1975.
17 Fair WR et al: Prostatic antibacterial factor: Identity and significance. *Urology* 7:169, 1976.
18 Meares EM Jr: Prostatitis syndromes: New perspectives about old woes. *J Urol* 123:141, 1980.
19 Fair WR, Wehner N: Antibacterial action of spermine: Effect on urinary tract pathogens. *Appl Microbiol* 21:6, 1971.
20 Fridlender B et al: Selective inhibition of herpes simplex virus type 1 DNA polymerase by zinc ions. *Virology* 84:551, 1978.
21 Tennican P et al: Topical zinc in the treatment of mice infected intravaginally with herpes genitalis virus (40922). *Proc Soc Exp Biol Med* 164:593, 1980.
22 Bedill GW, Soll DR: Effects of low concentrations of zinc on the growth and dimorphism of *Candida albicans:* Evidence for zinc-resistant and -sensitive pathways for mycelium formation. *Infect Immun* 26:348, 1979.
23 Soll DR et al: Zinc and the regulation of growth and phenotype in the infectious yeast *Candida albicans. Infect Immun* 32:1139, 1981.
24 Krieger JN, Rein MF: Canine prostatic secretions kill *Trichomonas vaginalis. Infect Immun* 37:77, 1982.
25 Krieger JN, Rein MF: Zinc sensitivity of *Trichomonas vaginalis:* In vitro studies and clinical implications. *J Infect Dis* 146:341, 1982.
26 American Society for Microbiology. Washington, D.C.: Zinc inhibits *Chlamydia trachomatis* (CT) infection in McCoy and human prostate cells [abstract 523], in *Programs and Abstracts of the Twentieth Interscience Conference on Antimicrobial Agents and Chemotherapy*, 1980.
27 Rozansky R et al: Studies on the antibacterial action of spermine. *J Gen Microbiol* 10:11, 1954.
28 Fair WR, Wehner N: Further observations on the antibacterial nature of prostatic fluid. *Infect Immun* 3:494, 1971.
29 Meares EM Jr: Serum antibody titers in urethritis and chronic bacterial prostatitis. *Urology* 10:305, 1977.
30 Meares EM Jr: Serum antibody titers in treatment with trimethoprim-sulfamethoxazole for chronic prostatitis. *Urology* 11:142, 1978.
31 Kumon H: Detection of a local prostatic immune response to bacterial prostatitis. *Infection* 3: 1992.
32 Albin RJ et al: Localization of immunoglobulins in human prostatic tissue. *J Immunol* 107:603, 1971.
33 Gray SP et al: Distribution of the immunoglobulins G, A, and M in the prostatic fluid of patients with prostatitis. *Clin Chim Acta* 57: 163, 1974.
34 Riedasch G et al: Antibody-coated bacteria in the ejaculate: A possible test for prostatitis. *J Urol* 118:787, 1977.
35 Thomas V et al: Antibody-coated bacteria in the urine and the site of urinary-tract infection. *N Engl J Med* 290:588, 1974.
36 Jones SR: Prostatitis as a cause of antibody-coated bacteria in urine. Letter to the editor. *N Engl J Med* 291:365, 1974.
37 Shortliffe L et al: Use of solid-phase radioimmunoassay and formalin-fixed whole bacterial antigen in the detection of antigen-specific immunoglobulin in prostatic fluid. *J Clin Invest* 67:790, 1981.
38 Shortliffe L et al: The detection of a local prostatic immunologic response to bacterial prostatitis. *J Urol* 125:509, 1981.
39 Wishnow KI et al: The diagnostic value of the immunologic response in bacterial and nonbacterial prostatitis. *J Urol* 127:689, 1982.
40 Fowler JE et al: Immunologic response of the prostate to bacteriuria and bacterial prostatitis: I. Immunoglobulin concentrations in prostatic fluid. *J Urol* 128:158, 1992.
41 Fowler JE Jr: Infections of the male reproductive tract and infertility: A selected review. *J Androl* 3:121, 1981.
42 Gray SP et al: Immunoglobulin levels in prostatitis. *Urol Nephrol* 73: 20, 1973.
43 Schaeffer AJ et al: Prevalence and significance of prostatic inflammation. *J Urol* 125: 215, 1981.
44 Harrison KL, Johnson DK: Chronic asymptomatic genital tract infection and semen quality. *Pathology* 11:289, 1979.
45 Krieger JN et al: Urinary tract infections in healthy university men. *J Urol* 149:1046, 1993.
46 Krieger J et al: Clinical manifestations of trichomoniasis in men. *Ann Intern Med* 118:844, 1993.
47 Krieger J et al: Evaluation of chronic urethritis: Defining the role for endoscopic procedures. *Arch Intern Med* 148:703, 1988.
48 Nishimura T et al: Macrophages in prostatic fluid. *Br J Urol* 52:381, 1980.
49 Wright ET et al: Prostatic fluid inflammation in prostatitis. *J Urol* 1994.
50 Clark RA, Klebanoff SJ: Generation of a neutrophil chemotactic agent by spermatozoa: role of complement and regulation by seminal plasma factors. *J Immunol* 117:1378, 1976.

51 Koehlef JK et al: Spermophagy, in *Atlas of Human Reproduction: By Scanning Electron Microscopy* ESE Hafez, P Kenemans (eds). Lancaster, UK, MTP Press, 1982, p. 213.
52 Kohnen PW, Drach GW: Patterns of inflammation in prostatic hyperplasia: A histologic and bacteriologic study. *J Urol* 121:755, 1979.
53 Doble A et al: Intraprostatic antibody deposition in chronic abacterial prostatitis. *Br J Urol* 65:598, 1990.
54 Doble A, Carter SS: Ultrasonographic findings in prostatitis. *Urol Clin North Am* 16:763, 1989.
55 Iunda IF, Varvashenia VV: Transrectal prostatic sonography as a useful diagnostic means for patients with chronic prostatitis or prostatodynia. *Br J Urol* 73:664, 1994.
56 Braeckman JG et al: Reproducibility of transrectal ultrasound of prostatic disease. *Scand J Urol Nephol* (suppl) 137:91, 1991.
57 Meares EM Jr, Stamey TA: Bacteriologic localization patterns in bacterial prostatitis and urethritis. *Invest Urol* 5:492, 1968.
58 Meares EM Jr: Prostatitis: Nephrology forum. *Kidney Int* 20:289, 1981.
59 Fritjofasson A et al: Chronic prostato-vesiculitis: Incidence and significance of bacterial findings. *Scand J Urol Nephrol* 8:173, 1973.
60 Drach GW: Problems in diagnosis of bacterial prostatitis: Gram-negative, gram-positive and mixed infection. *J Urol* 111:630, 1974.
61 Anderson RU, Weller C: Prostatic secretion leukocyte studies in nonbacterial prostatitis (prostatosis). *J Urol* 121:292, 1979.
62 Blacklock NJ: Some observations on prostatitis, in *Advances in the Study of the Prostate*, DC Williams, MH Briggs, M Stanford (eds). London, Heinemann, 1969, p. 37.
63 Jameson RM: Sexual activity and the variations of the white cell content of the prostatic secretion. *Invest Urol* 5:297, 1967.
64 Weidner W, Ludwig M: Diagnostic management in chronic prostatitis, in *Prostatitis Etiopathology, Diagnosis and Therapy*, W Weidner, PO Madsen, HG Schiefer (eds). Berlin, Springer-Verlag, 1994, p. 49
65 Krieger JN: Prostatitis, epididymitis, and orchitis, in Mandell, Douglas and Bennett's *Principle's and Practice of Infectious Diseases*, 4th ed, GL Mandell, JE Bennett, R Dolin (eds). New York, Churchill-Livingstone, 1995, vol. 1, p. 1098.
66 Dajani AM, O'Flynn JD: Prostatitic abscess: A report of 25 cases. *Br J Urol* 40:736, 1968.
67 Pai MG, Bhat HS: Prostatic abscess. *J Urol* 108:599, 1972.
68 Weinberger M et al: Prostatic abscess in the antibiotic era. *Rev Infect Dis* 10:239, 1988.
69 Meares EM Jr: Prostatic abscess. *J. Urol* 136:1281, 1986.
70 Chia JK et al: Computed axial tomography in the early diagnosis of prostatic abscess. *Am J Med* 81:942, 1986.
71 Cyton S et al: Value of transrectal ultrasonography for diagnosis and treatment of prostatic abscess. *Urology* 32:454, 1988.
72 Jacobsen JD, Kvist E: Prostatic abscess: A review of literature and a presentation of 5 cases. *Scand J Urol Nephrol* 27:281, 1993.
73 Granados EA et al: Prostatic abscess: Diagnosis and treatment. *J Urol* 148:80, 1992.
74 O'Dea MJ et al: Non-specific granulomatous prostatitis. *J Urol* 118: 58, 1977.
75 Carson CC et al: Bacterial prostatitis caused by *Staphylococcus saprophyticus*. *Urology* 19:576, 1982.
76 Shortliffe LM et al: Measurement of urinary antibodies to crude bacterial antigen in patients with chronic bacterial prostatitis. *J Urol* 141: 632, 1989.
77 Shortliffe LM et al: The characterization of nonbacterial prostatitis: Search for an etiology. *J Urol* 148:1461, 1992.
78 Winningham DG et al: Diffusion of antibiotics from plasma into prostatic fluid. *Nature* 19:139, 1968.
79 Winningham DG, Stamey TA: Diffusion of sulfonamides from plasma into prostatic fluid. *J Urol* 104:559, 1970.
80 Seppanen J: The penetration of sulfadiazine, sulfamethoxazole and trimethoprim into the prostate gland, epididymis and testis in man. *Ann Clin Res* 12(Suppl 25):47,1980.
81 Meares EM Jr: Long-term therapy of chronic bacterial prostatitis with trimethoprim-sulfamethoxazole. *Can Med Assoc J* (suppl) 112: 22, 1975.
82 Meares EM Jr: Observations on activity of trimethoprim-sulfamethoxazole in the prostate. *J Infect Dis* 129(suppl): S679, 1973.
83 Drach GW: Trimethoprim/sulfamethoxazole therapy of chronic bacterial prostatitis. *J Urol* 111:637, 1974.
84 McGuire EJ, Lytton B: Bacterial prostatitis: Treatment with trimethoprim-sulfamethoxazole. *Urology* 7:499, 1976.
85 Naber KG: Use of quinolones in urinary tract infections and prostatitis. *Rev Infect Dis* 11 (suppl 5):S1321, 1989.
86 Wolfson JS, Hooper DC: Fluoroquinolone antimicrobial agents. *Clin Microbiol Rev* 2:378, 1989.
87 Naber KG: The role of quinolones in the treatment of chronic bacterial prostatitis, in *Prostatitis: Etiopathology, Diagnosis and Therapy*, W Weidner, PO Madsen, HG Schiefer (eds). Berlin, Springer Verlag, 1994, p. 175.
88 Van Landuyt HW et al: The importance of the quinolones in antibacterial therapy. *J Antimicrob Chemother* 1990.
89 Montorsi F et al: Ciprofloxacin: An oral quinolone for the treatment of infections with gram-negative pathogens. Committee on Antimicrobial Agents. Canadian Infectious Disease Society. *Can Med Assoc J* 150:669, 1994.
90 Schaeffer AJ, Darras FS: The efficacy of norfloxacin in the treatment of chronic bacterial prostatitis refractory to trimethoprim-sulfamethoxazole and/or carbenicillin. *J Urol* 144:690, 1990.
91 Weidner W et al: Refractory chronic bacterial prostatitis: A re-evaluation of ciprofloxacin treatment after a median follow-up of 30 months. *J Urol* 146:350, 1991.
92 Oliveri RA et al: Clinical experience with geocillin in the treatment of bacterial prostatitis. *Curr Ther Res* 25:415, 1979.
93 Mobley DF: Bacterial prostatitis: Treatment with carbenicillin indanyl sodium. *Invest Urol* 19:31, 1981.
94 Ristuccia AM, Cunha BA: Current concepts in antimicrobial therapy of prostatitis. *Urology* 20:338, 1982.
95 Baumueller A et al: Rosamicin—A new drug for the treatment of bacterial prostatitis. *Antimicrob Agents Chemother* 12:40, 1977.
96 Sabath LD et al: Excretion of erythromycin and its enhanced activity in urine against gram-negative bacilli with alkalinization. *J Lab Clin Med* 72:916, 1968.
97 Mobley DF: Erythromycin plus sodium bicarbonate in chronic bacterial prostatitis. *Urology* 3:60, 1974.
98 Gimarellou H et al: A study of the effectiveness of rifaprim in chronic prostatitis caused mainly by *Staphylococcus aureus*. *J Urol* 128:321, 1982.
99 Baert L: A re-appraisal of treatment in chronic bacterial prostatitis. Letter to the editor. *J Urol* 123:606, 1980.
100 Baert L, Leonard A: Chronic bacterial prostatitis: 10 years of experience with local antibiotics. *J Urol* 140:755, 1988.
101 De la Rosette JJ et al: Ultrasonographic findings in patients with nonbacterial prostatitis. *Urol Int* 48:323, 1992.
102 Fox M: The natural history and significance of stone formation in the prostate gland. *J Urol* 89:716, 1963.
103 Eykyn S et al: Prostatic calculi as a source of recurrent bacteriuria in the male. *Br J Urol* 46:527, 1974.
104 Meares EM Jr: Infection stones of the prostate gland: Laboratory diagnosis and clinical management. *Urology* 4:560, 1974.
105 Meares EM Jr: Chronic bacterial prostatitis: Role of transurethral prostatectomy (TURP) in therapy, in *Therapy of Prostatitis*, W Weidner, H Brunner, W Krause, CF Rothauge (eds). Munich, Zuckschwerdt Verlag, p. 1986.
106 Phau A et al: The pH of the prostatic fluid in health and disease: Implications of treatment in chronic bacterial prostatitis. *J Urol* 119: 384, 1978.
107 Fair WR, Cordonnier JJ: The pH of prostatic fluid: A reappraisal and therapeutic implications. *J Urol* 120:695, 1978.
108 Fair WR et al: A re-appraisal of treatment in chronic bacterial prostatitis. *J Urol* 121:437, 1979.

109 Nickel JC et al: Bacterial biofilms: Influence on the pathogenesis, diagnosis and treatment of urinary tract infections. *J Antimicrob Chemother* 33(suppl A):S31, 1994.
110 Nickel JC, Costerton JW: Coagulase-negative staphylococcus in chronic prostatitis. *J Urol* 147:398, 1992.
111 Meares EM Jr: Prostatitis vs. "prostatosis": A clinical and bacteriological study. *JAMA* 224:1372, 1973.
112 Smart CJ, Jenkins JD: The role of transurethral prostatectomy in chronic prostatitis. *Br J Urol* 45:654, 1973.
113 Smart CJ et al: The painful prostate. *Br J Urol* 47:861, 1975.
114 Silber SJ: Transurethral resection, in: New York, Appleton-Century-Crofts, 1977, p. 133.
115 Mardh P-A, Colleen S: Search for urogenital tract infections in patients with symptoms of prostatitis. *Scand J Urol Nephrol* 9:8, 1975.
116 Mardh P-A et al: *Chlamydia* in chronic prostatitis. *Br Med J* 4:361, 1972.
117 Colleen S, Mardh P-A: Studies on non-acute prostatitis, clinical and laboratory findings in patients with symptoms of non-acute prostatitis, in *Genital Infections and Their Complications: Symposium Proceedings* D Danielsson, L Juhlin, P-A Mardh (eds). Stockholm, Almquist and Wiksell International, 1975, p. 121.
118 Colleen S, Mardh P-A: Effect of metacycline treatment on non-acute prostatitis. *Scand J Urol Nephrol* 9:198, 1975.
119 Mardh P-A et al: Role of *Chlamydia trachomatis* in non-acute prostatitis. *Br J Vener Dis* 54:330, 1978.
120 Berger RE et al: Case-control study of men with suspected chronic idiopathic prostatitis. *J Urol* 141:328, 1989.
121 Doble A et al: A search for infectious agents in chronic abacterial prostatitis using ultrasound guided biopsy. *Br J Urol* 64:297, 1989.
122 Bruce AW et al: The role of chlamydiae in genitourinary disease. *J Urol* 126:625, 1981.
123 Taylor-Robinson D: The role of chlamydiae in genitourinary disease. *J Urol* 128:156,1982.
124 Bruce AW, Reid G: Prostatitis associated with *Chlamydia trachomatis* in 6 patients. *J Urol* 142:1006, 1989.
125 Kuroda K et al: Detection of *Chlamydia trachomatis* in urethra of patients with urogenital infection. *Hinyokika Kiyo* 35:453, 1989.
126 Nilsson S et al: Isolation of *C. trachomatis* from the urethra and prostatic fluid in men with signs and symptoms of acute urethritis. *Acta Dermatol Venereol (Stockh)* 61:456, 1981.
127 Kennelly MJ, Osterling JE: Conservative management of a seminal vesicle abscess. *J Urol* 141:1432, 1989.
128 Weidner W et al: *Chlamydia trachomatis* in "abacterial" prostatitis: Microbiological, cytological, and serological studies. *Urol Int* 38: 146–149, 1983.
129 Poletti F et al: Isolation of *Chlamydia trachomatis* from the prostatic cells in patients affected by nonacute abacterial prostatitis. *J Urol* 134:245, 1985.
130 Abdelatif OM et al: *Chlamydia trachomatis* in chronic abacterial prostatitis: Demonstration by colorimetric *in situ* hybridization. *Hum Pathol* 22:41, 1991.
131 Shurbaji MS et al: Immunohistochemical demonstration of chlamydial antigens in association with prostatitis. *Mod Pathol* 1:348, 1988.
132 Kobayashi TK, Araki H: Immunocytochemical detection of chlamydial antigen in both the urethral scraping and prostatic aspirate in a case of abacterial prostatitis. *ACTA Cytol* 32:270, 1988.
133 Holland S et al: Demonstration of chlamydial RNA and DNA during a culture-negative state. *Infect Immun* 60:2040, 1992.
134 Weidner W et al: Quantitative culture of *Ureaplasma urealyticum* in patients with chronic prostatitis or prostatosis. *J Urol* 124:622, 1980.
135 Ohkawa M et al: Antimicrobial treatment for chronic prostatitis as a means of defining the role of *Ureaplasma urealyticum*. *Urol Int* 51: 129, 1993.
136 Isaacs JT: *Ureaplasma urealyticum* in the urogenital tract of patients with chronic prostatitis or related symptomatology. *Br J Urol* 72:918, 1993.
137 Krieger JN: Urologic aspects of trichomoniasis. *Invest Urol* 18:411, 1981.
138 Kuberski T: *Trichomonas vaginalis* associated with nongonococcal urethritis and prostatitis. *Sex Transm Dis* 7:135, 1980.
139 Drummand A: Trichomonas infestation of the prostate gland. *Am J Surg* 31:98, 1936.
140 Kawamura N: Trichomoniasis of the prostate. *Jpn J Clin Urol* 27: 335, 1973.
141 Gardner W Jr. et al: *Trichomonas vaginalis* in the prostate gland. *Arch Pathol Lab Med* 110:430,1986.
142 Kurnatowska A et al: Rare cases of prostatitis caused by invasion of *Trichomonas vaginalis* with *Candida albicans*. *Wiad Parazytol* 36: 229,1990.
143 Nielsen ML, Vestergaard BF: Virological investigations in chronic prostatitis. *J Urol* 109:1023,1973.
144 Nielsen ML, Justesen T: Studies on the pathology of prostatitis: A search for prostatic infections with obligate anaerobes in patients with chronic prostatitis and chronic urethritis. *Scand J Urol Nephrol* 8:1, 1974.
145 Meares EMJ: Prostatitis. *Med Clin North Am* 75:405, 1991.
146 Bergman B et al: *Staphylococcus saprophyticus* in males with symptoms of chronic prostatitis. *Urology* 34:241, 1989.
147 Sargent JC, Irwin R: Prostatic abscess: Clinical study of 42 cases. *Am J Surg* 11:334, 1931.
148 Danielsson D, Molin L: Demonstration of *N. gonorrhoeae* in prostatic fluid after treatment of uncomplicated gonorrheal urethritis. *Acta Derm Venerol (Stockh)* 51:73, 1971.
149 Doble A et al: Prostatodynia and herpes simplex virus infection. *Urology* 38:247, 1991.
150 Morrisseau P et al: Viral prostatitis. *J Urol* 103:767, 1970.
151 Corey L, Spear P: Infections with herpes simplex virus (second of two parts). *N Engl J Med* 314:749, 1986.
152 Benson PJ, Smith CS: Cytomegalovirus prostatitis. *Urology* 40:165, 1992.
153 Collier A et al: Cytomegalovirus infection in women attending a sexually transmitted disease clinic. *J Infect Dis* 162:46, 1990.
154 Ho M: Epidemiology of cytomegalovirus infection. *Rev Infect Dis* 12 (suppl):701, 1990.
155 Barbalias GA: Prostatodynia or painful male urethral syndrome? *Urology* 36:146, 1990.
156 O'Shauglinessy EJ et al: Chronic prostatitis fact or fiction? *JAMA* 160:540, 1956.
157 Segura JW et al: Prostatosis, prostatitis or pelvic floor tension myalgia? *J Urol* 122:168, 1979.
158 Mathur S et al: Clinical significance of sperm antibodies in infertility. *Fertil Steril* 36:486, 1981.
159 Bittinger A et al: Experimental autoimmune prostatitis (EAP): Enhanced release of reactive oxygen intermediates (ROI) in peritoneal macrophages. *Autoimmunity* 16:201, 1993.
160 Rosenbloom D: Chronic prostatitis—A psychosexual approach. *Calif Med* 82:454,1955.
161 Nilsson JK et al: Relationship between psychological and laboratory findings in patients with symptoms of non-acute prostatitis, in *Genital Infections and their Complications: Symposium Procedings*, D Danielsson, L Juhlin, PA Mardh (eds). Stockholm, Almquist and Wiksell International, 1975, p. 133.
162 Webster GD et al: The evaluation of bladder neck dysfunction. *J Urol* 123:196, 1980.
163 Siroky MB et al: Functional voiding disorders in men. *J Urol* 126: 200, 1981.
164 Barbalias GA: Prostatodynia or painful male urethral syndrome? *Urology* 36:146, 1990.
165 Towfighi J et al: Granulomatous prostatitis with emphasis on the eosinophilic variety. *Am J Clin Pathol* 58:630, 1972.
166 Lopatkin NA et al: The differential diagnosis of allergic prostatitis. *Urol Nefrol (Mosk)* Mar–Apr (2):17, 1990.
167 Messing EM: Interstitial cystitis and related conditions, in *Campbell's Urology*, 6th ed, PC Walsh, AB Retik, TA Stamey, E Darracott Vaughan, Jr. (eds). Philadelphia, W.B. Saunders, 1992, vol. 1, p. 982.
168 Servadio C, Leib Z: Chronic abacterial prostatitis and hyperthermia. A possible new treatment? *Br J Urol* 67:308, 1991.

169 Barbalas GA et al: Prostatodynia: Clinical and urodynamic characteristics. *J Urol* 130:514, 1983.
170 Hellstrom WJ et al: Neuromuscular dysfunction in nonbacterial prostatitis. *Urology* 30:183, 1987.
171 Miller H: Stress prostatitis. *Urology* 32:507, 1988.
172 Neal DEJ, Moon TD: Use of terazosin in prostatodynia and validation of a symptom score questionnaire. *Urology* 43:460, 1994.
173 Egan K, Krieger J: Psychological problems in chronic prostatitis patients with pain. *Clin J Pain* 10:218, 1994.
174 De la Rosette JJ et al: Personality variables involved in chronic prostatitis. *Urology* 42:654, 1993.
175 Darenkov AF et al: Transurethral electroresection in chronic prostatitis and its complications. *Urol Nefrol (Mosk)* Jan–Feb (1):18, 1989.
176 Lopatin WB et al: Retrograde transurethral balloon dilation of prostate: Innovative management of abacterial chronic prostatitis and prostatodynia. *Urology* 36:508, 1990.
177 Kumon H et al: Transrectal hyperthermia for the treatment of chronic prostatitis. *Nippon Hinyokika Gakkai Zasshi* 84:265, 1993.
178 Nickel JC, Sorenson R: Transurethral microwave thermotherapy of nonbacterial prostatitis and prostatodynia: Initial experience. *Urology* 44:458, 1994.
179 Wiseman LR, Balfour JA: Clinical experience with transurethral microwave thermotherapy for chronic nonbacterial prostatitis and prostatodynia. *J Endourol* 8:61, 1994.
180 Miroshnikov BI et al: Experience with the combined treatment of chronic prostatitis. *Vopr Kurortol Fizioter Lech Fiz Kult* May–Jun (3):38, 1990.
181 Vozianov AF et al: The laser reflexotherapy of patients with chronic prostatitis. *Vrach Delo* Feb (2):45, 1991.
182 Frazier HA et al: Total prostatoseminal vesiculectomy in the treatment of debilitating perineal pain [see comments]. *J Urol* 148:409, 1992.
183 Davis BE, Weigel JW: Adenocarcinoma of the prostate discovered in 2 young patients following total prostatovesiculectomy for refractory prostatitis. *J Urol* 144:744, 1990.
184 Clements R et al: Transrectal ultrasound appearances of granulomatous prostatitis. *Clin Radiol* 47:174, 1993.
185 Bryan RL et al: Granulomatous prostatitis: A clinicopathological study. *Histopathology* 19:453, 1991.
186 Miralles TG et al: Fine needle aspiration cytology of granulomatous prostatitis. *Acta Cytol* 34:57, 1990.
187 Servadio C: Wegener's granulomatosis presenting as lower back pain with prostatitis and uretheral obstruction. *J Rheumatol* 21:566, 1994.
188 Murty GE, Powell PH: Wegener's granulomatosis presenting as prostatitis. *Br J Urol* 67:107, 1991.
189 Hussain SF et al: Wegener's granulomatosis presenting as granulomatous prostatitis causing urinary retention. *Br J Urol* 65:104, 1990.
190 Bray VJ, Hasbargen JA: Prostatic involvement in Wegener's granulomatosis. *Am J Kidney Dis* 17:578, 1991.
191 Moore RA: Tuberculosis of the prostate gland. *J Urol* 37:372, 1937.
192 Venema RJ, Lattimer JK: Genital tuberculosis in the male. *J Urol* 78:65, 1957.
193 Brooker WJ, Aufderheide AC: Genitourinary tract infections due to atypical mycobacteria. *J Urol* 124:242, 1980.
194 Wetzel O et al: Tuberculous prostatitis: Nodularity may stimulate malignancy. *Br J Urol* 72:249, 1993.
195 Schwartz J: Mycotic prostatitis. *Urology* 19:1, 1982.
196 Bissada NK et al: Prostatic mycosis. *Urology* 9:327, 1977.
197 Schwarz J, Salfelder K: Blastomycosis. *Curr Top Pathol* 65:166, 1977.
198 Gritti EJ et al: Coccidioidomycosis granuloma of the prostate: A rare manifestation of the disseminated disease. *J Urol* 89:249, 1963.
199 Conner WT et al: Genitourinary aspects of disseminated coccidioidomycosis. *J Urol* 113:82, 1975.
200 Price MJ et al: Coccidioidomycosis of prostate gland. *Urology* 19: 653, 1982.
201 Brooks MH et al: Cryptococcal prostatitis. *JAMA* 192:639, 1965.
202 Hinchey WW, Someren A: Cryptococcal prostatitis. *Am J Clin* 75: 257; 1991.
203 Reddy PA et al: Progressive disseminated histoplasmosis seen in adults. *Am J Med* 46:629, 1990.
204 Campbell TB et al: Aspergillosis of the prostate associated with an indwelling bladder catheter: Case report and review. *Clin Infect Dis* 14:942, 1992.
205 Golz R, Mendling W: Candidosis of the prostate: A rare form of endomycosis. *Mycoses* 34:381, 1991.
206 Indudhara R et al: Isolated invasive candidal prostatitis. *Urol Int* 48: 362, 1992.
207 Thomson L: Syphilis of the prostate. *American Journal of Syphilis* 4:323, 1920.
208 Kelalis PP et al: Brucellosis of the urogenital tract: A mimic of tuberculosis. *J Urol* 88:347, 1962.
209 Clason AE et al: Urinary retention and granulomatous prostatitis following sacral herpes zoster infection: A report of 2 cases with a review of the literature. *Br J Urol* 54:166, 1982.
210 Miyashita H et al: BCG-induced granulomatous prostatitis: A comparative ultrasound and pathologic study. *Urology* 39:364, 1992.
211 Adams JR Jr. et al: Acquired immunodeficiency syndrome manifesting as prostate nodule secondary to cryptococcal infection. *Urology* 39:289, 1992.
212 Mikolich DJ, Mates SM: Granulomatous prostatitis due to *Mycobacterium avium* complex. *Clin Infect Dis* 14:589, 1992.
213 Krieger J: Evaluation and treatment of unconventional genitourinary tract infections. *Sem Urol* 3:193, 1985.
214 Wishnow KI et al: The diagnostic value of the immunologic response in bacterial and nonbacterial prostatitis. *J Urol* 127:689, 1982.

Section 4
Management of Dermatological and Extragenital Manifestations of STD/HIV

Chapter 63

Generalized cutaneous manifestations of STD/HIV infection: Typical presentations, differential diagnosis, and management

Roy Colven
David H. Spach

INTRODUCTION

Generalized skin lesions in any patient often can perplex both the patient and the practitioner. Evaluating generalized skin lesions in a patient who has a sexually transmitted disease (STD) or human immunodeficiency virus (HIV) infection can present special problems. The STD may be associated with, but not necessarily a cause of, the generalized rash. Patients infected with HIV may present with unique dermatoses, unusual infections, and atypical manifestations of common skin diseases. Among HIV-infected individuals, some type of skin disorder will develop in nearly 80 percent.[1] Certain common skin conditions—including herpes zoster, severe seborrheic dermatitis, persistent staphylococcal folliculitis, and generalized pruritus—occur with increased frequency in HIV-infected patients and thus may provide the first clue that an individual is HIV-infected.[2,3]

The first goal of this chapter is to outline a practical approach to the STD- and/or HIV-infected patient who presents with generalized skin disease (Fig. 63-1). Particularly important aspects of this approach are (1) to attempt to identify the primary lesion in a generalized skin condition, (2) to recognize any specific features or patterns of the primary lesion, and (3) to determine the distribution of the rash on the body surface. With this approach, the practitioner can usually generate a differential diagnosis. Evidence obtained from history and laboratory tests such as potassium hydroxide preparation or Gram stain can then be applied to narrow the differential-diagnosis list. If necessary, a skin biopsy can be easily performed to add more specific information. The second goal of this chapter is to familiarize the reader with the typical as well as atypical presentations of a number of STD- and/or HIV-related cutaneous manifestations. In addition, we discuss therapy of selected conditions.

APPROACH TO A GENERALIZED SKIN CONDITION

GENERAL APPEARANCE

One's first glance at a patient often consciously or unconsciously starts the dermatologic assessment. Is the patient obviously symptomatic with itching? Is there evidence of the skin condition on the face or scalp? Does the patient cover skin lesions with clothing or makeup? Does the patient have generalized edema? Vital signs, including the presence or absence of fever, are a critical part of this initial assessment. In order to examine the skin thoroughly, have the patient undress and put on a gown, thus exposing the skin. One also needs good lighting.

PRIMARY SKIN LESIONS

A "primary lesion" refers to the initial stage in the evolution of a skin lesion. Identifying the primary lesion in a patient with a generalized skin condition provides critical information in making an accurate dermatologic diagnosis. Moreover, characterizing the appearance of the primary lesion directs the practitioner to a category of conditions based on lesion morphology. "Secondary lesions" refer to skin lesions altered, either naturally over time or by outside forces, to the extent that the primary morphology becomes obscured. For example, a patient with pruritic papules (primary lesions) may intensely scratch these lesions and turn them into erosions (secondary lesions), likely misleading the practitioner to formulate a differential diagnosis that does not include generalized papules. Alternatively, one should not assume the presentation of certain lesions, such as erosions, always represent secondary lesions. Primary lesions are important in defining a generalized process and in communicating the appearance of a skin rash to another practitioner. A glossary of primary lesions is presented in Table 63-1.

SECONDARY FEATURES AND LESION PATTERNS

Unfortunately, relying solely on the primary-lesion morphology is often not sufficient to diagnose skin conditions accurately. The differential diagnosis of a papular eruption, for example, is extensive; knowing this information is not necessarily helpful when applied to an individual patient. If one can initially classify subsets of papular conditions based on other prominent features, the differential diagnosis quickly narrows. In Table 63-2, certain secondary features and lesion patterns are defined; these definitions can assist in further classifying cutaneous conditions. With the primary lesion and secondary features in mind, the clinician can better generate a differential diagnosis. Table 63-3 outlines generalized STD- or HIV-related cutaneous conditions based on the conditions' primary morphologies or predominant lesion patterns/distributions. Note that diagnoses, such as secondary syphilis and scabies, appear in multiple categories. Also, exceptions to the categorization will occur because syphilis and HIV can cause a wide range of cutaneous abnormalities. Though Table 63-3 distinguishes HIV- and STD-related conditions, this separation is arbitrary and is presented to help better organize one's differential diagnostic workup.

If the diagnosis cannot be established on clinical grounds, a skin biopsy often provides valuable information. Three- to 4-mm punch biopsies sent for routine histology and/or culture can be performed with minimal discomfort (Fig. 63-2). Performing a biopsy of an early lesion generally gives the best diagnostic yield.

SELECTED CONDITIONS

MACULAR AND PAPULAR CONDITIONS

Exanthem of acute HIV infection

During the period of viremia associated with acute HIV infection, a transient, evanescent, erythematous macular and papular ex-

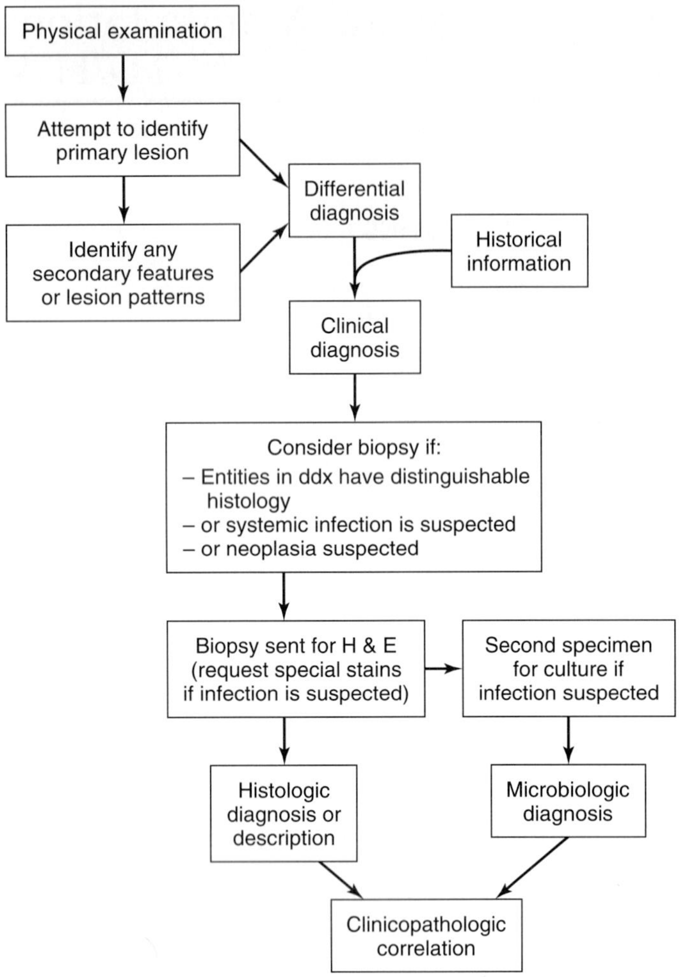

Figure 63-1. Approach to a patient with generalized rash.

Table 63-1. Definition of Primary Lesions

- **Macule:** a small (<0.5–1 cm diameter) area of color change without surface elevation
- **Patch:** a larger macular area
- **Papule:** a small (<0.5–1 cm diameter) solid elevation
- **Plaque:** a broad, solid elevation
- **Nodule:** a solid elevation distinguished from a papule by deeper penetration and larger diameter
- **Wheal:** a smooth-contoured, edematous elevation, which is often transient
- **Vesicle:** a small (<0.5–1 cm diameter), clear fluid-filled blister
- **Bulla:** a larger, clear, fluid-filled blister
- **Pustule:** a pus-filled blister
- **Abscess:** a collection of pus in the dermis and deeper tissues, often manifested by tenderness, fluctuance, warmth, and surrounding induration
- **Cyst:** a dermal sac with soft or fluid contents manifested by a soft, fluctuant, smooth-contoured elevation
- **Erosion:** moist or crusted, usually superficially depressed, area of partial or complete denudation of epidermis that generally heals without scarring
- **Ulcer:** depression in the skin surface caused by destruction of the epidermis (and at least part of the dermis) that generally heals without scarring
- **Atrophy:** a thinning of intact epidermis, dermis, or subcutaneous fat often resulting in wrinkling, translucency, or depression of the skin surface

- Other useful terms, though not considered primary skin lesions:
  - **Crust:** dried serous or serosanguinous transudate
  - **Eschar:** adherent, often black or gray product of coagulation necrosis of the dermis, typically found at the base of an ulcer
  - **Exanthem:** a generalized macular and papular rash on cutaneous surfaces mostly associated with a viral illness
  - **Enanthem:** a mucous membrane–limited erythematous eruption mostly associated with a viral illness

anthem may appear (see Color Plate 117). Although the subtle nature of this rash has made it difficult to determine its true incidence, some investigators have estimated that as many as 75 percent of symptomatic acutely infected patients will develop this rash.[4] Constitutional symptoms, namely fatigue, fever, and weight loss, often coexist with the rash and generally precede the exanthem by 2 days to 3 weeks.[5] The HIV-associated exanthem appears similar to those caused by other viruses, such as adenovirus or Epstein-Barr virus. In addition, patients may develop an enanthem.[6] Both the exanthem and enanthem generally resolve within 1 to 2 weeks, often within several days. At this early stage, patients will have a negative HIV antibody test, but tests for viral replication, such as an HIV RNA assay or a p24 antigen (in the setting of a negative antibody test), can confirm the diagnosis.

Scabies

Scabies classically manifests as linear papules distributed in finger web spaces, flexor wrists, axillae, nipples, waistline, ankles, and genitals, but usually sparing the head (see Plates 81 and 83). The linear lesions represent the burrowing of the adult mite into the epidermis (Plate 80). Burrows, however, appear relatively infrequently compared with eroded (usually excoriated) papules (see Plate 82). In general, one should consider the diagnosis of scabies in any patient with a generalized pruritic rash. Though described here under the category of papular rash, scabies may appear eczematous or papulosquamous, depending on the chronicity and immune status of the patient. The diagnosis of scabies is covered in Chap. 47.

Human immunodeficiency virus–infected patients have an increased incidence of atypical manifestations of scabies, particularly face and scalp involvement, nodular lesions, and hyperkeratotic (often referred to as crusted or Norwegian) scabies (Figure 63-3).[7] Because the diagnosis of scabies is often delayed in patients with atypical forms of the disease, community outbreaks and nosocomial infestations may result.

The treatment of choice for most cases of scabies is permethrin, 5% cream applied from the neck down, left on overnight, and rinsed off in the morning. Most patients do not need a second application at a later time, as is common practice in the use of other scabicides. Patients with crusted scabies, however, require

Table 63-2. Secondary Cutaneous Features Defined

- **Papulosquamous:** papules and plaques with prominent scale
- **Eczematous:** erythematous papules and plaques, often pruritic, with varying degrees of weeping, crust, and scale
- **Erythroderma:** <90 percent total body surface area involvement with erythema, usually with some degree of scale
- **Xerosis:** generalized dry skin
- **Hyperkeratosis:** thickening of the stratum corneum producing visible scale
- **Ichthyosis:** flaking of skin with a distinct fish-scale pattern
- **Purpura:** dermal or subcutaneous bleeding producing a violaceous macule or patch

Table 63-3. Differential Diagnosis Based on Lesion Morphology or Secondary Features

Lesion Morphology or Pattern	Possible HIV-Related Infections or Dermatoses	Possible STD or STD-Related Dermatoses
Macules/small papules	Exanthem of primary HIV infection, morbilliform drug eruption, measles, scabies	Morbilliform drug eruption, roseolar syphilis,* papular syphilis, Jarisch-Herxheimer reaction, prodrome of hepatitis B virus, viral exanthems (other than HIV), erythema multiforme (associated with HSV infection), scabies
Larger papules/nodules	Eosinophilic folliculitis, molluscum contagiosum, bacillary angiomatosis, papular syphilis, deep mycoses (disseminated cryptococcosis, histoplasmosis, coccidioidomycosis), scabies, Kaposi's sarcoma, verrucae, papular eruption of HIV	Scabies, nodular syphilis
Wheals/urticaria	Drug hypersensitivity, idiopathic	Drug hypersensitivity, prodrome of hepatitis B virus, idiopathic
Vesicles/bullae/erosions/crusts	Disseminated VZV, HSV, impetigo contagiosa, bullous impetigo, ecthyma, erythema multiforme, toxic epidermolytic necrolysis, porphyria cutanea tarda	Erythema multiforme, VZV (dermatomal or disseminated)
Ulcers	HSV, VZV, cytomegalovirus, ecthyma, fixed drug eruption, deep mycoses	Rupioid syphilis (lues maligna)
Pustules:		
hair follicle–based	Folliculitis (eosinophilic, staphylococcal, gram-negative, pityrosporum, demodex), acne	Folliculitis (especially staphylococcal), acne
not clearly hair follicle–based	Pustular psoriasis, Reiter's syndrome, disseminated HSV or VZV	Disseminated gonococcal infection, Reiter's syndrome (associated with chlamydial infection), pustular syphilis
Papules with scale (papulosquamous)	Seborrheic dermatitis, psoriasis, Reiter's syndrome, dermatophyte, scabies	Papulosquamous syphilis, Reiter's syndrome, pityriasis rosea, dermatophyte infection, seborrheic dermatitis
Eczematous	Seborrheic dermatitis, scabies, drug hypersensitivity, atopic dermatitis, dermatophyte	Scabies, atopic dermatitis, seborrheic dermatitis
Erythroderma	Seborrheic dermatitis, psoriasis, TEN, drug hypersensitivity	
Dry skin (xerosis), ichthyosiform	Ichthyosis, asteatosis, nutritional deficiencies, drug-related, atopic dermatitis	Atopic dermatitis
Purpura (including palpable purpura)	Kaposi's sarcoma, idiopathic thrombocytopenic purpura, vasculitis associated with hepatitis B or C virus	Disseminated gonococcal infection, vasculitic syphilis, vasculitis associated with hepatitis B or C virus
Pigmentary changes:		
hypo-/depigmentation	Postinflammatory hypopigmentation, vitiligo	Postinflammatory hypopigmentation with syphilis
hyperpigmentation	Postinflammatory hyperpigmentation, medication-related (zidovudine)	

[a] For any references to syphilis, assume the secondary stage unless otherwise specified.

repeated total body (and head) applications. For those patients with crusted scabies who develop hyperkeratosis, adding ammonium lactate (12% lotion applied bid) can help to diminish the scale, though it may temporarily irritate the skin. The use of single-dose oral ivermectin, 200 μg/kg, has shown promising results, even among patients with crusted scabies.[8]

Macular (roseolar) and papular secondary syphilis

An array of generalized rashes can develop in patients with secondary syphilis, including the macular (roseolalike) and papular variants. The macular lesions often appear as faint, pale, pink macules that do not have scale. In most instances, the rash requires good lighting (preferably daylight) to visualize adequately. Papular secondary syphilis occurs more frequently than the macular form and probably represents an evolution from undetected macular lesions. The papular lesions are typically distributed on the face, flexural folds, and trunk. Involvement of the palms and soles is characteristic, with lesions often appearing brownish in this location (see Plates 43 and 44). Several variants of papular syphilis have been described. Annular lesions, more commonly seen on the faces of Blacks with secondary syphilis, can resemble sarcoidosis or tinea. Corymbose ("flat-topped flower bouquet") lesions appear as a central large papule or nodule surrounded by small satellite papules. Papulosquamous secondary syphilis is discussed later in this chapter. Later in the course of secondary syphilis, papules may occur at certain sites, such as the corners of the mouth ("split papules"), angles of the nose, and body folds. Patchy, "moth-eaten," nonscarring alopecia is commonly present in secondary syphilis (Fig. 63-4). With all forms of secondary syphilis, patients develop varying degrees of generalized lymphadenopathy.

Jarisch-Herxheimer reaction

Two to eight hours after starting antimicrobial therapy for secondary syphilis, a febrile Jarisch-Herxheimer reaction associated with malaise, headache, tender adenopathy, pharyngitis, and leukocytosis can occur and will alarm the unprepared patient and the unsuspecting practitioner. During this reaction, the existing

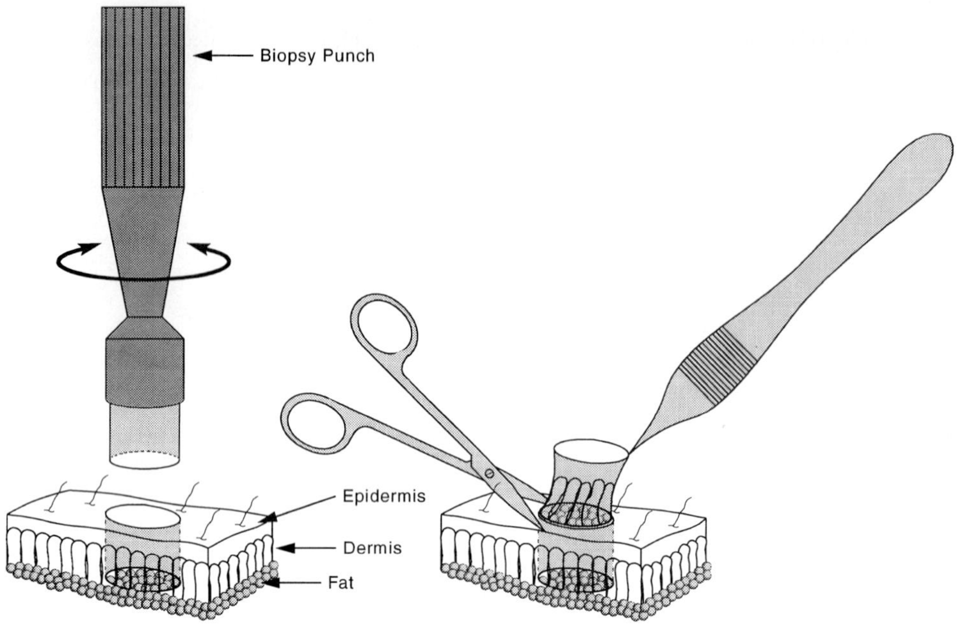

Figure 63-2. Technique of punch biospsy: After skin preparation and intradermal anesthesia, incises the skin with a twisting motion of a punch to the level of the subdermal fat. The specimen is then lifted carefully with teethed forceps, avoiding crushing, and the specimen is cut away from the fat using a fine scissors. A suture to close the wound is optional.

rash may become more prominent, or a previously unrecognized rash of secondary syphilis may appear. The incidence of the Jarisch-Herxheimer reaction is approximately 95 percent in patients with seropositive primary syphilis or secondary syphilis. The incidence decreases in late secondary syphilis and is frequently absent in latent syphilis.[9] This reaction is considered a therapy-associated response, not a drug-hypersensitivity reaction. The mechanism remains unknown (see Chap. 35). The sudden onset and associated systemic symptoms distinguish the Jarisch-Herxheimer reaction from most drug-associated eruptions, including the generalized rash observed with penicillins. Although the anaphylactic, urticarial reaction to penicillin has a rapid onset, one can easily distinguish it from the Jarisch-Herxheimer reaction on the basis of lesion morphology (a wheal in the case of urticaria). A similar Jarisch-Herxheimer reaction has been observed with the treatment of other spirochetal diseases, including Lyme disease and relapsing fever.

Drug hypersensitivity

Although cutaneous reactions to drugs can take many forms, the most common reaction is the generalized macular and papular eruption. Many authors have referred to this reaction as a "maculopapular" or "morbilliform" rash. Neither of these terms, however, is optimal—the former because true "maculopapules" do not exist and the latter because many medical providers in western countries have little experience diagnosing the "morbilliform" rash associated with measles. A generalized macular and papular drug hypersensitivity rash often begins on the trunk and spreads peripherally (Color Plate 118). Individual erythematous macules and papules will commonly coalesce and sometimes appear urticarial. Patients often complain of pruritus but generally not of fever or other constitutional symptoms. Although this type of drug

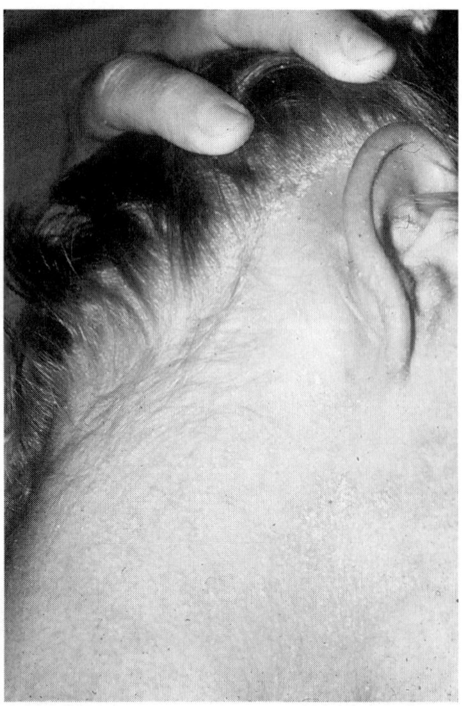

Figure 63-3. Hyperkeratotic scabies involving the scalp and face.

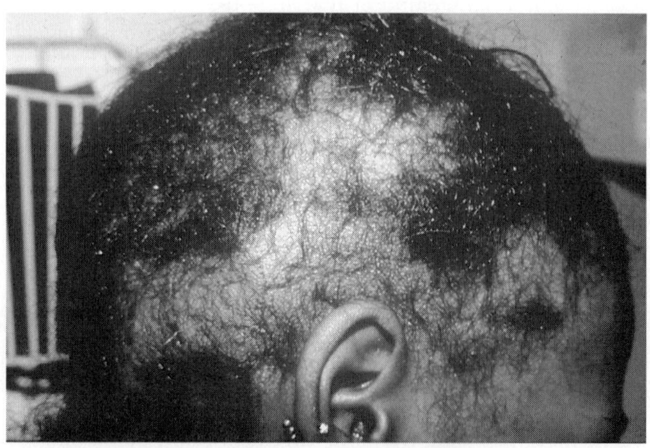

Figure 63-4. Patchy alopecia of secondary syphilis.

reaction most commonly appears within the first two weeks of introducing a new drug, it can occur after long-term use.

Some drug hypersensitivity eruptions are photodistributed; that is, they appear predominantly in ultraviolet (UV) light–exposed skin. Photosensitivity due to medications is divided into phototoxic and photoallergic reactions. Phototoxic reactions, which account for most photosensitive drug reactions, typically present as an exaggerated sunburn within 24 hours of UV light exposure and do not require prior sensitization. Photoallergic reactions are uncommon and present approximately 48 hours after UV light exposure. Photosensitizing drugs commonly used to treat STDs or HIV-related disorders include doxycycline (phototoxic) and trimethoprim-sulfamethoxazole (phototoxic or photoallergic).

Human immunodeficiency virus–infected individuals, when compared with HIV-negative persons, develop cutaneous manifestations of adverse drug reactions with increased frequency, even when controlling for the rate of usage of certain drugs, such as sulfonamides.[1] Moreover, the risk of drug hypersensitivity increases with advanced immune-system dysfunction. Proposed mechanisms for this apparent increased susceptibility to adverse drug reactions include enhanced T-cell susceptibility and/or decreased hepatic metabolism of drugs secondary to glutathione deficiency.[10]

The approach to a patient with a suspected drug-hypersensitivity reaction depends on the severity of the reaction, the need to continue use of the suspected drug, and the question of whether an equally effective alternative exists. In HIV-infected patients, approximately one-third of cutaneous reactions to sulfonamides spontaneously resolve and allow continued use for long-term *Pneumocystis carinii* pneumonia prophylaxis.[11] Symptomatic treatment with antihistamines and topical steroids can help relieve symptoms during the acute reaction. Close observation is recommended, however, because more severe reactions, such as Stevens-Johnson syndrome or toxic epidermal necrolysis, may ensue. Short courses of systemic steroids are occasionally needed with severe reactions; these severe reactions generally mandate stopping the suspected medication.

Erythema multiforme/Stevens-Johnson syndrome/toxic epidermal necrolysis

Erythema multiforme (EM) refers to an epithelial vascular reaction pattern and is traditionally considered to represent a spectrum of disorders. Erythema multiforme minor typically presents as acrally predominant papules that evolve to form classic target lesions, though atypical targets and urticarial plaques without targets sometimes form. Vesicles or bullae may develop within the center of these lesions (Fig. 63-5). Patients with EM minor generally do not have constitutional symptoms or mucosal involvement. Investigators have identified herpes simplex virus (HSV) infection, both genital and orolabial (including asymptomatic infection), as a precipitating event in some of cases of EM minor. In addition, recurrent EM minor can occur with recurrent herpetic outbreaks.

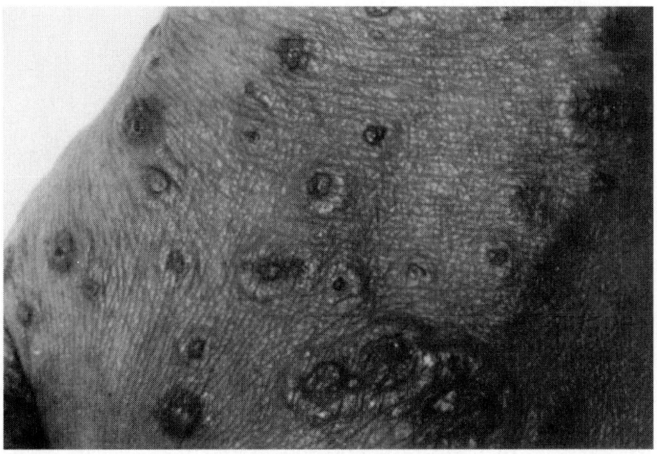

Figure 63-5. Typical target lesions in erythema multiforme on the wrist and hand. These lesions have central vesicles.

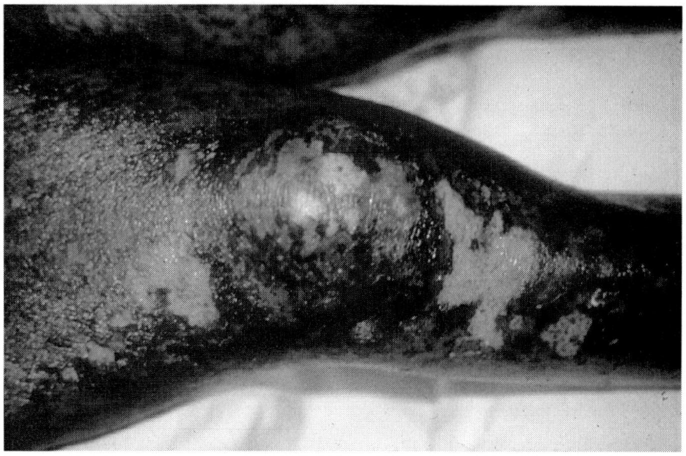

Figure 63-6. Toxic epidermal necrolysis due to trimethoprim-sulfamethoxazole. Initial confluent erythema progresses to epidermal sloughing.

Although most authors have traditionally equated EM major with Stevens-Johnson syndrome, recent investigation indicates these two disorders may be distinct. Stevens-Johnson syndrome is characterized by a sudden onset of fever, constitutional symptoms, rash, and mucosal erosions. The cutaneous lesions appear as erythematous or purpuric macules, sometimes with superficial vesicles or erosions, that tend to generalize with a truncal predominance. Mucosal involvement includes oral, ocular, or genital sites. Severe mucositis associated with acrally predominant target lesions is better termed EM major.[12] Investigators have attempted to distinguish Stevens-Johnson syndrome histologically from EM major, with more epidermal necrosis favoring Stevens-Johnson syndrome and more dermal inflammation suggesting EM major.[13] Most cases of Stevens-Johnson syndrome are drug-related, with sulfonamides and anticonvulsants most often incriminated, whereas most cases of EM major are HSV-related.[14]

Toxic epidermal necrolysis (TEN), conventionally considered to represent the most severe end of the EM spectrum, is characterized by the onset of erythroderma and painful skin, followed by widespread sloughing of the epidermis (Fig. 63-6). Mortality is approximately 20 percent. The initiators in toxic epidermal necrolysis are almost exclusively drugs, and most are the same as in Stevens-Johnson syndrome. An increased incidence of toxic epidermal necrolysis possibly exists among those with HIV infection,[15] but this may simply represent an increased use of medications, such as sulfonamides, known to cause toxic epidermal necrolysis.

GENERALIZED PAPULES AND NODULES

Molluscum contagiosum

The papules of molluscum contagiosum, caused by a pox virus, are distinctive. The lesions are generally 2 to 5 mm in size and may number from a few located on the face or genitals to numerous widely scattered lesions. They are flesh-colored to white-pink, domed, and centrally umbilicated (see Plate 84). Among HIV-infected individuals, the lesions tend to be more numerous and may be nodular ("giant molluscum") and disfiguring. Reports have described patients with disseminated cryptococcosis, coccidioidomycosis, or *Penicillium marneffei* presenting with multiple lesions that resemble molluscum contagiosum.[16–19] Treatment options for patients with molluscum include cryotherapy, electrodessication, gentle curettage, topical tretinoin (Retin-A), and superficial chemical peeling. Generally these therapies produce excellent cosmetic results. One report describes disfiguring molluscum contagiosum in an HIV-infected patient responding to combination antiretroviral therapy.[19a]

Kaposi's sarcoma

Kaposi's sarcoma lesions are usually easily recognized in the appropriate setting of patients with HIV disease. The lesions typically appear as violaceous papules and nodules that can be single, few, or multiple and widely scattered (see Plates 64 and 65). Incipient lesions commonly appear macular and may resemble a bruise. With isolated skin involvement, Kaposi's sarcoma lesions generally produce no symptoms; if, however, the lesions progressively extend into the subcutaneous and lymphatic tissues, edema may form.

Bacillary angiomatosis

Bacillary angiomatosis (BA) was first described in 1983 in HIV-infected patients with fever and subcutaneous nodules.[20] Since then, BA has been observed most commonly in the skin as solitary or multiple vascular lesions that clinically resemble Kaposi's sarcoma. Involvement of the liver (peliosis hepatis), spleen, lymph nodes, bones, lungs, and central nervous system (CNS) have all been attributed to BA. The causative organisms, *Bartonella henselae* and *B. quintana*, have been isolated using special culture techniques and identified with polymerase chain reaction techniques.[21,22] *Bartonella henselae* is the most common cause of cat-scratch disease in immunocompetent patients.[23] Exposure to cats, especially kittens, is associated with a higher risk of contracting BA and cat-scratch disease.[24]

Bacillary angiomatosis most often involves HIV-infected patients with advanced immunosuppression (CD4 count less than 100 cells/μl), though BA has rarely been reported in immunocompetent patients and organ transplant recipients.[25,26] The skin is most commonly involved. The lesions are red papules that progress to exophytic papules and nodules. These tend to be friable and are surrounded by a collarette of scale, resembling pyogenic granulomas. Subcutaneous lesions are flesh-colored, usually nontender, and mobile, similar to epidermoid cysts. Fever, night sweats, weight loss, and fatigue are common, though patients have variable degrees of constitutional illness.

Biopsy is very helpful, particularly when the clinical differential diagnosis includes Kaposi's sarcoma. Histologic appearance of BA lesions typically shows dermal vascular proliferation, with plump endothelial cells lining the vessels, as well as neutrophils aggregated around eosinophilic material.[27] With Warthin-Starry staining, innumerable black bacilli become evident. In some instances, cultures confirm the diagnosis. Treatment with erythromycin, 500 mg po qid, results in gradual improvement. Duration of therapy is not clear, though most recommend a minimum of 8 weeks of therapy for cutaneous lesions in HIV-infected patients.[28]

Systemic mycoses in HIV

Although the lesion morphology may vary, the cutaneous lesions of disseminated cryptococcus, histoplasmosis, and coccidioidomycosis generally appear as widely scattered papules or nodules. Indeed, these lesions often resemble molluscum contagiosum. Patients infected with HIV who have disseminated fungal infections almost always have a CD4 count less than 200 cells/μl (usually less than 100 cells/μl). Because primary cutaneous infections rarely occur with these deep mycoses, the disseminated cutaneous lesions presumably arise from a noncutaneous focus, such as the lungs. Other systemic mycoses that can rarely involve the skin in HIV-infected individuals include blastomycosis, disseminated sporotrichosis, aspergillosis, pneumocystosis, and penicilliosis (due to *Penicillium marneffei*).

Cryptococcus neoformans is found worldwide and is a major cause of morbidity and mortality among acquired immunodeficiency syndrome (AIDS) patients, primarily through CNS infection. Dissemination to the skin occurs in approximately 10 percent of immunocompromised patients and can be the presenting sign of cryptococcosis (Fig. 63-7).[29] The lesions usually appear as flesh-colored papules and nodules, often with central umbilication resembling molluscum contagiosum. The lesions are most often located on the face and neck, though they can be found anywhere on the body. Less frequently, the lesions can present as ulcers of the skin or mucous membranes, cellulitic plaques, palpable purpura, or Kaposi's sarcoma–like nodules.[29] The diagnosis of a disseminated fungal infection is confirmed by performing a biopsy and sending the specimen for histology and culture. In tissue, the yeast cells are found in the dermis, often within a gelatinous capsule. Special stains such as silver stain or mucicarmine will highlight the yeast cells or capsule, respectively. Initial therapy for HIV-infected patients with disseminated infection usually consists of amphotericin B with or without flucytosine. These patients generally require lifelong maintenance therapy with fluconazole.[30]

Histoplasmosis is acquired in endemic areas by inhaling *Histoplasma capsulatum* microconidia or hyphae.[31] Disseminated infection can occur with primary exposure or by reactivating an old infection; the latter explains how cases occur outside of endemic areas. Skin lesions, with no site predilection, develop in approximately 10 percent of HIV-infected patients with disseminated histoplasmosis. An array of lesions have been reported, including diffuse erythematous macules and papules, keratotic or ulcerated papules and nodules, and pustules. Ulcers of the oral and, rarely, rectal mucosa have been described. Biopsy with special stains offers a rapid, though relatively insensitive, method of diagnosis. Culture of the skin with other diagnostic methods (antigen detection, serology, and cultures of other tissues) will usually confirm

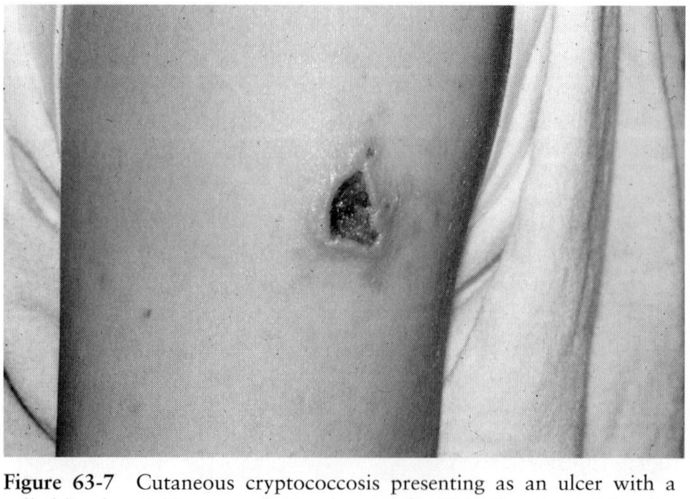

Figure 63-7 Cutaneous cryptococcosis presenting as an ulcer with a rolled border. A biopsy at the border sent for H & E and special stains for organisms and a second biopsy for culture is indicated here.

the diagnosis. Initial therapy consists of amphotericin B or itraconazole, followed by maintenance therapy with either itraconazole or weekly amphotericin B.[32]

Coccidioides immitis is endemic to the southwestern United States, northern Mexico, and Central America.[31] Infection occurs after inhaling arthroconidia, with subsequent hematogenous dissemination of endospores. Skin lesions occur in approximately 5 percent of patients with disseminated infection. The primary lesion usually begins as a papule that evolves to a nodule, plaque, pustule, or ulcer. The lesions have a predilection for the face and can resemble molluscum contagiosum.[18] The oral cavity is spared. Biopsy for histology and culture is indicated when considering the diagnosis. Histologic examination shows large (30–60 μm) spherules filled with endospores. Cultures, DNA probes, and serologic testing also help confirm the diagnosis. Most authors recommend initial therapy with amphotericin B, followed by lifelong maintenance therapy with either fluconazole or itraconazole.[33]

Cutaneous involvement in disseminated blastomycosis in HIV-infected individuals occurs less frequently than in immunocompetent patients.[31] Patients with disseminated blastomycosis typically present with papular and crusted lesions on the face or other regions of the body. Disseminated sporotrichosis can present as cutaneous papules and nodules, a papulosquamous eruption, ulcers, or subcutaneous nodules; the lesions appear in a generalized distribution, sparing the palms, soles, and mucosae.[18] Cutaneous aspergillosis in HIV-infected patients has occurred as part of an invasive infection and locally under adhesive tape. The former is associated with neutropenia, high-dose corticosteroids, or malignancy. The latter has occurred at intravenous catheter sites and produces papular lesions resembling molluscum contagiosum. Several case reports have described cutaneous pneumocystosis, including reports of widespread violaceous papules and nodules.[34] Moreover, direct extension of the organism from the eustachian tubes can produce polypoid papules of the external auditory canal. *Penicillium marneffei* has emerged as an important fungal pathogen in HIV-infected individuals in Southeast Asia.[19] The bamboo rat is the reservoir for this dimorphic fungus. Patients generally present with fever, cough, and a generalized skin eruption characterized by papules that have central necrosis or umbilication. These skin lesions have a predilection for the face, ears, upper trunk, and arms. Several reports have also described patients with genital and oral ulcers.

Papular eruption of HIV

There is controversy about the existence of the papular eruption of HIV as a distinct entity. As originally described, this condition consists of variably pruritic, waxing and waning skin-colored papules distributed over the head, neck, and upper trunk.[35] Most authors have grouped the papular eruption of HIV with various pruritic papular eruptions in HIV-infected patients and refer to them collectively as "itchy bump disease." Some authors have postulated that the pruritic papular eruption of HIV represents an exaggerated response to insect bites[36] or is a type of folliculitis,[37] despite the histologic lack of follicular involvement. Eosinophilic folliculitis is similar in its distribution and typical poor response to treatment with topical steroids, antihistamines, and most systemic antimicrobials. Ultraviolet light (UVB or psoralen with UVA) has been used with some success for the papular eruption of HIV as well as for eosinophilic folliculitis.

LESIONS WITH VESICLES, EROSIONS, OR CRUSTS

Impetigo/ecthyma

Impetigo can manifest in one of two forms: impetigo contagiosa or impetigo bullosa. Impetigo contagiosa is caused by *Staphylococcus aureus* or *Streptococcus pyogenes* (group A streptococci), though mixed infection with both of these organisms frequently occurs. Impetigo most often involves children, and the infection readily spreads via skin-to-skin contact. The primary lesion appears as a thin-roofed vesicle with an erythematous halo. Typically the lesion ruptures, leaving an erosion covered with a characteristic honey-colored crust. The lesions are painless but often pruritic. In most instances, they involve the exposed skin of the face and extremities, but they may also complicate other skin diseases (secondary impetigo). Patients with localized impetigo generally respond well to topical mupirocin ointment. For patients with more extensive disease, most authorities recommend treatment with an antistaphylococcal penicillin or first-generation cephalosporin. Poststreptococcal glomerulonephritis is a rare but serious complication of streptococcal impetigo.

Impetigo bullosa (bullous impetigo) is caused by infection with specific phage types of *S. aureus*. This infection is common in infancy, but it also occurs among adults with poor hygiene, especially in hot, humid conditions. Lesions appear as flaccid, thin-roofed vesicles and bullae, without an erythematous rim; they become cloudy and pustular over 1 to 2 days and rupture, leaving a dry, shiny, erythematous, "varnishlike" base. Lesions typically occur in the intertriginous areas of the axillae and groin and are pruritic. Oral antistaphylococcal antimicrobials are preferred for this form of impetigo.

Ecthyma represents a deeper version of impetigo, with eventual formation of a superficial ulcer (Fig. 63-8). Group A streptococcus is most often the causative agent. The lesions are typically located on the lower extremities. Even with an appropriate extended course of antimicrobial therapy, the lesions heal slowly. Autoinoculation is common, and poststreptococcal glomerulonephritis develops with a frequency similar to that following impetigo contagiosa.

Disseminated vesicular viral infections

Disseminated HSV infection rarely occurs among HIV-infected patients, even those with advanced immunosuppression. Disseminated varicella-zoster virus infection, however, is relatively more common in this patient population and may occur concurrently with or following dermatomal zoster. The disseminated lesions resemble localized (dermatomal) disease—vesicles or pustules on an erythematous base (Fig. 63-9). Clinical appearance and a positive Tzanck preparation (for detection of multinucleated epithelial cells) help to make a presumptive diagnosis (see Color

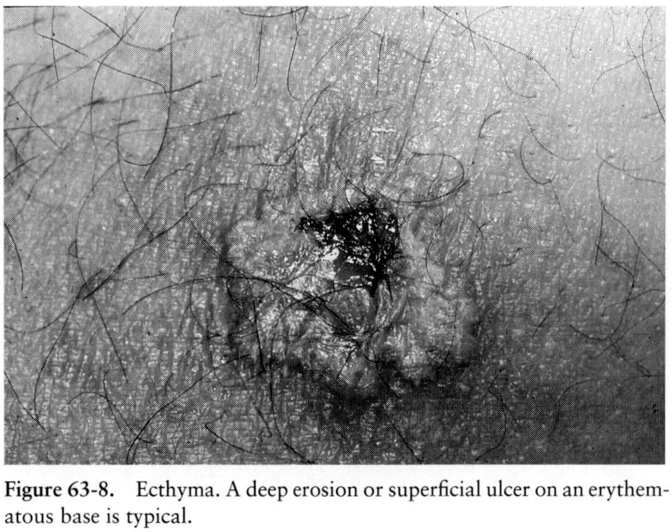

Figure 63-8. Ecthyma. A deep erosion or superficial ulcer on an erythematous base is typical.

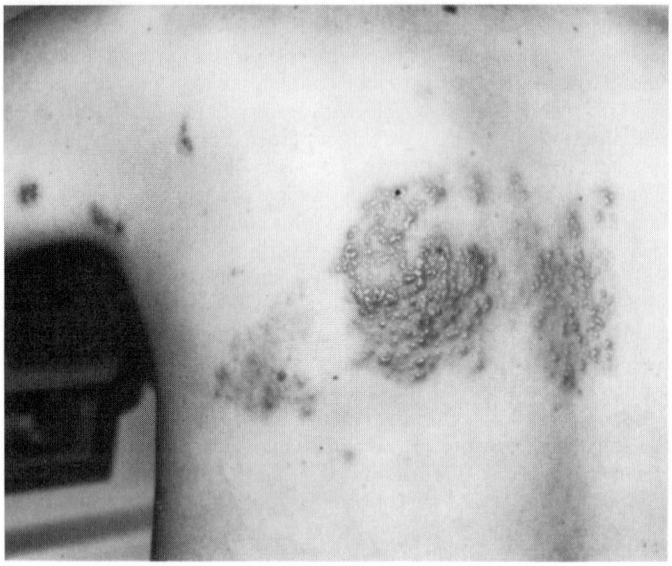

Figure 63-9. Dermatomal varicella-zoster virus infection.

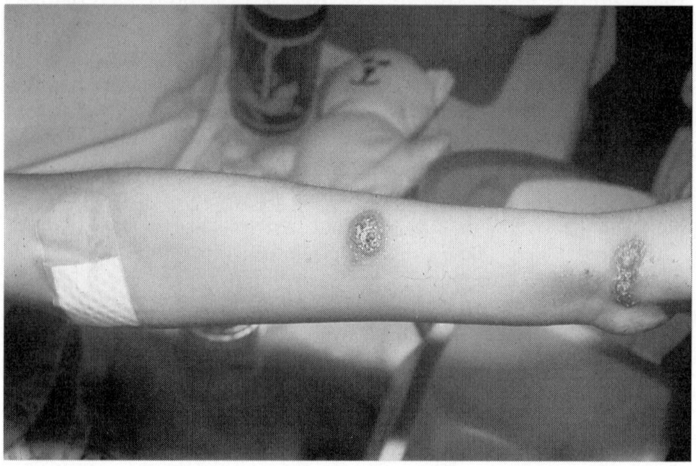

Figure 63-10. Chronic varicella-zoster infection in a child with AIDS. The lesions are difficult to distinguish from ecthyma.

Plate 29). A definitive diagnosis is best made using direct immunofluorescence and viral culture. If a patient presents with typical vesicles in a generalized distribution, the practitioner should presumptively treat for varicella-zoster virus until receiving results of direct immunofluorescence and viral culture tests.

Patients with advanced HIV disease may present with atypical ecthymatous or ulcerative varicella-zoster virus lesions (Fig. 63-10).[38] These lesions often have a chronic course, even if the patient receives appropriate therapy for varicella-zoster virus infection. Acyclovir and famciclovir are generally considered the drugs of choice for varicella-zoster virus infections in HIV-infected hosts.

Porphyria cutanea tarda

In recent years, investigators have increasingly recognized an association between porphyria cutanea tarda and viral infections, namely hepatitis C virus[39] and HIV.[40] The association with HIV, however, may simply result from co-risk factors for acquiring hepatitis C virus.[41] Porphyria cutanea tarda results from decreased activity of the hepatic enzyme uroporphyrinogen decarboxylase, either from acquired hepatic disease or from an inherited enzyme deficiency. This decreased enzyme activity leads to accumulation of intermediate substrates generated by heme synthesis, causing cutaneous photosensitivity and mechanical fragility. Skin lesions occur in sun-exposed areas, or in areas incurring even trivial trauma, and include erosions, bullae, and hypo- and hyperpigmentation (Fig. 63-11). In addition, patients often develop facial hypertrichosis. Treatment consists of discontinuing all potential liver toxins, particularly ethanol, as well as having the patient undergo weekly phlebotomy to induce a mild iron deficiency anemia (a relative iron overload exacerbates the condition). Antimalarial medications are also used to treat porphyria cutanea tarda.

FOLLICULITIS AND THE DIFFERENTIAL DIAGNOSIS OF PUSTULES

Folliculitis

Folliculitis refers to inflammation of the hair follicle and encompasses a number of disorders seen in STD patients and in HIV-infected individuals. A hair follicle–based pustule is the primary lesion that typifies this group of conditions. Folliculitis, however, can present as papules, sometimes with erosions and crusts. It can be difficult at times to determine whether a lesion is follicular.

Causes of folliculitis include infectious agents (*S. aureus*, gram-negative bacteria, pityrosporum, and demodex mites), chemical

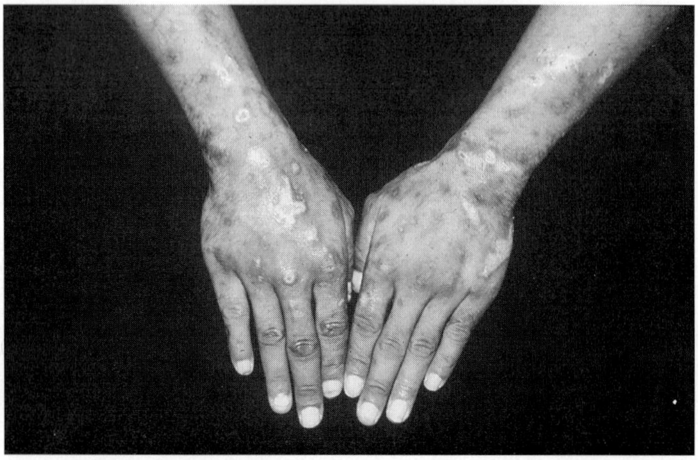

Figure 63-11. Porphyria cutanea tarda in a male with HIV and hepatitis C virus infection. Note erosions and hypo- and hyperpigmentation over the dorsal aspects of his hands and forearms.

irritation (chloracne), or physical injury. Examples of physical injury include occlusion of the skin, friction (e.g., "razor burn"), and pseudofolliculitis; the latter is a problem particularly in Blacks, in whom regrowth of tightly curled hair penetrates the nearby skin causing foreign-body inflammation. Other types of folliculitis that are of multifactorial or unclear cause include acne vulgaris, steroid acne, and eosinophilic folliculitis.

Staphylococcus aureus, a common cause of folliculitis, typically presents in areas of high hair density such as the scalp, buttocks, groin, thighs, forearms, or beard. The lesions often arise as painful pustules enclosing a central hair. The pustule is surrounded by erythema and induration that extends beyond the pustule. In patients who develop a cluster of folliculitis lesions, the involved area may become confluently indurated and very tender; in some instances, abscesses may form and require drainage. A Gram stain often reveals gram-positive cocci, either singly or in small clusters. If the patient has recently been hospitalized or recently taken antimicrobials, a culture with sensitivities would be indicated. Oral antistaphylococcal antimicrobials will usually clear the condition. Bathing with soap and water and replacing the blade of the razor used for shaving also helps to limit spread and decrease recurrences. In patients with recurrent staphylococcal folliculitis, eliminating nasal colonization with intranares application of 2% mupirocin ointment (bid × 5 days each month) may play an important role.[42]

In 1986, Soeprono first described HIV-associated eosinophilic folliculitis,[43] a disorder that resembles Ofuji's eosinophilic pustular folliculitis.[44] When this HIV-related condition occurs, it virtually always involves those with advanced stages of HIV disease (CD4 count less than 200 cells/μl). This disorder manifests as a chronic pruritic, papular, and pustular condition, with lesions typically distributed over the face and upper trunk. Patients may have peripheral eosinophilia. Cultures from the lesions are negative, and this type of folliculitis responds poorly to antibacterials. Biopsy shows follicular inflammation with a predominance of eosinophils. Although difficult to treat, this condition sometimes responds to a combination of ultraviolet-B light therapy, high-potency topical steroids, and nonsedating antihistamines such as cetirizine (5–10 mg po qd). One study showed relatively favorable results with oral itraconazole (200–300 mg po qd).[45] After 1 month of itraconazole therapy, 17 of 28 patients had complete responses, and 4 patients had a partial response; at 6 months follow-up, 31 percent of patients had inactive disease, 13 percent required only topical steroids for control, and 56 percent remained on itraconazole with benefit (complete or partial control). A recent report described the successful use of oral metronidazole (250 mg po tid × 3 weeks)[46]; this report involved two patients who had lesions that contained gram-negative organisms that resembled *Leptotrichia buccalis*, a normal oral anaerobe. Aerobic and anaerobic cultures were negative, however.

Nonfollicular pustules

The differential diagnosis of pustules also includes nonfollicular lesions, such as pustular secondary syphilis and pustular psoriasis. If one observes generalized pustules on areas such as the palms, soles, or lips, one may safely assume a nonfollicular process. The pustular eruption of secondary syphilis is typically located on the face and trunk (see Color Plate 42). The lesions begin as erythematous papules that subsequently develop a central pustule and finally erode with an overlying crust. Darkfield microscopy of a sample taken from a lesion shows treponemes; serologic tests generally confirm the diagnosis. Pustular psoriasis is an unusual form of psoriasis that mainly involves the palms and soles and may strongly resemble keratoderma blennorrhagicum (of Reiter's syndrome). Pustular psoriasis also includes a generalized form (von Zumbusch), which may follow tapering or cessation of corticosteroids used to treat severe plaque-type psoriasis.

Disseminated gonococcal infection initially appears as petechiae or palpable purpura, evolving to hemorrhagic pustules on an erythematous base (see Color Plates 70–72). The lesions are often tender, and typically they are few in number (less than 15) and acrally located, especially around the small joints. Cultures of material from the skin lesions of disseminated gonococcal infection are usually negative.

The natural evolution of many vesicular dermatoses includes a pustular stage. Thus, if one encounters a mixture of vesicular and pustular lesions, first consider the vesiculobullous infectious diseases, such as varicella, disseminated HSV, and disseminated varicella-zoster virus.

PAPULOSQUAMOUS CONDITIONS

Seborrheic dermatitis

Seborrheic dermatitis is an erythematous and scaly dermatosis that often involves the scalp (especially at the hairline), eyebrows, eyelash margins, nasal folds, beard area, and upper trunk. The scale often appears greasy, particularly on the scalp and face. Patients frequently complain of pruritus. This condition is common, with 10 to 15 percent of the normal, healthy population afflicted.[47] Seborrheic dermatitis afflicts up to 80 percent of HIV-infected individuals, depending on whether examination or history is used to determine incidence. In one study, 53 percent of HIV-infected patients examined in a military-based study had seborrheic dermatitis.[48] Although most persons tend to have a chronic course with seborrheic dermatitis, HIV-infected individuals generally have a more severe condition, especially those with advanced stages of HIV disease.[49] The pertinent differential diagnosis includes psoriasis and dermatophytosis, the latter readily diagnosed by a positive potassium hydroxide preparation. When seborrheic dermatitis involves the axillae and groin, some authors prefer the term "sebopsoriasis" (Fig. 63-12).

The exact cause of seborrheic dermatitis remains unknown, but both enhanced sensitivity to resident yeast on skin (*Malassezia furfur*) and overgrowth of this yeast within lesional skin appear to play an important role. For this reason, therapy usually consists of either a topical steroid (hydrocortisone 1 or 2.5% cream or lotion) and/or an antifungal preparation. Many HIV-infected patients respond better to topical antifungal regimens, such as

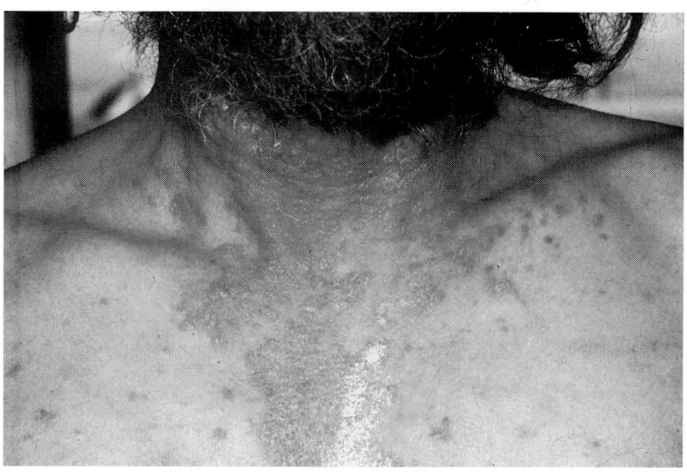

Figure 63-12. Sebopsoriasis. Erythematous papules and plaques with a greasy-appearing scale resembling seborrheic dermatitis.

2% ketoconazole cream. Those HIV-infected patients with severe seborrheic dermatitis, especially those with advanced immunosuppression, may require therapy with oral ketoconazole, 200 mg per day. Limited published experience exists with itraconazole and fluconazole for seborrheic dermatitis.

Psoriasis

Psoriasis is the prototype of papulosquamous diseases and affects 1 to 2 percent of the general population. The common plaque variety, psoriasis vulgaris, develops as salmon-colored plaques that have a silvery scale, typically located on the extensor surface of the elbows and knees, as well as on the trunk. Patients often have scalp and nail involvement, but only rarely do psoriasis lesions form on the face. Patients typically have minimal or no pruritus. One should always consider psoriasis in the differential diagnosis of a patient with scaly papules or plaques on the genitals. Lesions may appear in sites of skin trauma, such as linear plaques at sites of picking or scratching—the so-called Koebner phenomenon. Other forms of psoriasis exist, including guttate (droplike) psoriasis (see Color Plate 55). This form of psoriasis most often presents in young persons and may resemble papulosquamous secondary syphilis. An asymptomatic infection with *Streptococcus pyogenes* (group A streptococci) often precipitates guttate psoriasis.

Although one study found a psoriasis prevalence of 5 percent among HIV-infected individuals,[50] most studies have not shown HIV-infected individuals to have an increased prevalence of psoriasis when compared with the general population. Individuals infected with HIV do have an increased prevalence of arthritis associated with psoriasis, however, correlating with the presence of HLA B27 and C7 antigens. Some authors have placed HIV-associated psoriasis and Reiter's syndrome along the same spectrum of disease.[51]

The management of psoriasis is beyond the scope of this chapter, but therapy for HIV-related psoriasis has several unique aspects that warrant discussion. First, HIV-related psoriasis tends to respond to antiretroviral therapy. Although this was initially documented with zidovudine (AZT),[52] other antiretrovirals may produce similar responses. Second, despite initial reports of enhanced HIV replication and immune suppression caused by UV light treatment, subsequent studies have not found the use of UVB or PUVA (psoralen with UVA) to accelerate HIV disease progression. Third, many systemic agents for psoriasis, such as methotrexate, azathioprine, and cyclosporine A, cause nonspecific or specific T-cell immunosuppression and should be avoided, until studies indicate otherwise. Last, the retinoids, particularly etretinate, appear to help with moderate to severe psoriasis and do not cause immunosuppression.

Reiter's syndrome

Reiter's syndrome is a parainfectious reaction associated with urogenital infections (*Chlamydia trachomatis*) and enteric infections (*Shigella*, *Yersinia*, *Campylobacter*, and *Salmonella*). Reiter's syndrome usually involves individuals with the HLA B27 genetic marker, most often young men. The clinical syndrome is characterized by urethritis, conjunctivitis, and a seronegative spondyloarthritis. The cutaneous lesions keratoderma blennorrhagicum and circinate balanitis develop in 15 and 36 percent of patients, respectively (see Plates 67 and 68).[53] Mucocutaneous lesions may precede or follow the onset of extracutaneous illness (see Plate 69). The primary lesion of keratoderma blennorrhagicum begins as a dull red papule that rapidly forms a hyperkeratotic yellow surface. Lesions coalesce into plaques and may have a circinate collarette of scale. In some instances, pustular lesions form. Although keratoderma blennorrhagicum most often involves the soles of the feet, lesions may appear in other areas, such as the dorsa of the feet, legs, hands, fingers, nails, and scalp. Severe keratoderma blennorrhagicum can become generalized, especially in HIV-infected individuals; in this form, it resembles pustular psoriasis. On the penis, moist, red erosions merge to form circinate balanitis in the uncircumcised male; in the circumcised male, the lesions form hard crusts and plaques. Circinate vulvitis has been described.[54] Approximately 15 percent of patients with circinate balanitis have transient oral lesions, typically painless small vesicles that rapidly form superficial erosions, or a patchy erythema. Reiter's syndrome often recurs without obvious relationship to new infections, although one should consider reinfection from untreated partners.

Dermatophytosis

Dermatophyte (tinea) infections typically manifest as a localized reaction on the feet, intertriginous areas, trunk, or nails. The lesions generally appear annular with a relatively accentuated edge and scale. Infrequently, patients with tinea corporis present with a generalized rash. The fungus most commonly responsible is *Trichophyton rubrum*. Scraping a lesion and preparing a potassium hydroxide sample usually makes the diagnosis readily (Fig. 63-13).

With localized dermatophyte infections, topical antifungals, such as 1% clotrimazole or 2% ketoconazole, are generally sufficient. When large surfaces are involved, systemic treatment, at least initially, may be warranted. The systemic azole antifungals (ketoconazole, fluconazole, and itraconazole) and griseofulvin all have shown good efficacy. Systemic terbinafine, chemically distinct from the azoles, is fungicidal and also effective.

Patients infected with HIV who have dermatophytosis may present with lesions that do not have the typical annular appearance; in addition, they tend to have recurrent and more extensive involvement. Also, HIV-infected patients more commonly acquire proximal subungual onychomycosis, a dermatophyte infection of the nails that is rare in individuals with intact immune systems.[55]

Papulosquamous secondary syphilis

Patients with secondary syphilis often present with copper-colored discoid papules and plaques with varying degrees of scale (see Plate 45, 46, and 56). The lesions can mimic other papulosquamous dermatoses, namely psoriasis (see Color Plate 56) and

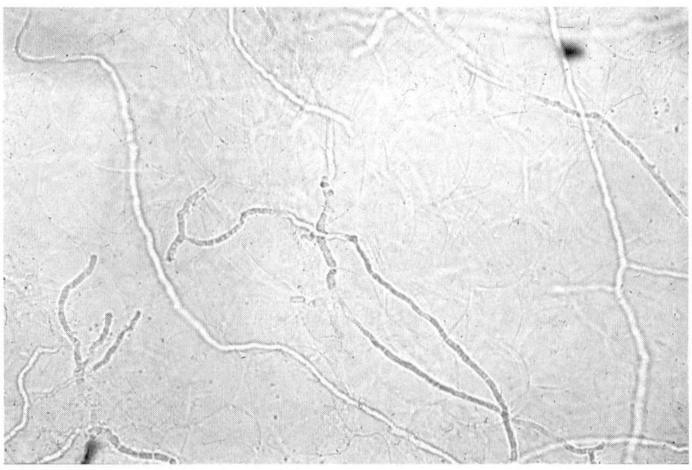

Figure 63-13. A potassium hydroxide preparation of scale from a patient with dermatophyte infection. Note abundant hyphae.

lichen planus. The color and generalized distribution (including the palms and soles) in a patient with generalized lymphadenopathy should cause one to suspect secondary syphilis.

Pityriasis rosea is a papulosquamous eruption morphologically similar to papulosquamous secondary syphilis but generally without lymphadenopathy or constitutional symptoms. Although the etiology is unknown, investigators suspect an infectious agent based on case-clustering and accounts of experimental transmission. Most cases occur in the winter months in persons 10 to 35 years of age. The first, and often the largest, lesion—referred to as the "herald patch"—usually appears on the thigh, upper arm, trunk, or neck. Initially, the lesion forms as an asymptomatic well-defined bright-red papule covered by a thin collarette of scale. After 5 to 15 days, crops of new lesions appear over a 7- to 10-day period. These lesions are oval, pale red with a dull, yellow-brown center; they are surrounded by a thin collarette of scale that points toward the center of the papule. The rash is distributed over the trunk, upper arms, thighs, neck, and, infrequently, the face. On the trunk, the long axes of the ovoid lesions follow the skin folds and give the typical "Christmas tree" appearance (see Color Plate 57). Infrequently, patients develop an inverse form of pityriasis rosea, with lesions found in intertriginous areas as opposed to convex surfaces. This variant may occur relatively more frequently in Blacks than Caucasians. Patients with pityriasis rosea do not have constitutional symptoms, except for a slight itch. Topical triamcinolone, 0.1% cream or ointment applied bid, will relieve the symptoms of itching. The lesions fade after 3 to 6 weeks, and usually no other therapy is required.

PURPURA

Vasculitis

Vasculitis is a general term used to describe the inflammatory reaction to endothelial deposition of antigen-antibody complexes. The local inflammation and hemorrhage produce the characteristic lesion of palpable purpura, a lesion that may progress to necrosis and ulceration. Lesions are commonly found in areas of venous hypertension, most often the lower legs (Fig. 63-14). In addition to cutaneous lesions, patients may have fever, arthralgias, gastrointestinal symptoms, and other constitutional manifestations. Vasculitis may develop as an acute disease, with hemorrhagic, necrotic lesions that appear in crops and persist for 2 to 3 weeks; or as a more indolent disease in which purpura, maculoerythematous lesions, urticaria, and papules predominate and crops appear over months or years. Known associations with vasculitis include streptococcal and staphylococcal infection, hepatitis B and C virus, tuberculosis, persistent bacterial infection (such as dental abscess), certain drugs, malignancy, collagen vascular diseases, and pregnancy. It is important to exclude infectious causes before attempts are made to use corticosteroids.

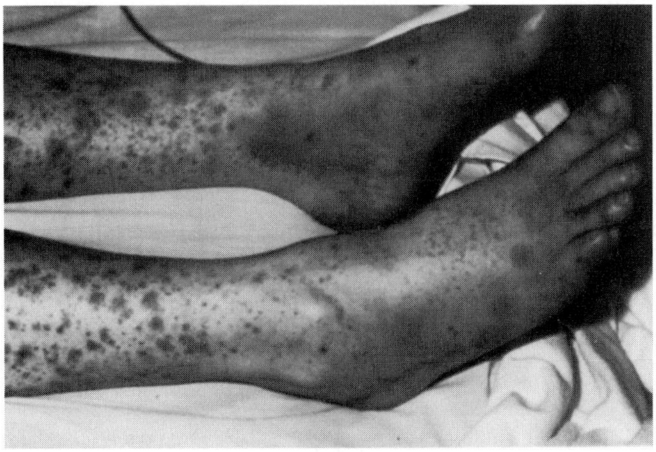

Figure 63-14. Purpuric papules and vesicles of vasculitis on the legs of a female intravenous drug user with the prodrome of hepatitis B.

In the prodromal stage of hepatitis B virus infection, patients can develop vasculitis and urticaria as well as macular and papular lesions. Hepatitis C virus (HCV) has been recognized as causing cryoglobulinemia-associated vasculitis.[56,57] This usually presents in the skin as palpable purpura, but livedo reticularis and urticaria have also been described. As opposed to the prodrome of hepatitis B, HCV-related vasculitis occurs during the course of active hepatitis. Rarely, patients with syphilis can develop cryoprecipitates that elicit a cutaneous vasculitis. Disseminated gonococcal infection, mentioned above in the section on nonfollicular pustules, often initially produces skin lesions that clinically and histologically suggest vasculitis, though this is not considered a true vasculitis.

PIGMENTARY CHANGES

Hyperpigmentation associated with HIV Infection

Treatment with zidovudine (AZT) can cause nail and, less commonly, cutaneous hyperpigmentation, especially among Blacks (Color Plate 119). Clofazimine, which has sometimes been used to treat disseminated *Mycobacterium avium*-complex infection in AIDS patients, can produce generalized orange or red-brown hyperpigmentation. Generalized hyperpigmentation, apparently independent of zidovudine or clofazimine therapy, has also been reported in AIDS patients.[58]

CONCLUSION

This chapter has attempted to introduce the health-care provider for patients with STDs or HIV to an approach to a patient presenting with a generalized cutaneous condition. Visual inspection of the skin, even before receiving any medical history, is often the most important diagnostic tool. Identifying the primary lesions, any secondary features, and the distribution of the rash are the keys to generating a differential diagnosis. This cannot be carried out without a thorough skin exam, which requires good lighting and adequate exposure of the skin.

The array of conditions that can present in patients with STDs or infected with HIV is vast and is certainly not restricted to those conditions listed in Table 63-3. It is critical to discern whether an infectious agent is the cause for the rash, since treatment is often specific and delay in treatment may result in significant morbidity. This is especially true in HIV-infected patients.

An interesting aspect of generalized dermatoses in STD-afflicted and HIV-infected patients is the significant proportion of noninfectious inflammatory cutaneous conditions. These include parainfectious phenomena such as HSV-related erythema multiforme, Reiter's syndrome, guttate psoriasis associated with streptococcal disease, and vasculitis associated with hepatitis B or C. In HIV-infected patients, the high frequency of inflammatory conditions such as drug hypersensitivity, seborrheic dermatitis, and eosinophilic folliculitis defies clear explanation and seems paradoxical within the simple paradigm of immunosuppression related to HIV infection. Perhaps immunodysregulation is a better term to explain the simultaneous risks of opportunistic infection and inflammatory skin conditions. Further investigation into these parainfectious phenomena and the "hyperimmune" conditions of

HIV-related skin disease will be needed to elucidate their pathogenesis.

References

1 Coopman SA et al: Cutaneous disease and drug reactions in HIV infection. *N Engl J Med* 328:1670, 1993.
2 Cockerall CJ: Cutaneous clues to HIV infection: Diagnosis and treatment. *Semin Dermatol* 13:275, 1994.
3 Hoover WD, Lang PG: Pruritus in HIV infection. *J Am Acad Dermatol* 6:1020, 1991.
4 Hulsebosch HJ et al: Human immunodeficiency virus exanthem. *J Am Acad Dermatol* 23:483, 1990.
5 Alessi E, Cusini M: The exanthem of HIV-1 seroconversion. *Int J Dermatol* 34:238, 1995.
6 Cooper DA et al: Acute AIDS retrovirus infection: Definition of a clinical illness associated with seroconversion. *Lancet* 1:537, 1985.
7 Sadick N et al: Unusual features of scabies complicating human T-lymphotropic type III infection. *J Am Acad Dermatol* 15:482, 1986.
8 Meinking TL et al: The treatment of scabies with ivermectin. *N Engl J Med* 333:26, 1995.
9 Brown ST: Adverse reactions in syphilis therapy. *J Am Ven Dis Assoc* 3:172, 1976.
10 Wolkenstein P et al: Metabolic predisposition to cutaneous adverse drug reactions. *Arch Dermatol* 131:544, 1995.
11 Gordin FM et al: Adverse reactions to trimethoprim/sulfamethoxazole in patients with the acquired immunodeficiency syndrome. *Ann Intern Med* 100:495, 1984.
12 Assier H et al: Erythema multiforme with mucous membrane involvement and Stevens-Johnson syndrome are clinically different disorders with distinct causes. *Arch Dermatol* 131:539, 1995.
13 Cote B et al: Clinicopathologic correlation in erythema multiforme and Stevens-Johnson syndrome. *Arch Dermatol* 131:1268, 1995.
14 Bastuji-Garin S et al: Clinical classification of cases of toxic epidermal necrolysis, Stevens-Johnson syndrome, and erythema multiforme. *Arch Dermatol* 129:92, 1993.
15 Saiag P et al: Drug-induced toxic epidermal necrolysis (Lyell syndrome) in patients with the human immunodeficiency virus. *J Am Acad Dermatol* 29:567, 1992.
16 Rico MJ, Penneys NS: Cutaneous cryptococcus resembling molluscum contagiosum. *Arch Dermatol* 121:901, 1985.
17 Jimenez-Acosta F et al: Cutaneous cryptococcus mimicking molluscum contagiosum in a haemophiliac with AIDS. *Clin Exp Dermatol* 12: 446, 1987.
18 Johnson RA, Dover JS: Cutaneous Manifestations of Human Immunodeficiency Virus Disease, in *Dermatology in General Medicine,* 4th edition, TB Fitzpatrick et al (eds). New York, McGraw-Hill, 1993, pp. 2637–89.
19 Hilsmarsdottir I et al: Disseminated *Penicillium marneffei* infection associated with human immunodeficiency virus and review of 35 published cases. *J Acquir Immune Defic Syndr* 6:466, 1993.
19a Resolution of intractable molluscum contagiosum in a human immunodeficiency virus-infected patient after institution of antiretroviral therapy with ritonavir. *Clin Inf Dis* 24:1023, 1997.
20 Stoler MH et al: An atypical subcutaneous infection associated with acquired immunodeficiency syndrome. *Am J Clin Pathol* 80:714, 1983.
21 Relman DA et al: The agent of bacillary angiomatosis: An approach to the identification of uncultured pathogens. *N Engl J Med* 323:1573, 1990.
22 Welch DF et al: *Rochalimaea henselae sp. nov.,* a cause of septicemia, bacillary angiomatosis, and parenchymal bacilary peliosis. *J Clin Microbiol* 30:275, 1992.
23 Zangwell KM et al: Cat scratch disease in Connecticut: Epidemiology, risk factors, and evaluation of a new diagnostic test. *N Engl J Med* 329:8, 1993.
24 Tappero JW et al: The epidemiology of bacillary angiomatosis and bacillary peliosis. *JAMA* 269:770, 1993.
25 Tappero JW et al: Bacillary angiomatosis and bacillary splenitis in immunocompetent adults. *Ann Intern Med* 118:363, 1993.
26 Black JR et al: Life-threatening cat-scratch disease in an immunocompromised host. *Arch Intern Med* 146:394, 1986.
27 LeBoit PE et al: Bacillary angiomatosis: The histopathology and differential diagnosis of a pseudoneoplastic infection in patients with human immunodeficiency virus disease. *Am J Surg Pathol* 13:909, 1989.
28 Adal KA et al: Cat scratch disease, bacillary angiomatosis, and other infections due to *Rochalimaea. N Engl J Med* 330:1509, 1994.
29 Durden FM, Elewski B: Cutaneous involvement with *Cryptococcus neoformans* in AIDS. *J Am Acad Dermatol* 30:844, 1994.
30 Paauw DS et al: Cryptococcosis, in *The HIV Manual,* DH Spach, TM Hooton (eds). New York, Oxford University Press, 1996, pp. 215–20.
31 Wheat J: Endemic mycoses in AIDS: A clinical review. *Clin Microbiol Rev* 8:146, 1995.
32 Panther LA, Skerrett SJ: Histoplasmosis, in *The HIV Manual,* DH Spach, TM Hooton (eds). New York, Oxford University Press, 1996, pp. 221–25.
33 Panther LA, Rosen H: Coccidioidomycosis, in *The HIV Manual,* DH Spach, TM Hooton (eds). New York, Oxford University Press, 1996, pp. 209–14.
34 Raviglione MC: Extrapulmonary pneumocystosis: The first 50 cases. *Rev Infect Dis* 12:1127, 1985.
35 James WD et al: A papular eruption associated with human T cell lymphotropic virus III disease. *J Am Acad Dermatol* 13:563, 1985.
36 Cockerall CJ: Cutaneous manifestations of HIV infection other than Kaposi's sarcoma: Clinical and histologic aspects. *J Am Acad Dermatol* 22:1260, 1990.
37 Berger TG: Dermatologic Manifestations of HIV Infection, in *The AIDS Knowledge Base,* PT Cohen, MA Sande, PA Volberding (eds). Boston, Little, Brown and Company, 1994, pp. 5.5:21–22.
38 Gilson IH et al: Disseminated ecthymatous herpes varicella-zoster virus infection in patients with acquired immunodeficiency syndrome. *J Am Acad Dermatol* 20:637, 1989.
39 Fargion S et al: Hepatitis C virus and porphyria cutanea tarda: Evidence of a strong association. *Hepatology* 16:1322, 1992.
40 Blauvelt A et al: Porphyria cutanea tarda and human immunodeficiency virus infection. *Int J Dermatol* 31:474, 1992.
41 McAlister F et al: Human immunodeficiency virus infection and porphyria cutanea tarda: Coexistence of risk factors or causative association? *Clin Infect Dis* 20:348, 1995.
42 Raz R et al: A 1-year trial of nasal mupirocin in the prevention of recurrent staphylococcal nasal colonization and skin infection. *Arch Intern Med* 156:1109, 1996.
43 Soeprono FF, Schinella RA: Eosinophilic pustular folliculitis in patients with the acquired immunodeficiency syndrome. *J Am Acad Dermatol* 14:1020, 1986.
44 Ofuji S et al: Eosinophilic pustular folliculitis. *Acta Derm Venereol (Stockh)* 50:195, 1970.
45 Berger TG et al: Itraconazole therapy for human immunodeficiency virus-associated eosinophilic folliculitis. *Arch Dermatol* 131:358, 1995.
46 Smith KJ et al: Metronidazole for eosinophilic pustular folliculitis in human immunodeficiency virus type 1-positive patients. *Arch Dermatol* 131:1089, 1995.
47 Johnson MLT, Roberts J: Prevalence of Dermatological Diseases Among Persons 1–74 Years of Age: United States. PHS Publication 79–1660. Washington, US Department of Health and Human Services, 1977.
48 Smith KJ et al: Cutaneous findings in HIV-1-positive patients: A 42-month prospective study. *J Am Acad Dermatol* 31:746, 1994.
49 Mathes BM et al: Seborrheic dermatitis in patients with acquired immunodeficiency syndrome. *J Am Acad Dermatol* 13:947, 1985.
50 Coldiron BM, Bergstresser PR: Prevalence and clinical spectrum of skin disease in patients infected with human immunodeficiency virus. *Arch Dermatol* 125:357, 1989.
51 Reveille JD et al: Human immunodeficiency virus (HIV)-associated, psoriatic arthritis, and Reiter's syndrome: A disease continuum. *Arthritis Rheum* 33:1574, 1990.

52 Duvic M et al: Remission of AIDS-associated psoriasis with zidovudine. *Lancet* 2:627, 1987.
53 Callen JP: The spectrum of Reiter's disease. *J Am Acad Dermatol* 1:75, 1979.
54 Thumbar IV et al: Circinate vulvitis in Reiter's syndrome. *Br J Vener Dis* 53:260, 1977.
55 Daniel CR et al: The spectrum of nail disease in patients with human immunodeficiency virus infection. *J Am Acad Dermatol* 27:93, 1992.
56 Ferri C et al: Association between hepatitis C virus and mixed cryoglobulinemia. *Clin Exp Rheumatol* 9:621, 1991.
57 Karlsberg PL et al: Cutaneous vasculitis and rheumatoid factor positivity as presenting signs of hepatitis C virus–induced mixed cryoglobulinemia. *Arch Dermatol* 131:1119, 1995.
58 Peter SA et al: Diffuse hyperpigmentation associated with acquired immunodeficiency syndrome. *J Nat Med Assoc* 84:977, 1992.

Chapter 64

Genital ulcer adenopathy syndrome

Ronald C. Ballard

Genital ulcer adenopathy syndrome is a frequent presentation of sexually transmitted diseases (STDs), especially in developing countries. The syndrome can be defined as a breach of the epithelium of the genital skin or mucous membranes, usually by sexually acquired organisms, resulting in the formation of open lesions. Under some circumstances the regional lymph nodes may become enlarged, and a combination of ulceration and inguinal and/or femoral lymphadenopathy is commonly encountered. In cases of lymphogranuloma venereum (LGV) the reason for consultation may be the lymphadenopathy alone, owing to the transient nature of the initial lesion. There are a number of different causes of genital ulcer disease, and since the clinical presentation of each may be variable and the treatment for each different, genital ulcer adenopathy syndrome creates considerable diagnostic and management problems for clinicians. The importance of genital ulcer disease and the need to provide prompt, effective treatment has increased considerably as a result of the finding that these lesions are a major cofactor in the transmission of the human immunodeficiency virus (HIV).

EPIDEMIOLOGY

Epidemiological data on the genital ulcer adenopathy syndrome are incomplete, because diagnostic tests for all causes of the syndrome are usually not available at services where treatment is provided. Even when comprehensive services are available, notably during research projects, it is often not possible to determine the etiology of the disease in a significant proportion of cases, owing to lack of sensitivity of the appropriate laboratory tests (Table 64-1).[1–7] Of all causes of the syndrome, the recording of cases is probably the most complete for syphilis, owing to widespread use of serological screening tests and the recognition of the potential consequences of the disease if it is left untreated. However, overreporting of syphilis may frequently occur in some settings, since many patients presenting with proven nonsyphilitic lesions may have positive serological tests for the disease.[8]

The National Health Service Genitourinary Medicine Clinics in England and Wales saw 27,439 cases of genital ulceration during 1995. Of these, 27,065 (98.6 percent) were cases of genital herpes, 283 (1.0 percent) were classified as infectious syphilis, and the remaining 91 cases were chancroid, LGV, or donovanosis (Public Health Laboratory Service Communicable Disease Surveillance Centre, London—personal communication). Unfortunately, genital herpes is not a reportable disease in the United States, and therefore comparable figures are not available. However, 16,500 cases of primary and secondary syphilis, 603 cases of chancroid, 186 cases of LGV, and no cases of donovanosis were reported to the Centers for Disease Control and Prevention (CDC) during the same year. This represents approximately one-fiftieth of the combined number of reported cases of gonococcal and chlamydial infection seen in the United States during the same period.

In contrast, genital ulcerations are seen relatively more frequently at STD clinics and primary health care facilities in developing countries. In sub-Saharan Africa and in Asia, genital ulcer disease may account for between 20 and 70 percent of STD clinic visits, whereas the comparable figure for Europe and North America is at most 5 percent.[9] In addition, the etiology of genital ulceration shows considerable geographical variability, with genital herpes the most frequent cause in North America and Europe, donovanosis the most frequent in Papua New Guinea, and chancroid the most frequent in sub-Saharan Africa and Southeast Asia (see Table 64-1). Chancroid has been recorded infrequently in the United States, where it has been associated with outbreaks of genital ulceration among minority populations, particularly in some eastern cities and in the South.[10,11] In 1994, five states (Florida, Georgia, Louisiana, New York, and Texas) accounted for more than 80 percent of all reported cases, and the disease appears to have become endemic in some communities.

Lymphogranuloma venereum and donovanosis appear to be restricted to geographical foci in tropical countries. LGV has been documented in sub-Saharan Africa, South America and the Caribbean, the Indian subcontinent, and Southeast Asia, while donovanosis has largely been restricted to India, Papua New Guinea and Northern Australia, southern Africa, and Brazil. These diseases are occasionally diagnosed in North America and Europe, largely as a result of importation from endemic areas, but LGV has been documented as a cause of severe proctocolitis and anorectal ulceration among gay men in the United States.[12] Overall, the proportion of STD patients with genital ulcerations and the causes of those ulcerations are probably dependent upon a number of factors, including geographical location, socioeconomic status, availability of diagnostic tests, sexual preference and practices, the relative importance of commercial sex in the spread of disease, the frequency of circumcision, and most recently, the prevalence of concomitant HIV infection.

Risk factors for genital ulceration inevitably vary according to etiology and population. The risk of acquisition of chancroid appears to be related to low socioeconomic status, geographic origin, commercial sex, and lack of circumcision.[13] In contrast, gay men account for the majority of cases of primary syphilis in some countries, while the disease has reemerged as a heterosexual problem in countries where women have turned to prostitution, sometimes to finance a drug habit.[14]

During the past few years a considerable body of evidence has accumulated linking genital ulceration with increased transmission of HIV.[15-17] These studies, conducted among gay men in the United States and among heterosexuals in developing countries, indicate not only that the presence of genital ulcers significantly enhances susceptibility to HIV infection but that the presence of genital ulcers in HIV-positive individuals results in increased transmission of the virus to others. Chancroid, in particular, has been identified as a significant cofactor in the heterosexual transmission of HIV in Africa and Southeast Asia, with cofactor effects per sexual exposure being estimated as high as 10–50 percent for male-to-female transmission, and 50–300 percent for female-to-male transmission in sub-Saharan Africa.[18] As a result, prompt management and prevention of genital ulcer disease has been identified as a priority within STD control programs aimed at reducing the incidence of HIV infection in developing countries.

ETIOLOGY

The most frequent infectious causes of genital ulceration include *Treponema pallidum*, herpes simplex virus (HSV), *Haemophilus ducreyi*, the L-serovars of *Chlamydia trachomatis*, and *Calymmatobacterium granulomatis*. In addition, *Phthirus pubis*–*Sarcoptes scabiei* pyoderma, *Trichomonas vaginalis*, *Entamoeba histolytica*, mixed nonsyphilitic spirochetes, and *Phthirus pubis*

Table 64-1. Etiology of Genital Ulcerations among Consecutive Patients in Different Populations

	% of patients with diagnosis							
Diagnosis	Detroit[1] N = 100	Antwerp[2] N = 100	Johannesburg[2] N = 102	Nairobi[3] N = 97	Rwanda[4] N = 109	Gambia[5] N = 104	Papua New Guinea[6] N = 101	Bangkok[7] N = 102
Syphilis	15	7	15	9	16	22	14	1
Herpes	37	61	8	4	15	6	0	10
Chancroid	0	5	58	62	18	52	0	36
Lymphogranuloma venereum	0	0	1	0	7	4	9	0
Donovanosis	0	0	1	0	0	0	22	0
Mixed etiology	5	3	3	2	8	44	37	2
Unsolved	43	24	14	23	36	12	18	51

or *Sarcoptes scabiei* infestation with secondary bacterial infection may cause breaks in the genital epithelium. While *Neisseria gonorrhoeae* may be isolated from genital ulcerations, this may represent transient contamination or colonization of the site rather than a causal relationship. The differential diagnosis of infectious genital ulceration includes trauma, malignancy, fixed drug eruption, and Behçet's and Reiter's syndromes.

CLINICAL MANIFESTATIONS

Superficially, the textbook descriptions of the clinical features of the individual causes of genital ulcer adenopathy syndrome appear to be characteristic (Table 64-2). However, in practice the clinical presentation of genital ulcerations often does not correspond to the classic description, and even experienced clinicians can be easily misled.[19–21] This situation is particularly evident in developing countries, where genital ulcerations are common and mixed infections are frequently encountered. In addition, other factors such as secondary bacterial infection; the local application of antiseptics, antibiotics, or corticosteroids; the systemic use of inappropriate or incomplete courses of antibiotics; and the influence of concomitant HIV infection with associated immunosuppression may all modify the clinical appearance of lesions.[11]

In general, the incubation period for chancroid and genital herpes is short (less than 7 days) whereas it is usually longer for syphilis, LGV, and donovanosis. Unfortunately, estimated incubation periods can often be misleading owing to the failure of patients to identify the correct source of the infection, especially when long incubation periods are involved.

Most genital ulcers in men are found on the prepuce (Fig. 64-1), near the frenulum, in the coronal sulcus, or on the penile shaft. In women, lesions may occur on the labia, on the vaginal walls and cervix, and on the inner thighs and fourchette. In both women and gay men, lesions may be found in the rectum and in the perianal region. Extragenital ulcers may be detected on the lips or in the throat as a result of orogenital contact. Classically, the lesions of primary syphilis and LGV are solitary, while those of chancroid, donovanosis, and genital herpes are multiple, but these and other features are often atypical as a result of secondary bacterial infection and mixed etiologies.

Although the characteristics of primary ulcerations may be misleading when one is endeavoring to establish a definitive diagnosis on clinical grounds, features of the associated regional lymphadenopathy, when present, may be helpful in differentiating the different diseases. In both sexes the lymphatic drainage of the external genitalia is primarily to the inguinal and to a lesser extent the femoral lymph nodes. However, the inner two-thirds of the vagina and cervix drain to the deep pelvic (sacral) and perirectal nodes. Regional lymphadenopathy is often associated with genital ulcer-

Table 64-2. Clinical Features of Genital Ulcers

	Syphilis	Herpes	Chancroid	LGV	Donovanosis
Incubation period	9–90 days	2–7 days	1–14 days	3 days–6 weeks	1–4 weeks (up to 6 months)
Primary lesions	Papule	Vesicle	Pustule	Papule, pustule, or vesicle	Papule
Number of lesions	Usually one	Multiple, may coalesce	Usually multiple, may coalesce	Usually one	Variable
Diameter	5–15 mm	1–2 mm	Variable	2–10 mm	Variable
Edges	Sharply demarcated, elevated, round, or oval	Erythematous	Undermined, ragged, irregular	Elevated, round, or oval	Elevated, irregular
Depth	Superficial or deep	Superficial	Excavated	Superficial or deep	Elevated
Base	Smooth, nonpurulent, relatively nonvascular	Serous, erythematous, nonvascular	Purulent, bleeds easily	Variable, nonvascular	Red and velvety, bleeds readily
Induration	Firm	None	Soft	Occasionally firm	Firm
Pain	Uncommon	Frequently tender	Usually very tender	Variable	Uncommon
Lymphadenopathy	Firm, nontender, bilateral	Firm, tender, often bilateral with initial episode	Tender, may suppurate, loculated, usually unilateral	Tender, may suppurate, loculated, usually unilateral	None; pseudobuboes

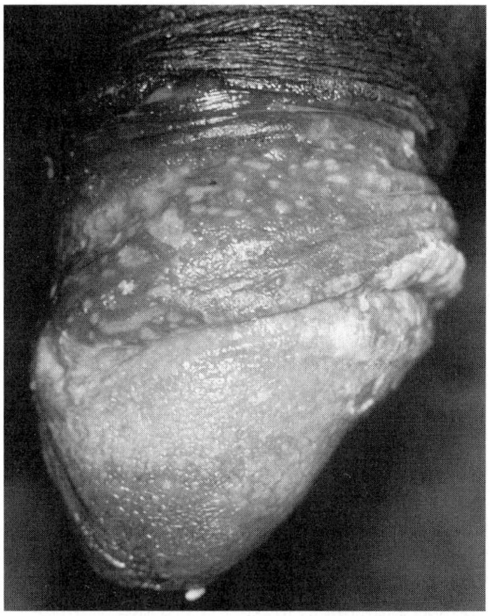

Fig. 64-1. Multiple, superficial, secondarily infected preputial lesions of genital herpes which mimic early chancroid ulcerations.

ation, which may be evident on the external genitalia or may be hidden within the vault of the vagina or in the urethra. Although there may be considerable overlap in the clinical characteristics of the lymphadenopathy, certain characteristics may aid the establishment of a diagnosis. Notably, the lymphadenopathy associated with primary syphilis is usually discrete, bilateral, firm, and painless, while the nodes associated with initial episodes of genital herpes are also bilateral but usually smaller and tender. In contrast, the lymphadenopathy associated with either chancroid or LGV is usually unilateral and painful and may frequently undergo suppuration to form inguinal abscesses, which may rupture.[22] Involvement of both inguinal and femoral glands separated by the inguinal ligament results in the formation of the classic "groove-sign," which was previously considered pathognomonic for LGV. However, many cases of chancroid may present with similar gland involvement (Fig. 64-2). Swellings in the groin associated with cases of donovanosis are not due to an adenitis; rather, they arise as a result of subcutaneous spread of the granulomas, resulting in pseudobubo formation.

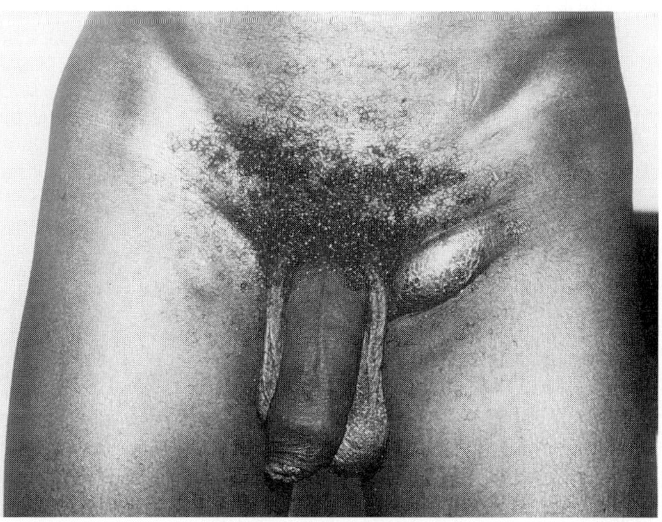

Fig. 64-2. Left inguinal and femoral lymphadenopathy separated by the inguinal ligament. *Haemophilus ducreyi* was isolated from a subpreputial lesion.

It should be noted that in developing countries, painful inguinal lymphadenopathy may be associated with nonsexually acquired lesions of the lower limbs and that chronic nontender lymphadenopathy in the absence of genital ulceration or associated with a persistent lesion may be suggestive of genital or lymphatic malignancy.

COMPLICATIONS AND SEQUELAE

Complications arising from sexually acquired genital ulcers include secondary infection, particularly with anaerobic bacteria, which may result in the formation of destructive or phagedenic ulceration, phimosis or paraphimosis, and local edema. Treatment of both chancroid and donovanosis may result in the formation of scars which, if sited on the foreskin, may cause a permanent phimosis which could require circumcision. In contrast, the lesions of primary syphilis and genital herpes usually heal spontaneously with no scarring within 6 weeks and 1 to 3 weeks, respectively. If left untreated, patients with primary syphilis may develop a secondary syphilitic rash and subsequently the sequelae associated with tertiary disease. Unfortunately, the majority of patients with primary genital herpes develop recurrent disease which, although less severe than the initial episode, may have considerable psychological consequences.

The most severe complications of chancroid and LGV are associated with lymph node involvement. Both chancroid and LGV may cause fluctuation and eventual ulceration of the inguinal and/or femoral glands, and autoinoculation of *H. ducreyi* may result in formation of satellite lesions in the inguinal region.

In LGV, the genitoanorectal syndrome may result in pelvic abscesses, perirectal abscesses, rectal strictures, and fistulae. The chronic manifestations of LGV may also result in blockage of the lymphatics draining the genitalia, causing edema. When the lymphatic edema is gross is termed elephantiasis or esthiomène. A pseudoelephantiasis occurs in advanced cases of donovanosis when scarring results in occlusion of the lymphatics.

LABORATORY DIAGNOSIS OF GENITAL ULCER ADENOPATHY SYNDROME

Ideally, appropriate treatment of genital ulcer disease should be guided by the determination of the etiology of the genital ulcer, using all relevant laboratory tests available. In industrialized countries, where the majority of ulcerations are attributable to genital herpes or syphilis, these should include either darkfield microscopy or direct immunofluorescence staining of genital ulcer material for *T. pallidum*; culture for herpes simplex virus or detection of HSV antigen with ELISA or direct immunofluorescence tests (DFA); and serological testing for syphilis. In developing countries, where other causes of genital ulcer adenopathy syndrome are frequently encountered and establishment of a diagnosis on clinical grounds may be even more difficult, addition of tests for *H. ducreyi*, LGV infection, or *Calymmatobacterium granulomatis* may be considered. However, in these situations laboratory facilities are usually either limited or not available at all. Under these circumstances syndromic management principles are often applied, but even so, serological tests for syphilis should be performed in each case.

A summary of laboratory tests used for diagnosis of genital ulcer adenopathy syndrome is outlined in Table 64-3. Specimens taken directly from the base of ulcerations should be obtained with small calcium alginate or rayon swabs following cleansing of the lesions with sterile saline. When small lesions are being sampled, care should be taken to overcome the inherent problems associated with reduction in sensitivity following multiple sampling. Specimens of ulcer exudate for darkfield microscopy or DFA for *T. pallidum* can be obtained by using a platinum scraper, loop, capillary tube, or glass coverslip following expression of exudate from a cleansed lesion. Specimens for herpes culture or HSV antigen detection are best obtained following disruption of vesicles and collection of vesicle fluid. Swabbings obtained from the bases of ulcerations are somewhat less sensitive for isolation of HSV but are generally the specimens of choice for isolation of *H. ducreyi* and *C. trachomatis*. Specimens of pus obtained from fluctuant lymph nodes should be obtained by aspiration of material with a wide-bore needle through healthy tissue in order to prevent fistula formation. Low rates of recovery of both *H. ducreyi* and/or *C. trachomatis* should be anticipated from such specimens.

MICROSCOPY

Darkfield microscopy has traditionally been recognized as the most appropriate technique for establishing a definitive diagnosis of primary or secondary syphilis. Unfortunately, the technique has major shortcomings, since it requires a suitably adapted microscope and considerable technical expertise to discriminate morphologically between *T. pallidum* and saprophytic spirochetes which may colonize genital lesions. In addition, a balanoposthitis associated with nontreponemal fusospirochetal infection has been described in tropical areas which may result in high rates of false-positive readings using this technique. Under these circumstances, direct immunofluorescence staining of ulcer material may represent a more convenient alternative. However, this technique requires immunofluorescence microscopy, an even more sophisticated technique. Scrapings obtained from the bases of ulcers or smears made from vesicle fluid may be examined for HSV infection by using immunofluorescence or immunoperoxidase techniques or by microscopic examination of Tzanck preparations; a less sensitive method which may reveal characteristic multinucleated giant cells.

Establishment of a definitive diagnosis of donovanosis is totally dependent upon the demonstration of intracytoplasmic encapsulated Donovan bodies within mononuclear cells in Giemsa- or Wright-stained smears or in sections made from scrapings obtained from the edges of active lesions or from punch-biopsy material. In contrast, microscopic examination of gram-stained smears obtained from genital ulcers exhibits both poor sensitivity and poor specificity for *H. ducreyi,* since many nonchancroidal lesions are colonized by gram-negative rods. As a result, this technique cannot be recommended for diagnosis of chancroid even in resource-poor settings.

ISOLATION OF CAUSATIVE AGENTS

Viral isolation remains the most frequent means of establishing a definitive diagnosis of genital herpes. The most frequently used cell lines are Vero cells and human diploid cells, such as MRC-5 cells or foreskin or lung fibroblasts.

The isolation of *H. ducreyi* has also emerged as the most frequent means of establishing a definitive diagnosis of chancroid. A number of solid, semiselective media have been developed which, when used either singly or in combination in biplates, have achieved sensitivities of approximately 80 percent. However, recovery of *H. ducreyi* from bubo aspirates is less efficient, with sensitivities of 40–50 percent.[11] Recently a transport medium has been developed which maintains the viability of *H. ducreyi* in swabs taken from clinical lesions for up to 1 week, provided the specimens are stored at 4°C.[23]

Isolation of the L-serovars of *C. trachomatis* from primary ulcers, the urethra, the endocervix, rectal lesions, or bubo aspirates is a common means of confirming a diagnosis of LGV. However, non-LGV strains of *C. trachomatis* associated with concomitant NGU or cervical infection may contaminate ulcerations and give false-positive results. If the vast majority of cells are infected in a tissue cell culture, it is highly likely to be a case of LGV. Despite frequent textbook references, bubo aspirates are probably the least appropriate source of material for chlamydial isolation, since few patients present with fluctuant glands. When patients do present, the organisms can rarely be demonstrated in bubo aspirates by culture, owing to the paucity of infectious organisms in bubo pus and the toxicity of this material for cell-culture monolayers.

SEROLOGICAL TESTS

Ideally, serological tests for syphilis should be performed routinely in all cases of sexually transmitted diseases, but particularly in cases of genital ulcer adenopathy syndrome. Cardiolipin (reagin) tests (RPR, VDRL) may be negative when a patient initially presents with primary syphilis, since seroconversion may occur as late as 6 weeks after infection. The fluorescent treponemal antibody absorption (FTA-Abs) test becomes positive earlier than the reagin tests (after about 3 weeks), but care in interpretation of a positive FTA-Abs test should be taken, since treponemal tests remain positive even after successful treatment of disease. In areas where syphilis is common, patients presenting with nontreponemal ulcerations may also present with reactive reagin and treponemal tests. These results may represent either concomitant untreated

Table 64-3. Laboratory Tests for the Diagnosis of Genital Ulcer Adenopathy Syndrome

	Syphilis	Herpes	Chancroid	LGV	Donovanosis
Microscopy	Darkfield or direct immunofluorescence	Antigen detection	Gram-staining has low sensitivity and specificity	Not available	Giemsa- or Wright-stained tissue smears and sections
Culture	Not available except by rabbit testicular inoculation	Cell culture	Sensitive, selective media available	Cell culture	Not available
Serology	RPR/VDRL, FTA-ABS, TPHA, MHA-TP	Rarely useful (primary herpes)	Experimental	Complement fixation and immunofluorescent antibody test	Experimental
Molecular techniques	PCR (experimental)	PCR (experimental)	PCR (experimental)	PCR/LCR	Not available

past syphilis or successfully treated but serofast cases.[8] Quantitative RPR or VDRL tests should also be used as a baseline against which responses to treatment can subsequently be measured. In regions where syphilis is uncommon, it is necessary to confirm the results of positive cardiolipin tests by performing an FTA-Abs or *T. pallidum* hemagglutination assay (TPHA) test, since false-positive reactions are frequently encountered. However, in regions where syphilis is commonly encountered the positive predictive value of the reagin (screening) tests is high, there are relatively few false-positive reactions, and there is therefore little value in confirming the results with a more specific test.

A variety of serological tests have been developed to detect antibody to herpes simplex virus. In general, significant rises in antibody titer are only detected in cases of first-episode genital herpes, and methods that are currently available commercially fail to distinguish between antibodies to HSV-1 and HSV-2. Recently a Western blot assay has been developed which can detect type-specific antibody to HSV glycoproteins G-1 and G-2,[24] and type-specific serology based upon ELISA is under commercial development. Unfortunately, these tests are not widely available.

The chlamydial complement-fixation test, which measures antibody to chlamydial group antigen, remains the most widely used serological test for diagnosis of LGV. Rising titers, or a single titer of $\geq 1/64$, usually have been considered diagnostic. A microimmunofluorescence (micro-IF) test which measures type-specific antibody to *C. trachomatis* has also been widely used, and broadly cross-reacting antibody titers of $\geq 1/256$ are frequently detected in cases of LGV.[25] Antibody to *H. ducreyi* may be detected in crude enzyme-linked immunoassays.[26] However, these tests are only useful for establishing lifetime exposure to the disease and are therefore only of value for epidemiological studies.

MOLECULAR TECHNIQUES FOR DIAGNOSIS

Although nucleic acid probes have been used to detect both HSV and *C. trachomatis* in clinical specimens, the development of amplified techniques such as the polymerase chain reaction (PCR) and ligase chain reaction (LCR) has resulted in methods which are both sensitive and specific for the detection of agents associated with genital ulcer adenopathy syndrome. Separate PCR assays have been used to detect the presence of *T. pallidum*,[27] *H. ducreyi*,[28] and HSV[29] in clinical specimens, and a multiplex PCR (M-PCR) amplification assay has recently been described which is able to detect the presence of these three organisms in a single ulcer specimen.[30,31] These techniques represent a significant increase in sensitivity of diagnostic tests for genital ulcer disease, which has resulted in only occasional cases remaining unsolved.

MANAGEMENT

In an ideal situation, treatment for genital ulcer adenopathy syndrome should be initiated only after establishment of a definitive diagnosis by using appropriate laboratory investigations. However, in order to provide appropriate treatment at the initial consultation, it is often necessary for clinicians to provide routine therapy for more than one infection. This approach, known as syndromic management, is necessary because no single antimicrobial agent affords reliable treatment for all causes of the genital ulcer adenopathy syndrome. In addition, the reliability of clinical signs is questionable, mixed infections are common, laboratory support for clinical services is limited, and there are few tests for these infections which can be provided on-site. Syndromic management is recommended by the World Health Organization, particularly for developing countries, and suitable flowcharts

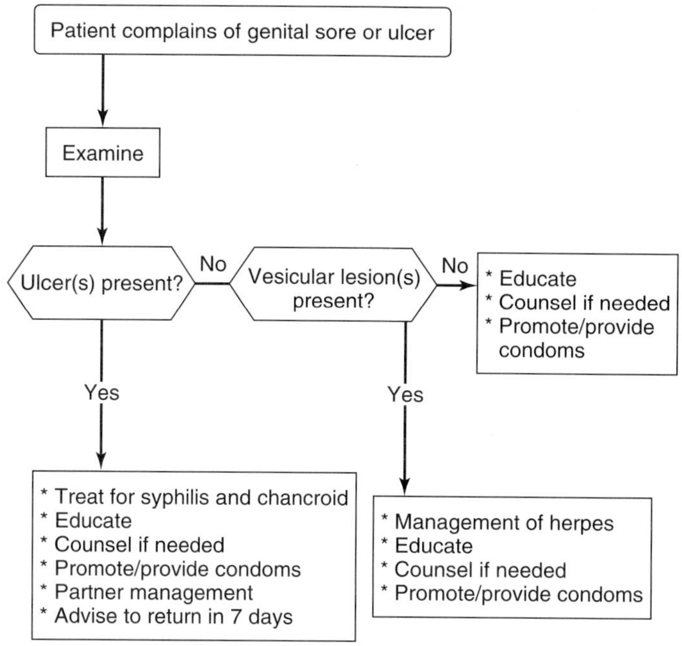

Fig. 64-3. Syndromic management of genital ulcerations.

representing appropriate management algorithms need to be developed on the basis of the patterns of disease presenting in a particular geographical location.[32] Two examples of flowcharts, the first for syndromic management of genital ulcerations and the second for management of inguinal buboes are shown in Fig. 64-3 and Fig. 64-4, respectively. It should be noted that these flowcharts should be validated in a particular setting by using the most sensitive laboratory tests available to establish the patterns of disease within the particular syndrome.[33]

Although all genital ulcers contain a mixed bacterial flora, it is usually not necessary to treat secondary infections in order to hasten healing. In cases that appear to be secondarily infected in developing country settings, some experts provide a nontreponemicidal antimicrobial such as cotrimoxazole. Topical antiviral or

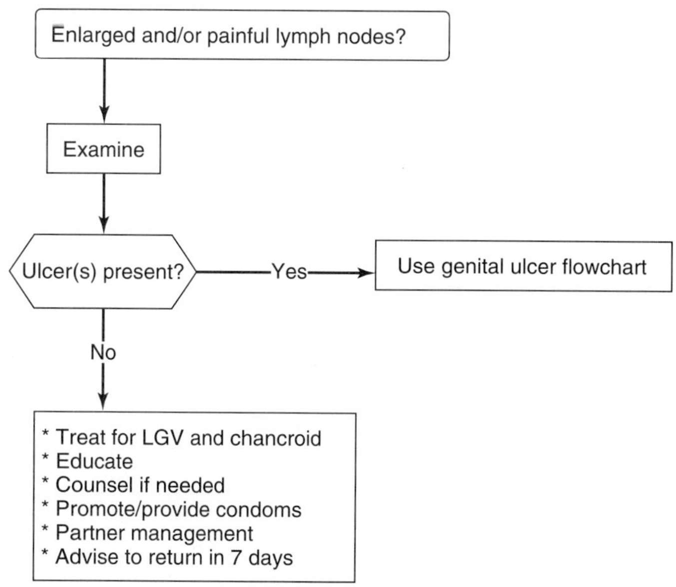

Fig. 64-4. Syndromic management of inguinal buboes.

antibacterial agents are sometimes used by clinicians, and topical agents are often dispersed in pharmacies without prescription or administered by traditional healers. Topical agents are not recommended, and corticosteroids should not be applied. Patients with genital ulcer adenopathy syndrome should be seen by clinicians because of the potentially serious consequences of such infections. Ulcerations usually commence healing within 48 hours of initiation of appropriate therapy, but fluctuant buboes, which are usually associated with chancroid or LGV, should be aspirated through healthy tissue to prevent spontaneous ulceration. Repeated aspiration may be necessary because the suppuration process may continue even in the presence of healing ulcers.

Although incision and drainage may be indicated in an industrialized country setting, aspiration may be more appropriate for resource-poor settings to prevent scarring and delayed healing. Aspiration should be performed with a large-bore needle because the initial exudate may be thick and purulent, while subsequent aspirates performed after initiation of effective therapy may be serous or serosanguineous.

The specific treatments for individual causes of genital ulcer adenopathy syndrome are discussed elsewhere in this book (Chaps. 21, 30, 35, 38, and 39). Antimicrobial resistance is a cause of treatment failure only in cases of chancroid, for which multiresistant strains of *H. ducreyi* have been recorded in most parts of the world. Concomitant HIV infection and its accompanying immunosuppression may influence responses to therapy in cases of genital ulcer adenopathy syndrome caused by any of the etiologic agents.

References

1 Chapel T et al: The microbiological flora of penile ulcerations. *J Infect Dis* 137:50–56,1978.

2 Duncan MO et al: The diagnosis of sexually acquired genital ulceration in black patients in Johannesburg. *S Afr J Sex Transm Dis* 1:20–23,1981.

3 Nsanze H et al: Genital ulcers in Kenya: Clinical and laboratory study. *Br J Vener Dis* 57:378–381,1981.

4 Bogaerts J et al: The etiology of genital ulceration in Rwanda. *Sex Transm Dis* 3:123–126,1989.

5 Mabey DCW et al: Aetiology of genital ulceration in the Gambia. *Genitourin Med* 63:312–315,1987.

6 Vacca A, MacMillan LL: Anogenital lesions in women in Papua New Guinea. *Papua New Guinea Med J* 23:70–73,1980.

7 Taylor DN: The role of *Haemophilus ducreyi* in penile ulcers in Bangkok, Thailand. *Sex Transm Dis* 11:148–151,1984.

8 Sichy A et al: Syphilis serology in patients with primary syphilis and non-treponemal sexually transmitted diseases in southern Africa. *Genitourin Med* 67:129–132,1991.

9 Piot P, Meheus A: Genital Ulcerations, in *Clinical Problems in Sexually Transmitted Diseases,* D Taylor-Robinson (ed). Boston, Martinus Nyhoff Publishers, 1985, p 207.

10 Schmid GP et al: Chancroid in the United States: Reestablishment of an old disease. *J Am Med Assoc* 258:3265,1987.

11 Trees DL, Morse SA: Chancroid and *Haemophilus ducreyi:* An update. *Clin Microbiol Rev* 8:357,1995.

12 Quinn TC et al: *Chlamydia trachomatis* proctitis. *N Engl J Med* 63: 195,1981.

13 Tyndall MW et al: Increased risk of infection with human immunodeficiency virus Type 1 among uncircumcised men presenting with genital ulcer disease in Kenya. *Clin Infect Dis* 23:449–453,1996.

14 Natashima AK et al: Epidemiology of syphilis in the United States, 1941–1993. *Sex Transm Dis* 23:16–23, 1996.

15 Holmberg SD et al: Prior herpes simplex virus type 2 infection as a risk factor for HIV infection. *J Am Med Assoc* 259:1048–1050,1988.

16 Wasserheit JN: Epidemiological synergy: Interrelationships between human immunodeficiency virus infection and other sexually transmitted diseases. *Sex Transm Dis* 19:61–77, 1992.

17 Laga M: Interrelationship of sexually transmitted diseases and HIV: Where are we now? *AIDS* 8:S5119-S5124, 1994.

18 Hayes RJ et al: The cofactor effect of genital ulcers on the pre-exposure risk of HIV transmission in sub-Saharan Africa. *J Trop Med Hyg* 98: 1–8, 1995.

19 Chapel TA et al: How reliable is the morphological diagnosis of penile ulcerations? *Sex Transm Dis* 4:150, 1977.

20 Dangor Y et al: Accuracy of clinical diagnosis of genital ulcer disease. *Sex Transm Dis* 17:184, 1990.

21 O'Farrell N et al: Genital ulcer disease: Accuracy of a clinical diagnosis and strategies to improve control in Durban, South Africa. *Genitourin Med* 70:7–11, 1994.

22 Viravan C et al: A prospective clinical and bacteriological study of inguinal buboes in Thai men. *Clin Infect Dis* 22:233–239, 1996.

23 Dangor Y et al: Transport media for *Haemophilus ducreyi. Sex Transm Dis* 20:5–9, 1993.

24 Sanchez-Martinez D et al: Evaluation of a test based on baculovirus-expressed glycoprotein G for detection of herpes simplex virus type-specific antibodies. *J Infect Dis* 164:1196, 1991.

25 Treharne JD et al: Modification of the microimmunofluorescence test to provide a routine serodiagnostic test for chlamydial infection. *J Clin Pathol* 30:510–517, 1977.

26 Museyi K et al: Use of an enzyme immunoassay to detect serum IgG antibodies to *Haemophilus ducreyi. J Infect Dis* 157:1039, 1988.

27 Burstain JM et al: Sensitive detection of *Treponema pallidum* by using the polymerase chain reaction. *J Clin Microbiol* 29:62–69, 1991.

28 West B et al: Simplified PCR for detection of *Haemophilus ducreyi* and diagnosis of chancroid. *J Clin Microbiol* 33:787–790, 1995.

29 Cone RW et al: Frequent detection of genital herpes simplex virus by polymerase chain reaction among pregnant women. *J Am Med Assoc* 272:792–796, 1994.

30 Orle KA et al: Simultaneous PCR detection of *Haemophilus ducreyi, Treponema pallidum* and Herpes Simplex Virus Type 1 and 2 from genital ulcers. *J Clin Microbiol* 34:49–54, 1996.

31 Morse SA et al: Comparison of clinical diagnosis and standard laboratory and molecular methods for the diagnosis of genital ulcer disease in Lesotho: Association with human immunodeficiency virus infection. *J Infect Dis* 175:583–589, 1997.

32 World Health Organization: Management of Patients with Sexually Transmitted Diseases, Report of a WHO Study Group. WHO Technical Report Series, no 810. Geneva, 1991.

33 Bogaerts et al: Simple algorithms for the management of genital ulcers: Evaluation in a primary health care centre in Kigali, Rwanda. *Bull WHO* 73:761–767, 1995.

Chapter 65
Genital dermatoses

Libby Edwards

The external genitalia are a common site for rashes, itching, and minor infections. This area is warm, moist, and occluded, and it is frequently exposed to irritating urine, feces, and vaginal secretions. In addition, concerns about hygiene and sexually transmitted diseases prompt some people to use overly vigorous cleaning regimens, deodorants, and specialized hygiene products. Abnormalities that, if they occurred elsewhere, would be considered trivial by the patient, suddenly become complicated by both the local environment and psychological factors. Prompt recognition of the cause or causes of visible genital abnormalities or uncomfortable sensations not only minimizes the duration of pain or itching but also helps to avoid damage to self-esteem and sexual relationships.

INFLAMMATORY PLAQUES AND PATCHES

The diseases in this section are characterized morphologically by large (generally >1.5 cm) areas of inflammation. Although these usually appear red, erythema is sometimes subtle and difficult to differentiate from the variable degree of normal background pinkness. Also, inflammation in black skin generally appears hyperpigmented rather than red. Whenever a patient complains of itching, burning, or pain, the skin is most likely inflamed, whether or not erythema is visible. In addition, normally scaly diseases such as eczema and psoriasis may lack visible scale owing to the damp nature of the skin in this area.

ECZEMA/NEURODERMATITIS

Eczema, also called neurodermatitis, is often called "the itch that rashes." Patients initially experience pruritus that may be caused by a yeast infection, heat, moisture, or any other irritant. Scratching produces inflammation that heightens the sensation of itching. As itching worsens, scratching increases until finally an itch–scratch cycle takes on a life of its own, even though the initial precipitating event may have resolved.

The morphology of eczema is consistent with skin that has been scratched or rubbed. Therefore, linear or angular erosions produced by fingernails are common. There is usually surrounding, poorly demarcated erythema, with or without visible scale (Color Plate 107).

Lichenification, or thickening of the skin as a result of rubbing, is extremely common (Color Plate 98). However, lichenification, usually detected by the thickened appearance of the skin with an accentuation of skin markings, can be difficult to appreciate over the scrotum and labia majora, where the skin normally can be thickened and rugated. When lichenification or significant inflammation occurs on the modified mucous membrane of the vulva, the skin frequently becomes white, a clue to subtle disease (Color Plate 99).

In men, eczema occurs most often on the posterior scrotum and relatively often in the crural crease and upper, inner thigh. The penis is a less common location for this condition. In women, the labia majora as well as the modified mucous membranes of the vulva often are affected.

The treatment of eczema requires attention to several specific facets of the disease. The most common cause of a poor response to therapy is the failure to address all factors simultaneously.

First, inflammation and itching should be treated with a topical corticosteroid preparation. Mild symptoms and mild itching often can be controlled with the safe, low potency corticosteroid, hydrocortisone 1 percent (over the counter) or 2.5 percent (available by prescription). More severe symptoms or marked skin findings often require a midpotency preparation such as triamcinolone 0.1 percent (Kenalog®), or, occasionally, even a limited trial of a high-potency medication such as fluocinonide 0.05 percent (Lidex®). Patients should be examined at least monthly to identify any early signs of adverse local effects, such as atrophy, and to decrease the potency of the topical corticosteroid as soon as this is warranted.

Second, any irritant should be discontinued. This begins with the appropriate choice of a vehicle for the corticosteroid. Creams contain alcohol, so that patients with significant inflammation and excoriation often are best treated with an ointment base. Occasionally, however, especially in obese patients or in hot weather, an ointment can be irritating by virtue of its occlusive properties, trapping warmth and moisture next to the skin. Other common irritants include over-washing, washing with harsh soaps, and the application of various borrowed and purchased medications. An extremely common irritant, especially in women, is secondary infection. This is most often caused by *Candida albicans,* but occasionally infection or colonization by *Staphylococcus aureus* or *Streptococcus* spp. produces irritation. Often, treatment of the secondary infection requires ongoing, suppressive therapy until the skin disease and symptoms are controlled, because recurrent infections are extremely common.

Finally, scratching must be stopped. Daytime itching can be minimized by the cited measures, but nighttime itching is often more severe. Sedation to produce deep sleep during the night can provide at least 8 hours of scratch-free time. This can be accomplished with oral diphenhydramine (Benadryl®) or hydroxyzine HCl (Atarax®), both at sedating doses of 25 to 100 mg. Some physicians prefer amitriptyline (Elavil®) at 10 to 100 mg because of the deeper and longer sleep induced.

Therapy should be continued until the patient looks and feels normal, although the potency of the corticosteroid can be decreased as the patient improves. Any remaining disease that is not treated will be scratched eventually, restarting the itch–scratch cycle. The patient should be warned that any future inflammation is also likely to induce itching and subsequent eczema.

IRRITANT CONTACT DERMATITIS

Inflammation produced by contact with irritating substances is a common problem. The patient usually describes irritation, soreness, stinging, or burning, although itching is present in some people. The most common irritants are soap and water, urine, feces, and infected or copious vaginal secretions. This mild chemical burn is manifested by erythema, sometimes with scale. More severe disease may exhibit edema, exudation, or even erosion (Color Plate 100).

The treatment for irritant contact dermatitis consists primarily of the identification and the elimination of irritants, which is sometimes surprisingly difficult. Patients must be asked specifically what they are using for any reason on their skin, including cleansing. Frequency is often important, because even clear water used multiple times daily serves as an irritant. In addition, a low-potency topical corticosteroid such as hydrocortisone 1 or 2.5 percent ointment can hasten improvement.

ALLERGIC CONTACT DERMATITIS

An allergic contact dermatitis is a pruritic inflammatory eruption occurring in response to contact of the skin with a specific allergen. This condition usually occurs 1 or 2 days, but sometimes up to 4 days following contact with the offending substance, unlike an irritant contact dermatitis, which occurs quickly.

An allergic contact dermatitis over the genitalia is usually indistinguishable morphologically from an irritant contact dermatitis and it often resembles eczema or neurodermatitis as well. This nonspecific picture is characterized by erythema, sometimes edema, and occasionally scale or desquamation (Color Plate 101). With a very strong allergic response, vesicles can be present and erosions may be formed as vesicles break.

The most common causes of genital allergic contact dermatitis are ingredients in topical medications, so that allergic contact dermatitis often complicates a pre-existing process.[1] Topical antibiotics, anticandidal agents, local anesthetics, and even corticosteroids sometimes produce allergic contact dermatitis. Preservatives and stabilizers can also cause allergic reactions, so that patch testing may be required to identify the specific allergen.

The treatment of allergic contact dermatitis includes the identification and elimination of the allergen. Topical corticosteroids, the elimination of irritants, and nighttime sedation as described for eczema/neurodermatitis are also necessary for maximal and rapid improvement.

LICHEN PLANUS

Lichen planus is believed to be an autoimmune disease of cell-mediated immunity. Antigens recognized by Langerhans cells, epidermal antigen-presenting cells, may initiate the recruitment of activated lymphocytes, with epidermal damage likely produced by cytokines and cytotoxic T cells. This disease exhibits extremely variable morphology, which is partially dependent on location. Although lichen planus has been long recognized as a common condition on the penis, the frequency of erosive vulvovaginal disease has only been appreciated recently.[2,3]

Patients with milder, papular disease generally report pruritus or no symptoms at all. Those with more severe, erosive disease generally describe pain, particularly with intercourse. These patients usually have associated mouth lesions.

On keratinized skin, such as the shaft of the penis, the circumcised glans, and the clinically hair-bearing portions of the genital area, lichen planus usually appears as well-demarcated, red or dusky, flat-topped papules (Color Plate 102). Although lichen planus is a scaly disease, scale is often very subtle. Sometimes, the surface of the papules shows a lacy or fern-like pattern of fine, white striate, a pathognomonic sign when present.

When occurring on moist skin, such as the uncircumcised glans, or the clinically non–hairbearing skin of the vulva, lichen planus is characterized by either white papules and plaques or erosions. Although the white lesions are occasionally well-formed, sharply demarcated and uniformly hypopigmented papules or plaques, much more often these are irregular, reticulate striae (Color Plate 103). Erosive lichen planus often appears as nonspecific, shallow erosions located most often at the introitus and inner labia minora of women and over the glans penis of men (Color Plate 104). Although a diagnosis based on the erosions alone is difficult, occasionally specific white, lacy papules of lichen planus are found on examination, or less specific coexisting white epithelium is present. These white lesions usually yield a definitive diagnosis of lichen planus on biopsy.

The white lesions of lichen planus are occasionally confused with Candida infection, but negative fungal smears and lack of response to anticandidal therapy distinguish these two entities. Erosive disease differs from a syphilitic chancre by its indolent nature and the superficial morphology of the erosion of lichen planus as compared to the indurated ulcer of syphilis. Unlike most skin diseases that affect the genitalia, other mucous membranes including the mouth and the vagina are often affected and may or may not cause symptoms. An examination of these areas can provide extremely valuable diagnostic information.

In the absence of erosions, genital lichen planus usually is treated satisfactorily with topical corticosteroids. Often, a mid-potency agent such as triamcinolone 0.1 percent is sufficient, but a high-potency medication such as fluocinonide 0.05 percent occasionally is required. Lichen planus does not resolve with these therapies, but symptoms abate and lesions improve. Because there is no cure for lichen planus, therapy must be restarted when symptoms recur. Some patients require chronic therapy, whereas other patients do well with intermittent treatment. Very mild papular lichen planus may not produce future symptoms, and further therapy is not required. Resolution of nonerosive disease generally occurs over months or years. However, patients should be followed carefully until remission occurs, to evaluate the patient both for local corticosteroid side effects and for transformation of the disease into progressive, erosive, and scarring lichen planus.

The management of erosive lichen planus is extremely difficult and often unrewarding. Moderate erosive lichen planus can be treated with a topical high potency or ultrapotent corticosteroid such as clobetasol propionate (with careful follow up to monitor local side effects, including atrophy). More severe disease may require oral prednisone at 40 to 60 mg each morning to induce healing so that topicals can then be used.

Erosive vulvar lichen planus is regularly accompanied by vaginal disease. Scrupulous treatment of secondary vaginal bacterial and fungal infections in conjunction with hydrocortisone acetate 25 mg suppositories used at bedtime can improve many patients. Unless the patient is having regular intercourse, she should insert a small vaginal dilator daily to prevent the formation of vaginal synechiae.

Other medications that have been used for unresponsive lichen planus, although not supported by definitive clinical trials, include oral griseofulvin, dapsone, hydroxychloroquine, retinoids, azathioprine, and cyclophosphamide, as well as topical and oral cyclosporine.[4,5]

PSORIASIS

Psoriasis is a red, scaling skin disease that occurs as a result of hyperproliferation of the epidermis. This disease tends to occur preferentially in areas of irritation or skin injury, such as the elbows and knees. Warmth, perspiration, irritating urine, and friction often precipitate psoriasis in the genital area.

Psoriasis is manifested by red, sharply demarcated, scaling plaques that occur primarily over the hairbearing skin of the vulva and the glans and shaft of the penis, as well as the crural creases (Color Plate 105). Because of the inherently moist nature of skin in the genital area, scale is often relatively inapparent as compared to the heavy, silvery scale of psoriasis in other locations. In addition, lesions are sometimes less well demarcated than in other areas.

Because the skin lesions of psoriasis in the genital area may not be classic for this disease, an examination of other areas of the body is warranted to make the diagnosis definitively. Most patients exhibit typical plaques on the elbows, knees, or scalp. Fingernails often show pitting or lifting of the nails from the nailbed, resembling a fungal infection.

Psoriasis is most often confused with eczema/neurodermatitis and tinea infection. Usually, the general body exam, and, when needed, microscopic smears to rule out fungus allow for the correct diagnosis.

The first-line treatment for genital psoriasis includes minimizing irritation and secondary infections and the application of topical corticosteroids. Genital skin is thin, so that long-term, potent topical steroids are generally avoided. However, psoriasis is only moderately steroid-responsive. Thus, low potency hydrocortisone cream 1 or 2.5 percent may not provide sufficient control. Patients with inadequate response to this low-potency medication can be treated with triamcinolone cream 0.1 percent, but careful follow up to evaluate for atrophy is very important.

More recently, calcipotriene ointment, or vitamin D_3, (Dovonex®), has become available for the treatment of psoriasis.[6] This medication may require several weeks to exert its effects, but it does not cause local atrophy.

Topical tar (Estar gel®, T-Derm®) applied twice a day is often beneficial for psoriasis, but this should be used with great care in the genital area because of the possibility of irritation.

Patient education is crucial in treating psoriasis. Patients should be made aware that psoriasis is a chronic disease without a cure. Should psoriasis become widespread or severe, the more aggressive therapies, such as ultraviolet light, weekly methotrexate, or oral retinoids, instituted by a dermatologist usually improve the genital area as well.

FUNGAL INFECTION

A classic and easily treatable cause of red plaques in the genital area is fungal disease.

Candida albicans, a yeast form, is the usual organism over the vulva or on the glans penis of uncircumcised men. *Dermatophyte fungi* (tinea cruris) produce the typical fungal infection over the proximal, medial thighs of men, and, less often, women.

Candida

Candida vulvitis can have several different morphologies (see also Chapter 45). Most often, there is simple, nonspecific erythema of the modified mucous membranes. Those with more severe or extensive disease, particularly obese women, may also have erythema and peeling of the hairbearing portion of their labia majora. Often, collarettes, a circular rim of scale, are found at the periphery of the involved skin. These represent very superficial pustules that have lost the blister roof. Candida vulvitis is regularly associated with Candida vaginitis unless the patient has treated her vagina without including the vulva. When occurring in men, Candida produces red papules or plaques over the glans of the uncircumcised penis. The shaft of the penis and the scrotum are generally spared since these areas are too dry to maintain a Candida infection.

The diagnosis of Candida is made on clinical grounds, generally with confirmation by a positive microscopic fungal preparation. In women, Candida can be confused (and sometimes coexist) with eczema, psoriasis, and lichen planus. Candida of the glans must be differentiated from psoriasis, lichen planus, and Bowen's disease. Therefore, any patient who does not respond to therapy should be referred to a dermatologist or undergo a skin biopsy.

Tinea

Dermatophyte (tinea) fungal infections occur on drier, keratinized skin. Manifested by scaling, well-demarcated, red plaques located primarily over the inner thighs, tinea cruris is far more common in men (Color Plate 106). The dermatophyte organism occasionally infects the stratum corneum of hair follicles, producing pustules or erythematous papules within the affected plaques. Unless the patient is immunosuppressed or using a topical corticosteroid on the area, a dermatophyte infection generally does not affect the scrotum or the penis.

Dermatophyte infections most closely resemble psoriasis, erythrasma, and eczema. Tinea cruris can be differentiated from these by a positive microscopic fungal preparation and the lack of psoriasis or eczema on other areas of the body.

The treatment of both Candida and dermatophyte infection usually can be achieved with topical antifungal agents. Azole creams such as miconazole, clotrimazole (both over the counter), ketoconazole, sulconazole, and econazole treat both forms of fungus. However, nystatin is only effective against Candida and terbinafine (Lamisil®) is primarily effective for dermatophyte infections.[7] A very convenient therapy, a single dose of fluconazole 150 mg, clears most vulvovaginal Candida infections.

Oral therapy is required for patients with a dermatophyte infection and evidence of follicular involvement. Oral griseofulvin 500 mg twice a day until clearing occurs is usually sufficient for therapy, but nausea and headache are common. Alternatively, but more expensive, is fluconazole 100 mg each day until the skin clears. Recurrences of fungal infections are common.

SQUAMOUS CELL CARCINOMA IN SITU

Squamous cell carcinoma in situ occurs in several settings, with morphology characteristic of each setting.

Bowen's disease

Classic Bowen's disease occurs in older patients and is usually manifested by an erythematous or hyperpigmented, scaling, sharply demarcated plaque (Color Plate 107). This is located anywhere over the vulva, perineum, or inguinal crease. In men, an additional common site is the glans penis. This form of Bowen's disease sometimes resembles a fungal infection, lichen planus, psoriasis, or eczema. Although most often an isolated finding, Bowen's disease sometimes is associated with urogenital malignancy.

Erythroplasia of Queyrat

Erythroplasia of Queyrat refers to squamous cell carcinoma in situ occurring over the glans of the uncircumcised penis. This disease presents as an inflammatory, moist plaque. Erythroplasia of Queyrat is believed to result from chronic irritation of smegma and retained secretions.

Bowenoid papulosis

When squamous cell carcinoma in situ occurs in younger patients, it is most often multifocal, occurring in the distribution and with general morphology similar to flat genital warts. Sometimes referred to as Bowenoid papulosis, these lesions are small, flat-topped, and either pink, pigmented, or sometimes skin-colored (Color Plate 108). These lesions occur as a result of infection with specific types of human papillomaviruses (HPV). They are most easily confused with genital warts, pigmented nevi, or seborrheic keratoses. Although this form of squamous cell carcinoma in situ is usually indolent without progression into invasive and metastatic disease, associated lesions on the cervix and in the anus have a strong propensity for invasion and metastasis.

The diagnosis of squamous cell carcinoma in situ is made by a high clinical suspicion confirmed by a skin biopsy. Management is by destruction or excision. However, any patient with areas of invasion should be managed by a gynecologic oncologist or a urologist.

EXTRAMAMMARY PAGET'S DISEASE

Extramammary Paget's disease is a malignancy of apocrine gland origin that appears as red, scaling, or glistening plaques. Usually occurring in older patients, extramammary Paget's disease is most common over the perineum and hairbearing portion of the labia majora. Morphologically, Paget's disease can be confused with Bowen's disease, eczema, tinea infection, or psoriasis. Diagnosis is by biopsy.

Extramammary Paget's disease is associated with underlying sweat gland carcinoma, or genitourinary, colon or breast malignancy in up to 20 percent of patients.[8]

Management includes an evaluation for associated malignancies, and local excision. Recurrence is usual.

PLASMA CELL (ZOON'S) MUCOSITIS

Plasma cell balanitis and vulvitis are uncommon, medically insignificant inflammatory plaques that may represent a variant of lichen planus. These lesions are located primarily over the glans penis or modified mucous membrane skin of the vulva. The plaques are red, nonscaling, well-demarcated, and moist. The diagnosis is made by a biopsy that reveals a plasma cell infiltrate. Circumcision often improves or obliterates the lesion in men, and topical corticosteroids, retinoids, and cyclosporine can be useful in others.[9]

RED PAPULES AND NODULES

ANGIOMAS

Cherry angiomas

Cherry angiomas are small, bright-red, sharply demarcated papules that are extremely common in older, white patients. Although most heavily distributed over the trunk, these can occur over the perineum as well. Angiokeratomas are similar in appearance but usually more purplish in color. Genetically predisposed patients may have uncountable numbers of these lesions over the labia majora or scrotum. Angiomas require no therapy.

Lichen planus

Lichen planus, particularly over the penis, is often papular (see previous section and Color Plate 102).

Pyogenic granulomas

Pyogenic granulomas are inflammatory vascular tumors that may be spontaneous or may occur at a site of injury. These are most common in pregnant women. Pyogenic granulomas are pedunculated, erythematous, often glistening tumors that require surgical removal. Histologic confirmation is essential since amelanotic melanomas can occasionally mimic this benign tumor.

Urethral caruncles

Urethral caruncles are red, polypoid, benign growths at the urethral meatus in postmenopausal women. These are generally asymptomatic and require no therapy. However, larger lesions can be excised and submitted for biopsy to rule out malignant change.

Urethral prolapse

Urethral prolapse occurs both in prepubertal children and in older women. This erythematosus lesion is generally annular as the distal urethra is extruded circumferentially. When asymptomatic, this may require no therapy. Otherwise, surgical removal is sometimes required.

Inflamed cysts

Cysts, including epidermal cysts, median raphe cysts, vestibular cysts, and Bartholin's duct cysts can sometimes become secondarily inflamed and appear red or cause tenderness. Although the inflammation is occasionally caused by infection (particularly with a Bartholin's abscess), most often the inflammation is due to friction or trauma. Incision and drainage, with a course of antibiotics is the obvious therapy for those cysts that are fluctuant and likely infected. However, most inflamed cysts are not infected and triamcinolone acetonide at a concentration of 5 mg per cc injected into the cyst decreases inflammation easily and quickly.

Inflamed tumors

Normally skin-colored tumors can become secondarily inflamed. Basal cell carcinomas, squamous cell carcinomas, intradermal nevi, and genital warts are more common lesions that sometimes appear red either owing to local friction or trauma or because of necrosis within a tumor that has outgrown its blood supply. The diagnosis of an inflamed tumor often requires a biopsy.

HIDRADENITIS SUPPURATIVA

Hidradenitis suppurativa is a relatively common condition that represents cystic acne of the axillae and/or genital area. Unlike acne, hidradenitis suppurativa does not generally remit after the teenage years.

This condition is manifested by nodules that represent apocrine pilosebaceous units with follicles distended by keratin and apocrine secretions. As these enlarge and rupture, nodules become very painful and red, occasionally draining to the surface with chronic sinus tract formation. The disease spans the spectrum from occasional, tender nodules to extensive, severe, deep scarring disease with frequent superinfection.

Most often confused with staphylococcal furuncles (boils), this diagnosis is made on the basis of its chronicity and location.

First-line therapy consist of oral antibiotics, partially for their antibacterial effect in eradicating secondary infection, but primarily for their antiinflammatory effects. Tetracycline and erythromycin at 500 mg twice a day, doxycycline and minocycline at 100 mg twice a day, and clindamycin at 150 mg twice a day as used for acne are all effective. However, more severe disease is rarely controlled with these regimens.

Antiandrogen therapy is used in more severe cases, including high-estrogen oral contraceptives and spironolactone.

Isotretinoin (Accutane®) produces good results, but, unlike for the therapy for acne, the disease rebounds after cessation of treatment so that ongoing therapy is required. The medication is generally too toxic for long-term therapy.

Although surgery is a treatment of choice for unresponsive axillary disease, the large area of apocrine glands over the genital area makes definitive surgery very difficult and sometimes mutilating.

WHITE LESIONS

LICHEN SCLEROSUS (ET ATROPHICUS)

Lichen sclerosus (hypoplastic dystrophy) is a skin disease of unknown etiology that preferentially affects the vulva and, less often, the penis and extragenital sites. The major symptoms are those of pruritus and eventual pain with more advanced disease. This disease occurs at all ages.

Lichen sclerosus is most often characterized by well-demarcated, hypopigmented plaques of fragile skin. Usually, at least some areas of the skin show fine crinkling, and fragility is often manifested by purpura or erosions (Color Plates 109, 110, 111). As lichen sclerosus progresses, scarring occurs, resulting in resorption of the labia minora and scarring of the clitoral hood to cover the clitoris. Narrowing of the introitus occasionally occurs, resulting in the nonspecific, late appearance of kraurosis vulvae, characterized by resorption of normal vulvar architecture and constriction of the vaginal opening. Uncircumcised males generally experience phimosis as a presenting abnormality. Men who are circumcised occasionally develop late scarring with a loss of the clear demarcation of the glans penis from the shaft. Although lichen sclerosus was once believed to spontaneously resolve at puberty when occurring in children, chronic disease is recognized now as a common occurrence.

Complicating factors in patients, particularly women, include superimposed eczema from rubbing and scratching and secondary bacterial infection, particularly in prepubertal and postmenopausal women who have normally thin skin in this area. About 5 percent of women with uncontrolled lichen sclerosus eventually develop an associated squamous cell carcinoma.[10]

Lichen sclerosus is sometimes confused with vitiligo, but vitiligo consists of otherwise asymptomatic color change, with no texture change, scale, or scarring. Eczema or neurodermatitis can occasionally appear white owing to hydrated, thickened skin from scratching, and sometimes a biopsy is required for diagnosis. The physician should also understand that endstage scarring can occur with several diseases, including cicatricial pemphigoid and erosive lichen planus, so that late vulvar scarring cannot be ascribed automatically to lichen sclerosus.

The treatment for lichen sclerosus consists of the topical application twice daily of an ultra-high potency corticosteroid such as clobetasol propionate (Temovate®) cream or ointment for two to four months, with careful monthly examinations.[11,12] Nighttime sedation and infection control are also important. Topical testosterone propionate was once the treatment of choice but has recently been shown to have no increased efficacy over placebo cream.[13,14] In addition, testosterone is often irritating and may produce increased libido, deepening of the voice, clitoromegaly, and hirsutism.

After lichen sclerosus has been controlled with a very potent corticosteroid, patients can be maintained with thrice weekly applications of the ultrapotent corticosteroid or more regular use of lower potency preparations. Patients should continue to receive occasional follow up both to monitor for local adverse reactions and to evaluate for the development of squamous cell carcinoma.

POSTINFLAMMATORY HYPOPIGMENTATION

Some inflammatory diseases, particularly eczema, can produce secondary color change in the genital skin. Especially visible in normally dark-complexioned patients, light skin can result from damage to melanocytes both by inflammation and by the trauma of scratching (Color Plate 98). Rarely, this white discoloration is sharply demarcated, so that lichen sclerosus and vitiligo should be included in the differential diagnosis as well. The diagnosis is made by the setting and response to therapy, although sometimes a skin biopsy is necessary.

VITILIGO

The pathogenesis of vitiligo is not known, but common theories include the autoimmune, antibody-mediated destruction of melanocytes, the eradication of melanocytes by neurochemical mediators, and the self-destruction of melanocytes by cytotoxic melanin precursors. Occurring first around orifices and over extensor surfaces of joints, the genital area sometimes is affected early. Vitiligo is characterized by sharply demarcated patches of milk-white skin that have no evidence of texture change, inflammation, or scale.

At times vitiligo can be difficult to distinguish from lichen sclerosus, or post-inflammatory hypopigmentation, particularly after the original inflammatory insult has resolved. The diagnosis can usually be made by an examination of other skin surfaces and by history. Therapy for vitiligo when occurring in the genital area is unnecessary although a mild topical corticosteroid occasionally induces some repigmentation.

ECZEMA/NEURODERMATITIS/LICHEN SIMPLEX CHRONICUS

Thickened, lichenified eczema in moist areas often appears white owing to hydrated, hyperkeratotic skin (Color Plate 99). Usually, the morphology is generally that of eczema (see the preceding discussion), which develops a whitish cast on thick, moist skin. Although the diagnosis can usually be made by the clinical appearance, a biopsy is occasionally required to differentiate between eczema superimposed on lichen sclerosus and eczema that is white simply because of hydrated, hyperkeratotic skin.

LICHEN PLANUS

Papular lichen planus or moist skin often appears white. White striae, sometimes in association with dusky red papules or plaques are most common (Color Plate 103). However, sometimes solid white epithelium occurs. (See discussion of lichen planus in the preceding discussion (or section).)

VESICULOBULLOUS/EROSIVE DISEASES

Most blisters on thin, genital skin quickly lose their blister roof and appear as round erosions. This is especially true of the moist, modified mucous membrane skin of the vulva, and the uncircumcised glans penis. The most common vesicular or erosive disease of the genitalia, herpes simplex virus infection, is discussed in Chapter 21.

EROSIVE LICHEN PLANUS

A very common cause of nonspecific, chronic erosions, primarily over modified mucous membranes of the vulva and the vagina, is erosive lichen planus (see also discussion in the preceding section and Color Plate 104). Most common, but not limited to middle-aged or older women, the primary symptom is one of irritation and dyspareunia, and sometimes itching. White epithelium or classic reticulate, white striae are occasionally present and provide clues to the diagnosis. More often, patients exhibit only introital erythema and erosions, frequently associated with a purulent vaginal discharge. These women usually have associated erosive, oral lichen planus that routinely affects the buccal mucosae and often involves the gingivae. Although erosive and scarring lichen planus occurs on the penis, especially the glans, this occurrence is much less common.

The diagnosis is made by the identification of classic associated lesions or by a biopsy of the edge of an erosion that includes some epithelial surface. Unfortunately, nondiagnostic biopsies are common.

The treatment of erosive genital lichen planus is discussed in the preceding section in this chapter.

CICATRICIAL PEMPHIGOID

Cicatricial pemphigoid is an uncommon autoimmune blistering disease of older individuals that produces scarring, particularly of mucous membranes. This diagnosis is relatively easy when non-mucous membrane surfaces are involved, because tense blisters are present and biopsies are generally diagnostic. However, the blistering nature is often not appreciated if only mucous membrane erosions are present. In addition, biopsies of these erosions are often nondiagnostic.

Cicatricial pemphigoid of the genitalia is manifested by nonspecific erosions, skin fragility, and sometimes intact blisters over clinically hairbearing skin.[15] As time progresses, scarring ensues and the clinical picture can be nearly identical to the more common erosive lichen planus (Color Plate 104). The labia minora are resorbed and the clitoris is buried under a scarred clitoral hood. Phimosis occurs in the uncircumcised male, and obvious scarring over the glans with loss of a sharp demarcation between the glans and shaft occurs in others. The severity of cicatricial pemphigoid spans the spectrum from mild, chronic, nonspecific inflammation to rapidly progressive erosions, scarring, and blindness from eye involvement. The diagnosis of cicatricial pemphigoid is made by the recognition and integration of multimucosal, scarring disease that includes the eyes, the mouth, and mucous membranes or modified mucous membranes of the genitalia. Disease is sometimes subtle so that a careful examination by an ophthalmologist may be required to identify conjunctival inflammation or scarring, and oral involvement may simply appear as mild gingivitis. The diagnosis often can be confirmed by routine biopsies from the edge of an erosion and an immunofluorescent biopsy from adjacent skin. If nonmucous membrane lesions are present, these usually are the easiest to biopsy and the most likely to yield a definitive diagnosis.

The therapy of cicatricial pemphigoid is oral corticosteroids. Careful local care to control infections is crucial, and a vaginal dilator inserted once a day may help to prevent vaginal adhesions. Occasionally, a topical steroid adds some additional benefits to systemic therapy.

PEMPHIGUS VULGARIS

Pemphigus vulgaris is an autoimmune, superficially blistering disease that usually begins over mucous membranes, most often the posterior mouth. Most common in younger adults, this disease progresses to affect other mucous membranes, and, ultimately, nonmucous membrane skin. Because of the very superficial nature of the blister, tense bullae are rarely encountered, even over hairbearing skin. Thinner, mucous membrane or modified mucous membrane skin displays erosions and keratinized skin shows flaccid bullae and areas of denuded skin. Although pemphigus vulgaris does not usually scar when occurring on keratinized skin or in the mouth, longstanding pemphigus vulgaris can cause genital scarring as described in the preceding section for cicatricial pemphigoid and lichen planus.

A routine skin biopsy from the edge of an erosion or the edge of a blister usually yields a diagnosis, which can be confirmed with biopsy for direct immunofluorescence from adjacent skin.

Therapy consists of systemic corticosteroids. Immunosuppressant agents such as azathioprine and cyclophosphamide are often used as adjunctive, steroid- sparing medications. Again, local care and attention to infection as discussed for lichen planus can minimize scarring and maximize comfort for the patient.

There is an 80 percent mortality for pemphigus vulgaris when untreated. Although pemphigus vulgaris treated aggressively rarely causes death, the high doses of prednisone required for remission of the disease carry their own morbidity. After the disease is controlled, most patients can be maintained on medication that is slowly tapered to safer dosing schedules, and medication sometimes can be discontinued altogether.

FIXED DRUG ERUPTION

The fixed drug eruption is a peculiar and uncommon but characteristic disease that occurs in some patients in response to certain medications. Although the list of offending drugs is very long, the most common medications responsible include acetaminophen, barbiturates, nonsteroidal antiinflammatory agents including salicylates, oral contraceptives, penicillins, tetracyclines, phenolphthalein, and sulfonamides.[16] One or a few blisters or erosions ranging from 1 to 3 cm appear within 1 to 2 days following ingestion of the offending medication. Subsequent exposure to the medication produces recurrence of lesions precisely at the same location, and occasionally additional areas as well. Fixed drug eruptions of the genitalia preferentially affect the glans penis and non–hairbearing skin of the vulva. On nonmucous membrane skin, lesions are very round edematous plaques or blisters, and, with recurrences, sharply demarcated, round patches of hyperpigmentation develop. Over mucous membranes, lesions tend to be smaller and they may lack their characteristic round shape (Color Plate 112). Because blisters are so short-lived on mucosal surfaces, well-demarcated, red erosions are usual. Hyperpigmentation generally does not occur on these areas.

The diagnosis of a fixed drug eruption is made by the characteristic appearance of these lesions that occur recurrently in the same area in conjunction with a compatible history of medication use. The most common disease mistaken for a fixed drug eruption is a herpes simplex virus infection because of the recurrent nature of both diseases. However, herpes simplex virus infection normally shows small, coalescing erosions rather than fewer, large, discrete erosions. In addition, most patients with a fixed drug eruption have either oral or classic nonmucous membrane lesions as well as genital lesions.

The treatment for fixed drug eruption is avoidance of the medication.

ERYTHEMA MULTIFORME

Erythema multiforme is a hypersensitivity reaction that, when occurring as mucous membrane erosions, is most often produced by medication allergy or occasionally by hypersensitivity to recurrent herpes simplex virus infection. Although uncountable numbers of different medications have been reported in association with erythema multiforme, a more limited number have a clinically significant association. These include penicillins, cephalosporins, sulfas, phenytoin, carbamazepine, phenobarbitol, hydrochlorothiazide, furosemide, procainamide, hydralazine, phenothiazines, allopurinol, nonsteroidal antiinflammatory medications, and any related medications, particularly those containing a sulfa ring.

Morphologically, there is a very wide range of severity and extent of disease. Sometimes, skin lesions are limited to erosions of the oral mucosa and modified mucous membranes of the vulva, the vagina, and the glans penis. Frequently there are associated erythematous, usually target-shaped red papules over the palms and soles. With more extensive disease, mucous membrane erosions are associated with red, nonscaling papules with central blisters scattered over the entire skin surface (Stevens-Johnson syndrome). Large areas of coalescing bullae and erosions occur with severe disease, producing the syndrome, toxic epidermal necrolysis, which has a 40 percent mortality rate (Color Plate 113).

Disease localized primarily to the genitalia and the mouth is most often confused with a herpes simplex virus infection or fixed drug eruption. Very extensive disease is more suggestive of pemphigus vulgaris. The diagnosis is made by the setting, the abruptness of onset, and a confirmatory skin biopsy.

Treatment consists of discontinuation of the offending medication. If there is a history of frequently recurring herpes simplex virus infection that is a likely cause, chronic suppression with oral acyclovir at 400 mg twice a day is indicated. Very early blistering erythema multiforme can possibly be ameliorated substantially by systemic corticosteroids for 2 or 3 days. Very severe disease can perhaps be minimized by intravenous corticosteroids in a hospital setting if instituted in the first 24 to 48 hours, but this quite controversial. It is clear that high doses of corticosteroids for widespread blistering after the first few days may worsen the prognosis owing to complications of systemic corticosteroids.

NONINFECTIOUS ULCERS

Ulcers are differentiated from erosions by their depth. Whereas erosions are simply lacking epithelium with most of the dermis intact, an ulcer extends well into, or, occasionally, even through the dermis.

The primary consideration in a patient who presents with a genital ulcer is a possibility of a sexually transmitted disease, especially primary syphilis, chancroid, granuloma inguinale, or herpes simplex virus infection occurring in an immunosuppressed patient. Infectious ulcers are discussed in Chapter 64 and noninfectious causes of erosions are discussed in the immediately preceding section of this chapter. However, there are several noninfectious diseases that can produce genital ulcers.

APHTHOUS ULCERS

Aphthous ulcers (sometimes called canker sores) are mucous membrane ulcerations that are extremely common on the oral mucosa, but less common over the genitalia. Although patients with genital aphthae nearly always report oral disease as well, oral and genital lesions do not necessary occur concurrently. Although oral aphthae are usually small, ranging from 1 to 2 mm, with an erythematous rim and a white fibrin base, genital aphthae are often larger and irregular. The base may be white, but deeper ulcerations may simply be red (Color Plate 114). These are often quite painful, and may heal with scarring. They are most common on the modified mucous membranes of the vulva and occasionally over the scrotum and penis.

When genital aphthae occur in patients who have systemic signs of disease such as inflammatory eye disease, arthritis, meningoencephalitis, or pustular vasculitis, the diagnosis of Behcet's disease should be considered. Patients with significant oral/genital aphthosis and gastrointestinal symptoms should be evaluated for inflammatory bowel disease, which can produce similar oral and genital ulcers.

Aphthae are diagnosed by appearance, the history of recurrent ulceration, and the exclusion of infectious and granulomatous causes, usually by skin biopsy.

For patients who have very occasional disease, oral prednisone at 40 to 60 mg for 3 to 7 days usually induces prompt alleviation of pain, and healing. Ongoing oral colchicine beginning at 0.6 mg three times a day or dapsone at 100 to 200 mg per day are sometimes useful in patients whose recurrences are too frequent for prednisone to be a safe and practical therapy.

CROHN'S DISEASE

Crohn's disease, a granulomatous disease of the small bowel, sometimes produces perineal ulcers or fistulas. Less often, Crohn's disease can produce infiltrated, red, granulomatous plaques.

Occasionally, this disease resembles hidradenitis suppurativa, which also produces sinus tracts, and in fact these diseases are sometimes seen together. The diagnosis of Crohn's disease is made by skin biopsy and the demonstration of intestinal disease. Therapy consists of oral corticosteroids, sulfones, and immunosuppressive agents.

PIGMENTED LESIONS

PIGMENTED NEVI

Pigmented nevi (moles) do not have a predisposition for the genital area, but they are found often in that area by virtue of their ubiquitous occurrence. In addition, nevi that occur on the vulva, particularly during pregnancy, sometimes have an atypical appearance on biopsy, although this does not necessarily portend malignant transformation. A benign nevus is a macule or papule that is smaller than 7 mm in diameter, with regular, sharply demarcated borders, and homogeneous, brown pigmentation. Although many nevi have some atypical features, several atypical features or one extraordinarily abnormal finding should prompt the physician to refer the patient to a dermatologist or to biopsy the lesion. Otherwise, therapy is unnecessary although nevi can be excised if desired.

SEBORRHEIC KERATOSES

Seborrheic keratoses are also benign tumors that do not exhibit a propensity for the genitalia, but they are so very common and sometimes so numerous that they may occur over this skin surface. Seborrheic keratoses are brown to skin-colored, keratotic, sharply demarcated, flat-topped papules. The firm, keratotic nature is sometimes not appreciated over the genitalia where the skin is damp. Seborrheic keratoses are most often confused with genital warts or nevi, and in fact some recent studies have reported finding HPV by polymerase chain reaction techniques in seborrheic keratoses. However, the extremely common background positivity for this virus sheds great doubt on HPV as an etiology for seborrheic keratoses. Seborrheic keratoses have no malignant predisposition, and therapy is unnecessary. The lesions can be removed by liquid nitrogen therapy or light curettage for cosmetic reasons or if the lesion becomes irritated.

SQUAMOUS CELL CARCINOMA IN SITU

Bowen's disease and Bowenoid papulosis (squamous cell carcinoma in situ, vulvar intraepithelial neoplasia, penile intraepithelial neoplasia) are sometimes hyperpigmented. Bowenoid papulosis results from the carcinogenic effects of some HPV types, and this condition is usually multifocal and resembles flat genital warts (Color Plate 108). Classic Bowen's disease is manifested as larger, single lesions. Individual lesions may be nearly macular or they may be infiltrated, with some erythema and scale. Diagnosis is by biopsy, and therapy consists of destruction or local excision. These diseases are discussed in the preceding section covering inflammatory patches and plaques.

PHYSIOLOGIC HYPERPIGMENTATION

Physiologic hyperpigmentation is noticeable primarily in patients who are naturally dark complexioned, and as a response to some hormones, especially sex hormones. Women experience hyperpigmentation of the perianal skin, and the edges of the labia minora. Less common in men, the hyperpigmentation primarily involves the scrotum and perianal skin. The diagnosis is by pattern and therapy is unnecessary.

MALIGNANT MELANOMA

Cutaneous melanoma is a malignant tumor of melanocytes. Arising in a pre-existing nevus or de novo, these lesions are not especially common in the genital area. However, melanomas located in this area are often diagnosed late and the prognosis grave.

Melanoma can occur anywhere over the genital area, including the modified mucous membranes and even within the vagina. Melanomas are usually greater than 7 mm in diameter with irregular and often poorly demarcated borders. The color is usually irregular and variegate. Most melanomas do not exhibit all of these clinical characteristics, but generally several are present.

Diseases in the differential diagnosis of melanoma include pigmented nevi, pigmented genital warts, pigmented squamous cell carcinoma in situ, benign genital lentiginosis, and hyperpigmentation associated with lichen sclerosus. The diagnosis is confirmed by biopsy, and therapy consists of local excision with margins determined by the thickness of the tumor. Thin melanomas (those <.86 mm thick) have a very good prognosis with most patients experiencing long-term, disease-free survival. However, as the lesions thicken, the risk of metastasis increases remarkably and metastatic melanoma is an extraordinarily aggressive disease.

BENIGN GENITAL LENTIGINOSIS

Benign genital lentiginosis is an uncommon, idiopathic cutaneous abnormality consisting of irregular, variegate patches and macules of hyperpigmentation. This totally flat hyperpigmentation sometimes displays frightening irregularity of browns, tans, and black that mimic cutaneous melanoma. Most common over the glans and shaft of the penis and the modified mucous membranes of the vulva, a biopsy is required to differentiate this condition from malignant melanoma. Although this condition is felt to be benign despite its worrisome appearance, there is one report of melanoma of the bladder in a patient with genital lentiginosis, so that at least occasional follow up is recommended by some.[17]

HYPERPIGMENTATION OF LICHEN SCLEROSUS

Patients with lichen sclerosus, particularly those with longstanding, treated lichen sclerosus, occasionally exhibit flat, irregular hyperpigmentation. Although the borders are irregular and poorly demarcated, and the color is irregular as well, the pigmentation is normally brown and tan, lacking the blue, black, and gray often seen with melanoma and genital lentiginosis. However, unless the patient is known to have or have had lichen sclerosus, a biopsy is definitely indicated to rule out both melanoma and squamous cell carcinoma in situ.

SKIN-COLORED PAPULES

Genital warts, the most common skin-colored papules found in the genital area, are usually sexually transmitted and are discussed in Chapter 25. Most other skin-colored papules are medically trivial but nonetheless important to the patient.

PEARLY PENILE PAPULES

Pearly penile papules are common, skin-colored, monomorphous, dome-shaped papules or papillae arranged in rows around the edge of the corona (Color Plate 115). These are most common in uncircumcised men. They are sometimes confused with genital warts, but the monomorphous nature and the arrangement in rows differentiate these from genital warts, and virologic studies have shown no evidence of HPV.[18] These are asymptomatic and require no therapy.

VESTIBULAR PAPILLOMATOSIS

Vestibular papillae are similar normal variants that occur over the modified mucous membrane of the introitus and medial labia minora. These tubular papillae are found in patches or lines that are bilaterally symmetrical. Like pearly penile papules, they are often mistaken for genital warts. However, these are very soft and monomorphous, and the papillae are discrete to the base, unlike genital warts that tend to be fused at the base.[19] In addition, the tips of the papillae are rounded rather than acuminate and keratotic. Although vestibular papillae often come to the patient's or physician's attention when vulvar itching or pain occur, these papillae are incidental findings present in about half of premenopausal women. They are asymptomatic and require no therapy.

CYSTS

Epidermal cysts

Cysts are common, benign tumors. Epidermal cysts (sometimes mistakenly called sebaceous cysts) are the most common. Although usually single or few in number, some patients exhibit large numbers of these firm, skin-colored to white, dermal nodules, particularly over the scrotum or the labia majora. These cysts generally represent hair follicles that have become blocked with keratin so that the proximal portion of the follicle has become distended with keratin and sebaceous material. Because pilosebaceous units are even found over the labia minora, epidermal cysts sometimes occur in this area. Epidermal cysts are usually asymptomatic and require no therapy. Surgical excision can be performed for those patients who wish removal.

Vestibular cysts

Vestibular cysts are skin-colored, slightly bluish, or slightly yellowish cysts found over the nonhairbearing portion of the vulva. These are usually asymptomatic and unnoticed by the patient. They are dome-shaped without surface change.

Median raphe cysts

Median raphe cysts are innocuous, skin-colored, dome-shaped papules over the midline underside of the shaft of the penis.

Pilonodal cysts

Pilonidal cysts are small, dome-shaped papules most often located over the sacrum, coccyx, and near the clitoris. These can become inflamed and occasionally drain and develop a sinus tract. Pilonidal cysts can be symptomatic and painful with chronic drainage. These may require excision.

SCLEROSING LYMPHANGITIS

Sclerosing lymphangitis consists of a firm, skin-colored cord located just proximal and parallel to the corona of the penis, sometimes encircling the shaft entirely. This asymptomatic, medically trivial, and self-resolving abnormality is believed to occur from trauma and friction.

FORDYCE SPOTS

Fordyce spots are enlarged sebaceous glands that occur primarily over the labia minora. Although usually subtle, at times these can be enlarged and may resemble small epidermal cysts or genital warts. However, Fordyce spots are usually monomorphous and slightly yellowish in color (Color Plate 116). Enlarged pilosebaceous units are sometimes present on the shaft of the penis also. These are small, scattered, skin-colored papules less than 1 mm in size. These are most often noticed when a patient has genital warts and the physician has difficulty discerning whether these pilosebaceous units are normal irregularities in the skin or extremely small warts. They are asymptomatic and require no therapy.

PRURITUS

Genital pruritus is a common symptom. In predisposed, atopic patients, any inflammation or irritant can produce itching. Often, the physical examination shows a specific abnormality. However, genital skin is often normally pink, and scale can be masked by moisture so that sometimes the genitalia can appear amazingly normal in the face of significant inflammation. Any patient with pruritus should be examined specifically for the following causes of pruritus.

INFECTION

The most common cause of acute pruritus is an infection, particularly in women. The vagina should be carefully evaluated, especially for yeast infection. However, trichomoniasis and bacterial infection occasionally produce pruritus. Pinworms, found primarily in children, can cause itching.

ECZEMA

The most common cause of chronic itching is eczema. Erythema and lichenification can be extremely subtle, so that in the absence of other abnormalities, the patient should be treated for eczema (see the preceding section).

OTHER SKIN DISEASES

Pruritus can occur with other skin diseases as well, including lichen sclerosus, lichen planus, and psoriasis. Itching often is caused or maintained by overwashing and the application of irritating or allergenic medication, colognes, or cleansers. Any irritation produces itching in predisposed, atopic patients.

DEPRESSION AND ANXIETY

Finally, depression and anxiety occasionally cause and very often exacerbate itching. Psychological factors should be recognized and addressed. Nighttime use of amitriptyline or doxepin sedates the patient, preventing awakening owing to pruritus, and provides antidepressant and anxiolytic effects.

GENITAL PAIN

SCROTODYNIA AND VULVODYNIA

Chronic genital pain, burning, or the sensation of irritation in the absence of obvious physical findings is an occasional but debilitating syndrome. Vulvodynia (burning of the vulva) is far more common than its counterpart in men, scrotodynia or penile pain. Because of the rarity of scrotodynia, this entity is poorly understood and there is little published information regarding causes and therapy. Some experienced clinicians feel that scrotodynia is usually a manifestation of psychosexual dysfunction.[20]

Although the vast majority of women with vulvodynia are extremely depressed and experience major disruption in their sexual functioning, vulvodynia is generally not believed to result primarily from psychosexual pathology. There are several known specific physical causes for vulvar burning, and directive therapy often produces major improvement in symptoms. Vulvodynia is often multifactorial.

Rarely, subtle skin disease produces vulvar irritation, soreness, and burning. Although eczema can be painful, this pain only occurs as a result of erosions from scratching, and the patient's primary complaint is one of pruritus. Very subtle lichen sclerosus sometimes produces pain, and erosive lichen planus is very often associated with pain. Occasionally, lichen planus can affect only the vagina, with irritating and superinfected vaginal secretions irritating the vulva secondarily.

Vaginal infections of any kind can sometimes produce secondary vulvar burning. Although *Candida albicans* usually produces itching, non-*albicans Candida* infections are more likely to produce burning, and often they are treated inadequately with the usual azole therapies. Vulvar burning can also result from a bacterial vaginitis, not to be confused with bacterial vaginosis. Vaginal secretions are purulent and alkaline rather than nonflammatory with clue cells, as occurs with bacterial vaginosis. This infection of the vaginal mucosa occurs most often when the mucosa is very thin and erosions develop, as occurs with postmenopausal vaginal atrophy, atrophic postpartum changes, or a primary skin disease of the vagina, especially lichen planus.

Finally, there are two patterns of vulvodynia that are not necessarily specific diseases, but rather help to classify idiopathic vulvar burning. Vulvar vestibulitis consists of entry dyspareunia and pain to any pressure applied to the introitus, or vestibule. Often, this is accompanied by erythema and many believe that this syndrome is a form of reflex sympathetic dystrophy. Dysesthetic vulvodynia occurs in older patients and consists of more generalized burning of the vulva, independent of touch. Many clinicians believe that this is also neuropathic pain, but more often a manifestation of pudendal neuralgia.

The therapy of vulvodynia consists of the identification and attempted correction of all observed vaginal and vulvar abnormalities, and a careful search for infection or inflammation. Also, tricyclic antidepressants such as amitriptyline or desipramine at a dose of 50 to 150 mg as therapy for neuropathic pain is beneficial in a majority of patients. Patients with vulvar vestibulitis who are recalcitrant to these conservative measures sometimes improve with local interferon alpha injections, although the mechanism is entirely unknown, or local excision of the painful area with advancement of the vaginal mucosa. Other therapies that have been used for vulvodynia include pelvic floor rehabilitation and a low oxalate diet in combination with oral calcium citrate. Although various forms of laser therapy have been used successfully at times, this therapy carries the risk of worsening the patient.

References

1 Marren P et al: Allergic contact dermatitis and vulvar dermatoses. *Br J Dermatol* 126:52, 1992.

2 Pelisse M: The vulvo-vaginal-gingival syndrome: a new form of erosive lichen planus. *Int J Dermatol* 28:381, 1989.

3 Eisen D: The vulvo-vagina-gingival syndrome of lichen sclerosus. The clinical characteristics of 22 patients. *Arch Dermatol* 130:1379, 1994.

4 Borrego L et al: Vulvar lichen planus treated with topical cyclosporine (Letter). *Arch Dermatol* 129:794, 1993.

5 Pelisse M: Treatment of vulvo-vaginal erosive lichen planus with topical cyclosporin A (CSA). Presented at the XIth World Congress of the International Society for the Study of Vulvar Disease, Oxford, England, September, 1991.

6 Kragballe K: Treatment of psoriasis with calcipotriol and other vitamin D analogues. *J Am Acad Dermatol* 27:1001, 1992.

7 Kagawa S: Clinical efficacy of terbinafine in 629 Japanese patients with dermatomycoses. *Clin Exp Dermatol* 14:114, 1989.

8 Paniel BJ et al: Paget's disease of the vulva: 46 cases (abstract). *J Reprod Med* 38:46, 1993.

9 Hautmann G: Vulvitis circumscripta plasmacellularis. *Int J Dermatol* 33:496, 1994.

10 Ridley CM: Dermatological conditions, in *The Vulva*, Ridley CM (ed). New York, Saunders, 1988, pp. 172–193.

11 Dalziel KL et al: Long-term control of vulval lichen sclerosus after treatment with a potent topical steroid cream. *J Reprod Med* 39:25, 1993.

12 Friedman M et al: Vulvar lichen sclerosus treated with super potent topical corticosteroid (clobetasol propionate 0.05%). *Cervix* 12:21, 1994.

13 Bracco GL et al: Clinical and histologic effects of topical treatments of vulval lichen sclerosus: A critical evaluation. *J Reprod Med* 38:37, 1993.

14 Sideri M et al: Topical testosterone in the therapy of vulvar lichen sclerosus: a randomized placebo-controlled evaluation. *Int J Obstet Gynecol* 46:53, 1994.

15 Edwards L et al Vulvar cicatricial pemphigoid: A lichen sclerosus imitator. *J Reprod Med* 37:561–564, 1992.

16 Sehgal VH et al: Genital fixed drug eruption. *Genitourin Med* 62:56, 1986.

17 Kerley SW et al: Multifocal malignant melanoma arising in vesicovaginal melanosis. *Arch Pathol Lab Med* 115:950, 1991.

18 Ferenczy A et al: Pearly penile papules: absence of human papillomavirus DNA by the polymerase chain reaction. *Obstet Gynecol* 78:118, 1991.

19 Moyal-Barracco M et al: Vestibular papillae of the vulva: lack of evidence for human papillomavirus etiology. *Arch Dermatol* 126:1594, 1990.

20 Lynch PJ et al: Anogenital pain, in *Genital Dermatology*. New York, Saunders, 1994, pp. 247–248.

Chapter 66

Ocular infections associated with sexually transmitted diseases and AIDS

John W. Chandler

INTRODUCTION

Many etiologic agents responsible for sexually transmitted diseases (STDs) are capable of causing external eye or intraocular infections. Blinding complications may result if these infections are not promptly recognized and appropriately treated. In other instances, these infections cause prolonged ocular symptoms. Ocular complaints and findings vary widely, and delays in conducting a comprehensive ophthalmologic examination may result in late recognition at a time when more advanced involvement and permanent visual loss occur.

Several chapters in this book mention ocular involvements as part of the clinical spectrum of STDs. This chapter emphasizes those ocular involvements, including their symptoms, signs, and local therapies. These involvements are seen in all age groups. Transmission method of STD agents to the eye includes transplacental, hematogenous, contamination of the ocular surface during birth, oculogenital contact, and direct or indirect contact by digits and fomites. While some clinical presentations are unique and indicate a specific diagnosis, many are less obvious and require laboratory diagnostic procedures. Frequently, the size of the inoculum for culture and cytology is small, and prompt, diligent specimen handling is important for the establishment of etiology.

Ocular and visual involvement in association with infections and other conditions in patients with acquired immunodeficiency syndrome (AIDS) are, in some cases, associated with blindness. Some of these conditions, especially retinal infections such as cytomegalovirus (CMV) retinitis, require careful monitoring and special therapeutic efforts. These ocular involvements are also described in this chapter, with special emphasis on detection and local therapy.

OCULAR MANIFESTATIONS OF SEXUALLY TRANSMITTED DISEASES IN ADULTS

Immunocompetent adults may present with a variety of ocular complaints and symptoms caused by microorganisms that are sexually transmitted. A majority of these complaints cause red eyes and ocular discomfort with little or no loss of vision. Most of these patients present to an ophthalmologist in a context that either minimizes or masks the information regarding STDs, and, in some instances, the ocular symptoms antedate genital-tract complaints. Patients with significant loss of vision are more apt to present to the ophthalmologist with the possible link to STDs already under consideration. In all clinical presentations, diligent searches for microorganisms in ocular tissues are warranted.

CHLAMYDIAL INFECTIONS

Adult ocular chlamydial infections that occur in the context of STDs are adult inclusion conjunctivitis (AIC), Reiter's syndrome, and ocular involvement in lymphogranuloma venereum.

Adult inclusion conjunctivitis is caused by serovars D, E, F, G, H, I, J, and K of *Chlamydia trachomatis* and appears as unilateral or bilateral follicular conjunctivitis 1 to 2 weeks after exposure to infected secretions (Fig. 66-1). The symptoms are variable in degree but typically include ocular irritation with redness and mucopurulent discharge. A subset of patients go on to develop corneal epithelial keratitis. Some will eventually have peripheral corneal subepithelial keratitis or corneal neovascularization. Conjunctival, but not corneal, scarring may occur. In experimental infections with serovars associated with AIC, the onset and degree of severity of conjunctivitis was dose-dependent.[1] Adult inclusion conjunctivitis is often detected together with clinical infections at nonocular sites. Because of the likelihood of multiple site infections, systemic rather than topical therapy is indicated, generally with 7 days of doxycycline or tetracycline given orally. Another therapeutic concern is the possibility of concomitant infection in sexual partners. Data from one study showed that one-half of the female partners of men with ocular chlamydial infections had genital chlamydial infections, and 80 percent of the male partners of women with ocular chlamydial infections had concomitant nongonococcal urethritis, a majority of which was due to *Chlamydia trachomatis*.[2] Sexual partners should therefore be referred for testing and treatment.

Reiter's syndrome was originally described as a condition in a young male with urethritis, arthritis, and conjunctivitis.[3] More recently, it is usually defined as reactive arthritis with various combinations of ocular, urogenital, and mucocutaneous inflammatory lesions.[4] A vast majority of these patients are positive for HLA-B27 and may be of either sex.[5] The endemic form of Reiter's syndrome appears to be sexually transmitted and generally involves infections with *Chlamydia trachomatis*. Ophthalmic involvement occurs in approximately one-half of Reiter's syndrome patients, and a few patients initially present because of ocular symptoms. Usually ocular involvement commences as a bilateral mucopurulent papillary conjunctivitis that is self-limited; there is no palpable preauricular node. In some cases, *Chlamydia trachomatis* has been detected in conjunctival specimens during the acute stage. A mild superficial keratitis, iritis, or iridocyclitis is seen in a few instances. Appropriately directed antibiotic therapy for chlamydial infection of the genital tract (see Chap. 29) in combination with topical anti-inflammatory medications are needed to manage the ocular component of Reiter's syndrome.

Lymphogranuloma venereum has on rare occasions involved the eye, presumably as a result of direct inoculation of the ocular surface. It is one of the causes of Parinaud's oculoglandular syndrome, which is characterized by an ulcerative conjunctival lesion, follicular conjunctivitis, and preauricular adenopathy.[6] Other involvements including superior corneal superficial neovascularization and iridocyclitis have been described.[7,8]

GONOCOCCAL OCULAR INFECTIONS

Gonococcal ocular infections usually begin suddenly and cause a severe, mucopurulent conjunctivitis with copious discharge, redness, and swelling of the conjunctiva.[9,10] Onset is typically 24 to 48 hours following exposure to urogenital secretions containing *Neisseria gonorrhoeae*. These infections are of particular concern because corneal involvement with subsequent perforation begins within 24 hours of onset. Unlike many microbes, this bacteria is capable of penetrating through an intact corneal epithelium. Prompt diagnosis along with rapid initiation of aggressive therapy are crucial to the prevention of corneal involvement and blindness. Treatment of uncomplicated gonococcal conjunctivitis can usually be accomplished with ceftriaxone, 250 mg IM. If there is corneal involvement, a 3- to 7-day course of ceftriaxone, 1 gm IV daily,

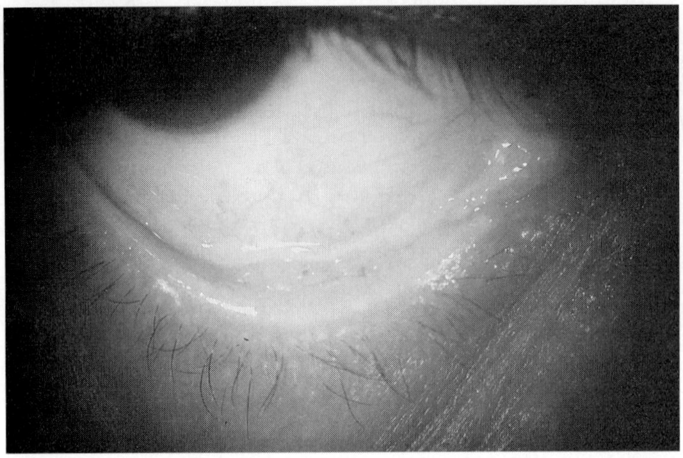

Fig. 66-1. Adult inclusion conjunctivitis with subconjunctival follicular response to chlamydial antigens.

is indicated. Although not part of the recommendations of the Centers for Disease Control and Prevention (CDC), many ophthalmologists add hourly topical applications of penicillin, 100,000 units per mL, because of the risk of perforation and subsequent blindness.

MOLLUSCUM CONTAGIOSUM

Molluscum contagiosum is often sexually transmitted in adults, and single or multiple lesions may be detected on the eyelid skin or at the eyelid margins. Some patients present to ophthalmologists complaining of chronic red eyes with irritation and mild discharge that have not responded to topical antibiotics. Examination reveals typical umbilicated epidermal lesions and follicular conjunctivitis. Most cases resolve following cryotherapy, excision, or curettage of the skin lesions.[11] Rarely, keratitis or corneal neovascularization occurs.

PHTHIRIASIS

Phthiriasis of the eyelids is usually caused by the pubic louse *Phthirus pubis*, and, to a much lesser extent, by head and body lice. *Phthirus pubis* preferentially tends to infest areas with widely spaced hairs such as the eyelashes as well as the hairs of the pubis, chest, axilla, and face. Acquisition of this infestation may be from sexual contact or fomites. The primary symptom of eyelash involvement is intense itching. The adult lice and their eggs are easily identified by slit-lamp examination (Fig. 66-2). The treatment of the eyelashes should be done in concert with treatment of other involved areas of the body (see Chap. 46). Lindane (Kwell) shampoo causes corneal toxicity and should not be used on the eyelashes; instead, trimming of the lashes and manual removal of the nits at the slit-lamp or smothering of the lice with applications of a bland ophthalmic ointment two to three times daily for a 10-day period will eliminate the infestation.

VERRUCA VULGARIS

Verruca vulgaris lesions due to papillomavirus can involve the skin of the eyelids and eyelid margins or the conjunctival epithelium (Fig. 66-3). The transmission of human papillomavirus to these sites occurs by a wide variety of modes, including oculogenital. Eyelid margin and conjunctival lesions cause papillary conjunctivitis and diffuse corneal epithelial erosions associated with superficial inflammation of the cornea. Surgical excision is utilized to remove these lesions on the skin of the eyelids, and cryotherapy is used to remove eyelid margin and conjunctival warts.

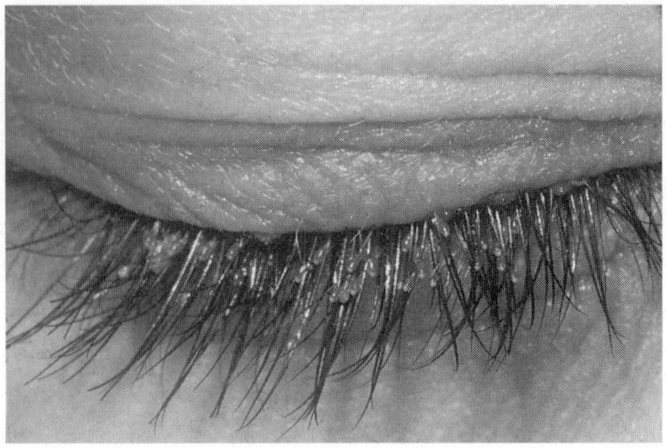

Fig. 66-2. Phthiriasis involving eyelashes and eyelid margins where adult lice and eggs are found.

HERPES SIMPLEX VIRUS

Herpetic keratitis, conjunctivitis, or keratoconjunctivitis are occasionally associated with oculogenital transmission of type 2 herpes simplex virus (HSV).[12,13] The vast majority of adult ocular herpetic disease is caused by type 1 HSV and is due to reactivation of latent infection of the trigeminal ganglion. Recurrent type 2 HSV ocular infections are also discovered when isolates are typed in the laboratory, however. The clinical courses and lesion appearances of keratitis caused by types 1 and 2 HSV are very similar (Fig. 66-4), but keratitis caused by type 2 HSV tends to last longer and responds less well to topical antiviral drugs.[14] Primary infections involving varying combinations of the eyelids, conjunctiva, and cornea of adults are uncommon. Careful attention to histories of possible exposure to someone with genital HSV infection or with other STD infections or exposures, or finding a type 2 HSV isolate, provide suggestive evidence of oculogenital transmission of type 2 HSV.

Corneal HSV infections are of particular concern because of the

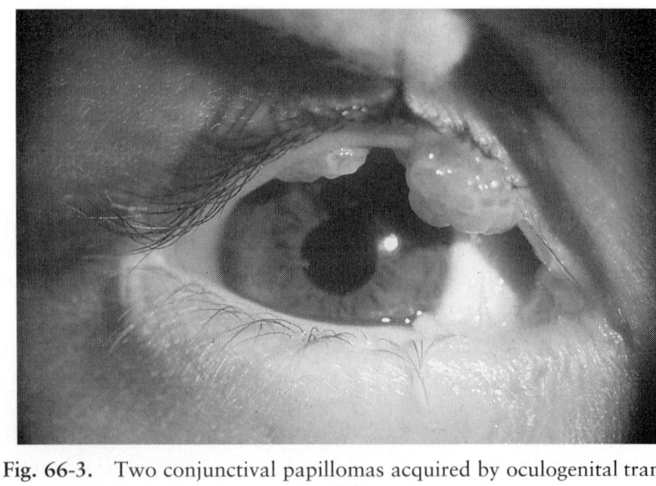

Fig. 66-3. Two conjunctival papillomas acquired by oculogenital transmission protrude past the upper eyelid margin.

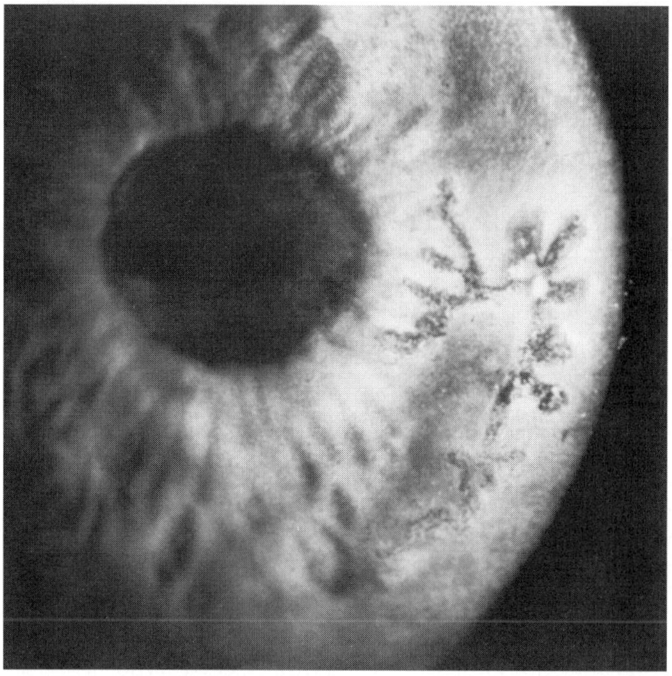

Fig. 66-4. Epithelial HSV keratitis with characteristic dendritic pattern seen after instillation of fluorescein.

risks of recurrent infections and subsequent visual loss due to corneal scarring. The recurrence rate after the initial bout of keratitis is approximately 10 percent at 1 year and 23 percent at 2 years.[15] After the first recurrence, the likelihood of further recurrences increases, and along with it the possibility of corneal scarring and significant visual loss is enhanced. Topical trifluridine, vidaribine, or idoxuridine speed the rate of healing of epithelial herpetic keratitis. Concomitant corneal inflammation is managed by judicious use of anti-inflammatory agents including topical corticosteroids. A recent multicenter trial studying the treatment of herpetic keratitis demonstrated a significant benefit of topical corticosteroid therapy in the management of corneal stromal inflammation.[16]

Because of the potential blinding consequences of ocular herpetic infections, prompt recognition in all settings, including oculogenital transmission, is important. The clinical appearances of ocular HSV infections can vary widely, and symptoms may range from slight visual reduction and foreign-body sensation to severe pain and marked visual loss. Every patient with HSV infection at any body site and complaints about his or her eyes should have a complete ophthalmologic examination.

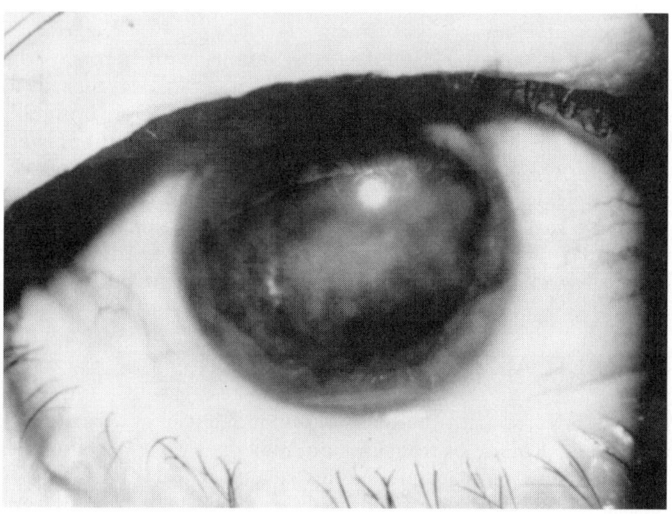

Fig. 66-5. Interstitial keratitis (old) due to congenital syphilis. Note patchy corneal clouding.

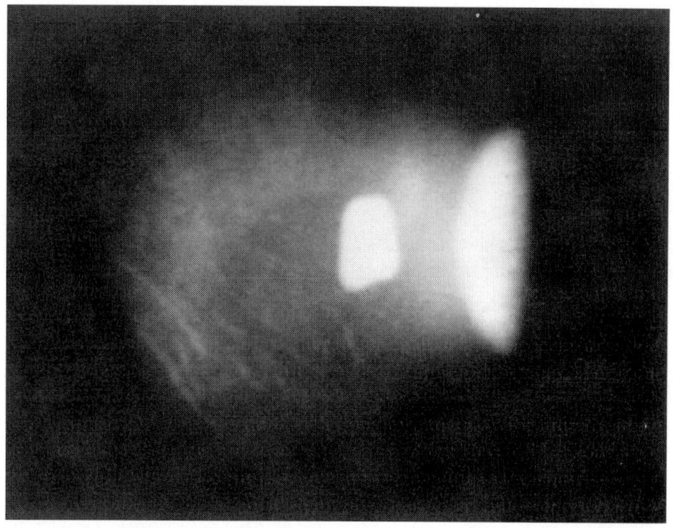

Fig. 66-6. Ghost vessels in the cornea due to old syphilitic interstitial keratitis, revealed by slit-lamp examination. Ghost vessels are residual vessels from earlier keratitis, no longer perfused by blood.

SYPHILIS

Almost all of the ocular manifestations of syphilis seen in adults are the result of congenital syphilis.[17] Between birth and 30 years of age, these individuals develop diffuse, bilateral interstitial keratitis with corneal stromal haze, white blood cell infiltration into the cornea, and neovascularization. A majority of these individuals are between 5 and 16 years of age when acute interstitial keratitis develops. Variable corneal scarring and ghost vessels no longer carrying blood can be detected by slit-lamp examination and are the life-long sequelae of this condition (Fig. 66-5 and Fig. 66-6). These findings warrant workup and treatment if the patient has not received adequate previous treatment. Other ocular manifestations of syphilis include chorioretinitis as a result of congenital or secondary syphilis, Argyl-Robinson pupillary abnormalities, episcleritis, scleritis, optic atrophy, and a conjunctival gumma in association with ipsilateral preauricular adenopathy (Parinaud's oculoglandular syndrome) (Fig. 66-7). All of these findings may also be caused by other infectious agents. If any of these clinical findings are detected, laboratory studies are indicated in order to determine the specific etiology.

OCULAR MANIFESTATIONS OF SEXUALLY TRANSMITTED DISEASES IN INFANTS

Infants exposed to STDs in utero or at the time of delivery may develop ocular infections in the early postnatal period. In some situations the ocular involvement is the initial presentation of the STD, and in others it is not evident unless careful examination is performed or a late, obvious, progressive manifestation develops. In each instance where an infant has possibly been exposed to any of the microorganisms associated with STDs, thorough exami-

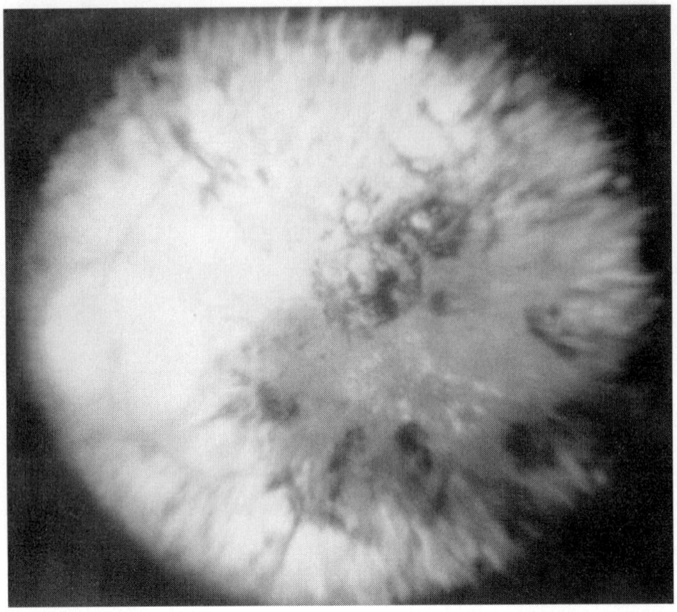

Fig. 66-7. Retinal scarring and pigmentary changes caused by healed syphilitic chorioretinitis.

nation of the eyes is warranted. The three most likely etiologies are *Chlamydia trachomatis*, herpes simplex virus, and *Neisseria gonorrhoeae*. In addition, the possibility of ocular involvements via transplacental transmission of *Treponema pallidum* and cytomegalovirus need to be considered.

CHLAMYDIA TRACHOMATIS

The serovars of *Chlamydia trachomatis* associated with sexual transmission infect the ocular surface (conjunctiva and cornea) of newborn infants. When mothers have untreated antepartum cervical infection with *Chlamydia trachomatis*, their infants have a 30 to 40 percent chance of developing chlamydial neonatal conjunctivitis along with involvements of other anatomic sites.[18] Neonatal inclusion conjunctivitis typically develops 5 to 14 days after birth, but infants may show clinical signs of infection beginning on the first day of life, especially when there has been premature rupture of membranes. Clinical signs of chlamydial conjunctivitis vary widely from scant mucoid discharge to the development of pseudomembranes of the conjunctiva and abundant purulent discharge that may be unilateral or bilateral. The ocular involvements are usually self-limited but corneal neovascularization can occur.[19] The involvements of other body sites are detailed in Chap. 83.

Prophylaxis of the ocular surface of newborns is an effective method for preventing neonatal chlamydial conjunctivitis.[20] Recent data indicate that instillation of povidone-iodine, 2.5% solution, is the least toxic and most efficacious prophylaxis agent.[21] Silver nitrate, 1% solution, tetracycline, 1% ointment, and erythromycin, 0.5% ointment, are also effective prophylaxis agents.[22,23] Because of simultaneous infection at other anatomic sites (pharynx, rectum, vagina), systemic rather than topical therapy is indicated for treatment of chlamydial conjunctivitis. Almost all chlamydial conjunctivitis episodes respond to a 14-day course of oral erythromycin syrup, 50 mg per kg per day in two to four doses. Evaluation and treatment of the mother and her sexual partners should also be undertaken. If conjunctivitis recurs, a repeat course of oral erythromycin should be given.[24]

GONOCOCCAL CONJUNCTIVITIS

Gonococcal ophthalmia neonatorum classically presents as a hyperacute conjunctivitis with onset by the second day of life. Inadequate prophylaxis at birth along with partial treatment of the mother prior to delivery may alter the clinical picture in terms of severity and time of onset. All cases of newborn conjunctivitis deserve appropriate microbiological workup in order to ascertain etiology and to select optimal treatment. Two major concerns are the capability of *Neisseria gonorrhoeae* to penetrate through intact corneal epithelium to cause perforation, scarring, and blindness, and the possibility of concomitant infection with two or more microorganisms.

Gonococcal conjunctivitis responds to parenteral antibiotics as described in Chap. 82, but the condition of the cornea must be constantly monitored. In any eye with a corneal epithelial defect or opacity, one should consider the addition of topical therapy with a solution of penicillin, 100,000 units per mL, every hour until the hyperacute phase subsides, in order to minimize the possibility of blindness due to a rapidly progressing corneal ulcer.

In populations where prenatal care includes detection and treatment of maternal gonococcal infections and where ocular prophylaxis of newborns is utilized, neonatal gonococcal eye infections are uncommon. For example, it is estimated that 2,000 cases occur annually in the United States.[25] In an area where these measures were not available, the frequency was 3.8 percent.[22] Health-policy decisions on requirements for ocular prophylaxis need to be formulated in the context of disease frequency and other confounding health issues.[20]

NEONATAL HERPES SIMPLEX VIRUS CONJUNCTIVITIS AND KERATITIS

Neonatal herpetic ocular surface infections may be unilateral or bilateral, and onset is usually in the first 2 weeks of life. Conjunctivitis or keratitis may occur alone or together with skin lesions. The corneal lesions include epithelial dendrites or geographic figures and stromal infiltrates and neovascularization. Sequelae include permanent corneal scarring and vascularization. Approximately 70 percent of all neonatal herpetic infections are caused by type 2 HSV, and it is likely that this is true for ocular involvements.[26]

Like all neonatal HSV infections, infants with herpetic conjunctivitis and keratitis should have systemic antiviral therapy as detailed in Chap. 85. Corneal HSV infections are likely optimally treated by the addition of topical 1% trifluridine solution, every 2 hours for 7 days or until re-epithelialization of the cornea occurs. Topical antiviral treatment should not exceed 21 days.[24]

A wide variety of other microorganisms exist which may cause neonatal conjunctivitis. These appear to be acquired after delivery, however, and are not due to STDs acquired during birth.[27]

HIV- AND AIDS-RELATED INFECTIONS

Persons infected with the human immunodeficiency virus (HIV), regardless of mode of transmission, may develop a large number of ocular complaints and findings related to HIV itself and to resulting opportunistic infections. Clinical ocular findings of some type are seen in more than 70 percent of patients with AIDS, and,

Table 66-1. Other Etiologic Causes of Ocular Involvements among Patients with AIDS

Eyelids and Conjunctiva
Molluscum contagiosum,[72,73] Kaposi's sarcoma,[74,75] conjunctival intraepithelial neoplasia,[76] *Cryptococcus neoformans*[77]

Cornea
Dry eye states[78,79]; microsporidiosis[80,81]; herpes simplex virus[82]; varicella-zoster virus[83,84]; cytomegalovirus[85]; bacterial, fungal, and parasitic corneal ulcers[86]; drug-induced lipidosis[87]

Retina and Uveal Tract (Iris, Ciliary Body, and Choroid)
Toxoplasma gondii,[88–91] *Pneumocystis carinii,*[92–94] *Cryptococcus neoformans,*[77,94,95] *Treponema pallidum,*[96] herpes simplex virus,[97] varicella-zoster virus,[98–101] *Histoplasma capsulatum,*[94] *Candida* sp.,[94] *Mycobacterium tuberculosis,*[94] *Mycobacterium avium* complex,[94] *Aspergillus fumigatus,*[94] *Fusarium* sp.,[102] primary intraocular lymphoma[103,104]

Neuroophthalmic Conditions
Optic neuropathy due to cytomegalovirus,[105] *Histoplasma capsulatum,*[106] *Treponema pallidum,*[96] *Cryptococcus neoformans*[107]

Orbit
Orbital infections due to *Pseudomonas aeruginosa, Staphylococcus aureus, Aspergillus fumigatus, Rhizopus arrhizus, Toxoplasma gondii,* and *Pneumocystis carinii*[108]; orbital lymphoma[109,110]

based on autopsy findings, approximately 90 percent of them have pathologic eye involvements.[28] While cytomegalovirus (CMV) retinitis, with its potential to cause blindness, is the most frequent severe ocular infection, there are a wide range of ocular problems that may occur. Additionally, opportunistic infections of the central nervous system (CNS) may cause ocular and visual system problems. The ocular manifestations of HIV and CMV infections are described below. Table 66-1 lists the other ocular and visual system infections seen in AIDS patients. Detailed descriptions of all the conditions and their management are beyond the scope of this chapter, but there are many references for this information.[28–30]

OCULAR INVOLVEMENTS CAUSED BY HIV

Human immunodeficiency virus alone is associated with some ocular findings in infected persons without other opportunistic infections. Among these findings are retinal cotton-wool spots,[31] decreased visual function detected by visual field measurements,[32] color vision and contrast sensitivity testing,[33] and marked loss of retinal ganglion cell nerve fibers.[34] These findings are detectable in patients with no evidence of ocular opportunistic infections or other CNS disorders. Their pathophysiologic bases are not completely elucidated, and several possibilities are under study. Macrophages that are HIV-positive are found in the retina, and HIV antigens have been detected in retinal microvascular endothelial cells.[35,36] Other possible causes include deposition of immune complexes or AIDS-associated hematologic abnormalities. The most common clinical ocular finding is cotton-wool spots—the clinical expression of infarcts of the ganglion cell nerve fibers—which are seen in a majority of AIDS patients and may be detected in those with asymptomatic infections (Fig. 66-8). The edematous state of cotton-wool spots after the occurrence of an infarct blocks visualization of retinal structures beneath them. They may be seen in association with retinal hemorrhages and microaneurysms, a constellation that is referred to as retinal microangiopathy. Cotton-wool spots usually are asymptomatic but may eventually result in decreases in visual function and numbers of nerve fibers on optic nerves seen in AIDS patients.[31–34]

Another ocular finding in HIV-infected adults and children is multiple well-circumscribed areas of depigmentation in the midperipheral retina in patients treated with dideoxyinosine.[37–39] Histopathologic evaluation shows areas of loss of retinal pigment epithelium (RPE), surrounded by RPE cell hypertrophy and hypopigmentation. The lesions appear to be related to cumulative dosage of dideoxyinosine and high peak levels. The macula appears to be spared, and central visual acuity is unaffected. All patients using dideoxyinosine should be monitored for the RPE changes.

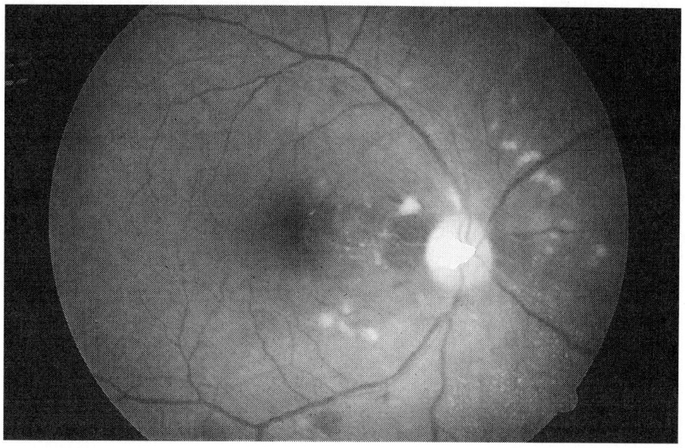

Fig. 66-8. Retinal microangiopathy of HIV infection with widespread cotton-wool spots and retinal hemorrhages.

Uveitis has been reported in AIDS patients who are receiving rifabutin for treatment of *Mycobacterium avium* complex infections.[40,41] The onset of the uveitis may not begin until several months after the initiation of rifabutin therapy. Failure to recognize the association may lead to unnecessary surgical diagnostic procedures. The uveitis may be intense and is effectively managed with topical corticosteroids. Rifabutin-associated uveitis will likely become more common with the increasing use of rifabutin as a prophylaxis agent in HIV patients with low CD4 cell counts.

CYTOMEGALOVIRUS RETINITIS

The most common causes of visual loss in HIV-infected individuals are CMV retinitis and its sequelae, including necrosis of retinal tissue and retinal detachment. While CMV infects many tissues, including lung, gastrointestinal tract, and brain, CMV retinitis accounts for 71 to 85 percent of all CMV infections in AIDS patients.[42,43] Depending upon the retinal location and extent of CMV retinitis, an infected patient's visual loss and symptoms may range from normal visual acuity (often associated with increased vitreous floaters) to profound blindness. It is especially important to recognize CMV retinitis in its early course in order to initiate therapy and protect against its blinding complications. Since CMV retinitis was relatively unknown until the 1980s, research over the past 15 years has been directed toward finding efficacious therapies in a setting where masking of clinicians and patients has been difficult and the natural history of the infection has not been fully described. Additional concerns are the method for measuring disease progression, CMV drug resistance, ocular side effects of therapy, and quality-of-life issues. Since virostatic therapies are now available, it is possible and necessary to conduct randomized trials to ascertain optimal treatment regimens. It is also clear that the optimal method for evaluating CMV retinitis therapies is with fundus photographs, which can be graded by masked observers using established criteria.[45] Serial fundus photographs are also valuable for following individual patients with CMV retinitis. Evidence of progression of infection is often subtle and may not be recognized as easily during an examination as it can be by comparisons of serial photographs. As CMV retinitis progresses, the destruction of neuroretinal layers and RPE appear clinically as areas of retinal necrosis and hemorrhage. Likewise, therapy may lead to involution of these overt clinical signs.

Typically, CMV retinitis occurs late in the course of AIDS, when CD4 counts have declined to 50 or less. It is estimated that up to 37 percent of AIDS patients will develop CMV retinitis.[46,47] Low CD4 counts or CMV infections at other sites are indications for monitoring for the development of CMV retinitis. Such patients need periodic eye examinations, regardless of the lack of symptoms, in addition to immediate examinations with the onset of decreased vision, floaters, or other unexplained visual system symptoms. These examinations must include thorough inspection of all regions of the retina. Table 66-2 lists the ocular symptoms and clinical findings associated with CMV retinitis, and Fig. 66-9 shows typical features of CMV retinitis and their response to antiviral therapy. Currently, all anti-CMV therapy is virostatic; relapse is seen following cessation of therapy, or occasionally during therapy if drug resistance occurs. Another major problem is the 50 to 60 percent probability that retinal detachment will occur within 1 year from the time that the diagnosis of CMV retinitis is made.[48,49] Anatomically successful surgical reattachment of the retina can be achieved in approximately 90 percent of cases, but visual improvement may not be satisfactory.[50,51]

At the time of the first recognized cases of CMV retinitis in AIDS patients 15 years ago, no effective therapies were available. Since that time a number of treatment options have become available, and several more are currently being evaluated. A number of investigative groups have reported that intravenous ganciclovir or intravenous foscarnet are effective in significantly delaying the time to progression of CMV retinitis. Additionally, the combination of intravenous ganciclovir and foscarnet is successful for relapsed disease.[48,52–55] Other trials have demonstrated the relative efficacy of oral ganciclovir as compared with intravenous ganciclovir.[56,57] A number of other reports indicate that intravitreal local therapies with ganciclovir or foscarnet provide options to systemic therapies.[58–62] Repeated intravitreal injections are feasible and tolerated,[63] and intravitreal injections also avoid systemic toxic effects of the drugs. Additionally, ganciclovir has been incorporated into an intraocular implant device that releases the drug for several months. The device is surgically placed into the peripheral vitreous and is sutured to the sclera.[64,65] Progression of CMV retinitis occurs after cessation of intravitreal injections and approximately 7 months after insertion of the ganciclovir implant device. Some patients have had additional devices surgically inserted, resulting in more prolonged control of CMV retinitis. Intravitreal injections of cidofovir have also been reported to stop progression of CMV retinitis.[66] An antisense drug is also in a controlled clinical trial to determine its safety and efficacy as an intravitreal drug against CMV retinitis. Fomivirsen sodium is a 21-

Table 66-2. Ocular Manifestations of CMV Retinitis in AIDS Patients

Symptoms	Decreased or hazy vision, loss of a portion of central or peripheral vision, multiple floaters, light flashes, sometimes asymptomatic
Clinical Findings	Keratic precipitates, iritis, vitritis, grayish retinal discoloration, retinal necrosis, retinal vascular sheathing, retinal hemorrhages, granular appearance of involved retina, disturbances of retinal pigment epithelium, retinal detachment

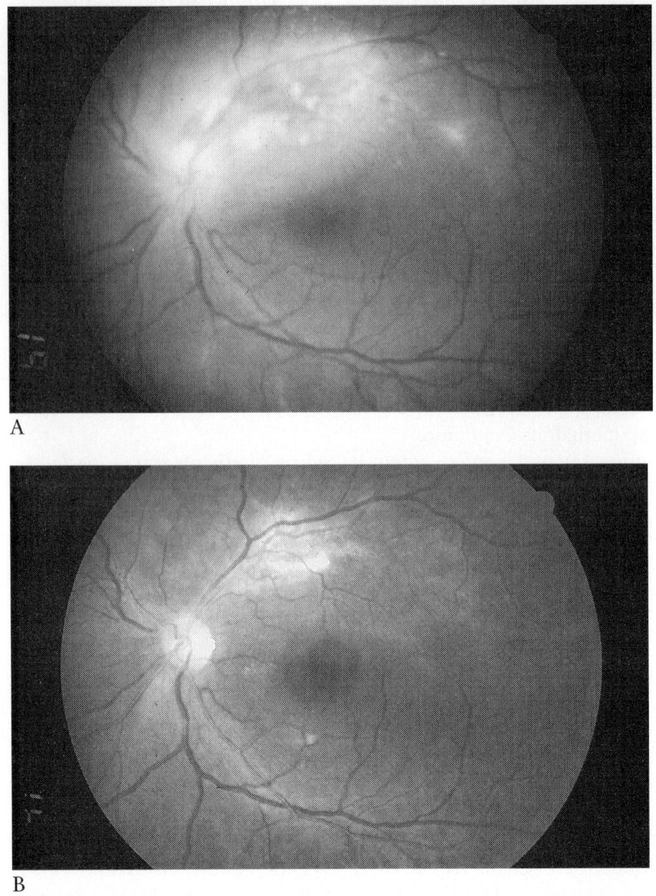

Fig. 66-9. *A*. Active, untreated CMV retinitis and papillitis with retinal hemorrhages, edema, and necrosis. *B*. Same eye 3 months later following repeated intravitreal injections of an anti-CMV drug demonstrating reduced activity of CMV retinitis.

base phosphothioate oligonucleotide designed to bind mRNA coding for two immediate early CMV proteins required for viral replication.[67] The drug is potent with an average EC_{50} of 0.5 μM against CMV isolates, some of which were resistant to ganciclovir, foscarnet, and cidofovir.[68,69] A phase-1b clinical study of intravitreally injected fomivirsen sodium in cases of refractory CMV retinitis demonstrated a dose response with safe and well-tolerated doses in the 150 to 330 μg injection range. The active drug appears to stay in the vitreous for reasonably long periods and allows maintenance dosing at every-other-week intervals with several patients receiving fomivirsen sodium for periods exceeding 11 months.[70]

A major shortcoming of any local therapy is the 50 percent risk of CMV retinitis in the other eye and the 31 percent risk of CMV infections at other sites.[65] The relative advantages and disadvantages of the various treatment options need to be considered in the selection of therapy for a specific patient. All of the current antiviral drugs directed against CMV fail to eliminate the virus from the retina. Once treatment is stopped, CMV again replicates and there is progression of the retinitis.[71]

OTHER OCULAR INFECTIONS ASSOCIATED WITH AIDS

A number of other ocular involvements have been reported in AIDS patients. Many have relentless, devastating effects on vision;

others, by the nature of their atypical presentations in immunocompromised individuals, may have delays in recognition and initiation of therapy. Table 66-1 outlines the sites of tissue involvements and the microorganisms that have been reported to cause infections in AIDS patients. This vast array of infections and their potential for causing blindness emphasize the importance of prompt ophthalmologic care in all AIDS patients with any visual system complaint. The role of routine eye examinations is still being determined.

References

1 Dawson CR et al: Experimental inclusion conjunctivitis: III. Keratitis and other complications. *Arch Ophthalmol* 78:341, 1967.

2 Patel HC et al: Chlamydial ocular infection: Efficacy of partner notification by patient referral. *Int J STD AIDS* 5:244, 1994.

3 Reiter H: Uber eine bisher unerkannte Spirochateninsektion. *Dtsh Med Wochenschr* 42:1535, 1916.

4 Lee DA et al: The clinical diagnosis of Reiter's syndrome: Ophthalmic and nonophthalmic aspects. *Ophthalmology* 93:350, 1986.

5 Martin DH et al: *Chlamydia trachomatis* infections in men with Reiter's syndrome. *Ann Intern Med* 100:207, 1984.

6 Koteen H: Lymphogranuloma venereum. *Medicine* 24:1, 1945.

7 Oliphant JW et al: Sulfadiazine in lymphogranuloma venereum ophthalmitis. *JAMA* 118:973, 1947.

8 Scheie HG et al: Keratitis associated with lymphogranuloma venereum. *JAMA* 35:333 1947.

9 Wan WL et al: The clinical characteristics and course of adult gonococcal conjunctivitis. *Am J Ophthalmol* 102:575, 1986.

10 Ullman S et al: *Neisseria gonorrhoeae* keratoconjunctivitis. *Ophthalmology* 94:525, 1987.

11 Gonnering RS et al: Treatment of periorbital molluscum contagiosum by incision and drainage. *Ophthalmic Surg* 19:325, 1988.

12 Oh JO et al: Acute ocular infection by type II herpes simplex virus in adults: Report of two cases. *Arch Ophthalmol* 93:1127, 1975.

13 Newman-Haeflin D et al: Herpes simplex virus type I and II in ocular diseases. *Arch Ophthalmol* 96:64, 1978.

14 Chandler JW: Genital herpetic infections and their associations with ocular herpetic *Ophthalmic Forum* 3:117, 1985.

15 Liesegang TJ: Epidemiology of ocular herpes simplex: Natural history in Rochester, Minn, 1950 through 1982. *Arch Ophthalmol* 107: 1160, 1989.

16 Wilhelmus KR, for the Herpes Eye Disease Study Group: Herpetic eye disease study: A controlled trial of topical corticosteroids for herpes simplex stromal keratitis. *Ophthalmology* 101:1883, 1994.

17 Oksala A: Studies on interstitial keratitis associated with congenital syphilis occurring in Finland. *Acta Ophthalmol (Copenh)* 30(suppl 138):1, 1952.

18 Harrison JR et al: *Chlamydia trachomatis* infant pneumonitis. *N Engl J Med* 298:702, 1978.

19 Forster RK et al: Late follow-up of patients with neonatal inclusion conjunctivitis. *Am J Ophthalmol* 69:467, 1970.

20 Chandler JW: Controversies in ocular prophylaxis of newborns. *Arch Ophthalmol* 107:814, 1989.

21 Isenberg SJ et al: A controlled trial of povidone-iodine as prophylaxis against ophthalmia neonatorum. *N Engl J Med* 332:562, 1995.

22 Laga M et al: Prophylaxis of gonococcal and chlamydial ophthalmia neonatorum: Silver nitrate versus tetracycline. *N Engl J Med* 318: 653, 1988.

23 Hammerschlag MR et al: Erythromycin ointment for ocular prophylaxis of neonatal chlamydial infection. *JAMA* 244:2291, 1980.

24 Chandler JW: Neonatal conjunctivitis, in *Duane's Clinical Ophthalmology,* W Tasman, EA Jaeger (eds). Philadelphia, Lippincott-Raven, 1955; vol 6, chap 6, pp 1–7.

25 Ullman S et al: Gonococcal keratoconjunctivitis. *Surv Ophthalmol* 32:199, 1987.

26 Whitley RJ et al: The natural history of herpes simplex virus infection of mother and newborn. *Pediatrics* 76:497, 1980.

27 Sandstrom KI et al: Microbiological causes of neonatal conjunctivitis. *J Pediatr* 105:706, 1984.

28 Pepose JS: Ophthalmic manifestations of HIV infection. *Curr Top AIDS* 2:191, 1989.

29 Stenson SM, Friedberg DN: *AIDS and the Eye.* New Orleans, Contact Lens Association of Ophthalmologists, Inc., 1995.

30 Orellana J, Lieberman RM, Teich SA: *Color Atlas of Ocular Manifestations of AIDS: Diagnosis and Management.* New York, Igaku-Shoin, 1995.

31 Freeman WR et al: Prevalence and significance of acquired immunodeficiency syndrome-related retinal microvasculopathy. *Am J Ophthalmol* 107:229, 1989.

32 Plummer DJ et al: Visual field loss in HIV-positive patients without infectious retinopathy. *Am J Ophthalmol* 122:542, 1996.

33 Quiceno JI et al: Visual dysfunction without retinitis in patients with acquired immunodeficiency syndrome. *Am J Ophthalmol* 113:8, 1992.

34 Tenhula WN et al: Optic nerve losses in AIDS: Morphometric comparisons. *Am J Ophthalmol* 113:14, 1992.

35 Pomerantz RJ et al: Infection of the retina by human immunodeficiency virus type I. *N Engl J Med* 317:1643, 1987.

36 Schmitt-Graff A et al: Evidence of cytomegalovirus and human immunodeficiency virus infection of the retina in AIDS. *Virchows Arch [A]* 416:249, 1990.

37 Whitcup SM et al: Retinal lesions in children treated with dideoxyinosine. *N Engl J Med* 326:1226, 1992.

38 Nguyen BY et al: A pilot study of sequential therapy with zidovudine plus acyclovir, dideoxyinosine, and dideoxycytidine in patients with severe human deficiency virus infection. *J Infect Dis* 168:810, 1993.

39 Whitcup SM et al: A clinicopathologic report of the retinal lesions associated with didanosine. *Arch Ophthalmol* 112:1594, 1994.

40 Shafran SD et al: Uveitis and pseudojaundice during a regimen of claritromycin, rifabutin, and ethambutol. *N Engl J Med* 330:438, 1994.

41 Saran BR et al: Hypopyon uveitis in patients with acquired immunodeficiency syndrome treated for systemic *Mycobacterium avium* complex infection with rifabutin. *Arch Ophthalmol* 112:1159, 1994.

42 Gallant JE et al: Incidence and natural history of cytomegalovirus disease in patients with advanced human immunodeficiency virus disease treated with zidovudine. *J Infect Dis* 166:1223, 1992.

43 Hoover DR et al: Occurrence of cytomegalovirus retinitis in human immunodeficiency virus immunosuppression. *Arch Ophthalmol* 114:821, 1996.

44 Kupfer C: General principles for AIDS research. *Arch Ophthalmol* 114:862, 1996.

45 The Studies of Ocular Complications of AIDS Research Group in Collaboration with the AIDS Clinical Trials Group: Assessment of cytomegalovirus retinitis: Clinical evaluation versus centralized grading of fundus photographs. *Arch Ophthalmol* 14:791, 1996.

46 Gross JG et al: Longitudinal study of cytomegalovirus retinitis in acquired immunodeficiency syndrome. *Ophthalmology* 97:681, 1990.

47 Jabs DA: Ocular manifestations of HIV infection. *Trans Am Ophthalmol Soc* 93:623, 1995.

48 The Studies of Ocular Complications of AIDS Research Group in Collaboration with the AIDS Clinical Trials Group: Foscarnet-ganciclovir cytomegalovirus retinitis trial: Visual outcomes. *Ophthalmology* 101:1250, 1994.

49 Jabs DA et al: Retinal detachments in patients with cytomegalovirus retinitis. *Arch Ophthalmol* 109:794, 1991.

50 Lim JL et al: Improved visual results after surgical repair of cytomegalovirus-related retinal detachments. *Ophthalmology* 101:264, 1994.

51 Kuppermann BD et al: A masked prospective evaluation of outcome parameters for cytomegalovirus-related retinal detachment surgery in patients with acquired immune deficiency syndrome. *Ophthalmology* 101:46, 1994.

52 Spector SA et al: A randomized, controlled study of intravenous ganciclovir therapy for cytomegalovirus peripheral retinitis in patients with AIDS. *J Infect Dis* 168:557, 1993.

53 The Studies of Ocular Complications of AIDS Research Group in Collaboration with the AIDS Clinical Trials Group: Mortality in patients with the acquired immunodeficiency syndrome treated with either foscarnet or ganciclovir for cytomegalovirus retinitis. *N Engl J Med* 326:213, 1992.

54 The Studies of Ocular Complications of AIDS Research Group in Collaboration with the AIDS Clinical Trials Group: Morbidity and toxic effects associated with ganciclovir or foscarnet therapy in a randomized cytomegalovirus retinitis trial. *Arch Intern Med* 155:65, 1995.

55 The Studies of Ocular Complications of AIDS Research Group in Collaboration with the AIDS Clinical Trials Group: Combination foscarnet and ganciclovir therapy vs monotherapy for the treatment of relapsed cytomegalovirus retinitis in patients with AIDS. *Arch Ophthalmol* 114:23, 1996.

56 Drews WL et al: Oral ganciclovir as maintenance treatment for cytomegalovirus retinitis in patients with AIDS. *N Engl J Med* 333:615, 1995.

57 The Oral Ganciclovir European and Australian Cooperative Study Group: European/Australian comparative study of efficacy and safety of oral ganciclovir in the prevention of cytomegalovirus retinitis recurrence in patients with AIDS. *AIDS* 59:471, 1995.

58 Ussery FM III et al: Intravitreal ganciclovir in the treatment of AIDS-associated cytomegalovirus retinitis. *Ophthalmology* 95:640, 1988.

59 Cantrill HL et al: Treatment of cytomegalovirus retinitis with intravitreal ganciclovir: Long-term results. *Ophthalmology* 96:367, 1989.

60 Heinemann MH: Long-term intravitreal ganciclovir therapy for cytomegalovirus retinopathy. *Arch Ophthalmol* 107:1767, 1989.

61 Cochereau-Massin I et al: Efficacy and tolerance of intravitreal ganciclovir in cytomegalovirus retinitis in acquired immune deficiency syndrome. *Ophthalmology* 98:1348, 1991.

62 Diaz-Llopis M et al: High-dose intravitreal foscarnet in the treatment of cytomegalovirus retinitis in AIDS. *Br J Ophthalmol* 78:120, 1994.

63 Engstrom RE Jr, Holland GN: Local therapy for cytomegalovirus retinopathy. *Am J Ophthalmol* 120:376, 1995.

64 Sanborn GE et al: Sustained-release ganciclovir therapy for treatment of cytomegalovirus retinitis: Use of an intravitreal device. *Arch Ophthalmol* 110:188, 1992.

65 Martin DF et al: Treatment of cytomegalovirus retinitis with an intraocular sustained-release ganciclovir implant: A randomized controlled clinical trial. *Arch Ophthalmol* 112:1531, 1994.

66 Kirsch LS et al: A phase I/II study of intravitreal cidofovir in the treatment of cytomegalovirus retinitis in patients with the acquired immunodeficiency syndrome. *Am J Ophthalmol* 119:466, 1995.

67 Anderson KP et al: Inhibition of human cytomegalovirus immediate-early gene expression by an antisense oligonucleotide complementary to immediate-early RNA. *Antimicrob Agents Chemother* 40:2004, 1966.

68 Azad RF et al: Antiviral activity of a phosphorothioate oligonucleotide complementary to RNA of the human cytomegalovirus major immediate-early region. *Antimicrob Agents Chemother* 37:1945, 1993.

69 Azad RF et al: Antiviral activity of a phosphorothioate oligonucleotide complementary to human cytomegalovirus RNA when used in combination with antiviral nucleoside analogs. *Antiviral Res* 28:101, 1995.

70 Palestine AG et al: Treatment of cytomegalovirus (CMV) retinitis with Isis 2922. *Invest Ophthalmol Vis Sci* 36:S181, 1995.

71 Pepose JS et al: Pathologic features of cytomegalovirus retinopathy after treatment with the antiviral agent ganciclovir. *Ophthalmology* 94:414, 1987.

72 Robinson MR et al: Molluscum contagiosum of the eyelids in patients with acquired immune deficiency syndrome. *Ophthalmology* 99:1745, 1992.

73 Charles NC, Friedberg DN: Epibulbar molluscum contagiosum in acquired immune deficiency syndrome. *Ophthalmology* 99:1123, 1992.

74 Shuler JD et al: Kaposi sarcoma of the conjunctiva and eyelids associated with the acquired immunodeficiency syndrome. *Arch Ophthalmol* 107:858, 1989.

75 Dugel PU et al: Ocular adnexal Kaposi's sarcoma in acquired immunodeficiency syndrome. *Am J Ophthalmol* 110:500, 1990.

76 Karp CL et al: Conjunctival intraepithelial neoplasia: A possible marker for human immunodeficiency virus infection. *Arch Ophthalmol* 114:257, 1996.

77 Muccioli C et al: Limbal and choroidal *Cryptococcus* infection in the acquired immunodeficiency syndrome. *Am J Ophthalmol* 120:539, 1995.

78 Geier SA et al: Sicca syndrome in patients infected with the human immunodeficiency virus. *Ophthalmology* 102:1319, 1995.

79 Lucca JA et al: Keratoconjunctivitis sicca in male patients infected with human immunodeficiency virus type I. *Ophthalmology* 97:1008, 1990.

80 Friedberg DN et al: Microsporidial keratoconjunctivitis in acquired immunodeficiency syndrome. *Arch Ophthalmol* 108:504, 1990.

81 Diesenhouse MC et al: Treatment of microsporidial keratoconjunctivitis with topical fumagillin. *Am J Ophthalmol* 115:293, 1993.

82 Young TI et al: Herpes simplex keratitis in patients with acquired immunodeficiency syndrome. *Ophthalmology* 96:1476, 1989.

83 Kestelyn P et al: Severe herpes zoster ophthalmicus in young African adults: A marker for HTLV-III seropositivity. *Br J Ophthalmol* 71: 806, 1987.

84 Engstrom RE, Holland GN: Chronic herpes zoster virus keratitis associated with the acquired immunodeficiency syndrome. *Am J Ophthalmol* 103:556, 1988.

85 Wilhelmus KR et al: Cytomegalovirus keratitis in acquired immunodeficiency syndrome. *Arch Ophthalmol* 114:869, 1996.

86 Stenson SM: Anterior segment manifestations of AIDS, in *AIDS and the Eye* SM Stenson, DN Friedberg (eds). New Orleans, Contact Lens Association of Ophthalmologists, Inc., 1995, chap 3, pp 35–63.

87 Wilhelmus KR et al: Corneal lipidosis in patients with the acquired immunodeficiency syndrome. *Am J Ophthalmol* 119:14, 1995.

88 Weiss A et al: Toxoplasmic retinochoroiditis as an initial manifestation of the acquired immunodeficiency syndrome. *Am J Ophthalmol* 101:248, 1986.

89 Holland GN et al: Ocular toxoplasmosis in patients with the acquired immunodeficiency syndrome. *Am J Ophthalmol* 106:653, 1988.

90 Cochereau-Massin I et al: Ocular toxoplasmosis in human immunodeficiency virus–infected patients. *Am J Ophthalmol* 114:130, 1992.

91 Berger B et al: Miliary toxoplasmic retinitis in acquired immunodeficiency syndrome. *Arch Ophthalmol* 111:373, 1993.

92 Shami MJ et al: A multicenter study of *Pneumocystis* choroidopathy. *Am J Ophthalmol* 112:15, 1991.

93 Koser MW et al: Treatment of *Pneumocystis carinii* choroidopathy. *Arch Ophthalmol* 108:1214, 1990.

94 Morinelli EN et al: Infectious multifocal choroiditis in patients with acquired immune deficiency syndrome. *Ophthalmology* 100:1014, 1993.

95 Carney MD et al: Cryptococcal choroiditis. *Retina* 10:27, 1990.

96 Becerra LI et al: Syphilitic uveitis in human immunodeficiency virus–infected and non-infected patients. *Ophthalmology* 96:1727, 1989.

97 Cunningham ET et al: Acquired immunodeficiency syndrome–associated herpes simplex virus retinitis: Clinical description and use of a polymerase chain reaction–based assay as a diagnostic tool. *Arch Ophthalmol* 114:834, 1996.

98 Kuppermann BD et al: Clinical and histological study of varicella zoster virus retinitis in patients with acquired immunodeficiency syndrome. *Am J Ophthalmol* 118:589, 1994.

99 Johnston WH et al: Recurrence of presumed varicella-zoster virus retinopathy in patients with acquired immunodeficiency syndrome. *Am J Ophthalmol* 116:42, 1993.

100 Sellitti TP et al: Association of herpes zoster ophthalmicus with acquired immunodeficiency syndrome and acute retinal necrosis. *Am J Ophthalmol* 116:297, 1993.

101 Engstrom RE et al: The progressive outer retinal necrosis syndrome: A variant of necrotizing retinopathy in patients with AIDS. *Ophthalmology* 101:1488, 1994.

102 Glascow BJ et al: Bilateral endogenous *Fusarium* endophthalmitis associated with acquired immunodeficiency syndrome. *Arch Ophthalmol* 114:873, 1996.

103 Schanzer MC et al: Primary ocular malignant lymphoma associated with the acquired immune deficiency syndrome. *Ophthalmology* 98: 88, 1991.

104 Stanton CA et al: Acquired immunodeficiency syndrome–related primary intraocular lymphoma. *Arch Ophthalmol* 110:1614, 1992.

105 Patel SS et al: Cytomegalovirus papillitis in patients with acquired immune deficiency syndrome. *Ophthalmology* 103:1476, 1996.

106 Yau TH et al: Unilateral optic neuritis caused by *Histoplasma capsulatum* in a patient with the acquired immunodeficiency syndrome. *Am J Ophthalmol* 121:324, 1996.

107 Cohen DB, Glascow BJ: Bilateral optic nerve cryptococcus in sudden blindness in a patient with acquired immunodeficiency syndrome. *Ophthalmology* 100:1689, 1993.

108 Kronish JW et al: Orbital infections in patients with human immunodeficiency virus infection. *Ophthalmology* 103:1483, 1966.

109 Matzkin DC et al: Simultaneous intraocular and orbital non-Hodgkin lymphoma in the acquired immune deficiency syndrome. *Ophthalmology* 101:850, 1994.

110 Reifler DM et al: Orbital lymphoma associated with acquired immune deficiency syndrome. *Surv Ophthalmol* 38:371, 1994.

Chapter 67

Treatment of chronic viral hepatitis

Ian Grimm
Nicholas Shaheen

INTRODUCTION

Prior to the development of interferon therapy in the mid-1980s, no drug had shown efficacy in treating chronic viral hepatitis. The demonstration that interferon alpha (IFN-α) could lead to a sustained remission in some patients with chronic hepatitis B and with non-A, non-B hepatitis (hepatitis C) was a major breakthrough in the treatment of liver disease. Today, IFN-α remains the only approved treatment for either chronic hepatitis B or hepatitis C. Unfortunately, not all affected patients are candidates for therapy, and many patients fail to respond to treatment. More effective approaches to treatment of chronic viral hepatitis are clearly needed.

The goals of therapy for chronic viral hepatitis are to terminate viral replication and to prevent the progression of chronic hepatic inflammation to fibrosis and end-stage liver disease. Approval of IFN-α therapy was based primarily on the drug's effect on intermediate markers of disease progression, such as serum aminotransferase levels and hepatic histology, but data regarding outcome measures such as morbidity and mortality from liver disease are scarce. Long-term follow-up will be required to assess the effect of IFN-α therapy on the development of cirrhosis, hepatocellular carcinoma, liver failure, or death.

This chapter summarizes current approaches to therapy in chronic viral hepatitis, focusing primarily on IFN-α. Because this is a rapidly evolving area, treatment recommendations are likely to change.

APPROACH TO THERAPY OF CHRONIC HEPATITIS

Chronic hepatitis is a syndrome defined by persistent necroinflammatory liver disease, typically lasting more than 6 months. In addition to the major viral causes—hepatitis B virus (HBV) and hepatitis C virus (HCV)—a diverse group of nonviral causes of chronic hepatitis must be considered in the differential diagnosis (Table 67-1). It is possible that additional, as yet unidentified, viral causes of chronic hepatitis exist. If so, these would account for only a small proportion of cases.

The histologic classification of chronic hepatitis has recently been revised to reflect advances in the understanding of the etiology and prognosis of chronic liver disease. Natural-history studies of HCV-infected patients have demonstrated that even a mild necroinflammatory lesion can eventually progress to cirrhosis. For this reason, older terms such as "chronic persistent" and "chronic active" hepatitis, which have prognostic implications, have been replaced with specific scales for grading necroinflammatory activity and for staging the degree of fibrosis present.[1]

The six-month definition of chronicity, while arbitrary, allows a reasonable time for spontaneous resolution of self-limited processes. In practice, nearly all patients diagnosed with hepatitis C have a chronic infection, particularly if a remote risk factor is identified. Acute hepatitis C is very rarely encountered, now that blood products are screened for antibodies to HCV. Patients with hepatitis B are likely to seek medical attention during a symptomatic flare of recurrent disease activity. Such an exacerbation of hepatitis can be a harbinger of spontaneous seroconversion and subsequent termination of the replicative state. Therefore, a six-month period of observation is advisable before recommending therapy for patients with chronic hepatitis B. Exacerbations of chronic hepatitis B can usually be distinguished from acute hepatitis B by the absence of IgM anti-HBc in chronic infection.

DIAGNOSIS

Chronic hepatitis is often discovered incidentally, with a positive serologic test during blood donation, or with elevated serum aminotransferase levels. Symptoms are frequently absent, even with advanced liver disease. Nonspecific complaints such as fatigue, weakness, or anorexia may occur, but these correlate poorly with the severity of the disease. Serologic diagnosis of chronic hepatitis B or hepatitis C is usually straightforward,but not all patients with persistently elevated aminotransferases and HBsAg or anti-HCV in serum have chronic hepatitis. An occasional patient with nonreplicative hepatitis B infection, or a false-positive serologic test for hepatitis C, may be mistakenly diagnosed with chronic viral hepatitis when his or her aminotransferase elevations are due to another cause, such as fatty liver or alcoholic liver disease. Because multiple potential causes of persistent liver inflammation or elevated serum aminotransferases can coexist, it is essential to arrive at a firm diagnosis before initiation of therapy. Thus, a liver biopsy and specific tests to document the presence of viremia (HBV-DNA, HCV-RNA) are often recommended prior to initiation of therapy. Consultation with a hepatologist is often appropriate.

IS A LIVER BIOPSY NECESSARY?

Previously, a liver biopsy had been considered essential before initiation of IFN-α therapy. With the recent development of accurate and sensitive assays for the presence of viremia (HBV-DNA, HCV-RNA), however, recommendations on pretreatment biopsies are now more variable. A liver biopsy prior to initiation of therapy allows for histologic confirmation of chronic viral hepatitis, and exclusion of other causes of liver inflammation. In addition, histologic grading and staging of hepatic inflammation and fibrosis are used to provide prognostic information and to establish the relative urgency for therapy. These benefits must be weighed against the costs and potential morbidity associated with the procedure. In patients with significant coagulopathy, such as hemophilia A, or coagulation defects associated with advanced liver disease, the risks of a biopsy may outweigh the benefit. In this situation, treatment without a biopsy may be appropriate.

The rationale behind performing a pretreatment liver biopsy may vary depending on the hepatitis virus involved. Some investigators feel that biopsies are unnecessary with chronic hepatitis B, because the decision to treat is not based on the histologic severity or stage of the disease. Rather, it is the presence of ongoing viral replication, and the associated risks of disease progression, hepatocellular carcinoma, and infectivity that provide the indication for therapy. By contrast, histologic criteria may play a greater role in guiding therapeutic recommendations for patients with chronic hepatitis C. Individuals with mild chronic hepatitis are more likely to respond to treatment with IFN-α than patients with cirrhosis. Once cirrhosis develops, IFN-α therapy appears to offer little benefit.

The availability of assays for the presence of viremia may di-

Table 67-1. Causes of Chronic Hepatitis

Viral
HCV
HBV ± HDV
Autoimmune liver disease
Drug-induced liver disease
Metabolic
Wilson's disease
alpha-1 anti-trypsin deficiency
hemochromatosis
Nonalcoholic steatohepatitis
Alcoholic liver disease

Table 67-2. Relative Contraindications to Interferon-α Therapy

Psychiatric
depression or suicidal ideation
other severe psychiatric disease
Hematologic
thrombocytopenia
leukopenia
Autoimmune
autoimmune hepatitis
other autoimmune diseases?
Cardiac
unstable angina
recent myocardial infarction
congestive heart failure
Pregnancy

minish the need for biopsies. Since antiviral therapy is indicated only for patients with ongoing viral replication, these markers provide a more rational basis for patient selection than surrogate markers such as serum aminotransferases or hepatic histology. While investigation continues in this area, most authorities continue to recommend a pretreatment liver biopsy.

BIOLOGY OF INTERFERONS

Despite many recent advances in understanding HBV and HCV, IFN-α remains the only approved treatment for these infections in the United States. Interferons are a group of naturally occurring cytokines that are released in response to viral infections. After binding to specific cell surface receptors, they induce profound antiviral, antiproliferative, and immunomodulatory effects. The viral life cycle is inhibited at several phases, including cell entry, uncoating, RNA synthesis, and protein synthesis. Induction of HLA class I antigens on the liver cell membrane by IFN-α promotes lysis of infected hepatocytes by CD8+ cytolytic lymphocytes.[2]

Many natural and recombinant interferons have been studied for the treatment of viral hepatitis. IFN-α and IFN-β both bind to the same cell receptor and thus have similar effects. Natural interferons (lymphoblastoid IFN, leukocyte IFN) and recombinant products of one or more IFN-α genes (r-IFN α_{2a}, r-IFN α_{2b}, r-IFN α_{2c}, consensus interferon) all appear to have similar efficacy in clinical trials.[2] Neutralizing antibodies to recombinant interferons may develop during therapy, and lead to loss of efficacy. Patients with chronic hepatitis C who develop a relapse during treatment with r-IFN α_{2a} are typically found to have IFN-α binding antibodies. Switching these individuals to natural lymphoblastoid interferon has been reported to rapidly restore a complete response.[3] Other studies have failed to find a significant correlation between the presence of neutralizing antibodies and a loss of IFN-α efficacy.

INITIATION OF INTERFERON-α THERAPY

CONTRAINDICATIONS

Depression and suicidal behavior have been reported in patients on IFN-α therapy, and therefore a history of a serious psychiatric disorder or depression is a relative contraindication to IFN-α. Patients with advanced liver disease and hypersplenism often have thrombocytopenia and leukopenia, which may limit tolerability of the drug. Other relative contraindications are listed in Table 67-2.

INTERFERON-α SIDE EFFECTS

Side effects of IFN-α therapy occur frequently, but most symptoms are tolerable (Table 67-3). Adverse effects are typically dose dependent and abate rapidly with reductions in dose or with temporary discontinuation. Only about 5 to 10 percent of patients need to stop IFN-α entirely.[4] Early side effects include fatigue, fever, chills, myalgias, and arthralgias. These flu-like symptoms occur almost universally after the first few doses,but administration at bedtime and use of acetaminophen help alleviate these effects, and they usually subside within several weeks. Fatigue and irritability are common late side effects. Dose reduction or discontinuation should be considered for significant neuropsychiatric side effects, or for symptoms that interfere with the patient's lifestyle. Bone marrow suppression and bacterial infections are potentially life threatening. Autoimmune thyroid disease develops in about 1 percent of patients and may be irreversible despite discontinuation of IFN-α.

MONITORING INTERFERON-α THERAPY

Regular follow-up visits are recommended to monitor for side effects and to obtain complete blood counts and liver tests. Visits are typically scheduled after the first and second weeks of therapy, and monthly thereafter. Dose reduction should be considered for platelet counts below 50,000/mL or granulocyte counts below 750/mL. For platelets less than 30,000/mL or granulocytes below 500/mL, treatment should be interrupted until counts return to their baseline levels. Thyroid-stimulating hormone (TSH) levels should be checked at baseline and every 3 to 6 months on therapy.

THERAPY OF CHRONIC HEPATITIS B

INTRODUCTION

Chronic hepatitis B is a major cause of cirrhosis and hepatocellular carcinoma worldwide. Thirty to 40 percent of patients with

Table 67-3. Side Effects of Interferon-α Therapy

Early	Late
Fever, chills, myalgias, fatigue, anorexia, nausea, arthralgias, headache, insomnia, seizures, hypotension, confusion	Fatigue, irritability, difficulty concentrating, depression, weight loss, hair loss, infections, myelosuppression, peripheral neuropathy, interstitial pneumonitis, retinopathy, thyroid disease, autoantibody production

persistent liver inflammation will progress to cirrhosis. Progressive liver injury occurs most rapidly during the phase of active viral replication, marked by the presence in serum of hepatitis B e antigen (HBeAg) and HBV-DNA. Many individuals with chronic hepatitis B eventually experience a spontaneous cessation of viral replication, which is followed by a histologic and biochemical remission of disease. Spontaneous clearance of HBV-DNA (by hybridization assay) and HBeAg from serum, with seroconversion to anti-HBe, occurs at a rate of 10–25 percent per year. Termination of viral replication is associated with a significant improvement in survival, even in patients with cirrhosis.[5,6] IFN-α therapy appears to hasten the rate of loss of viral replication. As with spontaneous remissions, successful IFN-α therapy leads to the loss of markers of viral replication, followed by biochemical and histologic improvement.

Table 67-4. Indications for Interferon-α Therapy of Chronic Hepatitis B

Chronicity (>6 months)
Elevated serum aminotransferases, and Serum HBsAG +
and
Viral Replication
HBeAG + (except in precore mutants), and/or
HBV-DNA + by hybridization assay
and
Compensated Liver Function
No ascites, encephalopathy, or variceal bleeding, and
Normal serum albumin and bilirubin, and
PT < 3 seconds prolonged

RESULTS OF CLINICAL TRIALS WITH INTERFERON-α

A recent meta-analysis of 15 randomized controlled studies (837 patients) concluded that about one-third of patients treated with IFN-α have a favorable outcome, defined as a sustained disappearance of HBeAg and HBV-DNA from serum. Loss of these markers of viral replication occurred significantly more often in those receiving IFN-α than in controls (33 percent versus 12 percent for loss of HBeAg, and 37 percent versus 17 percent for the loss of HBV-DNA). The absolute difference for disappearance of markers of viral replication was about 20 percent, indicating that only one of five patients benefited from treatment.[4] Higher IFN-α doses were more effective, but they were also associated with more side effects.

Because the pretreatment host characteristics associated with a response to IFN-α—such as a history of acute hepatitis, high alanine aminotransferase (ALT) levels, and low levels of HBV-DNA (see below)—are the same characteristics associated with spontaneous seroconversion, it is conceivable that many individuals who "responded" to IFN-α would have had the same eventual outcome without therapy. After adjusting for the effect of pretreatment variables on IFN-α response rates, a meta-analysis of 10 European trials (751 patients) found that the effect of treatment was less than previously assumed. The rate of disappearance of HBeAg in treated patients was increased, but only by a factor of 1.76.[7]

Long-term outcomes following IFN-α therapy have been analyzed retrospectively in a cohort of 103 patients followed for a mean of 5 years after treatment.[8] Cumulative clearance of HBeAg was estimated to be 56.0 percent after 5 years in IFN-α–treated patients, compared to 28.1 percent in a nonrandomized group of controls. Six of the treated patients died of liver failure, and two required liver transplantation; all eight had remained persistently positive for HBeAg. In contrast, none of the patients who lost HBeAg developed severe complications of cirrhosis or required transplantation. Overall survival, and survival without complications of cirrhosis, were significantly greater in patients who lost HBeAg following therapy. These data strongly suggest that IFN-α therapy improves the outcome of patients with chronic hepatitis B, even in the presence of cirrhosis.

PATIENT SELECTION FOR INTERFERON-α THERAPY

The decision to treat a patient with chronic hepatitis B is generally straightforward. Virtually all patients with compensated liver function who have had persistent elevation of serum aminotransferases and ongoing HBV replication should be considered candidates for therapy (Table 67-4). The risks of disease transmission and development of hepatocellular carcinoma in individuals with long-standing HBV infection provide a rationale for treatment regardless of the presence of symptoms or the degree of necroinflammatory activity on biopsy. Even patients with mild histologic liver injury are susceptible to spontaneous exacerbations and disease progression, and thus they should be treated. Carriers of hepatitis B surface antigen with persistently normal aminotransferase levels should not be treated. In the Western world, these individuals have an excellent prognosis and do not require therapy unless there is a reactivation of disease.[9] In general, patients with advanced cirrhosis or decompensated liver disease should not be treated with IFN-α.

PREDICTORS OF RESPONSE

Several patient characteristics correlate with the probability of success with IFN-α therapy (Table 67-5). Individuals with high aminotransferase levels, active liver disease, and relatively low levels of replicating virus in serum respond more frequently, presumably because these features are associated with a greater immune response to HBV infection. Poorer results are seen in patients with disease acquired during early childhood and in patients from areas of the world where perinatal transmission is common. Individuals infected early in life with HBV appear to have immune tolerance to the virus, often associated with very high levels of viral replication but normal aminotransferases and minimal necroinflammatory activity on biopsy. Patients with this pattern rarely respond to IFN-α. Similarly, treatment of individuals who are

Table 67-5. Factors Associated with Response to Interferon-α for Chronic Hepatitis B

Positive Predictors
HBV-DNA < 100 pg/mL
ALT > 100 IU/l
Active hepatitis on biopsy
Absence of HIV infection
Short duration of infection
History of acute hepatitis
Female sex
Negative Predictors
HBV-DNA > 200 pg/mL
ALT < 100 IU/l
Minimal inflammation on biopsy
Co-infection with HIV, HDV
Acquisition of HBV early in life
Immunosuppression

immunocompromised is rarely successful. In patients with favorable treatment characteristics, especially those with marked aminotransferase elevations, response rates of greater than 50 percent can be expected.

PRESCRIBING INTERFERON-α FOR HEPATITIS B

Recommended therapy consists of 5 million units of IFN-α daily, administered subcutaneously for 4 months. Alternatively, 10 MU of IFN-α can be administered three times weekly with equal efficacy. Larger doses appear to be marginally more effective, but they probably do not warrant the additional cost and side effects.[4] Pretreatment with a tapering dose of corticosteroids may induce an immunologic response to HBV antigens associated with elevations of ALT ("immunologic rebound") and may improve response rates in patients with low ALT levels.[10] This approach remains controversial, however, and is not recommended.[11]

PATTERNS OF RESPONSE TO INTERFERON-α THERAPY

An exacerbation of liver disease, with increases in serum aminotransferases to more than twice the baseline level, may occur during the second or third month of therapy. This flare-up is seen in up to two-thirds of responders and in about one-third of nonresponders. It is believed to indicate lysis of infected hepatocytes by an activated immune system, and it often precedes loss of HBV-DNA. Typically this "seroconversion hepatitis" is asymptomatic. It should be regarded as a favorable sign and should not prompt discontinuation of therapy, unless significant hepatic dysfunction occurs. Following the loss of HBV-DNA from serum (by hybridization assay), most responders have a clearance of HBeAg, seroconversion to anti-HBeAg, and eventual improvement in liver histology. All of these endpoints occur in 80–90 percent of responders, though loss of HBeAg may be delayed for several months following discontinuation of IFN-α.[12] Re-treatment of nonresponders is rarely effective. Only about 5–10 percent of responders lose HBsAg from serum in the first year after therapy with IFN-α. In a long-term follow-up study in the United States, however, 65 percent of patients who lost HBeAg eventually lost HBsAg a mean of 3 years later.[13] In endemic areas, rates of loss of HBsAg have been much lower.[14,15]

IFN-α responders can expect a durable remission of liver disease. Relapse may occur in 13–16 percent of patients, typically in the first year following therapy.[14] As long as HBsAg persists in serum, minute quantities of HBV-DNA are usually also detectable by the polymerase chain reaction (PCR). Following the disappearance of both HBsAg and HBV-DNA by PCR from serum, HBV-DNA may still be detectable in liver and in peripheral blood mononuclear cells. Thus, a potential for late relapse remains, especially in the setting of immunosuppression or chemotherapy.

SPECIAL PATIENT CATEGORIES

Hepatitis B Cirrhosis

Most studies of IFN-α for chronic hepatitis B have excluded patients with evidence of advanced cirrhosis, such as jaundice, hepatic synthetic dysfunction, ascites, encephalopathy, or variceal hemorrhage. Prescribing IFN-α for individuals with marginal liver function is hazardous, because seroconversion hepatitis can lead to decompensation and liver failure. Furthermore, these patients are susceptible to life-threatening infections and intolerable IFN-α side effects. These patients should generally be managed by experienced hepatologists at centers providing liver transplantation. Nonetheless, some Child's class A and B cirrhotics have been successfully treated with low-dose IFN-α, resulting in stabilization of disease and improved survival over nonresponders.[16,17] The nucleoside analogs lamivudine and famciclovir appear to be well tolerated in decompensated cirrhosis and may prove to be a safer alternative.

Precore mutants and delta hepatitis

The absence of detectable HBeAg in a patient who has high levels of serum HBV-DNA suggests the presence of a precore mutant, an HBV strain with a mutation in the upstream HBeAg reading frame that blocks the synthesis of HBeAg. These strains—which are often associated with severe liver disease—are prevalent in Mediterranean countries but are uncommon in the United States. Up to 50 percent of patients respond to IFN-α, but relapse rates are high.[2] Treatment of patients superinfected with the hepatitis delta virus (HDV) with high doses of IFN-α may lead to a gradual normalization of aminotransferase levels in up to one-half of treated patients. With cessation of therapy, however, relapse is also frequent.[18] Nonetheless, IFN-α therapy is generally advocated for delta hepatitis, as it is often rapidly progressive without therapy.

Human immunodeficiency virus co-infection

Because HBV and the human immunodeficency virus (HIV) share routes of transmission, coinfection with both viruses may occur in as many as 10 percent of HIV-infected individuals. Although responses to IFN-α are possible if CD4 counts are well preserved, a high level of HBV replication is common in the setting of immunosuppression, and responses to IFN-α are generally poor. Administration of lamivudine at doses of 300 to 600 mg daily as therapy for HIV infection markedly suppresses serum HBV-DNA to undetectable levels. During continued therapy for up to 1 year, breakthrough of viral replication appears uncommon. Mean ALT levels decline significantly, but the effect on disease progression has not been determined.[19] Thus, lamivudine should be included in HIV antiviral therapy for individuals co-infected with HBV.

OTHER ANTIVIRALS FOR CHRONIC HEPATITIS B

Many agents have been studied as possible treatments for chronic hepatitis B and have been found wanting. Recent progress in the development of animal models and cell culture systems for studying HBV replication has facilitated the identification of nucleoside analogs with activity against hepatitis B. The most promising of these agents are lamivudine and famciclovir. In addition, several newer and more potent inhibitors of the HBV reverse transcriptase have been identified in preclinical studies. Lamivudine (3-thiacytidine) is a potent inhibitor of HBV replication that causes termination of the nascent proviral DNA chain. During short-term therapy, HBV-DNA rapidly becomes undetectable in serum, but it rebounds promptly after discontinuation of the drug. In a three-month study, oral doses of either 100 or 300 mg daily led to a sustained suppression of HBV-DNA in 27 percent of patients, and loss of HBeAg in 18 percent.[20] Retreatment of nonresponders with 100 mg of lamivudine daily for up to 60 weeks resulted in a cumulative loss of HBeAg in an additional 39 percent of patients.[21] Mean ALT levels decline, and preliminary data suggest that liver histology improves during therapy.[22]

Sustained lamivudine therapy is well tolerated, but resistance to HBV may develop, resulting in a return of HBV-DNA levels. Mutations in the active site of the HBV polymerase account for the development of resistance.[23] Issues regarding the optimal duration of lamivudine therapy and the effect of combination therapy with IFN-α are under investigation. Pending the results of these studies and approval from the Food and Drug Administration (FDA), patients with serious liver disease and ongoing HBV replication who are not candidates for IFN-α or who have failed to respond to it should generally be offered enrollment in lamivudine treatment trials.

Famciclovir is a nucleoside analog developed to treat herpes viruses that also has activity against HBV. It is well tolerated, even in decompensated liver disease, but it may be less effective than lamivudine in suppressing viral replication.

No information is yet available concerning the cross resistance of HBV strains to different nucleoside analogs, but (as with HIV) it seems likely that combinations of antiviral therapies may prove most effective. Such combinations might include IFN-α.

SUMMARY

Treatment of chronic hepatitis B has advanced substantially in recent years. While there are still many patients who are not candidates for IFN-α therapy, or who fail to respond to treatment, at least one-third of treated patients enter a sustained remission, associated with a marked improvement in liver histology. The development of safe and effective oral nucleoside analogs that can chronically suppress HBV replication represents a major milestone in HBV therapy.

THERAPY FOR CHRONIC HEPATITIS C

INTRODUCTION

In contrast to hepatitis B, treatment strategies for hepatitis C are less well defined. IFN-α, the only approved treatment, usually fails to induce a sustained virologic remission. Selection of candidates for treatment is difficult, in part because the disease is indolent, and because its course is highly variable. Furthermore, clinicians differ widely in their views regarding IFN-α therapy and patients vary in their willingness to receive it. As additional data become available, treatment recommendations will continue to evolve.

RESULTS OF CLINICAL TRIALS WITH INTERFERON-α

The efficacy of IFN-α for treating transfusion-associated non-A, non-B hepatitis was demonstrated prior to the cloning of the HCV genome in 1989. Initial results led to a large controlled trial in which 46 percent of patients had a normalization or near-normalization of serum aminotransferase levels after treatment with 3 MU of IFN-α, three times weekly for 6 months.[24] This became the FDA-approved regimen. In a meta-analysis of numerous subsequent controlled trials, 45 percent of patients receiving this treatment were found to have had a complete response, defined as normalization of serum aminotransferase levels at the conclusion of 6 months of IFN-α therapy, while 55 percent had histological improvement.[25] Control subjects rarely improved. Unfortunately, sustained response rates, defined as persistently normal serum aminotransferase levels 6 months after completion of therapy, were only 21 percent.[25] Since about one-fourth of these sustained responders have persistence of HCV-RNA in serum, only about 15 percent of patients have a sustained virologic remission.[26]

These poor response rates have led investigators to increase both the dose and the duration of IFN-α therapy. Larger IFN-α doses do not substantially improve initial response rates, although sustained response rates are marginally better.[25,27] Unfortunately, the greater incidence of side effects requiring dose reduction limits this approach to therapy.[27] In contrast, prolongation of therapy from 6 to 12 months is associated with a 16-percent increase in sustained response rates.[25] These data suggest that therapy should be extended to 12, or even 18, months for patients who have an initial response.[28]

Long-term outcomes of IFN-α therapy have not been well studied, and it is unclear whether IFN-α can delay the development of hepatic fibrosis or hepatocellular carcinoma. One large trial showed that the incidence of cirrhosis was diminished in patients receiving prolonged therapy (18 versus 6 months), but this difference was not statistically significant.[28] Mortality has not been evaluated as an endpoint in clinical trials, in large part because the disease has such an indolent natural history. One large, retrospective study found that IFN-α therapy did not affect longevity among compensated cirrhotics with hepatitis C, compared to untreated patients.[29] Treatment of late-stage disease does not appear to improve survival.

PREDICTORS OF RESPONSE

Several pretreatment host factors are associated with increased rates of response to IFN-α therapy (Table 67-6). Younger age, lower serum HCV-RNA levels, HCV genotypes 2 or 3, shorter duration of infection, milder histologic lesions, and smaller body weight are positive prognostic indicators,[30–32] whereas high hepatic iron concentration, HCV genotypes 1a or 1b, and cirrhosis are negative indicators.[33,34] Of these variables, pretreatment levels of serum HCV-RNA and viral genotype appear to be the strongest independent predictors of sustained response.[30] Viral genotypes 1a and 1b, which together account for more than 70 percent of infected patients in the United States, show sustained response rates of less than 10 percent, whereas rates for genotypes 2 and 3 are more than 40 percent. While these factors are predictive of overall response rates, there is too much variability in individual responses to use any single predictor to exclude patients from treatment. The role of viral genotyping and quantification of viral load in selection of candidates for treatment remains unclear.

PATTERNS OF RESPONSE TO INTERFERON-α THERAPY

In patients who respond to therapy with IFN-α, there is typically a prompt decline in serum aminotransferases and HCV-RNA lev-

Table 67-6. Factors Associated with Response to Interferon-α for Chronic Hepatitis C

Positive Predictors
Low serum HCV-RNA levels
HCV genotypes 2, 3
Inflammation confined to portal tracts
Lower body weight
Short duration of infection
Negative Predictors
HCV genotype 1
Increased hepatic iron content
Co-infection with HIV?
Cirrhosis

Table 67-7. Efficacy of Interferon-α Therapy for Chronic Viral Hepatitis

	Hepatitis B	Hepatitis C
Initial response rate	40%	45%
Histologic improvement	most responders	55%
Relapse rate after IFN-α	13–16%	50–70%
No viremia after 1 year	35%	15–20%
Long-term remission	35%	few data
Improved natural history	probable	few data

els. Approximately 85 percent of patients who eventually respond have normalization of ALT levels by 8–12 weeks of therapy.[24] Unlike with HBV, an increase in aminotransferase levels shortly after initiation of IFN-α is not characteristic of HCV infection. Such a response should lead to discontinuation of therapy and a search for evidence of autoimmune hepatitis. Failure to attain complete normalization of aminotransferase levels is typically associated with persistence of viremia, and these patients are considered nonresponders. Similarly, an elevation of serum aminotransferase levels following an initial normalization indicates a resurgence of viremia.

Biochemical remission of hepatitis during IFN-α therapy has been shown to correlate well with histologic improvement, characterized by a reduction in lobular and periportal inflammation. A sustained normalization of ALT levels during therapy does not always indicate a virologic remission, however, as evidenced by the high relapse rate following discontinuation of IFN-α. Even individuals with persistently normal aminotransferase levels following IFN-α are at risk for late relapse. Up to one-fourth of such patients have persistence of HCV viremia by PCR, and many ultimately relapse.[26] Individuals with a negative HCV-RNA by PCR 12 months after completion of therapy appear to be cured; sustained remissions of greater than 5 years have been reported.[35] Late relapses have been observed even in these patients, however.[36]

PATIENT SELECTION FOR INTERFERON-α THERAPY

Consideration of IFN-α therapy is appropriate in all patients with persistently elevated aminotransferase levels and evidence of active HCV infection. Individuals with normal aminotransferase levels have poor response rates, and treatment is not currently recommended.[37] The decision to initiate therapy should be based on a candid discussion with the patient regarding the natural history of his or her disease, as well as the risks, contraindications, and benefits of IFN-α therapy. In addition to viral load and genotype, the patient's age, general health status, and the stage of fibrosis on biopsy are important. Symptoms of chronic hepatitis do not correlate with disease severity or prognosis and should not be used as a guide to treatment. Though initial efforts at treatment were focused on patients with severe chronic hepatitis on biopsy, patients with mild degrees of inflammation and no fibrosis on liver biopsy respond best to IFN-α therapy. Once cirrhosis has developed, IFN-α appears to have little effect on the course of the disease and rarely leads to a virologic remission. Young patients have the most potential life-years at stake, and treatment of this subgroup of patients may be most cost-effective.[38] Consideration of liver transplantation should not be postponed in favor of IFN-α therapy in the cirrhotic patient with decompensation.

PRESCRIBING INTERFERON-α FOR HEPATITIS C

The FDA-approved regimen of IFN-α for HCV is 3 MU given by subcutaneous injection three times a week for 6 to 12 months. Aminotransferase levels are the traditional means for monitoring therapy, but discrepancies between biochemical and virologic responses are not uncommon. Clearly, virologic markers provide a more accurate indication of the initial response to IFN-α and allow for earlier recognition of relapse; however, the appropriateness of using virologic markers to monitor and guide therapy remains controversial. An appropriate management strategy is to assess patients for a response to IFN-α therapy at 12 weeks by ALT or HCV-RNA PCR, and to continue those who have elimination of viral RNA or normalization of ALT on at least a 12-month course of IFN-α therapy.[25] There appears to be little benefit to increasing the IFN-α dose in individuals who have failed to demonstrate a response at 12 weeks of therapy. One study that assessed this issue found that 12 percent of patients responded after dose escalation to 5 or 10 MU, but none of these individuals had a sustained response.[27] Thus, dose escalation is unlikely to change long-term outcomes in initial nonresponders.

The appropriate treatment of patients who relapse after initial response to IFN-α therapy is not clear. Re-treatment with another 6–12 months of IFN-α may induce a second response in patients who had a transient viral clearance; however, relapse is likely to occur on withdrawal of the drug.[39] Few data justify continuing IFN-α in nonresponders. Although long-term therapy is associated with significant histologic improvement in the majority of treated patients, regardless of the persistence of viremia, insufficient data exist to advocate using IFN-α as a chronic suppressive therapy, outside of clinical trials. Conflicting data exist as to whether IFN-α therapy lowers the subsequent risk of hepatocellular carcinoma.[29,40] If cancer rates in treated patients are truly lower, this could provide an additional rationale for therapy.

COINFECTION WITH HIV OR HBV

There are few data on the natural history or appropriate treatment for HCV patients co-infected with either HIV or HBV. It appears that concurrent HIV disease portends a more aggressive course, especially in those with declining CD4 counts, as evidenced by cohort studies of both IV drug abusers[41] and hemophiliacs.[42] Additionally, patients with HCV and HIV have significantly higher viral loads than those with HCV alone.[43] Data concerning response to IFN-α therapy in patients with HCV/HIV co-infection are also scarce. One small trial suggests that response to IFN-α in co-infected patients was similar to that seen with HCV alone.[44] Alarming reports do exist, however, of rapid decline in CD4 counts after the initiation of IFN-α therapy.[45] While treatment of patients with early HIV infection may be reasonable, in later stages of HIV disease the potential benefits of IFN-α therapy decline.

Concomitant HCV infection occurs frequently in patients with chronic active hepatitis B, and liver disease may be more severe in co-infected individuals than those infected with a single virus.[46] Co-infection may lead to the suppression of one virus such that replication of the suppressed virus cannot be detected.[47] Both HCV and HBV viral loads should be measured prior to therapy in the co-infected patient. The specific IFN-α regimen should be targeted against the infection that is most active.

ACUTE HEPATITIS C INFECTION

Several studies suggest that IFN-α is effective in normalizing serum aminotransferase levels and in decreasing the rate of chronic infection after acute posttransfusion infection with hepatitis C. Meta-analysis of these trials demonstrated an increase in HCV-RNA clearance from 4 percent in controls to 41 percent in treated subjects.[25] Based on this study, patients with acute hepatitis C should receive 3 MU of IFN-α three times weekly for at least 3 months.

OTHER APPROACHES TO TREATING HEPATITIS C

A variety of agents has been tested for use in HCV, either alone or in combination with IFN-α, including corticosteroids, prednisone, nonsteroidal anti-inflammatory drugs (NSAIDS), acyclovir, ursodeoxycholic acid, and ribavirin. Although some of these drugs have shown promise in initial trials, none has emerged as a viable single-agent treatment strategy for HCV. The combination of IFN-α and ribavirin, however, appears more effective than IFN-α alone, based on several small trials. This combination led to a sustained response in 40 percent of patients who had previously failed or relapsed after initial IFN-α monotherapy,[48] and it appears to be about twice as effective as IFN-α alone as an initial treatment strategy.[49] Practice recommendations will be based on large trials in progress. The structure of the HCV protease enzyme has recently been elucidated.[50,51] This breakthrough should be able to facilitate development of more specific anti-HCV chemotherapeutic agents.

SUMMARY

IFN-α is currently the only approved treatment for chronic hepatitis C infection. Though results with this agent are often disappointing, a trial of therapy should be considered for all candidates, especially those with early-stage disease. Treatment of chronic hepatitis C prior to the development of significant fibrosis is probably necessary if the natural history of this condition is to be altered. Patient selection and treatment strategies continue to evolve as additional data become available. While the focus of current clinical research is on combination therapies, major therapeutic advances will likely require development of novel antiviral compounds.

References

1 Desmet VJ, Gerber M, Hoofnagle JH, et al: Classification of chronic hepatitis; diagnosis, grading and staging. *Hepatology* 19:513–20, 1994.

2 Wong DKH, Heathcote J: The role of interferon in the treatment of viral hepatitis. *Pharmacol Ther* 63:177–86,1994.

3 Roffi L, Colloredo G, Antonelli G, et al: Breakthrough during recombinant interferon alfa therapy in patients with chronic hepatitis C virus infection: Prevalence, etiology, and management. *Hepatology* 21:645–49, 1995.

4 Wong DKH, Cheung AM, O'Rourke K, et al: Effect of alpha interferon treatment in patients with hepatitis e antigen-positive chronic hepatitis B. A meta-analysis. *Ann Intern Med* 119:312–23, 1993.

5 De Jongh FE, Janssen LA, De Man RA, et al: Survival and prognostic indicators in hepatitis B surface antigen-positive cirrhosis of the liver. *Gastroenterology* 103:1630–35, 1992.

6 Realdi G, Fattovich G, Hadziyannis S, et al: Survival and prognostic factors in 366 patients with compensated cirrhosis type B: A multicenter study. *J Hepatol* 21:656–66, 1994.

7 Krogsgaard K, Bindslev N, Christensen E, et al: The European Concerted Action on Viral Hepatitis (Eurohep). The treatment effect of alpha interferon in chronic hepatitis B is independent of pre-treatment variables. Results based on individual patient data from 10 clinical controlled trials. *J Hepatol* 21:646–55, 1994.

8 Niederau C, Heintges T, Lange S, et al: Long-term follow-up of HBeAg positive patients treated with interferon alfa for chronic hepatitis B. *N Engl J Med* 334:1422–27, 1996.

9 de Franchis R, Meucci G, Vecchi M, et al: The natural history of asymptomatic hepatitis B surface antigen carriers. *Ann Intern Med* 118:191–94, 1993.

10 Perrillo RP, Schiff ER, Davis GL, et al: A randomized, controlled trial of interferon alfa-2b alone and after prednisone withdrawal for the treatment of chronic hepatitis B. *N Engl J Med* 323:295–301, 1990.

11 Krogsgaard K: Does corticosteroid pretreatment enhance the effect of alfa interferon treatment in chronic hepatitis B? *J Hepatol* 24:159–62, 1994.

12 Carreno V, Bartolome J, Castillo I: Long-term effect of interferon therapy in chronic hepatitis B. *J Hepatol* 20:431–35, 1994.

13 Korenman J, Baker B, Waggoner J, et al: Long-term remission of chronic hepatitis B after alpha-interferon therapy. *Ann Intern Med* 114:629–34, 1991.

14 Carreno V, Castillo I, Molina J, et al: Long-term follow-up of hepatitis B carriers who respond to interferon therapy. *J Hepatol* 15:102–106, 1992.

15 Lok AS, Chung H-T, Liu VWS, et al: Long-term follow-up of chronic hepatitis B patients treated with interferon alfa. *Gastroenterology* 105: 1833–38, 1993.

16 Perrillo R, Tamburro C, Regenstein F, et al: Low dose, titratable interferon alfa in decompensated liver disease caused by chronic infection with hepatitis B virus. *Gastroenterology* 109:908–16, 1995.

17 Hoofnagle JH, DiBisceglie AM, Waggoner JG, et al: Interferon alpha for patients with clinically apparent cirrhosis due to chronic hepatitis B. *Gastroenterology* 104:1116–21, 1993.

18 Farci P, Mandas A, Coina A, et al: Treatment of chronic hepatitis D with interferon alfa-2a. *N Engl J Med* 330:88–94, 1994.

19 Benhamou Y, Katlama C, Lunel F, et al: Effects of lamivudine on replication of hepatitis B virus in HIV-infected men. *Ann Intern Med* 125: 705–12, 1996.

20 Dienstag JL, Perrillo RP, Schiff ER, et al: A preliminary trial of lamivudine for chronic hepatitis B infection. *N Engl J Med* 333:1657–61, 1995.

21 Dienstag JL, Schiff ER, Mitchell M, et al: Extended lamivudine retreatment for chronic hepatitis B. *Hepatology* 24:188A, 1996.

22 Honkoop P, De Man RA, Zondervan PE, et al: Histological improvement in patients with chronic hepatitis B infection treated with lamivudine is associated with a decrease in HBV DNA by PCR. *Hepatology* 22:328A, 1995.

23 Ling R, Mutimer D, Ahmed M, et al: Selection of mutations in the Hepatitis B virus polymerase during therapy of transplant recipients with lamivudine. *Hepatology* 24:711–13, 1996.

24 Davis GL, Balart LA, Schiff E, et al: Treatment of chronic hepatitis C with recombinant interferon alfa: A multicenter randomized controlled trial. *N Engl J Med* 321:1501–1506, 1989.

25 Poynard T, Leroy V, Cohard M, et al: Meta-analysis of interferon randomized trials in the treatment of viral hepatitis C: Effects of dose and duration. *Hepatology* 24:778–89, 1996.

26 Chemello L, Cavalletto L, Casarin C, et al: Persistent hepatitis C viremia predicts late relapse after sustained response to interferon-α in chronic hepatitis C. *Ann Intern Med* 124:1058–60, 1996.

27 Lindsay KL, Davis GL, Schiff ER, et al: Response to higher doses of interferon alfa 2-b in patients with chronic hepatitis C: A randomized multicenter trial. *Hepatology* 24:1034–40, 1996.

28 Poynard T, Bedossa P, Chevallier M, et al: A comparison of three interferon alph-2b regimens for the long-term treatment of chronic non-A, non-B hepatitis. *N Engl J Med* 332:1457–62, 1995.

29 Fattovich G, Giustina G, Degos F, et al: Morbidity and mortality in compensated cirrhosis type C: A retrospective follow-up study of 384 patients. *Gastroenterology* 112:463–72, 1997.

30 Tsubota A, Chayama K, Ikeda K, et al: Factors predictive of response to interferon-alpha therapy in hepatitis C virus infection. *Hepatology* 19:1088–94, 1994.

31 Hino K, Sainokami S, Shimoda K, et al: Genotypes and titers of hepatitis C virus for predicting response to interferon in patients with chronic hepatitis C. *J Med Virol* 1994:42: 299–305.

32 Causse X, Godinot H, Chevallier M, et al: Comparison of 1 or 3 MU of interferon alpha-2b and placebo in patients with chronic non-A, non-B hepatitis. *Gastroenterology* 101:497–502, 1991.

33 Jouet P, Roudot-Thraval F, Dhumeaux D, et al: Comparative efficacy of interferon alpha in cirrhotic and noncirrhotic patients with non-A, non-B, C hepatitis. *Gastroenterology* 106:686–90, 1994.

34 Pagliaro L, Craxi A, Cammaa C, et al: Interferon-alpha for chronic hepatitis C: An analysis of pretreatment clinical predictors of response. *Hepatology* 19:820–28, 1994.

35 Shindo M, Di Bisceglie AM, Hoofnagle JH: Long-term follow-up of patients with chronic hepatitis C treated with α-interferon. *Hepatology* 15:1013–16, 1992.

36 Vento S, Cainelli F, Concia E, et al: Lack of sustained efficacy of interferon alpha in patients with chronic hepatitis C. *Hepatology* 24: 163A, 1996.

37 Serfaty L, Chazouilleres O, Pawlotsky J-M, et al: Interferon alfa therapy in patients with chronic hepatitis C and persistently normal aminotransferase activity. *Gastroenterology* 110:291–95, 1996.

38 Bennett WG, Inoue Y, Beck JR et al: Justification of a single six month course of interferon (IFN) for histologically mild chronic hepatitis C. *Hepatology* 22:A290, 1995.

39 Marcellin P, Boyer N, Pouteau M et al: Retreatment with interferon-α of chronic hepatitis C virus infection. *Lancet* 344:690–91, 1994.

40 Nishigushi S, Kuroki T, Nakatani S et al: Randomised trial of effects of interferon-α on incidence of hepatocellular carcinoma in chronic active hepatitis C with cirrhosis. *Lancet* 346:1051–55, 1995.

41 Di Martino V, Rufat P, Martinot M, et al: Influence of HIV infection on the outcome of chronic hepatitis C. *Hepatology* 24:382A, 1996.

42 Rockstroh KJ, Spengler U, Sudhop T, et al: Immunosuppression may lead to progression of hepatitis C virus-associated liver disease in hemophiliacs coinfected with HIV. *Am J Gastroenterol* 91:2563–68, 1996.

43 Bonacini M, Govindarajan S, Russell J, et al: Intrahepatic viral load in patients with hepatitis C with and without HIV infection. *Hepatology* 24:388A, 1996.

44 Boyer N, Marcellin P, Degott C, et al: Recombinant interferon-alpha for chronic hepatitis C in patients positive for antibody to human immunodeficiency virus. *J Infect Dis* 165:723–26, 1992.

45 Vento S, Di Perri G, Cruciani M, et al: Rapid decline of CD-4 + cells after interferon-alpha treatment in HIV-1 infection (letter). *Lancet* 341:958–59, 1993.

46 Crespo J, Lozano JL, de la Cruz P, et al: Prevalence and significance of hepatitis C viremia in chronic active hepatitis B. *Am J Gastroenterol* 89:1147–51, 1994.

47 Mimms LT, Mosley JW, Hollinger FB, et al: Effect of concurrent acute infection with hepatitis C virus on acute hepatitis B virus infection. *Br Med J* 307:1095–97, 1994.

48 Brillanti S, Garson J, Foli M, et al: A pilot study of combination therapy with ribavirin plus interferon alpha for interferon alpha-resistant chronic hepatitis C. *Gastroenterology* 107:812–17, 1994.

49 Lai MY, Kao JH, Yang PM, et al: Long term efficacy of ribavirin plus interferon alpha in the treatment of chronic hepatitis C. *Gastroenterology* 111:1307–12, 1996.

50 Love RA, Parge HE, Wickersham JA, et al: The crystal structure of hepatitis C virus NS3 proteinase reveals a trypsin-like fold and a structural zinc binding site. *Cell* 87:331–42, 1996.

51 Kim JL, Morgenstern KA, Lin C, et al: Crystal structure of the hepatitis C virus NS3 protease domain complexed with a synthetic NS4A cofactor peptide. *Cell* 87:343–55, 1996.

Chapter 68

Arthritis associated with sexually transmitted diseases

Peter A. Rice
H. Hunter Handsfield

INTRODUCTION

Acute arthritis is a common clinical problem, and in some settings disseminated gonococcal infection (DGI) and Reiter's syndrome together may account for more than one-half of all new cases of acute nontraumatic arthritis in sexually active young adults.[1,2] The association of acute arthritis with urethritis in men was recognized repeatedly from antiquity through the eighteenth century, and gonococcal arthritis and sexually acquired nongonococcal arthritis were characterized as distinct entities in the nineteenth and early twentieth centuries. The case described by Hans Reiter in 1916 was one of many such reports[3]; the syndrome that bears his name was "rediscovered" and definitively described in 1942.[4] Nevertheless, gonococcal arthritis and Reiter's syndrome often are confused with one another, and this lack of separation may have contributed to an apparent predominance of men over women in some reported series of gonococcal arthritis.

Reactive arthritis is the general term for inflammatory arthritis that follows a localized infection, which usually involves a mucosal surface.[5,6] The name *Reiter's syndrome* describes reactive arthritis that is associated with various combinations of inflammatory urogenital, ocular, and mucocutaneous manifestations. The classical presentation includes arthritis and nongonococcal urethritis (NGU), often but not universally accompanied or followed by conjunctivitis, the characteristic dermatitis, or both. Typically these manifestations follow a primary genital infection with *Chlamydia trachomatis* or lower gastrointestinal tract infection with one of a number of agents that cause infectious diarrhea. Reiter's syndrome includes the disorders commonly referred to as sexually acquired reactive arthritis, reactive spondyloarthropathy, reactive uroarthritis, postgonococcal arthritis, and postdysenteric arthropathy.[2,5,6] Reiter's syndrome and the other reactive arthritides occur in persons predominantly of the HLA-B27 haplotype, particularly in whites. Other sexually transmitted diseases (STDs) associated with acute arthritis include syphilis, lymphogranuloma venereum, hepatitis B virus infection, human immunodeficiency virus (HIV) infection, and, rarely, genital herpes, cytomegalovirus, and genital mycoplasma infections. Arthritis may also result from allergic reactions to drugs used in the treatment of sexually transmitted infections.

DISSEMINATED GONOCOCCAL INFECTION

ETIOLOGY AND PATHOGENESIS

Neisseria gonorrhoeae is the most common sexually transmitted pathogen that causes infective arthritis, and in parts of the United States it may have been the most common of all causes of infective arthritis during the 1970s and 1980s.[1,2,7,8] Septic monoarticular or oligoarticular gonococcal arthritis is commonly, but not always, associated with positive synovial fluid cultures for *N. gonorrhoeae*. This form of the disease accounts for somewhat less than 50 percent of cases of disseminated gonococcal infection (DGI). Most patients, however, present with polyarthralgias and sterile tenosynovitis and experience clinical courses that may resolve spontaneously. Although these features suggest an immunologic pathogenesis,[9,10] several lines of evidence indicate that this syndrome in fact results from direct synovial or periarticular infection: (1) Gonococcemia is commonly documented; positive blood cultures may occur in up to 50 percent of patients with tenosynovitis accompanied by polyarthralgias who are examined within 2 days of onset, providing an opportunity for synovial and periarticular seeding.[1,8,11–14] (2) Other common systemic manifestations of DGI, including cutaneous and visceral lesions, clearly are due to localized infection.[8,9,14–17] (3) *N. gonorrhoeae* occasionally has been identified histologically or by immunochemical methods in apparently sterile synovial fluid and periarticular tissues of patients with DGI or in skin lesions.[16,17] (4) The rapid response of polyarthralgias to antimicrobial therapy, usually resolving completely within 48 hours, is consistent with a direct therapeutic effect.[8,11,12,14,18–21] (5) Finally, searches for circulating immune complexes in patients with DGI have yielded conflicting results; consumption of complement to subnormal levels is uncommon, although less marked decreases in complement may be frequent.[8,22–24] The question of pathogenesis, however, still is not settled, and immune-complex deposition or other immunologic mechanisms may play pathogenic roles in some patients. For example, immune-complex synovitis early in the course of DGI may predispose to later entry of circulating gonococci into the joint space.[25] It is also possible that gonococcal cell wall constituents, such as peptidoglycan fragments, circulate from the site of a mucosal infection to initiate arthritis in the absence of viable gonococci.[26] Host factors and characteristics of *N. gonorrhoeae* that predispose to dissemination are discussed in Chap. 31.

EPIDEMIOLOGY

The overall risk of acquiring DGI in patients with gonorrhea has been estimated to be 0.5 to 3.0 percent, depending in part on the regional prevalence of specific strains of *N. gonorrhoeae* that possess features enabling them to disseminate,[8,14,15] as discussed in Chaps. 31 and 32. Such strains were endemic in Scandinavia and in the northwestern United States during the 1970s, when DGI apparently occurred in up to 3 percent of patients with gonorrhea.[27] During the preantibiotic era, DGI was documented primarily in men,[28] but studies in the 1960s and 1970s reported a female predominance of 78 to 97 percent.[1,8,11–14,27,29] A potential explanation for this change may be past misdiagnosis of Reiter's syndrome, which until recently was believed to be rare in women. In women, dissemination of *N. gonorrhoeae* may be most likely during menstruation. Possible explanations include hormonal factors and a more alkaline pH of genital secretions at the time of menses (conditions which are permissive to the growth of *N. gonorrhoeae*) and phenotypes of gonococci present during menses that may disseminate more readily. Gonococcal dissemination seems to be uncommon in homosexually active men, probably because infection with the strains of *N. gonorrhoeae* that are most likely to disseminate are uncommon in this population (Chap. 32).[30]

CLINICAL AND LABORATORY MANIFESTATIONS

The musculoskeletal manifestations of DGI are prominent. Whereas a single, hot, swollen joint is characteristic of nongonococcal bacterial arthritis, tenosynovitis and polyarthritis are more typical of DGI (Table 68-1). In a contemporary report, teno-

Table 68-1. Differential Features of Gonococcal and Nongonococcal Bacterial Arthritis

Gonococcal Arthritis	Nongonococcal Bacterial Arthritis
Usually healthy, young adults	Often compromised host, often very young or aged
Tenosynovitis often	No tenosynovitis
Polyarthritis common	Monoarthritis common
Skin lesions in two-thirds	No associated dermatitis
Wrists and small joints common	Large joints predominate
Migratory polyarthralgias	No prodromal joint symptoms
Synovial-fluid culture usually negative	Synovial-fluid culture usually positive
Blood cultures rarely positive, except in prodromal phase	Blood cultures positive in 50 percent of patients
Rapid and complete response to antibiotics; synovial-fluid drainage usually unnecessary	Slower response to antibiotics; synovial-fluid drainage important

synovitis was present in 68 percent of patients, polyarthritis in 52 percent, and monoarthritis in 48 percent.[29] In one series, 67 percent had tenosynovitis and 42 percent had arthritis.[8] The variable descriptions of these musculoskeletal manifestations may be related to differences in the definitions of arthritis and tenosynovitis among different authors. For example, a common criterion for arthritis requires the demonstration of purulent synovial fluid with >25,000 leukocytes/mm^3. Using this definition, frank arthritis may be less common than tenosynovitis accompanied by arthralgias.[8] It is not clear whether the increased frequency of tenosynovitis is related to a true change in the clinical manifestations or whether it is due to a greater appreciation and definition of tenosynovitis, as opposed to classifying all joint inflammation as arthritis. In the preantibiotic era, overt arthritis, confirmed by joint aspiration, was reported commonly and tenosynovitis less frequently.[28] Tenosynovitis usually involves multiple joints, especially the wrists, fingers, toes, and ankles.

Monoarthritis or oligoarthritis was reported in <50 percent of patients in recent series of DGI.[1,8,9] The knee has been the most commonly affected joint, which may reflect, in part, the ease of diagnosis and aspiration of a knee joint effusion. The synovial fluid leukocyte count has ranged between 40,000 and 60,000 cells/mm^3 (with >80 percent polymorphonuclear leukocytes) in most series that reported synovial-fluid analyses. The mean synovial-fluid leukocyte counts, however, have not been lower than those described in staphylococcal and other types of nongonococcal bacterial arthritis.[31] All joints, including the hip and shoulder, have been affected, but the sacroiliac, temporomandibular, and sternoclavicular joints rarely are involved.[32,33]

The second most frequent abnormality in DGI is dermatitis (Fig. 68-1; see Color Plates 70–72), which has been reported in about two-thirds of patients. The skin lesions usually are multiple, typically with 5 to 30 lesions; they occur most commonly on the extremities and sometimes on the trunk, but rarely on the face. They usually are painless and patients may be unaware of their presence, but occasionally they may be painful and appear pustular or resemble vasculitis. Small macules or papules are the most common lesions, but all forms of skin lesions have been associated with DGI; these include pustules, vesicles, bullae, and the lesions of erythema nodosum or erythema multiforme. *N. gonorrhoeae* usually cannot be recovered from skin lesions by culture, and lesions may occasionally appear after appropriate antibiotic therapy has been started.

Although most patients with DGI have fever and many have shaking chills, up to 40 percent have been reported to be afebrile. Most DGI patients deny local genitourinary, rectal, or pharyngeal

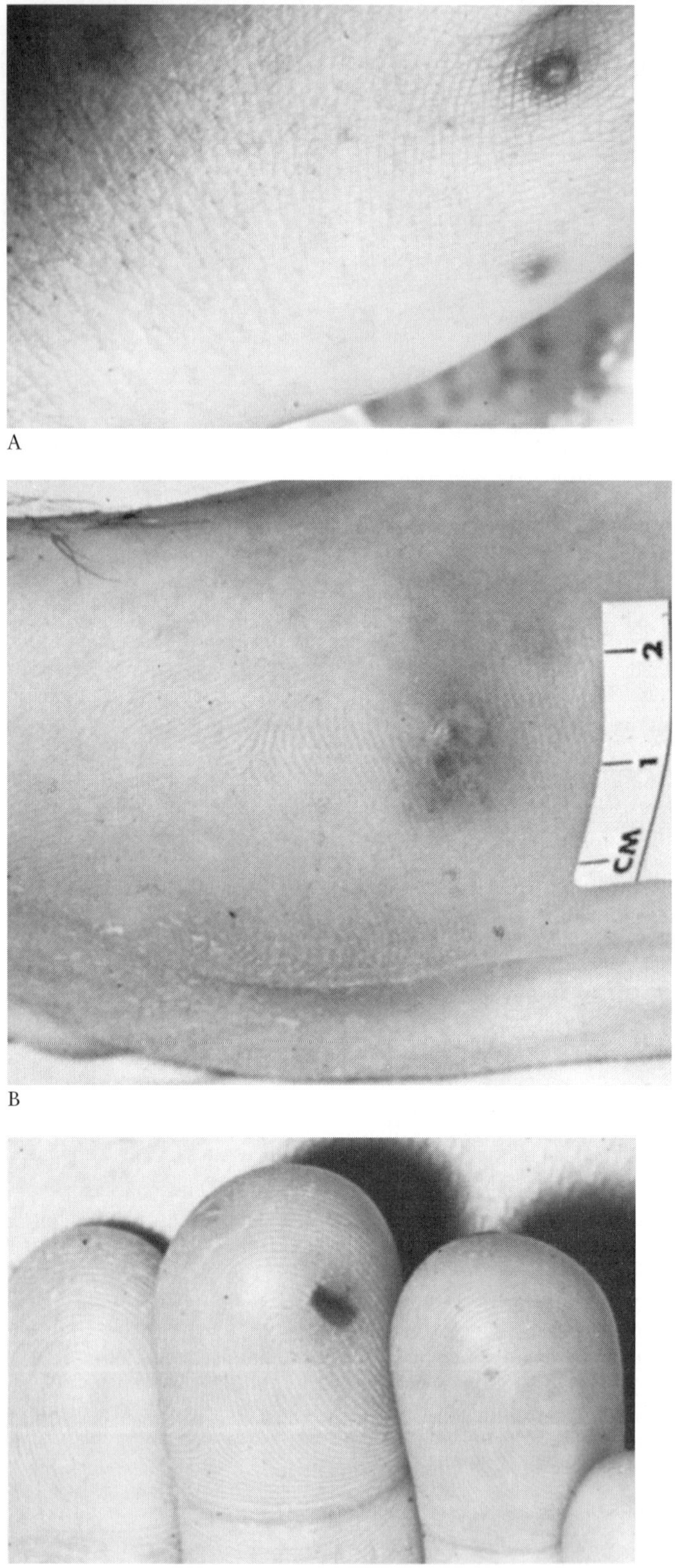

Fig. 68-1. Skin lesions in patients with disseminated gonococcal infection: (*A*) pustular and papular lesions of wrist and thumb; (*B*) large hemorrhagic pustule of foot; (*C*) petechial lesion of finger. (See also Color Plates.)

symptoms, despite the fact that *N. gonorrhoeae* is recovered from these local sites in about 80 percent of cases. The organisms can be recovered from the synovial fluid in about 25 percent of cases, but they are recovered from blood less commonly and rarely from skin lesions. Concurrently positive blood and synovial-fluid cultures are rare.[8,11–14,29,34] In the postantibiotic era, gonococcal meningitis and endocarditis have also been rare.[8,35] There have been a few reports of a presumed immune-mediated glomerulonephritis secondary to DGI.[36] Mild hepatitis has been reported in up to 50 percent of patients with DGI, but usually it is not clinically apparent.[14,37]

There has been a controversy regarding the concept of sequential clinical stages in DGI. Several investigators[1,11,14] have popularized the concept of an initial bacteremic phase that usually is associated with dermatitis and tenosynovitis ("arthritis-dermatitis syndrome"), followed by a joint localization (septic arthritis) stage. Other authors,[8] however, have suggested that there may be too much overlap in these manifestations to be consistently explained by such a temporal sequence of events. Although dermatitis is most common in patients with tenosynovitis (80 percent), fresh skin lesions also may be found in up to 30 percent of those with purulent arthritis. Therefore, many investigators now favor a continuum of DGI, during which signs of sepsis (fever accompanied by tenosynovitis and dermatitis) may be more prominent earlier in the disease. In addition, some patients have polyarticular involvement that resolves spontaneously, and others present with monoarticular septic arthritis without a preceding polyarticular syndrome or dermatitis. Thus, although the hypothesized sequential pathogenesis may occur, such clinical progression is by no means universal.

REITER'S SYNDROME

ETIOLOGY AND PATHOGENESIS

The pathogenesis of reactive arthritis is multifactorial and remains incompletely understood. A preceding infection, usually of a mucosal surface, likely serves as a trigger in a genetically predisposed host, and the disease may then persist or recur despite eradication of the infection.[2,5,6] Infectious agents that have been implicated include *Chlamydia trachomatis*, *Shigella flexneri*, *Salmonella* spp., *Yersinia enterocolitica*, and *Campylobacter* spp. and perhaps *N. gonorrhoeae*, the genital mycoplasmas, or other organisms. In several studies, genital *C. trachomatis* infection has been documented in approximately 50 percent of men with sexually acquired Reiter's syndrome.[5,6,38,39] Antichlamydial antibody is common in these patients, usually in higher titer than in patients with uncomplicated chlamydial infection.[5,39] Enhanced cellular immunity against *C. trachomatis* is also present, as evidenced by increases in lymphocyte-transformation responses to chlamydial antigen.[39]

A few reports have documented the occurrence of reactive arthritis after successful treatment of gonorrhea.[1,3,40–43] Often associated with postgonococcal urethritis, reactive arthritis is distinct from DGI and may be accompanied or followed by conjunctivitis or mucocutaneous lesions typical of Reiter's syndrome. Although simultaneous genital infection with *C. trachomatis* may occur in 10 to 40 percent of heterosexual patients with gonorrhea, chlamydial infection has not been sought in most reported cases of postgonococcal arthritis. In one report, three patients who developed typical Reiter's syndrome following gonococcal urethritis lacked both culture and serologic evidence of chlamydial infection. Thus, *N. gonorrhoeae* itself may initiate some cases of Reiter's syndrome.

The failure to demonstrate an immune response to *C. trachomatis* in one-fourth of patients or to isolate any sexually transmitted organism from urethral specimens of one-third to one-half of those who had sexually acquired Reiter's syndrome or reactive arthritis[38,39] suggests that other infectious agents may sometimes cause urethritis. In some cases of Reiter's syndrome, urethritis may be noninfective. For example, urethritis occurs in many patients with the enteric form of the disease,[5,44–46] and recurrence of urethritis may be a part of the late exacerbation of Reiter's syndrome in the absence of recent sexual exposure.[3]

How inflammation at a mucosal surface initiates a sustained systemic illness is not completely understood. Genetically susceptible individuals, however, particularly those who express the major histocompatibility-complex class 1 molecule HLA-B27, may develop an exaggerated or aberrant immune response that results in the inflammatory manifestations of Reiter's syndrome.[5,46,47] The HLA-B27 haplotype is found in 70 to 80 percent of white patients with Reiter's syndrome,[39,44,48,49] compared with 6 to 8 percent of whites in the general population. In African American persons with Reiter's syndrome, the reported prevalence of HLA-B27 has varied from 15 to 75 percent,[50–52] compared with about 2 percent in African Americans in the general population.[53] In one small study, 7 of 10 HLA-B27–negative patients with Reiter's syndrome possessed HLA antigens that cross-reacted with B27, such as B7, BW22, and BW42.[50]

It has been suggested[6,50] that HLA-B27, and perhaps cross-reacting antigens, induce recognition of B27 as a foreign antigen,[54,55] resulting in a self-perpetuating autoimmune process.[56] Alternatively, HLA-B27 or related antigens may present bacterial antigen to disease-causing CD8-positive cytotoxic T lymphocytes.[57–59] Another hypothesis suggests that the HLA-B27 antigen itself may be immunologically cross-reactive with certain bacterial proteins.[60,61] Several such proteins have been identified[61–63] (although not in *C. trachomatis*), and perhaps mapping of the human and the chlamydial genomes will reveal homologous sequences encoding for similar proteins. Heat shock proteins (HSP) are a family of peptides with considerable homology among bacteria, including *C. trachomatis*. These proteins may incite T-cell-mediated immunopathogenic responses involving local sites (e.g., endometrium and pelvic adnexa) as well as distal sites (e.g., the joints in Reiter's syndrome). The gene for HSP-60 of *Mycobacterium tuberculosis*, which shares homology with the HSP expressed by *C. trachomatis*, when transfected into an HLA-B27 cell line, resulted in the generation of peptide complexes that were recognized preferentially by antibodies present in HLA-B27–positive reactive patients with arthritis.[64]

The HLA-B27 haplotype is not the only determinant of disease expression, because no more than 25 percent of HLA-B27–positive individuals with NGU or shigellosis develop Reiter's syndrome. However, the initial manifestations of Reiter's syndrome and other forms of reactive arthritis tend to be more severe, and the natural course tends to be more aggressive in persons with the HLA-B27 haplotype than in those without it.[5,65] Recent experimental studies have directly implicated the B27 antigen in the disease process. Transgenic rats that overexpress the B27 gene spontaneously develop a disease characterized by diarrhea that is followed by arthritis. Clinical manifestations begin earlier in male rats than in females and are accompanied by genital inflammation.[66] Histopathologic examination has shown enthesitis (inflammation at tendon insertion sites) and anterior uveitis,[66] both of which are characteristic of Reiter's syndrome in humans. Adoptive transfer of bone marrow cells from transgenic rats to normal rats also transfers the disease. The disease cannot be reproduced in this model using athymic (nude) mice,[67] showing that T lymphocytes (probably CD8-bearing cytotoxic T cells) are critical to its pathogenesis.

Conflicting reports exist on the potential role of direct dissemination of the triggering pathogen in causing the arthritis and other inflammatory manifestations in humans with Reiter's syndrome. Initial reports of isolation of *C. trachomatis* from the synovial fluid in Reiter's syndrome[68] were inconclusive.[69,70] However, *C. trachomatis* was demonstrated by direct immunofluorescence (DIF) with monoclonal antibody in synovial fluid or biopsy tissue in five of eight patients (seven men and one woman) with sexually acquired reactive arthritis[71] and in five of nine women with nonrheumatoid arthritis.[72] More recently, chlamydial DNA has been identified in synovial fluid by polymerase chain reaction (PCR) when other methods to identify the organism have failed.[73] It has been speculated that *C. trachomatis* may be sequestered in synovial tissue and may cause "latent" infection. Antimicrobial therapy, though often used, however, has not generally been clinically beneficial in treating the articular manifestations in most patients with acute Reiter's syndrome, or in treating reactive arthritis that has flared long after the initial infection.[74] Nevertheless, prompt antimicrobial therapy of chlamydial infection may help prevent Reiter's syndrome, as suggested by a retrospective review of 224 patients with sexually acquired urethritis or cervicitis.[75] In that study, 68 patients were treated for presumed chlamydial infection with tetracycline or erythromycin; acute Reiter's syndrome developed in 7 (10 percent) of these patients. The other 156 patients had gonorrhea, or they had no identified pathogen, and were untreated or received only penicillin therapy; 57 (37 percent) of these patients developed Reiter's syndrome ($p > .001$).[75]

Immunologic studies in Reiter's syndrome

Many immunologic phenomena have been associated with Reiter's syndrome, but their importance and pathogenic roles are not always clear. Synovial-fluid lymphocytes from patients with Reiter's syndrome may be more reactive than peripheral-blood lymphocytes from the same patient when incubated with a variety of potential triggering agents, particularly *C. trachomatis*, but also with a number of enteric organisms, *N. gonorrhoeae*, and *Ureaplasma urealyticum*.[76,77] The ratio of T to B lymphocytes is higher in synovial fluid from patients with Reiter's syndrome than in synovial fluid from normal controls.[78] The blastogenic response of circulating lymphocytes to *C. trachomatis*[39] or *Y. enterocolitica*[79] in Reiter's syndrome associated with these pathogens is elevated relative to the response in patients who have chlamydial or yersinial infections without reactive arthritis. CD4-bearing (helper-inducer) lymphocytes outnumber CD8-positive (suppressor-cytotoxic) lymphocytes in the synovial fluids of patients with Reiter's syndrome, even though stimulation of CD8-positive cytotoxic-cell populations results from antigen presentation by, for example, HLA-B27 class 1 molecules. Further evidence favoring a pathogenic role of CD8-positive cytotoxic cells is represented by the occurrence of Reiter's syndrome in patients with acquired immunodeficency syndrome (AIDS) who have profound depletion of CD4-positive lymphocytes.[80] These observations are concordant with those in the athymic (nude) mouse model.[67] These observations suggest that an intact helper-inducer CD4 system may not be central to the pathogenesis of reactive arthritis.

Immune complexes of the IgG class are present in the blood of up to 76 percent of patients with Reiter's syndrome,[81] and synovial biopsies often reveal exudative synovitis with interstitial and intracellular deposits of IgG, IgA, and the third component of complement (C3).[82,83] Nonetheless, the clinical features of the arthropathy and the usual absence of glomerulonephritis, vasculitis, and other manifestations of immune-complex deposition suggest that this mechanism may not be central to the pathogenesis of reactive arthritis.

EPIDEMIOLOGY

Epidemiologically, Reiter's syndrome is characterized by an endemic form, usually sexually acquired, and a less common epidemic form, most often associated with enteric infection. Although endemic Reiter's syndrome commonly follows sexual contact with a new partner, clear evidence of sexual transmission of individual cases has been uncommon. One report[84] described the simultaneous occurrence of NGU and Reiter's syndrome in two HLA-B27–positive men after both had intercourse with the same woman. The enteric form of Reiter's syndrome typically follows shigellosis,[2,5,6,46,85] salmonellosis,[86,87] yersiniosis,[88–90] or infection with *Campylobacter* spp.[91] Although sexual transmission of enteric Reiter's syndrome has not been reported, such cases are likely to have occurred, because men who have sex with men are at increased risk for several of these infections (Chap. 69).

The incidence and prevalence of Reiter's syndrome are uncertain and may vary geographically.[2,5,65] In one series reported more than 20 years ago,[1] the diagnosis was made in 16 (11 percent) of 151 consecutively hospitalized adults with acute nontraumatic arthritis, second in frequency only to DGI as a cause of arthritis (Fig. 68-2). Septic arthritis related to injection drug use has become much more frequent in the past two decades and undoubtedly is now among the most common causes of acute arthritis in young adults. Because DGI cases have diminished in the past two decades, it is likely that Reiter's syndrome has become the most common cause of acute arthritis in young persons who are not injection drug users. The overall risk of acquiring Reiter's syndrome has been estimated to be 1 to 3 percent among men with sexually acquired NGU[73,92] and among patients with acute shigellosis,[45] rising to as high as 20 to 37 percent for individuals with the HLA-B27 haplotype.[45,74,92]

Although enteric Reiter's syndrome may occur in children (in whom infectious diarrhea is most common), most patients are adults. The modal age of patients with sexually acquired Reiter's syndrome is in the fourth decade, compared with the third decade for patients with DGI and most other STDs. This may be partly because some series included patients whose Reiter's syndrome was not sexually acquired or patients with recurrent disease. In most series, 80 to 90 percent of patients with Reiter's syndrome have been white, and most of the remainder have been African American.[6,51,52,73] Differences in racial susceptibility remain poorly defined because many studies do not report the racial compositions of the patients studied. It is likely that African Americans are less susceptible, however, in part because they have a lower prevalence of the HLA-B27 haplotype than whites.

Enteric Reiter's syndrome has been recognized to affect women somewhat less frequently than men, with reported male-to-female ratios that vary from 1 : 1 to 10 : 1.[5] Many series of patients with Reiter's syndrome have been drawn predominantly from male populations (e.g., from military installations, ships' companies, and military or veterans' hospitals). By contrast, few women have been included in most series of sexually acquired reactive arthritis; in one example, women accounted for only 20 (3.6 percent) of 557 contemporary cases.[5] In another series, however, 13 (52 percent) of 25 patients with Reiter's syndrome were women.[93] Clinical presentations of Reiter's syndrome described in 29 women, as well as their HLA haplotypes and their clinical courses, were reported to be similar to those in men.[94] Nonspecific rheumatic complaints and overt Reiter's syndrome have also been documented in women with histories of salpingitis, gonorrhea, bacterial urinary-tract infection, and trichomoniasis.[95] A high prevalence of musculoskeletal disorders in the sexual partners of men with Reiter's syndrome was found, and an association of salpingitis with radiologic evidence of sacroiliitis has been reported.[5,96] These observations suggest that reactive arthritis may be more

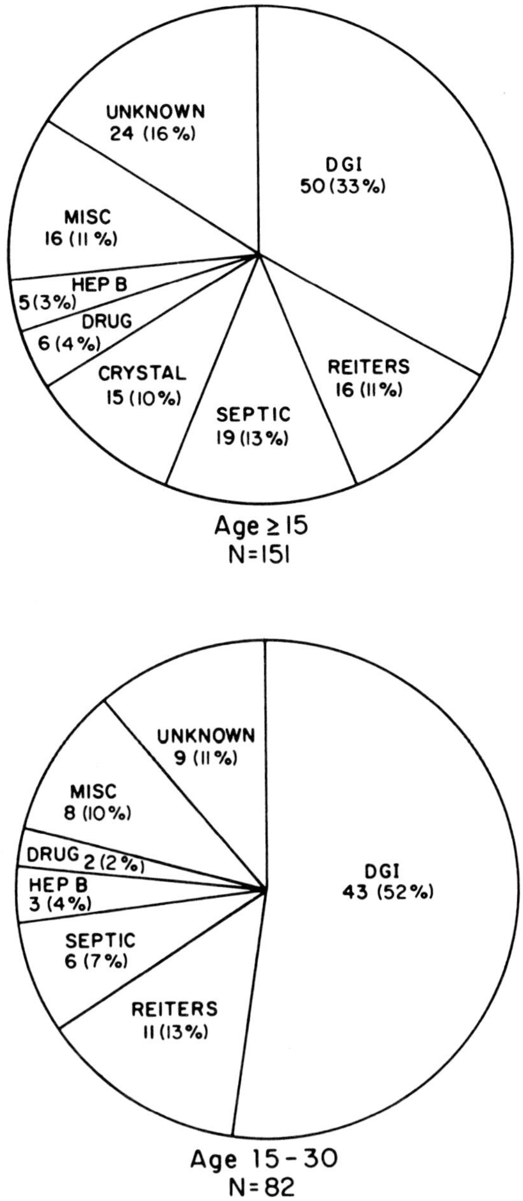

Fig. 68-2. Diagnoses in 151 consecutive adults (age ≥ 15 years) hospitalized in Seattle because of acute, nontraumatic arthritis of <14 days duration. REITERS includes postgonococcal arthritis; DRUG denotes drug-induced arthritis; HEP B denotes hepatitis B infection. (From HH Handsfield[1])

frequent in women than commonly realized, and that it may be sexually acquired.[97]

CLINICAL AND LABORATORY MANIFESTATIONS

The clinical manifestations of Reiter's syndrome include acute arthritis, lower-urogenital-tract inflammation, conjunctivitis, and mucocutaneous inflammatory lesions. Although it is uncommon for all of these manifestations to be observed at the time of presentation, most patients eventually develop all four features, especially if they are HLA-B27–positive.[44,49,70] The frequencies of these manifestations at presentation and during follow-up are shown in Table 68-2. The articular, mucocutaneous, and ocular manifestations usually follow onset of urethritis or diarrhea by 1 to 4 weeks, although delays of several months may be seen.[2,5,44,46,48]

Urogenital inflammation

Patients with Reiter's syndrome frequently give histories of recent sexual contact with a new partner, followed by the development of urethritis that is clinically indistinguishable from uncomplicated NGU.[44,49] Gonococcal urethritis has been reported in up to 20 percent of patients, but concomitant chlamydial infection has not always been excluded. Furthermore, culture and other tests for *C. trachomatis* may be insensitive.[44,98] Some studies have suggested that many patients with Reiter's syndrome had nonbacterial prostatitis,[42,44,99,100] but prostatitis was not always clearly differentiated from urethritis, cystitis, or other forms of lower-urogenital-tract inflammation.

Urethritis occurs in up to 90 percent of patients with enteric Reiter's syndrome[5,44,45,88,91]; it has also been documented in children[101] and in sexually inactive adults with enteric reactive arthritis, observations that imply an immunologic pathogenesis of urethritis. Therefore, genital inflammation in Reiter's syndrome should not always be assumed to be sexually acquired,[5,6] especially when reactive arthritis follows infectious diarrhea. Nevertheless, the possibility of sexual acquisition should be explored even in these cases, and the patient's sexual partner(s) should be examined. Symptoms or signs of urethritis or pyuria have been documented in 30 percent of women with Reiter's syndrome,[93,94] but standardized criteria for lower-genital-tract inflammation often were not used (Chap. 57). A number of studies[5,95–97] suggest that cervicitis, urethritis, cystitis, and salpingitis may all be important, but the spectrum of urogenital inflammation in women with Reiter's syndrome has not been clearly defined.

Arthritis

A wide range of articular disease occurs. Asymmetric polyarticular synovitis and tendinitis are often seen initially, followed by persistence of signs and symptoms usually referable to a few joints. Arthritis typically begins in the distal weight-bearing joints (knees,

Table 68-2. Frequencies of Clinical Manifestations in Patients with Reiter's Syndrome

	Percent of Patients	
	*Initial Attack**	*Entire Course†*
Urogenital inflammation		
Urethritis (criteria not specified)	85	87
Cervicitis (criteria not specified)	71	NA
Arthritis		
Monoarticular	14	3
Polyarticular	81	86
Arthralgia only	0	9
Sacroiliitis or back pain	49	21
Heel pain	40	Not recorded
Tendinitis or tenosynovitis	25	25
Fusiform dactylitis	17	Not recorded
Ocular involvement		
Conjunctivitis	57	50
Uveitis	0	12
Mucocutaneous involvement		
Balanitis/vulvovaginitis	39	69
Stomatitis	31	17
Keratoderma blennorrhagica	21	18
Nail changes	9	16
Other		
Cardiac	0	9
Neurologic	1	2
Diarrhea	14	12

* Data from RF Wilkens et al.[49] (N = 83).
† Data from M Kousa et al.[38] (N = 173).

ankles, feet), often with knee effusions and fusiform dactylitis ("sausage digits") (Fig. 68-3). Sacroiliitis (Fig. 68-4) is common, occurring in up to 10 percent of cases acutely and in higher proportions of those with chronic Reiter's syndrome; it often is detected as a subclinical radiographic abnormality, especially in sexually acquired cases.[5,44,102] Tendon-insertion sites (entheses) are common sites of inflammation, the basis for the rheumatologic classification of Reiter's syndrome as an enthesopathy.[65,103] Common enthesopathic sites include the insertion of the Achilles tendon and the plantar fascia. In contrast to ankylosing spondylitis and other spondyloarthropathies, spinal involvement is uncommon in Reiter's syndrome. Radiographic evidence of sacroiliitis has been reported in association with chronic prostatitis[99] and salpingitis[96,97] without other manifestations of Reiter's syndrome; it remains to be determined whether this represents a variant of the disease.

Mucocutaneous manifestations

Mucocutaneous lesions are common in sexually acquired Reiter's syndrome and in reactive arthritis following shigellosis, but apparently they are uncommon in reactive arthritis associated with *Salmonella*, *Campylobacter*, or *Yersinia* infections.[5] These lesions usually are painless and are easily overlooked. Circinate balanitis is the most common cutaneous manifestation, typically occurring in 20 to 40 percent[5] and perhaps up to 85 percent[44] of men with sexually acquired Reiter's syndrome. In uncircumcised men, circinate balanitis appears as a painless, serpiginous, "geographic" dermatitis of the glans penis and is diagnostic of Reiter's syndrome (see Color Plate 67). In circumcised men, circinate balanitis often takes the form of hyperkeratotic papules (Fig. 68-5) that, except for their location, closely resemble the other characteristic skin lesion, keratoderma blennorrhagica (Fig. 68-6). Erosive vulvitis, perhaps the female equivalent of circinate balanitis, has been documented in some women with Reiter's syndrome.[102]

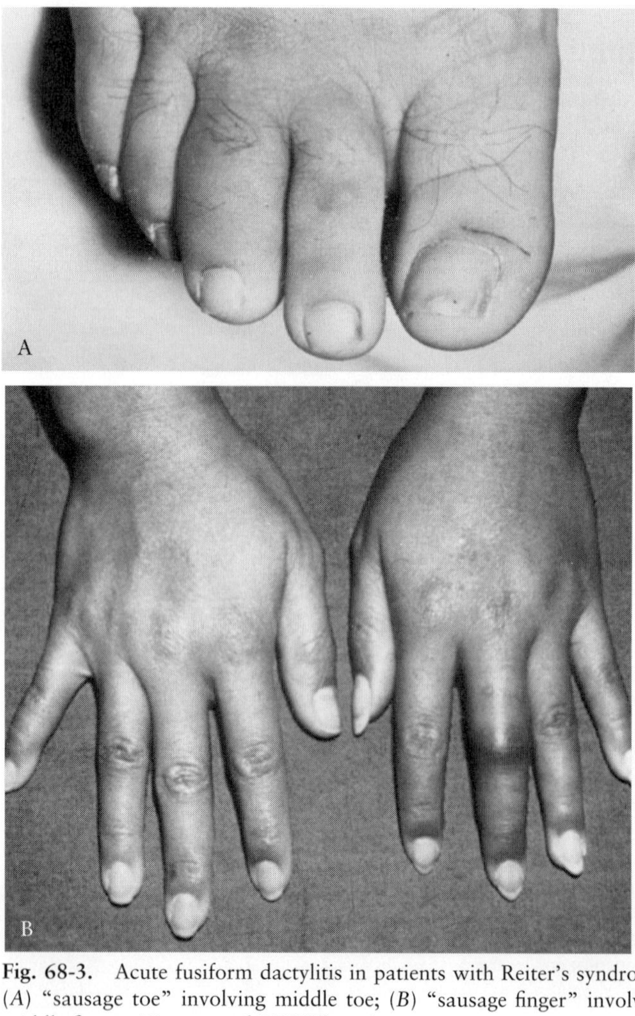

Fig. 68-3. Acute fusiform dactylitis in patients with Reiter's syndrome: (*A*) "sausage toe" involving middle toe; (*B*) "sausage finger" involving middle finger. (Courtesy of RF Wilkens.)

Lesions of keratoderma blennorrhagica (see Fig. 68-6 and Color Plate 68) begin as erythematous macules that gradually thicken and enlarge to form hyperkeratotic papules and plaques, sometimes with red halos and occasionally with central clearing. Keratoderma blennorrhagica resembles psoriasis both macroscopically and histologically, and some well-documented cases of Reiter's syndrome have evolved to become clinically indistinguishable from chronic psoriatic arthritis.[3,5,6,65,104,105] Keratoderma blennorrhagica most commonly involves the plantar surfaces of the feet (see Fig. 68-6) and occasionally the palms of the hands, but it may occur anywhere. Cutaneous manifestations have been reported to be more common (up to 20 percent) in patients with sexually acquired Reiter's syndrome than in those with the enteric form.[5]

In up to 30 percent of patients with Reiter's syndrome, especially those with the sexually acquired form, shallow, painless ulcers occur on the palate, tongue, buccal mucosa, lips, tonsillar pillars, or pharynx (Fig. 68-7; see Color Plate 69).[49,106] The nails are involved in up to 15 percent of patients, manifested by thickening and brown-yellow discoloration due to subungual hyperkeratosis.[2,3,38,44,49] Erythema nodosum occasionally occurs in reactive arthritis following yersiniosis but seems to be rare in other forms of the disease.[5]

Ocular inflammation

Ocular manifestations occur in up to half of patients with acute sexually acquired Reiter's syndrome and in up to 90 percent of cases following shigellosis.[5] Conjunctivitis, often sufficiently mild to escape detection in a cursory examination, is the most common ocular manifestation.[38,44,49] Iritis or more extensive uveitis ultimately develops in up to 10 percent of patients,[2,5,44,49] although these are uncommon at presentation.

Other systemic manifestations

Acute Reiter's syndrome is often accompanied by malaise, fever, anorexia, and weight loss. Transient and usually benign electrocardiographic abnormalities, including atrioventricular conduction disturbances, ST-segment elevation or depression, or nonspecific T-wave changes, occur during 9 to 30 percent of acute episodes.[44,107] Complete heart block, myocarditis, pericarditis, acute aortitis with aortic-valve incompetence, and congestive heart failure are rare but well-documented long-term sequelae, especially in sexually acquired cases.[108,109] Rare complications, each occurring in fewer than 1 percent of patients, include peripheral neuropathy, hemiplegia, meningoencephalitis, generalized lymphadenopathy, pleuritis, pneumonitis, thrombophlebitis, and amyloidosis.[2,44]

Laboratory features

Several nonspecific laboratory abnormalities are common. The erythrocyte sedimentation rate is elevated, exceeding 50 mm/hour in nearly one-half of patients,[44] but the degree of elevation does not correlate with the severity of the clinical manifestations. Leukocytosis, with up to 20,000 leukocytes/mm^3, and mild anemia

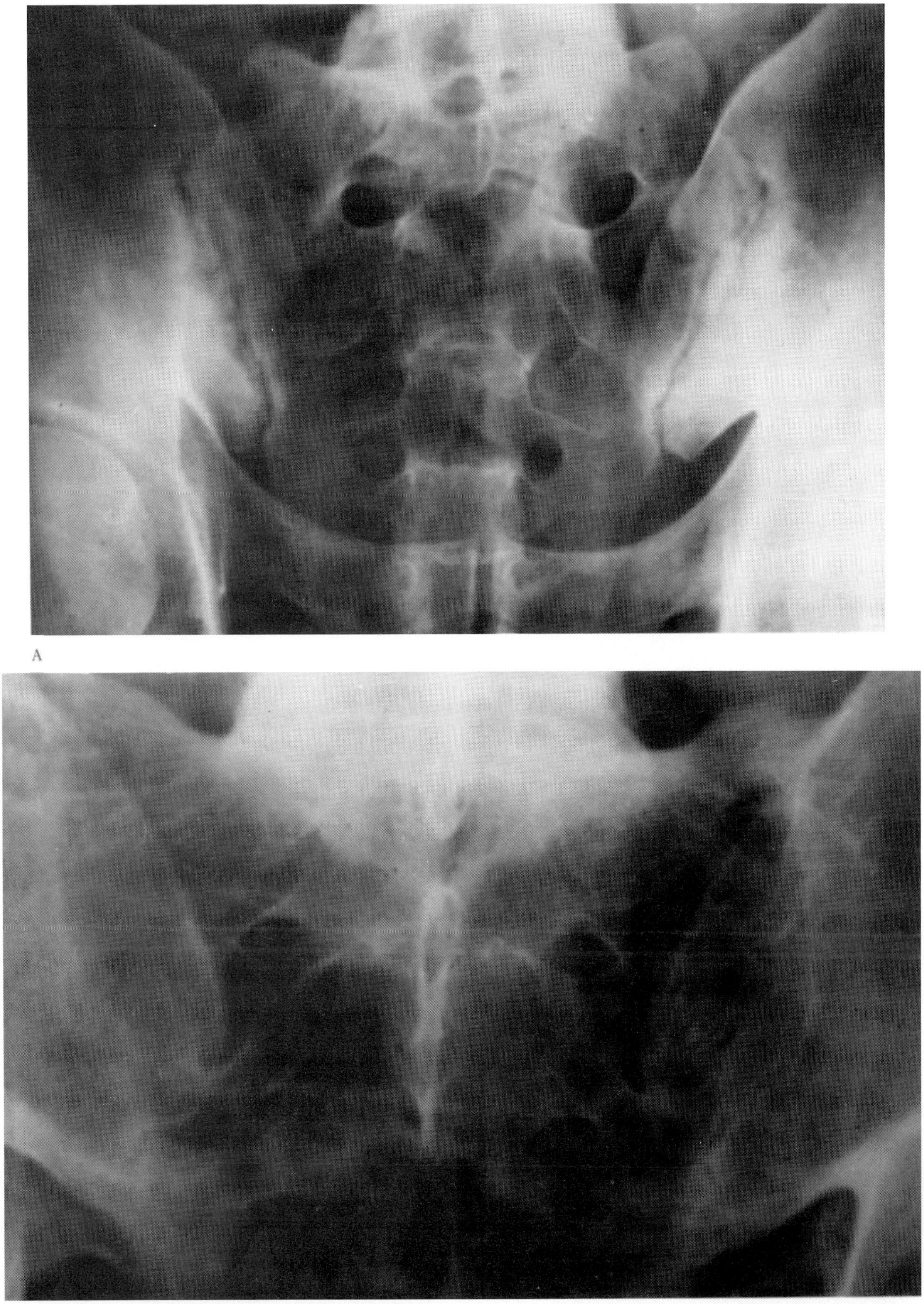

A

B

Fig. 68-4. Radiographs demonstrating bilateral sacroiliitis in patients with ankylosing spondylitis: (*A*) early sacroiliitis with subchondral bone resorption, sclerosis around joint, a "rosary bead" effect, and pseudowidening; (*B*) complete obliteration of sacroiliac joints with bony trabeculae across joints. (From the Clinical Slide Collection of the Arthritis Foundation.)

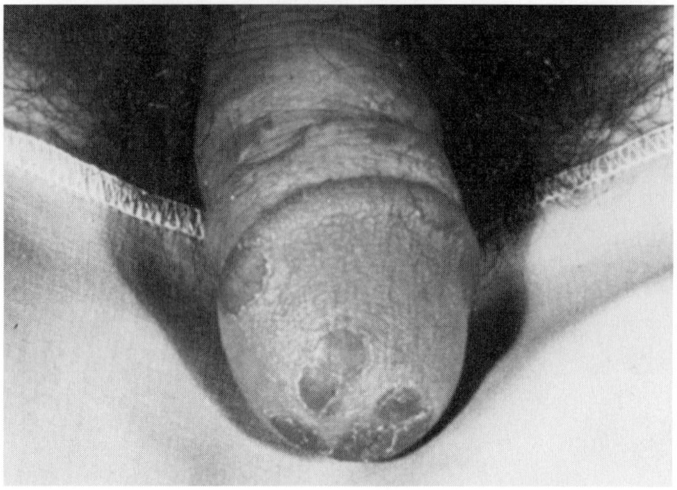

Fig. 68-5. Circinate balanitis in a circumcised man with Reiter's syndrome. (See also Plate 67.) (Courtesy of RF Wilkens.)

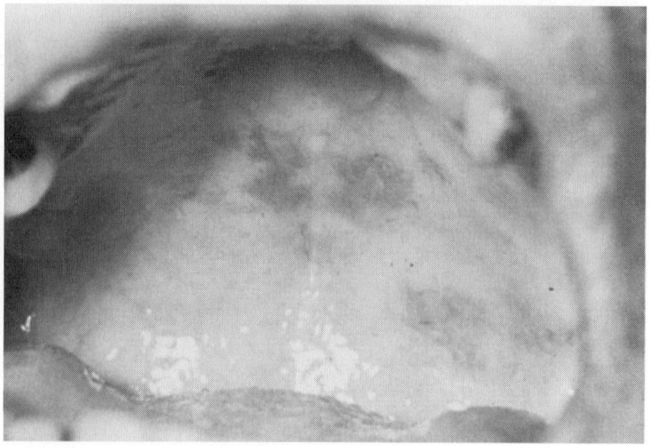

Fig. 68-7. Oral mucosal lesions in a patient with Reiter's syndrome. (See also Plate 69.)

are common. Antinuclear antibodies, rheumatoid factor, cryoglobulins, C-reactive protein, or circulating immune complexes are present occasionally.[2,5,44]

Synovial-fluid analysis is seldom specific. The results often mimic those of septic arthritis, with leukocyte counts that range from 500 to >50,000 cells/mm^3 and are >20,000/mm^3 in about 50 percent of patients; differential counts usually demonstrate >90 percent neutrophils. Decreased viscosity, normal or elevated complement levels, decreased ratio of synovial fluid to serum complement concentration,[82] and elevated protein levels are common. Synovial-fluid glucose levels usually are normal.

Clinical course

Most initial episodes of acute Reiter's syndrome resolve completely over 2 to 6 months, but recovery may be delayed for more than 1 year in up to 35 percent of patients and indefinitely in a few cases.[5,44] Subsequently, the annual risk of recurrent acute episodes has been estimated to be about 15 percent.[2,5,44,73] Recurrences may be manifested by any of the clinical features alone or in combination. In one series of 122 patients followed for a mean of 5.6 years, arthritis persisted or recurred in 83 percent, urethritis or cervicitis in 42 percent, ocular disease in 31 percent, circinate balanitis in 29 percent, and other mucocutaneous lesions in about 25 percent.[48] The severity of functional impairment caused by chronic Reiter's syndrome is variable. In one study, 34 percent of

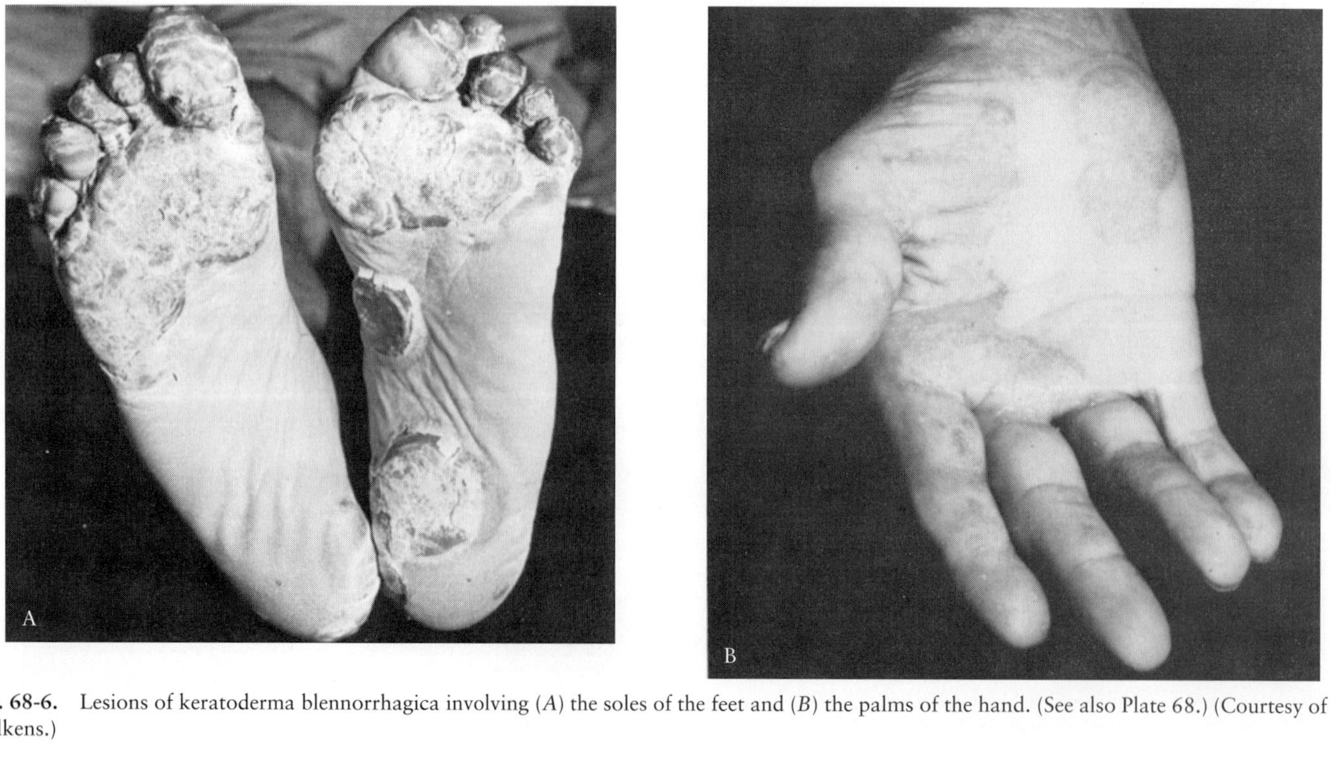

A

B

Fig. 68-6. Lesions of keratoderma blennorrhagica involving (*A*) the soles of the feet and (*B*) the palms of the hand. (See also Plate 68.) (Courtesy of RF Wilkens.)

patients had sustained disease activity, almost 16 percent required a change of job, and 11 percent were disabled for further employment.[48] Other investigators have reported similar rates of persistence or recurrence, but with substantially less functional impairment.[110] Death from Reiter's syndrome is rare, occurring primarily as the result of aortic valve incompetence,[108,109] amyloidosis,[111] or complications of drug therapy.[44]

HEPATITIS B VIRUS INFECTION

The occurrence of articular symptoms early in the course of viral hepatitis was first reported by Robert Graves in 1843 and was "rediscovered" in the 1970s.[112–117] Although hepatitis B virus (HBV) may invade the synovium,[113] several studies have confirmed the pathogenic role of immune-complex deposition in this syndrome. For example, complement levels are low in serum and synovial fluid during active joint inflammation and return to normal as the arthritis abates. Peak serum hepatitis B surface antigen (HBsAg) titers; synovial-membrane and fluid viral antigen; and cyroprecipitates containing HBsAg, complement components, IgA, and complement-fixing IgG antibodies have all been detected during acute arthritis.[114–116]

Generalized arthralgias occur in up to 50 percent of patients during the prodrome of hepatitis B. Ten to 20 percent of patients have overt polyarthritis, usually with symmetric involvement of the hands, knees, ankles, shoulders, wrists, and feet.[112–117] An urticarial rash, usually involving the lower extremities, occurs in about 25 percent of patients with arthralgias and in 50 percent of those with overt arthritis. The clinical syndrome closely parallels classical descriptions of serum sickness.[10] The onset of overt hepatitis usually coincides with resolution of the musculoskeletal and cutaneous manifestations. Many patients with hepatitis B are anicteric, however, and laboratory assessment of hepatic function and laboratory tests for HBV infection are indicated for all patients with acute polyarthritis, regardless of the presence or absence of jaundice or hepatomegaly.[117]

SYPHILIS

A small minority (probably <1 percent) of patients with secondary syphilis have overt osseous or synovial involvement.[118] Acute periostitis, sometimes mimicking acute arthritis, is the most common of these lesions, but some cases of true arthritis result from synovial invasion by *Treponema pallidum*, as demonstrated by darkfield examination.[119] Indirect immunologic mechanisms may be involved in some cases; complement consumption, circulating immune complexes, and immune-complex glomerulonephritis have all been documented in patients with primary, secondary, or congenital syphilis.[10,120] In late syphilis, acute or chronic arthritis usually is the result of direct spread into the synovial space from adjacent osteomyelitis or periostitis.[118] The Charcot joint is believed to be traumatic in origin, the indirect result of syphilitic neuropathy and, perhaps, microvascular disease.[118,121,122] Neuropathic joints almost always involve the lower extremities, but multiple neuropathic joints in the upper limbs and spine have been documented in a patient whose occupation required heavy use of the upper body.[122] A case of vertebral syphilitic osteitis in an adult has also been reported.[123]

LYMPHOGRANULOMA VENEREUM

Lymphogranuloma venereum (LGV) occasionally has been associated with a syndrome that resembles serum sickness, including polyarthritis, rash, cryoglobulinemia, and circulating rheumatoid factor.[124–127] It is uncertain whether direct synovial infection occurs; *C. trachomatis* antigen may have been demonstrated in synovial fluid of patients with LGV,[124] but isolation or antigenic detection of an LGV strain of *C. trachomatis* in synovial fluid has not been reported.

HUMAN IMMUNODEFICIENCY VIRUS INFECTION

Rheumatic manifestations occur frequently in persons with AIDS and earlier stages of infection with HIV.[128,129] Table 68-3 lists the most common conditions seen in these patients. Typical Reiter's syndrome and limited forms of reactive arthritis may be common; they have been documented both in HLA-B27–positive and –negative persons with AIDS.[130–132] In particular, seronegative spondyloarthropathy occurs in patients with advanced AIDS. This condition develops in the face of depletion of CD4-positive lymphocytes, indirectly emphasizing the possible role of CD8-positive cytotoxic T cells and their interaction with HLA-B27.[80] Most AIDS patients with Reiter's syndrome display an incomplete syndrome that usually lacks conjunctivitis and urethritis. Asymmetric oligoarthritis is usual, accompanied by enthesitis and other extra-articular features, including circinate balanitis, keratoderma blennorrhagica, and uveitis. In those who develop sacroiliitis or spondylitis, 70 percent are HLA-B27–positive.[129,132] The prevalence of rheumatologic manifestations thought to be Reiter's syndrome in HIV-infected persons varies in different reports and in different demographic groups, however, and it remains a matter of some disagreement. Reiter's syndrome has been reported to range from 0.1 percent to 11 percent in prevalence. In one prospective study, the prevalence of Reiter's syndrome was low to begin with (0.5 percent), and the incidence over the next 5 years was no different in HIV patients compared to an HIV-negative matched cohort.[133]

Patients with other HIV-associated arthropathies often present with oligoarticular or polyarticular asymmetric arthritis without extra-articular manifestations. These arthropathies may resemble those of Reiter's syndrome, rheumatoid arthritis, or psoriatic arthritis. These patients, who usually are men, are often HLA-B27–negative. Significant clinical improvement may occur in response to antiretroviral therapy. In HIV-infected women, the rheumatologic manifestations seem to be less frequent and clinically different than in men. Raynaud's phenomenon and livedo reticularis are the most common features in women, followed by vasculitis, lupuslike syndromes, and myositis.[134] The association of psoriasis and psoriatic arthritis with AIDS has also been well recognized.[135,136] The skin condition may precede AIDS or it may occur at any of its stages, and it may worsen as immunodeficiency progresses.

Massive parotid enlargement accompanied by xerostomia, resembling Sjögren's syndrome, has also been recognized in HIV-infected persons. CD8-positive lymphocytes infiltrate the parotid gland, other salivary glands, and other nonglandular tissues[137–139]

Table 68-3. Rheumatic Manifestations Associated with HIV Infections

- Reiter's syndrome, reactive arthritis, and spondyloarthropathy
- HIV-associated arthropathy
- Psoriatic arthritis
- Diffuse infiltrative lymphocytosis syndrome
- Myositis
- Nonspecific arthralgia
- Septic arthritis-bursitis

and may be associated with peripheral neuropathy.[140] This syndrome, termed *diffuse infiltrative lymphocytosis syndrome*, is not associated with circulating autoantibodies, unlike Sjögren's syndrome.[141,142] The syndrome may worsen when immunosuppressive therapy is given and may be more common in African American men.[138]

OTHER STDs ASSOCIATED WITH ARTHROPATHY

Mycoplasma hominis rarely has caused septic arthritis, often in association with postpartum fever and bacteremia.[143–145] *U. urealyticum* is an occasional cause of acute monoarticular or polyarticular septic arthritis in patients with hypogammaglobulinemia.[146–149] Herpes simplex virus, Epstein-Barr virus, and cytomegalovirus infections are rarely associated with acute monoarticular arthritis, perhaps due to direct synovial infection; they are more commonly associated with polyarthritis, probably related to circulating immune complexes.[150–154] Acute arthritis is a major manifestation of chronic meningococcemia and may also occur during or following acute meningococcemia, which rarely may be transmitted sexually[155]; the clinical picture may mimic that of DGI.[155–159] In addition, acute noninfective arthritis occasionally follows meningococcemia. This syndrome is not associated with the HLA-B27 haplotype and probably results from immune-complex deposition. Finally, therapy of sexually transmitted diseases with penicillin or other drugs occasionally causes allergic reactions manifested by serum sickness–like illnesses—with dermatitis, arthralgias, or arthritis—associated with high concentrations of circulating immune complexes.[10]

DIFFERENTIAL DIAGNOSIS

The differential diagnosis of acute arthritis is broad, but many cases are related to sexually transmitted infections. Figure 68-2 shows the diagnoses for 151 consecutive adults (age >15 years) who required hospitalization for acute, nontraumatic arthritis or tenosynovitis of <14 days duration.[1] Disseminated gonococcal infection was documented by isolation of *N. gonorrhoeae* from 38 patients (25 percent) and was suspected on the basis of clinical features and response to antibiotic therapy in 12 others (8 percent). Sixteen patients (11 percent) had Reiter's syndrome or post-gonococcal arthritis; none of these had symptoms or signs of enteritis. None of five patients who had arthritis associated with acute HBV infection gave histories of parenteral exposure, and two of six patients with arthritis that was attributed to drug reactions had been treated with penicillin or ampicillin for gonorrhea. Thus, 73 (48 percent) of the patients in this series had arthritis that was directly or indirectly related to an STD. Among the subset of 82 patients who were 15 to 30 years of age, 43 (52 percent) had DGI and 58 (71 percent) were related to sexually transmissible infections. In recent years, however, the decreasing incidence of gonorrhea and the declining prevalence of gonococcal strains that are likely to disseminate have reduced the frequency of DGI in many geographic areas.[155] Nevertheless, the proportion of acute arthropathy that is directly or indirectly due to an STD remains high. Infection with HIV also should be considered in all sexually active persons who present with acute arthritis.

Reiter's syndrome and disseminated gonococcal infection undoubtedly remain the two most common causes of sexually acquired arthritis, and either may present with a combination of arthropathy, genitourinary inflammation, dermatitis, and conjunctivitis or iritis. Sometimes this poses a diagnostic dilemma, but in most cases the correct diagnosis can be made readily using clinical criteria. The two syndromes usually can be differentiated from one another by their characteristic mucocutaneous lesions, if present. Several surveys have documented differing predilections of Reiter's syndrome and DGI for various joints or groups of joints, but the overlap in affected joints is considerable (Fig. 68-8). The pattern of joints involved also is nonspecific; the exceptions are sacroiliitis, typical fusiform dactylitis (see Fig. 68-3), or calcaneal enthesopathy, which are seen exclusively in Reiter's syndrome.[44,103] Tenosynovitis is often considered evidence for DGI, but it also may be the sole feature in Reiter's syndrome and does not reliably distinguish DGI from Reiter's syndrome or other acute arthritides. The presence of NGU, conjunctivitis, or radiographically confirmed sacroiliitis almost always indicates Reiter's syndrome rather than DGI.

Genital, anorectal, or pharyngeal gonococcal infection can be identified in 70 to 80 percent of patients with DGI or in their sex partners, but it has also been documented in up to 20 percent of patients with acute Reiter's syndrome.[44] All potential mucosal sites of infection should be tested for gonococcal infection, regardless of the presence or absence of local symptoms. *N. gonorrhoeae* was identified by culture or by the direct fluorescent antibody test in blood, synovial fluid, or skin lesions of 52 (51 percent) of 102 patients with DGI in a Seattle series[1] and in 23 (47 percent) of 49 patients studied in Boston.[8] Recent sex partners should also be examined; DGI sometimes is confirmed bacteriologically only by detection of gonorrhea in a partner.[1,160] Similarly, *C. trachomatis* should be sought in both patients with Reiter's syndrome and their sex partners.

Synovial-fluid analysis and tests for *N. gonorrhoeae* (ideally, both culture and DNA amplification) are important in identifying patients with crystal-induced arthritis and gonococcal septic arthritis. Other forms of septic arthritis also should be sought routinely with specific tests for pyogenic and other bacteria. Synovial-fluid leukocyte counts are useful in establishing the presence of

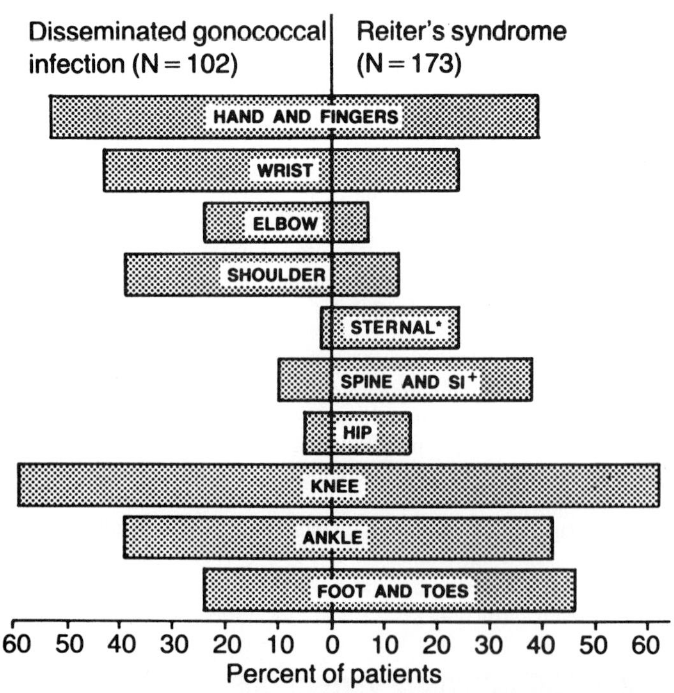

Fig. 68-8. Distributions of joints with arthritis in 102 patients with DGI[1] and 173 patients with Reiter's syndrome.[38] *Sternal includes the sternoclavicular joint. †SI denotes the sacroiliac joint.

inflammation, but not in establishing its cause. Protein, glucose, and complement levels provide nonspecific but sometimes useful information. Radiographs of peripheral joints, tests for serum uric acid levels, the erythrocyte sedimentation rate, and assays for rheumatoid factor, antinuclear antibodies, complement levels, and circulating immune complexes usually are not indicated as routine tests in acute arthritis, although they may be diagnostic in appropriate clinical settings. It has been argued that HLA typing is not diagnostically useful[161] because the diagnosis of Reiter's syndrome is more reliably based on clinical criteria and because the results of typing seldom affect therapy. On the other hand, a positive test may solidify an otherwise equivocal diagnosis of Reiter's syndrome.[162]

The diagnosis of DGI is unequivocal if *N. gonorrhoeae* is identified in blood, synovial fluid, a skin lesion, or cerebrospinal fluid. The diagnosis is also secure if a mucosal gonococcal infection is documented in the presence of a typical clinical syndrome that responds promptly to appropriate antimicrobial therapy,[1,20] especially if other causes of acute arthropathy are excluded. The presence of gonorrhea in a sexual partner also supports the diagnosis.

The American College of Rheumatology defines Reiter's syndrome as an episode of peripheral arthritis of >30 days duration occurring in association with urethritis or cervicitis.[49] These criteria will accurately classify the majority of patients with Reiter's syndrome. The occurrence of ocular inflammation or the typical mucocutaneous lesions, documentation of the HLA-B27 haplotype, and clinical or radiologic evidence of sacroiliitis help to confirm the diagnosis. The pattern of joint involvement and other clinical and laboratory features can help distinguish the reactive arthritides from rheumatoid arthritis and arthropathies due to immune-complex deposition.

Although most cases of DGI and Reiter's syndrome can be diagnosed by the above criteria, neither set of criteria is completely satisfactory for the initial evaluation of patients presenting with acute arthritis. The criteria for DGI require up to several days to obtain culture results, and those for Reiter's syndrome may require a month or more of clinical observation. The algorithm illustrated in Fig. 68-9 represents a diagnostic approach to reach a tentative diagnosis at the time of presentation of a sexually active patient with acute arthritis. The algorithm represents the logic used in analyzing the results of the initial clinical and laboratory examinations, rather than a flowchart for their performance. For example, evaluation for genital inflammation is indicated for all patients, regardless of whether a probable diagnosis is reached prior to the relevant branching point.

If synovial fluid is obtained, examination for crystals by wet preparation and for bacteria by Gram stain should be performed; occasionally these will lead to an immediate diagnosis. If no synovial fluid is present or its analysis is nondiagnostic, the results of a careful examination of the skin are considered. The presence of typical papular, pustular, or hemorrhagic lesions in various stages of evolution, located primarily on the extremities, is strong evidence of DGI. Similarly, keratoderma blennorrhagica or circinate balanitis in the patient with acute arthritis are diagnostic of Reiter's syndrome. In the absence of typical skin lesions, the results

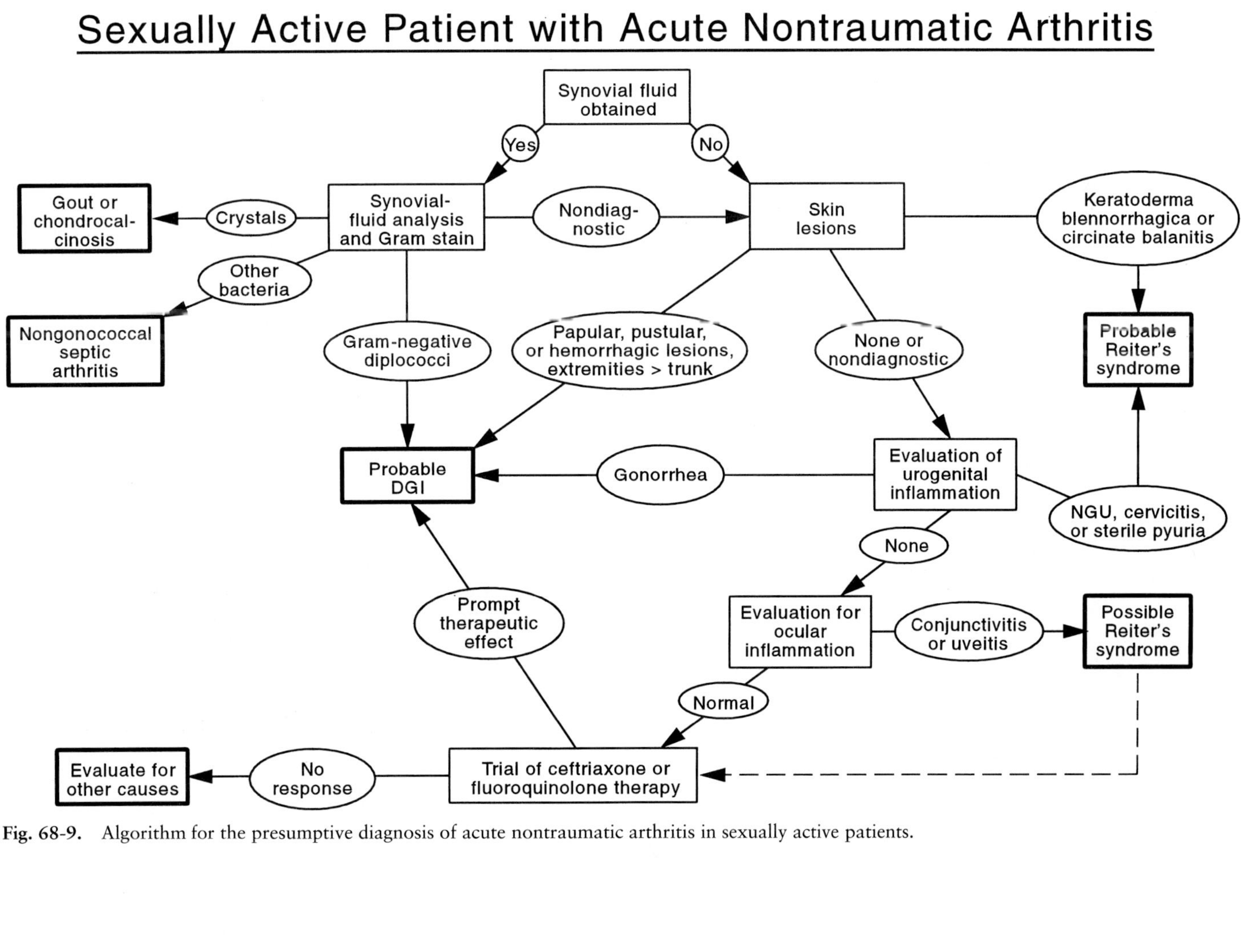

Fig. 68-9. Algorithm for the presumptive diagnosis of acute nontraumatic arthritis in sexually active patients.

of the evaluation for genital inflammation are considered. Gonococcal urethritis or cervicitis, identified by the presence of intracellular gram-negative diplococci, supports a tentative diagnosis of DGI. The presence of NGU or other nongonococcal genital-tract inflammation implies Reiter's syndrome. For patients who lack both diagnostic mucocutaneous lesions and urogenital inflammation, conjunctivitis, or uveitis suggests Reiter's syndrome, although absence of ocular inflammation is not diagnostically helpful. Regardless of the preliminary diagnosis, it is essential to obtain cultures or other sensitive and specific tests (e.g., DNA amplification assays) for *C. trachomatis* and *N. gonorrhoeae* from the cervix, urethra, and rectum, and for *N. gonorrhoeae* from the pharynx, blood, and synovial fluid. Other potentially useful tests, not reflected in the algorithm, include HLA typing, tests for HIV and HBV infection, and radiographic imaging of the sacroiliac joints.

In some cases a trial of antibiotic therapy is warranted; antibiotic-responsive, culture-negative acute arthritis in a sexually active young person often is due to DGI. Failure of response to treatment at this point necessitates further evaluation for an acute presentation of a rheumatic disease such as rheumatoid arthritis or systemic lupus erythematosus. Blood cultures must be obtained prior to the therapeutic trial not only to detect gonococcemia but also to help exclude other septic arthritides and infective endocarditis as a cause of arthritis. If monoarticular arthritis persists during continued observation, synovial biopsy may be required to exclude tuberculosis, fungal infection, or a synovial tumor.

MANAGEMENT

The treatment of DGI is discussed in Chap. 32. Ceftriaxone and the fluoroquinolones are now the mainstays of antibiotic therapy; bed rest, closed drainage of purulent synovial effusions, and anti-inflammatory drugs are adjuncts. In Reiter's syndrome, NGU or cervicitis should be treated, usually with doxycycline or azithromycin, as described in Chap. 29. Similarly, antimicrobial therapy is indicated for many cases of infectious enteritis, depending in part on the specific microbial etiology. Treatment of the triggering infection has not been shown to affect the course of established arthritis, mucocutaneous lesions, or ocular manifestations, however, and the mainstay of treatment is administration of anti-inflammatory drugs. The greatest published experience is with indomethacin, but several other nonsteroidal anti-inflammatory agents are effective for symptomatic control of the arthritis; aspirin and corticosteroids offer little benefit for most patients. Therapeutic trials with various drugs should be used as necessary to balance efficacy and tolerance in individual patients. For fulminant cases resistant to these drugs, methotrexate or immunosuppressive agents (e.g., azathioprine) have been used successfully. Most cases of Reiter's syndrome should be managed in consultation with a rheumatologist.

Arthritis due to HBV infection is self-limited and usually does not require drug therapy, although symptoms may be ameliorated by transient use of aspirin or other nonsteroidal anti-inflammatory drugs. Patients with arthritis due to syphilis, lymphogranuloma venereum, or other sexually transmitted infections should be treated with standard antibiotic regimens. Arthritis associated with HIV is managed with nonsteroidal anti-inflammatory drugs and may respond to antiretroviral therapy.

References

1 Handsfield HH: Disseminated gonococcal infection. *Clin Obstet Gynecol* 18:131, 1975.

2 Calin A: Reiter's Syndrome, in *Textbook of Rheumatology,* WN Kelly, ED Harris, S Ruddy, CB Sledge (eds). Philadelphia, WB Saunders, 1985, p 1007.

3 Reiter H: Ueber eine bisher unerkannte Spirochatern infektion (Spirochaetosis Arthritica). *Dtsche Med Wochenschr* 42:1535, 1916.

4 Bauer W, Engleman EP: A syndrome of unknown etiology characterized by urethritis, conjunctivitis and arthritis (so-called Reiter's disease). *Trans Assoc Am Physicians* 57:307, 1942.

5 Keat A: Reiter's syndrome and reactive arthritis in perspective. *N Engl J Med* 309:1606, 1983.

6 Calin A: Seronegative spondyloarthritides. *Med Clin North Am* 70: 323, 1986.

7 Manshady BM et al: Septic arthritis in a general hospital, 1966–1977. *J Rheumatol* 7:523, 1980.

8 O'Brien JP et al: Disseminated gonococcal infection: A prospective analysis of 49 patients and a review of pathophysiology and immune mechanisms. *Medicine* 62:395, 1983.

9 Shapiro L et al: Dermatohistopathology of chronic gonococcal sepsis. *Arch Dermatol* 107:403, 1973.

10 Williams RC: *Immune Complexes in Clinical and Experimental Medicine*. Cambridge, MA: Harvard University Press, 1980.

11 Keiser H et al: Clinical forms of gonococcal arthritis. *N Engl J Med* 279:234, 1968.

12 Brandt KD et al: Gonococcal arthritis: Clinical features correlated with blood, synovial fluid and genitourinary cultures. *Arthritis Rheum* 17:503, 1974.

13 Gelfand SC et al: Spectrum of gonococcal arthritis: Evidence for sequential stages and clinical subgroups. *J Rheumatol* 2:83, 1975.

14 Holmes KK et al: Disseminated gonococcal infection. *Ann Intern Med* 74:979, 1971.

15 Barr J, Danielsson D: Septic gonococcal dermatitis. *Br Med J* 1:482, 1971.

16 Tronca E et al: Demonstration of *Neisseria gonorrhoeae* with fluorescent antibody in patients with disseminated gonococcal infection. *J Infect Dis* 129:583, 1974.

17 Rothschild BM, Schrank GD: Histologic documentation of gonococcal infection in the absence of a culturable organism. *Clin Rheumatol* 3:389, 1984.

18 Gantz NM et al: Gonococcal osteomyelitis: An unusual complication of gonococcal arthritis. *JAMA* 236:2431, 1976.

19 Garcia-Kutzbach A et al: Gonococcal arthritis: Clinical features and results of penicillin therapy. *J Rheumatol* 1:210, 1974.

20 Handsfield HH et al: Treatment of the gonococcal arthritis-dermatitis syndrome. *Arch Intern Med* 84:661, 1976.

21 Cooke CL et al: Gonococcal arthritis: A survey of 54 cases. *JAMA* 217:204, 1971.

22 Walker LC et al: Circulating immune complexes in disseminated gonorrheal infection. *Ann Intern Med* 89:28, 1978.

23 Ludivicio CL, Myers AR: Survey for immune complexes in disseminated gonococcal arthritis-dermatitis syndrome. *Arthritis Rheum* 22: 19, 1979.

24 Martin DA et al: Identification of immune complexes in synovial fluids and sera of patients with disseminated gonococcal infections (DGI) using the Raji cell assay. *Arthritis Rheum* 24:S74, 1981.

25 Manicourt DH, Orloff S: Gonococcal arthritis-dermatitis syndrome: Study of serum and synovial fluid immune complex levels. *Arthritis Rheum* 25:574, 1982.

26 Flemming RJ et al: Arthropathic properties of gonococcal peptidoglycan fragments: Implications for the pathogenesis of disseminated gonococcal disease. *Infect Immun* 52:600, 1986.

27 Holmes KK et al. The gonococcal arthritis-dermatitis syndrome. *Ann Intern Med* 75:470, 1971.

28 Keefer CS, Spink WW: Gonococcal arthritis: Pathogenesis, mechanisms of recovery and treatment. *JAMA* 109:1448, 1937.

29 Brogadir SP et al: Spectrum of the gonococcal arthritis-dermatitis syndrome. *Semin Arthritis Rheum* 8:177, 1979.

30 Handsfield HH et al: Correlation of auxotype and penicillin susceptibility of *Neisseria gonorrhoeae* with sexual preference and clinical manifestations of gonorrhea. *Sex Transm Dis* 7:1, 1980.

31 Goldenberg DL, Cohen AS: Acute infection arthritis. *Am J Med* 60:369, 1976.

32 Wright V: Arthritis associated with veneral disease: A comparative study of gonococcal arthritis and Reiter's syndrome. *Ann Rheum Dis* 22:77, 1963.

33 Metzger AL: Gonococcal arthritis complicating gonorrheal pharyngitis. *N Eng J Med* 73:267, 1970.

34 Goldman JA: Patterns of gonococcal arthritis. *J Rheumatol* 8:707, 1981.

35 Cooke DB et al: Gonococcal endocarditis in the antibiotic era. *Arch Intern Med* 139:1247, 1979.

36 Ebright JR, Komorowski R: Gonococcal endocarditis associated with immune complex glomerulonephritis. *Am J Med* 68(5):793, 1980.

37 Fink CW: Gonococcal arthritis in children. *JAMA* 194:237, 1965.

38 Kousa M et al: Frequent association of chlamydial infection with Reiter's syndrome. *Sex Transm Dis* 5:57, 1978.

39 Martin DH et al: *Chlamydia trachomatis* infections in men with Reiter's syndrome. *Ann Intern Med* 100:207, 1984.

40 Rosenthal L et al: Aseptic arthritis after gonorrhea. *Ann Rheum Dis* 39:141, 1980.

41 Ford DK: Venereal arthritis. *Br J Vener Dis* 29:123, 1953.

42 Olhagen B: Chronic uropolyarthritis in the male. *Acta Med Scand* 168:339, 1960.

43 Cleuziou A et al: Reactive arthritis after gonococcal infection. *Rev Med Interne* 5:65, 1984.

44 Kousa M: Clinical observations on Reiter's disease with special reference to the venereal and nonvenereal aetiology: A follow-up study. *Acta Dermato Venereol (Stockh)* 58(Suppl 81):1, 1978.

45 Calin A, Fries JF: An "experimental" epidemic of Reiter's syndrome revisited: Follow-up evidence on genetic and environmental factors. *Ann Intern Med* 84:564, 1976.

46 Paronen I: Reiter's disease: A study of 344 cases observed in Finland. *Acta Med Scand* 130(suppl 212):1, 1948.

47 Repo H et al: Exaggerated inflammatory responsiveness plays a part in the pathogenesis of HLA-B27 linked diseases: Hypothesis. *Ann Clin Res* 16:47, 1984.

48 Fox R et al: The chronicity and disability in Reiter's syndrome. *Ann Intern Med* 91:190, 1979.

49 Wilkens RF et al: Reiter's syndrome: Evaluation of preliminary criteria for definite disease. *Arthritis Rheum* 24:844, 1981.

50 Arnett FC et al: Cross-reactive HLA antigens in B27-negative Reiter's syndrome and sacroiliitis. *Johns Hopkins Med J* 141:193, 1977.

51 Khan MA et al: Low association of HLA-B27 with Reiter's syndrome in blacks. *Ann Intern Med* 90:202, 1979.

52 Good AE et al: HLA-B27 in blacks with ankylosing spondylitis or Reiter's disease. *N Engl J Med* 194:166, 1976.

53 Khan MA et al: HLA-B27 in ankylosing spondylitis: Differences in frequency and relative risk in American blacks and Caucasians. *J Rheumatol* 4(supp 13):39, 1977.

54 Jardetzky TS et al: Identification of self-peptides bound to purified HLA-B27. *Nature* 353:326, 1991.

55 Schumacher TNM et al: Peptide selection by MHC class I molecules. *Nature* 350:703, 1991.

56 Schwimmbeck PL et al: Autoantibodies to HLA-B27 in the sera of HLA-B27 patients with ankylosing spondylitis and Reiter's syndrome: Molecular mimicry with *Klebsiella pneumoniae* as potential mechanism of autoimmune disease. *J Exp Med* 166:173, 1987.

57 McMichael AJ: Role of class I molecules of the major histocompatibility complex in cytotoxic T-cell function in health and disease. *Springer Semin Immunopathol* 14:1, 1992.

58 Kaufmann SHE: CD8+ T lymphocytes in intracellular microbial infections. *Immunol Today* 9:168, 1988.

59 Hassell AB, et al: MHC restriction of synovial fluid lymphocyte responses to the triggering organism in reactive arthritis: Absence of a class I-restricted response. *Clin Exp Immunol* 88:442, 1992.

60 Geczy AF, Yap J: A survey of isolates of *Klebsiella pneumoniae* which cross-react with HLA-B27-associated cell surface structure on the lymphocytes of patients with ankylosing spondylitis. *J Rheumatol* 9:97, 1982.

61 Ewing C et al: Antibody activity in ankylosing spondylitis sera to two sites on HLA-B27.1 at the MHC groove region (within sequence 65–85), and to a *Klebsiella pneumoniae* nitrogenase reductase peptide (within sequence 181–199). *J Exp Med* 171:1635, 1990.

62 Schwimmbeck PL, Oldstone MB: *Klebsiella pneumoniae* and HLA-B27 associated diseases of Reiter's syndrome and ankylosing spondylitis. *Curr Top Microbiol Immunol* 145:45, 1989.

63 Tsuchiya N et al: Studies of humoral and cell-mediated immunity to peptides shared by HLA-27.1 and *Klebsiella pneumoniae* nitrogenase in ankylosing spondylitis. *Clin Exp Immunol* 76:354, 1989.

64 Kellner H et al: Serum antibodies from patients with ankylosing spondylitis and Reiter's syndrome are reactive with HLA-B27 cells transfected with the *Mycobacterium tuberculosis* hsp60 gene. *Infect and Immun* 62:484, 1994.

65 Firestein GS, Zfaifler NJ: Reactive arthritis. *Annu Rev Med* 38:351, 1987.

66 Hammer RE et al: Spontaneous inflammatory disease in transgenic rats expressing HLA-B27 and human b2-m: An animal model of HLA-B27 associated human disorders. *Cell* 63:1099, 1990.

67 Breban M et al: Transmission of the inflammatory disease of HLA-B27 transgenic rats by bone marrow engraftment. *J Exp Med* 178:1607, 1993.

68 Dunlop EMC et al: Infection by TRIC agent and other members of the Bedsonia group, with a note on Reiter's disease: III. Genital infection and diseases of the eye. *Trans Opthalmol Soc UK* 86:321, 1966.

69 Schachter J: Can Chlamydial Infections Cause Rheumatic Disease? in *Infection and Immunology in the Rheumatic Diseases* DC Dumonde (ed). Oxford, Blackwell, 1976, p 151.

70 Reiter's syndrome [editorial]. *Lancet* 2:567, 1979.

71 Keat A et al: *Chlamydia trachomatis* and reactive arthritis: The missing link. *Lancet* 1:72, 1987.

72 Taylor-Robinson D et al: Evidence that *Chlamydia trachomatis* causes seronegative arthritis in women. *Ann Rheum Dis* 295:295, 1988.

73 Taylor-Robinson D et al: Detection of *Chlamydia trachomatis* DNA in joints of reactive arthritis patients by polymerase chain reaction. *Lancet* 340:81, 1992.

74 Csonka GW: The course of Reiter's syndrome. *Br Med J* 1:1088, 1958.

75 Bardin T et al: Antibiotic treatment of venereal disease and Reiter's syndrome in a Greenland population. *Arthritis Rheum* 35:190, 1992.

76 Ford DK et al: Cell-mediated immune responses of synovial mononuclear cells to sexually transmitted, enteric and mumps antigens in patients with Reiter's syndrome, rheumatoid arthritis, and ankylosing spondylitis. *J Rheumatol* 8:220, 1981.

77 Ford DK: Infectious agents in Reiter's syndrome. *Clin Exp Rheumatol* 2:273, 1983.

78 Bjelle A, Tarnvik A: Lymphocytes of synovial fluid and peripheral blood in reactive arthritis. *Scand J Infect Dis* 24(suppl):58, 1980.

79 Brenner MB et al: In vitro T lymphocyte proliferative responses to *Yersinia enterocolitica* in Reiter's syndrome. *Arthritis Rheum* 27:250, 1984.

80 Rowe IF, Keat ACS: Human immunodeficiency virus infection and the rheumatologist. *Ann Rheum Dis* 48:89, 1989.

81 Pereira AB et al: Detection and partial characterization of circulating immune complexes with solid-phase anti-C3. *J Immunol* 125:763, 1980.

82 Yates DG et al: Complement activation in Reiter's syndrome. *Ann Rheum Dis* 34:468, 1975.

83 Norton WL et al: Light and electron microscopic observations on the synovitis of Reiter's disease. *Arthritis Rheum* 9:747, 1966.

84 Paty JG: Reiter's syndrome: Occurrence in roommates. *Arthritis Rheum* 21:283, 1978.

85 Good AE, Schultz JS: Reiter's syndrome following *Shigella flexneri* 2a. *Arthritis Rheum* 20:100, 1977.

86 Jones RAK: Reiter's disease after *Salmonella typhimurium* enteritis. *Br Med J* 1:1391, 1977.

87 Warren CPW: Arthritis associated with *Salmonella* infection. *Ann Rheum Dis* 29:483, 1970.
88 Laitinen O et al: Relation between HLA-B27 and clinical features in patients with *Yersinia* arthritis. *Arthritis Rheum* 20:1121, 1977.
89 Ahvonen P: Human yersiniosis in Finland: II. Clinical features. *Ann Clin Res* 4:39, 1972.
90 Jacks JC: *Yersinia enterocolitica* arthritis. *Pediatrics* 55:236, 1975.
91 van de Putten LBA et al: Reactive arthritis after *Campylobacter jejuni* enteritis. *J Rheumatol* 7:531, 1980.
92 Keat AC et al: The role of *Chlamydia trachomatis* and HLA-B27 in sexually acquired reactive arthritis. *Br Med J* 1:605, 1978.
93 Neuwelt CM et al: Reiter's syndrome: A male and female disease. *J Rheumatol* 9:268, 1982.
94 Smith DL et al: Reiter's disease in women. *Arthritis Rheum* 23:335, 1980.
95 Yli-Kerttula UI et al: Urogenital involvements and rheumatic disorders in females: An interview study. *Clin Rheumatol* 4:170, 1985.
96 Hagenfeldt K, Szanto E: Sacroiliitis in women: A late sequela to acute salpingitis. *Am J Obstet Gynecol* 138:1039, 1980.
97 Vilppula AH et al: Musculoskeletal involvements in female sexual partners of males with Reiter's syndrome. *Clin Rheumatol* 2:347, 1983.
98 McCord WC et al: Acute venereal arthritis. *Arch Intern Med* 137: 858, 1977.
99 Catterall RD: Uveitis, arthritis and nonspecific genital infection. *Br J Vener Dis* 36:27, 1960.
100 Romanus R: Pelveospondylitis ossificans in the male and genitourinary infection. *Acta Med Scand* 280(suppl):53, 1963.
101 Singsen B et al: Reiter's syndrome in childhood. *Arthritis Rheum Dis* 30:213, 1971.
102 Daunt SD et al: Ulcerative vulvitis in Reiter's syndrome: A case report. *Br J Vener Dis* 58:405, 1982.
103 Ball J: Enthesopathy of rheumatoid and ankylosing spondylitis. *Ann Rheum Dis* 30:213, 1971.
104 Russell AS et al: The sacroiliitis of acute Reiter's syndrome. *J Rheumatol* 4:293, 1977.
105 Moll JMH et al: Association between ankylosing spondylitis, psoriatic arthritis, Reiter's disease, the intestinal arthropathies and Behçet's syndrome. *Medicine* 53:343, 1974.
106 Montgomery MM et al: The mucocutaneous lesions of Reiter's syndrome and keratosis blennorrhagica. *Ann Intern Med* 51:99, 1959.
107 Rossen RM et al: Atrioventicular conduction disturbances in Reiter's syndrome. *Am J Med* 58:280, 1975.
108 Block SR: Reiter's syndrome and acute aortic insufficiency. *Arthritis Rheum* 15:218, 1972.
109 Paulus HE et al: Aortic insufficiency in five patients with Reiter's syndrome. *Am J Med* 53:464, 1972.
110 Butler MJ et al: A follow-up study of 48 patients with Reiter's syndrome. *Am J Med* 67:808, 1979.
111 Caughey DE et al: A fatal case of Reiter's disease complicated by amyloidosis. *Arthritis Rheum* 16:695, 1973.
112 Alarcon GS, Townes AS: Arthritis in viral hepatitis. *Johns Hopkins Med J* 132:1, 1973.
113 Schumacher HR, Gall EP: Arthritis in acute hepatitis and chronic active hepatitis. *Am J Med* 57:655, 1974.
114 Alpert E et al: The pathogenesis of arthritis associated with viral hepatitis: Complement-component studies. *N Engl J Med* 285:185, 1971.
115 Onion DK et al: Arthritis of hepatitis associated with Australia antigen. *Ann Intern Med* 75:29, 1971.
116 Wands JR et al: The pathogenesis of arthritis associated with acute hepatitis-B surface antigen-positive hepatitis. *J Clin Invest* 55:930, 1975.
117 Schumaker JB et al: Arthritis and rash: Clues to anicteric hepatitis. *Arch Intern Med* 133:483, 1974.
118 McEwen C, Thomas EW: Syphilitic joint disease. *Med Clin North Am* 22:1275, 1938.
119 Reginato AJ et al: Synovitis in secondary syphilis: Clinical, light, and electron microscopic studies. *Arthritis Rheum* 22:170, 1979.
120 Tourville DR et al: Treponemal antigen in immunopathogenesis of syphilitic glomerulonephritis. *Am J Pathol* 82:479, 1976.
121 Floyd W et al: The neuropathic joint. *South Med J* 52:563, 1959.
122 Fishel B et al: Multiple neuropathic arthropathy in a patient with syphilis. *Clin Rheumatol* 4:348, 1985.
123 Moran SM, Mohr JA: Syphilis and axial arthropathy. *South Med J* 76:1032, 1983.
124 Koteen H: Lymphogranuloma venereum. *Medicine* 24:1, 1945.
125 Hickam JB: Cutaneous and articular manifestations in lymphogranuloma venereum. *Arch Dermatol Syphil* 51:330, 1945.
126 Lassus A et al: Auto-immune serum factors and IgA elevation in lymphogranuloma venereum. *Ann Clin Res* 2:51, 1970.
127 Keat A et al: Chlamydial infection in the etiology of arthritis. *Br Med Bull* 39:168, 1983.
128 Berman A et al: Rheumatic manifestations of human immunodeficiency virus infection. *Am J Med* 85:59, 1988.
129 Kaye BR: Rheumatologic manifestations of infection with human immunodeficiency virus (HIV). *Ann Intern Med* 111:158, 1989.
130 Forster SM et al: Inflammatory joint disease and human immunodeficiency virus infection. *Br Med J Clin Res* 296:1625, 1988.
131 Rynes RI et al: Acquired immunodeficiency syndrome-associated arthritis. *Am J Med* 84:810, 1988.
132 Muñoz Fernandez S et al: Rheumatic manifestations in 556 patients with human immunodeficiency virus infection. *Semin Arthritis Rheum* 21:30, 1991.
133 Hochberg MC et al: HIV infection is not associated with Reiter's syndrome: Data from the Johns Hopkins Multicenter AIDS Cohort Study. *AIDS* 4:1149, 1990.
134 Mendonca-Neto EC et al: HIV infection in women: Rheumatologic manifestations at the time of HIV diagnosis [abstr]. *Int Conf AIDS* 9:462, 1993.
135 Duvic M et al: Acquired immunodeficiency syndrome-associated psoriasis and Reiter's syndrome. *Arch Dermatol* 123:1622, 1987.
136 Reveille JD et al: Human immunodeficiency virus-associated psoriasis, psoriatic arthritis and Reiter's syndrome: A disease continuum? *Arthritis Rheum* 33:1574, 1990.
137 Talal N: AIDS and Sjogren's syndrome. *Bull Rheum Dis* 4:6, 1991.
138 Kazi S et al: The diffuse infiltrative lymphocytosis syndrome: Clinical and immunogenetic features in 35 patients. *AIDS* 10:385, 1996.
139 Itescu S et al: A diffuse infiltrative CD8 lymphocytosis syndrome in human immunodeficiency virus (HIV) infection: A host immune response associated with HLA-DR5. *Ann Intern Med* 112:3, 1990.
140 Moulignier A et al: Peripheral neuropathy in HIV-infected patients with diffuse infiltrative lymphocytosis syndrome (DILS). *Third Conference on Retroviruses and Opportunistic Infections*, Washington, DC, p.125, 1996.
141 Itescu S, Winchester R: Diffuse infiltrative lymphocytosis syndrome: A disorder occurring in human immunodeficiency virus-1 infection that may present as a sicca syndrome. *Rheum Dis Clin North Am* 18:683, 1992.
142 Itescu S: Diffuse infiltrative lymphocytosis syndrome in human immunodeficiency virus infection: a Sjögren's-like disease. *Rheum Dis Clin North Am* 17:99, 1991.
143 Verinder DGR: Septic arthritis due to *Mycoplasma hominis:* A case report and review of the literature. *J Bone Joint Surg* 60B:224, 1978.
144 Taylor-Robinson D et al: The association of *Mycoplasma hominis* with arthritis. *Sex Transm Dis* 10(suppl):341, 1983.
145 McDonald MI et al: Septic arthritis due to *Mycoplasma hominis. Arthritis Rheum* 26:2044, 1983.
146 Taylor-Robinson D et al: *Ureaplasma urealyticum* in the immunocompromised host. *Pediatr Infect Dis* 5(suppl):S236, 1986.
147 Roifman CM et al: Increased susceptibility to *Mycoplasma* infection in patients with hypogammaglobulinemia. *Am J Med* 80:590, 1986.
148 Webster ADB et al: *Mycoplasma* (*Ureaplasma*) septic arthritis in hypogammaglobulinemia. *Br Med J* 1:478, 1978.
149 Stuckey M et al: Identification of *Ureaplasma urealyticum* (T-strain mycoplasma) in patients with polyarthritis. *Lancet* 2:917, 1978.
150 Friedman HM et al: Acute monoarticular arthritis caused by herpes simplex virus and cytomegalovirus. *Am J Med* 69:241, 1980.

151 Sauter SVH, Utsinger PD: Viral arthritis. *Clin Rheum Dis* 4:225, 1978.
152 Brna JA, Hall RF Jr: Acute monoarticular herpetic arthritis. *J Bone Joint Surg* 66:623, 1984.
153 Remafedi G, Muldoon RL: Acute monoarticular arthritis caused by herpes simplex type 1. *Pediatrics* 72:882, 1983.
154 Ray CG et al: Acute polyarthritis associated with active Epstein-Barr virus infection. *JAMA* 248:2990, 1982.
155 Keys TF et al: Endocervical *Neisseria meningitidis* with meningococcemia. *N Engl J Med* 285:505, 1971.
156 Rompalo AM et al: The acute arthritis-dermatitis syndrome: The changing importance of *Neisseria gonorrhoeae* and *Neisseria meningitidis*. *Arch Intern Med* 147:281, 1987.
157 Fam AG et al: Clinical forms of meningococcal arthritis: A study of five cases. *J Rheumatol* 6:567, 1979.
158 Loebl DH: Acute joint infection with *Neisseria meningitidis*: A case of mistaken identity. *Milit Med* 143:777, 1978.
159 Muñoz AJ: Gonococcal and meningococcal arthritis. *Clin Rheum Dis* 4:169, 1978.
160 Mendelson J et al: Disseminated gonorrhea: Diagnosis through contact tracing. *Can Med Assoc J* 112:864, 1975.
161 Calin A: HLA-B27: To type or not to type. *Ann Intern Med* 92:208, 1980.
162 Khan MA, Khan MK: Diagnostic value of HLA-B27 testing in ankylosing spondylitis and Reiter's syndrome. *Ann Intern Med* 96:70, 1982.

Chapter 69

Sexually transmitted intestinal syndromes

Janice R. Verley
Thomas C. Quinn

Sexually transmitted intestinal syndromes involve a wide variety of pathogens involving multiple sites of the gastrointestinal tract. Infections of the anus and rectum are frequently sexually transmitted and occur primarily in homosexual men and heterosexual women who engage in anorectal intercourse. Anorectal infections with syphilis, gonorrhea, condyloma acuminata, lymphogranuloma venereum (LGV), and granuloma inguinale (donovanosis) have been recognized for many years, and more recently other common STD pathogens such as herpes simplex virus (HSV) and non-LGV strains of *Chlamydia trachomatis* have also been recognized as causing anorectal infection.[1–6] In addition, infections with pathogens that have traditionally been associated with food or waterborne acquisition or with foreign travel (for example, *Giardia lamblia*, *Entamoeba histolytica*, *Campylobacter*, *Shigella*, and hepatitis A) are known to occur via sexual transmission.

Over the past several years the array of sexually transmitted intestinal disorders has become even more complex, with the recognition of opportunistic infections within the gastrointestinal tract of patients with acquired immunodeficiency syndrome (AIDS).[7–9] Prominent among these infections are *Candida*, Microsporidia, *Cryptosporidium*, *Isospora*, *Cyclospora*, *Mycobacterium avium*–complex (MAC), and cytomegalovirus (CMV).[10–12] This diverse array of sexually transmitted infections responsible for intestinal disease remains a challenge to the clinician.

DEFINITIONS

Depending on the pathogen and the location of the infection, symptoms and clinical manifestations vary widely. The normal anorectal anatomy is illustrated in Figs. 69-1 and 69-2. The perianal area up to the anal verge is lined by keratinized, stratified squamous dermal epithelium. Thus, perianal lesions caused by syphilis, HSV, granuloma inguinale, chancroid, and condyloma acuminata generally resemble the corresponding lesions as they appear elsewhere in the genital area. The anal canal, which extends 2 cm from the anal verge internally to the anorectal (pectinate or dentate) line, is lined by epithelium which gradually changes from stratified squamous to stratified cuboidal epithelium and is supplied with one of the richest networks of sensory nerve endings in the body. Infection of this area is commonly very painful and results in constipation and tenesmus (ineffectual straining to defecate) due to spasm of the anal sphincter muscle. The external hemorrhoidal venous plexus surrounds the anal verge.

At the anorectal line, the separation of the anal canal from the rectum is indicated by the longitudinal folds called the columns of Morgagni. The internal hemorrhoidal venous plexus occurs at the level of the columns of Morgagni. In this area the epithelium consists of transitional cuboidal cells, mucus-producing columnar cells, and blind-end crypts.

From the anorectal line cephalad is the rectum, which is lined by columnar epithelium. The term *proctitis* refers to inflammation of the rectal mucosa. Symptoms include constipation, tenesmus, rectal discomfort or pain, hematochezia (passage of bloody stools), and a mucopurulent rectal discharge which is occasionally misinterpreted by the patient as diarrhea. Although stretching of rectal tissue causes pain, the area is insensitive to other direct stimuli such as a rectal biopsy. Hence, infections which involve the rectum but spare the anus are relatively painless. Sigmoidoscopic findings may range from normal mucosa with only mucopus present to diffuse inflammation of the mucosa with friability or discrete ulcerations. If these sigmoidoscopic findings are limited to the rectum and further passage of the sigmoidoscope reveals normal mucosa above 15 cm, the condition is properly termed proctitis; if the mucosa is abnormal as high as the sigmoidoscope is passed, the condition probably represents proctocolitis, which could be confirmed by colonoscopy. Proctitis and proctocolitis generally have different infectious etiologies. Rectal biopsy provides histologic confirmation of proctitis, and findings may reveal nonspecific inflammation or changes highly suggestive of certain infections such as LGV, HSV, or syphilis.[13]

Enteritis is an inflammatory illness of the duodenum, jejunum, and/or ileum. Sigmoidoscopy shows no abnormalities. Infectious enteritis is usually contracted either by ingestion of pathogens present in feces-contaminated water or food, or by certain sexual practices or other forms of human contact which result in fecal ingestion. Symptoms of enteritis consist of diarrhea, abdominal pain, bloating, cramps, and nausea. Additional symptoms may include flatulence, urgency, a mucous rectal discharge, and in severe cases melena. Systemic manifestations such as fever, volume depletion with orthostatic hypotension, acidosis, hypokalemia, malabsorption syndrome, weight loss, and myalgias may also be present. The presence of fecal leukocytes, as determined by Gram stain or methylene blue stain of stool or rectal swabs, usually implicates an invasive inflammatory process but does not differentiate between various sites of involvement of the intestinal tract.

Esophagitis is an inflammatory process of the esophagus which may or may not extend to involve the oral cavity. Infections of the esophagus are most commonly seen in immunocompromised individuals in whom opportunistic pathogens such as *Candida albicans*, CMV, and HSV infections proliferate and induce ulcerations. Symptoms of esophagitis typically consist of dysphagia and odynophagia. Esophograms may reveal irregularity of the mucosa, dilatation, and abnormal motility, and endoscopy frequently reveals either ulcerations or cottage-cheese exudates, depending upon the infecting organism.

ETIOLOGY AND EPIDEMIOLOGY

Microorganisms not requiring an intermediate host may be transmitted by the oral-anal or genital-anal routes.[14] Those pathogens which may cause gastrointestinal illness and which have been proved to be or have the potential to be sexually transmitted are shown in Table 69-1. Those enteric pathogens which are infectious at low inoculums, such as *Shigella* (10 to 100 organisms), *Giardia lamblia* (10 to 100 cysts), and *Entamoeba histolytica* (10 to 100 cysts), all occur commonly in homosexual men and are thought to be sexually transmitted, though the routes of transmission have not been defined. Hepatitis A virus appears to be transmitted by oral-anal sex.[15]

Sexual transmission of enteric pathogens which are shed in feces may be attributable to ingestion of feces during anilingus or during fellatio of a fecally contaminated penis or to direct intrarectal inoculation of organisms by a fecally contaminated penis. Anorectal infection with conventional STD pathogens in men is caused by rectal intercourse. Fomite transmission such as may occur with the shared use of unsterile equipment for rectal douching and co-

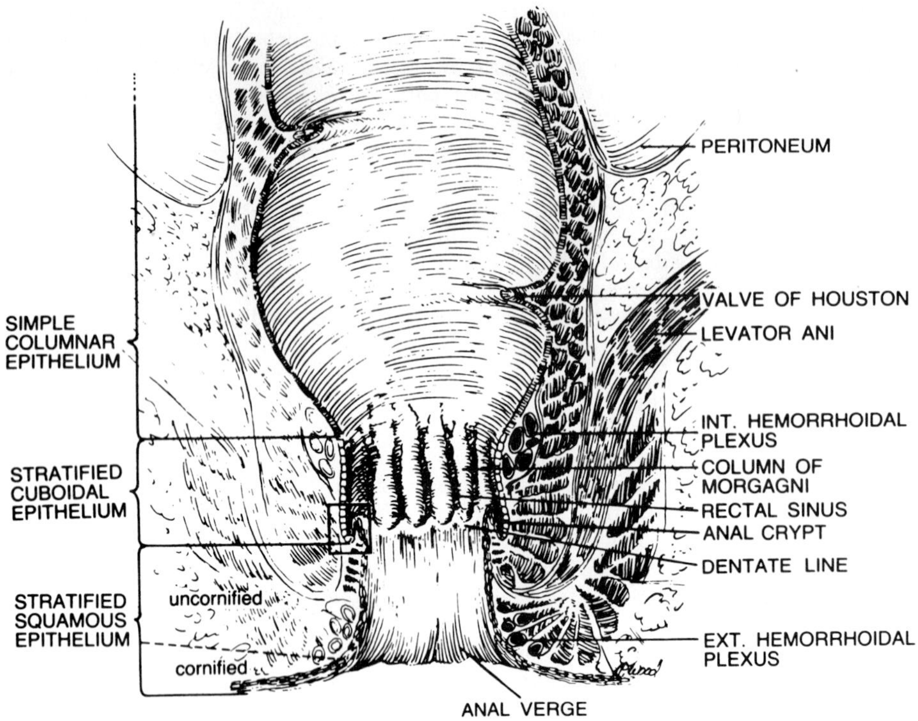

Fig. 69-1. Diagram of the rectum and anal canal, showing normal anal and rectal structures with the types of epithelium lining the anus and rectum. The box outlining the anal crypt is enlarged in Fig. 69-2.

lonic irrigation may be an additional mechanism. An outbreak of amebiasis has been traced to use of unsterile equipment for colonic irrigation.[16]

In the pre-AIDS era, the role of homosexual transmission of certain enteric infections was recognized with increasing frequency.[17] For example, in San Francisco between 1975 and 1977 the reported cases of amebiasis, shigellosis, hepatitis A, and hepatitis B showed a marked predominance in males between the ages of 20 and 39. Many of these individuals acknowledged homosexual contact, including anilingus and fellatio. Fecal cultures of homosexual contacts of men with *Shigella* infection revealed that their contacts were often asymptomatic carriers of *Shigella* of the same serotype. Similarly, several men with *Salmonella* infection had had sexual relations with men who were asymptomatic carriers of the same serotype.[18] A marked predominance of men in this age group was reported for these infections in other parts of the United States as well.[19–23]

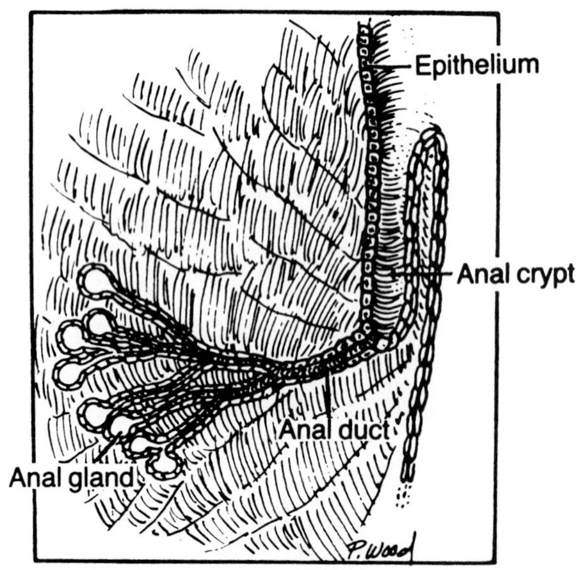

Fig. 69-2. Diagrammatic representation of the anal crypt. The anal crypts are located along the dentate line and consist of anal ducts which penetrate into muscle. These ducts are lined by both stratified squamous and mucus-secreting cells.

Heterosexuals could also be at risk for acquiring enteric infections by anilingus, and women can acquire anorectal STD by anal intercourse.[24] However, many sexually transmitted anorectal infections with *Neisseria gonorrhoeae*, *Chlamydia trachomatis*, HSV, and human papillomavirus in women probably result from contiguous spread of infection from the genitalia.

There are very few reports on the prevalence of anorectal infection with the infectious agents named above in patients seen in the STD clinic setting. In a study of 260 homosexual men with anorectal symptoms, specific infections, including gonorrhea, syphilis, hepatitis, amebiasis, *Shigella*, and LGV, were present in only 21 percent of the patients.[17] The remainder had condylomata acuminata, hemorrhoids, "nonspecific proctitis," and a variety of rectal conditions such as polyps, fissures, fistulas, perirectal abscesses, ulcers, and foreign bodies. However, in a more detailed microbiologic study of 194 homosexual men presenting to an STD clinic in the pre-AIDS era with anorectal and/or intestinal symptoms, specific anorectal or enteric infections with one or more pathogens were demonstrated in 80 percent.[25] In comparison, significantly fewer homosexual men without such symptoms who were seen in the same clinic were found to be infected with these pathogens. The prevalence of specific infections in each group is shown in Table 69-2.

The same study examined the association of specific pathogens with specific symptoms and signs (Table 69-3). Prominent pathogens in patients with symptoms and signs of proctitis were *N. gonorrhoeae*, HSV, *C. trachomatis* (non-LGV), and *Treponema pallidum*. The only pathogen associated with symptoms and signs of enteritis was *Giardia lamblia*. *Campylobacter* species, *Chla-*

Table 69-1. Sexually Transmissible Causes of Intestinal or Anal Infections in Homosexual Men

Bacterial pathogens
- *Neisseria gonorrhoeae*
- *Neisseria meningitidis*
- *Chlamydia trachomatis*
- *Haemophilus ducreyi*
- *Calymmatobacterium granulomatis*
- *Treponema pallidum*
- *Group A β-hemolytic streptococci*

Enteric bacterial pathogens
- *Shigella* sp.
- *Salmonella* sp.
- *Campylobacter* sp.

Fungus
- *Candida albicans*

Protozoa
- *Giardia lamblia*
- *Entamoeba histolytica*
- *Dientamoeba fragilis*
- *Cryptosporidium* sp.*
- *Isospora belli**
- Microsporidia*
- Cyclospora*
- "Nonpathogenic" protozoans

Helminths
- *Enterobius vermicularis*
- *Strongyloides stercoralis*

Viruses
- Herpes simplex virus
- Cytomegalovirus*
- Adenovirus*
- Human papilloma virus
- Human immunodeficiency virus
- Hepatitis A and B viruses

* Commonly seen in HIV-infected homosexual men; not necessarily sexually transmitted.

mydia trachomatis (LGV), and *Shigella flexneri* were associated with evidence of proctocolitis. In this study, 22 percent of symptomatic patients had multiple infections (see Table 69-2). For example, 48 percent of patients with anorectal gonorrhea were also found to have one or more additional pathogens present, and four or more pathogens were found in several patients. In the absence of a history of foreign travel, the demonstration of infections with multiple enteric pathogens, including "nonpathogenic" protozoa, should suggest sexual transmission. Histories of homosexual behavior have been recorded in other community outbreaks of shigellosis, giardiasis, and amebiasis.[21,22,26–28]

IMPACT OF HIV ON SEXUALLY TRANSMITTED INTESTINAL INFECTIONS

In recent years, studies have documented the interaction of HIV with other STDs. HIV transmission has been associated with a history of syphilis and HSV infections, antibodies to HSV-2[29–32] and *T. pallidum*,[33,34] anal warts,[35] *C. trachomatis*[36] and *N. gonorrhoeae* genital infection,[37] and rectal gonorrhea.[38] Law et al. recently demonstrated an independent association between HIV-seropositivity and histologically diagnosed proctitis in homosexual men.[39] Although the association between HIV and other STDs is clear, methodological variables have made it difficult to determine whether these infections truly facilitate HIV infection or serve as markers for other risk factors such as unprotected anal intercourse which have a significant impact on HIV transmission.[40]

Evidence is accumulating from in vitro data that STD pathogens may directly facilitate HIV transmission. Activation of HIV-1 from latency by coinfection with HSV-2 has been demonstrated. Recently Ho et al. showed that neutrophils from HIV-seronegative donors induced HIV-1 replication in chronically infected mononuclear cells in the presence of *C. trachomatis*.[41] Additionally, Moss et al. have shown that successful treatment of gonococcal urethritis is associated with a twofold reduction in urethral HIV-1 DNA, indicating that treatment of other STDs may decrease HIV-1 transmission.[42]

Other STDs may act as cofactors for HIV-1 transmission, and HIV infection may alter the clinical course of a variety of sexually transmitted gastrointestinal syndromes. Anorectal infections appear to have a more aggressive course in HIV-infected patients. Several studies have demonstrated failure of chancroid ulcers to respond to standard therapy,[43,44] more aggressive course of HSV-2 ulcers with development of giant ulcers,[45] more rapid progression to neurosyphilis,[46] atypical clinical and serologic response to syphilis,[47–49] failure to respond to standard syphilitic therapy,[50,51] and increased rates of anal intraepithelial neoplasia in patients coinfected with HPV and HIV-1.[52–55]

Table 69-2. Infectious Pathogens Identified in 194 Homosexual Men with and without Anorectal or Intestinal Symptoms

Anorectal and intestinal pathogens[a]	Symptomatic group, % (N = 119)	Asymptomatic group, % (N = 75)
Neisseria gonorrhoeae	31*	23
Herpes simplex virus	19*	4
Chlamydia trachomatis	10	5
Treponema pallidum	5	1
Entamoeba histolytica	29	25
Giardia lamblia	14	4
Campylobacter jejuni/C. fetus fetus	7	3
Shigella flexneri	3	1
Clostridium difficile cytotoxin	3	1
Enterovirus (Echovirus 11)	3	1
Patients with any of the above pathogens	80*	39
Patients with more than one of the above pathogens	22*	4

SOURCE: TC Quinn et al.[25]

[a] Other infectious agents identified were campylobacterlike organisms, nonpathogenic protozoans, *Candida albicans, Neisseria meningitidis, Ureaplasma urealyticum,* and *Mycoplasma hominis.*

* $p < .05$

Table 69-3. Microbial and Symptomatic Correlates of Proctitis, Proctocolitis, and Enteritis among 65 Homosexual Men with Intestinal Symptoms Who Underwent Sigmoidoscopy to a Distance above 15 cm

	Proctitis: sigmoidoscopic findings abnormal only below 15 cm (N = 41)	Proctocolitis: sigmoidoscopic findings abnormal beyond 15 cm (N = 15)	Enteritis: sigmoidoscopic findings normal (N = 9)
Sexually transmitted rectal pathogens:			
Neisseria gonorrhoeae	12	0	2
Herpes simplex virus	13	1	0
Chlamydia trachomatis (non-LGV)	8	1	0
Treponema pallidum	6	0	0
Total with any rectal pathogens	33*	2	2
Infectious causes of colitis:			
Campylobacter jejuni/C. fetus fetus	3	4	0
Shigella flexneri	0	2	0
Chlamydia trachomatis (LGV)	0	3	0
Entamoeba histolytica	5(26)[a]	4(11)	1(8)
Clostridium difficile cytotoxin	1	1	0
Total with any colitis pathogen	8	9	1
Infectious causes of inflammation limited to small intestine:			
Giardia lamblia	2(26)	2(11)	4(8)
Any three of the following four symptoms present: diarrhea, abdominal pain, bloating, nausea	3	8	9*
Any three of the following four symptoms present: constipation, rectal discharge, anorectal pain, tenesmus	38*	7	0

SOURCE: TC Quinn et al.[25]

[a] Figures in parentheses indicate the number of patients who submitted stools for examination for ova and parasites.

* $p < .05$, by multiple logistic regression analysis.

Several recent reports of HIV-infected patients referred to colorectal surgery clinics for anorectal diseases from 1983 to 1995 confirm the findings by Quinn et al.[25,56–59] The majority of these patients were homosexual men with AIDS. Approximately 63 percent of these patients had more than one lesion on presentation, and 20 percent had more than one pathogen identified.[56,57] The authors describe a wide variety of anorectal lesions, including ulcers, condylomas, fissures, fistulas, and abscesses. The most common etiologies were condylomas and CMV and HSV-2 ulcerations. Idiopathic anorectal ulcerations have also been described, usually in patients with CD4 counts of less than 20/mm^3. No etiology for the lesions was found after routine microbiologic, sigmoidoscopic, and histological examination. These ulcerations appear less responsive to steroid therapy than was previously reported for idiopathic esophageal ulcers.[60]

The gastrointestinal tract appears to be a major target organ in HIV infection.[61,62] In homosexual men the intestinal tract is a primary site of inoculation. Many reports have been recently published documenting intestinal pathology in HIV-infected patients, and the subject has been well reviewed by Smith.[63] HIV-infected mononuclear cells are found throughout the gastrointestinal tract, and in situ hybridization has detected HIV RNA in presumably neuroendocrine cells from the rectum, duodenum, and esophagus.[64,65] HIV infection is associated with villus atrophy, with or without crypt hyperplasia, decreased villus surface, dysmotility, decreased level of brush border enzymes, gastric acid secretory failure, and bacterial overgrowth.[63,66] It is believed that this is the pathogenesis of the chronic, nonbloody diarrhea with weight loss and malabsorption seen in some AIDS patients without detectable pathogens, which has been termed AIDS enteropathy.[63]

Recent studies indicate that a pathogen is identified in 50 to 85 percent of patients with HIV-associated diarrhea.[67–71] Limited studies evaluating the microbiology of HIV-associated gastrointestinal disease found oral-esophageal candidiasis was evident in 80 percent of cases, cryptosporidiosis in 30 percent, *Isospora* in 10 percent, and *E. histolytica*, *Strongyloides stercoralis*, *G. lamblia*, *Salmonella*, *Mycobacterium*, and CMV infections in approximately 5 to 10 percent of patients.[71–73] Evidence of CMV infection of the gastrointestinal tract by culture of biopsy is evident in 30 to 50 percent of AIDS patients.[70,71] Recent studies have suggested that in addition to CMV, other viruses such as adenovirus, astrovirus, and picornavirus may play an etiologic role in diarrhea in HIV-infected patients.[74–76] Janoff et al. identified adenovirus in 5 of 67 (7.4 percent) of infected patients with diarrhea compared with none of 10 AIDS patients without diarrhea.[74] Grohmann et al. identified astroviruses and picornaviruses in 35 percent of HIV-infected patients with diarrhea compared with 12 percent without diarrhea ($p < .001$).[75] Greenson et al. found that microsporidia and MAC are the pathogens most commonly identified following extensive evaluation for occult enteric infection in patients with AIDS.[68] Kotler et al. found 62 percent (27 of 43) of AIDS patients with chronic diarrhea of over 1 month's duration had partial villus atrophy with or without crypt hyperplasia on jejunal biopsy.[77] Seventy percent of these patients (19 of 27) had cryptosporidia or microsporidia identified. The villus architecture was normal in most of the AIDS patients without parasitic infection, even if they had other pathogens such as CMV, bacterial enteritis, or mycobacteria. Extensive *M. avium*–complex (MAC) infection was associated with villus atrophy. Malabsorption, as demonstrated by abnormal D-xylose and C14-glycerol-tripalmitin absorption, is likely due to this derangement of the villus architecture. In addition to protozoan parasites, MAC, and HIV-1, chronic bacterial enteropathy due to adherent bacteria alone may produce these symptoms in up to 17 percent of AIDS patients.[211]

The prevalence of gastrointestinal symptoms varies with the stage of disease as well as the population at risk for HIV infection.

In developed countries, 40 to 50 percent of homosexual men with AIDS have a history of a clinical prodrome characterized by progressive weight loss of >10 percent of body weight and diarrhea of unexplained origin, while this clinical presentation is much less frequent among intravenous drug users, transfusion recipients, hemophiliacs, and heterosexual partners of other groups at risk for AIDS. In developing countries gastrointestinal symptoms are observed in over 80 percent of AIDS patients, perhaps reflecting a greater exposure and susceptibility to gastrointestinal pathogens common to the specific geographic location, as well as less antibiotic therapy.[72,79,80] Because of the frequency of gastrointestinal complaints in many of these patients, AIDS has been commonly referred to as "slim disease" in many developing countries.

RECTAL GONORRHEA

Klein et al. reviewed the literature on gonococcal infection in women from 1966 to 1977. Rectal gonorrhea was documented in 26 to 63 percent (mean 44 percent) of women with gonorrhea, and in 0 to 20 percent (mean 4 percent) the rectum was the only site from which the organism was isolated.[81] Rectal gonococcal infection in women may sometimes be attributable to rectal intercourse,[82,83] but in most cases there is no history of rectal intercourse,[84,85] and the infection is thought to have resulted from contiguous spread of infected secretions from the vagina. The clinical manifestations of rectal gonococcal infection in women have not been well defined.

The prevalence of rectal infection in homosexual men attending steam bathhouses in the pre-AIDS era was between 6 percent and 8 percent, and among homosexual men seen at STD clinics it was between 13 percent and 45 percent.[82,85,86–88] In several studies the rectum was more commonly found to be infected than the pharynx or urethra.[89,90] Men who were identified as sexual contacts by homosexual men with gonococcal urethritis are usually found to have asymptomatic rectal gonorrhea. However, in homosexual men attending an STD clinic who have not been named as gonorrhea contacts, rectal gonorrhea is more often symptomatic. The concept that rectal gonorrhea in homosexual men is always asymptomatic is a misconception arising from sample biases in studies that used STD clinic populations. In such studies, men found to have rectal gonorrhea, like women found to have endocervical gonorrhea, were often asymptomatic chronic carriers called in to the clinic because they had been named as contacts of men with acute gonococcal urethritis. In a previous study in an STD clinic,[91] among men not named as gonorrhea contacts, *N. gonorrhoeae* was isolated from 11 of 23 with anorectal symptoms versus 11 of 55 without anorectal symptoms ($p = 0.016$). Among 14 men named as gonorrhea contacts, however, 13 had no anorectal symptoms and 12 of the 13 had rectal gonorrhea. The proportion of gonococcal infections which are asymptomatic is much higher for rectal infections than for urethral infections in male homosexual STD clinic patients.[90,92] Thus, asymptomatic infection of the rectum constitutes the main reservoir of gonococcal infection in homosexual men.

Symptoms, when present, develop 5 to 7 days after exposure. They are usually mild and include constipation, anorectal discomfort, tenesmus, and a mucopurulent rectal discharge which may cause secondary skin irritation resulting in rectal itching and perirectal erythema.[3] Occasionally, the patient may only notice strands of mucus on his stool or small amounts of blood commonly mistaken for hemorrhoidal bleeding. The relatively high rate of asymptomatic infection and coinfection suggest that isolation of *N. gonorrhoeae* from a homosexual man with anorectal symptoms does not prove causation. Although asymptomatic or mild local disease is common, complications such as fistulas, abscesses, strictures, and disseminated gonococcal infection (DGI) may occur. DGI is typically associated with isolation of arginine, hypoxanthine, and uracil (AHU)-auxotypes, and patients with terminal complement component deficiency are at increased risk.[93,94]

There is also evidence that specific gonococcal strains may cause preferential infection of the rectum. Compared with heterosexuals, homosexual men are more likely to be infected with strains with the *mtr* mutation, which confers antibiotic susceptibility and is associated with decreased membrane permeability.[95] These traits are believed to enhance the ability of this strain to survive in the rectum. A study from the United Kingdom evaluated gonococcal isolates from 383 episodes of infections in women and found one serovar, Bajk, isolated with significantly higher frequency in rectal (27 percent) than genital (17 percent) infections.[96]

Findings of rectal gonorrhea during proctoscopy are nonspecific and limited to the distal rectum.[97–99] The most frequent finding is the presence of mucopus in the rectum. The rectal mucosa may appear completely normal or demonstrate generalized erythema with localized areas of easily induced bleeding primarily near the anorectal junction. Histologically, abnormal findings are especially prominent at the anorectal junction around the anal crypts and columns of Morgagni.[97,100] However, only limited histologic studies of gonococcal infection of the distal rectum have been conducted because of the hazards of biopsy of this area with its surrounding venous hemorrhoidal plexus. With gonococcal infection there is patchy disorganization and derangement of these mucus-secreting cells, vascular engorgement, and an infiltration of neutrophils, plasma cells, and lymphocytes throughout the lamina propria.[97,98] These findings are not pathognomonic, and concomitant rectal infection with another pathogen may alter the proctoscopic and histopathologic findings.

Diagnosis is made by Gram stain and culture of material obtained by swabbing the epithelial mucosa of the distal rectal area. In men with anorectal symptoms the anoscope should be used to examine the rectum and obtain exudate for culture and gram staining. In a study of men with symptomatic rectal gonorrhea,[101] the sensitivity of the Gram stain of rectal exudate for identification of gonococci was 79 percent when obtained through an anoscope versus 53 percent for blindly inserted swabs. A positive smear showing intracellular gram-negative diplococci is usually reliable when the smear has been taken and analyzed properly, and therapy can be instituted while awaiting culture results. In men without anorectal symptoms, a sterile cotton swab can be inserted blindly 2 to 3 cm into the rectum. Cultures performed on material obtained in this way appear to be as sensitive as cultures performed on material obtained by anoscope.[102]

The actual sensitivity of a single rectal culture for gonorrhea is unknown and probably is no greater than the estimated 80 percent sensitivity of a single endocervical culture in women. Quinn et al. noted that the Gram stain missed 7 of 52 (14 percent) culture-positive infections in homosexual men. Selective media used to isolate *N. gonorrhoeae* contain antimicrobials active against other bacteria (for example, vancomycin and colistin). Since none of these antimicrobials inhibits swarming *Proteus* species, which are often present in feces, trimethoprim is commonly added to inhibit *Proteus* in selective media used for rectal cultures.[103]

DNA detection assays are now widely available for detection of gonorrhea in urogenital specimens, but they have not been extensively studied for rectal specimens.[104–108] A recent study evaluated the PACE-2 DNA probe assay for rectal and pharyngeal specimens in a population with a 4.7 percent (11 of 234) prevalence of rectal gonorrhea infection by culture.[109] The assay was able to detect all 11 infections detected by culture.

Present therapy for *N. gonorrhoeae* has focused on single-dose therapy effective against β-lactamase producing strains. A single dose of ceftriaxone 250 mg intramuscularly, cefixime 400 mg orally, ciprofloxacin 500 mg orally, or ofloxacin 400 mg orally is recommended regimens for uncomplicated anal infections.[110,111] These regimens cured over 95 percent of anal infections, and ceftriaxone and ciprofloxacin cured over 90 percent of pharyngeal infections, compared with 88 percent for ofloxacin. In contrast to ceftriaxone, the quinolones do not treat incubating syphilis and are not recommended for children less than 17 years old or for pregnant or nursing women. Alternative regimens include spectinomycin 2 gm IM in a single dose, but this regimen is relatively ineffective against pharyngeal infection. Other options include ceftizoxime 500 mg IM, cefotetan 1 gm IM, cefoxitin 2 gm IM, cefuroxime axetil 1 gm orally, cefpodoxime proxetil 200 mg orally, enoxacin 400 mg orally, lomefloxacin 400 mg orally, and norfloxacin 800 mg orally, all as a single dose.[110] Quinolone-resistant gonococcal isolates are increasing in prevalence, and clinical failures with these regimens have been reported (see Chap. 32).

ANORECTAL HERPES SIMPLEX VIRUS INFECTION

Although genital herpes infection is well recognized, and HSV is second only to *N. gonorrhoeae* in frequency of association with proctitis in homosexual men, there have been few descriptions of anorectal herpetic infections.[112–114] Clinical description of anal herpes was recorded in 1736 by Astruc, physician to the king of France.[115] He stated, "[It is] observed in catamites and pathics, if they contract foul ulcers in the anus by the unnatural use of venery; from these ulcers they are tormented by a grievous inflammation upon the extremity of the rectum . . . hence the evacuation of the faeces becomes difficult and painful." In one study, 236 homosexual men with anorectal herpes were seen in one genitourinary medicine clinic in England over a 2-year period.[5] In two Seattle studies, HSV was cultured from the anorectal area of 32 percent and 20 percent of homosexual men with anorectal symptoms.[116,117] Limited data are available on the risk of HSV anorectal infection in women. Koutsky et al. recently found serologic or virologic evidence of HSV-2 infection in 47 percent of 779 women seen at a Seattle STD clinic.[117] HSV-2 was isolated from the anus or rectum of 26 women (3 percent). In this study, a history of anorectal intercourse was not more common in women with anorectal HSV than in women with genital HSV infection or no infection. Anorectal herpes is usually acquired by anal intercourse, although oral-anal contact with an individual who has HSV type 1 (HSV-1) infection of the mouth or lips presumably could lead to anorectal infection with HSV-1. In the Seattle studies, 37 of 39 isolates from the rectum were HSV type 2 (HSV-2) and the remaining two isolates were HSV-1.[3,116]

Clinically, herpes infection may involve the perianal area, the anal canal, and/or the rectum. While symptoms are quite prominent in most cases, some individuals may be totally asymptomatic.[118] In one study, HSV was isolated from the anal canal of 3 of 75 asymptomatic homosexual men.[3] Thus, asymptomatic anorectal HSV shedding may contribute to transmission of the infection to other individuals.

Anorectal HSV infections are typically characterized by severe, often debilitating, anal pain, present in 94 percent of patients in one study.[116] Constipation, a nonspecific manifestation of proctitis, is usually present. The occurrence of constipation, anorectal pain, and urinary retention in a homosexual man strongly suggests herpetic proctitis.[116,118] Samarasinghe et al.[5] described 11 patients with herpetic proctitis, all of whom developed urinary difficulty of varying severity associated with sacral paresthesias, neuralgia, and impotence. Such symptoms are uncommon with HSV infection of the genitalia, which leads to latent infection of the S2 and S3 dorsal root ganglia. Urinary retention, constipation, and impotence in anorectal herpes are suggestive of a sacral radiculopathy, perhaps due to infection of lower-level sacral nerves and dorsal root ganglia; alternatively, urinary retention and constipation could be ascribed to a pain-induced reflex spasm of the anal and vesical sphincters caused by the severe anorectal pain associated with the syndrome. The dermatomic distribution of sacral dysesthesia or neuralgia has not been well characterized or compared in genital versus anorectal herpes.

Other symptoms of anorectal herpes include tenesmus, hematochezia, and rectal discharge. Constitutional symptoms such as fever, chills, malaise, and headache are common with primary anorectal HSV infection. Tender inguinal lymphadenopathy occurs in nearly one-half of men with primary anorectal herpes. Although initial attacks of genital herpes differ clinically from recurrent attacks (see Chap. 21), initial and recurrent attacks of anorectal herpes have not yet been carefully compared. However, clinical experience suggests that recurrent anorectal attacks are often mild, of shorter duration, and rarely associated with constitutional symptoms. The presence of concomitant HIV-1 infection can adversely affect the clinical course of HSV proctitis. Unlike immunocompetent hosts, who have spontaneous resolution of lesions, in the absence of treatment HIV-infected patients tend to develop chronic progressive disease leading to large, destructive perianal ulcers.[45] Chronic mucocutaneous HSV with positive HIV serology is diagnostic of AIDS.[119]

Clinically, many infected individuals will not have any visible ulcerative perianal lesions but instead will present with ulcerative findings deep in the anal canal or involving the rectal mucosa.[3,116] Quinn et al. noted only 4 of 15 (27 percent) patients with anorectal herpes had visible perirectal lesions.[3] When present externally, the initial lesion is a small vesicle or cluster of vesicles, each surrounded by a red areola. The vesicles soon rupture and may become confluent, particularly near or in the anal canal. With HSV infection of the rectum, the lower 10 cm of the rectum may appear edematous, with discrete focal vesicular or ulcerative lesions occasionally present (See Plates 73 and 74). HSV proctitis is more likely than other causes of proctitis to cause diffuse friability, primarily involving the distal 10 cm of the rectal mucosa. The rectal mucosa is characteristically normal above this level, although we have occasionally seen involvement above 10 cm. Histologic examination of rectal biopsies reveals acute nonspecific inflammation with focal ulcerative changes. The histologic findings which are characteristic of rectal herpes, though not found in all cases, are perivascular mononuclear cell infiltration, intranuclear inclusion bodies, and extensive nuclear debris (Fig. 69-3); multinucleated cells can also be seen occasionally but are not uniquely associated with this infection. Other rectal infections are commonly associated with HSV infection and may cause a more diffuse proctitis.

Diagnosis can often be made on clinical presentation, on the basis of typical herpetic lesions externally, or on the basis of proctitis with focal ulcerative changes of the distal rectum in a patient with severe anal pain, constipation, inguinal adenopathy, constitutional symptoms, and urinary retention. Cultures of external lesions, of rectal swabs, or of rectal biopsy are confirmatory. Immunofluorescent staining of tissue biopsy is also useful. If viral cultures are not available, the clinical diagnosis can be confirmed by serology utilizing a microneutralization technique only if paired sera are collected and demonstrate seroconversion or a fourfold or greater rise in antibody titer. Commercially available enzyme immunoassays (EIAs) do not distinguish well between antibody subtypes.[120] Recently, Western blot and immunodot assays for detection of glycoprotein G of HSV-2 have been shown to be highly specific and accurate for detection of these antibodies; however, these assays are not commercially available.[121] Isolation of HSV is the most specific means of confirming a first episode of infection, but detection of HSV-2-specific antibody is the most

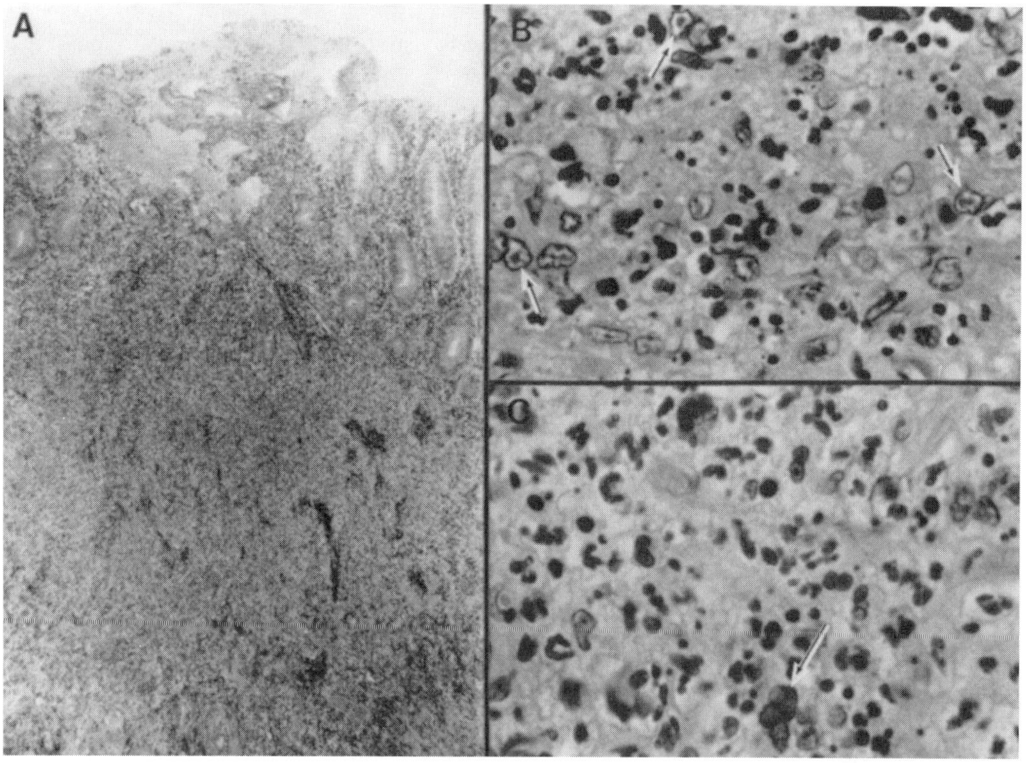

Fig. 69-3. Herpetic proctitis. *(A)* An ulceration and intense acute inflammation are present in the rectal mucosa. H&E stain, ×102 magnification. *(B)* Within this area of inflammation, intranuclear inclusions can be identified which are consistent with HSV infection (arrow). H&E stain, ×1360 magnification. *(C)* Multinucleated cells with a ground-glass appearance (arrow), a finding typical for HSV. H&E stain, ×1360 magnification. *(Courtesy of M. Schuffler.)*

sensitive way to confirm symptomatic reactivation and to detect asymptomatic infection.[117]

The clinical course of an initial attack of anorectal herpesvirus infection is self-limited, but manifestations may last for two to three weeks. Secondary bacterial superinfections, which are uncommon in genital herpes, may be more common in anorectal herpes, although this has not been determined. Treatment includes analgesics and sitz baths, and one study suggests that oral acyclovir may be efficacious in shortening the duration of symptoms and viral shedding of anorectal herpes.[122] Initial cases of infection should receive acyclovir orally 400 mg five times per day for 10 days. The newer antiviral agents famciclovir and valacyclovir have been used for genital HSV infection and may be efficacious for anorectal infection, although they have not been studied for this indication (see Chap. 21). Acyclovir 200 mg orally three to five times per day or 400 mg twice per day may be used to suppress clinical disease in patients with more than four symptomatic episodes per year.[110] Wald et al. recently showed that patients treated with acyclovir 400 mg twice daily for 70 days had subclinical shedding of HSV for 3 of 1,057 days (0.3 percent), compared with 64 of 928 (6.9 percent) with placebo ($p < 0.001$). This decreased asymptomatic shedding will likely decrease transmission.[123]

In AIDS patients with severe mucocutaneous herpes, 5 to 10 mg/kg of intravenous acyclovir should be administered every eight hours until clinical resolution is attained. The patient may then be placed on oral acyclovir 400 mg twice a day for suppression of recurrences, as these are more frequent and severe in AIDS patients.[110] Safety of daily dosing has been demonstrated in patients treated for up to five years; therapy can be stopped after one year to determine recurrences.[110,124]

ANORECTAL SYPHILIS

As with other STDs, the incidence of syphilis appears to be declining in homosexual men in industrialized countries, but a large percentage of early syphilis still occurs among homosexual men.[125] In 1990 the incidence of syphilis in the U.S. was 20 per 100,000 population; this has decreased to 8 per 100,000 in 1994, the lowest level in 35 years.[126,127] However, there were large differences in the rates in different demographic groups.[125,126] The high rate of syphilis among minority men and women has been attributed to limited access to health care and illegal drug use. In particular, the crack epidemic—with associated sex for drugs or money—seems to have fueled the epidemic by increasing transmission and impeding contact tracing.[128] The high rate of syphilis in this population puts minority men and women at a two- to ninefold greater risk for acquisition of HIV infection. In inner-city clinics in the United Kingdom, 80 percent of cases of primary anal syphilis are seen in homosexual men.[129] A study of homosexual men attending an STD clinic in the United States found 6 of 52 (12 percent) had anorectal syphilis.[3]

Treponema pallidum is commonly seen in its earliest infectious stages, with the primary anorectal lesion appearing two to six weeks after exposure by rectal intercourse. However, clinicians in the United States often fail to recognize anorectal chancres. Consequently, early syphilis in homosexual men is diagnosed in the secondary or early latent stage much more often than in the primary stage. It is not certain what proportion of anorectal chancres are asymptomatic. Careful perianal examination can reveal unsuspected perianal chancres, while digital rectal examination and anoscopy may be required to detect asymptomatic chancres higher in the anal canal or rectum. The variable appearance of the lesion accounts for the high rate of misdiagnosis. When anorectal syphilis causes symptoms, it is commonly misdiagnosed as a traumatic lesion, fissure, or hemorrhoiditis.[130]

Anorectal chancres due to syphilis have been recognized at least since the early 1900s. In 1925 Martin and Kallet found 20 patients (6.7 percent) with anorectal chancres among 300 proctologic cases.[131] Over the next 20 to 30 years there were several reports which stated that anorectal chancres represented 0 to 15 percent of extragenital chancres.[132,133] However, as STD clinicians have more frequently examined the anal area for chancres, the proportion of chancres found to involve the anorectal area has also increased.

As mentioned above, symptoms are commonly absent in the primary stage of anorectal syphilis, but when symptoms are present they include mild anal pain or discomfort, constipation, rectal bleeding, and occasionally a rectal discharge. Primary anorectal syphilis may appear as single or multiple eccentrically placed or mirror image ("kissing chancres") perianal ulcers.[134] It can also present as ulcerated masses, typically located on the anterior wall of the rectum.[134] Inguinal adenopathy with rubbery, nonsuppurative painless nodes may be associated with anorectal syphilis and helps distinguish it from fissures. Within the rectum, secondary syphilis may cause discrete polyps,[134,135] smooth lobulated masses,[135,136] mucosal ulcerations, and nonspecific mucosal erythema or bleeding, as well as submucosal irregularities with rubbery nodes which may be confused with lymphoma.[137,138] Syphilitic inflammation of the gastrointestinal tract is usually limited to the distal 15 cm but may be as high as 20 cm with secondary syphilis.

In secondary syphilis, condylomata lata may be found near or within the anal canal. These are smooth warty masses and must be differentiated from the more highly keratinized condylomata acuminata. Condylomata lata are often pruritic and produce a foul discharge which is highly infectious. The term condyloma latum has generally been limited to morphologically characteristic lesions involving stratified squamous epithelium, and we therefore do not use the term to include lesions of the columnar epithelial mucosa of the rectum. It is probable that secondary syphilis frequently involves the gastrointestinal tract, particularly the stomach. Constitutional symptoms, skin rash, and mucous patches can also occur. The lesions of primary and secondary syphilis may also coexist.[138,139]

Late syphilis may uncommonly involve the gastrointestinal tract, and the involvement can range from infiltrative, constrictive, or polypoid masses within the stomach to lesions of the lower bowel.[140,141] Anal sphincter paralysis and severe anal pain may develop with tabes dorsalis. Most past descriptions of gastrointestinal syphilis should be interpreted cautiously, since many of these lesions were ascribed to syphilis solely on the basis of serology, clinical responses to therapy, and compatible histology. Only a few reports have demonstrated *T. pallidum* in gastrointestinal lesions by silver stain or indirect immunofluorescence.[142–146]

Diagnosis of anorectal syphilis is based on serology, perirectal and digital rectal examination, and anoscopy. Detection of motile treponemes by darkfield examination is useful for evaluation of perianal and anal lesions but may be less specific for rectal lesions, since nonpathogenic treponemes can be found in the intestine. However, the number of species of nonpathogenic treponemes which have been described is greater in the mouth than in the intestine.[142] Additionally, since 10^5 treponemes/mL are required for visualization, a negative test does not rule out the diagnosis. Immunohistochemical stains of exudate from lesions may be useful in darkfield-negative specimens.[143] Biopsies of any rectal lesions or masses should be processed for silver staining, as well as routine histology, if syphilis is suspected. Although Nazemi et al.[137] described a case of syphilitic proctitis by demonstrating a spirochete on silver stain of a rectal biopsy, some investigators believe that silver stains are unreliable and recommend identification of *T. pallidum* by immunofluorescence using anti–*T. pallidum* antisera.[141,144] Fig. 69-4 illustrates a positive immunofluorescent stain for *T. pallidum* in a rectal mass lesion found in a homosexual man who had secondary syphilis associated with anorectal pain and discharge.

In addition, the histopathology of anorectal syphilitic lesions is also quite characteristic. As shown in Fig. 69-5, a hematoxylin and eosin preparation of the same tissue shown in Fig. 69-4 demonstrates at low magnification a uniform infiltrate of mononuclear cells throughout the submucosa and lamina propria. At higher magnification these are seen to be predominantly plasma cells, lymphocytes, and histiocytes. This degree of plasma cell infiltration is characteristic of gummas, syphilitic gastritis, condylomata lata, and syphilitic chancres.[141,145] Presumably, this intense plasma cell infiltrate in early syphilis represents an immune response to the large number of treponemes demonstrated throughout the tissue by immunofluorescent antibody staining.[145,146] These lesions often show an obliterative endarteritis with capillary proliferation and occasionally granulomas and crypt abscesses.[13,50]

Serologic diagnosis of syphilis is based on presence of antibodies to nontreponemal and treponemal antigens. A positive VDRL or RPR must be corroborated by a positive test specific for antibody to *T. pallidum* antigens, such as the fluorescent treponemal antibody absorption (FTA-ABS) test or the microhemagglutination (MHATP) test. Treponemal antibody titers do not correlate with disease activity and usually remain positive after the infection. The VDRL test detects approximately 50 to 70 percent of cases of primary syphilis, 100 percent of cases of secondary syphilis, and 85 to 100 percent of cases of tertiary syphilis. The FTA-ABS is the first serologic test to become positive and is present in 70 to 90 percent of patients with a chancre. This test is generally 100 percent sensitive in secondary and tertiary syphilis. The specificity of the VDRL varies with the population tested and is higher in healthy than in sick persons.[147]

Concomitant HIV-1 infection may alter the serologic manifestations of syphilis. There has been delayed or absent serologic test reactivity in patients infected with HIV-1 and proven secondary syphilis, particularly at a later stage of HIV infection.[47,48] Higher VDRL titers in patients with earlier-stage infection and secondary syphilis have also been noted.[49] Biological false-positive tests,

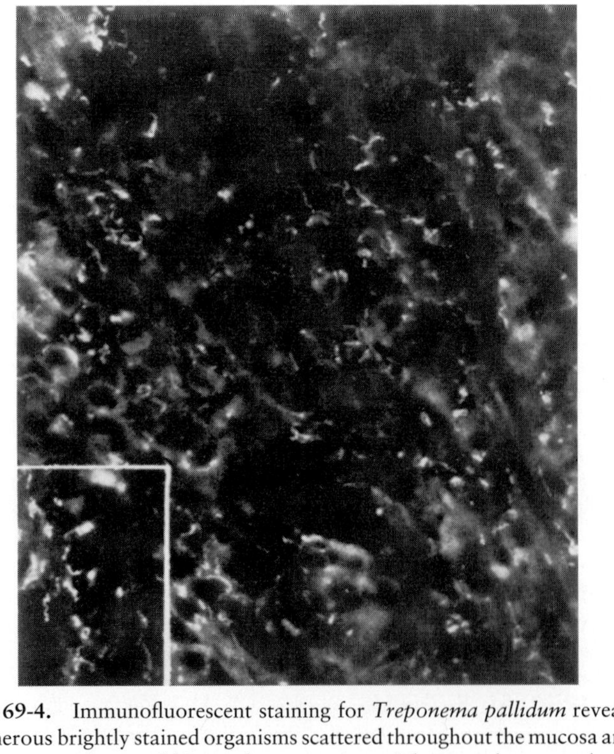

Fig. 69-4. Immunofluorescent staining for *Treponema pallidum* reveals numerous brightly stained organisms scattered throughout the mucosa and submucosa of a rectal biopsy from a patient with a rectal mass and secondary syphilis. *(Courtesy of S. Lukehart.)*

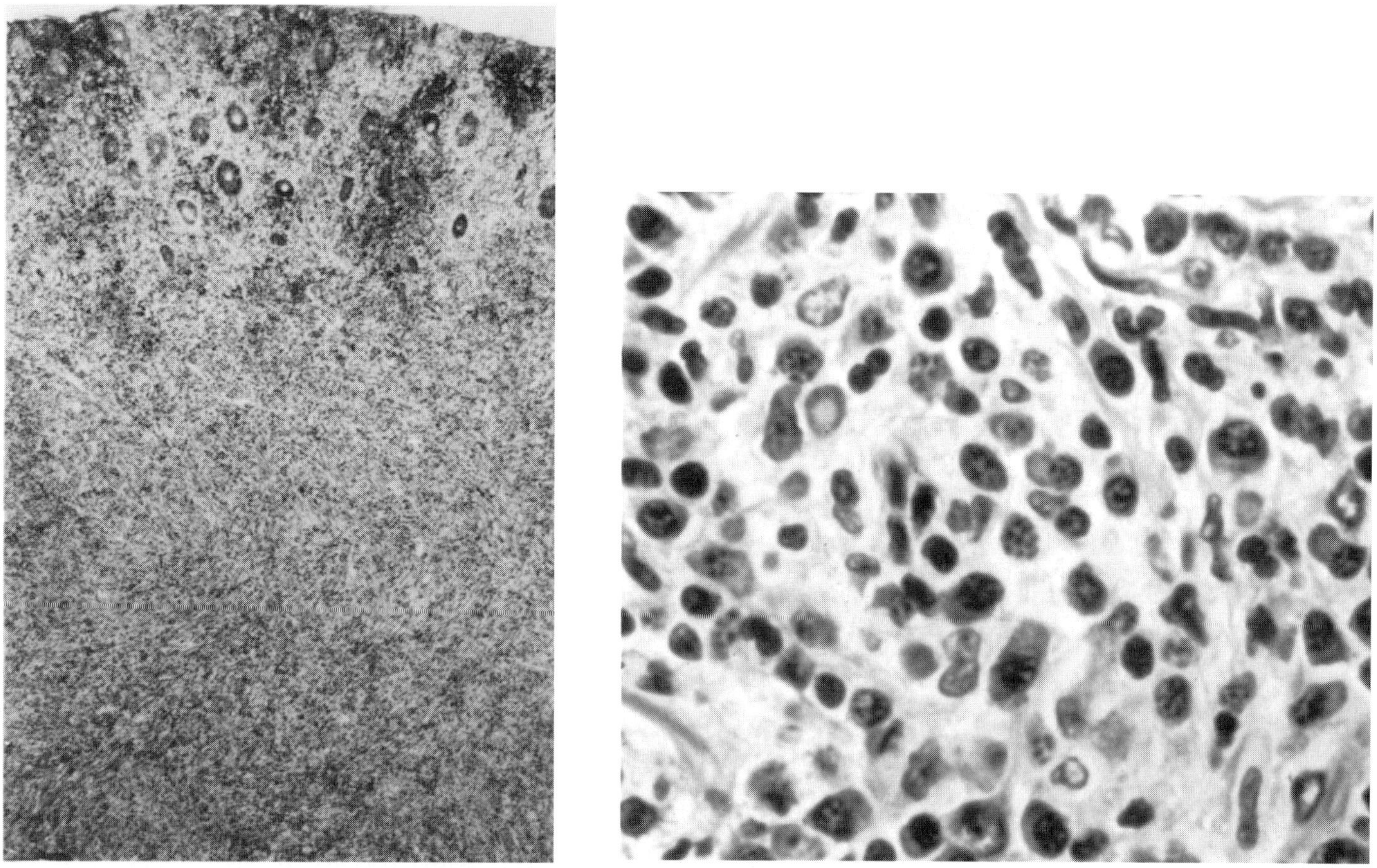

A B

Fig. 69-5. Biopsy of a rectal mass from a patient with secondary syphilis. *(A)* An extensive uniform cellular infiltrate has replaced the submucosa and lamina propria and has disrupted the muscularis mucosa. *(B)* The infiltrate consists of plasma cells, histiocytes, and lymphocytes.

VDRL- or RPR-positive and FTA-ABS- or MHATP-negative, which occur in a wide variety of infectious and noninfectious conditions, have been associated with HIV-1 infection.[148,149]

The differential diagnosis of anorectal syphilis includes ulcers due to HSV infection, chancroid, granuloma inguinale, LGV, trauma, and malignancy. Syphilitic lesions may be commonly misdiagnosed as anal fissures, fistulas, hemorrhoiditis, traumatic lesions, rectal polyps, condylomata acuminata, and even rectal carcinoma.[135–137] Indeed, there have been several reports of patients who underwent surgery for removal of lesions which were initially thought to be malignant but were later diagnosed as syphilitic lesions.[150]

Treatment for early syphilis is discussed in Chap. 35. Benzathine penicillin, in a single dose of 2.4 million units IM, remains the treatment of choice for early syphilis. Penicillin-allergic patients may be treated with a 15-day course of doxycycline, 100 mg orally given twice daily, or tetracycline 500 mg four times daily. Preliminary studies suggest azithromycin 500 mg daily for 10 days may be effective.[151] All patients should be offered HIV testing. All sexual contacts should be screened and treated.[110]

Although the standard regimen for early syphilis may be adequate for some patients coinfected with syphilis and HIV-1, several reports have documented poor response to standard therapy in this setting.[152,153] Syphilis may have a more aggressive course, and single-dose therapy with benzathine PCN for early syphilis has been associated with subsequent development of neurosyphilis.[152] Following treatment, the serologic titer may decrease more slowly in some HIV-infected patients.[154–156] These patients should have repeat serologic testing one, two, three, six, and twelve months after treatment to evaluate for response to therapy. Examination of CSF fluid is indicated in patients with neurological symptoms or if there is a rise or a less than fourfold decrease in the serologic titer following treatment.[110]

CHLAMYDIA TRACHOMATIS PROCTITIS

Several studies in the pre-HIV era demonstrated prevalences of 4 percent to 8 percent for anorectal *C. trachomatis* infection in men and 5 percent to 21 percent for anorectal infections in women.[157–161] Rates were higher for patients with symptoms of proctitis than for asymptomatic patients. In women with anorectal *C. trachomatis* infection, rectal intercourse was associated with the presence of symptoms. Barnes et al. compared serovars causing anorectal infection in homosexual and bisexual men with those causing cervical infections in heterosexual women in the same STD clinic.[162] They found D/D′ in 53 percent of rectal and 18 percent of cervical isolates, while serovar E was found in 32 percent of cervical and 6 percent of rectal isolates.[162] The highly significant difference in isolates from the two sites may be attributed to limited transmission between the two populations or to a decreased capability of certain serovars of surviving at one or the other mucosal site. Since the clinical manifestations and histopathology of *C. trachomatis* rectal infections differ according to the infecting immunotype, these will be discussed separately.

Rectal infections with LGV immunotypes of *C. trachomatis* have been recognized since 1936.[163] Infections with the LGV biovar of *C. trachomatis* are endemic in East and West Africa,

South America, and the Caribbean, but they have been seen only sporadically in the United States and Europe and more often in homosexual men than in heterosexual men or in women. Initially referred to as the anorectal syndrome of LGV, rectal involvement was generally believed to be a late, or secondary, manifestation of a genital infection. Secondary anorectal involvement does occur: after contact with an infected individual, a transient papule or ulcer sometimes appears on the genitalia, followed by systemic symptoms and prominent inguinal adenopathy; without treatment, the infection progresses to destructive granulomatous lesions of the lymph nodes and lower intestinal tract, which progresses to the formation of fistulas, strictures, and perianal abscesses and fistulas. The rectal strictures often form 2 to 5 cm above the anocutaneous margin, where there is a rich supply of lymphatics. Obstruction of lymphatic and venous drainage may cause perianal outgrowth of lymphatic tissue similar to hemorrhoids, called lymphorrhoids or perianal condylomas.[164]

More recently, primary anal or rectal infections have been described in women and homosexual men who practice anal intercourse. In these infections, rectal involvement is initially characterized by severe anorectal pain, a bloody mucopurulent discharge, and tenesmus. Inguinal adenopathy, which is characteristic of genital LGV, is often present. A recent study by Bauwens et al. suggests that the severity of infections may be associated with specific serovars and that infections with the L1 serovar may be less severe than those caused by L2.[165]

In both primary and secondary anorectal LGV, sigmoidoscopy reveals diffuse friability with discrete ulcerations in the rectum that occasionally extend to the descending colon.[166,167] Strictures and fistulas may become prominent and can be easily misdiagnosed clinically as Crohn's disease or carcinoma.[164,168] Histologically, rectal LGV may also be confused with Crohn's disease. Commonly, there is diffuse inflammation throughout the mucosa and submucosa, with plasma cells, neutrophils, and eosinophils, as well as giant cells, crypt abscesses, and granulomas (Fig. 69-6). Due to these similarities, Crohn[169] and others[170,171] speculated about a possible relationship between the two disorders. Schuller et al.[172] later demonstrated antibody to LGV strains in over 70 percent of patients with Crohn's disease and in less than 2 percent of healthy controls. At least three subsequent studies have failed to document such a relationship.[173–175] However, in our own analyses of rectal biopsies from homosexual men with proctitis, histopathologic findings were interpreted as consistent with Crohn's disease in two of three men from whom LGV immunotypes of *C. trachomatis* were isolated.[4] From these data, it appears that LGV infection should be suspected and ruled out in homosexual men with unexplained proctitis.

The non-LGV immunotypes of *C. trachomatis* are less invasive than LGV and cause a mild proctitis characterized by rectal discharge, tenesmus, and anorectal pain.[3] Anal lesions have not been described. Many infected individuals may be asymptomatic and can be diagnosed only by routine culturing. Data from Dean et al. suggests that serovar F may be associated with more severe female genital infections than serovar E.[176] This association of specific serovars and severity of infection has not been seen with non-LGV *C. trachomatis* anorectal infections. Even in asymptomatic cases, abnormal numbers of fecal leukocytes are usually present. Sigmoidoscopy may be normal or may reveal mild inflammatory changes with small erosions or follicles in the lower 10 cm of the rectum. Histology of rectal biopsies generally shows anal crypts and prominent follicles, as well as a neutrophilic infiltration of the lamina propria.

Diagnosis of chlamydial proctitis is best made by isolation of *C. trachomatis* from the rectum, together with response to appropriate therapy. Direct FA staining of rectal secretions using monoclonal antibodies can also be used to make the diagnosis.[177] Rompalo et al. used the direct fluorescent antibody technique to evaluate rectal swab samples for *C. trachomatis* and found a 90 percent sensitivity and 100 percent specificity for DFA compared with culture.[177] EIAs for chlamydial antigens have been attempted on rectal samples but give high false-positivity rates due to cross-reacting antigens on other fecal bacteria.[178] Serotyping by microimmunofluorescence[179] or monoclonal antibodies[180] can differentiate LGV from non-LGV isolates. Serology is useful for the diagnosis of LGV, particularly with the microimmunofluorescent (micro-IF) technique.[179] In consecutive cases of chlamydial proctitis, titers of 1:512 (all with broad immunotype specificity consistent with LGV) were found in three of three men with rectal LGV and in none of eight men with non-LGV chlamydial proctitis.[4] However, Schachter[181] found that among men with anorectal symptoms selected on the basis of having a high titer of micro-IF antibody (>1:1,000), four of six culture-positive men had non-LGV immunotypes isolated and the remaining two men had LGV immunotypes. Thus, the specificity of serodiagnosis of rectal LGV still requires further study. A complement-fixation titer of greater than 1:16 is also suggestive of LGV infection.

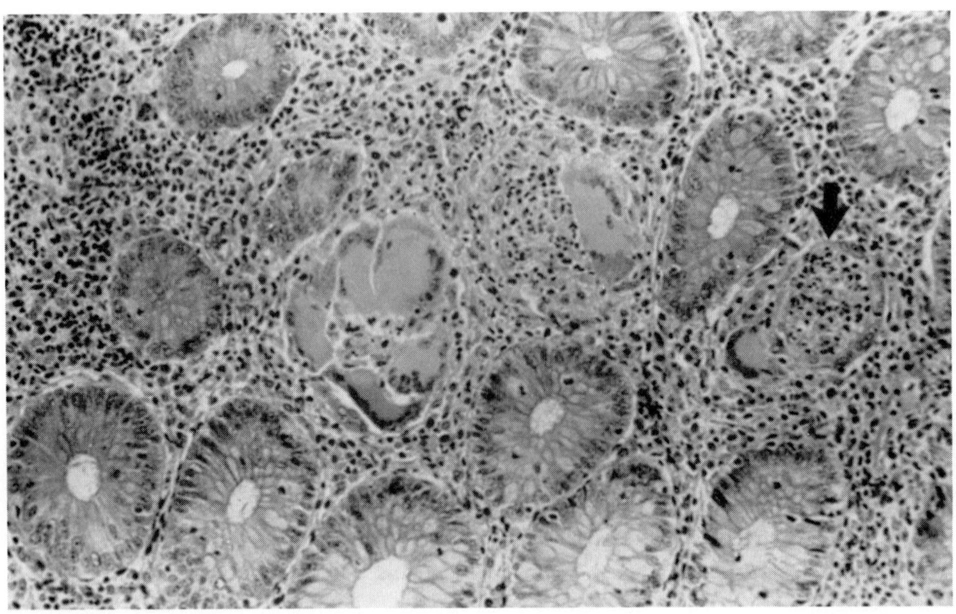

Fig. 69-6. Rectal biopsy from a patient with rectal LGV (*C. trachomatis*, LGV-2 immunotype). There is diffuse inflammation throughout the mucosa and submucosa. Giant cells, crypt abscesses (arrow), and granulomas are present.

Among men with non-LGV rectal chlamydial infection, serology has been less useful, since antibody titers are lower and in the range of antibody titers commonly found in men who are culture-negative, presumably reflecting previous infection. Demonstration of a fourfold rise in antibody titer in paired sera provides stronger evidence of chlamydial infection than does demonstration of a single elevated titer. Although widely studied and used for *C. trachomatis* urogenital infections, PCR and LCR tests have not been evaluated for anorectal infections.

Tetracycline, doxycycline, or azithromycin are the drugs of choice for infection with *C. trachomatis*. Doxycycline 100 mg twice daily for 7 to 10 days may be used[110]; azithromycin 1 gm as a single dose is effective for urethritis and cervicitis and has been recommended for uncomplicated rectal infections.[182,183] Patients should be followed carefully with repeat sigmoidoscopy, particularly when there is any question about the differential diagnosis of LGV versus inflammatory bowel disease. Therapy for LGV is discussed in Chap. 30.

PROCTOCOLITIS AND ENTERITIS DUE TO ENTERIC PATHOGENS

Epidemiologic and anecdotal reports have suggested the sexual transmission of several enteric pathogens, including *Shigella, Salmonella,* and *Campylobacter jejuni*.[185–188] Since these organisms are described in depth in Chap. 41, we will only briefly review some of the clinical and epidemiologic data concerning the role of these pathogens in homosexual men with symptoms and signs of enteritis or proctocolitis.

Although bacterial enteric infections account for fewer than 5 percent of opportunistic infections in AIDS patients in developed countries, these infections are significantly more common in AIDS patients than in similar patients without AIDS. Further, these infections tend to be more prolonged in AIDS patients and are associated with more frequent recurrences, more frequent bacteremia, and more antibiotic resistance than in non-AIDS patients. It is likely that the gastric hypoacidity which develops with AIDS predisposes to bacterial overgrowth and opportunistic enteric infections.[184]

Although several species of *Shigella* are responsible for human disease, *S. sonnei* and *S. flexneri* account for most infections in the United States. Since *Shigella* is highly infectious, transmission of the organism can occur rapidly and is commonly seen in children and travelers, in people in mental or penal institutions, and in populations where localized outbreaks are traced to contaminated food or water. The sexual transmission of *Shigella* was recognized in 1972, when reports from San Francisco and later from Seattle and New York documented that 30 to 70 percent of patients with *Shigella* were homosexual men.[185,188] Contact tracing demonstrated recovery of the same serotype from sexual partners, and no contaminated food or water source could be shown to be common to any of the cases.

Shigellosis presents with an abrupt onset of diarrhea, fever, nausea, and cramps. The diarrhea is usually watery but may contain mucus or blood. The infection may be complicated by the development of toxic megacolon. Sigmoidoscopy usually reveals an inflamed mucosa with friability not limited to the distal rectum, and histologic examination shows diffuse inflammation, with bacteria scattered through the submucosa and muscularis mucosa (Fig. 69-7). Diagnosis is made by culturing the organisms from the stool on selective media. Treatment is usually supportive, and antimotility agents should be avoided, but antibiotics are generally recommended to prevent complications in immunocompromised patients. Due to widespread development of resistance, selection of antibiotics should be based on regional antibiotic sensitivities. Ciprofloxacin 500 mg orally twice daily for 7 days is usually effective. As recurrences are common, antibiotic resistance may develop.[189] Repeat cultures of stool and blood are necessary to monitor response to therapy. Since asymptomatic carriers of *Shigella* exist, contact tracing is an important public health measure. Studies are needed on the value of tracing sexual contacts of homosexual men with shigellosis.

Campylobacter jejuni is one of the most commonly isolated bacterial agents from patients with acute diarrhea in the United States. In a recent survey of AIDS cases in Los Angeles from 1983 to1987, *Campylobacter* was reported in 29 of 4,433 (0.7 percent) AIDS cases. There was a 39-fold increased annual incidence in AIDS patients compared with other men ages 15 to 55 years.[190] It is believed that the 5 or 6 per 100,000 population rate reported to the CDC significantly underestimates the true incidence of 1,000 per 100,000 per year.[191] The underestimation is likely due to frequent asymptomatic infections and underutilization of the appropriate culture techniques. This pathogen is generally acquired by ingestion of contaminated water or food, particularly chicken and unpasteurized milk, or by close contact with infected animals.[192,193] Infection rates peak in the late summer and early fall. This is a significantly less infectious organism than *Shigella*, as 800–10^6 organisms are needed for infection in 10 to 50 percent of patients.

Sexual transmission has been documented in animals and was suspected in early reported cases of human abortion,[194] and a few reports have recently addressed the possible sexual transmission of *Campylobacter* in humans.[186,187,193,195] Campylobacter species or "atypical" campylobacter organisms have been recovered from the stools of 24 percent of symptomatic homosexual men and 10 percent of asymptomatic homosexual men.[25] In a subsequent study performed in 1986 in Baltimore, *Campylobacter* species were isolated from 4 percent of asymptomatic homosexual men, from 20 percent of homosexual men with intestinal symptoms, and from 9 percent of homosexual men with AIDS.[196] The most frequent isolates were *C. jejuni*, followed by campylobacterlike organisms.

These studies have clearly documented the frequent occurrence of "atypical" campylobacter organisms in homosexual men. In the AIDS era "atypical" campylobacter organisms have been recovered less often from rectal or stool cultures of homosexual men with diarrhea (Table 69-4) but have caused bacteremic illness in AIDS patients.[197] Although 99 percent of reported *Campylobacter* isolates in the United States are *C. jejuni* , there is a growing list of atypical *Campylobacter* and related species which have been

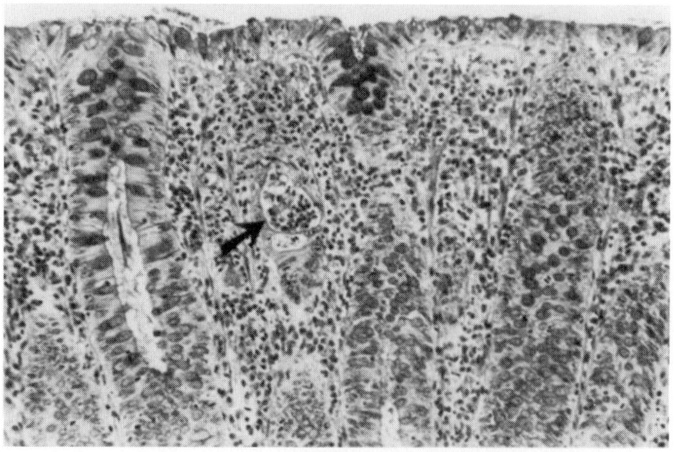

Fig. 69-7. *Campylobacter* colitis. The colonic mucosa is acutely inflamed, with polymorphonuclear leukocytes in the epithelium and lamina propria. A crypt abscess is also present (arrow). These findings are not specific for *Campylobacter* and may be found in the acute colitis caused by other invasive pathogens. H&E stain, ×340 magnification. *(Courtesy of M. Schuffler.)*

Table 69-4. Comparison of Gastrointestinal Infections among Homosexual Men Attending the Seattle STD Clinic in Two Time Periods

	% of patients positive for each pathogen*		
	1980–1981 (n = 119)	1983–1984 (n = 184)	p value
Neisseria gonorrhoeae	31	14	$p = .0003$
HSV	19	30	$p = .05$
Chlamydia trachomatis	10	14	NS
Treponema pallidum	5	6	NS
Entamoeba histolytica	29	15	$p = .02$
Giardia lamblia	14	7	$p = .07$
Campylobacter jejuni	7	7	NS
Campylobacterlike organisms	18	7	$p = .005$
Shigella	3	5	NS
Any pathogen	80	66	$p = .02$
≥2 pathogens	22	19	NS
HIV seroprevalence	14	58	$p < .001$

* Data from TC Quinn et al.[25] and WE Stamm (personal communication).

shown to cause diarrheal syndromes. These include *C. coli*, *C. upsaliensis*, *C. lari*, *Arcobacter cryaerophilia*, and *A. butzleri*. *Helicobacter fennelliae* and *H. cinaedi* (previously classified as *Campylobacter* species) have been associated with chronic mild diarrhea and proctitis in homosexual men.[191,197–199] Even when isolated from asymptomatic homosexual men these organisms are significantly correlated with the presence of neutrophils in rectal secretions, which suggests clinical disease.

Clinically, *C. jejuni* produces an acute diarrheal illness of several days duration, with fever, chills, myalgias, and abdominal pain. Gastrointestinal infections may mimic inflammatory bowel disease or acute appendicitis and may be complicated by pseudomembranous colitis, gastrointestinal hemorrhage, toxic megacolon, cholecystitis, and pancreatitis. Postinfectious complications include reactive arthritis[200] and Guillain-Barré syndrome.[201] Although the infection usually involves the small intestine, involvement of the colon and rectum has also been described.[202–204] The sigmoidoscopic and rectal biopsy findings are nonspecific and similar to those described for shigellosis (see Fig. 69-7). Fecal leukocytes are uniformly present, and diagnosis is confirmed by isolating the organisms from the stool by culture on selective media in a microaerophilic atmosphere.[192]

Although the need for antimicrobial therapy has not been fully established in human *Campylobacter* infection of the intestinal tract, treatment with azithromycin 500 mg daily for 3 days or erythromycin 500 mg four times daily for 1 week has been recommended for severely symptomatic cases and for immunocompromised patients.[191] Antimicrobial therapy started within the first 3 days of the illness reduces the duration of excretion of the organism in the stool. Ciprofloxacin- and azithromycin-resistant isolates from Thailand have recently been described.[205] Bacteremia and recurrent diarrhea following specific therapy have been reported.

There are several species of salmonella with more than 2,000 different serotypes that cause a variety of clinical entities in humans. There is an estimated twentyfold increased incidence of salmonellosis in AIDS patients.[206] These infections, which are primarily due to *S. typhimurium* and *S. enteritidis*, are often more severe and more frequently associated with bacteremia and relapse despite therapy in AIDS patients. *Salmonella* bacteremia in an HIV-infected individual is diagnostic of AIDS. Only anecdotal reports have commented on the possible sexual transmission of *Salmonella*; in one,[207] *S. typhi* was recovered from the stools of homosexual men and the same serotype was recovered from asymptomatic sexual partners with whom no housing, food, or water was shared. These organisms can survive in the environment for up to 30 months; therefore, fomite transmission may occur.[207] It appears that these organisms have different capabilities for invasiveness in different populations. A recent review of salmonellosis in New York City found that *S. enteritidis* was more competent in causing septicemia and less competent in causing gastroenteritis than *S. typhimurium* in HIV-infected patients, the reverse was true for HIV-uninfected patients.[208]

Diagnosis is made by culturing the organisms from the stool on selective media. Treatment must be individualized, depending on severity of symptoms and antibiotic sensitivity of the isolate. For AIDS patients with bacteremia, ciprofloxacin 750 mg twice daily for 14 to 30 days is generally recommended.[209] If relapse occurs, ciprofloxacin 500 mg twice daily is given indefinitely. Isolates sensitive to ampicillin and trimethoprim-sulfamethoxazole may be treated with these drugs. In immunocompetent patients with mild illness, supportive therapy without antibiotics is appropriate. Since asymptomatic carriers are common and may be employed as food handlers in public establishments (as were the reported cases), tracing of sexual partners of infected individuals is particularly important.

Recent reports suggest that enteroadherent bacteria may produce a chronic diarrheal syndrome in AIDS patients.[210] In one review these organisms were found in 17 percent of AIDS patients evaluated for chronic diarrhea in a 1-year period.[211] Typically these patients have less than 100 CD4 cells/mm^3 and present with diarrhea with malabsorption and weight loss. The right colon is most commonly involved. Histologically, three types of adherence patterns have been described: bacteria intercalated between microvilli, aggregates of bacteria loosely attached to damaged epithelium, and attaching and effacing lesions.[211,212] Cultures of biopsy samples have yielded *E. coli* in 67 percent of cases.[211] These infections have been described in homosexual men with AIDS, but the mechanism of transmission is not certain.

PARASITIC INFECTIONS

Although reports of cutaneous amebiasis of the penis, vulva, and cervix suggested sexual transmission of amebiasis,[213–215] it has only been within the last two decades that sexual transmission of certain parasitic infections has been fully appreciated.[21,22] In 1972 it was suggested that *Giardia lamblia*, *Iodamoeba bütschlii*, *Dientamoeba fragilis*, and *Enterobius vermicularis* were sexually transmitted among homosexuals.[216–219] In two separate surveys in New York City, the prevalence of infection with giardiasis and/or amebiasis was between 30 and 40 percent in selected homosexual men.[21,22] The presence of infection correlated better with a history of anilingus than with travel history.[21] In Seattle, 25 percent of homosexual men we have studied with anorectal or intestinal symptoms have had either *Giardia*, *Entamoeba histolytica*, or both present in their stools.[25] *G. lamblia* was associated with symptoms of enteritis, while *E. histolytica* was equally common in symptomatic and asymptomatic men. In addition, mixed infections with a variety of intestinal parasites, including other protozoans and nematodes, have also been described in homosexual men.[216–220] More recently Peters et al. found 48.5 percent (33 of 274) of homosexual men with symptomatic diarrhea in a community-based clinic in Chicago had at least one intestinal protozoan.[221] *E. histolytica* and *G. lamblia* were isolated from 26 percent and 8 percent, respectively, of these men and represented 53 percent and 16 percent, respectively, of positive isolates. Other parasites frequently isolated in this study were *E. nana* (39 percent), *E. coli* (14 percent), and *E. hartmanni* (9 percent). *D. fragilis*, *I. bütschlii*, *Chilomastix mesnili*, cryptosporidia, and *Isospora* were isolated in less than 1 percent of patients.

The etiologic agent of amebiasis is *E. histolytica*, although *D. fragilis* is believed by some authorities to be similarly pathogenic and closely related to *E. histolytica*. It is estimated that 10 percent of the world's population is infected with *E. histolytica*. High rates of infection occur in India, Africa, the Far East, and South and Central America; in the United States the prevalence is approximately 4 percent.[222] Although *E. histolytica* is primarily a waterborne agent, sexual transmission may be responsible for its high prevalence in homosexual men. In 1977, 40 percent of all reported cases of amebiasis in the United States were from New York City. Eighty percent of these cases were located in Manhattan, and its large male homosexual community had the highest morbidity rate.[23] Similarly, in San Francisco 89 percent of the reported cases of amebiasis were in males 20 to 39 years of age.[1] In a retrospective review of records of patients with *E. histolytica* infection seen at New York Hospital, Schmerin et al.[27] noted that 20 of 20 men who had not traveled were homosexual, while only 2 of 30 men who had traveled were homosexual. More recent studies have identified *E. histolytica* in 21 percent to 32 percent of selected homosexual male populations in North America and in 12 percent of homosexual men in the United Kingdom.[223–225]

The majority of infections are asymptomatic, and only 10 percent of those infected develop invasive disease with amebic dysentery or liver abscess. There has been considerable recent debate about whether, in most cases, *E. histolytica* actually causes illness in homosexual men who are positive by stool wet-mount exam.[226] The prevalence of *E. histolytica* is approximately equal in symptomatic and asymptomatic groups of homosexual men,[25] and many of those who are symptomatic have other pathogens in addition to *E. histolytica*. Additionally, AIDS patients do not seem to be at increased risk of invasive amebiasis.[227]

E. histolytica trophozoites have recently been divided into pathogenic and nonpathogenic zymodeme types using isoenzyme patterns.[227a] Most *E. histolytica* strains isolated from homosexual men are the nonpathogenic zymodemes, which are not usually associated with gastrointestinal symptoms, invasive disease,[224,228,229] or a serologic response.[230] Conversion from nonpathogenic to pathogenic zymodemes has been reported in culture but has not been seen in serial isolates from infected patients.[231] Pathogenicity of *E. histolytica* strains has been recently linked to the presence of a galactose-inhibitable adherence protein (GIAP). An ELISA which detects this antigen in serum and feces may be useful in distinguishing pathogenic and nonpathogenic strains.[232,233] The high rate of occurrence of asymptomatic infection facilitates transmission of infection within the male homosexual community, as inadvertent transmission occurs from patients unaware of their infection.

When present, symptoms may vary from mild diarrhea to fulminant bloody dysentery. Extension of the infection to the liver, lung, or brain occurs rarely. Amebic proctocolitis causes diffuse inflammation and ulceration of the distal colon, often clinically indistinguishable from inflammatory bowel disease, shigellosis, *Campylobacter jejuni* infection, or *Yersinia* enterocolitis.[234,235] These symptoms may wax and wane for weeks to months. Fulminant dysentery is uncommon and is associated with steroid use.[236] Amebomas, which are chronic localized amebic infections, may present as painful abdominal masses. They are usually located in the cecum and descending colon.[222] Complications of amebic colitis include peritonitis; hemorrhage; strictures of the anus, rectum, and sigmoid; and painful perianal ulcerations which are due to contiguous spread of intestinal infection.

Diagnosis is based on the demonstration of *E. histolytica* in the stool, in a wet mount of a swab, or in a biopsy of rectal mucosal lesions. Occasionally, multiple fresh stool examinations are necessary to demonstrate the cysts or trophozoites of *E. histolytica*. Barium, laxatives, antibiotics, and enemas should be avoided at the time of sample collection. Samples not evaluated immediately should be fixed with polyvinyl alcohol or refrigerated, to avoid disintegration of trophozoites. Sensitivity of stool examination can be increased with concentration techniques and with trichrome and iron hematoxylin stains.[222] Definitive diagnosis of amebic colitis is by colonoscopy with scraping or biopsy of the ulcer edge; however, there is a risk of perforation. Serology (indirect hemagglutination) is useful in acute amebic colitis because it is positive in 82 to 98 percent of infected patients.[222] Indirect hemagglutination tests may remain positive for years following infection.[222] Agar gel diffusion, counterimmunoelectrophoresis, and enzyme immunoassay (EIA) techniques are quite sensitive (87 to 95 percent for proctocolitis, 95 to 100 percent for amebic liver abscess) and have the benefit of becoming negative 6 to 12 months following infection.[236]

Treatment for amebiasis is discussed further in Chap. 44. Asymptomatic carriage of the organisms should be treated to prevent continued infection with a possible pathogenic strain and to prevent continued transmission of the infection. At present, three luminal amebicides are available to treat this type of infection. Iodoquinol 650 mg orally three times daily for 20 days is the regimen of choice.[237] Paromomycin 25 to 30 mg/kg/day in three doses for 7 days and diloxanide furoate 500 mg three times per day for 10 days are additional options.[238] Diloxanide furoate is presently only available from the CDC. Invasive intestinal disease should be treated with metronidazole 750 mg three times daily for 10 days.[237] This drug is well absorbed and does not eradicate organisms in the intestinal lumen, so iodoquinol 650 mg three times daily for 20 days should be given subsequently. Dehydroemetine 1.5 mg/kg/day (maximum 90 mg/day) IM, plus tetracycline 500 mg 4 times daily up to 5 days, may be used as an alternate regimen, followed by iodoquinol.

Giardia lamblia, another frequent waterborne disease, also appears to be sexually transmitted through oral-anal contact. In a review of giardiasis in men seen at New York Hospital, 19 (22 percent) had not traveled recently, and all were homosexual.[239] In 1977 Meyers et al. documented giardiasis in six of eight homosexual men who were sexual partners.[28] Giardiasis is typically an infection of the small intestine, although it is often found in association with amebiasis. Symptoms of giardiasis include diarrhea, abdominal cramps, bloating, and nausea. Multiple stool examinations are necessary to document infection with *G. lamblia*. Often, when stool examination has been negative, sampling of jejunal mucus by the Enterotest[240] or small bowel biopsy is necessary to confirm the diagnosis.

Metronidazole 250 to 500 mg three times a day for 7 days is presently recommended in the United States but is associated with a 10 to 20 percent failure rate.[237,241] Tinidazole, another 5-nitroimidazole available in Europe, given as a 2-gm single dose, may be more effective.[241] Paromomycin 500 mg orally three times daily or furazolidone 100 mg four times daily for 7 to 10 days may also be used as an alternative.[241] Quinacrine hydrochloride, previously used to treat giardiasis, is no longer available in the United States. Follow-up stool examinations are particularly important in management of *G. lamblia* and *E. histolytica* infection. Examination of sex partners of homosexual men may be important in reducing the reservoir of infection in the community; asymptomatic cyst passers should be treated.

Several reports have commented on the identification of *Enterobius vermicularis*, or pinworms, in homosexual men,[219,242] although this infection is commonly found in children. Adult pinworm infection is usually acquired by contact with an infected child or by sexual transmission via anilingus. Ova are deposited by the adult worm in the perianal area and are infective for several hours. Pruritus ani is a common symptom. Diagnosis is made by demonstrating the ova, collected on cellophane tape from the anal area. Ova are rarely seen in stool examinations. Mebendazole 100 mg, pyrantel pamoate 11 mg/kg orally, or albendazole 400 mg—all as a single dose, then repeated once after 2 weeks—are usually effective and well tolerated.[237]

Although many helminth infections cannot be transmitted person to person because of their particular life cycle, *Strongyloides stercoralis* could be transmitted sexually, since the infective filariform larvae are often found in the feces. However, there has been no published evidence as yet that this infection has been sexually transmitted.

Intestinal infection with three protozoan parasites—cryptosporidium, *Isospora*, and microsporidium—has been identified in homosexual men with AIDS.[243–246] Although there has been no documentation of sexual transmission of these parasites, this mode of transmission is highly suspect due to the relatively high frequency in homosexual men compared to other select populations with AIDS.

Cryptosporidium is a tiny protozoan parasite that primarily inhabits the microvillus region of epithelial cells. This parasite has been known to cause diarrhea in various animals, especially calves and other domestic animals.[247] In 1976 the first human infection with cryptosporidium was reported, and until 1983 this pathogen was identified only in immunosuppressed patients.[248,249] In 1983, however, investigators reported identification of this parasite in immunocompetent persons exposed to infected calves.[250] The prevalence of infection by stool samples is approximately 1 to 3 percent in Europe and North America; however serology suggests that 32 to 58 percent of European and North American adults may be infected. The prevalence is significantly higher (5 to 10 percent) in Asia and Africa.[251,252] Worldwide the organism can be isolated from the stool of 10 to 20 percent of patients with AIDS-associated diarrhea.[252]

Isospora belli is endemic in Africa, Asia, South America, and the Caribbean. The organism is isolated from 8 to 20 percent of Haitian and African AIDS patients; however, it has been associated with only 0.2 percent of cases of diarrhea in AIDS patients in the United States.[253] It is possible that *Isospora* is less frequently seen in the United States because drugs used for prophylaxis of *Pneumocystis carinii* and *Toxoplasma* are also effective against this organism.

Cryptosporidial infection may cause asymptomatic, transient, chronic, or fulminant infection.[252] The majority of immunocompetent patients develop profuse diarrhea with abdominal cramps, which is self-limited and subsides in 7 to 10 days. *Isospora* also can cause a self-limited diarrhea in immunocompetent hosts. Chronic, severe infection is associated with CD4 counts of less than 100 cells/mm^3.[254] In AIDS patients both infections can produce an illness characterized by intermittent episodes of abdominal cramps, bloating, and nausea in association with either steatorrhea or a profuse secretory diarrhea. Weight loss is usually profound, and the infection is unresponsive to any therapeutic attempts to eradicate it or to sustain nutritional status.[243,244] In addition to AIDS, IgA deficiency is an additional risk factor for severe cryptosporidial diarrhea.[255]

Diagnosis of either *Cryptosporidium* or *Isospora* can be rapidly established by a modified acid-fast stain or auramine stain of the stool or by concentration and identification of the organisms by the sugar-flotation method.[256] The large size of *Isospora* cysts helps differentiate them from the smaller *Cryptosporidium* cysts (4 to 5μm). A commercially available fluorescein monoclonal antibody assay increases the sensitivity for detection of cryptosporidia.[257] Intestinal biopsies are also useful in confirming the diagnosis. Primarily parasites of the small bowel, *Cryptosporidium* or *Isospora* can be present throughout the small bowel, colon, or both in AIDS. Mucosal biopsies usually reveal the organisms clustered on the surface epithelial cells of the villi with little or no mucosal destruction, ulceration, or inflammation. Consequently, fecal white blood cells are rarely seen in these protozoal infections as they are in infection with enteric bacteria. Improved diagnostic techniques will provide useful information on the epidemiology of these infections in homosexual populations and other populations at risk for infection.

Treatment of *Cryptosporidium* or *Isospora* infections in immunocompetent patients with self-limited diarrhea is rarely required. Despite numerous attempts to treat symptomatic infection in immunocompromised individuals, no drugs have been shown to be fully efficacious. In limited studies, the antiprotozoal drug spiromycin was reported to be effective in several AIDS patients with cryptosporidiosis,[258] but subsequent studies have not confirmed this finding. Paromomycin 500 mg four times daily for 14 to 28 days may improve symptoms; the response rate varies from 30 percent to 70 percent.[252,259,260] Azithromycin, roxithromycin, nitazoxanide, and atovaquone may also have some effect. *Isospora* infection does respond to antifolates, but the organism is rarely eradicated, and relapse occurs in 50 percent of treated AIDS patients. Trimethoprim-sulfamethoxazole 160 mg/800 mg (Bactrim DS), two tablets twice daily for 2 to 4 weeks followed by chronic suppressive therapy of one to two tablets daily is effective in these patients. An alternative regimen is pyrimethamine 50 to 75 mg daily with folinic acid for acute infection, then 25 mg daily for suppression.[252,261]

Like cryptosporidia and *Isospora*, *Cyclospora cayetanesis* is a cause of chronic diarrhea in immunocompetent and immunocompromised hosts. Previously called cyanobacteriumlike body (CLB), blue-green alga, and "Big Crypto," this organism is found worldwide.[252,262,263] The epidemiology of this infection is not fully elucidated; however, in the United States it has been identified as a cause of traveler's diarrhea[264] and has been associated with outbreaks due to ingestion of unwashed raspberries.[265] Evaluation of stool samples from patients with diarrhea in Chicago and Massachusetts found a prevalence of *Cyclospora* of 0.3 to 0.5 percent, similar to that of *Isospora*.[262,266] Pape et al. found cyclospora to be the cause of diarrhea in 11 percent of 450 HIV-infected Haitians but in no HIV-uninfected patients with diarrhea.[267] The clinical syndrome of watery nonbloody diarrhea is indistinguishable from cryptosporidiosis and isosporosis.

The diagnosis of *Cyclospora* infection can be made by identification of the 8- to 10-μm nonrefractile oocysts in fresh or preserved stool samples. The oocysts have variable acid-fast staining, and with UV epifluorescence they autofluoresce as neon blue circles. Bactrim DS four times daily for 10 days followed by suppressive therapy three times per week usually produces symptomatic improvement in AIDS patients.[267]

Microsporidia are obligate intracellular protozoa, and before AIDS only 10 cases of human infection had been documented. Since 1981 several hundred cases have been reported, most since 1991.[268,269] Of the five genera associated with disease in HIV-infected patients—*Enterocytozoon, Septata, Encephalitozoon, Pleistophora,* and *Nosema*—*E. bieneusi* and *S. intestinalis* have been associated with chronic diarrhea in HIV-infected patients.[246,269] The mode of transmission of these organisms is not known; however, they have been identified as a cause of diarrhea in homosexual men, and the majority of cases of infections are in adult males, suggesting sexual transmission.

Due to the small size of the organisms and subsequent difficulties with diagnosis the true prevalence of microsporidial infections is still unknown, but they may be the cause of diarrhea in over 25 percent of patients with negative stool studies.[269] At least eight cases of microsporidial disease in nonimmunocompromised patients have been described.[270] Recently, Sandfort et al. described the first case of *E. bieneusi* self-limited diarrhea in an HIV-negative patient.[271] In AIDS patients undergoing endoscopy for chronic diarrhea, the prevalence of microsporidial infection is 7 to 50 percent; however, ongoing prospective studies of chronic diarrhea in HIV-infected patients indicates that the prevalence of this infection in this population is 9 to 16 percent.[270]

Microsporidia cause a spectrum of disease from asymptomatic infection to severe diarrhea and malabsorption.[272] Rabeneck et al. recently identified *E. bieneusi* in the intestinal epithelial cells of HIV-infected patients without diarrhea. Self-limited diarrhea occurs in patients without severe immunodeficiency, and chronic watery diarrhea with malabsorption occurs with severe immunodeficiency.[273]

The diagnosis can be made by identification of the small (1 to 2μm) spores in stool and duodenal fluid by light- or electron microscopy. The organisms are well visualized by light microscopy with chromotrope staining.[274] Light- or electron-microscopic examination of semithin plastic sections of biopsy samples from the duodenum and jejunum demonstrates infection confined to enterocytes covering the villi, along with villous atrophy and cell degeneration. Electron microscopy is required for species identification.

At present there is no reliably effective therapy for microsporidial infection. Albendazole has been curative in some cases of infection with *Encephalocytozoon* and disseminated *Septata*.[275] Albendazole treatment of *E. bieneusi* may alleviate symptoms, but it does not seem to eradicate the organism and is associated with a high rate of relapse.[276] Symptomatic treatment with antidiarrheal agents such as lomotil, loperamide, octreotide, and nutritional supplements are helpful in refractory cases.[277]

CONDYLOMATA ACUMINATA

Anal warts due to human papillomaviruses are common in individuals who practice anal intercourse.[278] In one series of 260 homosexual men seen by proctologists, 134 (51.5 percent) had anal warts.[17] Warts due to papillomaviruses may occur anywhere in the anal or genital area but are particularly common in the anus in homosexual men. Of those individuals with warts in the study just cited, 6 percent had them in the perianal area, 10.5 percent had them only in the anal canal, and 83.5 percent had them in both areas. These warts rarely if ever extend beyond the pectinate line into the rectum. Perianal condylomata acuminata appear as raised pink-to-brown papules, usually in clusters, and occasionally as large cauliflowerlike masses. Patients immunocompromised due to malignancy or HIV infection are more likely to have frequent recurrences of extensive lesions which are recalcitrant to therapy.[279]

Diagnostically, warts should be differentiated from squamous cell carcinoma and from condylomata lata, the moist, flat papules of secondary syphilis. These may be diagnosed by a reactive serology for syphilis and by a darkfield demonstrating spirochetes in the lesions. Papanicolaou smears of mucosal lesions for dyskeratosis and koilocytes is less sensitive than DNA detection techniques such as dot blot and in situ hybridization.[280,281] These assays are less specific than Southern blot hybridization.

Therapy of genital warts is discussed in Chap. 25. Topical podophyllin (20% solution), commonly used for genital warts, is also effective in some cases of perianal warts; however, it can cause burns with subsequent stenosis when used intra-anally. A 0.5% podophyllin solution (podofilox) is effective and has the benefit of being able to be applied by the patient.[282] Cryotherapy with liquid nitrogen clears up to 90 percent of treated warts. Laser-beam therapy and surgical excision have been used in refractory cases. Interferons alpha, beta, and gamma have been successfully used as monotherapy and in combination with other modalities, such as surgical excision and laser therapy.[283–285]

There has been a recent increase in the number of cases of anal intraepithelial neoplasia (AIN) in homosexual men and a growing body of evidence to support the role of HPV in this malignancy. HPV types 16 and 18 have been found in 56 percent and 5 percent, respectively, of anal cancers.[286] Additionally, there appears to be an increased incidence of HPV infection and AIN in HIV-infected individuals. High-grade intraepithelial neoplasia has been found in 0.5 to 5.4 percent of HIV-seronegative homosexual men compared with 4–15.2 percent of HIV-seropositive men.[287] Risk of high-grade AIN was associated with HPV types 16 and 18 in both HIV-seronegative and seropositive men and was 2.9-fold higher for HIV-seropositive men with fewer than 500 CD4 cells/mm^3, compared with men with more than 500 CD4 cells/mm^3.[288]

MYCOBACTERIAL INFECTIONS

Mycobacterium avium–complex (MAC) is a group of "atypical" mycobacteria that has been identified in severely immunocompromised patients, including homosexual men with AIDS.[10] Ninety-eight percent of these isolates are *M. avium* (usually serovars 1, 4, and 8); the remainder include *M. intracelullare*. The gastrointestinal tract and lymph nodes appear to be the most common organs infected by this organism. Infections of the intestinal tract are usually part of disseminated infection which presents with fever, night sweats, abdominal pain, watery diarrhea, steatorrhea, and malabsorption. Both the clinical and the radiographic features of this disease may mimic Whipple's disease.[289] The major risk factor for this disease is severe immunocompromise, with less than 75 CD4 lymphocytes/mm^3 or previous opportunistic infection, especially cytomegalovirus disease.[289]

It has been postulated that the gastrointestinal symptoms of MAC infection are due to defective macrophage processing of the MAC pathogens, which leads to accumulation of macrophages and secondary malabsorption, as seen in Whipple's disease. The defective T-cell activation of macrophages has been proposed as a mechanism in the pathogenesis of Whipple's disease, an immunologic defect which is also characterized by depression of T-cell function.[289,290] The characteristic findings seen in MAC infection of AIDS patients, such as severe lymphopenia and anemia, reduction of circulating helper-T cells, skin test anergy, and polyclonal hypergammaglobulinemia, are not classically seen in Whipple's disease.

The diagnosis of MAC infection is based on stool culture, acid-fast staining of the organism in the stool, and histologic examination of small bowel biopsy specimens. Although some patients are asymptomatic excretors of MAC, histologic evidence of gastrointestinal involvement is indicative of disseminated infection. Fine, white mucosal nodules noted on endoscopy are highly suggestive of MAC disease.[291] The main histologic features on small bowel biopsy include increased numbers of macrophages filled with PAS-positive and acid-fast bacilli within the lamina propria, villous atrophy, and exudative enteropathy.[289] Blood and bone marrow cultures are positive in 85 to 90 percent of patients with gastrointestinal involvement. Blood cultures using the lysis centrifugation techniques for mycobacterial organisms are frequently positive in AIDS patients with disseminated MAC.[291]

The following combination drug regimes have been found to decrease bacteremia and improve symptoms: Clarithromycin 500 mg twice daily and ethambutol 15 to 25 mg/kg/day with or without ciprofloxacin 750 mg twice daily and rifabutin 300 mg daily, *or* azithromycin 500 mg daily and ethambutol 15 to 25 mg/kg/day with or without ciprofloxacin 750 mg twice daily and rifabutin 300 mg daily. Prophylaxis with clarithromycin 500 mg twice daily, azithromycin 1200 mg weekly, or possibly rifabutin 300 mg daily for AIDS patients with less than 50 CD4 lymphocytes/mm^3 is recommended to decrease the frequency of disseminated disease and improve survival.[292–294]

CYTOMEGALOVIRUS INFECTION

Gastrointestinal CMV disease may be sexually transmitted and can occur in immunocompromised and immunocompetent patients, involving any area from mouth to anus. Several case reports have described CMV proctitis or proctocolitis following sexual intercourse and as part of a primary CMV infection.[295–298] Gastrointestinal symptoms of CMV disease have been reported in 2 to 16 percent of organ transplant recipients, but AIDS patients are the immunocompromised population most at risk of developing CMV disease.[299] This is usually due to reactivation of latent infection, but a few cases may be due to primary infection or reinfection. AIDS patients with CMV disease, like those with MAC disease, usually have less than 100 CD4 lymphocytes/mm^3. In one autopsy series, gastrointestinal CMV was identified in 90 percent of AIDS patients, and in AIDS patients with intestinal symptoms CMV has been identified—in stool cultures or in rectal or intestinal biopsy samples at autopsy—in up to 50 percent.[7,12] CMV infection of the gastrointestinal tract may be associated with esophagitis, esophageal ulcerations, enteritis, colitis, or proctitis.

CMV most often presents as a diffuse colitis associated with fever, abdominal pain, anorexia, and watery or bloody diarrhea.[300–302] Occasionally, patients with CMV intestinal symptoms may present clinically with a solitary intestinal ulcer, occasionally resulting in toxic dilatation and rarely in intestinal perforation.[303] Barium enema may show a picture of segmental colitis or pancolitis.[304] Sigmoidoscopy or colonoscopy frequently shows erythema, ulceration, or occasionally plaques, nodules, polyps, or violaceous lesions resembling Kaposi's sarcoma. Biopsy of these lesions reveals CMV vasculitis giant cells with large pleomorphic nuclei containing basophilic intranuclear CMV inclusions; these are usually endothelial cells and fibroblasts. Biopsy also shows acute hemorrhage and inflammation in the lamina propria. The presence of intranuclear inclusion bodies suggests that CMV is present in the tissue, but its role in disease pathogenesis remains unclear, since its presence is documented in both inflamed and noninflamed tissue. Marked involvement of endothelial cells can be associated with frank vasculitis and secondary mucosal ischemic changes.

Diagnosis of CMV infection is confirmed by histologic demonstration of intranuclear inclusion bodies or by viral cultures or immunofluorescent stain of intestinal biopsies.[305] Abnormal cytopathology is more likely than isolation of the virus in culture to correlate with significant disease. Systemic cytomegalovirus can be determined by viral culture of the white blood cell buffy coat or urine.[304] New techniques using labeled nucleic acid probes and polymerase chain reaction (PCR) have been effective in detecting CMV in tissue and other specimens; however, detection of the organism by PCR does not distinguish infection from disease.[306,307]

Therapy for CMV disease has been best evaluated for CMV retinitis. Treatment with ganciclovir, foscarnet, and cidofovir have been effective in suppressing viral replication with subsequent negative cultures and stabilization of clinical disease, but relapses are common after therapy is discontinued.[308] Symptomatic improvement has been reported in 93 to 100 percent of solid organ transplant recipients with CMV gastrointestinal disease treated with ganciclovir. In AIDS patients, ganciclovir treatment of CMV esophageal ulcers produces improved symptoms in 75 percent; therapy for CMV colitis appears to be less effective.[306] Nelson et al. noted that while 15 of 18 (83 percent) patients with esophageal disease treated with foscarnet had complete response, only 11 of 18 (61 percent) patients with colitis had a complete response.[309] Pancytopenia is the major toxicity of ganciclovir; it may be alleviated with granulocyte colony–stimulating factor and erythropoietin. Nephrotoxicity is the major side effect of foscarnet and cidofovir.[308] Foscarnet also causes significant electrolyte wasting and may produce seizures. Without treatment and with continued immunosuppression, CMV may result in intestinal complications such as intestinal perforation, toxic megacolon, and acalculous gangrenous colitis.[306–310] Oral ganciclovir 1 gm three times daily may be effective in reducing the risk of CMV disease.[311]

INTESTINAL SPIROCHETOSIS

Spirochetes other than *T. pallidum* were documented in the human intestinal tract as early as the nineteenth century. However, the pathologic and clinical significance of this condition remains unclear.[312–315] McMillian and Lee reported the identification of intestinal spirochetes on biopsies of 36 of 100 homosexual men.[316] There was no attempt to correlate symptoms with the presence or absence of spirochetes, and a comprehensive search for other pathogens in these patients was not carried out. Surawicz et al. diagnosed intestinal spirochetosis in 15 percent of homosexual men and no heterosexual men. Rectal spirochetosis was not associated with other histopathologic abnormalities or symptoms.[314] Law et al. diagnosed rectal spirochetosis in 39 percent of healthy unselected homosexual men attending an STD clinic. Rectal spirochetosis was associated with a history of oral-anal contact (OR 3.45), detection of three to five different nonpathogenic protozoans in feces (OR 11.7), and positive HIV-1 serology (OR 4.48).[315]

The association of intestinal spirochetosis with symptomatic disease remains largely anecdotal. Kostman et al. described two AIDS patients with diffuse colitis who on histopathology had spirochetes overlying abnormal mucosa.[317] No other pathogen was identified. Both patients responded to metronidazole therapy. Gebbers et al. also report on two patients with mild intestinal symptoms in whom rectal spirochetosis was the only abnormality diagnosed.[318] Their histopathologic findings, as with the previous study, indicated invasion of the organism, with spirochetes within epithelial cells and subepithelial macrophages. They also found numerous partially degranulated mast cells and an increased proportion of IgE plasma cells, all suggesting an immune response to the infection. Antibiotic therapy was associated with clearance of the organisms and symptomatic improvement.[318] Additional studies have identified intestinal spirochetosis by biopsy in 28 of 100 symptomatic homosexual men[13] and by culture in 13 (39 percent) of 33 symptomatic and 33 (16 percent) of 203 asymptomatic men.[70] Identification of spirochetes by culture was more commonly associated with symptoms of diarrhea than with symptoms of proctitis. Although these data are not definitive, they suggest that intestinal spirochetosis is more prevalent in homosexual men and that it may be associated with diarrhea.

Intestinal spirochetosis is readily diagnosed histologically by the presence of a prominent hematoxophilic band adjacent to the luminal surface of mucosal epithelial cells.[13] Morphologically distinct from *T. pallidum*, intestinal spirochetes can be demonstrated by darkfield microscopy of fresh material or cultured anaerobically in selected medium. Serological tests for syphilis (VDRL and RPR) are negative.

Since the clinical significance of human intestinal spirochetosis remains in question, the treatment is controversial. No controlled trials have been undertaken to examine the efficacy of antibiotics and whether eradication of the spirochetes leads to resolution of symptoms. Anecdotal reports suggest that treatment with metronidazole 400 mg three times daily for 10 days is effective in eliminating spirochetes and may afford some symptomatic relief. Consequently, until adequate clinical antibiotic studies are performed, metronidazole should be recommended for the treatment of symptomatic human intestinal spirochetosis following the exclusion of other known pathogens. Treatment is not recommended for asymptomatic intestinal spirochetosis.

ORAL-ESOPHAGEAL CANDIDIASIS

Oral candidiasis, or thrush, is one of the more common signs of AIDS. It appears early in the symptomatic prodrome of AIDS and is part of the AIDS-related complex. Klein et al. found that oral candidiasis in homosexual men was a predictor of underlying immunosuppression and incipient AIDS.[11] In their study, 13 of 22 patients with oral candidiasis who were followed for 1 year acquired a major opportunistic infection or Kaposi's sarcoma. In contrast, none of 20 patients with generalized lymphadenopathy and immunodeficiency without oral candidiasis developed clinical evidence of AIDS.

Thrush is often associated with asymptomatic esophageal candidiasis. In a study by Tavitian et al. 10 of 10 patients with AIDS and oral candidiasis were found to have esophageal candidiasis on endoscopy.[319] Three of the 10 patients with esophageal candidiasis were symptom-free, whereas the remaining 7 were symptomatic. The authors concluded that the presence of oral candidiasis in patients with documented AIDS is invariably associated with esophageal candidiasis, which is often asymptomatic. Dilatation and abnormal motility of the esophagus on the esophagogram suggests the diagnosis of candidal esophagitis. The appearance of cottage-cheese exudates is frequently seen on endoscopy, often in association with deep esophageal ulcerations.[7,62] Biopsies of these lesions typically reveal invasive hyphae in the mucosa and submucosa. High-risk patients with odynophagia or dysphagia should be carefully examined by endoscopy to ascertain if esophagitis is present and due to *Candida albicans*.

Oral candidiasis can often be controlled with nystatin 500,000 units swish-and-swallow 4 to 6 times daily or with clotrimazole troches 10 mg 5 times daily. However, these regimens may be inadequate in the treatment of AIDS-associated esophageal candidiasis. Recent studies have shown fluconazole 100 mg daily to be more effective than ketoconazole 200 mg twice daily for candidal esophagitis. However, relapses following discontinuation of therapy are common.[320] Increased use of the azole antifungal drugs has been associated with increased isolation of candida isolates with in vitro and in vivo resistance to fluconazole.[321] Previous fluconazole use and severe immunosuppression are risk factors for resistance, but resistant isolates have been identified in patients without a history of fluconazole use.[321] This may be due to strain mutation or to acquisition of new strains by nosocomial or sexual transmission. Azole-resistant candida have generally been responsive to treatment with intravenous amphotericin B, but amphotericin-resistant strains are now being described.[322] The role of chronic suppressive therapy for candidal infection in AIDS patients is still uncertain, given concerns regarding emergence of resistant strains.

OTHER PERIANAL SEXUALLY TRANSMITTED DISEASES

Donovanosis (or granuloma inguinale) is a chronic ulcerative disease which generally involves the skin and subcutaneous tissue of the genital, inguinal, and anal regions. Described in Chap. 39, donovanosis is believed to be caused by *Calymmatobacterium granulomatis*, a bacterium which multiplies within tissue histocytes and monocytes.

Donovanosis is rare in industrialized countries but relatively common in tropical and subtropical countries such as New Guinea, India, central Australia, and the Caribbean. The disease occurs more often in males than in females, and it is more common in homosexual than in heterosexual men. Although donovanosis is probably sexually transmitted, the exact mechanism of transmission is still debated. Perianal lesions occur predominantly among those who practice anal intercourse,[323,324] although the disease can also spread contiguously from the genital area to the anal region. Very little is known concerning involvement of the rectum or gastrointestinal tract. Within the perianal and anal area, the infection starts as a small, commonly pruritic, papule and later ulcerates to form a granulomatous beefy-red ulcer. Opposing (kissing) lesions are common. Lesions can become hypertrophic, at which point they are similar in appearance to condylomata lata. Most of the lesions are painless. Lesions that are located in the anal canal may be associated with rectal bleeding, and they may lead to stenosis of the anal canal.

Diagnosis is based on demonstrating the intracellular organisms (Donovan bodies) on Giemsa-stained impression smears or sections of biopsies from a lesion. Treatment consists of doxycycline 100 mg twice daily for 10 days or longer.

Chancroid occasionally causes perianal lesions in women and homosexual men. Although anorectal chancroid has not been well studied, it is likely that the painful lesions produced by *Haemophilus ducreyi* would most closely resemble herpetic lesions in the anorectal area, as they do in the genital tract. Diagnosis and therapy of anorectal chancroid are analogous to the management of genital chancroid, which is discussed in Chap. 38.

ANORECTAL TRAUMA AND FOREIGN OBJECTS

Complications of anal intercourse include prolapsed hemorrhoids, fissures, rectal ulcers, tears, and foreign bodies.[19] Rectal tears, and occasionally rectal perforation, may be caused by rectal intercourse, by insertion of a closed fist and part of the forearm into the rectum, or by insertion of foreign bodies.[325,326] Typically, patients with anorectal trauma present with the acute onset of rectal bleeding, or with signs of an "acute abdomen" if rectal perforation has occurred above the peritoneal reflection. Medical attention may be sought because the patient is unable to remove a foreign object. Retained foreign bodies have included vibrators, rubber phalluslike devices, bananas, bottles, apples, billiard balls, light bulbs, a Bermuda onion, and a variety of other unusual objects.[326]

Management of such cases is based on the clinical history, evidence of an acute abdomen, the degree of rectal trauma, and the type of retained object. If an object is present, digital and radiographic examination should confirm the position of the object. The object may be removed through a proctoscope with biopsy forceps, snare, or Foley catheter. Occasionally, local or general anesthesia may be required to remove a foreign body manually or with obstetric forceps.[326]

DIFFERENTIAL DIAGNOSIS

Many agents that infect the gut in homosexual men cause similar pathology, and differentiation as to the causative agent is sometimes possible only by laboratory tests. Further, infection with several pathogens is not uncommon, and overlapping symptoms make differentiation on clinical grounds even more difficult. However, characteristic features of some infections are helpful in narrowing the diagnostic possibilities. It seems apparent that the majority of homosexual men with anorectal symptoms who consult an STD clinic have a specific infection, and diagnoses such as "idiopathic rectal ulcer," "nonspecific proctitis," or "trauma" are usually unwarranted unless specific infections are excluded. In general, it is clear that in homosexual men proctitis or discrete ulcerative lesions of the rectum are usually caused by conventional STD agents such as *N. gonorrhoeae*, *C. trachomatis*, HSV, and *T. pallidum* and are probably acquired by receptive rectal intercourse. Infections associated with proctocolitis are caused by enteric pathogens such as *E. histolytica*, *C. jejuni*, *Salmonella*, and *Shigella*, which may be acquired most often among homosexual men by anilingus. Symptoms of enteritis, without sigmoidoscopic evidence of proctocolitis, are most often attributable to *G. lamblia* infection in homosexually active men.[27]

In immunocompromised homosexual men with HIV infection, additional organisms should be considered, such as cryptosporidia, microsporidia, *Isospora, Cyclospora,* MAC, and cytomegalovirus, in addition to HIV-1. In these immunosuppressed patients, esophagitis may develop secondary to *Candida*, HSV, and CMV.

The constellation of fever, severe anorectal pain, constipation, urinary retention, and sacral neuralgias in a patient with ulcerative rectal mucosa strongly suggests HSV infection. The presence of nonpainful anorectal ulcers, rectal polyps, or nonspecific anorectal symptoms in a patient with a rash should suggest the possibility of anorectal syphilis. LGV proctitis or proctocolitis should be considered in homosexual men who have severe anorectal symptoms such as hematochezia, rectal discharge, diarrhea, and fever and who may have severe ulcerative rectal mucosa with granulomas present on rectal biopsy. LGV should also be considered in homosexual men who are suspected to have Crohn's disease of the rectum. Since *N. gonorrhoeae* and non-LGV *C. trachomatis* cause nonspecific anorectal symptoms without symptoms of enteritis and result in nonspecific pathology of the lower rectum, these pathogens should be considered in most individuals who present with anorectal symptoms, have only mild proctitis on sigmoidoscopy, and acknowledge receptive anorectal intercourse.

Campylobacter, *Salmonella,* and *Shigella* should be suspected in those individuals with a history of acute diarrhea associated with bloody stools and fecal leukocytes, especially if sigmoidoscopic findings are not limited to the distal rectum and if stools are negative for ova and parasites. *Giardia* infection will more often cause diarrhea which is more chronic and nonbloody and is associated with nausea and bloating. *E. histolytica* infection presents with symptoms ranging from acute bloody diarrhea to chronic diarrhea with intermittent exacerbations.

A heavy concentration of *Candida albicans* in stool has been associated with pruritus ani or rectal itching in homosexual men in our studies, and topical and oral therapy with appropriate antifungal agents may be beneficial in such patients. The presence of perianal dermatitis with or without pustulae may suggest anorectal candidiasis. However, perianal erythema extending over an area of several centimeters in diameter is commonly associated with rectal discharge caused by a variety of agents and is not specific for anorectal candidiasis. When symptoms of proctitis or enteritis occur during or after antimicrobial therapy, *C. albicans* infection or pseudomembranous enterocolitis with *Clostridium difficile* infection should be considered.

When the patient is known to be immunocompromised secondary to HIV infection or AIDS, a more extensive evaluation for opportunistic infections should be undertaken. *Candida*, HSV, and CMV should be evaluated in those patients with symptoms of esophagitis. Intestinal protozoans such as cryptosporidia, *Isospora*, and microsporidia, as well as MAC and CMV, should be considered in those immunocompromised patients presenting with a diarrheal illness of a chronic nature (longer than 2 to 3 weeks).

If no infectious etiology is demonstrated despite appropriate tests and a trial of antimicrobial therapy (see below) has no effect, then idiopathic inflammatory bowel disease, such as ulcerative colitis or Crohn's disease, or HIV-1 infection of the intestine should be considered. Because of clinical similarities between enteric infections (a common problem) and inflammatory bowel disease (much less common), all appropriate infectious agents should be ruled out before a diagnosis of inflammatory bowel disease is made. Additional noninfectious conditions that could be confused with enteric infections include radiation colitis, chemically induced colitis (due to drugs, gold therapy, soaps, lubricants, or other chemicals), and neoplasm.

MANAGEMENT

The large number of infectious agents which cause enteric and anorectal infections in homosexual men necessitate a systematic approach to the management of these conditions. The medical history should attempt to differentiate among proctitis, proctocolitis, and enteritis and should assess the constellations of symptoms that suggest one or another likely infectious etiology. The history should also investigate types of sexual practices and possible exposure to the pathogens known to cause proctitis, proctocolitis, or enteritis. Examination should include inspection of the anus, digital rectal examination, and anoscopy (avoiding or minimizing use of bacteriostatic lubricants, which might interfere with microbiologic studies) to identify general mucosal abnormalities. Such abnormalities, including easily induced bleeding and exudate and discrete polyps, ulcerations, or fissures, should be cultured and biopsied if appropriate. Anal warts are frequently detected, but if proctitis is present, therapy of these warts should usually be deferred until the proctitis is resolved.

Initial laboratory tests should include a Gram stain of any rectal exudate obtained with the use of an anoscope; if no exudate is seen, material should be obtained for the Gram stain from the rectal mucosa or from any abnormal appearing stool. The demonstration of leukocytes provides objective evidence for the presence of an infectious or inflammatory disease. Cultures for *N. gonorrhoeae* should be obtained from the rectum, urethra, and pharynx, and if possible a rectal culture for *C. trachomatis* should be performed. A serologic test for syphilis should be performed in all cases. If any external ulcers, rectal mucosal lesions, or suspected condylomata lata are seen, darkfield examination of these lesions and a rapid plasma reagin test should be performed in the clinic. HSV cultures should be performed if ulcerative lesions are present. If proctocolitis is likely on the basis of either symptoms or sigmoidoscopic exam, then additional cultures for *Campylobacter, Salmonella,* and *Shigella* and stool examination for *E. histolytica* are indicated.

If symptoms and signs suggest enteritis rather than proctitis or proctocolitis, stool should be cultured for *Campylobacter* and examined (in addition to jejunal aspirate, perhaps) for *Giardia*, cryptosporidia, *Isospora*, mycobacteria, and microsporidia. Additionally, endoscopy and biopsy can aid in diagnosis of HIV, microsporidia, CMV, and MAC enteropathy. Cultures for *Salmonella, Yersinia,* and *V. parahemolyticus* and attempts to demonstrate *C. difficile* toxin or enterotoxigenic *E. coli* are sometimes indicated in homosexual men, as in heterosexual men and women, although these agents have not been found with greater frequency in homosexual men.

If a diagnosis of gonorrhea is initially made by a positive Gram stain (see Plate 75), or if syphilis is confirmed by darkfield examination or rapid plasma reagin serology, appropriate treatment should be instituted promptly. Similarly, anyone with sexual contact with a person with known gonorrhea, syphilis, or chlamydial infection should be treated appropriately on an epidemiologic basis after complete physical examination, while results of cultures for *N. gonorrhoeae* and serology for syphilis are pending. A presumptive diagnosis of HSV can often be made initially on clinical appearance alone or by history, but laboratory confirmation of suspected herpetic lesions is always desirable unless the clinical appearance of vesicular lesions is diagnostic. If the patient remains symptomatic and a careful search reveals no pathogen, or if the patient remains symptomatic despite appropriate therapy for any pathogen found or after empiric therapy, then the patient should be evaluated by a specialist for the possibility of inflammatory bowel disease or other diseases which are not sexually transmitted.

In those patients found to be immunocompromised and infected with HIV, a more extensive evaluation of the intestinal tract is required. A careful oral examination should evaluate for the presence of thrush and/or oral lesions of Kaposi's sarcoma. Dysphagia or odynophagia may suggest the presence of esophageal candidiasis and/or esophageal involvement with cytomegalovirus or HIV infection. Systemic and/or abdominal lymphadenopathy and the presence or absence of gastrointestinal blood loss should suggest gastrointestinal neoplasms, including Kaposi's sarcoma and gastrointestinal lymphomas. Careful radiographic examinations of the esophagus, small bowel, and colon, as well as endoscopy and colonoscopy, may be warranted in these highly suspect patients. Stool examination should be carefully studied for the presence of cryptosporidia, *Isospora,* and mycobacteria, as well as the other enteric pathogens described above. Intestinal biopsies may be obtained of suspicious lesions and examined for cytomegalovirus, mycobacterium, intestinal protozoans, and other histologic features of infection or malabsorption.

Identification of any of the enteric pathogens should result in specific therapeutic regimens. Failure to respond to any specific antimicrobial regimens may represent drug resistance or, more commonly, the presence of additional pathogens, necessitating more comprehensive microbiologic and immunologic evaluation. If symptoms persist after eradication of infection or if no pathogens are identified, one must consider idiopathic inflammatory bowel disease, neoplastic lesions, or antibiotic-resistant opportunistic infections and institute diagnostic and therapeutic approaches to these diseases.

Because of the complexity of diagnosis and treatment of enteritis and proctitis in an STD population and the different levels of laboratory support at STD clinics and in office practice, we have outlined two algorithms. Algorithm A (Fig. 69-8) represents a systematic approach to diagnosis and treatment that is comprehensive and employs treatment only for identified pathogens. It basically represents a stepwise progression toward specific diagnosis and treatment of patient and exposed contacts. The major problem with this algorithm is that the microbiologic evaluation is expensive and time-consuming, factors which may indirectly allow continued discomfort of the patient and transmission of the pathogen before final diagnosis and treatment.

Algorithm B (Fig. 69-9) is based on empirical therapy, which

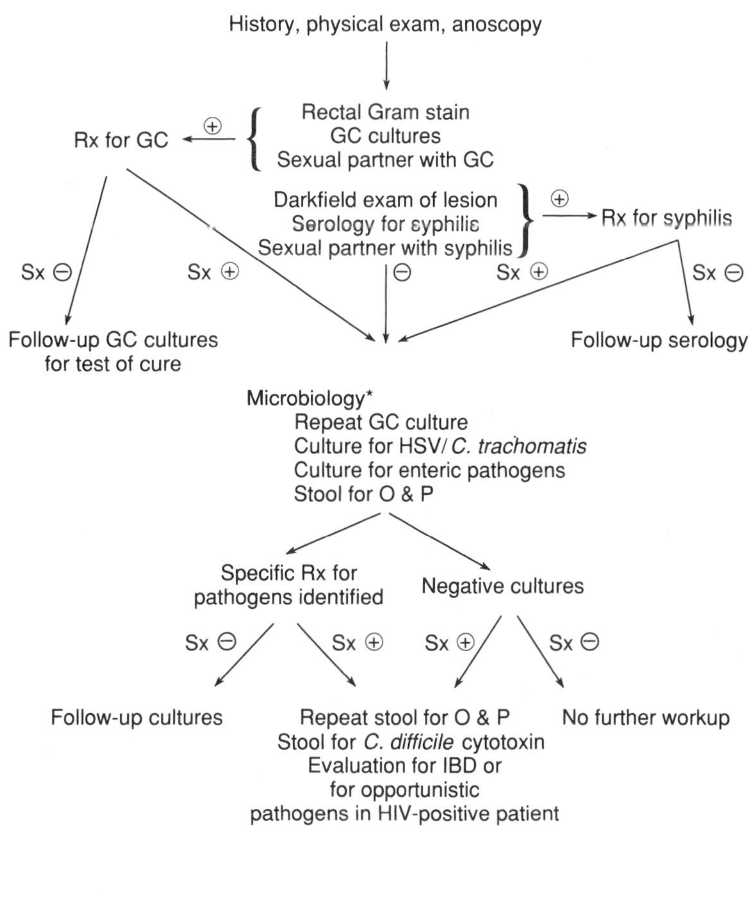

Fig. 69-8. Algorithm A: Evaluation and treatment of anorectal and/or intestinal symptoms in homosexual men. This algorithm emphasizes a full diagnostic evaluation and treatment for the specific pathogens identified. Ideally, microbiologic evaluation should be based on presenting symptoms and sigmoidoscopy findings. Rx = treatment, Sx = symptoms, GC = *N. gonorrhoeae,* O & P = ova and parasites, IBD = inflammatory bowel disease.

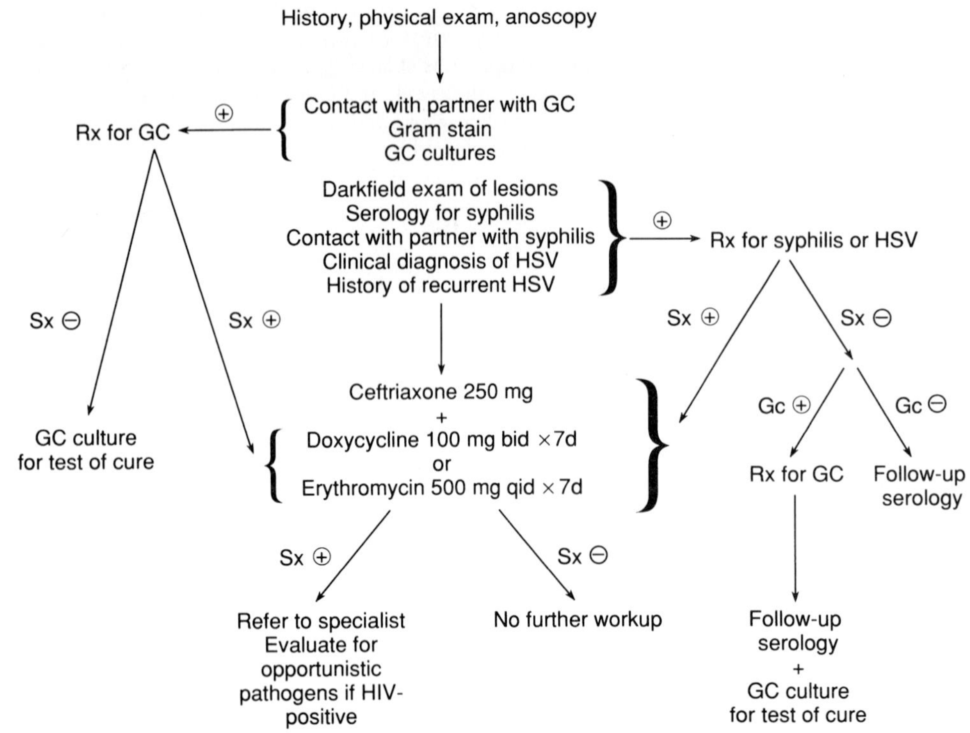

Fig. 69-9. Algorithm B: Evaluation and treatment of anorectal and/or intestinal symptoms in homosexual men. This algorithm emphasizes empirical therapy after an initial evaluation for gonorrhea and syphilis. Empirical therapy consists of intramuscular ceftriaxone 250 mg, followed by either azithromycin 1 gm, doxycycline, or erythromycin. If the patient remains symptomatic, he is referred for more complete evaluation. GC = *N. gonorrhoeae*, Rx = treatment, Sx = symptoms.

has the advantage of decreasing the cost of laboratory tests and provides immediate therapy to patients who may not return for follow-up visits. Such empirical therapy has recently been shown to produce more rapid resolution of the symptoms and signs of acute proctitis in homosexual men than specific therapy.[327] Empirical therapy has the disadvantage, however, of treating a patient before the diagnosis is known. In the study just cited, unrecognized HSV proctitis was the major reason for a failure of empiric therapy. The treatment may also convert the patient to an asymptomatic carrier, and most important, it interferes with public health efforts to trace contacts of the patient who may harbor a specific pathogen. Such public health efforts would be possible only if a specific diagnosis were made in the patient.

Selection between these two approaches must be based on clinic and public health priorities, budget, laboratory support, and patient population. Alternative approaches will undoubtedly become preferable as more is learned about the etiology and epidemiology of enteritis, proctitis, and proctocolitis in homosexual men.

PREVENTION

Because of the relatively high prevalence of asymptomatic anorectal carriage of pathogenic organisms in homosexual men, a concerted effort involving the clinician and public health authorities is necessary to control these infections. Examination and treatment of the sexual partners of homosexual men with STDs such as gonorrhea or syphilis is a conventional practice, yet similar management of the sexual contacts of homosexual men with enteric infection is not a routine procedure. Such an approach must be evaluated, not only for cases that come to medical attention through the STD clinic but also for those that are reported from other sources. We believe that when a specific pathogen is identified in a symptomatic homosexually active male patient, epidemiologic investigation of all sexual contacts within a time frame appropriate to the incubation period of the pathogen in question should be performed, and appropriate diagnostic tests for the pathogen(s) involved should be obtained from the contacts. This is especially important for those agents which can be eliminated by treatment, such as gonorrhea, *C. trachomatis*, syphilis, and the enteric pathogens. Because of the intermittent nature of virus shedding, HSV cultures in sex partners of men with rectal HSV infection is frequently unrewarding.

Most of the pathogens we have discussed should be reported to local public health workers, whose assistance in coordinating efforts to identify and examine culture contacts is helpful. Household as well as sexual contacts should be screened for infection when investigating the spread of enteric pathogens. After the acute infection subsides or following therapy, repeat laboratory tests should be performed to detect possible development of a carrier state. Infected individuals should abstain from sexual practices which might spread infection until repeat cultures are negative. Infected persons should also be educated regarding safe sex practices in the AIDS era.

Effective education of both physicians and patients about the different modes of transmission of these pathogens is necessary, along with more reliable and available laboratory techniques for diagnosis of certain of them. Recognition of the importance of sexual transmission in the spread of these infections is a prerequisite to designing public health programs that will effectively prevent their spread in the community at large. In addition, recognition of the role that some of these pathogens (especially HSV and syphilis) may play in facilitating the spread of HIV infection provides added incentive for their prevention.[328,329]

References

1 Dritz SK, Goldsmith RS: Sexually transmissible protozoal, bacterial, and viral enteric infections. *Comp Ther* 6:34, 1980.

2 Dritz SK: Medical aspects of homosexuality [Editorial]. *N Engl J Med* 302:463, 1980.

3 Quinn TC et al: The etiology of anorectal infections in homosexual men. *Am J Med* 71:395, 1981.
4 Quinn TC et al: *Chlamydia trachomatis* proctitis. *N Engl J Med* 305: 195, 1981.
5 Samarasinghe PL et al: Herpetic proctitis and sacral radiomyelopathy: A hazard for homosexual men. *Br Med J* 2:365, 1979.
6 Owen WF: Sexually transmitted diseases and traumatic problems in homosexual men. *Ann Intern Med* 92:805, 1980.
7 Gottlieb MS et al: The acquired immunodeficiency syndrome. *Ann Intern Med* 99:208, 1983.
8 Kotler DP et al: Enteropathy associated with the acquired immunodeficiency syndrome. *Ann Intern Med* 101:421, 1984.
9 Quinn TC: Gastrointestinal Manifestations of Human Immunodeficiency Virus, in *Current Topics in AIDS,* MS Gottlieb et al (eds). Chichester, Wiley, 1987, vol 1, p 155.
10 Gillin JS et al: Malabsorption and mucosal abnormalities of the small intestine in acquired immunodeficiency syndrome. *Ann Intern Med* 102:619, 1985.
11 Klein RS et al: Oral candidiasis in high-risk patients as the initial manifestation of the acquired immunodeficiency syndrome (AIDS). *N Engl J Med* 311:354, 1984.
12 Fauci AS et al: Acquired immunodeficiency syndrome: Epidemiologic, clinical, immunologic, and therapeutic consideration. *Ann Intern Med* 100:92, 1984.
13 Surawicz CM et al: Spectrum of rectal biopsy abnormalities in homosexual men with intestinal symptoms. *Gastroenterology* 91:651, 1986.
14 Noble RC: *Sexually Transmitted Disease: Guide to Diagnosis and Therapy*. Garden City, NY, Medical Examination Publishing, 1979, p 123.
15 Corey L, Holmes KK: Sexual transmission of hepatitis A in homosexual men: Incidence and mechanism. *N Engl J Med* 302:435, 1980.
16 Centers for Disease Control: Amebiasis associated with colonic irrigation: Colorado. *MMWR* 30:101, 1981.
17 Sohn N, Robilotti JG: The gay bowel syndrome: A review of colonic and rectal conditions in 200 male homosexuals. *Am J Gastroenterol* 67:478, 1977.
18 Dritz SK, Braff EH: Sexually transmitted typhoid fever. *N Engl J Med* 246:1359, 1977.
19 Bader M et al: Venereal transmission of shigellosis in Seattle—King county. *Sex Trans Dis* 4:89, 1977.
20 Drusin LM et al: Shigellosis: Another sexually transmitted disease? *Br J Vener Dis* 52:348, 1976.
21 William DC et al: High rates of enteric protozoal infections in selected homosexual men attending a venereal disease clinic. *Sex Trans Dis* 5:155, 1978.
22 Kean BH et al: Epidemic of amoebiasis and giardiasis in a biased population. *Br J Vener Dis* 55:375, 1979.
23 Felman YM, Ricciardi NB: Sexually transmitted enteric diseases. *Bull NY Acad Med* 55:533, 1979.
24 Boiling DR: Prevalence, goals, and complications of heterosexual anal intercourse in a gynecologic population. *J Reprod Med* 19:120, 1977.
25 Quinn TC et al: The polymicrobial origin of intestinal infections in homosexual men. *N Engl J Med* 309:576, 1983.
26 Dritz SK et al: Patterns of sexually transmitted enteric diseases in a city. *Lancet* 2:3, 1977.
27 Schmerin MJ et al: Amebiasis: An increasing problem among homosexuals in New York City. *JAMA* 288:1386, 1977.
28 Meyers JD et al: *Giardia lamblia* infection in homosexual men. *Br J Vener Dis* 53:54, 1977.
29 Holmberg SD et al: Prior herpes simplex virus type 2 infection as a risk factor for HIV infection. *JAMA* 259:1048–1050, 1988.
30 Nelson KE et al: Sexually transmitted diseases in a population of intravenous drug users: Association with seropositivity to the human immunodeficiency virus (HIV). *J Infect Dis* 164:457–463, 1991.
31 Stamm WE et al: The association between genital ulcer disease and acquisition of HIV infection in homosexual men. *JAMA* 260:1429–1433, 1988.
32 Quinn TC: Epidemiology and Serologic Evidence for Herpes Simplex Viruses in AIDS, in *Herpes Viruses, The Immune System, and AIDS,* L Aurelian (ed). Norwell MA, Kluwert Academic Publishers, pp 1–20, 1990.
33 Quinn TC et al: The association of syphilis with risk of human immunodeficiency virus infection in patients attending STD clinics. *Arch Intern Med* 150:1297–1302, 1990.
34 Darrow WW et al: Risk factors for HIV infections in homosexual men. *Am J Public Health* 77:479–483, 1987.
35 Quinn TC et al: Human immunodeficiency virus infection among patients attending clinics for sexually transmitted diseases. *New Engl J Med* 318:197–204, 1988.
36 Laga M et al: Non-ulcerative sexually transmitted diseases as risk factors for HIV-1 transmission in women: Results from a cohort study. *AIDS* 7:95–102, 1993.
37 Plummer FA et al: Cofactors in male-female sexual transmission of human immunodeficiency virus type 1. *J Infect Dis* 163:233–239, 1991.
38 Craib KJP et al: Rectal gonorrhoea as an independent risk factor for HIV infection in a cohort of homosexual men. *Genitourin Med* 71: 150–154, 1995.
39 Law CLH et al: Nonspecific proctitis: Association with human immunodeficiency virus infection in homosexual men. *J Infect Dis* 165: 150–154, 1992.
40 Weir SS et al: Gonorrhea as a risk factor for HIV acquisition. *AIDS* 8:1605–1608, 1994.
41 Ho JL et al: Neutrophils from human immunodeficiency virus (HIV)-seronegative donors induce HIV replication from HIV-infected patients' mononuclear cells and cell lines: An in vitro model of HIV transmission facilitated by *Chlamydia trachomatis*. *J Exp Med* 181: 1493–1505, 1995.
42 Moss GB et al: Human immunodeficiency virus DNA in urethral secretions in men: Association with gonococcal urethritis and CD4 cell depletion. *J Infect Dis* 172:1469–1474, 1995.
43 Tyndall MW et al: Single-dose azithromycin for the treatment of chancroid: A randomized comparison with erythromycin. *Sex Trans Dis* 21:231–234, 1994.
44 Tyndall MW et al: Ceftriaxone no longer predictably cures chancroid in Kenya. *J Infect Dis* 167:469–471, 1993.
45 Siegal FP et al: Severe acquired immunodeficiency in male homosexuals, manifested by chronic perianal ulcerative herpes simplex lesions. *N Engl J Med* 305:1439, 1981.
46 Johns DR et al: Alteration in the natural history of neurosyphilis by concurrent infection with the human immunodeficiency virus. *N Engl J Med* 316:1569–1572, 1987.
47 Hicks CB et al: Seronegative secondary syphilis in a patient infected with the human immunodeficiency virus (HIV) with Kaposi sarcoma: A diagnostic dilemma. *Ann Intern Med* 107:492–495, 1987. [Erratum, *Ann Intern Med* 107:946, 1987].
48 Tikjoh G et al: Seronegative secondary syphilis in a patient with AIDS: Identification of *Treponema pallidum* in a biopsy specimen. *J Am Acad Dermatol* 24:506–508, 1991.
49 Hutchinson CM et al: Characteristics of patients with syphilis attending Baltimore STD clinics: Multiple high-risk subgroups and interactions with human immunodeficiency virus infection. *Arch Intern Med* 151:511–516, 1991.
50 Hutchinson CM, Hook EW: Syphilis in Adults, in *Medical Clinics of North America,* vol 74(6):1389–1416, DH Martin (guest ed). Philadelphia, Saunders, 1990.
51 Musher DM et al: Effect of human immunodeficiency virus (HIV) infection on the course of syphilis and the response to treatment. *Ann Intern Med* 113:872–881, 1990.
52 Kiviat NB et al: Association of anal dysplasia and human papillomavirus with immunosuppression and HIV infection among homosexual men. *AIDS* 7:43–49, 1993.
53 Palefsky JM et al: Natural history of anal cytologic abnormalities and papillomavirus infection among homosexual men with group IV HIV disease. *J Acquir Immun Defic Syndr* 5:1258–1265, 1992.

54 Kiviat N et al: Anal human papillomavirus infection among human immunodeficiency virus-seropositive and seronegative men. *J Infect Dis* 163:358–361, 1990.
55 Caussy D et al: Interaction of human immunodeficiency and papilloma viruses: Association with anal epithelial abnormality in homosexual men. *Int J Cancer* 46:214–219, 1990.
56 Goldberg GS et al: Microbiology of human immunodeficiency virus anorectal disease. *Dis Colon Rectum* 37:439–443, 1994.
57 Orkin BA, Smith LE: Perineal manifestations of HIV infection. *Dis Colon Rectum* 35:310–314, 1992.
58 Schmitt SL, Wexner SD: Treatment of anorectal manifestations of AIDS: Past and present. *Int J STD AIDS* 5:8–10, 1994.
59 Safavi A et al: Anorectal surgery in the HIV+ patient: Update. *Dis Colon Rectum* 34:299–304, 1991.
60 Wilcox CM, Schwartz DA: Idiopathic anorectal ulceration in patients with human immunodeficiency virus infection. *Am J Gastroenterol* 89(4):599–604, 1994.
61 Dworkin B et al: Gastrointestinal manifestation of the acquired immunodeficiency syndrome: A review of 22 cases. *Am J Gastroenterol* 80:774, 1985.
62 Cone LA et al: An update on the acquired immunodeficiency syndrome (AIDS): Associated disorders of the alimentary tract. *Dis Colon Rectum* 29:60, 1986.
63 Smith PD: Intestinal Infections in HIV-1 Disease, in *Infections of the Gastrointestinal Tract,* MJ Blaser et al (eds). New York, Raven Press, 1995, p 763.
64 Nelson JA et al: Human immunodeficiency virus detected in bowel epithelium from patients with gastrointestinal symptoms. *Lancet* 1: 259–262, 1988.
65 Kotler DP et al: Chronic idiopathic esophageal ulceration in the acquired immunodeficiency syndrome. *J Clin Gastroenterol* 15(4):284–290, 1992.
66 Cummins AG et al: Quantitative histological study of enteropathy associated with HIV infection. *Gut* 31:317–321, 1990.
67 Bartlett JG et al: AIDS enteropathy. *Clin Infect Dis* 15:726–735, 1992.
68 Greenson JK et al: AIDS enteropathy: Occult enteric infections and duodenal mucosal alterations in chronic diarrhea. *Ann Int Med* 114: 366–372, 1991.
69 Smith PD et al: Gastrointestinal infections in AIDS. *Ann Int Med* 116: 63–77, 1992.
70 Laughon BE et al: Prevalence of enteric pathogens in homosexual men with and without acquired immunodeficiency syndrome. *Gastroenterology* 94:984–93, 1988.
71 Smith PD et al: Intestinal infections in patients with the acquired immunodeficiency syndrome (AIDS). *Ann Intern Med* 108:328, 1988.
72 Malebranche R et al: Acquired immunodeficiency syndrome with severe gastrointestinal manifestations in Haiti. *Lancet* 2:873, 1985.
73 Colebunders R et al: Persistent diarrhea, strongly associated with HIV infection in Kinshasa, Zaire. *Am J Gastroenterol* 82:859, 1987.
74 Janoff EN et al: Adenovirus colitis in the acquired immunodeficiency syndrome. *Gastroenterology* 100:976–978, 1991.
75 Grohmann GS et al: Enteric viruses and diarrhea in HIV-infected patients. *New Engl J Med* 329(1):14–20, 1993.
76 Cunningham AL et al: Gastrointestinal viral infections in homosexual men who were symptomatic and seropositive for human immunodeficiency virus. *J Infect Dis* 158(2):386–391, 1988.
77 Kotler DP et al: Small intestinal injury and parasitic diseases in AIDS. *Ann Int Med* 113:444–449, 1990.
78 Donovan RM et al: Changes in virus load markers during AIDS-associated opportunistic diseases in human immunodeficiency virus-infected persons. *J Infect Dis* 174:401–403, 1996.
79 Clumeck N et al: Acquired immune deficiency syndrome in African patients. *N Engl J Med* 310:429, 1984.
80 Pape JW et al: Characteristics of the acquired immune deficiency syndrome in Haitians. *N Engl J Med* 309:935, 1983.
81 Klein EJ et al: Anorectal gonococcal infection. *Ann Intern Med* 86: 340, 1977.
82 Pariser H, Marino AF: Gonorrhea: Frequently unrecognized reservoirs. *South Med J* 63:198, 1970.
83 Bhattacharyya MN, Jephcott AE: Diagnosis of gonorrhea in women. *Br J Vener Dis* 50:109, 1974.
84 Hetmans AL: Culture of gonococci from the rectum on Thayer and Martin's selective medium. *Dermatologica* 133:314, 1966.
85 Scott J, Stone AH: Some observations on the diagnosis of rectal gonorrhea in both sexes using a selective culture medium. *Br J Vener Dis* 42:103, 1966.
86 British Cooperative Clinical Group: Homosexuality and venereal disease in the United Kingdom. *Br J Vener Dis* 49:329, 1973.
87 Owen RL, Hill JL: Rectal and pharyngeal gonorrhea in homosexual men. *JAMA* 220:1315, 1972.
88 McMillan A, Young H: Gonorrhea in the homosexual man. *Sex Trans Dis* 5:146, 1978.
89 Judson FN et al: Screening for gonorrhea and syphilis in the gay baths: Denver, Colorado. *Am J Public Health* 67:740, 1977.
90 Merino HI, Richards JB: An innovative program of venereal disease case-finding, treatment, and education. *Sex Trans Dis* 4:50, 1977.
91 Weisner PJ et al: Gonococcal Anorectal Infection (abstract). Eleventh Interscience Conference on Antimicrobial Agents and Chemotherapy, 1971.
92 Handsfield HH et al: Correlation of auxotype and penicillin susceptibility of *Neisseria gonorrhoeae* with sexual preference and clinical manifestations of gonorrhea. *Sex Trans Dis* 7:1, 1980.
93 Eisenstein BI, Masi AT: Disseminated gonococcal infection (DGI) and gonococcal arthritis (GCA): I. Bacteriology, epidemiology, host factors, pathogen factors, and pathology. *Seminars Arthritis Rheumatism* 10(3):155–172, 1981.
94 McWhinney PHM et al: Disseminated gonococcal infection associated with deficiency of the second component of complement. *Postgrad Med J* 67:297–298, 1991.
95 McFarland L et al: Gonococcal sensitivity to fecal lipids can be mediated by an MTR independent mechanism. *J Clin Microbiol* 18:121–127, 1983.
96 Coghill DV, Young H: Genital gonorrhea in women: A serovar correlation with concomitant rectal infection. *J Infect* 18:131–141, 1989.
97 Harkness AH: The pathology of gonorrhea. *Br J Vener Dis* 24:132, 1948.
98 Kilpatrick ZM: Gonorrheal proctitis. *N Engl J Med* 287:967, 1972.
99 Babb RR: Acute gonorrheal proctitis. *Am J Gastoenterol* 61:143, 1974.
100 Catterall RR: Anorectal gonorrhoea. *Proc R Soc Med* 55:871, 1962.
101 William DC et al: The utility of anoscopy in the rapid diagnosis of symptomatic anorectal gonorrhea in men. *Sex Transm Dis* 8:16, 1980.
102 Deheragoda P: Diagnosis of rectal gonorrhea by blind anorectal swabs compared with direct vision swabs taken via a proctoscope. *Br J Vener Dis* 53:311, 1977.
103 Seth A: Use of trimethoprim to prevent overgrowth by proteus in the cultivation of *Neisseria gonorrhoeae. Br J Vener Dis* 46:201, 1970.
104 Ching S et al: Ligase chain reaction for detection of *Neisseria gonorrhoeae* in urogenital swabs. *J Clin Microbiol* 33(12):3111–3114, 1995.
105 Smith KR et al: Evaluation of ligase chain reaction for use with urine for identification of *Neisseria gonorrhoeae* in females attending a sexually transmitted disease clinic. *J Clin Microbiol* 33(2):455–457, 1995.
106 Iwen PC et al: Evaluation of nucleic acid-based test (PACE 2C) for simultaneous detection of *Chlamydia trachomatis* and *Neisseria gonorrhoeae* in endocervical specimens. *J Clin Microbiol* 33(10):2587–2591, 1995.
107 Stary A et al: Comparison of DNA-probe test and culture for the detection of *Neisseria gonorrhoeae* in genital samples. *Sex Trans Dis* 243–247, 1993.
108 Mahony JB et al: Multiplex PCR for detection of *Chlamydia trachomatis* and *Neisseria gonorrhoeae* in genitourinary specimens. *J Clin Microbiol* 33(11):3049–3053.

109 Lewis JS et al: Direct DNA probe assay for *Neisseria gonorrhoeae* in pharyngeal and rectal specimens. *J Clin Microbiol* 31(10):2783–2785, 1993.
110 Centers for Disease Control: 1993 sexually transmitted diseases treatment guidelines. *MMWR* 42:1, 1993.
111 Moran JS, Levine WC: Drugs of choice for the treatment of uncomplicated gonococcal infections. *Clin Infect Dis* 20(suppl 1):S47–65, 1995.
112 Waugh MA: Anorectal herpesvirus hominis infection in man. *J Am Vener Dis Assoc* 3:69, 1976.
113 Jacobs E: Anal infections caused by herpes simplex virus. *Dis Colon Rectum* 19:151, 1976.
114 Goldmeier D: Proctitis and herpes simplex virus in homosexual men. *Br J Vener Dis* 56:111, 1980.
115 Hutfield DC: History of herpes genitalis. *Br J Vener Dis* 42:263, 1966.
116 Goodell SE et al: Herpes simplex virus proctitis in homosexual men: Clinical, sigmoidoscopic, and histopathologic features. *N Engl J Med* 308:868, 1983.
117 Koutsky LA et al: Underdiagnosis of genital herpes by current clinical and viral-isolation procedures. *New Engl J Med* 326:1533–1539, 1992.
118 Goldmeier D et al: Urinary retention and intestinal obstruction associated with anorectal herpes simplex virus infection. *Br Med J* 1: 425, 1975.
119 Centers for Disease Control: Revision of the CDC Surveillance Case Definition for Acquired Immunodeficiency Syndrome. *MMWR* 36(suppl):15, 1987.
120 Ashley R et al: Inability of enzyme immunoassays to discriminate between infections with herpes simplex virus types 1 and 2. *Ann Intern Med* 115:520–526, 1991.
121 Ashley RL et al: Comparison of Western blot and IgG specific immunodot enzyme assay for detecting HSV-1 and HSV-2 antibodies in human sera. *J Clin Microbiol* 26:682, 1988.
122 Rompalo AM et al: Oral acyclovir vs. placebo for treatment of herpes simplex virus proctitis in homosexual men. *Clin Res* 33:58A, 1985.
123 Wald A et al: Suppression of subclinical shedding of herpes simplex virus type 2 with acyclovir. *Ann Int Med* 124(1, pt 1):8–15, 1996.
124 Goldberg LH et al: Continuous five-year treatment of patients with frequently recurring genital herpes simplex virus infection with acyclovir. *J Med Virol* 1(suppl):45–50, 1993.
125 Centers for Disease Control: Primary and secondary syphilis—United States, 1981–1990. *MMWR* 40:314, 1991.
126 Wasserheit JN, Aral SO: The dynamic topology of sexually transmitted disease epidemics: Implications for prevention strategies. *J Infect Dis* 174(suppl 2):S201–213, 1996.
127 Centers for Disease Control, Division of STD Prevention: Sexually Transmitted Disease Surveillance, 1994. Atlanta, U.S. Department of Health and Human Services, 1995.
128 DeHovitz JA et al: Sexually transmitted diseases, sexual behavior, and cocaine use in inner-city women. *Amer J Epidem* 140(12):1125, 1994.
129 British Cooperative Clinical Group: Homosexuality and venereal disease in the United Kingdom: A second study. *Br J Vener Dis* 56:6–11, 1980.
130 Blount JH, Holmes KK: Epidemiology of Syphilis and the Nonvenereal Treponematoses, in *The Biology of Parasitic Spirochetes,* RC Johnson (ed). New York, Academic Press, 1976, p 157.
131 Martin EG, Kallet HI: Primary syphilis of the anorectal region. *JAMA* 84:1556, 1925.
132 Jones AJ, Janis L: Primary syphilis of the rectum and gonorrhea of the anus. *Am J Syph* 28:453, 1944.
133 Smith D: Infectious syphilis of the anal canal. *Dis Colon Rectum* 6: 7, 1963.
134 Mirdel A et al: Primary and secondary syphilis, 20 years' experience: Clinical features. *Genitourin Med* 65:1–3, 1989.
135 Marino AWM: Proctologic lesions observed in male homosexuals. *Dis Colon Rectum* 7:121, 1964.
136 Lieberman W: Syphilis of the rectum. *Rev Gastroenterol* 18:67, 1951.
137 Nazemi MM et al: Syphilitic proctitis in a homosexual. *JAMA* 231: 389, 1975.
138 Akdamar K et al: Syphilitic proctitis. *Dig Dis Sci* 22:701–704, 1977.
139 Hutchinson CM et al: Altered clinical presentation of early syphilis in patients with HIV infection. *Ann Intern Med* 121:94, 1994.
140 Mitchell RD et al: Secretory and histologic changes after treatment of gastric syphilis. *Gastroenterology* 43:689, 1962.
141 Sachar DB et al: Erosive syphilitic gastritis: Darkfield and immunofluorescent diagnosis from biopsy specimen. *Ann Intern Med* 80:512, 1974.
142 Smibert RM: The Spirochetes, in *Bergey's Manual of Determinative Bacteriology,* 8th ed, RE Buchanan, NE Gibbons (eds). Baltimore, Williams and Wilkins, 1974, p 167.
143 Hook EW III et al: Detection of *Treponema pallidum* in lesion exudate with a pathogen-specific monoclonal antibody. *J Clin Microbiol* 22:241–244, 1985.
144 Jue R et al: Comparison of fluorescent and conventional darkfield methods for the detection of *Treponema pallidum* in syphilitic lesions. *Am J Clin Pathol* 47:809, 1967.
145 Johnson WC: Venereal Diseases and Treponemal infections, in *Dermal Pathology,* JH Graham et al (eds). New York, Harper and Row, 1972, p 371.
146 Quinn TC et al: Rectal mass caused by *Treponema pallidum:* Confirmation by immunofluorescent staining. *Gastroenterology* 82:135, 1982.
147 Larsen SA et al: Laboratory diagnosis and interpretation of tests for syphilis. *Clin Micro Rev* 8:1, 1995.
148 Rompalo AM et al: Association of biologic false-positive reactions for syphilis with human immunodeficiency virus infection. *J Infect Dis* 165:1124–1126, 1992.
149 Hook EW III, Mara CM: Acquired syphilis in adults. *New Engl J Med* 326:1060–1069, 1992.
150 Drusin LM et al: The role of surgery in primary syphilis of the anus. *Ann Surg* 185:65, 1976.
151 Verdon MS et al: Pilot study of azithromycin for treatment of primary and secondary syphilis. *Clin Infect Dis* 19:486, 1994.
152 Berry CD et al: Neurologic relapse after benzathine penicillin therapy for secondary syphilis in a patient with HIV infection. *N Engl J Med* 316:1587, 1987.
153 Romanowski B et al: Serologic response to treatment of infectious syphilis. *Ann Intern Med* 114:1005, 1991.
154 Yinnon AM et al: Serologic response to treatment of syphilis in patients with HIV infection. *Arch Intern Med* 156:321, 1996.
155 Musher DM et al: Effect of HIV infection on the course of syphilis and on the response to treatment. *Ann Intern Med* 113:872, 1990.
156 Rolfs RT: Treatment of syphilis. *Clin Infect Dis* 20:S23, 1995.
157 Stamm WE et al: *Chlamydia trachomatis* Proctitis in Homosexual Men and Heterosexual Women, in *Chlamydia Infections,* PA Mardh et al (eds). Amsterdam, Elsevier Biomedical, 1982, p 111.
158 Thompson CI et al: *Chlamydia trachomatis* infection in the female rectum. *Genitourin Med* 63:179–181, 1987.
159 McMillan A et al: Chlamydial infection in homosexual men: Frequency of isolation of *Chlamydia trachomatis* from the urethra, anorectum, and pharynx. *Br J Vener Dis* 57:47–49, 1981.
160 Goldmeier D, Darougar S: Isolations of *Chlamydia trachomatis* from throat and rectum of homosexual men. *Br J Vener Dis* 53:184, 1977.
161 Jones RB et al: *Chlamydia trachomatis* from the pharynx and rectum of heterosexual patients at risk for genital infection. *Ann Intern Med* 102:757, 1985.
162 Barnes RC et al: Comparison of *Chlamydia trachomatis* serovars causing rectal and cervical infections. *J Infect Dis* 156:953–958, 1987.
163 Bensaude R, Lambling A: Discussion on the aetiology and treatment of fibrous stricture of the rectum (including lymphogranuloma inguinale). *Proc R Soc Med* 29:1441, 1936.
164 Greaves AB: The frequency of lymphogranuloma venereum in persons with perirectal abscesses, fistula-in-ano, or both. *Bull WHO* 29: 797, 1963.

165 Bauwens JE et al: Infection with *Chlamydia trachomatis* lymphogranuloma venereum serovar L1 in homosexual men with proctitis: Molecular analysis of an unusual case cluster. *Clin Infect Dis* 20:576, 1995.
166 Coutts WE et al: Digestive tract infection by the virus of lymphogranuloma inguinale. *Am J Dig Dis* 7:287, 1940.
167 Miles RPM: Rectal lymphogranuloma venereum. *Br J Surg* 45:180, 1957.
168 Levin I et al: Lymphogranuloma venereum: Rectal stricture and carcinoma. *Dis Colon Rectum* 7:129, 1964.
169 Crohn BB, Yarnis H: *Regional Ileitis*. New York, Grune and Stratton, 1958.
170 Rodaniche EC et al: The relationship between lymphogranuloma venereum and regional enteritis: An etiologic study of 4 cases with negative results. *Gastroenterology* 1:687, 1943.
171 Tomenius E et al: Positive Frei tests in 7 cases of morbus Crohn (regional ileitis). *Gastroenterologica* 99:369, 1963.
172 Schuller JL et al: Antibodies against chlamydia of lymphogranuloma-venereum type in Crohn's disease. *Lancet* 1:19, 1979.
173 Mardh PA et al: Lack of evidence for an association between infections with *C. trachomatis* and Crohn's disease, as indicated by microimmunofluorescence antibody tests. *Acta Pathol Microbiol Scand [B]* 88:57, 1980.
174 Taylor-Robinson D et al: Low frequency of chlamydial antibodies in patients with Crohn's disease and ulcerative colitis. *Lancet* 1:1162, 1979.
175 Swarbrick ET et al: Chlamydia, cytomegalovirus, and yersinia in inflammatory bowel disease. *Lancet* 2:11, 1979.
176 Dean D et al: Major outer membrane protein variants of *Chlamydia trachomatis* are associated with severe upper genital tract infections and histopathology in San Francisco. *J Infect Dis* 172:1013, 1995.
177 Rompalo AM et al: Rapid diagnosis of *Chlamydia trachomatis* rectal infection by direct immunofluorescence staining. *J Infect Dis* 155: 1075, 1987.
178 Riordan T et al: False positive results with an ELISA for detection of chlamydial antigen. *J Clin Pathol* 39:1276–1277, 1986.
179 Wang SP et al: A simplified method for immunological typing of trachoma-inclusion conjunctivitis-lymphogranuloma venereum organism. *Infect Immun* 7:356, 1973.
180 Suchland RJ, Stamm WE: Simplified microtiter cell culture method for rapid immunotyping of *Chlamydia trachomatis*. *J Clin Microbiol* 29:1333–1338, 1991.
181 Schachter J: Confirmatory serodiagnosis of lymphogranuloma venereum proctitis may yield false positive results due to other chlamydia infections of the rectum. *Sex Trans Dis* 8:26, 1981.
182 Stamm WE et al: Azithromycin for empirical treatment of the nongonococcal urethritis syndrome in men. *JAMA* 274:545, 1995.
183 Centers for Disease Control: Recommendations for the prevention and management of *Chlamydia trachomatis* infections, 1993. *MMWR* 42:27–28, 1993.
184 Belitsos PC et al: Association of gastric hypoacidity with opportunistic enteric infections in patients with AIDS. *J Infect Dis* 166:277, 1992.
185 Dritz SK, Back AF: *Shigella* enteritis venereally transmitted [Letter]. *N Engl J Med* 291:1194, 1974.
186 Carey PB, Wright EP: *Campylobacter jejune* in a male homosexual. *Br J Vener Dis* 55:381, 1979.
187 Quinn TC et al: *Campylobacter* proctitis in a homosexual male. *Ann Intern Med* 93:458, 1980.
188 William DC et al: Sexually transmitted enteric pathogens in a male homosexual population. *NY State J Med* 77:2050, 1977.
189 Acheson DWK, Keusch G: Shigella and Enterinvasive *Escherichia coli*, in *Infections of the Gastrointestinal Tract*, MJ Blaser et al (eds). New York, Raven Press, 1995, p 763.
190 Sorvillo FJ et al: Incidence of campylobacteriosis among patients with AIDS in Los Angeles County. *J Acq Immune Def Syndr* 4:598, 1991.
191 Allos BM, Blaser MJ: *Campylobacter jejuni* and the expanding spectrum of related infections. *Clin Infect Dis* 20:1092, 1994.
192 Blaser MJ et al: *Campylobacter* enteritis: Clinical and epidemiologic features. *Ann Intern Med* 91:179, 1979.
193 Blaser MJ et al: Reservoirs for human campylobacteriosis. *J Infect Dis* 141:665, 1980.
194 Hood M, Todd JM: *Vibrio fetus:* A cause of human abortion. *Am J Obstet Gynecol* 83:506, 1960.
195 Simmers PD, Tabaqchali S: *Campylobacter* species in male homosexuals. *Br J Vener Dis* 55:66, 1979.
196 Laughon BE et al: Recovery of *Campylobacter* species from homosexual men. *J Infect Dis* 158:464, 1988.
197 Pasternak J et al: Bacteremia caused by campylobacter-like organism in two male homosexuals. *Ann Intern Med* 101:339, 1984.
198 Totten PA et al: *Campylobacter cinaedi* (sp. nov.) and *Campylobacter fennelliae* (sp. nov.): Two new *Campylobacter* species associated with enteric disease in homosexual men. *J Infect Dis* 151:131, 1985.
199 Fennell CL et al: Characterization of campylobacter-like organisms isolated from homosexual men. *J Infect Dis* 149:S58, 1984.
200 Bremell T et al: Rheumatic symptoms following an outbreak of campylobacter enteritis: A five-year follow up. *Ann Rheum Dis* 50:934–938, 1991.
201 Rees JH et al: *Campylobacter jejuni* infection and Guillain-Barré syndrome. *N Engl J Med* 333:1374, 1995.
202 Quinn TC et al: Infections with *Campylobacter jejune* and campylobacter-like organisms in homosexual men. *Ann Intern Med* 101: 187, 1984.
203 Blaser MJ et al: Acute colitis caused by *Campylobacter fetus* ss. *jejuni*. *Gastroenterology* 78:448, 1980.
204 Lambert ME et al: *Campylobacter* colitis. *Br Med J* 1:857, 1979.
205 DuPont HL: Antimicrobial-resistant *Campylobacter* species—a new threat to travelers to Thailand [Editorial response]. *Clin Infect Dis* 21:542, 1995.
206 Smith PD et al: *Salmonella typhimurium* enteritis and bacteremia in the acquired immunodeficiency syndrome. *Ann Intern Med* 102:207, 1985.
207 Morse EV, Duncan MA: Salmonellosis: An environmental health problem. *J Am Vet Med Assoc* 165:1015, 1974.
208 Gruenewald R et al: Relationship between HIV infection and salmonellosis in 20- to 59- year-old residents of New York City. *Clin Infect Dis* 18:358, 1994.
209 Pegues DA et al: *Salmonella* Including *S. typhi*, in *Infections of the Gastrointestinal Tract*, MJ Blaser et al (eds). New York, Raven Press, 1995, p 785.
210 Kotler DP, Orenstein JM: Chronic diarrheas and malabsorption associated with enteropathogenic bacterial infection in a patient with AIDS. *Ann Intern Med* 119:127, 1993.
211 Kotler DP et al: Chronic bacterial enteropathy in patients with AIDS. *J Infect Dis* 171:552, 1995.
212 Orenstein JM, Kotler DP: Diarrheogenic bacterial enteritis in AIDS: A light and electron microscopy study of 52 cases. *Hum Pathol* 26: 481, 1995.
213 Thomas JA, Antony AJ: Amoebiasis of the penis. *Br J Urol* 48:269, 1976.
214 Cooke RA: Cutaneous amoebiasis involving the anogenital region. *J Med Assoc Thai* 56:354, 1973.
215 Cohen C: Three cases of amoebiasis of the cervix uteri. *J Obstet Gynaecol Br Commonw* 80:476, 1973.
216 Abrahm PM: Snakes in the grass or, the worm turns on. *JAMA* 221: 917, 1972.
217 Shookhoff HB: Parasite transmission. *JAMA* 222:1310, 1972.
218 Lynch V de P: Parasite transmission. *JAMA* 222:1309, 1972.
219 Waugh MA: Threadworm infestation in homosexuals. *Trans St Johns Hosp Dermatol Soc* 58:224, 1972.
220 Most H: Manhattan: A "tropic isle?" *Am J Trop Med Hyg* 17:333, 1968.
221 Peters CS et al: Prevalence of enteric parasites in homosexual patients attending an outpatient clinic. *J Clin Microbiol* 24:684, 1986.
222 Ravdin JI: Amebiasis. *Clin Infect Dis* 20:1453, 1995.
223 Keyston JS et al: Intestinal parasitic infections in homosexual men: Prevalence, symptoms, and factors in transmission. *Can Med Assoc J* 123:512, 1980.

224 Sargeaunt PG et al: *Entamoeba histolytica* in male homosexuals. *Br J Vener Dis* 59:193, 1983.
224a Sargeant PG et al: The differentiation of invasive and non-invasive *Entamoeba histolytica* by isoenzyme electrophoresis. *Trans R Soc Trop Med Hyg* 72:519–521, 1978.
225 Chin ATL, Gerken A: Carriage of intestinal protozoal cysts in homosexuals. *Br J Vener Dis* 60:193, 1984.
226 Goldmeier D et al: Is *Entamoeba histolytica* in homosexual men a pathogen? *Lancet* 1:641, 1986.
227 Jessurun J et al: The prevalence of invasive amebiasis is not increased in patients with AIDS. *AIDS* 6:307, 1992.
228 Allason-Jones E et al: *Entamoeba histolytica* as a commensal intestinal parasite in homosexual men. *N Engl J Med* 315:353, 1986.
229 Reed SL, Wess DW: *Entamoeba histolytica* infection and AIDS. *Amer J Med* 90:269–270, 1991.
230 Sorvillo FJ et al: Amebic infections in asymptomatic homosexual men: Lack of evidence of invasive disease. *Public Health Briefs* 76: 1137, 1986.
231 Mirelman D et al: Changes in isoenzyme patterns of a cloned culture of nonpathogenic *Entamoeba histolytica* during axenization. *Infect Immun* 54:827–832, 1986.
232 Petri WA et al: Isolation of the galactose-binding lectin which mediates the in-vitro adherence of *Entamoeba histolytica*. *J Clin Invest* 80:1238–1244, 1987.
233 Haque R et al: Diagnosis of pathogenic *Entamoeba histolytica* infection using a stool ELISA based on monoclonal antibodies to the galactose-specific adhesin. *J Infect Dis* 167:347–349, 1993.
234 Pittman FE et al: Studies of human amebiasis: I. Clinical and laboratory findings in eight cases of acute amebic colitis. *Gastroenterology* 65:581, 1973.
235 Pittman FE et al: Studies on human amebiasis: II. Light and electron-microscopic observations of colonic mucosa and exudate in acute amebic colitis. *Gastroenterology* 65:588, 1973.
236 Reed SL: Amebiasis: An update. *Clin Infect Dis* 14:385–393, 1992.
237 Drugs for parasitic infections. *Med Letter* 37:99–108, 1995.
238 Sullam PM et al: Paromomycin therapy of endemic amebiasis in homosexual men. *Sex Trans Dis* 13:151–155, 1986.
239 Schmerin MJ et al: Giardiasis: Association with homosexuality. *Ann Intern Med* 88:801, 1978.
240 Beal CB et al: A technique for sampling duodenal contents: Demonstration of upper small bowel pathogens. *Am J Trop Med Hyg* 19: 349, 1970.
241 Farthing MJG: *Giardia lamblia*, in *Infections of the Gastrointestinal Tract*, MJ Blaser et al (eds). New York, Raven Press, 1995, p 1081.
242 McMillan A: Threadworms in homosexual males. *Br Med J* 1:367, 1978.
243 Soave R, Armstrong D: *Cryptosporidium* and cryptosporidiosis. *Rev Infect Dis* 8:1012, 1986.
244 Soave R, Johnson WD: *Cryptosporidium* and *Isospora belli* infections. *J Infect Dis* 157:225, 1988.
245 Orenstein JM: Microsporidiosis in AIDS. *Am Soc Parasitologists* 77: 843, 1991.
246 Weber R et al: Human microsporidial infections. *Clin Micro Rev* 7: 426, 1994.
247 Tzipori S et al: An outbreak of calf diarrhea attributed to cryptosporidial infection. *Vet Res* 107:579, 1980.
248 Nime FA et al: Acute enterocolitis in a human being infected with the protozoan *Cryptosporidium*. *Gastroenterology* 70:592, 1976.
249 Weinstein L et al: Intestinal cryptosporidiosis complicated by disseminated cytomegalovirus infection. *Gastroenterology* 81:584, 1981.
250 Current WL et al: Human cryptosporidiosis in immunocompetent and immunodeficient persons: Studies of an outbreak and experimental transmission. *N Engl J Med* 308:1252, 1983.
251 Current WL, Garcia LS: Cryptosporidiosis. *Clin Microbiol Rev* 4: 325–358, 1991.
252 Goodgame RW: Understanding intestinal spore-forming protozoa: *Cryptosporidia, Microsporidia, Isospora,* and *Cyclospora*. *Ann Intern Med* 124:429, 1996.
253 DeHovitz JA et al: Clinical manifestations and therapy of *Isospora belli* infection in patients with the acquired immunodeficiency syndrome. *New Engl J Med* 315:87–90, 1986.
254 Flanigan T et al: *Cryptosporidium* infection and CD4 counts. *Annals Intern Med* 116:840, 1992.
255 Jacyna MR et al: Protracted enteric cryptosporidial infection in selective immunoglobulin A and saccharomyces opsonin deficiencies. *Gut* 31:714–716, 1990.
256 Ma P, Soave R: Three-step stool examination for cryptosporidiosis in ten homosexual men with protracted watery diarrhea. *J Infect Dis* 147:824, 1983.
257 Grigoriew GA et al: Evaluation of the Merifluor immunofluorescent assay for the detection of *Cryptosporidium* and *Giardia* in sodium acetate formalin-fixed stools. *Diagn Microbiol Infect Dis* 19:89–91, 1994.
258 Portnoy D et al: Treatment of intestinal cryptosporidiosis with spiramycin. *Ann Intern Med* 101:202, 1984.
259 Bissuel F et al: Paromomycin: An effective treatment for cryptosporidial diarrhea in patients with AIDS. *Clin Infect Dis* 18:447–449, 1994.
260 White AC Jr et al: Paromomycin for cryptosporidiosis in AIDS: A prospective, double-blind trial. *J Infect Dis* 170:419–424, 1994.
261 Pape JW et al: Treatment and prophylaxis of *Isospora belli* infection in patients with the acquired immunodeficiency syndrome. *New Engl J Med* 320:1044–1047, 1989.
262 Soave R: *Cyclospora*: An overview. *Clin Infect Dis* 23:429, 1996.
263 Hale D et al: Diarrhea associated with cyanobacterialike bodies in an immunocompetent host. *JAMA* 271:144, 1994.
264 Berlin OGW et al: Recovery of *Cyclospora* organisms from patients with prolonged diarrhea. *Clin Infect Dis* 18:606, 1994.
265 Centers for Disease Control: Update: Outbreaks of *Cyclospora cayetanensis* infection—United States and Canada, 1996. *MMWR* 45: 611–618, 1996.
266 Huang P et al: The first outbreak of diarrheal illness associated with *Cyclospora* in the U.S. *Ann Intern Med* 123:409, 1995.
267 Pape JW et al: *Cyclospora* infection in adults infected with HIV. *Ann Intern Med* 121:654, 1994.
268 Orenstein J et al: A microsporidian previously undescribed in humans, infecting enterocytes and macrophages, and associated with diarrhea in an AIDS patient. *Hum Pathol* 23:722, 1992.
269 Bryan RT: Microsporidiosis as an AIDS-related opportunistic infection. *Clin Infect Dis* 21:S62, 1995.
270 Weber R, Bryan RT: Microsporidial infections in immunodeficient and immunocompetent patients. *Clin Infect Dis* 19:517, 1994.
271 Sandfort J et al: *Enterocytozoon bieneusi* infection in an immunocompetent patient who had acute diarrhea and who was not infected with HIV. *Clin Infect Dis* 19:514, 1994.
272 Lambl BB et al: Malabsorption and wasting in AIDS patients with microsporidia and pathogen-negative diarrhea. *AIDS* 10:739, 1996.
273 Rabeneck L et al: The role of Microsporidia in the pathogenesis of HIV-related chronic diarrhea. *Ann Intern Med* 119:895, 1993.
274 Weber R et al: Improved light-microscopical detection of microsporidia spores in stool and duodenal aspirates. *N Engl J Med* 326:161, 1992.
275 Dore GJ et al: Disseminated microsporidiosis due to *Septata intestinalis* in nine patients infected with HIV: Response to therapy with albendazole. *Clin Infect Dis* 21:70, 1995.
276 Blanshard C et al: Treatment of intestinal microsporidiosis with albendazole in patients with AIDS. *AIDS* 6:311, 1992.
277 Cello JP et al: Effect of octreotide on refractory AIDS-associated diarrhea. *Ann Intern Med* 115:705, 1991.
278 Krogh G: Clinical relevance and evaluation of genitoanal papilloma virus infection in the male. *Sem Derm* 11:229, 1992.
279 Bernard C et al: Viral co-infections in human papillomavirus-associated anogenital lesions according to the serostatus for the human immunodeficiency virus. *Int J Cancer* 52:731–737, 1992.
280 Velasco J et al: Diagnostic accuracy of the cytologic diagnosis of anal human papillomavirus infection compared with DNA hybridization studies. *Sex Trans Dis* 20:147–151, 1993.
281 Law CLH et al: Factors associated with clinical and subclinical anal human papillomavirus infection in homosexual men. *Genitourin Med* 67:92–98, 1991.

282 Bonnez W et al: Efficacy and safety of 0.5% podofilox solution in the treatment and suppression of anogenital warts. *Am J Med* 96: 420, 1994.
283 Abdullah AN et al: Treatment of external genital warts comparing cryotherapy (liquid nitrogen) and trichloracetic acid. *Sex Trans Dis* 20:334, 1993.
284 Fleshner PR, Freilich MI: Adjuvant interferon for anal condyloma: A prospective, randomized trail. *Dis Colon Rectum* 37:1255, 1994
285 Condylomata International Collaborative Study Group: Randomized placebo-controlled double-blind combined therapy with laser surgery and systemic interferon-alpha 2a in the treatment of anogenital condylomata acuminatum. *J Infect Dis* 167:824, 1993
286 Verley JR, Quinn TC: Sexually Transmitted Infections of the Anus and Rectum, in *Infections of the Gastrointestinal Tract,* MJ Blaser et al (eds). New York, Raven Press, 1995, p 411.
287 Critchlow CW et al: Prospective study of high grade anal squamous intraepithelial neoplasia in a cohort of homosexual men: Influence of HIV infection, immunosuppression, and human papillomavirus infection. *AIDS* 9:1255, 1995.
288 Kiviat NB et al: Association of anal dysplasia and human papillomavirus with immunosuppression and HIV infection among homosexual men. *AIDS* 7:43–49, 1993.
289 Gillin JS et al: Disseminated *Mycobacterium avium*–intracellulare infection in acquired immunodeficiency syndrome mimicking Whipple's disease. *Gastroenterology* 85:1187, 1983.
290 Hoover DR et al: An epidemiologic analysis of *Mycobacterium avium* complex disease in homosexual men infected with human immunodeficiency virus type 1. *Clin Infec Dis* 20:1250, 1995.
291 Horsburgh CR Jr: *Mycobacterium avium* complex infection in the acquired immunodeficiency syndrome. *N Engl J Med* 324:1332, 1991.
292 Shafran SD et al: A comparison of two regimens for the treatment of *Mycobacterium avium* complex bacteremia in AIDS: rifabutin, ethambutol, and clarithromycin versus rifampin, ethambutol, clofazimine, and ciprofloxacin. *New Engl J Med* 335:377, 1996.
293 Pierce M et al: A randomized trial of clarithromycin as prophylaxis against disseminated *Mycobacterium avium* complex infection in patients with advanced acquired immunodeficiency syndrome. *N Engl J Med* 335:384, 1996.
294 Havlir DV et al: Prophylaxis against disseminated *Mycobacterium avium* complex with weekly azithromycin, daily rifabutin, or both. *N Engl J Med* 335:392, 1996.
295 Spiller RC et al: Adult acquired cytomegalovirus infection with gastric and duodenal ulceration. *Gut* 29:1109, 1988.
296 Rabinowitz M et al: Sexually transmitted cytomegalovirus proctitis in a woman. *Amer J Gastroenterology* 83:885, 1988.
297 Cunningham M et al: Cytomegalovirus primo-infection in a patient with idiopathic proctitis. *Amer J Gastroenterol* 81:586, 1986.
298 Diepersloot RJA et al: Acute ulcerative proctocolitis associated with primary cytomegalovirus infection. *Arch Intern Med* 150:1749, 1990.
299 Buckner FS, Pomeroy C: Cytomegalovirus disease of the gastrointestinal tract in patients without AIDS. *Clin Infec Dis* 17:644, 1993.
300 Knapp AB et al: Widespread cytomegalovirus gastroenterocolitis in a patient with AIDS. *Gastroenterology* 85:1399, 1983.
301 Gertler SL et al: Gastrointestinal cytomegalovirus infection in a homosexual man with severe acquired immunodeficiency syndrome. *Gastroenterology* 85:1403, 1983.
302 Meiselman MS et al: Gastrointestinal colitis: Report of the clinical, endoscopic, and pathologic findings in two patients with the acquired immune deficiency syndrome. *Gastroenterology* 88:171, 1985.
303 Frank D, Raicht FF: Intestinal perforation associated with cytomegalovirus infection in patients with acquired immune deficiency syndrome. *Am J Gastroenterol* 79:201, 1984.
304 Balthazar EJ et al: Cytomegalovirus colitis in AIDS: Radiographic findings in 11 patients. *Radiology* 155:585, 1985.
305 Paya CV et al: Rapid shell vial culture and tissue histology compared with serology for the rapid diagnosis of cytomegalovirus infection in liver transplantation. *Mayo Clin Proc* 64:670–5, 1989.
306 Goodgame RW: Gastrointestinal cytomegalovirus disease. *Ann Intern Med* 119:924, 1993.
307 Emanuel D et al: Rapid immunodiagnosis of cytomegalovirus pneumonia by bronchoalveolar lavage using human and murine monoclonal antibodies. *Ann Intern Med* 104:476, 1986.
308 Danner SA: Management of cytomegalovirus disease. *AIDS* 9(suppl 2):3–8, 1995.
309 Nelson MR et al: Foscarnet in the treatment of cytomegalovirus infection of the esophagus and colon in patients with the acquired immune deficiency syndrome. *Amer J Gastroenterol* 86:876–881, 1991.
310 Kavin H et al: Acalculous cholecystitic and cytomegalovirus infection in acquired immunodeficiency syndrome. *Ann Intern Med* 104:53, 1986.
311 Spector SA et al: Oral ganciclovir for the prevention of cytomegalovirus disease in persons with AIDS. *New Engl J Med* 334:1491, 1996.
312 Laughon BD, Quinn TC: Intestinal Spirochetes, in *Enteric Infections,* MGJ Forthing, GT Keusch (eds). London, Chapman and Hall, 1989.
313 Nielsen RH et al: Colorectal spirochetosis: Clinical significance of the infestation. *Gastroenterology* 85:62–67, 1983.
314 Surawicz CM et al: Intestinal spirochetosis in homosexual men. *Amer J Med* 82:587–592, 1987.
315 Law CLH et al: Rectal spirochaetosis in homosexual men: The association with sexual practices, HIV infection, and enteric flora. *Genitourin Med* 70:26–29, 1994.
316 McMillian A, Lee FD: Sigmoidoscopic and microscopic appearance of the rectal mucosa in homosexual men. *Gut* 222:1035, 1981.
317 Kostman JR et al: Invasive colitis and hepatitis due to previously uncharacterized spirochetes in patients with advanced human immunodeficiency virus infection. *Clin Infec Dis* 21:1159–65, 1995.
318 Gebbers JO et al: Spirochaetosis of the human rectum associated with an intraepithelial mast cell and IgE plasma cell response. *Gut* 28:588–593, 1987.
319 Tavitian A et al: Oral candidiasis as a marker for esophageal candidiasis in the acquired immunodeficiency syndrome. *Ann Intern Med* 104:54, 1986.
320 Laine L et al: Fluconazole compared with ketoconazole for the treatment of candida esophagitis in AIDS, a randomized trial. *Ann Inter Med* 117:655–660, 1992.
321 Revankar SG et al: Detection and significance of fluconazole resistance in oropharyngeal candidiasis in human immunodificiency virus-infected patients. *J Infec Dis* 174:821–7, 1996.
322 Zipper RP et al: Resistance to fluconazole and amphotericin B in a patient with AIDS who was being treated for candidal esophagitis. *Clin Infec Dis* 23:649–50, 1996.
323 Marnell M: Donovanosis of the anus in the male: An epidemiologic consideration. *Br J Vener Dis* 34:213, 1955.
324 Goldberg J, Bernstein R: Studies on granuloma inguinale: VI. Two cases of perianal granuloma inguinale in male homosexuals. *Br J Vener Dis* 40:137, 1964.
325 Sohn N et al: Social injuries of the rectum. *Am J Surg* 134:61 1, 1977.
326 Barone JE et al: Perforations and foreign bodies of the rectum: Report of 28 cases. *Ann Surg* 184:601, 1977.
327 Rompalo AM et al: Empirical therapy for the management of acute proctitis in homosexual men. *JAMA* 260:348, 1988.
328 Holmberg SD et al: Prior herpes simplex virus type 2 infection as a risk factor for HIV infection. *JAMA* 259:1048, 1988.
329 Stamm WE et al: The association between genital ulcer disease and acquisition of HIV infection in homosexual men. *JAMA* 260:1429, 1988.

Chapter 70

Counseling and testing for HIV infection

Connie Celum
Susan Buchbinder

In this chapter we will cover several aspects of HIV counseling and testing of importance for clinicians and counselors, including (1) clinical guidelines for HIV counseling and testing; (2) trends in HIV testing in public and private sites over the past 10 years; (3) controversies over the efficacy of HIV counseling and testing in preventing HIV infection; and (4) new directions with home collection kits and rapid, on-site HIV tests.

CLINICAL GUIDELINES FOR HIV COUNSELING AND TESTING

HIV counseling and testing has four primary goals: (1) to identify HIV-infected persons for clinical interventions; (2) to provide counseling about risk reduction for HIV-negative persons at risk of HIV acquisition and for HIV-positive persons at risk of HIV transmission; (3) to provide referrals for medical and case management services for HIV-seropositives and for prevention interventions for those at high risk of HIV acquisition; and (4) to initiate partner notification with counseling and referral to prevention services for partners of HIV-positive clients. The efficacy of HIV counseling and testing as a primary HIV prevention strategy is controversial and will be summarized in the latter half of this chapter. However, the importance of HIV counseling and testing for early clinical intervention has been clearly established, as highly effective interventions such as prophylaxis against *Pneumocystis carinii* pneumonia have been identified.[1,2] There is also increasing evidence to support the role of early intervention in preventing other opportunistic infections, such as *Mycobacterium avium intracellularae* infections.[3]

The following discussion will describe three important aspects of HIV counseling and testing for providers conducting counseling: (1) clinical indications for HIV testing; (2) components of pre- and posttest counseling; and (3) issues in providing and documenting HIV antibody test results.

CLINICAL INDICATIONS FOR TESTING

In addition to offering counseling and testing to patients requesting an antibody test, HIV counseling and testing should be offered to patients in the following circumstances: symptoms compatible with an acute HIV-seroconversion syndrome; signs or symptoms suggestive of chronic HIV infection; confirmation of self-reported, undocumented positive HIV tests; risk behaviors associated with HIV acquisition; pregnancy; and potential occupational exposures (Table 70-1). Relative contraindications to HIV antibody testing include testing low-risk persons with high anxiety about HIV infection despite previous negative tests and testing persons with acute psychiatric illnesses or suicidal ideation. The pretest counseling session provides an important opportunity to counsel low-risk persons about the low predictive value of a positive HIV enzyme immunoassay (EIA) in low-prevalence populations and to probe the underlying etiology of their anxiety, which often can be better addressed by counseling referrals. Unless needed for medical evaluation of management, HIV testing of asymptomatic persons should be postponed for persons with acute psychiatric impairment or acute suicidal ideation until those issues can be addressed by appropriate providers.

The symptoms of acute HIV infection can be severe, often prompting newly infected individuals to seek medical care, but are also highly nonspecific, similar to symptoms attributable to other viral illnesses. In fact, the majority of persons presenting with acute HIV infection are misdiagnosed. In a series of individuals in Seattle referred to a primary HIV infection study who had a confirmed case of acute HIV infection within a 6-month period, only 5 of the 19 (26 percent) symptomatic seroconverters who sought medical care were accurately diagnosed as having acute HIV infection.[4] Newly infected individuals often have a high plasma viral load and are therefore potentially extremely infectious at a time when they are often unaware of their HIV status. Theoretically, secondary transmission of HIV during early HIV infection may fuel the HIV epidemic if the high viral load observed in early infection correlates with infectiousness.[6] Therefore, it is imperative that physicians have a low threshold for considering primary HIV infection and develop greater acumen in recognizing acute HIV infection. The usual serologic tests, the HIV EIA and Western blot, may not become positive for 1 to 2 months after acute HIV infection, whereas the more sensitive polymerase chain reaction (PCR) is usually positive during the acute symptomatic phase.[7,8] When acute HIV infection is suspected on clinical grounds in a person with reported HIV risk factors, the clinician should order supplemental assays, counsel the person about potentially high viral load during acute infection, stress the importance of safe sexual and injection drug use practices while awaiting laboratory confirmation, and arrange for close follow-up. PCR is more sensitive than the p24 antigen in the acute phase of infection and thus is the preferred diagnostic test.[7] A recent report of the efficacy of zidovudine in reducing viral load in acute HIV infection also has resulted in heightened interest in more timely diagnosis of primary HIV infection.[5,9] The long-term benefits of antiretroviral therapy and the role of monotherapy versus combination therapy in acute HIV infection are currently being studied in clinical trials in the United States and Europe.

The signs and symptoms of chronic HIV infection often are nonspecific, such as frequent or severe recurrences of vaginal candidiasis or genital herpes, herpes zoster, fever, and weight loss. Other earlier manifestations of HIV-related immunosuppression may be subtle, such as hairy leukoplakia, erythematous candidiasis, seborrheic dermatitis, or molluscum contagiosum lesions occurring in unusual locations, such as on the face. However, these nonspecific symptoms and subtle clinical findings should still prompt the clinician to obtain a thorough HIV risk history and to have a low threshold for recommending HIV testing.

As a result of the clinical and social importance of a positive HIV antibody test, it is advisable to document a positive test before providing HIV-related clinical or social services, particularly before beginning antiretroviral therapy. Occasionally individuals who believe they are HIV-positive may only be EIA-positive with either a negative or indeterminate Western blot. These individuals may have been tested in 1985 to 1987 when some HIV testing programs were accepting the high positive predictive value of a positive HIV EIA without confirmatory testing in high-risk per-

Table 70-1. Indications for HIV Counseling and Testing

Clinical indications
- Signs and symptoms of HIV (e.g., unexplained weight loss, fever, atypical pneumonia, or oral thrush)
- Acute HIV seroconversion symptoms*
- Confirmation, if prior reported positive test is not documented

Prior risk behavior
- Men who have had sex with men, injection drug use, transfusion between 1978 and 1985, hemophiliacs who received factor VIII before 1985, multiple sexual partners, sexual partner at risk, prior or recent STD diagnosis (especially early syphilis, chancroid, and gonorrhea)

Pregnant women

*Exposure to HIV**
- Occupational
- Sexual or drug use

Persons who request HIV testing

* In settings of recent exposure (i.e., less than 1 month) or symptoms compatible with an acute HIV seroconversion syndrome (i.e., fever, lymphadenopathy, papular rash, meningismus, sore throat), it may be necessary to order more sensitive diagnostic tests (e.g., polymerase chain reaction) in addition to the routine HIV EIA with confirmatory Western blot testing to identify HIV infection. If these diagnostic tests are not available or are initially negative, close clinical and serologic follow-up for 6 months is recommended.

sons. HIV testing and counseling programs and laboratories have subsequently required confirmatory testing with Western blot or immunofluorescence assay of all repeatedly reactive HIV EIA samples to differentiate those who have false-positive EIAs (those with negative confirmatory tests) from those with actual HIV infection (positive confirmatory tests). The recent advent of unlicensed home testing kits from overseas vendors may result in an increase in unconfirmed positive EIA results. Providers should inquire about the type and timing of prior positive HIV tests to identify individuals who have used home testing kits. The policy of routinely documenting HIV status will also occasionally identify persons who mistakenly believe they are positive because of a specimen mix-up or misinformation from a clinician and persons who falsely report being HIV-positive to obtain social service or medical benefits.[10]

The most common reasons HIV antibody tests are obtained in publicly funded HIV counseling and testing programs are because clients want to know their serostatus and to screen persons who have prior risks of exposure to HIV, either through sexual exposure or shared needles during injection drug use. In some communities, data suggest that the majority of gay and bisexual men have been tested for HIV at least once through public and private counseling and testing programs.[11,12]

Less is known about individuals who seek repeat testing and whether repeat testing should be encouraged. Several studies indicate that males who have sex with males (MSM) who have been repeatedly tested (e.g., tested three or more times) are at lower risk for being HIV-seropositive than first-time testers, although insufficient behavioral data were available to control for risk behavior between the first-time and repeat testers.[13,14] Some HIV counseling and testing programs recommend that persons at ongoing risk of HIV should be counseled and tested on a regular basis, such as every 6 months, to detect acute HIV infection if they are at high risk of seroconversion. However, HIV counseling and testing should not be viewed as a sufficient primary prevention intervention; some of the highest risk clients would also benefit from referral to other appropriate services, such as alcohol or drug abuse counseling, psychotherapy, risk reduction workshops or groups, or other services.

Several studies have documented the difficulty in identifying HIV-positive pregnant women based on HIV risk history alone.[15–18] Since prenatal use of zidovudine reduces vertical transmission of HIV by 66 percent, consensus has emerged that pregnant women should be counseled and voluntarily tested for HIV.[19–21] The U.S. Public Health Service recently published recommendations for counseling and voluntary HIV testing of pregnant women.[22] The rationale behind these recommendations is that knowledge of HIV status will enable HIV-infected pregnant women to make informed choices about their own health care. In addition, HIV-infected pregnant women should be counseled about the benefits of intrapartum zidovudine use and not breast-feeding in reducing the likelihood of transmitting HIV to the infant. Counseling pregnant women about HIV testing should include appropriate referrals for both infected and uninfected women to drug or alcohol treatment, prenatal care, and clinical and social services, as needed. Some experts have proposed an approach of near-universal but still voluntary HIV testing of pregnant women based on an informed "right of refusal."[20] HIV testing of pregnant women ideally should be voluntarily performed after obtaining informed consent early in pregnancy, and should include adequate counseling about the medical and social implications of a positive test. In the event of a positive HIV test result, options for intervention must be provided so that the pregnant woman can make decisions about pregnancy termination and zidovudine use and avoidance of breast-feeding.[20,21]

Occasionally persons will seek HIV counseling and testing after a possible exposure to HIV in an occupational setting. These persons are often highly distraught, and the clinician or interviewer must obtain detailed information about the event to assist in appropriate counseling. Transmission of HIV is essentially limited to percutaneous inoculation of HIV via a sharps or needlestick injury. Even here, the overall risk of HIV seroconversion from needlestick exposures to blood from a known HIV positive patient is only about 3 in 1,000. These data should be explained after assessing the specific characteristics of the individual's exposure.[23,24] Factors associated with an increased risk of transmission from needlesticks include larger-caliber needles, visible presence of blood on the needle before the percutaneous exposure, and advanced clinical stage of the index client.[25] Only four cases of HIV infection resulting from blood splashed on mucous membranes or prolonged contact of blood with nonintact skin have been reported, all in retrospective studies; prospective studies have failed to uncover any additional cases, confirming that the risk of infection from this type of exposure is very low. A recent case-control analysis suggested that the use of zidovudine for postexposure prophylaxis provided approximately 80 percent protection against HIV acquisition.[25] However, the caveat should also be made that several infections have occurred despite prompt initiation of zidovudine.[23] Guidelines for postexposure antiretroviral therapy have been developed by an expert advisory panel and the U.S. Public Health Service (Table 70-2). The U.S. Public Health Service is currently revising the guidelines for combination antiretroviral postexposure prophylaxis. The clinician should assist and support the health care worker in his or her decision about zidovudine use and ensure close medical follow-up for those who choose to take antiretrovirals. Appropriate safe sex practices should be encouraged in situations in which the exposure was nontrivial until the health care worker's HIV status can be determined. When providing HIV testing, a baseline antibody test should be drawn on all persons to document baseline seronegativity. Follow-up testing should include repeat serologies at 3 and 6 months, and can be supplemented by polymerase chain reaction, if available, at 6 weeks.

HIV testing is also requested by individuals based on their own perception of risk and concern about possible exposure to HIV. These requests should be probed by the clinician to determine whether they are based on substantial risk and proven modes of transmission. In general, testing should be performed in most sit-

Table 70-2. Summary of 1996 U.S. Public Health Service Recommendations for Post-exposure Prophyalxis of Occupational HIV Exposure

Type of exposure	Source material	Antiretroviral prophylaxis*	Antiretroviral regimen†
Percutaneous	Blood		
	Highest risk	Recommend	ADV plus 3TC plus IDV
	Increased risk	Recommend	ZDV plus 3TC, ± IDV#
	No increased risk	Offer	ZDV plus 3TC
	Fluid containing visible blood, other potentially infectious fluid,‡ or tissue	Offer	ZDV plus 3TC
	Other body fluid (e.g., urine)	Not offer	
Mucous membrane	Blood	Offer	ZDV plus 3TC, ± IDV#
	Fluid containing visible blood, other potentially infectious fluid,‡ or tissue	Offer	ZDV, ± 3TC
	Other body fluid (e.g., urine)	Not offer	
Skin, increased risk**	Blood	Offer	ZDV plus 3TC, ± IDV#
	Fluid containing visible blood, other potentially infectious fluid,‡ or tissue	Offer	ZDV plus 3TC, ± IDV#
	Other body fluid (e.g., urine)	Not offer	

* *Recommend*—Postexposure prophylaxis (PEP) should be recommended to the exposed worker with counseling.
Offer—PEP should be offered to the exposed worker with counseling.
Not offer—PEP should not be offered because these are not occupational exposures to HIV.

† Doses are zidovudine 200 mg tid, 3TC 150 mg bid, indinavir 800 mg tid and provided for 4 weeks.
Highest-risk exposure is defined as deep injury with large-diameter hollow needle containing blood from a known HIV-positive patient with possible high viral load.
Increased risk is defined as *either* exposure to large volume of blood or blood with a possible high titer of HIV.
No increased risk is defined as *neither* exposure to large volume of blood nor blood with a high titer of HIV.

\# Possible toxicity of additional drug may not be warranted. Decision about indinavir should be based on prior antiretroviral therapy use and concern about possible resistant virus.

** For skin, risk is increased for exposures involving a high titer of HIV, prolonged contact, an extensive area, or an area in which skin integrity is visibly compromised.
For skin exposures without increased risk, the risk for drug toxicity outweighs the benefit of PEP.

‡ Includes semen; vaginal secretion; cerebrospinal, synovial, pleural, peritoneal, pericardial, and amniotic fluids.

SOURCE: Adapted from *MMWR* 45:468–470, 1996.

uations when requested by a patient since some individuals may deny their risk, but still request HIV testing. However, some low-risk individuals have unfounded fears about HIV or believe in unproven modes of transmission, such as arthropod or airborne transmission of HIV. These fears and misperceptions should be addressed in the pre- and posttest counseling sessions. In addition, low-risk persons who repeatedly request HIV testing should be discouraged if no risk is identified in the pretest counseling session.

Clinicians may also be asked to provide HIV counseling and testing for social reasons that will not be covered in detail here. Examples include requirements for entry into the military, Job, and Peace Corps; immigration; visas; life and disability insurance; and employment. The same guidelines should be followed for informed consent and pre- and posttest counseling in these as in other situations, although questions have been raised about the meaning of informed consent in mandatory testing situations.

COMPONENTS OF PRE- AND POSTTEST HIV COUNSELING

Pretest counseling

The content of the pretest counseling visit should be tailored to the individual, taking into account whether the client has been counseled and tested for HIV previously, his or her knowledge about HIV diagnosis and transmission, and the client's level of reported risk (Table 70-3). For the clients who are being tested for HIV for the first time, the discussion of HIV transmission and natural history may need to be more detailed than for persons who have been counseled previously. Several recent publications detail methods of ascertaining HIV risk and providing pretest counseling in primary care settings.[26,27] In-depth counseling about risk behavior may be less feasible in busy office settings than in publicly funded clinics, but at a minimum should include informed consent and discussion of risk reduction.[28] Follow-up appointments for posttest counseling may provide additional opportunities for counseling about HIV transmission and the patient's risk behavior. The clinician should describe the difference between HIV (the virus) and AIDS (the clinical condition) and indicate that a positive antibody test indicates HIV infection but not the clinical syndrome of AIDS. The clinician should clarify that the antibody test can be either positive, negative, or indeterminate, and that the risk of false-positive or false-negative antibody tests is extremely low.[29] For clients with possible exposure to HIV in the past 6 months, the clinician should explain tests are generally positive within 3 months after exposure but may take up to 6 months to become positive (the "window period"). Therefore, repeat testing should be recommended 6 months after exposure, if the initial test is negative.

Table 70-3. Components of HIV Pretest Counseling

Ascertain risk
Discuss likelihood and meaning of positive, negative, and indeterminate test result
Assess understanding of HIV transmission and natural history; psychological stability; social support; impact of a positive result
Discuss confidentiality provisions. For states with name-based reporting of HIV, discuss options for anonymous testing if client refuses confidential testing
Ensure that follow-up is available (especially important when testing occurs in urgent care settings)
Emphasize the importance of obtaining test results
Discuss risk reduction plan and referral to other services (e.g., sexual safety counseling or support groups, drug treatment, needle exchange), if appropriate
Obtain informed consent for HIV antibody testing

For clients with ongoing risk behavior despite adequate knowledge of safe behaviors, the clinician should assist the client in identifying factors related to his or her continued risk behavior (e.g., substance use, new relationship, difficulties with communication or safe sex negotiation, low self-esteem, depression). The clinician may then either make appropriate referrals for more in-depth counseling or work with the client to develop a plan for risk reduction. Such a plan should pay attention to the triggers and context for high-risk behavior for that client. This client-centered approach to counseling is more likely to be effective than simply admonishing the client to follow safe sexual or drug use practices or repeating a summary of HIV transmission.[30] Chapter 54 and two recent reviews provide a more detailed discussion of behavioral intervention approaches.[31,32]

Many HIV testing programs have reported that a high proportion of persons who are tested for HIV do not return for their test results. In 1990, 37 percent of clients attending publicly supported HIV testing sites failed to return for test results, with lower rates among adolescents, persons of minority ethnicity, and those being tested at STD clinics.[33–35] Therefore, during the pretest counseling visit, it is critical that the clinician emphasize the importance of returning for posttest counseling and work with clients to develop a concrete plan for follow-up.

POSTTEST COUNSELING

During posttest counseling, the clinician should inform the client of the test result and its interpretation, reinforce the individualized risk reduction plan for both seronegative and seropositive individuals, and provide clinical and psychological follow-up for the newly identified HIV-seropositive person (Table 70-4). For the HIV-seronegative person, the clinician should reinforce the seronegative individual's plan for staying HIV-negative and determine the need for repeat HIV counseling and testing, depending on the time of the last possible exposure.

Table 70-4. Components of HIV Posttest Counseling

Ensure that client is ready to receive results
Disclose test results and provide interpretation (positive, negative, indeterminate) in the context of that person's risk of infection
For HIV seronegative persons:
- Readdress and reinforce risk reduction plan
- Discuss the need for repeat testing for those with recent (<6 months) exposure or ongoing risk behavior

For persons with indeterminate HIV-1 Western blots:
- Discuss prevalence of and risk factors for indeterminates
- For persons with p24 bands and for those with risk behavior, discuss the possibility of acute HIV infection; need for serologic follow-up at 1, 3, and 6 months; discuss safe sexual and drug use behavior until indeterminate is resolved
- Consider performing supplemental assays (e.g., polymerase chain reaction) to more quickly identify seroconverters and reassure those without HIV infection, particularly for pregnant women

For HIV seropositive persons:
- Counsel about the meaning of a positive HIV test (HIV-infected and thus potentially infectious)
- Differentiate between being HIV-infected and having AIDS (review natural history of HIV and immunosuppression)
- Emphasize the importance of early clinical intervention (ability to alter disease progression through antiretroviral therapy and prophylaxis against opportunistic infections)
- Discuss ways to avoid transmitting HIV to others (abstinence, condoms, not sharing needles if IDU)
- Assess need for psychological support
- Provide referrals for medical, psychological, or social services, if necessary
- Confirm HIV antibody test, if positive test is not consistent with risk history
- Schedule follow-up visit to assess psychological status, and to address partner notification issues

Occasionally clinicians will be faced with counseling individuals about indeterminate results, which occur in up to 10 percent of reactive EIA specimens.[29,36,37] Indeterminate HIV test results can occur during acute HIV seroconversion. In this situation, an initial p24 band develops on Western blot followed by additional envelope (gp41, gp120, and gp160) bands and then other anti-HIV bands over the next several weeks. This underscores the need for careful HIV risk assessment and serologic follow-up of high-risk persons with indeterminate Western blots.[8,38] However, the majority of persons with indeterminate HIV Western blots are not infected with HIV and have cross-reacting alloantibodies or autoantibodies.[39,40] Low-risk persons can be reassured of their very low likelihood of being infected and should be retested at 3 and 6 months to confirm the lack of seroconversion. Pregnant women with indeterminate Western blots are often understandably anxious about the significance of their tests; clinicians can explain the production of alloantibodies during pregnancy and obtain supplemental HIV tests (e.g., polymerase chain reaction) to resolve the indeterminate results more promptly.[36]

The clinician who is counseling a client about a new diagnosis of HIV infection must allot adequate time to handle potential emotional distress and to ensure that the client has had the opportunity to ask all questions and express his or her reaction to the test result. If the positive result is unexpected given the client's history, repeat serum should be drawn for confirmatory testing to rule out laboratory error. Some clinicians routinely confirm newly identified HIV-seropositive results, given the clinical and psychosocial importance of a positive test result. The clinician should again ensure that the client understands the difference between HIV infection and AIDS, discuss the natural history of HIV infection and immunosuppression, and emphasize the potential for slowing disease progression by early intervention with regular monitoring of the immune system and viral load, antiretroviral therapy, and prophylaxis against opportunistic infections. The provider should counsel the HIV-seropositive patient to follow safe sex practices, both to avoid HIV transmission to seronegative partners and to avoid acquisition of other STDs that theoretically may accelerate HIV disease. Medical referrals should be made if follow-up for HIV care is not available at that site, and the need for social and psychological services should be assessed. A follow-up appointment is advisable to reassess the client's ability to cope with the positive result, address the client's concerns, and discuss partner counseling and referral services. At this visit, the provider should ascertain the newly-diagnosed HIV positive person's reaction to the diagnosis, and discuss in more depth the importance and means to have partners of HIV unknown or negative status referred for HIV counseling and testing, and for HIV positive partners, clinical care and counseling. The rationale and methods for partner counseling and referral services are outlined in the new CDC Operational Guidelines for Partner Counseling and Referral Services, and discussed in more detail in Chapter 55.

HANDLING OF POSITIVE HIV TEST RESULTS

Most states have passed legislation that allow clinicians to chart positive test results and share test results with other clinicians, provided the disclosure is related to clinical care and the patient has signed a release of information form. The clinician should be familiar with the laws governing confidentiality of positive test results and name-based reporting in the state or jurisdiction in which they are practicing. As of November 1995, 29 states require name-based reporting of positive HIV antibody tests, whereas all states require reporting clinical or immunologic AIDS.

TRENDS IN HIV COUNSELING AND TESTING: 10 YEARS OF EXPERIENCE

The HIV antibody test was introduced in March 1985, and within 2 years, alternate testing sites were developed to provide high-risk persons with sites other than blood banks for HIV antibody testing. Over time, the alternate testing sites evolved to provide a greater emphasis on risk reduction counseling. After the first reports in 1989 of zidovudine's efficacy for HIV-positive persons with CD4 counts of less than 500, the focus of the counseling and testing sites (CTS) shifted to early detection of seropositive persons for clinical interventions. By 1990 HIV counseling and testing was provided in more than 5,000 sites, and CDC spent approximately $100 million in 1992 to support local HIV counseling and testing services.[42,43] The size of the CDC-funded CTS program led to more critical evaluations of the efficacy of counseling and testing, which will be described in the next section.[43,44]

Approximately 20 to 25 percent of the U.S. adult population has been tested for HIV, according to telephone-based surveys of households.[12,45] HIV testing was more common among respondents with reported risk behaviors (41.5 percent) than the general population (20.1 percent).[12] In spite of documented benefits of early intervention in HIV infection, late identification of HIV infection is still common. In a study of 2,441 persons in 11 U.S. cities diagnosed with AIDS between 1990 and 1992, 36 percent were first HIV-tested within 2 months of their AIDS diagnosis and 51 percent within 1 year.[46] Women, African American and Hispanic clients, injection drug users, and those who acquired HIV through heterosexual contact were more likely to have been HIV-tested less than 1 year prior to their AIDS diagnosis than other men and Caucasians. Reasons for late testing are complex and multifactorial, including a low index of suspicion on the part of the provider, client denial of risk, lack of awareness or of access to HIV testing, and limited confidence in the benefits of early clinical intervention.

Several studies have attempted to compare the characteristics of persons who have been tested for HIV to those never tested. An anonymous survey of 1,295 gay and bisexual men identified in gay bars and bathhouses in Toronto indicated that only 53 percent had been tested previously, 26 percent of whom previously tested positive. In this study, metropolitan residence and a history of anal intercourse were the strongest predictors of previous testing.[11] The major reasons for not previously being tested were the desire for anonymity, self-perceived good health status, denial of risk, and a lack of perceived benefit to learning one's serostatus. The 1991 National Health Interview Survey indicated that although rural and urban respondents reported a similar prevalence of risk behaviors (7.1 and 7.9 percent, respectively), the perceived risk of HIV was lower among the rural respondents and a significantly lower proportion had been tested (25.2 percent of rural and 33 percent of urban respondents had been tested for HIV, respectively).[47] Injection drug users (IDUs) are more likely to be tested if they are in drug treatment, but other characteristics and the overall proportion of IDUs who have been tested are not well-characterized. Notably, out of the 2.6 million HIV tests performed in public clinics in 1992, only approximately 100,000 of those tested were performed in drug treatment centers.[48]

The majority of HIV counseling and testing occurs in private settings, including private physicians' offices, hospitals, and outpatient clinics. The CDC's 1993 Behavioral Risk Factor Surveillance System (BRFSS) database on HIV counseling and testing indicates that 67 percent of HIV tests in 1990 were obtained in private provider settings and 33 percent were obtained in publicly funded sites.[45,49] The quality of risk reduction counseling is not well-characterized from most settings, including the publicly funded HIV testing sites. Data from the CDC 1993 Behavioral Risk Factor Surveillance System (BRFSS) indicated that 26 percent of the 84,039 respondents from 49 states and the District of Columbia had ever been tested for HIV outside of blood or plasma donation.[45] Of interest was the relatively low proportion who reported having received counseling with their last HIV test, which was reported by 61 percent of persons tested at publicly funded sites and 28 percent of those tested at a private site. These data are not definitive, are limited by recall, are based on self-reports about counseling, and provide no detail about the content or quality of the counseling. However, these data raise the concern that although three times as many HIV tests are performed in private settings, persons tested in private sites are three times less likely to report having received counseling with testing, underscoring the need for private providers to provide counseling at the time of HIV testing. The results from this survey also do not necessarily imply that the counseling provided in public sites is effective or appropriately client-centered. The external review of the CDC Counseling Testing Referral Partner Notification program in 1993 pointed to the deficiencies in client-centered counseling in many of the sites reviewed.[43] Risk reduction counseling was often limited to admonishments or reminders to use condoms and be tested again in 6 months, rather than client-centered counseling, as outlined in the previous section.

A 1992 survey of 4,011 primary care physicians by the American Medical Association indicated that 49 percent of primary care physicians always or usually ask their adult patients about sexually transmitted diseases, 31 percent about condom use, and 27 percent about sexual orientation compared to 94 percent who always or usually ask about cigarette smoking.[50] Over 90 percent of the primary care physicians surveyed would recommend HIV testing for gay men and injection drug users, but only 74 percent would recommend HIV testing for persons with a current or past STD, and 67 percent for heterosexual men with multiple sex partners. Thus, private providers may be underrecognizing HIV infection both by insufficiently obtaining HIV and STD risk assessments and not offering HIV testing to all risk groups. A recent review by Makadon and Silin summarized many of the obstacles and potential solutions to HIV prevention efforts by primary care providers.[51]

The demographics of clients tested in public settings differ from those tested in private settings. Clients who are tested in publicly funded HIV testing sites are often uninsured; in fact, approximately half of the 885,046 clients who had HIV tests performed at publicly funded sites in 1992 were uninsured.[52] Although some states have enacted programs to provide early basic diagnostic and therapeutic services to HIV-infected persons without insurance or Medicaid, this coverage is far from universal or adequate and must be addressed to ensure adequacy of referrals from publicly funded counseling and testing sites.

CONTROVERSIES IN HIV COUNSELING AND TESTING

EFFICACY OF COUNSELING AND TESTING IN AFFECTING CHANGES IN BEHAVIOR

One of the stated purposes of the HIV counseling and testing program has been to decrease risk behaviors in both HIV-positive and -negative persons. However, the efficacy of HIV counseling and antibody testing in reducing risk has been called into question. Interpretation of studies evaluating the impact of counseling and testing is difficult because of a number of methodologic issues. Many studies were conducted when counseling and testing was first available, and it may be difficult to extrapolate from these early studies to current practice. Some of the earliest studies evaluating the impact of HIV counseling and antibody testing among gay men were conducted in the 1980s at a time when unsafe sexual practices were declining dramatically for a variety of reasons unrelated to HIV counseling and testing. It is often difficult to separate the impact of public health campaigns to decrease unsafe activity from the impact of HIV antibody counseling and testing. In addition, most of these studies were not randomized trials, and individuals who chose to undergo HIV antibody testing may be different from those choosing not to be tested. Studies used different durations of follow-up, with many only evaluating the impact of counseling and testing on behavior change several weeks to months after an intervention. Thus, it is difficult to determine the long-term impact of counseling and testing on behavior change. It may be unrealistic to expect that a limited, two-session intervention such as pre- and posttest counseling should produce sustained behavior change. Last, most studies have evaluated the impact of counseling and testing on self-reported behaviors, rather than its impact on more objective measures, such as the incidence of sexually transmitted diseases, including HIV. The problem with using these less objective outcome measures is that self-reported high-risk behavior may be underreported, particularly when the same research staff conducts the risk reduction counseling and collects data about risk behavior measures.

Nonetheless, it appears that in selected situations, persons may decrease their risk owing to HIV antibody counseling and testing. The strongest evidence for the impact of counseling on risk comes from studies of HIV-serodiscordant heterosexual couples, in which one partner was found to be HIV-seropositive and the other HIV-seronegative.[53–56] Studies of heterosexuals recruited from other settings, including sexually transmitted disease clinics, have given conflicting results. One randomized controlled trial of HIV antibody testing in adult STD clinic patients in Los Angeles found that patients receiving counseling and testing were somewhat more likely to report avoiding unprotected sexual intercourse with their last sexual partner than patients randomized to the control arm, although this difference did not achieve statistical significance.[57] Two studies evaluated the incidence of sexually transmitted diseases in STD clinic patients who received HIV antibody posttest counseling. The first study from a Baltimore STD clinic found no significant difference between HIV-seropositive and -seronegative patients in the incidence of definitively diagnosed STDs (syphilis, gonorrhea, or trichomonas) 6 to 23 months after receipt of HIV antibody results and posttest counseling.[34] However, HIV-seropositive patients were significantly less likely to return with a "probable STD" diagnosis (nongonococcal urethritis or pelvic inflammatory disease) or to return having had an STD-infected sexual partner than HIV-seronegative patients. The overall rates of new STD acquisition were disturbingly high among both HIV-positive (14 percent) and HIV-negative (19 percent) patients. The second study from the Miami STD clinic evaluated the incidence of gonorrhea or other STDs in clinic patients in the 6 months before and 6 months after they received positive or negative HIV antibody test results. Patients counseled about a positive HIV antibody test were less likely to return to the clinic with gonorrhea in the 6 months after counseling than in the 6 months before HIV testing and counseling, whereas patients receiving a negative test result were somewhat more likely to return with gonorrhea; however, these differences were not statistically significant.[58]

The studies by Zenilman et al. and Otten et al. suggest that in some situations, learning about an HIV-positive test result may alter behavior, although it is also possible that these individuals were less likely to seek subsequent STD-related care where they had learned of their positive HIV result. These studies also raise important questions about the ability of a single counseling session to alter sexual behavior, particularly among the HIV-negative clients, and the potential for disinhibition from learning of one's HIV-negative status.[34,58] The efficacy of counseling and testing cannot be extrapolated from these descriptive studies in STD clinics with limited resources to track clients and poor follow-up rates, but these findings do emphasize the need to assess how well risk reduction messages are being delivered to or received by very high-risk individuals in these settings.[43]

Ickovics reported that the women recruited at community health clinics who requested HIV antibody counseling and testing reported less high-risk behavior at the first visit, but were no more likely to report behavior change over a 3-month period than women who did not receive counseling and testing.[60] This finding suggested that the women who sought counseling and testing may have reduced their high-risk behavior prior to testing, not as a result of the counseling. Heterosexual persons learning of their HIV-positive status may be somewhat less likely to report unsafe sexual practices or be diagnosed with certain sexually transmitted diseases compared to those who learned of their HIV-seropositivity. However, a similar decline in risk behaviors and incident STDs is not observed among persons learning they are seronegative.[60,61]

Studies of the impact of counseling and testing in homosexual men give conflicting results, with some finding no difference and others indicating a decline in reported risk activity in gay men receiving a positive test result compared with men who were seronegative or men declining to learn their results. However, many of these studies were conducted in the middle 1980s in the setting of profound behavioral changes in all three groups. In the studies that reported a decrease in risk behavior after counseling and testing, the reduction in risky sexual behavior was modest and limited to HIV-positive men; the impact was also generally only assessed in the first few months after antibody testing and posttest counseling. It is difficult to differentiate the effect of learning one's serostatus from the counseling intervention in many of these studies. Similarly, there is no evidence that HIV counseling and testing has a significant impact on unsafe injection or sexual practices among IDUs.[44] The effects of counseling without antibody testing have also been assessed, but the interventions in these studies were often considerably more intensive than typical HIV counseling and testing sessions in public clinics and provider offices and thus not geared to clinical practice settings.

NEW DIRECTIONS IN HIV TESTING: HOME COLLECTION AND RAPID, ON-SITE TESTS

HOME HIV COLLECTION AND TESTING KITS

In 1996 the U.S. Food and Drug Administration licensed home collection kits that made it possible for persons to receive HIV antibody testing and counseling at home.[62,63] The kits require the client to provide a blood specimen on filter paper by pricking his or her finger with a lancet. The specimen is then mailed to a laboratory for screening and confirmatory testing. After a prespecified interval, clients call into the testing service, provide a unique identifier code, and receive test results. Negative results may be given over the telephone by a prerecorded message, although clients may also have the option of speaking with a telephone counselor. Positive test results are generally provided by a counselor who conducts a standard posttest counseling session by telephone and provides referrals for both medical and psychosocial services. Persons receiving positive test results may have the option of receiving follow-up telephone counseling sessions. Oral fluid collection kits have been licensed for provider use for EIA and Western blot antibody testing, and the FDA is currently considering approval of this technology for home collection which will utilize a similar method of reporting test results. Although collection of urine specimen for EIA testing has been licensed for provider use, there is currently no FDA application for home collection.[64]

The role of home collection and testing in the United States and the potential for benefit and abuse through this system have been the subject of much debate.[63,65] Although some of the issues are specific to HIV testing, Bayer[63] points out that much of the debate raises broader policy issues about

"the role home-diagnostic techniques should have in the evolving practice of medicine in America and the extent to which federal regulatory bodies should protect people from technically accurate devices that may produce psychologically burdensome results."

Proponents of home collection and testing cite several potential benefits. Many persons at risk for HIV infection are unaware of their HIV status and home collection may increase access to HIV testing. Results from the 1992 National Health Interview Survey, a cross-sectional household interview survey of U.S adults, indicated that 63 percent of persons at risk for HIV infection had never been tested for HIV outside of blood donation.[65] Data from publicly funded clinics indicates that as many as one-third of persons who present for HIV antibody testing fail to return to receive test results.[33] As cited earlier in this chapter, a substantial proportion of HIV-infected persons only learn of their positive serostatus within several months of an AIDS-defining diagnosis, significantly limiting the period of time in which they would have access to early clinical interventions that may substantially decrease the risk of HIV disease progression or specific clinical outcomes. Home collection and testing could increase the proportion of at-risk persons who avail themselves of HIV antibody testing and potentially decrease the likelihood that persons would use blood donation as a mechanism for HIV antibody testing. Results from the 1992 National Health Interview Survey indicated that 42 percent of respondents at risk said they would be very or somewhat likely to use home test kits, and 31 percent said they would choose a home test over other testing alternatives.[65] Persons with less education, lower incomes, minority ethnicity, and less access to medical care were more likely to prefer home testing than other clients. Given that these groups traditionally have had less access to HIV prevention services, home collection for HIV testing may partially fill an unmet need.

Another argument in support of home testing is that HIV antibody testing can be provided in a more cost-efficient manner through home testing than other mechanisms. The retail costs for home testing are $30 to $40 per kit, whereas estimates for government costs at public clinics are $50 per test and for private physicians, $50 or more per test.[66] It has been argued that shifting testing from public clinics to home testing could shift costs from such clinics to the clients, freeing these public resources to be used for other prevention or treatment activities. However, it is unclear whether clients frequenting public clinics would have the resources or incentives to seek home testing if they were required to pay for these tests out of pocket. It should be noted that when respondents of the National Health Interview Survey were asked about the likelihood of using home test kits, they were not provided with information about cost. The potential resultant decrease in HIV tests and patient volume at publicly funded clinics could adversely affect their funding levels and consequently reduce their prevention activities and counseling and testing services for underserved clients.

Critics of home collection and testing cite a number of concerns. A concern raised initially was whether clients would be able to produce an adequate blood sample for testing. One study has shown that 88 percent of clients could obtain sufficient blood samples after instruction.[67] A greater concern that has been raised is whether telephone counseling is as effective as face-to-face counseling in assisting high-risk persons to decrease their risk behaviors. However, the efficacy of face-to-face counseling in promoting sustained risk reduction is under debate, as described previously. Moreover, data from the 1992 National Health Interview Survey suggest that a substantial proportion of persons currently being tested receive their HIV test results by telephone (17 percent) or mail (16 percent).[12,65] Moreover, data from the CDC's 1993 Behavioral Risk Factor Surveillance System suggests that nearly three-quarters of persons receiving HIV antibody testing from private settings report that they did not receive any counseling.[45] The quality of the counseling provided is likely to be more important rather than the setting in which counseling occurs.

Another concern raised about home collection is that inadequate resources or follow-up will be available for persons learning of HIV-positive test results, particularly if large numbers of HIV-seropositive persons are newly identified. However, Ryan White and other HIV care funding is linked to the number of HIV and AIDS cases, so increased detection could be accompanied by increased local resources for care services. Although there were early concerns that notification of positive test results may precipitate attempted suicides, data collected to date suggest that the risk of suicide in HIV-positive persons is related to the development of symptoms rather than notification of positive test results.[68,69] Vulnerable groups, such as adolescents, may need particular assistance when learning of positive test results. Mechanisms must be built into the counseling session to provide local referrals for clients, including crisis counseling.

Concerns have also been raised about the likelihood and mechanisms for dealing with false-positive test results. Data from dried blood spots collected from mothers and neonates suggests that dried blood spot testing should have similar sensitivity and specificity compared with venipuncture specimens, including specimens obtained around the time of seroconversion.[36] Less information is available on the sensitivity and specificity of the modified HIV-1 EIA and Western blot on oral fluids when compared with HIV-positive and HIV-negative serum specimens, although preliminary results imply that results may be comparable with a reported sensitivity of 99 percent and specificity of 97 percent.[70] The sensitivity of the oral fluid HIV-1 EIA for detection of antibodies during acute seroconversion is not known. Clearly, laboratories providing home testing must be subject to the same level of quality assurance in other HIV testing laboratories, and counselors providing positive test results must be aware of the possibility of false-positive tests and refer clients appropriately for confirmatory testing.

RAPID SCREENING TESTS FOR HIV

Tests also have been developed in which a clinician can perform a screening assay on a blood sample and provide preliminary test results within 20 minutes. The acceptability of these tests to both clients and providers appears high.[71] These assays must have very high sensitivity and specificity to ensure that a minimum number of clients leave the clinic with a false sense of security over false-negative results or unnecessary anxiety over false-positive results. Mechanisms must be in place to confirm positive rapid screening tests in as timely a manner as possible and to ensure adequate locator information is obtained to be able to track the occasional persons with false-positive rapid EIA tests. However, these potential problems must be weighed against the probable benefit that a much higher proportion of persons would undergo testing and receive their results than is currently observed.

The rapid HIV tests may be suitable for large-volume HIV testing sites with particularly poor follow-up rates, such as emergency rooms, STD clinics, hospitals with high HIV prevalence, and HIV testing sites in developing countries. Irwin and colleagues have tested the solid-phase HIV EIA in a busy urban hospital with HIV prevalence and found high sensitivity (100 percent), specificity (99.1 percent), and positive predictive value (87 percent) among a high HIV prevalence population.[72] Only 58 percent returned for posttest counseling for their HIV test results, underscoring the potential utility of rapid HIV tests in settings with poor follow-up rates. Rapid HIV tests may also be useful in labor and delivery suites to identify HIV-infected women who were not tested in pregnancy and who could benefit from interventions to reduce peripartum transmission of HIV. A study of the rapid Single Use Diagnostic System (SUDS) test in 2,000 consecutive samples from the Dallas STD clinic in 1993 indicated high sensitivity and specificity (100 and 99.5 percent, respectively) and positive predictive value (88 percent).[73] The study also identified technical issues that can reduce specificity of the SUDS with increased numbers of false-positive SUDS owing to insufficient speed of centrifugation. The investigators also assessed the acceptance of the rapid tests and found that 88 percent of STD clients who had previously been tested preferred the rapid test. Focus group results of the counselors found that although they had initial concerns about increased client and counselor stress, their final reaction to the protocol was favorable. The rapid testing protocol in the STD clinic was deemed practical, did not adversely affect patient flow during the clinic visit and counseling occurred while the test was performed, and was judged to be cost-effective.[71] Further studies are needed about the role of rapid test protocols in emergency rooms and other settings.

CONCLUSIONS

HIV counseling and testing provides an important function in terms of identification of HIV-seropositive persons for counseling about risk reduction and transmission, clinical interventions, and partner notification. Even though the HIV antibody test has been available since 1985, issues in the provision of confidential and quality counseling continue to be identified. Primary care providers need to do more thorough HIV/STD risk assessments in their adolescent and adult patients, provide accurate information about HIV infection in the pretest counseling session, ensure that clients return for their test results, and provide additional risk reduction counseling along with interpretation of the test results at the posttest counseling session.

The data about the efficacy of counseling and testing as a primary prevention intervention fail to show consistent evidence for significant and lasting behavioral change, especially among those persons who test HIV-negative. In those studies that show some effect on self-reported behavior, it is difficult to differentiate the impact of learning one's serostatus (HIV testing) from the pre- and posttest counseling. Unfortunately, many of these studies of the efficacy of HIV counseling and testing were not randomized, had small sample sizes, short follow-up, and relied on self-reported behavior change rather than harder outcomes, such as incident HIV and STDs. Overall, given the limitations of the studies, the data do not indicate that HIV counseling and testing alone suffice as effective interventions in achieving significant behavioral change. Additional research is needed to define the subpopulations who are at highest risk of HIV and STD acquisition and which interventions hold the most promise for reducing new HIV and STD infections in these persons.

New directions in HIV counseling and testing may include home collection kits for HIV testing of dried blood specimens and oral fluids. After these kits become widely available, it will be important to identify whether home collection kits provide increased access for persons traditionally underserved and to monitor the quality of the counseling and referral system. The attractiveness of the home collection kits might be reduced if testing sites are available to provide highly accurate and rapid, on-site screening tests in conjunction with individual in-person risk reduction counseling. The role of home collection kits and rapid on-site HIV tests will need to be carefully evaluated once these technologies become more widely available.

References

1 Centers for Disease Control: Recommendations for prophylaxis against *Pneumocystis carinii* pneumonia for adults and adolescents infected with human immunodeficiency virus. *MMWR* 41 (No-RR4), 1992.

2 Sande MA et al: Antiretroviral therapy for adult HIV-infected patients: Recommendations from a state-of-the-art conference. *JAMA* 270: 2583–2589, 1993.

3 Kaplan JE et al: USPHS/IDSA guidelines for the prevention of opportunistic infections in persons infected with the human immunodeficiency virus: An overview. *Clin Infect Dis* 21(Suppl 1): S1–11, 12–31, 1995.

4 Schacker T et al: The clinical and epidemiological presentation of primary HIV infection. *Ann Intern Med*, in press.

5 Kinloch-DeLoes SB et al: A controlled trial of zidovudine in primary HIV human immunodeficiency virus infection. *NEJM* 333:408–413, 1995.

6 Jacqucz JA et al: Role of the primary infection in epidemics of HIV infection in gay cohorts. *J AIDS* 7:1169–1184, 1994.

7 Busch MP et al: Time course of detection of viral and serologic markers preceding human immunodeficiency virus type 1 seroconversion: Implications for screening of blood and tissue donors. *Transfusion* 35: 91–97, 1995.

8 Celum CL et al: Indeterminate human immunodeficiency virus type 1 Western blots: Seroconversion risk, specificity of supplemental tests, and an algorithm for evaluation. *J Infect Dis* 164:656–664, 1991.

9 Ho DD: Time to hit HIV, early and hard. *NEJM* 333:450–452, 1995.

10 Tyson E: Fraudulent AIDS: A variant of Munchausen's syndrome (letter). *JAMA* 258:1889, 1987.

11 Myers T et al: Factors affecting gay and bisexual men's decisions and intentions to seek testing. *Am J Public Health* 83:701–704, 1993.

12 Anderson JE et al: HIV antibody testing and posttest counseling in the United States: Data from the 1989 National Health Interview Survey. *Am J Public Health* 82:1533–1535, 1992.

13 Langley CL et al: Increased risk for HIV infection among gay and bisexual men of color: Data from the national HIV counseling and testing system. *ISSTDR* 1995; abstract 049: New Orleans.

14 McFarland W et al: Repeat negative human immunodeficiency virus (HIV) testing in San Francisco: Magnitude and characteristics. *Am J Epidemiol* 142:719–723, 1995.

15 Fehrs LJ et al: Targeted HIV screening at a Los Angeles prenatal/family planning health center. *Am J Public Health* 81:619–622, 1991.

16 Barbacci MB et al: Human immunodeficiency virus infection in women attending an inner-city prenatal clinic: Ineffectiveness of targeted screening. *Sex Transm Dis* 17:122–126, 1990.

17 Ellerbrock TV et al: Heterosexually transmitted human immunodeficiency virus infection among pregnant women in a rural Florida community. *N Engl J Med* 327:1704–1709, 1992.

18 Lindsay MK et al: Determinants of acceptance of routine voluntary human immunodeficiency virus testing in an inner-city prenatal population. *Obstet Gynecol* 78:678–680, 1989.

19 Connor EM et al: Reduction of maternal-infant transmission of immunodeficiency virus type-1 with zidovudine treatment. *N Engl J Med* 31:1173–1180, 1994.

20 Minkoff H et al: Pediatric HIV disease, zidovudine in pregnancy, and unblinding heelstick surveys: Reframing the debate on prenatal HIV testing. *JAMA* 274:1165–1168, 1995.

21 Bayer R: Ethical challenges posed by zidovudine treatment to reduce vertical transmission of HIV. *N Engl J Med* 331:1223–12235, 1994.

22 Centers for Disease Control: U. S. Public Health Service Recommendations for Human Immunodeficiency Virus Counseling and Voluntary Testing for Pregnant Women. *MMWR* 44(RR-7):1–15, 1995.
23 Tokars JI et al: Surveillance of HIV infection and zidovudine use among health care workers after occupational exposure to HIV-infected blood. *Ann Intern Med* 118:913–919, 1993.
24 Gerberding JL: Incidence and prevalence of human immunodeficiency virus, hepatitis B virus, hepatitis C virus, and cytomegalovirus among health care personnel at risk for blood exposure: Final report from a longitudinal study. *J Infect Dis* 170:1410–1417, 1994.
25 Centers for Disease Control and Prevention: Case-control study of HIV seroconversion in health care workers after percutaneous exposure to HIV-infected blood—France, United Kingdom, and United States, January 1988–August 1994. *MMWR* 44:929–933, 1995.
26 Bor R et al: A testing time for doctors: Counseling patients before an HIV test. *Br Med J* 303:905–907, 1991.
27 Kassler WJ et al: Addressing HIV infection in office practice. *Prim Care* 19:19–33, 1992.
28 Kassler WJ et al: Sexually transmitted diseases, in *Health Promotion and Disease Prevention in Clinical Practice,* Woolf SH et al (eds). Baltimore, Williams & Wilkins, 1995, pp. 273–290.
29 Burke DS et al: Measurement of the false positive rate in a screening program for human immunodeficiency virus infections. *N Engl J Med* 319:961–964, 1988.
30 Centers for Disease Control: *HIV Counseling, Testing, and Referral: Standards and Guidelines.* Atlanta, GA: US Department of Health and Human Services, Public Health Service, CDC, 1994.
31 Oakley A et al: Behavioral interventions for HIV/AIDS prevention. *AIDS* 9:479–486, 1995.
32 Choi K-H et al: Prevention of heterosexual transmission through couple counseling. *J AIDS* 8:1371–1379, 1994.
33 Valdisseri RO et al: A study of clients returning for counseling after HIV testing: Implications for improving rates of return. *Pub Health Repts* 108:12–18, 1993.
34 Zenilman JM et al: Effect of HIV posttest counseling on STD incidence. *JAMA* 267:843–845, 1992.
35 Ilegbodu AE et al: Characteristics of teens tested for HIV in a metropolitan area. *J Adol Health* 15:479–484, 1994.
36 Granade TC et al: Factors influencing HIV-1 banding patterns in miniaturized Western blot testing of dried blood spot specimens. *J Immunol Meth* 154:225–233, 1992.
37 MacDonald KL et al: Performance characteristics of serologic tests for human immunodeficiency virus type 1 (HIV-1) antibody among Minnesota blood donors: Public health and clinical implications. *Ann Intern Med* 110:617–621, 1989.
38 Celum CL et al: Indeterminate HIV-1 Western blots: Implications and considerations for widespread HIV testing. *J Gen Intern Med* 7:640–645, 1992.
39 Dock NL et al: Evaluation of atypical human immunodeficiency virus immunoblot reactivity in blood donors. *Transfusion* 28:412–418, 1988.
40 Celum CL et al: Risk factors for repeatedly reactive HIV-1 EIA and indeterminate Western blots: A population-based case-control study. *Arch Intern Med* 154:1129–1137, 1994.
41 Drabick DL et al: A retrospective analysis of diseases associated with indeterminate HIV Western blot patterns. *Mil Med* 156:93–96, 1991.
42 Rugg DL et al: Evaluating the CDC program for HIV counseling and testing. *Pub Health Repts* 106:708–713, 1991.
43 External report on the CDC HIV counseling testing referral partner notification program, 1993.
44 Higgins DL et al: Evidence for the effects of HIV antibody counseling and testing on risk behaviors. *JAMA* 266:2419–2429, 1991.
45 Centers for Disease Control: HIV counseling and testing—United States, 1993. *MMWR* 44:169–173, 1995.
46 Wortley PM et al: HIV testing patterns: Where, why, and when were persons with AIDS tested for HIV? *AIDS* 9:487–492, 1995.
47 Mainous AG et al: Frequency of human immunodeficiency virus testing among rural U.S. residents and why it is done. *Arch Fam Med* 4: 41–45, 1995.
48 Gorsky RD et al: Prevention of HIV infection in drug abusers: A cost analysis. *Prev Med* 24:3–8, 1995.
49 Centers for Disease Control: HIV counseling and testing services from public and private providers—United States, 1990. *MMWR* 41:743, 749–752, 1992.
50 Centers for Disease Control: HIV prevention practices of primary care physicians—United States, 1992. *MMWR* 42:988–992, 1994.
51 Makadon HJ et al: Prevention of HIV infection in primary care: Current practices, future possibilities. *Ann Intern Med* 123:775–779, 1995.
52 Valdiserri RO et al: Clients without health insurance at publicly funded HIV counseling and testing sites: Implications for early intervention. *Pub Health Repts* 110:47–52, 1995.
53 Allen S et al: Effect of serotesting with counselling on condom use and seroconversion among HIV discordant couples in Africa. *Br Med J* 304:1605–1609, 1992.
54 Kamenga M et al: Condom use and associated HIV seroconversion following intensive HIV counseling of 122 married couples in Zaire with discordant HIV serology. Fifth International Conference on AIDS, June 6, 1989, Montreal.
55 DiVicenzi I et al: Heterosexual transmission of HIV: Follow-up of a European cohort of couples. Sixth International Conference on AIDS, June 28, 1990, San Francisco.
56 Padian NS et al: Prevention of heterosexual transmission through couple counseling. *J AIDS* 6:1043–1048, 1993.
57 Wenger NS et al: Reduction of high-risk sexual behavior among heterosexuals undergoing HIV antibody testing: A randomized clinical trial. *Am J Pub Health* 81:1580–1585, 1991.
58 Otten MW et al: Changes in sexually transmitted disease rates after HIV testing and posttest counseling, Miami, 1988 to 1989. *Am J Pub Health* 83:529–533, 1993.
59 Cohen DA: The efficacy of testing and counseling in limiting HIV transmission. *Am J Pub Health* 84:321, 1994.
60 Ickovics JR et al: Limited effects of HIV counseling and testing for women: A prospective study of behavioral and psychological consequences. *JAMA* 272:443–448, 1994.
61 Wenger NS et al: Effect of HIV antibody testing and AIDS education on communication about HIV risk and sexual behavior. *Ann Intern Med* 117:905–911, 1992.
62 Marwick C: Home testing kits for HIV apt to get FDA approval. *JAMA* 273:908–909, 1995.
63 Bayer R et al: Testing for HIV infection at home. *N Engl J Med* 332: 1296–1299, 1995.
64 Spielberg F et al: Rapid testing for HIV antibody: A technology whose time has come. *Ann Intern Med* 125:509–511, 1996.
65 Phillips KA et al: Who plans to be tested for HIV or could get tested if no one could find out the results? *Am J Prev Med* 11:156–162, 1995.
66 Phillips KA et al: Potential use of home HIV testing. *N Engl J Med* 332:1308–1310, 1995.
67 Feinberg J et al: Utility of a home test kit for the diagnosis of HIV infection. 35th ICAAC I232; 1995, San Francisco.
68 Cleary PD et al: Depressive symptoms in blood donors notified of HIV infection. *Am J Pub Health* 83:534–539, 1993.
69 Starace F: Suicidal behavior in people infected with human immunodeficiency virus: A literature review. *Int J Soc Psychiatry* 39:64–70, 1993.
70 Emmons WW et al: A modified ELISA and Western blot accurately determine anti-human immunodeficiency virus type 1 antibodies in oral fluids obtained with a special collecting device. *J Infect Dis* 171: 1406–1410, 1995.
71 Kassler WJ et al: HIV prevention counseling using an on-site, rapid HIV assay. Tenth International Conference on AIDS International Conference on STD; Yokohama, Japan, August 1994.
72 Irwin KL et al: Performance characteristics of a rapid HIV antibody assay in a hospital with a high prevalence of HIV infection. *Ann Intern Med* 125:471.5, 1996.
73 Kassler WJ et al: Performance of a rapid, on-site human immunodeficiency virus antibody assay in a public health setting. *J Clin Microbiol* 33:2899–2902, 1995.

Chapter 71

Clinical laboratory diagnosis of HIV-1 and use of viral RNA to monitor infection

Robert W. Coombs

Persons infected with HIV-1 are usually identified by the presence of antibodies reactive with the retrovirus. With recently developed techniques, however, HIV-1 infection can be detected by nucleic acid target or nucleic acid target-signal amplification assays of viral RNA or proviral DNA in nearly all HIV-1-seropositive persons.[1] The exquisite sensitivity of these nucleic acid assays must be balanced, however, against their specificity and concerns for amplicon contamination. It is generally fairly easy to develop a clinical suspicion of HIV infection given the appropriate signs and symptoms, such as prolonged fever, fatigue or weight loss, onset of opportunistic infections, and a history of membership in a high-risk group for HIV-1 infection: a participant in male-to-male sex, an IV drug user, a recipient of multiple blood-product transfusions, a person having heterosexual contact with a high-risk or HIV-seropositive partner, a resident of certain areas of Africa, Asia, or Haiti, a male or female prostitute, or a child born to parents who are members of these groups. However, physicians face a major challenge in diagnosing HIV infection in a person who may be acutely infected, who is asymptomatic, who has atypical signs and symptoms, or who denies being in a high-risk group.

Current recommendations are to treat HIV-infected pregnant women with zidovudine, to decrease vertical transmission,[2] as well as persons with primary HIV infection and otherwise asymptomatic HIV-1-infected persons who have CD4+ cell counts greater than 500 cells/μL but also viral RNA levels greater than 5,000 to 10,000 RNA copies/μL of plasma.[3] These recommendations raise additional challenges to the clinician and the clinical laboratory not only to diagnose infection as early as possible but also to assess quantitatively viral RNA, which provides prognosis for disease progression and the success or failure of therapy.

The current approach to the clinical management of HIV-1 infection is driven by the strong belief by many clinical investigators that plasma viral RNA level is the most suitable biological marker of clinical progression and therapy efficacy. Although the adequacy of viral RNA alone as a surrogate for clinical outcome has been questioned,[4–6] current expert opinion about the antiretroviral management of HIV-1 infection is based almost solely on monitoring viral RNA levels in plasma.[3,7,8] To understand the usefulness and limitations of this measurement in clinical practice, the reader must be aware of caveats that pertain to the use of plasma HIV-1 RNA as a marker of viral replication and clinical prognosis. These caveats will be discussed in this chapter.

For descriptive and technical purposes, laboratory detection of HIV-1 or HIV-2 infection can be stratified into assays that identify HIV-specific antibodies and those that identify infectious HIV virus, viral antigen, or viral nucleic acids. The reader is referred to several recent reviews for more technical detail of the detection methods used for the laboratory diagnosis of HIV infection.[9–13]

HIV ANTIBODY ASSAYS

GENERAL CONSIDERATIONS

The HIV-1 testing algorithm recommended by the United States Public Health Service comprises initial screening by a Federal Drug Administration (FDA)-licensed enzyme immunoassay (EI assay) followed by confirmatory testing of repeatedly reactive specimens with an FDA-licensed supplemental test, e.g., immunoblot (Western blot) or immunofluorescence assay (IFA).[14,15] Although the EI assays are highly sensitive and specific, the positive predictive value of the EI assay is highly dependent on the seroprevalence of HIV-1 antibody in the population to which the individual being tested belongs. Therefore, use of both the EI assay and a further supplementary test increases the accuracy of detecting HIV-1 infection. Clinical laboratory practice dictates that the results of a repeatedly reactive HIV EI assay should never be released to the clinician or patient by the clinical laboratory without the results of the more specific confirmatory testing.[16,17] For the maximum diagnostic accuracy, the laboratory HIV test results should be interpreted by the clinician in conjunction with the clinical and epidemiological history of the person being tested.[17]

ENZYME IMMUNOASSAYS

Enzyme immunoassays (EI assays) were first developed to detect HIV-1 antibodies in infected potential blood donors. These tests have now been adopted for screening high-risk groups for HIV infection. Following the initial screening procedure, more specific tests confirm the diagnosis.

There are three basic formats for commercially available EI assays. First generation assays use antigens derived from whole disrupted virus and an enzyme-conjugated anti-human IgG sandwich technique for capture and detection of anti-HIV antibodies. Second generation assays use recombinant (rDNA) viral protein (antigen) and conjugated anti-human IgG, or they use rDNA antigen for both capture of anti-HIV antibodies and detection of these antibodies, using enzyme-conjugated rDNA proteins as probe.[18,19] Third generation assays use synthetic peptides.[20,21] For example, the Genetic Systems™ HIV-1/HIV-2 Peptide EIA (Genetic Systems Corp., Redmond WA) is comprised of four highly conserved, immunodominant peptide sequences of envelope (env) and polymerase (pol) gene products for HIV-1 and HIV 2 that are adsorbed onto the surface of a microwell plate. If antibodies to either HIV-1 or HIV-2 are present, they bind to the adsorbed peptides and are recognized by an enzyme-conjugated anti-human IgG sandwich technique.

The median time interval between infection and confirmed seropositivity is approximately 3 months with the first and second generation EI assays, with 95% or more of subjects serconverting by 6 months.[22] However, the more sensitive third generation assays have shortened the estimated antibody-negative "window-period" of primary infection to approximately one month or less.[23] The specificities of the current commercial EI assays are above 99.5%.[24–27] False-positive reactivities result from nonspecific cross-reacting antibodies in persons with underlying immunological disease, gravidity, multiple transfusions, or recent immunization.[28,29] Several commercially available EI assays screen for both HIV-1 and HIV-2 antibody.

IMMUNOBLOT

As already mentioned, the positive predictive value of the EI assays are highly dependent on the seroprevalence of HIV antibody in the population from which the person being tested is from. Therefore, to prevent a false-positive diagnosis of HIV infection, confirmation of a reactive EI assay is required using an independent testing method with high specificity. The immunoblot (or Western blot) is the most commonly used confirmatory test in the United States.[15]

The Western blot detects the serum antibodies directed against specific HIV proteins of varying molecular weights following their separation by gel electrophoresis and blotting onto nitrocellulose paper. The Western blot detects antibodies to the following specific HIV-1 proteins: core (p17, p24, and the precursor p55); polymerase (p31, p51, p66); and envelope (gp41, gp120/160). The reported analytic specificity of the immunoblot assay is 97.8%.[15,24] The Western blot is interpreted as negative when no antibody-antigen band is present, positive when antibodies are present to core (p24) and envelope (gp41 or gp120/160) and, in some cases, polymerase proteins (p31). Although several organizations, including the World Health Organization[31] and Consortium for Retrovirus Serology Standardization,[31] have proposed criteria for interpreting Western blot reactivity, the Centers for Disease Control and Prevention (CDC) endorses interpretative criteria that require the presence of antibodies to two of p24, gp41, or gp120/160.[15,17,32]

Regardless of the HIV-1 antibody seroprevalence, a reactive EI assay and confirmatory Western blot together have a positive predictive value of greater than 99.99%.[33,34] In the blood donor population, approximately 10 of 10,000 persons (0.1%) without risk for HIV-1 infection will be repeatedly reactive by the HIV-1 EIA. Eight of those 10 low-risk persons with repeatedly reactive HIV-1 EI assays will be negative by the HIV-1 Western blot and 2 will be indeterminate.[34] False positive results for HIV-1 antibody, when both the EI assay and Western blot are reactive in a person who is not infected with HIV-1, are extremely rare (less than 1 in 100,000 persons screened).[33] Therefore, indeterminate Western blots are more common than false-positive Western blots in screening persons from populations with low HIV-1 antibody seroprevalence.[35]

The combination of HIV-1 EI assay and confirmatory immunoblot has clearly established evidence against the seroreversion of HIV-1 antibody in seroreactive individuals.[36] In a retrospective cohort study that reviewed the results of 5,446,161 HIV-1 antibody tests performed on 2,580,974 individuals (the U.S. Army HIV Data System) from 1985 through 1992, only 6 of 4,911 individuals were identified as potential seroreverters. Furthermore, in all 6 instances errors in specimen attribution or testing were identified.[37] Therefore, if seroreversion occurs, it is extremely rare.

OTHER CONFIRMATION METHODS

The indirect immunofluorescence assay (IFA) is also approved for confirmatory testing,[38] but it is used less commonly than the immunoblot confirmation method.[15,32] Other confirmation strategies have been reported.[39] For example, the use of a first or second generation EI assay as a screen followed by a native HIV-1 gp160 EI assay,[40] a recombinant DNA-derived antigen-based peptide EI assay,[41,42] or an immunoblot assay (RIBA),[43] have all reported comparable results but are not FDA approved for this purpose. Nevertheless, the combination of rapid tests, for example, could be a cheaper and faster alternative to the conventional testing algorithm in developing countries.[44]

INDETERMINATE IMMUNOBLOTS

With the increased use of HIV-1 antibody screening in low-risk populations, including health-care workers,[45] it is essential for the primary care provider to be able to interpret HIV-1 test results accurately.[35] Between 4% and 20% of serum samples that are repeatedly reactive by HIV-1 EI assay are interpreted as indeterminate by Western blot.[17,34,46] Indeterminate Western blots (IWBs) in HIV-1-infected persons may result from early antibody formation against viral core antigens during primary infection,[47] from early detection of HIV-1 antibody by the more sensitive third generation EI assays before there is confirmation by immunoblot,[48,49] and rarely, from the loss of core-specific antibody late in infection due to severe immunosuppression.[36,50,51] In HIV-1-negative persons, cross-reacting antibody to HIV-2 has been implicated.[52] False-positive immunoblots are extremely uncommon and occur with a frequency of <1 per 135,000 tests.[33,34]

In the only population-based case-control study (244 cases, 131 controls and 83 sexual partners of cases) to assess risk factors for IWBs, Celum and coworkers found that IWBs were associated with a low risk of HIV seroconversion (3.0%; 95% confidence interval, CI, 0.7% to 5.3%) for those with recent risk behaviors for HIV-1 acquisition, and that for low-risk persons, the major risk factors identified for IWBs related to alloimmunization (i.e., parity or recent immunization) or autoantibodies (i.e., antinuclear antibodies and rheumatoid factor).[53] Of interest, conditional logistic regression analysis indicated that an additional independent risk factor for IWBs among male cases and controls was a recent sexual contact with a prostitute (odds ratio, 3.0; 95% CI, 1.0 to 9.5). Contrary to other reports, however, no cross-reactivity was detected with HIV-2, human T-lymphotrophic virus type 1, feline immunodeficiency or feline leukemia, or bovine immunodeficiency viruses.

Celum and coworkers suggested four important principals for facilitating the management of IWBs for HIV-1 in the clinical setting.[53] First, approximately one-third of persons who present with IWBs will not be repeatedly reactive by EI assay and Western blot testing.[46] There is no need for further testing or follow-up of this group. Second, the most important factor for the association of seroconversion with an IWB was a p24 antibody band (approximately an 18% risk of seroconversion) and high-risk behavior which could be determined from the risk history.[46] Repeat Western blot and selective supplemental testing with HIV-1 culture, p24 antigen, HIV-1 DNA polymerase chain reaction amplification (and quite possibly RNA[49,54]) or third generation recombinant EI assays were also useful in identifying persons with no history of high-risk behaviors who proved to have false-positive Western blots. Third, no cross-reactivity with known human or animal retroviruses was shown. Fourth, in most cases the medical history is extremely important in identifying subjects with significant risk factors for IWBs (parity and autoantibodies among females, tetanus booster in the past 2 years and sexual contact with a prostitute since 1978 among males).[53]

In summary, the following recommendations are made for the clinical management of patients with an indeterminate Western blot. Low-risk individuals with a nonreactive EI assay upon repeat testing do not need further follow-up. High-risk individuals should be followed serologically for at least 6 months, especially those with a p24 band on Western blot. The early, selective use of supplemental tests such as HIV-1 p24 antigen, HIV-1 culture, HIV-1 proviral DNA, or plasma RNA may help determine the infectious status of high-risk individuals before full seroconversion occurs.[46,55,56] Negative supplemental tests may also help alleviate the anxiety associated with an indeterminate HIV-1 serology.

RAPID SEROLOGIC TESTING

Rapid, reliable, and less expensive alternatives to the EI assay with confirmatory immunoblot have been sought for use in acute care settings, emergency rooms, sexually transmitted disease clinics, medical field settings, and developing countries.[57] Testing formats have included latex agglutination[58,59] and solid-surface dot-blot EI assays.[60] However, only one, the Single Use Diagnostic System HIV-1 test (SUDS, Murex Corp., Norcross GA) is approved for diagnostic use in the United States.[60] The procedure takes 10 minutes, and negative results are available immediately. Positive tests must be confirmed with a Western blot or IFA. Generally the positive predictive value of these assays is comparable to the standard EI assays (>80%) and the negative predictive values approach 100% in some circumstances[59,61–64] but not others.[65] For the SUDS HIV-1 test, high temperature and inadequate separation of serum can lead to false positives.[60,62] The relative sensitivity (99.9%) and specificity (99.6%) of the SUDS HIV-1 test and its ability to detect both IgM and IgG antibody makes it particularly useful for detecting early infection.[61]

Consideration should be given to the introduction of rapid screening for HIV-1 antibody into certain clinical settings, such as sexually transmitted disease clinics, as this will greatly enhance testing programs by preventing the need for delayed counseling of seronegative patients and by providing preliminary results to seropositive patients.[66] These preliminary results may encourage patients to return for confirmatory test results and to adopt risk-reducing behaviors sooner than occurs using currently accepted testing algorithms.[67] In addition, the rapid HIV-1 screening of source contacts following occupational exposures to blood will minimize the duration of antiretroviral prophylaxis therapy for the exposed health care worker, thus minimizing cost and alleviating anxiety following the exposure sooner if the test is negative.

OVER-THE-COUNTER TESTING

Only one over-the-counter HIV-1 test kit is available for home collection (Home Access™, Home Access Health Care). The test is based on previous evaluations of blood collected on filter paper for stability and for detection of antibodies to HIV-1 by EI assay and confirmatory Western blot.[68–70] The kit consists of instructions and equipment for obtaining blood from a finger-stick. The blood-spot specimen is sent to a commercial laboratory for testing with an EI assay and confirmatory IFA. The results and counseling are provided over the phone; for positive results, patients are referred by a counselor to a physician for additional counseling and care.

DETECTION OF HIV-1 ANTIBODY IN SALIVA AND URINE

HIV-1 antibodies can be detected reliably in the oral fluids of HIV-1-infected persons.[71] There are a number of obvious advantages to collecting specimens for HIV-1 testing using a noninvasive specimen collection procedure.[72] For example, greater safety, increased patient compliance, and an alternative to phlebotomy.[73] Earlier problems with low sensitivity have been corrected by using special collection devices that concentrate and stabilize the salivary-associated immunoglobulins.[73] Modification of the EI assay and Western blot have increased the sensitivity to 97–100% and the specificity to 98–100% depending on the study.[71,73,74] For example, the Oral Fluid Vironostika HIV-1 Microelisa System (Organon Teknika, Durham NC) and the OraSure™ HIV-1 Western Blot Kit (Epitope Inc., Beaverton OR) in combination with the OraSure HIV-1 Collection Device (Epitope Inc., Beaverton OR) provided the correct result or triggered appropriate follow-up testing in 3,569 (>99.9%) of 3,570 cases.[73]

Early reports of discordant HIV-1 antibody results between antibody-negative blood serum and antibody-positive urine,[75] and the detection of the first case of HIV-1 group O in a patient who had urine antibody confirmed by Western blot but was serum Western blot sero-indeterminate,[76] has suggested a compartmentalized antibody response to early HIV-1 infection. As such, there has been an interest in using urine for HIV-1 antibody screening.[77] This has led to the testing of an experimental urine HIV-1 envelope-based EI assay, Calypte™ (Calypte Biomedical, Berkeley CA; also marketed as Sentinel™, Serdyn) which has demonstrated a positive predictive value of >99.2% and negative predictive value of >99.9% when combined with confirmatory immunoblot or immunofluorescence testing.[78,79] At this time, the absence of a FDA-licensed Western blot for urine testing requires that urine reactive for HIV-1 antibody be confirmed by testing of a blood specimen.

DETECTION OF HIV-1 SUBTYPES

The envelope protein of HIV-1 isolates from different geographic locations world-wide can differ in more than 35% of amino-acid positions (for a recent review, see Ref. 80). As a consequence of this diversity, HIV-1 strains are divided into two groups, M and O. Within the "major" group M, multiple subtypes (or clades) designated A-J have been documented. Group M and its subtypes are more clearly defined than others. Subtype B is the most common subtype in the United States and Europe, while subtypes A and E are prominent in Africa and Asia.[80]

There is as yet no obvious subtype pattern for viruses from the highly divergent "outlier" group O. Nevertheless, this virus stain has been isolated form persons of west-central African origins[81,82] with recent reports of group O virus from Europe[76,83,84] and most recently, the United States.[85] Because the commercial EI assays and confirmatory immunoblot assays are based on the predominant HIV-1 clade B virus, not all early commercially available diagnostic assays could detect the divergent group O strains.[86–88] Thereafter, diagnostic kit reagents were modified to ensure optimal sensitivity and specificity for group O virus antibody.[89,90]

Since most of the primer pairs for HIV-1 DNA polymerase chain reaction (PCR) amplification have been optimized for group B viruses (see below), it is not surprising that HIV-1 DNA PCR may also fail to detect HIV-1 group O and some group M subtypes.[91,92] To accommodate this deficiency, primer pair modifications have been incorporated into the recent Roche Amplicor™ HIV-1 DNA and Roche Monitor™ HIV-1 RNA assays. Because of the large number of *pol*-specific synthetic oligonucleotide target probes used by the bDNA assay (Chiron Quantiplex®, Emeryville CA), detection of group O and different group B subtypes has not been a problem for the bDNA assay.[93]

DETECTION OF HIV-2 ANTIBODIES

Although HIV-2 infection is less geographically dispersed than HIV-1, and the epidemic is primarily focused in western Africa, HIV-2 is present in the epidemic in India.[94,95] In the United States, only a relatively few cases of HIV-2 have been reported.[96] HIV-2 among United States blood donors is extremely rare, with only three cases detected from screening 74 million donations up to June, 1995.[97] Of the 62 persons reported with HIV-2 infection in the United States, 44 (77%) were born in, had traveled to, or had a sex partner from western Africa.[97] Nevertheless, diagnosis of HIV-2 infection will continue to be an emerging problem in the United States;[98] thus, antibody screening for both viruses is warranted.

HIV-1 and HIV-2 genomes share about 60% homology in conserved genes such as *gag* and *pol* and 35–45% homology in the *env* genes.[99] The core proteins of HIV-1 and HIV-2 display frequent cross-reactivity, whereas the envelope proteins are more type specific.[100] Despite this cross-reactivity, anti-HIV-1 EI assays used for screening blood donors in the United States are estimated to detect 55% to 91% of HIV-2 infections.[101] Western blots for HIV-1 antibodies may be positive, negative, or indeterminate with HIV-2-positive sera. (For the confirmation of HIV-2 EI assay reactivity, p26 and gp36 correspond to their HIV-1 counterparts p24 and gp41, respectively.)[102] Busch and coworkers tested 913 anti-HIV-1-reactive blood donor sera using an anti-HIV-2 screening EIA, with confirmation by an anti-HIV-2 env-peptide EIA and an anti-HIV-2 Western blot. These 913 sera were derived from anti-HIV-1 screening of approximately 242,000 donations over a three year period. No HIV-2 infections were identified.[101]

To examine HIV-2 seroprevalence in a higher risk population, a sentinel surveillance for HIV-2 was conducted by testing 31,533 anonymous blood specimens from patients at sexually transmitted disease clinics, injecting drug users at treatment centers, and clients at HIV counseling and testing sites in 14 US cities where West African immigrants often settle.[96] Specimens were tested by HIV-1 and HIV-2 whole virus and synthetic peptide enzyme immunoassay and confirmed by HIV-1 and HIV-2 Western blots. Nearly 10% of 31,533 sera were positive for HIV-1. In addition, two heterosexual male patients from West Africa were infected with HIV-2, and one of the HIV-2 positive specimens did not cross-react on HIV-1 enzyme immunoassay screening.[96]

When HIV testing is indicated, tests for antibodies to both HIV-1 and HIV-2 should be obtained if epidemiological risk factors for HIV-2 infection are present, if clinical evidence exists for HIV disease in the absence of a positive test for antibodies to HIV-1, or if HIV-1 immunoblot results exhibit the unusual indeterminate pattern of *gag* plus *pol* bands in the absence of *env* bands.[52,96,103] The following procedures are recommended if testing for both HIV-1 and HIV-2 is performed by means of a combination HIV-1/HIV-2 EI assay.[52] A repeatedly reactive specimen by HIV-1/HIV-2 EI assay should be tested by HIV-1 immunoblot (or another licensed HIV-1 supplemental test). A positive result by HIV-1 immunoblot confirms the presence of antibodies to HIV-1, and testing for HIV-2 is recommended only if HIV-2 risk factors are present. If the HIV-1 Western blot result is negative or indeterminate, an HIV-2 EI assay should be performed. If the HIV-2 EI assay is reactive, an HIV-2 supplemental test such as an HIV-1 specific Western blot should be performed.[52] In addition, HIV-2 DNA PCR has been used to determine infection with HIV-1, HIV-2 or both viruses[104,105] (see below).

DETECTION OF HUMAN IMMUNODEFICIENCY VIRUS

CULTURE

The detection of HIV-1 by mixed-lymphocyte coculture is a specialized procedure that has extremely high specificity but lower sensitivity in patients with high CD4+ cell counts[106–108] compared to viral nucleic acid detection methods (see below). HIV-1 coculture may be particularly useful as a supplemental test for assessing indeterminate immunoblots associated with primary infection where culture has a comparable specificity to viral RNA detection.[109] In the diagnosis of HIV-1 infection in perinatally exposed infants, a sequential-sample, combination assay algorithm comprising a HIV-1 DNA PCR on the first specimen followed by a culture of the second specimen was recommended over HIV-1 DNA PCR for diagnosis alone[110] by Paul and coworkers.[111] In a study of 208 HIV-1-exposed infants, they found that a positive HIV-1 DNA PCR result followed by a positive culture in the second sample confirmed infected status, while two consecutive negative PCR results reconfirmed as negative at 6 months of age established uninfected status.[111]

The lower sensitivity of HIV-1 coculture (other than for pediatric diagnosis) compared to currently available nucleic acid detection methods, as well as its greater cost, time requirements, and highly specialized technical nature, leaves HIV-1 culture restricted primarily to research laboratories. However, there may be a rekindled interest in using HIV-1 coculture for assessing viral containment following potent antiretroviral therapy[112,113] and for obtaining primary clinical HIV-1 isolates for viral syncytium-inducing and drug susceptibility phenotypes.[114]

HIV-1 P24 ANTIGEN

With the advent of nucleic acid amplification methods for monitoring HIV-1, the measurement of HIV-1 p24 antigen has a much more limited role than it once did. Now the primary use for p24 antigen detection is for identifying subjects in the antibody-negative window period of acute HIV-1 infection. Although antigen detection is a less expensive alternative to viral RNA detection in this setting, both viral RNA and peripheral blood mononuclear cell culture are significantly more sensitive than detection of p24 antigenemia,[48,49,109] even with the added sensitivity of p24 antigen acid dissociation.[115,116] The reactivity of the p24 antigen EI assay requires confirmation by a neutralization assay; this is similar to the HIV-1 specific antibody by the EI assay.[117]

Currently, the greatest use of p24 antigen testing is for screening the U.S. blood supply. Although this screening program was introduced in 1996 without a persuasive scientific rationale,[117,118] it is very likely that p24 antigen screening will be augmented by a plasma HIV-1 RNA screening assay to lower the residual risk of HIV-1 infection (now estimated to be <1 in 500,000 units) even further.

VIRAL NUCLEIC ACID

The detection of viral nucleic acid (proviral DNA or viral RNA) by commercially available amplification technologies provides a specific and sensitive direct detection method to identify persons who are infected but who have not seroconverted,[109,119] to identify infected infants,[120] and to resolve indeterminate HIV-1 antibody serologies.[46,48,121] In addition, the quantification of plasma viral RNA has assumed a critically important role in assessing disease prognosis and response to antiretroviral therapy.[122–127] Excellent technical reviews are presented by Ferré,[12] Holodniy,[13] and Clementi and coworkers.[10]

VIRAL DNA IN PERIPHERAL BLOOD MONONUCLEAR CELLS

Qualitative HIV-1 DNA polymerase chain reaction (PCR) amplification is the most commonly used assay method for the diagnosis of HIV-1 infection in neonates and infants.[128,129] The Roche Amplicor™ HIV-1 test (Roche Diagnostic Systems, Inc., Branchburg NJ.) is the only FDA-licensed commercial kit for clinical use.

The major advantages of HIV-1 DNA PCR over culture are its increased sensitivity and more rapid reporting time; that is, one day compared to 2–4 weeks. There is always a possible risk of false-positive reactivity due to contamination of the specimen with amplicons (so-called carry-over product contamination),[130] although this is decreased somewhat by the use of the uracil *N*-glycolsylase enzyme in the commercial assay.[131] False negatives can also occur because of inhibition of the PCR reaction by hemoglobin or heparin[132] or when there are fewer target cells in the assay than expected. To control for the latter, and to improve the precision of the assay, testing for HIV-1 DNA should also include concurrent amplification of a cell-associated host gene such as HLA-DQa or globin locus.[133] Participation in a quality assurance program will also ensure that problems with sensitivity and specificity are quickly identified.[134–137]

The use of HIV-1 DNA PCR for diagnosis was assessed recently for 96 studies for which reported sensitivities for HIV-1 DNA PCR range from 10% to 100% and specificities range from 40% to 100%.[139] The authors of this review concluded that the HIV-1 DNA PCR assay is not sufficiently accurate to be used for the diagnosis of HIV-1 infection without confirmation. Use of HIV-1 DNA PCR for the diagnosis of infection in adults should be limited to situations in which antibody tests are known to be insufficient.[46,138]

VIRAL RNA IN PLASMA

The detection of plasma HIV-1 RNA by reverse transcription-polymerase chain (RT-PCR) amplification is more sensitive than p24 antigen EI assay for detecting virus.[109,119,139–142] There is therefore much interest in using plasma HIV-1 RNA as a diagnostic test.[55,143] As mentioned above, HIV-1 RNA will likely be used to either replace or augment HIV-1 p24-antigen screening of all donor blood in the United States. However, the commercial HIV-1 RNA assays are not licensed for this screening purpose. To avoid false-positive diagnosis, the HIV-1 RNA assay should be used diagnostically only as a supplemental test for detecting antibody-negative acute infection.[55,138,144] Thus, in this particular diagnostic setting, a reactive HIV-1 RNA assay (particularly one with a low viral RNA copy number, <1,000 copies/mL)[55] should be confirmed by another nucleic acid technology (preferably HIV-1 DNA PCR), HIV-1 p24 antigen, HIV-1 culture, or the development of HIV-1 specific antibody, which should occur shortly after viral RNA is detected anyway.[109] The presence of HIV-1 RNA alone requires a correlation with the medical and epidemiological history and, importantly, a confirmatory repeat blood draw for HIV-1 testing.

HIV-1 RNA quantitative assays

Three different types of commercial assays are available to detect and quantify viral RNA in plasma; each approaches the quantification of viral RNA differently. A more detailed overview of the different methodologies may be found elsewhere.[10,12,13,145,146]

Briefly, the nucleic acid sequence-based amplification (NASBA, Organon Teknika Corporation, Advanced BioScience Laboratories, Inc., Kensington MD) assay involves first obtaining nucleic acid isolation by lysis and binding of the viral RNA to silicon dioxide (silica) microparticles, followed by isothermal amplification (so-called target amplification) using a reverse transcriptase, RNAse H, and T7 RNA polymerase.[147–149] Three internal calibrators are added to the specimen and adsorbed along with the specimen prior to the lysis step. Amplification covers approximately 1200 bases in *gag* and *pol*. Detection is by means of chemiluminescence. The sensitivity of the assay is approximately 100 RNA copies/mL, the quantitation limit is 500 copies/mL, and the dynamic range is up to 10,000,000 RNA copies/mL (NucliSens™ QT HIV-1 RNA assay). Acceptable whole blood anticoagulants include EDTA (lavender-top Vacutaner™ tubes [Becton Dickinson, Franklin Lakes NJ]), ACD (acid citrate dextrose, yellow-top tubes), and Heparin (green-top tubes).

The branched-chain DNA assay (Quantiplex® HIV RNA 2.0 Assay [bDNA], Chiron Corporation, Inc., Emeryville CA) is a nonisotopic sandwich nucleic acid hybridization assay that uses a series of *pol* target probes to hybridize the viral RNA target onto a series of capture probes on the surface of the microwell plate and also to the bDNA amplifier molecules.[150] Multiple alkaline phosphatase probes amplify the signal (so-called signal amplification); detection is by chemiluminescence. An external standard curve is used to calculate the HIV-1 RNA copy number. The detection and quantitation levels are at approximately 500 RNA copies/mL, with a dynamic range of up to 1,000,000 RNA copies/mL. A modification of the assay has increased the sensitivity to 50 RNA copies/mL of plasma.[151] The whole blood anticoagulant of choice is EDTA.

The only FDA-licensed assay for assessing HIV-1 disease prognosis at this time is the Roche Amplicor® HIV-1 Monitor™ Test (Roche Diagnostic Systems, Branchburg NJ). The assay uses the *Thermus thermophilus* rTth enzyme, which serves to catalyze both reverse transcription and DNA amplification of a 142-base *gag* sequence in a single reaction tube.[142] An internal quantitative standard is used to adjust for recovery and calculate the final HIV-1 RNA copy number. The assay has an analytic sensitivity of 200 RNA copies/mL and a quantitation limit of 400 RNA copies/mL, with a dynamic range of up to 750,000 RNA copies/mL. A centrifugation step (Amplicor HIV-1 Monitor™ Ultra Sensitive specimen preparation protocol, Roche Molecular Systems, Somerville NJ) can be used to concentrate virus and thus increase the sensitivity of the assay to approximately 50 RNA copies/mL, with a lower quantitation limit of 200 copies/mL.[152] The whole blood anticoagulant of choice is EDTA or ACD.

Specimen considerations for HIV-1 RNA quantitation

In order to minimize the variability of quantitative HIV-1 RNA test results, samples collected for a particular assay should be processed at the same time postdraw, using the same anticoagulant blood-draw tube type.[153] In general, EDTA is the preferred anticoagulant. Based on the work of Holodniy and coworkers,[153] the general recommendation has been to separate and store plasma at −70°C within 6 hours of collection. This rapid specimen processing may place a considerable burden on the laboratory. Moreover, a 6-hour processing requirement may be too stringent,[154] and a recent study is reassuring in this regard. For the Amplicor HIV-1 Monitor™ assay, viral RNA copy numbers were maintained within 0.5 $\log_{10}$ (3-fold) in both blood and plasma samples held at ambient temperature or 4°C for up to 3 days and remained stable despite limited freezing and thawing.[155]

As in the serologic diagnosis of HIV infection,[68–70] the use of filter paper to collect and store whole blood for later analysis of viral nucleic acid is an attractive alternative to phlebotomy. Studies by Cassol, Fiscus, and others have shown that both HIV-1 DNA and RNA can be detected reliably from blood dried on filter paper; moreover, RNA quantitation, corrected for the hematocrit, was comparable in terms of sensitivity and reproducibility to plasma.[156–158] This collection method appears to be suitable for both quantitation and sequencing of HIV specimens obtained under field conditions.[158,159]

ANTIRETROVIRAL SUSCEPTIBILITY GENOTYPE AND PHENOTYPE

Incomplete inhibition of HIV-1 replication in vivo may arise because of poor drug absorption, patient noncompliance with therapy, or infection with drug-resistant virus variants. This incomplete inhibition may result in the emergence of drug-resistant HIV-1 variants and thus is an important cause of therapy failure.[160] An assessment of drug resistance may be helpful in selecting subsequent antiretroviral therapy, but this has not been rigorously proven. A thoughtful review of the laboratory monitoring of HIV-1 drug resistance is given elsewhere.[161]Antiretroviral drug susceptibility is determined either phenotypically, by assessing for the susceptibility of the virus isolate ex vivo, or genotypically, by assessing for mutations that confer resistance. There are two phenotypic approaches: the first approach tests the sensitivity of the proviral population present in the peripheral blood mononuclear cells of the patient;[162] the second approach generates recombinant fragments of the virus that contain polymerase or protease genes obtained from the plasma- or serum-associated virus or from the cell-associated provirus.[163] There are several genotypic approaches: DNA sequencing of the entire viral population or clones,[164] selective polymerase chain reaction assay,[165] determination of point mutations,[166] differential probe hybridization;[167] enzyme-immunoassay modification of the oligoligase detection reaction assay;[168] and the commercially available HIV-1 reverse transcription line probe assay.[169] Genotypic changes may not correlate with changes in drug susceptibility of the clinical isolate;[170] much still needs to be learned about the genotype and phenotype correlation in patients who receive combination antiretroviral therapy before these techniques can be applied effectively in the clinic.[171] In the meantime, it is generally recommended that a patient's response to therapy be monitored by using the viral RNA level and CD4+ cell count.[3,172]

USE OF HIV-1 RNA TO MONITOR INFECTION

PROGNOSTIC ABILITY OF HIV-1 RNA IN INFECTED ADULTS

Natural history

Appreciation of the benefits and limitations of using viral RNA as a measure of disease progression requires understanding of a number of critical elements of viral pathogenesis. First, cell-free viral RNA in plasma represents a minority population of infectious virus and a majority population of noninfectious virus particles.[141] The ratio between these two depends on the replicative efficiency of the virus itself along with other factors such as the levels of HIV-1 specific p24 antibody.[173,174] Second, the level of plasma viral RNA may not reflect the level of cell-associated infectious virus. Cell-associated infectious virus can be recovered from the majority of patients who have had plasma viral RNA levels suppressed to below the level of detection after prolonged, potent antiretroviral therapy.[112,113] Third, the viral RNA level in plasma may not reflect the level of virus and kinetics of viral replication in other sites and compartments[175–178] such as latently infected cells in the lymph nodes,[179] central nervous system,[180] and genital tract.[181] Fourth, independent of viral RNA level, syncytium-inducing viral phenotype is strongly associated with disease progression.[124–126,172,182] Finally, patient attributes such as age[183] and immune status[184] may cause substantial variability in the level of viral replication.[185] Together these factors may explain, in part, the differences in disease progression among patients with similar plasma viral RNA levels, and they represent a limitation to the use of plasma viral RNA as the sole marker of therapeutic efficacy and clinical outcome.[4–6]

Nonetheless, one of the most important concepts to emerge from our understanding of HIV-1 disease pathogenesis is that the magnitude of HIV-1 replication in infected persons is associated with the rate of disease progression.[173,186,187] The level of plasma HIV RNA reflects the infected person's ability to contain viral replication such that the replication and clearance of virus reaches a quasi-steady state[175–178] and thus defines, in part, the subsequent rate of disease progression.[122,173,174,182,186,188,189] This quasi-steady state has been referred to as the viral "set-point" and appears to be established in the first 6 to 12 months following primary infection, during which time an HIV-specific humoral and cytotoxic lymphocyte response is established.[190–192] Interestingly, the plasma viral RNA level prior to the establishment of the steady state is not predictive of subsequent disease progression.[193] The viral steady state represents the nadir of viral containment, after which time the plasma viral RNA level may increase slowly,[190] conferring additional risk for the development of AIDS. However, some patients may continue to have a decline in plasma viral RNA from the steady state, conferring additional clinical benefit.[194]

The viral steady state is not absolute, and each plasma viral RNA level describes a range of times to the development of disease progression. To illustrate this point, Ioannidis and coworkers constructed a model to ascertain the predictive value of serum viral RNA in asymptomatic patients with >500 CD4 cells/μL, an unknown time since seroconversion, and no prior antiretroviral therapy.[185] They found that the minimum and maximum estimated time to progression to AIDS varied considerably at assigned serum viral RNA levels. For example, patients with a viral load of 10,000 (104) RNA copies/mL of serum could take from 2.8 to 19 years to develop AIDS, and those with 30,000 (104.5) RNA copies/mL could take anywhere from 1.9 to 8 years.[185]

In general, patients who are more likely to progress rapidly have a higher plasma viral RNA steady state than do those who progress more slowly. However, the predictive value of high plasma viral RNA levels decreases over time, while the predictive value of low CD4+ cell count and CD4+ cell function increases over time. Thus, in the later stages of infection, immune deficiency is most predictive of disease progression.[194] There is a monotonic relationship between the plasma viral RNA level and the rate of CD4+ cell decline, such that higher plasma viral RNA levels are associated with a greater rate of CD4+ cell decline.[122,186,189] For example, the Multicenter AIDS Cohort Study of the natural history of HIV-1 infection showed that the mean (95% confidence interval) decrease in CD4+ cell count per year was -36.3 (-42.3 to -30.4) cells for subjects with less than 500 viral RNA copies/mL of plasma compared to -76.5 (-82.9 to -70.5) cells for subjects with greater than 30,000 viral RNA copies/mL of plasma.[189]

In most untreated subjects the plasma viral RNA steady-state level lies within a relatively narrow range between 1,000 (10^3) to 100,000 (10^5) RNA copies/mL of plasma.[173,182,186,194] For example, in the largest cohort study, 74.3% of 1,531 untreated patients had plasma viral RNA levels of <30,000 RNA copies/mL by the bDNA assay.[189] Mellors and coworkers also defined five risk categories for disease progression based on the arbitrary distribution of 1,531 subjects into HIV-1 RNA level quintiles.[189] Highly significant differences in the proportion of patients who progressed to AIDS within 6 years of diagnosis were seen in these five risk categories: 500 copies/mL or less, 5.4% (95% CI, 0% to 17%); 501–3,000 copies/mL, 16.6% (12% to 21%); 3,001–10,000 copies/mL, 31.7% (7% to 43%); 10,001–30,000 copies/mL, 55.2% (25% to 84%); and more than 30,000 copies/mL, 80.0% (58% to 100%).[189]

Clinical trials

Importantly, because there is a continuous gradient of risk of disease progression associated with the viral RNA steady-state level, one of the objectives of antiretroviral therapy is to "reset" this plasma viral RNA steady-state level to one with a lower risk of disease progression. Results from HIV-1 therapy trials show that inhibition of HIV-1 replication (as assessed by plasma HIV-1 RNA level) is associated with a delay in clinical disease progression.[123–127] Although the relative clinical benefit of any given decline in plasma viral RNA does not depend on the baseline level of plasma viral RNA, the absolute risk of clinical disease progression remains higher in the patient with the higher pretherapy plasma viral RNA level.[172] In summarizing the data from seven large clinical trials involving 1,330 subjects who received primarily nucleoside therapies, Marschner and coworkers[72] showed that a 10-fold decrease in plasma viral RNA level from baseline to week 24 yielded a 72% reduction in the risk of progression (95% CI, 61% to 81%, $p < .001$) and that large reductions in plasma viral RNA level were the most desirable. Importantly, any reduction in excess of the natural variability of plasma HIV-1 RNA measurement (approximately 3-fold, or 0.5 $\log_{10}$) was associated with a delay in disease progression.[172] However, in this study and others the prognostic interpretation of any given plasma viral RNA reduction also depended on the treatment response of the CD4+ cell count.[172,195,196] Even though the change in plasma viral RNA is a better predictor of clinical progression than is the CD4+ cell response, together the viral RNA and CD4+ cell count responses more fully characterize the risk of disease progression than does either one alone.[172,195,197] These clinical trial data strongly suggest that a more complete assessment of a patient's prognosis can be achieved by monitoring the plasma viral RNA level and CD4+ cell count together.[172,195,197]

MONITORING INFECTION

In general, nadir responses in plasma viral RNA occur in most patients 4 to 12 weeks following initiation of potent antiretroviral therapy. With some potent antiretroviral regimens, plasma viral RNA values will decrease to less than 500 RNA copies/mL by 16 weeks in 60% to 80% of subjects and to less than 50 viral RNA copies/mL by 24 weeks in approximately 70%. The number of patients in these categories will depend on the study population and their prior antiretroviral experience.[127,198] With a stable response, continued monitoring at 3 to 4 month intervals seems warranted, with more frequent monitoring if a critical plasma viral RNA value is approached.[199] It is advisable to plot the plasma viral RNA values on a $\log_{10}$ scale and only repeat the plasma viral RNA measurement for values that are greater than the upper 95% confidence interval found for the expected variation in plasma viral RNA level (that is, 0.5 $\log_{10}$ above the mean nadir response value), thus ensuring that a change in plasma viral RNA level will lead to a change in therapy.[200–203]

The target of therapy must be a durable reduction in the plasma viral RNA by at least 3-fold (0.5 $\log_{10}$) from pretherapy levels[199,202] to below 1000 copies/mL[172] and, by current consensus guidelines, preferably to an "undetectable" level.[3] Although there are no published clinical trial data that carefully delineate the decrease in risk of disease progression associated with decreases in the plasma viral RNA to <1000 copies/mL,[172] a preliminary analysis of 1,083 patients from ACTG 320[127] showed that only 7 (5.6%) of 126 clinical events were associated with a preceding plasma HIV-1 level below 500 copies/mL, and for the remaining 119 clinical events the plasma viral RNA level was above 500 copies/mL.[204] Nevertheless, many investigators believe that the target for therapy should be at least one $\log_{10}$ value lower than this, i.e., <50 RNA copies/mL of plasma.

The "as-low-as-you-can-go" concept in HIV treatment[205] is appealing but has, by virtue of its repetition, been accepted for truth.[4] How this concept pertains to a chronic, persistent viral infection like HIV-1 still requires careful validation by controlled clinical trials, particularly in asymptomatic subjects with >500 cells/μL, since the long-term toxicities of the most potent protease-inhibitor-containing combinations are unknown but potentially worrisome.[206]

Importantly, therapy should also stabilize or increase the CD4+ cell count, at or above the expected level of biological variation, by more than 30% in the absolute cell number or by more than 3% in the proportion of cells.[200,208] Interpretation of any given plasma HIV-1 RNA reduction depends on the treatment response of the CD4+ cell count. Because of the interaction between viral RNA and CD4+ cell count, changes in both, along with a consideration of the clinical course, are necessary for defining therapeutic response. In an analysis of several clinical studies of primarily nucleoside therapy, for those subjects with no reduction in plasma HIV-1 RNA level, subjects with a reduction in CD4+ cell count had a 30% greater risk of clinical progression over 2 years compared to those who had an increase in CD4+ cells above pretherapy levels.[172]

Additionally, therapy should provide an improved sense of patient well-being with minimal side effects. In targeting for the lowest plasma viral RNA level, consideration must be given to prior antiretroviral drug exposure, balancing therapy compliance, tolerability of the regimen, and long-term toxicity of the therapy regimen.[3,7,8,209]

MONITORING HIV-1 RNA IN PREGNANT WOMEN

Monitoring of viral RNA levels in pregnant women is no different than for nonpregnant women or men.[2,7,8] Surprisingly, the natural history of plasma viral RNA during pregnancy is not well characterized. In two relatively small studies, the maternal viral load did not rise during pregnancy.[210,211] However, in a larger cohort study of 198 HIV-1-infected women, plasma HIV-1 RNA levels were higher at 6 months postpartum than during antepartum in many of the women.[212] Although both the plasma viral RNA level and the CD4 cell count are independently predictive of vertical transmission risk, the change in plasma viral RNA level only explains, at most, 50% of the benefit of zidovudine therapy.[213] These data strongly suggest that there is a prophylactic benefit from antiretroviral therapy on vertical transmission. Despite the association between vertical transmission and maternal plasma viral RNA level,[213,214] there are no data to support the use of plasma viral RNA levels as a guide to changing antiretroviral therapy to reduce the risk of vertical transmission during pregnancy. Furthermore, because transmission may occur when plasma HIV-1 RNA is not detectable,[212,213] plasma HIV-1 RNA levels should not be the determining factor when deciding when to use antiretroviral prophylaxis.[2]

USE OF PLASMA VIRAL RNA TO DEFINE VIROLOGICAL FAILURE

A precise definition of therapeutic failure based on viral RNA level is wanting. Such a definition should embrace as a minimum, the clinical status of the patient, the CD4+ cell count, and the plasma viral RNA level. The failure of plasma viral RNA to decline by at least 30-fold (1.5 $\log_{10}$) or more from baseline following 4 to 8 weeks of therapy is generally considered to represent a suboptimal virological response.[3,8,172] In addition, many clinicians would also consider the inability to achieve undetectable plasma viral RNA by 12 to 24 weeks of therapy as evidence for therapeutic failure.[3,7,8]

It is important to consider that the relative benefit of a decline in plasma viral RNA is the same no matter where the pretherapy viral RNA level started, although the pretherapy plasma viral RNA level itself confers an additional, independent risk of disease progression. For example, a decline from 100,000 (5.0 $\log_{10}$) viral RNA copies/mL of plasma to 10,000 (4.0 $\log_{10}$) viral RNA copies/

mL of plasma represents the same relative 72% reduction (95% CI, 61% to 81%, $p < .001$) in risk of disease progression as a change from 10,000 to 1,000 (4.0 $\log_{10}$ to 3.0 $\log_{10}$) viral RNA copies/mL.[172] However, each of the two pretherapy plasma viral RNA levels of 5.0 $\log_{10}$ and 4.0 $\log_{10}$ copies/mL confers a different relative hazard of disease progression, after controlling for the baseline CD4+ cell count and therapy assignment.[172] The target of reaching undetectable plasma viral RNA after 12 to 24 weeks of therapy is also affected by the pretherapy plasma viral RNA level. Achieving a detectable plasma viral RNA level of less than 5,000 (3.7 $\log_{10}$) copies/mL when starting with 1,000,000 (6.0 $\log_{10}$) copies/mL will confer clinical benefit and may be all that is obtainable given a patient's prior antiretroviral therapy experience.

It has been somewhat arbitrarily set that any sustainable 0.5 $\log_{10}$ (3-fold) rise in plasma viral RNA above the therapy-induced plasma viral RNA nadir that is not attributable to intercurrent infection, vaccination, incomplete adherence to the antiretroviral therapy regimen, decreased absorption of antiretroviral drugs, altered drug metabolism, drug-drug interactions, or testing methodology, likely represents viral failure due to the emergence of drug-resistant HIV variants.[7,8,199]. However, this must be viewed cautiously for the following reasons.

Viral resistance

Genotypic and phenotypic changes associated with drug resistance in vitro are not always synonymous with clinical drug failure.[215] For example, in a large clinical study,[216] persons who had received prior zidovudine therapy for more than six months benefited clinically after switching to didanosine, but the presence of high-grade phenotypic or genotypic zidovudine resistance at baseline independently predicted clinical progression and death regardless of therapy assignment.[114,217] Plasma viral RNA level, viral syncytium-inducing phenotype, and CD4+ cell response to therapy were each independently associated with the risk of clinical progression.[123–126,171] Thus, the independent association of zidovudine susceptibility suggests a more complex relationship between zidovudine susceptibility, these three variables, and other unidentified viral and host factors. Moreover, although there is a movement in clinical practice to use genotypic susceptibility patterns to adjust antiretroviral therapy, one clinical trial showed that viral genotype did not predict the subsequent plasma viral RNA response when patients were switched to a susceptible protease inhibitor drug.[218]

Clearly, the correct interpretation of viral genotype is complicated by the complexity of the mutational patterns observed, the potential for undetected subpopulations of mutant virus, and residual effects of prior antiretroviral therapy.[218] Thus, the clinician should approach the clinical management of patients using viral genotypic analysis cautiously until definitive clinical trial data are available.

Discordant viral RNA and CD4 cell responses

There may be discordant response between a rise in plasma viral RNA and either a sustained or a continued rise in CD4+ cell count.[196,219] This discordance occurs in approximately 14% of patients who receive antiretroviral therapy[172] The discordant response has been associated with a decrease in disease progression, raising questions about the wisdom of changing antiretroviral therapy based solely on the plasma viral RNA response.[5,6] Many clinical trials provide study patients with the endpoint measurement (i.e., plasma viral RNA level) on a real-time basis. This practice raises serious concerns about the introduction of selection bias and the ability to define a viral RNA-based therapeutic failure.

Thus, in the absence of clinical trials data, if the sustained rise in plasma viral RNA while on therapy is to either less than 0.5 $\log_{10}$ above the plasma viral RNA therapy nadir or less than 5,000 (3.7 $\log_{10}$) copies/mL, whichever is less, it might be prudent to observe carefully for a further deterioration in CD4+ cell count or clinical progression before considering a change of therapy. A sustained rise in plasma viral RNA that exceeds these criteria should warrant a reassessment of the antiretroviral regimen for adherence and possible therapy failure. A more aggressive approach would consider any detectable plasma viral RNA worthy of a switch in therapy. Neither approach, however, has received validation by a controlled clinical trial.

CAVEATS FOR THE CLINICAL USE OF HIV-1 RNA

Uncertainty in measuring HIV-1 RNA level

There is uncertainty in assigning a value to a single plasma viral RNA measurement.[137] This uncertainty arises from specimen handling, the performance characteristics of the assay, the technical variability of the assay, whether the different specimens are tested by batch or real-time, and the infected person's natural variation in virus level.[200,202] In total, these factors define, with 95% confidence, a variability in the estimated plasma viral RNA copy number of at least 5-fold (0.7 $\log_{10}$) for single RNA measurements.[200–202] Consequently, a single measurement of plasma viral RNA is associated with a defined range of values above or below the measured value at least 95% of the time (2.5% of the time values may be greater than and 2.5% of the time less than this 5-fold range). For example, a person with a plasma viral RNA value of 5,000 copies/mL obtained from a single plasma specimen taken today may have a measured viral RNA value anywhere from 1,000 to 25,000 copies/mL on repeat testing of another blood draw taken within the next few days to weeks, falling within this range 95% of the time.[181]

A rigorous virology quality assurance program has shown that the intra-assay standard deviation for these assays ranges from less than 0.1 to 0.2 $\log_{10}$ HIV-1 RNA copies/mL of plasma.[137,220] This precision enables the assays to distinguish reliably 3- to 8-fold changes in plasma viral RNA for batched testing and 4- to 19-fold changes for real-time testing. Obviously, the uncertainty in defining the true plasma viral RNA level contributes important *uncertainty* for changing antiretroviral therapy based on a single plasma viral RNA value.

In addition to the above considerations, variability in interpreting absolute plasma viral RNA levels across different clinical studies arises because of the patient population studied, the use of serum or plasma to assess the viral RNA level, different viral RNA assay methods, and different anticoagulants and storage conditions. For example, viral RNA levels are generally one-half log value less for serum than for plasma depending on the assay method used; bDNA values are generally 2-fold less than those for RT-PCR; and heparin interferes with the detection of viral RNA by both bDNA and RT-PCR assays but not for NASBA[137,154]

Thus, some patients could have successful therapy regimens inappropriately changed based on estimates of plasma viral RNA levels that are associated with considerable uncertainty both in their measurement and in the clinical meaning of the plasma viral RNA value, particularly when the plasma viral RNA and CD4+ cell responses are discordant.[172] This is of particular concern for aggressive therapy management decisions based on the detectability of viral RNA near the reliable limit of detection for an assay. Plasma viral RNA assessments by both the bDNA and RT-PCR assays are usually concordant for most patients below the level of quantitation. However, these assessments will be discordant in approximately 20% of patients, and the decision to either maintain or switch antiviral therapy based on the assay quantitation limit will be affected by the choice of the viral RNA assay used.[221]

Adequacy of plasma HIV-1 RNA level alone for explaining the clinical response to therapy

Much remains to be learned about how the favorable and relatively short-term laboratory responses to potent antiretroviral therapy translate into the long-term survival of the individual infected with HIV-1. Of particular concern is the recovery of infectious virus from the presumably longer-lived resting T-lymphocytes after prolonged, potent antiretroviral therapy.[112,113] Nevertheless, with continued suppression of viral replication, and failure to demonstrate the development of genotypic resistance to therapy drugs, the long-term outlook for many patients is encouraging,[112,113] providing the potent therapies are tolerated.

The use of plasma viral RNA to clinically monitor HIV-1 infection should be based on the following three critical validation points.[124] First, plasma viral RNA is detected in most infected persons, and the level of plasma viral RNA is associated with disease progression. Second, a decline in plasma viral RNA with therapy is associated with improved clinical outcome, and a rise in plasma viral RNA is associated with clinical progression. Third, the change in plasma viral RNA level completely explains the clinical benefit of antiretroviral therapy.[6]

Clearly, fulfillment of these three validation criteria is necessary to completely understand the limitations of plasma viral RNA as a substitute marker for disease progression in clinical trials.[6] The first two criteria for surrogacy have been fulfilled in several clinical studies, and the associations between plasma viral RNA level and disease progression are highly significant statistically.[123–125,172,187,189,197,222] On the basis of both natural history and clinical trial studies (mostly from adult-based studies), it is now widely accepted that the lower the plasma viral RNA level the better the clinical outcome.[172,189]

Importantly, the third criterion has not been completely fulfilled. Change in plasma viral RNA level explains only a portion of the clinical response to therapy (probably less than one-half, but the estimates are very imprecise at this time); thus, plasma viral RNA is only a partial surrogate marker for clinical outcome.[6,123,213] Although this may seem paradoxical given fulfillment of the first two validation criteria and the strong association between the change in plasma viral RNA and disease progression, the partial surrogacy of plasma viral RNA for clinical outcome means that other host and virus properties are necessary for a complete understanding of disease progression in the individual patient;[223] presumably, such information may eventually help to better define the individual management of patients in clinical practice.[224]

CONCLUSION

The diagnosis of HIV-1 infection by detecting and confirming the presence of specific antibodies is being augmented by more rapid antibody detection assays. These rapid assays have the potential for use in sexually transmitted disease clinics and urgent care settings. By providing a more rapid assessment of infection status, clinicians can offer better counseling for patients.

The application of molecular techniques, such as PCR and other nucleic acid amplification technologies, provides earlier supplementary confirmation for the serologic determination of HIV-1 infection and in particular a more definitive and timely resolution of indeterminate immunoblot results. With repeat specimen collection and testing, the nucleic acid amplification technologies have a defined role for diagnosing HIV infection in the absence of antibody (i.e., acute infection) or in the presence of acquired antibody (i.e., neonatal infection).

The direct quantitation of HIV-1 RNA in plasma has revolutionized the clinical management of HIV-1-infected patients over the past two years. However, there are other factors, such as the host's immune status and the viral phenotype and genotype, that contribute important prognostic information about disease progression which are not necessarily captured by a single viral RNA value. Further laboratory characterization of clinical viral isolates for viral resistance genotype or phenotype and syncytium-inducing phenotype are not warranted for general use until their role in clinical practice is better defined.

ACKNOWLEDGMENTS

I would like to thank Dr. Patricia Reichelderfer for thoughtful discussion and redaction, and Pam Easterling and Lorita Thykkuttathil for manuscript preparation. Grant support: NIH AI-27664, AI-27757, AI-30731; Social and Scientific Systems, Inc., 96VC002 and 97PVCL02.

References

1 Jackson JB et al: Human immunodeficiency virus type 1 detected in all seropositive symptomatic and asymptomatic individuals. *J Clin Microbiol* 28:16–19, 1990.

2 Centers for Disease Control and Prevention: Public health service task force recommendations for the use of antiretroviral drugs in pregnant women infected with HIV-1 for maternal health and for reducing perinatal HIV-1 transmission in the United States. MMWR *Morb Mortal Wkly Rep* 47 (No RR-2):1–30, 1998.

3 Carpenter CCJ et al: Antiretroviral therapy for HIV infection in 1997. *JAMA* 277:1962–1969, 1997.

4 Fessel WJ: Human immunodeficiency virus (HIV) RNA in plasma as the preferred target for therapy in patients with HIV infection: a critique. *Clin Infect Dis* 24:116–122, 1997.

5 Fleming TR, DeMets DL: Surrogate endpoints in clinical trials: are we being misled? *Ann Intern Med* 125:605–613, 1996.

6 De Gruttola et al: Validating surrogate markers—are we being naive? *J Infect Dis* 175:237–46, 1997.

7 Office of AIDS Research of the National Institutes of Health (NIH): Report of the NIH Panel to Define Principles of Therapy of HIV Infection *(www.hivatis.org/guide6.pdf)*. Washington DC: U. S. Public Health Service, 1997.

8 United States Department of Health and Human Services and the Henry J. Kaiser Family Foundation Panel on Clinical Practices for Treatment of HIV Infection: Guidelines for the Use of Antiretroviral Agents in HIV-Infected Adults and Adolescents *(ww.hivatis.org/guide6.pdf)*, 1997.

9 Schleupner CJ: Detection of HIV-1 Infection, in *Mandell, Douglas, and Bennett's Principles and Practice of Infectious Diseases*, Mandell GL et al (eds). New York, Churchill Livingston, 1996.

10 Clementi M et al: Clinical use of quantitative molecular methods in studying human immunodeficiency virus type 1 infection. *Clin Microbiol Reviews* 9:135–147, 1996.

11 Proffitt MR, Yen-Lieberman B: Laboratory diagnosis of human immunodeficiency virus infection. *Infect Dis Clin North Am* 7:203–219, 1993.

12 Ferré F: Polymerase chain reaction and HIV. *Clin Lab Med* 14:313–333, 1994.

13 Holodniy M: Clinical application of reverse transcription-polymerase chain reaction for HIV infection. *Clin Lab Med* 14:335–349, 1994.

14 Atkins D: Screening for Human Immunodeficiency Virus Infection, in *US Preventive Services Task Force: Guide to Clinical Preventive Services*, DiGuiseppi C et al (eds). Alexandria VA, International Medical Publishing, 1996, pp 303–323.

15 Centers for Disease Control and Prevention: Interpretive criteria used to report western blot results for HIV-1-antibody testing—United States. *MMWR Morb Mort Wkly Rep* 40:692–695, 1991.

16 Centers for Disease Control and Prevention: Update: Serologic testing for antibody to human immunodeficiency virus. *MMWR Morb Mort Wkly Rep* 36:833–845, 1988.

17 Centers for Disease Control and Prevention: Interpretation and use of the Western blot assay for serodiagnosis of human immunodeficiency virus type 1 infections. *MMWR Morb Mort Wkly Rep* 39 (Suppl 7):1–7, 1989.

18 Schochetman G: Diagnosis of HIV infection. *Clinica Chemica Acta* 211:1–26, 1992.

19 Farzadegan H: HIV-1 antibodies and serology. Clin Lab Med 14: 257–269, 1994.

20 Gnann JW, Jr et al: Synthetic peptide immunoassay distinguishes HIV type 1 and HIV type 2 infections. *Science* 237:1346–1349, 1987.

21 Fenouillet E et al: Early and specific diagnosis of seropositivity to HIVs by an enzyme-linked immunosorbent assay using env-derived synthetic peptides. *AIDS* 4:1137–1140, 1990.

22 Horsburgh CR, Jr et al: Duration of human immunodeficiency virus infection before detection of antibody. *Lancet* 2:637–640, 1989.

23 Zaaijer HL et al: Early detection of antibodies to HIV-1 by third-generation assays. *Lancet* 340:770–772, 1992.

24 Centers for Disease Control and Prevention: Update: serologic testing for HIV-1 antibody—United States, 1988 and 1989. *MMWR Morb Mort Wkly Rep* 39:380–383, 1990.

25 Ascher DP, Roberts C: Determination of the etiology of seroreversals in HIV testing by antibody fingerprinting. J Acq Imm Defic Syndr 6: 241–244, 1993.

26 Johnson JE: Detection of human immunodeficiency virus type 1 antibody by using commercially available whole-cell viral lysate, synthetic peptide, and recombinant protein enzyme immunoassay systems. *J Clin Microbiol* 30:216–218, 1992.

27 Parry JV et al: Sensitivity of six commercial enzyme immunoassay kits that detect both anti-HIV-1 and anti-HIV-2. *AIDS* 4:4355–4360, 1990.

28 MacKenzie WR et al: Multiple false-positive serologic tests for HIV, HTLV-1, and hepatitis C following influenza vaccination. *JAMA* 268:1015–1017, 1992.

29 Esteva MH et al:. False positive results to antibody to HIV in two men with systemic lupus erythematosus. *Ann Rheum Dis* 51:1071–1073, 1992.

30 World Health Organization: Proposed WHO criteria for interpreting results from Western blot assays for HIV-1, HIV-2, and HTLV-I/HTLV-II. *Wkly Epidemiol Rec* 37:281–283, 1990.

31 The Consortium for Retrovirus Serology Standardization: Serologic diagnosis of human immunodeficiency virus infection by Western blot testing. *JAMA* 260:674–679, 1988.

32 Centers for Disease Control and Prevention: Model performance evaluation program: testing for human immunodeficiency virus type-1 (HIV-1) infection. Washington DC, Department of Health and Human Services, 1991.

33 Burke DS et al: Measurement of the false-positive rate in a screening program for human immunodeficiency virus infections. *N Engl J Med* 319:961–964, 1988.

34 MacDonald KL et al: Performance characteristics of serologic tests of human immunodeficiency virus type-1 (HIV-1) antibody among Minnesota blood donors. *Ann Intern Med* 110:617–621, 1989.

35 Celum CL, Coombs RW: Indeterminate HIV-1 Western blots: implications and considerations for widespread HIV testing. *J Gen Intern Med* 7:640–645, 1992.

36 Farzadegan H et al: Loss of human immunodeficiency virus type 1 (HIV-1) antibodies with evidence of viral infection in asymptomatic homosexual men. A report from the Multicenter AIDS Cohort Study. *Ann Intern Med* 108:785–790, 1988.

37 Roy MJ et al: Absence of true seroreversion of HIV-1 antibody in seroreactive individuals. *JAMA* 269:2876–2879, 1993.

38 Sullivan MT et al: Evaluation of an indirect immunofluorescence assay for confirmation of human immunodeficiency virus type 1 antibody in U.S. blood donor sera. *J Clin Microbiol* 30:2509–2510, 1992.

39 Urassa WK et al: Alternative confirmatory strategies in HIV-1 antibody testing. *J AIDS* 5:170–176, 1992.

40 Nair BC et al: Enzyme immunoassay using native envelope glycoprotein (gp160) for detection of human immunodeficiency virus type 1 antibodies. *J Clin Microbiol* 32:1449–1456, 1994.

41 Fonseca K, Anand CM. Predicting human immunodeficiency virus type 1-positive sera by using two enzyme immunoassay kits in a parallel testing format. *J Clin Microbiol* 29:2507–2512, 1991.

42 Ng VL et al: Reliable confirmation of antibodies to human immunodeficiency virus type 1 (HIV-1) with an enzyme-linked immunoassay using recombinant antigens derived from the HIV-1 gag, pol, and env genes. *J Clin Microbiol* 27:977–982, 1989.

43 Busch MP et al: Reliable confirmation and quantitation of human immunodeficiency virus type 1 antibody using a recombinant-antigen immunoblot assay. *Transfusion* 31:129–137, 1991.

44 Sato PA et al: Strategies for laboratory HIV testing: an examination of alternative approaches not requiring Western blot. *Bull WHO* 72: 129–134, 1994.

45 Brennan TA: Transmission of the human immunodeficiency virus in the health care setting—time for action. *N Engl J Med* 324:1498–1500, 1991.

46 Celum CL et al: Indeterminate human immunodeficiency virus type 1 Western blots: seroconversion risk, specificity of supplemental tests, and an algorithm for evaluation. *J Infect Dis* 164:656–664, 1991.

47 Ranki A, et al: Long latency precedes overt seroconversion in sexually transmitted human-immunodeficiency-virus infection. *Lancet* 1:589–593, 1987.

48 Henrard DR et al: Detection of human immunodeficiency virus type 1 p24 antigen and plasma RNA: relevance to indeterminate serologic tests. *Transfusion* 34:376–380, 1994.

49 Clark SJ et al: Unsuspected primary human immunodeficiency virus type 1 infection in seronegative emergency department patients. *J Infect Dis* 170:194–197, 1994.

50 Montagnier L et al: Human immunodeficiency virus infection and AIDS in a person with negative serology. *J Infect Dis* 175:955–959, 1997.

51 Zaaijer HL et al: Temporary seronegativity in a human immunodeficiency virus type 1 infected man. *J Med Virol* 51:80–82, 1997.

52 O'Brien TR et al: Testing for antibodies to human immunodeficiency virus type 2 in the United States. *MMWR Morb Mort Wkly Rep* 41(No RR-12):1–9, 1992.

53 Celum CL et al: Risk factors for repeatedly reactive HIV-1 EIA and indeterminate Western blot. *Arch Intern Med* 54:1129–1137, 1993.

54 Coutlée F et al:. Absence of prolonged immunosilent infection with human immunodeficiency virus in individuals with high-risk behaviors. *Am J Med* 96:42–48, 1994.

55 Brown AE et al: Viral RNA in the resolution of human immunodeficiency virus type 1 diagnostic serology. *Transfusion* 37:926–929, 1998.

56 Eble BE, et al: Resolution of infection status of human immunodeficiency virus (HIV)-seroindeterminate donors and high-risk seronegative individuals with polymerase chain reaction and virus culture: absence of persistent silent HIV type 1 infection in a high-prevalence area. *Transfusion* 32:497–499, 1992.

57 Constantine NT. Serologic tests for the retroviruses: approaching a decade of evolution. *AIDS* 7:1–13, 1993.

58 Quinn TC et al: Rapid latex agglutination assay using recombinant envelope polypeptide for the detection of antibody to the HIV. *JAMA* 260:510–513, 1988.

59 Mitchell SW et al: Field evaluation of alternative HIV testing strategy with a rapid immunobinding assay and an agglutination assay. *Lancet* 337:1328–1331, 1991.

60 Kassler et al: Performance of a rapid, on-site human immunodeficiency virus antibody assay in a public health setting. *J Clin Microbiol* 33:2899–2902, 1995.

61 Samdal HH et al: Comparison of the sensitivity of four rapid assays for detection of antibodies to HIV-1/HIV-2 during seroconversion. *Clin Diag Virol* 7:44–61, 1996.

62 Malone JD et al: Comparative evaluation of six rapid serological tests for HIV-1 antibody. *J Acq Imm Def Synd* 6:115–119, 1993.
63 Spielberg et al: Field testing and comparative evaluation of rapid, visually read screening assays for antibody to human immunodeficiency virus. *Lancet* 1:580–584, 1989.
64 Spielberg et al: Performance and cost-effectiveness of a dual rapid assay system for screening and confirmation of human immunodeficiency virus type 1 seropositivity. *J Clin Microbiol* 28:303–306, 1990.
65 Starkey CA et al: Evaluation of the Recombigen HIV-1 Latex Agglutination Test. *J Clin Microbiol* 28:819–822, 1990.
66 Kassler WJ et al: On-site, rapid HIV testing with same-day results and counseling. *AIDS* 11:1045–1051, 1997.
67 Irwin K, et al: Performance characteristics of a rapid HIV antibody assay in a hospital with a high prevalence of HIV infection. CDC-Bronx-Lebanon HIV Serosurvey Team. *Ann Intern Med* 125:471–475, 1996.
68 Fortes P et al: Evaluation of blood collected on filter paper for detection of antibodies to human immunodeficiency virus type 1. *J Clin Microbiol* 27:1380–1381, 1989.
69 Beebe JL, Briggs LC: Evaluation of enzyme-linked immunoassay systems for detection of human immunodeficiency virus type 1 antibody from filter paper disks impregnated with whole blood. *J Clin Microbiol* 28:808–810, 1990.
70 Behets F et al: Stability of human immunodeficiency virus type 1 antibodies in whole blood dried on filter paper and stored under various tropical conditions in Kinshasa, Zaire. *J Clin Microbiol* 30:1179–1182, 1992.
71 Emmons WW et al: A modified ELISA and western blot accurately determine anti-human immunodeficiency virus type 1 antibodies in oral fluids obtained with a special collecting device. *J Infect Dis* 171: 1406–1410, 1995.
72 Malamud D: Oral diagnostic testing for detecting human immunodeficiency virus-1 antibodies: a technology whose time has come. *Am J Med* 102(Suppl 4A):9–14, 1997.
73 Gallo D et al: Evaluation of a system using oral mucosal transudate for HIV-1 antibody screening and confirmatory testing. *JAMA* 277: 254–258, 1997.
74 Emmons WW: Accuracy of oral specimen testing for human immunodeficiency virus. *Am J Med* 102(Suppl 4A):15–20, 1997.
75 Urnovitz HB et al: HIV-1 antibody serum negativity with urine positivity. *Lancet* 342:1458–1459, 1993.
76 Charneau P et al: Isolation and envelope sequence of a divergent HIV-1 isolate: definition of a new HIV-1 group. *Virology* 205:247–253, 1994.
77 Urnovitz HB, et al: Urine-based diagnostic technologies. *Trends Biotechnol* 14:361–364, 1996.
78 Berrios DC et al: Screening for human immunodeficiency virus antibody in urine. *Arch Pathol Lab Med* 119:139–141, 1995.
79 Urnovitz HB et al: Increased sensitivity of HIV-1 antibody detection. *Nat Med* 3:1258, 1997.
80 Korber B, Hoelsher M. HIV-1 subtypes: implications for epidemiology, pathogenicity, vaccines and diagnostics—Workshop report from the European Commission (DG XII, INCO-DC) and the joint United Nations programme on HIV/AIDS. *AIDS* 11:UNAIDS17-UNAIDS36, 1997.
81 Peeters M et al: Presence of HIV-1 group O infection in West Africa. *AIDS* 10:343–344, 1996.
82 Mauclere P et al: Serological and virological characterization of HIV-1 group O infection in Cameroon. *AIDS* 11:445–453, 1997.
83 De Leys R et al: Isolation and partial characterization of an unusual human immunodeficiency retrovirus from two persons of West-Central African origin. *J Virol* 64:1207–1216, 1990.
84 Hampl H et al: First case of HIV-1 subtype O infection in Germany. *Infection* 23:369–370, 1995.
85 Britvan L et al: Identification of HIV-1 group O infection—Los Angeles county, California. *MMWR Morb Mort Wkly Rep* 45:561–565, 1996.
86 Apetrei C et al: Lack of screening test sensitivity during HIV-1 non-subtype B seroconversions. *AIDS* 10:F57-F60, 1996.
87 Simon F et al: Sensitivity of screening kits for anti-HIV-1 subtype O antibodies. *AIDS* 8:1628–1629, 1994.
88 Schable C et al: Sensitivity of United States HIV antibody tests for detection of HIV-1 group O infections. *Lancet* 344:1333–1334, 1994.
89 Loussert-Ajaka I et al: HIV-1/HIV-2 seronegativity in HIV-1 subtype O infected patients. *Lancet* 343:1393–1394, 1994.
90 Gürtler L. Difficulties and strategies of HIV diagnosis. *Lancet* 348: 176–179, 1996.
91 Lefrère JJ et al: No evidence of frequent human immunodeficiency virus type 1 infection in seronegative at-risk individuals. *Transfusion* 31:205–211, 1991.
92 Arnold C et al: HIV type 1 sequence G transmission from mother to infant: failure of variant sequence species to amplify in the Roche Amplicor test. *AIDS Res Hum Retrovirus* 11:999–1001, 1995.
93 Coste J, et al: Comparative evaluation of three assays for the quantitation of human immunodeficiency virus type 1 RNA in plasma. *Med Virol* 50:293–302, 1996.
94 Pfützner A et al: HIV-1 ad HIV-2 infections in a high-risk population in Bombay, India: evidence for the spread of HIV-2 and presence of a divergent HIV-1 subtype. *J Acq Immun Defic Syndr* 5:972–977, 1992.
95 Grez M et al: Genetic analysis of human immunodeficiency virus type 1 and 2 (HIV-1 and HIV-2) mixed infections in India reveals a recent spread of HIV-1 and HIV-2 from a single ancestor for each of these viruses. *J Virol* 68:2161–2168, 1994.
96 Onorato IM et al: Sentinel surveillance for HIV-2 infection in high-risk US populations. *Am J Public Health* 83:515–519, 1993.
97 Centers for Disease Control and Prevention: Update: HIV-2 infection among blood and plasma donors—United States, June 1992-June 1995. *MMWR Morb Mort Wkly Rep* 44:603–606, 1995.
98 Hu DJ et al: The emerging genetic diversity of HIV. The importance of global surveillance for diagnostics, research, and prevention. *JAMA* 275:210–216, 1996.
99 Guyader M et al: Genome organization and transactivation of the human immunodeficiency virus type 2. *Nature* 326:662–669, 1987.
100 George JR et al: Efficacies of US Food and Drug Administration-licensed HIV-1-screening enzyme immunoassays for detecting antibodies to HIV-2. *AIDS* 4:321–326, 1990.
101 Busch MP et al: Monitoring blood donors for HIV-2 infection by testing anti-HIV-1 reactive sera. *Transfusion* 30:184–187, 1990.
102 Centers for Disease Control and Prevention:. Testing for antibodies to human immunodeficiency virus type 2 in the United States. MMWR Morb Mort Wkly Rep 41(R-12):1–8, 1992.
103 Kloser PC et al: HIV-2-associated AIDS in the United States: the first case. *Arch Intern Med* 149:1875–1877, 1989.
104 Rayfield M et al: Mixed human immunodeficiency virus (HIV) infection of an individual: demonstration of both HIV type 1 and HIV type 2 proviral sequences by polymerase chain reaction. *J Infect Dis* 158:170–176, 1988.
105 Pieniazek D et al: Identification of mixed HIV-1/HIV-2 infections in Brazil by polymerase chain reaction. *AIDS* 5:129–1299, 1991.
106 Nicholson JKA, et al:. Serial determinations of HIV-1 titers in HIV-infected homosexual men: association of rising titers with CD4 T cell depletion and progression to AIDS. *AIDS Res Hum Retrovirus* 5: 205–215, 1989.
107 Coombs RW et al:. Plasma viremia in human immunodeficiency virus infection. *N Engl J Med* 321:1626–1631, 1989.
108 Ho DD et al: Quantitation of human immunodeficiency virus type 1 in the blood of infected persons. *N Engl J Med* 321:1621–1625, 1989.
109 Schacker T et al: Clinical and epidemiologic features of primary HIV infection. *Ann Intern Med* 125:257–264, 1996.
110 Centers for Disease Control and Prevention: Public Health Service Task Force on use of zidovudine to reduce perinatal transmission of human immunodeficiency virus. *MMWR Morb Mort Wkly Rep* 43 (RR-11):1–21, 1994.

111 Paul MO et al: Laboratory diagnosis of infection status in infants perinatally exposed to human immunodeficiency virus type 1. *J Infect Dis* 173:68–76, 1995.

112 Finzi D et al: Identification of a reservoir for HIV-1 in patients on highly active antiretroviral therapy. *Science* 278:1295–1300, 1997.

113 Wong JK, et al: Recovery of replication-competent HIV despite prolonged suppression of plasma viremia. *Science* 278:1291–1295, 1997.

114 D'Aquilla RT et al: Zidovudine resistance and HIV-1 disease progression during antiretroviral therapy. *Ann Intern Med* 122:401–408, 1995.

115 Bollinger RC, Jr et al: Acid dissociation increases the sensitivity of p24 antigen detection for the evaluation of antiviral therapy and disease progression in asymptomatic human immunodeficiency virus-infected persons. *J Infect Dis* 165:913–916, 1992.

116 Quinn TC et al: Acid dissociation of immune complexes improves diagnostic utility of p24 antigen detection in perinatally acquired human immunodeficiency virus infection. *J Infect Dis* 167:1193–1196, 1993.

117 Alter HJ et al and the HIV-Antigen Study Group: Prevalence of human immunodeficiency virus type 1 p24 antigen in U.S. blood donors: an assessment of the efficacy of testing in donor screening. *N Engl J Med* 323:1312–1317, 1990.

118 Busch MP et al and the Transfusion Safety Study Group: Screening of selected male blood donors for p24 antigen of human immunodeficiency virus type 1. *N Engl J Med* 323:1308–1312, 1990.

119 Phair JP et al: Detection of infection with human immunodeficiency virus type 1 before seroconversion: correlation with clinical symptoms and outcome. *J Infect Dis* 175:959–962, 1997.

120 Shearer WT et al and the Women and Infants Transmission Study Group: Viral load and disease progression in infants infected with human immunodeficiency virus type 1. *N Engl J Med* 336:1337–1342, 1997.

121 Mariotti M et al: Failure to detect evidence of human immunodeficiency virus type 1 (HIV-1) infection by polymerase chain reaction assay in blood donors with isolated core antibodies (anti-p14 or -p17) to HIV-1. *Transfusion* 30:704–706, 1990.

122 Mellors JW et al: Prognosis in HIV-1 infection predicted by the quantity of virus in plasma. *Science* 272:1167–70, 1996.

123 O'Brien WA et al: Changes in plasma HIV-1 RNA and CD4+ lymphocyte counts and the risk of progression to AIDS. *N Engl J Med* 334:426–431, 1996.

124 Coombs et al for the AIDS Clinical Trials Group (ACTG) 116B/17 Study Team and the ACTG Virology Committee Resistance and HIV-1 RNA Working Groups: Association of plasma human immunodeficiency virus type 1 RNA level with risk of clinical progression in patients with advanced infection. *J Infect Dis* 174:704–712, 1996.

125 Welles SL et al for the AIDS Clinical Trials Group Protocol 116A/116B/117 Team: Prognostic value of plasma HIV-1 RNA levels in patients with advanced HIV-1 disease and with little or no zidovudine therapy. *J Infect Dis* 174:696–703, 1996.

126 Katzenstein DA et al: The relation of virologic and immunologic markers to clinical outcomes after nucleoside therapy in HIV-infected adults with 200 to 500 CD4 cells per cubic millimeter. *N Engl J Med* 335:1091–1098, 1996.

127 Hammer SM et al: A controlled trial of two nucleoside analogues plus indinavir in persons with human immunodeficiency virus infection and CD4 counts of 200 per cubic millimeter or less. *N Engl J Med* 337:725–733, 1997.

128 Owens KK, et al: A meta-analytic evaluation of the polymerase chain reaction for the diagnosis of HIV infection in infants. *JAMA* 275: 1342–1348, 1996.

129 Bremer JW et al: Diagnosis of infection with human immunodeficiency virus type 1 by a DNA polymerase chain reaction assay among infants enrolled in the Women and Infants Transmission Study. *J Pediatr* 129:198–207, 1996.

130 Kwok S, Higuchi R. Avoiding false positives with PCR. *Nature* 339: 237–238, 1989.

131 Longo MC et al: Use of uracil DNA glycosylase to control carry-over contamination in polymerase chain reactions. *Gene* 93:125–128, 1990.

132 Jackson JB. Detection and quantitation of human immunodeficiency virus type 1 using molecular DNA/RNA technology. *Arch Pathol Lab Med* 117:473–477, 1993.

133 Saiki RK et al: Analysis of enzymatically amplified beta-globin and HLA DQ alpha with allele-specific oligonucleotide probes. *Nature* 324:163–165, 1986.

134 Defer C et al: Multicenter quality control of polymerase chain reaction for detection of HIV DNA. *AIDS* 6:659–663, 1992.

135 Jackson BJ et al and the ACTG PCR Working Group and the ACTG PCR Virology Laboratories: Establishment of a quality assurance program for human immunodeficiency virus type 1 DNA polymerase chain reaction assays by the AIDS Clinical Trials Group. *J Clin Microbiol* 31:3123–3128, 1993.

136 Schuurman R, et al: Multicenter comparison of three commercial methods for quantification of human immunodeficiency virus type 1 RNA in plasma. *J Clin Microbiol* 34:3016–3022, 1996.

137 Brambilla R, et al: Absolute copy number and relative change in determinations of human immunodeficiency virus type 1 RNA in plasma: effect of an external standard on kit comparisons. *J Clin Microbiol* 36:311–314, 1998

138 Owens DK et al: Polymerase chain reaction for the diagnosis of HIV infection in adults. A meta-analysis with recommendations for clinical practice and study design. *Ann Intern Med* 124:803–815, 1996.

139 De Saussure P et al: HIV-1 nucleic acids detected before p24 antigenemia in a blood donor. *Transfusion* 33:164–167, 1993.

140 Piatak MJ et al: Viral dynamics in primary HIV-1 infection (Letter). *Lancet* 341:1099, 1993.

141 Piatak M et al: High levels of HIV-1 in plasma during all stages of infection determined by competitive PCR. *Science* 259:1749–54, 1993.

142 Mulder J et al: Rapid and simple PCR assay for quantification of human immunodeficiency type 1 RNA in plasma: application to acute retroviral infection. *J Clin Microbiol* 32:292–300, 1994.

143 Steketee RW et al: Early detection of perinatal human immunodeficiency virus (HIV) type 1 infection using HIV RNA amplification and detection. *J Infect Dis* 175:707–711, 1997.

144 Schwartz DH et al: Extensive evaluation of a seronegative participant in an HIV-1 vaccine trial as a result of false-positive PCR. *Lancet* 350:256–259, 1997.

145 Harrigan R. Measuring viral load in the clinical setting. *J Acq Immun Defic Syndr Hum Retrovirol* 10(Suppl 1):S34-S40, 1995.

146 Saag MS. Use of virologic markers in clinical practice. *J Acq Immun Defic Syndr Hum Retrovirol* 16(Suppl 1):S3-S13, 1997.

147 Kievits T et al: NASBA isothermal enzymatic in vitro nucleic acid amplification optimized for the diagnosis of HIV-1 infection. *J Virol Methods* 35:273–286, 1991.

148 Vandamme et al: Detection of HIV-1 RNA in plasma and serum samples using the NASBA amplification system compared to RNA-PCR. *J Virol Methods* 52:121–132, 1995.

149 Vandamme et al: Quantification of HIV-1 RNA in plasma: comparable results with NASBA HIV-1 RNA QT and the Amplicor HIV Monitor test. *J Acq Immun Defic Syndr* 13:127–139, 1996.

150 Todd J et al: Quantitation of human immunodeficiency virus plasma RNA by branched DNA and reverse transcription coupled polymerase chain reaction assay methods: a critical evaluation of accuracy and reproducibility. *Serodiagn Immunother Infect Dis* 6:233–239, 1994.

151 Collins ML et al: A branched DNA signal amplification assay for quantification of nucleic acid targets below 100 molecules/mL. *Nucleic Acids Res* 25:2979–2984, 1997.

152 Mulder J et al:. A rapid and simple method for extracting human immunodeficiency virus type 1 RNA from plasma: enhanced sensitivity. *J Clin Microbiol* 35:1278–1280, 1997.

153 Holodniy M et al: Comparative stabilities of quantitative human immunodeficiency virus RNA in plasma from samples collected in VA-

CUTAINER CPT, VACUTAINER PPT, and standard VACUTAINER tubes. *J Clin Microbiol* 33:1562–1566, 1995.

154 Lew J et al: Plasma HIV-1 RNA determinations: reassessment of parameters affecting assay outcome. *J Clin Microbiol,* 1998 (in press).

155 Sebire K et al: Stability of human immunodeficiency virus RNA in blood specimens as measured by a commercial PCR-based assay. *J Clin Microbiol* 36:493–498, 1998.

156 Cassol S et al: Stability of dried blood spot specimens for detection of human immunodeficiency virus DNA by polymerase chain reaction. *J Clin Microbiol* 30:3039–3042, 1992.

157 Comeau AM et al: Early detection of human immunodeficiency virus on dried blood spot specimens: sensitivity across serial specimens. *J Pediatr* 129:111–118, 1996.

158 Fiscus et al: Quantitation of human immunodeficiency virus type 1 RNA in plasma by using blood dried on filter paper. *J Clin Microbiol* 36:258–260, 1998.

159 Cassol et al: Detection of HIV type 1 env subtypes A, B, C, and E in Asia using dried blood spots: a new surveillance tool for molecular epidemiology. *AIDS Res Hum Retrovirus* 12:1435–1441, 1996.

160 Leigh-Brown AJ, Richman DD. HIV-1: Gambling on the evolution of drug resistance? *Nat Med* 3:268–271, 1997.

161 D'Aquila R. HIV-1 drug resistance. *Clin Lab Med* 14:393–422, 1994.

162 Japour AJ et al and the RV-43 Study Group and the AIDS Clinical Trials Group Virology Committee Resistance Working Group: Standardized blood mononuclear cell culture assay for determination of drug susceptibilities of clinical human immunodeficiency virus type 1 isolates. *Antimicrob Agents Chemother* 37:1095–1101, 1993.

163 Nijhuis M et al: Homologous recombination for rapid phenotyping of HIV. *Curr Opin Infect Dis* 10:474–479, 1997.

164 Schuurman R. State of the art of genotypic HIV-1 drug resistance. *Curr Opin Infect Dis* 10:480–484, 1997.

165 Larder BA et al: Zidovudine resistance predicted by direct detection of mutations in DNA from HIV-infected lymphocytes. *AIDS* 5:137–144, 1991.

166 Kaye S, et al: A microtiter format point mutation assay: application to the detection of drug resistance in human immunodeficiency virus type-1 infected patients treated with zidovudine. J *Med Virol* 37:241–246, 1992.

167 Eastman PS et al: Nonisotopic hybridization assay for determination of relative amounts of genotypic human immunodeficiency virus type-1 zidovudine resistance. *J Clin Microbiol* 33:2777–2780, 1995.

168 Frenkel LM et al: Specific, sensitive, and rapid assay for human immunodeficiency virus type 1 pol mutations associated with resistance to zidovudine and didanosine. *J Clin Microbiol* 33:342–347, 1995.

169 Stuyver L et al: Line probe assay for rapid detection of drug-selected mutations in the human immunodeficiency virus type 1 reverse transcription gene. *Antimicrob Agents Chemother* 41:284–291, 1997.

170 Larder BA et al: Potential mechanism for sustained antiretroviral efficacy of AZT-3TC combination therapy. *Science* 269:696–699, 1995.

171 Brun-Vézinet F et al: HIV-1 viral load, phenotype, and resistance in a subset of drug-naive participants from the Delta trial. *Lancet* 350: 983–990, 1997.

172 Marschner I et al: Use of changes in plasma human immunodeficiency virus type 1 RNA to assess the clinical benefit of antiretroviral therapy. *J Infect Dis* 177:40–47, 1998.

173 Henrard DR et al: Natural history of cell-free viremia. *JAMA* 274: 554–558, 1995.

174 Hogervorst E et al: Predictors for non and slow progression in human immunodeficiency virus (HIV) type 1 infection: low viral RNA copy numbers in serum and maintenance of high HIV-1 p24 specific but not V3-specific antibody levels. *J Infect Dis* 171:811–821, 1995.

175 Ho D et al: Rapid turnover of plasma virions and CD4 lymphocytes in HIV-1 infection. *Nature* 373:123–126, 1995.

176 Wei X et al: Viral dynamics in human immunodeficiency virus type 1 infection. *Nature* 373:117–122, 1995.

177 Perelson AS et al: HIV-1 dynamics in vivo: virion clearance rate, infected cell life-span, and viral generation time. *Science* 217:1582–1586, 1996.

178 Perelson AS et al: Decay characteristics of HIV-1-infected compartments during combination therapy. *Nature* 387:188–191, 1997.

179 Stellbrink H-J et al: Asymptomatic HIV infection is characterized by rapid turnover of HIV-RNA in plasma and lymph nodes but not of latently infected lymph-node CD4+ T cells. *AIDS* 11:1103–1110, 1997.

180 Peeters MF et al: Comparison of human immunodeficiency virus biological phenotypes isolated from cerebrospinal fluid and peripheral blood. *J Med Virol* 47:92–96, 1995.

181 Coombs RW, et al: Association between culturable human immunodeficiency virus type-1 (HIV-1) in semen and HIV-1 RNA levels in semen and blood: evidence for compartmentalization of HIV-1 between semen and blood. *J Infect Dis* 177:320–330, 1998.

182 Jurriaans S et al: The natural history of HIV-1 infection: virus load and virus phenotype independent determinants of clinical course? *Virology* 204:223–233, 1994.

183 Rosenberg et al and the Multicenter Hemophilia Cohort Study and the International Registry of Seroconverters: Effect of age at seroconversion on the natural AIDS incubation distribution. *AIDS* 8:803–810, 1994.

184 Kroner BL et al and the Multicenter Hemophilia Cohort and Hemophilia Growth and Development Studies: Concordance of human leukocyte antigen haplotype-sharing, CD4 decline, and AIDS in hemophilic siblings. *AIDS* 9:275–280, 1995.

185 Ioannidis JPA, et al: Predictive value of viral load measurements in asymptomatic untreated HIV-1 infection: a mathematical model. *AIDS* 10:255–262, 1996.

186 Mellors JW et al: Quantitation of HIV-1 RNA in plasma predicts outcome after seroconversion. *Ann Intern Med* 112:573–579, 1995.

187 O'Brien TR et al: Serum HIV-1 RNA levels and time to development of AIDS in the multicenter hemophilia cohort study. *JAMA* 276:105–110, 1996.

188 Saksela K et al: HIV-1 messenger RNA in peripheral blood mononuclear cells with an early marker of risk for progression to AIDS. *Ann Intern Med* 123:641–648, 1995.

189 Mellors JW et al: Plasma viral load and CD4+ lymphocytes as prognostic markers of HIV-1 infection. *Ann Intern Med* 126:946–954, 1997.

190 Schacker TW, et al: Biological and virological characteristics of primary HIV infection. *Ann Intern Med* 128, 1998 (in press).

191 Musey L et al: Cytotoxic-T-cell responses, viral load, and disease progression in early human immunodeficiency virus type 1 infection. *N Engl J Med* 337:1267–1274, 1997.

192 Rosenberg ES et al: Vigorous HIV-1-specific CD4+ T cell responses associated with control of viremia. *Science* 278:1447–1450, 1997.

193 Schacker T et al: Viral load in acute and very early HIV infection does not correlate with disease progression. Fourth Conference on Retroviruses and Opportunistic Infections, Washington DC, January 22–26, 1997, Abstract 475, p 152.

194 de Wolf F et al: AIDS prognosis based on HIV-1 RNA, CD4+ T-cell count and function: markers with reciprocal predictive value over time after seroconversion. *AIDS* 11:1799–1806, 1997.

195 Mofenson LM et al: The relationship between serum human immunodeficiency virus type 1 (HIV-1) RNA level, CD4 lymphocyte percent, and long-term mortality risk in HIV-1-infected children. *J Infect Dis* 175:1029–1038, 1997.

196 Reichelderfer PS, Coombs RW. Cartesian coordinate analysis of viral burden and CD4+ T-cell count in human immunodeficiency virus type-1 infection. *Antiviral Res,* 1998 (in press).

197 Hughes MD et al: Monitoring plasma HIV-1 RNA levels in addition to CD4+ lymphocyte count improves assessment of antiretroviral therapeutic response. *Ann Intern Med* 126:929–938, 1997.

198 Gulick RM et al: Treatment with indinavir, zidovudine, and lamivudine in adults with human immunodeficiency virus infection and prior antiretroviral therapy. *N Engl J Med* 337:734–739, 1997.

199 Saag MS et al: HIV viral load markers in clinical practice. *Nat Med* 2:625–629, 1996.
200 Raboud JM et al: Variation in plasma RNA levels, CD4 count, and p24 antigen levels in clinically stable men with human immunodeficiency virus infection. *J Infect Dis* 174:191–194, 1996.
201 Raboud JM, et al: Issues in the design of trials of therapies for subjects with human immunodeficiency virus infection that use plasma RNA level as an outcome. *J Infect Dis* 175:576–582, 1997.
202 Paxton WB et al: Longitudinal analysis of quantitative virologic measures in human immunodeficiency virus-infected subjects with ≥400 CD4 lymphocytes: implications for applying measurements to individual patients. *J Infect Dis* 175:247–54, 1997.
203 Deeks SG et al: Variance of plasma HIV-1 RNA levels measured by branched DNA (bDNA) within and between days. *J Infect Dis* 176: 514–517, 1997.
204 Demeter L et al: Predictors of virologic and clinical responses to indinavir (IDV)+ZDV+3TC or ZDV+3TC. Fifth National Conference on Retroviruses and Opportunistic Infections, Chicago IL, February 1–5, 1998, Abstract 509, p 175.
205 Ho DD. Time to hit HIV, early and hard. *N Engl J Med* 331:1173–80, 1995.
206 Dube MP et al: Protease inhibitor-associated hyperglycemia. *Lancet* 350:713, 1997.
207 Hengel RL et al: Benign symmetric lipomatosis associated with protease inhibitors. *Lancet* 350:1596, 1997
208 Stein DS, et al: CD4+ lymphocyte cell enumeration for prediction of clinical course of human immunodeficiency virus disease: a review. *J Infect Dis* 165:352–363, 1992.
209 BHIVA Guidelines Co-ordinating Committee. British HIV Association guidelines for antiretroviral treatment of HIV seropositive individuals. *Lancet* 349:1086–1092, 1997.
210 Weiser B et al: Quantitation of human immunodeficiency virus type 1 during pregnancy: Relationship of viral titer to mother-to-child transmission and stability of viral load. *Proc Natl Acad Sci USA* 91: 8037–8041, 1994.
211 Melvin AJ et al: Effect of pregnancy and zidovudine therapy on viral load in HIV-1-infected women. *J AIDS Hum Retrovirol* 14:232–236, 1997.
212 Cao Y et al: Maternal HIV-1 viral load and vertical transmission of infection. *Nat Med* 3:549–52, 1997.
213 Sperling RS, et al: Maternal viral load, zidovudine treatment, and the risk of transmission of human immunodeficiency virus type 1 from mother to infant. *N Engl J Med* 335:1621–29, 1996.
214 Dickover RE et al: Identification of levels of maternal HIV-1 RNA associated with risk of perinatal transmission: effect of maternal zidovudine treatment on viral load. *JAMA* 275:599–605, 1996.
215 Kuritzkes DR: Clinical significance of drug resistance in HIV-1 infection. *AIDS* 10(Suppl 5):S27-S31, 1996.
216 Kahn JO et al: A controlled trial comparing continued zidovudine with didanosine in human immunodeficiency virus infection. *N Engl J Med* 327:581–587, 1992.
217 Japour AJ, Welles et al: Prevalence and clinical significance of zidovudine resistance mutations in human immunodeficiency virus isolated from patients after long-term zidovudine treatment. *J Infect Dis* 171:1172–1179, 1995.
218 Para MF et al: Relationship of baseline genotype to RNA response in ACTG 333 after switching from long term saquinavir (SQVhc) to indinavir (IDV) or saquinavir soft gelatin capsule (SQVsgc). Fifth National Conference on Retroviruses and Opportunistic Infections, Chicago IL, February 1–5, 1998, Abstract 511, p 175.
219 Reichelderfer PS, Coombs RW. Cartesian coordinate analysis of viral burden and CD4+ cell count in HIV disease: implications for clinical trial design and analysis. *Antiviral Res* 29:83–86, 1996.
220 Lin HJ et al: Multicenter evaluation of methods for the quantitation of plasma HIV-1 RNA. *J Infect Dis* 170:553–62, 1994.
221 Yerkovich et al: Low HIV-1 RNA copy number assessed by bDNA and RT-PCR assays: implications for managing patients above or below the viral RNA quantitation limit. Fifth National Conference on Human Retroviruses, Chicago IL, February 1–5, 1998, Abstract 303, p 136.
222 O'Brien WA et al: Changes in plasma HIV RNA levels and CD4+ lymphocyte counts predict both response to antiretroviral therapy and therapeutic failure. *Ann Intern Med* 126:939–945, 1997.
223 Fauci AS: Host factors and the pathogenesis of HIV-induced disease. *Nature* 384:529–534, 1996.
224 Merigan TC: Individualization of therapy using viral markers. *J Acq Immun Defic Syndr Hum Retrovirol* 10:S41-S46, 1995.

Chapter 72

The psychosocial management of HIV disease in adults

Margaret A. Chesney
Susan Folkman

The biological course of HIV infection is accompanied by a psychosocial course that, like the biological course, is complicated and often unpredictable. The psychosocial course is particularly important in clinical management of HIV because, if unaddressed, it can have adverse effects on adherence to care, quality of life, and further transmission of HIV. The physical decline and uncertainties about future personal health associated with HIV infection are similar to those in other chronic illnesses, such as heart disease and cancer. What sets HIV disease apart from other diseases is that HIV infection is the result of a virus that, in most cases, is contracted by sexual and drug use behaviors that many cultures and policy making groups stigmatize and sanction. HIV disease differs from many other chronic illnesses also in that it usually strikes young people, forcing those infected to confront physical, financial, and social losses that are typically experienced later in one's lifetime. In addition, HIV infection is increasingly affecting marginalized, disadvantaged groups that do not have the resources to effectively manage the consequences associated with this illness.

The purpose of this chapter is to provide recommendations for the management of the psychosocial course of HIV infection. The presentation of these recommendations will follow the progression of HIV disease. The recommendations for the management of early HIV infection will cover issues that arise in conjunction with notification of a positive HIV antibody test, including disclosure of antibody status, modifying risk behaviors, and maintaining emotional and physical health. Recommendations for managing the intense psychosocial stressors that often arise over the course of illness will include details on a program to assist HIV-positive persons in coping. Effective psychosocial management of HIV-infected patients most often requires a collaborative physician–patient relationship that involves attention to adherence to jointly designed treatment plans. Managing the psychosocial course of HIV infection involves not only the patient–physician dyad but also the patient's informal caregivers and other formal care providers. The importance of these caregivers in the treatment of HIV-positive patients is often evident throughout the course of HIV disease, particularly as patients reach end of life decisions. Although broadening the physician's role to include psychosocial management and widening the physician–patient dyad to include other caregivers can pose challenges, these changes increase the likelihood of achieving effective clinical management.

The focus of this chapter is on the psychosocial management of HIV in the developed world. As will be evident, there has been little systematic study of this topic in developed countries, where the attention of policy makers and scientists has been on "finding a cure." Even less attention has been given to these issues in the developing world, where the focus has been on finding approaches to prevent infection. Persons living with HIV in the developing world confront all, and most likely more, of the challenges and needs as persons living with HIV in developed countries. As greater attention is paid to strategies for the psychosocial management of HIV in developed countries, a parallel effort could be launched in the developing world to conduct needs assessments and test approaches to addressing these needs. Some of these approaches might be based on the strategies that will be discussed in this chapter.

MANAGEMENT OF EARLY-STAGE HIV INFECTION

Early-stage HIV infection is an unfolding process that begins with notification of test results. This stage includes the psychological responses to test results and the identification of subsequent adaptive tasks. At the present time, HIV antibody test results are most often obtained at testing centers where people receive brief counseling to provide support and address the importance of obtaining medical care, notifying sex or drug partners who may also be HIV-infected, and practicing behaviors that reduce the risk of further HIV transmission. The immediate shock at the moment of notification of HIV infection is of such magnitude that people are unlikely to hear, process, or retain information given to them during posttest counseling.[1–3] This has important implications for psychosocial management. In order to lead to adaptive behavior change, important information covered in posttest counseling will need to be repeated in the context of a supportive, clinical environment.

An important development in the area of HIV testing involves home access testing. In the near future, in some countries, this alternative approach to clinic-based testing is likely to play an increasing role in identifying persons who are HIV-infected. Controversy has surrounded the introduction of those tests.[4] Kits currently available in the United States involve home collection of a blood specimen, depositing the blood specimen on a card, mailing the card for analysis, and calling a toll-free number for results after approximately 1 week. Code numbers on the card identify the participant so that personal identity is protected. People who call for their test results are given an option for hearing their results from a person or from a recorded message. Callers who are HIV-infected automatically hear their results from a counselor and are offered unlimited opportunities to call the toll-free number for additional counseling for up to 2 years. The counselors who speak to HIV-infected individuals have received specialized training, and they have manuals of referral resources for communities throughout the United States. There has been little research to date regarding the acceptability and psychological impact of learning results from home access testing. The experience with home testing will certainly be closely watched by other developed countries, such as France, that have not approved the testing kits. If home access testing is not accompanied by adverse psychological consequences, it and newer technologies such as rapid testing may prove helpful in increasing the timely HIV testing for certain populations.[5] Data from the National Health Interview Survey, for example, showed that people with less education and lower incomes and African American and Hispanic respondents were more likely to indicate that they would use home testing than others.[6]

PSYCHOSOCIAL RESPONSES TO A POSITIVE HIV TEST

Typical responses to a positive HIV test have changed over the course of the epidemic.[7,8] During the early years, the consequences of notification of a positive HIV antibody test included not only shock and denial, anxiety, and depression, but also somatic complaints and suicide ideation.[1,9–15] The incidence of severe psychological consequences of notification of HIV infection diminished after 1988, despite the rapid increase in the numbers of infected individuals.[8] This change has been attributed to more adequate pretest and posttest counseling and increased awareness on the part of at-risk individuals regarding the likelihood of their test results being positive.[16,17] Moreover, studies of distress reactions to notification of HIV infection indicate that the majority of those who become clinically depressed or attempt suicide have a previous history of psychiatric disorders.[18,19]

The psychological responses to a positive HIV antibody test are highly variable from one person to another. There is, however, a general time course to these initial reactions to HIV infection. Distress levels are most elevated immediately following notification and then decrease relatively quickly. In one study, distress levels had decreased significantly when assessed 2 and 10 weeks later, and in another study, they had decreased when assessed 5 weeks later.[16,20]

Patients seek HIV antibody testing in various disease stages. Some seek testing when they do not have symptoms but believe they may have been exposed to HIV. Others seek testing after symptoms appear. A recent study by the Centers for Disease Control of 2,441 individuals who had been diagnosed with AIDS in 11 states or cities from January 1990 through December 1992 indicates that approximately half of those testing positive for HIV had been infected years before testing.[21] Specifically, 51 percent of those reported with an AIDS diagnosis were first tested within 1 year of their diagnosis. Of these, 35 percent were tested for HIV within 2 months of receiving an AIDS diagnosis. This delay in testing, often until after symptoms appear, can complicate both medical and psychosocial case management. Health professionals' responses and responsibilities need to be tailored to the stage of disease at which the person first learns of infection.

Although the recent CDC study indicated alarming rates of testing late in disease, the current emphasis has not only shifted to earlier testing, but to testing for the presence of virus, prior to the development of antibodies. This new testing strategy will be accompanied by counseling regarding initiating aggressive triple-drug therapy.[22] Although the therapy may offer promise for longer-term prognosis, the rapidity with which it is begun, the complicated regimens it involves, the lack of information about the expected effects or duration of treatment, and the side effects of some of the drugs are likely to add to the stresses described in the preceding.

Women of childbearing age are encouraged to seek testing in order to decrease the rates of maternal–child HIV transmission. Pregnant women in particular are encouraged to learn their HIV serostatus in order to take advantage of antiviral regimens that can reduce the likelihood of HIV transmission.[23] Testing during pregnancy presents specific challenges for the clinician. Women who test positive face important decisions about continuing their pregnancy and starting antiviral treatment, in addition to adjusting to the personal knowledge of HIV infection. These issues require thoughtful counseling by the clinician.

IMPORTANT PSYCHOSOCIAL TASKS FOLLOWING HIV TESTING

HIV-infected persons need to address several important adaptive tasks. These include disclosing HIV status, modifying behaviors that could further transmit HIV, and maintaining physical and emotional health.

Disclosing HIV status

HIV-infected individuals must make a series of decisions about disclosing their HIV serostatus to each person or group of persons in their social network. A study of gay men revealed four considerations that influence decisions about disclosure: fear of rejection, desire to avoid others' pity, concern about causing loved ones emotional pain, and fear of discrimination.[24] These considerations may help explain why some individuals choose not to disclose their status even to their primary partner. In fact, in a survey of approximately 300 persons tested at an anonymous testing site, 12 percent said they would not tell their primary sexual partner their test results, and 27 percent said they would not tell their nonprimary partners.[25] These findings suggest that many of those who know they are HIV-infected may not disclose their HIV status to persons with whom they have engaged in risk behavior and who may be at risk for HIV acquisition. Research indicates that actual disclosure to persons at risk is selective. In a study of HIV-infected gay men, 96 percent reported disclosing their serostatus to primary sexual partners, but only 44 percent disclosed to regular but not primary partners, and none reported disclosing to casual and anonymous partners.[11] Similar findings have been reported in a study of HIV-infected Hispanic men.[26]

Psychosocial case management of HIV disease includes assisting HIV-infected persons in making decisions about who, when, and how to tell others of their status. To reduce further transmission of HIV, disclosure to others who need to be tested is critical. Health professionals, even though they have experience conveying "bad news" to patients, may not fully appreciate what HIV-infected persons experience when they disclose their "bad news"—their HIV status. Given the stigma associated with HIV infection, HIV-positive persons who disclose their status risk losing relationships that are important to them, including relationships with partners, family, and close friends. Knowledge that a person is HIV-infected can lead to loss of employment, friendships, denial of life and health insurance, loss of housing, dismissal from school, and denial of health care.[27,28]

Women represent an increasingly greater percentage of HIV-infected persons throughout the world, and their HIV testing is a priority. For HIV-infected women, as noted earlier, testing provides the opportunity for early prophylaxis and therapies, including prenatal regimens to reduce maternal–child HIV transmission.[23] Special considerations are necessary when counseling women about notifying sexual partners. The National Association of People with AIDS reports an association between AIDS and domestic violence.[29] A similar relationship was observed in a cohort of 921 women with steady partners in Kigali, Rwanda.[30] In the United States, a survey of women with AIDS found 17 percent who reported violence in the home. The risk of violence is directly linked to efforts by women to encourage partners to use condoms.[31,32] In an in-depth study of 20 HIV-infected mothers, 13 of the 20 had not told a single friend, and 5 (25 percent) had not told any members of their families about their HIV serostatus.[33] Reasons included the social stigma of HIV and a fear of rejection. Among those who did disclose their status, rejection was common. Compared to a matched control group of HIV-negative mothers, the infected mothers had a higher rate of separation (50 percent compared to 25 percent) from their partners.

Special considerations are also needed for assisting young people, including sexually active teens, in disclosing HIV status. Children who acquired HIV by perinatal transmission often do not know their HIV status. As children are living into young adulthood, reaching puberty, it is important that they be informed about their status and health practices so that they can help prevent further transmission.

Preventing further HIV transmission

Modifying behaviors that place others at risk for HIV infection is another important task for HIV-infected persons that needs to be addressed in psychosocial management of HIV. A proportion of those who are aware of their HIV infection continue to engage in risky sexual behaviors. In one study of 227 HIV-infected patients attending an outpatient HIV clinic, 179 patients reported sexual activity since testing positive.[34] These sexually active patients did not use condoms with 16 percent of their sexual partners who were known to be HIV-negative, 41 percent of partners of unknown HIV status, and 49 percent of HIV-positive partners. Although 71 percent of the partners were aware of the patient's HIV status, 29 percent of the partners were unaware, and 6 percent of the patients did not know if their partners were aware of their HIV infection.

There may be an important association between distress and high-risk behavior among HIV-infected persons. A study of 142 HIV-infected homosexual men found that 29 percent reported having engaged in unprotected intercourse in a 3-month period.[35] Recreational drug use and depression scores predicted this behavior. Similarly designed studies consistently report that approximately 25 percent of HIV-infected persons engage in behaviors that put others at risk.[36,37]

As noted in the preceding, HIV-infected women have special concerns about encouraging their partners to use condoms. In the in-depth study of 20 HIV-infected mothers, there was a high rate of unprotected sex, including encounters with known HIV-infected partners. Interviews revealed that the women viewed protection as their partner's choice. It is important to note, however, that many of the women did not inform others, including their partners, of their serostatus for fear of rejection.[33]

There has been very little attention paid to the issue of high-risk behavior among those who are aware of their HIV status. Psychosocial management of HIV disease needs to address the important issue of maintaining safe behavior for two compelling reasons: first, to reduce the further spread of HIV and second, to minimize risk to the HIV-infected person for sexually transmitted diseases that are known to adversely influence disease progression.[38] Health care providers have unique opportunities to influence the behavior of their HIV-infected patients. For example, a positive STD test provides an excellent reason to discuss the importance of safe sexual practices both for the health of the patient and the well-being of his or her partners.

Maintaining physical health

The most salient task for HIV-infected patients and their health care providers is maintaining physical health.[24] Interviews with HIV-positive patients reveal three sets of strategies. The first set involves actively seeking out medical treatment options, studying the efficacy and side effects of available treatments, and working to maintain health by avoiding tobacco, drugs, and alcohol; eating a well-balanced diet; and getting sufficient rest. The second set of strategies involves personal health monitoring, and keeping track of physical symptoms and CD4 counts. The third set of strategies focuses on making decisions about nonpharmacological treatments, including meditation, yoga, visualization, and various nutritious diets. Health care providers can support their patients' efforts to accomplish these goals, even though they may not fall within traditional medical practice.

Maintaining emotional health

Another important psychosocial task for HIV-infected persons and their providers is the maintenance of emotional health. Many HIV-infected persons cope effectively with their condition and continue to lead productive, meaningful lives. Unfortunately, others have difficulty managing the stresses associated with HIV illness, including the knowledge that they face a chronic, debilitating, and stigmatizing disease, with an unknown course and without a cure. Therefore an important feature of psychosocial case management for HIV-infected persons involves helping patients to cope with their condition by, for example, reassuring them that their worries and fears are normal, or when patients' distress appears to be debilitating, referring them to a mental health provider. We will outline a coping training program in the next section that is effective in assisting HIV-infected persons in managing the stress associated with HIV.

Failure to maintain emotional health can have serious consequences for the clinical management of HIV. In our research with HIV-infected gay men, we have found that psychological distress is often related to more frequently missed doses of zidovudine and other antiretroviral medications.[39] In addition, higher levels of depression are also significantly associated with fewer health-promoting behaviors.[40] The AIDS Cost and Service Utilization Survey (ACSUS), conducted by the U.S. Agency for Health Care Policy and Research, found that psychological distress is associated with greater health care utilization, even after controlling for stage of disease, level of symptoms, and insurance status.[41] The authors of this ACSUS evaluation pointed out that "in view of prior findings showing a direct effect of psychological distress on health care use, future studies should examine the combined effects of mood and symptoms on health care utilization among people with HIV infection." Coping interventions thus may not only help reduce risk behavior and serve the humanitarian goal of helping HIV-infected people maintain their emotional health, but they may also increase compliance or adherence and reduce unnecessary health care costs associated with HIV.

MANAGEMENT OF THE PSYCHOSOCIAL SEQUELAE OF HIV INFECTION

Theoretical and clinical research on coping with stress provides a valuable resource for health professionals working with patients who are faced with the challenge of living with HIV. Although physicians may lack the time to provide counseling, it is important for the well-being of their patients that they be familiar with the approaches described in this section. Others on their staff can carry out coping interventions or distressed patients can be referred to mental health professionals.

COPING WITH HIV: MANAGING EMOTIONS AND PROBLEM SOLVING

Coping effectively with a chronic, debilitating illness such as HIV disease involves coping to manage emotional distress (emotion-focused coping) and to solve problems related to HIV infection (problem-focused coping). Emotion-focused strategies include approaches such as relaxation and meditation, as well as maladaptive practices that are used to escape, such as alcohol and drug use. Problem-focused coping strategies include decision making, problem solving, and negotiation. Effective application of emotion-focused and problem-focused coping requires a "fit" between the choice of coping strategy and the extent to which the stressful situation is changeable. Emotion-focused strategies are more appropriate for situations that cannot be changed, whereas problem-focused coping strategies are more appropriate for situations that can be changed. When people fail to "fit" the coping strategy to the changeability of stressful situations, they are likely to experience increases in distress.[42–44]

These concepts of emotion- and problem-focused coping, and their fit to the changeability of stressors, are particularly appropriate to the cause of HIV infection, which is characterized by stressors that have both changeable and unchangeable aspects. Examples of unchangeable HIV stressors include an HIV-positive mother knowing that she transmitted the virus to her infant, the increasing need for caregiving of an HIV-positive person during the late stages of the disease, and the feelings experienced by an HIV-positive person associated with the likelihood of a premature death. Examples of changeable stressors include an HIV-positive person struggling with the decision to initiate a therapy or join a clinical trial, and fears about transmitting the virus associated with unsafe behaviors.

COPING EFFECTIVENESS TRAINING

We developed a program to teach adaptive coping to HIV-infected persons. Known as Coping Effectiveness Training (CET), this program focuses on teaching emotion- and problem-focused strategies specifically tailored to HIV stressors.[8,45] The primary approaches are presented in Table 72-1.

We conducted a clinical trial of CET to test whether persons could be trained to increase coping skills and whether doing so would decrease distress. We randomized 149 HIV-infected men to CET or to one of two control conditions. Men randomized to a CET program showed significantly greater increases in coping efficacy than men randomized to either an HIV-information group or to a waiting-list control group. We also found that men who received CET showed significantly greater decreases in distress and that these changes in distress were associated with changes in coping skills. Although in this trial CET was delivered in groups, the same concepts can be conveyed to patients individually as part of HIV care.

THE PHYSICIAN–PATIENT RELATIONSHIP

Balancing active involvement with hypervigilance

Research indicates that long-term survivors with HIV are typically involved in their medical care and participate actively with their physicians in making decisions about their care.[46] Persons who are HIV-infected should be encouraged to take an active role in maintaining their health, follow a healthy lifestyle, and maintain appropriate vigilance about their symptoms.[24] However, HIV-infected persons can become overly concerned and hypervigilant about their condition, which can lead to increases in distress.[24] Every laboratory test or minor symptom can become a source of anxiety and despair. Coping skills training can help patients view these tests and symptoms as "stressors" that can be effectively managed in the context of a positive physician–patient relationship.

One of the most significant sources of stress is the unknown. Therefore, providing information about the significance of symptoms or what patients may experience next is an important aspect of psychosocial management of HIV. However, it is important that this information be provided in "doses" that the patient can assimilate. Our clinical trial testing CET demonstrated the potential for the provision of HIV-related information to itself become a source of stress. The control group that received weekly sessions providing HIV information on such topics as clinical trials, disclosure of HIV status, maintaining low-risk behavior, and HIV medications, without any assistance in coping, reported *increases* in distress over time.[39]

Adhering to care

A critical task in the psychosocial management of HIV for patients and health providers is to pay particular attention to issues surrounding adherence to care. This includes supporting adherence or compliance, identifying potential barriers to adherence, and designing strategies to overcome them. The need for this attention is evident from reports of nonadherence from AIDS clinical trials and practice. In early clinical trials, approximately 30 percent of the patients were lost to follow-up or voluntarily withdrew from study medication.[47] More recent trials may report better adherence rates, but research at the Center for AIDS Research at the University of California, San Francisco suggests that this increase may be at the cost of allowing as many as 70 percent of those remaining in trials to deviate from the protocol regimen.[48] Similar reports have been made from clinical populations. In one study 70 percent of patients omitted drug doses and over 80 percent of patients reported adverse reactions, primarily attributable to zidovudine.[49] In another study of male hospitalized patients with AIDS, 90 percent of the patients refused some procedure or treatment.[50] This rate of refusal per hospital day was over four times greater than that in a control population of male leukemics. Other studies indicate that adherence to antiretroviral medication, over a short, 4-week period of time, ranges from 33 to 88 percent.[51,52] This wide range reflects differences across studies, including subject populations, as well as the manner in which adherence is assessed (33 percent using electronic pill containers compared to 88 percent relying on self-report).

These issues become all the more urgent now with the new

Table 72-1. Cognitive-Behavioral Interventions for Emotion- and Problem-Focused Coping

Emotion-focused coping	Problem-focused coping
Cognitive therapy—recognizing the association between thoughts and emotions, implementing strategies to modify thoughts in order to manage emotions.[36,37]	Problem-solving—focusing on problems apart from emotions; identify problem elements, generate and weigh alternatives, and implement plans.[38–41]
Cognitive restructuring—questioning irrational, dysfunctional beliefs and fears, helping individuals develop self-instructional thoughts to replace dysfunctional thoughts.[38,41,42]	Decision-making—strategically evaluating alternative solutions for problems, weighing costs and benefits so as to maximize positive outcomes while minimizing negative consequences.[38–41]
Relaxation—reducing the intensity of emotional distress, using progressive muscle relaxation, deep breathing exercise, meditation, and imagery.[43–49]	Social/communication skills—listening, acknowledging, establishing positive foundation for and conveying information.[43,44,47]
Humor—using laughter to distance individuals from emotionally laden situations and to introduce alternative perspectives from which to view problems. (Note: Humor must be used judiciously so as not to undermine the relationship with individual.)[40,50,51]	Negotiation—separating issues from problems, focusing on interests not positions, generating alternatives, and finding common ground.[43,44,47,52]
Positive morale and meaning—reflecting on positive moments in the day and identifying sources of positive meaning in day-to-day life.[22,42,53]	Health-promoting behavior—applying coping skills to make decisions about care, increase adherence to a treatment regimen developed jointly with health providers.[19,54,55]

highly effective protease inhibitors. Currently, high levels of adherence to frequent doses of these drugs is required to maintain suppression of viral replication and to prevent the development-resistant viral strains. Critical questions remain about whether the salugenic effects observed with protease inhibitors will persist under conditions of dose omission or drug termination. Clinicians, concerned about the potential for nonadherence-related resistance, are expressing reluctance to prescribe these new therapies to certain vulnerable, HIV-infected persons. Partnerships between biomedical and behavioral scientists with expertise in promoting and maintaining adherence are being forged to document the extent of the problem of adherence to protease inhibitors, to identify the factors that promote or deter adherence, and to develop interventions to promote adherence both in the context of clinical trials and care for persons with HIV. In the meantime, clinicians caring for persons living with HIV should give serious consideration to referring patients to a health professional with expertise in adherence so that patients would have an optimal opportunity to benefit from these new therapies.

In general, more research is needed to identify the factors that are associated with long-term adherence to care, especially as new treatment regimens are discovered that are expected to further lengthen life. Conversely, characteristics of these treatment regimens, clinical environments, and patients that are associated with nonadherence need to be identified because these characteristics may be amenable to change. To date, the studies of HIV-infected persons indicate that patients' perceptions of their study nurse as supportive is also associated with higher levels of adherence, whereas skipped doses of medication and failure to adhere to health-related regimens are associated with distressed mood.[39,53] These observations underscore the importance of using coping interventions that will help reduce distress and help maintain a positive physician–patient partnership as a strategy to address problems in the area of adherence to care.

SPECIAL DEMANDS OF LATE-STAGE DISEASE

As with any terminal illness, a number of issues become salient as HIV disease enters its most advanced stages. Among the most common issues are home care and hospice care and end of life decisions.

HOME AND HOSPICE CARE

Home caregivers become increasingly important as HIV disease advances and patients become less able to care for themselves. Often, the primary home caregiver is a family member, lover, or close friend, with other friends and family members playing support roles. These informal caregivers play a critical role in maintaining the patient's physical and emotional well-being. In addition to assisting with the basic activities of daily living—food preparation, eating, bathing, and toileting—they often supervise the treatment protocol, administer medications, including infusions, and provide critical emotional support.

Health care providers need to help ill patients recognize when they need home care and identify individuals who can assume care responsibilities. Although some friends, lovers, and family regard the provision of terminal care as their responsibility and their right, others may become deeply distressed and should not be expected to take on this responsibility.[54] Providers need to be sensitive to these possibilities. If the provider does not have time to discuss these issues, the patient should be referred to an appropriate counselor.

Health care providers can play an important role in the quality of home care through effective support of the home caregiver. As long as the caregiver's goals are consistent with the patient's and those of the provider, providers should include the caregiver in the triad of care by being attentive and responsive to his or her questions, apprehensions, and needs.[54] Often the home caregiver needs skills training, such as in the administration of medications, wound cleansing, and infection control. This training can help sustain the quality of life of the patient as well as the self-confidence of the caregiver. Such training can be provided by nursing staff, and in some regions, by community-based organizations that offer courses in home care for persons with AIDS.

In many instances formal caregivers, such as visiting nurses or personnel from home care agencies, are needed to assist patients who do not have an informal caregiver or to supplement the care provided by the informal caregiver. Providers can facilitate access to such care through direct referrals to community resources or through referrals to social workers.

Even under the best of home care circumstances, the management of the patient's disease at home can exceed the capacity of home caregivers. Hospice care is an alternative to home care that should be considered when home care is no longer effective, especially in regard to pain management. The provider should try to monitor the home care situation and when appropriate, provide access to information about hospice care.

END OF LIFE DECISIONS

Advance directives allow the patient's health care preferences to be known and respected, even after the patient is no longer capable of making decisions.[55] Written advance directives are generally more credible than are oral statements.[55] Two documents are important in this regard, the Durable Power of Attorney for Health Care and the Directive to Physicians, also known as the Living Will.[56]

The Durable Power of Attorney for Health Care is a document prepared in advance of an incapacitating illness. It enables individuals to designate a proxy to make health care decisions on their behalf in the event they become unable to participate in decisions about their care. The Durable Power of Attorney for Health Care can also include specific instructions. The designated individual is generally protected legally in acting on behalf of the patient. Decision-making responsibility is returned to patients if they regain their competency.[55,56] The Durable Power of Attorney for Health Care is especially important when the designated individual is not in a legally recognized relationship with the patient, as when the caregiver is the patient's lover.

The Directive to Physicians is completed after the patient is considered to be in the terminal phase of an illness. It allows patients to inform their doctors about preferences in regard to withholding or withdrawing "life-sustaining" procedures. This document has serious limitations.[56] It applies only in limited circumstances, and it allows patients to refuse only certain interventions. Further, a number of states do not permit patients to decline artificial nutrition and hydration.[56]

The terminal phase of AIDS is also likely to include discussions about aid-in-dying. These discussions commonly occur at home between the patient and his or her primary informal caregiver.[54] At times, patient or caregivers turn to the providers for advice. However, patients and their caregivers may be reluctant to broach these topics, so providers should be prepared to open the discussion. These discussions are important because they allow the patient to talk about fears of dying, concerns about pain, and anxieties about the burden of their care. Most importantly, these discussions allow providers to validate the patient's and caregiver's concerns and to listen and give support during the final stages of care.

CONCLUSION

In this chapter, we have provided recommendations for the management of the psychosocial course of HIV infection, from early HIV infection to discussion of the dying process. The psychosocial management of HIV involves a triad: the patient and both formal and informal care providers. Physicians or formal health care providers play a pivotal role in this care triad. Early in the epidemic, when HIV care was concentrated in AIDS epicenters, relatively few providers were directly involved in care of HIV-infected persons. However, as the epidemic aged, increasing numbers of providers have become involved in treating patients who are living with HIV. In a national random survey of primary care physicians conducted in 1990, 75 percent reported having cared for a patient with HIV infection.[57] Physicians with more experience treating HIV-infected persons report that although caring for HIV patients puts demands on their time, they find the experience personally rewarding.[57,58] An important aspect of the rewarding nature of providing care to HIV-infected persons involves the challenge of managing both the biomedical and psychosocial course of HIV, working with patients as partners in their care.

References

1 Grant D et al: Counseling AIDS antibody-positive clients: Reactions and treatment. *Am Psychol* 18:72–74, 1988.

2 Perry S et al: Counseling for HIV testing. *Hosp Commun Psychiatry* 39:731–739, 1988.

3 Perry S et al: Severity of psychiatric symptoms after HIV testing. *Am J Psychiatry* 150:775–779, 1993.

4 Bayer R et al: Testing for HIV infection at home. *New Engl J Med* 332:1296–1299, 1995.

5 Spielberg F et al: Rapid testing for HIV antibody: A technology whose time has come. *Ann Int Med* 125:509–511, 1996.

6 Phillips KA et al: The cost-effectiveness of HIV testing of physicians and dentists in the United States. *JAMA* 271:851–858, 1994.

7 Folkman S: Psychosocial effects of HIV infection, in Goldberger L et al (eds): *Handbook of Stress,* 2nd ed. New York, Free Press, 1993, pp. 658–681.

8 Chesney MA et al: Psychological impact of HIV disease and implications for intervention. *Psychiat Clin No Am* 17:163–182, 1994.

9 Miller D: Diagnosis and treatment of acute psychological problems related to HIV infection and disease, in Ostrow D (ed): *Behavioral Aspects of AIDS.* New York, Plenum, 1990, pp. 187–206.

10 Coates TJ et al: Behavioral consequences of AIDS antibody testing among gay men. *JAMA* 258:1889, 1987.

11 Huggins J et al: Affective and behavioral responses of gay and bisexual men to HIV antibody testing. *Social Work* 36:61–66, 1991.

12 Graham N et al: Zidovudine use in AIDS-free HIV-1-seropositive homosexual men in the multicenter AIDS cohort study (MACS) 1987, 1989. *J Acq Imm Defic Syndr* 4:267–276, 1991.

13 Moulton J et al: Results of a one-year longitudinal study of HIV antibody test notification from the San Francisco General Hospital cohort. *J Acq Imm Defic Syndr* 4:787–794, 1991.

14 Ostrow DG et al: HIV-related symptoms and psychological functioning in a cohort of homosexual men. *Am J Psychiatry* 146:737–742, 1989.

15 Ostrow DG et al: Disclosure of HIV antibody status: Behavioral and mental health correlates. *AIDS Educ Prev* 1:1–11, 1989.

16 Perry S et al: Psychological responses to serological testing for HIV. *AIDS* 4:145–152, 1990.

17 Kelly JA et al: Psychological interventions with AIDS and HIV: Prevention and treatment. *J Consult Clin Psychol* 60:576–585, 1992.

18 Dew A et al: Infection with human immunodeficiency virus and vulnerability to psychiatric distress. *Arch Gen Psychiatry* 47:737–744, 1990.

19 Hedge B: Psychosocial aspects of HIV infection. *AIDS Care* 3:409–412, 1991.

20 Ironson G et al: Changes in immune and psychological measures as a function of anticipation and reaction to news of HIV-1 antibody status. *Psychosom Med* 52:247–270, 1990.

21 Wortley PM et al: HIV testing patterns: Where, why, and when were persons with AIDS tested for HIV? *AIDS* 9:487–492, 1995.

22 Ho DD: Time to hit HIV, early and hard. *New Engl J Med* 125:450–451, 1995.

23 Zidovudine for the prevention of HIV transmission from mother to infant. *MMWR* 43:285–287, 1994.

24 Siegel K et al: Living with HIV infection: Adaptive tasks of seropositive gay men. *J Health Soc Behav* 32:17–32, 1991.

25 Kegeles SM et al: Intentions to communicate positive HIV-antibody status to sex partners [letter]. *JAMA* 259:216–217, 1988.

26 Marks G et al: Self-disclosure of HIV infection: Preliminary results from a sample of Hispanic men. *Health Psychol* 11:300–306, 1992.

27 Folkman S et al: Caregiver burden in HIV-positive and HIV-negative partners of men with AIDS. *J Consult Clin Psychol* 62:746–756, 1994.

28 Tross S et al: Psychological distress and neuropsychological complications of HIV infection and AIDS. *Am Psychol* 43:929–934, 1988.

29 HIV in America: A report by the National Association of People with AIDS. *Nat Assoc People AIDS.* Washington DC; 1992.

30 van der Straten A et al: Interpersonal violence and HIV infection among women in steady relationships in Kigali, Rwanda. (Unpublished manuscript.)

31 Weissman G: AIDS prevention for women at risk: Experience from a National Demonstration Research Project. *J Prim Prev* 12:49–63, 1991.

32 Worth D: Sexual decision-making and AIDS: Why condom promotion among vulnerable women is likely to fail. *Stud Fam Plan* 20:197–307, 1989.

33 Lester P et al: The consequences of a positive prenatal HIV antibody test for women. *J AIDS Hum Retrovirol* 10:341–349, 1995.

34 Wenger N et al: Sexual behavior of individuals infected with the human immunodeficiency virus: The need for intervention. *Arch Int Med* 154:1849–1954, 1994.

35 Kelly JA et al: Factors associated with severity of depression and high-risk sexual behavior among persons diagnosed with human immunodeficiency virus (HIV) infection. *Health Psychol* 12:215–219, 1993.

36 Wiktor SZ et al: Effect of knowledge of human immunodeficiency virus infection status on sexual activity among homosexual men. *J AIDS* 3: 62–68, 1990.

37 Catania JA et al: Changes in condom use among homosexual men in San Francisco. *Health Psychol* 10:190–199, 1991.

38 Chesney MA: Prevention of HIV and STD infection. *Prev Med* 23: 655–660, 1994.

39 Chesney MA et al: Coping effectiveness training for men living with HIV: Preliminary findings. *Int J STD AIDS* 7:75–82, 1996.

40 Berkman LF et al: *Health and Ways of Living: The Alameda County Study.* New York: Oxford University Press, 1983.

41 Fleishman JA et al: Correlates of medical service utilization among people with HIV infection. *Health Serv Res* 29:527–548, 1994.

42 Strentz T et al: Adjustment to the stress of simulated captivity: Effects of emotion-focused versus problem-focused preparation of hostages differing in locus of control. *J Personal Soc Psychol* 55:652–660, 1988.

43 Vitaliano PP et al: The ways of coping checklist: Revision and psychometric Properties. *Multivariate Behav Res* 20:3–26, 1985.

44 Folkman S: Personal control and stress and coping processes: A theoretical analysis. *J Personal Soc Psychol* 46:839–852, 1984.

45 Folkman S et al: Translating coping theory into intervention, in Eckenrode J (ed): *The Social Context of Stress.* New York, Plenum, 1991, pp. 239–260.

46 Remien RH et al: Coping strategies and health beliefs of AIDS long-term survivors. *Psychol Health* 6:335–345, 1992.

47 Volberding P et al: Zidovudine in asymptomatic human immunodeficiency virus infection: A controlled trial in persons with fewer than 500 CD4-positive cells per cubic millimeter. *New Engl J Med* 322: 941–949, 1990.
48 Chesney MA: Behavioral aspects of treatment and prevention for HIV-infected persons in care: Developing the research agenda, in *Improving Adherence and Retention in Care.* San Diego, 1995.
49 Chow R et al: Medication use patterns in HIV-positive patients. *Can J Hosp Pharm* 46:171–175, 1993.
50 Blumenfield M et al: Noncompliance in hospitalized patients with AIDS. *Gen Hosp Psychiatry* 12:166–169, 1990.
51 Wall TL et al: Adherence to zidovudine (AZT) among HIV-infected methadone patients: A pilot study of supervised therapy and dispensing compared to usual care. *Drug and Alcohol Depend* 37:261–269, 1995.
52 Samuels JE et al: Zidovudine therapy in an inner city population. *J Acq Imm Defic Syndr* 3:877–883, 1990.
53 Morse EV et al: Determinants of subject compliance within an experimental anti-HIV drug protocol. *Soc Sci Med* 32:1161–1167, 1991.
54 Cooke M et al: Dying of AIDS: The role of caregivers in intentionally hastened death. *JAMA,* in press.
55 Rubin SM et al: Increasing the completion of the durable power of attorney for health care. *JAMA* 271:209–212, 1994.
56 Lo B: *Resolving Ethical Dilemmas: A Guide for Clinicians.* Baltimore, Williams & Wilkins, 1995.
57 Gerbert B et al: Primary care physicians and AIDS: Attitudinal and structural barriers to care. *JAMA* 266:2837–2842, 1991.
58 McKusick L et al: The psychological impact of AIDS on primary care physicians. *West J Med* 144:751–752, 1986.

Chapter 73

Clinical management of HIV infection in primary health care

David H. Spach

As the human immunodeficiency virus (HIV) epidemic moves well into its second decade, the World Health Organization (WHO) has projected that more than 26 million persons will be infected with HIV, with approximately 800,000 of those persons living in the United States.[1] As antiretroviral therapy and opportunistic infection prophylaxis become increasingly more effective, it is essential that health care providers develop the skills to effectively identify and manage HIV-infected individuals. Moreover, the primary care of HIV-infected individuals has taken on greater complexity in recent years, especially given the multiple available antiretroviral therapies. The aim of this chapter is to provide health care providers with information particularly relevant to the primary care of HIV-infected individuals. Antiretroviral therapy, although an essential component of primary care management, is not discussed in this chapter since it is discussed in detail in Chapter 74. This chapter places particular emphasis on the initial evaluation as well as skin and oral manifestations. Manifestations of other organ systems are also covered, but in less detail.

CLASSIFICATION

In December 1992, the CDC published a revised classification system that factored in both CD4 status and clinical manifestations (Table 73-1); the most important change with this new classification system was that patients could be defined as having AIDS based on a CD4 count less than 200 cells/mm^3.[2] The shaded values in the table indicate an AIDS case based on this revised surveillance definition.

ACUTE HIV

Approximately 30 to 70 percent of individuals will develop an acute illness on acquiring HIV, typically 7 to 10 days after inoculation. The most common signs and symptoms associated with acute infection with HIV are fatigue, fever, sore throat, weight loss, and myalgia.[3] Less frequently observed signs and symptoms include headache, cervical lymphadenopathy, a diffuse morbilliform rash that mimics a drug rash (or measles), and ulcerations of the oral or genital region (Fig. 73-1).[3,4] The median duration of symptoms is 14 days. Some patients present with a constellation of symptoms—fever, headache, photophobia, and stiff neck—that suggest aseptic meningitis. Although most patients with symptomatic acute HIV infection seek medical care, the diagnosis is usually not made.

Individuals presenting with acute HIV infection generally have a high plasma HIV RNA level and thus are probably highly infectious.[3,4] Because patients have a negative HIV antibody test at the time they present with the acute HIV illness, correctly making the diagnosis requires using one of the newer assays that detect HIV RNA or by ordering a HIV p24 antigen test (analogous to detecting hepatitis B antigen before hepatitis B antibody develops). If neither of these confirmatory tests can be obtained, the patient with suspected acute HIV should undergo standard HIV antibody testing at 3 and 6 months following the suspected acute HIV illness. Regardless of what type of HIV test is ordered, the patient should undergo pre- and posttest counseling. Because those patients who test positive are probably highly infectious, it is critical to educate the patient about the modes of transmission of HIV, as well to inform them about safe sex and safe injection use practices and potential mother-to-fetus transmission of HIV.

One published study has shown possible benefit of using zidovudine (AZT) in the acutely infected patient.[5] Several unpublished studies that involved the use of potent combination regimens (including protease inhibitors) for acute HIV infection have shown profound virologic effects, but the long-term clinical impact of aggressive antiretroviral therapy for acute HIV infection remains unknown.[6] Most authorities recommend using an aggressive regimen if treatment is initiated in the acutely infected person.

INITIAL EVALUATION AND ROUTINE FOLLOW-UP

At the time of the initial evaluation, a critical interface occurs between the provider and the patient and this frequently sets the tone for subsequent interactions. Accordingly, the provider should have a well-thought-out approach to the initial evaluation. For practical purposes it is most reasonable to divide the initial evaluation into two visits that are spaced approximately 2 to 3 weeks apart. During the first of these two visits, the provider should, if possible, obtain extensive information regarding the patient's history, perform a thorough physical examination, and order relevant laboratory studies (Table 73-2). At the 2- to 3-week follow-up visit, the provider should review the laboratory results, discuss options for antiretroviral therapy (if indicated), start opportunistic infection prophylaxis (if indicated), and administer appropriate vaccinations. The follow-up visit also provides an opportune time to address any questions or concerns the patient may have, as well as to reinforce the importance of the patient not transmitting their HIV to anyone else.

MEDICAL HISTORY AND PHYSICAL EXAMINATION

Although many HIV-infected patients do not know when they acquired HIV, some can recall the acute HIV seroconversion illness, especially when a provider describes the signs and symptoms associated with acute HIV infection. Obtaining the approximate date of HIV acquisition may help in estimating the tempo of the patient's HIV disease progression. Other useful historical questions include when the patients first tested positive for HIV, what HIV-associated treatments they have received, which immunizations they have received, and whether they have a previous history of sexually transmitted diseases, hepatitis, pneumonia, or tuberculosis.[7] For HIV-infected patients, it is particularly important to obtain a history of adverse drug reactions as well as to determine what medications the patient currently takes, including nontraditional therapies. The patients should be asked whether they have any ongoing high-risk behaviors that place others at risk for HIV, as well as to place the patient at risk for acquiring infectious agents. Because HIV-infected patients may develop reactivation of infectious organisms previously acquired while residing in a region endemic for that organism, the provider should obtain a history of the patient's prior residence and previous travel.[8]

A complete review of systems and complete physical examination should be performed. Particular emphasis should be placed on the cutaneous, oral, lymph node, genital, and neurologic ex-

Table 73-1. 1993 Revised CDC Classification System for HIV Infection

	Clinical categories		
CD4 categories	(A) Asymptomatic, 1° HIV, or PGL	(B) Symptomatic, not A or C conditions	(C) AIDS-indicator conditions
(1) ≥500 cells/mm^3	A1	B1	C1
(2) 200–499 cells/mm^3	A2	B2	C2
(3) <200 cells/mm^3	A3	B3	C3

B conditions may include (listed in alphabetical order): bacterial endocarditis, meningitis, or sepsis; candidiasis (oral); candidiasis (persistent vulvovaginal); cervical dysplasia (or carcinoma in situ); constitutional illness (persistent unexplained fever or diarrhea or weight loss or disabling weakness); herpes zoster (multidermatomal); listeriosis; myelopathy; nocardiosis; oral hairy leukoplakia; pelvic inflammatory disease; peripheral neuropathy; and thrombocytopenic purpura (idiopathic).

C conditions (listed in alphabetical order): candidiasis (bronchial, esophageal, pulmonary, or trachea); cervical cancer (invasive); coccidioidomycosis (disseminated or extrapulmonary); cryptococcosis (extrapulmonary); cryptosporidiosis (intestinal, for longer than 1 month); cytomegalovirus (other than liver, spleen, or nodes); encephalopathy (HIV); herpes simplex (ulcers present for longer than 1 month or esophagitis or bronchitis or pneumonitis); histoplasmosis (disseminated or extrapulmonary); isosporiasis (intestinal, for longer than 1 month); Kaposi's sarcoma; lymphoma (Burkitt's, immunoblastic, or primary in brain); *Mycobacterium avium* complex (disseminated or extrapulmonary); *Mycobacterium kansasii* (disseminated or extrapulmonary); *Mycobacterium tuberculosis; Mycobacterium* of other or unidentified species (disseminated or extrapulmonary); *Pneumocystis carinii* pneumonia; recurrent pneumonia (two or more episodes in 1-year period); progressive multifocal leukoencephalopathy; salmonella (recurrent septicemia); toxoplasmosis (brain); wasting syndrome (>10% weight loss plus either chronic weakness or documented fever for at least 30 days in the absence of a concurrent illness that could explain this finding).

aminations. In addition, because HIV-infected women have an increased rate of cervical dysplasia and cervical cancer, all HIV-infected women should undergo a pelvic examination with Papanicolaou-smear testing.[9]

LABORATORY STUDIES

Among HIV-infected individuals, hematologic disorders frequently develop, particularly those patients with more advanced immunosuppression. Accordingly, a complete blood count and platelet count should be performed at the initial evaluation. In addition, since patients often receive marrow-toxic drugs, such as trimethoprim-sulfamethoxazole, zidovudine, or certain chemotherapeutic agents, the initial complete blood count serves as a useful baseline. Obtaining screening tests for serum electrolytes, blood urea nitrogen, and creatinine has a higher yield in HIV-infected patients compared with the general population and serves as a useful baseline. Given that hepatocellular and biliary complications occur with significant frequency among HIV-infected patients, screening with liver function tests is reasonable.

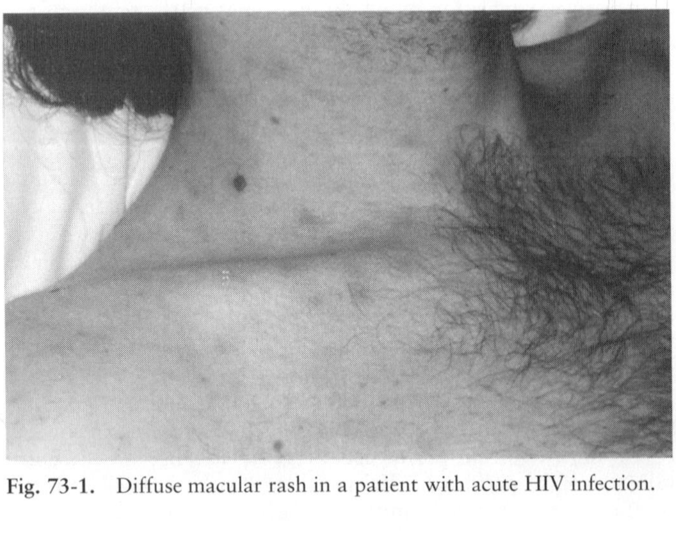

Fig. 73-1. Diffuse macular rash in a patient with acute HIV infection.

Several reports have described HIV-negative patients seeking care who claimed that they were HIV-infected when indeed they were not.[10,11] These factitious HIV cases were more likely to involve persons who had (1) a CD4 count greater than 700 cells/mm^3; (2) an HIV-infected sexual partner; and (3) a history of a suicide attempt.[11] Accordingly, if the patient does not have a documented positive HIV serology test from a reliable lab, one should perform HIV serologic testing to confirm that the patient is indeed infected with HIV. Serologic testing for syphilis—in all persons who acquired HIV infection through sexual contact or injection drug use—has been recommended by the CDC since 1988.[12] Several reports have described HIV-infected patients who developed syphilis, but had nonreactive serologic tests for syphilis; there are, however, no prospective studies to support the notion that the sensitivity of serologic tests for syphilis are altered in HIV-infected individuals.

Several recent studies have shown HIV RNA measurements (a quantitative measure of "viral load") provide the single best estimate of the rate at which a patient's HIV disease will progress.[13,14] In essence, the higher the HIV RNA level, the more rapid the HIV disease progresses. Moreover, measuring HIV RNA levels now plays an important role in deciding when to start antiretroviral therapy as well as following the response to therapy.[15,16] Measuring the CD4 cell count also provides valuable prognostic information.[17] In 1992, the CDC incorporated CD4 levels into the new definition for staging HIV-infected patients.[2] Moreover, these CDC revised staging guidelines included all patients with CD4 lymphocyte levels less than 200 cells/mm^3 (or <14 percent of total lymphocytes) in the AIDS case definition. Measurements of CD4 cells also have played a key role in determining when to initiate opportunistic infection prophylaxis or antiretroviral therapy. Since both the HIV RNA and CD4 cell count tests provide valuable information, they should be ordered on all patients at the time of initial evaluation. Other markers previously touted to have significant prognostic value, such as β_2-microglobulin, neopterin, and p24 antigen, have relatively little prognostic value compared with HIV RNA levels and CD4 cell counts and thus are not recommended.

All patient should have serologic tests to detect the presence of hepatitis B virus (HBV) antibodies and antigen(s). Testing will determine who should receive hepatitis B virus vaccination, as well

Table 73-2. Recommendations for Testing at the Time of Initial Evaluation

Test	Recommendation	Comment
Laboratory studies		
Complete blood count	Recommended	Abnormalities common, especially patients with AIDS
Platelet count	Recommended	Idiopathic thrombcytopenia is CDC category B disease
Serum chemistries	Recommended	Reasonable to screen for abnormalities, especially serum creatinine
Hepatitis B surface antigen	Recommended	Testing for hepatitis B mainly indicated for vaccine purposes
Hepatitis B surface antibody	Recommended	
Hepatitis C antibody	Optional	Would recommend testing if liver function tests abnormal; because no vaccine for hepatitis C virus, not as high priority as testing for hepatitis B virus
HIV serology	Recommended	Critical to document that patient is indeed HIV-infected
HIV RNA (viral load)	Recommended	Provides extremely valuable prognostic information
CD4 cell count	Recommended	Best reflector of current status of immune system; important for decisions on when to start opportunistic infection prophylaxis and antiretroviral therapy
p24 antigen	Not recommended	Inferior prognostic value compared with HIV RNA levels and CD4 cell count; may be useful in person with suspected acute HIV infection
β_2-microglobulin	Not recommended	Inferior prognostic value compared with HIV RNA levels and CD4 cell count
Neopterin	Not recommended	Inferior prognostic value compared with HIV RNA levels and CD4 cell count
Serologic testing for syphilis	Recommended	Syphilis rates increased among HIV-infected patients
Toxoplasma antibodies	Recommended	Useful test to have as baseline to determine if prophylaxis needed; also provides useful information if patient found to have brain mass lesion
Cytomegalovirus antibody	Optional	Generally not useful in homosexual men, since almost all are seropositive; would be more useful in other risk groups with lower cytomegalovirus prevalence; indicated in all groups if to receive blood products
Liver function tests	Optional	Reasonable considering increased hepatobiliary complications in HIV-infected persons
Cryptococcal antigen	Not recommended	Useful test for patient with suspected cryptococcal disease, but not useful as a screening test
Urinalysis	Optional	Screening generally low yield; most valuable test would be urine dipstick for protein
Radiographic studies		
Chest radiograph	Optional	Reasonable to obtain as baseline for later comparison; routine periodic screening not recommended
Brain computed tomography	Not recommended	Limited value as screening test, but often important in evaluating central nervous system disease
Chest computed tomography	Not recommended	Limited value as screening test
Abdominal computed tomography	Not recommended	Limited value as screening test

as identify patients with chronic hepatitis B virus infection. Testing for antibody to hepatitis C virus is also reasonable, but is not as high a priority as testing for hepatitis B virus infection, mainly because a vaccine for hepatitis C virus is not available and hepatitis C does not appear to be readily transmitted by sexual contact.

Among HIV-infected homosexual men, testing for cytomegalovirus antibodies generally has not been recommended, since more than 90 percent of homosexual males are cytomegalovirus antibody–positive.[18] The seropositivity rates among HIV-infected hemophiliacs, heterosexuals, and children, however, are significantly lower. Accordingly, performing routine cytomegalovirus antibody testing in those HIV-infected individuals who did not acquire HIV through homosexual contact appears to be a reasonable approach.

Many authorities recommend obtaining baseline IgG *Toxoplasma* titers for three major reasons: (1) cerebral toxoplasmosis is one of the most common opportunistic pathogens of the brain in HIV-infected patients; (2) almost all infections result from reactivation of prior *Toxoplasma* infection; and (3) without prophylaxis, about 30 percent of HIV-infected individuals with a positive antibody titer to *Toxoplasma gondii* will develop central nervous system toxoplasmosis.[19]

Although serum cryptococcal antigen is a highly sensitive marker for invasive cryptococcal disease in HIV-infected patients, routine screening has limited value since patients generally have negative titers unless they develop active cryptococcal disease.[20]

RADIOGRAPHIC STUDIES

A prospective study to determine the value of obtaining a routine chest radiograph in asymptomatic HIV-infected patients has not been performed.[21] Although a routine screening film is unlikely to show an abnormality in an asymptomatic patient, many clinicians obtain a baseline chest radiograph, mainly to have as a comparison film for the future. Routine periodic screening of asymptomatic patients with chest radiographs is not recommended, however.[22] As a baseline test for initial evaluation, computed tomographic studies of the brain, chest, or abdomen are not indicated, mainly based on their low yield and high cost.

TUBERCULIN SKIN TESTING

The initial evaluation of all HIV-infected patients should include tuberculin skin testing for three major reasons: (1) compared with incidence rates in the general population, the incidence of tuberculosis in HIV-infected individuals is significantly increased; (2) HIV-infected patients with active tuberculosis can spread this infection to persons in the community and within health care settings; and (3) effective chemoprophylactic regimens are available to prevent reactivation of tuberculosis. Testing for tuberculosis should be performed by administering five tuberculin units of purified-protein-derivative (PPD) tuberculin intradermally, and, 48 to 72 hours later, the skin induration (not erythema) should be measured.[23] For all HIV-infected patients, a tuberculin reaction ≥ 5 mm is considered positive, regardless of bacille of Calmette and Guérin (BCG) status. Individuals with a positive PPD should have active tuberculosis excluded with a chest radiograph and clinical evaluation. Assuming the patient has no evidence of active tuberculosis, they should receive chemoprophylaxis with isoniazid, 300 mg once daily, for 12 months.[24] The value of repeated PPD testing in this setting has not been evaluated; some have recommended yearly screening, especially in those patients who have ongoing risk factors for acquiring tuberculosis.

To perform anergy testing, two delayed-type hypersensitivity skin-test antigens, such as mumps, tetanus toxoid, or *Candida,* should be intradermally injected at the same time the PPD is placed.[23] Previously, the CDC has recommended that anergic patients should receive chemoprophylaxis if they are in a "high-risk" group in which the prevalence of tuberculosis is at least 10 percent; these groups include injection drug users, prisoners, homeless persons, migrant laborers, and persons born in countries (Asia, Africa, and Latin America) with high rates of tuberculosis. A recent study, however, found no difference in the incidence of tuberculosis among anergic "high-risk" individuals randomized to receive either isoniazid or placebo.[25] Based on this recent study, it is very likely that anergic testing will no longer be recommended.

VACCINATIONS

At the time of the initial evaluation, the provider should review the patient's vaccine history and administer appropriate vaccines. In general, HIV-infected patients produce inferior antibody responses to vaccines as compared with those produced by immunocompetent patients, but relatively good antibody response rates develop with most vaccines if the vaccine is given early in the course of the patient's HIV disease.[21] Recent studies have shown that vaccinations may upregulate HIV replication, as suggested by significant increases in HIV RNA levels shortly after vaccination. Such increases in HIV RNA, however, are transient and appear small compared with those observed during the actual infections one is trying to prevent with the vaccinations.[26] Presently, most experts do not consider the transient upregulation in HIV replication as a contraindication to vaccination.

Epidemiologic evidence strongly suggests that HIV-infected individuals have an increased risk of developing severe *Streptococcus pneumoniae* infections.[27] Accordingly, the CDC recommends that all HIV-infected patients receive the 23-valent pneumococcal polysaccharide vaccine as early in the course of the patient's HIV infection as possible.[28]

Although invasive *Haemophilus influenzae* infections occur with increased frequency among HIV-infected adults, those caused by *H. influenzae* type B are responsible for only about one-third of these cases.[29] At this time, a clear consensus on whether to administer *H. influenzae* type B vaccine to adults does not exist. Previous studies have shown that the polysaccharide *H. influenzae* type B vaccine produces good antibody responses for those patients vaccinated early in the course of their HIV infection, but among patients with AIDS, polysaccharide–protein conjugate vaccine produces the best responses.[30]

Although the risks of serious complications associated with influenza virus infection among HIV-infected persons remain unknown, many experts (including the CDC) recommend influenza vaccine.[31] In addition to trying to prevent influenza-associated morbidity and mortality, influenza pneumonia can resemble pneumonia caused by opportunistic infections and therefore lead to unnecessary diagnostic procedures. Moreover, HIV-infected patients have an increased risk of developing infection with pathogens, such as *S. pneumoniae*, that commonly complicate influenza pneumonia. Patients with early-stage HIV disease generally have good antibody responses to influenza vaccine, but those patients with advanced immunodeficiency often have poor responses.

Many HIV-infected patients belong to risk groups that also have a high rate of HBV infection. In addition, among HIV-infected patients who acquire HBV infection, a chronic carrier state develops approximately threefold more often than in HIV-negative patients. For these reasons, all HIV-infected individuals who lack evidence of protective anti-HBV antibodies should receive HBV vaccine. For HIV-infected patients, the recommendation for HBV vaccine is 40 μg of recombinant HBV vaccine in the deltoid muscle; if Recombivax HB is used, repeat the vaccine 1 and 6 months later and repeat at 1, 2, and 6 months with Engerix-B.[32] Unfortunately, HIV-infected patients often have suboptimal responses, even those with early-stage disease.[33]

For those HIV-infected patients who did not receive routine vaccinations during childhood, most recommend administering these routine vaccines, except for live oral polio vaccine.[28] In addition, most do not recommend giving measles vaccine to those patients with advanced immunosuppression. Vaccination with BCG in order to prevent tuberculosis is not recommended, mainly because this vaccination contains live mycobacteria and thus can cause active infection in immunocompromised individuals, even years after receiving BCG.[34]

ROUTINE FOLLOW-UP

The frequency of follow-up visits depends on the stage of the HIV disease and whether the patient has ongoing active problems. Most asymptomatic patients with a CD4 count greater than 500 cells/mm³ can be followed every 6 months, obtaining a CD4 cell count and HIV RNA measurement at each visit. Patients with a CD4 count less than 500 cells/mm³ or symptomatic HIV disease, as well as those taking antiretroviral therapy, should be followed at least every 3 months (obtaining CD4 cell count and HIV RNA measurements every 3 months). Patients with active major problems and those with a CD4 count less than 100 cells/mm³ generally need to be followed more frequently than every 3 months, typically every 4 to 6 weeks.

ORAL MANIFESTATIONS

Almost all HIV-infected persons will develop an oral disorder at some point in the course of their disease.[35,36] Several studies have shown that the type, frequency, and severity of oral lesions depends on the patient's stage of HIV disease, with more complications associated with more advanced HIV disease. The oral disorders can be classified on the basis of morphology or on the basis of the cause.

ORAL HAIRY LEUKOPLAKIA

Oral hairy leukoplakia occurs almost exclusively in HIV-infected patients (rare cases occur in cancer patients, solid organ transplant patients, or bone marrow transplant patients); one should consider the finding of oral hairy leukoplakia strongly suggestive of HIV infection. This disorder occurs with a frequency of approximately 20 percent in those with early-stage HIV disease and, with more advanced disease, increases to approximately 40 percent.[35] Although first described in homosexual HIV-infected persons, oral hairy leukoplakia has now been described in persons from all HIV risk groups and in all regions of the world.[36] The presence

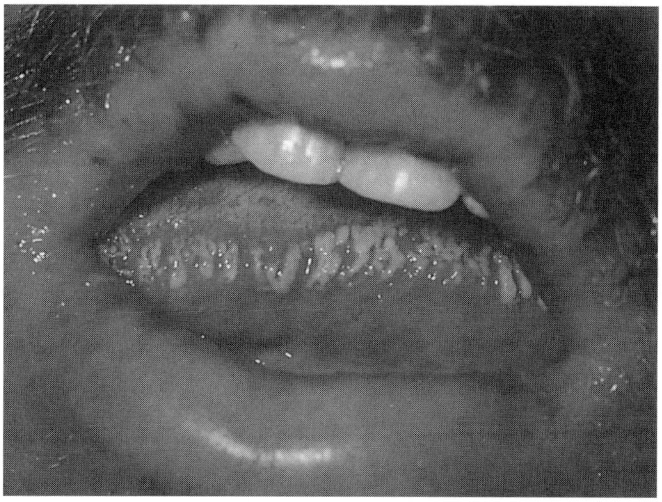

Fig. 73-2. Oral hairy leukoplakia in a patient with HIV infection.

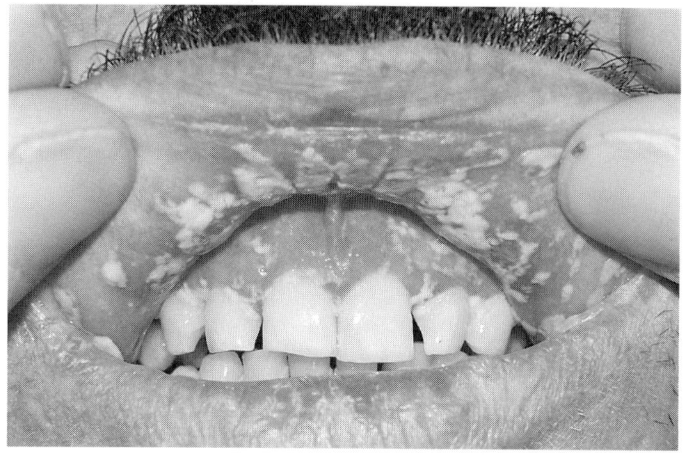

Fig. 73-3. Pseudomembranous oral candidiasis (thrush) in a patient with HIV infection.

of oral hairy leukoplakia reflects clinical immunodeficiency and predicts the development of AIDS independent of the patient's CD4 cell count. This abnormality is considered a CDC category B disease. Most evidence points to Epstein-Barr virus as the causative agent.[37]

Oral hairy leukoplakia typically appears as white, vertically oriented striations on the lateral aspect of the tongue (Fig. 73-2, See also Color Plate 61). In some patients, it may appear as a diffuse white film. The key to the presumptive diagnosis of oral hairy leukoplakia is the inability to remove lesions with scraping; almost all candida lesions will be removed with scraping, except for the rare cases of hyperplastic candidiasis (also known as candida leukoplakia). A definitive diagnosis can be made with a mucosal biopsy that shows Epstein-Barr virus, but this is rarely done. Although oral hairy leukoplakia rarely requires treatment, various topical and systemic agents have been effective. Reports with effective topical agents have included trichloroacetic acid, glycolic acid, and 25% podophyllum resin.[35] Systemic therapies with acyclovir and ganciclovir have also been shown to be effective.[38] All of the oral and systemic therapies, however, do not permanently eliminate Epstein-Barr virus, and the lesions may reoccur.

CANDIDIASIS

Oral candidiasis occurs very commonly among HIV-infected individuals, especially those with CD4 cells counts less than 300 cells/mm^3. Although the presence of oral candidiasis strongly suggests HIV infection, it can occur with other conditions, such as diabetes mellitus, cancer, and pregnancy, as well as with broad-spectrum antimicrobials and corticosteroids. Oral candidiasis in an HIV-infected person reflects clinical immunodeficiency and predicts progression to AIDS independent of the patient's CD4 cell count. This abnormality is considered a CDC category B disease. Although most cases of oral candidiasis are caused by *Candida albicans,* other distinct species, such as *C. tropicalis*, *C. glabrata*, and *C. krusei*, can occasionally cause clinical disease. All species of *Candida* are yeasts, not molds. Oral candidiasis can commonly appear in three different forms: pseudomembranous (thrush), atrophic (erythematous), and angular cheilitis. Pseudomembranous candidiasis appears as thick white plaques and can be present anywhere in the mouth, including the tongue, buccal mucosa, palate, gums, and the posterior pharynx; these lesions can readily be scraped off with a tongue blade (Fig. 73-3). The atrophic (erythematous) form, which is often underdiagnosed, appears as either patchy erythema on the hard palate or smooth slick areas on the tongue (Figs. 73-4 and 73-5). Patients with angular cheilitis have cracking and erythema at the corners of their mouth (Fig. 73-6). Symptoms associated with oral candidiasis often depend on the degree of candidiasis and may include pain, a burning sensation, or alterations in taste. Rarely, patients with oral candidiasis may develop nonremovable white patches (known as hyperplastic candidiasis); these lesions resemble oral hairy leukoplakia, especially since both are not easily removed with scraping. The hyperplastic candidiasis lesions, however, are homogeneous, do not have the typical vertical corrugations associated with oral hairy leukoplakia, and resolve with antifungal therapy.[36]

In most cases, a presumptive diagnosis is made on a clinical basis. A rapid confirmatory diagnosis can be made by scraping a suspected candida lesion and identifying yeasts under the microscope (either by Gram stain or potassium hydroxide staining). On Gram stain, the organisms appear bluish-purple and are much larger than bacteria. With Gram stain or potassium hydroxide staining, one may see budding yeasts or hyphae. Culture is generally not recommended unless fluconazole-resistant candidiasis is suspected.

In general, for mild oral candidiasis in a patient who does not have advanced HIV disease, initial therapy consists of topical

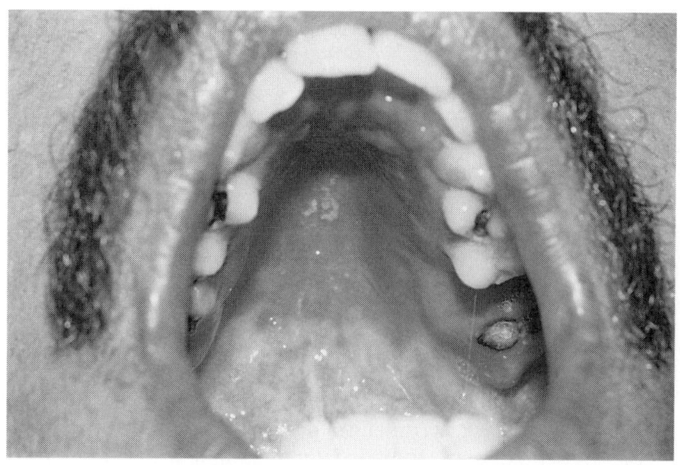

Fig. 73-4. Erythematous (atrophic) oral candidiasis in a patient with HIV infection.

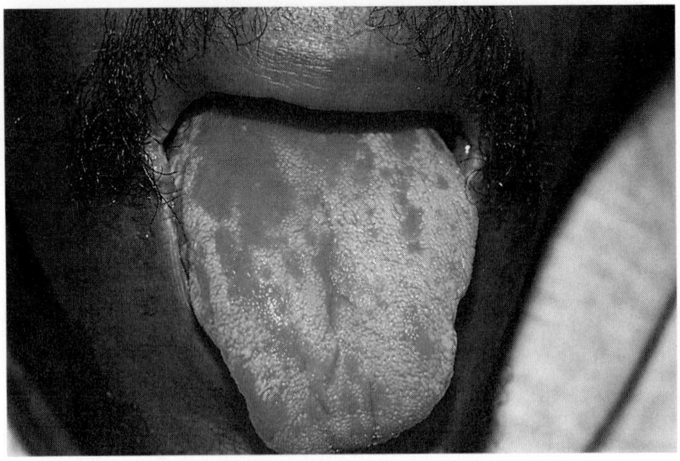

Fig. 73-5. Erythematous (atrophic) oral candidiasis in a patient with HIV infection.

agents, either clotrimazole troches, nystatin (pastilles, vaginal tablets, or solution), or amphotericin (tablets or solution). For the patient with moderate to severe oral candidiasis, as well as those who do not respond to topical therapy, systemic therapy is indicated, preferably with fluconazole or ketoconazole. Fluconazole is more expensive than ketoconazole, but is more effective, has fewer drug interactions, and does not have the problems of decreased absorption in nonacidic conditions in the stomach. The optimal approach for patients following their initial therapy, however, remains unknown. For angular cheilitis, topical antifungal agents, such as clotrimazole 1% cream or ketoconazole 2% cream, are often sufficient.

During the past several years, numerous reports have documented an increasing incidence of fluconazole-refractory oral candidiasis among HIV-infected patients who have a low CD4 count (generally less than 50 cells/mm^3).[39] For patients with oral candidiasis who do not respond to fluconazole, many authorities now recommend performing susceptibility testing on fungal isolates; an MIC of 64 or greater to fluconazole generally corresponds with clinical failure. The results from in vitro susceptibility testing, however, do not always correspond with clinical responses. Although the optimal therapy for fluconazole-refractory candidiasis remains to be determined, limited experience suggests that most patients will respond to intravenous amphotericin B (0.4 to 0.5 mg/kg/per day) when given two to four times per week. Other reasonable, but less reliable, options include amphotericin oral solution, oral itraconazole cyclodextrin solution, topical gentian violet, high-dose (600 to 800 mg/day) oral fluconazole, and 5-flucytosine (5-FC) combined with either fluconazole or amphotericin B.

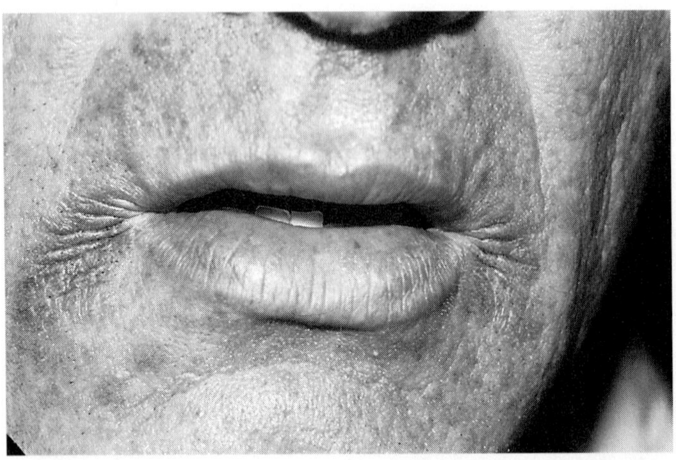

Fig. 73-6. Angular cheilitis caused by candidia infection in a patient with HIV infection.

HERPES SIMPLEX VIRUS

Herpes simplex virus (HSV) infections can present as primary or reactivation disease, although the latter is much more common as a cause of oral lesions in HIV-infected individuals. Chronic ulcerative HSV that persists for at least 1 month is an AIDS-defining diagnosis. Two types of HSV can cause oral lesions: HSV-1 (approx. 90 percent) and HSV-2 (approx. 10 percent). In contrast, genital HSV is caused by about 90 percent HSV-2 and only 10 percent HSV-1. Patients with early-stage HIV disease who develop oral HSV infection typically present with symptoms similar to those seen in immunocompetent individuals, namely, vesicular lesions on the lips or pharynx that resolve in 5 to 7 days. Individuals with advanced HIV disease, however, often develop nonhealing ulcerative lesions that may involve the tongue, gums, pharynx, or palate. In addition, patients with advanced HIV may develop extension of the lesions outside of the mouth onto the face. The presumptive diagnosis of HSV is not reliable, mainly because other oral disorders, such as aphthae, cytomegalovirus, and secondary syphilis, can appear similar to oral HSV.

The preferred method of diagnosis is to obtain a specimen for fluorescent antibody (FA) and culture. When obtaining a specimen, scrape the base of the lesion to obtain cells (the virus is an intracellular virus and thus it is critical to obtain cells). The FA results are often available within 24 hours; cultures typically turn positive in 2 to 3 days and 95 percent are positive within 5 days. When FA and culture is not available, the Tzanck preparation (Wright-Giemsa stain) should be used; this test is reasonably sensitive, but has poor specificity. Patients with early-stage HIV disease who develop oral HSV infection often have spontaneous resolution of the lesions in 7 to 10 days. Patients with more advanced disease generally require anti-HSV therapy with acyclovir 400 mg PO tid (or 200 mg PO 5×/day); therapy is generally given for 5 to 7 days, or until the lesions resolve. Long-term suppressive therapy remains controversial.

APHTHAE

Aphthae are painful ulcerations in the oral cavity of unknown cause. Although aphthae frequently occur among persons in the general population who are not HIV-infected, this disorder causes unique problems among those with HIV disease. Moreover, HIV-infected persons who have experienced aphthae in the past frequently develop an exacerbation of the condition after becoming infected with HIV. Patients with early-stage HIV disease who develop aphthae typically present with symptoms similar to those seen in immunocompetent individuals, namely small painful ulcers on the tongue, lips, or buccal mucosa that resolve in 5 to 7 days. Individuals with advanced HIV disease, however, generally develop nonhealing, progressively enlarging lesions that may involve the tongue, buccal mucosa, lips, pharynx, or palate (Fig. 73-7). In general, the diagnosis of aphthae is a diagnosis of exclusion. Infection with HSV should be ruled out in all patients.

Therapy for aphthae consists of pain relief and measures to heal the lesions. Viscous lidocaine (2% solution) rinsed in the mouth for 1 to 3 minutes every 3 to 6 hours provides effective pain relief, but breakthrough pain between treatments frequently occurs. Lo-

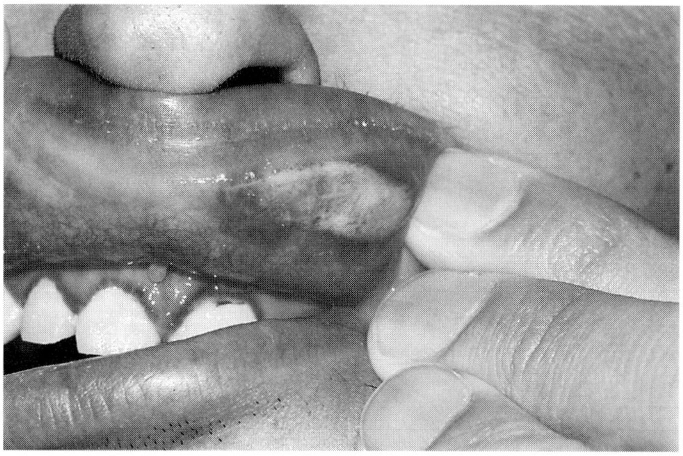

Fig. 73-7. Oral aphthae in a patient with HIV infection.

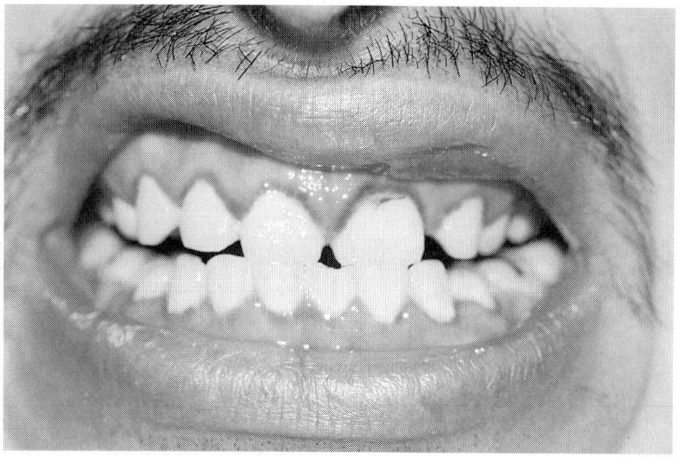

Fig. 73-8. Linear gingival erythema in a patient with HIV infection.

calized lesions in the oral cavity (mild to moderate disease) usually are best treated with topical steroid regimens, such as triamcinolone dental paste (0.1% applied to lesions 3×/day) or dexamethasone elixir (1/2 to 1 teaspoon of 0.5 mg/mL used as a 4- to 5-minute rinse 5×/day). Large, extensive oral lesions or ulcers distal to the mouth (severe disease) usually require systemic steroids; some have recommended prednisone 40 mg qd for 7 days, then taper by 10 mg every week. Recently, thalidomide (100 to 200 mg PO qd × 14 days) has shown promise as a therapy for aphthae; thalidomide, however, is not approved by the U.S. Food and Drug Administration.[40,41]

PERIODONTAL DISEASE

HIV-infected patients can develop one of four major forms of periodontal disease: linear gingival erythema (formerly HIV-associated gingivitis), acute necrotizing ulcerative gingivitis, necrotizing periodontitis (formerly HIV-associated periodontitis), and necrotizing stomatitis.[35] Linear gingival erythema refers to inflammation of the gingivae caused by oral microflora and presents as an intense erythematous band along the free gingival margin, often associated with mild to moderate gingival pain (Fig. 73-8). This involvement of the gums may become more severe and develop into an acute necrotizing ulcerative gingivitis. If this condition extends into the underlying alveolar bone, it is referred to as necrotizing periodontitis and patients present with halitosis, spontaneous gingival bleeding, a deep jaw ache, and increased tooth mobility; if not quickly recognized and treated it may lead to extensive tooth loss requiring extraction. In some instances, the gingival involvement progresses to involve adjacent soft tissues, a condition referred to as necrotizing stomatitis. The diagnosis of these conditions depends on the clinical appearance of the lesion. Routine bacterial cultures generally do not provide useful information and are not recommended on a routine basis. In patients with suspected necrotizing ulcerative gingivitis, however, cultures for herpes simplex virus should be obtained, mainly because herpetic gingivostomatitis can cause lesions that resemble necrotizing ulcerative gingivitis.

For very mild disease, patients should receive topical antiseptic mouth rinses, such as chlorhexidine 0.12% tid, as well as aggressive daily home oral hygiene (meticulous brushing and flossing). More extensive disease requires dental referral plus a 5- to 7-day course of systemic oral antimicrobial agents, such as penicillin (250 to 500 mg PO qid), metronidazole (250 to 500 mg PO tid), or clindamycin (300 to9 450 mg PO tid). Because these antimicrobial therapies have fairly potent killing of normal oral anaerobic flora, oral candidiasis frequently develops. With the more severe cases, a dentist should debride and curette all involved tissues. For prevention of periodontal disease, patients need to understand the importance of regularly brushing and flossing. Several devices that augment brushing and flossing, namely periodontal sulcular cleaning aids, proximal interdental brushes, and periodontal irrigators, have become commercially available.

CUTANEOUS MANIFESTATIONS

HIV-associated cutaneous disorders, both infectious and noninfectious, occur frequently throughout the course of HIV disease. The impairment of the skin immune system observed in HIV-infected individuals is believed to play an important role in causing these cutaneous disorders.[42] Common cutaneous disorders associated with HIV infection include infectious (viral, bacterial, fungal, and parasitic) as well as noninfectious causes (xerosis, eosinophilic folliculitis, and psoriasis).

MOLLUSCUM CONTAGIOSUM

Molluscum contagiosum, which is caused by a poxvirus, can develop at any stage of HIV disease, but is most often seen in patients with CD4 counts less than 200 cells/mm^3. Patients typically present with umbilicated flesh-colored, 2- to 5-mm papular lesions, most often located on the face, neck, and genital tract (Fig. 73-9).[43] If left untreated, the lesions can progress to several centimeters in size (giant molluscum) and can become widespread. In contrast with immunocompetent individuals who generally have a brief self-limited bout of molluscum, HIV-infected patients often have lesions that do not spontaneously resolve, especially if the person has advanced immunosuppression. The diagnosis is usually made clinically, based on the typical appearance. A definitive diagnosis can be made by shelling out the core of the lesion (or by performing a biopsy), and a Gram stain will show pathognomonic molluscum bodies that appear as large spherical homogeneous inclusion bodies within epidermal cells.

Although most patients do not describe problematic symptoms from molluscum, treatment is recommended for three reasons: (1) untreated lesions may progress to disfiguring lesions, which can be particularly distressing if they occur on the face; (2) treatment diminishes the likelihood of autoinoculation-induced widespread disease; and (3) treatment decreases the risk of person-to-person

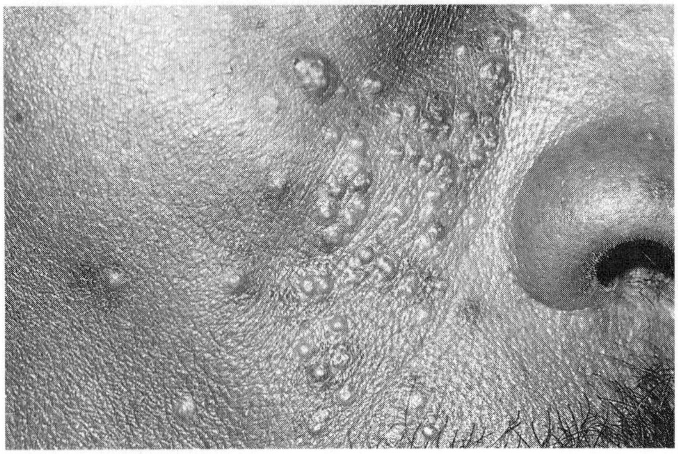

Fig. 73-9. Facial molluscum contagiosum in a patient with HIV infection.

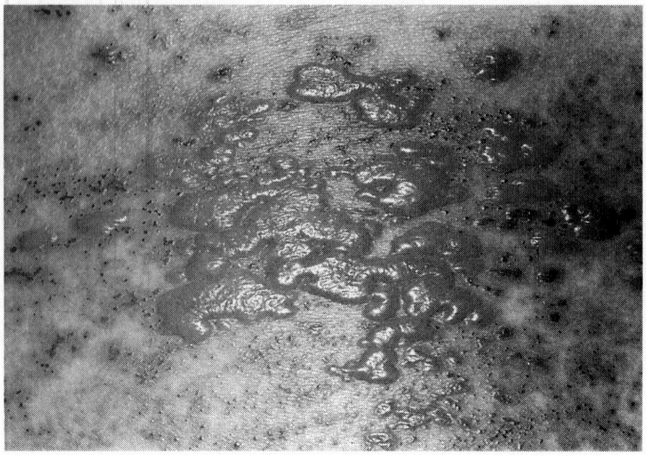

Fig. 73-10. Herpes zoster infection in a patient with HIV infection.

transmission of molluscum. The most realistic goal of treatment is to decrease the number and size of lesions. This goal can be accomplished with local destructive measures, such as liquid nitrogen cryotherapy (5- to 20-second liquid nitrogen freeze to each lesion repeated once after the lesion thaws); most patients require multiple treatments spaced several weeks apart, especially those with large lesions or widespread disease. Other local destructive measures include curettage and burning the lesions with a bifurcator needle or pen cautery. Ideally, repeat the treatment as often as needed to allow interval healing, but not significant regrowth of the lesion. Because local destructive measures may cause scarring and skin discoloration, patients should be warned about this complication. Topical tretinoin (0.025% cream to affected areas qhs), although not effective therapy for large lesions, often provides an excellent option for multiple small lesions (mild disease) and for the prevention of new lesions; topical tretinoin should not be applied to the genitals.

VARICELLA-ZOSTER VIRUS

Infection with varicella-zoster virus can develop at any stage of a patient's HIV disease, and, in some instances, it may be the first HIV-related manifestation. More than 90 percent of HIV-infected adults have a history of previous varicella (chicken pox); thus, in almost all cases, infections with this virus represent reactivation (zoster) in HIV-infected adults. HIV-infected patients have a much higher rate (about 15-fold) of zoster than age-matched persons who are not HIV-infected.[44] Patients typically develop painful grouped vesicles along a dermatomal distribution (Fig. 73-10). In some patients, dermatomal pain will precede the onset of cutaneous lesions. Although the initial clinical presentation of HIV-infected patients with zoster is usually similar to that in the immunocompetent patient, duration may be longer and the risk of dissemination higher.[45]

In most instances, zoster can be diagnosed on the basis of characteristic clinical findings. If the clinical diagnosis is uncertain and a confirmatory diagnostic test is needed, a lesion should be scraped to obtain a specimen for FA and culture. Performing a Tzanck test on the specimen is a reasonable alternative if the FA and culture are not available. It is critical to scrape the base of the lesion to obtain cells for any of these tests. The FA results usually become available within 24 hours, but cultures for varicella-zoster virus often take at least 7 days to turn positive. There have been no controlled studies regarding therapy of varicella or zoster in HIV-infected patients. For HIV-infected individuals, most recommend treatment with either acyclovir (800 mg PO 5 × per day × 10 to 14 days) or famciclovir (500 mg PO tid × 10 to 14 days), mainly to prevent dissemination and to decrease the duration and severity of the lesions. If lesions have not crusted or if new lesions continue to appear after 10 to 14 days of therapy, the therapy should be extended. Many authorities have shown reluctance to recommend valacyclovir because one study showed an increased incidence of a thrombotic thrombocytopenic purpura–like disorder in HIV-infected patients receiving long-term, high-dose valacyclovir for cytomegalovirus prophylaxis.[46] Among HIV-infected patients, no evidence exists that either acyclovir, famciclovir, or corticosteroid therapy decreases the incidence or duration of postherpetic neuralgia. Corticosteroids are not recommended for HIV-infected patients with zoster.

HERPES SIMPLEX VIRUS

Herpes simplex virus infections are common in HIV-infected patients.[47] In HIV-infected adults, most HSV infections result from reactivation disease. Chronic ulcerative HSV (present for longer than 1 month) is an AIDS-defining diagnosis. HIV-infected patients (especially those with more advanced HIV disease) often present with painful and ulcerative mucocutaneous HSV lesions, rather than classic vesicular lesions. These lesions can be chronic and are most often located on the face, penis, vulva, or perianal region. Patients may develop HSV in atypical locations, such as the ear, scalp, scrotum, or gluteal fold.

HSV is often misdiagnosed and clinicians need to have a high index of suspicion. Any unexplained ulcerative or vesicular lesion should be tested for HSV. The optimal tests for HSV are the FA and culture. Performing a Tzanck test on the specimen is a reasonable alternative if the FA and culture are not available. The FA results are usually available within 24 hours; with HSV, more than 90 percent of positive cultures will turn positive by 5 days. Therapy for recurrent oral or genital HSV generally consists of acyclovir (400 mg PO tid × 5 to 7 days) or famciclovir (125 mg PO bid × 5 to 7 days). Clinicians will often extend therapy past 5 to 7 days if lesions have not healed or if new lesions continue to appear while on therapy. Patients should receive intravenous acyclovir if they have severe mucocutaneous involvement, or if they fail conventional oral therapy. If a patient has a lesion that does not respond to high-dose oral or intravenous therapy, consider acyclovir resistance and obtain a viral culture specifically for acyclovir susceptibility testing.[48]

SEBORRHEIC DERMATITIS

This common problem is often an early manifestation of HIV infection. Although seborrheic dermatitis is a common problem in persons not infected with HIV, this disorder is more frequent and more severe in HIV-infected persons.[49] Seborrheic dermatitis is believed to result from both infection with the fungus *Pityrosporum* plus the host inflammatory response to this organism. Classically, the patient develops an erythematous scaly rash located on the forehead and sides of the face, with frequent involvement of the beard area. In addition, patients may have involvement of other areas, such as behind the ears, the central chest, and the axilla. The severity of seborrheic dermatitis often correlates with the degree of immunosuppression, and treatment may be more difficult in those individuals with a low CD4 cell count.

The diagnosis of seborrheic dermatitis is made on the basis of clinical findings; obtaining cultures or performing a skin biopsy is generally not necessary. Because cure of seborrheic dermatitis does not occur with therapy, the goal is to control the symptoms and manifestations. After control is achieved, therapy on an as-needed basis is generally sufficient. In general, ketoconazole cream (2% cream applied bid) is considered the preferred first-line therapy for facial seborrheic dermatitis in HIV-infected persons. For severe or refractory cases, ketoconazole cream should be combined with a topical steroid (1% hydrocortisone cream). For those patients who do not respond to topical ketoconazole plus hydrocortisone, systemic therapy with either ketoconazole (200 mg PO qd) or fluconazole (100 mg PO qd) should be used. After obtaining control with a systemic agent, attempt a switch back to topical therapy.

SCABIES

Scabies infection, caused by infestation with the mite *Sarcoptes scabeii*, is a common problem in HIV-infected individuals. This infection is spread via close person-to-person contact. Patients may develop two types of scabies: classic (typical) scabies or crusted (Norwegian) scabies. Classic scabies typically manifests as severe pruritus and with multiple urticarial papules and excoriations present on examination. Prominent areas of involvement include the the wrist, web spaces of the hands, the umbilicus, and the belt line. If burrows (long, slightly elevated, linear or tortuous lesions) are observed, they strongly suggest the diagnosis of scabies (Fig. 73-11, See also Color Plate 81). In addition, males often have involvement of the glans penis and buttocks (Fig. 73-12, See also Color Plate 82) as well as having indurated erythematous nodules (scabetic nodules) usually located on the scrotum. In HIV-infected patients, crusted scabies usually only occurs in patients with late-stage AIDS. Although patients with crusted scabies are infested with an extremely large number of mites, they amazingly often do not complain of pruritus. The lesions of crusted scabies typically appear as thick, grayish-white, hyperkeratotic crusts, often with fissuring and plaque formation.[50]

The diagnosis of scabies is usually suggested by the clinical appearance of the lesions. To make a definitive diagnosis, scrape a skin burrow and identify the scabies mite (or eggs) on microscopic examination (Fig. 73-13, See also Color Plate 80). The technique for skin scraping involves several steps. First, locate a burrow and apply a drop of mineral oil (the web spaces, fingers, wrists, and ankles provide the best locations). Second, scrape vigorously over the surface of the burrow with a number 15 scalpel blade held at an angle. Third, place the scraping onto a glass slide and place a coverslip on top of the specimen. (If you did not use mineral oil, apply a drop of potassium hydroxide.) For patients with crusted scabies, simply remove a small portion of an area with a thick hyperkeratotic crust, and microscopic examination typically shows abundant mites (and eggs).

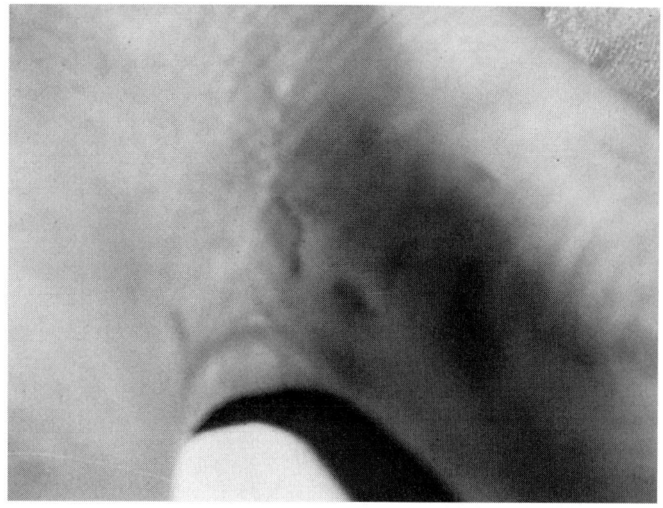

Fig. 73-11. Intradermal burrow of scabies demonstrated by coating the skin with ink, then wiping away surface ink, leaving the intradermal burrow filled with ink.

The treatment of choice is 5% permethrin cream (30 to 60 gm is typically required for each application); the patient should liberally apply the cream over the entire body from the neck down, leaving it on for 8 to 12 hours.[51] At the end of that time, the patient should wash the cream off. The patient should make sure to apply abundant cream to the nails, web spaces, genitalia, and intertriginous areas. Many experts recommend that patients with a CD4 count less than 100 cells/mm^3 also apply the cream to his or her head. The patient should repeat the treatment either the following night or 1 week later. Most consider lindane 1% lotion a reasonable alternative; it should be applied the same as with permethrin. All close contacts should be treated, even if asymptomatic. Some patients may have itching that persists longer than 10 to 14 days

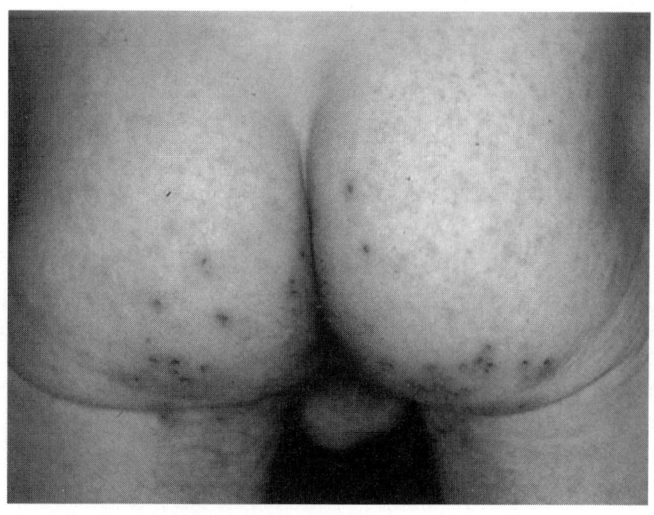

Fig. 73-12. Grouped excoriations caused by scabies on the lower buttocks, simulating dermatitis herpetiformis.

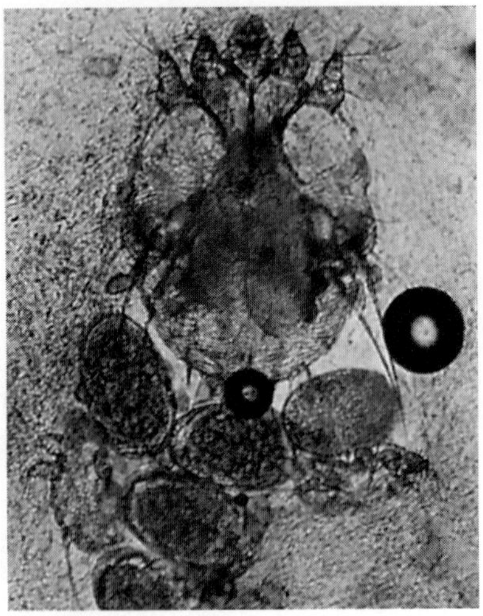

Fig. 73-13. *Sarcopus scabiei* mite with eggs in feces scraped from scabetic burrow.

after treatment; this may result from either reinfestation, inadequate treatment, or a slowly resolving hypersensitivity response. Patients with crusted scabies should receive repeated applications of permethrin for effective therapy.

FOLLICULITIS

HIV-infected patients frequently develop folliculitis, usually either bacterial folliculitis or eosinophilic folliculitis (also known as eosinophilic pustular folliculitis). Most cases of bacterial folliculitis are caused by *Staphylococcus aureus*, but other organisms, such as *Streptococcus* species, coagulase-negative *Staphylococcus*, *Pseudomonas aeruginosa*, or diphtheroids, occasionally can be involved. Patients with bacterial folliculitis present with a follicular eruption located in hair-bearing regions. In some instances, the lesion may extend deep into the soft tissues and form abscesses, furuncles, or carbuncles. The cause of eosinophilic folliculitis is unknown. Patients with eosinophilic folliculitis frequently complain of intense pruritus and present with follicular papules on the face, trunk, and upper extremities; involvement below the waist generally does not occur and suggests a diagnosis of bacterial folliculitis.[52] Patients with eosinophilic folliculitis usually vigorously scratch these lesions, thus obscuring the natural appearance of the lesion.

The diagnosis of folliculitis is made on a clinical basis, but differentiating the type of folliculitis often requires performing a punch biopsy. If bacterial folliculitis is suspected, as a first step, find a lesion that scratching has not altered and perform a Gram stain and culture. If the Gram stain and culture is not diagnostic, it is reasonable to give an empiric course of antistaphylococcal antimicrobial therapy to help clarify the cause. If the diagnosis remains in question, consider performing a punch biopsy of a lesion that scratching has not altered. Histologic findings with eosinophilic folliculitis typically show a perifollicular eosinophilic infiltrate and some follicular degeneration. Although not specific, many patients with eosinophilic folliculitis have a relative (or absolute) eosinophilia and increased IgE levels.

Bacterial folliculitis generally responds to appropriate systemic antimicrobial therapy, such as dicloxacillin (250 to 500 mg PO qid × 10 to 14 days) or cephalexin (250 to 500 mg PO qid × 10 to 14 days). More invasive lesion, such as furuncles, carbuncles, and abscesses, require incision and drainage. If a patient has recurrent bacterial folliculitis despite therapy, he or she may have sanctuary sites of infection, such as in the nares, rectum, or beneath the fingernails; these patients may benefit from treatment with nasal mupirocin (apply bid × 5 days); for refractory cases, consider adding rifampin (300 mg PO bid × 7 to 10 days). In general, treatment of eosinophilic folliculitis is problematic. Patients generally respond the best to ultraviolet light treatments (ultraviolet B therapy 3 to 5 × per week), although this type of therapy is expensive and inconvenient.[52] Recent success has also been reported in some patients with the use of high-dose itraconazole (200 to 400 mg/day).[53] Most patients do not respond well to treatment with antihistamines alone.

PULMONARY MANIFESTATIONS

HIV-infected patients can develop a myriad of pulmonary complications, including infectious and noninfectious causes. The details of the diagnosis and management of these disorders are given in Chaps. 75 and 76. HIV-infected individuals develop pneumonia with *S. pneumoniae* at an approximately tenfold increased rate when compared with the general population.[54] Although HIV-infected patients who develop pneumococcal pneumonia usually do so before they develop AIDS and most have clinical signs and symptoms similar to those in HIV-negative individuals, they have a 20-fold higher incidence of pneumococcal bacteremia and a higher relapse rate. Approximately 85 percent of the pneumococcal infections involve strains contained in the 23-valent pneumococcal polysaccharide vaccine; thus, patients should receive pneumococcal vaccination; responses to the vaccine are better if the vaccine is given early in the course of HIV disease. *Haemophilus influenzae* can also cause pneumonia in HIV-infected patients, but much less frequently than pneumococcal pneumonia.

Although the incidence of *Pneumocystis carinii* pneumonia (PCP) has decreased dramatically as a result of effective prophylaxis, it remains the most common AIDS-defining opportunistic infection. Patients with PCP generally have a CD4 count less than 200 cells/mm^3 and present with a subacute course that begins with nonspecific systemic symptoms, such as fever, night sweats, and malaise.[55] Subsequently, patients develop a nonproductive cough followed by varying degrees of dyspnea. In most instances, the pulmonary physical examination is not specific for PCP. Although up to 20 percent of patients with PCP may present with a normal chest radiograph, most patients have diffuse or perihilar interstitial infiltrates.

Tuberculosis, which is caused by *Mycobacterium tuberculosis*, can occur at any stage of HIV disease, but most often occurs in patients with a CD4 count less than 200 cells/mm^3. In general, tuberculosis in patients with early-stage HIV resembles the clinical presentation of tuberculosis in persons not infected with HIV, namely, involvement of the upper lobes of the lungs, frequent cavitation of upper lobes, and infrequent extrapulmonary disease.[24] In contrast, patients with AIDS often have an atypical presentation characterized by diffuse pulmonary infiltrates and frequent extrapulmonary disease.

Most HIV-infected patients with *Mycobacterium avium* complex (MAC) infection generally present with disseminated disease, but focal pulmonary disease can infrequently occur. In addition, isolation of MAC from the respiratory tract predicts the patient will subsequently develop disseminated MAC. Because screening of sputum for MAC has a low sensitivity, routinely obtaining respiratory cultures for MAC is not recommended.[56] Almost all patients who develop disseminated MAC have a CD4 count less than 75 cells/mm^3.[57] Currently, most experts believe that cytomegalovirus infrequently causes pulmonary disease in HIV-infected patients, although this virus frequently may be found in secretions in the respiratory tract. If cytomegalovirus is isolated from the respiratory tract, it does not accurately predict the presence or development of cytomegalovirus-induced disease of the retina or gastrointestinal tract. Among HIV-infected individuals, infection with *Cryptococcus neoformans* may infrequently present as pulmonary cryptococcosis.[58] Patients who develop pulmonary cryptococcosis usually have evidence of disseminated infection and present with nonspecific symptoms, such as fever, weight loss, cough, dyspnea, and headache. In patients with pulmonary cryptococcosis, abnormalities observed with chest radiography include interstitial infiltrates, nodular patterns, pleural effusions, and lymphadenopathy. In certain endemic regions, *Histoplasma capsulatum* can cause pulmonary disease. Only about 5 percent of patients with histoplasmosis, however, present with pulmonary disease.

Patients with pulmonary Kaposi's sarcoma typically develop cough and dyspnea; most have concomitant cutaneous involvement, but some may initially present with isolated pulmonary disease. Chest radiographic appearances vary, but most often consist of diffuse irregular-bordered reticular–nodular lesions and mediastinal enlargement. Less frequently, the chest radiograph may show evidence of a pleural effusion. A presumptive diagnosis can be made if characteristic endobronchial lesions are viewed during bronchoscopy; definitive diagnosis can be established by histologic examination of a transbronchial or open-lung biopsy specimen. Patients with pulmonary Kaposi's sarcoma have a poor prognosis. The management of these pulmonary opportunistic infections and malignancies are discussed in detail in Chaps. 75 and 76.

GASTROINTESTINAL MANIFESTATIONS

Among HIV-infected individuals, two major types of gastrointestinal manifestations predominate: (1) esophagitis and (2) diarrhea. The most common causes of esophagitis include candida, cytomegalovirus, idiopathic ulcers (aphthae), and herpes simplex virus.[59,60] These disorders typically involve patients with a CD4 count less than 100 cells/mm^3. Regardless of the cause, patients may develop severe malnutrition as a result of ingesting insufficient calories. Patients with esophagitis generally present with odynophagia and retrosternal chest pain. The recommended approach for HIV-infected patients with esophagitis is to first assess for characteristic symptoms of gastrointestinal reflux and if present, treat for reflux. If the patient does not have characteristic reflux symptoms, treat empirically for candida esophagitis, and if not improved in about 5 days, proceed to upper endoscopy with biopsy.

Although the causes of diarrhea in HIV-infected patients are extensive, patients generally develop symptoms characteristic of either small bowel enteritis or colitis.[61] Among HIV-infected patients with chronic diarrhea, a specific pathogen is identified about 80 percent of the time. HIV-infected patients with chronic diarrhea generally suffer significant morbidity, mainly from decreased absorption of food and resultant wasting. Because the differential diagnosis is extensive, a stepwise approach to the diagnosis is most often used. The first step in the evaluation of diarrhea should include cultures for bacterial enteric pathogens (*Salmonella* spp., *Shigella* spp., *Yersinia* spp., and *Campylobacter* spp.), special modified acid-fast stains of stool (cryptosporidiosis and isosporiasis), ova and parasite direct examination (giardiasis, amebiasis, strongyloidiasis), and, if recently hospitalized or recently on antimicrobial therapy, testing for *Clostridium difficile* culture and toxin. As a second step, it is reasonable to look for microsporidiosis using the modified trichrome stain (Weber stain). If these noninvasive tests remain negative and the patient persists with diarrhea, then proceed to gastrointestinal endoscopy with bowel biopsy; whether to first do upper or lower endoscopy would depend on the patient's symptoms. Endoscopy may occasionally reveal pathogens missed on stool examination, as well as other disorders, such as cytomegalovirus, gastrointestinal Kaposi's sarcoma, *Mycobacterium avium* complex, and lymphoma. The treatment of the specific disorders that cause esophagitis or diarrhea are discussed in Chaps. 69, 75, and 77.

OCULAR MANIFESTATIONS

HIV-infected individuals can present with various ocular manifestations. The most common nonserious disorder is cotton wool spots, which presumably result from direct retinal microvascular HIV infection. These cotton wool spots typically do not cause symptoms, but take on importance because some providers confuse them with cytomegalovirus retinitis, a serious complication of HIV disease.[62] Cytomegalovirus retinitis results from reactivation of cytomegalovirus in patients who almost always have CD4 counts less than 100 cells/mm^3, typically in those patients with less than 50 cells/mm^3. Unlike patients with HIV-related cotton wool spots, patients with cytomegalovirus retinitis generally have symptoms, such as seeing floaters or flashing lights. Examination often detects a visual field deficit. The diagnosis is suspected based on characteristic visual symptoms in a patient with a low CD4 cell count; a presumptive diagnosis can be made with fundoscopic evaluation performed by an ophthalmologist; the fundoscopic examination typically shows a mix of hemorrhage and exudates, often described as a "brush fire."[63] Treatment and prevention of cytomegalovirus retinitis is described in detail in Chap. 75. Several opportunistic infections, such as *T. gondii* or *Pneumocystis carinii*, can cause retinal lesions that mimic cytomegalovirus retinitis, but these occur much less often than cytomegalovirus retinitis and can be distinguished by an experienced ophthalmologist. Rarely, patients may develop Kaposi's sarcoma lesions on the eyelids or conjunctiva.

ENDOCRINE MANIFESTATIONS

Although no evidence proves that HIV directly infects cells of the endocrine system, HIV-infected patients develop a number of endocrine disorders.[64,65] Autopsy studies have shown that most late-stage AIDS patients demonstrate some type of adrenal pathology, most often as a result of infection with cytomegalovirus or *Mycobacterium avium* complex; the amount of tissue destruction, however, is generally insufficient to produce symptomatic adrenal insufficiency. In many patients, the diagnosis of adrenal insufficiency is suspected based on compatible clinical signs and symptoms, but fewer than 20 percent of such patients have a definitive diagnosis of adrenal insufficiency and require steroid replacement. Nevertheless, many HIV-infected individuals frequently have subtle disorders of cortisol secretion.

HIV-infected patients often develop hypogonadism, most often associated with marked weight loss. Patients frequently complain of fatigue, decreased libido, and impotence. Patients with low testosterone may have symptomatic improvement with testosterone replacement; recently therapy with testosterone has been suggested as a means to improve lean body mass in AIDS patients with wasting syndrome.

RENAL MANIFESTATIONS

The most common renal abnormality found among HIV-infected persons is HIV-associated nephropathy, a disorder characterized by nephrotic range proteinuria (>3.5 gm of protein/24 hours), enlarged kidneys, and rapid progression to end-stage renal disease.[66,67] For unexplained reasons, HIV-associated nephropathy predominantly occurs among African American males. Indeed, the cause of HIV-associated nephropathy remains unknown. HIV-associated nephropathy typically progresses from mild renal insufficiency to end-stage renal disease within 2 to 6 months, a more rapid progression than with other forms of nephrotic syndrome. By contrast, persons with heroin-associated nephropathy have a mean time to end-stage renal disease of 20 to 44 months.

Unfortunately, most patients who develop HIV-associated nephropathy do not have early signs or symptoms that would provide a clue to this diagnosis prior to the onset of progressive nephropathy. When HIV-associated nephropathy symptoms develop, patients may have mild hypertension, peripheral edema, anasarca, or symptoms of uremia. Because clinical findings are often absent until late in the course of this disorder, an abnormal urinalysis (nephrotic range proteinuria) or an increased serum creatinine level may provide the first evidence that a patient has HIV-associated nephropathy. The differential diagnosis of nephrotic range proteinuria includes diabetes mellitus, malignancy, multiple myeloma, hepatitis B virus infection, hepatitis C virus infection, and systemic lupus erythematosus. Most patients with HIV-associated nephropathy have findings of enlarged echogenic kidneys on renal imaging studies. In general, the diagnosis of HIV-associated nephropathy is presumptive, and biopsy is not performed (as long as other potentially treatable causes of nephropathy have been ruled out). If renal biopsy is performed, histologic findings most often show focal and segmental glomerulosclerosis, but investigators have reported a diverse array of histologic lesions. In general, the histopathologic findings of these lesions can be distinguished from that found with heroin-associated nephropathy. Although several case reports describe improvements in renal function with either zidovudine or corticosteroids, no controlled trials exist regarding therapy for HIV-associated nephropathy.[68,69]

CARDIAC MANIFESTATIONS

Among HIV-infected persons, myocarditis or dilated cardiomyopathy are the most common clinically significant cardiac abnormalities. These disorders, however, occur with much less frequency when compared with most other noncardiac HIV-related complications. Although uncommon overall, clinically significant HIV-related cardiac abnormalities have the highest rates among persons with CD4 counts less than 100 cells/mm^3.[70] The pathogenesis of HIV-related cardiac disease is not well understood and, in most cases, a specific cause is not identified. The prognosis of HIV-related dilated cardiomyopathy is generally poor: the median survival following the diagnosis of dilated cardiomyopathy was only 101 days.[71] Some patients, however, occasionally have reversal of their cardiomyopathy, and most patients die from noncardiac causes.

Patients with clinically significant myocarditis or cardiomyopathy typically present with fairly nonspecific symptoms, breathlessness, and fatigue. Diagnostic confusion may occur since these symptoms often resemble symptoms present in patients with pulmonary disease or anemia. If a patient progresses to overt heart failure, more cardiac-specific signs and symptoms become evident. Because HIV-related cardiac disease occurs with relatively low frequency, most experts do not recommend routine screening with electrocardiography or echocardiography. Other than supportive therapy, no specific recommendations exist for management of HIV-related cardiac disease.

References

1. Quinn TC: Global burden of the HIV pandemic. *Lancet* 348:99–106, 1996.
2. Centers for Disease Control and Prevention: 1993 revised classification system for HIV infection and expanded surveillance case definition for AIDS among adults and adolescents. *MMWR* 41(no. RR-17), 1992.
3. Schacker T et al: Clinical and epidemiologic features of primary HIV infection. *Ann Intern Med* 125:257–264, 1996.
4. Kinloch-de Lões S et al: Symptomatic primary infection due to human immunodeficiency virus type 1: Review of 31 cases. *Clin Infect Dis* 17: 59–65, 1993.
5. Kinloch-de Lões S et al: A controlled trial of zidovudine in primary human immunodeficiency virus infection. *N Engl J Med* 333:408–413, 1995.
6. Markowitz M et al: Triple therapy with AZT, 3TC, and ritonavir in 12 subjects newly infected with HIV, in Abstracts of the XI International conference on AIDS. Abstract Th.B.933. Vancouver, Canada. 1996.
7. Arditti DE et al: Initial evaluation and folow-up, in *The HIV Manual: A Guide to Diagnosis and Treatment,* 1st ed, DH Spach et al (eds.) New York: Oxford University Press, 1996, pp. 42–52.
8. Minamoto G, Armstrong D: Fungal infections in AIDS: Histoplasmosis and coccidioidomycosis. *Infect Dis Clin No Am* 2:447–456, 1988.
9. Centers for Disease Control. Risk for cervical disease in HIV-infected women: New York City. *MMWR* 39:846–849, 1990.
10. Zuger A, O'Dowd MA: The baron has AIDS: A case of factitious human immunodeficiency virus infection and review. *Clin Infect Dis* 14: 211–216, 1992.
11. Craven DE et al: Factitious HIV infection: The importance of documenting infection. *Ann Intern Med* 121:763–766, 1994.
12. Centers for Disease Control: Recommendations for diagnosing and treating syphilis in HIV-infected patients. *MMWR* 37:600–608, 1988.
13. Mellors JW et al: Prognosis in HIV-1 infection predicted by the quantity of virus in plasma. *Science* 272:1167–1170, 1996.
14. Mellors JW et al: Prognostic value of plasma HIV-1 RNA quantification in seropositive adult men, in Abstracts of the XI International conference on AIDS. Abstract We.B.410. Vancouver, Canada. 1996.
15. Saag MS et al: HIV viral load markers in clinical practice. *Nature Med* 2:625–629, 1996.
16. Carpenter CJ et al: Antiretroviral therapy for HIV infection in 1996. *JAMA* 276:146–154, 1996.
17. Stein DS et al: CD4+ lymphocyte cell enumeration for prediction of clinical course of human immunodeficiency virus disease: A review. *J Infect Dis* 165:352–363, 1992.
18. Drew WL et al: Prevalence of cytomegalovirus in homosexual men. *J Infect Dis* 143:188–192, 1981.
19. Luft BJ, Remington JS: Toxoplasmic encephalitis in AIDS. *Clin Infect Dis* 15:211–222, 1992.
20. Chuck SI, Sande MA: Infections with *Cryptococcus neoformans* in the acquired immunodeficiency syndrome. *N Engl J Med* 321:794–799, 1989.
21. Jewett JF, Hecht FM: Preventive health care for adults with HIV infection. *JAMA* 269:1144–1153, 1993.
22. Schneider RF et al: Lack of usefulness of radiographic screening for pulmonary disease in asymptomatic HIV-infected adults. *Arch Intern Med* 156:191–195, 1996.
23. Centers for Disease Control: Purified protein derivative (PPD)-tuberculin anergy and HIV infection: Guidelines for anergy testing and management of anergic persons at risk of tuberculosis. *MMWR* 40:27–33, 1991.
24. Barnes PF et al: Tuberculosis in patients with HIV infection. *N Engl J Med* 324:1644–1650, 1991.
25. Gordin FM et al: A prospective, double-blind, placebo-controlled trial of isoniazid (INH) for prevention of tuberculosis (TB) in anergic HIV-infected patients (pts) at high risk for TB, in Abstracts of the 36th Interscience Conference on Antimicrobial Agents and Chemotherapy. Abstract LB 11. New Orleans, LA, 1996.

26 Stanley S et al: Effects of immunization with a common recall antigen on viral expression in patients infected with human immunodeficiency virus type 1. *N Engl J Med* 334:1222–1230, 1996.

27 Rose DN et al: Influenza and pneumococcal vaccination of HIV-infected patients: A policy analysis. *Am J Med* 94:160–168, 1993.

28 Centers for Disease Control ACIP: General recommendations on immunization. *MMWR* 38:205–227, 1989.

29 Steinhart R et al: Invasive *Hemophilus influenza* infections in men with HIV infection. *JAMA* 268:3350–3352, 1992.

30 Steinhoff MC et al: Antibody responses to *Hemophilus influenza* type B vaccines in men with human immunodeficiency virus infection. *N Engl J Med* 325:1837–1842, 1991.

31 Centers for Disease Control: Prevention and control of influenza: Recommendations of the immunization practices advisory committee (ACIP). *MMWR* 41:1–17, 1992.

32 Centers for Disease Control: Protection against viral hepatitis: Recommendations of the immunization practices advisory committee (ACIP). *MMWR* 39:1–26, 1990.

33 Collier AC et al: Antibody to human immunodeficiency virus (HIV) and suboptimal response to hepatitis B vaccination. *Ann Intern Med* 109:101–105, 1988.

34 van Deutekom H et al: Bacille Calmette-Guérin (BCG) meningitis in an AIDS patient 12 years after vaccination with BCG. *Clin Infect Dis* 22:870–871, 1996.

35 Weinert M et al: Oral manifestations of HIV infection. *Ann Intern Med* 125:485–496, 1996.

36 Greenspan D, Greenspan JS: HIV-related oral disease. *Lancet* 348: 729–733, 1996.

37 Greenspan JS et al: Replication of Epstein-Barr virus within the epithelial cells of oral "hairy" leukoplakia, an AIDS associated lesion. *N Engl J Med* 313:1564–1571, 1985.

38 Newman C, Polf BF: Resolution of oral hairy leukoplakia during therapy with 9-(1,3-dihydroxy-2-propoxymethyl) guanine (DHPG). *Ann Intern Med* 107:348–350, 1987.

39 Newman SL et al: Clinically significant mucosal candidiasis resistant to fluconazole treatment in patients with AIDS. *Clin Infect Dis* 19: 684–686, 1994.

40 Bach MC et al: Odynophagia from aphthous ulcers of the pharynx and esophagus in the acquired immunodeficiency syndrome (AIDS). *Ann Intern Med* 109:338–339, 1988.

41 Patterson DL et al: Thalidomide as treatment of refractory aphthous ulceration related to human immunodeficiency virus infection. *Clin Infect Dis* 20:250–254, 1995.

42 Tschachler E et al: HIV-related skin disorders. *Lancet* 348:659–663, 1996.

43 Schwartz JJ, Myskowski PL: Molluscum contagiosum in patients with human immunodeficiency virus infection: A review of twenty-seven patients. *J Am Acad Dermatol* 27:583–588, 1992.

44 Buchbinder SP et al: Herpes zoster and human immunodeficiency virus infection. *J Infect Dis* 166:1153–1156, 1992.

45 Cohen PR et al: Disseminated herpes zoster in patients with human immunodeficiency virus infection. *Am J Med* 84:1076–1080, 1988.

46 Feinberg J et al: Phase III study of valaciclovir (VACV) for cytomegalovirus disease in patients with advanced HIV disease, in Abstracts of the 35th Interscience Conference on Antimicrobial Agents and Chemotherapy. Abstract 1215. San Francisco, CA, 1995.

47 Safrin S et al: Clinical and serologic features of herpes simplex virus infection in patients with AIDS. *AIDS* 5:1107–1110, 1991.

48 Erlich KS et al: Acyclovir-resistant herpes simplex virus infections in patients with the acquired immunodeficiency syndrome. *N Engl J Med* 320:293–296, 1989.

49 Mathes BM, Douglas MC: Seborrheic dermatitis in patients with acquired immunodeficiency syndrome. *J Am Acad Dermatol* 13:947–951, 1985.

50 Donabedian H, Khazan U: Norwegian scabies in a patient with AIDS. *Clin Infect Dis* 14:162–164, 1992.

51 Amer M, El Gharib I: Permethrin versus crotamiton and lindane in the treatment of scabies. *Int J Dermatol* 31:357–358, 1992.

52 Buchness MR et al: Eosinophilic pustular folliculitis in the acquired immunodeficiency syndrome: Treatment with ultraviolet phototherapy. *N Engl J Med* 318:1183–1186, 1988.

53 Berger TG et al: Itraconazole therapy for human immunodeficiency virus-associated eosinophilic folliculitis [letter]. *Arch Dermatol* 131: 358–360, 1995.

54 Janoff EN et al: Pneumococcal disease during HIV infection: Epidemiologic, clinical, and immunologic perspectives. *Ann Intern Med* 117:314–324, 1992.

55 Masur H: Prevention and treatment of *Pneumocystis carinii* pneumonia. *N Engl J Med* 327:1853–1860, 1993.

56 Havlik JA et al: Disseminated *Mycobacterium avium* complex infection: Clinical identification and epidemiologic trends. *J Infect Dis* 165: 577–580, 1992.

57 Horsburgh CR: *Mycobacterium avium* complex infection in the acquired immunodeficiency syndrome. *N Engl J Med* 324:1332–1338, 1991.

58 Cameron ML et al: Manifestations of pulmonary cryptococcosis in patients with acquired immunodeficiency syndrome. *Rev Infect Dis* 13: 64–67, 1991.

59 Wilcox CM: Esophageal disease in the acquired immunodeficiency syndrome: Etiology, diagnosis and management. *Am J Med* 92:412–421, 1992.

60 Wilcox CM et al: Esophageal ulceration in human immunodeficiency virus infection: Causes, response to therapy, and long-term outcome. *Ann Intern Med* 122:143–149, 1995.

61 Smith PD et al: Intestinal infections in patients with the acquired immunodeficiency syndrome (AIDS): Etiology and response to therapy. *Ann Intern Med* 108:328–333, 1988.

62 Pomerantz RJ et al: Infection of the retina by human immunodeficiency virus type I. *N Engl J Med* 317:1643–1647, 1987.

63 Bloom JN, Palestine AG: The diagnosis of cytomegalovirus retinitis. *Ann Intern Med* 109:963–969, 1988.

64 Grinspoon SK, Bilezikian JP: HIV disease and the endocrine system. *N Engl J Med* 327:1360–1365, 1992.

65 Dobs AS et al: Endocrine disorders in men infected with human immunodeficiency virus. *Am J Med* 84:611–616, 1988.

66 Bourgoignie JJ, Pardo V: HIV-associated nephropathies. *N Engl J Med* 327:729–730, 1992.

67 Glassock RJ et al: Human immunodeficiency virus (HIV) infection and the kidney. *Ann Intern Med* 112:35–49, 1990.

68 Babut-Gay ML et al: Zidovudine and nephropathy with human immunodeficiency virus (HIV) infection. *Ann Intern Med* 111:856–857, 1989.

69 Smith MC et al: Effect of corticosteroid therapy on human immunodeficiency virus-associated nephropathy. *Am J Med* 97:145–151, 1994.

70 Levy WS et al: Prevalence of cardiac abnormalities in human immunodeficiency virus infection. *Am J Cardiol* 63:86–89, 1989.

71 Currie PF et al: Heart muscle disease related to HIV infection: Prognostic implications. *Br Med J* 309:1605–1607, 1994.

Chapter 74

Antiviral therapy of human immunodeficiency virus infection

Joseph J. Eron Jr.
Martin S. Hirsch

Human immunodeficiency virus type 1 (HIV-1) causes a chronic viral illness that results in a gradual destruction in the host immune system manifested primarily as a loss in CD4+ lymphocytes and the occurrence of infections, malignancies, and other signs of immune impairment. The interaction between the infected host and HIV-1 is a complex interplay between viral replication and immune containment. Reduction, and perhaps eventually elimination, of HIV-1 replication is the goal of therapy. In specific populations of HIV-1–infected persons, antiretroviral therapy has been shown to improve the clinical course of HIV-1 disease and result in prolongation of survival.[1–5] These results have been achieved using agents with moderate in vivo activity, and benefit has generally not been prolonged or consistent across all HIV-1–infected populations.[6,7] Greater improvement in the clinical outcome resulting from antiretroviral therapy should result from more potent and sustained inhibition of HIV-1 replication.[8] The recent introduction of several new agents and combinations of agents with greater antiretroviral activity holds promise that significant improvement can be made in treatment outcomes.[9]

BRIEF OVERVIEW OF THE HIV-1 REPLICATION CYCLE

A retrovirus in the lentivirus subfamily, HIV-1 contains two single-stranded RNA molecules as its genome. The life cycle of this virus requires attachment to the host cell membrane (usually by an interaction between the viral envelope glycoproteins and the host cell CD4 receptor), fusion and entry into cell cytoplasm (mediated by co-receptors on the cell surface, CCR-5 or CXR-4),[10] and reverse transcription of HIV-1 RNA to DNA, which is then transported to the cell nucleus. Once in the nucleus, the double-stranded DNA is integrated into the host chromosome. The provirus can then remain latent and unexpressed, or RNA transcripts can be produced that allow replication to continue. The transcription of full-length HIV-1 RNA depends on interactions between host transcriptional factors (e.g., NFKB and others) and the products of viral regulatory genes (e.g., *tat* and *rev*). Once full-length transcripts are formed, they are transported out of the nucleus and translated into proteins. These proteins are processed by proteolytic cleavage, and the envelope protein is glycosylated. The gag, pol, and protease proteins are produced as one polyprotein that requires cleavage by the HIV-1 protease enzyme for appropriate assembly of the HIV-1 nucleocapsid. During the final assembly of the nucleocapsid around the genomic RNA molecules, the viral particle buds from the cell to complete the life cycle. Further details on the HIV-1 replicative cycle can be found in Chap. 16.

Any process in the viral replication cycle that can be inhibited in a relatively specific manner is a potential target for antiretroviral therapy. The interaction between the HIV-1 envelope and the CD4 molecule on the cell surface has been explored as a target for HIV-1 inhibition in the laboratory and in preliminary studies in HIV-1–infected individuals. Recombinant soluble CD4 has been shown to inhibit HIV-1 replication in vitro, though activity in HIV-1–infected individuals was disappointing.[11] This poor effect was probably due to decreased activity of rsCD4 against clinical isolates. Other agents that interfere with HIV-1 binding to CD4, or other steps in the binding or internalization of the virus, are under study.[12] The interactions between the HIV-1 and newly discovered second receptors on the cell surface—CCR-5 and CXR-4—may be additional targets for therapeutic agents.[13] The beta-chemokines RANTES, MIP-1alpha, and MIP-1beta, which are the natural ligands of CCR-5, inhibit HIV replication in vitro.[14]

Reverse transcription has until recently been the most successful target for antiretroviral therapy. Several compounds that are analogous to endogenous nucleosides and require phosphorylation to become active have activity against HIV-1. These compounds, which include zidovudine (ZDV), didanosine (ddI), zalcitabine (ddC), stavudine (d4T), and lamivudine (3TC), act as competitive inhibitors and chain terminators of the elongating DNA strand produced during reverse transcription. In addition to these nucleoside analog compounds, another class of compounds, collectively known as nonnucleoside reverse transcriptase inhibitors, interacts with the reverse transcriptase in a noncompetitive manner, does not require phosphorylation for activity, and has extremely potent inhibitory activity in vitro. Resistance develops rapidly, limiting activity in patients[15]; however, higher dosages, newer compounds in this class, and combinations with other agents may show greater activity.[16]

The movement of double-stranded HIV-1 DNA from the cellular cytoplasm to the nucleus may require specific nucleotide-binding sequences that interact with a transporter protein; these sites might be targets for specific inhibition. In addition, HIV-1 encodes an integrase that allows incorporation of HIV-1 DNA into the host chromosomal DNA. Inhibitors of HIV-1 DNA integration are being developed.[17] Control of transcription and translation of HIV-1 is a complex process that is influenced by cellular proteins and HIV-1 proteins such as *tat* and *rev*. Inhibitors of these HIV-1 proteins offer the theoretical promise of high specificity, although an early clinical trial of one putative *tat*-inhibitor showed no activity.[18]

As described above, HIV-1 proteins require posttranslational modification prior to their incorporation into viable HIV-1 particles. The *gag* structural proteins and enzymes are translated as one polyprotein that must be cleaved into smaller protein components by the HIV-1 protease. Several potent inhibitors of the HIV-1 protease are now available for clinical use or are under study. Later steps in the HIV-1 life cycle also may be amenable to inhibition, such as viral particle assembly[19] or modification of viral glycoproteins by cellular glycosidases.[20] As further information is gained about the replication cycle of HIV-1, newer or more precise targets for inhibition may be revealed.

HIV DISEASE PATHOGENESIS

Before discussing the clinical evaluation and application of antiviral therapies for HIV-1 infection, it is important to consider disease pathogenesis as it applies to therapeutic strategies. The duration of time from initial infection to onset of the defining symptoms of acquired immune deficiency syndrome (AIDS) can vary greatly, ranging from less than 3 years in some patients to potentially as long as several decades. Some infected individuals may become long-term nonprogressors, though this outcome is uncommon.[21]

PRIMARY INFECTION

Following exposure to HIV-1, newly infected individuals experience a high initial level of HIV-1 replication that may be detectable by blood culture, antigen detection assays, or measurement of plasma HIV-1 RNA. The level of viral replication and viremia is such that many patients experience an acute illness with lymphadenopathy and fever, sometimes accompanied by rash, pharyngitis, or aseptic meningitis. Viral replication results in destruction of host CD4 cells with detectable decreases in CD4+ lymphocyte counts in the peripheral blood that occasionally reach levels seen in later stages of the disease. These individuals may rarely become clinically immunocompromised, such that minor infections (thrush, herpes zoster, vaginal candidiasis) or AIDS-defining opportunistic infections (candida esophagitis, pneumocystis pneumonia) occur prior to the appearance of HIV-1 specific antibody detectable by standard enzyme-linked immunosorbent assay (ELISA) and Western blot testing. Whether therapeutic intervention during this period of intense viral replication would have either short- or long-term benefit is an open question.

Clinical studies evaluating therapy during seroconversion are ongoing. One study examined the use of ZDV compared to placebo during acute seroconversion in 77 subjects.[22] Over 15 months of follow-up, subjects treated with 6 months of ZDV had fewer minor opportunistic infections such as thrush and herpes zoster and on average had a slight increase in CD4 cell counts. Subjects receiving placebo had a decline in CD4 cell counts over time. No deaths or AIDS-defining opportunistic diseases occurred. Whether other, more potent therapies would result in more profound improvements in CD4 cell counts and in a delay in the appearance of HIV-1 disease–related symptoms or mortality is unknown at this time. Therapy of primary HIV-1 infection with more potent two- and three-drug regimens is currently under study.

LYMPH NODE DISSEMINATION AND DISEASE PROGRESSION

Following the primary infection period when HIV-1 is disseminated systemically, the human host produces a cellular and humoral immune response[23,24] that coincides with marked decreases in HIV-1 replication as measured by HIV-1 RNA levels in plasma, p24 antigen levels, or viral culture.[25] During this period of clinical quiescence, infected individuals may be completely asymptomatic or have only minor signs or symptoms. This period can vary markedly in length, though the median time from infection to first AIDS-defining symptom is approximately 8–10 years.[21,26] In most infected individuals, HIV-1 disease progression, involving progressive lymph node destruction and CD4 cell count decline and ongoing replication of HIV-1, occurs during this period. Particles of HIV-1 are detectable in blood plasma during all stages of HIV-1 disease in most infected individuals.[27,28] Lymphoid tissue appears to be the predominant site of HIV-1 replication and is the likely source of virions detectable in blood. Large numbers of viral particles and HIV-1–infected cells are present in lymphoid tissue, and there appears to be a gradual destruction of the lymph node as HIV-1 disease progresses, corresponding to the fall in peripheral blood CD4 lymphocyte counts.[28,29] As peripheral blood CD4 cell counts diminish, clinical signs and symptoms (fevers, malaise, weight loss, etc.) may develop and opportunistic infections or neoplasms may occur. These developments have had an impact on the design of clinical investigations of antiretroviral therapy and on the use of therapy in clinical practice.[30]

Recent studies have documented a surprisingly high level of HIV-1 replication that is ongoing in HIV-infected persons and rapid turnover of HIV-1 particles and CD4 lymphocytes in blood.[31,32] In individuals studied, an average of more than 10 billion virus particles were produced daily, and the half-life of HIV-1 particles in blood plasma was less than 1 day.[33] Destruction and replacement of CD4 lymphocytes occurred on a similar scale.[32] These observations have important implications for the use of antiretroviral therapy. Given the underlying mutation rate of the HIV-1 reverse transcriptase enzyme of approximately one error per 10,000 basepairs,[34] and the replication rate of HIV-1 in the human host, the likelihood of resistance development is high. This likelihood is especially high if single-drug therapies or even combination-drug therapies with only incomplete, modest suppression of HIV-1 replication are used. Given the underlying rate of replication and mutation of HIV, resistance mutations may exist at low levels even prior to therapy.[35] The close correlation between viral replication and CD4 cell destruction, however, suggests that effective inhibition of HIV-1 replication may result in a marked curtailment in CD4 cell destruction with partial or complete restoration of CD4 cell numbers.

Many questions remain concerning HIV-1 pathogenesis and therapy. How applicable are the results of these studies of replication dynamics to HIV-1–infected individuals with CD4 cell counts outside the range of the patients studied, such as individuals with CD4 cell counts >500 cells/μL or individuals with lower levels of HIV-1 RNA in their blood plasma? Are the CD4 cells produced to replenish ones destroyed by HIV-1 replication fully functional, and will the CD4 repertoire respond to a broad range of foreign antigens or remain limited despite return to higher CD4 cell numbers with effective therapy? When is the optimal time to begin therapy? As the answers to these questions become known, and as antiretroviral therapy becomes more potent, the time to initiate therapy may come early in the course of HIV-1 disease.[36] There is a marked variability among individuals in the rate of progression of HIV-1 disease, however, and there are persons with HIV-1 infection who have very low amounts of HIV-1 detectable in their peripheral blood and lymph nodes, who have stable CD4 cell counts over long periods of time, and who appear to have no disease progression in the absence of therapeutic intervention.[37] The study of these individuals may offer insights into effective immune control and the relative pathogenicity of different HIV-1 strains.[37] Alterations in the HIV-1 co-receptor CKR-5 may contribute to slower rates of progression in some individuals.[38] Therapeutic interventions that are developed in individuals with more rapid disease progression may not necessarily be applicable to these long-term nonprogressors. The pathogenesis of HIV-1 infection is considered in greater detail in Chap. 18.

CLINICAL EVALUATION OF ANTIRETROVIRAL COMPOUNDS AGAINST HIV-1

HIV-1 DISEASE MARKERS: THEIR SIGNIFICANCE FOR USE IN ASSESSING THERAPEUTICS

The uses of clinical and laboratory markers to define the stage of HIV-1 disease in an individual continue to evolve. Disease staging is important for epidemiologic and natural history studies and for estimating a prognosis for a given patient. Disease staging is also an integral part of the clinical study of antiretroviral therapy and the use of antiretroviral and prophylactic therapies. The evaluation of antiretroviral agents increasingly relies on the effect of the agent or agents being studied on a marker of HIV-1 disease such as CD4 cell count, HIV-1 RNA levels in blood plasma, or minor clinical endpoints. Changes in these markers may be used to measure the antiviral or immunologic effect of a particular therapy. A change in a marker may be a true surrogate for an ultimate effect on clinical endpoints such as progression to AIDS or survival. The applicability of a given marker to clinical trials may also carry over to clinical practice, where clinicians may be able to use changes in readily available markers to estimate the effect of the therapy for individual patients.

CD4 cell count

CD4 cell counts have been used as indicators of disease stage in HIV-1–infected patients for over a decade. CD4 cell counts that are below certain levels are predictors of disease progression independent of disease duration or clinical symptoms, and they can be used in conjunction with clinical symptoms to provide staging for an individual patient or a population of patients and to compare groups of patients across different studies. The likelihood of specific opportunistic infections varies depending on CD4 cell count (see Chap. 75).[39,40]

The extent to which changes in CD4 cell counts with therapy predict the clinical benefit of therapy is less clear. The change in CD4 cell count with initiation of ZDV, observed in a large prospective cohort study, predicted disease progression and mortality independent of baseline CD4 cell count, pneumocystis prophylaxis, and other antiretroviral therapy.[41,42] In two unrelated clinical trials of ZDV monotherapy in asymptomatic subjects, the change in CD4 cell count following therapy was demonstrated to underestimate the clinical benefit seen in one trial,[43] but it was shown to overestimate clinical benefit in the other trial.[7] In a more recent evaluation of surrogate markers during ZDV monotherapy, changes in CD4 cell counts were only partially predictive of clinical benefit.[44] In a trial comparing ZDV, ddI, and the combination of ZDV with ddI or ddC, the initial change in CD4 cell count produced by therapy was not predictive of clinical outcome when baseline RNA level and change in RNA level with treatment were taken into account.[45]

HIV-1 RNA levels in plasma

Recently, several methods have been developed to quantify the amount of HIV-1 RNA levels in blood plasma.[46,46a,46b] These assays are becoming widely available and are reproducible in repeated assays of the same sample within 0.3 $\log_{10}$ (twofold) (see Chap. 71). The ability to measure HIV-1 RNA levels in plasma has led to fundamental changes in the understanding of HIV-1 pathogenesis. Many HIV-1–infected persons have significant amounts of HIV-1 RNA in their plasma, even during the prolonged asymptomatic period that can occur during HIV-1 infection.[27] In contrast, persons with HIV-1 infection who have shown little or no progression of their disease over time usually have undetectable or low levels of HIV-1 RNA in their plasma.[37,47]

In addition to being a useful tool to investigate the pathogenesis of HIV-1 infection, HIV-1 RNA levels have been shown to be good predictors of disease progression. In a study of HIV-infected men with documented seroconversion, HIV-1 RNA levels within 1 year of seroconversion were shown be predictive of HIV-1 disease progression independent of CD4 cell counts and other HIV-1 disease parameters.[48] In another study of subjects with documented HIV-1 seroconversion who were a subset from a large prospective cohort of HIV-1–infected men, the ability to detect HIV-1 RNA consistently at levels greater than 10,000 copies per milliliter was strongly predictive of progression to AIDS. In a multivariate analysis that included CD4 cell count, acid-dissociated p24 antigen levels, neopterin, and β-2 microglobulin, an HIV-1 RNA level greater than 100,000 copies per milliliter was the strongest predictor of AIDS progression.[49] In a more extensive evaluation using subjects from the larger cohort (not just seroconverters), HIV RNA levels obtained after entry into the cohort were shown to have remarkable predictive value for progression to AIDS and survival independent of CD4 cell count and other markers.[50] Subjects with RNA levels in the lowest quartile at baseline had a greater than 10-year median AIDS-free survival, while subjects in the highest quartile had a 3.5-year median duration. Using information from an even larger number of subjects from this cohort, the prognostic power of employing both HIV RNA levels and CD4 cell counts has been demonstrated.[50a] Similar results have been observed in other cohort studies.[51] In the context of antiretroviral clinical trials, baseline RNA levels have been shown to be predictive of clinical disease progression independent of baseline CD4 cell count.[44,45] In a subset of subjects from a large prospective clinical trial, a 10-fold lower level of HIV-1 RNA at baseline was shown to correspond to a 65 percent reduction in the progression to AIDS or death.[45] The changes in HIV-1 RNA levels in plasma that occur as a result of effective antiretroviral therapy appear to be strong surrogate markers for the clinical benefit of treatment, and they appear to explain, at least partially, treatment benefits seen with therapy.[44,45,52–54] This predictive capacity appears independent of and provides additional information to changes in CD4 cell counts observed with treatment.[44] The improved understanding of HIV-1 pathogenesis, replication dynamics, and use of HIV disease markers should result in the development of more effective treatments and treatment strategies.[55]

SPECIFIC ANTIRETROVIRAL THERAPIES

Three classes of antiretroviral agents have been studied extensively. These classes are nucleoside analog reverse transcriptase inhibitors, nonnucleoside reverse transcriptase inhibitors, and HIV-1 protease inhibitors. Several reverse transcriptase (RT) and protease inhibitors have been approved for therapy in the United States and elsewhere (Table 74-1).

NUCLEOSIDE ANALOG REVERSE TRANSCRIPTASE INHIBITORS

Nucleoside analog reverse transcriptase inhibitors are phosphorylated intracellularly to triphosphorylated active metabolites; they inhibit viral replication by competing with endogenous nucleotides for incorporation into the elongating HIV-1 DNA that is being synthesized from the HIV-1 RNA genome by the viral reverse transcriptase. Once incorporated, these agents terminate chain elongation because the 3′ carbon lacks a hydroxyl group necessary for the addition of additional nucleotides.[56] Some of the toxicity seen with these agents results from their affinity for human DNA polymerases though the affinity is less than that for the HIV-1 reverse transcriptase. The relative affinity for specific human DNA polymerases of the agents varies for the different agents and may explain in part their differing toxicities.

Zidovudine

Zidovudine (3′-azido-2′,3′-dideoxythymidine—ZDV, AZT, or Retrovir) is a thymidine analog with an azido group at the 3′ location of the ribose ring. It enters the cell through passive diffusion, and after triphosphorylation by cellular kinases competes with deoxythymidine triphosphate for reverse transcriptase binding and then terminates HIV-1 DNA chain elongation. Zidovu-

Table 74-1. Antiretroviral Agents Approved for Use in the United States*

Class	Specific agent	Recommended dose for adults	Predominant toxicity
Nucleoside Reverse Transcriptase Inhibitors (NRTI)			
	zidovudine	200 mg every 8 hours or 300 mg twice daily	hematological
	didanosine	200 mg twice daily* (empty stomach)	gastrointestinal
	zalcitabine	0.75 mg every 8 hours	peripheral neuropathy, fever and stomatitis
	stavudine	40 mg twice daily*	peripheral neuropathy
	lamivudine	150 mg twice daily	neutropenia
Nonnucleoside RT inhibitors (NNRTI)	nevirapine	200 mg twice daily***	rash
	delaviridine (DLV)	400 mg three times daily	rash
Protease inhibitors			
	saquinavir	600 mg every 8 hours (with fatty meals)	gastrointestinal
	indinavir	800 mg every 8 hours (empty stomach)	nephrolithiasis, indirect hyperbilirubinemia
	ritonavir	600 mg every 12 hours∞ (with meals)	gastrointestinal, paresthesias, hypertriglyceridemia
	nelfinavir	750 mg 3 times daily	diarrhea

* as of July 1997
** for patients weight <60 kg dose is reduced; 125 mg BID for ddI, 30 mg BID for d4T
*** Nevirapine therapy should be initiated at 200 mg daily for 2 weeks to decrease incidence of rash
∞ Ritonavir should be dose-escalated starting at 200 to 300 mg BID to full dose over 7–14 days

dine is well absorbed orally (60–65 percent bioavailability). The serum half-life of ZDV is short (1–1.5 hours), but the intracellular half-life of ZDV-triphosphate may be up to 4 hours.[57] The activity of ZDV may correlate best with intracellular ZDV triphosphate levels.[58] Zidovudine penetrates the cerebrospinal fluid (CSF) well, with reported CSF/serum ratios of 0.1 to 1.35.[59] In early trials ZDV was administered every 4 hours up to 1,200 mg per day, but subsequent studies have shown that 500–600 mg/day have a similar effect on CD4 cell counts and clinical endpoints as the higher dose.[60] Many physicians now administer ZDV at 200 mg three times daily, and a dose of 300 mg twice daily is also being used. Zidovudine is metabolized predominantly by the liver via glucuronidation, and its one metabolite does not have antiretroviral activity. Approximately 10 percent of the parent drug is recovered in the urine. Probenicid decreases urinary excretion of ZDV.[61] Agents that affect glucuronidation may affect ZDV metabolism.[62]

The predominant long-term toxicity of ZDV is hematological, particularly causing anemia and neutropenia. Hematological toxicity was relatively frequent in earlier studies in patients with advanced disease when higher doses were used.[63] When ZDV is administered at 500–600 mg/day to patients with less advanced disease or who are asymptomatic, hematological toxicity occurs less frequently and may respond to dose reduction. Headache and nausea can occur early after initiation of therapy, though these symptoms will frequently subside with continued administration of ZDV. An additional toxicity seen in patients on prolonged ZDV therapy is myopathy, which is usually reversible with discontinuation of therapy.

Zidovudine monotherapy (at 1,500 mg/day) has been shown to improve survival in patients with AIDS or advanced AIDS-related complex who have not received previous therapy.[1,64] A reduced dose of 600 mg/day after 1 month of 1,500 mg/day improved estimated survival rates at 24 months over prolonged administration of 1,500 mg/day.[65] Zidovudine monotherapy has also been shown to decrease the rate of HIV-1 disease progression in patients with CD4 cell counts between 200 and 500 cells/μL who had minimal HIV-related symptoms.[66] There were only two deaths during this study, however, so no effect on survival was demonstrated. A study of early versus delayed initiation of ZDV therapy in symptomatic patients with the same CD4 cell count range gave similar results.[67] Volberding and colleagues demonstrated that ZDV decreased disease progression in HIV-1–infected individuals who were asymptomatic and had CD4 cell counts between 200 and 500/μL[68]; they also showed that the effect could be prolonged in some patients from this same study, particularly those individuals with CD4 cell counts greater than 300 cells/μL at the time of therapy initiation.[69] The number of deaths that occurred in this study was small, however, and no clear survival benefit of early treatment with ZDV could be observed when compared to initial treatment with placebo. For patients who began the study with CD4 cell counts greater than 500 cells/μL, clinical benefit of immediate ZDV therapy, compared to delaying initiation of therapy until CD4 cell counts fell below 500 cells/μL, could not be demonstrated.[70] A large study of immediate versus delayed initiation of ZDV monotherapy in asymptomatic HIV-1–infected patients was carried out in the United Kingdom, France, and Ireland.[7] Subjects were allowed entry with any CD4 cell count, and approximately 60 percent of counts were below 500 cells/μL. After 3 years of follow-up there were no significant differences in the rates of HIV-1–related clinical events, including progression to AIDS and death. These results conflict somewhat with previous studies, although some clinical benefit of immediate ZDV therapy was seen over the first 18 months of the study. Most recently, initial therapy with ZDV was compared to the combinations of ZDV and ddI, ZDV and ddC, and ddI monotherapy.[4] Initiation of therapy with nucleoside combinations was significantly more effective at preventing progression to the combined endpoint of AIDS or death than initial ZDV monotherapy.

Variants of HIV-1 resistant to ZDV have been isolated from many patients receiving ZDV therapy. The degree of phenotypic resistance increases with duration of ZDV therapy and occurs more rapidly and in a higher percentage of patients who begin therapy at a more advanced disease stage.[71] Approximately 15 percent of patients who had received more than 16 weeks of ZDV therapy were found to have high-level resistance, and 41 percent had some degree of ZDV resistance in one study of patients with advanced disease.[72] Amino acid changes at five separate codons of the HIV-1 reverse transcriptase have been associated with HIV-

1 resistance to ZDV.[73–75] In general, the greater the number of mutations, the higher the level of ZDV resistance in vitro. Resistance mutations while on ZDV therapy usually appear in an ordered pattern,[76] and mutations at two codons, 41 and 215, are associated with the highest levels of resistance and more rapid disease progression and death.[72] The appearance of an early mutation at codon 70 that confers a lower level of phenotypic ZDV resistance has been correlated with the loss of the initial antiretroviral effect.[77] Despite a large number of studies evaluating ZDV resistance, the exact clinical significance of ZDV resistance and how its presence should impact upon therapeutic decisions are not known. Variants of HIV-1 that are resistant to ZDV can be transmitted from one person to another,[78] and the prevalence of HIV-1 variants in the population that are resistant to ZDV may be increasing.[4]

Didanosine

Didanosine (2′,3′-dideoxyinosine—ddI or Videx) is an adenosine analog that lacks a hydroxyl group at the 3′ location. The active metabolite of ddI is dideoxyadenosine triphosphate (ddATP). Didanosine is absorbed poorly in an acid environment or in the presence of food and therefore needs to be administered in conjunction with an acid buffer either 30 to 60 minutes prior to eating or 2 hours after.[79] If administered correctly, ddI has a bioavailability of 40 to 50 percent,[80] but absorption is diminished if ddI is administered with any fluid other than water or water mixed with a small amount of apple juice. The half-life of ddI in serum ranges from 0.6 to 2.8 hours, and the intracellular half-life of ddATP is 12 to 24 hours, longer than that for ZDV triphosphate.[81] Didanosine is administered twice daily, and 60 percent is excreted unchanged in the urine. The rest is extensively metabolized in the liver.[82] Drugs that require an acid environment for absorption, such as itraconazole, should not be administered simultaneously with ddI.

The long-term toxicity of ddI may include idiosyncratic pancreatitis and dose-dependent peripheral neuropathy.[83–85] However, at doses equivalent to the currently recommended dose of 200 mg twice daily, reduced to 125 mg twice daily in patients who weigh less than 60 kilograms, the incidence of peripheral neuropathy and pancreatitis in large-scale clinical trials of ddI was no greater than in comparison groups taking ZDV.[4] Additional adverse effects seen with ddI include nausea, bloating, abdominal pain, and diarrhea that may be related to the antacid vehicle required for ddI absorption.

Didanosine monotherapy has been shown to have benefit in a variety of clinical situations. In patients with a broad range of disease stages who had previous ZDV therapy, a switch to ddI monotherapy resulted in delayed clinical progression and improved survival when compared to the continuation of ZDV.[2,4] In patients with very advanced disease, a change from ZDV to ddI produced results similar to a change from ZDV to ddC.[86]

Initiation of antiretroviral therapy with ddI has been studied and compared to initiation with ZDV or initiation with a combination of agents. In subjects with advanced disease and no previous treatment, ZDV appeared more effective than ddI in delaying disease progression or death.[85] The follow-up observation period in this study was short, and ddI appeared to have a more sustained positive effect on mean CD4 cell counts than ZDV monotherapy. In a large study of subjects with CD4 cell counts between 200 and 500 cells per cubic millimeter, initial ddI monotherapy was significantly more effective than ZDV monotherapy at delaying progression to the combined endpoint of AIDS, death, or a 50 percent fall from the baseline CD4 cell count.[4] If only clinical endpoints were examined, there were fewer endpoints in the ddI-treated group, but this difference did not reach statistical significance. When initiation of therapy with ddI was compared to initiation with ZDV plus ddI or ZDV plus ddC, there were fewer combined endpoints in the combination-treated subjects, although these did not reach statistical significance.

Isolates of HIV-1 resistant to ddI have been described.[87,88,89] HIV-1 from patients treated with ddI monotherapy usually has a mutation in the RT gene at codon 74. Virions with ZDV-resistant mutations that acquire the ddI-selected mutation at codon 74 may become sensitive to ZDV,[87] though this effect may not occur on all genetic backgrounds.[88] Patients treated with ZDV and ddI can develop HIV-1 resistant to both compounds,[89] and ddI resistance in this situation may be associated with reverse transcription mutations at codons other than 74.[90]

Zalcitabine

Zalcitabine (2′-3′-dideoxycytidine—ddC or Hivid) is an analog of cytidine and, like ddI, lacks the 3′ hydroxyl group. The active metabolite is ddCTP. Zalcitabine is rapidly absorbed orally, and absorption is decreased slightly by food.[91] Serum half-life is 1.5 hours, and intracellular half-life of ddCTP is 2–4 hours.[92] Zalcitabine is typically given three times daily, with a total daily dose of 2.25 milligrams. Seventy-five percent of ddC is excreted unchanged in the urine.[91]

Adverse events including fever, stomatitis, rash, and peripheral neuropathy were observed commonly at doses greater than currently recommended. These toxicities still occur in patients receiving 2.25 milligrams per day, though the incidence is less.[86] The peripheral neuropathy associated with ddC, if severe, may not always be reversible upon discontinuation of therapy. Therefore, most clinicians would discontinue ddC if neuropathy develops rather than pursue a course of dose reduction. In contrast, the fever, stomatitis, and rash syndrome may remit despite continued therapy.

Zalcitabine given as monotherapy has been evaluated in a limited number of studies. When compared to ZDV in patients with advanced AIDS-related complex or AIDS, there were more deaths over 1 year in patients treated with ddC (AIDS Clinical Trials Group [ACTG] 114). Zalcitabine was also compared to ddI in patients with advanced HIV-1 disease who had been previously treated with ZDV. There was no difference between ddI and ddC therapy in this study. The number of AIDS-related opportunistic illnesses and deaths in both arms of the study was high, and there was no placebo-treated group for comparison.[86] Currently ddC monotherapy is rarely used for treatment of HIV-1 infection.

Variants of HIV-1 resistant to ddC have been selected for by serial passage of virus in vitro in the presence of drug. A mutation at codon 65 of the reverse transcriptase confers approximately a fivefold decrease in susceptibility to ddC and cross-resistance to ddI.[93] This mutation is seen in patients treated with either ddC or ddI.[93] A mutation at codon 69 of the RT is also seen in vivo.[94] The frequency and clinical significance of ddC-resistant virus in patients treated with ddC has not been well delineated.

Stavudine

Stavudine (3′-deoxy-2′,3′-didehydrothymidine—d4T or Zerit) is a thymidine analog with an oral bioavailability of 60–80 percent,[95] a serum half-life of 1.5–2 hours,[96] and an intracellular half-life as the triphosphate metabolite of 3–4 hours.[97] Stavudine appears to have measurable CSF penetration.[95] It is excreted by both renal and nonrenal routes with approximately 40 percent of a dose excreted unchanged in the urine.[98] The standard dose of d4T is 40 mg twice daily, reduced to 30 mg twice daily in persons who weigh less than 60 kilograms. No significant drug-drug interactions have been described.

The initial administration of d4T is usually well tolerated. Long-term toxicity is predominantly sensory neuropathy. This adverse effect occurs in 10–15 percent of patients treated with d4T and may respond to dose interruption with resumption of therapy at a lower dose.

Stavudine has been studied as an alternative to continued therapy with ZDV in patients with a median of 88 weeks of ZDV experience.[3] In this study d4T therapy resulted in a statistically significant improvement in AIDS-free survival when compared to continued ZDV. There was also a trend toward improved overall survival using d4T in this setting. Stavudine as initial therapy for HIV-1 infection has been studied only on a limited basis.[99] The effect of d4T on CD4 cell counts in previously untreated patients appears similar to that of other nucleoside monotherapies in the same situation, but the effect of primary d4T monotherapy on HIV-1 RNA levels and on clinical disease progression is not yet well characterized.

Mutations in the reverse transcriptase gene associated with d4T resistance have been described but appear uncommon.[100] The clinical significance of these mutations is not known.

Lamivudine

Lamivudine (3TC or Epivir) is the (-)enantiomer of the cytosine analog 2′-deoxy-3′-thiacytidine, which contains a sulfur atom in the ribose ring. This compound also lacks a 3′ hydroxyl group. In addition to in vitro activity against HIV-1 and HIV-2, 3TC also inhibits hepatitis B virus and has antiviral activity in patients with chronic active hepatitis B (see Chap. 26).[101] Lamivudine has an oral bioavailability of greater than 80 percent in adults and greater than 60 percent in children.[102] The overall serum concentration is unaffected by food, and the intracellular half-life of 3TC triphosphate is in the range of 12 hours. The most commonly used dose is 150 mg twice daily; this dose is recommended in combination with ZDV. Lamivudine has been studied in monotherapy in a range of doses, including 300 mg twice daily in a relatively large clinical trial.[103–105] Lamivudine is excreted predominantly by the kidney.[102] Dose reduction is required in patients with moderate-to-severe renal failure.

In early studies of 3TC monotherapy, dose-limiting toxicity was not observed. At doses higher than currently recommended, neutropenia was observed in a minority of subjects.[102,105,106] Mild headache may occur with the use of 3TC, but the addition of 3TC to ZDV appeared to show no significant adverse effects other than those seen with ZDV alone.[103]

Lamivudine monotherapy resulted in a peak mean increase in CD4 cells of 35 cells/μL above baseline in subjects with CD4 cell counts between 200 and 500 cells/μL at study enrollment. Mean CD4 cell counts remained above baseline for approximately 8 months, an effect that was not different from that induced by ZDV monotherapy. HIV-1 RNA levels were decreased initially by a mean of 1.2 $\log_{10}$ and remained below baseline through 52 weeks of observation. These levels were reduced to a significantly greater extent with 3TC than with ZDV monotherapy.[103]

Resistance of HIV-1 to 3TC develops rapidly in vitro and is common in HIV isolates from patients treated with 3TC.[107–110] A single amino acid substitution at codon 184 of the reverse transcriptase results in a 100- to 1,000-fold decrease in activity of the drug in vitro. A virus that contains this mutation may also have a decreased replicative capacity.[111] When the 184 mutation is introduced into virions with high-level resistance to ZDV, these virions frequently regain sensitivity to ZDV.[108,111] The mutation that confers resistance to 3TC at codon 184 appears to result in a low level of cross-resistance to ddI and ddC.[112]

Other nucleoside analog reverse transcriptase inhibitors

Other nucleoside analog reverse transcriptase inhibitors are in development. These include the (-)enantiomer of 2′,3′-dideoxy-5-fluoro-3′-thiacytidine (FTC), carbovir[113]; there is also a related compound, 1592U89 succinate, a carbocyclic 2′,3′-ene nucleoside.[114] In a small trial, 1592U89 monotherapy produced substantial declines in HIV-1 RNA levels of 1.7 to 2.1 $\log_{10}$; these declines persisted through 12 weeks of therapy whether ZDV was added to 1592U89 or not.[115] Nucleotide analogs that contain a phosphate group are also being evaluated.[116]

NONNUCLEOSIDE REVERSE TRANSCRIPTASE INHIBITORS

Nonnucleoside reverse transcriptase inhibitors (NNRTI) are noncompetitive inhibitors of the HIV-1 reverse transcriptase that bind tightly and specifically[117] to the HIV-1 reverse transcriptase (RT).[118] The 50 percent inhibitory concentration (IC_{50}) in vitro for these compounds against wild-type HIV-1 is typically less than 50 n*M*.[118] Resistance emerges rapidly in vitro and in vivo in the presence of these inhibitors, however.[15,119–122] These observations suggest that the major use of these agents will be in combination with other agents. These agents have been shown to be synergistic in vitro with a variety of nucleoside analogs, alpha-interferon, and a protease inhibitor.[123] In addition, the selection of some but not all NNRTI resistance mutations in HIV-1 with high-level resistance to ZDV results in an increase in susceptibility of these variants to ZDV.[124] At the time of this writing, nevirapine and delavirdine are available in the United States.

Nevirapine

The pharmacokinetics of nevirapine (NVP or Virammune) are favorable with rapid, nearly compete absorption and a long half-life that supports once- or twice-daily dosing,[125] though twice-daily dosing may result in higher trough levels. The predominant adverse effect of nevirapine is rash, which occurs in approximately 30 percent of treated subjects; some instances may be severe.[126] The rash occurs more frequently with higher doses, though a dose-escalation strategy from 200 mg daily to 400 mg daily reduces the incidence. Stevens-Johnson syndrome has been observed, but rarely. Resistance develops rapidly to NVP, and characteristic mutations in the RT gene have been described.[121] The appearance of resistance is associated with rapid loss of antiretroviral activity. Higher doses of NVP (400 mg daily) may retain some antiretroviral effect even against resistant isolates.[122,127] Nevirapine is an inducer of the p450 enzyme system and may increase metabolism of other medications metabolized by this system, including HIV-1 protease inhibitors.

Delavirdine

Delavirdine (DLV or Rescriptor) is an NNRTI with potent activity against a broad range of HIV-1 variants in vitro, including isolates resistant to ZDV.[128] Delavirdine is rapidly absorbed, but significant variations in the pharmacokinetics have been observed among different individuals. The current recommended dose is 400 mg three times daily. The predominant side effect is rash, which occurs in approximately one-third of subjects and is usually mild. Delavirdine-resistant variants can be selected in vitro. The predominant mutation in the reverse transcriptase observed in vitro results in enhanced sensitivity to other NNRTI,[129] though other NNRTI resistance mutations also occur in vivo. In vivo DLV monotherapy selects rapidly for resistant variants with the loss of antiretroviral effect, likely limiting the usefulness of DLV monotherapy.[130] Delavirdine inhibits cytochrome p450 enzyme isoform 3A4 and may result in increased levels of medications metabolized by this enzyme. Levels of saquinavir and indinavir are increased when coadministered with delavirdine.

Loviride

Loviride is an α-anilinophenylacetamide (α-APA) NNRTI consisting of a positive and negative enantiomer, with all the antiretroviral activity residing in the (-)enantiomer. When compared to placebo, loviride had limited effects on HIV-1 RNA levels (a 0.3 $\log_{10}$ reduction at peak), and levels had returned to near baseline by 12 weeks. Total CD4 cell counts remained approximately 10 percent above baseline after 6 months. Adverse events requiring withdrawal were infrequent. The NNRTI resistance mutation at RT codon 103 was seen most commonly, though mutations at codon 181 and 188 were also seen.[131] In a large clinical trial, adding loviride and 3TC in subjects already receiving ZDV with or without other nucleosides resulted in no additional clinical benefit when compared to adding 3TC alone.[132]

HIV-1 VARIANTS RESISTANT TO MULTIPLE REVERSE TRANSCRIPTASE INHIBITORS

Recently HIV-1 variants resistant to multiple reverse transcriptase inhibitors have been isolated from individuals treated with more than one reverse transcriptase inhibitor typically for prolonged periods. Some subjects treated with ddI combined with ZDV were found to harbor isolates resistant to both agents and to ddC, and one isolate was also resistant to d4T. These isolates had RT mutations at one or more of the following codons: 62, 75, 77, 116, and 151.[90] The frequency with which these variants occur in individuals treated with multiple RT inhibitors is unknown.

PROTEASE INHIBITORS

Like other retroviruses, HIV expresses the products of its *gag* and *pol* genes as a single precursor polyprotein that must be cleaved by the HIV-encoded protease in order to produce infectious viral particles (see Chap. 16).[133] The amino acid cleavage sites for the HIV-1 aspartyl protease are specific and not similar to cleavage sites of human host proteases. Currently available protease inhibitors bind to the active site of the enzyme and are competitive inhibitors of the HIV-1 protease with K_i in the 1.0 n*M* range.

The HIV-1 protease is an enzyme that tolerates marked variability in amino acid sequence while still retaining function. Polymorphism has been shown to exist at almost half of the amino acid positions of this 99 amino acid homodimer.[134] Some of these amino acid substitutions also occur during protease inhibitor administration in vitro and in vivo and are thought to contribute to resistance to protease inhibitors.[135] Therefore, individuals who are treated with protease inhibitors already have HIV-1 variants with amino acid substitutions that may contribute to protease inhibitor resistance in those individuals.

Saquinavir

Saquinavir (Invirase) is a peptidomimetic HIV-1 and HIV-2 protease inhibitor with a molecular weight of 671. Saquinavir inhibits HIV-1 replication in both acutely and chronically infected cells with a 50 percent inhibitory concentration (IC_{50}) of 1 to 30 n*M*. Saquinavir in its current formulation has a bioavailability of approximately 4 percent when given with a high-fat meal, and concentrations are decreased approximately fivefold if saquinavir is given in the fasting state. The low bioavailability is due in part to first-pass metabolism in the intestinal wall and in the liver. Saquinavir was detected at low levels in the CSF in a small number of patients evaluated. It is metabolized in the liver by the cytochrome p450 system (CYP3A4). There appear to be no drug-drug interactions with ZDV and ddC. Ketoconazole increases saquinavir levels by about threefold, whereas rifampin and rifabutin decrease saquinavir levels by 80 percent and 40 percent, respectively. Ritonavir and delavirdine also increase saquinavir levels.

Saquinavir was studied as monotherapy in HIV-1-infected men who had minimal symptoms related to their HIV-1 disease, CD4 cell counts ≤500 cells/μL, and no previous antiretroviral therapy.[136] In this trial patients received either 25, 75, 200, or 600 mg three times daily for 16 weeks. The highest dose, 600 mg three times daily, produced an average median increase in CD4+ cells of 36/μL over the 16-week period, and the peak median percent decrease in HIV-1 RNA was 80 percent (or approximately 0.7 $\log_{10}$). Clinical toxicities were uncommon, with only one severe headache ascribed to the medication. Laboratory abnormalities occurred in all groups with no apparent dose relationship, and none was deemed clinically significant.[136] In a clinical trial in subjects with previous ZDV treatment, subjects who were switched to saquinavir monotherapy had no improvement in clinical progression when compared to subjects who were changed to ddC monotherapy.[137] Adverse gastrointestinal effects can occur with saquinavir, but these symptoms are usually mild and infrequently result in treatment discontinuation. Of note, small clinical trials of saquinavir given at two to three times the currently approved dose (1,800 mg per day) are being undertaken, and preliminary results suggest that these increased doses are well tolerated.[138] In addition, a formulation with a three- to fourfold increase in bioavailability is under study.

Resistance of HIV-1 to saquinavir has been demonstrated both in vitro and in vivo. Resistant isolates contain protease gene mutations at either codon 48 or codon 90 or both. Mutations that are associated with saquinavir resistance have been demonstrated in 30–50 percent of subjects treated with saquinavir, with the mutation at codon 90 occurring most commonly.

Indinavir

Indinavir (Crixivan) is a hydroxyaminopentane amide compound that is a potent inhibitor of the HIV-1 protease enzyme with a K_i of 0.34 n*M*.[139] This compound is highly active against laboratory and clinical isolates of HIV-1, including isolates resistant to ZDV and nonnucleoside RT inhibitors, with 95 percent inhibitory concentration (IC_{95}) values ranging from 12.0 to 100 n*M*. The toxic-to-therapeutic ratio in human cell lines in vitro is greater than 1,000.

In animal studies indinavir has a bioavailability of 14–72 percent, depending on the animal species tested. The agent is not tightly bound by human plasma, with the unbound fraction of the compound equal to 56 percent.[139] In HIV-1–infected subjects given 600 mg three times daily, the mean peak concentration was 4.9 μ*M*. The mean trough was 0.3 μ*M*, approximately 50 and 3 times the in vitro IC_{95} for clinical isolates.[140]

Indinavir has been studied in clinical trials both as a single agent and in combination with nucleoside analogs. Dose-escalation trials indicate that the optimal dose of IDV is 2,400 mg per day. When it was given at 600 mg four times daily at initiation of therapy, the mean maximal increase in CD4 cell count was 143 cells/μL in subjects with a mean baseline CD4 cell count of 66 cells per cubic millimeter. HIV-1 RNA levels fell by more than 1.5 $\log_{10}$ on average.[140] The current recommended dose of indinavir is 800 mg three times daily. Initiation of indinavir therapy at the maximal effective dose is important, as starting with suboptimal doses may select for resistant viruses that will not be suppressed by subsequent higher doses.[141]

Indinavir therapy is generally well tolerated. The most common serious side effect is nephrolithiasis, which occurs in approximately 2–5 percent of patients[9] and appears to be caused by precipitation of indinavir in the renal collecting system. This side effect may be reduced by vigorous hydration. Increases in indirect bilirubin are seen frequently. These increases are not usually accompanied by increases in serum aminotransferase activities and remain stable or decrease despite the continuation of indinavir therapy.[142]

Viral variants resistant to indinavir have been isolated from subjects treated with indinavir for 24–52 weeks.[143] These variants have a fourfold to greater than 30-fold increase in IC_{95} to indinavir. The establishment of high-level resistance appears to require multiple mutations in the protease gene, and these mutations appear to be acquired serially over time. Several of the mutations are at or near the active site of the protease enzyme, and one or two mutations at either codon 82 or 90 appear necessary but not sufficient for measurable resistance to indinavir.[143] Additional mutations at sites more distant to the active site may result in conformational changes in the enzyme that allow more efficient enzyme activity in the presence of the inhibitor. Some of the viral variants with high-level resistance to indinavir are broadly cross-resistant to other protease inhibitors.[143]

Ritonavir

Ritonavir (Norvir) is a transition state analog peptidomimetic with a molecular weight of 721. Ritonavir is very active in vitro against laboratory strains and clinical isolates of HIV-1 with IC_{50} ranging from 0.01 to 0.1 μM.[144,145] Cytotoxicity for human cells in vitro is in the 50 μM range.[145] Zidovudine-resistant isolates are sensitive to ritonavir.[146] Ritonavir has a bioavailability of 30–70 percent in animal models, depending on the species tested, and it is excreted in the stool after extensive hepatic metabolism by the p450 enzyme system. It binds extensively to human serum proteins, including human serum albumin and human alpha 1 acid glycoprotein (AAG), though the binding to AAG appears saturable. Ritonavir penetrates lymph node tissue in the rat, though it does not appear to cross the blood-brain barrier well. It is rapidly absorbed in humans with a high oral bioavailability,[146] and absorption is increased by food. The half-life is approximately 3 hours, and trough concentrations with twice-daily dosing support this dosing strategy.[147] Trough concentrations may decrease over 1–2 weeks[148] due to induction of the p450 liver enzyme metabolism. Over the first 7–10 days of therapy prior to the induction of the hepatic enzymes, the standard dose of ritonavir may result in very high blood levels, which are associated with nausea, vomiting, and paresthesias. Dose escalation of ritonavir over the initial 7–14 days appears to help avoid severe nausea and vomiting. Diarrhea is a common side effect, occurring in 20–45 percent of individuals, and nausea occurs commonly on therapy initiation. Patients may experience circumoral paresthesias, though this effect is not usually dose limiting.[148] Triglyceride levels have doubled in approximately 50 percent of patients on ritonavir.[148] Elevations in hepatic transaminases have also been seen in a minority of patients and have been reversible with discontinuation of the agent.

Because ritonavir is both an inducer and inhibitor of the human liver p450 cytochrome system, multiple drug-drug interactions exist. These interactions must be carefully considered when using this agent. As with other protease inhibitors, rifabutin and rifampin will lower serum concentrations of ritonavir. Ritonavir slows the metabolism of certain analgesics and anxiolytics and could potentially raise the level of terfenadine and hismanol, resulting in cardiac arrhythmias. Ritonavir may also induce glucuronidation by the liver and thereby lower ZDV and ethylene estradiol levels.

In initial studies ritonavir monotherapy produced a potent dose-response effect on HIV-1 RNA levels in plasma, with mean decreases greater than or equal to 1.0 $\log_{10}$ over 12 weeks and 0.8 $\log_{10}$ in a small number of patients through 32 weeks.[147] CD4 lymphocyte counts in peripheral blood increased a median of 80 cells over 12 weeks,[148] and in a high-dose cohort (600 mg twice daily) they increased a median of 230 cells over 32 weeks.

In a large placebo-controlled trial in which ritonavir was added in a blinded manner to patients on stable antiretroviral therapy, this agent demonstrated a significant effect on mortality and progression to AIDS-defining opportunistic illness over a 6- to 8-month period.[8] A total of 1,090 patients with CD4 cell counts $\leq$100 cells/μL who had received at least 9 months of previous antiretroviral therapy were randomized to receive their current therapy (no more than two approved nucleoside RT inhibitors) plus ritonavir or placebo. A nested virology substudy was performed on the first 159 patients who were enrolled and who had more than 15,000 copies of HIV-1 RNA per milliliter. In addition CD4 and CD8 cell count data were obtained from 215 subjects. After 16 weeks subjects could receive ritonavir if they had experienced an AIDS-defining illness. At the time of entry into the study, approximately 20 percent of subjects were on no therapy, and the majority of the remaining subjects were on either ZDV or d4T monotherapy. Approximately 10 percent of patients were receiving ZDV/ddC, and 5 percent were receiving ZDV/ddI. At baseline the median CD4 cell count of patients randomized was approximately 20 cells and the median HIV-1 RNA level was 5.4 $\log_{10}$/mL. The initial antiretroviral effect of ritonavir resulted in a 1.5 $\log_{10}$ decrease in HIV-1 RNA; this effect diminished to approximately 0.6 $\log_{10}$ at 16 weeks. CD4 cell counts rose 40 cells above baseline in the ritonavir-treated group and stayed at that level through 16 weeks. CD8 cell counts also rose by about 200 cells/μL over the initial 16 weeks of study. There were no significant changes from baseline in HIV-1 RNA levels or CD4/CD8 cell counts in the group treated with placebo. Over approximately 6 months of observation the progression to AIDS or death in subjects treated with ritonavir was significantly reduced, with 15.7 percent of subjects on ritonavir experiencing such endpoints compared to 33.1 percent of subjects who received placebo (relative hazard 0.44, CI 0.336-0.562). Survival alone was also improved by ritonavir therapy; there were 26 deaths in subjects treated with ritonavir (4.8 percent) and 46 deaths on placebo (8.4 percent, relative hazard 0.57). Risk reduction appeared to occur for most HIV-1–related opportunistic diseases. Adverse events related to ritonavir that required discontinuation of the therapy were predominantly gastrointestinal and occurred in approximately 15 percent of subjects.

Resistance of HIV-1 to ritonavir has been well documented, both in vitro and in vivo.[149] Loss of antiretroviral effect appears to correlate with the appearance of resistance.[148] Mutations appear to occur in a step-wise pattern in subjects treated with ritonavir, with mutations at codons 82 and 54 occurring in a significant number of variants.[150] Multiple additional mutations were described, some distant from the protease active site. These mutations may be compensatory mutations that improve protease function in an enzyme with mutations in the active site. Viruses with high-level resistance to ritonavir appear cross-resistant to indinavir and, to some degree, nelfinavir.[150] The rate of selection of ritonavir-resistant mutants was inversely correlated with trough ritonavir levels in these subjects.

Nelfinavir

Nelfinavir (Viracept) is a potent inhibitor of HIV-1 in vitro. The IC_{50} for this compound against a variety of ZDV-sensitive and ZDV-resistant laboratory and clinical isolates ranges from 9 to 60 n*M*. Fifty percent human serum does not change the IC_{50} in vitro. The cytotoxic-to-therapeutic ratios in these in vitro assays ranged from 500:1 to 1,000:1.[151]

This compound has an oral bioavailability of 17–47 percent in animals and is metabolized by the liver and excreted in the feces.[152] In animals nelfinavir has a wide tissue distribution and appears to be concentrated in the lymph nodes and the spleen.[152] This agent has been given to a small number of HIV-1–infected persons. To date the agent has been well tolerated, with the major side effect being diarrhea. It has shown antiretroviral activity with a decrease of HIV-1 RNA in plasma of approximately 1.0 $\log_{10}$ (10-fold) over a 12-week period.[153] The approved dose of nelfinavir is 750 mg three times daily, though the antiretroviral effect and the side-effect profile of more sustained therapy need to be evaluated. Nelfinavir, like other protease inhibitors, is likely to have the potential for drug-drug interactions with other medications that undergo hepatic p450 metabolism.

Resistance to nelfinavir has occurred with passage of HIV-1 in the presence of drug in vitro.[151] Isolates with 30-fold decrease in susceptibility contained mutations in the protease gene at codons 46 and 84. In vitro mutagenesis studies confirmed that these mutations conferred resistance when introduced into an HIV-1 laboratory isolate. These studies showed a threefold and fivefold decrease in susceptibility with mutations at codon 48 and 90, respectively. Cross-resistance in isolates resistant to indinavir and/or ritonavir may occur.[150] In vivo a mutation at codon 30 appears first on nelfinavir therapy; this mutation results in little cross-resistance with other protease inhibitors.[154]

Amprenavir

Amprenavir VX-478 (or 141W94) is an HIV-1 protease inhibitor that is in clinical development and has a high affinity for the HIV-1 protease (K_i of 0.60 n*M* against the HIV-1 protease) and an IC_{90} of 40 n*M* against a lab strain of HIV-1.[155] This compound has a hydroxyethylamino sulfonamide backbone with a low molecular mass (506 daltons),[155] limited effects of human plasma on IC_{90}, and good oral bioavailability in animal species.

Resistance of HIV-1 to amprenavir has been selected for in vitro by passage of HIV-1 in the presence of the drug.[156] A mutation in the protease gene that leads to an isoleucine-to-valine substitution at amino acid position 50 appears to be the pivotal mutation leading to resistance. High-level (14- to 20-fold) resistance occurs when additional mutations are selected for, and these mutations may be compensatory. Of note, some comprenavir-resistant HIV-1 variants remain sensitive to both saquinavir and indinavir or may have increased sensitivity to these agents,[157] suggesting the possibility that amprenavir and these other protease inhibitors could be used in combination or in sequence in patients infected with HIV-1. However, HIV-1 variants with multiple mutations in the protease gene cross-resistant to multiple inhibitors, including amprenavir, have been described.[143]

ENVELOPE ACTIVE AGENTS

Agents have been developed to interrupt the interaction between HIV-1 and its receptors on CD4+ cells. Recombinant soluble CD4 inhibits the replication of laboratory strains of HIV-1 in vitro. A randomized clinical trial showed limited activity of this therapy in patients, however.[11] The limited activity may be due to the failure of rsCD4 to neutralize wild-type HIV-1 isolates from patients.[158] Dextran sulfate was also shown to inhibit HIV-1 replication in vitro, but administration of dextran to HIV-1-infected patients was toxic and ineffective.[159]

Naphthalene sulfonate polymers interact with the CD4 molecule on the surface of CD4+ cells and block binding of gp120 to the CD4 molecule. These compounds are active against HIV-1 in vitro but are considerably toxic and have a relatively low therapeutic-toxic ratio.[160] Clinical testing of these compounds in humans is under way. An agent that blocks the interaction of HIV with the co-receptor CCR-5 has been recently described.[160a]

COMBINATION THERAPY

Given the limitations of antiretroviral monotherapy for HIV-1 infection, other strategies are needed to enhance the activity of the available agents. Resistance of HIV-1 to agents used in therapy may be one of the direct causes of drug failure. Given the underlying replication rate of HIV-1, the size of the virus population in an infected individual, and the error rate of the reverse transcriptase, mutant strains of HIV-1 containing amino acid substitutions that confer resistance to single agents are likely to be present in small numbers at the time of initiation of therapy. The presence in untreated patients of variants resistant to ZDV, protease inhibitors, and NNRTI has already been documented.[135,161] Such viral variants will be rapidly selected in the face of incomplete suppression of replication.[35]

Institution of therapy with a combination of agents, especially with agents that would require HIV-1 to have multiple separate mutations to develop resistance to all the agents in the combination, should reduce or delay the rate of treatment failure. The appearance of new mutations will be slowed significantly by drug combinations that result in very potent inhibition because of the reduction in number of replication cycles. The benefit of reduced heterogeneity should not be limited only to emergence of resistance to the agents used in therapy. In addition, the frequency of appearance of mutations in the envelope or other genes may be lowered in proportion to the decrease in number of replication cycles. This reduction in mutation frequency, in turn, would reduce the likelihood that mutants will arise which escape the immune response of the host. Alternatively, increased numbers of mutations or specific mutations may reduce the replication capacity of HIV variants in certain situations. Other potential advantages of combination therapy include additive-to-synergistic inhibition of HIV-1 replication, targeting of different tissue or cellular reservoirs, and targeting of cells at different states of activation.[162]

A specific combination may produce different results when given as initial therapy (Table 74-2) or when given to subjects who have had extensive previous treatment, especially if the past therapy included one of the agents in the combination. The underlying disease stage of the population under study may also influence the observed antiviral or clinical effects of therapy. Subjects with low initial CD4 cell counts may have less sustained rebound in their CD4 cell counts. The reasons for this observation may include: (1) higher rates of HIV-1 replication and therefore more rapid selection of resistant variants; or (2) depletion of the CD4 cell repertoire,[162a] resulting in an inability to restore CD4 cell counts to normal ranges despite the high rate of CD4 cell turnover that is ongoing in many individuals with HIV infection.[31,32] Conversely, despite the potential for a less vigorous improvement in immune response in subjects with advanced HIV-1 disease, com-

Table 74-2. Combination Antiretroviral Therapies with Documented Clinical Activity in Comparative Clinical Trials

Improvement in CD4 cell counts and/or HIV-1 RNA in plasma	Delayed progression to AIDS and/or prolonged survival
Initial therapy	
zidovudine and didanosine	zidovudine and didanosine
zidovudine and zalcitabine	zidovudine and zalcitabine
zidovudine and lamivudine	zidovudine and lamivudine*
stavudine and didanosine	
zidovudine and indinavir	
stavudine and lamivudine	
zidovudine, didanosine, and nevirapine	
zidovudine, lamivudine, nelfinavir	
ZDV or nucleoside experience patients	
zidovudine and didanosine	zidovudine and didanosine
zidovudine and lamivudine	ritonavir and nucleoside therapy
zidovudine, lamivudine, and indinavir	saquinavir and zalcitabine
zidovudine, didanosine, and nevirapine	lamivudine added to zidovudine (with or without didanosine or zalcitabine)
zidovudine, zalcitabine, and saquinavir	lamivudine, zidovudine, and indinavir
zidovudine, zalcitabine, and ritonavir	
ritonavir and saquinavir	

* Demonstrated by meta-analysis

bination therapy that produces significant decreases in HIV-1 replication may be more likely to result in changes in clinical disease progression or survival in patients with more advanced disease. In less advanced patients, the numbers of clinical endpoints such as progression to AIDS or death will occur less frequently and may be delayed.

COMBINATION NUCLEOSIDE THERAPY

By 1995 three large clinical trials had evaluated combinations of nucleoside analogs compared to nucleoside monotherapy. These trials included both subjects who had received and subjects who had not received previous therapy. The study population for each of the studies differed in their entry CD4 cell count range.

The AIDS Clinical Trials Group (ACTG) of the National Institute of Allergy and Infectious Diseases performed a large clinical endpoint study (ACTG 175) designed to evaluate the effect of antiretroviral therapy with combinations of nucleoside agents compared to therapy with ZDV or ddI as single agents.[4] Subjects entered the study with CD4 cell counts between 200 and 500/μL. The mean CD4 cell count at entry was 352 cells/μL, and 82 percent of the subjects were asymptomatic. In the group of patients who had received less than 1 week of previous antiretroviral treatment (N = 1,067), the initiation of therapy with the combination of ZDV and ddC significantly reduced progression to AIDS or death by 51 percent when compared to ZDV therapy alone. Initiating therapy with the combination of ZDV and ddI also reduced the rate of disease progression by 39 percent ($p = .08$). Zidovudine and ddC improved mortality in this subgroup of therapy-naïve patients with a trend toward statistical significance, $p = .08$, despite the relatively few deaths that occurred in the therapy-naïve group (49 total deaths). These results were obtained despite the fact that subjects were allowed to switch to combination therapy if their CD4 cell count fell below 50 percent of baseline or if they developed an AIDS-defining infection or malignancy. The median duration of follow-up for this group was 135 weeks, and 25 percent of patients were lost to follow-up. Didanosine monotherapy also appeared more active than ZDV alone in this treatment-naïve group, though the difference between ZDV and ddI was only significant when the aggregate endpoint of AIDS, death, and fall in CD4 cell count to below 50 percent of baseline was used.

This study also enrolled 1,400 subjects who had been treated previously with ZDV. Eighty percent of these subjects had received at least 6 months of ZDV therapy, and many (42 percent) had more than 2 years of previous therapy. In this group either adding or switching to ddI improved mortality by approximately 50 percent over continuing on ZDV therapy. The addition of ddC to ongoing ZDV therapy resulted in no improvement in survival or no improvement in the combined endpoints of survival or progression to AIDS over continued ZDV therapy.[4]

Overall numbers of adverse events in this trial differed in the treatment-naïve and treatment-experienced groups. In treatment-naïve patients, there were significantly fewer severe adverse events on initially assigned therapy with ddI combined with ZDV than on ZDV alone (13 vs. 22 percent). Subjects on ZDV combined with ddI had the fewest number of severe adverse events. The rates of severe adverse events in the treatment-experienced group did not differ significantly among treatment arms. Clinical pancreatitis did not appear to occur in greater frequency on the ddI-containing arms.

A similar trial was carried out in Europe and is referred to as the Delta trial.[163] The subjects in this trial were divided into treatment-naïve (Delta I) and treatment-experienced (Delta II) groups. The entry CD4 cell count range was lower than in the ACTG 175 trial, and only three treatment arms were evaluated: ZDV combined with ddI, ZDV combined with ddC, and ZDV given alone. Zidovudine was given in an unblinded fashion, and patients were randomized to either the ddI- (active or placebo) or ddC- (active or placebo) containing arms. Over 2,000 treatment-naïve subjects were enrolled in Delta I. The mean entry CD4 cell count was 212 cells/μL. Over 2 years of follow-up there was a highly significant difference in all-cause mortality, with an 84 percent overall survival for the subjects treated with ZDV/ddI compared to 73 percent survival on ZDV alone. In contrast to ACTG 175, ddI plus ZDV was significantly better than ddC plus ZDV in preventing progression to AIDS or death. In Delta II, approximately 1,000 subjects were studied who had received previous ZDV therapy. The mean baseline CD4 cell count of this group was 189 cells/μL. Differences between study treatments were less marked in this population, though the addition of ddI resulted in fewer clinical endpoints than if subjects remained on ZDV alone. The addition of ddC appeared to add no benefit, as was seen in the ACTG 175 trial. In Delta I and II the gastrointestinal adverse events associated with ddI or the ddI placebo, which contained equal amounts of buffer, were greater when compared to ZDV and ddC or the ddC placebo.

A third community-based trial examined the combination of ddI and ZDV and the combination of ddC and ZDV compared to ZDV alone in subjects with CD4 cell counts less than 200 cells/μL or in subjects who had had a previous AIDS-defining illness.[164] As in the Delta trial, ZDV was given in an unblinded fashion, and subjects were randomized to the ddI/ddI placebo or ddC/ddC placebo treatment arms. The mean CD4 cell count of the group was 119 cells/μL, and the majority of the patients had received prior ZDV therapy (77 percent; median duration 12 months). When all-cause mortality was analyzed in the entire study population, there were no significant differences between arms, with rates varying between 22 and 25 percent. When patients who were naïve to ZDV therapy were analyzed separately, the initial use of ddI plus ZDV resulted in a significant clinical improvement over 2 years compared to ZDV therapy.

A common thread among these three clinical trials of ZDV, ddI, and ddC appears to be that beginning therapy with a combination of either ddC or ddI with ZDV results in a decrease in mortality of approximately 40–50 percent in subjects with CD4 cell counts less than 500 cells/μL, compared to beginning therapy with ZDV alone. Though cross-study comparisons are difficult to interpret, the initiation of ddI and ZDV appears to be more effective in individuals with more advanced disease. The interpretation of the results of these three trials for individuals with previous ZDV experience is somewhat less clear, but the addition of ddI to ZDV or a switch in therapy to ddI appears beneficial. The addition of ddC to the therapy of individuals already receiving ZDV is not supported by these results.

Additional combinations of nucleoside analogs have been studied. The combination of 3TC and ZDV was evaluated in two studies of patients who had received little or no previous ZDV therapy, one conducted in North America and the other conducted in Europe. Both studies were randomized, double-blind, placebo-controlled multicenter studies comparing 3TC plus ZDV with ZDV monotherapy. Lamivudine monotherapy was also evaluated in the North American study. In that study, sustained CD4 cell increases were seen over 52 weeks for the combination of 3TC plus ZDV at two doses of 3TC, 150 mg and 300 mg twice daily, with a peak mean increase of 79 and 78 cells/μL, respectively, with little trend toward baseline over time.[103] By week 52, the difference between the mean CD4 cell count for either combination arm and ZDV monotherapy was >100 cells/μL. The median time-weighted change from baseline over 24 weeks was a decrease of 1.1 and 1.2 $\log_{10}$ for the low- and high-dose 3TC-plus-ZDV combinations, respectively, compared to a decrease of 0.3 $\log_{10}$ for ZDV monotherapy. Over the 52 weeks of the blinded-therapy phase, the combination of 3TC and ZDV had a persistent inhibitory effect on HIV-1 RNA levels of approximately 10-fold.

In the European study, the peak mean change in CD4 cell counts from baseline was 85 cells/μL at 8 weeks for ZDV plus 3TC and 34 cells/μL at 4 weeks for ZDV monotherapy.[165] At 24 weeks, the mean CD4 cell count was 78 cells above baseline for subjects on 3TC plus ZDV, while the mean CD4 cell count for subjects on ZDV monotherapy had decreased to 9 cells below baseline. Of the subjects who completed 24 weeks of study, 97 percent opted to continue on open-label 3TC and ZDV. Over the subsequent 24-week period, the positive effect of 3TC plus ZDV persisted, though it declined somewhat to a mean of 48 cells above baseline at week 48.

The combination of 3TC and ZDV has also been studied in patients with previous ZDV treatment. In a study that compared the addition of 3TC to ZDV to continuing ZDV alone, there was a significant increase in CD4 cell count in the patients treated with the combination; this effect persisted above baseline CD4 levels through 48 weeks.[166] An additional study in ZDV-experienced patients with CD4 cells between 100 and 300 cells/μL the addition of two doses of 3TC (150 and 300 mg twice daily) to ZDV were compared to the addition of ddC.[167] The addition of 3TC to ZDV resulted in significant increases in CD4 cell counts above baseline compared to the addition of ddC. The effects on HIV-1 RNA levels in plasma were similar in all three treatment arms. The number of CDC class B and C clinical endpoints was significantly greater in the ZDV-plus-ddC-treated group when compared to the 3TC/ZDV arms combined.

A meta-analysis of the clinical endpoints in these four trials has been performed. The combination of 3TC and ZDV was significantly more effective at delaying clinical endpoints when compared to the control arms in the combined studies.[168] When the clinical results were analyzed separately for subjects who were treatment-naïve and who had previous ZDV treatment, the combination of ZDV and 3TC resulted in an approximately 50 percent reduction in clinical disease progression. In addition, a large clinical endpoint trial (CAESAR Trial) was halted when an early analysis showed that subjects receiving either ZDV alone or ZDV in combination with ddI or ddC who had 3TC added to their treatment had an approximately twofold decrease in AIDS events or death when compared to subjects receiving 3TC placebo.[132]

The antiretroviral activity of the combination of 3TC and ZDV may be due in part to an interaction between the resistance mutations that occurs when individuals with HIV infection are treated with these agents. If HIV-1 containing some or all of the mutations conveying ZDV resistance acquires the mutation associated with high-level 3TC resistance—a methionine-to-valine substitution at reverse transcriptase codon 184—then these viruses regain their susceptibility to ZDV.[108] In individuals who have received no previous antiretroviral therapy, the initiation of ZDV and 3TC simultaneously results in a delay in the appearance of a mutation associated with ZDV resistance and early antiretroviral failure of ZDV monotherapy.[169] Whether 3TC in combination with other nucleoside analogs will have a similar effectiveness as ZDV plus 3TC is under study. In vitro studies suggest additive-to-synergistic interactions between 3TC and other agents.[170]

The combination of ddI and d4T has been studied in a small number of patients in an unblinded fashion.[171] Preliminary results of this study indicated that antiretroviral effects were potent and sustained through 1 year. There appeared to be no increase in the occurrence of peripheral neuropathy, an adverse event that has been described for both agents when given as monotherapy.

Multiple other potential combinations of nucleoside analogs exist but have had limited evaluation in HIV-1-infected individuals. The combination of d4T and ZDV is of some concern because both agents are phosphorylated by the same pathway. In vitro studies suggest an antagonism of these two agents against some HIV-1 isolates;[170] in a recent clinical trial of ZDV-experienced subjects, the ZDV/d4T treatment arm was prematurely discontinued when individuals receiving this treatment were found to have a more rapid decline in CD4 cell count than subjects receiving d4T alone.[172]

PROTEASE INHIBITOR AND REVERSE TRANSCRIPTASE INHIBITOR COMBINATION THERAPY

The combination of protease inhibitors with nucleoside or nonnucleoside reverse transcriptase inhibitors offers exciting prospects for greater inhibition of HIV-1 replication and potentially more durable clinical benefits. Combining agents that work at different sites in the life cycle of the pathogen may prolong inhibitory activity and delay resistance emergence. Precedence for this strategy exists for the treatment of other infectious diseases such as tuberculosis and enterococcal infection and for the treatment of malignancies. In vitro studies suggest additive-to-synergistic interactions between RT inhibitors and protease inhibitors against both ZDV-sensitive and ZDV-resistant isolates.[173] Toxicities of these agents may not overlap.

Studies of the combination of HIV-1 protease inhibitors and RT inhibitors have already been reported in populations of patients with extensive previous treatment with ZDV and in some cases other nucleoside RT inhibitors. In a clinical trial sponsored by the AIDS Clinical Trials Group (ACTG 229), the protease inhibitor saquinavir was combined with ZDV and with ZDV plus ddC. The combination of saquinavir, ddC, and ZDV was most effective at decreasing HIV-1 levels in plasma and at increasing CD4 cell counts.[174] In another study, saquinavir in combination with ddC also delayed progression to AIDS or death compared to ddC or saquinavir monotherapy.[175]

Indinavir has also been studied in combination with ZDV in patients naïve to previous therapy with CD4 counts less than 500 cells/μL and serum HIV-1 RNA levels greater than 20,000 copies per mL.[176] Through 24 weeks, the combination of indinavir and ZDV produced a median decrease from baseline in HIV-1 RNA of 2.5 $\log_{10}$ compared to 1.5 and 0.3 $\log_{10}$ decreases for ZDV and indinavir monotherapies, respectively. Increases in CD4 cell counts were not significantly different between the combination and indinavir monotherapy arms over 6 months of follow-up. The number of resistance mutations conferring ZDV or indinavir resistance observed with combination therapy was less than the number seen in either monotherapy arm, however.

Indinavir in combination with ZDV plus 3TC was evaluated in subjects with a mean CD4 cell count of approximately 170 cells/μL and who had received at least 6 months of previous ZDV therapy. This three-drug combination was compared to the protease inhibitor alone and to ZDV plus 3TC.[9] Despite a median previous treatment duration with ZDV of 30 months and the fact that 80 percent of subjects had HIV-1 isolates with ZDV-resistance mutations, subjects who received the three-drug combination had, on average, a greater than 100 fold decrease in the HIV-1 levels in plasma that persisted through 48 weeks of study. At 48 weeks 85 percent of subjects who received IDV plus 3TC plus ZDV had HIV-1 RNA levels below 500 copies per mL. This result occurred despite the fact that the median entry HIV-1 RNA level was 40,000 copies per mL. Approximately 40 percent of subjects treated with indinavir alone achieved this level of suppression at 48 weeks, while no subject who had only 3TC added achieved this result. The effect on CD4 cell counts appeared less dramatic, though the mean increase in CD4 cell count was greater than 100 cells/μL at 48 weeks in the subjects treated with the triple combination. A clinical endpoint trial, ACTG320, comparing ZDV and 3TC plus indinavir to ZDV plus 3TC, ended prematurely when the triple combination regimen was shown to result in a 50 percent decrease in disease progression and a 50 percent improvement in survival relative to the dual nucleoside arm.[177] The combinations of ritonavir combined with ZDV and ddC and ritonavir with ZDV and 3TC are in clinical study, as is nelfinavir, 3TC, and ZDV.[178] Treatment of HIV during or early after primary HIV infection may be advantageous if HIV has not disseminated fully to all potential tissue compartments or if the limited variant diversity that is theoretically present early in infection decreases the likelihood of resistant escape mutants. A study of ZDV monotherapy in primary infection gave suggestive results.[22] Further studies taking advantage of the combination of protease inhibitors with 3TC and ZDV have shown potent inhibition of HIV replication and immunologic evidence of decreased HIV-1 antigen presentation over time on therapy.[179]

PROTEASE INHIBITOR COMBINATIONS

Combinations of protease inhibitors might inhibit replication of HIV-1 more profoundly than monotherapy with these agents. Detailed in vitro studies of protease-protease interactions have not yet been reported, but antagonism has been seen between some protease inhibitors in preliminary in vitro studies.[180] Since initial resistance patterns differ between saquinavir and other approved agents, however, combinations of ritonavir or indinavir with saquinavir are worthy of study. By inhibiting cytochrome p450 enzyme activity, ritonavir inhibits the metabolism of saquinavir. Pharmacokinetic studies of ritonavir and saquinavir have shown marked increases in saquinavir level in HIV-1–infected subjects.[181] This pharmacokinetic interaction results in potent antiretroviral effect in the small number of patients studied. The durability of this effect and how it compares to the combination of nucleoside analogs and protease inhibitors is not known. The combination of ritonavir and saquinavir does not seem to have increased toxicity markedly, but the studies are small and of short duration.

Amprenavir also appears to select for a somewhat different pattern of resistance mutations than saquinavir, ritonavir, and indinavir, and combinations of amprenavir with these other inhibitors are also underway. However, prolonged exposure of a small number of subjects to indinavir not only selected for high-level resistance to indinavir but also some viral variants that were broadly cross-resistant to ritonavir, saquinavir, and amprenavir[143]; this observation raised the possibility that sequential or combination therapy with currently available protease inhibitors may have limited advantages over monotherapy with protease inhibitors.

NUCLEOSIDE-NONNUCLEOSIDE COMBINATION THERAPIES

Resistance develops rapidly in vitro and in vivo to NNRTI monotherapy, and the loss of antiretroviral activity correlates with appearance of resistance. However, NNRTI have been shown to be synergistic with nucleoside analogs in vitro, and the selection for NNRTI resistance in HIV-1 variants resistant to ZDV results in a decrease in phenotypic resistance to ZDV in these variants.[124] In a randomized, blinded study in subjects with ZDV treatment experience, the addition of NVP was compared to continued ZDV monotherapy.[182] The addition of NVP to chronic ZDV therapy resulted in significant improvements in average change in CD4 cell counts and HIV-1 RNA levels over 28 weeks of study. The treatment effect on HIV-1 RNA in plasma had returned to baseline after 4 months of combination therapy, however. A three-drug combination of ZDV, ddI, and NVP was compared to the combination of ZDV and ddI for 48 weeks in subjects previously treated with nucleoside analogs. The triple combination resulted in a greater antiretroviral effect as measured by HIV-1 RNA in plasma or peripheral blood mononuclear cell quantitative microcultures, and it resulted in a greater improvement in CD4 cell counts than ZDV/ddI. There was no significant difference in numbers of clinical endpoints, although the study was not powered to show such differences.[126] Therapy with ZDV, ddI, and NVP was also compared with ZDV/ddI and ZDV/NVP in previously untreated subjects.[16] Over 52 weeks the triple combination resulted in the suppression of HIV-1 RNA below the limit of detection in approximately 50 percent of subjects. If a more sensitive assay for HIV-1 RNA in plasma was used, the majority of these individuals still had levels below detectability;[16] similar suppression was not observed in the two-drug arms.

Delavirdine in combination with ZDV has been compared to ZDV monotherapy in patients who had not previously been treated with ZDV or who had less than 6 months of ZDV therapy.[183] Delavirdine at 900 and 1,200 mg per day in combination with ZDV resulted in a threefold fall in HIV-1 RNA for at least 60 weeks. Using these two doses in combination with ZDV resulted in mean CD4 cell counts approximately 20 cells above the baseline value for greater than 1 year. Treatment with delavirdine in combination with ddI in subjects who had received previous ZDV treatment and less than 4 months of ddI therapy resulted in no clinical benefit when compared to ddI monotherapy. Delavirdine has also been given in combination with two nucleoside agents in subjects with previous nucleoside inhibitor therapy, and it appears to add some additional antiretroviral effect.

OTHER COMBINATION THERAPIES

Hydroxyurea is an inhibitor of cell division that has been used for treatment of certain hematological malignancies, polycythemia vera, and sickle cell anemia. Hydroxyurea inhibits human ribonucleotide reductase, a human cellular enzyme that catalyzes the reduction of nucleotides (NTP) to deoxynucleotides (dNTP) needed for cellular DNA synthesis. The levels of deoxynucleotides within an HIV-infected cell influence the rate and amount of HIV-1 replication in that cell. In vitro, hydroxyurea reduces the level of HIV-1 replication in treated cells; hydroxyurea in combination with nucleoside analog RT inhibitors, especially ddI, synergistically inhibits HIV-1 replication in HIV-infected activated peripheral blood mononuclear cells (PBMC) and HIV-infected resting PBMC that become activated.[184,185] In vivo, the addition of hydroxyurea to ddI therapy has resulted in increased antiretroviral activity over ddI alone in trials evaluating small numbers of patients,[186,187] with prolonged potent antiviral effect observed in some patients.[188]

Interferon-alpha, a human protein with antiviral activity, has been shown to inhibit HIV replication in vitro and to be synergistic with a wide range of antiretroviral compounds including nucleoside and nonnucleoside RT inhibitors, protease inhibitors, and recombinant soluble CD4.[123,189–191] Interferon-alpha has been used in combination with ZDV to treat individuals with HIV,[192] and it appears to have increased antiviral effects as measured by effect on p24 antigenemia.[193] The utility of interferon-alpha is limited by the requirement for parenteral administration. Interferon-alpha has efficacy with ZDV in treatment of Kaposi's sarcoma[194–196] and possibly in HIV-related thrombocytopenia refractory to ZDV therapy.[197]

ZIDOVUDINE AND ACYCLOVIR

The concurrent use of ZDV and acyclovir, an agent with activity against herpes simplex viruses (HSV) and varicella zoster virus, has been associated with improved survival in individuals with HIV in some studies but not in others.[198,199] The mechanism for interaction between these agents is unclear, though active HSV infection has been shown to elevate transiently the levels of HIV-1 RNA in plasma. Some patients with frequently recurrent herpes infections might benefit from combinations that include acyclovir.

APPROACH TO PATIENT MANAGEMENT

In order to make decisions regarding antiretroviral therapy for an HIV-infected individual, the disease stage should be assessed. The rate of disease progression varies widely from patient to patient, and a careful history, physical exam, and laboratory assessment will provide information that allows an estimation of this rate of progression. The time of acquisition of HIV, documented by seroconversion, and the presence and severity of a primary infection syndrome can be useful in gauging HIV-1 disease progression. Clinical symptoms—for example, AIDS-defining illnesses and CDC class B symptoms/signs such as thrush and oral hairy leukoplakia—are predictors of disease progression independent of CD4 cell counts. The CD4 cell count provides information on the underlying degree of immunosuppression of a given patient, and it is also a predictor of disease progression. Levels of HIV-1 RNA in plasma have been shown to be strong predictors of survival and of progression to AIDS-defining illness in several cohort studies and studies of antiretroviral therapy.[44,48,49,50,50a,54] The predictive value of HIV-1 RNA levels is independent of CD4 cell count at the time the RNA level is measured, and it correlates with the rate of CD4 decline. The CD4 cell count and HIV-1 RNA level taken together offer a more accurate estimation of the likelihood of disease progression in an individual over time[50a,200,201] (see Appendix A). An important caveat from the studies of Mellors et al.[49,50,50a] is that because of sample storage in heparin for up to 8 to 10 years, RNA values are two- to fivefold lower than what would be expected from samples processed without prolonged storage or the presence of heparin.[201] Parameters such as HIV-1-related symptoms/signs, a CD4 cell count less than 500, an elevated HIV-1 RNA level, or a combination of two or three of these may be an indication to initiate antiretroviral therapy or to alter therapy in individuals who are already being treated (Table 74-3).[202]

A history of previous antiretroviral treatment impacts on the management of therapy. In patients who have not been previously treated, the first issue is when to initiate therapy. Currently no unanimity exists on when to initiate therapy; basing the initiation of therapy on a strict CD4 cell cut-off, such as less than 500 cells/μL, may be somewhat arbitrary, especially given the strong independent predictive value of HIV-1 RNA levels for survival and disease progression. Previously untreated patients with AIDS-defining opportunistic illnesses receive survival benefit from antiretroviral therapy. Asymptomatic patients with CD4 cell counts less than 500 cells/μL receive clinical benefit from combination antiretroviral therapy as evidenced by a delay in progression to AIDS or death.[4] Previously untreated patients who initiated therapy with the combination of ZDV and ddI had an improvement in all-cause mortality over that obtained with ZDV monotherapy.[163] The hypothesis that individuals with CD4 cell counts above 500 cells/μL who have either HIV-1-related symptoms or signs or high plasma HIV-1 RNA levels (<10,000–20,000 copies/mL) will benefit from potent antiretroviral therapy appears tenable but currently unproved (Table 74-3).[201–203]

A second issue for initial antiretroviral treatment is whether to begin therapy with a single agent or a combination of agents. Several studies now show that initial nucleoside combination therapy delays progression to AIDS and death when compared to ZDV monotherapy.[4,163] The availability of combinations with even more potent antiretroviral activity offers hope for more dramatic or prolonged clinical benefits.[9,177] Initiating therapy with multiple agents early in disease, however, means that patients will have to take large numbers of pills with potential side effects and over long periods of time while they are asymptomatic for their disease. Selection for HIV-1 variants resistant to medications within a patient's treatment regimen may occur. The appearance of HIV-1 variants with cross-resistance to multiple protease inhibitors in patients treated with indinavir[143] raises the concern that

Table 74-3. Indications for Initiation of Antiretroviral Therapy

Symptoms related to HIV-1
All patients regardless of CD4 cell count
(AIDS symptoms: Most experts would begin with combination therapy including a protease inhibitor)
Asymptomatic individuals with CD4 cell counts >500/μL
If HIV-1 RNA greater than 10,000–20,000 copies/mL (Some experts would begin therapy at any detectable level of HIV-1 RNA)
If CD4 cell counts are decreasing at more than 10 cells per month
Asymptomatic individuals with CD4 cell counts <500/μL
All patients (Some experts would defer therapy in patients with CD4 cell counts between 350 and 500/μL who have stable CD4 cell counts and low HIV-1 RNA levels [<5,000 copies/mL])

early initiation of treatment with one protease inhibitor could result in limited usefulness of this class of compound later in disease. Consensus appears to be emerging that the most appropriate initial therapy should consist of combinations of antiretrovirals, including potent agents such as protease inhibitors. Recommendations made by panels convened by the International AIDS society-USA and by the National Institutes of Health include several regimens as appropriate for initial consideration (Table 74-4).[201,203] For patients who present for initial antiretroviral therapy with symptomatic HIV-1 disease or elevated HIV-1 RNA levels, aggressive combination treatment that includes a protease inhibitor is recommended.[201,203]

For patients who have received previous antiretroviral therapy, therapeutic options will depend on what specific therapies were used in the past. For patients who have received only ZDV, the alternatives of switching to ddI or d4T or adding ddI or 3TC or adding 3TC plus indinavir appear to delay clinical progression to AIDS or death.[2,3,4,132,167,168,177] For patients with previous nucleoside treatment, the addition of ritonavir may also improve clinical outcome and survival.[8] The strategy of simultaneously adding a protease inhibitor while switching nucleoside therapies in patients previously treated with nucleoside analogs needs to be evaluated, but is recommended.[201,203] Currently there is no information on how to proceed with therapy in patients who have received extensive treatment with a protease inhibitor. The change in HIV RNA levels in response to antiretroviral therapy predicts at least in part the clinical benefit of the treatment,[44,45,54] and this fact may allow individualization of therapy, especially for patients who have had extensive previous treatment or who are intolerant to standard regimens.

An additional factor that will influence the choice of which agents to use for therapy in a given patient is the potential toxicity of specific agents and the medical history of the patient. The hematological toxicity of ZDV may limit its use in patients with diminished bone marrow reserve or who require treatment with other agents with hematological toxicity, including ganciclovir and certain chemotherapeutic agents. Didanosine should be used cautiously, if at all, in patients with a previous history of pancreatitis, heavy alcohol use, or an abnormal pancreatic amylase or lipase. Alternatives to ddC should be considered in patients with peripheral neuropathy, and d4T should be used cautiously in such patients, especially if neuropathy is severe enough to require treatment.

The protease inhibitor indinavir has been associated with kidney stones in 2–5 percent of patients treated with this agent. Patients with a history of kidney stones or who are at risk for dehydration may be at increased risk. Ritonavir is associated with nausea and vomiting and oral paresthesias, though patients at increased risk for these side effects have not yet been identified. The long-term effects of elevated triglyceride levels associated with ritonavir therapy are unknown, and whether patients with an abnormal lipid profile at baseline are at higher risk is also unknown. An additional factor that may influence selection of therapy for a given patient is the patient's ability to adhere to complex medication regimens. Indinavir, saquinavir, and ritonavir require taking 6, 9, and 12 pills per day. Indinavir can be taken only on an empty stomach, and saquinavir and ritonavir should be taken with food to enhance absorption. Ritonavir capsules require refrigeration, and care must be observed in using this agent with many other agents that undergo hepatic metabolism and that are commonly used in HIV-infected individuals. Nelfinavir also requires three pills three times daily and can result in significant diarrhea. Patients who have difficulty adhering to these regimens put themselves at increased risk for the emergence of HIV-1 resistant to the protease inhibitor they are taking. Once resistance develops, even close adherence to recommended doses may not result in an effective antiretroviral response.

Table 74-4. Recommended Initial Treatment Regimens

Most experts and expert panels[201,203] recommend initial therapy with potent combinations that are capable of sustained suppression of plasma viral load. Currently these combinations would include two NRTIs and a protease inhibitor or two NRTIs and an NNRTI. Recommended agents:

2 Nucleoside RT inhibitors	Protease inhibitors	Nonnucleoside RT inhibitors
ZDV plus ddI	indinavir	nevirapine
ZDV plus ddC	nelfinavir	delavirdine
ZDV plus 3TC	ritonavir	
d4T plus ddI		
d4T plus 3TC		

Two NRTIs may be appropriate in some circumstances especially in individuals who require therapy but in whom three-drug combination therapy is not possible due to lack of commitment to drug adherence, concern over potential side effects, cost, access, etc.

Therapeutic regimens combining two protease inhibitors and combining protease inhibitors with NNRTIs are under study.

SPECIAL CONSIDERATIONS

MOTHER-INFANT TRANSMISSION

In the absence of antiretroviral therapy, transmission of HIV-1 from infected mothers to their infants occurs approximately 15–30 percent of the time.[204–207] Factors that increase the risk of transmission include a more advanced disease stage in the mother, higher levels of viral replication, and possibly primary HIV-1 infection during pregnancy.[204] Treatment of pregnant HIV-1–infected women with ZDV beginning in the second or third trimester, including intravenous therapy during delivery and administration of ZDV to the infant, substantially reduced the risk of transmisson in pregnant women with > 200 CD4 cells/μL.[206] Recommendations for treatment of HIV-infected pregnant women are listed in Table 74-5.[208] It is unknown whether ZDV monotherapy will retain the observed level of efficacy as more HIV-infected women receive ZDV treatment prior to pregnancy and as the prevalence of ZDV resistance in the population increases.[209] Combination regimens that include ZDV and alternatives to ZDV are being studied. These issues are explored in greater detail in Chap. 80.

POSTEXPOSURE PROPHYLACTIC THERAPY

Percutaneous exposure to blood from an infected individual carries an approximately 0.3 percent chance of seroconversion. Mu-

Table 74-5. Antiretroviral Treatment in Pregnancy

After 14 weeks of pregnancy: Begin ZDV 200 mg PO three times a day
During labor: Administer ZDV intravenously; load 2 mg/kg over 1 hour then a continuous 1 mg/kg/hr infusion
Postpartum: Treat the infant with 2 mg/kg every 6 hours for 6 weeks

If the pregnant woman has had extensive pretreatment with ZDV, consideration should be given to an alternative regimen, including the addition of 3TC to ZDV; limited information is available about the efficacy or safety of other alternative strategies.

Table 74-6. CDC Recommendations for Post-exposure Prophylactic Antiretroviral Therapy

Type of exposure	Source of material*	Antiretroviral prophylaxis§
Percutaneous	Blood¶	
	Highest risk	Recommend ZDV/3TC/indinavir
	Increased risk	Recommend ZDV/3TC, ± indinavir**
	No increased risk	Offer ZDV/3TC
	Fluid containing visible blood, other potentially infectious fluid ++, or tissue	Offer ZDV/3TC
	Other body fluid (e.g., urine)	Do not offer
Mucous membrane	Blood	
	Fluid containing visible	Offer ZDV/3TC, ± indinavir**
	blood, other potentially infectious fluid ++, or tissue	Offer ZDV, ± 3TC
	Other body fluid (e.g., urine)	Do not offer
Skin, increased risk§§	Blood	Offer ZDV/3TC, ± indinavir**
	Fluid containing visible blood, other potentially infectious fluid ++, or tissue	Offer ZDV, ± 3TC
	Other body fluid (e.g., urine)	Do not offer

* Any exposure to concentrated HIV (e.g., in a research laboratory or production facility) is treated as percutaneous exposure to blood with highest risk.

§ Regimens: zidovudine (ZDV), 200 mg three times daily; lamivudine (3TC), 150 mg two times daily; indinavir, 800 mg three times daily (if indinavir is not available, saquinavir may be used, 600 mg three times daily). Prophylaxis is given for 4 weeks. For full prescribing information, see package inserts.

¶ Highest risk—BOTH larger volume of blood (e.g., deep injury with large-diameter hollow needle previously in source patient's vein or artery, especially involving an injection on source-patient's blood) AND blood containing a high titer of HIV (e.g., source with acute retroviral illness or end-stage AIDS; viral load measurements may be considered, but its use in relation to postexposure prophylaxis has not been evaluated). Increased risk—EITHER exposure to larger volume of blood OR blood with a high titer of HIV. No increased risk—NEITHER exposure to larger volume of blood NOR blood with a high titer of HIV (e.g., solid suture needle injury from source patient with asymptomatic HIV infection).

** Possible toxicity of additional drug may not be warranted.

++ Includes semen; vaginal secretions; cerebrospinal, synovial, pleural, peritoneal, pericardial, and amniotic fluids.

§§ For skin, risk is increased for exposures involving a high titer of HIV, prolonged contact, an extensive area, or an area in which skin integrity is visibly compromised. For skin exposures with increased risk, the risk for drug toxicity outweighs the benefit of postexposure prophylaxis.

cous membrane exposure to HIV-1-infected blood or other body fluids conveys substantially less risk. The use of ZDV as post-exposure prophylactic therapy has been controversial, but a retrospective, case-control study appears to document significant efficacy of ZDV following exposure.[210] Given the description of therapies with substantially more potent antiretroviral effect than ZDV monotherapy, recommendations from the CDC have been modified to incorporate these more potent alternatives (Table 74-6).[211]

CONCLUSIONS

The introduction of potent protease inhibitors and combination therapies that result in marked suppression of HIV-1 replication raises expectations for prolonged clinical benefits of these therapies. Combination therapy with nucleoside analogs alone has been shown to improve survival compared to ZDV therapy in patients who are asymptomatic. Therapies for HIV are constantly evolving, however. New agents are being introduced at a rapid rate, resulting in a large number of potential treatments and multiple potential treatment strategies that rely on different sequences and combinations of agents. The wide availability of HIV-1 RNA level testing that allows measurement of the antiretroviral effect of a specific regimen may allow the patient and his or her medical practitioner to alter therapy based on the individual's antiretroviral response.

ADDENDUM

Since this chapter has gone to press the field of HIV-1 antiretroviral therapy has continued to change rapidly. A new formulation of saquinavir in a soft gel capsule (saquinavir-SGC) is available. This formulation has an improved bioavailability and is also given at a higher dose (1200 mg three times daily), enhancing antiretroviral effect. Efavirenz (DMP-266), a potent non-nucleoside RT inhibitor, is also now available. This agent is administered as a 600 mg once daily dose. Studies of each of these agents in combination with nucleoside RT inhibitors have shown similar antiretroviral activity to other potent 3-drug regimens. The effects of potent antiretroviral combination therapy on progression to AIDS and survival has clearly been documented in large population-based studies.[212] New complications of potent antiretroviral therapy have been described including increases in blood triglycerides, redistribution of body fat stores (lipodystrophy) and insulin resistance. These side effects appear to have an association with protease inhibitor-containing regimens and complicate treatment decisions.

Comprehensive treatment guidelines have continued to be updated and recommendations for therapy now include the goal of suppressing HIV-1 RNA levels in plasma to below the limit of the most sensitive assay available.[201,213] Currently, the limit of the most sensitive assays is in the range of 50 copies/mL. The guidelines for the treatment of HIV-1 infected pregnant women to prevent vertical transmission have been updated. These guidelines focus both prevention of transmission and adequate treatment for the woman and center on the use of potent combinations to maintain maternal viral load as low as possible.[214] Guidelines for the use of antiretroviral therapy following exposure to HIV-1 have also been recently revised.[215] Resistance of HIV-1 to antiretroviral therapy has become a major focus of basic and clinical HIV research. An overview of the tests becoming available to assess resistance and the implication of these resistance tests for the clinical management of HIV-infected individuals has been published,[216] as has a case to transmission of a multi-drug resistant HIV-1 variant.[217]

References

1 Fischl MA, et al: The efficacy of azidothymidine (AZT) in the treatment of patients with AIDS and AIDS-related complex: A double-blind, placebo-controlled trial. *N Engl J Med* 1987; 317:185–91.

2 Kahn JO, et al, for the NIAID AIDS Clinical Trials Group: A controlled trial comparing continued zidovudine with didanosine in human immunodeficiency virus infection. *N Engl J Med* 1992; 327: 581–87.

3 Spruance S, et al: Clinical efficacy of monotherapy with stavudine compared with zidovudine in HIV-infected, zidovudine-experienced patients. *Ann Intern Med* 1997; 126:355–363.

4 Hammer S, et al: A trial comparing nucleoside monotherapy with combination therapy in HIV-infected adults with CD4 cell counts from 200 to 500 per cubic millimeter. *N Engl J Med* 1996; 335:1081–90.

5 Ioannidis JP, et al: Early or deferred zidovudine therapy in HIV-infected patients without an AIDS-defining illness. *Ann Intern Med* 1995; 122:856–66.

6 Lundgren JD, et al, for the AIDS in Europe Study Group: Comparison of long-term prognosis of patients with AIDS treated and not treated with zidovudine. *JAMA* 1994; 271:1088–92.

7 Concorde Coordinating Committee: MRC/ANRS randomised double-blind controlled trial of immediate and deferred zidovudine in symptom-free HIV infection. *Lancet* 1994; 343:871–81.

8 Cameron DW, et al: Randomized placebo-controlled trial of ritonavir in advanced HIV-1 disease: The advanced HIV disease ritonavir study group. *Lancet* 1998; 351:543–9.

9 Gulick RM, et al: Treatment with a combination of indinavir, zidovudine and lamivudine in HIV-1 infected adults with prior antiretroviral use. *N Engl J Med* 1997; 337:734–39.

10 Berson JF, et al: A seven-transmembrane domain receptor involved in fusion and entry of T-cell-tropic human immunodeficiency virus type 1 strains. *J Virol* 1996; 70:6288–95.

11 Schooley RT, et al: Recombinant soluble CD4 therapy in patients with the acquired immunodeficiency syndrome (AIDS) and AIDS-related complex. A phase I–II escalating dosage trial. *Ann Intern Med* 1990; 112:247–53.

12 Bristow CL, et al: Inhibition of HIV-1 by modification of a host membrane protease. *Intl Immunol* 1995; 7:239–49.

13 Deng H, et al: Identification of a major co-receptor for primary isolates of HIV-1. *Nature* 1996; 381:661–66.

14 Cocchi F, et al: Identification of RANTES, MIP-1 alpha, and MIP-1 beta as the major HIV-suppressive factors produced by CD8+ T cells. *Science* 1995; 270:1811–15.

15 Saag M, et al: A short-term clinical evaluation of L-697,661, a non-nucleoside inhibitor of HIV-1 reverse transcriptase. *N Engl J Med* 1993; 329:1065–72.

16 Montaner JSG: A randomized, double-blind trial comparing combinations of nevirapine, didanosine and zidovudine for HIV-infected patients: The INCAS trial. *JAMA* 1998; 279:930–37.

17 Dykstra C, et al: Identification of a new class of anti-HIV agents that inhibit integrase. *J Cell Biochem Suppl* 1994; 18B:161.

18 Haubrich RH, et al, for the AIDS Clinical Trials Group 213 Team: A randomized trial of the activity and safety of Ro 24–7429 (Tat antagonist) versus nucleoside for human immunodeficiency virus infection. *J Infect Dis* 1995; 172:1246–52.

19 Rice WG, et al: Inhibitors of HIV nucleocapsid protein zinc fingers as candidates for the treatment of AIDS. *Science* 1995; 270:1194–97.

20 Tierney M, et al, for the AIDS Clinical Trials Group (ACTG) of the National Institute of Allergy and Infectious Diseases: The tolerability and pharmacokinetics of N-butyl-deoxynojirimycin in patients with advanced HIV disease (ACTG 100). *J Acquir Immune Defic Syndr* 1995; 10:549–53.

21 Munoz A, et al: Long-term survivors with HIV-1 infection: Incubation period and longitudinal patterns of CD4+ lymphocytes. *J Acquir Immune Defic Syndr* 1995; 8:496–505.

22 Kinloch-De Loes S, et al: A controlled trial of zidovudine in primary human immunodeficiency virus infection. *N Engl J Med* 1995; 333: 408–13.

23 Moore JP, et al: Development of the anti-gp120 antibody response during seroconversion to human immunodeficiency virus type 1. *J Virol* 1994; 68:5142–55.

24 Koup RA, et al: Temporal association of cellular immune responses with the initial control of viremia in primary human immunodeficiency virus type 1 syndrome. *J Virol* 1994; 68:4650–55.

25 Daar ES, et al: Transient high levels of viremia in patients with primary human immunodeficiency virus type 1 infection. *N Engl J Med* 1991; 324:961–64.

26 Munoz A, et al, for the Multicenter AIDS Cohort Study Group: Acquired immunodeficiency syndrome (AIDS)–free time after human immunodeficiency virus type 1 (HIV-1) seroconversion in homosexual men. *Am J Epidemiol* 1989; 130:530–39.

27 Piatak MJ, et al: High levels of HIV-1 in plasma during all stages of infection determined by competitive PCR. *Science* 1993; 259:1749–54.

28 Pantaleo G, et al: HIV infection is active and progressive in lymphoid tissue during the clinically latent stage of disease. *Nature* 1993; 362: 355–58.

29 Embertson J, et al: Massive covert infection of helper T lymphocytes and macrophages by HIV during the incubation period of AIDS. *Nature* 1993; 362:359–62.

30 Pantaleo G, et al: New concepts in the immunopathogenesis of human immunodeficiency virus infection. *N Engl J Med* 1993; 328: 327–35.

31 Wei X, et al: Viral dynamics in human immunodeficiency virus type 1 infection. *Nature* 1995; 373:117–22.

32 Ho DD, et al: Rapid turnover of plasma virions and CD4 lymphocytes in HIV-1 infection. *Nature* 1995; 373:123–26.

33 Perelson A, et al: HIV-1 dynamic in vivo: Virion clearance rate, infected cell life-span and viral generation time. *Science* 1996; 271: 1582–86.

34 Mansky LM, et al: Lower in vivo mutation rate of human immunodeficiency virus type 1 than that predicted from the fidelity of purified reverse transcriptase. *J Virol* 1995; 69:5087–94.

35 Coffin JM, et al: HIV population dynamics in vivo: Implications for genetic variation, pathogenesis, and therapy. *Science* 1995; 267:483–89.

36 Ho DD, et al: Time to hit HIV, early and hard. [Editorial; comment.] *N Engl J Med* 1995; 333:450–51.

37 Cao Y, et al: Virologic and immunologic characterization of long-term survivors of human immunodeficiency virus type 1 infection. *N Engl J Med* 1995; 332:201–208.

38 Dean M, et al: Genetic restriction of HIV-1 infection and progression to AIDS by a deletion allele of the CKR5 structural gene. *Science* 1996; 273:1856–62.

39 Phair J, et al, for the Multicenter AIDS Cohort Study Group: The risk of *Pneumocystis carinii* pneumonia among men infected with human immunodeficiency virus type 1. *N Engl J Med* 1990; 322:161–65.

40 Nightingale SD, et al: Incidence of Mycobacterium avium-intracellulare complex bacteremia in human immunodeficiency virus-positive patients. *J Infect Dis* 1992; 165:1082–85.

41 Graham NM, et al: Prognostic value of combined response markers among human immunodeficiency virus-infected persons: Possible aid in the decision to change zidovudine monotherapy. *Clin Infect Dis* 1995; 20:352–62.

42 Graham NM, et al: CD4+ lymphocyte response to zidovudine as a predictor of AIDS-free time and survival time. *J Acquir Immune Defic Syndr* 1993; 6:1258–66.

43 Choi S, et al: CD4+ lymphocytes are an incomplete surrogate marker for clinical progression in persons with asymptomatic HIV infection taking zidovudine. *Ann Intern Med* 1993; 118:674–80.

44 O'Brien W, et al: Changes in plasma HIV-1 RNA and CD4+ lymphocyte counts and the risk of progression to AIDS. *N Engl J Med* 1996; 334:426–31.

45 Katzenstein D, et al: The relation of virologic and immunologic markers to clinical outcomes after nucleoside therapy in HIV-infected adults with 200 to 500 CD4 cells per cubic millimeter. *N Engl J Med* 1996; 335:1091–98.

46 van Gemen B, et al: A one-tube quantitative HIV-1 RNA NASBA nucleic acid amplification assay using electrochemiluminescent (ECL) labelled probes. *J Virol Methods* 1994; 49:157–67.

46a Mulder J, et al: Rapid and simple PCR assay for quantitation of human immunodeficiency virus type 1 RNA in plasma: application to acute retroviral infection. *J Clin Microbiol* 1994; 32:292–300.

46b Pachl C, et al: Rapid and precise quantification of HIV-1 RNA in plasma using a branched DNA signal amplification assay. *J Acquir Immune Defic Syndr* 1995; 8:446–54.

47 Pantaleo G, et al: Studies in subjects with long-term nonprogressive human immunodeficiency virus infection. *N Engl J Med* 1995; 332: 209–16.

48 Henrard DR, et al: Natural history of HIV-1 cell-free viremia. *JAMA* 1995; 274:554–58.

49 Mellors JW, et al: Quantitation of HIV-1 RNA in plasma predicts outcome after seroconversion. *Ann Intern Med* 1995; 122:573–79.

50 Mellors J, et al: Prognosis in HIV-1 infection predicted by the quantity of virus in plasma. *Science* 1996; 272:1167–70.

50a Mellors JW, et al: Plasma viral load and CD4+ lymphocytes as prognostic markers of HIV-1 infection. *Ann Intern Med* 1997; 126: 946–54.

51 O'Brien TR, et al: Serum HIV-1 RNA levels and time to development of AIDS in the Multicenter Hemophilia Cohort Study. *JAMA* 1996; 276:105–10.

52 Coombs R, et al: Association of plasma human immunodeficiency virus type 1 RNA level with risk of clinical progression in patients with advanced infection. *J Infect Dis* 1996; 174:704–12.

53 Welles SL, et al: Prognostic value of plasma human immunodeficiency virus type 1 (HIV-1) RNA levels in patients with advanced HIV-1 disease and with little or no prior zidovudine therapy. *J Infect Dis* 1996; 174:696–703.

54 Wathen L, et al: Viral burden at baseline or its reduction following antiretroviral therapy is highly correlated with reduced HIV-1 disease progression. Paper presented at the 3rd Conference on Retroviruses and Opportunistic Infections, Washington, DC, January 28–February 1, 1996.

55 Havlir DV, et al: Viral dynamics of HIV: Implications for drug development and therapeutic strategies. [Review.] *Ann Intern Med* 1996; 124:984–94.

56 Yarchoan R, et al: Clinical pharmacology of 3′-Azido-2′,3′-dideoxythymidine(zidovudine) and related dideoxynucleosides. *N Engl J Med* 1989; 321:726–38.

57 Stretcher BN, et al: Pharmacokinetics of zidovudine phosphorylation in peripheral blood mononuclear cells from patients infected with human immunodeficiency virus. *Antimicrob Agents Chemother* 1994; 38:1541–47.

58 Stretcher BN, et al: Correlates of zidovudine phosphorylation with markers of HIV disease progression and drug toxicity. *AIDS* 1994; 8:763–69.

59 Klecker R Jr, et al: Plasma and cerebrospinal fluid pharmacokinetics of 3′-azido-3′-deoxythymidine: A novel pyrimidine analog with potential application for the treatment of patients with AIDS and related diseases. *Clin Pharmacol Ther* 1987; 41:407–12.

60 Collier AC, et al: A pilot study of low-dose zidovudine in human immunodeficiency virus infection. *N Engl J Med* 1990; 323:1015–21.

61 McDermott J, et al: Pharmacokinetics of zidovudine plus probenecid. [Letter.] *J Infect Dis* 1992; 166:687–88.

62 Rajaonarison JF, et al: 3′-azido-3′-deoxythymidine drug interactions. Screening for inhibitors in human liver microsomes. *Drug Metab Dispos* 1992; 20:578–84.

63 Richman DD, et al: The toxicity of AZT in the treatment of patients with AIDS and AIDS-related complex: A double-blind, placebo-controlled trial. *N Engl J Med* 1987; 317:192–97.

64 Fischl MA, et al: Prolonged zidovudine therapy in patients with AIDS and advanced AIDS-related complex. *JAMA* 1989; 262: 2405–10.

65 Fischl MA, et al: A randomized controlled trial of a reduced daily dose of zidovudine in patients with the acquired immunodeficiency syndrome. *N Engl J Med* 1990; 323:1009–14.

66 Fischl MA, et al: The safety and efficacy of zidovudine (AZT) in the treatment of subjects with mildly symptomatic human immunodeficiency virus type I (HIV) infection: A double-blind, placebo-controlled trial. *Ann Intern Med* 1990; 112:727–37.

67 Hamilton JD, et al: A controlled trial of early versus late treatment with zidovudine in symptomatic human immunodeficiency virus infection. Results of the Veterans Affairs Cooperative Study. *N Engl J Med* 1992; 326:437–43.

68 Volberding PA, et al: Zidovudine in asymptomatic human immunodeficiency virus infection: A controlled trial in persons with fewer than 500 CD4-positive cells per cubic millimeter. *N Engl J Med* 1990; 322:941–49.

69 Volberding PA, et al: The duration of zidovudine benefit in persons with asymptomatic HIV infection. Prolonged evaluation of protocol 019 of the AIDS Clinical Trials Group. *JAMA* 1994; 272:437–42.

70 Volberding PA, et al, for the AIDS Clinical Trials Group: A comparison of immediate with deferred zidovudine therapy for asymptomatic HIV-infected adults with CD4 cell counts of 500 or more per cubic millimeter. *N Engl J Med* 1995; 333:401–407.

71 Richman D, et al: Effect of stage of disease and drug dose on zidovudine susceptibilities of isolates of human immunodeficiency virus. *J Acquir Immune Defic Syndrome* 1990; 3:743–46.

72 D'Aquila RT, et al, for the AIDS Clinical Trials Group Protocol 116B/117 Team and the Virology Committee Resistance Working Group: Zidovudine resistance and HIV-1 disease progression during antiretroviral therapy. *Ann Intern Med* 1995; 122:401–408.

73 Kellam P, et al: Fifth mutation in human immunodeficiency virus type 1 reverse transcriptase contributes to the development of high-level resistance to zidovudine. *Proc Natl Acad Sci USA* 1992; 89:1934–38.

74 Larder BA, et al: HIV with reduced sensitivity to zidovudine (AZT) isolated during prolonged therapy. *Science* 1989; 243:1731–34.

75 Larder BA, et al: Multiple mutations in the HIV-1 reverse transcriptase confer high-level resistance to zidovudine (AZT). *Science* 1989; 246:1155–58.

76 Boucher CA, et al: Ordered appearance of zidovudine resistance mutations during treatment of 18 human immunodeficiency virus-positive subjects. *J Infect Dis* 1992; 165:105–10.

77 de Jong M, et al: Host-parasite dynamics and outgrowth of virus containing a single K70R amino acid change in reverse transcriptase are responsible for the loss of human immunodeficiency virus type 1 RNA load suppression by zidovudine. *Proc Natl Acad Sci USA* 1996; 93:5501–6.

78 Erice A, et al: Brief report: Primary infection with zidovudine-resistant human immunodeficiency virus type 1. *N Engl J Med* 1993; 328: 1163–65.

79 Knupp CA, et al: Effect of time of food administration on the bioavailability of didanosine from a chewable tablet formulation. *J Clin Pharmacol* 1993; 33:568–73.

80 Drusano GL, et al: Impact of bioavailability on determination of the maximal tolerated dose of 2′,3′-dideoxyinosine in phase I trials. *Antimicrob Agents Chemother* 1992; 36:1280–83.

81 Morse GD, et al: Comparative pharmacokinetics of antiviral nucleoside analogues. [Review.] *Clin Pharmacokinet* 1993; 24:101–23.

82 Hartman NR, et al: Pharmacokinetics of 2′,3′-dideoxyadenosine and 2′,3′-dideoxyinosine in patients with severe human immunodeficiency virus infection. *Clinical Pharmacol Ther* 1990; 47:647–54.

83 Lambert JS, et al: 2′3′-dideoxyinosine (ddI) in patients with the acquired immunodeficiency syndrome or AIDS-related complex: A phase I trial. *N Engl J Med* 1990; 322:1333–40.

84 Cooley TP, et al: Once-daily administration of 2′,3′,-dideoxyinosine (ddI) in patients with the acquired immunodeficiency syndrome or AIDS-related complex. *N Engl J Med* 1990; 332:1340–45.

85 Dolin R, et al, for the AIDS Clinical Trials Group: Zidovudine compared with didanosine in patients with advanced HIV type 1 infection and little or no previous experience with zidovudine. *Arch Intern Med* 1995; 155:961–74.

86 Abrams DI, et al, for the Terry Beirn Community Programs for Clinical Research on AIDS: A comparative trial of didanosine or zalcitabine after treatment with zidovudine in patients with human immunodeficiency virus infection. *N Engl J Med* 1994; 330: 657–62.

87 St. Clair et al: Resistance to ddI and sensitivity to AZT induced by a mutation in HIV-1 reverse transcriptase. *Science* 1991; 253:1557–59.

88 Eron JJ, et al: pol mutations conferring zidovudine and didanosine resistance with different effects in vitro yield multiply resistant human immunodeficiency virus type 1 isolates in vivo. *Antimicrob Agents Chemother* 1993; 37:1480–87.

89 Shafer RW, et al, for the AIDS Clinical Trials Group 143 Virology Team: Drug resistance and heterogeneous long-term virologic responses of human immunodeficiency virus type 1-infected subjects to zidovudine and didanosine combination therapy. *J Infect Dis* 1995; 172:70–78.

90 Shirasaka T, et al: Emergence of human immunodeficiency virus type 1 variants with resistance to multiple dideoxynucleosides in patients receiving therapy with dideoxynucleosides. *Proc Natl Acad Sci USA* 1995; 92:2398–402.

91 Klecker R Jr, et al: Pharmacokinetics of 2′,3′-dideoxycytidine in patients with AIDS and related disorders. *J Clin Pharmacol* 1988; 28: 837–42.

92 Starnes MC, et al: Cellular metabolism of 2′,3′-dideoxycytidine, a compound active against human immunodeficiency virus in vitro. *J Biol Chem* 1987; 262:988–91.

93 Zhang D, et al: Resistance to 2′,3′-dideoxycytidine conferred by a mutation in codon 65 of the human immunodeficiency virus type 1 reverse transcriptase. *Antimicrob Agents Chemother* 1994; 38:282–87.

94 Fitzgibbon JE, et al: Human immunodeficiency virus type 1 pol gene mutations which cause decreased susceptibility to 2′,3′-dideoxycytidine. *Antimicrob Agents Chemother* 1992; 36:153–57.

95 Kline MW, et al: A phase I/II evaluation of stavudine (d4T) in children with human immunodeficiency virus infection. *Pediatrics* 1995; 96: 247–52.

96 Kaul S, et al: Dose proportionality of stavudine in HIV seropositive asymptomatic subjects: Application to bioequivalence assessment of various capsule formulations. *Biopharm Drug Dispos* 1995; 16:125–36.

97 Zhu Z, et al: Cellular pharmacology of 2′,3′-didehydro-2′,3′-dideoxythymidine (D4T) in human peripheral blood mononuclear cells. *Biochem Pharmacol* 1990; 39:R15–19.

98 Dudley MN, et al: Clinical pharmacokinetics of nucleoside antiretroviral agents. [Review.] *J Infect Dis* 1995; 171:S99–112.

99 Katlama C, et al: Stavudine (d4T) in HIV infected patients with CD4 > 350/mm³: Results of a double-blind randomized placebo controlled study. Paper presented at the 3rd Conference on Retroviruses and Opportunistic Infections, Washington DC, January 28–February 1, 1996.

100 Lin PF, et al: Genotypic and phenotypic analysis of human immunodeficiency virus type 1 isolates from patients on prolonged stavudine therapy. *J Infect Dis* 1994; 170:1157–64.

101 Dienstag JL, et al: A preliminary trial of lamivudine for chronic hepatitis B infection. *N Engl J Med* 1995; 333:1657–61.

102 van Leeuwen R, et al: The safety and pharmacokinetics of a reverse transcriptase inhibitor, 3TC, in patients with HIV infection: A phase I study. *AIDS* 1992; 6:1471–75.

103 Eron J, et al: Treatment with lamivudine, zidovudine or both in HIV-positive patients with 200–500 CD4+ cells per cubic millimeter. *N Engl J Med* 1995; 333:1662–69.

104 Schuurman R, et al: Rapid changes in human immunodeficiency virus type 1 RNA load and appearance of drug-resistant virus populations in persons treated with lamivudine (3TC). *J Infect Dis* 1995; 171: 1411–19.

105 van Leeuwen R, et al: Evaluation of safety and efficacy of 3TC (lamivudine) in patients with asymptomatic or mildly symptomatic human immunodeficiency virus infection: A phase I/II study. *J Infect Dis* 1995; 171:1166–71.

106 Pluda JM, et al: A phase I/II study of 2′-deoxy-3′-thiacytidine (lamivudine) in patients with advanced human immunodeficiency virus infection. *J Infect Dis* 1995; 171:1438–47.

107 Wainberg MA, et al: Development of HIV-1 resistance to (-)2′-deoxy-3′-thiacytidine in patients with AIDS or advanced AIDS-related complex. *AIDS* 1995; 9:351–57.

108 Tisdale M, et al: Rapid in vitro selection of human immunodeficiency virus type 1 resistant to 3′-thiacytidine inhibitors due to a mutation in the YMDD region of reverse transcriptase. *Proc Natl Acad Sci USA* 1993; 90:5653–56.

109 Schinazi RF, et al: Characterization of human immunodeficiency viruses resistant to oxathiolane-cytosine nucleosides. *Antimicrob Agents Chemother* 1993; 37:875–81.

110 Boucher CA, et al: High-level resistance to (-) enantiomeric 2′-deoxy-3′-thiacytidine in vitro is due to one amino acid substitution in the catalytic site of human immunodeficiency virus type 1 reverse transcriptase. *Antimicrob Agents Chemother* 1993; 2231–34.

111 Larder BA, et al: Potential mechanism for sustained antiretroviral efficacy of AZT-3TC combination therapy. *Science* 1995; 269:696–99.

112 Gao Q, et al: The same mutation that encodes low-level human immunodeficiency virus type 1 resistance to 2′,3′-dideoxyinosine and 2′,3′-dideoxycytidine confers high-level resistance to the (-) enantiomer of 2′,3′-dideoxy-3′-thiacytidine. *Antimicrob Agents Chemother* 1993; 37:1390–92.

113 Parker WB, et al. Metabolism of carbovir, a potent inhibitor of human immunodeficiency virus type 1, and its effects on cellular metabolism. *Antimicrob Agents Chemother* 1993; 37:1004–1009.

114 Saag M, et al: A Phase I/II study of a novel nucleoside reverse transcriptase inhibitor, 1592U89 monotherapy vs. 1592U89 + Zidovudine or placebo in HIV infected patients with CD4 counts 200–500/mm³. Paper presented at 3rd Conference on Retroviruses and Opportunistic Infections, Washington, DC, January 28–February 1, 1996.

115 Sonnerborg A, et al: The safety and antiviral effect of 1592U89 alone and in combination with zidovudine in HIV-1 infected patients with CD4 counts 200–500 cell/mm³. *AIDS* 1996; 10:S12.

116 Tsai CC, et al: Prevention of SIV infection in macaques by (R)-9-(2-phosphonylmethoxypropyl)adenine. *Science* 1995; 270:1197–99.

117 Cohen KA, et al: Characterization of the binding site for nevirapine (BI-RG-587), a nonnucleoside inhibitor of human immunodeficiency virus type-1 reverse transcriptase. *J Biol Chem* 1991; 266:14670–74.

118 Grob PM, et al: Nonnucleoside inhibitors of HIV-1 reverse transcriptase: nevirapine as a prototype drug. *AIDS Res Hum Retroviruses* 1992; 8:145–52.

119 Mellors JW, et al: A single conservative amino acid substitution in the reverse transcriptase of human immunodeficiency virus-1 confers resistance to (+)-(5S)-4,5,6,7-tetrahydro-5-methyl-6-(3-methyl-2-butenyl)imidazo[4,5,1-jk][1,4]benzodiazepin-2(1H)-thione (TIBO R82150). *Mol Pharmacol* 1993; 43:11–16.

120 Richman DD, et al: Nevirapine resistance mutations of human immunodeficiency virus type 1 selected during therapy. *J Virol* 1994; 68:1660–6.

121 Richman D, et al: Resistance of clinical isolates of human immunodeficiency virus to antiretroviral agents. *Antimicrob Agents Chemother* 1993; 37:1207–13.

122 Havlir D, et al, for the AIDS Clinical Trials Group Protocol 208: A pilot study to evaluate the development of resistance to nevirapine in asymptomatic human immunodeficiency virus–infected patients with CD4 cell counts of >500/mm³. *J Infect Dis* 1995; 172:1379–83.

123 Pagano PJ, et al: In vitro inhibition of human immunodeficiency virus type 1 by a combination of delavirdine (U-90152) with protease inhibitor U-75875 or interferon-alpha. *J Infect Dis* 1995; 171:61–67.

124 Larder BA, et al: 3′-Azido-3′-deoxythymidine resistance suppressed by a mutation conferring human immunodeficiency virus type 1 resistance to nonnucleoside reverse transcriptase inhibitors. *Antimicrob Agents Chemother* 1992; 36:2664–69.

125 Cheeseman SH, et al: Pharmacokinetics of nevirapine: initial single-rising-dose study in humans. *Antimicrob Agents Chemother* 1993; 37:178–82.

126 D'Aquila RT, et al: Nevirapine, zidovudine, and didanosine compared with zidovudine and didanosine in patients with HIV-1 infection: A randomized, double-blind, placebo-controlled trial. National Institute of Allergy and Infectious Diseases AIDS Clinical Trials Group Protocol 241 Investigators. *Ann Intern Med* 1996; 124:1019–30.

127 Havlir D, et al: High-dose nevirapine: Safety, pharmacokinetics, and antiviral effect in patients with human immunodeficiency virus infection. *J Infect Dis* 1995; 171:537–45.

128 Dueweke TJ, et al: U-90152, a potent inhibitor of human immunodeficiency virus type 1 replication. *Antimicrob Agents Chemother* 1993; 37:1127–31.

129 Dueweke T, et al: A mutation in reverse transcriptase of bis(heteroaryl)piperazine-resistant human immunodeficiency virus type 1 that confers increased sensitivity to other nonnucleoside inhibitors. *Proc Natl Acad Sci USA* 1993; 90:4713–17.

130 Para M, et al: Randomized phase I/II concentration-controlled trial of the anti-HIV activity of delavirdine. Paper presented at the 3rd Conference on Retroviruses and Opportunistic Infections, Washington, DC, January 28–February 1, 1996.

131 Staszewski S, et al: Evaluation of the efficacy and tolerance of R 018893, R 089439 (loviride) and placebo in asymptomatic HIV-1 infected patients. *Antiviral Ther* 1996; 1:42–50.

132 CAESAR Coordinating Committee: Randomised trial of addition of lamivudine or lamivudine plus loviride to zidovudine-containing regimens for patients with HIV-1 infection: the CAESAR trial. *Lancet* 1997; 349:1413–21.

133 Kohl NE, et al: Active human immunodeficiency virus protease is required for viral infectivity. *Proc Natl Acad Sci USA* 1998; 85:4686–90.

134 Kozal MJ, et al: Extensive polymorphisms observed in HIV-1 clade B protease gene using high-density oligonucleotide arrays. *Nat Med* 1996; 2:753–59.

135 Lech WJ, et al: In vivo sequence diversity of the protease of human immunodeficiency virus type 1: Presence of protease inhibitor-resistant variants in untreated subjects. *J Virol* 1996; 70:2038–43.

136 Kitchen VS, et al: Safety and activity of saquinavir in HIV infection. *Lancet* 1995; 345:952–55.

137 Salgo M, et al: Saquinavir vs. Hivid vs. combination as treatment for advanced HIV infection in patients discontinuing/unable to take retrovir. Paper presented at the XI International Conference on AIDS, Vancouver, Canada, July 7–12, 1996.

138 Schapiro JM, et al: The effect of high-dose saquinavir on viral load and CD4+ T-cell counts in HIV-infected patients [see comments]. *Ann Intern Med* 1996; 124:1039–50.

139 Vacca JP, et al: L-735,524: An orally bioavailable human immunodeficiency virus type 1 protease inhibitor. *Proc Natl Acad Sci USA* 1994; 91:4096–4100.

140 Stein DS, et al: A 24-week open-label phase I/II evaluation of the HIV protease inhibitor MK-639 (indinavir). AIDS 1996; 10:485–92.

141 Emini E: Infectious Disease Society of America: Protease Inhibitors. Paper presented at the 3rd Conference on Retroviruses and Opportunistic Infections, Washington DC, January 28–February 1, 1996.

142 Mellors J, et al: A randomized double blind study of the oral HIV protease inhibitor, L-735,524 vs. Zidovudine (ZDV) in p24 antigenemic, HIV-1 infected patients with less than 500 CD4 cells/mm³. Paper presented at the National Conference on Human Retroviruses and Related Infections. Washington, D.C., January 29–February 2, 1995.

143 Condra JH, et al: In vivo emergence of HIV-1 variants resistant to multiple protease inhibitors. *Nature* 1995; 374:569–71.

144 Kageyama S, et al: In vitro inhibition of human immunodeficiency virus (HIV) type 1 replication by C2 symmetry-based HIV protease inhibitors as single agents or in combinations. *Antimicrob Agents Chemother* 1992; 36:926–33.

145 Kempf DJ, et al: Antiviral and pharmacokinetic properties of C2 symmetric inhibitors of the human immunodeficiency virus type 1 protease. *Antimicrob Agents Chemother* 1991; 35:2209–14.

146 Kempf DJ, et al: ABT-538 is a potent inhibitor of human immunodeficiency virus protease and has high oral bioavailability in humans. *Proc Natl Acad Sci USA* 1995; 92:2484–88.

147 Danner SA, et al, for the European-Australian Collaborative Ritonavir Study Group: A short-term study of the safety, pharmacokinetics, and efficacy of ritonavir, an inhibitor of HIV-1 protease. *N Engl J Med* 1995; 333:1528–33.

148 Markowitz M, et al: A preliminary study of ritonavir, an inhibitor of HIV-1 protease, to treat HIV-1 infection. *N Engl J Med* 1995; 333: 1534–39.

149 Markowitz M, et al: Selection and analysis of human immunodeficiency virus type 1 variants with increased resistance to ABT-538, a novel protease inhibitor. *J Virol* 1995; 69:701–706.

150 Molla A, et al: Ordered accumulation of mutations in HIV protease confers resistance to ritonavir. *Nat Med* 1996; 2:760–66.

151 Patick A, et al: Antiviral and resistance studies of AG1343, an orally bioavailable inhibitor of human immunodeficiency virus protease. *Antimicrob Agents Chemother* 1996; 40:292–97.

152 Shetty BV, et al: Preclinical pharmacokinetics and distribution to tissue of AG 1343, an inhibitor of human immunodeficiency virus type 1 protease. *Antimicrob Agents Chemother* 1996; 40:110–14.

153 Markowitz M, et al: A preliminary evaluation of nelfinavir mesylate, an inhibitor of Human Immunodeficiency Virus (HIV)-1 protease, to treat HIV infection. *J Infect Dis* 1998; 177:1533–40.

154 Patrick A, et al: HIV-1 variants isolated from patients treated with the protease inhibitor, nelfinavir, are not cross-resistant to other protease inhibitors. *AIDS* 1996; 10:S18.

155 Kim E, et al: Crystal structure of HIV-1 protease in complex with VX-478, a potent and orally bioavailable inhibitor of the enzyme. *J Am Chem Soc* 1995; 117:1181–82.

156 Partaledis JA, et al: In vitro selection and characterization of human immunodeficiency virus type 1 (HIV-1) isolates with reduced sensitivity to hydroxyethylamino sulfonamide inhibitors of HIV-1 aspartyl protease. *J Virol* 1995; 69:5228–35.

157 Tisdale M, et al: Cross-resistance analysis of human immunodeficiency virus type 1 variants individually selected for resistance to five different protease inhibitors. *Antimicrob Agents Chemother* 1995; 39:1704–10.

158 Turner S, et al: Resistance of primary isolates of human immunodeficiency virus type 1 to neutralization by soluble CD4 is not due to lower affinity with the viral envelope glycoprotein gp120. *Proc Natl Acad Sci USA* 1992; 89:1335–39.

159 Flexner C, et al: Pharmacokinetics, toxicity, and activity of intravenous dextran sulfate in human immunodeficiency virus infection. *Antimicrob Agents Chemother* 1991; 35:2544–50.

160 Rusconi S, et al: Naphthalene sulfonate polymers with CD4-blocking and anti-human immunodeficiency virus type 1 activities. *Antimicrob Agents Chemother* 1996; 40:234–36.

160a Simmons G, et al: Potent inhibition of HIV-1 infectivity in macrophages and lymphocytes by a novel CCR5 antagonist. *Science* 1997; 276:276–9.

161 Najera I, et al: Natural occurrence of drug resistance mutations in the reverse transcriptase of human immunodeficiency virus type 1 isolates. *AIDS Res Hum Retroviruses* 1994; 10:1479–88.

162 Caliendo AM, et al: Combination therapy for infection due to human immunodeficiency virus type 1. *Clin Infect Dis* 1994; 18: 516–24.

162a Connors M, et al: HIV infection induces changes in CD4+ T cell phenotype and depletions within the CD4+ T cell repertoire that are not immediately restored by antiviral or immune-based therapies. *Nat Med* 1997; 3:533–40.

163 Delta Coordinating Committee: Delta: A randomized double-blind controlled trial comparing combinations of zidovudine plus didanosine or zalcitabine with zidovudine alone in HIV-infected individuals. *Lancet* 1996; 348:283–91.

164 Saravolatz L, et al: Zidovudine alone or in combination with didanosine or zalcitabine in HIV-infected patients with the acquired immunodeficiency syndrome or fewer than 200 CD4 cells per cubic millimeter. *N Engl J Med* 1996; 335:1099–1106.

165 Katlama C, et al: Safety and efficacy of lamivudine-zidovudine combination therapy in antiretroviral-naive patients: A randomized controlled comparison with zidovudine monotherapy. *JAMA* 1996; 276: 118–25.

166 Staszewski et al: Safety and efficacy of lamivudine-zidovudine combination therapy in zidovudine-experienced patients: A randomized controlled comparison with zidovudine monotherapy. *JAMA* 1996; 276:111–17.

167 Bartlett J, et al: Lamivudine plus zidovudine compared with zalcitabine plus zidovudine in patients with HIV infection. *Ann Intern Med* 1996; 125:161–72.

168 Staszewski S, et al: Reductions in HIV-1 disease progression AZT/3TC relative to control treatments: A meta-analysis. *AIDS* 1996; 10: S16.

169 Kuritzkes DR, et al: Drug resistance and virologic response in NUCA 3001, a randomized trial of lamivudine (3TC) versus zidovudine (ZDV) versus ZDV plus 3TC in previously untreated patients. AIDS 1996; 10:975–81.

170 Merrill DP, et al: Lamivudine or stavudine in two- and three-drug combinations against human immunodeficiency virus type 1 replication in vitro. *J Infect Dis* 1996; 173:355–64.

171 Pollard R, et al: Antiviral effect and safety of stavudine (d4T) and didanosine (ddI) combination therapy in HIV-infected subjects in an ongoing randomized double-blind trial. Paper presented at 3rd Conference on Retroviruses and Opportunistic Infections, Washington, DC, January 28–February 1, 1996.

172 Executive Summary ACTG 290: AIDS Clinical Trials Group, 1996.

173 Johnson VA, et al: Human immunodeficiency virus type 1 (HIV-1) inhibitory interactions between protease inhibitor Ro 31–8959 and zidovudine, 2′,3′-dideoxycytidine, or recombinant interferon-alpha A against zidovudine-sensitive or -resistant HIV-1 in vitro. *J Infect Dis* 1992; 166:1143–46.

174 Collier A, et al: Treatment of human immunodeficiency virus infection with saquinavir, zidovudine and zalcitabine. *N Engl J Med* 1996; 334:1011–17.

175 Executive Summary. NV 14256: Analysis of Clinical Endpoints: Roche, 1996.

176 Massari F, et al: A double-blind, randomized trial of Indinavir (MK-639) alone or with zidovudine vs zidovudine alone in zidovudine naive patients. Paper presented at the 35th ICAAC, San Francisco, September 17–20, 1995.

177 Hammer SM, et al: A randomized, placebo-controlled trial of indinavir in combination with two nucleoside analogs in human immunodeficiency virus infected persons with CD4 cell counts less than or equal to 200 per cubic millimeter. *N Engl J Med* 1997; 337:725–33.

178 Markowitz M, et al: Triple therapy with AZT and 3TC in combination with nelfinavir mesylate in 12 antiretroviral naive subjects chronically infected with HIV-1. Paper presented at the XI International Conference on AIDS, Vancouver, Canada, July 7–12, 1996. Vol. Suppl.

179 Markowitz M, et al: Triple therapy with AZT, 3TC and ritonavir in 12 subjects newly infected with HIV-1. Paper presented at the XI International Conference on AIDS, Vancouver, Canada, July 7–12, 1996. Vol. Suppl.

180 Merrill DP, et al: Antagonism between human immunodeficiency virus protease inhibitors indinavir and saquinavir in vitro. *J Infect Dis* 1997; 176:265–8.

181 Cameron W: Ritonavir plus saquinavir combination therapy. Paper presented at the 3rd International Congress on Drug Therapy in HIV Infection, Birmingham, UK, November 3–7, 1996.

182 Pollard R, et al: Surrogate marker response to NVP/ZDV or ZDV in a blinded clinical trial: Correlation to changes in HIV isolate phenotypic susceptibility to NVP and ZDV. Paper presented at 3rd Conference on Retroviruses and Opportunistic Infections, Washington, DC, January 28–February 1, 1996.

183 Freimuth W, et al: Delavirdine in combination with zidovudine causes sustained antiviral and immunological effects in HIV-1 infected individuals. Paper presented at the 3rd Conference on Retroviruses and Opportunistic Infections, Washington, DC, January 28–February 1, 1996.

184 Malley SD, et al: Synergistic anti-human immunodeficiency virus type 1 effect of hydroxamate compounds with 2′,3′-dideoxyinosine in infected resting human lymphocytes. *Proc Natl Acad Sci USA* 1994; 91:11017–21.

185 Lori F, et al: Hydroxyurea as an inhibitor of human immunodeficiency virus type-1 replication. *Science* 1994; 266:801–805.

186 Biron F, et al: Anti-HIV activity of the combination of didanosine and hydroxyurea in HIV-1-infected individuals. *J Acquir Immune Defic Syndr* 1995; 10:36–40.

187 Montaner JS, et al: A pilot study of hydroxyurea among patients with advanced human immunodeficiency virus (HIV) disease receiving chronic didanosine therapy: Canadian HIV trials network protocol 080. *J Infect Dis* 1997; 175:801–6.

188 Vila J, et al: 1-year follow-up of the use of hydroxycarbamide and didanosine in HIV infection. [Letter.] *Lancet* 1996; 348:203–204.

189 Hartshorn KL, et al: Synergistic inhibition of human immunodeficiency virus in vitro by azidothymidine and recombinant alpha interferon. *Antimicrob Agents Chemother* 1987; 31:168–72.

190 Johnson VA, et al: Three-drug synergistic inhibition of HIV-1 replication in vitro by zidovudine, recombinant soluble CD4, and recombinant interferon-alpha A. *J Infect Dis* 1990; 161:1059–67.

191 Johnson VA, et al: Two-drug combinations of zidovudine, didanosine, and recombinant interferon-alpha A inhibit replication of zidovudine-resistant human immunodeficiency virus type 1 synergistically in vitro. *J Infect Dis* 1991; 164:646–55.

192 Lane C, et al: Interferon-alpha in patients with asymptomatic human immunodeficiency virus infection. *Ann Intern Med* 1990; 112:805–11.

193 Mildvan D, et al: Synergy, activity and tolerability of zidovudine and interferon-alpha in patients with symptomatic HIV-1 infection: ACTG 068. *Antiviral Therapy* 1996; 1:77–87.

194 Krown S, et al: Interferon-alpha with zidovudine: Safety, tolerance, and clinical and virologic effects in patients with Kaposi sarcoma associated with the acquired immunodeficiency syndrome (AIDS). *Ann Intern Med* 1990; 112:812–21.

195 Kovacs J, et al: Combined zidovudine and interferon-alpha therapy in patients with Kaposi sarcoma and the acquired immunodeficiency syndrome (AIDS). *Ann Intern Med* 1989; 111:280–87.

196 Lane H, et al: Antiretroviral effects of interferon-alpha in AIDS-associated Kaposi's sarcoma. *Lancet* 1988; 2:1218–22.

197 Marroni M, et al: Interferon-alpha is effective in the treatment of HIV-1-related, severe, zidovudine-resistant thrombocytopenia. A prospective, placebo-controlled, double-blind trial. *Ann Intern Med* 1994; 121:423–29.

198 Cooper DA, et al, for the European-Australian Collaborative Group: The efficacy and safety of zidovudine alone or as cotherapy with

acyclovir for the treatment of patients with AIDS and AIDS-related complex: A double-blind randomized trial. *AIDS* 1993; 7:197–207.

199 Stein DS, et al: The effect of the interaction of acyclovir with zidovudine on progression to AIDS and survival. Analysis of data in the Multicenter AIDS Cohort Study. *Ann Intern Med* 1994; 121:100–108.

200 Phillips AN, et al: HIV-1 RNA levels and the development of clinical disease. North American Lamivudine HIV Working Group. *AIDS* 1996; 10:859–65.

201 Centers for Disease Control: Report of the NIH panel to define principles of therapy of HIV infection. Guidelines for the use of antiretroviral therapy in HIV-infected adults and adolescents. *MMWR* 1998; 47(No. RR-5):1–65.

202 Saag M, et al: HIV viral load markers in clinical practice. *Nature Med* 1996; 2:625–29.

203 Carpenter C, et al: Anitretroviral therapy for HIV infection in 1997: Updated Recommendations of the International AIDS Society-USA Panel. *JAMA* 1997; 277:1962–1969.

204 St Louis ME, et al: Risk for perinatal HIV-1 transmission according to maternal immunologic, virologic, and placental factors. *JAMA* 1993; 269:2853–59.

205 Lepage P, et al: Mother-to-child transmission of human immunodeficiency virus type 1 (HIV-1) and its determinants: A cohort study in Kigali, Rwanda. *Am J Epidemiol* 1993; 137:589–99.

206 Connor EM, et al, for the Pediatric AIDS Clinical Trials Group Protocol 076 Study Group: Reduction of maternal-infant transmission of human immunodeficiency virus type 1 with zidovudine treatment. *N Engl J Med* 1994; 331:1173–80.

207 European Collaborative Study: Children born to women with HIV-1 infection: natural history and risk of transmission. *Lancet* 1991; 337:253–60.

208 Centers for Disease Control and Prevention: Recommendations of the U.S. Public Health Service Task Force on the use of zidovudine to reduce perinatal transmission of human immunodeficiency virus. *MMWR* 1994; 43:1–20.

209 Mayers DL, et al: Prevalence and clinical impact of seroconversion with AZT- resistant (AZT R) HIV-1 between 1988 and 1994. *Natl Conf Hum Retroviruses Relat Infect* 1995; 125.

210 Centers for Disease Control and Prevention: Case-control study of HIV seroconversion in health-care workers after percutaneous exposure to HIV-infected blood—France, United Kingdom, and United States, January 1988–August 1994. *MMWR* 1995; 44:929–33.

211 Centers for Disease Control and Prevention: Update: Provisional Public Health Service recommendations for chemoprophylaxis after occupational exposure to HIV. *MMWR* 1996; 45:468–72.

212 Palella FJ, et al: Declining morbidity and mortality among patients with advanced human immunodeficiency virus infection. *N Engl J Med* 1998; 338:853–60.

213 Carpenter CCJ, et al: Antiretroviral therapy for HIV infection in 1998: updated recommendations of the International AIDS Society—USA panel. *JAMA* 1998; 280:87–86.

214 Centers for Disease Control and Prevention: Public Health Service task force recommendations for the use of antiretroviral drugs in pregnant women for maternal health and reducing perinatal transmission in the United States. *MMWR* 1998; 47(No. RR-2):1–30.

215 Centers for Disease Control and Prevention: Public Health Service Guidelines for management of health-care worker exposure to HIV and recommendations for post-exposure prophylaxis. *MMWR* 1998; 47(No. RR-7):1–28.

216 Hirsch MS, et al: Antiretroviral drug resistance testing in adults with HIV infection: implications for clinical management. International AIDS Society—USA panel. *JAMA* 1998; 279:1984–91.

217 Hecht FM, et al: Sexual transmission of an HIV-1 variant resistant to multiple reverse transcriptase and protease inhibitors. *N Engl J Med* 1998; 339:307–11.

Chapter 75

Management of opportunistic infections

Katherine M. Spooner
Henry Masur

The natural history of infection with the human immunodeficiency virus (HIV) is characterized by an inexorable decline in host immunity, which can be measured by a decline in CD4 cell counts. Since the acquired immune-deficiency syndrome (AIDS) epidemic was first recognized in the early 1980s, a great deal has been learned about what types of infections should be anticipated at various stages of the disease, and extensive research has led to improvements in prophylaxis, diagnosis, and treatment of such infections.

The circulating CD4 count is the best indicator of current susceptibility to opportunistic infection and to prognosis. The quantity of circulating HIV, or viral load, as measured by a nucleic acid amplification technique, is a valuable guide to the future slope of CD4 counts, i.e., whether they will be stable or decline. Because there is a characteristic relationship between the absolute CD4 count and the occurrence of opportunistic infections, this parameter is the standard reference for estimating when prophylactic regimens should be started and what opportunistic infections are likely when patients present with various clinical syndromes.[1,2] For example, *Pneumocystis carinii* pneumonia (PCP) rarely occurs when the CD4 count is above 200 cells/mm^3, *Mycobacterium avium* complex (MAC) disease rarely occurs when the CD4 cell count is above 50 cells/mm^3, and disease due to cytomegalovirus rarely occurs unless the CD4 cell count is below 50 cells/mm^3.[3]

One of the challenges in the management of HIV disease is that the epidemiology of opportunistic infections and complications from HIV is gradually changing due to the effects of antiretroviral therapy, prophylactic antimicrobial agents, and better therapy for acute complications. For example, in the beginning years of the epidemic, PCP was the most common opportunistic infection and occurred in 75 to 90 percent of HIV-infected individuals not receiving anti-*Pneumocystis* prophylaxis.[4] With widespread use of prophylaxis for PCP, the incidence has declined. In contrast, other infectious complications such as those due to cytomegalovirus and *M. avium* complex (MAC) are steadily increasing in frequency.[5,6] Furthermore, newer complications such as bartonellosis and microsporidiosis are increasingly recognized. This chapter will review the prophylaxis and management of opportunistic infections that are likely to be encountered during the care of HIV-infected individuals in North America.

PNEUMOCYSTIS CARINII

Until the late 1970s, PCP was a seldom diagnosed illness in immunocompromised hosts such as cancer patients, transplant recipients, and children with congenital immunodeficiencies. During the 1980s, diagnostic techniques were improved, and more cases were recognized, especially in patients who were receiving more potent immunosuppression. Since the AIDS epidemic began, it is estimated that 20,000 to 60,000 cases occur per year. Without prophylaxis, PCP occurs in 75 to 90 percent of patients at some time during the course of their illness. With prophylaxis, the incidence of PCP has declined, but the pulmonary disease remains a common complication. PCP is seen predominantly in those with CD4 cell counts of <200 cells/mm^3, although 5 to 15 percent of cases are seen in those with higher CD4 cell counts. In addition to data on CD4 cell counts, data from the prospective Multicenter AIDS Cohort Study (MACS) found that regardless of CD4 cell count, the presence of unexplained fevers or oropharyngeal candidiasis is independently associated with an increased risk of developing PCP.[7,8] Now that prophylaxis is recommended routinely for those patients at risk, the incidence of PCP has been declining, such that the lifetime risk of developing PCP in the MACS cohort decreased to 28 percent.[4]

DIAGNOSIS AND TREATMENT OF PCP

Disease due to *P. carinii* is almost exclusively pulmonary, although disseminated disease involving the skin, eye, ear, spleen, bone marrow, heart, lymph nodes, and thyroid can occur, especially in those receiving aerosolized pentamidine as prophylaxis.[9,10] PCP is often insidious in onset, with fatigue, weight loss, and fevers. As the disease progresses, dyspnea, substernal chest discomfort on inspiration, and a nonproductive cough characteristically occur. The chest radiograph characteristically demonstrates a diffuse bilateral interstitial pattern, although localized disease may be seen. In patients receiving aerosolized pentamidine as prophylaxis, upper lobe disease is often the initial presentation.[11,12] Diagnosis is generally established by demonstrating organisms in either induced sputum or bronchoalveolar lavage fluid. Evaluation of induced sputum can be diagnostic in up to 95 percent of cases.[13] Most laboratories rely on a Giemsa, methenamine silver, or immunoflourescent staining technique. Newer techniques such as polymerase chain reaction (PCR) are being evaluated in research settings. These techniques are quite sensitive for detecting organisms on pulmonary secretions and can detect organisms in peripheral blood as well.[14,15] The clinical utility of PCR for evaluating sputum, bronchoalveolar lavage fluid, or peripheral blood is currently being explored.

Treatment of PCP is summarized in Table 75-1. Some physicians treat PCP empirically in well-defined clinical settings.[16] When diagnostic facilities are not readily available, this may be appropriate in patients with typical presentations and mild disease. Trimethoprim-sulfamethoxazole (TMP-SMX) is the first choice for treatment for PCP and is the first choice even in patients with a history of mild toxicity or adverse reaction. Unless a severe toxicity such as Stevens-Johnson reaction, immediate hypersensitivity, or severe hematalogic compromise is seen, many experts recommend rechallenging the patient with TMP-SMX. Up to 30 to 40 percent of HIV-infected indivduals will develop an allergic reaction (fever, pruritus, and rash) or other toxicity such as nausea, anemia, or leukopenia.[17–19] Life-threatening toxicity is unusual. Mild adverse reactions do not necessitate discontinuation of therapy.

Pentamidine is equally effective as TMP-SMX but considerably less convenient because it must be given parenterally, and it is considerably more toxic. The predominant adverse effects of parenteral pentamidine are hypoglycemia, hypotension, renal impairment, and pancreatitis. Other agents effective for treating PCP include dapsone-trimethoprim, clindamycin plus primaquine, atovaquone, and trimetrexate with leucovorin.[20–22] Dapsone-trimethoprim is probably as effective as TMP-SMX but less toxic. It is only available as an oral preparation. Clindamycin plus primaquine is also quite effective, although the primaquine is only available orally. This regimen is associated with rash, hepatic dysfunction, and diarrhea. Atovaquone is a very well-tolerated oral

Table 75-1. Management of PCP in HIV-Infected Persons

Indication	Drug/dose	Alternative	Duration	Comments
Prophylaxis	TMP-SMX (double strength: 160 mg TMP, 800 mg SMX, or single strength: 80 mg TMP, 400 mg SMX) 1 PO QD	Dapsone 100 mg PO qd Aerosolized pentamidine 300 mg monthly	Lifelong	Initiate when CD4 < 200 cells/mm³, or after initial episode of PCP, or oral candidiasis, unexplained fevers, or wasting TMP-SMX 3 times weekly may be as effective for prophylaxis as daily adminsitration
Therapy: mild disease	TMP-SMX 2 DS PO tid Dapsone 100 mg PO qd with trimethoprim 20 mg/kg/day PO in 3 divided doses	Atovaquone 750 mg PO tid with food Pentamidine 4 mg/kg IV qd Primaquine 15 mg PO qd with clindamycin 600 mg IV qid	21 days	
Therapy: moderate to severe disease	TMP-SMX: 15 mg/kg TMP IV daily in 3 divided doses	Pentamidine 4 mg/kg IV qd Trimetrexate 30 mg/m² IV w/leukovorin 20 mg/m² IV quid	21 days	If arterial P_{O_2} < 70 mmHg, and oral prednisone taper: 40 mg bid × 5 days 40 mg qd × 5 days 20 mg qd × 11 days

regimen, but it is not as effective as TMP-SMX. It is appropriate for patients with mild PCP and no apparent gastrointestinal dysfunction.[23,24] Trimetrexate is available only as a parenteral agent and is very well tolerated when given with leucovorin. It is effective, although not as effective as TMP-SMX.

Moderate to severe disease, as defined by an increased room air arterial-alveolar oxygen gradient (>35 mmHg, and/or an arterial P_{O_2} of <70 mmHg), should be treated with adjunctive corticosteroids in addition to the specific anti-*Pneumocystis* regimen. The use of adjunctive corticosteroids substantially decreases morbidity and improves survival.[25]

PROPHYLAXIS FOR PCP

Primary prophylaxis for PCP is indicated once the CD4 cell count falls below 200 cells/mm³ or if the patient develops oral candidiasis or unexplained fever for more than 2 weeks. Secondary prophylaxis is indicated for all patients with a history of PCP, regardless of the CD4 cell count, since these patients have a risk of 66 percent of developing a second episode within 12 months.[26]

TMP-SMX is considered the agent of choice for both primary and secondary prophylaxis.[8,27,28] One trial assessing primary prophylaxis compared aerosolized pentamidine with daily oral TMP-SMX found that 11 percent in the pentamidine group had an episode of PCP as compared with no patients in the TMP-SMX group.[29] A study of secondary prophylaxis also compared TMP-SMX to pentamidine, with a recurrence rate of 4 percent in those given TMP-SMX and 18 percent in the pentamidine group.[30] In addition to enhanced efficacy, a further advantage of using TMP-SMX as prophylaxis is that this regimen also provides prophylaxis for toxoplasmosis and offers protection against respiratory bacterial pathogens, including *Hemophilus influenzae* and *Streptococcus pneumoniae.* Despite superior efficacy of TMP-SMX in PCP prophylaxis, a major drawback in its use is a significant rate of dose-limiting toxicities.[29–31] Bone marrow suppression is aggravated by the concomitant use of zidovudine but may be ameliorated by a dose reduction of the TMP-SMX. One double-strength tablet of TMP-SMX is probably of similar efficacy when given two or three times per week compared with daily administration. A single-strength tablet daily also is likely to give comparable efficacy compared with a double-strength tablet daily.

Monthly aerosolized pentamidine is quite effective prophylaxis, although not as effective as TMP-SMX, and is well-tolerated. Coughing or wheezing may occur in approximately one-third of the patients but can be ameliorated with beta-agonist inhalation therapy or prophylaxis and rarely requires discontinuation of the prophylaxis. It is important to screen patients for tuberculosis prior to initiation of aerosolized pentamidine, since this leads to risk of spread of tuberculosis among other patients and health care workers.[32] Dapsone is an effective alternative and has been shown to be comparable in efficacy to pentamidine.[33] Dapsone plus pyrimethamine is as effective as aerosolized pentamidine and has the advantage of anti-*Toxoplasma* acitivity as well.[34] Atovoquone is currently under investigation as a prophylactic agent. There are some data suggesting that azithromycin has some anti-*Pneumocystis* activity as well.

PROTOZOAL INFECTIONS

TOXOPLASMA GONDII

Toxoplasma gondii, an intracellular coccidian protozoan, is a zoonosis with felines as the definitive host. Infection in humans occurs after ingestion of raw or undercooked meat or ingestion of oocyst excreted by felines and usually causes asymptomatic or benign disease in immunocompetent hosts. Geographic prevalence is highly variable, with seroprevalence as high as 75 to 90 percent in western Europe, Latin America, and Africa, whereas in the United states seroprevalence is between 10 to 40 percent. Of those seropositive with concomitant HIV infection, up to 30 to 50 percent will develop disease due to *T. gondii.*[35,36] This rarely occurs until the CD4 count falls below 100 cells/mm³. In HIV-infected individuals, disease is presumed to represent the reactivation of latent infection.

The predominant clinical presentation of toxoplasmosis is encephalitis. Disease occasionally occurs in the gastrointestinal tract, skin, lung, heart, eye, liver, and pancreas.[37] Encephalitis can present with either focal or nonfocal symptoms, and the presence of constitutional symptoms such as fever and fatigue is variable. Toxoplasmosis is the most common treatable cause of multiple, ring-enhancing cerebral mass lesions, such that radiologic evaluation with computed tomography (CT) or magnetic resonance imaging (MRI) can lead to a presumptive diagnosis. In a patient with a compatible CD4 count (<100 cells/mm^3) and a presumptive radiologic diagnosis, it is appropriate to begin empirical treatment, especially if the patient is known to be seropositive for *Toxoplasma* infection. If there is not both clinical and radiologic improvement over 2 weeks, then a biopsy is indicated to establish the causative process. Other central nervous system (CNS) mass-occupying lesions in the differential diagnosis include lymphoma, tuberculoma, and cryptococcoma. The sensitivity of a IgG antibody to *Toxoplasma* is 80 to 85 percent in patients with confirmed toxoplasmosis[38]; however, almost all patients with proven cerebral toxoplasmosis are seropositive if their sera is assessed by a reference laboratory.

The preferred treatment of toxoplasmosis (Table 75-2) is the synergistic combination of pyrimethamine and sulfadiazine. Since the incidence of adverse reactions to sulfonamides in the setting of HIV infection is greater than 40 percent,[37] other regimens have been explored. A prospective study of clindamycin (initially given intravenously and then maintained with oral therapy) and pyrimethamine demonstrated comparable efficacy to standard therapy with pyrimethamine and sulfadiazine.[39] A European study comparing the two agents found similar results with acute therapy, but the pyrimethamine-clindamycin was associated with a higher rare of relapse in maintenance therapy.[40] Other agents that have shown efficacy in smaller trials include atovaquone[41] and azithromycin. These agents probably should be given in conjunction with pyrimethamine. As with many other opportunistic infections, treatment is continued lifelong.

Prophylaxis should be considered in seropositive individuals once the CD4 count falls below 100 cells/mm^3, and regimens could include TMP-SMX or dapsone-pyrimethamine.[31,42] Those who are seronegative may wish to reduce their likelihood of acquiring *T. gondii* infection by eliminating contact with cat feces and avoiding undercooked lamb and beef.

CRYPTOSPORIDIUM PARVUM

Cryptosporidium parvum is a coccidian protozoan that is present in the feces of cattle and some domestic pets and which can be present in rural or urban water supplies.[43] In immunocompetent hosts, infection generally leads to a mild, self-limited disease, in contrast to patients with AIDS, who develop a persistent chronic enteritis of variable severity. Severe disease occurs primarily in those with lower CD4 cell counts. In one study, those with counts above 180 cells/mm^3 had self-limited infections, while those with counts below 140 cells/mm^3 developed persistent diarrhea.[44,45] In addition to enteritis, biliary tract disease and even pulmonary or pleural disease can be seen in patients with AIDS. Diagnosis is based on direct microscopy of stool, small bowel biopsy, blood, or a respiratory specimen.

No drugs are clearly effective for therapy of cryptosporidiosis. The treatment of cryptosporidiosis (see Table 75-2) may require aggressive prolonged fluid support and antimotility agents in addition to anti-*Cryptosporidium* agents. Paromomycin, a nonabsorbable aminoglycoside, appears to have some activity. An open, uncontrolled study demonstrated a clinical response in 22 of 24 patients and complete remission in 18 of these.[46] A recent small, prospective, double-blinded trial also demonstrated modest success with paromomycin.[47] However, benefit due to paromomycin is usually brief. Azithromycin or atovaquone may have some efficacy. Patients with copious diarrhea often benefit from antimotility agents, intravenous hydration, or total parenteral nutrition.[48] To reduce exposure to *Cryptosporidium,* it is advisable to avoid consuming water from surface lakes and streams. Cats and dogs younger than 6 months of age and those from shelters or large breeders may shed oocysts. Whether avoiding urban water supplies in favor of boiled or bottled water is a useful preventive strategy is uncertain.

MICROSPORIDIA

Microsporidia are obligate, spore-forming intracellular protozoa. Five genera have been recognized as human pathogens (*Enterocytozoon, Septata, Nosema, Encephalitozoon,* and *Pleistophora*). *Enterocytozoon bienusi* has been most recognized as an emerging enteric pathogen in association with HIV infection.[49–52] Microsporidia are often but not invariably associated with diarrhea.[53]

Microsporidiosis can manifest as voluminous diarrhea, malabsorption, and wasting in patients with CD4 cell counts below 50 cells/mm^3. Similarly to cryptosporidia, Microsporidia can involve the biliary tract as well. Diagnosis is made by modified trichrome staining of stool or by light and electron microscopy of

Table 75-2. Management of Protozoal Infections in HIV-Infected Persons

Disease	Prophylaxis	Treatment	Maintenance	Comments
Toxoplasmosis	TMP-SMX 1 DS PO qd Dapsone 100 mg PO qd with pyrimethamine 50 mg PO weekly	Pyrimethamine 25–100 mg PO qd, *plus:* Sulfadiazine 1 g PO quid *or* Clindamycin 600 mg IV or 600 mg PO q6–8h	Pyrimethamine 50–100 mg PO qd, *plus:* Sulfadiazine 500–1000 mg PO qd, *or* Clindamycin 300 mg PO qid	Folinic acid 10 mg PO daily should be administered with pyrimethamine
Cryptosporidiosis	None effective	Paromomycin 25 mg/kg daily in 3 divided doses × 10 days has been reported to have some efficacy	Antimotility agents routinely administered for persistent diarrhea	May require parenteral nutrition if wasting occurs
Microsporidiosis	None effective	Anecdotal success with albendazole 100 mg bid	Antimotility agents routinely administered for persistent diarrhea	May require parenteral nutrition if wasting occurs
Isosporiasis	None recommended	TMP-SMX 1 DS PO quid × 10 days, then bid × 21 days Pyrimethamine 75 mg PO qd × 14 days	TMP-SMX DS PO 3 × weekly Pyrimethamine 25 mg PO qd	Folinic acid 10 mg PO daily should be administered with pyrimethamine

small bowel biopsy specimens.[50] Treatment (see Table 75-2) is often unsuccessful. Albendazole (400 mg orally twice daily) may be useful, especially for enteral *Septata* infections.[49,54]

ISOSPORA BELLI AND *CYCLOSPORA*

Isosporiasis is a disease due to the coccidian protozoa *Isospora belli,* which is commonly found in the tropical and subtropical climates. It is endemic in AIDS patients in Haiti and causes disease in the proximal small intestine leading to a severe diarrheal illness.[48,55] Diagnosis is made by identifying acid-fast oval oocysts in stool specimens. The disease is effectively treated with TMP-SMX (see Table 75-2). Pyrimethamine is also effective. In order to prevent relapse, patients require lifelong maintenance after the initial infection is controlled.[56]

Cyclospora infection in HIV-infected patients is similar to isosporiasis in that it is common in Haiti, responds to treatment with TMP-SMX, and has a high recurrence rate unless patients receive maintenance therapy. *Cyclospora* are water-borne and cause disease predominantly in the summer months.[57,58] Disease in immunocompetent hosts is self-limited, in contrast to the persistent enteritis seen in patients with HIV infection. Clinically, watery diarrhea is present with cramping, fatigue, and weight loss, and diagnosis is made by identifying acid-fast *Cryptosporidium*-like organisms in stool samples. Treatment appears to be effective with TMP-SMX.[59,60] Lifelong maintenace therapy is required to avoid relapse.

FUNGAL INFECTIONS

CANDIDA SPECIES

Candidiasis most often manifests as oral thrush, esophageal disease, or vaginitis in patients with HIV infection. While mucosal disease is common, invasive disease or hematogenous spread is unusual. Most candidiasis in patients with HIV infection has been due to *C. albicans,* although many other species have been described to cause disease. Oral candidiasis (thrush) is the most common fungal infection associated with HIV infection. In otherwise asymptomatic patients, it is predictive of clinical progression.[61] Thrush ultimately occurs in up to 90 percent of individuals infected with HIV and most often occurs when the CD4 count is below 100 cells/mm^3 but can occur at considerably higher counts. Esophagitis occurs in 10 to 20 percent of patients and may occur in the absence of obvious oral involvement. Esophagitis generally is seen when the CD4 count is less than 100 cells/mm^3.[62] HIV-infected women are susceptible to chronic or recurrent vulvovaginal candidiasis. Although other fungal infections such as those due to *Cryptococcus* and *Histoplasma* lead to fungemia, disseminated candidal infections are rarely seen even at advanced stages, unless there is a predisposing factor such as an indwelling venous catheter.

Oropharyngeal candidiasis presents with white plaques on the buccal mucosa and tongue that have a very characteristic appearance. Smears of lesions can be diagnostically useful if many yeast are seen. Esophagitis usually presents with dysphagia, odynophagia, or retrosternal discomfort. Because *Candida* is a much more likely cause of these symptoms than any other pathogen, an empirical course of antifungal therapy is usually reasonable.[63] Endoscopy for diagnosis is indicated only if there is no response to a 7- to 10-day course of empirical therapy.

Topical clotrimazole or nystatin may be effective for mild oral candidiasis (Table 75-3). Both are well tolerated and inexpensive. Many patients will have better compliance with oral fluconazole or itraconazole. Oral azole therapy is also effective for esophagitis or vaginitis. An increasing incidence of *Candida* species resistant to fluconazole and itraconazole is being recognized.[64] If patients fail to respond to oral therapy, especially those who have received recent courses of azoles or whose disease is due to *Candida* species other than *C. albicans,* a course of intravenous amphotericin may be necessary.

Prophylaxis is generally not given either to prevent initial disease or to prevent recurrences unless the recurrences are particularly frequent or severe. It is not recommended because of the cost, inconvenience, and potential drug interactions of fluconazole, as well as the potential for chronic prophylaxis to enhance the likelihood for azole-resistant strains.[64–67]

CRYPTOCOCCUS NEOFORMANS

Cryptococcosis occurs in 5 to 10 percent of patients with HIV infection in North America, where it is the most common invasive fungal disease.[68,69] Pigeons and other birds are most often considered the environmental source. Cryptococcosis rarely occurs until the CD4 cell count is below 50 cells/mm^3. Meningitis is the most common clinical manifestation, although pulmonary and cerebral disease, as well as disseminated disease, is well described. Meningitis often presents subtly with fatigue and headache. Meningismus is present in only 22 percent, and fever is present in 65 percent. Disease also may present with pulmonary or skin involvement and rarely involves the genitourinary tract or bone marrow. Diagnosis of cryptococcosis is established by the presence of the organism on stain or culture or by detection of cryptococcal antigen in the serum, cerebropinal fluid (CSF), or less often, some other tissue or fluid such as bone marrow, broncheoalveolar lavage fluid, or lymph node.[70,71]

Therapy (see Table 75-3) should be initiated with intravenous amphotericin B in preference to fluconazole. Treatment with amphotericin B requires close monitoring of its associated toxicites, such as fever, chills, nephrotoxicity, and myelosuppression, although mild toxicities can be tolerated through the course of treatment, and in general, toxicities resolve when the amphotericin is discontinued. Although traditional treatment of cryptococcosis in the non-HIV-infected population also had included flucytosine, it does not appear to offer a significant benefit in the setting of AIDS. A recent multicenter trial found similar clinical responses when comparing amphotericin 0.7 mg/kg for 14 days to amphotericin with flucytosine, although there was a trend to improved CSF sterilization with the addition of flucytosine.[72] This study also demonstrated that the higher dose of amphotericin (0.7 mg/kg) was reasonably well tolerated in this population.

The availability of oral triazole antifungal agents has led to several studies evaluating these as an alternative to amphotericin in the initial treatment of cryptococcal meningitis. The greatest experience has been with fluconazole, which has a high bioavailability, and adequate CSF levels are readily attained. Fluconazole has been found to be effective; however, it has been associated with a higher mortality in the first 2 weeks of treatment and a longer time to negative CSF cultures as compared with amphotericin.[73,74] Itraconazole is not an appropriate choice for initial management.

As with many opportunistic infections, treatment for cryptococcal disease is lifelong, since, without maintenance therapy, relapse rates as high as 60 percent can be expected.[75–77] Fluconazole has been shown to be effective and is the most commonly recommended choice for maintenance. Fewer relapses occur with fluconazole, although both agents were well tolerated.[78]

Prophylaxis of cryptococcal disease is controversial. Oral fluconazole has been shown to decrease the incidence of cryptococcal disease. However, chronic oral fluconazole has the disadvantages mentioned for candidiasis. No survival benefit has been shown, and thus many authorities do not recommend prophylaxis.[79]

HISTOPLASMA CAPSULATUM

Histoplasma capsulatum is a dimorphic fungus that grows as a mold in soil contaminated by bat or bird excreta. Primary infection occurs as microconidia are inhaled into the lungs, where they grow as the pathogenic yeast phase. Endemic areas include the Ohio and Mississippi river valleys and extend through Canada and down to South America. Cities such as Indianapolis, Kansas City, Memphis, and Houston have the highest incidence of histoplasmosis. In certain areas such as Indianapolis, as many as 25 percent of AIDS patients may develop histoplasmosis.[80] Disease may occur due to either primary infection or reactivation.[81,82] Clinical disease does not usually occur until the CD4 count is below 100 cells/mm^3, and in up to 95 percent of cases, patients present with disseminated disease.[83]

Histoplasmosis most often presents with fever, fatigue, and weight loss. Hepatosplenomegaly is usually present, and respiratory symptoms may or may not be reported. A severe syndrome resembling septicemia with hypotension and multiorgan system dysfunction is seen in 10 to 20 percent of cases; this is referred to as *progressive disseminated histoplasmosis* (PDH).[80] Other less common presentations include meningitis, encephalitis, chorioretinitis, or cutaneous ulcerations or rashes.[84,85]

Diagnosis of histoplasmosis is established either by recovery of the organism in culture or by visualization in histopathologic specimens. The detection of *H. capsulatum* polysaccharide antigen (HPA) has proved to be an excellent assay when performed in a reference laboratory, with a 95 percent sensitivity and 98 percent specificity for diagnosis of disseminated disease in patients with AIDS. Further, this has been shown to be useful in detecting relapse of histoplasmosis in AIDS patients.[80,86] This highly reliable test is not available in most laboratories.

The initial treatment of histoplasmosis (see Table 75–3) should be amphotericin B, at a dose of 0.6 to 1.0 mg/kg per day for 7 to 14 days, at which time therapy can be given every other day until a cumulative dose of 15 mg/kg is reached. This regimen has been reported to produce remission in 80 percent of patients.[87] Itraconazole has been used for induction but is not recommended by many experts, even in patients with mild disease. For maintenance, both itraconazole and fluconazole are effective.[88,89] Itraconazole (200 mg PO twice daily) prevents realpse with high efficacy and is the regimen of choice.[81,90] Fluconazole has some efficacy for maintenance.[88] Ketoconazole is generally not as effective.

COCCIDIOIDES IMMITIS

Coccidioidomycosis is endemic to the deserts of the southwestern United States, Mexico, and Central America and recently has been reported to be occurring at increasing rates in HIV- and non-HIV-

Table 75-3. Management of Fungal Disease in HIV-Infected Persons

Disease	Prophylaxis	Treatment	Maintenance	Comments
Oral and esophageal candidiasis	None recommended	Mild thrush only: Clotrimazole 10-mg troche 5× daily Systemic treatment: fluconazole 200 mg PD on day 1, then 100 mg qd × 10 days For resistant candidal disease, amphotericin B 0.25 mg/kg IV qd up to 100 to 200 mg total dose	For frequently recurrent disease, fluconazole 100 mg PO qd (may be effective less frequently)	
Cryptococcal meningitis	None recommended	Amphotericin B, 0.7 mg/kg IV qd × 2 weeks, then fluconazole 400 mg PO qd	Fluconazole 200–400 mg PO qd (preferred over itraconazole 200 mg qd) Amphotericin B 1 mg/kg IV weekly	For initial therapy, fluconazole not usually recommended Fluconazole is effective for prophylaxis but not routinely recommended Flucytosine as part of initial regimen (37.5 mg PO qid) appears to be associated with fewer relapses
Histoplasmosis	None recommended except in hyperendemic areas	Initially, amphotericin B 1 mg/kg IV qd × 2 weeks, then itraconazole 200 mg PO bid for 12 weeks acute treatment Mild disease: Itraconazole 200 mg PO tid × 3 days, then 200 mg bid for 12 weeks acute treatment		Fluconazole is also effective but less effective than itraconazole
Coccidioidomycosis	None recommended except in hyperendemic areas	Initially, amphotericin B 1 mg/kg IV qd until clinical response seen, then fluconazole 400 to 800 mg PO qd. Mild disease: Fluconazole 400 to 800 mg PO qd Itraconazole 200 mg PO qd	Fluconazole 200 to 400 mg PO qd	Itraconazole may be effective Either fluconazole or intrathecal amphotericin B must be used initially if meningismus present

infected populations in California.[91] Active disease may represent either reactivation of latent disease or recently acquired primary infection. A recent prospective study of coccidioidomycosis and HIV infection in an endemic area found that disease occurs primarily in those with a CD4 cell count below 250 cells/mm^3 and a previous diagnosis of AIDS.[92] This study also demonstrated that evidence of prior *Cocccidioides* infection (indicated by a positive skin test) was not predictive of the development of active disease.

Pulmonary disease is the most common manifestation and presents as cough, fever, night sweats, fatigue, and weight loss. Extrapulmonary disease also occurs in the meninges, skin, liver, peritoneum, and lymph nodes.[93] A reticulonodular pattern on chest radiograph should suggest the diagnosis, although definitive diagnosis is based on culture or histopathology. *C. immitis* can be cultured within 3 to 5 days from sputum, bronchoalveolar lavage fluid, or tissue. Blood cultures are rarely positive. Histopathologic examination of tissue specimens may reveal a distinctive appearance with spherules. IgG antibody is positive in the majority of cases, but it is not useful clinically because it may reflect latent, inactive infection and because 25 percent of active cases are seronegative.[94]

Treatment (see Table 75-3) of disseminated coccidioidomycosis in AIDS patients initially requires intravenous amphotericin B (0.6 to 1.0 mg/kg per day) until clinical response is seen. This usually requires a total of 1 to 2.5 g. In mild disease, oral fluconazole has been used, although this is not generally recommended, and data on this approach are limited. After acute therapy, maintenance therapy with fluconazole is preferred, although weekly amphotericin (0.5 mg/kg) can be used. Itraconazole may be an alternative for maintenance, but further data are needed to assess its efficacy relative to fluconazole.[80,95]

Prophylaxis, even in endemic areas, is generally not recommended, although it may be indicated in unusual epidemiologic circumstances.

VIRAL INFECTIONS

CYTOMEGALOVIRUS

Disease due to reactivation of latent cytomegalovirus (CMV) infection ultimately affects 40 percent of patients with AIDS.[96] Further, in autopsy series, up to 90 percent of AIDS patients have evidence of CMV infection, even if it was not apparent clinically prior to death in all cases.[97]

The majority of patients with HIV infection are seropositive for CMV, and homosexuals and intravenous drug users have very high seroprevalence rates: Up to 95 percent of homosexual men are seropositive. In patients whose only risk factor is heterosexual contact, the rate may be substantially less. Most CMV disease appears to be due to reactivation of latent disease, but primary infection or reinfection may be responsible for some cases.

Disease rarely occurs before the CD4 cell count falls below 100 cells/mm^3 and is seen most often in those with cell counts below 50 cells/mm^3. The most common manifestation is retinitis, although colitis and pneumonitis are seen frequently as well. Neurologic disease, especially polyradiculopathy, is being recognized with increased frequency. Other less common manifestations include encephalitis, hepatitis, adrenalitis, pancreatitis, and epididymitis.

Diagnosis of CMV retinitis is based on characteristic ophthalmalogic findings, while diagnosis of CMV disease elswhere, such as colitis, is based on histopathologic findings. Cultures have not proved to be useful, since many patients can have viremia or viruria without clinical disease.[98,99] Detection of CMV nucleic acid in peripheral blood has been useful in certain research laboratories for predicting the occurrence of disease in asymptomatic patients. PCR or branched DNA (BDNA) monitoring may become increasingly useful for deciding when to initiate prophylaxis, when to start therapy, or when to alter a treatment regimen, but it is not yet available or validated at most centers.[100]

CMV retinitis requires immediate treament (Table 75-4), since without appropriate care, it will progress rapidly and lead to blindness. Treatment of colitis and other manifestations of CMV disease is generally mandated when clinical manifestations are substantial, since therapy is often effective. Two agents, ganciclovir and foscarnet, have been evaluated extensively for the treatment of CMV disease.[98] Both agents are virustatic and not virucidal. Both ganciclovir and foscarnet have significant toxicities: Ganciclovir causes neutropenia, especially in patients on concomitant zidovudine, and foscarnet is nephrotoxic and neurotoxic and causes substantial derangement in electrolytes. Intravenous cidofovir (HPMPC) is approved for use in the treatment of CMV retinitis, although renal toxicity can be seen with this agent.[101] Other agents under evaluation for treatment of CMV disease include valacyclovir, a congener of acyclovir.

Both foscarnet and intravenous ganciclovir have been shown to slow the progression of CMV retinitis; however, despite acute plus maintenance treatment, retinitis eventually progresses. In one study of acute therapy followed by daily intravenous maintenance, the median time to progression after the initiation of ganciclovir was 58 days.[102] In noncomparative trials, foscarnet has been shown to have similar clinical activity. In one large multicenter trial comparing ganciclovir with foscarnet, the two drugs had equal clinical benefit in terms of time to halt progression and time to relapse. However, foscarnet also was found to produce a survival benefit, possibly due to instrinsic antiretroviral activity.[98,103]

A recent study has shown that for patients who relapse on either intravenous ganciclovir or foscarnet, switching to the other agent was no more effective than reinduction with the initial therapy. Combination therapy is more effective in controlling the retinitis in these patients; however, it has the disadvantage of combining the respective toxicities.[104–106] Resistant CMV strains have been documented,[107,108] and in this situation, switching agents may be appropirate.

Ganciclovir is also used in sustained-release intravitreal implants. These implants do not provide systemic treatment, which is important in patients with multiple end-organ involvement with CMV; however, there are minimal systemic toxicities, and the primary side effects are related to the surgical procedures. An early phase I study compared immediate treatment of peripheral retinitis using the implant with deferred treatment and found that the time to progression was 226 days for the treatment group and 15 days for the deferred group.[109] A more recent randomized study comparing the implant with intravenous ganciclovir found that the time to progression with the implant was 216 days compared with 104 days for the intravenous ganciclovir group.[110]

After induction therapy is given with either intravenous ganciclovir or foscarnet and clinical improvement is documented, maintenance treatment is necessary, since the natural course of the disease is for progression to blindness. Both intravenous ganciclovir and foscarnet are appropriate at lower doses for maintenance (see Table 75-4), and recently, oral ganciclovir has been shown to be effective.[111] Oral ganciclovir is appealing in that it is more convenient and alleviates the need for an indwelling venous catheter; however, due to the lower serum levels attained, there is concern for increased resistance.

Prophylaxis of CMV disease has been considered for susceptible patients with CD4 cell counts below 50 cells/mm^3. Oral ganciclovir has been shown to be associated with a 49 percent risk reduction for the development of CMV disease in one study.[112] However, there was no difference in vision or survival between the two groups. Moreover, in another study with a somewhat different design, oral ganciclovir showed no statistically significant benefit over placebo, although a trend favored oral ganciclovir in a few cases of retinitis. In addition to uncertainty about how effective oral ganciclovir is, consideration must be given to potential increased resistance as well as drug interactions in this advanced population. Valacyclovir also has been considered for prophylaxis.[113] It is not clear if valacyclovir (or acyclovir) provides benefit in the prevention of CMV disease.

HERPES SIMPLEX VIRUS

Infection with herpes simplex virus (HSV) types 1 and 2 is commonly associated with mucocutaneous involvement of the orolabial, genital, anorectal, and esophageal areas. Infection and reactivation disease can occur at any time during the course of HIV disease, but the most severe and chronic manifestations occur at CD4 cell counts below 100 cells/mm^3. HIV-infected individuals have a rate of seroprevalence of up to 77 percent.[114]

The diagnosis of HSV infection is often made empirically on the basis of characteristic vesicular lesions, although definitive diagnosis may be readily attained with cultures from affected areas or smears for viral inclusions.

Management of HSV disease (see Table 75-4) relies primarily on the use of acyclovir, which may be administered orally or intravenously.[115] Intravenous administration is indicated in severe disease, including patients in whom the use of oral medications is precluded by extensive oropharyngeal disease. Acyclovir is well tolerated and infrequently leads to renal impairment or CNS toxicity. Valaciclovir recently has been approved for the treatment of HSV disease and has been shown to be equally effective in initial management of HSV in an immunocompetent population. Valaciclovir is safe in immuocompetent patients and has an advantage of less frequent dosing intervals as compared with acyclovir.[116] In immunosuppressed patients, thrombotic thrombocytopenic purpura and hemolytic uremic syndrome have been reported, and the drug is labeled as contraindicated for patients with immunocompromise. Another related preparation, famciclovir, also has been shown to be effective in initial management for immunocompetent patients.[117] Although these newer agents will likely be useful in the management of HSV in HIV-infected individuals, they have not been evaluated extensively in patients with HIV infection, and acyclovir remains the most commonly recommended treatment.

The usual duration of acute treatment is 7 to 10 days, but in severe cases, acyclovir may need to be continued until clinical resolution is seen. If resolution is not seen, one also must keep in mind that acyclovir-resistant strains are encountered increasingly[118] and may require either higher doses of acyclovir or the use of foscarnet.[119] Foscarnet is given intravenously, although a topical preparation is being evaluated.[120] Cidofovir also may play a role in the treatment of resistant strains and has been used either intravenously or topically.[121] Since acyclovir resistance is usually due to altered thymidine kinase activity, ganciclovir generally is not useful in these patients.

Long-term maintenance therapy for HSV is not required, unlike most other opportunistic infections, although it should be considered in patients with frequent or severe outbreaks.[122]

VARICELLA-ZOSTER VIRUS

Varicella-zoster virus (VZV) disease in patients with HIV is almost always due to reactivation, although in the minority of individuals without childhood exposure to the disease, primary infection may occur. Reactivation disease is usually manifested by dermatomal lesions, which can occur at any stage of HIV infection, and is frequently the initial presentation of HIV. In most cases, reactivation disease is self-limiting. VZV disease rarely has been docu-

Table 75-4. Management of Viral Infections in HIV-Infected Persons

Disease	Treatment	Maintenance	Comments
CMV	Ganciclovir 5 mg/kg IV q12h × 14–21 days Foscarnet 90 mg/kg IV q12h × 14 days Ganciclovir intravitreal implant Cidofovir 5 mg/kg IV once weekly for 2 weeks	Ganciclovir 5 mg/kg IV qd or foscarnet 90 to 120 mg/kg IV qd Ganciclovir 1 gm PO tid Cidofovir 5 mg/kg IV every other week	Combination ganciclovir-foscarnet may be considered for refractory disease Cidofovir should be administered with probenicid: 2 g PO prior to each dose, 1 g PO 2 hours and 8 hours after each dose
HSV			
Mild mucocutaneous	Acyclovir 200 to 400 PO 5 × daily for 7 to 10 days Famciclovir 500–750 mg PO tid × 7 days	None	Prophylaxis for frequently recurrent VZV/HSV: consider acyclovir 200 to 400 mg PO bid to tid
Severe	Acyclovir 5 mg/kg IV q8h × 7 days	None	
VZV			
Zoster	Acyclovir 800 mg PO 5 × daily × 7 days Famciclovir 500–750 mg PO tid × 7 days Valaciclovir 1.0 gm PO tid × 7 days Sorivudine 40 mg qd × 10 days	None None	For severe or recurrent HSV or VZV disease with documented acyclovir resistance, treatment with foscarnet 60 mg IV q12h induction, then 60 mg daily maintenance
Disseminated	Acyclovir 10 mg/kg IV q8h × 7–10 days	None	

mented in patients with HIV infection to progress to dissemination of cutaneous lesions and visceral involvement. Other rarely encountered manifestations of VZV reactivation include sight-threatening acute retinal necrosis, which must be distinguished funduscopically from CMV retinitis.[123,124]

The treatment of shingles depends on the severity of the outbreak. In severe cases, such as cases where more than one dermatome or the ophthalmic division of the trigeminal nerve is involved or disseminated disease is present, the treatment should consist of intravenous acyclovir (see Table 75-4). Acyclovir should be continued for 7 to 14 days or longer if the clinical response is slow. Localized VZV disease in other locations can be treated with oral acyclovir or famciclovir. A recent study demonstrated that oral famciclovir (either 500 or 750 mg three times daily) is safe and effective in the treatment of shingles in immunocompetent hosts and decreased the duration of the disease's most common complication, postherpetic neuralgia.[125] Recently, sorivudine (BV-araU) has been approved and is more effective than acyclovir in accelerating cutaneous healing of herpes zoster in HIV-infected individuals.[126]

Acyclovir-resistant VZV disease has been documented in HIV-infected patients and has been reported to occur as disseminated disease in patients already receiving oral acyclovir.[127] Foscarnet should be used in these patients.

Maintenance regimens following acute therapy are generally not indicated. Dermatomal VZV disease may recur, but recurrences are rarely frequent enough to warrant chronic therapy.

BACTERIAL INFECTIONS

MYCOBACTERIUM AVIUM COMPLEX

Disseminated *Mycobacterium avium* complex (MAC) disease occurs in 40 percent of patients with AIDS in North America.[128] MAC is ubiquitous in the environment and has been found in water, food, and soil. Which environmental sources are most important for causing human disease is uncertain, since environmental subtypes do not always correlate with subtypes that cause disease.[129,130] Colonization occurs via the respiratory and gastrointestinal routes. Disseminated disease due to MAC is rarely seen until the CD4 cell count falls below 50 cells/mm^3.[131]

Fever, fatigue, night sweats, weight loss, and gastrointestinal symptoms are the most common clinical manifestations of disseminated MAC disease.[132] Elevated alkaline phosphatase levels and anemia are characteristically seen, but these are very nonspecific. Definitive diagnosis is based on blood cultures; bacteremia is often persistent, although colony counts can fluctuate substantially.[133] Diagnosis also can be made from cultures from normally sterile sites such as bone marrow, lymph node, or liver. Cultures of sputum or stool are diagnostically unhelpful because a positive result may indicate colonization rather than invasive disease. The positive predictive value of such cultures appears to be low.

Disseminated MAC disease requires lifelong treatment with combination regimens (Table 75-5). Single-agent therapy with clarithromycin, azithryomycin, rifabutin, rifampin, and ethambutol has been evaluated. Clarithromycin, azithromycin, rifabutin, and ethambutol each demonstrate microbiologic activity. The activity of clarithromycin and azithromycin is the most impressive, producing up to a 2 log fall in blood colony-forming units at 1 to 2 months. With monotherapy, however, this drop is not sustained: After 3 months, resistance often develops, and microbiologic and clinical relapses occur.[134–136]

Combination therapy in theory should be more potent and reduce the likelihood of resistance emerging. Rifabutin recently has been shown in a randomized study to be microbiologically effective in combination with clofazamine and ethambutol, as compared with the two latter agents in combination with placebo.[137] A combination of clarithromycin, clofazimine, and ethambutol has been shown to be more effective than the two-drug combination of clarithromycin and clofazimine.[138] Various other combinations have been used. A U.S. Public Health Service Task Force Report recommended the use of at least two agents, one of them being either azithromycin or clarithromycin. A logical second drug would be ethambutol; rifabutin and clofazimine are often used as a third drug.[139,140] Recent evidence suggests that clofazimine may not add much efficacy to these regimens.

Recent clinical trials have focused on the prevention of disease due to MAC in susceptible individuals with CD4 counts below 100 cells/mm^3. In two recent prospective, randomized trials, rifabutin at a dose of 300 mg daily was shown to decrease the incidence of MAC infection by 50 percent and delay the onset of fever and anemia.[141] Resistant organisms have not been documented as a consequence of rifabutin prophylaxis. Rifabutin leads to significant drug interactions because it induces hepatic cytochrome P450 and should be used cautiously, with appropriate dose adjustments with fluconazole and protease inhibitors, especially ritonavir and indinavir.

Clarithromycin (500 mg twice daily) has been shown to decrease the incidence of MAC infection by 68 percent and to produce a survival benefit.[142] Azithromycin, at a weekly dose of 1200 mg, also has been shown to be an effective alternative.[143] Two multicenter, randomized, controlled trials have assessed rifabutin versus a macrolide versus combination therapy. In one trial, azithromycin was more effective than rifabutin alone for preventing either disseminated MAC or bacterial respiratory infections. Azithromycin plus rifabutin was more effective than azithromycin alone.[144] In the other trial, clarithromycin alone was more effective than rifabutin alone. In this trial, the combination of clarithromycin plus rifabutin provided no additional benefit compared with clarithromycin alone.[145] A recent report suggests that dapsone and pyrimethamine at doses used for PCP prophylaxis may have some clinical utility in preventing MAC infection as well.[146] A decision to institute prophylaxis must be decided on a patient-by-patient basis. While rifabutin, clarithromycin, azithromycin, or combination drug prophylaxis can reduce the frequency of MAC bacteremia, and perhaps prolong life, these drugs also can be associated with toxicity, drug interactions, development of resistance, and substantial cost and add to compliance issues in terms of adding another drug to a potentially complex regimen.

MYCOBACTERIUM TUBERCULOSIS

Mycobacterium tuberculosis (TB) has been undergoing an epidemic of its own since the mid-1980s, coincident with the AIDS epidemic. Worldwide, up to one-third of the population is infected with *M. tuberculosis,* and a significant portion of these may have concomitant HIV infection. In the United States, more than one-quarter of new cases of tuberculosis have been diagnosed in patients infected concurrently with HIV,[147] and it is recommended that all patients with tuberculosis be tested for HIV infection.[148] HIV-infected individuals develop active disease after infection at a rate that is dramatically greater than the general population. The annual risk of active disease is 10 percent, compared with a lifetime risk of 10 percent in healthy individuals.[149,150] Skin reactions of >5 mm to a standard PPD are considered positive in HIV-infected individuals. A negative test is not useful for ruling out tuberculosis infection due to the frequency of anergy, especially in patients with low CD4 cell counts.[151] Twelve months of prophylaxis (see Table 75-5) is indicated for HIV-infected individuals with either a positive skin test or a significant exposure.

Active tuberculosis may occur at any level of immunosuppression and may be the presenting manifestation of HIV infection.[152,153] Although pulmonary involvement is present in 75 to 90 percent of cases, the radiographic appearances may be diverse. Extrapulmonary disease occurs in up to 60 percent of cases. Patients with higher CD4 cell counts tend to develop upper lobe disease with cavities, in contrast to those with lower CD4 cell counts, who develop lower lobe disease and adenopathy.[149,154,155] Virtually every organ system can be affected, and tuberculosis may present with lymphadenitis, miliary disease, or meningeal involvement. Other sites include the viscera, skin, and soft tissue.[156]

Diagnosis is based on identifying the acid-fast organism in any clinical specimen, which can include sputum, bronchoalveolar lavage washings or biopsy, blood, bone marrow, CSF, or urine. HIV-infected patients are more likely to have negative sputum stains than HIV-negative individuals,[149,157] warranting an aggressive approach to diagnosis in suspected cases. In respiratory samples, nucleic acid amplification systems can identify a smear-positive specimen within several hours as containing *M. tuberculosis* with a high degree of sensitivity and specificity. In smear-negative specimens, they also can document some specimens as positive long before culture results are available. If acid-fast organisms are present on smear of any clinical specimen, *M. tuberculosis* should routinely be considered as part of the differential diagnosis in addition to MAC disease, and the need for respiratory isolation should be considered. If the organisms are detected only by smear or PCR, the likelihood of transmission by a respiratory route is much less.

Culture of *M. tuberculosis* requires 10 to 21 days to detect growth using radiometric techniques, depending on the size of the inoculum and the specific strain involved. Identification is rapid (<24 hours) once adequate growth occurs using gene probe techniques. Drug susceptibility tests also can be available in 10 to 21 days.

Treatment of tuberculosis (see Table 75-5) relies on a standard three-drug regimen (isoniazid, rifampin, and pyrazinamide), with a fourth agent (ethambutol) commonly added if there is suspicion of possible drug resistance in the community or in an individual patient.[150] If the isolate is found to be sensitive, the ethambutol is not necessary. Three-drug therapy is continued for 2 months, and then two drugs are continued for 9 months or at least 6 months from conversion of the smear to negative. Although no data exist clearly defining the optimal length of treatment in the setting of HIV infection, therapy that is considered effective for non-HIV-infected patients is generally effective for HIV-infected patients.[158] A recent study in Zaire compared a 6-month regimen with a 12-month regimen and found that extending treatment from 6 to 12 months reduced the rate of relapse from 9 to 1.9 percent, although there was no difference in mortality.[159]

Multiple-drug-resistant tuberculosis (MDRTB) commonly is defined as resistance to isoniazid and rifampin, with or without resistance to other agents. The treatment depends on the resistance pattern but often includes agents such as fluoroquinolones, amikacin, and in some cases aminosalicylic acid and ethionamide. According to some experts, initiation of treatment should be done in the hospital setting. The optimal duration of treatment of MDRTB has not been clearly defined.[160]

Since a major contributor to resistance is noncompliance of therapy, directly observed therapy (DOT) should be emphasized, especially when patients have poor access to health care. For DOT, an appropriate intermittent regimen includes isoniazid (15 mg/kg), rifampin (10 mg/kg), pyrazinamide (50 to 70 mg/kg), and

Table 75-5. Management of Mycobacterial Disease in HIV-Infected Persons

Disease	Patient population	Initial regimen	Maintenance	Duration	Comments
M. tuberculosis	Positive skin test, no active disease	INH 300 mg PO qd For suspected INH resistance: add 2 drugs from: rifampin 600 mg PO qd, ethambutol 15 mg/kg PO qd, pyrazinamide 15–30 mg/kg PO qd		12 months	Defined as >5 mm induration: consider treating with 2 to 5 mm induration, and with suspected exposure in setting of anergy
	Active disease, sensitive strain	INH plus rifampin plus pyrazinamide and ethambutol × 2 months followed by INH and rifampin for 4 months		Total of 6 months, including 6 months after culture conversion	Pyridoxine 100 mg qd should be given concurrently with INH
	Active disease, resistant strain suspected or prevalent geographically	Determined by epidemiological data in geographic area		Total of 12 months after culture conversion; sometimes up to 24 months recommended	Alternatives include amikacin, ofloxacin
MAC	Stool or respiratory colonization: Prophylaxis for CD4 cell count <75	No treatment recommended Rifabutin 300 mg PO qd, or azithromycin 1200 mg PO 1 × week, or clarithromycin 500 mg PO bid			Rifabutin 300 mg PO qd is also effective, although less effective than macrolides
	Documented disseminated infection	Clarithromycin 500 mg PO bid or azithromycin 500 mg PO qd, plus 1–3 of the following: ethambutol 15 mg/kg PO qd, ciprofloxacin 750 mg PO bid, rifabutin 450 mg PO qd	Same as initial regimen	Lifelong	

streptomycin (25 to 30 mg/kg), each administered three times weekly by a health care provider (either in a clinic or in the field) for at least 6 months.[150]

BACTERIAL PNEUMONIA

Upper and lower respiratory infections that are commonly seen in the immunocompetent population, such as those due to the encapsulated organisms *S. pneumonia* and *H. influenzae,* are seen more frequently in HIV-infected persons.[161,162] Recent studies have found that, compared with HIV uninfected controls, HIV-infected individuals have a five times greater risk of developing bacterial pneumonia and a higher rate of sinusitis and bronchitis, and the risk increases as the CD4 cell count decreases. Further, intravenous drug abusers have a higher incidence of pneumonia. Among patients with lower CD4 cell counts, cigarette smoking was associated with an increased incidence of bacterial pneumonias.[163] In addition to pneumonia due to *S. pneumonia* and *H. influenzae,* pneumonia also may be caused by *Staphylococcus aureus, Escherichia coli,* and especially in nosocomial cases, gram-negative organisms such as *Klebsiella pneumoniae, Pseudomonas aeruginosa,* and *Enterobacter aerogenes.*[161] As of 1992, recurrent bacterial pneumonia has been included in the case definition of AIDS.[164]

Diagnosis of bacterial pneumonia is either made empirically by presentation and chest radiograph findings or definitively by culture methods. In the setting of advanced HIV infection, opportunistic etiologies other than *S. pneumoniae* and *Hemophilus* sp. should be considered, including uncommon pathogens such as *Rhodococcus equi.*

Conventional treatment of bacterial pneumonia in HIV-infected individuals is generally administered. Therapy of upper or lower lobe respiratory infections in patients with HIV infection need not differ from that for HIV-uninfected patients.

Prevention of infections due to *S. pneumonia* with the polysaccharide vaccine is currently recommended for all HIV-infected individuals, although no controlled clinical trial has demonstrated clinical efficacy. Antibody responses decrease as HIV disease progresses. PCP prophylaxis with trimethoprim-sulfamethoxazole has been shown to provide some protection against bacterial infections as compared with the use of pentamidine for PCP prophylaxis.[30] Further, the use of MAC prophyaxis with azithromycin decreases the incidence of bacterial infections.[144]

BARTONELLA

The AIDS epidemic has led to increased recognition of the *Bartonella* sp., some of which were classified previously as *Rochalimea.*[165,166] In immunocompetent hosts, *Bartonella* sp. have been shown to be the etiologic agent of cat-scratch disease, trench fever, and endocarditis. In patients with AIDS, *Bartonella* sp. are the etiologic agents of bacillary angiomatosis and peliosis hepatis. *B. henselae* is commonly associated with exposure to cats.[167] A similar association has not been found with *B. quintana. B. quintana* bacteremia has been reported often in HIV-negative populations such as inner-city alcoholic patients and as endocarditis in HIV-infected patients and may have a different epidemiologic source.[168,169]

Bacillary angiomatosis presents with subcutaneous and cutaneous vascular lesions that often appear similar to the lesions of Kaposi's sarcoma. Lesions often occur in the head and neck region,[170] although they can be found in lymph nodes, bone, brain, and mucosal surfaces. Histopathologically, vascular proliferation can be seen with bacillary organisms present on Warthin-Starry staining. Organisms also can be found in lesions of peliosis hepatis, although these are histopathologically different from cutaneous lesions with large, blood-filled spaces. Splenic lesions may occur with areas of fibrosis in the presence of organisms. Skin lesions may or may not be found in conjunction with hepatic or splenic disease, and CT scanning can help in the diagnosis.

Bacillary angiomatosis and peliosis hepatis can be treated with erythromycin. Courses for at least 8 to 12 weeks are recommended, since relapses occur, and some patients may require chronic suppressive antibiotics. Doxycycline is also effective, and azithromycin and ciprofloxacin may be effective.[171]

References

1 Crowe SM et al: Predictive value of CD4 lymphocyte numbers for the development of opportunistic infections and malignancies in HIV-infected persons. *J AIDS* 4:770–776, 1991.

2 Masur H et al: CD4 counts as predictors of opportunistic pneumonias in human immunodeficiency virus (HIV) infection. *Ann Intern Med* 111:223–231, 1989.

3 Decker CF, Masur H: Current status of prophylaxis for opportunistic infections in HIV-infected patients. *AIDS* 8:11–20, 1994.

4 Hoover DL et al: Clinical manifestations in the era of pneumocystis prophylaxis. *N Engl J Med* 329:1922–1926, 1993.

5 Farizo KM et al: Spectrum of disease in persons with human immunodeficiency virus infection in the United States. *JAMA* 267:1798–1805, 1992.

6 Katz MH et al: Temporal trends of opportunistic infections and malignancies in homosexual men with AIDS. *J Infect Dis* 170:198–202, 1994.

7 Phair J et al: The risk of *Pneumocystis carinii* pneumonia among men infected with HIV-1. *N Engl J Med* 322:161–165, 1990.

8 U.S. Public Health Service Task Force on Anti-*Pneumocystis* Prophylaxis in Patients with Human Immunodeficiency Virus Infection: Recommendations for prophylaxis against *Pneumocystis carinii* pneumonia for persons infected with human immunodeficiency virus. *J Acquir Immun Defic Syndr* 6:46–55, 1993.

9 Ravioglione MC: Extrapulmonary pneumocystosis: The first 50 cases. *Rev Infect Dis* 12:1127–1138, 1990.

10 Hughes WT: *Pneumocystis carinii* pneumonia, in *Infectious Diseases,* Gorbach SL et al (eds). Philadelphia, Saunders, 1992, pp 494–497.

11 Ognibene FP et al: The diagnosis of *Pneumocystis carinii* pneumonia in patients with the acquired immunodeficiency syndrome using subsegmental bronchoalveolar lavage. *Am Rev Respir Dis* 129:933–937, 1984.

12 Stover DE et al: Diagnosis of pulmonary disease in the acquired immunodeficiency syndrome (AIDS): Role of bronchoscopy and bronchoalveolar lavage. *Am Rev Respir Dis* 130:659–662, 1984.

13 O'Brien RF et al: Diagnosis of *Pneumocystis carinii* pneumonia by induced sputum in a city with a moderate incidence of AIDS. *Chest* 95:136–138, 1989.

14 Cartwright CP, Nelson NA, Gill VJ: Development and evaluation of a rapid and simple procedure for detection of *Pneumocystis carinii* by PCR. *J Clin Microbiol* 32:1634–1638, 1994.

15 Lipschick GY et al: Improved diagnosis of *Pneumocystis carinii* infection by polymerase chain reaction on induced sputum and blood. *Lancet* 340:203–206, 1992.

16 Masur H, Shelhamer J: Empiric outpatient management of HIV-related pneumonia: Economical or unwise. *Ann Intern Med* 124:451–453, 1996.

17 Sattler FR et al: Trimethoprim-sulfamethoxazole compared with pentamidine for treatment of *Pneumocystis carinii* pneumonia in the acquired immunodeficiency syndrome. *Ann Intern Med* 109:280–287, 1988.

18 Klein NC et al: Trimethoprim-sulfamethoxazole versus pentamidine for *Pneumocystis carinii* pneumonia in AIDS patients: Results of a

large prospective randomized treatment trial. *AIDS* 6:301–305, 1992.

19 Gordon FM et al: Adverse reactions to trimethoprim-sulfamethoxazole in patients with the acquired immunodeficiency syndrome. *Ann Intern Med* 100:495–499, 1984.

20 Sattler FR et al: Trimetrexate with leucovorin versus trimethoprim-sulfamethoxazole for moderate to severe episodes of *Pneumocystis carinii* pneumonia in patients with AIDS: A prospective, controlled multicenter investigation of the AIDS Clinical Trials Group 029/031. *J Infect Dis* 170:165–172, 1994.

21 Toma E et al: Clindamycin/primaquine versus trimethoprim-sulfamethoxazole as primary therapy for *Pneumocystis carinii* pneumonia in AIDS: A randomized, double-blind pilot trial. *Clin Infect Dis* 17: 178–184, 1993.

22 Medina I et al: Oral therapy for *Pneumocystis carinii* pneumonia in the acquired immunodeficiency syndrome: A controlled trial of trimethoprim-sulfamethoxazole versus trimethoprim-dapsone. *N Engl J Med* 323:776–782, 1990.

23 Falloon J et al: A preliminary evaluation of 566C80 for the treatment of *Pneumocystis* pneumonia in patients with the acquired immunodeficiency syndrome. *N Engl J Med* 325:1534–1538, 1991.

24 Hughes W et al: Comparison of atovaquone (566C80) with trimethoprim-sulamethoxazole to treat *Pneumocystis carinii* pneumonia in patients with AIDS. *N Engl J Med* 328:1521–1527, 1993.

25 Bozzette SA et al: A controlled trial of early adjunctive treatment with corticosteroids for *Pneumocystis carinii* pneumonia in the acquired immunodeficiency syndrome. *N Engl J Med* 323:1451–1457, 1990.

26 Fischl MA et al: A randomized controlled trial of a reduced daily dose of zidovudine in patients with the acquired immnodeficiency syndrome. *N Engl J Med* 323:1009–1014, 1990.

27 Centers for Disease Control and Prevention: Recommendations for prophylaxis against *Pneumocystis carinii* pneumonia for adults and adolescents infected with human immunodeficiency virus. *MMWR* 41(RR-4):1–11, 1992.

28 Fischl MA, Dickinson GM, La Voie L: Safety and efficacy of sulfamethoxazole and trimethoprim chemoprophylaxis for *Pneumocystis carinii* pneumonia in AIDS. *JAMA* 259:1185–1189, 1988.

29 Schneider MME et al: A controlled trial of aerosolized pentamidine or trimethoprim-sulfamethoxazole as primary prophylaxis against *Pneumocystis carinii* pneumonia in patients with human immunodeficiency virus infections. *N Engl J Med* 327:1836–1841, 1992.

30 Hardy WD et al: A controlled trial of trimethoprim-sulfamethoxazole or aerosolized pentamidine for secondary prophylaxis of *Pneumocystis carinii* pneumonia in patients with the acquired immunodeficiency syndrome. *N Engl J Med* 327:1842–1848, 1992.

31 Podzamczer D et al: Intermittent trimethoprim-sulfamthoxazole compared with dapsone-pyrimethamin for the simultaneous primary prophylaxis of pneumocystic pneumonia and toxoplasmosis in patients infected with HIV. *Ann Intern Med* 122:755–761, 1995.

32 Leoung GS et al: Aerosolized pentamidine for prophylaxis against *Pneumocystis carinii* pneumonia: The San Francisco community prophylaxis trial. *N Engl J Med* 323:769–775, 1990.

33 Slavin MA et al: Oral dapsone versus nebulized pentamidine for *Pneumocystis carinii* pneumonia prophylaxis: An open randomized prospective trial to assess efficacy and haematologic toxicity. *AIDS* 6:1169–1174, 1992.

34 Girard PM et al: Dapsone-pyrimethamine compared with aerosolized pentamidine as primary prophylaxis against *Pneumocystis carinii* pneumonia and toxoplasmosis in HIV infection. *N Engl J Med* 328: 1514–1520, 1993.

35 Luft BJ, Remington JS: Toxoplasmic encephalitis in AIDS. *Clin Infect Dis* 15:211–222, 1992.

36 Luft BJ, Remington JS: AIDS commentary: Toxoplasmic encephalitis. *J Infect Dis* 157:1–6, 1988.

37 Luft BJ et al: Toxoplasmic encephalitis in patients with the acquired immunodeficiency syndrome. *N Engl J Med* 329:995–1000, 1993.

38 Chaisson RE, Volberding PA: Clinical manifestations of HIV infection, in *Principles and Practice of Infectious Diseases,* 4th ed, Mandell GL, Bennett JE, Dolin R (eds). New York, Churchill-Livingstone, 1995, pp 1217–1253.

39 Dannemann B et al: Treatment of toxoplasmic encephalitis in patients with AIDS. *Ann Intern Med* 116:33–43, 1992.

40 Katlama C et al: Pyrimethamine-clindamycin vs pyrimethamine-sulfadiazine as acute and long-term therapy for toxoplasmic encephalitis in patients with AIDS. *Clin Infect Dis* 22:268–275, 1996.

41 Kovacs JA: Efficacy of atovaquone in treatment of toxoplasmosis in patients with AIDS: The NIAID-Clinical Center Intramural AIDS Program. *Lancet* 340:637–638, 1992.

42 Opravil M et al: Once-weekly administration of dapsone/pyrimethamine vs aerosolized pentamidine as combined prophylaxis for *Pneumocystis carinii* pneumonia and toxoplasmic encephalitis in human immunodeficiency virus-infected patients. *Clin Infect Dis* 20:531–541, 1995.

43 Petersen C: Cryptosporidium and the food supply. *Lancet* 345:1128–1129, 1995.

44 Peterson C: Cryptosporidiosis in patients infected with the human immunodeficiency virus. *Clin Infect Dis* 15:903–909, 1992.

45 Flanigan T et al: Cryptosporidium infection and CD4 counts. *Ann Intern Med* 116:840–842, 1992.

46 Bissuel F et al: Paromomycin: An effective treatment for cryptosporidial diarrhea in patients with AIDS. *Clin Infect Dis* 18:447–449, 1994.

47 White AC et al: Paromomycin for cryptosporidiosis in AIDS: A prospective, double blind trial. *J Infect Dis* 170:419–424, 1994.

48 Wittner M, Tanowitz HB, Weiss LM: Parasitic infection in AIDS patients. *Infect Dis Clin North Am* 7:569–586, 1993.

49 Weber R et al: Improved light-microscopical detection of Microsporidia spores in stool and duodenal aspirates. *N Engl J Med* 326: 161–166, 1992.

50 Asmuth DM et al: Clinical features of microsporidiosis in patients with AIDS. *Clin Infect Dis* 18:819–825, 1994.

51 Pol S et al: Microsporidia infection in patients with the human immunodeficiency virus and unexplained cholangitis. *N Engl J Med* 328:95–99, 1993.

52 Weber R et al: Detection of *Septata intestinalis* in stool specimen and coprodiagnostic monitoring of successful treatment with albendazole. *Clin Infect Dis* 19:342–345, 1994.

53 Rabeneck L et al: The role of Microsporidia in the pathogenesis of HIV-related chronic diarrhea. *Ann Intern Med* 119:895–899, 1993.

54 Dieterich DT et al: Treatment with albendazole for intestinal disease due to *Enterocytozoon bieneusi* in patients with AIDS. *J Infect Dis* 169:178–183, 1994.

55 Pape JW, Verdier RI, Johnson WD Jr: Treatment and prophylaxis of *Isospora belli* infection in patients with the acquired immunodeficiency syndrome. *N Engl J Med* 320:1044–1047, 1989.

56 Weiss LM et al: *Isospora belli* infection: Treatment with pyrimethamine. *Ann Intern Med* 109:474–475, 1988.

57 Wurtz R: *Cyclospora:* A newly identified pathogen of humans. *Clin Infect Dis* 18:620–623, 1994.

58 Ortega YR et al: *Cyclospora* species: A new protozoan pathogen of humans. *N Engl J Med* 328:1308–1312, 1993.

59 Pape JW et al: *Cyclospora* infection in adults infected with HIV: Clinical manifestations, treatment, and prophylaxis. *Ann Intern Med* 121: 654–657, 1994.

60 Madico G et al: Treatment of *Cyclospora* infections with cotrimoxazole. *Lancet* 342:122–123, 1993.

61 Kirby AJ et al: Thrush and fever as measure of immunocompetence in HIV-1 infected men. *J Acquir Immun Defic Syndr* 7:1242–1249, 1994.

62 Powderly WG: Fungi, in *Textbook of AIDS Medicine,* Broder S, Merigan TC Jr, Bolognesi D (eds). Baltimore, Williams & Wilkins, 1994, pp 345–357.

63 Porro GB, Parente F, Cernuschi M: The diagnosis of esophageal candidiasis in patients with acquired immune deficiency syndrome: Is endoscopy always necessary? *Am J Gastroenterol* 84:143–146, 1989.

64 Baily GG et al: Fluconazole-resistant candidosis in an HIV cohort. *AIDS* 8:787–792, 1994.

65 Laine L et al: Fluconazole compared with ketoconazole for the treatment of *Candida* esophagitis in AIDS: A randomized trial. *Ann Intern Med* 117:655–660, 1992.

66 Newman SL et al: Clinically significant mucosal candidiasis resistant to fluconazole treatment in patients with AIDS. *Clin Infect Dis* 19: 684–686, 1994.

67 Sangeorzan JA et al: Epidemiology of oral candidiasis in HIV-infected patients: Colonization, infection, treatment, and emergence of fluconazole resistance. *Am J Med* 97:339–346, 1994.

68 Powderly WG: Therapy for cryptococcal meningitis in patients with AIDS. *Clin Infec Dis* 14(suppl 1):S54–S59, 1992.

69 Currie BP, Casadevall A: Estimation of the prevalence of cryptococcal infection among patients infected with the human immunodeficiency virus in New York City. *Clin Infect Dis* 19:1029–1033, 1994.

70 Chuck SL, Sande MA: Infections with *Cryptococcus neoformans* in the acquired immunodeficiency syndrome. *N Engl J Med* 321:794–799, 1989.

71 Hernandez AD: Cutaneous cryptococcosis. *Dermatol Clin* 7:269–274, 1989.

72 Van Der Horst C et al: Randomized double blind comparison of amphotericin B plus flucytosine (AMB+FC) to AMB alone (step 1) followed by a comparison of fluconazole to itraconazole (step 2) in the treatment of acute cryptococcal meningitis in patients with AIDS, part 1 (abstract), in *Programs and Abstracts of the 35th Interscience Conference on Antimicrobial Agents and Chemotherapy, San Francisco, 1995*. p I216. American Society of Microbiology, Washington, DC, 1995.

73 Saag MS, Powderly WG, Cloud GA: Comparison of amphotericin B with fluconazole in the treatment of acute AIDS-associated cryptococcal meningitis. *N Engl J Med* 326:83–89, 1992.

74 Larsen RA, Leal ME, Chan LS: Fluconazole compared with amphotericin B plus flucytosine for cryptococcal meningitis in AIDS. *Ann Intern Med* 113:183–187, 1990.

75 Bozzette SA et al: A placebo-controlled trial of maintenance therapy with fluconazole after treatment of cryptococcal meningitis in the acquired immunodeficiency syndrome. *N Engl J Med* 324:580–584, 1991.

76 Powderly WG et al: A controlled trial of fluconazole or amphotericin B to prevent relapse of cryptococcal meningitis in patients with the acquired immunodeficiency syndrome. *N Engl J Med* 326:793–798, 1992.

77 Kovacs JA et al: Cryptococcosis in the acquired immunodeficiency syndrome. *Ann Intern Med* 103:533–538, 1985.

78 Saag M et al: Randomized double blind comparison of amphotericin B plus flucytosine (AMB+FC) to AMB alone (step 1) followed by a comparison of fluconazole to itraconazole (step 2) in the treatment of acute cryptococcal meningitis in patients with AIDS, part 2 (abstract), in *Programs and Abstracts of the 35th Interscience Conference on Antimicrobial Agents and Chemotherapy, San Francisco, 1995*. p I217.

79 Powderly WG et al: A randomized trial comparing fluconazole with clotrimazole troches for the prevention of fungal infections in patients with advanced human immunodeficiency virus infection. *N Engl J Med* 332:700–705, 1995.

80 Wheat LJ: Histoplasmosis and coccidioidomycosis in individuals with AIDS: A clinical review. *Infect Dis Clin North Am* 8:467–482, 1994.

81 Wheat LJ et al: Disseminated histoplasmosis in the acquired immunodeficiency syndrome: Clinical findings, diagnosis and treatment, and review of the literature. *Medicine* 69:361–374, 1990.

82 Wheat J: Histoplasmosis: Recognition and treatment. *Clin Infect Dis* 19(suppl1S):19–27, 1994.

83 Sarosi GA, Johnson PC: Disseminated histoplasmosis in patients with human immunodeficiency virus. *Clin Infect Dis* 14:S60–S67, 1992.

84 Wheat LJ, Batteiger BE, Sathapatayavongs B: *Histoplasma capsulatum* infections of the central nervous system: A clinical review. *Medicine* 69:244–260, 1990.

85 Eidbo J et al: Cutaneous manifestations of histoplasmosis in the acquired immunodeficiency syndrome. *Am J Surg Pathol* 17:110–116, 1993.

86 Wheat LJ et al: Histoplasmosis relapse in patients with AIDS: Detection using *Histoplasma capsulatum* variety capsulatum antigen levels. *Ann Intern Med* 115:936–941, 1991.

87 Nightingale SD et al: Disseminated histoplasmosis in patients with AIDS. *South Med J* 83:624–630, 1990.

88 Norris S et al: Prevention of relapse of histoplasmosis with fluconazole in patients with acquired immunodeficiency syndrome. *Am J Med* 96:504, 1994.

89 Wheat LJ et al: Itraconazole is effective treatment for histoplasmosis in AIDS: Prospective multicenter non-comparative trial (abstract 1206). Presented at the 32nd Interscience Conference on Antimicrobial Agents and Chemotherapy, American Society for Microbiology, Washington, DC, 1992.

90 Wheat JL et al: Prevention of relapse with itraconazole in patients with the acquired immunodeficiency syndrome. *Ann Intern Med* 118: 610–616, 1993.

91 Mischel PS, Vinters HV: Coccidioidomycosis of the central nervous system: Neuropathological and vasculopathic manifestations and clinical correlates. *Clin Infect Dis* 20:400–405, 1995.

92 Ampel NM, Dols CL, Galgiani JN: Coccidioidomycosis during human immunodeficiency virus infection: Results of a prospective study in a coccidioidal endemic area. *Am J Med* 94:235, 1993.

93 Fish DG et al: Coccidioidomycosis during human immunodeficiency virus infection: A review of 77 patients. *Medicine* 69:384, 1990.

94 Ampel NM et al: Fungemia due to *Coccidioides immitis:* An analysis of 16 episodes in 15 patients and a review of the literature. *Medicine* 65:312, 1986.

95 Galgiani JN et al: Fluconazole therapy for coccidioidal meningitis. *Ann Intern Med* 119:28–35, 1993.

96 Pertel P et al: Risk of developing cytomegalovirus retinitis in persons infected with the human immunodeficiency virus. *J Acquir Immun Defic Syndr* 5:1069–1074, 1992.

97 Drew WL: Cytomegalovirus infection in patients with AIDS. *Clin Infect Dis* 14:608–615, 1992.

98 Palestine AG et al: A randomized, controlled trial of foscarnet in the treatment of cytomegalovirus retinitis in patients with AIDS. *Ann Intern Med* 115:665–673, 1991.

99 Smith MA, Brennessel DJ: Cytomegalovirus. *Infect Dis Clin North Am* 8:427–438, 1994.

100 Bowen EF et al: Use of PCR to correlate virlogic parameters with progression of CMV retinitis (abstract), in *Program and Abstracts of the 3rd Conference on Retroviruses and Opportunistic Infections, Washington, DC, 1996*. p 162. American Society of Microbiology, Washington, DC, 1996.

101 Polis MA et al: Anticytomegaloviral activity and safety cidofovir in patients with human immunodeficiency virus infection and cytomegalovirus viruria. *Antimicrob Agents Chemother* 39:882–886, 1995.

102 Jacobson MA, Mills J: Serious cytomegalovirus disease in the acquired immunodeficiency syndrome (AIDS). *Ann Intern Med* 108: 585–594, 1988.

103 Mortality in patients with the acquired immunodeficiency syndrome treated with either foscarnet or gancyclovir for cytomegalovirus retinitis: Studies of the Ocular Complications of the AIDS Research Group, in collaboration with the AIDS Clinical Trials Group. *N Engl J Med* 326:213–220, 1992.

104 Studies of Ocular Complications of AIDS Research Group. Combination of foscarnet and ganciclovir therapy vs monotherapy for the treatment of relapsed cytomegalovirus retinitis in patients with AIDS (abstract), in *Program and Abstracts of the 3rd Conference on Retroviruses and Opportunistic Infections, Washington, DC, 1996*. p LB15. American Society of Microbiology, Washington, DC, 1996.

105 Manischewitz JF et al: Synergistic effect of gancyclovir and foscarnet on cytomegalovirus replication in vitro. *Antimicrob Agents Chemother* 34:373–375, 1990.

106 Dieterich DT et al: Concurrent use of ganciclovir and foscarnet to treat cytomegalovirus infection in AIDS patients. *J Infect Dis* 167: 1184–1188, 1993.

107 Flores-Aguilar M et al: Pathophysiology and treatment of clinically resistant cytomegalovirus retinitis. *Ophthalmology* 100:1022–1031, 1993.

108 Drew WL et al: Prevalence of resistance in patients receiving gancyclovir for serious cytomegalovirus infection. *J Infect Dis* 163:716–719, 1991.

109 Martin DF et al: Treatment of cytomegalovirus retinitis with an intraocular sustained-release ganciclovir implant. *Arch Ophthalmol* 112:1531–1539, 1994.

110 The Chiron Ganciclovir Implant Study Group: A randomized controlled multicenter clinical trial of a sustained-release intraocular ganciclovir implant in AIDS patients with CMV retinitis. Presented at the 35th Interscience Conference on Antimicrobial Agents and Chemotherapy, American Society for Microbiology, 1995.

111 Drew WL et al: Oral ganciclovir as maintenance treatment for cytomegalovirus retinitis in patients with AIDS. *N Engl J Med* 333: 615–620, 1995.

112 Wolitz R et al: Presentation and treatment outcome of CMV retinitis after oral ganciclovir prophylaxis (abstract), in *Program and Abstracts of the 3rd Conference on Retroviruses and Opportunistic Infections, Washington, DC, 1996.* p 9.

113 Feinberg J, Cooper D, Hurwitz S: Phase III study of valaciclovir (VACV) for cytomegalovirus (CMV) prophylaxis in patients with advanced HIV disease. Presented at the 35th Interscience Conference on Antimicrobial Agents and Chemotherapy, American Society for Microbiology, 1995.

114 Siegel D et al: Prevalence and correlates of herpes simplex infections: The population based AIDS in multiethnic neighborhoods study. *JAMA* 268:1702–1708, 1992.

115 Reichman RC et al: Treatment of recurrent genital herpes infections with oral acyclovir: A controlled trial. *JAMA* 251:2103–2107, 1984.

116 Fife KH, The International Valaciclovir HSV Study Group: Valaciclovir or acyclovir for the treatment of first episode genital herpes. Presented at the 35th Interscience Conference on Antimicrobial Agents and Chemotherapy, American Society for Microbiology, 1995.

117 Loveless LM, Harris W, Sacks S: Treatment of first episode genital herpes with famciclovir. Presented at the 35th Interscience Conference on Antimicrobial Agents and Chemotherapy, American Society for Microbiology, 1995.

118 Englund JA et al. Herpes simplex virus resistant to acyclovir: A study in a tertiary care center. *Ann Intern Med* 112:416–422, 1990.

119 Safrin S et al: A controlled trial comparing foscarnet with vidarabine for acyclovir-resistant mucocutaneous herpes simplex in the acquired immunodficiency syndrome. *N Engl J Med* 325:551–555, 1991.

120 Hardy D et al: Phase I, pilot study of the safety and efficacy of foscarnet (PFA) cream for treatment (Rx) of acyclovir-uunresponsive (ACV-R) herpes simplex (abstract), in *Program and Abstracts of the 3rd Conference on Retroviruses and Opportunistic Infections, Washington, DC, 1996.* p 167. American Society of Microbiology, Washington, DC, 1996.

121 Lalezari J et al: A randomized, double-blinded, placebo-controlled study of cidofovir topical gel for acyclovir-resistant herpes simplex virus infections in patients with AIDS (abstract), in *Program and Abstracts of the 3rd Conference on Retroviruses and Opportunistic Infections, Washington, DC, 1996.* p 174. American Society of Microbiology, Washington, DC, 1996.

122 Strauss SE et al: Oral acyclovir to suppress recurrent herpes simplex virus infections in immunodeficient patients. *Ann Intern Med* 100: 522–524, 1984.

123 Hellinger WC et al: Varicella-zoster virus retinitis in a patient with AIDS-related complex: Case report and brief review of the acute retinal necrosis syndrome. *Clin Infect Dis* 16:208–212, 1993.

124 Margolis TP et al: Varicells-zoter virus retinitis in patients with the acquired immunodeficiency syndrome. *Am J Ophthalmol* 112:119–131, 1991.

125 Tyring S et al: Famciclovir for the treatment of acute herpes zoster: Effects on acute disease and postherpetic neuralgia. *Ann Intern Med* 123:89–96, 1995.

126 Gnann J et al: Sorivudine (BV-araU) versus acyclovir for herpes zoster in HIV-infected patients (abstract), in *Program and Abstracts of the 3rd Conference on Retroviruses and Opportunistic Infections, Washington, DC, 1996.* p 12. American Society of Microbiology, Washington, DC, 1996.

127 Jacobson MA et al: Acyclovir-resistant varicella-zoster virus infection after chronic acyclovir therapy in patients with the acquired immunodeficiency virus sundrome (AIDS). *Ann Intern Med* 112:187–191, 1990.

128 Nightingale SD et al: Incidence of *Mycobacterium avium-intercellulare* complex bacteremia in human immunodeficiency virus-positive patients. *J Infect Dis* 165:1082–1085, 1992.

129 Fordham von Reyn C et al. Persistent colonization of potable water as a source of *Mycobacterium-avium* infection in AIDS. *Lancet* 343: 1137–1141, 1994.

130 Yajko DM et al: *Mycobacterium avium* complex in water, food, and soil samples collected from the environment of HIV-infected individuals. *J Acquir Immun Defic Syndr* 9:176–182, 1995.

131 Havlik JA Jr et al: Disseminated *Mycobacterium avium* complex infection: Clinical identification and epidemiologic trends. *J Infect Dis* 165:577–580, 1992.

132 Benson CA, Ellner JJ: *Mycobacterium avium* complex infection and AIDS: Advances in theory and practice. *Clin Infect Dis* 17:7–20, 1993.

133 Barnes PF, Arevado C: Blood culture positivity patterns in bacteremia due to *Mycobacterium avium-intercellulare. South Med J* 81:1059–1060, 1988.

134 Chaisson RE et al: Clarithromycin therapy for bacteremic *Mycobacterium avium* complex disease in patients with AIDS: A randomized, double blind, dose-ranging study in patients with AIDS. *Ann Intern Med* 121:905–911, 1994.

135 Young LS et al: Azithromycin for treatment of *Mycobacterium avium-intracellulare* complex infection in patients with AIDS. *Lancet* 338:1107–1109, 1991.

136 Kemper CA et al: The individual effect of three antimicrobial agents, clofazimine, ethambutol, and rifampin, on *Mycobacterium avium* complex bacteremia in patients with AIDS. *J Infect Dis* 170:157–164, 1994.

137 Sullam PM, Gordin FM, Wynne BA: Efficacy of rifabutin in the treatment of infection due to *Mycobacterium avium* complex. *Clin Infect Dis* 19:84–86, 1994.

138 Dube M et al: Prevention of relapse of MAC bacteremia in AID: A randomized study of clarithromycin plus clofazimine, with or without ethambutol (abstract), in *Program and Abstracts of the 3rd Conference on Retroviruses and Opportunistic Infections, Washington, DC, 1996.* p 206. American Society of Microbiology, Washington, DC, 1996.

139 Public Health Service Task Force on Prophylaxis and Therapy for *Mycobacterium avium* Complex: Recommendations on prophylaxis and therapy for disseminated *Mycobacterium avium* complex disease in patients infected with the human immunodeficiency virus. *N Engl J Med* 329:898–904, 1993.

140 Kemper CA et al: Treatment of *Mycobacterium avium* complex bacteremia in AIDS with a four-drug oral regimen: Rifampin, ethambutol, clofazimine, and ciprofloxacin. *Ann Intern Med* 116:466–472, 1992.

141 Nightingale SD et al: Two controlled trials of rifabutin prophylaxis against *Mycobacterium avium* complex infection in AIDS. *N Engl J Med* 329:828–833, 1993.

142 Pierce M et al: A placebo controlled trial of clarithromycin prophylaxis against MAC infection in AIDS patients (abstract A/2). Presented at the 34th Interscience Conference on Antimicrobial Agents and Chemotherapy, American Society for Microbiology, Washington, DC, Orlando, Fla, 1994.

143 Oldfield EC et al: Once weekly azithromycin for the prevention of *Mycobacterium avium* complex (MAC) infection in AIDS patients (abstract), in *Program and Abstracts of the 3rd Conference on Retroviruses and Opportunistic Infections, Washington, DC, 1996.* p 203. American Society of Microbiology, Washington, DC, 1996.

144 Havlir DV et al: A double-blind, randomized study of weekly azithromycin, daily rifabutin, and combination azithromycin and rifabutin for the prevention of *Mycobacterium avium* complex (MAC) in AIDS patients (abstract), in *Program and Abstracts of the 3rd Conference on Retroviruses and Opportunistic Infections, Washington, DC, 1996.* p 204. American Society of Microbiology, Washington, DC, 1996.

145 Benson CA et al: A phase III prospective, randomized, double-blind study of the safety and efficacy of clarithromycin (CLA) vs rifabutin (RBT) vs CLA+RBT for prevention of *Mycobacterium avium* complex (MAC) disease in HIV+ patients with CD4 counts <100 cells/μL (abstract), in *Program and Abstracts of the 3rd Conference on Retroviruses and Opportunistic Infections, Washington, DC, 1996.* p 205. American Society of Microbiology, Washington, DC, 1996.

146 Opravil M et al: Dapsone/pyrimethamine may prevent mycobacterial disease in immunosuppressed patients with the human immunodeficiency virus. *Clin Infect Dis* 20:244–249, 1995.

147 Theuer CP et al: Human immundeficiency virus infection in tuberculosis patients. *J Infect Dis* 162:8–12, 1990.

148 Centers for Disease Control and Prevention: Guidelines for preventing the transmission of tuberculosis in health-care settings, with special focus on HIV-related issues. *MMWR* 39(RR-17):1–27, 1990.

149 Barnes PF et al: Tuberculosis in patients with human immunodeficiency virus infection. *N Engl J Med* 324:1644–1650, 1991.

150 American Thoracic Society. Treatment of tuberculosis and tuberculosis infection in adults and children. *Am J Respir Crit Care Med* 149:1359–1374, 1994.

151 Markowitz N et al: Tuberculin and anergy testing in HIV-seropositive and HIV-seronegative persons. *Ann Intern Med* 119:185–193, 1993.

152 Barnes PF, Barrows SA: Tuberculosis in the 1990s. *Ann Intern Med* 119:400–410, 1993.

153 Centers for Disease Control and Prevention: Tuberculosis and AIDS—Connecticut. *MMWR* 36:133–135, 1987.

154 Fischl MA et al: Clinical presentation and outcome of patients with HIV infection and tuberculosis caused by multiple-drug-resistant bacilli. *Ann Intern Med* 117:184–190, 1992.

155 Chaisson RE et al: Tuberculosis in patients with the acquired immunodeficiency syndrome: Clinical features, response to therapy and survival. *Am Rev Respir Dis* 136:570–574, 1987.

156 Shafer RW: Tuberculosis, in *Textbook of AIDS Medicine,* Broder S, Merigan TC Jr, Bolognesi D (eds). Baltimore, Williams & Wilkins, 1994, pp 265–266.

157 Klein NC et al: Use of mycobacterial smears in the diagnosis of pulmonary tuberculosis in AIDS/ARC patients. *Chest* 95:1190, 1989.

158 Small PM et al: Treatment of tuberculosis in patients with advanced human immunodeficiency virus infection. *N Engl J Med* 324:289–294, 1991.

159 Perriens JH et al: Pulmonary tuberculosis in HIV-infected patients in Zaire. *N Engl J Med* 332:779–784, 1995.

160 Iseman MD: Treatment of multidrug-resistant tuberculosis. *N Engl J Med* 329:784–791, 1993.

161 Caiaffa WT, Graham NMH, Vlahov D: Bacterial pneumonia in adult populations with human immunodeficiency virus (HIV) infection. *Am J Epidemiol* 138:909–922, 1993.

162 Steinhart R et al: Invasive *Hemophilus influenzae* infections in men with HIV infection. *JAMA* 268:3350–3352, 1992.

163 Hirschtick RE et al: Bacterial pneumonia in persons infected with the human immunodeficiency virus. *N Engl J Med* 333:845–851, 1995.

164 Centers for Disease Control and Prevention: 1993 revised classification system for HIV infection and expanded surveillance definition for AIDS among adolescents and adults. *MMWR* 41(RR-17):1–19, 1992.

165 Tappero JW et al: The epidemiology of bacillary angiomatosis and bacillary peliosis. *JAMA* 269:770–775, 1993.

166 LeBoit PE: Bacillary angiomatosis. *Mod Pathol* 8:218–222, 1995.

167 Koehler JE, Glaser CA, Tappero JW: *Rochalimaea henselae* infection: A new zoonosis with the domestic cat as reservoir. *JAMA* 271:531–535, 1994.

168 Spach DH et al: *Bartonella (Rochalimaea) quintana* bacteremia in inner-city patients with chronic alcoholism. *N Engl J Med* 332:424–428, 1995.

169 Spach DH et al: Endocarditis caused by *Rochalimaea quintana* in a patient with human immunodeficiency virus. *J Clin Microbiol* 31: 692–694, 1993.

170 Hnatuk LAP, Brown DH, Snell GED: Bacillary angiomatosis: A new entity in acquired immunodeficiency syndrome. *J Otololaryngol* 23: 216–220, 1994.

171 Regnery RL, Childs JE, Koehler JA: Infections associated with *Bartonella* species in persons infected with human immunodeficiency virus. *Clin Infect Dis* 21(suppl 1):S94–S98, 1995.

Chapter 76

AIDS-related malignancies

Barbara Klencke
Paul Volberding

One in six HIV-positive patients also has cancer. The range of malignancies in these patients is relatively narrow, however, and the most common cancers in HIV-positive patients are not those most common in the general population. There is little evidence that any of the four most common cancers in this country—lung, colon, breast, and prostate—develop with increased frequency in HIV-infected patients. Other cancers are thousands-fold more common in these patients,[1,2] and the distribution of cancers in HIV-positive populations is skewed in much the same way as those of other immunosuppressed patient populations.

Kaposi's sarcoma (KS) was the first cancer to be recognized as AIDS-related[3,4] and was designated as such by the Centers for Disease Control (CDC).[5] The CDC subsequently added intermediate- and high-grade non-Hodgkin's lymphoma (NHL), primary central nervous system lymphoma (PCNSL), and cervical cancer to the list of AIDS-defining conditions.[6] The designation of cervical cancer is controversial because its high frequency may be on the basis of lifestyle rather than impaired immunity.[1] There are several other tumors for which data suggest an increased incidence but which have not yet been officially recognized by the CDC as AIDS-defining and thus do not result in a diagnosis of AIDS in an HIV-infected patient.[7] These include anal cancer,[7,8] Hodgkin's disease,[9] and benign and malignant smooth muscle tumors in children,[10–12] as well as skin cancers, oral mucosa and head and neck cancers, testicular cancer, and possibly lung cancer.[13–15]

To be designated as an AIDS-defining cancer by the CDC, a cancer must occur more frequently than expected even after adjusting for all factors such as shared risk factors; this is where the controversy exists. Through linkage of HIV and cancer data registries[16] or by comparing the observed rate of specific cancers in large cohorts of HIV individuals to the expected rate, epidemiologists can determine the relative risk for each cancer. Additional evidence useful in supporting or rejecting a direct relationship between a malignancy and the immune impairment of HIV includes clinical evidence of an unusual natural history for a tumor or knowledge of the pathogenesis of the cancer.

KAPOSI'S SARCOMA

Kaposi's sarcoma was first recognized and described by Moritz Kaposi in the late 1800s. It was rare in the United States before 1981, particularly in healthy young adults. When it did occur, it generally afflicted elderly men of Ashkenazi Jewish descent, most often affecting the feet and lower extremities. This variant, now referred to as classic KS, had an indolent course and was not accompanied by immune deficiency. Classic KS can be seen occasionally in gay men who remain HIV-negative.[17] Well before the AIDS epidemic, KS was known to be a common malignancy in Central Africa, where some of its variants were seen to be aggressive and infiltrating even in children and young adults without immune deficiencies.[18–20]

In the early 1970s, KS was reported to be associated with iatrogenic immune suppression, generally in the setting of organ transplantation. It has been reported most commonly in renal allograft recipients as well as in patients treated for various autoimmune diseases with corticosteroids.[21,22]

KAPOSI'S SARCOMA IN AIDS

Epidemiology and pathogenesis

KS is much more common in homosexual men with AIDS than in heterosexual AIDS patients.[23,24] It develops in 20 to 30 percent of HIV-infected gay men, compared with 1 percent of most other HIV-infected patients. The incidence has not changed significantly over the course of the HIV epidemic.[25] A co-infection has long been suspected based on the epidemiology of AIDS-related KS.[26,27] Then, in 1994, a newly recognized herpes virus, human herpes virus-8 (HHV-8), was discovered within KS lesions.[28] HHV-8 is found in endothelial spindle cells[29,30] of all types of KS including classic KS, African or endemic KS, transplant-associated KS, and AIDS-related KS.[31] The virus can also be found in peripheral blood mononuclear cells in many KS patients and not infrequently precedes the development of KS in AIDS patients.[32,33]

The HHV-8 virus is also associated with rare lymphoproliferative diseases most often seen in HIV-infected individuals, including Castleman's disease and a newly recognized form of NHL known as primary effusion lymphoma.[34] Multiple myeloma, a malignancy of mature B-cells that has not been described as occurring more frequently in AIDS patients, has an indirect association, in that nonmalignant dendritic cells in the bone marrow contain HHV-8.[35] It is speculated that an interleukin (IL)-6-like protein secreted by these HHV-8 infected dendritic cells contributes to myeloma oncogenesis.

Just how this virus may be transmitted is still unclear. It has been detected in semen and prostate tissue.[36] Results of serologic studies remain controversial, as HHV-8 antibody testing remains to be refined, but seropositive rates track as expected given the epidemiology of KS;[37] that is, gay men with HIV or other active sexually transmitted diseases have the highest seropositive rates. Others have reported evidence that exposure is more widespread and not only confined to HIV risk populations.[38] The report of an association with multiple myeloma raises the possibility that exposure may not be as highly restricted in this country as some suggest.

The pathogenesis of KS is complex, with multiple putative pathways involving HHV-8, HIV, cytokines, integrins, and altered apoptosis and cell cycle controls.[39,40] Some evidence supports KS being a monoclonal process,[41] although it may be a polyclonal proliferative process in other cases, especially in the initial phases of the disease process. Cytokines released from spindle cells and inflammatory cells stimulate the growth of the tumors in complex autocrine and paracrine pathways, as does the HIV *tat* gene product. Finally, the HHV-8 genome encodes cyclin-D1 and IL-6-like proteins, which may play a role.

Histopathology

The histopathology of KS is characterized by a proliferation of abnormal vascular structures. Three histologic variants have been reported: a spindle-cell form, an anaplastic form, and a mixed-cell form.[42–44] The spindle-cell variant consists of uniformly sized spindle cells with rare mitoses, whereas the anaplastic form is characterized by disordered, malignant-appearing cells with frequent mitoses. The mixed cellular variant is by far the most common of the three seen in AIDS patients. It is characterized by three features: a proliferation within the tumor of vascular structures and slits, often lined by abnormally large, malignant-appearing endothelial cells; a proliferation of surrounding spindle-shaped cells; and an extravasation of erythrocytes. The spindle cell appears to originate from lymphatic endothelium.[45]

Natural history

The natural history of AIDS-related KS is variable and incompletely understood.[46] The disease can manifest at a wide range of CD4 counts but becomes more common as the CD4 count drops. Although an occasional patient will have a spontaneous remission or long interval without disease progression, others have a rapid progression. It has been noted anecdotally that the initiation of highly active anti-retroviral therapy (HAART) is not infrequently associated with regression of KS lesions, although the association has not been well studied.[47] Patients with limited KS and no symptoms suggesting other underlying infectious disease (e.g., fevers, night sweats, weight loss) do reasonably well. More often, however, in the setting of uncontrolled HIV infection, KS progresses rapidly.

The clinical course of the newly diagnosed KS patient is difficult to predict, but several factors are associated with disease progression and shorter survival: previous opportunistic infections, night sweats, fever, weight loss, anemia, elevated erythrocyte sedimentation rate, a low helper to suppresser T-cell ratio, an absolute helper-cell count of less than 100 cells/mm^3, and gastrointestinal (GI) or pulmonary lesions.[48,49] Patients with the best prognosis have only a few small nodular lesions, no previous serious infections, and no recent weight loss, fevers, or night sweats. Neither the site of cutaneous involvement nor the presence or absence of lymph node involvement appears to be particularly important prognostically. Visceral KS, however, does imply a poor prognosis.

Clinical manifestations

Cutaneous KS. Most patients with AIDS-related KS have subcutaneous tumor nodules or lymphatic involvement.[50–52] Cutaneous lesions are typically pigmented red or purple, even early in the disease process. They are usually palpable, painless, and nonpruritic. Occasionally, surrounding ecchymosis is apparent, especially in cases of rapidly progressing disease. Lesions typically appear on the face and in the oral cavity or on the feet and lower legs, although they may affect almost any site. KS frequently involves the plantar surfaces of the foot, but rarely the palms. Other notable sites of disease include the tip of the nose, the region behind the ear, the conjunctiva, and the penis. Vascular sites devoid of lymphatic vasculature, such as the retina, rarely if ever develop KS. Lesions tend to be circular, but those on the back or around the neck can be linear, apparently following cutaneous lymphatic drainage patterns.

Exophytic tumor masses rarely occur in AIDS-related KS, but when they do they can necrose, bleed, and when present on the feet, be painful. With advanced disease, plaques of coalesced lesions are common, especially over the medial aspect of the inner thigh. Inactive, previously treated KS lesions may fade entirely but more commonly leave a permanent pigmentation due to hemosiderin-laden macrophages that have engulfed extravasated erythrocytes.

Lymphedema. Lymphedema, a common sequela of AIDS-related KS, is not unexpected, in that KS seems to arise from lymphatic endothelium. Lymphedema is often striking and is most typically seen in the face, where it causes disfiguration and can result in physical obstruction of vision and hearing. Involvement of the lower extremities is also common, with associated upper thigh, scrotal, and penile edema, which can be striking and rapidly progressive. In either location, lymphedema may be out of proportion to the extent of cutaneous tumors, reflecting obliteration of small cutaneous lymphatics. Once lymphedema is extensive it can be hard to reverse even with effective chemotherapy, and therefore therapy should begin early.

Mucosal and Visceral KS. Up to one-third of patients with AIDS-related KS have oral involvement at the time of diagnosis. KS lesions in the oral cavity commonly affect the mucosa of the hard and soft palate and less commonly the posterior pharyngeal wall or the tonsillar pillars.[53]

Visceral involvement is common in AIDS-related KS. Almost any organ can be involved, although CNS involvement is exceedingly rare.[54] The GI tract is affected in as many as 50 percent of patients, even early in the course of the disease.[55] Gastrointestinal involvement is often an incidental finding because it is most often asymptomatic. It can, however, produce obstructive symptoms, bleeding, and malabsorption. Pulmonary involvement tends to be progressive and can be rapidly fatal without treatment. A dry cough, intermittent hemoptysis, dyspnea, fevers, and an abnormal chest radiograph are typical.[56] Lymphadenopathic or visceral KS may occur in the absence of cutaneous manifestations.

Diagnosis

KS lesions are readily recognized. Irrespective of risk group or clinical appearance, biopsy should be performed to establish a histologic diagnosis. The differential diagnosis of KS includes other pigmented processes such as bacillary angiomatosis, dermatofibromas, granuloma annulare, insect bite reactions, pyogenic granuloma, stasis dermatitis, and cutaneous lymphoma. The biopsy can be performed at any site, but skin is most convenient. A small punch biopsy (2–4 mm) is usually adequate, but it is helpful to include unaffected adjacent skin in the punch specimen. Enlarged peripheral lymph nodes can also be biopsied. Aspiration cytology has also been used to diagnose KS.

If a biopsy shows KS in a patient without previously established HIV infection, a serologic test is necessary. Patients with a positive test are diagnosed with AIDS, no matter what their CD4 count. If the serologic test is negative, the KS is not considered to be AIDS-related, even if the patient is a member of an AIDS risk group.

In the initial evaluation of a KS patient, tumor extent should be determined by a complete skin examination. The oral cavity should also be carefully examined. However, clinically important visceral KS can occur in the absence of cutaneous or oral manifestations in approximately 15 percent of cases. If unexplained GI or pulmonary symptoms are present, endoscopy should be performed. The classic appearance of small submucosal vascular nodules establishes the diagnosis of visceral KS. Biopsies are diagnostic in only a minority of cases of GI KS because the tumors are generally submucosal, but biopsy specimens may exclude other diagnoses. Endobronchial biopsy is discouraged because of the risk of hemorrhage.

In all KS patients, associated symptoms such as fevers, night sweats, and weight loss should be recorded and immunologic status, including CD4 cell count and HIV viral load, assessed.

Therapy

The natural history of untreated KS is a pattern of waxing and waning disease activity. KS activity can flare during chemotherapy, and separating a flare due to presumed increased cytokine stimulation from the development of chemotherapy resistance is difficult. When disease activity increases, the treatment alternatives are to maximize the dose and frequency of the agent being used or to change to a new agent. When the disease is quiescent, the alternatives are to use a tolerable agent intermittently or to discontinue therapy until a clear progression is seen.

When to initiate treatment must be decided on a patient-by-patient basis. Even disease that does not appear to be medically complicated may raise difficult issues for the patient because KS may be so recognizable and socially stigmatizing.

The choice of therapy for AIDS-related KS is problematic for several reasons. (1) The natural history of KS is highly variable and thus unpredictable.[50] (2) Because of advances in HIV treatment, affected patients are living longer and may therefore have a more protracted course of KS. (3) Use of cytotoxic chemotherapy may impair cellular immunity and thus increase the risk of opportunistic infections. Other acute or cumulative toxicities include myelosuppression, allergic reaction, neuropathy, pulmonary fibrosis, and other risks depending on the agent used. (4) With initiation of HAART, lesions may regress without the use of cytotoxic chemotherapy. Concurrent initiation of HAART and chemotherapy in recent studies may make the response rate somewhat difficult to interpret. (5) Finally, studies that have used different response criteria are difficult to compare.

In recent years the AIDS Clinical Trials Group (ACTG) staging system and tumor response criteria have lead to better standardization among trials.[57] Unfortunately, the benefits experienced by patients are not well documented by this system. The AIDS Malignancy Clinical Trials Consortium is developing a clinical benefits scale which incorporates measures of edema, pain, and other components reflective of patient benefit rather than depending solely on size and number of lesions.

Therapeutic approaches may be classified as local or systemic. The disease is often systemic even if the manifestations seen are only localized, but patients with indolent disease activity and a limited number of lesions may be managed with local therapy for long periods.

Local therapy

Surgery, Cryotherapy, Intralesional Chemotherapy, and Laser Therapy. Several effective local control methods can be used for small, superficial, discrete cutaneous lesions. The usual role for surgery in KS is palliation of protuberant lesions that are uncomfortable or bleed with repeated friction against clothes or shoes. If the patient has only one or several such lesions, excision may be of temporary value. Cryotherapy generally leaves a hypopigmented area but can be effective for small, superficial lesions. Intralesional administration of vinblastine, a chemotherapy agent, causes necrosis of the KS, often accompanied by several days of pain, but the result may be good and possibly long-lasting.

Laser therapy is the newest addition to the list of local control measures. The pigmentation left after an active KS lesion has been controlled by chemotherapy or another intervention is often permanent. As with tattoo removal, this residual pigmentation can be removed effectively with laser therapy. Cosmetically, the outcome may be better than with other local therapies.

Radiation Therapy. Radiation therapy is very useful in managing AIDS-related KS, particularly if the tumor is locally symptomatic.[58,59] Superficial lesions are best treated with a low-energy electron beam, which only penetrates a short distance into tissues, sparing deeper structures. Facial lesions, especially those on the nose or eyelid, can be successfully treated this way, with good cosmetic results. Larger, plaque-like areas of disease or areas with considerable edema may require coverage with megavoltage photons. Even with low doses, brawny induration in the radiation field can develop, and radiation recall can occur when the patient moves on to systemic chemotherapy with anthracyclines. A single treatment at low dose (800 cGy) produces a complete response in approximately 50 percent of lesions so treated, but the duration of response is often shorter than if higher doses are given over a protracted course.

Systemic therapy

Chemotherapy. Many chemotherapy agents have been studied, either alone or in combination, as therapy for KS. These regimens were described in detail in a recent review.[60] Among the agents discussed are single agent or combined vinblastine, vincristine, bleomycin, doxorubicin, and etoposide. The most effective of these was a combination of doxorubicin (Adriamycin), bleomycin, and vincristine (ABV), which yielded response rates of nearly 80 percent.[61] These remain an effective treatment option for some cases. However, conventional chemotherapy has rarely produced durable remissions and has been associated with significant acute and chronic toxicity. For AIDS patients battling a number of chronic symptoms or intermittent infections, chemotherapy toxicity was often an excessive burden. Therefore, the goal of therapy was palliation of symptoms, and systemic chemotherapy was reserved for intermittent use during exacerbations of KS.

Recent advances in KS chemotherapy have changed the treatment of KS. Liposomal doxorubicin (Doxil) and liposomal daunorubicin (DaunoXome) are encapsulated anthracylines that are approved as single agents for the treatment of advanced KS. They differ both in the anthracycline and the liposome utilized, each component having therapeutic implications. Both drugs, however, are well tolerated and effective.

In a large randomized trial, Doxil produced a response rate nearly twice that of ABV.[62] In a similar study, a fourth of patients responded to either DaunoXome or ABV, but DaunoXome use was associated with a trend toward more opportunistic infections.[63] Even with long-term use, cardiotoxicity and other cumulative toxicity has not been seen. Mild myelosuppression is the most common side effect and generally develops after several cycles. The usual dose of Doxil is 20 mg/m^2 every 3 weeks or DaunoXome 40–60 mg/m^2 every 2 to 3 weeks, each given intravenously over 30 minutes.

Paclitaxel (taxol) appears to have significant amount of activity.[64] It is frequently used for patients whose disease has progressed during therapy with liposomal anthracyclines. It was recently approved as second-line treatment of KS. Two dosing schedules have activity, 100 mg/m^2 every 2 weeks and 135 mg/m^2 every 3 weeks. Side effects such as hair loss, myelosuppression, and neuropathy make it less appealing for some HIV infected patients. Given its high level of activity however, Paclitaxel might be therapeutic in smaller doses in combination with Doxil. This combination is being studied and may eventually be used in some manner as first-line therapy.

Biologic Agents and Experimental Therapies. Since the herpes virus that causes KS was identified, there has be a resurgence of interest in the pathogenesis of KS. It is a cytokine-driven proliferative process for which a number of theoretical approaches are being investigated.[65] The role of antiherpes viral medications as prophylaxis or treatment is unclear. While rare anecdotal cases have been reported of clinical benefit after the initiation of foscarnet, in general there is no effect.[66] Theoretically, there is more basis for expecting benefit with the use of these drugs in prophylaxis, but even here the data are mixed.[67–69] A protease inhibitor specific for HHV-8 is under development, but again, its role might best be in a preventive setting for patients who show evidence of HHV-8 infection but in whom KS has not yet developed.

Alpha-interferon is active against KS, especially in those patients with a relatively well-preserved immune system as measured by their CD4 count.[70] It is also one of the few agents that has been able to induce durable remissions, albeit in a minority of patients. Although neutropenia may develop, alpha-interferon has immune-enhancing and antiviral properties, including anti-HIV effects. The drawback is that it requires daily subcutaneous injections and is associated with toxicity such as a flu-like syndrome. Response rates are higher when alpha-interferon is given in combination with zidovudine, and studies are now ongoing to determine the response rates when it is combined with the newer, more effective antiviral agents.

Retinoids, which are vitamin A analogs, have shown benefit as a topical therapy for KS. Ongoing studies to identify an effective oral or intravenous formulation designed to provide systemic benefit seem to be limited by bothersome side effects. Anti-angiogenic compounds may have a greater chance of inducing a response in KS than with other solid tumors and represent an important direction of future clinical research. Hormonal therapies may have a potential role, given the dramatic male predominance of all variants of KS. Beta-human chorionic gonadotropin, given intralesionally, has some activity.[71] These and other novel agents may allow patients to avoid or minimize their use of chemotherapy for the control of KS.

Summary of Treatment Guidelines. Local therapy, alpha interferon, watchful waiting, HAART, and experimental agents are all reasonable approaches to the patient with limited disease or an indolent disease course. Effective control of HIV should be the first step.

Patients with associated B-symptoms (fevers, sweats, weight loss), edema, symptomatic visceral disease, or the rapid appearance of a number of new lesions should receive effective systemic therapy. Reasonable options include alpha interferon and chemotherapy with vincristine and bleomycin or with ABV, etoposide, Doxil, DaunoXome, or taxol. Doxil has become the most frequently used agent, followed by taxol if control is inadequate with Doxil.

No formal treatment guidelines have been published since the availability of liposomal anthracyclines. These are expensive agents but are so effective and well tolerated that there is a tendency to use them earlier in the disease course, with the goal of providing the most effective therapy to minimize the complications of the disease. Because the disease may be easiest to control at this time, it may also be a way to minimize the total amount of chemotherapy given. This presumes that we can alter the natural history of the disease, which has yet to be proven.

As durable remissions are possible, periodic trials off chemotherapy should be allowed to determine which patients may discontinue chemotherapy. More often, patients will require ongoing or intermittent chemotherapy to maintain the benefits that they achieved. However, any residual pigmentation, which may be permanent, needs to be distinguished from ongoing KS disease. Close observation during any period off chemotherapy, looking for progressive disease, may be the only way to determine if ongoing chemotherapy is still required.

NON-HODGKIN'S LYMPHOMA

Since the first cases of high-grade non-Hodgkin's lymphoma (NHL) were reported in the early 1980s,[72–74] many reports of aggressive lymphoma in patients at risk for AIDS have been published. In June 1985, the CDC amended their case definition of AIDS to include patients with high-grade, B-cell NHL in the setting of documented HIV infection.[6]

NHL IN IMMUNODEFICIENT NON-HIV-INFECTED POPULATIONS

It has been recognized for more than 30 years that in patients with congenital immune deficiency in which there is impaired cell-mediated immunity, such as the Wiskott-Aldrich syndrome, the incidence of cancer is 100 times greater than expected and malignant lymphomas comprise the majority of these malignancies.[75] Immunoblastic lymphoma is the most prevalent histologic pattern. Patients often have marked generalized lymphadenopathy for several years before the diagnosis of lymphoma.[76] Lymph node biopsies often show a pattern of reactive hyperplasia, as they do in renal transplant patients receiving immunosuppressive medications.[77,78] Renal transplant patients have a 35-fold increased risk of developing NHL, often in unusual sites.[79]

In one-third of patients with NHL associated with renal transplantation, the disease is confined to the central nervous system.[80] Lymphoproliferative disease may appear as a relatively benign polyclonal proliferation in renal transplant patients or as an invasive and aggressive monoclonal large-cell NHL.[77] A renal transplant recipient has been described in whom a high-grade immunoblastic lymphoma evolved from polyclonal lymphoproliferative process.

An etiologic role for Epstein-Barr virus (EBV) is supported by circumstantial evidence.[78] Serologic studies suggest either acute or reactivated EBV infection in most patients with post-transplant lymphoproliferative disease, and multiple copies of the EBV genome have been identified within the cells of many of these lymphomas.

NHL in AIDS

NHL in HIV-infected patients has many similarities to NHL seen in transplant patients. The rate of NHL among HIV-infected persons is about 200-fold greater than that in the general population and is fairly uniform throughout all HIV exposure risk groups.[81] About three percent of AIDS patients present with NHL, and it develops in another three percent subsequent to another AIDS-defining diagnosis.[1] NHL appears to be a relatively late manifestation of HIV infection, but whether HIV treatment advances such as HAART will reduce the risk remains to be determined. It is anticipated that the cumulative risk over the life of the individual may rise as other AIDS-related complications are controlled and patient survival is prolonged.

Systemic NHL comprises approximately 80 percent of all AIDS-related NHLs; the other 20 percent are confined to the CNS. The incidence of primary central nervous system lymphoma (PCNSL) is 1000-fold higher than that seen in the general population. The vast majority of systemic lymphomas are B-cell, intermediate- or high-grade, typically presenting with advanced disease and involving extranodal sites. The major histologic subtypes are small, non-cleaved Burkitt or Burkitt-like, immunoblastic, or large-cell lymphomas. EBV nuclear antigen (EBNA) has been identified in 40 to 50 percent of these tumors, and most patients have shown evidence of previous EBV infection. Virtually all PCNSLs contain EBV.

The pathogenesis of AIDS-related NHL is complex.[82,83] A state of chronic B-cell stimulation evidenced by polyclonal hypergammaglobulinemia and follicular (B-cell) hyperplasia typifies HIV infection. One-third of patients diagnosed with NHL have histories of persistent generalized lymphadenopathy (PGL). HIV appears to induce the production of a host of cytokines or growth factors that serve to induce a state of ongoing B-cell activation, differentiation, and proliferation. In the context of impaired T-cell immunity, ongoing EBV infection can drive polyclonal B-cell activation. The inherent genetic instability of EBV-infected and immortalized B-cell clones eventually leads to c-*myc* gene rearrangement, resulting in the emergence of a fully transformed, EBV-containing monoclonal B-cell lymphoma. AIDS-related NHL not infrequently carries c-*myc* rearrangements in the absence of EBV. A variety of other chromosomal translocations involving oncogenes have been described in AIDS-related NHLs, and multiple alternative molecular pathways likely contribute to lymphomagenesis in the setting of HIV.[84] In summary, major contributing factors are the immunosuppression, chronic antigenic stimulation, cytokine overproduction, and eventually genetic alterations in c-*myc*, *bcl*-6, *ras,* and/or p53.

In 1984, Ziegler et al. reported a retrospective, multi-institutional study of 90 homosexual men with HIV-associated NHL.[72] Of 77 patients diagnosed antemortem, 33 had a prodrome of generalized lymphadenopathy, 15 had previous opportunistic infections, and 9 had KS before NHL developed. All but 2 patients had evidence of extranodal disease; 42 percent of patients had central nervous system disease, and 33 percent had bone marrow involvement. Meningeal infiltration developed in two-thirds of patients by the time of death. The GI tract has become the most common extranodal site of involvement since CNS prophylaxis with intrathecal chemotherapy became standard practice. However, virtually any organ site may be infiltrated with NHL. The lungs and liver are also common sites.

The diagnosis is often elusive because the presentation can be so variable. Fevers and declining functional status, signs of organ compromise due to NHL infiltration, or the onset of asymmetric lymphadenopathy are common presentations. The differential diagnosis includes opportunistic infections, other malignancies such as KS, or benign lymphadenopathy. Fine needle aspiration is appropriate, but additional tissue may be required to confirm the diagnosis.

Recently, a rare type of NHL has been described in HIV-infected persons who present with ascites or with pleural or pericardial effusions.[34] This NHL is termed primary effusion lymphoma or body-cavity-based lymphoma. It appears to be especially aggressive and is often refractory to chemotherapy. Malignant cells universally contain HHV-8, often in conjunction with EBV.

High-grade B-cell NHL confined to the central nervous system (PCNSL) should be considered in any patient belonging to a risk group for AIDS who shows focal neurologic findings or evidence of increased intracranial pressure. The immune deficiency is more severe, with CD4 counts generally less than 50, in those in whom PCNSL develops.

Therapy

More than a decade ago, Ziegler and colleagues[72] reported that 53 percent of 66 evaluable patients achieved a complete response to combination chemotherapy, a rate substantially lower than that reported in immune-competent patients with the same high-grade lymphomas. Fifty-four percent of the complete responders subsequently relapsed. Although prognosis was generally poor, morbidity and mortality appeared to be directly related to the degree of previous HIV-related illness. Patients who were asymptomatic at the time of diagnosis showed the best treatment results. Only 2 of 21 patients with a previous AIDS diagnosis remained alive and well. Thirty-eight of 66 evaluable patients had died, half from progressive lymphoma and half from opportunistic infections.

Little has changed in the past decade.[85] The observations made early in the epidemic regarding presentation, histology, prognosis, low response rates, poor tolerance of chemotherapy toxicity, and relatively short survival still hold true.[86] A key prognostic factor is the immune function, as measured by the CD4 count at the time of diagnosis and history of a prior AIDS diagnosis. Others include the patient's performance status, the presence of extranodal disease, age, and response to therapy. Higher doses of cyclophosphamide have been associated with lower survival.

Data such as these prompted the use of attenuated doses of combination chemotherapy. Levine and colleagues initiated this approach with a study of low dose M-BACOD (methotrexate, calcium leucovorin, bleomycin, doxorubicin, cyclophosphamide, vincristine, and dexamethasone).[87] This led to a large multi-institutional trial of standard-dose versus low-dose M-BACOD. Kaplan et al. randomized 198 HIV patients with untreated intermediate- or high-grade NHL.[88] Prophylactic myeloid growth factors were added to the standard-dose arm and were used as needed in the low-dose arm. Complete responses were seen in half, and the median survival was 7 to 8 months. There was no difference between the two arms in overall survival, disease-free survival, and or the development of opportunistic infections. Toxicity was higher and quality of life was lower in those who received standard-dose therapy, although marginally so. No subgroup could be identified in whom standard-dose therapy was more beneficial. The investigators concluded that low-dose therapy should be the standard for most patients with AIDS-related NHL.

In summary, NHL is chemotherapy-sensitive enough that it almost always will offer at least palliation of cancer-related symptoms and clearly improves survival compared with no therapy at all, but the median survival and the proportion experiencing true long-term remissions are disappointingly small. Some investigators have suggested that the use of more aggressive chemotherapy in selected patients may improve survival.[89] No therapy has been effective in the setting of relapsed or refractory disease in the HIV patients. The current standard for non-HIV-associated NHL is high-dose therapy with stem-cell support, but this approach has been considered too risky before the development of HAART. Whether higher-dose therapy would be tolerated if the underlying HIV illness is well controlled has yet to be determined. Experimental approaches are truly needed, as not much has changed in the past decade and a half since this disease was first identified.

The prognosis for patients with PCNSL is extremely poor.[90,91] Most will die with recurrent disease within one year. Radiation therapy is the standard treatment approach, although combination chemotherapy followed by radiation is under study.[92] Responses are possible with systemic chemotherapy, as the blood-brain barrier is altered enough to allow drug penetration. However, chemotherapy is poorly tolerated by this patient population, and a survival advantage has not yet been demonstrated.

References

1 Biggar RJ, Rabkin CS: The epidemiology of AIDS-related neoplasms. *Hematol Oncol Clin North Am* 10:997–1010, 1996.

2 Rabkin CS, Yellin F: Cancer incidence in a population with a high prevalence of infection with human immunodeficiency virus type 1. *J Natl Cancer Inst* 86:1711–1716, 1994.

3 Ziegler JL et al: Kaposi's sarcoma: a comparison of classical, endemic, and epidemic forms. *Semin Oncol* 11:47–52, 1984.

4 Friedman-Kien AE et al: Disseminated Kaposi's sarcoma in homosexual men. *Ann Intern Med* 96:693–700, 1982.
5 Centers for Disease Control: The Case Definition of AIDS Used by CDC for National Reporting (CDC Reportable AIDS), Document 03125. Atlanta, Department of Health and Human Services, 1985.
6 Centers for Disease Control: Revision of the Case Definition of Acquired Immunodeficiency Syndrome for National Reporting—United States. Atlanta, Department of Health and Human Services, MMWR 4:373–374, 1985.
7 Melbye M et al: Changing patterns of anal cancer incidence in the United States, 1940–1989. *Am J Epidemiol* 139:772–780, 1994.
8 Melbye M et al: High incidence of anal cancer among AIDS patients. The AIDS/Cancer Working Group. *Lancet* 343:636–639, 1994.
9 Hessol NA et al: Increased incidence of Hodgkin disease in homosexual men with HIV infection [see comments]. *Ann Intern Med* 117:309–311, 1992.
10 Chadwick EG et al: Tumors of smooth-muscle origin in HIV-infected children. *JAMA* 263:3182–3184, 1990.
11 McClain KL et al: Association of Epstein-Barr virus with leiomyosarcomas in children with AIDS [see comments]. *N Engl J Med* 332:12–18, 1995.
12 McClain KL et al: Cancers in children with HIV infection. *Hematol Oncol Clin North Am* 10:1189–1201, 1996.
13 Lyter DW et al: Incidence of human immunodeficiency virus-related and nonrelated malignancies in a large cohort of homosexual men. *J Clin Oncol* 13:2540–2546, 1995.
14 Remick SC: Non-AIDS-defining cancers. *Hematol Oncol Clin North Am* 10:1203–1213, 1996.
15 Volm MD, Von Roenn JH: Non-AIDS-defining malignancies in patients with HIV infection. *Curr Opin Oncol* 8:386–391, 1996
16 Cote TR et al: AIDS and cancer registry linkage: measurement and enhancement of registry completeness. The National AIDS/Cancer Match Study Group. *Prev Med* 24:375–377, 1995.
17 Moore PS, Chang Y: Detection of herpes-like DNA sequences in Kaposi's sarcoma in patients with and without HIV infection. *N Engl J Med* 332:1181–1185, 1995.
18 Athale UH et al: Influence of HIV epidemic on the incidence of Kaposi's sarcoma in Zambian children. *J Acquir Immune Defic Syndr Hum Retrovirol* 8:96–100, 1995.
19 Chintu C et al: Childhood cancers in Zambia before and after the HIV epidemic. *Arch Dis Child* 73:100–104; discussion 104–105, 1995.
20 Patil P et al: Pattern of adult malignancies in Zambia (1980–1989) in light of the human immunodeficiency virus type 1 epidemic. *J Trop Med Hyg* 98:281–284, 1995.
21 Harwood AR et al: Kaposi's sarcoma in recipients of renal transplants. *Am J Med* 67:759–765, 1979.
22 Penn I: Kaposi's sarcoma in organ transplant recipients: report of 20 cases. *Transplantation* 27:8–11, 1979.
23 Guinan ME et al: Heterosexual and homosexual patients with the acquired immunodeficiency syndrome. A comparison of surveillance, interview, and laboratory data. *Ann Intern Med* 100:213–218, 1984.
24 Strathdee SA et al: The epidemiology of HIV-associated Kaposi's sarcoma: the unraveling mystery. *AIDS* 10 (suppl A):S51-S57, 1996.
25 Veugelers PJ et al: Is the human immunodeficiency virus-related Kaposi's sarcoma epidemic coming to an end? Insights from the Tricontinental Seroconverter Study. *Epidemiology* 6:382–386, 1995.
26 Beral V et al: Kaposi's sarcoma among persons with AIDS: a sexually transmitted infection? *Lancet* 335:123–128, 1990.
27 Jacobson LP, Armenian HK: An integrated approach to the epidemiology of Kaposi's sarcoma. *Curr Opin Oncol* 7:450–455, 1995.
28 Chang Y et al: Identification of herpesvirus-like DNA sequences in AIDS-associated Kaposi's sarcoma [see comments]. *Science* 266:1865–1869, 1994.
29 Boshoff C et al: Kaposi's sarcoma-associated herpesvirus infects endothelial and spindle cells. *Nat Med* 1:1274–1278, 1995.
30 Staskus KA et al: Kaposi's sarcoma-associated herpesvirus gene expression in endothelial (spindle) tumor cells. *J Virol* 71:715–719, 1997.
31 Schalling M et al: A role for a new herpes virus (KSHV) in different forms of Kaposi's sarcoma. *Nat Med* 1:707–708, 1995.
32 Whitby D et al: Detection of Kaposi's sarcoma associated herpesvirus in peripheral blood of HIV-infected individuals and progression to Kaposi's sarcoma. *Lancet* 346:799–802, 1995.
33 Humphrey RW et al: Kaposi's sarcoma (KS)-associated herpesvirus-like DNA sequences in peripheral blood mononuclear cells: association with KS and persistence in patients receiving anti-herpesvirus drugs. *Blood* 88:297–301, 1996.
34 Soulier J et al: Kaposi's sarcoma-associated herpesvirus-like DNA sequences in multicentric Castleman's disease. *Blood* 86:1276–1280, 1995.
35 Rettig MB et al: Kaposi's sarcoma-associated herpesvirus infection of bone marrow dendritic cells from multiple myeloma patients. *Science* 276:1851–1854, 1997.
36 Monini P et al: Kaposi's sarcoma-associated herpesvirus DNA sequences in prostate tissue and human semen. *N Engl J Med* 334:1168–1172, 1996.
37 Kedes DH et al: The seroepidemiology of human herpesvirus 8 (Kaposi's sarcoma-associated herpesvirus): distribution of infection in KS risk groups and evidence for sexual transmission. *Nat Med* 2:918–924, 1996.
38 Lennette ET et al: Antibodies to human herpesvirus type 8 in the general population and in Kaposi's sarcoma patients. *Lancet* 348:858–861, 1996.
39 Miles SA: Pathogenesis of AIDS-related Kaposi's sarcoma. Evidence of a viral etiology. *Hematol Oncol Clin North Am* 10:1011–1021, 1996.
40 Nickoloff BJ, Foreman KE: Charting a new course through the chaos of KS (Kaposi's sarcoma) [comment]. *Am J Pathol* 148:1323–1329, 1996.
41 Rabkin CS et al: Monoclonal origin of multicentric Kaposi's sarcoma lesions. *N Engl J Med* 336:988–993, 1997.
42 Green TL et al: Histopathologic spectrum of oral Kaposi's sarcoma. *Oral Surg Oral Med Oral Pathol* 58:306–314, 1984.
43 Dorfman RF: Kaposi's sarcoma revisited. *Hum Pathol* 15:1013–1017, 1984.
44 McNutt NS et al: Early lesions of Kaposi's sarcoma in homosexual men. An ultrastructural comparison with other vascular proliferations in skin. *Am J Pathol* 111:62–77, 1983.
45 Beckstead JH et al: Evidence for the origin of Kaposi's sarcoma from lymphatic endothelium. *Am J Pathol* 119:294–300, 1985.
46 Dezube BJ: Clinical presentation and natural history of AIDS-related Kaposi's sarcoma. *Hematol Oncol Clin North Am* 10:1023–1029, 1996.
47 Conant MA et al: Reduction of Kaposi's sarcoma lesions following treatment of AIDS with ritonavir. *AIDS* 11:1300–1301, 1997.
48 Cutler K et al: Prognostic Indicators at Presentation of Kaposi's Sarcoma. Third International Conference on AIDS, Washington, 1985.
49 Volberding PA et al: Prognostic factors in staging Kaposi's sarcoma in the acquired immune deficiency syndrome. *Abstract Proc Am Soc Clin Oncol* 3:51, 1984.
50 Mitsuyasu et al: Heterogeneity of epidemic Kaposi's sarcoma. Implications for therapy. *Cancer* 57:1657–1661, 1986.
51 Friedman-Kein AE et al: Disseminated Kaposi's sarcoma in homosexual men. *Ann Intern Med* 6:693–670, 1982.
52 Rogers MF et al: National case-control study of Kaposi's sarcoma and *Pneumocystis carinii* pneumonia in homosexual men: II. Laboratory results. *Ann Intern Med* 99: 151–158, 1983.
53 Lozada F et al: Oral manifestations of tumor and opportunistic infections in the acquired immunodeficiency syndrome (AIDS): findings in 53 homosexual men with Kaposi's sarcoma. *Oral Surg Oral Med Oral Pathol* 56:491–494, 1983.
54 Klatt EC et al: Evolving trends revealed by autopsies of patients with the acquired immunodeficiency syndrome. 565 autopsies in adults with the acquired immunodeficiency syndrome, Los Angeles, 1982–1993 [corrected]. *Arch Pathol Lab Med* 118:884–890, 1994. [Published erratum in Dec issue,118(12):1200].
55 Friedman SL et al: Gastrointestinal Kaposi's sarcoma in patients with acquired immunodeficiency syndrome. *Gastroenterology* 89:102–108, 1985.

56 Huang L et al: Presentation of AIDS-related pulmonary Kaposi's sarcoma diagnosed by bronchoscopy. *Am J Respir Crit Care Med* 153: 1385–1390,1996.

57 Krown SE et al: Kaposi's sarcoma in the acquired immune deficiency syndrome: a proposal for uniform evaluation, response, and staging criteria. AIDS Clinical Trials Group Oncology Committee. *J Clin Oncol* 7:1201–1207, 1989.

58 Swift PS: The role of radiation therapy in the management of HIV-related Kaposi's sarcoma. *Hematol Oncol Clin North Am* 10:1069–1080, 1996.

59 Stelzer KJ, Griffin TW: A randomized prospective trial of radiation therapy for AIDS-associated Kaposi's sarcoma. *Int J Radiat Oncol Biol Phys* 27:1057–1061, 1993.

60 Lee FC, Mitsuyasu RT: Chemotherapy of AIDS-related Kaposi's sarcoma. *Hematol Oncol Clin North Am* 10:1051–1068, 1996.

61 Gill PS et al: Advanced acquired immune deficiency syndrome-related Kaposi's sarcoma. Results of pilot studies using combination chemotherapy. *Cancer* 65:1074–1078, 1990.

62 Northfelt DW et al: Efficacy of pegylated-liposomal doxorubicin in the treatment of AIDS-related Kaposi's sarcoma after failure of standard chemotherapy. *J Clin Oncol* 15:653–659, 1997.

63 Gill PS et al: Randomized phase III trial of liposomal daunorubicin versus doxorubicin, bleomycin, and vincristine in AIDS-related Kaposi's sarcoma. *J Clin Oncol* 14:2353–2364, 1996.

64 Saville MW et al: Treatment of HIV-associated Kaposi's sarcoma with paclitaxel. *Lancet* 346:26–28, 1995.

65 Karp JE et al: AIDS-related Kaposi's sarcoma. A template for the translation of molecular pathogenesis into targeted therapeutic approaches. *Hematol Oncol Clin North Am* 10:1031–1049, 1996.

66 Morefeldt L, Torsander J: Long-term remission of Kaposi's sarcoma following foscarnet treatment in HIV-infected patients. *Scand J Infect Dis* 26:749–752,1994.

67 Jones JL et al: AIDS-associated Kaposi's sarcoma. *Science* 267:1078–1079,1995.

68 Costagliola D, Mary-Krause M: Can antiviral agents decrease the occurrence of Kaposi's sarcoma? Letter. *Lancet* 346:57, 1995.

69 Humphrey RW et al: Kaposi's sarcoma (KS)-associated herpesvirus-like DNA sequences in peripheral blood mononuclear cells: association with KS and persistence in patients receiving anti-herpesvirus drugs. *Blood* 88:297–301, 1996.

70 Krown SE: Interferon and other biologic agents for the treatment of Kaposi's sarcoma. *Hematol Oncol Clin North Am* 5:311–322, 1991.

71 Gill PS et al: The effects of preparations of human chorionic gonadotropin on AIDS-related Kaposi's sarcoma. *N Engl J Med* 335:1261–1269, 1996.

72 Ziegler JL et al: Non-Hodgkin's lymphoma in 90 homosexual men. Relation to generalized lymphadenopathy and the acquired immuno deficiency syndrome. *N Engl J Med* 311:565–570, 1984.

73 Kalter SP et al: Aggressive non-Hodgkin's lymphomas in immunocompromised homosexual males. *Blood* 66:655, 1985.

74 Levine AM et al: Retrovirus and malignant lymphoma in homosexual men. *JAMA* 254:1921–1925, 1985.

75 Knowles DM: Etiology and pathogenesis of AIDS-related non-Hodgkin's lymphoma. *Hematol Oncol Clin North Am* 10:1081–1109, 1996.

76 Frizzera G et al: Lymphoreticular disorders in primary immunodeficiencies: new findings based on an up-to-date histologic classification of 35 cases. *Cancer* 46:692–699, 1980.

77 Frizzera G et al: Polymorphic diffuse B-cell hyperplasias and lymphomas in renal transplant recipients. *Cancer Res* 41:4262–4279, 1981.

78 Hanto et al: Clinical spectrum of lymphoproliferative disorders in renal transplant recipients and evidence for the role of Epstein-Barr virus. *Cancer Res* 41:4253–4261, 1981.

79 Penn I: Cancers complicating transplantation. *N Engl J Med* 323: 1767–1769, 1990.

80 Hoover R, Fraumeni JF Jr: Risk of cancer in renal transplant recipients. *Lancet* 1:5, 1973.

81 Armenian HK et al: Risk factors for non-Hodgkin's lymphomas in acquired immunodeficiency syndrome (AIDS). *Am J Epidemiol* 143: 374–379, 1996.

82 Herndier BG et al: Pathogenesis of AIDS lymphomas. *AIDS* 8:1025–1049, 1994.

83 Knowles DM: Etiology and pathogenesis of AIDS-related non-Hodgkin's lymphoma. *Hematol Oncol Clin North Am* 10:1081–1109, 1996.

84 Kaplan LD et al: Influence of molecular characteristics on clinical outcome in human immunodeficiency virus-associated non-Hodgkin's lymphoma: identification of a subgroup with favorable clinical outcome. *Blood* 85:1727–1735, 1995.

85 Sandler AS, Kaplan LD: Diagnosis and management of systemic non-Hodgkin's lymphoma in HIV disease. *Hematol Oncol Clin North Am* 10:1111–1124, 1996.

86 Gill PS et al: AIDS-related malignant lymphoma: results of prospective treatment trials. *J Clin Oncol* 5:1322–1328, 1987.

87 Levine AM et al: Low-dose chemotherapy with central nervous system prophylaxis and zidovudine maintenance in AIDS-related lymphoma. A prospective multi-institutional trial. *JAMA* 266:84–88, 1991.

88 Kaplan LD et al: Low-dose compared with standard-dose m-BACOD chemotherapy for non-Hodgkin's lymphoma associated with human immunodeficiency virus infection. National Institute of Allergy and Infectious Diseases AIDS Clinical Trials Group. *N Engl J Med* 336: 1641–1648, 1997.

89 Gisselbrecht C et al: Human immunodeficiency virus-related lymphoma treatment with intensive combination chemotherapy. French-Italian Cooperative Group. *Am J Med* 95:188–196, 1993.

90 Forsyth PA, DeAngelis LM: Biology and management of AIDS-associated primary CNS lymphomas. *Hematol Oncol Clin North Am* 10: 1125–1134, 1996.

91 Gill PS et al: Primary central nervous system lymphoma in homosexual men. Clinical, immunologic, and pathologic features. *Am J Med* 78: 742–748, 1985.

92 Forsyth PA et al: Combined-modality therapy in the treatment of primary central nervous system lymphoma in AIDS. *Neurology* 44:1473–1479, 1994.

Chapter 77

Management of neurologic disease in HIV-1 infection

Christina M. Marra

Neurologic consequences of infection with human immunodeficiency virus type 1 (HIV-1) are common. Autopsy series have documented abnormalities in over 90 percent of brains from HIV-1-infected individuals,[1–3] in 33 percent of spinal cords,[2] and in 50 to 100 percent of peripheral nerves.[4–6] Clinically evident nervous system disease is estimated to develop in 40 to 60 percent of these persons,[7–9] most often when the peripheral blood CD4 cell count declines to <200 cells/μL. Dementia, toxoplasmosis, and cryptococcal meningitis are the most common central nervous system (CNS) disorders. In a recent study of 487 patients with acquired immune deficiency syndrome (AIDS) treated at San Francisco General Hospital, 35 percent developed one or more of these illnesses.[10] Distal sensory polyneuropathy is the most common peripheral nervous system disorder, and it occurs in 10 to 35 percent of HIV-1-infected persons.[11–15] Opportunistic nervous system infections and neoplasms are discussed in Chaps. 75 and 76. This chapter will focus on diagnosis and treatment of nervous system problems in adults that are associated with HIV-1 infection itself: dementia, myelopathy, and peripheral neuropathy.

DEMENTIA

CLINICAL FINDINGS

Dementia has been recognized as a complication of advanced HIV-1 infection since the early 1980s and originally was termed *subacute encephalitis* or *subacute encephalopathy*.[8,16,17] The disorder was characterized clinically by cognitive changes, psychomotor retardation, and social withdrawal that often was attributed to depression. Marked dementia ensued, accompanied in some patients by focal neurologic abnormalities and seizures.

In 1986, Navia et al.[9] introduced the concept of the *AIDS dementia complex* (ADC), so named because characteristic cognitive changes often were accompanied by motor or behavioral abnormalities. These workers reviewed the medical records of 70 autopsied AIDS patients and found that 46 (66 percent) met criteria for dementia. Table 77-1 details the neurologic symptoms in the 44 individuals seen early in their illness. The most common early symptoms were forgetfulness and loss of concentration. Motor difficulties, including loss of balance and leg weakness, also were prevalent and were the predominant complaints in 27 percent. Behavioral changes were noted in over one-third of patients and were the only initial complaint in 23 percent. Neurologic examination demonstrated slowed verbal and motor responses, ataxia, and hyperreflexia. Most patients developed global cognitive dysfunction and psychomotor retardation before death and typically were awake, mute, immobile, and incontinent. However, 7 (16 percent) of the 45 patients who were examined late in their illness exhibited an organic psychosis with delusions or visual hallucinations.

Price and Brew[18,19] subsequently proposed a staging system for the AIDS dementia complex (Table 77-2). This system is based on functional disability and ranges from normal cognitive and motor function (stage 0); to mild impairment (stage 1), characterized by ability to perform all but the more demanding tasks of work or daily activities; to end-stage disease (stage 4), distinguished by rudimentary comprehension and responses[18,19] (see Table 77-2).

This work[16–19] forms the foundation of our current notion of the cognitive changes associated with HIV-1 infection. However, problems with the definition of the AIDS dementia complex and with the staging system have been noted. For example, although most patients with this disorder have intellectual deficits in combination with motor or behavioral abnormalities, others may have psychiatric or motor symptoms alone.[9,20] In addition, not all patients with mild disease progress to more severe stages. A working group of the American Academy of Neurology AIDS Task Force attempted to deal with these issues by developing research case definitions for the cognitive disorders associated with HIV-1 infection.[21] They suggested that the term *HIV-1-associated dementia complex* exclude patients with primarily motor abnormalities and be reserved for patients with severe cognitive difficulties that impair all activities of daily living. This approach is consistent with the 1987 revised Centers for Disease Control and Prevention (CDC) guidelines in which *HIV-1 encephalopathy* is an AIDS-defining illness and is defined as " . . . disabling cognitive and/or motor dysfunction interfering with occupation or activities of daily living . . . in the absence of a concurrent illness or condition other than HIV-1 that could explain the findings. . . ."[22,23] Thus the CDC definition is similar to HIV-1-associated dementia complex[21] or to stage 2 AIDS dementia complex.[19]

EPIDEMIOLOGY

In the original descriptions, AIDS dementia complex was present in about one-third of the 46 patients prior to or at the time of an AIDS-defining diagnosis.[9] In a subsequent study of a larger sample of 112 patients with AIDS dementia complex, 29 (26 percent) developed dementia before or in the absence of a diagnosis of AIDS.[24] However, 23 of these 29 individuals had HIV-1-related symptoms and signs, including lymphadenopathy, malaise, and weight loss; only 6 (5 percent of the total) were medically well at the time they developed dementia. These data suggest that dementia uncommonly develops in the absence of significant HIV-1-related immunosuppression. Several other lines of evidence support this contention: reported mean peripheral blood CD4 cell counts for series of cases of HIV-1-associated dementia are consistently below 200 cells/μL[25–27]; data from the CDC document HIV-1 encephalopathy as the initial manifestation of AIDS in only 2.8 percent of adults[23]; and prospective longitudinal studies of neuropsychological function fail to show decline in performance in individuals without AIDS.[28–31]

Price et al.[9,18,20] initially suggested that at least 60 percent of patients with AIDS developed overt or subclinical AIDS dementia complex, but this may be an overestimate of prevalence due to referral bias. A study of 196 patients with AIDS from The Netherlands reported a prevalence of AIDS dementia complex of 39 percent in patients seen before the introduction of zidovudine and 6 percent after.[32] In a subsequent report of 536 symptomatic HIV-1-infected individuals, AIDS dementia complex was diagnosed in 7.5 percent.[25] Similarly, a multicenter European study of 6,548 adults with AIDS reported that AIDS dementia complex was diagnosed in 4.5 percent of patients at the time of AIDS diagnosis and in an additional 7.8 percent after an AIDS-defining illness.[27] An incidence study in 31 CDC stage IV patients defined an annual rate of dementia of 14 percent[33]; a larger incidence study of 492 men with AIDS from the Multicenter AIDS Cohort Study (MACS)[34] defined an annual rate of dementia of 7 percent during the first 2 years after development of AIDS.

Table 77-1. Early Symptoms of the AIDS Dementia Complex Seen in 44 Patients

Symptoms	Number of patients, (%)
Cognitive	29 (66%)
Forgetfulness	17 (39%)
Loss of concentration	11 (25%)
Confusion	10 (23%)
Slowness of thought	8 (18%)
Motor	20 (45%)
Loss of balance	15 (34%)
Leg weakness	9 (20%)
Deterioration in handwriting	6 (14%)
Behavioral	17 (39%)
Apathy, social withdrawal	16 (36%)
Dysphoric mood	5 (11%)
Organic psychosis	2 (4%)
Regressed behavior	1 (2%)

SOURCE: Modified from ref. 9, with permission.

In the largest prevalence study,[27] the risk of developing AIDS dementia complex was associated with increasing age, intravenous (IV) drug use, and decreased CD4 count. In the MACS incidence study, lower hemoglobin and body mass index 1 to 6 months before AIDS, more constitutional symptoms 7 to 12 months before AIDS, and older age at onset of AIDS were risk factors for more rapid development of dementia.[34] A subsequent report from the MACS shows that the incidence of HIV-1 dementia in the cohort did not change significantly between 1988 and 1992, with the highest rates among those with peripheral blood CD4 counts $\leq 200/\mu L$.[35]

PATHOGENESIS

HIV-1 encephalopathy, or HIV-1 encephalitis, as it was then termed, initially was attributed to human brain cytomegalovirus (CMV) infection because histologic examinations were consistent with viral encephalitis, showing nodular collections of microglial cells that sometimes contained cytomegalic inclusions within gray matter.[8,17]

However, several observations argue that HIV-1, rather than CMV, plays the primary role in causing dementia. Cytomegalovirus is rarely cultured from cerebrospinal fluid (CSF) or brain of demented patients.[8,17,36] In a study of 70 AIDS patients, 46 of whom had AIDS dementia complex, neuropathologic examinations demonstrated abnormalities primarily in the white matter and subcortical gray structures.[2] The most common findings were inflammatory infiltrates composed of lymphocytes and macrophages, including multinucleated giant cells in the more severe instances, and pallor, rarefaction, and vacuolation of white matter. Microglial nodules were seen in 41 (59 percent) of 70 brains and were almost always seen within gray matter. CMV inclusions were significantly more common in those brains with a greater number of microglial nodules. However, extent of CMV infection did not correlate with severity of cognitive and motor dysfunction, suggesting that CMV infection of brain was not the cause of AIDS dementia complex.[2] Finally, HIV-1 DNA, RNA, or viral antigen has been identified in CNS cells from individuals with dementia,[37–42] almost exclusively in macrophages, microglial cells, or multinucleated giant cells, and the distribution of these cells in white matter or deep gray structures parallels the location of the neuropathology seen in demented patients. Infected neurons appear to be uncommon,[37,39] although a single report identified HIV-1 DNA and RNA in 2 to 17 percent of neurons from three patients with dementia.[43] Similarly, oligodendroglial cells appear to be rarely infected by HIV-1.[44,45] Astrocytes have been demonstrated to be infected in some children and adults with dementia, but infection is usually nonproductive.[46–48] Vascular endothelium also may be infected.[39,49]

Studies of CSF HIV-1 RNA concentrations in adults and children with and without cognitive deficits further support the hypothesis that CNS HIV-1 infection causes dementia. Preliminary studies in adults have shown that CSF HIV-1 RNA concentration is proportional to the severity of dementia.[49a,49b] In an analysis of 41 CSF specimens from 30 children, CSF HIV-1 RNA copy number correlated with cognitive index scores ($R = -0.36, p = 0.04$), and children with CSF HIV-1 RNA concentrations greater than 10,000 copies per milliliter were more likely to have abnormalities on neuroimaging ($p = 0.04$).[49c] Similarly, in a study of CSF from 41 children, CSF HIV-1 RNA copy numbers were significantly higher in severely encephalopathic children compared with those who were mildly encephalopathic or not encephalopathic ($p = 0.007$).[49d]

Although the association between HIV-1 infection and dementia is now well established, HIV-1 does not appear to cause dementia by directly infecting neurons or other CNS elements. In many patients with dementia, neuropathologic examination fails

Table 77-2. Staging Scheme for the AIDS Dementia Complex (ADC)

ADC stage	Characteristics
Stage 0 (normal)	Normal cognitive and motor function
Stage 0.5 (equivocal)	Either minimal or equivocal symptoms of cognitive or motor dysfunction characteristic of ADC or mild signs (snout response, slowed extremity movements) but without impairment of work or capacity to perform activities of daily living (ADL); gait and strength normal
Stage 1 (mild)	Unequivocal evidence (symptoms, signs, neuropsychological test performance) of functional intellectual or motor impairment characteristic of ADC but able to perform all but the more demanding aspects of work or ADL; can walk without assistance
Stage 2 (moderate)	Cannot work or maintain the more demanding aspects of daily life but able to perform basic activities of self-care; ambulatory but may require a single prop
Stage 3 (severe)	Major intellectual incapacity (cannot follow news or personal events, cannot sustain complex conversation, considerable slowing of all output) or motor disability (cannot walk unassisted, requiring walker or personal support, usually with slowing and clumsiness of arms as well)
Stage 4 (end stage)	Nearly vegetative; intellectual and social comprehension and responses are at a rudimentary level; nearly or absolutely mute; paraparetic or paraplegic with double incontinence

SOURCE: Modified from ref. 19, with permission.

to show evidence of HIV-1 infection of brain either by identification of multinucleated giant cells (the histopathologic marker of productive HIV-1 infection, presumed due to fusion of infected macrophages or microglial cells) or by immunocytochemistry.[2,50,51] Conversely, abundant viral antigen may be identified in brains from nondemented individuals.[52] Nonetheless, several morphologic studies have documented loss of 30 to 50 percent of cortical neurons in demented and nondemented AIDS patients,[53–57] as well as neuronal vacuolization and changes in cortical dendrites and synapses.[55,57] Surprisingly, the degree of neuronal loss may not correlate with the degree of dementia.[58]

These observations have led to the hypothesis that HIV-1 causes brain injury and subsequent dementia via indirect mechanisms. Proposed models suggest that HIV-1-infected mononuclear phagocytes release toxic viral gene products such as gp120,[59–61] tat,[62–65] nef,[48] or rev[48] or release cell-derived toxins such as quinolinic acid,[66,67] cytokines including tumor necrosis factor alpha (TNF-α),[68–71] eicosanoids,[69,72] platelet-activating factor,[73] or nitric oxide.[74,75] These substances may then injure neurons directly, may injure astrocytes or oligodendrocytes and interfere with their supporting functions, or may stimulate astrocytes or oligodendrocytes to augment neurotoxicity.[76–80] The final common pathway in all models involves activation of glutamate receptors or voltage-dependent calcium channels or both, leading to increases in intracellular calcium concentrations and neuronal injury or death. In experimental systems, calcium channel-blocking agents and glutamate receptor antagonists protect neuronal cells from gp120-mediated death,[81–83] raising the possibility that neuronal injury in HIV-1-infected individuals may be preventable or reversible.

DIAGNOSIS

The diagnosis of HIV-1-associated dementia is based on clinical findings, with typical cognitive changes accompanied by motor or behavioral abnormalities, and remains a diagnosis of exclusion. Individuals with HIV-1-associated dementia show impaired performance on neuropsychological tests that target motor function, attention and concentration, speed of information processing, and visuospatial performance.[19,21,84] However, poor performance on these tests does not establish the diagnosis of HIV-1-associated dementia, nor does normal performance exclude the diagnosis.[19] Similarly, neuroimaging is useful in excluding other causes of cognitive change (see below) but does not establish the diagnosis of HIV-1-associated dementia. Cranial computed tomography (CT) may show atrophy or patchy white matter attenuation or may be normal.[9] Morphometric CT studies suggest that reduced basal ganglia volume, caudate atrophy, or increased ventricular volume around the caudate nuclei may distinguish demented from nondemented HIV-1-infected individuals.[85–87] Cranial magnetic resonance imaging (MRI) is more sensitive than CT for demonstration of white matter abnormalities and may show high T2-weighted signal in the periventricular regions and in the centrum semiovale (Fig. 77-1). However, atrophy and focal white matter abnormalities may be seen in HIV-1-infected individuals without cognitive changes.[88–90]

Conventional CSF analysis is useful in excluding opportunistic infections of the CNS but is not helpful in establishing the diagnosis of HIV-1-associated dementia. In fact, increases in CSF white blood cell (WBC) count and protein concentration and isolation of HIV-1 from CSF are common in early HIV-1 infection, even when there is no evidence of neurologic disease.[91,92] However, the concentration of a variety of other substances, such as p24 antigen,[93,94] neopterin,[95–97] and beta-2-microglobulin,[98–100] are elevated in CSF from HIV-1-infected patients with dementia; quantitation of CSF beta-2-microglobulin concentration has the greatest clinical utility. Data from the MACS suggest that a CSF beta-2-microglobulin concentration of >3.8 mg/dL in a CSF specimen with a normal WBC count is specific (but not sensitive) for the diagnosis of HIV-1-associated dementia.[100]

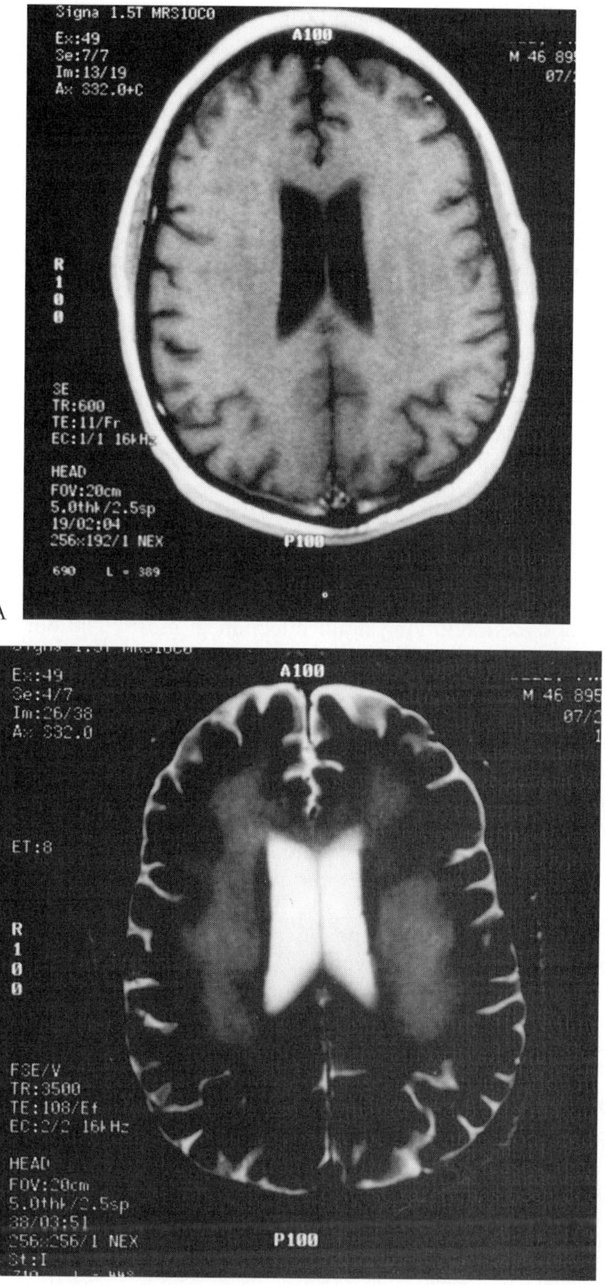

A

B

Fig. 77-1. MRI of brain from an HIV-1-infected patient with dementia. (*A*) The T1-weighted image shows atrophy, but no white matter changes are evident. (*B*) The T2-weighted image shows diffusely increased white matter signal.

DIFFERENTIAL DIAGNOSIS AND EVALUATION

HIV-1-infected individuals with peripheral blood CD4 counts of $\leq$200 cells/μL and cognitive changes should undergo neuroimaging and CSF analysis to exclude the possibility of CNS infection. A key consideration, particularly in individuals with very low CD4 counts, is CMV encephalitis. Brain CMV infection in HIV-1-infected individuals is identified in about one-quarter of autopsies,[2,101] but the clinical significance of this finding is not always obvious. In many instances, there are no clinical abnormalities,[102] and CSF or brain tissue often does not grow CMV, even when there is histologic evidence of brain infection.[36,102] As noted earlier, subacute encephalitis initially was attributed to CMV infection of brain, but the AIDS dementia complex was subsequently associated with brain HIV-1 infection.[2] A retrospective study of 14 histologically verified cases of CMV encephalitis and 17 demented AIDS patients without histologic evidence of brain CMV infection identified several clinical differences between the two groups[26] (Table 77-3). Patients with CMV encephalitis were more often confused and disoriented, were more likely to have focal findings on neurologic evaluation, had lower peripheral blood CD4 cell counts, and were more likely to have electrolyte abnormalities. Duration of symptoms before presentation and survival were shorter in the CMV encephalitis group. Periventricular inflammation by MRI or CT scan was present in 9 of 14 patients with CMV encephalitis but in none of the demented patients without brain CMV infection (Fig. 77-2).

The ability to identify brain CMV infection during life would help to further clarify its clinical correlates. Detection of CMV DNA in CSF by polymerase chain reaction (PCR) is sensitive and specific for identifying brain infection in most[103–105] but not all studies.[26,106] A drawback of the technique is that CMV DNA may be detected in CSF from patients with extensive as well as very limited brain infection. Quantitation of CMV DNA in CSF appears to circumvent this problem. A recent study shows that subjects with $>10^3$ CMV DNA molecules per 8 μL of CSF by semiquantitative PCR had more severe brain CMV infection and more severe clinical disease.[107] CSF CMV DNA concentration may decline with therapy directed against CMV.[108,109]

Besides CMV, other infections that should be considered and excluded in patients with suspected HIV-1-associated dementia are herpes simplex encephalitis,[8] the encephalitic form of toxoplasmosis,[110–112] neurosyphilis,[113] and cryptococcal meningitis[114] (Table 77-4). Patients with progressive multifocal leukoencephalopathy may have cognitive changes, but focal neurologic findings almost always distinguish them from patients with HIV-1-associated dementia.[115] Recent provocative reports suggest that dementia in some HIV-1-infected individuals may be associated with infection with *Bartonella* sp.[116,117] and human herpes virus type 6.[118] Further prospective study is required to clarify the role of these pathogens in HIV-1-associated dementia.

Early or mild HIV-1-associated dementia may be difficult to distinguish from metabolic encephalopathy, including the adverse effects of prescription or recreational drugs, and from psychiatric disease, particularly depression. In this situation, psychiatric consultation, neuropsychological testing, neuroimaging, and evaluation of CSF beta-2-microglobulin may be especially helpful.

Table 77-3. Clinical Findings in Patients with CMV Encephalitis and HIV-1-Associated Dementia without Histologic Evidence of Brain CMV Infection

	CMV encephalitis	HIV-1-associated dementia
Confused and disoriented, *n*	9/10	3/11
Focal signs, *n*	7/14	2/17
CD4 at presentation, mean cells/μL (range)	13 (0–24)	164 (0–517)
Serum electrolyte abnormalities	12/14	0/13
Duration of symptoms before presentation, mean (range)	3.5 weeks (1 day–13 weeks)	18 weeks (1 month–1 year)
Survival, median	5 weeks	22 weeks

SOURCE: Modified from ref. 26, with permission.

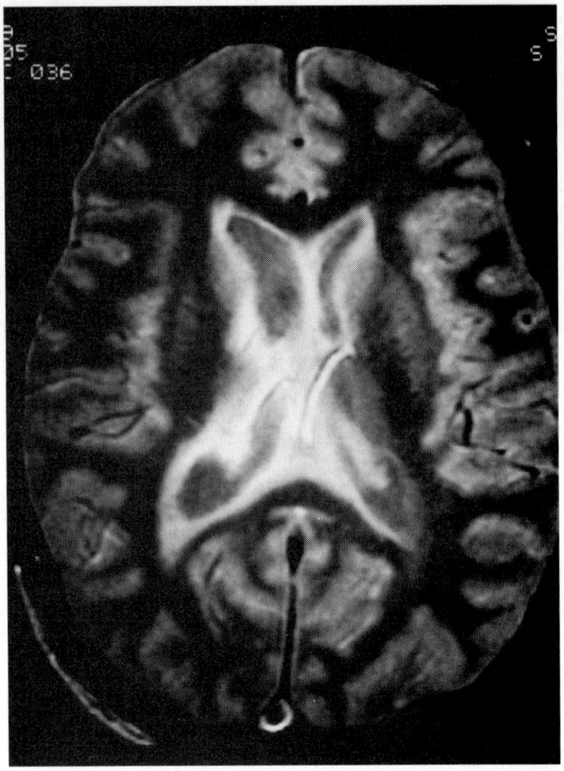

Fig. 77-2. MRI of brain from an HIV-1-infected patient with CNS cytomegalovirus infection showing increased signal intensity around the lateral ventricles.

PREVENTION

Several lines of evidence suggest that treatment with zidovudine (AZT, ZDV) may prevent dementia. Two retrospective studies from The Netherlands show that the incidence of dementia declined dramatically after zidovudine became widely available and

Table 77-4. Disorders That May Mimic HIV-1-Associated Dementia

Metabolic encephalopathy
- Psychoactive drugs (recreational or therapeutic)
- Dehydration
- Renal or hepatic failure

Psychiatric disease
- Depression
- Mania
- Psychosis

Infections
- Cytomegalovirus encephalitis
- Herpes simplex virus type 1 encephalitis
- Toxoplasmosis (encephalitic form)
- Neurosyphilis
- Crytococcal meningitis
- Progressive multifocal leukoencephalopathy (rare with nonfocal neurologic examination)
- ?*Bartonella henselae*
- ?Human herpes virus type 6

that dementia was significantly more likely in individuals who were not taking zidovudine.[25,119] The results of a prospective European study further support the contention that zidovudine therapy may prevent dementia and show a trend for reduced development of dementia with higher doses of zidovudine.[32] Thirteen (8 percent) of 160 subjects treated with 400 mg/day developed dementia, compared with 10 (6 percent) of 158 subjects given 800 mg/day and 5 (3 percent) of 156 subjects given 1,200 mg/day.[32] However, the results from the prospective MACS do not support the protective effect of zidovudine.[34,35] This difference may be explained in part by more advanced disease in the MACS subjects compared with those in the previously cited studies.

The influence of duration of zidovudine therapy on its potential protective effect has not been firmly established, and the results of currently available studies are contradictory. In one retrospective study, continuous therapy with zidovudine at a median dose of 500 mg/day for at least 12 months was associated with improved neuropsychological test performance,[120] while in a larger study the risk of development of dementia was reduced only in subjects who had taken zidovudine (at unspecified doses) for less than 18 months.[27] Similarly, the frequency of conventional HIV-1-related neuropathologic abnormalities is lower in patients treated until death with zidovudine,[121] but in one study the frequency of abnormalities increased after 12 months of therapy[122] and in another study the frequency of abnormalities decreased after 12 months of therapy.[50]

Strains of HIV-1 that are resistant to zidovudine have been identified in CSF,[123,124] and identification of zidovudine resistance in CSF HIV-1 is associated with progression of encephalopathy in children.[49d] Development of resistant strains might be a consequence of prolonged therapy or advanced HIV-1-related disease and could explain the differences observed in studies that have addressed prevention of dementia. Combination therapy might prevent development of resistance within the CNS and prolong the neuroprotective effects of zidovudine. However, little information is available regarding the ability of other antiretroviral agents to enter brain or to prevent dementia. A European randomized trial of didanosine failed to convincingly demonstrate a protective effect on development of dementia.[125] However, in an autopsy study, the frequency of conventional HIV-1-related neuropathologic abnormalities was lower in patients who received didanosine after zidovudine was discontinued compared with patients who stopped zidovudine within a month of death.[126] This observation suggests that, like zidovudine, didanosine may prevent HIV-1 replication within the CNS. In agreement with this conclusion, a small study showed that HIV-1 RNA levels in CSF declined in 12 of 13 patients after a mean of 8.9 months of zidovudine therapy; HIV-1 RNA levels in CSF declined in 3 of 3 antiretroviral-naive individuals treated with didanosine but increased in 3 of 3 didanosine-treated persons who had previously received zidovudine.[126a] Finally, preliminary data suggest that combination therapy with zidovudine plus lamivudine or stavudine plus lamivudine leads to a decline in CSF HIV-1 RNA concentration to below the limit of detection.[126b] Thus, in devising a combination antiretroviral regimen, it may be prudent to include zidovudine or stavudine in individuals with potential risk factors for dementia, such as older age, CD4 cell count below 200/μL, history of injection drug use, low hemoglobin, weight loss, or constitutional symptoms.

TREATMENT

Improvement in symptoms and signs of dementia in children and adults[127–132] and reduction in CSF neopterin and beta-2-microglobulin concentrations in adults have been documented after treatment with zidovudine.[96,99] A trial conducted by the Aids Clinical Trials Group(ACTG) compared placebo with treatment with zidovudine at 1,000 mg/day or 2,000 mg/day in individuals with mild to moderate dementia.[132] After 16 weeks of therapy, neuropsychological test performance in both zidovudine groups was better than in the placebo group; this difference was statistically significant only for the high-dose zidovudine group. It is difficult to assess whether there was continued improvement beyond 16 weeks because of loss of subjects to follow-up. Two small open studies that used lower zidovudine doses than used in the ACTG study also documented improvement in neuropsychological test performance and in symptoms and signs of dementia, but improvement waned after 6 to 12 months.[130,131] Improvement in symptoms and signs of dementia and in neuropsychological test performance also has been demonstrated in a small number of children and adults treated with didanosine,[133–135] with cognitive improvement in children maintained at 12 months.[134,135]

Potential adjunctive therapies, such as calcium channel and *N*-methyl-D-aspartate (NMDA) excitatory amino acid receptor blockers, are being investigated in HIV-1-associated dementia in adults. A small, placebo-controlled, phase I/II trial of the calcium channel blocker nimodipine showed that it was safe in patients with HIV-1-associated dementia and that patients receiving nimodipine tended to perform better on neuropsychological tests.[136] Other adjunctive therapies include vitamin B_{12},[137,138] levodopa or dopamine agonists,[139] antidepressants, antipsychotics, or psychostimulants.[140] Behavioral techniques that focus on compensation for lost abilities in early dementia and on providing a structured environment in late dementia may be helpful.[141]

COURSE

Not all patients with mild dementia will progress to more severe disease. Patients with moderate to severe dementia typically worsen, with survival ranging from 6 to 8 months.[25,27,34] In one study, median survival was 3 months in 20 demented patients not treated with zidovudine compared with 14 months in 10 demented patients treated with zidovudine ($p < 0.001$).[25] Patients with dementia should be treated with zidovudine at the highest tolerated dose. Demented patients who are not able to tolerate zidovudine should be treated with didanosine. The benefit of combination antiretroviral therapy in terms of increased efficacy or prevention of development of resistance in the CNS is not known.[142] Although it should be considered as an experimental therapy, nimodipine may be appropriate for patients with progression of dementia despite treatment with antiretroviral agents. An algorithm for treatment of HIV-associated dementia is shown in Fig. 77-3.

MYELOPATHY

CLINICAL FINDINGS

Vacuolar myelopathy in patients with AIDS was first described in 1983[17] and in more detail in 1985.[143,144] Petito et al.[144] found evidence of vacuolation of spinal white matter in association with lipid-filled macrophages in 20 (22 percent) of 89 consecutive autopsies. The white matter changes were located primarily in the lateral spinal cord at the middle to lower thoracic levels (cervical cord was not examined). These abnormalities resembled the changes seen in patients with subacute combined degeneration caused by vitamin B_{12} deficiency. Typically, individuals with

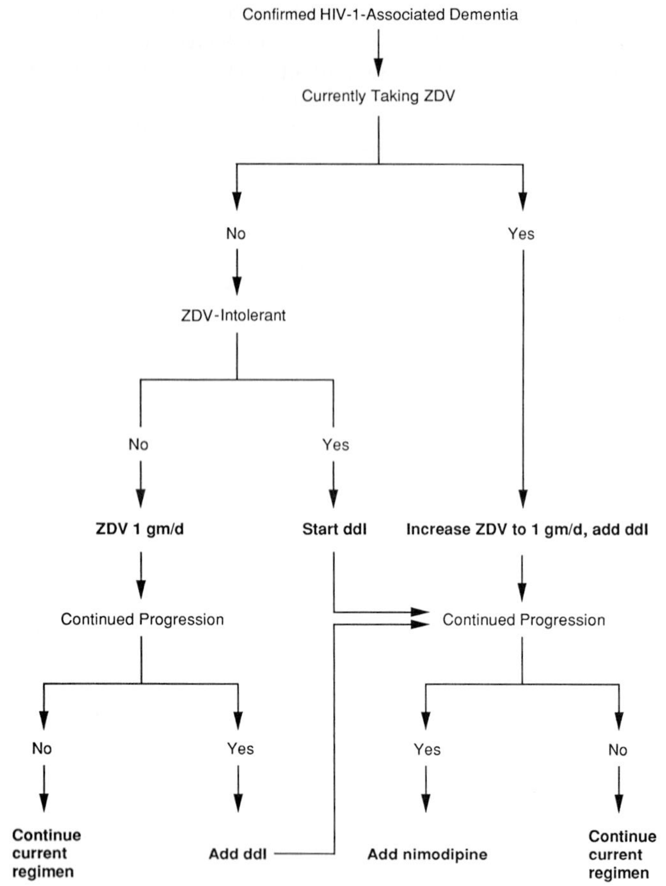

Fig. 77-3. Suggested treatment algorithm for HIV-1-associated dementia (*ZDV*, zidovudine; *ddI*, didanosine). In most instances, patients will already be taking a combination of antiretroviral agents. The recommendations in this algorithm are not meant to replace a patient's antiretroviral regimen but rather to augment it with agents known to be effective in treating HIV-1-associated dementia. Some experts recommend using stavudine (*d4T*) as an alternative to didanosine, particularly if patients are didanosine-intolerant.

moderate or severe pathologic changes had paraparesis with urinary incontinence that slowly developed over weeks to months, often accompanied by ataxia and spasticity. In contrast, weakness, ataxia, and spasticity were uncommon in individuals with mild pathologic changes, although urinary incontinence was seen in 3 (38 percent) of 8 patients. A more recent study showed that pathologic abnormalities predominate in the middle to lower thoracic cord in individuals with mild to moderate vacuolar myelopathy but that the severity of involvement is equivalent at the cervical and thoracic levels in individuals with severe vacuolar myelopathy.[145] A case-control study confirms that pathologic evidence of vacuolar myelopathy is more common than clinical abnormalities and that clinical finings are seen in individuals with more severe pathologic changes.[146] Of 100 subjects with autopsy evidence of vacuolar myelopathy, 15 (27 percent) of 56 patients who were examined by a neurologist within 3 months of death had clinical evidence of myelopathy; all had moderate or severe pathologic changes.

Similar clinical findings to those described in individuals with vacuolar myelopathy may be seen in individuals with HIV-1-associated dementia. In early series, vacuolar myelopathy and HIV-1-associated dementia were closely associated. In one autopsy-based report, almost half the demented patients had myelopathy, and 90 percent of patients with myelopathy were demented.[2] However, more recent series have not found an association between vacuolar myelopathy and HIV-1-associated dementia, perhaps because different criteria were used to establish the diagnosis of dementia or because of the influence of widespread use of antiretroviral agents.[50,146] Several studies have shown that peripheral neuropathy is commonly present in individuals with myelopathy.[146–148]

EPIDEMIOLOGY

Autopsy series document vacuolar myelopathy in up to 55 percent of AIDS patients,[2,144,146,149–152] with clinical evidence of myelopathy in approximately one-quarter to one-half.[144,146] A study of randomly selected Danish AIDS patients demonstrated that 16 (70 percent) of 23 had neurologic examination findings consistent with myelopathy.[147] All subjects had abnormal somatosensory evoked potential studies, with the greatest degree of abnormality seen in subjects with lower extremity weakness or ataxia. Vacuolar myelopathy occurs late in HIV-1 infection. In the case-control study described earlier, there was a strong association between more AIDS-defining illnesses and the likelihood of vacuolar myelopathy.[146]

PATHOGENESIS

Although an initial report suggested that vacuolar myelopathy may be caused by HIV-1 infection of the cord,[153] subsequent studies have not confirmed this hypothesis.[151,152,155] An autopsy study of 24 HIV-1-infected persons with vacuolar myelopathy and 15 HIV-1-infected individuals with similar brain pathology but without myelopathy showed that detection of HIV-1 in the spinal cord was not associated with the presence or severity of vacuolar changes.[154] A more recent autopsy study demonstrated activated macrophages in the posterior and lateral columns of spinal cords from HIV-1-infected individuals with and without vacuolar myelopathy.[155] The authors hypothesized that myelopathy occurs when these activated macrophages release toxins, such as cytokines, that damage myelin, oligodendrocytes, or neurons. This pathogenic hypothesis is similar to that proposed for HIV-1-associated dementia.

Because of the pathologic similarity between vacuolar myelopathy and myelopathy associated with vitamin B_{12} deficiency, nutritional or vitamin deficiencies also have been suggested as a cause of vacuolar myelopathy. In autopsy-based series, vitamin B_{12} levels in patients with vacuolar myelopathy are not low.[144,152,155] However, Kieburtz et al.[148] identified vitamin B_{12} deficiency in 6 (46 percent) of 13 patients with clinical evidence of myelopathy and in 6 (67 percent) of 9 patients with clinical evidence of both myelopathy and peripheral neuropathy. Although the patients with myelopathy alone did not improve with vitamin B_{12} replacement, those with combined myelopathy and neuropathy had symptomatic improvement within 1 week of initiating therapy. Vitamin E deficiency theoretically also could cause symptoms of myelopathy but has not been reported as a cause of this disorder in HIV-1-infected individuals.[156]

Vacuolar myelopathy has been documented in immunosuppressed HIV-1-uninfected individuals, some of whom had pathologic evidence of viral infection of the spinal cord, brain, or dorsal root ganglia.[157] These observations support theories of pathogenesis that implicate nutritional factors or indirect mechanisms of injury such as that caused by cytokines released from activated macrophages.

Table 77-5. Disorders That May Mimic Vacuolar Myelopathy

Compressive lesions
Epidural abscess
Hematoma
Tumor
Intramedullary infection
Cytomegalovirus
Herpes simplex virus types 1 and 2
Varicella-zoster virus
Toxoplasmosis
Mycobacteria
HTLV-I and HTLV-II
Neurosyphilis
Vitamin deficiencies
Vitamin B_{12}
Vitamin E

DIAGNOSIS

The diagnosis of vacuolar myelopathy is one of exclusion (Table 77-5). In the setting of back pain or a demarcated sensory level (both of which are uncommon in vacuolar myelopathy), an extradural compressive lesion such as tumor, hematoma, or abscess should be excluded by MRI. Intramedullary infection with herpes simple viruses,[158,159] varicella-zoster virus,[160,161] CMV,[162–165] *T. gondii*,[166–169] or mycobacteria[170] can be excluded by imaging and examination of CSF. HTLV-I and-II myelopathy[171] or syphilitic myelopathy[172] can be excluded by serologic tests and examination of CSF. MRI of the spinal cord in vacuolar myelopathy is usually normal, although enlargement of the thoracic cord with increased intramedullary signal intensity from the thoracic cord to the conus was described in one individual with myelopathy.[173] CSF is typically acellular with mild to moderate elevation of the protein concentration,[146] a profile characteristic of advanced HIV-1 infection.

THERAPY

Few data are available concerning therapy for vacuolar myelopathy. Case reports describe improvement in patients treated with zidovudine[174] and in patients treated with vitamin B_{12}.[148] An open pilot study of methionine, 3 gm PO bid, found that 7 of 10 individuals experienced mild to moderate improvement.[175]

COURSE

The clinical course of patients with vacuolar myelopathy is variable. Typically, patients remain stable or slowly worsen, but abrupt deterioration can occur. In the case-control study described earlier, mean survival in patients with vacuolar myelopathy was 12 months and was not different from survival of the control group with AIDS.[146]

PERIPHERAL NEUROPATHY

CLINICAL FINDINGS

Disorders of the peripheral nervous system are common in patients infected with HIV-1. Pathologic abnormalities of peripheral nerves can be demonstrated in 50 to 100 percent of individuals with advanced disease, even when they have no clinical evidence of a peripheral nervous system disorder.[4–6] Distal sensory polyneuropathy (DSPN) is the most common clinical syndrome. Patients with DSPN complain of symmetrical numbness or tingling of the toes that develops over weeks to months and gradually spreads proximally. Burning, aching, or lancinating pain in the toes and soles of the feet may be present in 8 to 60 percent.[13,14] Physical examination shows decreased or absent ankle reflexes and symmetrically decreased sensation to pinprick and vibration in the feet and legs. Position sensation is usually normal. Sensory symptoms and signs may develop in the fingers and hands, usually when similar lower extremity abnormalities have progressed to the knees. Weakness is not a prominent feature and, if present, is usually mild and involves the intrinsic muscles of the feet.

Histopathologic examination of peripheral nerves shows axonal loss, sometimes with demyelination.[5,15] Similarly, electrophysiologic studies are consistent with sensory and motor axonal neuropathy. The most common nerve conduction abnormality is reduction of the sural sensory action potential.[14,15] However, as many as 50 percent of patients with clinical evidence of neuropathy will have normal nerve conduction studies.[176,177]

EPIDEMIOLOGY

Distal sensory polyneuropathy is described in 10 to 35 percent of HIV-1-infected individuals with advanced disease[11–15] and is rare in persons with peripheral blood CD4 counts above 300/μL.[178] Data from the MACS show that the incidence of DSPN is highest in persons with CD4 counts below 100 cells/μL, with an incidence rate of 7.75 person-years in this group.[35] Furthermore, between 1988 and 1992, the yearly incidence of neuropathy in MACS participants increased 50 percent, more than any other neurologic condition.

PATHOGENESIS

The clinical findings, results of electrophysiologic studies, and evidence of gracile tract degeneration at autopsy[179,180] suggest that DSPN is caused by length-dependent axonal degeneration. However, the relationship to HIV-1 infection has not been established. Using PCR, Winer et al.[15] were unable to amplify HIV-1 proviral DNA from six sural nerve biopsies from HIV-1-infected patients with symptomatic neuropathy or from six patients without symptomatic neuropathy. Although virus has been cultured from some nerve biopsies and autopsy specimens, it is often not detected in the same specimens by immunocytochemistry[5,153] and is not identified in dorsal root ganglia,[179,180] although HIV-1 antigens could be identified in macrophages within ganglia in one study.[181] Researchers at Johns Hopkins University have shown that peripheral nerves from AIDS patients are infiltrated with macrophages that express several activation markers, such as MHC class II molecules, interleukin 1 (IL-1), IL-6, and TNF-α.[79,182] Furthermore, amounts of messenger RNA for TNF-α in peripheral nerves are significantly greater in HIV-1-infected patients with sensory neuropathy compared with those without sensory neuropathy, leading to the hypothesis that axonal degeneration in DSPN is caused by the toxic effect of TNF-α or some other cytokine or toxic cell product.[79]

Several other etiologies have been suggested for DSPN (Table 77-6). DSPN is seen more commonly in HIV-1-infected individuals with severe weight loss[14,15] and a longer history of systemic symptoms,[14] implicating nutritional factors. In some instances, DSPN may be associated with vitamin B_{12} deficiency.[148] An association between systemic CMV infection and painful sensory neuropathy has been suggested,[183] but pathologic evidence of CMV infection of nerve or dorsal root ganglia is uncommon in individuals with DSPN.[79,179,180] One study identified a significantly

Table 77-6. Disorders That May Mimic Distal Sensory Polyneuropathy Associated with HIV-1 Infection

Nucleoside antiretroviral toxicity
Zalcitabine (ddC)
Stavudine (d4T)
Didanosine (ddI)
Lamivudine (3TC) (rarely reported)
B_{12} deficiency or other nutritional factors
HTLV-II infection
?Cytomegalovirus infection

higher prevalence of antibodies to HTLV-II in HIV-1-infected individuals with peripheral neuropathy compared with those without neuropathy.[184]

DIAGNOSIS

The diagnosis of DSPN is based primarily on clinical findings. Electrophysiologic tests may confirm the diagnosis but may be normal.[14,15,176,177] CSF typically is normal or may show nonspecific abnormalities such as mild mononuclear pleocytosis and elevated protein concentration.[185,186] The nucleoside antiretrovirals didanosine, zalcitabine, and stavudine may cause a toxic neuropathy that is clinically indistinguishable from DSPN, although it may have a more acute onset, particularly in individuals given high doses of the offending agent[187–190]. Individuals with symptoms of neuropathy and other risk factors for neuropathy such as diabetes or alcohol abuse may be at increased risk for toxic neuropathy.[190–192] Definitive diagnosis of toxic neuropathy is established by documenting improvement in symptoms or signs after discontinuing or reducing the dose of the implicated agent. In some instances, patients may worsen clinically for the first 1 to 3 weeks after the agent is discontinued, a phenomenon called *coasting*. Improvement is usually seen within 8 weeks of discontinuation but may take longer; mean time to recovery in subjects treated with high-dose zalcitabine was 19 weeks in one study.[189] After symptomatic recovery, patients may tolerate reintroduction of the offending agent at a reduced dose without recurrence of symptoms.

TREATMENT

Suggested symptomatic therapy for painful DSPN includes vitamin B_{12} replacement,[148] nonsteroidal anti-inflammatory agents, tricyclic antidepressants, anticonvulsants, mexiletine, and narcotics.[13,187,193] The relative efficacy of these agents has not been established in large, controlled trials. Symptomatic improvement was attributed to therapy with zidovudine in one instance,[127] but subsequent experience has not confirmed this association.[13]

COURSE

Stabilization or improvement may be seen in one-half of patients with DSPN,[15,186] although slow progression of abnormalities is common in individuals with advanced disease.[13]

References

1 Petito CK: Review of central nervous system pathology in human immunodeficiency virus infection. *Ann Neurol* 23(suppl):S54-S57, 1988.

2 Navia BA et al: The AIDS dementia complex: II. Neuropathology. *Ann Neurol* 19:525–535, 1986.

3 Price RW et al: AIDS encephalopathy. *Neurol Clin* 4:285–301, 1986.

4 Griffin JW et al: Predominantly sensory neuropathy in AIDS: Distal axonal degeneration and unmyelinated fiber loss (abstract). *Neurology* 41(suppl 1):374, 1991.

5 de la Monte Su et al: Peripheral neuropathy in the acquired immunodeficiency syndrome. *Ann Neurol* 23:485–492, 1988.

6 Mah V et al: Abnormalities of peripheral nerve in patients with human immunodeficiency virus infection. *Ann Neurol* 24:713–717, 1988.

7 Levy RM et al: Opportunistic central nervous system pathology in patients with AIDS. *Ann Neurol* 23(suppl):S7-S12, 1988.

8 Levy RM et al: Neurological manifestations of the acquired immunodeficiency syndrome (AIDS): Experience at UCSF and review of the literature. *J Neurosurg* 62:475–495, 1985.

9 Navia BA et al: The AIDS dementia complex: I. Clinical features. *Ann Neurol* 19:517–524, 1986.

10 Wang F et al: Incidence proportion of and risk factors for AIDS patients diagnosed with HIV dementia, central nervous system toxoplasmosis, and cryptococcal meningitis. *J Acquir Immune Defic Syndr Hum Retrovirol* 8:75–82, 1995.

11 McArthur JC: Neurologic manifestations of AIDS. *Medicine* 66: 407–437, 1987.

12 de Gans J, Portegies P: Neurological complications of infection with human immunodeficiency virus type 1: A review of literature and 241 cases. *Clin Neurol Neurosurg* 91:199–219, 1989.

13 Cornblath DR, McArthur JC: Predominantly sensory neuropathy in patients with AIDS and AIDS-related complex. *Neurology* 38:794–796, 1988.

14 So YT et al: Peripheral neuropathy associated with acquired immunodeficiency syndrome. *Arch Neurol* 45:945–948, 1988.

15 Winer JB et al: A study of neuropathy in HIV infection. *Q J Med* 83:473–488, 1992.

16 Britton CB, Miller JR: Neurologic complications in acquired immunodeficiency syndrome (AIDS). *Neurol Clin* 2:315–339, 1984.

17 Snider WD et al: Neurological complications of acquired immune deficiency syndrome: Analysis of 50 patients. *Ann Neurol* 14:403–418, 1983.

18 Price RW, Brew BJ: The AIDS dementia complex. *J Infect Dis* 158: 1079–1083, 1988.

19 Sidtis JJ, Price RW: Early HIV-1 infection and the AIDS dementia complex (editorial). *Neurology* 40:323–326, 1990.

20 Price RW et al: The brain in AIDS: Central nervous system HIV-1 infection and AIDS dementia complex. *Science* 239:586–592, 1988.

21 Working Group of the American Academy of Neurology AIDS Task Force: Nomenclature and research case definitions for neurologic manifestations of human immunodeficiency virus-type 1 (HIV-1) infection: *Neurology* 41:778–785, 1991.

22 Centers for Disease Control and Prevention: Revision of the CDC surveillance case definition for acquired immunodeficiency syndrome. *Morb Mortal Wkly Rep* 36(suppl 1):1S-15S, 1987.

23 Janssen RS et al: Epidemiology of human immunodeficiency virus encephalopathy in the United States. *Neurology* 42:1472–1476, 1992.

24 Navia BA, Price RW: The acquired immunodeficiency syndrome dementia complex as the presenting or sole manifestation of human immunodeficiency virus infection. *Arch Neurol* 44:65–69, 1987.

25 Portegies P et al: Presentation and course of AIDS dementia complex: 10 years of follow-up in Amsterdam, The Netherlands. *AIDS* 7:669–675, 1993.

26 Holland NR et al: Cytomegalovirus encephalitis in acquired immunodeficiency syndrome (AIDS). *Neurology* 44:507–514, 1994.

27 Chiesi A et al for the AIDS in Europe Study Group: Epidemiology of AIDS dementia complex in Europe. *J Acquir Immune Defic Syndr Hum Retrovirol* 11:39–44, 1996.

28 Marra CM et al: Neurologic manifestations of HIV infection without AIDS: follow-up of a cohort of homosexual and bisexual men. *J Neuro-AIDS* 1:(2) 41–65, 1996.

29 Selnes OA et al and the Multicenter AIDS Cohort Study: HIV-1 infection: No evidence of cognitive decline during the asymptomatic stages. *Neurology* 40:204–208, 1990.

30 Selnes OA et al: HIV-1 infection and intravenous drug use: Longitudinal neuropsychological evaluation of asymptomatic subjects. *Neurology* 42:1924–1930, 1992.

31 McKegney FP et al: A prospective comparison of neuropsychologic function in HIV-seropositive and -seronegative methadone-maintained patients. *AIDS* 4:565–569, 1990.

32 Nordic Medical Research Councils' HIV Therapy Group: Double blind dose-response study of zidovudine in AIDS and advanced HIV infection. *Br Med J* 304:13–17, 1992.

33 Day JJ et al: Incidence of AIDS dementia in a two-year follow-up of AIDS and ARC patients on an initial phase II AZT placebo-controlled study: San Diego cohort. *J Neuropsychiatry Clin Neurosci* 4:15–20, 1992.

34 McArthur JC et al for the Multicenter AIDS Cohort Study: Dementia in AIDS patients: Incidence and risk factors. *Neurology* 43: 2245–2252, 1993.

35 Bacellar H et al: Temporal trends in the incidence of HIV-1-related neurologic diseases: Multicenter AIDS cohort study, 1985–1992. *Neurology* 44:1892–1900, 1994.

36 Nielsen SL et al: Subacute encephalitis in acquired immune deficiency syndrome: A postmortem study. *Am J Clin Pathol* 82:678–682, 1984.

37 Stoler MH et al: Human T-cell lymphotropic virus type III infection of the central nervous system: A preliminary in situ analysis. *JAMA* 256:2360–2364, 1986.

38 Shaw GM et al: HTLV-III infection in brains of children and adults with AIDS encephalopathy. *Science* 227:177–182, 1985.

39 Wiley CA et al: Cellular localization of human immunodeficiency virus infection within the brains of acquired immune deficiency syndrome patients. *Proc Natl Acad Sci USA* 83:7089–7093, 1986.

40 Koenig S et al: Detection of AIDS virus in macrophages in brain tissue from AIDS patients with encephalopathy. *Science* 233:1089–1093, 1986.

41 Pumarola-Sune T et al: HIV antigen in the brains of patients with the AIDS dementia complex. *Ann Neurol* 21:490–496, 1987.

42 Kure K et al: Cellular localization of an HIV-1 antigen in subacute AIDS encephalitis using an improved double-labeling immunohistochemical method. *Am J Pathol* 136:1085–1092, 1990.

43 Nuovo GJ et al: In situ detection of polymerase chain reaction-amplified HIV-1 nucleic acids and tumor necrosis factor-alpha RNA in the central nervous system. *Am J Pathol* 144:659–666, 1994.

44 Esiri MM et al: Fate of oligodendrocytes in HIV-1 infection. *AIDS* 5:1081–1088, 1991.

45 Esiri MM, Morris CS: Cellular basis of HIV infection of the CNS and the AIDS dementia complex: Oligodendrocyte. *J Neuro-AIDS* 1(1):133–160, 1996.

46 Tornatore C et al: HIV-1 infection of subcortical astrocytes in the pediatric central nervous system. *Neurology* 44:481–487, 1994.

47 Saito Y et al: Overexpression of *nef* as a marker for restricted HIV-1 infection of astrocytes in postmortem pediatric central nervous tissues. *Neurology* 44:474–481, 1994.

48 Ranki A et al: Abundant expression of HIV nef and rev proteins in brain astrocytes in vivo is associated with dementia. *AIDS* 9:1001–1008, 1995.

49 Moses AV et al: HIV infection of the brain microvasculature and its contribution to the AIDS dementia complex. *J Neuro-AIDS* 1(1): 85–99, 1996.

49a Lanier ER et al: CSF HIV RNA: Relationship to HIV-associated neurological disease (abstract We.B.3287). Presented at the XIth International Conference on AIDS, Vancouver, BC, Canada, July 7–12, 1996.

49b Brew BJ et al: Cerebrospinal fluid (CSF) HIV-1 RNA levels correlate with AIDS dementia complex (ADC) (abstract Mo.B.314). Presented at the XIth International Conference on AIDS, Vancouver, BC, Canada, July 7–12, 1996.

49c Pratt RD et al: Virologic markers of human immunodeficiency virus type 1 in cerebrospinal fluid of infected children. *J Infect Dis* 174: 288–293, 1996.

49d Sei S et al: Evaluation of human immunodeficiency virus (HIV) type 1 RNA levels in cerebrospinal fluid and viral resistance to zidovudine in children with HIV encephalopathy. *J Infect Dis* 174:1200–1206, 1996.

50 Glass JD et al: Clinical-neuropathologic correlation in HIV-associated dementia. *Neurology* 43:2230–2237, 1993.

51 Brew BJ et al: AIDS dementia complex and HIV-1 brain infection: Clinical-virological correlations. *Ann Neurol* 38:563–570, 1995.

52 Glass JD et al: Immunocytochemical quantitation of human immunodeficiency virus in the brain: Correlations with dementia. *Ann Neurol* 38:755–762, 1995.

53 Everall IP et al: Neuronal loss in the frontal cortex in HIV infection. *Lancet* 337:1119–1121, 1991.

54 Wiley CA et al: Neocortical damage during HIV infection. *Ann Neurol* 29:651–657, 1991.

55 Masliah E et al: Spectrum of human immunodeficiency virus-associated neocortical damage. *Ann Neurol* 32:321–329, 1992.

56 Oster S et al: Six billion neurons lost in AIDS: A stereological study of the neocortex. *APMIS* 103:525–529, 1995.

57 Masliah E et al: Patterns of neurodegeneration in HIV encephalitis. *J Neuro-AIDS* 1(1):161–173, 1996.

58 Asare E et al: Neuronal pattern correlates with the severity of human immunodeficiency virus-associated dementia complex: Usefulness of spatial pattern analysis in clinicopathological studies. *Am J Pathol* 148:31–38, 1996.

59 Brenneman DE et al: Neuronal cell killing by the envelope protein of HIV and its prevention by vasoactive intestinal peptide. *Nature* 335:639–642, 1988.

60 Dreyer EB et al: HIV-1 coat protein neurotoxicity prevented by calcium channel antagonists. *Science* 248:364–367, 1990.

61 Toggas SM et al: Central nervous system damage produced by expression of the HIV-1 coat protein gp120 in transgenic mice. *Nature* 367:188–193, 1994.

62 Sabatier JM et al: Evidence for neurotoxic activity of tat from human immunodeficiency virus type 1. *J Virol* 65:961–967, 1991.

63 Kolson DL et al: HIV-1 tat alters normal organization of neurons and astrocytes in primary rodent brain cell cultures: RGD sequence dependence. *AIDS Res Hum Retroviruses* 9:677–685, 1993.

64 Magnuson DSK et al: Human immunodeficiency virus type 1 tat activates non-*N*-methyl-D-aspartate excitatory amino acid receptors and causes neurotoxicity. *Ann Neurol* 37:373–380, 1995.

65 Nath A et al: Identification of a human immunodeficiency virus type 1 tat epitope that is neuroexcitatory and neurotoxic. *J Virol* 70: 1475–1480, 1996.

66 Heyes MP et al: Quinolinic acid in cerebrospinal fluid and serum in HIV-1 infection: Relationship to clinical and neurological status. *Ann Neurol* 29:202–209, 1991.

67 Sei S et al: Increased human immunodeficiency virus (HIV) type 1 DNA content and quinolinic acid concentration in brain tissues from patients with HIV encephalopathy. *J Infect Dis* 172:638–647, 1995.

68 Tyor WR et al: Cytokine expression in the brain during the acquired immunodeficiency syndrome. *Ann Neurol* 31:349–360, 1992.

69 Genis P et al: Cytokines and arachidonic metabolites produced during human immunodeficiency virus (HIV)-infected macrophage-astroglia interactions: Implications of the neuropathogenesis of HIV disease. *J Exp Med* 176:1703–1718, 1992.

70 Wesselingh SL et al: Intracerebral cytokine messenger RNA expression in acquired immunodeficiency syndrome dementia. *Ann Neurol* 33:576–582, 1993.

71 Wilt SG et al: In vitro evidence for a dual role of tumor necrosis

factor-alpha in human immunodeficiency virus type 1 encephalopathy. *Ann Neurol* 37:381–394, 1995.

72 Griffin DE et al: Elevated central nervous system prostaglandins in human immunodeficiency virus-associated dementia. *Ann Neurol* 35: 592–597, 1994.

73 Gelbard HA et al: Platelet-activating factor: A candidate human immunodeficiency virus type 1-induced neurotoxin. *J Virol* 68: 4628–4635, 1994.

74 Dawson VL et al: Human immunodeficiency virus type 1 coat protein neurotoxicity mediated by nitric oxide in primary cortical cultures. *Proc Natl Acad Sci USA* 90:3256–3259, 1993.

75 Bukrinsky MI et al: Regulation of nitric oxide synthase activity in human immunodeficiency virus type 1 (HIV-1)-infected monocytes: Implications for HIV-associated neurological disease. *J Exp Med* 181:735–745, 1995.

76 Epstein LG, Gendelman HE: Human immunodeficiency virus type 1 infection of the nervous system: Pathogenetic mechanisms. *Ann Neurol* 33:429–436, 1993.

77 Pulliam L et al: HIV-1 envelope gp120 alters astrocytes in human brain cultures. *AIDS Res Hum Retroviruses* 9:439–444, 1993.

78 Lipton SA, Gendelman HE: Dementia associated with the acquired immunodeficiency syndrome. *N Engl J Med* 332:934–940, 1995.

79 Tyor WR et al: Unifying hypothesis for the pathogenesis of HIV-associated dementia complex, vacuolar myelopathy, and sensory neuropathy. *J Acquir Immune Defic Syndr Hum Retrovirol* 9:379–388, 1995.

80 Price RW: The cellular basis of central nervous system HIV-1 infection and the AIDS dementia complex: Introduction. *J Neuro-AIDS* 1(1):1–29, 1996.

81 Lipton SA: Calcium channel antagonists and human immunodeficiency virus coat protein-mediated neuronal injury. *Ann Neurol* 30: 110–114, 1991.

82 Lipton SA: Memantine prevents HIV coat protein-induced neuronal injury in vitro. *Neurology* 42:1403–1405, 1992.

83 Perovic S et al: The triaminopyridine flupirtine prevents cell death in rat cortical cells induced by *N*-methyl-D-aspartate and gp120 of HIV-1. *Eur J Pharmacol* 288:27–33, 1994.

84 Tross S et al: Neuropsychological characterization of the AIDS dementia complex: A preliminary report. *AIDS* 2:81–88, 1988.

85 Dal Pan GJ et al: Patterns of cerebral atrophy in HIV-1-infected individuals: Results of a quantitative MRI analysis. *Neurology* 42: 2125–2130, 1992.

86 Aylward EH et al: Reduced basal ganglia volume in HIV-1-associated dementia: Results from quantitative neuroimaging. *Neurology* 43:2099–2104, 1993.

87 Hestad K et al: Regional brain atrophy in HIV-1 infection: Association with specific neuropsychological test performance. *Acta Neurol Scand* 88:112–118, 1993.

88 McArthur JC et al and the Multicenter AIDS Cohort Study: Incidental white matter hyperintensities on magnetic resonance imaging in HIV-1 infection. *J Acquir Immune Defic Syndr* 3:252–259, 1990.

89 Cohen WA et al: Prospective cerebral magnetic resonance study of HIV seropositive and seronegative men: Correlation of MR findings with neurological, neuropsychological, and cerebrospinal fluid analysis. *Am J Neuroradiol* 13:1231–1240, 1992.

90 Dooneief G et al: A prospective controlled study of magnetic resonance imaging of the brain in gay men and parenteral drug users with human immunodeficiency virus infection. *Arch Neurol* 49:38–43, 1992.

91 Appleman ME et al: Cerebrospinal fluid abnormalities in patients without AIDS who are seropositive for the human immunodeficiency virus. *J Infect Dis* 158:193–199, 1988.

92 Collier AC et al: Central nervous system manifestations in human immunodeficiency virus infection without AIDS. *J Acquir Immune Defic Syndr* 5:229–241, 1992.

93 Brew BJ et al: Cerebrospinal fluid HIV-1 p24 antigen and culture: Sensitivity and specificity for AIDS-dementia complex. *J Neurol Neurosurg Psychiatry* 57:784–789, 1994.

94 Royal W III et al: Cerebrospinal fluid human immunodeficiency virus type 1 (HIV-1) p24 antigen levels in HIV-1-related dementia. *Ann Neurol* 36:32–39, 1994.

95 Sönnerborg AB et al: Elevated neopterin and beta-2-microglobulin levels in blood and cerebrospinal fluid occur early in HIV-1 infection. *AIDS* 3:277–283, 1989.

96 Brew BJ et al: Cerebrospinal fluid neopterin in human immunodeficiency virus type 1 infection. *Ann Neurol* 28:556–560, 1990.

97 Griffin DE et al: Neopterin and interferon-gamma in serum and cerebrospinal fluid of patients with HIV-associated neurologic disease. *Neurology* 41:69–74, 1991.

98 Brew BJ et al: Cerebrospinal fluid beta-2-microglobulin in patients infected with human immunodeficiency virus. *Neurology* 39:830–834, 1989.

99 Brew BJ et al: Cerebrospinal fluid beta-2-microglobulin in patients with AIDS dementia complex: An expanded series including response to zidovudine treatment. *AIDS* 6:461–465, 1992.

100 McArthur JC et al for the Multicenter AIDS Cohort Study: The diagnostic utility of elevation in cerebrospinal fluid beta-2-microglobulin in HIV-1 dementia. *Neurology* 42:1707–1712, 1992.

101 Petito CK et al: Neuropathology of acquired immunodeficiency syndrome (AIDS): An autopsy review. *J Neuropathol Exp Neurol* 45: 635–646, 1986.

102 Morgello S et al: Cytomegalovirus encephalitis in patients with acquired immunodeficiency syndrome: An autopsy study of 30 cases and a review of the literature. *Hum Pathol* 18:289–297, 1987.

103 Cinque P et al: Cytomegalovirus infection of the central nervous system in patients with AIDS: Diagnosis by DNA amplification from cerebrospinal fluid. *J Infect Dis* 166:1408–1411, 1992.

104 Wolf DG, Spector SA: Diagnosis of human cytomegalovirus central nervous system disease in AIDS patients by DNA amplification from cerebrospinal fluid. *J Infect Dis* 166:1412–1415, 1992.

105 Gozlan J et al: Rapid detection of cytomegalovirus DNA in cerebrospinal fluid of AIDS patients with neurologic disorders. *J Infect Dis* 166:1416–1421, 1992.

106 Achim CL et al: Detection of cytomegalovirus in cerebrospinal fluid autopsy specimens from AIDS patients. *J Infect Dis* 169:623–627, 1994.

107 Arribas JR et al: Level of cytomegalovirus (CMV) DNA in cerebrospinal fluid of subjects with AIDS and CMV infection of the central nervous system. *J Infect Dis* 172:527–531, 1995.

108 Cinque P et al: Ganciclovir therapy for cytomegalovirus (CMV) infection of the central nervous system in AIDS patients: Monitoring by CMV DNA detection in cerebrospinal fluid. *J Infect Dis* 171: 1603–1606, 1995.

109 Cohen BA: Prognosis and response to therapy of cytomegalovirus encephalitis and meningomyelitis in AIDS. *Neurology* 46:444–450, 1996.

110 Gray F et al: Diffuse "encephalitic" cerebral toxoplasmosis in AIDS. *J Neurol* 236:273–277, 1989.

111 Arendt G et al: Two cases of cerebral toxoplasmosis in AIDS patients mimicking HIV-related dementia. *J Neurol* 238:439–442, 1991.

112 Artigas J et al: Anergic disseminated toxoplasmosis in a patient with acquired immunodeficiency syndrome. *Arch Pathol Lab Med* 117: 540–541, 1993.

113 Musher DM: Syphilis, neurosyphilis, penicillin, and AIDS. *J Infect Dis* 163:1201–1206, 1991.

114 Chuck SL, Sande MA: Infections with *Cryptococcus neoformans* in the acquired immunodeficiency syndrome. *N Engl J Med* 321:794–799, 1989.

115 Berger JR et al: Progressive multifocal leukoencephalopathy associated with human immunodeficiency virus infection: A review of the literature with a report of sixteen cases. *Ann Intern Med* 107: 78–87, 1987.

116 Schwartzman WA et al: *Rochalimaea* antibodies in HIV-associated neurologic disease. *Neurology* 44:1312–1316, 1994.

117 Schwartzman WA et al: *Bartonella (Rochalimaea)* antibodies, de-

mentia, and cat ownership among men with human immunodeficiency virus. *Clin Infect Dis* 21:954–959, 1995.

118 Knox KK, Carrigan DR: Active human herpesvirus (HHV-6) infection of the central nervous system in patients with AIDS. *J Acquir Immune Defic Syndr Hum Retrovirol* 9:69–73, 1995.

119 Portegies P et al: Declining incidence of AIDS dementia complex after introduction of zidovudine treatment. *Br Med J* 299:819–821, 1989.

120 Baldeweg T et al: Long-term zidovudine reduces neurocognitive deficits in HIV-1 infection. *AIDS* 9:589–596, 1995.

121 Gray F et al: Zidovudine therapy and HIV encephalitis: A 10-year neuropathological survey. *AIDS* 8:489–493, 1994.

122 Vago L et al: Reduced frequency of HIV-induced brain lesions in AIDS patients treated with zidovudine. *J Acquir Immune Defic Syndr* 6:42–45, 1993.

123 Wildemann B et al: In vivo comparison of zidovudine resistance mutations in blood and CSF of HIV-1-infected patients. *Neurology* 43:2659–2663, 1993.

124 Di Stefano M et al: Zidovudine-resistant variants of HIV-1 in brain. *Lancet* 342:865, 1993.

125 Portegies P et al: AIDS dementia complex and didanosine. *Lancet* 344:759, 1994.

126 Chrétien F et al: Protection of human immunodeficiency virus encephalitis by a switch from zidovudine to didanosine (letter). *Antimicrob Agents Chemother* 40:278, 1996.

126a Gisslén M et al: The effect on human immunodeficiency virus type 1 RNA levels in cerebrospinal fluid after initiation of zidovudine or didanosine. *J Infect Dis* 175:434–437, 1997.

126b Foudraine N et al: CSF and serum HIV-RNA levels during AZT/3TC and d4T/3TC treatment (abstract LB5). Presented at the 4th Conference on Retroviruses and Opportunistic Infections, Washington, DC, Jan 22–26, 1997.

127 Yarchoan R et al: Response of human immunodeficiency virus-associated neurological disease to 3′-azido-3′-deoxythymidine. *Lancet* 1:132–135, 1987.

128 Pizzo PA et al: Effect of continuous intravenous infusion of zidovudine (AZT) in children with symptomatic HIV infection. *N Engl J Med* 319:889–896, 1988.

129 Yarchoan R et al: Long-term administration of 3′-azido-2′,3′-dideoxythymidine to patients with AIDS-related neurological disease. *Ann Neurol* 23(suppl):S82-S87, 1988.

130 Reinvang I et al: Only temporary improvement in impaired neuropsychological function in AIDS patients treated with zidovudine (letter). *AIDS* 5:228–229, 1991.

131 Tozzi V et al: Effects of zidovudine in 30 patients with mild to end-stage AIDS dementia complex. *AIDS* 7:683–692, 1993.

132 Sidtis JJ et al and the AIDS Clinical Trials Group: Zidovudine treatment of the AIDS dementia complex: Results of a placebo-controlled trial. *Ann Neurol* 33:343–349, 1993.

133 Yarchoan R et al: Long-term toxicity/activity profile of 2′,3′-dideoxyinosine in AIDS or AIDS-related complex. *Lancet* 336:526–529, 1990.

134 Brouwers P et al: Effect of continuous-infusion zidovudine therapy on neuropsychologic functioning in children with symptomatic human immunodeficiency virus infection. *J Pediatr* 117:980–985, 1990.

135 Butler KM et al: Dideoxyinosine in children with symptomatic human immunodeficiency virus infection. *N Engl J Med* 324:137–144, 1991.

136 Lipton SA et al and the AIDS Clinical Trials Group: Double-blinded, randomized, placebo-controlled trial of the calcium channel antagonist nimodipine for the neurological manifestations of acquired immunodeficiency syndrome, including dementia and painful neuropathy (abstract). *Ann Neurol* 38:347, 1995.

137 Herzlich BC, Schiano TD: Reversal of apparent AIDS dementia complex following treatment with vitamin B_{12}. *J Int Med* 233:495–497, 1993.

138 Shor-Posner G et al: Plasma cobalamin levels affect information processing speed in a longitudinal study of HIV-1 disease. *Arch Neurol* 52:195–198, 1995.

139 Kieburtz KD et al: Excitotoxicity and dopaminergic dysfunction in the acquired immunodeficiency syndrome dementia complex: Therapeutic implications. *Arch Neurol* 48:1281–1284, 1991.

140 Brown GR: The use of methylphenidate for cognitive decline associated with HIV disease. *Int J Psychiatry Med* 25:21–37, 1995.

141 Boccellari A, Zeifert P: Management of neurobehavioral impairment in HIV-1 infection. *Psychiatr Clin North Am* 17:183–203, 1994.

142 Portegies P: HIV-1, the brain, and combination therapy (editorial). *Lancet* 346:1244–1245, 1995.

143 Goldstick L et al: Spinal cord degeneration in AIDS. *Neurology* 35:103–106, 1985.

144 Petito CK et al: Vacuolar myelopathy pathologically resembling subacute combined degeneration in patients with the acquired immunodeficiency syndrome. *N Engl J Med* 312:874–879, 1985.

145 Tan SV et al: AIDS-associated vacuolar myelopathy: A morphometric study. *Brain* 118:1247–1261, 1995.

146 Dal Pan GJ et al: Clinicopathologic correlations of HIV-1-associated vacuolar myelopathy: An autopsy-based case-control study. *Neurology* 44:2159–2164, 1994.

147 Helweg-Larsen S et al: Myelopathy in AIDS: A clinical and electrophysiological study of 23 Danish patients. *Acta Neurol Scand* 77:64–73, 1988.

148 Kieburtz KD et al: Abnormal vitamin B_{12} metabolism in human immunodeficiency virus infection: Association with neurological dysfunction. *Arch Neurol* 48:312–314, 1991.

149 Grafe MR, Wiley CA: Spinal cord and peripheral nerve pathology in AIDS: The roles of cytomegalovirus and human immunodeficiency virus. *Ann Neurol* 25:561–566, 1989.

150 Artigas J et al: Vacuolar myelopathy in AIDS: A morphological analysis. *Pathol Res Pract* 186:228–237, 1990.

151 Hénin D et al: Neuropathology of the spinal cord in the acquired immunodeficiency syndrome. *Hum Pathol* 23:1106–1114, 1992.

152 Petito CK et al: HIV antigen and DNA in AIDS spinal cords correlate with macrophage infiltration but not with vacuolar myelopathy. *J Neuropathol Exp Neurol* 53:86–94, 1994.

153 Ho DD et al: Isolation of HTLV-III from cerebrospinal fluid and neural tissues of patients with neurologic syndromes related to the acquired immunodeficiency syndrome. *N Engl J Med* 313:1493–1497, 1985.

154 Rosenblum M et al: Dissociation of AIDS-related vacuolar myelopathy and productive HIV-1 infection of the spinal cord. *Neurology* 39:892–896, 1989.

155 Tyor WR et al: Cytokine expression of macrophages in HIV-1-associated vacuolar myelopathy. *Neurology* 43:1002–1009, 1993.

156 Satya-Murti S et al: The spectrum of neurologic disorder from vitamin E deficiency. *Neurology* 36:917–921, 1986.

157 Kamin SS, Petito CK: Idiopathic myelopathies with white matter vacuolation in non-acquired immunodeficiency syndrome patients. *Hum Pathol* 22:816–824, 1991.

158 Tucker T et al: Cytomegalovirus and herpes simplex virus ascending myelitis in a patient with acquired immune deficiency syndrome. *Ann Neurol* 18:74–79, 1985.

159 Britton CB et al: A new complication of AIDS: Thoracic myelitis caused by herpes simplex virus. *Neurology* 35:1071–1074, 1985.

160 Gray F et al: Varicella-zoster virus infection of the central nervous system in the acquired immune deficiency syndrome. *Brain* 117:987–999, 1994.

161 Lionnet F et al: Myelitis due to varicella-zoster virus in two patients with AIDS: Successful treatment with acyclovir. *Clin Infect Dis* 22:138–140, 1994.

162 Jacobson MA et al: Failure of antiviral therapy for acquired immunodeficiency syndrome-related cytomegalovirus myelitis. *Arch Neurol* 45:1090–1092, 1988.

163 Mahieux F et al: Acute myeloradiculitis due to cytomegalovirus as the initial manifestation of AIDS. *J Neurol Neurosurg Psychiatry* 52:270–274, 1989.

164 de Gans J et al: Therapy for cytomegalovirus polyradiculomyelitis in patients with AIDS: Treatment with ganciclovir. *AIDS* 4:421–425, 1990.

165 Bélec L et al: Cytomegalovirus (CMV) encephalomyeloradiculitis and human immunodeficiency virus (HIV) encephalitis: Presence of HIV and CMV co-infected multinucleated giant cells. *Acta Neuropathol* 81:99–104, 1990.

166 Mehren M et al: Toxoplasmic myelitis mimicking intramedullary spinal cord tumor. *Neurology* 38:1648–1650, 1988.

167 Kayser C et al: Toxoplasmosis of the conus medullaris in a patient with hemophilia A-associated AIDS. *J Neurosurg* 73:951–953, 1990.

168 Overhage JM et al: Conus medullaris syndrome resulting from *Toxoplasma gondii* infection in a patient with the acquired immunodeficiency syndrome. *Am J Med* 89:814–815, 1990.

169 Resnick DK et al: Isolated toxoplasmosis of the thoracic spinal cord in a patient with acquired immunodeficiency syndrome. *J Neurosurg* 82:493–496, 1995.

170 Woolsey RM et al: Mycobacterial meningomyelitis associated with human immunodeficiency virus infection. *Arch Neurol* 45:691–693, 1988.

171 Rosenblum MK et al: Human T-lymphotropic virus type I-associated myelopathy in patients with the acquired immunodeficiency syndrome. *Hum Pathol* 23:513–519, 1992.

172 Berger JR: Spinal cord syphilis associated with human immunodeficiency virus infection: A treatable myelopathy. *Am J Med* 92:101–103, 1992.

173 Barakos JA et al: MR imaging of acute transverse myelitis and AIDS myelopathy. *J Comput Assist Tomogr* 14:45–50, 1990.

174 von Wichmann MA et al: Good response to azidothymidine in 3 patients with vacuolar myelopathy. *Med Clin Barc* 94:664–665, 1990.

175 Di Rocco A et al: Methionine treatment for AIDS-associated vacuolar myelopathy (abstract). *Neurology* (Suppl) 46:A464, 1996.

176 Hall CD et al: Peripheral neuropathy in a cohort of human immunodeficiency virus-infected patients: Incidence and relationship to other nervous system dysfunction. *Arch Neurol* 48:1273–1274, 1991.

177 Mehta P et al and the HIV Neurobehavioral Research Center, San Diego, CA: HIV-related distal sensorimotor polyneuropathy: Results from the HIV Neurobehavioral Research Center Study Cohort (abstract). *Ann Neurol* 36:286–287, 1994.

178 Barohn RJ et al: Peripheral nervous system involvement in a large cohort of human immunodeficiency virus-infected individuals. *Arch Neurol* 50:167–171, 1993.

179 Rance NE et al: Gracile tract degeneration in patients with sensory neuropathy and AIDS. *Neurology* 38:265–271, 1988.

180 Scaravilli F et al: The pathology of the posterior root ganglia in AIDS and its relationship to the pallor of the gracile tract. *Acta Neuropathol* 84:163–170, 1992.

181 Esiri MM et al: Sensory and sympathetic ganglia in HIV-1 infection: Immunocytochemical demonstration of HIV-1 viral antigens, increased MHC class II antigen expression and mild reactive inflammation. *J Neurol Sci* 114:178–187, 1993.

182 Griffin JW et al: Peripheral nerve disorders in HIV infection: Similarities and contrasts with CNS disorders. *Res Pub Assoc Res Nerv Ment Dis* 72:159–182, 1994.

183 Fuller GN et al: Association of painful peripheral neuropathy in AIDS with cytomegalovirus infection. *Lancet* 2:937–941, 1989.

184 Zehender G et al: High prevalence of human T cell lymphotropic virus type II infection in patients affected by human immunodeficiency virus type 1-associated predominantly sensory polyneuropathy. *J Infect Dis* 172:1595–1598, 1995.

185 Chaunu MP et al: The spectrum of changes on 20 nerve biopsies in patients with HIV infection. *Muscle Nerve* 12:452–459, 1989.

186 Miller RG: Neuropathies and myopathies complicating HIV infection. *J Clin Apheresis* 6:110–121, 1991.

187 Simpson DM, Tagliati M: Nucleoside analogue-associated peripheral neuropathy in human immunodeficiency virus infection. *J Acquir Immune Defic Synd Hum Retrovirol* 9:153–161, 1995.

188 Kieburtz KD et al: Extended follow-up of peripheral neuropathy in patients with AIDS and AIDS-related complex treated with dideoxyinosine. *J Acquir Immune Defic Syndr* 5:60–64, 1992.

189 Berger AR et al: 2′,3′-dideoxycytidine (ddC) toxic neuropathy: A study of 52 patients. *Neurology* 43:358–362, 1993.

190 Fichtenbaum CJ et al: Risk factors for dideoxynucleoside-induced toxic neuropathy in patients with the human immunodeficiency virus infection. *J Acquir Immune Defic Syndr Hum Retrovirol* 10: 169–174, 1995.

191 LeLacheur SF, Simon GL: Exacerbation of dideoxycytidine-induced neuropathy with dideoxyinosine. *J Acquir Immune Defic Syndr* 4: 538–539, 1991.

192 Blum AS et al: Low dose zalcitabine-related toxic neuropathy: Frequency, natural history, and risk factors. *Neurology* 46:999–1003, 1996.

193 Weissman JD: An open-label trial of mexiletine, nortriptyline, and capsaicin in HIV neuropathy (abstract). *Neurology* (Suppl) 46: A463, 1996.

PART VIII STD/HIV IN REPRODUCTIVE HEALTH AND PEDIATRICS

Chapter 78

Contraception, contraceptive technology, and STDs

Willard Cates, Jr.

INTRODUCTION

Using contraception has two main benefits[1–6]: prevention of unplanned pregnancies and protection against sexually transmitted diseases (STDs). Abstinence from sexual intercourse provides nearly absolute protection against both outcomes. For those choosing to be sexually active, contraception reduces, but does not eliminate, the risk of either pregnancy and/or STDs. Unfortunately, the contraceptives with the best record for pregnancy prevention provide minimal STD protection. Some contraceptives may even raise the risk of certain infections.

Moreover, the interaction of contraception and STDs cuts both ways: Not only does choice of contraception affect the risk of STDs, but also the perception of STD risk affects contraceptive choice. Thus, decisions about contraception by individuals, communities, and policymakers should involve balancing the relative need to prevent both unplanned pregnancies and STDs.

At the personal level, contraceptive *use* by couples is affected by the perceived risks and costs of STDs and/or pregnancy.[7] These involve such complex *individual* factors as rate of sex partner change, partner selection, coital frequency, timing of coitus within the menstrual cycle, safety of the contraceptive method, availability of the method, cost of the method, and acceptance of the method by the sex partner.[8]

At the community level, contraceptive *acceptance* is affected by the social norms of particular cultures.[9,10] This involves such complex *community* factors as the relative value of fertility within specific societies, local customs about sexual activity at early ages, community pressures on teenagers to bear children, societal norms about genital manipulation, and religious proscriptions against use of particular contraceptives.

At the policy level, contraceptive *emphasis* by policymakers is affected by the aggregate risks and costs of STDs and unplanned pregnancies in that particular society.[3] These involve such complex *public-health* factors as the local prevalence of sexually transmitted infections and unplanned pregnancies, the level of unprotected sexual activity, the political acceptance of individual choice over sexual and reproductive decisions, and the economic capacity of the society to support the existing population growth rate. Until the current pandemic of human-immunodeficiency virus (HIV), most national and international contraceptive policies had tended to downplay the risks of STD/HIV relative to those of unplanned pregnancy.

The choice of contraception is further complicated when considering its longer-range reproductive implications. Contraceptive use has an influence on not only the acute risks of STDs and unplanned pregnancy but also on the eventual reproductive capacity of those making contraceptive decisions. Therefore, personal choices, community programs, and/or policy decisions made in the short run to prevent STDs and unplanned pregnancies can simultaneously improve (or harm) chances of planned procreation in the long run.[11,12]

THE EFFECT OF STD/HIV ON CONTRACEPTIVE USE

Concerns about STDs can affect contraceptive choice and family planning services from a variety of perspectives.[13] At the clinical level, the impact of managing a client with a potential acute STD depends on whether the infection is symptomatic or asymptomatic, whether the infection is curable, and what STD services are available from the contraceptive provider. If the infection is symptomatic, it should be diagnosed and treated during the same patient visit in which contraceptive services are requested; in the absence of laboratory facilities, clinical algorithms (albeit imperfect) have been helpful.[13,14] If no symptoms are present, the visit by sexually active women to family planning providers offers an opportunity to screen for asymptomatic infections that can be treated in the lower genital tract before they result in complications.

In developed countries, contraceptive providers already play a key role in detecting STDs. More STD screening occurs during routine family planning visits in the United States than through any other type of health care.[15] The benefit-to-cost ratio of STD screening in family planning clinics, especially in areas where STDs have a low prevalence, can be improved by using a variety of factors to increase yield.[16–18] For example, if the patient has a new sex partner, this should trigger both screening for current lower-genital-tract infection and also counseling regarding safer sexual practices to reduce future risks of becoming infected. If the woman is found to have a current STD, not only should she be immediately treated, but also barrier contraceptive methods should be encouraged and intrauterine devices (IUDs) discouraged.

In resource-poor settings, the same criteria can be used to both initiate presumptive STD treatment and guide contraceptive choice (Fig. 78-1). The mix of demographic, behavioral, and clinical factors that predict STD risk form a continuum to aid family planning providers in managing their clients more appropriately.[13] For example, clients with a high likelihood of being currently infected (symptoms, recent exposure to an infected partner) can be treated on epidemiologic indications. Likewise, clients with a low probability of being infected could be considered candidates for an IUD.

At the operational level, the increasing provision of an array of STD services by family planning providers has squeezed limited budgets.[19] During the 1980s, those facilities in the United States offering contraceptive care using federal Title X funds saw their financial resources decline, while the spectrum of additional services required by their clients increased. By 1990, Pap smears for cervical cancer, risk assessment for HIV infection, and screening for bacterial STDs had become part of routine family planning care. For example, in 1990, more than 90 percent of family planning clinics reported screening for gonorrhea as well as treating infected patients and referring for partner notification. Two-thirds of family planning providers did the same for chlamydia.[20] Because of these pressures to offer more clinical services to the increasing number of patients with STDs, time and money available for contraceptive care declined proportionately.[19]

At the community level, some hypothesize that STDs may have a negative impact on family planning programs.[17] High prevalence of sexually transmitted infections can serve to decrease acceptance and/or continuation of family planning methods directly and indirectly. (1) Directly—STDs, if perceived as a complication of contraceptive methods, may result in nonuse or discontinuation of the methods. For example, trends in IUD use have been directly related to adverse publicity and litigation about its risks of upper-genital-tract infection. Likewise, in some countries use of hormonal methods has been affected by its potential association with HIV acquisition. (2) Indirectly—STDs, by compromising healthy childbearing in a community, may hinder any willingness

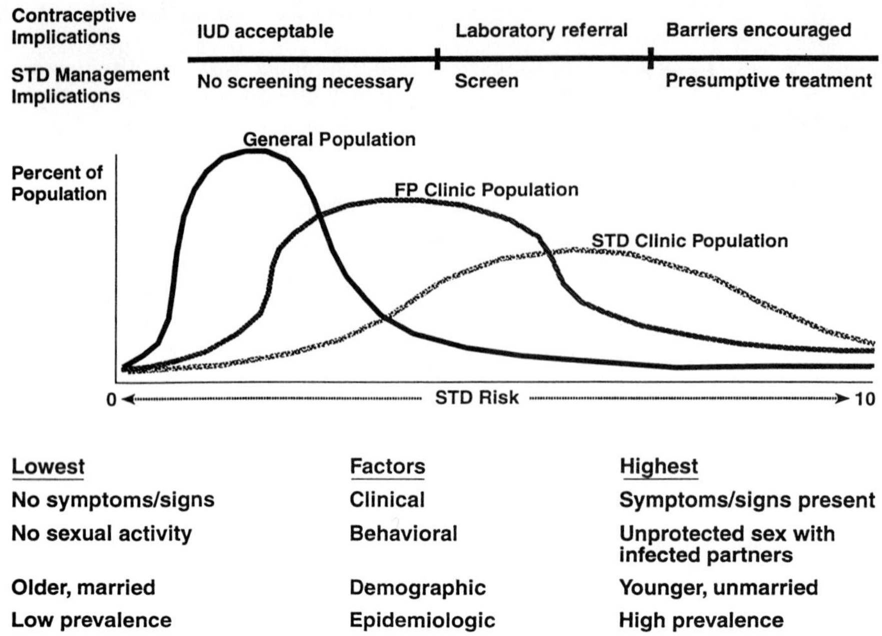

Fig. 78-1. Estimated levels of STD risk among different populations—implications on contraceptive and STD management. Adapted from Cates, 1997.[13]

to delay initial childbearing or space out live births.[9] In addition, in regions with high HIV prevalence, perceptions of shortened duration of life expectancy may accelerate desires to achieve the desired family size at an early age.

These direct and indirect perceptions of sexually transmitted infection can be addressed by effective community health/education programs and by improvements in the quality of family planning services. The 1994 International Conference on Population and Development in Cairo emphasized that provision of clinical services to reduce STDs in family planning settings will be regarded as essential for ensuring a healthy reproductive future.[21]

THE EFFECT OF CONTRACEPTIVE USE ON STD/HIV

The recent scientific literature has been replete with reviews of the effects of different contraceptives on the risk of STDs/HIV.[1–6,22–25] In general, they all come to the same conclusion (Table 78-1). Male condoms used correctly and consistently provide good protection against most STDs, both bacterial and viral. Spermicides alone and combinations of mechanical/chemical barrier methods can provide modest protection against bacterial STDs. Hormonal contraception may enhance some cervical infections, but its impact on *upper*-genital-tract infection and HIV is

Table 78-1. STD and Contraceptive Efficacy

Method	Effect on STD Acquisition	Contraceptive Effectiveness with Typical Use*
Barrier Methods:		
Male condom	Protects against STDs, including HIV	85–95%
Female condom	May protect against STDs; method under study	75–82%
Spermicide (nonoxynol-9 [N-9])	Protects modestly against bacterial STDs; no effect on HIV; effect on other viral STDs unknown	60–85%
Diaphragm with spermicide (N-9)	Protects against bacterial STDs; increased risk of bacterial vaginosis; effect on HIV unknown; protects against cervical neoplasia	80–95%
Hormonal Methods:		
Oral contraceptives	No protection against lower-genital-tract infections; protects against symptomatic PID; may increase risk of cervical chlamydia; effect on HIV under study	97%
Implant (Norplant)	No protection; added risk unknown	>99%
Injection (DMPA, NET-EN)	No protection; added risk unknown	>99%
Other Methods:		
Intrauterine device	No protection; increase of PID risk in first month after insertion	>97%
Surgical sterilization (vasectomy and tubal ligation)	No protection against lower-genital-tract infections; tubal ligation may reduce risk of PID	>99%

* Refers to the percentage of women relying on the method who will not become pregnant during first year of typical use (including inconsistent and incorrect use).

Adapted from Cates and Stone (1992)[1] and Trussel, Hatcher, Cates (1990).[45]

still unsettled. The IUD is associated with acute pelvic inflammatory disease (PID), albeit primarily during the interval after its insertion.

MALE CONDOMS

Condom quality, use, and effectiveness have been recently reviewed.[26–28] If men are willing to use them properly, condoms protect against transmission of STDs by preventing direct contact with semen, genital discharge, some genital lesions, or infectious secretions. To be effective, condoms must be applied prior to genital contact, must remain intact, and most important, must be used *consistently and correctly*.[26]

Laboratory studies confirm that latex and polyurethane condoms provide an impervious barrier to most STD pathogens. In experimental transmission models, condoms have been shown to be effective barriers against herpes simplex virus (HSV),[29] *Chlamydia trachomatis*,[29] HIV,[30] and low-molecular-weight dyes in aqueous solutions.[31] "Natural membrane" condoms, made of sheep intestinal membrane, may not be as effective as synthetic condoms. HIV, hepatitis B (HBV), and HSV may pass through natural membrane condoms,[32] whose permeability may relate to the size of pores in the membranes.

Men are protected, even against the more easily transmissible STDs, by using condoms. For example, among Australian soldiers returning from Vietnam, those who had used condoms were significantly less likely to have reported having had an STD than were those who had not.[33] In the Philippines,[34] no seamen who reported using condoms consistently while in port acquired gonorrhea or nongonococcal urethritis. In Sacramento, California,[35] men attending an STD clinic were given free condoms and then examined 3 months later. Those who always used condoms had less risk of gonorrhea than did men who never used them, although traditional statistical significance was not achieved. These data taken together are consistent with an increasing body of knowledge indicating that condoms are protective.

Epidemiologic studies show that women are protected by male condoms against some STDs as well, although the data are more equivocal. This may be due, in part, to the wider variety of organisms studied and the varying consistency of the partners' condom use. In Costa Rica, women whose partners used condoms had significantly lower risks of being infected with HSV-2 than those whose partners used other methods.[36] Among these women, longer duration of condom use was associated with an increasing protective effect against HSV-2 infection. For example, in Colorado, women attending STD clinics whose partners had used condoms during the previous month were less likely to have gonorrhea or trichomoniasis, but they were just as likely to have chlamydia or bacterial vaginosis.[37] In Kenya,[38] sex workers who reported using condoms all the time had less than one-fifth the risk of acquiring genital ulcers than those who never used condoms. Because HIV infection confounded the association, the protective impact of condoms on genital ulcer disease was not readily apparent until the data were adjusted for HIV status.

Much recent work has evaluated the male condom's influence in protecting against HIV (Fig. 78-2). Although low prevalence of infection has reduced the power of many studies to demonstrate statistically "significant" associations, the data are remarkably consistent. Regular use of male condoms reduces the risk of acquiring or transmitting HIV.[23] For example, in Kenya, consistent use of condoms by the clients of commercial sex workers led to lower HIV seroconversion rates in women.[39] In a French study, none of the female partners of HIV-seropositive men with hemophilia who always used condoms became infected with the virus.[40] In Rwanda, the rate of HIV seroconversion declined in a

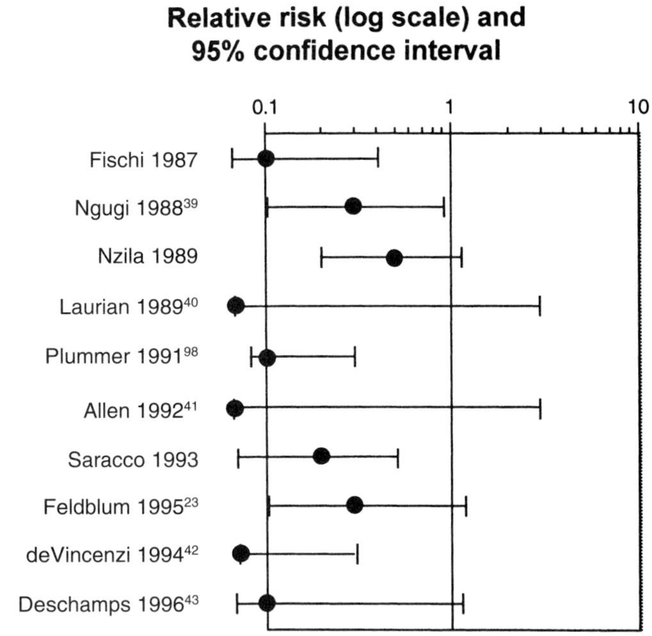

Fig. 78-2. Risk of HIV infection among heterosexual couples using condoms (selected cohort studies).

population of urban women who increasingly used condoms.[41] Finally, in the most definitive examples, the European and Haitian studies of HIV-discordant couples found those who reported consistent condom use had minimal or no HIV transmission after several years of observation.[42,43]

Taken together, these epidemiologic studies strongly support the protective effect of consistent condom use against many STDs. The variation in the data, however, implies that other factors also affect their impact. For example, the prevalence of particular STDs in populations and the risk of transmission per unprotected coital act affect the ability of scientific investigations to measure a protective effect. In addition, the quality of partner communication is apparently a strong predictor of consistent and correct use.[44] Future investigations will help clarify the behavioral determinants of more effective condom use at the population level.[12]

Condom failure

Condom failure may be due to nonuse, incorrect use, slippage, breakage, or leakage. In turn, breakage and leakage may be due to poor manufacture, improper storage, or incorrect use, especially of latex condoms.[23] Some researchers question the condom's effectiveness to prevent STDs, since the typical condom *contraceptive* unintended pregnancy rate is at least 12 percent.[45] However, much of this failure in both developed and developing countries is likely due to nonuse or incorrect use rather than poor condom quality.[46,47] At the present time, defective condoms manufactured in the United States are uncommon.[28]

In developing countries and tropical climates, latex-condom quality may be less reliable than in developed countries. Because of transportation difficulties, condom inventories may linger on shelves under less than ideal storage conditions. Temperature extremes, humidity, ultraviolet light, ozone, and other environmental factors are known to contribute to latex-condom deterioration.[48] Moreover, the quality of locally produced condoms may not conform to the standards in developed countries. During the past 10 years, numerous examples of advanced deterioration have been found in latex condoms stored in less developed countries.[48] To ensure high quality, a system for monitoring condom quality in the field is necessary. Moreover, the impact of plastic condoms—on both shelf life and product use—needs to be assessed.

Similarly, for more accurate comparison of condom effectiveness under typical situations, definitions for breakage and slippage need to be standardized.[49] Existing data show condom breakage is uncommon in developed countries. Self-reported breakage rates in a 6- to 12-month period ranged from 1 percent to 7 percent for anal intercourse.[26] In one survey, the 12-month condom-breakage rate during vaginal intercourse was 0.6 percent.[28] Among experienced Nevada brothel workers, none of 268 condoms consecutively examined after coitus showed evidence of breakage.[50]

Breakage rates in developing countries vary more widely.[46] Breakage does not appear to be strongly related to improper home-storage conditions or use of oil-based lubricants. Rather, high overall breakage rates are apparently associated with incorrect use or are disproportionately caused by certain characteristics of a few participants.[46,51,52] This suggests not only that culture-specific sexual practices may affect condom-breakage rates, but also that better analytic methods for comparing condom breakage need to be developed.

FEMALE CONDOMS

Several female condoms ("intravaginal pouches," "vaginal condoms") have been licensed in the United States and elsewhere.[53] These products are pouches made of polyurethane that line the vagina. As with male condoms, protection against STDs is likely only if these products are used consistently and stay properly positioned during intercourse. In vitro testing of the Reality™ female condom showed it to be an effective barrier to HIV and cytomegalovirus (CMV).[54] Moreover, it also provided significant in vivo protection against recurrent trichomonal infection.[55] However, the higher cost and lower acceptability of female condoms compared to male condoms are likely to limit usefulness, especially in developing countries.[56] Studies of the feasibility and safety of reusing the female condom after a soap-and-water wash are underway. Future products involving female physical barriers need to be less expensive and more available.

SPERMICIDES

In vitro studies have shown that contraceptive spermicides kill or inactivate most STD pathogens. The main spermicidal agent that has been evaluated in vivo is nonoxynol-9 (N-9), a nonionic surfactant that damages the cell walls of sperm and STD pathogens. Laboratory tests have documented activity against *Neisseria gonorrhoeae*, *Trichomonas vaginalis*, HSV, HIV, and *Treponema pallidum*.[23] Reports on the effect of spermicides on *Chlamydia trachomatis* are conflicting: Some researchers[57] found that nonoxynol-9 inactivated chlamydial organisms, while others[58] found no such effect.

In vitro microbicide activity, however, does not mean that spermicides can provide reliable in vivo protection. Data from epidemiologic studies of humans have been inconsistent regarding both the efficacy and safety of N-9. These studies have used different formulations and concentrations of spermicide and have been conducted in disparate populations. Thus, drawing clinically meaningful conclusions has been difficult. The best studies are randomized controlled trials (RCT). Through 1997, the four highest quality RCTs have compared three different products—a gel,[59,60] the film,[61,63] and the sponge.[62] Taken together, these studies have shown N-9 spermicide used alone reduces the risks of both gonorrhea and chlamydia infection, albeit at relatively low levels of protection (Fig. 78-3). In Alabama, regular use of N-9 gel by women attending an STD clinic reduced cervical gonorrhea by 24 percent, cervical chlamydial infection by 22 percent, trichomoniasis by 17 percent, and bacterial vaginosis by 14 percent.[59,60] In Thailand, women consistently using N-9 film were able to reduce the rates of cervicitis due to gonorrhea and chlamydia by 40 percent.[61] Other randomized trials,[64–66] albeit with greater methodologic problems, also found that spermicides protected against cervical gonorrhea and chlamydia.

No data suggest that spermicides alone, without any mechanical barriers, protect against HIV.[23,67] Published observational studies to date have produced conflicting results. Both RCTs have shown N-9 provides no protection against HIV.[62,63] Current ethical standards require that randomized controlled trials encourage study populations to use condoms as their primary method of HIV prevention. These designs will be able to assess only the *marginal* impact of adding spermicides to condoms as a means of protecting against HIV acquisition. Finally, methodologic issues such as the type of delivery system (e.g., film versus gel) and the population studied (e.g., sex workers versus family planning clients) also play a crucial role in allowing correct interpretation of studies involving spermicides and barriers.

A potential risk of spermicide users is chemical irritation of the vaginal epithelium, caused by nonoxynol-9's membrane-disrupting properties.[23] In Thailand, nearly half of sexually inactive women randomized to receive 150 mg nonoxynol-9 suppositories four times a day suffered epithelial disruption of their vaginal or cervical mucosa[68]; none of those receiving a placebo did. A second randomized clinical trial in Thailand showed that use of nonoxynol-9 vaginal film was associated with a small increase in genital irritation, but this did not vary with number of inserts used, nor was it related to clinical signs.[61]

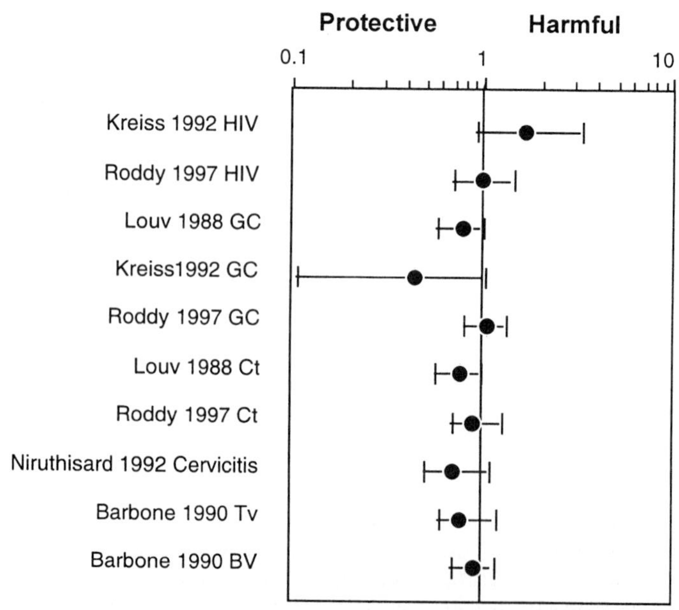

Fig. 78-3. Risk of STD among women using nonoxynol-9-containing spermicides, by organism, among the four highest quality randomized controlled trials.

COMBINED BARRIER CONTRACEPTIVES

Contraceptives for women that combine mechanical and chemical barriers apparently protect against the curable STDs. In three cross-sectional or case-control studies, diaphragm use was found to have more than a 50 percent reduction in cervical gonorrhea,[37] trichomoniasis,[37] hospitalization for PID,[69] and tubal infertility,[70] respectively. In Thailand, women at high risk of STDs who used the contraceptive sponge (soaked with spermicide) were protected against cervical gonorrhea and, to a lesser extent, against cervical *C. trachomatis*.[66]

Combined mechanical/chemical barrier methods may have harmful effects on normal genital flora. Vaginal infection with *Candida albicans* was more likely in sponge users,[66] possibly due to disruption to the normal lactobacilli. In addition, a cohort study of foam-condom users and diaphragm-spermicide users showed that both methods were associated with vaginal colonization and bacteriuria with *Escherichia coli*.[71] In addition, some studies have found that women using diaphragm-spermicide or spermicide-coated male condoms have higher risks of acute urinary tract infections.[72–74] Potential mechanisms for the *E. coli* colonization include alteration of the vaginal ecosystem by the spermicide and/or a mechanical effect of the diaphragm. Because facultative anaerobic microbial domination of vaginal flora (e.g., bacterial vaginosis) has been associated with both urinary- and upper-genital-tract infection,[73,75] the implications of this finding are of concern.

Carefully controlled studies need to assess the relative value of the different mechanical/chemical barrier methods used together in preventing transmission of all STDs, not just HIV. Moreover, the investigations need to compare these methods not only in the highest-risk situations but also in women who do not report unsafe behaviors. The "real world" effect of combination contraceptive methods on STD transmission remains to be seen.[76,77]

HORMONAL CONTRACEPTIVES

Combined oral contraceptives (OCs) have an array of noncontraceptive health benefits, but their influence on STDs, HIV, PID, and eventual reproductive sequelae remains unsettled. The majority of studies, but not all, have found an increased risk of cervical infections with *C. trachomatis* among users of OCs as compared with nonusers.[78–80] In Birmingham, OC users had higher rates of both *C. trachomatis* and *N. gonorrhoeae* detected in the cervix.[81] The association between OC use and cervical infection may be mediated through the cervical ectopy commonly induced by OCs.[81,82] *Chlamydia trachomatis* has been isolated more frequently among women with ectopy than among women without ectopy, regardless of the method of birth control used.[79]

The influence of OCs on the upper genital tract may be different than on the lower genital tract, however. Studies from Europe and the United States[83,84] have revealed that women using OCs are half as likely to be hospitalized for PID, compared with women who are sexually active but who do not use contraception. In a multicenter case-control study from the United States,[85] the protection was observed only among women who had been using OCs for more than 12 months. Past use of OCs conferred no protection. In Lund, Sweden,[86] OC use was associated with a significant reduction in the risk of gonococcal PID; the protective effect was not as strong for chlamydial PID. In Seattle, however, women using OCs apparently were differentially protected against chlamydial compared to gonococcal PID.[87]

Whether these findings are real, or whether they represent an artifact of clinical detection of PID, is unclear. Oral contraceptive users tend to have milder upper-genital-tract infection with *C. trachomatis*, as manifested by antibody response[88] and laparoscopy.[89] Oral contraceptive users also have increased risks of unrecognized endometritis.[90] In addition, data on the impact of previous OC use on primary tubal infertility are conflicting. In the United States,[68] among former users of low-estrogen OCs, tubal infertility was not reduced as might be expected if their use led to a decreased risk of PID. In fact, users of those OCs with estrogen levels higher than 50 μg had an increased risk of tubal infertility. In the Lund, Sweden cohort, however, women who had been using OCs at the time their salpingitis was diagnosed had a 70 percent lower risk of tubal infertility than women using other methods.[83] The reason for this discrepancy is unclear.

Possible mechanisms for the consistent protective effect of OCs on symptomatic PID remain speculative. The progestin component of combination OCs thickens the cervical mucus. Changes in either mucus composition or its immunologic properties might account for this protection. Likewise, the thinner endometrium and/or the decreased menstrual flow associated with OC use may play a role. Alternatively, if OC use tends to mask the symptoms of PID, they will appear protective even though unrecognized inflammation may be occurring.[90]

Consistent with this latter explanation, use of hormonal contraception seems to modify the acute clinical course of PID favorably. As judged by laparoscopic examination, women with PID who were using OCs had milder inflammation than women not using OCs.[89] Among women with chlamydial salpingitis, use of OCs protected against Fitz-Hugh-Curtis syndrome.[88] In addition, OC users had a significantly lower titer of antibodies against *C. trachomatis* than did nonusers.[88] Moreover, an IUD with progesterone protected against histologic salpingitis compared to nonhormonal IUDs.[91] In monkey models, however, OCs containing both estrogen and progesterone did not alter the course of experimentally induced chlamydial salpingitis.[92] Sex steroids can modify immunologic function,[93] so their impact on infectious inflammation is plausible, though still indefinite.

The effect of hormonal contraception use on HIV transmission, acquisition, or disease progression remains unsettled.[94,95] Animal models, using simian immunodeficiency virus (SIV) as the HIV surrogate, have raised concerns. Acquisition of SIV was increased nearly eightfold in monkeys with progesterone implants compared to monkeys challenged with SIV in the follicular phase of a normal menstrual cycle[96] and more than twofold compared to monkeys challenged randomly through a normal cycle.[97]

Epidemiologic studies in humans have produced equivocal results, however.[94] No RCTs have been performed. The initial cohort investigations examined use of *combined* oral contraceptives and HIV, while attempting to control for such intervening variables as cervical ectopy and infectious cervicitis (Fig. 78-4). Later observational studies have also been inconsistent regarding the use of progestin-only injectable contraceptives and HIV (Fig. 78-5). Investigations in sex workers in Kenya have provided support for the hypothesis that use of hormonal contraception could facilitate HIV acquisition.[98–101] However, a variety of other studies in Africa and on other continents have found little or no association between OC use and HIV seropositivity.[94,95]

Among women infected with HIV, use of hormonal contraception could also affect their risk of transmitting the virus to their partners. To date, human studies have been inconsistent on the role of hormonal contraception.[102] However, small numbers have limited their power. As with the risks for HIV acquisition, cervical ectopy associated with the use of COC may play an intermediate role in the causal pathway for potential cervical shedding.

Possible biologic mechanisms by which hormonal contracep-

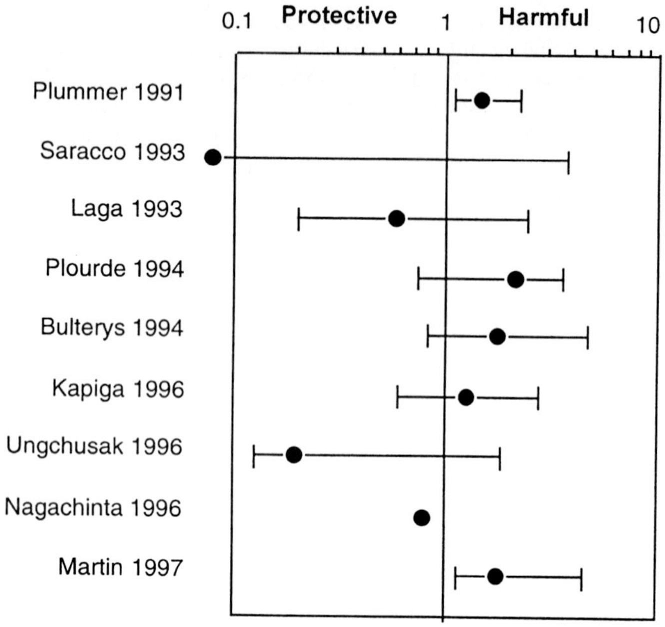

Fig. 78-4. Risk of HIV among women using oral contraceptives (selected cohort studies).

tion might facilitate HIV transmission include: (1) increased cervical ectopy (and associated friability) caused by OC use; (2) increased cervical chlamydial infection (and associated purulence), possibly associated with the ectopy; (3) systemic immunologic changes associated with some exogenous steroids; and (4) irregular uterine bleeding and/or thinning of the vaginal epithelium, if long-acting hormonal contraception is used. In addition, the particular type of estrogens and progestins contained in OCs or other long-term hormonal contraceptives may be important factors relating to any impact on HIV acquisition or transmission.[95]

A variety of biases could influence these inconsistent results of hormonal contraception and HIV, just as with any epidemiologic studies. Many problems exist in observational studies with the comparability either between cases (women infected with HIV) and controls (uninfected women) or between the exposed (users of hormonal contraception) and the unexposed (users or nonusers of other methods). Moreover, in most studies, a relatively small number of women used hormonal contraception. Thus, because of power limitations, the risk estimates are imprecise. Finally, the existing observational studies covered different populations, used differing designs, applied crude definitions of hormonal contraceptive use, had different hormonal mixes, and were unable to control for crucial confounders. Creative experimental designs, using randomized interventions, will probably be needed to answer definitively whether hormonal contraception and HIV are causally related. Because of the crucial role that OCs and other hormonal contraception play in international family planning programs, and because the HIV pandemic is the world's most important health problem, scientists must assign the highest research priority to resolving this issue.

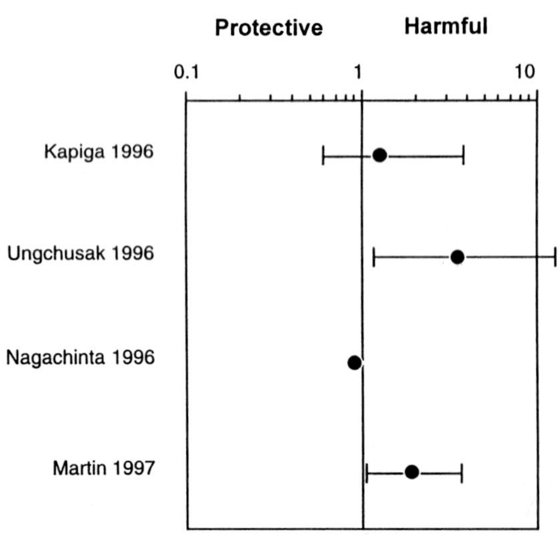

Fig. 78-5. Risk of HIV among women using injectable hormones (selected cohort studies).

INTRAUTERINE DEVICES

The precise risk of IUD use on STDs is also unclear. Few publications have objectively examined the effect of the IUD on *lower*-genital-tract infections. One review article concluded that the IUD was unrelated to cervical chlamydial infection.[103] However, an analysis of cross-sectional data from a population-based sample of Seattle women found that those who had used an IUD at some time had a significantly higher percentage of chlamydial antibodies than those who had never used an IUD, even after stratifying for number of sex partners.[104] In contrast, a prospective study in Antwerp found that IUD users had ninefold lower rates of chlamydia than OC users[105]; however, the same study showed that women using IUDs had nearly eight times higher rates of bacterial vaginosis.

The possible association between IUD use and the development of *upper*-genital-tract-infection remains a controversial topic in contemporary contraception. Epidemiologic evidence from the 1980s showed the initial association between IUD use and PID found in the 1970s to be overestimated.[106] Three particular methodologic problems in the early studies contributed to their overly pessimistic assessment. First, women using barrier or oral contraceptives served as the comparison group in most studies.[107] Since these methods *reduce* the risk of symptomatic PID, such comparisons artifactually elevated the apparent risk associated with IUD use. Second, the PID diagnosis often rests on highly subjective symptoms and signs that are difficult to assess.[108] Since the putative association between IUD use and PID has been recognized since the 1960s, PID "diagnostic bias" might occur among IUD users. Third, the early analyses did not adjust for type of IUD and the timing of its insertion. If either of these factors creates a disproportionate degree of PID risk, the overall crude risk for IUDs as a group is also spuriously elevated.

More sophisticated studies[109–112] have revised our understanding of the IUD-PID association. Current evidence suggests that the smaller, but still measurable, increased risk of PID associated with IUD use occurs around the time of insertion.[112] Thus, contamination of the endometrial cavity at insertion may be more responsible for IUD-related PID than the device itself. Because of the association of PID to the timing of IUD insertion, short-term antibiotics might help reduce the risks. In Kenya,[113] Nigeria,[114] and the United States,[115] randomized clinical trials of antibiotics given at the time of IUD insertion were limited by rates of IUD-associated PID that were much lower than expected, even among the placebo group. Because of the infrequency of IUD-related PID and because of the limited size of the studies, they had insufficient power to distinguish any statistically significant differences among treatment and placebo groups.

Many perceive the IUD's safety today as vastly different from that of a decade ago. With proper screening of clients, the IUD poses little, if any, added STD risk. For example, among women who had used copper IUDs and who had had only one sex partner, no increase occurred in the risk of either PID or tubal infertility.[110] Thus, the challenge for future researchers will be to establish criteria, based on a combination of demographic, behavioral, and clinical factors, that would expand the proportion of women for whom the IUD would be a good contraceptive choice.[13] Moreover, because newer IUDs containing levonorgesterol apparently are associated with even lower rates of PID,[116] they may be a more appropriate form of contraception in populations where the risk of STDs is unknown.

FERTILITY AWARENESS METHODS

Fertility awareness methods (FAM), also referred to as natural family planning, describe methods of planning or preventing pregnancy based on using naturally occurring signs and symptoms of the fertile and infertile phases of the menstrual cycle. Use of FAM for pregnancy prevention requires abstinence from intercourse on potentially fertile days. The pregnancy rates for this method vary widely, depending on the FAM approach used and the dedication of the users. No studies of the association between FAM and STD/HIV transmission have been conducted. Since these methods offer no obvious protection against infection, sexually active persons who wish to use FAM to prevent pregnancy and who are not having intercourse with partners known to be uninfected should be advised to use condoms for HIV/STD prophylaxis.

LACTATIONAL AMENORRHEA METHOD

Breast-feeding provides for another means of natural family planning, currently known as the lactational amenorrhea method (LAM). For some women, lactation-associated anovulation is a primary means of spacing births and avoiding pregnancies. Within the first 6 months following delivery, women who fully (or nearly fully) breast-feed have a low risk of pregnancy, 2 percent or less, prior to the return of menses.[117]

Breast milk may also be an avenue for transmission of infectious agents, however. The human immunodeficiency virus has been detected in breast milk, and postnatal transmission to the infant through breast milk has been well documented.[118] Several methods for reducing the risk of transmitting HIV through breast-feeding are being investigated. A complex trade-off exists between the contraceptive effect of LAM preventing an HIV-infected woman from becoming pregnant (and thus being at risk of transmitting HIV to her next child) versus the risk of transmitting HIV through breast milk to the child she is currently nursing.

For the mother who is uninfected, breast-feeding provides no protection against HIV or other STDs. Women who are using LAM as their contraceptive method, and who are at risk of STDs/HIV, should use condoms to protect themselves and, indirectly, their infants.

TUBAL STERILIZATION

Tubal sterilization protects against PID, but this protection is not absolute. Most typical cases of PID are thought to arise from ascent of cervical pathogens via the endometrial cavity; hence, disrupting the continuity of this passage should prevent inoculation of the distal fallopian tubes. Even though endometritis and proximal salpingitis are potentially possible, PID is rarely observed among women after tubal sterilization.[119] Anecdotal cases of PID and tubo-ovarian abscess continue to be reported. A more likely mechanism for poststerilization PID is iatrogenic contamination of the tubes during the operative procedure; in the less developed world, where sterile conditions are more difficult to maintain, this risk may be further elevated.

ABORTION

Women who have cervical infection with either *N. gonorrhoeae* or *C. trachomatis* have an increased risk of endometritis following induced abortion performed under proper hygienic conditions. The risk appears to be at least tripled with either organism.[120] A number of studies suggest that use of prophylactic antibiotics at the time of the abortion procedure reduces the risk of infection by one-half to two-thirds.[121] While preoperative screening for infection with these organisms is desirable, a brief perioperative course of an antibiotic such as azithromycin seems both safe and cost-effective. Women later found to be infected by *N. gonorrhoeae* and/or *C. trachomatis* can be followed up with a full course of recommended antibiotics, with notification and treatment of their sex partner(s).

The greatest risk of upper-genital-tract infection associated with induced abortion occurs in circumstances where sterile conditions are not maintained. In countries where abortion services are restricted by law or practice, and especially in resource-poor regions where, even if legal, access to sanitary procedures is limited, postabortion infection poses risks not only to future fertility but also to the woman's life.[122] More than half the estimated 100,000 annual abortion-related deaths worldwide occur in Southeast Asia, followed by sub-Saharan Africa, and then Latin America and the Caribbean.[123]

In both the developed and less-developed worlds, carrying a pregnancy to term leads to greater risks of infection and death than terminating it through induced abortion.[124,125] Under sterile conditions, abortion is five to ten times safer than childbearing. Under less hygienic conditions, the risks of adverse outcomes for *both* abortion and term delivery increase, and the gap between the infection risks from abortion and childbirth probably narrows. In these circumstances, use of any method of contraception to reduce pregnancy has simultaneous effects on reducing pregnancy-associated infection (see below).

CLINICAL AND POLICY IMPLICATIONS

CONTRACEPTIVE/STD PREVENTION TRADE-OFFS

In ideal circumstances, consistent and correct use of male or female condoms can prevent *both* pregnancy and STDs. In typical situations of inconsistent use, however, they provide lower rates of protection against these conditions. Moreover, if couples choose to use contraceptive methods other than condoms, those with the best record for pregnancy prevention provide little STD protection. Thus, trade-off choices are necessary.

For those whose families are not completed, yet who do not currently wish to become pregnant, hormonal contraceptives and the IUD remain the most effective reversible methods available to prevent unintended pregnancy. They provide no protection against vaginal or cervical infection, however, and inserting the IUD carries temporary risks to the upper genital tract. Hence, for persons who are not mutually monogamous, addition of a barrier method, such as a condom, will help reduce the risk of STDs as well as unplanned pregnancies. Under typical conditions, however, barrier methods are substantially less effective in preventing conception than hormonal methods, yet they offer important protection against STDs. To maximize protection against both unintended pregnancy and STD, a barrier method should be used in conjunction with a hormonal method or IUD.

Worldwide, for couples whose families are complete, male or female sterilization is an increasingly popular method of contraception.[126] While these operations protect against upper-genital-tract infections in sterilized persons, they confer no protection against lower-genital-tract infections. Alternatives to sterilization are hormonal implants or the IUD; both are effective methods of reversible contraception, but they offer no protection against cervical infection. Sterilized persons would still need to use barrier methods to protect against infections in the lower genital tract.

Because both mechanical and chemical barrier prophylaxes are coitally dependent, their efficacy in preventing either infection or unplanned pregnancy depends entirely on adherence by the couple. Some populations have demonstrated high levels of barrier-method use. For example, in Thailand, a "100 percent condom policy" in commercial sex facilities has led to widespread use among the workers and their clients; this, in turn, has been associated with marked reductions in HIV and other STDs.[127,128] In the United States, women working in Nevada brothels have had similar success.[50] Unfortunately, to date, most heterosexual populations worldwide have not reported the same magnitude of condom use and have not experienced decreases in the traditional STDs.[129]

The reasons for relatively low global condom use rates vary. In many settings, a woman cannot insist on a male-dependent method such as a male condom. For example, in South Africa, female sex workers serving male truck drivers were unable to persuade most of their customers to use condoms; fear of economic loss and personal violence limited any ability to negotiate.[130] However, in Cameroon, sex workers provided with condoms and regular counseling reported using condoms with their clients in nearly 90 percent of sexual acts.[63] Moreover, cultural taboos against discussing sex limit the practical negotiations that can take place. In some societies, use of condoms is associated with commercial sex, which makes them unacceptable for use in any primary relationship. Finally, in all surveys, men consider condom use to be a major inhibition to their sexual enjoyment.

Another important aspect to assessing trade-off concerns is whether conditions exist for safe, sterile childbirth and/or abortion. If pregnancy itself, regardless of whether it is terminated or continued, carries markedly high "iatrogenic" risks of genital infection, then the *pregnancy* prevention efficacy of the contraceptive choice takes on greater weight. By preventing undesired pregnancies, the contraceptive method(s) simultaneously protect against pregnancy-associated infections of the reproductive tract. In the developing world, postabortal and puerperal infections are important causes of tubal infertility. In Africa, where the infectious etiology of infertility was most evident,[131] genital infections occurring both before and after the first pregnancy were associated with tubal occlusion. In Asia, abortion appeared to play a larger role than childbirth in contributing to infectious infertility, whereas in Latin America the reverse was found.[132]

DUAL METHOD VERSUS DUAL PURPOSE

Another complex issue for reproductive-health providers serving clients at risk of STD/HIV is whether to encourage use of dual methods—one to prevent pregnancy and the other to prevent STD/HIV.[5] Clinicians promoting dual use must weigh interacting factors such as extra cost and effect on user adherence, as well as the level of STDs in particular client populations. Moreover, clients may attach differing priorities to preventing either pregnancies or infections, and these priorities may change over time and among various relationships.

Studies on dual-method use are limited and have focused on the use of the male condom added to other methods of contraception.[133–143] In general, based on investigations where participants were using primary methods other than the condom, the more effective the primary contraceptive method was in preventing pregnancy, the lower the level of consistent use of the male condom (Table 78-2). For example, in Baltimore and Philadelphia, respectively, 6 percent and 12 percent of women who were sterilized used condoms consistently to prevent STDs.[133,134] In Philadelphia, Norplant® users reported lower levels of condom use than those using daily OCs.[135] A higher percentage of HIV-infected women reported consistent condom use if sterilized (43 percent) or if using OCs as contraceptives (30 percent) than women unaware of their HIV-infection status.[136] Among HIV-infected women, however, those using the more effective methods of contraception were less likely to use condoms consistently than those using less effective contraceptive methods.

Several reasons can explain why concurrent condom use may decrease as perceived contraceptive effectiveness increases. First, many persons—even those with sexual behaviors putting them at risk of STDs—see pregnancy as a greater immediate threat. Thus, having taken proactive precautions against unintended pregnancies, they would be less motivated to undergo the extra effort and expense to use condoms. Second, situational differences in one's routine may exist between the compliance-independent contraceptive methods and the compliance-dependent methods, including both barriers and OCs. Those who are sterilized or who are using implantable or injectable hormones or IUDs do not have the coitally based requirements of barriers or the daily schedules of OCs to help keep them continually aware of, and prepared for, prophylactic needs. Without regular reminders of the need to protect against both pregnancy and STDs, individuals may be less likely to have condoms available when sexual opportunities arise.

Trends in dual-method use may be increasing. Among OC users, studies conducted in the 1990s have found higher levels of

Table 78-2. Studies of Condom Use in Conjunction with Other Contraceptive Methods

Primary Contraceptive/Study Location	Percent Reporting Consistent Condom Use/Reference
Sterilization	
Baltimore	6 (133)
Philadelphia	12 (134)
United States (HIV-infected women)	43 (136)
Norplant	
Houston	21 (137)
Atlanta	35 (138)
Philadelphia	17 (135)
Oral Contraceptives	
Baltimore—1988	16 (139)
Baltimore—1992	38 (140)
United States—1988	12 (141)
United States—1991	21 (142)
United States—1992	25 (142)
United States—1994	46 (142)
Philadelphia	29 (135)
United States (HIV-infected women)	30 (136)
Spermicides	
Mexico	75 (143)
Kenya	43 (143)
Dominican Republic	4 (143)
Condoms Only—Multiple studies	25–90

self-reported consistent condom use than in the 1980s.[142] Moreover, the way in which counselors and clinicians encourage dual methods apparently influences whether the message is effective. With spermicides as the primary contraceptive method, the percentage of consistent condom users varied dramatically among three countries.[143] This indicates that factors other than the method itself affect levels of concurrent condom use.

Finally, the percentage of people reporting consistent use of male condoms *alone* for both primary contraception and STD prophylaxis ranges from 25 percent to 95 percent among different populations.[126] As stated above, multiple factors affect consistent male condom use, including whether or not back-up female-controlled methods are recommended and available. Among Colombian sex workers, women randomized to a group counseled to use spermicides as a back-up method if their clients were unwilling to use male condoms were less likely to use them consistently than women encouraged to use only male condoms.[144] Similarly, among HIV-infected women, those using condoms as their sole contraceptive method were more likely to use them consistently than those using sterilization or hormonal methods as primary contraception.[136]

A recent creative approach to the use of dual methods is based on the availability of emergency contraception (EC), which describes contraceptive methods that people can use after intercourse to prevent pregnancy.[145] The most common method of EC includes a heightened dose of combined oral contraceptives; other approaches to EC involve using mefepristone, levonorgestrel, or danazol or inserting a copper IUD. While EC in itself provides no protection against HIV or other STDs, making EC more widely available as a backup to barrier contraception may cause more couples to choose (and use) barriers as a *dual-purpose* method.[146] This dual-purpose approach, namely using condoms to protect against both unplanned pregnancies and STDs/HIV, needs to be investigated through operational research designs. To the extent that the availability of EC increases overall barrier-method use, it would have a positive impact on the overall level of STDs/HIV within the community.

More research is clearly needed on the best mix of contraceptives. Studies that examine the use of the female condom, diaphragm, and/or spermicides in conjunction with long-term methods will help clarify this issue. In addition, the patterns of dual-method use with different sex partners needs to be evaluated. For example, if an individual uses one method with one partner and adds condoms with other partners, this might reduce risk, even if dual-method use is not consistent with the primary partner.

Service Integration

Even before the 1994 International Conference on Population and Development's Programme of Action highlighted the need for integrated reproductive-health services,[21] family planning and STD/HIV activities were being coordinated. However, most publicly supported family planning, maternal/child health, and STD clinics were begun as independent entities rather than one integrated reproductive-health unit. In contrast, the women being served by these clinics frequently had overlapping health needs.[14] For example, in family planning clinics in developed countries, risk-assessment surveys have found that approximately one-quarter of women report behaviors that put them at increased risk for HIV and the other STDs.[147] In STD clinics, up to half of reproductive-age, sexually active women report using no method of contraception,[148] despite most having histories of both STDs and unintended pregnancies.

In developing countries, the need for integrated care is even more acute. Since so few facilities are available for health care, they should not be fragmented.[14,149] Moreover, because access to health services is usually more cumbersome and time consuming in resource-poor settings, when patients make the effort to obtain one particular "categorical" service, the full range of clinical preventive care should be offered.

These overlapping needs have provided those interested in STDs and family planning with a unique opportunity to deliver more broad-based reproductive health care. In the United States, this collaboration was initiated in the early 1970s, when family planning clinics became crucial allies for the federal gonorrhea control program.[150] In the 1980s, half of all women receiving family planning services were simultaneously screened for STD, primarily gonorrhea; this screening appropriately targeted those women who had the highest infection risks.[15] Moreover, efforts to screen for chlamydia in family planning settings have also been productive, especially when selective criteria are applied, such as age younger than 24, more than one sex partner in the past 2 months, or signs of cervical infection.[151,152] The most successful of these has been the Region X chlamydia screening program, which led to a regional reduction of chlamydial prevalence between 1988 and 1993.[153] The extension of STD services in family planning clinics has had its costs, however,[17] because the proportion of time and resources available for contraceptive care decreased.

In a reciprocal manner, some STD clinics increasingly have been providing rudimentary contraceptive services, especially barrier methods. Recent concerns with incurable viral STDs, especially HIV, have provided the necessary social environment and financial resources both to emphasize condom use during client-counseling sessions and to increase advertising of condoms in the media. The development of women-controlled mechanical or chemical barrier contraceptives may be of further value in reducing STD risks.[154,155] For this reason, diaphragms (which protect only the cervical os), spermicides, and female condoms may play a wider role in upcoming efforts to prevent STDs/HIV.

The urgency of the HIV pandemic has hastened the need to integrate STDs and family planning services.[21] In the developing world, where heterosexual transmission predominates, family planning and maternal/child health facilities are increasing their HIV/STD roles.[156] Agencies have begun both to counsel women on how to reduce their risks and also to provide services to diagnose and treat those STDs that themselves may further facilitate acquisition/transmission of HIV.[157] If the client's HIV status is known, more specific counseling is warranted: for uninfected women, culturally sensitive messages regarding ways to protect themselves from STD/HIV exposure are essential; for HIV-infected women, family planning choices are even more complicated. Complex personal, ethical, and policy issues are involved in insuring the woman's right to determine her reproductive future, improving her quality and duration of life, decreasing the risk of perinatal HIV transmission, and decreasing the risk of further HIV transmission within the community.[158–160]

CONCLUSION

Because contraception affects not only the risk of unplanned pregnancies but also that of sexually transmitted infections, the choice of particular methods is important to future fertility. Important trade-offs exist, however. Contraceptives with the best record of preventing pregnancy provide little protection against sexually transmitted diseases (STDs). Moreover, epidemiologic studies are equivocal regarding the value of either recommending dual methods of contraception or relying on the condom alone to prevent both unplanned pregnancies and STDs. Use of emergency contraception as a backup to barrier methods is another approach that warrants evaluation. Continued biologic and behavioral research will be necessary to untangle these complex relationships.

References

1 Cates W Jr, Stone KM: Family planning, sexually transmitted diseases and contraceptive choice: A literature update—Part I and Part II. *Fam Plann Perspect* 24(2):75–84, 1992; 24(3):122–28, 1992.
2 Harlap S et al: *Preventing Pregnancy, Protecting Health: A New Look at Birth Control Choices in the United States.* New York: The Alan Guttmacher Institute, 1991.
3 DaVanzo J et al: Health consequences of contraceptive use and reproductive patterns. *JAMA* 265:2692–96, 1991.
4 Elias CJ, Leonard A: Family planning and sexually transmitted diseases: The need to enhance contraceptive choice. *Curr Issues in Public Health* 1:191–99, 1995.
5 Fox LJ et al: Improving reproductive health: Integrating STD and contraceptive services. *J AM Women's Med Assoc* 50:129–36, 1995.
6 Carlin EM, Boag FC: Women, contraceptives and STDs including HIV. *Int J STD AIDS* 6:373–86, 1995.
7 Luker K: Contraceptive risk taking and abortion. *Stud Fam Plann* 8:190–96, 1977.
8 Hatcher RA et al: *Contraceptive Technology,* 17th ed. New York: Irvington Press, 1998.
9 Caldwell JC, Caldwell P: The cultural context of high fertility in sub-Saharan Africa. *Pop Develop Rev* 13:409–37, 1987.
10 Caldwell JC et al: The social context of AIDS in sub-Saharan Africa. *Pop Develop Revc* 15:185–234, 1989.
11 Forrest JD: Timing of reproductive life stages. *Obstet Gynecol* 82: 105–11, 1993.
12 Cates W Jr: Contraception, unintended pregnancies, and sexually transmitted diseases: Why isn't a simple solution possible? *Am J Epidemiol* 143:311–18, 1996.
13 Cates W Jr: A risk assessment tool for integrated reproductive health services. *Fam Plann Perspect* 29:41–43, 1997.
14 Lande RE: Controlling sexually transmitted diseases. Popul Rep[L] No 9. Baltimore: Johns Hopkins University, Population Information Program, January 1993.
15 Mosher WD, Aral SO: Testing for sexually transmitted diseases among women of reproductive age: United States, 1988. *Fam Plann Perspect* 23:216–21, 1991.
16 Begley CE et al: The incremental cost of screening, diagnosis, and treatment of gonorrhea and chlamydia in a family planning clinic. *Sex Transm Dis* 16:63–67, 1989.
17 Donovan P: *Testing Positive: Sexually Transmitted Diseases and the Public Health Response.* New York: The Alan Guttmacher Institute, 1993.
18 Marrazzo JM et al: Performance and cost-effectiveness of selective screening criteria for *Chlamydia trachomatis* infection in women: implications for a National Chlamydia Control Strategy. *Sex Trans Dis* 24:131–141, 1997.
19 Donovan P: Family planning clinics: Facing higher costs and sicker patients. *Fam Plann Perspect* 23:198–203, 1991.
20 State Family Planning Administrators: *Family Planning Clinic Provision of STD and HIV Services: National Questionnaire Findings.* Seattle: Center for Health Training, 1991.
21 International Conference on Population and Development: *Programme of Action, Chapter VII, 7.2–7.6.* Cairo: International Conference on Population and Development, September 1994.
22 Anderson DJ, Voeller B: AIDS and contraception, in *Contraception,* D Soupe, FP Haseltine (eds). New York, Springer-Verlag, 1993, pp. 192–209.
23 Feldblum PJ et al: The effectiveness of barrier methods of contraception in preventing the spread of HIV. *AIDS* 9(suppl A):585–93, 1995.
24 Howe JE et al: Contraceptives and HIV. *AIDS* 8:861–71, 1994.
25 Cates W Jr: Contraceptive choice, sexually transmitted diseases, HIV infection, and future fecundity. *J Brit Fertil Soc* 1:18–22, 1996
26 Centers for Disease Control and Prevention: Update: barrier protection against HIV infection and other sexually transmitted diseases. *MMWR* 42:589–91, 1993.
27 Roper WL et al: Commentary: Condoms and HIV/STD prevention—clarifying the message. *Am J Public Health* 83:501–503, 1993.
28 Consumer Reports: How reliable are condoms? *Consumer Reports* May:320–25, 1995.
29 Judson FN et al: In vitro evaluation of condoms with and without nonoxynol 9 as physical and chemical barriers against *Chlamydia trachomatis*, herpes simplex virus type 2 and human immunodeficiency virus. *Sex Transm Dis* 16:51–56, 1989.
30 Conant M et al: Condoms prevent transmission of AIDS-associated retrovirus. *JAMA* 255:1706, 1986.
31 Voeller B et al: Gas, dye and viral transport through polyurethane condoms. *JAMA* 266:2986–87, 1991.
32 Van de Perre P et al: The latex condom, an efficient barrier against sexual transmission of AIDS-related viruses. *AIDS* 1:49–52, 1987.
33 Hart G: Factors influencing venereal infection in a war environment. *Br J Vener Dis* 50:68–72, 1974.
34 Cates W Jr, Holmes KK: Use of condoms and STD protection (letter). *Am J Epidemiol* 143:843–44, 1996.
35 Darrow WW: Condom use and use-effectiveness in high-risk populations. *Sex Transm Dis* 16:157–60, 1989.
36 Oberle MW et al: Herpes simplex virus type 2 antibodies: High prevalence in monogamous women in Costa Rica. *Am J Trop Med Hygiene* 41:224–29, 1989.
37 Rosenberg MJ et al: Barrier contraceptives and sexually transmitted diseases in women: A comparison of female-dependent methods and condoms. *Am J Public Health* 82:669–74, 1992.
38 Cameron DW et al: Condom use prevents genital ulcers in women working as prostitutes: Influence of human immunodeficiency virus infection. *Sex Transm Dis* 18:188–91, 1991.
39 Ngugi EN et al: Prevention of transmission of human immunodeficiency virus in Africa: Effectiveness of condom promotion and health education among prostitutes. *Lancet* 2:887–90, 1988.
40 Laurian Y et al: HIV infection in sexual partners of HIV seropositive patients with hemophilia. *N Engl J Med* 320:183, 1989.
41 Allen S et al: Effect of serotesting with counseling on condom use and seroconversion among HIV discordant couples in Africa. *Br Med J* 304:1605–1609, 1992.
42 De Vincenzi I: A longitudinal study of human immunodeficiency virus transmission by heterosexual partners. *N Engl J Med* 334:341–46, 1994.
43 Deschamps M-M et al: Heterosexual transmission of HIV in Haiti. *Ann Intern Med* 125:324–30, 1996.
44 Oakley D, Bogue EL: Quality of condom use as reported by female clients of a family planning clinic. *Am J Public Health* 85:1526–30, 1995.
45 Trussell J et al: Contraceptive failure in the United States: An update. *Stud Fam Plann* 21:51–54, 1990.
46 Steiner M et al: Condom breakage and slippage rates among study participants in eight countries. *Int Fam Plann Perspect* 20:55–58, 1994.
47 Vessey MP et al: Factors influencing use-effectiveness of the condom. *Br J Fam Plann* 14:40–43, 1988.
48 Free MJ, Hutchings J: Condom quality management, in *Heterosexual Transmission of AIDS*, NJ Alexander, HL Gabelnick, JM Spieler (eds). New York: Wiley-Liss, 1990, pp. 370–97.
49 Steiner M et al: Standardized protocols for condom breakage and slippage trials: A proposal. *Am J Public Health* 84:1897–1900, 1994.
50 Albert AE et al: Condom use among female commercial sex workers in Nevada's legal brothels. *Am J Public Health* 85:1514–20, 1995.
51 Steiner M et al: Can condom users likely to experience condom failure be identified? *Fam Plann Perspect* 25:220–6, 1993.
52 Sparrow MJ, Lavill K: Breakage and slippage of condoms in family planning clients. *Contraception* 50:117–29, 1994.
53 World Health Organization: The female condom: A review. Geneva: World Health Organization, 1997.

54 Drew WL et al: Evaluation of the virus permeability of a new condom for women. *Sex Transm Dis* 17:110–12, 1990.
55 Soper DE et al: Prevention of vaginal trichomoniasis by compliant use of the female condom. *Sex Transm Dis* 20:137–39, 1993.
56 Farr G et al: Contraceptive efficacy and acceptability of the female condom. *Am J Public Health* 84:1960–64, 1994.
57 Benes S, McCormack WM: Inhibition of growth of *Chlamydia trachomatis* by nonoxynol-9 in vitro. *Antimicrob Agents Chemother* 27:724–26, 1985.
58 Kappus EW, Quinn TC: The spermicide nonoxynol-9 does not inhibit *Chlamydia trachomatis* in vitro. *Sex Transm Dis* 13:134–37, 1986.
59 Louv WC et al: A clinical trial of nonoxynol-9 as a prophylaxis for cervical *Neisseria gonorrhoeae* and *Chlamydia trachomatis* infections. *J Infect Dis* 158:518–23, 1988.
60 Barbone F et al: A follow-up study of methods of contraception, sexual activity, and rates of trichomoniasis, candidiasis, and bacterial vaginosis. *Am J Obstet Gynecol* 163:510–14, 1990.
61 Niruthisard S et al: Use of nonoxynol-9 and reduction in rate of gonococcal and chlamydial infections. *Lancet* 339:1371–75, 1992.
62 Kreiss J et al: Efficacy of nonoxynol-9 contraceptive sponge use in preventing heterosexual acquisition of HIV in Nairobi prostitutes. *JAMA* 268:477–82, 1992.
63 Roddy RE et al: A randomized controlled trial of the effect of nonoxynol-9 film or male-to-female transmission of HIV-1. Presented at the National Institute of Allergy and Infectious Disease Ad Hoc Meeting, Bethesda, Maryland, April 9, 1997.
64 Cutler JC et al: Vaginal contraceptives as prophylaxis against gonorrhea and other sexually transmissible diseases. *Adv Planned Parent* 12:45–56, 1977.
65 Rendon AL et al: A controlled, comparative study of phenylmercuric acetate, nonoxynol-9 and placebo vaginal suppositories as prophylactic agents against gonorrhea. *Curr Ther Res* 27:780–83, 1980.
66 Rosenberg MJ et al: Effect of the contraceptive sponge on chlamydial infection, gonorrhea, and candidiasis. A comparative clinical trial. *JAMA* 257:2308–12, 1987.
67 Bird KD: The use of spermicide containing nonoxynol-9 in the prevention of HIV infection. *AIDS* 5:791–96, 1991.
68 Niruthisard S et al: The effects of frequent nonoxynol-9 use on the vaginal and cervical mucosa. *Sex Transm Dis* 18:176–79, 1991.
69 Kelaghan J et al: Barrier method contraceptives and pelvic inflammatory disease. *JAMA* 248:184–87, 1982.
70 Cramer DW et al: The relationship of tubal infertility to barrier method and oral contraceptive use. *JAMA* 257:244–50, 1987.
71 Hooton RM et al: *Escherichia coli* bacteriuria and contraceptive method. *JAMA* 265:64–69, 1991.
72 Foxman B et al: First-time urinary tract infection and sexual behavior. *Epidemiology* 6:162–68, 1995.
73 Hooten TM et al: A prospective study of risk factors for symptomatic urinary tract infection in young women. *N Engl J Med* 335:468–74, 1996.
74 Fihn SD et al: Association between use of spermicide-coated condoms and *Escherichia coli* urinary tract infection in young women. *Am J Epidemiol* 144:512–20, 1996.
75 Hillier SL et al: Role of bacterial vaginosis-associated microorganisms in endometritis. *Am J Obstet Gynecol* 175:435–41, 1996.
76 Stone KM, Peterson HB: Spermicides, HIV and the vaginal sponge. *JAMA* 268:521–23, 1992.
77 Feldblum PJ, Weir SS: The protective effect of nonoxynol-9 against HIV infection. *Am J Public Health* 84:1032–34, 1994.
78 Washington AE et al: Oral contraceptives, *Chlamydia trachomatis* infection, and pelvic inflammatory disease. *JAMA* 253:2246–50, 1985.
79 Cottingham J, Hunter D: *Chlamydia trachomatis* and oral contraceptive use: a quantitative review. *Genitourin Med* 68:209–16, 1992.
80 Park BJ et al: Contraceptive methods and the risk of *Chlamydia trachomatis* infection in young women. *Am J Epidemiol* 142:771–78, 1995.
81 Louv WC et al: Oral contraceptive use and risk of chlamydial and gonococcal infections. *Am J Obstet Gynecol* 160:396–400, 1989.
82 Critchlow CW et al: Determinants of cervical ectopia and of cervicitis: Age, oral contraception, specific cervical infection, smoking, and douching. *Am J Obstet Gynecol* 173:534–43, 1995.
83 Westrom L: Incidence, prevalence, and trends of acute pelvic inflammatory disease and its consequences in industrialized countries. *Am J Obstet Gynecol* 138:880–92, 1980.
84 Panser LA, Phipps WR: Type of oral contraceptive in relation to acute, initial episodes of pelvic inflammatory disease. *Contraception* 93:91–99, 1991.
85 Rubin GL et al: Oral contraceptives and pelvic inflammatory disease. *Am J Obstet Gynecol* 144:630–35, 1982.
86 Wölner-Hanssen P et al: Laparoscopic findings and contraceptive use in women with signs and symptoms suggestive of acute salpingitis. *Obstet Gynecol* 66:233–38, 1985.
87 Wölner-Hanssen P et al: Decreased risk of symptomatic chlamydial pelvic inflammatory disease associated with oral contraceptive use. *JAMA* 263:54–59, 1990.
88 Wölner-Hanssen P: Oral contraceptive use modifies the manifestations of pelvic inflammatory disease. *Br J Obstet Gynaecol* 93:619–24, 1986.
89 Svensson L et al: Contraceptives and acute salpingitis. *JAMA* 251:2553–55, 1984.
90 Ness RB et al: Oral contraception and the recognition of endometritis. *Am J Obstet Gynecol* 176:580–85, 1997.
91 Soderstrom RM: Will progesterone save the IUD? *J Reprod Med* 28:305–308, 1983.
92 Patton DL et al: Oral contraceptives do not alter the course of experimentally-induced chlamydial salpingitis in monkeys. *Sex Transm Dis* 21:89–92, 1994.
93 Grossman C: Possible underlying mechanisms of sexual dimorphism in the immune response: Fact and hypothesis. *J Steroid Biochem* 34:241–51, 1989.
94 Daly CC et al: Contraceptive methods and the transmission of HIV: Implications for family planning. *Genitourin Med* 70:110–17, 1994.
95 Taitel HF, Kafrissen ME: A review of oral contraceptive use and the risk of HIV-transmission. *Br J Fam Plann* 20:112–16, 1995.
96 Marx PA et al: Progesterone implants enhance SIV vaginal transmission and early virus load. *Nature Medicine* 2:1084–89, 1996.
97 Duerr A et al: Contraceptives and HIV transmission (letter). *Nature Medicine* 3:124, 1997.
98 Plummer FA et al: Cofactors in male-female sexual transmission of human immunodeficiency virus type 1. *J Infect Dis* 163:233–39, 1991.
99 Plourde PJ et al: Human immunodeficiency virus type 1 seroconversion in women with genital ulcers. *J Infect Dis* 170:313–17, 1994.
100 Sinei SKA et al: Contraceptive use and HIV infection in Kenyan family planning clinic attenders. *Int J STD AIDS* 7:65–70, 1996.
101 Nyange P et al: Cofactors for heterosexual transmission of HIV to prostitutes in Mombasa, Kenya [Abstract Tu.C.106]. Presented at IX International Conference on AIDS and STD in Africa, December 10, 1995.
102 Mostad SB, Kreiss JK: Shedding of HIV-1 in the genital tract. *AIDS* 10:1305–15, 1996.
103 Edelman DA: The use of intrauterine contraceptive devices, pelvic inflammatory disease, and *Chlamydia trachomatis* infection. *Am J Obstet Gynecol* 158:956–59, 1988.
104 Rossing MA et al: Past use of an intrauterine device and risk of tubal pregnancy. *Epidemiol* 4:245–51, 1993.
105 Avonts D et al: Incidence of uncomplicated genital infections in women using oral contraception or an intrauterine device: a prospective study. *Sex Transm Dis* 17:23–29, 1990.
106 Grimes DA: Intrauterine devices and pelvic inflammatory disease: Recent developments. *Contraception* 36:97–109, 1987.
107 Senanayake P, Kramer DG: Contraception and the etiology of pelvic inflammatory disease: New perspectives. *Am J Obstet Gynecol* 138:852–60, 1980.
108 Kahn JG et al: Diagnosing pelvic inflammatory disease: A comprehensive analysis and new algorithm. *JAMA* 266:2594–604, 1991.

109 Burkman RT, Women's Health Study: Association between intrauterine device and pelvic inflammatory disease. *Obstet Gynecol* 57: 269–76, 1981.

110 Lee NC et al: Type of intrauterine device and the risk of pelvic inflammatory disease. *Obstet Gynecol* 62:1–6, 1983.

111 Buchan H et al: Epidemiology of pelvic inflammatory disease in parous women with special reference to intrauterine device use. *Br J Obstet Gynaecol* 97:780–88, 1990.

112 Farley TMM et al: Intrauterine devices and pelvic inflammatory disease: An international perspective. *Lancet* 339:785–88, 1992.

113 Sinei SKA et al: Preventing IUD-related pelvic infection: The efficacy of prophylactic doxycycline at insertion. *Br J Obstet Gynaecol* 97: 412–19, 1990.

114 Ladipo OA et al: Prevention of IUD-related pelvic infection: The efficacy of prophylactic doxycycline at IUD insertion. *Adv Contracept* 7:43–54, 1991.

115 Walsh TL et al: Effect of prophylactic antibiotics on morbidity associated with IUD insertion: Results of a pilot randomized controlled trial. *Contraception* 50:319–27, 1994.

116 Luukkainen T, Toivonen J: Levonorgestrel-releasing IUD as a method of contraception with therapeutic properties. *Contraception* 52:269–76, 1995.

117 Kennedy KI et al: Lactational amenorrhea method for family planning. *Int J Gynaecol Obstet* 54:55–57, 1996.

118 John GC, Kreiss J: Mother-to-child transmission of human immunodeficiency virus type 1. *Epidemiol Rev* 18:149–57, 1996.

119 Vessey M et al: Tubal sterilization: Findings in a large prospective study. *Br J Obstet Gynaecol* 90:203–209, 1983.

120 Burkman RT et al: Untreated endocervical gonorrhea and endometritis following elective abortion. *Am J Obstet Gynecol* 126:648–51, 1976.

121 Sawaya GF et al: Antibiotics at the time of induced abortion: The case for universal prophylaxis based on a meta-analysis. *Obstet Gynecol* 87:884–90, 1996.

122 The Alan Guttmacher Institute: *Clandestine Abortion: A Latin American Reality*. New York: The Alan Guttmacher Institute, 1994.

123 Henshaw SK: Induced abortion: A world review, 1990. *Fam Plann Perspect* 22:76–89, 1990.

124 Cates W Jr: Legal abortion: The public health record. *Science* 215: 1586–90, 1982.

125 Tinker A, Koblinsky MA: *Making Motherhood Safe*, World Bank Discussion Papers, No. 202. Washington, DC: World Bank, 1993.

126 United Nations Family Planning Association: *Levels and Trends of Contraceptives Use as Assessed in 1993*. New York: United Nations, 1995.

127 Hanenberg RS et al: Impact of Thailand's HIV-control programme as indicated by the decline of sexually transmitted diseases. *Lancet* 344:243–45, 1994.

128 Nelson KE et al: Changes in sexual behavior and a decline in HIV infection among young men in Thailand. *N Engl J Med* 335:297–303, 1996.

129 World Health Organization: *Global Estimates of Curable Sexually Transmitted Diseases*. Geneva: World Health Organization, 1995.

130 Abdool Karim Q et al: Reducing the risk of HIV infection among South African sex workers: Socio-economic and gender barriers. *Am J Public Health* 85:1521–25, 1995.

131 Cates W Jr et al: The WHO Task Force on Infertility: Worldwide patterns of infertility: Is Africa different? *Lancet* 2:596–98, 1985.

132 WHO Task Force on Infertility: Infections, pregnancies and infertility: Perspectives on prevention. *Fertil Steril* 47:964–68, 1987.

133 Santelli JS et al: Surgical sterilization among women and use of condoms—Baltimore. *MMWR* 41:568–69, 575, 1992.

134 Armstrong KK et al: HIV-risk behaviors of sterilized and nonsterilized women in drug-treatment programs—Philadelphia, 1989–1991. *MMWR* 41:149–52, 1992.

135 Polaneczky M et al: The use of levonorgestrel implants (Norplant) for contraception in adolescent mothers. *N Engl J Med* 331:1201–206, 1994.

136 Diaz T et al: The relationship between use of condoms and other forms of contraception among human immunodeficiency virus-infected women. *Obstet Gynecol* 86:277–82, 1995.

137 Frank M et al: Characteristics and attitudes of early contraceptive implant acceptors in Texas. *Fam Plann Perspect* 24:208–13, 1992.

138 Humphries HO, Bauman KH: Condom use by Norplant users at risk for sexually transmitted diseases. *Sex Transm Dis* 21:217–19, 1994.

139 Weisman CS et al: Consistency of condom use for disease prevention among adolescent users of oral contraceptives. *Fam Plann Perspect* 23:71–74, 1991.

140 Santelli JS et al: Combined use of condoms with other contraceptive methods among inner-city Baltimore women. *Fam Plann Perspect* 27: 74–78, 1995.

141 Mosher WD, Pratt WF: Contraceptive use in the United States, 1973–88. Advanced Data. *Vital Health Stats* 182:1–12, 1990.

142 Brown S, Eisenberg L (eds): *The Best Intentions: Unintended Pregnancy and the Well-Being of Children and Families*. Washington, DC, National Academy Press, 1995, pp. 118–21.

143 Steiner M, Joanis C: Acceptability of dual methods use. *Fam Plann Perspect* 25:234, 1993.

144 Farr G et al: Use of spermicide and impact on prophylactic condom use among sex workers in Santa Fe de Bogota, Colombia. *Sex Transm Dis* 23:206–12, 1996.

145 Trussell J, Ellertson C: Efficacy of emergency contraception. *Fertil Control Revs* 4:8–11, 1995.

146 Cates W Jr, Raymond EG: Emergency contraception—Parsimony and prevention in the medicine cabinet. *Am J Public Health* 87:909–910, 1997.

147 Bowen GS et al: Risk behaviors for HIV infection in clients of Pennsylvania family planning clinics. *Fam Plann Perspect* 22:62–64, 1990.

148 Upchurch DM et al: Contraceptive needs and practices among women attending an inner city STD clinic. *Am J Public Health* 77: 1427–30, 1987.

149 Jamison DT, Mosley WM: Disease control priorities in developing countries: Health policy responses to epidemiological change. *Am J Public Health* 81:15–22, 1991.

150 Brown ST, Wiesner PJ: Problems and approaches to the control and surveillance of sexually transmitted agents associated with pelvic inflammatory disease in the United States. *Am J Obstet Gynecol* 138: 1096–1100, 1980.

151 Addiss DG et al: Selective screening for *Chlamydia trachomatis* infection in non-urban family planning clinics in Wisconsin. *Fam Plann Perspect* 19:252–56, 1987.

152 Katz AR: The Hawaii Chlamydia Network Project: A successful program incorporating close intra-agency cooperation. *Am J Public Health* 79:505–507, 1989.

153 Mosure DJ et al: Genital chlamydia infections in sexually active female adolescents: Do we really need to screen everyone? *Adolesc Health Care* 20:6–13, 1997.

154 Elias CJ, Heise LL: Challenges for the development of female-controlled vaginal microbicides. *AIDS* 8:1–9, 1994.

155 Stein ZA: More on women and the prevention of HIV infection. *Am J Public Health* 85:1485–88, 1995.

156 Mayhew S: Integrating MCH/FP and STD/HIV services: Current debates and future directions. *Health Pol and Plann* 11:339–353, 1996.

157 Wasserheit JN: Epidemiological synergy: Interrelationships between HIV infection and other STDs. *Sex Trans Dis* 19:61–77, 1992.

158 Bayer R: AIDS and the future of reproductive freedom. *Milbank Quart* 68(Suppl 2):179–204, 1990.

159 Levine C, Dubler NN: HIV and childbearing: 1) Uncertain risks and bitter realities: The reproductive choices of HIV-infected women. *Milbank Quart* 68:321–51, 1990.

160 Arras JD: HIV and childbearing: 2)AIDS and reproductive decisions: Having children in fear and trembling. *Milbank Quart* 68:353–82, 1990.

Chapter 79

Sexually transmitted diseases and infertility

Willard Cates, Jr.
Robert C. Brunham

Sexually transmitted diseases (STDs) affect human fertility primarily through infections of the female upper genital tract and their sequelae. Except for the rare bilateral epididymitis and obstruction of the male epididymis or vas deferens, STDs produce infertility in men less frequently. Therefore, this chapter will focus on infertility resulting from sexually acquired infections that ascend to produce endometritis and salpingitis. Chapter 58 examines the entity of pelvic inflammatory disease (PID); we will focus on sequelae to this condition.

DEFINITIONS

Infertility usually is defined clinically as the lack of recognized conception after 1 year of regular intercourse without the use of contraception. However, demographic surveys extend the interval to 2 years. In the general population, the conception rate is 10 to 15 percent per cycle (Fig. 79-1), whereas in couples who have been infertile for 1 year, it is 5 to 6 percent per cycle.[1] If infertility has persisted for 2 or more years, the conception rate falls markedly to about 1 to 3 percent per cycle.[2] In population-based studies of infertile couples, eventual pregnancy rates varied from 40 to 75 percent up to 10 years after the initial diagnosis.[2–6] Tubal infertility refers to infertility caused by damaged fallopian tubes, which can result from salpingitis, endometriosis, pelvic surgery, or congenital causes. We will address infertility only as it relates to salpingitis.

Salpingitis is an inflammation of the epithelial surfaces of the fallopian tubes caused by active infection with one or more of a number of organisms, most of which are sexually transmitted and ascend along mucosal surfaces from the cervix to the endometrium to the salpinx and, in some women, to the peritoneum.[7] PID is used to describe the symptoms and signs clinically associated with acute salpingitis. However, only about two-thirds of patients with a clinical diagnosis of PID actually have visual evidence of acute salpingitis by laparoscopy.[8] In the United States, the diagnosis of PID usually is made without laparoscopy. Many women with upper genital tract inflammation probably experience an asymptomatic or minimally symptomatic infection. In this chapter, we will use the term atypical PID to describe this condition (see Chap. 58).

HISTORY

An association between gonorrhea, PID, and tubal infertility was first reported in the pre-antibiotic era.[9,10] Upper genital tract infection, especially severe tubo-ovarian abscess, was a feared consequence of gonococcal infection, and rates of postgonococcal tubal obstruction of up to 70 percent were reported.[11] With the advent and use of sulfonamides and penicillin in the 1940s, both lower- and upper-genital tract infection caused by gonococci could be treated more effectively, and their sequelae were reduced.

The classic cohort studies of Weström and colleagues in Lund, Sweden in the 1960s demonstrated the impact of STD and salpingitis on subsequent tubal infertility.[12–14] These studies contributed data on such crucial topics as:

1. The clinical difference between PID and salpingitis;
2. The importance of chlamydia (in addition to gonorrhea) as a cause of tubal infertility;
3. The effects of different risk factors on fertility; and
4. The effects of different antibiotic regimens used for treatment of acute PID on fertility.

During the 1970s, the polymicrobial etiology of PID, and especially the role of *Chlamydia trachomatis* (CT), became increasingly appreciated.[15,16] More recently, the influence of contraceptives on both PID and tubal factor infertility has become clearer (Chap. 78). Intrauterine devices, especially the Dalkon Shield®, appeared to increase the risk of PID and infertility, whereas barrier methods—both mechanical and chemical—appeared protective.[17–19] Finally, an increased understanding of the role of atypical PID as a prelude to tubal obstruction has emerged from recent studies.[20]

DEMOGRAPHIC EFFECTS OF STD-RELATED INFERTILITY

In areas of the world where *Neisseria gonorrhoeae* and *C. trachomatis* infection are common, tubal infertility also is more frequent.[21,22] Particularly, strong data link the epidemiology of gonococcal infection with infertility. For instance, in Uganda, 15 districts recorded a significant inverse correlation between the annual reported incidence of gonococcal urethritis in men and the general fertility rate (Fig. 79-2).[23] A subsequent population-based study conducted in two rural districts of Uganda confirmed that gonococcal infection was the dominant determinant of fertility variation between the geographic districts, even after controlling for the effects of maternal nutrition and malaria.[24,25] Thus, STD-related infertility may be a major and under-recognized demographic factor affecting the rate at which populations expand.

To explore the potential relation between gonococcal and chlamydial infections and human population growth, mathematical models have been developed that combine epidemiologic and demographic data.[26,27] These models predict that in areas where untreated gonococcal and chlamydial infections are prevalent, STD-related infertility has a major impact on fertility and, concomitantly, on net population growth. Gonococcal infection was predicted to exert a greater demographic impact than chlamydial infection because of its greater incidence and higher prevalence of postinfection infertility.[27] Specifically, the models concluded that a 10 percent prevalence of gonorrhea in sexually active adults would result in a 25 percent reduction in net population growth; a 10 percent prevalence of chlamydia in sexually active adults would result in a 13 percent reduction in net population growth. Because demographers have raised valid questions regarding the assumptions underlying the mathematical models, additional demographic research into the recent expansion of world population is needed.[28]

Although data-based research will be required to provide compelling evidence to link STD-related infertility with demographic processes, the post-World War II demographic expansion may represent an "experiment-of-nature" that supports the notion that a reduction in gonorrhea incidence accelerates population growth.[29] In the United States in 1947, the incidence of gonococcal infection began to decline as penicillin treatment came into widespread clinical practice (Fig. 79-3). Simultaneously, the fertility rate rose and continued to rise until the early 1960s when newly introduced steroid contraceptives began to reduce the fertility

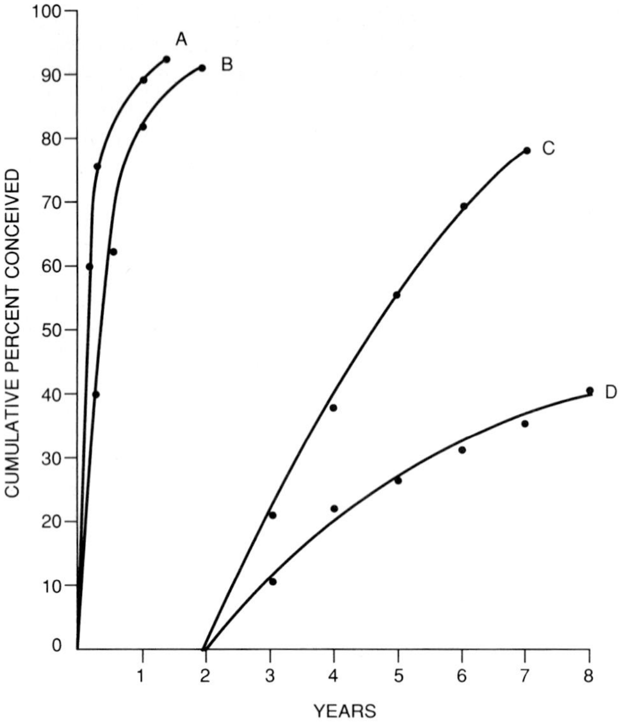

Fig. 79-1. The conception rates of a normal population of parous (A) and nulliparous (B) women are compared with the cumulative conception rates of apparently normal women with secondary infertility (C) and primary infertility (D). No conceptions occurred before the 2- to 3-year interval in the infertile groups as this was part of the selection criteria for these patients. From Lenton EA et al: Long-term follow-up of the apparently normal couple with a complaint of infertility. *Fertil Steril* 28:913, 1977. Used with permission.

rate.[30] The temporal correlations among the introduction of penicillin, declining incidence of gonorrhea and rising fertility are provocative.

The relation between STD-related infertility and demography is important to elucidate because of the major effect that population growth has on social and ecologic stability.[31,32] As developing countries strengthen health services, including those for STDs, accelerated population growth will occur and must be anticipated

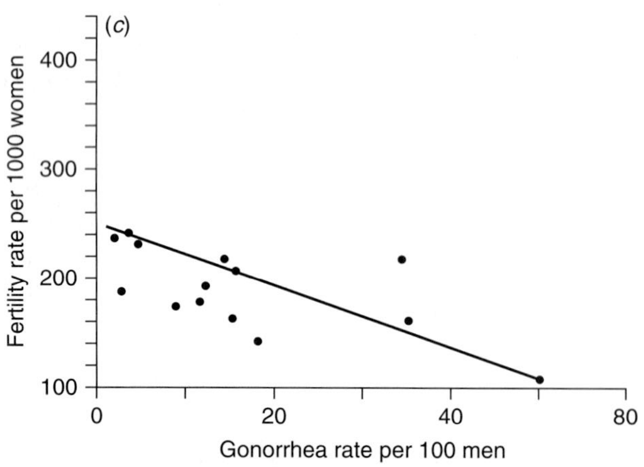

Fig. 79-2. Correlation between the annual reported incidence of gonococcal urethritis in men and the general fertility rate, Uganda health districts, 1960s. From Griffith HB: Gonorrhea and fertility in Uganda. *Eugen Rev* 55:103, 1963.

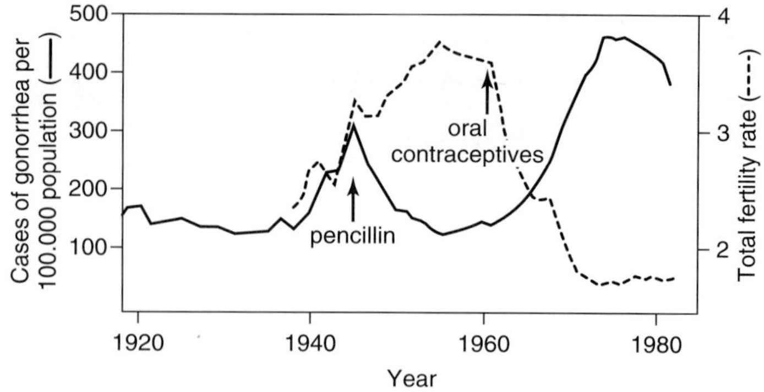

Fig. 79-3. The post-World War II decline in the incidence of gonorrhea in the United States was associated with the introduction of penicillin into clinical practice. This decline was associated with a rise in the fertility rate, which continued until 1962 when the fertility rate fell with the introduction of oral contraceptives into clinical practice. An equally precipitous ascent in the incidence of gonorrhea was also associated with the widespread use of oral contraceptives. GC continued to decrease by <200 in 1994 and TFR remains stable, through present. (Modified from Hook EW, Holmes KK. Gonococcal infections. *Ann Intern Med* 1985; 102:229–243; and Westoff CF. Fertility in the United States. *Science* 1986; 234:554–559.)

by those societies. In particular, as STD control programs are strengthened as part of HIV prevention strategies, the epidemiology of gonorrhea and chlamydia are likely to be substantially altered.[33] Thus, linkage of STD control programs with family planning initiatives will be important in achieving both short-term positive health benefits and a balanced longer-term social effect.[26,27,34]

PREVALENCE OF TUBAL INFERTILITY

From demographic surveys conducted worldwide, two yardsticks have generally been used to measure the prevalence of infertility: childlessness at older reproductive ages, and the absence of recent pregnancies in noncontracepting sexually active couples.[35,36] Using these definitions, rates of infertility have ranged from 1 to 16 percent of couples, with considerable regional variation.[37] When the denominator is confined to women who have actually attempted to become pregnant, about one in four had experienced infertility for at least 1 year and about 4 percent had never achieved a pregnancy.[5,38,39]

The presence of tubal damage can be identified only in women who are evaluated by a specialist. In the United States, couples in the middle to upper classes are more likely to seek such evaluation.[40] Because STD and salpingitis occur less frequently in these populations, the prevalence of tubal infertility is probably underestimated. In Bristol, England, where medical care is less subject to this bias, an average of 1.2 couples per 1000 population annually requested infertility advice from a specialist.[4] At this rate, approximately 1 in 6 couples (with an average length of infertility of 2.5 years) would seek help from a specialist at some time in their lives. Tubal damage was demonstrated in 14 percent of these infertile couples. In a representative Denmark population, nearly half of infertile couples had sought infertility services. One in five were diagnosed with tubal infertility, with older women (age >35 years) having higher rates.[5]

Internationally, the WHO multicenter study compared STD-related infertility in five different regions of the world.[41,42] More than 8000 infertile couples were enrolled in the study, and more than 6000 (71%) completed evaluation of the fallopian tubes. Almost two-thirds of infertility in African women was attributed

Table 79-1. Causes of Female Infertility, by Region

	Percent of cases associated with each cause			
Categories	Developed country	Africa	Asia	Latin America
No demonstrable cause	40	16	31	35
Bilateral tubal occlusion	11	49	14	15
Pelvic adhesions	13	24	13	17
Acquired tubal abnormalities	12	12	12	12
Anovulatory regular cycles	10	14	9	9
Anovulatory oligomenorrhea*	9	3	7	9
Ovulatory oligomenorrhea	7	4	11	5
Hyperprolactinemia	7	5	7	8
Endometriosis	6	1	10	3
Total†	115	128	114	113

*Includes amenorrhea.
†Total greater than 100 percent due to the presence of more than one factor in some women.
SOURCE: Adapted from Ref. 20.

to infection, including 49 percent with bilateral tubal occlusion and 24 percent with pelvic adhesions (Table 79-1). The prevalence of tubal occlusion in Africa was more than three times that of any other region. Developed countries had an 11 percent prevalence of tubal occlusion in infertile women. Non-African developing areas had higher rates of tubal occlusion than developed countries, although well below those of Africa.

Another approach to estimating the prevalence of tubal infertility utilizes extrapolation from the annual reported incidence of STDs. For example, approximately 3 million lower genital tract infections with chlamydia and/or gonorrhea occur in women each year in the United States.[43] Assuming 30 percent of these cause salpingitis, and that 17 percent of salpingitis leads to tubal occlusion, an estimated annual incidence of 125,000 cases of STD-related infertility occur each year.[44–46] Converting these to cumulative numbers, we estimate that approximately 2 million reproductive-age women (range 200,000 to 2.7 million) currently have tubal occlusion in the United States. However, only about one-half may desire more children, and a smaller percentage will seek infertility services.[47]

Although the preceding estimates are crude, they are internally consistent with the annually reported number of sexually transmitted infections, the number of ambulatory and hospitalized cases of PID, the number of infertility visits to private clinicians' offices, and the cross-sectional number of self-reported cases of PID and infertility in the American population of reproductive-age women.

SALPINGITIS AND TUBAL INFERTILITY

Tubal infertility is generally considered to be the direct result of acute salpingitis.[13] In long-term follow-up studies in Lund, Sweden, about 11 percent of women with laparoscopically documented acute salpingitis subsequently became infertile owing to tubal occlusion as compared with none of the control women with similar pelvic symptoms but noninflamed fallopian tubes.[12] The percentage of those with tubal infertility after PID was similar in women ages 25 years or older (12 percent) compared to younger women (11 percent) (Table 79-2).[12] Women who were using steroid contraceptives or IUDs at the time of the acute infection had lower rates of tubal infertility.[14]

The proportion who became infertile after a single episode of PID also varied directly with the severity of tubal inflammation

Table 79-2. Rate of Tubal Infertility among Women Trying to Conceive, by Age, Number of PID Episodes, and Severity of PID—Lund, Sweden, 1960–1984

Number of PID Episodes	Age <25		Age ≥25		Total	
One	7.7		9.1		8.0	
Mild		0.8		0.0		0.6
Moderate		6.4		5.6		6.2
Severe		20.1		25.0		21.2
Two	18.4		25.9		19.5	
Three or more	37.7		75.0		40.0	
Total	11.2		12.0		11.4	

Source: Adapted from Ref. 12.

(mild = 0.6 percent, moderate = 6.2 percent, severe = 21 percent).[12] Those women with symptomatic acute salpingitis who were taking steroid contraceptives generally had only mild tubal inflammation.[48] Women had an increasing risk of infertility with each episode of PID (one = 8 percent, two = 19 percent, three or more = 40 percent). Among the Lund cohort, the specific organism isolated from the cervix (*N. gonorrhoeae* vs. *C. trachomatis*) at the time of salpingitis made no discernible difference in subsequent infertility.

Most infertility following acute salpingitis presumably results from damaged fallopian tubes, since nearly all such women showed evidence of tubal obstruction by hysterosalpingography and/or surgery (Fig. 79-4).[14] Further evidence that obstruction of the fallopian tubes and peritubal adhesions are the sequelae of acute salpingitis is derived from animal models, especially monkeys and mice.[49–51] Although mechanical obstruction usually causes a hydrosalpinx, it leads to little residual damage.[52,53] In contrast, tubal infection with *C. trachomatis* results in necrosis of secretory cells and deciliation and eventually distal obstruction and hydrosalpinx (Figs. 79-5 and 79-6).[54]

Despite surgical lysis of adhesions and establishment of tubal patency, subsequent fertility rates are low. This probably results from the severe cellular and subcellular damage observed along the entire length of both fallopian tubes. For example, the tubes

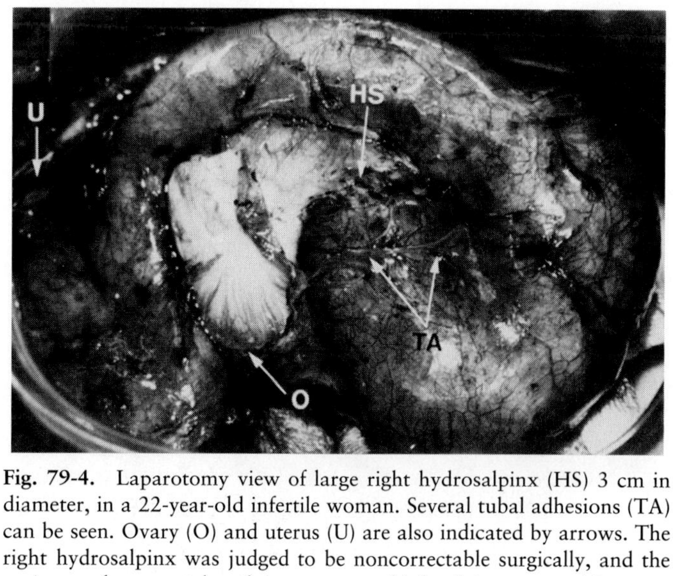

Fig. 79-4. Laparotomy view of large right hydrosalpinx (HS) 3 cm in diameter, in a 22-year-old infertile woman. Several tubal adhesions (TA) can be seen. Ovary (O) and uterus (U) are also indicated by arrows. The right hydrosalpinx was judged to be noncorrectable surgically, and the patient underwent right salpingectomy and left salpingostomy. (Courtesy of Dr. Michael R. Soules, Department of Obstetrics and Gynecology, University of Washington.)

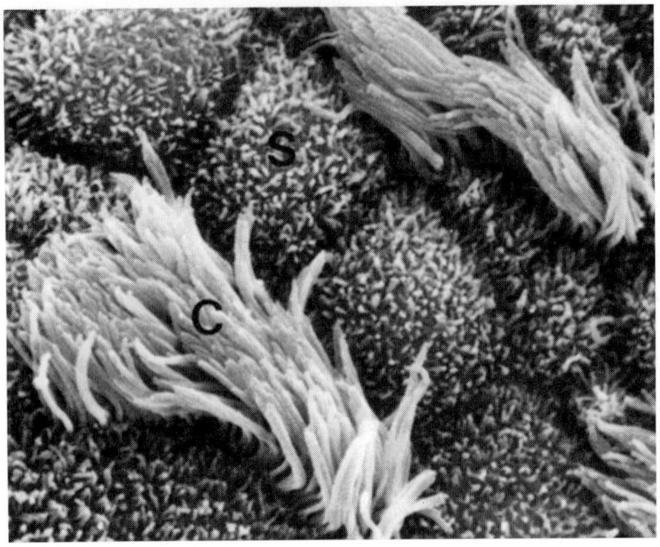

Fig. 79-5. Normal fallopian tube. Secretory cells (S) with abundant microvilli are surrounded by clumps of long, slender cilia (C) atop the ciliated cells. 4800×. (SEM provided by Dr. Dorothy L. Patton, Departments of Obstetrics and Gynecology and Biological Structure, University of Washington.)

of women undergoing surgical repair show marked deciliation. Physiologically, ciliary motion of such damaged epithelial cells is markedly reduced.[20] This reduction in ciliary activity is thought to be permanent.[54]

ETIOLOGY

Unraveling etiologic relationships among STDs, PID, and infertility is a complex exercise in causal reasoning (Fig. 79-7). We must

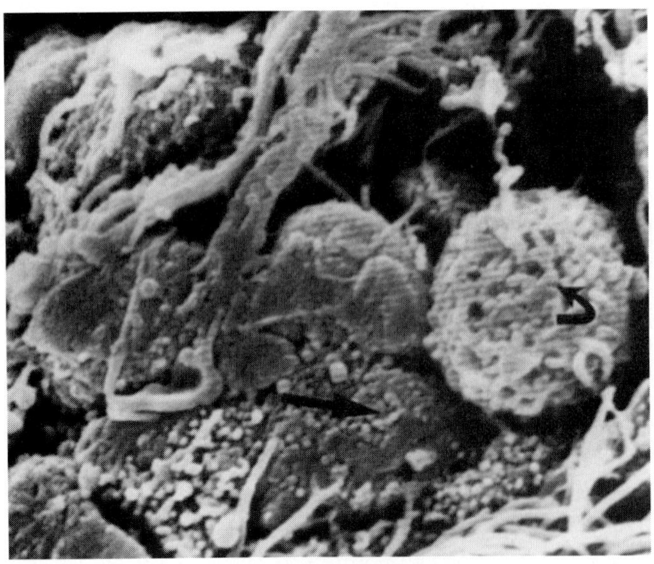

Fig. 79-6. Infertile fallopian tube following infection. Pronounced deciliation (straight arrow) of the ciliated cells and clubbing of the microvilli on the secretory (curved arrow) cells are evident in this biopsy taken from a distally occluded fallopian tube. 5200×. (SEM provided by Dr. Dorothy L. Patton, Departments of Obstetrics and Gynecology and Biological Structure, University of Washington.)

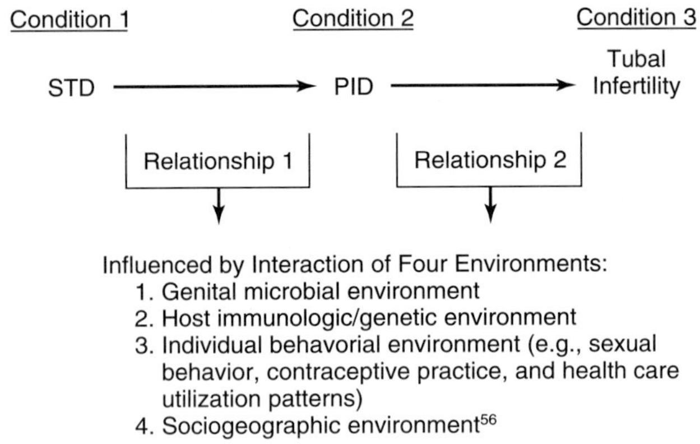

Fig. 79-7. Etiologic relationships among STD, PID, and tubal infertility as affected by four "environmental" influences.

examine correlations among variables with inconsistent definitions, imprecise diagnoses, and different microbial organisms.[55] The causal pathway includes three distinct links in the chain (lower genital tract STDs as the antecedent condition, upper genital tract PID as the intermediate condition, and eventual tubal infertility as the outcome). These conditions each have a temporal lag in clinical expression (STDs leading to PID, PID leading to tubal infertility). These relations in turn are influenced by the overlapping effects of four environments (Fig. 79-7).

All studies to date have found a strong association between STDs, PID, and tubal infertility. The cohort studies from Lund, Sweden, remain the best evidence for the link between salpingitis and infertility.[12–14] In addition, infertile women with a self-reported history of gonorrhea or nonspecific STD or PID were almost three times more likely to have tubal occlusion as a cause of their infertility.[57,58] Similarly, among American women with a history of PID, the proportion with fertility problems (44 percent) was twofold higher than among women without such a history (21 percent). This difference was found in both nulliparous and multiparous women.[59]

Salpingitis associated with either *N. gonorrhoeae* or *C. trachomatis* has been causally related to subsequent tubal infertility.[22] Prospective studies show the fertility prognosis is poor for women suffering symptomatic PID caused by either gonococcal or chlamydial agents.[12,22,60] Gonorrhea has been related to tubal infertility in studies using self-reported cervical infections, clinical diagnoses, laparoscopically proved salpingitis, and positive serology.[11,12,22,57,61,62] However, investigators from England have found gonococcal antibody less strongly associated with tubal occlusion than chlamydial antibody.[63]

The role that chlamydia plays in causing tubal infertility has been more exhaustively studied than the role of gonorrhea.[16] Investigators from at least 30 different cities around the world have documented that tubal occlusion is strongly associated with the presence of chlamydial antibody.[16,22,64–77] When these studies are combined, 70 percent of women with tubal infertility had antibodies to chlamydia versus 26 percent of control women.[16]

Despite the relatively benign symptoms and signs it produces, *C. trachomatis* apparently causes as much tubal inflammation—and ultimately tubal damage—as other agents.[78] The occurrence of severe tubal damage despite mild clinical signs is probably owing to the more subacute and prolonged nature of chlamydial salpingitis as compared with salpingitis caused by other organisms. This hypothesis is supported by the low prevalence of immunoglobulin M antibody to chlamydia among women with acute salpingitis.[77] As with trachoma, prolonged subacute chlamydial infection in the genital tract can lead to chronic inflammation and scarring in affected organs (Chap. 28).

CHLAMYDIAL HEAT SHOCK PROTEIN 60 AND TUBAL OBSTRUCTION

Seroepidemiologic study of women with tubal infertility has shown that women with CT-associated infertility have antibody to a distinctive chlamydial antigen of 57,000 daltons molecular mass.[67] Molecular study showed that this antigen was a highly conserved heat shock protein 60 (hsp60) whose homologs are widely found in both bacterial and eucaryotic cells.[79] Purified recombinant chlamydial hsp60 has been evaluated in animal models of chlamydial disease pathogenesis and shown to be a potent T-cell antigen capable of eliciting an intense inflammatory response when applied to the mucosal surfaces of the fallopian tube of immunologically primed animals.[80,81] These characteristics are highly suggestive of the hypothesized chlamydial hypersensitivity antigen implicated in chlamydial immunopathology and tissue fibrosis.[82]

The availability of recombinant chlamydial hsp60 also has facilitated detailed immunoepidemiological studies among CT-infected humans. Studies of antibodies to the chlamydial hsp60 antigen among women with different sequelae to chlamydial infection show a consistent gradient in seroprevalence to the hsp60 protein: 16 to 25 percent of microimmunofluorescent antibody-positive fertile women have chlamydial hsp60 antibody, as do 36 to 44 percent of women with CT cervicitis, 48 to 60 percent of women with CT PID, and 81 to 90 percent of women with CT-related fallopian tube obstruction (Fig. 79-8).[83–85] Furthermore, among women with laparoscopically visualized chlamydial PID, those with high antibody titers to chlamydial hsp60 have had significantly more severe inflammatory manifestations.[67] The enrichment for women with antibody responses to chlamydial hsp60 among those with the severest forms of CT infection suggests that hsp60 may induce the tissue damaging immune responses.

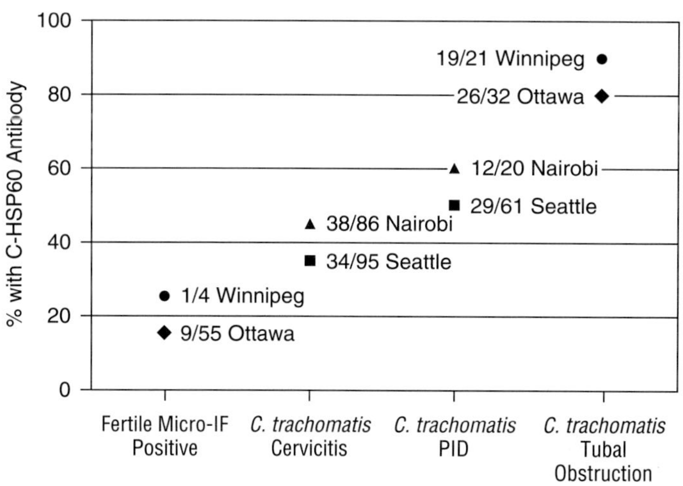

Fig. 79-8. Proportion of women with hsp60 antibody. From Brunham RC et al: *Chlamydia trachomatis*-associated ectopic pregnancy: Serologic and histologic correlates. *J Infect Dis* 165:1076, 1992; Stamm WE et al: Prevalence and correlates of antibody to chlamydial hsp-60 in *C. trachomatis* infected women. Presented at Eighth International Symposium on Human Chlamydial Infection, Chantilly, France, June 1994; Toye B et al: Association between antibody to the chlamydial heat-shock protein and tubal infertility. *J Infect Dis* 168:1236, 1993.

Hsp60 immune recognition may incite an autoimmune–inflammatory reaction because of molecular mimicry among shared peptide sequences between the chlamydial and human hsp60.[80] Relevant to this hypothesis, antibody responses to peptide epitopes from human hsp60 have been observed among women with CT-associated ectopic pregnancy.[86] Alternatively, antibody responses to chlamydial hsp60 may signal chronic persistent or repeated chlamydial infection with other chlamydial antigens sustaining the chronic inflammatory reaction.[87,88] Which of these mechanisms is operative in the pathogenesis of CT tubal infertility remains unclear at the present time.

Antibody responses to CT hsp60 are genetically determined in mice, and the same may be true in humans.[89] If immune responses to chlamydial hsp60 are central to the pathogenesis of chlamydial disease, it may be that genetic factors for chlamydial disease susceptibility exist and could explain the surprising heterogeneity in risk for chlamydial disease sequelae such as tubal infertility.

In aggregate, the clinical and experimental data are consistent with the hypothesis that CT disease pathogenesis is owing to immunologically mediated tissue injury. Immunopathological responses seem to occur in a subset of infected individuals who may be genetically predisposed. Although immune responses to chlamydial hsp60 correlate with disease severity and sequelae, the precise nature of immune-mediated tissue damage and its relation to hsp60 remains to be elucidated.

ATYPICAL PID

Studies of tubal infertility have reported that 39 to 81 percent (median 63 percent) of cases had no history of symptoms or signs of PID.[16] Demographically, women with tubal infertility who have no history of PID are similar to women with the same diagnosis who had a PID history.[20] By electron microscopy and by assessment of mucosal ciliary activity, the two groups also have identical cellular lesions. Both groups show severe ciliary denudation and decreased ciliary function. Moreover, using retrospective analyses, attempts to use clinical and epidemiological factors to identify women with atypical PID have been unsuccessful.[90]

An estimated 8 to 30 percent of women with cervical chlamydial infection will develop clinically apparent salpingitis if not treated with appropriate antibiotics.[45] The percentage that will develop atypical PID and tubal infertility is unknown. Although atypical PID is "asymptomatic" by the usual criteria, symptoms such as mild pelvic pain or abnormal uterine bleeding may signal ascending infection in some patients. In Seattle, 40 percent of women with cervicitis had endometritis demonstrated on biopsy; these women were either asymptomatic or had mild pelvic symptoms.[91] In Lund, Sweden, most women with laparoscopic evidence of previous chlamydial infection recollected having past pelvic symptoms, although never formally diagnosed as PID.[92] Collectively, these data suggest that unrecognized infection of the upper genital tract occurs frequently with CT. This chronic endometritis and cervicitis may serve to stimulate the immunologically mediated mechanism of tissue destruction described earlier.

PERSISTENCE OF ORGANISMS

Whether chlamydia or other microorganisms persist in the female genital tract for years after an initial episode of salpingitis is controversial. Since CT produces chronic subclinical infection of the eye (trachoma) that may persist and reactivate during periods of immunosuppression, a similar situation might occur with chlamydial PID.[93,94]

The most direct but controversial evidence for persistence of chlamydia in the fallopian tubes is isolation of the organism from the upper genital tract in women with tubal infertility. In Paris, women with tubal infertility often have had a yellowish, viscous effusion in the pelvis that is reported culture-positive for CT.[72] In Indianapolis, CT has been isolated from the endometrium of 32 percent of women with tubal infertility.[95] In Ontario, chlamydial antigen was demonstrated immunochemically in 1 of 16 tubal biopsy specimens in women with tubal factor infertility, despite negative endotubal cultures.[76] In Oslo, serologic evidence of active infection was found; IgM antibody to CT was found in 24 percent of infertile women with tubal occlusion compared with 2 percent of controls.[73] However, other centers have not been able to isolate chlamydia from women with tubal infertility using not only cervical cultures but also endometrial tissue and tubal swabs.[64,67,68,96]

This controversy remains unresolved. Molecular studies based on DNA hybridization suggest that noncultivatable chlamydial chronic infection that is not detectable by using cell culture or standard antigen detection techniques is commonly present in women with tubal infertility.[97,98] Further studies clearly are needed to resolve these important discrepancies.

RISK FACTORS FOR TUBAL INFERTILITY

Several factors affect the likelihood of the progression of PID to tubal occlusion. The first and most important variable is the number of previous PID episodes.[12] As noted in the preceding, each new acute salpingitis episode approximately doubles the rate of postsalpingitis infertility (Table 79-2).

Second, the severity of the pelvic inflammation, judged by laparoscopy, also influences the fertility outcome. Among those with only one PID episode, women with severe inflammatory changes had markedly higher rates of subsequent tubal infertility than those with mild disease; women with moderate changes are in between.[12]

Third, delaying seeking health care after pelvic symptoms occur affects future fertility.[99] Women who waited more than 3 days to see a clinician from the onset of their initial symptoms had a nearly threefold increased risk of impaired fertility compared to those who sought care promptly. Allowing inflammation a longer time to cause biologic damage apparently influences the prognosis of salpingitis, just as with other infections.

Fourth, contraceptive choice also affects the likelihood of tubal infertility. Women who had used IUDs in the past were found to have a higher risk of tubal factor infertility, with the Dalkon Shield® accounting for most of this risk.[17,18] Copper-containing IUDs had a lower, although still increased, risk of tubal infertility than that observed with the Dalkon Shield.® Barrier methods of contraception—including both condoms and spermicides—protected against eventual tubal infertility. Although the mechanical benefits of condoms provided only marginal protection, when coupled with the chemical benefits of spermicides, combination barrier methods provided a twofold protection against tubal infertility.[19]

The relation of oral contraceptive (OC) use to the risk of tubal infertility remains complicated. In one study, the use of oral contraceptives did not protect against tubal infertility, and OCs with higher levels of estrogen were associated with an increased risk of tubal infertility.[19] In contrast, a protective effect of OCs against symptomatic PID and tubal infertility has been reported by others despite *C. trachomatis* cervicitis being more common in OC users.[12,100–104]

A possible explanation for the findings is that OCs may mask the symptoms of acute PID without affecting the pathogenesis toward tubal obstruction. The sevenfold higher level of unrecognized endometritis, compared to symptomatic PID, among women using OCs supports this latter explanation.[105] Further studies are needed to clarify the relationship of OC use to acute PID and to its sequel tubal infertility.

Finally, smoking increases the risk of tubal infertility in nulligravid women, and the risk appears dose-related.[106,107] Women who both smoked and used an IUD were at greater risk than women who had either risk alone. Former smokers had no increased risk. Smoking may impair immune defenses that prevent ascent of STD organisms to the fallopian tubes. Lymphocytes of smokers show decreased humoral and cell-mediated immunity in vitro.[108–110]

PREVENTION

Preventing STD-related tubal infertility can take place on three levels—primary, secondary, and tertiary prevention. Primary prevention blocks acquisition of the infection, secondary prevention blocks progression of a lower genital tract infection to the upper genital tract, and tertiary prevention blocks the progression of upper genital tract infection to tubal obstruction and eventual infertility. Because of the excessive costs of treating "end stage" tubal infertility, investments in primary prevention have advantages over secondary and tertiary from the cost-benefit point of view.[111]

Primary prevention of STD has received a recent boost from the increased public awareness of the consequences of AIDS and HIV infections and is discussed in detail elsewhere in this volume. Secondary prevention of tubal infertility emphasizes the traditional STD control approaches of screening and partner notification. Although the fertility outcome of acute PID has been markedly improved in the antimicrobial era as compared to the pre-antimicrobial era, tertiary prevention using single antibiotics for PID has not been ideal.[112] In the Lund PID cohort, among women who were treated for PID with four different single antibiotic regimens, tubal infertility occurred among 10 to 13 percent regardless of the therapy used.[113] Antibiotics specifically directed against either *N. gonorrhoeae, C. trachomatis,* or predominantly facultative anaerobes were associated with virtually identical tubal infertility rates.

Currently recommended multiple antibiotic regimens may produce a better long-term fertility prognosis than single antibiotics.[112,114] However, even these regimens may have a limited effect on tubal damage that already existed before treatment was started or they may not eradicate smoldering chlamydia despite apparently negative cultures after treatment. This challenge is further complicated by the continuing and frequent use of inappropriate antibiotics to treat PID.[115] Future studies using fertility endpoints will help assess our current PID treatment guidelines.

It appears if we wish to have the greatest impact on STD-related tubal infertility, the infections will have to be prevented or treated before they reach the fallopian tubes. Recent evidence demonstrated widespread chlamydial screening, whether in regional family planning clinics or in HMO populations, can reduce levels of both lower and upper genital tract infections.[116,117]

DIAGNOSIS AND MANAGEMENT OF INFERTILITY

Most couples are unaware of tubal obstruction until they attempt to become pregnant. Usually after a predetermined length of time (such as 12 months), couples who have unsuccessfully attempted to conceive will seek infertility evaluation. Although economic, personnel, and laboratory resources in traditional STD or other reproductive health settings may be limited, some basic initial services should be provided by most outpatient facilities. For example, gathering pertinent historical information, especially about past STDs or PID, providing a thorough physical examination, and making a plan for diagnosis and treatment based on information gathered can be performed. Ultimately, tubal patency should be confirmed either by laparoscopy or by hysterosalpingogram. Tubal abnormalities may be amenable to corrective surgical procedures, in some cases requiring microsurgery. However, the delicate cilia and mucosa of the tubal lining cannot be surgically regenerated. Thus, surgery generally produces a low rate of tubal cure. In vitro fertilization may be the only way to bypass damaged fallopian tubes.

CONCLUSION

Sexually transmitted diseases are the main preventable cause of human infertility. Lower genital tract infections that ascend into the upper genital tract can produce inflammation and scarring that decreases the chances of intratubal fertilization and/or intrauterine implantation.

N. gonorrhoeae and *C. trachomatis* are the two sexually transmitted organisms most clearly associated with tubal infertility. Recent discovery of chlamydial hsp60 antigen may help explain the immunological reaction characteristic of chlamydial inflammation in the tubes. Atypical PID, possibly representing chronic endometritis, has become increasingly recognized as a major contributor to tubal infertility. To have the greatest impact on STD-related infertility, cervical infections will have to be prevented or treated before they reach the fallopian tubes.

References

1 Lenton EA et al: Long-term follow-up of the apparently normal couple with a complaint of infertility. *Fertil Steril* 28:913, 1977.
2 Collins JA et al: Treatment-independent pregnancy among infertile couples. *N Engl J Med* 309:1201, 1983.
3 Katayama KP et al: Computer analysis of etiology and pregnancy rate in 636 cases of primary infertility. *Am J Obstet Gynecol* 135:207, 1979.
4 Hull MG et al: Population study of causes, treatment, and outcome of infertility. *Br Med J* 291:1693, 1985.
5 Schmidt L et al: Infertility and the seeking of infertility treatment in a representative population. *Br J Obstet Gynaecol* 102:978, 1995.
6 Marchbanks PA et al: Research on infertility: definition makes a difference. *Am J Epidemiol* 130:259, 1989.
7 Kahn JG et al: Diagnosing pelvic inflammatory disease: A comprehensive analysis and considerations for developing a new model. *JAMA* 266:2594–2604, 1991.
8 Jacobson L et al: Objectivized diagnosis of acute pelvic inflammatory disease. *Am J Obstet Gynecol* 105:1088, 1969.
9 Noeggerath E: Latent gonorrhea, especially with regard to its fertility in women. *Trans Am Gynecol Assoc* 1292, 1976.
10 Brandt AM: *No Magic Bullet: A Social History of Venereal Disease in the United States Since 1880.* New York, Oxford University Press, 1985.
11 Falk V: Treatment of acute non-tuberculous salpingitis with antibiotics alone and in combination with glucocorticoids. *Acta Obstet Gynecol Scand* 44(suppl 6):85, 1965.
12 Weström L et al: Pelvic inflammatory disease and fertility: A cohort study of 1,844 women with laparoscopically verified disease and 657 control women with normal laparoscopic results. *Sex Transm Dis* 19:185–192, 1992.
13 Weström L: Effect of pelvic inflammatory disease on fertility. *Venerology* 8:219–224, 1995.
14 Weström L: Chlamydia and its effect on reproduction. *J Br Fertil Soc* 1:23–32, 1996.
15 Eschenbach DA et al: Polymicrobial etiology of acute pelvic inflammatory disease. *N Engl J Med* 293:166–170, 1975.
16 Cates W Jr et al: Genital chlamydial infections: Epidemiology and reproductive sequelae. *Am J Obstet Gynecol* 164:1777–1781, 1991.
17 Cramer DW et al: Tubal infertility and the intrauterine device. *N Engl J Med* 312:941, 1985.
18 Daling JR et al: Primary tubal infertility in relation to the use of an intrauterine device. *N Engl J Med* 312:937, 1985.
19 Cramer DW et al: The relationship of tubal infertility to barrier method and oral contraceptive use. *JAMA* 257:2446–2450, 1987.
20 Patton DL et al: A comparison of the fallopian tube's response to overt and silent salpingitis. *Obstet Gynecol* 73:622, 1989.
21 Belsey MA: The epidemiology of infertility: A review with particular reference to sub-Saharan Africa. *Bull WHO* 54:319, 1976.
22 World Health Organization Task Force on the Prevention and Management of Infertility: Tubal infertility: Serologic relationship to past chlamydial and gonococcal infection. *Sex Transm Dis* 22:71, 1995.
23 Griffith HB: Gonorrhea and fertility in Uganda. *Eugen Rev* 55:103, 1963.
24 Arya OP et al: Clinical, cultural, and demographic aspects of gonorrhoeae in a rural community in Uganda. *Bull WHO* 49:587, 1973.
25 Arya OP et al: Gonorrhea and female infertility in rural Uganda. *Am J Obstet Gynecol* 138:929, 1980.
26 Brunham RC et al: Gonococcal infection and human fertility in sub-Saharan Africa. *Proc R Soc Lond B* 246:173, 1992
27 Brunham RC et al: *Chlamydia trachomatis,* infertility, and population growth in sub-Saharan Africa. *Sex Transm Dis* 20:168, 1993.
28 Zaba B et al: The impact of eliminating sterility on population growth. *Sex Transm Dis* 21:289, 1994.
29 Westoff CF: Fertility in the United States. *Science* 234:554, 1986.
30 McFalls JA Jr et al: Disease and fertility. Orlando, Academic Press, 1984.
31 Rosenfield A: Population growth: Implications and problems. *Infect Dis Clin No Am* 5:277, 1991.
32 Bongaarts J: Population policy options in the developing world. *Science* 263:771–776, 1994.
33 Grosskurth H et al: Impact of improved treatment of sexually transmitted diseases on HIV infection in rural Tanzania: Randomised controlled trial. *Lancet* 346:530–536, 1995.
34 Cates W Jr: Family planning and sexually transmitted diseases: Strange or natural bedfellows, revisited. *Sex Transm Dis* 20:174, 1993.
35 Sherris JD et al: Infertility and sexually transmitted disease: A public health challenge. *Pop Rep* 4(L):L-114, 1983.
36 Schmidt L et al: Infertility, involuntary fecundity, and the seeking of medical advice in industrialized countries 1970–1992: A review of concepts, measurements and results. *Hum Reprod* 10:1407, 1995.
37 Cates W Jr et al: Patterns of infertility in the developed and developing world, in *Symposium on the Diagnosis and Treatment of Infertility,* Rowe PJ et al (eds). Bern, Switzerland, Hans Huber, 1988.
38 Page H: Estimation of the prevalence and incidence of infertility in a population: A pilot study. *Fertil Steril* 51:571, 1989.
39 Greenhall E, Vessey M:. The prevalence of subfertility: A review of the current confusion and a report of two new studies. *Fertil Steril* 54:978, 1990.
40 Hirsch MB et al: Characteristics of infertile women in the United States and their use of infertility services. *Fertil Steril* 47:618, 1987.
41 Cates W et al: Worldwide patterns of infertility: Is Africa different? *Lancet* 2:596, 1985.
42 World Health Organization: Infections, pregnancies, and infertility: perspectives on prevention. *Fertil Steril* 47:964, 1987.
43 Centers for Disease Control and Prevention: Division of STD Prevention Annual Report, 1996. Atlanta, GA: CDC, 1997.
44 Platt R et al: Risk of acquiring gonorrhea and prevalence of abnormal adnexal findings among women recently exposed to gonorrhea. *JAMA* 250:3205, 1983.
45 Stamm WE et al: Effect of treatment regimens for *Neisseria gonorrhoeae* on simultaneous infection with *Chlamydia trachomatis. N Engl J Med* 310:545, 1984.
46 Weström L: Influence of sexually transmitted diseases on sterility and ectopic pregnancy. *Acta Eur Fertil* 16:21, 1985.

47 Henshaw SK et al: The need and unmet need for infertility services in the United States. *Fam Plann Perspect* 19:180, 1987.
48 Svensson L et al: Infertility after acute salpingitis with special reference to *Chlamydia trachomatis. Fertil Steril* 40:322, 1983.
49 Patton DL et al: Host response to primary *Chlamydia trachomatis* infection of the fallopian tube in pig-tailed monkeys. *Fertil Steril* 40: 829, 1983.
50 Møller BR et al: Experimental pelvic inflammatory diseases provoked by *Chlamydia trachomatis* and *Mycoplasma hominis. Obstet Gynecol* 138:990, 1980.
51 Swenson CE et al: Infertility as a consequence of chlamydial infection of the upper genital tract in female mice. *Sex Transm Dis* 11:64, 1984.
52 Patton DL et al: Mechanically-induced hydrosalpinx: Long-term oviductal dilation does not impair ciliary transport function. *Fertil Steril* 36:808, 1981.
53 Halbert SA et al: Hydrosalpinx: Effect of oviductal dilation on egg transport. *Fertil Steril* 35:69, 1981.
54 Patton DL et al: Distal tubal obstruction induced by repeated *Chlamydia trachomatis* salpingeal infections in pig-tailed macaques. *J Infect Dis* 155:1292–1298, 1987.
55 Cates W Jr et al: Pelvic inflammatory disease and tubal infertility: the preventable conditions, in *Human Reproductive Ecology: Interactions of Environment, Fertility and Behavior. Annals of the New York Academy of Sciences,* Vol. 709, Campbell KL et al (eds). New York, New York Academy of Sciences, 1994, pp. 179–195.
56 Wasserheit JN: Effect of changes in human ecology and behavior on patterns of sexually transmitted diseases, including human immunodeficiency virus infection. *Proc Natl Acad Sci USA* 91:2430, 1993.
57 Sherman KJ et al: Sexually transmitted diseases and tubal infertility. *Sex Transm Dis* 14:12, 1987.
58 Cates W Jr et al: Sexually transmitted diseases, pelvic inflammatory disease, and infertility: An epidemiologic update. *Epidemiol Rev* 12: 219–220, 1990.
59 Aral SO et al: Contraceptive use, pelvic inflammatory disease, and fertility problems among American women: 1982. *Am J Obstet Gynecol* 157:59–67, 1987.
60 Plummer F et al: A comparison of doxycycline (DOX) and metronidazole (MET) with trimethoprim sulfamethoxazole (TMP/SMT) and metronidazole for treatment of pelvic inflammatory disease (PID): Assessment of effect on infertility (Abstract 65). Presented at the International Society for STD Research, Atlanta, Georgia, August 3, 1987.
61 Mabey DCW et al: Tubal infertility in the Gambia: Chlamydial and gonococcal serology in women with tubal occlusion compared with pregnant controls. *Bull WHO* 63:1107–1113, 1985.
62 Tjiam KH et al: Prevalence of antibodies to *Chlamydia trachomatis, Neisseria gonorrhoeae,* and *Mycoplasma hominis* in infertile women. *Genitourin Med* 61:175–178, 1985.
63 Robertson JN et al: Chlamydial and gonococcal antibodies in sera of infertile women with tubal obstruction. *J Clin Pathol* 40:377–383, 1987.
64 Moore DE et al: Increased frequency of serum antibodies to *Chlamydia trachomatis* in infertility due to distal tubal disease. *Lancet* 2: 574–577, 1982.
65 Guderian AM et al: Residues of pelvic inflammatory disease in intrauterine device users: A result of the intrauterine device or *Chlamydia trachomatis* infection? *Am J Obstet Gynecol* 154:497–503, 1986.
66 Quinn PA et al: Prevalence of antibody to *Chlamydia trachomatis* in spontaneous abortion and infertility. *Am J Obstet Gynecol* 154:291–296, 1987.
67 Brunham RC et al: *Chlamydia trachomatis:* Its role in tubal infertility. *J Infect Dis* 152:1275–1282, 1985.
68 Kane JL et al: Evidence of chlamydial infection in infertile women with and without fallopian tube obstruction. *Fertil Steril* 42:832–838, 1984.
69 Jones RB et al: Correlation between serum antichlamydial antibodies and tubal factor as a cause of infertility. *Fertil Steril* 38:553–558, 1982.
70 Gump DW et al: Evidence of prior pelvic inflammatory disease and its relationship to *Chlamydia trachomatis* antibody and intrauterine contraceptive device use in infertile women. *Am J Obstet Gynecol* 146:153–159, 1983.
71 Conway D et al: Chlamydial serology in fertile and infertile women. *Lancet* 1:191–193, 1984.
72 Henry-Suchet J et al: Microbiologic study of chronic inflammation associated with tubal factor infertility: Role of *Chlamydia trachomatis. Fertil Steril* 47:274, 1987.
73 Ånestad G et al: Infertility and chlamydial infection. *Fertil Steril* 48: 787–790, 1987.
74 Punnonen R et al: Chlamydial serology in infertile women by immunofluorescence. *Fertil Steril* 31:656–659, 1979.
75 Battin DA et al: *Chlamydia trachomatis* is not an important cause of abnormal postcoital tests in ovulating patients. *Fertil Steril* 42:233–238, 1984.
76 Sellors JW et al: Tubal factor infertility: An association with prior chlamydial infection and asymptomatic salpingitis. *Fertil Steril* 49: 451–457, 1988.
77 Gjonnaess H et al: Pelvic inflammatory disease: Etiologic studies with emphasis on chlamydial infection. *Obstet Gynecol* 59:550, 1982.
78 Svensson L et al: Differences in some clinical and laboratory parameters in acute salpingitis related to culture and serologic finding. *Am J Obstet Gynecol* 138:1017, 1980.
79 Cerrone MC et al: Cloning and sequence of the gene for heat shock protein 60 from *Chlamydia trachomatis* and immunological reactivity of the protein. *Infect Immun* 59:79, 1991.
80 Morrison RP et al: Chlamydial disease pathogenesis: The 57kD chlamydial hypersensitivity antigen is a stress response protein. *J Exp Med* 170:1271, 1989.
81 Patton DL: Demonstration of delayed hypersensitivity in *Chlamydia trachomatis* salpingitis in monkeys: A pathogenic mechanism of tubal damage. *J Infect Dis* 169:680, 1994.
82 Morrison RP et al: Immunology of *Chlamydia trachomatis* infections: Immunoprotective and immunopathogenetic responses. *Advances in Host Defense Mechanisms,* Vol 8. *Sexually Transmitted Diseases.* Raven Press, Ltd, 1992.
83 Brunham RC et al: *Chlamydia trachomatis*-associated ectopic pregnancy: Serologic and histologic correlates. *J Infect Dis* 165:1076, 1992.
84 Stamm WE et al: Prevalence and correlates of antibody to chlamydial hsp-60 in *C. trachomatis* infected women. Presented at Eighth International Symposium on Human Chlamydial Infection, Chantilly, France, June 1994.
85 Toye B et al: Association between antibody to the chlamydial heat-shock protein and tubal infertility. *J Infect Dis* 168:1236, 1993.
86 Yi Y et al: Continuous B-cell epitopes in *Chlamydia trachomatis* heat shock protein 60. *Infect Immun* 61:1117, 1993.
87 Beatty WL: Morphologic and antigenic characterization of interferon K-mediated persistent *Chlamydia trachomatis* infection in vitro. *Proc Natl Acad Sci USA* 90:3998, 1993.
88 Mueller BA et al: Detection of *Chlamydia trachomatis* deoxyribonucleic acid in women with tubal infertility. *Fertil Steril* 59:45, 1993.
89 Zhong GM et al: Antibody responses to the chlamydial heat shock proteins hsp60 and hsp70 are H2 linked. *Infect Immun* 60:3143, 1992.
90 Cates W Jr et al: Atypical pelvic inflammatory disease: Can we identify clinical predictors? *Am J Obstet Gynecol* 169:341–346, 1993.
91 Paavonen J et al: Prevalence and manifestations of endometritis among women with cervicitis. *Am J Obstet Gynecol* 152:280, 1985.
92 Wølner-Hanssen P: Silent pelvic inflammatory disease: Is it overstated? *Obstet Gynecol* 86:321, 1995.
93 Yang Y-S et al: Reactivation of *Chlamydia trachomatis* lung infection in mice by cortisone. *Infect Immun* 39:655, 1983.
94 Wang S-P et al: Trachoma in the Taiwan monkey, *Macaca cyclopis. Ann NY Acad Sci* 98:177, 1962.
95 Cleary RE et al: Recovery of *Chlamydia trachomatis* from the endometrium in infertile women with serum antichlamydial antibodies. *Fertil Steril* 44:233, 1985.

96 Cassell GH et al: Microbiologic study of infertile women at the time of diagnostic laparoscopy. *N Engl J Med* 308:502, 1983.
97 Campbell LA et al: Detection of *Chlamydia trachomatis* deoxyribonucleic acid in women with tubal infertility. *Fertil Steril* 59:445, 1993.
98 Cappuccio AL et al: Detection of *Chlamydia trachomatis* deoxyribonucleic acid in monkey models *(Macaca nemestrina)* of salpingitis by in situ hybridization: Implications for pathogenesis. *Am J Obstet Gynecol* 171:102, 1994.
99 Hillis SD et al: Delayed care for pelvic inflammatory disease as a risk factor for impaired fertility. *Am J Obstet Gynecol* 168:1503–1509, 1993.
100 Svensson L: Contraceptives and acute salpingitis. *JAMA* 251:2553, 1984.
101 Senanayake P et al: Contraception and the etiology of pelvic inflammatory disease: New perspectives. *Am J Obstet Gynecol* 138:852, 1980.
102 Rubin GL et al: Oral contraceptives and pelvic inflammatory disease. *Am J Obstet Gynecol* 144:630, 1980.
103 Wølner-Hanssen P et al: Laparoscopic findings and contraceptive use in women with signs and symptoms suggestive of acute salpingitis. *Obstet Gynecol* 66:233, 1985.
104 Washington AE et al: Oral contraceptives, *Chlamydia trachomatis* infection and pelvic inflammatory disease. *JAMA* 253:2246, 1985.
105 Ness RB et al. Oral contraception and the recognition of endometritis. *Am J Obstet Gynecol* 176:580–585, 1997.
106 Daling JR et al: Cigarette smoking and primary tubal infertility, in *Smoking and Reproductive Health*. PSG Publishing, 1987.
107 Phipps WR et al: The association between smoking and female infertility as influenced by cause of the infertility. *Fertil Steril* 48:377, 1987.
108 Hershey P et al: Effects of cigarette smoking on the immune system. Follow-up studies in normal subjects after cessation of smoking. *Med J Aust* 2:425, 1983.
109 Burton RC: Smoking, immunity, and cancer. *Med J Aust* 2:411, 1983.
110 Holt PG: Immune and inflammatory function in cigarette smokers. *Thorax* 42:241, 1987.
111 Potts M et al: STDs, IVF, and barrier contraception. *JAMA* 258:1729, 1987.
112 Brunham RC: Therapy for acute pelvic inflammatory disease. A critique of recent treatment trials. *Am J Obstet Gynecol* 148:235, 1984.
113 Weström L et al: Infertility after acute salpingitis: Results of treatment with different antibiotics. *Curr Ther Res* 26:752, 1979.
114 Walker CK et al: Pelvic inflammatory disease: Metaanalyses of antimicrobial regimen efficacy. *J Infect Dis* 168:969–978, 1993.
115 Grimes DA et al: Antibiotic treatment of pelvic inflammatory disease, trends among private physicians in the United States, 1966 through 1983. *JAMA* 256:3223, 1986.
116 Mosure DJ et al: Genital chlamydial infections in sexually active female adolescents: Do we really need to screen everyone? *J Adolesc Health Care* 20:6–13, 1997.
117 Scholes D et al: Prevention of pelvic inflammatory disease by screening for cervical chlamydial infection. *N Engl J Med* 334:1362–1366, 1996.

Chapter 80

Sexually transmitted diseases, including HIV infection in pregnancy

D. Heather Watts
Robert C. Brunham

As the spectrum of sexually transmitted diseases (STDs) has broadened, the medical and social consequences of STD in pregnancy have become more apparent. Ectopic pregnancy, spontaneous abortion and stillbirth, prematurity, congenital and perinatal infections, and puerperal maternal infections represent outcomes of pregnancy in which sexually transmitted infectious agents play important etiologic roles. The incidence of many STDs has increased during the last two decades, and the number of pregnancies per year is also again increasing; the superimposition of the one factor on the other can be expected to further amplify the effects of STD on pregnancy and neonatal morbidity.

In general, STD appears to pose a much greater problem in pregnant adolescents than in older pregnant women who are more sexually experienced and more likely to be involved in a stable monogamous sexual relationship at the time of conception. Adolescents have miscarriages more often than do older women—a difference that may be attributable in part to STD. Although the average age at which women first bear children is increasing, the average age at which women first initiate sexual activity has decreased, and teenage pregnancy remains common in many societies despite the availability of contraceptives. Among sexually active women, whether pregnant or nonpregnant, the prevalence of many STD agents, such as cytomegalovirus (CMV) and *Chlamydia trachomatis,* is highest among adolescents. The younger the patient, the greater is the likelihood that any given infection is a primary infection. Although immunity to most STD agents is not well defined, it is likely that, in general, primary infections in a nonimmune host cause the greatest morbidity.

The two classic venereal agents, *Neisseria gonorrhoeae* and *Treponema pallidum,* have pronounced effects on pregnancy, but measures for the diagnosis and management of these infections in pregnancy are readily available and routinely employed where appropriate at least in developed countries. Introduction of such measures still remains a major achievable goal in many developing countries and in subpopulations who do not seek prenatal care in developed countries. Certain of the recently recognized STD pathogens such as *C. trachomatis,* CMV, and herpes simplex virus (HSV-2) are even more common during pregnancy, are more difficult to diagnose and manage, and currently represent a greater dilemma to the obstetrical care provider in all countries. Finally, the prevention of in utero, intrapartum, and postpartum transmission of human immunodeficiency virus (HIV) has become one of the greatest public health challenges of our time.

Although the pregnant host is more susceptible to the effects of certain lower genital tract infections such as genital warts, it is the infections of the placenta, fetus, uterus, and tubes that make the effects of STDs on pregnancy particularly important. Infection prior to pregnancy can influence the process of implantation, causing ectopic pregnancy and infertility. Infection during pregnancy can produce spontaneous abortion, chorioamnionitis, prematurity, and congenital infection. Genital infection present at delivery can cause maternal puerperal infections and neonatal and infant infections.

Pregnancy modifies the manifestations of many STDs and presents unique problems for diagnosis and management. Some agents, such as *Candida albicans,* produce disease more commonly during pregnancy, and others, such as genital human papillomaviruses (HPVs), have enhanced virulence. The susceptibility of the pregnant host to infection may be enhanced, owing either to alterations in host defense mechanisms or to changes in anatomic structure.

ALTERATIONS OF HOST-PARASITE RELATIONSHIPS DURING PREGNANCY

IMMUNOLOGIC CHANGES

Immunologic rejection of the fetus does not normally occur during pregnancy, possibly in part because of suppression of maternal immunocompetence. Suppressed maternal immunocompetence may in turn affect the natural history of many infectious diseases. For instance, higher attack rates or more severe morbidity has been recorded for pneumococcal pneumonia,[1] smallpox,[2] influenza,[3] poliomyelitis,[4] candidiasis,[5] and malaria[6] in the pregnant host than in the nonpregnant host. Both the incidence and severity of viral hepatitis are also increased in pregnancy.[7] Immunologically mediated diseases caused by infectious agents may lessen in severity during pregnancy; for example, in the preantibiotic era it was observed that symptomatic syphilis was ameliorated during pregnancy.[8] Animal studies also support the notion that pregnancy interferes with maternal defense mechanisms through immune suppression.[9,10]

The bases for alterations in host immune response are likely multifactorial. Humoral substances that potentially suppress in vitro lymphocyte function are present in plasma from pregnant women.[11,12] T lymphocytes but not B lymphocytes are reduced in number in peripheral blood samples of pregnant women.[13] The decrease in T lymphocytes is entirely due to a decrease in the CD4+ T-helper subset, which is reduced nearly by half compared with values found in nonpregnant women (543 $\pm$ 169 versus 1,073 $\pm$ 441 CD4+ T lymphocytes per unit of peripheral blood, $p < 0.001$). No significant change occurs in the number of CD8+ T lymphocytes. The decrease in CD4+ T lymphocytes is maximal during the third trimester.[14]

In a large number of women evaluated during and after pregnancy we have noted impairment in the in vitro lymphocyte transformation (LT) response to a number of microbial antigens and phytohemagglutinin during pregnancy.[16] In vitro lymphocyte proliferation was significantly lower during pregnancy than in the postpartum period and was significantly lower for pregnant women than for nonpregnant women. Maximal suppression of the LT response was observed during the third trimester of gestation. Among women with current infection with *C. trachomatis,* the LT response was markedly suppressed in the third trimester in comparison with the LT response in the postpartum period or in nonpregnant women. These data support similar observations of suppressed LT response to microbial antigens made by Gehrz et al.[17]

Factors other than immunosuppression also may contribute to the increased maternal susceptibility to certain infections during pregnancy. For example, excessive mortality from bacterial pneumonia during pregnancy has been attributed to altered pulmonary mechanics,[18] and the increased susceptibility to renal infection during pregnancy may be related to changes in ureterovesicular muscular tone induced by high levels of progesterone or to partial ureteral compression by the gravid uterus.

ANATOMIC ALTERATIONS IN PREGNANCY

The anatomy of the genital tract changes dramatically during pregnancy. Figure 80-1 illustrates the relationship of the cervix and mucous plug, chorioamnion, and placental bed as seen in late pregnancy. Vaginal walls become hypertrophic and engorged with blood. The glycogen content of the vaginal epithelium increases, and the intravaginal pH significantly decreases during pregnancy.[19] These changes probably influence vaginal microbial flora. The cervix hypertrophies, and a larger area of columnar epithelium on the exocervix is exposed to microorganisms.[20] Similar cervical anatomic changes are evoked among nonpregnant women by oral contraceptives and have been associated with an increased prevalence of infection with *C. trachomatis* and *N. gonorrhoeae.*[21] It is not certain whether the higher prevalence of chlamydial and gonococcal infections in nonpregnant women with cervical ectopy is due to increased susceptibility to infection or enhanced cervical shedding among previously infected women or both. The increased area of cervical ectopy during pregnancy also may predispose the cervix to infection or reactivation of latent infection, but this has not been well studied. The cervix secretes highly viscid mucus during pregnancy, forming the so-called mucous plug. This mucus is generally believed to limit the access of microorganisms into the uterus, but little research has been done to study the actual effectiveness of cervical mucus as a physical or antimicrobial barrier.[22] Fetal growth is accommodated by uterine growth and by tremendous enlargement of uterine vessels. The risk of salpingitis decreases during pregnancy, especially after the twelfth week,[23] and the risk of chorioamnionitis increases after the sixteenth week of gestation.[24] After the twelfth gestational week, the uterine cavity becomes obliterated as the chorioamnion becomes juxtaposed with the decidua vera. The risk of infection of the uterine cavity and fallopian tubes is diminished by the elimination of this space. By the sixteenth week, the chorioamnion overlies the cervical os, which may be a factor in the increasing risk of chorioamnionitis during middle and late pregnancy.

The human placenta is of fetal origin and is directly perfused by maternal blood. The trophoblastic placental epithelium projects into the maternal vascular system. This trophoblastic layer regulates fetal uptake of many substances. Anatomically, two layers of trophoblastic epithelium are present, an inner multicellular stratified layer (cytotrophoblast or Langhan's layer) and an outer unicellular syncytial layer (syncytiotrophoblast). This is seen in Fig. 80-2. With advancing gestation, Langhan's layer becomes less noticeable but does not regress completely. Lying within the stroma of the mature placenta are placental macrophages (Hofbauer cells) that act as a first line of fetal defense to transplacental infection.

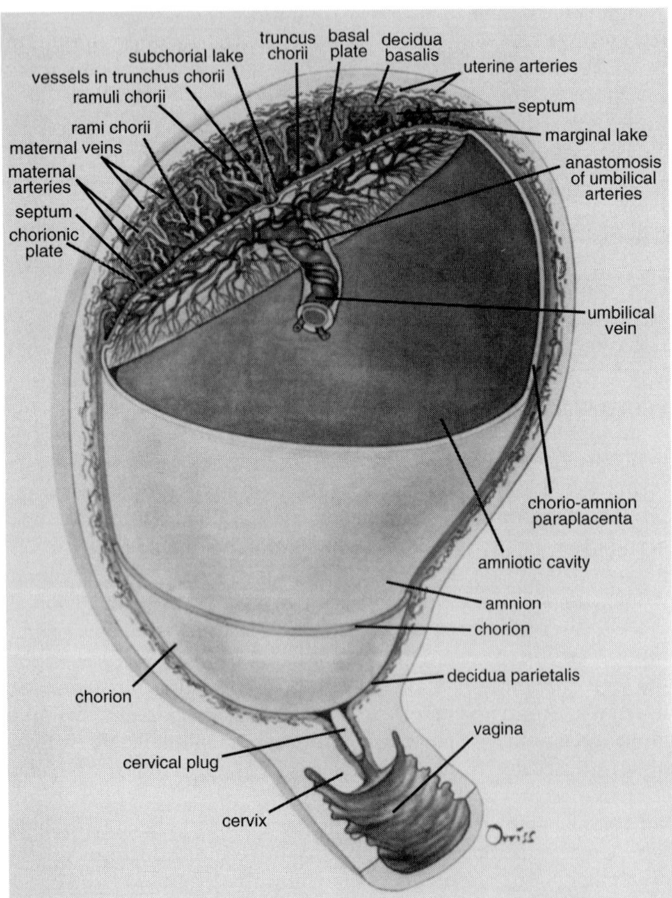

Fig. 80-1. The relationship within the gravid uterus of the mucous plug, fetal membranes (chorion and amnion), decidua, and placenta. *(From JD Boyd and WJ Hamilton: The Human Placenta. Cambridge, England: W. Heffer & Sons Ltd, 1970:111 & 143, by permission.)*

ALTERATIONS IN CERVICOVAGINAL MICROBIAL FLORA DURING PREGNANCY

The vaginal flora is a heterogeneous ecosystem of anaerobic and facultative bacteria.[25] Several studies have found that during pregnancy, the number of bacterial species present in the vagina decreases, particularly the number of anaerobic species, while the prevalence and the quantity of lactobacilli increase and the rate of carriage of Enterobacteriaceae, group B streptococci (GBS), and other facultative bacteria remains unchanged. Despite these data, we feel that the effects of pregnancy on vaginal bacterial flora of current interest have not been well defined. The mechanisms that may promote the reported changes in vaginal flora might include changes in the vaginal pH, glycogen content, and vascularity of the lower genital tract, as described above. Following delivery, an increase in rates of isolation of *Escherichia coli* and *Bacteroides* species (which may promote puerperal endomyometrial infections) has been reported, but this observation also requires confirmation.[26]

ECTOPIC PREGNANCY

Infertility and ectopic pregnancy are recognized consequences of salpingitis. Two sexually transmitted organisms, *N. gonorrhoeae* and *C. trachomatis,* produce the majority of cases of primary salpingitis (see Chap. 58). The risk of ectopic pregnancy increases about tenfold after an initial episode of salpingitis. The incidence of ectopic pregnancy has increased fivefold since 1970 in the United States, and this trend also has been observed in Sweden, Canada, and England.[27] It is likely that this rising incidence of ectopic pregnancy is due in part to an increasing incidence of gonococcal and chlamydial infections and of resulting tubal infections. Approximately 50 percent of operatively removed ectopic pregnancies are associated with histologic evidence of prior salpingitis.[28,29] One study correlated histology, *C. trachomatis* serology, and *C. trachomatis* cultures among 50 women with ectopic pregnancy.[30] Although no woman had *C. trachomatis* recovered from the fallopian tube, 22 percent had extensive subepithelial plasma cell infiltration in the tube and 47 percent had *C. trachomatis* antibody, with all women having plasma cell infiltration being seropositive.[30] These data document an associ-

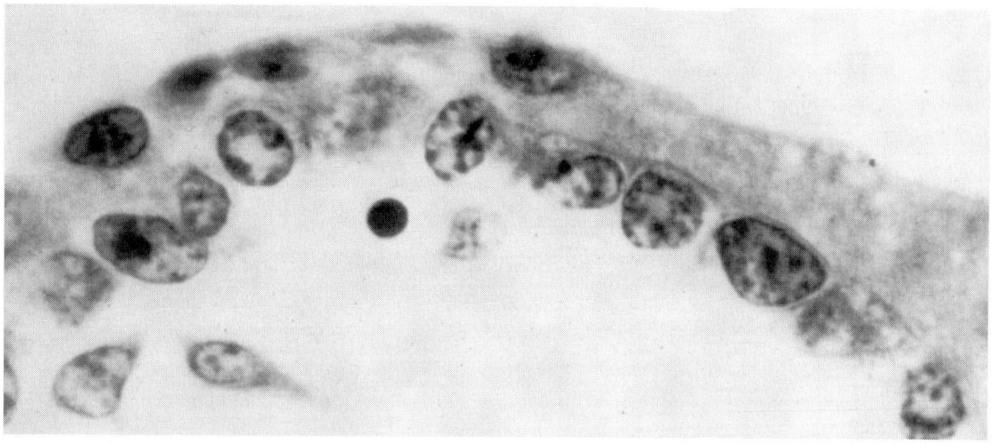

Fig. 80-2. Photomicrograph of the human trophoblast illustrating the outer (maternal) syncytiotrophoblast on the convex surface and the inner (fetal) cytotrophoblast of Langhan's layer. *(From JD Boyd and WJ Hamilton: The Human Placenta. Cambridge, England: W. Heffer & Sons Ltd, 1970:111 & 143, by permission.)*

ation of *C. trachomatis* infection with ectopic pregnancy. Based on these data, Kosseim et al.[31] estimated that approximately 30 percent of cases of ectopic pregnancy were due to prior *C. trachomatis* infection.

POSTABORTAL INFECTIONS

STDs and other vaginal infections are frequently detected among women presenting for elective termination of pregnancy.[32] *C. trachomatis, N. gonorrhoeae,* and bacterial vaginosis have each been associated with an increased risk of febrile morbidity after surgical abortion. In addition, infection rates after abortion were reduced with routine screening and treatment, if indicated, for both *C. trachomatis* and bacterial vaginosis.[33,34] Routine screening for *N. gonorrhoeae, C. trachomatis,* and bacterial vaginosis is indicated in most populations undergoing surgical abortion. Whether STDs are a risk factor for pelvic infections after medically induced abortions has not been studied,[35] but screening similar to that done before surgical abortion would seem reasonable, since suction procedures are still required in a small number of women after medical treatment.

INTRAUTERINE INFECTION

Intrauterine infection can result from either hematogenous or ascending microbial spread. Other routes of spread such as extension from infection in areas adjacent to the uterus occur rarely, although spread from infected foci within the endometrium to the placenta may be important for some pathogens such as CMV. A hematogenous origin appears to be the major route of spread for organisms present in maternal blood, such as *T. pallidum.* Hematogenous infection initially involves the placenta, producing the characteristic pathologic lesion of villitis. Placental mononuclear phagocytes (Hofbauer cells) likely serve as the initial antimicrobial defense in this situation.

Ascending infection by microorganisms present in the cervix or vagina can occur through intact or compromised fetal membranes, producing the characteristic pathologic lesion of chorioamnionitis and the syndrome of amniotic fluid infection. The integrity of the chorioamnion and the antimicrobial activity of amniotic fluid likely serve as the first line of fetal defense in this situation.

HEMATOGENOUS INFECTION

Only rarely does maternal bacteremia give rise to placental or fetal infection. The nature of the defense mechanisms responsible for protection of the developing placenta and fetus from bacteremic spread is not presently known. It appears that microbial agents inhibited primarily by a cell-mediated immune response are more likely to establish placental infection than are agents inhibited primarily by a humoral immune response, suggesting either that pregnant women are most susceptible to systemic spread of those agents that are inhibited by cellular immunity or that placental defense mechanisms are less effective against such microorganisms.

Microorganisms arrive at the placental bed within lymphocytes, monocytes, or neutrophils, or they may not be cell associated. The pathogenesis of fetal infection with CMV is particularly interesting, since this virus is able to establish latent infection in human mononuclear cells. Productive infection may be recalled during alloreactivity of infected lymphocytes.[36] It may be that alloreactions between maternal lymphocytes and foreign paternal histocompatibility or other antigens on the placenta contribute to the pathogenesis of recurrent congenital CMV infection. A similar pathogenetic mechanism may exist for in utero transmission of HIV.

Fetal defense mechanisms during placental infection include placental macrophages and local production of immune factors such as antibody and lymphokines. The immune role of the trophoblast is unknown, but since this epithelium possesses Fc receptors for immunoglobulin and unique antigenic determinants and secretory products that regulate lymphocyte reactivity in vitro, an important effect on the immune response seems likely.[37] Placental histopathology following infection with *T. pallidum* serves to illustrate the range of responses detectable in this tissue. *T. pallidum*–infected placentas are inappropriately large with focal proliferative villitis and vasculitis with areas of plasma cell infiltration and Langerhans' giant cell formation[38] (Fig. 80-3).

With hematogenous infection, placental infection generally precedes fetal infection, although theoretically it is possible for organisms to traverse the chorionic villi directly by pinocytosis or placental leaks or within maternal leukocytes. The fetal immune response to placental infection may be effective enough to limit infection to this site. Such circumscribed infection has been seen in cases of primary CMV infection[39] and in syphilis.[40] Often, however, spread from infected placental sites to the fetus occurs either by involvement of fetal blood vessels or by extension from placenta to fetal membranes with consequent infection of the amniotic fluid.

The manifestations of fetal infection depend to a great extent on the gestational age at which infection occurs. The STD agents capable of transplacental infection can produce similar effects. Abortion, stillbirth, prematurity, congenital disease, and persistent postnatal infection have all been described following infection

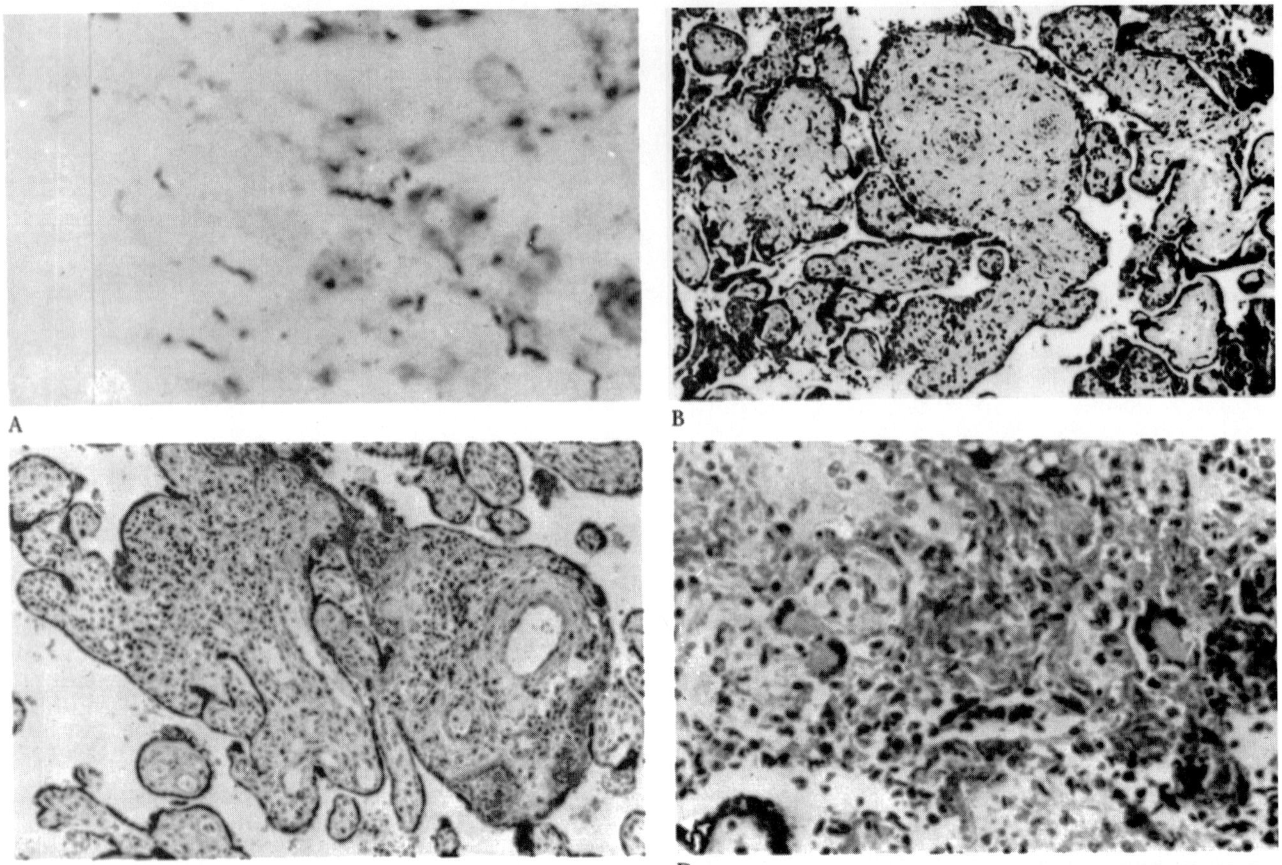
A B C D

Fig. 80-3. Placental abnormalities of congenital syphilis. (*A*) Typical corkscrew morphology of *T. pallidum* (Warthin-Starry stain; ×2000). (*B*) Endovascular proliferation and villitis (H&E stain; ×150). (*C*) Villitis with plasma cell infiltration (H&E stain; ×300). (*D*) Proliferative villitis with granulomatous and giant cell formation (H&E stain; ×400). *(Courtesy of G. Altshuler.)*

with CMV, HIV, *T. pallidum,* and herpes simplex virus (HSV). CMV also commonly causes developmental abnormalities.

ASCENDING INFECTION: CHORIOAMNIONITIS AND AMNIOTIC FLUID INFECTION

Acute inflammation of the fetal membranes (chorioamnionitis) and umbilical cord (funisitis) is seen even more frequently than hematogenous placentitis and often is associated with premature birth, prolonged rupture of the membranes (ROM), intrapartum fever, and perinatal sepsis. Chorioamnionitis is defined histologically by the presence of polymorphonuclear leukocytes (PMNs) in the membranes—usually within the chorion[41]; in some cases this acute inflammation is seen only on the fetal side of the discoid placenta. The migration of maternal PMNs from the intervillous spaces or of fetal PMNs through the amnion suggests transcervical infection of amniotic fluid rather than primary hematogenous infection. Figure 80-4 diagrammatically illustrates the patterns and stages of the maternal and fetal inflammatory response to amniotic fluid infection.

The etiology of acute chorioamnionitis is in many cases unknown. Delayed delivery following ROM, sometimes called *prolonged rupture of membranes,* is an important correlate of acute chorioamnionitis, but most cases of chorioamnionitis are not associated with prolonged ROM as an antecedent event.[24] The correlation of placental or chorioamnion culture results with histologic chorioamnionitis in several studies is shown in Table 80-1.[41–47] The varied rate of isolation of microorganisms among women with histologic chorioamnionitis can be accounted for by differences in patient populations and specimen handling and sampling, variable use of cultures for genital mycoplasmas, and antibiotic use before delivery. Limited microbiologic studies have strongly linked *Ureaplasma urealyticum* to chorioamnion inflammation. The organisms isolated from the chorioamnion are similar to those found in the vagina of women with bacterial vaginosis, and in fact, when evaluated, positive chorioamnionic cultures were associated with bacterial vaginosis.[41] Since microbial cultures of inflamed fetal membranes are often sterile, noninfectious causes such as meconium, anoxia, and decidual necrosis also have been proposed as eliciting inflammation within the membranes. However, studies in rabbits have shown clearly that only microorganisms are responsible for chorioamnionitis and that the suspected chemical factors did not produce chorioamnionitis.[48]

Perinatal bacterial infections, especially those occurring within the first 48 hours of life, are commonly acquired by ascending infection in utero. Russell[24] found evidence of neonatal sepsis in the first 48 hours of life in almost one-quarter of neonates whose placentas showed chorioamnionitis; neonatal sepsis was rare in the absence of placental inflammation. This study provides compelling data linking chorioamnionitis, prematurity, and perinatal sepsis.

Bacteria recovered from amniotic fluid of patients with chorioamnionitis include facultative organisms such as GBS, enteric gram-negative rods, *Haemophilus influenzae,* and strict anaerobic organisms such as peptostreptococci, *Fusobacterium* spp., *Bacteroides* spp., and *Prevotella bivia.*[49–51] These infections are often polymicrobial, resembling the spectrum of organisms found in the

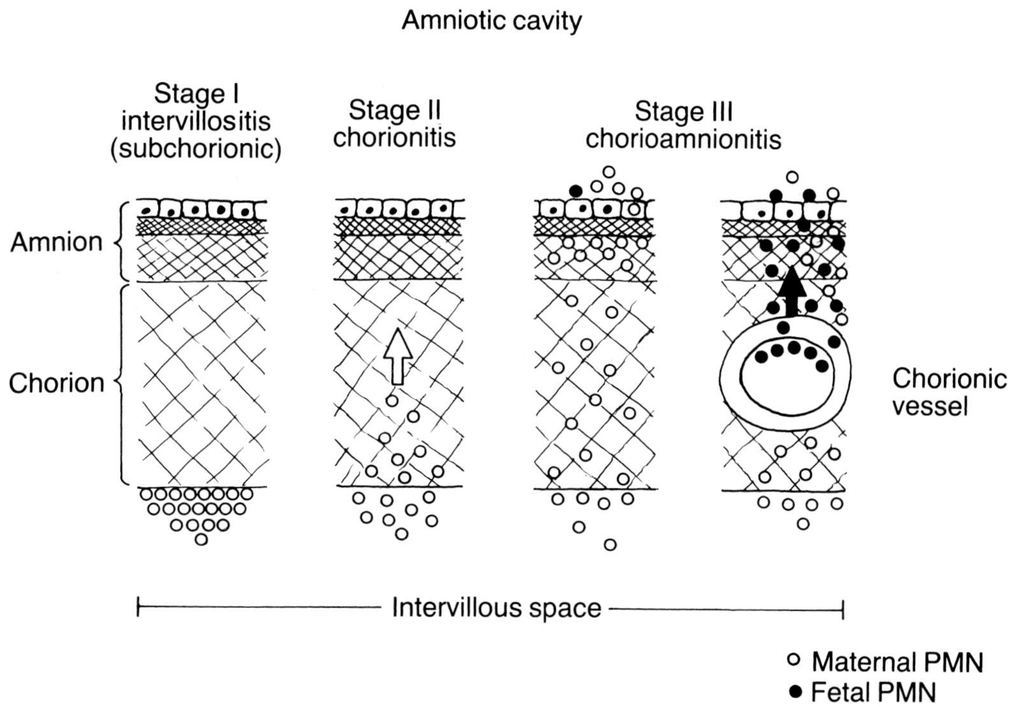

Fig. 80-4. The stages and patterns of maternal and fetal response to amniotic fluid infection. PMN = polymorphonuclear leukocytes.

upper genital tract of women with salpingitis or postpartum endometritis, and also include many of the organisms found in the vagina of women with bacterial vaginosis. The relationship of amniotic fluid infection, membrane infection, and histologic chorioamnionitis to preterm birth is discussed in more detail below.

The risk of chorioamnionitis is highest among nonwhite patients of low socioeconomic status who have not received prenatal care.[52,53] These demographic characteristics of patients with chorioamnionitis are similar to those of patients with STDs.

COITUS IN PREGNANCY

Approximately 40 percent of women studied in Durban, in Addis Ababa, and in Seattle had intercourse during the last 2 weeks of their pregnancy.[54] Naeye[55] reported that coitus during pregnancy was associated with low birth weight and an increase in the perinatal mortality rate. The U.S. Collaborative Perinatal Project showed the perinatal mortality rate (PMR) to be two- to fourfold higher when women continued coitus until near delivery than when they were sexually inactive. A large portion of the excess of perinatal deaths among those who had coitus was attributable to more frequent and severe amniotic fluid infections. At every gestational age, the proportion of fetuses and neonates dying with amniotic fluid infection was greater when coitus had occurred in the month before delivery. Abruptio placentae, the second most frequent cause of perinatal death in the collaborative study, was also 50 percent more frequent among sexually active than among sexually inactive pregnant women. Naeye[56] also has observed seasonal variations both in sexual activity and in the PMR rates and that these are virtually synchronous, peaking in May, June, and July. The incidence of gonococcal and chlamydial infections is also seasonal, peaking in August and September. Thus it is interesting that Keller and Nugent[57] observed an increase in perinatal mortality during July, August, and September, due mostly to an increase in infectious causes of perinatal death.

Table 80-1. Frequency and Relative Risk of Positive Placental Cultures with and without Histologic Chorioamnionitis

Author	Chorioamnionitis	No chorioamnionitis	Relative risk	95% CI*
Pankuch[42]	18/25 (72%)	6/39 (15%)	14.1	3.6–60
Hillier[41]	21/29 (72%)	14/65 (22%)	7.2	2.7–19
Quinn[43]	10/14 (71%)	8/29 (28%)	6.5	1.3–3.5
Kundsin[44]	32/84 (38%)	21/146 (14%)	3.7	1.8–7.3
Svensson[45]	7/10 (70%)	31/69 (45%)	1.6	0.5–5.0
Zlatnik[46]	26/51 (51%)	12/44 (27%)	3.4	1.2–10.0
Hillier[47]	32/101 (32%)	33/167 (20%)	1.9	1.1–3.5

* CI = confidence interval.

Naeye has speculated that coitus may cause amniotic fluid infection by introduction of a new sexually transmitted pathogen, by injury to the cervix or membranes, because seminal fluid may increase cervical mucus penetrability to vaginal bacteria or may inactivate antibacterial systems in the vagina, cervix, fetal membranes, or amniotic fluid.

However, not all studies support the concept that coitus in late pregnancy is dangerous. Mills et al.[58] reviewed nearly 11,000 pregnancies in Israel and observed no increased risk of low birth weight or perinatal death among women continuing coitus during the month prior to delivery when compared with women who abstained. Data from the Vaginal Infections and Prematurity Study group indicated that among women without *Trichomonas vaginalis, Mycoplasma hominis,* or bacterial vaginosis, the risk of preterm delivery was lower for those who had frequent intercourse during the third trimester than for those with less frequent intercourse.[59] However, *T. vaginalis* and *M. hominis* were risk factors for preterm delivery among women with, but not among those without, frequent intercourse in the third trimester. A recent study of 407 healthy, nulliparous women in Finland found a higher rate of preterm birth among women with less frequent or no intercourse in the third trimester than among those with more frequent intercourse.[60] A case-control study of perinatal deaths in Jamaica did not find an association between deaths from immaturity and coital frequency.[61] Reasons for these discordant findings are not readily apparent, but differences in time and population, including the prevalence of STDs in the populations studied, may have influenced the results. More recent data do not suggest a harmful effect from coitus in pregnancy among healthy women with normal genital flora.

FETAL WASTAGE, PREMATURITY, AND PRETERM RUPTURE OF MEMBRANES

Spontaneous abortion, stillbirth, and prematurity can each be caused by infection. However, the proportion of these events attributable to infection is not yet well defined and no doubt varies in different populations. Spontaneous abortion, defined as the delivery of a previable fetus before the twentieth week of gestation and weighing less than 500 gm, is a frequent outcome in pregnancy. It is estimated that 50 percent of fertilized ova fail to implant, and of those which do implant, at least 15 to 30 percent subsequently abort.[62] The majority of losses occur in the first trimester; less than 3 percent of women with a normal ultrasound at 7 to 12 weeks experience a loss by 20 weeks.[63] This distinction is clinically useful, since first-trimester abortions are usually associated with phenotypic or chromosomal fetal abnormalities. Second-trimester abortions and stillbirths (weight ≥500 gm, gestation ≥20 weeks) are more often associated with an otherwise normal fetus. Genital infections may thus be a relatively more important cause of fetal wastage in the second and third trimesters than in the first trimester. From 40 to 54 percent of pregnancies that terminated spontaneously in the second trimester have been associated with histologic evidence of chorioamnionitis.

Low birth weight, defined as birth weight less than 2,500 gm, usually results from a preterm birth but can be the result of intrauterine growth retardation. Both conditions have been associated with infectious agents. The proportion of cases of prematurity caused by infection versus that caused by noninfectious factors (e.g., diet, smoking, hypertension) remains to be defined. Among preterm births, approximately one-third are obstetrically indicated deliveries for maternal or fetal conditions such as hypertension or fetal distress, one-third are related to progressive preterm labor, and one-third are related to preterm rupture of the membranes. As discussed in this section, a high proportion of early preterm labor leading to delivery and a majority of cases of preterm rupture appear to be related to infection.

Despite a remarkable decline in the perinatal mortality rate in the United States in the last 30 years, the prematurity rate has remained essentially unchanged at approximately 6 to 8 percent[64] (Fig. 80-5). Between 70 and 80 percent of all perinatal deaths that are not attributable to congenital malformation occur following premature birth. Since prematurity and perinatal mortality are so strongly linked, it appears that the decline in perinatal mortality achieved during the last 30 years must be attributable to improvements in perinatal and neonatal care more than to improvements in prematurity rates.[65] The decline in perinatal mortality has thus been achieved as a result of enormously burgeoning costs of perinatal and neonatal intensive care. For instance, the average total cost of delivery and neonatal intensive care for an infant born at 25 to 27 weeks' gestation is $280,146 compared with $9,326 for a term infant.[66] The elucidation of treatable causes of prematurity will likely lead to preventive efforts that would further reduce both the perinatal mortality and the long-term morbidity rate seen in some infants who survive preterm delivery and substantially decrease health care costs.

Intriguing data implicating infectious agents in prematurity were serendipitously derived from studies by Elder et al.[67] In the course of investigating the role of urinary tract infection in prematurity, 279 nonbacteriuric women seen prior to 32 weeks of

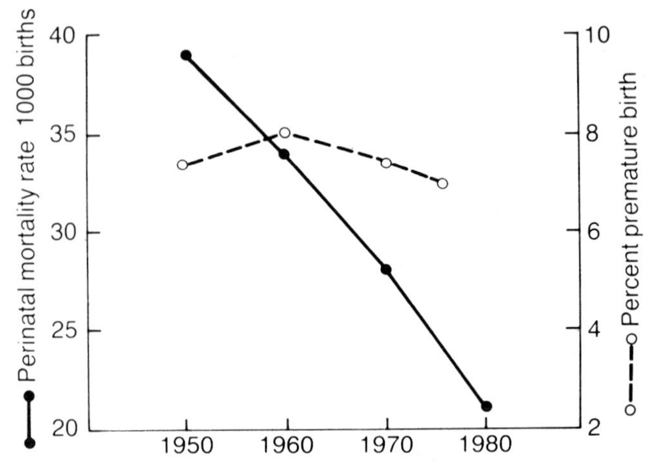

Fig. 80-5. Declining perinatal mortality rate that has occurred in the face of an unchanging prematurity rate in the United States. The perinatal mortality rate declined further to 10.7 per 100 live births for 1985, while the incidence of low birth weight (<2,500 gm) remained essentially unchanged at 6.8 per 100 live births for 1980 and 1985.

gestation were alternately allocated to treatment with 6 weeks of oral tetracycline at 1 gm per day or with placebo. The patients in both groups were of comparable age, gravidity, race, and marital status. As seen in Table 80-2, even in those without urinary tract infection, the tetracycline-treated group had significantly longer gestations, fewer premature live borns, fewer episodes of postpartum fever, and fewer neonatal complications than the placebo-treated group. The salutary effect of tetracycline suggested the presence of unidentified tetracycline-susceptible microorganism(s) that contributed to prematurity. In a subsequent treatment trial, Kass et al.[68] randomized 148 women to erythromycin therapy given for 6 weeks in the third trimester or to placebo. Infants in the placebo group weighed less than infants in the treatment group (3,187 versus 3,331 gm, $p = 0.04$). A more recent study in an African population with a high prevalence of STDs showed a reduction in low birth weight (4.0 versus 9.2 percent, $p = 0.08$) and postpartum endometritis (3.8 versus 10.4 percent, $p = 0.05$) and a higher mean birth weight (3,209 versus 3,056 gm, $p = 0.01$) among 200 women treated at 28 to 32 weeks' gestation with a single 250-mg intramuscular dose of ceftriaxone compared with 200 women randomly assigned to placebo.[69] These effects of antibiotics on birth weights suggest that prematurity may result from unrecognized maternal infection, perhaps STDs involving the lower genital tract.[70]

Many studies have been done comparing the rate of preterm birth and preterm ROM between women with or without specific lower genital tract infections either early in pregnancy or on admission for delivery. These studies will be discussed in detail below in sections dealing with specific infections. Conclusions from the studies are often limited because only one or a limited number of genital microorganisms were studied. Concomitant risk factors for preterm birth, such as smoking or drug use, that may be more prevalent among women with genital infections often were not considered in adjusting for these potential confounders, and gestational age at enrollment may have been later than the gestation age when complications sometimes occur. Despite these limitations, several lower genital tract infections, including *N. gonorrhoeae, C. trachomatis,* bacterial vaginosis, and *T. vaginalis* have been implicated in increasing the risk of preterm birth. In studies of women with gonorrhea, chlamydial infection, and bacterial vaginosis, rates of prematurity have been reduced among treated compared with untreated women, at least in some populations.

Table 80-2. Effect of 6 Weeks of Oral Tetracycline Given Prior to 32 Weeks on Outcome of Pregnancy in 279 Nonbacteriuric Women

Measurement	Tetracycline (n = 148)		Placebo (n = 131)		p
Mean gestation (weeks)	39.1		38.1		<0.025
Mean birth weight (gm)	3277		3141		NS*
	Number	%	Number	%	
Premature live born	8	(5.4)	20	(15.2)	<0.025
Stillborn	2	(1.4)	1	(0.8)	
	Number/total	%	Number/total	%	
Preterm ROM	14/142	(10)	16/128	(13)	NS
Postpartum fever	8/142	(6)	15/129	(12)	<0.001
Neonatal resuscitation	11/140	(8)	24/125	(19)	<0.005
Respiratory distress	1/140	(1)	9/125	(7)	<0.05

* Nonsignificant
SOURCE: Elder et al.[67]

Thus routine screening and treatment of certain genital infections in high-risk populations eventually may lead to a reduction in the rate of preterm birth. Primary viral infections such as CMV and HSV in pregnancy also may increase the risk of preterm delivery and neonatal infection. Prevention of primary viral infections and their complications in pregnancy will likely depend on development of effective vaccines.

Increased rates of chorioamnion inflammation and infection and amniotic fluid infection among preterm compared with term deliveries also imply an infectious etiology. The increased rate of neonatal sepsis among preterm infants may be related not only to a less mature immune system but also to frequent exposure to microorganisms in placental and amniotic fluid infection that caused the preterm delivery.

Russell[24] clearly documented the correlation of acute histologic chorioamnionitis with premature birth. Figure 80-6 illustrates the prevalence of chorioamnionitis by gestational age at delivery. Chorioamnionitis was found in 95 percent of pregnancies at less than 25 weeks' gestation, 35 to 40 percent of pregnancies from 25 to 32 weeks, 11 percent of pregnancies from 33 to 35 weeks, and only 3 to 5 percent of term pregnancies. The mean birth weight of neonates in the chorioamnionitis group was much lower than in a control group without chorioamnionitis (2,811 versus

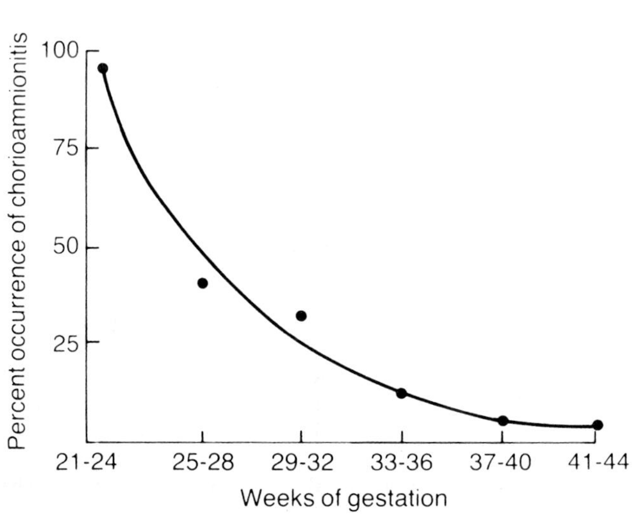

Fig. 80-6. Rate of chorioamnionitis among deliveries terminating at the stated intervals. The risk of chorioamnionitis is extremely high in very premature deliveries.

3,320 gm, $p < 0.001$). The lower birth weight of those with chorioamnionitis was appropriate for gestational age and not attributable to retarded intrauterine growth. Although chorioamnionitis frequently can be asymptomatic, especially when present near term, two-thirds of the group with chorioamnionitis had intrapartum fever, prolonged rupture of the membranes, and/or premature labor.

Several subsequent studies have confirmed the association between histologic chorioamnionitis and preterm birth and between membrane infection and preterm birth.[24,41,42,44,45,47,71–73] Results of these studies are summarized in Table 80-3. As discussed earlier, microorganisms are isolated more frequently from between the chorioamnionic membranes or from biopsy of placentas with histologic inflammation (see Table 80-1). The frequency of histologic chorioamnionitis decreases from over 90 percent of placentas delivered before 24 weeks' gestation to about 10 percent at term. Microorganisms isolated most frequently from the placental membranes are *U. urealyticum, Gardnerella vaginalis,* group B streptococci, *Escherichia coli,* anaerobic gram-positive cocci, *Bacteriodes* spp., *Prevotella bivia,* and *F. nucleatum.*

Among afebrile women presenting in preterm labor without other obvious cause, bacteria have been isolated from the amniotic fluid obtained by amniocentesis in 112 (11 percent) of a total of 1,017 women in several studies (range 0 to 19 percent).[50,74–87] The range of results can be explained by differences in enrollment criteria, interval from presentation to amniocentesis, gestational age distribution, and laboratory methods. The majority of women with positive amniotic fluid cultures delivered within 2 days (range 0 to 4 days) of admission despite tocolytic therapy, while women with negative cultures delivered on average 29 days (range 25 to 51 days) after amniocentesis. Women with positive cultures had a lower gestational age at amniocentesis than those with negative cultures. The curve of the frequency of amniotic fluid culture positivity by gestational age is similar to that of the frequency of histologic chorioamnionitis or positive membrane culture by gestational age, albeit at a lower level. The higher but parallel frequency of membrane infection or inflammation as compared with amniotic fluid infection suggests that infection ascends via the decidua and membranes with secondary infection of the amniotic fluid. Microorganisms most commonly isolated from the amniotic fluid include *F. nucleatum, Bacteroides* spp., *E. coli,* group B streptococci, *U. urealyticum, G. vaginalis,* and *Streptococcus viridans.* Bacteria isolated from the amniotic fluid are similar in distribution to those isolated from the chorioamnion, and in many cases, the same species are found in the vagina with bacterial vaginosis.

As the frequency of positive amniotic fluid cultures among

Table 80-3. Relationship of Positive Chorioamnion/ Placental Cultures or Histologic Chorioamnionitis to Preterm Birth

	No. with positive culture/total (%)			
Author	Preterm	Term	Odds ratio	95% CI*
Hillier[41]	23/38 (61%)	12/56 (21%)	3.8	1.5–9.9
Kundsin[44]	61/196 (31%)	40/312 (13%)	3.1	1.9–4.9
Pankuch[42]	27/53 (51%)	6/22 (27%)	2.8	0.8–9.4
Svensson[45]	8/16 (50%)	33/70 (47%)	1.2	0.3–3.8
Hillier[47]	36/112 (32%)	29/156 (19%)	2.1	1.1–3.8
	No. with histologic chorioamnionitis/total (%)			
Russell[24]	123/659 (19%)	269/6846 (4%)	5.6	4.4–7.1
Cooperstock[71]	287/1445 (20%)	817/17342 (5%)	5.0	4.3–5.8
Guzick[72]	80/244 (33%)	253/2530 (10%)	4.4	3.2–5.9
Fox[73]	16/34 (47%)	186/836 (22%)	3.1	1.5–6.5
Hillier[47]	66/112 (60%)†	35/156 (22%)	2.1	1.1–3.8

* CI = confidence interval.
† ≤34 weeks.

women in preterm labor became apparent, investigators began to evaluate the amniotic fluid and vagina for markers of inflammation. Macrophage products including tumor necrosis factor alpha (TNF-α), interleukin 1 (IL-1), and interleukin 6 (IL-6) in the amniotic fluid have been associated with preterm delivery, positive amniotic fluid culture, and histologic chorioamnionitis.[85,86,88–95] IL-6 is most consistent in predicting rapid delivery among women in preterm labor, even among those with negative amniotic fluid cultures, suggesting either insensitivity of the culture or infection that is limited to the membranes or decidua. In mice, systemic treatment of the mother with IL-1 led to preterm labor in all cases[96] that could be blocked by pretreatment with IL-1 receptor antagonist protein.[97] Interferon-gamma, a product of T lymphocytes, has not been elevated among women with preterm labor, even among those with high TNF-α, IL-1, and IL-6 levels.[86] Prostaglandin E_2 and $F_{2\alpha}$ levels also have been elevated among women with amniotic fluid infection, chorioamnionitis, and preterm birth, suggesting that the infection or the resulting inflammatory response leads to prostaglandin production from arachidonic acid in the fetal membranes.[98]

More recently, the presence of amniotic fluid cytokines has been associated with an increased frequency of complications in the neonate. Respiratory distress syndrome, intraventricular hemorrhage, and periventricular leukomalacia have all been detected significantly more frequently, even after adjusting for gestational age at delivery, among neonates born to women with, compared with those without, cytokines in the amniotic fluid.[99–101] Thus infection-related preterm birth may be doubly damaging, both because of the earlier gestational age of delivery and because of cytokine-mediated complications in the infant.

A monkey model for the study of infection-induced preterm labor has been employed to demonstrate a causal relationship between experimental intraamniotic infection and preterm delivery.[102] Findings from this model are consistent with observations in humans with preterm labor and amniotic fluid infection. Chronically catheterized pregnant rhesus monkeys were inoculated intraamniotically with group B streptococci, and amniotic fluid was sampled serially for levels of GBS, TNF-α, IL-1, IL-6, and prostaglandins E_2 and $F_{2\alpha}$. Intraamniotic cytokine levels rose between 9 and 18 hours after infection, with parallel increases in PGE_2 and $PGF_{2\alpha}$ levels. Increased uterine contractility occurred 10 to 20 hours after increased cytokine and prostaglandin levels were detected. This delay implies that when women present with preterm labor and amniotic fluid infection, they may have had elevated cytokine levels in the amniotic fluid for several hours or even days. Amniotic fluid and prostaglandin levels in the infected animals were severalfold higher than in control animals in spontaneous labor at term. None of the monkeys with intraamniotic

Table 80-4. Randomized, Placebo-Controlled Trials of Antibiotics for Preterm Labor with Intact Membranes ≤34 Weeks

Author	Antibiotic regimen	Total n	Prolonged gestational age	Reduced neonatal morbidity	Reduced maternal morbidity
McGregor[70]	Oral erythromycin	58	No*	No	No
Winkler[107]	Oral erythromycin	19	9 d ABX†	ND	ND
Newton[108]	IV ampicillin/oral erythromycin	103	No	ND	ND
McGregor[109]	IV clindamycin/po	103	10 d ABX	No	No
Romero[110]	IV ampicillin/oral erythromycin	277	No	No	No
Watts[111]	IV mezlocillin/oral erythromycin	56	No	No	Yes
Newton[112]	Amp/sulbactum IV indomethacin	86	No	No	ND
Gordon[113]	IV ceftizoxime	117	No	No	No
Cox[114]	IV amp/sulbactum oral amp/clavulanic acid	78	No	No	No

* Gestation prolonged by 10 days in antibiotic compared with placebo group among subset of women with cervical dilatation ≥1 cm at enrollment.
† ABX = antibiotic group.
ND = analysis not reported.

infection developed fever or leukocytosis during labor, consistent with observations in humans presenting in preterm labor with amniotic fluid infection. In a similar design, intraamniotic infusion of IL-1 without bacteria induced preterm labor in all treated animals.[103] This animal model appears to mimic infection-induced preterm labor in humans, allows serial sampling to determine the sequence and timing of cytokine and prostaglandin production, and should provide a valuable tool for evaluation of interventions such as cytokine inhibitors to arrest infection-induced preterm labor.

In addition to the infection-induced production of cytokines and prostaglandins leading to preterm labor and delivery, infection and the resulting inflammatory response may directly damage the fetal membranes leading to rupture. Preterm rupture of the membranes with resulting delivery accounts for up to one-third of preterm deliveries and frequently is associated with histologic chorioamnionitis. Pathogens commonly found in the genital tract, such as *Bacteroides* spp., GBS, and *T. vaginalis,* produce proteases that have been shown in vitro to reduce the strength and elasticity of the membranes.[104,105] In vitro addition of *E. coli* or GBS to cultured chorioamnion reduces the bursting pressure of the membranes.[106] Many bacteria produce phospholipases that may directly damage the membranes or lead to prostaglandin production. Thus exposure of the membranes near the cervical os to lower genital tract bacteria may lead to direct damage and rupture of the membranes or to ascending infection, causing similar resulting damage as well as an inflammatory response leading to cytokine and prostaglandin production and preterm labor.

Since data implicating infection as a cause of preterm labor and preterm rupture of the membranes are mounting, addition of antibiotics to standard treatments for these conditions might be expected to prolong pregnancy. However, placebo-controlled studies of antibiotics in addition to tocolytics for preterm labor with intact membranes have not shown prolongation of pregnancy[70,107–114] (Table 80-4). Since antibiotic levels in the amniotic fluid and the fetus approach or exceed maternal levels and the majority of microorganisms isolated are sensitive to the antibiotics, the infection should be eradicated. However, as shown in the monkey model, contractions are a late finding in the cascade, and antibiotics might not be expected to reverse the cytokine and prostaglandin response. Indeed, lysis of microorganisms during antibiotic treatment actually may increase the inflammatory response. Treatments aimed at blocking the cytokine and prostaglandin response while treating infection must be developed and tested in animal models.

Trials of antibiotic therapy after preterm rupture of the membranes have yielded more variable results in prolonging pregnancy, probably because the treatments used after preterm ROM have varied considerably[115–121] (Table 80-5). The use of steroids to enhance fetal lung maturity also may affect the fetal response to cytokines, and the use of steroids and of tocolytic agents is quite variable between institutions and between studies. The proportion of infants delivered more than 1 week after membrane rupture has been higher in the antibiotic treatment group than in the placebo group in several studies, although infant hospital stay was not necessarily shortened. The incidences of fever during labor and of postpartum endometritis also were reduced in the antibiotic treatment group in most studies, and infant sepsis and pneumonia were decreased. Because of the varied antibiotic regimens used and the variable results, no clear recommendations can be made for selections of antibiotic regimens in preterm ROM, except for the current recommendation to treat women with preterm ROM with an antibiotic active against GBS pending vaginal and rectal culture results.

Multiple lines of evidence including epidemiologic studies, data on upper genital tract infection, and animal models implicate lower genital tract infections in the early pathogenesis of a significant proportion of cases of preterm labor and preterm ROM. Since antibiotic treatment of infection-related preterm labor and preterm ROM to prolong pregnancy has been largely unsuccessful, the best strategy currently is prevention of these conditions by early detection and treatment of lower genital tract infections before complications occur. Pregnant women should be screened for bacterial vaginosis, *C. trachomatis, N. gonorrhoeae,* syphilis, and *T. vaginalis* on the first prenatal visit and treated if positive. Repeat screening later in pregnancy should be done for women in high-risk groups for STDs or with symptoms. Recently, additional tests have been evaluated for their ability to predict preterm delivery among populations at low or high risk for preterm delivery. Strategies evaluated include cervical or vaginal testing for fetal fibronectin, assessment of cervical length by ultrasound, and daily home uterine contraction monitoring. Fetal fibronectin is a basement membrane protein produced by the fetal membranes that appears important for binding the placenta and membranes to the decidua.[122] Fetal fibronectin is commonly present in the lower genital tract until 16 to 20 weeks of pregnancy but is detected thereafter in only 3 to 4 percent of cervical or vaginal specimens.[123] Fetal fibronectin was detected twice as often among pregnant women with compared with those without bacterial vaginosis at 23 to 24 weeks' gestation. Thus far, the clinical value of fetal fibronectin testing in screening patients at low risk for preterm delivery has been variable, although detection is clearly associated with a significantly increased risk of preterm birth.[123,124] Of interest, in the largest study of screening low-risk patients, fetal fibronectin was better at predicting preterm birth before 28 weeks' gestation,[123] the same period in gestation when infection is most often implicated as contributing to preterm labor. In the same study population, women with bacterial vaginosis and positive fetal fibronectin at 23 to 24 weeks had a 16-fold increase in clinical chorioamnionitis and a 6-fold increase in neonatal sepsis.[125] Fetal fibronectin testing has been better at predicting an increased risk of preterm birth among high-risk women such as those with

Table 80-5. Randomized, Placebo-Controlled Trials of Antibiotics in Patients with Preterm Rupture of Membranes

Author	Antibiotic regimen	Total *n*	Prolonged gestation	Reduced neonatal morbidity	Reduced maternal morbidity
Blanco[115]	Ceftizoxime	306	No	ND*	ND*
Johnston[116]	Mezlocillin, ampicillin	85	Yes	Yes	Yes
McGregor[117]	Erythromycin	55	No	No	No
Mercer[118]	Erythromycin	220	No	No	No
Kurki[119]	Penicillin	101	ND	No	No
Lockwood[120]	Piperacillin	75	Yes	No	No
Ernest[121]	Penicillin	148	No	No	Yes

* ND = analysis not reported.

previous preterm birth and multiple gestations.[126,127] However, no studies have evaluated interventions to reduce the risk of preterm birth among women with positive fetal fibronectin, so the clinical utility of screening is limited at present. Fetal fibronectin currently appears useful as a research tool to identify populations at increased risk of preterm birth who then can be targeted for intervention trials to reduce the risk of preterm birth. Fetal fibronectin also appears useful among women presenting with preterm contractions to identify those women more likely to deliver who can then be given aggressive tocolytic and other therapies compared with those with contractions unlikely to progress to preterm delivery.[128–130] Again, no studies have been reported evaluating altered treatment for fibronectin-positive women in preterm labor to attempt to decrease the rate of preterm birth.

Similarly, among women with preterm contractions, assessment of cervical length by ultrasound may help identify those at highest risk for progressive preterm labor, but its value in screening low-risk women to predict preterm birth remains unproven.[131,132] Home uterine activity monitoring appears to be of benefit in early detection of preterm labor in women with multiple gestations and other high-risk conditions but is not routinely recommended,[133,134] since the benefit of early detection of preterm labor and ability to intervene is not established. Women of reproductive age should be educated regarding the importance of early prenatal care, safer sexual practices, and STD screening. Pregnant women and their partners should be counseled on symptoms of preterm labor, safer practices, and avoidance of other partners during the pregnancy.

MATERNAL PUERPERAL INFECTION AS A COMPLICATION OF ANTENATAL SEXUALLY TRANSMITTED DISEASES

EPIDEMIOLOGY AND PATHOGENESIS

Puerperal endometritis, the most common maternal postpartum infection, can be divided into early infections occurring within the first 48 hours of delivery and late infections occurring from 2 days to 6 weeks after delivery.[135] Cesarean section greatly increases the risk of early postpartum infection. Without antimicrobial prophylaxis, 36 to 65 percent of women who undergo nonelective cesarean section develop infectious morbidity; women delivered by cesarean section are up to 20 times more likely to develop infectious morbidity than are women delivered vaginally. The high infection rate following cesarean section probably results from direct myometrial and peritoneal contamination by organisms present within the amniotic cavity at the time of cesarean section. Factors that increase microbial contamination of the uterus before delivery such as long duration of labor or rupture of membranes, chorioamnionitis, and number of vaginal examinations increase the risk of postpartum endometritis and puerperal sepsis.

In developed countries, most postpartum infections are related to cesarean section. In developing countries, where cesarean sections are performed less frequently and maternal STDs are more prevalent, postpartum upper genital tract infections after vaginal delivery are approximately 10 times more common than in developed countries.[136]

MICROBIAL ETIOLOGY OF POSTPARTUM ENDOMETRITIS AND PUERPERAL SEPSIS

Among women delivered vaginally in Nairobi, Kenya, Plummer et al.[136] noted that cervical gonococcal or chlamydial infection, prolonged labor (12 hours), and low socioeconomic status were the major determinants of puerperal pelvic infection. In pregnancies associated with maternal gonococcal infection, postpartum gonococcal pelvic infection and gonococcal ophthalmia neonatorum frequently occurred concomitantly. This association suggested that either uniquely virulent gonococcal strains were present or that shared host deficiency or perhaps early-stage maternal infection with large concentrations of gonococci in cervicovaginal secretions occurred in these mother-infant pairs. In this study, approximately 20 percent of mothers undergoing vaginal delivery developed postpartum pelvic infection, and approximately 35 percent of such cases were attributable to gonococcal and/or chlamydial infection.

Other microorganisms are undoubtedly involved in causing postpartum pelvic infections and puerperal sepsis and may be relatively more important causes in areas of low prevalence of maternal gonococcal and chlamydial infection. In particular, anaerobic bacteria (predominantly *Bacteroides* spp., *P. bivius*, and peptostreptococci) and *M. hominis* have been incriminated in postpartum pelvic infections after vaginal delivery.[137,139]

Wallace et al.[140] isolated *M. hominis* from the blood of 10 to 15 percent of women with postpartum fever. Women without antibody to *M. hominis* at the time of delivery had a higher rate of postpartum fever than women with antibody, and many febrile women acquired *M. hominis* antibody. None of the women with mycoplasmaemia was seriously ill; despite high temperatures, they had minimal uterine tenderness and no foul-smelling or purulent cervical discharge, and they improved rapidly following antibiotic administration.

The association of vaginal anaerobes and *M. hominis* with bacterial vaginosis suggests that bacterial vaginosis per se is a risk factor for puerperal infection after vaginal delivery. Similarly, early postpartum endometritis and bacteremia among women following cesarean delivery usually are due to the anaerobic and fac-

Table 80-6. Microorganisms Isolated from the Endometrium via Triple-Lumen Catheter and from Blood from 150 Febrile Women with Early Postpartum Endomyometritis

Microorganism	Endometrium (n = 150), number (%)	Blood (n = 150), number (%)
Facultatives:		
Streptococcus agalactiae (GBS)	12 (8)	5 (3)
Enterococci	18 (12)	1 (1)
Viridans streptococci	11 (7)	5 (3)
Staphylococcus aureus	3 (2)	0
Gardnerella vaginalis	57 (38)	10 (7)
Escherichia coli	12 (8)	2 (1)
Other Enterobacteriaceae spp.	9 (6)	0
Haemophilus influenzae	3 (2)	1 (1)
Anaerobes:		
Prevotella bivia	14 (9)	4 (3)
Bacteroides fragilis	3 (2)	0
Bacteroides spp.	27 (18)	2 (1)
Peptostreptococcus assacharolyticus	22 (15)	4 (3)
Other *Peptostreptococcus* spp.	43 (29)	5 (3)
Clostridium perfringens	4 (3)	0
Fusobacterium nucleatum	1 (1)	0
Mycoplasmas:		
Ureaplasma urealyticum	107 (71)	6 (4)
Mycoplasma hominis	36 (24)	4 (3)
Chlamydiae:		
Chlamydia trachomatis	10 (7)	0

SOURCE: Watts et al.[141]

ultative bacteria of the cervicovaginal flora, predominantly but not exclusively those associated with bacterial vaginosis[141] (Table 80-6). Indeed, the presence of bacterial vaginosis diagnosed by Gram stain on admission for delivery was an independent risk factor for postpartum endometritis (PPE) among women undergoing cesarean section (adjusted odds ratio 5.8, 95 percent confidence interval 3.0 to 10.9).[142] In a separate study assessing reasons for failure of antibiotic prophylaxis with cefoxiten or cefotetan to prevent PPE, only the presence of GBS or enterococci in the upper genital tract (amniotic fluid, decidua, chorioamnionic membranes) at delivery was associated with the development of PPE.[143] Among women without GBS or enterococci in the upper genital tract at delivery who developed PPE, microorganisms associated with bacterial vaginosis were isolated at the time of PPE.

In contrast, late postpartum endometritis, occurring 3 days to 6 weeks after delivery, has been correlated with *C. trachomatis* infection.[135] Wager et al.[144] found that approximately 30 percent of pregnant women with antepartum *C. trachomatis* developed puerperal infection. One-third of these cases had intrapartum fever attributed to chorioamnionitis, and two-thirds had late postpartum endometritis. Clinical manifestations of puerperal chlamydial endometritis, like those of nonpuerperal chlamydial endometritis and salpingitis, are generally mild. Patients are often afebrile, with mild uterine tenderness, and usually with no adnexal tenderness. Such minimally symptomatic postpartum chlamydial infections may contribute to the high rate of Chlamydia antibody among women with secondary infertility because of distal tubal obstruction (see Chap. 79).

The frequency of involvement of the fallopian tubes during postpartum pelvic infection is unknown, since no laparoscopic studies have been reported. The observation of Platt et al.[137] that peritoneal infection (as assessed by culdocentesis) commonly accompanies postpartum pelvic infection suggests that fallopian tube infection may not be rare. Similarly, the relationship of postpartum pelvic infection to secondary infertility due to tubal scarring is also unknown. Nevertheless, secondary infertility, usually due to tubal obstruction, is a major problem in Africa,[145] where the prevalence rates of maternal gonococcal and chlamydial infection and the incidence rates of postpartum pelvic infection are very high. However, in the United States, where the majority of postpartum infections occur after cesarean section, no evidence of an increased rate of impaired fertility has been seen after postpartum endometritis.[146]

NEONATAL CONSEQUENCES OF SEXUALLY TRANSMITTED DISEASES

Systemic perinatal bacterial infection is acquired in utero or during delivery in 1 to 5 per 1,000 live births.[147] Perinatal bacterial infections are two to three times more common than are perinatal viral and protozoal infections. Presently, about half of all neonatal bacterial infections in the United States are due to GBS, although marked regional variations occur. Temporal changes in the predominant pathogens found in perinatal infection also have occurred. The incidence of GBS neonatal infections increased at several medical centers during the 1960s and 1970s, more or less in parallel with the increase in other STDs. Group A beta-hemolytic streptococci, *Staphylococcus aureus,* Enterobacteriaceae spp., and, most recently, anaerobes also have been important neonatal pathogens.

Neonatal and pediatric STDs are discussed in detail in Chaps. 81 to 86. Table 80-7 summarizes the clinical manifestations and diagnostic findings that can occur with congenital or neonatal infection with STD agents.[148]

Table 80-7. Clinical Manifestations of Neonatal Infection with Sexually Transmitted Agents Acquired In Utero or at Delivery

	Microorganism				
Clinical sign	Cytomegalovirus	Herpes simplex virus	*Treponema pallidum*	*Chlamydia trachomatis*	*Neisseria gonorrhoeae*
Hepatosplenomegaly	+	+	+	−	−
Jaundice	+	+	+	−	−
Adenopathy	−	−	+	−	−
Pneumonitis	+	+	+	++	−
Lesions of skin or mucous membranes:					
Petechiae or purpura	+	+	+	−	+
Vesicles, ulcers	?	++	+	−	−
Maculopapular exanthem	−	+	++	−	−
Lesions of nervous system:					
Meningoencephalitis	+	+	+	−	+
Microcephaly	++	+	−	−	−
Intracranial calcifications	++	+	−	−	−
Bone lesions	+	+	++	−	−
Joint lesions	−	−	+	−	+
Eye lesions:					
Chorioretinitis	+	+	+	−	−
Conjunctivitis	−	+	−	++	++

NOTE: − = finding rare or not present; + = finding occurs in neonates during infection; ++ = finding has special diagnostic significance for this infection.
SOURCE: Modified from Nahmias and Visinthine.[148]

CONSEQUENCES, RECOGNITION, AND MANAGEMENT OF SPECIFIC SEXUALLY TRANSMITTED DISEASES DURING PREGNANCY

SYPHILIS

Epidemiology and manifestations

Syphilis remains a common complication of pregnancy, despite availability of cheap, accurate diagnostic tests and continued sensitivity of *T. pallidum* to penicillin. In the preantibiotic era, syphilis was estimated to be responsible for as many as 40 percent of stillbirths.[149] Presently, syphilis infrequently causes stillbirth in industrialized countries but remains a common cause in developing countries. Naeye[150] noted that 0.2 percent of perinatal deaths were attributable to syphilis among over 50,000 pregnancies studied in the U.S. Collaborative Perinatal Project between 1959 and 1966. From that time until 1978, the incidence of congenital syphilis in the United States steadily declined. However, from 1978 until 1990, the incidence of primary and secondary syphilis in women of childbearing age increased and, despite subsequent declines, remains at high levels, particularly in ethnic minority women, and this has been accompanied by high rates of congenital syphilis. A total of 16,491 cases of primary and secondary syphilis were reported to the Centers for Disease Control and Prevention in 1995, and 1,548 cases of congenital syphilis were diagnosed at less than 1 year of age,[151] representing a decline of over 50 percent in both forms of syphilis since 1992. Highest rates of primary and secondary syphilis in the United States were related to the epidemic of crack cocaine use and associated prostitution. Exact figures for the rate of primary and secondary syphilis among pregnant women are not available and vary depending on the population studied. In teaching hospitals in urban areas, prevalence rates of 2.2 to 3.9 percent in patients receiving prenatal care have been reported.[152,153] Rates of syphilis among women without prenatal care are consistently higher, with up to 11 percent of women not receiving prenatal care and 15 percent with positive cocaine screens at delivery having syphilis.[154] Eighty percent of women with infectious syphilis are within the 15- to 34-year age group, the peak reproductive years.

Congenital syphilis still remains a major problem in developing countries.[155] In past studies in Addis Ababa, Ethiopia, and in Durban, South Africa, congenital syphilis was the fifth and fourth leading cause of perinatal death, respectively. In a study of pregnant women in Zambia, serologic tests for syphilis were reactive in 43 percent of women who delivered stillborn babies, 19 percent who aborted, and 13 percent of normal women attending their first antenatal visit.[156]

Congenital syphilis is entirely preventable with appropriate case detection and treatment programs. In 1951, it was found that 50 percent of mothers of infants with congenital syphilis in Massachusetts had had inadequate or no prenatal care, 17 percent had been found infected during pregnancy but failed to complete antibiotic therapy, and 12 percent had become infected after an initially negative prenatal serologic test for syphilis.[157] During the outbreak of congenital syphilis in Texas in the early 1980s, 62 percent of mothers of infected infants had not received prenatal care.[158] The provision of adequate prenatal care to all pregnant women remains the foundation for prevention of congenital syphilis. The clinical manifestations of syphilis in adults are well described in Chaps. 33 to 36 and are not altered by pregnancy. The majority of pregnant women diagnosed with syphilis are asymptomatic, underscoring the need for routine serologic screening of all pregnant women as early as possible in pregnancy. Pregnant women in high-risk groups should have repeat serologic screening for syphilis in the third trimester in addition to their first visit. All patients diagnosed with syphilis should be counseled and tested for HIV infection as well. Women who have fetuses noted to have nonimmune hydrops on ultrasound or who experience stillbirth should always undergo serologic testing for syphilis. Darkfield examination of the amniotic fluid for spirochetes also may be helpful in the evaluation of stillbirth when syphilis is suspected but probably adds little to the evaluation of the patient with syphilis with a live infant.[159]

Pathogenesis

Placental infection with *T. pallidum* occurs during maternal spirochetemia, which is intense until resolution of the secondary stage. After resolution of the initial and secondary stages, the prevalence and intensity of spirochetemia are unknown except during secondary relapses. Whether pregnancy promotes recrudescence of spirochetemia, accounting for the congenital infections that occur occasionally in late syphilis, is uncertain. In the preantibiotic era, Moore[8] observed that the manifestations of primary and secondary syphilis were particularly mild in the pregnant woman. He speculated that pregnancy supplied "some substance which was able to suppress the manifestations of the disease."[11] *T. pallidum* infection produces less evident pathology among pregnant rabbits than among nonpregnant rabbits.[160] Since many of the manifestations of adult and congenital syphilis are thought to have an immunologic basis, the milder manifestations of syphilis during pregnancy are consistent with a relative state of immunosuppression during pregnancy. However, students of syphilis during the antibiotic era have not been impressed with an effect of pregnancy on the manifestations of syphilis.

Once the infection reaches the placenta, fetal infection usually follows. Dippel[149] showed that fetal infection with *T. pallidum* was not detectable until after 18 weeks of gestation. He examined abortuses and stillbirths delivered between the fourteenth and twenty-eighth week of gestation from 67 syphilitic women for the presence of *T. pallidum* by Levaditi's staining of fetal tissue. None of the 12 abortuses between 14 and 17 weeks' gestation, 3 of 29 (10 percent) abortuses between 18 and 22 weeks' gestation, and 13 of 26 (50 percent) stillbirths between 23 and 28 weeks' gestation were found to be infected. On this basis, he proposed that a placental barrier, perhaps Langhan's epithelial layer of cytotrophoblast, protected the fetus from infection prior to the eighteenth week of gestation. The validity of this hypothesis has been challenged by Harter and Benirschke,[161] who observed that fetal infection can occur as early as 9 weeks' gestation. These authors identified five untreated syphilitic women who were to undergo first-trimester therapeutic abortion. Fetal and placental tissue was studied by silver stain and immunofluorescence for spirochetes, and in two of the five cases fetal spirochetal infection was found. The authors comment on the paucity of organisms seen and the effort involved in their detection. Benirschke[162] subsequently pointed out that although Langhan's layer becomes less apparent after the eighteenth week of gestation, it does not totally disappear. Considered collectively, the data suggest that the fetus is susceptible to infection prior to the eighteenth week of gestation, but *T. pallidum* is more likely to be detectable in fetal tissue after the eighteenth week, for reasons not fully defined.

Silverstein[163] has proposed that the lesions of congenital syphilis do not become manifest until early manifestations of fetal immunocompetence appear at about the sixteenth week of gestation. He suggested that the pathogenesis of congenital syphilis may depend on the immune response of the fetus rather than on cytopathogenic effects of *T. pallidum*. This hypothesis (if true) also may explain why adequate therapy of maternal syphilis prior to the sixteenth week of gestation usually prevents fetal damage.

A detailed clinical description of congenital syphilis is provided in Chap. 84. Untreated primary or secondary syphilis during pregnancy affects virtually 100 percent of fetuses, with 50 percent of such pregnancies resulting in premature delivery or perinatal death.[157] Untreated early latent syphilis during pregnancy results in a 40 percent rate of prematurity or perinatal death. Ten percent of infants born to mothers with untreated late syphilis show signs of congenital infection, and the perinatal death rate is increased approximately tenfold. Whereas syphilis is rarely sexually transmissible longer than 2 years after acquisition, women with untreated syphilis apparently may remain infectious for their fetuses for many years, although the proportion of affected fetuses and the severity of fetal disease decrease with longer duration of untreated maternal infection. More recent reports have confirmed the abysmal prognosis with untreated syphilis in pregnancy. In a recent report of 56 cases, only 7 of whom received treatment during pregnancy, 34 percent were stillborn, and the mean gestational age at delivery was 32.3 weeks.[164] Other studies have shown a 28 percent incidence of preterm birth even among women with some treatment during pregnancy.[165] Presumptive evidence of congenital syphilis was seen in 15 (26 percent) of 57 women treated (not always adequately) by 24 weeks' gestation and in 41 (60 percent) of 70 women treated in the third trimester.[165]

Case detection

Congenital syphilis can be prevented by early prenatal diagnosis and treatment. Serology remains the most useful screening or diagnostic test for syphilis in women. Signs or symptoms are confirmatory but often are not demonstrable; of over 14,000 cases of early syphilis in women, only 11 percent had a primary lesion, 41 percent had secondary lesions, and 48 percent had no manifestations and were detected only by serology.[166]

Infected individuals will develop antibodies to *T. pallidum* by the time of chancre formation or within 2 to 3 weeks afterwards. Virtually all patients with secondary syphilis have a positive serologic test for syphilis, provided steps are taken to avert the prozone phenomenon. This phenomenon occurs when there is an overwhelming excess of antibody in the patient's serum that interferes with the binding to antigen in the flocculation test. If syphilis is strongly suspected and initial results are negative, the specimen should be diluted before retesting.[167] After lesions of secondary syphilis resolve, latent syphilis is detected serologically.

Despite the low prevalence of maternal syphilis in many developed countries, cost-benefit analysis still favors prenatal first-trimester serologic screening.[168] For instance, in Norway, with a 0.02 percent maternal prevalence rate, the cost-benefit ratio of the program was still 3.8. Only with an estimated prevalence of maternal syphilis of less than 1 per 20,000 would the costs of the screening program exceed the benefits. This analysis excluded intangible benefits of screening that cannot be measured in economic terms. The U.S. Centers for Disease Control and Prevention recommend serologic testing at the beginning of prenatal care, with repeat testing at the beginning of the third trimester (28 weeks and at delivery) for high-risk women.[169]

The many barriers to detection of syphilis early in pregnancy include those which lead to delayed prenatal care, particularly in developing countries and among poor and minority women in industrialized countries. Approximately one-fourth of pregnant women in the United States received no first-trimester prenatal care during 1985, with a disproportionately higher percentage among Medicaid recipients and uninsured women.[65] A recent publication outlines specific practical measures to improve early detection in pregnant women.[169] These measures include on-site pregnancy testing in STD clinics and drug-addiction programs of women whose menstrual periods are late, routine RPR testing whenever a positive pregnancy test is obtained in all pregnancy testing programs, and early testing by prenatal programs, before the regularly scheduled prenatal visit when the waiting time for the first scheduled visit is long. In developing country settings and in other settings where the system for testing and early return visit for test results and treatment is problematic, rapid clinic-based testing and treatment at the first prenatal visit is essential, even while confirmatory tests are pending.

Treatment

A positive screening test should be further evaluated with a quantitative nontreponemal test (VDRL) and a confirmatory treponemal test such as the fluorescent treponemal antibody-absorption test (FTA-ABS) or the microhemagglutination–*T. pallidum* (MHA-TP) test.

Women with a positive FTA-ABS test who do not have clear documentation of previous adequate treatment for syphilis require treatment. Women with an epidemiologic history of recent exposure to an individual with proven syphilis should be treated, regardless of serologic results.

It is not necessary to retreat women who have had documented adequate treatment for previous syphilis so long as no evidence of serologic or clinical relapse exists. If clinical or serologic relapse or reinfection occurs, therapy should, of course, be reinstituted. If doubt exists about the adequacy of previous therapy, retreatment should be given promptly.

Treatment of syphilis in the pregnant woman is generally the same as that in the nonpregnant patient and depends on the duration of infection and the presence or absence of central nervous system involvement. Some authors warn against performing a lumbar puncture in the pregnant patient for fear of precipitating preterm labor. Such concern does not appear justified if the lumbar puncture is performed properly.

Recommended choices and schedules of antimicrobials for the various clinical forms of syphilis are found in Chaps. 34 to 36 and 84. Pregnant women who develop a Jarisch-Herxheimer reaction after initiation of treatment for early syphilis may have precipitous onset of premature labor. In one report, 15 (65 percent) of 23 pregnant women with primary or secondary syphilis compared to none of 10 with latent syphilis experienced the Jarisch-Herxheimer reaction. Symptoms and signs developed within 2 to 8 hours of therapy, peaked at 6 to 12 hours, and abated by 16 to 24 hours after treatment.[170] Uterine contractions and decreased fetal movement or signs of fetal distress on fetal monitoring occurred in 67 percent of women with the Jarisch-Herxheimer reaction. We recommend hospitalization of women beyond 20 weeks' gestation who have early syphilis for close observation during initiation of therapy to permit fetal monitoring and early tocolytic therapy, if needed. Should penicillin allergy exist, no established recommendations for therapy are available. However, skin testing with penicillin G minor determinant mixture and penicylloyl polylysine is recommended.[171] The great majority of patients with a past history of penicillin allergy will have negative (nonreactive) skin tests and can be treated safely with penicillin G.[172] For pregnant women with positive immediate wheal and flare skin tests, desensitization can be achieved rapidly by oral administration of increasing doses of penicillin V. One desensitization schedule used in 15 pregnant women who had positive penicillin skin tests involved a starting oral dose of 100 units of penicillin V; the oral dose was doubled every 15 minutes, for a total of 14 doses, each diluted in 30 mL of water, given over a total elapsed time of 3 hours and 45 minutes, with the final dose equal to 640,000 units.[173] Women were desensitized in the hospital, with an intravenous line in place and a physician on hand at all times. After a further 30-minute observation period, parenteral penicillin was begun. Five patients had evidence of allergic reaction, one requiring epinephrine. After completion of the procedure, full doses of parenteral penicillin therapy can be instituted. Failures to prevent congenital syphilis following treatment of the mother during pregnancy with erythromycin, tetracycline, and chloramphenicol were summarized by Thompson.[174] Available data suggest that the failure rate with erythromycin is unacceptably high. Certain cephalosporins show good treponemacidal activity, but clinical trials are required to prove their safety and efficacy for syphilis in pregnancy. Pregnant women treated for early syphilis should have monthly quantitative serologies throughout pregnancy. Those who do not show a fourfold drop in titer at 3 months or who show a fourfold rise in titer should be retreated.

GONORRHEA

The recognition that maternal gonococcal infection posed a threat to the newborn's sight motivated Crede's prophylaxis: a major achievement of modern preventive medicine. In the 1880s, ophthalmia neonatorum was a frequent neonatal infection. In Crede's original series, 10 percent of newborns acquired ophthalmia neonatorum. Rothenberg[175] estimated that the maternal gonococcal infection rate among patients studied by Crede must have approached the astounding figure of 30 percent.

Epidemiology

The reported prevalence of gonococcal infection among pregnant women shows wide variations, determined by differences in populations studied. Generally, studies of indigent populations in the United States have shown higher prevalence rates than studies from other industrialized countries, and rates in most of the developing world are higher than rates in developed countries. Risk factors for infection remain the same in pregnancy as in the nonpregnant state. In North America, gonococcal recovery rates are highest in young, nonwhite, unmarried mothers of low socioeconomic status, particularly in large cities. Isolates resistant to penicillin and other antibiotics have increased in frequency, with 14.3 percent of isolates resistant to penicillin and 25.3 percent resistant to tetracycline in 1995 in the Gonococcal Isolate Surveillance Project.[151] Despite a decreasing incidence of gonococcal infection in men in most industrialized countries (presumably owing to behavioral changes due to AIDS), in childbearing women having the characteristics described above, the prevalence rate of gonorrhea remains high.[155,176,177]

Manifestations and pathogenesis

The manifestations and pathogenesis of gonococcal infection in the pregnant host have some unique features.[178] The rate of pharyngeal infection as the sole site of infection may be increased during pregnancy. In some studies, 15 to 35 percent of infected pregnant women have had *N. gonorrhoeae* isolated only from the throat and not from the endocervix or anal canal.[179,180] These findings suggest that endocervical cultures may be more apt to be falsely negative or that the frequency of oral sexual activity relative to vaginal intercourse may be increased during pregnancy. Pharyngeal colonization with gonococci may increase the risk of dissemination (see Chaps. 32 and 68), and some studies have suggested an increased risk of disseminated gonococcal infection (DGI) among pregnant women.[181]

The frequency of upper genital tract involvement following endocervical gonococcal infection during pregnancy is unknown. Among nonpregnant women, 10 to 20 percent with cervical gonorrhea have clinical evidence of pelvic inflammatory disease (PID), and up to 50 percent of women with recently acquired gonorrhea developed signs suggesting PID in one study.[182] In contrast, acute gonococcal PID appears to be a rare event during pregnancy. Positive prenatal cultures for *N. gonorrhoeae* are occasionally associated with fever and pain, and surgically verified cases of gonococcal salpingitis in pregnancy have been reported between 7 and 12 weeks' gestation (prior to obliteration of the endometrial cavity).[183] However, lower abdominal pain in pregnant women should not be ascribed to PID unless other causes of pain potentially requiring surgical treatment, such as ectopic pregnancy or appendicitis, have been ruled out.

Local cervical factors may decrease the risk for ascending gonococcal infection in pregnancy. Serum progesterone concentrations are greatly increased in pregnancy, and concentrations of progesterone 50 to 200 times that occurring during pregnancy are known to inhibit the growth of *N. gonorrhoeae* in vitro.[184] The menstrual cycle effects phenotypic changes in gonococci that may alter gonococcal virulence; the effects of pregnancy on phenotypic properties of *N. gonorrhoeae* have not been studied. Cervical mucus becomes impermeable to motile sperm (and perhaps to resistant ascent of microorganisms) under the influence of progesterone.[185] Perhaps most important, after the twelfth week of gestation, the chorion attaches to the endometrial decidua with obliteration of the intrauterine cavity, obstructing the route for ascending intraluminal spread of gonococci. All these factors may limit the spread of gonococci from the cervix to the endometrium and fallopian tubes during pregnancy.

We hypothesize that the chorioamnion itself may become the site of infection by ascending gonococci after the twelfth week of gestation. Among women hospitalized with gonococcal infection during pregnancy, in one study, 35 percent had septic abortion.[23] This observation has not been addressed subsequently.

In retrospective studies, data have been conflicting regarding the

Table 80-8. Pregnancy Outcome with Positive *N. gonorrhoeae* Cultures

Reference	No.	Preterm delivery	Perinatal mortality	Preterm PROM	Maternal morbidity
Positive any time					
Israel[186]	69	No increase over controls			
Amstey[187]	222	25%*	7.6%*	26%*	20%
Edwards[188]	178	12.3%	28%	28%	9.5%*
Stoll[189]	435	15.7%	2.2%		
Donders[190]	167	56%*			
Positive intrapartum					
Elliott[191]	166	OR = 2.9 (1.2–7.2)*			
Israel[186]	39	12.8%	2.6%		28.2%*
Edwards[188]	19	42.1%*	10.5%*	63%*	31.6%*
Maxwell[192]	11		9%		18%*

NOTE: PROM = preterm rupture of membranes; OR = odds ratio.
* Signification increase from controls ($p < 0.05$).

impact of gonococcal infection on prematurity[186–192] (Table 80-8). Edwards et al.[188] found an increased rate of prematurity among women with positive intrapartum, but not antepartum, gonorrhea cultures. Amstey and Steadman[187] found high preterm birth rates even in women treated for gonorrhea early in pregnancy who remained culture-negative after treatment, while Charles et al.[193] found no difference in outcome between women treated early in pregnancy and those who did not have gonorrhea in pregnancy. Likewise, the association between gonorrhea and increased perinatal mortality, premature rupture of the membranes, and maternal morbidity has been variable among retrospective studies. Overall, data from these studies suggest that cervical gonorrhea infection in the third trimester may be a risk factor for prematurity, rupture of the membranes before the onset of labor, and maternal febrile morbidity.

Data from recent prospective studies have been more consistent. In a case-control study of patients with preterm rupture of the membranes, *N. gonorrhoeae* was isolated from 13 percent of patients with preterm ROM and no term controls.[194] All patients in the study had been screened and, if positive, treated for gonorrhea early in pregnancy. Two studies from Africa showed a three- to sixfold increased risk of preterm birth and low birth weight among women with untreated gonorrhea, independent of other risk factors.[190,191]

In noncontrolled studies of maternal gonococcal infection, Berstine and Bland[195] reported that 32 percent of women with antenatal gonococcal infection had puerperal infectious morbidity. A related observation can be found in a matched-pair analysis of 228 cases of endometritis among 4,823 women following elective abortion.[196] These investigators found a threefold increased relative risk for endometritis in patients who had untreated gonococcal infection when compared with uninfected control subjects ($p < 0.05$).

In Nairobi, Kenya, Plummer et al.[136] found that postpartum upper genital tract infection (UGTI) was significantly correlated with intrapartum gonococcal and/or chlamydial infection. Forty-seven percent of women with intrapartum gonococcal infection developed postpartum UGTI; approximately 22 percent of postpartum UGTI was attributable to gonococcal infection in this setting, where the prevalence of maternal gonococcal infection was 6 percent.

These studies collectively provide convincing evidence that maternal gonococcal infection is detrimental to pregnancy. Gonococcal endocervicitis may cause preterm birth, premature ROM, and chorioamnionitis by infecting the lower pole of the chorioamnion. The effects of gonococcal infection on early pregnancy are less well studied than its effect on late pregnancy, but early infection may cause septic abortion. Acute salpingitis also occurs during the first trimester, but very infrequently. Disseminated gonococcal infection may occur more frequently during pregnancy. The risk of postpartum febrile morbidity is increased among women with cervical gonococcal infection, and neonatal gonococcal ophthalmia represents a frequent and severe complication.

Case detection and treatment

Because of these adverse effects on pregnancy, and because of the risk for neonatal infection, detection of *N. gonorrhoeae* by screening cultures during the initial antenatal visit is justified in most populations.[197] Repeat culture at 36 to 38 weeks' gestation is also indicated among high-risk individuals (young, nonwhite, single, primigravida, low socioeconomic status, current or past STD, especially gonorrhea earlier in pregnancy). Nearly 40 percent of pregnant women with gonorrhea give a past history of gonorrhea; therefore, past history of gonorrhea is a strong indicator for repeated screening cultures. In patients with premature ROM, intrapartum fever, or septic abortion, an endocervical swab for Gram stain and culture for *N. gonorrhoeae* also should be obtained.

In screening pregnant women for *N. gonorrhoeae*, culture on antibiotic-containing selective medium has long been the preferred method of detection. Gram stains are too insensitive in women to replace culture. Enzyme immunoassay methods and fluorescent antibody staining of direct smears lack consistent sensitivity and specificity in women, especially among populations with low gonococcal prevalence.[198–200] A DNA probe assay has been used increasingly for detection of cervical gonorrhea in pregnant and nonpregnant women.[201–203] The more sensitive nucleic acid amplification assays (see Chap. 92) for detection of *N. gonorrhoeae* and *C. trachomatis* require further evaluation in screening urine or cervical specimens from pregnant women but appear very promising.

Uncomplicated gonorrhea in the pregnant patient can be treated with ceftriaxone, 125 mg in a single intramuscular dose, or cefexime, 400 mg orally in a single dose.[171] In patients who cannot tolerate cephalosporins, spectinomycin, 2 gm in a single intramuscular dose, should be used. Tetracycline should not be used because of potential maternal and fetal toxic effects. Erythromycin or azithromycin, in dosages discussed below, can be added to treat possible coexisting *C. trachomatis* infections. Reinfection after treatment is common. Gonococcal reinfection rates of 11 to 30 percent have been reported despite efforts to treat partners. Notification and treatment of sexual partners should be pursued vigorously. If sexual partner therapy is not accomplished, repeat monthly cultures are appropriate.

For complicated gonococcal infection in pregnancy (e.g., septic abortion, chorioamnionitis), we recommend treatment for several days with ceftriaxone or cefoxitin plus an antibiotic effective against possible coexisting chlamydial infections, as recommended for pelvic inflammatory disease (see Chap. 58).

Neonatal gonococcal infection: implications for management of gonorrhea in pregnancy

In a recent study in Kenya, 42 percent of 67 newborns not receiving ocular prophylaxis who were exposed to maternal gonococcal infection acquired gonococcal ophthalmia neonatorum.[204] In addition to this well-recognized neonatal manifestation of exposure to maternal gonorrhea, infection at other body sites also can occur. *N. gonorrhoeae* has been recovered from orogastric aspirate samples from approximately 30 percent of neonates born of infected mothers.[188–205] Extraocular sites of neonatal gonococcal infection may be associated with a higher risk of disseminated infection.

The risk of gonococcal amniotic fluid infection syndrome and gonococcal ophthalmia appears to be increased after prolonged rupture of the membranes.[206,207] The failure of silver nitrate ocular prophylaxis to prevent gonococcal ophthalmia may result from in utero acquisition of *N. gonorrhoeae* in the setting of prolonged ROM.[208]

Gonococcal sepsis occurs in the newborn, although infrequently today. "Natural" bactericidal antibody to gonococci resides in the IgM fraction of serum and is absent from neonatal serum.[209] Whether neonates are at higher risk for gonococcal sepsis than are adults because of this is not established. More important, because neonates delivered of mothers with intrapartum gonococcal infection are more likely to be premature or to suffer prolonged labor, bacterial sepsis due to any etiology occurs more often.

For these various reasons, ophthalmic prophylaxis alone will not prevent all the manifestations and complications of gonorrhea in the neonate. Diagnostic screening and early treatment of infected women during pregnancy represent a more effective means of preventing neonatal gonococcal infection, as well as preventing complications in pregnancy itself.

In addition, in areas where the prevalence of maternal gonococcal infection is greater than 1 percent or where maternal screening is not undertaken, ophthalmic prophylaxis is useful and should be required.[175] The recommendations made by the Centers for Disease Control and Prevention for the prevention of gonococcal ophthalmia neonatorum (now endorsed by the American Academy of Pediatrics) state that ophthalmic ointment or drops containing 1% tetracycline, 0.5% erythromycin, or 1% silver nitrate are effective and acceptable. One randomized clinical trial of prophylaxis for gonococcal ophthalmia compared the effectiveness of 1% silver nitrate with 1% tetracycline ointment, and one study compared each of those agents to 0.5% erythromycin ointment.[210,211] Both studies found the agents studied to have similar efficacy in reducing the incidence of gonococcal ophthalmia. The prophylactic agents also were highly effective against multiresistant *N. gonorrhoeae*. However, the efficacy of topical 1% tetracycline in preventing gonococcal ophthalmia in neonates exposed to gonococci with resistance to tetracycline (25 percent of U.S. gonococcal isolates in 1995 and a much higher percentage of isolates from many developing countries) remains uncertain.

Neonates born to mothers with documented untreated antepartum or intrapartum gonococcal infection are at high risk for infection and should receive parenteral antibiotics in standard curative dosage (see Chap. 82) in addition to topical ocular prophylaxis.

CHLAMYDIA TRACHOMATIS INFECTIONS

Epidemiology

C. trachomatis infection rates for pregnant women have varied from 2 to 30 percent. Single marital status and young age, especially adolescence, are the major demographic correlates of chlamydial infections in pregnancy. Adolescents studied routinely have a prevalence of chlamydial infection of over 10 percent.[212] Although chlamydial infection rates have been highest among nonpregnant women in inner cities, higher rates of chlamydial infection have been reported among pregnant women in rural compared with urban areas in some parts of the country.[213] This difference may be related to lack of routine screening for chlamydia in nonpregnant women in rural areas with resulting underdiagnosing and underreporting.

Whether pregnancy per se influences shedding of *C. trachomatis* from the cervix is unknown. The rate of isolation of *C. trachomatis* has been reported to be higher during the third trimester than during the first or second trimester.[214,215] However, women who sought prenatal care in the first trimester in these cross-sectional studies may have had a lower risk of STDs than those who did not seek care until the third trimester. Shedding of *Chlamydia* might be influenced by the frequent development of ectopy in pregnancy, which is positively correlated with *C. trachomatis* isolation in nonpregnant women, or by alteration of the immune response to the organism. During pregnancy, the lymphocyte transformation (LT) response to *C. trachomatis* and other microbial antigens is significantly depressed, and a significant postpartum rise in the LT response occurs.[15] Whether the depressed cellular immunity influences susceptibility to shedding of *C. trachomatis* during pregnancy remains uncertain.

Maternal IgG antibody undergoes active transplacental transfer beginning as early as day 38.[216] The level of transfer remains fairly constant until the seventeenth week, at which time proportionate increases occur with advancing gestational age. Infants born to seropositive mothers with current or past *C. trachomatis* infection acquire antibody to this organism. Since about two-thirds of exposed neonates become infected (see Chap. 83), it is clear that passively acquired antibody is not completely protective. The influence of maternal antibody on the risk of acquisition of infection or on the severity of disease is unknown. The presence of antibody to *C. trachomatis* in breast milk or colostrum and the role of such colostral antibody in preventing or modifying neonatal chlamydial infection have not yet been evaluated.

Influence of *C. trachomatis* on reproduction and pregnancy

In some areas, up to two-thirds of cases of tubal infertility have been attributed to *C. trachomatis* infection.[31] If incomplete blockage of fallopian tubes occurs with infection, there is an increased risk of ectopic pregnancy (see Chaps. 58 and 79). In one study, 10 (59 percent) of 17 of patients with a history of ectopic pregnancy had antibodies to *C. trachomatis*.[217] In another case-control study, more women with ectopic pregnancy not related to intrauterine devices or previous tubal ligation had antibodies to *C. trachomatis* than did women with intrauterine pregnancies [18 of 32 (56 percent) versus 11 of 49 (22 percent), $p = 0.0021$].[30] Kosseim et al.[31] estimated that approximately one-third of cases of ectopic pregnancy may be attributable to chlamydial infection. Whether *C. trachomatis* infection can cause abortion is unknown. *C. psittaci* infection is an important cause of spontaneous abortion in lower mammals,[218] and Schachter[219] reported that *Chlamydia* were isolated from 4 of 22 first-trimester spontaneous abortuses in humans. Further work to define the relationship of chlamydial infection to abortion is needed.

The role of genital *C. trachomatis* infection in prematurity and

Table 80-9. Cohort Studies of the Effects of *Chlamydia trachomatis* on Pregnancy Outcome

Author	Gestational age at culture	No.	Adverse Outcome* Ct+	Adverse Outcome* Ct−	*p*
Martin[222]	<19 weeks	268	33%	8%	<0.01
Thompson[223]	1–2 trimester	433	14%	12%	N.S.
Harrison[139]	1–3 trimester	1185	14%	8%	<0.025†
Sweet[224]	1–3 trimester	540	19%	8%	0.03†
Gravett[225]	2–3 trimester	534	36%	12%	<0.01
Berman[226]	<24 weeks	781	9%	6%	N.S.
				5%	0.06†
Polk[227]	23–30 weeks	803		RR 1.7	0.01

NOTE: Ct = *Chlamydia trachomatis.*

* Includes abortion, low birth weight, stillbirth, neonatal death.

† Comparison of women with *C. trachomatis* and chlamydial IgM antibody with women without *C. trachomatis.*

in perinatal mortality is currently under active investigation. Examination of birth weights and gestational ages of infants with *C. trachomatis* infection has given conflicting results. Of infants with *C. trachomatis* ophthalmia neonatorum, 15 to 42 percent have had birth weights less than 2,500 gm.[207,220,221] Prospective studies of *C. trachomatis* and pregnancy outcome are summarized in Table 80-9.[139,222–227] Three separate studies at the University of Washington, each involving a different study design, have all shown a correlation of antenatal chlamydial infections with prematurity, defined by preterm delivery and/or low birth weight.[222,225,228] However, Frommell et al.[229] and Heggie et al.[230] found no association of antenatal *C. trachomatis* infection with prematurity. In a prospective study of 1,365 pregnant women, Harrison et al.[139] observed no significant correlation of *C. trachomatis* infection with prematurity but did find a significantly increased risk of low birth weight and of premature rupture of the membranes and a shorter gestation among women with serologically defined primary infection with *C. trachomatis* than among other culture-positive women or among culture-negative women. Similarly, Berman et al.[226] and Sweet et al.[224] confirmed the association of premature birth with IgM seropositivity among *C. trachomatis* culture-positive women. The biologic basis for these serologic correlations among *C. trachomatis*-infected women is not defined. Possibilities could include higher bacterial load and/or more extensive chlamydial infection or inflammation in a relatively nonimmune host. In an early study, Martin et al.[222] observed a correlation of antenatal *C. trachomatis* infection not only with prematurity but also with perinatal mortality. The latter observation has not been confirmed in other studies. Further prospective study of larger numbers of women is needed. A large multicenter study sponsored by the National Institute of Child Health and Human Development, still under analysis, should provide a more definitive assessment of the influence of *C. trachomatis* infection on pregnancy.

The role of *C. trachomatis* in maternal puerperal morbidity

Thygeson and Stone[231] noted in 1942 that 10 (26 percent) of 38 mothers whose infants had inclusion conjunctivitis developed puerperal infection.[231] Rees et al.[232] reported that 19 (61 percent) of 31 mothers of infants with *C. trachomatis* conjunctivitis developed postpartum infection after discharge from hospital (13 to 38 days postpartum).

Studies of pregnant women in Seattle and in Nairobi, Kenya, have confirmed that antepartum chlamydial infection, if not treated, is correlated with puerperal infection. Wager et al.[144] found that intrapartum fever (clinically ascribed to amnionitis) and late postpartum endometritis were both significantly correlated with untreated antepartum chlamydial infection (Table 80-10). Antenatal *C. trachomatis* infection was not associated with early postpartum fever, which was in the majority of instances associated with cesarean section. Overall, among women who delivered vaginally, puerperal infectious morbidity occurred in 10 (34 percent) of 29 women with and in 23 (8 percent) of 300 women without antenatal *C. trachomatis* infection ($p < 0.001$). Plummer et al.[136] subsequently reported from Nairobi that 24 percent of 183 women with intrapartum chlamydial infection developed postpartum upper genital tract infection (UGTI), a rate significantly greater than that observed in uninfected women (15 percent, $p = 0.02$). Chlamydial infection accounted for approximately 22 percent of postpartum UGTI in this setting; this rate may be representative of developing countries in Africa.

These studies collectively suggest that antepartum *C. trachomatis* infection causes amnionitis and postpartum endometritis, although attempts generally have not been made to isolate *C. trachomatis* at the time these complications have occurred.

Postabortal pelvic inflammatory disease

A syndrome related to postpartum pelvic infection is seen following therapeutic abortion. An excess rate of postabortal pelvic inflammatory disease has been seen among women with chlamydial infection at the time of the procedure.[33,233,234] In settings where gonococcal infection is much less prevalent than chlamydial infection, up to 60 percent of cases of postabortal PID may be attributable to chlamydial infection. In one study, the risk of postabortal PID among *Chlamydia*-infected women was inversely related to serum antibody titers to *Chlamydia*.[235] We recommend that women undergoing therapeutic abortion should be screened for chlamydial infection to prevent postabortal ascending infection. As noted below, bacterial vaginosis also has been associated with postabortal pelvic infection, and it is quite likely that in some populations gonococcal infection also contributes to this condition.

Current recommendations for diagnostic testing for chlamydial infection during pregnancy

The importance of detecting and treating chlamydial infection of the genital tract in pregnant women is certainly no less than in nonpregnant women. In fact, the unquestioned risk of intrapartum transmission to the neonate and the growing evidence that chlamydial infections cause complications of pregnancy and postpartum pelvic infection dictate that a very high priority be given to detecting and treating chlamydial infection in high-risk pregnant women. However, cell culture techniques currently available for isolation of *C. trachomatis* are highly tedious, labor-intensive, and expensive. Fortunately, the development of antigen and nucleic acid detection systems has substantially decreased the cost of identifying *C. trachomatis* infections and has made laboratory tests for *C. trachomatis* more widely available.

Although nonculture tests for *C. trachomatis* have been evaluated extensively in women, most studies have involved STD clinic populations or lower-prevalence populations of primarily nonpregnant women. Studies of pregnant women having prevalences

Table 80-10. Puerperal Infectious Morbidity in Patients with and without Antepartum *Chlamydia trachomatis* Infection, Matched for Demographic Characteristics and Parity

	C. trachomatis isolated ($n = 32$)		*C. trachomatis* not isolated ($n = 350$)		
Complication	Number	Percent	Number	Percent	*P*
Intrapartum fever >38°C	3	9	5	1	<0.025
Early postpartum fever <48 h	1	3	26	7	0.06
Late postpartum endometritis, 48 h to 6 weeks postpartum	7	22	18	5	<0.005
Total infectious morbidity	11	34	49	13	<0.01

SOURCE: Wager et al.[144]

of positive cultures ranging from 4.6 to 13.4 percent suggest that DNA probe assays and enzyme immunoassays have sensitivities of 67 percent or greater, but direct fluorescent antibody (DFA) testing was insensitive, possibly related to less adequate specimen collection from pregnant women.[202,236–239] Results from studies including both pregnant and nonpregnant women with culture-positive prevalences of 1.3 to 12.2 percent also indicate decreased sensitivity of DFA testing in pregnant women but reasonable sensitivity and specificity of DNA probe and enzyme immunoassays.[240–246] Ideally, if nonculture tests are used for screening in low-prevalence populations, they should be confirmed by culture, by a second nonculture test, or in the case of antigen-detection tests, by a blocking antibody test.[212] The potentially promising role of nucleic acid amplification tests for screening pregnant women is of considerable current interest.

As a minimum preventive intervention at present, we advocate selective diagnostic testing of pregnant women who are at high risk for chlamydial infection. Criteria for identifying women at high risk should be the same as for nonpregnant women, including screening of all pregnant women younger than 20 years of age, women 20 to 24 years of age with inconsistent use of barrier contraception or a new or more than one partner in the past 3 months, and women over 24 years of age with both these risk factors. Pregnant women should be screened at the first prenatal visit and again in the third trimester if at continued high risk of infection. Because of the increased number of white blood cells in the cervix in normal pregnant women, the diagnosis of mucopurulent cervicitis does not correlate well with the presence of *Chlamydia* in pregnancy and cannot be used as a screening tool.[247]

Treatment

Tetracyclines, the drugs of choice for *C. trachomatis* infection in nonpregnant adults, cannot be recommended for pregnant or nursing women. Erythromycin is considered the drug of choice in pregnant women. Acceptable options include erythromycin base, 250 mg four times daily for 14 days, erythromycin ethylsuccinate, 800 mg four times daily for 7 days or 400 mg four times daily for 14 days.[171] Erythromycin estolate is contraindicated in pregnant women because 10 percent of pregnant women receiving the drug developed elevated serum glutamate oxaloacetate transaminase activity.[248] Schachter et al.[249] reported that erythromycin ethylsuccinate, 400 mg four times a day for 7 days, given to pregnant women at approximately 36 weeks' gestation significantly reduced perinatal transmission of *C. trachomatis* from 50 percent among untreated mothers to 7 percent among treated mothers. Only 3 percent of pregnant mothers were intolerant of this regimen.

Because of frequent side effects, especially nausea and vomiting, with erythromycin therapy in pregnancy, several alternative treatments have been evaluated. Three randomized studies including a total of 395 pregnant women compared amoxicillin 500 mg three times daily to erythromycin 500 mg four times daily, each for 7 days.[250–252] In all studies, side effects were significantly more common among the erythromycin group, and cure rates were similar, suggesting that amoxicillin is a reasonable alternative therapy. Clindamycin 450 mg four times daily had a cure rate of 93 percent compared with a cure rate of 84 percent for erythromycin 333 mg four times daily, with significantly fewer side effects in the clindamycin group.[253] Retrospective reviews of azithromycin use in pregnancy indicate that it is well tolerated and at least as efficacious as erythromycin; randomized trials are in progress, but its use in pregnancy is not currently included in the indications for azithromycin.[254]

Prevention of neonatal *C. trachomatis* infections

Hammerschlag et al.[255] reported that erythromycin ocular ointment was significantly more effective than 1% silver nitrate in preventing neonatal chlamydial conjunctivitis. A later study found 0.5% erythromycin ointment to be of similar efficacy to 1% tetracycline ointment or 1% silver nitrate.[211] Others have been unimpressed with the use-effectiveness of topical erythromycin for this purpose in actual practice.[256] Laga et al.[210] compared 1% tetracycline ointment and 1% silver nitrate drops for the prevention of chlamydial ophthalmia. Both agents reduced the incidence of chlamydial conjunctivitis 68 to 77 percent in comparison with a historical control group of newborns who had not received ocular prophylaxis. Nonetheless, long-term follow-up of infants exposed to maternal chlamydial infection who received ocular prophylaxis revealed that 23 to 31 percent ultimately developed ocular *C. trachomatis* infection.[257] Most of these infections were subclinical. As with gonococcal infection, the detection and treatment of chlamydial infection during pregnancy, together with ocular prophylaxis, would be preferable to neonatal ophthalmic prophylaxis alone.

GENITAL MYCOPLASMAS

Many reproductive disorders have been ascribed to infection with the genital mycoplasmas, *U. urealyticum* and *M. hominis*. However, the ubiquity of these organisms and the high frequency of other coexistent risk factors for adverse pregnancy outcome and coinfection with other STD agents make it difficult to assess their etiologic roles in such disorders. Isolation of *M. hominis* is strongly associated with the presence of bacterial vaginosis, making it difficult to differentiate adverse effects related to *M. hominis* from the other bacteria found at increased levels in bacterial vaginosis. *M. hominis* has been linked to preterm birth, endometritis, and postpartum fever, while *U. urealyticum* has been associated with amniotic fluid infection, chorioamnionitis, low birth weight, and preterm birth.

Several studies have compared the rate of detection of genital mycoplasmas among women with spontaneous abortion compared with those with continuing pregnancies. The majority have shown no difference in recovery of either *U. urealyticum* or *M. hominis*,[223,258,259] with one study finding a lower rate of *U. urealyticum* recovery from women with spontaneous abortion.[139] All have been limited by the high frequency of *Mycoplasma* carriage, lack of testing for many other microorganisms, and poor characterization of other risk factors in the population. Harwick et al.[260] detected *M. hominis* bacteremia in 8 percent of women with febrile abortion versus none of those with afebrile abortion. Serologic evidence of infection with *M. hominis* was found in 50 percent of septic abortions versus 17 percent of afebrile abortions. These provocative data require confirmation, with studies of other relevant microbial species together with *M. hominis*. Several studies have found an increased frequency of isolation of genital mycoplasmas from spontaneous abortions than from induced first- and second-trimester abortions,[261,262] but it is unclear whether the infection was present before embryonic or fetal death or occurred as a consequence of nonviability of the pregnancy. In the most recent study, isolation of *U. ureaplasma* from products of conception did not correlate with the presence of histologic inflammation among specimens from spontaneous abortions.[263] Among women with recurrent miscarriage, the rate of isolation of genital *Mycoplasma* from the cervix was similar to the rate among control patients, but *Mycoplasma* were isolated from the endometrium more frequently among women with spontaneous abortion (28 percent) or infertility (50 percent) than among controls (7 percent).[264] Uncontrolled studies have suggested a benefit from treating women with recurrent abortion and genital *Mycoplasma* colonization with doxycycline or erythromycin, but controlled studies are lacking.[264,265] In summary, current data do not support a significant role for *M. hominis* or *U. urealyticum* in spontaneous first- or second-trimester abortion.

U. urealyticum and *M. hominis* must be considered individually when evaluating the potential role of genital mycoplasmas in prematurity. The isolation of *M. hominis* from the lower genital tract is strongly associated with the clinical or Gram stain diagnosis of bacterial vaginosis, making it difficult to assess the independent contribution of *M. hominis* to prematurity, if any.[266,267] Isolation of *U. urealyticum* from the lower genital tract during pregnancy is more common with young maternal age, black race, first pregnancies, low income, being unmarried or less educated, having more sexual partners, smoking, and use of marijuana or cocaine, all factors previously associated with an increased risk of preterm delivery.[268] Thus colonization with *U. urealyticum* may be a marker for other factors contributing to preterm birth. Studies of lower genital tract colonization and pregnancy outcome are summarized in Table 80-11.[139,226,258,268–277] Overall, the data do not suggest an increased risk of preterm delivery or low birth weight among women colonized in the lower genital tract with *U. urealyticum*, with prevalences ranging from 44 to 81 percent. Likewise, treatment studies using erythromycin in colonized women have not shown clear benefit in reducing prematurity. McCormack et al.[278] demonstrated higher birth weights among colonized women treated in the third trimester for at least 6 weeks with erythromycin compared with placebo but did not show benefit with second-trimester therapy.[278] In the large, multicenter NICHHD Collaborative Study of vaginal infections in pregnancy among 1,181 women with *U. urealyticum*, administration of erythromycin for up to 14 weeks during the third trimester had no effect on birth weight, gestational age at delivery, or neonatal outcome in comparison with women randomized to placebo.[279] The recovery rates of *U. urealyticum* at delivery were similar between the erythromycin- and placebo-treated groups, probably because erythromycin has minimal antimicrobial activity at the lower pH of the vagina. Reports of eradication of *U. ureaplasma* from the amniotic fluid with erythromycin suggest potential activity of erythromycin at that site,[280] although efficacy for treating chorioamnion infection has not been evaluated.

Table 80-11. Cohort Studies of *Ureaplasma urealyticum* in the Lower Genital Tract and Pregnancy Outcome

Author	UU+/total	%	Pregnancy outcome
Foy[258]	115/119	58	No difference
Braun[269]	388/485	80	Decrease BW in UU+
Harrison[270]	46/196	48	No difference
Ross[271]	71/162	44	Decreased preterm del in UU+
Harrison[139]	983/1365	72	No difference
Upadhyaya[272]	59/135	44	No difference
Minkoff[273]	151/233	65	More preterm labor, but not del in UU+
Berman[226]	942/1163	81	No difference
Carey[268]	3256/4934	66	No difference
McGregor[274]			No difference
McGregor[275]	112/176	64	No difference
Luton[276]	172/218	79	No difference
Choudhury[277]		40	No difference

NOTE: UU = *Ureaplasma urealyticum;* BW = birth weight; del = delivery.

Upper genital tract (amniotic fluid, chorioamnion) infection with several facultative or anaerobic bacteria has been strongly associated with preterm delivery and low birth weight, but isolation of *U. urealyticum* from the amniotic fluid is less clearly associated with preterm birth. In several studies of women in preterm labor with intact membranes, those with other bacteria in the amniotic fluid presented in preterm labor at 27 to 29 weeks' gestation and delivered within 1 day of admission. Women with negative amniotic fluid cultures presented with preterm labor at 31 to 32 weeks and delivered an average of 5 weeks after onset of preterm labor. Like those with negative cultures, women with *U. urealyticum* alone in the amniotic fluid also presented at 31 to 32 weeks' gestation, with an average interval to delivery of 4 to 5 weeks.[80,87] Chorioamnion infection with *U. urealyticum* has been found more commonly among women delivering preterm than among those delivering at term in case-control studies, but this has not been confirmed in cohort studies of prematurity. In fact, the presence of other bacteria in the chorioamnion was more consistently related to prematurity, as in the studies employing amniotic fluid cultures. However, isolation of *U. urealyticum* from the chorioamnion has been consistently associated with histologic chorioamnionitis in all studies.[43,44,47] These data suggest that *U. urealyticum* may induce a form of chorioamnionitis that is perhaps indolent and does not frequently lead to preterm delivery.

Whether or not *U. urealyticum* in the upper genital tract is a factor causing preterm delivery or a secondary finding, *U. urealyticum* has been implicated as a cause of congenital and neonatal pneumonia, especially in preterm infants.[281] In addition, *U. ureaplasma* infection among infants weighing less than 1,250 gm at birth appears to increase the risk of chronic lung disease by two- to threefold, possibly through an indolent, undiagnosed pneumonia.[281] Thus far, *M. hominis* has not been implicated as a cause of neonatal pneumonia or chronic lung disease.

Data link *M. hominis* to postpartum fever. Platt et al.,[138] in their follow-up study of 535 patients, found that 14 (50 percent) of 28 postpartum fevers were associated with rises in titers of antibody to *M. hominis*. Positive genital colonization and low predelivery antibody titer to *M. hominis* were predictive of postpartum fever. Harrison et al.[139] also reported a significantly increased risk of postpartum fever among women with antepartum *M. hominis* colonization who were delivered vaginally. However, given the strong association between vaginal *M. hominis* isolation and bacterial vaginosis, increased relative risk of postpartum endometritis with bacterial vaginosis,[142] and the almost uniform isolation of other microorganisms with *M. hominis* from the endometrium,[141] it is unclear which microorganisms are most important in the infection. Only a small proportion of colonized women developed this complication.

Current recommendations for management of genital *Mycoplasma* infection during pregnancy

Colonization of the lower genital tract with genital mycoplasmas does not appear to increase the risk of spontaneous abortion, preterm delivery, or preterm rupture of the membranes, and routine screening of pregnant women for these microorganisms is therefore not recommended. The presence of *U. urealyticum* in the upper genital tract is clearly related to histologic chorioamnionitis but not necessarily to preterm birth. Isolation of *U. urealyticum* alone from the amniotic fluid is not an indication for delivery, but treatment with erythromycin could be considered. Further study of the impact of Ureaplasma-induced inflammation on prematurity (chorioamnionitis) and chronic lung disease (pneumonitis) in preterm infants is required before routine treatment is recommended. Inclusion of antimicrobials with activity against genital mycoplasmas does not appear to be required in the antimicrobicidal treatment of women with postpartum endometritis but should be considered for women with recalcitrant infections or for those in whom other bacteria cannot be isolated.

BACTERIAL VAGINOSIS

Bacterial vaginosis (BV), formerly known as *nonspecific vaginitis* or *Gardnerella vaginitis,* is characterized by a nonpurulent, homogeneous, malodorous vaginal discharge, by an increase in vaginal pH, by the presence of characteristic amines and organic acids in vaginal fluid, and by changes in vaginal flora with a decrease in H_2O_2–producing facultative *Lactobacillus* and an increase in frequency and concentration of *Gardnerella vaginalis, M. hominis,* and several anaerobic species[282] (see Chaps. 14 and 42).

The prevalence and natural history of BV are similar in pregnant and nonpregnant women.[266,282,284] BV is detected in 12 to 23 percent of pregnant women depending on the population studied and the method of diagnosis.[266,282,284] Factors associated with an increased risk of BV among pregnant women have included black race, being unmarried, and not having used antibiotics recently.[284]

BV and pregnancy complications

A growing body of evidence links BV with an increased risk for pregnancy complications, including postabortal infections, preterm labor and delivery, preterm rupture of the membranes, fever during labor, and postpartum endometritis (see Chap. 42). In studies from Sweden, the risk of *postabortal infection* was found to be elevated among women with clue cells in the vagina,[285] and the elevated risk of infection was reduced among women with BV by treatment with metronidazole before and after the procedure.[34]

Among women with *clinically diagnosed intraamniotic infection* during labor, *G. vaginalis, M. hominis, P. bivia* (formerly *B. bivius*), and peptostreptococci were frequent isolates and frequently were isolated together.[286] Women with BV were significantly more likely to develop clinical manifestations of intraamniotic infection than those with normal vaginal flora on Gram stain.[142,286] In addition, detection of BV by Gram stain at delivery has been associated with an odds ratio of 5.8 for the development of postcesarean endometritis.[142] Microorganisms associated with BV are isolated in over 60 percent of women with *postcesarean endometritis*,[141] and these same bacteria have been associated with increased rates of *wound infection after cesarean section*.[287] BV clearly increases the risk of maternal morbidity during pregnancy.

Of even greater significance is the association of BV with *preterm labor, preterm rupture of the membranes,* and *preterm delivery.* Table 80-12 summarizes studies evaluating BV as a risk factor for preterm pregnancy complications.[225,228,266,288–294] BV consistently has been identified as a risk factor for preterm delivery, with odds ratios of 1.4 to 6.9. When preterm premature rupture of the membranes has been assessed, this also was increased by a factor of 2.1 to 7.3. The potential role of BV in initiating or continuing preterm labor leading to delivery is further indicated by the frequent detection of BV-associated bacteria in the amniotic fluid of women with preterm labor and intact membranes,[80,87] by isolation of BV-associated bacteria from the chorioamniotic membranes more commonly from women delivering preterm than from those delivering at term,[41] and by the association of such bacteria with histologic inflammation. Most important, systemic therapy for BV has decreased the rate of preterm birth in several studies[290,291,295–297] (Table 80-13). The lack of efficacy of topical clindamycin therapy in preventing BV-associated prematurity[290,296] may be related to a lack of effect on established, indolent upper tract infection or to effects related to vaginal overgrowth by *E. coli* and enterococcus.[267] Further studies comparing intravaginal metronidazole with systemic metronidazole are needed to answer this question.

G. vaginalis infrequently has caused *neonatal bacteremia, cutaneous abscess,* and *congenital pneumonia*.[298] Anaerobes, however, may be relatively important in *neonatal sepsis.* Neonatal anaerobic sepsis is often associated with prematurity, amniotic fluid

Table 80-12. Association of Bacterial Vaginosis with Preterm Labor (PTL), Preterm Delivery (PTD), and Preterm Rupture of the Membranes (PROM)

Author, year	Study design	GA at test	Reason for test	Method of diagnosis	Outcome odds ratio (95% CI)	Location
Kurki[288] 1992	Cohort $n = 790$	8–17	Screen	Culture	PTL 2.6 (1.3–4.9) PTD 6.9 (2.5–18.8) PROM 7.3 (1.8–29.4)	Sweden
Riduan[289] 1993	Cohort $n = 490$	16–20	Screen	Gram stain	PTD 2.0 (1.0–3.9)	Indoneisa
Hay[266] 1994	Cohort $n = 783$	9–24	Screen	Gram stain	PTD 2.8 (1.1–7.4) del 16–37 wks 5.5 (2.3–13.3)	U.K.
McGregor[290] 1994	Cohort $n = 271$	16–27	Screen	Gram stain	PTB 3.3 (1.2–9.1) PROM 5.7 (0.9–36.1)	Denver, CO
McGregor[291] 1995	Cohort $n = 559$	1st visit	Screen	Gram stain	PTD 1.9 (1.2–3.0) PROM 3.5 (1.4–8.9)	Denver, CO
Hillier[292] 1995	Cohort $n = 10397$	23–26	Screen	pH + GS	PTD of LBW 1.4 (1.1–1.8)	Multicenter U.S.A.
McGregor[293] 1990	Cohort $n = 202$	24	Screen	Gram stain	PTL 2.6 (1.1–6.5) PTD 1.5 (0.2–14.2)	Denver, CO
Gravett[225] 1986	Cohort $n = 534$	13–42	L & D	GLC	PML 2.1 (1.4–3.8) PROM 2.1 (1.4–4.2)	Seattle, WA
Martius[228] 1988	Case-control $n = 231$	20–42	L & D	Gram stain	PTD 2.3 ($p = 0.03$)	Seattle, WA
Holst[294] 1994	Case-control $n = 87$	23–42	L & D	Clue cells + Gram stain	PTD 2.1 (1.2–3.7)	Sweden

NOTE: GA = gestational age; CI = confidence interval; GS = Gram stain; L & D = admission to labor and delivery; GLC = gas liquid chromatography.

Table 80-13. Treatment of Bacterial Vaginosis in Pregnancy and Outcome

Author, year	GA at Rx	Rx	Method of diagnosis	Treatment efficacy	Preterm birth rate		
					Drug	Placebo	p
Morales[295] 1994	13–20	Oral metro 250 mg tid × 7 days	Clinical	89%	8/44 (18%)	16/36 (39%)	<0.05
McGregor[290] 1994	16–27	2% clindamycin vaginal cream	Gram stain	90%	9/60 (15%)	5/69 (7.2%)	0.26
McGregor[291] 1995	<22	Oral clindamycin 300 mg bid × 7 days	Gram stain	—	19/194 (10%)	31/165 (19%)*	0.02
Joesoef[296] 1995	14–26	2% clindamycin vaginal cream	Gram stain +pH > 4.5	86%	51/340 (15%)	46/341 (13.5%)	0.65
Hauth[297] 1995	22–24	Metro 250 mg tid × 7 days + Erythro base 333 mg tid × 14 days	3 of 4 clinical signs	86%	54/172 (31%)	42/86 (49%)	0.006

NOTE: GA = gestational age; Rx = treatment; Metro = metronidazole; tid = three times/day; bid = twice daily; Erythro = erythromycin.

* Patients were not randomized. Patients with bacterial vaginosis were not treated for the first 7 months of the study unless symptomatic; all patients with BV in the second 8-month phase of the study were offered treatment.

infection, and prolonged ineffective labor. Chow et al.[299] found that 26 percent of all cases of neonatal bacteremia observed at their institution were associated with anaerobes, with 1.8 episodes of anaerobic bacteremia per 1,000 live births. Anaerobic isolates were identified predominantly as species belonging to *Bacteroides, Peptococcus,* and *Peptostreptococcus.* The anaerobic flora associated with BV may provide a large inoculum and thus increased risk of anaerobic sepsis in the neonate.

Case detection and treatment

The sensitivity and specificity of methods available for the diagnosis of BV (see Chap. 42) do not seem to be altered by pregnancy. The two most practical methods for clinical use in pregnancy are the clinical criteria and vaginal Gram stain. BV is diagnosed clinically when at least three of the following criteria are present: (1) vaginal pH above 4.5, (2) thin, homogeneous white or gray vaginal discharge, (3) clue cells present on saline preparation of vaginal discharge, and (4) presence of fishy amine odor with addition of 10% potassium hydroxide to vaginal fluid. Diagnosis of BV by vaginal Gram stain is based on an absence or decrease of *Lactobacillus* morphotypes and an increase in small gram-variable or gram-negative rods (*G. vaginalis* and *Bacteroides* morphotypes) with or without the presence of curved gram-variable rods (*Mobiluncus* morphotypes).[300] Gram stain diagnosis may be especially helpful in the presence of bleeding or ruptured amniotic membranes when the pH and other clinical signs may be altered. Pregnant women with symptomatic vaginal discharge should undergo pelvic examination, pH testing, vaginal wet mount or Gram stain examination, and if indicated, testing for other STDs. Current data suggest that pregnant women with a previous preterm delivery after preterm labor or rupture of the membranes should be screened routinely and offered treatment for BV if it is present. Since the largest study thus far that showed a reduction in preterm birth included a combination of oral metronidazole and erythromycin therapy, it remains unclear whether treatment with metronidazole alone will prevent preterm birth in high-risk women with BV. Currently, the potential benefit in reducing preterm birth of screening low-risk pregnant women and treating those with BV remains unproven. A multicenter trial is in progress in the NICHHD-funded Maternal-Fetal Medicine Network to assess the value of routine screening and treatment for BV and *T. vaginalis* infection. If BV is diagnosed during pregnancy, women should be offered treatment with oral metronidazole, 250 mg three times daily for 7 days, or oral clindamycin, 300 mg twice daily for 7 days. Although topical therapy with intravaginal clindamycin or metronidazole has been found effective in eliminating BV[267,301] and would have seemed preferable to systemic therapy, these formulations have not been shown to reduce the preterm birth rate among women with BV, as the oral agents have. Routine treatment of sexual partners has not been shown to reduce rates of recurrent BV.

TRICHOMONAS VAGINALIS VAGINITIS

The prevalence of *T. vaginalis* infection in pregnancy has ranged from 3 to 48 percent depending on the population studied. Among 13,816 pregnant U.S. women studied between 23 and 26 weeks' gestation at six urban centers in the Vaginal Infections and Prematurity Study (VIP Study) during the late 1980s, the culture-positive rate was 12.6 percent.[302] Factors associated with having *T. vaginalis* in this study were black race, cigarette smoking, single marital status, less education, a history of gonorrhea, greater number of lifetime sexual partners, and lack of barrier or hormonal contraception in the 6 months before pregnancy. Many of these factors have been noted in other studies and are also associated with an increased risk of preterm delivery. Thus sociodemographic factors and coexisting infections also must be taken into account when assessing a possible role of *T. vaginalis* in preterm birth.

T. vaginalis has been associated with an increased risk of preterm delivery,[291,303–305] preterm rupture of the membranes,[273,306] and maternal puerperal morbidity.[307] The largest cohort study to evaluate lower genital tract infections and preterm birth, the VIP Study discussed above, has noted a 1.3-fold increased risk of preterm birth with *T. vaginalis* detected by culture at 23 to 26 weeks of pregnancy, even after adjustment for demographic, behavioral, and other infectious factors associated with preterm birth.[305] In this large study, while the attributable risk for low birth weight related to *T. vaginalis* infection was only 1.5 to 1.6 percent in white and Hispanic women, *T. vaginalis* accounted for 11 percent of low-birth-weight babies in black women. The potential role of *T. vaginalis* in preterm birth is further supported by in vitro studies showing that clinical *T. vaginalis* isolates and cell-free filtrates decrease the elasticity, the work to rupture, and the bursting tension of chorioamniotic membranes in an inoculum-dependent fashion.[308] This effect may be due to the organism itself, the proteases produced, the host inflammatory response, or a combination effect.

In 1931, Bland et al.[307] reported postpartum fever in 48 percent of 92 women with untreated antenatal trichomoniasis, compared with 25 percent of 110 women without trichomoniasis ($p = 0.001$). The difference was independent of race. Possible confounding by other STDs and bacterial vaginosis and by several other risk factors was not addressed, and the results were not subsequently confirmed by Trussell et al.,[309] who noted postpartum fever in 8.5 percent of 223 women with trichomoniasis compared with 8.3 percent of 657 women without trichomoniasis. It remains uncertain whether *T. vaginalis* might produce intra- or postpartum pelvic infections either on their own or through associated increases in anaerobic vaginal flora.

Neonatal infection with *T. vaginalis* is detected infrequently and causes little morbidity. Because of estrogenic influence during pregnancy, the vaginal mucosa of female neonates is susceptible to infection or colonization with *T. vaginalis*. This is reversed spontaneously within 3 to 4 weeks after delivery. The risk of neonatal infection with *T. vaginalis* overall is less than 1 percent and among exposed neonates is approximately 5 percent. Purulent vaginitis and urinary tract infection have been described as neonatal manifestations of infection.[310] Recently, *T. vaginalis* has been suspected as a cause of some cases of neonatal pneumonia.

Case detection

Whether totally asymptomatic pregnant women should undergo screening for *T. vaginalis* is unsettled. Vaginal culture is more sensitive than direct microscopy of vaginal secretions, but *T. vaginalis* can be detected by microscopy in most women with symptomatic disease.[311,312] Inoculation of vaginal secretions into commercial culture systems will detect the 25 to 50 percent of vaginal trichomonal infections that are asymptomatic (see Chap. 43). Vaginal fluid should be examined microscopically at any antenatal visit on all women with symptoms or signs of vaginitis; and in view of the association of *T. vaginalis* infections with preterm birth, screening of all pregnant women who are considered at increased risk for preterm birth or for *T. vaginalis* infection should be considered, using either wet-mount examination, culture, or DNA probe examination. Trichomonal infections suspected on Papanicolaou smears of the cervix should be confirmed by wet-mount examination or culture before treatment during pregnancy.

Treatment

Nitroimidazoles are mutagens of bacteria and carcinogenic in some animals.[313] Studies that have examined the frequency of congenital defects in infants born to mothers treated during pregnancy with metronidazole have not shown evidence of teratogenicity, although the numbers of patients examined preclude the exclusion of a small fetal risk.[314] Metronidazole is probably safe in pregnancy or the postpartum period, but as with any medication, treatment in early pregnancy should be deferred unless absolutely indicated. Because of the association of *T. vaginalis* with preterm birth and puerperal morbidity, treatment should be offered after the first trimester to women with documented infections. Clotrimazole, used intravaginally, has reportedly relieved symptoms in some women with *T. vaginalis* vaginitis and thus represents an alternative treatment. Other alternative treatments are discussed in more detail in Chap. 43.

CYTOMEGALOVIRUS INFECTION

Cytomegalovirus (CMV) is the most common cause of congenital viral infection of the fetus and is the most common infectious cause of mental retardation. The role of sexual transmission in the epidemiology of CMV is discussed in Chap. 22, and pediatric CMV infections are discussed in Chap. 85.

Epidemiology of CMV infection during pregnancy

Several studies have shown increasing rates of isolation of CMV from pregnant women with advancing gestation. Women with the highest prevalence of CMV infection may tend to seek care only later in pregnancy. Stagno et al.[315] isolated CMV from nonpregnant women at the same rate as from demographically similar pregnant women studied in the third trimester and suggested that lower rates of recovery in early pregnancy are actually due to suppression of CMV shedding in early pregnancy rather than to increased shedding in late pregnancy. Epidermal growth factor, which interferes with the tissue culture isolation of CMV, is present in urine during early pregnancy and may artificially suppress recovery of CMV early in pregnancy.[316]

Reynolds et al.[317] found that young primiparous women are the most likely to be cervical shedders of CMV. In one study, 17 percent of women 14 years of age or younger were culture-positive for CMV, compared with 0 percent of women 30 years of age or older.[315] Most women from whom CMV is isolated during pregnancy have chronic or recurrent infection rather than primary infection. Depending on the serologic technique employed and the population studied, up to 90 percent of pregnant women have had serum antibody to CMV. Stagno et al.[318,319] found that 36 percent of pregnant women in a middle- to high-income group and 77 percent of women in a low-income group were seropositive.

Among women who are seronegative at the beginning of pregnancy, primary infection occurs relatively frequently. In three studies, from 0.6 to 4.3 percent of seronegative women developed primary infection during pregnancy.[320–322] Currently, primary CMV infection is undoubtedly many times more common than primary rubella infection during pregnancy.

Fetal, neonatal, and infant infections with CMV all occur frequently. Congenital infection, as detected by isolation of CMV within the first week of life, occurred in 0.4 to 2.0 percent of liveborn infants studied in Western countries.[323,324] Prevalence rates of CMV shedding increase during the first few months of life and peak between 3 and 9 months of age at rates ranging from 5.8 to 56 percent of all infants. Some areas of the world have high rates despite relatively advanced economic development. Starr[325] studied epidemiologic characteristics of mothers whose neonates developed congenital infection. The mean maternal age of 19.0 ± 4.1 years was significantly younger than that of the general population of pregnant women (22.9 ± 5.9 years, $p < 0.01$), and the frequency of primiparity (62 percent) was significantly greater than that of the general population (31 percent, $p < 0.01$). These data are also consistent with the concept that primary CMV infection during pregnancy was most likely to lead to congenital CMV infection. Stagno et al.[318] found in a prospective study that congenital CMV infections were attributable to primary maternal CMV infection in about half the cases among high-income patients but were usually attributable to recurrent maternal infection among low-income patients (Fig. 80-7). Importantly, primary maternal infections were significantly more likely than recurrent maternal infection to result in clinically apparent congenital CMV infection during the neonatal period when infection occurred within the first half of gestation.

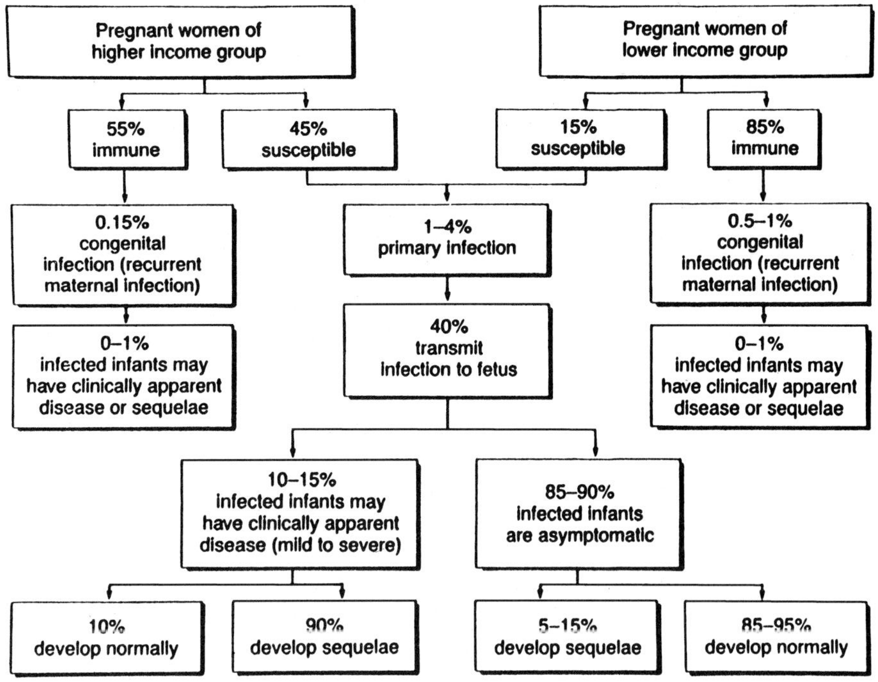

Fig. 80-7. Reactive frequency and consequences of cytomegalovirus infection in pregnancy. *(From Stagno S, Whitley RJ: Herpes virus infections of pregnancy: 1. Cytomegalovirus and Epstein-Barr virus infections. N Engl J Med 313:1271, 1985.)*

Manifestations in pregnant women and in the neonate

In the majority of pregnant women who develop primary CMV infection, no recognized clinical illness is discerned. Starr[325] could find no difference in the frequency or type of antenatal illness between 32 women who gave birth to congenitally infected infants and matched controls. All but 1 of 14 primary CMV infections observed by Griffiths et al.[322] in pregnant women were asymptomatic. Heterophile-negative mononucleosis occasionally is recognized in a mother undergoing a primary infection, and Bell's palsy accompanying primary CMV infection has been described during pregnancy.[326] A fetal ultrasound abnormality such as hydrocephalus,[327] intracerebral or hepatic calcifications,[328,329] or hyperechoic bowel[330] may be the first manifestation of primary CMV infection in the mother and fetus.

Women with recurrent (nonprimary) CMV infections almost always have no recognizable clinical abnormality. Cervicitis has not been clearly linked to cervical CMV shedding, but Paavonen et al.[331] described a striking association between isolation of CMV from the cervix and the presence of colposcopically visualized immature metaplasia involving the zone of cervical ectopy (odds ratio for the association 14.4, after adjustment for coinfections) among women attending an STD clinic. Thus the presence of immature metaplasia could be examined as a risk factor for perinatal transmission of CMV. Women shedding CMV from the genital tract often have simultaneous shedding in the urine and milk.[315] CMV has been isolated from placental tissue and infected placentas may show chronic villitis with mononuclear or plasma cell infiltrates. Typical cytoplasmic inclusion bodies are not always seen.[332] Amniotic fluid infection syndrome, histologic chorioamnionitis, and spontaneous abortion have not been recognized as manifestations of primary or recurrent maternal CMV infection, although CMV may be isolated frequently from the amniotic fluid of women with primary infections during pregnancy.[333]

Congenital infection is most common and most often associated with early clinical manifestations among neonates born to nonimmune mothers who developed primary CMV infection during pregnancy (see Fig. 80-7). In the largest study of congenitally infected infants born to mothers of known infection status in pregnancy, 24 (18 percent) of 125 infected infants born to mothers with primary infection were symptomatic at birth.[334] Findings among the symptomatic infants are summarized in Table 80-14. Ninety percent of infants with symptomatic CMV infection at birth will die or have serious sequelae, including microcephaly, mental retardation, developmental delay, seizures, sensorineural hearing loss, and ocular abnormalities.[334,335]

Congenital infection is less common and much less often clinically apparent among neonates born to mothers with preexisting CMV infection. Stagno et al.[336] noted that 7 (3.4 percent) of 208 seropositive women delivered congenitally infected neonates. None of these neonates had apparent clinical involvement. Nonetheless, given the high prevalence of seropositivity throughout the world, Stagno et al. suggested that recurrent rather than primary

Table 80-14. Sequelae in Children with Congenital CMV Infection According to Type of Maternal Infection

Sequela	Primary	Recurrent	*p* Value
Sensorineural hearing loss	(18/120) 15%	(3/56) 5%	0.05
Bilateral hearing loss	(10/120) 8%	(0/56) 0%	0.02
Speech threshold ≥ 60 dB*	(9/120) 8%	(0/56) 0%	0.03
IQ ≤ 70	(9/68) 13%	(0/32) 0%	0.03
Chorioretinitis†	(7/123) 6%	(1/54) 2%	0.20
Other neurologic sequelae‡	(8/125) 6%	(1/64) 2%	0.13
Microcephaly	(6/125) 5%	(1/64) 2%	0.25
Seizures	(6/125) 5%	(0/64) 0%	0.08
Paresis or paralysis	(1/125) 1%	(0/64) 0%	0.66
Any sequela	(31/125) 25%	(5/64) 8%	0.003

* For the ear with better hearing.

† Three of the seven children with chorioretinitis (43 percent) in the primary-infection group had visual impairment.

‡ Four of the eight children (50 percent) had more than one abnormality.

SOURCE: From Fowler et al.[334]

infection during pregnancy may be the leading cause of intrauterine CMV infection. Stern et al.[321,337] concluded that cellular immunity may play a role in preventing intrauterine transmission of CMV. In their small study of women with primary CMV infection, they found that the 8 women with positive lymphocyte transformation (LT) responses had unaffected infants in contrast with 4 congenitally infected infants born to the 6 women who had negative (LT) responses.

Transplacental infection producing cytomegalic placentitis is well recognized and likely occurs during viremia associated with primary infection of the pregnant woman. When congenital CMV infection complicates nonprimary CMV infection during pregnancy, either transplacental or transcervical spread is possible.

Intrapartum CMV infection and infection during infancy and childhood occur much more frequently than does congenital infection. By the end of the first year of life, 5 to 50 percent of infants have been infected. Intrapartum infection can result from exposure to maternal cervical CMV infection, while postpartum maternal-infant transmission can result from ingestion of infected maternal breast milk.[323] No short- or long-term ill-effects are known to result from intrapartum or early postpartum CMV infection, but further study is necessary.

Case detection and management

Although the incidence and clinical severity of congenital CMV infection are high following primary CMV infection during pregnancy, no recommendations currently exist for early identification of seronegative pregnant women who are at risk for primary infections. Women who develop a mononucleosis like illness during pregnancy probably should have serologic studies performed to exclude primary CMV, although most primary CMV infections in pregnancy are asymptomatic. Women at highest risk for seroconversion, e.g., women working in day-care centers with children under age 3,[338] may benefit from preconceptional testing, with follow-up testing in pregnancy if seronegative. In addition, women with abnormal findings on fetal ultrasound that may be related to congenital CMV infection (intracerebral or intrahepatic calcifications, hyperechoic bowel, hydrops, hydrocephaly, severe symmetric growth retardation) should have serologic testing. Often serum from serologic testing earlier in pregnancy for rubella, syphilis, or HIV may be available for testing to document seroconversion or preexisting immunity early in pregnancy. If earlier specimens are not available, then maternal primary infection can be documented by the presence of IgM by radioimmunoassay or enzyme-linked immunoassay. IgM antibody may be present for up to 4 months after primary infection and rarely with reactivation.[339] If maternal primary infection is confirmed, amniocentesis or fetal umbilical blood sampling may be helpful in determining the fetal infection status.[333,340–344] Amniotic fluid culture and polymerase chain reaction (PCR) testing appear to have a high specificity and a sensitivity of over 80 percent for the diagnosis of fetal infection status when performed after 20 weeks' gestation or at least 6 weeks after maternal infection. However, the presence of a positive culture in amniotic fluid does not predict the severity of infection in the fetus. In the presence of an abnormal ultrasound, a positive CMV culture suggests severe infection. Among women tested because of seroconversion, fetal umbilical blood sampling to evaluate for abnormal transaminase levels or thrombocytopenia may be helpful to detect severely affected infants, but these abnormalities may be transient. The patient needs to understand that normal ultrasound and fetal blood studies in the presence of a positive amniotic fluid culture do not rule out significant fetal damage. Although the risk to the fetus with recurrent CMV infection in pregnancy appears minimal, exceptions include immunosuppressed women, such as those with AIDS or after solid organ transplant, who may have symptomatic infant infection after reactivation of CMV.[345,346] Gancyclovir is showing promise as an effective drug for CMV infections in AIDS patients and may be useful for primary CMV infection in early pregnancy or in infants with symptomatic CMV infection. Further studies are needed to determine its safety and efficacy in pregnancy and in the newborn period before its use can be recommended.

Congenitally or perinatally infected infants often shed large amounts of the virus in saliva, respiratory secretions, and urine. Pregnant women should not be exposed to infants recognized to be shedding CMV. Ultimate prevention of severe congenital CMV infection will not occur until a safe and effective vaccine becomes available. Although several vaccines are in development, their potential for protection against congenital infection has not been evaluated. Ideally, pregnant women should avoid contact with toddler urine and saliva, because toddlers, especially those in day care, have a high rate of infection and shed high levels of virus. If pregnant women or fetuses require blood transfusion, CMV-negative blood should be used.

HERPES SIMPLEX VIRUS INFECTION

Herpes simplex virus (HSV) infection in pregnancy is of concern for two reasons: (1) primary HSV infection during pregnancy has been associated with spontaneous abortion and prematurity, and (2) maternal HSV shedding at delivery is associated with life-threatening neonatal infection. Congenital infections are unusual.

Epidemiology

The increase in incidence of genital HSV infection has been accompanied by an increase in neonatal HSV infection in some areas. The U.S. National Disease and Therapeutic Index Survey[347] showed more than a 10-fold increase in patient visits to physicians' offices for newly diagnosed infections from 1966 to 1995. In King County, Washington, the frequency of neonatal herpes rose from 2.6 to 11.9 cases per 100,000 live births between 1966 and 1981.[348] The point prevalence of HSV infection determined either cytologically or by culture among asymptomatic women seeking antenatal care is 0.5 to 1 percent. Antibody to HSV-2, which causes about 90 percent of cases of genital herpes, has been measured in the U.S. National Health and Nutrition Examination Survey (NHANES) of a random sample of U.S. adults. The prevalence of antibody to HSV-2 increased by 30 percent from the period 1976–1980 to the period 1988–1994[349,350] (see Chap. 21). Women were more likely than men to be HSV-2-seropositive, and African American women were more likely than Caucasian women to be HSV-seropositive. Among pregnant U.S. women, HSV-2-seroprevalence has ranged from 16.5 to 32 percent, with the majority being unaware of their genital herpes infection.[351,352] Interestingly, detailed questioning regarding signs and symptoms and past history of genital herpes did not increase the probability of seropositivity women.[353] In a U.S. study of neonatal herpes simplex virus infections, mothers of neonates acquiring HSV were most often young (mean age 21.2 years), white (63 percent), and primiparous (73 percent).[354]

Natural history and manifestations of genital HSV infection during pregnancy

Primary genital infection with HSV in women may be characterized by clinical illness averaging about 3 weeks in duration, with high concentrations of virus shed from vulvar and cervical lesions, inguinal adenopathy, and frequent systemic manifestations suggesting viremia. However, only about 25 percent of women with HSV-2 antibody are aware that they have had genital herpes, suggesting that most primary episodes must be asymptomatic or only produce mild or unrecognized symptoms. Further difficulty in recognizing primary infection in pregnancy was illustrated by a study of acyclovir for primary HSV in pregnancy. This study was terminated when it was found that of the 23 women enrolled with first clinical episodes of HSV, with symptoms suggestive of primary HSV (bilateral lesions, malaise, myalgia, or headache), only 1 (4 percent) was truly primary (seronegative for antibody to HSV-1 and HSV-2), while 3 (12 percent) had nonprimary first episodes (seropositive for antibody to HSV-1 at presentation) and 19 (84 percent) were recurrent (already seropositive at presentation).[355] Type-specific antibody testing, although not commercially available, is needed for women with their first clinical episode of genital HSV in pregnancy to identify those with true primary or initial infections. Among the 70 to 85 percent of women who are seronegative to HSV-2 or HSV-1 early in pregnancy, 0.25 to 1.3 percent will seroconvert by delivery.[351,356] In the largest study, 94 (1.3 percent) of 8,508 women seroconverted to HSV during pregnancy. Among women who were HSV-seronegative, HSV-1-seropositive, or HSV-2-seropositive at the first prenatal visit, adjusted rates of seroconversion were 3.4, 1, and 0 percent, respectively.[356] The rate of development of a primary genital HSV infection adjusted for the entire length of pregnancy (HSV-1 or HSV-2) was 1.8 percent.

Primary genital HSV infection in pregnancy has more potential for an adverse impact than nonprimary first-episode infection or recurrent infection, underscoring the benefit of serologic confirmation of the status of women with a first symptomatic episode of genital HSV in pregnancy. Transplacental infection with HSV during initial viremia appears to be rare, since congenital infection is diagnosed infrequently: Only 8 (4 percent) of 210 neonates with HSV infection enrolled in an antiviral trial were diagnosed as having congenital rather than neonatal infection.[357] Symptomatic primary genital HSV infection in pregnancy has been associated with a significant increase in spontaneous abortion, preterm labor, and low birth weight. Nahmias et al.[358] reported a spontaneous abortion rate of 54 percent among women with primary infection before 20 weeks' gestation. In that study, among women with symptomatic primary infection after 20 weeks' gestation, 35 percent of the infants had a birth weight below 2,500 gm and 50 percent developed neonatal herpes. In another study, among 15 episodes of primary HSV during pregnancy, 6 (40 percent) were associated with severe perinatal morbidity (preterm birth, growth retardation, or neonatal HSV infection).[359] Poor outcomes were observed among 4 (80 percent) of the 5 women with primary infection in the third trimester. Among the 14 women with nonprimary, first-episode disease in pregnancy, no cases of preterm delivery, growth retardation, or neonatal HSV occurred.[359] The lack of increase in preterm birth or fetal growth retardation among women with recurrent genital HSV has been confirmed recently in a larger study.[360] Among women with asymptomatic seroconversion in pregnancy, whether with or without preexisting antibody to the heterologous HSV type, the principal risk appears to be for preterm labor and increased risk of neonatal infection among those women without homologous antibody to the genital strain at delivery, e.g., with recent acquisition. Women with recent acquisition of HSV are also more likely to be shedding HSV, are more likely to shed both from the cervix and the vulva, and more likely to shed asymptomatically.[361] Asymptomatic cervical shedding of HSV-2 was detected by culture at 10.6 percent of visits among women with symptomatic primary genital HSV infection earlier in pregnancy and in 0.5 percent with nonprimary, first-episode disease earlier during the pregnancy.[359]

Data regarding the effects of pregnancy on recurrences of genital herpes are conflicting. Vontver et al.[362] followed with serial cultures 80 pregnant women with a history of recurrent genital HSV. Fifty-six (70 percent) had at least one positive culture during pregnancy. The proportion with positive cultures did not change with advancing gestation. A subsequent study of 147 women with a history of recurrent genital herpes detected an increase in the number of recurrences from a mean of 0.97 in the first trimester to a mean of 1.63 in the third trimester.[361] A recent study using daily home collection of vulvovaginal specimens for cultures and PCR testing among a small group of women in the third trimester of pregnancy with a history of recurrent genital herpes antedating pregnancy did not show a change in the rate of symptomatic recurrences, asymptomatic shedding, or PCR-positivity with advancing gestation.[363] Cultures were positive on 3.4 percent of days, and HSV was detected by PCR on 16.8 percent of days.

Taken together, the data suggest that women with symptomatic primary genital HSV infection in pregnancy are at increased risk for spontaneous abortion and preterm labor. This risk of preterm labor appears to be increased among women with asymptomatic seroconversion late in pregnancy as well. Both groups have increased risk of transmitting infection to the neonate, as described below.

Risk of neonatal transmission

Most neonatal herpes simplex viral infection is presumed attributable to intrapartum exposure to HSV-2 in the birth canal; up to 86 percent of HSV isolates from neonates are type 2. Few neonates are affected at birth, and most develop signs of infection in the second week of life. Up to one-half of neonates acquiring HSV infection have been exposed to mothers with primary infection occurring late in pregnancy. Whitley et al.[354] observed that 41 percent of neonates with HSV infection weighed less than 2,500 gm at birth and that 51 percent lacked antibody to HSV in the initial serum sample. Primary genital infection with HSV is likely the major risk factor for neonatal acquisition of HSV for several reasons. The association with prematurity makes delivery during the primary infection likely, at a time when the inoculum of virus present in the birth canal is large, cervical involvement is extensive, maternal viremia may occur, maternal antibody is absent, and the infant may be immunologically immature. Neonates born to mothers with recurrent HSV-2 infection appear to acquire protective immunity from the mother and are at low risk of acquiring HSV infection, particularly invasive disease.[364] Asymptomatic maternal genital HSV infection seems to be common among mothers of infants with perinatal HSV infection. Whitley et al.[354] observed that 70 percent of mothers with HSV-infected neonates had no signs or symptoms of HSV infection during pregnancy. Only 38 percent of these mothers had a history of genital herpes or had sexual partners with a history of genital lesions. This finding is probably related to both the higher risk of transmission with primary infection (which may not be apparent until after delivery) and to the frequency of asymptomatic primary infection, as demonstrated by the infrequent history of genital HSV among seropositive women.

As mentioned, the risk of neonatal HSV infection is much greater after first-episode infection than after reactivation during pregnancy. In five studies of infants born to women with first-episode genital infections at delivery, 19 (44 percent) of the 43 infants developed neonatal infection.[356,358,359,365,366] In the one study in which it was evaluated, transplacentally acquired HSV-1 antibody did not decrease the risk of neonatal HSV-2 infection.[366] Two large studies have found much lower rates of neonatal HSV among infants born to women with positive cultures at delivery related to reactivation: Neonatal HSV occurred among 1 (3 percent) of 34 infants and 0 of 34 infants born to women with recurrent HSV and positive cultures at delivery.[364,366] Given positive genital HSV cultures at delivery in 0 to 2.4 percent of asymptomatic women with history of recurrent genital herpes[352,362,367] and maximum rates of neonatal infection of 2 to 5 percent associated with recurrent maternal disease at delivery, the risk of neonatal herpes for an infant born to an asymptomatic woman with history of recurrent herpes can be estimated as approximately 2 to 5 per 100,000 deliveries. Given the higher neonatal attack rate (50 percent) for a positive culture related to primary HSV and the higher chance of viral shedding during or following primary infection, neonatal transmission after primary infection during pregnancy is much greater. Thus 35 to 50 percent of neonatal HSV infections are related to maternal primary infections, although only 1 percent of women have primary infection during pregnancy compared with 30 percent who have preexisting antibody to HSV-2. Therefore, any strategy directed at preventing neonatal HSV must address both prevention of primary infection in pregnant women and detection or prevention of reactivation of recurrent disease at delivery.

The route of delivery and duration of rupture of the membranes correlate with risk of neonatal infection when mothers have primary genital herpes at term. Approximately 50 percent of neonates exposed to such mothers during vaginal delivery acquired the disease. In contrast, only 1 (6 percent) of 16 neonates delivered by cesarean section within 4 hours of rupture of the membranes acquired the disease.[148,359] In cases where the membranes had been ruptured for more than 4 hours, 6 of 7 exposed neonates acquired the disease irrespective of the route of delivery. Among women with symptomatic recurrent disease at delivery, who have a much lower risk of transmitting HSV to the neonate during vaginal delivery, a further decrease in risk with cesarean section is assumed but not proven.

Whereas other neonatal viral infections are often subclinical, the majority of neonates with HSV infection have clinical manifestations of disease (see Chap. 85). The unique neonatal propensity to severe HSV infection, which persists for several months following delivery, is presumably related to a poor cellular immune response against HSV during this period.

Case detection and management

Since it is not practical to perform routine screening cultures for HSV on all women at delivery, prevention of neonatal HSV infection currently rests both on preventing primary HSV infection during pregnancy and on identifying high-risk women and defining a strategy for clinical and virologic monitoring of this high-risk group, as well as on recognizing clinical manifestations of genital herpes in any woman near delivery. Whitley et al.[354] analyzed the risk profile of mothers of neonates acquiring HSV and found that 57 percent had a history of genital herpes, a sex partner with genital lesions suggestive of herpes, or signs or symptoms of genital herpes during pregnancy. Unfortunately, Arvin et al.[365] reported that asymptomatic intrapartum shedding of HSV is not predictable from antepartum cultures for HSV. The risk of neonatal infection is very low among women with a history of genital herpes,[364,366] and cost-benefit analysis has documented the extremely high cost of weekly surveillance for asymptomatic HSV shedding in mothers near term.[368] Analysis showed that screening of 3.6 million women would avert 11.3 neonatal deaths and 3.7 cases of severe retardation, but 3.3 women would die as a result of cesarean delivery necessitated by culture results. The cost per case of neonatal HSV infection averted was approximately $1.8 million.

A rapid test for HSV shedding would allow timely detection of asymptomatic shedding and testing of suspicious but atypical genital lesions, thus targeting cesarean delivery for those actually shedding virus; unfortunately, none of the currently licensed rapid tests has adequate sensitivity for this use.[369] PCR testing has enhanced sensitivity to detect asymptomatic shedding, but this method has not been adapted for routine clinical use, and the risk of neonatal infection with low DNA copy numbers detectable by PCR has not been established.[370,371]

Thus we recommend the following approach: Clinicians should solicit and record in the prenatal record the presence or absence of a history of genital herpes in the patient or her partner(s) and should assess her current sexual behavior. Negative history in the patient (although insensitive for HSV-2-seropositivity), coupled with positive history in the partner (though nonspecific), or risky sexual lifestyle could prompt advice on use of condoms for any intercourse during pregnancy. Women at high risk for primary or recurrent infection should be observed carefully for clinical evidence of genital lesions and, in the absence of herpetic lesions during labor, should be delivered vaginally unless there are other indications for cesarean section. If recurrent herpetic lesions are present in the genital tract at the time of rupture of the membranes or during labor, cesarean section may reduce the risk of neonatal infection and ideally should be performed within 4 to 6 hours after membrane rupture. Although the value of routine cultures at delivery among women with a history of herpes but no visible lesions has not been established, women with a history of genital herpes or whose sex partner has a history should have a "sweep" culture of the vulva and cervix obtained on admission for delivery pooled for HSV culture to identify potentially exposed neonates.[369] Such infants, if clinically well, have a small risk of infection and should be followed closely. The benefit of weekly infant cultures to detect asymptomatic neonates after documented exposure at delivery is unproven but recommended by some experts.[369] If clinical deterioration occurs or vesicular lesions develop, acyclovir can be started.

For women with a first symptomatic episode of HSV infection in the second half of pregnancy, attempts should be made to determine whether the episode represents recurrent or true first-episode infection. If reliable testing for type-specific antibody is available (enzyme immunoassay using purified glycoprotein G of HSV-2 or Western blot analysis), then women with homologous antibody to the HSV strain isolated from the genital tract may be managed as discussed earlier for recurrent disease. Currently, available commercial serologic tests such as complement fixation, indirect immunofluorescence, or enzyme immunoassays not using HSV-2-specific glycoprotein G are not specific enough to prove recurrent infection. Thus, unless recurrent infection can be proven, women with first-episode genital HSV in the second half of pregnancy may still benefit from having weekly cervical and vulvar cultures performed in the last 6 to 8 weeks of pregnancy to detect the 10 to 15 percent of women with primary infection who will be persistently culture-positive. Women with persistent or frequent asymptomatic shedding may be advised of the high risk of shedding during labor and offered cesarean section. Women with repeatedly negative cultures without lesions at the onset of labor could be offered vaginal delivery, with cervical and vulvar cultures also done on admission.

Management of pregnant women with HSV lesions and early preterm rupture of the membranes must be individualized. If the pregnancy is at or beyond 34 weeks' gestation, then delivery by cesarean section as soon as possible is indicated. Before this time, risks of prematurity versus risks of in utero or neonatal infection based on gestational age, maternal antibody status, and other clinical factors must be weighed. Consideration should be given to the use of intravenous or oral acyclovir in the mother to shorten the maternal course and possibly decrease the risk of neonatal infection, though the value of acyclovir in this setting remains unproven.

Although primary genital HSV infection in early pregnancy may cause spontaneous abortion, congenital infection is considered uncommon. For this reason, therapeutic abortion is not recommended for pregnancies complicated by primary infection. If primary infection occurs at or near term and genital herpetic lesions are present at time of rupture of the membranes or during labor, there is general agreement that cesarean section should be performed if membranes have been ruptured for less than 4 hours, although the American Academy of Pediatrics has recommended this time be increased to 12 hours.[372] We favor the latter recommendation. Infants born vaginally to mothers with primary infection are at particular risk of invasive disease. Consideration should be given to the early empirical use of acyclovir in this situation, although controlled trials of this approach are needed.

Hospital infection control procedures for protection of workers and other patients reflect the mode of transmission by direct contact or droplet. Patients with active lesions or who are culture-positive should have private rooms and bathrooms. Standard body substance isolation procedures should be followed, with gowns and gloves used when handling contaminated articles; soiled linen and perineal pads should be handled as infected discharge and double-bagged.[373]

Future developments in management of herpes during pregnancy

Acyclovir has become available for treatment for herpes simplex infections and has been used successfully in pregnancy to treat disseminated herpes infections.[374] Use of this agent for primary or recurrent infections near term to prevent transmission to the neonate needs study. Two small studies have shown a reduction in symptomatic recurrences of HSV and cesarean section among women treated with acyclovir near term. The first was an observational study that showed a rate of cesarean section for HSV in 0 of 21 treated women compared with 9 (20 percent) of 46 untreated women ($p < 0.001$).[375] The second was a small, randomized, blinded, placebo-controlled study of women with first symptomatic episodes of HSV in pregnancy, although serologies were not done to distinguish primary, nonprimary, first-episode, or recurrent disease.[376] In this study, cesarean section for presumed HSV reactivation was done in 0 of 21 acyclovir-treated patients and 9 (36 percent) of the 25 placebo-treated patients ($p = 0.002$). Only 1 of the 9 patients in the placebo group undergoing cesarean section for HSV had a positive culture. Neither study adequately evaluated women receiving acyclovir for asymptomatic shedding, and the small total of 63 treated women makes any conclusions regarding the risk of neonatal infection impossible. Although the prophylactic use of acyclovir in late pregnancy among women with symptomatic genital HSV to suppress recurrences and decrease cesarean section seems logical, larger studies evaluating safety and efficacy in preventing both symptomatic and asymptomatic reactivation are needed before its routine use is recommended. Some persistent shedding of HSV even with acyclovir has been reported.[377,378]

Strategies aimed at decreasing recurrences among women entering pregnancy with history of genital herpes or HSV-2-seropositivity will only eliminate about half the cases of neonatal HSV. Up to 50 percent are related to acquisition of HSV, especially late in pregnancy. Strategies to decrease exposure and seroconversion in pregnancy would include development of a vaccine to be administered to teenagers before the onset of sexual activity, assessment of ongoing high-risk sexual exposures, and serotesting to identify discordant couples with an HSV-2-seronegative pregnant woman with a seropositive partner. Pregnant women at risk could be educated regarding prevention strategies, including abstinence, condoms, or potentially, acyclovir therapy for the partner.

HUMAN PAPILLOMAVIRUS INFECTION

From the 1960s through the mid-1980s, the number of initial office visits to physicians in the United States for condylomata acuminata, or genital warts, increased dramatically.[379] Since 1987, the number may have declined somewhat.[347] Genital human papillomaviruses (HPVs), the causative agents of genital warts and most cases of cervical, vaginal, and vulvar intraepithelial neoplasia and cancer, are of concern in pregnancy for three reasons: (1) warts may rapidly enlarge with advancing gestation and mechanically obstruct labor, (2) the most common form of therapy, podophyllin application, is contraindicated during pregnancy, and (3) perinatal exposure may result in laryngeal or genital papillomatosis in infancy or childhood. The worsening of cervical intraepithelial neoplasia (CIN) frequently observed during pregnancy also may be due to accelerated HPV replication.

Epidemiology

Neonatal exposure to HPV probably occurs during birth by aspiration of contaminated cervical, vaginal, or vulvar material. During pregnancy, genital warts may enlarge, with pronounced vascularity. During the puerperium, regression often follows. The responsible mechanism is unknown but may relate to depression of maternal immunocompetence during pregnancy.

Laryngeal papillomatosis, a form of recurrent respiratory papillomatosis (RRP), is the most frequent tumor of the larynx in children (see Chap. 86). There is a bimodal age distribution, with peaks in children between 2 and 5 years of age and in young adulthood. Twenty-eight percent of childhood cases were detected in infants under 6 months of age.[380] Studies using hybridization of labeled DNA probes prepared from various types of HPV, with cellular DNA from genital warts or from laryngeal papillomas, have shown that HPV types 6 and 11 account for the majority of genital warts and laryngeal papillomas.[381,382]

There is a strong relationship between maternal genital warts during vaginal delivery and infant laryngeal papillomatosis.[383] History of condylomata acuminata can be obtained from over 50 percent of mothers whose infants develop laryngeal papillomas. Subclinical genital HPV infection is presumably responsible for most of the remainder. Perinatal transmission during vaginal delivery is the likely mode of spread, since children born by cesarean section seem to have a lower risk of acquiring RRP.[384] Anal-genital warts in infants also may be related to maternal condylomata acuminata.[385]

The reported risk of transmission of HPV from mother to infant has varied considerably in different populations studied by various methods. Table 80-15 summarizes reports of HPV detection in the infant according to the HPV status of the mother.[386–394] Most studies have shown a high rate of detection of HPV in the neonatal period, although detection often was not significantly related to maternal HPV infection. Three recent studies evaluated infants beyond 6 weeks of age born to women of known HPV status in late pregnancy. In Finland, among 58 children ages 4 months to 11.5 years who underwent oral examinations and testing for HPV, 36 percent had evidence of oral HPV infection; the HPV detection rate was not related to detection of genital HPV infection in the mother during the pregnancy.[392] A second study of 16 infants found HPV type 16 or type 18 more often among infants born to women with HPV type 16 or type 18 in pregnancy, but the difference was not significant.[393] A University of Washington study that followed mothers prospectively during and after pregnancy and monitored children longitudinally for up to 3 years after delivery found no clear evidence of oral, genital, or anal HPV infection among a total of 143 infants, 74 percent of whom were born to mothers with clinical, cytologic, or PCR evidence of HPV

Table 80-15. Detection of Human Papillomavirus DNA in Asymptomatic Children

Author, year	Age at sample	Site	HPV method	Maternal HPV status* Positive	Negative
Sedlacek[387] 1989	Birth	NP	Southern blot	11/25 (44%)	4/20 (20%)
Roman[386] 1986	1–2 d	Foreskin	PCR	4/10 (40%)	—
Fredericks[388] 1993	6 wks	Oral	PCR	8/11 (72%)	1/19 (5%)‡
Pakarian[389] 1994	1 d	Oral	PCR	10/20 (50%)	1/11 (9%)‡
	6 wks	Genital	PCR	6/20 (30%)	2/11 (18%)
Smith[390] 1995	1–3 d	Oral/genital	PCR	1/25 (4%)	1/178 (0.6%)
St. Louis[391] 1993	3 yrs	Oral/anal	Virapap	10/81 (12%)	—
Puranen[392] 1996	4 mos–11 1/2 yrs	Oral	PCR	14/44 (32%)	7/14 (50%)
Cason[393] 1995	1 d	Oral/genital	PCR	28/42 (67%)	4/18 (22%)‡
	6 wks	Oral/genital	PCR	23/29 (79%)	2/9 (22%)‡
	6 mos	Oral/genital	PCR	9/12 (75%)	1/4 (25%)
Watts[394] 1996	0–3 yrs†	Oral/genital	PCR	3/80 (4%)	5/63 (8%)

NOTE: NP = nasopharynx; PCR = polymerase chain reaction.
* At delivery or ±3 months (except ref. 391); mothers tested when children tested at age 3 years.
† Infants sampled at birth (n = 34), 6 weeks (n = 145), 6 months (n = 122), 12 months (n = 93), 18 months (n = 37), 24 months (n = 51), and 36 months (n = 26).
‡ $p \geq 0.05$.

during pregnancy.[394] Thus data so far seem quite inconsistent and do not justify routine cesarean delivery for women with genital warts or certainly with asymptomatic HPV infection.

Case detection

All pregnant women should have Pap smears to detect CIN, and those with active or past genital warts should be observed to detect recurrence or excessive growth of wart lesions.

Treatment

In view of the potential complications of papillomavirus infection, removal of genital warts prior to delivery is desirable. The conventional techniques for treating genital warts in pregnancy include electrocoagulation, cryotherapy, and electrodesiccation. For large lesions, treatment of small areas in multiple sessions is recommended. Ferenczy[395] has reported successful treatment of pregnant women using laser therapy with a failure rate of only 5 percent and relatively few complications. Since both maternal and fetal deaths have resulted from podophyllin treatment of large vascular warts, this drug should not be used during pregnancy.[396]

Cesarean section is not currently recommended to prevent neonatal exposure to papillomavirus. However, it may be necessary in rare instances where extensive lesions obstruct the vaginal outlet.

HEPATITIS B

Hepatitis B is a small DNA virus containing three principal antigens: hepatitis B surface antigen (HBsAg), hepatitis B core antigen (HBcAg), and hepatitis Be antigen (HBeAg). Core antigen is present only in hepatocytes. Detection of HBeAg in blood indicates active viral replication and extremely high viral levels and infectiousness.

Acute hepatitis B virus (HBV) infection occurs in 1 to 2 per 1,000 pregnancies, and chronic infection is found in 5 to 15 per 1,000 pregnancies in the United States.[397] Risk factors for HBV infection include injection drug use, multiple sexual partners, history of other sexually transmitted diseases, work in a health care or public safety field, work or residence in an institution for the developmentally disabled, and receipt of clotting factor concentrates. Higher risks of infection are found among certain ethnic groups such as Native Alaskans and in immigrants from most developing countries. Despite the increased prevalence of HBV infection in patients with risk factors, screening in pregnancy based on risk factors alone will miss up to 75 percent of women with HBV infection.[398]

Clinical manifestations and natural history of HBV infection are described in Chap. 26. Symptoms of acute hepatitis B infection, if present, are similar in pregnant and nonpregnant individuals and include malaise, fatigue, anorexia, nausea, and right upper quadrant pain. Signs include jaundice, hepatomegaly, and dark urine. There is no evidence that pregnancy worsens the course of acute viral hepatitis. However, pregnant women with the signs and symptoms listed above, especially women in the third trimester, should be evaluated carefully for indications of preeclampsia (hypertension, proteinuria, edema) or acute fatty liver of pregnancy, since delivery is indicated if either of these is present.[397] Transaminase levels are usually less elevated (200 to 400 μm/mL range) with preeclampsia or acute fatty liver than with acute hepatitis B (over 1,000 μm/mL). The diagnosis of acute hepatitis B can be confirmed by the presence of HBsAg and anti-HBc IgM antibody in the serum (see Chap. 26). In pregnant women with hepatitis, testing acute and convalescent sera for CMV seroconversion is important because of the potential for fetal CMV infection. Pregnant women with acute liver disease should be evaluated for coagulopathy and hypoglycemia. Hospitalization is indicated for encephalopathy, coagulopathy, severe debilitation, or inability to maintain adequate nutrition.

With acute hepatitis B in pregnancy, the risk of perinatal transmission depends on the stage of gestation at time of infection. First-trimester infection is associated with transmission to the fetus in up to 10 percent of cases; third-trimester acute infection is associated with an 80 to 90 percent risk of transmission.[399] Since chronic HBV infection is more common than acute infection during pregnancy, 85 to 95 percent of cases of perinatal transmission of HBV are related to intrapartum exposure. The risk of perinatal transmission is 10 to 20 percent among women who are HBsAg-positive and HBeAg-negative but rises to 50 to 90 percent among HBeAg-positive women in the absence of infant immunization.[400–402] Because of the high risk of perinatal transmission of hepatitis B, the 25 percent risk of death in adulthood from chronic liver disease after infection during infancy, and the 85 to 95 percent efficacy of passive plus active immunization of exposed infants, all pregnant women should be screened at the first prenatal visit for HBsAg.[403] Sexual partners and children of HBsAg-positive women should be offered testing and vaccination. Determination of HBeAg status is important for care and follow-up of the mother but does not change the management of the infant. All infants born to HBsAg-positive women should receive hepatitis B immune globulin, 0.5 mL IM, and their first dose of hepatitis B vaccine (0.5 mL) at separate sites.[404] Vaccine doses should be repeated at 1 and 6 months of age. Infants born to HBsAg-negative mothers should receive vaccine on the same schedule or starting within 2 months of birth.

Both passive and active immunization against hepatitis B are safe in pregnancy. If a nonimmune pregnant woman has been exposed to hepatitis B, hepatitis B immune globulin should be given in standard doses followed by vaccine. Nonimmune pregnant women in high-risk groups for hepatitis B also should be offered vaccination.

Although the combination of immune globulin and vaccination in exposed infants prevents the majority of perinatal transmission, prudence suggests minimizing exposure to maternal blood and secretions during labor, as is currently recommended for HIV-seropositive women. Scalp electrodes or blood sampling and instrument deliveries should be avoided if possible. Artificial rupture of the membranes should be delayed as long as possible. Infants should be washed thoroughly before receiving shots or drawing blood.

HIV IN PREGNANCY

Women infected heterosexually represent the most rapidly increasing group of HIV-infected individuals in the United States. In 1994, women accounted for 18 percent of AIDS cases reported to the CDC and comprised an even higher proportion of all HIV-infected persons. Worldwide, the predominant mode of HIV transmission is heterosexual, and women make up at least half the HIV-infected population.[405] Over 85 percent of women with AIDS are in the reproductive years, so the combination of pregnancy and HIV-seropositivity is increasingly common. It is estimated that over 6,000 HIV-positive women deliver annually in the United States.[406] With growing public awareness that zidovudine therapy can decrease the perinatal transmission of HIV, with CDC recommendations encouraging HIV testing for all pregnant women in the United States, and with U.S. Congressional linkage of federal funding for AIDS programs to effective prevention of perinatal HIV transmission, a growing number of HIV-infected pregnant women are being identified, and the numbers of young children with AIDS is falling.[407a,407b]

In caring for the HIV-positive pregnant woman, the potential impact of the pregnancy on maternal health and on therapy and diagnosis of HIV-related conditions must be considered. The woman must consider the likely life-shortening impact of HIV and the long-term care needs of the child. The risk of perinatal transmission and interventions to minimize this risk must be discussed. The follow-up testing and course of pediatric HIV infection if it occurs must be addressed. Finally, the impact of HIV on pregnancy outcome should be discussed.

Impact of pregnancy on maternal health and on therapy of HIV

The question of whether or not pregnancy causes accelerated HIV replication and disease progression has not been clearly answered. Immunosuppression, including a fall in CD4 lymphocyte counts and percentage, occurs in both HIV-positive and HIV-negative pregnant women.[14] This drop in count could allow enhanced viral replication and disease progression. In addition, antigenic stimulation by fetal tissues during pregnancy could lead to T-cell activation and viral replication. Conversely, the relative immunosuppression of pregnancy could lead to decreased viral activity. Studies from Europe and United States do not show clearly that women with an intervening pregnancy have more rapid progression to an AIDS-defining illness or death,[408,409] while data from developing countries suggest a possible increased progression related to pregnancy.[410] No clear benefit from pregnancy termination on maternal health has been shown.

When counseling a pregnant woman with advanced HIV-related immunosuppression (CD4 lymphocyte count $\leq 200/mm^3$), she must understand the limited experience with use of most antiretrovirals and opportunistic infection therapies during pregnancy. Zidovudine (ZDV) is the only antiretroviral that has been used extensively in pregnancy, although other agents are currently under study. Trimethoprim-sulfamethoxazole is routinely recommended for *Pneumocystis carinii* pneumonia prophylaxis, but other agents for common opportunistic infections such as gancyclovir and fluconazole have not been studied in pregnancy.[411] Pregnancy also may confound the diagnosis of HIV-related conditions because the symptoms of pregnancy frequently resemble symptoms of HIV complications or of adverse drug effects such as nausea, headache, and dyspnea. In general, diagnostic procedures should be used as indicated regardless of pregnancy status.

When treating pregnant women with HIV infection, the physiologic changes of pregnancy must be considered.[412] Plasma volume increases by 45 percent, while red cell mass increases by only 20 to 30 percent, leading to dilutional anemia. Cardiac output and the glomerular filtration rate increase by 30 to 50 percent. Tidal volume increases by 200 mL, and increased pulmonary blood flow may lead to increased absorption of aerosolized medications. Albumin levels decrease by 20 percent. The effects of pregnancy on drug levels will vary depending on the type of clearance and method of administration.

Perinatal transmission

The risk of perinatal transmission of HIV has varied from 9.1 percent to over 50 percent in studies of women not receiving zidovudine routinely in pregnancy.[413] Factors consistently associated with transmission in untreated women include lower CD4 lymphocyte count or decreased CD4:CD8 ratio[414–423]; plasma viremia, p24 antigenemia, or high viral copy number[415–417,421,422,424–426]; AIDS-defining illness or symptomatic disease in the mother[417,427]; placental membrane inflammation[417,423]; prematurity; and prolonged breast-feeding.[417,428,429] Factors suggested but not consistently found to increase the risk of transmission or evaluated only in one study include female gender of infant,[423] higher maternal age,[422] maternal vitamin A deficiency,[430] and rupture of the membranes more than 4 hours before delivery.[431] Two small studies have detected no association between syncytium-inducing viral phenotype and vertical transmission.[432,433] One study suggested that women with monocytotropic HIV strains were more likely to transmit,[434] whereas another found that T-cell-line tropism was more likely in transmitters.[435] Results have been quite variable when evaluating the role of maternal antibodies, including anti-gp 120, anti-CD4 binding site, and autologous neutralizing antibody titers, in preventing vertical transmission.[425,428,432,433,435–439]

Zidovudine has decreased perinatal transmission of HIV in several studies.[424,440–442] The most striking effect was seen in a multicenter, randomized trial comparing maternal and infant placebo with prophylaxis with oral zidovudine during the second and third trimesters, plus intravenous ZDV during labor, plus oral therapy for 6 weeks in the infant among asymptomatic, predominantly ZDV-naive women with CD4 lymphocyte counts over $200/mm^3$.[440] Randomized groups were balanced with respect to

Table 80-16. Recommendations for Zidovudine (ZDV) Use in Pregnant Women and Their Infants to Reduce Vertical Transmission of HIV

Antepartum	ZDV 100 mg orally five times daily or 200 mg orally three times daily to start as soon as possible after 13 weeks' gestation
Intrapartum	Loading dose: ZDV 2 mg/kg IV over 1 hour followed by 1 mg/kg/hour until delivery
Infant	2 mg/kg orally every 6 hours (total 8 mg/kg/day) for 6 weeks, beginning 8 to 12 hours after birth

SOURCE: Connor et al.[440]

CD4 count, demographic characteristics, pregnancy history, and duration of study therapy. Perinatal transmission was reduced from 25.5 percent in the placebo group to 8.3 percent in the ZDV group ($p < 0.001$). Subsequent retrospective reviews of ZDV use in cohorts of women who were treated primarily for maternal indications (CD4 lymphocyte count $< 200/mm^3$ or symptomatic disease) have shown similar reductions in transmission despite the more advanced disease.[424,441,442] A recent placebo-controlled study from Thailand showed a reduction in vertical transmission from 18% to 9% with a regimen of oral zidovudine 300 mg twice daily from 36 weeks' gestation until labor and 300 mg orlly every three hours in labor until delivery, or placebo of each. No infant zidovudine was given, and all women were counseled against breast-feeding and were provided with infant formula. These results suggest that more limited courses of zidovudine, which may be able to be provided in countries unable to implement the full ACTG 076 regimen, may produce a substantial reduction in vertical transmission of HIV.[44a] Current recommendations for ZDV prophylaxis are summarized in Table 80-16.

The impact of cesarean delivery on reducing intrapartum transmission of HIV remains unclear. Two reports from an international registry of twins born to HIV-positive women demonstrate a significantly higher rate of infection in firstborn than in second-born twins when the twins' infection status was discordant, hypothetically attributable to longer exposure of the firstborn to the birth canal.[443,444] A recent review of studies evaluating the rate of transmission by mode of delivery suggests potential benefit of cesarean section[416,420,428,445–450] (Table 80-17). However, comparisons are tentative at best because of the variability between rates of transmission by center, the combining of cesarean sections done before labor with those done after prolonged labor, the variability in management of labor such as use of scalp electrodes and forceps, and lack of differentiation of antepartum from intrapartum transmission. Few of the women in any of the studies received ZDV, which may alter the risk of intrapartum transmission more than the mode of delivery. Transmission rates in the ACTG 076 trial did not vary by mode of delivery.[440] More recent analyses suggest that duration of ruptured membranes may be more important, at least in women not receiving ZDV, than mode of delivery.[431] Until results of a currently ongoing randomized trial in Europe of elective cesarean section compared with vaginal delivery become available, mode of delivery should be determined according to usual obstetrical indications. However, interventions such as internal fetal monitoring, artificial rupture of the membranes, and operative vaginal delivery that may increase the risk of fetal exposure to maternal blood and secretions and hence transmission should be avoided.

Transmission of HIV by breast-feeding has been well documented. Among women known to be HIV-negative at delivery who then seroconverted while breast-feeding, the risk of infant HIV infection is approximately 30 percent.[451–454] In studies of women with HIV infection antedating pregnancy and lactation, breast-feeding appears to confer an additional 15 to 20 percent risk above the risk of antepartum and intrapartum transmission.[414,415,447,450,454,455] The magnitude of risk may be related to the duration of breast-feeding.[429] In countries where safe alternatives exist, breast-feeding by HIV-infected women is not recommended at all. Currently in developing countries where HIV testing for pregnant women is not readily available and safe alternatives to breast-feeding are not available, breast-feeding by HIV-positive women is not discouraged. Studies are underway to evaluate the relative risks of bottle-feeding compared with breast-feeding by HIV-positive women with respect to HIV transmission, infant nutrition and diarrhea, and overall infant mortality. It may be that some limited period of breast-feeding will maximize nutritional and immunologic benefits while minimizing the risk of HIV transmission in developing countries. The contraceptive effects of breast-feeding also must be considered; when breast-feeding is discouraged to protect the current newborn, alternative contraceptives will prevent exposure of a future newborn child.

Many current and planned studies of interventions to decrease the risk of perinatal transmission of HIV are summarized in Table 80-18.[456] Possible strategies include maternal and infant antiretroviral therapy, immune modulators, vitamin A supplementation, vaginal cleansing, cesarean section, and bottle-feeding.

Case detection

All pregnant women deserve counseling regarding HIV testing procedures, potential benefits to themselves and their fetus, potential risks, and implications of a positive and negative test.[407]

Table 80-17. Mode of Delivery and Perinatal Transmission of HIV

Author, year	Study location	CS rate	Transmission Rate: Vaginal delivery	Transmission Rate: Cesarean section
ECS[446] 1994	Europe (ECS)	24%	136/773 (18%)	28/239 (12%)
Thomas[420] 1994	NYC	22%	56/170 (33%)	9/43 (19%)
Kind[447] 1992	Switzerland	31%	29/141 (21%)	9/64 (14%)
Goedert[428] 1989	Brooklyn	14%	39/151 (26%)	5/26 (19%)
Dunn[448] 1994	Newark	27%	17/96 (18%)	5/36 (14%)
Andiman[449] 1990	Connecticut	18%	25/105 (24%)	3/23 (13%)
Dunn[448] 1994	France	14%	141/708 (20%)	24/119 (20%)
Nair[445] 1993	Baltimore	17%	41/165 (25%)	11/34 (32%)
Hutto[450] 1991	Miami	23%	31/107 (29%)	11/31 (36%)
Dunn[448] 1994	Atlanta	22%	14/92 (15%)	5/26 (19%)
Dunn[448] 1994	Bronx	25%	6/36 (17%)	3/12 (25%)
Tibaldi[416] 1993	Turin, Italy	14%	6/25 (24%)	1/4 (25%)
			541/2569 (21%)	**114/657 (17%)**

NOTE: *OR* = 1.28 (1.02–1.16); ECS = European Collaborative Study; CS = cesarean section.
SOURCE: Dunn.[448]

Table 80-18. Current and Planned Trials for Reduction of Perinatal Transmission of HIV

Country	Study design	Target *n*	Antepartum	Intrapartum	Infant	Breastfeeding
Antiretrovirals						
Thailand (Harvard)	4-arm, factorial AC vs. AD vs. BC vs. BD	1200	ZDV start at 28 (A) vs. 36 wks (B)	Oral ZDV	ZDV 3d (C) vs. 6 wks (D)	No
Ivory Coast (CDC)	2-arm, placebo control	1534	ZDV start 34–36 wks	ZDV	None	Yes
Haiti (Hopkins)	3-arm, placebo control	940	ZDV start 31–34 wks	ZDV	ZDV mom & infant for 2 wks	Yes
			ZDV start 31–34 wks	ZDV	Placebo	
Uganda (HIV Net)	3-arm, placebo control	1200	None	ZDV	ZDV × 1 wk	Yes
			None	NVP	NVP 1 dose @ 3 days	
Africa/Brazil (WHO)	4-arm, placebo control	1900	ZDV/3TC 38 wks	ZDV/3TC	ZDV/3TC†/wk	Yes
			None	ZDV/3TC	ZDV/3TC* 1 wk	
			None	ZDV/3TC	None	
USA† (ACTG 316)	2-arm, ZDV control	900	ZDV start at 14–34 wks	ZDV	ZDV × 6 wks	
			ZDV start at 14–34 wks	ZDV/NVP	ZDV, 1 dose NVP @ 3 d	No
Ivory Coast	2-arm, placebo control, phase I/II	150	ZDV start 34–36 wks	oral ZDV	ZDV mom × 1 wk	Yes
Immune Modulators (HIV Ig)						
Uganda	2-arm, HIVIg vs. IgG	400	One infusion at 38 wks	None	One dose in newborn	Yes
Haiti	2-arm, HIVIg vs. IgG	576	None	None	One dose in newborn	Yes
USA (ACTG 230)	3-arm, 2 different gp 120 vaccines vs. adjuvant	120	None	None	Newborn	No
Vitamin A						
Malawi	2-arm, placebo control	960	10,000 IU vit. A	None	None	Yes
Tanzania	4-arm, placebo control, factorial design for micronutrients	960	5000 IU vit. A + 30 mg β-carotene	200,000 IU vit. A	None	Yes
South Africa	2-arm, placebo control	400	5000 IU vit. A + 20 mg β-carotene	200,000 IU vit. A	Mother 200,000 IU vit. A 1 ddpp	Yes
Zimbabwe	2-arm, placebo control	600	14 micronutrients	14 micronutrients	14 micronutrients in mom for 3 mos	Yes
Delivery mode						
Europe, South Africa, Brazil	2-arm, C-section vs. vag del	1500	None	CS vs. vag.	None	No
Vaginal cleansing						
Kenya	2-arm, wash vs. none	1000	None	Chlorhexidine wash vs. none	Baby wash	Yes
Ivory Coast	Phase I, BZK supp.	<100	Daily supp. start at 37 wks	Supp. in labor	Baby wash	Yes
Feeding mode						
Kenya	2-arm breast- vs. bottle-feeding	430	None	None	Bottle-feed vs. breastfeeding	—

NOTE: 3TC = lamivudine; ZDV = zidovudine; NVP = nevirapine; all ZDV and NVP dosing is oral; HIVIg and IgG dosing is intravenous; ACTG = AIDS Clinical Trials Group; BZK = benzalkoniumchloride, given as intravaginal suppository.

* ZDV and 3TC for both mother and infant for 1 week postpartum.

† Protocol in development, design, and antiretroviral agents may change.

** Closed April, 1997 because of lack of efficacy.

SOURCE: Modified from Fowler.[456]

All pregnant women of unknown HIV status should be encouraged to undergo HIV testing regardless of perceived risk factors for infection. Several studies have indicated that only half the women who test positive for HIV had identified potential risk factors for infection before testing.[457–459] Especially in areas of low prevalence where heterosexual transmission is the predominant risk factor among women, most women who test positive would not have identified themselves as being at risk. HIV testing and counseling including management of the patient with an indeterminate Western blot are discussed in Chap. 70.

Management

HIV-positive pregnant women should have a thorough history and physical examination on the first visit to allow early recognition and treatment of any complications and to document normal findings. Special attention should be given to the funduscopic, neurologic, and pelvic examinations to allow later comparison should symptoms develop. Pelvic examination should include cervical cytology to detect neoplasia and testing for *N. gonorrhoeae* and *C. trachomatis*. All HIV-positive women who have not had tuberculin skin testing within the past year should have an intermediate-strength purified protein derivative (PPD) placed. In areas or populations with a prevalence of tuberculosis above 10 percent or in women with a CD4 lymphocyte count below 400/mm^3, the role of concurrent anergy testing is debated.[411] Evaluation and management of pregnant women with positive skin tests for tuberculosis are the same as for nonpregnant individuals. Platelet count and lymphocyte subset determinations should be added to routine prenatal laboratory studies (complete blood count, blood type and antibody screen, hepatitis B surface antigen, rubella antibody, syphilis serology). Baseline antibody determination for CMV, *Toxoplasma gondii*, and herpes simplex virus should be obtained, and liver function testing should be done before starting ZDV therapy. Repeat lymphocyte subset determinations should be done each trimester to assess the need for PCP prophylaxis if the baseline CD4 lymphocyte count was below 500/mm^3.

ZDV therapy as outlined in Table 80 16 should be offered to all HIV-positive pregnant women. ZDV is clearly beneficial in ZDV-naive women with CD4 lymphocyte counts above 200/mm^3 and probably so in women with limited ZDV exposure and CD4 counts below 200/mm^3. However, the benefit in women with previous long-term ZDV use is unknown. Current studies of use of didanosine and nevirapine in the third trimester are underway, but experience with use of other antiretrovirals including protease inhibitors in pregnancy is limited. In general, as with other serious conditions in pregnancy, therapy in pregnancy should be the same as it would be if the woman were not pregnant, unless there are clear maternal or fetal contraindications to a specific therapy. Given that ZDV is the only drug that has been evaluated for reduction of perinatal transmission, ZDV should be included in the regimen unless the patient is intolerant. Reasonable initial regimens for therapy in pregnant women with CD4 counts below 500/mm^3 include ZDV with lamivudine or didanosine.[460] Viral load testing, if available, should be used to monitor the response to therapy, with a switch to another nucleoside analogue or addition of a protease inhibitor if pregnant women do not have a half-log or greater reduction in viral load on therapy. Although agents other than ZDV have not been evaluated for reducing perinatal transmission, given the correlation with maternal viral load and risk of transmission,[461a] agents that lower maternal viral load would be expected to also lower transmission rates. The relative benefit of maternal compared with infant therapy is unclear.[461b] In the woman who presents in early pregnancy on a stable antiretroviral regimen, the risk of rebound in viral load with potential increased risk of transmission with stopping therapy versus the unknown teratogenic risk of newer antiretroviral agents must be considered carefully. If the woman elects to continue her antiretroviral therapy and the pregnancy, detailed ultrasound for fetal anatomy at approximately 20 weeks' gestation and close surveillance for fetal growth in the third trimester should be performed and the pregnancy outcome reported to the Antiretroviral in Pregnancy Registry, Glaxo Wellcome, P.O. Box 12700, Research Triangle Park, NC 27709–9781 (919–248–2100). No data regarding the impact of any antiretroviral agent other than ZDV on perinatal transmission of HIV are currently available.

Prophylaxis for opportunistic infections in HIV-positive pregnant women should be considered using the guidelines for nonpregnant persons.[411] PCP prophylaxis should be given if the CD4 lymphocyte count is below 200/mm^3, if there is unexplained fever (100°F) for 2 weeks or more, or if there is a history of oropharyngeal candidiasis. The first choice for therapy is trimethoprim-sulfamethoxazole, one double-strength tablet daily. Alternatives include aerosolized pentamidine, 300 mg monthly via Respirgard II nebulizer, or oral dapsone, 100 mg daily. Patients at risk for glucose-6-phosphate dehydrogenase deficiency should be tested for this condition before starting sulfa or dapsone therapy. Prophylaxis for *Mycobacterium avium intracellulare* (MAI) should be considered after the first trimester when the CD4 lymphocyte count falls below 75/mm^3. Azithromycin, as recommended for nonpregnant individuals, would be the first choice for therapy, although rifabutin and clarithromycin would be acceptable also. If prophylaxis is not given, monthly MAI blood cultures should be done if the CD4 count is below 50/mm^3. If other opportunistic infections are suspected in the pregnant woman, diagnosis and therapy should then be determined on a case-by-case basis with collaboration of the maternal fetal medicine and infectious disease specialists.

Intrapartum management should include intravenous ZDV as outlined in Table 80-16. As discussed earlier, delivery should be vaginal unless there are obstetrical indications for cesarean section. Artificial rupture of the membranes, internal monitoring, and operative vaginal delivery should be avoided. Given the increased risk for both HSV-2-seropositivity and reactivation among HIV-positive women, careful vulvar and cervical examination and cultures for HSV should be done on admission for delivery.[462] The infant should be cleansed thoroughly before any blood drawing or injections are performed.

Studies on pregnancy outcome among HIV-positive women and their infants are summarized in Table 80-19.[414,463–471] In the United States and Europe, birth weight and gestational age do not differ between HIV-positive women and similar controls. However, in developing countries, the rates of low birth weight and preterm birth are increased among HIV-positive women, possibly related to concurrent infections or nutritional deficiencies. Of note, studies in the United States and Europe have primarily included drug-using women, with both HIV-infected and seronegative women having higher than average rates of low birth weight and prematurity.[472] Thus the concomitant substance abuse may mask subtle effects of HIV on outcome.

Postpartum, HIV-positive women and their infants require intensive psychosocial and medical follow-up. Management of infants at risk of HIV infection is discussed in Chap. 81. Although HIV-positive women should not breast-feed, lactation suppression is no longer used because of limited efficacy and potential complications of bromocriptine, including seizures and strokes. In addition to recommending routine use of condoms, contraceptive options should be discussed before hospital discharge. Hormonal contraceptive agents including combination estrogen-progesterone oral contraceptive pills, depomedroxyprogesterone acetate, and Norplant can be used by HIV-positive women, taking into account usual contraindications and potential interactions with other medications being taken. Intrauterine devices are not rec-

Table 80-19. Maternal HIV Status and Pregnancy Outcome

Site (reference), year	HIV status	n	Birth weight <2500 gm	<37 weeks or mean GA	Mean birth weight	Comments
USA, Europe						
UK (463) 1988	+	31	23%	16%	NA	More spontaneous
	−	54	22%	15%	NA	abortions in HIV+
USA (464) 1990	+	25	NA	32%	2760	More pneumonia,
	−	44	NA	32%	2760	breech in HIV+
USA (465) 1990	+	81	NA	38.2	2906	More STDs in HIV+
	−	115	NA	38.2	3014	
Italy (466) 1990	+	74	NA	15%	NA	No difference
	−	48	NA	29%	NA	
USA (467) 1993	+	101	27.7%	37.5	2824	More condylomata
	−	97	26.8%	37.8	2891	in HIV+
Africa, Haiti						
Zaire (414) 1989	AIDS	85	33%*	18%*	2698*	
	+	381	17%†	12%*	2931*	
	−	606	10%	3%	3107	
Haiti (468) 1990	+	199	19%*	7%*	2944*	
	−	1994	11%	2%	3111	
Kenya (469) 1990	+	177	9%*	NA	3090*	
	−	326	3%	NA	3220	
Rwanda (470) 1991	+	218	17%	35%	2840*	
	−	218	12%	30%	2970	
Kenya (471) 1994	+	315	24%*	21%*	2913*	More warts, syphilis,
	−	311	15%	9.4%	2072	PPE in HIV+

NOTE: GA = gestational age; STD = sexually transmitted disease; PPE = postpartum endometritis.
* $p < 0.05$ comparing HIV-positive to HIV-negative.
† $p < 0.01$.

ommended because of the potentially increased risk of pelvic infection. Tubal ligation is an option if the patient desires. The HIV-positive woman will need enhanced psychosocial support postpartum as she awaits determination of the infant's HIV infection status. No recommendations exist regarding the benefit versus risk of continuing antiretroviral therapy after delivery for women with CD4 lymphocyte counts above 500/mm^3 and low plasma viral load. Follow-up studies of viral load changes and disease progression among women receiving antiretroviral therapy solely for reduction of perinatal transmission are in progress to determine optimal therapy. Currently, postpartum antiretroviral therapy should be decided by the woman and her provider based on patient preference and changes in CD4 count.

SUMMARY: APPROACH TO MANAGEMENT OF SEXUALLY TRANSMITTED DISEASES IN PREGNANCY AND THE PERINATAL PERIOD

The most important approach to preventing STD morbidity related to pregnancy is to prevent STD infection in women of reproductive age through effective STD prevention programs. Another central prerequisite is ensuring prenatal care for all women; the potential for early detection and preventing STD-related morbidity in pregnancy represents one of the strongest arguments for extending prenatal care to all women. As an initial approach to the management of STD in pregnancy, a standard history concerning sexual behavior and past STDs should be obtained from all pregnant patients. Information on age, ethnicity, socioeconomic status, marital status, and health care behavior also may help identify those at highest risk of having an STD. Specific questions, for example, should include (1) prior modes of contraception including intrauterine device use, (2) previous history of gonorrhea, chlamydia, syphilis, HIV infection, vaginitis, genital warts, genital herpes, or pelvic inflammatory disease, (3) current sexual habits, number of current sexual partners (e.g., last 2 months), number of times of coitus per week, (4) past sexual experience (e.g., age at first coitus, lifetime number of sexual partners), and (5) intravenous drug abuse. Although it is not current practice to limit sexual activity during pregnancy, since data on the effects of coitus during pregnancy are conflicting, it may be wise to advise patients wishing to minimize risk that some studies have shown increased risk of prematurity and perinatal death with coital activity later in pregnancy. Pregnant women also should be appraised of the special risks of STDs acquired during pregnancy.

Pregnant women in most populations should routinely undergo cervical screening culture for gonorrhea and serologic testing for syphilis. Those with a history of past gonococcal infection or who have more than one current sex partner should be screened again in late pregnancy with both tests, and in the United States it has been recommended that all women be tested for syphilis in late pregnancy. A routine screening test for *C. trachomatis* is indicated in pregnant women who have risk factors for chlamydial infection, as outlined in Chap. 29, especially in adolescents, for whom the prevalence of chlamydial infection may exceed 25 percent. Schachter et al.[249] have argued that even culture testing (at $25 per test) is cost-effective in pregnant women when the prevalence of infection exceeds 6 percent. Tests for *C. trachomatis*, of course, also should be obtained from pregnant women with symptoms or signs consistent with chlamydial infection. Bacterial vaginosis or trichomoniasis should be managed as discussed earlier.

During pregnancy, a number of clinical situations occur in which the patient should be evaluated for selected STDs. Dysuria, a common complaint in pregnancy, should not be automatically attributed to urinary tract infection without excluding vaginitis, cervicitis, or urethritis as possible causes (see Chap. 57). Both gonorrhea and chlamydial infection can cause dysuria. Although it is not yet common practice, it seems advisable that women who suffer a syndrome consistent with cytomegalovirus (CMV) infection during pregnancy should be studied to exclude primary CMV infection in addition to other indicated studies. Women who have a history of genital herpes should be examined closely for recurrent clinical evidence of herpetic lesions late in pregnancy and during labor, as described earlier. Endocervical cultures for *N. gonorrhoeae* and *C. trachomatis* should be obtained from women at any stage of gestation who have signs of mucopurulent cervicitis or a history of exposure to a sex partner with urethritis. Neonatal chlamydial conjunctivitis or pneumonia dictates examination and treatment of mother and father for chlamydial infection. It is to be emphasized that in the setting of neonatal STD, both parents must be interviewed, examined, and treated where appropriate. Women with otherwise unexplained complications such as septic abortion, premature labor, premature rupture of the membranes, and intrapartum fever should be evaluated for sexually transmitted infection. Treatable infections (e.g., with *N. gonorrhoeae* and *C. trachomatis*) should always be excluded in women with these complications. Women with late-onset endometritis also should be evaluated for *C. trachomatis* infection.

Special surveillance of the neonate may be necessary when the mother is at high risk for STDs or develops puerperal infection or intrapartum fever. Such neonates may have to be closely monitored in the hospital for clinical evidence of sepsis and out of the hospital for evidence of ocular or respiratory infection. Neonates exposed during delivery to HSV require especially close surveillance, including frequent cultures from eye, throat, skin, rectum, and lesions, and antiviral treatment at the first clinical or virologic evidence of HSV infection.

Considerable controversy surrounds the use of neonatal ocular prophylaxis. To permit initial maternal-neonatal bonding, the American Academy of Pediatrics recommendations allow for prophylaxis to be delayed for up to one hour following birth. Presently, silver nitrate, erythromycin, and tetracycline ointment have all been recommended for the prevention of gonococcal ophthalmia neonatorum. An additional benefit of ocular prophylaxis may be the prevention of chlamydial conjunctivitis; the one-hour delay in applying prophylaxis may reduce the efficacy of prophylaxis for this purpose.

Neonatal prophylaxis for other STDs such as HSV requires further study. The efficacy of passive-active immunization for neonates exposed to hepatitis B has led to the recent recommendations that all women be tested early in pregnancy for HBsAg (later if clinically indicated) and that infants born to HBsAg-positive mothers receive both hepatitis B immunoglobulin, 0.5 mL intramuscularly, and hepatitis B vaccine in appropriate dosage (see Chap. 26).

In summary, as shown in Table 80-20, a spectrum of clinical events occurring during pregnancy is associated with infection by STD agents. The obstetrical consequences of antepartum STDs largely have been neglected until recently and, in fact, represent one of the most important areas for future research on STDs. Many studies have shown a relationship of individual STD agents to specific obstetrical complications, as reflected by the large number of citations in this relatively selective review of STDs in pregnancy. Many studies are sometimes difficult to interpret because coinfection with more than one STD agent is common and STD infection itself may be associated with other noninfectious risk factors for obstetrical morbidity. Primary or new infection with particular STD agents may carry a higher risk than chronic or recurrent infection with those same agents. It may be that coinfection with multiple STD agents is synergistic or additive in causing obstetrical morbidity. For example, primary infection with an agent such as *C. trachomatis, N. gonorrhoeae,* or HSV might produce chorioamnionitis and lead to premature rupture of the membranes, which in turn might lead to a particularly high risk of amniotic fluid infection syndrome in the presence of bacterial vaginosis or trichomonal vaginitis because of the increased concentration of anaerobic pathogens in the vagina in these types of vaginitis. Thus study of the impact, diagnosis, treatment, and prevention of STDs in pregnancy must remain a high priority.

Table 80-20. Disorders of Pregnancy and the Puerperium that Have Been Associated with Infection by STD Agents in One or More Studies

Clinical event	Associated STD agents
Ectopic pregnancy	Prior *C. trachomatis* infection; also, 50% of cases have histologic evidence of prior salpingitis
Spontaneous abortion	*N. gonorrhoeae,* herpes simplex virus
Posttherapeutic abortion–pelvic inflammatory disease	*C. trachomatis, N. gonorrhoeae,* bacterial vaginosis
Premature delivery, premature and prolonged rupture of membranes	*C. trachomatis, N. gonorrhoeae,* bacterial vaginosis, *M. hominis, U. urealyticum, T. pallidum,* herpes simplex virus, cytomegalovirus, *T. vaginalis*
Amniotic fluid infection	Bacterial vaginosis, *N. gonorrhoeae, U. urealyticum*
Congenital abnormalities	CMV, HSV, *T. pallidum*
Intrauterine growth retardation	CMV, HSV, *T. pallidum*
Puerperal endomyometritis:	
Early (<48 h postdelivery)	Bacterial vaginosis, *Strep. agalactiae, U. urealyticum, M. hominis, T. vaginalis*
Late (>48 h postdelivery)	*C. trachomatis*
Perinatal	
Stillbirth	*T. pallidum,* CMV, *C. trachomatis*
Neonatal death, neonatal infection	Herpes simplex virus, *N. gonorrhoeae, C. trachomatis,* CMV, *T. pallidum*

References

1 Finland M: Pneumonia and pneumococcal infections with special reference to pneumococcal pneumonia. *Am Rev Respir Dis* 120:481, 1979.

2 Rao AR et al: Pregnancy and smallpox. *J Ind Med Assoc* 40:353, 1963.

3 Greenberg M et al: Maternal mortality in the epidemic of Asian influenza, New York, 1957. *Am J Obstet Gynecol* 76:897, 1958.

4 Siegel M, Greenberg M: Incidence of poliomyelitis in pregnancy: Its relation to maternal age, parity and gestational period. *N Engl J Med* 253:841, 1955.

5 Odds FC: Factors that predispose the host to candidiasis, in *Candida and Candidiasis,* FC Odds (ed). Baltimore, University Park Press, 1979, p 75.

6 Gilles HM, et al: Malaria, anaemia and pregnancy. *Ann Trop Med Parasitol* 63:245, 1969.

7 Khuroo MS et al: Incidence and severity of viral hepatitis in pregnancy. *Am J Med* 70:252, 1981.

8 Moore JE: Studies on the influence of pregnancy in syphilis: 1. The course of syphilitic infection in pregnant women. *Johns Hopkins Med Bull* 34:89, 1923.

9 Hodes HL: Effect of pregnancy upon immunity of mice vaccinated against St. Louis encephalitis virus. *J Exp Med* 69:533, 1939.

10 Suzuki K, Tomasi TB: Immune responses during pregnancy: Evidence of suppressor cells for splenic antibody response. *J Exp Med* 150: 898, 1979.

11 St. Hill CA et al: Depression of cellular immunity in pregnancy due to a serum factor. *Br J Med* 1:513, 1973.

12 Stanley Y: Fetuin: An inhibitor of lymphocyte transformation. *J Exp Med* 141:242, 1975.

13 Sridama V et al: Decreased levels of helper T cells: A possible cause of immunodeficiency in pregnancy. *N Engl J Med* 307:352, 1982.

14 Biggar RJ et al: Immunosuppression in pregnant women infected with human immunodeficiency virus. *Am J Obstet Gynecol* 161:1239–1244, 1989.

15 Brunham RC et al: Depression of the lymphocyte transformation response to microbial antigens and to phytohemagglutinin during pregnancy. *J Clin Invest* 72:1629, 1983.

16 Sabahi F et al: Qualitative and quantitative analysis of T lymphocytes during normal human pregnancy. *Am J Reprod Immunol* 33:381–93, 1995.

17 Gehrz RC et al: A longitudinal analysis of lymphocyte proliferate responses to mitogens and antigens during human pregnancy. *Am J Obstet Gynecol* 140:655, 1981.

18 Finland M: Pneumonia, in *Obstetric and Perinatal Infections,* D Charles, M Finland (eds). Philadelphia, Lea & Febiger, 1973, p 167.

19 Singer A: The uterine cervix from adolescence to the menopause. *Br J Obstet Gynaecol* 82:81, 1975.

20 Ayra OP et al: Epidemiological and clinical correlates of chlamydial infection of the cervix. *Br J Vener Dis* 57:118, 1981.

21 Critchlow CW et al: Determinants of cervical ectopia and cervicitis: Age, oral contraception, specific cervical infection, smoking, and douching. *Am J Obstet Gynecol* 173:534–543, 1995.

22 Moghissi KS: Composition and function of cervical secretion, in *Handbook of Physiology,* sec 7: *Endocrinology,* vol 2: *Female Reproductive System,* part 2, RL Greep (ed). Washington, American Physiological Society, 1973, p 25.

23 Sarrell PM, Pruett KA: Symptomatic gonorrhea during pregnancy. *Obstet Gynecol* 32:670, 1968.

24 Russell P: Inflammatory lesions of the human placenta: 1. Clinical significance of acute chorioamnionitis. *Am J Diagn Gynecol Obstet* 1:127, 1979.

25 Larsen B, Galask RP: Vaginal microbial flora: Practical and theoretic relevance. *Obstet Gynecol* 55(suppl 5):1005, 1980.

26 Goplerud CP et al: Aerobic and anaerobic flora of the cervix during pregnancy and the puerperium. *Am J Obstet Gynecol* 126:858, 1976.

27 Centers for Disease Control and Prevention: Ectopic pregnancy—United States, 1990–1992. *MMWR* 44:46–48, 1995.

28 Bone NC, Greene RR: Histologic study of uterine tubes with tubal pregnancy. *Am J Obstet Gynecol* 82:1166, 1961.

29 Novak E, Darner HL: Correlation of uterine and tubal changes in tubal gestation. *Am J Obstet Gynecol* 9:295, 1975.

30 Brunham RC et al: *Chlamydia trachomatis* infection in women with ectopic pregnancy. *Obstet Gynecol* 67:721, 1987.

31 Kosseim M, Brunham RC: Fallopian tube obstruction as a sequela to *Chlamydia trachomatis* infection. *Eur J Clin Microbiol* 5:584, 1986.

32 Blackwell AL et al: Health gains from screening for infection of the lower genital tract in women attending for termination of pregnancy. *Lancet* 342:206–210, 1993.

33 Sorensen JL et al: Early- and late-onset of pelvic inflammatory disease among women with cervical *Chlamydia trachomatis* infection at the time of induced abortion: A follow-up study. *Infection* 22:242–246, 1994.

34 Larsson PG et al: Incidence of pelvic inflammatory disease after first-trimester legal abortion in women with bacterial vaginosis after treatment with metronidazole: A double-blind, randomized study. *Am J Obstet Gynecol* 166:100–103, 1992.

35 El-Refaey H et al: Induction of abortion with mifepristone (RU486) and oral or vaginal misoprostol. *N Engl J Med* 332:983–987, 1995.

36 Olding LB et al: Pathogenesis of cytomegalovirus infection: 1. Activation of virus from bone marrow-derived lymphocytes by in vitro allogenic reaction. *J Exp Med* 141:561, 1975.

37 McIntyre JA, Faulk WP: Antigens of human trophoblast: Effects of heterologous anti-trophoblast sera on lymphocyte responses in vitro. *J Exp Med* 149:824, 1979.

38 Russell P, Altshuler G: Placenta abnormalities of congenital syphilis: A neglected aid to diagnosis. *Am Dis Child* 128:160, 1974.

39 Haves K, Gibas H: Placental cytomegalovirus infection without fetal involvement following primary infection in pregnancy. *J Pediatr* 79: 401, 1971.

40 Dorman HB, Sahvun PF: Identification and significance of spirochetes in the placenta: A report of 105 cases with positive findings. *Am J Obstet Gynecol* 33:954, 1937.

41 Hillier SL et al: Case control study of chorioamnionic infection and chorioamnionitis in prematurity. *N Engl J Med* 319:972, 1988.

42 Pankuch GA et al: Placental microbiology and histology and the pathogenesis of chorioamnionitis. *Obstet Gynecol* 65:802–806, 1984.

43 Quinn PA et al: Chorioamnionitis: Its association with pregnancy outcome and microbial infection. *Am J Obstet Gynecol* 156:379–387, 1987.

44 Kundsin RB et al: Association of *Ureaplasma urealyticum* in the placenta with perinatal morbidity and mortality. *N Engl J Med* 310: 941–945, 1984.

44a Administration of zidovudine during late pregnancy and delivery to prevent perinatal HIV transmission-Thailand, 1996–1998. *Morb Mort Wkly Rep* 1998; 47:151–4.

45 Svensson L et al: Chorioamnionitis and the isolation of microorganisms from the placenta. *Obstet Gynecol* 67:403–409, 1986.

46 Zlatnik FG et al: Histologic chorioamnionitis, microbial infection, and prematurity. *Obstet Gynecol* 76:355–359, 1990.

47 Hillier SL et al: Microbiologic causes and neonatal outcomes associated with chorioamnion infection. *Am J Obstet Gynecol* 165:955–961, 1991.

48 Naeye R, Kissane JM: Perinatal diseases, a neglected area of the medical sciences, in *Perinatal Diseases,* RL Naeye et al (eds). International Academy of Pathology Monograph. Baltimore, Williams & Wilkins, 1980, p 1.

49 Bobitt JR, Ledger WJ: Unrecognized amnionitis and prematurity: A preliminary report. *J Reprod Med* 19:8, 1977.

50 Miller JM Jr et al: Bacterial colonization of amniotic fluid in the presence of ruptured membranes. *Am J Obstet Gynecol* 137:451, 1980.

51 Gibson M, Williams PP: *Haemophilus influenzae* amnionitis associated with prematurity and premature membrane rupture. *Obstet Gynecol* 52(suppl 1):70S, 1978.

52 Naeye RL, Blane WA: Relation of poverty and race to antenatal bacterial infections. *N Engl J Med* 283:555, 1970.

53 Naeye RL et al: Fetal and maternal features of antenatal bacterial infections. *J Pediatr* 79:733, 1971.

54 Naeye RL: Common environmental influences on the fetus, in *Perinatal Diseases,* RL Naeye (ed). International Academy of Pathology Monograph. Baltimore, Williams & Wilkins, 1980, p 52.

55 Naeye RL: Coitus and associated amniotic-fluid infection. *N Engl J Med* 301:1198, 1979.

56 Naeye RL: Seasonal variations in coitus and other risk factors and the outcome of pregnancy. *Early Hum Dev* 4:61, 1980.

57 Keller CA, Nugent RP: Seasonal patterns in perinatal mortality and preterm delivery. *Am J Epidemiol* 118:689, 1983.

58 Mills JL et al: Should coitus late in pregnancy be discouraged? *Lancet* 1:136, 1981.

59 Read JS, Klebanoff MA: Sexual intercourse during pregnancy and preterm delivery: Effects of vaginal microorganisms. The Vaginal Infections and Prematurity Study Group. *Am J Obstet Gynecol* 168: 514–519, 1993.

60 Kurki T, Ylikorkala O: Coitus during pregnancy is not related to bacterial vaginosis or preterm birth. *Am J Obstet Gynecol* 169:1130–1134, 1993.

61 Greenwood R, McCaw-Binns A: Does maternal behavior influence the risk of perinatal death in Jamaica? *Pediatr Perinat Epidemiol* 8(suppl 1):54–65, 1994.

62 Biggers JD: In vitro fertilization and embryo transfer in human beings. *N Engl J Med* 304:336, 1981.

63 Wilson RD et al: Risk of spontaneous abortion in ultrasonographically normal pregnancies. *Lancet* 2:920–923, 1984.

64 Centers for Disease Control and Prevention: Progress towards achieving the 1990 objectives for pregnancy and infant health. *MMWR* 37: 405, 1988.

65 Rush RW et al: Contribution of preterm delivery to perinatal mortality. *Br Med J* 2:905, 1976.

66 Luk B et al: The cost of prematurity: A case-control study of twins versus singletons. *Am J Public Health* 86:809–814, 1996.

67 Elder HA et al: The natural history of asymptomatic bacteriuria during pregnancy: The effect of tetracycline on the clinical course and the outcome of pregnancy. *Am J Obstet Gynecol* 111:441, 1971.

68 Kass EH et al: Genital mycoplasmas as a cause of excess premature delivery. *Trans Assoc Am Physicians* 94:261, 1981.

69 Temmerman M et al: Mass antimicrobial treatment in pregnancy: A randomized, placebo-controlled trial in a population with high rates of sexually transmitted diseases. *J Reprod Med* 40:176–180, 1995.

70 McGregor JA et al: Adjunctive erythromycin treatment for idiopathic preterm labor: Results of a randomized, double-blinded, placebo-controlled trial. *Am J Obstet Gynecol* 154:98–103, 1986.

71 Cooperstock M et al: Circadian incidence of labor onset hour in preterm birth and chorioamnionitis. *Obstet Gynecol* 70:852–855, 1987.

72 Guzick DS, Winn K: The association of chorioamnionitis with preterm delivery. *Obstet Gynecol* 65:11–15, 1985.

73 Fox H, Langley FA: Leukocytic infiltration of the placenta and umbilical cord. *Obstet Gynecol* 37:451–458, 1971.

74 Weibel DR, Randall HW Jr: Evaluation of amniotic fluid in preterm labor with intact membranes. *J Reprod Med* 30:777–780, 1985.

75 Duff P, Kopelman JN: Subclinical intraamniotic infection in asymptomatic patients with refractory preterm labor. *Obstet Gynecol* 69: 756–759, 1987.

76 Wallace RL, Herrick CN: Amniocentesis in the evaluation of preterm labor. *Obstet Gynecol* 57:483–486, 1981.

77 Hameed C et al: Silent chorioamnionitis as a cause of preterm labor refractory to tocolytic therapy. *Am J Obstet Gynecol* 149:726–730, 1984.

78 Leigh J, Garite T: Amniocentesis and the management of preterm labor. *Obstet Gynecol* 67:500–506, 1986.

79 Wahbeh CJ et al: Intra-amniotic bacterial colonization in premature labor. *Am J Obstet Gynecol* 148:739–743, 1984.

80 Gravett MG et al: Preterm labor associated with subclinical amniotic fluid infection and with bacterial vaginosis. *Obstet Gynecol* 67:229–237, 1986.

81 Bobitt JR et al: Amniotic fluid infection as determined by trans abdominal amniocentesis in patients with intact membranes in premature labor. *Am J Obstet Gynecol* 140:947–952, 1981.

82 Skoll MA et al: The incidence of positive amniotic fluid cultures in patients in preterm labor with intact membranes. *Am J Obstet Gynecol* 161:813–816, 1989.

83 Romero R et al: Infection and labor: V. Prevalence, microbiology, and clinical significance of intraamniotic infection in women with preterm labor and intact membranes. *Am J Obstet Gynecol* 161:317–324, 1989.

84 Harger JH et al: Low incidence of positive amniotic fluid cultures in preterm labor at 27–32 weeks in the absence of clinical evidence of chorioamnionitis. *Obstet Gynecol* 77:228–234, 1991.

85 Romero R et al: The diagnostic and prognostic value of amniotic fluid white blood cell count, glucose, interleukin-6, and gram stain in patients with preterm labor and intact membranes. *Am J Obstet Gynecol* 169:805–816, 1993.

86 Hillier SL et al: The relationship of amniotic fluid cytokines and prostaglandin E_2 with preterm delivery, anionic fluid infection, histologic chorioamnionitis and chorioamnion infection. *Obstet Gynecol* 81: 941–948, 1993.

87 Watts DH et al: The association of occult amniotic fluid infection with gestational age and neonatal outcome among women in preterm labor. *Obstet Gynecol* 79:351–357, 1992.

88 Romero R et al: Infection and labor: III. Interleukin-1: A signal for the onset of parturition. *Am J Obstet Gynecol* 160:1117–1123, 1989.

89 Romero R et al: Infection and labor: IV. Cachetin-tumor necrosis factor in the amniotic fluid of women with intraamniotic infection and preterm labor. *Am J Obstet Gynecol* 161:336–341, 1989.

90 Romero R et al: Tumor necrosis factor in preterm and term labor. *Am J Obstet Gynecol* 166:1576–1587, 1992.

91 Greig PC et al: Amniotic fluid interleukin-6 levels correlate with histologic chorioamnionitis and amniotic fluid cultures in patients in premature labor with intact membranes. *Am J Obstet Gynecol* 169: 1035–1044, 1993.

92 Matsuzaki N et al: Placental interleukin-6 production is enhanced in intrauterine infection but not in labor. *Am J Obstet Gynecol* 168: 94–97, 1993.

93 Lockwood CJ et al: Increased interleukin-6 concentrations in cervical secretions are associated with preterm delivery. *Am J Obstet Gynecol* 171:1097–1102, 1994.

94 Coultrip LL et al: The value of amniotic fluid interleukin-6 determination in patients with preterm labor and intact membranes in the detection of microbial invasion of the amniotic cavity. *Am J Obstet Gynecol* 171:901–911, 1994.

95 Inglis SR et al: Detection of tumor necrosis factor-alpha interleukin-6, and fetal fibronectin in the lower genital tract during pregnancy: Relation to outcome. *Am J Obstet Gynecol* 171:5–10, 1994.

96 Romero R et al: Systemic administration of interleukin-1 induces preterm parturition in mice. *Am J Obstet Gynecol* 165:969–971, 1991.

97 Romero R, Tartakousky B: The natural interleukin-1 receptor antagonist prevents interleukin-1-induced preterm delivery in mice. *Am J Obstet Gynecol* 167:1041–1045, 1992.

98 Romero R et al: Prostaglandin concentrations in amniotic fluid of women with intra-amniotic infection and preterm labor. *Am J Obstet Gynecol* 157:1461–1467, 1987.

99 Hitti J et al: Amniotic fluid tumor necrosis factor-alpha and risk of respiratory distress syndrome among preterm infants. *Am J Obstet Gynecol (in press)*.

100 Figueroa R et al: Elevated amniotic fluid interleukin-6 predicts neonatal periventricular leukomalacia and intraventricular hemorrhage. Abstract presented at the Society of Perinatal Obstetricians Annual Meeting, 1996.

101 Yoon BH et al: Amniotic fluid concentrations of interleukin-6 identify fetuses at risk for the development of periventricular leukomalacia. Abstract presented at the Society of Perinatal Obstetricians Annual Meeting, 1996.

102 Gravett MG et al: An experimental model for intraamniotic infection and preterm labor in rhesus monkeys. *Am J Obstet Gynecol* 171: 1660–1667, 1994.

103 Witkin SS et al: Induction of interleukin-1 receptor antagonist in rhesus monkeys after intraamniotic infection with group B streptococci or interleukin-1 infection. *Am J Obstet Gynecol* 171:1668–1672, 1994.

104 McGregor JA et al: Bacterial protease-induced reduction of chorioamniotic membrane strength and elasticity. *Obstet Gynecol* 69: 167–174, 1987.

105 Schoonmaker JN et al: Bacteria and inflammation cells reduce chorioamniotic membrane integrity and tensile strength. *Obstet Gynecol* 74:590–596, 1989.

106 Sbarra AJ et al: Effect of bacterial growth on the bursting pressure of fetal membranes in vitro. *Obstet Gynecol* 70:107–110, 1987.

107 Winkler M et al: Erythromycin therapy for subclinical intrauterine infections in threatened preterm delivery: A preliminary report. *J Perinat Med* 16:253–256, 1988.

108 Newton ER et al: A randomized, blinded, placebo-controlled trial of antibiotics in idiopathic preterm labor. *Obstet Gynecol* 74:562–566, 1989.

109 McGregor JA et al: Adjunctive clindamycin therapy for preterm labor: Results of a double-blind, placebo-controlled trial. *Am J Obstet Gynecol* 165:867–875, 1991.

110 Romero R et al: Antibiotic treatment of preterm labor with intact membranes: A multicenter, randomized, double-blinded, placebo-controlled trial. *Am J Obstet Gynecol* 169:764–774, 1993.

111 Watts DH et al: A randomized trial of antibiotics in addition to tocolytic therapy to treat preterm labor. *Infect Dis Obstet Gynecol* 1: 220–227, 1994.

112 Newton ER et al: Combination antibiotics and indomethacin in idiopathic preterm labor: A randomized double-blind clinical trial. *Am J Obstet Gynecol* 165:1753–1758, 1991.

113 Gordon M et al: A randomized, prospective study of adjunctive ceftizoxime in preterm labor. *Am J Obstet Gynecol* 172:1546–1552, 1995.

114 Cox SM et al: Randomized investigation of antimicrobials for the prevention of preterm birth. *Am J Obstet Gynecol* 174:206–210, 1996.

115 Blanco J et al: Multicenter, double-blind prospective random trial of ceftizoxime vs placebo in women with preterm premature rupture of membranes (PPROM). *Am J Obstet Gynecol* 168:378–382, 1993.

116 Johnston MM et al: Antibiotic therapy in preterm rupture of membranes: A randomized, prospective, double-blind trial. *Am J Obstet Gynecol* 163:743–747, 1990.

117 McGregor JA et al: Antimicrobial therapy in preterm premature rupture of membranes: Results of a prospective, double-blind, placebo-controlled trial of erythromycin. *Am J Obstet Gynecol* 165:632–640, 1991.

118 Mercer BM et al: Erythromycin therapy in preterm premature rupture of membranes: A prospective, randomized trial of 220 patients. *Am J Obstet Gynecol* 166:794–801, 1992.

119 Kurki T et al: Premature rupture of membranes: Effect of penicillin prophylaxis and long-term outcome of the children. *Am J Perinatol* 9:11–16, 1992.

120 Lockwood CJ et al: Double-blind, placebo-controlled trial of piperacillin prophylaxis in preterm membrane rupture. *Am J Obstet Gynecol* 169:970–976, 1993.

121 Ernest JM, Givner LB: A prospective, randomized, placebo-controlled trial of penicillin in preterm premature rupture of membranes. *Am J Obstet Gynecol* 1709:516–521, 1994.

122 Lockwood CJ et al: Fetal fibronectin in cervical and vaginal secretions as a predictor of preterm delivery. *N Engl J Med* 325:669–674, 1991.

123 Goldenberg RL et al: The preterm prediction study: Fetal fibronectin testing and spontaneous preterm birth. *Obstet Gynecol* 87:643–648, 1996.

124 Hellemans P, Verdonk P: Fetal fibronectin detection for prediction of preterm birth in low risk women. *Br J Obstet Gynecol* 102:207–212, 1995.

125 Goldenberg RL et al: The preterm prediction study: Fetal fibronectin, bacterial vaginosis, and peripartum infection. *Obstet Gynecol* 87: 656–660, 1996.

126 Leeson SC et al: Detection of fetal fibronectin as a predictor of preterm delivery in high risk asymptomatic pregnancies. *Br J Obstet Gynaecol* 103:48–53, 1996.

127 Bittar RE et al: Cervical fetal fibronectin in patients at increased risk for preterm delivery. *Am J Obstet Gynecol* 175:178–181, 1996.

128 Malak TM et al: Fetal fibronectin in cervicovaginal secretions as a predictor of preterm birth. *Br J Obstet Gynaecol* 103:648–653, 1996.

129 Bartnicki J et al: Fetal fibronectin in vaginal specimens predicts preterm delivery and very-low-birth-weight infants. *Am J Obstet Gynecol* 174:971–974, 1996.

130 Iams JD et al: Fetal fibronectin improves the accuracy of diagnosis of preterm labor. *Am J Obstet Gynecol* 173:141–145, 1995.

131 Iams JD et al: Cervical sonography in preterm labor. *Obstet Gynecol* 84:40–46, 1994.

132 Guzman ER et al: Sonography and transfundal pressure in the evaluation of the cervix during pregnancy. *Obstet Gynecol* 50:395–403, 1995.

133 American College of Obstetricians and Gynecologists Committee Opinion. American College of Obstetricians and Gynecologists, Washington DC, 1995.

134 Morrison JC et al: Prediction of spontaneous preterm birth by fetal fibronectin and uterine activity. *Obstet Gynecol* 87:649–655, 1996.

135 Hoyme UB et al: Microbiology and treatment of late postpartum endometritis. *Obstet Gynecol* 68:226–232, 1986.

136 Plummer FA et al: Postpartum upper genital tract infections in Nairobi, Kenya: Epidemiology, etiology and risk factors. *J Infect Dis* 156: 92, 1987.

137 Platt L et al: The role of anaerobic bacteria in postpartum endomyometritis. *Am J Obstet Gynecol* 135:814, 1979.

138 Platt R et al: Infection with *Mycoplasma hominis* in postpartum fever. *Lancet* 2:1217, 1980.

139 Harrison HR et al: Cervical *Chlamydia trachomatis* and mycoplasmal infections: Epidemiology and outcomes. *JAMA* 250:1721–1727, 1983.

140 Wallace RJ et al: Isolation of *Mycoplasma hominis* from blood cultures in patients with postpartum fever. *Obstet Gynecol* 51:181, 1978.

141 Watts DH et al: Early postpartum endometritis: The role of bacteria, genital mycoplasmas, and *Chlamydia trachomatis*. *Obstet Gynecol* 73:52–60, 1989.

142 Watts DH et al: Bacterial vaginosis as a risk factor for postcesarean endometritis. *Obstet Gynecol* 75:52–58, 1990.

143 Watts DH et al: Upper genital tract isolates at delivery as predictors of postcesarean infections among women receiving antibiotic prophylaxis. *Obstet Gynecol* 77:287–292, 1991.

144 Wager GP et al: Puerperal infectious morbidity: Relationship to route of delivery and to antepartum *Chlamydia trachomatis* infection. *Am J Obstet Gynecol* 138:1028, 1980.

145 Cates W et al: Worldwide patterns of infertility: Is Africa different? *Lancet* 2:596, 1985.

146 Hurry DJ et al: Effects of post cesarean section febrile morbidity on subsequent fertility. *Obstet Gynecol* 64:256–260, 1984.

147 Siegel JD, McCracken GH: Sepsis neonatorum. *N Engl J Med* 304: 642, 1981.

148 Nahmias AJ, Visinthine AM: Herpes simplex, in *Infectious Diseases of the Fetus and Newborn Infant,* JS Remington, JO Klein (eds). Philadelphia, Saunders, 1976, p 156.

149 Dippel AL: The relationship of congenital syphilis to abortion and miscarriage and the mechanisms of intrauterine protection. *Am J Obstet Gynecol* 47:369, 1944.

150 Naeye RL: Causes of perinatal mortality in the U.S. Collaborative Perinatal Project. *JAMA* 238:228, 1977.

151 Division of STD Surveillance: *Sexually Transmitted Disease Surveillance, 1995.* Atlanta, Centers fot Disease Control and Prevention, U.S. Department of Health and Human Service, Public Health Service, September 1996.

152 Chhabra RS et al: Comparison of maternal sera, cord blood and neonatal sera for detecting presumptive congenital syphilis: Relationship with maternal treatment. *Pediatrics* 91(1):88–91, 1993.

153 Klass PE et al: The incidence of prenatal syphilis at the Boston City Hospital: A comparison across four decades. *Pediatrics* 94:24–28, 1994.

154 Minkoff HL et al: The relationship of cocaine use to syphilis and human immunodeficiency virus infections among inner city parturient women. *Am J Obstet Gynecol* 163:521–526, 1990.

155 Brunham RC, Embree JE: Sexually transmitted diseases: Current and future dimensions of the problem in the third world, in *Reproductive Tract Infections: Global Impact and Priorities for Women's Reproductive Health,* A Germain et al (eds). New York, Plenum, 1992, pp 35–60.

156 Ratnam AV et al: Syphilis in pregnant women in Zambia. Presented at the First Sexually Transmitted Diseases World Congress, San Juan, Puerto Rico, 1981.

157 Fiumara NJ et al: The incidence of prenatal syphilis at the Boston City Hospital. *N Engl J Med* 247:48, 1952.

158 Mascuta L et al: Congenital syphilis: Why is it still occurring? *JAMA* 252:1719, 1984.

159 Wendel GD et al: Examination of amniotic fluid in diagnosing congenital syphilis with fetal death. *Obstet Gynecol* 74:967–970, 1989.

160 Brown WH, Pearce L: On the reaction of pregnant and lactating females to inoculation with *Treponema pallidum:* A preliminary note. *Am J Syph* 4:593, 1920.

161 Harter CA, Benirschke K: Fetal syphilis in the first trimester. *Am J Obstet Gynecol* 124:705, 1976.

162 Benirschke K: Syphilis: The placenta and the fetus. *Am J Dis Child* 128:142, 1974.

163 Silverstein AM: Congenital syphilis and the timing of immunogenesis in the human fetus. *Nature* 194:196, 1962.

164 Ricci JM et al: Congenital syphilis: The University of Miami/Jackson Memorial Medical Center experience, 1986–1988. *Obstet Gynecol* 74:687–693, 1989.

165 McFarlin BL et al: Epidemic syphilis: Maternal factors associated with congenital infection. *Am J Obstet Gynecol* 170:535–540, 1994.

166 Blount JH, Holmes KK: Epidemiology of syphilis and the nonvenereal treponematoses, in *The Biology of Parasitic Spirochetes,* RC Johnson (ed). New York, Academic, 1976, p 157.

167 Berkowitz K et al: False negative syphilis screening: The prozone phenomenon, non-immune hydrops and diagnosis of syphilis during pregnancy. *Am J Obstet Gynecol* 163:975, 1990.

168 Stray-Pederson B: Economic evaluation of maternal screening to prevent congenital syphilis. *Sex Transm Dis* 10:167, 1983.

169 Centers for Disease Control and Prevention: Guidelines for the prevention and control of congenital syphilis. *MMWR* 37(suppl l):l, 1988.

170 Klein VR et al: The Jarisch-Herxheimer reaction complicating syphilotherapy in pregnancy. *Obstet Gynecol* 75:375–380, 1990.

171 Centers for Disease Control and Prevention: 1993 Sexually transmitted diseases treatment guidelines. *MMWR* 42(RR 14):1–89, 1993.

172 Gadde J et al: Clinical experience with penicillin skin testing in a large inner-city STD clinic. *JAMA* 270:2456–2463, 1993.

173 Wendel GD Jr et al: Penicillin allergy and desensitization in serious infections during pregnancy. *N Engl J Med* 312:1229, 1985.

174 Thompson SE: Treatment of syphilis in pregnancy. *J Am Vener Dis Assoc* 3:159, 1976.

175 Rothenberg R: Ophthalmia neonatorum due to *Neisseria gonorrhoeae:* Prevention and treatment. *Sex Trans Dis* 6 (suppl 2):187, 1979.

176 Centers for Disease Control and Prevention: Declining rates of rectal and pharyngeal gonorrhea among men—New York City. *JAMA* 252:327, 1984.

177 Rice RJ et al: Gonorrhea in the United States 1975–1984: Is the giant only sleeping? *Sex Transm Dis* 14:83, 1987.

178 Goodrich JT: Treatment of gonorrhea in pregnancy. *Sex Transm Dis* 6:168, 1979.

179 Corman LC et al: The high frequency of pharyngeal gonococcal infection in a prenatal clinic population. *JAMA* 230:568, 1974.

180 Stutz DR et al: Oropharyngeal gonorrhea during pregnancy. *J Am Vener Dis Assoc* 3:65, 1976.

181 Holmes KK et al: Disseminated gonococcal infection. *Ann Intern Med* 74:979, 1971.

182 Platt R et al: Risk of acquiring gonorrhea and prevalence of abnormal adnexal findings among women recently exposed to gonorrhea. *JAMA* 23:3205, 1983.

183 Acosta AA et al: Intrauterine pregnancy and coexistent pelvic inflammatory disease. *Obstet Gynecol* 37:282, 1971.

184 Morse SA, Fitzgerald J: Effect of progesterone on *Neisseria gonorrhoeae. Infect Immun* 10:1370, 1974.

185 Moghissi KS: Cyclic changes of cervical mucus in normal and progestin-treated women. *Fertil Steril* 17:663, 1966.

186 Israel KS et al: Neonatal and childhood gonococcal infections. *Clin Obstet Gynecol* 18:143, 1975.

187 Amstey MS, Steadman KT: Asymptomatic gonorrhea and pregnancy. *J Am Vener Dis Assoc* 3:14, 1976.

188 Edwards L et al: Gonorrhea in pregnancy. *Am J Obstet Gynecol* 132: 637, 1978.

189 Stoll BJ et al: Treated maternal gonorrhea without adverse effect on outcome of pregnancy. *South Med J* 75:1236, 1982.

190 Donders GG et al: The association of gonorrhea and syphilis with premature birth and low birth weight. *Genitourin Med* 69:98–101, 1993.

191 Elliott B et al: Maternal gonococcal infection as a preventable risk factor for low birth weight. *J Infect Dis* 161:531–536, 1990.

192 Maxwell GL, Watson WJ: Preterm premature rupture of membranes: Results of expectant management in patients with cervical cultures positive for group B streptococcus or *Neisseria gonorrhoeae. Am J Obstet Gynecol* 166:945–949, 1992.

193 Charles AG et al: Asymptomatic gonorrhea in prenatal patients. *Am J Obstet Gynecol* 108:595, 1970

194 Alger LS et al: The association of *Chlamydia trachomatis, Neisseria gonorrhoeae,* and group B streptococci with preterm rupture of membranes and pregnancy outcome. *Am J Obstet Gynecol* 159:397–404, 1988.

195 Berstine JB, Bland GW: Gonorrhea complicating pregnancy and its relation to ophthalmia neonatorum. *Urol Cutan Rev* 52:464, 1948.

196 Burkman RT et al: Untreated endocervical gonorrhea and endometritis following elective abortion. *Am J Obstet Gynecol* 126:648, 1976.

197 Goddeiris JH, Bronken TP: Benefit-cost analysis of screening: A comparison of tests for gonorrhea. *Med Care* 23:1242, 1985.

198 Schachter J et al: Enzyme immunoassay for diagnosis of gonorrhea. *J Clin Microbiol* 19:57, 1984.

199 Thomason JL et al: Effectiveness of gonozyme for detection of gonorrhea in low-risk pregnant and gynecologic populations. *Sex Transm Dis* 16:28, 1989.

200 Thin RNT et al: Direct and delayed methods of immunofluorescent diagnosis of gonorrhea in women. *Br J Vener Dis* 47:27, 1971.

201 Panke ES et al: Comparison of Gen-Probe DNA probe test and culture for the detection of *Neisseria gonorrhoeae* in endocervical specimens. *J Clin Microbiol* 29:883, 1991.

202 Hosein IK et al: Detection of cervical *Chlamydia trachomatis* and *Neisseria gonorrhoeae* with deoxyribonucleic acid probe assays in obstetric patients. *Am J Obstet Gynecol* 167:588, 1992.

203 Lewis JS et al. Direct DNA probe assay for *Neisseria gonorrhoeae* in pharyngeal and rectal specimens. *J Clin Microbiol* 31:2783–2785, 1993.

204 Laga M et al: Epidemiology of ophthalmia neonatorum in Kenya. *Lancet* 2:1145, 1986.

205 Handsfield HH et al: Neonatal gonococcal infection: 1. Orogastric contamination with *Neisseria gonorrhoeae. JAMA* 225:697, 1973.

206 Rothbard MJ et al: Intrapartum gonococcal amnionitis. *Am J Obstet Gynecol* 121:565, 1975.

207 Armstrong JH et al: Ophthalmia neonatorum: A chart review. *Pediatrics* 57:884, 1976.

208 Thompson TR et al: Gonococcal ophthalmia neonatorum: Relationship of time of infection to relevant control measures. *JAMA* 228: 186, 1974.

209 Schoolnik GK et al: Immunoglobulin class responsible for gonococcal bactericidal activity of normal human sera. *J Immunol* 122:1771, 1979.

210 Laga M et al: Prophylaxis of gonococcal and chlamydial ophthalmia neonatorum: A comparison of silver nitrate and tetracycline. *N Engl J Med* 318:653, 1988.

211 Hammerschlag MR et al: Efficacy of neonatal ocular prophylaxis for the prevention of chlamydial and gonococcal conjunctivitis. *N Engl J Med* 320:769–772, 1989.

212 Centers for Disease Control and Prevention: Recommendations for the prevention and management of *Chlamydia trachomatis* infections. *MMWR* 42(RR-12):1–39, 1993.

213 Ferris DG, Litaker M: Chlamydial cervical infections in rural and urban pregnant women. *South Med J* 86:611–614, 1993.

214 Khurana CM et al: Prevalence of *Chlamydia trachomatis* in the pregnant cervix. *Obstet Gynecol* 66:241, 1985.

215 Harrison HR et al: The prevalence of genital *Chlamydia trachomatis* and mycoplasmal infections during pregnancy in an American Indian population. *Sex Transm Dis* 10:184, 1983.

216 Githin D: Development and metabolism of the immune globulins, in *Immunologic Incompetence,* B Kagen, ER Stiehm (eds). Chicago, Year Book Medical, 1971, p 3.

217 Rowland GF, Moss TR: In vitro fertilization, previous ectopic pregnancy, and *Chlamydia trachomatis* infection. *Lancet* 2:830, 1985.

218 Page LA, Smith PC: Placentitis and abortion in cattle inoculated with *Chlamydia* isolated from aborted human placental tissue. *Proc Soc Exp Biol Med* 146:269, 1974.

219 Schachter J: Isolation of *Bedsoniae* from human arthritis and abortion tissue. *Am J Ophthalmol* 63:1082, 1967.

220 Chandler JW et al: Ophthalmia neonatorum associated with maternal chlamydial infections. *Trans Am Acad Ophthalmol Otolaryngol* 83: 302, 1978.

221 Rowe DS et al: Purulent ocular discharge in neonates: Significance of *Chlamydia trachomatis*. *Pediatrics* 63:628, 1979.

222 Martin DH et al: Prematurity and perinatal mortality in pregnancies complicated by maternal *Chlamydia trachomatis* infections. *JAMA* 247:1585, 1982.

223 Thompson S et al: A prospective study of *Chlamydia* and *Mycoplasma* infection during pregnancy: Relation to pregnancy outcome and maternal morbidity, in *Chlamydial Infections,* March PA et al (eds). Amsterdam: Elsevier Biomedical, 1982.

224 Sweet RL et al: *Chlamydia trachomatis* infection and pregnancy outcome. *Am J Obstet Gynecol* 156:824, 1987.

225 Gravett MG et al: Independent associations of bacterial vaginosis and *Chlamydia trachomatis* infections with adverse pregnancy outcome. *JAMA* 256:1899, 1986.

226 Berman SM et al: Low birth weight, prematurity, and postpartum endometritis: Association with prenatal cervical *Mycoplasma hominis* and *Chlamydia trachomatis* infections. *JAMA* 257:1189, 1987.

227 Johns Hopkins Study of Cervicitis and Adverse Pregnancy Outcome: Association of *Chlamydia trachomatis* and *Mycoplasma hominis* with intrauterine growth retardation and preterm delivery. *Am J Epidemiol* 129:1247–1257, 1989.

228 Martius J et al: Relationship of vaginal *Lactobacillus* species, cervical *Chlamydia trachomatis,* and bacterial vaginosis to preterm birth. *Obstet Gynecol* 71:89, 1988.

229 Frommell GT et al: Chlamydial infection of mothers and their infants. *J Pediatr* 95:28, 1979.

230 Heggie AD et al: *Chlamydia trachomatis* infection in mothers and infants. *Am J Dis Child* 135:507, 1981.

231 Thygeson P, Stone W: Epidemiology of inclusion conjunctivitis. *Arch Ophthalmol* 27:91, 1992.

232 Rees E et al: Chlamydia in relation to cervical infection and pelvic inflammatory disease, in *Non-Gonococcal Urethritis and Rectal Infections,* K Hobson, KK Holmes (eds). Washington, American Society for Microbiology, 1977, p 140.

233 Qvigstad E et al: Therapeutic abortion and *Chlamydia trachomatis* infection. *Br J Vener Dis* 58:182, 1982.

234 Moller BR et al: Pelvic infection after elective abortion associated with *Chlamydia trachomatis*. *Obstet Gynecol* 59:210, 1982.

235 Osser S, Persson K: Postabortal pelvic infection associated with *Chlamydia trachomatis* and the influence of humoral immunity. *Am J Obstet Gynecol* 150:699, 1984.

236 Ferris DG, Martin WH: A comparison of three rapid chlamydial tests in pregnant and nonpregnant women. *J Fam Pract* 34:593–597, 1992.

237 Grossman JH III et al: Diagnosis of chlamydial infection in pregnant women using the testpack chlamydia diagnostic kit. *Obstet Gynecol* 77:801–803, 1991.

238 Grossman JH III et al: Pathfinder direct fluorescent antigen test for diagnosing maternal chlamydial infections: An evaluation. *J Reprod Med* 37:170–172, 1992.

239 Klufio CA et al: Endocervical *Chlamydia trachomatis* infection in pregnancy: Direct test and clinicosociodemographic survey of pregnant patients at the Port Moresby General Hospital antenatal clinic to determine prevalence and risk markers. *Aust NZ J Obstet Gynaecol* 32:43–46, 1992.

240 Bass CA et al: Clinical evaluation of a new polymerase chain reaction assay for detection of *Chlamydia trachomatis* in endocervical specimens. *J Clin Microbiol* 31:2648–2653, 1993.

241 Gann PH et al: Accuracy of *Chlamydia trachomatis* antigen detection methods in a low-prevalence population in a primary care setting. *J Clin Microbiol* 28:1580–1585, 1990.

242 Lee HH et al: Diagnosis of *Chlamydia trachomatis* genitourinary infection in women by ligase chain reaction assay of urine. *Lancet* 345: 213–216, 1995.

243 Mercer L et al: Test pack chlamydia for chlamydial detection in physicians' offices. *J Reprod Med* 35:1141–1144, 1990.

244 Skulnick M et al: Use of polymerase chain reaction for the detection of *Chlamydia trachomatis* from endocervical and urine specimens in an asymptomatic low-prevalence population of women. *Diagn Microbiol Infect Dis* 20:195–201, 1994.

245 Woods GL et al: Evaluation of a nonisotopic probe for detection of *Chlamydia trachomatis* in endocervical specimens. *J Clin Microbiol* 28:370–372, 1990.

246 Yang LI et al: Detection of *Chlamydia trachomatis* endocervical infection in asymptomatic and symptomatic women: Comparison of deoxyribonucleic acid probe test with tissue culture. *Am J Obstet Gynecol* 165:1444–1453, 1991.

247 Nugent RP, Hillier SL: Mucopurulent cervicitis as a predictor of chlamydial infection and adverse pregnancy outcome. *Sex Transm Dis* 19:198–202, 1992.

248 McCormack WM et al: Hepatoxicity of erythromycin estolate during pregnancy. *Antimicrob Agents Chemother* 12:630, 1977.

249 Schachter J et al: Experience with the routine use of erythromycin for chlamydial infections in pregnancy. *N Engl J Med* 314:276, 1986.

250 Magat AH et al: Double-blind randomized study comparing amoxicillin and erythromycin for the treatment of *Chlamydia trachomatis* in pregnancy. *Obstet Gynecol* 81:745–749, 1993.

251 Silverman NS et al: A randomized, prospective trial comparing amoxicillin and erythromycin for the treatment of *Chlamydia trachomatis* in pregnancy. *Am J Obstet Gynecol* 170:829–832, 1994.

252 Alary M et al: Randomized comparison of amoxycillin and erythromycin in treatment of genital chlamydial infection in pregnancy. *Lancet* 26:1461–1465, 1994.

253 Alger LS, Lovchik JC: Comparative efficacy of clindamycin versus erythromycin in eradication of antenatal *Chlamydia trachomatis*. *Am J Obstet Gynecol* 165:375–381, 1991.

254 Johnson RB: The role of azalide antibiotics in the treatment of chlamydia. *Am J Obstet Gynecol* 164:1794–1796, 1991.

255 Hammerschlag MR et al: Erythromycin ointment for ocular prophylaxis of neonatal chlamydial infections. *JAMA* 244:2291, 1980.

256 Bell TA et al: Comparison of ophthalmic silver nitrate solution and erythromycin ointment for prevention of natally acquired *Chlamydia trachomatis*. *Sex Transm Dis* 14:195, 1987.

257 Datta P et al: Infection and disease after perinatal exposure to *Chlamydia trachomatis* in Nairobi, Kenya. *J Infect Dis* 158:524–528, 1988.

258 Foy HM et al: Isolation of *Mycoplasma hominis,* T-strains and cytomegalovirus from the cervix of pregnant women. *Am J Obstet Gynecol* 106:635–638, 1970.

259 Dimusto JC et al: *Mycoplasma hominis* type I infection and pregnancy. *Obstet Gynecol* 41:33, 1973.

260 Harwick HJ et al: *Mycoplasma hominis* and abortion. *J Infect Dis* 121:260, 1970.

261 Caspi E et al: Early abortion and mycoplasma infection. *Isr J Med Sci* 8:122, 1972.

262 Sompolinsky D et al: Infection with *Mycoplasma* and bacteria in induced midtrimester abortion and fetal loss. *Am J Obstet Gynecol* 121:610, 1975.

263 Joste NE et al: Histology and *Ureaplasma urealyticum* culture in 63 cases of first trimester abortion. *Am J Clin Pathol* 102:729–732, 1994.

264 Stray-Pedersen B et al: Uterine T-mycoplasma colonization in reproductive failure. *Am J Obstet Gynecol* 130:307, 1978.

265 Quinn PA et al: Efficacy of antibiotic therapy in preventing spontaneous pregnancy loss among couples colonized with genital mycoplasmas. *Am J Obstet Gynecol* 145:239, 1983.

266 Hay PE et al: A longitudinal study of bacterial vaginosis during pregnancy. *Br J Obstet Gynecol* 101:1048–1053, 1994.

267 Hillier SL et al: Microbiologic efficacy of intravaginal clindamycin cream for the treatment of bacterial vaginosis. *Obstet Gynecol* 76(1): 407–413, 1990.

268 Carey JC et al: Antepartum cultures for *Ureaplasma urealyticum* are not useful in predicting pregnancy outcome. *Am J Obstet Gynecol* 164:728–733, 1991.

269 Braun P et al: Birthweight and genital mycoplasmas in pregnancy. *N Engl J Med* 284:167–171, 1971.
270 Harrison RF et al: Genital mycoplasmas and birth weight in offspring of primigravid women. *Am J Obstet Gynecol* 133:201–203, 1979.
271 Ross JM et al: The effect of genital mycoplasmas on human fetal growth. *Br J Obstet Gynaecol* 88:749–755, 1981.
272 Upadhyaya M et al: The role of mycoplasmas in reproduction. *Fertil Steril* 39:814–818, 1983.
273 Minkoff H et al: Risk factors for prematurity and premature rupture of membranes: A prospective study of vaginal flora in pregnancy. *Am J Obstet Gynecol* 150:965–972, 1984.
274 McGregor JA et al: Cervicovaginal microflora and pregnancy outcome: Results of a double-blind, placebo-controlled trial of erythromycin treatment. *Am J Obstet Gynecol* 163:1580–1591, 1990.
275 McGregor JA, French JI: *Chlamydia trachomatis* infection during pregnancy. *Am J Obstet Gynecol* 164:1782–1789, 1991.
276 Luton D et al: Prevalence and influence of *Mycoplasma hominis* and *Ureaplasma urealyticum* in 218 African pregnant women and their infants. *Eur J Obstet Gynaecol Reprod Biol* 56:95–101, 1994.
277 Choudhury MR et al: Prevalence of genital *Mycoplasma* and *Ureaplasma* infections in pregnancy and their effect on pregnancy outcome. *Ind J Med Res* 100:15–18, 1994.
278 McCormack WM et al: Effect on birth weight of erythromycin treatment of pregnant women. *Obstet Gynecol* 213:202, 1987.
279 Eschenbach DA et al: A randomized placebo-controlled trial of erythromycin for the treatment of *Ureaplasma urealyticum* to prevent premature delivery. *Am J Obstet Gynecol* 164:734–742, 1991.
280 Romero R et al: Eradication of *Ureaplasma urealyticum* from the amniotic fluid with transplacental antibiotic treatment. *Am J Obstet Gynecol* 166:618–620, 1992.
281 Cassell GH et al: *Ureaplasma urealyticum* intrauterine infection: Role in prematurity and disease in newborns. *Clin Microbiol Rev* 6:69–87, 1993.
282 Hillier SL et al: The role of bacterial vaginosis and vaginal bacteria in amniotic fluid infection in women in preterm labor with intact fetal membranes. *Clin Infect Dis* 20(suppl 2):S276-S278, 1995.
283 Paavonen J et al: Prevalence of nonspecific vaginitis and other cervicovaginal infections during the third trimester of pregnancy. *Sex Transm Dis* 13:5, 1986.
284 Hillier SL et al: Characteristics of three vaginal flora patterns assessed by gram stain among pregnant women. Vaginal Infections and Prematurity Study Group. *Am J Obstet Gynecol* 166:938–944, 1992.
285 Larsson P-G et al: *Mobiluncus* and clue cells as predictors for PID after first trimester abortion. *Acta Obstet Gynaecol Scand* 68:217–220, 1989.
286 Silver HM et al: Evidence relating bacterial vaginosis to intraamniotic infection. *Am J Obstet Gynecol* 161:808–812, 1989.
287 Emmons SL et al: Development of wound infections among women undergoing cesarean section. *Obstet Gynecol* 72:559–564, 1988.
288 Kurki T et al: Bacterial vaginosis in early pregnancy and pregnancy outcome. *Obstet Gynecol* 80:173–177, 1992.
289 Riduan JM et al: Bacterial vaginosis and prematurity in Indonesia: Association in early and late pregnancy. *Am J Obstet Gynecol* 169: 175–178, 1993.
290 McGregor JA et al: Bacterial vaginosis is associated with prematurity and vaginal fluid mucinase and sialidase: Results of a controlled trial of topical clindamycin cream. *Am J Obstet Gynecol* 170:1048–1060, 1994.
291 McGregor JA et al: Prevention of premature birth by screening and treatment for common genital tract infections: Results of a prospective controlled evaluation. *Am J Obstet Gynecol* 173:157–167, 1995.
292 Hillier SL et al: Association between bacterial vaginosis and preterm delivery of a low-birth-weight infant. The Vaginal Infections and Prematurity Study Group. *N Engl J Med* 333:1737–1742, 1995.
293 McGregor JA et al: Antenatal microbiologic and maternal risk factors associated with prematurity. *Am J Obstet Gynecol* 163:1465–1473, 1990.
294 Holst E et al: Bacterial vaginosis and vaginal microorganisms in idiopathic premature labor and association with pregnancy outcome. *J Clin Microbiol* 32:176–186, 1994.
295 Morales WJ et al: Effect of metronidazole in patients with preterm birth in preceding pregnancy and bacterial vaginosis: A placebo-controlled, double-blind study. *Am J Obstet Gynecol* 171:345–349, 1994.
296 Joesoef MR et al: Intravaginal clindamycin treatment for bacterial vaginosis: Effects on preterm delivery and low birth weight. *Am J Obstet Gynecol* 173:1527–1531, 1995.
297 Hauth JC et al: Reduced incidence of preterm delivery with metronidazole and erythromycin in women with bacterial vaginosis. *N Engl J Med* 333:1732–1736, 1995.
298 Platt MS: Neonatal *Haemophilus vaginalis* infection. *Clin Pediatr* 10: 513, 1971.
299 Chow AW et al: The significance of anaerobes in neonatal bacteremia: Analysis of 23 cases and review of the literature. *Pediatrics* 54: 736, 1974.
300 Nugent RP et al: Reliability of diagnosing bacterial vaginosis is improved by a standardized method of gram stain interpretation. *J Clin Microbiol* 29:297–301, 1991.
301 Hillier SL et al: Efficacy of intravaginal 0.75% metronidazole gel for the treatment of bacterial vaginosis. *Obstet Gynecol* 81:963–967, 1993.
302 Cotch MF et al: Demographic and behavioral predictors of *Trichomonas vaginalis* infections among pregnant women. *Obstet Gynecol* 78:1087–1092, 1991.
303 Hardy PH et al: Prevalence of six sexually transmitted disease agents among pregnant inner-city adolescents and pregnancy outcome. *Lancet* 2:333–337, 1984.
304 Meis PJ et al: The preterm prediction study: Significance of vaginal infections. *Am J Obstet Gynecol* 173:1231–1235, 1995.
305 Cotch MF et al: *Trichomonas vaginalis* associated with low birth weight and preterm delivery. *Sex Transm Dis* 24:1–8, 1997.
306 Grice AC: Vaginal infection causing spontaneous rupture of the membranes and premature delivery. *Aust NZ J Obstet Gynaecol* 14:156–158, 1974.
307 Bland PB et al: Vaginal trichomoniasis in the pregnant woman. *JAMA* 96:157, 1931.
308 Draper D et al: *Trichomonas vaginalis* weakens human amnio chorion in an in vitro model of premature membrane rupture. *Infect Dis Obstet Gynecol* 2:267–274, 1995.
309 Trussell RE et al: Vaginal trichomoniasis: Complement fixation, puerperal morbidity, and early infection of newborn infants. *Am J Obstet Gynecol* 44:292, 1942.
310 Bramley M: Study of female babies of women entering confinement with vaginal trichomoniasis. *Br J Vener Dis* 52:58, 1976.
311 Fouts AC, Kraus SJ: *Trichomonas vaginalis:* Reevaluation of its clinical presentation and laboratory diagnosis. *J Infect Dis* 141:137, 1980.
312 Krieger JN et al: Diagnosis of trichomoniasis: Comparison of conventional wet-mount examination with cytologic studies, cultures, and monoclonal antibody staining of direct specimens. *JAMA* 259: 1223–1227, 1988.
313 Goldman P: Metronidazole. *N Engl J Med* 303:1212, 1980.
314 Burtin P et al: Safety of metronidazole in pregnancy: A meta-analysis. *Am J Obstet Gynecol* 172:525–529, 1995.
315 Stagno S et al: Cervical cytomegalovirus excretion in pregnant and nonpregnant women: Suppression in early gestation. *J Infect Dis* 131: 522, 1975.
316 Knox GG et al: Alteration of the growth of cytomegalovirus and herpes simplex virus type I by epidermal growth factor, a contaminant of crude human chorionic gonadotropin preparation. *J Clin Invest* 61:1635, 1978.
317 Reynolds DW et al: Maternal cytomegalovirus infection and perinatal infection. *N Engl J Med* 289:1, 1973.
318 Stagno S et al: Congenital cytomegalovirus infection: The relative importance of primary and recurrent maternal infection. *N Engl J Med* 306:945, 1982.

319 Stagno S et al: Primary cytomegalovirus infection in pregnancy: Incidence, transmission to fetus, and clinical outcome. *JAMA* 256: 1904, 1986.

320 Monif GRG et al: The correlation of maternal cytomegalovirus infection during varying stages in gestation with neonatal involvement. *J Pediatr* 80:17, 1972.

321 Stern H, Tucker SM: Prospective study of cytomegalovirus infection in pregnancy. *Br Med J* 2:268, 1973.

322 Griffiths PD et al: A prospective study of primary cytomegalovirus infection in pregnant women. *Br J Obstet Gynaecol* 87:308, 1980.

323 Stagno S et al: Breast milk and risk of cytomegalovirus infection. *N Engl J Med* 302:1073, 1980.

324 Starr JG et al: Inapparent congenital cytomegalovirus infection: Clinical and epidemiologic characteristics in early infancy. *N Engl J Med* 282:1075, 1970.

325 Starr JG: Cytomegalovirus infection in pregnancy. *N Engl J Med* 282: 50, 1970.

326 Walters BNJ, Redman CWG: Bell's palsy and cytomegalovirus mononucleosis in pregnancy. *J R Soc Med* 77:429, 1984.

327 Twickler DM et al: Congenital cytomegalovirus infection presenting as cerebral ventriculomegaly on antenatal sonography. *Am J Perinatol* 10(5):404–406, 1993.

328 Fakhry J, Khoury A: Fetal intracranial calcifications: The importance of periventricular hyperechoic foci without shadowing. *J Ultrastruct Med* 10:51–54, 1991.

329 Achiron R et al: Prenatal ultrasonographic diagnosis of fetal cerebral ventriculitis associated with asymptomatic maternal cytomegalovirus infection. *Prenat Diagn* 14:523–526, 1994.

330 Dechelotte PJ et al: Pseudo-meconium ileus due to cytomegalovirus infection: A report of three cases. *Pediatr Pathol* 12:73–82, 1992.

331 Paavonen J et al: Colposcopic manifestations of cervical and vaginal infections. *Obstet Gynecol Surv* 43:373, 1988.

332 Mostocefi-Zadeh M et al: Placental evidence of cytomegalovirus infection of the fetus and neonate. *Arch Pathol Lab Med* 108:403, 1984.

333 Donner C et al: Prenatal diagnosis of 52 pregnancies at risk for congenital cytomegalovirus infection. *Obstet Gynecol* 82:481–486, 1993.

334 Fowler KB et al: The outcome of congenital cytomegalovirus infection in relation to maternal antibody status. *N Engl J Med* 326:663–667, 1992.

335 Pass RF et al: Outcome of symptomatic congenital cytomegalovirus infection: Results of long-term longitudinal follow-up. *Pediatrics* 66: 758, 1980.

336 Stagno S et al: Congenital cytomegalovirus infection: Occurrence in an immune population. *N Engl J Med* 296:1254, 1977.

337 Stern H et al: An early marker of fetal infection after primary cytomegalovirus infection in pregnancy. *Br Med J* 292:718, 1986.

338 Pass RF et al: Increased rate of cytomegalovirus infection among day care center workers. *Pediatr Infect Dis J* 9:465–470, 1990.

339 Demmler GJ et al: Enzyme-linked immunosorbent assay for the detection of IgM-class antibodies to cytomegalovirus. *J Infect Dis* 153: 1152–1155, 1986.

340 Catanzarite V, Dankner WM: Prenatal diagnosis of congenital cytomegalovirus infection: False-negative amniocentesis at 20 weeks' gestation. *Prenat Diagn* 13:1021–1025, 1993.

341 Donner C et al: Accuracy of amniotic fluid testing before 21 weeks' gestation in prenatal diagnosis of congenital cytomegalovirus infection. *Prenat Diagn* 14:1055–1059, 1994.

342 Hogge WA et al: Prenatal diagnosis of cytomegalovirus (CMV) infection: A preliminary report. *Prenat Diagn* 13:131–136, 1993.

343 Watt-Morse ML et al: The natural history of fetal cytomegalovirus infection as assessed by serial ultrasound and fetal blood sampling: A case report. *Prenat Diagn* 15:567–570, 1995.

344 Weiner CP, Grose C: Prenatal diagnosis of congenital cytomegalovirus infection by virus isolation from amniotic fluid. *Am J Obstet Gynecol* 163:1253–1255, 1990.

345 Schwebke K et al: Congenital cytomegalovirus infection as a result of nonprimary cytomegalovirus disease in a mother with acquired immunodeficiency syndrome. *J Pediatr* 126:293–295, 1995.

346 Laifer SA et al: Congenital cytomegalovirus infection in offspring of liver transplant recipients. *Clin Infect Dis* 20:52–55, 1995.

347 Division of STD Prevention: *Sexually Transmitted Disease Surveillance, 1995.* Atlanta, Centers for Disease Control and Prevention, U.S. Department of Health and Human Services, Public Health Service, September 1996.

348 Sullivan-Bolyai J et al: Neonatal herpes simplex virus infection in King County, Washington: Increasing incidence and epidemiologic correlates. *JAMA* 250:3059, 1983.

349 Johnson RE et al: A seroepidemiologic survey of the prevalence of herpes simplex virus type 2 infection in the United States. *N Engl J Med* 321:7–12, 1989.

350 Siegel D et al: Prevalence and correlates of herpes simplex infections. *JAMA* 268:1702–1708, 1992.

351 Boucher FD et al: A prospective evaluation of primary genital herpes simplex virus type 2 infections acquired during pregnancy. *Pediatr Infect Dis J* 9:499–504, 1990.

352 Frenkel LM et al: Clinical reactivation of herpes simplex virus type 2 infection in seropositive pregnant women with no history of genital herpes. *Ann Intern Med* 118:414–418, 1993.

353 Brown ZA et al: A comparison between detailed and simple histories in the diagnosis of genital herpes complicating pregnancy. *Am J Obstet Gynecol* 172:1299–1303, 1995.

354 Whitley RJ et al: The natural history of herpes simplex virus infection of mother and newborn. *Pediatrics* 66:489, 1980.

355 Hensleigh P et al: Genital herpes during pregnancy: Inability to distinguish primary and recurrent infections clinically. *Obstet Gynecol* 89:891–895, 1997.

356 Brown ZA et al: HSV seroconversion during pregnancy: Its frequency and impact on pregnancy outcome. *N Engl J Med (in press).*

357 Whitley R et al: A controlled trial comparing vidarabine with acyclovir in neonatal herpes simplex virus infection. *N Engl J Med* 324: 444–449, 1991.

358 Nahmias AJ et al: Perinatal risk associated with maternal genital herpes simplex virus infection. *Am J Obstet Gynecol* 100:825, 1971.

359 Brown ZA et al: Effects on infants of a first episode of genital herpes during pregnancy. *N Engl J Med* 317:1246–1251, 1987.

360 Brown ZA et al: Asymptomatic maternal shedding of herpes simplex virus at the onset of labor: Relationship to preterm labor. *Obstet Gynecol* 87:483–8, 1996.

361 Brown ZA et al: Genital herpes in pregnancy: Risk factors associated with recurrences and asymptomatic viral shedding. *Am J Obstet Gynecol* 153:24–30, 1985.

362 Vontver L et al: Recurrent genital herpes simplex virus infections in pregnancy: Infant outcome and frequency of asymptomatic recurrences. *Am J Obstet Gynecol* 143:75, 351.

363 Boggess K et al: HSV-2 detection by culture and polymerase chain reaction and relationship to genital symptoms and cervical antibody status during the third trimester of pregnancy. *Am J Obstet Gynecol* 176:443–51, 1997.

364 Prober CG et al: Low risk of herpes simplex virus infection in neonates exposed to the virus at the time of vaginal delivery to mothers with recurrent genital herpes simplex virus infection. *N Engl J Med* 316:240, 1987.

365 Arvin A et al: Failure of antepartum maternal cultures to predict the infant's risk of exposure to herpes simplex virus at delivery. *N Engl J Med* 315:796–800, 1986.

366 Brown ZA et al: Neonatal herpes simplex virus infection in relation to asymptomatic maternal infection at the time of labor. *N Engl J Med* 324:1247–1252, 1991.

367 Catalano PM et al: Incidence of genital herpes simplex virus at the time of delivery in women with known risk factors. *Am J Obstet Gynecol* 164:1303–1306, 1991.

368 Binkin N et al: Preventing neonatal herpes: The value of weekly viral cultures in pregnant women with recurrent genital herpes. *JAMA* 251:2816, 1984.

369 Prober CG et al: The management of pregnancies complicated by genital infections with herpes simplex virus. *Clin Infect Dis* 15:1031–1038, 1992.

370 Hardy DA et al: Use of polymerase chain reaction for successful identification of asymptomatic genital infection with herpes simplex virus in pregnant women at delivery. *J Infect Dis* 162:1031–1035, 1990.
371 Cone RW et al: Frequent detection of genital herpes simplex virus DNA by polymerase chain reaction among pregnant women. *JAMA* 272:792–796, 1994.
372 American Academy of Pediatrics: Perinatal herpes simplex virus infections. *Pediatrics* 66:147, 1980.
373 Gibbs RS: Infection control of herpes simplex virus infections in obstetrics and gynecology. *J Reprod Med* 31:395, 1986.
374 Cox SM et al: Treatment of disseminated herpes simplex virus in pregnancy with parenteral acyclovir: A case report. *J Reprod Med* 31:1005, 1986.
375 Stray-Pedersen B: Acyclovir in late pregnancy to prevent neonatal herpes simplex (letter). *Lancet* 336:756, 1990.
376 Scott LL et al: Acyclovir suppression to prevent cesarean delivery after first-episode genital herpes. *Obstet Gynecol* 87:69–73, 1996.
377 Haddad J et al: Oral acyclovir and recurrent genital herpes during late pregnancy. *Obstet Gynecol* 82:102–104, 1993.
378 Straus SE et al: Effect of oral acyclovir treatment on symptomatic and asymptomatic virus shedding in recurrent genital herpes. *Sex Transm Dis* 16:107–113, 1989.
379 Centers for Disease Control and Prevention: Condyloma acuminatum—United States, 1966–1981. *MMWR* 32:306, 1983.
380 Cohen SR et al: Papilloma of the larynx and tracheobronchial tree in children: A retrospective study. *Ann Otol Rhinol Laryngol* 89:497, 1980.
381 Gissmann L et al: Human papillomavirus types 6 and 11 DNA sequences in genital and laryngeal papillomas and in some cervical cancers. *Proc Natl Acad Sci USA* 80:560, 1983.
382 Steinberg BM et al: Laryngeal papilloma virus infection during clinical remission. *N Engl J Med* 308:1261, 1983.
383 Haliden C, Maimundar B: The relationship between juvenile laryngeal papillomatosis and maternal condylomata acuminata. *J Reprod Med* 31:804, 1986.
384 Shah K et al: Rarity of cesarean delivery in cases of juvenile-onset respiratory papillomatosis. *Obstet Gynecol* 68:795, 1986.
385 DeJong A et al: Condyloma acuminata in children. *Am J Dis Child* 136:704, 1982.
386 Roman A, Fife K: Human papillomavirus DNA associated with foreskins of normal newborns. *J Infect Dis* 153:855, 1986.
387 Sedlacek TV et al: Mechanism for human papillomavirus transmission at birth. *Am J Obstet Gynecol* 161:55–59, 1989.
388 Fredericks BD et al: Transmission of human papillomavirus from mother to child. *Aust NZ J Obstet Gynaecol* 33:30–32, 1993.
389 Pakarian F et al: Cancer associated human papillomaviruses: Perinatal transmission and persistence. *Br J Obstet Gynaecol* 101:514–517, 1994.
390 Smith EM et al: Perinatal transmission and maternal risks of human papillomavirus infection. *Cancer Detect Prev* 19:196–205, 1995.
391 St Louis ME et al: Genital types of papillomavirus in children of women with HIV-1 infection in Kinshasa, Zaire. *Int J Cancer* 54: 181–184, 1993.
392 Puranen M et al: Vertical transmission of human papillomavirus from infected mothers to their newborn babies and persistence of the virus in childhood. *Am J Obstet Gynecol* 174:694–699, 1996.
393 Cason J et al: Perinatal infection and persistence of human papillomavirus types 16 and 18 in infants. *J Med Virol* 47:209–218, 1995.
394 Watts DH et al: Risk of perinatal transmission of human papillomavirus (HPV) is low: Results from a prospective cohort study. *Am J Obstet Gynecol (In press).*
395 Ferenczy A: Treating genital condyloma during pregnancy with the carbon dioxide laser. *Am J Obstet Gynecol* 148:9, 1984.
396 Chamberlain MJ et al: Toxic effect of podophyllum application in pregnancy. *Br Med J* 1:391, 1972.
397 Hepatitis in pregnancy. *ACOG Technical Bulletin,* November 1992.
398 Greenspoon JS et al: Necessity for routine obstetric screening for hepatitis B surface antigen. *J Reprod Med* 34:665–668, 1989.
399 Sweet RL: Hepatitis B infection in pregnancy. *Obstet Gynecol Rep* 2:128–139, 1990.
400 Margolis HS et al: Hepatitis B: Evolving epidemiology and implications for control. *Semin Liver Dis* 11:84–97, 1991.
401 Beasley RP et al: Efficacy of hepatitis B immunoglobulin for prevention of perinatal transmission of the hepatitis B virus: Final report of a randomized double-blind, placebo-controlled trial. *Hepatology* 3: 135–141, 1983.
402 Zu ZY et al: Prevention of perinatal acquisition of hepatitis B virus carriage using vaccine: Preliminary report of a randomized double-blind placebo-controlled and comparative trial. *Pediatrics* 76:713–718, 1985.
403 Margolis HS et al: Prevention of hepatitis B virus transmission by immunization. *JAMA* 274:1201–1208, 1995.
404 Centers for Disease Control and Prevention: Hepatitis B virus: A comprehensive strategy for eliminating transmission in the United States through universal childhood vaccination: Recommendations of the Immunization Practices Advisory Committee (ACIP). *MMWR* 40(RR-13):1–20, 1990.
405 Holmes KK, Kreiss J: Heterosexual transmission of human immunodeficiency virus: Overview of a neglected aspect of the AIDS epidemic. *J AIDS* 1:602, 1989.
406 Gwinn M et al: Prevalence of HIV infection in childbearing women in the United States. *JAMA* 265:1704–1708, 1991.
407a Centers for Disease Control and Prevention: U.S. Public Health Service recommendations for human immunodeficiency virus counseling and voluntary testing for pregnant women. *MMWR* 44:1–15, 1995.
407b Fiscus SA et al. Perinatal HIV infection and the effect of zidovudine therapy on transmission in rural and urban counties. *JAMA* 275: 1483–8, 1996.
408 Berrebi A et al: Influence of pregnancy on human immunodeficiency virus disease. *Eur J Obstet Gynaecol Reprod Biol* 37:211–217, 1990.
409 Johnstone FD et al: Survival time of AIDS in pregnancy. *Br J Obstet Gynaecol* 99:633–636, 1992.
410 Deschamps MM et al: A prospective study of HIV-seropositive asymptomatic women of childbearing age in a developing country. *J Acquir Immun Defic Syndr* 6:446–451, 1993.
411 Centers for Disease Control and Prevention: USPHS/IDSA guidelines for the prevention of opportunistic infections in persons infected with human immunodeficiency virus: A summary. *MMWR* 44:5–22, 1995.
412 Cruikshank DP, Hayes PM: Maternal physiology in pregnancy, in *Obstetrics: Normal and Problem Pregnancies,* SG Gabbe et al (eds). New York, Churchill-Livingstone, 1991, pp 125–146.
413 Paz I et al: Maternal transmission of human immunodeficiency virus-1. *Obstet Gynecol Surv* 49:577–584, 1994.
414 Ryder RN et al: Perinatal transmission of the human immunodeficiency virus type 1 to infants of seropositive women in Zaire. *N Engl J Med* 320:1637–1642, 1989.
415 European Collaborative Study: Risk factors for mother-to-child transmission of HIV-1. *Lancet* 339:1007–1012, 1992.
416 Tibaldi C et al: Asymptomatic women at high risk of vertical HIV-1 transmission to their fetuses. *Br J Obstet Gynaecol* 100:334–337, 1993.
417 St Louis ME et al: Risk for perinatal HIV-1 transmission according to maternal immunologic, virologic, and placental factors. *JAMA* 269:2853–2859, 1993.
418 Hague RA et al: Maternal factors in HIV transmission. *Int J STD & AIDS* 4:142–146, 1993.
419 Burns DN et al: Cigarette smoking, premature rupture of membranes, and vertical transmission of HIV-1 among women with low CD4+ levels. *J Acquir Immun Defic Syndr* 7:718–726, 1994.
420 Thomas PA et al: Maternal predictors of perinatal human immunodeficiency virus transmission. *Pediatr Infect Dis J* 13:489–495, 1994.

421 Bredberg-Raden U et al: Predictive markers for mother-to-child transmission of HIV-1 in Dar es Salaam, Tanzania. *J Acquir Immun Defic Syndr* 8:182–187, 1995.

422 Mayaux M-J et al: Maternal factors associated with perinatal HIV-1 transmission: The French cohort study: 7 years of follow-up observation. *J Acquir Immun Defic Syndr* 8:188–194, 1995.

423 Temmerman M et al: Risk factors for mother-to-child transmission of human immunodeficiency virus-1 infection. *Am J Obstet Gynecol* 172:700–705, 1995.

424 Boyer PJ et al: Factors predictive of maternal-fetal transmission of HIV-1. *JAMA* 271:1925–1930, 1994.

425 Khouri YF et al: Vertical transmission of HIV-1: Correlation with maternal viral load and plasma levels of CD4 binding site anti-gp120 antibodies. *J Clin Invest* 95:732–737, 1995.

426 Roques P et al: Correlation between HIV provirus burden and *in utero* transmission. *AIDS* 7:S39–S43, 1993.

427 Lallemant M et al: Mother-to-child transmission of HIV-1 in Congo, central Africa. *AIDS* 8:1451–1456, 1994.

428 Goedert JJ et al: Mother-to-infant transmission of human immunodeficiency virus type 1: Association with prematurity or low anti-GP 120. *Lancet* 2:1351–1354, 1989.

429 Datta P et al: Mother-to-child transmission of human immunodeficiency virus type 1: Report from the Nairobi study. *J Infect Dis* 170: 1134–1140, 1994.

430 Semba RD et al: Maternal vitamin A deficiency and mother-to-child transmission of HIV-1. *Lancet* 343:1593–1597, 1994.

431 Minkoff H et al: The relationship of the duration of ruptured membranes to vertical transmission of human immunodeficiency virus. *Am J Obstet Gynecol* 173:585–589, 1995.

432 Husson RN et al: Vertical transmission of human immunodeficiency virus type 1: Autologous neutralizing antibody, virus load, and virus phenotype. *J Pediatr* 126:865–871, 1995.

433 Kliks SC et al: Features of HIV-1 that could influence maternal-child transmission. *JAMA* 272:467–474, 1994.

434 Ometto L et al: Viral phenotype and host-cell susceptibility to HIV-1 infection as risk factors for mother-to-child HIV-1 transmission. *AIDS* 9:427–434, 1995.

435 Devash Y et al: Vertical transmission of human immunodeficiency virus is correlated with the absence of high-affinity/avidity maternal antibodies to the gp120 principal neutralizing domain. *Proc Natl Acad Sci USA* 87:3445–3449, 1990.

436 Lallemant M et al: Maternal antibody response at delivery and perinatal transmission of human immunodeficiency virus type 1 in African women. *Lancet* 343:1001–1005, 1994.

437 Markham RB et al: Maternal IgG1 and IgA antibody to V3 loop census sequence and maternal-infant HIV-1 transmission. *Lancet* 343:390–391, 1994.

438 Robertson CA et al: Maternal antibodies to gp120 V3 sequence do not correlate with protection against vertical transmission of human immunodeficiency virus. *J Infect Dis* 166:704–709, 1992.

439 Rossi P et al: Presence of maternal antibodies to human immunodeficiency virus 1 envelope glycoprotein gp120 epitopes correlates with the uninfected status of children born to seropositive mothers. *Proc Natl Acad Sci USA* 86:8055–8058, 1989.

440 Connor EM et al: Reduction of maternal-infant transmission of human immunodeficiency virus type 1 with zidovudine treatment. Pediatric AIDS Clinical Trials Group Protocol 076 Study Group. *N Engl J Med* 331:1173–1180, 1994.

441 Matheson PB et al: Efficacy of antenatal zidovudine in reducing perinatal transmission of human immunodeficiency virus type 1 (HIV). *J Infect Dis* 172:353–358, 1995.

442 Frenkel LM et al: Effects of zidovudine use during pregnancy on resistance and vertical transmission of human immunodeficiency virus type 1. *Clin Infect Dis* 20:1321–1326, 1995.

443 Goedert JJ et al: High risk of HIV-1 infection for first-born twins. *Lancet* 338:1471–1475, 1991.

444 Duliege AM et al: Birth order, delivery route, and concordance in the transmission of human immunodeficiency virus type 1 from mothers to twins. International Registry of HIV-Exposed Twins. *J Pediatr* 126:625–632, 1995.

445 Nair P et al: Maternal and neonatal characteristics associated with HIV infection in infants of seropositive women. *J Acquir Immun Defic Syndr* 6:298–302, 1993.

446 European Collaborative Study: Cesarean section and risk of vertical transmission of HIV-1 infection. *Lancet* 343:1464–1467, 1994.

447 Kind C et al: Epidemiology of vertically transmitted HIV-1 infection in Switzerland: Results of a nationwide prospective study. *Eur J Pediatr* 151:442–448, 1992.

448 Dunn DT et al: Mode of delivery and vertical transmission of HIV-1: A review of prospective studies. J *Acquir Immun Defic Syndr* 7: 1064–1066, 1994.

449 Andiman WA et al: Rate of transmission of human immunodeficiency virus type 1 infection from mother to child and short-term outcome of neonatal infection. *Am J Dis Child* 144:758–766, 1990.

450 Hutto C et al: A hospital-based prospective study of perinatal infection with human immunodeficiency virus type 1. *J Pediatr* 188:347–353, 1991.

451 VanderPerre P et al: Mother-to-infant transmission of human immunodeficiency virus by breast milk: Presumed innocent or presumed guilty? *Clin Infect Dis* 15:502–507, 1992.

452 Hira SK et al: Apparent vertical transmission of human immunodeficiency virus type 1 by breast-feeding in Zambia. *J Pediatr* 117:421–424, 1990.

453 Palasanthrian P et al: Breast-feeding during primary maternal human immunodeficiency virus infection and risk of transmission from mother to infant. *J Infect Dis* 167:441–444, 1993.

454 Colebunders R et al: Breastfeeding and transmission of HIV. *Lancet* 2:1487, 1988.

455 Blanche S et al: A prospective study of infants born to women seropositive for human immunodeficiency virus type 1. HIV Infection in Newborns French Collaborative Study Group. *N Engl J Med* 320: 1643–1648, 1989.

456 Fowler MG, Mofenson LM: Progress in prevention of perinatal HIV-1. *Acta Pediatr (in press).*

457 Barbacci MB et al: Human immunodeficiency virus infection in women attending an inner-city prenatal clinic: Ineffectiveness of targeted screening. *Sex Transm Dis* 17:122–126, 1990.

458 Fehrs LJ et al: Targeted HIV screening at a Los Angeles prenatal/family planning health center. *Am J Public Health* 81:619–622, 1991.

459 Lindsay MK et al: Determinants of acceptance of routine voluntary human immunodeficiency virus testing in an inner-city prenatal population. *Obstet Gynecol* 78:678–680, 1989.

460 Carpenter CC et al: Antiretroviral therapy for HIV infection in 1996. Recommendations of an international panel. International AIDS Society USA. *JAMA* 276:146–154, 1996.

461a Sperling RS et al: Maternal viral load, zidovudine treatment, and the risk of transmission of human immunodeficiency virus type 1 from mother to infant. *N Engl J Med* 335:1621–1629, 1996.

461b Frenkel LM et al: Analysis of the maternal components of the AIDS clinical trial group 076 zidovudine regimen in the prevention of mother-to-infant transmission of human immunodeficiency virus type-1. *J Infect Dis* 175:971–974, 1997.

462 Hitti J et al: Herpes simplex virus seropositivity and reactivation in labor among pregnant women infected with human immunodeficiency virus-1. *Am J Obstet Gynecol* (in press).

463 Johnstone FD et al: Does infection with HIV affect the outcome of pregnancy? *Br Med J* 296:467, 1988.

464 Selwyn PA et al: Prospective study of human immunodeficiency virus infection and pregnancy outcomes in intravenous drug users. *JAMA* 261:1289–1294, 1989.

465 Minkoff HL et al: Pregnancy outcomes among mothers infected with human immunodeficiency virus and uninfected control subjects. *Am J Obstet Gynecol* 163:1598–1604, 1990.

466 Semprini AE et al: Perinatal outcome in HIV-infected pregnant women. *Gynecol Obstet Invest* 30:15–18, 1990.

467 Alger LS et al: Interactions of human immunodeficiency virus infection and pregnancy. *Obstet Gynecol* 82:787–796, 1993.
468 Halsey NA et al: Transmission of HIV-1 infections from mothers to infants in Haiti: Impact on childhood mortality and malnutrition. The CDC/JHU AIDS Project Team. *JAMA* 264:2088–2092, 1990.
469 Braddick MR et al: Impact of maternal HIV infection on obstetrical and early neonatal outcome. *AIDS* 4:1001–1005, 1990.
470 Lepage P et al: Perinatal transmission of HIV-1: Lack of impact of maternal HIV infection on characteristics of livebirths and on neonatal mortality in Kigali, Rwanda. *AIDS* 5:295–300, 1991.
471 Temmerman M et al: Maternal human immunodeficiency virus-1 infection and pregnancy outcome. *Obstet Gynecol* 83:495–501, 1994.
472 European Collaborative Study: Perinatal findings in children born to HIV-infected mothers. *Br J Obstet Gynaecol* 101:136–141, 1994.

Chapter 81

Pediatric HIV infection

Wilma Lim
Martha Rogers

EPIDEMIOLOGY OF HIV AMONG WOMEN AND CHILDREN

Over the two past decades, human immunodeficiency virus (HIV) infection has spread worldwide. Although most transmissions in developed countries occur via male-to-male sexual contact or injecting drug use, heterosexual transmission is increasing in these countries and accounts for most infections in the developing world. As a result, the World Health Organization (WHO) estimates that as of December 1996, over 11 million women had become infected with HIV worldwide. Because HIV can be readily transmitted from women to their infants during pregnancy, delivery, and through breast feeding, an estimated 2.6 million children have also become infected worldwide.

In the United States, women and children constitute the fastest growing populations with AIDS. As of December 31, 1996 over 85,000 cases of AIDS in women and nearly 8000 cases in children under 13 years of age had been reported to the Centers for Disease Control and Prevention (CDC).[1] The percentage of AIDS cases that are women has increased from 7 percent of all cases in 1985 to 20 percent of all cases in 1996. AIDS is now the third leading cause of death in young women aged 25 to 44 and the sixth leading cause of death in children aged 1 to 4 years.

Through the national HIV Survey of Childbearing Women, a blinded HIV seroprevalence survey that utilizes blood left over from routine metabolic screening of infants in 44 states, the prevalence of HIV among childbearing women and the number of HIV-infected infants can be estimated based on the last year for which these data were available (1994). Since the survey began in 1989, an estimated 6000 to 7000 HIV-infected women have given birth each year. In other words, approximately 1 of every 625 women giving birth to a liveborn infant each year in the United States is infected with HIV.[2] Although prevalence rates tend to be highest in large urban metropolitan areas, some states, particularly in the Southeast, have prevalence rates in smaller urban and even rural areas that are similar to those in large urban areas.[3]

Data from the survey have been used in statistical models to estimate the cumulative incidence of HIV infection in children since 1978. Approximately 14,920 HIV-infected infants were born in the United States between 1978 and 1993, of which 12,240 children were living at the beginning of 1994.[4] Of the total 14,920 HIV-infected children, about one-third (36 percent) had developed AIDS as indicated by cases reported to the CDC national AIDS surveillance system.

AIDS cases among women and children have been reported from all 50 states and four U.S. territories. States with the highest cumulative number of AIDS in children are New York, New Jersey, and Florida. These states also have the highest cumulative number of cases in women. Most cases in women and children are concentrated in states along the East Coast and Southeastern part of the United States.[1]

HIV infection among women and children in the United States has disproportionately affected African Americans and Hispanic Americans. The cumulative incidence of AIDS is nearly 20 times higher among African American children and about seven times higher in Hispanic children compared to the incidence in white children. Overall, 85 percent of children with AIDS and 76 percent of women with AIDS are African American or Hispanic.

TRANSMISSION OF HIV AMONG WOMEN AND CHILDREN

TRANSMISSION MECHANISMS

Transmission of HIV among women occurs primarily through heterosexual contact (40 percent of all AIDS cases in women reported in 1996) and injecting drug use (34 percent of female AIDS cases reported in 1996).[1] Among women with heterosexually acquired AIDS, at least one-third had partners who were injecting drug users, emphasizing the major role drug use plays in spreading HIV infection among women. Crack, a smokable form of cocaine, also plays a role in the spread of HIV because of the frequent exchange of sex for drugs or money to purchase drugs. A study involving street-recruited young men and women from inner city neighborhoods found that HIV prevalence was significantly higher among regular users of crack compared with nonusers from the same neighborhoods (15.7 versus 5.2 percent). Among crack smokers, women who had recently exchanged sex for money or drugs had the highest prevalence of HIV infection: 40.9 percent, a prevalence similar to that found in male homosexuals (42.9 percent).[5]

Women are often unaware of their risk and exposure to HIV through male sexual partners. In one study of pregnant women attending an antenatal clinic in a south Florida community, 21 percent of the HIV-infected women had only two to five lifetime sexual partners, no known high-risk sexual partners, had never used crack cocaine, and had no positive tests for sexually transmitted diseases.[6] This finding emphasizes the fact that many HIV-infected women, especially those who are unaware of their risk, do not seek HIV testing and are often not diagnosed until after symptoms develop. Thus, they are not able to take advantage of interventions that preserve their own health (e.g., PCP prophylaxis, early antiretroviral therapy) and those that reduce their risk of perinatal transmission (e.g., zidovudine use during pregnancy), emphasizing the importance of HIV counseling and voluntary testing among young women.

Transmission to children occurs predominantly through perinatal transmission (also known as vertical transmission, mother-to-child transmission). Among the 7629 children under 13 years of age reported to CDC as of December 1996, 90 percent acquired their infection perinatally.[1] The remaining children acquired their infection largely via transfusion of blood or blood products: 5 percent from transfusions and 3 percent as a result of treatment for clotting disorders (e.g., hemophilia). Rarely, transmission to children has occurred through sexual abuse.

Other rare modes of transmission to children include close, person-to-person contact involving extensive and repeated exposure to blood or exposure to injection equipment. Only a handful of cases involving child-to-child, child-to-mother, or mother-to-child transmission have been reported.[7] No cases of transmission within school or day care settings have been reported; however, universal precautions should be used to prevent exposure to blood or body fluids in these settings.[8] No isolation procedures are necessary for HIV-infected children attending school or day care and screening of children for HIV infection prior to entry is unnecessary.

Perinatal transmission of HIV can occur during pregnancy, labor and delivery, and through breast feeding. HIV has been detected in fetal tissue as early as 8 weeks gestation and several studies have found an increased rate of fetal demise among HIV-infected pregnant women versus noninfected women.[9] However, increasing evidence indicates that most perinatal transmission to liveborn infants probably occurs late in gestation or during delivery. Using a working definition for non–breast feeding women of in utero transmission (virus detectable by culture or polymerase chain reaction [PCR] in the first few days of life) and intrapartum transmission (no virus detectable until after the first week of life), studies indicate that about 60 to 70 percent of all perinatal transmissions were intrapartum and 30 to 40 percent occur in utero. Among breast feeding women, a study of infants followed in a cohort in Zaire found that 23 percent of transmissions occur in utero, 65 percent intrapartum, and 12 percent via breast feeding.[10] A meta-analysis of studies comparing transmission rates in breast feeding vs non–breast feeding women found that breast feeding contributed an additional 14 percent risk, consistent with these estimates.[11]

The overall rate of perinatal transmission has varied from as low as 13 percent in untreated European populations to as high as 45 percent in some untreated African populations.[9] These differences are probably attributable to differences in factors that either facilitate or inhibit transmission. One of the most consistent findings is that women with advanced disease, low CD4 counts, and high viral titers transmit at higher rates when compared with women with less advanced disease. Maternal immunologic factors, including neutralizing antibody to HIV, may also play a role. Placental factors are also important in that women with chorioamnionitis have been shown to transmit at higher rates. Obstetrical factors including increased fetal exposure to maternal blood, prolonged rupture of membranes, and premature delivery have been associated with higher transmission rates. Cesarean section delivery has been associated with lower rates of transmission in some studies, but not others. More recently, the role of micronutrients has been examined. One study in Malawi found that vitamin A deficiency was associated with higher rates of perinatal transmission.[12] Vitamin A has been associated with increased morbidity in other diseases, such as measles, and may effect HIV transmission because of the vitamin's essential role in immune function and in maintaining membrane integrity. Other studies are needed to corroborate these findings.

PREVENTION OF TRANSMISSION OF HIV TO INFANTS

Based on our understanding of perinatal transmission of HIV, several strategies for interrupting transmission have been hypothesized and many are currently under study. These strategies may differ depending on whether they are aimed at interrupting in utero, intrapartum, or postpartum transmission, as both timing, safety concerns, and mechanisms of protection may differ. Most strategies, however, are aimed at achieving one or more of the following: (1) lowering maternal viral titer either in blood, the genital tract, or both; (2) boosting maternal, fetal, placental, or infant immunity; (3) prophylaxing the infant during or prior to delivery; and (4) avoidance of breast feeding. The use of zidovudine during pregnancy, labor and delivery, and in the newborn has been shown to significantly decrease the risk of perinatal transmission and may involve one of more of these mechanisms. AIDS Clinical Trials Group Protocol 076, a randomized, placebo-controlled clinical trial, found a reduction in transmission from 25 percent in the untreated group to 8 percent in the zidovudine-treated group.[13] These findings led the U.S. Public Health Service (USPHS) to issue clinical guidelines on the use of zidovudine in HIV-infected pregnant women and their newborns and to recommend that all pregnant women in the United States be routinely counseled and voluntarily tested for HIV during pregnancy.[14,15] USPHS recently updated the antiretroviral treatment guidelines for HIV-infected pregnant women recommending the current standard of care using combination antiretroviral therapy to be considered during pregnancy, since monotherapy is now considered suboptimal treatment for HIV infection.[16] In a clinical trial in Thailand, a short course zidovudine regimen given to non–breast feeding HIV-infected pregnant women (oral ZDV given at 36 weeks gestation and every 3 hours during labor to the mothers but none to infants) resulted in a 51 percent reduction in perinatal HIV transmission.[17] The regimen in this study is more easily implemented in developing countries because it is less expensive and simpler than the current regimen used in the United States. The USPHS has recommended against breast feeding for infected women in the United States since 1985. Breast feeding is recommended, however, in those countries where safe alternatives to breast feeding are not available. As feasible intervention becomes available in developing nations, prevention of the infection occurring by breastfeeding must also be considered as part of the programs.

Other methods for reducing the risk of perinatal transmission are under study. The use of topical microbicides in an attempt to reduce the viral load in the genital tract during labor have been proposed. However, a recent study found that cleansing the vagina during labor with a solution of chlorhexidine did not lower the rate of transmission in the treated group vs the untreated group although it decreased the bacterial infections in the neonates.[18] Possible reasons for failure of this approach include the following possibilities: (1) that transmission occurs prior to passage through the birth canal; (2) that some mechanism other than exposure to genital tract virus is responsible for transmission; or (3) that the agent failed to lower genital tract viral load. No virologic studies of the effectiveness of this agent in lowering the genital tract viral load have been done.

C-section has been hypothesized to reduce the risk of perinatal transmission by preventing exposure of the infant to genital tract virus. The effect of mode of delivery on transmission has been examined in several observational studies with conflicting results. A meta-analysis of these studies indicated a modest protective effect of C-section when compared with vaginal delivery, although the odd's ratio did not reach statistical significance.[19] No recommendations for C-section have been made; however, a clinical trial randomizing HIV-infected women to C-section versus vaginal delivery is underway in Europe. A meta-analysis of several large prospective studies is ongoing.

Randomized controlled trials of HIV immuneglobulin (HIVIG) given to the mother, baby, or both are also underway, as are trials of shorter (2 to 3 weeks) antenatal courses of zidovudine than were used in the ACTG 076 study. Virologic and safety studies of other antiretrovirals are also in progress. A recent study (ACTG 185) did not show an additional protective effect of HIVIG when used in women who were already taking zidovudine prophylaxis for prevention of perinatal transmission.[20]

Results from a study of HIV-exposed health care workers suggest that prophylaxis of the infant exposed at the time of delivery might be effective in preventing transmission. A case-control study comparing HIV-exposed health care workers who seroconverted to HIV with those who did not found that postexposure use of zidovudine was associated with a lower risk for HIV transmission.[21] To address the postexposure prophylaxis hypothesis in infants, studies of the use of antiretrovirals, HIV vaccines, or hyperimmune globulin given to the mother during labor or to the infant immediately postpartum are being planned or are under way.

The role of genital tract infections in perinatal transmission of

HIV is not well defined. It has been hypothesized that genital tract infections may increase the viral load in the vagina and thereby increase the likelihood of intrapartum transmission. Several studies have found that women with sexually transmitted diseases during pregnancy had higher rates of transmission of HIV when compared with women without these infections; however, this has not been a consistent finding in all studies. Chorioamnionitis has also been associated with higher rates of transmission that may occur as a result of disruption of the placental membranes serving as a maternal–fetal barrier.

Concerns have been raised about obstetrical and perinatal procedures that may increase the infant's exposure to maternal blood and vaginal secretions during labor and delivery. Although most studies of individual procedures have not shown an association with increased transmission, few of these studies have had sufficient power to detect small risks. One study did find that mothers with events involving fetal exposure to maternal blood, including abruption or fetal scalp electrodes were more likely to transmit to their infants when compared with mothers who did not have these events.[22] Given the concerns about transmission, the American College of Obstetricians and Gynecologists has recommended that direct contact between maternal blood and vaginal secretions and fetal blood be avoided whenever possible. To avoid injuring the mucosa of the infant during suctioning after birth, wall suction device pressure should be kept at under 140 mm Hg.

DIAGNOSIS OF PERINATAL HIV INFECTION

Identification of HIV-exposed infants and young children is optimally accomplished by recognizing HIV infection in their mothers before or during pregnancy. Detection of HIV infection in a pregnant woman allows timely and optimal care for the infected woman herself and earlier recognition and appropriate management of the HIV-exposed or HIV-infected child. Delays in diagnosis and treatment of HIV-infected children are associated with substantially poorer patient outcomes.

Definitive diagnosis of perinatal HIV infection can be achieved by using sensitive virologic methods.[23] Definitive diagnosis is possible by 6 months of life, and in most cases by 1 to 2 months of life. HIV-exposed infants should have HIV virologic testing (PCR or HIV culture) performed within the first 48 hours of life and again at around 2 weeks of life. If these tests are negative, repeat testing should be done at 1 to 2 months of age and at 3 to 6 months of age.[23] A positive virologic test is a presumptive indication of HIV infection and should be confirmed by a second virologic test. HIV infection can be reasonably ruled out after obtaining two or more negative HIV virologic tests at greater than 1 month of age, at least one of which was performed at greater than 4 months of age.[24]

Serologic tests for HIV-specific IgG antibodies are the mainstay of laboratory diagnosis of HIV infection in adults, adolescents, and children older than 18 months of age. The most common antibody tests are the enzyme-linked immunosorbent assays (ELISA) with supplemental western blot or immunofluorescence assay to confirm positive ELISA reactions.[25] Owing to the presence of maternal anti-HIV IgG antibodies that passively cross the placenta to the fetus, virtually all HIV-exposed infants are HIV antibody positive at birth. Perinatally-exposed infants are defined as "seroreverters" if they have become HIV antibody negative after 6 months of age, have no laboratory evidence suggesting HIV infection (i.e., immunodeficiency), and have not met any AIDS surveillance case definitions. In uninfected children, the median age of seroreversion is ten months, although HIV antibody may persist until 18 months of age in a few children. Standard HIV antibody tests, therefore, cannot be used for the definitive diagnosis of HIV infection before 18 months of age (see Table 81-1).

Table 81-1. Diagnosis of Human Immunodeficiency Virus (HIV) Infection in Children

Diagnosis: HIV infected

a) A child < 18 months of age who is known to be HIV seropositive or born to an HIV-infected mother **and:**
  has positive results on two separate determinations (excluding cord blood) from one or more of the following HIV detection tests:
    HIV culture,
    HIV polymerase chain reaction,
    HIV antigen,

or

  meets criteria for acquired immunodeficiency syndrome (AIDS) diagnosis based on the 1987 AIDS surveillance case definition.

b) A child ≥ 18 months of age born to an HIV-infected mother or any child infected by blood, blood products, or other known modes of transmission (e.g., sexual contact) who:
  is HIV-antibody positive by repeatedly reactive enzyme immunoassay (EIA) and confirmatory test (e.g., Western blot or immunofluorescence assay [IFA]);
  meets any of the criteria in the preceding.

Diagnosis: Perinatally exposed

A child who does not meet the preceding criteria who:
  is HIV seropositive by EIA and confirmatory test (e.g., Western blot or IFA) and is < 18 months of age at the time of test;

or

  has unknown antibody status, but was born to a mother known to be infected with HIV.

Diagnosis: Seroreverter

A child who is born to an HIV-infected mother and who:
  has been documented as HIV-antibody negative (i.e., two or more negative EIA tests performed at 6–18 months of age or one negative EIA test after 18 months of age);

and

  has had no other laboratory evidence of infection (has not had two positive viral detection tests, if performed);

and

  has not had an AIDS-defining condition.

Modified from: CDC: 1994 Revised classification system for human immunodeficiency virus infection in children less than 13 years of age. *MMWR* 43(no. RR-12):1–10; 1994.

HIV DIAGNOSTIC METHODS AND FINDINGS IN CHILDREN

Detecting directly the presence of HIV or its components denotes HIV infection and is a useful tool in making the diagnosis in children who are less than six months of age. Definitive diagnosis of perinatal HIV infection can therefore be made by virus isolation (HIV culture), or by tests that detect viral nucleic acids (HIV DNA or RNA amplified by the polymerase chain reaction method [PCR] or reverse transcription-PCR [RT-PCR]) and viral proteins (p24 antigen capture assay). PCR-based assays and viral culture are the most sensitive and specific assays to detect HIV infection in HIV-exposed children.

HIV culture

A sensitive technique for isolation of HIV involves coculturing patients' peripheral blood mononuclear cells (PBMC) with phytohemagglutinin-stimulated PBMC feeder cells from a healthy uninfected individual.[26] At least 2×10^6 patient cells are cocultivated with an equal number of donor cells. Cultures are supplemented with fresh media and feeder cells every 3 to 5 days and supernatants are periodically sampled for the presence of HIV by detection of p24 antigen or the activity of the HIV reverse transcriptase enzyme using an enzymatic assay. HIV culture is a complex procedure, expensive, takes longer to perform than PCR, and requires a specialized laboratory, making it impractical in many settings as well as inaccessible to many physicians.

HIV RNA or DNA by RT-PCR and PCR

PCR is a very sensitive diagnostic tool for detecting HIV infection. PCR is a method for amplifying proviral DNA[27] or HIV RNA[28] (after a reverse transcription step) up to 1 million times or more, to increase the probability of detection. PCR can be used for diagnosing HIV infection by detecting the presence of HIV proviral DNA in patients' PBMCs. This is the preferred virologic method for diagnosing HIV infection in infancy owing to the inherent technical difficulties in HIV culture assays. PCR also avoids the problem of persistent maternal antibody, requires less volume of blood, and can be performed in a few days.[29] Several studies evaluating the use of DNA PCR for early diagnosis of perinatal HIV infection have shown that approximately 30 to 50 percent of HIV-infected infants test positive around birth, and this percentage increases to nearly 100 percent by 3 months of life.[29,30] From a meta-analysis of published data involving 271 infected children, 38 percent of infected children had positive PCR tests within the first week of life and 93 percent by 14 days of age.[31] RT-PCR can also be used to measure active virus replication by detecting HIV RNA in plasma, and is the most useful tool for monitoring circulating virus and in assessing response to anti-HIV therapies. However, RT-PCR should not be used in place of HIV DNA PCR for routine diagnostic purposes in infants. Administration of antiretroviral agents (especially therapy with potent combination agents during the prenatal and early postnatal period) can theoretically result in little or no detectable HIV replication in the infected neonate. Although a positive RT-PCR is presumptive evidence of HIV infection, a negative result can not rule out HIV infection in an infant.

HIV p24 antigen

The standard assay for the detection of viral protein is the p24 antigen capture assay. In early studies of infants born to HIV-infected mothers, few infants were found to be p24 antigen positive, most likely owing to low levels of antigen in the first few months of life and the presence of excess maternal HIV antibody that complexes with p24 antigen present in the infants' blood.[29,32] The low sensitivity of the standard p24 antigen assay may be increased if the sample is first treated with a weak acid to dissociate antigen–antibody complexes.[33] Despite its limitations in early diagnosis, the p24 antigen test can be helpful in settings where virus is present but specific antibody is low or absent, such as hypogammaglobulinemic infants with HIV infection.[34] Despite its high specificity, p24 antigen tests (standard or immune-complex dissociated) have low sensitivity compared to the other HIV virologic tests and should not be routinely utilized as a primary tool in diagnosing HIV infection in infants.[35]

HIV virologic findings in children

Viral burden in perinatally infected infants is generally higher than in HIV-infected adults. A large prospective study showed that the median HIV RNA level was below the detectable level at birth, but increased dramatically to median values of 318,000 and 256,000 copies/ml at 1 and 2 months of age, respectively.[36] These values then slowly declined to 34,000 copies/ml by 24 months of age. Interestingly, the average viral burden and the slope of decline during the first year were similar in infants believed to have early infection (in utero transmission) and late infection (peripartum transmission). Infants whose disease progressed rapidly tended to have higher HIV RNA levels in the first 2 months of life than those without rapid progression, although there was considerable overlap in the values between the two groups. There were no infants with an RNA level of less than 70,000 copies/mL and rapidly progressive disease. Levels of viremia have also been correlated with HIV disease progression and survival in other studies of HIV infection in infants and young children.[37,38] Unfortunately, however, there is considerable overlap in the HIV RNA levels in children with rapid or slow disease progression, precluding a precise clinical predictive value for any given level of HIV viremia.

In another study, a wide range of baseline plasma HIV RNA levels, from undetectable (<4000 copies/mL) to 32,000,000 copies/mL, was noted in a group of HIV-infected children enrolled in the NICHD Intravenous Immunoglobulin (IVIG) clinical trial. The RNA levels were highest among infants less than 1 year of age, with a geometric mean of greater than 400,000 copies/ml.[39] Mean HIV RNA levels did not decline to less than 100,000 copies/ml until 3 years of age, with a subsequent slower decline to less than 70,000 copies/ml around 4 to 5 years of age. This study also showed that CD4 lymphocyte percent of less than 15 percentage was predictive of mortality risk.

As compared to adults, the collective HIV RNA data in children indicate a unique pattern of viral replication and viral containment. The slow decline in the viral load in children most likely reflects lower efficiency of the immature or developing neonatal immune system in containing viral replication.[23] The available data indicate that both HIV RNA levels and CD4+ cell percentage independently correlate with mortality risk in HIV-infected children, and both can be used to predict survival in children.[39,40]

CLINICAL MANIFESTATIONS, PROGRESSION, AND SURVIVAL IN CHILDREN WITH HIV INFECTION

Perinatally acquired HIV infection is associated with a wide spectrum of clinical manifestations. These range from asymptomatic infection to full-blown AIDS with considerable variation in rates of disease progression, from slow to rapid. Until recently, reported series of AIDS cases have mostly involved severely ill children. Disease progression and survival can be best summarized from data of longitudinal prospective studies of perinatally infected children identified soon after birth. However, availability of such studies is sparse owing in part to delays in the systematic identification of many infants, some of whom are recognized only after HIV symptoms have developed, and the relatively small number of pediatric HIV exposures. Information regarding the natural history of perinatally acquired HIV infection continues to evolve, and difficulties in understanding the natural history of infection are compounded by rapid changes in supportive care (e.g., *Pneumocystis carinii* pneumonia prophylaxis) and the aggressive administration of HIV antiretroviral therapies that clearly modify the course of HIV infection in children. Most information in the following discussion is derived from studies that were completed before protease inhibitors were used in clinical trials.

Most infected children are completely asymptomatic at birth and lack appreciable clinical or laboratory signs of HIV disease.[41] Thus, timely diagnosis of HIV infection in infants and young children depends largely on the appropriate identification of HIV-exposed children, rather than on clinical stigmata, since there is no conclusive evidence of a congenital HIV syndrome. In 1987, the CDC established a classification system that described the clinical manifestations of HIV in children based on limited data available early in the HIV epidemic.[42] As more knowledge evolved of HIV disease among children, a revised HIV classification system was published in 1994. The new system classified HIV-exposed children according to the level of documentation of HIV infection, and the clinical and immunologic features of the child.[43] This classification lists, but is not limited to, signs and symptoms commonly seen in HIV-infected children less than 13 years of age. Category N includes children with no HIV signs or symptoms. Category A includes children with evidence of mild disease, such as lymphadenopathy, hepatomegaly, splenomegaly, parotitis, or recurrent or persistent upper respiratory infection, sinusitis, or otitis media. Category B (Table 81-2) includes children with signs and symptoms considered representative of moderate disease and that are not included in categories A and C. Category C includes all AIDS-defining clinical conditions (Table 81-3) except lymphoid interstitial pneumonitis (LIP), which is included in category B. LIP has been separated from the other AIDS-defining conditions in Category C because it is associated with substantially better prognosis than the other AIDS defining conditions.[43]

The Pediatric Spectrum of Disease (PSD) project, coordinated by CDC, has been conducting active surveillance for HIV disease among children since 1988. In a recent report of PSD data collected from 2148 children from seven geographic regions (Los Angeles County, New York City, three cities in Texas, Massachusetts, Washington, DC, Puerto Rico, and the San Francisco Bay area) who were perinatally infected with HIV, the natural history of HIV infection was divided into five groups using the CDC 1994 pediatric HIV classification system: stage N (no signs or symptoms), stage A (mild signs or symptoms), stage B (moderate signs or symptoms), stage C (severe signs or symptoms), and stage D (death).[44] It was estimated that a child with perinatally acquired HIV infection had a 75 percent probability of surviving to 5 years of age and a mean survival time (birth to death) of 9.4 years. The study indicated a 50 percent chance of developing severe signs or symptoms by 5 years of age. For a child with severe signs or symptoms, the estimated mean time from stage C to death was 2.8 years and the chance of surviving 5 years was 17 percent. Children who entered stage B had a 60 percent chance of developing severe signs or symptoms within the next 5 years and the estimated mean time to death was 8.2 years. The overall estimated mean time from birth to AIDS was 4.8 years.[44] The results of Markov modeling of pediatric data suggest a more rapid disease progression in children when compared with a similar Markov model performed in a cohort of adults. Results of the adult model indicated that adults remained asymptomatic for 4.4 years and AIDS developed after 9.8 to 15 years.[45]

Although available studies indicate that HIV infection in children follows a more accelerated course compared with adults, estimates of disease progression in infected individuals change over time as more therapeutic interventions and early prophylactic interventions are made available. However, if untreated, HIV-related symptoms usually develop by 18 to 24 months of age in perinatally infected children. Two different patterns of disease expression have been described. One group of children develop profound immune deficiency, often with multiple opportunistic infections and other AIDS-related symptoms within the first 6 months of life. This group is characterized by rapid progression of the disease and high mortality in the first 2 years of life.[46–48] The other pattern of disease expression is evident in children who develop immune deficiency and HIV-related symptoms at a much slower rate, with usually only nonspecific clinical signs and symptoms in the first few years of life. This group generally survives for a substantially greater number of years, with a small proportion first developing HIV symptoms only during their teen years.

Table 81-2. Clinical Categories for Children with HIV Infection

Category N: Symptomatic
Children who have no signs or symptoms considered to be the result of HIV infection or who have only one of the conditions listed in Category A.
Category A: Mildly symptomatic
Children with two or more of the conditions listed below but none of the conditions listed in Categories B and C. Lymphadenopathy (≥0.5 cm at more than two sites; bilateral = one site) Hepatomegaly Splenomegaly Dermatitis Parotitis Recurrent or persistent upper respiratory infection, sinusitis, or otitis media
Category B: Moderately symptomatic
Children who have symptomatic conditions other than those listed for Category A or C that are attributed to HIV infection. Examples of conditions in clinical Category B include but are not limited to: Anemia (<8 gm/dl), neutropenia (<1000/mm^3), or thrombocytopenia (<100,000/mm^3) persisting ≥30 days Bacterial meningitis, pneumonia, or sepsis (single episode) Candidiasis, oropharyngeal (thrush), persisting (>2 months) in children >6 months of age Cardiomyopathy Cytomegalovirus infection, with onset before 1 month of age Diarrhea, recurrent or chronic Hepatitis Herpes simplex virus (HSV) stomatitis, recurrent (more than two episodes within 1 year) HSV bronchitis, pneumonitis, or esophagitis with onset before 1 month of age Herpes zoster (shingles) involving at least two distinct episodes or more than one dermatome Leiomyosarcoma Lymphoid interstitial pneumonia (LIP) or pulmonary lymphoid hyperplasia complex Nephropathy Nocardiosis Persistent fever (lasting >1 month) Toxoplasmosis, onset before 1 month of age Varicella, disseminated (complicated chickenpox)
Category C: Severely symptomatic
Children who have any condition listed in the 1987 surveillance case definition for AIDS with the exception of LIP (see Table 81-3).

Modified from: CDC: 1994 Revised classification system for human immunodeficiency virus infection in children less than 13 years of age. *MMWR* 43(no. RR-12):1–10; 1994.

The age of first AIDS-related symptoms and the pattern of the primary and secondary disease manifestations provide a consistent indicator of disease progression in children.[46,49–53] Multiple studies have consistently reported a poor prognosis in children who have early onset of HIV symptoms or full-blown AIDS.[47–49,51,52,54,55] Emerging data suggest that infants who develop symptoms early have high HIV DNA copy numbers in PBMCs, lower CD4+ cell numbers, and higher mortality rates.[56,57]

Table 81-3. Conditions Included in Clinical Category C for Children Infected with Human Immunodeficiency Virus (HIV)

Category C: Severely symptomatic
Serious bacterial infections, multiple or recurrent (i.e., any combination of at least two culture-confirmed infections within a 2-year period), of the following types: septicemia, pneumonia, meningitis, bone or joint infection, or abscess of an internal organ or body cavity (excluding otitis media, superficial skin or mucosal abscesses, and indwelling catheter-related infections)
Candidiasis, esophageal or pulmonary (bronchi, trachea, lungs)
Coccidioidomycosis, disseminated (at site other than or in addition to lungs or cervical or hilar lymph nodes)
Cryptococcosis, extrapulmonary
Cryptosporidiosis or isosporiasis with diarrhea persisting >1 month
Cytomegalovirus disease with onset of symptoms at age >1 month (at a site other than liver, spleen, or lymph nodes)
Encephalopathy (at least one of the following progressive findings present for at least 2 months in the absence of a concurrent illness other than HIV infection that could explain the findings): a) failure to attain or loss of developmental milestones or loss of intellectual ability, verified by standard developmental scale or neuropsychological tests; b) impaired brain growth or acquired microcephaly demonstrated by head circumference measurements or brain atrophy demonstrated by computerized tomography or magnetic resonance imaging (serial imaging is required for children <2 years of age); c) acquired symmetric motor deficit manifested by two or more of the following: paresis, pathologic reflexes, ataxia, or gait disturbance
Herpes simplex virus infection causing a mucocutaneous ulcer that persists for >1 month; or bronchitis, pneumonitis, or esophagitis for any duration affecting a child >1 month of age
Histoplasmosis, disseminated (at a site other than or in addition to lungs or cervical or hilar lymph nodes)
Kaposi's sarcoma
Lymphoma, primary, in brain
Lymphoma, small, noncleaved cell (Burkitt's), or immunoblastic or large cell lymphoma of B-cell or unknown immunologic phenotype
Mycobacterium tuberculosis, disseminated or extrapulmonary
Mycobacterium, other species or unidentified species, disseminated (at a site other than or in addition to lungs, skin, or cervical or hilar lymph nodes)
Mycobacterium avium complex or *Mycobacterium kansasii,* disseminated (at site other than or in addition to lungs, skin, or cervical or hilar lymph nodes)
Pneumocystis carinii pneumonia
Progressive multifocal leukoencephalopathy
Salmonella (nontyphoid) septicemia, recurrent
Toxoplasmosis of the brain with onset at 1 month of age
Wasting syndrome in the absence of a concurrent illness other than HIV that could explain the following findings: a) persistent weight loss >10% of baseline OR b) downward crossing of at least two of the following percentile lines on the weight-for-age chart (e.g., 95th, 75th, 50th, 25th, 5th) in a child ≥1 year of age OR c) <5th percentile on weight-for-height chart on two consecutive measurements, 30 days apart PLUS a) chronic diarrhea (i.e., at least two loose stools per day for ≥30 days) OR b) documented fever (for ≥30 days, intermittent or constant)

Modified from: CDC: 1994 Revised classification system for human immunodeficiency virus infection in children less than 13 years of age. *MMWR* 43(no. RR-12)1–10; 1994.

Other studies have provided additional information regarding survival of perinatally infected children. In a prospective study of infants born to HIV-infected women in New York City, more than 80 percent of HIV-infected children were symptomatic with at least two nonspecific HIV-related findings, whereas 36 percent progressed to AIDS or death in the first year of life.[58] The European Collaborative Study reported that 70 percent of infected children were symptomatic although only 23 percent progressed to AIDS within the first year of life.[59] Other prospective studies in different European populations have reported AIDS-defining diagnoses in about one-third of infants within the first year of life, and in greater than 50 percent by 2 years of life.[48,60] In a multicenter and prospective study carried out by the French Pediatric HIV Infection Study Group, the incidence of category C disease was 17 percent during the first year of life.[57] The risk of developing AIDS was 38 percent if there were associated adenopathies, spleen, and liver enlargement at birth, compared to 15 percent when these signs were absent.

OPPORTUNISTIC INFECTIONS AND OTHER AIDS-DEFINING CONDITIONS COMMONLY SEEN AMONG HIV-INFECTED CHILDREN

Opportunistic infections (OIs) are the most significant causes of morbidity and mortality in HIV-infected children. OIs may be caused by viruses, fungi, and parasites. Most of these OIs are considered elsewhere in this volume in the context of HIV infection in adults. Only those aspects of these AIDS-defining conditions that are uniquely relevant to pediatric HIV infection will be considered here.

PNEUMOCYSTIS CARINII PNEUMONIA (PCP)

PCP is the most common AIDS-identifying OI in children. PCP is characterized by a tetrad of signs: tachypnea, dyspnea, fever, and cough. Chest radiograph often reveals bilateral diffuse interstitial markings. Its clinical course is often progressive and if untreated patients develop marked tachypnea, dyspnea, and severe hypoxemia. PCP most often occurs around 3 to 6 months of age and is preventable by early institution of antibiotic prophylaxis before 2 months of age, when the risk of acquiring primary PCP infection begins to increase dramatically.[61] The effectiveness of this prevention modality is entirely dependent on identifying infants who are HIV-exposed, which is dependent in turn on the recognition of HIV infection on mothers. According to the revised PCP prophylaxis guideline, all HIV-exposed infants and children should receive PCP prophylaxis beginning at 4 to 6 weeks of life regardless of CD4+ cell count.[24] Since definitive diagnosis (or reasonable exclusion of HIV infection) may not be achieved until 4 to 6 months of age or later, it is frequently necessary to commence PCP prophylaxis in HIV-exposed children whose infection status is not clear. Table 81-4 shows the PCP prophylaxis and CD4+ monitoring guidelines for HIV-exposed and HIV-infected children. Adherence to these guidelines should contribute to a reduction in PCP incidence. New cases of PCP can usually be attributed to delay or failure in identifying infants at risk of HIV infection in sufficient time to initiate PCP prophylaxis. Trimethoprim-sulfamethoxazole is the preferred prophylactic agent, although alternative agents may be used in children intolerant to TMP-SMX. Alternate prophylactic regimens include dapsone and aerosolized pentamidine.[24]

LYMPHOID INTERSTITIAL PNEUMONITIS (LIP)

LIP is an AIDS-defining condition commonly described in HIV-infected children. LIP is associated with a better prognosis than other AIDS-defining conditions; thus, it is included in Category B (moderately symptomatic) of the revised pediatric HIV classification (see Table 81-2). Its evolution typically follows a chronic and more indolent pattern than that of most opportunistic (e.g.,

Table 81-4. Recommendations for PCP Prophylaxis and CD4+ Monitoring for Human Immunodeficiency Virus-exposed Infants and HIV-infected Children, by Age and HIV-infection Status

Age/HIV infection status	PCP Prophylaxis	CD4+ Monitoring
Birth to 4–6 weeks, HIV-exposed	No prophylaxis	1 month
4–6 weeks to 4 months, HIV exposed	Prophylaxis	3 months
4–12 months		
HIV infected or indeterminate	Prophylaxis	6, 9, and 12 months
HIV infection reasonably excluded	No prophylaxis	None
1–5 years, HIV infected	Prophylaxis if: CD4+ <500 cells/μl or CD4+ <15%	Every 3–4 months
6–12 years, HIV infected	Prophylaxis if: CD4+ <200 cells/μl or CD4+ <15%	Every 3–4 months

Modified from: CDC. 1995 Revised guidelines for prophylaxis against Pneumocystis carinii pneumonia for children infected with or perinatally exposed to human immunodeficiency virus. *MMWR* 44(RR-4):1–11; 1995.

PCP) and bacterial infections of the lungs. Its etiology and pathogenesis are not well understood. Various studies have failed to demonstrate any evidence of infection (e.g., virus, fungi, parasite, bacteria or acid-fast bacilli) with a specific etiologic agent.[62,63] Primary infection of the lung with HIV, Epstein-Barr virus (EBV) or both, or by another agent yet to be identified or an exaggerated immunologic response to inhaled or circulating antigens are suggested etiologies of LIP.[64] Although the definitive diagnosis of LIP can only be made by histopathology, chest x-ray is often the initial diagnostic procedure used to evaluate a child with suspected LIP.[65] The presence of a reticulonodular pattern pneumonia, with or without hilar adenopathy, that persists on chest x-ray for 2 or more months and is unresponsive to antimicrobial therapy is considered presumptive evidence and an acceptable radiographic diagnosis of LIP.[64] In clinical practice, care must be taken to exclude other possible etiologies, especially those that may present in a subacute or chronic manner (e.g., CMV pneumonitis or pulmonary tuberculosis) mimicking the presentation of LIP. LIP initially presents as chronic infiltration of the lungs with minimal clinical symptoms. Pulmonary worsening occurs as a result of progressive infiltration of the lung and superimposed recurrent infections. Clinical deterioration is often accompanied with progressive changes on chest x-ray and sometimes may be associated with bronchiectasis. In contrast to PCP, LIP is often described in older (>1 year old) children. Patients may have normal levels of alkaline phosphatase, and affected children may only have minimal respiratory symptoms. LIP may be the first clinical manifestation of HIV infection. Often, generalized lymphadenopathy, hepatomegaly, splenomegaly, or parotid enlargement are present as well as elevation of serum immunoglobulins.

BACTERIAL INFECTIONS

These contribute significantly to morbidity in HIV-infected children. The importance of serious bacterial infections was highlighted by their inclusion in the 1987 and 1994 revised Pediatric HIV Classification system.[42,43] In the most recent revised classification, a single episode of invasive bacterial infection (meningitis, pneumonia, sepsis) is considered as a Category B (moderate) symptom. Multiple or recurrent invasive bacterial infections (i.e., any combination of culture-confirmed infections within a 2-year period) are considered as severe symptoms.[43] The increased susceptibility to bacterial infections appears to be related to multiple immune abnormalities, including abnormal T-helper lymphocyte function, altered B-lymphocyte function resulting in dysfunctional antibody production, and defects in chemotactic and bactericidal functions of neutrophils and macrophages.[66–68]

The true incidence of bacterial disease in HIV-infected children is likely underestimated. Most reports of bacterial infections in HIV-infected children are based on retrospective reviews resulting in skewed representation of the true incidence of bacterial infection. Many clinical syndromes are not adequately diagnosed as bacterial infections because of limitations in confirming a bacteriologic etiology. For example, the evaluation of pneumonias is often bacteriologically inconclusive since invasive procedures (e.g., needle biopsy of the lung) are rarely used in routine practice. In addition, anaerobic cultures are not often obtained in many clinical settings. OI prophylaxis and use of other medical interventions may also modify the incidence of bacterial infections or confound bacteriologic evaluations.

The most common serious bacterial infections in HIV-infected children involve staphylococci, pneumococci, enterococci, salmonella species, and *Pseudomonas aeruginosa*, which establish serious systemic infections through respiratory, gastrointestinal, or cutaneous portals of entry. Occasionally, other respiratory pathogens are implicated (e.g., other streptococci or *Hemophilus influenzae*), and children with endstage disease can become systemically infected with a broad range of bacterial commensals, for example, *Staphyloccocus epidermidis* spp., viridans streptococci, and various gut flora (Enterobacter, Klebsiella, *Escherichia coli*, Citrobacter, Acinetobacter, etc.). In a retrospective study of 204 bacterial infections (excluding otitis media) in HIV-infected children during a 3-year period, soft tissue infection, bacteremia, pneumonia, and sinusitis were encountered most frequently.[69] Staphylococcal infections were most common in children with central venous catheters, whereas *Streptococcus pneumoniae* was the most frequent organism recovered in children without catheters. This study also suggested that the use of antiretroviral therapy resulted in a lower frequency of bacterial infections. In another retrospective and prospective study using data from a population-based pediatric HIV surveillance project, a high cumulative incidence of invasive pneumococcal infection (6.1 cases per 100 patient-years, through age 7) was noted.[70] In the general population, children are at increased risk for invasive pneumococcal infection in the first 2 years of life, but incidence rates drop significantly thereafter.[71] Among HIV-infected children, the incidence of invasive pneumococcal disease remained high through age 7.

A randomized, double-blind, placebo-controlled trial demonstrated that monthly infusions of intravenous immunoglobulin (IVIG) helped reduce serious bacterial infections, particularly invasive pneumococcal disease, in HIV-infected children with CD4 cell counts greater than 200/mm^3, but not in children with lower CD4 cell counts.[72] A similar randomized study failed to show additional benefit from administration of IVIG in children receiving trimethophrim-sulfamethoxazole prophylaxis for PCP.[73] Although the role of preventive IVIG administration is not clearly defined in HIV-infected children, it appears reasonable to use IVIG in hypogammaglobulinemic patients and patients with recent histories of multiple serious infections. Antibiotic treatment of suspected bacterial infections in HIV-infected children with relatively intact immunity can generally await culture confirmation of the infection, but antibacterial therapy should be initiated presumptively in children with advanced HIV disease, leukopenia, hypotension, or severe cardiopulmonary compromise.

NEUROLOGIC DYSFUNCTION

Neurologic disease is a significant problem in children with HIV infection. However, the true incidence of HIV-related central nervous system (CNS) disease in infants and children is unknown. Although earlier reports estimated a much higher prevalence rate of progressive encephalopathy, later studies that included asymptomatic to mildly symptomatic HIV-infected children reported a much lower prevalence rate. CNS involvement in HIV-infected children may range from progressive encephalopathy to a more static or subacute progressive course followed by either improvement or deterioration.[74,75] Encephalopathy is included in Category C of the revised pediatric HIV classification (see Table 81-3) and is manifested by varying degrees of cognitive, motor, and behavioral impairment. The HIV disease stage and age of the child seem to be the two factors that most influence the incidence of encephalopathy. The incidence of progressive encephalopathy is greater for infants and young children. CNS disease progression is further influenced by genetic, environmental, and other factors. Developmental delay is a frequent neurologic manifestation in symptomatic HIV-infected children.[76] Comprehensive psychological assessment should be employed to evaluate the different neurodevelopmental abnormalities seen in HIV-infected infants and children. Head CT scan may show varying degrees of cerebral atrophy and decreased attenuation of the white matter in patients with encephalopathy. Basal ganglia calcification may also be noted. Improvements on serial CT scans have been reported after antiretroviral therapy.[77] As more aggressive and earlier antiretroviral therapies are initiated, changes in the natural history and incidence of HIV encephalopathy are also expected.

ANTIRETROVIRAL THERAPY IN CHILDREN

Early clinical trials demonstrated that antiretroviral therapy provided clinical benefit to HIV-infected children with immunologic or clinical symptoms of HIV disease.[23,77,78] These studies have shown significant improvements in neurodevelopment, growth, and virologic and immunologic parameters with an antiretroviral monotherapy regimen. Recently, combination therapies with either ZDV and 3TC or ZDV and ddI have been found to be superior as initial therapy compared to monotherapy with ZDV or ddI.[79,80] Another trial involving combination therapy with a protease inhibitor showed a superior response when compared to dual nucleoside combination therapy.[81] A Pediatric Working Group on Antiretroviral Therapy recently provided guidelines for the treatment of HIV-infected infants and children (Tables 81-5 and 81-6).[23] As new information and clinical experience become available in the future, these guidelines will need to be modified. Therefore, these recommendations should be regarded as flexible guidelines and should not supersede the clinical judgment of experienced health care providers.

One should consider changing antiretroviral therapy when there is failure of the current regimen with evidence of disease

Table 81-5. Indications for Initiation of Antiretroviral Therapy in Children with Human Immunodeficiency Virus (HIV) Infection

Clinical symptoms associated with HIV infection (i.e., clinical categories A, B, or C [Tables 81-2 and 81-3]).
Evidence of immune suppression, indicated by CD4+ T-lymphocyte absolute number or percentage.
Age <12 months—regardless of clinical, immunologic, or virologic status.
For asymptomatic children aged ≥1 year with normal immune status, two options can be considered:
- Preferred Approach
  - Initiate therapy—regardless of age or symptom status.
- Alternative Approach

Defer treatment in situations in which the risk for clinical disease progression is low and other factors (e.g., concern for the durability of response, safety, and adherence) favor postponing treatment. In such cases, the health care provider should regularly monitor virologic, immunologic, and clinical status. Factors to be considered in deciding to initiate therapy include the following:
- High or increasing HIV RNA copy number.
- Rapidly declining CD4+ T lymphocyte number or percentage to values approaching those indicative of moderate immune suppression (Category B [Table 81-2]).
- Development of clinical symptoms.

Modified from: CDC. Guidelines for the Use of Antiretroviral Agents in Pediatric HIV Infection. *MMWR* 47(no. RR-4):1–43, 1998.

Table 81-6. Recommended Antiretroviral Regimens for Initial Therapy for Human Immunodeficiency Virus (HIV) Infection in Children

Preferred Regimen
Evidence of clinical benefit and sustained suppression of HIV RNA in clinical trials in HIV-infected adults; clinical trials in HIV-infected children are ongoing.
- One highly active protease inhibitor plus two nucleoside analogue reverse transcriptase inhibitors (NRTIs)
  - Preferred protease inhibitor for infants and children who cannot swallow pills or capsules: nelfinavir or ritonavir. Alternative for children who can swallow pills or capsules: indinavir.
  - Recommended dual NRTI combinations; the most data on use in children are available for the combinations of zidovudine (ZDV) and dideoxyinosine (ddI) and for ZDV and lamivudine (3TC). More limited data are available for the combinations of stavudine (d4T) and ddI, d4T and 3TC, and ZDV and Zalcitabine (ddC).

Alternative Regimen
Less likely to produce sustained HIV RNA suppression in infected adults; the combination of nevirapine, ZDV, and ddI produced substantial and sustained suppression of viral replication in two of six infants first treated at age <4 months.
- Nevirapine and two NRTIs

Secondary Alternative Regimen
Clinical benefit demonstrated in clinical trials involving infected adults and/or children, but initial viral suppression may not be sustained.
- Two NRTIs

Not Recommended
Evidence against use because of overlapping toxicity and/or because use may be virologically undesirable.
- Any monotherapy
- d4T and ZDV
- ddC and ddI
- ddC and d4T
- ddC and 3TC

Modified from: CDC. Guidelines for the use of antiretroviral agents in pediatric HIV infection. *MMWR* 47(no. RR-4)1–43; 1998.

progression, toxicity or intolerance, and when new information shows that a new drug or regimen is superior to the current regimen.[23] Patients with progressive neurodevelopmental deterioration, growth failure, or disease progression (advancement from one clinical category to another, Tables 81-2 and 81-3) constitute clinical criteria warranting change in antiretroviral therapy. CD4+ lymphocyte count and percentage decline should be validated by at least another measurement before considering changing antiretroviral therapy. HIV RNA levels should be obtained every 3 months to monitor response to therapy but at least two measurements (1 week apart) should be performed before considering a change in therapy. If one has to discontinue antiretroviral therapy for an extended period of time, it is recommended to stop all antiretroviral agents simultaneously to minimize the risk of developing drug resistance.

The choices of antiretroviral agents in infants and children are still limited when compared to those available for adults, and studies of antiretroviral agents in children often lag behind studies in adults delaying development of pediatric drug formulations. Therefore, one should bear in mind that the choice of a new regimen will have an impact on future treatment options. Education regarding medicine adherence should be incorporated in any clinical setting to achieve better compliance.

SOCIAL CONSIDERATIONS IN MANAGING HIV-EXPOSED OR HIV-INFECTED CHILDREN

In most settings, identification of HIV exposure in an infant is preceded by either initial recognition of HIV infection in the mother during the pregnancy or even after delivery.[82] The future impact of the mother's HIV diagnosis is enormous for her and her family. If not yet accomplished, testing of the father should be strongly recommended. There should be an effort to make sure that the mother is receiving proper health care. In some instances, the HIV-infected mother is already seriously ill and may have partners or other children who are ill or have died from AIDS. Psychosocial issues often faced in this setting include poverty, single parenthood, lack of health care insurance or fear of losing existing health insurance coverage, substance abuse involving alcohol, crack, cocaine, or other illicit drugs, domestic violence, housing issues, denial, hostility, and depression. All of these factors require a team approach to ensure that social services are accessible to the patients and the families, and to facilitate proper care of the infant. If the social situation necessitates removal of the child from the home setting, the primary care of the child may need to be placed in a foster care setting.

The parents or foster parents should be appropriately counseled regarding the need for frequent medical follow-up of their HIV-exposed child, the necessity of HIV testing to determine infection status in infants, neonatal prophylaxis with zidovudine to reduce the risk of HIV infection in the infant, the need for PCP prophylaxis to be started as early as 4 to 6 weeks of age, the avoidance of breast feeding, and adherence to universal precautions in the home setting.[82] Once HIV infection is diagnosed in the neonate, the parents or caregivers should be appropriately counseled regarding symptoms and clinical presentations related to HIV infection in children (e.g., recurrent otitis media, failure to thrive, neurologic manifestations, etc.). Sufficient information about the child's HIV status should be provided to the caregiver to ensure appropriate health care for the child. The pediatrician should also discuss the need for permanency planning for children, so that alternative child care arrangements can be planned in advance when the HIV-infected parent(s) become too ill to care for the child.

References

1 Centers for Disease Control and Prevention: *HIV/AIDS Surveillance Report* 8(2); 1996.

2 Davis SF et al: HIV Prevalence among US childbearing women 1989–1994. 11th International Conference on AIDS, Vancouver, Canada. July 1996 Abs Mo.C.331.

3 Wasser SC et al: Urban-nonurban distribution of HIV infection in childbearing women in the United States. *J Acquir Immundef Syndr* 6:1035–1042; 1993.

4 Davis SF et al: Prevalence and incidence of vertically acquired HIV infection in the United States. *JAMA* 247:952–955; 1995.

5 Edlin BR et al: Intersecting epidemics—crack cocaine use and HIV infection among inner-city young adults. *N Engl J Med* 331:1422–1427; 1994.

6 Ellerbrock TV et al: Heterosexually transmitted human immunodeficiency virus infection among pregnant women in a rural Florida community. *N Engl J Med* 327:1704–1709; 1992.

7 Centers for Disease Control: Human immunodeficiency virus transmission in household settings—United States. *MMWR* 43:347–356; 1994.

8 Chanock S et al: Medical issues related to provision of care for HIV-infected children in hospital, home, day care, school, and community, in Pizzo P et al (eds): *Pediatric AIDS*, 2nd ed. Baltimore, Williams & Wilkins, 1994, chap 48, pp. 889–906.

9 Mofenson LM: Mother-child HIV-1 transmission: Timing and determinants. *Obstet Gynecol Clinics NA* 24:759–784, 1997.

10 Bertolli J et al: Estimating the timing of mother-to-child transmission of human immunodeficiency virus in a breast feeding population in Kinshasa, Zaire. *J Infect Dis* 174:722–726; 1996.

11 Dunn DT et al: Risk of human immunodeficiency virus type 1 transmission through breast-feeding. *Lancet* 340:585–588; 1992.

12 Semba RD et al: Maternal vitamin A deficiency and mother-to-child transmission of HIV-1. *Lancet* 343:1593–1597; 1994.

13 Connor EM et al: Reduction of maternal-infant transmission of human immunodeficiency virus type 1 with zidovudine treatment. *N Engl J Med* 331:1173–1180; 1994.

14 Centers for Disease Control and Prevention: Recommendations for the use of zidovudine to reduce perinatal transmission of human immunodeficiency virus. *MMWR* 43(RR-11):1–20; 1994.

15 Centers for Disease Control and Prevention. U.S. Public Health Service recommendations for human immunodeficiency virus counseling and voluntary testing for pregnant women. *MMWR* 44(No. RR-7): 1–15; 1995.

16 Centers for Disease Control and Prevention: Recommendations for the use of antiretroviral drugs in pregnant women and for reducing perinatal HIV-1 transmission in the United States. *MMWR* 47(RR-2):1–30; 1998.

17 Centers for Disease Control and Prevention: Administration of zidovudine during late pregnancy and delivery to prevent perinatal HIV transmission—Thailand, 1996–1998. *MMWR* 47:151–154; 1998.

18 Biggar RJ et al: Perinatal intervention trial in Africa: Effect of a birth canal cleansing intervention to prevent HIV transmission. *Lancet* 347:1647–1650; 1996.

19 Dunn DT et al: Mode of delivery and vertical transmission of HIV-1: A review of prospective studies. *J Acquir Immune Defic Syn* 7: 1064–1066; 1994.

20 Pediatric ACTG Protocol 185 Executive Summary: National Institute of Child Health and Human Development, National Institutes of Health. Bethesda, MD, March 25, 1997.

21 Centers for Disease Control and Prevention: Case-control study of HIV seroconversion in health-care workers after percutaneous exposure to HIV-infected blood—France, United Kingdom, and United States, January 1988–August 1994. *MMWR* 44:929–933; 1995.

22 Boyer PJ et al: Factors predictive of maternal-fetal transmission of HIV-1: Preliminary analysis of zidovudine given during pregnancy and/or delivery. *JAMA* 271:1925–1930; 1994.

23 Centers for Disease Control and Prevention: Guidelines for the Use

of Antiretroviral Agents in Pediatric HIV Infection. *MMWR* 47(RR-4):1–43; 1998.
24 Centers for Disease Control: 1995 Revised guidelines for prophylaxis against Pneumocystis carinii pneumonia for children infected with or perinatally exposed to human immunodeficiency virus. *MMWR* 44(No.-RR-4):1–11; 1995.
25 Centers for Disease Control: Interpretation and use of the Western Blot results for serodiagnosis of human immunodeficiency virus type 1 infection. *MMWR* 38:S1–S7; 1989.
26 Hammer S et al: Use of virologic assays for detection of human immunodeficiency virus in clinical trials: Recommendations of the AIDS clinical trials group virology committee. *J Clin Microbiol* 31:2557–2564; 1993.
27 Ou CY et al: DNA amplification for direct detection of HIV-1 in DNA of peripheral blood mononuclear cells. *Science* 239:295–297; 1988.
28 Bagnerilli P et al: Detection of human immunodeficiency virus type 1 genomic RNA in plasma samples by reverse transcription polymerase chain reaction. *J Med Virol* 34:89–95; 1991.
29 Rogers MF et al: Use of the polymerase chain reaction for early detection of the proviral sequences of human immunodeficiency virus in infants born to seropositive mothers. *N Engl J Med* 320:1649–1654; 1989.
30 Krivine A et al: HIV replication during the first weeks of life. *Lancet* 339:1187–1189; 1992.
31 Dunn DT et al: The sensitivity of HIV-1 DNA polymerase chain reaction in the neonatal period and the relative contributions of intrauterine and intra-partum transmission. *AIDS* 9:F7-F11; 1995.
32 Borkowsky W et al: Human immunodeficiency virus type 1 antigenemia in children. *J Pediatr* 114:940–945; 1989.
33 Miles SA et al: Rapid serologic testing with immune-complex-dissociated HIV p24 antigen for early detection of HIV infection in neonates. *N Engl J Med* 328:297–302; 1993.
34 Borkowsky W et al: Human-immunodeficiency-virus infections in infants negative for anti-HIV by enzyme-linked immunoassay. *Lancet* 1:1168–1171; 1987.
35 Nesheim S et al: Diagnosis of perinatal human immunodeficiency virus infection by polymerase chain reaction and p24 antigen detection after immune complex dissociation in an urban community hospital. *J Infect Dis* 175:1333–1336; 1997.
36 Shearer WT et al for The Women and Infants Transmission Study Group: Viral load and disease progression in infants infected with human immunodeficiency virus type 1. *N Engl J Med* 336:1337–1342, 1997.
37 Zaknun D et al: Correlation of ribonucleic acid polymerase chain reaction, acid dissociated p24 antigen, and neopterin with progression of disease. *J Pediatr* 130:898–905; 1997.
38 Palumbo PE et al: Viral measurement by polymerase chain reaction-based assays in human immunodeficiency virus-infected infants. *J Pediatr* 126:592–595; 1995.
39 Mofenson LM et al for the National Institute of Child Health and Human Development Intravenous Immunoglobulin Clinical Trial Study Group: The Relationship between serum human immunodeficiency virus type I (HIV-1) RNA level, CD4 lymphocyte percent, and long-term Mortality risk in HIV-infected children. *J Inf Dis* 175:1029–1038; 1997.
40 Palumbo PE et al: Disease progression in HIV-infected infants and children: Predictive value of quantitative plasma HIV RNA and CD4 lymphocyte count. *JAMA* 279:756–761; 1998.
41 Blanche S et al: A Prospective Study of Infants born to women seropositive for human immunodeficiency virus type I. *N Engl J Med* 320:1643–1648, 1989.
42 Centers for Disease Control and Prevention: Classification system for human immunedeficiency virus (HIV) infection in children under 13 years of age. *MMWR* 36:225–230; 1987.
43 Centers for Disease Control and Prevention: 1994 Revised classification system for human immunodeficiency virus infection in children less than 13 years of age. *MMWR* 43(RR–12):1–10; 1994.
44 Barnhart HX et al and the Pediatric Spectrum of Disease Clinical Consortium: Natural History of human immunodeficiency virus disease in perinatally infected children: An analysis from the Pediatric Spectrum of Disease Project. *Pediatrics* 97:710–716; 1996.
45 Longini IM, Jr et al: Estimating the stage-specific numbers of HIV infection using a Markov model and back-calculation. *Stat Med* 11:831–843; 1992.
46 Auger I et al: Incubation periods for paediatric AIDS patients. *Nature* 336:575–577; 1988.
47 Scott GB et al: Survival in children with perinatally acquired human immunodeficiency type 1 infection. *N Engl J Med* 26:1792–1796; 1989.
48 Blanche S et al: Longitudinal study of 94 symptomatic infants with perinatally acquired human immunodeficiency virus infection: Evidence for a bimodal expression of clinical and biological symptoms. *AJDC* 144:1210–1215; 1990.
49 Krasinski K et al: Prognosis of human immunodeficiency virus infection in children and adolescents. *Pediatr Infect Dis J* 8:216–220; 1989.
50 European Collaborative Study: Children born to women with HIV-1 infection: Natural history and risk of transmission. *Lancet* 337:253–260; 1991.
51 Newell M-L, European Collaborative Study: The natural history of vertically acquired HIV infection. *J Perinat Med* 19 (suppl 1):257–262; 1991.
52 Tovo PA et al: Prognostic factors and survival in children with perinatal HIV-1 infeciton. *Lancet* 339:1249–1252; 1992.
53 Duliege A-M et al: Natural history of human immunodeficiency virus type 1 infection in children: Prognostic value of laboratory tests on the bimodal progression of disease. *Pediatr Infect Dis J* 11:630–635; 1992.
54 Rogers MF et al: Acquired immunodeficiency syndrome in children: report of the Centers for Disease Control National Surveillance, 1982 to 1985. *Pediatrics* 79:1008–1014; 1987.
55 Turner BJ et al: Survival experience of 789 children with the acquired immunodeficiency syndrome. *Pediatr Infect Dis J* 12(4):310–320; 1993.
56 Bryson YJ et al: Proposed definitions for in utero versus intrapartum transmission of HIV-1. *N Engl J Med* 327:1246–1247; 1993.
57 Mayaux M-J et al: Neonatal characteristics in rapidly progressive perinatally acquired HIV-1 disease. *JAMA* 275:606–610; 1996.
58 Bamji M et al: Prospective study of human immunodeficiency virus-1 related disease among 512 infants born to infected women in New York City. The New York City Perinatal HIV Transmission Collaborative Study Group. *Pediatr Infect Dis J* 15(10):891–898, 1996.
59 The European Collaborative Study: Natural history of vertically acquired human immunodeficiency virus-1 infection. The European Collaborative Study. *Pediatrics* 94:815–819; 1994.
60 Ader AE et al: Children born to women with HIV-1 infection: Natural history and risk of transmission. *Lancet* 337:254–260: 1991.
61 Simmonds RJ et al: Pneumocystis carinii pneumonia among U.S. children with perinatally acquired HIV infection. *JAMA* 270:470–473; 1993.
62 Rubenstein A et al: Pulmonary disease in children with acquired immune deficiency syndrome and AIDS-related complex. *J Pediatr* 108:498–503; 1986.
63 Scott GB et al: Acquired immunodeficiency syndrome in infants. *N Engl J Med* 310:76–81; 1984.
64 Connor EM et al: Lymphocytic interstitial pneumonitis, in Pizzo P, Wilfert C (eds). *Pediatric AIDS,* 2nd ed. Baltimore, Williams & Wilkins, 1994, chap 25, pp 467–481.
65 Anderson VM et al: Lymphocytic interstitial pneumonitis in pediatric AIDS. *Pediatric Pathol* 8:417–421; 1988.
66 Roilides E et al: T helper cell responses in children infected with human immunodeficiency virus type 1. *J Pediatr* 118:724–730; 1991.
67 Pahwa S et al: Pediatric acquired immunodeficiency syndrome; demonstration of B lymphocyte defects in vitro. *Diagn Immunol* 4:24–30; 1986.
68 Roilides E et al: Impairment of neutrophil chemotactic and bactericidal function in HIV-infected children and partial reversal after in

vitro exposure to granulocyte-macrophage colony-stimulating factor. *J Pediatr* 117:531–540; 1990.

69 Roilides E et al: Bacterial infections in human immunodeficiency virus type 1-infected children: The impact of central venous catheters and antiretroviral agents. *Pediatr Inf Dis J* 10:813–819; 1991.

70 Mao C et al: Invasive pneumococcal infections in human immunodeficiency virus-infected children. *J Infect Dis* 173:870–876; 1996.

71 Musher DM: Infections caused by Streptococcus pneumoniae: Clinical spectrum, pathogenesis, immunity, and treatment. *Clin Infect Dis* 14:801–809; 1992.

72 National Institute of Child Health and Human Development Intravenous Immunoglobulin Study Group: Intravenous immunoglobulin for the prevention of bacterial infections in children with symptomatic human immunodeficiency virus infection. *N Engl J Med* 325: 73–80; 1991.

73 Spector SA et al: A controlled trial of intravenous immune globulin for the prevention of serious bacterial infetions in children receiving zidovudine for advanced human immunodeficiency virus infection. *N Engl J Med* 331:1181–1187; 1994.

74 Epstein LG et al: Progressive encephalopathy in children with acquired immune deficiency syndrome. *Ann Neurol* 17:488–496; 1985.

75 Belman A et al: Pediatric acquired immunodeficiency syndrome: Neurologic syndromes. *Am J Dis Child* 142:29–35; 1988.

76 Epstein L et al: Neurologic manifestations of human immunodeficiency virus in children. *Pediatrics* 78:678–687; 1986.

77 Pizzo et al: Effect of continuous intravenous infusion of zidovudine (AZT) in children with symptomatic HIV infection. *N Engl J Med* 319:889–896; 1988.

78 McKinney RE et al: A multicenter trial of oral zidovudine in children with advanced human immunodeficiency virus disease. *N Engl J Med* 324:1018–1025; 1991.

79 Englund JA et al: Zidovudine, didanosine or both as the initial treatment for symptomatic HIV-infected children. *N Engl J Med* 336: 1704–1712; 1997.

80 McKinney RE, for the PACTG Protocol 300 Team: Pediatric ACTG Trial 300: clinical efficacy of ZDV/3TC vs ddI vs ZDV/ddI in symptomatic HIV-infected children, in Program and abstracts of the 37th Annual Meeting of the Infectious Disease Society of America; Sept 13–16, 1997; San Francisco, Abstract 768.

81 Yogev R et al for the PACTG 338 Protocol Team: Virologic efficacy of ZDV+3TC vs d4T+Ritonavir (RTV) vs ZDV+3TC+RTV in stable antiretroviral experienced HIV-infected children (Pediatric ACTG Trial 338), in 37th Interscience Conference on Antimicrobial Agents and Chemotherapy program addedum, Sept 28–Oct 1, 1997; Toronto, Ontario, Canada. [Abstract LB-6].

82 Committee on Pediatric AIDS: Evaluation and medical treatment of the HIV exposed infant. *Pediatrics* 99:909–917; 1997.

Chapter 82

Gonococcal diseases in infants and children

Laura T. Gutman

GONOCOCCAL INFECTIONS IN CHILDREN

The worldwide epidemic of *Neisseria gonorrhoeae* infections has been widely publicized, but the increasing risk of infection in children has gained public recognition only slowly. In the United States, the age-specific incidences of gonococcal disease in children from birth to 9 years was rising until 1980. Since then the rates have plateaued; in this age range, in both 1980 and 1985, the rate was 6.5 per 100,000 population, although some geographic areas have much higher rates.[1] The majority of gonococcal disease is reported in young female children, but increases in the number of infected males occur during the teens and early adult years.[2]

Retrospective reviews and case reports based on detection of symptomatic infection provide us with the estimates of infection in preadolescent children and early adolescent youths. Presenting complaints of symptomatic children who are subsequently established to have *N. gonorrhoeae* infection are primarily vaginal or urethral discharge. Some infected children present for evaluation of sexual abuse or assault, and a number of children have a variety of complaints not related to the genitalia. Gonococcal infection in prepubertal children is particularly important because it may be an indicator of child abuse. Identification of infection in children should lead to a search for adult contacts. When such contact investigations are performed, the results include identification of significant numbers of adults, often family members, who are also infected.[3,4] Unfortunately, investigation of contacts of infected adults very rarely includes child contacts.

Gonococcal infections in children may produce a variety of syndromes that are age related. Extensive investigation of adult gonococcal disease syndromes (disseminated disease, localized symptomatic genital disease, localized asymptomatic genital disease, etc.) have demonstrated that there is a very extensive interaction and accommodation between gonococcal surface structures and the host milieu.[5] There have been no studies of gonococcal infections of infants or prepubertal children to investigate host-microbe interactions, and consequently nothing is known. The means of transmission of infection varies by age; thus, newborn gonococcal infection will be considered separately from infection with *N. gonorrhoeae* in prepubertal children. For further discussion of issues of sexual abuse and STDs of children, see Chap. 87.

MATERNAL AND PERINATAL *N. GONORRHOEAE* INFECTION

Since the 1970s, health clinics have encouraged the routine screening of sexually active women for gonorrhea. This is especially important during pregnancy, and rates of gonorrhea in pregnant women range from rare to about 10 percent. Pregnant teenagers in specific settings may have a high prevalence of gonorrhea. In 1995 the reported rate of gonorrhea in U.S. females of all races age 10–14 years was 73 per 100,000 and for females age 15–19 was 840 per 100,000. Rates have been very much higher in some populations, however, and the overall rate in African-American females age 15–19 years in 1995 was approximately 4,433 per 100,000 population. Recognition of gonorrhea early in pregnancy identifies a population at risk that should be followed sequentially throughout pregnancy, since re-infection rates may be high.

Gonococcal infections present several unique problems during pregnancy, some of which have important consequences for the fetus or neonate. Ascending infection of the mother's upper genital tract may occur with gonococcal infection of pregnancy and have an adverse effect on the pregnancy. From 10 to 20 percent of nonpregnant women with gonorrhea have had clinical evidence of pelvic inflammatory disease (PID) in many studies (see Chap. 58), and the rate increases in women with recently acquired gonorrhea. Pelvic inflammatory disease probably occurs less often in pregnant women with gonorrhea, although surgically verified gonococcal salpingitis has been reported between 7 and 12 weeks' gestation, prior to obliteration of the endometrial cavity.[6] Local host defense factors may decrease the risk for ascending gonococcal infection during pregnancy. Under the influence of progesterone, cervical mucus becomes impermeable to motile sperm and possibly to microorganisms. Most important, after the twelfth week of gestation the chorion attaches to the endometrial decidua with obliteration of the intrauterine cavity, obstructing the route for ascending intraluminal spread of gonococci.

The chorioamnion itself may become the site of ascending gonococcal infection after the twelfth week of gestation,[7,8] and the clinical spectrum of symptomatic gonococcal infection in pregnant patients thus included septic abortion and premature rupture of membranes in 22 and 26 percent of cases in two studies.[9,10] Several other retrospective studies have analyzed the relationship of antepartum gonococcal infection to the course of late pregnancy. Charles et al. reported that premature rupture of membranes occurred in 43 percent of 14 women with untreated gonorrhea at the onset of labor, as opposed to 3 percent of 144 women with gonococcal infection that was identified and treated during pregnancy.[11] Handsfield and colleagues reported that prematurity and delayed delivery after rupture of membranes were significantly correlated with intrapartum gonococcal infection.[12] Edwards and colleagues matched 19 pregnant women who had intrapartum gonococcal infection with 41 uninfected controls on the basis of age, race, parity, socioeconomic status, and date of delivery.[13] Patients with intrapartum gonococcal infection were significantly more likely than controls to have chorioamnionitis, premature rupture of membranes, delayed delivery after rupture of membranes, and prematurity.

The effects of untreated gonococcal disease of the mother on the health of the fetus and infant have been reviewed by several authors, and the results are shown in Table 82-1. In these six studies, rates of premature delivery were between 13 and 67 percent, rates of perinatal distress were 5 to 10 percent, and rates of perinatal deaths were 2 to 11 percent. The rates of apparently normal or term deliveries were only 35 to 77 percent of the reported pregnancies. The studies of Charles, Amstey, Edwards, and Handsfield included the outcomes of pregnancy of mothers who were not infected with *N. gonorrhoeae,* and the outcomes of uninfected mothers were significantly more favorable for the infant. In Amstey's study, the risk of these adverse outcomes was the same in women who were treated for gonorrhea during pregnancy as in those who were not treated prior to delivery.

These studies provided scant information on other associated conditions or genital infections. However, there is increasing evidence that many or most infections of the lower genital tract of women (including *M. hominis, Ureaplasma urealyticum*, and *Chlamydia trachomatis*[15–18]), when they occur during pregnancy, carry a significant burden of adverse outcomes to the pregnancy, including premature rupture of membranes, spontaneous abortions, perinatal mortality, and prematurity.

Table 82-1. Outcome of Pregnancy in Mothers Who Were Infected with *N. gonorrhoeae* at Delivery

Outcome	Charles[11] (n = 14)	Sarrell[9] (n = 37)	Isreal[14] (n = 39)	Amstey[10] (n = 222)	Edwards[13] (n = 19)	Handsfield[12] (n = 12)
Normal or term infant	—	13 (35%)	30 (77%)	142 (64%)	7 (37%)	—
Aborted	—	13 (35%)	1 (2%)	24 (11%)	—	—
Perinatal death	—	3 (8%)	1 (2%)	15 (8%)	2 (11%)	—
Premature	—	6 (17%)	5 (13%)	49 (22%)	8 (42%)	8 (67%)
Perinatal distress	—	—	2 (5%)	—	2 (10%)	—
Premature rupture of membranes	6 (43%)	8 (21%)	—	52 (26%)	12 (63%)	9 (75%)

* Data is provided showing that the outcomes of pregnancies of mothers not infected with *N. gonorrhoeae* were significantly more favorable than for infected mothers.

A final demonstration of ascending infection of the fetus prior to delivery is found in a report of an infected stillborn infant who was found at autopsy to have multiple submucosal foci of the esophagus and upper respiratory tracts containing Gram-negative diplococci.[19] The location of the lesions indicated that infection had been contracted in utero during swallowing and respiration. Chorioamnionitis of the placenta was an accompanying finding.

NEONATAL GONOCOCCAL OPHTHALMIA

An association of neonatal conjunctivitis with vaginal discharge in the mother was noted by Quelimaltz in 1750, but gonococcal ophthalmia neonatorum was not recognized as a distinct entity until 1881. Inclusion conjunctivitis was subsequently differentiated from gonococcal ophthalmia by Lindner in 1909.

The incidences of various forms of neonatal gonococcal disease in exposed infants are listed in Table 82-2. Exposed infants who have had ocular silver nitrate prophylaxis have been reported to experience incidences of gonococcal ophthalmia of 0 to 5 percent, while exposed infants who have not had prophylaxis have had incidences of 2 to 30 percent. Oropharyngeal infection occurs in 35 percent of infants with gonococcal ophthalmia.

Ophthalmia neonatorum occurred in 1 to 15 percent of infants born in U.S. and European hospitals during the nineteenth century, and the great majority of cases were presumably gonococcal. In 1881, Crede reported the topical use of silver nitrate to prevent ophthalmia neonatorum.[29] He reported a reduction in the rate of neonatorum from 10 to 0.3 percent with this method of prophylaxis, which consisted of cleansing the eyes with ordinary water, after which the eyelids were held open and a single drop of silver nitrate was instilled in each eye. This was later modified by substituting 1 percent silver nitrate in individual dispensers in place of the higher-strength solution. The prevention of ophthalmia neonatorum with increasing use of Crede's method was reflected in a reduction in the importance of this syndrome as a cause of blindness. In the United States, the proportion of new entrants to schools for the blind with blindness attributable to ophthalmia neonatorum decreased from 28 percent in 1908 to 11 percent by 1933. When sulfonamides and penicillin became available for antepartum care and for treatment of gonococcal ophthalmia neonatorum, this proportion of new entrants to schools for the blind attributable to ophthalmia neonatorum further decreased to 1 percent by 1950, and to less than 0.1 percent by 1959.[30]

Etiology and differential diagnosis

The resurgence of gonorrhea during the 1960s and 1970s was associated with a reappearance of gonococcal ophthalmia neonatorum in the United States.[31–33] In a 1969 report from Glasgow, Scotland,[34] *N. gonorrhoeae* was the most common cause of ophthalmia neonatorum in children who required hospitalization for this condition. Recent data concerning the relative frequency of microbiologic etiologies of conjunctivitis in early infancy are presented in a study published in 1992 from Seattle.[35] The case-control study identified, in order of prevalence, disease due to the pathogens *Haemophilus influenzae, Streptococcus pneumoniae, Neisseria cinerea, Klebsiella pneumoniae,* and *Chlamydia trachomatis.* In addition, isolation of *Streptococcus mitis* was associated with an increased risk of conjunctivitis, and cultures from cases of conjunctivitis were more likely to yield diphtheroids than were controls. Finally, viral causes include herpes simplex virus and adenovirus. In most areas, gonococcal infection remains a rela-

Table 82-2. Incidences of Neonatal Gonococcal Disease in Exposed Infants

Site of neonatal infection	Reported incidences of infection, %	Population	References
Conjunctiva	5; 0; 2	Exposed infants who had $AgNo_3$ ocular prophylaxis	Edwards[13] Allen[20] Armstrong[21] Chen[22]
	2; 30	Exposed infants who had no ocular prophylaxis	Rothenberg[23] Fransen[24]
Orogastric fluid	40; 26	Infants of infected mothers	Handsfield[12] Edwards[13]
Oropharynx	43/122 (35)	Infants with gonococcal ophthalmia	Laga[25]
Disseminated disease as a proportion of all neonatal gonorrhea	0–1 (rare)	Reported series of neonatal gonococcal disease	Folland[26] Tomeh[27] Wald[28] Edwards[13] Fransem[24]

tively infrequent, albeit the most serious, cause of bacterial conjunctivitis in the newborn. In developed countries, *C. trachomatis* is among the most common causes of neonatal conjunctivitis, and *N. gonorrhoeae* is among the least common.

A mild chemical conjunctivitis can be expected after instillation of 1 percent nitrate drops. Evidence of epithelial desquamation and polymorphonuclear leukocytic exudate appears usually within 6 to 8 h and disappears usually within 24 to 48 h.

Conjunctival infection caused by *N. gonorrhoeae* in the newborn usually produces an acute purulent conjunctivitis that appears from 2 to 5 days after birth. The initial course is occasionally indolent, however, and onset can occur later than 5 days after birth,[21,33] perhaps because of partial suppression of infection by ophthalmic prophylaxis, because of small inoculum size, or because of strain-to-strain variations in gonococcal virulence. Cases with incubation periods up to 19 days have been reported after inoculation of the eye with contaminated urine,[6] and gonococcal conjunctivitis infection without any signs of inflammation has been detected by routine screening of neonates. Chronic mild, intermittent gonococcal conjunctivitis of 3 months' duration has been reported in a 4-month-old child.[38] Prolonged incubation after perinatal acquisition is hard to distinguish from delayed onset due to postnatal acquisition. Therefore, *gonococcal infection must be ruled out in every case of conjunctivitis in infants,* regardless of severity or time of onset. At the opposite extreme, gonococcal ophthalmia neonatorum has also been detected at birth or during the first few hours of life in infants born after a prolonged interval between rupture of membrane and delivery,[21,39] and infection in utero may have also occurred in an infant who developed gonococcal ophthalmia following a cesarean section that was performed after membrane rupture.[39,40]

As already noted, the risk of disease in the newborn by *N. gonorrhoeae* may be increased by premature rupture of membranes and by prematurity.[21,41,42] Brown et al.[33] noted prematurity in 19 (83 percent) of 23 infants with gonococcal ophthalmia, perhaps because infants who are premature also have often been delivered after premature rupture of membranes, and therefore the infection was established before delivery. Ocular silver nitrate is not efficacious for therapy of established gonococcal ophthalmia.[21] Gonococcal ophthalmia neonatorum has been more common in male than in female infants in some studies.[33] In contrast, in older children gonococcal conjunctivitis is more common in girls, who usually have associated vulvovaginitis.

Although gonococcal conjunctivitis is usually less severe and less rapidly progressive in the newborn than in the adult, permanent corneal damage following gonococcal ophthalmia neonatorum was usual in the preantibiotic era. The infant typically develops tense edema of both lids, followed by chemosis and a progressively purulent and profuse conjunctival exudate, which literally pours or squirts out of the lids when they are separated. If treatment is delayed, the infection extends beyond the superficial epithelial layers, reaching the subconjunctival connective tissue of the palpebral conjunctivae and, more significantly, the cornea. Corneal complications include ulcerations that may leave permanent nebulae or may cause perforation and lead to anterior synechiae, panophthalmitis (rarely), and loss of the eye. In the past, systemic spread occasionally caused peripheral manifestations of gonococcemia and death. Such local and systemic complications of gonococcal conjunctivitis are now more in the newborn, if treatment is begun promptly, while the cornea is still intact.

In addition to ocular complications of neonatal gonococcal ophthalmia, the disease may spread locally, cause primary disease at other mucous membrane sites, or cause systemic disease. The ocular disease serves as a signal that the infant has been infected. Examples of extension of gonococcal disease beyond the eye include the observation that 35 percent of infants with gonococcal ophthalmia also yield *N. gonorrhoeae* from pharyngeal culture and the description of gonococcal meningitis[43] and arthritis[44] in infants with ophthalmia.

GONOCOCCAL ARTHRITIS IN THE NEONATE

Septic arthritis has been the most commonly recognized manifestation of gonococcemia in the neonatal period. The association of arthritis in the newborn with ophthalmia neonatorum was noted by Lucas in 1885. Holt[45] reported 26 cases of gonococcal arthritis in children, including two infants who developed arthritis within the first month of life. One of these children also had ophthalmia neonatorum, most had no recognized focus, and rectal cultures were not taken. It is remarkable that ophthalmia neonatorum has often been absent in subsequent reported cases of neonatal gonococcal arthritis. The primary focus of infection in most of the 53 infants with gonococcal arthritis reported by Cooperman[46] was uncertain; only one had ophthalmia neonatorum. All of the females were said to have had vulvovaginitis, while several infants had proctitis. Bacteremia in some other cases has been attributed to infection of the mouth, nares, and umbilicus, while the source of bacteremia has been inapparent in many cases reported in the English language since the 1940s.[44,47–52]

The onset of clinical evidence of gonococcal arthritis in the newborn usually occurs from 1 to 4 weeks after delivery. One cannot distinguish between perinatal and postnatal acquisition of infection in most cases. The efficacy of ophthalmic prophylaxis, together with prompt recognition and treatment of gonococcal ophthalmia neonatorum when it occurs despite prophylaxis, may explain the absence of conjunctivitis in most cases of neonatal gonococcal arthritis reported since 1940. The pustular and necrotic skin lesions that characteristically appear during gonococcemia in the adult[53] have not yet been described in the newborn. The natural history of gonococcal arthritis in the infant is uncertain. Of the 53 cases in newborns who were presumably infected by a single epidemic strain of *N. gonorrhoeae,* described by Cooperman, none had a fatal outcome, and permanent impairment of function was uncommon, even without antibiotic therapy.[54] In contrast, 14 of 26 cases that occurred in a series of outbreaks described by Holt[45] in 1905 were fatal.

Infants with neonatal gonococcal arthritis share several important characteristics with neonates whose arthritis is of other etiologies (see Table 82-3).[55] Polyarticular involvement is the norm.[44] The primary presentation is refusal to move the involved limb, leading to the appearance of paralysis. Of particular concern is the difficulty in providing an early diagnosis of bacterial infection of the hip in neonates and young children. Inflammatory disease of the hip does not present a visible external swelling, and

Table 82-3. Presentations of Gonococcal Disease of the Newborn

Associated mucosal sites:
- Conjunctivitis, ophthalmia
- Asymptomatic pyuria
- Urethritis, vaginitis, proctitis, pharyngitis, rhinitis
- Scalp abscess
- Contaminated orogastric contents

Systemic findings:
- Multiply involved joints
- Pseudoparesis of involved joints
- "Sepsis of the newborn"
- Onset age 3–21 days

the hip-joint capsule of an infant is relatively distensible so that pain on movement may fail to provide a diagnosis. Nevertheless, infants with bacterial infections of the hips have a high incidence of subsequent development of aseptic necrosis of the head of the femur, and the physician must examine the child with particular care for this condition. If the infant with gonococcal disease fails to show normal spontaneous movement of a leg, a full workup, often including arthrocentesis, is indicated.

OTHER MANIFESTATIONS OF NEONATAL GONOCOCCAL INFECTION

Until recently, the recognized clinical spectrum of neonatal gonococcal infection essentially included only ophthalmia neonatorum and the systemic complications of gonococcemia, although other localized forms of neonatal gonococcal infection such as vaginitis,[56] rhinitis,[57] anorectal infection,[24] funisitis, and urethritis[58] have also been reported. More recent are case reports of gonococcal scalp abscesses attributed to intrauterine fetal monitoring.[59–63]

N. gonorrhoeae may be an indirect or a direct cause of early neonatal sepsis in the absence of gonococcal arthritis. As noted, intrapartum gonococcal infection has been associated with premature delivery and premature rupture of membranes, which may lead to amniotic fluid infection with a variety of vaginal organisms capable of causing neonatal sepsis. Premature infants have increased susceptibility to sepsis. *N. gonorrhoeae* was the third most common pathogen (after *E. coli* and group B streptococci) recovered from nasogastric aspirates in one study, usually in association with suspected neonatal sepsis.[12] *N. gonorrhoeae* has been isolated from blood of newborn infants with clinical sepsis without arthritis.[44,63] The incidence of neonatal complications with *N. gonorrhoeae* will reflect, of course, the incidence of disease in that community and the success or failure of maternal screening and treatment programs.

PREVENTION OF NEONATAL GONOCOCCAL DISEASE

Prevention of ophthalmia neonatorum is a principal goal of medical care of the newborn. The optimal method is the prevention and treatment of the disease in the mother, so that exposure of the newborn does not occur. In this regard, it is recommended that endocervical cultures for gonorrhea should be taken in the first and third trimester, since populations of women with gonorrhea in early pregnancy have shown a high incidence of recurrence during the pregnancy.[64]

Most states require ocular prophylaxis of some form, and silver nitrate has been the single recommended agent for many decades. Because of the high incidence of chemical conjunctivitis with silver nitrate and the importance of eye contact in mother-infant bonding, interest has developed in the use of other agents.[65] Recent recommendations by the American Academy of *Pediatrics* state that effective prophylaxis may be given with topical installation of either 1 percent silver nitrate (in single-dose ampules), 1 percent tetracycline, or 0.5 percent erythromycin.[66] It should be noted that chemical prophylaxis of the newborn conjunctivae provides excellent but not perfect protection. Silver nitrate does not provide effective therapy for an established infection, and some infants with failure of prophylaxis were born after prolonged rupture of the membranes, when the infection may already have been established. The advantages of using silver nitrate, however, include absence of development of microbial resistance to the preparation. For example, a recent outbreak of erythromycin-resistant staphylococcal conjunctivitis in newborns occurred in a nursery that was using topical erythromycin for ocular gonococcal prophylaxis.[67]

MICROBIOLOGIC DIAGNOSIS OF *N. GONORRHOEAE* INFECTION IN INFANTS AND CHILDREN

The microbiologic diagnosis of gonococcal infection and disease in infants and children must be made using techniques that are highly specific. This is because the societal response to such infections, in addition to the medical implications, often also includes considerations of abuse and neglect. Because of these medical/legal issues, as well as special aspects of the diseases in the young, the following principles and approaches should be observed:

1. Testing for *N. gonorrhoeae* in infants and children should use only standard culture systems for the isolation of *N. gonorrhoeae.* Rapid, nonculture tests, which have been studied in adults, have not been adequately evaluated in children and are not approved for diagnosis. These nonapproved methods include direct Gram-stained smear, enzyme immunoassay (EIA) tests, and DNA probes.
2. It appears that in order to achieve satisfactory results from cultures, specimens for culture from children may require particularly meticulous handling. First, specimens should immediately be placed into *prewarmed* media. Second, in many pediatric gonococcal infections the *N. gonorrhoeae* organisms are sparse or are a minority of the flora. It appears to improve isolation rates when two separate chocolate agar plates (one with inhibitory antibiotics, one without) are used rather than a biplate. The larger surface area provided by full-sized plates appears to enable technicians to recognize colonies more completely. Third, plates must be *promptly* introduced into a 36°C incubator with enhanced CO_2 environment, such as a candle jar. This implies that the clinician must arrange for the appropriate triage of specimens, often to distant laboratories and through inclement weather.
3. The clinician should have a policy regarding the identification of specimens and establish a chain of custody so that results can be supported in court procedures when/if issues of the child's safety are being considered.
4. The identification of *N. gonorrhoeae* from a pediatric specimen should be confirmed with at least two tests that employ different principles. Currently used identification models are biochemical, serologic, and enzyme substrate. The standard biochemical tests demonstrate a positive oxidase test and utilization of glucose, but not matose, sucrose, or lactose. There have been reports of the misidentification of related organisms to be *N. gonorrhoeae.*[68–70] Because of the societal responses, such occurrences bring the child into risk of loss of home and social chaos.
5. Finally, the diagnosis of gonococcal infection or disease in a child requires an evaluation for the source of infection and of other children who may also have been exposed to the perpetrator. In one study of 244 persons who were family members and associates of children with gonorrhea, 18 percent had gonorrhea.[3]

Although direct culture is the only appropriate means of diagnosing *N. gonorrhoeae* infections in children, in some circumstances a Gram stain of exudate provides a preliminary diagnosis. Conjunctival exudate should be directly examined by Gram stain for the presence of gram-negative intracellular bean-shaped diplococci typical of *N. gonorrhoeae,* for gram-negative coccobacilli typical of *Hemophilus sp,* or for gram-positive cocci suggestive of infection with gram-positive pathogens. The presence of one or more polymorphonuclear leukocytes per oil-immersion field in a conjunctival smear supports the diagnosis of conjunctivitis. Detection of typical gram-negative diplococci by Gram stain warrants the presumptive diagnosis of gonococcal conjunctivitis, although other *Neisseria* species, such as *N. meningitidis,* have also been associated with purulent ophthalmia neonatorum. If gonococcal conjunctivitis is suspected on the basis of examination of the Gram-stained smear of conjunctival exudate, cultures for *N. gonorrhoeae* should also be obtained from the oropharynx and anal canal, since concomitant infection of these sites has been demonstrated in association with gonococcal ophthalmia neonatorum.

GONOCOCCAL DISEASE BEYOND INFANCY

VAGINITIS

Gonococcal vaginitis is the most common form of gonorrhea in children, excluding the neonatal period. In contrast to adults, in prepubertal girls the nonestrogenized alkaline vaginal mucosa may be colonized and infected with *N. gonorrhoeae.* Transmission of gonorrhea from an infected male to a prepubertal female occurs efficiently. In one study in an orphanage, 53 of 95 abused girls were infected.[71] Gonococcal vaginitis is often a mild disease, perhaps because it is restricted to the superficial mucosa. Prepubertal vaginitis has been attributed not only to *N. gonorrhoeae* but also to numerous irritative and infectious agents, such as pinworms, foreign bodies, streptococci, *T. vaginalis*, shigella, Group A streptococci, and other bacteria.

The incidences of gonorrhea in several studies of children who were known or suspected to have been sexually abused, or in adolescents who were sexually active, are tabulated in Table 82-4. Gonococcal vaginitis was the most frequently recognized of these. Not all children were symptomatic; Hein and associates[77] demonstrated a 7 percent prevalence of asymptomatic gonorrhea in sexually active adolescent females and a 1.9 percent rate in males. Asymptomatic disease is probably common in prepubertal children also, and it is usually recognized when a child is undergoing an evaluation for suspected sexual abuse.[78] In a study of 266 asymptomatic prepubertal girls who were examined for gonorrhea because of suspected sexual abuse, 14 (5.3 percent) were found to be infected.[79] Some authors advocate restricting the collection of clinical samples to children who are symptomatic.[80] When attempting to enhance the safety of the child, however, it is very valuable for the clinician to recognize gonococcal infection when present. Consequently, strong consideration should be given to obtaining cultures, even when the child is asymptomatic, if child abuse is seriously suspected.

The majority of symptomatic children have vaginal itching and minor crusting discharge that may discolor the underwear; other signs may be minimal to absent, or they may point to systemic infection. Dysuria and polymorphonuclear leukocytes in the urine may accompany this infection. A Gram stain of the vaginal secretions may lead to suspicion of the diagnosis.[81]

A review of reported complications of 1232 cases of gonococcal vaginitis in the preantibiotic era revealed that 35 percent had urethritis, 19 percent had proctitis, and 6 percent had peritonitis.[82] Although ascending infection is uncommon, it may result in salpingitis or peritonitis. Ten percent of girls with gonorrhea have signs compatible with peritonitis, including fever, diffuse abdominal pain, leukocytosis, and decreased bowel sounds—findings that are similar to those of appendicitis. For these reasons, a perineal examination for vaginal irritation, discharge, or both is important prior to abdominal surgery in young girls.

PELVIC INFLAMMATORY DISEASE AND SALPINGITIS

Vaginal infection of females who are adolescent or younger may progress to involve the fallopian tubes or may disseminate to the pelvis, leading to perihepatitis and PID; in adolescents, the latter may be particularly likely to result in infertility and ectopic pregnancy, and it is the single most common cause of infertility in young women.[83,84] Between 1970 and 1989 the rate of ectopic pregnancies per 1,000 live births in the United States increased from 4.5 to 16. Between 1975 and 1981 the rate of hospitalization for salpingitis of females age 15–19 was 4 per 100,000.[85]

The identification of the cause of PID is complicated by the difficulty of obtaining fallopian-tube specimens prior to therapy. Although gonococcal infections are a very common cause of acute PID in adolescents, other major causes include *C. trachomatis, M. hominis, Haemophilus influenzae,* and mixed aerobic and anaerobic flora.[86]

Risk factors for PID and acute salpingitis have been shown to include young age at acquisition of gonococcal disease, a history of previous PID, multiple sexual partners, and use of an IUD for contraception. Approximately 15 percent of teenagers who develop gonorrhea will progress to PID.

Diagnosis of PID may be difficult, and the differential diagnosis in the adolescent includes numerous other conditions of the lower abdomen, including appendicitis, ectopic pregnancy, mesenteric adenitis, pyelonephritis, and septic abortion. Misdiagnosis of PID is common and is one of the more common causes of laparotomy. Recommendations by Shafer and associates suggest that a clinical diagnosis of PID be supported by the presence of lower abdominal pain and tenderness with motion of the cervix, and adnexal tenderness.[87] Fever, leukocytosis, elevated sedimentation rate, and adnexal mass on abdominal ultrasonography support the diagnosis but may be absent. Culdocentesis, if performed, may reveal evidence of purulent reaction in the peritoneal cavity. It is probable that the outcome for fertility is improved with prompt and vigorous therapy.

Indications for parenteral therapy for therapy of PID include adolescence; they are listed in Table 82-5.

URETHRITIS

Gonococcal urethritis in prepubertal males is much less common than is vaginitis in girls. When recognized, the disease is usually symptomatic and resembles gonococcal urethritis in the adult male. As with vaginitis, asymptomatic pyuria is a presentation with which the pediatrician should be familiar.[88] In children with

Table 82-4. Prevalence of *Neisseria gonorrhoeae* in Abused or Sexually Active Children and Adolescents

Author, date, ref	Age (years), sex	Number % infected	Population	Special risk, etc.
Ingram, 1984[61]	1–12, F	10/50 (20%)	North Carolina	Known sexual contact or abuse
Fraser, 1983[62]	Adolescent, F	15/125 (12%)	Oklahoma	Sexually active
Dejong, 1986[63]	1–14, M and F	25/532 (4.7%)	Pennsylvania	Known sexual abuse
Jamison, 1995[25]	Adolescent, F	45/632 (7.1%)	Colorado	Urban clinic
Ingram, 1992[76]	Children	41/1469 (2.8%)	North Carolina	Suspected sexual abuse

Table 82-5. Indications for Hospitalization of Children with Suspected Salpingitis

Adolescence
Diagnostic uncertainty
Failure to respond to prior regimen
Pregnancy
Fever, peritoneal signs
Adnexal mass
IUD use
Noncompliance with medical regimen

gonococcal infection of the genitourinary tract, concomitant anorectal and tonsillopharyngeal colonization is common. This colonization is usually asymptomatic, as in adults, but it may also be symptomatic.[89]

DISSEMINATED DISEASE

Gonococcal arthritis in older children resembles that of adults and may be accompanied by cutaneous lesions.[90] Multiple septic involvement of joints is not as common as in the newborn period, although a migratory polyarthritis may be part of the prodrome.[91] More typically a single, severely affected joint and myositis and tenosynovitis predominate.

Treatment of gonococcal arthritis depends on prompt recognition of the disease. Cultures of all mucous membranes (nasopharynx, rectal, vaginal or endocervical, conjunctival), blood culture, and aspiration of the involved joint should be performed. In the newborn period, the gastric aspirate may be cultured to determine contamination from a material source. A history for an adult contact should be taken. If the contact has not responded to therapy, the possibility of a penicillinase-producing strain may be considered.

Each patient must be evaluated for the need for drainage of an involved joint. Sincc complete response to medical therapy may not occur for several days, most physicians attempt to avoid an open drainage procedure and manage the pyarthrosis with needle aspirations if possible. An exception is purulent arthritis of the hips, in which early drainage may be necessary to prevent necrosis of the femoral head.

OTHER FORMS OF GONOCOCCAL DISEASE

Other complications of gonorrhea are rarely, if ever, reported in the pediatric literature. Gonococcal sepsis, meningitis, endocarditis, myocarditis, conjunctivitis, and hepatitis occur in adults; they may be expected to occur in children and may be fatal.[92,93], The pediatric experience with these conditions is too minimal for comment, however.

GONORRHEA AS AN INDICATOR OF SEXUAL ABUSE IN CHILDREN

Gonorrhea in children beyond the newborn period is an infection that, with very rare exceptions, is definitive evidence that the child has been sexually assaulted or abused.[94] Gonococcal infection may be the major factor for the clinician to suspect abuse. In a study of 75 children in Kansas City who acquired gonorrhea during sexually abusing contact, in 83 percent the abuse was recognized because of the infection.[4] All children with acquired gonorrhea should be reported by the examining clinician to the agency designated by that community to receive reports of suspected child abuse. Child abuse and evaluations for sexually transmitted diseases (STDs) are discussed in greater detail in Chap. 87, but a clinician who is examining a prepubertal child for a possible STD should be aware of the following points:

1. In the 1980s, gonorrhea was the most common of the STDs isolated from children who were being evaluated for suspected abuse. Among 744 children evaluated in three reported series, 7 to 20 percent had gonorrhea.[95–97] More recent data suggest declining prevalence rates.[76] After any event, the clinician should ensure high-quality diagnostic techniques when dealing with children.
2. Children may have compelling reasons to refrain from disclosing abuse, even when a defining infection has been identified. In one study of the rate of disclosure among children who presented with physical complaints related to gonococcal infection, only 43 percent were able to provide valid verbal disclosure during the first interview.[98]
3. Gentle coaching of most children will enable the clinicians to visualize the genitalia adequately and to obtain necessary culture material. Introital and intravaginal specimens may be required in prepubertal children, intracervical are not. The child should never be restrained. If necessary, anesthesia may be used to facilitate an examination. A speculum or other intravaginal devices should never be attempted in an awake prepubertal female. The hymen in prepubertal females is very sensitive to touch, and manipulation may cause extensive pain.
4. Contrary to adults, it is not necessary to obtain a specimen from the cervical canal in order to provide culture material from a prepubertal child for gonorrhea. A specimen from the vaginal canal suffices.
5. Sexual abuse of children is usually a chronic and recurring condition. Consequently, if the child remains unprotected, reabuse is likely. If the perpetrator has a sexually transmitted disease, the child may present with recurrent STD infection.[99]

TREATMENT

Recommendations for therapy of childhood gonorrhea based on guidelines from the U.S. *Centers for Disease Control*[100] are as follows:

Pediatric patients encompass children from birth to adolescence. When a child is postpubertal or weighs more than 45 kg (100 lb.), he or she should be treated with dosage regimens as defined for adults (see Chap. 32).

Studies of the efficacy of many therapeutic regimens for uncomplicated and complicated gonococcal infections of prepubertal children are sparse or nonexistent. In the United States, about one-third of gonococcal isolates during 1994 were resistant to the penicillins and/or the tetracyclines. It is therefore recommended that physicians treat all children with gonococcal disease with a regimen suitable for therapy of tetracycline- or penicillin-resistant strains. Thus, ceftriaxone is the preferred drug for gonococcal infection in children.

NEONATAL DISEASE

Gonococcal ophthalmia: The patient should be hospitalized until the infection has been controlled. Recommended therapy is ceftriaxone, 25–50 mg IV or IM in a single dose, not to exceed 125 mg. Topical antimicrobial therapy is optional but probably not beneficial.

Complicated infection: Arthritis, abscess, and septicemia should be treated by hospitalization and administration of ceftriaxone, 25–50 mg/kg/day in a single dose for at least 7 days. Meningitis should be treated for at least 10 to 14 days.

CHILDHOOD DISEASE BEYOND INFANCY

Children who weigh less than 45 kg and have uncomplicated localized gonococcal disease (vulvovaginitis, urethritis, pharyngitis, proctitis, conjunctivitis) may receive ceftriaxone, 125 mg in a single dose, or spectinomycin, 40 mg/kg in a single dose (Table 82-6). Children who weigh less than 45 kg and have disseminated gonococcal disease (bacteremia, arthritis, meningitis, perihepatitis) may receive ceftriaxone, 50 mg/kg IM or IV in a single daily dose for 7 to 14 days. Note that only parenteral cephalosporins are recommended for therapy in children; oral cephalosporins have not been adequately evaluated. *All children with gonococcal disease should also be evaluated for syphilis, chlamydial infection, and HIV infection.*

Treatment of pelvic inflammatory disease

Co-infection with both chlamydia and gonococci is common in children as well as adults. In female adolescents, treatment of gonococcal cervicitis with drug regimens that are effective against gonococci but not chlamydia has led to a high incidence of residual salpingitis in females, and of urethritis in males, both of which are associated with continued disease due to chlamydia. Optimal therapy for known or possible co-infection with both pathogens has not been explored in children. Ceftriaxone and spectinomycin alone fail to eradicate chlamydia. The following regimen may be employed, pending further data:[101] **For children under 45 kg in weight,** treat with ceftriaxone *plus* erythromycin, 50 mg/kg/day divided into four doses for 10–14 days. **For children weighing ≥45 kg but age <8 years,** treat with ceftriaxone *plus* erythromycin base, 500 mg orally four times a day for 7 days *or* erythromycin ethylsuccinate 800 mg orally four times a day for 7 days. **For children ≥8 years of age,** treat with ceftriaxone *plus* doxycycline, 100 mg orally twice daily for 7 days *or* azithromycin, 1 gm orally in a single dose.

PREVENTION OF NEONATAL INFECTION

All pregnant women should have endocervical culture examinations for gonococci as an integral part of prenatal care at the first prenatal visit. A second culture late in pregnancy should be obtained from women who are at high risk of gonococcal infection.

Table 82-6. Recommendations for Treatment of Gonococcal Infections in Children Who Weigh <45 kg.

Uncomplicated Vulvovaginitis, cervicitis, urethritis, pharyngitis, proctitis
Treatment of choice: ceftriaxone 125mg in a single IM dose
Alternative: spectinomycin 40mg/kg (maximum 2g) IM in a single dose
Complicated infection-bacteremia, arthritis, meningitis, peritonitis
Recommended regimen: ceftriaxone 50 mg/kg (maximum 1 g) IM or IV in a single dose daily for 7 days (for meningitis increase maximum dose to 2 g, duration of treatment to 10–14 days)
Complicated infection-pelvic inflammatory disease
See text.

Routine prevention of gonococcal ophthalmia

Studies of the treatment of most forms of gonorrhea in children are very sparse and are derived from experiences in adults. A notable contrast is the prevention of gonococcal ophthalmia of the newborn, for which prevention trials have been conducted.[102] Silver nitrate instillation at delivery reduces infection rates by approximately 83 percent. Tetracycline reduces rates by similar or slightly greater amounts.

Recommended regimens are: 1 percent $AgNO_3$ in a single application (do not irrigate with saline), *or* erythromycin (0.5 percent) in a single application, *or* tetracycline ophthalmic ointment (1 percent) in a single application. Bacitracin ointment (not effective) and penicillin drops (sensitizing) should not be used.

Management of asymptomatic infants born to a mother with untreated gonococcal infection

The infant born to a mother with untreated gonorrhea should have orogastric and rectal cultures taken routinely. It is recommended that the child receive ceftriaxone, 25–50 mg/kg IV or IM as a single dose.

References

1 Desenclos J-CA, Garrity D, Wroten J: Pediatric gonococcal infection, Florida, 1984 to 1988. *Am J Public Health* 82:426, 1992.
2 Centers for Disease Control and Prevention: Special focus: Surveillance for sexually transmitted diseases. *MMWR* 42(SS-3):1, 1993.
3 Alexander WJ, Griffith H, Housch JG, et al: Infections in sexual contacts and associates of children with gonorrhea. *Sex Transm Dis* 11:156, 1984.
4 Geidinghagen DH, Hoff GL, Biery RM: Gonorrhea in children: Epidemiologic unit analysis. *Pediatr Infect Dis J* 11:973, 1992.
5 Cohen MS, Sparling PF: Mucosal infection with *Neisseria gonorrhoeae. J Clin Invest* 89:1169, 1992.
6 Acosta AA et al: Intrauterine pregnancy and coexistent pelvic inflammatory disease. *Obstet Gynecol* 37:282, 1971.
7 Rothbard MJ et al: Intrapartum gonococcal amnionitis. *Am J Obstet Gynecol* 121:565, 1975.
8 Quinn PA et al: Chorioamnionitis: Its association with pregnancy outcome and microbial infection. *Am J Obstet Gynecol* 156:378, 1987.
9 Sarrell PM, Pruett KA: Symptomatic gonorrhea during pregnancy. *Obstet Gynecol* 32:670, 1968.
10 Amstey MS, Steadman KT: Symptomatic gonorrhea and pregnancy. *J Am Vener Dis Assoc* 3:14, 1976.
11 Charles AG et al: Asymptomatic gonorrhea in prenatal patients. *Am J Obstet Gynecol* 108:595, 1970.
12 Handsfield HH et al: Neonatal gonococcal infection. 1. Orogastric contamination with *Neisseria gonorrhoeae. JAMA* 225:697, 1973.
13 Edwards L et al: Gonorrhea in pregnancy. *Am J Obstet Gynecol* 132:637, 1978.
14 Israel KS et al: Neonatal and childhood gonococcal infections. *Clin Obstet Gynecol* 18:143, 1975.
15 Kass EH et al: Genital mycoplasmas as a cause of excess premature delivery. *Trans Assoc Am Physicians* 94:261, 1981.
16 Kundson RB et al: Association of *Ureaplasma urealyticum* in the placenta with perinatal morbidity and mortality. *N Engl J Med* 310:941, 1984.
17 Gravett MG et al: Independent associations of bacterial vaginosis and *Chlamydia trachomatis* infection with adverse pregnancy outcome. *JAMA* 256:1899, 1986.
18 Berman SM et al: Low birth weight, prematurity, and postpartum endometritis. Association with prenatal cervical *Mycoplasma hominis* and *Chlamydia trachomatis* infections. *JAMA* 257:1189, 1987.

19 Oppenheimer EH, Winn KJ: Fetal gonorrhea with deep tissue infection occurring in utero. *Pediatrics* 69:74, 1982.

20 Allen JH, Barrere LE: Prophylaxis of gonorrheal ophthalmia of the newborn. *JAMA* 141:522, 1949.

21 Armstrong JH et al: Ophthalmia neonatorum: A chart review. *Pediatrics* 57:884, 1976.

22 Chen J-Y: Prophylaxis of ophthalmia neonatorum: Comparison of silver nitrate, tetracycline, erythromycin, and no prophylaxis. *Pediatr Infect Dis J* 11:1026, 1992.

23 Rothenberg R: Ophthalmic neonatorum due to *Neisseria gonorrhoeae:* Prevention and treatment. *Sex Transm Dis* 6(suppl 2):187, 1979.

24 Fransen L et al: Ophthalmia neonatorum in Nairobi, Kenya: The roles of *Neisseria gonorrhea* and *Chlamydia trachomatis. J Infect Dis* 153:862, 1986.

25 Laga M et al: Single-dose therapy of gonococcal ophthalmia neonatorum with ceftriaxone. *N Engl J Med* 315:1382, 1986.

26 Folland DS et al: Gonorrhea in preadolescent children: An inquiry into source of infection and mode of transmission. *Pediatrics* 60:153, 1977.

27 Tomeh MO, Wilfert CM: Venereal diseases of infants and children at Duke University Medical Center. *North Carolina Med J* 34:109, 1973.

28 Wald ER et al: Gonorrheal disease among children in a University Hospital. *Sex Transm Dis* 7:41, 1980.

29 Forbes G, Forbes GM: Silver nitrate and the eyes of the newborn. *Am J Dis Child* 121:1, 1971.

30 Hatfield EM: Causes of blindness in school children. *Sight Sav Rev* 33:218, 1963.

31 Friendly DS: Gonococcal conjunctivitis in the newborn. *Clin Proc Child Hosp DC* 25:1, 1969.

32 Snowe RJ, Wilfert CM: Epidemic reappearance of gonococcal ophthalmia neonatorum. *Pediatrics* 51:110, 1973.

33 Brown WM et al: Gonococcal ophthalmia among newborn infants at Los Angeles County General Hospital, 1957–1963. *Public Health Rep* 8 1:926, 1966.

34 Smith JA: Ophthalmia neonatorum in Glasgow. *Scott Med J* 14:272, 1969.

35 Krohn MA, Hillier SL, Bell JA et al: The bacterial etiology of conjunctivitis in early infancy. *Am J Epidemiol* 138:326, 1993.

36 Valenton MJ, Abendanio R: Gonorrheal conjunctivitis. *Can J Ophthalmol* 8:421, 1973.

37 Podgore JK, Holmes KK: Ocular gonococcal infection with minimal or no inflammatory response. *JAMA* 246:242, 1981.

38 Fivush B et al: Gonococcal conjunctivitis in a four-month-old infant. *Sex Transm Dis* 7:24, 1979.

39 Thompson TR et al: Gonococcal ophthalmia neonatorum. Relationship of time of infection to relevant control measures. *JAMA* 228: 186, 1974.

40 Diener B: Cesarean section complicated by gonococcal ophthalmia neonatorum. *J Fam Pract* 13:739, 1981.

41 Dundas GHG: Ophthalmia neonatorlini before birth. *Lancet* 1:122, 1921.

42 Pearson HE: Failure of silver nitrate prophylaxis for gonococcal ophthalmia neonatorum. *Am J Obstet Gynecol* 73:805, 1857.

43 Bradford WL, Kelley HW: Gonococcic meningitis in a newborn infant. *Am J Dis Child* 46:543, 1933.

44 Kohen DP: Neonatal gonococcal arthritis: Three cases and review of the literature. *Pediatrics* 53:436, 1974.

45 Holt LE: Gonococcus infections in children with especial reference to their prevalence in institutions and means of prevention. *NY Med J* 81:521, 1905.

46 Cooperman MB: Gonococcus arthritis in infancy. *Am J Dis Child* 33:932, 1927.

47 Parrish PP et al: Gonococcic arthritis of a newborn treated with sulfonamide. *JAMA* 114:241, 1940.

48 Jones JB, Ramsey RC: Acute suppurative arthritis of hip in children. *US Armed Forces Med J* 7:1621, 1956.

49 Sponzilli EE, Calabro JJ: Gonococcal arthritis in the newborn. *JAMA* 177:919, 1961.

50 Glaser S et al: Gonococcal arthritis in the newborn. *Am J Dis Child* 112:185, 1966.

51 Gregory JE et al: Gonococcal arthritis in an infant. *Br J Vener Dis* 48:306, 1972.

52 Kleiman MB, Lamb GA: Gonococcal arthritis in a newborn infant. *Pediatrics* 52:285, 1973.

53 Holmes KK et al: Disseminated gonococcal infection. *Ann Intern Med* 74:979, 1971.

54 Cooperman MB: End results of gonorrheal arthritis: Review of 70 cases. *Am J Surg* 5:241, 1928.

55 Gutman LT: Acute, subacute and chronic osteomyelitis and pyogenic arthritis in children. *Curr Probl Pediatr* 15:1, 1985.

56 Barton LL, Shuja M: Neonatal gonococcal vaginitis. *J Pediatr* 98: 171, 1981.

57 Kirkland H, Storer RV: Gonococcal rhinitis in an infant. *Br Med J* 1:263, 1931.

58 Hunter GW, Fargo ND: Specific urethritis (gonorrhea) in a male newborn. *Am J Obstet Gynecol* 38:520, 1939.

59 Plavidal FJ, Welch A: Gonococcal fetal scalp abscess: A case report. *Am J Obstet Gynecol* 127:437, 1977.

60 Reveri M, Krishnamurthy C: Gonococcal scalp abscess. *J Pediatr* 94: 819, 1979.

61 Brook I et al: Gonococcal scalp abscess in a newborn. *South Med J* 73:396, 1980.

62 D'Auria A et al: Gonococcal scalp wound infection. *MMWR* 24: 115, 1975.

63 Thadepalli H et al: Gonococcal sepsis secondary to fetal monitoring. *Am J Obstet Gynecol* 126:510, 1976.

64 Jones DED et al: Gonorrhea in obstetric patients. *J Am Vener Dis Assoc* 2:30, 1976.

65 Rothenberg R: Ophthalmia neonatorum due to *Neisseria gonorrhoeae:* Prevention and treatment. *Sex Transm Dis* 6:187, 1979.

66 Committee on Infectious Diseases of the American Academy of Pediatrics: *1994 Red Book,* 23rd ed. AAP, Elf Grove Village Ill, 1994, pp 533–535.

67 Hedberg K, Ristinon TL, Solor JT et al: Outbreak of erythromycin-resistant staphylococcal conjunctivitis in a newborn nursery. *Pediat Infect Dis J* 9:268, 1990.

68 Denison MR, Perlman S, Anderson RD: Misidentification of Neisseria species in a neonate with conjunctivitis. *Pediatrics* 81:877, 1988.

69 Dossett JH, Appelbaum PC, Knapp JS et al: Proctitis associated with *Neisseria cinerea* misidentified as *Neisseria gonorrhoeae* in a child. *J Clin Microbiol* 21:575, 1985.

70 Whittington WL, Rice RJ, Biddle JW et al: Incorrect identification of *Neisseria gonorrhoeae* from infants and children. *Pediatr Infect Dis J* 7:3, 1988.

71 Ahmed HJ, Ilardi I, Antognoli A et al: An epidemic of *Neisseria gonorrhoeae* in a Somali orphanage. *Int J STD and AIDS* 3:52, 1992.

72 Ingram DL et al: Vaginal *Chlamydia trachomatis* infection in children with sexual contact. *Pediatr Infect Dis* 3:97, 1984.

73 Fraser JJ et al: Prevalence of cervical *Chlamydia trachomatis* and *Neisseria gonorrhoeae* in female adolescents. *Pediatrics* 71:333, 1983.

74 Dejong AR: Sexually transmitted diseases in sexually abused children. *Sex Transm Dis* 13:123, 1986.

75 Jamison JH, Kaplan DW, Hamman R et al: Spectrum of genital human papillomavirus infection in a female adolescent population. *Sex Transm Dis* 22:236, 1995.

76 Ingram DL, Everett NO, Lyna PR et al: Epidemiology of adult sexually transmitted disease agents in children being evaluated for sexual abuse. *Pediatr Infect Dis J* 11:945, 1992.

77 Hein K et al: Asymptomatic gonorrhea: Prevalence in a population of urban adolescents. *J Pediatr* 90:634, 1977.

78 Loney LC et al: Silent gonorrhea in siblings. *Missouri Med* 80:18, 1983.

79 Bogaerts J, Lepage P, DeClorcq A et al: *Shigella* and gonococcal vulvovaginitis in prepubertal central African girls. *Pediatr Infect Dis J* 11:890, 1992.
80 Sicoli RA, Losek JD, Hudlett JM et al: Indications for *Neisseria gonorrhoeae* cultures in children with suspected sexual abuse. *Arch Pediatr Adolescent Med* 149:86, 1995.
81 Wald ER: Gonorrhea diagnosis by Gram stain in the female adolescent. *Am J Dis Child* 131:1094, 1977.
82 Benson RA, Weinstock E: Gonorrheal vaginitis in children. A review of the literature. *Am J Dis Child* 59:1083, 1940.
83 Mueller BA, Luz-Jimenez M, Daling JR et al: Risk factors for tubal infertility. *Sex Transm Dis* 92:28, 1992.
84 Brunham RC, Binns B, Guijon F et al: Etiology and outcome of acute pelvic inflammatory disease. *J Infect Dis* 158:510, 1988.
85 Washington AE et al: Hospitalization for pelvic inflammatory disease. *JAMA* 251:2529, 1984.
86 Eschenbach DA et al: Polymicrobial etiology of acute pelvic inflammatory disease. *N Engl J Med* 293:166, 1975.
87 Shafer MAB et al: Acute salpingitis in the adolescent female. *J Pediatr* 100:339, 1982.
88 Dawar S, Hellerstein S: Gonorrhea as a cause of asymptomatic pyuria in adolescent boys. *J Pediatr* 81:357, 1972.
89 Abbott SL: Gonococcal tonsillitis-pharyngitis in a 5 year old girl. *Pediatrics* 52:287, 1973.
90 Angevine CD et al: A case of gonococcal osteomyelitis. A complication of gonococcal arthritis. *J Dis Child* 130:1013, 1976.
91 Coulter K: Migratory polyarthritis in a nine-year old girl. *Pediatr Infect Dis J* 9:856, 1990.
92 Pasquariello CA et al: Fatal gonococcal septicemia. *Pediatr Infect Dis J* 4:204, 1985.
93 Lewis LS, Glauser TA, Joffe MD: Gonococcal conjunctivitis in prepubertal children. *Amer J Dis Child* 144:546, 1990.
94 Committee on Child Abuse Neglect: Guidelines for the evaluation of sexual abuse of children. *Pediat* 87:254, 1991.
95 Rimsza ME, Niggemann EH: Medical evaluation of sexually abused children: A review of 311 cases. *Pediatrics* 69:8, 1982.
96 White ST et al: Sexually transmitted diseases in sexually abused children. *Pediatrics* 72:16, 1983.
97 Ingram DL et al: Vaginal *Chlamydia trachomatis* infection in children with sexual contact. *Pediatr Infect Dis* 3:97, 1984.
98 Lawson L, Chaffin M: False negatives in sexual abuse disclosure interviews. *J Interpersonal Violence* 7:532, 1992.
99 Laras L, Craighill M, Woods ER et al: Epidemiologic observations of adolescents with *Neisseria gonorrhoeae* genital infections treated at a children's hospital. *Adolesc Pediatr Gynecol* 7:9, 1994.
100 Centers for Disease Control and Prevention: 1998 Guidelines for Treatment of Sexually Transmitted Diseases. *MMWR* In press, 1998.
101 Burnakis TG, Hildebrandt NB: Pelvic inflammatory disease: A review with emphasis on antimicrobial therapy. *Rev Infect Dis* 8:86, 1987.
102 Laga M, Plummer FA, Piot P et al: Prophylaxis of gonococcal and chlamydial ophthalmia neonatorum. *N Engl J Med* 318:653, 1988.

Chapter 83

Chlamydial infections in infants and children

Margaret R. Hammerschlag

The biology and spectrum of *Chlamydia trachomatis* infection in adults are discussed in Chaps. 28 and 29. This chapter covers perinatally acquired *C. trachomatis* infection in infants, including conjunctivitis and pneumonia, and infection in older children, including the relationship with sexual abuse.

HISTORY

At the turn of the twentieth century, there was no screening of expectant mothers for sexually transmitted diseases (STDs), no instillation of prophylactic eyedrops, no antibiotic treatment for established infections. In this period, the term *ophthalmia neonatorum* was for all practical purposes synonymous with gonococcal conjunctivitis. As neonatal conjunctivitis came under control with silver nitrate prophylaxis, the importance of another form of ophthalmia neonatorum, termed *inclusion blennorrhea,* was noted. The relationship between maternal genital infection and conjunctivitis of the newborn associated with inclusion bodies within epithelial cells was established by Lindner, Halberstader, Von Prowazek, and others.[1] It was not until the 1950s that *Chlamydia trachomatis* was isolated from an infant with inclusion blennorrhea.[2] In 1967, Schachter and colleages further emphasized the relationship of sexual transmission of the infection in the parents of infants with inclusion conjunctivitis.[3]

Respiratory infection in infants due to *C. trachomatis* was probably first reported in 1941 by Botsztejn, who described an entity he called *pertussoid eosinophilic pneumonia.*[4] It was not until 1975, however, that Schachter and colleagues isolated *C. trachomatis* from the respiratory tract of an infant with pneumonia.[5] The syndrome of infantile chlamydial pneumonia was further characterized by Beem and Saxon in 1977.[6]

EPIDEMIOLOGY

Epidemiologic evidence strongly suggests that the infant acquires chlamydial infection from his or her mother during parturition.[7–14] This is based on a number of well-controlled prospective studies of maternal-infant infection, where infection essentially occured only in those infants born to infected mothers (Table 83-1). There is no convincing evidence of horizontal transmission from mother to infant, other family members to infant, or from infant to infant after delivery. Infection after cesarean delivery or through intact membranes is rare but may occur.[15] In the former, there has usually been early rupture of the amnionic membranes. Depending on the population examined, cervical infection with *C. trachomatis* has been reported in 2 to 30 percent of pregnant women attending prenatal clinics (see Table 83-1). In most studies, chlamydial infection was far more prevalent than gonococcal infection.

The pregnant woman with chlamydial infection is most likely to be young. Hammerschlag et al. found cervical chlamydial infection in 8 percent of pregnant women in an inner-city hospital.[14] Among a subgroup of adolescents (up to 18 years of age) attending the Teen Prenatal Clinic at Kings County Hospital, Brooklyn, however, the prevalence was 14 percent. This inverse relationship with age has been reported by other investigators.[16,17]

If the infant is delivered to a mother with active chlamydial infection, the overall risk of acquiring infection at any anatomical site has been approximately 50 to 75 percent in various studies (see Table 83-1). Infants are often infected at more than one site, including the conjunctiva, nasopharynx, rectum, and vagina.

The most frequent clinical manifestation of neonatal chlamydial infection, inclusion conjunctivitis, has been reported to occur in 15 to 37 percent of infants born to mothers with cervical chlamydial infection. The most frequent site of infection, however, is the nasopharynx, with 78 percent of infected infants having positive nasopharyngeal cultures in one study.[18] Approximately one-half of infants with inclusion conjunctivitis will also be infected in the nasopharynx. It appears that a minority of infants with nasopharyngeal infection go on to develop chlamydial pneumonia; Hammerschlag et al. found only 4 of 12 (33 percent) infants with isolated nasopharyngeal infection subsequently developed pneumonia.[18] The overall risk of developing pneumonia among infants born to chlamydia-positive mothers has been reported to range from 1 to 22 percent (see Table 83-1).

Data on the risk of acquiring rectal or vaginal infection are more limited. Schachter et al. found vaginal and rectal infection in 13.9 and 13.5 percent, respectively, of infants born to chlamydia-positive mothers. The vaginal and rectal infections were detected later than those at other sites—between 70 and 154 days after birth, compared to within 22 days for conjunctival infections.[7] Nasopharyngeal infections were detected throughout the first 3 months of life, earlier with conjunctivitis and later with pneumonia. The rectal and vaginal infections were asymptomatic. A subsequent study by Bell and colleagues demonstrated that perinatally acquired infection may persist for months to years.[19] Twenty-two infants born to women with culture-documented chlamydial infection were followed, and positive cultures from the nasopharynx and oropharynx in the infants were detected as late as 28.5 months after birth. Rectal and vaginal infection persisted for at least 1 year. This becomes an important confounding variable when young children are tested for the presence of *C. trachomatis* during evaluation for suspected sexual abuse.

NATURAL HISTORY AND CLINICAL MANIFESTATIONS OF INFECTION DURING PREGNANCY

The majority of women, including pregnant women, with chlamydial infection will be asymptomatic. Preliminary results from a multicenter, National Institutes for Health (NIH)–sponsored study of 8,000 pregnant women (Vaginal Infection and Prematurity [VIP] Study Group) found that cervical polymorphonuclear leukocytes (PMN) were poor predictors of the existence of chlamydial infection.[20] The predictive values of cervical mucopus and cervical PMNs were lower than those reported in nonpregnant women. Cervical friability was also an insensitive indicator.

Infection with *C. trachomatis* in pregnancy has been inconsistently linked to prematurity. A major problem with several of these studies has been the confounding presence of other infections, especially the genital mycoplasmas (*Mycoplasma hominis* and *Ureaplasma urealyticum*), which also may have adverse effects on the pregnancy and fetus.[16,17] Results from the VIP study found an increased risk of low birth weight among children of women who were colonized with genital mycoplasmas and *Trichomonas*.[20] Chlamydial infection was associated with a nonsignificant increase in risk for low-birth-weight infants following ad-

Table 83-1. Prospective Studies of Chlamydial Infection in Mothers and Infants

Study	Location	Mothers positive/total, (%)	Infants followed positive/total, (%)				
			Conjunctivitis	Pneumonia	NP	Rectum	Vagina
Schachter[7]	San Francisco	262/5531 (5)	23/131 (18)	21/131 (16)	—	17/126 (14)	5/36 (14)
Chandler[8]	Seattle	18/42 (13)	8/18 (44)	—	—	—	—
Frommell[9]	Denver	30/340 (9)	8/18 (44)	2/18 (22)	—	—	—
Hammerschlag[10]	Boston	6/322 (2)	2/6 (33)	1/6 (17)	—	—	—
Hammerschlag[11]	Seattle	67/572 (12)	12/60 (20)	4/60 (7)	8/60 (14)	—	—
Mardh[12]	Lund	23/273 (9)	5/23 (22)	—	—	—	—
Datta[13]	Nairobi	49/223 (22)	18/47 (37)	6/49 (12)	—	—	—
Hammerschlag[14]	Brooklyn	341/4357 (8)	35/230 (15)	2/230 (1)	8/230 (4)	—	—

justment for these other risk factors. Women with mucopurulent cervicitis defined as ≤30 polymorphonuclear cells per 1,000 × field were twice as likely to deliver a low-birth-weight infant. Mucopurulent cervicitis had very poor sensitivity, specificity, and positive predictive value as an indicator of chlamydial infection in pregnant women, however.

CONJUNCTIVITIS

C. trachomatis is the most frequent identifiable infectious cause of neonatal conjunctivitis and the major clinical manifestation of neonatal chlamydial infection. Approximately 30 to 50 percent of infants born to chlamydia-positive mothers will develop conjunctivitis.[7–14] Studies have identified *C. trachomatis* in 10 to 40 percent of infants less than 1 month of age who present with conjunctivitis.[21–25] The incubation period is 5 to 14 days after delivery, or earlier if there has been premature rupture of membranes. At least 50 percent of infants with chlamydial conjunctivitis will also have nasopharyngeal infection. The presentation is extremely variable, ranging from mild conjunctivitis with scant mucoid discharge to severe conjunctivitis with copious purulent discharge, chemosis, and pseudomembrane formation.[21,22] The conjunctiva can be very friable and may bleed when stroked with a swab. Eyelid erythema and edema are frequently present. A gram-stained conjunctival smear may initially reveal a predominance of PMNs. Chlamydial conjunctivitis needs to be differentiated from gonococcal ophthalmia in some infants, especially those born to mothers who did not receive any prenatal care, had gonorrhea during pregnancy, and/or abused drugs. There can be overlap in both incubation periods and presentation. Bilateral infections are present in two-thirds of cases. Asymptomatic eye infection with *C. trachomatis* has been reported in several European and African studies; in one study from Kenya, for example, many of these ocular infections were detected when the infants were more than 2 months of age.[25] This is at variance with the experience in the United States, where asymptomatic ocular chlamydial infection has been uncommon.[14] A follicular reaction is not seen because infants less than 3 months of age do not have the requisite lymphoid tissue present in the conjunctiva. Although uncommon, chlamydial neonatal conjunctivitis has been noted to induce the long-term sequelae of corneal neovascularization and scarring. However, Hammerschlag and colleagues did not detect micropannus at 1 year of age in seven infants who had culture-documented neonatal *C. trachomatis* conjunctivitis.[18]

Table 83-2. Clinical Characteristics of Infant Pneumonitis

	Infants	
	Chlamydia-positive/total	Chlamydia-negative/total
Presentation at 3–11 weeks	53/57 (93%)	19/42 (45%)
Prodrome more than 1 week	45/57 (79%)	17/42 (40%)
Conjunctivitis	26/57 (46%)	5/39 (13%)
Ear abnormalities	24/41 (59%)	0/15 (0%)
Staccato cough	24/41 (59%)	4/15 (27%)
Wheeze	9/57 (16%)	14/32 (44%)
Rales	14/16 (88%)	14/27 (52%)

SOURCE: After Harrison et al.[27] and Tipple et al.[28]

PNEUMONIA

As stated earlier, the nasopharynx is the most frequent site of perinatally acquired chlamydial infection. Approximately 70 percent of infected infants will have positive cultures at that site. The majority of these nasopharyngeal infections are asymptomatic and may persist for 3 years or more, but chlamydial pneumonia develops in only about 30 percent of infants with nasopharyngeal infection. There has been some debate as to whether the nasopharynx becomes infected secondary to infection of the conjunctiva or through direct infection of the nasopharynx during delivery, probably from the aspiration of infected cervical secretions. The results of prospective studies of maternal-infant infection have documented that pneumonia can develop in infants who never had chlamydial conjunctivitis, which suggests that the latter mechanism is more likely.[7–14]

Table 83-3. Laboratory Characteristics of Infant Pneumonitis

	Infants	
	Chlamydia-positive/total	Chlamydia-negative/total
Radiography		
Diffuse infiltrates	47/57 (82%)	20/42 (48%)
Hyperinflation	47/57 (82%)	15/42 (36%)
Eosinophilia		
>300/mm³	29/41 (71%)	1/15 (7%)
>400/mm³	12/16 (75%)	3/27 (11%)
Immunoglobulins		
IgG		
Elevated	38/41 (93%)	3/15 (20%)
>500 mg/dL	13/15 (87%)	9/20 (45%)
IgM		
Elevated	41/41 (100%)	8/15 (53%)
>110 mg/dL	14/15 (93%)	1/21 (5%)
IgA		
Elevated	34/41 (83%)	4/15 (27%)
>30 mg/dL	11/15 (73%)	8/21 (38%)

SOURCE: After Harrison et al.[27] and Tipple et al.[28]

In those infants who develop pneumonia, the presentation and clinical findings are very characteristic,[27,28] (Tables 83-2, 83-3). The children usually present between 4 and 12 weeks of age. A few cases have been reported presenting as early as 2 weeks of age, but no cases have been seen beyond 4 months. The infants frequently have a history of cough and congestion with an absence of fever. On physical examination the infant is tachypneic, and rales are heard on auscultation of the chest; wheezing is distinctly uncommon. There are no specific radiographic findings except hyperinflation (Fig. 83-1). Significant laboratory findings include

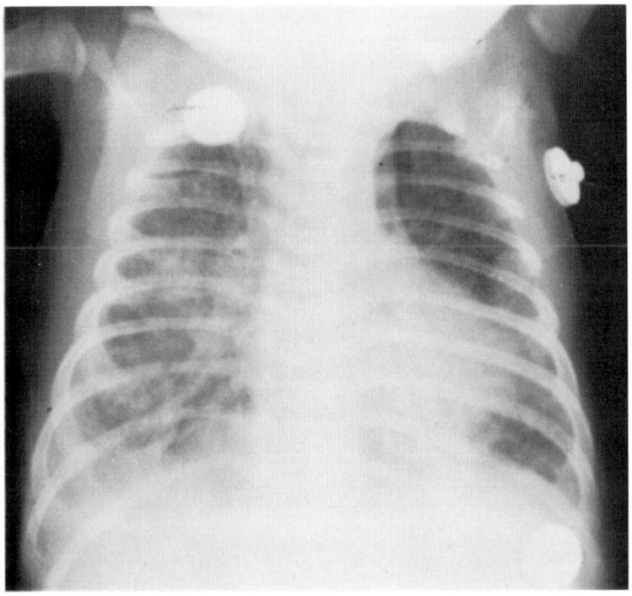

A

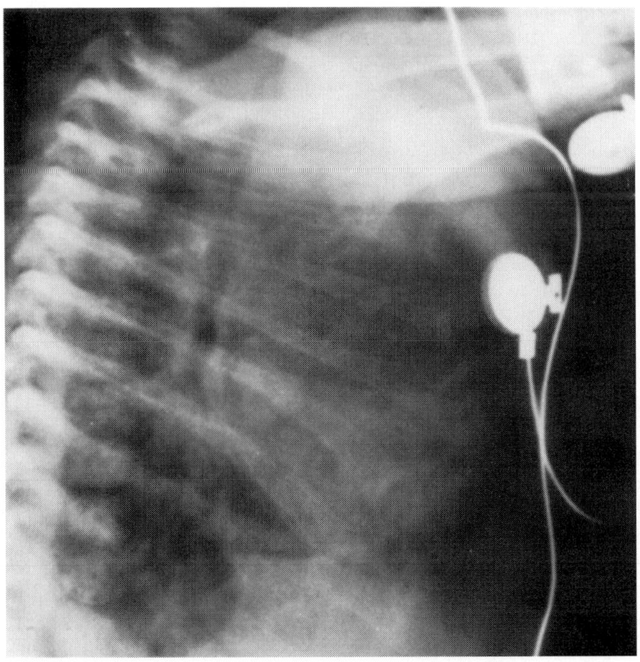

B

Fig. 83-1. (a) Anteroposterior and (b) lateral chest radiographs of a severely ill one-month-old male infant with chlamydial pneumonitis. Diffuse interstitial infiltrates and hyperaeration with flattened diaphragms are prominent.

peripheral eosinophilia (>300 cells/cm^3) and elevated serum immunoglobulins. If cultured, infants with *C. trachomatis* pneumonia may remain symptomatic and shed the organism from the nasopharynx for protracted periods.[18,27,28] Generally, infantile pneumonia due to *C. trachomatis* appears to be self-limited. Most infants can be managed as out-patients although there are a few reports of severe disease requiring hospitalization and assisted ventilation. *C. trachomatis* pneumonia in infants also appears to be associated with few sequelae, although data are limited. In 1983 Ringel et al. reported a case of infantile *C. trachomatis* pneumonia complicated by myocarditis.[29] No significant antiviral antibodies developed.

Harrison et al. studied 10 infants with serologic evidence of *C. trachomatis* infection determined retrospectively.[30] Clinically, the infants had bronchiolitis or pneumonia. Four of the infants were followed for an average duration of five and a half years; another four were followed for an average of one year after the acute illness. The results demonstrated that infants who were hospitalized with presumed chlamydial lower-respiratory-tract infection had a higher incidence of chronic respiratory symptoms than infants with non-chlamydial respiratory infection or controls. The parameters studied were cough, wheeze, and abnormal functional residual capacity (FRC). Subsequently, Weiss and coworkers evaluated the pulmonary status of 18 children, 7 to 8 years after hospitalization for chlamlydial pneumonia at 4 to 10 weeks of age.[31] *C. trachomatis* infection was diagnosed by serology and by isolation of *C. trachomatis* from nasopharyngeal secretions. Infants with concurrent viral infection were excluded. The authors found that chlamydial pneumonia of infancy was associated with abnormal pulmonary function tests (including FRC) and, in some cases, with subsequent obstructive lung disease. How specific this is for *C. trachomatis* is not clear, however, especially given the long interval after the acute infection in infancy. Viral infection in infants, especially respiratory syncytial virus, has also been associated with pulmonary abnormalities in later childhood, specifically reactive airway disease. Recently, *C. pneumoniae* has also been reported to be associated with reactive airway disease in children.[32]

OTHER INFECTIONS

Otitis media

Isolation of *C. trachomatis* from middle-ear fluid was first reported by Tipple et al.[28] The organism was isolated from the middle-ear aspirates of 3 of 11 infants with chlamydia pneumonia. These infants were all under 3 months of age and had the typical infantile chlamydial pneumonia and what was described as "serous" otitis media. This may not imply a causal relationship, as the middle ear is contiguous with the nasopharynx and the organism is present in the mucosa of the nasopharynx. Infants with chlamydial pneumonia have a significant degree of nasal congestion, which can lead to eustachian-tube dysfunction, and thus the presence of serous otitis media may not be directly attributable to the presence of *C. trachomatis* in middle-ear fluid. However, subsequent studies that have examined middle-ear fluids from older infants and children with acute and chronic otitis media have not found convincing evidence of *C. trachomatis* as an etiologic agent of otitis. Four studies examined middle ear fluids from a total of 337 children ranging in age from 5 months through 12 years.[33–36] *C. trachomatis* was isolated from ear fluids from five of these children enrolled in two of the studies.[33,34]

Chang et al. isolated *C. trachomatis* from ear aspirates of 3 of 26 (11.5 percent) children, but the age of only 1 of these children, a 10-month-old, was given.[34] The culture method used was IUDR-treated McCoy cells with iodine staining. In the other study, Dawson and colleagues isolated presumptive *C. trachomatis* from two ear aspirates from 217 Australian aboriginal children.[33] The positive children were 4 and 8 years of age. The researchers used McCoy cells but confirmed the isolates with a genus-specific monoclonal antibody, and thus it is possible that both isolates may have actually been *C. pneumoniae*. Considering that perinatally acquired nasopharyngeal *C. trachomatis* infections may persist for at least 2 years, it is possible that the organism may be isolated from middle-ear fluids beyond early infancy, but a causal relationship has not been established. *C. pneumoniae* is a more likely candidate as a cause of otitis media in older children.

Rectogenital infection in older children

C. trachomatis has not been associated with any specific clinical syndrome in older infants and children. Most attention to *C. trachomatis* infection in these children has concentrated on the relationship to child sexual abuse. It has been suggested that the isolation of *C. trachomatis* from rectal or genital sites in children without prior sexual activity may be a marker of sexual abuse.[37] Although evidence for other modes of spread, such as through fomites, is lacking for this organism, perinatal maternal-infant transmission resulting in vaginal and/or rectal infection has been documented with prolonged infection for periods up to 3 years.[19] This is an important confounding variable.

Before 1980, vaginal infection with *C. trachomatis* was reported uncommonly in prepubertal children, and the possibility of sexual contact was frequently not even discussed. In 1981, Rettig et al. reported concurrent or subsequent chlamydial infection in 9 of 33 (27 percent) episodes of gonorrhea in a group of prepubertal children.[38] This compares with rates of concurrent infection in men and women of 11 to 62 percent, depending on the study. *C. trachomatis* was not found in any of 31 children presenting with urethritis or vaginitis that was not gonococcal, however. No information was given about possible sexual activity.

Recent studies have identified rectogenital chlamydial infection in 2 to 13 percent of sexually abused children, when these children were routinely cultured for the organism.[37,39,40] The majority of those with chlamydial infection were asymptomatic. In two early studies that had control groups, similar percentages of control patients were also infected. The control group in one study consisted of children who were also referred for evaluation of possible sexual abuse, but were found to have no history of sexual contact, and siblings of abused children.[39] The mean age of this group was 4.5 years as compared to 7.5 years for the group with a history of sexual contact, thus suggesting a bias related to the inability to elicit a history of sexual contact from young children. In the second study the control group was selected from a well-child clinic.[37] Three girls in this group were found to have positive chlamydial cultures; two who had positive vaginal cultures were sisters who had been sexually abused 3 years previously and had not received interim treatment with antibiotics. The implication of this observation was that these children were infected for at least 3 years and were totally asymptomatic. The remaining control child had *C. trachomatis* isolated from her throat and rectum; no history of sexual contact could be elicited. A subsequent larger study by Ingram and colleagues found a stronger association between vaginal chlamydial infection and a history of sexual abuse, but not with pharyngeal infection, which was found in a similar number of controls.[40] Rectal infection was detected in only 1 of 124 children. The possibility of prolonged vaginal or rectal carriage in the sexually abused group was minimized in the study of Hammerschlag and coworkers,[37] since the chlamydial cultures obtained at the initial examination were negative and the infection was only detected at follow-up examination 2 to 4 weeks later. However, the two abused girls who developed chlamydial infection were victims of a single assault by a stranger. In the setting of repeated abuse by a family member, over long periods of time, development of infection would be difficult to demonstrate. Even among adolescents and adults who are victims of sexual assault, acquisition of *C. trachomatis* is uncommon, less than 2 percent over the rate found at baseline.[41] The 1993 Centers for Disease Control and Prevention (CDC) STD Treatment Guidelines has dropped the recommendation that cultures for *C. trachomatis* be obtained routinely from the pharynx and urethra in children who are suspected victims of sexual abuse,[42] primarily because of the low yield from the urethra and the tendency for longer persistence of perinatally acquired pharyngeal infection. *C. pneumoniae* may also be confused with *C. trachomatis* in pharyngeal cultures.[43] Asymptomatic nasopharyngeal infection with *C. pneumoniae* occurs in as many as 5 percent of asymptomatic children.[32]

PATHOLOGY/HISTOPATHOLOGY

Data on pathology of *C. trachomatis* infections in infants are limited mostly to the pneumonia. The pathology of *C. trachomatis* infant pneumonitis has not been thoroughly elucidated. What is known has been gained mainly from lung biopsy material in a few patients who underwent that procedure for diagnosis and from data obtained in animal models. Beem and Saxon noted only an interstitial pneumonia without unusual histologic features in two lung specimens obtained by open biopsy.[6] They did not, however, recover organisms. Harrison and colleagues reported another case with similar lung biopsy histology, but again without recovery of *C. trachomatis*.[44] A number of other unpublished attempts to recover the organism at biopsy have been unsuccessful. Frommell later isolated *C. trachomatis* and cytomegalovirus by culture of the lung biopsy of an infant with pneumonitis.[45] Microscopic examination revealed a diffuse interstitial and alveolar infiltrate of monocytes and neutrophils. Intranuclear inclusions characteristic of cytomegalovirus infection were present in the tissue, while chlamydial inclusions could not be seen. Arth and colleagues, in another culture-positive lung biopsy specimen, found pleural congestion and nearly total alveolar and partial bronchiolar consolidation with a mononuclear exudate containing occasional eosinophils.[46] No other pathogens were found by culture or microscopic examination. Again, no chlamydial inclusions were found in the tissue. Notably absent were significant interstitial or neutrophilic infiltrates. Harrison and colleagues, in an experimental model, induced chlamydial pneumonitis in two of three baboons.[44] All three animals developed prolonged nasopharyngitis, including one that was not inoculated at that site. This development supports the observation that *C. trachomatis* infection appears to be favored at the nasopharynx. These investigators noted marked similarities in histopathology between the baboon lungs and a biopsy specimen from a human infant with chlamydial pneumonitis: (1) patchy and nodular areas of interstitial, peribronchiolar, and perivascular infiltration with lymphocytes, plasma cells, eosinophils, and neutrophils; (2) germinal centers within nodules; and (3) airway plugs of mucus and inflammatory cells that lead to atelectasis. In the baboons, inclusions were seen in airway tissue, and chlamydia could be cultured from central but not peripheral lung tissue. They were neither seen nor cultured in high titer, however. The baboon experiments provided corroborative evidence for a *C. trachomatis*–produced pneumonitis and allowed more immunopathologic investigation than had been available in human infants.

Even before the animal-model stimulus was provided by the discovery of *C. trachomatis*–induced human pneumonitis, the organism had been found to produce lung infection in mice. Graham found that both lymphogranuloma venereum and oculogenital strains of *C. trachomatis* reliably induced pneumonitis in TO mice.[47,48] This was characterized by early patchy consolidation with hyperactive airway epithelium, luminal exudate, and a peribronchiolar cellular infiltrate. Inclusions were found both in bronchiolar epithelial cells and in alveoli. By the fifth day after inoculation, alveolar and peribronchiolar exudates had become predominantly lymphocytic and histiocytic. Chen and Kuo developed a model for *C. trachomatis* pneumonitis in Swiss-Webster white mice using intranasal inoculation.[49] On pathologic examination, the lungs showed congestion and patchy consolidation. Interstitial pneumonitis with intense infiltration of neutrophils was seen, with areas of alveoli filled by exudate. Bronchioles were spared even though they were often filled with the inflammatory exudate. Chlamydial inclusions were seen in the interstitium and in bronchial epithelial cells. Inflammation was most intense on days 2 and 3 after inoculation, gradually changed to mononuclear cells after day 3, and was gone by days 10 to 14. Organisms could be recovered from lung tissue on days 1 to 7, with highest yields on day 2. Antichlamydial antibody appeared between days 7 and 10 and was sustained. Furthermore, delayed hypersensitivity was present from days 5 to 21, with a maximum on day 7. Harrison and coworkers have developed a second mouse pneumonitis model using C57 black mice and a smaller intranasal dose.[50] They too found a patchy interstitial process with bronchial plugging and an early polymorphonuclear response changing to lymphocytes, plasma cells, and eosinophils. Very little consolidation was seen, however, and the intensity of the acute response was not as great, which leads to the possibility that some of the acute changes seen in the Swiss-Webster mice were due to the direct toxic effect of the high-titer inoculum. In the C57 mice, organisms could be seen by immunofluorescence on days 3 to 6 in airways but not in interstitial space, and they could be recovered from tissue during that time. The lung infiltrates were maximal on days 7 to 10 and consisted predominantly of peribronchial infiltrates of mononuclear cells. By immunofluorescence, the mononuclear cells appear to be complement IgM- and IgG-bearing lymphocytes. Antibody and cell-mediated immunity (CMI) to chlamydia (as measured by blastogenic response of splenic lymphocytes to specific antigen) appeared on day 7, and CMI was maximal on day 10.

In summary, despite minor differences, a consistent picture of the histopathology of chlamydial pneumonitis has emerged. Organisms infect the bronchial epithelium and replicate within it in a patchy fashion and perhaps also replicate within alveoli and interstitial spaces. The acute cellular response is interstitial, alveolar, bronchial, and peribronchial, and predominantly polymorphonuclear; this leads to some consolidation, interstitial thickening, plugging of airways, and atelectasis. The second stage of the response seems to be a combined humoral and cellular one, with the appearance of antibody and mononuclear phagocytic cells, lymphocytes, plasma cells, and cell-mediated immunity. The response appears to slow the multiplication of organisms, is maximal after organisms disappear, and persists for some time (in the baboons, 3.5 weeks after infection). These results support the hypothesis that many of the prolonged pulmonary findings in infants are due to the host response. The difficulty in recovering or seeing organisms in tissue (i.e., negative lung biopsies) may be due to the fact that tissue is obtained during the chronic phase when chlamydial replication has been limited by host defenses. It should also be noted that lung biopsies may be negative for the organism because the biopsies are peripheral whereas the focus of the disease is in the small airways.

Only a small proportion (25 to 30 percent) of infants who have *C. trachomatis* isolated from the nasopharynx actually go on to develop pneumonia.[18] The limitation of the occurrance of *C. trachomatis*–related pneumonia to early infancy could be due in part to possible maturational or functional differences between alveolar macrophages of infants and adults. At birth, a function of the alveolar macrophage is to clear the alveolar surface of fetal lung fluid, which contains large amounts of surfactant-related lipids. Studies have suggested that phagocytosis of this surfactant-related material may reduce the microbicidal activity of alveolar macrophages in newborn animals.[51]

Nakajo and colleagues demonstrated that alveolar macrophages from healthy, non-smoking adults were capable of killing both human biovars of *C. trachomatis,* with complete killing observed within 48 hours of inoculation.[52] Preincubation of alveolar macrophages from adults with surfactant did not reduce the capacity of the cells to kill *C. trachomatis.*

Another important question in chlamydial pneumonitis is that of respiratory infection mixed with another pathogen. In 41 infants with chlamydial pneumonitis, Tipple et al. isolated cytomegalovirus from 9 infants (22 percent), respiratory syncytial virus from 4 infants (10 percent), as well as miscellaneous rhinoviruses (4 infants), adenovirus (1 infant), and enterovirus (1 infant).[28] Of 19 infants observed, Harrison and colleagues demonstrated concurrent infection with respiratory syncytial virus in 3 (16 percent) and enterovirus and adenovirus in 1 infant each.[27] Frommell et al. saw cytomegalic inclusions in the lung biopsy of the infant on which they reported.[45] Brasfield et al., in studying pneumonitis in infants of less than 3 months, found other potentially pathogenic infections in half of them. However, one-third of these infants were identified by serology only.[53]

The high prevalence of cytomegalovirus infection in infants with chlamydial pneumonia may be a consequence of the fact that both agents are sexually transmitted and often appear together in other epidemiologic situations. The presence of other viruses in these hospitalized patients is not entirely surprising. *C. trachomatis* pneumonitis is clearly a chronic illness (see below) with, in many cases, only mild to moderate symptoms. It is possible that acute or chronic viral coinfection increases the respiratory dysfunction to the point where a mildly symptomatic infant develops more severe disease and requires hospitalization.

DIAGNOSIS

It is difficult to make an etiologic diagnosis of neonatal conjunctivitis on clinical grounds alone. There can be significant overlap in both incubation period and clinical findings with infections due to other organisms, especially *N. gonorrhoeae*. In a high-risk population, gonococcal ophthalmia must be seriously considered. Chemical conjunctivitis secondary to being treated with silver nitrate usually occurs in the first day of life and disappears spontaneously within 3 to 4 days. The incubation period for gonococcal conjunctivitis is usually 3 to 5 days, but it can be longer. The incubation period for chlamydial conjunctivitis is approximately 5 to 14 days. Most cases will present by 2 weeks of age, which is after the infant leaves the hospital. Data from Fransen et al., from Kenya, suggest that the incubation period and duration of symptoms observed with infants with nongonococcal, nonchlamydial conjunctivitis was longer, and the severity of the symptoms was significantly less, than was observed with either gonococcal or chlamydial conjunctivitis.[54]

Epidemiologic clues can help the physician decide whether gonococcal ophthalmia needs to be considered. Hammerschlag and colleagues noted that seven of the eight infants who presented with gonococcal conjunctivitis were born to mothers who had not received any prenatal care.[14] Five of these women were abusers of crack cocaine. Another epidemiologic clue is a history of gonorrhea or other sexually transmitted disease during pregnancy.

Table 83-4. Performance of Antigen Detection Tests Compared to Culture for the Diagnosis of Neonatal Chlamydial Conjunctivitis

Author, city	Test	No. infants	% with chlamydial infection	% sens.	% spec.
Hammerschlag et al, Brooklyn[24]	EIA[a]-Chlamydiazyme	90	44	93	98
Rapoza et al, Baltimore[25]	DFA[b]-MicroTrak	100	43	100	94
Roblin et al, Brooklyn[55]	DFA-MicroTrak	56	32	94	88
Stenberg et al, Uppsala[56]	EIA-Chlamydiazyme	117	47	88	99
	DFA-Chlamyset	107	43	81	98
	MicroTrak	118	47	87	97
Hammerschlag et al, Brooklyn[57]	EIA-Chlamydiazyme	97	30	97	100
	Pathfinder			97	100
Hammerschlag et al, Brooklyn[58]	EIA-SureCell	75	40	97	100
Dumornay et al, Brooklyn[59]	CIA[c]-MagicLite	71	31	84	100
Roblin et al, Brooklyn[61a]	PCR[d]-AMPLICOR	75	17.3	92.3	100

[a]EIA—enzyme immunoassay, [b]DFA—direct fluorescent antibody, [c]CIA—chemiluminometric immunoassay, [d]PCR—polymerase chain reaction.

The clinical presentation of C. *trachomatis* pneumonitis in infants is fairly characteristic, and one may be able to make a clinical diagnosis with a degree of certainty. The "gold standard" for diagnosis of C. *trachomatis* infections in infants and children remains isolation by culture from the conjunctiva, nasopharynx, vagina, or rectum.

The conjunctiva may be one of the best sites for culture due to accessibility, high number of organisms present, and lack of other bacteria that may interfere with culture.

USE OF NONCULTURE TESTS

Classically, the diagnosis of chlamydial ophthalmia may be made by examining a Giemsa-stained conjunctival scraping for the characteristic basophilic intracytoplasmic inclusions. The correlation of cytology and chlamydia culture in chlamydial ophthalmia ranges from 39 percent to more than 90 percent. This method has been replaced by culture and antigen detection tests.

Several nonculture methods have approval from the Food and Drug Administration (FDA) for diagnosis of chlamydial conjunctivitis. These methods include enzyme immunoassays (EIA)—specifically Chlamydiazyme (Abbott Diagnostics), Pathfinder (Sanofi-Pasteur), and SureCell (Kodak)—and direct fluorescent antibody tests (DFA), including Syva MicroTrak (Genetic Systems) and Pathfinder (Sanofi-Pasteur). These tests appear to perform very well with conjunctival specimens with sensitivities ≥90 percent and specificities ≥95 percent compared to culture (Table 83-4).[24,25,55–59] Unfortunately, the performance with nasopharyngeal specimens has not been as good (Table 83-5). Although sensitivities for detecting C. *trachomatis* in nasopharyngeal specimens in infants with pneumonia have been over 90 percent, the sensitivities at this site in infants with conjunctivitis ranges from 33 to 91.7 percent.[60,61] Although a commercially available DNA probe, Pace II (GenProbe), has become perhaps the most widely used nonculture test for the diagnosis of chlamydial infections in many parts of the country, it has FDA approval only for cervical and urethral sites in adults, where its performance has been similar to most of the approved EIAs. It does not have approval for any site in children, including the conjunctiva, vagina, or rectum. The recently approved polymerase chain reaction (PCR) assay, Amplicor® (Roche Diagnostic Systems, Branchburg, NJ), also has approval only for genital sites in adults. Roblin et al. evaluated Amplicor for the detection of C. *trachomatis* in ocular and nasopharyngeal specimens from 75 infants with suspected chlamydial conjunctivitis.[61a] Amplicor was equivalent to culture for eye specimens with sensitivity and specificity of 92.3 and 100 percent, respectively. The sensitivity and specificity for nasopharyngeal specimens was 100 and 97.2 percent, respectively, which is dramatically better than the performance of available EIAs at this site. Polymerase chain reaction was also able to detect C. *trachomatis* in the urine of 12 of 12 mothers of culture-positive infants.

Use of these tests for vaginal and rectal specimens in the evaluation of children suspected of being sexually abused has been associated with positive tests.[62,63] Fecal material can give false-positive reactions with any EIA, and no EIAs are even approved for this site in adults. Common bowel organisms, including *E. coli*, Group B streptococcus, and even some respiratory flora such

Table 83-5. Performance of Antigen Tests Compared to Culture for the Detection of *Chlamydia trachomatis* in Nasopharyngeal Specimens from Infants with Pneumonia and Conjunctivitis

Author, city	Test	No. infants	% with chlamydial infection	% sens.	% spec.
Roblin et al, Brooklyn[55]	DFA-MicroTrak	56**	5	33	89
	Pathfinder			50	93
Paisley et al, Denver[60]	DFA-MicroTrak	125+	23	93	98
Hammerschlag et al, Brooklyn[61]	EIA-Chlamydiazyme	131**	24	87	92
		16+	37.5	100	100
Hammerschlag et al, Brooklyn[57]	EIA-Chlamydiazyme	111**	16.2	67	96
	Pathfinder			78	95
Dumornay et al, Brooklyn[59]	CIA-MagicLite	85*	14	91.7	100
Roblin et al, Brooklyn[61a]	PCR-AMPLICOR	75*	4	100	97.2

** Conjunctivitis and pneumonia
* Conjunctivitis only
+ pneumonia only

as Group A streptococcus can also give false-positive reactions with EIAs.[19] Another potential problem can occur with use of an EIA for respiratory specimens. As all of the available EIAs use genus-specific antibodies, if used for respiratory specimens, these tests will also detect *C. pneumoniae*.[43] It should be reemphasized that nonculture tests should never be used for rectal or vaginal sites in children. This is stated clearly in the 1993 STD Treatment Guidelines and the 1993 Chlamydia Guidelines.[42,64] Even though culture is considered the gold standard, culture of *C. trachomatis* is not regulated in any way, and sensitivity may vary from laboratory to laboratory. The methods used for culture confirmation became an issue when several large commercial laboratories started using an EIA instead of FA staining and visual identification of inclusions for culture confirmation. This has resulted in at least one "outbreak" of *C. trachomatis* infection in the evaluation of suspected sexual abuse among residents and staff of an institution for the mentally retarded in Ohio in 1990.[65] All the "positive" cultures, mostly rectal specimens, were subsequently determined to be false-positives resulting from carryover of fecal material and bacteria in the culture specimens. The major advantage of culture is that it is 100 percent specific. When cultures are obtained for *C. trachomatis* in the evaluation of suspected sexual abuse, one should pay careful attention to the laboratory used. Unlike Canada, the United States does not have a system of designated reference laboratories to be utilized for evaluation of sexual abuse or assault.

TREATMENT OF CHLAMYDIAL CONJUNCTIVITIS AND PNEUMONIA IN INFANTS

Although topical sulfonamides have been the traditional treatment for neonatal inclusion conjunctivitis, the findings of several studies have conclusively demonstrated that any type of topical therapy, including sulfacetamide drops, erythromycin, tetracycline, and chloramphenicol ointments, is often inadequate.[18,66,67] As more than 50 percent of infants with chlamydial conjunctivitis will also be infected at other sites, including the nasopharynx, vagina, or rectum, systemic therapy is indicated. The only antibiotics that have been investigated so far are erythromycin estolate and erythromycin ethylsuccinate suspensions. Studies have demonstrated that a 10- to 14-day course of either preparation of erythromycin at the above dosage administered either two or four times a day will eliminate both conjunctival and nasopharyngeal infection in approximately 80 percent of infants.[18,66,67] A Swedish study demonstrated a 100 percent cure rate following a twice-daily dosing schedule.[68] The CDC recommends a 14-day course of erythromycin at a dose of 50 mg/kg/day orally, four times a day. The efficacy of this dosing regimen was evaluated in a U.S. inner-city population, which found a 19 percent treatment-failure rate.[25] There are no data to support the use of topical therapy in addition to the oral therapy. Patients not responding to the first course of erythromycin should be adminstered a second course at the same dosage.

Data on treatment of pneumonia are even more limited. Beem et al. compared sulfisoxazole (150mg/kg/day) and erythromycin ethylsuccinate (40mg/kg/day) for approximately 14 days in 32 infants with chlamydial pneumonia.[69] Although all infants became culture-negative from the nasopharynx within several days of beginning of treatment, two infants, each of whom had received sulfisoxazole and erythromycin, became culture-positive again 1 to 5 days after treatment was stopped.

Treatment failure may be due to poor compliance with antibiotic adminstration, insufficient absorption of the drug, reinfection, or resistance of the organism to the antibiotic. If treatment failure again occurs, consider trimethoprim sulfamethoxazole pediatric suspension, 0.5 mL in two doses a day for 2 weeks. The patient should be examined and retested following the conclusion of treatment.

Several new macrolide and azalide antibiotics have recently been introduced. Single-dose azithromycin is recommended by the CDC as a first-line drug for chlamydial infections of adults in the United States.[42] Others, including roxithromycin, are available in Europe and Japan. These drugs have superior tissue penetration and improved pharmacokinetic profiles and patient tolerance as compared to erythromycin. In addition, they are more active against *C. trachomatis* in vitro. Roxithromycin can be administered twice a day, but it requires a 10-day course of therapy. Azithromycin has a 30-hour half-life in serum and a greater than 5-day half-life in tissue, which allows for single-dose treatment. These drugs may prove to be very effective for the treatment of neonatal chlamydial conjunctivitis, offering improved efficacy and shorter courses of treatment. Only roxithromycin has been studied so far and appears to be equivalent to erythromycin for the treatment of neonatal chlamydial conjunctivitis.[70] Roxithromycin is not available in the United States.

PREVENTION AND CONTROL STRATEGIES

Since *C. trachomatis* infections are transmitted vertically from mother to infant during delivery, there are several possible options for intervention. One of the first to be considered was neonatal ocular prophylaxis. Prophylaxis to prevent ophthalmia neonatorum due to *Neisseria gonorrhoeae* has been standard practice in many developed countries for at least a century.[71] Although neonatal ocular prophylaxis with silver nitrate is specified by law in most of the United States, it is not common practice in many developing countries and in some European nations. It has generally been assumed, based on the results of prospective studies of mother-to-infant transmission of *C. trachomatis*, that neonatal ocular prophylaxis with silver nitrate does not prevent the development of chlamydial conjunctivitis. These studies had found that the risk of conjunctivitis among infants born to infected women ranged from 18 to 50 percent. As erythromycin and tetracycline ophthalmic ointments were also approved and used for ocular prophylaxis, it was suggested that they might also be effective for prevention of chlamydial conjunctivitis.

In 1980, Hammerschlag and coworkers found that not one of 24 infants in Seattle born to chlamydia-positive women and who received topical erythromycin developed chlamydial conjunctivitis, compared to 33 percent (12 of 36) of those who received silver nitrate drops.[11] There was no effect on the incidence of nasopharyngeal infection or on the subsequent development of chlamydial pneumonia. Alexander and Harrison found that chlamydial conjunctivitis developed in 25 percent of infants who received erythromycin ophthalmic ointment and in 49 percent who received tetracycline ointment.[72] Initially, a delay in application of the ointments was thought to have contributed to these results, since the preparations were given to the infants when they arrived in the nursery, often 1 hour after delivery. A subsequent report by Bell et al. found that erythromycin prophylaxis lacked efficacy as compared with silver nitrate; the cumulative proportion of infants in whom chlamydial conjunctivitis developed was 25 percent in each group.[73] These researchers did not conduct a randomized trial, however. Both prophylactic preparations were used in the delivery room and given on an ad-hoc basis as requested by the parents. The application of the preparations was delayed for as long as 1 hour after delivery in some infants.

A study by Laga et al. in Nairobi, Kenya, compared tetracycline ointment with silver nitrate drops.[26] Of the infants born to women with cultures positive for chlamydia, chlamydial ophthalmia developed in 10.1 percent who received silver nitrate drops as prophylaxis and in 7.2 percent who received tetracycline ointment. The authors initially concluded that both preparations were efficacious when compared with a historical cohort in which the disease developed in 31.3 percent of the infants who were not treated prophylactically and who were born to infected women. Most of the infants in this study were followed only for the first 4 weeks of life, however, and the follow-up rate was less than 50 percent. When these authors examined a smaller group of infants who were followed for at least 6 months, 23 and 31 percent of those who received silver nitrate and tetracycline, respectively, ultimately acquired an ocular infection with *C. trachomatis*. What is especially interesting about these results is that many of these ocular infections were detected when the infants were more than 2 months of age and were asymptomatic. This is very different from the experience in the United States, where asymptomatic ocular infection has been uncommon.

In 1989, Hammerschlag et al. compared silver nitrate, erythromycin, and tetracycline as neonatal ocular prophylaxis in a large urban hospital in Brooklyn, New York.[14] The prophylaxis preparations were given within 30 minutes of birth. Chlamydial conjunctivitis developed in 20 percent (15 of 76) of infants born to infected mothers who received silver nitrate drops, 14 percent (13 of 92) of those who received erythromycin, and 11 percent (7 of 62) of those who received tetracycline. There was no effect on the incidence of nasopharyngeal infection and pneumonia. A subsequent study from Taiwan compared silver nitrate, the two antibiotics, and no prophylaxis.[74] This study, in contrast to previous studies, did not specifically follow infants born to women with culture-documented chlamydial infection, but instead followed all infants delivered during the period of the study—for 4 weeks or until they developed conjunctivitis. Again, there was no difference in the incidence of neonatal chlamydial conjunctivitis among the 4 groups. The incidences of chlamydial conjunctivitis in the tetracycline, erythromycin, silver nitrate, and no prophylaxis group were 1.3, 1.5, 1.7, and 1.6 percent, respectively. Diagnosis of *C. trachomatis* was by DFA rather than culture. No data were given as to the prevalence of maternal infection with *C. trachomatis* or *N. gonorrhoeae*. Differences in the prevalence of maternal infection among the four groups could lead to different rates of *C. trachomatis* conjunctivitis in the infants that were unrelated to prophylaxis. Respiratory infection was not assessed.

A similar study from a clinic in Kenya was reported by Isenberg et al. comparing povidine-iodine, erythromycin ophthalmic ointment, and silver nitrate drops as neonatal ocular prophylaxis.[75] Povidine-iodine was selected because, in vitro, it has a broad antibacterial spectrum; it is also antiviral and is very inexpensive compared to the other prophylaxis agents. As with the study from Taiwan, the pregnant women were not screened for *C. trachomatis* prenatally, and chlamydial conjunctivitis in the infants was diagnosed by DFA. Mothers were told to bring their infants back if conjunctivitis developed. Use of povidine-iodine appeared to result in a 50 percent reduction in *C. trachomatis* conjunctivitis compared to silver nitrate (5.5 versus 10.5 percent of infants) and an approximately 30 percent reduction compared to erythromycin (7.4 percent). There was no difference in the proportions of infants who developed gonococcal ophthalmia. Because of the structure of the study, one cannot be sure if every infant who developed conjunctivitis returned to the clinic. As the prevalence of chlamydial infection among the pregnant women in the population was unknown, the investigators did not know how many cases of chlamydial ophthalmia to expect. Use of povidone-iodine for neonatal ocular prophylaxis may be appropriate in some populations, mainly because of cost. It would still appear that neonatal ocular prophylaxis should be directed primarily toward preventing gonococcal ophthalmia, as it is the agent that poses the greatest risk of eye injury.

Given the apparent ineffectiveness of ocular prophylaxis with silver nitrate or antibiotics for the prevention of neonatal chlamydial conjunctivitis, the most effective method of control may be screening and treatment of pregnant women. This would also have the advantage of preventing chlamydial respiratory infection, including pneumonia and infection of the vagina and rectum. Although the CDC recommends four different treatment regimens (three erythromycin regimens and amoxicillin) for treatment of chlamydial infection in pregnant women, data on the efficacy of any of these regimens, as well as the effects on infection in the infant, are limited. Unlike gonorrhea, treatment of *C. trachomatis* infection requires multiple-dose regimens, and tolerance and compliance are frequent problems.

In 1986, Schachter et al. reported on the effect of the routine use of erythromycin for treating chlamydial infections in pregnancy on the outcome of infection in the infants.[76] Treatment with erythromycin ethylsuccinate (400 mg, qid for 7 days) was offered to 184 pregnant women with cervical chlamydial infection at 36 weeks gestation. Thirty-two women refused treatment, and 24 of their infants were followed as controls. A large number of treated women were lost to follow-up. Chlamydial infection developed in only 4 (7 percent) of 59 infants of treated mothers, however, compared to 12 (50 percent) of the 24 infants of untreated mothers. Of five published, controlled studies comparing erythromycin to amoxicillin or clindamycin for treating chlamydial infection in pregnant women,[77–81] only two followed infants born to these women for the development of chlamydial infection.[77,81] In both studies the development of chlamydial conjunctivitis was significantly reduced compared to historical data (1 to 2 versus 30 to 50 percent). Single-dose azithromycin is not approved for use in pregnancy,[42,64] but azithromycin is being used for this indication although the data on safety and efficacy in pregnancy are extremely limited. Bush and Rosa[82] compared 1 gm azithromycin as a single dose to erythromycin, 500 mg four times a day for 7 days in 30 pregnant women (15 in each treatment group). Azithromycin was well tolerated with less gastrointestinal side effects than erythromycin, but safety was not assessed by monitoring serum chemistries. The "cure" rates were 100 percent for erythromycin and 93 percent for azithromycin; chlamydial cultures were not done, however. *C. trachomatis* was detected by DFA, and bacterial eradication was also based on DFA. The infants were not followed.

Reasons for failure of maternal treatment to prevent infantile chlamydial infection include poor compliance and reinfection from untreated sexual partners. Even with effective screening, some infected women will be missed, depending on the methods used. There are also women who do not seek prenatal care. There is a need for additional treatment studies of chlamydial infection during pregnancy, especially evaluation of azithromycin.

References

1 Thygeson P, Stone W: Epidemiology of inclusion conjunctivitis. *Arch Ophthalmol* 27:91, 1942.

2 Jones BR et al: Isolation of virus from inclusion blennorhea. *Lancet* 1: 902, 1959.

3 Schachter J et al: The venereal nature of inclusion conjunctivitis. *Am J Epidemiol* 85:445, 1967.

4 Botsztejn A: Die pertossoide eosinophile pneumoniae des sauglings. *Ann Paediatr (Basel)* 157:28, 1941.

5 Schachter J et al: Pneumonitis following inclusion blennorrhea. *J Pediat* 87:779, 1975.

6 Beem MO, Saxon EM: Respiratory-tract colonization and a distinctive pneumonia syndrome in infants infected with *Chlamydia trachomatis*. *N Engl J Med* 296:306, 1977.

7 Schachter J et al: Prospective study of perinatal transmission of *Chlamydia trachomatis*. *JAMA* 255:3374, 1986.

8 Chandler FW et al: Ophthalmia neonatorum associated with maternal chlamydia infections. *Trans Acad Ophthalmol Oto* 83:302, 1977.

9 Frommell GT et al: Chlamydial infection of mothers and their infants. *J Pediatr* 95:28, 1979.

10 Hammerschlag MR et al: Prospective study of maternal and infantile infection with *Chlamydia trachomatis*. *Pediatrics* 64:142, 1979.

11 Hammerschlag MR et al: Erythromycin ointment for ocular prophylaxis of neonatal chlamydial infection. *JAMA* 244:2291, 1980.

12 Mardh PA et al: Colonisation of pregnant and puerperal women and neonates with *Chlamaydia trachomatis*. *Br J Vener Dis* 56:980, 1980.

13 Datta P et al: Infection and disease after perinatal exposure to *Chlamydia trachomatis* in Nairobi, Kenya. *J Infect Dis* 158:524, 1988.

14 Hammerschlag MR et al: Efficacy of neonatal ocular prophylaxis for the prevention of chlamydia and gonococcal conjunctivitis. *N Engl J Med* 320:769, 1989.

15 Bell TA et al: Risk of perinatal transmission of *Chlamlydia trachomatis* by mode of delivery. *J Infect Dis* 29:165, 1994.

16 Harrison HR et al: Cervical *Chlamydia trachomatis* and mycoplasmal infections in pregnancy. *JAMA* 250:1721, 1983.

17 Berman SM et al: Low birth weight, prematurity and postpartum endometritis. *JAMA* 257:1189, 1987

18 Hammerschlag MR et al: Longitudinal studies on chlamydial infections in the first year of life. *Pediatr Infect Dis* 1:395, 1982.

19 Bell TA et al: Chronic *Chlamydia trachomatis* infections in infants. *JAMA* 267:400, 1992.

20 Nugent RP, Hillier SL: Mucopurulent cervicitis as a predictor of chlamydial infection and adverse pregnancy outcome. *Sex Transm Dis* 19: 198, 1992.

21 Rowe DS et al: Purulent ocular discharge in neonates: Significance of *Chlamydia trachomatis*. *Pediatrics* 63:628, 1979

22 Sandstrom KI et al: Microbial causes of neonatal conjunctivitis. *J Pediatr* 105:706, 1984.

23 Barry WC et al: *Chlamydia trachomatis* as a cause of neonatal conjunctivitis. *Arch Dis Child* 61:797, 1986.

24 Hammerschlag MR et al: Enzyme immunoassay for diagnosis of neonatal chlamydial conjunctivitis. *J Pediatr* 107:741, 1985

25 Rapoza PA et al: Assessment of neonatal conjunctivitis with a direct immunofluorescent monoclonal antibody stain for *Chlamydia*. *JAMA* 255:3369,1986.

26 Laga M et al: Prophylaxis of gonococcal and chlamydial ophthalmia neonatorum: A comparison of silver nitrate and tetracycline. *N Engl J Med* 318:653,1988.

27 Harrison HR et al: *Chlamydia trachomatis* infant pneumonitis: Comparison with matched controls and other infant pneumonitis. *N Engl J Med* 298:702, 1978.

28 Tipple MA et al: Clinical characteristics of the afebrile pneumonia associated with *Chlamydia trachomatis* infection in infants less than 6 months of age. *Pediatrics* 63:192, 1979.

29 Ringel RE et al: Myocarditis as a complication of infantile *Chlamydia trachomatis* pneumonitis. *Clin Pediatr* 22:631, 1983.

30 Harrison R et al: *Chlamydia trachomatis* and chronic respiratory disease in childhood. *Pediatr Infect Dis* 1:29, 1982.

31 Weiss SG et al: Pulmonary assessment of children after chlamydial pneumonia of infancy. *J Pediatr* 108:659, 1986.

32 Emre U et al: The association of *Chlamydia pneumoniae* infection and reactive airway disease in children. *Arch Pediatr Adolesc Med* 143: 727, 1994.

33 Dawson VM et al: Microbiology of chronic otitis media with effusion among Australian aboriginal children: Role of *Chlamydia trachomatis*. *Aust J Exp Biol Med Sci* 63:99, 1985.

34 Chang MJ et al: *Chlamydia trachomatis* in otitis media in children. *Pediatr Infect Dis* 1:95, 1982.

35 Hammerschlag MR et al: Role of *Chlamydia trachomatis* in middle ear effusions in children. *Pediatrics* 66:615, 1980.

36 Blackston ML et al: Presence of *Chlamydia trachomatis* in tympanocentesis fluid assessed by immunofluorescence microscopy and cell culture. *Otolaryngol Head Neck Surg* 100:348, 1989.

37 Hammerschlag MR et al: Are rectogenital chlamydial infections a marker of sexual abuse in children? *Pediatr Infect Dis* 3:100, 1984.

38 Rettig PJ, Nelson JD: Genital tract infection with *Chlamydia trachomatis* in prepubertal children. *J Pediatr* 99:206, 1981.

39 Ingram DL et al: Vaginal *Chlamydia trachomatis* infection in children with sexual contact. *Pediatr Infect Dis* 3:97, 1984.

40 Ingram DL et al: Childhood vaginal infections: Association of *Chlamydia trachomatis* with sexual contact. *Pediatr Infect Dis* 5:226, 1986.

41 Glaser JB et al: Epidemiology of sexually transmitted diseases in rape victims. *Rev Infect Dis* 11:246, 1989.

42 Centers for Disease Control and Prevention: 1993 Sexually Transmitted Diseases Treatment Guidelines. *MMWR* 42:(RR-14)1, 1993.

43 Bauwens JE et al: *Chlamydia pneumoniae* (strain TWAR) isolated from two symptom-free children during evaluation for possible sexual assault. *J Pediatr* 119:591, 1991.

44 Harrison HR et al: Experimental nasopharyngitis and pneumonia caused by *Chlamydia trachomatis* in infant baboons: Histopathological comparison with a case in a human infant. *J Infect Dis* 139:141, 1979.

45 Frommell GT et al: Isolation of *Chlamydia trachomatis* from infant lung tissue. *N Engl J Med* 296:1150, 1977.

46 Arth C et al: Chlamydial pneumonitis. *J Pediatr* 93:447, 1978.

47 Graham DM: Growth and neutralization of the trachoma agent in mouse lungs. *Nature* 207:1379, 1965.

48 Graham DM: Growth and immunogenicity of TRIC agents in mice. *Am J Ophthalmol* 63:1173, 1967.

49 Chen WJ, Kuo C-C: A mouse model of pneumonitis induced by *Chlamydia trachomatis*: Morphologic, microbiologic and immunologic studies. *Am J Pathol* 100:365, 1980.

50 Harrison HR et al: *Chlamydia trachomatis* pneumonitis in the C57BL/KsJ mouse: Pathologic and immunologic features. *J Lab Clin Med* 100: 953, 1982.

51 Zeligs BJ et al: Chemotactic and candidacidal responses of rabbit alveolar macrophages during post-natal development and the modulating roles of surfactant in these responses. *Infect Immun* 44:379, 1984.

52 Nakajo MN et al: Chlamydicidal activity of human alveolar macrophages. *Infect Immun* 58:3640, 1990.

53 Brasfield DM et al: Infant pneumonitis associated with cytomegalovirus, *Chlamydia, Pneumocystis,* and *Ureaplasma*: Follow-up. *Pediatrics* 79:76, 1987.

54 Fransen L et al: Ophthalmia neonatorum in Nairobi, Kenya: The roles of *Neisseria gonorrhoeae* and *Chlamydia trachomatis*. *J Infect Dis* 153:862, 1986.

55 Roblin PM et al: Comparison of two rapid microscopic methods and culture for detection of *Chlamydia trachomatis* in ocular and nasopharyngeal specimens from infants. *J Clin Microbiol* 27:968, 1989.

56 Stenberg K et al: Culture, ELISA and immunofluorescence tests for the diagnosis of conjunctivis caused by *Chlamydia trachomatis* in neonates and adults. *APMIS* 98:514, 1990.

57 Hammerschlag MR et al: Comparison of two enzyme immunoassays to culture for the diagnosis of chlamydial conjunctivitis and respiratory infections in infants. *J Clin Microbiol* 28:1725, 1990.

58 Hammerschlag MR et al: Office diagnosis of neonatal chlamydial conjunctivitis. *Pediatr Infect Dis J* 10:540, 1991.

59 Dumornay W et al: Comparison of a chemiluminometric immunoassay with culture for diagnosis of chlamydial infections in infants. *J Clin Microbiol* 30:1867, 1992.

60 Paisley JW et al: Rapid diagnosis of *Chlamydia trachomatis* pneumonia in infants by direct immunofluorescence microscopy of nasopharyngeal secretions. *J Pediatr* 109:653, 1986.

61 Hammerschlag MR et al: Comparison of enzyme immunoassay and culture for diagnosis of chlamydial conjunctivitis and respiratory infections in infants. *J Clin Microbiol* 25:2306, 1987.

61a Hammerschlag MR et al: Use of polymerase chain reaction for the detection of *Chlamydia trachomatis* in ocular and nasopharyngeal specimens from infants with conjunctivitis. *Pediatr Infect Dis J* 16:293, 1997.

62 Hammerschlag MR: False-positive results with the use of chlamydial antigen detection tests in the evaluation of suspected sexual abuse in children. *Pediatr Infect Dis J* 7:11, 1988.

63 Porder K et al: Lack of specificity of chlamydiazyme for detection of vaginal chlamydial infection in prepubertal girls. *Pediatr Infect Dis J* 8:358, 1989.

64 Centers for Disease Control and Prevention: Recommendations for the prevention and management of *Chlamydia trachomatis* infections, 1993. *MMWR* 42:RR-12, 1993.

65 Centers for Disease Control and Prevention: False-positive results with use of chlamydia tests in the evaluation of suspected sexual abuse—Ohio, 1990. *MMWR* 39:932, 1991.

66 Patamasucon P et al: Oral vs topical erythromycin therapies for chlamydial conjunctivitis. *Am J Dis Child* 136:817, 1982.

67 Heggie AD et al: Topical sulfacetamide vs oral erythromycin for neonatal chlamydial conjunctivitis. *Am J Dis Child* 139:564, 1985.

68 Sandstrom I: Treatment of neonatal conjunctivitis. *Arch Ophthalmol* 105:925, 1987.

69 Beem MO et al: Treatment of chlamydial pneumonia of infancy. *Pediatrics* 63:198, 1979.

70 Stenberg K, Mardh PA: Treatment of chlamydial conjunctivitis in newborns and adults with erythromycin and roxithromycin. *J Antimicrob Chemother* 28:301, 1991.

71 Rothenberg R: Ophthalmia neonatorum due to *Neisseria gonorrhoeae*: Prevention and treatment. *Sex Transm Dis* 6:187, 1979.

72 Alexander ER, Harrison HR: Role of *Chlamydia trachomatis* in perinatal infection. *Rev Infect Dis* 5:713, 1983.

73 Bell TA et al: Comparison of ophthalmic silver nitrate solution and erythromycin ointment for prevention of natally acquired *Chlamydia trachomatis. Sex Transm Dis* 14:195, 1987.

74 Chen JY: Prophylaxis of ophthalmia neonatorum: Comparison of silver nitrate, tetracycline, erythromycin and no prophylaxis. *Pediatr Infect Dis J* 12:1062, 1992.

75 Isenberg SJ et al: A controlled trial of povidone-iodine as prophylaxis against ophthalmia neonatorum. *N Engl J Med* 332:562, 1995.

76 Schachter J et al: Experience with the routine use of erythromycin for chlamydial infections in pregnancy. *N Engl J Med* 314:276, 1986.

77 Crombleholme WR et al: Amoxicillin therapy for *Chlamydia trachomatis* in pregnancy. *Obstet Gynecol* 75:752, 1990.

78 Alger LS, Lovchik JC: Comparative efficacy of clindamycin vs erythromycin in eradication of antenatal *Chlamydia trachomatis. Am J Obstet Gynecol* 165:375, 1991.

79 Magat AH et al: Double-blind randomized study comparing amoxicillin and erythromycin for the treatment of *Chlamydia trachomatis* in pregnancy. *Obstet Gynecol* 81:745, 1993.

80 Silverman NS et al: A randomized, prospective trial comparing amoxicillin and erythromycin for the treatment of *Chlamydia trachomatis* in pregnancy. *Am J Obstet Gynecol* 170:829, 1994.

81 Alary M et al: Ramdomised comparison of amoxycillin and erythromycin in treatment of genital chlamydial infection in pregnancy. *Lancet* 344:1461, 1994.

82 Bush MR, Rosa C: Azithromycin and erythromycin in the treatment of cervical chlamydial infection during pregnancy. *Obstet Gynecol* 84: 61, 1994.

Chapter 84

Congenital syphilis

Justin D. Radolf
Pablo J. Sánchez
Kenneth F. Schulz
F. Kevin Murphy

HISTORY

EARLY OBSERVATIONS

Congenital syphilis is the oldest recognized congenital infection. The transmission of syphilis to infants was described in the earliest medical writings on "the French disease" (*morbus gallicus*). Among the first treatises on syphilis was that of Garpar Torella, written in 1497—within four years of the first known outbreaks of syphilis in Spain. Torella noted that syphilis was "often seen" in nursing children, first appearing on the face or in the mouth. Although early writers clearly recognized the possibility of congenital transmission,[1–3] they usually presumed that the wet nurse was the source of infection. The first measure advocated for the prevention of congenital syphilis was proscription of the use of wet nurses who had "the French disease," even if apparently cured. Ambroise Paré, the eminent French surgeon, displayed the same prejudice in a chapter on syphilis among his collected works.[4] Paré described a good family of Paris, all of whom allegedly were infected from a syphilitic wet nurse, even the nursing child's two siblings. He concluded by advocating that the nurse be whipped, naked, through the streets of the city.

The German alchemist and physician Paracelsus was the first to state (in 1529) that congenital syphilis is a hereditary illness that passes from father to son.[5] In 1565 Simon de Vallembert described a case of "hereditary syphilis" in the first French text on pediatrics.[6] After apparent recovery from syphilis, a goldsmith of Tours fathered several afflicted children over a 14-year period, although their mother remained unaffected.

In the novel *Moll Flanders*,[7] Daniel Defoe demonstrated that a basic understanding of syphilis transmission from adult to neonate had been achieved by the eighteenth century. Recalling an encounter with a drunken baronet who had paid for her services, Moll imagines the baronet's regret on arriving home to his family:

> How would he be trembling for fear he had got the pox. . . . how would he, if he had any principles of honour, abhor the thought of giving any ill distemper, if he had it, as for aught he knew he might, to his modest and virtuous wife, and thereby sowing the contagion in the life-blood of his posterity!

In spite of lingering misconceptions about its mechanisms of transmission, several important empirical observations regarding congenital syphilis were made during the nineteenth century, which, in that simpler time, were accorded the status of "laws." Colles's law (1837) stated that syphilitic infants could transmit the disease to previously healthy wet nurses but never to their own mothers.[8] Profeta's law (1865) stated that a healthy infant born to a syphilitic mother is immune to the disease. Kassowitz's law (1876) stated that the toll of the mother's syphilis diminishes with successive pregnancies. Both Paul Diday (1854) and Jonathan Hutchinson (1863) had made this same observation.[9,10] Although neither Colles nor Profeta understood the basis for their observations, their laws illustrated the principle that infection with syphilis confers immunity to reinoculation. The essential character of congenital syphilis finally was clarified in 1906 with Wasserman's development of a serologic test that made it possible to demonstrate that transmission of syphilis to a fetus required an infected, albeit sometimes asymptomatic, mother.[11]

EARLY CLINICAL DESCRIPTIONS

Actual clinical descriptions of congenital syphilis were sparse during the sixteenth through the eighteenth centuries. Lenoir, in 1780, established a lying-in hospital in Paris for syphilitic mothers, the first facility for specialized care of neonates and high-risk pregnancies. Bertin wrote his classic monograph (1810) on congenital syphilis based upon the large accumulated experience at this institution.[12] He recognized several cutaneous lesions; mucous-membrane lesions involving eyes, nose, urethra, and anus; adenopathy; and bone lesions, including epiphysitis. Bertin and others recognized the importance of the skeletal examination, although many later authorities, including Trousseau and Diday, considered skeletal lesions rare in congenital syphilis. Diday's major text, originally published in 1854,[9] described most of the cutaneous and visceral manifestations of congenital syphilis known today and characterized the general appearance of the infant as that of "a little, wrinkled, pot-bellied old man with a cold in his head."[5] Jonathan Hutchinson's writings dominated nineteenth-century British clinical descriptions of congenital syphilis just as Diday's dominated French literature.[13,14] His presentation, in 1857, before the Pathological Society of London, of the characteristic dental malformations, the first description of late sequelae of infant syphilis, was received with "expression of incredulity." Hutchinson is best known for this work as well as for his association of the dental deformities of late congenital syphilis with interstitial keratitis and deafness (Hutchinson's triad).[13,14]

Working without the benefit of x-rays, Parrot[15] and Wegner[16] provided clear descriptions of the osteochondritis of congenital syphilis; Parrot went so far as to declare that every bone of the infantile syphilitic skeleton is affected. His name is applied to both the cranial nodes ("hot cross bun" skull) and the pseudoparalysis that he described. Unfortunately, Parrot also mistakenly believed that rickets was a later lesion of congenital syphilis, an error subsequently corrected by the American Robert Taylor.[17] Between 1900 and 1907 a succession of bright young radiologists proved that bony lesions were the most sensitive indication of clinical disease and that these lesions could be demonstrated in infants without other clinical manifestations.

The risks of delivering a congenitally infected infant were well described in the landmark Oslo study of untreated syphilis conducted from 1891 to 1910. Boeck observed that 26 percent of babies born to syphilitic mothers remained free of disease or recovered spontaneously with conversion to seronegativity, 25 percent were seropositive but remained clinically unaffected, and 49 percent displayed manifest disease.[18]

MILESTONES IN PREVENTION

Fournier, a student of Diday, wrote a detailed treatise on the prevention of congenital syphilis[19]; his concepts influenced premarital counseling for almost a century. Before marriage or resumption of intercourse, he required (1) that the syphilitic patient have no active lesions, (2) that the patient wait 3 to 4 years after onset of disease, (3) that the patient wait at least 18 to 24 months after the last sign of disease, (4) that the form of syphilis not be grave, and (5) that an "adequate" course of potassium iodide and mercury be completed (3 to 4 years). After 1906, serological testing for syphilis was added as a further pre-marital requirement.

Several observations made in rapid succession during the early twentieth century became cornerstones of strategies to curtail the spread of congenital syphilis.[5] The experimental transmission of syphilis to apes by Roux and Metchnikoff[5] and the microscopic demonstration of *Treponema pallidum* by Schaudinn and Hoffmann[5] established the microbiologic etiology of venereal syphilis. Wassermann's development of a complement fixation test using syphilitic fetal liver as a source of antigen enabled physicians, for the first time, to identify individuals with asymptomatic syphilitic infection.[5] Within a year Levaditi[5] demonstrated both the presence of spirochetes in syphilitic fetal tissue and the suitability of uninfected liver as an antigen source for the Wassermann test. It was soon recognized that identification of cases of maternal syphilis with the Wassermann test and arsenical treatment of the mother could prevent neonatal syphilis. With the introduction of penicillin in 1943 by Mahoney,[5] all of the essential clinical tools for the control of congenital syphilis were available.

EPIDEMIOLOGY

GENERAL TRENDS

The introduction of penicillin as syphilotherapy resulted in a dramatic decline in acquired and congenital syphilis incidence in the United States and Europe. The incidence of syphilis began to rise again in 1959, despite the fact that inexpensive therapy was readily available. It was not until 1978 that the incidence again reached the 1957 low of 3.8 cases per 100,000 live births. From 1986 through the early 1990s, there was a dramatic increase in the number of cases of congenital syphilis, partly reflecting the increases in primary and secondary syphilis among inner-city heterosexual minorities during this same period[20] and partly reflecting a revision of the surveillance definition.[21–23] Interestingly, during this same period, syphilis incidence rates decreased steadily in other industrialized countries.[24,25]

INCIDENCE AND PREVALENCE PRIOR TO PENICILLIN

Osler observed in 1917 that syphilis accounted for 20 percent of all stillbirths and 18 to 22 percent of infant deaths in the United States.[26] In Edinburgh, in 1922, Browne found that 35 of 153 neonatal deaths were syphilitic in origin.[27] The overwhelming importance of perinatal syphilis in that period was a reflection of the prevalence of the disease in adults; 10 percent of women of the "hospital class" and 4.5 percent of umbilical cord blood samples in Glasgow's Royal Maternity & Women's Hospital had positive Wassermann tests.[28] School examinations in 1922 and 1923 in Plymouth, England, indicated an 8-percent prevalence of manifest congenital syphilis among school-age children. Between 1922 and 1937, the prevalence of syphilis declined steadily, with prenatal seropositivity falling to 1.8 percent in Glasgow and from 12 to 4 percent in Kansas City.[29] A 1936 U.S. Public Health Service survey indicated, however, that 2 percent of U.S. children and 5.6 percent of U.S. infants were syphilitic, with striking disparities between whites and African Americans (1.7 versus 12.2 percent) and between public and private patients (5.3 versus 1 percent). Investigations of families of an index case revealed latent or manifest syphilis in about one-fourth of family members.[30] A major upsurge in syphilis incidence during World War II in Europe and the United States was associated with a corresponding two- to threefold increase in the number of cases of congenital syphilis.[31] However, this effect was blunted somewhat in areas such as Glasgow where comprehensive prenatal screening programs were well established.[30]

CURRENT INCIDENCE AND DEMOGRAPHICS

Syphilis is the only congenital infection with national surveillance data. Infections during the perinatal period comprise the vast majority of new cases of congenital syphilis. Consequently, the incidence of congenital syphilis closely follows that of primary and secondary syphilis among women in the peak childbearing age group (15 to 29 years) (Fig. 84-1); this is also the peak age group in which early syphilis occurs. From 1970 to 1979, men with male sexual partners accounted for an increasing share of syphilis morbidity, and the ratio of male to female cases of infectious syphilis rose during those same years, peaking at 3.5 : 1 in 1980 (Fig. 84-2).[24] Congenital syphilis rates, accordingly, declined steadily during this period (Fig. 84-1 and 84-3). With changing sexual behavior among male homosexuals in response to the threat of acquired immune deficiency syndrome (AIDS), the male-to-female ratio of early syphilis cases has decreased since 1980; by 1993 the ratio had fallen to 1.1 : 1, reflecting the fact that new cases were occurring predominantly in heterosexuals (Fig. 84-2). During this same period, congenital syphilis rates increased markedly (Figs. 84-1 and 84-3).

Two factors are responsible for the dramatic increase in congenital syphilis observed in the United States from 1990 through 1994. The first was the adoption in 1989 of revised reporting guidelines that broadened the surveillance definition for congenital syphilis (Table 84-1).[23,32] Previous criteria for reporting cases of congenital syphilis were based on a clinical case definition; only infants who had clinically apparent disease or laboratory findings

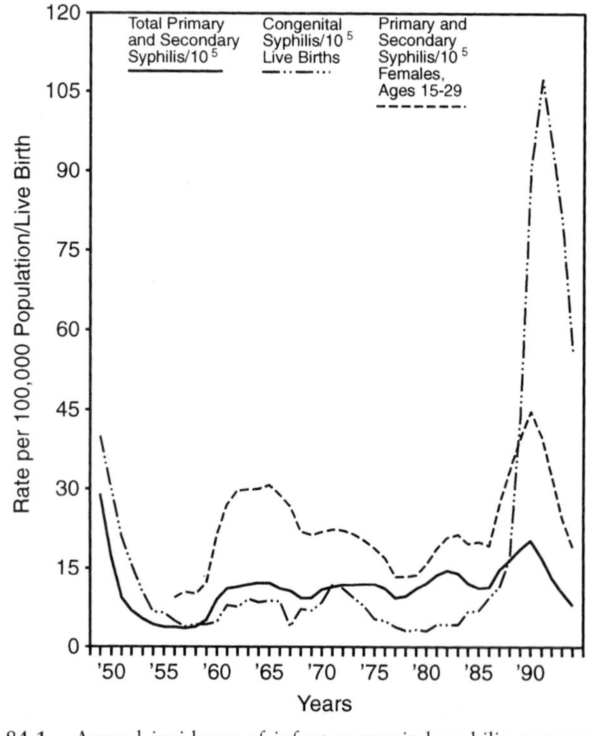

Fig. 84-1. Annual incidence of infant congenital syphilis compared to that of primary and secondary syphilis, United States, 1949 to 1994. The trend for congenital syphilis follows that of women in the childbearing age group by approximately 12 to 18 months. *(Courtesy of Kathy Dry, Division of STD Prevention, NCHSTP, CDC, Atlanta.)*

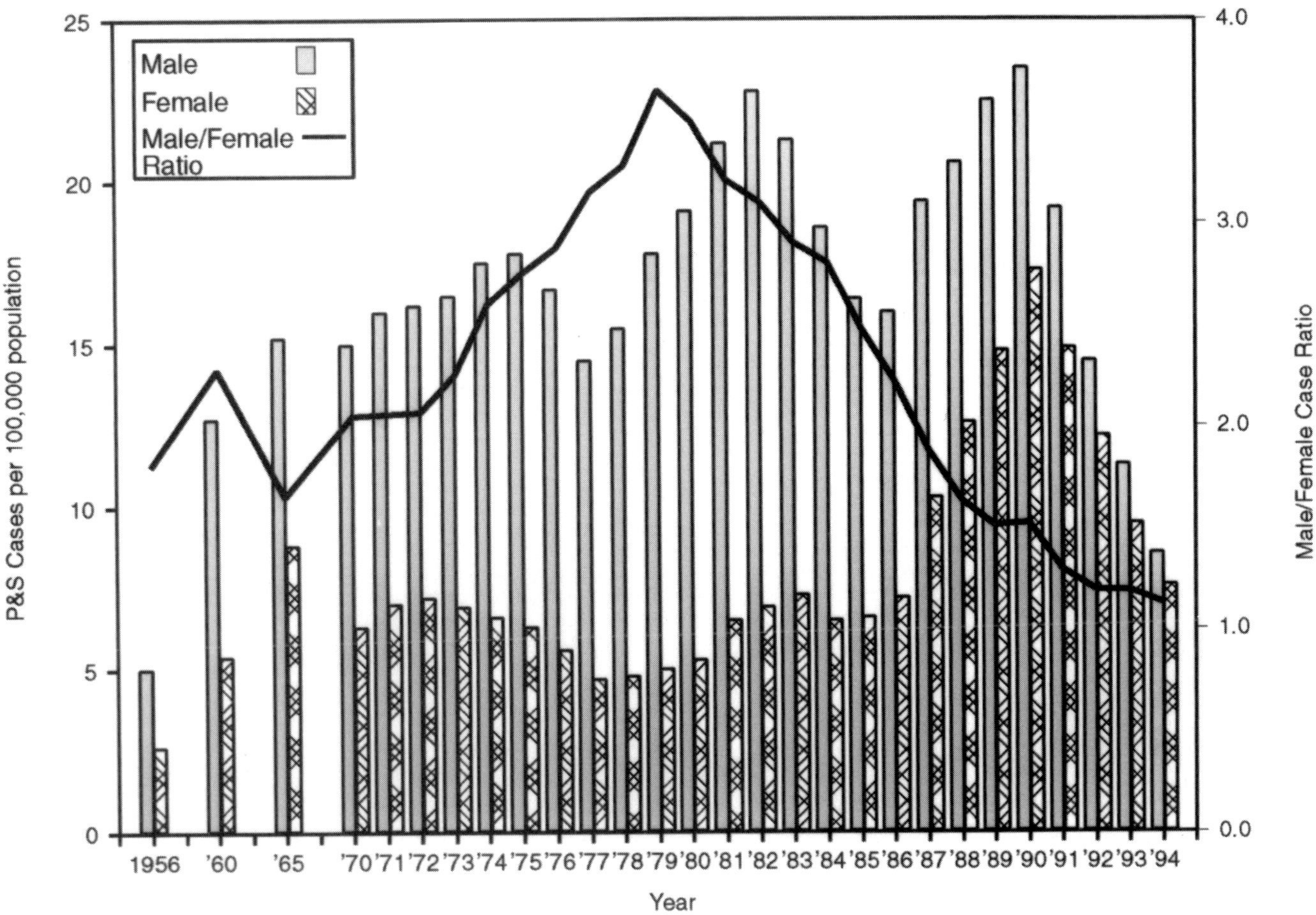

Fig. 84-2. Incidence rates of early infectious syphilis for men and women, with the male-to-female case ratio, in the United States from 1956 to 1994. *(Courtesy of Kathy Dry, Division of STD Prevention, NCHSTP, CDC, Atlanta.)*

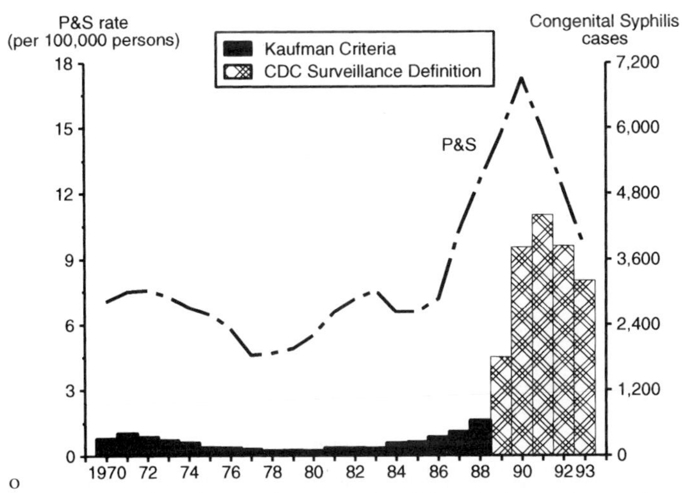

Fig. 84-3. Reported cases of congenital syphilis in infants <1 year of age and rates of primary and secondary syphilis among women, United States, 1970–1993. *(Courtesy of Kathy Dry, Division of STD Prevention, NCHSTP, CDC, Atlanta.)*

suggestive of congenital syphilis were reported.[23] A confirmed case represented an infant or stillbirth in whom *T. pallidum* was identified by either dark-field microscopy or specific stains in specimens from lesions. A probable case was that of an infant or stillbirth who had a reactive test for syphilis and an abnormal physical examination, abnormal long-bone radiograph, abnormal cerebrospinal fluid (reactive CSF-VDRL and/or elevated CSF cell count or protein without other cause), a nontreponemal serologic test titer fourfold higher than the mother's, a rising nontreponemal test titer during follow-up, or a persistently reactive treponemal test beyond one year of age. Although relatively specific, two problems with this definition were that it did not include infected liveborn infants without evidence of congenital syphilis and it depended in many cases upon follow-up serologic data to make a diagnosis (Table 84-1). The new surveillance case definition includes all infants with clinical evidence of active syphilis, as well as normal appearing neonates and stillbirths delivered to women with untreated or inadequately treated syphilis (Table 84-1).[21,23] Use of these guidelines increases the sensitivity for reporting cases of congenital syphilis, albeit by including at-risk but truly uninfected cases. Studies have shown that the new surveillance definition results in a four- to five-fold increase in the number of reported cases.[22,32,33]

The second factor responsible for the recent upsurge in congenital syphilis cases was the near-epidemic increase in the incidence of primary and secondary syphilis among young females in the United States (Figs. 84-1 and 84-2), particularly among inner-city minorities in New York, California, Florida, Texas, and Michigan

Table 84-1. Summary of the Modified Kaufman and Revised Centers for Disease Control and Prevention (CDC) Criteria for Congenital Syphilis Surveillance

Kaufman criteria	Revised CDC criteria
Definite	**Confirmed**
Treponema pallidum by dark-field or histologic examination	Laboratory demonstration of *Treponema pallidum*
Probable	**Presumptive**
Rising Venereal Disease Research Laboratory (VDLR) titer over 3 months or a reactive serologic test for syphilis (STS) that does not revert to nonreactive within 4 months	Any infant whose mother had untreated or inadequately treated syphilis during pregnancy†
One major or two minor criteria* and either a reactive STS or fluorescent treponema antibody (FTA) test	Any infant with a reactive STS and one of the following
One major and one minor criteria	Evidence of congenital syphilis on physical examination‡
Possible	Reactive CSF VDRL or CSF cell count ≥5 or CSF protein ≥50 without other cause
A reactive STS or FTA test without clinical criteria	Reactive FTA-ABS-19S-immunoglobulin M antibody test
	Syphilitic stillbirth
	A fetal death occuring after 20 weeks gestation or weighing ≥500g, in which the mother had untreated or inadequately treated syphilis at delivery

CSF = cerebrospinal fluid. ABS = absorption.
* Major criteria: condyloma lata, osteochondritis, periostitis, snuffles, hemorrhagic rhinitis. Minor criteria: fissures of lips, cutaneous lesions, mucous patches, hepatomegaly, splenomegaly, generalized lymphadenopathy, central nervous signs, hemolytic anemia, CSF cell count ≥20, CSF protein ≥100.
† Inadequate therapy defined as nonpenicillin therapy or penicillin given ≤5 days before delivery.
‡ Signs in infants (≤2 years old) are snuffles, hepatosplenomegaly, characteristic skin rash, condyloma lata, anemia, jaundice (nonviral hepatitis), pseudoparalysis, or edema (nephrotic syndrome and/or malnutrition).
SOURCE: Thompson et al. [22]

and among rural African Americans throughout the Southeast.[21,24,34–36] A major contributor to the increase in urban areas was the use of crack cocaine and the exchange of illegal drugs for sex among multiple sexual partners.[20,37–39] The use of spectinomycin, which is not effective against incubating syphilis,[40,41] for the treatment of penicillinase-producing *Neisseria gonorrhoeae* also may have been contributory. Fortunately, the past several years have seen substantial decreases in the incidence of both infectious syphilis in females and congenital syphilis (Figs. 84-1 and 84-2).[42] These decreases have been attributed to the implementation of innovative, community-based outreach methods that facilitate identification and serologic testing of persons at high risk for syphilis by focusing on sex-for-drugs locations rather than on contact tracing of named sexual partners of persons with early syphilis.[43,44]

Women who deliver syphilitic babies are more likely than the general population to be adolescent, unmarried, and African American or Hispanic; of lower socioeconomic status; and to use crack cocaine.[42,45,46] Of the 3,209 cases of congenital syphilis reported to the Centers for Disease Control and Prevention (CDC) in 1993, 71 percent were African American, 20 percent were Hispanic, 5 percent were white, and 4 percent were of other or unknown race.[47] A number of studies have identified inadequate prenatal care as the leading predisposing factor.[22,31,46,48,49] In the United States, one-third of the mothers of syphilitic babies who do receive prenatal care attend three or fewer clinical visits, and, overall, mothers of affected neonates average only six prenatal visits.[49] By contrast, pregnant women in the United States overall average 11 of the 13 visits recommended by the American College of Obstetrics & Gynecology.[50] Overall, African-American mothers are twice as likely to receive delayed or no care for their pregnancies. Thompson et al. recently emphasized how these "missed opportunities" to diagnose and treat syphilis during pregnancy contribute to neonatal infection.[22]

SUB-SAHARAN AFRICA

In parts of the world where traditional "venereal diseases" are poorly controlled, such as sub-Saharan Africa, the problems associated with syphilis during pregnancy are strikingly reminiscent of those faced by the Western world in the early 1900s. According to available data, the incidence of adverse outcomes attributed to syphilis appears to be higher in sub-Saharan Africa than almost anywhere else in the world.[51]

Syphilis during pregnancy

With the intense research activity related to infection from the human immunodeficiency virus (HIV), many seroprevalence surveys undertaken over the past decade have included serologic examination for syphilis. In the surveys in sub-Saharan Africa that estimated rates of active syphilis (positive results for both *T. pallidum* hemagglutination [TPHA] and rapid plasma reagin [RPR] or Venereal Disease Research Laboratory [VDRL] tests) in pregnant women, the median reported prevalence was 6 percent, with areas in Kenya, Cameroon, Tanzania, Gabon, and Malawi all reporting rates of greater than 10 percent.[52] Based on these studies from major African cities, as well as unpublished reports from other countries in Africa demonstrating seroprevalences in excess of 10 percent, one can conclude that syphilis during pregnancy is prevalent throughout much of Africa. One potential problem with the use of serologic tests to assess the prevalence of syphilis is that these tests cannot distinguish between venereal syphilis and yaws, a nonvenereal treponematosis endemic to parts of equatorial Africa. Presently, however, yaws in Africa is confined to rural tribal populations and is not found in the large urban areas in which venereal syphilis is prevalent.[53]

The most common outcome of syphilis during pregnancy is probably spontaneous abortion during the second and early third trimester; the precise magnitude of this problem is difficult to measure because African women usually do not come for prenatal care until the third trimester.[54] Furthermore, compliance with syphilis treatment is poor; only 10 percent of women completed their prescribed treatment at a teaching hospital, hindering both patient management and data acquisition.[55] In Ethiopia, an estimated 5 percent of all pregnancies are lost each year as a result of syphilis-induced abortions (75,000 pregnancy losses).[56] In another study from Ethiopia, pregnant women who were seroreactive for syphilis were five times more likely to have a spontaneous abortion or stillbirth than women who were seronegative.[57] In Zambia, 19 percent of miscarriages were attributed to syphilis.[54] The spontaneous abortion rate among pregnant African women with syphilis is estimated to be as high as 50 percent.[58]

Perinatal, neonatal, and infant deaths

In Africa, as elsewhere, a strong relationship exists between syphilis during pregnancy and stillbirth. A case-control study from Zambia demonstrated a 28-fold increased risk (95 percent confidence interval, 12 to 63) in stillbirths among women with high-titer RPR card test seroreactivity.[59] In the University Teaching Hospital in Lusaka, Zambia, 42 percent of stillbirths were attributed to syphilis during pregnancy.[54] In Zambia, congenital syphilis was implicated in 20 to 30 percent of total perinatal infant deaths (50 per 1,000 births).[60] One to 1.5 percent of all Zambian pregnancies that extend beyond 20 to 27 weeks end in death due to syphilis. This statistic underestimates the magnitude of the problem because it does not include postneonatal infant deaths and because many stillborn infants lack clinical evidence of congenital syphilis. In Ethiopia, syphilis was the fourth most common cause of perinatal death, accounting for 10 percent of the approximately 70 perinatal deaths per 1,000 births; syphilis also caused nearly 5 percent of all postneonatal infant deaths.[61] Thus, at least 1 percent of Ethiopian pregnancies extending beyond 20 to 27 weeks end in a perinatal or postneonatal infant death due to syphilis. In absolute numbers, each year 15,000 fetal and infant deaths in Ethiopia are directly attributable to syphilis.[56]

Incidence of congenital syphilis

Compared with data from Africa on acquired syphilis during pregnancy, much less information is available on congenital syphilis. A study in Zambia established that nearly 1 percent of the babies delivered at the University Teaching Hospital in Lusaka had signs of congenital infection at birth, and as many as 6.5 percent were seroreactive at birth and thus considered at risk.[62] In another study from Zambia, seroreactivity among infants under 6 months of age was 2.9 percent.[60] Half the seroreactive infants had two or more clinical features suggestive of early congenital syphilis and, of these, 60 percent required hospitalization. Further confirmation of the incidence and morbidity associated with early congenital syphilis in Zambia comes from two treatment studies. Early congenital syphilis was diagnosed in nine percent of admissions to one nursery ward and in eight percent of admissions to the intensive care unit.[63] These data also suggest that in sub-Saharan Africa congenital syphilis often is not diagnosed until weeks or months after birth.[64] While one might anticipate that the revised CDC criteria will be useful for obtaining more precise incidence data, Meyer has pointed out that their lack of specificity could be particularly problematic in Africa, where a high proportion of mothers have reactive syphilis serologies, infants often have other congenital disorders that produce physical findings similar to syphilis, and sophisticated laboratory and radiological studies are unavailable.[65]

Model of outcomes of pregnancy in sub-Saharan Africa

The best estimates of the outcome of pregnancies of women with syphilis in Africa that continue to the third trimester come from earlier Western data, which present African conditions appear to simulate.[64] To estimate adverse outcomes associated with syphilis in pregnancy, we assumed a 10-percent seroreactivity rate in pregnant women and followed 1,000 women in a simple deterministic model (Table 84-2). We then compared the results from the model with actual reported data from Africa.[58] The estimate that 5 percent of all pregnancies in Ethiopia are lost to spontaneous abortion caused by syphilis during pregnancy appeared to be plausible inasmuch as the model yielded a consistent estimate of 3.5 percent. The model estimated that of pregnancies extending beyond 20 to 27 weeks, 1.7 percent would result in a perinatal death caused by syphilis. This was consistent with, though slightly higher than, the 1- to 1.5-percent estimates from Ethiopia and Zambia. Using the model, we estimated that 20 percent of perinatal deaths were caused by syphilis, which was consistent with the 10 to 30 percent reported from Zambia and Ethiopia. In the model, 2.1 percent of pregnancies that extended into the perinatal period resulted in infants with syphilis, which was consistent with results from Zambia of 1 percent of infants with signs of congenital syphilis at birth and 2.9 to 6.5 percent seroreactive at birth or shortly thereafter.

Table 84-2. Reproductive Outcome Model Assuming 10 Percent Seroreactivity in 1,000 Pregnant Women

	Seroreactive	Nonseroreactive
Pregnancies	100	900
Pregnancies lost to spontaneous abortion in the second or early third trimester	50 (50%)	135 (15%)
Excess spontaneous abortion due to syphilis	35	—
Pregnancies extending beyond 20 to 27 weeks	50	765
Perinatal deaths	17 (34%)	54 (7%)
Excess perinatal deaths due to syphilis	14	—
Syphilitic infants	17	—

SOURCE: Schulz et al.[58]

PATHOGENESIS AND PATHOLOGY

TRANSMISSION OF SYPHILIS DURING PREGNANCY

Although a mother can transmit syphilis to her infant at the time of delivery,[66,67] the vast majority of cases are believed to arise from *in utero* infection. In fact, no form of syphilis better exemplifies the remarkable invasiveness of *T. pallidum* than congenital syphilis. Studies with cultured human umbilical vein endothelial cells have documented that *T. pallidum*, but not nonpathogenic treponemes, efficiently penetrates endothelial cells via intercellular junctions,[68,69] and it is likely that a similar, if not identical, process underlies the traversal of maternal and fetal tissues *in utero*.[68,69] The finding of spirochetes in the placenta and umbilical cord in association with typical histopathologic changes supports transplacental invasion during maternal spirochetemia as the major route of transmission.[70–74] Alternatively, *T. pallidum* may gain access to the fetal circulation by first traversing the fetal membranes and infecting the amniotic fluid.[75–78]

The risk of congenital syphilis is directly related to the stage of maternal syphilis during pregnancy. It is extremely high during the first four years after acquisition, when spirochetemia is common, and then decreases during late syphilis, when spirochetemia becomes a rare event. Harman (in 1917) followed obstetric events in 150 syphilitic women and 150 healthy women of similar social status (Table 84-3).[79] Sixty-one percent of the pregnancies of the syphilitic women were attended by accidents of pregnancy or the birth of an infected child, compared to a complication rate of 20.4 percent in healthy women. In 1951, Ingraham reported that following untreated maternal early syphilis of four years or less duration, 41 percent of infants were liveborn with congenital syph-

Table 84-3. Prospective Observations of Obstetric Events in Syphilitic Women

Event	150 syphilitic women	150 controls
Pregnancies	1001	826
Miscarriages	9.2%	7.4%
Stillbirths	8.0%	2.1%
Infant deaths	22.9%	11.4%
Infant syphilis	21.0%	0.0%
Healthy child	38.9%	79.1%

SOURCE: Harman[79]

ilis, 25 percent were stillborn, 14 percent died in the neonatal period, 2 percent were premature but without evidence of congenital syphilis, and only 18 percent with normal full-term living infants.[80] In contrast, only 2 percent of infants born to mothers with untreated late syphilis of over four years duration had congenital syphilis.[80] Subsequently, in 1952, Fiumara and colleagues reported that among infants born to mothers with primary or secondary syphilis, approximately half of the infants were premature, stillborn, or died in the neonatal period; the other 50 percent developed congenital syphilis (Table 84-4).[48] With early latent syphilis, the transmission rate decreased to approximately 40 percent, while 20 percent were premature, 4 percent died in the neonatal period, and 10 percent were stillborn; 20 percent of infants were normal and full term (Table 84-4). With late latent syphilis, approximately 10 percent of infants had congenital syphilis and another 10 percent were stillborn, but there was no increase in premature births or neonatal deaths beyond the expected rate among women without syphilis (Table 84-4).[48] Sánchez et al.[81] documented similar rates in a small cohort of 19 infants. In that series, two of two infants born to mothers with primary syphilis had laboratory evidence of infection (reactive serum IgM immunoblot, positive serum/CSF polymerase chain reaction, or positive rabbit infectivity testing) as did six of six infants born to mothers with secondary syphilis. In contrast, only 6 of 11 (55 percent) infants born to mothers with early latent infection had evidence of infection.

In the past, it was a commonly held obstetric principle that infection of the fetus does not occur before 18 weeks. In 1938, Beck and Dailey proposed that the prominence of the Langhans' cell layer of the cytotrophoblast prior to midgestation explained the rarity of early transplacental infection, and its regression thereafter left the fetus vulnerable to spirochetal invasion.[82] This belief was supported by Dippel's series and his review of more than 200 fetal autopsies culled from the literature.[83] He found no cases of infected abortuses prior to 18 weeks, and the proportion of abortuses that were infected rose steadily with advancing gestation to a peak at 8 months. Dippel also noted that only 19 percent of syphilitic abortuses showed delayed regression of the Langhans' layer, whereas 50 percent of uninfected abortuses had an intact Langhans' layer.[83] This theory, however, was disproved by electron microscopic demonstration of the persistence of the Langhans' cell layer throughout pregnancy and by the detection of spirochetes by silver staining and immunofluorescent techniques in fetal tissue from spontaneous abortions at nine and ten weeks of gestation.[70,84] Recently, Nathan and coworkers demonstrated spirochetes in amniotic fluid as early as 17 weeks of pregnancy, further proving that *T. pallidum* can gain access to the fetal compartment early in gestation.[77] It is now believed that congenital syphilis can occur following maternal infection at any time in gestation, with the risk of fetal infection increasing as the stage of pregnancy advances. Failure to appreciate syphilis as a cause of first-trimester stillbirth, and therefore to seek treponemes in tissues, is due to the fetus's inability to mount a characteristic histopathologic response within the first 18 to 20 weeks of gestation.[85]

Table 84-4. Outcome of Pregnancy in Relation to Stage of Maternal Syphilis

Outcome	Primary and secondary, %	Early latent, %	Late latent, %	Normal, %
Prematurity	50%	20%	9%	8%
Perinatal death	0	20%	11%	1%
Congenital syphilis	50%	40%	10%	0
Healthy child	0	20%	70%	90%

SOURCE: Fiumara et al.[48]

HISTOPATHOLOGY

General features

Congenital syphilis can involve almost any and every fetal organ, with liver, kidneys, bone, pancreas, spleen, lungs, heart, and brain being the most frequently affected.[86] As with acquired syphilitic infection, the fundamental histologic lesion of congenital syphilis is an obliterative endarteritis typically consisting of mononuclear and plasma cell infiltrates surrounding blood vessels with intimal hyperplasia (of larger vessels) and swollen, hyperplastic endothelial cells.[87–89] Based upon our current understanding of endothelial cell biology[90] as well as recent immunohistochemical analyses of cutaneous biopsies from patients with secondary syphilis,[91] it is reasonable to presume that the endothelial cells in these lesions are activated and expressing adhesion receptors, cytokines, and other molecules that initiate and sustain the inflammatory response.[90] Moreover, recent studies have shown that both motile *T. pallidum* and *T. pallidum* lipoproteins can activate vascular endothelium.[69]

Fibrosis and gummas are also frequently observed in congenitally infected tissues. Fibrosis may be relatively fine in character, consisting primarily of collagen deposition about affected blood vessels, or it may substantially distort and replace the parenchyma in affected organs, such as the liver, pancreas, bone and lung.[86] Microscopic gummas are common, especially in skin, mucous membranes, bone, and liver. They typically consist of a thin peripheral rim of mononuclear cell infiltration, central coagulation ("gummy" necrosis), and fibrosis, but any of these three features may predominate. Unlike the staged histopathology of acquired syphilis, a distinctive feature of congenital syphilis is that these tissue reaction patterns may be present, to various extents, as part of a single syndrome.

Placenta and umbilical cord

Inflammatory changes in the placenta are often more striking than those of the fetus. Grossly, the infected placenta is large, thick, and pale, weighing up to one-third of fetal weight.[70,92,93] Microscopic changes include (1) focal proliferative villitis with necrosis and focal infiltrations of maternal lymphocytes and plasma cells, (2) endothelial and adventitial proliferation of villous vessels leading to obliteration, (3) villi which are immature, large, clubbed, and crowded, (4) extensive stromal hyperplasia and deposition of granulation tissue, and (5) occasionally, multiple small ("miliary") gumma (Fig. 84-4).[89,92,94] Spirochetes can often be visualized by silver stain or with more specific immunohistochemical methods (Fig. 84-4). The umbilical cord also may be involved. A deeply seated inflammatory process within the matrix of the umbilical cord, termed *necrotizing funisitis*, has been described,[71] although

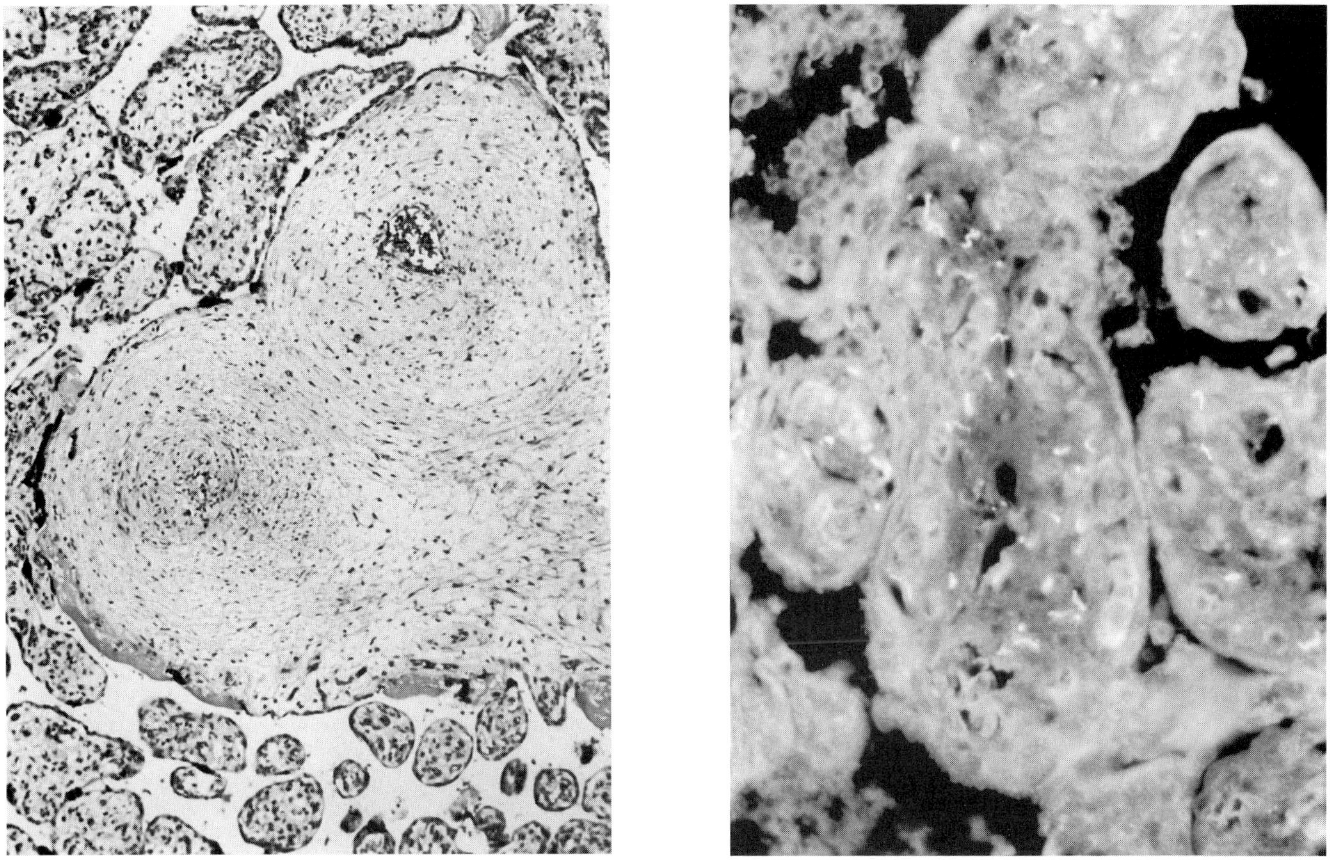

Fig. 84-4. Syphilitic placentitis. (left) Blood vessels within the enlarged, clubbed villi exhibit endothelial and adventitial proliferation resulting in near vascular obliteration (×150). *(Courtesy of G. Wendel.)* (right) Detection of *T. pallidum* by indirect immunofluorescence with rabbit anti-*T. pallidum* antiserum. *(Courtesy of S. Norris.)*

there is disagreement as to whether this lesion is specific for syphilis.[73] Macroscopically, the umbilical cord resembles a "barber pole"; the edematous portions have a spiral-striped zone of red and pale blue discoloration interspersed with streaks of chalky white (Fig. 84-5). On cross-section, abscess-like foci of necrosis located within Wharton's jelly are centered around the umbilical vessels (Fig. 84-5).

Skeletal system

Characteristic bony lesions are present in 97 percent of autopsied infants by 6 months of age.[89] Membranous bones are less involved than endochondral (long) bones, in which the pathological process is concentrated at the metaphyseal-epiphyseal junction. Grossly, an irregular yellow line is found at the zone of provisional calcification.[95] When membranous bone is involved, it is generally a periostitis, which leads to localized exostosis and osteoporosis. A perivascular inflammatory infiltrate, found in both types of bone, erodes the trabeculae and eventually gives way to fibrosis.[96,97] A debate persists regarding the relative importance of inflammatory and trophic influences ("syphilitic dystrophy") on the production of these lesions.[98,99] Caffey attributes the transverse striping of the metaphyses to nutrition and argues that any severe disease of the fetal and neonatal period may produce it.[98] Others have made careful pathoradiologic correlations, describing the sequential development of an "osteochondritis."[100,101] When fully developed, the epiphyseal plate is destroyed, the end of the diaphysis is destroyed, and fragments of bone and cartilage separate to produce a "pseudo-Charcot's joint." The diaphysis acquires a worm-eaten appearance resembling fibrocystic disease. Marrow is trapped between thick layers of periosteum, and islands of cartilage are trapped within metaphyseal bone. Epiphyseal ossification centers are usually spared.

In surviving infants, healing occurs over the first six months, usually without residual lesions, and seems little influenced by penicillin.[102,103] This suggests that much of the pathogenesis of these lesions may be trophic rather than directly infectious and that the severely ill infant who comes to autopsy may not be representative of the survivors whom radiologists and clinicians most commonly encounter. Marked inflammation and exuberant fibrosis may be hallmarks of more profoundly affected infants.

Liver, spleen, pancreas, intestines, and lungs

Liver involvement typically takes the form of inflammation confined to the portal triads with rings of collagen deposited about portal ducts and blood vessels. In some cases, focal inflammation and scarring irregularly replace hepatic parenchyma. In the most severe cases, the inflammatory infiltrates produce a diffuse hepatitis with separation of liver plates and, eventually, extensive scarring. Though not specific for syphilis, excessive extramedullary hematopoiesis within hepatic sinusoids and portal triads often accompanies these changes. Diffuse gumma also may be seen. Silver stains of hepatic tissue often show heavy infiltration with treponemes even in the absence of pronounced histologic abnormalities.

Splenic sinusoids are widened and crammed with masses of blood-forming cells, explaining the characteristic splenomegaly. Deposition of granulation tissue about splenic blood vessels can

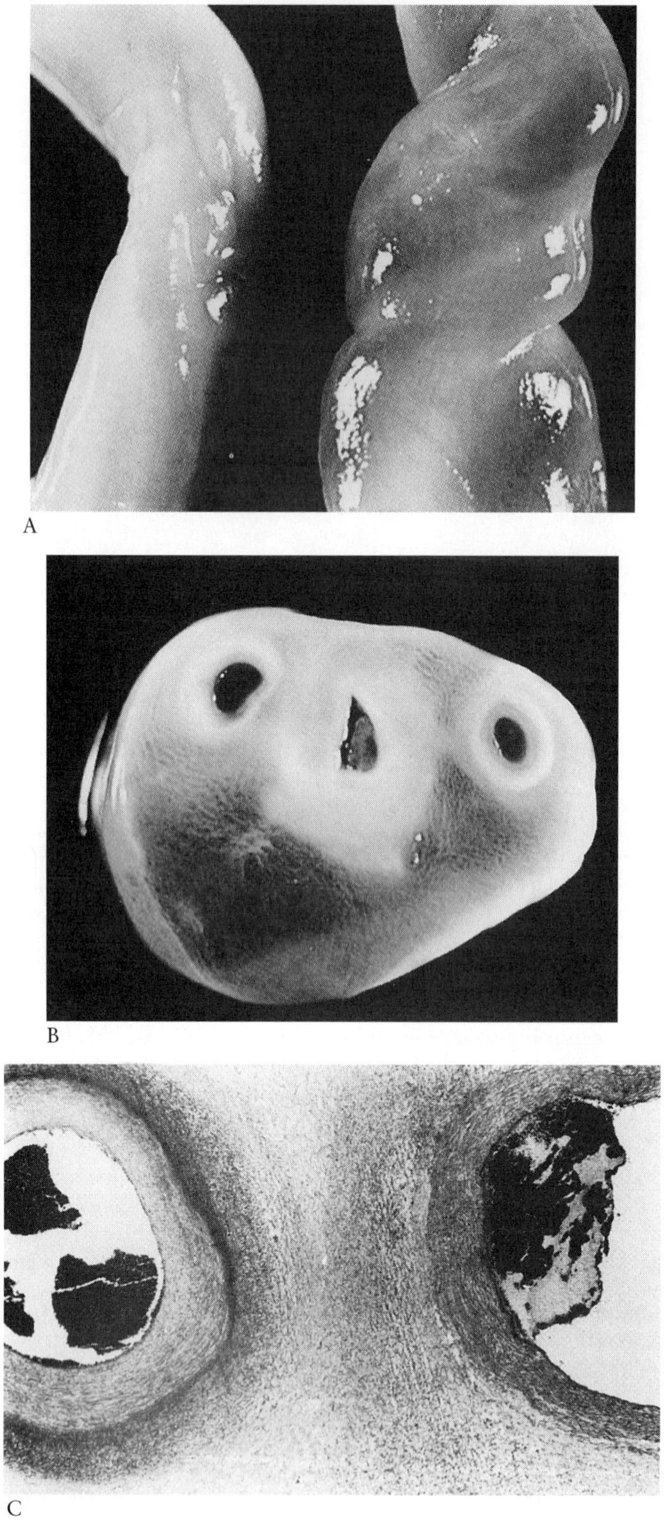

Fig. 84-5. Necrotizing funisitis. (A) Umbilical cord in congenital syphilis. A normal segment is at the left of the segment with necrotizing funisitis. (B) Cross section showing opaque white lesions surrounding blood vessels and venous thrombosis. (C) Histological section showing perivascular inflammation and necrosis corresponding to white lesions surrounding blood vessels. *(From Fojaco et al.*[71]*)*

be severe enough to cause "onion skinning." Pancreatitis, which may be intense, consists of isolation and obliteration of ductules as well as acini by inflammatory infiltrates and perivascular deposition of rings of collagen.[86] In the gastrointestinal tract, mucosal and submucosal infiltration with mononuclear and plasma cells is associated with a striking fibrotic response and increase in the width of the submucosa. Though now rare,[86] the classical "pneumonia alba" of congenital syphilis is characterized by grossly enlarged, firm, yellowish-white lungs; these changes are due to an intense obliterative fibrosis in the interalveolar septae.[89]

Nervous system

Meningeal involvement is grossly apparent as a discoloration and thickening of the basilar meninges, especially around the brainstem and optic chiasm.[89] The microscopic changes consist of endarteritis with various degrees of infarction and neuronal damage.[89] Fibrosis during healing may result in obstructive hydrocephalus and/or entrapment of cranial nerves. Parenthymatous forms of late congenital neurosyphilis (e.g., general paresis, tabes dorsalis), now extremely rare, are pathologically indistinguishable from those of acquired syphilis in adults.[104]

Kidneys

An epimembranous glomerulopathy is associated with two different forms of immune complex injury. One involves deposition of IgA, IgG, and IgM with complement and the other involves immune complex deposition without complement along the glomerular basement membrane.[105] Elution studies have demonstrated that the complexes consist of treponemal antigens and anti-treponemal antibodies.[106] Interstitial perivascular infiltrates consisting of mononuclear and plasma cells also are present.

Teeth

The late dental consequences of neonatal syphilis are abnormalities of form, structure, and size. There is apical notching, the amelodentinal junction is irregular, enamelization is defective, and the affected teeth are small. The pathogenesis of dental stigmata has been a long-standing controversy. Although Hutchinson himself at first regarded the changes as a part of the syndrome of mercurial stomatitis, he subsequently attributed them to trophic changes.[13,14] Early difficulty in confirming the presence of spirochetes in developing dental tissue contributed to the notion that hypoplasia and malformation were due to the general nutritional state of syphilitic infants, to local impairment of nutrition due to endarteritis, or even to rickets.[107] Indeed, as Hutchinson emphasized, it is the first (6-year) molars and central incisors of the permanent set that are specifically affected. These begin to calcify just before and just after birth, respectively. Therefore, perinatal injury would be expected to produce malformation of these teeth, particularly if a disturbed process of calcification is the major mechanism of pathogenesis. From 1932 to 1953, however, a series of observations suggested that direct treponemal invasion of the developing permanent tooth and the resulting inflammation are the cause of dental stigmata.[108]

The tooth is formed by mesenchymal protrusion into an ectodermal tooth bud, which invaginates to receive it (Fig. 84-6). A dental papilla of mesenchymal origin gives rise to an outer layer of odontoblasts that ultimately produce dentin abutting the ectodermal enamel organ. An enamel epithelium on the inner aspect of the enamel organ consists of ameloblasts that ultimately produce a layer of enamel rods, lining the outer aspect of the dentin. Interactions between ameloblasts and the underlying mesenchymal odontoblasts initiate the apposition of enamel and dentin. This is followed by calcification of both enamel and dentin and finally by eruption. When the jaws of newborn infants dying of congenital syphilis are examined, the tooth germs of the permanent teeth are inflamed and spirochetes can be found throughout the enamel organ and dental papilla. There is endarteritis and

Fig. 84-6. Development of the permanent incisor, illustrating the effect of treponemal infection or morphogenesis.

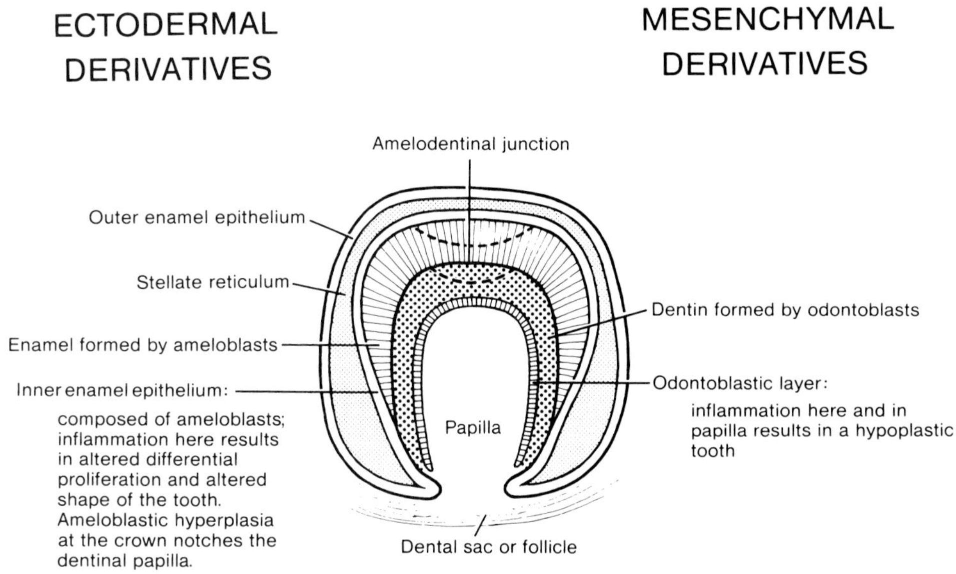

perivascular inflammation in the dental papilla, and spirochetes are found in vessel walls. This results in a complex pathological process culminating in a failure to lay down enamel at the center of the notch and an irregular amelodentinal junction in the mature tooth. Radiographs of syphilitic incisors suggest that the irregular amelodentinal junction is the internal counterpart to the external deformity. The impaired growth of the dentinal papilla, on the other hand, is the precursor of the small size of the incisors and first molars.

CLINICAL MANIFESTATIONS

PREMATURITY AND INTRAUTERINE GROWTH RETARDATION

Intrauterine growth retardation, a commonly cited feature of congenital syphilis, is thought to reflect inadequate nutrition of the fetus as a result of syphilitic placentitis.[109–111] Until recently, however, there were no clear criteria for distinguishing between premature infants and those who are small for gestational age. Furthermore, Naeye's study of 36 syphilitic perinatal deaths seemed to show that, in contrast to rubella and cytomegalovirus infection, syphilis did not affect fetal growth.[112] The difficulty in sorting out the contribution of syphilis to fetal-growth retardation is compounded by the fact that gestational syphilis disproportionately affects the same population in which other causes of fetal-growth retardation, such as maternal use of intravenous drugs and poor nutritional status, are prevalent. Recent controlled studies, however, strongly support the association between intrauterine infection with *T. pallidum* and prematurity, low birth weight, and small size for gestational age.[113,114]

EARLY CONGENITAL SYPHILIS

Similar to acquired syphilis in adults,[115,116] congenital syphilis traditionally is divided into early and late disease. Those features that typically appear within the first two years of life comprise early congenital syphilis, while those that occur after 2 years of age, most often near puberty, comprise late congenital syphilis. In current practice, the vast majority of cases present within the perinatal period.

The clinical manifestations of early congenital infections are a consequence of active infection with *T. pallidum* and the resultant inflammatory response induced in various organs and tissues. The severity of these manifestations is extremely variable, ranging from life-threatening involvement of multiple organs and body systems, as is seen in fetal hydrops, to radiologic or laboratory abnormalities in an otherwise normal-appearing newborn.[109] Indeed, most infected infants are entirely asymptomatic at birth.[30,117–120] In a recent study from Detroit, only 16 (22 percent) of 72 infants born to mothers with untreated syphilis had clinical, laboratory, or radiologic evidence of congenital syphilis.[114] When syphilis is not identified in normal appearing infants, the diagnosis is delayed until the patient presents weeks later with such nonspecific complaints as rhinitis, pneumonia, or failure to thrive.[66,67,121,122] In two-thirds of untreated cases, the clinical signs of early congenital syphilis begin to appear in the third to the eighth week of life; in nearly all cases, the signs appear within three months.[121,123]

Neonates born with manifest syphilis are often severely affected and carry a worse prognosis. Among these are the infants who display the classic picture of marasmic syphilis: the "wizened, pot-bellied, hoarse old man with withered brown skin and runny fissured nose . . . senescent decrepitude in miniature."[30] In an earlier era, a number of signs were very suggestive of syphilis, especially when seen together (e.g., snuffles, certain skin eruptions, pseudoparalysis, and epitrochlear lymphadenopathy).[117] Marfan (as cited by Stokes) considered snuffles, palmar and plantar bullae, splenomegaly, pseudoparalysis, and cutaneous syphilids to form a diagnostic pentad[121]; Bueno suggested that the first three of these signs comprise a triad.[124] None can be considered entirely pathognomonic, however.

Mucocutaneous lesions

Among those infants who have clinical evidence of congenital syphilis, 15 to 60 percent will manifest mucocutaneous lesions consisting of rash and/or rhinitis (Table 84-5). Nasal discharge is the earliest sign of congenital syphilis, occurring 1 to 2 weeks before the rash (Fig. 84-7). It was reported in 68 to 86 percent of older series,[102,107,123] but has been much less common in recent years (Table 84-5).[125,126] The discharge, which contains spirochetes in high concentration, is initially watery and indistinguishable from that of viral or allergic rhinitis, but then it becomes progressively thicker and purulent and then hemorrhagic. Resulting nasal obstruction interferes with feeding. Ulceration leads to

Table 84-5. Clinical Presentations of Early Congenital Syphilis

Total number	Hepatomegaly	Splenomegaly	Anemia	Jaundice	Skin rash	Petechiae	Snuffles	Abnormal bone x-ray	Lymphad-enopathy	Pseudo-paralysis	Ref.
15	13/15	15/15	13/15	6/15	11/15	8/15	—	6/7	—	—	131
18	17/18	14/18	7/8	6/18	6/18	—	3/18	13/15	—	1/18	125
102	21/102	21/102	13/102	21/102	21/102	—	11/102	43/102	—	16/102	99
16	16/16	16/16	8/16	7/16	8/16	4/16	8/16	11/16	6/16	—	86
21	12/21	12/21	—	—	12/21	—	11/21	21/21	—	21/21	120
6	2/6	4/6	4/6	1/6	2/6	—	1/6	—	1/6	3/6	129
10	10/10	10/10	—	—	5/10	—	2/10	—	—	—	130
24	18/24	12/24	14/22	13/24	9/22	10/23	9/21	14/17	—	—	224
Total (%)	104/212 (51)	104/212 (49)	60/179 (34)	54/181 (30)	74/210 (35)	22/54 (41)	45/194 (23)	108/178 (61)	7/22 (32)	41/147 (28)	

deeper involvement, including chondritis with necrosis, and eventually to the septal perforation or saddle-nose deformity of late congenital syphilis. Extension into the throat produces laryngitis and either a hoarse or an aphonic cry.

As with secondary syphilis in adults, there are myriad cutaneous lesions in congenital syphilis. The most common lesion is a large round pink macule that fades to a dusky or coppery hue, lasts one to three months without treatment, and leaves a residual pigmentation.[30,121] These lesions are typically distributed over the back, perineum, extremities, palms, and soles, sparing the anterior trunk; they develop slowly over a period of weeks. They may be covered with a fine, silvery scale and may mingle with indurated plaques of similar size and color. The corymbiform lesion consists of a grouped papule around a large central plaque, like a "hen and chicks"; annular lesions occur but are less common than in acquired secondary syphilis.[29] The vesiculobullous eruption, known as *pemphigus syphiliticus*, is highly distinctive when present.[121] Intraepidermal edema leads to spongiotic midepidermal blisters that are most prominent on the palms and soles; the blister fluid teems with spirochetes.[89] When the bullae rupture, they leave a macerated, dusky red surface that readily dries and crusts (Fig. 84-8). Even in the absence of frank bulla formation, desquamation is common and may be generalized or confined to the periungual areas of fingers and toes. Palmar and plantar desquamation is preceded by subcutaneous edema underlying a shiny erythema and sometimes accompanied by shedding of the nails.[3,30] Paronychia also leads to narrow, atrophic nails, producing a claw-nail deformity, particularly of the fourth and fifth digits. Hair may be brittle and sparse; infantile alopecia, especially affecting the eyebrows, is considered very suggestive of syphilis.[30]

The face, perineum, and intertriginous sites are particular targets of syphilitic lesions that may be eczematoid, impetiginous, or even gangrenous (Fig. 84-9).[3,30,121] The facial eruption preferentially affects the middle third of the face, from the medial portions of the supraorbital ridges in the chin.[127] At the nares, lips, and anus, the initial lesions may be indistinguishable from the mucous

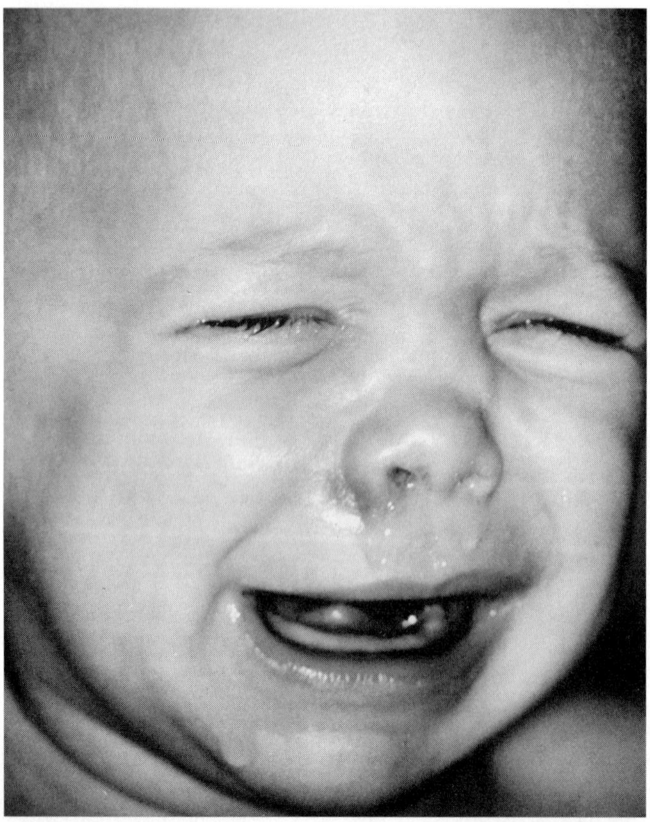

Fig. 84-7. Snuffles: a persistent, often sanguinous, nasal discharge. Treponemes abound in the discharge, providing a definitive means of diagnosis. *(Courtesy of C. Ginsburg.)*

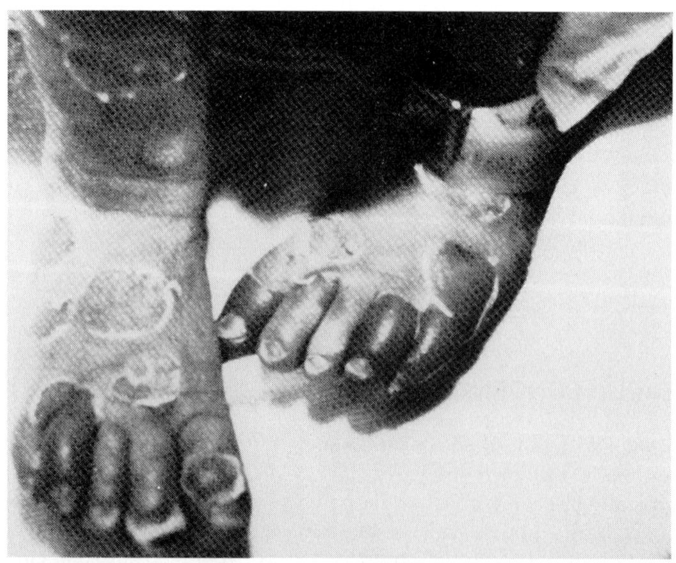

Fig. 84-8. Typical bullae and desquamation of congenital syphilis. *(Courtesy of C. Ginsburg.)*

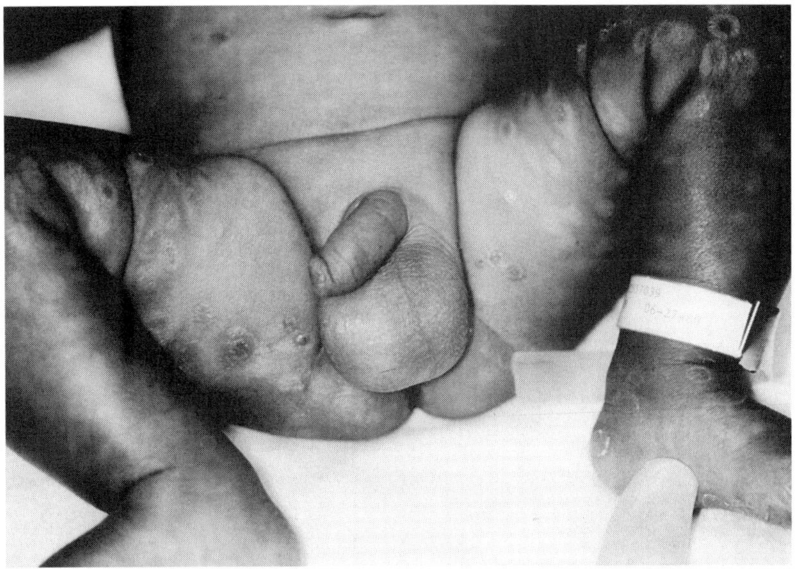

Fig. 84-9. Scaling, annular rash of congenital syphilis. *(Courtesy of C. Ginsburg.)*

patches of secondary syphilis but then become deeply fissured and hemorrhagic, leading to Parrot's radial scars of late congenital syphilis, known as rhagades.[30] Mucous patches are also found on the tongue and palate.

Condylomata lata affect the same mucocutaneous and intertriginous areas and are raised, flat, moist verrucae that are seen in recurrences of untreated congenital syphilis.[30] They are seen typically toward the end of the first year of life,[3] and, together with the furuncle of Barlow, may be regarded as an intermediate manifestation between early and late congenital syphilis. The syphilitic furuncle is a deep violaceous nodule, usually on the upper outer thigh, that occurs after nine months and before three years of age.[30]

Reticuloendothelial system

Syphilis was once the most common cause of hepatosplenomegaly in infancy.[128] The majority of infants with clinical evidence of early congenital syphilis will manifest hepatosplenomegaly (Table 84-5).[86,99,120,125,129–131] Hepatomegaly may occur as an isolated manifestation,[125] but splenomegaly without hepatic enlargement occurs rarely, if ever. Both hepatic and splenic enlargement are caused by subacute inflammation and by compensatory extramedullary hematopoiesis.[86,132] Hypersplenism also may contribute to spleen size.[121,133] Up to one-third of infants with hepatic involvement will manifest both direct and indirect hyperbilirubinemia as well as elevated transaminase, γ-glutamyltransferase, and alkaline phosphatase levels.[134] For unknown reasons, the liver dysfunction may actually worsen with the initiation of penicillin therapy, before gradually improving weeks to months later.[134] On occasion, the liver abnormalities may require as long as a year to resolve; permanent hepatic sequelae (e.g., cirrhosis) are rare, however. Generalized lymphadenopathy is found in 20 to 50 percent of cases.[102,126,129,135] The nodes are firm, rubbery, and nontender. Epitrochlear adenopathy, found in 20 percent of those with adenopathy, is considered especially characteristic of congenital syphilis.[109,121,126,136]

Skeletal involvement

Among syphilitic infants under one year of age studied by Nabarro,[30] more than 30 percent had physical evidence and more than 80 percent had radiographic evidence of osteochondritis. In an unpublished series from Texas, 70 percent of infants with probable or definite congenital syphilis had osteochondritis,[137] a figure similar to those in other reports (Table 84-5). The majority of affected infants do not have any symptomatology from skeletal involvement; on occasion, however, the bony lesions may be painful or have superimposed fracture resulting in pseudoparalysis of the affected limb, termed *pseudoparalysis of Parrot*.[109] The physical signs of skeletal syphilis in infants are limited to the signs of epiphysitis. Epiphyses of the radius, femur, humerus, and fibula, in descending order of frequency, are involved. There may be periarticular swelling, and the end of the bone is tender on passive motion of the adjacent joint. When the proximal humerus is affected, the arm hangs in flaccid immobility, internally rotated with the forearm in pronation. Pain elicited by passive motion of the shoulder, however, and development of the condition after birth distinguish this pseudoparalysis from intrapartum brachial plexus injury. When the femur is involved, the leg is held in rigid flexion. Dactylitis (tender, fusiform swelling of the fingers) was observed in 2 to 6 percent of older series,[107] but it has been uncommon in recent experience, probably because it was typically seen in recurrences of untreated congenital syphilis.[26] Osteitis of the skull, particularly of the central margins of the occipital and parietal bones, produces softening (craniotabes) that indents or yields on pressure, "like stiff parchment."[30,121] Parrot's nodes are focal, bilateral, frontoparietal swellings, typically separated by a cruciform furrow.

Roentgenographic methods have been used diagnostically in congenital syphilis for more than 80 years. Because the radiographic changes are relatively specific, x-ray formerly rivaled serology in importance for diagnosis and is still highly useful in distinguishing active infection from transplacental transfer of maternal antibodies.[117] The proliferative and destructive changes in bone tissue produce a "celery stick" appearance of increased density alternating with rarefaction on x-ray.[100,138] Radiographic changes are most readily observed in the areas of rapid bone growth, such as in the provisional zone of calcification and in the periosteum (Fig. 84-10). Syphilitic osteochondritis requires approximately 5 weeks to become roentgenographically demonstrable, while periostitis—multiple layers of new periosteal bone formation in response to diaphyseal inflammation—requires 16 weeks. This corresponds to the clinical observation that osteochondritis is usually manifest perinatally, whereas periostitis sometimes is not seen until four to five months later.[117] When both

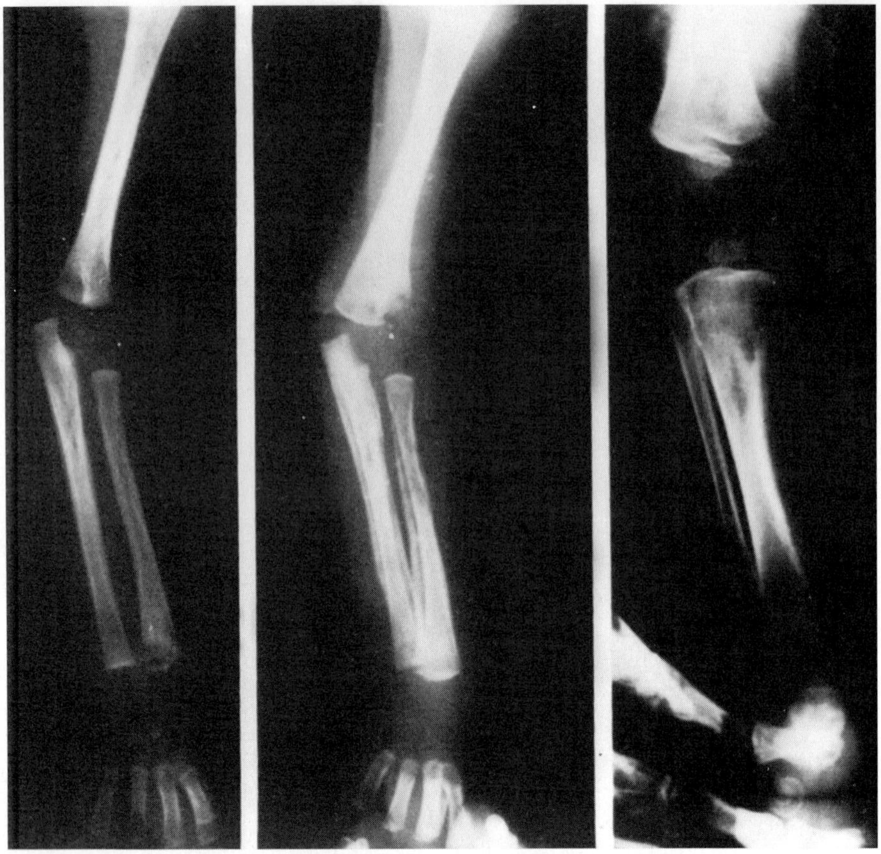

Fig. 84-10. *(Left)* Focal metaphyseal destruction of the lateral aspect of the distal radius; faint metaphyseal banding of distal ulna; longitudinal lines of rarefaction and density extend into the ulnar diaphysis proximally. *(Middle)* Extensive mottling of diaphysis and periostitis. Dense periosteal new bone formation encasing ulna and radius (periosteal cloaking); complete encasement is called the *sarcophagus sign.* Focal lateral metaphyseal defect of distal humerus; erosion of sigmoid notch of ulna (Levin's sign). *(Right)* Focal metaphyseal defect of proximal tibia (Wimberger's sign). *(Courtesy of G. Currarino.)*

lesions are present perinatally, it suggests that the infant was infected during the second trimester[139]; the combination of these lesions makes a diagnosis of syphilis very likely. When periostitis is present by itself, it usually means that an earlier osteochondritis has already healed. Although single bone lesions can occur,[140] such a finding should suggest another diagnosis.

A skeletal survey is required to evaluate infants for congenital syphilis. Widespread lesions involve multiple, symmetrical sites of the long bones and occasionally involve the cranium, spine, and ribs. The tibia and ulna are most commonly followed by fibula, radius, humerus, and femur. Lower extremities are more commonly affected than upper extremities; the femur is more often affected distally, the tibia and humerus proximally.[30] The earliest changes occur in the metaphysis, consisting of a transverse sawtooth radiodense band below the epiphyseal plate; this widened and enhanced zone of provisional calcification is accompanied by an underlying zone of osteoporosis, evident as a radiolucent band. A series of alternating dense and lucent bands may extend into the diaphysis.[97] This process may be followed by radiolucent mottling and finally by fragmentation of the metaphysis itself. Focal defects with cortical destruction may be seen on the lateral aspect of the metaphysis; in the tibia, such lesions occur on the medial aspect of the proximal metaphysis and are usually bilateral, giving rise to the distinctive "cat bit" or Wimberger's sign in 21 percent of cases of infant syphilis.[141] Erosion of the sigmoid notch of the ulna may be of similar significance.[103] Though also seen in hyperparathyroidism, infantile generalized fibromatosis, and bacterial osteomyelitis, the "cat bite" sign is most suggestive of syphilitic osteitis. Later, longitudinal lines of rarefaction may also extend into the diaphysis; in serial array, these linear lucencies resemble a "celery stick," a sign also seen in rubella and cytomegalovirus infection.[97] Irregular, patchy focal lucencies may appear in the diaphysis, sometimes containing sequestra that invite confusion with suppurative osteomyelitis.[142] The epiphysis is relatively spared of radiographic changes, except that it may separate as a result of minor trauma.

Fractures through the degenerating metaphysis occur readily, followed by exuberant callus formation, resulting in a cap over the metaphysis called the "bucket handle" sign.[141] Periostitis is found in 71 percent of cases of infant syphilis and consists of multiple layers of periosteal new bone formation ("onion peel periosteum") in response to diaphyseal inflammation[141]; when exuberant, this process leads to hypertrophic "periosteal cloaking" of the bone, with layers of marrow trapped between layers of subperiosteal bone, thus encasing the entire shaft and producing a radiographic "sarcophagus sign" (Fig. 84-10).

Hematologic manifestations

The major hematologic features of early congenital syphilis are anemia, leukocytosis or leukopenia, and thrombocytopenia. Whitaker et al. found anemia to be the most common laboratory finding in 24 out of 25 cases (96 percent).[133] The anemia of congenital syphilis is Coombs' test–negative, normochromic and normocytic or macrocytic with polychromasia, and often striking reticulocytosis and erythroblastosis.[30] Severe anemia may be associated with replacement of marrow by granulation tissue in syphilitic osteitis or with maturation arrest in the erythroblastoid line.[30,143] Autoimmune hemolysis, however, is a more common mechanism,[133,144] and it may be associated with cryoglobulinemia, macroglobulinemia, or circulating immune complexes.[105,106,145,146] Hemolysis may persist for some time following treatment and can be sufficient, if prolonged or complicated by bleeding, to lead to iron-deficiency anemia.

Neutrophilic leukocytosis occurs in over 70 percent of cases, and congenital syphilis is one of the classic causes of leukemoid reactions in infancy.[147] Leukopenia and monocytosis also have been described.[148] Thirty percent of babies with syphilis develop significant thrombocytopenia.[131,133] Bleeding complications occur in 60 percent of those who are thrombocytopenic. Thrombocytopenia is believed to be due to diminished platelet survival mediated by immune complexes or hypersplenism.[131,133]

Nephropathy

Syphilitic nephrotic syndrome in infancy is an uncommon complication that has, nevertheless, been recognized since the end of the nineteenth century.[127] Nephrosis was found in 5 percent of cases of infant syphilis at the Hospital for Sick Children, in London, between 1917 and 1939,[30] which is similar to recent series[97,144]; glomerulonephritis, with hematuria and cylindruria, is less common.[149] Evidence of nephrotic syndrome appears at 2 to 3 months of age with the onset of edema, ascites, hypoproteinemia, and proteinuria.

Central nervous system involvement

Neurologic involvement in congenital syphilis ranges from asymptomatic CNS invasion by *T. pallidum* to acute syphilitic leptomeningitis. Traditionally, asymptomatic involvement of the CNS is inferred from abnormal CSF indices (pleocytosis, elevated protein content, reactive CSF-VDRL test). In 1949, Platou reported a 60 percent incidence of congenital neurosyphilis based upon diagnostic criteria consisting of >5 wbc/mm^3, a protein content >45 mg/dl, and a reactive CSF-VDRL test.[102] These criteria are relatively insensitive and nonspecific, however; in neonates, as many as 25 to 32 wbc/mm^3 and a protein content as high as 170 mg/dl in CSF can be within the normal range.[150,151] Furthermore, the significance of a reactive CSF-VDRL test in the absence of other diagnostic evidence of congenital syphilis is suspect, inasmuch as nontreponemal IgG antibodies can pass from the serum to the CSF.[152,153] More recently, investigators have analyzed neonatal CSFs utilizing immunoblotting for *T. pallidum*–specific IgM antibodies and rabbit infectivity testing (RIT)[154] to arrive at a more precise estimate of the frequency of asymptomatic CNS involvement. Both of these modalities indicated that the likelihood of CNS involvement correlates with the degree of clinical severity. Among infants with clinical and laboratory evidence of congenital syphilis, CNS involvement by IgM immunoblotting ranged from 44 percent (11 of 25) to 82 percent (14 of 17).[81,153,155,156] In contrast, only 10 to 20 percent of normal-appearing infants with congenital infection had detectable IgM antibodies in CSF.[155,156] By RIT, the prevalence of central nervous system invasion by *T. pallidum* was 86 percent (6 of 7) in infants with symptomatic congenital syphilis, but only 8 percent (1 of 12) among infants with normal physical examination and laboratory evaluation.[81]

The neurosyphilitic syndromes described in early congenital syphilis essentially represent diverse clinical expressions of a single pathogenic process—basilar meningitis and meningovascular syphilis. Acute syphilitic leptomeningitis, with meningismus, bulging fontanelles, and intractable vomiting, carries a grave prognosis.[109] Patients who survive this syndrome untreated or inadequately treated are usually left with obstructive hydrocephalus, seizure disorders, and impaired intellectual development. Cerebrovascular accidents occur in the neonatal period, probably as a combined consequence of cerebral arteritis and thrombocytopenia.[131] Untreated neurosyphilis can lead to a chronic meningovascular process that results in hydrocephalus, cranial nerve palsies, and cerebral infarction late in the first year. Hypopituitarism manifested by persistent neonatal hypoglycemia has been observed among some infants with congenital syphilis.[157] Autopsy specimens have demonstrated interstitial inflammation, fibrosis, and occasionally focal necrosis of the anterior lobe.[86,157] The neurohypophysis is usually normal. Magnetic resonance imaging (MRI) of the pituitary, combined with evaluation of pituitary function, has aided in its diagnosis.

Ocular involvement

Three ocular lesions are associated with early congenital syphilis: chorioretinitis, glaucoma, and uveitis. Syphilitic chorioretinitis typically produces a "salt and pepper" pattern of pigmentary patches at the periphery of a granular fundus.[158] Proptosis, blepharospasm, corneal clouding and edema, and excessive tearing should suggest the possibility of glaucoma. Uveitis usually occurs as an extension of choroiditis. Interstitial keratitis and optic neuritis have been described in infantile syphilis,[30] but they are generally regarded as lesions of late congenital syphilis.

Other manifestations

Syphilitic pneumonitis (pneumonia alba) is uncommon. Radiographically it produces bilateral, streaky infiltrates that can progress to widespread consolidation and may be confused with respiratory distress syndrome (Fig. 84-11).[30,159] Diarrhea in early congenital syphilis may be due to either pancreatitis with malabsorption or direct involvement of the intestinal mucosa. Approximately 10 percent of infants dying of syphilis have myocarditis.[160] The clinical importance of myocardial involvement in living infants is unknown; there is no convincing evidence of myocardial sequelae in surviving adolescents and adults with congenital syphilis.

LATE CONGENITAL SYPHILIS

The malformations or stigmata of late congenital syphilis represent the delayed consequences of the localized inflammatory processes established at sites of treponemal infection during the early stage of disease.[111,161,162] Thus, late congenital syphilis can be prevented simply by appropriate treatment of early infection. Late congenital syphilis in the child or adolescent corresponds to tertiary syphilis in the adult, and, as with tertiary syphilis, late con-

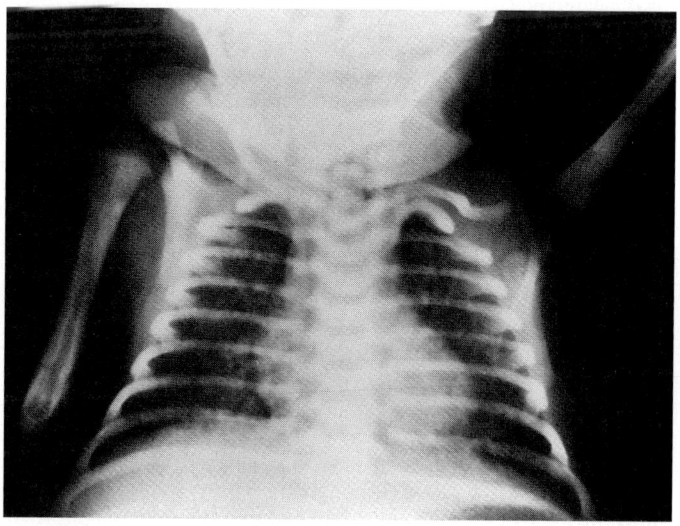

Fig. 84-11. Syphilitic pneumonitis ("pneumonia alba") consisting of patchy interstitial infiltrates. Long bone involvement in the same x-ray is highly suggestive of congenital syphilis.

genital syphilis is not infectious. Although the cardiovascular system is usually spared in the child, other target organs (e.g., bone and soft tissue, eyes, ears, and the central nervous system) are similar in late adult and congenital syphilis. Moreover, in both instances, gummatous (i.e., granulomatous) lesions tend to supplant the mononuclear and plasmacytic perivascular infiltrates of early syphilis.

Malformations (stigmata)

Chondritis and focal osteitis in infancy may lead to the craniofacial malformations that classic writers on congenital syphilis found so fascinating. The most common is frontal bossing, which occurs in some form in 30 to 87 percent of symptomatic cases.[107,121,162,163] Involvement of the parietal bone produces squaring of the cranium or occasionally a "hot cross bun" deformity. Other variations of this malformation include supraorbital thickening (Olympian or beetled brow), a high cranium or "tower skull," and, with parietal bossing alone, a sloping skull.[29] Robinson attributed the absence of bossing among his own cases to the disappearance of rickets.[164] By ascribing cranial bossing to associated, unrecognized rickets, he revived the nineteenth-century confusion between rickets and congenital syphilis. Since bossing was common in the only other modern series of cases,[162] the controversy may outlive the disease.

Deep necrotizing nasal chondritis in infancy produces a collapsed saddle-nose deformity in 10 to 30 percent of patients with late congenital syphilis.[121,126] Involvement of adjacent structures may also lead to a short maxilla and a high palatal arch. The resulting facies has a flat, "dished out" look, with a relatively prominent mandible. Circumoral radiating furrows (rhagades) complete the syphilitic facies in 5 to 10 percent. Laryngeal scarring may leave the child hoarse.[30]

Sequelae of periostitis of long bones affect primarily the tibia, clavicle, and scapula, in that order. Anterior bowing of the tibia (saber shin) occurred in 30 to 40 percent of older series but is now uncommon (Fig. 84-12).[162,164] Particularly in these children, recurrent acute periostitis of the tibia, ulna, fibula, or femur sometimes followed trauma or febrile illness, and it might be heralded by local tender nodules resembling erythema nodosum.[30] Thickening of the clavicle in its medial third is called Higoumenakis' sign and occurs preferentially on the side of the patient's handedness.[121] Robinson doubted its authenticity as a sign of syphilis.[164] Affected scapulae assume a scaphoid shape, concave medially.

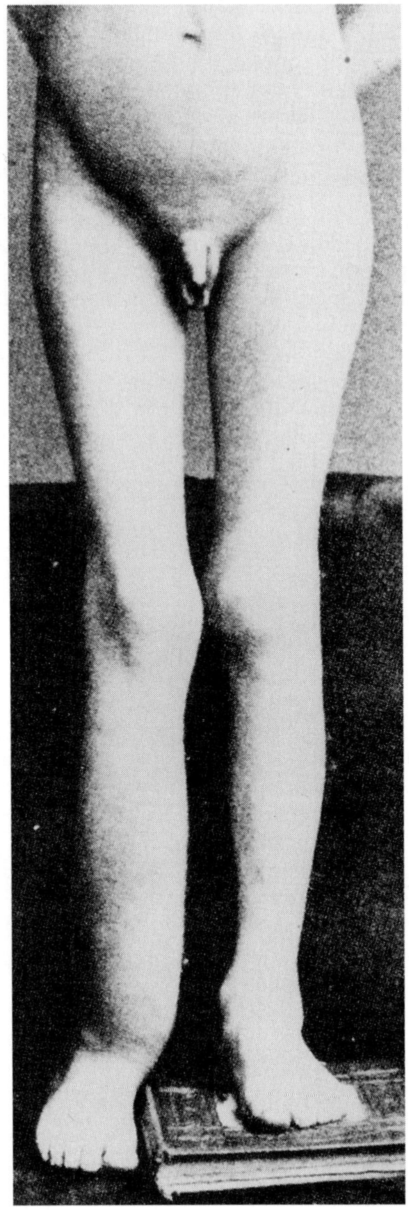

Fig. 84-12. Tibial thickening (saber shin) due to periostitis in late congenital syphilis; one of Hutchinson's cases. *(From J. Hutchinson.[14])*

Teeth. Syphilis affects morphodifferentiation and apposition, rather than the later stage of calcification as in rickets. There are no consistent abnormalities in deciduous teeth, but when affected they are misshapen and hypoplastic. The permanent teeth that develop later than the central incisors and first molars are much less commonly affected. If the mesenchymal progenitor cells have been destroyed in the newborn period, later developing permanent teeth may be missing. Hutchinson described small canines and incisors that were widely spaced and peg- or screwdriver-shaped.[13] They were tapered from the gingival bases toward a notched biting edge and were rough, dull, and dirty gray in color due to insufficient enamel (Fig. 84-13). These changes most often affect the upper central incisors but they may also affect the upper, lower, and lateral incisors. They are changes of the permanent, not the deciduous, teeth, although the latter are believed to be more prone to caries than normal in late congenital syphilis. In the first year of life, the diagnosis can be made by x-ray of the unerupted central incisors.[165] Variations of the classic Hutchinson tooth also occur. The lower incisors may have parallel sides and lack a notch but are otherwise small, round, and spaced, resembling little tombstones or top hats projecting from the gum.[30] The upper incisors are sometimes pointed (cannibal teeth) rather than notched.[3] Henry Moon described more completely the molars whose peculiar "tubercular projections" Hutchinson had mentioned; the characteristic 6-year (first lower) molars are dome-shaped with diminutive cusps arrayed in a tight circle at the top of the dome (Fig. 84-13).[165a] Moon's molars have been variously likened to a mulberry, a *bouton de fleur*, a cow's udder, or a string purse. Poorly enamelized, they are highly prone to decay and are rarely present beyond puberty; they are strongly indicative of congenital syphilis when found.

Inflammatory lesions

Inflammatory lesions produce a variety of clinical manifestations, as described below.

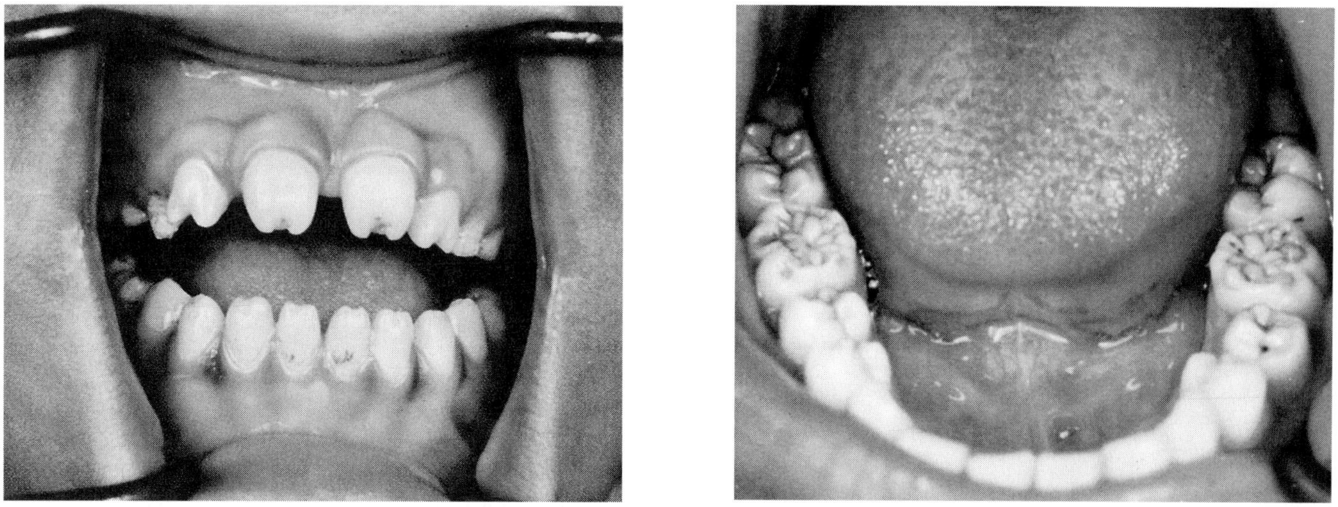

Fig. 84-13. (left) Hutchinson's teeth: the upper and lower incisors are conical, tapered toward the apex, and notched; the canine teeth are hypoplastic and poorly enamelized. (right) Mulberry molars: the 6-year molars are dome-shaped with a circle of small nob-shaped cusps at the apices. *(From HBG Robinson and AS Miller, Color Atlas of Oral Pathology, Philadelphia, Lippincott, 1990.)*

Interstitial Keratitis. Interstitial keratitis, when accompanied by neural deafness and typical dental abnormalities, forms Hutchinson's triad. Taken alone, keratitis is the most common late manifestation (20 to 50 percent).[121,164] The onset, between 5 and 16 years of age, is heralded by unilateral photophobia, pain, excess tearing, and blurred vision. Neovascularization may be so marked as to give the cornea a "salmon patch" appearance. The second eye is involved within two months in 80 to 90 percent of patients. Keratitis occurs more commonly in females than males and pursues a self-limited, sometimes relapsing, course that ends in corneal clouding (syphilitic nebulae) (Fig. 84-14) or secondary glaucoma. Chorioretinitis and iritis may be found, but less commonly than in congenital syphilis of infancy.

Deafness. Deafness is the least common of Hutchinson's triad. The primary lesion is osteochondritis affecting the otic capsule and leading to cochlear degeneration. The ossicles occasionally may be affected, so that an associated conduction defect does not exclude syphilis as a cause of sensorineural hearing loss. Karmody and Schuknecht distinguished between the abrupt onset of bilateral deafness without vertigo in childhood and a more gradual asymmetric pattern in adults associated with tinnitus and vertigo.[166] Congenital leutic involvement of the otic capsule leads to fibrous adhesion between the medial surface of the stapedial foot plate and the membranous labyrinth (vestibulofibrosis). The result is Hennebert's positive "fistula sign without a fistula"; this consists of nystagmus and vertigo, despite an intact tympanic membrane, when positive and negative pressure are alternately applied to the external canal. Once considered a classic sign of syphilis, Hennebert's sign also occurs in Ménière's disease and vestibular Schwannoma.[167] Hearing loss begins at high frequencies and often progresses to complete bilateral loss of cochlear and vestibular function.

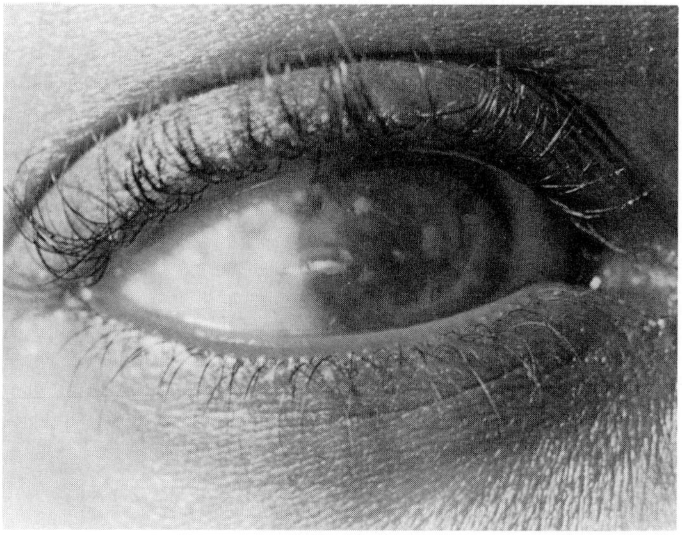

Fig. 84-14. Interstitial keratitis causing blindness. *(From Syphilis: a synopsis. Public Health Service publication No. 1660.)*

Clutton's Joints. Between the ages of 8 and 15, 1 to 3 percent of children with congenital syphilis develop symmetrical, painless swelling of the knees (occasionally elbows), with preservation of mobility, often following trauma.[168,169] Adjacent bone erosion (von Gie joint) is rarely seen. Synoviocentesis reveals 10,000 to 30,000 leukocytes, predominantly lymphocytes. This hydrarthrosis is believed to be due to perisynovitis and resolves spontaneously over several months.

Palatal Deformations. Gummata of the palate, throat, and nasal septum begin in late childhood or even adulthood as a gray, sharply defined "raucous patch." These lead painlessly to perforation of the septum and of the soft palate, usually in the midline. Deep ulcers of the throat and tongue occur in a similar fashion.

Neurosyphilis. As many as one-fourth to one-third of patients over the age of two years have asymptomatic neurosyphilis.[126] Symptomatic neurosyphilis, on the other hand, is quite rare, is usually delayed until adolescence, and fits the adult patterns of tabes dorsalis, syphilitic encephalitis (general paresis), and local gummata.[104] Juvenile paresis is the most common of these, occurring in 1 to 5 percent of congenital syphilitics, and is generally more severe than the acquired variety.[30,126,164] It typically begins around puberty with deteriorating school performance, bizarre behavior, emotional inappropriateness, and inattention. Over the ensuing 6 to 12 months, the child develops ataxis, tremor, and dysarthria; half of these patients have seizure disorder, and nearly all have pupillary findings.[170,171] Sequelae of untreated neurosyphilis in infancy, including hydrocephalus, convulsive disorders, and cranial neuropathies, were once common.

Paroxysmal Cold Hemoglobinuria. Late congenital and acquired syphilis were once the leading cause of paroxysmal cold hemoglobinuria.[172] Only half of these syphilitic patients had other manifestations of disease. About 8 hours following immersion of hands or feet into ice water (Rosenbach test) or other cold exposure, the patient experiences a myalgic, shaking chill and voids dark red or black urine. Many of the syphilitic cases have associated Raynaud's phenomenon.[30] The Coombs' test, Donath-Landsteiner (cold hemolysin) test, and VDRL are all positive. In the syphilitic cases, the attacks cease following penicillin therapy.

DIAGNOSIS

ANTEPARTUM DIAGNOSIS AND STILLBIRTHS

Ultrasonography can be used to diagnose fetal syphilis. The sonographic findings of nonimmune fetal hydrops due to syphilis include skin thickening, placental thickening, serous cavity effusions, hepatosplenomegaly, and hydramnios.[78,173–176] At Parkland Memorial Hospital, hepatomegaly has been a reliable sonographic sign of fetal infection and has correlated with detection of treponemes in amniotic fluid by RIT.[78] Hill and Maloney also reported noncontinuous gastrointestinal tract obstruction in association with hepatosplenomegaly and placentomegaly in a syphilitic fetus.[176]

As noted earlier, stillbirth is a common outcome of gestational syphilis. According to CDC criteria, a syphilitic stillbirth is defined as a death of a fetus weighing >500 g or having a gestational age >20 weeks in which the mother had untreated or inadequately treated syphilis (Table 84-1). Whenever possible, this diagnosis should be supported by long-bone radiography or xeroradiography or confirmed by detection of spirochetes in fetal tissues at autopsy.[23,177]

DIAGNOSIS IN THE LIVEBORN INFANT

As noted previously, in 1989 the CDC issued revised criteria for congenital syphilis surveillance (Table 84-1). Although intended primarily to help assess the public-health impact of congenital syphilis, these same guidelines also are used by practicing clinicians to determine which infants need further evaluation and treatment. The strength of these criteria lies in their recognition that the diagnosis of congenital syphilis is problematic for three reasons: (1) *T. pallidum* is noncultivatable and often difficult to demonstrate in clinical specimens, (2) serologic analysis of the infant is complicated by the presence of transplacentally acquired maternal antibodies (i.e., absence of a serologic "gold standard"), and (3) a majority of liveborn, infected infants have no evidence of infection.[23,178]

CONFIRMED CONGENITAL SYPHILIS

A confirmed diagnosis of congenital syphilis requires laboratory demonstration of *T. pallidum* (Table 84-1). In current practice, this involves detection of live treponemes in body fluids by dark-field microscopy or visualization in body fluids and tissue specimens by silver staining, immunofluorescence, or immunocytochemistry. Dark-field microscopy or immunofluorescence should be performed whenever nasal discharge, mucous patches, vesiculobullous lesions, or condylomata are present. Treponemes abound in such lesions, so definitive diagnosis can be achieved in most cases that exhibit these signs. Unfortunately, conventional methods for detection of *T. pallidum* in clinical specimens are insensitive and/or inapplicable because they require an invasive procedure. For this reason, a confirmed diagnosis is achieved only in the small proportion of infants with florid infection. This situation may change in the future with the application of gene amplification methodologies (e.g., [PCR]) for detection of *T. pallidum* DNA in clinical specimens.[179,180]

Histopathologic Examination of the Products of Conception. Since the earliest descriptions of syphilitic placentitis, pathologic examination of placentas and umbilical cords has been recognized as a readily available and yet underutilized tool for diagnosing congenital syphilis in at-risk infants.[181,182] Placentas from infants with clinical and/or laboratory evidence of congenital syphilis have very high incidence of histopathological abnormalities, including presence of spirochetes by silver staining.[113,114] Immunohistochemical methods can facilitate detection of *T. pallidum* in placental tissues.[183] Stoll and coworkers emphasized the importance of a multidisciplinary approach involving close cooperation among obstetricians, neonatololgists, and pathologists to assure that placentas are obtained for routine pathologic evaluation.[113]

Presumptive diagnosis

Congenital syphilis is diagnosed presumptively in the absence of direct demonstration of *T. pallidum* in clinical specimens. The descriptor "presumptive" encompasses a wide spectrum ranging from the floridly symptomatic infant, in whom the diagnosis is essentially certain, to normal-appearing infants without clinical or laboratory evidence of infection.

When a child is born to a woman with reactive syphilis serologies, physical examination should be performed and the infant's nontreponemal test tier should be compared to the mother's. (Treponemal tests generally are not performed on the neonate because they are not titered and infant reactivity merely reflects the transplacental passage of maternal anti-treponemal antibodies.) The CDC no longer recommends obtaining umbilical cord blood because of the potential for contamination with maternal blood. Moreover, there also has been concern that RPR testing of umbilical cord blood is prone to false-positives due to contamination with Wharton's jelly.[109] In our experience, however, both RPR and VDRL testing of umbilical cord blood are acceptable provided that the specimens are properly collected. Because titers measured by the RPR test are usually two- to fourfold higher than those obtained by VDRL testing,[184] it is important that maternal and infant sera be analyzed with the same nontreponemal test. A guide for the interpretation of maternal and infant syphilis serologies and an algorithm for the evaluation of infants born to mothers with reactive syphilis serologies are presented in Table 84-6 and Fig. 84-15, respectively.[47,185] A diagnosis of congenital syphilis can be made with confidence if the mother has reactive nontreponemal and treponemal serologies and the infant manifests classic signs of disease. Congenital syphilis also is highly likely when the infant's nontreponemal antibody titer is fourfold or greater than the mother's serum, even in the absence of physical findings. In both of the above instances, infants should undergo further evaluation consisting of lumbar puncture, and complete blood cell

Table 84-6. Guide for Interpretation of the Syphilis Serology of Mothers and their Infants

Nontreponemal test		Treponemal test		
Mother	Infant	Mother	Infant	Interpretation*
–	–	—		No syphilis or incubating syphilis in the mother and infant
+	+	—		No syphilis in mother (false-positive nontreponemal test with passive transfer to infant)
+	+ or –	+		+Maternal syphilis with possible infant infection; or mother treated for syphilis during pregnancy; or mother with latent syphilis and possible infection of infant†
+	+	+		+Recent or previous syphilis in the mother; possible infection in infant
–	–	+		+Mother successfully treated for syphilis before or early in pregnancy; or mother with Lyme disease, yaws, or pinta (i.e., false-positive serology)

* Presents a guide and not the definitive interpretation of serologic tests for syphilis in mothers and their newborn infants. Other factors that should be considered include the timing of maternal infection, the nature of timing of maternal treatment, quantitative maternal and infant titers, and serial determination of nontreponemal test titers in both mother and infant.

† Approximately 20 percent of mothers with latent syphilis have nonreactive nontreponemal tests.

SOURCE: Stoll[47]

count to determine the extent of disease and establish a baseline for follow-up. Other tests such as long bone radiographs, liver function tests, audiologic and ophthalmologic examination should be performed as clinically indicated. Most commonly, the maternal and infant serologic titers are similar or the infant's titer is lower than the mother's.[47,114] Further evaluation is dependent on the maternal stage of disease and treatment status and the infant's physical findings. The following are the most frequently encountered scenarios (Fig. 84-15):

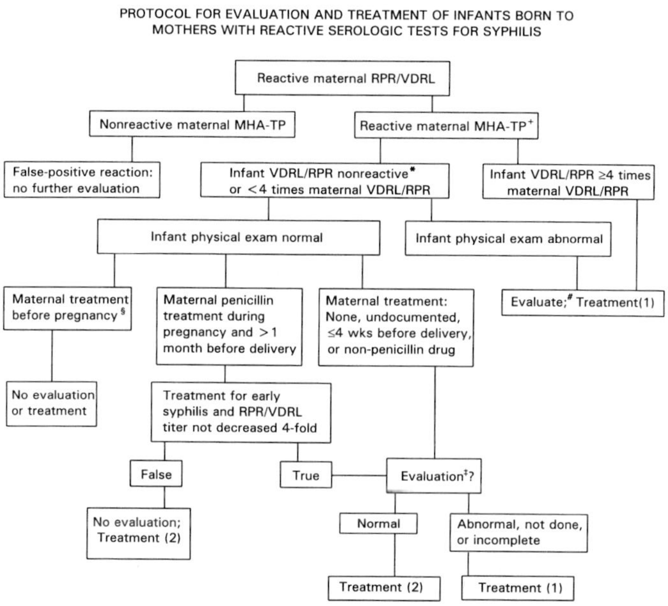

Fig. 84-15. Approach for evaluation of infants born to mothers with reactive serologic tests for syphilis. + Testing for HIV antibody. Infants of HIV-Ab ⊕ mothers do not require different evaluation or treatment. * Infant's VDRL may be nonreactive due to low maternal VDRL titer or recent maternal infection. If the mother has untreated or inadequately treated syphilis and infant's physical exam is normal, some experts would not perform diagnostic evaluation but would treat infant with a single IM injection of benzathine penicillin (50,000 U/kg). # Evaluation consists of CBC, platelet count; CSF examination for cell count, protein, and quantitative VDRL; Other tests as clinically indicated (eye exam, long-bone films; chest x-ray; liver function tests; cranial ultrasound; auditory brainstem response). § Women who maintain a VDRL titer ≤1:2 beyond 1 year following successful treatment a considered serfast. ‡ CBC, platelet count; CSF examination for cell count, protein, and quantitative VDRL; Long bone films. TREATMENT: (1) Aqueous penicillin G 50,000 U/kg IV q 12 hr (≤1 wk of age), q 8 hr (>1 wk), or procaine penicillin G 50,000 U/kg IM single daily dose × 10 days. (2) Benzathine penicillin G 50,000 U/kg IM × 1 dose.

1. The mother was treated *before* pregnancy and her nontreponemal test titer is decreasing appropriately or she is known to be serofast. No further evaluation is required if the infant is asymptomatic.
2. The mother was treated for early syphilis *during* pregnancy more than 30 days prior to delivery and her nontreponemal titer decreased fourfold or more prior to delivery. No further evaluation is necessary if the infant is asymptomatic, particularly if follow-up can be assured.
3. The mother was treated appropriately for early syphilis *during* pregnancy more than 30 days prior to delivery but her titer did not decrease at least fourfold. Full diagnostic evaluation of the infant (lumbar puncture, complete blood count, long bone radiographs) should be performed to determine appropriate therapy.
4. The mother was untreated, treated during pregnancy with an antimicrobial other than penicillin, or treated appropriately less than 30 days prior to delivery. These all constitute inadequate therapy for the fetus, and the infant should be fully evaluated as in 3 above.
5. The mother was treated *during* pregnancy for late latent syphilis and maintained a low, stable titer through delivery. The infant does not require further evaluation if asymptomatic.

Evaluation for *T. pallidum*–Specific IgM Antibodies. Serodiagnosis of congenital syphilis poses a difficult problem because of the presence of transplacentally acquired maternal IgG in newborn sera. IgM, on the other hand, does not cross the placenta and is actively synthesized by the third-trimester fetus in response to infection. An early approach to the diagnosis of congenital syphilis was the measurement of serum IgM levels at or shortly after birth. In addition to lacking sensitivity,[186] however, elevated total IgM levels are nonspecific and may result from intrauterine infection with other common pathogens including cytomegalovirus, *Toxoplasma gondii*, and rubella.[23] A diagnosis of presumptive congenital syphilis can be made in an infant with normal physical examination and laboratory/radiologic studies if *T. pallidum*–specific IgM antibodies are detected in the infant's serum. In 1968, Scotti and Logan described an indirect immunofluorescence test for the detection of IgM antibody against *T. pallidum* (fluorescent treponemal antibody–absorption [FTA-ABS] IgM test) as a means of distinguishing infant from maternal antibody.[187] Unfortunately, despite some early successes,[119,188] the FTA-ABS IgM test has been shown to lack both sensitivity and specificity and has fallen into disuse.[189] Chromatographic separation of IgM in neonatal sera to remove maternal blocking antibodies and rheumatoid factor has been used to improve the performance of the FTA-ABS test; this improved version of the FTA-ABS IgM test has been designated the FTA-ABS-19S-IgM test.[190] Though more sensitive than the original FTA-ABS IgM test[113], the FTA-ABS-19S-IgM test is technically demanding and available at only a handful of centers and, therefore, is no longer recommended. Stoll et al.[113] evaluated a commercial IgM capture enzyme-linked immunosorbent assay (ELISA) for *T. pallidum*–specific antibodies but found a sensitivity of only 88 percent among infants with clinical and laboratory findings consistent with congenital syphilis. Both the FTA-ABS-19S-IgM test and the IgM capture ELISA appear to have poor sensitivity for detecting infection in at-risk infants with normal clinical and laboratory findings.[113]

Novel molecularly based diagnostic tests for asymptomatic neonates

The major dilemma in the diagnosis of early congenital syphilis is to differentiate normal-appearing, infected infants from uninfected at-risk infants with reactive serologies due to transplacentally acquired maternal antibodies. Unfortunately, none of the currently available serologic tests can do this with high degrees of sensitivity and specificity in asymptomatic neonates. To address this critical issue, several investigators have utilized immunoblotting techniques to detect and characterize the neonatal IgM response to *T. pallidum*.[81,155,191–195] IgM antibodies directed against *T. pallidum* antigens with apparent molecular masses ranging from 93- to 15-kDa have been detected in sera from infants with clinical and laboratory evidence of congenital syphilis. IgM immunoblot analysis of asymptomatic infants born to mothers with untreated syphilis has documented that as many as 20 to 42 percent of at-risk infants possess IgM anti-treponemal antibodies and can be considered actively infected. Fractionation of neonatal sera into IgM and IgG components by high-performance liquid chromatography has confirmed that IgM reactivities obtained with whole sera are not due to rheumatoid factor and are not diminished by maternal IgG antibodies.[191] Dobson and colleagues showed that the serum IgM reactivity disappears one to three months after appropriate penicillin treatment of neonates, further supporting the validity of IgM antibody detection as a marker for active infection.[192] Recently, Sánchez and co-workers showed that immunoblot analysis with recombinant forms of two highly immunogenic *T. pallidum* lipoproteins (47-kDa and 17-kDa lipoproteins) appeared to be even more sensitive than immunoblotting with native *T. pallidum* antigens.[196]

Detection of *T. pallidum* is the most definitive means of proving that an asymptomatic child has active infection. Given the cost and difficulties inherent in RIT, PCR has emerged as a highly attractive alternative. Grimprel et al.[180] and Sánchez et al.[81,156] have shown that PCR results for neonatal sera and CSF correlate quite closely with those obtained by RIT. In our experience, virtually all symptomatic at-risk infants have positive PCR and IgM serum studies.[81] In contrast, only 2 of 12 asymptomatic at-risk infants had positive PCR results on serum, while 5 of 12 had *T. pallidum*–specific IgM serum antibodies detectable by immunoblotting.[81] The PCR results presumably reflect low spirochetal burdens and spirochetemia rates in asymptomatic infected infants. Interestingly, one asymptomatic at-risk infant with a negative immunoblot had a positive serum PCR. These data suggest that a comprehensive strategy involving both IgM immunoblotting and PCR of serum will be needed for maximal sensitivity to distinguish infected from uninfected asymptomatic neonates.

DIAGNOSIS OF LATE CONGENITAL SYPHILIS

Diagnosis of late congenital syphilis is almost always presumptive and based on the typical clinical findings in association with reactive serologic tests. In the absence of a maternal history of syphilis, serologic testing of the mother can be helpful for distinguishing between acquired and congenital infection.

TREATMENT

Penicillin remains the drug of choice for the treatment of both acquired and congenital syphilis.[116,197,198] A serum concentration of 0.018 mcg/mL is required to ensure adequate killing of the organism and must be maintained for 7 days in early cases and up to 3 weeks in late disease.[199] In contrast to erythromycin,[200] penicillin resistance has not been confirmed among any isolates.

TREATMENT DURING PREGNANCY

Pregnant women with reactive serologic tests for syphilis should be counseled concerning the risks of HIV infection, tested for HIV antibody, and treated with the penicillin regimen appropriate for the stage of syphilis (Table 84-7).[197,198] Tetracycline and doxycycline are contraindicated in pregnancy because both can result in staining of decidual teeth and impairment of long-bone growth. Moreover, tetracycline use during pregnancy has been associated with hepatic toxicity when there is concomitant renal dysfunction. Erythromycin also should not be used because of reports of infants born with clinical findings of congenital syphilis after their mothers received erythromycin treatment during pregnancy.[201–203] Patient noncompliance with erythromycin therapy due to gastrointestinal side-effects also is a major problem. Moreover, there remains concern over unpredictable maternal serum levels and erratic transplacental transfer of the drug.[204] Insufficient data exist on ceftriaxone to recommend its use in the treatment of syphilis during pregnancy.[198]

Table 84-7. Treatment Guidelines for Acquired Syphilis During Pregnancy

Stage of infection	Regimen
Primary	Benzathine penicillin G, 2.4 mU IM × 1
Secondary	
Early latent (≤1 yr)	
Late latent (>1 yr)	Benzathine penicillin G, 2.4 mU IM q week × 3
Unknown duration	
Neurosyphilis	Aqueous penicillin G 2-4 mU IV q 4 hr × 10–14 d* or Procaine penicillin G 2.4 mU IM and Probenicid 500 mg PO qid × 10–14 d*

* Some authorities recommend following this regimen with benzathine penicillin 2.4 mU IM q wk × 3.
SOURCE: Centers for Disease Control[198]

Table 84-8. Oral Desensitization Protocol for Patients with a Positive Skin Test

Penicillin V suspension dose*	Amount† (units/mL)	mL	Units	Cumulative dose (units)
1	1,000	0.1	100	100
2	1,000	0.2	200	300
3	1,000	0.4	400	700
4	1,000	0.8	800	1,500
5	1,000	1.6	1,600	3,100
6	1,000	3.2	3,200	6,300
7	1,000	6.4	6,400	12,700
8	10,000	1.2	12,000	24,700
9	10,000	2.4	24,000	48,700
10	10,000	4.8	48,000	96,700
11	80,000	1.0	80,000	176,700
12	80,000	2.0	160,000	336,700
13	80,000	4.0	320,000	656,700
14	80,000	8.0	640,000	1,296,700

Observation period: 30 minutes before parenteral administration of penicillin.

* Interval between doses, 15 minutes; elapsed time, 3 hours and 45 minutes; cumulative dose, 1.3 million units.

† The specific amount of drug was diluted in approximately 30 mL of water and then administered orally.

SOURCE: Wendel et al.[205]

Approximately 5 to 10 percent of pregnant women with syphilis report a history of penicillin allergy. Wendel and colleagues have shown that those individuals who are at risk for acute allergic reactions to penicillin can be identified by skin testing; if the skin test is positive, they can undergo oral penicillin desensitization, which makes them temporarily tolerant to a course of parenteral penicillin.[205] No serious adverse reactions were observed, and this regimen is currently recommended so that all pregnant women with syphilis can receive penicillin therapy (Table 84-8).

The Jarisch-Herxheimer reaction commonly occurs after treatment of acquired early syphilis in adults.[116] It consists of fever, chills, myalgias, headache, hypotension, tachycardia, and transient accentuation of the cutaneous lesions; it typically begins within several hours of treatment and resolves within 24 to 36 hours. The etiology is not fully known; however, since *T. pallidum* lacks lipopolysaccharide,[206,207] the release of treponemal lipoproteins that possess proinflammatory activities from dead or dying organisms recently has been implicated as the likely inducer of this clinical phenomenon.[208,209] Klein and coworkers have shown that another manifestation of the Jarisch-Herxheimer reaction in pregnant women is uterine contractions, possibly mediated secondarily by prostaglandins.[210] By fetal monitoring during the episode, they demonstrated evidence of fetal stress with tachycardia and decelerations, along with a marked decrease in fetal activity (Fig. 84-16). For this reason, we sonographically evaluate the fetuses of all third-trimester early syphilis patients prior to initiating therapy. If hepatomegaly or other signs of hydrops are detected, the patient is hospitalized for fetal monitoring during the first 24 hours following the administration of penicillin therapy. If there is evidence of fetal compromise prior to the initiation of therapy, the infant is first delivered by cesarian section and then mother and infant are treated.[211]

Concern also exists that presumably adequate maternal treatment for syphilis in the final four weeks of pregnancy may be inadequate fetal therapy.[212] A possible explanation is that altered penicillin pharmacokinetics leading to lower serum and CSF levels of penicillin in both the mother and fetus may occur due to increases in renal clearance and plasma volume that are normal adaptations as pregnancy progresses.[213] Moreover, maternal treatment in the final weeks of pregnancy may not allow sufficient time for the fetus to be adequately treated, thus necessitating penicillin therapy for the newborn infant.[214] Because currently available methodologies for diagnosis of congenital syphilis do not accurately identify infants with active infection, the majority of these so-called "treatment failures" probably reflect resolving abnormalities from treated fetal infection. It is well known that the clinical and laboratory abnormalities seen in infants infected with *T. pallidum* may require months for complete resolution, even after prolonged intravenous penicillin therapy. Nonetheless, some treatment failures do occur, as evidenced by autopsy findings of stillborn infants.

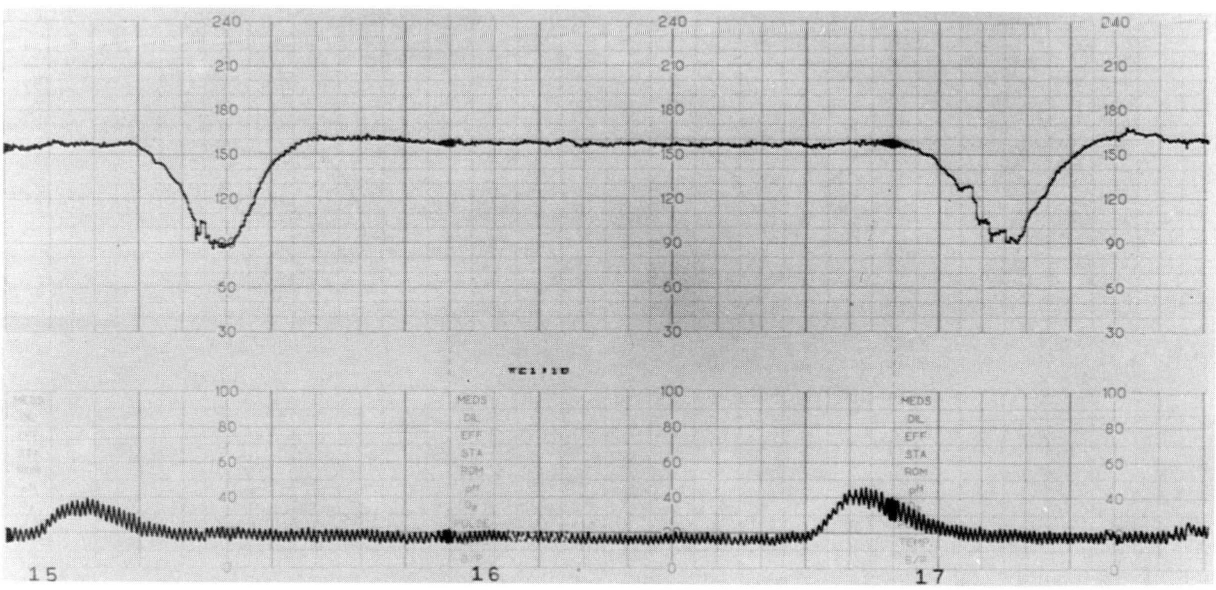

Fig. 84-16. Fetal heart rate pattern, uterine contractions, and late decelerations occurring during a maternal Jarisch-Herxheimer reaction. Maternal blood pressure was 110/72 mm Hg, temperature 37.2°C, and pulse 84 beats per minute. *(From Klein et al.[210])*

TREATMENT OF THE INFANT

Given the current absence of a diagnostic "gold standard" and the fact that untreated congenital syphilis is potentially devastating, CDC guidelines recommend treatment of all infants who fit the surveillance-case definition to avoid undertaking the difficult task of determining which at-risk asymptomatic infants are truly infected.[198] Treatment, therefore, is required for infants (1) with clinical, laboratory, and/or radiographic findings consistent with congenital syphilis; (2) with nontreponemal test titers fourfold or greater than their mothers'; (3) born to mothers whose treatment before delivery cannot be documented, is unknown, was inadequate, or occurred 30 days or less prior to delivery; (4) born to seronegative mothers with suspected incubating syphilis; (5) whose nontreponemal test titers increase fourfold or more during follow-up, (6) whose treponemal test remains reactive beyond 15 months of age, or (7) who have specific anti-treponemal IgM antibodies detected by an approved method. Furthermore, treatment should be considered for infants born to mothers treated for syphilis during pregnancy, particularly if follow-up cannot be ensured. Additionally, low-risk infants should be treated if adequate follow-up is uncertain. Treatment should not be delayed until a definitive clinical or serologic diagnosis is made.

Infants 4 weeks of age or less who have confirmed or presumptive disease should be treated for 10 to 14 days with either: (1) aqueous crystalline penicillin G, 50,000 U/kg administered intravenously every 12 hours for the first 7 days of life and every 8 hours beyond 1 week of age; or (2) aqueous procaine penicillin G, 50,000 U/kg administered intramuscularly once daily (Table 84-9).[198] In our experience, 10 days of either form of penicillin is sufficient. All patients who received aqueous crystalline penicillin G, but only 82 percent of those who received procaine, had treponemicidal levels in the CSF at the time of testing.[215] Although the significance of this finding is uncertain given that both regimens are curative,[81] some authorities believe that the aqueous crystalline penicillin G regimen is the preferred therapy, particularly in extremely ill infants or infants with neurosyphilis.[47]

An infant with normal physical examination, CSF, radiographic, and laboratory studies and whose nontreponemal test titer is the same or less than the maternal titer can be treated with a single intramuscular injection of benzathine penicillin G (50,000 U/kg) under the following circumstances (Table 84-9):[198,216] (1) the mother received erythromycin during pregnancy; (2) the mother was treated with the appropriate regimen 30 days or less prior to delivery; (3) the mother received the recommended penicillin therapy for the stage of infection during the pregnancy, but the nontreponemal titer has not yet decreased fourfold; (4) the mother has untreated syphilis or her treatment status is undocumented.

After the newborn period, children diagnosed with syphilis should have a CSF examination to exclude neurosyphilis and records should be reviewed to assess whether the child has congenital or acquired syphilis. Any child thought to have congenital syphilis (or having neurologic involvement) should receive aqueous crystalline penicillin G administered as 50,000 U/kg IV or IM every 4 to 6 hours for 10 to 14 days.[198] Procaine penicillin for this age group has not been fully evaluated and, therefore, is not recommended. Children with acquired syphilis who have a normal CSF examination can receive IM benzathine penicillin G, 50,000 U/kg per dose as dictated by the stage of infection; the amount of penicillin should not exceed that recommended for adults.[198]

Infants born to women coinfected with syphilis and HIV may be at higher risk of acquiring infection with both syphilis and HIV.[217,218] It is not known whether infants coinfected with syphilis and HIV respond to treatment for congenital syphilis differently from other infants not infected with HIV. Nonetheless, there are no data to support more aggressive or prolonged penicillin ther-

Table 84-9. Treatment Guidelines for Congenital Syphilis Surveillance

Physical examination and/or evaluation*	Maternal stage/treatment	Regimen
Abnormal	Any or none	Aqueous penicillin G, 50,000 U/kg IV q 12 hr (≤1 wk), q 8 hr (>1 wk, ≤4 wk), q 6 hr (>4 wk) × 10–14 d or Procaine penicillin G, 50,000 U/kg IM × 10–14 d (≤4 wk)
Normal	Early syphilis and/or no or undocumented treatment	Aqueous penicillin G, 50,000 U/kg IV q 12 hr (<1 wk), q 8 hr (>1 wk, ≤4 wk), q 6 hr (>4 wk) × 10–14 d or Procaine penicillin G, 50,000 U/kg IM × 10–14 d (≤4 wk) or Benzathine penicillin G,† 50,000 U/kg IM × 1
	Late latent syphilis Erythromycin or non-penicillin treatment Adequate therapy ≤4 wks before delivery Adequate therapy >1 month before delivery but maternal nontreponemal titers have not decreased fourfold	Benzathine penicillin G, 50,000 U/kg IM × 1
	Adequate therapy >1 month before delivery and maternal nontreponemal titers have decreased fourfold	Clinical and serologic follow-up only or Benzathine penicillin G, 50,000 U/kg IM × 1 if follow-up uncertain
	Adequate therapy before pregnancy and stable titers (VDRL ≤1:2) throughout pregnancy	Clinical and serologic follow-up only

* CSF examination, bone radiographs, CBC, platelets, cord/serum VDRL/RPR
† If follow-up ensured
SOURCE: Centers for Disease Control[198]

apy beyond the regimens recommended for infants not exposed to maternal HIV infection. The necessity of serologic follow-up of these high-risk infants cannot be over emphasized.[198]

Less than 1 percent of infants who are treated for presumed congenital syphilis develop, within several hours of initiation of penicillin therapy, a Jarisch-Herxheimer reaction, consisting of fever, tachypnea, tachycardia, hypotension, accentuation of the cutaneous lesions, and/or death due to cardiovascular collapse.[109] Other than supportive care, there is not specific treatment or prophylaxis.

FOLLOW-UP MANAGEMENT

Infants who have reactive serologic tests for syphilis should have serial quantitative nontreponemal tests performed until nonreactivity is documented.[109,214] Follow-up for these infants can be incorporated into routine pediatric care at 2, 4, 6, 12, and 15 months.[185] Among infants with congenital syphilis, nontreponemal serologic tests become nonreactive within 12 months after appropriate treatment.[216] Uninfected infants usually become seronegative by six months of age. A reactive treponemal test beyond 15 months of age, when the infants has lost all maternal antibody, confirms the diagnosis of congenital syphilis.[216] Infants with abnormal CSF findings should have a repeat lumbar puncture performed six months after therapy.[185,198] A reactive CSF VDRL test, unexplained persistent pleocytosis, or abnormal protein at that time is an indication for retreatment.[198] Infants who maintain persistently low, stable titers of nontreponemal tests also require retreatment.

PREVENTION AND CONTROL

DETECTION OF SYPHILIS DURING PREGNANCY

The mainstay of prevention of congenital syphilis involves identifying and treating infected pregnant women; penicillin therapy during pregnancy is 98-percent effective in preventing congenital infection.[102,219] Maternal treatment regimens and follow-up are discussed in detail in the 1998 Guideline for Treatment of Sexually Transmitted Diseases published by CDC,[198] and in Chap. 80. The obstetrician must be alert to the signs and symptoms of syphilis in the pregnant woman. In addition to looking for evidence of active syphilis during prenatal visits, syphilis serologic testing should be performed at the mother's first prenatal visit and, in high-risk populations, at 28 weeks and at delivery.[51,220] Repeat-testing of high-risk populations is essential to identify women with incubating syphilis as well as women infected later in pregnancy. False-negative nontreponemal tests also may result from the prozone phenomenon that occurs when an excess of nontreponemal antibodies prevents the flocculation reaction required for a reactive test. Experienced laboratories routinely dilute serum specimens to identify prozones. Screening tests at delivery should be performed on maternal blood specimens rather than on umbilical cord blood; nontreponemal test titers in umbilical cord blood are usually lower than the mother's and may even be nonreactive in the face of a low maternal titer.[114]

Pregnancy occasionally produces a false-positive nontreponemal test (i.e., a reactive nontreponemal test with a nonreactive treponemal test).[221] A cautionary note must be sounded here, however, because an isolated low nontreponemal test titer may be seen with very early syphilitic infection and have disastrous consequences for the fetus if untreated.[114] A detailed sexual history, careful physical examination (looking for evidence of primary syphilis), and serologic follow-up of the mother are required to distinguish false-positive reactivity from early infection. Treatment is warranted if follow-up serologic testing cannot be assured. Women who have previously received standard therapy for syphilis may remain seropositive with a low nontreponemal test titer; these women are designated "serofast." Because it can be difficult to distinguish the serofast state from reinfection, our practice is to re-treat asymptomatic women whose nontreponemal test titers are greater than 1:2 at the first screening. Women considered to be serofast are followed with serial serologic testing and re-treated if the titer increases fourfold or more.

PUBLIC-HEALTH STRATEGIES FOR PREVENTION

While the cause of congenital syphilis, strictly speaking, is *Treponema pallidum*, the network of social and economic factors that fosters the transmission of syphilis during pregnancy and then allows it to go untreated also must be considered as part of its etiology. From a public-health standpoint, congenital syphilis can be regarded as a "sentinel health event" whose occurrence reflects a failure of delivery systems for prenatal care as well as syphilis control programs.[47] The tragedy of congenital syphilis is that it is a completely preventable disease.

The lines of public-health defense against congenital syphilis can be seen as a series of demographic circles around the fetal population at risk (Fig. 84-17). The first line of defense is the treatment of cases of primary and secondary syphilis and case detection through contact investigations. As noted earlier, this activity is now being supplemented, in many instances, by location-based epidemiologic case finding and treatment. The fewer the total number of cases of primary and secondary syphilis, the fewer the number of cases that joins the pool of early and late latent syphilis, and therefore the fewer the number of latent syphilitics among women in the childbearing age group. The second line of defense is follow-up of positive serologic tests reported to the health department by clinical laboratories, supplemented by routine screening of high-risk populations. By assuring adequate therapy of cases so detected, this strategy is designed to reduce the pool of women who begin gestation with untreated syphilis. Routine prenatal screening is the last major line of defense against congenital syphilis.

Syphilis screening optimally should be performed at the ante-

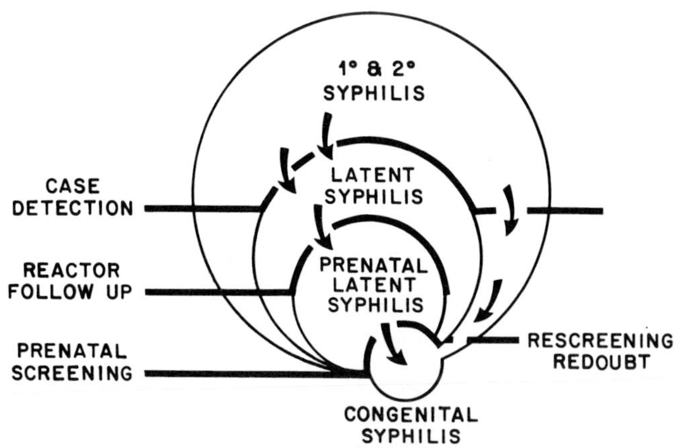

Fig. 84-17 Sequential lines of defense against congenital syphilis consist of (i) case detection to decrease the population of transmitters of early syphilis, (ii) reactor follow-up to decrease the residual pool of latent syphilis, and (iii) the last line of defense, prenatal screening. In addition, a redoubt is needed to protect the flank (i.e., rescreening to detect acquisition of syphilis during pregnancy).

natal care site, and women found to be seroreactive should be treated on the same visit.[51] This on-site testing approach recommended by the World Health Organization (WHO) could avoid the major difficulties that materialize with laboratory-based testing. On-site testing appears feasible in many situations, particularly since a recent study showed that electricity is not needed to implement the procedure.[222] The investigators found that hand rotation for the rapid plasma reagin (RPR) test for syphilis serology yielded the same result as mechanical rotation in 98.8 percent of the cases in a sample of 327 sera.[222] Moreover, they found that RPR antigen stored at room temperature yielded the same results as the antigen stored in a refrigerator.[222] These results confirm the applicability and feasibility of on-site testing in virtually any setting in the world. A syphilis-intervention study in Zambia used this on-site testing and treatment approach in three intervention centers and compared the outcomes to those in three control centers in which the approach was not used.[223] The investigators found that the adverse outcomes attributable to syphilis were reduced to 28.3 percent, which was almost a two-thirds reduction when compared with the 72.4 percent adverse outcome rate at the control centers ($p > .001$).[223] This substantial effect was achieved despite suboptimal implementation of screening and treatment.

Prevention of congenital syphilis appears to be cost-effective as well as feasible. The WHO group found that at seroprevalences of 15, 10, and 1 percent, respective expenditures of only $9.30, $12, and $70 would avert one adverse outcome.[51] With an appropriate commitment of resources, control of the adverse effects of syphilis during pregnancy would be within the grasp of the international health community.

References

1 Mettler CC: *History of Medicine*. Philadelphia, Blakiston, 1947.

2 Goodman H: *Notable Contributions to the Knowledge of Syphilis*. New York, Froben Press, 1943.

3 Dennie CC: *A History of Syphilis*. Springfield, IL, Charles C. Thomas, 1962.

4 Paré A: *The Works*. London, J. Hindemarsh, 1691.

5 Oriel JD: *The Scars of Venus*. London, Springer-Verlag, 1994.

6 de Vallembert S: *Cinq Livres, de la Manière de Nourrir et Gouverner les Enfants dès leur Naissance*. Poitiers, Marnefs, and Bouchetz, 1565.

7 Defoe D: *Moll Flanders*. New York, Modern Library, 1950.

8 Colles A: *Practical Observations on the Venereal Disease and on the Use of Mercury*. London, Sherwood, Gilbert, and Piper, 1837.

9 Diday PE: *A Treatise on Syphilis in Newborn Children and Infants at the Breast*. New York, Wm Wood and Co., 1883.

10 Hutchinson J: *A Clinical Memoir on Certain Diseases of the Eye and Ear Consequent on Inherited Syphilis*. London, 1863.

11 Wasserman A, et al: Eine serodiagnostische reaktion bei syphilis. *Dtsch Med Wochenschr*, 32:745, 1906.

12 Bertin M: *Traité de la Maladie Vénérienne chez les Enfants Nouveau—nés, les Femmes Enceintes et les Nourrices, etc.* Paris, Gabon, 1810.

13 Hutchinson J: Clinical lecture on heredito-syphilitic struma: And on the teeth as a means of diagnosis. *Br Med J* 1:515, 1861.

14 Hutchinson J: *Syphilis*, London, Cassell, 1909.

15 Parrot J: *La Syphilis Herreditaire et la Rachitis*. Paris, Masson, 1886.

16 Wegner FRG: Ueber hereditare Knochensyphilis bei jungen Kindern. *Virchows Arch*, 50:305, 1870.

17 Taylor RW: *Syphilitic Lesions of the Osseous System in Infants and Young Children*. New York, Wm Wood and Co., 1875.

18 Danholt N, et al: The Oslo study of untreated syphilis: A restudy of the Boeck-Brunsgaard material concerning the fate of syphilitics who receive no specific treatment. *Acta Dermatologica Venereologica* 34: 34, 1954.

19 Fournier A: *Lectures Delivered at the St. Louis Hospital, Paris*. New York, Appleton and Co., 1881.

20 Dunn RA, Rolfs RT: The resurgence of syphilis in the United States. *Curr Opin Infect Dis* 4:3, 1991.

21 Centers for Disease Control: Congenital syphilis—New York City, 1986–1988. *MMWR*, 38:825, 1989.

22 Thompson BL, et al: Congenital syphilis in Maryland, 1989–1991: The effect of changing the case definition and opportunities for prevention. *Sex Transm Dis* 22:364, 1996.

23 Zenker PN, Berman SM: Congenital syphilis: Trends and recommendations for evaluation and management. *Pediatr Infect Dis J*, 10:516, 1991.

24 Nakashima AK, et al: Epidemiology of syphilis in the United States, 1941–1993. *Sex Transm Dis*, 23:16, 1996.

25 Hook EW III: Biomedical issues in syphilis control. *Sex Transm Dis*, 23:5, 1996.

26 Osler W: The anti-venereal campaign. *Trans Med Soc Lond*, 40:290, 1917.

27 Browne FJ: Neonatal death. *Br Med J*, 2:590, 1922.

28 Cruickshank JT: Maternal syphilis as a cause of death of the foetus and of the newborn child. *Medical Research Council Special Report Series* no 82, 1924.

29 Dennie CC, Pakula SF: *Congenital Syphilis*. Philadelphia, Lea & Febiger, 1940.

30 Nabarro D: *Congenital Syphilis*. London, E. Arnold, 1954.

31 Laird SM: Elimination of congenital syphilis. *Br J Vener Dis*, 35:15, 1959.

32 Cohen DA, et al: The effects of case definition in maternal screening and reporting criteria on rates of congenital syphilis. *Am J Public Health*, 80:316, 1990.

33 Sánchez PJ, et al: Congenital syphilis: The Dallas experience. *Pediatr Res* 29:286A, 1991.

34 Centers for Disease Control: Syphilis and congenital syphilis—United States, 1985–1988. *MMWR*, 37:486, 1988.

35 Centers for Disease Control: Continuing increase in infectious syphilis—United States. *MMWR*, 37:35, 1988.

36 Rawstron SA, et al: Maternal and congenital syphilis in Brooklyn, NY. Epidemiology, transmission, and diagnosis. *Am J Dis Child*, 147: 727, 1993.

37 Marx R, et al: Crack, sex, and STD. *Sex Transm Dis*, 18:92, 1991.

38 Rolfs RT, et al: Risk factors for syphilis: Cocaine use and prostitution. *Am J Public Health*, 80:853, 1990.

39 Greenberg MS, et al: The association between congenital syphilis and cocaine/crack use in New York City: A case-control study. *Am J Public Health*, 81:1316, 1991.

40 Petzoldt D: Effect of spectinomycin on *T. pallidum* in incubating syphilis. *Br J Vener Dis*, 51:305, 1975.

41 Schroeter AL, et al: Therapy for incubating syphilis. Effectiveness of gonorrhea treatment. *JAMA*, 218:711, 1971.

42 Evans HE, Frenkel LD: Congenital syphilis. *Clin Perinatol*, 21:149, 1994.

43 Centers for Disease Control: Alternative case-finding methods in a crack-related syphilis epidemic—Philadelphia. *MMWR*, 40:77, 1991.

44 Centers for Disease Control: Selective screening to augment syphilis case-findings—Dallas, 1991. *MMWR*, 42:424, 1993.

45 National Center for Health Statistics, U.S. Department of Health and Human Services: *Vital Statistics of the US, 1997*. Vol. 2, *Natality*. Washington, D.C., U.S. Government Printing Office, 1981.

46 Webber MP, et al: Maternal risk factors for congenital syphilis: A case-control study. *Am J Epidemiol*, 137:415, 1993.

47 Stoll BJ: Congenital syphilis: Evaluation and management of neonates born to mothers with reactive serologic tests for syphilis. *Pediatr Infect Dis J*, 13:845, 1994.

48 Fiumara N, et al: The incidence of prenatal syphilis at the Boston City Hospital. *N Engl J Med*, 247:48, 1952.

49 Kaufman RE, et al: Questionnaire survey of reported early congenital syphilis: Problems in diagnosis, prevention, and treatment. *Sex Transm Dis*, 4:135, 1977.

50 Taffel S: *Prenatal Care in the US, 1969–75*. Ser 21, no 33. Data from the National Vital Statistics System. Washington, D.C., US Department of Health, Education and Welfare, Publication no PHS 78-1911, 1978.

51 World Health Organization: *Maternal and perinatal infections: Report of a WHO consultation*. Geneva, World Health Organization, WHO/MCH/91.10, 1991.

52 Stanecki KA, et al: *Sexually transmitted diseases in sub-Saharan Africa and associated interactions with HIV*. Washington, D.C., U.S. Bureau of the Census, IPC Staff Paper No. 75, 1995.

53 Meheus A, Antal GM: The endemic treponematoses: Not yet eradicated. *World Health Stat Q*, 45:228, 1992.

54 Ratnam AV, et al: Syphilis in pregnant women in Zambia. *Br J Vener Dis*, 58:355, 1982.

55 Manning B, et al: Syphilis in pregnant black women. *S Afr Med J*, 67:966, 1985.

56 Bishaw T, et al: Prevention of Congenital Syphilis, in *Proceedings of the Third African Regional Conference on Sexually Transmitted Diseases*, H Nsanze, et al (eds). Basle, Switzerland, Ciba Geigy, 1983, p. 148.

57 Larsson Y, Larsson U: Congenital syphilis in Addis Ababa. *Ethiop Med J*, 8:163, 1970.

58 Schulz KF, et al: Pregnancy loss, infant death, and suffering: legacy of syphilis and gonorrhoea in Africa. *Genitourin Med*, 63:320, 1987.

59 Watts TE, et al: A case-control study of stillbirths at a teaching hospital in Zambia, 1979–80: Serological investigations for selected infectious agents. *Bull World Health Organ*, 62:803, 1984.

60 Hira SK: *Epidemiology of Maternal and Congenital Syphilis in Lusaka and Copperbelt Provinces of Zambia*. Republic of Zambia, Lusaka, Zambia, 1984, p 1.

61 Naeye RL, et al: Causes of perinatal mortality in an African city. *Bull World Health Organ*, 55:63, 1977.

62 Bhat CJ, et al: Congenital syphilis in Lusaka—ii. Incidence at birth and potential risk among hospital deliveries. *East Afr Med J*, 59:306, 1982.

63 Hira SK, et al: Congenital syphilis in Lusaka—i. Incidence in a general nursery ward. *East Afr Med J*, 59:241, 1982.

64 Rosenberg MJ, et al: Sexually transmitted diseases in sub-Saharan Africa. A priority list based on Family Health International's Meeting. *Lancet*, 2:152, 1986.

65 Meyer MP: Criteria for early congenital syphilis—A perspective from Africa. *Genitourin Med*, 68:290, 1992.

66 Sánchez PJ, et al: Congenital syphilis associated with negative results of maternal serologic tests at delivery. *Am J Dis Child*, 145:967, 1991.

67 Dorfman DH, Glaser JH: Congenital syphilis presenting in infants after the newborn period. *N Engl J Med*, 323:1299, 1990.

68 Thomas DD, et al: *Treponema pallidum* invades intercellular junctions of endothelial cell monolayers. *Proc Natl Acad Sci (USA)*, 85: 3608, 1988.

69 Riley BS, et al: Virulent *Treponema pallidum* activates human vascular endothelial cells. *J Infect Dis*, 165;484, 1992.

70 Benirschke K: Syphilis—The placenta and the fetus. *Am J Dis Child*, 128:142, 1974.

71 Fojaco RM, et al: Congenital syphilis and necrotizing funistis. *JAMA*, 261:1788, 1989.

72 Qureshi F, et al: Placental histopathology in syphilis. *Human Pathol*, 24:779, 1993.

73 Jacques SM, Qureshi F: Necrotizing funisitis: A study of 45 cases. *Human Pathol*, 23:1278, 1992.

74 Bromberg K, et al: Diagnosis of congenital syphilis by combining *Treponema pallidum*-specific IgM detection with immunofluorescent antigen detection for *T. pallidum*. *J Infect Dis*, 168:238, 1993.

75 Wendel GD Jr., et al: Identification of *Treponema pallidum* in amniotic fluid and fetal blood from pregnancies complicated by congenital syphilis. *Obstet Gynecol*, 78:890, 1991.

76 Wendel GD, et al: Examination of amniotic fluid in diagnosing congenital syphilis with fetal death. *Obstet Gynecol*, 74:967, 1989.

77 Nathan L, et al: In utero infection with *Treponema pallidum* in early pregnancy. *Prenat. Diagn*, 17:119–123, 1997.

78 Nathan L, et al: Fetal syphilis: Correlation of sonographic findings and rabbit infectivity testing of amniotic fluid. *J Ultrasound Med*, 12: 97, 1993.

79 Harman N: *Staying the Plague*. London, Methuen, 1917.

80 Ingraham NR: The value of penicillin alone in the prevention and treatment of congenital syphilis. *Acta Derm Venereol (Stockh)*, 31 (suppl 24):60, 1951.

81 Sánchez PJ, et al: Evaluation of molecular methodologies and rabbit infectivity testing for the diagnosis of congenital syphilis and neonatal central nervous system invasion by *Treponema pallidum*. *J Infect Dis*, 167:148, 1993.

82 Beck AC, Dailey WT: Syphilis in pregnancy. *Pub Am Assoc Adv Sci*, 6:101, 1938.

83 Dippel AL: The relationship of congenital syphilis to abortion and miscarriage and the mechanism of intrauterine protection. *Am J Obstet Gynecol*, 47:369, 1976.

84 Harter C, Benirschke K: Fetal syphilis in the first trimester. *Am J Obstet Gynecol*, 124:705, 1976.

85 Silverstein AM: Congenital syphilis and the timing of immunogenesis in the human fetus. *Nature*, 194:196, 1962.

86 Oppenheimer EH, Hardy JB: Congenital syphilis in the newborn infant: Clinical and pathological observations in recent cases. *Johns Hopkins Med J*, 129:63, 1971.

87 Fraser JF: The pathology of congenital syphilis. *Acta Dermatol Syph*, 38:491, 1920.

88 Hoffmann E: Congenital syphilis in light of 30 year's investigation of the spirochete and 25 year's experience with salvarsan. *J Pediatr*, 9: 569, 1936.

89 Stowens D: *Pediatric Pathology*. Baltimore, Williams & Wilkins, 1959.

90 Pober JS, Cotran RS: Cytokines and endothelial cell biology. *Physiol Rev*, 70:427, 1990.

91 Radolf JD, McBroom R: Unpublished observations, 1996.

92 Russell P, Altshuler G: Placental abnormalities of congenital syphilis. *Am J Dis Child*, 128:160, 1974.

93 Malan AF, et al: Relative placental weight in congenital syphilis. *Placenta*, 11:3, 1990.

94 McCord JR: Syphilis of the placenta. The histologic examination of 1,085 placentas of mothers with strongly positive Wasserman reactions. *Am J Obstet Gynecol*, 28:743, 1934.

95 Turnbull HM: Recognition of congenital syphilis inflammation of the long bones. *Lancet*, 1:239, 1922.

96 Park EA, Jackson DA: The irregular extensions of the end of the shaft in the x-ray photograph in congenital syphilis, with pertinent observations. *J Pediatr*, 13:748, 1938.

97 Cremin BJ, Fisher RM: The lesions of congenital syphilis. *Br J Radiol*, 43:333, 1970.

98 Caffey J: *Pediatric X-ray Diagnosis*. Chicago, Yearbook, 1978.

99 Engeset A, et al: On the significance of growth in the roentgenological skeletal changes in early congenital syphilis. *Am J Roentgenol*, 69: 542, 1953.

100 Pendergrass EP, Bromer RS: Congenital bone syphilis. Preliminary report: Roentgenologic study with note on the histology and pathology of the condition. *Am J Roent Ther*, 22:1, 1929.

101 McLean S: The roentgenographic and pathologic aspects of congenital osseous syphilis. *Am J Dis Child*, 41:130, 1931.

102 Platou RV: Treatment of congenital syphilis with penicillin. *Adv Pediatr*, 4:39, 1949.

103 Levin E: Healing in congenital osseous syphilis. *Am J Radiol*, 110: 591, 1970.

104 Swartz MN: Neurosyphilis, in *Sexually Transmitted Diseases, 2d ed*, KK Holmes et al (eds). New York, McGraw-Hill, 1990.

105 Kaplan BS, et al: The glomerulopathy of congenital syphilis—An immune deposit disease. *J Pediatr*, 81:1154, 1972.

106 Losito A, et al: Membranous glomerulonephritis in congenital syphilis. *Clin Nephrol*, 12:32, 1979.

107 Jeans PC, Cooke JV: *Prepubescent Syphilis*. New York, Appleton-Century, 1930.
108 Bradlaw R: The dental stigmata of prenatal syphilis. *Oral Surg*, 6; 147, 1953.
109 Ingall D, et al: Syphilis, in *Infectious Diseases of the Fetus and Newborn Infant*, JS Remington, JD Klein (eds). Philadelphia, Saunders Company, 1994.
110 Budell JW: Treatment of congenital syphilis. *J Am Venereol Dis Assoc*, 3:168, 1976.
111 Rathbun KC: Congenital syphilis. *Sex Transm Dis*, 10:93, 1983.
112 Naeye RL: Fetal growth with congenital syphilis: A quantitative study. *Am J Clin Pathol*, 55;228, 1971.
113 Stoll BJ, et al: Clinical and serologic evaluation of neonates for congenital syphilis: A continuing diagnostic dilemma. *J Infect Dis*, 167: 1093, 1993.
114 Reyes MP, et al: Maternal/congenital syphilis in a large tertiary-care urban hospital. *Clin Infect Dis*, 17:1041, 1993.
115 Lukehart SA, Holmes KK: Syphilis, in *Harrison's Principles of Internal Medicine*, E Braunwald, et al (eds). New York, McGraw-Hill Book Company, 1994.
116 Hook EW III, Marra CM: Acquired syphilis in adults. *N Engl J Med*, 326:1060, 1992.
117 Ingraham NR: The diagnosis of congenital syphilis during the period of doubt. *Am J Syph Neurol*, 19:547, 1935.
118 Brown JW, Moore BM: Congenital syphilis in the United States. *Clin Pediatr*, 2:220, 1963.
119 Mamunes P, et al: Early diagnosis of neonatal syphilis. Evaluation of a gamma M–fluorescent treponemal antibody test. *Am J Dis Child*, 120:17, 1970.
120 Bwibo NO: Congenital syphilis. *East Afr Med J*, 48:185, 1971.
121 Stokes JH, et al: *Modern Clinical Syphilology*. Philadelphia, W.B. Saunders, 1934.
122 McDonald R: Congenital syphilis has many faces. *Clin Pediatr*, 9: 110, 1970.
123 Findlay L: *Syphilis in Childhood*. Oxford, Oxford Medical Publications, 1919.
124 Bueno M, et al: Congenital syphilis. *Paediatrician*, 8:17, 1979.
125 Saxoni F, et al: Congenital syphilis: A description of 18 cases and re-examination of an old but ever-present disease. *Clin Pediatr*, 6:687, 1967.
126 Wile U, Mundt LK: Congenital syphilis: A statistical study with special regard to sex incidence. *Am J Syph Gon Vener Dis*, 26:70, 1942.
127 Still FG: Hereditary syphilis, in *System of Syphilis, Vol. 1*, DA Power, JK Murphy (eds). Oxford: Oxford University Press, 1909.
128 Sylvester PH: Observations on congenital syphilis. *South Med J*, 193: 392, 1925.
129 Teberg A, Hodgman JE: Congenital syphilis in newborn. *California Medicine*, 118:5, 1973.
130 Tan KL: The re-emergence of early congenital syphilis. *Acta Paediatr Scand*, 62:601, 1973.
131 Freiman I, Super M: Thrombocytopenia and congenital syphilis in South African Bantu infants. *Arch Dis Child*, 41:87, 1966.
132 Murphy K, Patamasucon P: Unpublished observations, 1981.
132 Brooks SE, Audretsch JJ: Hepatic ultrastructure in congenital syphilis. *Arch Pathol Lab Med*, 102:502, 1978.
133 Whitaker JA, et al: Hematological aspects of congenital syphilis. *J Pediatr*, 66:629, 1965.
134 Shah MC, Barton LL: Congenital syphilitic hepatitis. *Pediatr Infect Dis J*, 8:891, 1989.
135 Roberts MH: Congenital syphilis. *Am J Dis Child*, 45:461, 1933.
136 Hill RM, Knox JM: Syphilis, in *Brennerman's Practice of Pediatrics*, New York, Harper & Row, 1970.
137 Masola A: Personal communication, 1983.
138 Whipple DV, Dunham EC: Congenital syphilis. I: incidence, transmission, and diagnosis. *J Pediatr*, 12:386, 1938.
139 Rosen EU, Solomon A: Bone lesions in early congenital syphilis. *S Afr Med J*, 50:135, 1976.
140 Dzebolo NN: Congenital syphilis: An unusual presentation. *Radiology*, 136:372, 1980.
141 Solomon A, Rosen E: The aspect of trauma in the bone changes of congenital lues. *Pediatr Radiol*, 3:176, 1975.
142 Solomon A, Rosen E: Focal osseous lesions in congenital lues. *Pediatr Radiol*, 7:36, 1978.
143 Josephs HW: Anemia of infancy and early childhood. *Medicine*, 15: 307, 1936.
144 Sartain P: The anemia of congenital syphilis. *South Med J*, 58:27, 1965.
145 Marchi AG, et al: An isolated case of congenital luetic cryoglobulinemia. *Minerva Pediatr*, 18:1155, 1966.
146 Wiggelinkhuizen J, et al: Congenital syphilis and glomerulonephritis with evidence for immune pathogenesis. *Arch Dis Child*, 48:375, 1973.
147 Hilts SV, Shaw CC: Leukemoid blood reactions. *N Engl J Med*, 249: 434, 1953.
148 Karayalcin G, et al: Monocytosis in congenital syphilis. *Am J Dis Child*, 131:782, 1977.
149 Yampolsky J, Mullins DF: Acute glomerular nephritis in an infant with congenital syphilis. *Am J Dis Child*, 69:163, 1945.
150 Berry MC, Dajani AS: Resurgence of congenital syphilis. *Infect Dis Clin North Am*, 6:19, 1992.
151 Klein JO, Marcy SM: Bacterial sepsis and meningitis, in *Infectious Diseases of the Fetus and Newborn Infant*, JS Remington, JD Klein (eds). Philadelphia, W.B. Saunders.
152 Thorley JD, et al: Passive transfer of antibodies of maternal origin from blood to cerebrospinal fluid in infants. *Lancet*, 1:651, 1975.
153 Sánchez PJ, et al: IgM antibody to *Treponema pallidum* in cerebrospinal fluid of infants with congenital syphilis. *Am J Dis Child*, 146; 1171, 1992.
154 Turner TB, et al: Infectivity tests in syphilis. *Br J Vener Dis*, 45;183, 1969.
155 Lewis LL, et al: Evaluation of immunoglobulin M western blot analysis in the diagnosis of congenital syphilis. *J Clin Microbiol*, 28:296, 1990.
156 Sánchez PJ: Unpublished observations, 1996.
157 Daaboul JJ, et al: Neonatal hypoglycemia caused by hypopituitarism in infants with congenital syphilis. *J Pediatr*, 123:983, 1993.
158 Contreras F, Pereda J: Congenital syphilis of the eye with lens involvement. *Arch Ophthalmol*, 96:1052, 1978.
159 Edell DS, et al: A common presentation of an uncommon cause of neonatal respiratory distress: pneumonia alba. *Pediatr Pulmonol*, 15: 376, 1993.
160 McCulloch H: Congenital syphilis as a cause of heart disease. *Am Heart J*, 6:136, 1930.
161 Digre KB, et al: Late-onset congenital syphilis. A retrospective look at University of Iowa Hospital admissions. *J Clin Neuro Ophthalmol*, 11:1, 1991.
162 Fiumara NJ, Lessell S: Manifestations of late congenital syphilis. An analysis of 271 patients. *Arch Dermatol*, 102:78, 1970.
163 Cooperative Clinical Group: Late prenatal syphilis. *Arch Dermatol*, 35:563, 1937.
164 Robinson RCV: Congenital syphilis. *Arch Dermatol*, 99:599, 1969.
165 Putkonen T, Paaero YV: X-ray photography of unerupted permanent teeth in congenital syphilis. *Br J Vener Dis*, 37:190, 1961.
165a Moon H: On irregular and defective tooth development. *Trans Odont Soc Gr Br* (new series), 9:223–243, 1876.
166 Karmody CS, Schuknecht HF: Deafness in congenital syphilis. *Arch Otolaryngol*, 83:18, 1966.
167 Nadol JB Jr.: Hearing loss of acquired syphilis: diagnosis confirmed by incudectomy. *Laryngoscope*, 85:1888, 1975.
168 Clutton HH: Symmetrical synovitis of the knee in hereditary syphilis. *Lancet*, 1:391, 1886.
169 Gray SM, Philp T: Syphilitic arthritis. *Ann Rheum Dis*, 22:19, 1963.
170 Kauder JV, Solomon HC: Juvenile paresis. *Am J Med Sci*, 166:545, 1923.
171 Meninger, WC: *Juvenile Paresis*. Baltimore, Williams & Wilkins, 1936.
172 MacKenzie GM: Paroxysmal cold hemoglobinuria: A review. *Medicine*, 8:159, 1929.

173 Barton JR, et al: Nonimmune hydrops fetalis associated with maternal infection with syphilis. *Am J Obstet Gynecol*, 167:56, 1992.

174 Hallak M, et al: Nonimmune hydrops fetalis and fetal congenital syphilis. A case report. *J Reprod Med*, 37:173, 1992.

175 Satin AJ, et al: Congenital syphilis associated with dilation of fetal small bowel. A case report. *J Ultrasound Med*, 11:49, 1992.

176 Hill LM, Maloney JB: An unusual constellation of sonographic findings associated with congenital syphilis. *Obstet Gynecol*, 78:895, 1991.

177 Cox SM, Wendel GD: Xeroradiography and skeletal survey in the diagnosis of congenital syphilis following fetal death. *Abstract 42, Society of Perinatal Obstetricians*, 1987.

178 Taber LH, Huber TW: Congenital syphilis, in *Infections of the Fetus and the Newborn Infant*. S Krugman, AA Gershon (eds). New York, Liss, 1975.

179 Burstain JM, et al: Sensitive detection of *Treponema pallidum* by using the polymerase chain reaction. *J Clin Microbiol*, 29:62, 1991.

180 Grimprel E, et al: Use of polymerase chain reaction and rabbit infectivity to detect *Treponema pallidum* in amniotic fluids, fetal and neonatal sera, and cerebrospinal fluids. *J Clin Microbiol*, 29:1711, 1991.

181 Dorman HG, Sahyun PF: Identification and significance of spirochetes in the placenta. *Am J Obstet Gynecol*, 33:954, 1937.

182 McCord JR: A study of two hundred autopsies made on syphilitic fetuses. *Am J Obstet Gynecol*, 33:954, 1937.

183 Ohyama M, et al: Syphilitic placentitis: Demonstration of *Treponema pallidum* by immunoperoxidase staining. *Virchows Arch [A]*, 417: 343, 1990.

184 Hambie EA, et al: Comparison of a new rapid plasma reagin card test with the standard rapid plasma reagin 18-mm circle card test and the venereal disease research laboratory slide test for serodiagnosis of syphilis. *J Clin Microbiol*, 17:249, 1983.

185 American Academy of Pediatrics: Syphilis, in *Report of the Committee on Infectious Diseases (Red Book)*, 1997.

186 Ackerman BD: Congenital syphilis: Observations on laboratory diagnosis of intrauterine infection. *J Pediatr* 74:459, 1969.

187 Scotti AT, Logan L: A specific IgM antibody test in neonatal congenital syphilis. *J Pediatr*, 73:242, 1968.

188 Alford CA Jr., et al: Gamma-M–fluorescent treponemal antibody in the diagnosis of congenital syphilis. *N Engl J Med*, 280:1086, 1969.

189 Kaufman RE, et al: The FTA-ABS (IgM) test for neonatal congenital syphilis: A critical review. *J Am Vener Dis Assoc*, 1:79, 1974.

190 Muller F, Sinzig G: Specificity and sensitivity of immunological diagnosis of congenital neonatal syphilis by the 19S(IgM)-FTA-ABS test. *Zeitschrift fur Hautkrankheiten*, 57:983, 1982.

191 Sánchez PJ, et al: Molecular analysis of the fetal IgM response to *Treponema pallidum* antigens: Implications for improved serodiagnosis of congenital syphilis. *J Infect Dis*, 159:508, 1989.

192 Dobson SR, et al: Recognition of *Treponema pallidum* antigens by IgM and IgG antibodies in congenitally infected newborns and their mothers. *J Infect Dis*, 157:903, 1988.

193 Lewis LL: Congenital syphilis. Serologic diagnosis in the young infant. *Infect Dis Clin North Am*, 6:31, 1992.

194 Sánchez PJ, et al: Fetal IgM response to *Treponema pallidum* antigens in asymptomatic infants with suspected congenital syphilis. *Pediatr Res*, 25:281A, 1989.

195 Schmitz JL, et al: Laboratory diagnosis of congenital syphilis by immunoglobulin M (IgM) and IgA immunoblotting. *Clin Diagn Lab Immunol*, 1:32, 1994.

196 Sánchez PJ, et al: IgM immunoblotting utilizing recombinant 47- and 17-kDa antigens for the diagnosis of congenital syphilis. *35th ICAAC, San Francisco, CA*, 1995.

197 Wendel GD: Gestational and congenital syphilis. *Clin Perinatol*, 15: 287, 1988.

198 Centers for Disease Control and Prevention: 1998 Guidelines for Treatment of Sexually Transmitted Diseases. *MMWR*, 1998, in press.

199 Rein MF: Biopharmacology of syphilotherapy. *J Am Vener Dis Assoc*, 3:109, 1976.

200 Stamm LV, et al: In vitro assay to demonstrate high-level erythromycin resistance of a clinical isolate of *Treponema pallidum*. *Antimicrob Agents Chemother*, 32;164, 1988.

201 Fenton LJ, Light IJ: Congenital syphilis after maternal treatment with erythromycin. *Obstet Gynecol*, 47:492, 1976.

202 South MA, et al: Failures of erythromycin estolate therapy in utero syphilis. *JAMA*, 190:70, 1964.

203 Hashisaki P, et al: Erythromycin failure in the treatment of syphilis in a pregnant woman. *Sex Transm Dis*, 10:36, 1983.

204 Philipson A, et al: Transplacental passage of erythromycin and clindamycin. *N Engl J Med*, 288:1219, 1973.

205 Wendel GD Jr, et al: Penicillin allergy and desensitization in serious infections during pregnancy. *N Engl J Med*, 312:1229, 1985.

206 Hardy PH Jr., Levin J: Lack of endotoxin in *Borrelia hispanica* and *Treponema pallidum*. *Proc Soc Exp Biol Med*, 174:47, 1983.

207 Young EJ, et al: Studies on the pathogenesis of the Jarisch-Herxheimer reaction: Development of an animal model and evidence against a role for classical endotoxin. *J Infect Dis*, 146:606, 1982.

208 Radolf JD, et al: Lipoproteins of *Borrelia burgdorferi* and *Treponema pallidum*, activate cachectin/tumor necrosis factor synthesis: Analysis using a CAT reporter construct. *J Immunol*, 147:1968, 1991.

209 Radolf JD, et al: *Treponema pallidum* and *Borrelia burgdorferi* lipoproteins and synthetic lipopeptides activate monocytes/macrophages. *J Immunol*, 154:2866, 1995.

210 Klein VR et al: The Jarisch-Herxheimer reaction complicating syphilotherapy in pregnancy. *Obstet Gynecol*, 75:375, 1990.

211 Wendel GD Jr: Personal communication, 1996.

212 Mascola L, et al: Inadequate treatment of syphilis in pregnancy. *Am J Obstet Gynecol*, 150:945, 1984.

213 Nathan L, et al: Penicillin levels following the administration of benzathine penicillin G in pregnancy. *Obstet Gynecol*, 82:338, 1993.

214 Sánchez PJ: Syphilis, in *Gellis and Kagan's Current Pediatric Therapy*, FD Burg, JR Ingelfinger, ER Wald (eds). New York: W.B. Saunders, 1993.

215 Azimi PH, et al: Concentrations of procaine and aqueous penicillin in the cerebrospinal fluid of infants treated for congenital syphilis. *J Pediatr*, 124:649, 1994.

216 Sánchez PJ, et al: Serologic follow-up in congenital syphilis: What's the point? 34th Interscience Conference on Antimicrobial Agents and Chemotherapy, Abstract L22, Orlando, FL, 1994.

217 Sánchez PJ, et al: Congenital syphilis and HIV infection. *Pediatr Res*, 27:276A, 1990.

218 Pollack H, et al: Maternal syphilis is associated with enhanced perinatal HIV transmission. 30th Interscience Conference on Antimicrobial Agents and Chemotherapy, 1990.

219 Ingraham NR, Beerman H: The present status of penicillin in the treatment of syphilis in pregnancy and infantile congenital syphilis. *Am J Med Sci*, 219:433, 1950.

220 Opai-Tetteh ET, et al: Re-screening for syphilis at the time of delivery in areas of high prevalence. *S Afr Med J*, 83:725, 1993.

221 Miller JN: Value and limitations of nontreponemal and treponemal tests in the laboratory diagnosis of syphilis. *Clin Obstet Gynecol*, 18: 191, 1975.

222 Van Dyck E, et al: Rapid plasma reagin card test: Evaluation of hand-rotation procedure and stability of the RPR antigen. *Bull World Health Organ*, 741:743, 1994.

223 Hira SK, et al: Syphilis intervention in pregnancy: Zambian demonstration project. *Genitourin Med*, 66:159, 1990.

224 Murphy K, Patamasucon P: Unpublished observations, 1981.

Chapter 85

Herpesvirus infections in neonates and children: cytomegalovirus and herpes simplex virus

Sergio Stagno
Richard J. Whitley

CONGENITAL AND PERINATAL CYTOMEGALOVIRUS INFECTIONS

Cytomegaloviruses (CMV) comprise a group of agents in the herpesvirus family known for their ubiquitous distribution in humans and in numerous other mammals. These viruses thus share a number of biologic attributes in common with herpes simplex virus and other members of the herpesvirus family (see Chapter 20). Both in vivo and in vitro, the infection is highly species-specific.[1] The first description of cells containing intranuclear and cytoplasmic inclusions dates from 1881 when Ribbert found them in the kidneys of a stillborn infant with congenital syphilis.[2] In 1954, Smith succeeded in propagating murine CMV in explant cultures of mouse embryonic fibroblasts.[3] Utilization of similar techniques led to the independent isolation of human CMV shortly thereafter by Smith, Rowe, et al., and Weller et al.[4–6] The term cytomegalovirus was proposed in 1960 by Weller, Hanshaw, and Scott to replace the names cytomegalic inclusion disease and salivary gland virus, which were misleading, since the virus usually involved other organs and the term salivary gland virus had been used to designate unrelated agents obtained from bats.[7]

The propagation of CMV in vitro led to the rapid development of serologic methods and the ability to isolate the virus from clinical specimens. It became quickly apparent that CMV is a significant human pathogen.[8] The natural history of human CMV infection is very complex. Following a primary infection, viral excretion (occasionally from several sites) persists for weeks, months, or years before becoming latent. Asymptomatic episodes of recurrent infection with renewed viral shedding are common, even years after primary infection. Most maternal CMV infections are subclinical. However, although infection may be without consequences for the mother, it can have serious repercussions for the fetus.[9]

EPIDEMIOLOGY

GENERAL

Humans are the only reservoir for CMV. The infection is endemic and without seasonal variation.[1–8] Climate does not affect the prevalence of infection, and there are no known vectors in the natural transmission cycle. Seroepidemiologic surveys have found CMV infection in every human population that has been tested. The prevalence of antibody to CMV increases with age, but according to geographic, ethnic, and socioeconomic backgrounds, the patterns of acquisition of infection vary widely among populations. In general, the prevalence of CMV infection is higher in developing countries and among the lower socioeconomic strata of developed nations. These differences are particularly striking during childhood.

The level of immunity among women of childbearing age also varies widely in different populations. In the United States and eastern Europe, seropositivity rates in young women range from less than 50 to 85 percent.[9] In contrast, in the Ivory Coast, Japan, and Chile the rate of seropositivity is greater than 90 percent by the end of the second decade of life.[10–12] Prospective studies of pregnant women in the United States indicate that the rate of CMV acquisition for childbearing age women of middle to higher socioeconomic background is approximately 2 percent per year, whereas it is 6 percent among women of lower socioeconomic background.[13]

The modes of transmission from person to person are incompletely understood.[8] The following features of CMV infection make it difficult to study the modes of acquisition. In the majority of individuals, CMV infections are subclinical, including those acquired in utero and during the perinatal period. Virus excretion persists for years following congenital, perinatal, and early postnatal infections. Prolonged viral shedding is also a feature of primary infection in older children and adults. These infected persons continue to expose other susceptible people. Since recurrent infections are fairly common, intermittent excretion of virus can be anticipated in a significant proportion of seropositive adults. It is clear that a large reservoir of CMV exists in the population at all times. Transmission occurs by direct or indirect person-to-person contact. Sources of virus include urine, oropharyngeal secretions, cervical and vaginal secretions, semen, milk, tears, blood, and transplanted organs.[14,15]

The spread of infection requires close or intimate contact with infected secretions. Sexual contact contributes to the spread of CMV. Higher rates of seropositivity have been observed among males and females with multiple sex partners and histories of sexually transmitted diseases.[14,16–21]

Certain child-rearing practices influence the spread of CMV among children. Because seropositive women often excrete CMV in milk, the incidence of perinatal CMV infection is high where breast feeding is a common practice.[15] As breast feeding regains popularity in the United States, the incidence of perinatal transmission of CMV will increase, thus creating an even larger pool of infected children.

In 1971, Weller suggested that the high rate of seropositivity among Swedish children was probably due to the frequent use of daycare centers.[1] Swedish children had a rate of infection that was three to four times higher than that observed in London or Rochester, New York. High rates of CMV infection among children attending daycare centers were later confirmed in the United States.[22–24] Pass et al. reported that in a group of 70 children of middle- to upper-income background whose ages ranged from 3 to 65 months, the rate of CMV excretion in urine and saliva was 50 percent.[22] The lowest rate of excretion (9%) occurred in infants less than 1 year of age, and the highest rate (88%) among toddlers in their second year of life. Infants younger than 12 months of age in group daycare who excrete CMV are more likely to have acquired CMV congenitally or perinatally from maternal cervical secretions or breast milk. Twelve children whose mothers were seronegative excreted CMV, which indicated that their infection was not perinatally acquired. The findings of Pass et al. subsequently have been confirmed by other investigators.[23–26] There is now compelling evidence that the high rate of CMV infection among children in group daycare is caused by horizontal transmission from child to child. The route of transmission that appears most likely is the transfer of virus that occurs through saliva on hands and toys.[27,28] The strongest evidence supporting child-to-child transmission was obtained by Adler by analysis of the restriction enzyme digestion patterns of CMV DNA of the isolates obtained from infected children attending daycare.[29] His findings have been confirmed by others and demonstrate that CMV is very efficiently transmitted from child to child in the daycare setting, and that it is not unusual to find excretion rates as high as 20 to 40 percent in young toddlers. In many instances, these rates of infection are substantially higher than the seroprevalence rates for the parents of the children and young adults in the cities where the studies were done. No data have indicated CMV transmission via respiratory droplets.

With the changes in childrearing practices now occurring in the United States and the resurgence of breast feeding, the epidemiology of CMV will undergo significant changes.

An important issue is whether children excreting CMV can become a source of infection for serosusceptible child care personnel and parents, particularly women of childbearing age. This mode of transmission has been confirmed by restriction endonuclease mapping of CMV DNA.[30,31] Seroepidemiologic studies suggest that parents often acquire CMV from their children who became infected outside the family.[32–34] Adler and Pass et al. have presented compelling evidence linking the acquisition of CMV by children in daycare with subsequent infection in their mothers and caretakers. Pass et al. followed seronegative parents whose children attended a daycare center and seronegative parents whose children did not attend daycare.[26] The groups were followed for a mean of 17 and 21 months, respectively. The study revealed that 14 of 67 seronegative parents with children in daycare centers acquired CMV, compared with none of 31 serosusceptible parents whose children did not attend daycare. More significant, all 14 parents of the daycare group who seroconverted had a child who was shedding CMV in saliva or urine. In fact, seroconversion occurred in 14 of 48 parents of children who shed CMV, compared with none of 21 whose children did not excrete CMV. The highest risk of seroconversion (45%) was for parents with a child shedding CMV who was 18 months of age or less at enrollment. In two of the 14 cases, DNA analysis indicated the child as the source of CMV infection. In a subsequent study, this group of investigators also demonstrated by means of restriction enzyme analysis that infections acquired by a mother from a child can be transmitted to her fetus.[25] In a very similar study, Adler observed that of 18 seronegative mothers whose children shed CMV strains associated with daycare, six seroconverted and excreted CMV strains identical to the strains shed by their children.[35] On average, these mothers acquired the infection within 4.2 months (range, 3–7 months) after their children became infected.

In assessing the risk to caretakers working with young children in daycare centers, Adler has reported an annual seroconversion rate of 11 percent among 202 seronegative women employed at 33 daycare centers in Richmond, Virginia.[36] This rate was significantly higher than the 2 percent annual rate occurring among a group of 229 female hospital employees matched for age, race, and marital status. The restriction endonuclease DNA patterns of 17 of 31 isolates of CMV obtained from daycare workers were compared with the DNAs of isolates shed by the children cared for by these women. Nine of the 17 isolates were identical to the DNAs of isolates shed by one or more children. These observations provide compelling evidence that serosusceptible women who work with children in daycare have an occupational risk of acquiring CMV.

From the data generated from these studies, it is reasonable to expect that approximately 50 percent of susceptible children between the ages of 1 and 3 years who attend group daycare will acquire CMV from their playmates and become an important potential source of infection for susceptible parents and caretakers. Of particular concern is the risk to seronegative mothers who have children in group daycare and who become pregnant.

Fomites may also play some role in transmission because CMV has been shown to retain infectivity for hours on plastic surfaces and CMV has been isolated from randomly selected toys and surfaces in a daycare center.[27,28]

MATERNAL INFECTION AND VERTICAL TRANSMISSION

Maternal CMV infection is the origin of congenital infections and of most perinatal infections. As used here, vertical transmission implies mother-to-infant transmission.

Congenital infection

Congenital infection is assumed to be the result of transplacental transmission. In the United States, congenital CMV infection occurs in between 0.2 and 2.2 percent (average 1%) of all newborn infants. The natural history of CMV infection during pregnancy is particularly complex and has not been fully explained. With infections such as rubella and toxoplasmosis, transmission in utero occurs only as a result of a primary infection acquired during pregnancy, whereas the in utero transmission of CMV can occur as a consequence of both primary and recurrent infections.[37] Far from being a rare event, congenital infection resulting from recurrent CMV infection has been shown to be quite common, especially in highly immune populations. The initial clue was provided by three independent reports of congenital CMV infections that occurred in consecutive pregnancies.[38–40] In all three instances, the first infant was severely affected or died and the second born in each case was subclinically infected. More convincing evidence came from a prospective study of women known to be seroimmune before conception.[37] The rate of congenital CMV infection was 1.9 percent among 541 infants born to these seropositive women. Clearly these congenitally infected infants were not infected as a result of primary maternal CMV infection since all of the mothers were known to have been infected with CMV from one to several years before the onset of pregnancy. This remarkable phenomenon of intrauterine transmission that occurs in the presence of humoral immunity has been attributed to reactivation of endogenous virus but reinfection has not been included as a possibility. This unique characteristic (intrauterine transmission in immune women) accounts for the high incidence of congenital CMV infection in populations with the highest rate of seroposivity.[41] At present, it is impossible to define by either virologic or serologic markers which patient may reactivate CMV, neither is it possible to define the time of intrauterine transmission with such reactivation during pregnancy. The sites from which CMV reactivates to produce congenital infection are not known. Although CMV excretion is a relatively common event during and after pregnancy, simple isolation of virus from the cervix or urine or both is a poor indicator of the risk of intrauterine infection.[42,43]

Virus can be shed at variable rates from single or multiple sites following primary or recurrent infections in both pregnant and nonpregnant women. Pregnancy per se has no discernible effect on the overall prevalence of viral shedding. However, gestational age has a significant influence on the rate of CMV excretion, with the rate of viral shedding being significantly lower in the first trimester.[44]

The rates of CMV excretion in the genital and urinary tract of women are inversely related to age after puberty.[45]

Perinatal infection

In contrast to the poor correlation that exists between CMV excretion during pregnancy and congenital infection, there is good correlation between maternal shedding in the genital tract and milk and perinatal acquisition. In one study, the two most efficient sources of transmission in the perinatal period were infected breast milk (which resulted in a 63% rate of perinatal infection) and the infected genital tract, particularly in late gestation, which was associated with transmission in 57 percent of the cases (natal infection).[15] Viral shedding from the pharynx and urinary tract of the mother late in gestation and during the first months of postpartum has not been associated with perinatal transmission.

There is considerable variability in perinatal transmission of CMV throughout the world. The age of the mother and her prior experience with CMV, which in turn influence the frequency of viral excretion into the genital tract and breast milk, certainly are important factors. Younger seropositive women who breast feed are at a greater risk for transmitting virus in early infancy, especially in lower socioeconomic groups. It is remarkable that in Japan, Guatemala, Finland, and Thailand, where the rates of CMV excretion within the first year of life are extremely high (39–56%), the practice of breast feeding is almost universal, and the majority of women of childbearing age are seroimmune for CMV.

SEXUAL TRANSMISSION

In general, in developing areas of the world, 90 to 100 percent of the population is infected during childhood, even as early as 5 years of age. Sexual transmission in these populations plays a minor role as a source of primary CMV infection, and its importance in reinfection is unclear. In developed countries, the infection is acquired at a lower rate and in some population groups there is a marked increase in prevalence of infection after puberty.

Several lines of evidence indicate that sexual transmission of CMV is at least partly responsible for this increase in seroprevalence. CMV is frequently recovered from semen and cervical secretions.[14,16–21] Increased seroprevalence of CMV and excretion of virus has been found in women attending sexually transmitted disease clinics and in young male homosexuals. Chretien et al. reported a cluster of cases with CMV mononucleosis that occurred in sex partners, but not in persons who shared living quarters but did not engage in sexual contact.[46] Handsfield et al. showed that, in two pairs of sex partners with CMV infections attending a sexually transmitted disease clinic, strains of virus were identical by restriction endonuclease analyses of DNA.[45] Evidence has also been provided for sexual transmission in less promiscuous populations.[18,19] Among the many variables investigated, a significant correlation was found between seropositivity to CMV and greater numbers of lifetime sexual partners and past or present infection with *Chlamydia trachomatis*. Although the evidence for sexual transmission of CMV is thus compelling, the fact that CMV is frequently shed in saliva indicates that oral contact may also be an important route of transmission.

TRANSMISSION VIA TRANSFUSION OF BLOOD AND BLOOD PRODUCTS

Nosocomial CMV infection is an important hazard of blood transfusion and organ transplant. In compromised hosts, such as small premature newborns and bone marrow transplant recipients, transfusion acquired CMV has been associated with serious morbidity and even fatal infection. The association between the acquisition of CMV infection and blood transfusion was first suggested in 1960 by Kreel et al., who described a syndrome characterized by fever and leukocytosis occurring 3 to 8 weeks after open heart surgery.[47] Reports that followed expanded the syndrome to include fever, atypical lymphocytosis, splenomegaly, rash, and lymphadenopathy.[48–55] The term "postperfusion mononucleosis" was then proposed. Prospective studies incriminated blood transfusion as the major risk factor and demonstrated that while the clinical syndrome occurred in approximately 3 percent of the patients receiving transfusion, inapparent acquisition of CMV infection occurred in 9 to 58 percent. It has been estimated that blood donors capable of transmitting CMV range from 2.5 to 12 percent. In a study of seronegative children receiving blood for cardiac surgery, the risk of acquiring CMV was calculated to be 2.7 percent per unit of blood.[51] There is a significant correlation between the risk of acquisition of CMV by seronegative patients and the total volume of blood transfused.[56] Studies have demonstrated that seronegative immunocompromised patients receiving prophylactic white blood cell (WBC) transfusions from multiple donors (of whom 50% are expected to be seropositive) are also at increased risk of acquiring CMV.[56]

The observation that two newborn infants who received large volumes of fresh blood subsequently developed symptomatic CMV infections led McCracken et al. to suggest an association between blood transfusion and clinically apparent postnatal CMV infection.[57] Subsequent reports indicated an association between postnatal CMV infection and exchange transfusions.[58] With exchange transfusions, the probability of a seropositive infant receiving seropositive blood becoming infected is 20 percent, whereas for a seronegative infant receiving seropositive blood, the probability is 50 percent. This remarkably high incidence after exchange transfusions is most likely owing to the fact that infants who receive the transfusions usually receive large volumes (150–200 mL/kg) of fresh whole blood from a single donor. Intrauterine transfusions were implicated by King-Lewis and Gardner as the source of CMV in two pregnant women who subsequently seroconverted and whose infants developed viruria between 2 and 8 weeks of postnatal life.[59]

Two prospective studies have presented compelling evidence that seropositive blood is the source of acquired CMV in neonates undergoing multiple transfusions. In the study of Yeager et al., 10 of 74 infants of seronegative mothers who were exposed to one or more seropositive blood donors acquired CMV.[60,61] The risk of infection increased to 24 percent for patients who received more than 50 mL of packed red cells from at least one seropositive donor. The use of solely seronegative blood completely eliminated the acquisition of CMV by seronegative infants. A subsequent study by Adler confirmed these findings and proved further that significant risk factors for transmission of CMV and subsequent disease included transfusions from multiple seropositive donors, lack of passively acquired maternal antibody to CMV, and low birth weight (<1250 g).[48,62]

TRANSMISSION TO HOSPITAL WORKERS

Because hospital workers are often women of childbearing age, there has been concern about occupational risk through contact with patients shedding CMV. Yeager reported a higher seroconversion rate for neonatal (4.1%/year) and pediatric nurses (7.7%/year) than for non-nurse hospital employees (0%), but these differences were not statistically significant.[63] Friedman et al. noted higher seroconversion rates in a pediatric hospital among workers with patient contact compared with those without such contact.[64] Although the difference in rates was not statistically significant, when "high-risk" employees (intensive care nurses and an IV team) were compared with others, a significantly higher rate of CMV infection was found in the former. Dworsky studied nurses in newborn nurseries and other health care workers and found no difference when the seroconversion rate in these women was compared with that of a large group of pregnant women in the community.[33] Balfour and Balfour measured incidence of CMV infection among transplant/dialysis nurses, neonatal intensive care nurses, student nurses, and a control group; neither the initial rate of seropositivity nor the annual seroconversion rate differed significantly among any of the groups.[65] Their annualized seroconversion rate of 1.84 percent was very close to rates determined for middle-income pregnant women in Birmingham, Alabama.[13]

The risk for hospital personnel is a function of the prevalence of CMV excretion among patients, the prevalence of seronegative health care workers, and the degree of their exposure to infected patients. In general, among hospitalized infants and children, viruria occurs in approximately 1 percent of newborn infants, 13 percent of premature infants hospitalized for 1 month or longer, and 5 to 10 percent of older infants and toddlers. The rate of viral excretion in premature infants depends on the rates of perinatal transmission from mother to infant, breast feeding practices, and blood transfusion policies. In toddlers and older children, viral excretion depends on factors like crowding, socioeconomic status, and childrearing practices (breast feeding, attendance at daycare centers). On the other hand, age, race, and, to some extent, sex, influence the prevalence of seronegative hospital personnel.

Working with hospitalized children will inevitably lead to contact with a child shedding CMV. However, it is important that workers who develop primary infection not assume that their occupational exposure or contact with a specific patient is the source of infection.[66–68] Two case reports illustrate this point well. Yow et al. and Wilfert et al. described health care workers who acquired CMV while pregnant and after attending a patient known to be excreting CMV.[69,70] In each of these reports, restriction endonuclease analysis of DNA from CMV isolates indicated that the source of CMV for the worker and her aborted fetus was not the patient under suspicion. Adler et al. used restriction enzyme methods to study CMV strains from 35 newborns and a nurse who seroconverted.[67] All 35 strains were different, supporting the conclusion that nosocomial spread of CMV to workers or among newborns was not occurring in their nursery. Although hospital workers, particularly those who attend children or immunocompromised patients, will likely have occupational exposure to CMV, there is no convincing evidence that their risk of infection is increased. There is little information about the risk of CMV acquisition by house officers and medical students. In one study, the annual rate of seroconversion for 25 seronegative pediatric residents was 2.7 percent, which differed little from nursery nurses (3.3%) but was higher than the risk (0.6%) for 89 serosusceptible students completing their clinical rotations.[65]

PATHOGENESIS

Of the women who acquire CMV infection during pregnancy, 30 to 40 percent transmit the virus to their fetuses.[13] The risk for those who reactivate the infection is less than 2 percent. Acute and/or long-term morbidity occurs in a small number (5–15%) of infected offspring. Generalized cytomegalic inclusion disease is generally the result of primary maternal infection.

Although not clearly established, intrauterine infection is assumed to result from maternal viremia with subsequent placental infection and hematogenous dissemination to the fetus. Since intrauterine transmission occurs in only 30 to 40 percent of pregnant women with primary CMV infection, a mechanism(s) that is not understood, but is generally referred to as the placental barrier, must operate to prevent fetal infection.

Boppana and Britt examined CMV specific antibody responses after primary maternal infection to determine if specific deficits in antibody response were associated with in vitro uterine transmission.[71] They reported that anti-glycoprotein B IgG antibodies were significantly higher at delivery in women who transmitted the infection compared to the nontransmitters. This observation suggests that the amount of antiviral antibody was not reflective of protection from transmission. They also examined the qualitative antibody response and found lower neutralizing antibody titers in transmitters, suggesting an association between neutralizing activity and in utero transmission. They also found that a higher antibody avidity index (≥2.0) occurred in the majority of nontransmitters but in less than 20 percent of transmitters. Antibody avidity correlated with neutralizing titers, suggesting that antibody affinity maturation is critical for production of high levels of neutralizing antibodies during primary CMV infection. This defect in affinity maturation may indicate that subtle abnormalities in cellular immune mechanisms were present in this group. Previous studies of pregnant women suggested that abnormalities in CMV-specific T-lymphocyte responses occurred in some women. Gehrz showed a transient reduction of the blastogenic response during the second and third trimester.[72] The defect was not generalized, moreover none of the women with the defect excreted CMV, nor did they transmit the infection in utero. Stern showed that women with recently acquired infection who had depressed blastogenic responses had a greater risk of delivering a congenitally infected infant.[73]

In immune pregnant women with recurrent infection, it is difficult to postulate that congenital infection results from cell-free virus in plasma causing placental infection with subsequent spread to the fetus.[74] In this circumstance, the virus could evade the immune system within leukocytes, or local reactivation of infection within the endometrium, myometrium, or cervical canal could occur.

Once intrauterine infection has occurred, the incidence of harmful effects is higher than at any other time in life, with the exception of severely immunocompromised patients (see Chapter 21). The clinical manifestations of congenital CMV infection are very different from the signs and symptoms associated with infection acquired at delivery or soon after, even in immature infants, suggesting the importance of the intrauterine environment itself.

Why some infants are severely affected and others remain free of symptoms is not clear. The most obvious, but not necessarily the most important, pathogenic mechanism is continuous viral replication in affected organs. Longitudinal studies of infants with congenital and perinatal infections have demonstrated that excretion of CMV into urine and saliva persists for years. It is likely that chronic viral replication also occurs at other sites that are less accessible to virologic examination. Many cells are susceptible to the direct cytocidal effect of CMV, but differences in the intrinsic susceptibility of various tissues to CMV-mediated injury may determine the frequency with which different organs are involved during the course of CMV infection. Another possible factor is vasculitis, which may occur in utero or after birth. Infants with serious congenital CMV who die soon after birth usually have disseminated intravascular coagulopathy.[75] Proliferating endothelial cells within inflamed tissue are susceptible to CMV infection. Injury mediated by immunologic factors also has been studied. The humoral immune system of infected infants is generally intact and responds normally to antigenic stimulation.[41]

Perinatal infection results mainly from recurrent (mostly reactivated) infection in immune women. However, transplacental maternal antibody protects only 50 percent of exposed infants from becoming infected.[76] The ensuing infection, although chronic, remains subclinical in the vast majority of infants, indicating that the passive transfer of maternal antibody is more protective for virulence than for transmission. Studies show transfusion-acquired infection is more virulent in seronegative than in seropositive infants irrespective of underlying diseases or gestational age.

Congenitally and perinatally infected infants have also been noted to have impaired specific cell-mediated immunity as assessed by the lymphocyte transformation response to CMV antigen (LTR).[77–80] This test measures only the recognition, not the effector function, of T-lymphocytes and does not require other techniques like the use of syngeneic target cells. Another defect consistently observed is the inability of the lymphocytes of these infants to induce interferon production in vitro when challenged with CMV antigens. The impairments are not a reflection of a generalized disturbance, since it is restricted to a blastogenic response to CMV and is highly virus specific. CMV-infected patients who have antibodies to herpes simplex virus, for example, have a normal blastogenic response to this virus. Infants with impaired LTRs respond normally to both killed and live vaccines. The impairment has no relation to the clinical presentation and outcome, but it is more intense and longer lasting in patients with symptomatic CMV infection. As patients grow older, the impairment disappears together with viral replication. It is possible that subtle alterations of host defense mechanisms could contribute to disease, in conjunction with persistent viral replication.

NATURE OF MATERNAL INFECTION

The nature of the maternal infection is a major pathogenetic factor for congenital CMV infection. Primary infections are more likely to be transmitted to the fetus and are likely to cause more fetal injury than recurrent infections.[81] Intrauterine transmission following primary infection occurs in approximately 30 to 40 percent of cases. Current information suggests that gestational age has no apparent influence on the risk of transmission of CMV in utero. However, several studies suggest that infection at an earlier gestational age produces the worst outcome.

Congenital infection may also result from recurrences of infection. A recurrence is used here to represent either reactivation of infection or reinfection with the same or a different strain of CMV during pregnancy. Evidence to date indicates that despite the inability of maternal immunity to prevent transmission of this virus to the fetus, congenital infections that result from recurrent infections are less likely to affect the offspring than those resulting from primary infections.[81] The risk of congenital CMV infection resulting from a recurrence of infection during pregnancy ranges from a high of 1.5 percent for an American population of low socioeconomic background to 0.19 percent for women of middle or upper socioeconomic extraction in the United States or from Britain and Sweden.[13,70,82]

In recurrent infection, it is likely that preexisting immunity partially inhibits the occurrence of viremia. Maternal IgG antibodies are transmitted to the fetus but their precise role has not been elucidated. It is conceivable that cellular immunity may be more important than humoral immunity.

PERINATAL INFECTION

Naturally acquired perinatal CMV infections result from exposure to infected maternal genital secretions at birth or to breast milk during the first months of postnatal life. The presence of CMV in these two sites may be the result of either primary or recurrent maternal infection. Iatrogenic CMV infections are acquired predominantly from transfusions of blood or blood products and breast milk from CMV-infected donors. Exposure to CMV in the maternal genital tract has resulted in a 30 to 50 percent rate of perinatal infection. During delivery the infant is literally bathed in genital secretions that may contain high titers of CMV. The transmission from mother to infant via breast milk occurs in 30 to 70 percent if nursing lasts for over 1 month. Following ingestion, CMV infection is presumably established at a mucosal surface (buccal, pharyngeal, or esophageal mucosa) or in the salivary glands for which CMV is known to have a special tropism.

Transmission of CMV by blood transfusion is more likely to occur when larger quantities of blood are transfused. The failure to isolate CMV from the blood or blood elements of seropositive healthy blood donors suggests that the virus exists in a latent state, presumably within leukocytes. It has been suggested that following transfusion, when infected cells encounter the allogeneic stimulus, CMV becomes reactivated.

CLINICAL MANIFESTATIONS

CONGENITAL INFECTION

Symptomatic infection

Acute Manifestations. Cytomegalic inclusion disease, or CID, is characterized by involvement of multiple organs, in particular the reticuloendothelial and central nervous system (CNS), with or without ocular and auditory damage. Weller and Hanshaw defined the abnormalities found most frequently in infants with symptomatic congenital infection as hepatomegaly, splenomegaly, microcephaly, jaundice, and petechiae.[83] As illustrated in Table 85-1, a combination of petechiae, hepatosplenomegaly, and jaundice is the most frequently noted presentation. In addition, the magnitude of the prenatal insult is reflected in the occurrence of

Table 85-1. Clinical and Laboratory Findings in 106 Infants with Symptomatic Congenital CMV Infection in the Newborn Period*

Abnormality	Positive/Total Examined (%)
Prematurity (<38 wk)	36/106 (34)
Small for gestational use	53/106 (50)
Petechiae	80/106 (76)
Jaundice	69/103 (67)
Hepatosplenomegaly	63/105 (60)
Purpura	14/105 (13)
Neurologic findings	
One or more of the following	72/106 (68)
Microcephaly	54/102 (53)
Lethargy/hypotonia	28/104 (27)
Poor suck	20/103 (19)
Seizures	7/105 (7)
Elevated alanine aminotransferase (>80U/L)	46/58 (83)
Thrombocytopenia	
$<100 \times 10^3/mm^3$	62/81 (77)
$<50 \times 10^3/mm^3$	43/81 (53)
Conjugated hyperbilirubinemia	
Direct serum bilirubin >4 mg/dL	47/68 (69)
Hemolysis	37/72 (51)
Increased cerebrospinal fluid protein (>120 mg/dL)†	24/52 (46)

* From Boppana S et al. Symptomatic congenital cytomegalovirus infection: neonatal morbidity and mortality. *Pediatr Infect Dis J* 11:93–99, 1992, with permission.[87]

† Determinations in the first week of life.

microcephaly with or without cerebral calcification, intrauterine growth retardation, and prematurity.[84] Inguinal hernia in males and chorioretinitis with or without optic atrophy are less common. Occasionally clinical findings include hydrocephalus, hemolytic anemia, and pneumonitis. Among the most severely affected infants, mortality may be as high as 30 percent. Most deaths occur in the neonatal period. Mortality during the neonatal period is usually owing to multiorgan disease with severe hepatic dysfunction, bleeding, disseminated intravascular coagulation, and secondary bacterial infections. When death occurs after the first month but during the first year, it is usually owing to progressive liver disease with severe failure to thrive. Death after the first year is usually restricted to the severely neurologically handicapped children and is owing to malnutrition, aspiration pneumonia, and overwhelming infections.

Hepatomegaly. This sign, along with that of splenomegaly, is probably the most common abnormality found in the newborn period in infants born with symptomatic congenital CMV infection. Liver function tests are often abnormal but usually not markedly so. The persistence of hepatomegaly is variable. In some infants liver enlargement disappears by the age of 2 months. In others, significant enlargement persists throughout the first year of life. However, massive hepatomegaly extending beyond the first 12 months of life is uncharacteristic of CID.

Splenomegaly. Enlargement of the spleen is especially frequent in congenital CMV infections. It may be the only abnormality present at birth. In some instances splenomegaly and a petechial rash coexist as the only manifestations of the disease. Occasionally the enlargement is such that the spleen may be felt 10 to 15 cm below the costal margin. Splenomegaly usually persists longer than hepatomegaly.

Jaundice. Jaundice is a common manifestation of CID. The pattern of hyperbilirubinema may take several forms, ranging from high levels on the first day to undetectable jaundice on the first day with gradual elevation of the bilirubin level to clinically apparent jaundice. In some instances jaundice is a transient phenomenon, beginning on the first day and disappearing by the end of the first week. More often, however, it tends to persist beyond the time of physiologic jaundice. Occasionally, transient jaundice may occur in early infancy with pronounced elevation of bilirubin levels during the third month. Bilirubin levels are high in both the direct and indirect components. Characteristically, the direct component increases after the first few days of life and may constitute as much as 50 percent of the total bilirubin level. It is rare for the indirect bilirubin component to rise high enough to require exchange transfusion, but this has been reported.

Petechiae and Purpura. There is evidence that CMV has a direct effect on the megakaryocytes of the bone marrow that results in a depression of the platelets and a localized or generalized petechial rash. In some patients the rash is purpuric in character, not unlike that observed in the expanded rubella syndrome. Unlike the latter infection, however, pinpoint petechiae are a more common manifestation of congenital CMV infection. The rash usually appears within a few hours of birth; it may be transient, disappearing within 48 h. The petechiae may be the only clinical manifestation of CMV infection. More often, however, enlargement of the liver and spleen is associated. The petechiae may persist for weeks after birth. Crying, coughing, the application of a tourniquet, a lumbar puncture, or restraints of any kind may result in the appearance of petechiae even months after birth. Platelet counts in the first week of life range from less than 10,000 to 125,000, with a majority in the 20,000 to 60,000 range. Some infants with petechial rashes do not have associated thrombocytopenia.

Microcephaly. Microcephaly, usually defined as a head circumference of less than the fifth percentile occurs in approximately 50 percent of patients with symptomatic congenital infection. Not all infants remain microcephalic. This is especially true if the head measurement is close to the fifth percentile in an infant of low birth weight. If intracranial calcifications are present, the growth of the brain is invariably impaired.

Ocular Defects. The principal abnormality related to the eye in CMV infection is chorioretinitis, with strabismus and optic atrophy being uncommon. Microphthalmia, cataracts, retinal necrosis and calcification, blindness, anterior chamber and optic disk malformations, and pupillary membrane vestige have also been described in association with generalized congenital CID. Chorioretinitis occurs in approximately 14 percent of infants born with symptomatic congenital infection. CMV chorioretinitis cannot be differentiated from the lesions produced by toxoplasmosis on the basis of location or appearance. Both *Toxoplasma gondii* and cytomegalovirus can induce central retinal lesions. Chorioretinitis caused by CMV differs from that caused by toxoplasmosis in that it rarely progresses postnatally, becoming inactive in early infancy.

Pneumonitis. Pneumonitis, a common clinical manifestation of CMV infection following bone marrow and renal transplant in adults, is not usually a part of the clinical presentation of congenital CMV infection in newborn infants. In the author's experience, diffuse interstitial pneumonitis occurs in less than 1 percent of congenitally infected infants, even when the most severely affected cases are considered. CMV-associated pneumonitis is more likely to develop in infants with perinatally acquired CMV infections.

Deafness. Sensorineural deafness is the most common handicap caused by congenital CMV infection. Medearis was the first investigator to call attention to the presence of deafness in symptomatic congenitally infected infants.[85] Subsequent reports confirmed this association and provided evidence that CMV can also cause sensorineural hearing loss in children with subclinical infection.[86]

Because hearing is not commonly assessed within the first month of life, it is difficult to say how many congenitally infected infants, whether symptomatic or not, are born with hearing impairments. This handicap, however, becomes significant in infancy and early childhood. In general, the frequency and severity of the hearing impairment is worse in patients with symptomatic infection.[84] Of 104 surviving patients with symptomatic CMV infection we have prospectively followed over the past 20 years, 100 have had adequate audiometric evaluations and 58 of them (58%) suffer from some degree of hearing impairment.[84] Among the 330 patients with subclinical infection, 299 have received at least one adequate audiometric evaluation and 22 (7.4%) manifest some degree of hearing loss. The sensorineural hearing loss is bilateral in over half the cases and of significant magnitude (50 to 100 dB) to produce serious difficulties with verbal communication and learning.

Long-Term Outcome. The long-term clinical manifestations of symptomatic congenital CMV infection are highly variable. It is clear that the infection is usually not recognized in infants, espe-

Table 85-2. Sequelae in Children after Congenital CMV Infection*

Sequelae	Percent Symptomatic (No.)	Percent Asymptomatic (No.)
Sensorineural hearing loss	58 (58/100)	7.4 (22/299)
Bilateral hearing loss	37 (37/100)	2.7 (8/299)
Speech threshold moderate to profound (60–90 dB)†	27 (27/100)	1.7 (5/299)
Chorioretinitis	20.4 (19/93)	2.5 (7/281)
IQ < 70	55 (33/60)	3.7 (6/159)
Microcephaly, seizures or paralysis	51.9 (54/104)	2.7 (9/330)
Microcephaly	37.5 (39/104)	1.8 (6/330)
Seizures	23.1 (24/104)	0.9 (3/330)
Paresis/paralysis	12.5 (13/104)	0 (0/330)
Death‡	5.8 (6/104)	0.3 (1/330)

* Adapted from Pass RR, Fowler KB and Boppana S. Progress in cytomegalovirus research. In Landini MP (ed), *Proceedings of the Third International Cytomegalovirus Workshop*, Bologna, Italy, June 1991. London, Excerpta Medica, 1991, pp. 3–10.[88]
† For the ear with better hearing.
‡ After newborn period

cially when it is marked by minor signs such as failure to thrive, mild splenomegaly, and neonatal jaundice. In some cases, psychomotor retardation, neurologic dysfunction, hearing loss, and other delayed complications may take years to identify. The medical significance of congenital CMV derives primarily from the adverse effects that this infection has on the developmental potential of children. The likelihood of survival with normal intellect and hearing following symptomatic congenital CMV infection is small. The most common long-term complications are hearing loss, mental retardation, microcephaly, chorioretinitis, optic atrophy, seizures, paraparesis, diplegia, language delay, and learning disabilities (Table 85-2).

Asymptomatic infection

As indicated in the previous section, nearly 90 percent of infants with congenital CMV infections have no early clinical manifestations and their long-term outcome is much better. Nevertheless, anywhere from 5 percent to perhaps as many as 15 percent, are at risk for developing a multitude of developmental abnormalities, such as sensorineural hearing loss, microcephaly, motor defects such as spastic diplegia or quadriplegia, mental retardation, chorioretinitis, and dental defects. These abnormalities usually become apparent within the first 2 years of life. Table 85-2 illustrates results based on our prospective longitudinal study of 330 patients with asymptomatic congenital infection and followed by using serial clinical, psychometric, audiometric, and visual assessments.[88] Follow-up studies of patients with inapparent congenital CMV infection have also been done by Kumar et al., Saigal et al., Melish and Hanshaw, and Pearl et al.[89–92] In general their findings resemble the results of our study presented in Table 85-2.

In summary, these observations underscore the need for longitudinal follow up of patients with congenital CMV infection regardless of its clinical presentation at the outset. Careful assessments of perceptual functions (hearing, visual acuity), psychomotor development, and learning abilities must be made in order to recognize the full impact of CMV. With early identification of a problem, corrective measures can be instituted to reduce psychosocial and learning problems.

PERINATAL INFECTION

In order to establish the diagnosis of perinatal CMV infection, one must first exclude congenital infection by showing absence of viral excretion during the first 2 weeks of life. The incubation period of perinatal CMV infection ranges between 4 and 12 weeks. Although the quantity of virus excreted by infants with perinatal infection is less than that seen with intrauterine acquisition, the infection is also of a chronic nature, with viral excretion persisting for years. The vast majority of otherwise healthy infants with naturally acquired perinatal infections remain asymptomatic and the infection does not appear to have an adverse effect on growth, perceptual functions, or motor or psychosocial development.

CMV has been incriminated as a cause of pneumonitis in infants less than 4 months of age.[85,93,94] CMV-associated pneumonitis is clinically and radiographically indistinguishable from other causes of afebrile pneumonia in this age group.

In premature and sick term infants, naturally acquired CMV infection may pose a greater risk. Yeager et al. found that premature infants weighing less than 1500 g at birth who acquired CMV from a maternal source often developed hepatosplenomegaly, neutropenia, lymphocytosis, and thrombocytopenia coinciding with the onset of virus excretion.[95] Frequently, these patients required longer treatment with oxygen. In a later prospective study, Paryani et al. suggested that there may be a propensity for an increased incidence of neuromuscular impairments, particularly in premature infants with onset of CMV excretion during the first 2 months of life. However, sensorineural hearing loss, chorioretinitis, and microcephaly occurred with similar frequency in both groups.

Transfusion-acquired perinatal CMV infection can cause significant morbidity and mortality, particularly in premature infants with a birth weight of less than 1500 g born to CMV seronegative mothers.[58–62] The syndrome of posttransfusion CMV infection in premature newborn infants has been characterized by Ballard and coworkers and consists of deterioration of respiratory function, hepatosplenomegaly, unusual gray pallor with disturbing septic appearance, both an atypical and absolute lymphocytosis, thrombocytopenia, and hemolytic anemia.[96] The syndrome was more severe in low-birth weight infants and occurred approximately 4 to 12 weeks posttransfusion, at a time when the infants were progressing satisfactorily. Although the course of the disease was generally self-limited (lasting 2–3 weeks), death occurred in 20 percent of the sick infants. Subsequent work by Yeager and Adler has confirmed these observations.[48,61] Yeager demonstrated that the risk of infection is related to the serologic status of the donor and that these infections could be prevented by transfusing seronegative newborns with blood from seronegative donors.

TREATMENT AND PREVENTION

ANTIVIRAL THERAPY

There is as yet no safe, effective treatment for symptomatic congenital CMV infection. Therapeutic trials with systematically administered antiviral agents have yielded little or no clinical benefit and have been hampered by moderate to severe toxicity.[97,98] The most encouraging results have been obtained with Ganciclovir in a Phase II study that compared dosages of 8 and 12 mg/kg daily in divided doses at 12-hour intervals for 6 weeks. A total of 47 infants with symptomatic congenital CMV infection were evaluated. In 19 percent of these patients, therapy was discontinued because of toxicity. Absolute neutropenia (≥500 mm^3) was the most common adverse experience (34%). Other events which occurred in one patient each included necrotizing enterocolitis, diarrhea, elevated liver function tests, and anemia. Quantitative excretion of CMV in the urine decreased; however, after cessation of therapy, viruria returned to pretreatment levels. The most encouraging result is that 3 of 20 patients with hearing loss at baseline, had normal hearing on follow up. However, normal hearing which became abnormal occurred in 11 babies. A controlled clinical trial of symptomatic congenital CMV infection with Ganciclovir at 12 mg/kg/day is now underway. Confounding factors to verify clinical efficacy are the wide spectrum of disease resulting from symptomatic congenital CMV infection, the unpredictable natural course of the disease, and the fact that many patients incur irreversible damage before birth.

VACCINES

Two live attenuated vaccines have undergone efficacy trials in both immune and susceptible normal hosts and renal transplant recipients.[99,100] Immunization of susceptible kidney transplant recipients with Towne strain (live attenuated) CMV vaccine significantly reduced the morbidity of primary CMV infection although it did not prevent acquisition of infection. No evidence of reactivation of vaccine virus was found when the patients were immunosuppressed.[101] An important objective for the development of a CMV vaccine is to prevent the serious consequences of congenital infection. A candidate vaccine should be able to prevent primary infection in pregnant women without inducing latent infection. In a very small study of 22 young females immunized with the AD-169 attenuated strain followed up for 8 years, antibody and lymphocyte antigenic responses induced by the vaccine disappeared in 50 percent of the cases. In eight women immunized at different intervals prior to pregnancy, congenital infection was not detected.[102] Although the AD-169 and the Towne strain vaccines have not been shown to reactivate, the possibility that reactivations might occur during pregnancy with transmission to the fetus raises concern about their use, even in vaccine trials.

A more attractive approach is to use a subunit vaccine that contains surface glycoproteins. The best candidate is glycoprotein gB because it is the most abundant protein complex of the viral envelope, is exposed on the surface of infected cells and contains the majority of viral neutralizing epitopes. A glycoprotein gB vaccine formulation has been shown to be immunogenic in a mouse model. Phase I–II trials in humans are now underway and preliminary results have demonstrated both humoral and cell mediated immune response with minimal or no side effects. We must now await further studies on the protective efficacy of such subunit vaccines.

PREVENTION OF CONGENITAL INFECTION

CMV is not very contagious and its horizontal transmission requires close direct contact with infected material, namely, secretions that contain the virus and, less likely, fomites. With the exception of a few small studies that were designed to prevent infection via blood and blood products and grafted organs, no broad-based strategies for preventing the transmission of this virus have been tested. Although there are still no effective means of preventing congenital CMV infection, or most perinatally acquired CMV infections, a few common sense recommendations can be made.

An average of 2 percent of susceptible pregnant women acquire CMV infection during pregnancy in the United States; the majority have no symptoms and only 40 percent of the episodes result in fetal infection. With no effective antiviral therapy and a low risk of fetal morbidity, serologic screening of pregnant women searching for primary CMV infections during pregnancy is of limited value.

Primary CMV infection should be suspected in pregnant women with symptoms compatible with a heterophil-negative mononucleosis-like syndrome. At present the sensitivity of intrauterine diagnosis before the 22nd week of gestation is only 50 percent.[103–107] Thus, there is inadequate information to serve as a basis for recommendations regarding termination of pregnancy after a primary CMV infection. Similarly, there is no information regarding how long conception should be delayed after primary infection.

The data on which to base recommendations for prevention of congenital CMV infection after recurrent maternal infection are even more inadequate.[73,108–111] At present, there are no techniques for identifying women with reactivation of CMV that result in intrauterine transmission. Since the risk of transmission is very low and the risk of fetal disease even lower, women known to be seropositive before conception do not need to be virologically or serologically tested, nor do they need to be unduly worried about the very low risk of transmitting the virus to the fetus.

The principal sources of CMV infection among women of childbearing age are exposure to children excreting CMV and sexual contacts. Sexual transmission of CMV can probably be prevented by barrier methods (condoms, spermicides) that reduce the transmission of more common sexually transmitted infections, although no data have been published to specifically assess the effectiveness of such methods for CMV. Concerning the risk from exposure to children, those at greatest risk are susceptible pregnant mothers of CMV-infected children who attend day care centers. Hand washing and simple hygienic measures that are routine for hospital care can be recommended, but it is unrealistic to expect many mothers to comply.

Although hospital workers do not appear to be at increased risk for CMV infection, personnel who work in day care centers certainly are. In the hospital, vigorous adherence to routine infection control procedures such as hand washing and gloving should make nonparenteral acquisition of CMV less likely than in the community. Since the majority of patients who shed CMV are asymptomatic and unrecognized, universal precautions should be emphasized to prevent transmission from unrecognized infected patients as well as from known CMV-excreting patients. In the daycare setting, where hygiene is difficult at best, preventive measures may be more difficult to implement. Although there is still debate about the need for routine screening of female hospital personnel and daycare workers, we believe it should be recommended for potentially childbearing women whose occupation exposes them to CMV. Those found seropositive can be strongly reassured. Those found to be serosusceptible should be provided with information and reassured that common sense measures, such as hand washing and avoiding contact with secretions, should reduce the risk of acquisition of CMV. Attempts to identify all CMV-excreting patients or children in the workplace so that seronegative workers can avoid contact with them is totally unreasonable.

NEONATAL HERPES SIMPLEX VIRUS INFECTIONS

HISTORY

Infections caused by herpes simplex viruses (HSV) have been recognized since the era of the ancient Greeks. Greek scholars defined the word *herpes* to mean to creep or crawl in reference to the visualized skin lesions. The Greek historian Herodotus associated mouth ulcers and lip vesicles with fever and called this event *herpes febriles*.[112] Genital herpetic infections were first described by a physician to the eighteenth century French court, Astruc.[113] Over the ensuing two centuries, the infectious nature of HSV was delineated. The transmissibility of these viruses was unequivocally established by passage of virus from lip and genital lesions of humans to either the cornea or the scarified skin of the rabbit.[114]

Only 50 years ago, the first written descriptions of neonatal HSV infections were attributed nearly simultaneously to Hass, when he described the histopathologic findings of a fatal case, and to Batignani, who described a newborn child with HSV keratitis.[115,116] Subsequently, histopathologic descriptions of the disease demonstrated a broad spectrum of involvement in infants.

In the mid 1960s, Nahmias and Dowdle demonstrated two antigenic types of HSV.[117] The differentiation of HSV into two types resulted in the development of viral typing methods, which were critical in clarifying the epidemiology of these infections. Herpes simplex virus infections "above the belt," primarily of the lip and oropharynx, were found in most cases to be caused by HSV-1. Those infections "below the belt," particularly genital infections, were usually caused by HSV-2. With the finding that both genital herpes infections and neonatal HSV infections were most often caused by HSV-2, a natural cause-and-effect relationship developed between these two disease entities. This causal relationship was strengthened by the finding of viral excretion in the maternal genital tract at the time of delivery, suggesting that acquisition of the virus by the infant occurs by contact with infected genital secretions during birth.

Over the past 20 years, our knowledge of the epidemiology, natural history, and pathogenesis of neonatal HSV infections has expanded greatly (see Chapter 21). The development of antiviral therapy represents a significant advance in the management of infected children, providing the opportunity to decrease mortality and improve the morbidity associated with these infections. Of all the herpesvirus infections, neonatal HSV infection represents the one that should be most amenable to prevention and treatment because it is acquired most often at birth rather than early in gestation. As our knowledge of the epidemiology of HSV infections has increased, it has become apparent that there are modes of infection other than contact with infected maternal genital secretions during delivery. Postnatal acquisition of HSV-1 has been documented from nonmaternal sources. These issues, as well as the management of hospital personnel with HSV infections, will be the focus of this section. The changing presentation of neonatal HSV infection, particularly the increasing difficulty of diagnosing infection, and the success of antiviral therapy, will be stressed.

EPIDEMIOLOGY OF NEONATAL HSV INFECTION

NATURE OF INFECTION

Transmission of HSV most often occurs in association with intimate, personal contact, as reviewed.[118] Virus must come in contact with mucosal surfaces or the abraded skin of a susceptible individual for infection to be initiated. After viral replication at the site of infection, either an intact virion or the nucleocapsid is transported by neurons to the ganglia where latency is established. Infection with HSV-1, generally limited to the oropharynx, can be transmitted by respiratory droplets or through direct contact of a susceptible individual with infected secretions (such as virus-containing labial vesicular fluid). Acquisition often occurs during childhood.

Primary HSV-1 infection in the young child is usually asymptomatic. If present, clinical illness is manifested by gingivostomatitis. Primary infection in young adults has been associated with pharyngitis and with a mononucleosis-like syndrome. Like other herpesvirus infections, seroprevalence studies have demonstrated that acquisition of HSV-1 infection is related to socioeconomic factors. Antibodies, indicative of past infection, are found early in life among individuals of lower socioeconomic groups and are presumed to be the consequence of crowded living conditions that provide a greater opportunity for direct contact with infected individuals.

As many as 75 to 90 percent of individuals from lower socioeconomic populations develop antibodies by the end of the first decade of life. In comparison, in middle and upper socioeconomic groups only 30 to 40 percent are seropositive by the middle of the second decade of life.[119–122] A declining seroprevalence of HSV-1 may account, in part, for the increased clinical awareness of HSV-2 infections, since HSV-1 antibodies may be partially protective against type 2 infection.[123,124]

Because infections with HSV type 2 are usually acquired through sexual contact, antibodies to this virus are rarely found until adolescence. Thereafter, progressive increase in seroprevalence of HSV type 2 develops in all populations.[125] The risk of acquisition of infection with HSV-2 appears related to both socioeconomic factors and the number of sexual partners. Utilizing nonspecific serologic assays, as many as 50 to 60 percent of lower socioeconomic populations have antibodies to HSV-2. In contrast, 10 to 20 percent of individuals in higher socioeconomic groups are seropositive.[126,127] Utilizing a type-specific assay for HSV-2 (glycoprotein (g) G-2), antibodies were identified in 35 percent of middle-class women receiving care through an Atlanta health maintenance organization.[128] Similarly, there are differences in seroprevalence between blacks and Caucasians of childbearing age, 65 versus 35 percent overall, respectively.[129]

MATERNAL INFECTION

The epidemiology and clinical nature of genital HSV infection do not appear to be greatly influenced by pregnancy (see Chapter 21). Infection during gestation can manifest in a variety of ways. The most serious but fortunately uncommon problem encountered with HSV infections during pregnancy is that of widely disseminated disease. Infection has been documented to involve multiple visceral sites, in addition to cutaneous dissemination.[130–135] In a limited number of cases, dissemination after primary oropharyngeal or genital infection has led to such severe manifestations of disease as necrotizing hepatitis with or without thrombocytopenia, leukopenia, disseminated intravascular coagulopathy, and encephalitis. Although only a small number of patients have suffered from disseminated infection, the mortality among these pregnant women is reported to be greater than 50 percent. Fetal deaths have also occurred in more than 50 percent of cases, although mortality did not necessarily correlate with the death of the mother. Surviving fetuses were delivered by cesarean section either during the acute illness or at term and none had evidence of neonatal HSV infection.

Localized genital infection is the most common form of HSV infection during pregnancy. Overall, prospective investigations utilizing cytologic and virologic screening indicate that genital herpes occurs with a frequency of about 1 percent at any time during gestation.[136] Most of these infections are recurrent, although a few are primary. Those factors that influence the frequency of both primary and recurrent infection in pregnancy are not well defined.

Maternal primary infection prior to 20 weeks gestation has been associated with spontaneous abortion.[137,138] Although the original estimate of spontaneous abortion following a symptomatic primary infection during gestation was thought to be as high as 25 percent, it is likely that this calculation is erroneously high because of the very small number of women followed. Unfortunately, precise data, indicating the true risk of spontaneous abortion following primary infection during gestation, are not available. Infection that develops later in gestation was not associated with the termination of pregnancy.[138–140]

The frequency of HSV recurrences during gestation should be of concern for women with a known history of infection. Transmission of infection to the fetus is most frequently related to the actual shedding of virus at the time of delivery. Since HSV infection of the fetus is usually the consequence of contact with infected maternal genital secretions at the time of delivery, the determination of viral excretion at this time is of utmost importance. The actual incidence of viral excretion at delivery ranges from 0.39 to 1.0 percent.[118,136,141–145] Utilizing polymerase chain reaction (PCR) detection of viral DNA, the prevalence of viral shedding is even higher.[146] Several prospective studies have evaluated the frequency and nature of viral shedding in pregnant women with a known history of genital herpes. In a predominantly white, middle-class population, documented recurrent infection occurred in 84 percent of pregnant women.[143] Moreover, asymptomatic viral shedding occurred in at least 12 percent of the recurrent episodes. Viral shedding from the cervix occurred in 0.56 percent of symptomatic and 0.66 percent of asymptomatic infections, data similar to the nonpregnant state.[142,144] The incidence of cervical shedding in asymptomatic pregnant women has been reported to be as high as 3 percent.[140] However, the observed rate of shedding among asymptomatic pregnant women has varied more than that among nonpregnant women (0.2–7.4 percent), depending on the study population and trial design.[140,142,144,147–150] Overall, these data indicate that the frequency of cervical shedding is low, rendering the risk of transmission of virus to the infant similarly low when the infection is recurrent in nature.[136] The frequency of shedding does not appear to vary by trimester during gestation.[140,151] Overall, no increased incidence of premature onset of labor is apparent in these prospective studies. Regardless, given the high seroprevalence of infection, a significant degree of protection for the fetus must exist or else the incidence of neonatal disease should be significantly higher. Importantly, most infants who develop neonatal disease are born to women who are completely asymptomatic at the time of delivery and have neither a past history of genital herpes nor a sexual partner reporting a genital vesicular rash.[136,149,151,152] These women account for 60 to 80 percent of all women whose infected children develop infection.

Only 27 percent of women delivering children who developed neonatal HSV infection have had either a history of or evidence of recurrent lesions indicative of HSV infection during the current pregnancy.[152] Furthermore, only half of these women reported genital HSV infection in their sexual partners. The majority of women were without signs or symptoms of genital herpetic infection.

FACTORS THAT INFLUENCE TRANSMISSION OF INFECTION TO THE FETUS

The type of maternal genital infection at the time of delivery influences the incidence of neonatal herpes.[145] The duration and quantity of viral excretion and the time to total healing vary with primary, initial (first episode at the nonprimary site) and recurrent (HSV-1 and -2) maternal genital infection (See Chapter 21).[153,154] Primary infection is associated with larger quantities of virus replicating in the genital tract ($>10^6$ viral particles/0.2 mL of inoculum) and a period of viral excretion which may persist for an average of 3 weeks. In contrast, virus is shed for an average of only 2 to 5 days and at lower concentrations (approx 10^2–10^3/0.2 mL of inoculum) in women with recurrent genital infection. The difference in the natural history of primary and recurrent disease is likely a major factor that influences the frequency of transmission and, perhaps, the severity of neonatal disease.

Paralleling the type of maternal infection, the mother's antibody status to HSV at delivery appears to be an additional factor that also influences the severity of infection as well as the likelihood of transmission. Transplacental maternal neutralizing antibodies appear to have a protective, or at least an ameliorative, effect on acquisition of infection for babies inadvertently exposed to virus.[141,155,156] Maternal primary infection late in gestation may not result in significant passage of maternal antibodies across the placenta to the fetus. The distinction between symptomatic and asymptomatic disease whether primary, initial, or recurrent remains poorly defined at present in relation to the risks of transmission of infection to the infant.

The duration of ruptured membranes is also a risk factor for acquisition of neonatal infection. Observations by Nahmias and colleagues indicate that prolonged rupture of membranes (>6 hours) increases the risk of acquisition of virus, probably the consequence of ascending infection from the cervix.[136,138] Based on this observation, it is recommended that women with active genital lesions at the time of onset of labor be delivered by cesarean section, as discussed in the following. There may be benefits associated with cesarean section beyond 6 hours of ruptured membranes, but this has not been proven at the present time. It should be recognized that infection of the newborn has occurred in spite of delivery by cesarean section.[152,157]

Fetal scalp monitors can be a site of inoculation of virus, and may increase the risk of neonatal HSV infection.[158,159] Such devices are contraindicated in women with a history of recurrent genital HSV infections.

INCIDENCE OF NEWBORN INFECTION

The estimated incidence of neonatal HSV infection is approximately 1 in 2000 to 1 in 5000 deliveries per year.[136] A progressive increase in the number of cases of neonatal HSV infection has been noted in some areas with rates approaching 1 in 1500 deliveries (see Chapter 21).[160] Neonatal HSV infection occurs far less frequently than genital HSV infections in the adult childbearing population. Several countries do not appear to recognize a significant number of cases of neonatal HSV in spite of the high prevalence of antibodies to HSV-2. Serologic studies in central Africa indicate that women have a high frequency of antibodies to HSV-2, but the first case of neonatal herpes was reported only relatively recently.[161,162] The United Kingdom presents a similar dilemma. Genital herpetic infection is relatively common in the United Kingdom, but very few cases of neonatal HSV infection are recognized in that country. This may reflect a low number of primary HSV infections in pregnant women. Overall, the United States has approximately 4 million deliveries a year and an estimated 2500 to 5000 cases of neonatal infection.

TIME OF TRANSMISSION OF INFECTION

Herpes simplex virus infection of the newborn can be acquired at one of three times: in utero, intrapartum, or postnatally. The mother is the source of infection for the first two routes of transmission. For postnatal acquisition of HSV infection, the mother may be the source of infection from a genital or nongenital site, or other environmental or patient sources of virus can lead to infection of the child. Nevertheless, a maternal source should be suspected when herpetic lesions are discovered promptly after the birth or when the baby's illness is caused by HSV-2. Although intrapartum transmission accounts for 80 to 90 percent of cases, the other two routes must be recognized and identified in a child with suspect disease for both public health and prognostic purposes.

Although it was originally presumed that intrauterine infection resulted in either a totally normal baby or premature termination of gestation, intrauterine acquisition of infection can lead to the clinical symptomatology of congenital infection.[138,142,163–165] Utilizing stringent diagnostic criteria (namely, identification of infected babies within the first 48 hours of life who have virologic confirmation of infection) and excluding other pathogens with similar clinical findings such as congenital cytomegalovirus infection, rubella, syphilis, or toxoplasmosis, over 100 babies have been identified in the world's literature to date with symptomatic congenital disease.[165] The manifestations of disease in this group of children range from significant neurologic abnormalities to simply the presence of skin vesicles at the time of delivery.

Intrauterine infection can occur as a consequence of either transplacental or ascending infection. Examination of the placenta in cases of neonatal herpes thought to be the consequence of in utero transmission has helped to clarify the route of transmission. A placenta showing evidence of necrosis and inclusions in the trophoblasts suggests a transplacental route of infection and can result in a baby with hydraencephaly at birth or may be associated with spontaneous abortion following intrauterine herpes simplex viremia.[166–168] Virus has been isolated from the products of conception in such circumstances.[166] Histopathologic evidence of chorioamnionitis, suggestive of ascending infection, has been identified as an alternative route for in utero infection as compared with transplacental spread.

Risk factors associated with intrauterine transmission are not known. However, both primary and recurrent maternal infection can result in infection of the fetus in utero. Although it might be convenient to assume that only primary maternal infection is associated with transmission of virus in utero, it has been documented that women with recurrent genital infection can transmit HSV to the fetus as well, leading to disease.

The second, and most common, route of infection is that of intrapartum contact of the fetus with infected maternal genital secretions. Approximately 80 to 90 percent of infected babies acquire HSV infection by this route. Those factors that favor intrapartum transmission of infection have been described in the preceding text.

The third route of transmission is postnatal acquisition. Even though HSV-1 has been associated with genital lesions, postnatal transmission of HSV has been increasingly suggested because 15 to 20 percent of neonatal HSV infections are caused by this virus type.[136]

In fact, more recent data from the National Institutes of Allergy and Infectious Diseases (NIAID), Collaborative Antiviral Study Group indicate that the proportion of babies with neonatal herpes simplex infections owing to HSV-1 has increased to nearly 30 percent.[152] This observation, in light of the recognition that genital HSV-1 infections appear to account for only approximately 5 to 15 percent of all genital HSV infections, creates greater concern for postnatal acquisition of infection. However, data recently suggest an increasing number of genital herpes cases caused by HSV-1 in the United States, as occurs in Japan.

Relatives and hospital personnel with orolabial herpes may be a reservoir of virus for transmission to the newborn. The recent documentation of postnatal transmission of HSV has focused attention on such sources of virus for neonatal infection.[169–176] Postnatal transmission from mother to child has been documented. Maternal–infant postpartum transmission has been reported as a consequence of nursing on an infected breast.[172–175] Furthermore, father-to-baby transmission has been documented.[176]

Many individuals asymptomatically excrete HSV from the oropharynx and, therefore, represent a potential source of infection for the newborn. The occurrence of fever blisters in various groups of adults has ranged from 16 to 46 percent.[177,178] Population studies in two hospitals indicated that 15 to 34 percent of hospital personnel had a past history of nongenital herpetic lesions.[179–181] In both hospitals surveyed, at least 1 in 100 individuals had a recurrent cold sore each week. No cases of neonatal HSV infection were documented in these nurseries.[179,182] However, the demonstration in other studies of identical viruses (utilizing restriction endonuclease analyses of viral DNA) in babies with different mothers leaves little doubt of the possibility of spread of virus in a high-risk nursery.[170,171] The sources of virus and vectors for transmission have been inadequately studied. The potential legal implications for HSV infections acquired in a nursery are obvious. There is significant variation in the United States regarding both the concern for nosocomial transmission of infection in the hospital as well as infection control policies for its prevention.

Various individuals and committees have recommended that personnel with cold sores not work in the nursery. If such a policy were followed, the estimated medical costs would be nearly 20 million dollars annually in the United States if calculated just on the basis of estimates of lost work days.[181] Likely, vigorous hand washing procedures and continuing education of personnel in newborn nurseries has helped contribute to the low frequency of transmission in this environment. The existence of a herpetic whitlow in staff providing patient care should preclude direct patient contact, irrespective of nursing unit.

IMMUNOLOGIC RESPONSE TO HSV INFECTION

The host response to HSV in newborns must be distinguished from that of older individuals. Impairment of host defense mechanisms has been implicated as a cause of the increased severity of some infectious agents in the fetus and the newborn. Factors that must be considered in defining host response include the mode of transmission of the agent (viremia vs mucocutaneous infection), time of acquisition of infection, and the potential of increased virulence of certain strains, although this last point remains purely speculative. Two broad issues are of relevance: protection of the fetus by transplacental antibodies and definition of host response of the newborn.

Host responses to HSV infection influence the likelihood of disease, severity of infection, and the development, maintenance, and reactivation of HSV.[183–185] Clearly, humoral immune responses do not prevent either recurrences or exogenous reinfection. Thus, not surprisingly, transplacentally acquired antibodies from the mother are not totally protective against newborn infection. The key issue, then, is to what extent these antibodies protect and whether specific antibody classes confirm greater protection than others. Transplacentally acquired neutralizing antibodies seem to either prevent or ameliorate infection in exposed newborns.[155,156] Nevertheless, the presence of antibodies at the time of clinical presentation with disease does not appear to influence the subsequent outcome.[149,152,186]

Infected newborns produce IgM antibodies, as detected by immunofluorescence, specific for HSV within the first 3 weeks of infection. These antibodies increase rapidly in titer during the first 2 to 3 months of life and persist for as long as 1 year. The most reactive immunodeterminants include the viral surface glycoproteins, particularly gD and gB. Humoral antibody responses have been studied using immunoblot technology.[186,187] These studies indicate that the severity of infection correlates directly with the number of antibody bands to defined polypeptides. Children with more limited infection, namely, infection of the skin, eye, and/or mouth, have fewer antibody bands as compared with those children with disseminated disease. The quantity of neutralizing antibodies in babies with disseminated infection is lower.[187]

Cellular immune responses have been considered important in the resolution of primary herpetic infections. Newborns with HSV infections have a delayed T-lymphocyte proliferative response compared with older individuals.[187] Most infants studied in a recent evaluation had no detectable T-lymphocyte responses to HSV 2 to 4 weeks after the onset of clinical symptoms, as noted previously by other investigators.[78,187,188] The delayed response to T-lymphocyte antigens in children who have disease localized to the skin, eye, or mouth at the onset of disease may be an important determinant of the frequency of disease progression.[187,189]

Infected newborns have decreased production of alpha interferon in response to HSV antigen when compared to adults with primary HSV infection.[187] The importance of alpha interferon in the maturation of host responses, particularly the elicitation of natural killer cell responses, remains to be defined. Infected babies have decreased gamma interferon production during the first month of life.[187,190,191] Taken together, the data indicate that the newborn has a delayed cell-mediated immune response and lymphokine generation.

Antibodies plus complement and antibodies with killer lymphocytes, monocytes, macrophages, or polymorphonuclear leukocytes will lyse HSV infected cells in vitro.[192] Antibody-dependent cell-mediated cytotoxicity is an important component of the development of host immunity to infection.[193] However, the total population of killer lymphocytes in the newborn is lower than that in older individuals. Thus, certain cell-mediated immune factors do appear relevant in neonatal disease. Both the type and quantity of antibodies present as well as the immaturity of monocyte and macrophages of human neonates are of greater importance than in adults.[192,194–200] These findings are supported by animal model data.[192,199,200]

NEONATAL HSV INFECTION

PATHOGENESIS

Following direct exposure, the newborn will either limit viral replication to the portal of entry (namely, the skin, eye, or mouth) or viral replication will progress and cause more serious disease, including involvement of the brain (causing encephalitis) or multiple other organs. Host mechanisms responsible for control of progression of viral replication at the site of entry are unknown. For central nervous system disease, intraneuronal transmission of viral particles provides a privileged site that may be immune to circulating humoral and cell-mediated defense mechanisms. Thus, transplacental maternal antibodies may be of less value under such circumstances. In contrast, disseminated infection may be the consequence of viremia or secondary to extensive cell-to-cell spread as occurs with pneumonitis following aspiration of infected secretions.

CLINICAL PRESENTATION

The clinical presentation of babies with neonatal HSV infection is a direct reflection of the site and extent of viral replication. Neonatal HSV infection is almost invariably symptomatic and frequently lethal. Although reported cases of asymptomatic infection in the newborn exist, they are most uncommon, and long-term follow up of these children to document absence of subtle disease or sequelae has not been carefully performed. Classification of newborns with HSV infection is mandatory for prognostic and therapeutic considerations. Babies with congenital infection should be identified within the 48 to 72 hours following birth. Babies who are infected intrapartum or postnatally can be divided into three categories: (1) disease localized to the skin, eye, or mouth; (2) encephalitis with or without skin, eye, and/or mouth involvement; and (3) disseminated infection which involves multiple organs, including central nervous system, lung, liver, adrenals, skin, eye, and/or mouth. Prospectively acquired data obtained through the NIAID Collaborative Antiviral Study Group will be reported here.

INTRAUTERINE INFECTION

In the most severely afflicted group of babies, intrauterine infection is apparent at birth and is characterized by a triad of findings, including skin vesicles or skin scarring, eye disease, and the far more severe manifestations of microcephaly or hydranencephaly. Often chorioretinitis alone or in combination with other eye findings, such as keratoconjunctivitis, is a component of the clinical presentation. Serial ultrasound examination of the mothers of those babies infected in utero has demonstrated the presence of hydranencephaly. Chorioretinitis alone can be a presenting sign and should alert the pediatrician to the possibility of this diagnosis, albeit HSV infection is a less common cause than other congenital infections. Severe disease can follow acquisition of infection virtually at any time in gestation. The frequency of occurrence of these manifestations has been estimated to be between 1 in 100,000 to 1 in 200,000 deliveries.[165]

A small group of children will have skin or eye lesions that are present at the time of delivery. These children are frequently born to women who have had prolonged rupture of membranes, sometimes for as long as 2 weeks prior to delivery. The babies have no other findings of invasive multiorgan involvement, including chorioretinitis, encephalitis, or evidence of other diseased organs. The prognosis for successful antiviral therapy in this group of babies is far better than in the children who are born with hydranencephaly.

DISSEMINATED INFECTION

Table 85-3 summarizes the disease classification of 291 babies with neonatal HSV from the NIAID Collaborative Antiviral Study Group. Babies with disseminated infection have the worst prognosis in terms of both mortality and morbidity. Children with disseminated infection usually present to tertiary care centers for therapy between 9 and 11 days of life. However, signs of infection are usually present on an average for 4 to 5 days earlier. Prior to antiviral therapy, this group of babies accounted for approximately one-half to two-thirds of all children with neonatal HSV infection. The principal organs involved following disseminated infection are the liver and adrenals. However, infection can involve multiple other organs including the larynx, trachea, lungs, esophagus, stomach, lower gastrointestinal tract, spleen, kidneys, pancreas, and heart. Encephalitis appears to be a common component of this form of infection, occurring in about 60 to 75 percent of children. Constitutional signs and symptoms include irritability, seizures, respiratory distress, jaundice, bleeding diatheses, shock, and frequently the characteristic vesicular exanthem that is often considered pathognomonic for infection. The vesicular rash, as described in the following, is particularly important in the diagnosis of HSV infection. However, over 20 percent of children

Table 85-3. Demographic and Clinical Characteristics of Infants Enrolled in NIAID Collaborative Antiviral Study

	Disease classification		
	Disseminated	CNS	SEM†
Number of babies	93 (32)	96 (33)	102 (35)
Male/female	54/39	0/46	51/51
Race: Caucasian/other	60/33	73/23	76/26
Premature (<36 weeks)	33 (35)	20 (21)	24 (24)
Gestational age	36.5 ± 0.4	37.9 ± 0.4	37.8 ± 0.3
Enrollment age	11.6 ± 0.7	17.4 ± 0.8	12.1 ± 1.1
Maternal age	21.7 ± 0.5	23.1 ± 0.5	22.8 ± 0.5
Clinical findings			
Skin lesions	72 (77)	60 (63)	86 (84)
Brain involvement	69 (74)	96 (100)	0 (0)
Pneumonia	46 (49)	(4)	3 (3)
Mortality: 1 year	56 (60)	13 (14)	0 (0)
Neurologic impairment of survivors:			
Total	15/34* (44)	45/81† (56)	10/93† (11)
Ara-A	13/26† (50)	25/15† (49)	3/34† (9)
Acyclovir	1/6† (17)	18/27† (67)	4/5† (8)
Placebo	1/2† (50)	2/3† (67)	3/8† (38)

* Irrespective of therapy.
† Inspections localized to skin, eye, and/or mouth.
Denominators vary according to number with follow up available.

having disseminated infection never develop skin vesicles during the course of illness.[152,201] In the absence of skin vesicles, the diagnosis becomes exceedingly difficult, since other clinical signs are often vague and nonspecific, mimicking those of neonatal sepsis. Mortality in the absence of therapy exceeds 80 percent; all but a few survivors are impaired. The most common cause of death in babies with disseminated disease is either HSV pneumonitis or disseminated intravascular coagulopathy.

Evaluation of the extent of disease is imperative, as with all cases of neonatal HSV infection. The clinical laboratory should be utilized to define hepatic enzyme elevation (SGOT and GGT), direct hyperbilirubinemia, neutropenia, thrombocytopenia, and bleeding diatheses, among others. Cerebrospinal fluid (CSF) examination and use of noninvasive neurodiagnostic tests, as defined in the following, will help assess the extent of brain disease. In addition, chest roentgenograms, abdominal x-rays, electroencephalography, and computed tomography of the head all can be judiciously and serially employed to determine the extent of disease. The radiographic picture of HSV lung disease is characterized by a diffuse, interstitial pattern that progresses to a hemorrhagic pneumonitis. Not infrequently, pneumatosis intestinalis can be detected when gastrointestinal disease is present.

ENCEPHALITIS

Infection of the central nervous system occurs alone or in combination with disseminated disease and presents with the findings indicative of encephalitis in the newborn. Overall, nearly 90 percent of babies with dissemination or encephalitis have evidence of acute brain infection. Brain infection can occur either as a component of multiorgan disseminated infection or as encephalitis with or without skin, eye, and mouth involvement. Nearly one-third of all babies with neonatal HSV infection only have encephalitis. The pathogenesis of these two forms of brain infection is likely different. Babies with disseminated infection probably seed the brain by a blood-borne route, resulting in multiple areas of cortical hemorrhagic necrosis. In contrast, babies who present with encephalitis alone are likely to develop brain disease as a consequence of retrograde axonal transmission of virus to the central nervous system. Two pieces of data support this contention. First, babies with disseminated disease have documented viremia and are hospitalized earlier in life (at 9–10 days vs 16–17 days) than those with encephalitis. Second, babies with encephalitis are more likely to receive transplacental neutralizing antibodies from their mothers, which may not prevent intraneuronal transmission of virus to the brain.

The clinical manifestations of encephalitis include seizures (both focal and generalized), lethargy, irritability, tremors, poor feeding, temperature instability, bulging fontanelle, and pyramidal tract signs. Although babies with disseminated infection often have skin vesicles in association with brain infection, the same is not true for the baby with encephalitis alone. The latter group of children have skin vesicles in only 60 percent of cases at any time in the disease course.[152,201–203] Cultures of CSF yield HSV in 25 to 40 percent of all cases. Anticipated findings on CSF examination include pleocytosis and proteinosis (as high as 500–1000 mg/dL). Although a few babies with central nervous system infection proven by brain biopsy have been reported to have no abnormalities of their CSF, this occurs very rarely. Serial CSF examination is useful diagnostically as the infected child with brain disease will demonstrate progressive increases in the CSF protein content. The importance of CSF examinations in all infants is underscored by the finding that even subtle changes have been associated with significant developmental abnormalities. Furthermore, as discussed in Diagnosis, CSF provides an essential biologic specimen for diagnostic evaluation by PCR.[204,205]

Electroencephalography and computed tomography can be very useful in defining the presence of central nervous system abnormalities.[206] Death occurs in 50 percent of babies with localized central nervous system disease who are not treated and is usually related to brain stem involvement. With rare exceptions, survivors are left with severe neurologic impairment.[201,203]

The long-term prognosis, following either disseminated infection or encephalitis, is poor. As many as 50 percent of surviving children have some degree of psychomotor retardation, often in association with microcephaly, hydranencephaly, porencephalic cysts, spasticity, blindness, chorioretinitis, or learning disabilities. It is unclear at this time whether visceral or central nervous system damage can be progressive after initial clearance of the viral infection, a possibility suggested by long-term assessment of children with skin, eye, or mouth disease and more recently, in a group of babies with more severe disease.[136,152,207,208]

Despite the presumed difference in pathogenesis, the clinical manifestations of encephalitis alone are virtually identical to those that occur with brain infection in disseminated cases. Only two of three babies with encephalitis will develop a vesicular rash characteristic of HSV infection. Thus, a newborn with pleocytosis and proteinosis of the CSF but without a rash can easily be misdiagnosed as having a bacterial or other viral infection unless HSV infection is carefully considered. In such circumstances, a history of genital lesions in the mother or her sexual partner may be very important in suggesting HSV as a cause of illness.

SKIN, EYE, AND/OR MOUTH INFECTION

Infection localized to the skin, eye, and/or mouth is associated with lower mortality, but it is not without significant morbidity. When infection is localized to the skin, the presence of discrete vesicles remains the hallmark of disease. Clusters of vesicles often appear initially on the presenting part of the body that was in direct contact with the virus during birth. With time, the rash can progress to involve other areas of the body as well. Vesicles occur in 90 percent of children with skin, eye, and/or mouth infection. Children with disease localized to the skin, eye, or mouth generally present at about 10 to 11 days of life. Those babies with skin lesions invariably will suffer from recurrences over the first 6 months (and longer) of life, regardless of whether therapy was administered or not. Although death is not associated with disease localized to the skin, eye, and/or mouth, approximately 30 percent of these children eventually develop evidence of neurologic impairment.[139,152,206]

Vesicles usually erupt from an erythematous base and are usually 1 to 2 mm in diameter. They can progress to larger bullous lesions greater than 1 cm in diameter. Although discrete vesicles on various parts of the body are usually encountered, crops and clusters of vesicles have also been described. For most babies with neonatal HSV infection localized to the skin, eye, and/or mouth, the vesicular skin rash involves multiple and often distant cutaneous sites. However, a limited number of babies have had infection of the skin limited to one or two vesicles and no further evidence of cutaneous disease. This group of babies warrants careful evaluation because many have developed encephalitic involvement when antiviral therapy was not administered. Other manifestations of skin lesions have included a zosteriform eruption.

Infections involving the eye may manifest as keratoconjunctivitis or, later, chorioretinitis. The eye can be the only site of HSV involvement in the newborn.[202] These children present with keratoconjunctivitis or, surprisingly, evidence of microphthalmia and retinal dysplasia. In the presence of persistent disease and no therapy, chorioretinitis can result, caused by either HSV-1 or -2.[209–211] Keratoconjunctivitis, even in the presence of therapy, can progress to chorioretinitis, cataracts, and retinal detachment. Cataracts have been detected on long-term follow-up in three infants with proved perinatally acquired HSV infections.[212]

Localized infection of the oropharyngeal cavity is found in approximately 10 percent of neonates with HSV infection.

Long-term neurologic impairment including spastic quadriplegia, microcephaly, and blindness has been encountered in children whose disease appeared localized to the skin, eye, and/or mouth. Important questions regarding the pathogenesis of delayed-onset neurologic debility are raised by such clinical observations. Despite normal clinical examinations, neurologic impairment develops between 6 months and 1 year of life. The clinical presentation occurs in a manner similar to that associated with congenitally acquired toxoplasmosis or syphilis. As noted in the following, two factors appear to predict neurologic outcome in babies with disease localized to the skin, eye, or mouth. These are: (1) frequency of recurrent skin lesions over the first 3 months of life and (2) detection of HSV DNA by PCR in the CSF at the end of therapy.

SUBCLINICAL INFECTION

Although it has been suggested that two newborns had evidence of HSV infection proved by culture isolation of virus but without evidence of symptoms, it has been difficult to document such cases through the serial evaluation in over 1000 infants evaluated in multiple centers around the United States. Because of the propensity of the newborn to develop disease, any evidence of infection should be considered potentially serious and an indication for antiviral therapy.

DIAGNOSIS

CLINICAL EVALUATION

The clinical diagnosis of neonatal HSV infection has become increasingly difficult because of the apparent decrease in the incidence of skin vesicles as an initial component of disease presentation. A variety of other infections of the newborn can masquerade as neonatal HSV infections, including hyaline membrane disease, intraventricular hemorrhage, necrotizing enterocolitis, and various ocular or cutaneous disorders. Bacterial infections of newborns can mimic neonatal HSV infection. It is not uncommon for some babies infected by HSV to also experience a concomitant bacterial infection, particularly those caused by the group B streptococcus, *Staphylococcus aureus, Listeria monocytogenes,* and Gram-negative bacterial infections.

As with other vesicular rashes, alternative causes of such exanthems should be excluded. Such diseases include varicella-zoster virus infection, enteroviral disease, and disseminated cytomegalovirus infection. With the aforementioned clinical findings in a child presenting to the hospital during the first 3 weeks of life, consideration of neonatal HSV infection is necessary. The presence of skin vesicles provides a natural site for attempted isolation of virus in order to rapidly determine if the etiology of the vesicular rash is HSV as opposed to varicella-zoster virus. Simultaneously, serologic specimens and other virologic cultures should be obtained to exclude other common causes of perinatal infection, including toxoplasmosis, cytomegalovirus infection, rubella, and syphilis. Such cutaneous disorders as erythema toxicum, neonatal melanosis, or acrodermitis enteropathica often confuse physicians who suspect neonatal HSV infections. Lesions associated with these diseases can be rapidly distinguished from those caused by HSV by the presence of eosinophils on a Wright stain of a tissue scraping and by appropriate viral cultures.

The most difficult clinical diagnosis to make is that of HSV encephalitis, as nearly 40 percent of children with central nervous system infection will not have a vesicular rash at the time of clinical presentation. Herpes simplex virus infection of the central nervous system should be suspected in the child who has evidence of acute neurologic deterioration with the onset of seizures and in the absence of intraventricular hemorrhage and metabolic causes. Serial increases in CSF fluid cell counts and protein concentrations, negative bacterial cultures of the CSF, and negative CSF antigen studies help suggest the diagnosis of HSV infection of the central nervous system. A maternal genital culture or history of genital herpes in either the mother or a sexual partner reinforces the suspicion of neonatal HSV infection. As noted previously, noninvasive neurodiagnostic studies can be used to define the sites of involvement.

LABORATORY ASSESSMENT

Every effort should be made to confirm infection by viral isolation, the definitive diagnostic method. If skin lesions are present, a scraping of skin vesicles should be transferred in appropriate virus transport media to a diagnostic virology laboratory. Clinical specimens should be shipped on ice for inoculation into appropriate cell culture systems. Shipping of specimens and their processing should be expedited. In addition to skin vesicles, other sites from which virus may be isolated include the cerebrospinal fluid, stool, urine, throat, nasopharynx, and conjunctivae. It may also be useful in infants with evidence of hepatitis or other gastrointestinal abnormalities to obtain duodenal aspirates for HSV isolation. The virologic results of cultures from these sites along with clinical findings should be used in conjunction with clinical findings to establish a disease classification. Typing of a HSV isolate may be done by one of several techniques.

Over the past several years, PCR detection of HSV-DNA in CSF has become the diagnostic method of choice for central nervous system disease, replacing brain biopsy. It has proved both sensitive and specific when properly performed.[205,213–216]

The serologic diagnosis of HSV infection is not of great clinical value. Therapeutic decisions can not await the results of serologic studies. Further, the inability of the commonly available serologic assays to distinguish between antibodies to HSV-1 or 2 as well as to denote the presence of transplacentally acquired maternal IgG, as opposed to endogenously produced antibodies, makes the assessment of the neonate's antibody status difficult during acute infection. Serial antibody assessment may be useful if a mother without a prior history of HSV infection has a primary infection late in gestation and transfers very little or no antibody to the fetus.

TREATMENT OF NEONATAL HSV INFECTIONS

BACKGROUND

Since most babies acquire HSV infection at the time of delivery or shortly thereafter, successful antiviral therapy should decrease mortality and improve long-term outcome. Inherent in this presumption is the recognition that diagnosis shortly after the onset of clinical illness is essential, as is the case with other perinatally acquired infections. Children presenting with disease localized to the skin, eye, and/or mouth progress to either involvement of the central nervous system or disseminated infection in approximately 70 percent of cases when no therapy is administered.[149] When such occurs, the likelihood of an adequate outcome, even with established drugs, is not optimal as many of these children will either die or be left with significant neurologic impairment. Such factors must be considered in the development of any treatment strategy.

ANTIVIRAL THERAPY

Vidarabine was the first drug proven effective for treatment of infants with disseminated or localized central nervous system disease, being associated with a decline in mortality rate from 75 to 40 percent.[207] However, vidarabine has been replaced by acyclovir as the treatment of choice for neonatal HSV infection. When outcome was examined according to each of the three disease classifications, the best therapeutic result was achieved in babies with either encephalitis or skin, eye, and/or mouth infection.

Acyclovir is the treatment of choice for neonatal HSV infections of the central nervous system. It is a selective inhibitor of HSV replication, representing one of the most important advances in antiviral therapy (see Chapter 21). Acyclovir is a synthetic acyclic purine nucleoside analog which selectively inhibits HSV-1 and HSV-2.[217,218] Acyclovir is converted to its monophosphate derivative by virus encoded thymidine kinase, an event that does not occur to any significant extent in uninfected cells. Subsequent di- and triphosphorylation is catalyzed by cellular enzymes and results in acyclovir triphosphate concentrations 40- to 100-fold higher in HSV infected cells than in uninfected cells. Acyclovir triphosphate inhibits viral DNA synthesis by competing with deoxyguanosine triphosphate as a substrate for viral DNA polymerase.[219,220] DNA synthesis is then terminated because acyclovir triphosphate lacks the 3′ hydroxyl required for DNA chain elongation. The viral polymerase has greater affinity for acyclovir triphosphate than cellular DNA polymerase, resulting in little incorporation of acyclovir into cellular DNA. In vitro, acyclovir is active against HSV-1 (average $ED_{50} = 0.04\ \mu g/mL$), HSV-2 (0.10 μg/mL), and varicella-zoster virus (0.50 μg/mL).

Acyclovir has been established as efficacious for the treatment of primary genital HSV when administered by intravenous, oral, and topical routes (see Chapter 21).[221–223] Furthermore, the oral and intravenous administration of acyclovir to the immunocompromised host decreases both the frequency of reactivation following immunosuppression and disease duration.[224,225] Acyclovir is superior to vidarabine for the treatment of HSV encephalitis.[226] Because this compound is a selective inhibitor of viral replication, it has a low frequency of side effects. Acyclovir has become a preferred treatment for all serious HSV infections.

In the treatment of neonatal HSV infections, intravenous acyclovir has been shown to be as effective as vidarabine treatment; but it is not superior.[227] No infant with disease localized to skin, eye, or mouth died, but the mortality rate of infants with encephalitis or disseminated infection overall was 18 and 55 percent, respectively. Importantly, even though HSV infection appeared to be localized to the skin, eye, and mouth, neurologic impairment developed beyond 2 years in children who received vidarabine and acyclovir, accounting for morbidity in 10 and 2 percent of patients, respectively. Following encephalitis, 50 percent of survivors treated with vidarabine and 43 percent of survivors treated with acyclovir were developing normally. Infants who survived disseminated infection, developed normally at rates of 62 and 57 percent following vidarabine and acyclovir treatment, respectively. The dosage of acyclovir which was employed in these studies was 10 mg/kg intravenously every 8 hours for 10 to 14 days. Unlike other studies comparing vidarabine and acyclovir, these two drugs had identical effects on outcome for the treatment of this disease. Nevertheless, viral clearance in infants who received acyclovir was accelerated compared to vidarabine recipients. Parenthetically, approximately 10 percent of babies with either encephalitis or disseminated disease with brain involvement relapsed 5 to 15 days after completing a course of antiviral therapy. Unfortunately, CSF for PCR detection of HSV DNA at the completion of therapy, as opposed to the time of relapse, was not available for laboratory evaluation.

To improve outcome, more active drugs that have greater activity in the CNS must be developed. Importantly, therapy must prevent progression of infection to the CNS or disseminated disease. Ideally, prevention of neonatal HSV infection, including CNS involvement, by either immunization of the mother at risk or immunoprophylaxis and therapy of the newborn delivered to the mother with asymptomatic primary or initial infection would be far more desirable. Although the currently recommended intravenous dose is 10 mg/kg three times daily, higher dosages and for longer period of time are being investigated.

Recognizing that disease is often present in these babies for 4 or 5 days prior to diagnosis, a window for administration of therapy earlier in life does exist. This point must be reiterated as earlier therapeutic intervention for any microbial infection will lead to improved outcome, particularly when a vital organ such as the brain is involved. Furthermore, when therapy is instituted early, fewer children will progress from localized skin involvement to more serious forms of infection. Therapy decreases the frequency of progression.

Infants with ocular involvement caused by HSV should receive topical antiviral medication in addition to parenteral therapy. At the present time, few safety and tolerance data are available for topical ophthalmic antiviral drugs. In older patients, viroptic (trifluorothymidine) has the greatest antiviral activity and is the treatment of choice for HSV infection of the eyes. Vidarabine ophthalmic and Stoxil (idoxuridine) have been utilized for a longer period of time. There is more experience regarding their safety in both adults and children, but they are less active.

During the course of therapy, careful monitoring is important in order to assess therapeutic response. Even in the absence of clinical evidence of encephalitis, the central nervous system should be examined serially for prognostic purposes. Evaluation of certain hepatic (increased SGPT or SGOT) and bone marrow parameters (decreased platelets) may indicate viral involvement of these organs or drug toxicity.

As for all drugs, a consideration of the therapeutic index for a ratio of efficacy to toxicity is important. Experience with vidarabine and acyclovir, thus far, has indicated little toxicity when used appropriately. However, the possibility of both acute and long-term toxicity should be considered in any child receiving parenteral antiviral therapy and assessed by serially evaluating bone marrow, renal, and hepatic function. The potential for long-term harm from these drugs remains to be defined. Since these compounds act at the level of DNA replication, physicians responsible for follow up of these children should be aware of the possibility of mutagenic or even teratogenic effects that may not appear until decades later. A recent topic of debate is the possibility of the development of viral resistance to a drug (see Chapter 21); the clinical significance remains to be defined, although it has occurred in the newborn.[228]

Continuing discussion surrounds the administration of oral acyclovir following intravenous therapy. Oral therapy appears to decrease the frequency of cutaneous recurrences but has been associated with absolute neutropenia.[228] The significance of this finding is under investigation.

Since the child with neonatal HSV infection, particularly with skin vesicles, will excrete virus in large quantities, isolation of the newborn is important in order to decrease the potential for nosocomial transmission of infection.

FACTORS PREDICTIVE OF NEUROLOGIC OUTCOME

Table 85-4 summarizes the risk factors for mortality and morbidity even with therapy of neonatal HSV infection.[229] Mortality is best predicted by disease classification, level of consciousness, and disseminated intravascular coagulopathy for the entire study population. As it relates to morbidity, disease classification, virus type (HSV-2), and the presence of seizures predict a poor neurologic outcome.

Notably, for babies with disease localized to the skin, eye or mouth, risk of neurologic impairment increases with the frequency of recurrent cutaneous lesions within three months of the completion of therapy. Additionally, infection caused by HSV-2 appears more likely to cause neurologic impairment.

OTHER THERAPEUTIC APPROACHES

At present there is no indication that administration of immune globulin or hyperimmune globulin is of value in therapy of neonatal HSV infection. Although a series of studies have suggested that high levels of transplacental neutralizing antibodies will ameliorate neonatal HSV infections at the time of presentation with clinical disease, the presence or absence of antibodies does not influence the subsequent course of infection.[152,155,156] At present no other form of therapy is useful for treating neonatal HSV infection. Various experimental modalities including BCG, interferon, immune modulators, and immunization have been used, but none have produced demonstrable effects.

LONG-TERM MANAGEMENT OF HSV-INFECTED BABIES

With the advent of antiviral therapy, an increasing number of newborns who suffer from HSV infection survive and require careful long-term follow up. Three areas of follow-up warrant attention from a medical standpoint. First, it is not infrequent that parents of children with neonatal HSV infection have significant guilt feelings. A once stable marriage can suffer and require interventive support from psychologists, psychiatrists, or marriage counselors. The family physician or pediatrician in this situation can provide support to the family. Second, the most common complications of neonatal HSV infection include neurologic and ocular sequelae which are detected only on long-term follow up. Therefore, these children should receive serial long-term evaluations from qualified pediatric specialists in these areas, including neurodevelopmental, ophthalmologic, and hearing assessments. Third, skin vesicles will recur with time. These vesicles provide a potential reservoir for transmission of infection to other children who have direct contact with these infants. The increasing use of daycare for children in this country, including children surviving neonatal HSV infections, has stimulated many questions concerning how these children should receive care. Certainly, there is some risk that children with recurrent HSV skin lesions will transmit the virus to other children in this environment. The most reasonable recommendation in this situation appears to be simply to cover the lesions to prevent direct contact with them. More likely, HSV-1 is present in the daycare environment in the children with symptomatic or asymptomatic gingivostomatitis. In both cases, virus is present in the mouth and pharynx, so that the frequent

Table 85-4. Prognostic Factors Identified by Multivariate Analyses for Neonates and HSV Infection*

	Relative Risk	
	Mortality	Morbidity
Total group (n = 202)		
Extent of disease		
Skin, eyes, or mouth	1	1
CNS	5.8†	4.4†
Disseminated	33†	2.1†
Level of consciousness		
Alert or lethargic	1	NS
Semicomatose or comatose	5.2†	NS
Disseminated intravascular coagulopathy	3.8†	NS
Prematurity	3.7†	NS
Virus type		
HSV-1	2.3‡	1
HSV-2	1	4.9†
Seizures	NS	3.0†
Infants with disseminated disease (n = 46)		
Disseminated intravascular coagulopathy	3.5†	NS
Level of consciousness		
Alert or lethargic	1	1
Semicomatose or comatose	3.9†	4.0†
Pneumonia	3.6†	NS
Infants with CNS involvement (n = 71)		
Level of consciousness		
Alert or lethargic	1	NS
Semicomatose or comatose	6.1†	NS
Prematurity	5.2†	NS
Seizures	NS	3.4†
Infants with infection of the skin, eyes, or mouth (n = 85)		
No. of skin-vesicle recurrences		
<3	NA	1
≥ 3	NA	21†
Virus type		
HSV-1	NA	1
HSV-2	NA	14‡§

* CNS denotes central nervous system, NS not statistically significant ($p > 0.05$), and NA not applicable. (No baby with disease confined to the skin, eyes, or mouth died.)

† $p < 0.01$.

‡ $p < 0.05$.

§ Because of the correlation between virus type and skin-vesicle recurrence, virus type was not significant in the multivariate model; however, it was significant as a single factor. Adapted by permission of the *N Engl J Med* from Whitley et al.[229]

exchange of saliva and other respiratory droplets that occurs among children in this setting makes this route of transmission much more likely. Education of daycare workers and the general public concerning herpesvirus infections, their implications, and the frequency with which they occur would do much to calm fears and correct common misconceptions concerning infections with this virus.

PREVENTION OF NEONATAL HSV INFECTION

BACKGROUND

In spite of the progress that has been made over the last 15 years in the development of antiviral therapy for treatment of neonatal HSV infection, the best approach is that of prevention. It is not surprising that because of the attention of the lay press to the devastating outcome of neonatal herpes, many women with known genital herpetic infection elect to be delivered by cesarean section rather than undergo the potential risks of exposure of the fetus to the virus at the time of vaginal delivery. As a consequence, an unnecessarily high frequency of cesarean infections is believed to occur in these individuals. All individuals involved in the care of pregnant women and their offspring should individualize the care of mother and child to optimize patient management. Cultures obtained for HSV prior to delivery do not predict neonatal infection and, therefore, are not indicators.[230–232]

Several questions regarding the value of cesarean section in the prevention of neonatal HSV infections remain unresolved. Although surgical abdominal delivery has been associated with the decreased transmission of infection when membranes are ruptured less than 4 hours, cesarean section has not proved efficacious when membranes are ruptured for longer periods of time. Nevertheless, it has been recommended that when membranes are ruptured up to 24 hours, cesarean section will be of value. Although these recommendations are predicated on logic, no data from adequately performed clinical trials are available (see also Chapter 21).

For women with a past history of genital HSV infection, a careful vaginal examination at presentation to the delivery suite is of paramount importance. Although visualization of the cervix is often difficult, speculum examination for documentation of recurrent lesions is extremely important and should be attempted in these women. A culture for HSV obtained at the time of delivery may be of great importance in establishing whether transmission of infection to the fetus is likely.

The fact that predelivery cultures not only fail to predict the woman who excretes virus at delivery but are also an unnecessarily large health care cost burden places their value in further question. Thus, alternative management approaches will have to be developed.[231]

Clearly, identifying the woman who excretes HSV at delivery and then optimizing either prophylactic protocols with safe and acceptable antivirals or delivery by cesarean section is the optimal way to manage genital infection at the time of delivery. Unfortunately, at present isolation of virus in tissue culture is the only commonly available test capable of documenting the excretion of virus. Alternative, rapid non-culture-based diagnostic approaches are being developed in order to expedite identification of women at risk for delivering an infected baby.[233]

An alternative strategy is evolving for women with a history of recurrent genital herpes. The administration of acyclovir during the last 6 weeks of gestation has resulted in a lower frequency of cesarean sections and viral shedding. However, the safety of this approach for the fetus has not been established.[234]

For infections that occur in the first half of gestation, no specific recommendations regarding the termination of pregnancy can be made at this time. It appears that the frequency of infection acquired in utero is approximately 1 in 200,000 deliveries and can occur as a consequence of either maternal primary or recurrent infection. Nevertheless, detailed prospective studies to document this occurrence have yet to be performed. Thus, no specific recommendation regarding termination of pregnancy with such findings can be made.

Serious forms of neonatal HSV infections will continue to be associated with significant mortality and morbidity, even with acyclovir therapy. As a consequence, some investigators have suggested that acyclovir may be useful in preventing the occurrence of neonatal HSV infections in infants who are delivered unknowingly through an infected birth canal. Since the incidence of neonatal HSV infection following maternal recurrent disease is low, the risks and costs will likely outweigh the benefits. However, with a suspected maternal primary infection and a vaginal delivery intravenous acyclovir therapy may be indicated.

Specifically, the pharmacokinetics and metabolism of acyclovir in the human fetus is totally unknown at the present time. The possibility of acyclovir fetal nephrotoxicity, a potential risk of drug administration, must be considered. In addition, it must be recognized that the women who are at greatest risk for delivering babies who develop neonatal HSV infection are those least likely to have a history of recurrent genital HSV infection.[234]

MANAGEMENT OF HIGH-RISK WOMEN AND THEIR OFFSPRING

Infants delivered either vaginally or by cesarean section when membranes are intact to mothers who have no evidence of active genital herpetic infection are at low risk for acquiring neonatal HSV infection. These children need no special evaluation in the nursery other than initial isolation until results of maternal genital cultures are available. With negative maternal genital cultures, these children can be discharged at the time the mother leaves the hospital.

Infants delivered vaginally to mothers with active genital herpes should be isolated if medically possible, and appropriate cultures obtained between 24 and 48 hours after delivery. If possible, these cultures should be repeated at 2- to 3-day intervals during the period of time when infection is usually detectable—the first 4 weeks of life but especially the first 2 weeks. Sites from which virus should be sought include eye, oronasopharynx, and suspect lesions. These recommendations should serve only as guidelines until formal data are available. It should be emphasized that if any site is positive, a thorough virologic and clinical examination must be performed and therapy instituted. Other sites to be considered for viral isolation include the cerebrospinal fluid, urine, and buffy coat of the blood. In addition, neurodiagnostic evaluation by electroencephalogram and a computed tomographic scan, if indicated, is essential.

POSTNATAL INFECTION

Isolation of mother from baby

An issue of frequent concern is whether the mother with active genital HSV infection at delivery should be isolated from her child after delivery. Women with recurrent orolabial HSV infection as well as cutaneous herpes simplex infections at other sites (breast lesions) are at similar risk for transmission of virus to their newborn. The risks presented to the newborn by other family members, medical personnel, and friends remain unknown but are low and do not justify removal of personnel from the nursery at this time. Since transmission occurs by direct contact with the virus, appropriate precautions by the mother, including careful hand washing before touching the infant, should prevent the necessity of separation of mother and child. Similarly, breast feeding is contraindicated only if the mother has vesicular lesions involving the breast. We do not isolate babies born to infected women unless they themselves become infected. Hospitalization is not prolonged in the uninfected child.

Parental education

At the time of discharge, it is essential to educate parents with known recurrent herpetic infection regarding the possibility that their child may become infected. The parental stigma of a diagnosis of genital herpes and the monitoring procedures associated with evaluating the newborn can create excessive fear and anxiety in the family. The parents and responsible family members must be educated in order to relieve anxiety and provide prompt access to the health care delivery system should evidence of infection appear. Information regarding infection should include an overview of HSV infection, the risks associated with transmission of infection to the newborn, the necessity for monitoring, the anticipated consequences of positive and negative viral cultures, planned approaches to treatment, and the potential for postnatal acquisition of infection at home.

Hospital staff

At many institutions, a policy that requires transfer or provision of medical leave for nursing or other personnel in nurseries with a labial HSV infection is impractical and causes an excessive burden in those attempting to provide adequate care. Temporary removal of personnel with cold sores has been advocated on some clinical services. As noted previously, individuals with herpetic whitlows carry a high risk of viral shedding. These individuals should be removed from care of newborns at risk for acquiring neonatal HSV infection since even gloves may not prevent transmission of infection. Education regarding the risk of transmission of virus and the importance of hand washing when lesions are present should be repeatedly emphasized to health care workers. In addition, hospital personnel should wear masks when active lesions are present.

SUMMARY

Neonatal HSV infection remains a life-threatening infection for the newborn in the United States today. With an increasing incidence of genital herpes and an increase in the incidence of neonatal HSV infections, it is important that pediatricians, neonatologists, obstetricians, and family practitioners continue to maintain a high index of suspicion in infants whose symptoms may be compatible with HSV infections so that early identification leads to prompt treatment. Hopefully, over the next decade, the development of safe and efficacious vaccines as well as a better understanding of factors associated with transmission of virus from mother to baby will allow ultimate prevention of neonatal HSV infection.

ACKNOWLEDGMENTS

The cytomegalovirus portion of this chapter was supported in part by grants from the National Institutes of Health, NICHD (HD10699), and General Clinical Research Center (MOI RROO32). Dr. Whitley is indebted to the members of the National Institute of Allergy and Infectious Diseases Collaborative Antiviral Study Group for their support and assistance in developing the database that provided the basis for this report, in particular Drs. C.A. Alford, Jr. and A.J. Nahmias. In addition, he is exceedingly grateful for the assistance of Arlene Abrams and Rhonda Morrow.

Studies performed by Dr. Whitley and reported in this chapter were supported in part by research grant RR-032 from the Division of Research Resources, National Institutes of Health, grant CA-13148 from the National Cancer Institute, a contract, NOIA1-62554, from the Development and Applications Branch from the National Institute of Allergy and Infectious Diseases, and a grant from the state of Alabama.

References

1 Weller TH: The cytomegaloviruses: Ubiquitous agents with protean clinical manifestations. *N Engl J Med* 285:203, 1971.
2 Ribbert D: Uber protozoenartige Zellen in der Niere eines syphilitischen Neugeborenen und in der Parotis von Kindern. *Zentralbl Allg Pathol* 15:945, 1904.
3 Smith MG: Propagation of salivary gland virus of the mouse in tissue culture. *Proc Soc Exp Biol Med* 86:435, 1954.
4 Smith MG: Propagation in tissue cultures of a cytopathogenic virus from human salivary gland virus disease. *Proc Soc Exp Biol Med* 92: 424, 1956.
5 Rowe WP et al: Cytopathogenic agent resembling human salivary gland virus recovered from tissue cultures of human adenoids. *Proc Soc Exp Biol Med* 92:418, 1956.
6 Weller TH et al: Isolation of intranuclear inclusion producing agents from infants with illnesses resembling cytomegalic inclusion disease. *Proc Soc Exp Biol Med* 94:4, 1957.
7 Weller TH et al: Serologic differentiation of viruses responsible for cytomegalic inclusion disease. *Virology* 12:130, 1960.
8 Gold et al: Cytomegalovirus. p. 143. In Evans, AS (Ed): *Viral infections of humans: epidemiology and control.* Plenum Publishers, New York, 1976.
9 Alford CA et al. Epidemiology of cytomegalovirus. In *The human herpesviruses: an interdisciplinary perspective,* Nahmias, A, Dowdle, W & Schinazi, R (eds): New York, Elsevier Publishers, 1981, p. 159.
10 Schopfer K et al: Congenital cytomegalovirus infection in newborn infants of mothers infected before pregnancy. *Arch Dis Child* 53:536, 1978.
11 Numazaki Y et al: Primary infection with human cytomegalovirus: Virus isolation from healthy infants and pregnant women. *J Epidemiol* 91:410, 1970.
12 Vial P et al: Serological study of cytomegalovirus, herpes simplex and rubella virus, hepatitis B and toxoplasma gondii in 2 populations of pregnant women in Santiago, Chile. *Bol Oficina Sanit Panam* 99:528, 1985.
13 Stagno S: Primary cytomegalovirus infection in pregnancy: Incidence, transmission to fetus and clinical outcome in two populations of different socioeconomic backgrounds. *JAMA* 256:1904, 1986.
14 Lang DJ et al: Cytomegalovirus in semen: Observations in selected populations. *J Infect Dis* 132:472, 1975.
15 Stagno S et al: Breast milk and the risk of cytomegalovirus infection. *N Engl J Med* 302:1073, 1980.
16 Jordan MC et al: Association of cervical cytomegaloviruses with veneral disease. *N Engl J Med* 288:932, 1973.
17 Willmott FE: Cytomegalovirus in female patients attending a VD clinic. *Br J Vener Dis* 51:278, 1975.
18 Drew WL et al: Prevalence of cytomegalovirus infection in homosexual men. *J Infect Dis* 143:188, 1981.
19 Chandler SJ et al: The epidemiology of cytomegaloviral infection in women attending a sexually transmitted disease clinic. *J Infect Dis* 152:597, 1985.
20 Collier AC et al: Cytomegalovirus infection in homosexual men. *Am J Med* 82:493, 1987.
21 Kingsley LA et al: Risk factors for seroconversion to human immunodeficiency virus among male homosexuals. *Lancet* 2:345, 1987.

22 Pass RF et al: Cytomegalovirus infection in day care center. *N Engl J Med* 307:477, 1982.

23 Adler SP et al: Cytomegalovirus transmission among children attending a day care center. *Pediatr Res* 19:285A, 1985.

24 Murph JR et al: The prevalence of cytomegalovirus infection in a midwest day care center. *Pediatr Res* 19:205A, 1985.

25 Pass RF et al: Increased rate of cytomegalovirus infection among parents of children attending day care centers. *N Engl J Med* 314:1414, 1986.

26 Adler SP: Molecular epidemiology of cytomegalovirus: evidence for viral transmission to parents from children infected at a day care center. *Pediatr Infect Dis* 5:315, 1986.

27 Hutto C et al: Isolation of cytomegalovirus from toys and hands in a day care center. *J Infect Dis* 154:527, 1986.

28 Faix RG: Survival of cytomegalovirus on environmental surfaces. *J Pediatr* 106:649, 1985.

29 Adler SP: The molecular epidemiology of cytomegalovirus transmission among children attending a day care center. *J Infect Dis* 152: 760, 1985.

30 Spector SA et al: Molecular epidemiology of cytomegalovirus infection in premature twin infants and their mother. *Pediatr Infect Dis* 1:405, 1982.

31 Dworsky ME et al: Cytomegalovirus transmission within a family. *Pediatr Infect Dis* 3:236, 1984.

32 Yeager AS: Transmission of cytomegalovirus to mothers by infected infants: another reason to prevent transfusion-acquired infections. *Pediatr Infect Dis* 2:295, 1983.

33 Dworsky ME et al: Occupational risk for primary cytomegalovirus infection among pediatric health-care workers. *N Engl J Med* 309: 950, 1983.

34 Taber LH et al: Acquisition of cytomegaloviral infections in families with young children: a serological study. *J Infect Dis* 151:948, 1985.

35 Adler SP: Molecular epidemiology of cytomegalovirus: viral transmission among children attending a day care center, their parents, and caretakers. *J Pediatr* 112:366, 1988.

36 Adler SP: Cytomegalovirus and child daycare. Evidence for an increased infection rate among day-care workers. *N Engl J Med* 321: 1290, 1989.

37 Stagno S et al: Congenital cytomegalovirus infection. *N Engl J Med* 296:1254, 1977.

38 Embil JA et al: Congenital cytomegalovirus infection in two siblings from consecutive pregnancies. *J Pediatr* 77:417, 1970.

39 Stagno S et al: Congenital cytomegalovirus infection: consecutive occurrence due to viruses with similar antigenic compositions. *Pediatrics* 52:788, 1973.

40 Krech U et al: Congenital cytomegalovirus infection in siblings from consecutive pregnancies. *Helv Paediatr Acta* 26:355, 1971.

41 Stagno S et al: Maternal cytomegalovirus infection and perinatal transmission. *Clin Obstet Gynecol* 25:563, 1982.

42 Stern H et al: Prospective study of cytomegalovirus infection in pregnancy. *Br Med J* 2:268, 1973.

43 Nankervis A et al: Primary infection with cytomegalovirus during pregnancy. *Pediatr Res* 8:487, 1974.

44 Knox GE et al: Comparative prevalence of subclinical cytomegalovirus and herpes simplex virus infections in the genital and urinary tracts of low-income, urban women. *J Infect Dis* 140:419, 1979.

45 Handsfield HH et al: Cytomegalovirus infection in sex partners: evidence for sexual transmission. *J Infect Dis* 151:344, 1985.

46 Chretien JH et al: Veneral causes of cytomegalovirus mononucleosis. *JAMA* 238:1644, 1977.

47 Kreel I et al: A syndrome following total body prefusion. *Surg Gynecol Obstet* 111:317, 1960.

48 Adler SP: Transfusion-associated cytomegalovirus infections. *Rev Infect Dis* 5:977, 1983.

49 Seaman AJ et al: Febrile postcardiotomy lymphocytic splenomegaly: a new entity. *Ann Surg* 156:956, 1962.

50 Onorato JM et al: Epidemiology of cytomegalovirus infections: recommendations for prevention and control. *Rev Infect Dis* 7:479, 1988.

51 Armstong JA et al: Cytomegalovirus infection in children undergoing open-heart surgery. *Yale J Biol Med* 49:83, 1976.

52 Prince AM et al: A serologic study of cytomegalovirus infections associated with blood transfusions. *N Engl J Med* 284:1125, 1971.

53 Rinaldo CR et al: Interaction of cytomegalovirus with leukocytes from patients with mononucleosis due to cytomegalovirus. *J Infect Dis* 136:667, 1977.

54 Stevens DP et al: Asymptomatic cytomegalovirus infection following blood transfusion in tumor surgery. *JAMA* 211:1341, 1970.

55 Kaariainen L et al: Rise of cytomegalovirus antibodies in an infectious mononucleosislike syndrome after transfusion. *Br Med J* 1:1270, 1966.

56 Lang DJ et al: Reduction of postperfusion cytomegalovirus-infections following the use of leukocyte depleted blood. *Transfusion* 17:391, 1977.

57 McCracken GJ, Jr. et al: Congenital cytomegalic inclusion disease. A longitudinal study of 20 patients. *Am J Dis Child* 117:522, 1969.

58 Kumar A et al: Acquisition of cytomegalovirus infection in infants following exchange transfusion: a prospective study. *Transfusion* 20: 327, 1980.

59 King-Lewis PA et al: Congenital cytomegalic inclusion diseases following intrauterine transfusion. *Br Med J* 2:603, 1969.

60 Yeager AS: Transfusion-acquired cytomegalovirus infection in newborn infants. *Am J Dis Child* 128:478, 1974.

61 Yeager AS et al: Prevention of transfusion-acquired cytomegalovirus infection in newborn infants. *J Pediatr* 98:281, 1981.

62 Adler SP et al: Cytomegalovirus infections in neonates acquired by blood transfusions. *Pediatr Infect Dis* 2:114, 1983.

63 Yeager AS: Longitudinal, serological study of cytomegalovirus infections in nurses and in personnel without patient contact. *J Clin Microbiol* 2:448, 1975.

64 Friedman HM et al: Acquisition of cytomegalovirus infection among female employees at a pediatric hospital. *Pediatr Infect Dis* 3:233, 1984.

65 Balfour CL et al: Cytomegalovirus is not an occupational risk for nurses in renal transplant and neonatal units. *JAMA* 256:1909, 1986.

66 Brady MT et al: Cytomegalovirus infection in pediatric house officers: susceptibility and risk of primary infection. *Pediatr Res* 19:179A, 1985.

67 Adler SP et al: Molecular epidemiology of cytomegalovirus in a nursery: lack of evidence for nosocomial transmission. *J Pediatr* 108:117, 1986.

68 Demmler GJ et al: Nosocomial transmission of cytomegalovirus in a children's hospital. *Pediatr Res* 20:308A, 1986.

69 Wilfert CM et al: Restriction endonuclease analysis of cytomegalovirus deoxyribonucleic acid as an epidemiologic tool. *Pediatrics* 70: 717, 1982.

70 Ahlfors K et al: Congenital cytomegalovirus infection and disease in Sweden and the relative importance of primary and secondary maternal infections: preliminary findings from a prospective study. *Scand J Infect Dis* 16:129, 1984.

71 Boppana SB et al: Antiviral antibody responses and intrauterine transmission after primary maternal cytomegalovirus infection. *J Infect Dis* 171:1115, 1995.

72 Gehrz RC et al: Cytomegalovirus-specific humoral and cellular immune responses in human pregnancy. *J Infect Dis* 143:391, 1981.

73 Stern H et al: An early marker of fetal infection after primary cytomegalovirus infection in pregnancy. *Br Med J Clin Res (Clin Res Ed)* 292:718, 1986.

74 Griffiths PD: Cytomegalovirus, in *Principles and practice of clinical virology*, Zuckerman, AJ, Banatvala, JR & Pattison (eds), New York, Wiley, 1987, p. 75.

75 Stagno S et al: Congenital and perinatal cytomegalovirus infections. *Semin Perinatol* 7:31, 1983.

76 Reynolds DW et al: Maternal cytomegalovirus excretion and perinatal infection. *N Engl J Med* 289:1, 1973.

77 Pass RF et al: Specific cell-mediated immunity and the natural history of congenital infection with cytomegalovirus. *J Infect Dis* 148:953, 1983.

78 Pass RF et al: Specific lymphocyte blastogenic responses in children with cytomegalovirus and herpes simplex virus infections acquired early in infancy. *Infect Immunol* 34:166, 1981.

79 Reynolds DW et al: Specific cell-mediated immunity in children with congenital and neonatal cytomegalovirus infection and their mothers. *J Infect Dis* 140:493, 1979.

80 Starr SE et al: Impaired cellular immunity to cytomegalovirus in congenitally infected children and their mothers. *J Infect Dis* 140:500, 1979.

81 Fowler KB et al: The outcome of congenital cytomegalovirus infection in relation to maternal antibody status. *N Engl J Med* 326:663, 1992.

82 Griffiths PD et al: A prospective study of primary cytomegalovirus infection during pregnancy: final report. *Br J Obstet Gynecol* 91:307, 1984.

83 Weller TH et al: Virologic and clinical observations on cytomegalic inclusion disease. *N Engl J Med* 266:1233, 1962.

84 Pass RF et al: Outcome of symptomatic congenital CMV infection: Results of long-term longitudinal follow-up. *Pediatrics* 66:758, 1980.

85 Medearis DN, Jr: Observations concerning human cytomegalovirus infection and disease. *Bull Johns Hopkins Hosp* 114:171, 1964.

86 Stagno S et al: Auditory and visual defects resulting from symptomatic and subclinical congenital cytomegalovirus and Toxoplasma infection. *Pediatrics* 59:669, 1977.

87 Boppana SB et al: Symptomatic congenital cytomegalovirus infection: neonatal morbidity and mortality. *Pediatr Infect Dis J* 11:93, 1992.

88 Adapted from Pass RF et al. Outcome of symptomatic congenital cytomegalovirus infection: results of long term longitudinal follow up. In *Proceedings of the Third International Cytomegalovirus Workshop,* Bologna, Italy, Landini, MP (ed): London, Excerpta Medica, 1991, p. 3.

89 Kumar ML et al: Inapparent congenital cytomegalovirus infection: a follow-up study. *N Engl J Med* 288:1370, 1973.

90 Saigal S et al: The outcome in children with congenital cytomegalovirus infection: a longitudinal follow-up study. *Am J Dis Child* 136: 896, 1982.

91 Melish ME et al: Congenital cytomegalovirus infection: developmental progress of infants detected by routine screening. *Am J Dis Child* 126:190, 1973.

92 Pearl KN et al: Neurodevelopmental assessment after congenital cytomegalovirus infection. *Arch Dis Child* 61:323, 1986.

93 Stagno S et al: Infant pneumonitis associated with cytomegalovirus, chlamydia, pneumocystis, and ureaplasma: A prospective study. *Pediatrics* 68:322, 1981.

94 Whitley RJ et al: Protracted pneumonitis in young infants associated with perinatally acquired cytomegaloviral infection. *J Pediatr* 80:10, 1976.

95 Yeager AS et al: Sequelae of maternally derived cytomegalovirus infections in premature infants. *J Pediatr* 102:918, 1983.

96 Ballard RB et al: Acquired cytomegalovirus infection in pre-term infants. *Am J Dis Child* 133:482, 1979.

97 Whitley RJ et al: Ganciclovir treatment of symptomatic congenital cytomegalovirus infection: Results of a phase II Study. *J Infect Dis,* in press.

98 Nigro G et al: Ganciclovir therapy for symptomatic congenital cytomegalovirus infection in infants: A two-regimen experience. *J Pediatr* 124:318, 1994.

99 Elek SD et al: Development of a vaccine against mental retardation caused by cytomegalovirus infection in utero. *Lancet* 1:1, 1974.

100 Plotkin SA et al: Candidate cytomegalovirus strain for human vaccination. *Infect Immunol* 12:521, 1975.

101 Plotkin SA et al: CMV: *Pathogenesis and prevention of human infection.* New York, Alan R. Liss, Inc., 1984.

102 Stern H: Live cytomegalovirus vaccination of healthy volunteers: Eight year follow-up studies. *CMV: pathogenesis and prevention of human infection.* In Plotkin, SA, Michelson, S, Pagano, JS et al (eds), New York, Alan R. Liss, Inc., 1984.

103 Donner C et al: Accuracy of amniotic fluid testing before 21 weeks' gestation in prenatal diagnosis of congenital cytomegalovirus infection. *Prenat Diagn* 14:1055, 1994.

104 Nicolini U et al: Prenaatal diagnosis of congenital human cytomegalovirus infection. *Prenat Diagn* 14:903, 1994.

105 Donner C et al: Prenatal diagnosis of 52 pregnancies at risk for congenital cytomegalovirus infection. *Obstet Gynecol.* 72:481, 1993.

106 Pass RF: Commentary: Is there a role for prenatal diagnosis of congenital cytomegalovirus infection? *Pediatr Infect Dis J* 11:608, 1992.

107 Grose C et al: Prenatal diagnosis of congenital cytomegalovirus infection by virus isolation after amniocentesis. *Pediatr Infect Dis J* 11: 605, 1992.

108 Rutter D et al: Cytomegalic inclusion disease after recurrent maternal infection. *Lancet* 2:1182, 1985.

109 Morris DJ et al: Symptomatic congenital cytomegalovirus infection after maternal recurrent infection. *Pediatr Infect Dis J* 13:61, 1994.

110 Portolani M et al: A fatal case of congenital cytomegalic inclusion disease following recurrent maternal infection. *New Microbiolog* 18: 427, 1995.

111 Schwebke K et al: Congenital cytomegalovirus infection as a result of nonprimary cytomegalovirus disease in a mother with acquired immunodeficiency syndrome. *J Pediatr* 126:293, 1995.

112 Mettler C: *History of medicine.* New York, McGraw-Hill (Blakiston), 1947.

113 Astruc J: *De morbis venereis libri sex.* Paris, 1736.

114 Gruter W: Das herpesvirus, seine atiologische und klinische bedeutung. *Munch Med Wschr* 71:1058, 1924.

115 Hass M: Hepatoadrenal necrosis with intranuclear inclusion bodies: report of a case. *Am J Pathol* 11:127, 1935.

116 Batignani A: Conjunctive da virus erpetico in neonato. *Boll Ocul* 13: 1217, 1934.

117 Nahmias AJ et al: Antigenic and biologic differences in herpesvirus hominis. *Prog Med Virol* 10:110, 1968.

118 Whitley RJ: Herpes simplex virus. In *Fields virology.* Fields, BN, Knipe, DM, Howley, PM, et al (eds): Philadelphia, Lippincott-Raven Publishers, 1996, p. 2297.

119 McClung H et al: Relative concentrations in human sera of antibodies to cross reacting and specific antigens of herpes simplex virus types 1 and 2. *Am J Epidemiol* 104:192, 1976.

120 Smith IW et al: The incidence of herpesvirus hominis antibodies in the population. *J Hyg* (Lond) 65:395, 1967.

121 Wentworth BB et al: Seroepidemiology of infections due to members of herpesvirus group. *Am J Epidemiol* 94:496, 1971.

122 Nahmias AJ et al: Antibodies to herpesvirus hominis type 1 and 1 in humans. I. Patients with genital herpetic infections. *Am J Epidemiol* 91:539, 1970.

123 Allen WP et al: Concept review of genital herpes vaccines. *J Infect Dis* 145:413, 1982.

124 Brown ZA et al: Effects on infants of a first episode of genital herpes during pregnancy. *N Engl J Med* 317:1246, 1987.

125 Nahmias AJ et al: Sero-epidemiological and sociological patterns of herpes simplex virus infection in the world. *Scand J Infect Dis* 69:19, 1990.

126 Stavaraky NM et al: Sexual and socioeconomic factors affecting the risk of past infections with herpes simplex virus type 2. *Am J Epidemiol* 118:109, 1983.

127 Mann SL et al: Prevalence and incidence of herpesvirus infections among homosexually active men. *J Infect Dis* 149:1026, 1984.

128 Nahmias AJ et al: *Prevalence of herpes simplex virus (HSV) type-specific antibodies in a USA prepaid group medical practice population.* London, England. 1985.

129 Johnson RE et al: A seroepidemiologic survey of the prevalence of herpes simplex virus type 2 infection in the United States. *N Engl J Med* 321:7, 1989.

130 Flewett TH et al: Acute hepatitis due to herpes simplex virus in an adult. *J Clin Pathol* 22:60, 1969.

131 Anderson JM et al: Herpes encephalitis in pregnancy. *Br Med J* 1: 632, 1972.

132 Goyette RE et al: Fulminant herpesvirus hominis hepatitis during pregnancy. *Obstet Gynecol* 43:191, 1974.

133 Young EJ et al: Disseminated herpesvirus infection associated with primary genital herpes in pregnancy. *JAMA* 235:2731, 1976.

134 Hensleigh PA et al: Systemic herpesvirus hominis in pregnancy. *J Reprod Med* 22:171, 1979.
135 Peacock JE et al: Disseminated herpes simplex virus infection during pregnancy. *Obstet Gynecol* 61(Suppl 3):13S, 1983.
136 Nahmias AJ et al: Herpes simplex. In *Infectious diseases of the fetus and newborn infant,* Remington, JS, and Klein, JO (eds): Philadelphia, WB Saunders Company, 1983, p. 636.
137 Hutto C et al: Intrauterine herpes simplex virus infections. *J Pediatr* 110:97, 1987.
138 Nahmias AJ et al: Perinatal risk associated with maternal genital herpes simplex virus infection. *Am J Obstet Gynecol* 110:825, 1971.
139 Grossman JH et al: Management of genital herpes simplex virus infection during pregnancy. *Obstet Gynecol* 58:1, 1981.
140 Harger JH et al: Characteristics and management of pregnancy in women with genital herpes simplex virus infection. *Am J Obstet Gynecol* 145:784, 1983.
141 Tejani N et al: Subclinical herpes simplex genitalis infections in the perinatal period. *Am J Obstet Gynecol* 135:547, 1979.
142 Bolognese RJ et al: Herpesvirus hominis type-2 infections in asymptomatic pregnant women. *Obstet Gynecol* 48:507, 1976.
143 Vontver LA et al: Recurrent genital herpes simplex virus infection in pregnancy: infant outcome and frequency of asymptomatic recurrences. *Am J Obstet Gynecol* 143:75, 1982.
144 Rattray MC et al: Recurrent genital herpes among women: Symptomatic versus asymptomatic viral shedding. *Br J Vener Dis* 54:262, 1978.
145 Brown ZA et al: Neonatal herpes simplex virus infection in relation to asymptomatic maternal infection at the time of labor. *N Engl J Med* 324:1247, 1991.
146 Cone RW et al: Frequent detection of genital herpes simplex virus DNA by polymerase chain reaction among pregnant women. *JAMA* 272:792, 1994.
147 Adams HG et al: Genital herpetic infection in men and women: Clinical course and effect of topical application of adenine arabinoside. *J Infect Dis* 133:151, 1976.
148 Guinan ME et al: The course of untreated recurrent genital herpes simplex infection in 27 women. *N Engl J Med* 304:759, 1981.
149 Whitley RJ et al: The natural history of herpes simplex virus infection of mother and newborn. *Pediatrics* 66:489, 1980.
150 Whitley RJ et al: The natural history, pathogenesis, and treatment of neonatal herpes simplex virus infections. *Sem Pediatr Infect Dis* 5: 56, 1994.
151 Whitley RJ et al: Neonatal herpes simplex virus infection: follow-up evaluation of vidarabine therapy. *Pediatrics* 72:778, 1983.
152 Whitley RJ et al: Changing presentation of neonatal herpes simplex virus infection. *J Infect Dis* 158:109, 1988.
153 Corey L et al: Genital herpes simplex virus infections: clinical manifestations, course and complications. *Ann Intern Med* 98:958, 1983.
154 Corey L: The diagnosis and treatment of genital herpes. *JAMA* 248: 1041, 1982.
155 Yeager AS et al: Relationship of antibody to outcome in neonatal herpes simplex infections. *Infect Immunol* 29:532, 1980.
156 Prober CG et al: Low risk of herpes simplex virus infections in neonates exposed to the virus at the time of vaginal delivery to mothers with recurrent genital herpes simplex virus infections. *N Engl J Med* 316:240, 1987.
157 Stone KM et al: Neonatal herpes: results of one year's surveillance. Interscience Conference on Antimicrobial Agents and Chemotherapy, Minneapolis, Minnesota, 1985.
158 Parvey LS et al: Neonatal herpes simplex virus infection introduced by fetal monitor scalp electrode. *Pediatrics* 65:1150, 1980.
159 Kaye EM et al: Neonatal herpes simplex meningoencephalitis associated with fetal monitor scalp electrodes. *Neurology* 31:1045, 1981.
160 Sullivan-Bolyai J et al: Neonatal herpes simplex virus infections in King County, Washington: Increasing incidence and epidemiologic correlates. *JAMA* 250:3059, 1983.
161 Adam E et al: Seroepidemiologic studies of herpesvirus type-2 and carcinoma of the cervix. II. Uganda. *J Natl Cancer Inst* 48:65, 1972.
162 Templeton AC: Generalized herpes simplex in malnourished children. *J Clin Pathol* 23:24, 1970.
163 Florman AL et al: Intrauterine infection with herpes simplex virus: resultant congenital malformation. *JAMA* 225:129, 1973.
164 South MA et al: Congenital malformation of the central nervous system associated with genital type (type 2) herpesvirus. *J Pediatr* 75: 13, 1969.
165 Baldwin S et al: Intrauterine herpes simplex virus infection. *Teratology* 39:1, 1989.
166 Garcia A: Maternal herpes simplex infection causing abortion: histopathologic study of the placenta. *Hospital* 78:1267, 1970.
167 Witzleben CL et al: Possible transplacental transmission of herpes simplex infection. *Pediatrics* 36:192, 1965.
168 Gagnon RA: Transplacental inoculation of fetal herpes simplex in the newborn. *Obstet Gynecol* 31:682, 1968.
169 Light IJ: Postnatal acquisition of herpes simplex virus by the newborn infant: A review of the literature. *Pediatrics* 63:480, 1979.
170 Linnemann CC Jr et al: Transmission of herpes simplex virus type-1 in a nursery for the newborn: identification of viral species isolated by DNA fingerprinting. *Lancet* 1:964, 1978.
171 Hammerberg O et al: An outbreak of herpes simplex virus type 1 in an intensive care nursery. *Pediatr Infect Dis* 2:290, 1983.
172 Sullivan-Bolyai JZ et al: Disseminated neonatal herpes simplex virus type 1 from a maternal breast lesion. *Pediatrics* 71:455, 1983.
173 Dunkle LM et al: Neonatal herpes simplex infection possibly acquired via maternal breast milk. *Pediatrics* 63:250, 1979.
174 Kibrick S: Herpes simplex virus in breast milk. *Pediatrics* 64:390, 1979.
175 Yeager AS et al: Transmission of herpes simplex virus from father to neonate. *J Pediatr* 103:905, 1983.
176 Douglas J et al: Acquisition of neonatal HSV-1 infection from a paternal source contact. *J Pediatr* 103:908, 1983.
177 Rawls WE et al: Epidemiology of herpes simplex virus type 1 and 2. In *The human herpesviruses: an interdisciplinary perspective.* Nahmias A, Dowdle W, Schinazi R (eds), Amsterdam, Elsevier/North-Holland, 1981, p. 137.
178 Nahmias AJ et al: *Viral infections of humans.* New York, Plenum, 1981.
179 Hatherley LI et al: Herpesvirus in an obstetric hospital. II. Asymptomatic virus excretion in staff members. *Med J Aust* 2:273, 1980.
180 Schreiner R et al: Maternal oral herpes: Isolation policy. *Pediatrics* 63:247, 1979.
181 Hatherley LI et al: Herpesvirus in an obstetric hospital I: Herpetic eruptions. *Med J Aust* 2:205, 1980.
182 Hatherley LI et al: Herpesvirus in an obstetric hospital. III: Prevalence of antibodies in patients and staff. *Med J Aust* 2:325, 1980.
183 Notkins LA: Immune mechanisms by which the spread of viral infections is topped. *Cell Immunol* 11:478, 1974.
184 Lopez C: The herpesviruses. In *Immunobiology and prophylaxis of human herpesvirus infections,* Roizman B, Lopez C (eds), New York, Plenum, 1985.
185 Oakes JE et al: Lymphocyte reactivity contributes to protection conferred by specific antibody passively transferred to herpes simplex virus-infected mice. *Infect Immunol* 29:642, 1980.
186 Kahlon J et al: Antibody response of the newborn after herpes simplex virus infection. *J Infect Dis* 158:925, 1988.
187 Sullender WM, et al: Humoral and cell-mediated immunity in neonates with herpes simplex virus infection. *J Infect Dis* 155:28, 1987.
188 Rasmussen L et al: Role of T-lymphocytes in cellular immune responses during herpes simplex virus infection in humans. *Proc Natl Acad Sci USA* 75:3957, 1978.
189 Chilmonczyk BA et al: Characterization of the human newborn response to herpesvirus antigen. *J Immunol* 134:4184, 1985.
190 Burchett SK et al: Ontogeny of neonatal mononuclear cell transformation and interferon gamma production after herpes simplex virus stimulation. *Clin Res* 34:129, 1986.
191 Taylor S et al: Impaired production of gamma interferon by newborn cells in vitro is due to a functionally immature macrophage. *J Immunol* 134:1493, 1984.

192 Rouse BT: Immunobiology and Prophylaxis of Human Herpesvirus Infections. In *The herpesviruses.* Roizman B, Lopez C (eds), New York, Plenum Press, 1985, p. 103.
193 Kohl S et al: Normal function of neonatal polymorphonuclear leukocytes in antibody-dependent cellular cytotoxicity to herpes simplex virus infected cells. *J Pediatr* 98:783, 1981.
194 Kohl S et al: Human neonatal and maternal monocyte-macrophage and lymphocyte mediated antibody dependent cytotoxicity to herpes simplex infected cells. *J Pediatr* 93:206, 1978.
195 Zisman B et al: Selective effects of anti-macrophage serum, silica and anti-lymphocyte serum on pathogenesis of herpes virus infection of young adult mice. *J Immunol* 104:1155, 1970.
196 Trofatter KJ et al: Growth of type 2 herpes simplex virus in newborn and adult mononuclear leukocytes. *Intervirology* 2:117, 1979.
197 Mintz H et al: Age dependent resistance of human alveolar macrophages to herpes simplex virus. *Infect Immunol* 28:417, 1980.
198 Lopez C et al: Marrow dependent cells depleted by Sr mediate genetic resistance to herpes simplex virus type 1 infection in mice. *Infect Immunol* 28:1028, 1980.
199 Armerding D et al: Induction of natural killer cells by herpes simplex virus type 2 in resistant and sensitive inbred mouse strains. *Immunobiology* 158:369, 1981.
200 Hirsch MS et al: Macrophages and age-dependent resistance to herpes simplex virus in mice. *J Immunol* 104:1160, 1970.
201 Arvin AM et al. Neonatal herpes simplex infection in the absence of mucocutaneous lesions. *J Pediatr* 100:715, 1982.
202 Whitley RJ et al: Neonatal herpes simplex virus infections. *Pediatr Rev* 7:119, 1985.
203 Yeager AS et al: Reasons for the absence of a history of recurrent genital infections in mothers of neonates infected with herpes simplex virus. *Pediatrics* 73:188, 1984.
204 Kimberlin DK et al: Application of the polymerase chain reaction to the diagnosis and management of neonatal herpes simplex virus disease. *J Infect Dis* 174:1162, 1996.
205 Lakeman FD et al: Diagnosis of herpes simplex encephalitis: Application of polymerase chain reaction to cerebrospinal fluid from brain biopsied patients and correlation with disease. *J Infect Dis* 171:857, 1995.
206 Mizrahi EM et al: A unique electroencephalogram pattern in neonatal herpes simplex virus encephalitis. *Neurology* 31:164, 1981.
207 Whitley RJ et al: Vidarabine therapy of neonatal herpes simplex virus infection. *Pediatrics* 66:495, 1980.
208 Guttman LT et al: Herpes simplex virus encephalitis in children: analysis of cerebrospinal fluid and progressive neurodevelopmental deterioration. *J Infect Dis* 154:415, 1986.
209 Nahmias AJ et al: Eye infections. *Surv Ophthalmol* 21:100, 1976.
210 Nahmias A et al: Ocular manifestations of herpes simplex in the newborn. *Int Ophthalmol Clin* 12:191, 1972.
211 Reested P et al: Chorioretinitis of the newborn with herpes simplex type 1: Report of a case. *Acta Ophthalmol* 57:1096, 1979.
212 Cibis A et al: Herpes simplex virus induced congenital cataracts. *Arch Ophthalmol* 85:220, 1971.
213 Rowley A et al: Rapid detection of herpes simplex virus DNA in cerebrospinal fluid of patients with herpes simplex encephalitis. *Lancet* 335:440, 1990.
214 Aurelius E et al: Rapid diagnosis of herpes simplex encephalitis by nested polymerase chain reaction assay of cerebrospinal fluid. *Lancet* 337:189, 1991.
215 Aurelius E et al: Encephalitis in immunocompetent patients due to herpes simplex virus type 1 or 2 as determined by type-specific polymerase chain reaction and antibody assays of cerebrospinal fluid. *J Med Virol* 39:179, 1993.
216 Field JH et al: Isolation and characterization of acyclovir-resistant mutants of herpes simplex virus. *J Gen Virol* 49:115, 1980.
217 Schaeffer HJ et al: 9-(2-hydroxyethoxymethyl) guanine activity against viruses of the herpes group. *Nature* 272:583, 1978.
218 Elion GB et al: Selectivity of action of an antiherpetic agent, 9-(2-hydroxyethoxymethyl)guanine. *Proc Natl Acad Sci USA* 74:5716, 1977.
219 Fyfe JA et al: Thymidine kinase from herpes simplex virus phosphorylates the new antiviral compound, 9-(2-hydroxyethoxymethyl) guanine. *J Biol Chem* 253:(24)8721, 1978.
220 Derse D et al: Inhibition of purified human and herpes simplex virus-induced DNA polymerase by 9-(2-hydroxyethoxymethyl)guanine [acyclovir] triphosphate: effect on primertemplate function. *J Biol Chem* 256:11447, 1981.
221 Corey L et al: Treatment of primary first episode genital herpes simplex virus infections with acyclovir. Results of topical, intravenous, and oral therapy. *J Antimicrob Chemother* 12:79, 1983.
222 Bryson YJ et al: Treatment of first episodes of genital herpes simplex virus infection with oral acyclovir: A randomized double-blind controlled trial in normal subjects. *N Engl J Med* 308:916, 1983.
223 Corey L et al: A Trial of topical acyclovir in genital herpes simplex virus infections. *N Engl J Med* 306:1313, 1982.
224 Saral R et al: Acyclovir prophylaxis of herpes simplex virus infections: A randomized, double-blind, controlled trial in bone-marrow-transplant recipients. *N Engl J Med* 305:63, 1981.
225 Meyers JD et al. Multicenter collaborative trial of intravenous acyclovir for treatment of mucocutaneous herpes simplex virus infection in immunocompromised host. *Am J Med* 73:229, 1982.
226 Whitley RJ et al: Vidarabine versus acyclovir therapy in herpes simplex encephalitis. *N Engl J Med* 314:144, 1986.
227 Whitley RJ et al: A controlled trial comparing vidarabine with acyclovir in neonatal herpes simplex virus infection. *N Engl J Med* 324: 444, 1991.
228 Kimberlin D et al: Administration of oral acyclovir suppressive therapy following neonatal herpes simplex virus disease limited to the skin, eyes, and mouth: results of a Phase I/II trial. *Pediatr Infect Dis J* 15:247, 1996.
229 Whitley RJ et al: Predictors of morbidity and mortality in neonates with herpes simplex virus infections. *N Engl J Med* 324:450, 1991.
230 Arvin AM et al: Failure of antepartum maternal cultures to predict the infant's risk of exposure to herpes simplex virus at delivery. *N Engl J Med* 315:796, 1986.
231 Prober CG et al: The management of pregnancies complicated by genital infections with Herpes simplex virus. *Clin Infect Dis* 15:1031, 1992.
232 Prober CG et al: Use of routine viral cultures at delivery to identify neonates exposed to herpes simplex virus. *N Engl J Med* 318:887, 1988.
233 Richman D: *Immunobiology and prophylaxis of human herpesvirus infection.* New York, Raven Press, 1986.
234 Scott LL et al: Acyclovir suppression to prevent cesarean delivery after first-episode genital herpes. *Obstet Gynecol* 87:69, 1996.

Chapter 86

Recurrent respiratory papillomatosis

Haskins Kashima
Keerti Shah
Phoebe Mounts

INTRODUCTION

Recurrent respiratory papillomatosis (RRP) is a condition in which histologically benign epithelial growths—papillomata—occur at sites in the respiratory tract from the nasal vestibule to the peripheral lung. The larynx is the site most often diseased. The growths exhibit patterns of regrowth after surgical removal, hence the designation *recurrent respiratory papillomatosis*.

The syndrome of RRP is most often identified on the basis of laryngeal lesions that cause hoarseness and upper-airway obstructive symptoms (Fig. 86-1). Other common sites of papillomatous growths include the nasal vestibule, the nasopharyngeal surface of the soft palate, the midsection of the laryngeal surface of epiglottis (Fig. 86-2), the vocal folds, the upper and under surface of vocal folds, carina, bronchi and bronchioles (particularly at the sites of bifurcation), and the peripheral lung fields. The foregoing sites have squamo-ciliary junctions that appear to have particular predilection for papillomatous growths.[1] When tracheotomy has been performed, the junction of tracheal mucosa to the stomal lining and the tracheal mucosa at the level of the distal tip of the tracheotomy tube become iatrogenic squamo-ciliary junctions. Isolated papilloma of the oral cavity most often occurring on the palate, tonsils, tongue dorsum, and the buccal mucosa typically have human papillomavirus (HPV) etiology, but the specific HPV type may differ from those associated with RRP.

Recurrent respiratory papillomatosis occurs among two distinct age groups. Approximately one-half of the cases are designated *juvenile onset recurrent respiratory papillomatosis* (JO-RRP), with symptoms beginning shortly after birth, during infancy, or in the preschool years. Newly diagnosed cases may occur as late as 12 to 13 years of age; it is unusual to diagnose new cases between 12 and 20 years of age. *Adult onset recurrent respiratory papillomatosis* (AO-RRP) RRP occurs and has peak incidence during the third and fourth decades; occasionally new cases may be diagnosed in patients as old as 60 or 70 years of age. Juvenile onset disease, particularly during the first several years of life, exhibits rapid regrowth and requires frequent, repeated surgical excisions because of severe hoarseness and because the lesions may obstruct the upper airway. In childen, even a small growth can produce respiratory distress because of their small laryngotracheal dimensions. The inter-operative intervals lengthen with age. The papilloma regrowth rate appears to be slower in adults; this may be attributable to their full-sized larynges, which are less susceptible to airway compromise by tumor regrowth.

HISTORICAL BACKGROUND

The essential features of laryngeal papillomatosis, encompassing the clinical and histologic appearance as well as the tendency to recur, were recognized by Sir Morell Mackenzie in 1871.[1] The first reference to "warts" was by Marcellus Donatus in the early seventeenth century. (Cited by Mackenzie.[2])

Virchow, Mackenzie,[3] and others attributed the papillomatous growths to chronic inflammation and catarrh, whereas Fauvel, in 1876, suggested excessive voice use as the primary factor in the development of the lesions. A report by Dunbar Roy in 1902 incriminated alcohol and tobacco, in addition to voice abuse, as important factors in the development of papillomata. In addition, Roy recognized that papillomata occurred in adults as well as in children, and he considered that these might have differing etiologies. Baumgarten (cited by Roy) made the interesting speculation that maternal gonorrheal discharge at birth could have etiologic relevance.[4]

In 1853 Buck recognized the similarity of laryngeal papillomata, condylomata acuminata and epidermal verrucae (cited by Geopfert, 1982).[5] Jadasshon in 1895 identified a filterable virus as the causative agent for skin warts. Ullman performed a series of experiments using cell-free filtrate of laryngeal papilloma and succeeded in producing papillomas on his own arm and on the arm of an associate.[6] In a 1956 case report, Hajek linked the presence of maternal condyloma with the occurrence of RRP in the child.[7]

The history of the treatment of RRP begins with the first successful peroral excision of laryngeal papillomata by Koderik in 1750. Surgical excision by thyrotomy was first performed by Brauers in 1883. Subsequent development of the laryngoscope caused Mackenzie to advocate endoscopic excision as the most effective means for papilloma removal, surpassing the more invasive methods of thyrotomy and laryngofissure. Endoscopic excision has been the cornerstone of therapy ever since, and the major improvements to this method have been the utilization of the operating microscope and the surgical laser.[8] Surgical excision, even with refinements, has not been successful in permanent eradication of this troublesome disorder. A wide variety of adjuvant agents have been used, including "causticum, sanguinaria, thuja, belladonna, calcerea phosphate, conium silicea."[9] Podophyllum has enjoyed long-standing favor as an adjuvant to surgical excision; it has proven efficacy in condylomata acuminata, but its adverse reactions have included growth stimulation of papilloma and possible carcinogenicity in mice, raising a note of caution in its use.[10]

CLINICAL MANIFESTATIONS

Juvenile onset RRP is diagnosed on basis of hoarseness, often present in the first year of life, perhaps from the time of birth. Upper-airway obstructive symptoms of varying severity are aggravated during intercurrent respiratory-tract infection, and the initial presentation may be as an airway emergency (Fig. 86-1). Endoscopic excision of the papillomatous growths restores a safe airway and improves the voice, but rapid regrowth of papilloma may require repetition of endoscopic excisions at intervals as often as weekly. For the most severely affected patients, as many as 100 or more endoscopic excisions may be necessary to maintain a safe and adequate airway.

As the patient enters puberty, the intervals between operations generally become longer due to the combination of increased laryngeal dimensions and reduced rate of papilloma regrowth. An undetermined number of patients continue to experience papilloma regrowth, and the lesions may extend from the larynx into the trachea (see Fig. 86-1, C), to the bronchi, and eventually to the lungs (Fig. 86-3).[11] The risk of extension into the trachea and lower respiratory tract appears to be increased in patients who have had tracheotomy performed; hence, experienced laryngolo-

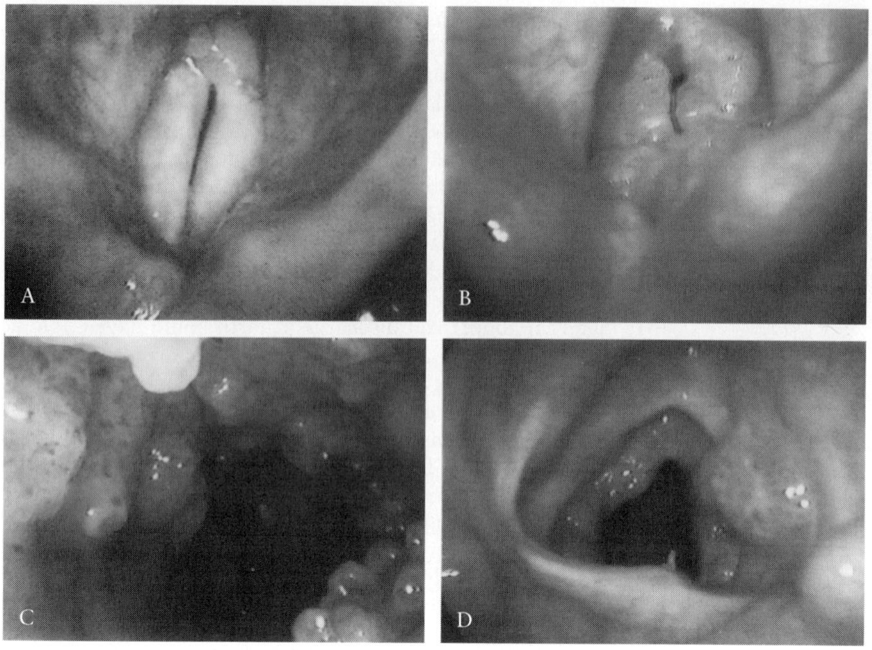

Fig. 86-1. *Laryngeal papilloma. A.* Lesions at anterior commissure. *B.* Lesions on vocal folds, bilaterally. *C.* Tracheal lesions producing marked dyspnea. *D.* Lesions on right false cord and circumferentially in subglottis.

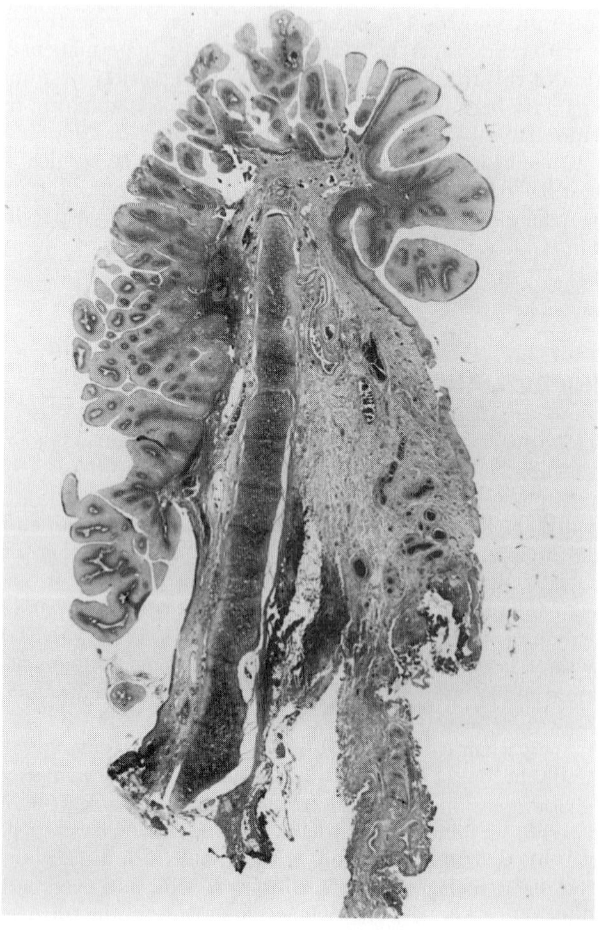

Fig. 86-2. *Epiglottic lesion.* Fern-like lesion arising from laryngeal surface of epiglottis and producing severe airway obstruction.

gists advocate repeated and meticulous endoscopic excision and *avoidance of tracheotomy.*

Among AO-RRP patients the usual initial symptom is persistent hoarseness. The clinical appearance evaluation may suggest a benign polyp, but histologic examination of the excised specimen reveals the growth to be a papilloma. Widespread papillomatosis occurs in a minority of the adult onset patients.

In 3 to 5 percent of RRP patients, malignant transformation to squamous cell carcinoma occurs.[12,13] Irradiation therapy and tobacco usage have been implicated as factors predisposing to malignant transformation of respiratory papillomatosis, but carcinomas have also developed in long-standing papillomas in individuals who do not have these risk factors.

The issue of spontaneous remission of respiratory papillomatosis is unsettled. In 1964, Majoros and colleagues reported that a 56-year review of 77 patients at the Mayo Clinic showed that 85 percent of the patients became "free of disease."[14] Bjork and Holinger, in reviewing separate clinical experiences, agreed that AO-RRP patients were more likely to attain remission than JO-RRP patients.[15,16] However, Dedo and Jackler described 10 patients with a *normal* indirect laryngoscopic examination in whom the presence of papilloma was found upon suspension microlaryngoscopy on the following day. Underscoring that clinical detection and recognition of papilloma in early or limited lesions may be difficult—even for those with extensive clinical skills and experience.[17] Steinberg et al. have demonstrated the presence of HPV DNA in histologically normal laryngeal epithelium, in specimens from patients with papillomatosis elsewhere in the respiratory tract.[18] These sites should be regarded as latent disease with potential for new or recurrent growth. The high frequency of subclinical latent disease underscores the necessity to accept with caution the report of complete remission from papillomatosis.

DIAGNOSIS

A diagnosis of respiratory papillomatosis begins with a history of hoarseness often accompanied by upper airway obstruction of variable severity. The essential examination is laryngoscopy to document any abnormal growths or impaired motion of one or

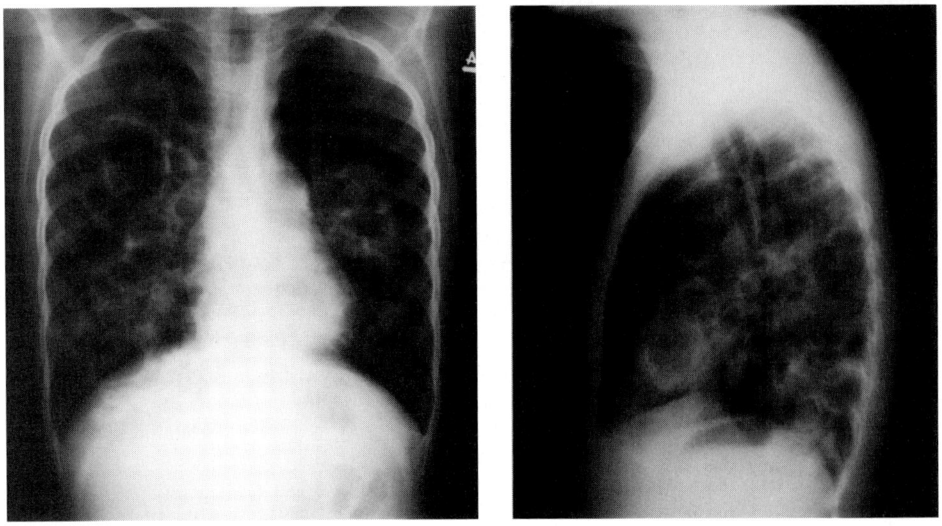

Fig. 86-3. *Pulmonary papilloma in 10 year old.* Papilloma enlarge, cavitate centrally, and produce respiratory failure.

both vocal folds. Laryngoscopy is traditionally performed using laryngeal mirrors, rigid or flexible laryngoscopy, which provide illumination and magnified imaging. The typical papilloma is a papillary (moist wart) most often on the vocal folds where it interferes with normal closure during phonation and results in hoarseness. The vestibular fold and epiglottis are other sites commonly diseased with papilloma. The papillomas have characteristic clinical appearance of multinodular growths with a small centered subepithelial vascular tuft. The lesions may be sessile and widespread or exophytic and arising from a narrow stalk (Fig. 86-2). Varying degrees of epithelial atypia have been observed, and these cases, particularly, require careful follow-up. Inasmuch as malignant transformation has been noted in the larynx, trachea, and lungs, the specimens obtained at each operation should be carefully labeled to identify the site of biopsy so that any histologic change of concern can be precisely identified.

ETIOLOGY

The viral etiology for respiratory papillomatosis had been long suspected, and precise identification of human papillomavirus types 6 and 11 (HPV-6 and HPV-11) as the etiologic agents was achieved simultaneously in several laboratories. They are also implicated as the causative agents in genital condyloma. Infection by HPV-11 (also described as HPV-6C) has been correlated with the most severe form of the disease including extension into the trachea and lungs.[20]

PATHOGENESIS

Using immunohistochemical and *in situ* hybridization techniques, the presence of HPV in tissue sections of RRP has been demonstrated. Inasmuch as the identical HPV types are associated with genital condyloma, it has been commonly assumed that viral transmission of JO-RRP occurs at the time of delivery. The observed low rate of clinical respiratory papillomatosis is imperfectly understood. Cases of self-limited papillomatosis, manifested only by hoarseness, may escape diagnosis. It has been speculated that some cases of neonatal and infantile asphyxia may be attributable to unsuspected papillomatous growths in the airway.

AO-RRP has been presumed to be transmitted by sexual contact, namely oral-genital exposure. In some cases of papillomatosis initially diagnosed in adulthood, a lifelong history of hoarseness suggests the possibility that the initial viral transmission may have occurred at childbirth and remained latent until adulthood.

Transmission of viral infection through infected oropharyngeal secretions has not been documented. There are no documented cases of papillomatosis occurring in family members who have been constantly exposed to secretions from patients with papillomatosis. There are, however, numerous anecdotal reports of surgeons who developed warty growths on the face and upper body, presumably from exposures occurring at the time of surgical excisions. In spite of the precise virological techniques currently available, HPV transmission from mother-to-child or between intimate adults, or inadvertent HPV transmission during medicosurgical encounters, has not been conclusively documented.

CLINICAL COURSE

The clinical course of recurrent respiratory papillomatosis is predictably unpredictable. Initial presentation of the disorder is usually as a solitary lesion which, after excision, follows one of several courses: 1) the lesion may be permanently eradicated, never to recur; 2) the lesion recurs after variable intervals, often at the precise site of the original growth, hence, the designation *recurrent* laryngeal papillomatosis; 3) papilloma distribution extends to previously nondiseased sites in growth sites in the larynx/tracheobronchial tree and/or lung; 4) papilloma at any of the growth sites may undergo malignant transformation into squamous carcinoma; 5) in rare instances, established papilloma may undergo spontaneous regression. Neither the determinate factors nor the probability of these various alternative outcomes are known and await precise documentation based on long-term outcome studies on a population of patients with juvenile onset and adult onset recurrent respiratory papillomatosis.

Because of the smaller size of the larynx, the pediatric patients, particularly infants, have significant risk for critical upper airway obstruction. Patients with adult onset papillomatosis are generally more troubled by their voice impairment, rather than airway compromise. Adolescent aged patients usually require operative intervention at less frequent intervals when at a younger age, for the same reason.

RRP SEVERITY ASSESSMENT

The clinical course of RRP is predictably unpredictable. Accordingly, evaluation as to the efficacy of any treatment modality requires objective and reproducible description and staging.

Historically, severity of RRP has been based on the total numbers of operations (per lifetime or per unit time, e.g.,per year). Alternatively, inter-operative intervals have been used (equating longer intervals to indicate clinical improvement and shorter intervals to indicate clinical worsening). As there is no objective standard to specify the necessity for surgical excision, severity assessment, based on total numbers of operations or on intervals between operations, is an imperfect index of disease severity.

In order to standardize severity assessment during a multi-institutional randomized clinical trial to evaluate interferon efficacy in RRP, a numerical severity scoring system was devised.[21] This lesion-based score took into account the numbers of specific anatomic sites in the respiratory tract diseased with papilloma, the extent of surface area at each anatomic site diseased with papilloma, and the extent of airway encroachment at each anatomic site, as determined by the degree of cross-sectional airway compromise at each anatomic site. The resulting composite score correlated with the symptom severity as reported by patients, and showed remarkable consistency of scores reported by surgeon-investigators at different institutions. *Complete remission* is defined as total absence of papilloma for six consecutive months, and *partial remission* as a 50-percent reduction in composite score of at least six-months duration. This scoring system, with minor modifications, has been successfully adopted by investigators in several subsequent clinical studies and could become the basis of a uniform severity assessment system. A valid and reproducible severity scoring system is necessary to improve understanding of the natural history and course of disease in this imperfectly understood disorder, and to evaluate objectively the efficacy of new treatment options.

EPIDEMIOLOGY

Laryngeal papilloma is recognized as the most common benign neoplasm in the larynx; it is, however, an uncommon disorder. On the basis of a 1979 mail survey, with a 62 percent response rate, it was estimated that 1,500 new cases of RRP were diagnosed in the United States in 1976, an average of 7.1 new cases per year per million population.[22]

Derkay and the Task Force on Recurrent Respiratory Papillomas conducted a mail survey in 1994; they estimated that more than 2,000 new JO-RRP and approximately 3,500 new AO-RRP cases were diagnosed in the United States during the preceding 12 months.[23] The incidence of JO-RRP is estimated to be 4.3 per 100,000 children under age 14 and 1.8 per 100,000 adults above age 15. Among JO-RRP subjects, 31 percent showed extralaryngeal papilloma extension; 16 percent of AO-RRP subjects experienced extralaryngeal spread. Tracheostomies had been performed in 14 percent of JO-RP and in 6 percent of AO-RRP patients.

Buck in 1853 and Hajek in 1956 are generally credited as having described maternal condyloma in association with a newborn subsequently diagnosed as having RRP.[6] Hajek's case is particularly noteworthy in that the maternal condylomata underwent spontaneous regression shortly after the woman gave birth; this pattern of rapid accelerated growth during pregnancy and swift postpartum regression of maternal condylomata may account for the infrequent recognition of the probable association of these two conditions. Maternal condyloma is present in 30 to 50 percent of mothers who give birth to childen who develop JO-RRP.

It is not irrelevant that, among RRP clinical populations, as many as 20 percent of JO-RRP patients are adopted. This conforms to the recognized pattern that the juvenile-onset disease is predominantly observed in the first-born child of young (teenaged) pregnant women. The triad of a first born delivered vaginally to a teenaged pregnant woman with condyloma describes a high-risk profile for JO-RRP. An unexplained observation is that there is only rare documentation of siblings having RRP. The wider availability of sensitive and accurate testing methods, including viral typing of the RRP lesion matched to tissue specimens from the mother's birth canal, may provide more conclusive evidence as to the mechanism of transmission.

A 30- to 50-percent prevalence of genital condyloma has been observed among women giving birth to patients with JO-RRP.[24] If it is assumed that 5 percent of women of child-bearing age are infected with HPV-6 or HPV-11, then of the 4.0 million live births occurring in the United States each year, 200,000 pregnancies occur in women so affected. Presently 20 percent of deliveries are by cesarean section, so 160,000 women with HPV-6 or HPV-11 infection give birth vaginally.[25] If one accepts that 1,500 new cases of JO-RRP occur each year, the risk of papillomatosis for a newborn from an HPV-infected mother can be estimated at about 1 in 100. Alternative assumptions can vary this risk. The risk may be greater when the mother has clinical disease (condylomata) than when the mother has subclinical infection. The apparent discrepancy between the small numbers of juveniles (new borns) developing papilloma versus the large number at risk may be attributable to features of the maternal genital-tract infection, including the duration of infection, status of treatment, and host immune factors. The immune status of the newborn as well as the period of exposure (time in labor, premature rupture of membranes, and other obstetrical considerations) may be decisive. The relevance of the host immune status is underscored in the reports of papillomavirus infections (skin warts and respiratory papilloma) occurring in individuals whose immune status is compromised as a result of immune suppression for organ transplantation or while receiving chemotherapy.

In a recent review that combined the clinical experiences from two major medical centers, 1 of 109 patients with JO-RRP was found to have been delivered by cesarean section. Hence, the recommendation for cesarean section in women with condylomata does not guarantee that an offspring will not develop RRP.[26] It has been presumed that AO-RRP is a sexually transmitted disorder, but epidemiological verification has not been established.

TREATMENT

A long list of escharotics, antimitotic agents, hormonal preparations, and antibiotics have been examined but all were ultimately found ineffective in treating RRP. Autogenous vaccines, prepared from the patient's own lesions, were used by Holinger and coworkers with variable benefit.[27] Gross and Hubbard reported favorable responses in 9 of 22 patients receiving autogenous vaccine.[28]

Haglund and colleagues reported that seven patients with recurrent respiratory papillomatosis were treated with interferon (IFN). Their promising results at the Karolinska Institute stimulated numerous pilot studies; virtually all reported favorable outcomes, including some with complete remissions of short duration.[29] Two multi-institutional randomized studies have been completed in the United States; one study, utilizing New York Blood Center interferon at 2 MU/m^2 for one year, concluded that interferon was ineffective in treating RRP.[30] A second study, utilizing IFN alpha n1 at 5 MU/m^2 for 6 months, observed statistically significant benefit, with 8 of 57 patients achieving complete remission (CR) and 19 achieving partial remission (PR). Most patients, however, relapsed when IFN was discontinued.[31] Longer-term sustained administration (median duration of treatment 200 days, range up to 1,850 days) produced 22 CR and 25 PR in the 60 patients enrolled in the study. The duration of response was up to 2,400 days for CR and 1,400 days for PR. Interferon doses of 2 MU/m^2 and 4 MU/m^2, three times per week yielded comparable responses.[32]

Zenner et al. have reported 11 CR and 7 PR in 20 patients treated with IFN alpha-2C.[33] With increased interest in antiviral therapy, Retinoids, specifically 13-cis-retinoic acid, have been under investigation in pilot studies. There is continuing interest in photodynamic therapy, in which a hematoporphyrin derivative is activated by argon laser to release singlet oxygen and destroy the papilloma lesion.[34] Extreme photosensitivity prohibits subjects from being exposed to sunlight. The search for the most suitable hematoporphyrin continues.

In 1922 Crowe and Breitstein[19] advocated the careful use of radium in the treatment of papillomatosis, particularly in adults. Subsequent experience with the use of irradiation therapy led to the recognition of growth disturbance in the laryngeal cartilages of pediatric patients and, more important, of malignant degeneration of previously benign laryngeal papillomatosis. These developments have relegated irradiation therapy to a management option used only in exceptional circumstances.

PREVENTION

The optimum obstetrical management of women with HPV infection deserves careful study (see Chap. 80). Neither the specific clinical lesion (whether cervical, vaginal, or vulvar) nor the cofactors predisposing to an increased risk of offspring developing papillomatosis have been identified. Given the present state of indefinite knowledge regarding the incidence of RRP, the precise risk of developing papillomatosis cannot be defined. The risk rates as presently estimated do not justify the recommendation for delivery by cesarean section in all pregnant women infected with HPV-6 or HPV-11, particularly given the several instances in which papillomatosis has developed in children delivered by cesarean section. Extensive maternal condylomas at the time of birth or in a young woman in her first pregnancy describes the high-risk profile, for a newborn with papilloma and should be considered an for cesarean delivery.

THE FUTURE

The history of the search for an effective adjuvant in RRP management reveals that, with few exceptions, the published reports are of pilot studies that inevitably share one or more of the following flaws: lack of defined criteria for advising adjuvant; lack of objective description of disease severity at study entry; and lack of criteria for measuring response—including duration of response. Given that RRP is an uncommon condition, the undertaking of a meaningful Phase III trial with adequate numbers of subjects necessitates multi-institutional collaboration.

References

1 Kashima H, Mounts P, Leventhal B, et al: Sites of predilection in recurrent respiratory papillomatosis. *Ann Otol Rhinol Laryngol,* 102: 580–84, 1993.

2 Mackenzie GH: The treatment of laryngeal growths in children. *Br Med J* 2:883–885, 1901.

3 Mackenzie GH: *Essay on Growths in the Larynx: With Reports and an Analysis of One Hundred Consecutive Cases Treated by the Author.* Philadelphia, Lindsay and Blakiston, 1871.

4 Roy D: The treatment of laryngeal papillomata with report of a case. *Ann Otol Rhinol Laryngol,* 11: 482–90, 1902.

5 Goepfert H, Sessions RB, Gutterman JU, et al: Leukocyte interferon in patients with juvenile laryngeal papillomatosis. *Ann Otol Rhinol Laryngol,* 91: 431–36, 1982.

6 Ullman EV: On the aeitology of the laryngeal papilloma. *Acta Otolaryngol (Stockh),* 5:317–34, 1923.

7 Hajek EF: Contribution to the etiology or laryngeal papilloma in childen. *J Laryngol Otol,* 70:166–68, 1956.

8 Alberti PW, Dykun R: Adult laryngeal papillomata. *J Otolaryngol,* 10: 463–70, 1981.

9 Al-Saleem T, Peale AR, Norris CM: Multiple papillomatosis of the lower respiratory tract. *Cancer,* 22:1173–84, 1968.

10 Leventhal BG: Cytotoxic and Antiviral Drugs for the Treatment of Papillomatosis. Presented at the UCLA Symposia on Papilloma-Viruses, 1985.

11 Weiss MD, Kashima HK: Tracheal involvement in laryngeal papillomatosis. *Laryngoscope,* 93:45–48, 1983.

12 Solomon D, Smith RL, Kashima HK, et al: Malignant transformation in non-irradiated recurrent respiratory papillomatosis. *Laryngoscope,* 95:900–904, 1985.

13 Kashima HK, Wu T-C. Mounts P, et al: Carcinoma ex-papilloma: histologic and virologic studies in whole-organ sections of the larynx. *Laryngoscope,* 98:619, 1988.

14 Majoros M, Parkhill EM, Devine KD: Papilloma of the larynx in children. *Am J Surg,* 108:470–75, 1964.

15 Holinger PH, Schlid JA, Maurizi DG: Laryngeal papilloma: Review of etiology and therapy. *Laryngoscope,* 78:1462–74, 1968.

16 Bjork H, Teir H: Benign and malignant papilloma of the larynx in adults. *Acta Otolaryngol (Stockh),* 47:95–104, 1957.

17 Dedo HH, Jackler RK: Laryngeal papilloma: Results of treatment with CO_2 laser and podophylium. *Ann Otol Rhinol Laryng,* 91:425–430, 1982.

18 Steinberg BM, Topp WC, Schneider PS, et al: Laryngeal papillomavirus infection during clinical remission. *N Engl J Med,* 388:1261–64, 1983.

19 Crowe SF, Breitstein ML: Papilloma of the larynx in children. *Arch Surg,* 4:275–99, 1922.

20 Mounts P, Kashima H: Association of human papillomavirus subtype and clinical course in respiratory papillomatosis. *Laryngoscope,* 94: 28–33, 1984.

21 Kashima H, Leventhal BG, Clark K, et al: Scoring system to assess severity and course in recurrent respiratory papillomatosis. In: *Papilloma viruses:* Molecular and clinical aspects. *UCLA Symposia on Molecular and Cellular Biology, New Series Vol. 32,* PM Howley, TR Broker (eds). New York, A.R. Liss, Inc., 1985, p. 125.

22 Strong MS, Vaughn CW, Healy GB: Recurrent respiratory papillomatosis, in *Laryngo-Tracheal Problems in the Pediatric Patient,* GB Healy, TGI McGill, (eds). Springfield, IL, Charles C. Thomas, 1979.

23 Derkay C: Task force on recurrent respiratory papillomas—A preliminary report. *Arch Otolaryngol Head Neck Surg,* 21:1386–1391, 1995.

24 Quick CA, Kryzyzek RA, Watts SL, et al: Relationship between condylomata and laryngeal papilloma. *Ann Otol Rhinol Laryngol,* 89: 467, 1980.

25 Kashima H, Shah F, Lyles A, et al: A comparison of risk factors in juvenile-onset and adult-onset recurent respiratory papillomatosis. *Laryngoscope,* 102:9–13, 1992.

26 Shah K, Kashima H, Polk BF, et al: Rarity of Caesarean delivery in cases of juvenile onset recurrent respiratory papillomatosis. *Obstet Gynecol,* 68:795, 1986.

27 Holinger PH, Shipkowitz NL, Holper JC, et al: Studies of etiology of laryngeal papilloma and an autogenous laryngeal papilloma vaccine. *Acta Otolaryngol,* 65:63–69, 1968.

28 Gross CW, Hubbard R: Management of juvenile laryngeal papilloma: Further observations. *Laryngoscope,* 84:1090–97, 1974.

29 Haglund S, Lundquist PG, Cantell K, et al: Interferon therapy in juvenile laryngeal papillomatosis. *Arch Otolaryngol Head Neck Surg,* 107:327–32, 1981.

30 Healy GB, Gelber RD, Trowbridge AL: Treatment of recurrent respiratory papillomatosis with human leukocyte interferon: Results of a multi-center randomized clinical trial. *N Engl J Med,* 319:401, 1988.

31 Leventhal BG, Kashima HK, Weck PW, et al: Randomized surgical adjuvant trial of inteferon alfa-n1 in recurrent papillomatosis. *Arch Otolaryngol Head Neck Surg,* 114:1163–69, 1988.

32 Leventhal BG, Kashima HK, Mounts P, et al: A long-term study of lymphoblastoid interferon in recurrent respiratory. Papillomatosis. *N Engl J Med,* 325:613, 1991.

33 Zenner HP, Kley W, Claros P, et al: Recombinant interferon alpha-2c in laryngeal papillomatosis: preliminary results of a prospective multicenter trial. *Oncology,* 42 (suppl 1): 15, 1985.

34 Abramson AL, Shikowitz MJ, Mullooly VM, et al: Clinical effect of photodynamic therapy on recurrent laryngeal papillomas. *Arch Otol Head Neck Surg,* 118:25, 1992.

Chapter 87

Child sexual abuse and sexually transmitted diseases

Nyssa Matson
Laura T. Gutman

DEFINITIONS

Child sexual abuse represents one facet of the far-wider spectrum of *child maltreatment.* Child maltreatment includes any physical injury, sexual abuse, psychological or emotional harm, or general medical or educational neglect that is inflicted onto a child by someone acting in the role of a caretaker. The acts of abuse may vary in nature, frequency, intensity, or duration, and each state has statutes to help define what is considered injurious to children. Although there is considerable consensus on the definition of child abuse, each state may vary on the required response to recognized maltreatment. Clinicians should be aware of the mandates and child protecting agencies in the state in which the child resides. To recognize sexual abuse, clinicians caring for children must recognize presentations of all forms of child maltreatment, since there is very wide overlap between sexual abuse and other forms of maltreatment. Children who have been maltreated in any way should be considered for evaluation of sexual abuse, and vice versa.

Within the wide range of child maltreatment, neglect has been reported to occur most frequently and is probably the most life-threatening. Neglect makes up 47 percent and sexual abuse makes up 15 percent of maltreatment cases. Child abuse and neglect frequently occur together with other forms of interfamilial violence, including spouse battering and violence between siblings.[1]

Definitions of child sexual abuse vary among state statutes and medical opinions. The three primary foci of definitions of abuse include age differences between child and perpetrator, the acts that are perpetrated, and the caretaking relationship between the child and the assailant. Regarding age differences, many states exclude acts between peers who have less than 5 years difference in ages, where the perpetrator is not age 13 or greater and where the victim is not age 13 or less. Regarding the acts performed, attention is often given to circumstances involving force, threat, coercion, fear, and exploitation of authority. Statutes of many states regarding criminal acts with minors include penile penetrative anal, vaginal, or oral contact; digital penetrative acts; involvement of the child in any act for sexual gratification; allowing a child to be a witness of adult sexual activity, either in person or on film; involvement of a child in the production of child pornography; use of a child for child prostitution; and general statutes such as contributing to the moral degeneration of a child, allowing a child to enter an environment that is injurious to the child's welfare, and contributing to the delinquency of a child. Regarding caretaking relationships, it is usual to categorize a sexual assault on a child by a caretaker as "abuse" and to categorize an assault by a noncaretaker under the legal definitions of "assaults" also pertaining to adult victims. Common statutes include rape, indecent liberties, and assault on a female. In most aspects, the medical issues of abuse and of assault are similar, although the agency responses may differ widely. In this chapter, the term *abuse* is used to include both categories, unless otherwise specified.

PREVALENCE

Information on the prevalence of child sexual abuse is difficult to obtain because it is usually a hidden offense, surrounded by secrecy, criminality, and shame. It was first described by Kempe[2] as a "hidden pediatric problem" and remains so to the present. The available statistics include only the cases disclosed to the child protection agencies or to law enforcement. A 1994 national study of violence in U.S. homes conducted by the Institute of Justice omitted data on children under the age of 12 years, thus omitting from the report those children who were in the age range for child sexual abuse. An estimate of U.S. national incidence in 1993 found 330,000 reports of child sexual abuse, of which 150,000 were substantiated. A recent study by the Bureau of Justice Statistics evaluated female rape victims under age 12 years and whose perpetrators were reported under the FBI's Uniform Crime Reporting Program in 1991 and 1992.[4] An estimated 17,000 girls under age 12 were raped in 1992, representing 16 percent of all female rape victims and not including unreported rapes. Studies of convicted rapists and victims indicated that 20 percent of victims under age 12 had been raped by their fathers and 46 percent by a family member. Studies of adults give varying results but conclude that approximately 1 percent of female children in North America experience sexual abuse yearly,[5] with cumulative rates of 6 to 24 percent by age 18.[6–8] This statistic is suggested to be low, again due to the shame and secrecy involved. Only approximately 5 percent of cases are reported to police.[9]

Although the peak age of vulnerability for sexual abuse for both girls and boys has been thought to be between 7 and 13 years of age, the mean age of confirmed cases of sexual abuse in the authors' clinic is 4 years of age. In studies by Finkelhor on adult survivors, 90 percent of the diagnosed cases of sexual abuse involved male perpetrators, 70 to 90 percent of whom were known to the child.[10,11] The abuse of boys more frequently involves penetrative oral or anal abuse than is the case for girls.[12] Boys are reportedly abused at one-third to one-quarter the rate of girls.[10,11] One-third of reported offenders are under age 18.[13,14] Of all child sexual abuse cases, 20 to 25 percent involve anal or vaginal penetration or oral-genital contact.

Although there are profound legal and psychosocial differences between consequences of sexual assault by a noncaretaker and sexual abuse by a caretaker, this chapter incorporates both situations into the term *sexual abuse* unless otherwise specified.

Compared with the general population, children who experience poverty, parental inadequacy, unavailability, conflict, harsh discipline, and emotional deprivation experience elevated risks of abuse.[15–17] Substance-abusing parents, chaotic home environments, spousal abuse, other felonies on the part of household members, and high levels of stress are also commonly noted. All the above-named factors decrease the quality and quantity of supervision and protection, leaving the children more needy, emotionally deprived, and at higher risk.[18] Race appears not to be a risk factor. There are concerns that given the changing demographics observed in today's families, with dispersion of responsibility for care and safety of children, increasing proportions of children are potentially at risk.[19]

CONSEQUENCES

The effects of sexual abuse on the behaviors of a child may vary widely, and there is no "sexual abuse syndrome" that a child develops once sexually abused. How a child internalizes a trauma and then copes with it depend on many factors. Issues that worsen the impact of sexual abuse on the emotional well-being of the child include the extent of familial denial; abuse that is longer in duration; type and frequency of abuse; closer relationships to the perpetrator; the use of violence, threats, force, or penetration; lack of maternal support; and the child's overall functioning before the abuse began. Posttraumatic stress disorder is one of the most commonly cited aftereffects of child sexual abuse.[20–22] Attention deficit hyperactivity disorder (ADHD) and oppositional behaviors also appear more frequently in children who have been sexually abused.[23] One study of preschoolers suggested that overt sexualized behaviors (public masturbation; compulsive sexual curiosity; acting out of adult sexualized themes on toys, other children, or themselves; and exposure of genitals) comprise behaviors that are relatively specific for sexual abuse.[24] However, sexual behavior is also related to a number of variables other than sexual abuse. These include family nudity, the boundaries displayed in the home, stress, exposure to sexual activity, and exposure to both pornography and sexually explicit materials.

Although there are no universal behavioral consequences of sexual abuse, there are commonly seen symptoms.[1,25] Absence of or presence of a given symptom cannot automatically rule in nor rule out sexual abuse. Symptoms in abused males often differ from those in females.[26] The severity of symptoms is influenced by numerous factors, including the protective response of the mother or lack thereof, use of force during the assault, duration of time during which the child experienced repetitive assaults, the relationship of the perpetrator to the child (in which assault by trusted family members is more severe), and penetrative trauma.[27–29] Table 87-1 lists common symptoms.

PERPETRATORS

Perpetrators of sexual assault or abuse of children often appear to be otherwise normally functioning citizens and may be without history of other criminal behaviors. However, higher rates of perpetrators come from populations of persons who have histories of inflicting domestic violence on any family member, have sexually assaulted other children, are alcoholic or use illicit drugs, or have criminal records of felonies. Approximately 90 percent of perpetrators are males. Caretakers appear to perpetrate more frequently than do biologic parents.[30]

Substantial numbers of offenders are juveniles, and several studies of incarcerated adult offenders have reported accounts of perpetration against children that began while the adult was a juvenile.[31,32] Juvenile offenders can be any age between 5 and 19, with the median age being 14 or 15 years of age.[33,34] Adolescent sexual offenders frequently penetrate or attempt penetration of the victim, and the offending behavior often escalates over time if untreated.[35,36] Juveniles may offend peers, children, and at times, adults. It appears that the prior experience of the adolescent as an abused or nonabused child may influence his or her behaviors as a perpetrator.[37] Some commonly seen behaviors noted in juvenile offenders are listed in Table 87-2.

REPORTING OF SEXUAL ABUSE

Every state has formal child abuse reporting laws.[38] When a clinician suspects sexual abuse, reporting that suspicion is mandated. Persons making good faith reports are protected from liability. Most state statutes specify that this reporting requirement supersedes all claims of professional-client privilege. Sexual assault of a child is a crime in all 50 states and the District of Columbia. Almost all states have specific criminal penalties for failure of a "mandated reporter" to report a suspected child abuse situation. Mandated reporters include persons in positions of responsibility over the child such as physicians and teachers.

The laws regarding reporting indicate that any person or institution having cause to suspect that any child is abused, neglected, or has died as the result of maltreatment must report to the child protection agency of the county in which the child resides. The report may be made orally, by telephone, or in writing.

Laws are often vague concerning how much evidence regarding abuse must be available to a clinician in order to require that a report be made. Since abuse of children is highly prevalent in the United States, most pediatricians consider the possibility that abuse may play a role in the condition of many of their patients. Similarly, laws are often silent about the timing of a required report, and the clinician must use his or her best judgment. All clinicians who provide medical care for children should familiarize themselves with the laws and practices of their community regarding resources for evaluating children suspected of being abused. The agency that receives reports of suspected abuse or neglect is usually the county department of social services. Some communities have agencies that are very activist in the protection of children, while others require a greater level of evidence before an investigation is initiated. A high level of mutual respect and education between clinicians and agencies is essential for optimal evaluation and protection of endangered children.

Although the rate of reporting has increased, only a minority of cases are actually reported. One 1989 publication indicated that only 6 percent of cases had been reported.[9] One reason for failure to report is fear of lack of adequate evidence.[39] Despite reporting mandates for professionals, the largest category of reports is made primarily by victims (30 percent), followed by school personnel (16 percent), legal professionals and social service providers (each at 12 percent), and medical professionals (11

Table 87-1. Common Behaviors and Symptoms of Sexually Abused Children

Perpetration of abuse of other children
Posttraumatic fear, anxiety
Concentration difficulty
Impaired sense of self
Depression
Anger, aggressiveness toward others
Social isolation
Avoidant behaviors
Sexually acting out
Promiscuity in adolescents
Cruelty to animals
Self-mutilation
Indiscriminate sexual behaviors
Fire-setting

Table 87-2. Behaviors and Histories Commonly Noted in Juvenile Offenders

Lack of social skills
Low academic performance
Learning disorders
Lack of impulse control
Depression
Low self-esteem
Unstable home environment
Sexual pathology in a parent
Violence in the home
Parental loss or separation
Child viewing of sexual interactions between parents
History that juvenile was sexually abused

percent).[40] In surveying physicians, 24 percent indicated that they had failed to report a suspected case because they felt that the child protective services were of poor quality or overreacted to reports.[39]

MEDICAL DIAGNOSIS OF SEXUAL ABUSE

The basic elements of the medical evaluation of a child for child sexual abuse may include the following components:

1. An intake process to coordinate the components of the evaluation
2. Gathering documentation and information about the relevant other services concerned with the child (teachers, physician)
3. Interview of primary caretaker for child's medical history and review of systems
4. Diagnostic interview with child's caretaker(s)
5. Separate diagnostic interview with the child
6. Physical examination of the child (general physical, genital, and anal examinations)
7. Laboratory tests as indicated by examination and history
8. Review of case with relevant agencies
9. Documentation of the findings

An interview with the primary caretaker gathers information on the child's medical and behavioral symptoms and history, family constellation, family history for risk factors for sexual deviancy and violence, family dynamics, caretaking arrangements, household boundaries, and prior traumatic events.

The diagnostic interview of the child (one or several) is taken of children who are verbal (approximately age 3 years) and capable of participating. Children suspected of having experienced sexual abuse often will be referred to a professional agency that specializes in evaluating children for suspected sexual abuse. The purpose of the interview is to determine the child's perception of trauma and safety. In cases where abuse is suspected, descriptions of specific acts with contextual detail and identification of specific perpetrator(s) with identifying details constitute information that, when present, may lead to protection. Diagnostic interviewing of a sexually abused and/or traumatized child is a specially service that requires specific skills. The majority of sexually abused children are abused chronically and do not come to diagnostic attention at the first assault. Only the minority of diagnoses are for one-time assaults that the child discloses and of which the caretaker is believing. There are many well-studied reasons why a child may not disclose sexual abuse or will disclose sexual abuse initially but subsequently will recant their statements[41] (Table 87-3). As many as one-quarter of the children who have been confirmed to have been sexually abused, as evidenced by admission of the perpetrator, recant their disclosure at some time in the interviewing procedure. Most often the reason for a child to recant is pressure from the family to protect the alleged perpetrator. Disclosure is a function of the child's safety and developmental level and is a reflection of the child's environment. Disclosure is often a process rather than a one-time event and often occurs in stages rather than as an initially complete account.[42]

Standards for training diagnostic interviewers and for conducting a diagnostic interview have been formulated by the American Professional Society on the Abuse of Children. Reaching those standards should be the goal of clinicians who provide these services to children.[43]

Clinicians interviewing children need to create a safe atmosphere that will encourage disclosure and not further traumatize the child. The child should not be accompanied to the interview by a suspected perpetrator. The child should be interviewed alone. Never interview a child in front of his or her parents, since the child may internalize the parents' reaction to his or her statements. In addition, there is often no guarantee that one or both of the parents are not perpetrators involved in some way in facilitating the abuse. A child will rarely disclose sexual abuse if he or she is living with the perpetrator.

At the beginning of an interview, an interviewer must assess the child's developmental level and then proceed interviewing using the child's language and developmental abilities. Open-ended questions are the most commonly used technique, since the legal validity of any information from the child might be jeopardized by use of leading questions. An interview needs to be done in a neutral manner with no suggestion that the interviewer knows what the child should feel or what has happened. The interviewer should make no personalized comments or react strongly to what the child states, since this may cause the child to withdraw. The interviewer may state that the child is doing a good job talking and that the interviewer will listen to everything he or she has to say.

In a professional interview, the goal is to obtain information regarding many aspects of their environment, especially if sexual abuse is suspected but the child is unable to provide a disclosure. Questions about violence in the home, substance abuse, who takes care of the child, neglect issues, bathing and sleeping arrangements, domestic violence, and who is currently residing in the home are all factors that are important in determining a child's safety and risk. In a professional interview, techniques are used to determine a child's credibility by attempting to obtain contextual details, consistency, and validity to the statements. Many children state things that appear or sound fantastic but may indeed have validity. The interviewer avoids discounting or believing a child's statement until there is substantial reason to do so.

When a disclosure of abuse is given by a child, it is useful to have the child express this disclosure in more than one medium, since consistency helps to assess the child's validity. Useful tools that both help assess validity and facilitate communication include play telephones, doll houses, art supplies, writing paper, stuffed animals, and anatomic dolls.

Anatomic dolls are used frequently in interviewing children for

Table 87-3. The Child Sexual Abuse Accommodation Syndrome

1. *Secrecy.* Secrecy is both the source of fear and the promise of safety. "Everything will be OK if you don't tell." Most children never tell.
2. *Helplessness.* The adult expectation of child self-protection and immediate disclosure ignores the basic subordination and helplessness of children within authoritarian relationships. The child often has no choice but to submit quietly to the overpowering adult and to keep the secret.
3. *Entrapment and accommodation.* Often, the only option for the child is to learn to accept the situation and survive. The child is given the power to destroy the family (by telling the secret) and the responsibility to keep it together (by keeping the secret).
4. *Delayed, conflicted, and unconvincing disclosure.* Many adults, including parents, teachers, doctors, social workers, and attorneys, cannot believe that a normal adult could be capable of repeated, unchallenged sexual molestation of a child. Disclosure generally is an outgrowth either of overwhelming family conflict, incidental discovery by a third party, or outreach and education by child protective agencies. Disclosure may occur months or years after the initial abuse. It may contain details and descriptions that seem distorted or fanciful and therefore appear to lack credibility.
5. *Retraction.* The child's retraction is often readily accepted by authorities and relatives as the truth, whereas the child's detailed disclosure of abuse is considered doubtful. Unless there is consistent support for the child and immediate intervention to force responsibility on the perpetrator, the child will follow the "normal" course and retract his or her complaint.

sexual abuse. There has been considerable controversy about the use of anatomic dolls and their role in evaluating sexually abused children. Anatomic dolls have a unique purpose in certain situations but should only be used by trained professionals who are making distinct decisions about the specific use of the dolls in each case. The use of anatomic dolls alone is not an adequate diagnostic tool, and no determination of child sexual abuse can be made based on the child's play or nonplay with the dolls. An initial concern regarding the use of such dolls was that they might be overly suggestive. However, research indicates that this is not the case.[44–46] Guidelines on the use of anatomic dolls have been developed by professional organizations such as the American Professional Society on the Abuse of Children (APSAC).

Methods of recording the professional interview include videotaping of the interview, transcription of verbatim notes, and audiorecording. Methods used vary widely with each state and agency or clinic. Each of the techniques mentioned is supported by APSAC, and each technique has advantages and limitations or disadvantages. Because the issues of credibility and suggestibility of the child are often raised, the use of videotaping or transcription of verbatim notes provides a means of ensuring an accurate and complete record of the interview.

Table 87-4. General Policies Regarding the Physical Examination

The genital examination of an awake prepuberal female should not include use of devices inserted through the hymen such as a speculum, otoscope, or ureteroscope; if the child requires an invasive examination, general anesthesia is often indicated.
A child should not be examined if he or she is unable to fully cooperate. Conscious sedation may be required for very fearful children. Physical restraint should *not* be used.
The child should have as much decision making as possible during the examination. He or she may be asked by whom he or she wishes to be accompanied, draping or gowning wishes, etc. Books should be available should the child's caretaker wish to distract the child.
The accompanying caretaker should be instructed to remain at the head of the table, assisting and reassuring the child. Out of respect for the child's privacy, the caretaker should not view the child's anal or genital findings.
When sexual abuse is strongly suspected for any reason, the clinician should attempt to ensure that the child leaves the clinic to go to a safe environment. This may require urgent services from the police or department of social services.
Results of assays of clinical specimens may have legal implications. Specimens must be labeled, delivered to a laboratory, and processed in a manner that allows a chain of custody to be supported.

PHYSICAL EXAMINATION

The general physical examination should include all the usual and expected components. The clinician should be alert to evidence of dermal injuries and scars, bite marks, whipping marks, burn injuries, mucosal lesions, pain and tenderness, other conditions that have not received usual medical attention, and the child's response to the examination. Lesions of concern are documented in the record and, where possible, photographed. It is the authors' general policy that children are asked about how injuries occurred and, for current lesions, if they are painful. Careful, specific, and detailed documentation must be taken when a child states to a clinician a disclosure of abuse. All relevant statements concerning the abuse or injury must be documented accurately to help ensure the safety of the child in the future. Many children will only state the abuse once. If this disclosure is not documented carefully, the child may not receive adequate protection subsequently. Many clinicians elect to refrain from asking detailed questions about sexual abuse during the physical examination. The reason to restrict questioning to the diagnostic interview is that a caretaker is usually present during the physical examination and the child may be inhibited from disclosing in the presence of the caretaker. If this is the case, the child also may fail to disclose to the diagnostic interviewer during subsequent interviews.

Adequate examination, documentation, and interpretation require education and experience. See references 47 to 57 for further descriptions.

Following the general physical examination, the child receives an examination of the anal and genital areas. See Table 87-4 for important general policies regarding these examinations. A goal is that the child cooperates with this aspect of the examination and not perceive that he or she is assaulted by the clinician. Gentle and careful coaching will allow most children to reach a level of trust. For some reluctant children, a practice examination with their clothes on or an examination of a doll, a return home to be reassured and encouraged by a caretaker, and later a return to complete the examination are successful.

Female children are examined for genital findings in both the supine and the knee-chest positions. The knee-chest position is important in order to visualize the hymenal margins while gravity assists in unrolling the margins. The knee-chest position also is very helpful in both genders in obtaining an optimal view of the anal and perianal tissues and in assessing the child for anal dilatation.

During the physical examination, the child's behavior should be noted. Children who have been sexually traumatized may complete the general examination without difficulty and display various trauma symptoms when the genital or anal examination is initiated. Common trauma symptoms include a fearful inability to endure a visual examination, sexualized behaviors during the examination, and dissociative symptoms.

The physical examination may be classified as to the significance of the findings. Findings that are often accepted as proof of sexual abuse in most instances include the presence of semen, pregnancy, acute injuries, healed injuries that are diagnostic of prior penetrative trauma, and the presence of acquired gonorrhea or syphilis. Findings that are often accepted as confirming evidence of penetrative sexual trauma include healed injuries to the hymen that result in a hymenal width of less than 1 mm laterally or posteriorly and significant changes over time of genital examinations when there is not an acceptable explanation. It should be noted that a large proportion (approximately half) of children confirmed to have been sexually assaulted have normal physical examinations, and a normal examination does not provide evidence that abuse has not occurred.[57–59] The definitions of abnormal and normal anal and genital findings are a subject of rapid and intense research.

EVALUATION FOR SEXUALLY TRANSMITTED DISEASES

An integral component of the physical examination of a child for suspected sexual abuse is the evaluation of the child for sexually transmitted diseases (STDs). The results of assessments for STDs are critical for the welfare of the child because the evaluation pertains not only to the physical health of the child and any required therapy but also may provide evidence that the child has been abused and is therefore in need of protection from further assault. Unfortunately, large numbers of clinical questions pertaining to pediatric STDs remain unaddressed because of inadequate data or resources. Clinical services specializing in pediatric STDs have not been developed in the United States. Consequently, most children are examined in facilities with marginal or inadequate provisions for the microbiologic handling of specimens. In addition, absence of support from funding agencies has retarded research, retarded the development of clinical expertise, and discouraged interest in the field.

Prevalences of STDs among children being evaluated for possible sexual abuse have been relatively low in most studies. Table 87-5 presents extracted results from four recent studies of prepuberal children. Prevalences of gonorrhea were between 2 and 4 percent, with other infections less frequently recognized. It should be noted that not all children were evaluated for each condition. In some instances, only clinically symptomatic children had diagnostic testing performed. It is likely that the proportion of abused children with STDs will vary and depend in part on the rates in the perpetrators to whom the children are exposed.

Identification of prevalences of pediatric STDs requires an understanding of normal genital flora in nonabused prepuberal children. Unfortunately, sexual abuse is so common a condition that a given child cannot be assumed to be nonabused unless an evaluation has been made. Even after an evaluation, abuse often cannot be excluded. Instances in which sexually transmitted organisms were recovered from children who had been assumed to be nonabused and had been enrolled in studies of normal genital flora provide examples of the difficulties of defining normal flora in prepuberal children.[64,65]

Adequate studies of normal pediatric genital flora require that a nonabused population be studied and also that the obstacles inherent in attempts to obtain pediatric genital samples be overcome.[62,66,67] Results of recent studies that have achieved both requirements have shown that the common adult STDs (*Chlamydia trachomatis, Neisseria gonorrhoeae, Trichomonas vaginalis*, human papillomavirus) were not identified.[62,66,67] Some questions remain regarding whether or not other organisms or conditions whose STD status is uncertain in adults are sexually transmitted when identified in children. There is some evidence that *Gardnella vaginalis, Mycoplasma hominis, Ureaplasma urealyticum,* and bacterial vaginosis in children may represent results of traumatic genital injury resulting from sexual abuse, but at the present time they are not considered to be reportable pediatric STDs.[68–71]

Children may or may not have genital or anal signs or symptoms when infected with STDs.[61,72,73] Reasons that many services may examine only selected children for STDs include the relatively low yield from asymptomatic children, the pain caused by contact with the prepubertal hymen during specimen collection, the difficulty of coaching a young child into allowing a specimen to be obtained, and financial considerations. The decision of whether to collect cultures for STDs should be made individually and may take the following factors into consideration:

1. The child's physical signs or symptoms.
2. The prevalence of an STD in the community.
3. The policies of the clinical service regarding the appropriate level of thoroughness for an abuse investigation.
4. Information (if any) available to the clinician regarding the medical condition of the perpetrator and contact with the child.
5. If decisions regarding examination for STDs depend on knowing that penetrative contact with the child has occurred, it is relevant that many children minimize the disclosure and disclose only less humiliating or painful acts. Therefore, the abuse may have been more intrusive than the clinician is aware of.

Children may be at *highest priority* for evaluation for acquired STDs when they present with the following circumstances:

1. The child has symptoms or signs of anal, vaginal, urethral, and/or oral disease.
2. The child is known or suspected to have acquired any infection that is associated with sexual contact.
3. The perpetrator is known or suspected to have an STD or is at high risk of having an STD.
4. The child shares an environment (sibling, common caretaking arrangements) with another child who has an STD.
5. The child and/or parents request testing.

Children may be at *intermediate priority* for evaluation for acquired STDs when they present with the following circumstances:

1. The child or witness discloses abuse that included genital-mucosal contact.
2. The child has physical findings that represent acute injuries or residue of penetrative trauma.
3. The assailant is unidentified or there are multiple assailants.[74]

Finally, numerous services provide STD evaluations for all children referred for abuse evaluations. Such a policy is compatible with good medical practice.

SCHEDULING SEXUALLY TRANSMITTED DISEASE EVALUATIONS

The 1998 Guidelines for Treatment of STDs (in preparation) are expected to recommend that children being examined for STDs be evaluated according to the schedule found in Table 87-6. The following issues should be noted:

The majority of children who are evaluated for suspected sexual abuse and for whom a diagnosis of abuse is made have been victims of repeated abuse, or there was an appreciable delay between the last probable incident and the evaluation. Only infrequently is the child first examined for an acute and single assault. For this reason, in many instances the child can be examined for STDs and serologic specimens may be taken without a need to repeat the assays at a later time. Nevertheless, the child who is seen after a single and recent assault may require follow-up serologic assays and physical examinations.

Treatment guidelines for each of the conditions can be found

Table 87-5. Sexually Transmitted Diseases in Prepubertal Children Being Evaluated for Suspected Sexual Abuse

		Number of children who had diagnosis of					
Author, date	No. of children evaluated	Gonorrhea	Chlamydia	Syphilis	BV	Trichomonas	Condylomata acuminatum
Ingram,[61] 1992	1469	41 (2.8%)	17 (1.2%)	1 (0.1%)	7 (.5%)	3 (.2%)	28 (2%)
Gardner,[62] 1992	160	2 (2%)	1 (.75%)	ND	9 (6%)	0	ND
DeJong,[60] 1986	532	25 (4.7)	1 (.25%)	1 (0.2%)	2 (.5%)	0	3 (0.6%)
Siegel,[63] 1995	249	6 (3.1%)	2 (0.8%)	0 of 127		0 of 119	3 (1%)

Table 87-6. Schedule of STD Evaluations

	Males	Females
Initial examination:		
N. gonorrhoeae	Pharynx Anus Meatus	Pharynx Anus Vagina
C. trachomatis	Anus	Anus Vagina
T. vaginalis	—	Vagina
Bacterial vaginosis	—	Vagina
HIV, syphilis, HBV	Serologic	Serologic
12 Weeks after assault:		
HIV, syphilis, HBV	Serologic	Serologic

in the "1998 Guideline for Treatment of STDs" and in the "1994 Red Book" (American Academy of Pediatrics). Periodic updates of both these sources should be noted by clinicians caring for children with relevant problems.

N. GONORRHOEAE

See Chap. 92 for further information on the processing of these specimens. Only standard culture methods should be used.

C. TRACHOMATIS

Rapid assays for *C. trachomatis,* when used with pediatric specimens, have had a dismal record of frequent rates of false-positive and false-negative results. Only standard cell culture systems should be used. The clinic must be prepared to maintain the specimen on wet ice following inoculation into transport medium. It should be noted that prolonged shedding of *C. trachomatis* may occur after contamination of the infant in the perinatal process and may last until age 3 years; consequently, genital *C. trachomatis* is a confirming STD only in children older than 3 years of age.

BACTERIAL VAGINOSIS AND TRICHOMONIASIS

A wet prep of a vaginal swab should be examined for clue cells, odor with 10% KOH, and motile trichomonads.[76] A culture should be taken for *T. vaginalis* when disease is suspected, since the culture method is more sensitive than is direct examination. Although each of the conditions has been the subject of very little pediatric study, bacterial vaginosis (BV) appears to be a common cause of symptomatic disease in young abused females, and diagnosis and therapy are frequently helpful to the patient.[71] Both conditions may first cause recognizable discharge and symptoms after a delay of days or even weeks beyond the last assault. The child's caretakers should be aware that itching, discharge, and discomfort with a delayed onset are reasons to have the child reevaluated.

HUMAN PAPILLOMAVIRUS DISEASE

Genital human papillomavirus (HPV) disease may be recognized clinically as classic genital warts or, as in adults, as flat mucosal lesions in any body site (mouth, eye, anus, urethra, introitus). As in adults, an exfoliative cytologic examination of mucosal lesions may yield a diagnosis, or a biopsy may be indicated.[77] HPV disease of the genital area is a relatively common STD of children and is usually, although certainly not invariably, transmitted during abusive contact.[78] In early childhood (usually age 2 or less), some cases may have resulted from passive transfer during delivery through an infected birth canal. Limitations in diagnosis of preverbal children have led to uncertainty regarding the means of transmission, especially in this age group.

HUMAN IMMUNODEFICIENCY VIRUS (HIV)

Much more information is needed to formulate a data-based policy regarding selective HIV testing of subpopulations of children suspected of having been sexually abused. There are no substantive data regarding the HIV status of subpopulations of child assailants, the forms of abuse that transmit HIV to children, or the prevalence of abuse-transmitted HIV infection in children. Child protection teams seldom are in a position to know with useful certainty the risk factors for HIV that a given assailant may have, whether the assailant acted alone, the HIV status of the assailant(s), or even with certainty the acts that were committed. Until very recently, child sexual abuse was not an exposure category for the national reporting forms for pediatric HIV/AIDS. Above all, there has been and continues to be a reluctance to report sexual abuse as an exposure category if any other possible category coexists. For all these reasons, the medical community is not close to a formulation of policies for testing of children, and there are no widely accepted guidelines to which clinical services adhere. Nevertheless, it is clear from the very limited data available that sexual abuse contributes to the pool of pediatric HIV infection, and the contribution may be considerable.[25,79–84]

Because of these limitations of information and concerns, each service must construct its own policies. The authors have elected to test relatively widely the children coming to their clinic for evaluation of sexual abuse. A large majority of the children identified above to be "highest priority" have serologic assays for HIV, as well as for syphilis and hepatitis B virus (HBV). Pre- and posttest counseling should be provided. In some states, children may be tested if medically indicated even if the parent is reluctant to permit it.

A major challenge to clinicians is to obtain repeat assays for HIV at 12 weeks after the assault for those children believed to have been acutely assaulted. A tickler file may be helpful.

In instances in which a perpetrator is reported to the police, it is occasionally possible to obtain serologic assays from that person. A negative result from the perpetrator appears to provide some measure of reassurance to the parents and should be encouraged.[85]

A form of child abuse is Munchausen's syndrome by proxy. This condition occurs when a parent manipulates a child to simulate medical illness for gain to the parent. Adults have simulated HIV infection for gain,[86] and factitious infection of a child also has occurred. Clinicians caring for children with a diagnosis of HIV infection should ensure adequate documentation of infection.

SYPHILIS

Many of the comments regarding the paucity of data for acquired HIV infection could be repeated regarding acquired syphilis in childhood. Relatively few cases attributable to sexual abuse in the preteenage years are recognized or described.[87] We recommend that children at both highest and intermediate priority be tested for syphilis. The authors have cared for two young children with acquired syphilis who had progressed to tertiary disease of the central nervous system and permanent neurologic sequelae. Both these experiences provide incentives for an activist policy for assessment.

HEPATITIS B

We recommend that children who are being examined for HIV and/or syphilis also should be considered for testing for hepatitis B.

GENITAL HERPES

Herpes simplex virus (HSV) infection of the genitalia may present with typical multiple vesicles or may present with a more generalized erythema of varying severity. HSV type 1 and HSV type 2 have been recovered from the genital area in children who appear to have been sexually abused[88,89]; conversely, most children with recognized HSV infection of the genital tract also have evidence of sexual abuse. In a seroepidemiologic study of the prevalence of HSV-2 type-specific antibody, only 2 of 785 children in the United States were seropositive, and only 1 of the 2 children was less than 10 years of age.[90] (Note, however, that commercially available serologic tests do not distinguish HSV-1 antibody from HSV-2 antibody, so serologic testing for antibody to HSV-2 is not recommended for children with suspected sexual abuse.) It appears, therefore, that type 2 infection is very infrequent in the general population of children. Certainly, any child with HSV disease of the genitalia should have safety carefully assessed.

REPORTING CHILDREN WITH SEXUALLY TRANSMITTED DISEASES FOR SUSPECTED ABUSE

Each state mandates that persons who suspect that a child has been the victim of abuse must make a report to an authority that is constituted to receive and investigate such reports. In many states, these laws specify that persons who are in positions of authority over children must make such reports, and clinicians are usually included as "mandated reporters." For the clinician who has diagnosed a child with an STD, two major decisions must be made. First, he or she must decide the strength of the evidence, based on the diagnosis of the STD, that the child has been abused. Second, he or she must decide if the child should be reported to the agency constituted by that community to receive reports of suspected child abuse. Recommendations on these two issues as they pertain to the major STDs are found in Table 87-7 and represent recommendations formulated by the American Academy of Pediatrics.[5] Only two acquired STDs, gonorrhea and acquired syphilis, are accepted to provide a confirmed diagnosis of sexual abuse for which no other supportive findings are necessary. Diagnosis of *C. trachomatis,* genital warts, *T. vaginalis,* and HSV-2 provides the clinician with a "probable" diagnosis of sexual abuse or is confirming in only certain circumstances. Diagnosis of these conditions should result in a report to the investigative agency and thorough evaluation of the child for safety and for other evidence of possible abuse. The significance of bacterial vaginosis and several other organisms, including genital moluscum contagiosum, is uncertain, and their presence usually is not evidence, when seen alone, that requires a report. However, a child with bacterial vaginosis should be evaluated for other STDs.

Table 87-7. Special Significance of Genital Pediatric STDs and Recommendations Regarding Reporting of Suspected Abuse to the Relevant Community Agency (from Ref. 5).

Infection	Evidence of abuse	Recommended action
N. gonorrhoeae	Certain	Report
Acquired syphilis	Certain	Report
C. trachomatis	Probable (age restrictions)	Report
T. vaginalis	Probable	Report
Genital warts	Probable (age restrictions)	Report
Bacterial vaginosis	Uncertain	Evaluate for abuse
Herpes simplex virus type 2	Probable	Report
Herpes simplex virus type 1 (genital)	Possible	Report

COORDINATION OF FINDINGS

The final diagnosis of sexual abuse may be derived from information from numerous sources. These may include the medical evaluation, school information, home evaluation, police investigation, witnesses, and acknowledgment by a perpetrator. The medical evaluation for abuse should summarize the results of the findings and the medical conclusions. The conclusions should include a statement of the level of certainty of the diagnosis and whether or not the evaluation was completed. For example, the report may state that the diagnosis of sexual abuse was confirmed, suspected, or unknown or that there was no evidence of abuse. The basis of the conclusion should be clearly stated. The report should state whether or not a report of suspected abuse was made or had already been made. If safety measures are indicated, the report should clarify who is responsible for planning and implementing these services.

If abuse is confirmed or strongly suspected and a perpetrator identified, other siblings or children closely exposed to the perpetrator should receive an evaluation for abuse.[91] If no perpetrator is identified, other children sharing the same environment as the abused child should be evaluated.

Following the examination, most caretakers wish to know the results. The clinician should coordinate with any involved agencies as to whether or not a report should go to the caretakers. If a child has disclosed abuse or neglect by a family member, decisions must be made regarding the distribution of the information to the family. In addition, for most instances of suspected or confirmed sexual abuse, a mental health evaluation of the child should be scheduled. In many abusive/neglectful homes, parental compliance with treatment interventions is poor, and the child may require extensive monitoring in order to ensure safety and recovery. This is especially the case in families of sexually abused children.[92]

The evaluation and management of problems resulting from sexual abuse of a child require the most skilled personnel from numerous intersecting services and agencies. These commonly include physicians, other medical examiners, social workers, police, guardians ad litem, other court personnel, and mental health evaluators and therapists. Care of the child is likely to "fall through the cracks" without continuous and excellent levels of communication between the agencies. The medical record is one of the components of this communication. Multiagency review of cases also may facilitate improved care of sexually abused children.[93] Reabuse is common even when high-quality services have been provided.[94] Advocacy for the child and tracking to ensure continued safety are services that clinicians may bring to the situation.[95] It is likely that the most important means of preventing sexual abuse of children is the prompt recognition and treatment of abused and/or perpetrating children and identification and control of their assailants.

References

1 Wissow LS: Child abuse and neglect. *N Engl J Med* 332:1425–1431, 1995.

2 Kempe CH: Sexual abuse, another hidden pediatric problem. *Pediatrics* 62:382–389, 1978.

3 McCurdy K, Daro D: Child maltreatment: A national survey of reports and fatalities. *Journal of Interpersonal Violence* 9(1):75, 1994.

4 Langan PA, Harlow CW: *Child Rape Victims, 1992*. Washington, U.S. Dept. of Justice, NCJ-147001, June 1994.

5 American Academy of Pediatrics: Guidelines for the evaluation of sexual abuse of children. *Pediatrics* 87:254–260, 1991.

6 Wyatt GE, Peters SD: Methodological considerations in research in the prevalence of child sexual abuse. *Child Abuse Negl* 10:241–251, 1986.

7 Siegel JM et al: The prevalence of childhood sexual assault. *Am J Epidemiol* 126:141–153, 1987.

8 Russell DEH: The incidence and prevalence of intrafamilial and extrafamilial sexual abuse of female children. *Child Abuse Negl* 7:133–146, 1983.

9 Fuller AK: Child molestation and pedophilia. *JAMA* 261:602–605, 1989.

10 Finkelhor D et al. Sexual abuse in a national survey of adult men and women: Prevalence, characteristics, and risk factors. *Child Abuse Negl* 14:19–28, 1990.

11 Finkelhor D: The international epidemiology of child sexual abuse. *Child Abuse Negl* 18:409–417, 1994.

12 Pierce R, Pierce LH: The sexually abused child: A comparison of male and female victims. *Child Abuse Negl* 8:191–199, 1985.

13 Krugman R: Recognition of sexual abuse in children. *Pediatr Rev* 8: 25–30, 1986.

14 National Center on Child Abuse and Neglect: *Study Findings: Study of National Incidence and Prevalence of Child Abuse and Neglect, 1988*. Washington, U.S. Dept. of Health and Human Services, 1988.

15 Cappelleri JC et al: The epidemiology of child abuse: Findings from the second national incidence and prevalence study of child abuse and neglect. *Am J Public Health* 83:1622–1624, 1993.

16 Margolin L: Child abuse by mothers' boyfriends: Why the overrepresentation? *Child Abuse Negl* 16:541–551, 1992.

17 Moore KA, Nord CW, Peterson JL: Nonvoluntary sexual activity among adolescents. *Fam Plann Perspect* 21:110–114, 1989.

18 Finkelhor D: Risk factors in the sexual victimization of children. *Child Abuse Negl* 4:265–273, 1980.

19 Alexander PC: Application of attachment theory to the study of sexual abuse. *J Consult Clin Psychol* 60:185–195, 1992.

20 McLean SV et al. Sexually abused children at high risk for posttraumatic stress disorder. *J Am Acad Child Adolesc Psychiatry* 31:875–867, 1992.

21 Deblinger E et al: Posttraumatic stress in sexually abused, physically abused, and nonabused children. *Child Abuse Negl* 13:403–408, 1989.

22 Briere J, Runtz M: Post sexual abuse trauma: Data and implications for clinical practice. *J Interpers Violence* 2:367–369, 1987.

23 Famular R et al. Psychiatric diagnosis of maltreated children: Preliminary findings. *J Am Acad Child Adolesc Psychiatry* 31:863–867, 1992.

24 Friedrich WN et al: Normative sexual behavior in children. *Pediatrics* 88:456–464, 1991.

25 Gutman LT: Sexually transmitted diseases in children and adolescents with HIV infection, in *Infection in Infants, Children and Adolescents*, 2d ed, Pizzo PA, Wilfert CM (eds). Baltimore, Williams & Wilkins, 1994, pp 269–287.

26 Faller KC: Characteristics of a clinical sample of sexually abused children: How boy and girl victims differ. *Child Abuse Negl* 13:281–291, 1989.

27 Mennen FE, Meadow D: The relationship of abuse characteristics to symptoms in sexually abused girls. *J Interpers Violence* 10:259–274, 1995.

28 Faller KC: *Child Sexual Abuse*. New York, Columbia University Press, 1988.

29 Friedrich WH et al. Psychotherapy outcome of sexually abused boys. *J Interpers Violence* 7:396–409, 1992.

30 Russell DEH: The prevalence and seriousness of incestuous abuse: Stepfathers vs biological fathers. *Child Abuse Negl* 8:15–22, 1984.

31 Becker JV et al: Characteristics of adolescent incest sexual perpetrators. *J Fam Violence* 1:85–97, 1986.

32 Longo R, Groth AN: Juvenile sexual offenses in the histories of adult rapists and child molesters. *Int J Offender Ther Comp Criminol* 27: 150–155, 1983.

33 Becker J: Offenders: Characteristics and treatment, in *Future of the Children: The Sexual Abuse of Children*, Behrman R-E (ed). Center for the Future of Children, Los Altos, CA. 1995, pp 176–197.

34 Becker J: Treating adolescent sexual offenders. *Prof Psychol Res Pract* 528:215–222, 1990.

35 Wasserman J, Kappel S: *Adolescent Sex Offenders in Vermont*. Burlington, Vermont Dept. of Health, 1985.

36 Abel GG et al: Self-reported sex crimes of nonincarcerated parophiliacs. *J Interpers Violence* 2:3–25, 1987.

37 Kaufman KL et al: Subgroup differences in the modus operandi of adolescent sexual offenders. *Child Maltreat* 1:17–24, 1996.

38 Myers J (ed): *Evidence in Child Abuse and Neglect Cases*, 2d ed. New York, Wiley, 1992.

39 Kerns DL et al: The role of physicians in reporting and evaluating child sexual abuse cases, in *Future of Children: The Sexual Abuse of Children*, Behrman R-E (ed). Center for the Future of Children, Los Altos, CA. 1994, pp 119–134.

40 Pence DM, Wilson CA: Reporting and investigating child sexual abuse, in *The Future of Children: The Sexual Abuse of Children*, Behrman R-E (ed). Center for the Future of Children, Los Altos, CA. 1994, pp 70–83.

41 Summit R: The child abuse accommodation syndrome. *Child Abuse Negl* 7:177–193, 1983.

42 Sorenson T, Snow B: How children tell: The process of disclosure in child sexual abuse. *Child Welfare* 70:3–15, 1991.

43 American Professional Society on the Abuse of Children: *Guidelines for Psychosocial Evaluation of Suspected Sexual Abuse of Young Children*. Chicago APSAC, 1991, pp 1–7.

44 Teer L: Anatomicly correct dolls: Should they be used as a basis for expert testimony? *J Am Acad Child Adolesc Psychiatry* 27:254–257, 1988.

45 Boat BW, Everson M: Use of anatomic dolls among professionals in sexual abuse evaluations. *Child Abuse Negl* 12:171–179, 1988.

46 Everson M, Boat BW: Putting the anatomic dolls controversy in perspective: An examination of the major uses and criticisms of the dolls in child sexual abuse evaluations. *Child Abuse Negl* 18:113–129, 1994.

47 Levitt CJ: Medical evaluation of the sexually abused child. *Primary Care* 2:343–354, 1993.

48 Reece RM: *Child Abuse Medical Diagnosis and Management*. Philadelphia, Lea & Febiger, 1994.

49 Paradise JE: The medical evaluation of the sexually abused child. *Pediatr Clin North Am* 37:839–862, 1990.

50 McCann J et al: Perianal findings in prepubertal children selected for non-abuse: A descriptive study. *Child Abuse Negl* 13:179–193, 1989.

51 McCann J et al: Genital findings in prepubertal girls selected for non-abuse: A descriptive study. *Pediatrics* 86:428–439, 1990.

52 St Claire K et al (eds): *Duke University Medical Center Child Protection Team Manual 1996*. Durham, Duke University Press, 1996.

53 McCann J, Voris J, Simon M: Genital injuries resulting from sexual abuse: a longitudinal study. *Pediatrics* 89:307–317, 1992.

54 Herman-Giddens ME et al: Prepubertal females genitalia: Examination for evidence of sexual abuse. *Pediatrics* 80:203–208, 1987.
55 Bays J, Chadwick D: Medical diagnosis of the sexually abused child. *Child Abuse Negl* 17:91–110, 1993.
56 Bays J, Jenny C: Genital and anal conditions confused with child sexual abuse trauma. *Am J Dis Child* 144:1319–1322, 1990.
57 Muram D: Child sexual abuse: Relationship between sexual acts and genital findings. *Child Abuse Negl* 13:211–216, 1989.
58 Adams JA et al: Examination findings in legally confirmed child sexual abuse: It's normal to be normal. *Pediatrics* 94:310–317, 1994.
59 DeJong AR, Rose M: Legal proof of child sexual abuse in the absence of physical evidence. *Pediatrics* 88:506–511, 1991.
60 DeJong AR: Sexually transmitted diseases in sexually abused children. *Sex Transm Dis* 13:123–126, 1986.
61 Ingram DL et al: Epidemiology of adult sexually transmitted disease agents in children being evaluated for sexual abuse. *Pediatr Infect Dis J* 11:945–950, 1992.
62 Gardner JJ: Comparison of the vaginal flora in sexually abused and nonabused girls. *J Pediatr* 120:872–877, 1992.
63 Siegel RM et al: The prevalence of sexually transmitted diseases in children and adolescents for sexual abuse in Cincinnati: Rationale for limited STD testing in prepubertal girls. *Pediatrics* 96:1090–1094, 1995.
64 Hammerschlag MR et al: Microbiology of the vagina in children: Normal and potentially pathogenic organisms. *Pediatrics* 62:57–62, 1978.
65 Hammerschlag MR et al: Colonization of sexually abused children with genital mycoplasmas. *Sex Transm Dis* 14:23–25, 1987.
66 Hill GB et al: Anaerobes predominate among the vaginal microflora of prepubertal girls. *Clin Infect Dis* 20(suppl 2):S269–270, 1995.
67 Gutman LT et al: Evaluation of intravaginal specimens from sexually abused and nonabused girls for human papillomavirus infection. *Am J Dis Child* 146:694–699, 1992.
68 Bartley DL et al: *Gardnerella vaginalis* in prepubertal girls. *Am J Dis Child* 114:1014–1017, 1987.
69 Hammerschlag MR et al: Anaerobic microflora of the vagina of children. *Am J Obstet Gynecol* 131:853–856, 1978.
70 Ingram DL et al: *Gardnerella vaginalis* infection and sexual contact in female children. *Child Abuse Negl* 16:847–853, 1992.
71 Hammerschlag MR et al: Nonspecific vaginitis following sexual abuse of children. *Pediatrics* 75:1028–1031, 1985.
72 Bogaerts J et al: *Shigella* and gonococcal vulvovaginitis in prepubertal Central African girls. *Pediatr Infect Dis J* 11:890–892, 1992.
73 Folland DS et al: Gonorrhea in preadolescent children: An inquiry into source of infection and mode of transmission. *Pediatrics* 60:153–156, 1977.
74 Herman Giddens ME et al: Association of coexisting sexually transmitted diseases and multiple abusers in female children with genital warts. *Sex Transm Dis* 15:63–67, 1988.
75 Centers for Disease Control and Prevention: 1998 Guideline for Treatment of STDs. *MMWR* 1998.
76 Jones JG et al: *Trichomonas vaginalis* infestation in sexually abused girls. *Am J Dis Child* 139:846–847, 1985.
77 Gutman LT et al: Cervical-vaginal and intra-anal human papillomavirus infection of young girls with external genital warts. *J Infect Dis* 170:339–344, 1994.
78 Gutman LT et al: Transmission of genital human papillomavirus disease: Comparison of data from adults and children. *Pediatrics* 91:31–38, 1993.
79 Gutman LT et al: Human immunodeficiency virus transmission by child sexual abuse. *Am J Dis Child* 145:137–141, 1991.
80 Gutman LT et al: Sexual abuse of human immunodeficiency virus-positive children: Outcomes for perpetrators and evaluation of other household children. *Am J Dis Child* 146:1185–1189, 1992.
81 Gutman LT, Herman-Giddens M, McKinney RE Jr: Pediatric AIDS: Barriers to recognizing the role of child sexual abuse. *Am J Dis Child* 147:775–780, 1991.
82 Gellert GA et al: Situational and sociodemographic characteristics of children infected with HIV from pediatric sexual abuse. *Pediatrics* 91:39–44, 1993.
83 Oleske J: Human immunodeficiency testing of sexually abused children and their assailants. *Pediatr Infect Dis J* 9:67, 1990.
84 Siegel R et al: Incest and *Pneumocystis carinii* pneumonia in a twelve-year-old girl: A case for early human immunodeficiency virus testing in sexually abused children. *Pediatr Infect Dis* 11:681–682, 1992.
85 Gostin LO et al: HIV testing, counseling and prophylaxis after sexual assault. *JAMA* 271:1436–1444, 1994.
86 Craven DE et al: Factitious HIV infection: The importance of documenting infection. *Ann Intern Med* 121:763–766, 1994.
87 Gutman LT: Congenital syphilis, in *Atlas of Infectious Diseases*, vol 5: *Sexually Transmitted Diseases*, Mandell GL (ed). Philadelphia, Current Medicine, 1996, pp 11.2–11.14.
88 Gardner M, Jones JG: Genital herpes acquired by sexual abuse of children. *J Pediatr* 101:243–244, 1984.
89 Kaplan KM et al: Social relevance of genital herpes simplex to children. *Am J Dis Child* 138:872–874, 1984.
90 Johnson RE et al: A seroepidemiologic survey of the prevalence of herpes simplex virus type 2 infection in the United States. *N Engl J Med* 321:7–12, 1989.
91 Muram D et al: Genital abnormalities in female siblings and friends of child victims of sexual abuse. *Child Abuse Negl* 15:101–110, 1991.
92 Famularo R et al: Parental compliance to court-ordered treatment interventions in cases of child maltreatment. *Child Abuse Negl* 13:507–514, 1989.
93 Kolbo JR, Strong E: Multidisciplinary team approaches to the investigation and resolution of child abuse and neglect: A national survey. *Child Maltreat* 2:61–72, 1997.
94 Faller KC: What happens to sexually abused children identified by child protective services? *Child Youth Serv Rev* 13:101–111, 1991.
95 Jellinek MS et al: Protecting severely abused and neglected children: An unkept promise. *N Engl J Med* 323:1628–1630, 1990.

PART IX PREVENTION AND CONTROL OF STD/HIV

Chapter 88

Individual, group, and population approaches to STD/HIV prevention

Nancy Padian
Sevgi O. Aral
King K. Holmes

Whoever wishes to investigate medicine properly, should proceed thus: in the first place to consider the seasons of the year, and what effects each of them produces (for they are not at all alike, but differ much from themselves in regard to their changes). Then the winds, the hot and the cold, especially such as are common to all countries, and then such as are peculiar to each locality. We must also consider . . . the mode in which the inhabitants live, and what are their pursuits, whether they are fond of drinking and eating to excess, and given to indolence, or are fond of exercise and labor, and not given to excess in eating and drinking. . . .

For if one knows all these things well, or at least the greater part of them, he cannot miss knowing, when he comes into a strange city, either the diseases peculiar to the place, or the particular nature of common diseases, so that he will not be in doubt as to the treatment of the diseases, or commit mistakes, as is likely the case provided one had not previously considered these matters. And in particular....he can tell what epidemic diseases will attack the city . . . and what each individual will be in danger of experiencing from the change in regimen.[1]

Hippocrates was clearly focusing on risk factors for disease that can only be considered on a population level. Perhaps in his day the contribution of an individual to his or her own health was given less consideration. In contrast, today, many would argue that more attention is paid to the individual and less to the population. More recently, partly in response to this focus on the individual, Geoffrey Rose introduced into public health the importance of differences between "sick individuals" and "sick populations," and the need for different prevention strategies for the control of individual and population level health problems.[2] In this chapter we hope to reinforce this notion, and focus on STDs and HIV as multilevel problems.

Table 88-1 presents examples of how the individual, the group, and the population can be considered in epidemiologic and prevention research. For epidemiologic research, risk factors can be measured on an individual, group, or population level, and likewise, the disease of interest may be measured in individuals, groups, or across populations. Similarly, in prevention research, the mechanism or vehicle or agent of change may be considered on an individual, group, or population level, whereas the beneficiary or target of the intervention may be an individual, group, or a population. For example, peer-led interventions (that use individuals to implement change) and that target groups of commercial sex workers benefit not only the individual prostitutes but also their clients, and the wives and other sex partners of their clients, so that ultimately the general population benefits. Indeed, the benefit to the population may exceed the benefit to the individual sex workers. For example, in areas such as Thailand or Kenya, characterized by high occurrence of HIV infection, many individual female sex workers eventually become infected, because of repeated high-risk exposures, despite continuously striving toward consistent condom use, even though incident infection is reduced in the population.[3–5]

Although the concepts displayed on Table 88-1 apply to all diseases and health outcomes, special attention must be given to their application to communicable diseases. After a discussion of such applications as they pertain to individual and population approaches to etiologic and methodologic research on STDs, we then spend the majority of the chapter on these principles as they apply to prevention and intervention research.

ETIOLOGIC RESEARCH AND METHODOLOGICAL CONSIDERATIONS

Preventive interventions target those risk factors revealed in etiologic research that influence both the probability of acquiring infection for individuals and the possibility of transmission within the population. Table 88-2 provides examples of two possible risk factors for HIV infection, hormonal contraception and the presence of the penile foreskin, and the kinds of research needed at individual and population levels to support development of interventions addressing these risk factors for STDs and HIV. For risk factor research, the difference between individual and population levels may sometimes be one of measurement, because all individual variables may be assessed by summarizing the results across several individuals, for example, an individual's age, versus the average age of a population, or an individual's infection status versus the prevalence of infection in a population. Alternatively, factors that affect morbidity in the population may not be reducible to the individual level. For example, higher levels of social inequality in populations are correlated with higher syphilis rates.[6] Other examples of factors that only apply to the population include degree of urbanization, political factors such as the amount of governmental funds spent on public health or war, or social factors such as cultural norms.

The differences between communicable and noncommunicable diseases have methodological implications as well. For chronic, noncommunicable diseases, the relative risk, risk difference, and attributable risk together with the pattern of distribution of a particular risk factor in the population measure the overall importance of the factors as a cause of the diseases in the population. If the attributable risk for a particular factor is low, then only a small proportion of the chronic disease attributable to that factor could be prevented if the risk factor were eliminated. However, for communicable disease in general, and STDs in particular, because they are transmitted by intimate person-to-person contact, the infection status of one individual with many exposures can cause infection of many others. Thus, traditional measures of effect that are static in nature may be less straightforward for STD than for chronic noncommunicable diseases.[7,8] More complex mathematical models are required to predict the proportion of communicable disease prevented by elimination of risk factor.

One additional complication is that with communicable diseases, risk factors measured on an individual level can contribute to either increased individual susceptibility or to increased infectiousness. For example, infection with an STD may increase both the infectiousness of an HIV-infected individual and the susceptibility of an uninfected person to HIV and thus, such individual level factors may amplify the spread of infection in the population. Therefore, it may be inappropriate to use purely individual level study models when assessing such risk factors for STD/HIV

Table 88-1. Examples of Individual, Group, and Population-level Approaches in STD/HIV Preventive Interventions

Level of intervention	Risk factor	Target of intervention	Beneficiary of intervention	Mechanism of change	Measure of disease
Individual	Unprotected intercourse with partner(s)	Women attending family planning clinics	Individual woman and her partner(s)	Counsel women to use condoms	Individual infection
Group	Unprotected intercourse with clients	Female sex workers (FSW)	Clients of sex workers subsequent female partners of these clients	Peer leader mediated condom promotion with FSW	Prevalence or incidence of infection in population
Population	Social status of women	School-aged female children	Women; whole population	Education of school-aged female children	Prevalence or incidence of infection in population

infection.[9] Another level of complexity involves sexual contact patterns and networks. The pattern of sexual mixing, which can only be measured at the population level, may be the most important determinant of disease spread.

PREVENTION RESEARCH

Although Rose's work has helped to stimulate a growing awareness of differences in individual and population perspectives on the epidemiology and prevention of STD/HIV, he concentrated more on chronic and environmental health problems (as it appears did Hippocrates). For example, in preventive medicine for noncommunicable diseases, the term "primary prevention" generally refers to prevention of the first occurrence of disease, and secondary prevention refers to prevention of complications or reoccurrence of disease among those who already are affected. At the individual level, primary prevention encompasses health education and counseling coupled with risk assessment to promote healthy life styles and reduce risk behaviors, as well as screening for modifiable risk factors and evidence of subclinical manifestations of diseases (e.g., elevated blood pressure, intraocular pressure, blood cholesterol). At the population level, "primary prevention" encompasses interventions that protect entire populations of individuals (e.g., fluoridation of water, reducing environmental pollution).

In contrast, interventions for STDs including HIV differ from those developed for chronic disease largely because occurrence of communicable diseases is determined by transmission between individuals. For diseases that are communicable by person-to-person contact, early detection and treatment of infected individuals also can prevent further transmission to others, and thus provides primary prevention of infections at the population level, in addition to offering secondary prevention of complications of infection in the individual patient. In fact, for STDs, the greatest primary prevention impact at the population level may be the early detection and treatment provided to those most likely to transmit infection.

Finally, because of the social stigma attached to diseases transmitted via sexual contact, prevention of STDs also has powerful political, social, and related economic consequences. In communicable diseases, individuals "at risk" for acquiring disease (the uninfected) are often perceived by society as differing markedly from those likely to transmit it (i.e., the former may be perceived as potential victims, the latter as threats), whereas for chronic noncommunicable diseases, because exposure does not depend on contact with other individuals, society generally does not differentiate between those with and without disease (obviously, exceptions could include those with behavioral or emotional disorders which could pose a threat to others).

The distinction between acquisition and transmission is not trivial. Interventions focused on infected individuals and designed to limit transmission benefit the population. Alternatively, interventions focused on susceptible individuals limit acquisition and more directly benefit the individual. Thus, emphasis on preventing acquisition of infection among all susceptible individuals in the community versus emphasis on preventing transmission of infection from a relatively small number of infected individuals, produces differing distributions of costs and benefits across the population.[10] In the United States, by the time the HIV/AIDS epidemic was recognized, a large proportion of men having sex with men and IV drug users had become infected, and prevention emphasized changing the behaviors of all susceptible members of high risk groups, and even on changing behaviors of the general population. In contrast, in Sweden, where only a small proportion of individuals in these highest risk groups had become infected by the time the HIV/AIDS epidemic was recognized, a much greater emphasis was placed on identifying and changing the behaviors of the few who had become infected. When the emphasis is on prevention of acquisition for all susceptibles (a universal prevention strategy), the whole population incurs the financial costs of interventions and the intangible costs of undergoing preventive behavior change, and they collectively receive the benefits of avoiding acquisition of infection. With emphasis on prevention of transmission by a relatively small proportion of the population, a more targeted approach would be justified; the general population

Table 88-2. Individual and Population Perspectives on Objectives of Research on Risk Factors for HIV Infections*

	Individual perspective	Population perspective
Objective of research	Assess individual risk factors associated with susceptibility or progression to disease	Consider risk factors measured across groups or populations associated with transmission.
Contraception	Study OCP** use and other forms of contraception, as risk factors for an individual's acquiring HIV	Study OCP use and other forms of contraception as risk factors for mucosal shedding and transmission of HIV
Male circumcision	Determine association of circumcision with reduced risk of an individual's acquiring HIV	Assess the proportion of circumcised men and correlate with prevalence of HIV in populations

*With two current examples of research on possible risk factors.
**OCP = oral contraceptive pill

still receives the benefit of avoiding acquisition and associated future health costs, and may again incur the financial costs of implementing the intervention. However, these financial costs may be less and fewer people incur the major burden of behavior change. It has become apparent that many countries have selectively avoided developing prevention efforts specifically designed to prevent transmission by individuals with chronic viral STD, because targeting prevention efforts to infected individuals carries the risk of stigmatization and discrimination. Researchers, clinicians, and public health programs are belatedly turning increased attention to this approach.

PREVENTIVE INTERVENTIONS

Prevention strategies may also be conceptualized on different levels depending on who is the target of the intervention, who is the beneficiary of the intervention, and what is the mechanism or agent which delivers the intervention (Fig. 88-1). Interventions may be directed (targeted) primarily toward individuals, groups, or populations. The benefits of the intervention may extend primarily to the individual, a specific group, or the population as a whole. The mechanism of the intervention and the messenger, or the vehicle of delivery of that intervention, may involve an individual (e.g., an individual counselor), group (e.g., group of activists) or a population level mechanism (e.g., changes in the legal or economic structure). Interventions directed toward individuals or groups may primarily benefit the individual, the group or population (e.g., promotion of condom use by sex workers and clients benefits the entire population); and conversely interventions that target the population ultimately benefit the individual. Use of screening tests in asymptomatic women in family planning clinics to identify those needing treatment for infection primarily benefits the individual woman, but also may contribute somewhat to decreasing transmission to future partners. Such screening also defines the prevalence of infection within that group, thereby guiding decisions to implement widescale population-level prevention interventions, such as mass condom promotion. This separation of levels is not always straightforward or distinct; these various approaches should be viewed as complementary and overlapping both in implementation and impact, but it is conceptually important to clarify the meanings of the terms "individual," "group," and "population" level interventions.

Table 88-3 provides individual and population perspectives on the objective of STD/HIV preventive interventions, examples of specific types of interventions, and examples of behavioral and biomedical prevention research. Note that the distinction between biomedical and behavioral prevention research, although commonly made, is misleading because biomedical interventions require supportive behavioral intervention components. In addition, biomedical outcomes are needed in the more definitive behavioral intervention research; and multiple (biomedical plus behavioral) interventions are of growing interest in prevention research (as in the Masaka, Uganda study that combined behavioral and STD treatment intervention for HIV prevention). The principles here are similar to those that apply to research on etiology of disease. From an individual perspective, interventions may prevent initial acquisition of infection and prevent subsequent development of associated sequelae, whereas the most important principle from the population perspective is to prevent transmission. Depending on whether the focus is on the beneficiary or the target, some of the interventions listed here could be classified either as population- or individual-level interventions. Further, risk factors defined on a population level can influence interventions directed toward individual risks. For example, accepted social norms defined on a population level can constrain and shape behavioral interventions targeted toward individuals.[11]

The next section of the chapter describes particular interventions in greater detail, and reviews interventions that occur among progressively larger units of analysis: couples, groups, communities, populations, and the networks that link individuals and

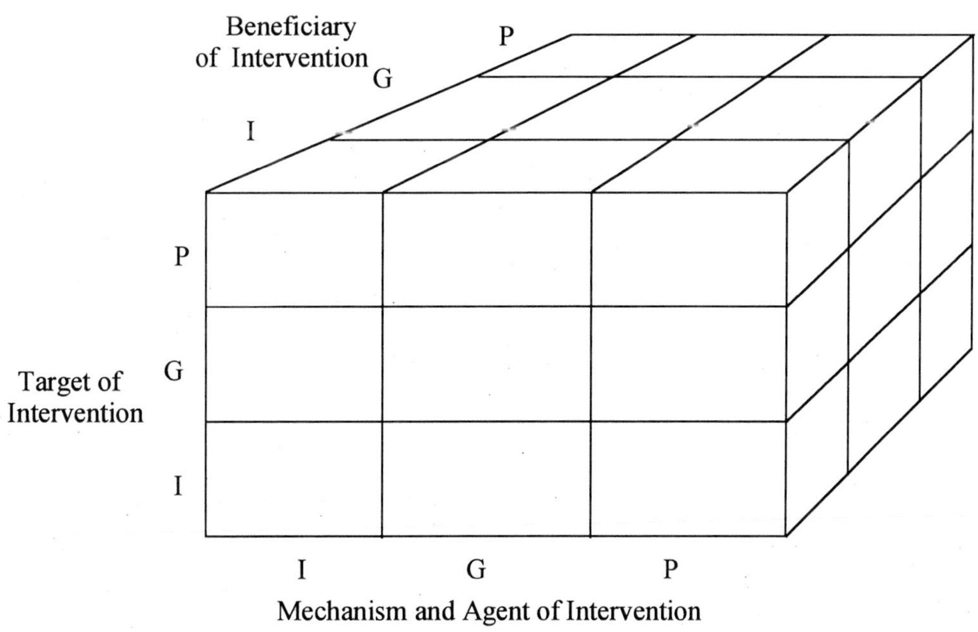

Fig. 88-1. Multi-dimensional taxonomy of interventions. I = individual, G = group, P = population. (Modified from Ehrhardt AA, Fishbein M, Washington E, Smith W, Holmes KK, and the NIAID Study Group on Integrated Behavioral Research for Prevention and Control of Sexually Transmitted Diseases. Part II: Issues in designing behavioral interventions. In: *Research Issues in Human Behavior and Sexually Transmitted Diseases in the AIDS Era.* Wasserheit JN, Aral SO, Holmes KK (eds). Washington D.C., American Society for Microbiology, pg. 364, 1991.)

groups. Examples of the strengths and weaknesses of approaches at each level are discussed, as are relevant methodological issues.

We contend that STDs and HIV infection represent multilevel health problems that may be considered on progressively larger units of analysis. Specialists who narrowly focus on interventions at the individual level (e.g., clinicians providing diagnosis and treatment to symptomatic patients), could have more impact by considering chains and networks of transmission, and interventions that impact larger groups.

Although we advocate this kind of multilevel approach, limited resources may constrain choice. Several other factors could also contribute to selection of the appropriate strategy. For example, choice of the level on which to target an intervention might also depend on the stage of an epidemic. In general, at the early stages of an epidemic in settings where small core groups of high risk individuals are the first to acquire disease and account for most transmissions, core group interventions may be most feasible and cost effective; in later stages of a mature epidemic when prevalence is more widespread, interventions directed toward core groups may remain most cost effective but no longer sufficient to rapidly contain the epidemic.[12] Although a multilevel approach may not always be feasible or cost effective, clearly more can be gained from simultaneous consideration of multiple levels than from the traditional medical model, which focuses on diagnosis and treatment of individual cases of infection.

Table 88-3. Individual and Population-level Perspectives on Objectives of STD/HIV Preventive Interventions*

	Individual perspective	Population perspective
A. Objectives of preventive interventions	Prevent acquisition Relieve symptoms and prevent progression to complications or death	Prevent transmission Intervene in those most likely to transmit, to achieve maximum effect with minimum expense
B. Examples of interventions		
Partner notification, treatment	Treat exposed partner	Treat source partner
Screening	Screen individuals and treat those found to be infected Screening based on risk factors for having infection, or developing a complication; for example, screen all younger females, regardless of number of partners Detect, treat late syphilis	Establish subpopulation specific prevalences, and mass treat subgroups depending on prevalence Screening based on risk factors for spreading infection, for example, screen males with many partners Detect, treat infectious syphilis
Condom promotion	Promote use of condoms by male with spouse	Promote use of condoms by men during sex with sex workers
Improve access to STD/HIV services	Provide STD services in managed care organizations for employed, insured individuals Provide treatment for early chlamydial or gonococcal infection in women, to prevent tubal factor infertility	Provide free access to STD services for uninsured inner city crack-cocaine users Provide treatment for early chlamydial or gonococcal infection in men, to prevent tubal infertility in women
Counseling/education risk reduction	Counsel or educate susceptibles on decreasing acquisition	Counsel or educate infecteds on decreasing transmission
C. Prevention research		
Vaccine programs	Evaluate therapeutic vaccine to reduce progression of HIV	Evaluate preventive HIV vaccine to reduce acquisition or mucosal shedding and thus prevent subsequent transmission
STD treatment to prevent HIV infection	Randomized trial of selective routine treatment of STD in sex workers to lower their risk of acquiring HIV	Community randomization trial of syndromic management of STD (Mwanza trial) or of mass treatment of STD (Rakai trial) to lower community-wide incidence of HIV infection
HIV antiretroviral treatment	Evaluate impact of antiretroviral therapy on progression of immunodeficiency	Evaluate impact of antiretroviral therapy on mucosal shedding or transmission to partners
Microbicides	Evaluate existing spermicides and new microbicides on prevention of acquisition of HIV and other STDs	Evaluate impact of spermicide and microbicide use on preventing transmission of STD/HIV
Needle exchange/drug treatment	Evaluate impact of needle exchange program on incidence of HIV in exchange participants Randomized trial of impact of increased access of uninfected IDU to drug treatment programs on individual risk of acquisition of HIV, HBV, HCV, or HTLV-II	Evaluate impact of needle exchange program on incidence of HIV in the general population of IDU who don't use the exchange Community randomization trial of the impact of improved access of infected IDU to drug treatment programs on incidence of HIV, HBV, HCV, and HTLV-II among community cohorts of IVDU
Behavioral research	Evaluate individual behaviors associated with risk of acquiring infection Randomized trial of impact of individual, small group, or work site information, education, or counseling on rate of acquisition of STD/HIV	Evaluate individual behaviors associated with transmission of infection Evaluate characteristics of risky sexual networks Community randomization trial of impact of population-wide information education, and communication for STD/HIV prevention on incidence of STD/HIV

*With examples of preventive intervention, and of biomedical and behavioral prevention research.

INDIVIDUAL INTERVENTIONS

Examples of individual approaches to prevention include programs that seek to alter the modifiable individual-level factors. Individual-level risk factors include factors related to host susceptibility in susceptibles (or factors that increase infectiousness in the infecteds), and include biological factors such as cervical ectopy, vaginal flora, immunological competence and viral load; behavioral risks including sexual practices, number, and choice of partners; and preventive behaviors such as use of condoms and microbicides. The mechanism of change involves: vaccination, counseling and testing, contact tracing, or case finding (either clinic-based or active outreach screening programs) and subsequent treatment.

Using the individual as a target for an intervention allows tailoring the intervention to the needs of particular individuals. Because of the communicable nature of STDs, an additional benefit to this kind of program may be that prevention or treatment of infection in one individual may break a chain of transmission, preventing further spread. Individual risk profiles may be developed, and appropriate interventions can then be selected. Prochaska's stages of change model is an example of this kind of approach where individuals are "staged" according to their readiness to adopt a prevention strategy and then the intervention is tailored to this stage.[13] One weakness of this kind of approach is that it fails to take into account potential differences in the staging of different members of the couple, that is, one partner may be more ready to change than the other. Another weakness is that the time and labor involved can make the intervention costly because accurate staging requires an individual assessment. In addition, it may be difficult to identify those individuals at-risk who would benefit most from the intervention. Finally, interventions that work for particular individuals may not work as well when applied to larger social units.

COUPLE-BASED INTERVENTIONS

As mentioned, because STDs by definition are transmitted between individuals, it may be more appropriate to use couples rather than individuals as the smallest unit of analysis for epidemiologic study. This would enable simultaneous examination of factors related to infectiousness and susceptibility, including those individual factors delineated in the preceding. The mechanism of change in couple-based interventions may parallel those identified for individual interventions, such as case finding, counseling, and testing.

Interventions directed toward couples discordant either based on their infection status or their risk status provide excellent examples of prevention strategies directed towards couples. In one study, Kamenga et al. studied 149 HIV serodiscordant couples in Zaire.[14] At entry into the study fewer than 5 percent of the couples consistently used condoms, compared to 77 percent of couples 18 months later. They detected a seroconversion rate of three new infections per 100 person years of follow-up. In a similar study in Rwanda, Allen et al. counseled and followed 60 serodiscordant couples.[15] Condom use was reported by 3 percent of couples at baseline and by 57 percent at 12 months follow-up. They reported an HIV seroconversion rate of four per 100 man years of follow-up, and nine per 100 women years of follow-up. As a comparison, based on rates observed over time among individuals who were not identified and counseled as part of their study, they determined that in the absence of their couples program, they would have expected 22 new infections among serodiscordant couples. Finally, Padian et al. followed 175 such couples in California.[16] Among these couples, 32 percent reported consistent condom use at entry into the study, and 75 percent reported consistent condom use as many as 9 years later. In this study, which had no control group, no new seroconversions were observed during greater than 3000 couple-months of follow-up. Although these studies have focused on behavior change and condom promotion among HIV-discordant couples, discordance on other STDs may merit other approaches. For example, if herpes transmission is enhanced during symptomatic episodes, a possible intervention that would not require testing, could be based on lesion identification in the infected partner.

The strengths of the "couples" approach are apparent. Because transmission events are associated with sexual activity between individuals, targeting interventions toward couples is obviously appropriate. A weakness of this approach is that these interventions are only appropriate for couples who are in relationships that remain stable at least for the duration of the intervention. Interventions delivered to couples may be less effective for individual members of the couple following the break-up, and selection of couples likely to remain together throughout the research trial may require very restrictive eligibility criteria. Finding couples who meet all eligibility criteria can be difficult and costly, requiring intensive outreach to identify participants. In addition, including serostatus as part of eligibility adds complexity because not all individuals know or want to know their serostatus and because these parameters, such as the status of the partnership itself, change over time. Identifying concordant seronegative couples who become discordant can be difficult, although extending the definition of discordance to discordance on *any* as opposed to all outcomes (enabling eligible couples to include some who are jointly infected by one STD (e.g., HSV-2), whereas discordant on another [e.g., HIV]) can facilitate identification of such couples. In fact, interventions directed toward coinfection with other STDs that may further enhance infection may prove very effective in preventing HIV.

"CORE" GROUP INTERVENTIONS

Groups may be thought of as clusters of individuals and couples. One type of such a group that is considered central to STD epidemiology is the "core group," first described by Heathcote and Yorke.[17] Although the definition of core groups varies somewhat, they are generally characterized by individuals connected to each other through social and sexual networks, who display risk behaviors and high infection rates, and who sustain transmission of an STD pathogen within the population. The theory is that population rates of STDs are driven by spread among groups of individuals that are characterized by high rates of exposure to an STD (often related to frequent concurrent exposure versus others who are also at high risk), longer duration of infection (often related to poor access to acceptable health care) and highly efficient transmission of infection per exposure (often related to undiagnosed or untreated coinfection with other STDs, young age, risky practices, lack of male circumcision, etc.). These groups act as foci for STD spread so that a pathogen newly introduced into the community soon becomes concentrated in these groups. By virtue of mixing (or "bridging") with individuals outside of the group, they may also be responsible for seeding infection among individuals who are not identified as being part of the core group.[18] Examples of groups that have been considered as core groups include men and women involved in commercial sex, migrant workers, or truckers, STD clinic attendees who have repeat infections, or individuals who have many sexual partners over a defined period of time.

One strategy for interventions targeting core groups employs peer individuals as the agents of change, since peer leaders such as opinion leaders, role models, or peer educators, can best influence the behavior of the entire group.[19,20] Their objective is to change social norms. Another strategy involves population-based actions such as changes in laws or health codes as they apply to such groups. These approaches, characterized by removal of barriers to implementation of prevention interventions or creation of barriers that prevent risky behavior, have been called "enabling" approaches because they enable the desired behavior change to occur.[21]

One example of interventions targeted at core groups are the many condom distribution programs aimed at female sex workers. In both Kenya and Zimbabwe, such programs increased rates of condom use and decreased rates of STDs both among the women and the larger community.[20] Here the major part of the intervention was delivered by peer educators and counselors who distributed condoms and provided information about safe sex along existing social networks linking at-risk women. In Kenya, 1 year after initiation of this program, sex during menstruation and the number of clients during the week before the study was undertaken decreased, the charge per client increased, and the frequency of condom use with all clients increased from 4.6 to 36.5 percent. Similar results were reported in Zimbabwe where condom use increased form 18 to 66 percent within 2 years of the program.

In the condom promotion program among sex workers implemented in Thailand, individuals educated other individuals, as in the programs described herein, but governmental sanctions were added to insure behavior change.[22] Here, the government required condom use at brothels, and free condoms were distributed. This was supplemented by mass advertising, interviews of brothel workers to insure that condoms were used, and identification of particular customers when a worker was diagnosed with an STD. Over 2 years, reported condom use in brothels increased from 14 to 94 percent, and five major STDs (syphilis, gonorrhea, nongonococcal urethritis, lymphogranuloma venereum, and chancroid) decreased in men by 79 percent over 5 years. Nevertheless, although rates of these STDs were reduced, HIV incidence among young men initially remained high. Eventually, in military conscripts who were also targeted by HIV prevention programs, HIV rates did fall subsequently, but the enduring effects of this program remain to be seen.[4,5]

The benefits of targeting interventions at core groups extend beyond the core to the larger community in which such groups reside.[23,24] In addition, targeting many individuals within the core group simultaneously provides a stronger chance that behavior change programs could result in changes in social norms than if such programs were targeted at individuals. Such interventions could also be cost-effective because they do not require assessment of infection status or behavioral risks among individuals. Weaknesses of this kind of program include the potential for stigmatization where core group identification becomes a kind of labeling. Likewise, because core group membership is ill-defined and individuals may move in and out of such groups, they can represent a kind of moving target, making it difficult to successfully identify members.

COMMUNITY-BASED INTERVENTIONS

Groups of individuals who live or work together or who have similar life styles represent another kind of group characterized by more heterogeneous behavioral risks than in core groups, as described in the preceding. Examples of these kinds of communities include minority, urban teens of low socioeconomic status, gay men of diverse risk status, or geographic or work site clusters. Here, the strategy for promotion can resemble that described for core groups.

One example of an intervention that used the community as the unit of analysis was the community intervention among gay men implemented by Kelly et al.[25] The intervention began with selection of opinion leaders who then engaged community members in bars in peer conversations about the benefits of safe sex, resulting in so-called "diffusion" of the intervention into the community. The intervention, conducted in a staggered, serial fashion in three cities, resulted in a 15 to 24 percent decrease in unprotected anal intercourse, insertive anal intercourse decreased by 14 to 29 percent, and unprotected receptive anal intercourse decreased by 26 to 28 percent.

The Mwanza study of improved syndromic management of STD in rural communities in Tanzania represents another example of a successful community-based intervention.[26] Six intervention villages were paired with six control villages. The intervention included training of clinic staff in syndromic diagnosis and treatment of sexually transmitted diseases, provision of necessary antimicrobial drugs, and dose supervision. After a 2-year period, HIV seroconversion rates were 1.2 percent in the intervention communities, compared to 1.9 percent in the control communities (relative risk = .58, 95 percent confidence interval = .42 to .79); a 42 percent decrease in HIV incidence. Adjustment for differences on baseline prevalence of infection lowered the impact only slightly, to a 38 percent decrease in HIV incidence.

The strengths of these community-level interventions are similar to those that result from targeting core groups of sex workers. The communities chosen—gay men frequenting bars and rural Tanzanians with STDs—were likely engaging in risky sex behaviors. It is easier to change social norms when several individuals are being targeted at once.

POPULATION-BASED INTERVENTIONS

As with group or community level interventions, changing of social norms may also be a goal of interventions targeting entire societies. Programs that operate at this level may include structural mechanisms to restrict risky behaviors and encourage healthy behavior. Mechanisms of change employed may include use of mass media for health education, modifications in the environment, institution of laws or regulations, taxation of alcoholic beverages, service delivery (clinical guidelines for HIV or chlamydia screening). Examples have included legalizing needle exchanges, outlawing bath houses or closing brothels, providing routine selective screening and treatment for STDs, mandating 100 percent condom use in brothels, and providing training and economic opportunities for women. The Thai condom promotion distribution programs described in the preceding used a structural mechanism of change but targeted a core group rather than the whole population even though the whole population might benefit from the intervention.[22]

In the HIV control program in Cuba, government regulations resulted in a ban on all imported blood and blood derivatives; enforced widespread screening of travelers, blood donors, pregnant women with STDs, prisoners, and individuals identified in certain neighborhoods where infection rates were prevalent; imposed quarantine of infected individuals; and recommended abortions among HIV-infected pregnant women.[27] Although this program has not been objectively evaluated by an external group, infection rates remain low, and unlike many of its Caribbean neighbors, Cuba does not seem to have a major HIV epidemic. On the other hand, it has been argued that segregation of high-risk individuals away from the rest of the population could accelerate the spread of infection within the high risk group, so that occasional contact with others outside the group through so-called "bridge populations" could continue to spread infection.[4]

One strength of population-level programs is that the cost of strategies employing use of mass media may be lower than the cost of individual and group outreach. In addition, the potential for social stigma could be avoided if universal prevention strategies are employed, even though particular individuals may be more affected by the strategy than others. For example, outlawing bath houses applies to everyone, although frequent patrons may be more likely to feel the effects of this change. Although Rose and others have argued that prevention must be universal so that shifts in the distribution of risk can be made for the entire population, many individuals not at risk are targeted.[2] Such programs may curtail individual rights and privileges to benefit the health of the population.

NETWORK ANALYSES

Prevention approaches that seek to identify social and sexual networks to characterize patterns of mixing between individuals combine considerations of individual, group, and population approaches. Both the overall rate and the extent of spread of STDs depend on the structure of sexual networks.[28] Frequent rates of concurrent sexual interactions among people lead to rapid rates of STD spread. Greater numbers of sexual linkages among subgroups can lead to extensive dissemination of infection between subgroups and throughout the population. Conversely, if a population is divided into isolated subpopulations with low rates of sexual interaction within each, STDs entering the population tend to be confined primarily to one subpopulation and to spread slowly in that subpopulation.[29]

The sexual networks that fuel the spread of STDs do not tend to overlap greatly with the social networks that channel the spread of prevention information and preventive behaviors. Sexual networks that spread STD are most frequently located in subpopulations at the lowest levels (tails) of the education, income, power, and prestige distributions, whereas networks responsive to prevention efforts are generally located within subpopulations at the highest levels of these distributions. In addition, although sex partners are usually chosen from among those with whom social linkages already exist, particular types of sexual linkage, for example, commercial or casual sex, take place between individuals less likely to be socially linked to each other.[30]

Just as the structure of sexual networks and sexual mixing patterns determine routes of transmission of STDs, the structure of social networks and social mixing patterns determine routes of the diffusion of attitudes, beliefs, life styles, and behavior patterns through a society.[32,33] Social networks tend to be more open than sexual networks, and are marked by higher rates of interchange within population subgroups, greater numbers of social contacts, and greater numbers of linkages across population subgroups. Thus, attitudes, beliefs, and behavior patterns, including preventive patterns, would spread more rapidly and extensively throughout the population. Moreover, the responsiveness of individuals to prevention information and interventions varies across population subgroups. For example, population subgroups marked by higher levels of education would be more accessible to prevention programs and more responsive to prevention messages. Similarly, population subgroups with lower prevalences of risk behaviors may respond more effectively to prevention efforts owing to their higher levels of education and their health-seeking orientation.[33] In summary, prevention efforts first reach and affect subpopulations that are least likely to contain sexual networks that spread STD. Furthermore, the nature of social networks within subpopulations having high STD rates may hinder diffusion of prevention information and interventions into the sexual networks within these subpopulations.

Although health education and health promotion interventions utilize the social network concept, contact tracing or partner notification, mentioned previously under couple-based interventions (where infected individuals name sexual partners and these partners are then identified, tested, and treated or counseled), is a public health intervention based on the sexual network notion. Attempts have been made to identify more extensive sexual networks that trace partners of partners and so on. The technique known as "cluster contact tracing," in which serologic screening for syphilis was extended to social contacts of persons with infectious syphilis, was an interesting experiment in extending disease control efforts from sexual networks to social networks. However, behavioral and other prevention interventions that target this more complex type of network have been given little attention. Probably the closest approximation are those interventions based on social diffusion where few individuals who are integrally bound into the community initiate and model social change, described in community-based interventions.[19] Such diffusion models are theoretically capable of changing social norms throughout the community while identifying and targeting sexual networks. This is clearly an area that merits additional research.

CONCLUSION

The acknowledgment of differentiation within the population with respect to infection status, risk behaviors, incurring of intangible and financial costs, as well as receipt of benefits, has led to the formulation of a series of questions related to the political economy of STD epidemiology and prevention and related issues of policy. Who is at risk? Should prevention strategies be targeted or universal? Who should pay for the intervention? All of these concerns may underlie the unfortunate subconscious distinction between noncommunicable diseases, where the disease is too often viewed as the enemy, and communicable diseases, where the infected individual is viewed by some as the enemy. In this chapter we have highlighted only a few examples of successful interventions applied using targets and levels of intervention at various units of analysis. Our goal was to illustrate individual, group, and population perspectives on STD/HIV prevention. Glib references to "individual level" or "population-level" interventions, without distinguishing between the target of the intervention, the beneficiary of the intervention, and the mechanism and agent or vehicle of the intervention, has often led to confused communications, and poorly conceived design and evaluation of STD/HIV interventions. We do not advocate any one approach over another, but suggest that STD/HIV is a multilevel problem. In the same way that risk factors can be defined on multiple levels, interventions need to be designed and evaluated appropriately for multiple levels.

References

1 Hippocrates: *The Genuine Works of Hippocrates.* Adams F (trans). New York, William Wood & Company, 1891, vol. 1, pp. 156,157.

2 Rose G: Sick individuals and sick populations. *Intl J Epid,* 14:32–35; 1985.

3 Kilmarx PH et al: Declining prevalence of gonorrhoeae and chlamydia in female sex workers, Chiang Rai, Thailand, 1991–1994. Abstract

presented at the XI International Conference on AIDS, Vancouver, 1996.

4 Morris M et al: Bridge populations in the spread of HIV/AIDS in Thailand. *AIDS* 10:1265–1271; 1996.

5 Celantano DD et al: Risk factors for HIV-1 seroconversion among young men in northern Thailand. *JAMA* 275:122–127; 1996.

6 Aral SO: The social context of syphilis persistence in the Southeastern United States. *Sex Trans Dis* 23(1):9–15, 1996.

7 Vittinghoff E et al: Attributable risk of exposures associated with sexually transmitted disease. *J Infect Dis* 174 (Suppl 2):S182–187, 1996.

8 Koopman JS et al: The ecological effects of individual exposures and nonlinear disease dynamics in populations. *Am J Public Health* 84(5): 836–842; 1994.

9 Shiboski S et al: Population and individual based approaches to the design and analysis of epidemiological studies of STD transmission. *J Infect Dis* 174 (Suppl 2):S188–200; 1996.

10 Aral SO et al: Overview: Individual and population level approaches to the epidemiology and prevention of STD. *J Infect Dis* 174 (Suppl 2):S127–233; 1996.

11 Anderson RM et al: The significance of sexual partner contact networks for the transmission dynamics of HIV. *J Acquir Immune Defic Syndr* 3:417–429 1990.

12 Ainsworth M et al: Confronting AIDS: Public priorities in a global epidemic. World Bank Policy Research Report. Oxford, Oxford University Press, 1997.

13 Grimley DM et al: Contraceptive and condom use adoption and maintenance: A stage paradigm approach. *Hlth Educ Quar* 22(1):20–35; 1995.

14 Kamenga M et al: Evidence of marked sexual behavior change associated with low HIV-1 seroconversion in 149 married couples with discordant HIV-1 serostatus: Experience at an HIV counseling center in Zaire. *AIDS* 5:61–67; 1991.

15 Allen S et al: Effect of serotesting with counseling on condom use and seroconversion among HIV-discordant couples in Africa. *Br Med J* 304:1605–1609; 1992.

16 Padian NS et al: Prevention of heterosexual transmission of human immunodeficiency virus through couple counseling. *J Acquir Immune Defic Syndr* 6:1043–1048; 1993.

17 Heathcote H et al: Gonorrhea transmission dynamics and control. Lecture Notes in Biomathematics. New York, Springer-Verlag, 1984; no. 56.

18 Handsfield H et al: Localized outbreak of penicillinase-producing Neisseria gonorrhoeae: Paradigm for introduction and spread of gonorrhea in a community. *JAMA* 261:2357–2361; 1989.

19 Kelly JA et al: HIV risk behavior reduction following intervention with key opinion leaders of population: An experimental analysis. *Am J Public Health* 81:168–171; 1991.

20 Ngugi EN et al: Focused peer-meditated educational programmes to reduce STD and HIV transmission in Kenya and Zimbabwe. *J Infect Dis* 174 (Suppl 2):S240–247; 1996.

21 Tawil O et al: Enabling approaches for HIV/AIDS prevention: Can we modify the environment and minimize the risk? *AIDS* 9:1299–1306; 1995.

22 Hanenberg RS et al: Impact of Thailand's HIV-control programme as indicated by the decline of sexually transmitted diseases. *Lancet,* 344: 243–245; 1994.

23 Laga M et al: Condom promotion, sexually transmitted diseases treatment, and declining incidence of HIV-1 infection in female Zairian sex workers. *Lancet* 344:246–248; 1994.

24 Over M et al: HIV infection and other sexually transmitted diseases in developing countries: Public health importance and priorities for resource allocation. *J Infect Dis* 174 (Suppl 2):S162–175; 1996.

25 Kelly JA et al: Community AIDS/HIV risk reduction: The effects of endorsements by popular people in three cities. *Am J Public Health* 82(11):1483–1489; 1992.

26 Grosskurth H et al: Impact of improved treatment of sexually transmitted diseases on HIV infection in rural Tanzania: Randomized controlled trial. *Lancet* 346(8974):530–536; 1995.

27 Scheper-Hugher N: AIDS, public health, and human rights in Cuba. *Lancet* 342(8877):965; 1993.

28 Klovdahl AS: Social networks and the spread of infectious disease: The AIDS example. *Soc Sci Med* 21:1203–1216; 1985.

29 Wasserheit JN et al: The dynamic topology of STD epidemics: Implication for STD prevention. *J Infect Dis* 174 (Suppl 2):S201–213; 1996.

30 Laumann E et al: *The Social Organization of Sexuality.* Chicago: University of Chicago Press, 1994.

31 Aral SO: Patterns of sex partner recruitment and types of mixing as determinants of STD transmission: Limits to the spread of sexually transmitted infections. *Vernerology* 8:240–242; 1995.

32 Rogers EM: *Diffusion of Innovations*, 3rd ed. New York, The Free Press, 1983.

33 Fisher ED, Jr: Editorial: The results of the COMMIT trial. *Am J Public Health,* 85:159–160, 1995.

Chapter 89

Conceptual framework for STD/HIV prevention and control

Michael E. St. Louis
King K. Holmes

Local, state, national, and international programs for prevention of STD/HIV differ in how they organize diverse prevention elements, strategies, and available resources into their own distinctive public health approaches. This chapter considers principles on which a comprehensive public health approach to HIV and STD prevention might be designed or improved, reviews some examples of such approaches, and proposes a framework for weighing alternatives to increase the public health impact of a particular program or approach to prevention. Principles and frameworks appropriate for prevention of communicable diseases necessarily differ from those for prevention of chronic diseases and should consider both individual and population-level aspects of disease prevention and health promotion. Public health approaches to different STDs can be compared within the same population, and approaches to the full range of HIV and other STDs can be compared between countries or other geopolitical jurisdictions.

AN EPIDEMIOLOGIC FRAMEWORK FOR HIV AND STD PREVENTION AND CONTROL EFFORTS

The core functions of public health have been described as consisting of assessment, policy development, and assurance.[1] Translated into the domain of the communicable disease control practitioner, these functions constitute an epidemiologic framework for *assessing* needs, *analyzing* opportunities to enhance prevention, *guiding* implementation policy, and continuously refining program design by *evaluating* the impact on disease rates of specific activities as well as the overall program (Fig. 89-1).

Assessing the burden or health impact of an STD is generally the first step in development of an organized prevention and control program. In the 1930s, the dramatic human and economic impact of syphilis in the United States fueled its recognition as a preeminent health problem in the United States and led to the first major sexually transmitted disease campaign in the United States.[2] Later, an analysis of the health impact—and especially of the economic burden—of pelvic inflammatory disease (PID) and its associated sequelae in the United States in 1987 catalyzed development of national guidelines for control and prevention of chlamydial infections in 1993, with ensuing legislation and federal funding specifically allocated for chlamydia control in 1994.[3,4] The direct medical costs of selected STDs, exclusive of HIV/AIDS and of pregnancy-related and perinatal morbidity, have recently been estimated at approximately $7.5 billion for 1995 in the United States (See Chap. 99). HIV infection continues to generate direct, lifetime medical costs of greater than $100,000 per infected person, and sexually transmitted HIV infections resulted in direct medical costs estimated at approximately $5.0 billion in 1994.[5,6] These estimates do not include indirect costs related to loss of productivity (often approximated at two to three times the direct medical costs) and do not yet take into account the amount of disability-adjusted or quality-adjusted life years lost owing to STDs.

In addition to the cost and other public health impacts of a particular STD, the *current* ongoing costs and benefits of prevention need to be considered, since these represent potential savings if a specific communicable disease can be sufficiently suppressed or eliminated. For example, routine smallpox vaccination was terminated in the United States even before the disease was eradicated worldwide, once the risk for domestic acquisition had become sufficiently remote. Furthermore, the cost of maintaining worldwide smallpox vaccination established a cost-benefit benchmark for the costs of an elimination effort.[7] Although data exist for many of these parameters, a systematic approach to comparing these factors for individual STDs has not been employed. At present, only dracunculiasis and polio are currently targeted for global eradication.[7] Because none of the STDs has been designated for global eradication, reduced STD transmission should lead to a shift in prevention priorities, and probably to reduced costs of prevention, but not to cessation of all prevention efforts in the foreseeable future. An important advance in the assessment of the burden of STDs was made in the 1993 World Bank Books *Disease Control Priorities in Developing Countries,* which estimated the disability-adjusted life years lost due to STDs and concluded that targeted STD prevention was one of the most cost-effective health interventions of any type available to the developing world.[8] The report singled out operational research in STD prevention as the highest research priority.[9]

A second step in a broad epidemiologic approach to disease control involves analysis of the prevention opportunities (see Fig. 89-1). This begins with the basic descriptive epidemiology of time, place, and person but continues on with analysis of risk factors for acquiring infection, delayed treatment, and progression to adverse sequelae. One special and often productive approach is the analysis of "missed opportunities" for prevention and of the settings or venues where interventions might have been or could be cost-effectively delivered. Wherever feasible, this should culminate in prevention research trials of the intrinsic efficacy of a potential intervention and in estimates of the potential cost-benefit or cost-utility of the intervention.

These first two steps from Fig. 89-1, assessments of burden of disease and analyses of prevention opportunities, exist in a dynamic equilibrium that may change with a reassessment of either the burden of the disease or with technological or other advances in prevention opportunities.[10] For example, increasing recognition of the long-term reproductive health impact of *C. trachomatis* infections in women, combined with development of nonculture diagnostic tests feasible for large-scale screening programs, has recently led to greater interest in and resources for chlamydia prevention activities in the United States.[11]

The third step in the basic epidemiologic approach to prevention involves guidance of the implementation efforts through development or adaption of prevention guidelines to local circumstances and establishment and use of surveillance and other data to set prevention objectives (see Fig. 89-1). This step corresponds to the second basic function of public health, policy development, but emphasizes the use of local data to establish jurisdictional guidelines or other policy statements and standards. The use of local data to adapt general guidelines to local circumstances and to establish program objectives is an especially powerful principle that (1) reinforces the importance of using surveillance and other data reflecting the actual occurrence of disease, rather than only attending to the process measurements and idiosyncratic experiences and agendas of individuals and public health organizations; (2) continually redirects program efforts toward the geographic areas and subpopulations at high risk of disease;

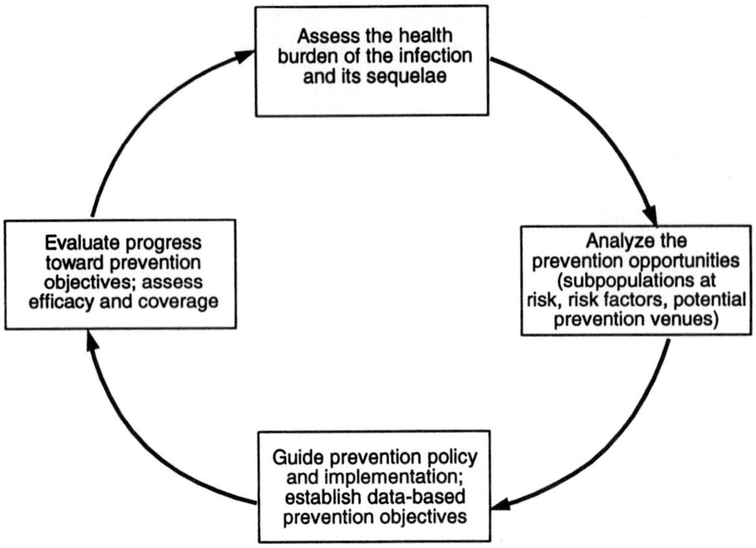

Fig. 89-1. Epidemiologic approach to STD/HIV prevention iterative uses of data.

and establishes the basis for program evaluation and redesign in an intrinsic, iterative, natural way.[12] At a national level in the United States, this process is reflected in the Healthy People 2000 Objectives, but this process of establishing program objectives based on local data is scalable down through states to local health units, where its potential impact is greatest.[13]

In the fourth step, the evaluation of the process of implementation, one assesses the real-world effectiveness of the intervention in terms of population coverage or uptake, compliance outside the research setting, the targeting of the intervention in relation to the distribution of disease (are those at highest risk of acquiring or transmitting infection included?), and the impact of the prevention activities in the local program on disease morbidity. If local disease surveillance and other data have been incorporated into the first three steps of this epidemiologic approach to prevention, especially the third step, program evaluation follows naturally and iteratively in the manner of "continuous quality improvement" efforts.

Much of the following discussion of a conceptual framework for STD/HIV prevention is somewhat abstract, and its applicability is not evident to all public health workers. However, this basic epidemiologic model or approach to STD/HIV prevention is usually readily understood and can be applied to any STD and any of the facets of STD prevention discussed in the remainder of this chapter. Tools for self-assessment of the capacity of local health departments to conduct data-based planning and program evaluation have also been developed.[14] Although we call the outline and conceptual framework represented in Fig. 89-1 an "epidemiologic approach" because each step involves assessment of disease rates in populations or subpopulations, the activities themselves—particularly the development of interventions and the evaluation process—are highly interdisciplinary, and optimal execution involves skills of laboratory, behavioral, health services, statistical, and other scientists, along with public health professionals.

DETERMINANTS OF HIV AND STD TRANSMISSION IN POPULATIONS

Public health efforts to enhance HIV and STD prevention strategies should be considered in the context of the general determinants of STD transmission in populations. The basic model for the reproductive rate of new infections in a population holds that

$$R_0 = D \times c \times \beta,$$

where R_0, the reproductive rate, represents the average number of secondary cases that arise from any new case of infection (see Chap. 3).[15] If R_0 exceeds 1, the infection will spread, and incidence increases. The objective is to reduce and maintain R_0 below 1, so that the infection will die out in the population. This can be accomplished by influencing the determinants of R_0: D represents the duration of transmissible infections in persons already infected; c is a complex factor, representing the average rate of exposure of susceptible to infectious people in the population; and β represents the average likelihood of transmission of infection, given such exposure.

This dynamic model and its predecessors establish the theoretical basis for essentially all current STD/HIV control efforts.[16] In a sense, the rest of this chapter constitutes an examination of the implications of this model for STD prevention and control efforts under the diverse biologic, epidemiologic, sociologic, and technologic circumstances of different STDs in different societies. The public health science of STD prevention lies in trying to identify the most cost-effective ways to decrease transmission by influencing one or more of these three transmission determinants, translating theoretical insights and empirical data into specific tasks to be incorporated into the work plans of public health practitioners.

A further general concept that follows from this model is that the higher the value of R_0 for any given STD within any particular population, the greater will be the reduction in D, c, or β that is required to reduce R_0 below 1. This will likely require a more intensive effort when R_0 is very large than when the value of R_0 is at or just above 1. There is an obvious need to balance the *intensity* of the prevention efforts to the "force of infection" in the particular population for a particular STD (the force of infection is defined as the per capita rate at which susceptibles acquire infection, which typically varies by age and other subpopulation characteristics).[17]

THE BASIC ACTIVITIES OF STD/HIV PREVENTION

In the past, the basic prevention activities (e.g., screening, contact tracing, or health education) in STD/HIV prevention programs

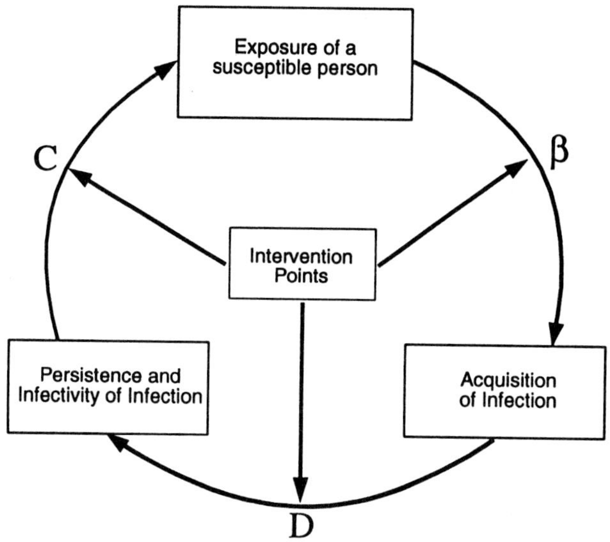

Fig. 89-2. Intervention points according to the determinants of STD/HIV transmission. Reprinted with permission from reference 6.

have often been classified into primary and secondary prevention strategies. This follows a chronic disease paradigm in which diseases can either be prevented from developing (primary prevention) or treated effectively once acquired to prevent complications (secondary prevention). This paradigm, although convenient and familiar, is best not applied to the communicable diseases, since early diagnosis and treatment of communicable disease constitutes secondary prevention at the individual level, but primary prevention (by reducing D, the duration of infectivity) at the population level, prevents spread to subsequent sex partners through sexual networks.[18]

A more explicit and useful approach to classifying the basic STD and HIV prevention efforts is to categorize them according to the principal determinants of STD transmission D, c, and β, which can be targeted by specific types of intervention activities (Fig. 89-2). One such classification of the basic strategies of STD prevention is shown in Table 89-1. Of note, many public health interventions may simultaneously influence more than one of these general determinants of transmission. For example, partner notification that leads to treatment contributes to shortening duration of infectivity for treatable infections, but it also may reduce exposure or efficiency of transmission if partner notification and associated counseling have an impact on subsequent sexual behavior and partner selection (impact on exposure, c) or on condom use or sexual practices (impact on efficiency of transmission, β).

Examples of specific preventative intervention activities are classified in Table 89-2 according to the three determinants of transmission. Interventions that could shorten duration of infectivity (D) include: active case-finding through widespread access to acceptable and good quality clinical care, screening, and contact tracing; prompt and effective diagnosis and treatment for symptomatic persons; clinical practice that emphasizes *timeliness* of treatment (e.g., by use of syndromic diagnostic algorithms and rapid diagnostic tests) rather than placing greatest priority on very high specificity of diagnosis; screening practices for asymptomatic infections; promoting awareness among potentially infected persons of the symptoms of STDs and the need to seek care in a timely way; and other supporting strategies or tactics, such as "epidemiologic treatment," selective mass treatment, and so on. Outbreak identification, investigation, and control are functions that

Table 89-1. Basic Strategies of STD/HIV Prevention According to Determinants of the Reproductive Rate of Infection

Decrease duration of infectivity (to prevent further transmission and complications)
Early detection (case-finding)
Treatment (curative or suppressive)
Decrease exposures of susceptibles to infectious persons
Modify behavior of susceptibles
Modify behavior of known infected persons (especially for persistent infections)
Modify behavior of potentially infected persons
Decrease acquisition of infection by susceptibles, if exposed
Decrease efficiency of transmission per exposure

address duration of infectivity, particularly in the special circumstance when a disease has become relatively rare. Most of the more traditional clinically oriented activities of STD control programs principally function to reduce mean duration of infectivity in the population.

Interventions that reduce exposure to STDs (c) may target any of the determinants of sexual behavior, sexual mixing, and sexual decision-making in a society, a highly complex and value-laden matrix of factors. Potential activities to reduce exposure include: promotion of delayed initiation of sexual intercourse among young adolescents, abstinence, monogamy, reduced rates of sex partner change, and avoidance of concurrent sexual partnerships; HIV counseling and testing to reduce unprotected sexual contact between HIV-infected and HIV-seronegative persons (e.g., the efficacy of Project Respect is described in Chap. 54); clinic-level health education for risk reduction; and focused, community-level interventions to modify community norms toward less acceptance of specific, high–risk behaviors.[19] A critical area for long-term impact on exposure is through school health education programs, which having been shown to generally increase abstinence rates and reduce rates of sexual activity and pregnancy in sexually-active teens, nonetheless remain highly controversial in the United States.[20]

Intervention activities that decrease efficiency of transmission of STD (β) during sexual exposure include those that increase consistent and correct use of barrier contraceptive methods (e.g., condoms, spermicides) during sex; decrease specific risky sexual practices (e.g., avoidance of unprotected anal intercourse, adoption of "outercourse" and other nonpenetrative sexual interaction styles); biomedical measures that decrease or lower transmissibility (e.g., early detection and treatment of other STDs to reduce transmission of HIV in Mwanza, Tanzania); antiretroviral treatment to prevent perinatal HIV transmission; postexposure antiretroviral prophylaxis; intercurrent suppressive antiviral therapy in the infected partner with HIV or genital herpes; and measures that lower host susceptibility (e.g., hepatitis B vaccines).[21–24]

There is no dearth of effective interventions to reduce transmission and sequelae of STD, including HIV infection. This is evidenced by the success of the Mwanza, Tanzania study; of postexposure antiretroviral prophylaxis for needle-stick exposure to HIV infection; of perinatal antiretroviral prophylaxis; of Project RESPECT; the effectiveness of chlamydia screening in preventing PID and probably in lowering prevalence of *C. trachomatis* infection; the known efficacy of hepatitis B vaccine and of many approaches to detection and treatment of curable STD; and the probable effectiveness of many other interventions, such as needle exchange.[21,22,25–29] The challenge now is to develop systems of public health and clinical medicine to effectively deliver these other interventions at the operational level.

Interventions that decrease exposure to infectious persons, or decrease efficiency of transmission of many or all STDs (e.g., by

Table 89-2. Examples of Specific Intervention Activities of STD/HIV Prevention Programs*

Determinant of Transmission	Potential Activities or Interventions to Address the Determinant
D (Duration of infectivity)	Monitor† the *prevalence* and *duration* of infections and subcategories of infections (such as antimicrobial resistance) in diverse subpopulations Conduct active case finding through screening, surveillance, and partner notification Improve effective access to medical care (cost, quality, location, timeliness, etc. of medical services) Increase awareness of STDs; improve symptom recognition and health care-seeking behavior Implement strategies (e.g., syndromic management, use of rapid tests) to shorten or eliminate time delay between first medical encounter and definitive treatment Shorten duration of infection among latently or potentially infected persons by epidemiologic treatment or selective mass treatment Rapidly detect and control outbreaks of diseases for which endemic transmission within the jurisdiction has been eliminated
c (Exposure of susceptible to infectious persons)	Monitor† the prevalence of high-risk exposures (e.g., sex for drugs, needle-sharing among IDUs, unprotected anal intercourse) in specific populations or facilities (e.g., detention facilities) Promote delayed sexual debut, abstinence, monogamy, or reduced rates of sex partner change Reduce *concurrent* (as opposed to sequential) sex partnerships that may involve an infected and an uninfected person Develop and promote messages about selection of *safer* partners Promote widespread testing, such as HIV testing and counseling, if undertaken so that identified HIV-seropositive persons will reduce sex with uninfected persons Promote selection of sex partnerships between persons concordant (either both infected or both uninfected) for persistent viral infections (e.g., HSV, HIV) Develop and promote media messages and norms targeted toward infected or potentially infected persons to protect partners (e.g., "avoid sex if any symptoms exist"; "avoid unprotected sex with regular partner soon after sex with risky partner") Promote healthy genital hygiene (e.g., regular washing; avoidance of unsafe foreign substances, drying agents, etc.) Reduce community exposures to settings of very high risk sex (crack houses, bath houses, brothels) and establish prevention efforts in such settings
β (Efficiency of transmission during exposure between susceptible and infectious partners)	Monitor† *transmissibility* of infections (e.g., through systematically collected data on partner notification and testing) and on key behaviors or other factors influencing transmissibility, such as condom use, practice of anal intercourse, etc. Hepatitis B immunization Increase condom use, especially for nonmonogamous and risky (e.g., casual, commercial) sexual interactions Reduce risky sexual practices (e.g., unprotected anal intercourse) or other risk behavior (e.g., needle-sharing) that increases likelihood of infection if exposure occurs Reduce a critical cofactor that increases infectivity (e.g., reduce other STD to reduce HIV transmission) Reduce sexual exposure in particularly critical *stages* of infection (e.g., very early and late HIV infection; primary HSV-2 infection) Promote genital hygiene (e.g., pre- and postcoital washing) Consider local or systemic chemoprophylactics Provide suppressive chemotherapy that reduces infectivity in infected partner (e.g., AZT in pregnant women, potentially acyclovir in genital herpes) Provide postexposure prophylaxis (e.g., antimicrobials, antivirals, or immune serum globulin after known exposure to STD)

* Classified according to the three general determinants of STD transmission.
† Assessment objectives.

adoption of safer sexual practices or barrier prophylaxis), are particularly important for at least three reasons. First, the growing importance of STDs for which treatment is not curative, especially HIV, but also human papillomavirus (HPV) infections and herpes simplex virus (HSV) infections, calls for such interventions. Second, such strategies would have impact across all or many STDs, rather than being pathogen-specific, in contrast to use of a screening test or a vaccine for a specific infection. Third, to the extent adoption of healthier behaviors can become normative, these behaviors may become increasingly sustainable.

Unfortunately, these are the domains of Table 89-2, in which public health departments have generally had the least experience, compared to reducing the *duration* of infection through screening and treatment. Further, for various reasons, the vast majority of prevention research trials designed to reduce exposure, reduce unsafe practices, or promote barrier prophylaxis have not measured impact on disease acquisition at either the individual or population level—not even for a single STD, much less for the broad spectrum of STDs that theoretically could be prevented by such interventions. Whether outcomes such as reported behavior change represent adequate surrogates or predictors of an impact on disease acquisition remains a matter of debate.[30] Thus, with few notable exceptions (Project RESPECT[26]), the impact of such interventions on disease acquisition remains uncertain.[30] Topical (vaginal) microbicides represent another potential intervention broadly applicable against a full range of STDs. However, where controlled trials have been undertaken of topical microbicides, results have differed between studies and for different STD agents (see Chap. 78). Of note, it is also theoretically possible that some short- or medium-term *increase* in transmission could arise from behavioral interventions that lead to differential decline in availability to "core group" members of sex partnerships with lower-risk persons, resulting in increased sexual contact rates within the core group. Analogously, certain strategies for promotion of one type of prophylaxis (e.g., topical microbicides) could decrease reliance on a more effective barrier prophylaxis (e.g., condom use).[31] In addition, increased attention to reducing risky exposure as a prevention objective will likely have implications for other aspects of the prevention approach, such as the "venues" or settings at which interventions may be most effectively implemented or the types of staff who may be most effective in message and program delivery.

INDIVIDUAL AND POPULATION AND COMMUNITY PERSPECTIVES

Exposure, transmission, and persistence of STDs may each be addressed through interventions fundamentally targeted at either the individual or the population levels.[18] Viewed differently, HIV and STD prevention activities may have different ramifications for individuals and for populations. In general, the individual level addresses the *personal health* and *personal responsibility* issues, whereas at the population level, macroepidemiologic effect focuses on the contribution to limiting transmission and persistence of pathogenic organisms in communities and on the social or collective responsibility for establishing the community structures, practices, and norms that will tend to reduce or eliminate dissemination of the organism in the community. Chapters 88 and 90 address this important distinction in detail.

SYSTEMS FOR STD/HIV PREVENTION

The determinants of transmission in the reproductive rate equation constitute the theoretical basis of STD/HIV control. However, specific preventive intervention activities described in Table 89-2 depend on a limited number of *systems* or domains in which prevention activities are implemented (Table 89-3 and see Chap. 90). These systems, for example, the system of clinical services, may exist completely within public health departments, completely outside of the domain of the public health departments, or—most commonly—represent a complex mixture of health department activities with those of other institutions or agencies, with different blends in different jurisdictions. Although it is well recognized that the "system" of health care services differs dramatically in the United States, for example, and other industrialized countries,[32] it is less widely appreciated that there currently exists extraordinary diversity in the blend and composition of public and private medical care across and within states and local areas within the United States, requiring great flexibility and creativity on the part of STD/HIV prevention authorities to optimally mobilize clinical care for STD prevention across diverse jurisdictions. Also, importantly, the public health systems listed in Table 89-3 often correspond more closely than the basic determinants of transmission, c, β, and D, to how health and public health services are organized within departments or divisions of agencies. Optimal STD/HIV prevention requires proper functioning of each of these systems. Thus, public health authorities need to *assess* and *assure* effective function of these systems, whether or not they are directly involved in carring out the activities that constitute parts of the systems. This is the case, for example, when an important part or all of the clinical care for STD/HIV is provided in the private medical sector.

In the setting of the broad social forces that truly drive public health, the *prevention programs* of local, state, regional, national, or international agencies consist of the public health sector components suspended in these broader systems of preventive intervention activities (see Chap. 90). Thus, the impact of public health programs and their specific preventive interventions result not only from the intrinsic efficacy of the interventions in isolation but from how they influence the entire system. With the rapid growth of managed care organizations for delivery of clinical care in the United States, for example, which widely use the performance measures described in the Health Plan Employer Data and Information Set (HEDIS) "report card," incorporation into HEDIS 3.0 of a performance measure related to chlamydia screening has the potential to dramatically influence an important clinical STD preventive service throughout a wide range of organizations.

Health promotion and behavioral intervention is one such system and a necessary, integral component of any disease control and prevention program (Table 89-4). Even for diseases for which highly effective therapy (all of the bacterial STDs) or vaccination (HBV) exist, health education and promotion remain critical prevention elements in order, for example, to ensure timely health care–seeking behavior or high rates of HBV vaccination in communities at high risk. Thus, it is paradoxical that little effort until now has been given in the United States or many other countries to promoting utilization of effective clinical services. It is as if the providers of limited, inadequately funded services don't want them promoted or more heavily utilized. Perhaps the wide technical and organizational gap between health promotion and clinical service represents a formidable barrier to closer collaboration that must be overcome. For some STDs, health education and promotion represent potentially the only component, as is currently the case for prevention of subclinical genital HPV infections, since no specific therapeutic or preventive modalities are in operation other than general promotion of less unsafe sex, including lower rates of partner change and of unprotected sex.

Listed second among the STD/HIV prevention systems is assurance of access to high-quality clinical care to persons voluntarily seeking clinical care for STD or other health concerns (see Table 89-4). First, relevant and appropriate clinical practice guidelines are needed at the national level. These should include not only treatment guidelines (consistent with, although potentially differing from, WHO guidelines, depending on epidemiology and drug availability) but also guidelines for testing and other prevention activities.[33,34] These guidelines may serve as a standard by which to assess quality, coverage, and accessibility of care for STD. Provider training is important, with the definition of providers including all those who actually encounter and treat patients with STDs in the jurisdiction, which may include paraprofessionals and pharmacists in some settings. High-quality, timely STD laboratory services are important, at least in reference centers and "centers of excellence." It is hard to maintain quality in a clinical system based on syndromic diagnosis alone, or on less sensitive or specific laboratory tests such as Gram's stains or microscopy, without feedback and quality control from a reliable laboratory. Also,

Table 89-3. Public Health Systems for STD/HIV Prevention

Health promotion and behavioral intervention
Clinical and laboratory services
Partner services
Outbreak response
Surveillance, information systems, and epidemiologic analysis
Professional training
Research and evaluation
Leadership and management

measurement of the prevalence of HIV and other STDs, at least on the basis of periodic surveys, is necessary to assess prevention impact and revise treatment guidelines and intervention priorities.

Management of the intervention program, systems, and activities is essential, requiring leadership, clearly articulated policies and guidelines, and supportive laws and regulations. Partnerships and linkages to other institutions are an important element in accomplishing HIV/STD prevention at a societal level. Professional and other provider groups are obviously necessary partners, who can easily confound specific strategies (such as syndromic algorithms for STD management) about which they are not convinced. With the shift in incidence of syphilis in the United States from homosexual or bisexual men and female prostitutes to substance abusers, agencies such as correctional health facilities and drug treatment centers take on a more central role as necessary participants in STD control in the United States. The development of a strong advocacy group for AIDS prevention in the United States has been promoted not only by the severity of the epidemic but by the preexisting cohesiveness of the community of homosexual men in the United States and by the inclusion of affected groups in the priority-setting and design of prevention programs, a model is now being followed in prevention research programs for other STDs in the United States.[35,36] In Colombia and Brazil, recent campaigns to eliminate congenital syphilis have involved special efforts to bring maternal child health programs together with STD control programs for joint planning and implementation (Claudio Betts and Paulo Naud, personal communication). In the United States, the CDC, Office for Population Affairs, and the Infectious Diseases Society of America have led an effort to jointly develop reproductive health guidelines for family planning and STD prevention.

IMPORTANCE OF PREVENTION IN GROUPS AT HIGHEST RISK FOR ACQUIRING AND TRANSMITTING STD/HIV

The appropriate interventions and target populations vary for different diseases in different settings, but programs must prioritize high-risk groups and high-risk venues or institutional settings. The impact on incidence of STD/HIV in the general population is much greater by preventing a case of STD among those likely to transmit to others than by preventing a case of STD in the general population.[37,37a] Assuming comparable costs and feasibility of prevention per case in high-risk groups and in the general population, this can translate into much greater cost-effectiveness of intervention focused on those most likely to transmit infections. However, such interventions might be more expensive than routine, "passive" provision of services—for example, to patients who present voluntarily seeking care. Therefore, the prioritization of interventions should be based on data and strategically chosen. A community-based intervention to change behavioral norms, attitudes, and motivations for HIV prevention among persons at high risk for sexual or injection-related HIV transmission in the United States is one example of such an intervention, as are the several examples of specialized clinical services for commercial sex workers (CSWs) in developing countries and in the one state in the United States with legalized prostitution.[38–41] Intensive contact tracing, assessment of social and sexual networks, and expanded epidemiologic treatment of sexual contacts and "associates" (persons identified during so-called "cluster investigation" of the individuals who are closely associated with a patient with syphilis) may be considered types of focused intervention.[42] Surveillance for HIV and STD may include universal notifiable case reporting of STD in settings with capacity for such activity. At a minimum (and perhaps optimum for certain highly prevalent conditions, even in industrialized countries), monitoring the prevalence of infection in certain high-risk or vulnerable subpopulations or institutional settings can assist in evaluating and retargeting intervention efforts. As mentioned, some basic laboratory capacity is essential in this regard.

STAGES IN THE PREVENTION AND CONTROL OF STDS

Table 89-4 describes a classification of STD/HIV prevention efforts into stages, according to the extent to which the strategies, intervention activities, and public health systems outlined in Tables 89-1, 89-2, and 89-3 have been adopted or brought into play in the service of disease prevention, as well as the extent of population coverage by the program. This classification builds on other useful schemas that have recently been proposed, including a schema for "staging" epidemic or emergent STDs and a schema to facilitate an economic assessment of STD/HIV prevention strategies.[8,10] "Stages" of intervention in case management also have been described, but we emphazise stages in application of the available strategic intervention activities, derived from the epidemiologic models of transmisstion (see Chap. 48). We classify disease-specific prevention efforts into three rather distinct categories, based on three criteria: (1) Are the prevention strategies (see Table 89-1) and related activities (see Table 89-2) sufficiently comprehensive, relative to the average force of infection for a specific infection in the population? In general, comprehensive strategies will be needed to control infections characterized by a high force of infection (e.g., gonorrhea and chlamydial infection in most populations), whereas less comprehensive strategies may suffice for infections which seem to have lower force of infection (e.g., chancroid, LGV, donovanosis, which have been eliminated from most populations). (2) Have strong public health systems (see Table 89-3) and infrastructures been developed to effectively implement strategic intervention activities? (3) Is the coverage of the population appropriate? Specifically, are all populations at high risk for acquiring and transmitting infection effectively covered by strategic intervention activities?

Different countries vary in their levels of effort (i.e., stage) of prevention for different STDs; within one country, the stage of prevention of different STDs also typically varies substantially. There are several reasons for this. For any given STD, the force of infection differs between countries and between populations, largely because of differing patterns of sexual behavior and perhaps because of differing determinants of efficiency of transmission. Conversely, for any given population, the force of infection differs between STDs, because of differing efficiencies of transmission and differing natural histories between STDs. Further, the package of strategies and activities available to prevent various STDs differs, depending, for example, on whether diagnostic tests are accurate and inexpensive and whether they are preventable by vaccination or by barriers or other methods and whether they are curable, suppressible, or largely unaffected by treatment. Finally, populations may give higher or lower priority to health or to STD/HIV prevention among health priorities, and they may give higher priority for prevention to some STDs (e.g., HIV, chlamydia) than to others (e.g., HSV, HPV). These intersecting factors have been explored recently in a sophisticated way that addressed the multidimensional interface (the "topology") between the forces promoting disease transmission and persistence in the prevention programs installed to counter those forces.[10]

As outlined in Table 89-4, at the least developed level, Stage I, with essentially no effective preventive efforts, an STD reaches an equilibrium determined by baseline patterns of exposure, efficiency of transmission, and the natural history of that infection.

Table 89-4. Stages in Control and Prevention of Sexually Transmitted Diseases

Stages	Stages in Prevention and Control	Typical Corresponding Epidemiologic Setting	Examples of Pathogen-Jurisdiction Combinations That Reflect the Particular Stage in Various Settings*: US and Other Industrialized Countries	Less Industrialized Countries
I	No *specific* control or prevention guidelines or focus; very limited personal preventive care (screening, etc.)	Hyperendemic or unknown epidemiology	HPV in United States; and most European countries; chlamydia in United States before 1987	Chlamydia in Southeast Asia, Africa, and Latin America; bacterial STD in many sub-Saharan African countries
II	Moderate access to personal preventive health care services; limited to no surveillance and specific intervention	Highly prevalent infections	HSV in United States	Gonorrhea in Latin American capital cities
III	Coordinated screening and other preventive services; some disease surveillance; some health education and communication	Declining, but still widely prevalent	Chlamydia in United States	Syphilis in Latin American capital cities
IV	Widespread access to *clinical* preventive services; *careful* surveillance; implementation of *specific prevention initiatives* (e.g., rigorous outbreak investigation and partner notification)	Limited, focal, endemic transmission within core groups	Syphilis in United States; chlamydia in Sweden	—
V	Prevention focus on outbreak investigation and control; heightened surveillance, with careful investigation of each infectious case	Elimination or near-elimination status, with limited endemic transmission and importation-type epidemiology; occasional small outbreaks	Chancroid and LGV in United States; syphilis in United Kingdom; gonorrhea in Sweden; HIV in Sweden	—

*Examples pertain to 1998 unless otherwise stated.

In Stage II, prevention efforts have begun, but some of the prevention strategies required to reduce the incidence at the population level (i.e., to reduce R_o to <1) either do not exist or have not been adopted; or if adopted, have not been strongly pursued with strategic intervention activities orchestrated by strong public health systems and infrastructure; or if adopted and strongly pursued, have not achieved adequate coverage of the populations that experience the highest force of infection; thus, infection rates remain high.

Stage III represents a more advanced prevention effort, in which the strategies and activities necessary to reduce transmission to an acceptable level have been adopted and implemented, orchestrated by strong public health systems and infrastructure(s), with populations appropriately covered by these intervention activities. In Stage III, rates of the STI are falling, or have fallen, to an acceptable target level of endemic transmission. Criteria for "acceptable" incidence or prevalence rates of an STI remain to be defined and could be based on formal cost-benefit analyses, which depend on the morbidity per case associated with the STI and the reduction in morbidity expected with incremental increases in cost; or—as for the targets set in the United States for the year 2000—targets can be based upon expert opinions of what is feasible.[13]

In Stage IV, prevention efforts are sustained and pursued with sufficient intensity and coverage with respect to the force of infection that persists in only marginal geographic, demographic, or behavioral subsets of the population. Localized elimination may be considered as a strategy. Intensified community interventions may be undertaken in foci of persisting endemic transmission.

In Stage V, prevention programs as described for Stage III have been sufficient to eliminate sustained endemic transmission, so that morbidity is now limited to imported infections, with secondary cases or outbreaks arising from these imported infections. Assuming efforts to prevent exposure and to reduce efficiency of transmission have been sustained, the emphasis in Stage V is to contain outbreaks by early detection and early treatment of imported and secondary cases.

ASSESSING TRENDS IN STAGES OF STD/HIV PREVENTION AND CONTROL

In general, as disease prevention and control advance toward Stage V, prevention activities can increasingly focus on smaller geographic areas and high risk populations that continue to sustain endemic transmission. A similar point has been made by Brunham and colleagues, who noted that the general direction of STD prevention and control was to progressively restrict transmission from broad social groups to specific subpopulations, mathematically describable as core populations.[43] A potential danger is that as prevalence of a specific STD declines and the intensity of control efforts shifts toward intensive, highly argeted interventions in small residual core groups in the population, the broader systems of health education and promotion, clinical recognition and services, and surveillance may erode for what in that jurisdiction has become a rare disease. This is the current situation for chancroid in the United States, with a dramatic recent decline in awareness, dismantling of clinical laboratory detection capacity, and deterioration of surveillance; as a result, major outbreaks that occur can escape recognition and control efforts for prolonged periods.[44–48] A similar rationale has been invoked for the current difficulties in dealing with resurgent STDs in China, after decades of no reported STD transmission.[49]

Applying the preceding STD-specific criteria for classifying STD/HIV prevention and control efforts, the stages of a national program can be evaluated. In the United States, the 37-year interval that followed World War II and continuing until recognition of the HIV/AIDS pandemic spanned much of the antibiotic era, when STD prevention efforts shifted away from the social hygiene movement to focus on reducing the duration of infectivity through diagnosis and treatment of bacterial STDs (other than chlamydial infection) and trichomoniasis. The brief period of genital herpes hysteria during the 1970s, and the growing incidence and awareness of other viral STDs, including genital warts and hepatitis B had already led to some public discussion of decreasing exposure and use of condoms, which was greatly expanded by the advent of HIV/AIDS. These HIV/AIDS-related behavioral interventions to decrease exposure and transmission, when added to the existing diagnosis and treatment prevention programs, produced a more comprehensive prevention strategy against the bacterial STDs and undoubtedly contributed to the continuing decline in rates of gonorrhea and syphilis (although this has not been documented). This was interrupted transiently in parts of the United States by an upswing in the late 1980s, associated with and perhaps attributable to the crack cocaine epidemic. Thus, as of the late 1990s, the gonorrhea prevention and control efforts are in Stage III in most of the United States, and syphilis prevention efforts are in Stage III or IV in most areas (with about three-quarters of U.S. counties reporting no P&S syphilis in 1997). Trichomoniasis has been substantially reduced in most middle-class populations in the United States. However, in much of the southeastern United States, prevention and control of bacterial STDs and trichomoniasis should be classified as Stage II because of weak public health systems for STD prevention (especially relative to the force of infection in the southeastern U.S. populations) and exceptionally poor coverage of high-risk populations; even chancroid still undergoes sustained transmission in this area. Nationally, efforts to prevent chlamydial infection vary from Stage II (in areas where screening for chlamydia is just beginning) to Stage III (e.g., in the Pacific Northwest and Wisconsin, where screening programs have been in place for a decade, and the incidence of chlamydial infections has been falling). Currently, the major national effort for chlamydia prevention is expansion of clinical services for case detection and treatment, encouraged by national guidelines and funding, and on improved surveillance (chlamydia was made nationally reportable in 1995).

For the viral STDs, the continuing very high incidence of HSV-2 and of genital HPV infection in the general population indicates lack of effectiveness of current prevention efforts (Stage I in Table 89-4). Essentially no HPV-specific prevention is underway in the United States other than the basic health education, health promotion, and condom promotion fundamentally targeted to HIV and other STDs, supplemented by the use of cervical Pap smears to detect premalignant cytologic effects of HPV. Similarly, specific efforts to prevent HSV-2 are largely limited to prevention of perinatal HSV-2 transmission and limited use of antiviral drugs to suppress recurrent HSV infections.

For HIV infection, the U.S. prevention efforts could be assessed as Stage II as of early 1997; age-appropriate sex education programs are not widely implemented, efforts to decrease exposure have largely ignored those who are HIV-infected and have not included expansion of harm reduction programs, such as better access to treatment for users of illicit drugs or federal funding for needle exchange; efforts to decrease efficiency of transmission by condom promotion have been actively resisted by some conservative groups; and programs to strengthen early detection and treatment of other STDs (and thereby decrease efficiency of sexual transmission of HIV) have been minimally endorsed at a policy level and inadequately funded.[6] Populations with persisting high rates of STDs and heterosexual HIV transmission have been inadequately covered by these intervention activities.

Generally, as discussed by Wasserheit and Aral, specific advances in prevention first await identification of the organism and understanding of its epidemiology, advances in diagnosis, and characterization of its consequences.[10] These allow for application of the first two steps in the epidemiologic approach to prevention (see Fig. 89-1): accurate assessment of the burden of disease and consideration of the applicability of possible prevention activities and opportunities within the context of the STD transmission model (see Table 89-2). Even when disease syndromes have been recognized and clinical epidemiologic patterns of disease have emerged before identification of the causal pathogen (e.g., AIDS in gay men, nongonococcal urethritis in men after new sexual exposures, cervical dysplasia and cancer in women with multiple sex partners), the discovery of the causal pathogen(s) has led to improved understanding of clinical epidemiology and improving insights into prevention. Improved understanding of etiology, pathogenicity, detection of infection, and treatment all can potentially and progressively lead new prevention activities to be incorporated into the basic public health infrastructure and prevention systems already in place (Tables 89-3 and 89-4).

THE STD EPIDEMIOLOGIC TRANSITION

As a direct result of the relative balance between the stage of STD prevention and control efforts versus the force of infections for various STDs in different populations, a characteristic (but not necessarily universal) "STD epidemiologic transition" occurs in individual countries, regions, or districts, as measured by the approximate levels of control of bacterial genital ulcer diseases; gonorrhea and chlamydia; and the viral STDs. This STD epidemiologic transition is analogous to the well-known demographic transition that typically occurs as birth rates fall, life spans increase, and communicable diseases of young people give way to chronic diseases of older people.[9,9b] Generally, bacterial genital ulcer diseases are brought under control first, followed by gonorrhea, and then chlamydia, leaving the common viral STDs, such as HSV-2 and HPV infection, as the predominant STD. A crude system for classifying countries in their STDs prevention and control evolution could be identified, for example, by classifying a country (or region or district) according to its progress along this STD epidemiologic transition. Many developing countries of Africa and Asia would not yet be undergoing this transition, reflected in bacterial genital ulcer diseases, such as syphilis and chancroid and even LGV and donovanosis, remaining highly endemic. Latin America, the Caribbean, and parts of the southeastern United States would be in an early phase of this transition, with low rates of some of the more exotic bacterial genital ulcer diseases but persisting high rates of syphilis, gonorrhea, and chlamydial infection. However, large areas of the United States, particularly rural and relatively affluent areas, are more advanced, with no endemic syphilis and rapidly declining rates of gonorrhea.[50] Sweden and a small number of other northern European countries have progressed the furthest along this STD epidemiologic transition, having eliminated endemic transmission of all the curable STDs except chlamydia, which has been declining for several years. Assessment of the importance of different STDs, as well as the choice of different potential strategies and approaches, will be strongly influenced by the extent of progress along the STD epidemiologic transition in a particular jurisdiction and population.

SOCIETAL CONTEXT FOR STD/HIV PREVENTION APPROACHES

The theoretical discussions in the preceding sections were unconstrained by social and societal factors, the divergent structure of medical care in different countries and states, social norms, laws, economics, and details of organization of governments and of public and private organizations that play a role in determining the opportunities and constraints for HIV and STD prevention. Policy makers and communicable disease control practitioners do not have this option. The set of optimal or even the feasible approaches to HIV/STD prevention are highly dependent on societal factors that constitute opportunities or barriers. Among the most important are: population structures and diversity; social norms and values; and the health care system in which the prevention program is set.

Critical population structural issues include the age of the population, especially the presence of a high proportion of young adults in age groups where sexual activity and sex partner change rates are characteristically highest. Gender imbalance is a population-level rather than a personal characteristic associated with high STD prevalence rates, possibly associated with higher partner change rates and other more subtle changes in STD transmission dynamics. High levels of poverty and especially disparity in incomes, wealth, or access to care are associated with high STD rates. Ethnic diversity is a factor often associated with higher STD rates, though for reasons that may be reducible to other, more truly causative factors. However, ethnic diversity, especially when accompanied and amplified by sharply unequal socioeconomic status, certainly complicates the possible prevention approach. Patient-provider interactions may be complicated in clinical settings, and targeting of prevention efforts to high-risk persons becomes substantially more complex and subject to interpretation as discriminatory when ethnic differentials exist in disease rates. An intangible, rarely mentioned, but often ultimately determining factor is the degree of social cohesiveness, trust, and distrust in a society in general, as well as between various subpopulations and public health authorities in particular. Mandatory partner notification for all STDs and mandatory behavior change for persons recognized to have transmitted HIV infection to others may be a more feasible strategy in Sweden, with its homogeneous population, universal access to health care, and extensive social welfare system than in the United States, where none of these properties characterize the sociologic situation.[51]

Social norms and values are another critical determinant of STD rates as well as a contextual factor strongly influencing the potential prevention approach. Key domains of social norms applicable to HIV and STD prevention include: normative attitudes and beliefs concerning sexual behavior, condoms and their dissemination, substance use, STDs and persons who acquire STDs, and so on. Social norms may vary substantially between populations in different settings: In one study, homosexual men in the United States were more likely to use condoms (decreasing efficiency of transmission) than a comparable cohort in Denmark, but the Danish homosexual men were more likely to inform each other of their HIV serostatus and to form seroconcordant partnerships (decreasing exposure).[52] Americans may have a peculiar limitation in being able to discuss sexual matters frankly and openly, including STDs, and this normative constraint may be most pronounced in the southeastern part of the United States with the highest rates of STDs.[53] Understanding and designing interventions according to prevailing patterns of such norms among communities at risk can have a major impact on the ultimate effectiveness of the program.

HIV/STD prevention approaches must obviously be designed differently to fit into the local system(s) of medical services. At one extreme, some countries in sub-Saharan Africa have limited ability to provide even the most basic preventive health services, and the provision of high-quality curative care for treatable, symptomatic STDs is erratic and a function of the patient's financial means and sophistication in seeking care. At the other extreme, in Scandinavian countries, comprehensive systems of medical care are accessible to all persons, including attractive STD clinics, with few financial or social barriers to care. In between are countries like the United States, Brazil, and South Africa, with highly sophisticated care available to subsets of the population but with many persons moderately to severely underserved. In the case of Brazil, a legislative commitment to universal access to comprehensive services is not backed by sufficient resources to make such a commitment a reality; in such a situation, partial solutions such as Brazil's efforts to establish Integrated Assistance to Women's Health (PAISM), including family planning, antenatal and obstetric care, and gynecologic cancer screening, may provide an appropriate intermediate-term platform for incorporating STD prevention activities into relevant clinical service delivery structures within the health care system.[54]

MATCHING THE PREVENTION APPROACH TO THE CURRENT PREVENTION OPPORTUNITIES

The determinants of transmission of STDs/HIVs reflected in the transmission model in the preceding underpin our theoretical approach. Nonetheless, our ability is limited to sufficiently defined, deterministic mathematical models and parameters to characterize a "local" (including state or national) situation to permit us to reliably predict the marginal impact on prevention of STDs/HIVs likely to result from a marginal change in an STD/HIV prevention strategy. In such a setting, it may be useful to consider a single qualitative "prevention impact model" constructed from parameters that may be more accessible. This prevention impact model is very similar to the "impact fraction" developed by Morgenstern and others to estimate the potential impact of a prevention program on the incidence of certain noninfectious disease conditions in a population, but with the intent to adapt that concept to the setting of communicable diseases.[55] Certain of these parameters might be further exploitable as potential indicators to evaluate the successful implementation of a new preventive intervention activity:

$$\text{Prevention impact} = \begin{array}{c}\text{Efficacy of the proposed intervention}\\ \text{in the specific target population}\end{array} \times \begin{array}{c}\text{Proportional contribution to the outcome}\\ \text{in question of the specific target population}\end{array} \times \begin{array}{c}\text{Achieved } \textit{effective coverage} \text{ of the}\\ \text{intervention in the target population}\end{array}$$

This can be more simply but less completely stated as:

$$\text{Prevention impact} = \text{Efficacy} \times \begin{array}{c}\text{Transmission contribution}\\ \text{of targeted population}\end{array} \times \begin{array}{c}\text{Coverage of}\\ \text{targeted population}\end{array}$$

In this qualitative model, the population-specific efficacy of a proposed innovation (e.g., enhanced HIV counseling and testing among persons at high risk in STD clinics or screening for chlamydia in a managed care setting) either is known to be efficacious or may have been subjected to careful scientific research, or can be estimated from mathematical models.[27,56–58]

Estimating the specific contribution of the population being addressed in the intervention to the outcome in the general population is often the most difficult element. This latter element is the aspect that most clearly distinguishes the "impact" model proposed in the preceding, intended to represent the special situations and dynamics of infectious diseases, from better known chronic disease models.[59] The "transmission contribution" in the short form of the impact model is highly volatile and dependent on characteristics of the subpopulation being addressed, the characteristics of other subpopulations within the society, the nature and extent of interactions between those populations, and the nature and extent of the current control and prevention programs in place in the relevant jurisdiction at a particular point in time. One recent review summarized this multidimensional interface as the "dynamic typology" of STDs, defined by transmission dynamics and control program elements.[10] For example, if a behavioral intervention increased condom use by 50 percent or even 100 percent among clients of sex workers, what would be the impact on total HIV transmission in the United States? How much do sex workers actually contribute to syphilis transmission in the United States in the late 1990s? To gonorrhea? To HIV infection? What then would be the total population-level impact of a program to register sex workers, require regular screening for HIV and other STDs, and insist on and assure consistent condom use by their clients, as has been undertaken in the United States only in the state of Nevada? Another classic example of the importance of "transmission contribution" of the target population concerns partner notification. In general, it is easier to notify and treat regular partners exposed to a person with an STD (e.g., the spouse of a man with gonorrhea) than to notify and treat the suspected source contact who gave the man the gonorrhea. Although the transmission contribution of the source contact should be much greater than that of the exposed partner, little effort is currently made to focus partner notification on suspected source contacts or to differentiate and privatize the type of partners who are reached based on their potential for contributing to ongoing transmission in the community.

The contribution of chlamydia screening in an HMO to prevention of PID in the screened population has recently been quantified.[27] However, the quantitative effect of a more widespread screening effort to a different outcome, such as lowered prevalence or incidence of chlamydial infections within a population for chlamydia transmission, has not been estimated. Moreover, given the current level of screening for chlamydia in the United States, what would be the marginal impact of expanding screening among men versus women? Use of this heuristic model for considering the potential impact of different intervention strategies prompts consideration of key parameters at the interface between transmission dynamics of the STD and our disease prevention efforts.

The effective *coverage* of a prevention activity is an important parameter that deserves more frequent consideration. Partner notification for syphilis, given the epidemiologic parameters of that disease, should theoretically have very high efficacy in eliminating syphilis from populations.[60] However, in recent years, the effective coverage of partner notification has been low, and the sociologic and contextual setting in which syphilis is transmitted may have shifted in a way that makes it unlikely that traditional partner notification for syphilis can reach sufficient coverage in the individuals who most contribute to ongoing transmission to achieve its potential impact.[61,62] Other, community-oriented approaches proposed for syphilis prevention may plausibly achieve higher coverage in the specific subpopulations that are critical to sustaining ongoing transmission, but these new approaches need to be evaluated for empirical efficacy as well as their theoretical advantages.[63]

This "prevention impact" model applies to specific interventions being considered, but in reality it needs to be considered in the context of all ongoing prevention activities, other interventions, and the status of the critical prevention systems, yielding an assessment of the *marginal* impact of any proposed new effort (see Table 89-4). For example, if a substantial information, education, and communication (IEC) campaign to promote condom use for HIV prevention is underway in a community, supplementary new interventions against gonorrhea that focus on condom promotion may add relatively little to the aggregate impact across gonorrhea and HIV prevention, whereas interventions promoting more timely health care–seeking behavior for gonorrhea might have a substantial, additional impact on both diseases, attacking duration of infectivity (D) for gonorrhea and efficiency of transmission (β) for HIV.[64]

CRITERIA FOR ASSESSING POTENTIAL PREVENTION ACTIVITY

The preceding discussion suggests a number of criteria that might be used to assess proposed new public health activities or approaches (Table 89-5).

1. The importance of a disease and its sequelae, as perceived by the public, public health and medical experts, and health economists, set the context for consideration of its rank in disease prevention priorities.
2. The potential impact of proposed new activities or redesign of current activities on the epidemiology of transmission and persistence of the infection at the population level, as reflected in the prevention impact model, will help separate higher from lower priority activities. This type of disease transmission analysis has not necessarily been explicitly or effectively incorporated into prevention program components in the past, for example, in prioritization of partner notification activities. Good empirical data on transmission patterns, linked to mathematical modeling of prevention impact, would support a continuous, critical review of resource allocation to different disease prevention activities. A rethinking of epidemiologic analysis appropriate to communicable disease transmission is needed in this regard.[65]
3. Empirical or projected cost-effectiveness are essential criteria for decision-making. Good data on cost linked to effectiveness or yield have seldom been collected for many prevention program elements, but these will be needed to guide prevention efforts. This will not be a one-time effort, since both cost and yield for many or most interventions are likely to change, perhaps dramatically, as the epidemiology and sociology of the STD evolve.

Table 89-5. Potential Criteria for Assessing A Proposed STD/HIV Prevention Approach or Strategy

- Importance of the targeted condition
- Potential impact of a proposed new strategy on the epidemiology of transmission and persistence of the infection at the population level
- Cost and cost-effectiveness
- Logistical feasibility
- Consonance with culture and politics of the broader society as well as with the culture of specific organizations; acceptability to affected communities, as well as to sponsoring and implementing agencies
- Synergy, interdependence, or conflict with activities to address other health or social problems (such as teen pregnancy or infant mortality); capacity or likelihood to stimulate or to enhance community support and policymaker support for STD/HIV prevention programs rather than elicit a negative reaction and lead to decreased support

4. The logistical feasibility of an approach or strategy within the health care and public health infrastructure constitutes a fundamental criterion of successful implementation.
5. Explicitly evaluating the acceptability of new prevention activities to communities affected by HIV or STDs has largely been introduced into the field in response to the HIV epidemic. Baseline formative research combined with active, bona fide participation in and contribution to the prevention effort by community representatives may create good will needed to implement prevention activities in those communities, while technically improving the interventions. Assessment of community response to and participation in new prevention strategies is increasingly being attempted in the United States, through approaches such as HIV Prevention Community Planning and through new approaches to syphilis control.[35,36]
6. The degree of synergy, alignment, or potential conflict with activities to address other public health or social problems will influence public support and public health consensus for ongoing HIV and STD prevention; this may be a relatively intangible but important element of new strategies and approaches.

Recognition and articulation of the relationship between STD/HIV prevention and diverse health goals such as women's health, infant health, minority health, and adolescent health including prevention of teen pregnancy, has been increasingly established in recent years.[44,66–69] Linkage of STD programs to family planning in a unified approach to women's reproductive health was a critical factor that finally led to a federal chlamydia control effort in the early 1990s.[28] The first new federal funding in several decades specifically for syphilis prevention in 1998 in the United States was promoted syphilis prevention as an explicit goal for minority health and was incorporated into a set of activities explicitly designed to reduce racial disparities in health outcomes, since such disparities have been so severe for syphilis in the United States.[70] Attention to these alignment issues and to the need to generate a broad base of support and platform for advocacy may substantially affect the selection of the basic activities of prevention, if some of these stimulate and reinforce community support for the prevention efforts more than other alternative strategies or activities (see Table 89-2). This influence of political factors on program content may often be construed by program staff as "political" interference in their efficient pursuit of disease prevention unless the long-term, strategic perspective is clearly articulated to all.

PUBLIC HEALTH APPROACHES TO DIFFERENT STDs

It is impossible to consider priorities for prevention of different STDs separately from the specific strategies and intervention activities available for the individual STDs, because a high feasibility and cost-effectiveness of available strategies for a particular STD may elevate its priority within a comprehensive prevention program even though it does not cause as much overall morbidity as another condition, if that second condition is less preventable or the cost-benefit ratio for its available strategy is worse or if a special issue of time-urgency exists, such as a disease elimination or eradication effort.

The conceptual considerations in the preceding sections may be clarified by considering the implications for prevention strategies and approaches toward specific STDs. The characteristics of STDs and of the corresponding prevention tools that define the prevention priority and approach are listed in Table 89-6 and discussed in the following.

Table 89-6. Characteristics of Specific STDs and of the Corresponding Prevention Tools That Define the Prevention Priority

Epidemiologic Characteristics
- Overall incidence, prevalence, and public health impact
- Homogeneous vs. focal distribution of infections and of key sequelae

Clinical Characteristics
- Symptomatic vs. asymptomatic infection
- Factors influencing susceptibility to infection
  - Age-specific susceptibility
  - Cofactors (e.g., other infections, douching, contraceptives)
- Natural history of infectivity
- Natural history of important sequelae

Status of Prevention Tools and Technologies
- Availability of prompt, accurate diagnostic tests
- Availability of inexpensive, preferably single-dose treatment
- Technologies for reducing efficiency of transmission (including vaccines, condoms, microbicides)
- Recognition of specific risk or protective sexual or other behaviors (e.g., needle-sharing) *and* proven interventions to changing those behaviors
- Availability of surveillance data or other information to adequately characterize the scope of the problem and to develop data-based prevention objectives

CHARACTERISTICS OF DIFFERENT STDs THAT INFLUENCE PREVENTION PRIORITIES AND APPROACHES

In addition to the importance of overall public health impact, the distribution of an STD by geographic, demographic, or risk-group characterization may determine prevention strategies and intervention activities. Homogeneously distributed, broadly prevalent diseases such as *C. trachomatis* infections may be addressed most cost-effectively through screening and treatment in primary care settings that reach very broad segments of the at-risk population. In most industrialized countries, chlamydia prevalence is determined more by age and intensity of screening efforts than by geography, race, socioeconomic status, or individual risk behaviors, such as multiple sex partners or substance abuse. Conversely, for diseases in Stage III or IV of prevention and control, such as syphilis in the United States, characterized by a limited, highly focal distribution, any large-scale screening effort not highly targeted to the few high-risk areas is not likely to be very cost-effective.[71] Targeted intervention efforts highly focused in areas where endemic transmission persists, or in areas with patterns of risk factors that would likely support dissemination whenever syphilis is inevitably reintroduced, are likely to be much more cost-effective. Where an STD has become quite rare and disease-specific prevention resources are limited (e.g., screening, treatment, partner notification), a decision is needed about whether to pursue an aggressive disease elimination strategy on the one hand or to shift such resources toward other, more prevalent infections on the other hand. In effect this would allow the currently lower-prevalence condition to rise somewhat to a higher steady-state level of prevalence and incidence.[72] Coordination is important in this regard. One state or county that elects to pursue a syphilis elimination strategy is unlikely to be successful if its neighboring jurisdictions decide to shift resources from syphilis control to chlamydia screening. Since every commitment of resources to one or more strategies against a particular disease represents an opportunity lost to do something else with those resources, implicit decisions of this type are made constantly, even if, as is usually the case, such prioritizations and trade-offs are not explicitly made or even explicitly considered.

Clinical characteristics of infection and the status of the biomedical tools available for diagnosis and treatment may determine the overall prevention approach. For example, approaches to PID and associated infertility have been modified by better appreciation for the importance of atypical or asymptomatic PID, which shifted the emphasis of prevention toward detecting and preventing asymptomatic cervical infections with gonorrhea and especially chlamydia, rather than relying solely on detection and timely treatment of early PID.[4,73] Symptoms associated with a particular infection may vary by gender or other population characteristics. For example, gonorrhea is generally symptomatic in men but largely asymptomatic in women. Therefore, improved health-seeking behavior in response to symptoms in men, plus effective notification of partners of symptomatic men may improve detection and treatment of gonorrhea; screening for asymptomatic infection in women may also have an important role. Because chlamydial infection is often asymptomatic in both genders, screening and partner notification of both genders may be important. Pregnant women symptomatic for genital herpes infection have a higher risk for perinatal herpes infection of their infants, but most serious perinatal HSV infections occur in infants delivered from women who do not report genital symptoms or even a past history of recognized genital herpes.[74] The cost-benefit of an intervention could be highest when targeting women with symptomatic herpes in the third trimester, but such an intervention would not prevent most perinatal herpes; on the other hand, the requirements for an intervention targeting all asymptomatically infected women are very large, making a comprehensive prevention strategy very costly for unit impact.

The relationship between the clinical characteristics of infection and the capacity and responsiveness of the health care system to properly diagnose and manage infection can be represented by a pyramid adapted from Waller and Piot to characterize the health service response to infection with *Mycobcterium tuberculosis* (see Fig. 48-2). This figure shows not only the potential reasons why infected persons may not be cured, but also the various levels at which interventions could be targeted to ensure that all infected persons are cured. All of the characteristics of different STDs and of the readiness of the available prevention tools that influence the design of the prevention approach can be reflected in a similar diagram.

The shape of this inverted pyramid differs dramatically for different STDs, reflecting the interaction of the natural history of infection and disease with the capacity of the health education, clinical, diagnostic, and treatment services that ensure prevention of exposure, prevention of transmission, detection, and management of the specific STD. For example, chancroid and gonorrhea in men: (1) are thought to be nearly always symptomatic; (2) generate painful symptoms likely to consistently drive health care–seeking behavior; (3) yield relatively characteristic and distinctive clinical syndromes; (4) have available diagnostic tests (although capacity for chancroid diagnosis by culture is generally very limited in the United States); and (5) have definitive therapies available; hence, it may be likely that the natural history/health services pyramids for chancroid and gonorrhea in men are fairly steep (Fig. 89-3). By contrast, chlamydial infection in women: (1) is often asymptomatic or underrecognized; (2) seldom results in health care seeking; and (3) diagnostics have not been widely available until recently. Although treatment is effective, subclinical infection in untreated sex partners presents a high risk of reinfection. These dramatic differences in the natural history and health services pyramids for chancroid or gonorrhea in men on the one hand, and chlamydial infection in women on the other, contribute to the different prevention approaches to these STDs, such as the relatively greater importance of screening for chlamydial infection in women versus the importance of providing prompt access to diagnostic testing and treatment for genital ulcer disease and for gonorrhea in men.

Experience in concerted public health control and prevention efforts for sexually transmitted viral STDs for which vaccines are not available has been much more limited than for the treatable bacterial infections and is dominated by the response to the HIV epidemic, for which the full range of potential public health strategies and activities has not been completely explored in the United States, both because of human rights concerns and because of opposition to harm-reduction programs.[75] This is less properly construed as "interference" by political factors than as a product of distrust of some components of public health from both ends of the political spectrum, requiring not only skills in communication and negotiation, but a clear common understanding of the prevention strategies, activities, and systems needed, as well as a transparent process of defining prevention priorities and cost-benefits. Such processes are greatly facilitated by collaboration with affected communities and with institutions that are in a position to either facilitate or block any strategy, approach, or intervention developed without their explicit or implicit input.

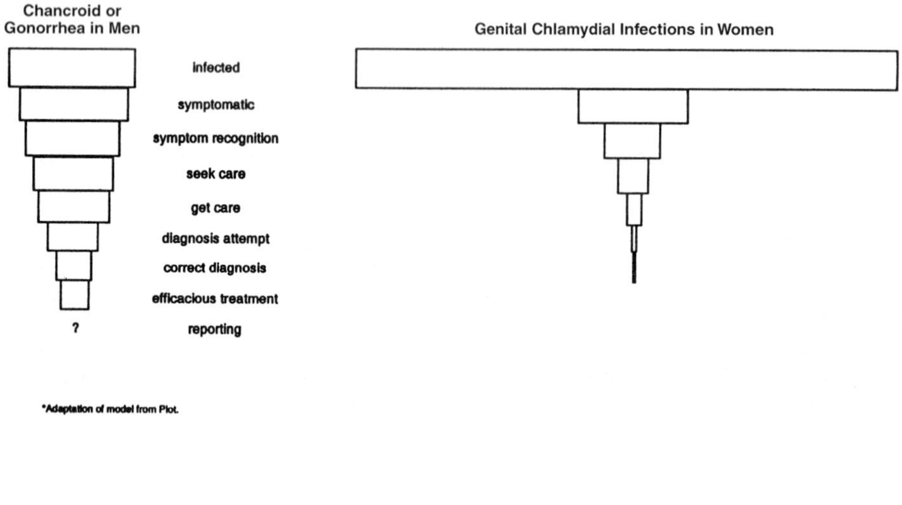

Fig. 89-3. Examples of diversity in the awareness, health care–seeking behavior, and detection of STDs in a community. Chancroid and gonorrhea in men and chlamydial infections in women.

EFFECTIVENESS AND COST OF PREVENTION STRATEGIES, ACTIVITIES, AND TOOLS

The strategies and activities for prevention of different STDs cannot be considered independently of the efficacy, cost, and feasibility for delivery of the available prevention interventions. The performance, cost, and convenience of diagnostic tests strongly influences feasibility of a variety of prevention activities. Implementation of a national gonorrhea control program in the United States in the 1970s, HIV counseling and testing in the 1980s, and a national chlamydia prevention program in the 1990s each followed the development and commercialization of relatively inexpensive, good quality, diagnostic tests suitable for large-scale screening programs. With increasing availability of testing for HPV infection, interest in HPV prevention is also increasing. By contrast, type-specific serologic tests for HSV-2 infection were still not available commercially in the United States as of early 1998, handicapping any concerted public health initiative to prevent genital herpes infections. There is a paucity of careful efficacy evaluation of behavioral interventions despite their acknowledged importance, especially for HIV infection and other viral STDs.[76]

The efficacy, simplicity, and cost of treatment also strongly influence the choice of prevention activities. This is most starkly represented by the distinction between the suppressible but incurable viral infections and the curable bacterial infections and trichomoniasis. Mandatory prenatal screening for syphilis has gone unchallenged for decades, whereas promotion of even voluntary screening for HIV infection in pregnant women remains surprisingly controversial in the United States; the potential for curative treatment for syphilis defines substantially the difference in societal response to this particular prevention activity. "Part-way technologies," such as suppressive therapy for genital herpes infections and AZT for reduction of perinatal, occupational, or conceivably, sexual transmission of HIV, are increasingly used.[22–25] The plausibility that aggressive early therapy for HIV infection might improve long-term outcomes may finally align the personal health and public health interests in early detection and treatment. If early and aggressive chemotherapy also lowers transmissibility of infection, as well as progression of disease, the population-level or public health impact of the current movement toward earlier, more aggressive antiretroviral therapy might be multiplied.[75] Although HIV vaccine research has not yet yielded grounds to expect a practical prevention tool within 5 to 10 years, that might be reversed with a single new breakthrough in knowledge. Other advances in basic science could provide new biomedical and other tools that rapidly change the prevention dynamic.[10]

Other prevention technologies and approaches differ in their relevance to different STDs. Among STDs, vaccination is currently available only for hepatitis B and hepatitis A, [a pathogen increasingly associated in the United States. with sex-related outbreaks among men who have sex with men (MSMs)]. Although a recent trial of a subunit glycoprotein HSV-2 vaccine showed no efficacy in preventing acquisition of infection, other HSV-2 vaccines are still under evaluation, trials of HPV vaccines are now underway, and naked-DNA vaccine technology is now being applied in efforts to develop vaccines against several STD pathogens. On the other hand, although reduction in rates of sex partner change is theoretically applicable to prevention of all STDs, a substantial number of women with syphilis in the United States and the majority of women with HIV infection in Rwanda or Thailand report only one long-term, stable sex partner, so that alternative interventions are clearly needed for these risk groups.[77] Condoms are highly effective for preventing most STDs, particularly those STDs that infect the urethra and endocervix, but have unproven efficacy for prevention of HSV-2 and HPV infection. Spermicides such as nonoxynol-9 also may have a heterogeneous effect, being more effective for agents for which the cervix is the portal of entry or for pathogens most susceptible to surfactants than for other pathogens (see Chap. 78). Modification in specific sexual practices, such as a shift among homosexual men away from unprotected anal intercourse, may have been an important factor contributing to declining HIV and HBV incidence among such men in the United States. Ironically, such positive behavior change may contribute to unmasking inherently less risky behavior that nevertheless becomes more salient in contributing to disease transmission when more risky behaviors are reduced, such as the increasing prominence of oral sex in HIV transmission among MSMs in areas where unprotected anal sex has declined substantially.[78]

FUTURE PROGRESS IN DEVELOPMENT OF PREVENTION PROGRAM STRATEGIES AND APPROACHES

The development and growing acceptance of the basic STD transmission model of Anderson and May constituted a conceptual breakthrough, establishing a theoretical basis that links many different determinants of HIV and STD incidence and prevalence in a society. This chapter has outlined the ways in which this model helps to define: (1) the broad strategies for reducing transmission; (2) the intervention activities useful in pursuing these strategies; (3) the public health systems needed to implement these interventions; and (4) the importance of targeting interventions to achieve effectiveness, while neglecting no population at high risk for acquiring or transmitting infection. A system is described for staging the level of prevention efforts deployed against different STDs. This staging system then provides objective criteria for comparing the prevention efforts mounted by different national, regional, or local programs and for evaluating whether the type of prevention efforts adopted and the level of effort expended on prevention is sufficient to overcome the force of infection for the disease and populations concerned. Outcomes will be reflected in the resulting trends in incidence and prevalence of specific infections and their sequelae and in progress along an "STD epidemiologic transition." During this transition, each of the more preventable STDs should sequentially come under control, bacterial STDs may be eliminated from an increasing range of jurisdictions, and strategies developed and implemented to limit transmission of the pathogens most challenging for prevention, such as HSV-2 and HPV.

References

1 Institute of Medicine: *The Future of Public Health.* Washington, DC, National Academy Press; 1988.
2 Parran T: *Shadow on the Land.* New York, Reynal and Hitchcock; 1937.
3 Washington AE et al: *Chlamydia trachomatis* infections in the United States. What are they costing us? *JAMA* 257:2070–2072, 1987.
4 Centers for Disease Control and Prevention: Recommendations for the prevention and management of *Chlamydia trachomatis* infections, 1993. *MMWR* 42:1–39, 1993.
5 Holtgrave DR, Pinkerton SD: Updates of cost of illness and quality of life estimates for use in economic evaluations of HIV prevention programs. *J Acquir Immun Defic Syndr Hum Retrovir* 16:54–62, 1997.
6 Institute of Medicine: *The Hidden Epidemic. Confronting Sexually Transmitted Diseases.* Washington, DC, National Academy Press, 1997, pp. 1–54.
7 Centers for Disease Control and Prevention: Recommendations of the International Task Force for Disease Eradication. *MMWR* 42:1–38, 1993.

8 Over M, Piot P: HIV infection and sexually transmitted diseases, in *Disease Control Priorities in Developing Countries*, DT Jamison et al (eds). New York, Oxford University Press, 1993, pp. 455–527.

9 Mosley WH et al: The health transition: implications for health policy in developing countries, in *Disease Control Priorities in Developing Countries*, DT Jamison et al (eds). New York, Oxford University Press, 1993, pp. 673–699.

9b Holmes KK, Aral SO: Behavioral interventions in developing countries. In: Wasserheit JN, Aral SO, Holmes KK, Hitchcock PJ (eds). Research issues in human behavior and sexually transmitted diseases in the AIDS era. American Society for Microbiology, Washington DC, 1991.

10 Wasserheit JN, Aral SO: The dynamic topology of sexually transmitted disease epidemics: implications for prevention strategies. *J Infect Dis* 174:S201-S213, 1996.

11 Hillis S et al: New opportunities for chlamydia prevention: applications of science to public health practice. *Sex Transm Dis* 22:197–202, 1995.

12 Berwick DM: Developing and testing changes in delivery of care. *Ann Intern Med* 128:651–6, 1998.

13 U.S. Department of Health and Human Services, Public Health Service: *Healthy People 2000: Midcourse Review and 1995 Revisions.* Washington, DC, 1995.

14 National Association of County Health Officials: APEX-PH: Assessment protocol for excellence in public health. Washington, DC, 1991.

15 Anderson RM, May RM: Epidemiological parameters of HIV transmission. *Nature* 333:514–519, 1988.

16 Hethcote HW, Yorke JA: *Gonorrhea Transmission Dynamics and Control.* New York, Springer-Verlag, 1984.

17 Anderson RM, May RM: *Infectious Diseases of Humans. Dynamics and Control.* Oxford, Oxford University Press; 1992.

18 Aral SO et al: Overview: individual and population approaches to the epidemiology and prevention of sexually transmitted diseases and human immunodeficiency virus infection. *J Infect Dis* 174:S127-S133, 1996.

19 Kelly JA et al: Community AIDS/HIV risk reduction: The effects of endorsements by popular people in three cities. *Am J Public Health* 82:1483–1489, 1992.

20 Kirby D et al: School-based programs to reduce sexual risk behaviors: A review of effectiveness. *Public Health Reports* 109:339–359, 1994.

21 Grosskurth H et al: Impact of improved treatment of sexually transmitted diseases on HIV infection in rural Tanzania: Randomised controlled trial. *Lancet* 346:530–536, 1995.

22 Connor EM et al: Reduction of maternal-infant transmission of human immunodeficiency virus type 1 with zidovudine treatment. *N Engl J Med* 331:1173–1180, 1994.

23 Katz MH, Gerberding JL: Postexposure treatment of people exposed to the human immunodeficiency virus through sexual contact or injection-drug use. *N Engl J Med* 336:1097–1100, 1997.

24 Wald A et al: Suppression of subclinical shedding of herpes simplex virus type 2 with acyclovir. *Ann Intern Med* 124:8–15, 1996.

25 Cardo DM et al: A case-control study of HIV seroconversion in health care workers after percutaneous exposure. *N Engl J Med* 337: 1485–1490, 1997.

26 Kamb ML et al: Efficacy of risk-reduction counseling to prevent human immunodeficiency virus and sexually transmitted diseases: a randomized controlled trial. Project RESPECT Study Group. *JAMA* 280: 1161–1167, 1998.

27 Scholes D et al: Prevention of pelvic inflammatory disease by screening for cervical chlamydial infection. *N Engl J Med* 334:1362–1366, 1996.

28 Britton TF et al: STDs and family planning clinics: A regional program for chlamydia control that works. *Am J Gynecol Health* 6:24–31, 1992.

29 Des Jarlais DC et al: HIV incidence among injecting drug users in New York City syringe-exchange programmes. *Lancet* 348:987–991, 1996.

30 Fishbein M: Editorial: Great expectations, or do we ask too much from community-level interventions? *Am J Public Health* 86:1075–1076, 1996.

31 Farr G et al: Use of spermicide and impact of prophylactic condom use among sex workers in Santa Fe de Bogota, Colombia. *Sex Transm Dis* 23:206–212, 1996.

32 Anonymous: Health care in America. Your money or your life: Patients or profits? *The Economist* 15:23–26, 1998.

33 Centers for Disease Control and Prevention: 1998 guidelines for treatment of sexually transmitted diseases. *MMWR* 47(no. RR-1), 1–116, 1998.

34 Centers for Disease Control and Prevention: USPHS/IDSA guidelines for the prevention of opportunistic infections in persons infected with human immunodeficiency virus: a summary. *MMWR* 44(no. RR-08): 1–34, 1995.

35 Valdiserri RO et al: Community planning: A national strategy to improve HIV prevention programs. *J Community Health* 20:87–100, 1995.

36 Centers for Disease Control and Prevention: Innovations in syphilis prevention in the United States: Reconsidering the epidemiology and involving communities (Announcement 523). *Fed Reg* 60:19943, 1995.

37 Over M, Piot P: Human immunodeficiency virus infection and other sexually transmitted diseases in developing countries: Public health importance and priorities for resource allocation. *J Infect Dis* 174: S162-S175, 1996.

37a World Bank Policy Research Report: Confronting AIDS: Public priorities in a global epidemic. Oxford, Oxford University Press, 1997.

38 Centers for Disease Control and Prevention: Community-level prevention of human immunodeficiency virus infection among high-risk populations; the AIDS Community Demonstration Projects. *MMWR* 45 (no. RR-06):1–24, 1996.

39 Laga M et al: Condom promotion, sexually transmitted diseases treatment, and declining incidence of HIV-1 infection in female Zairian sex workers. *Lancet* 344:246–248, 1994.

40 Plummer FA et al: The importance of core groups in the epidemiology and control of HIV-1 infection. *AIDS* 5:S169-S176, 1991.

41 Albert AE et al: Condom use among female commercial sex workers in Nevada's legal brothels. *Am J Public Health* 85:1514–1520, 1995.

42 Engelgau MM et al: Control of epidemic early syphilis: The results of an intervention campaign using social networks. *Sex Transm Dis* 22:203–209, 1995.

43 Brunham RC, Plummer FA: A general model of sexually transmitted disease epidemiology and its implications for control. *Med Clin North Am* 74:1339–1352, 1990.

44 Centers for Disease Control and Prevention: Pregnancy, sexually transmitted diseases, and related risk behaviors among U.S. adolescents. Adolescent Health: State of the Nation monograph series, no. 2, CDC publication no. 099–4630. Atlanta, 1994.

45 Beck-Sague CM et al: Laboratory diagnosis of sexually transmitted diseases in facilities within the United States. *Sex Transm Dis* 23: 342–349, 1996.

46 Centers for Disease Control and Prevention: Chancroid in the United States, 1981–1990: Evidence for underreporting of cases. *MMWR* 41:57–61, 1992.

47 Centers for Disease Control and Prevention: Chancroid detected by polymerase chain reaction— Jackson, Mississippi, 1994–1995. *MMWR* 44:567–574, 1995.

48 Mertz KJ et al: An outbreak of chancroid in Mississippi: Implications for HIV prevention. *Infect Dis* 178:1060–1066, 1998.

49 Cohen MS et al: Successful eradication of sexually transmitted diseases in the People's Republic of China: Implications for the 21st century. *J Infect Dis* 174:S223-S229, 1996.

50 Division of STD Prevention: Sexually Transmitted Diseases Surveillance, 1996. U.S. Department of Health and Human Services, Atlanta: Centers for Disease Control and Prevention, Sept. 1997.

51 Cronberg S: The rise and fall of sexually transmitted diseases in Sweden. *Genitourin Med* 69:184–186, 1993.

52 Wiktor SZ et al: Effect of knowledge of human immunodeficiency

virus infection status on sexual activity among homosexual men. *AIDS* 3:62–68, 1990.

52a Michael RT et al: Private sexual behavior, public opinion, and public health policy related to sexually transmitted diseases. *Am J Public Health* 88:749–754, 1998.

53 Centers for Disease Control and Prevention: Assessment of STD prevention program responses to the early syphilis epidemic in the southern United States (BSRC 700/96/003), 1996.

54 Faundes A, Tanaka AC: Reproductive tract infections in Brazil: solutions in a difficult economic climate, in *Reproductive Tract Infections: Global Impact and Priorities for Women's Reproductive Health*. A Germain et al (eds). New York, Plenum, 1992, pp. 253–273.

55 Morgenstern H, Bursic ES: A method for using epidemiologic data to estimate the potential impact of an intervention on the health status of a target population. *J Community Health* 7:292–309, 1982.

56 Kamb ML et al: Efficacy of risk-reduction counseling to prevent human immunodeficiency virus and sexually transmitted diseases: a randomized controlled trial. Project RESPECT Study Group. *JAMA* 280: 1161–1167, 1998.

57 Kamb ML et al: Quality assurance of HIV prevention counseling in a multi-center randomized controlled trial. *Public Health Rep* 111: 99–107, 1996.

58 Boily M, Brunham RC: The impact of HIV and other STDs on human populations. Are predictions possible? *Infect Dis Clin North Am* 7: 771–792, 1993.

59 Teutsch SM: A framework for assessing the effectiveness of disease and injury prevention. *MMWR* 41:1–12, 1997.

60 Cates W et al: Syphilis control: The historical context and epidemiologic basis for interrupting sexual transmission of *Treponema pallidum*. *Sex Transm Dis* 23:68–75, 1996.

61 Andrus JK et al: Partner notification: Can it control epidemic syphilis? *Ann Intern Med* 112:539–543, 1990.

62 Oxman GL, Doyle L: A comparison of the case-finding effectiveness and average costs of screening and partner notification. *Sex Transm Dis* 23:51–57, 1996.

63 St. Louis ME et al: Untangling the persistence of syphilis in the South. *Sex Transm Dis* 23:1–4, 1996.

64 Cohen MS et al: Reduction of concentration of HIV-1 in semen after treatment of urethritis: Implications for prevention of sexual transmission of HIV-1. *Lancet* 349:1868–1873, 1997.

65 Koopman JS: Comment: Emerging objectives and methods in epidemiology. *Am J Public Health* 86:630–632, 1996.

66 Aral SO, Wasserheit JN: Interactions among HIV, other sexually transmitted diseases, socioeconomic status, and poverty in women, in *Women at Risk: Issues in the Primary Prevention of AIDS*. A O'Leary, LS Jemmott (eds). New York: Plenum, 1995 pp. 13–41.

67 Goldenberg RL et al: Sexually transmitted diseases and adverse outcomes of pregnancy, in *Clinics in Perinatology*. BJ Stoll, LE Weisman (eds). Philadelphia, PA, Saunders, 1997, pp. 23–41.

68 Centers for Disease Control and Prevention: Update: AIDS among women—United States, 1994. *MMWR* 44:81–84, 1995.

69 Hauth JC et al: Reduced incidence of preterm delivery with metronidazole and erythromycin in women with bacterial vaginosis. *N Engl J Med* 333:1732–1736, 1995.

70 St. Louis ME: Strategies for syphilis prevention in the 1990s. *Sex Transm Dis* 23:58–67, 1996.

71 Nakashima AK et al: Epidemiology of syphilis in the United States, 1941–1993. *Sex Transm Dis* 23:16–23, 1996.

72 Yekutiel P: Lessons from the big eradication campaigns. *World Health Forum* 1:465–490, 1981.

73 Cates W et al: Atypical pelvic inflammatory disease: Can we identify clinical predictors? *Am J Obstet Gynecol* 169:341–346, 1993.

74 Brown ZA et al: The acquisition of herpes simplex virus during pregnancy. *N Engl J Med* 337:509–515, 1997.

75 Francis DP: Every person infected with HIV-1 should be in a lifelong early intervention program. *Sex Transm Dis* 23:351–352, 1996.

76 Oakley A et al: Sexual health education interventions for young people: A methodological review. *Br Med J* 310:158–162, 1995.

77 Allen S et al: Confidential HIV testing and condom promotion in Africa. Impact on HIV and gonorrhea rates. *JAMA* 268:3338–3343, 1992.

78 Schacker T et al: Clinical and epidemiologic features of primary HIV infection. *Ann Intern Med* 125:257–264, 1996.

Chapter 90

Assessment of STD/HIV prevention programs in the United States: national, local, and community perspectives

Judith N. Wasserheit
Ronald O. Valdiserri
Robert W. Wood

Effective prevention efforts for sexually transmitted diseases (STDs), including human immunodeficiency virus (HIV) infection, are among the most powerful determinants of the community prevalence and distribution of risk factors, morbidity, and mortality related to these diseases. Yet critical analysis of the design, implementation, and impact of comprehensive STD/HIV prevention efforts is difficult and, therefore, quite limited. This is true, at least in part, because, to be effective and sustainable at the community level, prevention efforts must weave a complex array of behavioral and biomedical interventions through a variety of societal structures to form multifaceted prevention "programs" grounded in local epidemiology and sociocultural context. Their scope, complexity, heterogeneity, and history have often confounded our ability to plan, successfully implement, and evaluate these programs. Indeed, at both the national and local levels in the United States, STD/HIV prevention programs have rarely been explicitly defined or well documented, and most analyses of determinants of STD patterns do not even mention prevention programs.

In this chapter, we define an STD/HIV prevention program and discuss its population and individual health goals and essential components. Building on the conceptual framework described in the previous chapter, which emphasizes the reproductive rate model of STD/HIV transmission, and the related dynamic topology model of phase-specific STD/HIV prevention efforts, we examine the system that currently exists in the United States, highlighting emerging and ongoing issues in STD/HIV prevention policy, practice, and program-relevant research.[1–3]

DEFINING STD/HIV PREVENTION PROGRAMS

An STD or HIV prevention program refers to *a set of synergistic intervention and support components linked by a conceptual framework based on epidemiologic and contextual assessment.* Although there is substantial agreement on the goals of these programs, little attention has been given to defining precisely which components represent essential functions.

POPULATION AND INDIVIDUAL HEALTH GOALS OF STD/HIV PREVENTION PROGRAMS

The goals of STD/HIV prevention programs focus on two levels and are complementary, but distinct. At the population or public health level, the goal is to reduce transmission to the point that the infection cannot sustain itself in the community. At the individual or personal health level, the goals are to prevent acquisition, eliminate symptoms, and prevent complications. Most STD/HIV interventions do not serve all of these goals equally well.[4] For a specific type of infection, the potential contribution to each goal will depend, primarily, on the population to which the intervention is targeted and the effectiveness of behavioral and biomedical interventions in that population, particularly the availability of curative therapy (Table 90-1). One of the central challenges in designing and implementing effective prevention programs lies in achieving appropriate balance among interventions that address these multiple goals.

Strategies to achieve that balance are resource-dependent, and differ depending on the phase and subpopulation structure of an STD or HIV epidemic.[3] Recent theoretical and empiric work in this area has built on two key concepts in STD transmission dynamics. In 1978, Yorke and colleagues introduced the concept that all endemic and epidemic transmission of curable STDs is sustained by small subsets of the population called "core groups" (more recently dubbed "spread networks") that, therefore, represent an epidemiological "bull's-eye" for prevention programs.[5,6] A decade later, May and Anderson developed an elegantly simple formula that defines the basic reproductive rate of a sexually transmitted infection (R_0) in a susceptible population as a function of the average transmission efficiency of the pathogen (β), the rate of exposure of susceptible individuals to infectious sex partners (c), and the average duration of infectiousness (D).[2] Together, these concepts suggest that effective STD/HIV prevention efforts can be expected, over time, to concentrate disease in precisely those subpopulations that are most difficult to reach with and least responsive to prevention efforts.[3,7,8] This is because STDs can spread ($R_0 > 1$) or persist ($R_0 = 1$) only if reductions in one parameter of the May-Anderson model (e.g., "D" by increasing access to therapy) are offset by increases in another (e.g., "c").

Communicable disease epidemics are shaped by a dynamic interplay among the pathogen, the behaviors of the subpopulations in which it emerges, and the prevention efforts that are developed to limit its impact. They typically move from an initial phase of unbridled (and often unrecognized) *growth*, through *hyperendemic* phases (first in the absence of coordinated prevention efforts and then marked by initiation of early prevention activities), to a phase characterized by a *decline* in prevalence and incidence that leads either to *elimination* or to a phase in which infection persists at low *endemic* levels. In the case of STD and HIV epidemics, evolution through these phases has been shown to be paralleled by predictable changes in the sexual and social networks that fuel these epidemics so that the networks become located in subpopulations characterized by progressively higher rates of sex partner change or less effective contact with the health care system, that is, core groups or spread networks.[9–15]

This changing subpopulation structure or dynamic topology of STD and HIV epidemics has important implications for the mix of strategies that should be deployed to address both the population and individual level goals of prevention programs. It implies that a two-pronged approach is critical, and that as these infections move from the hyperendemic phase toward low endemicity or elimination, programs should shift not only the balance between strategies primarily targeting spread networks (with $R_0 > 1$) and those primarily targeting maintenance networks (sexual and social networks in which infection persists but has a marginal hold because $R_0 = 1$), but also the combination of interventions within each of these strategies (Fig. 90-1).[3] For example, during the hyperendemic phase, simultaneous initiation of public and private sector prevention efforts, both in subpopulations that contain spread networks and in those that contain maintenance networks, may be important in achieving rapid, sustained reductions in mor-

Table 90-1. Potential Contribution of Essential Intervention Components to STD/HIV Prevention Goals

	Population health goal	Individual health goals		
	Reduce transmission	Prevent acquisition	Eliminate symptoms	Prevent complications
General population				
Health promotion				
Healthy sexual behavior	+	+++	NA	NA
Early, effective health care behavior	+	NA	++/+*	+++/+*
Clinical and laboratory services	+	NA	++/+*	+++/+*
Partner services	+	++	+	++/+*
Spread networks*†**				
Health promotion				
Healthy sexual behavior	+++	++	NA	NA
Early, effective health care behavior	+++/++*	NA	++/+*	++/+*
Clinical and laboratory services	+++/++*	NA	++/+*	++/+*
Partner services	+++/++*	+	+	++/+*
Outbreak response	+++/++*	++	+	++/+*

*Curable STDs/currently incurable STDs, including HIV infection
†Spread networks have previously been called "core groups." See reference 3 for more detailed discussion.

bidity and potentially in partially preempting stigmatization and late phase concentration of disease in groups that are inaccessible or resistant to prevention efforts. Mass media campaigns to promote public awareness of the "new"disease and what to do about it; provision of detection and treatment (or vaccination) services by public and private providers, linked with risk-reduction counseling; and patient-initiated partner notification leading to related partner services will reduce infection in subpopulations containing maintenance networks. However, to limit disease spread in subpopulations containing spread networks (and, therefore, ultimately eliminate the infection in all groups), a complementary approach must be implemented. It should include strategies such as targeted health promotion, frequently through one-on-one encounters at the community level; screening and treatment (or vaccination) services offered in outreach formats (e.g., mobile vans, housing projects, schools, storefronts, parking lots) linked with peer risk-reduction counseling; provider-assisted partner notification and related partner services; and community-level behavioral interventions to change sexual and health care behaviors within relevant social networks. These efforts must be tailored to the educational, socioeconomic, cultural, and, often, linguistic realities of these populations.

Throughout subsequent phases, this balance and intervention mix should shift. In the public sector, repeatedly retargeting ac-

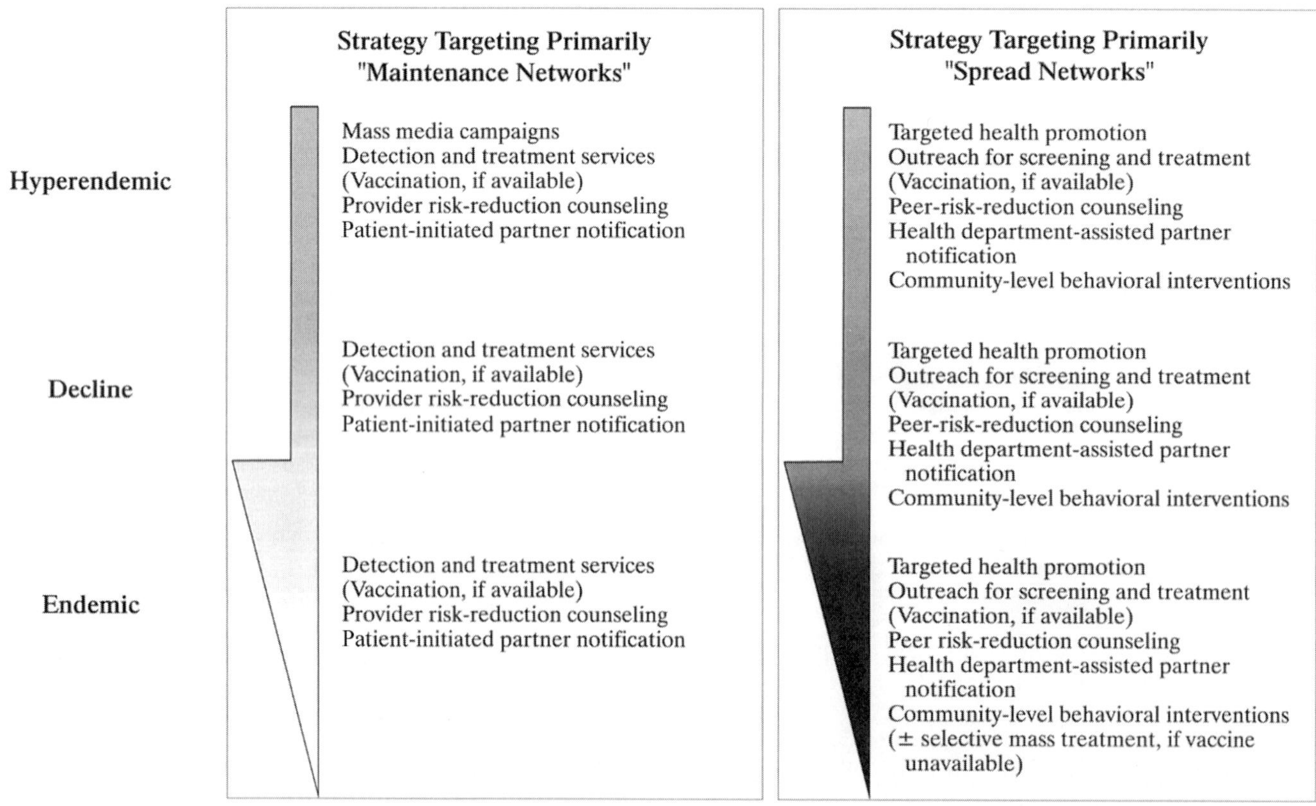

Fig. 90-1. Example of two-pronged, phase-appropriate STD prevention strageties. *Modified and reprinted with permission from reference 3.*

tivities to focus increasingly on groups in which spread networks are located becomes progressively more essential and more feasible. Although there is an ongoing need and ethical imperative to meet the personal health goals of STD/HIV prevention by continuing to provide services to subpopulations in which maintenance networks are located, the participation of private providers should increase to fill much of this need. Furthermore, in decline and low endemic phases, mass media campaigns are usually of limited value because basic knowledge about the STD, approaches to risk reduction, and sources of care have reached high levels in these groups. With increased participation of private providers, the reduced need for mass media campaigns, and shrinking morbidity in subpopulations containing maintenance networks, public health programs should place greater emphasis on achieving the population level goal of reduced transmission through spread network strategies, particularly targeted outreach approaches that bridge the increasingly apparent differences between service providers and people who are at highest risk for infection.

ESSENTIAL COMPONENTS OF STD/HIV PREVENTION PROGRAMS

The Centers for Disease Control and Prevention (CDC), the World Health Organization (WHO), and the U.S. Agency for International Development-sponsored international AIDS Control and Prevention (AIDSCAP) Project of the early 1990s have each conceptualized the fundamental "building blocks" of STD/HIV prevention programs in slightly different ways.[16–19] In this chapter, we will use a formulation that builds on these three approaches and characterizes STD/HIV prevention programs as consisting of four essential intervention components (health promotion, clinical and laboratory services, partner services, and outbreak response) buttressed by four essential support components (leadership and management, surveillance and data management, professional training, and research and evaluation).

Within each of these categories, as is discussed in the following, a range of approaches is currently being used. Unfortunately, STD/HIV program managers at the state and local levels must frequently choose among these approaches, both within and across categories, in the face of evidence for effectiveness that is limited in quality and quantity. At the present time, these limitations are particularly notable for approaches to health promotion, partner services, and outbreak response. Even when data are available and strongly suggest that interventions or support strategies "work," there are usually caveats with respect to population, sociocultural context, measurement approaches, and cost. These caveats mean that rational program planning and resource allocation must link knowledge of the "menu" of options within each essential component and the limited effectiveness data for alternative approaches with systematic assessment of local epidemiology and context, *and* with local evaluation. The further challenge is to move beyond evaluation of individual approaches to develop methods to examine the joint effects of the "packages" of intervention and support approaches that truly constitute STD/HIV prevention programs.

Intervention and support components differ in their strategic foci (Table 90-2). As is highlighted in the previous chapter, a useful approach is to think of the four intervention components as working in combination to reduce STD/HIV transmission by reducing the three determinants of the reproductive rate (R_0), that is, the efficiency of transmission during STD/HIV exposure (β), the exposure of susceptible individuals to infectious individuals (c), or the duration of infectivity (D).[1,2] The support components, on the other hand, combine to define direction, and ensure capacity and quality in provision of essential STD/HIV prevention services and related activities.

STD/HIV prevention programs have traditionally operated within the health sector, particularly the public health sector. STD prevention has long been a primary responsibility of public health agencies because, as is the case with other communicable diseases, these efforts result in a *public* good. They protect multiple mem-

Table 90-2. Essential Components of National, State, and Local STD/HIV Prevention Systems: Strategic Foci, Component Systems, and Relevant Sectors

			Health sector		Non–health sector			
Components	Strategic foci	Systems	Public	Private	Community Leaders (lay and religious)	Education	Entertainment and news media	Legislative and public policy
Intervention	• Reduce efficiency of transmission during STD/HIV exposure (β) • Reduce exposure of susceptible persons to infectious persons (c) • Reduce duration of infectivity (D)	• Health promotion	✓	✓	✓	✓	✓	✓
		• Clinical and laboratory services	✓	✓				
		• Partner services	✓	✓				
		• Outbreak response	✓					
Support	• Define direction to achieve goals	• Leadership and management	✓	✓	✓	✓	✓	✓
	• Ensure essential prevention capacity	• Surveillance and data management	✓	✓				✓
	• Ensure quality of prevention services and related activities	• Professional training	✓	✓		✓		
		• Evaluation and research	✓	✓				

bers of the community from costly adverse health consequences by reducing their risk of exposure to infection. However, as was recently highlighted in the U.S. by the Institute of Medicine (IOM), to be optimally effective, almost all of the intervention and support components of STD/HIV prevention efforts must be provided through a "coherent, comprehensive, and coordinated" system that includes non-health sectors (e.g., education, entertainment, etc.), as well as health sectors, and involves both private and public agencies within these various sectors.[20] Therefore, in this chapter, we will use the term *system* when we discuss *sets of synergistic intervention and support components aggregated across sectors at the national, state, or community level.* Thus, an effective STD or HIV prevention *system* at each of these levels includes the public health program, but goes beyond it to encompass essential components involving both private and public agencies in other sectors (see Table 90-2).

CRITICAL ASSESSMENT OF STD/HIV PREVENTION EFFORTS IN THE UNITED STATES

In the real world of finite resources, any prevention effort should be designed and assessed on the basis of characteristics of the disease, the interventions or activities, and the people who are most affected by both. In assessing how well current STD/HIV prevention priorities and strategies in the United States meet the population and individual health goals discussed in the preceding, it is useful to consider at least five factors: (1) the importance of these diseases in terms of their health and economic impact; (2) the feasibility of and support for preventive and curative interventions; (3) the effectiveness, cost, cost-effectiveness, and acceptability of prevention activities, particularly in communities in greatest need of services; (4) the selection and coverage of target populations; and (5) the synergy of efforts across STDs and with other efforts to improve health. The first two, disease impact and intervention feasibility (or, conversely, disease vulnerability) provide the foundation for rational prioritization of prevention efforts among the STDs. The remaining three determine the quality, likely impact, and sustainability of specific prevention strategies for prioritized diseases, and must be examined in light of the phase of the epidemic and the extent of intersectoral involvement in prevention efforts. Unfortunately, data limitations plague each of these areas, especially the last three, when one tries to examine "prevention packages," rather than individual interventions.

HEALTH AND ECONOMIC IMPACT OF STDS IN THE UNITED STATES

STD rates in the United States are high, both in comparison to STD rates in other countries and in comparison to rates of other notifiable diseases in this country. Reported rates of curable STDs are the highest in the industrialized world, with reported gonorrhea rates, for example, approximately 50 times those in Sweden and eight times those in Canada.[20] In 1995 and 1996, STDs accounted for 87 percent of the ten most frequently reported nationally notifiable diseases in the United States and 85 percent of all such diseases.[21,22] In fact, the true health burden of STDs is manyfold higher than reported morbidity because the majority of STDs are asymptomatic, the most common STDs (genital herpes, human papillomavirus infection, and trichomoniasis) are not nationally notifiable, and substantial underreporting persists, even for notifiable STDs (Table 90-3).[23,24] An expert panel convened by the American Social Health Association (ASHA) recently reviewed and updated published estimates of STD incidence and prevalence, and assessed the strength of the evidence supporting those estimates. The panel estimated that in 1997 the cumulative number of incident STDs in the United States was more than 15 million cases annually, with a wide range of 10 to 20 million cases because of the poor quality of the surveillance data for the most common of these diseases.[25] Roughly two-thirds of these incident cases are STDs for which no coordinated prevention efforts currently exist, and almost half are viral STDs other than HIV infection.

A related dimension of the health impact of these diseases is reflected in the phase and distribution of the multiple STD epidemics that coexist in this country (Table 90-3). From a national perspective, after 60 years of public sector prevention efforts in the United States, in 1997 syphilis has fallen to historically low levels as an endemic disease with a highly focal geographic distribution that makes it vulnerable to elimination.[23,26,27] Gonorrhea continues in the decline phase that began in 1975, 3 years after a nationwide prevention program was established, and is somewhat more widely distributed than syphilis both geographically and across sexual and social networks.[23] Following the more recent initiation of national HIV and hepatitis B (HBV) prevention efforts in 1985 and 1990, respectively, these diseases have also begun to decline.[22,28] In contrast, chlamydia, for which national prevention efforts were launched in 1994, and trichomoniasis, genital herpes (HSV), and human papillomavirus (HPV) infection, for which coordinated prevention efforts have yet to be established, remain hyperendemic with broader distributions not only geographically, but also across sexual and social networks, socioeconomic status, and race and ethnicity.[3,23,29,30] Although at the local level and for subpopulations both locally and nationally, disease-specific patterns may differ, these national trends provide a dynamic "snapshot" of the relative health impact of the major STDs in the United States, as well as insights into the most appropriate combination of phase-appropriate prevention approaches.

The long-term complications of STDs are another key consideration in setting prevention priorities, particularly because the majority of uncomplicated STDs are asymptomatic or resolve even in the absence of therapy in immune-competent hosts. Were it not for the severe, costly consequences of these diseases, from a health and economic perspective, most would fall into the same category as the common cold. It is major sequelae such as involuntary infertility, potentially fatal tubal pregnancy, congenital infection, malignancies (genital, anal, hepatocellular, and other opportunistic tumors), increased risk of HIV infection, and life-threatening opportunistic infections that truly define the health importance of STDs/HIV and drive their economic costs, which conservatively total almost $17 billion annually (see Table 90-3).[20] Indeed, many would argue that much of the recent increased interest in STDs is the result of growing appreciation of the impact of other STDs on HIV transmission. Similarly, recent data suggesting that trichomoniasis may not only facilitate HIV transmission, but also be associated with a 30 percent increase in low birth weight and prematurity has stimulated new commitment to addressing this STD.[31]

FEASIBILITY OF PREVENTIVE AND CURATIVE INTERVENTIONS IN THE UNITED STATES

To prioritize diseases rationally for coordinated prevention and control efforts at the national, state, or local level, the feasibility of interventions must be considered in parallel with the magnitude of the health and economic burden. These considerations should also influence the design of disease-specific intervention strategies. For example, the availability of inexpensive, rapid, diagnostic tests and curative therapy or effective vaccines has repeatedly been a key stimulus in launching national STD prevention programs in

Table 90-3. Health and Economic Impact of STDs in the United States

STD	Reported 1997 incidence*	Estimated 1997 incidence/prevalence†	Phase/focality	Major sequelae in the United States	Estimated annual direct cost (1994 $ in millions)§
Bacterial and protozoal					
Chancroid	243	NA	Low endemic/High	↑ HIV transmission	N/A
Syphilis	45,387	50,000–70,000/NA	Low endemic/High	Congenital infection and stillbirth, neurosyphilis, ↑ HIV transmission	$46–79**
Gonorrhea	324,901	650,000–700,000/NA	Decline/Medium	Infertility and ectopic pregnancy, congenital infection, ↑ HIV transmission	$790–1050††
Chlamydia	526,653	3,000,000/NA	Hyperendemic, early prevention efforts/Low	Infertility and ectopic pregnancy, congenital infection and low birth weight, ↑ HIV transmission	$670–1,510§§
Trichomoniasis	NNN	3,000,000–5,000,000/NA	Hyperendemic, no coordinated prevention efforts/Low	Low birth weight/prematurity, ↑ HIV transmission	NA
Viral					
HIV	NNN	40,000/560,000	Decline/High	Opportunistic infections and malignancies	$5,030***
HBV	8,656	82,000/417,000	Decline/Medium	Chronic hepatitis, cirrhosis, liver cancer	$110†††
HSV-2	NNN	1,000,000/45,000,000	Hyperendemic, no coordinated prevention efforts/Low	Congenital infection, ↑ HIV transmission	$178§§§
HPV	NNN	5,500,000/≥20,000,000	Hyperendemic, no coordinated prevention efforts/Low	Anogenital cancer	$3,510****

NNN = not nationally notifiable.
NA = not available.
* See reference 12.
† See reference 14; prevalence estimates refer to currently infected or seropositive individuals.
§ Siegel JE: The economic burden of sexually transmitted diseases in the United States, in Holmes KK et al. (eds): *Sexually Transmitted Diseases,* 3rd ed. New York, McGraw-Hill, 1998.
** Includes only treatment costs for adult syphilis plus global cost estimates for congenital syphilis (see reference 3 for further discussion).
†† Includes costs for gonococcal PID, infertility, and ectopic pregnancy.
§§ Includes costs for chlamydial PID, ophthalmia neonatorum, and infant pneumonia.
*** Sexually transmitted HIV or chronic HBV infection only.
††† Does not include costs for sequelae of HBV infection
§§§ Based on HSV-2 prevalence in late 1970s (~25.4 million cases rather than 1990s estimate of ~45 million cases. See reference 3 for further discussion).
**** Includes treatment costs for genital warts, and for cervical dysplasia and invasive cervical cancer owing to HPV infection.

the United States (Table 90-4). Factors such as high proportions of symptomatic disease, reliability of syndromic diagnosis, and single dose, oral treatment regimens have further facilitated and shaped prevention efforts.

HIV prevention efforts are the striking exception to this pattern. In that case, the high case-fatality ratio and extremely effective constituent advocacy not only triggered establishment of a national prevention program in the absence of both curative therapy and an effective vaccine, but also halved the 8- to 10-year lag that occurred between the advent of detection and intervention tools, and the initiation of national prevention programs for other STDs, such as gonorrhea, chlamydia, and HBV infection. One of the most important legacies of HIV prevention efforts is that it expanded the range of primary interventions considered sufficient to mount a nationwide STD prevention program beyond the traditional biomedical alternatives of antimicrobials and vaccines to include behavioral "virtual vaccines" to increase condom use and promote other healthy sexual behaviors. This paradigm shift is particularly relevant for nascent efforts to address genital herpes and HPV infection, although condom efficacy, per se, may be more limited for these STDs than for HIV infection. An equally profound lesson is the pivotal role of advocacy in creating and sustaining the political will and resources to address diseases such as STDs that are linked with politically sensitive behaviors or concentrated in marginalized groups.

CURRENT STD/HIV PREVENTION EFFORTS IN THE UNITED STATES

Disease priorities

As in most other industrialized countries, in the United States joint consideration of health and economic impact, and intervention feasibility has led public sector prevention programs to place highest priority on the common, bacterial STDs (syphilis, gonorrhea, and chlamydial infection) and on AIDS/HIV infection. The U.S. prevention approach for each of these diseases has emphasized early detection and treatment, not only through diagnosis of patients specifically seeking STD or HIV/AIDS care, but also, in recognition of the frequency of asymptomatic infection, through case finding in individuals seeking health care for other reasons and screening in settings unrelated to health care (e.g., premarital syphilis testing). Although initial HIV prevention efforts emphasized assuring a safe blood supply, promotion of condoms and other safer sexual behaviors, and risk reduction approaches for injection drug users, as soon as effective antiretroviral regimens

Table 90-4. Feasibility of Preventive and Curative Interventions in the United States

STD	Percent symptomatic at any time	Utility of syndromic diagnosis	Availability of cheap, rapid, accurate etiologic tests	Availability of therapy			Vaccine efficacy	Condoms efficacy	Constituent advocacy
				Curative	Single-dose	Oral			
Bacterial & protozoal									
Chancroid	80–90	High	Medium	Yes	Yes	Yes	No	High	None
Syphilis	60–90	Medium	High	Yes	Yes[1]	Yes[1]	No	Probably high; data inadequate[2]	None
Gonorrhea	F 10–70 M 80–95	F-Low M-High	High	Yes	Yes	Yes	No	High	None
Chlamydia	F ~ 25 M ~ 50	F-Low M-Medium	Medium	Yes	Yes	Yes	No	Probably high; data inadequate	Medium
Trichomoniasis	F 50–90 M 10–50	F-Medium M-Low	Medium	Yes	Yes	Yes	No	Probably high; data inadequate	None
Viral									
HIV[3]									
1°infection	60–80	Low	High	No	No	Yes	No	High	High
Non1°HIV/AIDS	Variable	Low/Medium	High	No	No	Yes	No	High	High
HBV	25–50	Low	High	No[4]	No	No[4]	Yes	Probably high; data inadequate	Low–medium
HSV-2	10–25	Medium	Medium	No	No	Yes	No	Probably medium; data inadequate[2]	Medium
HPV									
6 and 11	50	High	Low	No	No	No	No	Probably medium;	Low
Other	<5	Low	Low	No	No	No	No	data inadequate[2]	Low–medium

[1] Azithromycin appears promising, but data are preliminary and are for incubating syphilis.
[2] Condom effectiveness depends on whether condom covers ulcer or lesion.
[3] Depends on stage of infection.
[4] Interferon may result in 10 to 15% of patients; 3TC/Lamividine is used in a small portion of patients.

became available, early detection and treatment became a cornerstone of HIV prevention programs. The intensive serological screening campaigns for syphilis that began in the 1940s were followed by an aggressive gonorrhea screening program that began in the 1970s, massive HIV screening efforts that began in the 1980s, and an expanding chlamydia screening program that began in the 1990s. These nationwide casefinding or screening mobilizations have been extraordinary public health feats that have dramatically reduced rates of infection with bacterial STDs and have been cost-effective in many settings during the hyperendemic phase (as is the case currently for chlamydial infection).[32,33] However, failure to recognize the phase-specific nature of broad-based disease detection policies and to reassess screening criteria with declining prevalence have frequently limited the long-term cost effectiveness of these efforts.

Surveillance of morbidity trends has been another cornerstone of the approach to each of these diseases. As is highlighted by the results of a modified Delphi survey conducted among CDC staff and these authors, the strategies for these "big four" diseases have been more variable in their emphasis on other essential prevention components, such as health promotion (both for infected and uninfected individuals), partner services, outbreak response, and research and evaluation (Table 90-5). For example, as is discussed in the following, HIV prevention programs that initially had few treatment options to offer have focused heavily on clinic- and community-based interventions to reduce risky sexual behaviors, whereas many local STD prevention programs have made far more nominal commitments to clinic-based risk reduction counseling and community STD education. Instead, the latter programs often focused on provider-assisted partner notification and epidemiological treatment as a way to augment early detection and treatment efforts.

In contrast, chancroid and hepatitis B infection, the two remaining STDs for which national prevention programs have been mounted, have received lower priority (see Table 90-5). Chancroid, a rare disease in the United States with less than 5000 cases reported annually since 1950 and no recognized sequelae prior to the HIV pandemic, has been addressed primarily through outbreak investigation with limited diagnosis and treatment, partner services, surveillance, training, and basic research efforts.[23] Hepatitis B infection is the first vaccine-preventable STD. HBV prevention efforts, therefore, provide yet a third model that focuses primarily on maximizing vaccine coverage of individuals at risk for sexual transmission who, over the last 10 years, have constituted approximately 30 to 60 percent of new HBV infections in this country.[34] This is part of a comprehensive HBV vaccination strategy that now also includes antenatal screening and routine vaccination of all newborns, older children at high risk for HBV infection, and 11- to 12-year-old children who have not previously been vaccinated. The vaccine strategy has been supported by limited health promotion activities, clinical and laboratory services, surveillance, training, and research and evaluation. To date, however, HBV vaccine coverage has been low, particularly among those at high risk for sexual transmission.[35]

The other STDs that are common in the United States, trichomoniasis, genital herpes, and HPV infection, have not yet been addressed by coordinated, national or local public health programs, even though, in aggregate, they represent the vast majority of disease. Although clinical and laboratory services for these diseases are currently offered by some private providers and in selected public clinics, they are not linked with other essential activities that have high population impact, such as partner services and surveillance. Until recently, disinterest in trichomoniasis has been owing to the limited data suggesting significant health or economic impact, whereas the barrier to addressing herpes and HPV infection has been limited feasibility of interventions. In both

Table 90-5. Current Emphasis in U.S. Prevention Approach: Modified Delphi Survey Results* and Federal Research and Evaluation Expenditures

STD	Health promotion	Clinical and laboratory services: Diagnosis	Screening	Vaccination	Partner services	Outbreak response	Leadership and management	Surveillance	Training	Research and evaluation (1997 $ in millions)†
Bacterial and protozoal										
Chancroid	0	1+	0	0	1+	2+	0	1+	1+	$1.5
Syphilis	2+	3+	3+	0	3+	3+	3+	3+	2+	$4.9
Gonorrhea	1+	3+	2+	0	2+	2+	2+	2+	2+	$13.9
Chlamydia	2+	3+	2+	0	1+	0	3+	2+	2+	$14.4
Trichomoniasis	0	1+	0+	0	0	0	0	0	1+	$1.0
Viral										
HIV/AIDS	3+	3+	3+	0	2+	2+	3+	3+	3+	$720.3
HBV	1+	1+	1+	1+	0	0	1+	1+	1+	$2.8
HSV-2	1+	1+	0	0	0	0	0	0§	1+	$18.8§§
HPV	1+	1+**	0††	0	0	0	0	0	1+	$6.2

* Respondents were asked to rate, within each column, the relative current emphasis of the specific prevention components for each disease.
† NIAID and CDC expenditures in 1997
§ Although nationally representative seroprevalence data are available for HSV-2 from the National Health and Nutrition Examination Survey (NHANES), HSV-2 infection is not a notifiable disease in any state.
§§ Includes basic research on HSV-1 and HSV-2.
** Refers to genital warts.
†† Although screening for HPV-related premalignant lesions by Papanicolau smears is a central part of cervical cancer prevention programs; screening for HPV infection is rare.

cases, recent research advances warrant reassessment of our public health approach to prevention of these STDs.

Critique of essential program or system components

Within the context of these disease priorities, it is useful to consider the nature and quality of each of the essential components of the U.S. STD/HIV prevention program or system.

Health Promotion to Improve Sexual, Substance Use, and Health Seeking Behaviors. Before the advent of HIV/AIDS, effective community- and individual-targeted methods to promote healthier sexual behaviors, reduce substance use, and improve health-care related behaviors played minimal roles in U.S. STD prevention efforts. Recognizing that communicable diseases are unique in that elimination of infection in index patients *is* prevention of infection transmission to future partners, STD experts and program managers focused more on biomedical than behavioral interventions. They knew relatively little about how best to provide the knowledge and skills to change risk behaviors with the generalizability needed to be useful in prevention programs, and few behavioral scientists were sufficiently involved in STD prevention efforts to provide this expertise. Although the lethality and untreatable nature of HIV infection and AIDS greatly increased national efforts to reduce risky behaviors, even these expanded attempts continue to fall far short of what is necessary to achieve population and individual health goals, particularly for prevention of STDs other than HIV infection. Furthermore, progress has been even more limited in understanding the determinants of early and effective health care behaviors, and translating those insights into interventions to help people strengthen these behaviors. In addition, substantial barriers to health care access persist in the United States for large numbers of persons, particularly those at greatest risk of acquiring STDs or HIV infection, such as persons with lower than average education, marginalized people of color, the homeless, and the disenfranchised.[36]

Although many have convincingly argued that sexual and substance use behaviors can and should be changed for society's benefit, the use of federal or other governmental funds and policy methods for these purposes has remained controversial and underutilized.[37,38] At the community level, the United States has been slow and conflicted in employing health communication and promotion strategies for STD/HIV prevention, despite compelling evidence that behavioral interventions can reduce risk of infection transmitted through sex or injection drug use.[39] This ignores the hard-won lessons of other prevention efforts, such as those to limit smoking that have successfully combined aggressive, multi-pronged antismoking campaigns with legislative interventions.[40] It also contrasts sharply with many Western European countries that, for example, in response to the AIDS pandemic, took early steps to develop large, comprehensive campaigns to promote safer sex, including national mailouts of information about HIV/AIDS.[41,42] The first mention of HIV/AIDS by a U.S. president (Ronald Reagan) did not occur until 1987, and Surgeon General C. Everett Koop's mailing on "Understanding AIDS" to every American household occurred in 1988, 7 years after the first AIDS case report.[43] State and local mass media campaigns promoting sexual and drug-related risk reduction have been small in number and scope. The quantity, quality, and support for sex education in the United States also lags substantially behind that in many Western European countries.[44–46] Despite public support documented in national polls, there is continuing reluctance to address sexual behavior and risk-taking in school settings using comprehensive, science-based, developmentally appropriate curricula.[47,48]

Finally, even in the face of strong scientific evidence, many national and local policymakers and opinion leaders (both secular and religious) in this country have been deeply ambivalent and confused about providing leadership and resources for STD/HIV prevention, and particularly for promotion of healthy sexual behaviors and substance use harm-reduction strategies. Perhaps this is, in part, because these efforts operate in a public health domain that some believe conflicts with fundamental religious tenents.[49,50] For example, although there is no clear evidence that abstinence-based STD/HIV prevention works long-term, such programs have recently received increased federal funding.[51–54] Yet, needle exchange programs that have repeatedly been shown to reduce HIV transmission without increasing drug use still cannot be funded using federal dollars.[39,55–57] Similarly, although condoms are highly effective for prevention of HIV infection and many other STDs when used consistently and correctly, in many communities, condom availability has been restricted even in STD clinics, and mention (let alone promotion) of condom use in the public media has been problematic.[58,59] This is especially disturbing in light of the barrage of sexual messages that surrounds Americans and ranges from mass media advertisements to entertainment. For example, recent analyses have documented an average of 10 incidents of sexual behavior each hour on prime-time network television, with approximately 25 for every one instance of preventive behavior shown or mention of consequences, such as STDs or unintended pregnancy.[20] Not surprisingly, knowledge about STDs is low among Americans, with about a third being unable to name a single STD other than HIV/AIDS, more than half believing that all STDs except HIV/AIDS are curable, and two-thirds of adolescent and young adult women reporting little or no knowledge about these diseases.[20,60] Americans also have less tolerant attitudes about sexual behavior and have lower condom use than, for example, the British.[61]

Health promotion strategies that work at the individual level are often inadequately operationalized and supported. In busy STD/HIV clinical settings, one-on-one or group counseling to reduce risky sexual behaviors is constrained by time pressures, limited expertise, and reimbursement issues. Furthermore, "counseling" often largely consists of provision of information in ways that are not tailored to the educational, linguistic, or sociocultural needs of the client. Assessment of clients' readiness to change behaviors, and assistance in building the necessary skills are rarely offered. Even when relatively brief "client-centered" counseling models have been developed and shown to be effective in increasing condom use and reducing incident STDs, these approaches have not been widely implemented.[62,63] Other one-on-one or small group interventions, such as those involving popular members of social networks or peer volunteers in community-based venues have been shown to be effective, but have not been replicated extensively.[64–67] Limited expertise and resources again seem to be barriers to broader implementation. Finally, there is a growing appreciation of the need for more intermediate strategies targeting persons who find safer behaviors hard to achieve and sustain, particularly men who have sex with men (MSM), and users of illicit and licit (i.e., alcoholic) substances. Drug treatment capacity for injection drug users (IDUs) is available in most locales for fewer than one in five injectors, and waiting lists are long and discouraging to anyone who is eager and ready for healthier alternatives.[68] University of Washington investigators, through simple advertising, in an effort to reduce HIV risk behaviors, attracted substantial numbers of men, mostly MSM, who reported feeling sexually "out of control, as if addicted."[69,70] Through 2-month group interventions, including relapse prevention methods, and programs ultimately expanded to 1–800 phone line groups nationwide, substantial numbers of clients reported persistently reduced risk.[71]

In summary, the central importance of health promotion as part of an effective STD prevention program has long been recognized in the United States, and HIV prevention research and development have greatly expanded the science-base for and use of interventions to reduce risky sexual and substance use behaviors, harnessing approaches that are acceptable to populations most in need of these services. However, particularly in efforts to prevent STDs other than HIV/AIDS, the health promotion component often remains underutilized and poorly integrated with other components of comprehensive STD/HIV prevention programs. Synergy among STD, HIV, and pregnancy prevention health promotion efforts is rarely optimized. When health promotion activities are implemented, they frequently focus on providing "one-size-fits-all" information, without assessing epidemic phase or clients' needs, tailoring the information to those needs, and linking it with other key elements of behavior change interventions, such as skill building. Particularly with the growing options for highly active antiretroviral therapy (HAART), the focus on promoting early and effective health care-related behaviors should be greatly expanded. Finally, in an area in which intersectoral participation is essential, there has been stunningly little involvement of groups beyond the public health sector, such as educators, the entertainment industry, and faith communities.

Clinical and Laboratory Services. The clinical and laboratory services component of STD/HIV prevention programs in the United States presents remarkable contrasts. As indicated, historically this has been an area of primary focus and relative strength in public sector programs. Etiologic testing for some STD pathogens and effective antimicrobials have been widely available onsite through many public clinics providing STD or HIV services. In several cities, strong linkages between university-based researchers and health department staff have resulted in STD and HIV care that ranks with the finest in the world. Furthermore, with the advent of STD/HIV detection methods that use urine or saliva specimens, and single-dose, oral therapy for almost all of the curable STDs, these services are beginning to move out of clinics into community venues, such as schools, recreation centers, housing projects, and parking lots, in attempts to serve those who traditionally have been among the hardest to reach.[67,67a,72] For example, in a pilot project for high-risk youth in Denver, peer volunteers and project outreach workers provided chlamydia screening using urine nucleic acid amplification tests. Almost 7 percent of the 486 urine specimens collected during the first 20 months of the project were positive, with chlamydia positivity rates being approximately three times higher (11.9% vs 4.4%, $p < 0.05$) among youth screened in field settings (i.e., alleys, parking lots, parks, and residences) than in facility-based settings (i.e., community/recreation centers, high schools, and an STD/HIV prevention storefront).[67] Particularly impressive is the fact that 97 percent of infected male adolescents were treated in the field within a median of 8 days. Finally, home testing has made anonymous (although somewhat costly) HIV testing available in most of the country, even in the remotest rural areas, and home test kits have been used in some public health settings to relieve the pressure from low-risk populations seeking subsidized HIV testing often provided in public health testing sites. Home testing for other STDs may well be on the horizon.[73]

At the system level, one of the most successful and cost-effective models for collaboration in public health today is the delivery of chlamydia detection and treatment services in Title X family planning clinics through the joint efforts of federally funded STD and family planning programs.[32,74–76] In managed care settings, selective screening and treatment for chlamydia have also been demonstrated to reduce the incidence of pelvic inflammatory disease (PID) by almost 60 percent.[77] Furthermore, these well-documented and dramatic reductions in both lower and upper genital tract infections in women have resulted in the development of a chlamydia screening measure that is being evaluated for inclusion in the Health Plan Employer Data and Information Set (HEDIS), the "report cards" used by purchasers of private health care to assess the performance of capitated managed care organizations.[78,79]

Yet, simultaneously, profound problems pervade provision of STD/HIV clinical and laboratory services in the United States. In the public sector, access and acceptability issues are the greatest problems, whereas in the private sector quality of care is often the primary concern. A nationally representative survey of local health departments conducted in 1995 indicated that only half of

U.S. health departments provide STD services, and that only 61 percent of those could see a new patient the same day that the individual sought services.[80] Fifteen percent could not see these potentially infected and infectious patients for 3 days or more. In health department clinics, patients who are able to obtain care frequently must wait for many hours in physically and socially uncomfortable surroundings prior to seeing a clinician. Overburdened or inadequately trained staff may compound these barriers by failing to communicate with patients in ways that are respectful, culturally sensitive, and nonstigmatizing. Provider and facility shortages, inconvenient hours of clinic operation, cost, lack of transportation, and limited numbers of trained minority staff have been specifically cited as programmatic factors contributing to the persistence of high levels of syphilis in the southern states.[81] Routine STD testing and treatment are also rare in settings such as correctional institutions and drug treatment centers, where prevalence of infection is frequently high and sexual behaviors following release often facilitate transmission.[82,83]

In the public sector, HIV clinical and laboratory services have evolved over the course of the AIDS epidemic. With the advent of HIV testing in 1985, most local public health departments, with federal support from CDC, implemented HIV counseling and testing for high-risk populations, partly to provide testing site alternatives to blood and other tissue banks, which immediately began routine screening for HIV. For the first decade of the epidemic, the majority of federal prevention resources were used for counseling and testing, linked with referral of patients to care and partner notification (CTRPN).[84] In 1986, the Robert Wood Johnson Foundation, followed in 1987 by the Health Services and Resources Administration (HRSA), provided funds for care services to persons with HIV infection, some of which were used through secondary prevention programs to help assure continued linkage with "Early Intervention" care programs to help infected persons prevent transmission to others.[85] Other support for prevention and care services, including HIV counseling and testing for IDUs and their sex partners, eventually came from other Department of Health and Human Services (DHHS) agencies.

Public health STD/HIV laboratory services have primarily consisted of serologic tests for syphilis and HIV, and culture or antigen detection tests for gonorrhea, chlamydia, and, in some larger facilities, chancroid, along with screening for HIV-related diseases such as tuberculosis. A number of local public health departments have also funded limited immunologic testing (i.e., CD4 cell counts), and more recently viral load tests for HIV-infected persons. In Seattle, these services have been funded by the HRSA Ryan White Title I community care planning process as a way to help "bridge" the transition of HIV-infected persons into the care system. At the same time, particularly in smaller facilities, the 1988 Clinical Laboratory Improvement Act (CLIA) certification requirements have limited the ability of many public clinics to provide "on-site," "STAT" laboratory tests for STDs.[86] This latter change coupled, in some cases, with resource constraints, has recently resulted in several STD programs reverting to syndromic management for initial treatment pending results of etiologic testing.

In the public sector, clinical and laboratory services are often fragmented. Although chlamydia screening is increasingly available in Title X family planning clinics, and HIV counseling and testing are offered in more than 95 percent of STD clinics, STD and HIV public sector care in more than half of the 50 states and six largest cities in the United States continues to be offered through categorical clinics that do not integrate STD, HIV, and pregnancy prevention clinical services at the client level. For example, STD services are currently provided in less than 20 percent of HIV clinics in these areas.[87] Recent guidelines on "HIV prevention through early detection and treatment of other STDs" and forthcoming reproductive health guidelines may help programs better link these services in the future.[88] In addition, despite the documented effectiveness and cost-effectiveness of chlamydia screening and treatment, federal resources are currently sufficient to cover only about half of women in need of these clinical services in 20 states. In the remaining 30 states, in which 75 percent of at-risk women reside, federal funds cover less than 15 percent of women attending public clinics who should be screened for chlamydia.

The majority of STD/HIV care in this country is sought in the private sector.[89,90] Although state-of-the-art, comprehensive HIV/AIDS care is available from private providers in the United States, its cost precludes many infected Americans from accessing its benefits.[91,92] In addition, many private providers do not routinely conduct appropriate risk assessments or screening tests for other STDs.[93–96] A recent Kaiser Family Foundation/Glamour Magazine national survey of 18- to 44-year-old women visiting a new provider for gynecologic or obstetric care revealed that at the initial visit a sexual history was elicited by only about one-third of clinicians.[96] HIV/AIDS and other STDs were discussed by 19 and 12 percent of providers, respectively.[96] Among private providers, awareness and utilization of STD treatment guidelines may also be low.[97] As an ever-increasing proportion of U.S. health care, including that for Medicaid patients, is provided by managed care organizations, the limited availability and quality of STD services offered by these providers is particularly problematic. In some parts of the country, divestiture of STD clinical services by public health departments in anticipation of health care market shifts to managed care or other types of health care reform has resulted in substantial declines in clinic visits, laboratory testing, and reported morbidity.[98]

Thus, STD/HIV clinical and laboratory services are one of the strongest components within U.S. prevention programs, with evidence for effectiveness and, in some cases, for cost-effectiveness of many practices. Nevertheless, access to these services is grossly inadequate in the public sector, and strategies to reach those who are most important to transmission (e.g., in correctional institutions or through outreach approaches) remain underutilized. Service quality is often limited by patient volume, provider attitudes and training, and failure to offer STD services that are integrated with other related essential health services. In the private sector, and particularly among managed care providers, there is limited expertise and interest in STD care. Linkages across public and private sectors are still minimal.

Partner Services. The third essential component of STD/HIV prevention programs, partner services originated in Europe in the 19th century as "contact tracing," and has been a central strategy of U.S. public health programs for more than 50 years.[99–102] Contact tracing, or "partner notification (PN)" as it was renamed in the late 1980s in response to the concerns of the gay community and others affected by the HIV epidemic, is, fundamentally, the confidential, voluntary behavioral outreach intervention designed to link sexual and needle-sharing partners of STD- or HIV-infected people with a comprehensive set of services both to limit further spread of infection and to prevent sequelae. Although there has been little debate about the concept that partners exposed to infected individuals should have access to clinical services and counseling about how to protect themselves from future STD/HIV risk, PN itself has been controversial because of ethical issues that arise when the health needs and human rights of index patients, partners, and society at large must be balanced.[103] These issues have been particularly complex for HIV/AIDS prevention programs because of the frequency of discrimination and, until recently, the limited treatment options for this disease.

In the United States, PN is a voluntary process that is conducted using two basic approaches. "Provider referral" means that the infected person's partners are informed of their potential STD/

HIV exposure and advised by a health care worker to obtain care. In public clinics, this advice is usually provided by a Disease Intervention Specialist [DIS] specifically trained in a standardized interviewing and contact tracing process originally developed in the late 1940s. Confidentiality is maintained by not revealing the identity of the original patient. "Patient referral" relies on index patients to inform their own partners. In practice, a third option, "conditional referral," has evolved. In this case, health care workers notify partners if the index patient has not done so within a specified time period.

In terms of federal financial and human resources for non–HIV STD prevention programs, historically, partner notification has been a high priority and one of the single largest expenditure categories. For many years federally trained DIS assigned to state and local health departments supervised and trained local counterparts, creating a wealth of expertise based on a combination of epidemiological principles and real-world experience. Meticulous attention is paid to confidentiality, and breeches have been stunningly rare. A cadre of unusually dedicated, field-savvy public health professionals (called public health advisors) developed from this background, and many have formed the backbone of other public health programs.[100]

Most STD/HIV experts agree that PN is an effective means of identifying previously undetected cases. However, there are few prospective data from well-designed studies to indicate which approach is most effective (and cost-effective) for each STD and for HIV infection in specific populations.[99,102,104] In the United States, programmatic indices and limited observational data suggest that effectiveness may have declined as caseloads mushroomed with the addition of gonorrhea, chlamydia, and in some areas, HIV infection, with increases in anonymous sex, and with contraction of the core groups or spread networks into hard-to-read populations. Furthermore, although investigators have recently begun to examine such options as home urine sampling and partner-delivered therapy as alternative models for partner services, in general there has been little exploration of innovative PN approaches that might capitalize on new technology or other research advances to improve effectiveness.[105] PN is also unusual among behavioral interventions in that decisions about which approach to apply have been based primarily on the disease diagnosed in the index patient, rather than on patient or partner characteristics. Thus, in most states provider referral is the rule for primary and secondary (P&S) syphilis, whereas patient referral is the standard procedure for chlamydial infection, regardless of the sociocultural and behavioral characteristics of the individuals involved.

Acceptability of PN is determined primarily by two factors, assurance of confidentiality and availability of effective treatment.[99,106] Although most patients and partners appear to be receptive to PN, acceptability probably varies by subpopulation, with greatest concerns being raised in communities that have experienced profound and persistent discrimination, such as MSM and communities of color.[99,101] Provider referral for HIV infection remains particularly controversial. It is much less frequently employed than patient referral in most states and other jurisdictions, despite the fact that PN is a requirement for eligibility for federal funding through CDC and HRSA. However, as HIV has become a more treatable infection with more potent antiretroviral combination regimens, public health officials, health care providers, and some HIV advocates are arguing that provider referral should be more routinely applied to HIV-infected persons.

Yet there are several special challenges in implementing HIV PN. These include the fact that a large proportion of HIV-infected Americans are MSMs and IDUs whose partners are frequently anonymous, unidentifiable, and not locatable. Additionally, many partners of IDUs and MSM may already be aware of their risk, and may even know that they harbor HIV. Thus, notification efforts may produce relatively fewer new cases or little added awareness of risk and risk reduction. In Seattle, for example, in 1996 some 200 HIV-infected persons (mostly MSM) estimated they had had about 3500 partners in the preceding 12 months, but of these only about 200 partners could be identified, and only 50 could be located and notified of their exposure. Of 1045 index clients interviewed in 1997 at the LA County Health Department (E. Harvey, personal communication), 412 patients provided the names of 806 partners, and of these 494 were located. This resulted in counseling and testing of 160 HIV seropositives, 42 percent of whom were unaware of their serostatus. Consistent with other such data, partners of HIV-infected persons typically have high rates of infection but less than half are unaware of their status.[107] Partner notification is particularly cost-effective in lower HIV seroprevalence settings in locating and counseling unknowingly seropositive persons, who constitute as many as 10 to 35 percent of partners contacted and tested.[108–115] Also potentially worth targeting are the partners of persons with primary HIV infection who may be most infectious.[116–119]

Another problem in employing provider referral (which appears to be more effective in HIV case-finding than patient referral) stems from the fact that the states with the most cases of HIV have not made HIV reportable to local public health authorities, although this situation is gradually changing.[101,120–123] Since providers in states without HIV reporting are generally prohibited from identifying cases to local public health authorities, they cannot turn over the task of identifying and notifying partners to their public health partners, who generally perform this function for other STDs. Private providers are not trained or skilled at performing this function, yet they may see most of the HIV cases. Therefore, they tend to pay lip service to the need to assure notification of partners, and deal with the responsibility by asking patients to notify partners themselves, often without follow-up or assurance. Not only for HIV infection, but for all STDs, this is likely to be an important issue in the transition to Medicaid-managed care.

In summary, partner notification is a longstanding, central component of U.S. public sector STD prevention programs that is strongly supported by epidemiological concepts and observational evidence. However, the narrow paradigm within which it has been implemented and data limitations on the effectiveness, cost-effectiveness, and acceptability of alternative approaches have made PN a controversial area, particularly with respect to incurable or highly stigmatizing diseases in key subpopulations. There is poor uptake by private sector providers, including managed care providers. The Institute of Medicine recommended that PN activities for curable STDs be "redesigned to improve outreach, mobilize public health staff in new ways, and enlist support from community groups or other programs that provide services to high risk populations."[20] Although there are tremendous opportunities and need for cross-fertilization between the STD prevention and HIV prevention communities in this arena, philosophical and historical differences have made progress extremely slow. Yet with the advent of improved HIV treatment regimens, PN is beginning to be reframed as part of a comprehensive set of partner services, examined in rigorous studies, and implemented more widely for HIV, as well as for other STDs.

Outbreak Response. Outbreak response is the final and most neglected of the essential intervention components. It is the only component that is the unique responsibility of the public health sector, and it becomes increasingly important as diseases move from the hyperendemic phase toward elimination because outbreaks become responsible for a growing proportion of the disease burden (see Table 90-2). Outbreak response capacity is closely tied to the strength of surveillance and epidemiological analysis, but goes beyond these routine, ongoing activities. It requires a rapid, time-limited emergency response capability that mobilizes support of the affected community and is triggered by changes in STD/HIV patterns that reach a specific, preestablished magnitude.

Currently, in the United States, STD/HIV outbreak response preparedness is weak. Although syphilis and HIV/AIDS surveillance capacities are relatively strong, surveillance for the other STDs ranges from mediocre to nonexistent (see the following). At the state and local levels, STD programs have a median of half a full-time equivalent (FTE) epidemiologist, and one-quarter of programs have no epidemiologists.[124] Less than 5 percent of public STD prevention programs have written outbreak response plans in place (Jack Spencer, personal communication). This is particularly disturbing as the nation considers embarking on an initiative to eliminate domestic transmission of syphilis.[125]

Because of the intense stigma and fear that may be associated with STD, and particularly HIV outbreaks, these epidemics and the public health response often become highly political. Some of these cases, such as the one that occurred in Chattaqua, New York in 1997, have received widespread attention, and have evoked public rage, sometimes catalyzing changes in public health laws or policies.[126–128]

Leadership and Management. Effective leadership and sound management are central to weaving the four intervention components discussed into functional programs and systems to prevent STDs, including HIV infection. Although management can be characterized by processes such as planning, budgeting, organizing, and staffing, leadership is more likely to embrace those direction-setting activities that create organizations and successfully adapt them to a myriad of environmental changes.[129] Leadership and management of STD/HIV prevention programs take place within the larger system that has public and private, governmental and nongovernmental dimensions (see Table 90-2).

In the United States, public health functions are the primary responsibility of state and local authorities. Federal financial, direct personnel, and technical assistance are provided by CDC to state and local health departments, particularly for communicable diseases such as STDs, which pose health threats that cross jurisdictional boundaries. STD prevention programs are the most longstanding example of this federal–state partnership and reflect both the benefits and the unintended liabilities of this system. Federal support for STD prevention began in 1918 as "Grants-in-Aid" to the states to control syphilis and, starting in 1948, was coupled with the assignment of federal "field staff" (called public health advisors) to assist state and local health departments in the management and implementation of these programs.[130,131] Over the subsequent 50 years, the number of federal assignees grew to over 600, and this system not only provided stability and quality assurance to politically sensitive STD prevention programs across the country, but also built a cadre of field-savvy individuals with exceptional program management expertise who became the backbone of a broad range of public health programs at the local, state, and federal levels. The system has facilitated communication between CDC and state programs, and probably has expedited the implementation of many national initiatives. Unfortunately, the infusion of federal personnel may have also inadvertently marginalized STD prevention efforts in some states. Some have argued that overburdened and under-resourced local health officials have often seen STD prevention as a "federal program" that could get by with more limited local financial and personnel support than other programs.[20] Furthermore, in some areas, tensions have arisen between federal and state personnel because of salary differentials and perceptions that federal staff may be given preference in promotion to management positions.[20] In the 1990s, with downsizing of federal staff and reassessment of the federal role in public health programs, this model is shifting to one in which federal field assignees will increasingly serve as "capacity builders" to help develop necessary skills among local staff.

A key leadership and management function is effective program planning. At a national level, the United States initiated a landmark experiment in January 1994 when it undertook a major change in the way federally funded HIV prevention programs are planned. HIV Prevention Community Planning is an ongoing cyclical, evidence-based planning process in which the authority for identifying fundable HIV prevention priorities is vested in one or more planning groups composed of community representatives (particularly representing communities affected by the HIV epidemic), scientists and other technical experts (especially epidemiologists and behavioral scientists), and program staff from nongovernmental organizations as well as departments of health, education, and substance abuse.[132] A survey conducted at the end of the effort's second year documented substantial increases in the priority given to health education and risk reduction efforts, community level interventions, capacity building, and evaluation.[133] This finding was validated in a subsequent multivariate analysis that demonstrated that the relative allocation of HIV prevention funding changed substantially after the implementation of community planning, with fewer resources directed toward clinic-based HIV counseling and testing activities and more resources directed toward community-based health education and risk reduction activities.[134]

Differences between HIV and STD prevention programs, such as budget disparity, the greater reliance on biomedical approaches to interrupt the transmission of certain STDs, and the greater use of nongovernmental organizations to deliver publicly funded HIV prevention services, may require specific adjustments or changes, should health departments wish to apply a community planning process to their STD prevention and control efforts. The practice of involving representatives of the groups for whom the programs are intended during the planning and implementation of these activities is especially demanding, given the time commitment involved and the fact that many of the community representatives may not have a technical background in the scientific issues being discussed.[135] Epidemiological, biomedical, and behavioral data must be translated from professional and scientific jargon into understandable, nontechnical terms.

When dealing with representatives from racial, ethnic, and other minority communities, it is especially important to address proactively barriers to participation, including mistrust of government and health authorities, resulting from a legacy of racism and other forms of discrimination. However, as reported by the National Alliance of State and Territorial AIDS Directors (NASTAD) in a survey of 55 of the 65 state, territorial, and local health departments that receive federal HIV prevention funds, by 1997, 27 percent of responding jurisdictions stated that their community planning groups were providing health departments with recommendations on STD prevention priorities as well as on HIV prevention priorities.[136] Fifty-one percent of the respondents indicated that the issue of coordinated HIV and STD prevention planning was of concern to their planning groups. This same report cited barriers to coordinated HIV and STD prevention planning that included separate bureaucratic structures for HIV and STD at both the state and federal levels; concerns about diversion of resources; and the time and resource intensity of the HIV Prevention Community Planning model.

Two leadership issues that are intimately related to planning and priority setting are targeting resources based on epidemiological data and creating incentives for innovation. These are both areas in which U.S. STD prevention efforts could be strengthened. For example, an internal CDC review of federally funded STD prevention programs conducted in 1996 revealed that about half reported little or no screening or health promotion to high risk groups outside of clinic facilities (S. Moses, personal communication). It was not until 1994 that federal resources were routinely provided on a competitive basis for pilot projects to evaluate locally relevant, innovative approaches to STD prevention. However, since it was established, this program, which requires local matching funds (one dollar of local resources for every two dollars of federal funds), has been highly successful in that it has demonstrated the feasibility and effectiveness of new approaches and has galvanized considerable local interest in STD control in several parts of the country.[137]

Particularly for STD prevention efforts, mobilizing vocal advocacy and effective communitywide participation is a pivotal leadership function. HIV advocates, primarily from the gay community, have been a driving force in every aspect of U.S. HIV prevention and research efforts. They have clearly contributed to the high visibility of HIV as an issue for policy makers and the general public. In contrast, the constituency for prevention of other STDs has been far more limited in number and influence, and STDs have rarely emerged "on the radar screen" for policy makers or the public at large.[20,138] At the federal, state, and local levels, there have been few proactive, strategic attempts to develop a broader constituency for STD prevention, in part because of regulations restricting government employees from activities that could be interpreted as lobbying. Fortunately, several important new governmental and nongovernmental groups have formed recently, including the National Coalition of STD Directors (consisting of directors of state STD prevention programs), the STD Prevention Partnership (consisting of representatives of more than 50 national organizations working in fields related to STD Prevention), and the National STD Action Forum (an intersectoral group convened to provide national leadership on STD prevention). These groups also reflect a growing synergy in leadership across STD, HIV, and pregnancy prevention efforts.

A particular leadership challenge of STD and HIV prevention systems at the end of the 20th century is the widespread adoption of managed health care delivery models and their potential to alter communicable disease control practices.[139,140] It is essential that STD/HIV prevention leadership develop strong and proactive relationships with managed care organizations "to optimize patient care and protection of the public health while minimizing cost."[140] These changes in the U.S. health care delivery system provide new opportunities for communitywide, population-oriented STD/HIV prevention efforts that crosscut public and private sectors.[141] Local public health and government leaders also have important roles to play in this relationship, especially in terms of negotiating relationships with managed care organizations that minimize cost-shifting from health plans to public health clinics.

Surveillance and Data Management. The sixth essential component of STD/HIV prevention programs, surveillance and data management, is critical in focusing and monitoring prevention activities. In the United States, national STD/HIV surveillance capacity ranges from a highly sophisticated and well-resourced AIDS surveillance system, through relatively strong, but far more limited syphilis and gonorrhea surveillance capabilities, to evolving, but still incomplete systems for HIV and chlamydia reporting.[24] As indicated, the most common STDs, genital herpes, genital HPV infection, and trichomoniasis, are not currently nationally notifiable. The routine collection of STD/HIV-related behavioral risk factor and health services data are beginning to receive increased attention as important parts of a comprehensive surveillance system.

Surveillance for AIDS has been in place in every U.S. jurisdiction since 1984, with local health departments collecting standard identifying information, source of exposure, opportunistic disease diagnoses, and other relevant information (e.g., CD4 count, date of HIV test). After HIV testing became possible in 1985, three states (Colorado, Minnesota, and Wisconsin) immediately made HIV infection reportable. As of 1998, 29 additional states have implemented this requirement; however, several of the states with the largest numbers of HIV-infected persons have not begun HIV reporting (e.g., California). Among those states with both HIV and AIDS case reporting, the discrepancies between HIV and AIDS trends are considerable and growing, as highly effective treatments to delay the onset of AIDS have become the standard of care, and have further uncoupled AIDS detection and reporting from initial HIV infection.[142,143] Because of these limitations, reliance on AIDS surveillance data alone is increasingly problematic for public health and community partners in planning how best to target prevention messages to those at highest risk for incident HIV infection.

In 1988, CDC supplemented AIDS surveillance with blinded HIV serosurveys to augment understanding of the spread of HIV using multiple convenience samples, including sentinel hospitals, STD clinics, tuberculosis clinics, drug treatment facilities, and women's clinics.[24] The most comprehensive and only population-based survey, the Survey of Childbearing Women, which was terminated in 1995, provided insights into HIV trends in the general population of women through blinded monitoring of newborns for maternal HIV antibodies. Additional HIV/AIDS data have been collected in many states through surveillance for HIV-related mortality and through other surveys, such as the Supplement HIV/AIDS Surveillance (SHAS), the adult AIDS Spectrum of Disease (ASD) studies, and HIV incidence studies. Finally, alternative HIV testing sites in some cities have routinely collected data on risk behaviors, self-reported STDs, and HIV serostatus for large numbers of persons presenting for HIV counseling and testing.[144,145] Using these data and applying "detuned" assays (less sensitive, thus able to recognize more recently infected persons who are seronegative on the detuned assay, but seropositive on the standard test) to stored sera from HIV seroconverters, may permit such HIV C/T sites to better estimate the movement of new HIV infections into new populations.[146] Thus, despite a lack of HIV reporting in many of the most heavily affected areas, arguably HIV/AIDS surveillance data are among the most comprehensive available for any disease of public health significance.

The infrastructure for surveillance of other STDs is much more limited at all levels and varies by disease. As of 1998, some line-listed syphilis data are reported electronically to CDC by most federally funded STD prevention programs, and the gap between reported incidence and the true incidence of P&S syphilis is probably small (see Table 90-3). Electronic, line-listed gonorrhea and chlamydia data, on the other hand, are reported by fewer programs, and probably represent roughly only one-half and one-sixth of the true burden for each of these diseases, respectively. Chlamydia reporting is compromised by the fact that routine screening is usually limited to women, and many symptomatic chlamydia-infected men are never reported because if they also have gonorrhea, they are treated for both STDs without chlamydia testing. The surveillance system that forms the foundation of national notifiable disease reporting may be particularly problematic for STDs because reporting for these stigmatizing diseases is far more complete from public clinics than from private providers. This reporting pattern biases the sociodemographic profile of reported STD rates and artificially inflates racial and ethnic differentials because poor or uninsured patients, a larger proportion of whom are African-American or Hispanic than Caucasian, tend to seek care from public facilities.[20,24,147] This basic STD surveillance system has been complemented by a strong sentinel surveillance system to monitor trends in gonococcal antibiotic resistance, by chlamydia prevalence monitoring in selected family planning clinics, by evolving efforts to monitor STD prevalence in jails and juvenile detention facilities, and by intermittent nationally representative, population-based surveys of HSV-2 seroprevalence (and potentially chlamydia prevalence in urine specimens).[23,29,30,148]

Several cross-cutting surveillance and data management challenges confront STD/HIV prevention programs. Behavioral risk factor surveillance is being developed through the addition of questions about STD/HIV risk behaviors to surveys such as CDC's Behavioral Risk Factor Surveillance System (BRFSS), the Youth Risk Behavior Surveillance System (YRBS), and the National Survey of Family Growth (NSFG).[149] Routine monitoring of STD/HIV care and prevention services has not yet progressed to a similar point, but awareness of its importance is growing, particularly in light of the tremendous changes that are occurring in the U.S. health care system. The advent of managed care, itself, has generated new opportunities to improve STD reporting from private providers, utilizing the excellent information systems that are in place in many large HMOs. Finally, technological advances in hardware and software are making feasible the development of integrated surveillance systems that ultimately may streamline the burden of disease reporting for state and local health departments, facilitate analyses across diseases, and permit linkages among morbidity, behavioral, and health services data.

Professional Training. Training and education of health care professionals and others involved in STD/HIV prevention in the skills needed for each of the essential prevention components is a prerequisite for any effective program or system. The caliber and reach of current training efforts define the quality and scope of future prevention efforts. Unfortunately, many aspects of current training efforts are far from optimal.

STD/HIV training in the United States has focused primarily on clinicians. Yet, even these efforts have fallen far short of the need. Of 127 U.S. and Canadian medical schools surveyed in 1981, 70 percent offered no STD clinical training to students and three-quarters provided no clinical experience to residents.[150] When STD rotations were offered, participation was low and students received an average of only 6 hours of instruction. A follow-up survey of 126 U.S. medical schools conducted in 1991 found that over the intervening decade, STD clinical training had increased in 77 percent of schools, decreased in 6 percent, and was unchanged in the remainder.[151] Nevertheless, only 37 percent of institutions offered students clinical electives in STDs or HIV/AIDS. The Institute of Medicine has noted that "inadequate professional training no doubt also contributes to the widespread tendency of clinicians to oversimplify and underestimate the importance of STDs."[20] One survey of family practitioners, gynecologists, and urologists in an urban setting found significant practice variations from recommended clinical management guidelines for vaginitis and pelvic inflammatory disease.[152] Even more disturbing are documented variations in mortality; a group of investigators from New York state found that among Medicaid-enrolled women, those women receiving HIV care in "high experience clinics" had a nearly 50 percent reduction in their relative hazard of death compared with women in "low experience clinics."[153]

Postgraduate care providers are often in need of STD training, and investigators have strived to meet these needs using alternatives to the traditional conference or training venues. A randomized controlled trial conducted among office-based primary care physicians demonstrated that mailed educational materials combined with an office visit by a simulated patient instructor, improved the recipient's performance of risk assessment and risk reduction counseling for STDs, including HIV infection.[154]

Although much of the published literature deals with STD training inadequacies in medical school, nursing school, and postgraduate settings, it should also be noted that public sector investments in STD training are likewise often inadequate. In 1993, when the Public Health Foundation measured expenditures for core public health functions in eight states, they found that training and education accounted for the lowest per capita investment of each of the 10 core functions assessed.[155] Furthermore, training is minimal in nonclinical areas such as community-based behavioral interventions, surveillance and program evaluation, and for other types of professionals, such as those working in community-based organizations.

Fortunately, there are some exceptions that provide examples of far-reaching, national efforts to improve the STD/HIV prevention and management skills of both practicing providers and those who are still in training. The regional AIDS Education and Training Centers supported by the Health Resources and Services Administration (HRSA) provide a national network to augment the skills of providers, particularly primary care providers, caring for persons living with HIV. CDC's regionalized network of ten STD/HIV Prevention Training Centers (PTCs) also focuses primarily on practicing clinicians and public health professionals. These PTCs provide education and training in the clinical diagnosis and management of STDs, individual and community-level behavioral interventions to promote risk reduction, and disease intervention activities such as partner notification. With the advent of managed care, and especially Medicaid managed care, the STD/HIV training needs of primary care providers have been thrown into relief. This has stimulated discussion of the potential role of public sector training networks, such as the ones outlined in the preceding, in working with health plans to improve the knowledge and skills of large numbers of private providers who do not perceive that their patients are at risk for these infections.

Two additional CDC training programs focus on health professionals who are currently in postgraduate fellowships or medical school, and attempt to strengthen linkages between academic institutions and public health departments. Each year, up to six postdoctoral STD Public Health Fellowships are awarded to individuals who plan to specialize in STD prevention research and practice. In recognition of the fact that many of the most effective STD prevention programs in the United States are grounded in close, formalized collaborations between health departments and university-based researchers, the goal of these fellowships is to create a cadre of STD experts who have the skills to forge health department-university links by serving in jointly appointed positions. The two-year university-based fellowships include training in clinical care, research, and public health program development through extended rotations with the state or local health department and with CDC in Atlanta. To expand the number of medical schools that are centers of excellence in STD training and research, and augment the STD training of graduating physicians who will *not* specialize in STDs or AIDS, CDC has also initiated an "STD Faculty Expansion Program." This program assures 5-year start-up support for junior faculty with STD expertise through a phased commitment of federal and university funds. It requires the participating medical school to increase the number of curriculum hours devoted to STDs, and mandates a joint appointment of the faculty member with the state or local health department.

Finally, a variety of STD/HIV training activities are publicly funded at the state and federal levels and target midlevel practitioners and program support staff. Among the most innovative of these efforts is the Graduate Certificate Training Program developed by CDC in collaboration with several nationally prominent academic centers. This program targets the existing and evolving skill base of program field staff (i.e., nonmedical staff who are responsible for various management and other functions in federally funded state and local prevention programs) and includes areas such as program planning and evaluation, health systems management, health policy analysis, community health promotion, epidemiology, information management, and communication skills.[156] The program is carried out through a combination of on-site and distance-based learning and could serve as a model for similar efforts targeting postgraduate providers of HIV and STD prevention and care services. However, it should be noted that there remain numerous opportunities to better coordinate STD/HIV training efforts across agencies and disciplines, including primary care and reproductive health. Even when they are exceptional in quality, current STD and HIV training efforts tend to be delivered along categorical lines.

Research and Evaluation. The final essential component of STD/HIV prevention programs, research and evaluation, is fundamental to sustaining high quality efforts that operate at the cutting edge of science-based practice and policy. Ironically, although the United States has developed one of the finest basic biomedical research capacities in the world, investments in applied research related to prevention programs have been limited. Resources for research on and evaluation of STDs other than HIV/AIDS have consistently been severely constrained (see Table 90-5). When applied epidemiological, behavioral, or health services research has been conducted, STD/HIV program staff have often not informed or participated in the process. Partially owing to resource constraints, research and, to a lesser extent, rigorous program evaluation are often viewed by program managers as sophisticated luxuries that compete with, rather than support, prevention activities. Finally, rapid and effective translation of research results into routine practice remains a tremendous challenge. Investigators in Wisconsin are currently examining several approaches to community-level HIV behavioral intervention "technology transfer" in a groundbreaking randomized controlled trial involving 75 AIDS service organizations in 44 states.[157]

Program evaluation capacity is even more limited than applied, program-relevant research capacity. Expertise and resources are thin at all levels in this area, and few training options are in place. Nevertheless, with the growing emphasis on accountability across public and private sectors, and methodological developments in evidence-based medicine, there is increased interest in performance measurement and program evaluation. At CDC, in 1999, updated STD Program Operations Guidelines will form the foundation for development of performance indicators through a collaborative process involving state and local partners. In addition, state and local health departments delivering HIV prevention services are being provided with detailed, new guidance and increased resources to improve their capacity to track budget expenditures at the client level and to implement outcome evaluation of their prevention activities. The HEDIS "report cards" used by health plan purchasers to assess the performance of managed care organizations have begun to reshape the thinking of many public health professionals about program evaluation. Conversely, the testing of a HEDIS chlamydia measure, as mentioned above, has been an influential first step in focusing private health plans on STD prevention issues.

FUTURE STD/HIV PREVENTION EFFORTS IN THE UNITED STATES

As was highlighted by the Institute of Medicine, the overarching challenge for U.S. STD prevention efforts and, to a lesser extent, HIV prevention efforts in the 21st century is the forging of a comprehensive, well-coordinated system that is seamless at the client level and utilizes a broad array of community resources.[20] Currently, the essential components of STD and HIV public sector programs are in place in most parts of the country, but vary tremendously in capacity. In many communities, these components must be strengthened, and better linked with each other and with the analogous components of other prevention programs, particularly those addressing pregnancy prevention, antenatal care, and substance abuse. Public health programs must become the coordinating focus for a coherent set of prevention activities that includes the active participation of private providers and nonhealth sectors, as outlined in Table 90-2. Research advances must be harnessed to move detection and treatment services out of clinics to community venues and to complement these clinical services with more widely available, science-based behavioral interventions. Finally, methodologically sound program evaluation must become a routine, high priority element of STD/HIV prevention efforts. This will require an explicit, ongoing resource and training commitment at all levels.

References

1 St. Louis ME et al: Conceptual framework for STD/HIV prevention and control, in *Sexually Transmitted Diseases*, 3rd ed, Holmes KK et al (eds). New York, McGraw-Hill, 1998.

2 May RM et al: Transmission dynamics of HIV infection. *Nature* 326: 137–142, 1987.

3 Wasserheit JN, Aral SO: The dynamic topology of sexually transmitted disease epidemics: Implications for prevention strategies. *J Infect Dis* 174 (suppl 2):S201–213, 1996.

4 Aral SO et al: Overview: Individual and population approaches to the epidemiology and prevention of sexually transmitted diseases and human immunodeficiency virus infection. *J Infect Dis* 174(suppl 2): S127–133, 1996.

5 Yorke JA et al: Dynamics and control of the transmission of gonorrhea. *Sex Transm Dis* 5:51–57, 1978.

6 Thomas JC et al: The development and use of the concept of a sexually transmitted disease core. *J Infect Dis* 174(suppl 2):S134–43, 1996.

7 Brunham RC et al: A general mode of sexually transmitted disease epidemiology and its implications for control. *Med Clin North Am* 74:1339–1352, 1990.

8 Brunham RC: Core group theory: A central concept in STD epidemiology. *Venereology* 10:28–31, 1997.

9 Stoner BP et al: Variation in frequency of sex partner change within sexually transmitted disease networks (abstract 5), in *Program and Abstracts of the 33rd Interscience Conference on Antimicrobial Agents and chemotherapy (New Orleans)*. Washington, DC: American Society for Microbiology, 1993.

10 Hook EW et al: Comparative behavioral epidemiology of gonococcal and chlamydial infections among patients attending a Baltimore, Maryland sexually transmitted disease clinic. *Am J Epidemiol* 136: 662–672, 1992.

11 Potterat JJ: "Socio-geographic space" and sexually transmissible diseases in the 1990s. *Today's Life Sci* December:16–31, 1992.

12 Rice RJ et al: Sociodemographic distribution of gonorrhea incidence: Implications for prevention and behavioral research. *Am J Pub Health* 81:1252–1258, 1991.

13 Potterat JJ et al: Gonorrhea as a social disease. *Sex Transm Dis* 12: 25–32, 1984.

14 Centers for Disease Control and Prevention. Gang-related outbreak of penicillinase-producing *Neisseria gonorrhoeae* and other sexually transmitted diseases—Colorado Springs, Colorado. 1989–1991. *Morb Mort Week Rep* 42:25–28, 1993.

15 Blanchard JF et al: The evolving epidemiology of chlamydial and gonococcal infections in response to control programs in Winnipeg, Canada. *Am J Pub Health* 1998, in press.

16 Centers for Disease Control: Guidelines for STD Control Program Operations. Atlanta, Centers for Disease Control, 1985.

17 Centers for Disease Control and Prevention: Program Guidance for Comprehensive STD Prevention Systems. Atlanta, Centers for Disease Control, 1998.
18 World Health Organization: *Control of Sexually Transmitted Diseases*. Geneva, Switzerland, World Health Organization, 1985.
19 Dallabetta GA et al: *Control of Sexually Transmitted Diseases: A Handbook for the Design and Management of Programs*. Arlington, Virginia, AIDSCAP/Family Health International, 1996.
20 Eng T et al: *The Hidden Epidemic: Confronting Sexually Transmitted Diseases*. Washington, DC, National Academy Press, 1997.
21 Centers for Disease Control: Ten leading nationally notifiable infectious diseases—United States, 1995. *Morb Mort Week Rep* 1996;45: 883–4.
22 Centers for Disease Control: Summary of notifiable diseases, United States 1996. *Morb Mort Week Rep* 45:1–87, 1997.
23 Division of STD Prevention: *Sexually Transmitted Disease Surveillance, 1997* .U.S. Department of Health and Human Services, Public Health Service. Atlanta: Centers for Disease Control and Prevention, 1998.
24 Ward JW et al: STD/HIV Surveillance, in *Sexually Transmitted Diseases*, 3rd ed, Holmes KK et al (eds). New York, McGraw-Hill, 1998.
25 Cates W Jr, ASHA Panel to Estimate STD Incidence and Cost: Incidence and prevalence of STD in the United States. *Sex Transm Dis*, in press.
26 Centers for Disease Control: *Primary and secondary* syphilis—United States, 1997. *Morb Mort Week Rep* 47:493–497, 1998.
27 St. Louis ME, Wasserheit JN: Elimination of syphilis in the United States. *Science* 281:353–354, 1998.
28 Centers for Disease Control and Prevention: *HIV/AIDS Surveillance Report* 9(2), 1997.
29 Mertz KJ et al: A pilot study of the prevalence of chlamydial infection in a national household survey. *Sex Transm Dis* 25:225–228, 1998.
30 Fleming DT et al: Herpes simplex virus type 2 in the United States, 1976 to 1994. *N Engl J Med* 337:1105–1111, 1997.
31 Cotch MF et al: Trichomonas vaginalis associated with low birth weight and preterm delivery. The vaginal infections and prematurity group. *Sex Transm Dis* 24(6):353–360, 1997.
32 Centers for Disease Control: *Chlamydia trachomatis* genital infections—United States, 1995. *Morb Mort Week Rep* 46:193–198, 1997.
33 Marrazzo JM et al: Performance and cost-effectiveness of selective screening criteria for *Chlamydia trachomatis* infection in women: Implications for a notional chlamydia control strategy. *Sex Transm Dis* 24(6):131–141, 1997.
34 Centers for Disease Control: 1998 Guidelines for Treatment of Sexually Transmitted Diseases. *Morb Mort Week Rep* 47(RR-1):1–116, 1998.
35 Staat MA et al: Susceptibility to vaccine-preventable diseases in a sexually transmitted disease clinic population. *Sex Transm Dis* 25(7): 331–334, 1998.
36 National Research Council, Panel on Monitoring the Social Impact of the AIDS Epidemic Staff: The Social Impact of AIDS in the United States. National Academy Press, 1993.
37 Skinner BF: *Beyond freedom and dignity*. New York, Bantam, 1972.
38 Fishbein M et al: Using information to change sexually transmitted disease-related behaviors: An analysis based on the theory of reasoned action, in *Research Issues in Human Behavior and Sexually Transmitted Diseases in the AIDS Era*, Wasserheit JN et al (eds). Washington, DC, American Society for Microbiology, 1991.
39 Expert Panel: *Interventions to Prevent HIV Risk Behaviors*. NIH Consensus Development Conference Statement 15(2)1–41, Feb 11–13, 1997.
40 Siegel M: Mass media antismoking campaigns: A powerful tool for health promotion. *Ann Intern Med* 129:128–132, 1998.
41 Dubois-Arber F et al: Increased condom use without other major changes in sexual behavior among the general population in Switzerland. *Am J Pub Health* 87:558–566, 1997.
42 Spira A et al: Cross-national comparisons of sexual behavior surveys-methodological difficulties and lessons for prevention (Editorial). *Am J Pub Health* 88(5):730–731, 1998.
43 Davis D: "Understanding AIDS"—the national AIDS mailer. *Pub Health Rep* 106(6):656–662, 1991.
44 Rotheram-Borus MJ: Annotation: HIV Prevention challenges—realistic strategies and early detection programs. *Am J Pub Health* 87(4):544–546, 1997.
45 Merson MH: Returning home: Reflections on the USA's response to the HIV/AIDS epidemic. *Lancet* 347:1673–1676, 1996.
46 Cotton P: US sticks head in the sand on AIDS prevention. *JAMA* 272(10):756–757, 1994.
47 *Messages that work: sexually transmitted diseases as a health issue*. New York, EDK Associates, 1998, in press.
48 Kirby D: School-based programs to reduce sexual risk-taking behaviors. *J School Health* 62(7):280–286, 1992.
49 DesJarlais DC: Harm reduction—a framework for incorporating science into drug policy (Editorial). *Am J Pub Health* 85:10–11, 1995.
50 Springer E: Effective AIDS prevention with active drug users: The human reduction model. *J Chem Depend Treat* 4(2):141–157, 1991.
51 Collins C, Stryker J: Should we teach only abstinence in sexuality education? Center for AIDS Prevention Studies, Fact sheet #30E, September 1997.
52 DiClemente RJ: Preventing sexually transmitted infections among adolescents: A clash of ideology and science. *JAMA* 279:1574–1575, 1998.
53 Jemmott JB et al: abstinence and safer sex HIV risk-reduction interventions for African-American adolescents: A randomized controlled trial. *JAMA* 279:1529–1536, 1998.
54 U. S. Congress: Welfare Reform Act (Pub law No. 104–193, section 510).
55 Hurley SF et al: Effectiveness of needle exchange programmes for prevention for HIV infection. *Lancet* 349:1797–1800, 1997.
56 Wren C: White House drug and AIDS advisers differ on needle exchange. *New York Times*, March 23, 1998.
57 Stolberg SG: President decides against financing needle programs. *The New York Times*, April 21, 1998.
58 Stone KM et al: Barrier methods for the prevention of sexually transmitted diseases, in *Sexually Transmitted Diseases*, 3rd ed, Holmes KK et al (eds). New York, McGraw-Hill, 1998.
59 Roper WL et al: Commentary: Condoms and HIV/STD prevention: Clarifying the message. *Am J Pub Health* 83:501–504, 1993.
60 Lowry DT et al: Prime time TV portrayals of sex, "safe sex" and AIDS: A longitudinal analysis. *Journalism Q* 70:628–637, 1993.
61 Michael RT et al: Private sexual behavior, public opinion, and public health policy related to sexually transmitted diseases: A US-British Comparison. *Am J Pub Health* 88:749–754, 1998.
62 Kamb ML et al: Quality assurance of HIV prevention counseling in a multicenter randomized controlled trial. *Pub Health Reports* 111 (suppl 1):99–107, 1996.
63 The National Institute of Mental Health (NIMH) Multisite HIV Prevention Trial Group: the NIMH Multisite HIV Prevention Trial: Reducing HIV Sexual Risk Behavior. *Science* 280;1889–1894, 1998.
64 Kelly JA et al: Randomized, controlled, community-level HIV prevention-intervention for sexual-risk behavior among homosexual men in US cities. *Lancet* 350:1500–1505, 1997.
65 O'Reilly KR et al: AIDS community demonstration projects for HIV prevention among hard-to-reach groups. *Pub Health Reports* 106: 714–720, 1991.
66 Centers for Disease Control and Prevention: Community-level prevention of human immunodeficiency virus infection among high-risk populations: The AIDS community demonstration projects. *Morb Mort Week Rep* 45:2–24, 1996.
67 Rietmeijer CA et al: Feasibility and yield of screening urine for chlamydia trachomatis by polymerase chain reaction among high-risk male youth in field-based and other nonclinic settings. *Sex Transm Dis* 24(7);429–435, 1997.
67a Marrazzo JM et al: Community-based urine screening for *Chlamydia trachomatis* with a ligase chain reaction assay. *Ann Intern Med* 127: 796–803, 1997.

68 Expert Panel: Effective medical treatment of heroine addiction. NIH Consensus Statement Nov 17–19; 15(6), 1997.
69 Roffman RA et al: Relapse prevention as an interventive model for HIV risk-reduction in gay and bisexual men. *AIDS Educ Prev* 10:1–18, 1998.
70 Roffman RA et al: Cognitive-behavioral group counseling to prevent HIV transmission in gay and bisexual men: Factors contributing to successful risk reduction. *Res Soc Work Pract* 7:165–186, 1997.
71 Roffman RA et al: HIV prevention group counseling delivered by telephone: An efficacy trial with gay and bisexual men. *AIDS Behav* 1:137–154, 1997.
72 Cohen DA et al: A school-based chlamydia control program using DNA amplification technology. *Pediatrics* 1:101(1), 1998.
73 STD Diagnostic Initiative reference
74 Britton TF et al: STDs and family planning Clinics: A regional program for chlamydia control that works. *Am J GYN Health* VI(3): 24–31, 1992.
75 Hillis S et al: New opportunities for chlamydia prevention: Applications of science to public health practice. *Sex Transm Dis* 22(3):197–202, 1995.
76 Hillis S et al: Screening for chlamydia—a key to the prevention of pelvic inflammatory disease (Editorial). *N Engl J Med* 34(21):1399–1401, 1996.
77 Scholes D et al: Prevention of pelvic inflammatory disease by screening for cervical chalmydial infection. *N Engl J Med* 334(21):1362–1366, 1996.
78 Harris JR et al: Measuring the public's health in an era of accountability: Lessons from HEDIS. *AM J Prev Med* 14(3S);9–13, 1998.
79 McGlynn EA et al: Developing a clinical performance measure. *Am J Prev Med* 14(3S):14–21, 1998.
80 Landry DJ, Forrest JD: Public health departments providing sexually transmitted disease services. *Fam Plan Perspect* 28:261–266, 1996.
81 Liebow EB et al: Syphilis in the South: A case study assessment in eight southern communities (Final report). Battelle Centers for Public Health Research and Evaluation, April 28, 1997.
82 Centers for Disease Control and Prevention. Assessment of sexually transmitted diseases services in city and county jails—United States, 1997. *Morb Mort Week Rep* 47(21):429–431, 1998.
83 Hammett TM: National Institute of Justice, Centers for Disease Control and Prevention: Research in Brief: Public health/corrections collaborations: Prevention and treatment of HIV/AIDS, STDs, and TB, July 1998.
84 Valdiserri RO: Managing system wide change in HIV prevention programs. *Pub Admin Rev* 56(6):545–553, 1996.
85 Francis DP et al: Targeting AIDS prevention and treatment toward HIV-1-infected persons: The concept of early intervention. *JAMA* 262(18):2572–2576, 1989.
86 Centers for Disease Control and Prevention: CLIA Compliance and Phlebotomy Assessment. Unpublished survey of the impact on clinical services in prevention programs of the 1988 Clinical Laboratory Improvement Act.
87 Spencer JN et al: Cost comparison of alternatively structured STD and HIV prevention programs in the US (Abstract #13288), in *Conference Record of the 12th World AIDS Conference (Geneva)*, June 28–July 3, 1998, p 143.
88 Centers for Disease Control and Prevention: HIV prevention through early detection and treatment of other sexually transmitted diseases—United States. *Morb Mort Week Rep* 47(RR-12):1–24, 1998.
89 Centers for Disease Control: HIV counseling and testing services from public and private providers—US, 1990. *Morb Mort Week Rep* 41(40):743–752, Oct 9, 1992.
90 Family Planning Perspectives, Jan. 1999, in press.
91 Hellinger FJ: Forecasts of the costs of medical care for persons with HIV: 1992–1995. *Inquiry* 29(3):356–365, 1992.
92 Bozzette S et al: Characteristics of HIV infected patients receiving regular care in the U.S.: Results from the HIV cost and services utilization (HCSUS). International conference on AIDS 1998; 12:131 (Abstract #13229).
93 Rabin DL et al: Improving office-based physicians' prevention practices for sexually transmitted diseases. *Ann Intern Med* 121:513–519, 1994.
94 Centers for Disease Control: HIV prevention practices of primary-care physicians—United States, 1992. *Morb Mort Week Rep* (January 7) 42:988–992, 1994.
95 ABT survey.
96 Kaiser Family Foundation/Glamour National Survey on STDs: Talking about STDs with health professionals: Women's experiences, 1997.
97 Hessol NA et al: Management of pelvic inflammatory disease by primary care physicians. A comparison with Centers for Disease Control and Prevention guidelines. *Sex Transm Dis* 23(2):157–163, 1996.
98 Kimball AM et al: The impact of health care market changes on local decision making and STD care: Experience in three counties. *Am J Prev Med* 13(suppl):75–84. 1997, Nov–Dec.
99 Cowan FM et al: The role and effectiveness of partner notification in STD control: A review. *Genitourin Med* 72(4):247–252, 1996.
100 Potteratt JJ et al: Partner notification early in the AIDS Era: Misconstruing contact tracers as bedroom police. *Res Soc Pol* 6:1–15, 1998.
101 West GR, Stark KA: Partner notification for HIV prevention: A critical review. *AIDS Edu Prev* 9 (suppl):68 –78, 1997.
102 Rothenberg R et al: Partner notification for STD/HIV, in *Sexually Transmitted Diseases*, 3rd ed, Holmes KK et al (eds). New York, McGraw-Hill, 1998.
103 Bayer R, Toomey KE: HIV prevention and the two faces of partner notification. *Am J Pub Health* 82(8):1158–1164, 1992.
104 Oxman AD et al: Partner notification for sexually transmitted diseases: An overview of the evidence. *Can J Pub Health* 85(suppl 1): S41–47, 1994.
105 Andersen B et al: Home sampling versus conventional contact tracing for detecting chlamydia trachomatis infection in male partners of infected women: Randomised study. *Br Med J* 316(7128):350–351, 1998.
106 Fenton KA, Peterman TA: HIV partner notification: Taking a new look *AIDS* 11:1535–1546, 1997.
107 Makadon HJ, Silin JG: Prevention of HIV infection in primary care: Current practices, future possibilities. *Ann Intern Med* 123(9):715–719, 1995.
108 Giesecke J et al: Efficacy of partner notification of HIV infection. *Lancet* 338:1096 1100, 1991.
109 Rutherford GW et al: Partner notification and the control of human immunodeficiency virus infection. Two years experience in San Francisco. *Sex Transm Dis* 18:107–110, 1991.
110 Wykoff RF et al: Contact tracing to identify human immunodeficiency virus infection in a rural community. *JAMA* 259:3563–3566, 1988.
111 Pavia AT et al: Partner notification for control of HIV: Results after 2 years of a statewide programme in Utah. *Am J Pub Health* 83: 1418–1424, 1993.
112 Pattman RS, Gould EM: Partner notification for HIV infection in the United Kingdom: A look back on seven years experience in Newcastle upon Tyne. *Genitourin Med* 69:94–97, 1993.
113 Wells KD, Hoff GL: Human immunodeficiency virus partner notification in a low incidence urban community. *Sex Transm Dis* 22:377–379, 1995.
114 Marks C et al: HIV-infected men's practices in notifying past sexual partners of infection risk. *Pub Health Rep* 107:100–103, 1992.
115 Rothenberg KH, Paskey SJ: The risk of domestic violence and women with HIV infection: Implications for partner notification, public policy, and the law. *Am J Pub Health* 85:1569–1546, 1995.
116 Giesecke J et al: Partner notification for HIV in Sweden (letter). *Lancet* 366:508, 1990.
117 Jacquez JA et al: Role of primary infection in epidemics of HIV infection in gay cohorts. *J Acq Immune Def Syndr* 7:1169–1184, 1994.
118 Schacker T et al: Clinical and epidemiologic features of primary HIV infection. *Ann Int Med* 125(4): 257–264, 1996.
119 Koopman JS et al: The role of early HIV infection in the spread of HIV through populations. *J Acq Im Def Synd Hum Retrovirol* 14(3): 249–258, 1997.

120 Landis S et al: Results of a randomized trial of partner notification in cases of HIV infection in North Carolina. *N Engl J Med* 326:101–106, 1992.

121 Katz BP et al: Efficiency and cost-effectiveness of field follow-up for patient with chlamydia trachomatis infection in a sexually transmitted diseases clinic. *Sex Transm Dis* 15:11–16, 1998.

122 Ramstedt K et al: Contact tracing for human immunodeficiency virus (HIV) infection. *Sex Transm Dis* 17:47–51, 1990.

123 Jones JL et al: Partner acceptance of health department notification of HIV exposure, South Carolina. *JAMA* 264:1284–1286, 1990.

124 Finelli L et al: Epidemiologic support to state and local sexually transmitted disease control programs. Perceived need and availability. The Field Epidemiology Network for STDs (FENS). *Sex Transm Dis* 25(3):132–136, 1998.

125 CDC's Report to congress on syphilis elimination.

126 Wypijewski J: The Secret Sharer: Sex, race and denial in an American small town. *Harper's Magazine*, 1998.

127 Altman LK: Sex, privacy and tracking HIV infections. *The New York Times,* Nov 4, 1997.

128 State of New York: Title III, Human immunodeficiency virus, Section 2130. AIDS and HIV infection; duty to report. 4422-B, Cal No. 337, 97–98 regular session in Senate, April 11, 1997.

129 Kotter JP: *Leading Change.* Boston, Harvard Business School Press, 1996.

130 Merrill MH: Responsibility of public health in a program for syphilis eradication, in U.S. Department of Health, Education, and Welfare, Public Health Service. *Proceedings of the World Forum on Syphilis and other Treponematoses.* Washington, DC, September 1962, pp 45–50.

131 Centers for Disease Control: CDC: Forty years of prevention. *Dateline: CDC* 18(5, Rev), 1986.

132 Valdiserri RO et al: Community planning: A national strategy to improve HIV prevention programs. *J Comm Health* 20:87–100, 1995.

133 United States Conference of Mayors: *HIV Prevention Community Planning Profiles: Assessing the Impact.* Washington, DC, 1996.

134 Valdiserri RO et al: Determining allocations for HIV-prevention interventions: Assessing a change in federal funding policy. *AIDS Pub Pol* 12(4):138–148, 1997.

135 Haviland ML: The enduring myth of power to the people: Community participation in public health. *Curr Issues Pub Health* 1:156–159, 1995.

136 National Alliance of State and Territorial AIDS Directors: *Community Planning and Prevention: 1997 Status Report.* Washington, DC, October 1997.

137 DeLisle S, Wasserheit JN: Accelerated campaign to enhance STD services (ACCESS) for youth: Successes, challenges and lessons learned. (Prepared for Kaiser Family Foundation, STD Forum: Conspiracy to Innovate, Menlo Park, CA, 1998) *Sex Transm Dis,* in press.

138 *In search of a public conversation about STDs: Getting beyond denial.* New York, EDK Associates, 1998.

139 Association of Territorial Health Officials: *Introduction to Managed Care for State Health Agencies.* Washington DC, November 1995.

140 Association of State and Territorial Health Officials: *Communicable Disease Control in a Managed Care Environment.* Washington, DC, November 1995.

141 Gunn RA et al: The changing paradigm of sexually transmitted disease control in the era of managed health care. *JAMA* 279(9):680–684, 1998.

142 Centers for Disease Control and Prevention: Diagnosis and reporting of HIV and AIDS in states with integrated HIV and AIDS surveillance—United States, January 1994–June 1997. *Morb Mort Week Rep* 45(15):309–314, 1998.

143 Carpenter et al: Antiretroviral therapy for HIV infection in 1996: Recommendations of an international panel. *JAMA* 276:146–154, 1996.

144 Wood RW et al: HIV Transmission: Womens' risk from bisexual men. *Am J Pub Health* 83:1757–1759, 1993.

145 Goldbaum G et al: Changes at an HIV testing clinic in the prevalence of unsafe sexual behavior among men who have sex with men. *Sex Transm Dis* 23:109–113, 1996.

146 Janssen RS et al: New testing strategy to detect early HIV-1 infection for use in incidence estimates and for clinical and prevention purposes. *JAMA* 280(1):42–48, 1998.

147 Anderson JE et al: Factors associated with self-reported STDs: Data from a national survey. *Sex Transm Dis* 21(6):303–308, 1994.

148 Fox KK et al: Antimicrobial resistance in *Neisseria gonorrhoeae* in the United States, 1988–1994: The emergence of decreased susceptibility to the fluoroquinolones. *J Infect Dis* 175:1396–1403, 1997.

149 Centers for Disease Control and Prevention: Youth risk behavior surveillance—United States, 1997. *Morb Mort Week Rep* (47 SS-3):1–89, 1998.

150 Stamm WE et al: Clinical training in venereology in the United States and Canada. *JAMA* 248(16):2020–2024, 1982.

151 MacKay et al: Survey of clinical training in STD and HIV/AIDS in the United States. *Proceedings of the IDSA Annual Meeting*; September 16–18, 1995, San Francisco (abstract no. 281).

152 Sellors JW et al: Factors associated with appropriate physician management of sexually transmitted diseases in an urban Canadian center. *Sex Tranms Dis* 24:393–397, 1997.

153 Laine C et al: The relationships of clinic experience with advanced HIV and survival of women with AIDS. *AIDS* 12:417–424, 1998.

154 Rabin DL et al: Improving office-based physicians' prevention practices for sexually transmitted diseases. *Ann Intern Med* 121:513–519, 1994.

155 Public Health Foundation: Measuring state expenditures for core public health functions. *Am J Prev Med* 11 (suppl 2):58–73, 1995.

156 *Proceedings of the Government Learning Technology Symposium.* Washington DC, January 21–22, 14–19, 1998.

157 Kelly JA et al: Bridging the gap between science and service: A randomized trial of technical assistance methods to transfer research-based HIV prevention approaches to CBOs. Presented at the global program on AIDS, Geneva, Switzerland, July 1998.

Chapter 91

Sexually transmitted disease and reproductive health clinical services: Categorical clinics and integrated programs

Edward W. Hook, III
Jacqueline E. Darroch
David Landry
David Mabey

Ideally, all facets of health care, especially prevention-related services, should be available to all clients from single providers or from well-integrated groups with broad capacities and abilities. Such services could provide males and females with fully integrated reproductive health care that would be beneficial for clients in addressing multiple needs and beneficial for providers because of the efficiencies in provision of care, record keeping, and resource allocation. In fact, however, despite the variety of systems that have evolved to deliver health care, reproductive health services, including clinical and prevention services for sexually transmitted diseases (STDs), are often provided by specialized clinics that focus primarily on STD- or family planning–related services.

In terms of efficiency, there are a number of potential benefits to integration of reproductive health care services. Areas of potential overlap between family planning and STD clinical services include the following: that risks addressed by the two (unintended pregnancy and STDs) covary and are each unintended consequences of sexual activity; that both disciplines are focused primarily on the reproductive tract, with care often requiring pelvic examination for women; that risks for both unplanned pregnancy and STDs are most common in the unmarried, who typically are young; and that risk for nearly every STD or STD complication is modified by contraceptive measures (see Chap. 94).

Yet publicly funded clinics providing STD and family planning services usually have evolved separately to reflect their different origins, different primary subject emphasis, different gender distribution of patient populations, different sources of funding, and different social pressures (e.g., STD-related stigma, concerns about teen pregnancy, controversy over abortion). In the past 15 to 20 years, increasing appreciation of the substantial overlap in populations at risk for STDs and unplanned pregnancy, as well as the numerous interactions between contraceptive measures and STD risk, has led to increased discussion and efforts to better integrate these and other types of clinical care. Emerging from the International Conference on Population and Development held in Cairo, Egypt, in 1994, the Cairo Agenda has redirected focus for women's health from contraception to a broader view of reproductive health (including prevention and management of STDs).[1] In addition, in the United States, in part due to actual and anticipated changes in health care financing and delivery, experts who traditionally focused on STDs or on family planning have increasingly begun to interact and collaborate.

Systems for provision of STD and other reproductive health care worldwide also have evolved to address local needs and priorities and to complement other available health services. Consequently, there are nearly as many different variations on provision of publicly funded reproductive health care as there are health care models. Thus clear, comprehensive descriptions of how STD, family planning, or general reproductive health care is provided are not available. Finally, no single model is likely to be optimal for all settings. Within countries, the scope of services may vary from clinic to clinic based on differences in local needs and resources.

This chapter will examine current provision of reproductive health care in categorical STD and family planning clinics in the United States, describe examples of the categorical STD services provided in other developed nations, and briefly describe examples of STD care and interventions carried on in developing nations. Finally, the chapter will attempt to discuss potential benefits and limitations of efforts to more fully integrate all aspects of reproductive health care for men and women.

THE UNITED STATES

In the United States, health care needs and opportunities differ for men and for women. For women, the concept of regular visits to health care providers for reproductive health services such as Papanicolaou (PAP) smear screening is often tied to medical contraceptives such as the pill, while there are few analogous links for men. As a result, opportunities for STD screening are more common for women. Similarly, symptomatic women generally have more potential locations for seeking evaluation and care than men with genitourinary symptoms. In 1988, although the proportion of women seeking health care of any sort was unclear, data from the National Survey of Family Growth indicated that 26 percent of sexually active women of reproductive age reported being tested for an STD.[2] This estimate is likely to be conservative. Many women are unaware that STD screening is sometimes a part of their routine reproductive health care. Conversely, some (albeit probably fewer) women may assume that they were comprehensively tested for STDs when, in fact, they were not or were tested for only one or two.[3,4] Of those who reported being tested, the majority (55 percent) were tested at the time of family planning visits.[2] Reported testing was higher for women attending family planning clinics (54 percent) than for women who had family planning visits with private doctors (34 percent) or for women who reported no family planning visits (16 percent). While similar data on the prevalence of STD testing for males is lacking, it is clear that there is less emphasis on routine STD screening for males and that there are fewer facilities other than STD clinics where routine testing for men is likely to be performed.

STD CLINICS

In the United States, current systems for provision of STD care evolved out of publicly funded syphilis treatment clinics[5] that were developed, in part, to provide weekly therapeutic injections for syphilis in the prepenicillin era. These units operated nationwide through public health departments to provide therapy and surveillance figures that could be assembled to provide national data. In addition, public health officials often worked out of these clinics to coordinate and carry out other syphilis intervention strategies such as screening and partner notification/management. In the 1960s, early syphilis had become less common, and a federally funded gonorrhea control campaign, which utilized many of the same control strategies (free, observed treatment; free STD screening, partner notification, and management), led to development of more comprehensive, public health department–operated STD clinics, the services of which have expanded further in recent years to address management of a broader spectrum of STDs. Such clinics see higher proportions of men than women, attempt to see clients on relatively short notice, primarily provide clinical management for symptomatic patients, and tend to emphasize diagnostic testing and treatment for bacterial STDs such as gonorrhea (*Neisseria gonorrhoeae*), chlamydia (*Chlamydia trachomatis*), syphilis (*Treponema pallidum*), and chancroid (*Haemophilus ducreyi*).

In the United States, over 4,000 STD clinical services sites other than physician offices have been identified.[6] These include health department clinics, family planning clinics, student health centers, and hospitals. In 1995, a sample survey of 587 local health departments found that specialized STD clinics are almost uniformly present in large and medium-sized cities as well as in most smaller communities. The care provided is often influenced by local factors such as population size, density, and available resources. About half (49 percent) of local health departments providing STD clinical services offered both dedicated STD management sessions and sessions where STD services were integrated with other services (most often family planning).[6] In another 37 percent of health departments, STD sessions were always integrated into other clinic services, whereas in the final 14 percent, STD services were only provided in the context of dedicated clinic sessions.[6] These clinics are generally open during business hours, 5 days weekly, with little after-hours (23 percent of clinics) or weekend (5 percent of clinics) care (Fig. 91–1). In these clinics, STD services were reported to be available from 61 percent of health departments on the same day that clients contact the service site, whereas 24 percent indicated that it would take 1 to 2 days, and 15 percent, 3 or more days, before being seen for STD diagnosis and treatment.[6] Four percent indicated that clients would need to wait 6 or more days in order to obtain STD diagnosis and treatment.

The spectrum of services provided by such clinics varies substantially, based on factors such as the availability of funding, local demand for services, and whether or not the clinics are associated with university-based teaching or research programs. At a minimum, however, they serve as local centers for management and reporting of gonorrhea and syphilis. In general, dedicated, publicly funded STD clinics attempt to provide low-cost (or free) STD-related health care on a walk-in or same-day appointment basis and emphasize risk-based, syndromic management and rapid (where possible, observed), single-dose therapy for bacterial STDs. Consistent with the focus on bacterial STDs, over 80 percent of public health laboratories supporting these clinics offer etiologic (e.g., culture or nonculture) testing for *N. gonorrhoeae* and syphilis serologic testing, whereas about 71 percent provide diagnostic testing for *C. trachomatis* for at least some patients.[7] Testing and therapy for viral STDs such as genital herpes or human papillomavirus infections are less readily available and more variable from clinic to clinic than for management of bacterial STDs.

Both because bacterial STDs are more common in socially or financially disadvantaged minority groups and because reporting of STD morbidity is more complete from public clinics than from private health care providers, patients attending public STD clin-

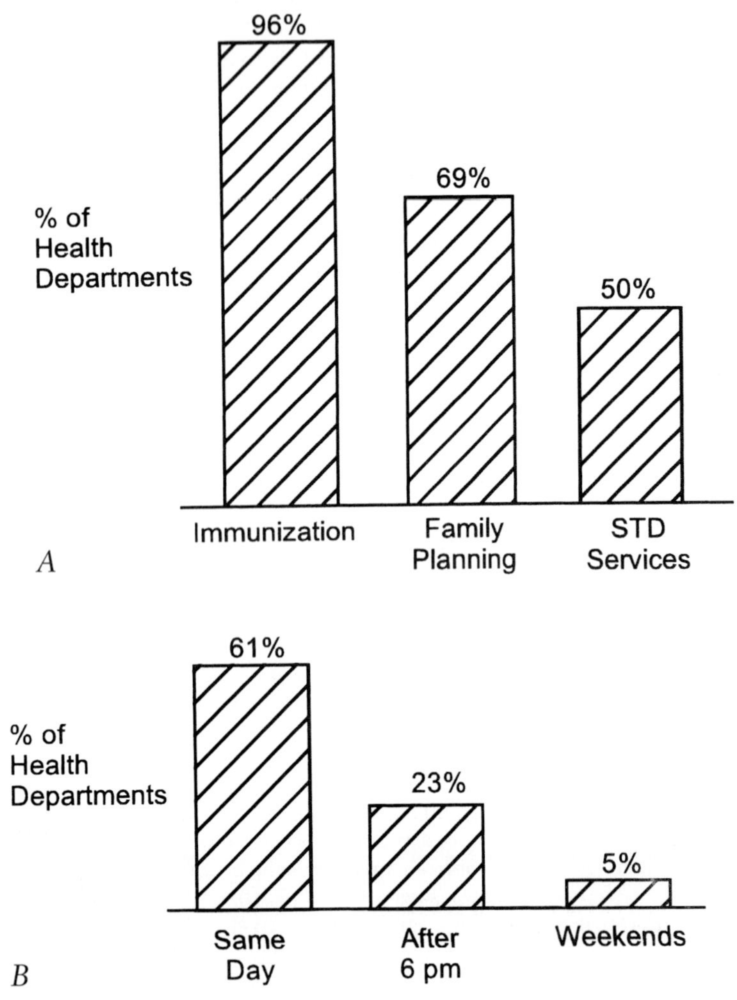

Fig. 91-1. In 1995, a sample survey of 587 local health departments found that specialized STD clinics are almost uniformly present in large and medium-sized cities. *A*. Graph of services provided on-site and *B*. timing for provision of clinical services.

ics (and therefore racial and social minority groups) are disproportionately represented in reported STD morbidity. In a recent survey, those receiving STD services from public health clinics are disproportionately young (36 percent less than 20 years of age and only 15 percent over age 30) members of racial/ethnic minorities (34 percent African Americans, 9 percent Hispanic) with limited financial resources (45 percent with incomes below the official poverty level and 38 percent between 100 and 200 percent of poverty)[6] (Table 91–1). A majority (60 percent) of persons receiving STD services at health departments were female; agencies providing sessions solely devoted to STDs had the lowest proportion (46 percent) of female clients as compared with health departments that offered both separate and integrated STD sessions (59 percent females) or only provided STD care in sessions integrated with other services such as family planning or maternal and child health (69 percent female).

The proportion of reported U.S. STD morbidity generated by STD clinics also varies from disease to disease. In 1995, 69 percent of reported primary and secondary syphilis, 54 percent of gonorrhea, and 28.6 percent of *C. trachomatis* infections reported to the Centers for Disease Control and Prevention were recorded by public STD clinics. The proportions of infections detected in STD clinics also vary by gender. For each disease listed above, STD clinics generated a higher proportion of all reported infections in males than in females. In 1995, for males 73.1 percent primary and secondary syphilis, 66 percent of gonorrhea, and 46 percent of chlamydia cases were reported by STD clinics as compared with 64.9, 40.4, and 27.5 percent of the same diseases, respectively, in women.[8]

A recent survey conducted in five urban STD clinics (Birmingham, Alabama; St. Paul, Minnesota; San Francisco, California; Seattle, Washington; and Raleigh, North Carolina) provides data on selected demographic characteristics and STD morbidity typically seen in large, urban, university-affiliated U.S. STD clinics.[9] Patients attending these five clinics predominantly attended the clinics for symptom evaluation (Table 91–2). In addition, despite substantial variation in the prevalence of specific diseases across sites, overall, 75 percent of participants were diagnosed with at least one STD at their clinic visit[9] as compared with 57 percent among all health departments that provide STD services.[6] Thus patients attending publicly funded STD clinics are not representative of the larger U.S. population but use STD services because they are at increased risk and have a higher prevalence of STDs.

Despite their relatively young age, clients attending publicly funded STD clinics in the United States tend to have a number of health care needs. Many have other health risks and needs such as illegal drug use, failure to use contraception effectively, and increased risks for tuberculosis, hepatitis B, cervical cancer, and human immunodeficiency virus (HIV) infection.[10–15] While efforts to expand the scope of services in dedicated STD clinics are by no means universal, in a number of instances STD programs have chosen to broaden their scope of services to address these unmet health care needs for their clients.

Among women attending dedicated STD clinics, a particularly common problem is that a significantly higher proportion than in the general population are not practicing effective family planning to reduce their risk for unplanned pregnancy.[10] Despite the numerous parallels and the fact that public funding partially supports both types of service, funding streams are largely separate, and each service has its own advocates and infrastructure. Thus only recently have administrators of STD control programs begun to invest in family planning or, conversely, have family planning providers begun to emphasize STD diagnosis and management.[16] The most clear-cut example of the benefits of STD screening in family planning clinics is the highly successful national STD-related Infertility Prevention Program, which supports chlamydia screening.[17] There have been fewer, less well documented instances of provision of noncondom family planning services in STD clinics. Clearly, however, without such integration, many health care opportunities are missed. For instance, data from a Baltimore, Maryland, STD clinic demonstrated that only 17 percent of patients who were not practicing family planning at the time of STD clinic attendance and who stated that they were interested in pursuing the opportunity to obtain family planning services actually kept referral appointments at family planning clinics.[10]

Almost all (98 percent) health departments providing STD ser-

Table 91-1. Percentage Distribution of STD Clients' Demographic Characteristics by Type of STD Clinic Session Integration

Demographic Characteristic	Total	STD Clinic Session Integration: Separate	Mixed	Integrated
Total	100.0	14.0	48.7	37.3
Percent of visits	100.0	37.1	52.0	10.0
Age (years)				
<15	2.9	2.2	3.5	2.5
15–17	13.3	10.9	13.4	14.3
18–19	19.4	16.1	19.9	20.2
20–24	29.5	29.0	29.3	30.0
25–29	20.1	21.4	19.1	20.7
>29	14.8	20.4	14.8	12.3
Total	100.0	100.0	100.0	100.0
Sex				
Female	60.4	46.4	59.3	68.0
Male	39.6	53.6	40.7	32.0
Total	100.0	100.0	100.0	100.0
Poverty status				
<100% of poverty	45.4	41.9	42.8	49.2
100–249% of poverty	37.5	39.4	39.7	34.5
250%+ of poverty	17.1	18.7	17.5	16.3
Total	100.0	100.0	100.0	100.0
Race/ethnicity				
Non-Hispanic white	55.0	50.5	50.5	62.9
Hispanic	8.7	11.1	8.9	7.4
Non-Hispanic black	34.5	36.4	38.2	28.8
Non-Hispanic other	1.8	2.0	2.4	0.9
Total	100.0	100.0	100.0	100.0

Table 91-2. Selected Characteristics of Clients Attending Five Urban U.S. STD Clinics

	Percent	Range
Age ≤25 years	51	30–72%
Race/ethnicity		
White	36	8–55%
African American	48	23–92%
Hispanic	5	0–15%
Other	11	0–20%
Unemployed	43	28–52%
Insurance status		
Uninsured	58	44–73%
Medicaid	14	7–18%
Private	27	18–38%
Reason for clinic attendance		
Symptoms	63	51–71%
Contact to partner with STD	18	13–21%
STD screening/checkup	17	15–19%
Other	16	5–32%

vices distribute male condoms, whereas about three-quarters offer oral contraceptives, spermicides, and other methods in at least some sites providing STD care.[6] Agencies that provide STD care in separate sessions are unlikely to offer methods other than condoms to clients. For example, only 22 percent provide oral contraceptives as compared with 80 to 88 percent of agencies where STD management is sometimes or always offered together with services such as family planning.[6]

In a number of instances, local health departments have initiated pilot projects to explore the feasibility of expanding the scope of services offered by STD clinics. In each instance, these projects represent a locally derived response to perceived needs. With regard to contraceptive measures other than condoms, in some clinics, noncontracepting women are provided with several-month "starter packs" of oral contraceptive pills and referred to local family planning services. In a more ambitious pilot project conducted in Baltimore's STD clinics, clients who were not currently contracepting were offered free contraceptive supplies (oral contraceptive pills, diaphragms, spermicides, condoms; intrauterine devices were not recommended for this high-risk population, and injectable contraceptives were not fully available) and follow-up in the STD clinic. The specific aims of this pilot project were to provide both effective contraceptive care and increased STD screening opportunities for high-risk women, as well as to promote use of reversible contraceptive measures that would reduce risk for STD acquisition (alone or in combination with the oral contraceptive pill). Overall, cumulative follow-up rates in this project were comparable with rates for local, dedicated family planning clinics (approximately 53 percent), and over 80 percent of clients at least expressed an interest in utilizing dual methods of contraception. In addition, the project did prove to provide STD screening opportunities for a group at high risk of STD acquisition. In 147 (22.7 percent) of 648 follow-up visits, new, treatable STDs were diagnosed. The success of this project has led the Baltimore City Health Department to continue provision of contraceptive care and follow-up for a subset of women seen in its STD clinics.

Similarly, U.S. STD clinics have become an important focus of counseling and testing for HIV infection. Patients with STDs have clearly been identified as being at increased risk for both prevalent and incident HIV infections.[11,14] In addition HIV-infected patients identified in STD clinics often have little or no health insurance yet have infections that have progressed to the point where therapy is recommended.[18] HIV and STD services are integrated in 74 percent of health departments that provide STD care, separately administered in 21 percent, and there are no HIV services in 5 percent.[6]

In response to such needs, some U.S. STD control programs have begun to expand their services to include at least some HIV staging and/or management. In some clinics, initial assessments such as determination of CD4 lymphocyte concentrations and tuberculosis skin testing are provided for patients found to be HIV-seropositive, and in a few, initial provision of antiretroviral therapy is also available[12,13] (C. Celum, Seattle–King County Health Department, personal communication). The benefits of provision of HIV-related management in STD clinics may go beyond the benefits for individual patients themselves and contribute to reduction of likelihood of spread of HIV within communities. For instance, a number of studies have shown that coexistent STDs may potentiate HIV shedding and hence transmission of HIV to uninfected individuals. Thus STD diagnosis and provision of therapy for the up to 15 percent yearly incidence of new STDs among HIV-infected individuals seen in STD clinics[13,15,19] may reduce their likelihood of transmitting HIV to sexual partners. While there are few data to suggest that the limited posttest counseling provided for patients found to be HIV-seropositive through STD clinic-based screening reduces risk for STD acquisition (a sentinel event indicating continued high-risk behavior), more comprehensive continuing care may accomplish this goal. In Baltimore, analysis of gonorrhea incidence in patients enrolled in the Health Department's STD clinic-based HIV early intervention program indicates that continued behavioral counseling provided in the context of the program may have contributed to a reduction in gonorrhea incidence as well as increased screening and treatment opportunities.[13] More recently, however, as management of HIV infection has evolved to include viral-load determinations and polydrug therapy for HIV infection, STD programs providing such services have begun to reevaluate their ability to provide HIV management (J. Zenilman, C. Celum, personal communication).

FAMILY PLANNING AGENCIES AND CLINICS

In the United States, a system of family planning clinics originated and evolved separately from the publicly funded, specialized STD clinics described above. In the 1930s and 1940s, there were a small number of clinics that were privately owned, organized, and operated. In the 1960s, as new medical contraceptives such as the oral contraceptive pill and the intrauterine device (IUD) became available, the numbers of clinics increased. In the 1970s, major federal funding for family planning services became available through Title X of the Public Health Service Act, leading to expansion of existing organizations, creation of new organizations, and development of free or subsidized family planning clinics in public health departments. Influenced by funding that focused on family planning and reproductive health for women and operating in an environment where agencies were competing for available funds, these clinics have emphasized provision of reversible contraception for women. In general, family planning clinics are designed to provide long-term care with infrequent but periodically scheduled visits and client-centered, nondirective service emphasizing choice of contraceptive methods and client counseling and education to promote effective use. Since effective, reversible medical contraceptive methods are only available for women, family planning clinics provide relatively little care for men. Often related to contraceptive method choice, such clinics also have incorporated elements of basic health screening (e.g., blood pressure testing) but, until recently, have tended to carry out little STD screening other than Pap smears or health department–funded screening for *N. gonorrhoeae*.

In the United States, family planning services are provided by approximately 2,614 agencies in at least 7,122 clinics.[20] Unlike publicly funded STD clinics, which are usually affiliated with health departments, clinic sites for family planning are quite varied and in 1994 included health departments (44 percent), Planned Parenthood affiliates (13 percent), hospitals (11 percent), and a variety of other agencies (32 percent). While many of these agencies also provide a variety of other services, most have separate clinic sessions devoted to family planning. Finally, in addition to being provided by multiple agencies and again in distinction to STD clinics, a variety of sources provide funding for family planning sources. The federal Title X program provides part of the budgets for family planning clinics in over 60 percent of agencies. Family planning services are also supported by state and local governments (68 percent of agencies), by client fees (88 percent), and by Medicaid (91 percent), among other sources.[21]

The level and focus of STD testing performed in family planning clinics also vary substantially. For instance, all family planning agencies routinely include annual Pap smear screening[21] and 82 percent offer HIV testing.[22] In contrast, routine testing for bacterial STDs is less common and varies from organism to organism; 64 percent of agencies include routine testing for gonorrhea, 42 percent for syphilis, and 54 percent for chlamydia.[21]

A particularly noteworthy example of effective integration of STD services into family planning agencies has been the campaign initiated by the CDC in 1988 to support and promote screening for *C. trachomatis* in family planning clinics. In 1988 this program began as a demonstration project in the Pacific Northwest (Region X) to provide support for increased chlamydia screening in family planning clinics.[17] As would be anticipated, chlamydia test positivity was initially relatively high (9.3 percent) among women attending these clinics and over a period of 7 years declined by 65 percent to 3.3 percent.[8] The success of this program has led to additional federal support enabling initiation of similar STD-related infertility-prevention programs in the remainder of the nation.

CLINICAL SERVICES: INTEGRATED APPROACHES

EXAMPLES FROM OUTSIDE THE UNITED STATES

In many parts of the world, including most of Europe, Asia, and South America, STD services are provided by dermatovenereologists with combined training and expertise in both dermatology and STDs. For clients, this has the advantage of avoiding the stigma attached to attendees at categorical STD clinics, but on the other hand, the emphasis of dermatovenereology clinics tends to be more on clinical features than on the public health aspects of STD control or on interrelationships with other reproductive health activities such as family planning. Partner notification and counseling services are sometimes neglected. In some countries (e.g., France and certain Francophone countries in Africa), compulsory registration and regular examination of commercial sex workers have been advocated as a strategy for STD control, but there is no evidence that it is effective, and it may exacerbate the problem by driving commercial sex underground.

In the United Kingdom, for example, a network of public categorical STD clinics was established by the Venereal Disease Act of 1917. These are now known as genitourinary medicine *(GUM)* clinics. They are free and accessible to all without prior appointment, and confidentiality is enforced in them by law. Traditionally, like U.S. STD clinics, GUM clinics have concentrated their efforts on the treatable bacterial STDs and have adopted a disease-based approach emphasizing laboratory diagnosis before treatment, testing patients for other STDs, follow-up to ensure clinical and microbiologic cure, and tracing and investigation of contacts. Considerable importance is attached to partner notification, which has, in the past, traditionally been performed by health advisers. However, in recent years, patient referral has been increasingly encouraged, leaving health advisers more time to concentrate on health education and counseling of patients.

In recent years, as the incidence of bacterial STDs has declined in the United Kingdom and appreciation of the importance and prevalence of the incurable viral STDs has increased, a more holistic concept of sexual health has been adopted, with increasing emphasis on primary prevention through health education and the promotion of condom use. HIV tests are available on demand, and screening for cervical dysplasia, colposcopy, and immunization against hepatitis B are often also available. An increasing number of GUM clinics are providing family planning services, and following the example of other European countries (e.g., the Netherlands),[23] some clinics are implementing innovative outreach programs for groups who are perceived to underutilize existing services (e.g., intravenous drug users, commercial sex workers). There is an STD clinic in almost every health district in England and Wales, often more than one in large towns, but they seldom open outside normal working hours, limiting their accessibility. In 1993–1994, 45,000 new episodes of STDs were reported in the 225 STD clinics in England and Wales, corresponding to 1 in 50 of the adult population aged 16 to 64 years. In family planning clinics, apart from Pap smears, no STD screening tests are performed routinely. Most clinics have facilities for chlamydia testing that, because of funding constraints, are generally limited to individuals perceived to be at high risk, e.g., those with a recent partner change and those with symptoms of vaginal discharge or menstrual irregularity. Screening tests or presumptive therapy for chlamydial infection generally are performed before termination of pregnancy or IUD insertion; women found to be infected are referred to the nearest STD clinic for partner notification. There are only two clinics in the United Kingdom that offer truly integrated STD and family planning services, sharing facilities and medical records (John Guillebaud, personal communication). As in the United States, it is not possible to say how many cases were treated outside these clinics by general practitioners, gynecologists, urologists, or family planning providers.[24]

In general, this system has worked well. The incidence and prevalence of the treatable STDs remain low in the United Kingdom (in 1995 unlinked studies found HIV seroprevalence to be 0.8 and 0.5 percent, respectively, for male and female GUM clinic clients in London and 0.1 percent for both groups seen in GUM clinics outside London), the incidence of HIV infection is low in the heterosexual population, and antibiotic-resistant strains of *N. gonorrhoeae* are not prevalent. Screening for syphilis is mandatory in antenatal clinics in the United Kingdom, but there are no screening programs for other bacterial STDs, and the prevalence of infection with *C. trachomatis* remains higher than in some other European countries, such as Sweden, where there is an aggressive partner notification program and screening is more widely practiced.

DEVELOPING COUNTRIES

In developing countries, until recently, STD services have been accorded low priority. In some large cities in Africa and Asia, categorical STD clinics are run by municipal public health departments, but due to a lack of resources and poor staff motivation, the service they offer is often less than optimal. Moreover, these clinics are often inaccessible and, as in industrialized nations, are often unpopular with patients because of the stigma attached to them. The result has been that many patients with STDs, especially women, prefer to seek treatment in the private sector or from unqualified pharmacists, quacks, or traditional healers, who offer a more user-friendly service but usually provide inappropriate treatment and are rarely concerned with counseling, health education, or the treatment of sexual partners.[25] This has contributed to a high prevalence of STDs, the spread of multiply resistant strains of *N. gonorrhoeae* and *H. ducreyi* in many parts of the developing world, and accelerated heterosexual transmission of HIV.

Recently, with growing recognition that the treatable bacterial STDs facilitate heterosexual transmission of HIV infection, their control has been given higher priority. Given the higher prevalence of STDs and the more profound lack of resources in many developing countries, it frequently has not been possible to provide service using categorical STD clinics modeled after programs in industrialized nations. Instead, STD programs integrated within the existing primary health care structure have been implemented successfully in several countries, particularly in Africa. In Zimbabwe, for example, syndromic management of STDs by nurses was introduced in primary health care clinics in the early 1980s.[26] This decentralized service was essential, since there was a high incidence of STDs and a lack of medical staff in Zimbabwe, with only two trained venereologists in the government service. To address the problem, nursing staff from the 14 primary care clinics and 9 polyclinics in Harare were trained at the central STD clinic. Primarily using in-service training rather than formal lectures, nurses were trained to take a proper history and to conduct a thorough examination, to obtain appropriate specimens for laboratory diagnosis, to administer appropriate treatment, to discuss the nature of the disease and its possible sequelae with patients, and to detect and manage treatment side effects. They also were taught to counsel patients about the importance of referring their sexual partners for treatment, of refraining from sex until cured, and of compliance and attendance for follow-up. Finally, they were trained to record the diagnosis for later analysis and evaluation. This decentralized service has proved highly successful, with less than 5 percent of cases requiring referral to the central clinic.

Despite an economy and health services that had been devastated by a long war, decentralized STD management services also have been established successfully in Mozambique, within the national AIDS Control Program.[27] An important contributor to this success is an expert training unit that included representatives covering the fields of clinical management, training, laboratory techniques, health education, and epidemiology and developed a national STD control plan. In addition, a referral clinic was established at the central hospital in the capital, Maputo, where staff from 20 primary health care centers was trained, national treatment guidelines were developed based on the few epidemiologic data available, the essential drugs list was adapted to include appropriate STD treatment regimens, and laboratory equipment was supplied for Gram stain and syphilis serology. In addition to training staff from health centers in syndromic STD management, a program of syphilis screening was established in antenatal clinics, and midwives and traditional birth attendants were trained to provide ocular prophylaxis to neonates. Regular supervisory visits were made to health centers where staff had been trained. Measures of this program's success include a reduction in the percentage of STD patients referred to the central clinic from 8 percent to less than 5 percent and a low cost per case treated (U.S.—$1.08). Of 38,867 patients treated in the program's first year, more than half were female, in marked contrast with the high male-female ratio usually seen in categorical STD clinics in other developing countries.

In the Mwanza Region of Tanzania, a similar program, with a central clinic for training and operational research and a decentralized service based on syndromic management in rural health centers and dispensaries, reduced the incidence of HIV infection by approximately 40 percent over a 2-year period.[28] As in Mozambique, it was found that a short training course (1 week of classroom teaching and 2 weeks in the clinic) was sufficient but that regular (two monthly) supervisory visits also were essential to ensure the continuing success of the program.

Encouraging though these results are, certain weaknesses of these programs are also apparent. First, although the STD services are decentralized, the management and supervision of the programs are vertical rather than fully integrated within the management structure of the health service; this raises doubts about their sustainability in the long term. Second, the syndromic approach to STD treatment probably will have little impact on STD prevalence unless supplemented by an effective system of partner referral and/or screening to detect asymptomatic cases, particularly among women. Screening of antenatal clinic attenders for syphilis often has failed in developing countries for logistic reasons,[29] and screening for other STDs (e.g., gonorrhea or chlamydial infection) requires relatively expensive laboratory tests that are unlikely to become available at the peripheral level in developing countries. Attempts to implement screening for these infections through risk assessment in antenatal or family planning clinics have not been very successful, with sensitivities and specificities of, at best, 70 percent. The application of syndromic treatment in such female populations is likely to lead to considerable overtreatment when the prevalence of STDs is low, with a consequent waste of scarce resources.[30,31] Finally, although there is general agreement that it is important to provide targeted STD services for high-risk and vulnerable groups in developing countries, it has proved extremely difficult to do this effectively in practice.

Continuing financial support for such programs is also a concern. In Zimbabwe and Tanzania, STD treatment has been provided free of charge, whereas in Mozambique, a cost-recovery scheme was implemented. It was found that, at least in urban areas, most patients could afford to pay a small fee designed to cover the cost of drugs. However, a marked decline in the number of patients attending the main STD clinic in Nairobi, Kenya, was noted after the imposition of user charges.[32] A strong case can be made for providing free treatment for STDs on public health grounds, in the same way as it has been made for other communicable diseases such as tuberculosis, but this would need to be supported by the international donor community in the poorest countries.

SUMMARY

Specialized clinics for provision of services such as STD, HIV, and contraceptive care are common throughout the world. These clinics represent an important "safety net" for clients with acute needs for service. In addition, clinics with specialization in management of STD, HIV, and family planning may serve as useful sites for training and with which providers can consult regarding particularly difficult or complex cases. For most persons, however, it is likely that more inclusive care, which integrates STD and other reproductive health care into comprehensive care, has benefits for patients, providers, and systems of health care delivery. In the United States, where categorically organized clinics provide a greater proportion of HIV and reproductive health services than in other developed nations, the feasibility of integrated approaches has been demonstrated by the successes of demonstration projects conducted in family planning and STD clinics, by the success of the CDC's STD-related Infertility Prevention Program, and by the choices made disproportionately by individuals with more options for seeking health care. To expand such a model of health care, however, will require, at a minimum, less concern about "turf" in publicly funded STD and family planning programs, more comprehensive training of health care providers, and a shift in emphasis in some clinics from definition of program success in terms of numbers of clients and/or visits provided to a definition of success that includes the quality of care (as defined using client input, cost-effectiveness analyses, and minimum standards of care) as well as qualitative evaluations.

Similarly, certain recommendations can be made concerning the provision of services for the management of STDs in resource-poor settings such as developing nations. For instance, at a minimum, STD control programs should be fully integrated with AIDS control programs, since this will ensure that duplication of effort is avoided: A central referral clinic, with laboratory facilities, is needed in each country and perhaps in every region of larger countries for training and operational research, but treatment services should be decentralized as far as possible. Treatment in peripheral clinics should be based on the syndromic approach, but there is also a pressing need for validation of syndromic management algorithms and for screening services—in particular for syphilis screening in antenatal clinics. Operational research is needed to identify how best to deliver this service and how to deliver appropriate services to high-risk groups. Finally, there is a great need for simple, cheap, and reliable screening tests for gonorrhea and chlamydial infection that could be applied at antenatal, family planning, or maternal and child health clinics in developing countries.

References

1 International Conference on Population and Development: Programme of Action, Chapter VII, 7.2–7.6. Cairo, International Conference on Population and Development, Sept. 1994.

2 Mosher WD, Aral SO: Testing for sexually transmitted diseases among women of reproductive age: United States, 1988. *Fam Plann Perspect* 23:216–221, 1991.

3 Sawyer JA et al: Accuracy of women's self report of their last Pap smear. *Am J Public Health* 79:1036–1037, 1989.

4 Horn JE et al: Reproductive health practices in women attending an inner-city STD clinic. *Sex Transm Dis* 17:133–137, 1990.

5 Brandt AM: *No Magic Bullet: A Social History of Venereal Disease in the United States Since 1880.* New York, Oxford University Press, 1985.

6 Landry DJ, Forrest JD: Public Health departments providing sexually transmitted disease services. *Fam Plann Perspect* 28:261–266, 1996.

7 Beck-Saque CM et al: Laboratory diagnosis of sexually transmitted diseases in facilities within the United States: Results of a national survey. *Sex Transm Dis* 23:342–349, 1996.

8 Centers for Disease Control and Prevention: *Chlamydia trachomatis* genital infections—United States, 1995. *MMWR* 46(9):193–198, 1997.

9 Celum CL et al: Demographic characteristics, STD morbidity, insurance status, and preferences for source of STD care. *Sex Trans Dis* (in press).

10 Upchurch DM et al: Contraceptive needs and practices among women attending an inner-city STD clinic. *Am J Public Health* 77:1427–1430, 1987.

11 Quinn TC et al: Human immunodeficiency virus infection among patients attending clinics for sexually transmitted diseases. *N Engl J Med* 318:197–203, 1988.

12 Zuckerman RD et al: Tuberculosis screening in a sexually transmitted diseases clinic. *Sex Transm Dis* 23:299–303, 1996.

13 Golden MR et al: Early intervention for human immunodeficiency virus in Baltimore sexually transmitted disease clinics: Impact on gonorrhea incidence in patients infected with HIV. *Sex Transm Dis* 23:370–377, 1996.

14 Kassler WJ et al: Seroconversion in patients attending sexually transmitted disease clinics. *AIDS* 8:351–355, 1994.

15 Otlen MW Jr et al: Changes in sexually transmitted diseases rates after HIV testing and posttest counseling, Miami 1988 to 1989. *Am J Public Health* 83:529–533, 1993.

16 Stein Z: Family planning, sexually transmitted diseases and the prevention of AIDS: Divided we fail? *Am J Public Health* 86:783–784, 1996.

17 Britton TF et al: STDs and family planning clinics: A regional program for chlamydia control that works. *Am J Gynecol Health* 6:24–30, 1992.

18 Hutchinson CM et al: CD4 lymphocyte concentrations in patients with newly identified HIV infection attending STD clinics: Potential impact on publicly funded health care resources. *JAMA* 266:253–256, 1991.

19 Zenilman JM et al: Effect of HIV post-test counseling on STD incidence. *JAMA* 267:843–845, 1992.

20 Frost J: Family planning clinic services in the United States, 1994. *Fam Plann Perspect* 20:90–100, 1996.

21 Frost J, Bolzan M: The provision of public sector services by family planning agencies in 1995. *Fam Plann Perspect (in press).*

22 Henshaw SK, Torres A: Family planning agencies: Services, policies and funding. *Fam Plann Perspect* 26:52–59, 1994.

23 Coutinho RA et al: Influence of special surveillance programs and AIDS on declining influence of syphilis in Amsterdam. *Genitourin Med* 63:210–213, 1987.

24 Renton A et al: Health care needs assessment, in *Genitourinary Medicine Services,* A Stevens, J Raftery (eds). London, Radcliffe Medical Press, 1996.

25 Kantharaj K et al: Sexually transmitted disease services in Madras: Could their role in AIDS prevention be strengthened. *Ind J Public Health* 39:93–98, 1995.

26 Latif AS et al: The decentralization of the sexually transmitted diseases service and its integration into primary health care. *Afr J Sex Transm Dis* 2:85–88, 1986.

27 Bastos dos Santos R et al: Reproductive tract infections in Mozambique: A case study of integrated services, in *Reproductive Tract Infections,* A Germain et al (eds). New York, Plenum Press, 1992.

28 Grosskurth H et al: Impact of improved treatment of sexually transmitted diseases on HIV infection in rural Tanzania: Randomized controlled trial. *Lancet* 346:530–536, 1995.

29 Temmerman M et al: Syphilis prevention in pregnancy: An opportunity to improve reproductive and child health in Kenya. *Health Policy Plan* 8:122–127, 1993.

30 Vuylsteke B et al: Clinical algorithms for the screening of women for gonococcal and chlamydial infection: Evaluation of pregnant women and prostitutes in Zaire. *Clin Infect Dis* 17:82–88, 1993.

31 Mayaud P et al: Risk assessment and other screening options for the identification of gonorrhea and chlamydial infection in rural Tanzanian antenatal clinic attenders. *Bull WHO* 73:621–630, 1995.

32 Moses S et al: Impact of user fees on attendance at a referral centre for sexually transmitted diseases in Kenya. *Lancet* 340:463–466, 1992.

Chapter 92

Laboratory services for sexually transmitted diseases: Overview and recent developments

Max A. Chernesky

This chapter reviews various aspects of specimen collection and transport and laboratory procedures available for the diagnosis of sexually transmitted diseases (STDs). The microorganisms causing signs or symptoms in genitourinary sites and others that can be transmitted easily through sexual behavior are listed in Table 92-1.

HISTORY

Although the concept of providing comprehensive laboratory services for the diagnosis of STDs has surfaced relatively recently, many of the landmark discoveries of STD etiology, pathogenesis, and epidemiology were facilitated through discovery and refinement of diagnostic techniques many years ago. The coming together of microscopy, culture, serology, and antigen and nucleic acid detection into the discipline of clinical microbiology alongside clinical chemistry, hematology, and pathology has taken place in the last 40 years. Early use of the microscope and cytology stains enabled Edwin Klebs to observe *Treponema* spirochetes as early as 1875 and Albert Neisser to describe the gonococcus in 1879 in clinical specimens even before Hans Gram described his famous stain in 1884. During this era of great discovery, Ducrey described the chancroid bacterium in 1889, and Donovan provided the first description of gram-negative tissue-encapsulated bodies of *Calymmatobacteria* in 1905. Five years later Heymann demonstrated chlamydia inclusions in epithelial cells from a cervical specimen collected from a woman whose infant had inclusion conjunctivitis, and Linder demonstrated similar inclusions in urethral epithelial cells from men with nongonococcal urethritis. Further microscopic refinements, such as darkfield viewing by Lansteiner in 1906 and silver staining by Noguchi and Moore in 1913, took place for syphilis diagnosis. At this time, Wasserman described his version of the complement-fixation (CF) serologic test that led to the development of modern-day syphilis serology. Muller and Oppenheim adapted the CF technique for the diagnosis of gonorrhea. Although the earliest culture of an STD was reported by Leistikow and Loeffler in 1882 for the gonococcus, it was not until the middle of the century that STD organisms began to be isolated routinely from clinical specimens on artificial media, and Schubert propagated *Neisseria gonorrhoeae* in 1947 by inoculating clinical exudates onto agar.

Throughout the 1940s and 1950s, immunofluorescence (IF) was applied to both antigen and antibody assays. Coons introduced the fluorescent treponemal antibody test (FTA) in 1950, and Deacon demonstrated IF gonococcal antigens in clinical exudates in 1959. The techniques of immobilization by Nelson and Mayer in 1949, immune adherence by Nelson in 1953, and agglutination by McLeod and Magnu in 1953 all became adaptable to syphilis diagnosis. It also was during this decade that Jones, Collier, and Smith propagated chlamydia by inoculating the yolk sac of embryonated hens' eggs with cervical scrapings.

During the 1960s, cell cultures were being used extensively to isolate viruses, including herpes simplex virus, from genital lesions. In 1965, Gordon and Quan reported that centrifugation of clinical specimens onto cell cultures that were metabolically arrested allowed the formation of large intracytoplasmic inclusions of *C. trachomatis* to be seen under the microscope after staining with iodine.

During the 1970s, most STDs were being diagnosed clinically and by microscopy, culture, or serology. The discovery of monoclonal antibodies by Kohler and Milstein in 1975 ushered in an era of antigen detection for STDs either by solid-phase enzyme immunoassays (EIA) or by direct fluorescent antibody (DFA).

During the 1980s, STD diagnostic tests moved forward largely due to assay commercialization and the realization that rigorous evaluations of the new assays were required. Effective antibiotic treatments also stressed the need for accurate diagnosis. During this time, nucleic acid detection became a feasible diagnostic approach for the diagnosis of *C. trachomatis* and human papillomavirus, and in the past 7 years this has been extended even further into the ultrasensitive nucleic acid amplification techniques such as polymerase chain reaction (PCR), ligase chain reaction (LCR), and several others. This ability to detect and amplify single genes has led to the discovery that less traditional specimen types such as urine or vaginal swabs can be applied to the diagnosis of urethral and cervical infections in the 1990s.

COLLECTION OF SPECIMENS

The following principles should be considered concerning the collection of specimens:

1. The user of a laboratory facility should communicate with the laboratory staff to discuss matters about collection, transportation, and testing of specimens.
2. All specimen-collection procedures should be performed while wearing appropriate protective clothing.
3. Contamination from indigenous commensal flora should be avoided to ensure representative sampling of the infectious process.
4. Adequate volumes of each specimen should be collected.
5. Each specimen should be labeled with the patient's name, identification number, and source and the date and time of collection.
6. All specimen containers should be leakproof and transported within a sealable, leakproof plastic bag having a separate compartment for paperwork.
7. Sexually transmitted pathogens are usually fastidious and fragile, and thus cultures and techniques that detect viable organisms may give false-negative results unless transport conditions are optimal.
8. In general, transport must be as rapid as possible for the recovery of infectious organisms, with excesses of temperature avoided; e.g., for *C. trachomatis,* the ideal transportation temperature is 4°C; for specimens to detect *N. gonorrhoeae*, nutritive and nonnutritive systems are commonly used, and ambient room temperature is recommended for transport. When the test used is based on the detection of products of organisms or on antigen detection, conditions for transport are usually less stringent.

BLOOD

For serologic diagnosis, a clotted specimen is needed.

Table 92-1. A List of Microorganisms Transmitted Through Sexual Behavior According to the Presence or Absence of Signs or Symptoms

Disease	Microorganisms
Genital ulcers	*T. pallidum*
	H. ducreyi
	HSV
	LGV serovars of *C. trachomatis*
Urethral or cervical discharge	*N. gonorrhoeae*
	C. trachomatis
	M. hominis
	M. genitalium
	U. urealyticum
Vaginal discharge	*T. vaginalis*
	C. albicans
	G. vaginalis
	N. gonorrhoeae, C. trachomatis
Dysplasia, granuloma, or none	HPV
	C. granulomatis
	LGV
	Group B streptococci
	HIV
	HBIV, HCV
	CMV

CERVIX

Cervical specimens should not be taken from prepuberal girls, since sexually transmitted infections in this age group involve the vagina, not the cervix. In puberal and postpuberal females, a speculum is inserted to view the cervix. To diagnose gonorrhea, it is not necessary to clear cervical mucus, but it should be removed before swabbing for the diagnosis of chlamydial infections. To obtain a cervical specimen, the swab or cytobrush is inserted 2 to 3 cm into the endocervical canal, rotated for 10 to 30 seconds, and then withdrawn.

PHARYNX

Swab the posterior pharynx and the tonsillar crypts for chlamydial and gonococcal infections. In a young infant a nasopharyngeal aspirate is used for the collection of specimens for *C. trachomatis*.

RECTUM

To obtain a rectal specimen by blind swabbing, the appropriate swab is inserted 2 to 3 cm into the anal canal and pressed laterally to try to avoid fecal material and, in the case of *C. trachomatis*, to obtain columnar epithelial cells. If there is visible fecal contamination of the specimen, it should be discarded and another swab used. With anoscopy, in symptomatic patients, specimens can be taken under direct visualization, avoiding fecal material.

ULCERS

Remove scabs or overlying debris, and gently debride the lesion to induce exudation relatively free of blood. Collect fluid into a capillary tube or small-bore syringe. Alternatively, a swab should be obtained from the base of the lesion.

URETHRA

Urethral material is obtained with meatal or intraurethral swabs, and the choice depends on the organism and the amount of urethral discharge. In males, detection of urethral discharge can be enhanced by milking the penis from the base to the glans. The meatal discharge is an appropriate specimen for testing for *N. gonorrhoeae*. If there is no meatal exudate, an intraurethral swab should be used by using a thin swab with a flexible-wire shaft. Ideally, the patient should not have voided for at least 2 hours, since voiding reduces the amount of exudate and may decrease the ability to detect organisms. Introduce the swab slowly 2 to 3 cm, rotate slowly, and withdraw gently. Moistening the swab with sterile nonbacteriostatic saline before insertion will help reduce discomfort. For prepuberal boys, the swab should be rotated in the meatal opening rather than introduced further into the urethra.

Swabbing the urethra is only recommended for routine use in women with a surgically removed cervix. As for males, a thin swab on a flexible-wire shaft should be inserted 1 to 2 cm and rotated. In prepuberal girls, a meatal specimen should be obtained.

URINE

To obtain a first-void urine (FVU), provide the patient with a sterile plastic container that has a large enough opening, and ask the patient to collect only the first 10 to 15 mL into the container. The specimen can be collected at any micturition.

VAGINA

Collection of vaginal swabs from adolescents and adults is usually done as part of a speculum examination. Pooled vaginal secretions can be collected or the vaginal wall in the posterior fornix swabbed. Vaginal specimens can be taken without a speculum in prepubescent girls, with swabs that have been moistened with sterile nonbacteriostatic saline. In very young children, collection of secretions with eye droppers or very thin swabs is more appropriate.

VESICLES

For the detection of herpes simplex virus from vesicles, collect fluid into a small-bore syringe or capillary tube for electron microscopy. Alternatively, vesicles should be broken and fluid collected onto a swab and the base of the lesion vigorously rubbed or scraped. The swab should be placed in viral transport media for culture or into an appropriate container for specific nonculture tests. If vesicles are not present, the urethra and meatus of males can be swabbed. For asymptomatic women, use one swab premoistened with saline to rub the clitoral hood, labia minora, labia majora, perineum, and perianal region. For asymptomatic neonates, use one swab premoistened with saline, and gently apply to conjunctiva; insert into the mouth, and gently rub around the lips, external ear canal, umbilicus, axillae, and groin.

DIAGNOSTIC APPROACHES

Table 92-2 summarizes the various approaches to the diagnosis of any STD.

Table 92-2. Approaches to Diagnosis of STDs

1. Microscopy
2. Culture
3. Antigen detection
4. Nucleic acid detection
5. Serology
6. Measurement of enzymes or metabolites

MICROSCOPY

If microscopy is to be used for diagnosis, the choices will be light microscopy, darkfield microscopy, or electron microscopy. Light microscopy may be used routinely for the diagnosis of *N. gonorrhoeae, Haemophilus ducreyi,* or *C. trachomatis* for certain clinical conditions.

Light microscopy

Gram staining is used routinely for examining exudates. The swab is rolled onto the slide, which is air-fixed or passed through a flame. The slide is flooded with crystal violet (10 gm 90% dye in 500 mL absolute methyl alcohol) and after 10 seconds gently washed with water. It is then flooded with iodine (6 gm iodine crystals, 12 gm KI, and 1,800 mL distilled water) and after 10 seconds washed with water. The slide is then decolorized with acetone-alcohol (400 mL acetone with 1,200 mL 95% ethyl alcohol) and washed immediately with water. It is then flooded with safranine (10 gm 99% safranine dye in 100 mL distilled water) for 10 seconds, rinsed with water, blotted dry with filter paper, and examined under oil immersion (×1000). The direct microscopic examination of swabs and identification of gram-negative intracellular diplococci are presumptive for *N. gonorrhoeae.* The presence of gram-negative diplococci outside polymorphonuclear leukocytes (PMNLs) is not highly predictive and should be confirmed by culture. PMNLs without diplococci are a negative finding in the diagnosis of gonococcal infection. Gram stain of urethral specimens from symptomatic adolescent and adult males has a sensitivity and specificity of >95 percent; endocervical specimens from adult females have a sensitivity of 45 to 65 percent and a specificity of >90 percent. Gram stain for specimens collected from other sites has low accuracy and is not recommended.

Direct examination of gram-stained smears taken from ulcers has been used with varying degrees of success as an aid in the diagnosis of chancroid. The identification of *H. ducreyi* is based on characteristics of cell morphology, staining, and arrangement. When visualized on smears, the gram-negative *H. ducreyi* rods may be situated intracellularly, but more often organisms are observed extracellularly either singly or in small clusters. Direct examination of clinical material by a Gram stain may be misleading because of the polymicrobial flora of most genital ulcers. Specific immunochemical staining with fluorescent antibody may be of help in preliminary identification of the organism, but every attempt should be made to confirm the diagnosis by culture procedures.

For a complete description of the laboratory diagnosis of bacterial vaginosis (BV), refer to Chap. 42. In typical Gram smears from patients with BV, squamous vaginal epithelial cells covered with vaginal bacteria (clue cells) are accompanied by a mixed flora consisting of very large numbers of small gram-negative and gram-variable rods and coccobacilli (predominantly *Gardnerella vaginalis*) in the absence of larger gram-positive rods. When the clinical examination is normal, *Lactobacillus* morphotypes are found alone or in the presence of small numbers of *G. vaginalis* morphotypes.

Mycoplasmas are gram-negative but do not take up counterstain sufficiently well for the small individual organisms to be recognized on microscopic examination of Gram-stained clinical specimens.

The Gram stain cannot be used to detect chlamydia because they are gram-negative and do not take counterstain. An alternative approach is the use of Giemsa stain. Elementary bodies (EB) of chlamydia are approximately 0.3 μm in diameter and stain purple or bluish with Giemsa stain. Reticulate bodies (RB) (measuring 0.5 to 1.0 μm), which are the replicating unit in eukaryotic cells, stain blue also. Intracytoplasmic inclusions of *C. trachomatis* stain dark purple with Giemsa stain, but microscopy of clinical genital samples has a very low sensitivity compared with cultures, particularly in asymptomatic, nonacute cases, and are thus not recommended. However, in acute chlamydial eye infections, light microscopy is of diagnostic value.

Cells from herpes simplex virus (HSV) lesions show cytopathology of enlarged and intranuclear inclusions, fusion of cells, and multinucleated giant cells. Scraping of oral-labial or genital HSV lesions and staining of the cells with Wright-Giemsa (Tzanck preparation) stain provides a rapid, inexpensive, and simple test for the detection of infections caused by the herpes group of viruses, but with a sensitivity of only about 50 percent. Examination of these stained smears does not discriminate between HSV and varicella-zoster virus (VZV). More specific techniques, such as IF, can be used to differentiate HSV from VZV infections when necessary. The Papanicolaou (Pap)-stained smear containing both endo- and exocervical cells may show Tzanck-type inclusions due to HSV or intracytoplasmic inclusions due to *C. trachomatis* by light microscopy. Although trichomonads are often reported on Pap smears, the sensitivity is only 60 percent, and findings are often nonspecific.

Wet mount preparations can be used to examine unstained clinical specimens. One can determine the morphology of organisms, gross structure, and biologic activity, including motility, reaction to certain chemicals, and serologic reactivity. The specimens are examined under bright-field, phase-contrast, or darkfield microscopy depending on the microorganisms sought. In the basic wet mount procedure, 1 drop of 0.85% warm (37°C) aqueous NaCl is added to the slide, and then 1 drop of specimen is added and mixed with the NaCl. A coverslip is overlaid, and the slide is examined at 100× to 1000×. The diagnosis of trichomoniasis is made by observing the parasites, which are ovoid and slightly larger than PMNLs; they are best recognized by their motility. By phase-contrast or darkfield microscopy, the individual flagella and undulating membrane are easily recognized. Observation of a single motile trichomonad establishes the diagnosis, but the wet mount reveals trichomonads in only approximately 40 to 80 percent of cases. It is more difficult to demonstrate *Trichomonas vaginalis* directly in male urine or genital secretions. The diagnosis of bacterial vaginosis is suggested by the presence of vaginal epithelial cells that appear granular with obscured margins because they are heavily coated with adherent bacteria. Vulvovaginal candidiasis is likely when fungal hyphal elements are seen.

Wet mounts prepared in 10% KOH are used to help distinguish fungal elements in thick mucoid specimens or in specimens with keratinous material. The proteinaceous components of the host cells are partially digested, leaving the polysaccharide-containing fungal cell wall intact and more apparent. An aliquot of specimen is simply added to a drop of 10% KOH, which can be preserved with 0.1% thimerosal. A wet mount or saline preparation should be done routinely not only to identify the presence of yeast cells and mycelia but also to exclude the presence of "clue cells" and motile trichomonads. Large numbers of neutrophils should suggest trichomoniasis or cervical infection with *N. gonorrhoeae, C. trachomatis,* or herpes simplex virus.

Microscopy performed on freshly crushed granulomatous tissue stained with Wright's or Giemsa stain may show Donovan bodies in clusters of blue- or black-staining organisms within the cytoplasm of large histiocytic cells. The *Calymmatobacterium granulomatis* organisms usually can be differentiated easily from debris with inflammatory cell infiltrates.

Darkfield microscopy

Direct microscopic examination of lesion material by darkfield microscopy permits the most definitive diagnosis of treponemal infection. The ideal specimen is serous fluid rich in *Treponema pallidum* and free of red blood cells and other lesion constituents. Darkfield microscopy has long been the standard test of choice when the patient has moist ulcerative lesions to rule out syphilis as the cause of lesions associated with other STDs such as HSV, *H. ducreyi,* and LGV (although direct fluorescent antibody testing and PCR testing represent increasingly attractive alternatives for detection of *T. pallidum*). A diagnosis of syphilis in the primary and secondary stages can be made by demonstrating *T. pallidum* in suspected lesions or regional lymph nodes; *T. pallidum* is recognized by its morphologic characteristics: length 6 to 14 μm, thickness 0.25 to 0.30 μm, spiral amplitude 0.5 to 1.0 μm, and characteristic movement.

The direct fluorescent antibody–*T. pallidum* (DFA-TP) test is a practical alternative to direct darkfield examination when smears cannot be examined immediately and when examining oral lesions. The collection methods for darkfield microscopy are applicable to the DFA-TP. Slides and/or coverslips are air dried and heat-fixed or air-dried and fixed with acetone or 10% methanol before staining. For the DFA-TP, lesion material also may be collected in heparinized microhematocrit capillary tubes, sealed with plasticine or like material, and stored at 4 to 8°C until slides are prepared. The lesion material fixed to the slide is stained with fluorescein-labeled anti–*T. pallidum* globulin. The test offers the advantage of specifically detecting *T. pallidum,* thereby eliminating confusion with other spiral organisms, especially in oral lesions. Motile organisms and experience with darkfield microscopy are not required. The demonstration of treponemes with characteristic morphology and motility for *T. pallidum* by darkfield microscopy or a reactive DFA-TP test result constitutes a positive diagnosis of syphilis in primary, secondary, early congenital, and infectious relapse stages regardless of the outcome of serologic testing. Failure to find the organism does not exclude a diagnosis of syphilis.

Electron microscopy

Demonstration of herpesvirus particles in vesicular lesions by electron microscopy (EM) is a rapid diagnostic technique. Its utility is limited by the specialized equipment required and the apparent low sensitivity of this technique in genital herpes compared with culture. The technique is most successful when pure vesicular fluid can be collected in a small-bore syringe or capillary tube and examined in the EM undiluted using a negative stain such as phosphotungstic acid (PTA).

CULTURE

Not all STD agents can be cultured, and those which can usually have special conditions needed for their growth.

Calymmatobacterium granulomatis

C. granulomatis, considered the causative agent of donovanosis, has not been consistently cultured on artificial medium in the laboratory.

Candida albicans

As with most STDs, diagnosis requires a correlation between clinical conditions and more than one laboratory test. Vaginal cultures are done on selective media such as Sabouraud agar or Nickerson's, Microstix, or chloramphenicol-treated artificial medium.

Chlamydia trachomatis

McCoy cells are the most widely used cell line for the isolation of *C. trachomatis.* Other cell types used include HeLa 229 cells and baby hamster kidney cells (BHK 21). Cycloheximide is a glutaramide antibiotic that reduces the metabolic activity of eukaryotic cells and is added to the culture medium. DEAE-dextran may be used to transform the physicochemical properties of the surfaces of cells, enhancing attachment and phagocytosis of *C. trachomatis.* For primary isolation, centrifugation of cell cultures after inoculation with chlamydiae is required in order to obtain optimal culture results. Centrifugation forces of 300*g* pellet the organisms onto the cell monolayer, increasing the chlamydiae-cell contact. Chlamydial inclusions develop within 48 to 72 hours after incubation at 36°C and can be identified using Giemsa, iodine, or immunofluorescence staining. Giemsa staining is not widely used for purposes of routine isolation because the inclusions are more difficult to visualize. Iodine staining produces dark brown inclusions that are readily seen against a yellow background. However, compared with iodine or Giemsa, fluorescein-conjugated monoclonal antibody staining is more sensitive, identifying three- to eightfold more inclusions.

Laboratories will make a decision to use shell vials with cells grown on coverslips or cells grown on the bottom of 96-well culture plates according to the number of specimens processed on a daily basis. The decision also will be influenced by populations sampled. The larger volume of sample inoculated into shell vials may facilitate more positive isolations from patients without symptoms and with lower numbers of elementary bodies in the samples. Blind passage of initial negatives also may increase the number of positive specimens, depending on the culture and staining systems used.

Cytomegalovirus (CMV)

CMV can be isolated from urine and genital swabs by inoculation into human fibroblasts. These cells are most sensitive for showing CMV cytopathic effect (giant cells and syncytium) in freshly seeded vessels with cells early in passage ($<$15). Conjugated monoclonal antibodies to CMV early antigens can be used to speed up the detection of CMV in cell cultures as early as 1 to 2 days after inoculation.

Gardnerella vaginalis (vaginal cultures)

Direct microscopic examination of vaginal secretions is more relevant for the diagnosis of bacterial vaginosis than is isolation, because low concentrations of *G. vaginalis* represent a normal part of the endogenous flora, and because the overall pattern of bacterial morphotypes seen rather than detection of any single organism, is most useful for the diagnosis. However, for isolation of *G. vaginalis,* semiselective human blood bilayer Tween agar may be inoculated by rolling a swab across a sector of the plate.

This inoculum should be streaked with a loop to allow a semi-quantitative estimate of the growth of the isolate, and the plates may be incubated at 35°C in a candle jar or in a humid atmosphere containing 5% CO_2. After 48 hours of incubation, the plates may be examined for colonies exhibiting diffuse beta-hemolysis. A presumptive identification of *G. vaginalis* may be based on the typical cell morphology on the Gram stain, beta-hemolysis with diffuse edges on the Tween agar, and a negative catalase test.

Haemophilus ducreyi

Currently, accurate clinical diagnosis of chancroid depends on isolation of *H. ducreyi*. Various medium formulations have been used for isolation. GC agar base containing 1% to 2% hemoglobin, 5% fetal bovine serum, and 3 μg of vancomycin per milliliter appears to have the highest sensitivity for the isolation of *H. ducreyi* from clinical specimens. Several investigators have observed that the use of two different types of media significantly increases the sensitivity of culture for *H. ducreyi*. The two media can be incorporated into a single biplate to facilitate their use. The size and appearance of colonies of *H. ducreyi* vary depending on the growth medium and length of incubation. Colonies are generally pinpoint size at 24 hours (0.5 mm) and increase to 1 to 2 mm in 48 to 72 hours. The colonies are nonmucoid, raised, compact, and granular and have a tan, yellowish, or grayish yellow color. A zone of hemolysis is seen on plates containing rabbit blood. A water-saturated atmosphere containing 5% to 10% CO_2 and a reduced incubation temperature of 33 to 35°C are important for primary cultivation of this organism. Presumptive identification can be made by demonstrating short, gram-negative bacilli with occasional streptobacillary chaining from solid media and by the inability of isolates to produce porphyrin from L-aminolevulinic acid by the porphyrin test. Confirmatory identification requires the demonstration of a hemin (X factor) requirement for growth and the absence of a requirement for NAD (V factor) on media otherwise nutritionally enriched. The porphyrin test is the preferred method of demonstrating hemin requirement, and the oxidase test requires tetramethyl-*p*-phenylenediamine. Starch aggregation may be a useful property for the presumptive identification of *H. ducreyi* colonies in a mixed culture.

Hepatitis B virus (HBV)

There is no cultivation system for HBV. Diagnosis is performed by testing serum or plasma for viral antigens, antibodies, or nucleic acids.

Herpes simplex virus (HSV)

HSV will grow in a variety of tissue culture cells of both human and animal origin. Human diploid and amnion cells are often used. Commonly used animal cells include rabbit kidney, guinea pig embryo, continuous African green monkey kidney (Vero) cells, and BHK cells. The earliest manifestation of HSV replication is rounding of cells in several areas of the monolayer. The cells later become swollen and refractile and eventually will die and detach from the surface of the culture vessel. With a large inoculum, a cytopathogenic effect (CPE) can be seen as early as 18 to 24 hours after infection. Eighty percent of positive specimens are identified within 4 days.

Isolates can be confirmed as HSV by neutralization using type-specific antisera, by specific immunologic methods such as immunofluorescence (IF), or by nucleic acid hybridization. IF is the most popular method. Cells from cultures exhibiting a CPE are scraped off the glass and spotted onto glass slides and fixed in acetone. Fluorescein-conjugated anti-HSV antiserum allows identification of HSV. Conjugated monoclonal reagents may allow typing of the HSV isolate as type 1 or 2. A shell vial technique combines culture and immunologic detection by inoculating cells growing on microscope slides with the specimen to be tested, incubating the culture for 24 (or 48) hours, and then removing the slide and staining with antibody to HSV. The cultured cells usually will contain detectable HSV antigens before CPE is evident.

Human immunodeficiency virus (HIV)

See Chap. 70.

Human papillomavirus (HPV)

There are no culture systems available for HPV. Diagnostic approaches have developed using nucleic acid hybridization and polymerase chain reaction performed on tissue and some body fluids.

Mycoplasma hominis, M. genitalium, Ureaplasma urealyticum

The most sensitive method for the isolation of mycoplasmas consists of inoculation of specimens into liquid medium that is diluted serially, followed by subculture to liquid or agar medium. Color changes in liquid medium due to metabolic activities may indicate growth when colonies fail to develop on agar. *M. hominis* produces such a change within a week, and *U. urealyticum* does so usually within 24 to 48 hours or less. Aliquots of medium from the cultures that are just changing color are subcultured into fresh broth medium and/or onto agar medium. The medium used is comprised of beef heart infusion broth, available commercially as PPLO broth, supplemented with 10% fresh yeast extract and 20% horse serum. Fetal calf serum may improve the medium. Colonies of the genital mycoplasmas develop best in an atmosphere of 95% N_2 plus 5% CO_2. The colonies are about 200 to 300 μm and have the classic fried-egg appearance. Colonies of *M. genitalium* are often much smaller, and many do not have the typical appearance. As an aid to detecting *Ureaplasma* colonies, an aliquot of urea-containing broth medium that has just changed color is subcultured to agar medium containing urea, buffer, and a sensitive indicator of ammonia. The ureaplasmas form dark brown colonies that are slightly larger and more easily recognizable. Kits to isolate and identify *M. hominis* and *U. urealyticum* are available commercially. *M. genitalium* is best diagnosed by a PCR test.

Neisseria gonorrhoeae

Selective media for *N. gonorrhoeae*, such as modified Thayer-Martin (MTM) and Martin-Lewis (ML) media, contain ingredients to inhibit gram-positive and gram-negative bacteria, most commensal *Neisseria* species, swarming *Proteus* species, and fungi. New York City (NYC) medium is a clear medium that also permits the growth of large-colony mycoplasmas and *U. urealyticum*. Certain strains that require arginine, hypoxanthine, and uracil (AHU) are susceptible to the concentrations of vancomycin used in selective media. Other gonococci may be susceptible to trimethoprim. It is advisable to periodically assess the adequacy of isolation of fastidious strains of *N. gonorrhoeae* from urethral and endocervical specimens from men and women on selective and nonselective media. Cultures for the isolation of *N. gonorrhoeae* are always incubated at 35 to 37°C in a CO_2-enriched, humid atmosphere for up to 72 hours, examining plates at 24-hour intervals. Colonies of *N. gonorrhoeae* vary in diameter from 0.5 to 1 mm owing to the formation of different colony types. The oxidase reaction aids the search for gonococcal colonies in mixed cultures. A drop of tetramethyl- or dimethyl-paraphenylene-diamine is poured over suspected gonococcal colonies, which quickly turn pink and then dark blue. A Gram stain of oxidase-positive colonies is essential. In urogenital specimens, oxidase-positive organisms containing gram-negative diplococci provide a presumptive diagnosis of gonococci. Carbohydrate degradation tests are the reference confirmatory tests to differentiate gonococci from other *Neisseria* spp. and related organisms.

Group B streptococci

To isolate group B streptococci (GBS), one or two swabs of the vaginal introitus and anorectal canal should be placed into an appropriate transport tube and inoculated at the laboratory into selective enriched broth medium. This is usually a Todd-Hewitt type of broth supplemented with nalidixic acid and colistin or gentamicin. The broth culture is subcultured to a sheep blood agar plate after 18 to 24 hours. GBS colonies will be gram-positive, catalase-negative, and beta-hemolytic or nonhemolytic after 24 hours on the plate.

Treponema pallidum

Limited success has been achieved in growing *T. pallidum* in cell cultures. Specimens for in vivo isolation in rabbits can be collected from lesions in heparinized capillary tubes, frozen, and transported to a reference laboratory. The lesion material is injected intratesticularly into rabbits. The treponemes are harvested from the testicles and passed to a second animal after 2 to 3 weeks. Because of these difficulties, diagnostic procedures have been concentrated on serology.

Trichomonas vaginalis

Because of the low sensitivity of direct microscopy for detecting trichomonads in specimens from men, culture is used to isolate the parasite from urethral swabs, urine sediment, or prostatic fluid. Culture is also more sensitive than direct microscopy for detecting trichomonads in vaginal specimens. A number of media have been used (see Chap. 43), and some (e.g., Trichosel broth) are available commercially for routine use. The cultures are incubated anaerobically, and growth may be seen within days. Cultures generally are performed only in reference laboratories, which should be contacted about special procedures for specimen collection and storage.

ANTIGEN DETECTION

Detection of microbial antigens in clinical specimens has done much to increase the number of patients identified with STDs and to provide us with a greater understanding of the natural history of disease. Organisms such as HBV (which is noncultivable) and others such as *N. gonorrhoeae* and *C. trachomatis* (which can be fastidious) have been identified with sensitive and specific antigen-detection methods.

The earliest antigen-detection tests used antibodies conjugated with fluorescein isothiocyanate to enhance microscopic methods of identification. Other approaches used erythrocytes or latex particles linked to antibodies to demonstrate specific antigens in clinical specimens. The most popular approach has been the construction of solid-phase immunoassays (SPIA) using reaction indicators that employ an enzyme acting on a substrate and producing a chromogenic, chemiluminescent, or fluorescent end product (also known as enzyme immunoassay, or EIA technology).

Most SPIAs for the detection of antigen employ one of three methods: (1) competitive, (2) direct (double-antibody sandwich method), or (3) indirect (double-antibody sandwich-antiglobulin method) (Fig. 92-1). In competitive assays, labeled antigen is mixed with the test sample that may contain antigen, and these antigens compete for a limited amount of antibody attached to the solid phase. A negative control sample containing only labeled antigen is included. Unbound antigen is washed away, and the

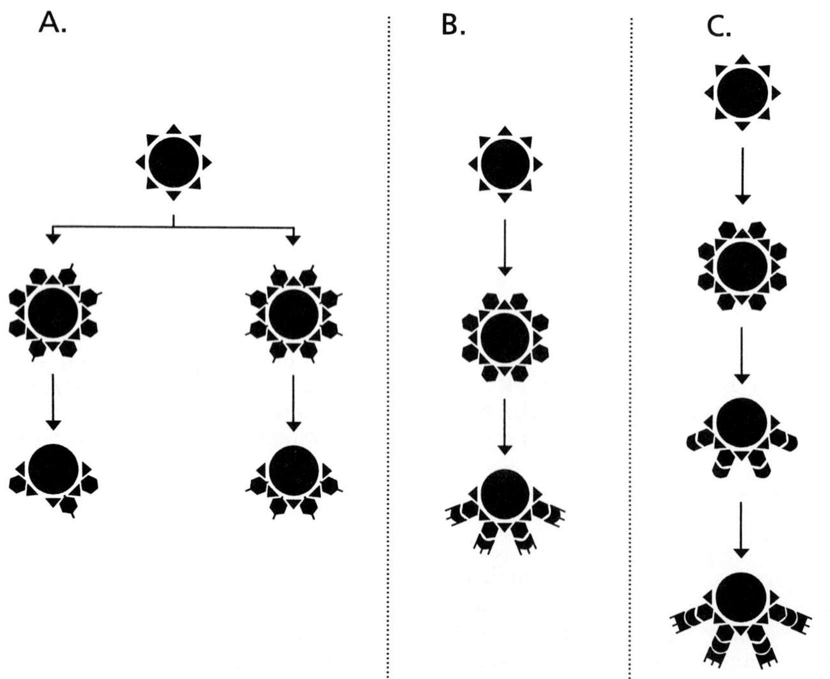

Fig. 92-1. Solid-phase immunoassays: (A) Competitive. (B) Direct. (C) Indirect. ● Solid phase; ▲ capture antibody or antigen put onto solid phase; ⬢ antibody or antigen trapped from clinical specimens; ◖ detector antibody; conjugated detector antibody; conjugated indicator antibody; conjugated competitive antibody or antigen.

difference in indicator activity between the specimen and control is measured. A direct SPIA for detection of antigen involves adding the clinical specimen to a capture antibody (CA) attached to the solid phase. Unbound antigen is washed away before the addition of a substrate-labeled detector antibody (DA). The DA is measured, and the more substrate label that is detected, the more antigen is present in the sample. The indirect test is similar to the direct assay employing a CA and DA, but the DA is not labeled. Instead, a third indicator antibody (IA) that is antispecies to DA is labeled; the remainder of the assay is similar to the direct procedure. This approach has become the most popular because of the availability of IA conjugates from commercial sources. The indirect test also provides some amplification of the binding reactions. They may create some problems, however, because they are very sensitive, and antispecies antisera may cross-react nonspecifically.

Antigen-detection methods have had variable utility in diagnosing the following STDs: *C. trachomatis,* HBV, HSV, *N. gonorrhoeae, T. pallidum, H. ducreyi,* and *T. vaginalis.*

Commercial kits for laboratory use to detect *C. trachomatis* lipopolysaccharide (LPS) or major outer membrane protein (MOMP) were introduced in the early 1980s in the form of direct fluorescent antibody (DFA) or SPIA tests. Most of these tests were evaluated originally for sensitivity and specificity compared with cell culture for swabs and first-void urine (FVU). These types of "one-way" comparisons with a single reference standard showed sensitivity ranges of 75 to 100 percent.[1–6] Generally speaking, when patients were symptomatic with high levels of organism present, the antigen positivity rates were higher. It soon became apparent that false-positive results could be seen with SPIA, which led to the development and routine use of supplementary or confirmatory testing by a neutralization or blocking test or another nonculture test identifying a different antigen than that detected by the initial screening test.[7–9]

Adoption of this procedure helped to reduce the reporting of false-positive results but also identified a problem of using culture as the sole reference standard for comparison. Further expansion of the reference standard through use of the ultrasensitive amplified genetic probes[10–12] has provided a better understanding of the overall sensitivity and specificity of antigen detection, which range from 50 to 75 percent and 95 to 100 percent, respectively.

A few "rapid" and simple antigen-detection tests (i.e., Clearview, Testpak, Surecell) have been developed for clinic use and evaluated for diagnosis of *C. trachomatis* infection. Where the comparisons have been made to an expanded standard, these tests generally have been 10 to 15 percent less sensitive than the laboratory-based SPIAs and have lacked sufficient specificity to be useful for routine diagnosis, especially in low-prevalence populations.

The DFA procedure[13,14] has been very successful for laboratories testing small numbers of specimens on a daily basis, whereas laboratories with large numbers of specimens have been able to use automated SPIAs to cope with the workload.

A SPIA for the detection of gonococcal antigens (Gonozyme) was introduced to the market by Abbott Laboratories in the early 1980s and has been evaluated by comparing it to Gram stain and/or culture on male and female clinical specimens. The Gonozyme test was shown to be as sensitive and specific as the Gram stain for male urethral swabs and FVU but less sensitive for endocervical swabs.[15–17]

EIAs for hepatitis B surface antigen (HBsAg) have evolved from previous generations of antigen tests that used counter immunoelectrophoresis and radioimmunoassays. Since the late 1970s, these highly sensitive EIAs have virtually eliminated the risk of HBV transmission by blood transfusion. In most developed countries, transmission of HBV now most often happens through unprotected sex or intravenous drug use. Most of the commercially available HBsAg detection kits are close to 100 percent sensitive and specific when performed on serum or plasma.

DFA reagents and EIA kits are available commercially for direct testing of clinical specimens for HSV antigens. These provide a rapid diagnosis but are only 65 to 85 percent sensitive compared with culture and are prone to false-positive reactions.[18,19] They become even less sensitive in detecting asymptomatic shedding of virus. Thus their usefulness is limited to screening and confirming positives. Negatives in these tests need to be further tested in more sensitive assays such as culture or PCR.

Detection assays for HIV p24 antigens have had limited success in the diagnosis of HIV infection. The EIA or DFA kits have been used to detect antigenemia in early infection or reactivation.

DFA tests for *T. pallidum* can be performed on body fluids, secretions, lesion exudates, and tissue. These polyclonal or monoclonal fluorescent reagents detect pathogenic treponemes, differentiating them from those which are nonpathogenic.[20,21] Although experience with these tests remains surprisingly limited, the sensitivity and specificity of DFA tests for diagnosing early and later stages of syphilis appear very promising.

SPIAs have been described for the detection of *H. ducreyi* antigens in clinical specimens.[22,23] They have shown some promise in limited evaluations.

Limited studies have been performed on the use of antigen detection for *T. vaginalis*. DFA tests using monoclonal reagents have been reported as 86 percent sensitive.[24] EIA capturing the 65-kDa surface polypeptide was shown to be 89 percent sensitive and 97 percent specific in detecting *T. vaginalis* in clinical specimens compared with culture.[25] Large-scale studies have not yet been reported.

Group B streptococci (GBS) diagnosis by antigen detection has been focused mainly on diagnosing GBS neonatal infection. When multiple specimens (blood, trachea, rectum, urine, etc.) were tested by counterimmunoelectrophoresis (CIE), approximately 95 percent of cases were detected.[26–28] Latex agglutination and immunofluorescence tests also have been used with good success to identify infected neonates and mothers who are heavily colonized.[29–31] These procedures are not as sensitive in identifying pregnant women who are lightly colonized.

Antigen-detection assays for the rest of the STD organisms have either not been developed or are under research protocols at the present time.

NUCLEIC ACID DETECTION

Hybridization

In the solid-phase DNA probe hybridization procedure, intact cells are lysed, and DNA is denatured and then directly fixed onto a nylon membrane in a dot or slot configuration. The membrane is immersed in a hybridization solution containing a DNA reporter probe and allowed to hybridize. The unbound reporter probes are then washed away, and the bound probe is detected. A variation on the dot- or slot-blot utilizes sandwich or capture hybridization. This procedure uses two probes that bind to different sites on the target nucleic acid. One probe is attached to the membrane and serves to capture the target nucleic acid in the sample. The second probe is labeled and serves as the detector.

The Southern blot is a solid-phase hybridization assay that allows determination of size of DNA fragments bound by the reporter probe. In the Northern blot, the reporter probe is used to detect RNA instead of DNA. In both types of blots, the nucleic acids are transferred to a nitrocellulose or nylon membrane for hybridization with a specific probe. Because of their complexity, the requirement for large amounts of sample nucleic acids, and the time required for completion of the assay, these procedures are not used routinely in clinical microbiology.

In solution-phase hybridization, both the target nucleic acid and the probe are free to interact in an aqueous reaction mixture that speeds the rate at which hybridization occurs. The key to successful solution-phase hybridization is a single-stranded DNA probe that does not hybridize with itself. Hybridization in solution can be detected by nuclease digestion of single-stranded DNA and recovery of remaining double-stranded reporter probe hybrids. The method in routine use for detecting probe hybridization in solution is the hybridization protection assay, where an acridinium ester moiety attached to a DNA probe is hybridized to target DNA and treated with alkali, emitting detectable light.

In situ hybridization assays involve the same general principles as solid- and solution-phase hybridizations. However, hybridization occurs within infected tissue. In clinical settings, formalin-fixed paraffin-embedded tissue sections frequently form the starting material for in situ hybridization assays. The sensitivity of in situ hybridization is limited by the accessibility of target nucleic acids within the cell.

Signal-amplification procedures have been designed to increase the signal generated by the probe hybridized to a specific sequence of target DNA or RNA. Signal-amplification procedures can detect a minimum of 10^3 to 10^5 nucleic acid targets, still well below the sensitivity of highly optimized nucleic acid target or probe amplification procedures. A branched DNA (bDNA) probe system (developed by Chiron Corp.) isolates the nucleic acid sequence of interest, which is then followed by hybridization with an unlabeled target-binding probe. An advantage of the bDNA probe system is the ease with which several different capture and target-binding probes can be incorporated into a single test system that is capable of detecting nucleic acid targets with significant sequence heterogeneity, as is the case for human immunodeficiency virus (HIV). These bDNA probe systems are also being developed for hepatitis B and C and CMV.

Nucleic acid amplification

The technology of nucleic acid amplification methods falls into one of three general categories: (1) target amplification such as polymerase chain reaction (PCR), self-sustaining sequence replication (3SR), or strand displacement amplification (SDA), (2) probe-amplification systems, which include Qβ replicase or the ligase chain reaction (LCR), and (3) signal amplification, in which the signal generated from each probe molecule is increased by using compound probes or branched-probe technology.

Polymerase chain reaction (PCR)

This method is based on the ability of DNA polymerase to copy a strand of DNA by elongation of complementary strands initiated from a pair of closely spaced oligonucleotide primers (Fig. 92-2). Each cycle of the reaction doubles the amount of target DNA, resulting in millionfold or more levels of amplification. A commonly used set of cycling temperatures includes denaturation of double-stranded DNA at 94°C for less than 1 minute, hybridization of oligonucleotide primers at 52°C for 15 seconds to 2 minutes, and extension (polymerase-mediated complementary-strand synthesis) from the primers at 72°C for 15 seconds to 3 minutes. These three steps are repeated for 25 to 40 cycles.

Numerous modifications of the standard PCR procedure have been developed. Nested PCR uses two sets of amplification primers, with one set targeted within the amplification product of the other set and two rounds of amplification in order to amplify specific target DNA. The procedure is designed to increase the sensitivity of PCR by directly reamplifying the product from a primary PCR with a second PCR. Two common nested PCR procedures are in use. A two-tube procedure uses a primer set 1 added to a PCR reaction mixture and cycled. The tube is then opened, and the product is transferred to a second tube containing primer set 2, which is complementary to the product from the first reaction but binds 3′ internal to primer set 1. The second reaction is then cycled, and the product is analyzed by standard methods. A single-tube procedure is also in vogue, where the tube does not have to be opened, so the chance of aerosol release of amplified DNA into the laboratory environment is reduced. However, it is much more complex. Because of the high level of target amplification with nested PCR, a single target molecule frequently can be detected by direct DNA staining, thus eliminating the additional steps involved in postamplification hybridization with a labeled probe.

Multiplex PCR detects two or more unique target DNA sequences in a specimen and amplifies them simultaneously. Multiplex PCR probably will be used most frequently in diagnostic assays that use one set of primers to amplify an internal control to verify the integrity of the PCR, while the second set of primers is targeted to the DNA sequence of interest. Multiplex PCR also may be used in the clinical microbiology laboratory to simultaneously probe a specimen for several different organisms in a single PCR tube. The primers are designed so that each amplification product is a unique size, allowing the detection and identification of a specific organism in the specimen even though primers to several different organisms are present in the reaction mixture.

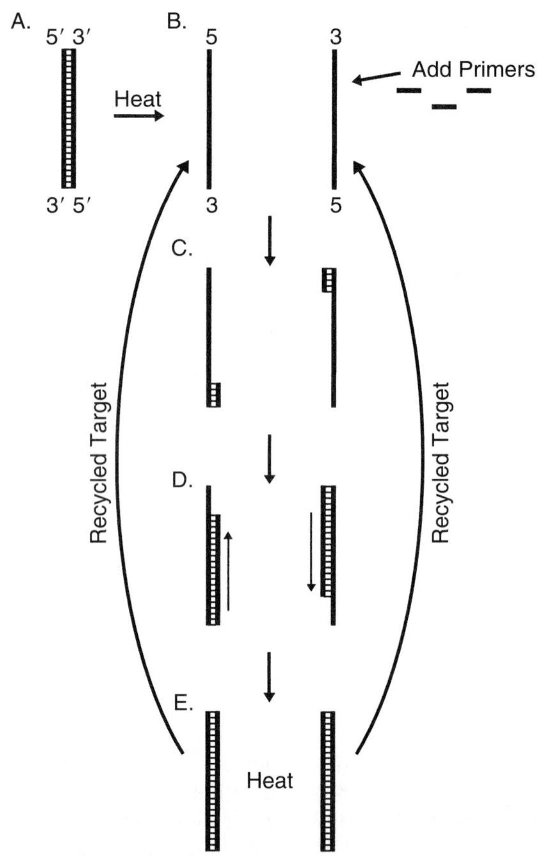

Fig. 92-2. Polymerase chain reaction. *(A)* Addition of target; *(B)* heat strand separation; *(C)* primer annealing; *(D)* primer extension; *(E)* next cycle of heat strand separation.

The ability to detect RNA by using a sensitive procedure such as PCR would be useful for the identification of organisms that contain thousands of copies of specific rRNA molecules, further enhancing the sensitivity of PCR. Some viruses only have RNA and do not undergo reverse transcription into a DNA intermediate during their life cycles. A recombinant DNA polymerase derived from *Thermus thermophilus* has become commercially available and possesses efficient reverse transcriptase activity in the presence of manganese, allowing PCR amplification of RNA.

Self-sustaining sequence replication (3SR)

This method utilizes the collective activities of three enzymes to isothermally amplify an RNA target. Up to a 10-million-fold amplification occurs within a 1- to 2-hour incubation.

While 3SR is well suited for amplification of single-stranded RNA, it is a more complicated procedure when it comes to the amplification of double-stranded DNA. For DNA amplification, heat denaturation steps are required in the initial stages of the reaction in order to generate the necessary amplification intermediates.

Strand displacement amplification (SDA)

This procedure is an isothermal DNA amplification method that uses specific primers, a DNA polymerase, and a restriction endonuclease to achieve exponential amplification of target. Published reports claim approximately 10^7-fold amplification of target following a 2-hour reaction. With the exception of an initial 95°C denaturation step, SDA is isothermal and requires no specialized laboratory equipment other than a temperature-controlled environment of 37°C. SDA can be applied to either single- or double-stranded DNA. Compared with PCR, SDA may be more difficult to decontaminate because the shorter target sequences (50 to 100 base pairs) generated are more difficult to inactivate. A unique isothermal transcription-mediated amplification (TMA) technique for rRNA target amplification is similar in some aspects to SDA. The use of two primers and two enzymes enables transcription of DNA and subsequent RNA amplicons with built-in degradation (Fig. 92-3).

Qβ replicase

The Qβ replicase method is a probe-amplification procedure based on the incorporation of a single-stranded oligonucleotide probe into an RNA molecule that can be amplified exponentially after target hybridization by the enzyme Qβ replicase. The kinetics of the Qβ replicase reaction are very rapid. Theoretically, a 200-nucleotide RNA target will yield 10^{12} progeny strands in only 13 minutes at 37°C. Target DNA is first heated to 85°C to denature it into single strands. As the reaction mixture is cooling, the midivariant-1 reporter probe, a naturally occurring template for Qβ replicase into which the probe oligonucleotide has been inserted, and specific capture probes are added. The reaction mixture is incubated for 30 minutes at 37°C to allow hybridization to take place, and Qβ replicase is added to initiate the amplification reaction. The amplified product can be detected by any one of a number of techniques. Probe hybridization, amplification, and detection of amplified product can be completed in 2 to 3 hours. The procedure involves isothermal reaction conditions that require no specialized laboratory equipment except a temperature-controlled environment. If the problem of background noise can be solved, the simplicity and tremendous amplifying power of Qβ replicase will make it an attractive technology for the diagnostic laboratory.

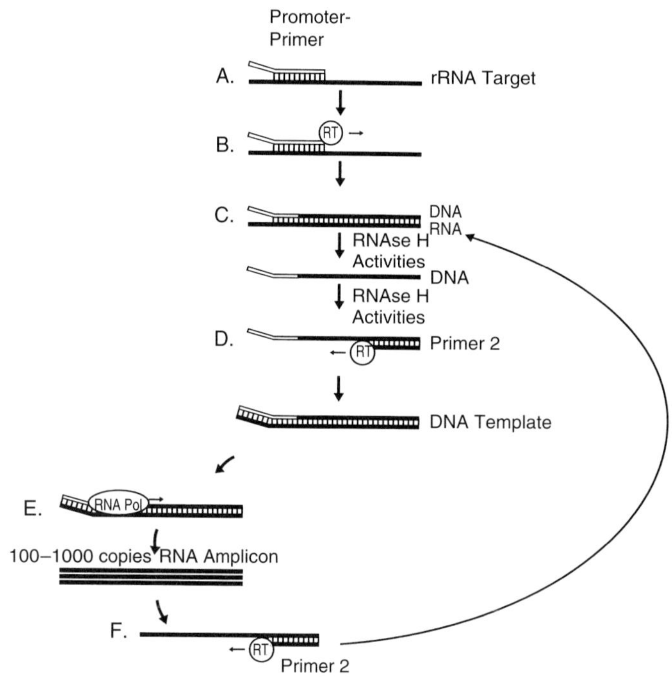

Fig. 92-3. Transcription-mediated amplification (TMA). *(A)* Promoter-primer binds to rRNA target; *(B)* reverse transcriptase (RT) creates DNA; *(C)* RNAse degrades rRNA from the DNA-RNA duplex; *(D)* RT creates new DNA, forming double-strand template; *(E)* RNA polymerase transcribes RNA copies; *(F)* second primer restarts the cycle.

Ligase chain reaction (LCR)

The LCR is a probe-amplification technique based on sequential rounds of template-dependent ligation of four oligonucleotide probes. Linear amplification of the specific probes is achieved when a single pair of oligonucleotides is ligated. Exponential amplification is achieved when two pairs of oligonucleotides, one complementary to the upper strand of target DNA and one complementary to the lower strand, are used. In the first step of LCR, two sets of oligonucleotide pairs are allowed to anneal to their target DNA at 65°C (Fig. 92-4). When complementary base pairing exists at the ligation junction, the ligase joins the pair, forming a longer product that is bound to the template. Any mismatch at the pair junction prevents ligation between the two oligonucleotides, which determines the specificity of the detection reaction. The reaction mixture is then heated to 94°C to denature the ligated product from the target and cooled to 65°C to allow annealing and ligation, and the cycle is then repeated. Newly formed ligation products are used as templates for ligation. Once ligated products form, subsequent cycles increase the amounts of products at exponential rates. Two pairs of oligonucleotide primers are annealed to opposite strands of target DNA but are spaced so that a polymerase is required to fill the gap between the primers; the ligase then connects the filled gap. This modified procedure is called *gapped LCR*.

Specimen preparation for nucleic acid assays

An ideal specimen preparation procedure would accomplish the following: release the nucleic acids from the target organism, prevent degradation of the free nucleic acids, remove any substances inhibitory to nucleic acid amplification or hybridization, and concentrate the nucleic acids into a small volume of appropriate buffer. Characteristics of the target nucleic acid will influence the preparation procedure, since RNA is much more susceptible to

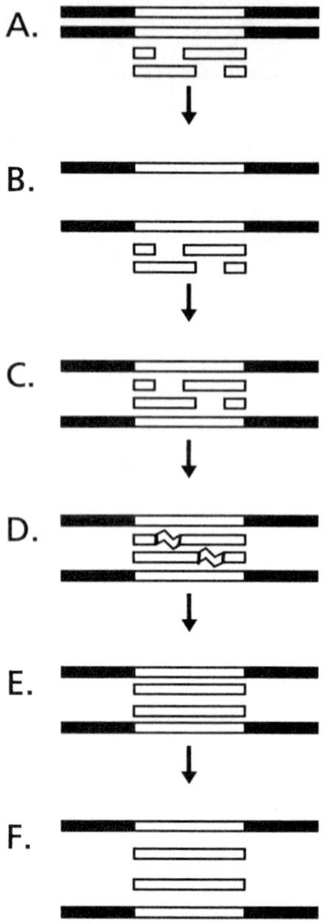

Fig. 92-4. Gapped ligase chain reaction (LCR) amplification of DNA. *(A)* Specimen with target, *(B)* heat to separate strands *(C)* cool to allow probes to bind, *(D)* PCR to fill gaps, *(E)* ligase links two adjoining probes, *(F)* heat to separate new targets.

degradation than DNA. Because of the limited sensitivity of hybridization procedures compared with nucleic acid amplification, specimen preparation for use in hybridization must be capable of processing and concentrating larger amounts of specimens. The number of suspected organisms in a specimen dictates the sensitivity requirements for the assay and the volume of specimen required. However, in nucleic acid amplification, the final reaction volume is restricted to between 20 and 100 μl, so factors such as the size of the specimen and the ease of concentration of organisms in the specimen are variables that must be considered when the optimal specimen preparation procedure is being selected. If nucleic acid amplification is the basis of the diagnostic procedure, the procedure selected must contain steps designed to remove or neutralize potential inhibitors. Several nucleic acid extraction procedures have been evaluated for specimen preparation. The basis of a successful genital swab preparation procedure involves separation of the DNA from the inhibitors. Phenol-chloroform extraction of the DNA followed by ethanol precipitation has been used successfully. Use of silica matrices that bind DNA and allow the contaminants to be washed away and repetitive washing of the specimen pellet with detergents also have yielded amplifiable DNA. Numerous lysis and nucleic acid extraction procedures have been reported for use with urine specimens. Like most specimen sources, urine is known to contain uncharacterized inhibitors of Taq polymerase.

Clinical utility of DNA assays

As was the case for antigen-detection procedures, the major thrust to develop STD nucleic acid hybridization and amplification assays focused initially on *C. trachomatis*. A single-stranded DNA probe, PACE-2 (Genprobe, San Diego, CA), was developed to detect *C. trachomatis* ribosomal RNA. The probe is labeled with an acridinium ester, and the presence of DNA-RNA hybrids is measured in a chemiluminometer. The assay has been used extensively on cervical and urethral swab specimens. The initial comparisons were made with culture or antigen detection, which showed good sensitivity and specificity of the probe assay. More recently, PACE-2 comparisons have been made to culture, antigen detection, and PCR, which have shown its sensitivity and specificity performance to be in the same range as good EIAs.[32–34] As with EIAs, the fear of false-positive results in low-prevalence populations has led to a consideration for confirmation of positives. A probe competition assay (PCA) has been developed for this purpose. It uses competitive nucleic acid hybridization to differentiate a true-positive signal from a false-positive one.[35]

Amplification assays for *C. trachomatis* detection in clinical specimens include PCR, LCR, Qβ replicase, and transcription-mediated amplification (TMA).

In PCR, primers have been developed to amplify (1) the *C. trachomatis* plasmid DNA, (2) chromosomal DNA fragments coding for the major outer membrane protein (MOMP), and (3) ribosomal RNA. Plasmid DNA amplification has become the most popular approach because of its inherent theoretically higher sensitivity, which is due to the presence of 7 to 10 plasmids per *C. trachomatis* elementary body. The PCR procedure also has been used to do direct gentopying of *C. trachomatis* strains by performing restriction fragment length polymorphism analysis (RFLPA) or DNA sequencing on products of PCR amplification.[36–38] Using an increased number of primers in a "nested" PCR and RFLPA improved the sensitivity of this genotyping procedure.[38] The commercially available PCR called *Amplicor* (Roche Molecular Systems, Branchburg, NJ) targets the *Chlamydia* cryptic plasmid for amplification and has received extensive evaluation on female swab and male urine specimens. On both these specimens the sensitivity of the assay has been reported to be approximately 20 percent higher than culture or antigen-detection methods.[39–45] Because of this, several approaches to confirming the extra positives have been developed. This usually has been done by performing a second PCR whose primers are directed against a totally different gene or to a different fragment of the same gene.[10,11,43] This has demonstrated a remarkable lack of false-positive results with amplification technology. PCR rarely demonstrates a sensitivity of 100 percent because of inhibitors of amplification found in clinical specimens. The rate of appearance of these yet-to-be-identified substances probably varies according to specimen type and also may be different according to gender. Inhibitors of Taq polymerase have been found that disappear on storage[41,43] and can be concentrated by centrifugation.

The clinical evaluation experience with LCR (Abbott Laboratories, Chicago, IL) has had some similarities to PCR. Female cervical specimens have ranged in sensitivity from 87 to 97 percent,[46] and LCR testing of female first-void urine (FVU) specimens has identified as many positive patients as cervical cultures in the limited number of studies reported thus far.[47–50] LCR also has proved to be an effective assay performed on male FVU.[47,50,51] The test has identified most infected men, and the presence or absence of symptoms of urethritis has not affected the positivity rate. Effective protocols using small amounts of male or female FVU, centrifuged and washed, may lead to screening programs in high-risk populations. Inhibitors also play a role in LCR, but the rate seems to be lower than for PCR.

Gene-Trak, Inc. (Framingham, MA), has developed a Q-beta replicase-amplified hybridization assay that detects and amplifies *C. trachomatis* rRNA or rDNA. The company has performed studies on a limited number of clinical specimens, reporting a sensitivity of 83 percent and a specificity of 96 percent compared with culture.[52,53] The company also has done a comparison with a 16S rRNA PCR. The study showed the PCR to be inhibited in 13 clinical specimens that were not inhibitory for Qβ replicase.

A fourth nucleic acid amplification assay for *C. trachomatis* has been developed by Gen-Probe (San Diego, CA). This TMA assay is isothermal. Performed on a limited number of swabs and urine specimens from men and women, the assay performed as well as PCR when compared with an expanded "gold standard."

N. gonorrhoeae and *C. trachomatis* are the major bacteria causing urethral or cervical discharge. Both separate and combined hybridization or amplification assays have been developed for their diagnosis. The PACE-2 test for *N. gonorrhoeae* has been used in the field for a number of years, detecting rRNA in greater than 90 percent of cervical or urethral culture-positive specimens with few false-positive results.[54–56] The company also has a test that can do a combined detection of *N. gonorrhoeae* and *C. trachomatis*. PCR has been developed for *N. gonorrhoeae*. Primers for gene fragments encoding the gonococcal outer membrane protein, rRNA, or the pJD cryptic plasmid *CppB* gene have been used in creating PCR assays. Evaluation of these assays has shown them to be as sensitive as culture.[57,58] Abbott Laboratories has elected to develop LCR for *N. gonorrhoeae* in a separate assay from *C. trachomatis*. In field evaluations it has performed very well, with high sensitivity and specificity.[59] In contrast, Roche Molecular Systems has developed a coamplification PCR that amplifies DNA from both the major causes of urethritis. It has performed well in preclinical evaluations on male urine specimens and urethral swabs and female cervical swabs. Mahony et al.[60] have published their findings on the performance of their multiplex *C. trachomatis* and *N. gonorrhoeae* PCR. The assay was 100 percent specific and detected all *C. trachomatis*- and 92.3 percent of *N. gonorrhoeae*-infected men by testing FVU.

A similar multiplex approach has been taken to use amplification technology to diagnose the potential causes of genital ulcers. Individual PCR assays have been developed for *H. ducreyi*,[61–63] but their reported sensitivities on clinical specimens have been less than desirable, ranging from 62 to 83 percent. Treponemal PCRs using primers to amplify a fragment of the gene encoding the 47-kDa membrane lipoprotein immunogen have been described but were found to be too susceptible to inhibitors of PCR to be clinically useful.[64,65] PCR for HSV DNA amplification has been shown to be more sensitive than culture or antigen detection on ulcer specimens.[66] An attempt has been made to construct a multiplex genital ulcer PCR containing primers for gene fragments from *T. pallidum, H. ducreyi,* and HSV. On limited numbers of specimens this approach has been more than 90 percent sensitive for each agent and very specific.

The other syndrome for which single or multiplex probe assays have been developed is vaginal discharge or bacterial vaginosis. A commercial kit (Affirm VP Microbial Identification) for *T. vaginalis, Candida* species, and increased concentrations of *G. vaginalis* in a single assay has shown promising results on limited evaluation.[67] Individual slot-blot hybridization assay and a PCR amplifying the nucleotide sequence of the internal transcriber spacer region of *G. vaginalis* DNA have been described[68,69] and await appropriate clinical evaluation.

Commercial hybrid capture tests have been available and continue to be used to identify HPV DNA in tissue and secretions. A comparison of a Southern blot (Oncor, Inc., Gaithersburg, MD) and a viral-type dot-blot (Digene Diagnostics, Inc., Silver Springs, MD) has been published.[70] Compared with a Pap smear and selected risk factors, both assays were effective in identifying HPV positives and negatives using cervical and penile biopsy tissues. The Digene kit identifies 14 HPV types in two groups (high or low risk) and yields quantitative data reflecting viral concentration. The test was accurate and reliable in an interlaboratory agreement study.[71] More recently, HPV PCRs have been described that are more sensitive than hybrid capture.[72–74] The presence of more than 70 viral types, including at least 20 found in the genital mucosa, has led investigators to design consensus primers that amplify highly conserved viral gene fragments in a single reaction. The amplified products can then be typed. Biopsy tissue, genital swabs, and urine have yielded positive findings in HPV PCR. These tests will soon be commercialized and then used more extensively in at-risk populations.

Nucleic acid amplification tests are available to detect HIV. A PCR is available (Roche Molecular Systems) to detect proviral DNA and has been used to detect pediatric infection.[75] RNA tests are also available to quantitate viral RNA in plasma. Viral RNA quantitation can be used to complement the measurement of changes in lymphocyte subset levels and viral phenotype predominance as an index of the success or failure of anti-HIV chemotherapy. At the present time, there are three commercial kits available. The assays are as follows: reverse-transcriptase PCR (Roche Molecular Systems), NASBA (Organon-Teknika), and branched DNA (Chiron Corporation). Some of the characteristics of these three amplification assays are summarized in Table 92-3. Although all three tests are capable of providing measurements in creating response curves before and after drug therapy, the lower limits of detection of nucleic acid are still not below 350 copies of RNA per milliliter (Roche), 400 copies of HIV-1 RNA (Organon-Teknika), and 10 kEq (about 10 times that of the other two tests) in the Chiron quantiplex branched DNA test. A recent comparative study of the three assays demonstrated that they could be used to measure HIV-1 RNA copy number without significant differences in sensitivity or RNA levels in plasma in response to therapy in 36 infected patients.[76] If measured within 6 months

Table 92-3. Comparison of Several Aspects of Three Quantitative Commercial Assays for HIV

AMPLICOR HIV-1 monitor (Roche Molecular Systems)	NASBA HIV-1 RNA QT (Organon-Teknika)	QUANTIPLEX HIV-1 RNA (Chiron Corporation)
Frozen plasma or serum (0.2 mL)	Plasma, whole blood, leukocytes, or CSF (0.1 mL)	Frozen plasma 2.0 mL
Sample lysis	Sample lysis, RNA purification on silica	Centrifugation, lysis, RNA capture hybridization of bDNA amplifier molecules
Target amplification by RT-PCR	RNA coamplification (WT RNA and three internal standards)	Signal amplification by branched DNA
Immobilized capture probe (Microwell)	Isothermal amplification	Multiple probes to each bDNA molecule
Colorimetric label	Electrochemiluminescent probes	Chemiluminescent label
A–E subtypes	Detects all known subtypes	A–E subtypes
Lower limit of detection 200 copies/mL	Detection limit 4000 copies/mL	10,000 equivalent (lower limit of detection)
6 hours per 10 samples	5-hour assay, 10 samples per run	1.5 days per 42 samples

after seroconversion, the plasma RNA level is predictive of progression to AIDS.[77] In this review by Schooley, greater than 10^5 equivalents of RNA per milliliter showed a high likelihood ratio for progression of 10.8 compared with 1.7 when the RNA level was a log lower. Generally, elevation of the plasma HIV RNA level correlates with increases in infectious virus and proviral DNA in plasma and a fall in CD4 cells.[78] Increases in viral load (plasma HIV RNA) also can be correlated with the presence of the viral codon 215 mutation as opposed to wild-type HIV: there is also a correlation with increases in p24 HIV immune-complex-dissociated antigen and decreases in CD4 counts in patients treated with a second drug or placebo.[79]

SEROLOGY

For most STD-related microorganisms, some form of serologic test has been used to identify infected individuals. These tests include neutralization, complement fixation (CF), hemagglutination inhibition, passive hemagglutination, immunoassays, precipitation, latex agglutination, and protein-specific blotting (Western blot). They have all had some success in determining past experience with particular organisms.

Of all the microorganisms listed in Table 92-1, only *T. pallidum, C. trachomatis,* HIV, HBV, and HSV have been shown to have an immune serologic response useful for the diagnosis of current infection. Serologic methods for some of these have only been of value in certain specific situations.

Serodiagnosis of neonatal chlamydial pneumonia has been a good approach,[80] with both microimmunofluorescence and EIA IgM tests being 100 percent sensitive and specific. Elevated titers to *C. trachomatis* by EIA or complement fixation are found in most cases of *C. trachomatis*–associated tubal factor infertility, but also in some fertile women. Lymphogranuloma venereum is usually associated with microimmunofluorescence antibody titer ≥ 256. Other lower genital tract syndromes have not been diagnosed successfully by serology.

HSV antigens in a clinical specimen may exhibit antiprotein profiles in a Western blot.[81] Antibody to the glycoprotein G2 is specific for infection by HSV-2 and can be detected with high sensitivity and specificity by Western blot or ELISA. Such testing is currently available only in reference laboratories.

In patients infected with HBV, the presence of anti-HBc IgM without HBsAg may be useful in identifying recent infection.[82]

For HIV, serologic SPIAs have become the method of choice for screening tests of sera or plasma. Some success also has been experienced by measuring antibodies in saliva or whole blood. Most recent generations of SPIAs combine recombinant or synthetic antigens to detect infection with either HIV-1 or HIV-2. These assays are close to 100 percent sensitive but need to be confirmed with other methods such as WB, IF, or RIBA. Some of the newer recombinant and synthetic peptide SPIAs have been designed to detect HIV IgM and therefore provide an earlier serologic diagnosis than the earlier generations of tests.[83]

Of all the STDs, serology has been most useful for diagnosing syphilis. The approach for routine serologic screening of patients without lesions for *T. pallidum* infection involves an initial screening for antibodies in a nontreponemal test. At the present time, these include the following: Venereal Disease Research Laboratory (VDRL) slide test, unheated serum reagin (USR) test, rapid plasma reagin (RPR) 18-mm-circle card, Visuwell reagin (VR) test, and toluidine red unheated serum test (TRUST). All these tests have alcohol-derived amounts of cardiolipin, cholesterol, and lecithin. The VDRL and USR tests are flocculation tests requiring microscopic examination. The RPR and TRUST are visual agglutination tests. Both IgG and IgM responses to lipoidal and lipoprotein antigens of treponemes and damaged host cells are measured.

Positive nontreponemal tests should be confirmed by a treponemal test, particularly in low-prevalence populations. These tests are as follows: fluorescent treponemal antibody absorption (FTA-ABS), microhemagglutination assay for antibodies to *T. pallidum* (MHA-TP), IgG or IgM enzyme immunoassays (EIA), and WB. Approximately 30 percent of patients with early primary syphilis may have negative nontreponemal results. The tests are close to 100 percent sensitive in secondary and latent syphilis. Some false-positive results are seen in all tests in any of the stages of syphilis. The treponemal tests are used effectively as confirmatory tests on samples positive by nontreponemal testing, and in late syphilis, specimens negative in the nontreponemal tests may still be positive in one of the treponemal tests.

ENZYMES OR METABOLITES IN CLINICAL SPECIMENS

Gas chromatographic analysis of vaginal fluid from patients with bacterial vaginosis (BV) will detect bacterial metabolic by-products. When lactobacilli are predominant, lactic acid is the primary short-chain fatty acid found. In women with BV, acetate, succinate, proprionate, butyrate, isobutyrate, and valeric acids can be found in increased amounts. Ratios of the relative amounts of these short-chain fatty acids have been used to establish diagnostic criteria for BV,[84] although certain specimens will lack fatty acid peaks in the chromatograph. A thin-layer chromatograph test also has been used to diagnose BV.[85] It measures putrescine and cadaverine in vaginal fluid and is suitable for screening large numbers of specimens. A microtiter plate proline aminopeptidase test has been used to measure this enzyme in vaginal fluid. The color change after adding an appropriate substrate can be diagnostic because lactobacilli lack the enzyme. The test has been shown to possess good sensitivity and specificity, as defined by clinical criteria for BV.[86] A rapid diagnostic diamine spectrophotometric test for BV has been compared with culture of *G. vaginalis,* clue cells, and the amine (Whiff) test in general practice and family planning clinics.[87] The sensitivity ranged from 86 to 97 percent, but the specificity was only 81 to 84 percent.

The leukocyte esterase (LE) dipstick test, which is an indicator of inflammatory cells being present, generally has had sensitivities for diagnosing chlamydial or gonococcal infection ranging between 40 and 100 percent depending on the specimen assayed (usually male urethral swabs or FVU) and whether symptoms were present.[88,89] In these and other evaluations, a considerable number of false-positive results have been reported. The studies are difficult to compare because different levels for LE positivity are used, and assays for specific organisms with different sensitivity levels for specific organisms have been used for comparison. Also, not all the organisms causing urethral inflammation have always been considered. This more generic approach to testing patients for STDs together with the selection of patient risk factors may reduce the number of patients who would need to be tested by the other diagnostic approaches in certain populations.

CONCLUSION

Diagnostic laboratory services for STDs may range from highly specialized methods such as fragment-length polymorphism typing or antibiotic susceptibility assays to rapid and simple self-administered tests. The modern laboratory should attempt to provide the appropriate technology for the clinical situation, which will demand accurate diagnosis, management, and treatment of patients. This can be accomplished through the use of any or all of the approaches listed in Table 92-2. Test accuracy needs proficiency test monitoring both in the highly specialized central laboratory and in satellited services closer to the patient. The challenge for the millennium will be to determine the meaning of detecting organism gene fragments in clinical specimens in relation to transmission and disease.

References

1 Chernesky MA et al: Detection of *Chlamydia trachomatis* antigens by enzyme immunoassay and immunofluorescence in genital specimens from symptomatic and asymptomatic men and women. *J Infect Dis* 154:141–148, 1986.

2 Lefebre J et al: Comparison of three techniques for detection of *Chlamydia trachomatis* in endocervical specimens from asymptomatic women. *J Clin Microbiol* 26:726–731, 1988.

3 Lebar WD et al: Comparison of IDEIA III and cell culture for the detection of *Chlamydia trachomatis* in endocervical specimens. *J Clin Microbiol* 28:1447–1448, 1990.

4 Leonardi GP et al: Evaluation of three immunoassays for detection of *Chlamydia trachomatis* in urine specimens from asymptomatic males. *J Clin Microbiol* 30:2793–2796, 1992.

5 Moncada J et al: Evaluation of Syva's enzyme immunoassay for the detection of *Chlamydia trachomatis* in urogenital specimens. *Diagn Microbiol Infect Dis* 15:663–668, 1992.

6 Clark A et al: Multicenter evaluation of the antigEnz *Chlamydia* enzyme immunoassay for diagnosis of *Chlamydia trachomatis* genital infection. *J Clin Microbiol* 30:2762–2764, 1992.

7 Mahony J et al: Diagnosis of *Chlamydia trachomatis* genital infections by cell culture and two enzyme immunoassays detecting different chlamydial antigens. *J Clin Microbiol* 27:1934–1938, 1989.

8 Schwebke JR et al: Use of sequential enzyme immunoassay and direct fluorescent antibody tests for detection of *Chlamydia trachomatis* infections in women. *J Clin Microbiol* 28:2473–2476, 1990.

9 Chernesky MA et al: Confirmatory testing demonstrates that false-positive rates in the Chlamydiazyme assay are influenced by gender and genital specimen type. *Sex Transm Dis* 20:301–306, 1993.

10 Mahony JB et al: Confirmatory polymerase chain reaction testing for *Chlamydia trachomatis* in first-void urine from asymptomatic and symptomatic men. *J Clin Microbiol* 30:2241–2245, 1992.

11 Mahony JB et al: *Chlamydia trachomatis* confirmatory testing of PCR-positive genitourinary specimens using a second set of plasmid primers. *Mol Cell Probes* 6:381–388, 1992.

12 Thejls H et al: Expanded gold standard in the diagnosis of *Chlamydia trachomatis* in a low prevalence population: Diagnostic efficacy of tissue culture, direct immunofluorescence, enzyme immunoassay, PCR and serology. *Genitourin Med* 70:300–303, 1994.

13 Tam M et al: Culture-independent diagnosis of *Chlamydia trachomatis* using monoclonal antibodies. *N Engl J Med* 310:1146–1150, 1984.

14 Stamm WE et al: Diagnosis of *Chlamydia trachomatis* infections by direct immunofluorescence staining of genital secretions. *Ann Intern Med* 101:638–641, 1984.

15 Danielson D et al. Diagnosis of urogenital gonorrhea by detecting gonococcal antigen with a solid phase enzyme immunoassay (Gonozyme). *J Clin Pathol* 36:674, 1983.

16 Schachter J et al: Enzyme immunoassay for diagnosis of gonorrhea. *J Clin Microbiol* 19:57, 1984.

17 Stamm WE et al: Antigen detection for the diagnosis of gonorrhea. *J Clin Microbiol* 19:399, 1984.

18 Moseley RC et al: Comparison of viral isolation, direct immunofluorescence, and indirect immunoperoxidase for the detection of genital herpes simplex virus infection. *J Clin Microbiol* 13:913, 1981.

19 Lafferty WE et al: Diagnosis of herpes simplex virus by direct immunofluorescence and viral isolation from samples of external genital lesions in a high-prevalence population. *J Clin Microbiol* 25:323, 1987.

20 Larsen SA et al: *A Manual of Tests for Syphilis,* 8th ed. Washington, American Public Health Association, 1990.

21 Ito FR et al: Specific immunofluorescent staining of pathogenic treponemes with a monoclonal antibody. *J Clin Microbiol* 30:831–838, 1992.

22 Roggen EL et al: Antigen detection and immunological typing of *Hemophilus ducreyi* with a specific rabbit polyclonal serum. *J Clin Microbiol* 31:1820–1825, 1993.

23 Schalla WO et al: Use of dot-immunobinding and immunofluorescence assays to investigate clinically suspected cases of chancroid. *J Infect Dis* 153:879–887, 1986.

24 Kreiger JN et al: Diagnosis of trichomoniasis: Comparison of conventional wet-mount examination with cytologic studies, cultures and monoclonal antibody staining of direct specimens. *JAMA* 259:1223–1227, 1988.

25 Lisi PJ et al: Monoclonal-antibody-based enzyme-linked immunosorbent assay for *Trichomonas vaginalis*. *J Clin Microbiol* 26:1684–1686, 1988.

26 Hill HR et al: Rapid identification of group B streptococci by counterimmunoelectrophoresis. *J Clin Microbiol* 1:188, 1975.

27 Rhodes PG et al: Countercurrent immunoelectrophoresis (CIE) of urine: A rapid diagnostic tool for group B streptococcal (GBS) sepsis in the neonate. *J Pediatr* 91:833, 1977.

28 Stechenberg BW et al: Countercurrent immunoelectrophoresis in group B streptococcal disease. *Pediatrics* 64:632, 1970.

29 Bromberger PI et al: Rapid detection of neonatal group B streptococcal infections by latex agglutination. *J Pediatr* 96:104, 1980.

30 Ingram DL et al: Detection of group B streptococcal antigen in early-onset and late-onset group B streptococcal disease with the Wellcogen Strep B latex agglutination test. *J Clin Microbiol* 16:656, 1982.

31 Wald ER et al: Rapid detection of group B streptococci directly from vaginal swabs. *J Clin Microbiol* 25:573, 1987.

32 Lebar W et al: Comparison of DNA probe, monoclonal antibody enzyme immunoassay, and cell culture for the detection of *Chlamydia trachomatis*. *J Clin Microbiol* 27:826–828, 1989.

33 Clarke LM et al: Comparison of Syva Microtrak enzyme immunoassay and Gen-Probe PACE 2 with cell culture for diagnosis of cervical *Chlamydia trachomatis* infection in a high-prevalence female population. *J Clin Microbiol* 31:968–971, 1993.

34 Altwegg M et al: Comparison of Gen-Probe PACE 2, Amplicor Roche, and a conventional PCR for the detection of *Chlamydia trachomatis* in genital specimens. *Med Microbiol Lett* 3:181–187, 1994.

35 Kluytmans JA et al: Improved performance of PACE 2 with modified collection system in combination with Probe competition assay for detection of *Chlamydia trachomatis* in urethral specimens from males. *J Clin Microbiol* 32:568–570, 1994.

36 Gaydos CA et al: Gene typing of *Chlamydia trachomatis* by polymerase chain reaction and restriction endonuclease digestion. *STD* 19:303–308, 1992.

37 Lan J et al: Direct detection and genotyping of *Chlamydia trachomatis* in cervical scrapes by using polymerase chain reaction and restriction fragment length polymorphism analysis. *J Clin Microbiol* 31:1060–1065, 1993.

38 Lan J et al: Improved PCR sensitivity for direct genotyping of *Chlamydia trachomatis* serovars by using a nested PCR. *J Clin Microbiol* 32:528–530, 1994.

39 Bass CA et al: Clinical evaluation of a new polymerase chain reaction assay for detection of *Chlamydia trachomatis* in endocervical specimens. *J Clin Microbiol* 31:2648–2653, 1993.

40 Jaschek G et al: Direct detection of *Chlamydia trachomatis* in urine specimens from symptomatic and asymptomatic men by using a rapid polymerase chain reaction assay. *J Clin Microbiol* 31:1209–1212, 1993.

41 Bauwens JE et al: Diagnosis of *Chlamydia trachomatis* endocervical infections by a commercial polymerase chain reaction assay. *J Clin Microbiol* 31:3023–3027, 1993.

42 Bauwens JE et al: Diagnosis of *Chlamydia trachomatis* urethritis in men by polymerase chain reaction assay of first-catch urine. *J Clin Microbiol* 31:3013–3016, 1993.

43 Mahony JB et al: Role of confirmatory PCRs in determining performance of *Chlamydia* Amplicor PCR with endocervical specimens from women with a low prevalence of infection. *J Clin Microbiol* 32:2490–2493, 1994.

44 Skulnick M et al: Use of the polymerase chain reaction for the detection of *Chlamydia trachomatis* from endocervical and urine specimens in

an asymptomatic low-prevalence population of women. *Diagn Microbiol Infect Dis* 20:195–201, 1994.

45 de Barbeyrac B et al: Evaluation of the Amplicor *Chlamydia trachomatis* test versus culture in genital samples in various prevalence populations. *Genitourin Med* 70:162–166, 1994.

46 Schachter J et al: Ligase chain reaction to detect *Chlamydia trachomatis* infection of the cervix. *J Clin Microbiol* 32:2540–2543, 1994.

47 Chernesky MA et al: Diagnosis of *Chlamydia trachomatis* infections in men and women by testing first-void urine by ligase chain reaction. *J Clin Microbiol* 32:2682–2685, 1994.

48 Lee HH et al: Diagnosis of *Chlamydia trachomatis* genitourinary infection in women by ligase chain reaction assay of urine. *Lancet* 345: 213–216, 1995.

49 Bassiri M et al: Detection of *Chlamydia trachomatis* in urine specimens from women by ligase chain reaction. *J Clin Microbiol* 33:898–900, 1995.

50 vanDoornum GJ et al: Detection of *Chlamydia trachomatis* infection in urine samples from men and women by ligase chain reaction. *J Clin Microbiol* 33:2042–2047, 1995.

51 Chernesky MA et al: Diagnosis of *Chlamydia trachomatis* urethral infection in symptomatic and asymptomatic men by testing first-void urine in a ligase chain reaction assay. *J Infect Dis* 170:1308–1311, 1994.

52 Shah JS et al: Novel, ultrasensitive, Q-beta replicase-amplified hybridization assay for detection of *Chlamydia trachomatis*. *J Clin Microbiol* 32:2718–2724, 1994.

53 An Q et al: Comparison of characteristics of $Q\beta$ replicase-amplified assay with competitive PCR assay for *Chlamydia trachomatis*. *J Clin Microbiol* 33:58–63, 1995.

54 Granato PA et al: Use of the Gen-Probe PACE system for the detection of *Neisseria gonorrhoeae* in urogenital samples. *Diagn Microbiol Infect Dis* 13:217–221, 1990.

55 Panke ES et al: Comparison of Gen-Probe DNA probe test and culture for the detection of *Neisseria gonorrhoeae* in endocervical specimens. *J Clin Microbiol* 29:883–888, 1991.

56 Stary A et al: Comparison of DNA-probe test and culture for the detection of *Neisseria gonorrhoeae* in genital samples. *STD* 20:243–247, 1993.

57 Ho BS et al: Polymerase chain reaction for the detection of *Neisseria gonorrhoeae* in clinical samples. *J Clin Pathol* 45:439–442, 1992.

58 Liebling MR et al: Identification of *Neisseria gonorrhoeae* in synovial fluid using the polymerase chain reaction. *Arthritis Rheum* 37:702–709, 1994.

59 Smith KR et al: Evaluation of ligase chain reaction for use with urine for identification of *Neisseria gonorrhoeae* in females attending a sexually transmitted disease clinic. *J Clin Microbiol* 33:455–457, 1995.

60 Mahony JB et al: Multiplex PCR detection of *Chlamydia trachomatis* and *Neisseria gonorrhoeae* in genitourinary specimens. *J Clin Microbiol* 33:3049–3053, 1995.

61 Grimprel E et al: Use of polymerase chain reaction and rabbit infectivity testing to detect *Treponema pallidum* in amniotic fluid, fetal and neonatal sera and cerebrospinal fluid. *J Clin Microbiol* 29:1711–1718, 1995.

62 Johnson SR et al: Development of a polymerase chain reaction assay for the detection of *Hemophilus ducreyi*. *STD* 21:13–23, 1994.

63 West B et al: Simplified PCR for detection of *Hemophilus ducreyi* and diagnosis of chancroid. *J Clin Microbiol* 33:787–790, 1995.

64 Grimprel E et al: Use of polymerase chain reaction and rabbit infectivity testing to detect *Treponema pallidum* in amniotic fluid. *J Clin Microbiol* 29:1711–1718, 1991.

65 Sanchez PJ et al: Evaluation of molecular methodologies and rabbit infectivity testing for the diagnosis of congenital syphilis and neonatal central nervous system invasion by *Treponema pallidum*. *J Infect Dis* 167:148–157, 1993.

66 Cone RW et al: Extended duration of herpes simplex DNA in genital lesions detected by the polymerase chain reaction. *J Infect Dis* 164: 757, 1991.

67 Briselden AM et al: Evaluation of affirm VP microbial identification test for *Gardnerella vaginalis* and *Trichomonas vaginalis*. *J Clin Microbiol* 32:148–152, 1994.

68 Sheiness D et al: High levels of *Gardnerella vaginalis* detected with an oligonucleotide probe combined with elevated pH as a diagnostic indicator of bacterial vaginosis. *J Clin Microbiol* 30:642–648, 1992.

69 van Belkum A et al: Development of a species-specific polymerase chain reaction assay for *Gardnerella vaginalis*. *Mol Cell Probes* 9:167–174, 1995.

70 Halstead DC et al: Evaluation of two commercially available DNA tests for detection of human papillomavirus. *Infect Dis Obstet Gynecol* 2:255–262, 1995.

71 Schiffman MH et al: Accuracy and interlaboratory reliability of human papillomavirus DNA testing by hybrid capture. *J Clin Microbiol* 33: 545–550, 1995.

72 Villa LL et al: An approach to human papillomavirus identification using low stringency single specific primer PCR. *Mol Cell Probes* 9: 45–48, 1995.

73 Coutlee F et al: Detection of human papillomavirus DNA in cervical lavage specimens by a nonisotopic consensus PCR assay. *J Clin Microbiol* 33:1973–1978, 1995.

74 Vossler JL et al: Evaluation of the polymerase chain reaction for the detection of human papillomavirus from urine. *J Med Virol* 45:354–360, 1995.

75 Cassol SA et al: Diagnosis of vertical HIV-1 transmission using the polymerase chain reaction and dried blood spot specimens. *J Acquir Immune Defic Syndr* 5:113–119, 1992.

76 Revets H et al: Comparative evaluation of NASBA HIV-1 RNA QT, Amplicor-HIV monitor, and Quantiplex HIV RNA assay, three methods for quantification of human immunodeficiency virus type 1 RNA in plasma. *J Clin Microbiol* 34:1058–1064, 1996.

77 Schooley RT: Correlation between viral load measurements and outcome in clinical trials of antiviral drugs. *AIDS* 9:S15–19, 1995.

78 Lin HJ: Laboratory tests for human immunodeficiency viruses. *JIFCC* 7:61–66, 1995.

79 Merigan, TC et al: The prognostic significance of serum viral load, codon 215 reverse transcriptase mutation and CD4+ T cells on progression of HIV disease in a double-blind study of thymopentin. *AIDS* 10:159–165, 1996.

80 Mahony JB et al: Accuracy of immunoglobulin M immunoassay for diagnosis of chlamydial infections in infants and adults. *J Clin Microbiol* 24:731–735, 1986.

81 Ashley RL et al: Comparison of Western blot and gG-specific immunodot enzyme assay for detecting HSV-1 and HSV-2 antibodies in human sera. *J Clin Microbiol* 26:662, 1988.

82 Chernesky MA et al: Diagnostic significance of anti-HBcIgM prevalence related to symptoms in Canadian patients acutely or chronically infected with hepatitis B virus. *J Med Virol* 20:269–277, 1986.

83 Spiegel CA et al: Anaerobic bacteria in nonspecific vaginitis. *N Engl J Med* 303:601, 1980.

84 Chen KSS et al: Biochemical diagnosis of vaginosis: Determination of diamines in vaginal fluid. *J Infect Dis* 145:337, 1982.

85 Thomason JL et al: Proline aminopeptidase as a rapid diagnostic test to confirm bacterial vaginosis. *Obstet Gynecol* 71:607, 1988.

86 Shafer MA et al: Evaluation of urine-based screening strategies to detect *Chlamydia trachomatis* among sexually active asymptomatic young males. *JAMA* 270:2065–2070, 1993.

87 O'Dowd TC et al: Evaluation of a rapid diagnostic test for bacterial vaginosis. *Br J Obstet Gynecol* 103:366–370, 1996.

88 Sellors JW et al: Screening urine with a leukocyte esterase strip and subsequent chlamydial testing of asymptomatic men attending primary care practitioners. *STD* 20:152–157, 1993.

89 Tyndall MW et al: Leukocyte esterase urine strips for the screening of men with urethritis: Use in developing countries. *Genitourin Med* 70: 3–6, 1994.

Chapter 93

STD-related health care seeking and health service delivery

Sevgi O. Aral
Judith N. Wasserheit

Timely treatment of sexually transmitted infections plays a central role in the prevention of sequelae of sexually transmitted diseases (STD), and in limiting their spread. Treatment of STD cases constitutes primary prevention of that STD for other members of the population, and secondary prevention of complications for infected individuals. To the extent that the encounter between infected individuals and the health care system delivers effective primary prevention messages, treatment of STD cases may also constitute primary prevention of repeat infections with the same organism, or future infections with other sexually transmitted organisms, for the infected individual him- or herself.

Three large categories of social and behavioral factors contribute to the timely treatment of STDs. These are health care seeking behaviors of members of the population, behaviors of health care providers who deliver STD care, and the organization of STD-related health service delivery. Each of these three components can be conceptualized at both the individual and the population levels, and is influenced by and, in turn, influences factors at both levels.

Currently, an STD-specific paradigm that integrates the relevant conceptual frameworks and empirical findings in the areas of health care seeking, health care provision and health service organization, is not available. However, general conceptual frameworks that can be adopted to the STD area have been formulated, and discrete research findings are beginning to shed light on several aspects of the many factors that influence the timely treatment of STDs. This chapter summarizes the conceptual frameworks that may be applicable to STD-related heath care seeking, the provision of STD services, and the behaviors of health care providers. It proposes an STD-specific conceptual framework based on integration and adaptation of the general conceptual models, through the consideration of selected additional factors that are specific to STDs. These factors include characteristics of the STDs and the populations affected by them; phase of the particular STD epidemic; the detection strategies and technologies employed; the therapeutic regimens and sex partner management approaches utilized; providers who see STD patients (e.g., their skill levels); and the health system (e.g., availability, accessibility and acceptability of services, the availability of patient management guidelines, and the extent to which compliance with such guidelines is assured).

Research findings relevant to STD-related health care seeking, behaviors of STD care providers, and organization of STD services are summarized in separate sections. The conclusion discusses implications of available conceptual frameworks and empirical findings for future directions in STD research and prevention efforts.

Throughout the discussion, the underlying integrating focus is provided by the health outcome of interest, which is defined as the timely and appropriate treatment of individuals infected with sexually transmitted pathogens to achieve cure of bacterial and parasitic STDs, and suppression of incurable viral STDs. Cure of bacterial or parasitic STDs stops symptoms and infectiousness, and prevents complications. Suppression of incurable viral STDs, in general, decreases severity of symptoms, decreases viral shedding (thereby decreasing infectiousness), and may slow disease progression. Both cure of bacterial STDs and suppression of incurable viral STDs decrease duration of infectiousness, which intervenes in the transmission dynamics of the infection and slows the rate of spread of infection in the population. To the extent that infection with some STDs increases infectiousness of and susceptibility for other STDs, decreases in the duration of infectiousness with one STD will also decrease the transmissibility (and therefore the rate of spread) of other STDs.

CONCEPTUAL FRAMEWORK

Several theoretical approaches have dealt with the issues of health service utilization and health care seeking, in general, at both the population and individual levels of analysis. These are helpful in understanding STD-related health care seeking and provision.

POPULATION-LEVEL, GENERAL CONCEPTUAL MODELS

At the population level, two general conceptual models that deal with implications of health policy decisions in the health service utilization area are relevant. McKinlay's Major Approaches to Characterizing Predictors of Health Services Utilization is an inductively constructed model based on integration of research findings.[1] The Behavioral Model of Health Services Utilization is a systems model originally formulated by Ronald Andersen in 1968 and further developed by Aday, Andersen, and other colleagues between 1974 and 1987.[2,3]

According to McKinlay, the six approaches to health service utilization are the demographic; social structural; social psychological; economic; organizational; and systems approaches.[1] The demographic approach focuses on age, sex, marital status, family size, and residence as predictors; the social structural approach emphasizes social class, ethnicity, education, and occupation; the social psychological approach considers health beliefs, values, attitudes, norms, and culture; the economic approach covers family income, insurance coverage, price of services, and provider:population ratios; the organizational approach looks at the organization of physicians practices, referral patterns, and regular source of care. The systems approach adopted by McKinlay includes all or most of the predictors mentioned in the preceding in the context of a set of relationships.

The Behavioral Model of Health Services Utilization assumes that health policy decisions, whether they deal with issues of financing or organization, will have an effect on utilization of health services, consumer satisfaction, and the characteristics of both the population at risk and the health delivery systems, which in turn affect each other.[3a] The characteristics of the population, including demographic, social structural, and belief variables, are predisposing factors that describe the propensity of individuals to use services. The means individuals have available to them to use services, such as income and insurance are enabling factors. Finally, health status, or need for health services is a key determinant of utilization in this model. These factors may be alterable by health policy, that is, mutable, or biological or social givens, not open to alteration by health policy. The latter factors are termed immutable.

This model has been applied to evaluate whether services are equitably distributed. To the extent that differences in utilization are explained by need variables and demographic correlates of need such as age or sex distribution of services is considered equitable. If other factors such as income or insurance coverage are the most important predictors of who gets care, then the system is considered to be inequitable.

Research results, in general, support this model, at least in the United States.[4] Of the population characteristics, age is curvilinearly related to health service utilization, with the young and the old having higher utilization than those in the middle. Utilization is higher among women than men; among whites than non-whites (although the gap is narrowing); among whites and non-whites than Hispanics; among those living in metropolitan and urban areas than those living outside metropolitan areas and in rural areas; and among those in poor health than those in good health.

Education and income are related to health service utilization in more complex ways. People with higher education tend to utilize preventive services more than those with less education, whereas people with less education have higher rates of hospitalization. Prior to Medicare and Medicaid, persons with greater income tended to utilize health services to a greater extent; however, following the enactment of Medicare and Medicaid, lower income persons have started using certain health services at higher rates than persons with high incomes.

Focusing on the characteristics of the health care delivery system, regular source of medical care consistently emerges as a strong, consistent predictor of health service utilization, particularly the utilization of preventive services. Moreover, the directionality of this association has been explored and availability of regular source of medical care appears to have a direct and causally prior impact on health services utilization.[4]

INDIVIDUAL-LEVEL, GENERAL CONCEPTUAL MODELS

At the individual level, there are at least four conceptual models of patient decision making regarding health care seeking. One of these is Suchman's sociological five-stage decision making model that focuses on an illness episode and describes the stages of decision making as experience of symptoms; assumption of the sick role; establishment of contact with medical care; assumption of the dependent patient role; and recovery and rehabilitation.[5] According to Suchman's model, persons with traditional, parochial affiliations and a popular orientation to medical care would tend to delay assuming the sick role and seeking medical care, and would not comply with therapeutic recommendations.[5–7]

Kossa and Robertson's psychological stage model of patient decision making describes four stages, including assessment of disturbance; anxiety arousal; application of the person's own medical knowledge to address the problem; and an attempt to alleviate anxiety either through rational therapeutic activities or through gratifying activities that facilitate denial.[8]

A third conceptual model of patient decision making was developed by David Mechanic.[9] According to this model, the social and psychological factors that affect perception of need to seek care are symptom recognizability; perceived seriousness of symptoms; the extent to which symptoms disrupt regular activity; the frequency, persistence, and recurrence of symptoms; the tolerance level of persons evaluating the symptoms; the information, knowledge, and cultural assumptions of the evaluator; basic needs that lead to denial; needs that compete with illness responses; competing interpretations for symptoms; and finally the availability of care and financial and psychological costs of taking action, including issues of stigma, social distance, and humiliation.[9]

The fourth conceptual model that has focused on patient decision making regarding health care seeking is Marshall Becker's health belief model.[10] This model focused on the individual's subjective state of readiness based on perceptions of susceptibility and severity of consequences of illness; the individual's evaluation of the costs and benefits of seeking care; and a cue to action that may be "internal" (e.g., symptoms) or "external" (e.g., coverage of the issue in the mass media).

More recent conceptual work focusing on individual level factors that affect health care seeking behaviors has viewed health care seeking as a continuous variable. These recent approaches focus on delays in seeking care.[11] Such conceptualization represents a departure from earlier models, discussed in the preceding, which have constructed health care seeking as a dichotomous variable measuring a decision either to seek or not seek health care.

These recent models propose that appraisal of whether an unusual bodily condition is, indeed, a symptom typically accounts for the major portion of the delay in seeking care.[11] Expectations lengthen this period of appraisal in various ways, including the attribution of the cause of the condition to factors in the environmental context; an unrealistic optimism regarding the risk of contracting disease (optimistic bias); denial that a threat exists; and biased monitoring of bodily changes.[12–14] In addition, "lay theories of disease" also contribute to delays in seeking care.[15]

One recent STD-specific conceptualization, recognizing that the process of problem identification differs from the process of resolving barriers to seeking care, used the timing of the decision to seek care to distinguish two intervals: an "appraisal interval" defined as the time between recognition of a problem and the decision to seek clinical care, and a "procrastination interval" defined by the interval between the decision to seek care and actual care.[16] As would be expected, factors that influence the appraisal interval are different from the factors that influence the procrastination interval.

At the health systems level, how care is organized and financed has a great impact on both health care seeking behaviors and health care providers' behaviors. The most immediate operational indicators for the individual patient of how care is organized and financed are whether one has a regular source of care and insurance coverage, and the particular type of care and coverage. Currently, in the United States, these factors are in flux, as they relate to STD care.

Person-time of infectiousness (PTI): a behavioral model

The conceptual model being proposed here has several important characteristics. First, the outcome being focused on is a health outcome rather than a behavioral outcome. Second, the health outcome of interest here is jointly determined by factors at the individual, population (or societal), and health system levels, and the interactions among these factors. Third, this health outcome is influenced, perhaps equally, by the behaviors of infected individuals and providers, and properties of the health system.

As mentioned earlier, the health outcome of interest is the timely and appropriate treatment of individuals infected with sexually transmitted pathogens to achieve the cure of bacterial and parasitic STDs and suppression of incurable viral STDs. This particular health outcome translates into duration of infectiousness (D), one of the three determinants of the reproductive rate in infectious disease transmission dynamics. Therefore, it is a key parameter in the epidemiology of STDs.[17,18]

The timely and appropriate treatment of STDs is a function of four basic detection and treatment components (11 subcomponents) and one additional prevention component. These components may be viewed both in terms of the proportion of the infected population that never successfully complete the component (percent of individuals experiencing delay) *and* the time spent in each component by those who are able to move to the next one (duration of infectiousness) (Fig. 93-1). Although, in the final analysis, both types of concepts are reducible to the single measurement of "infectious person days" or "person days of infectiousness" (referred to as Person Time of Infectiousness [PTI]), conceptually differentiating between proportions of the population who never complete a component, and the time it takes to complete the component for those who do, facilitates the identification of individual, population, and system level factors and the behaviors of infected individuals and providers that influence the components and the outcome of interest. The four components of the model follow.

Component I: Lost to Detection and Resolution of Infectiousness. This component refers to the proportion of infected individuals (both symptomatic and asymptomatic) who never receive treatment. It translates into PTI terms as the time elapsed from infection to resolution of infectiousness (if applicable) as determined purely by biological dynamics between the pathogen and the host. It includes symptomatic individuals who never seek health care, symptomatic or asymptomatic infected individuals who are not detected through testing, and symptomatic or asymptomatic individuals who are not brought to treatment through partner notification. Individuals may not be brought to treatment because they are never detected or because they are lost to follow up during components III or IV.

Component II: Health Care Seeking Delays. This component focuses on time elapsed from infection to initial contact with the health care provider who makes the diagnosis and recommends therapy. It is composed of five subcomponents: (1) Time elapsed in symptom or risk appraisal, during which the individual attempts to interpret symptoms, often by gathering additional information regarding the symptoms and their significance. Individuals may wait and see if the symptoms resolve on their own or they may attempt to treat themselves during this period. Asymptomatic individuals, who suspect exposure, may gather information regarding their potential risk of infection and wait to see if symptoms occur; (2) Time elapsed from decision that symptoms (or risk of exposure) require attention from a health care provider to decision regarding where to seek care, often involving information gathering regarding types of providers and accessible service sites; (3) Time elapsed from decision to seek care from a specific provider or clinic to making the call or the visit to make the appointment, referred to as the procrastination period; (4) Time elapsed from making the appointment until the time of the appointment, which may range from minutes to days or weeks depending, often, on the health care provider and system; and (5) Time elapsed from arriving at the health care facility to initial contact with the provider, which generally would not be longer than a few hours.

Component III: Diagnostic Delays. Time elapsed from initial contact with the health care provider to diagnosis constitutes this component. It is conceptually composed of two subcomponents: time elapsed from initial contact with provider to establishment of a laboratory diagnostic test result; and time elapsed from establishment of a laboratory diagnosis to the infected individual's return to the health facility to receive the test result. The first subcomponent includes the time it takes to send the specimen to the laboratory, the laboratory processing of the specimen, and the communication of the test result to the provider. In situations in which individuals are treated presumptively, providers rely on clinical diagnosis based on signs and symptoms, or rapid tests are available on site, one or both components of diagnostic delays may not apply. On the other hand presumptive treatment and clinical diagnosis may lead to coinfections being missed or misdiagnosed.

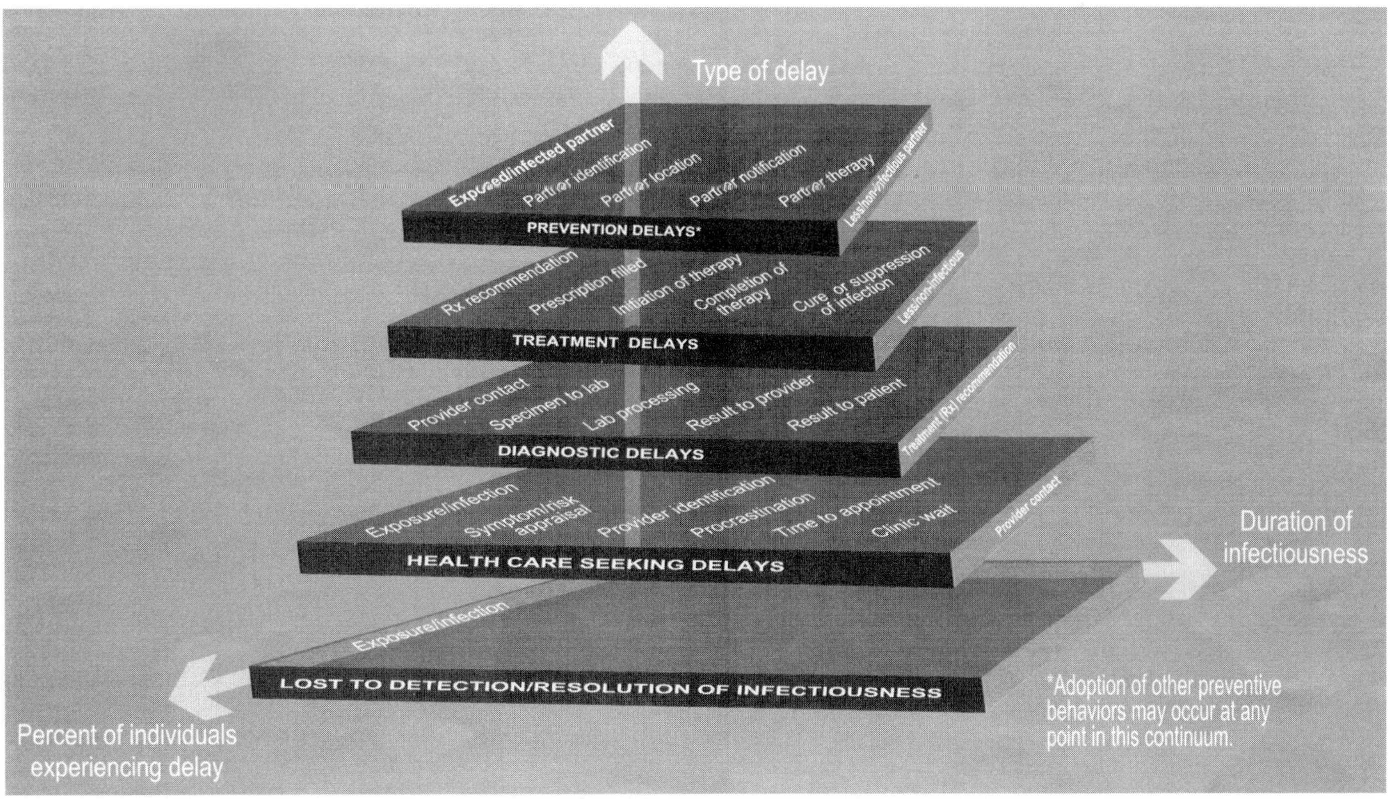

Fig. 93-1. The Person-Time of Infectious Model.

Table 93-1. Factors Influencing PTI: Lost to Detection

Properties of the pathogen and host	Proportions symptomatic; proportions with signs
Individual behavior parameters	Gender, risk recognition, symptom recognition, symptom description, extent of routine contact with health care
Provider behavior parameters	Risk assessment practices, screening practices, counseling practices, PN practices, compliance with programmatic and diagnostic guidelines
Health system parameters	Existence and quality of guidelines on risk assessment, screening, counseling, PN and diagnosis; existence and quality of STD health-education/health promotion programs; extent of reinforcement for provider compliance with existing guidelines; extent and quality of provider training, cost of care
Societal parameters	Level of education, level of overall health, available diagnostic technologies, availability, acceptability, accessibility of health care, cultural factors affecting sexuality, health, and disease, phase of epidemic, and stage of program

Component IV: Treatment Delays. This component consists of time elapsed from therapy recommendation to cure of bacterial and parasitic infections and suppression of viral infections. It is composed of four subcomponents: (1) Time elapsed from the infected individual receiving the therapy recommendation to filling the prescription; (2) Time elapsed from the individual filling the prescription to actually starting the medication; (3) Time elapsed from initiation of therapy to completion of therapy; and (4) Time elapsed from completion of therapy to actual cure or suppression. In some cases cure or suppression may occur prior to completion of therapy; however, data on the frequency of this occurrence are scarce. Multidose therapy regimens pose problems in that individuals may not complete the recommended course. On the other hand, single dose, directly observed therapy may also pose problems in that individuals may assume they are cured instantaneously and may resume sexual activity while still infectious.

Component V. An additional, post-PTI component in the model, referred to as *prevention delays*, includes time elapsed to the treatment of partners and adoption of preventive behaviors to prevent reinfection and infection with other sexually transmitted pathogens.

FACTORS THAT INFLUENCE PERSON-TIME OF INFECTIOUSNESS

A certain proportion of individuals infected with sexually transmitted pathogens are never identified as cases and are never treated (component I, Fig. 93-1). Properties of the pathogen and host, health seeking behaviors of the infected individuals, behaviors of providers, health system, and societal parameters all contribute to this component (Table 93-1). Some STDs tend to be more frequently asymptomatic compared to others. For example, only one out of ten individuals who had serologic evidence of infection with herpes simplex virus Type 2 reported ever having had genital herpes.[19] Whether or not a particular infection is symptomatic also varies by gender. Many STDs tend to be more frequently asymptomatic among women than men. Persons with asymptomatic infections do not have a reason for seeking STD-specific health care. The STD prevention program may successfully identify these persons as being infected if effective screening initiatives are in place. Whether or not wide-scale screening is conducted depends on the stage of the particular prevention program and the phase of the particular epidemic.[20] In addition, if the prevention program has effective health education initiatives for the general population in place, individuals who have been exposed to risk of acquiring infection may recognize their risk and seek screening. Another element of a prevention program that identifies infected persons (whether they are symptomatic or not) is partner notification. Provider behaviors also contribute to component I. Providers who do effective risk assessment help identify infected individuals even if the person is not seeking STD care. Thus, those STDs that tend to be asymptomatic; those providers who do not conduct effective STD risk assessment; and those prevention programs that do not include effective screening, partner notification, and health education for the general population all contribute to higher proportions of infected individuals who never get treated.

At a more global or societal level, the availability, accessibility, and acceptability of health care may contribute to the proportion of infected individuals who are never identified as cases and treated. Acceptability of available STD services may be a major issue for members of particular subpopulations. High levels of overall poor health may be associated with persons not seeking care even for severely symptomatic STDs. For example, observations in South Africa indicate that this may be the case for some parts of the population in that country (Ronald Ballard, personal communication). The quality of existing clinical and laboratory STD diagnoses is another system level factor that may contribute to the proportion of infected individuals who may never be detected and treated, even if they are seen in a clinic setting. For example, in Morocco, some women with vaginal infections are not diagnosed as such (Caroline Ryan, personal communication).

Table 93-2. Factors Influencing PTI: Health Care Seeking Delays

Explosure/infection			Contact with provider	
Symptom/risk appraisal	Identification of provider	Procrastination	Time to appointment	Clinic wait
Properties of the pathogen and host	Proportions with symptoms			
Individual behavior parameters	Gender,* risk recognition, symptom recognition, symptom description, extent of routine contact with health care, awareness of availability, and properties of STD specific health services			
Provider behavior parameters	Clinical and referral practices, partner notification practices			
Health system parameters	Availability, accessibility, acceptability *and* visibility of services, clinic overload, hours of operation, waiting time to clinic appointment, waiting time in the clinic (after clinic arrival)			
Societal parameters	Organization of STD health services; organization of funding for STD health services; cultural factors influencing STD, STD services, and sexuality stigma			

* This demographic parameter is included here because it is so strongly associated with symptom status and health care behaviors.

Table 93-3. Factors Influencing PTI: Diagnostic Delays

Provider contact		Treatment recommendation	
Specimen to laboratory	Lab processing	Result to provider	Result to patient
Properties of the pathogen and host	Proportions with symptoms; proportions with signs; the extent to which signs and symptoms are differentiating		
Individual behavior parameters	Risk recognition and reporting; symptom recognition and reporting		
Provider behavior parameters	Risk asessment practices; clinical diagnostic practices; laboratory diagnostic choices; specimen collection practices		
Health system parameters	Availability of and choice for diagnostic technologies; availability and quality of diagnostic guidelines and protocols; quality and timeliness of laboratory procedures; extent and quality of training for clinicians and laboratory personnel; sanctions association with compliance with clinical and laboratory guidelines		
Societal parameters	Phase of epidemic; stage of program; technological, societal, and economic development stage		

Thus, among infected individuals who do seek care or get screened, a certain proportion may not be identified as cases. All infected individuals, whether asymptomatic or symptomatic, who are never identified as STD cases are considered to contribute to component I in the model proposed here. That is, component I refers to all infected individuals who are never identified as cases.

For those who are ultimately identified, there may be a variable period of delay before they are identified as infected. Such delays increase the probability of complications following infection and may contribute to further transmission of infection in the population. Properties of the pathogen and host, in combination with the symptom recognition and description behaviors of infected individuals and risk-assessment behaviors of providers contribute to health care seeking delays (Table 93-2).

Some STDs are easier to detect than others. Ease and rapidity of detection may be affected by the diagnostic approach employed, including clinical versus laboratory diagnosis, choice of diagnostic test, and laboratory in which the testing is performed. Some laboratory tests take longer than others. The prevention program and the health care system affect these parameters both directly and indirectly through availability of screening guidelines, systems for timely reporting of laboratory results, and specific training for health care providers and laboratory workers. Thus, factors that affect detection delays include properties of the infection that influence severity and duration of symptoms; symptom recognition and reporting behaviors of infected individuals; risk assessment, clinical diagnosis, and specimen collection behaviors of providers; and their test and laboratory choices (Table 93-3). At the health system level, diagnostic delays are affected by the availability of diagnostic technologies, availability and quality of screening guidelines, quality and timeliness of laboratory processing and reporting procedures, and the extent and quality of required training for clinicians and laboratory personnel. At a more global societal level, the levels of economic and technological development and the phases of the program and the STD epidemic influence the choices of diagnostic protocols, the levels of training, the availability of appropriate guidelines, and the extent to which provider compliance with guidelines is assured.

Many factors contribute to treatment delays once a therapy recommendation has been made by the provider (Table 93-4). Properties of the infecting pathogen affect responsiveness or resistance to therapy. Therapy compliance (or adherence) behaviors of the infected individual determine whether the patient takes all of the prescribed medication at the prescribed times. Patients' nonadherence may be owing to misunderstanding or forgetting, or may be intentional—the patient may experience a side effect, or decide the drug dosage is too much, or that he or she is already cured. Therapy delays are also influenced by the providers' compliance with treatment guidelines and choice of therapy, including the timing and duration of therapy, the number of medications to be taken, and consideration of whether the patient can adhere to the recommended therapy regimen. The providers' communication behaviors, including counseling the patient on the importance of taking the full course of medication at the recommended times, and assessing the patient's ability and willingness to comply with the recommendations, are also important. Finally, health system properties including the availability, accessibility, and affordability of medications; quality and dissemination of treatment guidelines; and existence of an effective surveillance system that detects emerging resistant strains in a timely manner are important in this context.

Factors that influence prevention delays or adoption of preventive behaviors also include those at individual, provider, and health system levels (Table 93-5). At the individual level, motivation to reduce risk; current behaviors; current social environment; extent of control over social environment; ability and will-

Table 93-4. Factors Influencing PTI: Treatment Delays

Treatment recommendation		Less/noninfectious	
Prescription filled	Initiation of therapy	Completion of therapy	Cure of suppression of infection
Characteristics of the pathogen and host	Proportions symptomatic, severity of symptoms, responsiveness to medication, existence of resistant strains		
Individual behavior parameters	Adherence with dosage and recommendations; patient nonadherence may be owing to misunderstanding, forgetting, or intention (person may decide the dosage is too much or they are cured and do not need to continue medication)		
Provider behavior parameters	Therapy choices of providers, including number, dosage, timing of medications, and side effects provider compliance with treatment guidelines, consideration of patients' adherence to recommended therapy in therapy choices, communication behaviors in explaining the need for compliance.		
Health system parameters	Availability, accessibility, affordability of medications; availability, quality, extent of dissemination of treatment guidelines; availability of effective surveillance or resistant strains, emerging and reemerging infections; phase of the epidemic and stage of the program.		
Societal parameters	Overall level of education, level of development, level of health, relative importance of health		

Table 93-5. Factors Influencing PTI: Prevention Delays

Exposed/infected partner			Less/noninfectious partner
Partner identification	Partner location	Partner notification	Partner therapy adoption of preventive behaviors
Individual behavior parameters	Level of motivation, current behaviors, social environment, control over social environment; ability and willingness to help with the identification, location, and notification of partners or to offer medication to partners		
Provider behavior parameters	Counseling patients on adoption of preventive behaviors; counseling patients on partner management issues, partner notification practices, partner management behaviors		
Health system parameters	Availability of a variety of partner management procedures; effective triaging of patients to the partner management procedures most appropriate to their situation; availability of continuous and effective health education/ health promotion; existence of good relationships that encourage trust between health agencies and population; stage of epidemic, stage of program		
Societal parameters	Overall level of education, level of development, level of health; relative importance of prevention; the extent to which social networks are conducive to diffusion of interventions		

ingness to help with the identification, location, and notification of partners or to offer medication to partners all influence prevention delays. Providers' counseling behaviors, including counseling patients on adoption of preventive behaviors and on partner management issues are important in this context. Health system characteristics, including the availability of continuous and effective health education and health promotion initiatives, maintenance and reinforcement of good relationships that encourage trust between health agencies and the populations they serve, availability of a variety of partner management procedures, effective triaging of patients to the partner notification and management procedures most appropriate to their needs, and well-trained staff to assist with partner notification and management, when appropriate, may be the factors with the greatest impact on prevention delays.

The model described in the preceding is influenced by at least two conceptual approaches formulated earlier, namely, the force-of-infectivity concept, and the application of Piot's public health model on tuberculosis to STDs, by Fransen.[21,22] However, this particular conceptualization is new. Thus, the existing literature in this area does not lend itself to an organization exclusively by the components of our conceptual model. On the other hand, each component of the model is influenced by factors related to patients, providers, and the health system. In the following, we review the available data on STD care seeking behaviors, provision of health services, provider behaviors, and health care system characteristics.

STD CARE SEEKING BEHAVIORS

WHERE CARE IS SOUGHT

Available data on STD-specific care seeking behaviors are limited. However, interest in empirical investigations in this area has increased drastically within the past decade. Recent data from the United States indicate that the majority of people seek care for bacterial STDs at private physicians' offices (53%) or non-STD public facilities (35%), and only a minority (12%) report seeking care at dedicated STD clinics.[23] The proportions seeking care for viral STDs are even more skewed (80, 15, and 5%, respectively). The proportion of adolescents and women seeking care at STD clinics are still lower.[23] Similar patterns are observed in health care seeking for pelvic inflammatory disease (PID). Women with acute PID often seek care in emergency rooms (ERs). In 1992, according to data from the National Hospital Ambulatory Medical Care Survey (NHAMCS), 316,308 cases of PID were treated in ERs.[24] Only 36 percent of these patients were treated with Centers for Disease Control and Prevention (CDC) recommended dual antibiotic regimens. High proportions of ER visits for PID occur among adolescents.

A somewhat different picture is gleaned from a focus on STD clinic attendees in a study that sought to characterize the demographic characteristics, STD morbidity, insurance status, reasons for attending the STD clinic, and preferences for where clients would seek STD services under universal access to STD care.[25] Responses of 2,490 clients attending five STD clinics for new problem visits indicated that walk-in services, confidentiality, and low cost were the major reasons why clients sought care at STD clinics. Even if they had unlimited choice, two-thirds of clients surveyed would still prefer to be seen at STD clinics in the future.

One study sought to determine how often STD clinic patients use other health care sources and whether choice of other sources of care differed by gender and STD diagnosis.[26] Among STD clinic patients who reported treatment for an STD within the past year, 14 percent of men and 35 percent of women treated for STDs reported receiving care only in non-STD clinic settings. Women were significantly more likely to have received care in non-STD clinic settings, including doctor's offices (19.9 vs 6.1%); emergency rooms (10.0 vs 4.9%), family planning clinics (4.7 vs 0.5%), and other sites (3.7 vs 0.7%).

Results of a nationally representative general population survey conducted in the United Kingdom indicate that health care seeking behaviors of people living in England are, in general, similar to those of people living in the United States.[27] Of the respondents, 8.3 percent of men and 5.6 percent of women had attended an STD clinic in their lifetime, and, 3.4 percent of men and 2.6 percent of women had done so within the last 5 years. Behaviors, but not the attitudes, of STD clinic attenders differed markedly from those of nonattenders. As in the United States, clinics appear to attract primarily those with high-risk lifestyles but only a minority of those reporting risk markers for STD transmission attend STD clinics.[27]

DELAYS IN CARE SEEKING

At the individual level, the first delay in receiving treatment for STDs relates to the time elapsed between the perception of STD-related symptoms by the patient and health care utilization. A common response to illness is to "wait and see" if symptoms subside, persist, or worsen.[5] This is apparently the case with STDs. For example, symptoms of gonococcal and chlamydial cervicitis are often mild, inconspicuous, or completely absent, and syphilitic chancres are not only painless, but resolve spontaneously, which presumably contributes to delayed health care seeking. Apparently many women interpret their STD symptoms as part of normal variation in their menstrual cycle.[28] Uncertainty regarding genital symptoms ultimately leads to health care seeking, but only

45 percent of women motivated to seek care do so immediately.[28] In another study, about 25 percent of individuals with STD-related symptoms waited longer than 4 weeks before seeking care.[29] Delay in seeking care was particularly long among women living with one "permanent" partner, perhaps reflecting their perception of low STD risk associated with their own monogamous sexual behavior.[29] These data also suggested that the stigma concerning STDs may act as a barrier to prompt care seeking. Moreover, neither higher perception of vulnerability resulting from having sex with more than one partner without using a condom, nor being a recurrent attender at STD clinics with STD-related symptoms resulted in less delay in seeking health care.[29] In fact, previous delayed health care seeking may be a predictor of delayed health care seeking in the present and future.[30]

Apparently, prior to health seeking, compared to adolescent men, adolescent women spend a longer period of time on symptom appraisal, whereas time spent seeking social support, seeking information, and self-treating are common to both men and women.[16] The average total care seeking interval (the interval from presumed infection to seeking care) was 9.6 days for symptomatic women, 5.8 days for asymptomatic women, 6.3 days for symptomatic men, and 7.3 days for asymptomatic men. Low income and perception of stigma related to STD were associated with longer delays in health care seeking for adolescent women.[16]

These findings highlight the importance of differentiating between symptomatic and asymptomatic infection with respect to delays in detection. In the case of symptomatic infection, the most important social and behavioral factors contributing to delays in detection are factors related to the client. In the case of asymptomatic infections, factors related to the behaviors of health care providers and those related to the health system may play a more important role. Asymptomatic women may recognize that they are at risk following a risky sexual encounter, and seek screening. Alternatively, health care providers may recognize risky behavioral patterns through history taking, or respond to demographic characteristics associated with risk for infection and screen asymptomatic women for a particular STD. Finally, the health system may provide guidelines that result in routine screening of asymptomatic women on the basis of individual or population level markers that may not be recognized by either the client or provider.

On the other hand, the difference between symptomatic and asymptomatic infections should not be overemphasized. In some populations, response to symptoms of STD may be minimal and may in fact be associated with considerable delays in seeking health care. In one investigation of a chancroid outbreak in Mississippi, an assessment of health care seeking behavior of male patients with ulcers showed long delays in seeking treatment and a substantial amount of unprotected sex with untreated ulcers during this delay.[31] The median time from onset of symptoms to clinic visit was significantly longer for syphilis (14 days) and chancroid patients (10 days) than for HSV patients (4 days); for 65 percent of all male ulcer patients there was at least a 1-week delay in receiving care.

Similarly, in one multisite study of delay in care seeking, of 1,621 patients with genitourinary symptoms, over one-third (35% of men and 37% of women) presented to STD clinics only after 1 week or more of symptoms.[32] Men with genital warts (73%), with nongonococcal urethritis (23.1%) or symptomatic men who were recent contacts to sex partners with STDs were significantly more likely to delay clinic attendance more than 1 week than men with gonorrhea (6.5%—$p < 0.001$ for each). Overall, 43.8 percent of women receiving specific clinical diagnoses other than genital warts delayed clinic attendance for more than 1 week. When asked why they delayed clinic attendance respondents were most likely to respond that they hoped their symptoms would "go away" (48.5% of men and 49.4% of women who waited 1 week or more before seeking care).

An additional issue related to health care seeking among adolescents involves confidentiality. In a recent survey, a majority (58–69%) of adolescents indicated that they had health concerns they wished to keep confidential and that they would not seek health services because of these concerns.[33] Confidentiality concerns may constitute an equally important (or perhaps more important) issue for persons of all ages in smaller or rural communities or among some minorities.

Perhaps related to issues of confidentiality, seeking to cure symptoms through self-treatment is one specific reason why men and women delay health care seeking after onset of symptoms. In one recent study, women were almost two times more likely to self-treat than men, and the average incremental delay in health care seeking associated with self-treatment was 2 days.[34] In another study conducted in Kenya, self-treatment was the most important factor contributing to delayed care seeking.[35]

COMPLIANCE WITH THERAPY RECOMMENDATIONS

Noncompliance with therapy recommendations on the part of infected individuals is another factor that contributes to delays in cure and some proportions of infected persons not being cured. The literature suggests that among women with PID who seek care, noncompliance with multidose regimens may exceed 65 percent.[36] Among women with asymptomatic gonococcal or chlamydial infections, noncompliance rates may be even higher.

PROVISION OF STD SERVICES

SOURCES OF CARE

As is the case in the health care seeking area, data on STD-related health care provision issues are scant. Often available data are not specific to particular population subgroups or particular STD diagnoses. Nevertheless, in order to minimize time elapsed between infection and treatment for cure of curable bacterial or parasitic STD and suppression of incurable viral STD, it is important that information on where to seek care for STD related symptoms (or suspicion of exposure to STD) is available to the population; STD services are accessible and acceptable to the population being served; communication between providers and patients is effective; and, where necessary, outreach services are available for hard-to-reach populations.

According to the first survey ever of a nationally representative sample of public health department STD programs, in 1994, public sector STD services in the United States are limited in distribution, clinic hours and outreach capacities and address a limited range of STDs. An estimated 1437 local health departments—half of all local health departments in the country provided STD diagnosis and treatment to clients, through 2 million visits, at 2587 clinic locations.[37] Of those clients who received these services, 16 percent were under 18 years of age, 19 percent were 18 to 19, and 30 percent were 20 to 24; six out of ten clients were women; 45 percent had incomes below the official poverty level, and 38 percent were between 100 percent and 250 percent of the poverty level; 55 percent were non-Hispanic whites, 35 percent were African Americans, and 9 percent were Hispanic. On average, 43 percent of these clients did not have any STDs. Among those who had a STD, 40 percent had chlamydia, 22 percent had gonorrhea, 5 percent had early syphilis, and 32 percent had some other sexually transmitted disease. Almost all agencies offer testing and treatment for gonorrhea and syphilis but only 82 percent offer testing for chlamydia.

Only 14 percent of local health departments that offer STD services do so in clinic sessions solely devoted to STDs. These health departments are much more likely to be in large metropolitan areas, and to have large client caseloads; they provide 37 percent of all STD visits annually, and most of their clients are men. Most local health departments that offer STD services integrate STD and other health services, such as family planning, in the same clinic session (37%), or offer both integrated sessions and sessions devoted to STDs (49%). Providers that integrate STD services and other health care in the same clinic sessions tend to serve nonmetropolitan areas, serve smaller number of STD clients, and have women as the majority of their clients.[37]

The findings from the survey also indicate that 40 percent of the half of the local health departments that do provide STD services cannot see a new patient on the same day that he seeks care and 15 percent report that new clients have to wait 3 days or longer before being diagnosed and treated. Only 23 percent of STD clinics are open evenings, and only 5 percent are open on weekends. These data are consistent with those from a 1993 study of STD clinics in 24 metropolitan areas demonstrating that up to 46 percent of patients cannot be seen on the same day that they present for care.[38] In aggregate, these data are remarkable in that they document the overburdening of public health department STD clinics serving clients living in metropolitan areas. An average of 3 days' delay in diagnosis and treatment would significantly add to the duration of infectiousness, and in the ecologic setting of metropolitan areas may greatly accelerate the spread of STD.

Public health departments provide only one portion of all STD services. However, information on STD services provided by other sources is even more limited. Preliminary results from a pilot study being conducted in four states in the United States indicate that STD clinics report the greatest numbers of new STD cases diagnosed within the past 2 weeks: 46 percent report five or more new STD cases; followed by family planning clinics, 36 percent; colleges, 16 percent; hospitals, 15 percent; and abortion clinics, 12 percent (Abt. associates, personal communication). Of the specialties surveyed, those in emergency medicine and general practice reported the greatest numbers of new STD cases.

STD HEALTH CARE PROVIDER BEHAVIORS

Health care provider behaviors constitute a major contributing factor in determining the proportions of STD-infected individuals who never get detected or who are not treated even if detected. Provider behaviors also contribute to the delay between infection and cure. Provider behaviors that are important in this context include conducting STD risk assessment, arriving at a clinical or laboratory diagnosis, providing a therapy recommendation, providing counseling for preventive behaviors, and providing partner referral counseling and management. Available data on provider behaviors are limited; however, in recent years a few studies of provider behaviors have been conducted both in the United States and in developing countries.

A recent national survey of health care providers conducted in the United States indicated that most providers do not actively assess patients' risk for STDs, but rely on patients to mention STD symptoms or concerns.[39] STD risk assessments are not a routine part of care by physicians or other office-based health care staff. Only 16 percent of physicians indicated that they evaluate all new adult patients for STD risk, and only 27 percent of other health care professionals assess STD risk in all new adult patients. Fifty-five percent of physicians and 43 percent of other health care providers stated that they conduct a risk assessment only when prompted by patients' symptoms or complaints. Only 65 percent of physicians and 63 percent of other providers collect information on a patient's prior history of STDs. A 1992 national survey of primary care physicians found that although the majority of these providers routinely asked about cigarette, alcohol, and contraceptive use, the percentage of physicians who would "usually" or "always" assess STD risk by asking about condom use, number and type of sex partners, or sexual orientation ranged from 27 to 31 percent with new adult patients and 27 to 52 percent with new adolescent patients.[40] These risk assessment behaviors on the part of providers may lead to underdiagnosis and undertreatment, or at a minimum, delayed detection and treatment of STDs.

Other provider behaviors related to STD detection are perhaps more difficult to study and data on these behaviors are not available. However, at a population level, whether providers use clinical diagnostic approaches, based on signs and symptoms, or laboratory diagnostic approaches may have a great effect on the proportion of infected individuals who are appropriately diagnosed, and on the length of time that elapses between the infected individual's initial contact with the provider and the identification of a cause of infection and, ultimately, effective treatment. Indeed, there are tradeoffs between the more timely detection and treatment of a larger number of patients using clinical diagnosis and the more accurate detection of a smaller number of patients whose treatment may be delayed. Symptoms and signs for some STDs may not be reliable for diagnostic purposes. Many STDs are asymptomatic, particularly in women; moreover most populations do not receive adequate STD-related health education to provide them with symptom recognition skills. As mentioned earlier, in a nationally representative serologic survey, only one out of ten individuals with serologic evidence of HSV-2 reported having genital herpes.[19] Signs for STDs may also be misleading, particularly in women and particularly for nonulcerative STDs. However, even clinical diagnosis of genital ulcers may be problematic if providers fail to recognize that multiple etiologies are common in their population and do not tailor treatment regimens accordingly. For example, in a recent chancroid outbreak in Mississippi, cases of ulcers that were not clinically diagnosed as being caused by chancroid were found to be caused by *Hemophilis ducreyi* on testing with the polymerase chain reaction (PCR) technique.[31] In South Carolina, a 1993 to 1994 trial of STD diagnosis using clinical signs and symptoms with only Clinical Laboratory Improvement Act (CLIA)-waived laboratory test (vaginal pH and endocervical swab test) instead of "moderately complex" CLIA tests (RPR, dark fields, Gram stains, and wet mounts) resulted in substantial increases in misdiagnosis, particularly for genital ulcers and discharge syndromes in women (Greene and Lindman, personal communication). Moreover, signs may vary across populations, depending on the phase of the particular epidemic and whether infections being diagnosed are predominantly incident infections or longstanding prevalent infections (Ryan, personal communication).[20]

Choice of laboratory test may be associated with other issues. The type of specimen that is required for a given test will determine not only patient acceptance of testing, but also ease of specimen collection, storage, and transport by the provider. Furthermore, ease of specimen processing is often offset by reduced sensitivity and specificity, contributing to underdiagnosis of STDs. Time elapsed between specimen collection and receipt of the test result is another consideration in choosing between alternative diagnostic tests. Delay in receipt of test results contributes to longer durations of infectiousness in infected individuals and, in addition, may result in lower proportions of infected individuals being treated since some persons do not return to get their results and therapy recommendations. In one study that compared a rapid office-based test with standard cell culture for screening of women for chlamydia infections, the median interval between testing and therapy for women with positive screening cultures was 14 days. Nearly 25 percent of the women with positive screening cultures did not return for therapy.[41]

Another study evaluated treatment outcomes of patients with positive cultures who had not received presumptive treatment at their initial visit, using retrospective chart reviews of computerized medical records. The findings indicated that overall, 20 percent of patients with positive screening cultures for gonorrhea and chlamydia failed to return to the clinic for treatment within 30 days of screening. Of those who did return, 30 percent did so only after at least 2 weeks had elapsed.[42]

Although recommendations for detection and treatment are important factors influencing provider behaviors in these areas, some providers do not adhere to such recommendations. A recent study compared PID screening, diagnosis, treatment, and reporting practices among primary care physicians with the CDC guidelines for PID.[43] Fifty-five percent of primary care physicians surveyed had treated at least one case of PID during the preceding 12 months. Of these, 52 percent were unsure of, or did not follow, the CDC guidelines for PID, and only 44 percent reported that they consistently followed the CDC guidelines. Among the physicians who reported treating PID during the past year, only 3 percent answered all of the PID management questions in accordance with the CDC guidelines. Major deviations from the guidelines occurred in the areas of diagnosis (11%), overtreatment (11%) and undertreatment (12%).[43] The largest number of PID patients was seen by emergency physicians.

Based on findings from the national survey of providers, counseling behaviors of health care providers could also be improved. Only 35 percent of physicians and 38 percent of other providers routinely discuss safer sex or condom use with their herpes patients. Only 31 percent of physicians and 29 percent of other providers discuss telling sex partners about STDs.[39] Available findings also indicate that STD patient–provider interactions may be problematic at best, and perhaps are counterproductive.[44] Patient and provider expectations of the clinical encounter may vary significantly. Patients expect to be examined in a timely fashion, and excessive waiting times or early clinic closures tend to frustrate and distance patients from the health service delivery system. Lack of privacy and confidentiality in the clinical encounter create further problems. In one study, in St. Louis, Missouri, 55 percent of women and 44 percent of men were dissatisfied with the amount of time they had to wait to be seen; and 26 percent of women and 34 percent of men stated that their privacy was not preserved in interactions with clinical staff.[44]

STD HEALTH CARE SYSTEM CHARACTERISTICS

Several properties of the health system have important effects on the time elapsed between infection and cure of bacterial or parasitic STD or suppression of viral STD. These include education and training of providers, availability and distribution of diagnostic tests, availability and distribution of medications, and program and practice guidelines, organization and funding of basic services necessary for effective STD prevention including laboratory diagnostic services, screening services, and partner management services.

Education and training of health care providers in STD and HIV/AIDS is often inadequate. In 1991, 126 medical schools in the United States and Puerto Rico were queried to determine the extent of clinical training for medical students in the areas of sexually transmitted diseases (STD) and HIV/AIDS. Responses were received from 102 medical schools. The median number of hours of clinical training in STD, by department, ranged from 1 hour (dermatology, urology, and psychiatry) to 5 hours (internal medicine and obstetrics and gynecology). The median number of hours of clinical training in HIV ranged from 1 hour (dermatology, urology, and family practice) to 4.5 hours (internal medicine). The departments most likely to have STD training as an explicit objective were obstetrics and gynecology (87%) and internal medicine (73%), whereas the least likely were dermatology (26%), urology (26%), and psychiatry (21%). Clinical training in HIV/AIDS was most likely to be an explicit objective in internal medicine (86%) and obstetrics and gynecology (68%), and was least likely in dermatology (23%) and urology (15%). A clinic specifically devoted to STD existed at 42 percent of institutions, and one devoted to AIDS existed at 73 percent, but an exclusive elective for medical students in STD or HIV/AIDS existed at 37 percent of the institutions. In comparison to other topics in the curriculum, the amount of attention devoted to STD/HIV/AIDS was judged to be excessive (1%), adequate (67%) or less than adequate (32%). In the 10 years prior to 1991, the amount of clinical training in STD had decreased at 6 percent of the institutions, remained the same at 17 percent, and increased at 77 percent.[45] Particularly in the areas of STD diagnosis, treatment, and prevention, new technologies and knowledge accumulate rapidly. Thus, there is an additional need for continuing education of health care providers. However, national data on the numbers and proportions of health care providers who receive continuing education in the STD area are not available. Moreover, a formal assessment of provider education, training, and continuing education needs has not been conducted.

Since many STDs are asymptomatic or have nonspecific symptoms, laboratory diagnosis is required for their detection. Underuse of laboratory testing, owing to lack of availability of reagents or other resources, may limit appropriate detection, reporting, and treatment of STDs. No national data are available to assess the facilities that offer testing for various STDs, identify trends in testing, or estimate training and support needs for the future.[46] A recent study analyzed responses to a survey inquiring about range of tests offered, changes in testing, and reasons for changes.[46] Results indicated that, in recent years, the number of facilities testing for *C. trachomatis* has increased with increased funding and availability of nonculture tests; the number of facilities testing for chancroid and gonorrhea has decreased; and that the implementation of the Clinical Laboratory Improvement Act (CLIA) may be associated with a decrease in the number of facilities performing tests for STDs. Most of the 405 responding facilities collected specimens for nontreponemal tests for syphilis (86.9%). Since each facility's information was last updated, the number reporting testing for *Chlamydia trachomatis* rose from 39.5 to 71.1 percent, but testing for gonorrhea and chancroid decreased from 90.1 to 81 percent, and from 44.9 to 7.9 percent, respectively. Of 364 responses to a question on changes in tests performed in the last 2 years, 249 (68.4%) reported no change, 81 (22.3%) reported an increase, and 37 (10.2%) reported a decrease. The most frequently added tests were nonculture tests for *C. trachomatis* (34 of 81 [42%]), and the most frequent reasons for adding tests was targeted funding (25 of 81 [30.9%]). The most frequently discontinued tests were cultures and Gram stains for gonorrhea (15 of 37 [40.5%]) and other in-house tests (9 of 37 [24.3%]). Most facilities that discontinued testing cited the Clinical Laboratory Improvement Act as the reason.

An additional aspect of laboratory diagnosis that affects the timely and appropriate treatment of STDs relates to the timeliness of laboratory testing and reporting of positive test results. Many health system level factors may contribute to timeliness of laboratory services, including inadequate resources, overburdening of particular facilities owing to absolute overload or uneven distribution of demand for laboratory services, and characteristics of diagnostic technology. In a recent study of completeness and timeliness of laboratory surveillance for syphilis, timeliness was found to be a much more serious problem than completeness, especially for laboratories outside public clinics.[47]

Availability of up-to-date program and practice guidelines for the prevention, detection, and treatment of all STDs is an important health system parameter with great potential impact on timely and appropriate STD management. However, such availability does not assure provider compliance with guidelines. In fact, recent data indicate that compliance levels may be quite low, even in the United States, where higher levels of compliance with practice guidelines would be expected in the light of malpractice legislation.[43]

Organization and funding of STD services may be the most important health system parameter influencing timely treatment of STDs. In the United States, the evolution toward managed care has accelerated dialogue between public health and private medicine regarding the mutual responsibilities of these sectors. In general, the public health sector is more narrowly defining its responsibilities to encompass population level health services, including health planning, disease surveillance, and primary prevention activities (such as health promotion and education, partner notification, vaccines, and regulatory strategies). It will rely on the private medical sector to accept more of the responsibility for providing individual level detection and treatment services.

For STDs, the private sector can play an important and expanded role in disease prevention. However, those without insurance for private care include many of the economically and socially marginalized persons most likely to acquire and transmit STDs. Furthermore, with the advent of Medicaid managed care, some of the distinctions between private and public sector are beginning to blur. Because early detection and curative treatment represent primary prevention for communicable diseases, the public health sector must ensure that accessible, acceptable services for STD prevention are available to both the uninsured and insured alike.[48]

STD health system characteristics in the United States are probably not as favorable to minimizing time elapsed from infection to cure or suppression of STDs as those in other developed countries. The limited data available from developing countries indicate that health system characteristics in many of these countries also greatly compromise the timely and appropriate treatment of STDs.

A recent initiative undertaken by AIDSCAP, called targeted intervention research (TIR), has brought to light many aspects of STD health system characteristics as well as health seeking and provider behaviors in several developing countries, including Malawi, Senegal, Ethiopia, Zambia, and the Phillippines.[49] Findings point to the importance of lack of knowledge regarding STDs, lay theories regarding STD etiology, perceptions of stigma, seeking of health care through inappropriate sources such as pharmacies and traditional healers, inadequate knowledge and training regarding STD diagnosis and treatment among health care providers, lack of resources for appropriate diagnostic technologies, and inadequate communication between patients and providers as the main factors impeding appropriate and timely diagnosis and treatment of STDs in many developing countries.[49] A survey of STD case management conducted in Malawi in 1994 found that the prevention indicator rate for correct assessment and treatment of STD patients was 11 percent (81% for history taking, 46% in physical examination, and 13% in current antibiotic treatment according to national guidelines).[50] In the same study, the prevention indicator rate for overall patient counseling was 29 percent (65% for partner notification and 40% for condom advice). Only 16 percent of patients with genital ulcers were treated effectively for chancroid and 56 percent were treated effectively for syphilis. Female STD patients were treated less comprehensively than male STD patients, and only 20 percent of STD patients were offered condoms.[50] These findings reflect the net effects of inadequacies in the prevention and control of STDs resulting from a multiplicity of problems in the interface of health seeking behaviors, provider behaviors, and health system characteristics related to STDs.

IMPLICATIONS FOR FUTURE RESEARCH AND PREVENTION EFFORTS

The AIDS epidemic has resulted in far-reaching advances in our understanding of and ability to change risky sexual behavior. In contrast, empiric work on the prevalence and determinants of timely and effective STD-related health care, and on the development and evaluation of interventions to achieve it remains extremely limited. Future research in this critical area must bridge factors operating at the client, provider, and health system levels in considering each of the components and subcomponents contributing to "person-time of infectiousness." Research to define and address factors shaping component I (lost to detection) is likely to be particularly important because of the large numbers of infected individuals that fall into this category, especially in subpopulations and communities with the highest STD rates. New STD and HIV detection technologies, including urine and saliva tests, will facilitate the kinds of population-based studies that are needed to answer questions about component I. Research on factors shaping components III and IV (diagnostic delays and treatment delays) is even more limited than that on health care seeking. Such research is critical to conduct since provider behaviors and health system variables may prove more responsive to interventions than behaviors of the general population. Advances in STD and HIV detection technologies, prevention technologies, and the organization of health services in the United States also suggest that, in many communities, STD/HIV-related health care behaviors may be uniquely vulnerable to intervention or in transition already. This makes the need for both descriptive and intervention research in this area particularly urgent and relevant to prevention of all STDs, including HIV infection.

The PTI conceptual framework and the data summarized in the preceding also have profound implications for STD prevention efforts. They highlight the need for interventions that promote early and effective STD-related health care behaviors to go beyond the traditional focus on partner notification, and, in some settings, clinic-based counseling. STD prevention programs must build on local assessment of the PTI components and subcomponents not only to target improvements in clinical prevention services to those provider and health system factors responsible for the greatest delays, but also to incorporate into health promotion efforts tailored messages that will reduce loss to detection, health care seeking delays, and noncompliance with management recommendations in high-risk subpopulations. Partner notification approaches should also be re-examined in light of the concepts discussed here. Finally, available data clearly indicate that the majority of STD care is not sought through public sector categorical clinics. To optimize STD-related health care, STD services must also be offered as part of routine primary health care by both public and private sector providers. This means that, in the future, efforts directed at provider behaviors, such as guideline development, training, and evaluation, must extend to providers in these settings, and stronger linkages must be forged across these health system components.

References

1 McKinlay JB: Some approaches and problems in the study and use of services—an overview. *J Health Soc Behav* 13:115, 1972.

2 Andersen R: *A Behavioral Model of Families' Use of Health Services.* Research Series No. 25. Chicago, IL, Center for Health Administration Studies, The University of Chicago, 1968.

3 Aday LA et al: Indicators and predictors of health services utilization, in Williams SJ et al (eds): *Introduction to Health Services*, 3rd ed. Albany, New York, Delmar Publishers, 1988.

3a Aday LA et al: *Access to Medical Care in the U.S.: Who Has It, Who Doesn't.* Chicago, Pluribus Press, 1984.

4 Williams SJ et al: *Introduction to Health Services.* Albany, New York, Delmary Publishers, 1988.

5 Suchman EA: Social patterns of illness and medical care. *J Health Soc Behav* 6:2, 1965.

6 Suchman EA: Stages of illness and medical care. *J Health Soc Behav* 6:114, 1965.

7 Suchman EA: Health orientation and medical care. *Am J Public Health* 56:97, 1966.

8 Kosa J et al: The social aspects of health and illness, in Kosa J et al (eds): *Poverty and Health: A Sociological Analysis.* Cambridge, MA, Harvard University Press, 1975, pp. 40–79.

9 Mechanic D: *Medical Sociology: A Comprehensive Text.* New York, The Free Press, 1978.

10 Becker MH (ed): *The Health Belief Model and Personal Health Behavior.* Thorofare, NJ, Charles B. Slack, 1974.

11 Jones RA: Expectations and delay in seeking medical care. *J Soc Iss* 46:81, 1990.

12 Prohaska TR et al: Impact of symptoms and aging attribution on emotions and coping. *Health Psychol* 6:495, 1987.

13 Weinstein ND: Why it won't happen to me: perceptions or risk factors and susceptibility. *Health Psychol* 3:431, 1984.

14 Pennebaker JW et al: Selective monitoring of physical sensations. *J Personality Soc Psychol* 41:213, 1981.

15 Leventhal H et al: Illness representations and coping with health threats, in Baum A et al (eds): *A handbook of psychology and health*, vol 4. Hillsdale, NJ, LEA, 1984, pp. 219–252.

16 Fortenberry JD: Health care seeking behaviors related to sexually transmitted diseases among adolescents. *Am J Public Health* 87:417, 1997.

17 Anderson RM et al: *Infectious Diseases of Humans: Dynamics and Control.* Oxford, Oxford University Press, 1991.

18 Anderson RM: The transmission dynamics of sexually transmitted diseases in Wasserheit JN et al (eds): *Research Issues in Human Behavior and Sexually Transmitted Diseases in the AIDS Era.* Washington, DC, American Society for Microbiology, 1991.

19 Fleming D et al: The evolving epidemiology of herpes simplex virus type 2 in the United States, 1976 to 1994. Forthcoming, 1997.

20 Wasserheit JN et al: The dynamic topology of sexually transmitted disease epidemics: implications for prevention strategies. *JID* 174(Suppl 2):S201, 1996.

21 Rothenberg RB et al: Temporal and social aspects of gonorrhea transmission: the force of infectivity. *Sex Transm Dis* 15:88, 1988.

22 Pamela Rao IR: Safe sex operational model: a tool for planning & monitoring safe sex activities in developing countries. Abstract presented at the IUVDT World STD/AIDS Congress Meeting. Singapore, March 19–23, 1995.

23 Brackbill RM et al: Where do people go for treatment of sexually transmitted diseases (STDs) in the U.S.? Unpublished abstract; 1995.

24 Southwick KL et al: Management of pelvic inflammatory disease in emergency rooms: findings from the national hospital ambulatory medical care survey. EIS Conference, April 22–26, 1996, Atlanta, GA.

25 Celum C et al: Patients attending STD clinics in an evolving health care environment: demographic, insurance coverage, preferences for STD services, and STD morbidity. *STD*, in press, 1997.

26 Lawrence JM et al: Additional sources of care for STD clinic patients: implications for HIV/STD prevention efforts (abstract).

27 Johnson AM et al: Who goes to sexually transmitted disease clinics: results from a national population survey. *Genitourin Med* 72:197, 1996.

28 Harrisson RM: Women's treatment decisions for genital symptoms. *J Roy Soc Med* 75:23, 1982.

29 Leenaars PEM et al: Seeking medical care for a sexually transmitted disease: determinants of delay-behavior. *Psychol Health* 8:17, 1993.

30 Timko C: Seeking medical care for a breast cancer symptom: determinants of intentions to engage in prompt or delay-behavior. *Health Psychol* 6:305, 1987.

31 Mertz KJ et al: An outbreak of chancroid in Mississippi: implications for HIV prevention *NEJM*. Forthcoming, 1997.

32 Hook EW III et al: Delayed presentation to clinics for sexually transmitted diseases by symptomatic patients: a potential contributor to continuing STD morbidity. Forthcoming 1997.

33 Cheng TL et al: Confidentiality in health care. A survey of knowledge, perceptions, and attitudes among high school students. *JAMA* 269: 1404, 1993.

34 Irwin DE: Self-treatment patterns and medical-care seeking behavior in STD patients. (Abstract #20). Eleventh Meeting of the International Society for STD Research. New Orleans, LA, August 30, 1995.

35 Moses S et al: Health care seeking behavior related to the transmission of sexually transmitted diseases in Kenya. *AJPH* 84:1947, 1994.

36 Brookoff D: Compliance with doxycycline therapy for outpatient treatment of pelvic inflammatory disease. *So Med J* 87:1088, 1994.

37 Landry PJ et al: Public health departments providing STD services. *Family Planning Perspectives,* 1996, forthcoming.

38 Hare ML et al: Evaluation of STD Clinic Flow and Utilization. Battelle Report for CDC. Arlington, VA, December 2, 1993.

39 Barbour D et al: Evaluation of physician practices in counseling patients with sexually transmitted diseases (STDs). (Abstract #423). Eleventh Meeting of the International Society for STD Research. New Orleans, LA, August 30, 1995.

40 HIV Prevention Practices of Primary-Care Physicians—United States, 1992. *MMWR* 42:988–992, 1994.

41 Hook EW III et al: Use of cell culture and a rapid diagnostic assay for *chlamydia trachomatis* screening. *JAMA* 272:867–870, 1994.

42 Schwebke JR et al: Positive screening tests for gonorrhea and chlamydia fail to lead to treatment of patients attending an STD clinic. *Sex Transm Dis* 24:181, 1997.

43 Hessol NA et al: Management of pelvic inflammatory disease by primary care physicians: a comparison with centers for disease control and prevention guidelines. *Sex Transm Dis* 23:157–163, 1996.

44 Stoner BP: The health care consumer-health care provider interface: facilitators and impediments to STD care. Paper presented at the American Public Health Association Annual Meeting, November 2, 1995, San Diego, CA.

45 Mackay HT et al: Survey of clinical training in STD and HIV/AIDS in United States Medical Schools. Presented at IDSA September 16–18, 1995, San Francisco.

46 Beck-Sague CM et al: Laboratory diagnosis of sexually transmitted diseases in facilities within the United States. Results of a national survey. *Sex Transm Dis* 23:342, 1996.

47 Fleming DT et al: Rapid assessment of laboratory-based syphilis surveillance, Fulton County, Georgia. EIS Conference, April 22–26, 1996. Atlanta, GA.

48 Aral SO et al: Overview: individual and population approaches to the epidemiology and prevention of sexually transmitted diseases and human immunodeficiency virus infection. *JID* 174(Suppl 2):S127, 1996.

49 Field ML: Listening to patients: targeted intervention research to improve STD programs. *AIDScaptions* 3:16, 1996.

50 Chilongozi DA et al: Sexually transmitted diseases: a survey of case management in Malawi. *Int J STD-AIDS* 7:269, 1996.

Chapter 94

Barrier methods for the prevention of sexually transmitted diseases

Katherine M. Stone
Judith Timyan
Elizabeth L. Thomas

Prevention of HIV infection and other sexually transmitted diseases (STDs) is a global public health emergency. The AIDS pandemic and the recognition that STDs greatly facilitate HIV transmission have fueled a worldwide campaign to develop new biomedical prevention technologies or refine currently existing ones, yet we are not using our available technology to its fullest potential.[1] In addition to raising awareness of the need to conduct long-overdue basic science research on the genital tract and STD pathogenesis, this campaign has ushered in a new societal paradigm that increasingly involves consumers in research and development and attempts to meet the special needs women have in protecting their sexual health. However, development of new prevention methods that are safe, effective, and acceptable to consumers is a long, arduous process that can take decades, and we must capitalize on what is available now. Many physical and chemical barrier methods are available worldwide, effective against a wide variety of STDs, and acceptable to many sexually active persons, yet are not in widespread use for STD prevention or contraception. This chapter presents an overview of these methods in terms of their clinical effectiveness, advantages and disadvantages, and user acceptability. The barrier methods discussed include the male condom, the female condom, the sponge, the diaphragm, the cervical cap, spermicides, and microbicides. New products currently being developed are also presented.

MALE CONDOM

Male condoms protect the wearer and his partner by covering the penile glans and shaft, which are the major portals of entry and exit for STD pathogens. To be effective, condoms must be placed on the penis prior to any genital contact, must remain intact, and, most important, must be used consistently. Most research has focused on latex condoms, although condoms made from other materials are now widely available.

LATEX CONDOM

Clinical effectiveness and adverse effects of the latex condom

Laboratory and clinical studies have shown that latex condoms are effective against a variety of STDs, including HIV infection.[2] Several laboratory studies, some of which attempted to simulate the mechanical friction of coitus, have clearly demonstrated that a latex condom is a continuous, impervious barrier to sexually transmitted bacteria and viruses, including HIV and the much smaller hepatitis B surface antigen.[3–12] One laboratory study that found detectable leakage of HIV-size particles in 29 out of 89 condoms tested has been widely misinterpreted as showing that latex condoms are porous.[13] However, the study conditions were extremely harsh and included concentrations of particles up to 100 million times the concentration of HIV in semen, suspension of the particles in a fluid medium much less viscous than semen, and exposure of the condoms to physical conditions equivalent to 10 minutes of vigorous thrusting after ejaculation. The authors and other researchers, therefore, concluded that latex condoms provide an effective mechanical barrier to the fluid transfer necessary for HIV transmission.[13–15]

Multiple studies conducted on sexually active persons have shown that condoms protect users and their partners against HIV and a wide variety of other STDs including gonorrhea, ureaplasma infection, and herpes simplex virus infection. Several recent review articles have tabulated these studies and quantified the protective effects of condom use.[2,16] Effectiveness varies among studies. Several studies show 100 percent effectiveness, whereas others show that some individuals became infected despite their reported condom use. Methodologic differences in studies may easily explain these disparities. Individuals may have become infected prior to consistent condom use, hence the limited usefulness of cross-sectional and case-control studies to assess magnitude of protection. Some individuals may overreport condom use; such overreporting is likely to bias the study toward finding a falsely low protective effect.[17] Differences in effectiveness across studies may also be explained by differences in user compliance, which was not measured in most studies conducted prior to the 1990s.[18] Both consistent use and correct use are critical in order to achieve a high degree of effectiveness.

Compelling clinical evidence that consistent use of condoms is highly effective for prevention of HIV infection is available from prospective studies of discordant couples in whom one partner is infected with HIV and the other is not (Table 94-1).

In one large study, none of the 123 consistent condom users seroconverted over a 2-year period, despite repeated sexual exposure to their HIV-infected partners.[26] Of the couples who did not use condoms consistently, 12/122 (9.8 percent) partners became infected. In the other large study, 3/171 (1.8 percent) of consistent condom users became infected over a 2-year period, whereas 16/134 (11.9 percent) of inconsistent condom users became infected.[25] A metanalysis of studies of discordant couples has been widely cited and misinterpreted as evidence that condoms do not offer strong protection.[30] This metanalysis did not include the DeVincenzi[26] and Saracco[25] studies and did not take compliance into account.[18] Other prospective studies have found a strong protective effect for condoms against HIV infection and are summarized in recent reviews and Table 94-1.[2,16] One prospective study found no protective effect for condoms among commercial sex workers who also were using nonoxynol-9 (N-9) during the study period.[28]

Data on condom protection from STDs other than HIV are more limited, and no discordant couples studies are available. Cross-sectional and case-control studies have shown protective effects against a variety of STDs, including gonorrhea, chlamydia, ureaplasma, trichomoniasis, and herpes simplex virus (HSV).[2] Several prospective cohort studies clearly show a strong protective effect against gonorrhea in men and women (Table 94-2). In one of these studies, men who acquired gonorrhea despite condom use reported incorrect use (genital contact prior to condom use) on reinterview.[33] This points to a basic problem in accurately assessing the protective effect of condoms because of the lack of clarity in the best way to measure consistent and correct condom use.

A prospective cohort study of incident STDs found no protective effect of condom use in men and women and the authors

Use of trademarks is for identification purposes only and does not imply endorsement by the Department of Health and Human Services.

Table 94-1. Prospective Studies of Barrier Methods for Prevention of HIV Infection

Study	Design	Population	Method	Use	RR, (95% c.i.)
Fischl et al., 1987[19]	Cohort	Partners of AIDS patients, Florida	Condom	Regular	0.1 (0.0–0.40)
Ngugi et al., 1988[20]	Cohort	CSW, Kenya	Condom	Any vs. none	0.3 (0.13–0.92)
Laurian et al., 1989[21]	Cohort	Partners of hemophiliacs, France	Condom	Always vs. other	0.0 (p = 0.15)
Moss et al., 1991[22]	Cohort	Discordant couples, Kenya	Condom	Not specified	"Not associated"
Plummer et al., 1991[23]	Cohort	CSW, Kenya	Condom	Any vs. none	0.11 (0.05–0.27)
Allen et al., 1992[24]	Cohort	Discordant couples, Rwanda	Condom	Always/sometimes vs. never	Men 0.0 (0.0–0.6) Women 0.17 (0.1–1.6)
Saracco et al., 1993[25]	Cohort	Discordant couples, Italy	Condom	Always vs. other	Women 0.1 (0.0–0.5)
DeVincenzi et al., 1994[26]	Cohort	Discordant couples, Europe	Condom	Always vs. other	0.0 (0.0–3.8)
Kreiss et al., 1992[27]	RCT	CSW, Kenya	N9 sponge		1.7 (0.9–3.0)
Zekeng et al., 1993[28]	Cohort	CSW, Cameroon	N9 100-mg suppositories + condom	N9 ≥ 67% use Condom > 63% use	0.1 (0.1–0.6) 1.1 (0.4–2.9)
Feldblum et al., 1995[29]	Cohort	Discordant couples, Zambia	N9 film, foam, suppositories + condom	Consistent N9 use Consistent condom use	Couples 0.8 (0.2–2.8) Women 0.5 (0.1–3.8) Couples 0.2 (0.0–1.6)

CSW = Commercial sex worker.
RCT = Randomized clinical trial.
SOURCE: Updated from Cates/Stone.[2]

speculate that condom use may have been overreported.[17] However, several other methodologic limitations could easily explain why this study found no protective effect.[36,37] When incident chlamydia was analyzed separately, a strong protective effect for consistent condom use was found for men but not women.

A randomized clinical trial found a strong protective effect of condoms for gonorrhea and chlamydia among commercial sex workers who were also using N-9 film.[38] Concurrent use of condoms and N-9 limits the ability to assess the magnitude of protection offered by either method alone.

Protection against trichomoniasis, HSV, human papillomavirus (HPV), and hepatitis B virus (HBV) has not been assessed in cohort studies. A cross-sectional study reported that college students who consistently used condoms had a lower risk for prevalent HPV infection.[39] Previous studies have not found a protective effect for condom use and HPV infection, but they did not assess consistency of condom use. Moreover, HPV infection may well have preceded condom use.

Consistent and correct condom use should protect against almost all cases of STDs. Condoms cover the male urethral opening and therefore should protect against infections (gonorrhea, chlamydia, trichomoniasis, HIV, HBV) that are transmitted from men via semen/urethral fluids or to men via urethral contact with a partner's infectious fluids. Moreover, condoms also should protect against most cases of STDs (HSV, HPV, chancroid, syphilis, LGV) that are transmitted by skin-to-skin contact, since the large majority of these infections clearly involve areas of the penis typically covered by the condom.

No clinical studies have been conducted to determine whether spermicidally lubricated condoms are more effective than those with nonspermicidal lubricants. The amount of N-9 contained in most prelubricated condoms is fairly low at the time of packaging and decreases over time as the N-9 leaches into the latex.[40,41]

Adverse effects of latex condoms include latex allergy or sensitivity, the estimated prevalence of which is 1 to 3 percent in the general U.S. population and 6 to 7 percent for individuals who have frequent exposure to latex, such as health care workers.[42] Laboratory data suggest that the N-9 lubricant on commercially available spermicidally lubricated condoms may cause allergenic proteins to leach out of latex condoms.[43] One well publicized

Table 94-2. Prospective Studies of Male and Female Condoms to Prevent STD

Study	Design	Population	Outcome	Method	Use	RR, (95% c.i. or p value)
Hart, 1974[31]	Cohort	Australian soldiers, Vietnam	Self-reported STD	Condom	Always vs. never	Men 0.00
Cates/Holmes, 1996[32]	Cohort	Naval crewmen, Philippines	Gonorrhea Gonorrhea/NGU	Condom	Users vs. nonusers Users vs. nonusers	Men 0.00 ("not significant") Men 0.00 (p = 0.02)
Darrow, 1989[33]	Cohort	STD clinic, California	Gonorrhea	Condom	Always vs. never	Men 0.34 (0.10–1.13)
Cameron et al., 1991[34]	Cohort	CSW, STD clinic, Kenya	Genital ulcers	Condom		Women 0.18 (0.10–0.88)
Zenilman et al., 1995[17]	Cohort	STD clinic, Maryland	Gonorrhea/chlamydia/ syphilis/trichomoniasis Chlamydia	Condom	Always vs. never	Men 1.4 (0.6–3.3) Women 0.6 (0.2–1.4) Men 0.0 (p = 0.015) Women "not significant"
Soper et al., 1993[35]	NRCT	Gyn clinics, United States	Trichomoniasis	Female condom	Always vs. controls Users vs. controls	Women 0.0 (0.0–1.7) Women 0.6 (0.2–2.5)

CSW = Commerical sex worker.
NGU = Nongonococcal urethritis.
NRCT = Nonrandomized clinical trial.
SOURCE: Updated from Cates/Stone.[2]

study reported adverse effects in commercial sex workers who used spermicidally lubricated condoms, but since no control group was studied it is difficult to conclude that the effects were due to the spermicidal lubricant.[44] Alterations in vaginal flora have been studied only in condom users who also use N-9.

Advantages and disadvantages of using the latex condom

Latex condoms are safe, easy to use, and readily available in a wide range of retail outlets. In addition to protection from STDs, they are highly effective against pregnancy when used properly.[45] Condoms can prolong an erection and prevent premature ejaculation, thus enhancing pleasure for some couples. They decrease the messiness of intercourse, because the semen is contained within the condom itself. This containment of semen also offers "proof of protection," which provides some couples greater confidence in the method.[42]

Unlike the female-controlled barrier methods, condoms may not be a protection option for some women. Many men do not like condoms because they interrupt intercourse and decrease sensitivity and sensation. If not used properly, they can break or slip off and, unlike the diaphragm or cervical cap, a new condom must be used for each sex act. Some latex condoms have an unpleasant smell, and latex condoms cannot be used with oil-based lubricants. In addition, they should not be used at the same time as oil-based, vaginal yeast infection medications (e.g., butoconazole, miconazole, and terconazole).[46] Attention must be paid to condom storage conditions, as harsh environments may cause the latex to deteriorate.[45]

Acceptability of the latex condom

The acceptability of condoms is complex, encompassing social as well as product-related factors. There are two major barriers to condom acceptability: they have a bad or embarrassing reputation, and they are not enjoyable to use. Condoms have long been associated with disease, promiscuity, and distrust of one's sex partner. Some people may feel that suggesting condom use to their partner is offensive or insulting. Actual and perceived social norms are important influencers of condom acceptability. The extent to which a person perceives that people who are important to him or her approve of condom use is an important determinant of how acceptable that person finds condoms and whether or not condoms are used by that person. A study in the eastern Caribbean found that social norms imposed by friends, sex partners, and parents were important predictors of condom use. In Uganda, an intervention designed to change social norms in the workplace resulted in an increase in actual condom use.[47]

The 1991 U.S. National Survey of Men found that almost 75 percent of respondents felt that using a condom shows that you are a concerned and caring person, which suggests that the condom's negative image may be changing in some subgroups of the American population. At the same time, an almost identical percentage felt that condoms reduced sensation. Approximately one-quarter of the respondents said that condoms were embarrassing to buy, and one-quarter said that they were difficult to put on.[48]

Specific condom characteristics play a large role in condom choice. In the 1991 survey mentioned earlier, respondents preferred those condoms that stayed on during sex, were easy to don, had the right amount of lubrication, and were easy to obtain. Only small percentages of men said that color, ribbing, and low cost were important characteristics.[48]

In a Danish study comparing different types of latex condoms, over 80 percent of respondents preferred lubricated condoms, and over half preferred condoms with reservoir tips. Color was not an important characteristic for most couples.[49] Similarly, respondents in a 1989 *Consumer Reports* study revealed that lubrication and a reservoir tip were the most popular condom characteristics. Only about one-quarter of women in this study favored textured condoms, and about 35 to 40 percent of respondents preferred spermicidally lubricated condoms.[50] In a study of two different spermicidally lubricated condoms in five countries, researchers at Family Health International found that both were well-liked, and that the vast majority of participants preferred them to their normal lubricated condoms.[51]

A recent attempt to combat some of the device-related complaints about condoms has resulted in the introduction of the Pleasure Plus® latex condom from Reddy Labs. Unlike the traditional snug and form-fitting condom, this model is loose at the tip of the condom and snug at the base. The movement of the loose material during intercourse is designed to provide more friction and therefore more pleasure. Designed to make safe sex more enjoyable, Pleasure Plus® has gotten rave reviews in the popular press.[52,53]

Natural membrane condom

Natural membrane condoms, also known as lambskin condoms, are one alternative for the 1 to 3 percent of the U.S. population who are latex-sensitive.[42] Unlike latex condoms, however, natural membrane condoms are naturally porous, and leakage of small viruses such as HBV and phage X174 and the larger HIV and HSV has been demonstrated in laboratory tests.[7–9,12,54] However, the likelihood that semen or other fluids containing infectious particles (or sperm) could leak through a natural membrane condom during intercourse cannot be predicted from these studies, since they did not simulate the fluid dynamics of coitus. No contraceptive or STD prevention efficacy data are available for natural membrane condoms.

Natural membrane condoms are considerably stronger than latex (although less elastic), and reportedly feel more natural and provide better sensation than latex condoms, although no scientific data are available. They tend to be significantly more expensive than latex condoms.[50]

Polyurethane (plastic) condom

The latest breakthrough in condom technology is polyurethane, or plastic, condoms such as the Avanti® condom. Made of a thinner material than latex, polyurethane condoms are reported to be twice as strong as latex. In addition, they reportedly allow for more sensitivity and greater sensation, although no scientific data are available. They are odorless and colorless and can be used with oil-based lubricants.[55] In addition, they are more resistant to deterioration during storage.[56] There are, however, a few disadvantages to using polyurethane condoms. They cost about twice as much as latex condoms, they may be "noisy" during sex, and they may require more lubrication.[57,58]

Family Health International is in the process of developing two new thermoplastic condoms. The first one, which is awaiting FDA approval, is rolled on like a latex condom, but is loose fitting, transparent, and odorless. In a preliminary acceptability study, 70 percent of couples gave the condoms average to excellent ratings in terms of comfort and use. The second condom, which has received patent approval and is in the human testing stage, is slipped, not rolled, onto the penis. Like the first condom, it is loose fitting, transparent, and odorless. One small-scale study revealed that couples found the condom easy to use, sensitive to heat and touch, and comfortable.[45] Studies of the effectiveness of the plastic condom for prevention of STDs and pregnancy are in progress.

A new product due on the market sometime in 1998 is the Tactylon® condom. It is made of the same material used in nonallergenic examination gloves, known as a synthetic thermoplastic elastomer, and it is an effective alternative for those sensitive to latex. A preliminary study in an Atlanta family planning clinic yielded promising acceptability results. Participants compared the Tactylon® to latex condoms and gave both condoms similar ratings for several characteristics.[59]

CONDOM PROMOTION

Of the barrier methods, condoms are the most widely and most consistently promoted for prevention of STD/HIV transmission. Most of this promotion is carried out by public health programs; however, increasingly condom manufacturers have taken up STD/HIV prevention messages in an open way. They are generally prohibited from advertising on the three major TV networks in the United States, although smaller networks, such as Fox and MTV, have agreed to run condom ads.[60] Ansell, the manufacturer of Lifestyles® condoms, has taken advantage of the opportunity to use music television to reach younger audiences by running a series of innovative condom ads that they started in 1994. One Lifestyles® ad featured a group of young women talking about characteristics they find attractive in men. It ended with one woman saying that she would never have sex with a guy who would not wear a condom. In 1995, Ansell also sponsored a nationwide video contest that asked participants to create their own commercials about safer sex in the 1990s.[60] In another example of innovative condom promotion, Ansell sponsored a sweepstakes that was advertised in popular women's magazines and awarded trips to various destinations. All sweepstakes entrants were sent packets on condom use.[61] Ansell has also been the first manufacturer to develop packaging in Spanish in an effort to make condoms more accessible to Latino populations.[62]

Other manufacturers, such as Carter-Wallace (manufacturer of Trojan® condoms), are reportedly following Ansell's lead and negotiating with the smaller networks for advertising space.[63] In addition, Carter-Wallace has successfully launched a new line of condoms targeted at price-conscious shoppers. Named Class Act®, the condoms come in packs of 13 instead of the traditional 12.[64]

Schmid Laboratories, manufacturer of Ramses® condoms, is attempting to increase sales by offering discount coupons for condom purchases in conjunction with Wyeth-Ayerst birth control pills. Sagami, a Japanese manufacturer, has targeted women shoppers by making its packaging more appealing to them. The U.S. manufacturer Safetex has tried to increase sales by marketing trial-size packs and has also concentrated on the development of niche products, geared toward young, "hip" audiences (e.g., Gold Circle Coin® condoms, packaged in foil).[64,65]

In addition to advertising efforts by manufacturers, public service announcements such as those produced by the Centers for Disease Control and Prevention are playing an increasingly large role in condom promotion for the prevention of STDs, including HIV infection. Community-based projects, such as Project Action in Portland, Oregon, have developed innovative strategies for promoting condom use by sexually active youth. The project's activities have included development of a condom brand targeted toward youth that sells for 25 cents apiece, installation of condom vending machines in popular youth hangouts, development of condom promotion ads shown on local television as public service announcements, and training of young adults to be peer educators.[66] (Refer to Chap. 99 for a more in-depth discussion of condom promotion and health education in the United States.)

Fewer restrictions have been put on condom promotion in developing countries than in the United States, partially because HIV has taken such a devastating toll in these areas. Condom promotion programs in these countries often are seen as an essential component in the national fight against AIDS and are typically funded by large international aid agencies. Social marketing organizations, such as Population Services International (PSI) and The Futures Group, have used international aid funding to create new and innovative condom promotion strategies. Condom ads are found on large billboards in the center of Abidjan, Cote d'Ivoire; on the sails of river boats in Dhaka, Bangladesh; on the walls of public buildings in Conakry, Guinea; on the backboards of sports stadiums in Port-au-Prince, Haiti and La Paz, Bolivia; on the sides of public buses in Durban, South Africa; and on parade horses in Burkina Faso. Condom use demonstration and promotion are common events at rock concerts, dance contests, and sports events in many countries of Africa, Asia, and Latin America. Information on condom use as protection from HIV and other STDs is printed in school notebooks in Zaire, school pencil boxes in Cambodia, on matchboxes in Cote d'Ivoire, in comic books in Haiti and Bolivia, on shopping bags in Cameroon, and on calenders in Zambia and Nigeria.[67,68] In religiously conservative countries, such as Niger and Mali, social marketing organizations have been able to promote condoms successfully by educating and gaining the support of religious leaders.[69]

FEMALE CONDOM

The Reality® female condom is a loose-fitting, prelubricated polyurethane sheath that fits into the vagina, lining it from labia to cervix. Flexible rings at both ends help in positioning the sheath; the one at the closed end fits behind the pubic bone, whereas the open end lies flat against the labia, outside the body. Insertion is similar to that of a diaphragm.

Clinical effectiveness and adverse effects of the female condom

Laboratory studies have shown that the Reality® female condom is an effective mechanical barrier to sexually transmitted viruses, including HIV.[70,71] One study showed that all 20 consistent users were protected from trichomoniasis reinfection; inconsistent users had a reinfection rate (14.7 percent) similar to that of controls (14 percent).[35] Other studies of effectiveness for STD/HIV prevention are underway.[72]

No adverse effects have been reported for the Reality® female condom. One study demonstrated that use of the female condom does not alter vaginal flora.[73]

Advantages and disadvantages of using the female condom

The Reality® female condom has features that have the potential to provide increased sexual pleasure for both men and women: The device does not constrict the man's penis, and therefore does not prevent the pleasurable sensation of friction, and the polyurethane material allows transfer of body heat. Additional advantages of the device are that it covers the introitus, thus providing additional protection, and it can be used with oil-based lubricants, unlike latex male condoms. Despite these technologic features, the device also has the potential to make sex less enjoyable. Since the outer ring of the device hangs outside of the vagina, it can be aesthetically unappealing, and women may not want to insert it well in advance of intercourse. In that case, sexual foreplay must be interrupted for insertion, as with the male condom.[45] In addition, movement of the penis inside the condom can be noisy, which some couples may find disagreeable.[74] The device has been promoted as a female-controlled method but in fact, because men are aware of its presence, their cooperation is needed for its use.[45] Therefore, using the device requires its own set of negotiation skills.

Other disadvantages have been reported in the use of this device. As it comes in only one size, it may slip out during intercourse if the woman's vagina is small.[74] Care must be taken during intercourse so that the penis does not penetrate the vagina outside the outer ring. The device can be difficult to insert because of the slipperiness of the lubricant and the awkwardness of manipulating the inner ring. In addition, the two rings may cause discomfort during intercourse for one or both partners.[45] In terms of cost, the female condom is significantly more expensive than the male condom, costing approximately $2.50 per condom in commercial retail outlets.[45] There are special rates for public sector organizations, however, ranging from 50 to 90 cents per device, depending on the quantity purchased.[75]

Acceptability of the female condom

Numerous acceptability studies of the Reality® female condom have been conducted in a variety of contexts in both developed and developing countries (Table 94-3). Results have been mixed, and clear trends have been hard to distinguish. The overall percentage of women who reported liking the female condom has ranged from 32 percent in a Dutch study to 95 percent in a study conducted in Cameroon.[81,87] In some studies, the percentage of women saying that they would use the condom again has been greater than the percentage who reported liking it, suggesting that other factors are at play in the decision-making process besides a comfort level with the product.[83,85] For example, it may be more important for women to have a method that they can control than to have a method that is 100 percent comfortable. In other cases, however, more women have said that they liked the condom than reported that they would use it again.[78,86] These results suggest that either the physical discomforts of the female condom outweigh the benefits, or perhaps that partner resistance plays a stronger role in some women's use of the device than the woman's personal preference.

The main features that women have liked about the condom are very similar across the studies. Many have liked the fact that the device is a form of protection over which they have some control, and that it provides protection against both pregnancy and sexually transmitted diseases.[76,78,82,83,86] Women have also liked the fact that it is stronger than male (latex) condoms.[82,83,85] Some women have reported that the female condom feels good and makes sex more enjoyable.[86]

Things that women have not liked about the female condom

Table 94-3. Female Condom Acceptability Studies

Study	Participants enrolled/ completed	Type of participants	Percent who liked FC	Percent who would use again	Percent who preferred to male condom	Percent whose partner liked	Percent finding insertion easy
Gollub et al. (U.S.)[76]	52/41 (79%) (2 weeks)	Hospital patients and staff	Avg. score of 1.1†	n/a	73%	49%	Avg. score of 1.2§
Ashery et al. (U.S.)[77]	37/28 (76%) (3 weeks)	IDU and crack-using women	n/a	71%	n/a	14%	20%
Ford and Mathie (U.K.)[78]	214 66% (1 use) 31% (3 months)	FP* clinic and general practice patients and partners	52% (after 3 mos)#	44% (after 3 mos)#	n/a	n/a	25% (1st use) 70% (10 uses)
Masters et al. (U.K.)[79]	79/60 (76%) (2 months)	Genitourinary patients	n/a	83% (after 3 uses)	n/a	26%	49% (after 3 uses)
Bounds et al. (U.K.)[80]	110/10 (9%) (12 months)	FP patients	43% (all users)	82% (study completers)	n/a	42% (all users)	29% (all users)
Patent et al. (Holland)[81]	300/116 (39%) + 166 partners (3 uses)	FP* patients, CSWs, magazine readers, partners	32%	31%	25% (women) 53% (men)	Avg. male score = 5.3‡	71%
Jenkins (Papua New Guinea)[82]	336/224 (67%) (incl. 15 men) (6 uses)	Urban men and women	100% (M) n/a (F)	97.6% (if sold at good price)	57% (women)	n/a	87% (women)
Blogg and Blogg (Malawi)[83]	160/153 (96%) (2 months)	CSWs and couples	91%—CSWs 56%—F 54%—M	96% (all women) 94% (men)**	81% (all women) 67% (men)	n/a	n/a
Chan and Soon (Singapore)[84]	29/21 (72%) (1 week)	CSWs	52%	n/a	24%	Less than 50%	43%
Sakondhavat and Joanis (Thailand)[85]	22/21 (95%) (2 weeks)	CSWs	9.5% (a lot) 62% (a little)	48%	n/a	81% (said some liked)	14%
Ruminjo et al. (Kenya)[86]	48 95% (Phase I) 25% (Phase II) (6 weeks)	Ob/gyn staff and patients	18%—very much, 66%—fairly well (Phase I)	55% (Phase I)	39% (Phase I)	29%	47% (Phase I) 92% (Phase II)
Monny-Lobe et al. (Cameroon)[87]	40 95% (Phase I) 85% (Phase II) (4 weeks)	CSWs	61%—very much, 34%—fairly well (Phase I)	87% (Phase I)	63% (Phase I)	68% (fairly well) 11% (very much)	53% (Phase I) 74% (Phase II)

NOTES: * FP = family planning.
† Average score based on a scale of 0–4, where 0 = liked very much and 4 = disliked very much.
§ Average score based on a scale of 0–4, where 0 = very easy and 4 = very difficult.
# Includes male partners.
‡ Average score based on a scale of 1–10, where 1 = very bad and 10 = excellent.
** Assuming that modifications were made.

include difficulty of insertion, messiness, and discomfort caused by the inner and outer rings.[79,82,85–88] Others have complained about noisiness during intercourse, ugliness of the device, and high cost.[78,84–89] Several studies also have reported incidences of the condom being pushed into the vagina during intercourse and the penis being inserted in between the condom and the vagina.[76,78,80]

In general, the percentages of women who have said their partners like the female condom have been lower than the percentages of women who have liked the device themselves. Several studies have mentioned problems of partner resistance to the condoms.[78,84,90] Interestingly, two studies that asked men whether or not they preferred the female to the male condom yielded generally positive results, with over half of the men responding "yes" in both cases.[82,83] Women's responses when asked this same question have been mixed. The percentage saying "yes" has ranged from 24 percent in a Singapore study to 81 percent in a Malawi study.[83,84]

SPONGE

THE TODAY® SPONGE

Note: In March 1995, the Today® sponge was taken off the market because of the inability of its manufacturer, Whitehall-Robins, to comply with FDA manufacturing regulations.[91] Since the discontinuation was not the result of any feature of the product itself, it is possible that the same or a similar device could be manufactured again in the future (such as the new Protectaid® sponge, discussed in the following).

Clinical effectiveness and adverse effects of the sponge

Two randomized trials have shown that the sponge protects women from some STDs, but not from HIV infection (see Table 94-4). One randomized trial involving female commercial sex workers in Thailand showed a strong protective effect against chlamydia and a moderate protective effect against gonorrhea.[98] A highly publicized randomized clinical trial showed that frequent use of the Today® sponge did not protect commercial sex workers in Kenya from HIV infection.[27] The study found a strong protective effect against gonorrhea, and a moderate protective effect against chlamydia. A strong protective effect against gonorrhea and trichomoniasis also was demonstrated in a cross-sectional study; however, this same study showed a weak protective effect against chlamydia and no effect on bacterial vaginosis.[100] The effects of sponge use on trichomoniasis and bacterial vaginosis have not been addressed in prospective cohort studies.

One randomized trial showed that sponge use increases the risk of candidiasis.[98] Another randomized trial showed that sponge use appeared to increase risk for genital ulcers (mostly vaginal) and vulvitis, and users had higher rates (although not statistically significantly higher) of HIV seroconversion than placebo users.[27] However, these findings of adverse effects for the Today® sponge should not be generalized to other spermicidal products containing N-9, since the sponge contains 1,000 mg of N-9 and most other products contain 100 mg or less. Furthermore, the sex workers in this randomized trial used the sponges very frequently, averaging 14 weekly.[101]

Advantages and disadvantages of using the sponge

Sponges are less expensive than diaphragms or cervical caps, because they are one-size-fits-all and do not require a clinical fitting. They are available over-the-counter and are easier to insert than either the cervical cap or the diaphragm. Sponges come already impregnated with spermicide, making them less messy to use than other barrier methods and allowing for the possibility of multiple coital acts without the insertion of additional spermicide. Because they are made of soft material, they are more comfortable to wear than either the diaphragm or cervical cap. Sponges can be inserted ahead of time, so that intercourse does not need to be interrupted.[45] The sponge is disposable and thus, unlike the diaphragm or cervical cap, does not need to be washed or stored after each use.

Sponges have several disadvantages, however. They may be difficult to remove because of the necessity of locating the string. Like the diaphragm and cervical cap, they must be left in for 6 hours after intercourse. They are not recommended for use during menstruation and are more expensive than other disposable barrier methods, such as condoms and spermicides.[45] The cost for one sponge ranges from $1.25 to $1.50.[42] Some men may find the string uncomfortable during intercourse.[102] In addition, the fact that they are one-size-fits-all means that they may not fit snugly in all women (especially those who have already borne children).[103]

Acceptability of the sponge

Results from acceptability studies on the Today® sponge are mixed. A U.S. clinical trial involving 51 women revealed high rates of vaginal infections, odor problems, irritation, and difficulty with removal. Over three-quarters of the women experienced at least one of these problems.[104] A four-site international study comparing use of the sponge with vaginal foaming tablets by 1,299 women concluded that women found the tablets to be more acceptable than the sponge. At the site in Bangladesh, almost half of the women had problems with the sponge staying in place, and women at all sites reported problems with insertion and removal.[105]

A study of 50 women in Malaysia produced more positive results, however. Very few women in this study had problems with insertion or removal and there were almost no reports of discomfort or difficulties with use. This could have been because the Malaysian women received more detailed training on correct use of the device than did the women in the multisite study.[106]

A U.S. telephone survey of 800 current and past Today® sponge users revealed moderate to high levels of satisfaction with the device. Current sponge users gave it an average rating of 4.4 on a scale of 1 to 5, where 1 represented extremely dissatisfied and 5 represented extremely satisfied. Women chose to use the device because they perceived it to be effective, comfortable, and convenient.[107]

THE PROTECTAID® SPONGE

A new sponge device, Protectaid®, is being developed by AXCAN (Mont St. Hilaire, Quebec, Canada). The sponge is impregnated with a combination of sodium cholate, N-9, and benzalkonium chloride (BZK). In vitro, sodium cholate and F5 gel (N-9 combined with BZK) have been shown to have a dose-dependent inhibitory effect on HIV reverse transcriptase and on infectivity of HIV.[108] N-9 and BZK have been shown to inactivate a broad range of STD pathogens.[2,109] A small study of 20 women who used the Protectaid® sponge showed 100 percent contraceptive effectiveness, but studies to assess STD/HIV protection have not yet been conducted.[102]

The Protectaid® sponge has a new, flexible shape that adapts to fit the individual woman, thus making it a better fit than the

Table 94-4. Prospective Studies of Vaginal Spermicides, Antiseptics, and Condoms to Prevent STD in Women

Study	Design	Population	Method	Outcome	Use	RR (95% c.i.)
Edwards, 1973[92]	NRCT	CSW, Nevada	Vaginal orthoiodobenzoic acid	Gonorrhea		0.08 (0.02–0.37)
Cutler et al., 1977[93]	RCT	STD clinic, Pennsylvania	N-9 foam	Gonorrhea		0.11 (0.02–0.55)
Limsuwan et al., 1978[94]	NRCT	CSW, Thailand	Vaginal providone-iodine	Gonorrhea		0.25 (0.15–0.42)
Rendon et al., 1980[95]	RCT	Outpatient clinic, Mexico	Phenylmercuric acetate suppositories	Gonorrhea		0.30 (0.08–1.14)
			N-9 suppositories	Gonorrhea		0.60 (0.21–1.73)
Louv et al., 1988[96]	RCT	STD clinic, Alabama	N-9 suppositories	Gonorrhea		0.76 (0.59–0.98)*
				Chlamydia		0.78 (0.64–0.96)*
Barbone et al., 1990[97]	RCT	STD clinic, Alabama	N-9 gel	Trichomoniasis		0.83 (0.61–1.12)
				Bacterial vaginosis		0.86 (0.69–1.12)
Rosenberg et al., 1987[98]	RCT	CSW, Thailand	N-9 sponge	Gonorrhea		0.67 (0.42–1.07)
				Chlamydia		0.31 (0.16–0.60)
Kreiss et al., 1992[27]	RCT	CSW, Kenya	N-9 sponge	Gonorrhea		0.4 ($p < 0.001$)
				Chlamydia		0.6 (not significant)
				Genital ulcers		3.3 ($p < 0.0001$)
Niruthisard et al., 1992[38]	RCT	CSW, Thailand	N-9 film + condoms	Gonorrhea/chlamydia	N-9 any	0.75 (0.5–1.1)
					N-9 > 75%	0.6 (0.3–1.0)
					Condoms > 75% use	0.5 (0.3–0.7)
Weir et al., 1994[99]	RCT	CSW, Cameroon	N-9 suppositories + condoms	Gonorrhea	N-9 > 75%	0.14 (0.07–0.29)
					N-9 51–75%	0.23 (0.12–0.46)
					Condoms > 90%	0.05 (0.01–0.39)
					Condoms 76–90%	0.2 (0.1–0.39)

* 90% confidence interval.
CSW = Commercial sex worker.
NRCT = Nonrandomized clinical trial.
RCT = Randomized clinical trial.
SOURCE: Updated from Cates/Stone.[2]

Today® sponge. Protectaid® has no strings; built-in grooves make it easy to insert and remove. The low-dose combination of spermicides used (sodium cholate, BZK, and N-9) is less likely to be irritating than the relatively high concentration of N-9 found in the Today® sponge. A preliminary study of 20 young women yielded high levels of acceptability and no side effects or irritation (cervical cultures were conducted after 6 months and 12 months).[102]

DIAPHRAGM

Clinical effectiveness and adverse effects of the diaphragm

No prospective studies have assessed the protective effects of the diaphragm on HIV infection or other STD.[2] Case-control and cross-sectional studies have found a protective effect against gonorrhea, chlamydia, trichomoniasis, PID, and infertility, but not against bacterial vaginosis.[100–113] Because the diaphragm covers the cervix and is almost always used with spermicides that have an effect on many STD pathogens, protection against certain STDs that primarily involve the cervix (gonorrhea and chlamydia) is biologically plausible and should be explored in prospective studies.

Diaphragm use is associated both with alterations in normal vaginal flora and with an increased risk for urinary tract infections.[114–117] The causal mechanisms are not completely understood, but are most likely related to the direct chemical effects of the spermicides usually used with diaphragms. Specific alterations in vaginal flora include increased colonization with *E. coli* and uropathogens, but no dramatic effect on lactobacilli or yeast.[117,118] Whereas a small prospective study reported that diaphragm use was associated with increased colonization with *Candida* species and decreased colonization with lactobacilli, a more recent and much larger prospective study reported no effect on lactobacilli, yeast, *Gardnerella vaginalis*, Group B streptococci, or anaerobic gram-negative rods.[117,118]

Advantages and disadvantages of using the diaphragm

The diaphragm is reusable, needing to be replaced only every 3 years.[42] It can be inserted up to 6 hours before intercourse and thus can be used without the partner's knowledge. Although it can be left in place for 24 hours, thus offering protection for multiple coital acts, spermicide must be reapplied every time intercourse occurs.[45]

There are disadvantages to this method, however. Male partners can feel the ring and therefore may experience discomfort. Some women find the diaphragm difficult to insert and remove. If not inserted properly, the device may become dislodged during intercourse, which compromises its effectiveness. If a woman gives birth or experiences a weight gain or loss of more than 5 kg, the device must be refitted. Diaphragms are made of latex, which absorbs odors, resulting in user complaints of unpleasant odors with extended use.[45] Additionally, diaphragms cannot be used with oil-based lubricants or oil-based vaginal yeast infection medications (e.g., butoconazole, miconazole, and terconazole).[45,46] The device must be washed and properly stored after each use.

Diaphragms must be fitted by clinicians, a factor that increases the cost of obtaining this device. The combined cost can range from $50 to $150, depending on the fee charged by the provider for the fitting. The diaphragm itself costs approximately $22; the cost of the accompanying spermicidal cream or gel is approximately 25 cents per application.[42]

Acceptability of the diaphragm

Acceptability of the diaphragm has been mixed. In general, it has been most successfully used among older, highly motivated women. Ortho Pharmaceutical's 1992 Birth Control Study of U.S. women aged 15 to 44 showed that only 33 percent of all respondents and 76 percent of diaphragm users had a favorable opinion of the method. These percentages were significantly lower than ratings received for other barrier methods, such as the condom and the sponge.[119] In a recent study of diaphragm acceptability among women of low socioeconomic status in Brazil, there was a high discontinuation rate after only 1 to 3 months. One of the most common reasons for discontinuation was difficulty with insertion and removal of the device.[120] A survey among middle-class adolescent diaphragm users in the northeastern United States revealed that only about one-third of respondents used their diaphragm during every act of intercourse, and the main reason for nonuse was that it was "too much trouble." Over half (53 percent) of these diaphragm users disliked the messiness and preparation of the method.[121]

Other studies have shown more positive attitudes toward the device, such as a study conducted involving 85 Israeli women. The rate of continuation after 2 years was high (87 percent), and side effects were reported in less than 1 percent of women.[122] Another study of 158 German family planning clients yielded a 76 percent continuation rate after an average of 19 months. A large majority of women (82 percent) reported either improvement or no change in their sexual feelings with use of the device.[123]

CERVICAL CAP

Clinical effectiveness and adverse effects of the cervical cap

No data on the effectiveness of the cervical cap for HIV/STD prevention are currently available. Use of cervical caps with nonoxynol-9 increases vaginal colonization by *E. coli* and *Enterococcus*, but has no adverse effect on vaginal lactobacilli.[118]

Advantages and disadvantages of using the cervical cap

Cervical caps are smaller and more durable than diaphragms and can be left in place for 48 hours. They require only a small amount of spermicide and, unlike the diaphragm, do not require additional spermicide with repeated acts of intercourse. Theoretically they can be used without the partner's knowledge but, like the diaphragm, they must be left in place for 6 hours after intercourse.[45]

Like diaphragms, cervical caps must be fitted by a clinician. They come in only four sizes, which means that not all women are able to be fitted. Dislodgement of the device during intercourse is a frequently reported problem, perhaps owing to the fact that the device cannot be fitted precisely. Insertion of the device requires instruction and practice, and removal also can be difficult. One of the most frequently reported problems has been an unpleasant odor produced with extended use. Like the diaphragm, the cervical cap must be washed and stored properly after each use.[45] Correct use of the cap requires extensive touching of the genitalia and an ability to determine the exact location of the cervix, which may be unappealing or difficult for some women.[42]

The cost of obtaining a cervical cap ranges from $50 to $150, depending on the fee charged by the provider for fitting the device. Cervical caps by themselves cost approximately $22, and must be replaced every 3 years.[42]

Acceptability of the cervical cap

No acceptability research has been published on this method since the mid-1980s, when it was introduced into the U.S. market. In one Canadian study, 84 percent of respondents were satisfied with the cap, whereas in another, 54 percent of women were very satisfied and 23 percent were somewhat satisfied with the method.[124,125] A U.S. study did not inquire about satisfaction explicitly, but found that 75 percent of women did not experience any discomfort or difficulties with insertion of the device, and the vast majority (83 percent) said that they would recommend it to a friend.[126] Major complaints about the method included unpleasant odor, dislodgement, and partner discomfort.[124–126]

New developments for the cervical cap

Two new devices are on the horizon. The first is a newly designed device, called Femcap®, which has many advantages over the traditional cervical cap. Made of silicone, it is more resistant to light and heat and does not absorb odors. In addition, its unique "sailor's hat" shape results in a snugger fit because it stays in place through a suction mechanism.[45] Femcap® comes in two sizes: one for women who have had a vaginal birth, and one for women who have not. The device has a built-in strap to facilitate removal.[127] Like the traditional cervical cap, Femcap® must be used with a spermicide.[128] Sparse data are available on contraceptive efficacy and none on STD prevention efficacy.

Results of a 2-year clinical trial showed a high level of acceptability among users, with respondents giving Femcap® high ratings on a number of features. Over 90 percent of the women were very satisfied with the lack of dislodgement, the absence of discomfort, and with the spontaneity and health safety. Ease of removal received the lowest ratings, however, with only 16 percent of respondents claiming that they were highly satisfied.[128] (Note: This study was conducted before the modification of the device to include the removal strap.)

The second product, Lea's Shield®, is still being tested. This is a cup-shaped device that covers the cervix through a suction mechanism. It has a one-way valve that allows vaginal secretions and menstrual fluid to flow from the vagina. The device will be sold over the counter and will come in one-size-fits-all. Like Femcap®, it is made of silicone rubber, making it safe for use by women with latex allergies.[129] Lea's Shield® can be worn for up to 48 hours and requires only 2 cc of spermicide.[130] Preliminary studies in the United States and Europe have yielded high levels of safety and acceptability. In a U.S. study of 184 women, 87 percent said that they would recommend Lea's Shield® to a friend. In an Austrian study, 69 percent of women and their partners were satisfied with the product, and 52 percent chose the device as their new method of contraception. Twenty-four women in a German study were asked to rate the device on a scale of 1 to 10 (with 10 being the highest). The device received average scores of 9.3 for snugness of fit, 8.2 for lack of disturbance during intercourse, 7.8 for removal, and 7.6 for disturbance during intercourse.[131]

SPERMICIDES

The term "spermicide" as used here refers to chemicals used for contraception whose mechanism for killing sperm also kills STD pathogens. Commonly available spermicides include N-9, octoxynol, chlorhexadine, benzalkonium chloride, and menfegol. Most STD prevention studies have evaluated N-9. Laboratory, animal, and human studies demonstrate varying levels of protection by spermicides against HIV infection and certain STDs.

Clinical effectiveness and adverse effects of spermicides

Nonoxynol-9. Laboratory studies show that small concentrations of N-9 kill or inactivate HIV, *T. pallidum, N. gonorrhoeae, H. ducreyi*, and HSV.[2,109] All except one in vitro study showed that N-9 inactivates *C. trachomatis*.[132,133] One laboratory study showed that N-9 markedly reduced infectivity of CMV but did not inactivate bovine papillomavirus (BPV-1) or BK virus, both of which are nonenveloped viruses.[134] No in vitro studies have assessed effects of N-9 on HPV or HBV. Because N-9 is a nonionic surfactant that disrupts lipid envelopes, it is likely that it inactivates viruses with a lipid envelope (HBV) but not necessarily nonenveloped viruses such as HPV.

Studies using various animal models have demonstrated a protective effect of vaginally applied N-9 against infection with the simian immunodeficiency virus (SIV), the feline immunodeficiency virus (FIV), HSV, and chlamydia.[135–138] One study also demonstrated that rectal application of N-9 protected cats against HSV infection.[137]

Clinical studies of women show various levels of protection against some STDs; protection against HIV infection is unclear (see Tables 94-1 and 94-4). Most randomized clinical trials and cohort studies have demonstrated a protective effect against gonorrhea and chlamydia in women, and one study suggested a protective effect against trichomoniasis and bacterial vaginosis (see Table 94-4). Another randomized trial involving commercial sex workers in Thailand showed that compliant use ($\geq$76 percent) of N-9 film reduced risk for gonorrhea or chlamydia by 40 percent, after controlling for concurrent use of condoms.[38]

One cohort study of commercial sex workers in Cameroon showed that compliant use of N-9 at least two-thirds of the time conferred strong protection against HIV infection after controlling for concurrent condom use.[139] A study in Zambia showed a slight reduction in risk for HIV seroconversion among discordant couples who reported consistent N-9 use, and a moderate protective effect for women.[29] However, the concurrent use of condoms by participants in both of these studies limits the ability to draw conclusions about the level of protection afforded by N-9 used alone. A randomized trial of N-9 film currently underway in Cameroon may further clarify the protective effect of N-9 on HIV infection among women.

The effect of anorectal use of N-9 on STD transmission risk has not been assessed in men or women, nor has the effect of vaginal N-9 on female-to-male STD transmission.

The frequency of adverse effects of vaginal spermicides used for contraception is generally low.[140] However, concerns have been raised that women using them for STD/HIV prevention may use them more frequently and in larger doses than is common for contraceptive use. Frequent use could potentially lead to inflammation and microscopic ulceration of vaginal tissue or render natural mucosal defense mechanisms less protective (e.g., alterations of beneficial vaginal flora), and thereby theoretically increase the risk for HIV infection and other STDs. Concerns about adverse effects of N-9 rose to a fever pitch after a randomized trial of the Today® sponge showed no protective effect against HIV and an increased risk for genital ulcers; however, these concerns are not justifiable for other, lower-dose formulations of N-9 or less frequent users of this sponge.[101]

Two recent studies provide evidence that harmful effects on the cervicovaginal mucosa are related to dose and frequency of use, involve mainly the cervix and vagina, and are often asymptomatic. One study of high-dose use conducted in Thailand in 1991 found that six of 14 (43 percent; 95 percent confidence interva[l] 71 percent) women had colposcopic evidence of cervico[vaginal] epithelial disruption, bleeding, or both after 14 consecutiv[e days] of using one vaginal suppository (each containing 150 mg [ac]tive ingredient) hourly for 4 hours.[141] A larger study in the [Do]minican Republic found that women who used 150-mg N-9 v[agi]nal suppositories at high frequencies had a rate of colposcopic[ally] diagnosed epithelial disruption five times that of placebo users. Women using the suppositories every other day had rates simil[ar] to placebo users. Women who used the suppositories daily o[r] twice daily had rates of epithelial disruption that were 2.5 time[s] higher than that of placebo users.

A large study to assess the protective effect of 100-mg N-9 suppositories on HIV infection in a cohort of sex workers in Cameroon found that increased use of N-9 was not associated with an increase in cervical and vaginal ulcers diagnosed clinically without a colposcope and may have had a protective effect.[143] The clinical relevance of colposcopically identified microtrauma after N-9 use is questionable, since intercourse itself is commonly associated with microabrasions and broken capillaries.[144] A recent small randomized trial showed that an increased dose of N-9 in condom lubricants was associated with increased numbers of vaginal polymorphonuclear leukocytes but not with clinical signs of inflammation; however, the clinical relevance of this finding is unclear.[145]

Another concern is the effect of N-9 on the vaginal ecosystem, especially the vaginal flora, since N-9 is a nonselective detergent that, in vitro, kills a broad range of microorganisms. In vitro, low concentrations of N-9 kill lactobacilli (with a selective effect on the beneficial H_2O_2-producing lactobacilli) and *Gardnerella*, but not *Candida* or *E. coli* and other uropathogens.[117,146] However, owing to the complexity of the vaginal ecosystem, in vitro data cannot adequately predict the effects of N-9 on human vaginal flora (or STD pathogens) and clinical sequelae. Potential clinical consequences of altered vaginal flora include bacterial vaginosis, candidiasis, *E. coli* bacteriuria, and urinary tract infection. The relationships between N-9 use, decreased vaginal colonization with lactobacilli or other alterations of flora, and bacterial vaginosis are not well understood. Indeed, results of clinical studies generally have not correlated well with the results of in vitro studies. Clinical studies have not shown dramatic adverse effects of N-9 on vaginal lactobacilli.[118] Prospective studies have shown that the incidence of bacterial vaginosis or candidiasis is no higher in vaginal N-9 users than in controls.[38,96,97] Vaginal colonization with *E. coli* and *E. coli* bacteriuria is associated with N-9 use and also with sexual intercourse in women who use N-9 with diaphragms or condoms.[115,117,118] The role of concomitant mechanical barrier use is not clear; indeed, a small study suggested that alterations in flora among a small number of users of vaginal N-9 alone were similar (and included decreased lactobacilli) but not identical to those observed in users of N-9 with diaphragms or cervical caps.[117] Moreover, the interrelationships between vaginal colonization with *E. coli*, lactobacilli, intercourse, vaginal pH, and N-9 use are complex.[147,148] Another issue to consider is the effect of N-9 itself versus the effects of the vehicles used in commercially available vaginal preparations.[149,150]

Novel N-9 Products. New delivery systems for N-9 are being developed and evaluated.[151,152] Studies are currently underway to assess the effectiveness of a commercially available controlled-release gel, Advantage 24 Bioadhesive Contraceptive Gel®, for HIV prevention.[153,154] A previous multisite randomized placebo-controlled trial to evaluate safety of the product showed that the prevalence of genital ulcers and abrasions was similar for women using the product, placebo, or neither.[153]

Two new products are not yet commercially available. One controlled-release product, called Triad®, combines a fast-releasing layer of N-9 on the outer surface with intermediate-releasing granules and slow-releasing pellets on the inside. Another product in development is a lipid that becomes a gel on contact with vaginal secretions and provides a physical and chemical barrier.

Other Spermicides. In vitro, many other spermicidal compounds kill STD pathogens.[2,109,155] These include octoxynol, chlorhexadine, benzalkonium chloride, gramicidin, gossypol, and povidone-iodine. Clinical studies to evaluate the effectiveness for STD/HIV protection have not been conducted with most of these compounds. A randomized placebo-controlled study to evaluate the safety of menfegol foaming vaginal suppositories (Neosampoon®) in commercial sex workers was stopped because the incidence of genital lesions was high in study subjects who used the tablets more than once daily; however, the similarly high incidence of lesions in women using placebo tablets suggested that the irritant effects may have been due to the vehicle rather than the active ingredient.[150]

Advantages and disadvantages of using spermicides

Spermicides have several advantages over other barrier methods. They are easy to use and available over the counter. They can be inserted ahead of intercourse and typically are not felt by either partner, making them ideal for women who want to use a method without the knowledge of their partners. In addition, there are no long-term side effects.[45] Some couples may also enjoy the extra lubrication provided by spermicides.

Spermicides also have several disadvantages. Some women may feel uncomfortable touching their genitalia in order to insert them, although in the case of gels and creams, insertion can be done with an applicator, minimizing genital contact. Some formulations, such as foams and creams, can be messy to insert and may leak out of the vagina. This extra lubrication may be unappealing to some couples, especially in parts of the world where "dry sex" is very popular.[45,156]

If sexual activity is unplanned and insertion is not done ahead of time, intercourse may need to be interrupted for use of this method. Some spermicidal formulations, such as film, suppositories, and tablets, require that the couple wait 10 minutes for the spermicide to dissolve before engaging in intercourse. Although spermicides have no long-term side effects, they may cause irritation and discomfort in one or both partners; some women report an unpleasant sensation of warmth when foaming tablet spermicides dissolve.[45]

Despite these drawbacks, some spermicides, such as the vaginal contraceptive film (VCF), have experienced a gain in popularity during the past several years. Clinicians in some family planning clinics and state health departments have found that women prefer the film over spermicidal foam, owing to the fact that it is discreet, easy to carry, and less messy.[157] The new controlled-release product, Advantage 24 Bioadhesive Contraceptive Gel®, also promises to be popular. It is reportedly effective for 24 hours and, because of bioadhesive technology that allows it to stick to the cervix, it can be inserted long before intercourse. It is odorless and flavorless and is sold in prefilled applicators, which make insertion less messy. In addition, it contains a lower dose of N-9 than other spermicidal formulations, resulting in a smaller likelihood of irritation.[158]

In general, spermicides are more expensive than condoms, but less expensive than the cost of being fitted for a diaphragm or cervical cap. A 12-pack of spermicidal suppositories can cost as little as $4.00, whereas spermicidal film can cost twice as much at $9.00 for 12 sheets.[42] Advantage 24® sells at approximately $8.00 for a 3-pack, making it prohibitively expensive for low-income women.[158]

Acceptability of spermicides

Studies have shown overall acceptability of spermicides to be high, with most of the variance depending on the formulation used. In a study among low-income Latino women in the United States, three-quarters of respondents said that spermicidal foam made sex more comfortable and enjoyable than sex with no method, and almost all of them said they would use it again the next time they had intercourse.[159] Similarly, a Thai study of menfegol and N-9 foaming tablets over a 12-month period found that the vast majority of respondents reported using the tablets for every act of intercourse, with an increasing number reporting no problem with use as the study progressed. Very few women complained about either tablet being messy or inconvenient and very few cases of male discomfort were reported. The most frequently reported problems were burning, stinging, or itching.[160]

An Egyptian clinical trial comparing menfegol foaming tablets with N-9 spermicidal foam reported very few complaints of burning or discomfort and very few women complained that either formulation was troublesome or messy. As in the Thailand study, a very high percentage of women used the spermicides at every intercourse (90 percent of those returning for at least one follow-up visit), indicating high acceptability levels.[161] A multisite study conducted in Yugoslavia, Taiwan, and Bangladesh found that menfegol foaming tablets compared favorably with the sponge in two sites and were more acceptable than the sponge in two others. Although more women complained of burning and itching problems with the tablets than with the sponge, this discomfort seemed to be tolerable, as very few women discontinued use because of it.[105]

A study of spermicidal foam, suppositories, and foaming tablets involving male and female STD patients in Zambia showed high levels of satisfaction with all three methods. Of the three, women preferred the foaming tablets best and rated them highest in terms of sexual satisfaction, whereas men gave all of the methods equally high ratings. The percentage of coital episodes unprotected by any method was highest among foam users, suggesting a lower acceptability level for this method.[162]

Another study conducted in Kenya, Mexico, and the Dominican Republic compared the acceptability of vaginal contraceptive film with foaming tablets and found that both women and their partners in all three countries preferred the film. Women reported that they liked the feel of the film better, which coincides with many women's complaint that the tablets were messy or wet. The main complaint about the film was that it stuck to women's fingers during insertion.[163]

A study of family planning clinic patients in the United Kingdom compared the acceptability of diaphragm use with both contraceptive film and spermicidal cream or jelly. Although both groups reported high rates of satisfaction with their methods, women in the film group were more likely to give positive comments about their method, especially regarding lack of messiness.[164]

A recent multisite study comparing three formulations of N-9 (suppository, gel, and film) showed a wide variation in acceptability of the different formulations. Factors affecting the women's preferences included the amount of lubrication provided, the "messiness" of the product, ease of storage and disposal, and perceptions of the product's association with sexual pleasure and health. Communication with male partners also played an important role in product preference.[165]

MICROBICIDES

The term "microbicides" has recently been used to connote chemicals that could be used topically to prevent infection with STD

Table 94-5. Potential Targets and Mechanisms for Agents that Prevent Pregnancy and/or STD

Target	Agent	Mechanism	Intended effect
Sperm	Nonoxynol-9	Surfactant	Spermicidal
	C31G	Surfactant	Spermicidal
	Chlorhexidine	Surfactant	Spermicidal
	Peroxides	Membrane-active	Spermicidal
	Antibody (MAb)	Agglutination	Decreases forward motility
		Shaking phenomenon	Decreases forward motility
	Magainin	Pore formation	Spermicidal
	Decapacitation factor	Blocks capacitation	No acrosome reaction
	Progesterone	Activates calcium channels	Premature acrosome reaction
	AGB	Acrosin inhibitor	Blocks fertilization
	Sulfonated polystyrene	Acrosin inhibitor	Blocks fertilization
		Agglutination	Decreases forward motility
	ZP mimics	Blocks ZP binding	Blocks fertilization
	Acidic buffer	Maintains low pH	Spermicidal
	Zinc	Blocks capacitation	Blocks fertilization
	Neem	Membrane-active	Spermicidal
	Squalamine	Membrane-active	Microbicidal
Pathogens	Nonoxynol-9	Disrupts membrane/envelope	Microbicidal
	C31G	Disrupts membrane/envelope	Microbicidal
	Chlorhexidine	Disrupts membrane/envelope	Microbicidal
	Milk fatty acids	Disrupts membrane/envelope	Microbicidal
	Peroxides	Membrane-active	Microbicidal
	Antibody	Agglutination	Immune exclusion
	Docosanol	Disrupts membrane/envelope	Microbicidal (enveloped viruses)
	CAM mimic	Decoy	Blocks adhesion
	Sulfated polymer	Coats cells	Blocks adhesion
		Coats virus	Blocks fusion
	AGB	Protease inhibition	Blocks adhesion
	Protegrins	Pore-formation	Microbicidal
	Acidic buffer	Maintains low pH	Microbicidal
	Zinc	Binds proteins	Microbicidal
	Neem	Membrane-active	Microbicidal
	Squalamine	Membrane-active	Microbicidal
	PMPA	Inhibits reverse transcriptase	Anti-HIV
Cervicovaginal environment			
Mucus	Acidic buffer	Lowers or maintains pH	Microbicidal
	Lactoferrin	Fe binding	Inhibits Fe-dependent pathogens
	Lysozyme	Enzymatic bacteriolysis	Bactericidal
	Zinc	Protein binding	Microbicidal
	Sulfonated polystyrene	Increases viscosity	Decreases sperm migration
	Chlorhexidine	Increases viscosity	Decreases sperm migration
	Inhibits mucopolysaccharidase	Increases viscosity	Decreases sperm migration
	Lubricating gels	Increases lubricity	Reduces trauma
Epithelium	Docosanol	Membrane-active	Microbicidal
	β-lactoglobulin	Blocks HIV receptors	Anti-HIV
	Squalamine	Inhibits Na^+/H^+ exchange	Anti-HIV
	C31G	Fibrin formation	Trauma repair
	Lubricating gels	Prevents abrasions	Blocks pathogen entry
	Zinc sulfate	Promotes wound healing	Blocks pathogen entry
Immune system	Cytokines	Activates macrophages	Phagocytosis
	Antibodies	Interacts with mucus	Immune exclusion
		Agglutination	Immune exclusion
		Blocks adhesion	Immune exclusion
Commensals	Acidic buffers	Decreases acid-intolerant bacteria	Increases lactobacilli
	Peroxides	Decreases peroxide-intolerant bacteria	Increases lactobacilli
	Lactobacillus	Microbial competition	Decreases pathogens

SOURCE: Adapted with permission from Contraceptive Research and Development. Copyright 1996 by the National Academy of Sciences. Courtesy of the National Academy Press, Washington, D.C.

pathogens.[109,155,166,168] The term is also used to describe chemicals that do not necessarily kill pathogens, but otherwise interfere with some mechanism necessary for infection to occur (e.g., epithelial attachment).

Clinical effectiveness and adverse effects of microbicides

A wide variety of global research and development activities is currently taking place under the auspices of several agencies, including the World Health Organization, Family Health International, Contraceptive Research and Development Program (CONRAD), the Medical Research Council, the Population Council, the National Institutes of Health, the Food and Drug Administration, and the Centers for Disease Control and Prevention.[72,151,152,155,168,169]

Compounds with a potentially broad spectrum of STD/HIV prevention include products designed to augment natural host defense mechanisms, such as acid-buffering agents, lactobacilli preparations, and antimicrobial peptides, such as magainins, protegrins, and defensins. Other compounds would interfere with the entry of a virus into susceptible epithelial or other target cells. These include monoclonal antibodies, sulfated polysaccharides, and sulfonated polymers. After candidate compounds are tested in vitro and in animal models, they will be evaluated for safety and effectiveness in women and men. Most research is focused on developing a compound that can be used vaginally to protect women from STD/HIV, although some efforts are currently underway to explore rectal use of microbicides.

Several products are currently being evaluated (Table 96-5).[151,152,155,169] Praneem® polyherbal cream and suppositories are potential contraceptive and microbicidal products that have three active ingredients: extracts from the neem tree, the reetha nut (soapnut), and quinine hydrochloride.[170,171] Several safety and acceptability studies have been completed on these products, and additional studies are underway in India, Nigeria, Kenya, China, Dominican Republic, and Brazil.[170–172] A new surfactant spermicide, C31G, inactivates a broad spectrum of bacteria and viruses but seems to cause less vaginal irritation than N-9 and, unlike N-9, diffuses into cervical mucus. Sulfated polysaccharides such as dextrin sulfate prevent adherence of HIV and chlamydiae to cells in vitro. *N*-docosanol is actively antiviral and may inhibit nonenveloped and enveloped viruses. Preliminary studies show that vaginal application of *N*-docosanol protected five of six rhesus macaques from SIV infection. Researchers at Reprotect (Baltimore, Maryland) have developed a buffering gel (BufferGel®) that will maintain low vaginal pH and not disturb vaginal flora. Squalamine is a steroid-based compound that has been shown to inhibit gonococci, chlamydiae, HIV, and HSV in vitro and appears to have a prolonged duration of activity.

With the advent of inexpensive manufacturing methods, monoclonal antibodies are being explored as a means for protecting genital mucosal surfaces against a broad range of STD pathogens.[173,174] Vaginal application of monoclonal antibodies has been shown to protect against HSV-2 infection in mouse models.[174,175]

Acceptability of microbicides

There are no product acceptability data currently available for microbicides. As new compounds are developed and tested for safety and effectiveness, they will also be tested for acceptability. Several advocacy projects are underway to ensure that women's needs and perspectives are integrated into all phases of microbicide development. The Microbicide Research Advocacy Project, jointly sponsored by the Center for Women Policy Studies and the Reproductive Health Technologies Project, has garnered wide support in the medical research and political arenas to ensure that clinical trials of new microbicides will include adequate measures of consumer acceptability.[176,177] The Health Development Policy Project and Women's Health Advocates for Microbicides are also working on the international level to facilitate development of prevention methods that are safe, effective, and meet the needs of women.[178]

CONCLUSION

Condoms have long been the only barrier method recommended and used as protection against the transmission of STDs. However, for a variety of reasons, many people do not or cannot use condoms for protection of their sexual health. The reasons given include they reduce pleasure, they inconveniently interrupt the sex act, and they don't allow a man to deposit his semen inside his partner. An additional barrier for women is the difficulty or impossibility of getting a reluctant partner to wear a condom. Other barrier methods effective against STD transmission that address these condom use issues are obviously needed. Most of the methods discussed in this chapter provide protection against STDs, albeit not always as safely or effectively as condoms. Efforts must be made to make them more widely available to those that need them while the research is being conducted to develop new prevention methods that are safe, highly effective, and have none of the user acceptability drawbacks of condoms.

References

1 Quinn TC: Association of sexually transmitted diseases and infection with the human immunodeficiency virus: Biological cofactors and markers of behavioral interventions. *Int J STD & AIDS* 7(Suppl. 2): 17, 1996.

2 Cates W et al: Family planning, STD, and contraceptive choice: A literature update—Part I. *Fam Plann Perspect* 24:75, 1992.

3 Conant MA et al: Condoms prevent transmission of AIDS-associated retrovirus. *JAMA* 255:1706, 1986.

4 Conant MA et al: Herpes simplex virus transmission: Condom studies. *Sex Transm Dis* 11:94, 1984.

5 Judson FN et al: In vitro evaluations of condoms with and without nonoxynol 9 as physical and chemical barriers against *Chlamydia trachomatis*, herpes simplex virus type 2, and human immunodeficiency virus. *Sex Transm Dis* 16:51, 1989.

6 Katznelson S et al: Efficacy of the condom as a barrier to the transmission of cytomegalovirus. *J Infect Dis* 150:155, 1984.

7 Minuk GY et al: Condoms and the prevention of AIDS [letter]. *JAMA* 256:1443, 1986.

8 Minuk GY et al: Condoms and hepatitis B virus. *Ann Intern Med* 104:584, 1986.

9 Minuk GY et al: Efficacy of commercial condoms in the prevention of hepatitis B virus infection. *Gastroenterology* 93:710, 1987.

10 Reitjmeijer CAM et al: Condoms as physical and chemical barriers against human immunodeficiency virus. *JAMA* 259:1851, 1988.

11 Scesney SM et al: Impermeability of condoms to HIV and inactivation of HIV by the spermacide nonoxynol-9 [abstract WP171]. *Third International Conference on AIDS*, Washington, DC, 1987.

12 Van de Perre P et al: The latex condom, an efficient barrier against sexual transmission of AIDS-related viruses. *AIDS* 1:49, 1987.

13 Carey RF et al: Effectiveness of latex condoms as a barrier to human immunodeficiency virus-sized particles under conditions of simulated use. *Sex Transm Dis* 19:230, 1992.

14 Carey RF: Condom safety and HIV [letter]. *Sex Transm Dis* 21:60, 1994.

15 Vail JG et al: Comments from PATH [letter]. *Sex Transm Dis* 21:61, 1994.

16 d'Oro LC et al: Barrier methods of contraception, spermicides, and sexually transmitted diseases: A review. *Genitourin Med* 70:410, 1994.

17 Zenilman JM et al: Condom use to prevent incident STDs: The validity of self-reported condom use. *Sex Transm Dis* 22:15, 1995.

18 Warner DL et al: A meta-analysis of condom effectiveness in reducing sexually transmitted HIV [letter]. *Soc Sci Med* 38:1169, 1994.

19 Fischl MA et al: Evaluation of heterosexual partners, children, and household contacts of adults with AIDS. *JAMA* 257:640, 1987.

20 Ngugi EN et al: Prevention of transmission of human immunodeficiency virus in Africa: Effectiveness of condom promotion and health education among prostitutes. *Lancet* 2:887, 1988.

21 Laurian Y et al: HIV infection in sexual partners of seropositive patients with hemophilia. *N Engl J Med* 320:183, 1989.

22 Moss G et al: Despite safer sex practices after counseling, seroconversion is high among HIV serodiscordant couples in Nairobi, Kenya [abstract W.C.3119]. *VII International Conference on AIDS*, Florence, June 17, 1991.

23 Plummer FA et al: Cofactors in male-female sexual transmission of human immunodeficiency virus type 1. *J Infect Dis* 163:233, 1991.

24 Allen S et al: Effect of serotesting with counselling on condom use and seroconversion among HIV discordant couples in Africa. *Br Med J* 304:1605, 1992.

25 Saracco A et al: Man-to-woman sexual transmission of HIV: Longitudinal study of 343 steady partners of infected men. *J AIDS* 6:497, 1993.

26 DeVincenzi I et al: A longitudinal study of human immunodeficiency virus transmission by heterosexual partners. *N Engl J Med* 331:341, 1994.

27 Kreiss J et al: Efficacy of nonoxynol 9 contraceptive sponge use in preventing heterosexual acquisition of HIV in Nairobi prostitutes. *JAMA* 268:477, 1992.

28 Zekeng L et al: Barrier contraceptive use and HIV infection among high-risk women in Cameroon. *AIDS* 7:725, 1993.

29 Feldblum P et al: Condom and nonoxynol-9 use and HIV incidence in serodiscordant couples in Zambia [abstract 62]. Eleventh Meeting of the International Society for STD Research, New Orleans, August 1995.

30 Weller SC: A meta-analysis of condom effectiveness in reducing sexually transmitted HIV. *Soc Sci Med* 36:1635, 1993.

31 Hart G: Factors influencing venereal infection in a war environment. *Br J Vener Dis* 50:68, 1974.

32 Cates W, Holmes KK: Re: Condom efficacy against gonorrhea and nongonococcal urethritis [letter]. *Am J Epidemiol* 143:843–844, 1996.

33 Darrow WW: Condom use and use-effectiveness in high-risk populations. *Sex Transm Dis* 16:157, 1989.

34 Cameron DW et al: Condom use prevents genital ulcers in women working as prostitutes: Influence of HIV infection. *Sex Transm Dis* 18:188, 1991.

35 Soper DE et al: Prevention of vaginal trichomoniasis by compliant use of the female condom. *Sex Transm Dis* 20:137, 1993.

36 Weir SS et al: Condom use to prevent incident STDs [letter]. *Sex Transm Dis* 23:76, 1996.

37 Galavotti C et al: Condom use to prevent incident STDs [letter]. *Sex Transm Dis* 23:77, 1996.

38 Niruthisard S et al: Use of nonoxynol-9 and reduction in rate of gonococcal and chlamydial infections. *Lancet* 339:1371, 1992.

39 Kotloff K et al: Outcome of genital human papillomavirus (HPV) infection among college students [abstract H1]. 35th Interscience Conference on Antimicrobial Agents and Chemotherapy, San Francisco, September 1995.

40 Trap R et al: Evaluation of the amount of nonoxynol available in condoms for the inhibition of HIV using a method based on HPLC. *Int J STD AIDS* 1:346, 1990.

41 Smith N: Nonoxynol in condoms. *Int J STD AIDS* 1:449, 1990.

42 Hatcher R et al: *Contraceptive Technology*. New York, Irvington Publishers, 1994.

43 Stratton P et al: Nonoxynol-9 lubricated latex condoms may increase release of natural rubber latex protein [abstract Th.C.433]. *XI International Conference on AIDS*, Vancouver, July, 1996.

44 Rekart ML: The toxicity and local effects of the spermicide nonoxynol-9. *J AIDS* 5:425, 1992.

45 Feldblum P et al: *Modern Barrier Methods: Effective Contraception and Disease Prevention*. Research Triangle Park, NC: Family Health International, 1994.

46 Centers for Disease Control and Prevention: 1993 Sexually transmitted disease treatment guidelines. *MMWR* 42(RR-14):72, 1993.

47 Middlestadt S: Field Note#1: AIDSCOM research lessons learned. In *AIDSCOM Lessons Learned: AIDS Prevention in Africa*. Washington, DC: Academy for Educational Development, 1993.

48 Grady WR et al: Condom characteristics: The perceptions and preferences of men in the United States. *Fam Plann Perspect* 25:67, 1993.

49 Boldsen JL et al: Aspects of comfort and safety of condom. *Scandinavian J Soc Med* 20:247, 1992.

50 Consumers Union: Can you rely on condoms? *Consumer Reports* March:135, 1989.

51 Potter LS et al: Multicountry study of acceptability of spermicidally-lubricated condoms: preliminary report, in *Selected Proceedings of Southern Regional Conference on International Health in the 1990s: Directions in Research and Development, Chapel Hill, NC, October 29–31, 1987*. Washington, DC: National Council for International Health, 1988.

52 Roman M: What to wear to bed. *Men's Health* July/August:35, 1994.

53 Schachter P et al: The condom test. *The Boston Phoenix* March 18: 4, 1994.

54 Lytle CD et al: Virus leakage through natural membrane condoms. *Sex Trans Dis* 17:58, 1990.

55 London International U.S Holdings: Launch of first polyurethane male condom introduces a new sensation. Undated press release.

56 Rosenberg MJ et al: The male polyurethane condom: A review of current knowledge. *Contraception* 53:141, 1996.

57 Condomania Mail Order Division Catalog, Los Angeles, CA, 1995.

58 Connell C et al: New technology for contraception and prevention of STDs, in *Family Planning: Meeting Challenges, Promoting Choices. Proceedings of the IPPF Family Planning Congress, October 1992, New Delhi*, PL Senanayake et al (eds). New York, Parthenon, 1993.

59 Trussell J et al: Condom performance during vaginal intercourse: Comparison of Trojan-Enz® and Tactylon™ condoms. *Contraception* 45:11, 1992.

60 Anonymous: Condom sales continue to lag. *Chain Drug Review*, May 9:35, 1994a.

61 Lynn Peterson: Personal communication. Tarkenton & Addams, January, 1996.

62 Addams JF: Ansell breaks new advertising ground with reciprocal ads for Lifestyle condoms. Press release. 1995.

63 Ansell Consumer Products: And the walls come tumbling down. *Condom Sense*, p. 1, undated.

64 Brookman F: Condoms: Enticing female shoppers. *Non-Foods Merchandising* July:55, 1994.

65 Miller C: Condom sales cool off; carefree attitudes of youth, poor marketing are blamed. *Marketing News* February 28:8, 1994.

66 Project Action: Promotional video: Population Services International, 1995.

67 Population Services International: *Summary of IEC Activities*. Internal report. 1995.

68 Population Services International (PSI): *1995/1996 Annual Report*.

69 Futures Group: SOMARC launches five new condom campaigns. *SOMARC Highlights* 3:3, 1995.

70 Drew WL et al: Evaluation of virus permeability of a new condom for women. *Sex Transm Dis* 17:110, 1990.

71 Voeller B: Gas, dye, and viral transport through polyurethane condoms. *JAMA* 266:2986, 1991.

72 Anonymous: Programs conducting/sponsoring female-controlled barrier research. *J Women's Health* 3:309, 1994b.

73 Soper DE et al: Evaluation of the effects of a female condom on the female lower genital tract. *Contraception* 44:21, 1991.

74 Williamson NE et al: Acceptability of barrier methods for prevention of unwanted pregnancy and infection, in *Barrier Contraceptives: Current Status and Future Prospects*, CK Mauck et al (eds). New York: Wiley-Liss, 1994.

75 The Female Health Company: Reality female condom news flash: Price cuts! Two cases for the price of one! Promotional Flyer, 1996.

76 Gollub E et al: Short-term acceptability of the female condom among staff and patients at a New York City hospital. *Fam Plann Perspect* 27:155, 1995.

77 Ashery RS et al: Female condom use among injection drug- and crack cocaine-using women. *Am J Public Health* 85:736, 1995.

78 Ford N et al: The acceptability and experience of the female condom, Femidom among family planning clinic attenders. *Br J Family Plan* 19:187, 1993.

79 Masters L et al: How acceptable is the female condom to attenders of a department of genitourinary medicine? Department of Genitourinary Medicine, King's College Hospital. Unpublished report. 1994.

80 Bounds W et al: Female condom (Femidom): A clinical study of its use-effectiveness and patient acceptability. *Br J Family Plan* 18:36, 1992.

81 Parent JM et al: The female condom in the Netherlands: The results of an initial investigation. The Rutgers Foundation. Unpublished report. 1990.

82 Jenkins C: A study of the acceptability of the female condom in urban Papua New Guinea. Papua New Guinea Institute of Medical Research. Unpublished report. 1995.

83 Blogg S et al: Acceptability of the female condom (Femidom) within a population of commercial sex workers and couples in Salima and Nkhotakota, Malawi. Unpublished report, 1994.

84 Chan R et al: Report on an acceptability survey of Femidom (female condoms) among female sex workers in Singapore. Unpublished report. 1993.

85 Sakondhavat C et al: Consumer preference study of a modified female condom in a sexually active population at risk of contracting AIDS. Family Health International. Unpublished report. 1993.

86 Ruminjo J et al: Consumer preference and functionality study of the Reality female condom in a low risk population in Kenya. Family Health International. Unpublished report. 1991.

87 Monny-Lobe T et al: Acceptability of the female condom among a high risk population in Cameroon. Family Health International. Unpublished report. 1991.

88 Family Planning Association of Hong Kong: Preliminary findings of female condom survey 1993–1994. Unpublished report. 1994.

89 Klapholz J: Reality-brand condoms: How realistic are they? AIDS Project Los Angeles. Unpublished report. 1995.

90 Farr G et al: Contraceptive efficacy and acceptability of the female condom. *Am J Pub Health* 84:1960, 1994.

91 American Health Consultants: FDA inspection sounds death knell for sponge. *Contraceptive Technology Update* 16:43, 1995.

92 Edwards WM: A study of Progonasyl using prostitutes in Nevada's legal houses of prostitution. *J Reprod Med* 11:81, 1973.

93 Cutler JC et al: Vaginal contraceptives as prophylaxis against gonorrhea and other sexually transmissible diseases. *Adv Planned Parent* 12:45, 1977.

94 Limsuwan A et al: A clinical trial of a vaginal preparation regimen for the prophylaxis of gonorrhea. *J Med Assoc Thai* 61:435, 1978.

95 Rendon AL et al: A controlled, comparative study of phenylmercuric acetate, nonoxynol-9 and placebo vaginal suppositories as prophylactic agents against gonorrhea. *Curr Ther Res* 27:780, 1980.

96 Louv WC et al: A clinical trial of nonoxynol-9 as a prophylaxis for cervical *Neisseria gonorrhoeae* and *Chlamydia trachomatis* infections. *J Infect Dis* 158:518, 1988.

97 Barbone F et al: A follow-up study of methods of contraception, sexual activity, and rates of trichomoniasis, candidiasis, and bacterial vaginosis. *Am J Obstet Gynecol* 163:510, 1990.

98 Rosenberg MJ et al: Effect of the contraceptive sponge on chlamydial infection, gonorrhea, and candidiasis. *JAMA* 257:2308, 1987.

99 Weir SS et al: The use of nonoxynol-9 for protection against cervical gonorrhea. *Am J Public Health* 84:910, 1994.

100 Rosenberg MJ et al: Barrier contraceptives and sexually transmitted diseases in women: A comparison of female-dependent methods and condoms. *Am J Public Health* 82:669, 1992.

101 Stone KM et al: Spermicides, HIV, and the vaginal sponge. *JAMA* 268:521, 1992.

102 Psychoyos A: Protectaid, a new vaginal contraceptive sponge with anti-STD properties, in *Barrier Contraceptives: Current Status and Future Prospects,* CK Mauk et al (eds). New York, Wiley-Liss, 1994.

103 Diaz A et al: Frequency of use, knowledge and attitudes toward the contraceptive sponge among inner-city Black and Hispanic adolescent females. *J Adol Health Care* 11:125, 1990.

104 Kass-Annese B et al: A study of the vaginal contraceptive sponge used with and without the fertility awareness method. *Contraception* 40: 701, 1989.

105 Chi I et al: Clinical acceptability, use-patterns and use-effectiveness of the vaginal contraceptive sponge and Neo Sampoon tablets: An international multi-center randomized clinical trial. *Contraception* 36:499, 1987.

106 Ismail MTM et al: A prospective study of the acceptability of Today™ vaginal contraceptive sponge among Malaysian women. *Malaysian J Reprod Health* 5:17, 1987.

107 Beckman LJ et al: The contraceptive sponge: Factors in initiation and use. *Contraception* 40:481, 1989.

108 Psychoyos A et al: Spermicidal and antiviral properties of cholic acid: Contraceptive efficacy of a new vaginal sponge (Protectaid®) containing sodium cholate. *Hum Reprod* 8:866, 1993.

109 Elias CJ et al: *The Development of Microbicides: A New Method of HIV Prevention for Women.* Programs Division Working Paper No. 6. New York, The Population Council, 1993.

110 Magder LS et al: Factors related to genital *Chlamydia trachomatis* and its diagnosis by culture in a sexually transmitted disease clinic. *Am J Epidemiol* 128:298, 1988.

111 Bradbeer CS et al: Prophylaxis against infection in Singaporean prostitutes. *Genitourin Med* 64:52, 1988.

112 Kelaghan J et al: Barrier-method contraceptives and pelvic inflammatory disease. *JAMA* 248:184, 1982.

113 Cramer DW et al: The relationship of tubal infertility to barrier method and oral contraceptive use. *JAMA* 257:2446, 1987.

114 Hooton TM et al: A prospective study of risk factors for symptomatic urinary tract infection in young women. *N Engl J Med* 335:468, 1996.

115 Hooton TM et al: *Escherichia coli* bacteriuria and contraceptive method. *JAMA* 265:64, 1991b.

116 Fihn SD et al: Association between diaphragm use and urinary tract infection. *JAMA* 254:240, 1985.

117 Hooton TM et al: Effects of recent sexual activity and use of a diaphragm on the vaginal microflora. *Clin Infect Dis* 19:274, 1994.

118 Hillier SL et al: Effect of contraceptive method on vaginal flora [abstract]. Presented at Infectious Diseases Society for Obstetrics and Gynecology (IDSOG), 1996.

119 Forrest JD et al: Women's contraceptive attitudes and use in 1992. *Fam Plann Perspect* 25:175, 1993.

120 Di Giacomo do Lago T et al: Acceptability of the diaphragm among low-income women in Sao Paolo, Brazil. *Int Fam Plann Perspect* 21: 114, 1995.

121 Fisher M et al: Comparative analysis of the effectiveness of the diaphragm and birth control pill during the first year of use among suburban adolescents. *J Adol Health Care* 8:393, 1987.

122 Dicker D et al: The vaginal contraceptive diaphragm and the condom—a reevaluation and comparison of two barrier methods with the rhythm method. *Contraception* 40:497, 1989.

123 Schätzler TG: Contraception with the diaphragm: A 2-year follow-up study, in *Sexology,* W Eicher, G Kockott (eds). Heidelberg, Springer-Verlag, 1988.

124 Johnson J: The cervical cap: A retrospective study of an alternative contraceptive technique. *Am J Obstet Gynecol* 148:604, 1984.
125 Powell MG et al: Contraception with the cervical cap: Effectiveness, safety, continuity of use and user effectiveness. *Contraception* 33: 215, 1986.
126 Lauerson NH et al: The cervical cap: Effectiveness, safety, and acceptability as a barrier contraceptive. *Mount Sinai J Med* 53:233, 1986.
127 FEMCAP®, Inc: How to use the Femcap®. Undated brochure.
128 Shihata A et al: Acceptability of a new intravaginal barrier contraceptive device (Femcap). *Contraception* 46:511, 1992.
129 Yama Inc: Comparison between the diaphragm and Lea's Shield®. Unpublished information sheet.
130 Yama Inc: Concept statement for Lea's Shield®. Unpublished information sheet.
131 Yama Inc: Lea® Contraceptivum: New "one-size-fits-all" female barrier contraceptive. Unpublished abstract. 1995.
132 Kappus EW et al: The spermicide nonoxynol-9 does not inhibit *Chlamydia trachomatis* in vitro. *Sex Transm Dis* 13:134, 1986.
133 Ehret JM et al: Activity of nonoxynol-9 against *Chlamydia trachomatis*. *Sex Transm Dis* 15:156, 1988.
134 Hermonat PL et al: The spermicide nonoxynol-9 does not inactivate papillomavirus. *Sex Transm Dis* 19:198, 1992.
135 Miller CJ et al: The effect of contraceptives containing nonoxynol-9 on the genital transmission of simian immunodeficiency virus in rhesus macaques. *Fertil Steril* 57:1126, 1992.
136 Moench TR et al: The cat/feline immunodeficiency virus model for transmucosal transmission of AIDS: Nonoxynol-9 contraceptive jelly blocks transmission by an infected cell inoculum. *AIDS* 7:797, 1993.
137 Whaley KJ et al: Nonoxynol-9 protects mice against vaginal transmission of genital herpes infections. *J Infect Dis* 168:1009, 1993.
138 Lyons JM et al: Reducing the risk of *Chlamydia trachomatis* genital tract infection by evaluating the prophylactic potential of vaginally applied chemicals. *Clin Infect Dis* 21(Suppl w):S174, 1995.
139 Feldblum PJ et al: The protective effect of nonoxynol-9 against HIV infection. *Am J Public Health* 84:1032, 1994.
140 Sherris JD et al: New developments in vaginal contraception. *Pop Reports* Series H, No. 7, 1984.
141 Niruthisard S et al: The effects of frequent nonoxynol-9 use on the vaginal and cervical mucosa. *Sex Transm Dis* 18:176, 1991.
142 Roddy RE et al: A dosing study of nonoxynol-9 and genital irritation. *Int J STD AIDS* 4:165, 1993.
143 Weir SS et al: Nonoxynol-9 use, genital ulcers, and HIV infection in a cohort of sex workers. *Genitourin Med* 71:78, 1995.
144 Norvell MK et al: Investigation of microtrauma after sexual intercourse. *J Reprod Med* 29:269, 1984.
145 Ward H et al: Nonoxynol-9 in lubricated condoms: Results of a study in female prostitutes. *Sex Transm Dis* 23:413, 1996.
146 McGroarty JA et al: Hydrogen peroxide production by Lactobacillus species: Correlation with susceptibility to the spermicidal compound nonoxynol-9. *J Infect Dis* 165:1142, 1992.
147 Klebanoff SJ: Effects of the spermicidal agent nonoxynol-9 on vaginal microbial flora. *J Infect Dis* 165:19, 1992.
148 Jones BM et al: The in vivo effects of nonoxynol-9 contraception on vaginal microbial flora and colonization with *Escherichia coli* [letter]. *J Infect Dis* 167:777, 1993.
149 Larsen B: *Microbiology. Basic Science Monograph in Obstetrics and Gynecology*. Washington, DC: Council on Resident Education in Obstetrics and Gynecology, 1991.
150 Goeman J et al: Frequent use of menfegol spermicidal vaginal foaming tablets associated with a high incidence of genital lesions. *J Infect Dis* 171:1611, 1995.
151 Alexander NJ: Barriers to sexually transmitted diseases. *Sci Am* 3:32, 1996.
152 Cohen J: Women: Absent term in the AIDS research equation. *Science* 269:777, 1995.
153 World Health Organization: A randomized, placebo-controlled clinical trial to evaluate the safety of COL-1492 in healthy women at low risk of HIV infection. WHO, Global Programme on AIDS, Final Report, 4 October 1995.
154 Ghys PD et al: Acceptability and feasibility of a clinical trial to assess the efficacy of a microbicide-containing vaginal gel to prevent HIV infection among female sex workers in Abidjan, Cote D'Ivoire [abstract Th.C.321]. *XI International Conference on AIDS*, Vancouver, July 1996.
155 Harrison PF et al (eds): *Contraceptive Research and Development: Looking to the Future*. Washington, DC: National Academy Press, 1996.
156 Civic D et al: Dry sex in Zimbabwe and implications for condom use. *Soc Sci Med* 42:91, 1996.
157 American Health Consultants: The switch is on from contraceptive foam to film. *Contraceptive Technology Update* 14:169, 1993.
158 Lake Pharmaceutical Inc: Advantage 24 bioadhesive contraceptive gel: You've got 24 hours. Take advantage of it. Brochure. 1995.
159 Cohen D et al: Influencing spermicide use among low-income minority women. *J Am Med Women's Assoc* 50:11, 1995.
160 Chompootaweep S et al: A comparative study of the safety, effectiveness and acceptability of two foaming vaginal tablets. *Contraception* 41:507, 1990.
161 Youssef H et al: A clinical trial of Neo Sampoon vaginal tablets and Emko foam in Alexandria, Egypt. *Contraception* 35:101, 1987.
162 Hira S et al: Spermicide acceptability among patients at a sexually transmitted disease clinic in Zambia. *Am J Public Health* 85:1098, 1995.
163 Steiner M et al: Acceptability of spermicidal film and foaming tablets among women in three countries. *Int Fam Plann Perspect* 21:104, 1995.
164 Loudon NB et al: A comparative study of the effectiveness and acceptability of the diaphragm used with spermicide in the form of C-film or a cream or jelly. *Br J Fam Plann* 17:41, 1991.
165 Elias CJ et al: Women's preferences regarding the formulation of over-the-counter vaginal spermicides [abstract Th.C.322]. *XI International Conference on AIDS*, Vancouver, July 1996.
166 Stone AB et al: Vaginal microbicides for preventing the sexual transmission of HIV. *AIDS* 8(suppl):S285, 1994.
167 Elias CJ et al: Challenges for the development of female-controlled vaginal microbicides. *AIDS* 8:1, 1994.
168 International Working Group on Vaginal Microbicides: Recommendations for the development of vaginal microbicides. *AIDS* 10: UNAIDS1, 1996.
169 Voelker R: Scientists zero in on new HIV microbicides. *JAMA* 273: 979, 1995.
170 Talwar GP et al: Praneem polyherbal cream and suppositories, in *Barrier Contraceptives: Current Status and Future Prospects*, CK Mauk et al (eds). New York, Wiley-Liss, 1994.
171 Lapido OA: South to south experience with polyherbal cream in the treatment of vaginal infection, in *Barrier Contraceptives: Current Status and Future Prospects*, CK Mauk et al (eds). New York, Wiley-Liss, 1994.
172 Garg S et al: Praneem polyherbal cream Phase I clinical trials in India, in *Barrier Contraceptives: Current Status and Future Prospects*, CK Mauk et al (eds). New York, Wiley-Liss, 1994.
173 Cone RA et al: Monoclonal antibodies for reproductive health: Part I. Preventing sexual transmission of disease and pregnancy with topically applied antibiotics. *Am J Reprod Immunol* 32:114, 1994.
174 Whaley KJ et al: Passive immunization of the vagina protects mice against vaginal transmission of genital herpes infections. *J Infect Dis* 169:647, 1994.
175 Sherwood JK et al: Controlled release of antibodies for long-term topical passive immunoprotection of female mice against genital herpes. *Nat Biotechnol* 14:468, 1996.
176 Reproductive Health Technologies Project: *Review of Programs, Activities, and Accomplishments* (monograph). Reproductive Health Technologies Project, Washington, DC.
177 Allina A: Personal communication. Microbicide Research Advocacy Project, Washington, DC. October 1996.
178 Heise L: Personal communication. Health Development Policy Project, Takoma Park, Maryland, April 1996.

Chapter 95

Community outreach and education

Jeffrey A. Kelly
Kathleen J. Sikkema
David R. Holtgrave

Community outreach and education programs have a long history of use in many public health primary prevention, early disease detection, and health care interventions. Within the primary prevention arena, community-level approaches have been widely used—with varying degrees of effectiveness—to address issues such as cigarette smoking cessation, cancer and cardiovascular risk reduction, and alcohol and other drug abuse prevention. Community-level early disease detection methods have been used to encourage care-seeking behaviors related to screening and early diagnosis of breast cancer, hypertension, prostate cancer, and other diseases where early intervention is critical. Community outreach methods have also been widely used in both developing and developed countries to promote other health care-related behaviors such as pre- and postnatal care, child immunizations, and HIV testing among persons at risk for AIDS. These interventions have in common their focus on using community-level interventions to encourage behavior change on the part of population members, particularly those at risk for negative health outcomes. Similar community outreach and prevention methods, targeted toward sexual behavior change, are pertinent to efforts to prevent and control sexually transmitted diseases (STDs).

People contract STDs in the community, not inside STD clinics, physicians' offices, or other clinical and health care settings. Communities, therefore, are appropriate venues for STD prevention interventions. Although secondary prevention efforts often need to take place within settings that treat people who have already contracted STDs, primary prevention efforts to reduce the incidence of STDs may have their greatest potential effect when they are undertaken in communities, not just in clinics. To the extent that it is possible to reduce levels of sexual risk behavior in population segments presently vulnerable to STDs, it should also be possible to reduce the number of new disease cases arising in those communities.

The beneficial impact of community-level sexual behavior change on STD incidence is most clearly evident in data on STD rates among gay or bisexual men in major AIDS epicenters. In the early- to mid-1980s and in response to AIDS, there were substantial reductions in rates of high-risk sexual behavior practices and substantial increases in condom use among gay men in many large cities.[1,2] In addition to a leveling of HIV infection prevalence—albeit often at very high levels—there were significant declines in the incidence of other sexually transmitted diseases among gay men in these epicenters, including reduction in hepatitis B infection, gonorrhea, and other STDs.[3–5] These data provide convincing evidence that widescale sexual behavior change in a population can produce decreases in the incidence of STDs. A key research question in the primary prevention of STDs is how to develop interventions that can promote and hasten such important behavioral changes.

In this chapter, we will consider how community-level and community outreach interventions can be used in the primary prevention of STDs. We will organize this discussion around three major issues: (1) psychosocial characteristics of community or population members associated with high levels of sexual risk behaviors, and that therefore are characteristics that can serve to define the nature and targets for community interventions; (2) the goals of community intervention; and (3) models and examples of community-level STD prevention interventions undertaken to date.

PSYCHOSOCIAL CHARACTERISTICS RELATED TO SEXUAL RISK BEHAVIOR IN STD-VULNERABLE POPULATIONS

Community-level STD prevention interventions—and, indeed, behavior change interventions of any kind—are effective only when they are focused on changing psychological and social characteristics that presently "drive" risk-taking behavior. Understanding the determinants of high-risk sexual behavior within populations vulnerable to STDs provides information needed to tailor interventions to change those relevant determinants. Fortunately, behavioral and social science research, guided by several theoretical frameworks concerning behavior and its change, has identified a set of psychosocial factors that predict levels of sexual risk behavior in a variety of STD-vulnerable populations, including ethnic minority heterosexual adolescents, sexually active college students, heterosexual men and women, and gay and bisexual men.[6–10] The fact that a relatively consistent set of sexual risk-taking behavioral determinants has been identified across multiple and diverse community populations attests to the salience of these psychosocial factors.

There are at least six key elements and objectives of community-level sexual risk behavior change interventions (Table 95-1). Normative perceptions concerning whether peers and sexual partners use condoms and practice safer sex are highly predictive of an individual's own level of risk behavior. To the extent that peers or members of one's social reference group, as well as one's own sexual partners, are believed to subscribe to the norm that condom use is accepted and expected, individuals are more likely to use condoms themselves.[11–15] Strength of behavior change intentions, a robust predictor of behavior change enactment in many health-related areas, also predicts condom use.[7,13,15–17] Positive attitudes toward condoms, including perceived benefits of condom use and positive outcome expectancies, are associated with greater likelihood of engaging in STD preventive behavior.[18–19] Individuals high in perceived self-efficacy for enacting risk reduction behavior change—those who are confident in their ability to take risk reduction steps in relevant personal situations—are more likely to exhibit behavior change than persons low in self-efficacy.[20–21] Well-developed sexual communication skills, including assertiveness skills for refusing high-risk sexual coercions and sexual negotiation skills for initiating discussion with potential partners about condom use, have been associated with lower levels of sexual risk behavior.[18,22] Finally, and recognizing that different members of a population are at different stages of contemplating, attempting, making, and maintaining change, an individual's present stage or readiness for change has proven to be a useful heuristic for understanding the type of intervention that may best meet the needs of given populations and population members.[8,23–25]

These are not the only determinants shown in the literature to predict STD high-risk behavior or success in behavior change efforts. A number of situational factors—including substance use, relationship status and familiarity of sexual partners, positive HIV serostatus knowledge, and presence of competing life stressors—also influence levels of sexual risk behavior in some populations.[26–29] Although AIDS risk knowledge does not frequently ap-

Table 95-1. Key Elements and Objectives of Community-Level Sexual Risk Behavior Change Interventions

Element	Community change objective
Sexual behavior normative perceptions	Creation of social reference group norms, especially among peers and sexual partners, that encourage and support behavior changes to reduce or avoid STD/HIV risk
Behavior change intentions	Strengthening population members' intentions and personal commitment to reduce or avoid sexual risk behavior
Attitudes toward condoms	Creating positive attitudes toward condoms including perceived benefits, positive outcome expectancies, and connotation of condom use with positive attributes (concern, caring, pride, and responsibility)
Perceived risk reduction self-efficacy	Instilling confidence that individuals can successfully enact personal risk reduction or risk avoidance behavior change strategies
Risk reduction behavioral skills	Providing opportunities to observe, model, and rehearse behavioral skills needed to reduce risk including technical skills (such as condom use) and sexual assertiveness, negotiation, and communication skills
Readiness for change	Tailoring messages that encourage movement along a continuum from behavior change contemplation to preparation to action to maintenance of action in reducing risk

pear as a strong determinant of sexual risk behavior, probably because basic factual knowledge about AIDS is now quite high in most populations, there are likely to be more widespread misconceptions about STDs other than HIV, and it is possible that these misconceptions contribute to STD risk-taking behavior. For example, women's use of oral contraceptives protects against pregnancy, but oral contraceptive use not only increases risk of cervical chlamydial infection, but also predicts non-use of barrier methods that protect against STDs.[30] Perhaps this is owing, in part, to misconceptions about the protective effects of birth control pills.

The body of research identifying determinants of sexual risk behavior in populations is critical to the development of community-level and outreach-based STD prevention interventions because it identifies domains in which those intervention efforts should focus their attention. Based on research conducted to date and summarized here, important targets for community-level STD prevention programs include changing population normative perceptions about the social desirability risk reduction steps; strengthening behavior change intentions, attitudes, and perceived efficacy of change; and increasing population member skills (and motivation to use those skills) to resist coercions to engage in unwanted or unsafe sex and to negotiate safer sex practices.

DEFINING A COMMUNITY FOR INTERVENTION AND IDENTIFYING THE GOALS OF INTERVENTION

It is possible to conduct mass (and usually mass media) sexual behavior change encouragement programs directed toward the entire population of a city, state, or county. "American Responds to AIDS" is an example of a broadly focused press media campaign directed, especially in its earlier years, toward the American population as a whole. Evaluations of such untailored educational campaigns indicate that they can increase public awareness of a problem, can increase public knowledge and correct misconceptions, and may influence general attitudes but rarely have been shown to impact on actual sexual risk behavior especially among hard-to-reach and high-risk population segments.[31–32] This may be owing to what is usually the very general and nontailored nature of mass campaign messages directed toward the public as a whole, messages likely to be especially nonexplicit in a potentially controversial area such as sexual behavior. The preponderance of both theory and research literature indicates that community-level risk reduction behavior change interventions, whether undertaken using mass media or other community and outreach intervention approaches, are most successful when they are directed toward a particular and identifiable segment or subpopulation of a community; when the community intervention is carefully tailored to the culture, attitudes, beliefs, and change readiness that characterize that population segment; when the intervention is sustained and uses multiple channels of delivery; and when the intervention is based on psychological, motivational, and social principles rather than factual information provision alone.[33–35]

The ultimate public health goal of STD prevention interventions is to reduce the incidence and prevalence of sexually transmitted diseases. However, community-level STD prevention behavioral intervention trials rarely have been designed to examine change in disease rates in a population as a primary intervention outcome endpoint. Instead, most community interventions tested to date have sought to change population risk behavior characteristics or, even less proximal to the disease change outcome, to change population psychological or motivational characteristics related to risk behavior. Examples of behavior change outcomes relevant to STD prevention are reducing rates of multiple-partner sexual contacts, reducing sexual network "mixing" between members of presently low-STD prevalence population segments and members of high-STD prevalence population segments (such as reducing contacts with commercial sex workers), or increasing rates of condom use in sexual encounters that might otherwise confer STD risk. Less proximal endpoints in community-level interventions are promoting changes in population member risk behavior knowledge, attitudes, or change intentions. Although much less convincing as a sole endpoint than outcomes that demonstrate change in population risk behavior levels or STD rates, it is possible to make the case that attitudinally "moving" a presently condom-resistant population toward greater acceptance of condom use, for example, is an intervention goal not without merit.

Community-level and outreach-based interventions may also have behavior change goals other than sexual risk behavior change. Examples of such goals might be encouraging greater HIV or STD testing within the population, or encouraging population members to access more intensive and personalized risk behavior change assistance resources in their community. The key point here is that community and outreach-based STD prevention refers to a modality for delivering prevention services to population members in the community; the behavioral objectives of these programs may vary, and the elements to be incorporated in a given program need to be defined by what kind of change—sexual risk behavior change, attitude or motivation change, or other kinds of prevention help-seeking—the intervention is meant to bring about.

Finally, community-level interventions may be critical for promoting not just the initiation of risk reduction behavior change but also its successful maintenance in STD-vulnerable populations. Traditional one-on-one and clinic-based counseling—even when intensive, culturally-tailored, and guided by sound behavior change principles—is based on the presumption that persons will be able to carry forth successfully their risk reduction efforts in the real world when they "leave" counseling, and that they will be able to do this for long periods. However, the real world does not always, and perhaps does not often, reinforce persons' risk avoidance efforts. Resisting coercion to have sex or insisting on condom use are actions that may elicit negative reactions from sexual partners or potential partners, and risk reduction behavior changes are not yet accepted norms within many of the populations segments at greatest risk for STDs. It is possible to view STD prevention as the task of attempting to change an individual's attitudes, motivations, and skills, and then hoping that the individual will be able to sustain change when confronting unsupportive real-life relationships and risk pressures. Alternatively, it is possible to take a boarder social learning perspective, in which behavior change maintenance is viewed not only as a function of an individual's efforts but also of peer group social norms that may either help to reinforce change efforts or contribute to relapse over time.[6] Community and outreach-based interventions that change norms and behavioral expectations within at-risk populations to support risk avoidance efforts can play an important role in creating social environments that promote behavior change maintenance.

EXAMPLES OF COMMUNITY AND OUTREACH-BASED INTERVENTIONS TO REDUCE SEXUAL RISK BEHAVIOR

A number of investigations and program descriptions of community-level risk behavior change interventions have appeared in the literature and have advanced our knowledge concerning how to produce population-level risk reduction. Most of these interventions have been cast primarily as AIDS/HIV prevention efforts. Because many of the same behavior changes that afford protection from HIV also reduce risk for other STDs, we will consider HIV and STD sexual risk reduction interventions together. Three types of community-level intervention have most commonly been reported in the literature. These are: (1) approaches that use community opinion leaders to redefine sexual norms and safer sex expectations within this peer groups; (2) outreach-based risk reduction workshops offered in community settings; and (3) multifaceted community mobilization and activation risk reduction programs.

OPINION LEADER COMMUNITY NORM CHANGE INTERVENTIONS

Peers—and, in particular, those members of one's own social reference group who are considered popular, influential, and likable—are potentially important models of behavior. From a social learning, well-liked peers can serve to influence the behavior standards of those who observe their actions.[6] From the perspective of diffusion of innovation theory, popular individuals within a community social network often function as opinion leaders who can set new trends that are observed by others, that are then copied by "early adopters," and that gradually diffuse throughout the social network until the new trends become accepted and normative.[36] From either theoretical framework, the implication for behavior change promotion is that cadres of well-liked, popular opinion leaders or peer models can—through endorsement and modeling processes—influence the social norm perceptions and behavior of the larger population segment or social network in which they are influential.

In a community-level trial, Kelly and colleagues evaluated whether interventions based on diffusion of innovation principles can produce population-wide reductions in the level of HIV high-risk sexual behavior among gay men who lived in three small cities and patronized gay bars in those cities.[37–39] The project focused on gay men in small cities because prior research had revealed that many small-city gay men, unlike their counterparts in major AIDS epicenters, continue to engage frequently in high-risk sexual behavior and do not perceive safer sex as a socially accepted peer norm.[40] To establish baseline levels of population risk behavior, all men entering all gay bars in each study city were administered anonymous surveys eliciting information on their sexual behavior practices in the past 2 months and on their perceptions concerning the safer sex norms held by friends. Although there was some variability across city populations, about one-third of men reported engaging in unprotected anal intercourse in the past 2 months, usually not with an exclusive partner of known HIV serostatus.[37,38,40]

When the intervention was ready to be initiated sequentially in the three cities, bartenders were trained to observe the crowd of people in a city's clubs and to identify those persons who were most popular, most sought out for conversations by others, and most frequently seen to interact with others. About 15 percent of the total number of persons in the bars were identified as popular opinion leaders by multiple, independent bartender observers. These key opinion leaders were then contacted and invited to attend a series of four group sessions that taught them how to communicate effective risk reduction behavior change endorsement messages to their friends and acquaintances, provided guidance and problem solving in how to initiate norm change conversations with others, and systematically engaged each opinion leader to seek out opportunities to have peer conversations following each group session. Some opinion leaders self-monitored up to 100 risk reduction endorsement conversations with friends over a 6-week period. The opinion leaders also wore distinctive buttons that visually demonstrated their personal involvement and support of risk reduction efforts.

To determine the effectiveness of the intervention in changing population-wide sexual risk behavior, all men patronizing bars in each intervention city were again surveyed 3 months following the intervention. In each city population, reduction of between 15 and 29 percent from baseline levels were found in the proportion of population members who reported engaging in any unprotected anal intercourse in the past 2 months. In a subsequent expansion of the trial to 16 additional cities, half of which received the same opinion leader intervention and half of which served as comparison cities, a similar magnitude of population behavior change effects was found at 1-year followup.[41] Taken together, these findings indicate that interventions that actively engage a sufficient number of key opinion leaders to endorse and recommend behaviors change to their peers can produce reductions in population sexual risk behavior levels.

OUTREACH-BASED RISK REDUCTION WORKSHOPS OFFERED IN COMMUNITY SETTINGS

A number of randomized clinical outcome trials have demonstrated the efficacy of intensive small-group intervention programs based on cognitive-behavioral change principles for producing reductions in HIV risk behavior among gay and bisexual men, at-risk inner-city women, and disadvantaged adolescent males and females.[22,42–48] Although tailored in content to the different risk circumstance confronting each population, these interventions—delivered in workshops or in multiple-session programs—have all combined such elements as risk education, sexual assertiveness and negotiation skills training, teaching condom use and risk behavior self-management skills, enhancing positive attitudes and motivations toward behavior change, and reinforcing efforts to change risk behavior.[27,39] All of these intervention trials produced effect sizes indicative of moderate to large reductions in sexual risk behavior, usually reflected by reductions in rates of unprotected sex and increases in condom use. Behavior change self-reports have often been corroborated by change in other indices of risk reduction such as condom redemption or purchase, improvement in objectively assessed sexual assertiveness skills, and other validation measures.

For the most part, research evaluations of these small-group and workshop interventions have taken place in clinic or institutional settings. However, a number of projects have utilized outreach methods to "market" and recruit participants in AIDS-vulnerable communities to attend the workshops or small-group programs, and, in this sense, the interventions can be viewed as prevention resources available for at-risk community members who are identified through community outreach.[42,45]

Another form of workshop intervention widely used by community-based organizations in the United States and abroad is the "Stop AIDS" program.[49–51] Originating in the gay community but extended more recently to other HIV-vulnerable populations, Stop AIDS consists of workshop programs usually led by trained volunteer facilitators that involve discussion about risk behavior, promotion of positive attitudes toward behavior change, and skills training exercises in areas related to the successful implementation of changes. The 3- to 4-hour workshops are often conducted in community members' homes, and frequently include members of entire social networks and friendship circles who participate together in the same session. Because Stop AIDS originated as a grassroots, community-based HIV prevention program to deal with a health emergency, it was implemented directly without planning for scientifically controlled or randomized evaluation methods. Nonetheless, outcome evaluations have shown that participants exhibit change in sexual risk behavior knowledge, attitudes, change intentions, and behavior following attendance at Stop AIDS groups.[50,51]

MULTIFACETED COMMUNITY MOBILIZATION AND ACTIVATION INTERVENTIONS

Several community-level interventions focused on shifting population risk behavior utilizing multiple components have recently been described in the literature. Those interventions differ from those described earlier because they rely on a combination of different programs and levels of effort in order to mobilize or activate population behavior change.

Because young gay men continue to contract HIV and other STDs at high rates and have been less influenced by AIDS prevention efforts than their older counterparts, young men who have sex with men constitute a population of importance in HIV/STD prevention efforts.[52] Kegeles and colleagues evaluated a community intervention in a small California city that combined risk reduction workshops with ongoing community social events that included risk reduction endorsement messages disseminated by opinion leaders identified in the populations of young gay men.[53] The intervention also included distribution of safer sex education materials, t-shirts, and logos among young men in the cities' bars, clubs, and other socializing areas. Cross-sectional population member and cohort followup surveys revealed reductions in rates of risk behavior of about 20 percent from preintervention levels to followup in each city.

Sikkema and colleagues have undertaken a community mobilization intervention focused on women who live in 18 housing developments within inner-city census tracts with high rates of STDs.[54] In nine housing developments that received the HIV prevention intervention, women identified by their neighbors as key opinion leaders were invited to attend workshop programs offered in the developments; the workshops focused on women's health concerns, HIV and STD, risk education, risk reduction skills building, and strategies for "networking" HIV prevention messages to other women in the development. The opinion leader women also recruited successive "waves" of their neighbors to attend the same program, and the key group of women initially identified as opinion leaders formed "Women's Health Councils" in each development to plan ongoing social events organized around AIDS prevention and awareness themes. The program was evaluated by conducting anonymous risk behavior surveys of all women in the nine intervention and nine control condition housing developments before and again 3 months and 9 months after intervention. Preliminary findings of the study indicate that condom use among women in the intervention housing developments increased from about 24 percent of intercourse occasions at baseline to approximately 43 percent of intercourse occasions at followup, with the effects most pronounced among those women who both attended risk reduction workshops and were also exposed to the community-level AIDS awareness events. No significant change was found over time in rates of unprotected sex or condom use among women in the control condition housing developments.

Finally, and in a large multisite demonstration project, investigators at the Centers for Disease Control and Prevention (CDC) have evaluated the impact of community-level and population-focused HIV prevention interventions for a variety of AIDS-vulnerable but hard-to-reach populations, including men who have sex with men, youth in high-risk situations, female partners of IDUs, and female commercial sex workers.[23,55] The interventions tested in these AIDS community demonstration projects include community educational outreach by lay prevention educators, the use of culturally tailored "role model" portrayals used in "small media" campaigns to illustrate how peers have changed risk behavior, and intervention elements intended to increase population member readiness or stage of change for enacting risk reduction steps. Evaluated with street intercept interviews conducted with targeted population members before and following intervention, outcome findings of the project indicate evidence of attitude, change readiness, and risk behavior change in a number of the population. In neighborhoods in which the interventions were delivered and among community members who reported exposure to the intervention elements, consistent condom use with nonprimary partners significantly improved relative to rates of risk behavior found in comparison neighborhoods. Greater behavior change readiness was also was observed in the intervention area populations.[55]

GAPS IN OUR KNOWLEDGE, ABOUT COMMUNITY-LEVEL INTERVENTIONS

Although the programs described here have demonstrated the effectiveness of community outreach interventions in promoting sexual behavior change in some populations, there remain important unanswered questions about how best to apply these approaches to other STD-vulnerable groups. Most community-level sexual behavior change interventions have been developed from the perspective of HIV prevention, and the populations targeted by intervention often have been gay men. With the exception of the Sikkema et al. community-level intervention and several reports describing risk reduction small group programs undertaken in community settings with at-risk women, there have still been very few applications of community outreach sexual behavior change interventions tailored expressly for women, even though women are, in many respects, the population most affected by non-HIV STDs.[22,44,45,54]

Related to this, most conceptualizations of factors related to sexual risk behavior change appear to be based on the premise that sexual behavior decisions are volitional and determined primarily by an individual's own wishes, attitudes, intentions, skills, and normative perceptions. However, these models do not adequately take into account the behavior change barriers; social, economic, and cultural factors; and relationship pressures faced by women who are in coercive and power-imbalanced relationships with high-risk men resistant to condom use. Until further advances are made in female-controlled STD and HIV prevention methods, special obstacles will continue to be faced by women in dependent relationships with high-risk men. Finally, and given the present likelihood that men's attitudes substantially influence whether or not condoms will be used during sex, community-level outreach interventions focused on changing the attitudes, norm perceptions, and behavior practices of high-risk heterosexual men are essential. To date, little intervention attention has been directed to this critical population.

CONCLUSIONS

Community and outreach-based interventions to encourage population member reduction in sexual risk activities hold considerable promise for the primary prevention of STDs. Such approaches to intervention have the potential for bringing culturally-tailored prevention services to hard-to-reach population members and for changing the risk awareness, social norm perceptions, attitudes and change readiness, and sexual risk behavior of populations presently vulnerable to STDs. A specific and unique benefit of community interventions for STD prevention is their potential for creating social norm changes in populations that encourage the maintenance of sexual risk behavior changes. The field of community-level interventions to prevent STDs is still new, and many issues concerning how best to tailor, implement, and evaluate the effectiveness of these programs still require attention and study. Nonetheless, community and outreach programs are important components of comprehensive approaches to STD primary prevention.

References

1 Martin JL: Impact of AIDS on gay male sexual behavior patterns in New York City. *Am J Pub Health* 77:578–581, 1987.

2 McKusick L et al: AIDS and sexual behavior reported by gay men in San Francisco. *Am J Pub Health* 75:493–496, 1985.

3 Judson FN: Fear of AIDS and gonorrhea rates in homosexual men. *Lancet* 2:159–160, 1983.

4 Carne CA et al: Prevalence of antibodies to human immunodeficiency virus, gonorrhea rates, and changed sexual behavior in homosexual men in London. *Lancet* 1:656–658, 1987.

5 Sorvillo FJ et al: Declining rates of amebiasis in Los Angeles County: A sentinel for decreasing acquired immunodeficiency syndrome (AIDS) incidence? *Am J Pub Health* 79:1563–1564, 1989.

6 Bandura A: *Social Leaning Theory.* Englewood Cliffs, NJ, Prentice-Hall, 1977.

7 Fishbein M et al: *Belief, Attitude, Intention, and Behavior: An Introduction to Theory and Research.* Reading, MA, Addison-Wesley, 1975.

8 Prochaska JO et al: Stages and processes of self-change of smoking: Toward an integrative model of change. *J Consult Clin Psychol* 51: 287–305, 1983.

9 Catania Ja et al: Towards an understanding of risk behavior: An AIDS risk reduction model (ARRM). *Health Educ Quart* 17:53–72, 1990.

10 Fisher JD et al: Changing AIDS risk behavior. *Psychol Bull* 111:455–474, 1992.

11 Jemmott LS et al: Applying the theory of reasoned action to AIDS risk behavior: Condom use among Black women. *Nurs Res* 40:228–233, 1991.

12 Fisher JD et al: Social influence and AIDS preventive behavior, in *Social Influence Processes and Prevention,* Edwards J et al (eds). New York, Plenum, 1990, pp. 39–70.

13 Kelly JA et al: Factors predicting continued high-risk behavior among gay men in small cities: Psychological, behavioral, and demographic characteristics related to unsafe sex. *J Consult Clin Psychol* 63:101–107, 1995.

14 Kelly JA et al: Psychological factors that predict AIDS high-risk and AIDS precautionary behavior. *J Consult Clin Psychol* 58:117–120, 1990.

15 Joseph JB et al: Magnitude and determinants of behavioral risk reduction: Longitudinal analysis of a cohort at risk for AIDS. *Psychol Health* 1:73–96, 1987.

16 Sikkema K et al: Prevalence and predictors of HIV risk behavior among women living in low-income, inner-city housing developments. *Am J Pub Health,* 86:1123–1128, 1996.

17 Heckman TG et al: Predictors of condom use and HIV test seeking among women living in inner-city public housing developments. *Sex Trans Dis,* 23:357–365, 1996.

18 Catania JA et al: Condom use in multiethnic neighborhoods of San Francisco: The population-based AMEN (AIDS in multiethnic neighborhoods) study. *Am J Pub Health* 82:284–287, 1992.

19 Sacco W et al: Attitudes about condom use as an AIDS-relevant behavior: Their factor structure and relation to condom use. *Psychol Assess* 3:265–272, 1991.

20 Aspinwall LG et al: Psychosocial predictors of gay men's risk reduction behavior. *Health Psychol* 10:432–444, 1991.

21 Sikkema KH et al: Levels and predictors of HIV risk behavior among women living in low-income public housing developments. *Pub Health Rep* 110:707–713, 1995.

22 Kelly, JA et al: The effects of HIV/AIDS intervention groups for high-risk women in urban clinics. *Am J Pub Health* 84:1918–1922, 1994.

23 O'Reilly KR et al: AIDS Community Demonstration Projects for HIV prevention among hard-to-reach groups. *Pub Health Rept* 106:714–720, 1991.

24 Community-level prevention of human immunodeficiency virus infection among high-risk populations: The AIDS Community Demonstration Projects. *MMWR* 45:1–24, 1996.

25 Grimley DM et al: Assessing the stages of change and decision-making for contraceptive use for the prevention of pregnancy, sexually transmitted disease, and acquired immune deficiency syndrome. *Health Educ Quart* 20:455–470, 1993.

26 Kelly JA: Advances in HIV/AIDS education and prevention. *Fam Rel* 44:345–352, 1995.

27 Kelly JA et al: Psychological interventions to prevent HIV infection are urgently needed: New priorities for behavioral research in the second decade of AIDS. *Am Psychol* 48:1023–1034, 1993.

28 Mays VM et al: Issues in the perception of AIDS risk and risk reduction activities by Black and Hispanic/Latina women. *Am Psychol* 43:949–957, 1988.

29 Kelly JA et al: Increased attention to human sexuality can improve HIV/AIDS prevention efforts: Key research issues and directions. *J Consult Clin Psychol* 63:907–918, 1995.

30 Centers for Disease Control: Childbearing and contraceptive use plans among women at high risk for HIV infection: Selected U.S. sites, 1980–1991. *MMWR* 41:35–141, 1992.

31 Caron SL et al: "American Responds to AIDS" but did college students: Differences between March, 1987 and September, 1988. *AIDS Educ Prev* 4:18–28, 1992.

32 Gerbert B et al: Public acceptance of the Surgeon General's brochure on AIDS. *Pub Health Rep* 104:130–133, 1989.

33 Maibach E et al: Advances in public health communication. *Annu Rev Pub Health* 16:219–238, 1995.

34 Atkin C et al: *Mass Communication and Public Health.* Newbury Park, CA, Sage, 1990.

35 Andreasen AR: *Marketing Social Change.* San Francisco, Jossey-Bass, 1995.
36 Rogers EM: *Diffusion of Innovations.* New York, Free Press, 1983.
37 Kelly JA et al: HIV risk behavior reduction following intervention with key opinion leaders of a population: An experimental community-level analysis. *Am J Pub Health* 81:168–171, 1991.
38 Kelly JA et al: Community AIDS/HIV risk reduction: The effects of endorsements by popular people in three cities. *Am J Pub Health* 82: 1483–1489, 1992.
39 Kelly JA: *Changing HIV Risk Behavior: Practical Strategies.* New York, Guilford, 1995.
40 Kelly JA et al: AIDS/HIV risk behavior among gay men in small cities: Findings of a 16-city national sample. *Arch Intern Med* 152:2293–2297, 1992.
41 Kelly, JA et al: Social diffusion models can produce population-level HIV risk behavior reduction: Field trial results and mechanisms underlying change. Paper presented to the IX International Conference on AIDS, Berlin, June, 1993.
42 Kelly JA et al: Behavioral intervention to reduce AIDS risk activities. *J Consult Clin Psychol* 57:60–67, 1989.
43 Valdiserri R et al: AIDS prevention in homosexual and bisexual men: Results of a randomized trial evaluating two risk reduction interventions. *AIDS* 3:341–346, 1989.
44 Hobfoll SE et al: Reducing inner-city women's AIDS risk activities. *Health Psychol* 13:397–403, 1994.
45 DiClemente RJ et al: A randomized controlled trial of an HIV sexual risk reduction intervention for young African American women. *JAMA* 274:1271–1276, 1995.
46 Rotheram-Borus MA et al: Reducing HIV sexual risk behaviors among runaway adolescents. *JAMA* 266:1237–1241, 1991.
47 Jemmott JB et al: Reductions in HIV risk-associated sexual behaviors among Black male adolescents: Effects of an AIDS prevention intervention. *Am J Pub Health* 82:372–377, 1992.
48 St. Lawrence JS et al: Cognitive-behavioral intervention to reduce African American adolescents' risk for HIV infection. *J Consult Clin Psychol* 63:221–237, 1995.
49 Bye LL: Moving beyond counseling and knowledge-enhancement intervention: A plea for community-level AIDS prevention strategies, in *Behavioral Aspects of AIDS,* Ostrow DG (ed). New York, Plenum, 1990, pp. 157–167.
50 Flowers JV et al: Comparison of the results of a standardized AIDS prevention program in three geographic locations. *AIDS Educ Prev* 3: 189–196, 1991.
51 Miller TE et al: Changes in knowledge, attitudes, and behavior as a result of a community-based AIDS prevention program. *AIDS Educ Prev* 2:12–23, 1990.
52 Lemp GF et al: Seroprevalence of HIV and risk behaviors among young homosexual and bisexual men: The San Francisco/Berkeley Young Men's Survey. *JAMA* 272:449–454, 1994.
53 Kegeles SD et al: The M-Powerment project: A community-level HIV prevention intervention for young gay men. *Am J Pub Health* 86: 1129–1136, 1996.
54 Sikkema KJ et al: HIV risk behaviors among inner-city women: Intervention issues. Paper presented to the Fourth International Congress of Behavioral Medicine and Health, Washington DC, March, 1996.
55 Centers for Disease Control and Prevention: Community-level prevention of human immunodeficiency virus infection among high-risk populations: The AIDS Community Demonstration Projects. *MMWR* 45: 1–24, 1996.

Chapter 96

Marketing, communication, and advocacy for large-scale STD/HIV prevention and control

William A. Smith
Robert Hornik

This chapter focuses on large-scale behavior change using marketing, communication, and/or advocacy to influence the behavior of individuals at risk of disease. It defers discussion of individual and small group approaches that have been characteristic of counseling and testing, for example, in favor of a better understanding of community and/or mass approaches to influencing human behavior. In practice, individual and large-scale approaches often go hand-in-hand (e.g., a mass media program can be used to increase the number of individuals volunteering for counseling and testing). In this chapter, however, we focus on the unique problems and opportunities of large-scale behavior change.

Figure 96-1 contrasts large-scale and small-scale interventions. Note that small-scale interventions (individual and group counseling) are characterized by immediate, intimate, and interactive response to the client that permit corrective change in the provider's communication over a short span of time. The factors necessary to effective small group approaches include the face-to-face meeting, listening skills, and immediate responsiveness tailored to a specific individual's needs. A large-scale program of behavior change (a campaign to increase the number of people coming for STD testing or an advocacy program to promote funding of needle exchange programs among injecting drug users) has low immediacy with the target audience. Its intimacy is inhibited by societal and political norms and its interactivity is low or delayed over long periods of time. Large-scale approaches, however, offer tremendous public health advantages in scale of effect if they can overcome these differences.

The influential approaches most commonly used by large-scale programs are quite different than those used by small-scale programs. They include three broad approaches that can be managed, changed, or integrated in different ways to create comprehensive programs of large-scale change. The influential approaches are the following.

SERVICE APPROACHES

Service approaches that make it easier for people to make healthy choices by increasing the access and attractiveness of services that make prevention and control more viable (longer operating hours, services closer to home, ensured confidentiality, etc.).

MESSAGE APPROACHES

Message approaches that help ensure that people are both aware of and believe in the control and prevention choices opened to them. Message approaches ensure that information is clear, accurate, and persuasive, and then selects channels of communication that reach the audience frequently, appropriately, and with great credibility to the audience.

CONTROL APPROACHES

Control approaches that use law, regulation, and enforcement actions to provide disincentives for unhealthy behavior and its supports (criminalize sex with minors, criminalize prostitution, close bath houses, tax pornography, etc.), or provide positive incentives for healthy behavior (lower insurance premiums, tax breaks, antidiscriminatory legislation).

The practice of large-scale behavior change is the story of how these three approaches are combined by different practitioners to produce effective programs. Practitioners tend to fall into one of three categories that reflect a bias toward one of the three approaches. Marketing professionals tend to stress the design and delivery of better products and services as a way to influence behavior. Communication professionals tend to emphasize the role of messages in the support of new behavior. Advocates tend to stress the role of control through the formulation of policy and regulations that support behavior change. This chapter will discuss the strengths of each approach and argue that the most effective programs are those that take a strategic, comprehensive look at behavior, organizing interventions that provide for creating new services, persuasive messages, and changes in policy as required by a given population. These programs are referenced here as population-oriented interventions that are defined as large-scale interventions that reflect both the objective needs of a population and the subjective perception of need that often influences a population's willingness to adopt and sustain health behavior.

This chapter will discuss three specific population-oriented intervention strategies (marketing, communication, and advocacy) that help program managers understand and influence the relationship of *people's perceptions* of the problem, and the actions or behaviors they choose to take. Marketing, communication, and program advocacy strategies have contributed significantly to our understanding of how service, message, and control approaches work together to produce effective behavior change. Each of the three strategies has tended to specialize in one of the three approaches—marketing in service delivery, communication in message development, and advocacy in policy reform. However, as we will demonstrate, the biggest gains have been made through programs that integrate and sustain combinations of the three approaches strategically over time.

Although different in many important ways, all three program strategies also share a common belief that interventions should be designed based on the perceived desires, the real world barriers, and the objective health needs of the at-risk population. They are based on a fundamental recognition that behavior is influenced by people's perceptions, as well as objective scientific fact. They begin by asking what do people *want* in order to act in a healthy manner, not only what do people *need* in order to act in a healthy manner. The complementary focus of *want* and *need* is a fundamental shift from a clinical/medical model to a marketing/behavioral model. If we were to ask what does an individual need, versus what does she want, we would identify quite different, although possibly complementary, answers. An individual may *need* to understand STDs better; she may need to use a condom or go for a STD check-up. However, she *wants* to feel supported; she *wants* to keep her disease a secret; and she *wants* it to go away. The success of population-oriented interventions lies in their ability to satisfy both the individual's health needs and as many of her human wants as necessary to gain her participation and control over her own condition and to do so on a scale that is epidemiologically

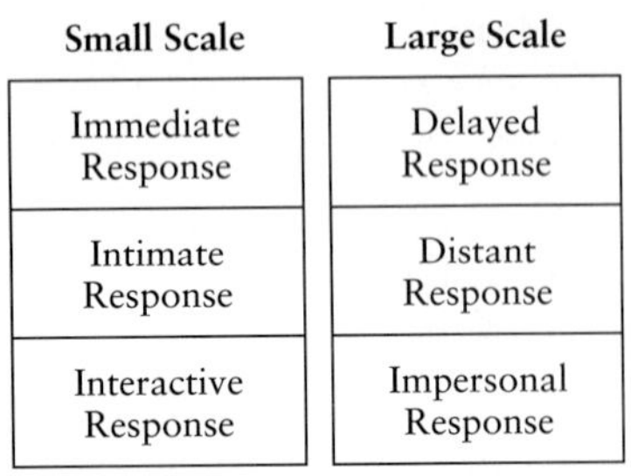

Fig. 96-1. Large-scale and small-scale interventions.

significant. The basic assumptions underlying this chapter are the following.

1. Behavior of both providers and at-risk populations is a critical aspect of any STD/HIV prevention and control program.
2. People's perceptions of what service, messages and control offer, as well as the offerings themselves, influence their behavior.
3. Behavior is best influenced by integrated programs of service, message, and control approaches.
4. Policy's role is to allocate resources strategically to service, message, and control approaches in order to influence behavior.
5. Marketing, communication, and advocacy are three ways to implement those resource allocations strategically.

In the following section we define and briefly discuss three population-oriented intervention strategies—social marketing, health communication, and advocacy. Figure 96-2 summarizes the three approaches and strategies. Note that it illustrates that although each strategy emphasizes a particular approach, all these strategies take other approaches into account.

DEFINITIONS

SOCIAL MARKETING

Social marketing can be defined as a program-planning process that promotes the voluntary behavior of target audiences by offering benefits they want, reducing barriers they are concerned about, and using persuasion to motivate their participation in program activity leading toward improved personal and social welfare.[1] Social marketing uses in-depth information about both consumers and the health system to (1) define products, services, and behaviors that are most acceptable to users; (2) organize delivery systems or places that ensure easy access and facilitate adoption of products and behaviors; (3) establish a price in terms of barriers (dollars, time, social status, or convenience) that users are willing to accept; and (4) create and promote messages about those products and behaviors that motivate and persuade.[2]

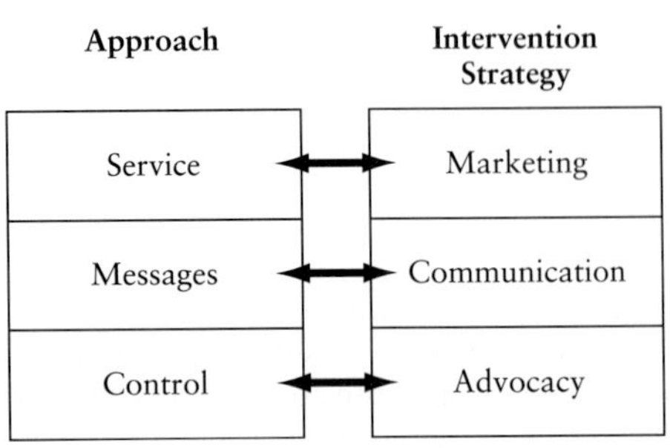

Fig. 96-2. The three population-oriented intervention strategies.

Social marketing differs substantially from both communication and advocacy when they are applied individually to the problem of behavior change. In a communication strategy the basic assumption is that an individual lacks information, awareness, or "understanding" of a problem. In an advocacy strategy the basic assumption is that people must be prevented through sanctions from doing harm to themselves or others. Marketing uses a structured, staged process for program decision making that interrelates action with research. Decision making moves through a process of listening to audiences, planning interventions, pretesting plans, developing test markets, going to scale, and then monitoring and changing programs as they progress.[3]

Social marketing programs often stress the provision of services in innovative ways to overcome access and awareness barriers. Programs such as Project ACTION[4] in Portland, Oregon have used an innovative condom distribution network not only to reach youth at risk of STDs and HIV but also to build an entire campaign around condom distribution.[4] Highly visible advertising, community organizing, promoting prevention messages among community leaders in both the public and private sector, along with marketing a branded condom targeted at the youth market, have used marketing as a paradigm to address service, message, and control needs of this population. The Centers for Disease Control and Prevention (CDC) is using a social marketing model in five cities throughout America to test the transferability of key social marketing technology to community control. In a program entitled the Prevention Marketing Initiative, these five communities are using social marketing to create a community-based HIV prevention program for youth.[5] This test represents an effort to determine whether these technologies can be adapted successfully by paraprofessional community groups. Success in this program will open the field to much wider application and reduce reliance on highly trained marketing professionals.

Internationally, the experience with social marketing—particularly condom social marketing—is perhaps even more extensive. The family planning community, and more recently the AIDS prevention community, has demonstrated conclusively the ability of social marketing programs to increase the availability of condoms, increase condom usage among lower socioeconomic consumers, and contribute to declines in fertility rates. In Zaire, a program supported by a private sector company, PSI, in conjunction with USAID, increased condom sales from a low in 1988 of 300,000 condoms sold to a high in 1991 of over 18 million condoms.[6] Experiences in Switzerland with a branded condom for gay men, in Zaire with a branded condom for AIDS, in India with specific branded condoms for lower SES consumers have all demonstrated that several aspects of social marketing are robust across culture: (1) target marketing to specialized segments of the population; (2) audience research; (3) an emphasis given to distribution outlets and pricing; and (4) positioning of condoms to meet a felt need of audiences rather than a health need of the society.

HEALTH COMMUNICATIONS

Health communications can be defined as a process for the development and diffusion of messages to specific audiences in order to influence their knowledge, attitudes, and beliefs in favor of healthy behavioral choice.[7] Health communications is largely an educational approach to behavior change. It recognizes that education alone is often insufficient to influence behavior change, but health communications, unlike marketing, does not assume responsibility for the organization and management of services and control. Health communications is developed within a different professional community than social marketing, but shares many of its characteristics, for example, an emphasis on consumer research and a commitment to consumer-centered program development. Health communications programs in developing countries have been particularly effective as catalysts for the creation of comprehensive consumer-based programs, especially programs addressing issues such as breast-feeding, for which packaged products are not a viable alternative. The social marketing of breast-feeding in third-world countries has relied heavily on communication strategies to organize communities, influence social norms, and publicize new services.[8] Again, some of the most effective health communications programs have integrated changes in services (e.g., the availability of day care for working mothers), messages (e.g., broad campaigns on the benefits and acceptability of breast-feeding), and control (e.g., policy prohibiting promotion of bottle feeding in hospitals) into an integrated, long-term program of behavior change.[9] Similar examples are found in the literature on the development of HIV prevention programs in the Caribbean, East Africa, the Philippines.[10]

SOCIAL ADVOCACY

Social advocacy, often referred to as media advocacy, is defined as a process for influencing public policy and institutional structures leading to improved health behavior and health outcomes.[11] To address the increasing need for new policy and regulatory controls, social advocacy programs emerged as an approach to behavior change. Much of the legislative support for antismoking and drunk driving, and indeed HIV/AIDS support, has come from the determined, strategic, and creative work of social advocates. Advocates often are frustrated by social marketing and communications approaches, which they argue "blame the victim." Advocates place primary emphasis on public policy and institutional change rather than on individual behavior. They focus on the behavior of policymakers who control the structural elements of programs that make it easier for individuals to avoid high-risk behavior. Typically, advocates are interested in making it more difficult for manufacturers to market harmful substances (e.g., controls on advertising and distributing cigarettes) or in reducing barriers to healthy choices (e.g., reducing discriminatory employment policies which make at-risk populations reluctant to disclose their STD or HIV status and, thus, get proper treatment). Important examples of successful advocacy efforts include the 20-year fight for controls on the tobacco industry and the nation's effort to reduce drunk driving accidents and fatalities.[12]

Important differences among marketing, communication, and advocacy should be understood. Marketers, for example, have traditionally been interested in the provision of consumer-oriented services, communicators in the promotion of effective messages, and advocates in the development of effective control strategies. The growing complexity of social problems has fostered a growing specialization within each community. However, many of the specific program tools, such as awareness campaigns, public advertising, public relations, demonstrations, audience segmentation, consumer research, and policy research are used by marketers, communicators, and advocates alike. More important, the central organizing approach shared by all three strategies remains an in-depth understanding of their consumer (e.g., high-risk individual, influential family and friends, community, general public, or policymaker) based on strategic consumer research and driven by a desire to satisfy what that consumer wants in order to make the right decision—whether that decision is to use a condom, talk supportively to a friend, or pass a law closing bath houses. All three action strategies are fundamentally consumer-centered and focus on social change and human behavior.

Social psychology is strengthening audience research by adding a set of key measures of the determinants of human behavior. A new look at social norms and their importance in large-scale change is providing a solid theoretical foundation for many of the empirical lessons emerging from the practice of marketing, communication, and advocacy.

Today there is a growing belief that comprehensive programs that strategically combine marketing, communication, and advocacy strategies do better than piecemeal and opportunistic efforts.[13] These comprehensive models suggest ways to assess opportunities for all three intervention points—services, messages, and control. Several of these new models reflect a growing role for behavioral science.[14] For example, models such as the Applied Behavior Change (ABC) Framework that integrate experiences and techniques emerging from all three intervention approaches now are visible in the literature.[15] The ABC Framework has been developed at the Academy for Educational Development to integrate all these streams of knowledge into a straightforward approach to program design. The ABC Framework helps prevention program managers answer the practical questions: Where do I start? What do I worry about at each stage of development? and, What milestones should I measure and evaluate? The framework uses five phases—assess, plan, pretest, implement, and monitor—to guide program managers through both marketing and advocacy issues. It is important because it shows that the integration of these disciplines provides benefits far in excess of any one approach in isolation.

Marketing, communication, and advocacy can be best characterized by the assertion that behavior is the key to success and that people's perceptions of services, messages, and control are as important as the services, messages, and controls themselves. Although these approaches use operations research to define specific tactics and understand their selected audiences, these are not research models but intervention models. Their purpose is to influence behavior, not just understand it. Considerable research has been done on all three approaches. Despite the serious limitations of this research, the following section reviews what works and, to some degree, why it works.

HEALTH STATUS AND BEHAVIORAL EFFECTS ON A LARGE SCALE

Although there is evidence for the effectiveness of large-scale social marketing, health communication, and advocacy programs, the evidence does not, and could not, conform to rigorous standards for evidence of effects. One way that effective social marketing, health communication, and advocacy programs work is to reach their target audiences directly with services and messages. However, a complementary path of effect, one often deliberately incorporated into the best population-oriented programs, is to stimulate the activities of other channels that reach audiences, including the general mass and news media. The level and characteristics of these activities are beyond the control of the marketer or advocate. A program can direct its public service announcements (PSAs), but the occurrence of unintended news events (such as an announcement by Magic Johnson that he is HIV-positive) is uncontrolled. A social program is no less happy if an unplanned, breaking news event stimulates attention to AIDS on a national talk show or a network news broadcast or through a local newspaper or television station. Despite the benefit to social programs of unplanned events, measurement of their effects cannot be easily distinguished from the effects of the planned events. In this context, it serves no purpose to separate the effects of a deliberate social marketing PSA from those resulting from operations of the rest of the news media. Deliberate stimulation of the news media has, in fact, become a major strategy that many population-oriented interventions now use regularly. Definition of effects and causality, however, is hampered by our inability to isolate the size or importance of the inputs.

CDC's America Responds to AIDS (ARTA) campaign has depended, in part, on public service announcements. Evidence for the reach of that campaign includes estimates of the value of media time made available ($67 million between 1987–1991) and the number of times the average adult between 18 and 54 had the opportunity to view an ARTA PSA during the period (56 times per month).[16] However, it is likely that other elements of CDC's efforts to stimulate attention to HIV/AIDS, including a flood of press releases and video and audio format materials for use by local television and radio stations, were also responsible for a great deal of exposure. Similarly, the announcements by Rock Hudson, Magic Johnson, and Arthur Ashe of their personal HIV status—events not planned by CDC—had significant impact on public attention given to AIDS. Efforts by other agencies, including community organizations, state health departments, and national nonprofit organizations, along with expanded commercial marketing of condoms, operated simultaneously and with similar purposes.

We know that there have been substantial changes in knowledge, attitudes, and behavior among Americans during this period, with resulting health benefits. For example, condom use during the last intercourse is reported to have increased from 25 percent to over 50 percent among young people since the onset of the epidemic, and gonorrhea rates have declined from 324/100,000 in 1987 to 247/100,000 by 1991 and 150/100,000 in 1995.[17–19] Similarly, in other countries with major public communication and social marketing programs, the evidence for a shift toward safer behavior is even stronger. The Swiss Stop AIDS campaign and the Netherlands AIDS program used mass media heavily to reach audiences believed to be at risk of infection with HIV. Nongovernment community groups created and marketed some of the first gay AIDS condoms, called the Hot Rubber. Government authorities carefully developed television and radio advertisements, as well as billboards and newspaper inserts, the content of which was quite explicit in encouraging the use of condoms for protection. At the same time, as in much of the rest of the world, mass media were full of AIDS coverage. In both countries, the operation of these programs was associated with a period of substantial change in use of condoms. Self-reported use of condoms with all "casual" partners in the previous 6 months increased from 8 percent to over 60 percent among 17- to 30-year-olds in Switzerland between 1987 and 1992, and from 9 percent to over 40 percent in the Netherlands between early 1987 and late 1989.[20,21]

Although all of these programs have operated inseparably from the broader mass media environment, there are a few cases where the possibility of attributing effects to a more limited social marketing or health communication effort is plausible. Harvey provides evidence about 1991 condom sales in 24 condom social marketing programs in less developed countries, where condoms had relatively little usage before the introduction of these programs and where sales data refer specifically to the brands of condoms promoted by the social marketing efforts.[22] The sales vary a great deal across sites, but among those 12 programs where the cost of 100 condoms per year was less than 1 percent of GNP per capita, sales were between 0.2 and 1.0 condoms per capita. One condom per capita represents sales equivalent to 5 percent of the population using condoms for contraception, but a much larger percentage use them on an irregular basis.[22] So, if a large proportion of condom use already achieved was focused on men who were having sex outside of marriage, a great deal of protection from HIV transmission could be achieved. This was the pattern in some contexts.[23,24]

Another type of evidence that allows direct attribution to specific social marketing efforts has to do with promotion of AIDS hotlines. There is evidence, for example, that the use of such hotlines is directly affected by increased promotion. In 1988, the number of calls monthly to the Surgeon General's AIDS hotline tripled (from 70,000 to 210,000) during the period when the Surgeon General's pamphlet, including the hotline phone number, was mailed out.

There are also important data on large-scale effects of social marketing, health communication, and advocacy programs from work done in other health areas. The National High Blood Pressure Education Program (NHBPEP) was a prototype for such efforts. Begun in 1972, it included institutional consensus building, education of health professionals, some public education through community organizations, and major efforts in mass media education. These media efforts included distribution of public service announcements for broadcast on radio and television and stimulation of coverage of hypertension by various media outlets. The effects associated with this program were very great. Between 1960 and 1972, before the initiation of the NHBPEP, the age-adjusted stroke mortality rate was declining at 1.6 percent per year for all U.S. whites; from 1972 to 1984 the rate declined at 5.9 percent per year.[25] There is some controversy about the attribution of all of this decline to improvements in hypertension control associated with the NHBPEP. Nonetheless, the sheer volume of the effect precisely timed to the introduction of the NHBPEP is impressive. The National Cholesterol Education Program appears to have been associated with sharp declines in cholesterol consumption in an analogous fashion, as much because it changed the public agenda concerning cholesterol as because of its direct educational programs.

Warner made a case for a substantial effect of the original televised smoking counter-advertising campaign between 1967 and 1970.[26] The networks were required by the "Fairness Doctrine," then in force, to match cigarette manufacturers' commercials with anti-smoking commercials. The period of broadcast of frequent anti-smoking commercials was associated with a reduction of 10 percent in per capita consumption of cigarettes. Attribution of this change to the counter-advertising effort is strengthened by the finding that when the counter-advertising effort was eliminated, per capita consumption increased 5 percent, returning to a trend present before the counter-advertising began.

A study by Hu and colleagues suggested that the current anti-smoking campaign in California has produced large effects on cigarette consumption, substantially associated with both policy change (tax increases) and a mass media campaign.[27] They suggest that a $20 million media campaign produced a decline of about 232 million packs of cigarettes smoked over a 2-year period, or about $1 spent per 11 packs not smoked. They estimate that the effect of the combined strategy campaign was such that each 10 percent increase in media time purchased (or about $2 million) would produce an additional decline of 0.5 percent in cigarette sales.

Interventions often need to stimulate demand for services provided by the health system. The 1989 to 1990 Communication for Child Survival campaign in the Philippines used heavy television and radio advertising along with improvements in the system to encourage early immunization. The number of children with timely, complete coverage increased from 32 to 56 percent in one year. Much of the effect of this program was to reduce delay in coming for vaccination, with a smaller effect in reaching children who otherwise would have remained unvaccinated.[28]

Thus, in other areas of health, as well as STD-specific work, there is good evidence for association between the large outreach operations of social marketing, health communication, and advocacy programs and effects on behavior and even health outcomes. Although causal attribution of effects to integrated marketing, communication, and advocacy efforts are better studied in other areas than STD control, the evidence suggests continued efforts in this area are justified.

APPLICATIONS TO HIV/STD CONTROL AND PREVENTION

The first problem that any effort at changing HIV/STD behavior must face is understanding why some people are engaging in the recommended behavior and some people are not. For example, Fishbein et al. wanted to understand the determinants of condom use in two Caribbean islands prior to the development of a comprehensive intervention.[29] There were many possibilities for the intervention: the program might address the availability of condoms, the perception that AIDS was not a personal risk to the at-risk population, or the perception that there was a widely shared social norm not favoring condom use in risky sexual contact.

The results of a preprogram audience survey were clear: Condom access was not a problem for this population, and the perception of the risk of AIDS was shown to be unrelated to whether or not an individual used condoms frequently.

In contrast, three types of reports of normative pressure to use condoms (talking with friends about condom use, reporting that friends used condoms, and reporting that sexual partners had ever requested the respondent to use a condom) were each substantially related to frequency of condom use. The authors recommended that the program focus on increasing the perception of normative pressure to use condoms, and not waste resources on personal risk messages, or new condom distribution systems.

This approach to analysis is totally situation specific. Its relevance relates entirely to particular audiences at particular times for particular behaviors. For example, if STD clinics are inaccessible and ordinary clinics are ineffective at diagnosing or treating STDs, public education to increase treatment-seeking alone may be counterproductive. An intervention, in this case, might better target providers whose skills are problematic or legislators who must allocate funds for expanded STD facilities. In another situation, if knowledge about the negative outcomes of a particular disease is low (e.g., infertility associated with untreated chlamydia), yet those who know about the risks are much more likely to obtain treatment, an information campaign to increase knowledge of the risks of untreated STDs makes sense.

The principle is clear: Before the program is designed, the nature of the behavior problem must be well understood in its complexity. This information guides the definition of audience(s) to be reached (legislators, medical providers, individuals engaging in high-risk behaviors, and the social networks that surround those individuals) and suggests strategies to best influence their behavior.

Any strategy also must be well-executed to be effective. Many programs fail despite good messages and good definition of target audiences, because they do not achieve the exposure they need in order to affect the thinking and behavior of those audiences. For example, Hingson et al. found that children who had spoken to physicians about AIDS were more likely to have adopted condom use to avoid HIV exposure.[30] Of the 80 percent of adolescents in that survey who reported seeing a physician in the past year, however, only 13 percent were counseled about AIDS. Chang et al. interviewed STD clinic clients in 1988 and found that they were quite knowledgeable about AIDS.[31] However, only 30 percent said they acquired information from the clinics. Similarly, poorly implemented provider training, poorly supplied condom distributors, or poorly positioned advocacy approaches produce poor results.

A particularly striking example of this issue of gaining audience exposure to messages comes from the National Cancer Institute–sponsored Community Intervention Trial for Smoking Cessation (COMMIT).[32] This was a major smoking education intervention that tried to affect the smoking cessation rates among heavy smokers. Twenty-two cities were randomly assigned to receive the intervention or be in a control condition. At completion, there was very little difference between intervention and control cities in cessation rates (both were around 18%). This apparent failure of outcome belied a more fundamental failure: there was virtually no difference between the intervention and control communities in the level of reported exposure to messages on any of the five major channels used. The intervention communities did not do any *better* than the control communities because they did not do any *more* than the control communities. Success involves both choosing appropriate strategies and using them with sufficient intensity and competency to influence the audience. The most effective way to do this will vary with the audience and the nature of the behavior. These questions must be answered through empirical research for each intervention, setting, and behavior.

THE IMPORTANCE OF COMPETENCY AND INTENSITY OF IMPLEMENTATION

The Centers for Disease Control and Prevention (CDC) has often supported intensive face-to-face outreach efforts as the best way to reach those socially marginalized and at highest risk, for example, female sex workers (FSWs) or intravenous drug users (IDUs). Thus, in Colorado Springs, street outreach to prostitutes by county health workers included HIV/STD education plus condom distribution and encouragement for regular testing and screening. The program, implemented between 1987 and 1991, was associated with a threefold drop in the number of FSWs testing positive for STDs and a 16 percent decline in reported gonorrhea rates for the entire population of the county. Gonorrhea among FSWs in Denver, where there was no parallel program, showed no consistent decline in the same period. Quasi-experimental results from other CDC-sponsored programs have suggested success for theory-based, resource-intensive street outreach programs for IDUs and for FSWs across a number of cities.[33] The replicability of these successes is often questioned owing to the resource- and management-intensive efforts required. Other outreach programs—programs with less intense interventions—have been less successful in reaching the relevant populations. In Connecticut, for example, a survey of members of the target audience for community outreach programs noted that more than 30 percent had heard of them, but only 6 percent of those who described themselves as at medium or high risk of AIDS had actually made use of the services of those agencies.[34] The problem in some communities has been assuring contact with the audience on a continuing basis. This has led some experts to argue that these socially marginalized groups might be reached through mass media–based programs, both to encourage safer sexual and needle-use behavior and to encourage involvement with available outreach programs.[35]

Evidence exists that some of these populations are commonly exposed to the mass media and do not conform to the stereotypes of street people isolated from common channels of communication. Jason et al. reports that among a sample of Baltimore IDUs, the median television viewing was 4 hours a day in a home setting.[36] Ross et al. found that among Australian IDUs, general media habits looked much like those of the general population.[37] Mak and Plum found that 98 percent of prostitutes in Ghent, Belgium reported television as their primary source of information about AIDS.[38] Chang et al. found that 70 percent of their STD clinic attendees reported mass media as their major source of AIDS information.[31]

Although exposure to AIDS information through the mass media is apparently as common for these groups as for others, there is only tentative evidence about the effect of organized mass media–based programs on the behavior of these groups. Some mass media–based programs have developed messages specifically for one or another audience. Other campaigns assumed that the IDU and prostitute/client audiences were likely to be influenced by general messages about safer sex. Some of these have shown evidence of behavior change. The examples that follow show evidence of effects of general campaigns and general messages on groups frequently targeted in narrowly focused campaigns. We do not discuss the large number of campaigns that address narrowly focused groups alone. Van den Hoek et al. reported on the changes in sexual behavior among a cohort of intravenous drug users in Amsterdam before (1988–1989) and after (1989–1990) a large national AIDS prevention campaign.[39] They found some increases in regular condom use for casual sex and a reduction in the number of female IDUs working as FSWs. Similarly, de Fine Olivarius et al. found substantial declines in gonorrhea (but not other STDs) at an "inner city STD clinic" in Copenhagen, Denmark, comparing women studied before (1984) and after (1988) a general campaign for safer sex.[40] Neaigus et al. find evidence in New York that behavior changes among IDUs enrolled in an outreach program are partly attributable to the outreach intervention and partly attributable to external trends, including, presumably, the general education efforts then prevalent.[41] Similarly, Swiss researchers found in a 1989–1990 study that "drug users and ex-drug users use condoms more often than the rest of the population," with the implication that the several years of campaigning prior to that study had produced that effect.[20]

These studies provide evidence of behavior changes among IDUs or FSWs and their clients consistent with the operation of communication, marketing, and advocacy programs. Clearly, there may have been other influences on these reported behavior changes besides the deliberate efforts at public education that have occurred, including most importantly, general press coverage of AIDS and its risks. At best, current evidence suggests, but does not establish, the possible value of large-scale media programs in affecting these audiences.

There are several conclusions that may be drawn from this and other evidence about social marketing, health communication, and advocacy for STDs. Crucial to program success is the need for planners to understand their audience well: what the audience is doing now and how it perceives the relevant behavior; what the major determinants of current behavior are; promising routes to influencing those behaviors; and what channels of outreach are likely to reach and influence them. Appropriate research approaches for investigating these issues will reflect the resources available and the scale of the program. Informal interviewing may be all a small individual clinic can justify before launching a program for its clientele. Major surveys, multiple focus groups, continuous monitoring of exposure to messages, and effects on knowledge and behavior can easily be justified, however, by national programs with a long-term agenda.

No less central is a clear plan for assuring adequate exposure to messages to affect behavior. There is, unfortunately, little systematic evidence about dose-response to exposure; that is, how much exposure is required to produce how much behavior change. It is clear that programs that achieve high levels of exposure have shown substantial effects. Programs with little or no exposure have little or no effects. The dose-response curve surely is a reflection of the presence of countervailing influences, the quality of the messages to which an individual is exposed, and the complexity of the behavior change being addressed. Cigarette smoking has yielded only slowly to growing exposure from multiple sources. This slow yield is in the context of an addictive behavior and an extensive promotion of cigarettes. In the area of STD-relevant behavior, it appears that condom use in casual sex has proved susceptible to comprehensive broad-based programs, but behavior favoring abstinence has been slow to change.

Finally, there is the difficulty of organizing these programs and keeping them operating over time. The smoking programs have been effective because the antismoking effort has remained on the public agenda for many years. The effects in any one year have been minimal. The NHBPEP was an extraordinary success, but it benefited from maintaining the work on many fronts over many years. Similarly, the substantial success in reducing the risk of HIV infection in past years can be attributed partly to the central place it has had on the public agenda. The risk that the place will be lost is large, as the public agenda shifts and as the epidemic focuses more on the disenfranchised. It is sometimes suggested that the major work of public awareness is done and that future shifts in behavior will all reflect work done locally and directed specifically to high-risk individuals and their communities. Thus, the role for large-scale social marketing programs is over. An alternative view is that this shift will have a major cost. If the national social marketing effort ends, the support it provides for maintaining and increasing the patterns of safer behavior that have been adopted in the general population will be lost. The COMMIT study suggests not that the target intervention was weak but that the control intervention was strong. The strength of that control intervention was owing largely to a broad national effort. A national effort provides for continued attention in the national media. A critical issue is that STD/AIDS continue to be legitimized/supported as an area of political and thus budgetary concern. If the national focus is softened, the funds and political will that underpin local programs also may be lost.

FUTURE APPLICATIONS TO STD/HIV CONTROL AND PREVENTION

STD/HIV control and prevention programs are already using social marketing, communication, and advocacy extensively. Social marketing of condoms, for example, is now a widespread enterprise with significant documented success (as in Portland, the Caribbean, India, and Switzerland, among others).[42] Communication approaches, including the management of the news media, have greatly increased the world's understanding of HIV/AIDS. Polls consistently indicate high levels of AIDS knowledge. Advocacy has been successful in the United States in protecting funding for HIV prevention in a period of political skepticism about prevention. Other STDs might well benefit from a strategic review of program goals using a broad marketing, communication, and advocacy framework. In addition, the application of specific intervention techniques, such as: (1) integrating targeted audience research; (2) developing lifestyle profiles for high-risk populations; (3) long-range planning and integrating service, messages, and control targeted to a narrow, high-priority problem; (4) maintaining program intensity levels that could incorporate all tactics into existing and new programs; and (5) increasing attention to policy change and advocacy approaches.

FUTURE RESEARCH NEEDS

Social marketing, communication, and advocacy research continue to be dominated by a vaccine paradigm that attempts to establish the "efficacy" of various interventions so those interventions can be discarded, improved, or replicated in other communities. Studies continue to compare different interventions (peer education vs. mass media approaches) as though these were competing "vaccines" or they attempt to establish the efficacy of a particular intervention in a real-world setting (community trials of smoking cessation interventions). This vaccine approach to intervention research has led to disappointing results because behavioral interventions are not like biological vaccines. The variability of hosts (social groups vs. human anatomy) over time is much greater in social institutions than biological entities. Thus, the replicability of interventions is much less achievable in social communities than in biological laboratories. New forms of research are needed that respect the characteristics of effective behavioral interventions, such as: (1) the importance of multiple interacting forces; (2) the need for responsive changes in interventions to meet unpredictable changes in the social environment; and (3) the importance of both intensity and long-term durability of interventions to produce measurable effect. Behavioral intervention research might better turn to marketing research models, where a set of best practices are applied by highly trained and experienced practitioners and adapted by them to meet the needs of different patients or clients. Research, in this case, is formative as well as evaluative. It helps shape programs as well as document their apparent success or failure.

References

1 Kotler P et al: *Social Marketing: Strategies for Changing Public Behavior.* New York, The Free Press, 1989, p. 24.

2 Andreasen AR: *Marketing Social Change: Changing Behavior to Promote Health, Social Development, and the Environment.* San Francisco, Jossey-Bass Publishers, 1995, pp. 15–16.

3 Andreasen AR: *Marketing Social Change: Changing Behavior to Promote Health, Social Development, and the Environment.* San Francisco, Jossey-Bass Publishers, 1995, p. 73.

4 Hedberg K et al: From Baseline Phase November 1992–January 1993 of PSI/Project ACTION Outcome Evaluation Conducted by the Oregon Health Division and The Kaiser Permanente Center for Health Research, May 1993.

5 Decentralized Plan for Technical Assistance in Second Year of HIV Prevention Community Planning. *CDC HIV/AIDS Prev* 5(4):11, 1995.

6 Social Marketing and Communications for Health, PSI, 1994, Country Programs in Africa, Zaire, p. 23.

7 Rasmuson M et al: *Communication for Child Survival* 7. 1988.

8 Marin P et al: The breast-feeding programme in Brazil, in *Programmes to Promote Breast-feeding,* Jelliffe DB et al. (eds). Oxford, Oxford University Press, 1988, chap 20, pp. 153–160.

9 Jelliffe DB et al: *Programmes to Promote Breast-feeding.* Oxford, Oxford University Press, 1988, pp. 344–371.

10 Smith WA et al: Building skills for condom use, in *A World Against AIDS: Communication for Behavior Change,* Smith et al (eds). Washington DC, 1993, pp. 71–89.

11 Wallack L et al: *Media Advocacy and Public Health: Power for Prevention.* Newbury Park, SAGE Publications, 1993, pp. 2–3.

12 Pertschuk M: *Giant Killers.* New York, W.W. Norton & Company, 1986, p. 31.

13 Wasserheit JN et al: *Research Issues in Human Behavior and Sexually Transmitted Diseases in the AIDS Era.* Washington, DC, American Society for Microbiology, 1991.

14 Leviton L: Theoretical Foundations of AIDS-Prevention Programs, in *Preventing Aids: The Design of Effective Programs,* Valdiserri RO (ed). New Brunswick, Rutgers University Press, 1989, pp. 42–91.

15 Smith WA et al: The Applied Behavior (ABC) Framework, in *A World Against AIDS: Communication for Behavior Change,* Smith WA et al. (eds). Washington, DC, Nov 1993, pp. 19–37.

16 Woods DR et al: "America Responds to AIDS": Its content, development process and outcome. *Pub Health Rpts* 106(6):616–622, 1991.

17 Sonenstein FL et al: Sexual activity, condom use and AIDS awareness among adolescent males. *Fam Plann Perspect* 21(4):152–158, 1989.

18 Forrest JD et al: The sexual and reproductive behavior of American women, 1982–1988 [published erratum appears in *Fam Plann Perspect* 1990 Nov–Dec;22(6):285] [see comments]. *Fam Plann Perspect* 22(5):206–214, 1990.

19 Division of STD Prevention: *Sexually Transmitted Disease Surveillance, 1995.* U.S. Department of Health and Human Services, Public Health Service. Atlanta: Centers for Disease Control and Prevention, September 1996.

20 Kocher KW: The stop AIDS story. Bern: Stop AIDS Campaign of the Swiss AIDS Foundation and the Federal Office for Public Health, 1993.

21 deVroome EM et al: AIDS in The Netherlands: The effects of several years of campaigning. *Int J STD AIDS* 1(4):268–275, 1990.

22 Harvey PD: "The impact of condom prices on sales in social marketing programs." *Stud Fam Plan* 25(1):52–58, 1994.

23 Ferreros C: Social Marketing of Condoms for AIDS Prevention in Developing Countries: The Zaire Experience. Washington, DC: Population Services International, 1990.

24 Population Services International: Condom User Intercept Study in the Cameroons. Washington, DC: Population Services International, 1991.

25 McGovern PG et al: Trends in mortality, morbidity, and risk factor levels for stroke from 1960 through 1990: The Minnesota Heart Survey. *JAMA* 268(6):753–759, 1992.

26 Warner KE: Cigarette smoking in the 1970s: The impact of the antismoking campaign on consumption. *Science* 211(4483):729–731, 1981.

27 Hu TW et al: Reducing cigarette consumption in California: Tobacco taxes vs. an anti-smoking media campaign. *Am J Pub Health* 85:1218–1222, 1995.

28 Zimicki S et al: Improving vaccination coverage in urban areas through a health communication campaign: The 1990 Philippines experience. *Bull WHO* 72(3):409–422, 1994.

29 Fishbein M et al: Using an AIDS KAP survey to identify determinants of condom use among sexually active adults from St. Vincent and the Grenadines. *J Appl Soc Psychol* 25(1):1–20, 1995.

30 Hingson R et al: Acquired immunodeficiency syndrome transmission: Changes in knowledge and behaviors among teenagers: Massachusetts statewide surveys, 1986 to 1988. *Pediatrics* 85(1):24–29, 1990.

31 Chang HG et al: Assessment of AIDS knowledge in selected New York State sexually transmitted disease clinics. *NY State J Med* 90(3):126–128, 1990.

32 I. Cohort Results from a four year intervention. *Am J Pub Health* 85: 183–192, 1995.

33 Centers for Disease Control and Prevention: Community-level prevention of human immunodeficiency virus infection among high-risk population: The AIDS community demonstration projects. *MMWR* (RR-6):1–16, 1996.

34 Checko PJ et al: Community awareness and use of HIV/AIDS prevention services among minority populations—Connecticut, 1991. *MMWR* 41(43):825–829, 1992.

35 HIV-infection prevention messages for injecting drug users: Sources of information and use of mass media—Baltimore, 1989. *MMWR* 40(28):465–469, 1991.

36 Jason J et al: Potential use of mass media to reach urban intravenous drug users with AIDS prevention messages. *Int J Addict* 28(9):837–851, 1993.

37 Ross MW et al: Media sources of HIV/AIDS information in injecting drug users. *Austral J Pub Health* 16(3):324–327, 1992.

38 Mak R et al: Do prostitutes need more health education regarding sexually transmitted diseases and the HIV infection? Experience in a Belgian city. *Soc Sci Med* 33(8):963–966, 1991.

39 van den Hoek JAR et al: Little change in sexual behavior in injecting drug users in Amsterdam. *J Acq Imm Def Syn* 5(5):518–522, 1992.

40 de Fine Olivarius F et al: Sexual behaviour of women attending an innercity STD clinic before and after a general campaign for safer sex in Denmark. *Gen Med* 68:296–299, 1992.

41 Neaigus A et al: Effects of outreach intervention on risk reduction among intravenous drug users. *AIDS Educ Prev* 2(4):253–271, 1990.

42 *AIDS Prevention Through Health Promotion: Facing Sensitive Issues.* Geneva, World Health Organization, 1991.

Chapter 97

Public health surveillance for HIV/AIDS and other STDS: guideposts for prevention and care

John W. Ward
Joel R. Greenspan

For the proper treatment of clinical disease, a health care provider requires information to diagnose the nature and location of the condition, gauge its severity, and monitor the response to therapy. This clinical information is gathered through patient interview, physical examination, laboratory and radiologic studies, and other procedures conducted in the health care setting. A public health practitioner also needs information to assess the risks to the public's health posed by a condition, the number and characteristics of persons with the condition, and the efficacy of community-based prevention programs. Public health surveillance systems gather this information to guide community health programs.

Public health surveillance is defined as the systematic and ongoing collection, analysis, and dissemination of information to monitor the occurrence of specific health problems in populations.[1] Because surveillance systems function as information loops, the analysis and dissemination of surveillance data are as important as data collection (Fig. 97-1). The surveillance process provides disease prevention program staff with information that helps them decide the strategies and resources needed to halt the spread of disease and determine the impact of the program on the public's health. Thus, the information needs of prevention programs should guide the type of data collected by surveillance. First and foremost, surveillance systems help to define the size of a public health problem and the changes in the size of that problem over time by tracking morbidity and mortality. This surveillance function is essential for effective public health planning. Surveillance systems also typically collect demographic, geographic, transmission mode, and other data to describe disease burdens in subpopulations and in specific geographic areas to permit the strategic targeting of prevention efforts. Beyond these traditional data-gathering efforts, which are focused on health outcomes, surveillance systems are increasingly called on to respond to additional programmatic needs. These needs are diverse and include behavioral data to document risk behaviors that may lead to sexually transmitted diseases (STDs), health services data to track access to and utilization of STD treatment services, and laboratory data to monitor the changing patterns of drug resistance or genomic characteristics that may influence the quality of detection and treatment. Thus, surveillance program directors must remain responsive to prevention program and treatment needs and adapt surveillance efforts to these needs as resources permit. Regardless of the surveillance data collected, the greatest usefulness of surveillance systems comes from periodic or ongoing data collection that affords the opportunity to describe temporal trends in disease patterns and to assist in the evaluation of the impact of prevention efforts.

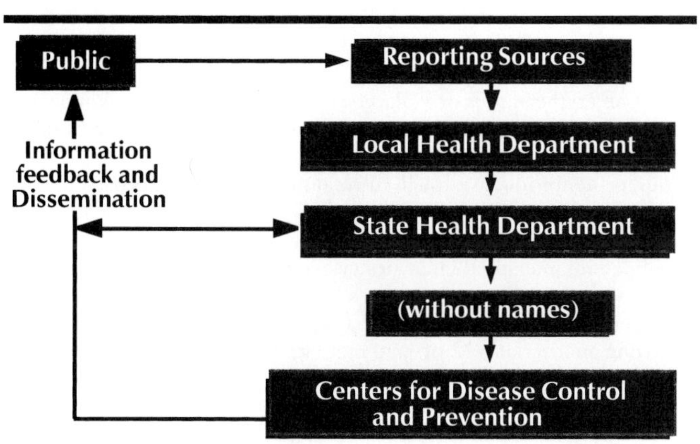

Fig. 97-1. HIV/STD surveillance system flow of information.

A variety of surveillance systems are used to monitor HIV/AIDS and other STDs. The most common methods are notifiable diseases registries, laboratory and clinic-based sentinel surveillance systems, and vital records. The type of surveillance used for HIV/AIDS and other STDs is guided by the type of information needed for disease prevention and control, the community's acceptance of the surveillance methodology, and the availability of human and technologic resources. Surveillance systems are typically evaluated for timeliness, representativeness, and completeness of case reporting. Each surveillance approach has strengths and limitations that should be taken into account when reviewing surveillance data.

DISEASE REGISTRIES

HIV/AIDS and other STD disease registries in states are based on the legal authority of states to mandate reporting of these and other conditions by health care providers and laboratories according to standardized surveillance case definitions. Standardized case definitions allow disease tracking and reporting measures to be compared across time and place. Case finding for public health surveillance is closely tied to the health care system, and case definitions for HIV/AIDS and other STDs comprise both laboratory and clinical reporting criteria (Tables 97-1 and 97-2).[2,3] To ensure the comparability of data from state to state in national comparisons, the U.S. Public Health Service and states have agreed on and published surveillance case definitions for HIV infection, AIDS, chancroid, chlamydia, genital herpes, genital warts, gonorrhea, granuloma inguinale, hepatitis B, lymphogranuloma venereum, nongonococcal urethritis, pelvic inflammatory disease (PID), and syphilis (all stages, including neurosyphilis, congenital syphilis, and syphilitic stillbirth).[2] In the United States, each of the main public health jurisdictions (principally states) determines which diseases and conditions pose a sufficient public health threat to require reporting to local public health authorities. Only AIDS, gonorrhea, hepatitis B, and syphilis (including congenital syphilis) are reportable in all states. As of late 1996, HIV infection (not AIDS) was reportable in 29 states, including three states that have HIV reporting for children only. In 1996, chlamydia was reportable in 49 states. Only 42 states require the reporting of chancroid.

Health department disease registries for HIV/AIDS, gonorrhea, hepatitis B, and syphilis are based on confidential case reports by name from clinicians, laboratories, and other sources. The confidentiality of case registries must be ensured by state and local health authorities. The release of names from disease registries is protected by a variety of state and local laws and regulations, and public health surveillance systems have an excellent record of protecting the confidentiality of case information. If confidentiality is compromised, potential reporters will be hesitant to forward case

Table 97-1. Case Definitions for Public Health Surveillance: Acquired Immune Deficiency Syndrome (AIDS)

Definitive Diagnostic Methods for Diseases Indicative of AIDS

Diseases	Diagnostic Methods
Cryptosporidiosis Isosporiasis Kaposi's sarcoma Lymphoma Pneumocystis carinii pneumonia Progressive multifocal leukoencephalopathy Toxoplasmosis Cervical cancer	Microscopy (histology or cytology)
Candidiasis	Gross inspection by endoscopy or autopsy or by microscopy (histology or cytology) on a specimen obtained directly from the tissues affected (including scrapings from the mucosal surface), not from culture
Coccidioidomycosis Cryptococcosis Cytomegalovirus Herpes simplex virus Histoplasmosis	Microscopy (histology or cytology), culture, or detection of antigen in a specimen obtained directly from the tissues affected or a fluid from those tissues
Tuberculosis Other mycobacteriosis Salmonellosis	Culture
HIV encephalopathy (dementia)	Clinical findings of disabling cognitive or motor dysfunction interfering with occupation or activities of daily living, progressing over weeks to months, in the absence of a concurrent illness or condition other than HIV infection that could explain the findings. Methods to rule out such concurrent illness and conditions must include cerebrospinal fluid examination and either brain imaging (computed tomography or magnetic resonance) or autopsy
HIV wasting syndrome	Findings of profound involuntary weight loss of >% of baseline body weight plus either chronic diarrhea (at least two loose stools per day for >30 days), or chronic weakness and documented fever (for >30 days, intermittent or constant) in the absence of a concurrent illness or condition other than HIV infection that could explain the findings (e.g., cancer, tuberculosis, cryptosporidiosis, or other specific enteritis).
Pneumonia, recurrent	Recurrent (more than one episode in a 1-year period), acute (new x-ray evidence not presented earlier) pneumonia diagnosed by both: (a) culture (or other organism-specific diagnostic method) obtained from a clinically reliable specimen of a pathogen that typically causes pneumonia (other than *Pneumocystis carinii* or *Mycobacterium tuberculosis*), and (b) radiologic evidence of pneumonia; cases that do not have laboratory confirmation of a causative organism for one of the episodes of pneumonia will be considered to be presumptively diagnosed.

Suggested guidelines for presumptive diagnosis of diseases indicative of AIDS

Diseases	Presumptive Criteria
Candidiasis of esophagus	a. Recent onset of retro sternal pain on swallowing; AND b. Oral candidiasis diagnosed by the gross appearance of white patches or plaques on an erythematous base or by the microscopic appearance of fugal mycelial filaments from a noncultured specimen scraped from the oral mucosa.
Cytomegalovirus retinitis	A characteristic appearance on serial ophthalmoscopic examinations (e.g., discrete patches of retinal whitening with distinct borders, spreading in a centrifugal manner along the paths of blood vessels, progressing over several months, and frequency associated with retinal vasculitis, hemorrhage, and necrosis). Resolution of active disease leaves retinal scarring and atrophy with retinal pigment epithelial mottling.
Mycobacteriosis	Microscopy of a specimen from stool or normally sterile body fluids or tissue from a site other than lungs, skin, or cervical or hilar lymph nodes that shows acidfast bacilli of a species not identified by culture.
Kaposi's sarcoma	A characteristic gross appearance of an erythematous or violaceous plaque-like lesion on skin or mucous membrane. (*Note:* Presumptive diagnosis of Kaposi's sarcoma should not be made by clinicians who have seen few cases of it.)
Pneumocystis carinii pneumonia	a. A history of dyspnea on exertion or nonproductive cough of recent onset (within the past 3 months); AND b. Chest x-ray evidence of diffuse bilateral interstitial infiltrates or evidence by gallium scan of diffuse bilateral pulmonary disease; AND c. Arterial blood gas analysis showing an arterial pO2 of <70 mm Hg or a low respiratory diffusing capacity (<80% of predicted values) or an increase in the alveolar-arterial oxygen tension gradient; AND d. No evidence of a bacterial pneumonia.

Table 97-1. Case Definitions for Public Health Surveillance: Acquired Immune Deficiency Syndrome (AIDS) *(Continued)*

Suggested guidelines for presumptive diagnosis of diseases indicative of AIDS

Diseases	Presumptive Criteria
Pneumonia, recurrent	Recurrent (more than one episode in a 1-year period), acute (new symptoms, signs, or x-ray evidence not present earlier) pneumonia diagnosed on clinical or radiologic grounds by the patient's physician.
Toxoplasmosis of brain	a. Recent onset of a focal neurologic abnormality consistent with intracranial disease or a reduced level of consciousness; AND b. Evidence by brain imaging (computed tomography or nuclear magnetic resonance) of a lesion having a mass effect or the radiographic appearance of which is enhanced by injection of contrast medium; AND c. Serum antibody to toxoplasmosis or successful response to therapy for toxoplasmosis.
Tuberculosis, pulmonary	When bacteriologic confirmation is not available, other reports may be considered to be verified cases of pulmonary tuberculosis if the criteria of the Division of Tuberculosis Elimination, National Center for Prevention Services, CDC, are used. The criteria in use as of January 1, 1993, are available in *MMWR* 1990; 39(No. RR-13):39–40.

Table 97-2. Case Definitions for Public Health Surveillance: Other Sexually Transmitted Diseases (STDs)

Diseases	Case Definition
Chancroid	*Clinical Description:* A sexually transmitted disease characterized by painful genital ulceration and inflammatory inguinal adenopathy. The disease is caused by infection with *Haemophilus ducreyi.* *Laboratory Criteria for Diagnosis:* Isolation of *H. ducreyi* from a clinical specimen *Case Classification:* **Probable**—A clinically compatible case with one or more painful genital ulcers and both a) no evidence of *Treponema pallidum* infection by darkfield examination of ulcer exudate or by a serologic test for syphilis performed at least 7 days after onset of ulcers, and b) the clinical presentation of the ulcer(s) is not typical of disease caused by herpes simplex virus (HSV), or HSV culture is negative **Confirmed**—A case that is laboratory confirmed
Chlamydia trachomatis, genital infections	(revised March 1995) *Clinical Description:* Infection with sexually transmitted *Chlamydia trachomatis* may result in urethritis, epididymitis, cervicitis, acute salpingitis, but is often asymptomatic in women. Perinatal infections may result in inclusion conjunctivitis and pneumonia among newborns. Other syndromes caused by *C. trachomatis* include lymphogranuloma venereum and trachoma. *Laboratory Criteria for Diagnosis:* Isolation of *C. trachomatis* by culture, or demonstration of *C. trachomatis* in a clinical specimen by detection of antigen or nucleic acids *Case Classification:* **Confirmed**—A case that is laboratory confirmed
Genital Herpes (Herpes Simplex Virus)	*Clinical Description:* An illness characterized by visible, painful genital or anogenital lesions *Laboratory Criteria for Diagnosis:* Isolation of herpes simplex virus from cervix, urethra, or anogenital lesion, or demonstration of virus by antigen detection technique in clinical specimens from cervix, urethra, or anogenital lesion, or demonstration of multinucleated giant cells on a Tzanck smear of scrapings from an anogenital lesion *Case Classification:* **Probable**—A clinically compatible case (in which primary and secondary syphilis have been ruled out by serology and darkfield microscopy, when available) with either a diagnosis of genital herpes based on clinical presentation (without laboratory confirmation) or a history of one or more previous episodes of similar genital lesions **Confirmed**—A clinically compatible case that is laboratory confirmed *Comment:* Herpes should be reported only once per patient. The first diagnosis for a patient with no previous diagnosis should be reported.
Genital Warts	*Clinical Description:* An infection characterized by the presence of visible, exophytic (raised) growths on the internal or external genitalia, perineum, or perianal region *Laboratory Criteria for Diagnosis:* Histopathologic changes characteristic of human papillomavirus (HPV) infection on biopsy or exfoliative cytology *Case Classification:* **Probable**—A clinically compatible case without histopathologic diagnosis and without microscopic or serologic evidence that the growth is due to secondary syphilis **Confirmed**—A clinically compatible case that is laboratory confirmed

Table 97-2. Case Definitions for Public Health Surveillance: Other Sexually Transmitted Diseases (STDs) *(Continued)*

Diseases	Case Definition
Gonorrhea	*Clinical Description:* A sexually transmitted infection commonly manifested by urethritis, cervicitis, or salpingitis. Infection may be asymptomatic. *Laboratory Criteria for Diagnosis:* Isolation of Neisseria gonorrhoeae from a clinical specimen, or Observation of Gram-negative intracellular diplococci in a urethral smear obtained from a man *Case Classification:* **Probable**—Demonstration of gram-negative intracellular diplococci in an endocervical smear obtained from a woman, or a written (morbidity) report of gonorrhea submitted by a physician **Confirmed**—A case that is laboratory confirmed
Granuloma Inguinale	*Clinical Description:* A slowly progressive ulcerative disease of the skin and lymphatics of the genital and perianal area caused by infection with *Calymmatobacterium granulomatis.* A clinically compatible case would have one or more painless or minimally painful granulomatous lesions in the anogenital area. *Laboratory Criteria for Diagnosis:* Demonstration of intracytoplasmic Donovan bodies in Wright or Giemsa-stained smears or biopsies of granulation tissue *Case Classification:* **Confirmed**—A clinically compatible case that is laboratory confirmed
Hepatitis B	*Clinical Case Definition:* An illness with a) discrete onset of symptoms and b) jaundice or elevated serum aminotransferase levels *Laboratory Criteria for Diagnosis:* IgM anti-HBc-positive (if done) or HBsAg-positive, and IgM anti-HAV-negative (if done) *Case Classification:* **Confirmed**—Case that meets the clinical case definition and is laboratory confirmed *Comment:* Chronic carriage or chronic hepatitis should not be reported.
Lymphogranuloma Venereum Infection	*Clinical Description:* Infection with L1, L2, or, L3 serovars of *Chlamydia trachomatis* may result in a disease characterized by genital lesions, suppurative regional lymphadenopathy, or hemorrhagic proctitis. The infection is usually sexually transmitted. *Laboratory Criteria for Diagnosis:* Isolation of *C. trachomatis,* serotype L1, L2, or L3, from clinical specimen, or demonstration of inclusion bodies by immunofluorescence in leukocytes of an inguinal lymph node (bubo) aspirate, or positive microimmunofluorescent serologic test for a *lymphogranuloma venereum* strain of *C. trachomatis* (in a clinically compatible case) *Case Classification:* **Probable**—A clinically compatible case with one or more tender fluctuant inguinal lymph nodes or characteristic proctogenital lesions with supportive laboratory findings of a single *C. trachomatis* complement fixation (CF) titer of greater than 64 **Confirmed:** A case that is laboratory confirmed
Nongonococcal Urethritis	*Clinical Description:* Urethral inflammation that is not the result of infection with *Neisseria gonorrhoeae.* Urethral inflammation may be diagnosed by the presence of one of the following criteria: A visible abnormal urethral discharge (excludes scant amounts of clear mucus); a positive leukocyte esterase test from men less than 60 years of age without a history of kidney disease or bladder infection, prostate enlargement, urogenital anatomic anomaly; or recent urinary tract instrumentation; microscopic evidence of urethritis (greater than or equal to 5 WBC per high-power field) on a Gram stain of a urethral smear *Laboratory Criteria for Diagnosis:* No evidence of *N. gonorrhoeae* infection by culture or Gram stain *Case Classification:* **Confirmed**—A clinically compatible case among males in whom gonorrhea is not found, either by culture or Gram stain *Comment:* Nongonococcal urethritis (NGU) is a clinical diagnosis of exclusion. The syndrome may result from infection with several agents (see *Chlamydia trachomatis* genital infections). A clinically compatible case excluding gonorrhea and chlamydia should be classified as NGU. An illness among men that meets the case definition of NGU and *C. trachomatis* infection should be classified as chlamydia.
Pelvic Inflammatory Disease	*Clinical Case Definition:* A clinical syndrome resulting from the ascending spread of microorganisms from the vagina and endocervix to the endometrium, fallopian tubes, and/or contiguous structures. All of the following clinical criteria must be present: Abdominal direct tenderness; and tenderness with motion of the cervix; and adnexal tenderness. In addition to all of the above criteria, at least one of the following findings must also be present: Meets the surveillance case definition of *Chlamydia trachomatis* infection or gonorrhea; or temperature greater than 38 C; or leukocytosis greater than 10,000 WBC/cu mm; or purulent material in the peritoneal cavity obtained by culdocentesis or laparoscopy; or pelvic abscess or inflammatory complex on bimanual examination or by

Table 97-2. Case Definitions for Public Health Surveillance: Other Sexually Transmitted Diseases (STDs) ***(Continued)***

Diseases	Case Definition
	sonography; or patient is a sexual contact of a person known to have gonorrhea, chlamydia, or nongonococcal urethritis *Case Classification:* **Confirmed**—A case that meets the clinical case definition
Syphilis	Syphilis is a complex, sexually transmitted disease with a highly variable clinical course. Classification by a clinician with expertise in syphilis may take precedence over the following case definitions developed for surveillance purposes.
Primary Syphilis	*Clinical Description:* The characteristic lesion of primary syphilis is the chancre, but atypical primary lesions may occur. *Laboratory Criteria for Diagnosis:* Demonstration of *Treponema pallidum* in clinical specimens by darkfield, fluorescent antibody, or equivalent microscopic methods *Case Classification:* **Probable**—A clinically compatible case with one or more ulcers (chancres) consistent with primary syphilis and a reactive serologic test **Confirmed**—A clinically compatible case that is laboratory confirmed
Secondary Syphilis	*Clinical Description:* A stage of infection due to *Treponema pallidum,* characterized by localized or diffuse mucocutaneous lesions and generalized lymphadenopathy. Constitutional symptoms are common, and clinical manifestations are protean. The primary chancre may still be present. *Laboratory Criteria for Diagnosis:* Demonstration of *T. pallidum* in clinical specimens by darkfield, fluorescent antibody, or equivalent microscopic methods *Case Classification:* **Probable**—A clinically compatible case with a reactive nontreponemal (VDRL, RPR) test titer of greater than or equal to 4 **Confirmed**—A clinically compatible case that is laboratory confirmed
Latent Syphilis	*Clinical Description:* A stage of infection due to *Treponema pallidum* in which organisms persist in the body of the infected person without causing symptoms or signs. Latent syphilis is subdivided into early, late, and unknown syphilis categories based upon the length of elapsed time from initial infection. *Case Classification:* **Presumptive**—No clinical signs or symptoms of syphilis and the presence of one of the following: No past diagnosis of syphilis and a reactive nontreponemal test, and a reactive treponemal (fluorescent treponemal; or antibody-absorbed [FTA-ABS], microhemagglutination assay for antibody to *Treponema pallidum* [MHA-TP]) test; or a past history of syphilis therapy and a current nontreponemal test titer demonstrating fourfold or greater increase from the last nontreponemal test titer
Early Latent Syphilis	*Clinical Description:* A subcategory of latent syphilis. When initial infection has occurred within the previous 12 months, latent syphilis is classified as early. *Case Classification:* **Presumptive**—Latent syphilis (see above) of a person who has evidence of having acquired the infection within the previous 12 months based on one or more of the following criteria: A nonreactive serologic test for syphilis or a nontreponemal titer that has dropped fourfold within the past 12 months; or a history of symptoms consistent with primary or secondary syphilis without a history of subsequent treatment in the past 12 months; or a history of sexual exposure to a partner with confirmed or presumptive primary or secondary syphilis, or presumptive early latent syphilis, and no history of treatment in the past 12 months; or reactive nontreponemal and treponemal tests from an individual whose only possible exposure occurred within the preceding 12 months
Late Latent Syphilis	*Clinical Description:* A subcategory of latent syphilis. When initial infection has occurred greater than 1 year previously, latent syphilis is classified as late. *Case Classification:* **Presumptive**—Latent syphilis (see above) of a patient who shows no evidence of having acquired the disease within the past 12 months (see Early Latent Syphilis) and whose age and titer do not meet the criteria specified for unknown latent syphilis
Unknown Latent Syphilis	*Clinical Description:* A subcategory of latent syphilis. When the date of initial infection cannot be established as occurring within the previous year, and the patient's age and titer meet criteria described below, latent syphilis is classified as unknown latent. *Case Classification:* **Presumptive**—Latent syphilis (see above) that does not meet the criteria for early latent syphilis, and the patient is 13–35 years of age with a nontreponemal test serologic titer of greater than or equal to 32
Neurosyphilis	*Clinical Description:* Evidence of CNS infection with *Treponema pallidum* *Laboratory Criteria for Diagnosis:* A reactive serologic test for syphilis and reactive VDRL in cerebrospinal fluid (CSF)

Table 97-2. Case Definitions for Public Health Surveillance: Other Sexually Transmitted Diseases (STDs)

Diseases	Case Definition
	Case Classification: **Presumptive**—Syphilis of any stage, a negative VDRL in CSF, and both of the following: Elevated CSF protein or leukocyte count in the absence of other known causes of these abnormalities; and clinical symptoms or signs consistent with neurosyphilis without other known causes for these clinical abnormalities **Confirmed**—Syphilis, of any stage, that meets the laboratory criteria for neurosyphilis
Congenital Syphilis	*Clinical Description:* A condition caused by infection in utero with *Treponema pallidum.* A wide spectrum of severity exists, and only severe cases are clinically apparent at birth. An infant (<2 years) may have signs such as hepatosplenomegaly, characteristic skin rash, condyloma lata, snuffles, jaundice (nonviral hepatitis), pseudoparalysis, anemia, or edema (nephrotic syndrome and/or malnutrition). An older child may have stigmata such as interstitial keratitis, nerve deafness, anterior bowing of shins, frontal bossing, mulberry molars, Hutchinson teeth, saddle nose, rhagades, or Clutton joints. *Laboratory Criteria for Diagnosis:* Demonstration of *T. pallidum* by darkfield microscopy, fluorescent antibody, or other specific stains in specimens from lesions, placenta, umbilical cord, or autopsy material *Case Classification:* **Presumptive**—The infection of an infant whose mother had untreated or inadequately treated syphilis at delivery (inadequate treatment consists of any nonpenicillin therapy or penicillin given less than 30 days before delivery), regardless of signs in the infant; or the infection of an infant or child who has a reactive treponemal test for syphilis and any one of the following: Any evidence of congenital syphilis on physical examination; or any evidence of congenital syphilis on long bone x-ray; or a reactive cerebrospinal fluid (CSF) VDRL; or an elevated CSF cell count or protein (without other cause); or a reactive test for fluorescent treponemal antibody absorbed-19S-IgM antibody **Confirmed**—A case (among infants) that is laboratory confirmed *Comment:* Congenital and acquired syphilis may be difficult to distinguish when a child is seropositive after infancy. Signs of congenital syphilis may not be obvious, and stigmata may not yet have developed. Abnormal values for CSF VDRL, cell count, and protein, as well as IgM antibodies, may be found in either congenital or acquired syphilis. Findings on long bone x-rays may help, since x-ray changes in the metaphysis and epiphysis are considered classic for congenitally acquired disease. The decision may ultimately be based on maternal history and clinical judgment. The possibility of sexual abuse should be considered. For reporting purposes, congenital syphilis includes cases of congenitally acquired syphilis among infants and children, as well as syphilitic stillbirths.
Syphilitic Stillbirth	*Clinical Case Definition:* A fetal death that occurs after a 20-week gestation or in which the fetus weighs greater than 500 g, and the mother had untreated or inadequately treated syphilis at delivery (inadequate treatment consists of any nonpenicillin therapy or penicillin given <30 days before delivery). *Comment:* For reporting purposes, syphilitic stillbirths should be reported as cases of congenital syphilis.

information, and the completeness of reporting will decrease. Although case reporting is legally mandated, the completeness of case reporting from those required to report may differ depending on the ease of reporting, the number of cases to be reported, availability of staff to report cases, and other factors. Active surveillance systems, whereby health department specialists actively solicit case reports from health care providers or laboratories, provide more complete reporting than passive reporting systems.[4,5] The most recent evaluation of AIDS surveillance, an active case-finding system, found that 85 to 90 percent of persons with AIDS-defining opportunistic illnesses were reported to the AIDS surveillance system.[6]

Disease registries are used to construct unduplicated case counts of disease occurrences, conduct follow-up investigations of cases of particular epidemiologic importance, and as a starting point to ensure that reported persons are receiving prevention and treatment services. Because registries comprise mandated reports from all reporting sources in a state or other geographic area, these surveillance data are used to calculate disease rates for the population. Periodically, states voluntarily send HIV/AIDS and other STD surveillance data without personal identifiers (such as name or address) to CDC, where national and regional analyses are performed. Based on these analyses, CDC issues a variety of national surveillance reports.

HIV/AIDS SURVEILLANCE

From 1981, when the AIDS epidemic was first recognized and surveillance began, through June 1996, 548,102 adults and children with AIDS have been reported to CDC.[7–9] Over this period, AIDS surveillance data documented the rapid increase in case rates through the early to mid-1980s and a slowing of the growth of the epidemic through the first half of 1996 (Fig. 97-2). In 1995, estimated AIDS incidence was 29 per 100,000 population and increased less than 2 percent from the rate in 1994, suggesting that the national AIDS epidemic reached a plateau in 1995 and decreased in 1996. This decline in 1996 is related to treatment advances which have slowed the progression of HIV disease and

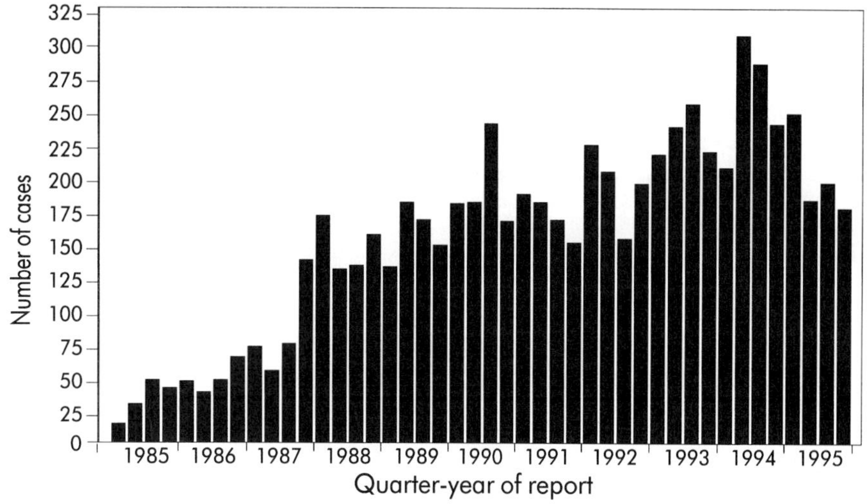

Fig. 97-2. AIDS cases by quarter-year of report through December 1995.

this decline is observed in several sub-populations of persons with HIV disease.[10] As the growth of the AIDS epidemic slowed, AIDS surveillance data have revealed the changing characteristics of persons with AIDS.[10–16] During 1990 to 1996, for men, the estimated incidence of AIDS was approximately level for homosexual and bisexual men compared with increases in AIDS incidence for male injecting drug users and men with heterosexually-acquired AIDS (Fig. 97–3). Accordingly the proportion of cases related to male homosexual activity decreased from 64% of 39,400 AIDS cases diagnosed among men in 1990 to 56% of 45,200 diagnosed among men in 1996. Simultaneously, for women, the proportionate increase in AIDS incidence during 1990 through 1996 was approximately 13 times that for men (91 vs 7%), and the number of annual cases in women related to heterosexual transmission has surpassed the number related to injecting drug use (Fig. 97-4). In 1996, AIDS rates for black adults were seven times greater than for whites and four times greater for Hispanic adults than for whites—a disparity that has widened in the most recent years.[10] From 1990 through 1996, AIDS incidence for blacks and Hispanics increased 54 percent for blacks and 9 percent for Hispanics compared with a 9% decline in AIDS cases among whites (Fig. 97-5). AIDS surveillance data have also signaled a decrease in perinatally acquired AIDS temporally related to guidelines for zidovidine therapy to interrupt transmission and an increase in the rates of AIDS in small and medium-sized metropolitan areas and rural areas, particularly in the South.[10,17]

Confidential HIV infection reporting is also an important way to complement AIDS surveillance data to monitor the HIV epidemic since it examines HIV-infected persons at an earlier stage of disease than it does persons with AIDS. For the 29 states that have adopted this surveillance system, HIV infection reporting provides a minimum estimate of the number of persons diagnosed with HIV infection in the area. For example, in 1995, New Jersey received 2,565 reports of HIV infection in addition to the 4,409 case reports of AIDS.[10] HIV infection reporting data have been used to anticipate trends that have been later verified by AIDS surveillance.[18] HIV infection reporting may be particularly useful in describing the extent of HIV infection in adolescents and young persons who are under-represented in AIDS case reports because of the long latency from HIV infection to AIDS (Fig. 97-6). HIV reporting also provides an opportunity to conduct more in-depth epidemiologic investigations among adolescents and other persons with evidence of recent HIV infection.[19] However, the interpretation of HIV infection reporting data is limited by the variability of HIV testing practices and the test-seeking behaviors of individuals across areas and over time. Thus, the characteristics of persons reported with HIV infection are not necessarily representative of all persons with HIV infection. In addition, HIV infection surveillance has not been more widely adopted, in part, because of concerns about the possibility that HIV infection reporting by name deters persons from seeking HIV counseling and testing.[20]

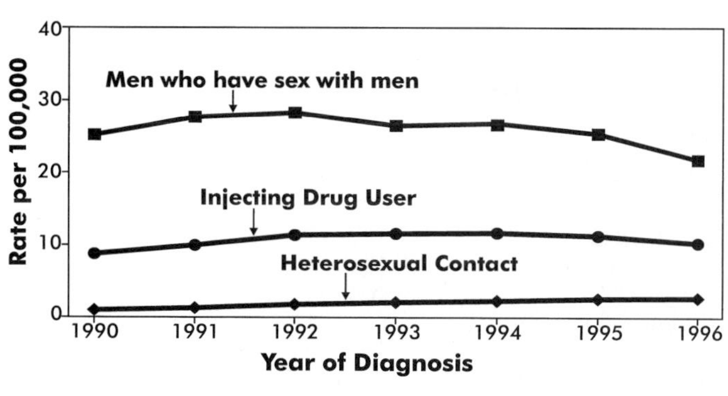

Fig. 97-3. Estimated AIDS incidence rate by risk exposure among men per 100,000 population 1990–1996, United States.

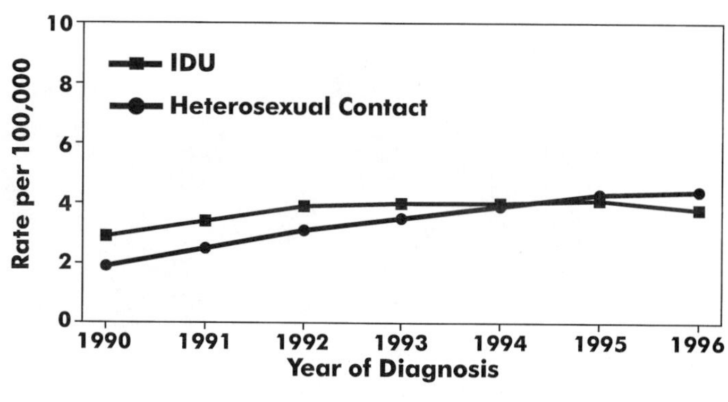

Fig. 97-4. Estimated AIDS incidence rate by risk exposure among women per 100,000 population, 1990–1996, United States.

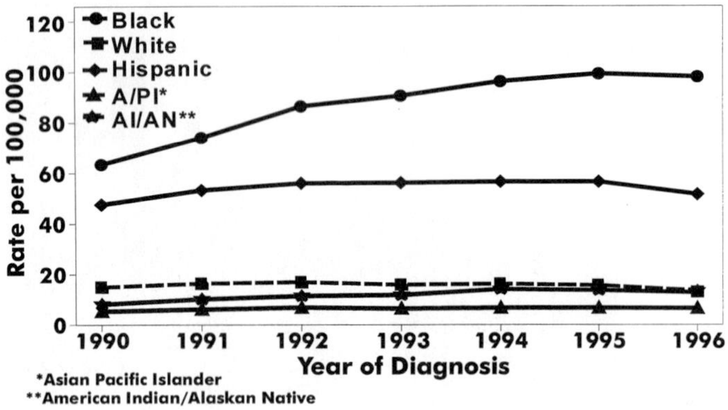

Fig. 97-5. Estimated AIDS incidence by race/ethnicity per 100,000 population, 1990–1996.

Chlamydia trachomatis surveillance

Although the surveillance of chlamydia infections is improving, it remains incomplete in many areas of the country. A combination of factors limits documentation of the incidence and prevalence of genital chlamydia infection, such as variable compliance with public health laws and regulations that require health care providers and laboratories to report cases to local health authorities; large numbers of asymptomatic persons who can be identified only through screening; limited resources for screening activities; and incomplete information management infrastructures for collecting, maintaining, and analyzing morbidity data. Thus, for most areas, the number of chlamydia cases reported to CDC by state health departments reflects both the degree of local interest in chlamydia as a public health problem and initial attempts to resolve reporting limitations, rather than true disease burden or trends.

In 1996, 490,080 chlamydia infections were reported to CDC from 49 states, the District of Columbia, and New York City, making chlamydia the most commonly reported notifiable disease in the United States for the third consecutive year.[21] This was the third consecutive year that chlamydia cases exceeded the number of reported cases of gonorrhea.[22] Surveillance trends demonstrating progressive increases in chlamydia rates continue to reflect primarily increased screening for and recognition of asymptomatic infection (mainly in women) and improved reporting capacity rather than true trends in disease incidence. Although this surveillance system measures cases detected, measures of the percentage of positive test results for women screened for chlamydia is a more useful gauge of disease burden. Trends in percentage of positive tests are steadily decreasing in areas where chlamydia screening has been widely implemented, suggesting that screening is playing a major role in reducing the amount of infection in these populations (Fig. 97-7). Differential screening practices are believed, for the most part, to explain the higher 1996 rate of chlamydia for women (321.5 per 100,000 population) compared with that for men (60.4 per 100,000 population) (Fig. 97-8). In 1996, the chlamydia case rate was highest in the South, reflecting a recent expansion of screening activity in this Region. Prior to 1996, chlamydia rates were highest in the West and Midwest, where substantial resources had been initially committed for organized screening programs, especially in family planning clinics. In the areas where these screening programs are in place, chlamydia rates far exceed gonorrhea rates. During a 9-year demonstration project in the Pacific Northwest, family planning clinic screening programs have consistently demonstrated both the highest chlamydia positivity rates for adolescents (Fig. 97-9) and higher positivity rates for black and Native American women than for women of other races.[22] The large number of reported cases of chlamydia and the serious sequelae that may result from chronic infection emphasize the need for standardized surveillance to target screening and treatment resources.

Neisseria gonorrhoeae surveillance

In 1996, 325,883 cases of gonorrhea were reported to CDC.[22] The rate of gonorrhea has declined in the United States since 1975; from 1995 through 1996, the rate decreased 17% from 149.4 cases to 124.0 cases per 100,000 population (Fig. 97-10). The 1996 gonorrhea rate is the lowest rate since national reporting began. Gonorrhea rates decreased between 1995 and 1996 in 32 of the 35 states reporting more than 1,000 cases in 1996. The geographic distribution of gonorrhea is similar to that of primary and secondary syphilis and of HIV in childbearing women (Fig. 97-11). The general decrease in regional gonorrhea rates continued in 1996, although the South continued to exhibit the

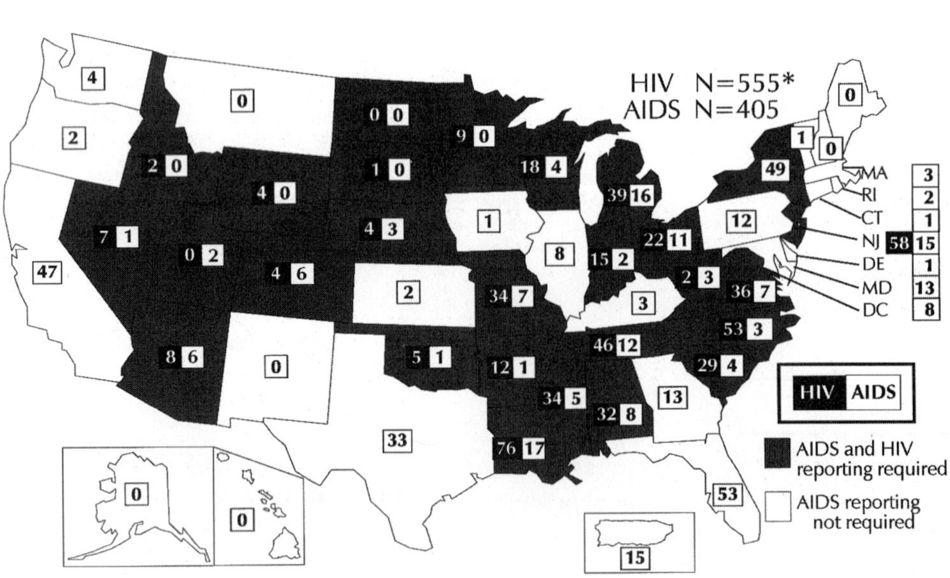

Fig. 97-6. HIV infections (not AIDS) and AIDS in adolescents (13–19 years) reported in 1995.

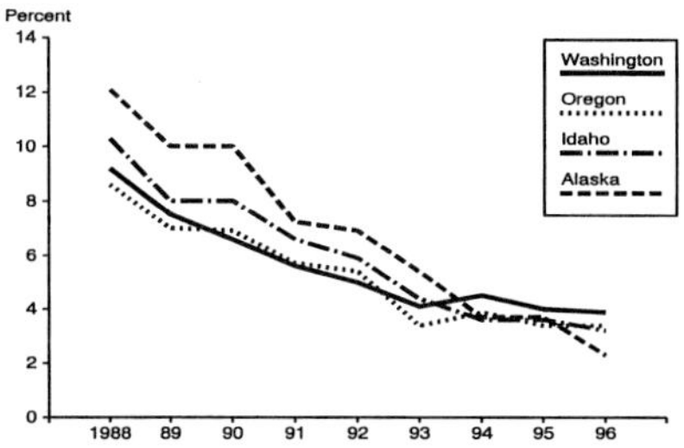

Note: Women who met screening criteria were tested.

Source: Region X Chlamydia Project (Alaska, Idaho, Oregon and Washington)

Fig. 97-7. Chlamydia—percent positivity among women tested in family planning clinics by state: region X, 1988–1996.

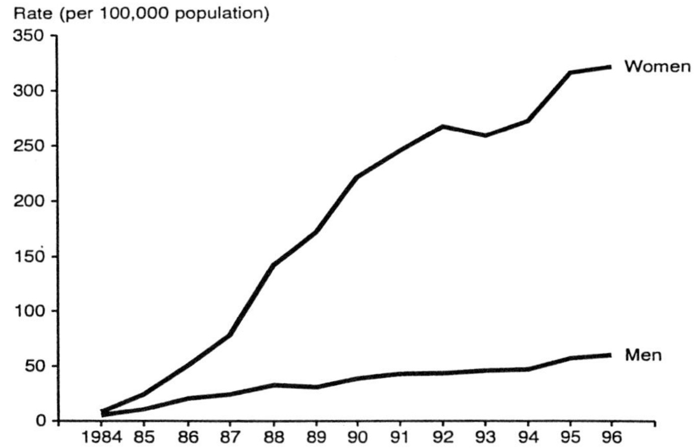

Fig. 97-8. Chlamydia—rates by gender: United States, 1984–1996.

highest regional rate. The gonorrhea rate for men continued to decline in 1996, as did the rate for women. In 1996, gonorrhea rates decreased for all racial and ethnic groups except American Indians/Alaska Natives for whom the rate increased 12.6 percent, from 92.9 in 1995 to 105.6 in 1996. The gonorrhea rate for blacks decreased from 1045.5 cases per 100,000 population in 1995 to 825.5 in 1996, but remained 31-fold higher than for whites (Fig. 97-12). Gonorrhea is also a major health problem for adolescents. The highest rates of gonorrhea for women (756.8 per 100,000) and the second highest rates for men (394.3 per 100,000) in 1996 occurred for adolescents (15 to 19 years old). Between 1995 and 1996, the gonorrhea rate for 15- to 19-year-old adolescents decreased by 14.9 percent from 670.7 to 570.8 cases per 100,000 population. Gonorrhea is a particular problem among black adolescents for whom the rates were 24-fold higher than for white adolescents (3063.6 vs 129.7).

SYPHILIS SURVEILLANCE

Syphilis surveillance is primarily conducted at the local level in conjunction with notification, screening, and therapeutic services for infected persons and their sexual contacts. Syphilis surveillance data have been used to examine national and regional trends and rate disparities among racial/ethnic groups. The well-circumscribed geographic distribution of syphilis cases is used to allocate STD prevention resources to high incidence areas.[22,23] After an increase in the late 1980s, the syphilis rate declined during the 1990s. In 1996, the 4.3 cases of diagnosed primary and secondary (P&S) syphilis per 100,000 population was 32 percent less than the 1995 rate of 6.3 per 100,000. The 11,387 reported P&S cases was the lowest number reported since 1959. The rate of congenital syphilis also decreased from 47.4 cases per 100,000 live births in 1995 to 30.4 cases in 1996. In 1996, the highest regional rate of syphilis occurred in the South (8.7 cases per 100,000 population). P&S syphilis rates differ widely and 73 percent of U.S. counties reported no cases, whereas many other counties reported very few cases (Fig. 97-13). In 1996 the geographic distribution of syphilis was highly concentrated: 50 percent of all reported P&S syphilis cases came from less than 1.2 percent of U.S. counties. Since 1990, the rates of P&S syphilis have declined for all racial and ethnic groups. However, the 1996 rate for blacks (30.2 cases per 100,000 population) was 50 times greater than the rate for whites.

Some caution is warranted in interpreting both gonorrhea and syphilis trends. There are often differences among reporting areas in the methods used to collect surveillance data and the degree to which uniform case definitions are adhered to, both within and among reporting areas. In many areas reporting from publicly supported institutions such as STD clinics is more complete than from private providers. In many areas, minority populations are

Fig. 97-9. Chlamydia—percent positivity among women tested in family planning clinics by age group: region X, 1988–1996.

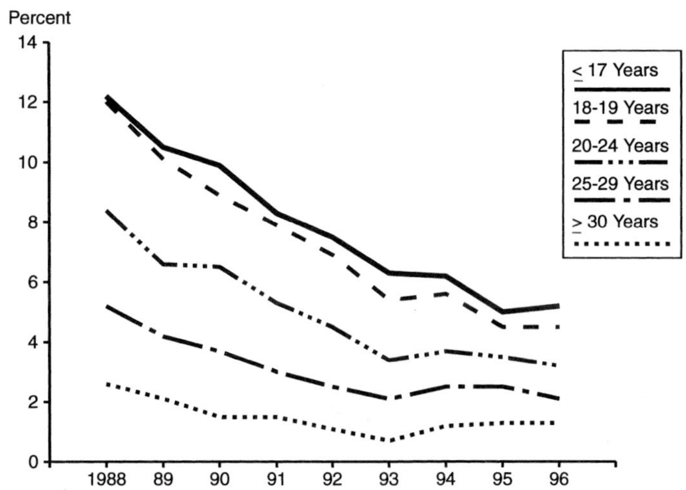

Note: Women who met screening criteria were tested.
Source: Region X Chlamydia Project (Alaska, Idaho, Oregon and Washington)

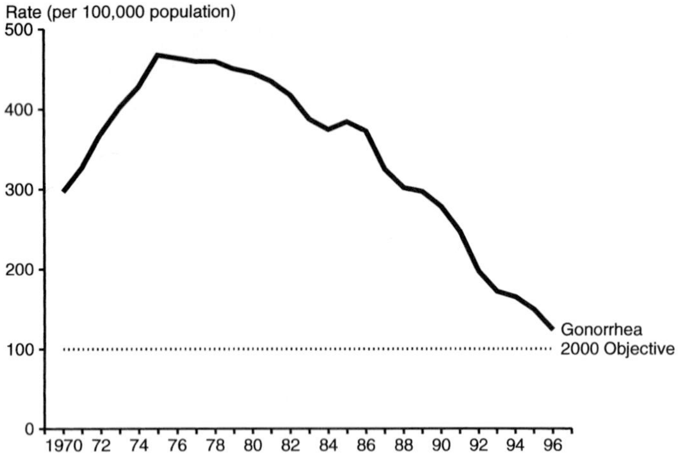

Fig. 97-10. Gonorrhea—reported rates: United States, 1970–1996 and the Healthy People year 2000 objective.

disproportionately served in these types of public health clinic sites. Another concern that could affect the interpretation of public health surveillance data is the drive toward cost containment in private health services. In some instances the decision to treat common STDs syndromically (without laboratory confirmation) could lead to reports of decreasing STD rates when rates may actually be stable or even increasing. Even when laboratory confirmation is sought by a provider, the use of large, centralized commercial laboratories in another state may interfere with timely, complete reporting of STDs by that laboratory to the health department in the patient's home of record.

SENTINEL SURVEILLANCE

Sentinel surveillance systems may work as early warning systems, but more frequently they monitor health markers in a defined population or setting. Sentinel surveillance systems collect data that are not generally available in disease registries. These data may range from risk exposures and health-seeking behaviors, such as screening information, to information about related illnesses and characteristics of the causative organisms. Three examples of sentinel surveillance systems for STDs and HIV/AIDS are those that are used to characterize changes in the antibiotic susceptibility of *Neisseria gonorrhoeae,* to determine trends in chlamydia prevalence in selected subpopulations, and to determine trends in HIV infection through blinded serologic testing in selected clinical and screening settings. Although sentinel surveillance does not typically allow disease rates to be calculated for the general population, the use of standardized survey methods and laboratory test procedures permit data to be compared across sites and time. However, changes in the population served by a clinic or laboratory, or changes in the screening practices for a targeted population must be taken into account when sentinel surveillance data are analyzed.

Gonococcal isolate surveillance project

This laboratory-based system collects antibiotic susceptibility data for *Neisseria gonorrhoeae* in 26 U.S. STD clinics and five laboratories that analyze approximately 400 gonococcal isolates each month.[22] Antimicrobial resistance remains an important consideration in the treatment of gonorrhea, and temporal changes in susceptibility must be detected to reduce the likelihood of treatment failures. Overall, 29.0 percent of isolates collected in 1996 by the Gonococcal Isolate Surveillance Project (GISP) were resist-

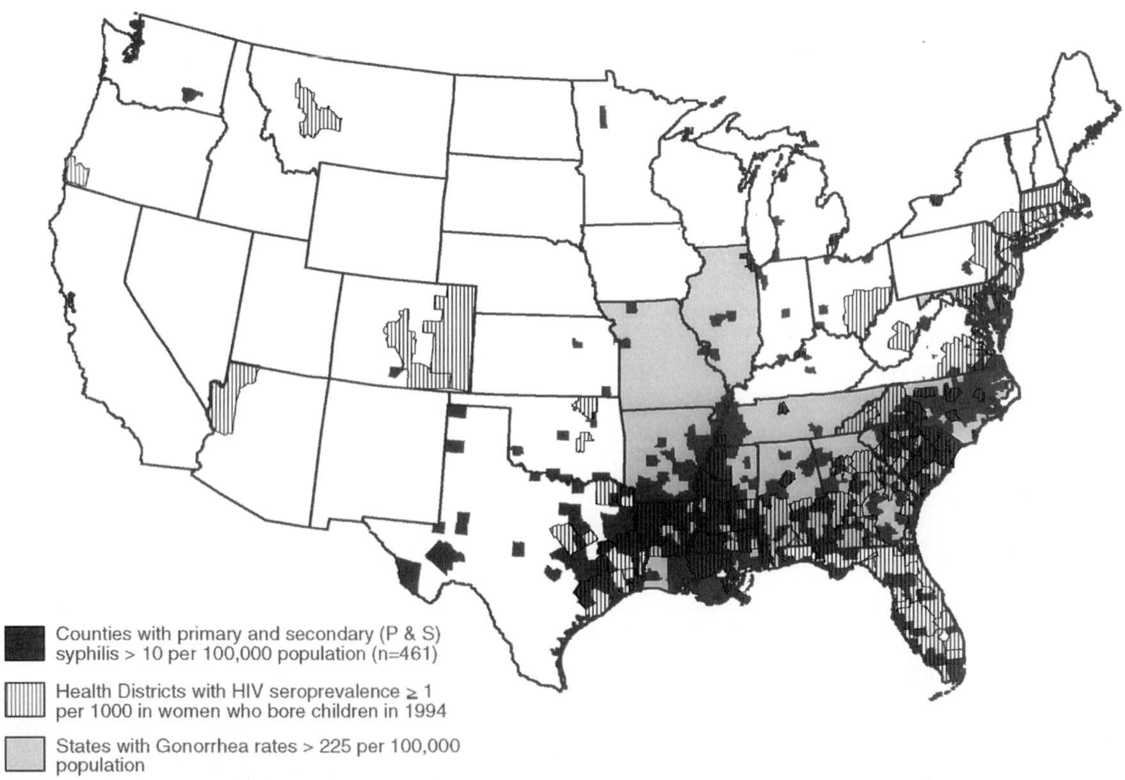

Fig. 97-11. Health districts with the highest HIV seroprevalence in women who bore children in 1994, counties reporting the highest primary and secondary syphilis rates (1993), and states reporting the highest gonorrhea rates (1993), United States.

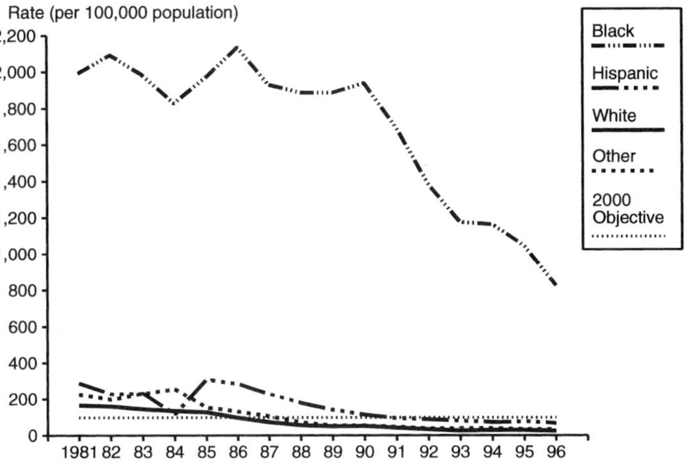

Fig. 97-12. Gonorrhea—rates by race and ethnicity: United States, 1981–1996 and the Healthy People year 2000 objective.

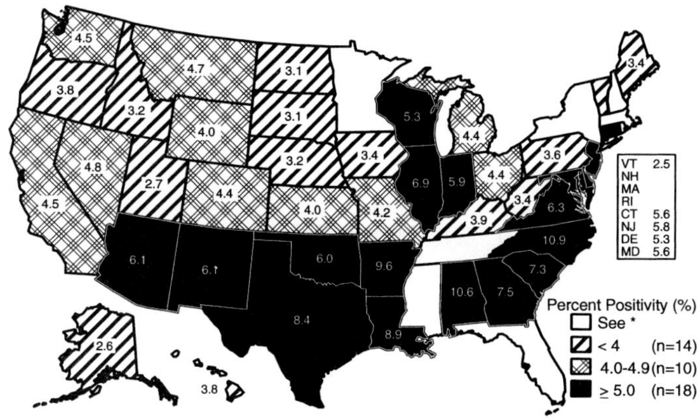

Fig. 97-14. Chlamydia—percent positivity among 15- to 24-year-old women tested in selected family planning clinics by state, 1996. (*These states did not report chlamydia positivity data or reported on fewer than 1,000 women screened during 1996.)

ant to penicillin or tetracycline or both; this rate is similar to that observed in earlier years. Fortunately, this sentinel surveillance system has yet to demonstrate clinically significant resistance to the antimicrobial agents currently recommended for therapy of gonorrhea. However, some gonococcal isolates have begun to demonstrate decreased levels of susceptibility to some of these agents, suggesting that the emergence of resistant strains may be forthcoming.

Chlamydia prevalence monitoring

Surveillance systems that monitor chlamydia prevalence (number of positive tests/number screened times 100) in populations are established in areas where STD screening is done. The populations under surveillance in this type of system are generally those sampled by convenience where large-scale, ongoing screening has already begun, such as in family planning clinics. These data supplement disease registry data from case reports and help clarify the dynamics of chlamydia in a community or region.

Beginning in 1994, with funds provided by the Preventive Health Amendments of 1992, regional clinical screening networks were established across the country, mainly in family planning clinics, to provide chlamydia screening for adolescent girls and young adult women. Each regional network agreed on standard screening criteria, pertinent data elements, and data collection methods. Chlamydia prevalence data from this system are used to document geographic differences and trends in disease burden (Fig. 97-14).

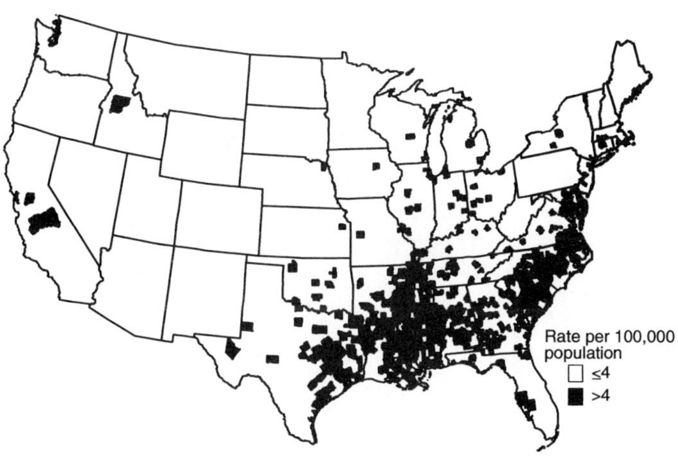

Fig. 97-13. Primary and secondary syphilis—counties with rates above and counties with rates below the Healthy People year 2000 objective: United States, 1996.

HIV serologic surveys

Because of the long interval between infection with HIV and the development of AIDS, additional HIV serologic surveys have been used to supplement the information obtained through AIDS surveillance. These serologic surveys can be used to ascertain the prevalence rate of HIV infection in certain populations. Since 1988, blinded HIV serologic surveys have been conducted in STD clinics, tuberculosis clinics, drug treatment clinics, sentinel hospitals, and other clinical settings.[24–32] Blinded testing avoids self-selection, which may bias estimates of the HIV seroprevalence rate.

Blinded serologic surveys conducted in STD clinics in many metropolitan areas provide a measure of temporal trends in HIV prevalence for persons with new STDs.[28,32] Of the homosexual and bisexual men seen in these clinics in 1993, 30 percent were HIV antibody positive and the rate of HIV infection ranged from 9 to 51 percent. From 1988 to 1995, HIV seroprevalence decreased among homosexual and bisexual men with STDs regardless of race or ethnicity, suggesting that HIV incidence may have decreased as well (Fig. 97-15).[28] The HIV prevalence rate for women in STD clinics has remained at approximately 2.3 percent. Studies in these same clinics have described HIV seroprevalence rates of approximately 8 percent for heterosexual men who reported injecting drug use and 2 percent for heterosexual men who did not report injecting drug use. For each of these risk categories, regardless of behavioral risks, HIV infection rates tend to be higher for blacks than whites.[28]

HIV seroprevalence studies of entrants to drug treatment clinics have demonstrated very high rates of HIV infection for injecting drug users, particularly in the Northeastern United States, and the highest rates of HIV infection continue to be observed for injecting drug users along the Atlantic Coast (Fig. 97-16).[31–33] In 1993, the median seroprevalence was 42 percent in New York City and New Jersey as compared with only 2 percent HIV seroprevalence

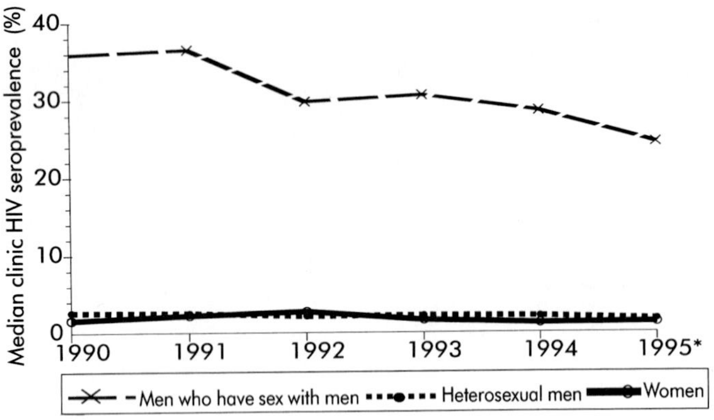

Fig. 97-15. Median HIV seroprevalence among patients attending sexually transmitted disease clinics, 1990–1995.

among injecting drug users in Los Angeles, and a 5 percent seroprevalence in San Francisco. The prevalence of HIV infection for persons in these clinics has been level since 1990, suggesting that the prevalence of HIV infection is not increasing for injecting drug users.

The Survey of Childbearing Women estimates the HIV infection rate for this population through HIV antibody testing of newborn specimens collected as part of metabolic screening.[32,34–35] HIV antibody testing of the infant measures infection in the mother because of the placental transfer of maternal antibodies. These data provide a precise estimate of the number of infections in and the rate of HIV infection for women of childbearing age and have been used to project the size of the epidemic as a whole.[35,36] Information about the childrens infection status is less direct because fewer than one-third of children whose mothers are infected acquire HIV infection. This proportion of infected infants born with perinatal exposure to HIV is further reduced by about two-thirds when zidovidine is used during the perinatal period.[37] In 1994, the Survey of Childbearing Women was conducted in 45 states, the District of Columbia, and the Virgin Islands; the HIV seroprevalence for childbearing women in the United States was 1.5 per 100 live births.[32,38] This rate was similar to the 1.6 per 1000 of the specimens collected in 1989 to 1990.[31] However, the prevalence of HIV for childbearing women has changed during this time in different areas of the country. In the Northeast, the HIV seroprevalence rate decreased from 4.1 per 1,000 live births in 1989 to 2.1 per 1,000 in 1994, whereas the seroprevalence in the South increased from 1.6 per 1,000 in 1989 to 2.0 per 1,000 in 1991; in 1994, the seroprevalence rate in the South decreased to 1.9 per 1000.[38] Childbearing women in some areas of the rural South have rates of HIV infection that approach those for similar women in metropolitan areas of the Northeast.[34] Based on these serosurveillance data, in 1995, nationally, an estimated 6,300 HIV-infected women gave birth and (assuming a 25% rate of maternal (child transmission) 1600 children were born with HIV infection. Approximately 14,000 perinatally infected children are living in the United States.[35,36]

Large groups of persons who are tested routinely provide unique opportunities for sentinel surveillance. These sources are valuable, but they are biased if they represent populations from which persons at high risk for HIV infection are excluded. Among 3.7 million civilian applicants for military service screened from October 1985 through December 1992, the crude prevalence of HIV infection was 0.11 percent, and higher rates were observed for men than for women and for blacks and Hispanics than for whites.[32] However, the HIV seroprevalence rate has decreased over time for all applicants.[39,40] A decrease in HIV seroprevalence

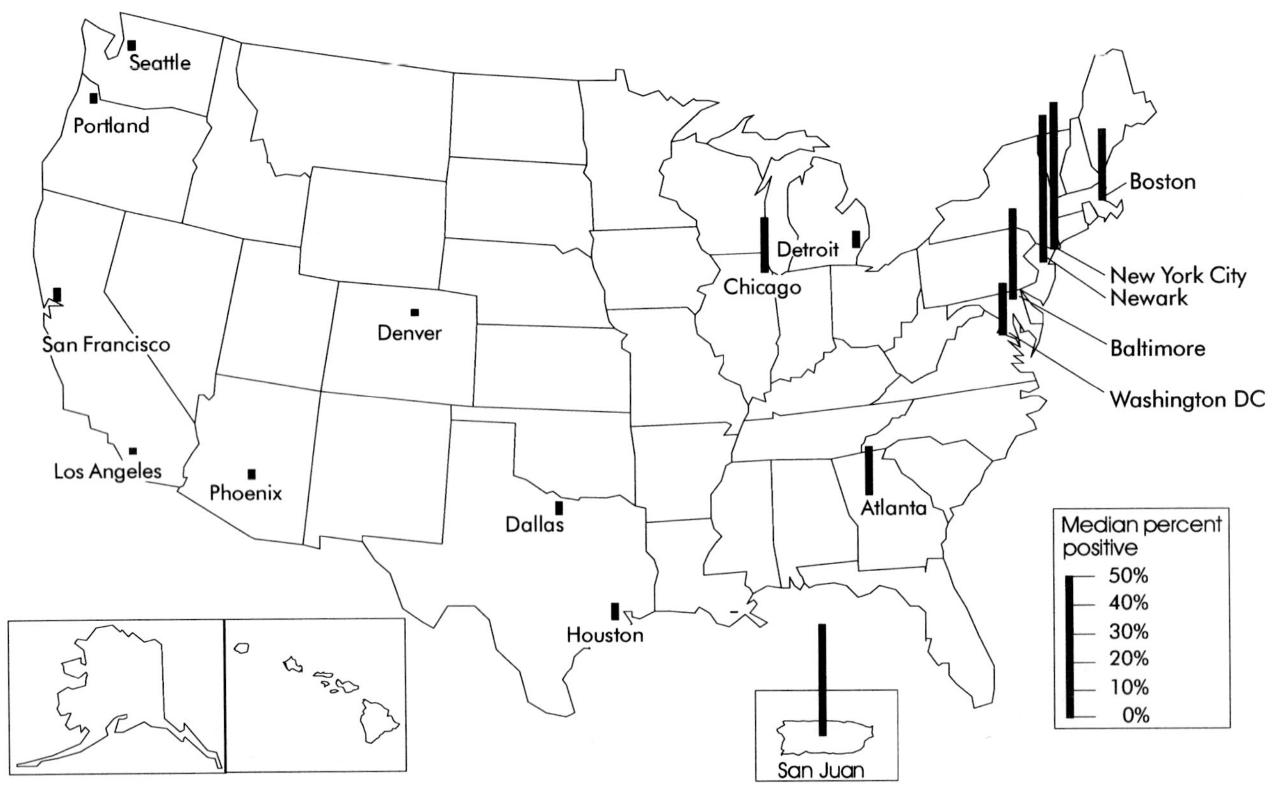

Fig. 97-16. HIV seroprevalence among injecting drug users, drug treatment center surveys, 1993.

has not been readily interpretable because at-risk applicants have been actively discouraged in some settings.

Students who enter Job Corps training programs tend to be economically disadvantaged, African American and Hispanic youths drawn both from urban and rural areas.[27] For students 16 to 21 years of age who entered the program from October 1987 through 1992, three of every 1000 students were infected with HIV.[32] This rate was almost three times the rate for applicants for military service. The rate of HIV infection increased over time for female students and was highest for older students and students from the large urban areas in the Northeast and from rural areas and smaller cities in the South.[27] In 1993, the HIV infection rate decreased for women and remained unchanged for men.

VITAL STATISTICS

Mortality statistics are collected independently of other surveillance systems, are very complete because of compulsory reporting of deaths in all areas, and are an ongoing low-cost source of information that includes age, gender, race or ethnicity, date of death, and other useful information.[41] For an infection with a high case fatality rate, such as HIV infection, vital registries data clearly illustrate the severity of the HIV/AIDS epidemic. In 1994, HIV infection or AIDS was reported as an underlying condition for approximately 42,000 deaths. HIV was the leading cause of death for men and women 25 to 44 years of age (Fig. 97-17).[42] In 1994, of persons 25 to 44 years of age at diagnosis, the cause of death was HIV-related for 32 percent of black men (mortality rate, 178/100,000) and 22 percent of black women (mortality rate 51/100,000). From 1995 to 1996, HIV deaths plateaued and then declined reflecting the increased survival for persons with AIDS who receive effective antiretroviral therapy. Vital registries have also been used to monitor the various AIDS-defining opportunistic illnesses as causes of mortality.[43] Public health mortality registries are limited in that the reporting delay may be quite long and final statistics for a specific time period may not be available for 1 to 2 years after that period has ended. Because of the systematic under reporting of some HIV-related causes of death, the number of reported HIV-related deaths represents a minimum estimate. In addition, vital registries are less useful for other STDs that cause significant morbidity but little mortality. For example, in 1992, only 91 deaths related to syphilis and 24 deaths related to gonorrhea were reported in the United States.

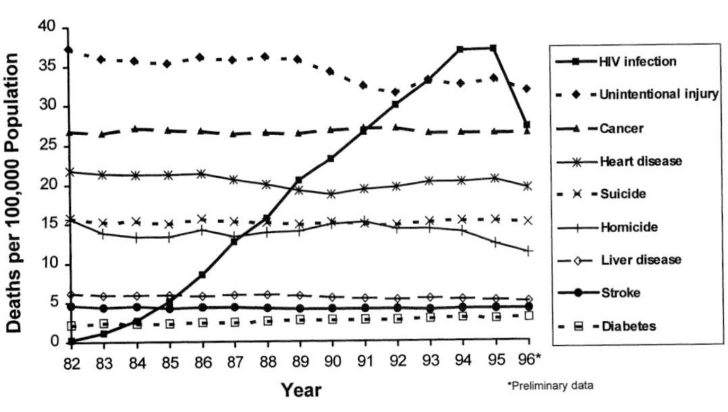

Fig. 97-17. Death rates from leading causes of death in persons aged 25–44 years, United States, 1982–1996.

USE OF SURVEILLANCE DATA

Surveillance data answer the basic questions—"Who? Where? When? and How Many?"—in a way that detects temporal trends. Most analyses of surveillance data focus on these temporal trends in the general population and subpopulations identified by gender, race or ethnicity, age, or risk of disease. Surveillance data may also be used as a basis for statistical projections or mathematical modeling. For example, AIDS surveillance data have been used in a statistical back-calculation model to estimate HIV prevalence. Using this method, researchers recently estimated that 630,000 to 897,000 adults and adolescents were living with HIV as of January 1993.[44] National PID data were used in a cost-analysis to estimate that the direct and indirect costs associated with PID were $4.2 billion in 1990.[45] AIDS surveillance data have also been used to estimate the relative frequency of AIDS-defining conditions and the characteristics of persons with specific AIDS-defining opportunistic illnesses such as tuberculosis and to estimate the survival time from the diagnosis of AIDS-defining conditions to death for various subpopulations.[16,46–48]

The power and usefulness of surveillance data to target populations at greatest need for prevention services are enhanced at the local level by linkages with other population-based data systems. A linkage of AIDS surveillance data and vital records, conducted in 23 states, found that approximately 30 percent of persons dying with AIDS in rural areas of the United States were residents of larger metropolitan areas at the time of diagnosis.[49] This linkage provided a more complete estimate of the number of persons with AIDS in some rural areas because AIDS surveillance is based on residence at the time of initial AIDS diagnosis and does not usually account for the location of treatment sites or residence at death. A comparison of AIDS and other surveillance data by postal zone or census tract provides additional data to more completely describe high-risk communities. For example, studies that compared AIDS case rates in areas of Newark, New Jersey, and Los Angeles by sociodemographic factors in the U.S. census data found that the highest rates of AIDS were in communities that had the lowest socioeconomic indicators.[50,51] Similar studies in Seattle showed that areas with the lowest socioeconomic status, where approximately 25 percent of the city population resided, accounted for 60 percent of gonorrhea cases.[52] In Colorado Springs, mapping has also been used to identify core census tracts for gonorrhea and to demonstrate the relationship of these areas to the main sites of social aggregation.[53]

A comparison of STD and HIV/AIDS surveillance data may also be useful for targeting prevention resources and evaluating prevention efforts. STDs are a marker for sexual behaviors that lead to the acquisition of HIV infection, and STDs are also cofactors that biologically facilitate the transmission of HIV.[54] High rates of STDs observed in STD surveillance may predict increases in HIV infection rates in the same areas. Areas with the highest HIV rates for childbearing women also tend to have high rates of primary and secondary syphilis (see Fig. 97-11). The distribution of HIV infection in childbearing women is strongly correlated with syphilis and gonorrhea patterns 4 to 5 years earlier.[55] For example, in Houston, an increase in HIV infection rates for African American women 15 to 19 years of age was preceded by an increase in P&S syphilis in this same population.[56] Conversely, a decrease in STD rates for white homosexual and bisexual men in many areas of the country heralded a decrease in HIV infection and AIDS rates for these men.[57] However, the rates of syphilis and other STDs are also affected by the quality of detection and treatment services for those curable diseases. Thus, behavioral risks for HIV in a community may not change, even though STD rates drop or are low.

DATA DISSEMINATION

No laws or regulations govern which diseases are reportable to the CDC for the purpose of compiling national statistics. Instead, state health departments and CDC agree on a list of reportable conditions for which state data will be shared voluntarily and regularly with CDC for national analysis and dissemination.[58] At the request of state health departments, CDC agrees to receive data without personal identifiers from all states in which AIDS, HIV infection, chancroid, chlamydia, gonorrhea, hepatitis B, and syphilis are reportable. National HIV/AIDS surveillance data and other STD surveillance data are disseminated through regular surveillance summaries, *Morbidity and Mortality Weekly Report (MMWR),* peer-reviewed journals, and other publications. Surveillance data may also be published in press releases and as part of public presentations. The regular surveillance publications and the *MMWR* articles are available on the Internet (CDC home page, http//www.cdc.gov), and the HIV/AIDS surveillance data are also available from the National AIDS Clearinghouse (1-800-458-5231). For persons who wish to conduct independent analyses, CDC makes available an electronic HIV/AIDS surveillance public information data set. Local surveillance data are also available through state health departments. Local surveillance programs should periodically review their methods of data dissemination to ensure that the information is reaching the persons most in need of it.

CHALLENGES FOR THE FUTURE

Surveillance systems for HIV/AIDS and other STDs have been very effective in tracking STD incidence, HIV and chlamydia prevalence, severe HIV disease or AIDS, and HIV-related deaths. The current patchwork of different systems and data sources that is used to gather, process, and interpret trends and disease burden of HIV/AIDS and other STDs is far from complete or ideal. In fact, the National Academy of Science's Institute of Medicine has recently acknowledged some of the limitations of the current system and has recommended that a comprehensive evaluation of the national system be conducted and that findings be applied to future improvements. In particular, improvements should be made in completeness and timeliness of reporting from private sector providers and laboratories and from other public sector venues where STD services are delivered.[59]

In a revised national system, the scope of information collected about reported cases would be expanded beyond demographic and risk factor characteristics. Information is needed to track health care utilization for the treatment of STDs and HIV and the locations where persons receive STD care to ensure that the proper treatment and prevention services are received and that these cases are reported. HIV/AIDS surveillance will also need to continue to adapt to changes in HIV medical knowledge and practice. For example, the appropriate place in surveillance activities for the tracking of viral load measurements as a predictor of severe HIV disease, the impact of new antiretroviral therapies on the rate of progression to AIDS and death, the increasing need for HIV case surveillance to provide population-based trends not affected by treatment practices, and the role of surveillance in identifying the prevalence of HIV strain variation and drug resistance are just some of the challenges.

Interest is also increasing in the development of sexual behavior monitoring systems that detect temporal changes in these behaviors or the adoption of protective behaviors, which herald a change in HIV/AIDS and other STD rates. Efforts to prevent HIV/AIDS and other STDs are directed toward infected and uninfected persons whose sexual behaviors place them at risk for future morbidity, but traditional public health case registries include only documented infections. Ideally, a behavioral surveillance system for HIV/AIDS and other STDs should monitor the behaviors of the general population as well as subpopulations at high risk.

Behavioral surveys of a representative sample of the general population have demonstrated the ability to collect reliable data to monitor the number of sexual partners, condom use, and other sexual behavior information. The Youth Risk Behavior Survey is conducted in 44 states to collect data on in-school youth 15 to 19 years of age and has included sexual behavior questions for several years.[60] For example, the survey has found that among adolescents in schools, the use of condoms at most recent sexual intercourse increased from 46 percent in 1991 to 53 percent in 1995, whereas the proportion who had ever had sexual intercourse remained stable at 53 percent.[61] The Behavior Risk Factor Surveillance System collects information on a variety of health indicators through telephone interviews of a scientific sample of households in a state, but this system has typically not included sexual behavior questions.[62] General population-based surveys conducted in Europe have successfully documented changes in sexual behavior, such as a large increase in condom use by Swiss young adults.[63] A sexual behavior module is now an optional part of the Behavior Risk Factor Surveillance System and more than half the states received federal funds to add these questions to their 1997 surveys.

Subpopulation surveys supplement data from general population surveys. General surveys may not adequately represent persons with high-risk behaviors for HIV/AIDS and other STDs because these persons represent a small, nonuniformly distributed proportion of the general population. Surveys of subpopulations such as homosexual and bisexual men have yielded valuable information, such as the extent of receptive anal intercourse and HIV test history, but tend not to be conducted so that temporal trends can be addressed.[64] Some investigators have attempted to conduct surveys that would be representative of homosexual and bisexual men in a given area.[65] Identifying the most efficient means of conducting these behavioral surveillance activities, particularly among subpopulations, while following surveillance tenets to ensure interpretable data, will be just one of the challenges in this effort.

Surveillance practices must also adapt to changes in health care delivery, advances in information systems, and the availability of public health resources. Electronic information transfer using established procedures to protect the confidentiality of medical records could greatly increase the efficiency of case finding and expand our understanding of health care utilization. The growth of managed care organizations and the increasing automation of medical records hold promise that data can be made more readily available to assess health outcomes, risk behaviors, and health care utilization. To realize the potential of electronic reporting and paperless surveillance will require that potential reporters recognize a benefit to their organizations, that modern electronic information-gathering systems be available in public health agencies, and that surveillance staff receive training to conduct electronic surveillance effectively and confidentially. All these efforts will have potential cost-saving benefits in the long term but will require a commitment of substantial resources in the immediate future.

SUMMARY

Public health surveillance is conducted under the authority of states and provides the information foundation for local and state planning. Through a federal-state partnership that uses standardized surveillance practices to safeguard confidentiality, these data also are used for national program planning and evaluation. These systems must be flexible to gather new types of information through innovations in surveillance systems. Regardless of the type of information collected, effective public health surveillance depends on the work of thousands of dedicated clinicians, infection control practitioners, public health workers, laboratory workers, and others. Keeping all participants in these surveillance systems properly trained, informed, and motivated must be a public health priority.

References

1 Thacker SB et al: Public health surveillance in the United States. *Epidemiol Rev* 10:164–190, 1988.

2 Centers for Disease Control and Prevention: Case definitions for public health surveillance. *MMWR* 39(No.RR-13):1–43, 1990.

3 Centers for Disease Control and Prevention: 1993 revised classification system for HIV infection and expanded surveillance case definition for AIDS among adolescents and adults. *MMWR* 41(RR-17):1–19, 1992.

4 Conway GA et al: Under reporting of AIDS cases in South Carolina, 1986 and 1987. *JAMA* 262:2859–2863, 1989.

5 Modesitt SK et al: Evaluation of active versus passive AIDS surveillance in Oregon. *Am J Pub Health* 80:463–464, 1990.

6 Rosenblum LS et al: The completeness of AIDS case reporting, 1988: A multisite collaborative surveillance project. *Am J Pub Health* 82: 1495–1499, 1992.

7 Centers for Disease Control and Prevention: Pneumocystis pneumonia—Los Angeles. *MMWR* 30:250–252, 1981.

8 Centers for Disease Control and Prevention: Kaposis sarcoma and *Pneumocystis* pneumonia among homosexual men(New York City and California. *MMWR* 30:305–308, 1981.

9 Centers for Disease Control and Prevention: First 500,000 AIDS cases—United States, 1995. *MMWR* 44:849–853, 1995.

10 Centers for Disease Control and Prevention: Update: Trends in AIDS Incidence-United States, 1996. *MMWR* 1997; 46:861–867.

11 Chamberland ME et al: Epidemiology and prevention of AIDS and HIV infection, in *Principles and Practice of Infectious Diseases,* Mandell GL et al (eds). New York, Churchill and Livingstone, 1994, pp. 1174–1203.

12 Centers for Disease Control and Prevention: Heterosexually acquired AIDS—United States, 1993. *MMWR* 43:155–160, 1994.

13 Centers for Disease Control and Prevention: AIDS among racial/ethnic minorities—United States, 1993. *MMWR* 43:644, 1994.

14 Centers for Disease Control and Prevention: Update: Trends in AIDS among men who have sex with men—United States, 1989–1994. *MMWR* 44:401, 1995.

15 Centers for Disease Control and Prevention: Update: HIV-2 infection among blood and plasma donors—United States, June l992(June l995. *MMWR* 44:603, 1995.

16 Slutsker L et al: Epidemiology of extrapulmonary tuberculosis among persons with AIDS in the United States. *Clin Infect Dis* 1993;16:513.

17 Centers for Disease Control and Prevention: AIDS in children—United States, 1996. *MMWR* 45:1005–1010, 1996.

18 Fleming PL et al: Mandatory HIV reporting: characteristics of adults reported with HIV compared to AIDS in the United States [Abstract WS-C17–2] IX International Conference on AIDS, Berlin, Germany, June 6–11, 1993.

19 Sweeney P et al: Monitoring current HIV transmission to promote prevention: Supplementing AIDS surveillance. *AIDS* 9:645–647, 1995.

20 Ward JW et al: Annotation: What will be the role of HIV infection reporting? *Am J Pub Health* 84;1923–1928, 1994.

21 Centers for Disease Control and Prevention: Ten leading nationally notifiable infectious diseases. *MMWR* 45:883–884, 1996.

22 Centers for Disease Control and Prevention, Division of STD Prevention: *Sexually Transmitted Disease Surveillance, 1996.* Atlanta, U.S. Department of Health and Human Services, Public Health Service, September 1997.

23 Nakashima AK et al: Epidemiology of syphilis in the United States, 1941–1993. *Sex Trans Dis* 23(1):1–8, 1996.

24 Dondero TJ et al: Monitoring the levels and trends of HIV infection: The Public Health Services HIV surveillance program. *Public Health Rep* 103:213, 1988.

25 Pappaioanou M et al: The family of HIV seroprevalence surveys: objectives, methods, and uses of sentinel surveillance for HIV in the United States. *Pub Health Rep* 105:113, 1990.

26 St. Louis ME et al: Seroprevalence rates of human immunodeficiency virus infection at sentinel hospitals in the United States. *N Engl J Med* 323:213–218, 1990.

27 Conway GA et al: Trends in HIV prevalence in disadvantaged youth: Survey results from a national job training program, 1988–1992. *JAMA* 269:2887, 1993.

28 Weinstock HS et al: Trends in HIV seroprevalence among persons attending sexually transmitted disease clinics in the United States, 1988–1992. *J Acquire Immune Def Synd, Hum Retroviral* 9:514, 1995.

29 Onorato IM et al: Prevalence of human immunodeficiency virus infection among patients attending tuberculosis clinics in the United States. *J Infect Dis* 165:87, 1992.

30 Allen DM et al: Human immunodeficiency virus infection in intravenous drug users entering drug treatment, United States, 1988–1989. *Am J Pub Health* 82:541, 1992.

31 Centers for Disease Control and Prevention: National HIV Serosurveillance summary: results through 1992, vol. 3. Atlanta, U.S. Department of Health and Human Services; 1994.

32 Centers for Disease Control and Prevention: National HIV Serosurveillance summary: Update—1993, vol. 3. Atlanta, U.S. Department of Health and Human Services, 1995.

33 Prevots DR et al: Trends in HIV seroprevalence among injection drug users entering drug treatment centers, United States, 1988–1993. *Am J Epidemiol* 143:733–742, 1996.

34 Wasser SC et al: Urban-nonurban distribution of HIV in childbearing women in the United States. *J Acquir Immune Defic Syndr* 6:1035, 1993.

35 Davis SF et al: Prevalence and incidence of vertically acquired HIV infection in the United States. *JAMA* 274:952, 1995.

36 Karon JM et al: Prevalence of HIV infection in the United States, 1984 to 1992. *JAMA* 276:126–131, 1996.

37 Conner EM et al: Reduction of maternal-infant transmission of human immunodeficiency virus type 1 with zidovidine treatment. *N Engl J Med* 331:1173–1180, 1994.

38 Davis SF et al: HIV prevalence among U.S.childbearing women 1989–1994. XI International Conference on AIDS. Vancouver, Canada, July 7–12, 1996. Abstract WeC.331.

39 Withers BG et al: A brief review of the epidemiology of HIV in the US Army. *Mil Med* 157:80–84, 1992.

40 McNeil JG et al: Trends of HIV seroconversion among young adults in the US Army, 1985 to 1989. *JAMA* 265:1709–1714, 1991.

41 Centers for Disease Control and Prevention: National Center for Health Statistics: Annual summary of births, marriages, divorces, and deaths: United States, 1994. Hyattsville, Maryland; U.S. Department of Health and Human Services, Public Health Service, CDC: 1995, P18 (monthly vital statistics report; vol 43, no 13).

42 Centers for Disease Control and Prevention: Update: Mortality attributable to HIV infection among persons aged 25–44 years—United States, 1994. *MMWR* 45:121, 1996.

43 Selik RM, Chu SY et al: Trends in infectious diseases and cancers among persons dying of HIV infection in the United States from 1987 to 1992. *Ann Intern Med* 123:933, 1995.

44 Rosenberg PS: Scope of the AIDS epidemic in the United States. *Science* 270:1372–1375, 1995.

45 Washington AE et al: Cost of and payment source for pelvic inflammatory disease: Trends and projections, 1983 through 2000. *JAMA* 266:2565–2569, 1991.

46 Jones JL et al: Surveillance of AIDS defining conditions in the United States. *AIDS* 8:1489–1493, 1994.

47 Lemp GF et al: Survival trends for patients with AIDS. *JAMA* 263: 402–406, 1990.

48 Neal JJ et al: Survival among heterosexuals with AIDS, United States, 1988–1990 [Abstract 1096], in *Abstracts of the 122nd Annual Meeting of the American Public Health Association.* Washington D.C., October 30–November 3, 1994, 45.

49 Buehler JW et al: The migration of persons with AIDS: Data from 12 states, 1985 to 1992. *Am J Pub Health* 85(11):1552–1555, 1995.

50 Hu DJ et al: Geographical AIDS rates and socio-demographic variables in the Newark, New Jersey metropolitan area. *AIDS Pub Policy J* 9(1): 20–25, 1994.

51 Simon PA et al: Income and AIDS in Los Angeles County. *AIDS* 9(3): 281–284, 1995.

52 Rice RJ et al: Sociodemographic distribution of gonorrhea incidence: implications for prevention and behavior research. *Am J Pub Health* 81;1252–1258, 1991.

53 Potterat JJ et al: Gonorrhea as a social disease. *Sex Trans Dis* 12:25–32, 1985.

54 Laga M et al: Non-ulcerative sexually transmitted diseases as risk factors for HIV transmission in women: Results from a cohort study. *AIDS* 7:95–102, 1993.

55 St Louis ME et al: Covariation of HIV infection among childbearing women with other sexually transmitted diseases (STD) in the United States. [Abstract 050]—Eleventh meeting of the International Society for STD Research. New Orleans, Louisiana, August 27–30, 1995.

56 Levine WC et al: Dual epidemics of syphilis and HIV infection among adolescent African American women in Houston, 1988–1993 [Abstract 051]—Eleventh meeting of the International Society for STD Research. New Orleans Louisiana, August 27–30, 1995.

57 Centers for Disease Control and Prevention: Declining rates of rectal and pharyngeal gonorrhea among males—New York City. *MMWR* 33:295–297, 1984.

58 Centers for Disease Control and Prevention: Summary of notifiable diseases, United States, 1994. *MMWR* 43(53):1–80, 1994.

59 IOM (Institute of Medicine): *The Hidden Epidemic: Confronting Sexually Transmitted Diseases.* Eng TR et al (eds). Washington DC: National Academy Press, 1997.

60 Kann L et al: HIVrelated knowledge, beliefs, and behaviors among high school students in the United States: Results from a national survey. *J Sch Health* 61:397–401, 1991.

61 Collins JL et al: Five-year trends in HIV risk behaviors among youth. XI International Conference on AIDS. Vancouver, Canada, July 7–12, 1996. [Abstract Tu.D.471].

62 Centers for Disease Control and Prevention: State- and sex-specific prevalence of selected characteristics—behavioral risk factor surveillance system, 1992 and 1993. *MMWR* 1996;45(No. SS-6).

63 Jeannin A et al: General population in Switzerland: improvements in condom use without other major changes in sexual activity. XI International Conference on AIDS. Vancouver, Canada, July 7–12, 1996. [Abstract Mo.D.1703].

64 Osmond DH et al: HIV infection in homosexual and bisexual men 18 to 29 years of age: The San Francisco young mens study. *Am J Pub Health* 84:1933–1937, 1994.

65 Stall R et al: A comparison of younger and older gay mens HIV risk-taking behaviors: The Communication Technologies 1989 Cross-Sectional Survey. *J Acquir Immune Defic Syndr* 5:682–687, 1992.

Chapter 98

Evaluation of sexually transmitted diseases and HIV/AIDS prevention programs

Thierry E. Mertens
William J. Kassler

Although evaluation may appear to some to be a luxury, it is a crucial resource for program reorientation. Unless plans for evaluation are made early, programs run the risk of generating unfulfilled expectations, frustration and even disillusionment, owing to lack of feedback on the impact of the work carried out.[1,2] In many instances, evaluation is tied to future funding, with further support being conditional on the success of present activities.

There are several reasons why evaluation is important. First, it enables health planners and workers to identify more clearly the consequences of their actions. Second, evaluation can identify the processes by which particular outcomes are brought about. Strategies and intervention approaches then can be replicated, taking into account the differences of context, in the hope that the benefits that accrue in one context may do so in others. Third, monitoring and evaluation can enhance the accountability of service providers. It can indicate when perceived needs are being met, identify the factors that facilitated or prevented a particular intervention, bringing about the desired outcomes, point to alliances between different groups that led to successful developments and, in the final instance, aid decision making about whether or not resources have been well allocated.[1,3]

Evaluation has a strong tradition in some fields of social sciences, such as politics, economics, public administration, psychology, or education. This tradition has highlighted some of the challenges of evaluation. As Michael Quinn Patton summarized, these difficulties result from "multiple methods, multiple audiences, multiple funding sources, multiple perspectives, multiple paradigms, multiple roles, and multiple solutions to multiple problems."[4] Indeed, to some people, evaluation calls for complex experimental studies. To others, it means pausing at the end of an activity to sort out what was successful and what was not successful. There is little consensus about the best way to evaluate health projects and programs. Some favor a rigorous quantitative approach in which the emphasis is on measuring selected outcomes in relation to the interventions that have taken place. Others focus more qualitatively on the processes by which results are brought about.[5] Some attempt to include both. Increasing emphasis is also being placed on the cost-effectiveness of the program. Figure 98-1 illustrates the most important concerns of evaluation. Each of the emphases is associated with very different research methods.

There are two main purposes of evaluation: (1) to provide feedback to the project (small scale) or program (large scale) itself on performance primarily by comparing *initial* objectives and *actual* achievement; and (2) to provide feedback to the planning process by comparing project achievements with the goals of *current policy*.[6]

An evaluation thus may take many forms. It may concentrate on macro, sector, or program problems (e.g., the planning process, the resource allocation mechanism, the health impact for the general population); project/program organization (e.g., outreach methods, form of service delivery, sustainability); specific problems (e.g., cost overruns, message contents); particular policy issues (e.g., tariff policy of services); or specific outcomes in the target population (e.g., reduction of risk behaviors or level of HIV or STD infection).

This chapter describes a variety of possible approaches for the evaluation of STD and HIV/AIDS programs and projects, with illustrative examples focusing on health care delivery and community-based prevention. Guidance is given on how to select the appropriate evaluation design and methods. It is anticipated that managers will realize that, despite existing pressures on time, the results of well-conducted evaluations ease the workload of policy makers, program administrators, and project implemetors, and attract additional resources.

TYPES OF EVALUATION

Evaluation has been defined as the "critical assessment, on as objective a basis as possible, of the degree to which activities, entire services or their component parts fulfill stated goals."[7,8] It is useful to approach the whole evaluation process in terms of the question, Does it work? and if so, How much does it work? The four main types of evaluation usually are described as formative, process, outcome, and impact (Fig. 98-2).[9] This classification suggests that any program, project, or activity can be evaluated at one or more stages in its life cycle, and that these types of evaluations may employ significantly different methods.

FORMATIVE EVALUATION

Formative evaluation assists in the design, development, or refinement of interventions and usually is conducted at the beginning of a program to inform about the possible options for interventions.[10] It includes the assessment of the relevance of policy, and the adequacy of the program's plan in meeting specified needs. The determination of the relevance of a program's goals and objectives requires a definition of the health status of populations, the target populations, and their needs in their specific context (Fig. 98-3). This typically involves conducting an assessment such as an epidemiologic profile, needs assessment, situation analysis, or audience segmentation.

Determining the adequacy of a program's strategies in meeting its objectives implies verifying the soundness of the program's logic within its context (the external factors likely to affect performance). The context encompasses the social, environmental, and epidemiological situation, the overall political support to the program, the implementor's comparative advantages and capacity to deliver the intervention, and the level of (human and financial) resource allocation.

Formative evaluation requires multilevel approaches using broad and flexible methodologies; qualitative such as focus group discussions, open-ended interviews, ethnographic analysis, message analysis or the screening of different intervention options for feasibility; or mixed quantitative and qualitative methods such as scoring observations.

Sometimes, when programs and expected outcomes are complex, or when resources are limited, an evaluability assessment is conducted to determine the feasibility of evaluating the outcomes of the program. These assessments examine potential design and measurement issues, and the soundness of the program's logic, goals, and objectives.

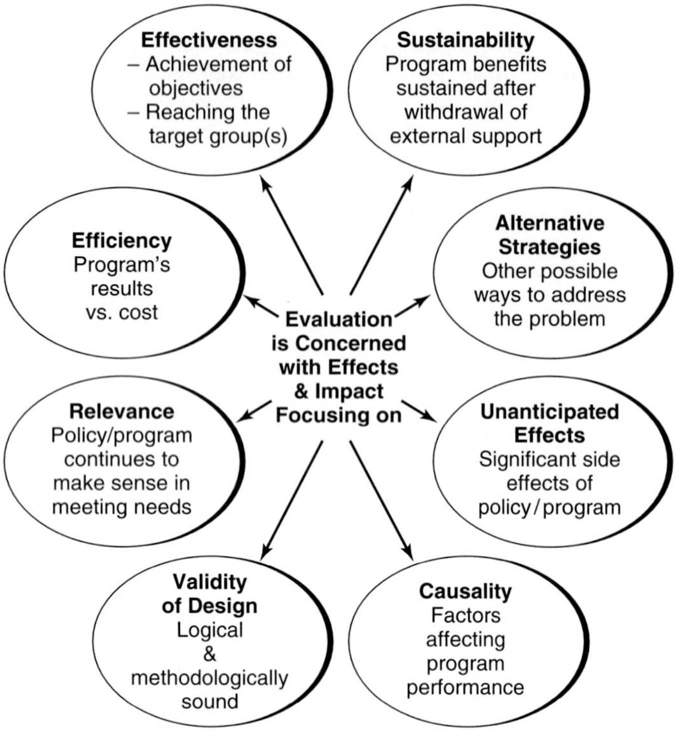

Fig. 98-1. Concerns of evaluation.

PROCESS EVALUATION

Process evaluation can be defined as the continuous oversight of the program's implementation to ensure that its activities are proceeding according to plan.[7] This type of evaluation is a descriptive process that examines the quality, volume, and nature of intervention delivery, in terms of expected goods and services. Questions include: How is the intervention implemented? What services are delivered, at what frequency and coverage? What is the quality of services? How much does it cost? Process evaluation therefore is concerned with the comparison of actual and scheduled activities, the identification of reasons for achievements or shortcomings, and the indication of remedies for any shortcomings. To do this, a core set of indicators and methods to measure them need to be developed, which may relate to staff performance, timeliness, appropriateness, and quality of services delivered. Common methodologies used for process evaluation often include direct standardized observation, record reviews, organizational records, written questionnaires, activity or participation log, client surveys, and simulated patients. Progress reviews keeps track of milestones achieved, personnel matters, supplies and equipment, and money spent in relation to budgets allocated. It should also include a review of the equity of program's distribution.

Knowing why and where a program succeeds or is inadequate is as important as knowing whether it is succeeding or failing. Failure or delays may be linked to inappropriate human resource management or to over-ambitious objectives. Qualitative methods usually are used to document the reasons for success and failure.[2,3]

Efficiency is an expression of the relationship between the results obtained from a program and the efforts expended in terms of human, financial, and other resources. The assessment of efficiency is aimed at improving implementation with respect to cost, and adds to the progress review.

Increasingly, because of the need to use resources as economically and effectively as possible, evaluation includes economic analysis. Economic choices are made on the basis of cost and the expected benefits from that cost. Choices generally will be made that optimize the benefits in relation to the cost. Economic analyses will allow the different options to be compared, either in terms of the quality of the outcome for a given cost or in terms of the costs for a desired outcome. When calculating the cost of a program, due attention should be given to all costs involved, direct and indirect, including labor, supplies, training, infrastructure, and time for people to attend.

Process evaluation usually is reflected in regular progress reports that are put together using appropriate management information systems (MIS). Process evaluation should be conducted by those who implement the program. Regular supervision by program managers is key to the success of process evaluation.

OUTCOME EVALUATION

Outcome evaluation attempts to determine if there were changes in behaviors or health outcomes as a result of the intervention. Questions generally asked during this type of evaluation include: Did the program make a difference? What was the effect of the program on participants? What alternative approaches would work better? These questions involve the underlying determination of what would have happened to program participants, had they not received the intervention. This must be inferred from studies using methods allowing the assessment of cause and effect (i.e., experimental or quasiexperimental methods). Demonstrating changes in outcomes, itself, is difficult. The challenge in outcome

	Formative ➡	Process ➡	Outcome ➡	Impact
Primary purpose	Needs assessment Program planning	Oversight & monitoring Compares actual with planned Identify reasons for success/failure Quality assurance	Demonstrate changes in outcomes Attribute outcome to the program - Did the program work? - What alternatives work better?	Assess overall program effect on the population
Key methods	Qualitative methods: - focus groups - interviews - participant observation - document reviews	Descriptive methods: - standardized observation - record review - surveys - cost identification Process indicators	Research assessing causality: - randomized controlled trials - quasi-experimental studies - techniques to control for bias Cost-effectiveness Outcome indicators	Trend analysis of societal-level outcomes: - behavioral data - socio-cultural responses - morbidity data
Timing	Early stages	Continuous	Periodic intervals	Later stages

Fig. 98-2. Relationship between different types of evaluation.

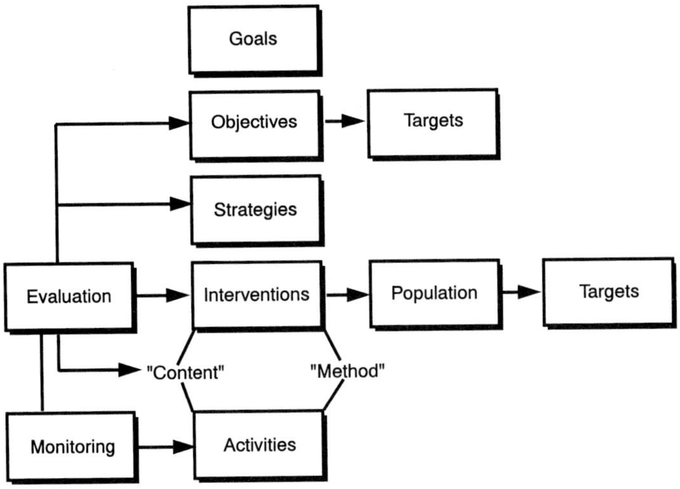

Example:

Goal	- Prevent STD/HIV Transmission
Objectives:	- Prevent Sexual Transmission of HIV
Strategy:	- STD Treatment + Prevention
Intervention:	- Promote Health Seeking Behaviour for Women aged 15 - 49 - Improve Diagnosis + Treatment Procedures for Men Working in Factories
Activities:	- Develop Messages for Family Planning Clinics for Posters and Peer Counseling - Increase Drug + Laboratory Supplies in STD Treatment Facilities

Fig. 98-3. Objectives, strategies, interventions, and the evaluation feedback.

evaluation is to attribute those changes to the intervention under evaluation.

The efficacy of interventions—whether they can, in ideal circumstances, produce the desired outcomes—can be most reliably ascertained by randomized controlled trials. Once efficacy has been formally evaluated, the interventions are implemented in circumstances that differ from those existing during experimental testing. The resources, the level of staffing, the degree of human motivation, and the level of auxiliary support are typically more limited when programs are implemented in real-world settings than during the conduct of formal intervention trials. It is commonly found that the outcomes of health interventions are more favorable during trials than during routine practice.[2]

Therefore, it is necessary to evaluate the effectiveness of programs, that is, the degree to which the potential benefits demonstrated in trials, are realized in usual practice. Effectiveness measures the degree of attainment of the predetermined objectives or targets of a program, service, institution, or support activity in reducing the problem.

In general, efficacy is tested for single interventions carried out within a specific "project," whereas effectiveness applies to a "program" made of a number of interventions and activities (Fig. 98-3). Although efficacy usually will be assessed by experimental methods (trials), the evaluation of the effectiveness of programs more often will use quasi-experimental and sometimes observational designs that combine expertise from multiple disciplines, including epidemiology, health services research, and social sciences. Quasi-experimental and purely observational methods usually are considerably less costly than experimental designs and are the only feasible methods in many field settings.

In summary, there is a need to make a clear distinction between evaluation of national (or subnational) program evaluation and the evaluation of specific discrete interventions or projects. Although at the national level it is often appropriate to combine contextual and policy analyses with observational methods measuring at repeated intervals a set of predefined indicators, the evaluation of specific interventions must be an integral part of a project's design, and ideally starts with efficacy trials.

Impact is an expression of the overall effect of a program, service, or institution on the health and related socioeconomic development of the population concerned. One expression of impact thus is the effectiveness of the interventions of a program, taking into account the number of people the program has reached. In the case of HIV and some other STDs prevention programs, the ultimate impact (disease reduction and increased life expectancy), can be measured only after a relatively long period of time. In the short term, such programs often are evaluated on the basis of their intermediate outcomes, such as improved knowledge about prevention and care in a given population. Since evaluation of programs and projects are carried out to inform choices between alternative courses of action, it is also important that the data required for supporting medium or long-term decision making are collected.[10]

There is debate around the question of what is sufficient evidence that a health program "has made the difference."[11–14] The limitations of evaluations focusing exclusively on health impact can be summarized as follows. First, it is important to establish the degree to which the program was implemented prior to seeking evidence of outcomes or impact. Second, there is likely to be an important time lag between program initiation and detectable outcomes or impact. Third, the complexities of health program evaluation often lead to problems of interpretation: What is actually making the difference?[14] Factors that contribute to the difficulties of conducting and interpreting evaluations include the logistics of prospective studies to determine changes in behavior or incidence, the challenge of validating self-reported behaviors, the lack of adequate comparison groups, and the difficulties of measuring and accounting for intervening variables, such as exposure to other interventions or temporal trends. Finally, a frequent objection relates to the use of resources in evaluating interventions already widely believed to be efficacious. In the context of STD and HIV prevention, for example, it can be argued that the question is not whether the use of condoms prevents transmission, but rather how to encourage people to use condoms.[2]

An additional serious difficulty in assessing the impact of HIV/AIDS prevention programs arises because the prevalence of chronic infections such as HIV is a poor indicator of incidence.[2,15] Similarly, where serological markers of past infection persist, as in syphilis, changes in prevalence of such markers may be hard to interpret. For these infections, it can be argued that in the peripubertal age group, changes in prevalence closely reflect changes in incidence among those just beginning sexual activity. For example, it is reasonable to hypothesize that HIV or TPHA seroprevalence in 15 year olds closely parallels HIV or syphilis incidence in 15 year olds. In a public health context, however, a community-based survey of (only) 15 year olds would be extremely difficult. On the other hand, the underlying hypothesis may not be sufficiently robust to allow extrapolation to 15 to 24 year olds (a 10-year age band), which is more feasible.[2]

The difficulty may be illustrated by modeling the expected changes in HIV prevalence in a hypothetical high incidence population. In these conditions, a consistent and gradual decrease in HIV incidence from 100,000 infections to 30,000 over 7 years owing to a successful prevention program would hardly be detectable using HIV prevalence after a period of 4 years (Fig. 98-4). Indeed, in many circumstances, programs are likely to face the problem of confronting a rise in seroprevalence for some years, even if the incidence is decreasing. Arguing that a program has had an impact may then become problematic, as one would have to compare the observed rise in prevalence with a hypothetically greater one, had there been no effective intervention. Conversely, the situation could occur where an apparent decrease in prevalence is misinterpreted as the result of program efforts. In the initial years of the epidemic the vast majority of HIV-infected persons are asymptomatic. Later, an increasing proportion develop AIDS, and mortality increases. Therefore, with a 10-year 15 to 24 age band, even if HIV incidence remains high, a fall in HIV prevalence may be seen as mortality rates increase among those of the 15 to 24 year olds with longer-term HIV infection.[2,17]

Finally, when HIV infection is introduced for the first time into a country or region, the age and sex distribution of new infections is predominantly determined by age- and sex-specific patterns of sexual behavior. With the passage of time, this distribution of new HIV infection changes, as adolescents and other newly sexually active age groups begin to predominate in the pool of individuals who are uninfected with HIV and possess HIV-associated risk behaviors and practices.[18] Therefore, if HIV prevalence in adolescents and young adults (e.g., 15–24 year olds) is monitored, under such conditions a rise in prevalence in 15 to 24 year olds may be observed, whether or not overall HIV incidence was on the increase.[2,15]

However, the complexities of interpreting HIV prevalence trends do not preclude the cautious use of surveillance data for evaluation purposes. In fact, surveillance data may be the first indication of a change in the dynamic of a particular epidemic and is invaluable as a starting point for in-depth investigations of the determinants of such changes.[19] Similarly, STD surveillance data, although not exempt from interpretation problems, can be a very useful adjunct to other data for the purpose of outcome evaluation. For example, routine gonorrhea surveillance data recorded from STD clinics in Thailand provided the first indications of STD/HIV program success.[15,20] In developing a framework for evaluation, one must balance the problems inherent in using prevalence data as an indicator of program success against the logistic difficulties of obtaining incidence data.[2,21]

OUTCOME MEASURES

Outcomes research is concerned with the end result of STD and HIV prevention and care interventions, the effect of programs on the health of populations. Meaningful and measurable outcomes are useful in the evaluation of a program's effectiveness because they provide a measure that can be compared across various treatment and prevention interventions. These outcome measures can also be used for planning, to evaluate policy options, and to answer questions such as which interventions work best and for whom.

Criteria for selecting and using outcomes for evaluation include that the outcomes must be: (1) objective, in that it can be observed; (2) measurable in ways that are reliable and valid; (3) attributable to the intervention delivered; and (4) sensitive to the degree of change anticipated by the intervention. Table 98-1 summarizes potential biological, behavioral, cognitive, economic, and health status outcomes that may be used in evaluating STD programs. The challenge is in selecting the appropriate outcomes for the circumstances of the evaluation.

BIOLOGIC MEASURES

Health outcomes data from most research studies or data gathered by public health agencies traditionally use physiologic measurements such as numbers of positive lab tests, numbers of infections, complication rates, or death. With some exceptions (as discussed in the preceding text), routine public health surveillance data are not appropriate for program evaluation because surveillance data cannot differentiate who has or has not been exposed to the intervention. In addition, general surveillance systems may not have the degree of sensitivity necessary for evaluating specific programs. Traditional STD rates, calculated using reported cases as the numerator and total population as the denominator, are subject to several forms of bias. First, using total population in the denominator underestimates the magnitude of risk since the denominator includes individuals who are not at risk because they are not having sex, and sexually active individuals who are not at risk because they are in mutually monogamous relationships.[22] Second, unbiased numerator estimates often are difficult to obtain. Reporting from public sector sources is typically far better than reporting from private sector sources, and, in some settings, racial

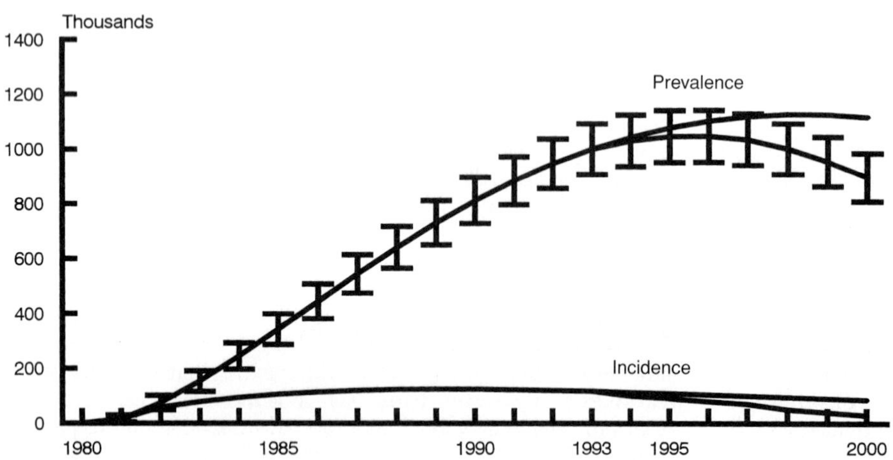

Fig. 98-4. How soon can we detect impact on HIV incidence, using prevalence data? Modeling of HIV incidence and prevalence was made for an adult population of 10 million using epimodel and assuming the epidemic began in 1980. An estimated prevalence of 10 percent was assumed in 1993. Confidence intervals were calculated at 90 percent level for a sample size of 3000 blood samples to determine prevalence. (See text for explanations.)

Table 98-1. Summary of Possible Evaluation Outcome Measures

Biological outcomes
Incidence of HIV infection
Fertility rate
Incidence of sexually transmitted diseases
Behavioral outcomes
Primary prevention behaviors
Elimination of risk behaviors
Abstinence from all sexual contact
Abstinence from all IV drug use
Avoidance of anal and vaginal intercourse
Avoidance of unsterilized IV drug injection equipment
Avoidance of pregnancy by HIV-positive women
Reduction of risk behaviors
Monogamy
Avoidance of anonymous and extradomestic sex
Avoidance of "shooting galleries"
Protective skills and behaviors
Use of condoms
Use of spermicides
Use of bleach for cleaning IV drug paraphernalia
Participation in needle exchange program
Complementary prevention behavior
Behavioral counseling
STD detection (including HIV testing) and treatment
Enrolling in drug treatment programs
Determining HIV status of sexual or drug partners
Providing names of contacts to public health agents
Using family planning services
Personal involvement in prevention program
Cognitive outcomes
Awareness and attitudes toward STDs and HIV
Knowledge of disease transmission modes
Intentions toward protective behaviors
Economic outcomes
Direct medical costs
Direct nonmedical costs
Indirect costs
Intangible costs
Health status and quality of life outcomes
Functional status
Physical function
Social function
Emotional and psychological functioning and well-being
Mental health (depression/anxiety)
Cognitive functioning
Health perceptions (includes a general sense of well-being)
Pain
Vitality (energy/fatigue)
Satisfaction with care
Access
Convenience
Financial coverage
Quality

* Adapted from Coyle et al., 1991 and Patrick and Erickson, 1993.[11,35]

and ethnic minority populations seek care in public sector clinics more often than wealthy populations, resulting in biased numerators.

For some STD such as HIV, there are additional challenges to using surveillance (prevalence) data in evaluating prevention programs. The incidence of AIDS (in the form of newly reported cases) or the prevalence of HIV are poorly sensitive outcome measures. Because of the long interval between acquisition of HIV and development of AIDS, incidence of AIDS (e.g., newly reported AIDS cases) does not accurately reflect programmatic outcomes. Similarly, because HIV-infected persons may have been infected for widely variable periods of time, prevalence cannot determine when the infection occurred. An American study of STD clinics with a high but decreasing HIV seroprevalence documented that the decreasing prevalence hid a high HIV incidence.[23] Similarly, in Zaire, the same observation was made among antenatal clinic attenders.[17] Individuals who seroconvert represent recently infected persons, and evaluation of seroconverters is likely to be a more sensitive indicator of interventions than are studies of AIDS incidence or HIV seroprevalence.[2,24]

Incidence rates generally are the most useful biological outcome measure for program evaluation, since the overall goal of most programs is the prevention of new infections. However, for some STDs the incidence rate is often too low to be useful for evaluation purposes. For example, HIV seroconversion in the United States, even among high risk, high prevalence groups, is sufficiently rare that most evaluations using HIV incidence would require enrolling thousands of participants and following them for many years before a statistically significant difference could be shown.

Incidence of selected STDs is a useful surrogate for HIV incidence as a biological outcome to evaluate HIV prevention programs.[15,25] Incident STDs can provide a proxy for HIV incidence because they reflect situations where at-risk sexual behavior occurs that results in documented disease transmission. However, caution must be applied to the interpretation of different STD rates as proxies for HIV-related outcomes, because the epidemiological patterns of these diseases are still poorly understood. For example, researchers in Miami found that, in spite of a high degree of clustering of syphilis and gonorrhea in similar geographic and demographic subgroups, the incidence rates for these diseases showed different trends in the subgroups examined.[26]

Finally, biologic measures cannot adequately capture the true burden of illness. Simple morbidity rates understate the burden of disease because counting rates of infection ignores entire dimensions of the health problem. Sequelae such as social and psychological complications, chronic pain, infertility, ectopic pregnancy, adverse pregnancy outcomes, infant morbidity and mortality, and cancer are ignored in traditional rates. Because the long-term consequences of most STDs are more serious for women than for men, and because of societal values and stigmatization, STD rates, in particular, grossly underestimate the social and psychological burden of disease in women.

BEHAVIORAL MEASURES

Although the ultimate goal of an STD/HIV intervention may be to prevent new infections, many prevention programs are designed to produce changes in behavior as a strategy to achieve that goal. Compared with biological measures, behavioral outcomes have the advantage of being more proximal to the intervention, and more common. Thus, evaluations using behavioral outcomes can be completed in a more timely manner and with a smaller sample size than evaluations using seroconversion. Much is known about what behaviors lead to STD/HIV infection, and the choice of which behavioral outcomes to measure is, in part, determined by which behaviors are targeted by the intervention being evaluated.

However, most STD and HIV risk behaviors cannot be directly observed or objectively measured. Therefore, most behavioral outcomes rely on self-reports of these behaviors. Both reliability and validity of measures of self-reported behaviors are difficult to determine.[27–29] Self-reported behaviors may be subject to systematic biases such as inaccurate recall or giving socially desirable responses.[30,31] This response bias is particularly worrisome in the context of evaluating interventions where the intervention is targeted toward changing a participant's behaviors. In this context, there can be substantial pressure on participants to answer with a desired response.

Another issue with behavioral outcomes is lack of standardization in the field. Although standards for behavioral measures are common in other fields (e.g., smoking cessation), they have been slow to develop in STD/HIV prevention. Evaluation data are most useful if outcome data are collected in a consistent way such that interventions can be compared with each other. For policy makers and those charged with allocating resources among effective programs, it is necessary to link resources expended with "units" of behavior change and estimates of how many cases of STD/HIV could be averted. Unless a core set of behavioral outcomes are agreed on, and the surveys and questionnaires used to measure these outcomes are worded in a consistent manner, it becomes difficult to interpret and compare results from different evaluations.[2]

ECONOMIC MEASURES

The costs of the health outcome being averted and costs associated with any side effects of the intervention are both important outcomes measures. The cost of the actual program being evaluated is essential for economic evaluation and will be discussed later with the research designs of economic evaluation. Cost of illness is one measure that researchers use to assess the burden of disease.

There are three basic types of cost outcomes that can be measured: direct, indirect, and intangible. Direct medical costs are the resources expended on illness. They include drugs, physicians fees, tests, and procedures. Direct nonmedical costs include food, travel, and lodging associated with medical treatment.

Indirect costs are the resources forgone as a result of illness, and can be measured as lost productivity. There are two ways of measuring indirect costs. The human capital approach measures productivity loss as the value of the future earnings that may be lost owing to premature morbidity or mortality from the illness. The challenge with this method is that not everyone works, and some people work for no money, so the human capital approach tends to value outcomes less for women, elderly, disabled, minorities, and others with low incomes or children. The willingness to pay approach is an alternative method that determines how much people are willing to pay to decrease their risk of illness or death. The results of this method are influenced by how much money the respondent has, and increases with increased income, so the willingness to pay approach yields relatively low estimates for those with low incomes.

Intangible costs are nonfinancial outcomes such as pain, suffering, or grief. Since intangible costs are difficult to measure, and even more difficult to translate into economic terms, they are often ignored in economic analyses.

In the cost-of-illness approach to measure the burden of disease, the outcomes are quantifiable (in monetary terms), can often be validated, and can be standardized across diseases. However, the weaknesses of this approach are that it relies on estimates, excludes intangibles, only counts earnings, and is biased because it undervalues some groups relative to others, thus underestimating the value of preventing STDs. Thus, such analyses must be interpreted with caution, recognizing that they represent the lower bound estimate of the true human cost of illness.

HEALTH STATUS AND QUALITY OF LIFE MEASURES

Health status and quality of life measures attempt to broadly capture not only participants' physical health but their functional status, well-being, and satisfaction with care, to compliment the traditional biologic and economic outcomes measures. These health status measures can assess the end result on overall health and quality of life in contrast to death or infection rates by emphasizing more common elements of health that are important to patients and families. Furthermore, such measures can provide a single indicator that can cut across populations and compare various diseases, and can provide a comparable measure of output for program evaluation.

One measure of fatal outcomes that is frequently used is years of potential life lost. The number of years of life lost can be calculated in several ways, but a common way is to use the difference between the actual age at death and the life expectancy of individuals in that age group. As we have seen, only looking at years of potential life lost underestimates the burden of disease, because it does not take into account pre-death illness, or illness that does not result in a fatal outcome. Several composite measures have been developed to include both nonfatal outcomes and premature mortality.

One common outcome of cost-utility analyses is the quality adjusted life year (QALY). The QALY measures health improvement in terms of individual preferences for time spent in different health states. The results of such analyses are often expressed as the number of QALYs gained and the cost per QALY gained as a result of the intervention. QALYs are calculated by combining life expectancy with a preference-based estimate of the quality of life. Methods used to measure these preferences are complex, and involve various techniques of assessing the value that individuals or society places on specific health states. However, there are currently no standardized methods for measuring quality. Thus, those using or interpreting QALY outcomes cannot assume that all QALY are comparable, a major handicap given the objective of comparison.

A second way to measure nonfatal outcomes, developed by the World Bank and the World Health Organization, is the disability adjusted life year (DALY), which focuses on impairments, disabilities, and handicaps resulting from illness.[32,33] The DALY is an estimate of the number of years of healthy life lost, which combines the number of years lost owing to premature death with an estimate of the expected duration of disability. The incidence, age of onset, and duration of each specific disease is estimated on the basis of community-based epidemiological data, and other available sources. Six disability classes are defined and relative weights of severity are assigned. The time lived in each class is multiplied by the disability weight. Finally, death and disability are discounted so future years of healthy life are valued less than present health; and age weights are applied so years of life at different ages are given different values.

DALYs have been featured most prominantly in the World Bank's World Development Report of 1993.[33] Here, STD-related DALYs were compared with DALYs from different diseases, and among different populations. Use of this method clearly shows the heavy burden of STDs on women compared to other diseases, and compared to the burden on men. Although the DALY is quite useful for comparisons across disease categories, it is still not sensitive to the burden of disease for most STDs, because the calculation only includes the most crude measures of disability (e.g., loss of procreative function from PID). Finally, analyses using DALY provide a picture of the burden of disease smoothed across social classes. Since between social classes the age structure of the population may be different, it is recommended to stratify the data by at least age and other variables related to socioeconomic status.[34] Because the burden of illness is not equally distributed across all communities, and among all people within a community, such measures should equitably value life across ethnic, age, gender, and class groups.

A third way to measure nonfatal outcomes involves placing a value on duration of life lost or gained, as modified by dimensions of health such as pain, emotional and psychological well-being, physical, social, cognitive, and reproductive functioning.[35] These "health-related quality of life" (HRQOL) measures define the dimensions of health status, measure them, and summarize these dimensions as outcomes of programs.

HRQOL measures have been quite useful in evaluating HIV related treatment regimens. For example, in one randomized controlled trial of zidovudine (ZDV) versus zalcitabine (ddC) in advanced HIV infection, whereas there was no obvious clinical advantage to taking ddC versus ZDV, ZDV had a clear advantage in improving quality of life, as measured in a self-administered survey assessing disability, symptom impact, health status, and function.[36] In a placebo-controlled trial of ZDV in early symptomatic disease, the drug was shown to delay progression to AIDS by a few months; however, at the high doses given, not only did the drug not improve functional status and well-being compared to the placebo, but the quality of life in the placebo group was better. Subsequently, the study was repeated using lower doses and demonstrated that, for asymptomatic patients taking lower dose ZDV, the reduction in quality of life owing to medication side effects was about equal to the increase in quality of life associated with a delay in progression of the disease.[37] Recent advances in antiviral therapy makes these regimens obsolete, yet the precedent of including HRQOL outcomes in clinical trials is well established.

Health outcomes from most evaluation studies, and outcomes collected by public health departments understate the burden of STDs, and researchers in the field need to adopt more sophisticated STD-related outcomes measures that capture not only infection rates, but broader measures of patient welfare. If we continue to define the value of medical treatment and prevention activities in terms of simply preventing infections or postponing death, then we undervalue those interventions.

RESEARCH DESIGNS AND METHODS

Non-experimental Designs

Perhaps the most common non-experimental design in the literature on program evaluation is the one group pretest–posttest, also called before/after design.[38] This design has no separate comparison group, and compares pre- and post-intervention observations on the same group. Another common design is the one-group posttest only design, which lacks both pre-intervention observations and a comparison group. The posttest-only design with nonequivalent groups has a comparison group, but no pre-intervention observation. The latter is common where a policy or program was initiated before a researcher could collect baseline data. In all three of these designs the outcome can be attributed either to the intervention or to the selection of who gets the intervention, or to a variety of other historical or environmental factors. There is no way of determining what the true effect of the intervention really is. Such evaluations, although they may be useful for formative research, are generally uninterpretable for program evaluation.[38,39]

QUASI-EXPERIMENTAL DESIGNS

Quasi-experimental designs use a separate, non-randomized control group. The control group(s) is usually separated temporally or spatially. There are two common designs for quasi-experimental studies: interrupted time series and the nonequivalent groups design. In an interrupted time series, the effects of the treatment are inferred by comparing measures taken at many time periods before and after the treatment. This design can be improved by adding a control group that, although not randomized, is comparable. In the matched design, the response of an experimental group is compared to that of a control group before and after the intervention. Variants also include having proxy preintervention measures when baseline data was not collected, and using preintervention measures at more than one time interval (such as a wait-list control), which strengthens the design.[39]

The advantages of quasi-experimental designs are that they achieve some control when randomization is not possible. This situation occurs frequently because it is difficult to randomize the receipt of services. Furthermore, it is often too late to randomize in the context of a program evaluation. The primary disadvantage of these designs is that comparisons are being made on nonequivalent groups that differ in many ways in addition to presence or absence of intervention. This leads to numerous threats to the validity of the study that would not exist were there random assignment. Because of the nonequivalent comparison groups, treated and nontreated groups may differ in outcome even if treatment has no effect. Because the researcher cannot rely on randomization to rule out bias, strategies must be adopted to address the noncomparability of groups. The first is to measure all known differences in groups and to have sufficient knowledge of the population to explain why subjects are selected into the different groups. These known and measured factors can be controlled for by matching in the design, and by adjustment in the analysis. For unknown and unmeasured, or frequently unknowable and unmeasurable differences, one must still attempt to estimate the magnitude of potential biases and relate that to the observed effect size.

This reflects best practice in most applied evaluation research. The use of data from multiple sources (sometimes called triangulation) can serve to enhance these designs. When these data confirm the results of the quasi-experimental analysis, causal inference can be strengthened.[40]

RANDOMIZED CONTROLLED TRIALS

Randomized controlled trials represent true experiments, and provide the strongest evidence for (or against) a program's effectiveness. In this design, program participants are randomized to receive either the intervention or to become a control group. Properly done randomized controlled trials assure that the intervention and control groups are probabilistically equivalent except for the intervention. This provides for much stronger inference that any differences in outcome between the groups can be attributed to the effects of the intervention and not to some other extraneous cause. This design can also be modified to ask the question: What works better? Program participants can be randomized into different comparison groups, each receiving a different intervention or a different level of intensity of the same intervention to compare intervention strategies.

Randomized trials have the disadvantages of being costly, time-consuming, and subject to some methodological flaws such as differential dropout. They can present legal and ethical challenges and are sometimes subject to community and political opposition.

Nevertheless, the U.S. National Academy of Sciences Panel on Evaluation of AIDS Programs has stated that, "to improve interventions that are already broadly implemented the panel recommends the use of randomized field experiments of alternative or enhanced interventions." And, "before a new intervention is broadly implemented, the panel recommends that it be pilot tested in a randomized field experiment."[11]

STD and HIV prevention programs, because they often take place on a community-wide scale, are suited to be evaluated using community-based randomized control trials.[16] The unit of randomization in such trials is the community (rural area, village, town, city) and trials should include several communities (at least 12) for comparison purposes.[16] A recent application of such a trial in Tanzania to assess the effect of STD case management on HIV incidence has documented spectacular reductions in HIV incidence rates in the six intervention communities.[41] Such trials, although expensive to undertake, have an important impact on health policy.

QUALITATIVE METHODS

Although qualitative methods such as ethnographic assessment, focus groups, in-depth interviews, direct observation, and document reviews cannot contribute to determinations of causality and efficacy, these methods are an indispensable part of evaluation as they allow the evaluator to put results in their context and interpret them. Qualitative methods are used constantly to frame the research questions, and in the development of data collection instruments. During an evaluation, qualitative techniques can provide detailed information about program operation; help to determine the quality of services; identify unintended outcomes, benefits, or harms of a program; help to interpret quantitative data by providing context and explanations; and provide important information to those wanting to replicate or scale-up an intervention.[2,3,27,42] Content analysis frequently is used to analyze qualitative data. This method involves the use of predetermined categories to code participants' responses, and examine frequencies, sequences, and other patterns in the data.

ECONOMIC EVALUATION

How can we use the available prevention resources to avert the maximum number of infections? Traditional behavioral and epidemiological techniques and outcome measures cannot answer this question. Economic evaluations allow comparisons that consider both the costs and outcomes of alternative prevention strategies to assess whether the benefits gained from a program are worth the resources expended. Specifically, these evaluations can answer several types of questions that may be of importance to policy makers: What are the financial resources necessary to establish and run a program? Does the program's benefits outweigh its costs? If a program is not cost-saving, how does its costs compare to what society is willing to pay to achieve similar benefits? Even if a program is beneficial, could the financial resources be better spent by funding a different program? Which combination among all of the potentially beneficial programs, funded at what levels, represents the most efficient allocation of scarce prevention resources?

To answer these questions, six basic data elements are needed.[43]

1. The program description;
2. The health outcome averted through the program (e.g., cases of PID or HIV infections averted);
3. The rates and societal burden of the health outcome;
4. The proportion of this health outcome potentially averted as a result of the program (e.g., the preventable fraction);
5. The program's cost; and
6. The cost of the health outcome prevented.

Once these basic data elements are obtained, several analytic techniques can be used to address policy questions. Cost-effectiveness analysis is the most commonly used model to combine the cost of implementing a prevention program with the effectiveness of that intervention. Cost-effectiveness analysis measures the money expended (in monetary units) per health outcome achieved (e.g., cost per case of HIV infection averted). Another term, cost-efficiency, refers to how well a program's resources are being used in terms of the level of services provided in relation to the cost. Additional models include cost-benefit analysis and cost-utility analysis. Cost-benefit is the relationship between the cost of an activity and the benefits that accrue from it, expressed in monetary terms. Cost-benefit analysis converts health outcomes into a monetary value, based on how much society values the outcome or is willing to pay for it, expressing the results as money expended per monetary value of the benefit achieved and is typically expressed as a single cost:benefit ratio. A common use of cost-benefit analysis is to evaluate whether, from a societal perspective, the benefits of a program outweigh its costs. Cost-utility analysis is a form of economic evaluation in which the costs are expressed in monetary terms but health outcomes are expressed in units of utility, for example, quality-adjusted life-years (QALYs), or healthy days of life, or disability adjusted life-years (DALYs). Cost-utility analyses are useful in comparing programs with different health outcomes.

Because these models tend to be simple, static models, they cannot capture the complexity of population level transmission dynamics. For example, a model of partner notification of chlamydia for prevention of PID may adequately estimate the program effects on reinfection rates, and first generation partners, but cannot include the population-level effects from second or subsequent level infections.[44] Furthermore, these models frequently do not include intangible costs, such as quality of life. Thus, they underestimate the burden of STDs, and undervalue the benefits of prevention. However, for many policy questions, and for cases which demonstrate a clear cost-effectiveness of a strategy, these models may be quite sufficient.[10,45,46] Additionally, because economic analyses distribute costs and consequences equally across society, these models often do not (or cannot) address issues of resource inequity that arise because STDs and HIV infection are not equally distributed across society.[34] The costs and benefits to specific communities and sociodemographic groups may be of importance to decision makers when assessing program impact. This is related to an additional limitation of these quantitative models, in that they cannot address unstated goals of a program, such as com-

Table 98-2. Criteria for Economic Evaluations*

Does the study:

1. Have a well-defined question or objective?
2. Provide a complete description of the alternative strategies being compared?
3. Clearly state the perspective of the analysis (e.g., societal, individual, government)?
4. Establish evidence of the program's effectiveness?
5. Specify costs and consequences of each alternative?
6. Measure costs and consequences accurately?
7. Use discounting?
8. Include sensitivity analysis for key variables?

* Adapted from Drummond et al., 1987.[60]

munity empowerment, which may only peripherally be linked to the health outcome averted.

Table 98-2 summarizes the main criteria for conducting economic evaluations.

EVALUATING PREVENTION, CARE, AND SUPPORT FOR LARGE-SCALE PROGRAMS

THE EXAMPLE OF GLOBAL HIV/STD PREVENTION INDICATORS

Indicators are observable measures of the progress toward goals, objectives, and performance targets (see Fig. 98-3). For the selection of indicators, consideration must be given to ease of assessment, and to the feasibility, accuracy, reliability, and validity of the measurements taken. Based on these considerations, ten indicators of progress and outcomes of prevention activities were developed in 1993 to 1994 by the World Health Organization (WHO) (Table 98-3).[2,21] The reasoning behind the formulation of these prevention indicators, and the practical issues surrounding methods for their measurement have been discussed extensively elsewhere.[2,21] Five indicators are measured during a population survey: reported knowledge of preventive practices (PI1), condom availability at peripheral level (PI3), reported frequency of nonregular sexual partners (PI4), reported condom use during nonregular sexual encounters (PI5), and reported STD incidence among men (PI9). Condom availability at central level (PI2) is assessed through a record review and key-informant interviews with major distributors. Structured observations during a health facility survey allow assessment of the appropriateness of STD case management (PI6 and PI7). These two indicators will be discussed with the assessment of care quality. Finally a serosurvey among antenatal clinic attenders aged 15 to 24 years allows the measurement of HIV and syphilis seroprevalence in that population (PI8 and PI10). Such surveys should be repeated after a period of 1 to several years, depending on the type of survey, the available resources, and the level of program implementation.

Table 98-3. List of Prevention Indicators (PI)

PI1: Knowledge of preventive practices
- Number of people citing at least two acceptable ways of protection from HIV infection
- Total number of people aged 15 to 49 surveyed

PI2: Condom availability (central level)
- Total number of condoms available for distrubition during the preceding 12 months
- Population aged 15 to 49

PI3: Condom availability (peripheral level)
- Number of people who can acquire a condom
- Population aged 15 to 49

PI4: Reported nonregular sexual partners
- Number of people aged 15 to 49 who report having had at least one sex partner other than a regular sex partner(s) in the last 12 months
- Total number of people aged 15 to 49 who report having been sexually active in the last 12 months

PI5: Reported condom use with nonregular sex partners
- Number of people aged 15 to 49 reporting the use of a condom during the most recent act of sexual intercourse with a nonregular sex partner
- Total number of people aged 15 to 49 reporting sexual intercourse with a nonregular sex partner in the last 12 months

PI6: STD case management
- Number of individuals presenting with STD in health facilities assessed and treated in an appropriate way (according to national standards)
- Number of individuals presenting with STD in health facilities

PI7: STD case management
- Number of individuals presenting with STD or for STD care in health facilities who received basic advice on condoms and on partner notification
- Number of individuals presenting with STD or for STD care in health facilities

PI9: Reported STD incidence, men
- Number of reported episodes of urethritis in men aged 15 to 49 in the last 12 months
- Number of men aged 15 to 49 surveyed

Under development

PI8: STD prevalence, women
- Number of pregnant women aged 15 to 24 with positive serology for syphilis
- Total number of pregnant women aged 15 to 24 attending antenatal clinics whose blood has been screened

PI10: HIV prevalence, women
- Number of pregnant women aged 15 to 24 seropositive for HIV
- Total number of pregnant women aged 15 to 24 attending antenatal clinics whose blood has been screened

The prevention indicators provide a quantitative but incomplete picture of some of the efforts to prevent HIV transmission through modification of patterns of sexual behavior and through comprehensive management of STD. A comparison of all the PI estimates can aid interpretation of both STD and HIV program effectiveness. To infer an association between, for example, an increase in PI1 (knowledge of preventive practices), and a decrease in PI10 (HIV prevalence in antenatal clinic attenders aged 15–24) is invalid unless an analysis of the scores of all the PIs and their trends over time, combined with a contextual analysis, is performed.[47]

A full understanding is required of the context within which programs operate, to interpret results provided by PIs. This (formative and process) evaluation necessitates multilevel approaches using broad and flexible field research methodologies. The first step is to collect relevant published data, at national and subnational levels, on the political and administrative context, demography, economy, and health sector system. Emphasis should be on factors relevant to sexual behavior and situations enhancing risk during sexual encounters, as well as on health and social services infrastructure. A second key area is the documentation of program targets and level of implementation. Data that may be relevant here relate to the content and quantity of information, education and communication materials, educational efforts by various sectors, resource allocation, and availability of condoms and drugs to treat STDs. Finally it is essential that a thorough analysis of each of the surveys is conducted, beyond the simple computation of indicators. Breakdowns by sex, age, and geographical location are an essential component of the interpretation of each PI.

Following an extensive WHO training program in different regions of the world, surveys for the assessment of prevention indicators are being performed and analyzed in 22 countries. Results from a variety of baseline evaluation have been or are being published, including collaborative evaluations between governments and WHO.[48–52] Furthermore, some work has been completed relating to the validity of the population survey method proposed for some of the PIs.[28] The challenge is now to repeat the surveys to provide trends over time in a variety of settings. The conduct of evaluations using PI indicators has, in virtually all cases, mobilized program managers, clinicians and other participating sectors to plan for improved efforts in the area of condom supply, STD case management, and interventions for behavioural change.

EVALUATING THE QUALITY OF STD CARE

Control and prevention of STDs are important goals in their own right, and also constitute a major strategy in the prevention of HIV infection. Medical consultations for STDs can contribute in several ways to reducing the risk of STD and HIV transmission. First, treatment will reduce duration and incidence of STDs. Second, since existing STDs increase the probability of HIV transmission during a sexual encounter between an HIV infected and non-HIV infected person, successful treatment of STDs is likely to decrease the frequency sexual transmission of HIV occurs, as was recently demonstrated in a community level randomized trial.[16,41,53,54] Third, attenders at STD clinics form a group among whom health promotion aimed at increasing the practice of safer sexual behavior is important. Optimal clinical management of STDs therefore has several components. First, accurate diagnosis and successful treatment of the existing STD. Second, health education and counseling with respect to safer sex, in particular condom use. Finally, partner notification followed by partner referral, to facilitate targeting of STD treatment and health education.

In recognition that appropriate clinical management of STDs is of such importance for STD/HIV/AIDS prevention, the World Health Organization (WHO) has developed a protocol for the surveillance of the clinical management of STDs (PI6, PI7; Table 98-3) as part of a global set of indicators.[2,10,21,50] PI6 measures the proportion of individuals who are assessed and treated for STDs in an appropriate way; PI7 measures the proportion who receive advice on condom use and partner notification.

A survey is conducted of a sample of health care facilities providing care to people presenting with STD complaints, with the following methods of data collection: enumeration of all health care facilities providing STD care; interviews with health care providers; and observation of the practices of health care providers with individual patients. These methods provide an overview of the facilities that deliver STD care to a significant part of the population (enumeration), allow the identification of constraints in supplies and areas for improvement in health care provision (interviews), and the evaluation of the quality of case management (observation). During the observation a score (positive or negative) is given for each consultation between a patient and a health care provider, in order to assess the quality of case management. Up to 300 observations are required to compute PI6 and PI7 and detect an improvement of 50 percent in the original score on repeating the survey, taking into account the fact that observations made on the same health care provider are not independent. (The sample size is increased by a factor of at least 1.5.) Such surveys are best undertaken at a regional level and can be repeated at an interval of 1 to 2 years, depending on the results of the baseline survey and the resources available.

"Appropriate STD assessment and treatment" are defined in terms of the health care provider's adherence to certain standards in history taking, examination and treatment. Clinicians may diagnose and treat on a presumptive (based on symptoms and syndromes), a clinical (based on signs) or an etiologic (with laboratory confirmation of the diagnosis) basis. Since the diagnosis cannot be independently confirmed during observation, it does not contribute to the scoring of PI6, but the way diagnosis is made (using a presumptive, clinical, or an etiologic approach) and its results are recorded in order to assess the appropriateness of treatment. The criteria for appropriate treatment will have a big impact on the outcome score. In South India, using minimum treatment criteria the PI6 score revealed that 67 percent of observed health care provider-patient encounters met the requirement of "appropriate case management." But a more strict interpretation for PI6 is that all patients be given presumptive (syndromic) treatment, unless a positive etiological diagnosis is made, because this approach ensures that the patient is treated for most pathologies making up a syndrome. Using such a strict scoring method, the PI6 was positive in only 10 percent of the observations in South India.[2,50]

For PI7, "basic" advice refers to the promotion of condom use, and a request that partners be informed and referred for treatment. The provision of condoms at the clinic is recorded but is not part of the scoring. Health care providers are expected to discuss the use of condoms in preventing STD and also to provide basic instructions on condom use. If this were included in the PI7 score it appears that most clinicians would score very poorly.[2,49,50] Figure 98-5 shows the percentage of observed encounters in four major cities of Ethiopia in which different aspects of clinical management were handled appropriately, whereas Fig. 98-6 shows the result of observation for prevention.[47]

The process of observation is likely to influence the behavior of clinicians who will pay more attention to their behavior than on a routine basis. Even if the scored PIs are overestimates owing to such "Hawthorne effect," the exercise is useful in identifying that even the maximal standard is low. To investigate the problem of the Hawthorne effect, it is proposed to use persons with fictitious symptoms (simulated patients) in a few settings, perhaps on a subsample basis, to obtain an estimate of the quality of STD case management with the potential bias of known observation removed. This technique has been used in the evaluation of health care for children and family planning services.[50,55,56]

It is recognized that patients with symptomatic STD consult a wide range of health care providers, including public, private, in-

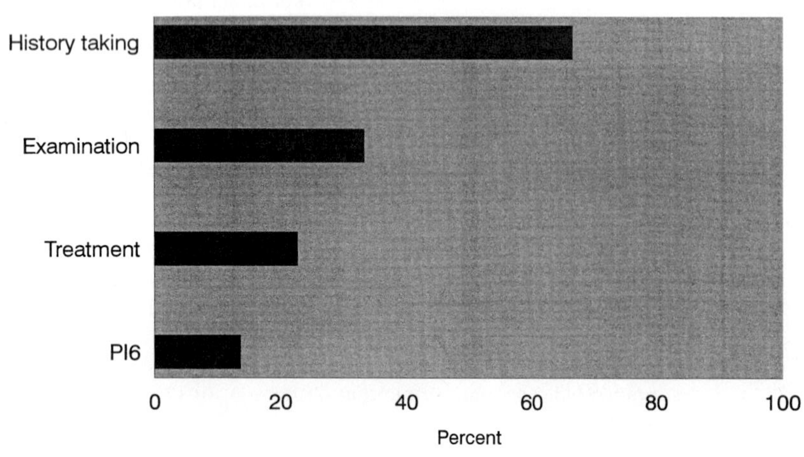

Fig. 98-5. STD case management, Ethiopia. Percentage of observed encounters in which different aspects of STD clinical management were handled appropriately.[47]

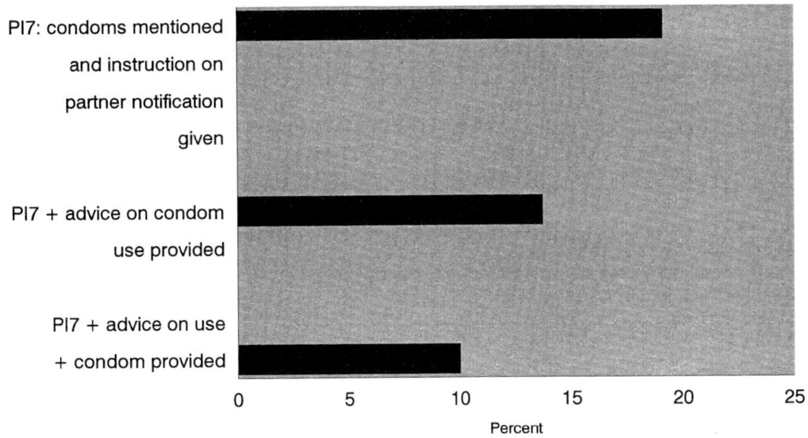

Fig. 98-6. STD case management, Ethiopia. Percentage of observed encounters in which different aspects of STD prevention were handled appropriately.[47]

formal, and traditional sources of care. For logistic reasons, however, the protocol for assessing STD care explicitly focuses on the measurement of the indicators in health facilities (public and private) and does not address the quality of care provided by other health care providers such as traditional healers and pharmacists.

EVALUATING CARE OF HIV/AIDS

Quality care of HIV related conditions not only alleviates suffering but can also improve life expectancy of HIV-infected persons. In addition, prevention and care are strongly interrelated. Since resources are limited, especially in developing countries, strategies need to be developed to provide an acceptable standard of care at an affordable price.

Two indicators have been developed to assess whether the basic conditions for HIV/AIDS care could be met.[10] The first Care and Support indicator (CSI) assesses the availability as well as the capacity of a health care structure to deliver standard services of care for HIV-infected persons. Facilities should offer the five following standard services; they must

1. Be adequate to provide nursing and medical care;
2. Have the appropriate level of diagnostic facilities;
3. Have the required medications;
4. Have the capacity to provide counselling and prevent discrimination; and
5. Have measures in place to prevent nosocomial transmission of HIV, including through use of screened blood transfusions.

Every health care structure should have the capacity to manage and/or appropriately refer three major conditions potentially related to HIV infection: lower respiratory tract infections (including pulmonary tuberculosis), chronic diarrhea, and oral candidiasis.[10,57]

The second indicator evaluates directly the quality of HIV/AIDS case management in assessing the proportion of patients with potentially HIV-related conditions who are appropriately managed in health facilities. For a number of reasons one is unlikely to be able to evaluate patients with proven HIV-related conditions; not all patients will have been tested for HIV infection, testing facilities are not available everywhere, and some patients may not wish to have their HIV infection status disclosed. These problems are partially overcome by assessing the management of patients suffering from conditions that are frequently, but not always, HIV-related. In contrast to CSI1, only one condition predicitve of HIV infection is selected: lower respiratory tract infections (including pulmonary tuberculosis, pleural effusion, and bacterial infiltrates).

Data for CSI1 are collected by interview of specific persons using a standard questionnaire as well as by standardized recording of observations. For CSI2, medical records of in-patients with lower respiratory tract infection are reviewed with the physician, medical assistant, and/or nurse. The information is also collected by a standardized recording of observations, and structured interviews of in-patients.

ASSESSING PROGRESS TOWARD ELIMINATION OF DISCRIMINATION AGAINST PEOPLE WITH HIV

Since the effectiveness of a prevention policy will depend to a great extent on the feelings of acceptance experienced by individuals, it is essential to combat discrimination. Two indicators have been developed in this area.[10,58]

From a practical standpoint, discrimination may be found at three levels: in legislative texts; in the internal regulations of institutions; in practice, both legal and institutional, for which there is no official written basis. Bringing discrimination to light will pose different problems for the three sources. The difficulty in detecting it will be inversely proportional to the degree to which the forms of discrimination are public and official. Moreover, in the case of indirect discrimination, measures may not mention seropositivity or AIDS and yet may effectively be aimed at persons who are seropositive (e.g., measures of health control imposed on sex workers on the basis that they are, or may be persons at risk).

To enable programs to identify and then monitor the evolution of rules and practices that discriminate against persons with HIV/AIDS, the following indicator is proposed as CSI3: Proportion of nondiscriminatory practices/rules identified in relation to the total number of practices/rules that may be discriminatory with respect to HIV/AIDS.

A list of forms of discrimination has been developed that should enable AIDS programs to apprehend and to combat situations where there is discrimination based on HIV serostatus, taking into account the legal system of their countries. Thirty nine situations in nine major areas of social life in which distinctions, exclusions, or restrictions for persons with HIV and AIDS may occur have been listed. The list has been structured around the principal areas of social life: Health; Employment; Administration; Justice/Legal process; Social welfare; Housing; Education; Family life; Insurance.[10,58]

Information should be systematically gathered in the nine areas from persons with special knowledge of each of these areas. The investigators should therefore systematically interview key informants, such as all the persons professionally concerned with people with HIV/AIDS: doctors, social workers, nursing and paramedical personnel, teachers, and lawyers.

Finally, societal responses or reactions can cause considerable harm to those with HIV or subpopulations thought to be implicated in HIV transmission, and may hinder efforts national and community efforts to minimize HIV transmission. For these reasons, positive action against discrimination and negative public perceptions of AIDS are an important component of national HIV/AIDS programs strategies and progress towards change should be evaluated. The fourth indicator therefore assesses the proportion of people aged 15 to 49 years who report nondiscriminatory attitudes towards individuals with HIV/AIDS. The indicator is derived from answers to a sequence of four questions (e.g., "would you be willing or not to take care of a family member with AIDS?"), in the interview schedule for the general population survey used to measure prevention indicators.

The protocols for the assessment of HIV/AIDS case management have been field-tested in Kenya and Uganda and the protocol for assessing discriminatory practices in Cote d'Ivoire and the Philippines and are in the process of being finalized.[10]

EVALUATING HEALTH PLANS: THE HEDIS EXAMPLE

Another example of tools that can be used to evaluate clinical and preventive care are performance indicators. In the United States, HEDIS (Health Plan Employer Data and Information Set) is a set of over 60 standardized performance measures used to evaluate the quality of managed care plans. HEDIS forms the basis of most health plan "report cards," and is used by many health plans for their own quality improvement efforts, or because the purchasers with whom they do business (consumers, corporations, and public purchasers) require the reporting of HEDIS.[59] By using standard definitions, specific methodologies and a common set of reporting standards for assessing health plan performance, HEDIS enables tracking of plan performance over time, and allows evaluators to make comparisons across health plans.

There are eight "domains," into which HEDIS is organized.

1. Effectiveness at achieving appropriate clinical results;
2. Access and availability of care to patients;
3. Patient satisfaction with the care they receive;
4. Effectiveness with which plans educate and inform their patients;
5. Attributes and operating characteristics of the plan and its management;
6. Cost of care;
7. Stability of a plan's finances and of its network of providers; and
8. Efficiency with which a plan uses its resources.

Although there are currently no STD or HIV-related HEDIS measures, a measure on chlamydia screening has been proposed, and is currently being tested for potential inclusion in 2000. The proposed measure would assess the extent to which health plans are successful in implementing existing guidelines for chlamydia testing of sexually active women. This would be measured as the number of women between the ages of 15 to 25 tested for chlamydia divided by the number of sexually active women between the ages of 15 to 25 enrolled in the health plan. To report the numerator, health plans will need to know the total number of women tested which will mean extracting data from a laboratory data base. To report the denominator, plans will need to know the total number of sexually active women between the ages of 15 to 25 enrolled in the plan. This may mean extracting data from several administrative and clinical data sets.

In the United States, inclusion of a chlamydia screening measure in HEDIS will most likely drive health plans to improve their screening rates. Because the HEDIS project represents an evaluation tool targeted at a health system, it encompasses a diverse set of measures and cannot evaluate STD-related performance in more detail. A set of similar measures focused on the more limited scope of STD clinical and preventive care can and should be developed for use by STD managers to evaluate their programs' activities.

CONCLUSION

In general, the evaluation of comprehensive STD and HIV/AIDS prevention programs must combine several of the evaluation types, designs and methods discussed in this chapter. There is a need to integrate the different components of evaluation. First, to assess the appropriateness of efforts, evaluators must understand the context in which these efforts are taking place to slow the spread of STD and HIV and to manage patients with these infections. Second, once activities are underway, there is a need to examine whether they are being carried out as planned, are on schedule and are within budget. Third, the outputs and outcome of these activities should be examined against their stated objectives. Fourth, costing of activities must be done and the costs compared to the outcomes. In practice, however, each of these components is closely interlinked and the sequence may change over time. Monitoring of implementation is a continuous process, while contextual analysis and outcome evaluation, for example, are conducted at particular times.

Evaluation usually begins by identifying a clear statement of the objectives of the program. The evaluation planning process often further clarifies the objectives, making them more specific, measurable, and time-phased. For a specific set of activities, the specific objectives must be clearly defined. For a community outreach activity, for example, the objectives may include reducing the incidence of STD in local sex workers, increasing their access to local health care, reducing unsafe sexual practices, and increasing the number of trained peer educators.

Next follows the identification of qualitative assessments or quantitative indicators to be measured. These should relate to the stated overall objectives, but may also include "process measures," such as the number of pharmacies invited to take part in condom distribution or the number of staff trained in STD case management, as well as qualitative assessments of facilitators and barriers to program implementation.

Finally, decisions are made about how these assessments or indicators are to be conducted or measured, which methods to use for qualitative assessments and how often this will be done, through routine monitoring or special surveys.

Ultimately, what distinguishes evaluation research from other forms of scientific research is the objective of providing information to decision makers. The evaluation should be guided by the important program-relevant decisions and policy questions, and should recognize the interests of the various stakeholders. The success and relevance of the evaluation process is thus tied to the involvement in the process of program staff, participants, and other stakeholders. It follows that those conducting the evaluation then have a responsibility to communicate their findings, and to help decision makers use these findings to inform policy, improve programs, and to advocate for more resources.

To ensure optimal use of the evaluation process and its results and to learn from experience a participatory approach is required.[60] A participatory approach leads to ownership of evaluation results by all stakeholders and, therefore, leads to increased action taken on the results. The adoption of this principle does not preclude the complementary use of methods such as peer review or the involvement of external experts. The participatory approach implies that the evaluation team should include planners, program officers, and program members. Involvement of representatives of those who participated in the program is also key to the full utilization of the evaluation process.

A number of reviews have emphasized the shortcomings of current evaluation designs for most intervention projects for STD/HIV/AIDS and some have recommended that projects should use randomized controlled trials.[16,38,41,62,63] A lot more attention is also required to the way large scale (national or subnational) programs are evaluated to make full use of the multiple experiences, within and between counties. The appropriate conduct and use of evaluation requires a change in culture among implementors, researchers, and policy makers who must agree that the primary purpose of evaluation is to prove the worth of or improve program.

References

1 Stecher BM et al: *How to focus an evaluation?* London, Sage publication, New Delhi, 1987.
2 Mertens T et al: Prevention indicators for evaluating the progress of national AIDS programs. *AIDS* 8:1359–1369, 1994.
3 Aggleton P et al (eds): *Does it work?* London, Health Education Authority, 1992.
4 Quinn Patton M: *Utilization focused evaluation.* New Delhi, Sage Publications, 1986.
5 St. Leger AS et al: *Evaluating health services" effectiveness; a guide for health professionals, service managers and policy makers.* Open University Press, Milton Keynes, 1992.
6 Cairncross S et al: *Evaluation for village water supply planning.* Chichester, John Wiley and Sons, 1978.
7 Last J (ed): *A dictionary of epidemiology.* Oxford University Press, New York, 1983.
8 Rhodes T et al: *Hard to reach or out of reach, an evaluation of an innovative model of HIV outreach health education.* London, Tuffnell Press, 1991.
9 World Health Organization: *Evaluation of family planning in health services.* Report of a WHO Expert Committee. Technical Report Series 569, 1975.
10 Mertens TE et al: Evaluation of HIV/AIDS prevention, care and support: an update. *AIDS Education and Prevention* 9:133–145.
11 Coyle SL et al (eds): *Evaluating AIDS Prevention Programs.* Washington DC, National Academy Press, 1991.
12 Tuomilehto J et al: The changing role and legitimate boundaries of epidemiology: community-based prevention programs. *Soc. Sci. Med* 25:589–598, 1987.
13 Van Noren B et al: Simplifying the evaluation of primary health care programs. *Soc. Sci. Med* 26:1091–1097, 1989.
14 Schrettenbrunner A et al: different approach to evaluating PHC projects, in developing countries: how acceptable is it to aid agencies? *Health Policy and Planning* 8:128–135, 1993.
15 Mertens TE et al: Global estimates and epidemiology of HIV and AIDS: further heterogeneity in spread and impact. *AIDS* 9(suppl A): S259–S272, 1995.
16 Mertens TE et al: Epidemiological methods to study the interaction between HIV infection and other sexually transmitted diseases. *AIDS* 4:57–65, 1990.
17 Batter V et al: High HIV incidence in young women masked by stable overall seroprevalence among childbearing women in Kinshasa, Zaïre: estimating incidence for serial seroprevalence data. *AIDS* 8:811–818, 1994.
18 Mertens TE et al: Global estimates and epidemiology of HIV infections and AIDS. *AIDS* 8(Suppl 1):S361–S372, 1994.
19 Mertens TE et al: HIV and AIDS: where is the epidemic going? *Bull. WHO* 74:121–129, 1996.
20 Mertens T et al: Global aspects of HIV/AIDS epidemiology: general consideration, in De Vita V et al (eds): *AIDS, etiology, diagnosis, treatment and prevention.* Philadelphia, Lippincott, 103–118, 1996.
21 World Health Organization/GPA/TCO/SES/94.1: *Evaluation of a National AIDS Program, a methods package.*, WHO, Geneva, 1994.
22 Kassler WJ et al: Gonorrhea rates among US men, adjusted for sexual activity. *Am J Public Health* 84:(9)1524–1525, 1994.
23 Peterman TA et al: Decreasing prevalence hides a high HIV incidence: Miami *AIDS* 9:965–970, 1995.
24 Kassler WJ et al: Seroconversion in patients attending sexually transmitted disease clinics. *AIDS* 8:351–335, 1994.
25 Kamb ML et al: Designing a multicenter, randomized trial to evaluate the efficacy of HIV prevention counseling: Project RESPECT. *Prev Med,* in review.
26 Hammers FF et al: Syphilis and gonorrhea clustering in Miami: similar clustering, different trends. *Am J. Public Health* 85:1104–1108, 1995.
27 Report of the NIAID Study Group on Integrated Behavioral Research for Prevention and Control of Sexually Transmitted Diseases, in Wasserheit JN et al (eds): *Research issues in human behavior and sexually transmitted diseases in the AIDS era.* Washington DC, American Society for Microbiology, 353–371, 1991.
28 Konings E et al: Validating population surveys for the measurement of HIV/STD prevention indicators. *AIDS* 9:375–382, 1995.
29 Aral SO et al: Measuring outcomes of behavioral interventions for STD/HIV prevention. *Int J STD AIDS* 7(suppl 2):30–38, 1996.
30 Catania JA et al: Methodological problems in AIDS behavioral research: influences on measurement error and participation bias in studies of sexual behavior. *Psycho Bull* 108:339–362, 1990.
31 Zenilman JM et al. Condom use to prevent incident STDs: the validity of self-reported condom use. *Sex Trans Dis* 22:15–21, 1995.
32 Murray CJ: Quantifying the burden of disease: the technical basis for disability-adjusted life years. *Bull. WHO* 72:429–445, 1994.
33 The World Bank: *World Development Report 1993.* New York, Oxford University Press.
34 Gwatkin DR: Distributional implications of alternative strategic responses to the demographic-epidemiological transition-an initial inquiry, in *The Epidemiological Transition,* 1996.
35 Patrick D et al: *Health status and health policy.* New York, Oxford University Press, 1993.
36 Bozzette SA et al: Relative effects of ddC or ddI versus zidovudine on health status, function and disability in N3300 (ACTG 114) and ACTG 116b/117. *Int Conf AIDS,* 1992.
37 Wu AW et al: Functional status and well-being in a placebo-controlled trial of Zidovudine in early symptomatic HIV infection. *J. AIDS* 6: 452–458, 1993.
38 Choi KH et al: Prevention of HIV infection. *AIDS* 8:1371–1389, 1994.
39 Cook TD et al: *Quasi-experimentation: design and analysis isues for field settings.* Boston, Houghton Mifflin, 1979.
40 Rietmeyer K et al: Increasing the use of bleach and condoms among injecting drug users in Denver: outcomes of a targeted, community-level HIV prevention program. *AIDS* 10:291–298, 1996.
41 Grosskurth H et al: Impact of improved treatment of sexually transmitted diseases on HIV infection in rural Tanzania: randomised controlled trial. *Lancet* 346:530–536, 1995.
42 Gilliam A: Evaluating HIV prevention programs using qualitative methods, in *CDC handbook for evaluating HIV education.* Washington DC, USPHS, 1994.
43 Centers for Disease Control: Assessing the effectiveness of disease and injury prevention programs: costs and consequences. *MMWR* 44:(RR-10), 1995.
44 Howell MR et al: Partner notification to prevent pelvic inflammatory disease in women: cost-effectiveness of two strategies. *Sex Trans Dis* 24(5)287–292, 1997.
45 Haddix AD et al: The cost effectiveness of azithromycin for Chlamydia trachomatis infections in women. *Sex Trans Dis* 22:(5)274–280, 1995.
46 Watts C et al: Quantifying the impact of HIV prevention strategies. Why use DALYs? *Health Policy,* under review.

47 Mehret M et al: Baseline for the evaluation of an AIDS program: a case study in Ethiopia. *Bull WHO,* 74:25–33, 1996.

48 Bryce J et al: Quality of sexually transmitted disease services in Jamaica: evaluation of a clinic-based approach. *Bull WHO* 72:239–247, 1994.

49 Khantaraj K et al: Sexually transmitted disease services in Madras: could their role in AIDS prevention be strengthened? *Indian J Pub Health* 23(3):93–99, 1995.

50 Mertens TE et al: Observations of sexually transmitted disease consultations in Madras. *Public Health,* in press.

51 Watts C et al: Estimating the impact of five HIV prevention strategies. *IX-th International Conference on AIDS and STD in Africa,* Kampala, 10–15 December 1995.

52 Mertens TE et al: Evaluation of STD case management in Cote d'Ivoire, Ethiopia and Tanzania. How can we improve standards? *IX-th International Conference on AIDS and STD in Africa,* Kampala, 10–15 December 1995.

53 Cameron DW et al: Female to male transmission of human immunodeficiency virus type 1: risk factors for seroconversion in men. *Lancet* 2:403–407, 1989.

54 Laga M et al: Non ulcerative sexually transmitted diseases as risk factors for HIV-1 transmission in women. Results from a cohort study. *AIDS* 7:95–102, 1993.

55 Goodburn E et al: Management of childhood diarrhoea by pharmacists and parents: is Britain lagging behind the third world? *Br Med J* 302: 440–443, 1991.

56 Huntington D et al: The simulated client method: evaluating client-provider interactions in family planning clinics. *Studies in family planning* 24:187–193, 1993.

57 Kahindo M et al: Evaluation of case management of HIV/AIDS patients. Lessons learned from a field test in Kenya. *IX-th International Conference on AIDS and STD in Africa,* Kampala, 10–15 December 1995.

58 Carael M et al: Tools to evaluate AIDS care. *Global AIDS News* 4: 10–11, 1995.

59 The National Committee for Quality Assurance: *HEDIS 3.0: circulation draft for review and comment.* Washington DC, July 1996.

60 Rossi PH et al: *Evaluation. systematic approach.* London, Sage, 1993.

61 Drummond MF et al: *Methods for the economic evaluation of health care programs.* Oxford, Oxford University Press, 1987.

62 Oakley A et al: Behavioural interventions for HIV/AIDS prevention. *AIDS* 9;479–486, 1995.

63 De Zoysa I et al: Role of HIV counselling and testing in changing risk behavior in developing countries. *AIDS* 9(suppl A):S95–S101, 1995.

Chapter 99

The economic burden of sexually transmitted diseases in the United States

Joanna E. Siegel

Cost-of-illness measures provide a sense of the magnitude of the impact of an illness, as well as a point of reference for the consideration of program budgets and intervention priorities. Estimates of the economic cost of illness have been developed for many of the major causes of morbidity and mortality in the United States.[1–3] However, although the health burden imposed by the classical sexually transmitted diseases (STDs) is large, little research has been devoted to quantifying the economic impact of these diseases in the United States.

The lack of attention given to the cost of STDs may result from underrecognition of the prevalence and the consequences of STDs. Conversely, greater appreciation of the costs of STDs may focus greater attention on interventions to reduce their prevalence and consequences. Surveys have shown a lack of public awareness of STDs, and health care practitioners are frequently reluctant to discuss or evaluate their patients' sexual risks.[4] Both biologic factors, such as asymptomatic illness and delayed symptom onset, and social factors, such as the stigma associated with STDs, contribute to what the Institute of Medicine has termed a "hidden" epidemic.[4] As a result, many aspects of these diseases, including prevalence, incidence, and cost, are not well documented.

This chapter outlines a framework for considering the costs of STDs and presents available information on the costs of gonorrhea, chlamydia, syphilis, genital herpes, human papilloma virus (HPV), chancroid, hepatitis B, and human immunodeficiency virus (HIV). This information is intended to establish the groundwork for more extensive research in this area and to provide a basis for expanding the policy dialogue.

THE ECONOMIC BURDEN OF ILLNESS

The economic burden of an illness to society reflects the opportunity cost of resources consumed as a result of the illness; that is, the value of resources in their preferred alternative use. A measure of the economic burden of STDs thus indicates the value of resources that would be available for other purposes if they were not required to address STDs. The costs of STDs are covered by diverse sources: federal programs, private insurers, providers (physician, clinic, and hospital services that are not reimbursed), and patients themselves. The economic burden reflects the sum of resources devoted to STDs, regardless of the site of service or the source of payment.

The costs associated with disease, including STDs, are often divided into "direct" costs and productivity costs. Direct costs are those for services and materials, both medical and nonmedical. Major categories of direct costs include the costs of health care workers' services (those of physicians, nurses, technicians, and others), pharmaceuticals, medical equipment and supplies, and other resource inputs to outpatient treatment or hospital admissions. The costs of transportation, home care, special schooling, and other such resources are also direct costs.

Productivity costs are also incurred by illness. These costs, often termed "indirect" costs, reflect the value of productive time the affected individual (and society) lose because of illness. Productivity costs include both time spent sick, when an individual is unable to engage in the activities in which he or she otherwise would, and premature mortality. The impact of an illness on a person's productive ability is also included. The time an individual invests in treatment—traveling to obtain care, waiting in the clinic waiting room, filling a prescription, undergoing a procedure—could be categorized either as a direct cost or a productivity cost, but it entails an opportunity cost regardless of how it is catalogued.

The economic burden of disease can be demonstrated by calculating either the prevalent costs (the annual costs of cases prevalent during a given year) or the lifetime costs of incident cases. This chapter focuses on the former measure of economic burden, often termed the "cost-of-illness." This approach seeks to capture the costs associated with the cross section of existing cases—including current costs for cases that occurred previously—but does not reflect future costs associated with a disease. Prevalent costs provide an estimate of economic burden that is useful for comparisons in an annual context, for example, with federal, state, or institutional budgets. Incident costs, in contrast, demonstrate the full impact of an illness over time on a cost-per-case basis. They include the present value of future costs associated with the cases occurring during a given year.

For some illnesses, the distinction between prevalent and incident costs is of minimal importance, as the primary costs of the disease relate to the acute infection and occur during the first year of the disease. For most illnesses, however, costs occur over a longer period of time. This is clearly true for debilitating congenital illnesses, for which costs of care may extend over a lifetime. It is also true for STDs that have long-term consequences, such as pelvic inflammatory disease (PID) and infertility. When long-run costs of a disease are significant, prevalent and incident costs of illness will generally provide different measures of the impact of the disease.

This effort focuses on the collection and adjustment of existing estimates. It estimates prevalent costs (costs-of-illness) for the year 1994. The emphasis is on direct costs, although productivity loss estimates are reported where they exist. It should also be noted that this cost-of-illness approach does not evaluate the distribution of costs; that is, the differential burden of costs on payers or population groups.

WHY ASSESS THE COST OF ILLNESS?

Policy makers solicit and researchers undertake cost-of-illness studies to demonstrate the importance of an illness to society. As noted earlier, these studies place the burden of illness in the context of annual spending related to a specific cause. Consumers of this information then have some basis for assessing the priority of a problem or the appropriateness of the level of spending. So, for example, the Senate Appropriations Committee recently requested that the National Institutes of Health compile a table of annual costs of illness for leading causes of morbidity and mortality, which includes a column indicating NIH support for disease-specific research.[3]

Annual spending does not necessarily provide a good reflection of the impact of a disease. In the early 1980s, for example, annual costs for HIV represented only a very small portion of the eventual total costs for the cases prevalent at that time. Neither is the annual burden of an illness directly related to its priority for intervention. For that, cost-effectiveness information, which gives an indication of the impact of dollars expended on preventive or curative measures, is a better guide. Nonetheless, the annual figure gives a broad indication of the importance of the problem at a point in time. As a result, federal offices and congressional committees have demonstrated interest in clarifying the methodology for these studies, in conducting them, and in assembling their results.[5,6]

CHALLENGES TO ASSESSING ECONOMIC IMPACT

There are numerous obstacles to accounting accurately for resource use associated with disease and to assigning dollar values to these resources. Some problems are specific to assessing the cost of STDs, whereas others apply equally to STDs and other illnesses.

A basic problem in assessing the cost of STDs is the difficulty in establishing incidence and prevalence. Counts of cases are critical, as cost estimates are often based on an annual cost per case that is multiplied by the estimated total number of cases. Because the United States has no integrated and comprehensive medical data system, incidence of illnesses must be estimated. Many STDs are reportable, which should make their incidence easier to ascertain than that of many other diseases. However, the government does not require the reporting of some important STDs (particularly viral diseases), and even reportable STDs are under reported.

The extent of STD under reporting is not well understood. Surveys completed more than two decades ago demonstrated that private physicians reported only 25 to 50 percent of the gonorrhea cases they treated.[7,8] Updated information on reporting is currently being gathered. Meanwhile, the Centers for Disease Control and Prevention (CDC) assume that only half of all gonorrhea cases are reported. Reported syphilis cases, in contrast, are believed to provide a good indicator of the incidence of that disease.[8]

Other factors complicating the determination of STD counts are errors in the communication of reported statistics, obstacles to clinical diagnosis, and errors in laboratory testing.[9,10] In addition, some infected persons never engage the health care system and therefore are not counted in data systems. This is true, for example, for genital herpes, where primary infection is asymptomatic or at least unrecognized in more than half of cases.[10,11] Patients may also seek treatment long after the initial infection. Sequelae of STDs that motivate treatment, such as PID, may occur years later.

The valuation of resources used in the identification and treatment of illness, which links counts of events and medical interventions to final estimates of cost, can also be problematic. In most analyses, market price (the amount of money required to purchase a good) is used to approximate opportunity cost (the underlying value of a good). Although price and resource cost are not the same thing, prices are an adequate reflection of the opportunity cost of resources in competitive markets according to economic theory. The use of prices is generally the most tractable method of estimation. However, health care markets are generally acknowledged to diverge from the standard criteria for competitive markets, so prices may deviate significantly from resource costs. For example, hospital costs for most patients have long been covered by health insurance, creating a market in which the consumer and the seller of hospital services have had no direct contact. As a result, consumers have exhibited little price sensitivity. Health care markets have become dramatically more competitive in recent years owing principally to the buying power of managed care organizations and other large purchasers. However, it is unclear whether these changes have caused "prices," that is, fees and charges, to become more reflective of costs.

Many of the prices used to estimate costs in the literature are administrative prices, established more or less arbitrarily by a payer or a provider. Administrative prices, such as per diem rates or reimbursement rates based on diagnostic categories, are likely to be only rough surrogates for cost. It is difficult to obtain full information with which to compute administrative prices. In addition, these prices inevitably lag behind changes in health care technology.

A particular problem affecting the estimation of STD-related costs is that a large proportion of patients are treated in public STD clinics. Little is known about the units of service provided in these settings and their costs, because the clinics are allocated budgets and do not generate case-by-case claims records for purposes of reimbursement. A problem common to cost estimates of a range of diseases is that treatment patterns and costs vary geographically and by care settings. Studies using a variety of data sets would be required to accurately assess the distribution of costs.

The estimation of the economic burden of illness suffers further from the virtual lack of information on some categories of resource use. In general, there is little information on the "out-of-pocket" costs paid by patients and family members. Similarly, the amount of time spent pursuing treatment is not usually documented, nor is the amount of sick time owing to a particular disease. The valuation of productive time lost, once it is identified, is complicated both by practical and ethical issues. For example, the wage rates most frequently used to value time lost to illness generally do not reflect the replacement of labor by unemployed workers, and they do not apply readily to some categories of individuals affected by illness, such as the unemployed, children, homemakers, and the retired.

The obstacles to obtaining adequate measures of cost are reflected in the estimates of economic impact presented in this chapter. In some cases, the estimates are carefully developed, subject to the broader constraints of the field. In other instances, estimates are rough; these are usually intended to provide policy makers and the research community with a general gauge of costs.

COST ESTIMATES FROM THE LITERATURE

LITERATURE METHODS

This chapter provides the results of a review of the literature to identify existing estimates of the economic impact of sexually transmitted diseases in the United States. The MEDLINE and Health databases were the primary means of identifying literature. MEDLINE covers the international biomedical literature, including the allied health fields, the biological and physical sciences, humanities, and information services as they relate to medicine and health care. The Health database contains references from the Hospital Literature Index and other selected journals in addition to MEDLINE information.

The following headings were used as keywords in both titles and abstracts: acquired immunodeficiency syndrome, cervical cancer, cost and cost analysis, chlamydia, chancroid, economics, genital herpes, gonorrhea, health expenditures, herpes simplex, hepatitis B, HIV-1, human papilloma, pregnancy, sexually transmitted diseases, and syphilis. These headings were used separately and in combinations. Additional information was obtained from the Centers for Disease Control and Prevention (CDC), from members of the Institute of Medicine (IOM) Committee on Prevention and Control of Sexually Transmitted Diseases, and through citations in journals and textbooks.

ADJUSTMENTS

Two primary adjustments are made to cost estimates from the literature in order to present annual costs for 1994. The first is an adjustment for inflation: All cost estimates are converted to 1994 dollars. This adjustment is made using the general medical component of the Consumer Price Index (CPI), except in a few cases where another conversion factor is more specific to the cost being considered. In those cases, the specific category is identified (e.g., the Hospitals component of the CPI). In most of the literature containing cost estimates, the year of costs is given in the study. When it is not, it is assumed that costs in the original literature were collected for the year prior to the year of publication.

The second major adjustment to estimates in the literature is for changes in the incidence or prevalence of illness. Many of the estimates in the literature reflect incidence rates from the early 1980s, which were higher in many cases than 1994 incidence rates. In adjusting an overall cost estimate for current trends, the assumption is made that the cost per case has remained constant. For example, if estimated 1994 incidence was 60 percent as high as an earlier year, the cost estimate was adjusted to 60 percent of the original figure.

In some cases, estimates for STD treatment costs are calculated. The recommended treatment regimens are obtained from the CDC Treatment Guidelines.[12] Costs for a physician visit are estimated at $61, based on a survey of physician fees charged to privately insured patients.[13] This is the estimated charge for a new patient office visit for a general/family practice physician. New patient visits for other types of physicians can be much higher (e.g., the comparable fee for an internist is $122). However, fees for established patients are in this range for most relevant physician specialties (general/family: $44; internal medicine: $62; all physician average: $56). In addition, Medicaid fees and costs of physicians at public clinics are likely to be lower. Thus, the $61 fee seems a reasonable approximation for a majority of visits. Costs of drug treatments are obtained from the Drug Topics Red Book.[14]

To estimate costs consistently for STDs, a standard set of cost categories should be employed. Many categorizations would be reasonable. For example, Bowie divides resource use associated with STDs as follows:[15]

- Routine STD laboratory testing (screening, diagnosis): diagnostics, specimen collection and transport, laboratory resources, reporting
- Nonroutine diagnostic testing
- Physician costs: counseling, acute management, follow-up evaluations, complications
- Other health care providers
- Medication-associated costs for treatment: drug costs, prescribing fees, equipment for packaging
- Hospitalization
- Costs to affected individuals
- Preventive medications/ barrier methods
- Administration: collection of statistical data, control programs, accounting

Ideally, costs should be counted for all STDs in all relevant categories. In the estimates presented in this chapter, this type of consistency is not attempted. For example, in some cases, an estimate of treatment costs included costs of personnel, laboratory testing, and contact tracing, whereas in other estimates, some of these costs were purposely excluded. In far more cases, there was simply no detailed assessment of many categories of the relevant costs in the literature.

In this chapter, all available information is presented, and the limited number of adjustments listed in the preceding are used. Because many components of cost are missing, the totals calculated should be considered a lower bound for estimates of the economic burden of most STDs individually and of STDs as a group.

EXISTING ESTIMATES OF ECONOMIC IMPACT

There are several types of studies in the literature that bear on economic impact. The first, and most relevant for the purpose of this review, are studies evaluating the overall, or global, annual cost of an illness. Global studies seek to capture the full range of costs resulting from an illness and its sequelae. For example, a cost-of-illness study of human papilloma virus (HPV) would include costs for diagnosis, treatment, and nursing care associated with cancers caused by HPV, as well as diagnosis and treatment of genital warts and other manifestations of HPV infection. In the area of STDs, there are global studies on gonorrhea, chlamydial infection, herpes simplex virus, and HIV.

A second type of study assesses costs for a component of an illness, that is, for some subset of the resource use associated with the STD. The articles reviewed here focus either on relatively narrow subsets, such as drug treatment of an STD, or on larger subsets, such as the costs of congenital syphilis or PID. These studies are useful building blocks for estimates of overall economic burden.

Finally, there are cost-effectiveness and cost-benefit studies, often termed economic evaluations. These studies are of limited use in assessing economic burden, although they may contain information relevant to calculating annual costs. They are often prescriptive, assessing costs for medical technologies that are not yet used or only partially implemented. Their assessment of economic impact is (appropriately) almost always based on an analysis of lifetime costs of an illness.

Studies containing cost estimates or data used in the estimates presented in Tables 99–1 and 99–2 are reviewed herein. This chapter seeks to be comprehensive in its inclusion of global cost-of-illness estimates. However, only cost-effectiveness analyses from which specific data have been obtained for estimates are described; there are many others in the literature.

Global studies of STDs

A global study on the costs of gonorrhea was conducted as part of the IOM report, *New Vaccine Development: Establishing Priorities*.[7] The study sought to demonstrate the cost of vaccine-preventable gonorrhea, which required development of an estimate of the total economic burden of disease.

The authors of the IOM study estimate annual cases of gonorrhea, adjusting for underreporting and misdiagnosis. They divide symptomatic cases into morbidity categories, assigning costs based on treatment profiles for each of these categories. Costs attributable to sequelae of gonorrhea (PID and ectopic pregnancy) are included, based on estimates of the annual occurrence of these conditions. Costs of infertility resulting from PID are also included; these appear to be calculated using an incident cost-of-illness approach, rather than the annual estimates otherwise used in their calculations. Incidence of epididymitis, ophthalmia neonatorum, and disseminated infection are assumed to be negligible and are not included.

The IOM estimates exclude productivity costs. In addition, they exclude the costs of public health measures to prevent further spread of gonorrhea, such as contact tracing. The advantages of these estimates relate to their comprehensiveness: all major components of cost attributable to the illness, from acute infection to sequelae, are included. The disadvantages stem from the lack of detail in cost calculation and lack of data to verify treatment protocols and cost estimates used in the calculations. The IOM estimate is clearly intended to provide a "ballpark" figure, rather than a precise estimate.

In the same report and using the same general procedures, the IOM estimates costs for herpes simplex viruses (HSV) 1 and 2.

Table 99-1. Estimates of Cost of Illness in the Literature (in millions of U.S. dollars)

STD	Original estimate (direct costs)	Original estimate (indirect costs)	Original year	Source	Estimate in 1994 dollars
Gonorrhea*	$937	§	1984	IOM, 1985	$1,980
Chlamydial infection*	$727	$687	1985	Washington et al., 1987	$1,350 (direct) $1,280 (indirect)
PID*	$2,730	$1,510	1990	Washington and Katz, 1991	$3,540 (direct) $1,950 (indirect)
PID*	$699	$557	1980	Curran, 1980	$2,230 (direct) $1,780 (indirect)
Syphilis	§	§			
Congenital syphilis	$12.4 (first-year costs only)	§	1990	de Lissovoy et al., 1995	$16.1
Herpes simplex† (genital)	$84.5	§	1984	IOM, 1985	$178
Human papilloma virus (HPV)	§	§			
Chancroid	§	§			
Hepatitis B virus infection	§	§			
HIV	$13,500		for 1994 in 1991$ (direct)	Hellinger, 1992 (direct)	$16,100 (direct)
		$38,582	for 1991 in 1984$ (indirect)	Scitovsky and Rice, 1988 (indirect)	$76,225 (indirect)
	$5,030#	$6,680#	1994	IOM, 1997	$5,030 (direct) $6,680 (indirect)

NOTE: Cost estimates are reported using three significant digits.
* Cost estimates for chlamydial infection and gonorrhea contain costs for PID resulting from these infections; overall PID costs reflect cases resulting from infection by either gonorrhea or chlamydia. See text for further discussion of these estimates.
† The IOM estimate for all types and sequelea of herpes simplex virus is $452.20 million (1984$) or $954.56 million (1994$).
§ No published estimate found.
# For sexually transmitted HIV only.

The same basic strengths and weaknesses apply. Owing to a striking lack of information on such components of cost as the number of annual recurrent cases of herpes and the frequency and extent of treatment of these cases, important aspects of these costs estimates are based (unavoidably) on relatively crude estimates. Similarly, the judgment of experts is used to categorize cases in terms of severity (and likely treatment) and treatment protocols. However, the estimates are ambitious, broad, and comprehensive, and often cited in the literature.[16,17] It should be noted in using the IOM's unadjusted estimate that it is for both HSV-1 and HSV-2.

Costs of herpes in the IOM document are estimated separately for primary and recurrent cases of genital and labial herpes, as well as herpes keratitis. A substantial proportion (40%) of the total costs calculated for herpes are associated with herpes keratitis, including costs for medical treatment, corneal transplants, and blindness. Costs for other sequelae reflect encephalitis, immunocompromized and disseminated HSV, and long-term costs associated with central nervous system impairment. Neonatal herpes and its prevention are also included, although costs associated with HSV cultures during pregnancy are now outdated as a result of changes in obstetrical practice. Costs incorporated into estimates are annual, with the exception of those associated with central nervous system impairment. Annual cost estimates for this outcome are available in the report, but the global cost estimates use total costs per case rather than using the costs on an annualized basis.

Washington and others provide a global cost estimate for chlamydial infection.[18] Their estimates of chlamydia incidence are based on gonorrhea incidence, using ratios of diagnosed gonorrhea to chlamydial infection among men and women at sentinel sites and in published reports. They obtained estimates of epididymitis from national data sets and from this information estimated a proportion of physician visits and hospital admissions attributable to chlamydial epididymitis. Similarly, costs of uncomplicated infection among women and of PID are estimated nationally and a proportion assigned to chlamydia. Incidence of conjunctivitis among infants is based on a CDC estimate of births to chlamydia-infected women and an attack rate estimated from published sources (A. Eugene Washington, University of California at San Francisco, personal communication, 1996).

Cost data are based on national average physician fees, a survey of bills from two hospitals (for epididymitis), and published estimates. The authors base their estimates for conjunctivitis on assumptions regarding hospitalization rates, diagnostic related group (DRG) rates, and physician fees. Indirect costs are based on assumptions about work loss and loss of homemaking services resulting from illness. Indirect costs for infants are included as the cost of lost work for parents. This is an unusual interpretation of the indirect cost for infants, which would ordinarily seek to capture the value of the infant's time; the parents' caretaking time would be included additionally.

The authors note exclusion of a number of cost sources, such

Table 99-2. Derived and Adjusted Estimates of Direct Cost of STDs (in millions of U.S. dollars)

STD	Original estimate (1994$)*	Adjusted estimate (1994$)†	Components	
			Treatment§	Other
Gonorrhea#	$1,980	$791–1,050	$72.9–96.4	
Chlamydial infection#	$1,350	$668–$1,510	$138–189	
PID#	$3,560	$3,120		
Syphilis	—	—	$35.8–67.0	
Congenital	$16.1	$10.1–12.4		
Herpes simplex	$178	—		$20.9–31.3** (induced Cesarean)
Neonatal HSV	—	—	$10.5 (first year treatment)	$2.47 (care for existing cases)
Human papilloma virus			$2,880 (drug treatment, follow up and treatment of abnormal pap smears)	$633‡ (cervical cancer)
Chancroid	—	—	$0.053–0.066 (drug treatment)	
Hepatitis B virus infection	—	—	$111 (acute infection)	
HIV	$5,030§§–16,100	$5,030§§–16,100##		

SOURCE: See Table 99-1.
NOTE: Cost estimates are reported using three significant digits.
* Original estimate adjusted to 1994 dollars (see Table 99-1).
† Original estimate recalculated to account for changes in incidence and other changes.
§ This column contains costs for treatment only and does not reflect costs of long-term care, effects of sequelae, or other types of costs that may be included in global cost estimates.
\# Cost estimates for chlamydial infection and gonorrhea contain costs for PID resulting from these infections; overall PID costs reflect cases resulting from infection by either gonorrhea or chlamydia. See text for further discussion of these estimates.
** Lower estimate based on Randolph and others, 1993; higher estimate based on IOM 1985.
‡ Estimate assumes that cervical cancer attributable to STDs is responsible for 80 percent of total cervical cancer costs.
§§ For sexually transmitted HIV only.
\## Estimate was projected for 1994; not adjusted.

as adverse pregnancy outcomes and some sequelae of infection. However, probably the most important sources of uncertainty relate to disease incidence. Cost data, because they reflect only private practice physicians and not clinics, may also pose a source of error. PID costs comprise a substantial proportion of the costs attributed to chlamydia. These estimates are taken from the literature; their limitations are discussed in the preceding.[19]

The cost of HIV/AIDS has attracted attention since the early days of the epidemic, centering on the concentration of costs in specific population groups, geographic locations, and particular payers as well as on the absolute magnitude of costs attributable to HIV.[20,21] As a result of the apprehension concerning the economic impact of HIV, more, and more diverse, studies of AIDS costs have been undertaken than of costs of other STDs. These include evaluations of lifetime costs for persons with AIDS, assessments of the impact of costs on Medicaid and public hospitals, and costs of AIDS in specific cities and states. Studies have assessed indirect as well as direct costs.[20,22–29]

The first major cost-of-illness study addressing annual costs of AIDS in the United States was conducted in the mid-1980s by Scitovsky and Rice.[30] This study estimated direct medical costs in 1985 and 1986 and projected costs for 1991. These estimates included expenditures for hospital services, physician services, outpatient ancillary services, nursing home care, home care, and hospice. They were based on data for AIDS patients at San Francisco General Hospital, considering three expense groups based on survival during the year, and, within these groups, three diagnostic groups differentiated by their initial diagnosis. Additional data were obtained from the literature. This study estimated indirect costs for morbidity and mortality associated with AIDS using wage data.

A more recent estimate of the national cost of HIV infection was conducted by Hellinger based on the AIDS Cost and Service Utilization Survey (ACSUS), the Multicenter AIDS Cohort Study (MACS), and several additional sources.[23] This study includes costs for HIV-infected persons without AIDS as well as for people with AIDS. It includes costs for hospital, physician, drug, nursing home, and home health care utilization, but does not include indirect costs. Since the total costs of AIDS care reflect changing treatment patterns as well as increases in prevalence, these recent estimates provide the most useful estimates of the costs associated with AIDS.

Component studies

De Lissovoy and others constructed a model to estimate the direct medical costs of congenital syphilis cases during 1990.[31] The study generated a case severity distribution for true and presumptive cases and estimated costs for five treatment protocols, assuming treatment would be based on severity. The cost of hospital care was obtained from Maryland hospital per diems; Resource Based Relative Value Scale (RBRVS) rates were used for outpatient visits and procedures, using a Maryland conversion factor. Only direct, first-year medical costs are estimated. The study does not attempt to account for costs of stillbirths resulting from congenital syphilis, nor does it consider the annual costs associated with long-term disability after the first year of life. The authors test their model for sensitivity to the assumptions contained in the model, reporting that the cost estimates are significantly sensitive to the assumed severity of cases.

Hibbs and Gunn examined an on-site syphilis control intervention conducted during a cocaine-related syphilis outbreak in Chester, Pennsylvania.[32] The program involved screening and treatment, targeting cocaine users and sex workers. The study reports costs and cases identified by the program, as compared to routine syphilis identification and treatment activities at public STD clinics. Its purpose was to assess the viability of this type of targeted intervention, and it does not address issues of generalizability to other populations, situations, or intervention strategies.

Washington and others, Washington and Katz, and Curran have conducted studies of costs of pelvic inflammatory disease.[19,33,34] The Curran study is not reviewed here, because it is based on data from the early 1970s, now quite dated. However, estimates from this study appear in Table 99–1.

The methodology used in the remaining two studies, Washington and others and Washington and Katz, was similar, although incidence and cost data were updated in the 1991 study. Both studies calculated indirect as well as direct costs.[19,33] Costs were estimated separately for hospitalized cases of PID, outpatient visits, ectopic pregnancies, and infertility.

Data on hospitalized cases of PID and ectopic pregnancy were from the Hospital Discharge Survey in both cases. Data on outpatient visits were obtained from the National Ambulatory Medical Care Survey for the earlier study and from the National Disease Therapeutic Index for the later study. Both studies used the National Health Survey of Physician Visits to estimate costs of clinic and emergency room visits.

Data were collected to estimate costs of PID hospitalization for both studies. The later study is more detailed, including a longer time period and statewide discharge data as well as individual hospital data. Costs for outpatient physician visits are more approximate. The number of physician visits per case (2.5) does not appear to be based on data. Outpatient expenses included an estimate of laboratory tests and medications in addition to physician charges, but these estimates were derived from national average private practice data on physician costs and, in the case of the 1991 study, from information on a specific hospital physician group. The alternative to these approximations would have been to survey these costs, as no obviously better sources of data were available.

Indirect cost calculations were based on assumptions regarding work loss and regarding the distribution of occupation for affected women. There are few data available on which to base this type of calculation.

These studies confronted problems of inadequate data regarding outpatient services including those for treatment of PID, ectopic pregnancy, and infertility. The extent of bias introduced by the assumptions used is not clear. For example, the ratio of initial physician visits to office-based practices versus clinics or emergency departments is 2.27 to 1 in the 1986 study, whereas in the 1991 study this ratio was assumed to be the reverse (1:2 physician offices to clinics and emergency departments). As no explanation is given for this difference, the data available and the authors' interpretation of them (rather than changes in utilization of medical services) may be responsible for the discrepancy. All data on ectopic pregnancy pertain to hospitalization. These data are likely to exclude an increasing number of cases, since more than half of all ectopic pregnancies are now treated on an outpatient basis rather than requiring hospital admission.[35]

For infertility, both studies used estimates of the number of cases of PID as the basis for estimating the number cases of infertility owing to PID treated annually. This method is approximate; it assumes that cases of PID occurring in a given year are associated with infertility treatment the same year (or, alternatively, that the annual incidence of PID is constant). Because of the delay between occurrence of PID and desired childbearing, it is conceivable that the current costs of infertility are more closely related to the higher incidence of PID in the 1980s. Costs of infertility treatment are based on a 1989 study, and, owing to the rapid change in technology and insurance coverage in this field, these costs may have changed significantly in the past 5 years.

Cost-effectiveness analyses and related studies

Randolph and others conducted a cost-effectiveness analysis examining the practice of cesarean delivery for women presenting with genital herpes lesions.[36] The analysis estimates the cost per case averted and cost per quality adjusted life year (QALY) of this practice. It was conducted for the purpose of demonstrating the excess cost associated with cesarean sections, given evidence of a low attack rate for women with recurrent HSV (who comprise the majority of women undergoing cesarean section for genital herpes). The analysis is model-based. It considers a cohort of one million pregnant women. No national figures are presented. Some cost data are included, but no aggregate costs are calculated.

ADJUSTED COST ESTIMATES FOR STDS

Gonorrhea

During 1994, a total of 418,738 cases of gonorrhea were reported to the CDC. Assuming a stable incidence in the state of Georgia, which did not report cases that year, an estimated 450,221 cases occurred in the United States and outlying areas. This total reflects a significant decrease in gonorrhea incidence since the 1980s. The peak numbers of reported cases occurred earlier, but even since 1990, the number of cases decreased by about 35 percent. The decreasing trend has been less marked in the last few years, and the number of cases in 1993 and 1994 was similar.

As noted earlier, reported cases are likely to underestimate the actual number of cases, although the true extent of current under reporting is not well-documented. Assuming, as the CDC does, that only half of cases are reported, the 1994 reported cases represent an actual number of cases closer to 900,442. In a recent publication, however, the CDC estimated an incidence of 800,000.[16]

Global Cost Estimate. The 1985 Institute of Medicine study estimated the total direct cost of gonorrhea at $936.68 million (1984$).[7] This estimate was based on 960,933 *reported* cases. The 238,730 cases reported in private physicians' offices were assumed to represent only 25 percent of the caseload, so that after adjustment for both under reporting and misdiagnosis, the total cases were estimated to number two million. A subset of these cases—those estimated to be symptomatic—were assumed to receive care according to a treatment profile. The estimate includes costs for primary infection, PID, ectopic pregnancies, and infertility.

If the 1994 estimate of 900,442 cases were adjusted for misdiagnosis in the same manner, the true figure would be closer to 1,059,345 total cases. Keeping all other aspects of the cost estimate constant, the IOM estimates would imply a current cost of $496.13 million (1984$), or 1,046.84 million (1994$). Alternatively, using the CDC estimated incidence of 800,000, the annual cost estimate is $790.56 million (1994$).

Although a more recent detailed review of the cost of gonorrhea is not available in the literature, there are more recent estimates of some of the major components of the cost of gonorrhea.

Treatment of Uncomplicated Gonorrhea. Begley and others reviewed the treatment costs of uncomplicated gonorrhea in a family planning clinic serving high-risk adults.[37] For symptomatic patients, they estimated a cost of $46 in 1987 for diagnosis, treatment, and contact-tracing activities. This cost, adjusted for inflation and to reflect changes in the current treatment of gonorrhea (Table 99–3), is $81 (1994$). The majority of the STDs treated in this study were identified through the screening of family planning patients. Whereas the marginal cost was lower for each of these cases, total costs reflect the screening of negative patients. The cost per case of gonorrhea or chlamydial infection found was $66 in 1987, or $107 in 1994 dollars. (Because more than twice as many patient had chlamydial infection than gonorrhea, the cost per case found of gonorrhea alone is higher than this estimate.)

Based on these estimates and current incidence of 900,442, and assuming these costs apply to all reported cases, the cost of treatment of uncomplicated gonococcal infection is an estimated $72.94 million to $96.35 million annually (1994$).

Chlamydial infection

Chlamydia screening and reporting are increasing rapidly with the advent of easier and less expensive tests and with congressional support to build a national chlamydia prevention program. However, testing for chlamydia remains far more limited than for gonorrhea, and reporting of *Chlamydia trachomatis* is not consistently mandated across the United States. The 451,752 cases reported to the CDC in 1994, representing 47 states and the District of Columbia, clearly understate the incidence of chlamydial infection.[35] In an article estimating the impact of chlamydial infection, Washington and others used case ratios from sentinel sites to estimate the incidence of chlamydial infection relative to gonorrhea.[18] If those 1983 to 1985 rates applied today (1.4 chlamydia cases for each case of gonorrhea for men and 2.6 for women), current annual incidence would be closer to 1,765,539 adult cases (Table 99–4).

Table 99-3. Treatment Costs for Gonorrhea in a Family Planning Clinic and Adjustment for Current Recommended Treatment

	Gonorrhea		Chlamydia	
	Screening visit	Diagnostic visit	Screening visit	Diagnostic visit
Visit	$ 9.74	$19.92	$ 9.74	$19.92
Treatment-related costs				
Contact letters	$ 3.32	$ 3.32	$ 3.32	$ 3.32
Treatment visit	$ 6.64	$ 6.64	$ 6.64	$ 6.64
Test of cure (includes lab)	$12.84	$12.84	$16.14	$16.14
Medications	$ 1.92*	$ 1.92*	$ 5.10†	$ 5.10†
Pharmacist	$ 1.19	$ 1.19	$ 1.19	$ 1.19
Total (1987$)	$35.65	$45.84	$40.94	$51.16
Total (1994$)	$57.82	$74.33	$66.40	$82.97
Adjustment				
Cost of current medication (1994$)	$ 9.72§	$ 9.72§	$ 3.78#	$ 3.78#
Total without medication (1987$)	$33.73	$43.91	$35.84	$46.06
Total without medication (1994$)	$54.70	$71.21	$58.13	$74.70
Adjusted total (1994$)	$64.42	$80.93	$61.91	$78.48

* Ampicillin + probenecid.
† Tetracycline and erythromycin (weighted average of costs).
§ Ceftriaxone 125mg plus doxycycline (for chlamydial infection) 1400 mg.
# Doxycycline 100mg po × 2 per day × 7 days.
Cost per Case Found: $65.82 (1987$) for 96 cases of gonorrhea and chlamydial infection. ($106.75 (1994$)). (No adjustment for changes in treatment.)
SOURCE: Begley et al., 1987.

Table 99-4. Calculation of 1,765,539 Cases of Chlamydial Infection Using Estimates of Gonorrhea Incidence

Estimate of total gonorrhea
- CDC total reported cases of gonorrhea: 450,221
  - Adds 1993 state estimate for Georgia (31,483) to total (418,738).
- Total estimated cases of gonorrhea accounting for underreporting: 900,442

Estimate of ratio of chlamydial infections in men and women
- Ratio of men to women cases of gonorrhea*: 1.14
- Ratio of 1.14 applied to total gonorrhea cases gives:
  - 479,675 cases of gonorrhea among men
  - 420,767 cases of gonorrhea among women
- Using chlamydial/gonorrhea case ratio†
  - Men: 479,675 × 1.4 = 671,545 case of chlamydia
  - Women: 420,767 × 2.6 = 1,093,994 cases of chlamydia
- Estimate of total chlamydia cases: 1,765,539 cases chlamydia

* CDC, DSTDP (Division of STD Prevention) 1995.
† Washington et al., 1987.

Global Cost Estimate. This annual incidence is about one-half of the 3,570,000 adult cases estimated for 1985, which was the basis for an overall cost estimate for chlamydial infection of $727 million in direct cost (1985$) (Table 99–5).[18] This estimate includes costs for an estimated 73,800 cases of conjunctivitis and 37,100 cases of pneumonia among infants. Without accounting for changes in costs associated with treatment of chlamydial infection and its complications, but accounting for inflation, the change in incidence would imply that 1994 costs should have been in the range of $668.39 million (1994$). A recent CDC estimate of chlamydia incidence, however, is much higher—4,000,000—implying 1994 costs of $1513.87 million (1994$).[16]

Treatment of Pelvic Inflammatory Disease (PID) and Its Sequelae. PID is an important complication of both gonorrhea and chlamydial infection, resulting from the spread of these or other microorganisms to the fallopian tubes and other reproductive organs. PID can cause chronic pelvic pain and recurrent infection. The resultant scarring can cause ectopic pregnancy and/or impaired fertility. In a long-term study of pregnancy rates, about 20 percent of women were unable to conceive following PID.[38] STDs appear to be responsible for up to 80 percent of all cases of PID.[38]

In their study of the costs of PID, Washington and Katz estimated annual direct medical costs of this infection and its sequelae at $2.73 billion (1990$), or $3.54 billion in 1994 dollars.[33] This figure is based on an estimated 200,000 hospitalizations (average

Table 99-5. Estimate of Chlamydia Cases

Number of gonorrhea cases times multiplier (chlamydia to gonorrhea):
- 1,107,200 × 1.4 = 1,550,080 cases among men
- 776,200 × 2.6 = 2,018,120 cases among women

Total: 3,568,200 cases, excluding children

SOURCE: Washington et al., 1987.

of 1987–1988), 1,277,000 outpatient cases (average of 1985–1989), 44,000 ectopic pregnancies, and 25,500 new cases of infertility annually.

Table 99–6 revises this cost calculation based on 1994 incidence data, reflecting a decreasing trend in hospitalization but a relatively constant rate of initial outpatient visits for PID. In 1993, the number of PID hospitalizations was 115,670 (including admissions for both acute and chronic PID), and there were 386,860 PID-related initial visits to physicians' offices in 1993.[35] Assuming, as Washington and Katz did, that initial visits occur in clinics and hospital emergency rooms twice as often as in private offices, these data suggest 1,160,580 total initial outpatient visits for PID. There were 51,687 hospitalizations for ectopic pregnancy in 1993, half of which may be attributed to PID.[33,35] However, these cases do not reflect the estimated half of all cases that are treated on an outpatient basis. The CDC estimates that a total of 108,800 ectopic pregnancies occurred in 1992, implying that an estimated 57,000 women were treated as outpatients.[39] Costs for these individuals are an estimated $1,200–1,500 lower per case (Table 99–6).[40] Assuming that 20 percent of women with PID become infertile each year and that 25 percent of those seek treatment, the incidence of infertility would have been an estimated 232,116 cases in 1993, with 58,029 seeking treatment.[33] Adjusting the 1991 estimates for inflation and for current incidence, the 1994 estimate of the total cost of PID is $3,118.79 million (Table 99–6).

Owing to differences in methodology of the studies calculating the costs of gonorrhea, chlamydial infection, and PID, the PID cost estimate is higher than the combined estimates for chlamydial infection and gonorrhea, when it should be a subset of this total.[7,18,33] (The total costs for gonorrhea and chlamydial infection should include costs for treatment of uncomplicated gonorrhea and chlamydial infection among both men and women and other costs such as neonatal infection, in addition to PID costs). The PID study is the most recent and likely provides the most accurate estimate of PID costs.[33] Incidence estimates in this study do not differ substantially from those in the other studies; it is the costs per case that drive the higher estimate of PID costs. An additional source of discrepancy is that the studies of gonorrhea and chlamydial infection each include 40 percent of PID cases; thus the sum of the cost estimates in these two studies do not account for the costs of 20 percent of PID cases.

Table 99-6. Original and Adjusted Direct Costs of Pelvic Inflammatory Disease

	Original estimate in millions (1991)	Adjusted to 1994*
Hospitalized PID†	$1850.40	$1476.64
Outpatient PID§	$ 249.15	$ 734.07
Ectopic Pregnancy# (PID-related)	$ 392.18	$ 317.82 (hospitalized) $ 312.01 (outpatient)
Infertility** (PID-related)	$ 236.34	$ 278.25
Total Direct Costs	$2728.07	$3118.79

* 1991 Estimates adjusted for incidence and inflation.

† Original: $1,850.40 million (200,000 admissions × $9252 (1990$)); Adjusted: $1,476.6 million (115,670 admissions × $12766 (1994$)) (Hosp CPI).

§ Original: $249.15 million (1,277,000 × $195 (1990$)); Adjusted: $734.07 million 1994$ (1,160,580 initial visits × 2.5 visits/case = 2,901,450 visits) (2,901,450 × $253 (1994$)).

Hospitalized: Original: $392.18 million (44,000 × 8913 (1990$)). Assumes 0.5 of total ectopic pregs related to PID; Adjusted: $317.82 million (1994$) (0.5 × 51,687 × $12,298 (1994$) (Hosp CPI)). *Outpatient* Original: (No estimate); Estimate: $312.02 million (1994$) (0.5 × 57,000 × $10,948 (1994$)) Costs estimated to be $1,350 less than hospitalized costs.

** Original: $236.34 (255,000 cases × $3700 (1990$) × 0.25). Assumes 25 percent of cases of PID-related infertility seek treatment. Adjusted: $278.25 (232,116 × $4795 (1994$) × 0.25).

SOURCE: Washington et al., 1991.

Syphilis

The recent incidence of primary and secondary syphilis peaked in 1990 and has declined consistently since then. In 1994, the CDC reported a total of 83,751 cases of syphilis (all stages). This included 20,947 cases of primary and secondary syphilis; 32,970 cases of early latent syphilis; and 27,597 cases of late and late latent cases. Adjusting for under reporting, the estimated incidence is higher, 101,000 (16). No reports of the overall cost of syphilis are available in the literature.

Treatment of Early Syphilis. Hibbs and Gunn estimated costs for the identification and treatment of patients at STD clinics at $469 per case treated in 1989 dollars ($663 per case in 1994$).[32] This estimate, from an area of high incidence (Chester, Pennsylvania), includes investigator hours, practitioner wages, and diagnostic and treatment costs. If applied to the 1994 reported cases of primary, secondary, and early latent syphilis (53,917 cases), this estimate would amount to some $35.75 million (1994$) in treatment costs. The implied treatment costs would be $66.96 million (1994$) using the higher CDC incidence estimate.

Congenital Syphilis and Its Treatment. Mirroring the incidence of primary and secondary syphilis, the incidence of congenital syphilis rose during the late 1980s, peaked in 1991, and has since declined. Some 2,224 cases were reported in 1994 in the United States.[35]

In a model of congenital syphilis costs, de Lissovoy and others assigned a treatment protocol to patients as a function of estimated level of severity of illness.[31] According to their estimates, 75 percent of patients required hospitalization for treatment, with a median charge of $3,171 (1990$). They estimate direct, first-year medical costs (charges) of $12.4 million (1990$) for 1990, based on 3,484 reported cases and an assumed 916 (20%) unreported cases.

Using the estimates of de Lissovoy and others and adjusting for current incidence, the current estimated cost of congenital syphilis is $7.8 million (1990$), or $10.1 million (1994$). This assumes, as did de Lissovoy and his colleagues, that 20 percent of current cases go unreported.[31] Using a higher CDC estimate of 3,400 cases this figure is 12.4 million (1994$).[16] These figures do not reflect nonmedical costs and do not reflect annual costs for infants who were infected in earlier years.

Genital herpes

Studies from the early and mid-1980s indicate that an estimated 200,000 to 500,000 primary episodes of genital herpes were occurring each year.[41] The IOM estimate was higher: 724,000 new cases annually.[7] Because herpes is an incurable viral STD, this high annual incidence has resulted in growing HSV prevalence.[10] A nationally representative sero-survey found that the prevalence of HSV-2, the predominant causative agent for genital herpes, was 16.4 percent among United States adults in the late 1970s, translating into an estimated 25.4 million cases of HSV-2.[11] A decade later, prevalence is estimated to be 22 or 23 percent, corresponding to about 44.9 million infected persons.[10,42]

Recent counts of initial physician visits for genital herpes demonstrate the general upward trend in incidence since the 1970s. In 1993, estimates based on data from the National Disease and Therapeutic Index (NDTI) indicated that there were 171,565 initial visits to private physicians' offices for genital herpes.[35,43] The incidence of herpes simplex is clearly much higher than this figure, because the infection is often asymptomatic, and even when symptoms are present, patients may not seek medical treatment. The utilization of medical services is also clearly much higher; the NDTI estimate does not reflect visits to STD clinics and other types of practices, and it does not reflect visits for treatment of recurrent infection.

The IOM's estimates of the costs of herpes simplex include $84.5 million (1984$) attributable to genital herpes.[7] This figure, adjusted for inflation, is $178.3 million (1994$). The estimate incorporates estimated costs in the following categories: primary genital herpes, recurrent genital herpes, neonatal HSV, costs associated with culturing during pregnancy, and cesarean section (Table 99–7). It does not include costs for keratitis or encephalitis, some cases of which may be due to HSV-2. This IOM cost calculation is based on the estimated 724,000 new infections, plus an estimated 4,826,667 annual recurrences.

The IOM figure is clearly dated; however, a revised cost calculation is beyond the scope of this review. A simple proportional adjustment to reflect the increased prevalence of HSV-2 will not provide an adequate estimate of the current impact of genital herpes. Most importantly, a revised estimate must address the frequency and cost of treating symptomatic recurrences of genital herpes—factors not readily derived from current literature. Recurrent cases comprised the largest component of the 1984 IOM cost estimate and, because of their numbers, are likely the largest contributor to current cost.[7]

Recurrence rates have been estimated for the period following initial infection, and there are some indications of the trends in recurrence over the subsequent (early) years of infection.[44,45] These estimates could be used to model the annual number of recurrences, although virtually no incidence information is available with which to estimate time from infection (which appears to affect recurrence).[44] An equally important gap is the dearth of information describing longitudinal treatment patterns either during the initial years of infection or over the longer term. The IOM model of costs associated with herpes infection, although it provides the best available estimate, is based on rough estimates of these rates. Revised estimates of cost would require a revised model, or, preferably, empirical analyses or surveys of medical expenditures.

Table 99-7. Costs of Genital Herpes

Primary genital	
Severity A	$5,680,00
Severity B	$5,287,000
Recurrent genital	$25,581,000
Nenatal HSV	$7,156,000
Neonatal HSV	
Mild CNS impairment	$702,000
Serious CNS impairment	$1,495,000
Very severe CNS impairment	$15,982,000
Cultures during pregnancy	$5,391,000
Cesarean sections	$17,250,000
TOTAL	$84,524,000 (1984$) ($178.3 million (1994$))

NOTE: This estimate does not include costs of encephalitis or herpes keratitis. Some cases of these complications are owing to genital herpes, and should be included. It includes present value of future costs attributable to central nervous system impairment.
SOURCE: IOM, 1985.

Induced Cesarean Sections. An important cost generated by genital herpes is that of Cesarean deliveries performed to reduce the risk of viral transmission from the mother to the newborn. Studies have questioned the necessity and wisdom of an aggressive approach; however, Cesarean delivery in the presence of herpetic lesions during labor is currently standard practice.[36,41,46]

In their study of the cost-effectiveness of Cesarean section to prevent neonatal herpes, Randolph and others estimated the cost of excess Cesarean sections in hypothetical cohorts of pregnant women with and without a history of HSV infection.[36] Costs for Cesarean among women with recurrent HSV were $22.3 million (1992$) ($24.7 million in 1994$) *per million pregnant women*, and costs for women with a negative history are $341,000 (1992$) ($378,000 in 1994$) *per million pregnant women.* These calculations were based on the assumption that the incremental cost of a Cesarean section instead of vaginal delivery is $3725 in 1992$ ($4135 in 1994$). The estimate of 20 percent prevalence of HSV-2 infection among pregnant women implies that current costs for excess Cesareans are about $20.9 million (1994$) annually.[36]

The IOM estimated the total costs of Cesarean at a higher figure of $17.3 million (1984$), or $36.4 million in 1994 dollars.[7] This total cost estimate would be somewhat lower—$31.3 million (1994$)—if Randolph's estimate of the incremental cost of a Cesarean were used.[36] However, the IOM estimate is still higher than the $20.9 million figure, despite a lower assumed prevalence of HSV-2 of 5 percent (Table 99–8). This difference may reflect the number of Cesarean sections attributed to herpes infection. Under current policy, it is no longer recommended to perform a Cesarean section based on a series of prenatal viral cultures, but only if a herpetic lesion is present at the time of delivery.

Neonatal HSV. Neonatal herpes is not reported to the CDC, so most estimates of incidence depend on surveys. Based on a review of surveys, Chuang estimated incidence to be between 1/7,500 births and 1/30,000 births, depending on the geographic location and the population included in the survey.[47] Chuang gives 1/15,000 as potentially the most likely incidence. With 3.979 million births in 1994, this estimate suggests a 1994 incidence of 265 cases.[48]

The 1985 IOM study estimates first-year treatment costs for neonatal herpes to be $7.156 million (1984$). If adjusted to reflect 265 cases, this figure would suggest costs of $10.530 million (1994$). The IOM estimates were computed by determining the present value of future spending for cases involving central nervous system impairment. Using the IOM estimates of mild, severe, and very severe impairment and their corresponding annual care costs, the cost for 1994 cases would be an estimated $2.47 million (1994$) (Table 99–9). Thus, in 1994, total annual costs of neonatal HSV would have been an estimated $13.00 million (1994$).

Table 99-8. Estimated Cost of Excess Cesareans for Women with Genital Herpes

Proportion of live births receiving medical attention: 95%
Proportion of these that have a history of genital herpes: 5%
Proportion of women with positive history who will have HSV cultures: 20%
Proportion of those screened who will have cesarean section: 21%

SOURCE: IOM, 1985.

Table 99-9. Calculation of Annual Costs for Central Nervous System Impairment Secondary to Neonatal HSV Infection

IOM (1985) estimates:
- 7% of cases mild CNS impairment, $2000 per year (1984$), for 20 years ($4220 in 1994$)
- 6% of cases serious CNS impairment, $5000 per year (1984$), for 20 years ($10,550 in 1994$)
- 16% of cases very severe CNS impairment, 20,000 per year (1984$), for 20 years ($42,200 in 1994$)

Assume average incidence of 322 per year (between the IOM's estimate (380) and current estimates (265)). Total: $2.47 million (1994$)

SOURCE: IOM, 1985.

Human Papilloma Virus (HPV)

Although routine surveillance is not conducted for HPV in the United States, surrogate measures suggest that, like many other STDs, the incidence of HPV rose through the 1970s and 1980s and appears to have decreased since 1987. In that year, there were 351,370 initial visits to physicians' offices to seek care for genital warts, in contrast to 166,796 initial visits to physicians' offices in 1993.[35] However, estimates of HPV incidence are several times higher than these figures suggest. The CDC estimates an annual incidence of 500,000 to 1,000,000 cases of HPV infection.[16] Prevalence estimates range from 10 million to 40 million; CDC's estimate is 24 million.[16,49]

Treatment. An estimated 20 to 30 percent of genital warts resolve without treatment.[12] For those that are treated, the CDC recommends a range of therapies, although some expensive regimens are specifically not recommended. Treatment often entails multiple office visits, adding to its cost.

No studies of treatment costs for genital warts have been published in the literature. However, Koutsky estimates these costs at $2,878 million (1994$), based on an estimated prevalence of 1.3 million warts and using Medicaid data to obtain costs of diagnosis and treatment (Laura Koutsky, University of Washington, personal communication, 1997).[4] This estimate includes costs for the follow up and treatment of precancerous cervical lesions associated with HPV detected by Pap smears; it does not include costs associated with cervical cancer.

Cancer. HPV infection is associated with the risk of genital and anal cancers. One recent study found HPV to be responsible for about three-fourths of invasive cervical cancer.[50] Others have concluded that HPV infection is associated with a minimum of 80 percent of invasive cervical cancer.[4]

The National Institutes of Health estimated the direct cost of cervical cancer to be $610 million in 1990 (1990$), or $791 million in 1994$.[3] Assuming that 80 percent of this cost is attributable to HPV, this would imply an annual cost burden of $633 million (1994$).

Other cancer costs attributable to HPV include those for cancers of the vulva, vagina, anus, and penis. Sixty to 90 percent of these cancers are associated with HPV.[4] No estimates of the costs of these cancers are available in the literature.

Chancroid

A total of 773 cases of chancroid were reported to the CDC in 1994.[35] This number represents a decrease from the mid-1980s, when the occurrence of chancroid reached its highest levels since the 1950s.[9] Chancroid is difficult to diagnose because of the complexity of laboratory testing procedures. Reliance on clinical diagnosis may result in either under reporting or over reporting.[9]

The treatments recommended by CDC are azithromycin, ceftriaxone, or erythromycin.[12] The current cost for these drugs range from $7 to 24 per treatment regimen. The cost of treatment, with physician visit, for all reported cases would be $53,000 to 66,000 (1994$).

Hepatitis B

Some 200,000 to 300,000 cases of hepatitis B virus (HBV) infection are estimated to occur annually in the United States, and approximately one million individuals are chronic carriers.[51,52] Most (90%) of cases occur among adults. Although drug abuse and occupational exposure are important modes of transmission, sexual activity appears to be responsible for more cases than any other single mode of transmission—34 percent of cases according to one source 38 percent according to another.[41,51] In at least an additional 30 percent of cases, the mode of transmission is unknown.[51] In 1994, CDC estimated an incidence of 53,000 cases of sexually transmitted hepatitis B virus infection.[16]

The cost of hepatitis B has been a subject of relatively strong interest in the literature; however, no estimates that can reasonably be considered to reflect global costs are available. Cost estimates for hepatitis B virus infection prepared by the IOM attribute $146.22 million (1984$) to acute infection.[7] Using 36 percent (the midpoint of the preceding estimates) as the proportion attributed to sexual activity, this would imply $111.07 (1994$) in annual costs for acute sexually transmitted hepatitis B.

The sequelae of HBV infection (chronic persistent hepatitis, chronic active hepatitis, cirrhosis, and primary hepatocellular carcinoma) are clearly responsible for a large proportion of the costs of this disease. The IOM attributes an additional $138.38 million (1984$) to these sequelae. However, this estimate reflects the discounted present value of treatment for these conditions and thus is not an annual cost. More recent studies have focused on the calculation of lifetime costs of hepatitis B virus infection for the purpose of assessing the cost-effectiveness of hepatitis B vaccine.[53–55] Like the 1985 IOM report, these do not present annual costs for sequelae.

HIV

HIV is currently estimated to infect from 630,000 to 897,000 Americans, and 79,897 cases of AIDS were reported in 1994.[4] The Hellinger study, as noted earlier, provides the most current estimates of HIV/AIDS costs.[23] This study employs data available through 1991, to project costs for 1992 through 1995. Direct cost estimates, all in 1991 dollars, are $10,301 million for 1992, $13,488 million for 1994, and $15,199 million for 1995. The 1994 figure translates into $16,079 million in 1994 dollars.

Because this study projects future costs—as is the rule for AIDS cost-of-illness studies—it contains an adjustment for predicted increases in AIDS incidence. The Hellinger estimates are based on an estimated 86,800 cases of AIDS in 1994, about 7,000 more than were actually reported. This error biases the 1994 cost estimate upwards, but the rising trend in costs for AIDS treatment may offset this error to some extent.[23] Nonetheless, estimates of annual HIV/AIDS costs conducted for the Institute of Medicine are lower, in the range of $7 billion (James G. Kahn, University of California at San Francisco, personal communication, 1997). The IOM report estimates the costs of HIV/AIDS that are attributable to sexual transmission, rather than transmission via intravenous drug use or other modes, is $7.48 billion.[4]

Indirect costs

Although most of the cost-of-illness studies reviewed do not undertake the estimation of indirect costs, morbidity and mortality are clearly an important part of the burden of STDs. In a recent study, Ebrahim and others estimated the number of STD-related deaths occurring among women to be 9,179 in 1992.[56] This total represents a relatively stable number of STD-related deaths from non-HIV-related causes (approximately 6,500 deaths per year) and a rapidly increasing annual number of deaths from HIV/AIDS. Cervical cancer is by far the most common cause of STD-related deaths, representing 5,210 deaths in 1992 (57% of the total). (This estimate assumes that sexually transmitted agents are responsible for all deaths from cervical cancer.) The next most common causes of death are HIV/AIDS (2,665 cases, 29% of the total), hepatitis B and C virus infection (960 deaths, 10% of the total) and PID (220 deaths, 2% of the total). An earlier study estimated that in 1975, STDs were responsible for 20 percent of reproductive mortality among women in the United States.[57] However, this precedes HIV infection and does not include cervical cancer.

Indirect costs reflect the quantification of health effects—both morbidity and mortality—in terms of their monetary value. With the exception of studies on HIV/AIDS, few studies have examined indirect costs of STDs. Those that have done so have *assumed* quantities of work loss owing to STD morbidity, including both formal employment and household management.[18,19,33,34] These assumptions are particularly important in the computation of indirect costs of STDs, because productivity costs related to morbidity appear to dwarf those related to mortality for most STDs.[19] A preferable option would be to obtain survey data describing the work time lost to STDs, as has been done for other illnesses (Rice et al., 1985); however, this has not yet been attempted. It should also be noted that the value of leisure time is not included in these estimates.

Indirect costs associated with AIDS morbidity and mortality have been investigated in several studies.[20] Scitovsky and Rice estimated indirect costs to be $3,626 million in 1985, $6,556 million in 1986, and $52,280 million in 1991 (1984$).[30] Their study found indirect costs to comprise about 80 percent of the total costs attributable to AIDS. At the time of the study, however, there were few costs associated with HIV for people without AIDS (so direct costs were lower), and people with AIDS had significantly shorter survival (so productivity costs were higher). As a result, indirect costs are now likely a lower proportion of total AIDS costs (James G. Kahn, University of California at San Francisco, personal communication, 1997).

The studies assessing indirect cost use gender-specific average wages to place a value on morbidity time. Because many STDs disproportionately affect people earning below average wages—that is, the poor, certain racial and ethnic groups, and younger people—it can be argued that a lower wage should be used.[35] However, it can also be argued that the use of gender-specific wages for women, because they are lower than those of men, undervalues the economic burden.[34]

OTHER IMPORTANT COSTS

COSTS FOR SURVEILLANCE

The costs of STD surveillance are not included in the estimates of disease burden in this review. Such costs are not traditionally included in cost-of-illness estimates, which focus on personal medical and productivity costs. However, surveillance costs can be substantial, and it is useful to consider the extent to which government surveillance and reporting systems are part of the burden imposed by STDs.

Although surveillance costs are incurred as a result of STDs, it would not be correct to attribute their entire cost to a specific disease (or disease grouping). To an important extent, surveillance costs are fixed. The need for surveillance will continue as long as there are STDs anywhere in the world or the risk of new infections developing. Thus, although surveillance in the United States would not be necessary if STDs were entirely eliminated, practically, surveillance is a part of the public health infrastructure.

A conservative assessment of the sexually transmitted disease burden should consider the incremental costs of surveillance that are related to increases in incidence or prevalence of an STD. These incremental costs are directly attributable to the occurrence of disease, rather than to the preventive or informational roles of government agencies.

PREVENTION OF STDS

The costs of national public health STD prevention efforts, such as educational programs, or partner notification, are not included in most of the estimates reviewed, nor are clinical preventive services for STDs. Like surveillance, prevention is not a standard component of disease burden calculations. When the incidence and/or prevalence of a disease is high or increasing, it stands to reason that medical practitioners and public health officials increase preventive interventions. However, if these services are effective, the investment of increased resources in preventive services will be associated with decreased burden of illness: decreased incidence and/or prevalence, and decreased direct and indirect costs associated with the illness, including costs for diagnosis, treatment of acute illness, and treatment of sequelae. In this manner, society trades costs of preventive services against the economic burden of illness.

Current prevention outlays, however, should not be weighed against current costs of illness. The size of a prevention effort should relate to the benefit of that effort, not to the remaining burden of illness. For example, if the economic burden of a disease is $50 million, a $75 million prevention effort might nonetheless be warranted; that campaign might be preventing a still larger illness burden. The benefit of many preventive measures—those targeting the risky sexual behaviors responsible for the transmission of STDs—includes not only a reduction in the burden of STDs, but reductions in abortions and other consequences of unwanted pregnancy.

RESEARCH

The costs of research generally are not included in cost-of-illness studies but can be a major investment of resources. This is the case for HIV research, which, in 1994, consumed $1.3 billion of support from the National Institutes of Health, in addition to other public and private research sources.[3]

The unrecognized costs of adverse outcomes of pregnancy

Adverse outcomes of pregnancy clearly contribute to the economic burden of STDs. Some of these costs are reflected in the literature reviewed. For example, existing estimates reflect the burden of neonatal HSV, congenital syphilis, and ectopic pregnancies associated with gonorrhea and chlamydial infection. However, STDs are now suspected of having an even greater impact on the infants of infected mothers. Bacterial vaginosis has recently been associated with premature delivery of low-birthweight infants.[4] Chlamydia, gonorrhea, early syphilis, primary genital herpes, and trichomonias also appear to be associated with low birthweight, prematurity, and fetal wastage.[58,59] The economic impact of these effects has not been studied but is likely to include long-term medical and educational costs in addition to costs for hospitalization and treatment of affected infants.

STDs as a risk factor for HIV transmission

The presence of STDs increases the risk for transmission of HIV.[4] Seroconversion studies from developing and industrialized countries have shown that both genital ulcers and nonulcerative STDs facilitate HIV transmission. In two United States studies, the attributable risk of syphilis and gonorrhea for HIV seroconversion has been estimated to be 2 to 18 percent.[60,61] A recent community-level randomized trial of STD treatment to prevent HIV transmission demonstrated a 40 percent reduction in HIV seroconversion.[62]

Although the exact number of additional HIV infections that occur because of the presence of other STDs—or occur earlier than they otherwise would—is not clear, the evidence now suggests that the number is likely to be substantial in populations with high STD rates. The costs are included in the annual costs of AIDS. However, these additional cases and case-years of HIV are easily overlooked when considering the burden of the classical STDs.

CONCLUSION

The cost estimates reviewed here demonstrate the limited amount of research that has been conducted to quantify the current annual economic burden imposed on society by sexually transmitted diseases in the United States. The primary sources of information in this area are the IOM study conducted a decade ago, and a series of studies conducted by the Institute for Policy Studies at the University of California at San Francisco.[18,19,33] Far more research has assessed the cost-effectiveness of specific policies related to sexually transmitted disease—both proposed and realized—but these studies do not contribute to an assessment of the economic burden of disease. This review also demonstrates the limitations of national estimates of the incidence and prevalence of sexually transmitted diseases.

As described earlier, the estimates compiled in this report only partially describe the economic burden of STDs. Important effects of some STDs—for example, some of the adverse outcomes of pregnancy described earlier—have only recently been recognized, and cost implications have not yet been considered. Much of the actual resource use associated with STDs is not documented in the literature, because collection of the data necessary to accurately describe these categories of cost would require new and large research efforts. It should also be noted that this chapter reviews costs only for a subset of STDs. There are others, some of which may impose a significant economic burden.

Despite the limits of the present review, it is clear that STDs exact a substantial cost. Conservatively, the subset of classical STDs examined here (excluding HIV) cost the nation $7 billion annually in direct cost. This estimate places STDs in the ranks of diseases such as asthma, atherosclerosis, or prostate cancer.[3] With HIV, the annual total increases to at least $12 billion in direct costs. The full impact of these diseases, which includes the cost to society of premature death and time lost to ill health, is considerably greater.

ACKNOWLEDGMENTS

Thanks are due the following individuals for their assistance with this project: James Ida (research assistant), Kate Crowley, Melinda Flock, Alan Friedlob, Mike St. Louis, Tom Eng, John Graham, Gene Washington, and Judy Wasserheit.

References

1 Brown ML et al: The economic burden of cancer, in *Cancer Prevention and Control,* Greenwals P et al (eds). New York, Marcel Dekker, 1995 pp. 69–81.

2 Rice DP et al: The economic costs of alcohol and drug abuse and mental illness, 1985 and 1988. DHHS Publication #ADM90-1694. Washington DC, U.S. DHHS.

3 NIH (National Institutes of Health), Public Health Service: Disease-specific estimates of direct and indirect costs of illness and NIH support. November 1995.

4 IOM (Institute of Medicine): *The Hidden Epidemic: Confronting Sexually Transmitted Diseases,* Eng TR et al (eds). Washington DC, National Academy Press, 1997.

5 Rice DP et al: The economic costs of illness: A replication and update. *Health Care Financing* Rev 7:61–80, 1985.

6 Hodgson TA et al: Cost-of-illness methodology: A guide to current practices and procedures. *Milbank Memorial Fund Quarterly* 60(3): 429–462, 1982.

7 IOM: *New Vaccine Development: Establishing Priorities.* Washington DC, National Academy Press, 1985.

8 Moran JS et al: Survey of health care providers: who sees patients needing STD services, and what services do they provide? *Sexually Trans Dis* 22:67–69, 1995.

9 Schmid GP et al: Chancroid in the United States: reestablishment of an old disease. *JAMA* 258:3265–3268, 1987.

10 Corey L: The current trend in genital herpes: progress in prevention. *Sexually Trans Dis* March–April 21:2 Suppl S38–S44, 1994.

11 Johnson RE et al: A seroepidemiologic survey of the prevalence of herpes simplex virus type 2 infection in the United States. *N Engl J Med* 321:7–12, 1989.

12 CDC (Centers for Disease Control and Prevention): 1993 Sexually transmitted diseases: treatment guidelines. *MMWR* 42(No. RR-14)56–66, 1993.

13 AMA (American Medical Association): *Physician Marketplace Statistics 1994.* Center for Health Policy Research 1994.

14 *Drug Topics Red Book.* Montvale, NJ, Medical Economics Company, Inc. 1995.

15 Bowie WR: Drug therapies for sexually transmitted diseases: Clinical and economic considerations. *Drugs* 4:496–515, 1995.

16 CDC, DSTD/HIVP (Division of STD/HIV Prevention): Annual Report 1994. U.S. Department of Health and Human Services, Public Health Service. Atlanta: Centers for Disease Control and Prevention. 1995.

17 Cates Jr W: The "other STDs": Do they really matter? *JAMA* 259:24: 3606–3608, 1988.

18 Washington AE et al: Chlamydia trachomatis infections in the United States: what are they costing us? *JAMA* 257:2070–2072, 1987.

19 Washington AE et al: The economic cost of pelvic inflammatory disease. *JAMA* 255:13:1735–1738, 1986.

20 Sisk JE: The costs of AIDS: A review of the estimates. *Health Affairs* 6(2):5–21, 1987.

21 Siegel JE et al: AIDS in the mid-1990s, in *System in Crisis: The Case for Health Care Reform,* Blendon RJ et al (eds). New York, Faulkner and Gray, 1991.

22 Hardy AM et al: The economic impact of the first 10,000 cases of acquired immunodeficiency syndrome in the United States. *JAMA* 255: 209–211, 1986.

23 Hellinger FJ: Forecasts of the costs of medical care for persons with HIV: 1992–1995. *Inquiry* 29:356–365, 1992.

24 Hellinger FJ: The lifetime cost of treating a person with HIV. *JAMA* 270:474–478, 1993.

25 Andrulis DP et al: The 1987 US hospital AIDS survey. *JAMA* 262: 784–794, 1989.

26 Andrulis DP et al: The provision and financing of medical care for AIDS patients in US public and private teaching hospitals. *JAMA* 258: 1343–1346, 1987.

27 Scitovsky AA et al: Medical care costs of patients with AIDS in San Francisco. *JAMA* 256:3103–3106, 1986.

28 Seage GR et al: Medical care costs of AIDS in Massachusetts. *JAMA* 256:3107–3109, 1986.

29 Bennett CL et al: The costs of AIDS in Los Angeles. *J Acq Immune Def Synd* 4:197–203, 1991.

30 Scitovsky AA et al: Estimates of the direct and indirect costs of acquired immunodeficiency syndrome in the United States, 1985, 1986, and 1991. *J Med Pract Man* 3:234–241, 1988.

31 de Lissovoy G et al: The cost of a preventable disease: estimated U.S. national medical expenditures for congenital syphilis. 110:403–409, 1995.

32 Hibbs JR et al: Public health intervention in a cocaine-related syphilis outbreak. *Am J Pub Health* 81:1259–1262, 1991.

33 Washington AE et al: Cost of and payment source for pelvic inflammatory disease: Trends and projections 1983 through 2000. *JAMA* 266:2565–2569, 1991.

34 Curran JW: Economic consequences of pelvic inflammatory disease in the United States. *Am J Obstet Gynecol* 138:848–851, 1980.

35 CDC, DSTDP (Division of STD Prevention): Sexually transmitted disease surveillance, 1994. U.S. Department of Health and Human Services, Public Health Service. Atlanta: Centers for Disease Control and Prevention, September 1995.

36 Randolph AG et al: Cesarean delivery for women presenting with genital herpes lesions: efficacy, risks, and costs. *JAMA* 270:77–82, 1993.

37 Begley CE et al: The incremental cost of screening, diagnosis, and treatment of gonorrhea and chlamydia in a family planning clinic. *Sexually Trans Dis* April–June, 63–67, 1989.

38 Westrom L et al: Acute pelvic inflammatory disease (PID), in *Sexually Transmitted Diseases. 1990.* Holmes KK et al (eds). New York, McGraw-Hill, pp. 593–613.

39 CDC. Ectopic pregnancy: United States, 1990–1992. *MMWR* 44:46–48, 1995.

40 Creinin MD et al: Cost of ectopic pregnancy management: surgery versus methotrexate. *Fertil Steril* 60:963–969, 1993.

41 U.S. Preventive Services Task Force: *Guide to Clinical Preventive Services,* 2nd ed. Baltimore, Williams & Wilkins, 1996.

42 Fleming DT et al: The evolving epidemiology of herpes simplex virus type 2 in the United States, 1978 to 1991. National STD Conference [abstract], Tampa. Dec 9–12, 1996.

43 IMS America: National disease and therapeutic index (NDTI). IMS America. Plymouth Meeting, PA, 1993.

44 Corey L et al: Genital herpes, in *Sexually Transmitted Diseases,* 3rd ed. Holmes KK et al (eds). New York, McGraw-Hill, 1995.

45 Reeves WC et al: Risk of Recurrence after first episodes of genital herpes: Relation to HSV type and antibody response. *N Engl J Med* 305:315–319, 1981.

46 Chang TW et al: Cesarean section and genital herpes. *N Engl J Med* 296:573, 1977.

47 Chuang TY: Neonatal herpes: incidence, prevention, and consequences. *Am J Prev Med* 4:47–53, 1988.

48 Singh GK et al: Annual summary of births, marriages, divorces, and deaths: United States, 1994. Centers for Disease Control and Prevention, National Center for Health Statistics. *Monthly Vital Statistics Report* 43:13. Oct 23, 1995.

49 Fish RM: Herpes simplex, in *Sexually Transmitted Diseases: Problems in Primary Care.* Fish RM et al (eds). Los Angeles, Practice Management Information, 1992.

50 Schiffman MH et al: Epidemiologic evidence showing that human papillomavirus infection causes most cervical intraepithelial neoplasia. *J Nat'l Cancer Inst* 85:958–964, 1993.

51 Margolis HS et al: Hepatitis B: Evolving epidemiology and implications for control. *Semin in Liver Dis* 11:2:84–92.

52 Hall CB et al: Control of hepatitis B: to be or not to be? *Pediatrics* 274–277, 1992.

53 Margolis HS et al: Prevention of hepatitis B virus transmission by immunization. *JAMA* 274:15:1201–1208, 1995.

54 Arevalo JA et al: Cost-effectiveness of prenatal screening and immunization for hepatitis B virus. *JAMA* 259:3:365–369, 1988.

55 Bloom BS et al: A reappraisal of hepatitis B virus vaccination strategies using cost-effectiveness analysis. *Ann Int Med* 118:298–306, 1993.

56 Ebrahim SH et al: Mortality related to sexually transmitted diseases in women, US, 1973–1992. 11th meeting of the International Society for STD Research, August 27–30, 1995, New Orleans, LA [abstract no. 343].

57 Grimes DA: Deaths due to sexually transmitted diseases: The forgotten component of reproductive mortality. *JAMA* 255:1727–1729, 1986.

58 Wasserheit JN et al: Reproductive tract infections: Challenges for international health policy, programs, and research, in *Reproductive Tract Infections.* Germain A et al (eds). New York: Plenum Press, 1992, pp. 7–33.

59 Watts H et al: Sexually transmitted diseases including HIV infection in pregnancy, in *Sexually Transmitted Diseases,* 3rd ed. Holmes KK et al (eds): New York, McGraw-Hill, 1995.

60 Otten MW et al: High rate of HIV seroconversion among patients attending urban sexually transmitted disease clinics. *AIDS* 8:549–553, 1994.

61 Kassler WJ et al: Seroconversion in patients attending sexually transmitted disease clinics. *AIDS* 8:351–355, 1994.

62 Grosskurth H et al: Impact of improved treatment of sexually transmitted diseases on HIV infection in rural Tanzania: Randomised controlled trial. *Lancet* 346(8974):530–536, 1995.

Section 2

Special Aspects of STD/HIV Prevention and Control in Developing Countries and Resource Poor Settings in Industrialized Countries

Chapter 100

Prevention and control of sexually transmitted diseases in developing countries

C. Johannes van Dam
Gina Dallabetta
Peter Piot

This chapter highlights some of the epidemiological differences between STD in the industrialized and the developing world. A section on Policies and Principles of STD Control lists briefly the objectives of STD control programs, and describes aspects of behavioral preventive interventions, case management, and support components, such as training, surveillance, research, and laboratory services. Particular attention is paid to the syndromic approach as a feasible and cost-effective way of providing STD care to symptomatic patients and their partners. In the last section, Practical Steps in STD Control, a sequence of steps is described that are considered essential for the development and successful implementation of an effective and public health–oriented STD control program.

SEXUALLY TRANSMITTED DISEASES (STDs): A PUBLIC HEALTH PRIORITY

The epidemiology of sexually transmitted diseases differs substantially in the industrialized and the developing world. A number of sociocultural and economic conditions contribute to making STD one of the main public health priorities in most countries in the developing world. The World Bank has estimated that, in 1990, STDs, excluding HIV infection, rank second, after all maternal causes, as a cause for healthy life lost in women, aged 15 to 44. HIV infection was the most important cause for healthy life lost in men, aged 15 to 44, whereas HIV infection combined with traditional STD was responsible for 15 percent of all healthy life lost in this age group.[1] Figure 100-1 shows the burden of disease in the developing world for adults aged 15 to 44 years by gender.

Six unique features of the STD situation in the developing world are described in the following.

Incidence and prevalence rates of STD are generally high, both in urban and rural populations, although there is considerable variation (Chap. 4).[2–5] Table 100-1 presents data reported during the 1990s on the prevalence of gonococcal and genital chlamydial infection and positive serological tests for syphilis for pregnant women in the developing world. Rates of sexually transmitted HIV infection, and consequently rates of AIDS, in most developing countries are much higher than in the industrialized world. The presence of STD is a marker for behavior that predisposes for HIV infection, and STDs have been found to facilitate the acquisition and transmission of HIV infection.[6]

Rates of complications and long-term sequelae are high as well, because diagnosis and effective treatment often are delayed. These complications affect mostly women and children, and include pelvic inflammatory disease, ectopic pregnancy, and chronic abdominal pain in women; adverse pregnancy outcomes, including abortion, intrauterine death, and premature delivery; neonatal and infant infections, and blindness in infants owing to gonococcal ophthalmia neonatorum; infertility in both men and women; urethral strictures in men; and genital malignancies, such as cancer of the cervix uteri and penile cancer.[7]

Substantial gender inequalities exist in most developing countries, which render women more vulnerable to sexually transmitted infections and reduce access by women to information and to health care services. This increased vulnerability is biological, cultural, and socioeconomic. Biologically there is greater transmissibility of some STDs from males to females than from female to male, and women are more likely to be asymptomatic. Young women are especially vulnerable, until several years after menarche, owing to the large zone of cervical ectopy, which regresses slowly as a result of squamous metaplasia with increasing age. Culturally, women tend to marry or have sexual intercourse with older men, who usually are sexually more experienced and thus more likely to be infected and carry the cumulative experience of chronic viral STD. Low awareness of the burden of STD in women, and the impact on general and reproductive health, the stigmatizing nature of STD, and the cultural unacceptability of undergoing a genital examination all contribute to insufficient access to health care services for women. In most parts of the world women have little or no control over decisions relating to sexuality or the use of condoms, whereas lack of economic opportunities forces many women to enter into prostitution.[8]

STD care is provided by a large variety of health care providers. In many developing countries the public sector caters only to a small proportion of all STD patients, whereas the majority make use of private health care providers, many of whom are unqualified and not certified, or resort to self-medication. The range of providers includes allopathic private physicians as well as pharmacists, drug vendors, injectionists, herbalists, quacks, and practitioners of various forms of traditional medicine. Many of these providers are poorly trained in STD case management, and the quality of care is questionable.[9,10]

Health care–seeking behavior is often inadequate, especially but not only among women, owing to the frequently asymptomatic nature of STD in women, the generally low awareness of genital health, and the stigma associated with genital symptoms.[8] A study in Nairobi, Kenya, found that 42 percent of patients had been symptomatic for more than 1 week before coming to a clinic, and 23 percent had been symptomatic for more than 2 weeks.[10] In Douala and Yaounde, Cameroon, the mean time between onset of symptoms and seeking medical care from a pharmacist was 7 and 6 days, respectively.[11]

Public sector resources are limited, and most developing countries have seen their health care budgets shrink. Per capita health expenditure in the developing world is only 2 percent of that in the industrialized world, yet the burden of disease in the developing world is more than seven times that of the industrialized world.[1] In this situation, vertical programs frequently compete for limited resources, personnel are underpaid and overworked, and effective medication often is unavailable or unaffordable. Clinical facilities commonly lack privacy for history taking or examination, electricity and water supplies may be absent or erratic, and budgets are insufficient to sustain laboratory services.

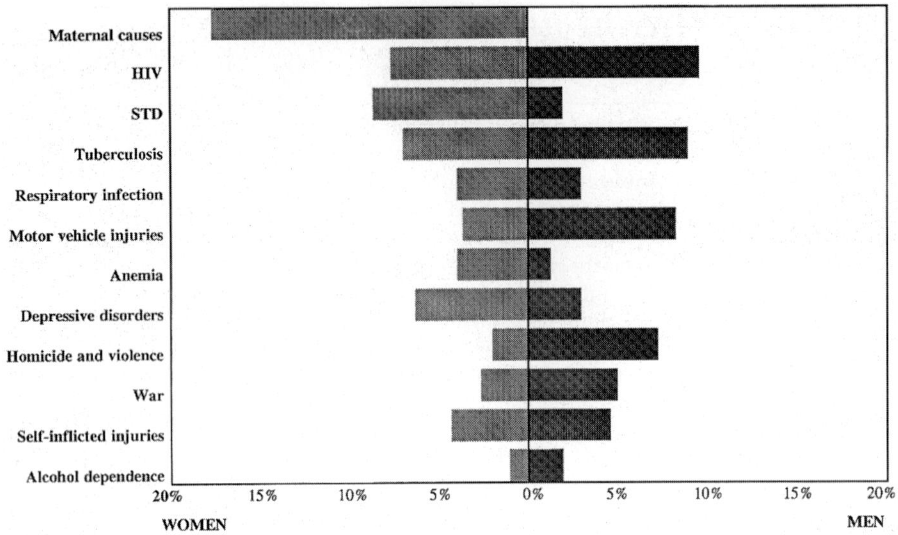

Fig. 100-1. Burden of disease in the developing world for adults aged 15 to 44 years by gender, 1990. Source: World Bank: *World Development Report 1993: Investing in Health.* New York, Oxford University Press, 1993, pp. 215–223.

It should be noted that the situation described in the preceding occurs equally in some underprivileged and resource-poor settings in the industrialized world.[12]

PRINCIPLES AND PRIORITIES FOR STD CONTROL

The main objectives of STD control are: (1) to interrupt the transmission of sexually transmitted infections; (2) to prevent the development of complications and sequelae; and (3) to reduce the incidence of HIV infection.

This can be achieved through a combination of the following core intervention strategies: (1) promotion of behavioral changes that reduce exposure to infection, including promotion of the use of protective barriers such as condoms and avoidance of risky sexual practices; (2) promotion of appropriate health care–seeking behavior; (3) provision of services for the comprehensive management of people infected with STD; and (4) provision of condoms. Comprehensive management involves prompt diagnosis and treatment, together with education and counseling of patients on treatment compliance and risk reduction, partner notification, and provision of condoms. For the effective implementation of these strategies a number of support activities need to be developed. These include: training, development of laboratory services, research, and surveillance. Other support components that are usually outside the direct influence of an STD control program are: a commodities procurement and distribution system for drugs, condoms, and laboratory supplies; a health education unit that supplements and reinforces clinic messages for behavioral change and appropriate health care–seeking behavior; and a health statistics unit to process and analyze surveillance data.

Table 100-1. Prevalence of *N. gonorrhoeae* (NG), *C. trachomatis* (CT), and Positive Syphilis Serology (VDRL or RPR) among Pregnant Women in Selected Developing Countries

Country	Syphilis (%)	NG (%)	CT (%)
Botswana[53]	16.8	14	
Cameroon[54]	15.8		
Congo[55]	9		26.8
Ethiopia	13.7[56]		29[57]
Gabon[58]			19
Gambia[59]	9.3		
Haiti[60]	11	4	10.1
Jamaica[61]	4.9		
Kenya[62]	5.3	7.1	
	6.5[63]		
Lesotho[64]	12	5	14
Rwanda[65]		7	
HIV +ve	6.3	2.4	3.4
HIV −ve	3.7		5.5
South Africa[66]	6.7		
Tanzania[67]	10.1	2.1	6.6
Zimbabwe[68]	11		

Guidelines for the development of comprehensive national STD control programs have been developed and revised regularly by the World Health Organization.[9,13,14] Growing emphasis is placed on behavioral interventions to reduce exposure, in view of the growing importance of incurable viral STD, including HIV infection. A comprehensive priority public health package for STD control in developing countries includes the following:

1. Health promotion to reduce risk of exposure to infection and adoption of "safer sex" practices, including the use of condoms and the maintenance of these safer behaviors.
2. Adequate management of patients with STD and their partners.
3. Intensified interventions in population groups with highest rates of risk behaviors.
4. Case finding and treatment of syphilis in antenatal populations.
5. Prophylaxis of gonococcal ophthalmia neonatorum.

For the implementation of this package, it is essential that a supportive national policy be adopted that endorses and elaborates on these components. National guidelines for patient management and STD treatment must be developed and widely disseminated. This will facilitate development of training materials and training programs. Specification of selected recommended essential STD treatments will simplify STD drug logistics and monitoring of antimicrobial sensitivity. An essential aspect of national policy and guidelines development is obtaining wide-ranging consensus. National consensus greatly facilitates the implementation of an STD policy. It is of particular importance in countries where the STD program is evolving toward a public health-oriented approach, often against initial resistance from established and influential STD clinicians. For instance, the introduction of flowcharts for syndromic management of STD patients at the peripheral level of the health care system is greatly facilitated if support from STD specialists can be obtained. A broad-based national technical or advisory STD committee involving experts from different fields, such as STD specialists; microbiologists; public or community health specialists; information, education and communication (IEC) experts and social scientists; and representatives from the private and nongovernmental sectors, will facilitate the process of obtaining peer approval for the national policy and strategies, and is more likely to generate political commitment to STD control.[15]

STDs are not evenly distributed through a population, and some individuals contribute disproportionately to further spread of infection. Individuals with a higher number of sexual partners, and especially those with multiple concurrent partners per unit of time, contribute more significantly to the spread of STD than those with fewer serially spaced partners.[16,17] Interventions to prevent the spread of STD are particularly cost-effective when targeted to groups of high-frequency transmitters.[5] Such interventions should be multipronged and combine strategies for health education and promotion with structural interventions to improve delivery of services for the management of STD and for condom programs. Specific approaches to reach these groups should involve members of the group and their natural leaders, as well as different partners in intervention development, such as nongovernmental organizations (NGOs) and the private and informal sectors. The success of a targeted intervention with sex workers in Calcutta, India, has been attributed to a combination of a multipronged approach as described in the preceding, with STD services integrated into a general health facility to reduce stigmatization and meet other health care needs as well, and the involvement of sex workers and NGOs in all phases of intervention development and implementation.[18]

BEHAVIORAL INTERVENTIONS FOR PREVENTION

The current dimensions of the STD problem, which include many incurable viral infections, increasing rates of antibiotic resistance in bacterial infections, and above all the advent of HIV infection and AIDS, have greatly increased the importance of health education strategies. The objectives of behavioral strategies for prevention of STD and sexually transmitted HIV infection are similar: a reduction of the number of sexual partners, avoidance of risky sexual practices, and where indicated, the consistent use of barrier methods, such as condoms, and a change toward appropriate healthcare–seeking behavior, where infection is suspected.

Many populations in the developing world have only limited awareness of the seriousness of STD and of the signs and symptoms of STD. Mass media can be used to raise general awareness, but a combination of mass media and interpersonal communication, with approaches to modify community norms, and supported by services seems most promising to maintain safe behavior or prevent and change unsafe behavior.[19] In addition, there is a need for sustained health promotion and education strategies targeted at specific groups at increased risk of sexually transmitted infections. Such approaches need to be tailored to the needs and sensitivities of the group, and should be developed and pretested in close collaboration with members of the target group. The content of health promotion messages should be appropriate and, in general, offer options. For young adolescents, for instance, the message could be to abstain from sexual intercourse until one is in a stable relationship or to explore nonpenetrative forms of intercourse, but to use condoms when penetrative intercourse takes place.

Examples of specific groups that should be targeted with health education and health promotion approaches are: STD patients and their contacts, sex workers and their clients, long-distance truck drivers, street children, adolescents, and students. It is important that the necessary conditions are created for people to take the desired steps to prevent and control STD. For instance, where condoms are promoted for the prevention of STD and HIV infection, good quality, affordable condoms should be readily available, and where appropriate health care–seeking behavior is promoted, good quality, effective, and acceptable services should be available to people with STD.

The rapid global spread of sexually transmitted HIV infection has focused attention of health planners and international donors on the urgent need for implementation of behavioral change strategies. However, HIV infection continues to spread, and especially in Asia prevalence rates are increasing dramatically, whereas STD rates remain high in most developing countries.[2,3] Many societies are reluctant to openly address issues involving sex and sexuality and to recognize the realities of the sometimes widespread existence of pre- and extramarital sexual intercourse. Both for STD control as well as for prevention and control of HIV infection, it is essential that health education and promotion efforts be intensified and sustained to achieve an urgently needed change in risk-taking behaviors, to maintain safe behaviors, and to develop an environment that enables people to adopt and sustain safe behavior.

CASE MANAGEMENT

Clinical case management of people with STD is an essential component of STD control. Early diagnosis and treatment prevents further transmission, the development of complications and late sequelae, and has the potential to greatly reduce sexual transmission of HIV. Improved STD treatment was found to reduce HIV incidence by 42 percent in a study in Mwanza, Tanzania, whereas in Kinshasa, Zaire, a clinic-based intervention, consisting of STD care and condom promotion, resulted in a decline of HIV-1 incidence from 11.7 to 4.4 per 100 women-years.[20,21]

Asymptomatic infections, low awareness of genital health and of the symptoms of STD, and the stigma associated with genital symptoms all contribute to poor health care–seeking behavior. For those who do seek health care, effective and adequate services often are not available (see Chap. 48). The model in Fig. 100-2 lists the operational steps required for an effective STD case management program and the cumulative effect of poor health care–seeking behavior and ineffective STD services.[22]

Comprehensive case management consists of the following:

- Diagnosis and treatment of people with STD
- Education and counseling of patients, including their partners, on:
  - treatment compliance
  - risk reduction, including condom use
  - partner notification
- Provision of condoms

Laboratory facilities to confirm a clinical diagnosis or to screen patients for other STDs are not available to the vast majority of STD patients in the developing world, with the possible exceptions of a Gram stain to diagnose gonorrhea in the urethral exudate and a serological screening test for syphilis. Even these tests, however, are not available in many peripheral areas in many developing countries. Management of STD patients is thus largely based on clinical grounds, that is, history and physical examination, supported by simple laboratory tests, if available.

Syndromic approach

Several major STD syndromes are common in developing countries, and often caused by pathogens that can be cured with an-

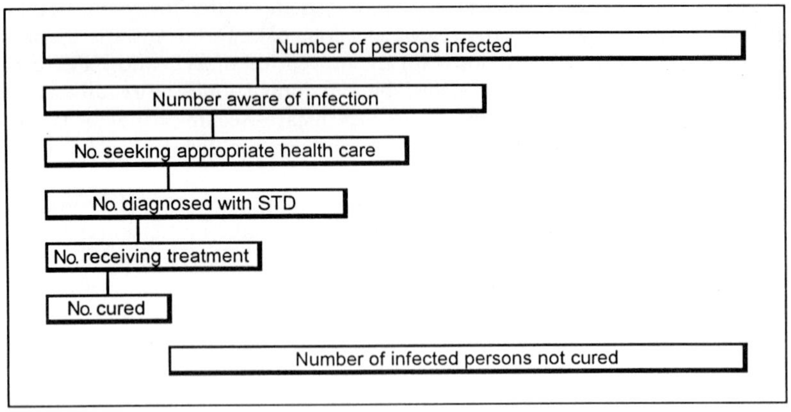

Fig. 100-2. The effect of poor health care–seeking behavior and ineffective STD services on STD prevalence. Source: World Health Organization: *Policies and Principles for Prevention and Care of Sexually Transmitted Diseases.* Geneva, WHO, 1996, in press.

timicrobial treatment. Patients with symptomatic STD usually present with one of the following syndromes presented in Table 100-2.

Syndromic approaches to management of patients with STD have been developed and evaluated during the last 20 years. The principles have been described elsewhere (see Chap. 102)[9,14] The syndromic approach is based on (1) the recognition of relatively consistent and characteristic combinations of signs and symptoms (syndromes) with which STDs commonly present; (2) knowledge of the most common local etiologies of the different syndromes; (3) knowledge of the antimicrobial susceptibility pattern of these organisms; and (4) knowledge of the behavioral and demographic characteristics of people with STD. Cure of STD patients is achieved through recognition of the presenting syndrome and provision of effective antibiotics against the most important causative organisms.[23] Knowledge of health care–seeking behavior of STD patients will assist in identifying the existing range of providers and may identify barriers and constraints to utilization of some of these providers. This, in turn, will assist decisions on which providers should be involved in STD service delivery, and what can be done to improve existing services and make these more acceptable to potential users.

Flowcharts have been developed that illustrate the steps taken to arrive at a treatment recommendation. These flowcharts ideally should be adapted and validated for local conditions, and can be used for training health care providers and as a reminder for those who see STD patients infrequently.

In Fig. 100-3 an example is given of a flowchart to address the syndrome of urethral discharge, in a situation where microscopy is not possible.[14] A more detailed description of a flowchart-based, syndromic approach can be found in Chap. 102.

Pelvic inflammatory disease and epididymitis are largely managed on the basis of symptoms, signs, and risk assessment even in industrialized countries, as in developing countries. To a lesser extent, urethritis is also managed on a syndromic basis in many settings in industrialized countries. In developing countries, the syndromic approach has been found to be highly effective when applied to the syndromes of urethral discharge and genital ulcer. Validation studies in Côte d'Ivoire and Kigali, Rwanda, for instance, showed, respectively, cure rates of 100 and 99 percent for genital ulcers with the syndromic approach.[24,25] Disadvantages of the syndromic approach are the inevitable overtreatment, since it is necessary to provide antimicrobial coverage against all of the major etiologies of a particular syndrome. Essentially, the syndromic approach has high sensitivity, at the cost of specificity, and usually requires treatment with more than one antimicrobial drug. In the developing world the relatively expensive antimicrobials recommended for STD syndromic management are currently often not easily available. These disadvantages should be seen against current practices of (self-) medication and the costs of inadequate or nontreatment of STD. Antibiotics are freely available over the counter or from drug peddlers in most developing countries. However, the cost of medicines leads to a situation where people usually fill prescriptions only partially or buy suboptimal dosages for self-treatment or prophylactic purposes. Even though the syndromic approach involves a higher cost for drugs, the overall cost per patient cured following the syndromic approach is considerably less than either a specialist- or laboratory-based approach.[26] The cost-effectiveness of the syndromic approach increases further when applied to populations with high STD prevalence rates,[43] or when the long-term costs of chronic STD, continued transmission of STD, or increased HIV transmission owing to chronic STD are taken into account.[5,27] The problem of antimicrobial resistance and the degree to which this is promoted by either the syndromic approach or current treatment practices, including self-treatment and prophylaxis, requires further research.

Table 100-2. Major STD Syndromes Commonly Caused by Pathogens that Can Be Cured with Antimicrobials

Urethral discharge
Vaginal discharge
Lower abdominal pain
Genital ulceration
Inguinal bubo
Painful swollen epididymis
Conjunctivitis in a newborn

Patients with symptomatic STD

One of the first priorities of an STD case management program is the provision of effective services for patients with symptomatic STD and their partners. Symptomatic patients are usually aware of being infected and some promptly seek health care, but many defer health care seeking if affordable, acceptable care is not accessible, and others wait until symptoms subside. A program that offers effective treatment not only meets a perceived need, it also establishes the facilities providing this treatment as effective and credible sources of health care. This in turn is likely to lead to greater utilization of these facilities, as well as greater receptiveness to health promotion activities. There is also a pragmatic aspect to the initial focus on symptomatic patients: The syndromic approach works well, for males with urethritis and for patients with genital ulcer disease, and is the standard of care for PID and

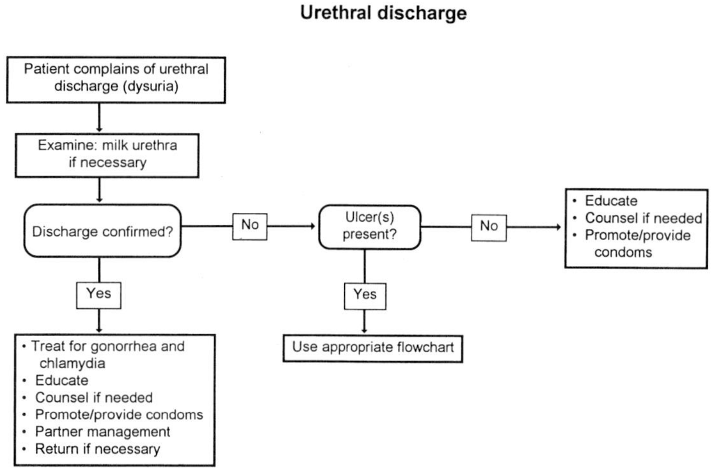

Fig. 100-3. Flowchart for the management of urethral discharge in the absence of microscopy. Source: World Health Organization: *Management of Sexually Transmitted Diseases.* WHO/GPA/TEM/94.1, WHO, Geneva, 1994.

epididymitis syndromes; besides, diagnostic tests to establish an etiological diagnosis are not available in the large majority of health care facilities where STDs are managed.[28,29]

Patients with asymptomatic infections

Identification of people with asymptomatic infections, through case finding or screening, is constrained by the absence of simple, rapid, and inexpensive diagnostic tests that can be used in resource-poor settings. The only exception to this are serological screening tests for syphilis, such as the rapid plasma reagin (RPR) test and the leukocyte esterase test, which is used in some settings to detect urethritis in men.[30,31] The development of simple STD diagnostics is of prime importance for the management of asymptomatic patients, and development of tests for the diagnosis of cervical gonococcal and chlamydial infection and for diagnosis of chlamydial infection of the male urethra is a high priority for the global STD Diagnostics Initiative.[28,44] Asymptomatic infection can be suspected in sexual partners of people with STD, but as diagnostic tests will not be available for the majority of such contacts, infection can rarely be confirmed. In this case epidemiological treatment, that is, treatment without a diagnosis, but based on the likelihood of being infected, is recommended for partners of patients presenting with the syndromes of urethral discharge, genital ulcer disease, and pelvic inflammatory disease, as well as those diagnosed with gonorrhea, chlamydial infection, syphilis, and chancroid.[14] Treatments for partners generally should be the same as those used for the index patient.

Where laboratory tests are available and where indicated, because of suspected high rates of infection, case finding and screening could be implemented. Such programs should focus on cervical gonococcal and chlamydial infection and on syphilis in men and women. The cost-effectiveness can be increased by concentrating on individuals at higher risk for these infections. Individuals at increased risk of infection can also be identified by applying an epidemiological risk profile as a selection tool, which can contribute to savings in screening cost.[32] In Nairobi, Kenya, the most important predictor of infection with an STD in women was the number of reported partners in the preceding 3 months.[33]

The cost-effectiveness of syphilis screening among antenatal clinic attenders has been well established. A demonstration project in Lusaka, Zambia, found that in an area with a prevalence of positive syphilis serology among pregnant women of 8 percent, adverse pregnancy outcomes attributable to syphilis could be reduced by two-thirds, at a total cost per averted adverse outcome of U.S.$12.[34] Even in countries with low rates of maternal syphilis, this is a cost-effective intervention. For example, in Norway, with a maternal prevalence rate of 0.02 percent, the benefits of a screening program outweigh the costs by a factor of 3.8. The benefits of a screening program will equal the costs if the prevalence of infection in mothers is 1:20,000.[35] Although maternal syphilis screening and treatment of seroreactive mothers is clearly a highly cost-effective public health intervention, programs are absent or highly ineffective in many countries. In Nairobi, Kenya, logistical and managerial constraints led to a situation where only 1 out of 11 women with reactive serology received treatment, whereas for 92 percent of ANC attenders, blood was not taken, or if it was taken, no results were available.[36] Maternal syphilis screening programs should be developed urgently where they do not exist, or strengthened where they do not cover all ANC attenders or where treatment is not provided to all those who were found to be seroreactive to syphilis screening tests.

Empiric periodic selective mass treatment

Under certain circumstances, mass treatment of a selected population group within a community or region can be contemplated, for instance in situations where prevalence rates of STD are high and where laboratory facilities are insufficient or absent or when dealing with highly mobile populations.[37] Prevalence rates can be reduced rapidly with mass treatment, but in many if not all instances some infected individuals within the community and region are not treated, and reintroduction of infection from outside the community or region remains likely (except in very unusual situations, such as China during the 1960s and 1970s). Furthermore, baseline sexual behaviors in those populations with high enough prevalence to warrant consideration of mass treatment are likely to lead to rapid spread when infections are reintroduced. In Greenland, community-based mass treatment, supplemented by mass laboratory examinations and contact tracing, resulted in a 50 to 75 percent decline in gonorrhea rates. However, within 3 to 6 months after discontinuation of the program gonorrhea prevalence was at preintervention levels.[38] High rates of reinfection as can be expected, for instance, in sex workers, would necessitate periodic treatment, supplemented with intensive behavioral change interventions particularly condom promotion to reduce rates of reinfection. Occasional or more regular mass treatment of sex workers is done in some countries, but it is poorly evaluated and thus remains controversial.[6,39] The feasibility of mass treatment at the community level is currently being investigated in several studies in Africa.[40]

Health education and counseling

Diagnosis and treatment of STD patients by itself is not sufficient to control STD. People with one diagnosed or suspected sexually transmitted infection are clearly at risk for future infections, including HIV infection. They have been infected by a sexual partner, and they may already have infected others. Health education and counseling of individual patients (see Chap. 88) and distribution of condoms (see Chap. 94) are integral parts of comprehensive patient management. The specific objectives of health education and counseling of individual patients with STD are: (1) to effect a behavioral change to reduce the risk of future infections; (2) to ensure treatment compliance, and a return visit if symptoms persist; and (3) to ensure that the partner(s) of the patient be evaluated and treated. Health education and counseling usually are accomplished by a variety of providers, including physicians, nurses, social workers, and attendants, with varying degrees of training and skills in interpersonal communication and counseling. People with STD need to be informed about STDs, their modes of transmission, and ways to prevent infection. They also should be informed about the need for compliance with treatment, to return for follow-up visits if indicated, and to collaborate in partner notification. However, risk reduction may be outside the control of the patient, as is the case for many women in the developing world, and partner notification, especially of the spouse, may lead to considerable marital discord. Ideally, people with STD should be assisted to explore ways in which they can reduce their personal risk of infection and collaborate with health professionals in the notification of their partner(s). Such counseling of patients requires specific skills and considerable time, both of which are usually absent in facilities where STD patients are managed. Moreover, limited staff resources and time constraints will, in many settings, reduce even health education to the bare minimum.

For communication, however brief, to be effective at all, it is essential that staff have nonjudgmental and supportive attitudes, privacy and confidentiality are strictly maintained, and interpersonal communication be supported by appropriate visual materials. Leaflets can provide patients with essential information, which can be referred to at a later stage and be shared with others. Last, condoms should be made available to patients, and proper use should be demonstrated on a model or other suitable object. The success of health education, and indeed the degree to which services attract patients, depend to a large extent on the attitudes of health care workers. The development of appropriate attitudes, in turn, requires health care workers to examine and be aware of their own sensitivities and attitudes toward sex and sexuality. Interpersonal skills development should be part of all STD case management training.

Partner notification

Evaluation and, if indicated, treatment of the sexual contact(s) of STD patients is an important aspect of STD case management, to prevent reinfection of the patient, to prevent development of sequelae and long-term complications in the partner(s), and to prevent further spread of the infection. Notification of partners can be done by health care providers, acting on the information provided by the patient (also called provider referral or active notification); by the patients themselves (patient referral or passive notification); or by a combination of both.[41] Provider referral is labor intensive and costly, and can be difficult or impossible where stigma associated with STD is high, where patients are highly mobile, or where no formal addresses exist, such as, for instance, in urban slums.[42,43] Patient referral can take the following forms: (1) the patient informs his or her contact(s); (2) The patient hands contact card(s) to his or her contact(s); and (3) the patient accompanies his or her contact(s) to a health facility. The use of contact cards, which offered free treatment at any public health facility, led to a 27 percent return rate of partners in Botswana in a relatively mobile population (van Dam, unpublished data). In Rwanda, 45 percent of the partners indicated by index patients as accepting referral coupons in primary health care facilities came for treatment.[44] In Haiti a combination of patient and provider referral for antenatal clinic attenders diagnosed with STD resulted in 41.5 percent of the partners attending the facility.[45] In Lusaka, Zambia, 65 percent of male partners of antenatal clinic attenders with positive syphilis serology presented for treatment as a result of patient referral in 1994 (Islam, personal communication). Although patient referral is the most feasible strategy in most resource-constrained settings, this requires motivation and cooperation of patients. Whether this can be obtained depends on the general level of awareness of STDs, the degree to which people with STDs are stigmatized, and the attitudes of health care staff.

A strategy that is currently being evaluated in the United States is to provide the index patient with treatment for the contact(s).[46] Alternatively, a health care worker could deliver medication during home visits. Further evaluation of the cost-effectiveness of different approaches to partner notification in different settings is required.

As most of the people seeking STD care in developing countries are males, treatment of their frequently asymptomatic female partners may be one of the very few feasible strategies for the management of women with STD.

Partners with symptomatic infection should be managed according to the management protocol for that particular infection. In most countries, this implies syndromic management and use of the appropriate flowchart. For asymptomatic partners the ideal approach would be to confirm infection through laboratory tests, and follow with treatment if the partner is confirmed to be infected. In most developing countries, however, laboratory facilities are minimal or absent, and case detection will not be possible. In view of the seriousness of long-term complications of gonococcal and chlamydial infection, and of syphilis and chancroid, it is recommended that epidemiological treatment be given to the sexual contact(s) of patients treated for either of these conditions.

SUPPORT COMPONENTS

For the development and implementation of effective STD control programs a number of support components need to be developed, such as: training; supervision and quality assurance; surveillance; laboratory services; and research, both sociobehavioral and biomedical. Other support components are usually not under the direct control of a national STD program. These include: a commodity procurement and logistics program and the national health information, education, and communication (IEC) or health education program. It is crucial that STD program managers establish good working relationships with those responsible for the procurement and distribution of drugs, diagnostic reagents, and condoms to ensure that STD drugs, condoms, and relevant diagnostics are made available to facilities where STD patients are managed. Similarly, collaboration with the national health education program is essential to creating a supportive environment for behavioral change messages and for appropriate health care–seeking behavior.

Training

Training is a key component of any STD control program. Program managers at national, provincial, and municipal levels need training in the planning and management of STD programs. This involves the development of skills in situation assessment, prioritization and resource allocation, a good understanding of the public health package for STD control, and skills to collaborate with and involve different partners in the public and private sector. Service providers need to be trained in effective case management, education and communication on sex, sexuality, STDs, HIV, prevention, condom use, treatment compliance and partner notification, and the development of nonjudgmental and open attitudes. Laboratory technicians may require refresher training in the use of STD diagnostics.

For training to be effective, and to use limited resources in as optimal a way as possible, training must be need-based, skills-oriented, and targeted. Thus, the skills required by a particular group of health care workers or program managers should be carefully defined, and an assessment should be made of the training needs. The theoretical part of any training should be kept to a minimum, and emphasis should be on skills building. A set of STD Case Management Training Modules has been developed by WHO and follows a workbook approach to train health care workers in the use of the syndromic approach, patient education, partner notification, and reporting.[47]

Supervision and quality assurance

Regular supervision, with the objectives of providing positive feedback on performance and solving problems, is important to maintain quality of care. A methodology for the evaluation of national AIDS programs, based on a combination of population- and facility-based studies, has been developed by the World Health Organization (see Chap. 98).[48] Two of the 10 indicators used measure the quality of STD case management through a combination of direct observation of health provider–patient interaction and health provider interviews. Although relatively labor-intensive, the results of field tests showed that it is possible to obtain information on the maximum standards of STD case management and that these were generally low. Integration of evaluation into STD programs can draw attention to shortcomings in the current practices and standards of service delivery and has the potential to serve as a quality assurance tool.

Surveillance

One of the reasons for the generally low priority allocated to STD control in many countries was undoubtedly a lack of data to convince policy makers and health planners of the extent and seriousness of the problem.[49] The HIV/AIDS epidemic has contributed to a greater emphasis on and resource allocation to STD prevention and control, in addition to considerable efforts to effect behavioral change. STD incidence and prevalence rates are more sensitive indicators for behavioral change than HIV incidence and prevalence rates, and are major indicators to measure the impact of STD prevention and control. For example, the effect of a massive condom promotion program in Thailand, in brothels and among clients of sex workers, contributed to a 79 percent decrease in incidence of the five classic STDs in men between 1989 and 1993.[50]

Routine reporting of new cases is the usual form of surveillance for many conditions including STD in most countries (see Chap. 97). However, reports are typically only submitted by public sector health facilities, whereas in developing countries a majority of people with STD seek care outside the public sector, from a variety of providers. Thus, it is not possible to infer incidence data from routine reporting, and this is compounded by the lack of a confirmed etiological diagnosis for most patients and erratic reporting even by public sector health facilities. A reduction or increase in the reported number of cases is difficult to interpret. Any change in health care–seeking behavior could cause a reduction (for instance, when facilities run out of drugs or when user charges are introduced) or an increase (when accessible and affordable care, including effective drugs, is offered).[3]

The objectives of surveillance are: (1) to measure the magnitude of the STD problem; (2) to measure disease trends and patterns of disease distribution over time and by region; and (3) to monitor program implementation and the efficacy of case management, including monitoring the distribution of pathogens, drug sensitivity, drug availability, and clinic utilization. These objectives can be met by a surveillance system that is based on sentinel site reporting, complemented by surveys in specific population groups and by studies of antimicrobial susceptibility. Sentinel sites included in the reporting system ideally should represent all sectors delivering STD care, and reporting should be done by syndrome or by etiological diagnosis, depending on the level of sophistication of the site. A maternal and congenital syphilis control program could provide additional data on the prevalence of positive syphilis serology in women in the reproductive age group, although these data should be carefully interpreted, taking into account the proportion of women participating in antenatal care and the effectiveness of the syphilis control program.

Laboratory services

Laboratory services are important for the development and implementation of STD control programs in the following areas: (1) program management; (2) patient management; (3) research, such as the development of new diagnostic tests, new drugs, and new control methodologies. In terms of program management, the laboratory plays an essential role in epidemiological and microbiological surveys, antimicrobial susceptibility studies, and the validation of treatment and STD case management approaches, such as the syndromic approach.

Even though the syndromic approach to STD case management enables health care workers to successfully treat most patients with STD, there are limitations to this approach. First there is considerable overtreatment. In general, overtreatment is clearly preferable and more cost-effective than undertreatment for many curable STDs.[5,27] Nonetheless, the approach could be made more specific, and thus reduce overtreatment, by the judicious use of laboratory tests. Second, diagnostic tests are essential for the diagnosis of asymptomatic patients, such as in screening of pregnant women for syphilis.

The underlying principles are that test results must contribute to better patient management, and that tests should be cost-effective. Until rapid, simple, and inexpensive STD diagnostic tests are developed, most patients with STD in the developing world will be managed without the benefit of a laboratory to support a presumptive diagnosis or to diagnose asymptomatic infections.[27] Depending on the size of individual countries, one or more laboratories should, however, be strengthened to conduct essential epidemiological and microbiological research, to monitor antimicrobial sensitivity and to validate patient management approaches, or to adapt these to the local situation. Where operationally feasible, simple tests could be incorporated in the syndromic approach, such as, for instance, the use of a Gram stain to exclude infection with *N. gonorrhoeae* in urethral discharge. Results of such tests should be available within a short period of time to ensure that these contribute to patient management.

Research

In addition to the clinical and microbiological research mentioned above, there is a need for sociobehavioral research in the development and implementation of STD control programs. Such research will normally employ a combination of qualitative and quantitative research methodologies to describe the spread and extent of risk behavior in communities, to describe and understand community and individual perceptions of sexuality and STD, and health care–seeking behavior in relation to reproductive and sexual health. In India, a study was undertaken in all state and union territory capitals and cities with a population of half a million or more, 65 cities in all, to map risk behavior patterns and to identify potential partners for intervention development.[51]

To develop appropriate and effective prevention and control programs, a better understanding is needed of the perception of STDs, their causative mechanisms and transmissibility, as well as related health care–seeking behaviors and the reasons for behavioral choices. A rapid assessment methodology has been developed and pretested, which involves the community and local health care workers in assessing the STD situation and developing an understanding of the community perspective on STD and STD services and in developing relevant and focused programs which incorporate this understanding.[52]

Last, operational research on the development of indicators for monitoring and evaluation of STD programs is urgently required.

A PRACTICAL APPROACH TO STD CONTROL

The following steps should be taken urgently, or existing efforts be strengthened where indicated, to develop and implement an effective STD control and prevention program.

1. An initial assessment of the STD situation should use existing databases supplemented by rapid surveys to define what is known locally about prevalences of STD in specific population groups, patterns of high-risk sexual behaviors, and sources of STD prevention and treatment services. Following an initial rapid assessment, the program will provide more detailed information over time. Sources of information are: available literature, results of syphilis screening in antenatal clinic attenders and blood donors, data from neighboring countries, and results of surveys in specific population groups. These data help convince policy makers and health planners of the public health importance of STD and help ensure allocation of resources. Data on STD prevalence also provide a baseline to measure future program impact.
2. Specific groups in need of intensive intervention development need to be identified. These can include those at increased risk of infection, such as STD patients, sex workers and their clients, and possibly others, like truck drivers, adolescents, and students. Qualitative methodologies should be employed to rapidly collect information on the location and size of such groups, as well as identify potential partners for intervention development.
3. A national body should develop or update existing patient management and treatment guidelines. These can be based on the WHO recommendations and should take into account local factors, such as the relative frequency of causative organisms, the susceptibility of these organisms, and the availability of STD drugs. National guidelines and recommendations provide a means to standardize case management and guide training, supervision, drug logistics, and monitoring of drug resistance.
4. This should be followed by the development and implementation of well-targeted interventions. These should have the following components: health education and health promotion to reduce risky sexual behaviors and to improve health care–seeking behavior; condom promotion and distribution; and STD case management. It is recommended that services for STD care be integrated into existing services, although development of specific facilities for some groups may be indicated. Such facilities should meet the health care needs of the target population, which are usually not restricted to STD. As categorical STD clinics are often perceived as stigmatizing, it is recommended that clinics be developed as general health facilities, but that staff be well trained in STD case management.[22] Initially clinical services should focus on symptomatic patients and, if possible, their partners. Depending on the prevalence and incidence of asymptomatic STD and the availability of laboratory diagnostic tests, screening and case-finding programs may be indicated. Another option in situations where rates of STD are high is selective mass treatment. Because there is little information supporting the benefit of such approaches, however, this should be regarded as experimental, and should be carefully evaluated for cost-effectiveness and adverse effects during initiation and implementation.
5. STD care services for the general population should be strengthened in both the public and the private sectors. The initial focus should be on approaches to identify, treat, and educate symptomatic patients and their partners. This component of the program usually will be implemented in a phased approach, and should start in those areas where STD rates are relatively high, for instance, in cities or along major highways. Major prerequisites for effective STD case management are training of health care workers and the availability of effective drugs. An assessment of the expected drug requirements should be made, followed by development of a logistics program to ensure drug availability.
6. Mass media should be employed to increase awareness of STD and sexual and reproductive health, to create an environment that is more conducive to behavioral change. This must be supplemented with educational programs prioritizing specific groups.
7. A syphilis screening and treatment program for pregnant women attending antenatal clinics should be implemented or strengthened.
8. A program for prophylaxis of ophthalmia neonatorum should be implemented or strengthened. For successful syphilis screening and treatment and prophylaxis of ophthalmia neonatorum programs there should be close collaboration between the STD control program and the mother and child/reproductive health program.
9. Development of a research capability, with the following objectives: (1) to conduct basic epidemiological studies on STD, including monitoring the prevalence of STDs in antenatal clinic populations; (2) to monitor antimicrobial susceptibility; (3) to intermittently assess the efficacy of syndromic approaches through clinical trials; and (4) to further develop and validate diagnostic procedures, including the syndromic approach. This type of research can usually be conducted from one or more centrally located research, training, and referral centers. However, development and maintenance of such centers is usually costly, and although essential, should not be done at the expense of strengthening STD case management through integrated services.

References

1 World Bank: *World Development Report 1993: Investing in Health.* New York, Oxford University Press, 1993, pp. 215–223.

2 Laga M: Epidemiology and control of sexually transmitted diseases in developing countries. *Sex Transm Dis* 21(Suppl 2):S45–50, 1994.

3 Piot P et al: Sexually transmitted diseases in the 1990s—global epidemiology and challenges for control. *Sex Transm Dis* 21(Suppl 2): S7–13, 1994.

4 De Schryver A et al: Epidemiology of sexually transmitted diseases: The global picture. *Bull WHO* 68:639–654, 1990.

5 Over et al: HIV infection and sexually transmitted diseases, in *Disease Control Priorities in Developing Countries,* DT Jamison et al (eds). New York, Oxford University Press, 1993, pp. 455–527.

6 Laga M et al: Inter-relationship of sexually transmitted diseases and HIV: Where are we now? *AIDS* 8(Suppl 1):S119–124, 1994.

7 Meheus A et al: Development of prevention and control programs for sexually transmitted diseases in developing countries, in *Sexually Transmitted Diseases,* 2nd ed, KK Holmes et al (eds). New York, McGraw-Hill, 1990, pp. 1041–1046.

8 van Dam CJ: HIV, STD and their current impact on reproductive health: The need for control of sexually transmitted diseases. *Int J Gynecol Obs* 50(Suppl 2):S121–S129, 1995.

9 World Health Organization: Management of patients with sexually transmitted diseases. Report of a WHO study group. *Technical Report Series* 810, WHO, Geneva, 1991.

10 Moses S et al: Health care-seeking behavior related to the transmission of sexually transmitted diseases in Kenya. *Am J Pub Health* 84;12: 1947–1951, 1994.

11 Trebucq A et al: Treatment regimens of STD patients in Cameroon: A need for intervention. *Sex Transm Dis* 21;2:124–126, 1994.

12 Aral S et al: Sexually transmitted diseases in the AIDS era. *Sci Am* 264; 2:62–69, 1991.

13 World Health Organization and Pan American Health Organization: *Control of Sexually Transmitted Diseases.* WHO, Geneva, 1985.

14 World Health Organization: *Management of Sexually Transmitted Diseases.* WHO/GPA/TEM/94.1, WHO, Geneva, 1994.

15 van Dam CJ et al: Guidelines for the Management of STD Programs, in *Control of Sexually Transmitted Diseases: A Handbook for the Design and Management of Programs,* 1st ed, G Dallabetta et al (eds). FHI, North Carolina, 1996, Chapter 2.

16 Yorke AY et al: Dynamics and control of the transmission of gonorrhea. *Sex Transm Dis* 5;2:51–56, 1978.

17 Brunham RC: The concept of core and its relevance to the epidemiology and control of sexually transmitted diseases. *Sex Transm Dis* 18;2:67–68, 1991.

18 Jana S et al: An integrated intervention strategy and its effect on STD/ HIV transmission. Abstract presented at the *11th meeting of the International Society for STD Research,* New Orleans, LA, August 27–30, 1995. Abstract 411.

19 Choi K-H et al: Prevention of HIV infection. *AIDS* 8:1371–1389, 1994.

20 Grosskurth H et al: Impact of improved treatment of sexually transmitted diseases on HIV infection in rural Tanzania: Randomized controlled trial. *Lancet* 346:530–536, 1995.

21 Laga M et al: Condom promotion, sexually transmitted diseases treatment, and declining incidence of HIV-1 infection in female Zairian sex workers. *Lancet* 344:246–248, 1994.

22 World Health Organization: *Policies and Principles for Prevention and Care of Sexually Transmitted Diseases.* Geneva, WHO, 1996, in press.

23 van Dam CJ: Syndromic management of genital ulcer disease: A reply. *Genitourin Med* 72;1:75–76, 1996.

24 La Ruche et al: Therapeutic algorithms for the management of sexually transmitted diseases at the peripheral level in Côte d'Ivoire: Assessment of efficacy and cost. *Bull WHO* 73;3:305–313, 1995.

25 Bogaerts J et al: Simple algorithms for the management of genital ulcers: evaluation in a primary health care centre in Kigali, Rwanda. *Bull WHO* 73;6:761–767, 1995.

26 Islam QM et al: Analysis of the cost-effectiveness of approaches to STD case management. *Sex Transm Dis* 21(Suppl 2):S138, 1994.

27 Piot P et al: Economic impact of reproductive tract infections and resources for their control, in *Reproductive Tract Infections: Global Impact and Priorities for Women's Reproductive Health,* A Germain et al (eds). New York, Plenum Press, 1992, pp. 227–249.

28 Hitchcock PJ et al: Sexually transmitted diseases in the AIDS era: Development of STD diagnostics for resource-limited settings is a global priority. *Sex Transm Dis* 18;2:133–135, 1991.

29 Anyangwe S et al: STD management in Zambia: Making a case for the syndromic approach. *Presented at the 11th meeting of the International Society for STD Research,* New Orleans, LA, August 27–30, 1995, Abstract 055.

30 Shafer M-A et al: Evaluation of urine-based screening strategies to detect chlamydia trachomatis among sexually active asymptomatic young males. *JAMA* 270;17:2065–2070, 1993.

31 Tyndall MW et al: Leukocyte esterase urine strips for the screening of men with urethritis: Use in developing countries. *Genitourin Med* 70; 1:3–6, 1994.

32 Addiss DG et al: Decreased prevalence of chlamydia trachomatis infection associated with a selective screening program in family planning clinics in Wisconsin. *Sex Transm Dis* 20;1:28–35, 1993.

33 Moses S et al: Sexual behaviour in Kenya: Implications for sexually transmitted disease transmission and control. *Soc Sci Med* 39;12: 1649–1656, 1994.

34 Hira SK et al: Syphilis intervention in pregnancy: Zambian demonstration project. *Genitourin Med* 66; 3:159–164, 1990.

35 Stray-Pederson B: Economic evaluation of maternal screening to prevent congenital syphilis. *Sex Transm Dis* 10;4:167–172, 1983.

36 Temmerman M et al: Syphilis prevention in pregnancy: An opportunity to improve reproductive and child health in Kenya. *Health Pol Plan* 8;2:122–127, 1993.

37 World Health Organization: *WHO Expert Committee on Venereal Diseases and Treponematoses,* Sixth Report, Geneva, Switzerland. WHO, 1986, 87–88.

38 Olson GA: Epidemiological measures against gonorrhea: experience in Greenland. *Br J Vener Dis* 49;2;130–133, 1973.

39 Mugrditchian D et al: Innovative Approaches to STD Control, in *Control of Sexually Transmitted Diseases: A Handbook for the Design and Management of Programs,* 1st ed, G Dallabetta et al (eds). FHI, North Carolina, 1996, chapter 13.

40 Karim SSA: Editorial: Challenges to the control of sexually transmitted diseases in Africa. *Am J Pub Health* 84;12:1891–1893, 1994.

41 Potterat JJ et al: Partner notification: Operational considerations. *Int J STD & AIDS* 2:411–415, 1991.

42 Asuzu MC et al: Contact tracing in the control of STDs in Ibadan, Nigeria. *Br J Vener Dis* 60;2:114, 1984.

43 Asuzu MC et al: The use of mail reminders in STD contact tracing in Ibadan, Nigeria. *E Afr Med J* 67:75–78, 1990.

44 Steen R et al: Partner referral as a component of integrated sexually transmitted disease services in two Rwandan towns. *Genitourin Med* 72;1:56–59, 1996.

45 Desormeaux J et al: Introduction of partner referral and treatment for control of sexually transmitted diseases in a poor Haitian community. *Tenth International Conference on AIDS,* Yokohama, Japan, 7–12 August 1994, Abstract 365C.

46 Handsfield HH: Design and implementation of a successful Chlamydia control program. *35th Interscience Conference on Antimicrobial Agents and Chemotherapy,* 17–20 September, 1995, Abstract S65.

47 World Health Organization: STD Case Management Workbook, modules 1–7, WHO, Geneva, 1995.

48 Mertens T et al: Prevention indicators for evaluating the progress of national AIDS programmes. *AIDS* 8;10:1359–1369, 1994.

49 Willcox RR: VD Education in developing countries: A comparison with developed countries. *Br J Vener Dis* 52;2:88–93, 1976.

50 Hanenberg RS et al: Impact of Thailand's HIV-control programme as indicated by the decline of sexually transmitted diseases. *Lancet* 344: 243–245, 1994.

51 Sethi G et al: Effective training for researchers of high risk behaviour. *Third International Conference on AIDS in Asia and the Pacific,* 17–21 September 1995, Abstract B505.

52 Helitzer-Allen DL et al: *The Manual for Targeted Intervention Research on Sexually Transmitted Illnesses with Community Members.* AIDSCAP, FHI, Hubert Allen & Associates, Baltimore, MD, 1994.

53 Pedersen Sheller J et al: HIV-infection, syphilis og genitale laesioner i Maun, Botswana (HIV infection, syphilis and genital lesions in Maun, Botswana). *Ugeskr Laeger* 152;20:1441–1443, 1990.
54 Ndumbe PM et al: Seroprevalence of hepatitis and HIV infection among rural pregnant women in Cameroon. *APMIS* 102:662–666, 1994.
55 Yala F et al: Enquête virologique et bactériologique sur l'infection materno-foetale à Brazzaville. *Bull Soc Path Ex* 84:627–634, 1991.
56 Azeze B et al: Seroprevalence of syphilis amongst pregnant women attending antenatal clinics in a rural hospital in north west Ethiopia. *Genitourin Med* 71;6:347–350, 1995.
57 Duncan ME et al: Seroepidemiological and socioeconomic studies of genital chlamydial infection in Ethiopian women. *Genitourin Med* 68; 4:221–227, 1992.
58 Fassassi-Jarretou A et al: Impacts de *Chlamydia trachomatis* sur les femmes enceintes au Gabon. *Bull Soc Path Ex* 84:620–626, 1991.
59 Greenwood AM et al: Treponemal infection and the outcome of pregnancy in a rural area of the Gambia, West Africa. *JID* 166;4:842–846, 1992.
60 Behets FM-T et al: Control of sexually transmitted diseases in Haiti: Results and implications of a baseline study among pregnant women living in Cité Soleil shantytowns. *JID* 172;3:764–771, 1995.
61 Prabhakar P et al: Seroprevalence of toxoplasma gondii, rubella virus, cytomegalovirus, herpes simplex virus (TORCH) and syphilis in Jamaican pregnant women. *W Ind Med J* 40;4:166–169, 1991.
62 Temmerman M et al: Rapid increase of both HIV-1 infection and syphilis among pregnant women in Nairobi, Kenya. *AIDS* 6;10:1181–1185, 1992.
63 Jenniskens F et al: Syphilis control in pregnancy: Decentralisation of screening facilities to primary care level, a demonstration project in Nairobi, Kenya. *Int J Gynaecol Obstet* 48(Suppl):S121–S128, 1995.
64 Fehler HG et al: STD among women attending STD family planning and antenatal clinics in Maseru, Lesotho. Abstract presented at the *11th Meeting of the International Society for STD Research,* New Orleans, LA, August 27–30, 1995, Abstract 344.
65 Leroy V et al: Should screening of genital infections be part of antenatal care in areas of high HIV prevalence? A prospective cohort study from Kigali, Rwanda, 1992–1993. *Genitourin Med* 71;4:207–211, 1995.
66 Delport SD: On-site screening for maternal syphilis in an antenatal clinic. *S Afr Med J* 83;10:723–724, 1993.
67 Mayaud P et al: Risk assessment and other screening options for gonorrhoea and chlamydial infections in women attending rural Tanzanian antenatal clinics. *Bull WHO* 73;5:621–630, 1995.
68 Aiken CGA: The causes of perinatal mortality in Bulawayo, Zimbabwe. *C Afr J Med* 38;7:263–281, 1992.

Chapter 101

Approach to the management of HIV/AIDS in developing countries

Kevin M. De Cock
Elly T. Katabira

In the early days of the HIV/AIDS pandemic, before the full demographic and social impact had become manifest in resource-poor countries, the emphasis of public health officials and international agencies was on prevention of HIV infection. Care for persons with AIDS was perceived as an infinite demand yielding no public health benefit. By the early 1990s attitudes concerning the need for HIV/AIDS care had changed, although the nature of care in developing countries, and the appropriate level of resources for care, remain topics of debate. This chapter considers the need and justification for care for HIV/AIDS in resource-poor settings, and discusses possible approaches. Since antiviral drugs are inaccessible to most HIV-infected persons in developing countries, they are not considered further in this discussion.

THE NEED AND JUSTIFICATION FOR HIV/AIDS CARE IN RESOURCE-POOR COUNTRIES

By mid-1996 approximately 27.9 million persons were estimated to have been infected by HIV, over 7.5 million cases of AIDS were judged to have occurred, and 21.8 million persons were believed to be living with HIV infection.[1] By the end of the century the cumulative total of HIV-infected persons is expected to reach at least 40 million, 90 percent of whom will be citizens of countries that are not industrialized.[2] The greatest burden of disease to date has been in Africa, which supports less than 10 percent of the world's population but has seen approximately two-thirds of global AIDS cases. The overwhelming importance of heterosexual transmission in the spread of HIV infection in sub-Saharan Africa is demonstrated by the fact that 90 percent of the world's AIDS cases in women and children have occurred in this region. The recent but rapid spread of HIV infection in India and Southeast Asia will result in an increasing proportion of future AIDS cases occurring in this most densely populated part of the world; in Africa, HIV spread has been especially rapid in the southern part of the continent in recent time.

Justifications for investment in AIDS care in countries with limited resources are both ethical and practical (Table 101-1).[3] It is ethically unacceptable to have clinical services for a disease of global dimensions available only in those parts of the world that are economically developed. Ministries of health in all countries have to provide clinical services for their populations, and in heavily affected African cities as many as half of medical hospital beds are now filled by HIV-infected patients. Persons infected with HIV will continue to present to health care structures with the complications of immune deficiency, many of which may not be obviously indicative of HIV disease. Some of the complications of HIV infection are potentially life-threatening but may respond well to treatment. HIV/AIDS has become just another disease process that overburdened health care systems have to deal with, making it all the more important to ensure resources on HIV/AIDS care are spent rationally and effectively. Irrational HIV/AIDS care, whether inappropriately sophisticated or neglectful, will ultimately detract from the quality of services provided to all persons, irrespective of their HIV status.

For several conditions, including some associated with HIV infection, the distinction between prevention and care is unclear. For sexually transmitted diseases and tuberculosis, for example, prevention of transmission requires identification and treatment of ill, infected persons. A clinical trial showed that treatment of pregnant women late in pregnancy with zidovudine lowered HIV transmission to their infants by two-thirds.[4] Experience in industrialized countries has shown that behavior change and acceptance of responsibility for one's own health are more likely in an environment providing respect and assistance in time of need. Whatever the socioeconomic context, access to care when sick should be seen as a basic right.

The question facing heavily affected, resource-poor countries, therefore, is not whether to invest in prevention or care for HIV/AIDS, but how to use the limited resources available for a comprehensive approach that will prevent new HIV infections, limit suffering, and prolong life in those already infected. One of the aims of providing diagnosis, counseling, and care is to allow affected persons to plan as best as possible for the future of their families, especially their children, and to transfer technical, practical, or theoretical skills and knowledge on to survivors. Defining a minimum standard of care to which all HIV-infected persons could aspire is central to this challenge.

THE SPECTRUM OF HIV/AIDS IN ADULTS IN RESOURCE-POOR COUNTRIES

The delivery of rational care for HIV/AIDS requires basic understanding of the disease process. Surprisingly, knowledge concerning the natural history of HIV infection in developing countries and its associated spectrum of disease is limited. The widely held belief that progression of HIV-induced immune deficiency is more rapid in Africa than in industrialized countries is not substantiated by data, since so few natural history studies have been done in representative African populations. Short survival has been reported in rural Uganda, for example, but this could theoretically result from early death from aggressive conditions such as tuberculosis at relatively sustained CD4+ lymphocyte counts, from lack of access to treatment, from more rapid progression of immune deficiency following specific infections (as has been suggested for tuberculosis), or from genuine faster progression of immune depletion in Africans infected with HIV.[5]

No evidence to date suggests that different subtypes of HIV-1 are associated with different outcomes. Although HIV-2 infection is associated with similar opportunistic diseases as infection with HIV-1, the rate of development of immune deficiency is slower in HIV-2-infected persons; long-term natural history and survival in persons with HIV-2 infection are consequently more favorable.[6–8] A retrospective cohort study in London comparing HIV-infected Africans (virtually all assumed to have been infected in Africa with non-B subtypes of HIV-1, with a median duration of residence outside of Africa of less than 2 years) with non-Africans showed significant differences in the frequency of different opportunistic infections, but no differences in survival (Del Amo; unpublished). A cautious conclusion from this work was that access to treatment in an environment carrying a lower risk of exposure to acute infectious diseases erased any differences in natural history.

The spectrum of disease associated with HIV infection differs in different regions of the world (Table 101-2). Although mucocutaneous abnormalities such as oral candidiasis, varicella zoster,

Table 101-1. Justifications and Aims for HIV/AIDS Care in Resource-Poor Countries

Justifications
- Care enhances prevention
- Care is ethically necessary
- Well-organized care offers most efficient use of resources
- Well-organized care can help limit the socioeconomic impact of HIV/AIDS

Aims
- Prolong life
- Control symptoms
- Enhance HIV/AIDS prevention
- Limit social impact of HIV/AIDS
- Provide counseling, psychosocial support, and material assistance
- Enhance transfer of knowledge and resources to survivors

and pruriginous dermatitis can occur at levels of modest immune deficiency (CD4+ lymphocyte count 200–500/mm^3), in most cases major opportunistic illnesses occur when immune deficiency has advanced, as indicated by a CD4+ lymphocyte count of less than 200/mm^3. Tuberculosis and pneumococcal infection may occur with relatively preserved immune function (median CD4+ lymphocyte count >200/mm^3).[9–12]

In Africa, tuberculosis, bacterial infections, and parasitic diseases such as toxoplasmosis and those associated with diarrhea are especially prevalent. An autopsy study conducted in Abidjan, Cote d'Ivoire, showed that tuberculosis was the leading cause of death in HIV-infected patients, responsible for 32 percent of deaths.[6] Toxoplasmosis and bacterial infections were the next most important diseases demonstrated; together, these three conditions accounted for over half of deaths in patients infected with HIV. Cross-sectional, hospital-based studies have shown that *Streptococcus pneumoniae* and nontyphoid species of *Salmonella* are frequent pathogens in patients with bacteremia.[13,14] Infectious causes of diarrhea include *Salmonella* infection, cryptosporidiosis, isosporiasis, and microsporidiosis. Cryptococcal infection, mostly presenting as meningitis, probably varies in frequency across the African continent, as does Kaposi's sarcoma; the latter seems most prevalent in East and Central Africa, where endemic Kaposi's sarcoma is commonest. Cryptococcal disease is probably more frequent in East, Central, and Southern Africa than in West Africa. Important clinical presentations in patients with AIDS include wasting with chronic diarrhea and fever ("slim disease," the HIV wasting syndrome), respiratory disease, and chronic fever without an obvious localizing source.[15] Mucocutaneous disease is frequent and can cause distressing symptoms.

Table 101-2. Regional Variation in the Spectrum of HIV-Associated Disease

Disease	Europe, North America	Africa	South America	Asia
Tuberculosis	+	+++	++	+++
Toxoplasmosis	+/++	++	++	?
Pneumocystosis	+++	+	++	?
Bacterial infections	++	+++	++	?
Kaposi's sarcoma	++	++	++	?
Cryptococcosis	+	++	+	++
MAC	++	+	+	?
HIV wasting	+	+++	++	?
HIV encephalopathy	++	+	?	?
CMV disease	++	+	+	?
Lymphoma	++	+	?	?
Penicilliosis	–	–	–	++

Tuberculosis also seems to be the dominant pathogen in patients with HIV/AIDS in Latin America and South and Southeast Asia.[16] Parasitic infections such as those causing diarrhea as well as toxoplasmosis are prevalent in Latin American patients, but there also seems to be a higher prevalence than in African patients of diseases indicative of very advanced immune deficiency, such as cytomegalovirus disease and disseminated *Mycobacterium avium* complex (MAC) infection.[16] Infections with a number of parasites endemic to parts of Latin America, including *Trypanosoma cruzi,* the cause of Chagas' disease, and the agents of visceral and cutaneous leishmaniasis, have been reported to cause unusual disease patterns in patients infected with HIV.[17,18] Cryptococcosis has been reported to be a frequent opportunistic infection in HIV-infected patients in Asia, and penicilliosis, disseminated infection with *Penicillium marneffei,* has been a common disease in several Southeast Asian countries.[19,20]

Limited information is available concerning survival once patients have AIDS-defining illnesses in the developing world. Recent data from Thailand indicated a median survival in patients with AIDS of 7 months.[19] Similarly, survival in patients in different sub-Saharan African countries is short after an AIDS diagnosis.[21] As would be expected, survival from the initial onset is longer. In Kampala, Uganda, the mean duration of illness from onset of symptoms to death was 30 months, with some patients surviving for many years; approximately one-quarter of patients survived at least 4 years after developing first symptoms (Katabira E; unpublished observations).

African patients living in London who presented with AIDS had no significant differences in survival or CD4+ decline compared with non-Africans after adjustments had been made for CD4+ counts at presentation (Del Amo et al.; in preparation). Although the CD4+ lymphocyte count in most patients dying with AIDS in industrialized countries is now well under 50/mm^3, a recent study in Abidjan, Cote d'Ivoire, showed it to be between 50 and 100/mm^3.[21] The impression, therefore, is that survival with AIDS is worse in developing than in industrialized countries, largely because of late presentation and limited facilities for care and support; nevertheless, some patients with HIV/AIDS in developing countries can live for a surprisingly long time.

THE SPECTRUM OF HIV/AIDS IN CHILDREN IN RESOURCE-POOR COUNTRIES

Understanding of the spectrum of HIV disease in children in developing countries is very limited.[22] Recent studies showed that similarities in the pathology of HIV disease between children in West Africa and Europe or North America were greater than for adults from these different regions.[23] In addition, HIV-infected African children share many of the frequent diseases of childhood with their HIV-negative siblings. Autopsy studies in Cote d'Ivoire showed that *Pneumocystis carinii* pneumonia accounted for 22 percent of deaths in HIV-positive children aged less than 15 months.[23] Other major pathologies included bacterial pneumonia, bacterial meningitis, and, in children aged 15 months or more, measles.

In clinical studies in West Africa, six clinical syndromes dominated hospital admissions for both HIV-infected and HIV-negative children; these were acute respiratory infections, malnutrition, diarrheal diseases, malaria, anemia, and meningitis.[24] In the HIV-infected children, respiratory infections and malnutrition predominated. Tuberculosis was strikingly infrequent in both clinical and pathologic evaluations.[23,24] Since the annual risk of infection with *Mycobacterium tuberculosis,* even in countries with the highest incidence rates in the world, is of the order of 2 percent, it is likely that most HIV-infected children in developing countries die without ever having been exposed. Although there is some evidence from cross-sectional clinical studies of an increased frequency of tuberculosis in children with HIV infection, this disease does not occupy the dominant position it does in AIDS in adults in the developing world.

TUBERCULOSIS AND HIV INFECTION IN DEVELOPING COUNTRIES

The impact of the HIV pandemic on the global tuberculosis situation justifies special mention of HIV-associated tuberculosis. By the year 2000, when the annual incidence of tuberculosis is expected to reach 11 million cases, approximately 14 percent of cases are expected to be attributable to HIV infection.[25] In some countries of sub-Saharan Africa tuberculosis case rates have increased two- to threefold as a result of the HIV epidemic; in many African cities today half of new tuberculosis patients are HIV-infected. Similar effects must be expected in countries of South and Southeast Asia, where tuberculosis is prevalent and HIV infection is spreading in epidemic fashion.

Persons with HIV infection are at increased risk for tuberculosis from reactivation of previously acquired infection, from reinfection, or from rapid progression following first exposure.[26] The clinical expression of tuberculosis is heavily influenced by the severity of underlying immune deficiency.[26,27] Early in the course of HIV disease, when immune function is relatively well preserved, clinical differences between HIV-positive and HIV-negative tuberculosis patients are minimal. With a decline in immune function, the mycobacterial burden increases, extrapulmonary disease becomes more frequent, pulmonary disease is less likely to be cavitary in nature, and miliary spread becomes more likely.[27,28] Patients with advanced HIV disease frequently have widely disseminated, multibacillary tuberculosis, the histology of which is nonreactive in nature.[6]

HIV infection influences the diagnosis and response to treatment. Diagnosis may be more difficult because HIV-infected patients, compared with HIV-negative persons, more often have smear-negative pulmonary tuberculosis or extrapulmonary disease, and tuberculin skin tests are frequently negative from cutaneous anergy. Although bacteriologic response to treatment is similar to that in HIV-negative patients provided treatment with a rifampicin-containing regimen is completed, the mortality is greatly increased, both during and after treatment.[10,29] HIV-positive tuberculosis patients have a mortality rate of approximately 20/100 person years after diagnosis. The causes of death include tuberculosis, especially in those dying early in treatment; however, it is generally believed that most patients die from other HIV-associated illnesses such as bacterial infections.[30] Relapse rates following treatment do not appear to be increased in HIV-infected patients treated with rifampicin-containing regimens, although they may be in persons receiving old style regimens that do not include rifampicin in the initiation phase.[29,31,32]

THE ROLE OF HIV TESTING

Considerable controversy surrounds the issue of testing for HIV infection in developing countries. In many cultures people prefer not to know future problems they cannot influence, and the benefits of knowing one's HIV status when services for HIV-infected persons are lacking may be very theoretical. Discrimination against HIV-infected persons may be particularly extreme in its consequences in resource-poor countries, affecting all aspects of an individual's life. For example, women who have been identified as infected with HIV have suffered abandonment, expulsion from the marital home, dispossession, and domestic violence in different countries.[33] On the other hand, potential advantages include accurate diagnosis of medical problems, assessment of prognosis, counseling about HIV infection and its consequences, prophylaxis against specific opportunistic infections, prevention of HIV transmission to others, and social and legal planning for the future.[16,34,35] HIV testing should not be considered in isolation from the question of services and assistance available to the HIV-infected; if the result of a person's HIV test is not going to influence future management, caution may be indicated before proceeding. International consensus now is that HIV testing should not be performed without informed consent and pre- and post-test counseling.

THERAPY AND CARE

Any approach to HIV/AIDS treatment must take into account the limited resources available in developing countries for therapy, and must be realistic in goals and expectations.[36] Appropriate aims in treating patients suffering from HIV/AIDS are to prolong life maximally, reduce suffering, promote prevention, and assist in reducing the social and economic damage from the disease (see Table 101-1).

As elsewhere, treatment should be oriented to specific diagnoses. An essential part of HIV/AIDS care is the provision of counseling, defined as "a confidential dialogue between a client and a care provider aimed at enabling the client to cope with stress and make personal decisions related to HIV/AIDS. The counseling process includes an evaluation of personal risk of HIV transmission and facilitation of preventive behavior" (Global Programme on AIDS, WHO). Counseling provides initial psychological support for an infected person to accept his or her serostatus and plan for the future. Although counseling is aimed at individuals, it should encourage involvement of the infected person's family or other close contacts. Counseling provides essential information for the prevention of further transmission of infection, and can assist the infected person's family or support system in facing and managing the future.

In most developing countries, and certainly outside of major hospitals, diagnostic facilities may be very limited. WHO has developed diagnostic and treatment algorithms that take account of the level of sophistication of the facility (university hospital, district hospital, dispensary) and have been modified in individual countries; Figs. 101-1 and 101-2 show the algorithms for patients with chronic diarrhea and lymphadenopathy, respectively, from the guidelines in Botswana.[37] In major hospitals, facilities may be available for full investigation, including clinical microbiology and diagnostic imaging such as cerebral CT scanning for suspected toxoplasmosis; in district hospitals, investigation may be limited to chest x-rays and light microscopy; in dispensaries, virtually no investigation may be possible.

The approach to therapy must also take account of what is known about the spectrum of HIV disease in the country concerned and what diseases are curable. A list of essential drugs for HIV/AIDS care should be available, incorporating medicines for treating curable diseases as well as for providing symptomatic relief (Table 101-3).

Since the most common opportunistic infection in HIV-infected persons is tuberculosis, a particularly high index of suspicion is required for this diagnosis.[6,27] All patients with respiratory presentations, especially those with chronic symptoms (>3 weeks), should have three sputum specimens examined for acid-fast bacilli. Patients with smear-negative pulmonary disease should receive treatment with broad-spectrum antibiotics for the treatment of possible bacterial pneumonia before a diagnosis of smear-neg-

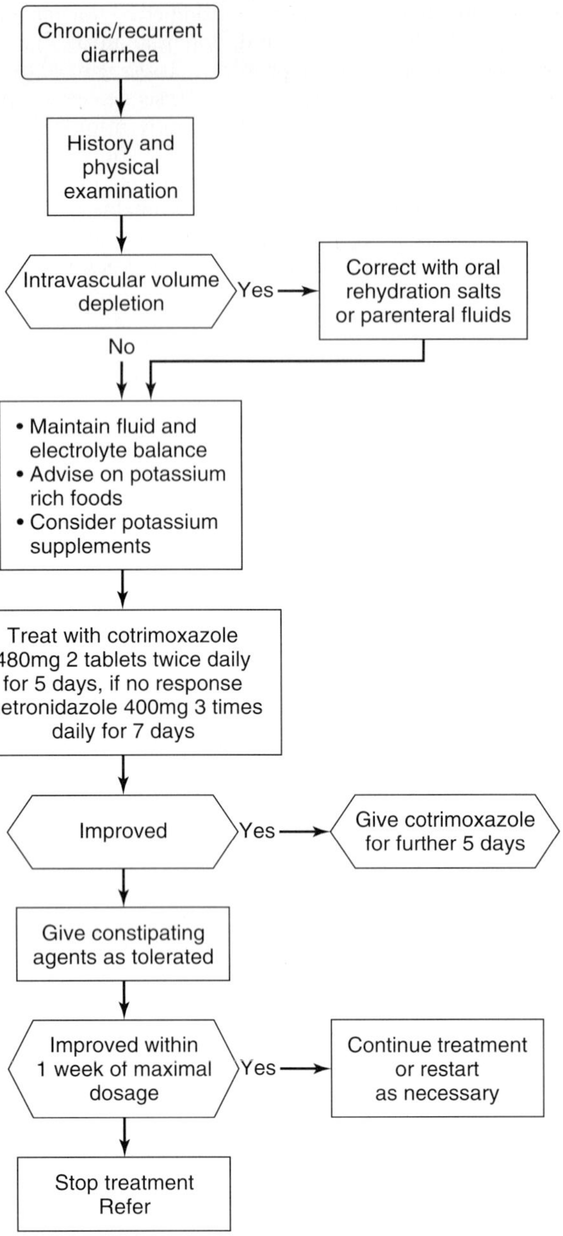

Fig. 101-1. Algorithmic approach to chronic diarrhea, Botswana. Adapted from Clinical Management of HIV Infection in Adults, Vol. II, Botswana Guidelines for Health Posts, Clinics, and Primary Hospitals. AIDS/SID Unit, Ministry of Health P. Bag 00451, Gaborone, Botswana.

ative tuberculosis is entertained. Although ideally this diagnosis would be supported by mycobacterial culture, this is not possible in most situations. A diagnosis of nocardiosis should be considered in patients with chest radiographs suggestive of tuberculosis but with sputum smears negative for acid-fast bacilli.[38] Bronchoscopy with bronchoalveolar lavage is also not possible in most settings, but is especially useful for the diagnosis of pneumocystosis and Kaposi's sarcoma in patients with pulmonary infiltrates not responding to antibiotic therapy; even among such patients, however, tuberculosis is a more frequent diagnosis.[39]

Patients presenting with a febrile syndrome who do not have tuberculosis will most often be suffering from bacterial infections with nontyphoid *Salmonella* organisms or Gram-positive organisms such as pneumococci or staphylococci. Appropriate antibiotics for these infections should be available, although in some countries high levels of resistance may pose constraints. A very frequent presentation is with the HIV wasting syndrome; underlying common diagnoses include tuberculosis, *Salmonella* septicemia, and cryptosporidiosis. Diagnosis of disseminated tuberculosis may be difficult, although histologic examination of bone marrow may be helpful. The treatment of cryptosporidiosis is unsatisfactory and essentially symptomatic.

The two most important causes of neurologic disturbance are toxoplasmosis and cryptococcal meningitis. The latter is easily diagnosed on lumbar puncture, although this investigation is potentially dangerous in patients whose differential diagnosis includes a space-occupying lesion of the brain unless a cerebral scan has been performed first. Specific treatment is available for both conditions.

Apart from drugs for specific infections, a variety of drugs for the control of symptoms of HIV disease should be available, in-

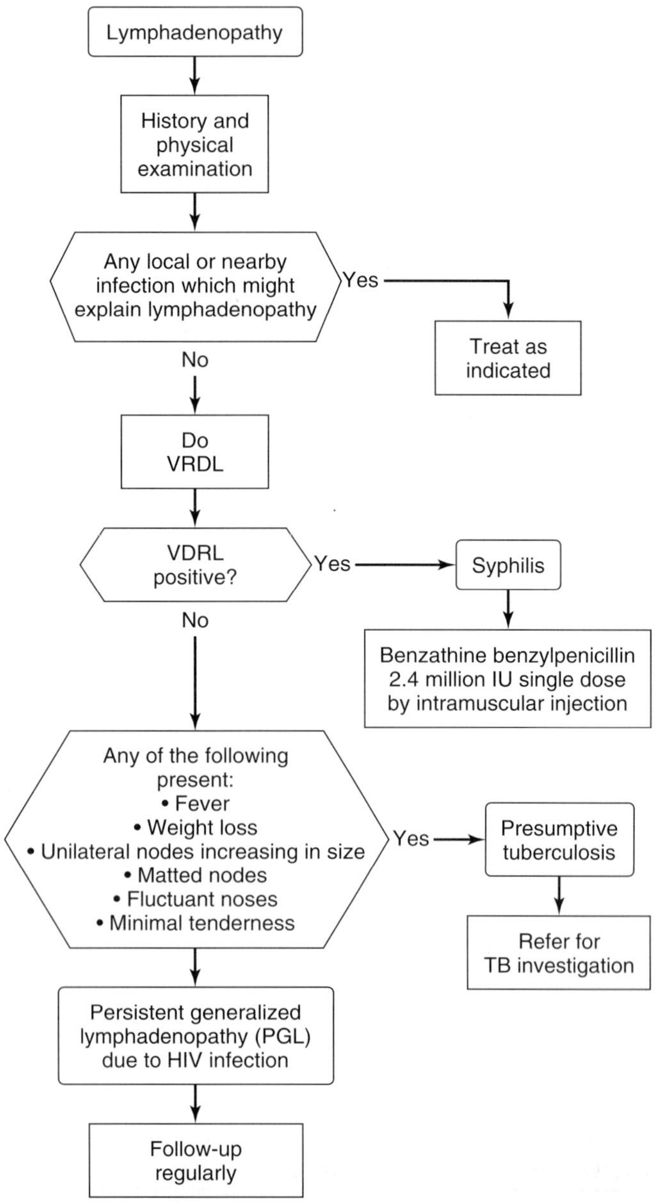

Fig. 101-2. Algorithmic approach to lymphadenopathy, Botswana. Adapted from Clinical Management of HIV Infection in Adults, Vol. II, Botswana Guidelines for Health Posts, Clinics, and Primary Hospitals. AIDS/SID Unit, Ministry of Health P. Bag 00451, Gaborone, Botswana.

Table 101-3. Example of an Essential Drugs List for HIV/AIDS in Resource-Poor Countries

Antituberculosis drugs	Codeine
Cotrimoxazole	Morphine
Ketoconazole (or fluconazole)	Paracetamol
Metronidazole	Aspirin
Broad-spectrum antibiotic (e.g. ampicillin)	Chlorpromazine
Nystatin	Diazepam
Gentian violet	Multivitamin
Hydrocortisone cream	Calamine lotion

After Katabira and Goodgame, Uganda, 1989.

cluding for the care of those who are terminally ill. Especially important are medicines for pain, itching, diarrhea, and cough. Inadequate use has been made in developing countries of opiates for palliation of symptoms in patients with advanced disease. There has been a tendency in many areas to automatically hospitalize all patients with severe immune deficiency, whereas many could in fact be managed as outpatients or at home. To avoid overcrowding of hospitals, it is important to clearly define indications for hospitalization; essentially, these are for the provision of diagnostic or treatment services that cannot be provided otherwise (Table 101-4).

Finally, it should be remembered that care constitutes much more than simply medical intervention. Persons with HIV/AIDS may have many more immediate requirements than accurate diagnosis and specific treatment, including pain control, psychosocial support, and material needs taken for granted in industrialized countries (Table 101-5). Any comprehensive approach to HIV/AIDS care, no matter who undertakes it, must address these basic ingredients for patients' survival. Social complications of HIV/AIDS will also need addressing, such as the welfare of children whose parents are dying, the education of orphans, and the disposal of possessions of those who have died to spouses and children in a fair manner.

OPPORTUNITIES FOR PROPHYLAXIS

Although the gap between clinical services in industrialized and developing countries is wide, most patients with HIV/AIDS in resource-poor countries die at relatively low CD4+ lymphocyte counts.[21] Since several of the major causes of death in persons with HIV/AIDS are preventable, an urgent question is whether prophylaxis could improve life expectancy in HIV-infected persons in developing countries.[16,40] The major diseases for which prophylaxis is available are tuberculosis, toxoplasmosis, pneumococcal and other bacterial infections, pneumocystosis, and fungal infections (Table 101-6).[16,40]

Several placebo-controlled trials have shown that preventive therapy with isoniazid can reduce the incidence of tuberculosis in HIV-infected persons.[41,42] International recommendations are that HIV-infected persons who have a positive tuberculin skin test should receive 6 to 12 months of isoniazid.[43–46] Uncertainties around this intervention are the duration of protection, and thus whether treatment should be continued lifelong, and the best practice in persons who are anergic. Although the risk of tuberculosis in HIV-infected persons is highest in persons with the lowest CD4+ lymphocyte counts, preventive therapy is recommended at first diagnosis of HIV infection.[47] Best practice concerning secondary prophylaxis (after persons have been cured of tuberculosis) is not established.

Table 101-4. Indications for Hospitalization for Patients with HIV/AIDS in Resource-Poor Settings

Special investigations (e.g., lumbar puncture)
Special treatment (e.g., intravenous fluids)
Special nursing (e.g., for altered consciousness)
Special social reasons (e.g., for respite for caregivers)

Table 101-5. Social and Medical Requirements of Persons with HIV/AIDS in Resource-Poor Settings

Food and drink	Psychosocial support
Clothing	Symptom control
Shelter	Diagnosis
Personal hygiene	Treatment for OI
Nursing	Palliative care
	Terminal care

OI = opportunistic infection.

Data concerning the prevention of toxoplasmic encephalitis come largely from observations made from trials assessing preventive interventions for pneumocystosis.[48] For the prevention of toxoplasmic encephalitis, trimethoprim-sulfamethoxazole is generally considered the drug of choice, with dapsone and pyrimethamine an alternative. Secondary prophylaxis for toxoplasmic encephalitis is with continuation of the drugs used for specific therapy, either sulfadiazine and pyrimethamine or clindamycin and pyrimethamine.

There have been no clinical trials assessing different regimens for the prevention of bacterial infections, but a reduced incidence of such infections has been reported in persons receiving trimethoprim-sulfamethoxazole for the prevention of *Pneumocystis carinii* pneumonia.[49,50] A concern about extensive use of this drug, however, is widespread acquisition of resistance by organisms such as *Streptococcus pneumoniae* and *Salmonella* species. Prophylactic penicillin has not been evaluated in HIV-infected persons, and is considered of low priority in view of increasing penicillin resistance, including resistance in strains recovered from HIV-infected persons. Although data are lacking on vaccine efficacy in HIV-infected persons with different levels of immune deficiency, administration of a single dose of 23-valent polysaccharide pneumococcal vaccine is recommended in the United States as soon as possible after diagnosis of HIV infection.[51] Prophylaxis against fungal infections is rarely practiced but may merit consideration in circumstances where incidence is unusually high.[52]

Table 101-6. Approaches to Prophylaxis against Opportunistic Infections in Resource-Poor Countries

Disease	Prophylaxis	Status
Tuberculosis	Isoniazid	Recommended*
Toxoplasmosis	Cotrimoxazole	Under study†
Pneumococcal infection	Vaccination ? Cotrimoxazole	Recommended; under study§
Other bacterial infections (salmonellosis, nocardiosis)	? Cotrimoxazole	Under study**
Fungal infections	? Fluconazole or ketoconazole	Under discussion‡

* Internationally recommended after exclusion of active tuberculosis in HIV-infected persons with positive tuberculin skin test. See refs. 41 to 46.
† Recommended in industrialized countries in HIV-infected persons at risk for toxoplasmosis; usually given as prophylaxis against *Pneumocystis carinii* pneumonia.
§ Pneumococcal vaccine is recommended in industrialized countries, but efficacy in advanced HIV disease uncertain. Cotrimoxazole is under study.
** See ref. 30.
‡ See ref. 52.

Candidiasis (oropharyngeal, vaginal, esophageal) is very common in advanced HIV disease but is easily treated and has low morbidity; its prevention, therefore, is outweighed by factors of cost and the risk of inducing drug resistance. Observational data as well as the results from controlled trials suggest that the incidence of cryptococcal disease is reduced in persons taking long-term azole therapy, usually fluconazole; the effect is most obvious in the most immunosuppressed patients.[53] Improved survival has not been demonstrated. Since the incidence of cryptococcal disease seems to vary regionally, use of preventive therapy may be more relevant in some areas than others. For the prevention of penicilliosis, itraconazole may be more useful.

From a research standpoint, evaluation of a prevention package combining some or all of the discussed preventive measures is required.[16] Operational questions must not be overlooked, especially the issues of cost and adherence. Experience in the field in Uganda with preventive therapy for tuberculosis in HIV-infected persons highlighted numerous problems in drug delivery and adherence, so that few persons actually eligible benefited from the intervention.[54] For the time being it is likely that prophylaxis against opportunistic infections will be applicable only in selected populations such as the military, the police, workers enrolled in industrial health schemes, and individuals with access to private health care. If it can be shown that interventions are useful in such groups, attention should be given later to attempting to provide them on a broader basis.

CONCLUSIONS

No matter how limited resources are, addressing the burden of clinical HIV disease has to be part of any society's response to HIV/AIDS; this is inescapable for ethical as well as practical reasons. Attempts are needed to define the minimum standard of care to which any HIV-infected person should have access within developing countries, and which should be tailored to the specific spectrum of HIV disease seen in that region. Counseling, psychosocial support, and assistance with basic material needs form part of HIV/AIDS care, in addition to diagnosis and specific treatment. For the time being, antiviral drugs play little role in the management of HIV disease in resource-poor settings. For the future, research into prophylactic interventions and their evaluation should be a priority but pilot studies of their rational use are planned.

References

1 UNAIDS and WHO. The HIV/Aids situation in mid 1996: Global and regional highlights. UNAIDS Fact Sheet, Geneva, July, 1996.

2 The HIV pandemic: status and trends, in *AIDS in the World,* JM Man et al (eds). Cambridge, MA, Harvard University Press, 1992, pp. 11–108.

3 De Cock KM et al: Clinical research, prophylaxis, therapy and care for HIV disease in Africa. *Am JPH* 83:1385–1389, 1993.

4 Connor EM et al: Reduction of maternal-infant transmission of human immunodeficiency virus type 1 with zidovudine treatment. *N Engl J Med* 331:1174–1180, 1994.

5 Mulder DW et al: HIV-1 incidence and HIV-1-associated mortality in a rural Ugandan population cohort. *AIDS* 8:87–92, 1994.

6 Lucas SB et al: The mortality and pathology of HIV infection in a West African city. *AIDS* 7:1569–1579, 1993.

7 Marlink R et al: Reduced rate of disease development after HIV-2 infection as compared to HIV-1. *Science* 265:1587–1590, 1994.

8 Kanki PJ et al: Epidemiology and transmission of HIV-2. *AIDS* 8(Suppl 1):S85–S93, 1994.

9 Mukadi Y et al: Spectrum of immunodeficiency in HIV-1-infected patients with pulmonary tuberculosis in Zaire. *Lancet* 342:143–146, 1993.

10 Ackah A et al: Response to therapy, mortality, and CD4+ lymphocyte counts in HIV-infected persons with tuberculosis in Abidjan, Cote d'Ivoire. *Lancet* 345:607–610, 1995.

11 Martin DJ et al: CD4+ lymphocyte count in African patients co-infected with HIV and tuberculosis. *J Acquir Immun Def Synd* 8:386–391, 1995.

12 Gilks CF et al: Invasive pneumococcal disease in a cohort of predominantly HIV-1 infected female sex workers in Nairobi, Kenya. *Lancet* 347:718–723, 1996.

13 Gilks CF et al: Life-threatening bacteraemia in HIV-1 seropositive adults admitted to hospital in Nairobi, Kenya. *Lancet* 336:545–549, 1990.

14 Vugia DJ et al: Pathogens and predictors of fatal septicemia associated with human immunodeficiency virus infections in Ivory Coast, West Africa. *J Infect Dis* 168:564–570, 1993.

15 Gilks CF et al: The presentation and outcome of HIV-related disease in Nairobi. *Q J Med* 82:25–32, 1992.

16 Kaplan J et al: Preventing opportunistic infections in HIV-infected persons: Implications for the developing world. *Am J Trop Med Hyg* 55: 1–11, 1996.

17 Rocha A et al: Pathology of patients with Chagas' disease and acquired immunodeficiency syndrome. *Am J Trop Med Hyg* 50:261–268, 1994.

18 Rosenthal E et al: Visceral leishmaniasis and HIV-1 co-infection in southern France. *Trans Roy Soc Trop Med Hyg* 89:159–162, 1995.

19 Kitayaporn D et al: Survival of AIDS patients in the emerging epidemic in Bangkok, Thailand. *J Acquir Immun Defic Syndr* 11:77–82, 1996.

20 Supparatpinyo K et al: Disseminated *Penicillium marneffei* infection in Southeast Asia. *Lancet* 344:110–113, 1994.

21 Grant A et al: Spectrum of clinical disease and immunosuppression in HIV-infected adults admitted to an infectious disease unit in Abidjan, Cote d'Ivoire. *Ninth International Conference on AIDS and STD in Africa, Kampala,* Abstract TuB166, 10–14 December 1995.

22 Lepage P et al: Natural history and clinical presentation of HIV-1 in children. *AIDS* 5:S117–S125, 1991.

23 Vetter KM et al: Clinical spectrum of HIV disease in children in a West African city. *Ped Infect Dis J* 1:438–442, 1996.

24 Lucas SB et al: Disease in children infected with HIV in Abidjan. *BMJ* 312:335–338,1996.

25 Raviglione MC et al: Global epidemiology of tuberculosis: Morbidity and mortality of a world-wide epidemic. *JAMA* 273:220–226, 1995.

26 De Cock KM: Impact of interaction with HIV, in *Tuberculosis: Back to the Future,* JDH Porter et al (eds). Chichester UK, J Wiley and Sons, 1994, pp. 35–49.

27 De Cock KM et al: Tuberculosis and HIV infection in sub-Saharan Africa. *JAMA* 268:1581–1587, 1992.

28 Abouya L et al: Radiologic manifestations of pulmonary tuberculosis in HIV-1 and HIV-2 infected patients in Abidjan, Cote d'Ivoire. *Tub Lung Dis* 76:436–440, 1995.

29 Kassim S et al: Two year follow-up of persons with HIV-1- and HIV-2-associated pulmonary tuberculosis treated with short course chemotherapy in West Africa. *AIDS* 9:1185–1191, 1995.

30 Greenberg AE et al: Autopsy-proven causes of death in HIV-infected patients treated for tuberculosis in Abidjan, Cote d'Ivoire. *AIDS* 9: 1251–1254, 1995.

31 Nunn P et al: Cohort study of human immunodeficiency virus infection in patients with tuberculosis in Nairobi, Kenya: Analysis of early (6-month) mortality. *Am Rev Respir Dis* 146:849–854, 1992.

32 Hawken M et al: Increased recurrence of tuberculosis in HIV-1-infected patients in Kenya. *Lancet* 342:332–337, 1993.

33 Temmerman M et al: The right not to know HIV test results. *Lancet* 345:969–970, 1995.

34 Kamenga M et al: Evidence of marked sexual behavior change associated with low HIV-1 seroconversion in 149 married couples with discordant HIV-1 serostatus: Experience at an HIV counseling center in Zaire. *AIDS* 5:61–67, 1991.

35 Allen S et al: Confidential HIV testing and condom promotion in Africa: Impact on HIV and gonorrhea rates. *JAMA* 268:3338–3343, 1992.

36 Goodgame RW: AIDS in Uganda: Clinical and social features. *N Engl J Med* 323:383–389, 1990.

37 AIDS/STD Unit: Clinical management of HIV infection in adults. Volume II. Botswana Guidelines for Health Posts, Clinics and Primary Hospitals. Ministry of Health, Gaborone, Botswana, 1993.

38 Lucas SB et al: Nocardiosis mimicking tuberculosis in HIV-positive patients: An autopsy study in West Africa. *Tub Lung Dis* 75:301–307, 1994.

39 Malin AS et al: *Pneumocystis carinii* pneumonia in Zambia. *Lancet* 346:1258–1261, 1995.

40 Kaplan JE et al: Prevention of opportunistic infections in persons infected with human immunodeficiency virus. *Clin Infect Dis* 21(Suppl 1):S1–141, 1995.

41 Pape JW et al: Effect of isoniazid prophylaxis on incidence of active tuberculosis and progression of HIV infection. *Lancet* 342:268–272, 1993.

42 Nsubuga P et al: Preventive therapy for tuberculosis in HIV-infected Ugandans. *Ninth International Conference on AIDS and STD in Africa. Kampala*, Abstract MoB010, 10–14 December 1995.

43 Purified protein derivative (PPD)-tuberculin and HIV infection: Guidelines for anergy testing and management of anergic persons at risk of tuberculous infection. *MMWR* 40:27–33, 1991.

44 WHO: Tuberculosis preventive therapy in HIV-infected individuals. *Wkly Epidemiol Rec* 68:361–368, 1993.

45 De Cock KM et al: Preventive therapy for tuberculosis in HIV-infected persons: International recommendations, research, and practice. *Lancet* 345:833–836, 1995.

46 O'Brien RJ et al: Preventive therapy for tuberculosis in HIV infection: The promise and the reality. *AIDS* 7:665–673, 1995.

47 Antonucci G et al: Risk factors for tuberculosis in HIV-infected persons: A prospective cohort study. *JAMA* 274:143–148, 1995.

48 Richards FO et al: Preventing toxoplasmic encephalitis in persons infected with human immunodeficiency virus. *Clin Infect Dis* 21(Suppl1):S49–56, 1995.

49 Hardy WD et al: A controlled trial of trimethoprim-sulfamethoxazole or aerosolized pentamidine for secondary prophylaxis of *Pneumocystis carinii* pneumonia in patients with human immunodeficiency virus infection. *N Engl J Med* 327:1836–1841, 1992.

50 Mayer HB et al: The effect of *Pneumocystis carinii* pneumonia prophylaxis regimens on the incidence of bacterial infections in HIV-infected patients. *AIDS* 7:1687–1689, 1993.

51 Keller DW et al: Preventing bacterial respiratory tract infections among persons infected with human immunodeficiency virus. *Clin Infect Dis* 21(Suppl1): S77–83, 1995.

52 Clumeck N: Primary prophylaxis against opportunistic infections in patients with AIDS. *N Engl J Med* 332:739–740, 1995.

53 Powderly WG et al: A randomized trial comparing fluconazole with clotrimazole troches for the prevention of fungal infections in patients with advanced human immunodeficiency virus infection. *N Engl J Med* 332:700–705, 1995.

54 Aisu T et al: Preventive chemotherapy for HIV associated tuberculosis in Uganda: An operational assessment at a voluntary counseling and testing centre. *AIDS* 9:267–273, 1995.

Chapter 102

Approach to management of STDs in developing countries

Bea Vuylsteke
Marie Laga

WHAT MAKES CASE MANAGEMENT OF STDS DIFFERENT IN DEVELOPING COUNTRIES?

In theory, appropriate management of STDs is based on the same criteria worldwide. However, in practice, the approach taken to STD case management may differ according to the realities of a specific setting. We will consider three aspects of STD management that differ between developing and developed countries, including the aspect of the provision of treatment, the characteristics of the patients, and the disease profile. Some of these features concern health care in general, whereas others are specific for STD care itself.

THE PROVIDER

Whether STD case management is provided by a primary health care worker or a clinician in a categorical STD clinic, logistic problems often are similar. An obvious hurdle for any health care provision is the poor infrastructure in many developing countries. Bad roads and poor transport facilities make accessibility to the services difficult. In many places, a consultation room is not available or is underequipped, and privacy often is lacking. Laboratory facilities may not exist and, where they do, they may not be efficient or capable of performing the relevant tests. Clinicians who can provide comprehensive case management often must work without the help of health educators, contact tracers, counselors, or administrative personnel. The maximum time that can be spent per patient is often not more than 5 to10 minutes.

Another, and probably a most important, problem is the lack of a continuous and sufficient supply of drugs or the absence of effective, in general more expensive, drugs for the treatment of STD.

THE PATIENT

The patient's belief in the efficacy of treatment by a formal Western-type health service is, in general, weaker in developing countries than in the industrialized world. Many patients continue to consult traditional healers, especially for STD, and self-medication is common.[1] Some may first go to the informal sector, and only later, when this treatment does not appear to work, present at a clinic.[2] Seeking treatment in an appropriate health service and compliance with treatment are also related to other social, economic, and cultural factors.[3] Many people may simply be too poor to pay for the transport to and from the health service or for a consultation or for the drugs (full-treatment regimen). However, in many developing countries, the dependence of women on men and their inferior social status may also play a major role.[1] For example, women may not have the time to go to the health center, and STD clinics often are stigmatizing for them. Many women cannot afford informing their husband of the presence of a STD for fear of being blamed for infidelity and hence, of being chased away from the family. In some societies, women need the permission of their husband to consult a health service. Some women may thus wait too long or never seek treatment.[4]

Another aspect that may complicate effective STD management is the patient's capacity to recognize the symptoms correctly. A good example is provided by Rwanda, where high production of vaginal flow during sex is much appreciated.[5] Vaginal discharge may thus be perceived not as a sign of disease but as an indication of sexual health. However, seeking treatment for STDs presupposes the perception of a problem. In sum, the patient's capacity to seek timely treatment in an appropriate health service is directly affected not only by the availability, accessibility, and affordability of such services but also by his or her capacity to recognize the symptoms correctly, his or her belief in the efficacy of the health service, and by his or her social, economic, and cultural environment. In developing countries, these factors are certainly different from the industrialized world and many remain poorly understood.

THE DISEASE

Although the remainder of this chapter deals in detail with case management of STDs, a few general points are highlighted here.

Both the prevalence and the incidence of STDs tend to be considerably higher in developing countries than in the industrialized world. The relative distribution of the various STDs takes on a different disease spectrum, such as higher relative frequency of chancroid as a cause of genital ulcer or *N. gonorrhoeae* as an etiological agent in urethritis.[2,6] Some STDs, such as granuloma inguinale, are virtually only seen in developing countries. The high rates of HIV infection in many geographic areas may have repercussions on the natural history and response to treatment of STDs.[7,8]

In many parts of the developing world, resistance to drugs, such as penicillins and tetracyclines, increased rapidly over the past two decades. This results in the need for more expensive effective drugs for the treatment of gonorrhea and chancroid.[9,10]

Finally, in developing countries, patients with STDs tend to present with more severe and a higher frequency of STD-related complications, which is largely a result of delayed treatment or lack of effective treatment.

STD SYNDROMIC CASE MANAGEMENT

STD case management should be completed during one patient visit, using simple diagnostic methods that are neither time-consuming nor expensive. A clinical approach has the advantage of offering prompt diagnosis and hence prompt treatment. However, a clinical "etiological" guess may be highly inaccurate for STD. It is, for instance, very difficult to differentiate between gonococcal, nongonococcal urethritis, and mixed etiology, on the basis of clinical observation only. Similarly, the "typical" clinical presentations of primary syphilis, chancroid, and genital herpes, have a low diagnostic accuracy.[6,11,12] Moreover, it is impossible to identify clinically dual or mixed infection, which are both very common. Many laboratory tests for STD diagnosis are too sophisticated, and generally are not available in most settings. Simple, rapid, and affordable tests for the diagnosis of chlamydia infection or chancroid have been on the priority list for STD research for years, but as yet remain unavailable.

The "syndromic" approach does not require identification of the underlying etiology. Instead, it is based on the identification of a syndrome, that is, a group of symptoms and easily recognized signs associated with a number of well-defined etiologies. Treatment is provided for the majority of the organisms locally responsible for the syndrome.

Many developing countries have adopted the syndromic approach in their national STD guidelines. These guidelines have been adapted to the local infrastructure and examination possibilities (e.g., possibility of a speculum examination) and to the regional epidemiological situation. Sometimes, adaptation to local circumstances will require a validation of the diagnostic approach used in the flowcharts. This validation consists of a comparison of the diagnostic outcome of the flowchart to a "gold standard." As such the sensitivity, specificity, and predictive value of the approach for the different STDs will be determined.

COMPREHENSIVE CASE MANAGEMENT

A syndromic approach should offer more than a diagnosis and treatment alone. Compliance, counseling, condoms, and contact notification and treatment are the four keys to comprehensive case management.

Compliance with treatment is very important not only for cure, but also for preventing transmission of infection to a sexual partner, although single-dose therapy should be used whenever possible. Explaining the mechanisms of transmission and the complications of no or incomplete treatment will help to motivate the patient to take the full course of antibiotics and to refrain from sex during treatment.[13]

During the contact with the patient, the opportunity should not be missed to provide health education about STD and HIV prevention, and this should include a demonstration of correct condom use. An STD patient is, by definition, a person who is at increased risk for HIV because of his or her high-risk behavior. In addition, his or her vulnerability to HIV infection is increased by the very presence of STD, which increases the risk for acquisition of HIV. More comprehensive counseling (e.g., for HIV testing) will not be possible in most situations in developing countries, because of limitations in time and personnel.

Condoms should be available in every health service that provides STD case management. Whether they should be handed out free or sold depends on local policy.

Asymptomatic partners who would not seek treatment can be reached by partner notification and treatment. However, some of the problems associated with partner notification are more apparent in developing countries. Active contact tracing by telephone, mail, or home visits often is not possible. The use of contact cards, which are handed over by the index patient, is a simple and cheap way to bring in partners for treatment, as was illustrated in Zimbabwe.[14] Moreover, a large proportion of STD are contracted during commercial sex activities, which further complicates contact notification and treatment. Thus, in Nairobi, 37 percent of male STD patients named a prostitute as the source of their infection, and another 27 percent named a casual pickup.[3] In Blantyre, 64 percent of the men with urethritis had sex with a bar girl in the previous month.[2]

Another problem in developing countries is the social inequality between men and women, which makes it extremely difficult for a woman to inform her husband of a STD. In such situations, many women are blamed for the disease and face violence or even expulsion by their husbands. On the other hand, experience from Zambia and Kenya shows that a large proportion of male partners of pregnant women with syphilis were willing to come to the antenatal clinic for treatment for syphilis.[15]

In conclusion, every contact between a STD patient and a health care worker is a unique opportunity to give preventive messages, promote condom use, and, where possible, promote treatment of at least one partner.

COMMON STD SYNDROMES IN DEVELOPING COUNTRIES

URETHRAL DISCHARGE

Urethritis is probably the most common STD syndrome in men in developing countries.[3,16] In many parts of the developing world, the estimated incidence of urethritis is considerably higher than in developed countries. For example, in a population-based study in two cities in Cameroon, 10 percent of the interviewed men reported at least one episode of urethritis during the past 6 months.[17] This proportion was even higher (20%) among male bar clients.[17] In a similar study in a rural area of Tanzania, the annual incidence was 7 percent.[18] These figures stand in sharp contrast with those reported for Europe and North America, where the annual incidence of urethritis in men is less than 1 percent.[19,20]

Another striking difference in the epidemiology of urethritis in developed and developing countries relates to its etiology (Fig. 102-1). Although *Chlamydia trachomatis* and *Ureaplasma urealyticum* are the major causes of urethritis in the developed world, *N. gonorrhoeae* continues to be the major cause of urethritis in many developing countries.[2,16,21] However, owing to the many difficulties surrounding the diagnosis of chlamydial infection, the presence of multiple etiological agents tends to be underestimated in these countries. Given these etiological patterns, a syndromic approach of urethritis requires a treatment for both gonorrhea and nongonococcal urethritis (NGU).

Figure 102-2 gives examples of flowcharts for the management of urethral discharge. In the first example, a simple syndromic approach is adopted, whereby every patient complaining of urethral discharge and/or dysuria is treated for both gonorrhea and nongonococcal urethritis. It is important to rely on patients' reports rather than on the clinical sign of urethral discharge, since discharge is not always visible. This approach is of particular relevance in large parts of Africa, where many people combine treatment from a variety of places. In Malawi, for instance, 53 percent of patients with urethral syndrome reported to have sought treatment elsewhere before consulting the formal health sector.[2] As such, if urethritis is only treated when discharge is visible during physical examination, many infections may be missed and remain untreated.

To decrease overtreatment and diminish consumption, some countries have adopted a policy of sequential treatment, that is, first treatment for gonorrhea and, failing this, treatment for NGU. The success of sequential treatment obviously depends on the patients' compliance to return to the health service if initial treatment has failed. In reality, such compliance is low and sequential treatment, therefore, is no longer recommended.[13]

An alternative method to decrease the cost of a syndromic treatment consists in including simple laboratory tests for detecting gonococci, as shown in the second example in Fig. 102-2. A Gram stain is used for the detection of intracellular diplococci in urethral discharge. Including a Gram stain in a diagnostic flowchart for urethritis should be advised only when appropriate laboratory facilities are available and results can be given within reasonable time delays, that is, no return visit is necessary for treatment. However, gonococcal infection cannot always be excluded by Gram stain.

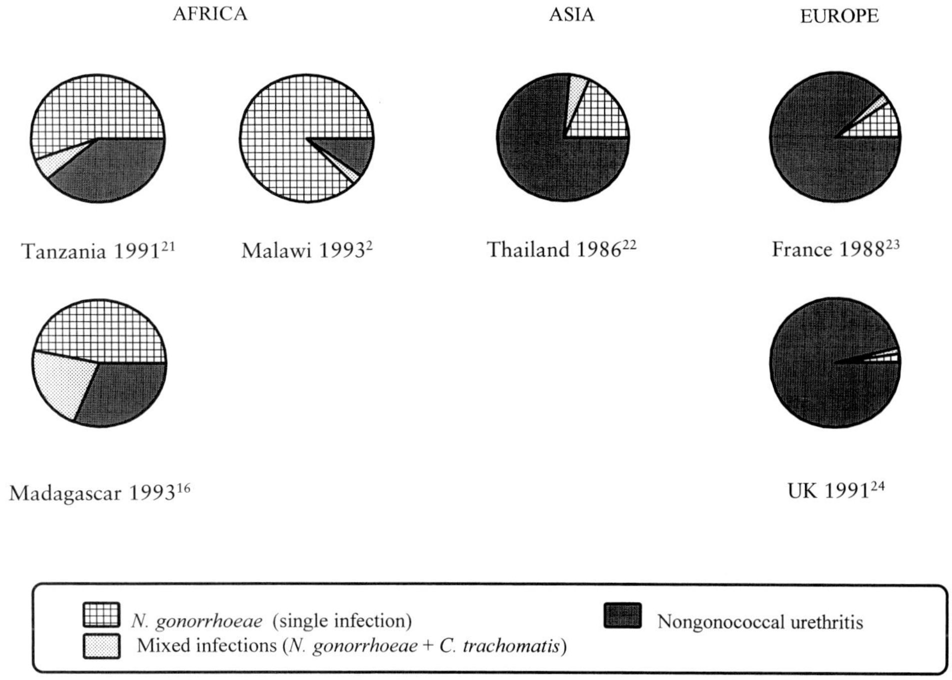

Fig. 102-1. Etiologies of urethritis in selected developing and industrialized countries.

In optimal conditions, the Gram stain has a sensitivity of 90 to 95 percent and a specificity of 95 to 100 percent for the detection of intracellular diplococci.[26] However, its validity, and hence the validity of a diagnostic flowchart, including Gram stain (see Fig. 102-2), varies substantially with the experience of the laboratory technician and the field conditions within countries.[27]

A syndromic approach of urethritis requires a treatment for both gonorrhea and nongonococcal urethritis. In recent years, antimicrobial resistance to the commonly available antibiotics such as penicillin, trimethoprim/sulfamethoxazole, thiamphenicol, and the tetracyclines has been increasing in many parts of the developing world (Table 102-1). These relatively inexpensive antibiotics, therefore, no longer can be recommended as a first choice treatment option in many countries. However, antibiotics with 95 percent efficacy, such as spectinomycin, ciprofloxacin, and azithromycin, are much more expensive and often not affordable in many populations. In practice, drug choices therefore are often a trade-off between drug efficacy and the cost of treatment.

Establishing appropriate treatment strategies is further complicated by the fact that resistance patterns are changing rapidly. In Hong Kong, for example, the proportion of penicillinase-producing *N. gonorrhoeae* (PPNG) declined from 25 to 4 percent in less than 2 years. In this same period, the 4-fluoroquinolone resistance increased from 0.5 to 10.5 percent.[34] This illustrates the importance of monitoring of drug resistance patterns at regular intervals within countries.

In contrast to gonorrhea, infections caused by *C. trachomatis* can be cured using the classic treatment with tetracyclines (doxycycline, tetracycline). However, compliance may be a problem as 7 days of uninterrupted treatment is required.

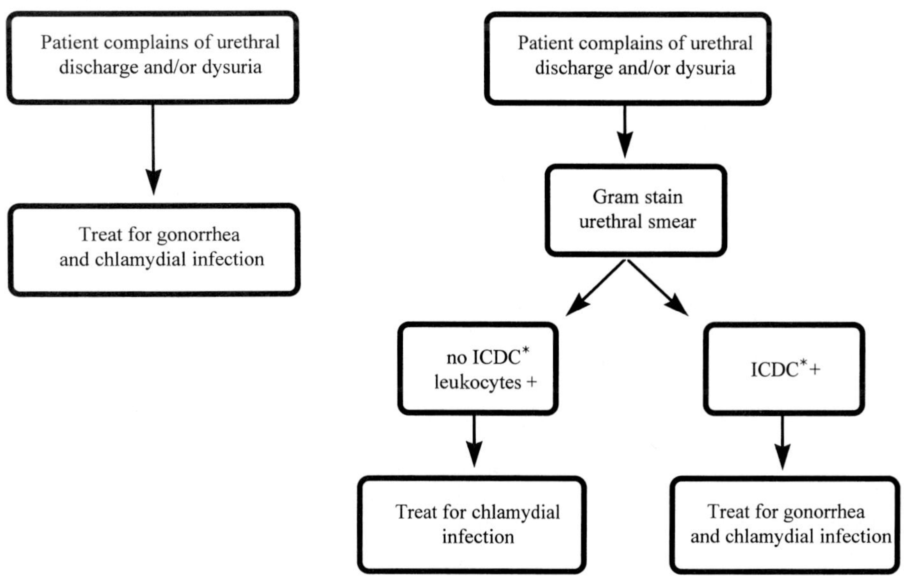

Fig. 102-2. Examples of flowcharts for the management of urethral discharge. *ICDC: Intracellular diplococci

Table 102-1. In Vitro Resistance of *N. gonorrhoeae* against Selected Antibiotics in Africa (1988–1994)

	Percentage of strains resistant to						
	Penicillin		Tetracycline				
Site, year (ref.)	PPNG, %	CMRNG, % (non-PPNG)	TRNG, %	CMRNG, %	TMP/SMZ, %	Kanamycine, %	Thiamphenicol, %
Ethiopia 1990[28]	73	19		0	77	13	0
Ghana 1991–1993[29]	94		0	68	100		
Rwanda 1989[30]	41	39	64	60		0	60
Senegal 1988[31]	24	4		7		0	2
The Gambia, 1990[32]	49	52	0	92			51
Zaire (1988–1990[90]	67	20	45	38			37
Zimbabwe 1988[33]	67	53		16		0	3

PPNG: Penicillinase-producing *N. gonorrhoeae.*
CMRNG: Chromosomally mediated resistant *N. gonorrhoeae.*
TRNG: Tetracycline-resistant *N. gonorrhoeae.*
TMP/SMZ: Trimethoprim/sulfamethoxazole.

SWOLLEN SCROTUM

Acute infectious epididymitis in men aged between 15 and 35 years is usually sexually acquired.[35] It is a common complication of urethritis, with which it shares the same etiological agents. In a study conducted in South Africa, 78 percent of the urine samples of men with acute epididymitis tested positive for *N. gonorrhoeae* and/or *C. trachomatis*.[36] Furthermore, men with swollen scrotum often have also signs of urethritis and, as a study in Malawi showed, 1.8 percent of men with urethral symptoms have scrotal swelling.[2]

A syndromic STD management of swollen scrotum includes treatment similar to the treatment of urethritis syndrome (Fig. 102-3). However, prior to applying a syndromic approach, a non-infectious origin of the syndrome must be excluded. A traumatic cause can be identified from the patient's medical history. Simple clinical examination does not always ensure a correct diagnosis since it is sometimes difficult to differentiate between epididymitis and testicular torsion. However, in prepubertal boys, testicular torsion tends to be more common than epididymitis.[35]

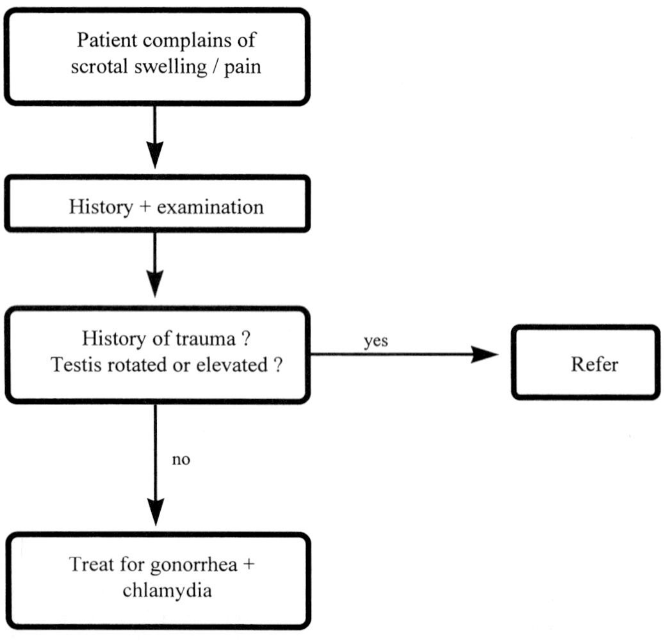

Fig. 102-3. Example of a flowchart for the management of scrotal swelling.

GENITAL ULCERS

Like urethritis, genital ulcers are much more common in developing countries than in industrialized countries. However, considerable regional variation exists. There appears to be a higher prevalence of genital ulcer disease (GUD) in Southern African countries compared to West and Central African countries. In rural Zimbabwe, for instance, 63 percent of the male STD patients presented with genital ulcers.[37] In this clinic, genital ulcers were the main reason for consultation. Similarly, in rural Mozambique, genital ulcers were the primary reason for consultation in 38 percent of all STD cases.[38] In addition to high levels of GUD in STD patients, patients with a genital ulcer tend to wait a long time before presenting themselves at a health center. Thus, in a study in Rwanda, 36 percent of GUD patients had waited for more than 2 weeks.[6] Similarly, in South Africa, this proportion corresponds to 35 and 36 percent among men and women, respectively, whereas in Gambia, 52 percent of all patients had waited for over 2 weeks.[39–41] In many cases, patients continued to have sex before consultation.

Table 102-2 illustrates the different etiologies of GUD in different geographical areas. Although their relative distribution may differ within countries, the most common causes of genital ulcers in virtually all developing countries are *Haemophilus ducreyi* (chancroid), syphilis, and genital herpes. It should be noted that the proportion of syphilis shown in the table is probably an overestimate of current infection as the diagnosis of syphilis in the selected studies is based on a positive serology (RPR and TPHA). In studies conducted after 1985, the proportion of GUD accounted for by herpes simplex virus appears to be higher than in earlier studies. It is not known to what extent the AIDS epidemic has played a role in this phenomenon. In Rwanda, for instance, a study in one health center showed that in 1986, herpes simplex virus was the third and second most important cause of genital ulcers in men and women, respectively.[46] By 1992, herpes simplex virus had become the second cause of genital ulcers in men and the leading cause in female patients.[6] During that same period, HIV prevalence among patients with genital ulcers increased from 43 to 67 percent in men, and from 77 to 83 percent in women.[6,46]

Table 102-2. Etiology of GUD in Different Countries

Country	*H. ducreyi* (culture +), %	Syphilis (darkfield or serology +), %	*H. ducreyi* and syphilis, %	Genital herpes (culture HSV +), %	No. etiology identified, %
Rwanda (n = 95) 1992[6]	29	28	7	22	32
South Africa (n = 200) 1989[11]	17	43	5	14	19
Malaysia (n = 249) 1990[42]	9	7	1	19	60
Swaziland (n = 155) 1979[43]	44	19	2	12	15
The Gambia (n = 104) 1986[41]	52	22	10	6	27
Kenya (n = 120) 1980[44]	48	10	?	6	36
Thailand (n = 120) 1982[45]	38	4	2	12	50

These data suggest that widespread HIV infection may change etiological patterns of GUD.

Two rather rare causes of GUD are lymphogranuloma venereum (LGV) and donovanosis. In its primary stage, LGV may present as an ulceration. LGV was detected in 6, 7, 14, and 0 percent of patients with a genital ulcer, in South Africa, Gambia, Rwanda, and Kenya, respectively.[11,41,46,44] Donovanosis as a cause of genital ulceration is limited to certain regions, such as Papua New Guinea. Because the disease is extremely rare in most parts of the world, and often is not associated with genital ulcer disease, donovanosis is not considered in most flowcharts. The role of sexual transmission of this disease is still controversial.

In most developing countries, a syndromic approach to the genital ulcer syndrome includes treatment for syphilis and chancroid, but not for herpes, as antiherpetic chemotherapy is rarely available in developing countries (Fig. 102-4).

Determining the underlying causes of GUD is extremely difficult. Clinical diagnosis is unreliable.[6,11,12] For example, typical vesicles were seen or reported in only 4 percent of confirmed cases in Rwanda.[6] Adding a rapid plasma reagin (RPR) test for syphilis to a diagnostic flowchart may be considered if the results of the test are readily available. However, the test cannot exclude chancroid as a possible cause of GUD. Therefore, patients with a reactive RPR test should be treated for syphilis as well as chancroid. An additional difficulty is that the RPR test is negative in 30 to 50 percent of patients with a primary syphilitic ulcer.[47] However, in developing countries, where patients may wait longer before seeking care, the test is probably more sensitive at presentation. In Rwanda, for example, only one patient seroconverted during follow-up, the other 109 syphilis patients were positive at the first visit.[6]

Because of the high proportion of unidentified etiology, it is difficult to validate a diagnostic approach for genital ulcers. In Table 102-3, the results of a validation study for genital ulcers in Rwanda are presented. Three approaches for the diagnosis of syphilis or chancroid were compared: a syndromic approach, a clinical diagnosis, and a diagnosis based on the RPR test result.[6] The proportion of correctly managed patients amounted to 99 percent with the syndromic approach, 82 percent with the laboratory approach, and 38 percent with the clinical diagnosis.

In many parts of the world, patients with syphilis often are coinfected with HIV. Whereas standard treatment of early syphilis and early latent syphilis in patients with HIV infection may be less effective, a few studies did not find a different clinical or serologic response after one dose of benzathin penicillin in HIV-positive as compared to HIV-negative patients.[48,49]

Antimicrobial resistance of *H. ducreyi* is another recently observed problem. In one study in Kenya, failure of a single intramuscular injection of 250 mg of ceftriaxone was strongly associated with HIV infection.[50] Increasing resistance to trimethoprim/sulfamethoxazole (TMP/SMZ) and treatment failure have also been documented in Rwanda, but HIV infection and the degree of CD4+ cell depletion were unrelated to clinical and bacteriologic outcomes.[10] Because of such emerging antimicrobial resistance, treatment of chancroid ideally should be based on local antimicrobial susceptibility data.

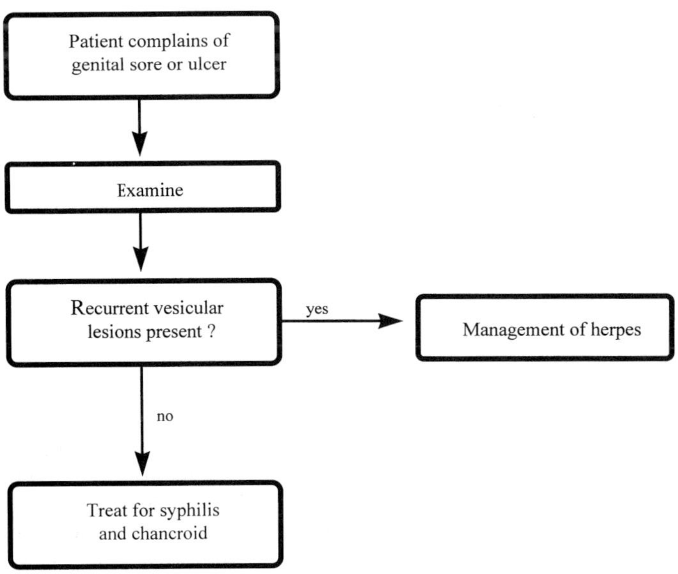

Fig. 102-4. Example of a flowchart for the management of genital ulcers in developing countries.

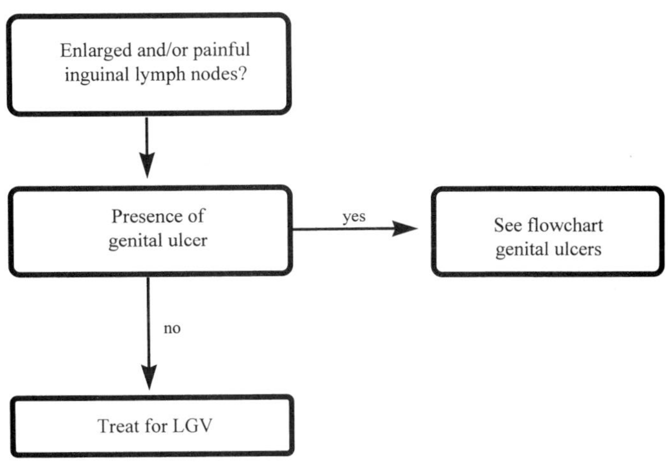

Fig. 102-5. Example of a flowchart for the management of inguinal lymphadenopathy.

Table 102-3. Number of Patients with Chancroid and/or Syphilis Correctly Managed When Applying Three Different Diagnostic Strategies in Rwanda

	Confirmed syphilis	Confirmed chancroid	Confirmed syphilis and chancroid	Total
Number of GUD patients	81	86	29	196
Number of these patients correctly managed (%)				
Syndromic approach*	79 (97.5)	86 (100)	29 (100)	194 (99.0)
Diagnosis based on RPR test results†	78 (96.3)	83 (96.5)	0 (0)	161 (82.1)
Clinical diagnosis	18 (22.2)	57 (66.3)	0 (0)	75 (38.3)
Mixed approach: clinical diagnosis + syndromic approach§	41 (50.6)	69 (80.2)	5 (17.2)	115 (58.7)

* See Fig. 102-4.
† Patients with RPR+ received treatment for syphilis, patients with RPR− received treatment for chancroid.
§ Patients with clear-cut clinical diagnosis were treated accordingly. Patients with undetermined clinical diagnosis received syndromic treatment for chancroid *and* syphilis.

INGUINAL LYMPHADENOPATHY

STDs are important causes of inguinal lymphadenopathy in developing countries. For example, 8.5 percent of male and 4.7 percent of female STD patients in Kenya were complaining of genital or inguinal swelling.[3]

Lymph nodes that are 2 cm or larger, and become fluctuant, are considered buboes. The main causes of buboes are chancroid and lymphogranuloma venereum (LGV). In Zimbabwe, 20 percent of men and 6 percent of women with genital ulcers presented with buboes.[37] In Rwanda, these proportions were, respectively, 12.4 and 4 percent.[6]

LGV is usually seen in a secondary stage of acute lymphadenitis with bubo formation, without a sign of the primary ulcer.

As proposed in the diagnostic flowchart shown in Fig. 102-5, a practical way to manage buboes is to consider them as LGV when no ulcer is visible, and to manage them as a genital ulcer syndrome when an ulcer is present. Aspiration of the bubo (through the healthy skin) may be required.

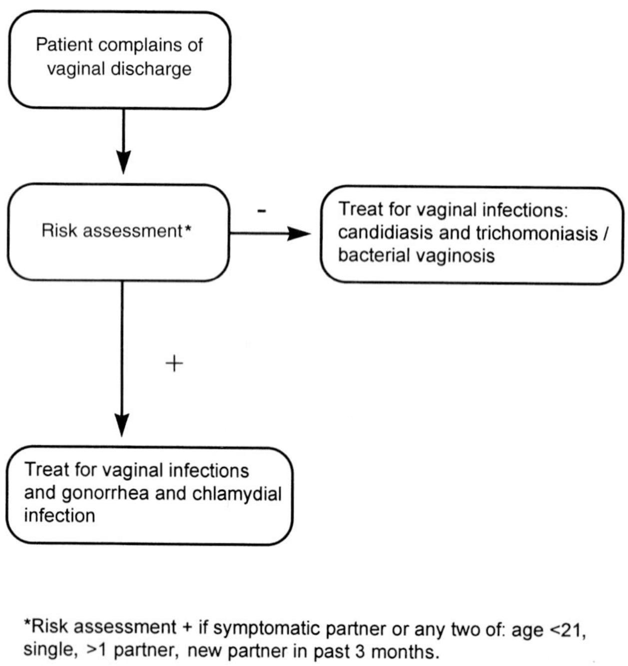

Fig. 102-6. Example of a flowchart for the management of vaginal discharge.

VAGINAL DISCHARGE

Abnormal vaginal discharge is a very common complaint among women, in both developing and industrialized countries.[3,37,51] It is the main symptom of both cervicitis and vaginitis. The underlying causes of cervicitis in women are gonococcal or chlamydial infection, which are usually localized in the endocervix and urethra. If cervicitis remains untreated, it may cause serious complications such as acute pelvic inflammatory disease, ectopic pregnancy, and infertility.[52] The failure of many infected women, including those who are symptomatic, to seek medical care, may explain the high prevalence of gonococcal and chlamydial infections, and particularly of their complications in some developing countries. For example, among pregnant women in a rural area in Mozambique, 7 percent had gonorrhea and 8 percent had chlamydial infection.[38]

The most frequent causes of vaginal infection are candidiasis, bacterial vaginosis, and trichomoniasis. The possible complications of vaginal infection are much more limited except for a potential, but not proven, role in facilitating acquisition of HIV, as well as a role in causing premature birth. As they are a very common reason why women consult health services, the quality of care for vaginal discharge may have a great impact on the confidence that women have in the health service.

In three surveys among women presenting with vaginal discharge at an STD clinic (in Jamaica) or at a primary health care center (in Tanzania and Zimbabwe), the most common causes of their complaints were related to vaginitis (Table 102-4). Nevertheless, a syndromic approach to vaginal discharge should also take cervicitis into account, because of the public health importance of gonococcal or chlamydial infections.

Designing a flowchart that addresses the problem of cervicitis adequately is difficult because of the poor validity of symptoms and clinical signs. None of the symptoms (vaginal discharge, lower abdominal pain, or dysuria) or clinical signs (vaginal discharge, cervical mucopus, friability, or pain on mobilization of the cervix) is both sufficiently sensitive and specific for cervicitis. Asymptomatic gonococcal and chlamydial infections are very common. Thus, in a rural area in Mozambique, up to 89 percent of infected pregnant women did not report any symptoms, and among prostitutes in Zaire, newly acquired infections remained asymptomatic in 69 percent of all cases.[38,55] However, even in symptomatic women, the predictive value of symptoms and signs for cervicitis remains low. For example, in a study among symptomatic women

Table 102-4. Etiology of Vaginal Discharge Complaints in Different Clinical Settings in Developing Countries

Country (ref)	Total number of women with vaginal discharge	Vaginitis: Candidiasis, %	Vaginitis: Bacterial vaginosis, %	Vaginitis: Trichomoniasis, %	Cervicitis: Gonorrhea, %	Cervicitis: Chlamydial infection, %
Jamaica[53]	609	35	41	25	17	25
Tanzania[54]	395	38	NA	25	12*	
Zimbabwe[37]	65	42	15	39	17	15

* Gonorrhea and/or chlamydial infection, %.
NA: Not available.

in Jamaica, the symptom of vaginal discharge was 83 percent sensitive but only 19 percent specific for cervicitis.[53]

Several studies have demonstrated that risk markers are more predictive for gonococcal or chlamydial cervicitis than signs and symptoms (Fig. 102-6).[53,56] This management strategy ensures that a woman with a complaint of vaginal discharge will systematically be treated for vaginitis, but her risk for cervicitis will also be assessed. When her risk assessment is positive, she should receive additional treatment for both gonococcal and chlamydial infection. Risk markers such as a symptomatic partner, being younger than 21 years of age, being single, having more than one or having a new sexual partner in the last 3 months have been successfully validated and the feasibility of asking these questions has been tested in some settings, including Jamaica and rural Tanzania.[53,54] In other cultures, especially in parts of Asia and Latin America, the acceptability and feasibility of asking such questions may prove more difficult.

Moreover, simple laboratory tests, such as Gram stain or a leukoesterase test, which are useful in detecting urethritis in men, are not specific and sensitive enough to detect cervical infections.[56,57]

The recommended treatment for vaginitis is shown in Fig. 102-6. It includes treatment for both candidiasis and trichomoniasis, which also covers bacterial vaginosis. Cervicitis should be treated with antibiotics for gonorrhea and chlamydia infection.

LOWER ABDOMINAL PAIN

Pelvic inflammatory disease (PID) is a common complication of untreated cervicitis, *N. gonorrhoea* and *C. trachomatis* are its main causes as was shown from different studies in Africa, whereas data from most other continents are lacking.[58,59]

The most common symptom of PID is lower abdominal pain that may or may not be accompanied by signs such as fever, cervical motion tenderness, palpable mass, and vaginal discharge.[58,60] Simple flowcharts for PID or postpartum endometritis have not been evaluated (Fig. 102-7).

Lower abdominal pain in sexually active women can also be a symptom of ectopic pregnancy or of other causes of acute abdomen. These emergencies must be excluded before treating for PID. Recommended treatment regimens and indications for hospitalization are discussed in Chapter 58.

NEONATAL CONJUNCTIVITIS

Both gonococcal and chlamydial ophthalmia neonatorum are still common in many developing countries. Although gonococcal ophthalmia tends to be more severe, more purulent, and with an earlier onset than ophthalmia caused by chlamydial infection, the

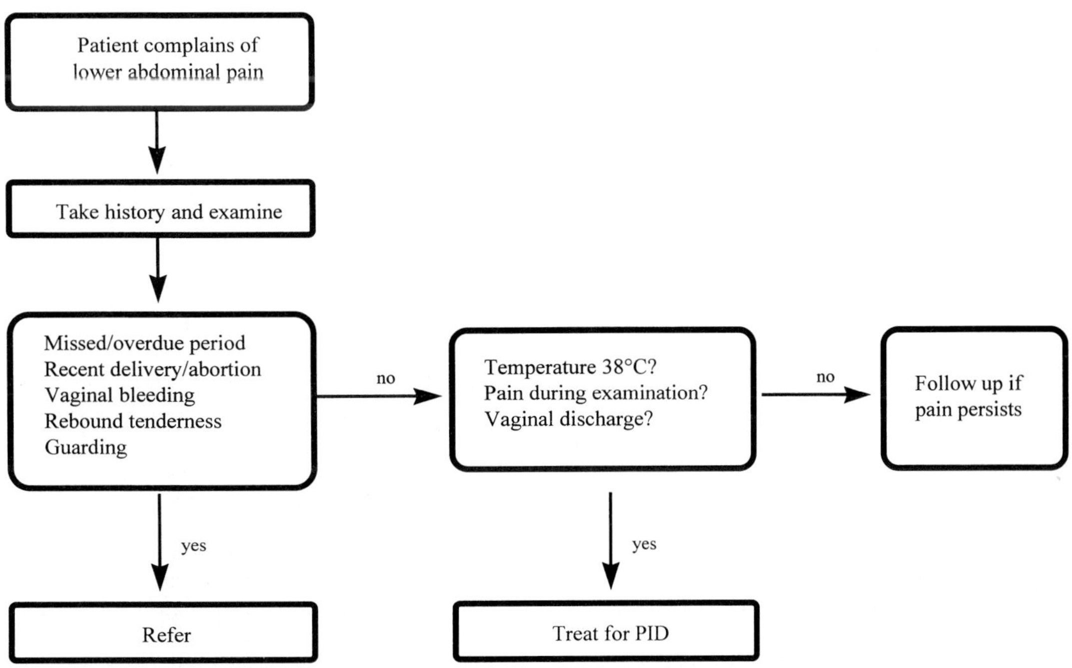

Fig. 102-7. Example of a flowchart for the management of abdominal pain.

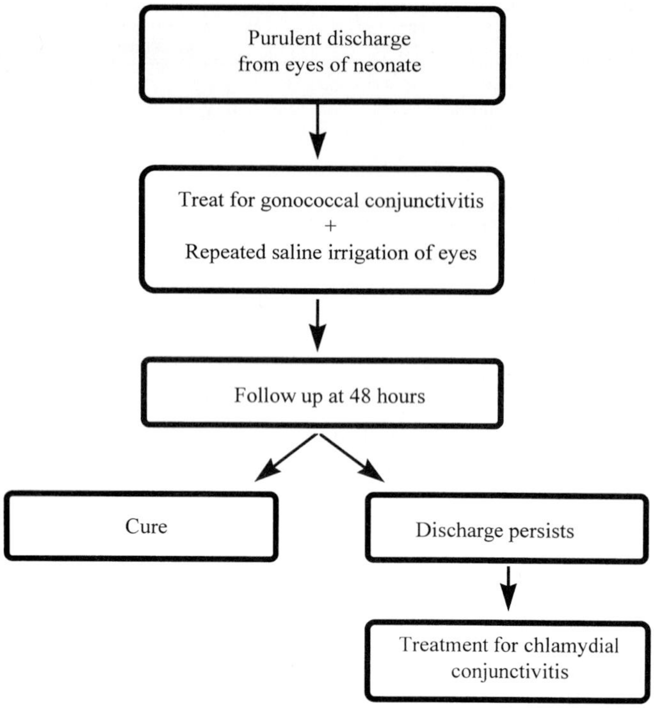

Fig. 102-8. Example of a flowchart for the management of ophthalmia neonatorum.

etiological cause (gonococcal or chlamydial) cannot be assumed on the basis of clinical signs only.

An example of a diagnostic flowchart for ophthalmia neonatorum is provided in Fig. 102-8. The rationale behind the flowchart is that every case of purulent ophthalmia neonatorum should be considered and treated as gonococcal ophthalmia, because this infection may rapidly lead to blindness. Effective treatment dramatically changes the course and outcome of the disease, usually with noticeable improvement within 24 hours. The eyes of the baby should be washed with frequent saline irrigations. Unfortunately, the availability of recommended drugs such as ceftriaxone IM or spectinomycin IM for pediatric preparations is a problem in many developing countries. Kanamycin (25 mg/kg as a single IM dose) can be given as a suboptimal alternative.

Management should also include the treatment of the mother and her partner(s).

CASE FINDING FOR STD IN DEVELOPING COUNTRIES

Because of the asymptomatic nature of many infections, particularly in women, and of the serious complications resulting from untreated infections, active case finding or screening for STD is an obvious public health strategy.

Case finding refers to the detection of infection among individuals consulting for another reason than a STD, for example, for an antenatal visit. Mother and child health clinics and family planning clinics are often women's primary and only contact with the health care system. They are, therefore, ideal places to reach a very high number of sexually active women.

The lack of a simple and valid diagnostic tool is the main technical obstacle for case finding. Furthermore, STD service delivery strategies have to be evaluated for acceptability and feasibility in various populations.

TECHNICAL ASPECTS OF STD CASE FINDING

With the exception of the RPR test (or equivalent) for syphilis screening, no simple, valid, affordable tests are available for detecting STD in asymptomatic patients.

Case finding on the basis of symptoms and clinical signs has proven difficult, because of the very low sensitivity of symptoms and signs for infection. The validity of signs and symptoms for detecting gonococcal and/or chlamydial cervicitis has been summarized in Table 102-5, for two groups of women not spontaneously complaining of STD symptoms. The prevalence of cervicitis varied from 6.5 to 16 percent in pregnant women and from 31 to 45 percent in prostitutes.[56,61]

The sensitivity of the symptoms of vaginal discharge for gonococcal or chlamydial infection is not higher than 36 and 42 percent, for pregnant women and prostitutes, respectively. Because of these low sensitivities, case finding on the basis of symptoms or clinical signs is not recommended. Moreover, the combination of low prevalence of infection and poor specificity results in a very low positive predictive value.

As was mentioned in the preceding, several studies have demonstrated that risk markers rather than symptoms and signs are predictive for gonococcal or chlamydial cervicitis. However, preliminary evaluations have shown that including risk markers in case-finding strategies do not dramatically improve the positive predictive value.[54,56]

In conclusion, an acceptable case-finding strategy, without laboratory tests and that combines a high sensitivity with a specificity, is not available. Defining a diagnostic strategy will always be a trade-off between an acceptable sensitivity and specificity, depending on the population for which the strategy is meant. In vulnerable groups with a high prevalence of STDs, such as prostitutes, the sensitivity will be more important than the specificity, in order not to miss infections. In some situations, where prevalences are extremely high, periodic mass treatment could be an

Table 102-5. Sensitivity of Selected Symptoms and Signs for Gonococcal and/or Chlamydial Infection in Pregnant Women and Prostitutes in Africa

Symptom/sign	Sensitivity in pregnant women, percent(ref.)	Sensitivity in prostitutes, percent(ref.)
Symptoms		
Vaginal discharge	29[61]	27[56]
	36[56]	42
		33†
Lower abdominal pain	39[61]	44[56]
	43[56]	39†
Dysuria	7[56]	12†
	11[61]	11[56]
Clinical signs		
Vaginal discharge	36[61]	55†
	67[56]	63[56]
Cervical mucopus	25[61]	48*
	1[56]	13[56]
Cervical friability	7[56]	7[56]
	43[61]	47*
Pain on mobilization of cervix	9[56]	10[56]
		41†

* Côte d'Ivoire (P Ghys, abstract presented at Xth International Meeting ISSTDR, August 1993, Helsinki).

† Benin (M. Alary, abstract presented at IXth International Conference on AIDS and STD, December 1994, Marrakech).

option. One example is São Paulo, Brazil, where as many as 66 percent of the prostitutes were infected with syphilis.[62] In contrast, in low prevalence groups, such as pregnant women or family planning visitors, specificity and predictive value of the decision to treat will play a major role, in order to avoid the costs of overtreatment and its complications, especially in pregnant women.

In conclusion, a syndromic approach that offers prompt and effective treatment is the preferable option for the management of symptomatic patients. Case-finding strategies for asymptomatic STDs in developing countries, however, are still hindered by the unavailability of a simple and inexpensive test for the diagnosis of gonococcal and chlamydial infection.

References

1 Crabbé F et al: Why do men with urethritis in Cameroon prefer to seek care in the informal health sector? *Genitourin Med* 72:220–222, 1996.

2 Lule G et al: STD/HIV control in Malawi and the search for affordable and effective urethritis therapy: a first field evaluation. *Genitourin Med* 70:384–388, 1994.

3 Moses S et al: Health care-seeking behavior related to the transmission of sexually transmitted diseases in Kenya. *Am J Pub Health* 84(12): 1947–1951, 1994.

4 Puentes-Markides C: Women and access to health care. *Soc Sci Med* 35(4):619–626, 1992.

5 Taylor CC: The concept of flow in Rwandan popular medicine. *Soc Sci Med* 27(12):1343–1348, 1988.

6 Bogaerts JV et al: Simple algorithms for the management of genital ulcers: evaluation in a primary health care centre in Kigali, Rwanda. *Bull WHO* 73(6):761–767, 1995.

7 Kamenga MC et al: The impact of human immunodeficiency virus infection on pelvic inflammatory disease: A case-control study in Abidjan, Ivory Coast. *Am J Obstet Gynecol* 172(3):919–925, 1995.

8 Ghys PD et al: Genital ulcers associated with human immunodeficiency virus-related immunosuppression in female sex workers in Abidjan, Ivory Coast. *J Infect Dis* 172:1371–1374, 1995.

9 Van Dyck E et al: Epidemic spread of plasmid-mediated tetracycline resistant *Neisseria gonorrhoeae* in Zaire. *Int J STD AIDS* 6:577–579, 1995.

10 Bogaerts J et al: Failure of treatment for chancroid in Rwanda is not related to human immuodeficiency virus infection: In vitro resistance of *Haemophilus ducreyi* to trimethoprim-sulfamethoxazole. *Clin Infect Dis* 20:924–930, 1995.

11 O'Farrell N et al: Genital ulcer disease: Accuracy of clinical diagnosis and strategies to improve control in Durban, South Africa. *Genitourin Med* 70:7–11, 1994.

12 Chapel TA et al: How reliable is the morphological diagnosis of penile ulcerations? *Sex Transm Dis* 4(4):150–152, 1977.

13 Homedes N et al: Patients' compliance with medical treatments in the third world: What do we know? *Hlth Pol Plan* 8(4):291–314, 1993.

14 Winfield J et al: Tracing contacts of persons with sexually transmitted diseases in a developing country. *Sex Transm Dis* 12(1):5–7, 1985.

15 Hira SK et al: Syphilis intervention in pregnancy: Zambian demonstration project. *Genitourin Med* 66:159–164, 1990.

16 Harms Get al: Pattern of sexually transmitted diseases in Malagasy population. *Sex Transm Dis* 26(6):315–320, 1994.

17 Louis JP et al: Prise en charge des maladies sexuellement transmissibles au Cameroun, en milieu urbain, en 1992. *Ann Soc Belge Méd Trop* 73:267–278, 1993.

18 Mosha F et al: A population-based study of syphilis and sexually transmitted disease syndromes in north-western Tanzania: 1. Prevalence and incidence. *Genitourin Med* 69:415–420, 1993.

19 Treurniet HF et al: Sexually transmitted diseases reported by STD services in the Netherlands, 1984–1990. *Genitourin Med* 69:434–438, 1993.

20 Meyer L et al: Surveillance of sexually transmitted diseases in France: Recent trends and incidence. *Genitourin Med* 70:15–21, 1994.

21 Mayaud P et al: The value of urine specimens in screening for male urethritis and its microbial aetiologies in Tanzania. *Genitourin Med* 68:361–365, 1992.

22 Kuvanont K et al: Etiology of urethritis in Thai men. *Sex Transm Dis* 16(3):137–140, 1989.

23 Lefèvre JC et al: Clinical and microbiologic features of urethritis in men in Toulouse, France. *Sex Transm Dis* 18(2):76–79, 1991.

24 Zelin JM et al: Chlamydial urethritis in heterosexual men attending a genitourinary medicine clinic: Prevalence, symptoms, condom usage and partner change. *Int J STD AIDS* 6:27–30, 1995.

25 World Health Organization: Management of sexually transmitted diseases. GPA/TEM/94.1.

26 Hook EW III et al: Gonococcal infections in the adult, in *Sexually Transmitted Diseases*, 2nd ed, Holmes KK et al (eds). New York, McGraw-Hill, 1990, pp. 149–165.

27 Goodhart ME et al: Factors affecting the performance of smear and culture tests for the detection of *Neisseria gonorrhoeae*. *Sex Transm Dis* 9:63–69, 1982.

28 Geyid A et al: Isolates of STD causative agents from sex workers Addis Ababa (a preliminary report). *Ethiop J Health Dev* 4(2):155–162, 1990.

29 Addy PAK: Susceptibility of *Neisseria gonorrhoeae* isolated at the Komfo, Anokye Teaching Hospital, Ghana to commonly prescribed antimicrobial agents. *East African Med J* 71(6):368–372, 1994.

30 Bogaerts J et al: Effectiveness of norfloxacin and ofloxacin for treatment of gonorrhoea and decrease of in vitro susceptibility to quinolones over time in Rwanda. *Genitourin Med* 69:196–200, 1993.

31 Van de Velden L et al: *Neisseria gonorrhoeae* à Pikine (Sénégal): Surveillance de la sensibilité aux antibiotiques. *Ann Soc Belge Méd Trop* 70:99–103, 1990.

32 Ison CA et al: The dominance of a multiresistant strain of *Neisseria gonorrhoeae* among prostitutes and STD patients in The Gambia. *Genitourin Med* 68:356–360, 1992.

33 Mason PR et al: Antimicrobial susceptibility of *Neisseria gonorrhoeae* in Harare, Zimbabwe. *Sex Transm Dis* 17(2):63–66, 1990.

34 Kam KM et al: Rapid decline in penicillinase-producing *Neisseria gonorrhoeae* in Hong Kong associated with emerging 4-fluoroquinolone resistance. *Genitourin Med* 71:141–144, 1995.

35 Berger RE: Acute epididymitis, in *Sexually Transmitted Diseases*, 2nd ed, Holmes KK et al (eds). New York, McGraw-Hill, 1990, pp. 641–651.

36 Hoosen AA et al: Microbiology of acute epididymitis in a developing community. *Genitourin Med* 69:361–363, 1993.

37 Le Bacq F et al: HIV and other sexually transmitted diseases at a rural hospital in Zimbabwe. *Genitourin Med* 69:352–356, 1993.

38 Vuylsteke B et al: High prevalence of sexually transmitted diseases in a rural area in Mozambique. *Genitourin Med* 69:427–430, 1993.

39 O'Farrell N et al: Genital ulcer disease in men in Durban, South Africa. *Genitourin Med* 67:327–330, 1991.

40 O'Farrell N et al: Genital ulcer disease in women in Durban, South Africa. *Genitourin Med* 67:322–326, 1991.

41 Mabey DCW et al: Aetiology of genital ulceration in the Gambia. *Genitourin Med* 63:312–315, 1987.

42 Zainah S et al: A microbiological study of genital ulcers in Kuala Lumpur. *Med J Malaysia* 46(3):274–282, 1991.

43 Meheus A et al: Etiology of genital ulcerations in Swaziland. *Sex Transm Dis* 10(1):33–35, 1983.

44 Fast MV et al: The clinical diagnosis of genital ulcer disease in men in the tropics. *Sex Transm Dis* 11(2):72–76, 1984.

45 Taylor DN et al: The role of *Haemophilus ducreyi* in penile ulcers in Bangkok, Thailand. *Sex Transm Dis* 11(3):148–151, 1984.

46 Bogaerts J et al: The etiology of genital ulceration in Rwanda. *Sex Transm Dis* 16(3):123–126, 1989.

47 Larsen SA et al: *Sexually Transmitted Diseases*, 2nd ed, Holmes KK et al (eds). New York, McGraw-Hill, 1990, pp. 927–934.

48 Levine WC et al: Development of sexually transmitted diseases treat-

ment guidelines: New methods, recommendations, and research priorities. *Sex Transm Dis* 21(2):S96–S101, 1994.
49 Goeman J et al: Similar serological response to conventional therapy for syphilis among HIV-positive and HIV-negative women. *Genitourin Med* 71:275–279, 1995.
50 Tyndall M et al: Ceftriaxone no longer predictably cures chancroid in Kenya. *J Infect Dis* 167:469–471, 1993.
51 Lefèvre JC et al: Lower genital tract infections in women: Comparison of clinical and epidemiologic findings with microbiology. *Sex Transm Dis* 15(2):110–113, 1988.
52 Wasserheit JN: The significance and scope of reproductive tract infections among third world women. *Int J Gynaecol Obstet* 3:145–168, 1989.
53 Behets F et al: Effective use of algorithms for management of vaginal discharge in women attending a Jamaican STD clinic: Use of diagnostic algorithms versus laboratory testing. *Clin Infect Dis* 21:1450–1455, 1995.
54 Mayaud P et al: Risk assessment and other screening options for gonorrhea and chlamydial infections in women attending rural Tanzanian antenatal clinics. *Bull WHO* 73(5):621–630, 1995.
55 Alary M et al: Signs and symptoms of prevalent and incident cases of gonorrhea and genital chlamydial infection among female prostitutes from Kinshasa, Zaire. *J Infect Dis* 22:477–484, 1996.
56 Vuylsteke B et al: Clinical algorithms for the screening of women for gonococcal and chlamydial infection: Evaluation of pregnant women and prostitutes in Zaire. *Clin Infect Dis* 17:82–88, 1993.
57 Knud-Hansen C et al: Surrogate methods to diagnose gonococcal and chlamydial cervicitis: Comparison of leukocyte esterase dipstick, endocervical Gram stain, and culture. *Sex Transm Dis* 18(4):211–216, 1991.
58 De Muylder X et al: The role of *Neisseria gonorrhoeae* and *Chlamydia trachomatis* in pelvic inflammatory disease and its sequelae in Zimbabwe. *J Infect Dis* 162:501–505, 1990.
59 Mabey DCW et al: Tubal infertility in the Gambia: Chlamydial and gonococcal serology in women with tubal occlusion compared with pregnant controls. *Bull WHO* 63(6):1107–1113, 1985.
60 Weström L et al: Acute pelvic inflammatory disease (PID), in *Sexually Transmitted Diseases*, 2nd ed, Holmes KK et al (eds). New York, McGraw-Hill, 1989, pp. 593–613.
61 Braddick MR et al: Towards developing a diagnostic algorithm for *Chlamydia trachomatis* and *Neisseria gonorrhoeae* cervicitis in pregnancy. *Genitourin Med* 66:62–65, 1990.
62 Lurie P et al: Socioeconomic status and risk of HIV-1, syphilis and hepatitis B infection among sex workers in Sao Paulo State, Brazil. *AIDS* 9(suppl 1):S31–S37, 1995.

Chapter 103

Laboratory diagnosis of sexually transmitted diseases in resource-limited settings

Milton R. Tam

The control and prevention of sexually transmitted diseases (STDs) remain a major global public health problem.[1,2] Although control of STDs has essentially been achieved in some regions, the incidence of STDs is high or still increasing in others, especially in parts of the developing world and other regions where the resources needed to provide prompt, effective STD diagnosis are limited.[3,4] The 1993 *World Development Report: Investing in Health*, published by the World Bank, recommends the immediate development and use of appropriate STD diagnostic technology to improve the efficacy of AIDS control programs.[5] Development, integration, and effective use of simple and rapid STD diagnostic tests should lead to decreased HIV/AIDS transmission, since a link between STDs and increased transmission or acquisition of HIV infection has been identified.[6,7] Where concentrated efforts to control STDs have been made, as in Rakai, Tanzania, a significant decrease in the incidence of new cases of HIV infection has resulted.[8]

In addition to HIV/AIDS control, prompt diagnosis and effective treatment of STDs is needed to reduce its overall transmission. The need for simple and rapid diagnostic tests is especially urgent for women, since the health consequences and complications of unrecognized, untreated disease may be severe and can result in pelvic inflammatory disease, infertility, complications in pregnancy, and low birth weights and congenital infections in their children.[9] Appropriate laboratory test methods for diagnosis of STDs also are needed for case-finding to identify and treat asymptomatic individuals in core groups capable of transmitting disease. STD control must continue to be a high priority for international health programs.

A clinical laboratory for diagnosis of STDs should be an integral part of STD control programs. This is not often possible, however, because many health care systems and providers lack adequate facilities, resources, personnel, and time needed to perform effective laboratory diagnosis.[9,10] In addition, since laboratory diagnosis often takes hours or even days to obtain results, many patients can not or do not return for their results, and are lost to therapy and follow-up. Therefore, providers are forced to rely on clinical symptoms, risk assessment, or syndromic algorithms for diagnosis. Unfortunately, many clinical signs and syndromic protocols, especially in women, lack sufficient accuracy to be effective, result in patient overtreatment, and do not address the greater pool of asymptomatic patients that may represent the core transmitters of disease.[11]

BASIC DIAGNOSTIC APPROACHES

Health care providers have used one or a combination of approaches for diagnosis of STDs depending on their available resources: (1) etiologic diagnosis based on laboratory testing; (2) presumptive etiologic diagnosis based on clinical findings; and (3) syndromic diagnosis.

ETIOLOGIC DIAGNOSIS BASED ON LABORATORY TESTING

Microscopy or specific laboratory diagnostic methods are used in presumptive and confirmatory testing for STD pathogens. This is the preferred and most clinically accurate method to identify specific pathogens so that the correct therapeutic regimen can be assigned to the patient. The feedback from laboratory test results also can be essential in honing and improving the diagnostic skills of clinicians. Unfortunately, in many resource-limited settings, tests have generally been unavailable; therefore, development of these essential clinical skills often may be limited.

Etiologic diagnosis relies on a well-functioning laboratory; accurate and timely return of results; systems for quality control and quality assurance; dependable supplies of test kits, reagents, and disposables; a system of patient recall for test results; and adequate to abundant technical personnel and financial resources. Some presumptive diagnostic methods are relatively simple and accurate, such as microscopy (Gram stain) on urethral exudates for detection of gonorrhea in men. Other test methods can be relatively expensive, technically complex, or time-consuming, often demanding sophisticated protocols, differential culture media, tissue culture facilities, complex confirmatory testing methods, or several days to obtain a result.

PRESUMPTIVE ETIOLOGIC DIAGNOSIS BASED ON CLINICAL FINDINGS

The accuracy of clinical etiologic diagnosis depends on the specificity and positive predictive value of syndromes and signs for particular infections (e.g., herpetic vesicles or curdlike vaginal discharge are reasonably specific for diagnosis of herpes and vulvovaginal candidiasis, respectively); on the experience and expertise of the clinical staff examining the patient; and on knowledge of the usual etiologies of clinical syndromes in the local population. When a diagnosis is made, immediate treatment can be administered to the patient. This is an advantage in many resource-limited clinics where the examination time for each patient, by necessity, is moderately to severely limited. Although this method can be rapid, inexpensive, and does not depend on laboratory diagnosis, it can be relatively inaccurate for some STDs, and often results in underdiagnosis or prescription of ineffective therapy.[11–13]

SYNDROMIC DIAGNOSIS

In general, syndromic management aims to provide treatment for the majority of curable etiologies of a particular syndrome, whereas presumptive etiologic diagnosis based on clinical findings aims to narrow the treatment to the most probable cause of the syndrome. Thus, syndromic management can lead to overtreatment, whereas presumptive etiology in diagnosis can lead to undertreatment and erroneous treatment of disease.

In order to improve STD management in settings where resources are limited, generalized flowcharts have been published by the World Health Organization and other local and regional health care providers for the major STD syndromes, such as genital ulcer disease, urethritis, cervicitis, lower abdominal or pelvic pain, and vaginal discharge (see Chap. 102).[14] When these flowcharts are followed, the accuracy of some clinical diagnoses, such as for male urethritis, can be improved, but for other common syndromes, such as vaginal discharge or lower abdominal pain, accuracy may still be relatively low and therefore still not satisfactory.

For both presumptive clinical etiologic and syndromic diagnosis, however, asymptomatic infections cannot be addressed, multiple infections can easily be overlooked, and partner notification is more problematic than when etiologic diagnoses are confirmed by laboratory testing.[15] In some cases, microscopy and simple, nonspecific tests such as the leukocyte esterase dipstick or pH indicators may be successfully integrated into presumptive clinical etiologic or syndromic protocols to enhance their accuracy.

PERIPHERAL, REGIONAL, AND CENTRAL LABORATORY SUPPORT SYSTEMS

A typical national system is a three-tier, interlocking system of laboratories starting with central laboratories, typically located in major cities or population areas, which radiate into a network of regional and peripheral laboratories.[16] For the system to perform effectively, specimens, test results, epidemiologic data, and recommendations for therapy must travel freely and quickly back and forth through this network. *Central* laboratories have the best equipped facilities. They must have access to the most sophisticated and accurate diagnostic tests available, possess culture facilities (including tissue culture), and perform antibiotic susceptibility testing. They must also communicate information, including trends in STD epidemiology and common etiologies of STD syndromes and cost-effective laboratory diagnostic protocols, to laboratories in their network. Central laboratories should also share available information with local private-sector health care providers, since in many developing countries the majority of STD patients may initially present themselves at pharmacies or private practitioners. The *intermediate*-level or regional laboratories should have many, but not all, of the capabilities of the central laboratories, including presumptive diagnostic testing and the responsibility for quality control and quality assessment for peripheral laboratories and for participating STD control programs. The intermediate laboratories need to serve as key links between the central and peripheral facilities. *Peripheral* clinics, which are often (but not always) found in rural areas, usually provide care for the majority of patients, and serve as the points of first patient contact. The laboratories attached to these clinics are most always overburdened, since they need to provide as much diagnostic information as possible, but usually have the least capabilities and resources.

The effectiveness of peripheral laboratories therefore is critical to overall STD control, and they must diagnose disease as accurately as possible. Since peripheral, or even regional, laboratories in many resource-limited areas do not perform cultures or use sophisticated or expensive diagnostic tests to improve the accuracy of presumptive clinical or syndromic diagnosis, they must rely on information and test results from reference or central laboratories to resolve diagnostic problems, reinforce clinical etiologic diagnosis, and make recommendations for the most accurate diagnosis and treatment of disease at the lowest possible cost.

DIAGNOSTIC TESTS APPROPRIATE FOR RESOURCE-LIMITED SETTINGS

Simple, rapid, and inexpensive diagnostic tests for STDs should be used in all resource-limited facilities wherever possible in order to strengthen and expand existing clinical diagnosis and improve syndromic algorithms. In order to effectively perform on-site testing and more rapidly return results to patients, a laboratory should be established within or proximal to the STD clinic. This clinical laboratory in turn needs support by regional and central reference laboratories that, although perhaps distant from the local laboratory, can evaluate specimens from patients with more accurate, technically complex, or higher-volume diagnostic methods.

The primary application of diagnostic testing in low-resource settings is for presumptive identification of STDs by testing greater numbers of samples and screening for STDs in high-risk groups at major STD clinics and testing of lower numbers of samples at peripheral health care facilities. If multiple tests can be economically performed, and the sensitivity and specificity of these tests is appropriate, the result will be less waste and more effective use of available therapeutic drugs. If results of testing can be returned within minutes, therapy can be started at once and with fewer patients lost to follow-up.

For diagnostic technologies to be appropriate and useful in resource-limited settings, they should be: (1) relatively inexpensive or cost-effective; (2) simple to use; (3) rapid, so that results can be returned to patients in the same day; (4) convenient and socioculturally acceptable for the collection of specimens; (5) stable so that they can be used in the field; and (6) reasonably accurate for their intended use. The specific characteristics of appropriate diagnostic tests needed for use in resource-limited settings are presented in Table 103-1.

The value of simple and appropriate methods such as microscopy and syphilis screening tests has been well-established. These basic diagnostic laboratory procedures are relatively inexpensive to perform and have their strengths and weaknesses, some of which are summarized in the following. There is now evidence that simple, rapid, and nonspecific methods such as the leukocyte esterase dipstick (LED) are useful. Other newer, rapid tests are available, but are still relatively expensive, which currently makes their expanded use problematic in laboratories and clinics that are resource-limited.

MICROSCOPY

Despite its initial cost (U.S.$1,000–$1,500), a good-quality binocular microscope is an essential tool for all basic STD laboratories. Supplies and reagents such as stains, glass slides, coverslips, and immersion oil for microscopic analysis are inexpensive. A trained microscopist can effectively identify a range of STD organisms and make presumptive diagnoses of infection with a binocular microscope. Microscopic analysis of wet mounts and stained patient specimens are simple and rapid, but sensitivity may be limited by the adequacy and type of specimens used. In many resource-poor settings, the cost and need for maintenance of a high-quality binocular microscope and availability of an experi-

Table 103-1. Characteristics of Appropriate Diagnostic Tests for Use in Resource-Limited Settings

Inexpensive: The assay must be affordable, with a cost to the provider of U.S.$0.10 to $1.00 per test when used in large volumes.

Simple: Minimal training necessary, and only easy-to-use equipment or no equipment needed.

Rapid: Results available before the patient leaves the clinic, and preferably in 10 to 15 minutes or less. Distances traveled, limited transportation, limited access to clinicians, and other constraints make follow-up much more problematic in resource-limited settings.

Convenient: Specimens simple to collect, socioculturally acceptable, and with minimal preparation or pretreatment.

Stable: For potential use in the field or in rural clinics, the assay reagents should have a long shelf life (1–2 years) at ambient temperature (≥30°C).

Accurate: Appropriately sensitive and specific, discriminates past from present (acute) infection.

enced microscopist for the best interpretation of slides have been significant barriers to its effective use. Several common STD pathogens can be reliably identified by their characteristic morphologies, motility, or staining properties.

GONORRHEA

Microscopic examination of gram-stained urethral exudate specimens have proven to be sensitive and specific (>90 percent), for example, for detection of *Neisseria gonorrhoeae* infection in men. Gram stain is much less sensitive (50–60 percent vs. culture) for detection of gonococcal infection in women.[17] A rapid Gram-stain procedure using small quantities of stains and decolorizing reagents can be effectively employed in which reagents are sequentially applied to and, seconds later, washed off the slide. In examination of the slide, pairs of gram-negative (saffranin red stained) kidney bean shaped diplococci found intracellular or extracellular to polymorphonuclear neutrophils are indicative of infection. Other rapid, one-step staining methods using methylene blue or saffranin are sometimes used. Their cost is even lower, and preparation of reagents is relatively simple, but one-color staining methods cannot be recommended unless the microscopist is very experienced and familiar with gonococcal morphology.

SYPHILIS

Microscopy can be used to identify *Treponema pallidum* in genital ulcer lesion scrapings. Serous exudate expressed from a cleaned, abraded lesion is preferentially used since it is often rich in organisms. Other specimens can be used such as lymph node aspirates or even cerebrospinal fluid. Silver staining has been used experimentally to identify treponemes directly from lesions, but was found to be relatively low in accuracy and could not be dependably used for the diagnosis of primary syphilis.[18] A darkfield microscope attachment to provide incident light to illuminate treponemes in specimens can be more dependable for diagnosis. However, because it must be carefully adjusted, and considerable experience is necessary to identify *T. pallidum* by its characteristic morphology and motility without confusing it with nonpathogenic treponemes, dark-field microscopy is best performed only at reference laboratories and clinics.[19]

GENITAL HERPES

Microscopy of Papanicolaou- or Giemsa-stained skin and mucosal scrapings (Tzanck preparations) is an affordable, but somewhat insensitive, method for detection of genital herpes infection, usually characterized by the presence of abnormally large, multinucleate cells with abundant cytoplasm. Individual virus particles are too small to be seen by light microscopy, but viral inclusions occasionally can be resolved in specimens that have been stained with hematoxylin and eosin.

VAGINITIS

For vaginal discharge, wet mounts or stained preparations can be effectively used for identification of trichomonads, yeasts, or clue cells associated with bacterial vaginosis (BV), but they are lower in sensitivity for diagnosis of gonorrhea and chlamydia. *Trichomonas vaginalis* infections can be reliably determined by wet mount observation of vaginal fluid and identified by their characteristic tumbling motion, polar flagellae, undulating membrane, and their size and shape. The morphological details of wet mounts can be enhanced for microscopy with the addition of very dilute buffered methylene blue solution.[20] Gram stains and acridine orange also have been effectively used for detection of trichomonads with a sensitivity equivalent to wet mounts. Trichomonads can also be detected in Giemsa- and Papanicolaou-stained specimens, but with less sensitivity and specificity compared to wet mounts. Microscopy can also be useful for detection of trichomonads in urethral exudates from men.[21]

For vaginal candidiasis, a 10% KOH (potassium hydroxide) solution can be added to a wet mount of vaginal fluid (with or without heating the slide) to dissolve clumps of epithelial cells and to more completely reveal budding fungal cells and pseudohyphae. The addition of KOH to the wet mount marginally increases sensitivity compared with a standard saline preparation.[22] For BV, wet mounts are also used to detect "clue" cells, squamous epithelial cells to which the small, coccobacillary *Gardnerella vaginalis* associated with BV are attached.

Despite its effective use in recognizing some of the organisms responsible for sexually transmitted infections, microscopy is limited in that only a presumptive diagnosis can be made. Also, some infections, including those that are deep, complicated, or in which only few organisms are typically present, are often difficult to detect by microscopy. Sensitivity for detection of STD organisms by microscopy may also be limited in inherent variations in sampling and specimen adequacy. Other STD organisms, such as those that cause chlamydia, genital herpes, and chancroid, cannot be routinely identified by simple light microscopy because the organisms are either too small to be resolved or do not possess a characteristic and therefore a definitive staining morphology.

In summary, microscopy can be effectively used in STD clinics in resource-poor settings in industrialized countries to rapidly test and prescribe therapy for some STDs based on the results. In developing countries, however, the initial cost of the microscope, its maintenance, need for quality control and quality assessment, availability of a technician, and the lack of opportunities to compare the results of microscopy versus results of other diagnostic methods are all difficulties that make even this approach all too often limited to central or intermediate referral centers and not at the primary health care level.

SIMPLE BIOCHEMICAL INDICATORS

Simple, inexpensive single-indicator tests that have high predictive values when used may improve the accuracy of clinical or syndromic diagnosis of STDs so that proper therapy can be more consistently assigned. One example is the leukocyte esterase dipstick (LED) test that was originally developed for presumptive diagnosis of urinary tract infections. The majority of investigators have found the LED test to be useful as a general indicator for urethritis (pyuria) in symptomatic and asymptomatic men and as a case-finding tool for detection of chlamydial or gonococcal infection.[23–26] The LED test was found to improve diagnostic accuracy and reduce indiscriminate use of antibiotics in symptomatic men presenting at a developing world STD clinic in Kenya.[27] Other reports, however, indicated that the sensitivity of the LED was relatively low and in need of improvement.[28,29] Use of the LED with noninvasive specimens such as urine and urine sediments has also been encouraging and should be more thoroughly investigated.[25,30] The LED therefore is of potential value for use in peripheral STD clinics in many developing world countries that cannot offer a full range of diagnostic services, and it can be a cost-effective screening tool to select patients for subsequent etiologic diagnostic testing for gonorrhea or chlamydia.[26,31,32] At the same time, however, other researchers have cautioned the use of

LED tests with cervical specimens since sensitivity or specificity was found to be less than optimal, and false-positive LED tests may occur in patients with neoplasms or patients treated with commonly used antibiotics.[33,34]

Additional simple, inexpensive, and rapid indicators like the LED test are urgently needed for use in resource-limited settings. For example, for diagnosis of BV in basic laboratories, a 10% potassium hydroxide (KOH) solution may be simple, effective, and may be an alternative to microscopy. KOH added to vaginal exudates will release amines, producing a "fishy" odor characteristic of BV. Alternatively, a simple but accurate test strip to measure pH could be used, which, if found to be greater than 4.5, is indicative of BV infection.[22] In addition a lactoferrin agglutination test indicating the presence of inflammatory cells has recently been described and may be of use in identifying inflammatory genital infections.[35]

Swab tests have been commercially marketed that claim to identify specific *biochemical* markers for rapid diagnosis of chlamydia or gonorrhea. These tests have not been shown to be reliable and acceptable for use. Were such methods ever to be proven feasible, they would be ideally suited for use in resource-poor settings.

RAPID AND SIMPLE TESTS

A few simple, culture-independent, and rapid immunological techniques are commercially available, including tests for syphilis, chlamydia, and bacterial vaginosis. However, no rapid and simple commercial tests for the etiologic diagnosis of gonorrhea, trichomoniasis, or chancroid yet exist.

SEROLOGICAL TESTS FOR SYPHILIS

The rapid plasma reagin (RPR) or the toluidine red unheated serum test (TRUST) are serological tests used to screen blood samples for syphilis. Both are stable, particle-agglutination tests using a nonspecific cardiolipin antigen to detect an acute immune response to infection. The older, lower-cost Venereal Disease Research Laboratory (VDRL) slide method is still used in some higher-volume central reference laboratories. It is a relatively economical method, but for best results, test reagents must be freshly made every day. The Pan American Health Organization views the VDRL test as an essential tool to monitor quality control in laboratories in Latin America because its effective use depends on several simple steps in preparation that laboratories should be able to consistently carry out. All screening tests for syphilis are agglutination tests, and as such, are subjectively interpreted and require an experienced reader in order to obtain the best results. Because there will be some biological false-positive results from screening tests, all positives should then be evaluated with one of several confirmatory tests using specific *T. pallidum* antigens.[19,36]

Although screening tests for syphilis are reasonably accurate, inexpensive, and simple to perform, their current test protocols for specimen preparation are not especially rapid, simple, or practical. For example, protocols often call for venipuncture using sterile needles and syringes (or vacutainer tubes) to obtain a specimen and a basic laboratory for specimen processing, including a centrifuge and a mechanized rotary platform on which to perform the assay. Since processing of samples for testing takes time and is most efficiently done in batches, test results may not be available on the same day as they are submitted, and some patients may therefore be lost to therapy and follow-up. To address this problem, plasma separator cards have been successfully used with peripheral (finger-stick) blood to prepare plasma within 15 minutes of specimen collection for use in RPR tests.[37] Other potential problems associated with syphilis testing include improper disposal of used materials and risk of disease transmission by misuse or reuse of blood-drawing equipment. "Teardrop" cards for hand-agitation of RPR tests have been evaluated; however, the general consensus is that if mechanical rotator platforms are used, they produce more consistent and accurate results.[38]

Since screening tests use cardiolipin, a nonspecific, cross-reactive antigen, all positives should be confirmed with specific tests such as the *T. pallidum* hemagglutination (TPHA) or fluorescent treponemal antibody absorption (FTA-ABS) test. Because these tests are usually performed in a reference laboratory, in most cases far from where the sample was collected, the timely return of results is seldom possible. In the developing world, confirmatory testing may take several additional days—or even weeks—for results to be returned. A simple and rapid confirmatory test (or a single test that can be used for both screening and confirmation) using a relatively noninvasive specimen such as peripheral blood or saliva and a specific *T. pallidum* antigen therefore is urgently needed for use at peripheral clinics.

RAPID TESTS FOR CHLAMYDIAL INFECTION

Commercial simple and rapid tests for chlamydia are currently formatted for developed world markets and therefore can be relatively expensive (U.S.$5.00–$8.00 or more per test) when purchased in small volumes. However, some manufacturers have established a concessionary price for their use in regional and state laboratories in the United States. Their price has decreased considerably in recent years to approximately U.S.$1.50 apiece, indicating that they may yet become more affordable for routine use in low-resource settings. These rapid tests all recognize chlamydial lipopolysaccharide antigen and employ immunochromatographic or optical refraction principles to provide a specific reaction.[39–42] The tests require specimen extraction as preparatory steps, which may require heating, and some basic technical expertise to perform. For highest accuracy, positives may need to be confirmed by another method or by specific antibody inhibition to rule out false-positives in low-prevalence areas or in non-STD clinic settings. Relative sensitivities for rapid, simple chlamydia tests have been reported as 60 to 90 percent compared with culture results, but in reality may be somewhat lower if new sensitivity standards are established using DNA amplification tests (see the following).[39–42] A parallel rapid, simple test for diagnosis of both chlamydia and gonorrhea on the same format and using a common specimen extraction method is very much needed, especially for etiologic diagnosis of cervicitis; however, currently this does not exist.

BACTERIAL VAGINOSIS

For rapid diagnosis of BV, a commercial test recently has been introduced in which the bacterial amines are specifically recognized by a biochemical reaction resulting in a colored readout. If this product proves to have adequate accuracy, and can be produced and distributed at reasonable cost, it could prove to be a practical alternative for resource-limited clinics.

REFERENCE LABORATORY–BASED TESTS

Because of their relatively high level of technical complexity; reliance on and need to maintain sophisticated equipment; need for highly trained, highly motivated technicians to perform testing; and competing priorities for use of financial and personnel resources in public health programs, many existing diagnostic tests cannot be used or sustained in intermediate and peripheral clinics in resource-limited settings. These diagnostic techniques nevertheless are important to have available and should be performed routinely in central reference laboratories to support secondary health care facilities in which resources are more limited. Key roles of the reference laboratory at the central or intermediate levels should include the provision of: (1) a referral service for diagnosis of STDs in patients with complicated disease or infections that cannot be resolved at the next lower level; (2) current information on prevalence and trends of selected STDs; (3) recommendations for antibiotic therapy based on the local or regional prevalence of resistant strains of *N. gonorrhoeae* and *H. ducreyi*; and (4) specimen panels to assess laboratory quality control and the consistency of their diagnostic protocols.

A summary of the diagnostic tests and techniques available for reference laboratories is given in the following; however, greater detail is given in Chaps. 52 and 92.

DIRECT FLUORESCENT ANTIBODY (DFA) TESTS

Diagnostic DFA test reagents for chlamydia and genital herpes have been developed that utilize specific monoclonal antibodies conjugated to fluorescein isothiocyanate. Organisms or infected cells can be detected in specimens taken directly from patients.[43,44] A characteristic staining intensity and morphology is used to identify pathogens and differentiate positive from negative specimens. The DFA test is relatively rapid (15–30 minutes), but its main drawback is a requirement for an expensive (U.S.$7,000–$10,000), high-quality, fluorescence microscope; oil-immersion lenses for best resolution of organisms; and well-trained microscopists to interpret results. It is also a relatively low-volume assay, because operator fatigue may reduce test accuracy and throughput. The DFA has been used to resolve discrepant results from other assays and as a confirmatory method to improve the accuracy of testing.[45,46] Specimen adequacy is also a concern, since, for chlamydia diagnosis, best results are obtained when columnar and transitional epithelial cells are included in the specimen.[47,48] Sensitivity and specificity of DFA tests can be good, and the cost of reagents is low to moderate. The DFA for diagnosis of genital chlamydial infections can also be used for diagnosis of conjunctival infections in children and should be effective for diagnosis of extragenital chlamydia and LGV in genital ulcer disease.[49] Although there have been research studies reported, as well as a culture confirmation test for gonorrhea developed using fluorescein-conjugated monoclonal antibodies, commercial DFA tests are not yet available for diagnosis of chancroid, gonorrhea, or syphilis directly from clinical specimens.[50–53]

ENZYME-LINKED IMMUNOSORBENT ASSAY (ELISA) METHODS

Microwell plate ELISA antigen-detection test kits for chlamydia, syphilis, and genital herpes are commercially available and may provide adequate sensitivity and specificity equal to or higher than rapid test methods.[39,45,46,54,55] ELISA test kits for gonorrhea have been available, although they are not currently.[56] Their cost is reasonable and enables central or intermediate-level laboratories to perform batched, higher-volume testing. ELISAs, especially in microtest plate formats, in general are inappropriate for rapid diagnosis. Applications for use of ELISAs are in referral laboratories performing batched testing or for surveillance and research studies. Disadvantages include the facts that ELISA kits have a limited shelf life, require refrigeration, and can be used effectively only in appropriately equipped testing sites, since ELISA methods require electricity, dedicated equipment, and trained personnel. Other disadvantages include required maintenance of equipment, and "gray zone" equivocal results may be common in some ELISA tests.

For syphilis, plate ELISAs are commercially available with cardiolipin antigen (reagin) or with specific treponemal antigens.[57–60] Such tests are best used with large numbers of specimens in the clinical laboratory or for blood bank testing when serum is used.

ELISA-based tests for the routine detection of antibodies for STDs other than syphilis have not been considered useful.[61] Serologies can be effectively applied only in regions where the prevalence of infection or reinfection is very low, and if titers can be determined to identify possible complicated or invasive infections in women.[62] Serological testing therefore is of limited value in STD endemic or epidemic areas, since past (treated) as well as current infections will test as positive. Serological tests would be much more useful for diagnosis of STDs if specific antigens were found that would only bind those antibodies produced in acute phase, but not in previously treated infections.

NUCLEIC ACID–BASED TESTS

Nucleic acid probe assays show considerable promise for use as reference laboratory–based assays. Sensitivity and specificity can be adequate with nonamplified probe methods that detect ribosomal RNA specific for chlamydia.[63] Both chlamydial and gonococcal infections can be detected with nonamplified probes using a single specimen, a clear advantage over current immunological test methods.[41,42] Amplified probe methods such as the polymerase chain reaction (PCR) test and ligase chain reaction (LCR) test are setting new standards, as they appear to be more sensitive than culture for diagnosis of chlamydial infection, have also been used for diagnosis of gonorrhea, and show promise when used with minimally invasive specimens such as vaginal fluids or first-void urines.[64–69] Some specimens possess inhibitors to amplification; therefore, despite their inherently high sensitivity, PCR or LCR methods can still produce false-negative results.[70] Other types of probes, such as the Q-beta replicase system, are currently under development.[71] ELISA-type readouts using amplified probes are becoming standard and are leading to easier processing of assays and interpretation of results. Probe methods are now commercially available, but costs are still high (U.S.$5.00–$20.00 per test), and the tests are highly equipment dependent and technically demanding to perform.

Probe tests are not currently suited for use in peripheral or intermediate laboratories in resource-poor settings, but rather, are most effective if used in sophisticated central reference laboratories. Nevertheless, some nucleic acid amplification technologies, such as Q-beta replicase, are relatively stable and can be performed under isothermal conditions independent of expensive thermocycling equipment (see Table 103-1). If technical developments and improvements continue, and if a low test cost is maintained, such tests may eventually be well-suited for use in laboratories in resource-limited settings.

CULTURE

Culture using selective media has in the past been considered the "gold standard" reference method for diagnosis of many organisms, including chlamydia and gonococci.[72] As indicated, this view may be modified by recent reports that indicate that some nucleic acid amplification tests such as PCR or LCR may be even more sensitive than culture. Culture, however, is unlikely to be phased out in the near future since it allows for isolation, subculturing, and purification of organisms for confirmatory testing, determination of qualitative or quantitative antibiotic sensitivity or resistance, and epidemiological studies such as determination of auxotrophy or typing of strains. Production of some selective media (e.g., for culture of gonococci) is relatively straightforward and possible in many better equipped facilities. Media are also widely available for purchase if financial resources are available. However, adequate facilities for preparation, supplies of media, petri dishes, and quality control for gonococcal culture plates often are unavailable or unsustainable in resource-poor settings, thus limiting their availability. Table 103-2 describes the basic resources for materials and facilities needed for culture of gonococci.

Some culturable organisms, including *C. trachomatis*, *H. ducreyi*, *T. vaginalis*, and genital herpes viruses are quite fastidious in their growth, requiring tissue culture or complex media, and incubation under CO_2; they are essentially culturable only in well-equipped central reference laboratories since facilities and media for culture are expensive. Immunofluorescent antibody tests have been developed for the culture confirmation of gonorrhea, chlamydia, and genital herpes infections.[44,50,73] *T. pallidum* is considered essentially unculturable.

METHODS TO DETERMINE ANTIBIOTIC RESISTANCE

Development of bacterial resistance has been linked to many factors, including excess prescription of, and easy access to, common antibiotics, and incomplete, often prophylactic self-treatment in high-risk groups such as commercial sex workers. In the past few years, microbial resistance to bacterial STDs, especially *N. gonorrhoeae*, has become a rapidly increasing problem that has created new challenges in the treatment of bacterial infections and has added the significant expense of more costly antibiotics.[74]

Antimicrobial resistance studies currently cannot be effectively performed outside well-equipped reference laboratories with facilities for bacterial isolation and culture. Antimicrobial resistance is usually determined on selected isolates of bacteria from patients in the community or from the region. The surveillance data from these studies must then be transmitted back to regional and provincial laboratories accompanied by guidelines and recommendations for effective antibiotic therapy.

Presumptive beta-lactamase resistance to penicillin, such as is found in penicillinase-producing *N. gonorrhoeae* (PPNG) strains, may be determined by using commercially available nitrocefin (chromatogenic cephalosporin) strips or discs. For use, the strips or discs can be placed directly on pure cultures of gonococci on agar plates, or a drop of gonococcal suspension can be placed on

Table 103-2. Requirements for Equipment and Supplies for Culture of *Neisseria gonorrhoeae**

Activity and requirements	Equipment and glassware	Reagents and expendables
Specimen collection		
Trained clinical personnel	Speculum	Swabs
Private examination area	Sterilization facilities	Gloves
Electricity	Examination table and light	
Culture media production		
Laboratory facilities	Water bath	GC base medium
Trained technicians	Various-sized beakers or flasks	Distilled, deionized water
Electricity	Heat source	VCN inhibitor (trimethoprim may be included at greater cost)
	Autoclave	XV-like supplement
	Refrigerator	Hemoglobin
		Petri dishes†
Specimen transport		
Motor vehicle or other means of rapid delivery to culture lab	CO_2-enriched atmosphere—e.g., "candle jars" (commercial glass jars are suitable)	Candles (without coloring or scent) and matches
Specimen processing and culture		
Laboratory facilities	Incubator§—able to maintain 36 (±1)°C with moist CO_2-enriched atmosphere, with thermometer	Oxidase reagent
Trained technicians		Gram stain reagents
Electricity		Glass slides
		Immersion oil
	Microscope#	
Susceptibility testing		
Laboratory facilities	CO_2 incubator or incubator with candle jars	GC base medium
Trained technicians		XV-like supplement
Electricity		Petri dishes†
		Antibiotic discs or E-test strips**

* Culture for urogenital and ocular specimens; specimens from the pharynx (and anorectum) require additional steps to confirm isolation of *N. gonorrhoeae*.

† *Petri dishes:* Glass dishes may be substituted for plastic dishes, if glassware washing structure is in place. Petri dishes of 100 mm diameter are recommended, because of their greater surface area and possible ability to ensure separation of colonies.

§ *Incubator:* If candle jars are utilized, its size must be sufficient to house jars upright; smaller incubators may be used with "zip-lock" plastic bags and CO_2-generating tablets.

Microscope: Should be binocular with illuminator.

** SOURCE: Courtesy of Dr. Wil Whittington, University of Washington, Seattle, WA.

a nitrocefin strip. Beta-lactamase is detected by observing a rapid color change from light yellow to red in the strip or disc by the enzymatic cleavage of an amide bond. Nitrocefin discs or strips cannot be recommended for use directly on clinical specimens, since pure cultures need to be used.

Semiquantitative resistance to penicillin, including non-PPNG resistance, and resistance to other antibiotics is commonly determined by disc diffusion studies on agar culture plates (Fig. 103-1). To perform this test, an agar plate is inoculated with pure bacterial culture, and filter paper discs impregnated with different antibiotics are then placed in a pattern on the plate. After an overnight incubation, the areas of bacterial growth or nongrowth by that isolate around the discs indicate relative resistance or susceptibility to the antibiotics.

Often, a minimal inhibitory concentration (MIC), a more quantitative determination, is determined to identify newly introduced strains, monitor progressive acquisition of resistance, and advise client clinics of the relative efficacy of an available antibiotic. This may be accomplished by a number of methods including dilutions of antibiotics on agar plates or commercial antibiotic gradient strips for individual antibiotic sensitivity determinations.

The agar plate dilution method incorporates progressive dilutions of antibiotics into individual plates to determine the MIC within a selected range of antibiotic concentrations. The accuracy of quantitation can be high. For the most cost-effective use, several strains of bacteria are applied to the plates in a consistent pattern, and resistance to only one antibiotic at a time can be tested using each series of plates.

Antibiotic gradient strips such as the E-test (AB Biodisc, Solna, Sweden) present an alternative to MIC testing which is suitable for use in less well-equipped laboratories. The E-test is highly quantitative and easy to perform since strips are provided with a very wide dynamic range of antibiotic concentrations. Figure 103-2 illustrates the use of the E-test to provide a highly quantitative determination of sensitivity of gonococcal strains to a given antibiotic. A wide variety of antibiotics is available. There is a relatively high cost per test, however ($2.50–$5.00 for *each* antibiotic), and availability could be low in developing countries since there is only a single global supplier. Figure 103-3 illustrates a close correlation of MIC versus E-test results for ciprofloxacin obtained from a panel of gonococcal strains isolated from the Philippines.

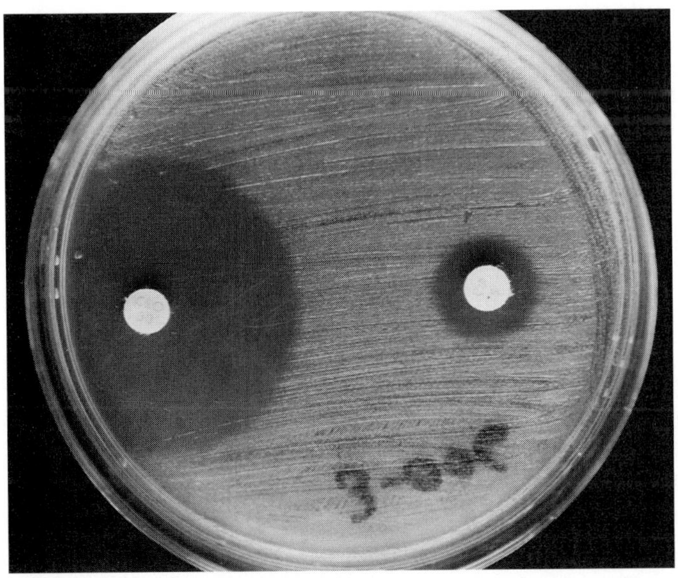

Fig. 103-1. Disc antibiotic diffusion test. Zone diameters of inhibition for ciprofloxacin is 8.0 mm (right side) and for ceftriaxone is 48.0 mm (left side) tested on *N. gonorrhoeae* strain 3-006. Illustration provided by Dr. W. Whittington, University of Washington, Seattle, WA.

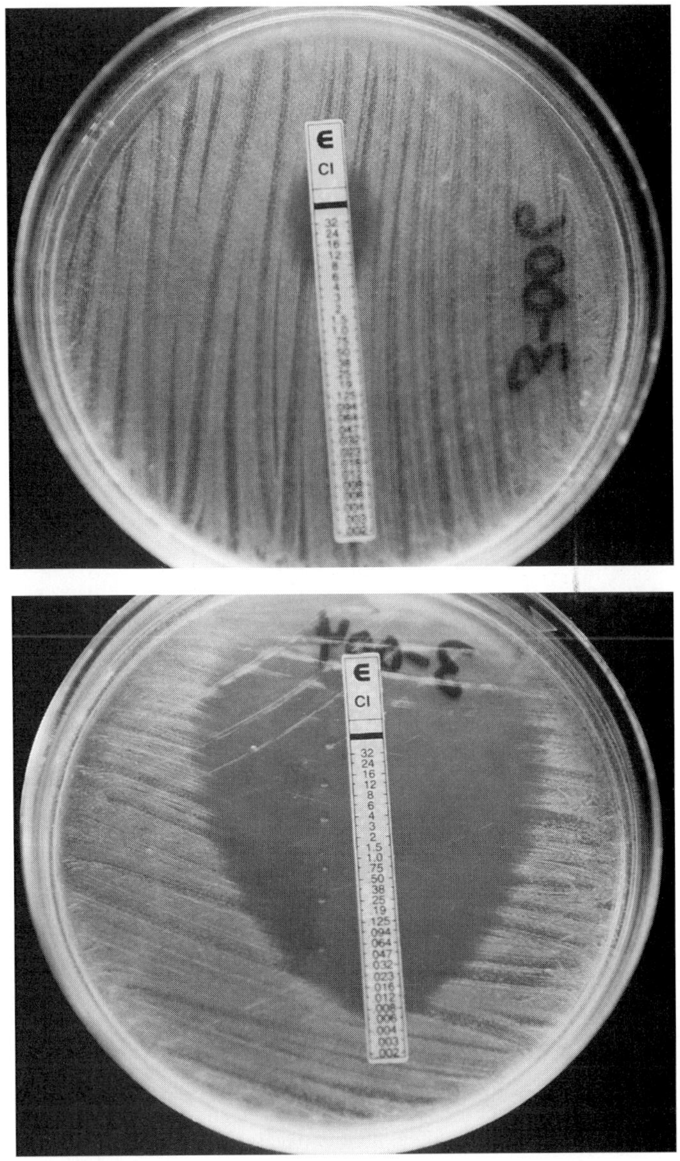

Fig. 103-2. The E-test for ciprofloxacin. *N. gonorrhoeae* strain 3-006 tested on ciprofloxacin yielding an E-test value of 8 mg/mL (upper panel) and *N. gonorrhoeae* strain 3-004 yielding an E-test value of 0.008 mg/mL (lower panel). Illustrations provided by Dr. W. Whittington, University of Washington, Seattle, WA.

THE NEED FOR NEW OR MORE EFFECTIVE DIAGNOSTIC TESTS

The control of STDs demands effective diagnostic interventions at the point of the patient's first contact with the health care system, a minimal delay between diagnosis and treatment, and identification and treatment of all contacts. Treatment of partners is guided by specific laboratory diagnosis, and positive laboratory tests may help to motivate partner referral. As indicated in the preceding, the use of syndromic management protocols can im-

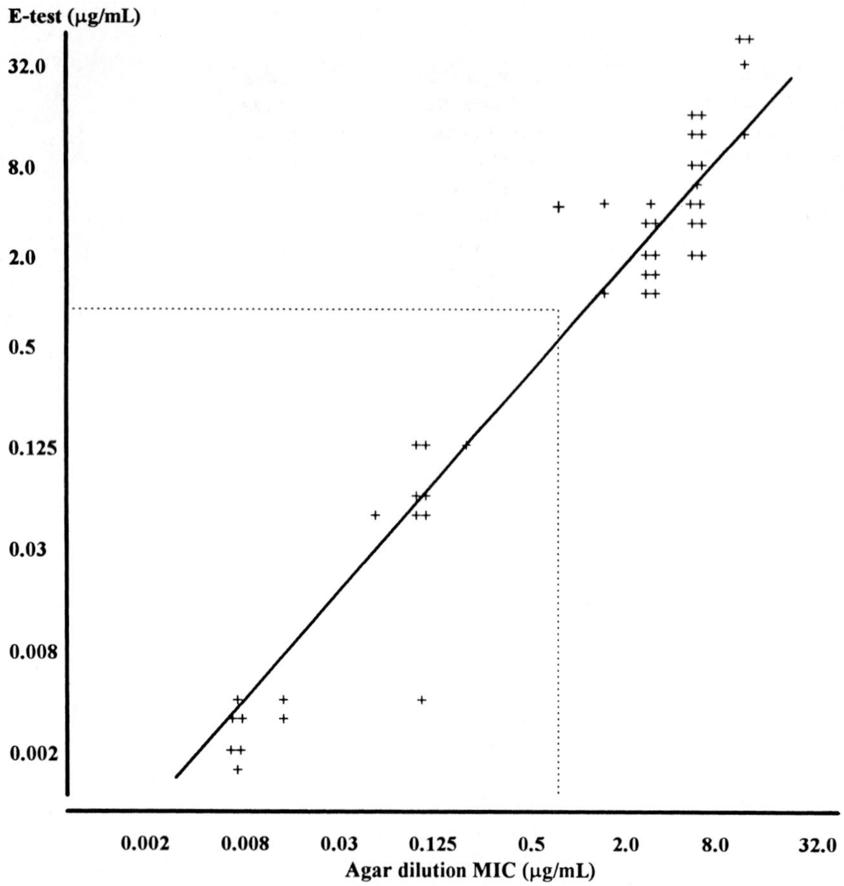

Fig. 103-3. Correlation of the MIC test (x-axis) versus the E-test (y-axis). This scattergram includes 55 clinical isolates and three reference strains of *N. gonorrhoeae*. The dotted vertical and horizontal lines indicate proposed criteria for interpretation of resistance to ciprofloxacin. Graph provided by Dr. W. Whittington, University of Washington, Seattle, WA.

prove clinical diagnosis, but still results in overtreatment with drugs and does not address the population with asymptomatic disease.

Existing laboratory tests for the major, curable STDs can be highly sensitive and specific, but because of required equipment and/or relatively high cost, they cannot effectively be used at intermediate or peripheral clinics in developing countries and in other resource-limited settings. Additional simple and rapid tests, for example, for diagnosis of syphilis, gonorrhea, and chancroid, therefore are still urgently needed. These needs are summarized in Table 103-3. New tests could utilize newly developed technologies, or alternatively, they can be built on existing diagnostic platforms. For example, rapid and simple chlamydia tests using the immunochromatographic strip (ICS) format have been commercially available for some time, but still require further simplification and reformatting to reduce production costs. Their current levels of sensitivity also need to be improved. The ICS is a potentially valuable, one-step, "walk-away" test after the specimen is applied to the strip. Most ICS tests contain a procedural control, and results can be read directly from the strip a few minutes later.

Table 103-3. Priorities for STD Diagnostic Development

Priorities	Available tests	Tests needed
Screening, identification of male urethritis	Microscopy, leukocyte esterase dipstick (LED) on first-void urines	Better and wider training of microscopists; LED and/or other simple tests with higher specificity
Differential diagnosis of gonococcal versus nongonococcal urethritis	Microscopy, LED, oxidase indicators on urethral discharge specimens	Rapid, simple test for etiologic diagnosis of chlamydia and gonorrhea
Screening/identification of cervicitis	None	Test for leukocytes with better specificity than LED that identifies both chlamydia and gonococci
Differential diagnosis of gonorrhea and chlamydia in women	ELISA, some rapid chromatographic strip tests for chlamydia; none for gonorrhea	Rapid, simple test for etiologic diagnosis of gonorrhea and chlamydia
Differential diagnosis of genital ulcer disease	None	Serological or antigen detection test for *H. ducreyi;* differential rapid test for *T. pallidum* versus *H. ducreyi*
Screening, identification of syphilis	RPR, TRUST, TPHA, FTA-ABS, others	Improve existing tests; simplify blood collection methods; develop rapid and inexpensive strip test using specific *T. pallidum* antigen as screening and confirmatory test
Diagnosis of congenital syphilis	None	Rapid IgM/IgA method; simple strip or Western blot test

Packaged and sealed with desiccant, the ICS test can be stable for months at ambient temperatures, is simple to interpret, and manufacturing costs are low when produced in volume, making it a potentially ideal format. ICS tests have already been developed for detection of hepatitis B surface antigen (HBsAg). With a claimed detection level of 1 to 2 ng HBsAg/mL, sensitivity of this ICS test approaches that of standard ELISA test kits. A diagram of the ICS test format is presented as Fig. 103-4.

In addition, a reliable source of high-quality, durable binocular microscopes should be identified and made available for resource-limited laboratories at or near their manufacuturing cost. Microscopes could be made available to resource-limited STD control programs through special arrangements or through international agencies willing to purchase them in bulk. Training programs in microscopy should be developed or expanded. Effective quality control and quality assessement programs also need to be developed to evaluate existing laboratories that routinely use microscopy for STD diagnosis.

DESIGNING A "CLIENT-CENTERED" APPROACH

Too often, because resources may be moderately to severely limited, clinical and diagnostic laboratory services may be created in a haphazard manner, and often with minimal concern or thought for the patients seeking medical examination and treatment. In addition, the overall management of these services may not be as effective or efficient as necessary. As a result, patients may experience unnecessary delays in seeking or receiving treatment and in obtaining results of laboratory testing. There can be significant hardship for the patient in terms of lost income or time away from home during the period in which care is being sought. Shortcomings to the current clinical and laboratory "systems" which have been observed and which need to be corrected have been described in Chap. 88 as: (1) "the pinball effect;" (2) the "supposed-to" syndrome; and (3) the "don't-fire-until-you-see-the-whites-of-their-eyes" strategy.

The "pinball effect" describes situations commonly found in poorly *integrated* laboratories and clinical systems that put unreasonable demands on the patient, who may be bounced around town like the ball in a pinball game, from a clinician for examination, to a laboratory for tests, back to a clinician for results of tests and a prescription, and finally to a pharmacy for medication. This can be controlled by offering a "one-stop shopping" approach, where examination, tests, and dispensing of directly observed treatment are provided at the same place and time.

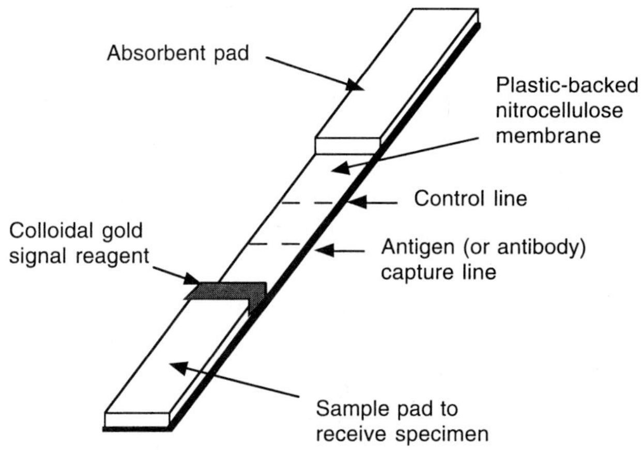

Fig. 103-4. Diagram of the immunochromatographic strip (ICS) test. Existing ICS tests are rapid and simple, and the technology has considerable promise for the further development of diagnostic tests for STDs.

The "supposed-to" syndrome is the name given to a poorly *managed* clinical and diagnostic system that is "supposed-to" hand off responsibilities for diagnostic testing and patient management from clinic to laboratory and back, but may not perform its duties in an effective, coordinated, or timely manner. This operational malaise may develop through a gradual erosion in resources and services, rather than as a result of any established policies. Because the operational systems may be too complex, they present ample opportunities for disconnects and misunderstandings among the people who work within the system. This system is a chain that is only as strong as its weakest link; any breakdown in specimen handling, testing, flow of information, or patient compliance interferes with treatment. The "supposed-to" syndrome can be corrected by implementing a "top-down" system of clinical and laboratory management, with supervisors establishing individual responsibility and accountability, and a "client-centered" training program for clinic and laboratory personnel.

The "don't-fire-until-you-see-the-whites-of-their-eyes" strategy, made famous by a United States Civil War general, takes its name from the conservative strategy of withholding therapy until a diagnosis is confirmed. For example, in some resource-poor clinics, treatment of genital ulcer disease is withheld until primary syphilis is excluded with certainty. In a patient presenting with genital ulcer disease, the patient may be required to have three consecutive negative darkfield examinations and serological screening tests that are negative in 1 or 2 weeks before treatment can be initiated. This involves multiple visits to the clinic. Meanwhile, if significant time has passed between the patient's first visit and receipt of therapy, the patient may have infected additional partners, or worse yet, may not return to the clinic and therefore may be lost to follow-up. Also, if the inherent sensitivity of a diagnostic test is low (e.g., Gram stains and microscopy for diagnosis of gonorrhea in women), or if quality control is poor, the reliance on inaccurate laboratory results is often worse than having no laboratory at all and may impair rather than assist in the effective control of disease. To be most effective, a STD service should establish a relatively low diagnostic threshold for syphilis as well as "reasonable" diagnostic thresholds for other STDs that neither overprescribe drugs nor unnecessarily withhold treatment, especially if supplementary syndromic diagnostic protocols indicate that infection is likely.

In summary, to improve control of STDs, laboratory testing should be client-centered. Ideally, laboratories capable of performing basic diagnostic procedures must be physically integrated within or proximal to each clinic, even at peripheral levels, and a pharmacy must be identified or established within easy reach of the clinic and laboratory in order to create a "one-stop shopping" approach. Basic diagnostic laboratories should also be considered in clinical facilities such as antenatal or family planning clinics that do not usually offer these services. Creation of integrated service systems in clinics that may not presently offer on-site diagnosis and treatment of STDs will very likely result in improved, expanded patient care, with fewer patients lost to follow-up.[75] Management of STD clinics may need strengthening, improvement, and operational protocols established to prevent or discourage the "supposed-to" syndrome. Clear responsibilities must be established to maintain rapid and reliable processing and testing of specimens and the return of those results to the patient. Finally, for laboratories to be an effective part of an STD control program, they must provide consistently accurate results. Laboratories need to be periodically and continuously evaluated through quality control and quality assessment programs administered through the central or intermediate levels of the laboratory service. As a last resort, national STD control authorities should be prepared to shut down laboratories that are found to perform poorly until those laboratory personnel undergo a program of retraining or requalification.

THE ROCKEFELLER FOUNDATION SCIENCE FOR DEVELOPMENT PRIZE (THE STD DIAGNOSTICS CHALLENGE)

The specific and immediate needs identified by international agencies for appropriate tests for gonococcal and chlamydial diagnosis were highlighted in the 1994 announcement by The Rockefeller Foundation of a one-million-dollar prize to be awarded to developers of a novel, low-cost, rapid diagnostic test (or tests) for detection and diagnosis of gonorrhea and chlamydia in resource-limited settings. The winning entry must be capable of reliably detecting chlamydial and gonococcal infection, even in asymptomatic individuals, and must meet a set of predetermined technical criteria addressing test sensitivity and specificity, suitability for use in developing countries, and a low projected cost. Adequate assurances must also be given to ensure that the diagnostic device(s) will be available for use in developing countries under appropriate licensing and distribution agreements. For further information about and the rules governing the STD Diagnostics Challenge contact The Rockefeller Foundation, 420 Fifth Avenue, New York, NY 10018 (phone) 212-869-8500 (fax) 212-764-3468.

THE STD DIAGNOSTICS INITIATIVE (SDI)

The SDI was established in 1990 by a voluntary group of agencies, clinical specialists, and public health experts who were concerned about the apparent lack of appropriate STD laboratory diagnostic tests available for use at primary health care facilities in the developing world and in other resource-limited settings.[5,10] The goal of the SDI is to identify appropriate and affordable diagnostic tools, to ensure they are developed, and to introduce those tools into laboratories in STD prevention and control programs. Where appropriate commercial products exist but are not accessible or affordable because of a lack of market information or to a high pricing structure, the SDI's role is to provide information and identify expanded commercial opportunities. Where no appropriate products currently exist, the SDI's role is to foster product adaptation, evaluation, and new developments. The SDI is currently headquartered at UNAIDS in Switzerland. For more information contact the Executive Director, STD Diagnostics Initiative, UNAIDS, World Health Organization, 20 Via Appia, 1211 Geneva 27, Switzerland.

CONCLUSIONS

Microscopy and some rapid, simple, and specific diagnostic tests are currently available for use in basic STD laboratories at the periphery of the health care system. The variety of tests is not large, but those that are available can be reasonably accurate and useful for presumptive diagnosis of some STDs in resource-poor settings. Other nonspecific indicators, such as the LED test, can be used to supplement syndromic diagnosis, assist in case-finding in asymptomatic individuals, and function as a cost-effective tool for prescreening specimens for further etiologic diagnostic testing. Many more accurate, simple, rapid, and inexpensive tests are still needed, however, to fill the considerable gaps in the diagnostic capabilities of resource-limited laboratories to improve the quality of their service.

The types of tests most urgently required for resource-limited laboratories include the following: (1) etiologic diagnosis of gonorrhea versus chlamydia, especially for use with cervicitis and vaginal discharge in women; (2) etiologic diagnosis of chancroid versus syphilis in genital ulcer diseases; (3) combined screening and confirmatory syphilis testing; and (4) congenital syphilis. In addition, specimen collection procedures require simplification and to be as noninvasive as possible compared with current methodology, for example, collection of urine rather than cervical specimens in women, or finger-sticks rather than venipuncture for sampling blood. Existing diagnostic platforms such as the ICS technology may be used to develop some needed tests; however, the longer-term, significant investments in academic research and commercial product development need to be sustained in order to produce true "breakthough" technologies that will fulfill the criteria for appropriate diagnostic tests outlined in Table 103-1. National governments and the international donor community must also consider providing incentives to industry, including guaranteed markets for useful and appropriate diagnostic tests.

References

1 *World Health Organization*: An overview of selected curable sexually transmitted diseases. WHO website: ⟨http://www.who.ch/stds/akagmer.htm⟩, 1997.

2 Over M et al: Infection and STD: Disease control priorities. Washington, DC, World Bank Publication, 1991.

3 Aral SO et al: Sexually transmitted diseases in the AIDS era. *Sci Amer* 262:62–69, 1991.

4 Cates W et al: Sexually transmitted diseases in the 1990's. *N Engl J Med* 325:1368–1379, 1991.

5 *World Development Report 1993: Investing in Health*. Published for the World Bank. New York, Oxford University Press, 1993, p. 154.

6 Laga M et al: The interrelationship of sexually transmitted diseases and HIV infection: Implications for the control of both epidemics in Africa. *AIDS* 5:55–63, 1991.

7 Wasserheit J: Epidemiological synergy: Interrelationships between HIV infection and other STDs. *Sex Trans Dis* 19:61–77, 1992.

8 Grosskurth H et al: A community trial of improved treatment of sexually transmitted diseases in rural Tanzania: Randomized controlled trial. *Lancet* 346:530–536, 1995.

9 Wasserheit JN: The significance and scope of reproductive tract infections among Third World women. *Int J Gyn Obst* (suppl 3):145–168, 1989.

10 Hitchcock P et al: Sexually transmitted diseases in the AIDS era: Development of STD diagnostics for resource-limited settings is a global priority. *Sex Trans Dis* 18:133–135, 1991.

11 Dangor Y et al: Accuracy of clinical diagnosis of genital ulcer disease. *Sex Trans Dis* 17:184–189, 1990.

12 Ndinya-Achola J et al: Presumptive specific diagnosis of genital ulcer disease (GUD) in a primary health care setting in Nairobi. *Int J STD AIDS* 7:201–205, 1996.

13 Rothenberg R et al: The clinical diagnosis of urethral discharge. *Sex Trans Dis* 10:24–28, 1983.

14 Liskin L: Sexually transmitted diseases, syndromic and laboratory diagnosis, treatment, and follow-up. Supplement to: Population Reports, *Controlling Sexually Transmitted Diseases*, series L, Volume XXI, No. 1.

15 *World Health Organization:* Management of patients with sexually transmitted diseases. WHO Technical Report no. 810. WHO, Geneva, 1991.

16 Sng EH. Necessary laboratory support for the peripheral, regional, and national level, in *Sexually Transmitted Diseases,* 1st ed. Holmes KK et al. (eds). New York, McGraw-Hill, 1984, pp. 992–997.

17 Judson FN: A clinic-based system for monitoring the quality of techniques for the diagnosis of gonorrhea. *Sex Trans Dis* 5:141–145, 1978.

18 Bogaerts J et al: The etiology of genital ulceration in Rwanda. *Sex Trans Dis* 16:123–126, 1989.

19 Larsen SA et al: Laboratory diagnosis and interpretation of tests for syphilis. *Clin Microbiol Rev* 8:1–21, 1995.

20 Van Dyck E et al: Bench-level laboratory manual for sexually transmitted diseases. *World Health Organization.* WHO/VDT/89.443, 1989.

21 Kreiger JN et al: Diagnosis of trichomoniasis: Comparison of conventional wet mount examination with cytologic studies, cultures, and monoclonal antibody staining of direct specimens. *JAMA* 259:1223–1227, 1988.

22 Spiegel C: Vaginitis, in *Laboratory Methods for the Diagnosis of Sexually Transmitted Diseases,* Wentworth BB et al (eds). Washington, DC, American Public Health Association, 1994, pp. 151–168.

23 Kusumi RK et al: Rapid detection of pyuria by leukocyte esterase activity. *JAMA* 245:1653–1655, 1981.

24 Sheer WD: The detection of leukocyte esterase activity in urine with a new reagent strip. *Am J Clin Pathol* 87:86–93, 1987.

25 Domeika MA et al: Non-invasive sampling for detection of genital infection with *Chlamydia trachomatis* in males utilizing urinary leukocyte esterase tests and immunoassays. *Infect Immunol* 22:65–68, 1994.

26 Shafer MA et al: Urinary leukocyte esterase screening test for asymptomatic chlamydial and gonococcal infections in males. *JAMA* 262: 2562–2566, 1989.

27 Tyndall MW et al: Leukocyte esterase strips for the screening of men with urethritis: Use in developing countries. *Genitourin Med* 70:3–6, 1994.

28 McNagny SE et al: Urinary leukocyte esterase test: A screening method for the detection of asymptomatic chlamydial and gonococcal infections in men. *J Infect Dis* 165:573–576, 1992.

29 Patrick DM et al: Evaluation of leukocyte esterase test of first void urine in male STD clinics and street-involved clients. *Sex Transm Dis* 21:s154, 1994.

30 Sellors JW et al: Screening urine with a leukocyte esterase strip and subsequent chlamydial testing of asymptomatic chlamydial and gonococcal infections in males. *Sex Trans Dis* 20:152–157, 1993.

31 Genc M et al: An economic evaluation of screening for *Chlamydia trachomatis* in adolescent males. *JAMA* 270:2057–2064, 1993.

32 Grosskurth H et al: The use of urine leukocyte esterase dipstick test as a screening tool for the detection of gonorrhea in asymptomatic male patients in a rural population in Mwanza region, Tanzania. *Sex Trans Dis* 20:s161, 1994.

33 Knud-Hansen CR et al: Surrogate methods to diagnose gonococcal and chlamydial cervicitis: Comparison of leukocyte esterase dipstick, endocervical Gram stain, and culture. *Sex Trans Dis* 17:211–216, 1991.

34 Beer JH et al: False positive results for leukocytes in urine dipstick test with common antibiotics. *Br Med J* 313:25, 1996.

35 Rein MF et al: Use of a lactoferrin assay in the differential diagnosis of female genital tract infections and implications for the pathophysiology of bacterial vaginosis. *Sex Trans Dis* 23:517–521, 1996.

36 Nandwani R et al: Are you sure it's syphilis? A review of false positive serology. *Int J STD AIDS* 6:241–248, 1995.

37 Ndinya-Achola J et al: Evaluation of a plasma separator card used with the rapid plasma reagin (RPR) test in the diagnosis of syphilis. *Abstracts of the XI International Conference on AIDS*, Vancouver, BC, Canada (abstr) B.1049.

38 Van der Sluis JJ: Laboratory techniques in the diagnosis of syphilis: A review. *Genitourin Med* 68:413–419, 1993.

39 Stratton NJ et al: Evaluation of the rapid Clearview chlamydia test for direct detection of chlamydiae from cervical specimens. *J Clin Microbiol* 29:1551–1553, 1991.

40 Young H et al: Preliminary evaluation of "Clearview Chlamydia" for the rapid detection of chlamydial antigen in cervical secretions. *Genitourin Med* 67:120–123, 1991.

41 Kluytmans JAJW et al: Performance of nonisotopic DNA probe for detection of *Chlamydia trachomatis* in urogenital infections. *J Clin Microbiol* 29:2685–2689, 1991.

42 Wells A: Evaluation of the BioStar chlamydia OIA assay for *Chlamydia trachomatis* in an outpatient setting, in Abstr 35th ICAAC, American Society for Microbiology, Washington, DC, p. 305, abstr. K84.

43 Tam MR et al: Culture-independent diagnosis of *Chlamydia trachomatis* using monoclonal antibodies. *N Engl J Med* 310:1146–1150, 1984.

44 Nowinski RC et al: Monoclonal antibodies for diagnosis of infectious diseases in humans. *Science* 219:637–644, 1983.

45 Fonseca K et al: Detection of *Chlamydia trachomatis* antigen by enzyme immunoassay: Importance of confirmatory testing. *J Clin Pathol* 48:214–217, 1995.

46 Gaydos CA et al: Evaluation of Syva enzyme immunoassay for detection of *Chlamydia trachomatis* in genital specimens. *J Clin Microbiol* 28:1541–1544, 1990.

47 Howard C et al: Correlation of the percent of positive *Chlamydia trachomatis* direct fluorescent antibody detection tests with the adequacy of specimen collection. *Diag Microbiol Inf Dis* 14:233–237, 1991.

48 Moncada J et al: Cytobrush in collection of cervical samples for detection of *Chlamydia trachomatis. J Clin Microbiol* 27:1863–1866, 1989.

49 Bell TA et al: Direct fluorescent monoclonal antibody stain for rapid detection of infant *Chlamydia trachomatis* infections. *Pediatrics* 74: 224–228 1984.

50 Cavicchini S et al: Monoclonal antibody direct immunofluorescence for the identification of *Neisseria gonorrhoeae* strains grown on selective culture media. *Sex Trans Dis* 4:195–197, 1989.

51 Schalla WD et al: Use of dot-immunobinding and immunofluorescence assays to investigate clinically suspected cases of chancroid. *J Infect Dis* 153:879–887, 1986.

52 Hook III EW et al: Detection of *Treponema pallidum* in lesion exudate with a pathogen-specific monoclonal antibody. *J Clin Microbiol* 22: 241–244, 1985.

53 Ito F et al: Specific immunofluorescent staining of pathogenic treponemes with monoclonal antibody. *J Clin Microbiol* 30:831–838, 1992.

54 Wu TC et al: Evaluation of the DuPont HERPCHEK herpes simplex virus antigen test with clinical specimens. *J Clin Microbiol* 27:1903–1905, 1989.

55 Thomas BJ et al: Limited value of two widely used enzyme immunoassays for detection of *Chlamydia trachomatis* in women. *Eur J Clin Microbiol Inf Dis* 13:651–655, 1994.

56 Martens MG et al: Rapid gonococcal detection in low-risk pregnant women using the solid-phase enzyme immunoassay, Gonozyme. *Am J Gyn Health* 6:27–31, 1992.

57 Pedersen NS et al: Enzyme-linked immunosorbent assay for detection of antibodies against venereal disease research laboratory (VDRL) antigen in syphilis. *J Clin Microbiol* 25:1711–1716, 1987

58 Moyer NP et al: Evaluation of the Bio-EnzaBead test for syphilis. *J Clin Micro* 25:619–623, 1987.

59 Lefevre JC et al: Evaluation of the Captia enzyme immunoassays for detection of immunoglobulins G and M to *Treponema pallidum* in syphilis. *J Clin Microbiol* 28:1704–1707, 1990.

60 Nayar R et al: Evaluation of the DCL syphilis-G enzyme immunoassay test kit for the serologic diagnosis of syphilis. *Am J Clin Pathol* 99: 282–285, 1993.

61 Schachter J et al: Failure of serology in diagnosing chlamydial infections in the genital tract. *J Clin Microbiol* 10:647–649, 1979.

62 Thejls H et al: Diagnosis and prevalence of persistent chlamydia infection in infertile women: Tissue culture, direct antigen detection, and serology. *Fertil Steril* 55:304–310, 1991.

63 Clarke LM: Comparison of Syva MicroTrak enzyme assay and Gen-Probe PACE-2 with cell culture for diagnosis of cervical *Chlamydia trachomatis* infection in genital specimens. *J Clin Microbiol* 32:568–570, 1994.

64 Birkenmeyer L et al: Preliminary evaluation of the ligase chain reaction for specific detection of *Neisseria gonorrhoeae. J Clin Microbiol* 30: 3089–3094, 1992.

65 Lee HH et al: Diagnosis of *Chlamydia trachomatis* genitourinary infections in women by ligase chain reaction assay of urine. *Lancet* i: 213–216, 1995.
66 Quinn TC: Recent advances in diagnosis of sexually transmitted diseases. *Sex Trans Dis* (suppl 2) 21:19–27, 1994.
67 Haase AM et al: Improved detection of *Chlamydia trachomatis* in cervical specimens by using a new polymerase chain reaction assay. *NZ Med J* 106:292–294, 1995.
68 Ho BSW et al: Polymerase chain reaction for the detection of *Neisseria gonorrhoeae* in clinical samples. *J Clin Pathol* 45:439, 1992.
69 Stary A et al: Comparison of ligase chain reaction and culture for detection of *Neisseria gonorrhoeae* in genital and extragenital specimens. *J Clin Microbiol* 35:239–242, 1997.
70 Mahony JB et al: Role of confirmatory PCRs in determining performance of Amplicor PCR with endocervical specimens from women with a low prevalence of infection. *J Clin Microbiol* 32:2490–2493, 1994.
71 Shah JS: Novel, ultrasensitive Q-beta replicase-amplified hybridization assay for detection of *Chlamydia trachomatis. J Clin Microbiol* 32: 2718–2724, 1994.
72 Ison CA: Methods for diagnosing gonorrhea. *Genitourin Med* 66:453–469, 1990.
73 Stephens RS et al: Sensitivity of immunofluorescence for detection of *Chlamydia trachomatis* inclusions in cell culture utilizing monoclonal antibodies. *J Clin Microbiol* 16:4–7, 1982.
74 Handsfield HH: Old enemies: Combating syphilis and gonorrhea in the 1990s. *JAMA* 264:1451–1452, 1990.
75 Kitabu MZ et al: Quality control assessment in an ongoing syphilis screening programme in 8 Nairobi clinics from June to Dec 1992. *IX International Conference on AIDS*, Berlin, Germany. Abstr. B44–2551, p. 560.

Chapter 104

Sexual behavior and behavioral interventions in the developing world

Kevin R. O'Reilly
Monir Islam
Werasit Sittitrai

Although it has long been seen as the key exposure in sexually transmitted diseases, sexual behavior, the most intimate of human interactions, was little studied and even less understood worldwide until recently. The relative ease of treatment of the bacterial STDs diverted attention from prevention through sexual behavior change to prevention through timely treatment of infected individuals to stop continued spread. The increase in the chronic, incurable viral STDs in the late 1970s began to change the focus somewhat, but it wasn't until the advent of HIV/AIDS with its high case fatality ratio that the study of sexual behavior received serious attention. Now our understanding of sexual behavior throughout the world has grown significantly thanks to the many studies that have been conducted in the last decade. More important, perhaps, has been the increase in our understanding of how to change sexual behavior or establish safe sexual behavior patterns, a field about which virtually nothing was known a decade ago. Although far from perfect, our knowledge of these two areas has advanced enormously as the scientific community has addressed the inadequacies of the past.

In this chapter, we focus our attention on the developing world, where the problem of STDs and their control is that much more complex. We first review what is now known about sexual behavior around the world, and then what is known about other important behaviors relevant to the transmission of STD. We then review what has been done to change these behaviors, on both a small and a large scale.

ISSUES IN PREVENTION AND CONTROL OF STD/HIV

The basic reproductive rate of STD has been modeled as a function of the efficiency of transmission, the rate of new partner acquisition, and the duration of infectiousness.[1] Each of these components can be addressed by interventions. In the first case, condom use or sexual practices that do not include penetration can decrease the transmissibility of STD. In the second case, reducing the number of sex partners through the promotion of monogamy can also affect the basic reproductive rate of STD. Finally, early treatment of STD can affect the duration of infectiousness in the case of the bacterial STDs.

Additional actions can also help. Partner notification can affect the duration of the symptoms and infectiousness for those sex partners of individuals who seek treatment and are infected with bacterial STDs. In the clinical setting, counseling for condom use, partner referral, partner reductions, and timely treatment seeking that includes compliance with treatment recommendations and abstinence until cured can all affect STD spread by decreasing the duration of symptoms in the infected and the efficiency of transmission to the uninfected. These activities can also take place in the community, where interventions to decrease the transmissibility of STD/HIV through condom promotion, the rate of new partner acquisition, and the duration of infectiousness can all be addressed.

Risk of STD is considered to be largely but not exclusively determined by individual behavior.[2] Other factors outside the control of the individual (the populational determinants) are also important, but these factors, such as sociogeographic factors that include economic and other social characteristics, for example, poverty and role and status of women, are seen as immune to intervention. If we restrict our thinking about intervention to the traditional clinically based approaches, this implication is accurate. The traditional STD intervention approach, focused on clinic-based activities and treatment, has been unable to address the populational determinants of STD. Since the advent of the AIDS epidemic, however, the prevalence of condom use in the general and the at-risk population and the economic empowerment of women are now being explored as potential ways to decrease STD/HIV transmission. Interventions now exist to address these more distal determinants of STD prevalence as well. In our review of interventions, we will consider these approaches as well.

SEXUAL BEHAVIOR IN THE DEVELOPING WORLD

A decade of study, driven by the needs to address the AIDS epidemic, has helped erase the ignorance about sexual behaviors that decades or more of inattention had caused. These studies have ranged from international multisite comparisons to operational studies conducted by national AIDS programs. Starting in the middle of the 1980s, a series of studies of sexual behavior was planned and undertaken in many developing countries. These studies, some of which have been summarized in a recent book, have clearly shown that sexual behavior indeed varies in degree around the world.[3] It is not a matter of whether a certain behavior takes place at all in a certain country or region of the world, as all sexual behaviors appear to take place virtually everywhere. Some cultures hold strong beliefs about the morality or cultural acceptability of certain behaviors and assume that these beliefs prevent those behaviors from occurring. In fact, it appears more likely that such strong cultural proscriptions may decrease the frequency with which the behaviors occur, and even more important, the freedom with which people admit or discuss those behaviors; however, the behaviors themselves do exist. In the following, we review some of the research published in recent years from a variety of countries and regions around the world.

Not all sexual behavior poses equal risk for STD; in fact, some sexual behaviors pose no risk at all. The sexual behaviors that deserve consideration for STD prevention are listed in Table 104-1. The variables at the top of the table, those addressing partners, are the most important for consideration. Type of sexual activity (i.e, vaginal, oral, or anal) is relatively unimportant for the more infectious bacterial STDs, except for the implications for clinical examination, but is important for the transmission of the less infectious agents, particularly HIV. All these behaviors pose much less risk and perhaps no risk at all, however, when condoms are used appropriately. In the case of unprotected sex, however, which is still the norm throughout most of the developing world, the frequency with which these variables occur in a population largely determines the prevalence and incidence of STD in that population.

Throughout the world, the key variables that drive the epidemic of HIV/STD certainly are partner numbers and frequency of partner change. In the sections that follow, we address these variables directly and examine groups that are characterized by these behaviors.

Table 104-1. Key Sexual Behaviors in STD/HIV Transmission

Partner variables
Number of sexual partners
Frequency of acquiring sexual partners
Concurrence of sexual partners
Types of partners (i.e., commercial, unknown)
Sexual act variables
Age at first sexual intercourse
Type of sex (vaginal, oral, anal)
Use of drying agents?
Less or unimportant variables
Frequency of sex
Nonpenetrative sex

NUMBER OF PARTNERS

Studies from the developing world have shown clearly that what are sometimes referred to in the literature as "extramarital sexual relationships," but are perhaps better thought of in epidemiologic terms as multiple sexual partner behaviors, are widespread and frequent in countries of Africa and Asia.[3–6] In some places, this behavior is culturally acceptable for both men and women, but predominantly expectations for male sexual behavior are different from those for women.[4] In almost all cases, men engage in these behaviors more frequently than women. For example, studies of sexual behavior in nine African, four Asian, and one Latin American country revealed wide variations in levels of extramarital sex.[7] In all studies, however, men reported the behavior with much higher frequency than women. Men consistently report higher partner numbers.[8–11] In part, this can be due to the greater hesitance of women to admit those behaviors to interviewers, making the real difference in men's and women's behavior perhaps smaller than the levels reported in many surveys. It is also true, however, that cultural expectations for men are usually more lenient and often even endorse multipartner behavior as a proof of virility, as has been reported in Thailand, for example.[6,11]

Not only extramarital sexual behaviors or multipartner behaviors vary for men and women, but also premarital sex varies. In most places, single men are also more likely to have had sex than are single women and to have had their initial sexual experience at an earlier age than women.[9,12] This also increases the number of lifetime sex partners and can contribute to the epidemic spread of STD/HIV.

Perhaps in response to intervention efforts to slow the epidemic, or to the epidemic itself, it appears that many people in the most affected areas of Africa have been limiting the numbers of their partners. In Uganda, for example, survey data collected in 1988 revealed that the overwhelming majority of respondents knew that practicing monogamy effectively reduced HIV risk and more than half of male respondents claimed to be doing so.[13]

In addition to numbers of partners, the concurrence of sexual relationships has also received attention.[14] Although the issue may not be as important for the more infectious bacterial STDs, concurrence of relationships may be particularly important in enhancing the transmissibility of HIV by increasing the probability of transmission during the elevated state of viremia following infection.[15] In some studies, the existence of simultaneous sexual relationships has been shown to facilitate the passage of infection across the partnerships and explain more variance in HIV prevalence than numbers of partners alone.[16] Even relatively low numbers of sexual partners in a lifetime could still pose significant risk of STD, particularly HIV, in areas of high prevalence.

HOMOSEXUAL BEHAVIOR

Although the frequency of partner change and numbers of partners are undoubtedly the most important variables to consider in modeling an epidemic of STD in a population, the types of sex one engages in can increase the risk for some STDs. Although the predominant mode of transmission of STD and HIV throughout the world is heterosexual sex, usually defined as vaginal intercourse, it is important to recognize that unprotected anal sex among men who have sex with men takes place around the world as well. Although studied less and reported in the literature with less frequency, reports on homosexual behavior from South America and Asia do exist.[17–20] In the Asia-Pacific region and in Latin America, it is not uncommon for men who identify as heterosexual to report having had anal sex with other men. A study of military recruits in Thailand found that 11 percent of otherwise heterosexual men had tried this behavior.[21] Even in Africa, where male homosexual behavior has commonly been thought of as unthinkable and nonexistent, reports of such behavior in special circumstances such as prisons are now beginning to come to light.[22] Discounting the possibility of such behavior in any cultural setting could seriously hamper the quality of STD services offered.

CORE GROUPS

Just as the levels of multiple partner behaviors vary from country to country, they also vary within countries. Even in countries where it is common to have multiple partners, the practice does not distribute uniformly in populations. The concept of core group transmitters, long a feature in epidemiologic and modeling studies of STD in industrialized countries, appears to be important in developing countries as well.[23–25] Although the concept can be seen as stigmatizing or criticized for facilitating a blaming of the victims, it is difficult to explain the epidemiologic patterns of STD and HIV in many countries without acknowledging the importance of core groups.

Perhaps singular among core groups in most countries are those involved in sex work, both as sex workers and as clients. In fact, it is the latter group, the men who use the services of sex workers, who transmit STD/HIV to other sex workers in other locales and to wives and partners who may have no other risk factors or knowledge of the behaviors of their partners' sexual behavior. The frequency of this behavior is supported by the fact that, in many parts of the world, it is socially and culturally acceptable for men to regularly visit sex workers.[11] Because of the central role of sex work in the epidemic of STD/HIV worldwide, this core group has been more studied and examined than any other. Because of the greater ease of research among sex workers, many of whom may be nearly a captive audience, much more is known about the behavior of sex workers than of their clients. Although it is not exclusive to that region, sex work in Asia has strong cultural and economic roots and may have contributed more to the epidemic of HIV/STD there than in any other region.[11] In Asia, the frequency of sexual contact and of STD/HIV infection among sex workers has been extensively studied in India, Hong Kong, Nepal, China, Thailand, and Indonesia.[26–33] In all these settings, the rate and frequency of partner change were high, as is characteristic of sex work, but rates of condom use were in general low and insufficient to prevent substantial incidence of STDs. In Africa, studies of sex workers have revealed similar levels of risk behavior, although perhaps in a context of a less organized or structured working environment.[34] Sex work has also been widely studied in Latin America, where similar behavior patterns have been found.[35] In general, sex work appears to be ubiquitous and, as practiced around the world today, a substantial risk for the continued spread of STD/HIV.

Clients of sex workers have also been studied, although the greater difficulty in identifying them outside of sex work areas makes this research more difficult to conduct. Some studies have identified visiting sex workers as the primary risk factor for HIV infection and have discovered high rates of patronage of sex workers.[36] In Cambodia, more than 40 percent of sexually experienced men reported visiting a sex worker in the previous year.[11] Numerous studies have focused on men attending STD clinics, many of whom attribute their infections to sex workers. In India, Somalia, and Thailand, for example, the sexual behavior of men attending STD clinics who claim to have visited sex workers has been studied.[37–39] As could be expected, condom use was infrequently reported. In some parts of the world, clients' knowledge of condoms and their protective effect for STD/HIV was low, as was the case in Indonesia.[40] Occupational groups of men likely to use the services of sex workers have also been studied, with attention focused particularly on men who must leave their families for work.[19] This economically driven separation is usually seen as contributing to the likelihood and the frequency of visits to sex workers and hence to continued transmission of STD/HIV.[41]

Young people are also seen as an important focus of study for sexual behavior and STD/HIV. Earlier age at sexual debut has been reported to be a risk factor for STD, particularly compounded in girls by the possible existence of cervical ectopy. For both sexes, patterns of sexual risk-taking behaviors established in adolescence may be difficult to change and the STDs acquired then may be chronic or even fatal. The sexual behavior of young people has been well documented in the developing world, both in terms of age at sexual debut and of the numbers of partners young people have. Early age at first intercourse is seen as an important risk for HIV in Uganda, especially for young girls, who often have their first sexual encounters with older men likely to be infected with HIV.[9,42]

UNDERSTANDING THE DETERMINANTS OF SEXUAL BEHAVIOR

Largely driven by concerns about the epidemic of HIV/AIDS, the understanding of the qualitative aspects of sexual behavior has grown enormously. Understanding the frequency with which sexual behaviors take place helps to assess the magnitude of the potential for epidemic spread of STD/HIV. However, it is generally not sufficient information on which to base the design of interventions to decrease those frequencies and to decrease the risk for STD/HIV. To accomplish that, it is necessary to understand the determinants and motivations for sexual behavior, apart from just the physical.[43] Although this understanding has generally lagged behind descriptions of the quantitative aspects of sexual behavior, important studies have been conducted and important thinking has shed light on the individual and other (i.e., social and socioeconomic) determinants.[2] It is now clearer than ever that sexual behavior is one of the most complex human social behaviors. For example, studies in recent years have focused attention on the economic aspects of much of the sexual exchange that takes place, particularly for women, who may need the financial support as much as the emotional support in many parts of the world. Development strategies that create surplus cash but also inequalities between more highly paid men and more lowly paid women also exacerbate this problem.[33] Studies in Asian sites seem to indicate that this phenomenon may be more important there than elsewhere, but studies in Africa also identify this theme.[7,34] In some cases, as in Zimbabwe, the economic principle involved is straightforward: Women expect to receive rewards for sex outside marriage.[45] In other cases, such as Thailand, the principle is compounded by additional considerations: Women involved in sex work are expected to comply with traditional family support roles by sending money home to their families.[46] In many cases, the choice women face is between a long-term threat of disease with unknown probabilities and a short-term threat of poverty with which they are too familiar.[47] Interventions that ignore this complex reality face little chance of success.

The economic aspects of sexual behavior are intimately wrapped up in issues of migration in much of the developing world. Migration has been associated with the spread of STD/HIV in much of the developing world.[48] In Lesotho, women's need to engage in extramarital sexual relations for financial considerations is compounded by migration: Men in Lesotho commonly migrate to South Africa for work and leave women in need of money and basic necessities.[49] Such absences for labor additionally put men at risk for commercial or other casual sexual encounters. In Kenya, males with STD were more likely to be single or, if married, to be living away from their spouses and to have had more sex partners than men with other non-sexually transmitted health complaints.[50] In Senegal, local HIV epidemics are thought to be fueled by the migration of men for seasonal labor.[51,52] Labor camps for migrant males in Asia have also been seen as likely to increase chances of commercial sex encounters.[53]

The discrepancy between cultural expectations for men's and women's roles in sexual behavior in developing countries has also been studied. These expectations, which often demand sexual acquiescence from women but allow sexual experimentation for men, make it difficult if not impossible for women to implement many of the prevention suggestions and guidance they receive.[54] In Africa and in Asia, the latitude afforded men for extramarital relationships and the limitations placed on women's ability to refuse sex, even to partners suspected of HIV, is a serious cultural constraint on prevention efforts.[4,6] In some areas of Asia, going to a brothel has been identified as a social activity for groups of men, not just a sexual activity for an individual man.[55] This sort of power discrepancy does not characterize women only. It also exists for street youth in Brazil, who must support themselves through the sale of sex and are in no position to demand safer sexual practices.[56] As our understanding of the power relationships, economic exchange, and other determinants of risky sexual behavior increase, so too does our understanding of how to develop interventions to help those who most need it avoid risky sexual behavior.

BEHAVIORAL INTERVENTIONS

The field of behavioral interventions for HIV/AIDS prevention has come under criticism for not demonstrating sufficient results or not demonstrating those results clearly enough.[57] However, in recent times, the number and quality of the interventions to change sexual and other behaviors for STD/HIV have both increased. In the section that follows, we focus our attention on intervention trials and evaluations of their effect, particularly measured by behavior change or changes in disease transmission. Although the quantity of reports from developing countries may be somewhat limited, the creativity of what is attempted there can be encouraging. We focus our attention on interventions for individuals, couples, groups, and communities.

INTERVENTIONS FOR INDIVIDUALS, COUPLES, AND GROUPS

The traditional approach to STD prevention has been the prompt treatment of infected individuals (the index case) in clinical settings and the identification and treatment of any individuals identified as sexual contacts of the index case during the infectious period. This strategy was basically effective in controlling the epidemic of syphilis in the United States and Western Europe in the 1960s and early 1970s. With the advent of the epidemic of viral STDs, including HIV, the effectiveness of this prevention and control strategy became more limited because the infections were not treatable and perhaps worse, the infectious period was not known or was unlimited. Reliance on treatment alone was no longer effective. In developing countries, assessments of service capabilities to address the growing epidemic of STD and HIV often revealed serious inadequacies.[58]

What was needed were serious attempts to assist individuals in their ability to change risky sexual behaviors. Counseling was one of the first methods attempted. It has been used in STD clinics and other health care settings to address issues of avoiding reinfection and referring partners for treatment. In the developing world, this approach has shown promising results in Zimbabwe.[59] Counseling is most commonly provided with HIV antibody testing to first reduce psychological stress and anxiety and leading to self-assessment of risk and the decision to change risk behaviors. This approach is becoming increasingly common in the developing world. Counseling has been defined for HIV prevention purposes as an interactive process in which a trained counselor assists a client in developing and rehearsing a personal risk reduction strategy, including, if necessary, role playing of important steps that might be required. Topics typically addressed in counseling for HIV prevention include informing partners and introducing condom use into new and existing relationships. Counseling is one of the most common interventions used for individuals in clinical settings.

HIV antibody testing and counseling (VCT) has been the cornerstone of the HIV prevention effort in the United States since the mid-1980s. Extensive reviews of the literature on VCT have revealed variable effectiveness for the different risk groups and the different risk behaviors for which it could be evaluated.[60,61] Clinical trials of the effectiveness of VCT in assisting individuals in developing countries to change behavior are under way.[62] In a number of earlier studies in Africa, counseling and knowledge of HIV antibody status did not seem to have a significant effect on condom use.[63,64] In Uganda, which has perhaps counseled a higher percentage of its sexually active adult population than any other country, an evaluation of VCT revealed the majority of clients seeking VCT were sexually abstinent at the time.[65] Those who tested seronegative were likely to return to sexual activity but with very high levels of condom use. The majority of those seropositive remained abstinent, with the minority resuming sexual activity monogamously and with condoms. Less striking results were reported previously from a study in the same setting.[66]

The greatest potential effect of VCT may be when it is used with couples, when the issue of condom use in an established relationship can be addressed with the help of a professional counselor. In Rwanda, VCT for discordant couples resulted in an increase in condom use from 3 to 57 percent in 1 year.[67] In Zaire, condom use following counseling for discordant couples increased from less than 5 percent to more than 70 percent very quickly.[68]

Interventions for groups, long popular in the United States, have also been tried in the developing world. At times, counseling for discordant couples has been provided in group settings.[68] Group counseling in the workplace has been used as well. Recent evidence from a trial of a group counseling and educational intervention for Thai military personnel has shown effectiveness in increasing condom use, decreasing visits to sex workers, and curbing of HIV transmission.[69] Group interventions have also been used for those at highest risk, such as sex workers in Kenya, where the percentage of women reporting at least occasional condom use increased from 7 percent before to 58 percent 12 months after one intervention.[70]

PARTNER NOTIFICATION AND MANAGEMENT

Preventing spread of infection from the index case and preventing reinfection of the treated index case are important variables to address to change the basic reproductive rate of STD. To accomplish this, partners who are likely to have been exposed must be notified and referred to treatment. Partner notification can either be passive, as when an individual with a sexually transmitted infection is expected to inform his or her partners about the possibility of exposure and the need for treatment (i.e., partner referral), or active, in which clinic staff elicit names of sexual contacts and search for them.

Although it is recognized as important for control of STD and HIV in the developing world, experience with partner notification in developing countries is limited and yields mixed results.[71,72] A study in Zimbabwe demonstrated good cooperation with active partner notification, with successful follow-up of 40 percent of partners named.[73] In another Zimbabwean study, the inclusion of partner referral in counseling for STD patients was felt to increase the concern for sex partners.[59] A Kenyan study was able to demonstrate that more than two-thirds of STD patients in primary health care clinics who returned for follow-up 1 week after initial treatment had referred their partners for treatment of STD; women referred more often than men.[74] A Nigerian study, on the other hand, found that passive partner referral was more productive and that postal reminders to contacts who failed to seek treatment were unsuccessful.[75] In Kenya, pregnant women who were syphilis-seroreactive were counseled and given a contact slip, without any name, describing the need and availability of treatment for their partners. More than 60 percent of partners came for treatment, with an expressed concern for the unborn baby being the reason most commonly given.[76] In another area of the world, studies among people of Mexican origin in California indicated that partner notification is acceptable for both men and women.[77]

Under the rubric of counseling, advice about and assistance for partner notification given to patients in primary care facilities seeking STD treatment are an essential intervention for STD/HIV prevention. Given the experiences described in the preceding, it is difficult to recommend whether a more active or passive approach to partner notification is preferable in developing countries. It appears that both approaches, partner notification and partner referral, perform fairly well under some, but perhaps not all, circumstances. Experience has shown, however, that as the prevalence of substance use in relation to sex and the frequency of anonymous partner or commercial sex increases, neither strategy functions very successfully. Given the greater cost for active partner notification, it is tempting to consider possible avenues to increase the effectiveness of partner referral through counseling programs for individuals who seek treatment in STD clinics. Cost should not be the only consideration in deciding this strategy, however, as the cultural acceptability of the different courses of action is also important.

HEALTH CARE SEEKING FOR STD

The timely and effective treatment of individuals with bacterial STDs is one of the more powerful ways to affect the basic reproductive rate of STD. However, motivating individuals to seek treatment from trained medical practitioners at the first sign of STD is a difficult task. Health care seeking for any reason is an understudied and misunderstood concept. The literature on health care seeking in general is scant; on the specific topic of STD health care seeking, it is virtually nonexistent. Nonetheless, greater attention is now being paid to promotion of health care seeking for STDs as an important component of STD/HIV prevention. A manual designed to help program managers and designers understand existing patterns of care seeking has been developed, and studies are being conducted throughout the world.[78] In this section we will review what little has been published on this topic and include the unpublished observations and experiences of those working in the area of STD treatment in the developing world.

The predominant belief among those designing and providing STD services seems to be that a natural demand for services exists. The mere establishment of competent services is sufficient; promoting those services is not necessary. In fact, there is some evidence that this belief may be justified. In Kenya, an attempt to promote care seeking for STD infection was planned, with the first step being the improvement of the clinical services offered. Once this step was concluded, however, clinic attendance increased to such an extent that the subsequent steps of promoting the services were abandoned (S. Moses, personal communication). In Uganda, however, a different reaction was encountered. In preparation for establishing a competent, state-of-the-art STD facility in a rural underserved area, a survey of people in Masaka district was conducted and included questions about health care seeking for STD.[79] The study revealed that only about 40 percent of people with symptoms of STD had sought treatment from the formal health sector for their last STD. An additional 30 percent had sought help from the informal health care sector and 30 percent had not taken any action at all. Two years later, after a new clinic was established offering up-to-date diagnostics and treatment with a well-trained staff and a ready availability of drugs, a resurvey was done. Once again, about 40 percent of respondents had sought treatment from the formal sector, half at the program's new STD clinic. The remaining 60 percent continued to seek treatment in the informal sector or take no action at all. The temptation to view use of formal clinics for treatment of STD as a function of availability, accessibility, and competence of the clinics must be resisted, therefore. Clearly, these issues are important, however, as no one can expect that people will attend clinics that are inaccessible or incompetent, either in the quality of technical services provided or of the personal interactions. Addressing these issues alone, however, may only result in diverting that proportion of the STD population that already seeks care in the formal sector to a new and improved location, while leaving what may be the majority of cases that seek care in the informal sector or those that seek no care at all untouched.

Attendance at clinics is not the only important indicator of STD care seeking. Even for those people who do come to STD or other primary health care clinics for a sexually transmitted infection, the duration of symptoms before treatment is sought is important in determining the basic reproductive rate of STD. This delay can greatly enhance the chances of complications of the infection and of secondary spread if sexual activity is continued. Timely treatment seeking is not the norm in many developing countries. In Zimbabwe, for example, the delay in seeking treatment was compared for men with genital ulcers and men with headache or cough. On average, men with genital ulcers waited 10 days before coming to clinics for treatment; men with headaches or cough waited only 3 days.[80] Delays in seeking treatment for STD can be long. In Masaka district, the median delay in seeking treatment for the minority of men who did eventually attend clinics was 6 and a half weeks for those with urethral discharge, 5 and a half for those with dysuria, and 1 and a half weeks for those with GUD. The range for urethral discharge and dysuria extended to more than 1 year. For females, the average delays in seeking treatment were shorter: 3 weeks for those with vaginal discharge, 2 weeks for those with dysuria, and 1 and a half weeks for those with GUD, with the range extending up to 28 weeks for dysuria and 12 weeks for vaginal discharge.[79] The opportunity for continued spread of infection is great if people infected with STD delay treatment and continue to be sexually active during that time.

Unfortunately, the evidence seems to indicate the people with untreated STD continue to have sex before seeking treatment. In the Zimbabwe study cited in the preceding, even men with painful genital ulcers continued to engage in penetrative sexual activity. Although this may seem like irrational behavior given our knowledge of what causes STD, other people have different explanations for disease occurrence. In Mwanza, Tanzania, local descriptions of STD symptoms and explanations for disease occurrence were investigated. In the case of urethral discharge, more than a dozen different types were identified, each with its own native etiology. Only three of these types of discharge were related to sexual activity (H. Grosskurth, personal communication). In the Masaka district of Uganda, women did recognize some symptoms of STD: vaginal discharge that was yellow in color, foul smelling, or accompanied by pain was considered abnormal. Other types of vaginal discharge, however, were seen as unrelated or even normal.[79] Obviously, efforts to promote abstinence from sexual contact during symptoms and improved care seeking behavior for STD must be based on an understanding of local beliefs and explanatory models of disease and should accommodate, rather than supplant, them.

An example where promotion of STD health care seeking has been promoted with success is in Tanzania.[81] In a large controlled trial of the effect of STD management on HIV incidence, the intervention provided included frequent visits to the villages in the study to alert people to the symptoms of STD and the availability of treatment and to stress the need for timely treatment seeking. The study reported a 40 percent reduction in HIV incidence; part of that effect is probably owing to the change in care seeking behavior by the people in the study.[82]

Competent clinical care is an essential component of any STD/HIV prevention strategy. However, clinical care alone cannot control the epidemic of STD/HIV that now exists in many countries of the world. Other approaches to prevention should be considered for the synergistic effect they can have with clinic-based interventions.

INTERVENTIONS FOR COMMUNITIES

In developing countries, where often only a minority of individuals with sexually transmitted infections seek treatment in the formal health sector and then only after long delays, the potential to control STD/HIV transmission through clinical interventions alone is certainly more limited than it is in developed countries. Effective prevention anywhere, but particularly in developing countries, requires a mix of interventions that address all of the operative variables that influence the reproductive rate of STD: increasing condom use in the general population and the highest risk or core groups and decreasing the rate of partner change. In this section, we review attempts to promote condom use or partner reduction in the developing world.

BASIC PREMISES BEHIND COMMUNITY APPROACHES

The term "community" is often used but little defined. The term can be used to connote a physical area. For epidemiology, this meaning is useful when location is important, as in the study of point-source outbreaks or exposures to toxic substances. The term "community" can also be used to describe groups of people who interact in a substantive way with each other. This interaction can imply shared behaviors or norms, beliefs, and values that influence behaviors. In epidemiology, this definition can be useful when behaviors and social interactions are important, as is the case with STD and AIDS. The weakness of this definition is the inability to locate or enumerate exactly what the "community" is, as community identity is a product of ideology, not geography. The study of assortative mating and core groups in the epidemiology of STD/HIV is, to some degree, an attempt to identify the socially defined community within the context of the physically defined community.

Armed with a better understanding of what drives or determines the behaviors of people, modern community-level interventions have focused their efforts not just on the behaviors that place people at risk but on the social, cultural, psychological, and environmental factors that characterize socially defined communities at risk. These intervention approaches not only target members of communities but also use elements of the organizational structure of the community to facilitate behavior change. Evaluations of such efforts, then, include measurement of changes in key beliefs and perceptions, as well as changes in behavior and, in rarer cases, changes in disease transmission. In our review of community interventions, we give preference to those published studies that report behavior change and disease transmission.

COMMUNITY APPROACHES FOR STD/HIV PREVENTION IN THE GENERAL POPULATION

Some community interventions have been broad in scope, not specifically limited to those at highest risk. Because of its reach and power to influence knowledge and attitudes, mass media has been used for STD/HIV prevention efforts. Although many of these efforts are merely short announcements that aim to inform, mass media interventions also have taken the form of long-running soap operas or serials. In these approaches, the goal is to educate and influence social norms for large segments of the population while providing entertainment.[83] In some developing countries, these soap operas have been able to attract enormous audiences, making them commercially viable. Evidence of social norm change has been documented in some of these cases, but only after long exposure to the interventions—more than 200 installments.[84] Documented behavior change is much more difficult to measure or attribute to mass media interventions.

Social marketing has also been extensively used for HIV prevention. Applying basic principles of marketing, and offering a subsidized product at low or affordable prices, this approach has contributed to enormous increases in condom sales and distribution in Africa, with Zaire perhaps being the best example.[85] Social marketing has also been used for other commodities, such as STD drugs in Cameroon, where the availability of drugs and the stigma associated with STD were identified as barriers to seeking treatment in clinics.[86] The innovative program encountered resistance from physicians and other barriers that have slowed its implementation and possibly lessened its effect. Other attempts to involve more peripheral health workers in the promotion and distribution of condoms have also been tried. An attempt to dispense information and condoms through pharmacists in Mexico was found to be only partially successful, however.[87]

COMMUNITY APPROACHES FOR HIGH-RISK GROUPS

Interventions for sex workers have been given a high priority in the areas hardest hit by HIV but few community interventions have been evaluated. In Nigeria, sex workers were trained to be peer educators to work with clients and sex workers. Consistent condom use reportedly doubled in 1 year.[88] Larger increases in condom use were reported from a similar intervention in Zimbabwe and Ghana, both using trained peer educators.[89,90] On a larger scale, an intervention in Cote d'Ivoire includes frequent large community meetings in all areas of sex work in Abidjan. The evaluation, which used lagged implementation for comparison, found that condom use at the last sexual contact was 90 percent for the intervention area, compared to 67 percent for the comparison areas.[91] Less significant increases in knowledge about STD/HIV were also found.

Interventions for sex workers have also been evaluated in Asia. In Calcutta, an intervention in a larger red-light area uses community outreach workers to bring risk-reduction education and condoms to all brothels each week and a community clinic to provide STD treatment and primary care to sex workers and their children. This intervention is distinctive for addressing STD/HIV prevention in the context of women's other social and health needs. Evaluation has shown significant increases in condom use, significant reductions in syphilis, and only a minor increase in HIV prevalence at a rate much lower than that of sex workers in other Indian cities.[92] In Kinshasa, Zaire, an intervention for sex workers included regular STD examination and treatment, promotion of condom use by sex workers, and the support and collaboration of bar owners where sex work was practiced. Regular use of condoms increased fivefold over 3 years, to nearly 70 percent. HIV incidence among women reporting regular condom use was one-third that of irregular users or nonusers.[93]

Community approaches can decrease the prevalence of STD/HIV risk behaviors. In developing countries, where the provision of services can be limited, expensive, and fraught with other difficulties, the opportunity to decrease the burden STD clinics face by decreasing the prevalence of risk behaviors in a community would seem well worth the investment.

STRUCTURAL AND ENVIRONMENTAL APPROACHES FOR STD/HIV PREVENTION

The bulk of HIV prevention and much of STD prevention as well relies on choices individuals make about their sexual behavior. The use of a condom, however, must be negotiated with another individual, placing that choice outside any one individual's exclusive control. For this and other reasons, the issue of choice in sexual behavior is not simple or equally the province of both women and men. In many regions of the world, discrepancies exist in the relative power of women and men to make decisions about sexual behavior, both for cultural and economic reasons, as we have seen. What is needed is a way to minimize risk of STD/HIV without relying on individual choices about sexual behavior alone.

In other areas in public health, interventions are not restricted only to those approaches that rely on influencing individual behavior and choice, as vitamin supplementation of foods, taxes on harmful products, and laws requiring protective measures such as immunizations and seat belt use indicate. The possibility and even the existence of such approaches for STD/HIV prevention have been proposed.[94–96] Focusing on structural and environmental changes, two principal areas present themselves for consideration: policy and economic approaches. In the first case, policy approaches can include both removing restrictive policies to enable reduced risk behaviors to be practiced (as in legalizing the sale and possession of sterile injection equipment) and erecting barriers to continued risk taking. In the second case, economic approaches can include taxation or pricing mechanisms that make risky behavior economically less attractive than reduced risk behavior, that make means of risk reduction truly affordable, or that offer economic empowerment to women. Approaches such as these offer the possibility of shaping and influencing behavior even in areas where it is difficult to influence and persuade all people at risk to change. For women in the developing world, these types of approaches may be important adjuncts to the approaches outlined previously.

Some examples of the application of policy approaches to STD/HIV prevention do exist. A policy approach to HIV prevention has been successfully implemented in Thailand and appears to be effective.[97,98] Beginning with a pilot program in the north, the government instituted a policy of mandatory condom use in brothels. The policy was designed to make condom use the responsibility of the customer and the brothel owner, not of the women, who are usually not in a position to demand or negotiate. The police are charged with assuring the compliance of the brothel owners. Public health clinics, which continue to screen the sex workers for STD regularly, use incident STD among sex workers as evidence of lax enforcement at a particular brothel. The policy has been evaluated and appears to be successful. Surveys of sex workers indicate high rates of condom use (exceeding 90% using on the last commercial sex encounter in most provinces), greatly decreased rates of STD among both sex workers and males who patronize them, and decreasing HIV prevalence among young males, as indicated by surveys among Thai military recruits. Although the policy allows the high-risk behavior (i.e., multipartner sex) to continue, it mandates sufficient changes (i.e., condom use) apparently to remove much of the risk.

Another policy approach has been tried in some places. This entails the mandatory placement of condoms in short-term stay hotels, where risky sexual behavior is likely to take place. An evaluation of such an approach was conducted in the Dominican Republic.[99] The effect of that policy on condom use was measured by randomly selecting hotels that were compliant with the policy and those noncompliant hotels and comparing condom use by observing used condoms and wrappers in the room after checkout. The ready availability of condoms doubled the rate of usage, from 12 to 24 percent. Clearly, a simple policy on condom placement appears to be a useful element in a comprehensive STD/HIV prevention effort.

Economic approaches may also be helpful in STD/HIV prevention. To date, these approaches have usually focused on income-generating alternatives to sex work, a difficult challenge given the potential wages of sex work compared to other wage labor available to women.[100] However, an example from family planning may be illustrative of a different approach. In Bangladesh, the Grameen Bank has been operating revolving loan schemes for rural women. Through this cooperative, women can borrow money to finance the development of self-employment activities. The loan schemes have been successful, with high rates of repayment, and have been associated with women's economic and social empowerment.[101] Participation in the cooperative was also associated with increased use of contraception, even for women who lived in villages where the Grameen Bank scheme operated but who did not themselves participate in the scheme, compared to women in villages without the scheme. Based on this study, it would appear that economic empowerment facilitates women's ability to control their personal decisions, including use of contraception. The evidence also suggests a diffusion of new norms from the successful participating women to other women in their villages who did not participate. The inclusion of economic approaches that assist women in developing power over certain areas of their lives may be useful in assisting them to exert the necessary control of their sexual behavior that they need to avoid STD/HIV.

The preceding examples argue that interventions that address the structure or the environment in which risk behavior takes place are not only feasible but also can be effective in a relatively short time. They may well represent an additional approach to STD/HIV that has received entirely too little attention and that could be used with other more individual and community approaches.

CONCLUSIONS

After a decade of essential research on sexual behavior and interventions to change it, we are now better able to address the epidemic of STD/HIV than we have ever been before. Our understanding of sexual behavior, the varieties of forms it takes, and how ubiquitous those behaviors are has been refined through the research and the gradual accretion of empirical evidence that has characterized the response to the AIDS epidemic. Our understanding of how to change these sexual behaviors has also improved, from an initial focus on the behaviors themselves to a more refined focus on the determinants of those behaviors. Most encouraging, perhaps, has been the widening of thinking about possible ways to address the epidemic of STD/HIV, away from single-action interventions and toward more complex mixes of interventions at all levels. Some of the most creative examples of prevention thinking have come from the developing world, and the interchange of ideas and approaches between the developed and the developing world can only improve prevention efforts everywhere.

References

1 Anderson RM et al: Epidemiologic parameters of HIV transmission. *Nature* 333:514–519, 1988.

2 Holmes, KK: Human ecology and behavior and sexually transmitted bacterial infections. *Proc Natl Acad Sci USA* 91:2448–2455, 1994.

3 Cleland J et al: Sexual behaviour and AIDS in the developing world. London, Taylor and Francis, 1995.

4 Orubuloye IO et al: Sexual networking and the risk of AIDS in southwest Nigeria, in *Sexual Behaviour and Networking: Anthropological and Sociocultural Studies on the Transmission of HIV,* T Dyson (ed). Liege, Belgium, Editions Derovaux-Ordina, 1992, pp. 283–301.

5 Anarfi JK et al: Experimental research on sexual networking in some selected areas of Ghana. *Health Trans Rev* 3(suppl):29–43, 1993.

6 Asavaroegchai S: Double standard, double threat: HIV and reproductive health in Thailand, in *Private Decisions, Public Debate: Women, Reproduction and Population,* J Mirsky et al (eds). London, Panos Publications, 1994, pp. 107–120.

7 Carael M et al: Extramarital sex: Implications of survey results for STD/HIV transmission. *Health Trans Rev* 4(suppl):153–172, 1994.

8 Zuloaga-Posada L et al: Sexual behaviour and health problems in university students, University of Antioquia, 1991. *Bull Pan Am Health Org* 29:299–311, 1995.

9 Agyei WA et al: Teenage life: Sex education should start early. *African Women Health* 1:15–21, 1993.

10 Patullo AL et al: Survey of knowledge, behaviour and attitudes relating to HIV infection and AIDS among Kenyan secondary school students. *AIDS Care* 6:173–181, 1994.

11 Brown T et al: Heterosexual risk behaviour in Asia: The implication for HIV/AIDS. *Curr Sci (Ind Acad Sci)* 69:840–848, 1995.

12 Kane TT et al: Grossesse de l'adolescente et contraception dans l'agglomeration de Banjul: Les jeunes ont besoin d'une information precise. *Pop Sahel* 13:28–34, 1990.

13 Konde-Lule JK et al: Focus group interviews about AIDS in Rakai District of Uganda. *Soc Sci Med* 37:679–684, 1993.

14 Hudson CP: Concurrent partnerships could cause AIDS epidemics. *Int J STD AIDS* 4:349–353, 1993.

15 Phanuphak P: Concurrent relationships could cause AIDS epidemics: Thailand's point of view (letter). *Int J STD AIDS* 5:155–156, 1994.

16 Watts CH et al: The influence of concurrent partnerships on the dynamics of HIV/AIDS. *Math Biosci* 108:89–104, 1992.

17 Santos BR et al: Changing patterns of HIV-1 transmission in southern Brazil 1985–1991. *Int J STD AIDS* 5:202–206, 1994.

18 Beyrer C et al: Same-sex behavior, sexually transmitted diseases and HIV risks among young northern Thai men. *AIDS* 9:171–176, 1995.
19 Singh YN et al: Long-distance truck drivers in India: HIV infection and their possible role in disseminating HIV into rural areas. *Int J STD AIDS* 5:137–138, 1994.
20 Sittitrai W et al: Levels of HIV risk behaviour and AIDS knowledge in Thai men having sex with men. *AIDS Care* 5:261–271, 1993.
21 Nopkesorn T et al: HIV prevalence and sexual behaviours among Thai men aged 21 in northern Thailand. Program on AIDS, Thai Red Cross Society, 1991: Research Report No.3.
22 Vaz RG et al: Syphilis and HIV infection among prisoners in Maputo, Mozambique. *Int J STD AIDS* 6:42–46, 1995.
23 Lamptey P: An overview of AIDS interventions in high-risk groups: Commercial sex workers and their clients, in *AIDS and Women's Reproductive Health,* L Chen et al (eds). New York, Plenum Press 1991, pp. 151–163.
24 Plummer FA et al: The importance of core groups in the epidemiology and control of HIV-1 infection. *AIDS* 5(suppl 1):S169–S176, 1991.
25 Ronald A et al: Social epidemiology in Africa: Slowing the heterosexual transmission of AIDS. *AIDS Soc* 2:7–8, 1991.
26 Jana S et al: Community-based survey of STD/HIV infection among commercial sex workers in Calcutta, India: Part II. Sexual behaviour, knowledge and attitudes towards STD. *J Comm Dis* 26:168–171, 1994.
27 Pal N et al: Community-based survey of STD/HIV infection among commercial sex workers in Calcutta, India: Part IV. Sexually transmitted diseases and related risk factors. *J Comm Dis* 26:197–202, 1994.
28 Das A et al: Community-based survey of STD/HIV infection among commercial sex workers in Calcutta, India: Part III. Clinical findings of sexually transmitted diseases (STD). *J Comm Dis* 26:192–196, 1994.
29 Wong KH et al: Condom use among commercial sex workers and male clients in Hong Kong. *Int J STD AIDS* 5:287–289, 1994.
30 Bhatta P et al: Commercial sex workers in Kathmandu Valley: Profile and prevalence of sexually transmitted diseases. *J Nepal Med Assoc* 32:191–203, 1994.
31 Gil VE et al: Prostitutes, prostitution and STD/HIV transmission in mainland China. *Soc Sci Med* 42:141–152, 1996.
32 Bonhomme MG et al: Incidence of sexually transmitted diseases among massage parlor employees in Bangkok, Thailand. *Int J STD AIDS* 5:214–217, 1994.
33 Jones GW et al: Prostitution in Indonesia. Working Papers in Demography #52, Research School of Social Sciences, Australian National University, Canberra, 1995.
34 Nkya WM et al: Sexually transmitted diseases in prostitutes in Moshi and Arusha, Northern Tanzania. *Int J STD AIDS* 2:432–435, 1991.
35 Uribe-Zuniga P et al: La prostitucion et SIDA en la Ciudad de Mexico. *Salud Publica Mex* 37:592–601, 1995.
36 Celentano DD et al: Risk factors for HIV-1 seroconversion among young men in northern Thailand. *JAMA* 275:122–127, 1996.
37 Kaur V et al: Sexual and treatment behaviour of STD patients. *Ind J Sex Trans Dis* 13:83–86, 1992.
38 Ismail SO et al: Sexually transmitted diseases in men in Mogadishu, Somalia. *Int J STD AIDS* 1:102–106, 1990.
39 Turner R: HIV infection rate, use of prostitutes are both high among young military recruits in northern Thailand. *Int Fam Plann Perspect* 1994, 20: 35–6.
40 Fajans P et al: AIDS knowledge and risk behaviors among domestic clients of female sex workers in Bali, Indonesia. *Soc Sci Med* 41:409–417, 1995.
41 Bwayo J et al: Human immunodeficiency virus infection in long-distance truck drivers in east Africa. *Arch Intern Med* 154:1391–1396, 1994.
42 Agyei WK et al: Contraception and prevalence of sexually transmitted diseases among adolescents and young adults in Uganda. *Int J Epidemiol* 21:981–988, 1992.
43 Aggleton P et al: Risking everything? Risk behavior, behavior change and AIDS. *Science* 265:341–345, 1994.
44 Meursing K et al: Condoms, family planning and living with HIV in Zimbabwe. *Reprod Health Matt* (May):56–67, 1995.
45 Vos T: Attitudes to sex and sexual behaviour in rural Matabeleland, Zimbabwe. *AIDS Care* 6:193–203, 1994.
46 Wawer MJ et al: Origins and working conditions of female sex workers in urban Thailand: Consequences of social context for HIV transmission. *Soc Sci Med* 42:453–462, 1996.
47 Schoepf B: Women at risk: case studies from Zaire, in *The Time of AIDS*, Herdt G et al (eds). London, Sage Publications, 1992, pp. 259–286.
48 Quinn TC: Population migration and the spread of types 1 and 2 human immunodeficiency viruses. *Proc Natl Acad Sci USA* 91:2407–2414, 1994.
49 Romero-Daza N: Multiple sexual partners, migrant labor and the makings for an epidemic: Knowledge and beliefs about AIDS among women in Lesotho. *Hum Org* 53:192–205, 1994.
50 Moses S et al: Sexual behaviour in Kenya: Implications for sexually transmitted disease transmission and control. *Soc Sci Med* 39:1649–1656, 1994.
51 Pison G et al: Seasonal migration: A risk factor for HIV infection in rural Senegal. *J Acq Imm Def Synd* 6:196–200, 1993.
52 Kane F et al: Temporary expatriation is related to HIV-1 infection in rural Senegal. *AIDS* 7:1261–1265, 1993.
53 Moodie R et al: Confronting the HIV epidemic in Asia and the Pacific: Developing successful strategies to minimize the spread of HIV infection. *AIDS* 7:1543–1551, 1993.
54 Gupta GR et al: Women's lives and sex: Implications for AIDS prevention. *Cult Med Psychiatr* 17:399–412, 1993.
55 Havanon N et al: Sexual networking in a provincial Thai setting. *Stud Fam Plann* 24:1–17, 1993.
56 Filguerias A: Taking health promotion onto the streets. *AIDS ACT* 1992, (June):7.
57 Aral SO et al: Defining behavioral methods to prevent sexually transmitted diseases through intervention research. *Infect Dis Clin No Am* 7:861–873, 1993.
58 Kantaraj K et al: Sexually transmitted disease services in Madras: Could their role in AIDS prevention be strengthened? *Ind J Pub Health* 39:93–99, 1995.
59 Wynendaele B et al: Impact of counselling on safer sex and STD occurrence among STD patients in Malawi. *Int J STD AIDS* 6:105–109, 1995.
60 Higgins, DL et al: Evidence for the effects of HIV-antibody and testing on risk behaviors. *JAMA* 266:2419–2429, 1991.
61 Choi K-H et al: Prevention of HIV infection. *AIDS* 8:1371–1389, 1994.
62 de Zoysa I et al: Role of HIV counseling and testing in changing risk behavior in developing countries. *AIDS* 9(suppl A):S95–S101, 1995.
63 Pickering H et al: Effects of post-test counselling on condom use among prostitutes in the Gambia. *AIDS* 7:271–273, 1993.
64 Heyward WL et al: Impact of HIV counseling and testing among child-bearing women in Kinshasa, Zaire. *AIDS* 7:1633–1637, 1993.
65 Moore M et al: Impact of HIV counseling and testing (CT) in Uganda. IV International Conference on AIDS/IV STD World Congress. Berlin, June 1993.
66 Muller O et al: HIV prevalence, attitudes and behaviour in clients of a confidential HIV testing and counselling centre in Uganda. *AIDS* 6:869–874, 1992.
67 Allen S et al: Effect of serotesting with counselling on condom use and seroconversion among HIV-discordant couples in Africa. *BMJ* 304:1605–1609, 1992.
68 Kamenga M et al: Evidence of marked sexual behavior change associated with low HIV-1 seroconversion in 149 married couples with discordant HIV-1 serostatus: Experience at an HIV counselling center in Zaire. *AIDS* 5:61–67, 1991.
69 Celentano DD et al: HIV prevention in the Royal Thai Army reduces HIV risks among conscripts. Paper presented at the Third International Conference on AIDS in Asia and the Pacific, Chiang Mai, Thailand, September 17–21, 1995.

70 Ngugi EN et al: Prevention of HIV transmission in Africa: Effectiveness of condom promotion and health education among prostitutes. *Lancet* 2(8616):887–890, 1988.
71 Pinto I: Guidelines for partner notification. *AIDS Bull* 2(suppl):1–4, 1993.
72 World Health Organization: Consensus statements on HIV transmission. *Lancet* 1(8634):396, 1989.
73 Winfield J et al: Tracing contacts of persons with sexually transmitted diseases in a developing country. *Sex Trans Dis* 12:5–7, 1985.
74 Njeru EK et al: STD partner notification and referral in primary level health centers in Nairobi, Kenya. *Sex Trans Dis* 22:231–235, 1995.
75 Asuzu MC et al: The use of mail reminders in STD contact tracing in Ibadan, Nigeria. *East African Med J* 67:75–78, 1990.
76 Jenniskens F et al: Syphilis control in pregnancy: Decentralization of screening facilities to primary care level, a demonstration project in Nairobi, Kenya. *Int J Gynaecol Obstet* 48(suppl):S121–128, 1995.
77 Carrier JM et al: Use of ethnosexual data on men of Mexican origin for HIV/AIDS prevention programs. *J Sex Res* 28:189–202, 1991.
78 Helitzer-Allen DL et al: *The Manual for Targeted Intervention Research on Sexually Transmitted Diseases with Community Members.* Arlington, VA, AIDSCAP/Family Health International.
79 Mulder DW: Disease perception and health seeking behaviour for sexually transmitted diseases. Paper presented at Workshop on Sexually Transmitted Diseases of the Network of AIDS Researchers of Eastern and Southern Africa, Mwanza, Tanzania, 7–12 November 1993.
80 Mbengeranwa L: Pilot study on the evaluation of the effectiveness of genital ulcer disease control and its impact on HIV transmission in Harare, Zimbabwe: Report to GPA.
81 Hayes R et al: A community trial of the impact of improved sexually transmitted disease treatment on the HIV epidemic in rural Tanzania: 1. Design. *AIDS* 9:919–926, 1995.
82 Grosskurth H et al: Impact of improved treatment of sexually transmitted diseases on HIV infection in rural Tanzania: Randomized controlled trial. *Lancet* 346:530–536, 1995.
83 Brown WJ et al: Pro-development soap operas: A novel approach to development communication. *Media Dev* 4:43–47, 1989.
84 Chandran et al: Using entertainment for development: Viewer identification with a pro-social Indian soap opera. Paper presented at the Intercultural and Development Communication Division, Communication Association, June 1993, Washington, DC.
85 Global Programme on AIDS. Effective approaches to AIDS prevention: Report of a meeting (Geneva). Geneva: World Health Organization, 1992.
86 Dadian MJ: Public health approaches to STD control: New challenges in the era of AIDS. *AIDS Cap* 3:24–28, 1996.
87 Pick S et al: AIDS prevention training for pharmacy workers in Mexico City. *AIDS Care* 8:55–69, 1996.
88 Williams E et al: Implementation of an AIDS prevention program among prostitutes in the Cross River State of Nigeria (Letter). *AIDS* 6:229–230, 1992.
89 Wilson D et al: A Community-Level AIDS Prevention Programme among Sexually Vulnerable Groups and the General Population in Bulawayo, Zimbabwe. Harare: University of Zimbabwe; 1993.
90 Asamoah-Adu A et al: Evaluation of a targeted AIDS prevention intervention to increase condom use among prostitutes in Ghana. *AIDS* 8:239–246, 1994.
91 Kale K et al: Evaluating a behavioural intervention in high risk settings in Abidjan, Cote d'Ivoire. Xth International Conference on AIDS/International Conference on STD, Yokohama, Japan, August 1994.
92 Jana S et al: Changes in sexual behavior of prostitutes in Calcutta. Xth International Conference on AIDS/International Conference on STD, Yokohama, Japan, August 1994.
93 Laga M et al: Condom promotion, sexually transmitted diseases treatment and declining incidence of HIV-1 infection in female Zairian sex workers. *Lancet* 344:246–248, 1994.
94 Tawil O et al: Enabling approaches in HIV/AIDS prevention: Can we modify the environment and minimize the risk? *AIDS* 9:1299–1306, 1995.
95 Sweat MD et al: Reducing HIV incidence in developing countries with structural and environmental interventions. *AIDS* 9(suppl A):S251–257, 1995.
96 O'Reilly KR et al: International perspectives on individual and community approaches to the prevention of sexually transmitted diseases and human immunodeficiency virus infection. *J Infect Dis* 174(suppl 2):S214–S2122, 1996.
97 Rojanapithayakorn W: The one hundred percent condom programme in Thailand: An update. Xth International Conference on AIDS/Vth STD World Congress. Yokohama, Japan, August 1994.
98 Nelson KE et al: Changes in sexual behavior and a decline in HIV infection among young men in Thailand. *N Engl J Med* 335(5):343–345, 1996.
99 Guerrero E et al: Disponibilidad y uso de condones en hoteles/moteles de paso, Santa Domingo 1994. Final report to GPA.
100 Ford N et al: The socio-cultural context of transmission of HIV in Thailand. *Soc Sci Med* 33:405–414, 1991.
101 Schuler SR et al: Credit programs, women's empowerment and contraceptive use in rural Bangladesh. *Stud Fam Plan* 25:65–76, 1994.

PART X SPECIAL MEDICAL/LEGAL/SOCIAL ISSUES

Chapter 105
Sexual assault and STD

Consuelo M. Beck-Sague
Carole Jenny

Sexual assault is defined as an act of sexual intimacy performed without the consent of the victim through use, or threat of use, of force, or when the victim is unable to give consent because of physical or mental disability.[1]

Sexually transmitted diseases (STDs) are among the most common medical problems complicating sexual assault. STDs diagnosed at the time of a sexual assault can add to the emotional problems experienced by victims, whether or not the disease was acquired as a result of the assault. In addition, victims often express severe anxiety about the possibility of contracting an STD from the assailant. This anxiety can accentuate the emotional trauma they experience, aggravate any posttraumatic stress, and delay their recovery. The possibility of HIV transmission during the sexual assault has further added to the panic and stress related to sexual victimization.[2]

INCIDENCE AND PREVALENCE OF SEXUAL ASSAULT

The true incidence and prevalence of sexual assault is unknown. For over 20 years, the incidence of reported sexual assault steadily increased from 17/100,000 for women 12 years of age or older to 80/100,000 in 1990.[3,4] Sexual assault remained the "fastest growing violent crime" in the United States until 1993, when a slight decline was observed.[5]

From nine to over 24 percent of U.S. women will be sexually assaulted at least once in their lifetimes.[6,7] Extrapolating from surveys, in a 1-year period, it is estimated that more than 683,000 acts of forced vaginal, anorectal or oral, genital, digital, or foreign object penetration are experienced by U.S. women over the age of 18[8]; of all sexual assaults, approximately 22 percent, are committed by strangers and 16 percent are reported to the police.[8] The U.S. rate has been and continues to be many times higher than that of other Western countries during peacetime.[9] Among the studies that suggest this high prevalence of sexual assault is a study of 930 randomly selected San Francisco households, in which 24 percent of adult women reported having experienced a sexual assault.[10]

Sexual assault of males is probably less common, although comparable community-based studies to determine its prevalence have not been reported. Men do experience sexual harassment, ranging from sexual coercion to violent sexual assault.[11] In the United States, 5 to 10 percent of reported sexual assaults are against men, and 10 to 23 percent of persons seeking assistance in sexual assault victim support centers are male.[12–14] Because of multiple concerns, including fear of being labeled or stigmatized as homosexuals, male sexual assault may be even more underreported than sexual assault of female victims. The sexual orientation of men who sexually assault men and male children has been an object of some debate. Some studies have indicated that sexual assault is rarely committed by homosexual men, and that the majority of assailants (75%) in noninstitutional assaults of male victims were total strangers.[15,16] In noninstitutional assaults, male victims sustained considerable trauma, were held captive for prolonged time, multiple assailants participated, and most victims regarded the assault as an act of violence and humiliation perpetrated by self-identified heterosexuals. However, there is evidence that in studies where victims are recruited from sources other than police, hospital, and victim-support settings by methods designed to yield a large proportion of self-identified homosexual and bisexual victims, only 18 percent were assaulted by strangers and 29 percent of victims had had previous consensual homosexual relations with the assailant.[17,18] Men and male children in prisons, juvenile detention and custody centers, correctional facilities, and other such institutions, including military environments, appear to be at greatly elevated risk of sexual assault, generally from assailants who self-identify as heterosexuals.[19]

Statistics collected by law enforcement agencies are low estimates of the occurrence of sexual assault, since many, if not most, victims, regardless of age or gender, are reluctant to report the crime.[20] Because sexual assaults occur frequently, medical practitioners who treat STD are likely to see sexual assault victims in their practices.

EPIDEMIOLOGY OF SEXUAL ASSAULT

The epidemiology of sexual assault is similar in some ways to the epidemiology of most STDs. Several risk factors have been defined, some of which are the same for both situations.

AGE

Young people are at increased risk of sexual assault. The highest incidence occurs in female older adolescents and young adults.[21] Young age is an important risk factor for male victims as well; in one study, only 16 percent of male victims were over the age of 15 at the time of the assault.[22] Although sexual assault is primarily a problem of young persons, more than 60,000 sexual assaults of women older than 50 years of age are reported each year; victims over the age of 50 accounted for 2.2 to 7 percent of reported cases and sustain considerably more genital trauma from the assaults than did younger victims.[23–25]

GENDER

Despite the increasing recognition of male victimization, regardless of how victims are recruited, female victims predominate in all surveys of noninstitutional sexual assault.[22,25]

MARITAL STATUS

Single people report sexual assault in disproportionately high numbers compared to married people.[21] Some of these assaults are "date rapes" that occur after social encounters.

SOCIOECONOMIC STATUS

Sexual assault is more frequently reported among low-income populations.[26] Poor people are more likely to live in unsafe or overcrowded housing; to live in high-crime, relatively less police-protected neighborhoods; and to have less safe means of transportation. Risk factors for sexual assault identified in recent studies include some strongly associated with low socioeconomic status, including homelessness, dependence on drugs such as crack cocaine, and commercial sex work, including exchange of sex with numerous partners for drugs, food, or shelter.[27–29] Nevertheless, studies that actively sought participants in middle-class populations have indicated that over 14 percent of employed, middle-class women reported sexual assault and 25.7 percent of women in college campuses reported nonconsensual sexual activity.[30–32]

RACE

Many studies of sexual assault report a higher incidence in racial and ethnic minorities; such women report sexual assault twice as frequently as white women.[26] When populations are closely matched for socioeconomic status, however, this association tends to be much weaker; in fact, in one such study of indigent prenatal patients, white patients reported a lifetime prevalence of sexual assault of 51/409 (13%), compared to 29/768 (3.8%), among black patients and 40/1181 (3.4%) among Hispanic patients ($p < .001$).[33]

SEASONALITY AND HOURS OF THE DAY

More sexual assaults occur during the summer months than during other times of the year. Fewest occur during the winter months.[34] The hours between midnight and 6:00 AM appear to be particularly high-risk times for assaults.

SUBSTANCE ABUSE

Urban sexual assault survivors are significantly more likely to report substance abuse than are women who do not report sexual assault.[27,29] Alcohol abuse plays a role in a substantial proportion of sexual assault, both among victims and assailants.[35]

DISABILITY

Physical and mental disabilities may place both men and women at significantly higher risk of sexual victimization, presumably because of the greater vulnerability of disabled persons in resisting assault, communicating effectively to elicit the belief or assistance of others, and/or other factors.[36,37]

The preceding factors are somewhat interrelated. For instance, young people and minorities are more likely to be poor and single. All of these factors may also be affected by different rates of reporting of sexual assault to law enforcement agencies.[38] During war time and other social upheavals, such as revolutions, mass migrations, and forced detention, sexual victimization may greatly increase, and actually become widely disseminated in a society, even among persons otherwise at low risk.[39]

Victims are more likely to report sexual assault if they believe the reporting leads to arrest and conviction of the offender.[38] The perceptions by different groups of the effectiveness of law enforcement could lead to different rates of reporting. It is essential to appreciate that the limited data on both domestic and other types of victimization suggest that reporting of the abuse, acknowledgment of the assailant's responsibility, and particularly, apprehension of the offender, may greatly reduce subsequent risk of further abuse to the victim and aids in the emotional recovery from the victimization.

FACTORS AFFECTING THE RISK OF STD AFTER SEXUAL ASSAULT

Several factors make the diagnosis and treatment of STD in victims of sexual assault different from managing STD in other sexual relationships. Although sometimes well known to the victim, often the assailant is a stranger or casual acquaintance. Since the health status of the offender is likely to be unknown, it may be difficult to estimate the risk of contracting an STD in any individual case. Moreover, male sex offenders may be at higher risk for STD than the general population. In surveys of sexual behaviors of sex offenders, they report multiple sexual behaviors that would expose them to sexually transmitted organisms, including sexual contact with numerous consenting and nonconsenting male and female partners.[40] Moreover, the following have been reported in men in correctional facilities: very high prevalence of HIV infection, with rates exceeding 20 percent in some prison systems; high prevalence of STDs and AIDS; and risk factors for STDs and HIV infection, particularly drug use.[41–43] Although there are insufficient data to establish this, it is believed that sex offenders are overrepresented in prison populations.

Often, sexual assault victims are seen after a single episode of sexual contact. Little is known about the infectivity of most STDs after a single episode of intercourse, although the relative infectivity of some organisms has been determined; among regular partners of male patients with gonorrhea and *Chlamydia trachomatis* infection, studies employing culture diagnosis found rates of 80 and 45 percent, respectively.[44] The risk of transmission of *N. gonorrhoeae* from an infected female prostitute in a single sexual exposure has been estimated to be 22 to 25 percent; although equivalent data from single male to female exposure are not available, the risk would be expected to be at least that high.[45,46] Up to 20 to 27 percent of monogamous partners of patients with hepatitis B infection are found to be infected;[47,48] the risk of infection after a single exposure is probably less, but is likely to vary with factors such as bleeding during the exposure and presence of hepatitis B antigen in the infected partner. Similarly, 30 percent of sexual partners of patients with syphilis are found to be infected, but again, the risk of infection after a single exposure doubtless varies by stage of syphilis and aspects of the encounter.[49] Upper limits of risk for transmission of HIV per single anal or genital exposure have been estimated to range from up to 3.2 to 5.6 percent.[49–51] Many factors can affect the HIV transmission risk, and may elevate it above this level of risk; these include assailant infectiousness, which can vary by stage of infection, other infections, including STDs, in either the assailant or the victim, and strain infectivity and virulence.[50,52] Factors particularly relevant to the sexual assault setting itself, such as trauma during sex, particularly that which results in bleeding, may greatly increase risk of transmission.

It is generally difficult, among victims with prior consensual sexual activity, to determine if an STD diagnosed after a sexual assault predated the assault or resulted from the assault. Even if a positive culture or nucleic acid amplification test is obtained shortly after the assault, it is possible that the test represents bacteria or viruses found in infected semen rather than a previously undiagnosed asymptomatic infection. With some organisms, such as herpes simplex virus, hepatitis B virus, or HIV, highly specific serologic tests exist to detect seroconversion in the victim, which may indicate whether or not infection was recently acquired.[53] Reliable tests for immune responses to many sexually transmitted organisms, such as *Neisseria gonorrhoeae,* do not exist. Others, such as *Chlamydia trachomatis,* may be difficult to interpret in relation to the acquisition of repeated infections. However, once an organism is isolated, molecular subtyping may be useful in establishing the source of infection (see the following).

The anatomic site of the assault may also affect the likelihood of contracting an STD. For example, because of their ability to infect cervical columnar epithelium, *N. gonorrhoeae* and *C. trachomatis* may be more readily transmitted by vaginal intercourse than by anal or oral intercourse, whereas human immunodeficiency virus (HIV) may be most likely to be transmitted by anal intercourse.[50,51]

Although it has been suspected that the risk of postassault infections is higher among victims assaulted by more than one assailant, it has not been possible to consistently prove this association. Finally, whether or not the male assailant ejaculates during a sexual assault may affect the likelihood of the victim's contracting certain STD. A survey of sexual functioning during episodes of assault reported by male sex offenders in prisons showed that 34 percent were sexually dysfunctional.[55] In a more recent study, 20 percent of 50 victims of sexual assault reported that their assailant experienced erectile insufficiency at some point during the assault, and another 12 percent reported retarded ejaculation or failure to ejaculate by their attacker.[56] Sexual dysfunction during the assault prohibiting intromission and ejaculation may decrease the victim's risk of STD or pregnancy resulting from the assault, but there is some suggestion that it may increase the risk of intra-assault physical violence and degrading sexual activity related to the sexual assault.[56,57] Violent behavior that produces severe bleeding of the victim may increase the risk of transmission of such pathogens as HIV or hepatitis B from relatively low-risk fluids, such as pre-ejaculatory fluid. Moreover, in 7 (44%) of 16 cases of sexual assault where the victim denied penetration or ejaculation, seminal fluid was detected.[58] This is particularly important to appreciate in cases where decisions regarding diagnosis or prophylaxis may be affected by the victim's report that the assailant failed to penetrate or ejaculate during the assault.

DATA ON SPECIFIC DISEASES AFTER SEXUAL ASSAULT

Of the series articles published from 1976 through 1997, most were evaluations of STDs after sexual assault primarily of female victims (Table 105-1); only one small series reported on a series of assaulted men.[59–73] Only a relative few articles report on anal, rectal, or pharyngeal cultures obtained after anal or oral assault, including one series that reported the first anal transmission of *C. trachomatis*.[64,66–69] Relatively few studies have attempted to determine the frequency of STDs resulting specifically from the sexual assault instead of pre-existing STD or STD acquired after the assault; even in these, the rates of return for followup among victims examined initially have been relatively low.[64,65,68,71,72] Treatment with prophylactic antimicrobials and the low rates of medical followup after assault make the determination of risk of STD associated with the assault difficult.

Each study is influenced by the underlying prevalence of disease in the population in the community at the time the data were collected. Most studies have examined the prevalence of gonorrhea, *C. trachomatis* infections, and syphilis. Fewer data are available on viral STDs or vaginitis in this group.

GONORRHEA

The rate of cervical infections with *N. gonorrhoeae* detected after sexual assault in female victims varied at initial examination from

Table 105-1. Surveys of Sexually Assaulted Women and Men Published 1976–1997

Author	City	Number of Participants	NG	CT	TV	BV	CA	TP	HSV	HIV
Kaufman[59]	Albuquerque	50	3 (6.0)	—	—	—	—	0	—	—
Everett[60]	Oklahoma	117	14 (12.0)	—	—	—	—	3 (2.9)	—	—
Soules[61]	Denver	110	(9.0)	—	—	—	—	0	—	—
Evrard[62]	Providence	126	7 (5.0)	—	—	—	—	0	—	—
Tintinalli[63]	Royal Oak	372	19 (5.1)	—	—	—	—		—	—
Forster[64]	London	<8 days 46	3 (6.5)	4 (8.7)	4 (8.7)	7 (15.0)	1 (2.2)	0	0	—
		>7 days	0	2 (4.8)	2 (4.8)	0	—	0	0	—
Jenny[65]	Seattle	Initial 203	13 (6.4)	20 (10.1)	30 (14.7)	70 (34.3)	—	0	4 (2.4)	1 (0.8)
		F/U 109	3 (4)	1 (2)	10 (12)	15 (19)	—	0	0	0
Estrich[66]	London	124	15 (12.1)	6 (4.8)	15 (12.1)	—	11 (8.9)	—	2 (1.6)	1 (2.3)
Lacey[67]	Manchester	90	10 (4.8)	7 (7.7)	6 (6.6)	17 (18.8)	2 (2.2)	0	—	—
Sturm[68]	St. Paul	Initial 232	10 (4.8)	13 (6.1)	—	—	—	—	—	—
		F/U 62	0	1 (1.9)						
Hillman[69]	Edinburgh	5	1 (20.0)	0	—	—	1 (20)	—	0	1 (20)
Ross[70]	Edinburgh	43	1 (2.3)	2 (4.7)	1 (2.3)	1 (2.3)	1 (2.3)	—	1 (2.3)	—
Glaser[71]	Brooklyn	Initial 76	2 (2.6)	13 (17.1)	15 (19.7)	29 (38.2)	—	0	0	—
		F/U 37–58	0	7 (9.0)	2 (2.3)	9 (12.0)	—	0	0	—
Rambow[72]	Portland	Initial 177	18 (10.7)	—	—	—	—	1 (.6)	—	—
		F/U 44–100	1 (1.1)	—	—	—	—	1 (3.6)	—	—
Davies[73]	Birmingham	110	2 (1.8)	9 (8.2)	6 (5.5)	14 (12.7)	2 (1.8)	0	3 (2.7)	—

* NG = *Neisseria gonorrhoeae*
CT = *Chlamydia trachomatis*
TV = *Trichomonas vaginalis*
BV = Bacterial vaginosis
CA = Condyloma-acuminata/or human papilloma virus infection
TP = *Treponema pallidum*
HSV = Herpes simplex virus
HIV = Human immunodeficiency virus
F/U = Follow-up

1.8 to 20.1 percent (see Table 105-1). Rates of gonorrhea at follow-up examination of previously culture-negative victims were 4.0 to zero percent in prospective studies.[64,65,66,68,72]

SYPHILIS

Rates of positive serologic tests for syphilis in sexual assault victims ranged from zero to 3.6 percent (see Table 105-1). Most of these studies did not differentiate between previously treated and newly diagnosed cases of syphilis. Only one serologic conversion suggested a new case of syphilis.[72]

CHLAMYDIA

In 11 studies, the prevalence of *C. trachomatis* infection at initial exam of female victims ranged from 4.7 to 17.1 percent; at followup, the rate of infection in women whose initial cultures were negative and who had not had prophylactic antibiotics ranged from 1.9 to 9 percent (see Table 105-1).

VAGINITIS

Female sexual assault victims have shown rates of trichomonal vaginitis (TV) and bacterial vaginosis (BV) at initial examinations, as high or higher than the rates of infection with *N. gonorrhoeae* or *C. trachomatis* (see Table 105-1). *Candida albicans* infections were found less frequently.

VIRAL STD

The prevalence and rate of acquisition of viral STD have been lower than rates of vaginal bacterial and trichomonal infections in sexual assault victims (see Table 105-1). The prevalence at initial examination of condylomata acuminata in series of female victims where these were explicitly mentioned ranged from 1.8 to 8.9 percent. However, there are few data available on prevalence or acquisition of HPV using DNA amplification tests; or on cytomegalovirus infection; and studies of HSV-2 and HBV seroconversion are limited.

Rates of abnormal Papanicolaou (Pap) smears of the cervix as high as 27.2 percent have been observed in sexual assault victims, reflecting both inflammatory changes associated with the high rates of other infections, as well as neoplastic and preneoplastic changes associated with human papilloma virus infection.[64]

In summary, STDs are frequently diagnosed in sexual assault victims and are common enough to warrant a thorough diagnostic workup for STD as part of a sexual assault evaluation. *N. gonorrhoeae* and *C. trachomatis* are less frequently found than trichomoniasis and bacterial vaginosis among female victims. Syphilis and viral STDs are relatively rarely reported after assault. Nevertheless, in one recent study, HIV infection was extraordinarily common (23.3%) among urban women in the United States who reported having been sexually assaulted in their lifetime.[27] Moreover, HIV infection has been reportedly transmitted through sexual assault.[69,74,75] Hepatitis B has occurred after sexual assault by multiple assailants.[76]

STDs AS EVIDENCE IN SEXUAL ASSAULT CASES

STDs are often a factor in sexual assault cases tried in courts of law in the United States. They have been recognized by criminal courts as proof that sexual contact has occurred, especially where the victim is a child or young adolescent.[77,78] STD has been upheld as evidence of sexual assault when both the defendant and the victim were infected with the same disease.[79,81] Even in an incident when a child victim was infected without evidence that the accused rapist was infected, the Alabama Court of Appeals held that "such . . . evidence was competent to show the corpus delicti" (that a crime had been committed).[82]

When an STD is found in the victim and is thought to be the result of sexual contact with the accused, positive cultures or blood tests for antibodies from the defendant can be helpful as corroborative evidence. The collection of those specimens, however, must be done without violating the defendant's rights. Compulsory physical examinations and blood tests for diagnosis of a sexually transmitted disease without permission of the accused or without a court order to obtain such evidence were once held by some courts to violate witnesses' immunity from testifying against themselves.[83,84] A ruling in 1853 said "that an accused person cannot be compelled to exhibit those portions of his body which are usually covered, for the purpose of securing his identification, or in other ways affording evidence against him."[85]

However, under the modern federal rules of evidence for criminal proceedings, cultures, blood tests, and physical examinations for STD can be done on the defendant, after court hearings are held before a judge to determine "probable cause" that evidence will be recovered. The defendant's fourth amendment rights to protection from unreasonable search and seizure must be respected.[86] Despite multiple legal protections, testing assailants for STDs, particularly HIV, has been extremely controversial. Human rights abuses have been anticipated against both assailant and victim, including breeches in confidentiality and use of HIV serostatus to reduce the credibility of the victim.[87,88]

The interpretation of STD evidence requires a thorough knowledge of the epidemiology, natural course of infection, infectivity, and response to treatment of the STD in question. For instance, if a victim is found to be infected with an STD at the time of a sexual assault, the accused may or may not become infected after a single act of intercourse. Negative cultures obtained from the defendant will not necessarily prove he did not commit the crime.

If positive diagnostic studies are obtained from both the victim and the assailant, matching the organisms for various biologic properties could theoretically be useful in linking the assailant to the crime. Matching of victim and assailant strains by molecular and other techniques, such as serologic typing,[77] and techniques that have established the relatedness of strains of *C. trachomatis* and *N. gonorrhoeae* among sexual partners and the putative source HIV strain in a dentist and patients who subsequently were infected, may be used for forensic purposes.[89–92] Such matching can be used if the characteristics studied are stable from generation to generation in *in vivo* and *in vitro* systems. In one case, HIV gene sequencing using the pol and gag genes instead of the env gene used in the dentist case, was decribed; this sequence may be even more stable.[93] Potentially, these techniques could provide very specific matching of organisms to trace the path of transmission between assailant-victim pairs.

DIAGNOSIS AND TREATMENT OF STD IN VICTIMS OF SEXUAL ASSAULT

DIAGNOSTIC TESTS FOR STD

Initial management

Because of the high prevalence of STDs among adolescents and adults who have been sexually assaulted, their identification following assault may be more important for the medical management of STDs, and for assisting in the psychological and physical recovery of the victim, than for forensic purposes.[94] Diagnostic tests recommended by the Centers for Disease Control and Prevention include cultures for *N. gonorrhoeae* and *C. trachomatis* collected from any sites of penetration or attempted penetration.[94] If chlamydial culture is not available, presumptive nonculture tests for *C. trachomatis* are an acceptable substitute, particularly the nucleic acid amplification tests; if a nonculture test is used, a positive test result should be verified with a second test based on a different diagnostic principle. Nucleic acid amplification tests may offer advantages of increased sensitivity and possible medicolegal use if confirmation is available. Wet mount and culture of a vaginal swab specimen for *T. vaginalis* infection should be performed, and if the vaginal discharge has abnormal characteristics consistent with BV (increased amount, homogeneous, and adherent to vaginal walls, malodorous), then further evaluation for BV is warranted (see Chapter 42). Serum samples for syphilis, hepatitis B (if the patient does not have a history of immunization) and HIV (after counseling) should be collected.

Follow-up examinations

Very often, sexual assault victims do not comply with instructions to return for follow-up examinations weeks after an assault. Symptoms of posttraumatic stress disorder, reactive depression and anxiety may interfere with compliance. Even a victim who is otherwise very knowledgeable about health care issues, may find that repeated visits recommended at 2, 6, 12 and 24 weeks (Table 105-2), prompt recall of a highly traumatic event he or she is trying to forget.[94] Moreover, use of prophylactic antimicrobials, or even treatment for BV or trichomoniasis, may be seen by victims as sufficient management. Nevertheless, follow-up examinations are essential to detect new infections acquired during or after the assault; to complete hepatitis B immunization, if indicated; to complete counseling and treatment for other STDs, injuries, and HIV; and to participate in activities intended to assist in rapid recovery.

At the visit 2 weeks after the assault, examination for bacterial STDs and trichomoniasis, including culture(s) and wet mount, should be repeated, unless prophylactic treatment has been provided. Even if prophylactic treatments have been provided, sexual activity since the assault may warrant repeating the examination.

Table 105-2. Centers for Disease Control and Prevention Recommendations for Prophylaxis and Follow-Up Examinations for Adolescent and Adult Victims of Sexual Assault, 1997[94]

Prophylaxis*
Ceftriaxone 125 mg IM in a single dose
PLUS
Metronidazole 2 g orally in a single dose
PLUS
Azithromycin 1 g orally in a single dose OR doxycycline 100 mg orally two times a day for 7 days
Follow-up Examinations
2-Week Examination
Culture for *Neisseria gonorrhoeae, Chlamydia trachomatis, Trichomonas vaginalis*
Wet-mount and pH determination for bacterial vaginosis
6, 12, 24-Week Examinations
Serologic tests for syphilis, HIV infection, if initial tests were negative

* There are no data to support the effectiveness of these regimens when used prophylactically. For patients requiring alternative treatments, refer to the appropriate sections of the CDC STD Treatment Guidelines.[94]

Serologic tests for syphilis and HIV infection should be repeated 6, 12, and 24 weeks after the assault if initial tests were negative. If positive, the patient should be managed according to published guidelines.[94]

Prophylaxis

Although controversial, most victims probably benefit from prophylaxis because followup is very often difficult and victims may be reassured if offered treatment or prophylaxis for possible infection. Emergency hormonal treatment to prevent pregnancy is an essential part of vaginal sexual assault management.[95] Antiemetics may be of value in assuring compliance, especially with specific drug combinations (e.g., postexposure metronidazole, antiretrovirals [see the following], and contraceptives), although they are not routinely prescribed for any of those agents when used alone. Measures addressing the more common microorganisms are summarized in Table 105-2.[94]

At the initial examination and, as needed in follow-up examinations, patients should be counseled regarding symptoms of STDs and the need for immediate examination if symptoms occur. They should be advised to refrain from sexual intercourse until STD prophylactic treatment is completed.

Since HIV-antibody seroconversion has been reported among persons whose only known risk factor was sexual assault or abuse, HIV infection is clearly a possibility, although the risk is probably minimal in most instances. The risk of transmission of HIV infection may vary by type of sexual exposure (vaginal, anal, oral), presence of trauma, site of exposure to ejaculate and many other factors. Postexposure prophylaxis (PEP) for HIV with zidovudine was associated with reduced risk of HIV infection in a small study of health care workers percutaneously exposed.[96] In a large prospective study of pregnant women treated with zidovudine, a direct protective effect of zidovudine on the fetus and/or infant may have contributed to the two-thirds reduction in perinatal HIV transmission, independent of effects of treatment on maternal viral load.[97] It is not yet known whether these findings can be extrapolated to other HIV exposure situations, such as sexual assault. In many sexual assaults, timely determination of the HIV-infection status of the assailant is not possible. The decision to consider PEP in these situations depends on the nature of the assault, availability of information about assailant HIV risk behaviors (including injection drug or "crack" use), and the local epidemiology of HIV/AIDS.

When the assailant is known to be HIV positive, the assault history suggests a significant risk of HIV transmission (e.g., no condom used, ejaculation, vaginal tears/bleeding, or other factors facilitating potential transmission) and the patient presents for care within 24–36 hours after the assault, antiretroviral PEP should be considered, along with information about the unknown efficacy and known toxicities of antiretrovirals in this situation. The discussion with the victim should also include the need for frequent dosing implicit in prophylactic treatment, the fact that close followup and compliance are essential, and that the treatment must be initiated immediately.[50] At this time, the Public Health Service is developing guidelines for PEP; when these are available, the PEP regimen and HIV counseling and testing should be implemented according to those Public Health Service guidelines, with consideration for drug interactions with concurrently prescribed drugs for STDs or pregnancy prevention.[98] The decision to continue the PEP once it is initiated depends on the results of the victim's test, and whether she or he can tolerate it.

If the testing related to the sexual assault reveals an unsuspected HIV infection in the patient, the extremely sensitive multidisciplinary management of the victim needs to include ensuring that she or he promptly accesses support and therapy. Regardless of the infection status of the victim, it is essential that measures to aid the patient's recovery—the chances for effective prosecution, if the victim at that time or later decides that it should be pursued; and to prevent further abuse of the patient and reduction of risk—be effectively implemented.[11,99,100] The management of sexual assault, a catastrophic act of violence, should be approached within the context of a public health crisis as well as a personal tragedy, with emphasis on reduction of risk of rape, and prevention of sequelae in victims of rape.[101]

References

1 Rodabaugh BJ, Austin M: *Sexual Assault.* New York, Garland STPM Press, 1981, pp. 6–10.

2 Baker TC et al: Rape victims' concerns about possible exposure to HIV infection. *J Interpersonal Violence* 5;49, 1990.

3 U.S. Bureau of the Census: Statistical Abstract of the United States: 1986, 106th Ed. Government Printing Office, Washington DC, 1986, pp. 166.

4 U.S. Department of Justice: *Uniform Crime Reports for the United States.* Washington, DC, Government Printing Office, 1985.

5 U.S. Bureau of the Census: Statistical Abstract of the United States: 1995, 115th ed. Government Printing Office, Washington DC, 1995, pp. 199.

6 Koss MP: Detecting the scope of rape: A review of prevalence research methods. *J Interpersonal Violence* 8;198, 1993.

7 Council on Scientific Affairs, American Medical Association. Violence against women: Relevance for medical practitioners. *JAMA* 267;3184, 1992.

8 National Victim Center, Crime Victims Research and Treatment Center. National Women's Study. In: *Rape in America: A Report to the Nation.* Charleston, SC: Medical University of South Carolina, 1992.

9 Schiff AF: Rape in other countries. *Med Sci Law* 11:3, 1971.

10 Russell DEH: *Sexual Exploitation: Rape, Child Sexual Abuse, and Workplace Harassment.* Beverly Hills, CA, Sage, 1985, p. 35.

11 King M: Sexual assaults on men: Assessment and management. *Br J Hosp Med* 53;245, 1995.

12 Kaufman A et al: Male rape victim: Noninstitutionalized assault. *Am J Psychiatry* 137;221, 1980.

13 Anderson CL: Males as sexual assault victims: Multiple levels of trauma. *J Homosex* 7;145, 1982.

14 Forman BD: Reported male rape. *Victimology* 7:235, 1982.

15 McMullen R. *Male Rape: Breaking the Silence on the Last Taboo.* London, Gay Men's Press, 1990.

16 Groth N, Burgess W: Male rape: Offenders and victims. *Am J Psychiatr* 137;806, 1980.

17 Mezey G, King M: The effects of sexual assault on men: A survey of 22 victims. *Psychol Med* 19;205, 1989.

18 Hickson FCI et al: Gay men as victims of nonconsensual sex. *Arch Sex Behavior* 23;281, 1994.

19 King M: Male rape in institutional settings. In: Mezey G, King MB (eds). *Male Victims of Sexual Assault.* Oxford, Oxford University Press, 1992, p. 67.

20 Holmstrom LL: The criminal justice system's response to the rape victim. In: *Rape and Sexual Assault,* Burgess AW (ed). New York, Garland Publishing, 1985, pp. 189–191.

21 Amir M: *Patterns in Forcible Rape.* Chicago, University of Chicago Press, 1971, pp. 51–52.

22 Dunn SFM, Gilchrist VJ: Sexual assault. *Primary Care* 20;359, 1993.

23 United States Department of Justice, Federal Bureau of Investigation, United States Government Printing Office: Uniform Crime Reports for the United States, 1988, pp. 46–48.

24 Ramin S et al: Sexual assault in postmenopausal women. *Obstet Gynecol* 80;861, 1992.

25 Ruckman LM: Victims of rape: The physician's role in treatment. *Curr Opinion Obstet Gynecol* 5;721, 1993.

26 *Report to the Nation on Crime and Justice: The Data.* Washington, DC, U.S. Department of Justice, NCJ-87068, 1983, p. 20.

27 Irwin KL et al: Urban rape survivors: Characteristics and prevalence of human immunodeficiency virus and other sexually transmitted diseases. *Obstet Gynecol* 85;330, 1995.

28 Peterson RD, Bailey WC: Forcible rape, poverty and economic inequality in US metropolitan communities. *J Quant Criminol* 4;99, 1988.

29 Bourgois P, Dunlap E: Exorcising sex-for-crack: An ethnographic perspective from Harlem. In: Ratner MS (ed). *Crack Pipe as Pimp: An Ethnographic Investigation of Sex-for-Crack Exchanges.* New York, Lexington Books, 1993, pp. 97–132.

30 Smikle CB et al: Physical and sexual abuse. A middle-class concern? *J Reproductive Med* 40;347, 1995.

31 Koss MP et al: The scope of rape: Incidence and prevalence of sexual aggression and victimization in a national sample of higher education students. *J Consult Clin Psych* 55;162, 1987.

32 Sorensen SB et al: The prevalence of adult sexual assault: The Los Angeles Epidemiologic Catchment Area Project. *Am J Epidemiol* 126; 1154, 1987.

33 Satin AJ et al: The prevalence of sexual assault: A survey of 2404 puerperal women. *Am J Obstet Gynecol* 167;973, 1992.

34 Katz S, Mazur MA: *Understanding the Rape Victim: A Synthesis of Research Findings.* New York, Wiley, 1979, pp. 132–133.

35 Koss MP, Harvey MR: *The Rape Victim: Clinical and Community Interventions,* 2nd Ed. *Newbury Park, CA, Sage, pp. 36, 120, 160, 1991.*

36 Furey FM: Sexual abuse of adults with mental retardation. *Mental Retardation* 32;173, 1994.

37 Rinear EE: Sexual assault and the handicapped victim. In: Burgess AW (Ed). *Rape and Sexual Assault: A Research Handbook.* New York, Garland Publishing, 1985, pp. 139–145.

38 Lizotte AJ: The uniqueness of rape: Reporting assaultive violence to the police. *Crime Delinquency* 31:169, 1985.

39 Swiss S, Giller JE. Rape as a crime of war. *JAMA* 270;612, 1993.

40 Abel GG et al: Self-reported sex crimes of nonincarcerated paraphiliacs. *J Interpersonal Violence* 2:3, 1987.

41 National Commission on AIDS. HIV disease in correctional facilities. National Commission on AIDS. Washington, DC, 1991, p. 10.

42 Heimberger TS et al: High prevalence of syphilis detected through a jail screening program: A potential measure to address the syphilis epidemic. *Arch Intern Med* 153;1799, 1993.

43 vanHoeven KH et al: Drug use among New York City prison inmates: a demographic study with temporal trends. *Int J Addiction* 26;1089, 1991.

44 McCutchan JA: Epidemiology of venereal urethritis: Comparison of gonorrhea and nongonococcal urethritis. *Rev Infect Dis* 6:669, 1984.

45 Holmes KK et al: An estimate of the risk of men acquiring gonorrhea by sexual contact with infected females. *Am J Epidemiol* 91:170, 1970.

46 Hooper RR et al: Cohort study of venereal disease. I. The risk of gonorrhea transmission from infected women to men. *Am J Epidemiol* 108;136, 1978.

47 Judson FN: Epidemiology of sexually transmitted hepatitis B infections in heterosexuals: A review. *Sex Transm Dis* 8(suppl);336, 1981.

48 Mosley JW: The epidemiology of viral hepatitis: An overview. *Am J Med Sci* 270;253, 1975.

49 Holmberg SD: Biologic factors in the sexual transmission of human immunodeficiency virus. *J Infect Dis* 160;116, 1989.

50 Katz MH, Geberding JL: Postexposure treatment of people exposed to the human immunodeficiency virus through sexual contact or injection drug use. *N Engl J Med* 336; 1097, 1997.

51 Royce RA et al: Sexual transmission of HIV. *N Engl J Med* 336;1072, 1997.

52 Laga M et al: Non-ulcerative sexually transmitted diseases as risk factors for HIV-1 transmission in women: Results from a cohort study. *AIDS* 7;95, 1993.

53 Cunningham AL et al: Herpes simplex virus type 2 antibody in patients attending antenatal or STD clinics. *Med J Austral* 158;525, 1993.

54 Winkelstein W et al: Sexual practices and risk of infection by the human immunodeficiency virus: The San Francisco Men's Health Study. *JAMA* 257:321, 1987.
55 Groth AN, Burgess AW: Sexual dysfunction during rape. *N Engl J Med* 297:764, 1977.
56 Bownes IT, O'Gorman EC: Assailants' sexual dysfunction during rape reported by their victims. *Med Sci Law* 31;322, 1991.
57 Grubin D: Sexual murder. *Br J Psych* 165;624, 1994.
58 Hook SM et al: Penetration and ejaculation: Forensic aspects of rape. *NZ Med J* 105;87, 1992.
59 Kaufman A et al: Follow-up of rape victims in a family practice setting. *So Med J* 69:1569, 1976.
60 Everett RB, Jimerson GK: The rape victim: A review of 117 consecutive cases. *Obstet Gynecol* 50:88, 1977.
61 Soules et al: The spectrum of alleged rape. *J Reprod Med* 20;33, 1978.
62 Evrard JR, Gold EM: Epidemiology and management of sexual assault victims. *Obstet Gynecol* 53:381, 1979.
63 Tintinalli JE, Hosizer M: Clinical findings and legal resolution in sexual assault. *Ann Emerg Med* 14:447, 1985.
64 Forster GE et al: Incidence of sexually transmitted diseases in rape victims during 1984. *Genitourin Med* 62:267, 1986.
65 Jenny C et al: Sexually transmitted diseases in victims of rape. *N Engl J Med* 322;713, 1990.
66 Estreich S et al: Sexually transmitted diseases in rape victims. *Genitourin Med* 66;433, 1990.
67 Lacey HB: Sexually transmitted diseases and rape: The experience of a sexual assault centre. *Int J STD AIDS* 1;405, 1990.
68 Sturm JT et al: The prevalence of *Neisseria gonorrhoeae* and *Chlamydia trachomatis* in victims of sexual assault. *Ann Emerg Med* 19; 587, 1990.
69 Hillman RJ et al: Sexual assault of men: A series. *Genitourin Med* 66;247, 1990.
70 Ross JDC et al: Rape and sexually transmitted diseases: Patterns of referral and incidence in a department of genitourinary medicine. *J Roy Soc Med* 84;657, 1991.
71 Glaser JB et al: Sexually transmitted diseases in postpubertal female rape victims. *J Infect Dis* 164;726, 1991.
72 Rambow B et al: Female sexual assault: Medical and legal implications. *Ann Emerg Med* 21:78, 1992.
73 Davies AG, Clay JC: Prevalence of sexually transmitted disease infection in women alleging rape. *Sex Transm Dis* 19;298, 1992.
74 Murphy S et al: Rape and subsequent seroconversion to HIV. *Br Med J* 299;718, 1989.
75 Hillman R et al: Rape and subsequent seroconversion to HIV. *Br Med J* 299;1100, 1989.
76 Crowe C et al: A case of acute hepatitis B occurring four months after multiple rape. *Int J STD AIDS* 7;133, 1996.
77 Ahmed HJ et al: An epidemic of *Neisseria gonorrhoeae* in a Somali orphanage. *Int J STD AIDS* 3;52, 1992.
78 Giedinghagen DH. Gonorrhea in children: Epidemiologic unit analysis. *Ped Infect Dis J* 11;973, 1992.
79 *Poe* v *State,* 95 Ark 172, 129 SW 292, 1910.
80 *Long v State,* 84 Ga App 638, 66 SE 2d 837, 1951.
81 *State* v *Mason,* 152 Minn 306, 189 NW 452, 1922.
82 *State* v *Oliver,* 78 ND 398, 49 NW 2nd 564, 1951.
83 *Malone* v *State,* 37 Ala App 432, 71 So 99, 1953.
84 *State* v *Horton,* 247 Mo 663, 153 SW 1051, 1912.
85 *State* v *Nordstrom,* 7 Wash 506, 35 P 382, 1853.
86 *Schmerber* v *California,* 384 US 757, 16 L Ed 2d 908, 86 S CT 1826, 1966.
87 Gostin LO et al: HIV testing, counseling, and prophylaxis after sexual assault. *JAMA* 271;1436, 1994.
88 Herbert B et al: HIV testing, counseling and prophylaxis after sexual assault. *JAMA* 272;1577, 1994.
89 O'Rourke M et al: Opa-typing: A high-resolution tool for studying the epidemiology of gonorrhea. *Mol Microbiol* 17;865, 1995.
90 Poh CL et al: Genetic diversity of *Neisseria gonorrhoeae* IB-2 and IB-6 isolates revealed by whole-cell repetitive element sequence-based PCR. *J Clin Microbiol* 34;292, 1996.
91 Lan J et al: Genotyping of *Chlamydia trachomatis* serovars derived from heterosexual partners and a detailed genomic analysis of serovar F. *Genitourin Med* 71;299, 1995.
92 Ou CY et al: Molecular epidemiology of HIV transmission in a dental practice. *Science* 256;1165, 1992.
93 Albert J et al: Analysis of a rape case by direct sequencing of the the human immunodeficiency virus type 1 pol and gag genes. *Virology* 68;5918, 1995.
94 Centers for Disease Control and Prevention. 1998 Guidelines for treatment of sexually transmitted diseases. *MMWR* 47:108, 1998.
95 Hatcher RA et al: Chapter 16. Emergency contraception: Postcoital options. In: *Contraceptive Technology,* 16th Rev Ed. New York, Irvington Publishers, 1994, p. 415.
96 Cardo DM et al: A case-control study of HIV seroconversion in health-care workers after percutaneous exposure. Centers for Disease Control and Prevention Needlestick Surveillance Group. *N Engl J Med* 337:1542, 1997.
97 Sperling RS et al: Maternal viral load, zidovudine treatment and the risk of transmission of human immunodeficiency virus type 1 from mother to infant. *N Engl J Med* 335;1621, 1996.
98 CDC: Provisional Public Health Service recommendations for chemoprophylaxis after sexual exposure to HIV, in preparation, 1998.
99 Schafran LH. Topics for our times: Rape is a major public health issue. *Am J Public Health* 86;15, 1996.
100 Hamptom HL: Care of the woman who has been raped. *N Engl J Med* 332;234, 1995.
101 D'Onofrio G et al: Care of the victim of rape. *N Engl J Med* 332; 1714, 1995.

Chapter 106

Legal and political aspects of STD prevention: public duties and private rights

Edward P. Richards
Donald C. Bross

The success of public health is determined by law and politics as much as by medical science. All traditional public health triumphs—vaccinations, pasteurization of milk, pure food and drug laws, drinking water sanitation, the eradication of smallpox, and all basic epidemiology that depends on the systematic reporting of communicable diseases—require the coercive power of the government and the consent of the public in democratic societies. Although education and voluntary behavioral change are key parts of public health, they are not enough. Public health cannot be maintained entirely as a voluntary action by enlightened citizens.

STD prevention is the most legally and politically complex public health problem. STDs involve the most intimate human behaviors and are intertwined with deeply held religious and moral beliefs. In our modern "age of the condom," issues of STD control are easily obscured by the rhetoric of personal protection. This chapter outlines the legal and political issues involved in STDs as a public, rather than a private, health issue. It is a guide for both lawmakers and public health professionals.

The political and legal dimensions of STD prevention have prevented any jurisdiction from employing the full range of effective control strategies for STDs. In the United States, which has the resources to support proper STD prevention, short-sighted political expediency has been a problem.[1] In Africa and other third world countries, limited health care and financial resources further complicate STD prevention. It would be a tragedy if legal scholars and public health professionals confuse political expediency with law and morality, and attempt to graft the political choices of the United States onto other countries. Mistakes that can be largely overcome in developed counties might prove devastating to countries whose lack of resources allows for little error in setting STD prevention priorities. The objective of this chapter is to identify the key legal and human rights issues that must be considered in STD prevention programs.

CURRENT TRENDS

The previous version of this chapter was written in 1989, about 8 years into the HIV epidemic. At that time the special issues of HIV were overshadowing other STD prevention efforts, and the hasty reactions to the need for special HIV laws was threatening to undermine both STD prevention programs and disease prevention measures in general. As of this writing in 1996, these trends have continued.

HIV has continued to spread in Africa, and is growing explosively in Asia. The demographics of HIV in the United States are broadening to make it a disease of the disadvantaged, both men and women, as well as of gay men. The fastest increases are in persons of color, drug addicts, and inner-city adolescents.[2] The success of HIV education in the gay community is being questioned as young gay men revert to the dangerous sexual practices of the 1970s, raising the issue of whether decreases in unsafe sex were owing as much to behavioral changes as to the deaths of those who did not change.[3,3a] Some cities are even allowing gay bathhouses to reopen, threatening to repeat the cycle of infection that so devastated the gay community in the early 1980s.[4]

Changes in traditional patterns of travel and land use are resulting in the emergence of new agents and the reemergence of old ones.[5] Urban homelessness, emigrations driven by war and famine, and other dislocations in the human environment are fostering the spread of communicable diseases and hampering control efforts. More fundamentally, the ecology of communicable diseases is changing. The golden age of magic bullets is over. Bacteria and viruses often develop resistance to antimicrobial agents and we should not rely entirely on the development of new agents.

Antimicrobial resistance poses several difficult problems. First, it often drives up the costs of treatment because newer agents are much more expensive. This can make treatment impossible in developing countries. Second, it may shift therapy toward more toxic agents, increasing the risks of treatment and making it more problematic to do epidemiologic treatment. Finally, it may make the disease untreatable. The specter of pan-drug resistant strains of gonorrhea has worried STD prevention programs for years. Although this is not yet a problem, some easily treated STDs, such as gonorrhea, are becoming relatively drug resistant. Given the special difficulties of controlling STDs through behavior modification, and the recognized link between preexisting STD infection and susceptibility to HIV transmission, STD prevention depends on the rational use of antibiotics throughout society.

These trends make it critical that public health and disease control again become a central focus for society. Yet this is complicated by a final trend: the shift from community-oriented public health jurisprudence to a focus on individual rights. This has undermined all aspects of disease control, from the management of tuberculosis to the reporting and investigation of STDs. A paradox addressed in this chapter is why many persons in leadership positions in public health now put the privacy rights of individuals over the health of their community. It has been this shift in the attitudes of public health professionals, rather than a shift in the United States' legal system or international law, that has undermined public health jurisprudence.

INTERNATIONAL LAW AND NATIONAL DEFENSE

The proper exercise of public health authority is grounded in international law and in the laws of the specific country where the control measures are applied. Until recently, international law was concerned only with the relations between states. The first right of a nation state is self-preservation, whether from external attack or internal threat. These threats may be military, demographic, economic, or environmental.[6] Historically, the prime environmental threat was disease. The black plague destroyed the fabric of European society in the Middle Ages. The diseases carried by Western missionaries and sailors did more to destroy indigenous cultures than did their religious and cultural imperialism.[7] Epidemic disease has been resisted with quarantines, embargoes, and limitations on travel since the earliest days of international commerce, making the right to close one's borders to outside threats fundamental to international law.

National defense concerns have also driven both general communicable disease and STD prevention efforts. Disease control is fundamental to maintaining an army in the field. It has only been in the last 75 years that munitions have outstripped disease as a killer of soldiers. STDs have always followed military campaigns. Even in the United States, the only serious political commitments to controlling gonorrhea and syphilis grew out of a concern with military readiness.[8]

NATIONAL LAW

A central role of a nation is to protect its citizens from harms that they, individually, are unable to fend off.[9] Nations with Anglo-American legal systems discuss this right in terms of *parens patria*, police powers, and other formulations that recognize the authority of the state to protect its citizens, even from themselves. Since these labels have less meaning in nations that do not have Anglo-American legal systems, we will also discuss legal roles from a more general human rights perspective. Although the rules may differ in other countries, the public policy issues in the U.S. cases are universal.

A nation may choose to act as a parent and prevent a citizen from harming him- or herself. Laws against suicide are a clear example of this protection from self-harm. Although some cultures view this protection from self as contrary to their societal norms, many endorse it as a valid concern to protect society by preserving its productive citizens. The broadest consensus on the necessity to prevent self-harm is the protection of minors from personally harmful behavior, such as smoking and drinking.

A nation may choose not to protect its citizens from self-harm, without necessarily creating a serious threat to general public safety. A nation must, however, exercise a police function to protect citizens from other citizens. Again, the basic motivation of this protection is the preservation of the nation itself, with the citizen's individual welfare a secondary concern. The crime that best illustrates this motivation is mayhem, which was the crime of injuring a person so that he would not be an effective soldier.[10] The mayhem law protected individual citizens from injury, both the immediate injury and the possibility of future injury derivative of the inability to protect oneself, but the intent was to protect the king's ability to raise an army.

U.S. CONSTITUTIONAL STATUS OF PUBLIC HEALTH LAWS

There are many philosophical differences between public health and criminal laws, but the legal distinction in the United States is rooted in the Constitution. The U.S. Constitution requires that before individuals may be punished, their guilt must be determined by a jury under procedural rules designed to protect their rights. The Constitution does not require that these same protections be provided when the person is being restricted to protect the public health and safety. This distinction was present in the colonial period, was recognized by the drafters of the Constitution, and was consistently upheld until the 1960s.

In 1967, the United States Supreme Court called this distinction into question with the decision of In re Gault, and rejected it in large part with In re Winship.[11,12] Both of these cases dealt with minors in trouble with the law, who had been sent to juvenile facilities. Both boys had a court hearing, but in neither case did the state law give them the same procedural protections required to convict an adult and send the adult to prison. Since these laws were not intended to punish the minors, but to remove them from the community and maintain them in a disciplined, structured environment, they passed the traditional test for a public health or *parens patria* measure. The U.S. Supreme Court disagreed, looking instead at the conditions of confinement rather than the stated intent of the law. The Court held that if the offender was locked up, then it must be a criminal law and the person was entitled to criminal law due process protections.

These holdings implicitly questioned much of public health jurisprudence involving the restriction of individuals. Interpreted one way, they would have justified the assumption of some legal scholars that traditional public health law would not stand modern Constitutional review. In a series of decisions involving sexual predators, the mentally ill, pretrial detainees, the refusal to release a prisoner after a successful habeas corpus petition, and the pretrial detention of a defendant to prevent the defendant from committing crimes, the U.S. Supreme Court limited In re Gault and In re Winship, and explicitly rejected them in part.[13–17] The Court forcefully stated that individuals could be restricted to protect the public health and safety without full criminal law due process protections, as long as the intent of law was prevention rather than punishment.

THE PROPER SCOPE OF PUBLIC HEALTH LAW

Public health laws may be used only to prevent future harmful conduct, not to punish past behavior, compensate injured persons, or as a subterfuge for impermissible medical experiments.[18] Although criminal laws are concerned with the state of mind of the defendant, public health laws are only concerned with the threat posed by the individual. Active (infectious) tuberculosis is a good illustration of the difference between public health and criminal laws. Assume that a man has active tuberculosis and is at large in the community, under no public health isolation orders. (This is a common occurrence in jurisdictions that require extensive court hearings before allowing disease carriers to be restricted.) This tuberculosis carrier infects a fellow passenger on a bus, and the passenger eventually dies from the infection.

The causation is clear—the bus passenger died because of the actions of the disease carrier. This would not be a crime because there was no evil intent or reckless disregard of societal rules, thus it would be impermissible to incarcerate the tuberculosis carrier as a punishment for spreading the disease. In contrast, it would be a proper exercise of public health authority to restrict this tuberculosis carrier to prevent the spread of disease.[19] When the carrier is successfully cured and rendered noninfectious, the health department's authority to hold him would end.

PUBLIC HEALTH PROCEDURAL DUE PROCESS

The authority of the public health officer to take certain actions against individuals without having to go to court first is a special case of the general right of individuals and society to act against immediate threats. Fire departments routinely break into buildings and destroy their contents as part of their efforts to prevent the spread of fire. Many times this is without the consent of the owner, and they have the right to proceed even if the owner does not want the fire extinguished. Governmental officials are permitted to take emergency actions without legal process because society recognizes that the delay necessary for even rudimentary court supervision would make effective action impossible. These actions are subject to review after the fact by both the government and private citizens.[20]

Some public health actions are emergencies in that minutes or hours matter. These actions mostly involve contaminated food, accidental spills of toxic chemicals, and certain communicable disease outbreaks. In these situations, governmental action would be ineffective if it required prior court approval. Most public health actions, including STD prevention, are done on longer time frames. Although it might be theoretically possible to get court review for these actions, this is not constitutionally mandated. These actions are reviewed under the standards for administrative law, the branch of law that governs the actions of noncriminal justice governmental agencies.

Boards of health were among the first governmental agencies and figure in many historic constitutional cases. As applied to public health actions, administrative law has two major tenets. First, decisions should be made by experts, not lay judges and juries. Administrative law recognizes that decisions that involve technical or scientific information must be made by persons with proper educational training and experience. The agency will be required to show that it has an expert justification for its decision, and a procedure to assure that the regulatory process is carried out in a consistent and even-handed manner. The court will defer to the agency's decision unless it finds that it is arbitrary or capricious, that is, that it did not follow that agency's procedures or that it was not consistent with the agency's rationale. The court will not allow litigants to contest whether the agency made the correct choice from acceptable alternatives.[21]

The second tenet is that agencies must be free to act with the minimum of judicial involvement so that they can make routine decisions without incurring huge costs. These transaction costs for decision making are called "agency costs." As an example, the Social Security Administration of the United States processes millions of benefits claims each year. If every determination that affected a citizen's rights required court review, the costs of providing a court hearing would be more than many of the claims the agency is asked to pay. It would also increase the cost of making a claim beyond the means of most claimants.

Agency costs are very critical to the functioning of the agency. If the agency costs are too high, the agency cannot act. A common political strategy to destroy an agency's ability to regulate is to raise its costs with procedural requirements. The group demanding the higher procedural requirements claims that it is just protecting the rights of the regulated entities, not attempting to paralyze the agency. The efforts to require agencies to pay landowners for any diminished value of their property owing to regulation is an attempt to raise agency costs to a prohibitive level. Civil libertarian groups have been very successful in crippling public health agencies by demanding extensive legal procedural protections before the agency can impose any restrictions on individuals. The agencies lose their ability to act because they do not have the resources to litigate each case. (This is further complicated in the United States because health departments are usually not allowed to have their own lawyers. They must depend on the city, county, or state attorneys to act for them, and these attorneys are often disinterested in public health enforcement.)

Public health authority must be broad and flexible to meet the challenges of new diseases and new knowledge about old diseases. Until recently this was the rule. Even in the United States, with its suspicion of unconstrained public authority, state laws generally gave health officers the authority to do whatever was necessary to protect the public health. These statutes specified the broad outlines of disease control programs, leaving to the discretion of the health officer the specific details on which diseases will be reported, within what time frame, in what form, and how the infected individuals will be managed. The health officer then promulgated regulations to detail the specifics of the disease control strategies. These administrative regulations give notice of a citizen's obligations, but may be quickly changed to reflect changes in disease dynamics. Courts have struck down laws that used unfounded public health arguments to support discriminatory actions against racial or ethnic groups, but in general the courts defer to the expertise of local health officers.[22]

The United States Supreme Court has found few limits on the authority of public health officials to take whatever actions are, in their expert opinion, necessary to protect the public's health. These have included imposing quarantines on large geographic areas, holding persons infected with communicable diseases in custody to prevent the spread of the disease, the forced treatment of disease carriers, and the seizure and destruction, without compensation, of any property that threatens the public health.[23] Most countries have done the same.

Historically, the Court's deference to expert decision making and the political process in public health jurisprudence resulted in a bias toward the community's health and the prevention of communicable disease. Unfortunately, as the public lost its fear of communicable diseases, the societal consensus on public health has broken down. Its consequences are profound for public health because public health professionals themselves have abandoned their support for disease control measures. Since courts look to public health professionals to set the acceptable limits of public health authority, it is critical to understand why these professional have abandoned their willingness to exercise that authority on the behalf of the community.

THE SHIFT TO PERSONAL HEALTH SERVICES

Nations support disease control measures in proportion to the citizenry's fear of communicable diseases. In the United States and other industrialized countries, the fear of communicable diseases has diminished greatly since the polio epidemics of the 1950s.[24] With the advent of broad-spectrum antimicrobials and effective vaccines, the medical establishment and the general public shifted its interest to the treatment and prevention of chronic diseases, especially cancer and cardiovascular diseases. This was appropriate for a developed country such as the United States where the vast majority of premature deaths were no longer owing to infectious disease. The problem came in the pursuit of these avenues to the neglect of maintaining the disease control programs and public health–related research and training necessary to keep communicable diseases in check.

In addition to the emphasis on chronic diseases, the 1960s also saw dramatic expansions of federal and state programs to provide medical care to indigent persons. As this federal money flowed into communities, health departments began to be centers for providing personal medical care and social services. Many state health departments became the intermediary, distributing federal and state personal health services dollars. Since the cost of personal health services dwarfs those of disease control services, often at 100:1 ratios in personnel and dollars, public health disease control became a very minor part of health department activities. (Perhaps the only significant exception was the overreaction to the outbreak of Swine flu in the 1970s, a reflection of the politicization of public health decision making that had occurred by that time.)[25] As the health departments became personal health services centers, health directors and health officers who were professionals skilled in communicable disease control were replaced with persons whose expertise was in the delivery in personal health services.

Unfortunately, public health and personal health services have profoundly different professional and legal paradigms. The "client" in public health is society, not the individual disease carrier. It is not that the infected individual's rights do not matter, it is that they may be secondary to the rights of society. A public health focus also assumes that an individual should no more be allowed to choose to carry or be exposed to a communicable disease than a person should be allowed to consent to being the victim of a crime.

This difference in paradigms has many manifestations. Effective public health management and planning depends on knowing the prevalence of communicable diseases in the community, whether the demographics of known diseases are shifting, and whether new diseases are emerging. Such epidemiologic information demands systematic testing for communicable diseases, reporting of positive tests, and the investigation of the reports. These activities are carried out irrespective of the wishes of the infected person. In contrast, personal health services are based on the informed consent of the patient. Since the core legal requirement defining informed consent is the right to refuse, patients have an almost unlimited right to refuse personal medical services.[26] This includes refusing to be tested and treated for communicable diseases.

The core difference is the psychology of the relationship between public health professional and the client. Well-run indigent health care and social service programs encourage a trusting relationship between the client and the professional, with the professional often becoming personally invested in the concerns of the client. This is exacerbated in programs such as family medicine clinics that have long-term dealings with the client. Disease prevention professionals have many concerns in addition to the patient's own care. Although they should not be dishonest with patients, they must resist the temptation to the interests of the clinic patients above those of society.

As traditional disease prevention professionals were replaced with personal health services professionals, health departments began to be advocates for their patients rather than for society. They incorporated patient empowerment rhetoric from the bioethics movement into health department policies, ignoring the conflict with their traditional role as protectors of society. When HIV fueled public fears of contagion in the early 1980s, health departments were in the forefront with education campaigns stressing that HIV is only a problem for people who do not take precautions to protect themselves. Although this was a useful step in reducing discrimination against HIV-infected persons, it was carried to the extreme of denying the value of traditional disease control measures such as reporting and contact tracing.[27–27d]

POLITICAL PRESSURES IN PUBLIC HEALTH

The metamorphosis from protecting the public to seeing the primary clients of the health department as the patients in its clinics was encouraged by political realities: Politicians decide the merits of programs based on their political support. With no public clamor for public health, politicians only see the special interest groups most affected by the health department rules. These include restaurateurs who do not want to meet food inspection standards, developers who want to use septic tanks rather than sanitary sewers, and persons with communicable diseases who do not want to restrict their lifestyles to prevent the spread of disease. For example, with no public opposition to their operation, and gay political groups lobbying to keep them open, the bathhouses were not closed in the 1970s when their role in the explosive transmission of STDs was first documented. Although the courts found no constitutional right to frequent bathhouses, most cities did not close them until the mid-1980s, after most of their patrons were dead or dying.[28]

Health directors who did not bend to the demands of special interests found their programs thwarted.[29] Eventually most found themselves out of office, replaced with more politically malleable individuals. In many instances, public health physicians were replaced with nonphysicians, and in some cases with persons with neither disease prevention nor medical care training. The result in the United States has been to demoralize and deprofessionalize public health. This was documented in the most detailed study of the United States public health, the Institute of Medicine's (IOM) 1988 Report, The Future of Public Health, which described the system as ". . . a hodgepodge of agencies, and well-intended but unbalanced appropriations without coherent direction by well-qualified professionals."[30] When the IOM's Committee on Emerging Microbial Threats to Health revisited the issue in 1992, it reported:

> It is the committee's view that there has been little positive change in the U.S. public health system since the release of that [the 1988 IOM] report. The recent rapid increases in the incidence of measles and tuberculosis are evidence of these continuing problems. . . . Steps have been taken to address inadequacies in these programs, but these responses are reactive, not proactive. It is the committee's belief that the *prevention* of infectious diseases must be stressed if the health of this nation's inhabitants is to be maintained or improved.[31]

With the public health establishment increasingly unwilling to support disease prevention programs, it is not surprising that public health laws became a low priority with the city and county prosecutors charged with enforcing them. Murder cases and other criminal law prosecutions drive the headlines necessary for reelection and promotion. Public health cases usually go to the lawyer with the least seniority, who moves on to other matters as soon as possible. Successes are largely impossible, and failures, as represented by disgruntled "victims" of efforts to prevent disease, can use laws on confidentiality to present only a partisan view of the issues. With few governmental attorneys with either experience or institutional memory of public health enforcement as a counterweight, legal scholars who are opposed to disease prevention measures have been very influential in shaping the media's views on public health law.

PRIVATE LAW AND STD CONTROL

The state's role in disease prevention law is to prevent the spread of disease. There is also a private law remedy to compensate persons injured by disease carriers who do not take proper precautions to prevent the spread of their disease. This is called tort law, and it is most extensively developed in the United States because attorneys in the United States may prosecute a case for a percentage of the ultimate recovery and are not required to pay the attorney's fees and costs of the winning party.

The United States has well-articulated liability theories that will be applied to the three types of communicable disease compensation cases: (1) infectees suing infectors; (2) infectees suing physicians for failing to warn them that a patient of the physician was a disease carrier; and (3) patients suing their physicians for medical malpractice. There have been cases awarding compensation for infecting an unsuspecting person with an STD and for malpractice in treating a STD.[32] A physician who fails to report HIV in a state that attempts to warn persons at risk will be sued for negligence per se: the tort remedy for breaking a law.[33] These are difficult lawsuits to defend because the reporting law sets the standard of behavior.

In general, tort law has not been an effective incentive for disease prevention. There has been little litigation over the negligent transmission of STDs because there is no one to pay the compensation and the attorney's fees: Few STD carriers are wealthy enough to pay a court-ordered award, and all insurance policies exclude coverage for STD transmission. There have been a few awards against physicians for failing to take proper disease control measures, but most litigation involving physicians has been over patient privacy issues. These lawsuits generally attempt to limit the access to information about STDs, creating an incentive for physicians to not conduct proper disease reporting, testing, and disease control. Physicians should expect to see more litigation over failing to made a timely diagnosis of HIV as antiviral therapies become more effective. (One court has already awarded in excess of one million dollars in such a case.[34])

DISEASE REPORTING

The importance of incidence, prevalence, and population data make reporting of STDs a logical foundation for a STD prevention program. High-quality data on disease epidemiology may be obtained by large-scale surveys of randomly sampled practitioners, without requiring routine individual disease reports. This type of survey is expensive and time-consuming, making it virtually impossible to detect short-term changes in disease dynamics. Surveys that preserve the anonymity of those surveyed also fail to address the duty to warn, which requires the identification of individual infected patients.

Requiring physicians to report each infected individual for selected STD has been a component of STD prevention for many years in the United States. Unfortunately, epidemiologic information about STDs has been very difficult to collect even with legal persuasion, in part because of the health care providers concerns with protecting their patients' privacy.[35] Such legislation should recognize the three functions served by reporting: (1) statistical assessment of disease epidemiology; (2) direct disease control interventions; and (3) discharge of the physician's duty to warn persons at risk of contracting a disease from the patient.

Requiring individual reporting of STDs (passive surveillance) does not assure adequate epidemiologic data. The most effective approach is a combination of mandated reporting with active surveillance by the health department (e.g., polling by the designated practitioners most likely to diagnose and treat STDs). Many physicians do not comply with their statutory reporting duties, but will supply information on request. Other approaches to surveillance are discussed in Chap. 97.

STD RISK ANALYSIS

Disease reporting is minimally intrusive and has been used for many STDs, mostly without controversy. Although politics have prevented most states from requiring the reporting of HIV, those that do require it to be reported have not experienced any problems. Disease reporting is just the beginning of STD prevention. Contact tracing, screening, and treatment pose more difficult legal questions as to balance between individual and community rights. This balance must be based on a scientific analysis of benefits of the proposed intervention, not on its political popularity. An ineffective strategy is not justifiable, even if constitutionally permitted.

The simplest way to express this analysis of benefits from an intervention is in terms of the magnitude of the disease burden to society in the absence of the intervention, and the extent of reduction in the magnitude of risk that can be achieved by the intervention. One way of expressing the magnitude of the disease burden is to estimate the direct and indirect costs, as well as the noneconomic social costs of the various STDs. Another way is to express the magnitude of the "risk" (R) to society for a communicable disease as determined by the severity (S) of the disease, its transmissibility (T), and the number of persons at risk (P): (R) = (S)(T)(P). Although these factors are difficult or impossible to reduce to meaningful numeric values, (R) increases as any or all of the three factors increase.

Severity may range from very low (the common cold) to high (HIV). Transmissibility may range from high (gonorrhea) to extremely low (leprosy). The population at risk may range from the entire population (a complete new strain of influenza, to which no one has immunity) to all sexually active individuals involved in sex and networks not exclusively monogamous (gonorrhea) to persons with defects in their immune systems (e.g., communicable opportunistic infections).

It is obvious that the time frame for the spread and progression of the disease could greatly affect societal perception of the magnitude of risk (R). Diseases that spread rapidly and cause immediate illness are most likely to be recognized as a great threat to society. They can overwhelm the health care system. The obviousness of the threat prompts the mobilization of the resources necessary to contain the threat. HIV is more insidious; although it can spread relatively rapidly through vulnerable societies (e.g., reaching high, stable prevalence in 5 years or less), acquisition of the infection is on average disassociated from symptomatic illness and death by many more years. The 1997 Institute of Medicine report on sexually transmitted diseases emphasizes that this disassociation between acquisition of infection and onset of severe sequelae (e.g., infertility, cancers) is true of many STDs.[36]

GONORRHEA AS A MODEL

Gonorrhea is an extremely common disease, which makes it readily susceptible to statistical analysis. It is a disease that afflicts industrialized countries, countries that have the money to invest in medical and sociological research. It is also, unlike HIV, a disease without a political constituency. These factors result in gonorrhea being among the best understood of the STDs.[37]

Yet for all of this understanding, gonorrhea is still a scourge, causing significant morbidity from pelvic inflammatory disease and sterility. This is true, despite the ease with which gonorrhea is treated. Gonorrhea is also a useful model for the transmission of other STDs. Political considerations aside, there are strong parallels between the epidemiology of gonorrhea and sexually transmitted components of HIV infections. Both are sexually transmitted diseases, both have a substantial prevalence in the community (gonorrhea because carriers rapidly become reinfected, and HIV because carriers remain infected), and they share the dynamics that contacts with a relatively small group of infected individuals account for a disproportionate fraction of new infections. For these reasons, insights from the risk calculus of gonorrhea should be useful in evaluating legal strategies for the prevention of all STDs.

Although gonorrhea has been eliminated as an endemic disease in some industrialized regions of the world, and the incidence continues to decline in the United States, the disease is sufficiently far from the extinction point, and incremental changes in the resources available for gonorrhea control might well result in proportional declines in gonorrhea incidence. The gonorrhea equilibrium is rapidly responsive in that changes in sexual behaviors or prevention resources are reflected in changes in gonorrhea rates in less than 2 months.[36] In the United States, many states and local programs have chosen to allocate only enough resources to gonorrhea control programs to set the incidence point at levels many times higher than that of virtually all other industrialized countries. Assuming that this resource allocation has been rationally determined, then it reflects the amount of money that these states and localities in the United States are willing to invest in a disease that poses the risk (R) of gonorrhea to their societies.

A legally significant characteristic of gonorrhea is that it is a disease whose incidence and prevalence in the general population are driven by core groups of transmitters. Although there may be mixing between core groups and the general population, it is the incidence and prevalence of gonorrhea in this core group that largely determines gonorrhea dynamics. Thus, core group members pose a disproportionate threat to the community, justifying legal strategies that disproportionately focus on members of this core group. These strategies are good law precisely because they flow from good science.

Core group transmission is possible for diseases that do not induce solid, lasting immunity, thus allowing members of a subpopulation to remain infectious for months if not treated, and to acquire multiple reinfections. Thus, core group members cycle between uninfected (susceptible) and infected with gonorrhea. This results in what is termed a susceptible, infected-susceptible, or SIS dynamic.[38] Since infection with gonorrhea renders a person infectious essentially at once, the probability that a core group member will be infectious at a given time is determined by three intervals: the delay between infection and treatment; the duration of infection without treatment; and the delay between treatment or spontaneous cure of infection and reinfection. Increased numbers of sexual partners in a given time increases the reinfection rate, asymptomatic disease increases the delay between infection and treatment. The role of core groups in transmission of other STD has been extremely discussed elsewhere; and is assessed in Chaps. 3 and 4.[38]

IDENTIFYING CORE GROUP MEMBERS

Core group members can be identified on the basis of behavioral, sociodemographic, and medical criteria.[38,39] Social demographic and medical (e.g., past or current STD) factors are valuable in determining which groups to target for prevention measures, including screening and contact tracing.

CASE-FINDING

Screening is the process of testing persons for a sexually transmitted infection. Screening may be nonselective, or it may be selective based on identified risk factors. Contact tracing also is a subset of the general class of case-finding strategies. Because gonorrhea is spread by core groups, blind screening of the general population is not as effective as screening persons with certain risk factors for acquiring or transmitting gonorrhea. For example, previous infection with gonorrhea increases the probability that a given person is a core group member. Seeking out and testing these previously infected persons is rescreening: ". . . rescreening is approximately four times as effective per number of individuals tested as screening in reducing incidence. The intuitive reason why rescreening is more effective than screening is that since rescreened individuals were infected before, they are more likely to be infectious again when rescreened."[40]

Thus for gonorrhea, limited screening resources are best spent monitoring the infectious status of known core group members. To the extent that there are privacy concerns about screening, the legal rationale for rescreening known core group members is stronger than the rationale for de novo screening of the general population.

CONTACT TRACING

Contact tracing is used in the investigation of all communicable diseases. Despite its effectiveness in controlling diseases such as tuberculosis, measles, hepatitis, and bringing persons with curable STDs to treatment, contact tracing is one of the most controversial issues in HIV prevention.[41] It has been criticized because of coercion, because it is not perfectly effective, and because it might increase the chance of violence toward infected women.[42] Even the term is being abandoned in favor of partner notification.[43]

Partner notification is a very narrow concept, properly limited to intentional voluntary relationships. It is appropriate for a spouse or lover, but not for rapists or pederasts, for medical personnel, or other nonconsensual exposures. We continue to use contact tracing because it is the more general term and because it stresses that HIV prevention must be part of an overall public health approach to communicable disease prevention.

The fears of contact tracing are ungrounded. First, no jurisdiction in the United States coerces individuals to divulge the names of their contacts. This would not be justified in contact tracing for STDs because effective contact tracing does not depend on perfect reporting. The overlapping sexual networks make it likely that the individuals with the most contacts will be identified by at least one contact. Most people infected with an STD cooperate in identifying their contacts.[44] The identity of the reporter of the contact is never divulged: The contact is only told that he or she has been exposed to a STD. By investigating the named contacts to identify their spouses and other individuals at high risk, most of the persons at risk can be identified. The contact is usually approached by a public health investigator, but in some circumstances the reporter may prefer personally to give his or her partner a "contact slip" that explains the risk of infection with an STD and provides information on how to contact the public health department for medical testing or treatment. The contacts that are missed will be those at lowest risk, and although it would be ideal to identify all contacts, the risk to the community is lower, even if there are still some individuals at risk.

The finding that contact tracing puts women at risk for domestic violence is real and troubling, but it is neither new nor limited to HIV. The typical scenario is the woman who is screened as part of her prenatal care and found to be HIV-infected. The investigator then notifies her husband, who is often the source of the disease, who assaults his wife for involving him with the public health officers. This same problem has always plagued STD prevention. Before HIV, the problem was syphilis, which is also subject to prenatal screening because of the risk of congenital syphilis.[45] (It was not so long ago that infection with syphilis also carried a harsh social stigma.) Although there is the risk of violence, this threat may be owing to the absence of systematic contact tracing. In a community that has HIV reporting requirements, enforces these requirements, and traces all cases of HIV, there should be few cases of HIV first identified as women seek medical care.

This is a critical problem to solve because, with the proven efficacy of antiviral therapies in preventing most cases of perinatal infection, some believe it is morally unacceptable not to screen pregnant women for HIV. It also has profound legal implications because physicians are legally liable for preventable injuries to the babies born to the women for whom they provide care. As cases involving other medical tests have demonstrated, juries tend to assume that patients only refuse simple tests because the physician was negligent in informing the patient of the benefits of the test.[46] With an innocent baby as the plaintiff, and the mother likely dead by the time of trial, these will be very difficult cases to defend.

It is also morally questionable to not warn sexual contacts of a person with newly diagnosed HIV infection of their risk of infection because of the potential for interrupting the spread of the HIV through directed informing and counseling. The United States now requires states seeking federal grant money for HIV-related services to make a good faith to notify the spouses of HIV-infected persons that they are at risk of HIV infection and should seek testing.[47] It seems discriminatory to deny this same protection to unmarried couples and to homosexual partners.

The most fundamental criticism of contact tracing for HIV is that the only justification for tracing HIV carriers is to treat them, and that since there is as yet no cure for HIV, there is not reason to identify contacts. However, the advent of more effective antiretroviral combination therapies, growing interest in early therapy, and the benefits of intervention for preventing opportunistic infections, all rebut this criticism. Further, the relatively lower transmissibility of HIV (compared with that of gonorrhea) means that (1) contact tracing for HIV can warn persons as yet uninfected that they are being exposed to HIV by one of their partners; and (2) for persons unaware of their infection, it provides an early warning so that they may take measures to protect their loved ones. (These self-imposed restrictions will be most critical for women of childbearing potential.) If individuals with early HIV infection are most likely to spread the infectious disease, identification by contact tracing of those with new infections may be important in interrupting transmission.[48] Treatment may also reduce infectivity, which could have significant impact in reducing the spread of HIV.[47] Finally, for any STD, contact tracing allows the identification of the small but epidemiologically significant number of persons who may know they are infected yet continue to act in a socially irresponsible manner.

INVOLUNTARY SCREENING, TREATMENT, AND RESTRICTIONS

Informed consent to all medical treatment and testing has become a fundamental tenet of the international medical and bioethics communities. It is a laudable goal, but it poses three difficult questions for STD prevention: (1) What if the patient refuses lifesaving treatment? (2) What if the patient refuses treatment that would make him or her noninfectious? and (3) If it is impossible to "fully" inform every patient, should that alone deny the affected person effective treatment that might otherwise not be provided in a timely manner?

The first question poses few problems and most courts allow mentally competent adults to refuse medical treatment if the only risk is to themselves. The second is much more difficult because it implies a choice to endanger others. For communicable diseases, as opposed to most noncommunicable diseases, this is always a consideration. The courts in the United States uphold orders requiring involuntary treatment to avoid putting the public at risk. The patient is usually given a choice between incarceration and treatment, and it is very unusual for the court to order the use of physical force to overcome the patient's objections to treatment. However, international disease control programs, such as the smallpox eradication program, have found it necessary to use aggressive strategies, including involuntary immunization and bribing villagers to report hidden cases of disease.[49]

The third question deals with a special case of no informed consent; the patient would be willing to accept the treatment, but for language, educational, cultural, or medical reasons, it is not possible to get a full informed consent. In these cases it is very important to differentiate between research and care that is intended to benefit the patient or the community. If the goal of the intervention is solely research, with no potential benefits to the patient, then the international treaties on medical research apply. In these cases, consent is mandatory before testing or treatment.

For most STDs, the patient and the community benefit from testing and treatment. Even acquisition of useful epidemiologic information is of sufficient value to override the patient's privacy interests.[50] In these cases it would be proper to test or treat a willing patient or a mentally incompetent or unresponsive patient who otherwise might not have been able to give an effective consent to research.[51] It would also be proper to treat people based on the epidemiologic risk of STD exposure, without proof of infection. Such strategies will be very important in developing countries where American-style "informed consent" may be impossible. For example, a program that treats STDs to determine if this reduces HIV infection could be justified as beneficial treatment, rather than as research.

Isolation and quarantine are venerable techniques to public health officials.[52] The use of confinement in the case of STDs, however, seems to have little practical use. Unlike many diseases, intimate contact is required for the spread of STDs. In effect, drawing a blood sample or administering an antibiotic under medically indicated circumstances is a less restrictive means of state intervention in the control of STDs than isolation.

The fatal and thus far incurable nature of HIV infection may force attention to isolation as a remedy in rare cases. Depending on the factual situations that arise with HIV infection, for example, associated dementia or an independent mental illness, the courts may well have to consider mental health law and public health law measures for isolating an individual with HIV who is clearly a danger to others or who is gravely disabled and unable to obtain treatment.

Given that isolation is a very restrictive approach to STD control, some comparable mechanism that will ensure participation in examinations and agreements not to expose others is needed. The alternative of health hold orders should be considered. As used here, a health hold order means a specific order issued by an authorized public health official to a named individual to cooperate with examination, treatment, or to behave within certain limits necessary to protect the public health.[53] Such an order could be appealed to the courts in a confidential proceeding. The health hold also might be in the form of a voluntary agreement subject to enforcement by court order, and result in a very brief detention for examination or a "show cause" contempt proceeding if the voluntary agreement is not likely to be kept or in fact is not being kept. Health holds might also be administered conveniently to persons detained in institutional settings for alleged sexual crimes. Health authorities can avoid having the health hold used for nonhealth matters, such as to compel cooperation in criminal matters, by focusing strictly on what is required for individual and epidemiologic treatment of STD.

IMMUNIZATIONS

Currently the only STD with an effective vaccine is hepatitis B. As discussed in Chap. 80, CDC and other U.S. guidelines now call for routine prenatal screening for hepatitis B surface antigen, HBsAg vaccination of all infants (with hepatitis B immunoglobulin for those exposed to HBsAg-positive mothers at birth), as well as vaccination of high-risk teens and adults.[54,55] Lawmakers could require all third-party payers to pay for the vaccine, and should consider mandating the screening of pregnant women for HBsAg. If a pregnant woman is infected, then the law should require that her baby be vaccinated.[56] Given that these babies are not detected where physicians do not comply with the CDC guidelines for screening, HBV could pose nearly as serious a medical malpractice threat as HIV infection in this context.

CONCLUSIONS

Effective laws to prevent STDs are based on accurate understanding of available resources, legal and cultural traditions, and intelligent shaping of legislation to meet sound, and probably narrow, disease prevention goals. Laws to organize the reporting of STDs, the screening of persons at greatest risk, and the tracing of the contacts of disease carriers should be a priority of lawmakers concerned with preventing STDs. Personal privacy and liberty must be protected to the greatest extent possible, consistent with the protection of society from STDs. As demonstrated by the contrast between the magnitude of societal risks for gonorrhea and for HIV infection, the milder the disease, the more it can be tolerated for the sake of preserving personal liberties.

Public and private professionals involved in STD prevention must conform their actions to laws governing diagnosis, treatment, reporting, quarantine, and isolation. Law is an effective device in the prevention of STDs to the extent that it is wielded as one tool in a comprehensive prevention, diagnosis, treatment, and management strategy. Many traditions of public health and legal precedents are valuable standards against which responses to new conditions such as HIV infection must be measured.

References

1 Shilts R: *And the Band Played On: Politics, People, and the AIDS Epidemic.* New York, Penguin Books; 1988 (hereinafter Shilts).

2 Centers for Disease Control: Update: mortality attributable to HIV infection among persons aged 25–44 years: United States, 1994. *MMWR* 45(6):1,1996.

3 Lemp GF et al: Seroprevalence of HIV and risk behaviors among young homosexual and bisexual men: The San Francisco/Berkeley Young Men's Survey. *JAMA* 272(6):449(6), 1994.

3a Van Griensven GJP et al: Changes in sexual behaviour and the fall in incidence of HIV infection among homosexual men. *Br Med J* 298: 218–221, 1989.

4 Neal J: Sex Clubs and Bathhouses again with Some Gay Men, *All Things Considered* (NPR 4:30 PM Et) June 1, 1995, Transcript # 1865–10.

5 Morse SS: Factors in the emergence of infectious diseases. *EID* 1:7, 1995.

6 International Nuclear Safety Advisory Group, Summary Report on the Post-Accident Review Meeting on the Chernobyl Accident, 1 (Safety Series No. 75-INSAG-1, IAEA 1986).

7 McNeill WH: *Plagues and Peoples.* New York, Doubleday, 1976.

8 Cutler JC et al: Venereal disease control by health departments in the past: Lessons for the present. *Am J Pub Health* 78:372, 1988.

9 Hobbs T: *Leviathan*, 1651.

10 Blackstone W: *Commentaries on the Laws of England, Book the Fourth* (1769). Oxford, Clavendon Press.

11 In re Gault, 387 U.S. 1, 1967.

12 In re Winship, 397 U.S. 358, 1970.

13 Allen v. Illinois, 478 U.S. 364, 1986.

14 Addington v. Texas, 441 U.S. 418, 1979

15 Bell v. Wolfish, 441 U.S. 520, 1979.

16 Hilton v. Braunskill, 107 S.Ct. 2113, 1987

17 United States v. Salerno, 481 U.S. 739, 1987.

18 Jones J: Bad Blood: The Tuskegee Syphilis Experiment. New York, Free Press, 1981.

19 Application of Halko, 54 Cal Rptr 661, 2d Dist, 1966.

20 North American Cold Storage Co. v. Chicago 211 U.S. 306, 1908.

21 Jacobson v. Massachusetts 197 U.S. 11 (1905); New York v. New St. Mark's Baths, 130 Misc. 2d 911, 497 N.Y.S.2d 979, 1986.

22 Yick Wo v. Hopkins, 118 U.S. 356, 1886.

23 Richards EP: The jurisprudence of prevention: The right of societal self-defense. *16 Hastings Const LQ* 16:329, 1989.

24 Wain H: *A History of Preventive Medicine.* Springfield, Thomas, 1970.

25 Neustadt RE et al: *The Epidemic That Never Was: Policy-Making and the Swine Flu Scare.* New York, Random House, 1983.

26 Application of President and Director's of Georgetown College, 331 F2d 1000, App DC, 1964.

27 Landis SE et al: Results of a randomized trial of partner notification in cases of HIV infection in North Carolina. *N Engl J Med* 326:101–106, 1992.

27a Potterat JJ et al: Partner notification: Operational considerations. *Int J STD AIDS* 2:411–5, 1991.

27b Rothenberg RB et al: Strategies for management of sex partners, in *Sexually Transmitted Diseases*, 2nd ed, Holmes KK et al (eds). New York, McGraw-Hill, 1990, pp. 1081–1086.

27c Toomey KE et al: Partner notification for the prevention of HIV infection. *AIDS* 3:(Suppl 1):S57–S62, 1989.

27d Adler MW et al: Contact tracing for HIV infection. *Br Med J* 296: 1420–1421, 1988.

28 City of New York v. New Saint Mark's Baths, 130 Misc.2d 911, 497 N.Y.S.2d 979 (Supp.), 1986.

29 Joseph SC: *Dragon Within the Gates.* New York, Carroll & Graf Publishers, Inc., 1992.

30 Institute of Medicine: *The Future of Public Health.* Washington, DC, National Academy Press, 1988.

31 Lederberg J et al (eds): *Emerging Infections: Microbial Threats to Health in the United States.* Washington, DC, National Academy Press, 1992.

32 Molien V: Kaiser Foundation Hospitals, 616 P.2d 813 (1980); B.N. v. K.K., 538 A.2d 1175 Md., 1988.

33 Colo. Rev. Statutes, § 25-4-1401, et seq., (suppl.), 1987.

34 Doe v. McNulty, 630 So. 2d 825 (La. Ct. App. 4th Cir.), 1993.

35 Potterat JJ et al: Gonorrhea in street prostitutes: Epidemiologic and legal implication. *Sex Trans Dis* 6:58, 1979.

36 Institute of Medicine: *The Hidden Epidemic: Confronting Sexually Transmitted Diseases.* TR Eng et al (eds). Washington DC, National Academy Press, 1996.

37 Hethcote HW et al: *Gonorrhea Transmission Dynamics and Control.* Springer-Verlag, 1984.

38 Holmes KK et al: Impact of a gonorrhea control program, including selective mass treatment, in female sex workers. *J Infect Dis* 174(suppl2):S230–S239, 1996.

39 Thomas JC et al: The development and use of the concept of a sexually transmitted disease core. *J Infect Dis* 174(suppl2):S134–S143, 1996.

40 Hethcote at 41.

41 Judson FN et al: The impact of AIDS and HIV on state and local health departments. *Am J Pub Health* 78:387, 1988.

42 Cates W et al: AIDS and absolutism: The demand for perfection in prevention. *N Engl J Med* 327:492–494, 1992.

43 Joseph SC et al: *Dragon within the Gates.* New York, Carroll & Graf, 1992, pp. 99–100.

44 Potterat JJ et al: Partner notification in the control of human immunodeficiency virus infection. *AJPH* 79(7):874–876, 1989.

45 Rathbun KC: Congenital syphilis: a proposal for improved surveillance, diagnosis, and treatment. *Sex Trans Dis* 10:102–107, 1983.

46 Truman v. Thomas, 611 P.2d 902 (Cal.), 1980.

47 The Ryan White Act, as amended in 1996: 42 USCS § 300ff-27a (1996).

48 Koopman JS et al: The role of early HIV infection in the spread of HIV through populations. *J Acq Imm Defic Synd Hum Retrovirol* 14:249–259, 1997.

49 Brilliant LB: *The Management of Smallpox Eradication in India.* Ann Arbor, MI, The University of Michigan Press, 1985.

50 Whalen v. Roe 429 U.S. 589, 1977.

51 Reynolds v. McNichols, 488 F.2d 1378 (10th Cir.), 1973.

52 People v. Victor, 398 P.2d 391 (1965); Ex Parte Woodruff, 210 P.2d 191 (Crimm App. 1949); Ex Parte Kilbane, 67 N.E.2d 22, 22–23 (1945); People v. Robertson, 302 Ill. 422, 1922.

53 Application of Halko, 246 Cal. App. 2d 553, 54 Cal. Rptr. 661, 1966.

54 Margolis HS et al: Prevention of hepatitis B virus transmission by immunization. *JAMA* 274:1201–1208, 1995.

55 Centers for Disease Control: Hepatitis B virus: A comprehensive strategy for eliminating transmission in the United States through universal childhood vaccination: Recommendations of the Immunization Practices Advisory Committee (ACIP). *Morb Mortal Wkly Rept* 40(RR-13):1–20, 1990.

56 Centers for Disease Control: Prevention of perinatal transmission of hepatitis B virus: prenatal screening of all pregnant women for hepatitis B surface antigen. *MMWR* 37:341, 1988.

Chapter 107

Ethical issues

Ronald Bayer

AIDS, the first serious epidemic disease to strike advanced industrial nations in more than a generation, has posed an extraordinary array of ethical challenges. Some are akin to those posed by other sexually transmitted diseases. Others are starkly different, reflecting the fatal nature of AIDS, the burdens it has imposed on already stigmatized populations, gay and bisexual men and intravenous drug users. Among the ethical issues that AIDS has compelled us to confront are: the duty of the state to prevent the spread of disease; the obligation of physicians to care for those who are in need, the limits and significance of medical confidentiality, the obligation to seek informed consent before testing and commencing treatment, the functions of counseling infected individuals about their duties to partners and of assisting women who are infected as they are compelled to make reproductive decisions, the clash between the canons of research and the canons of care, the limits of acceptable underwriting by insurance companies, the rights of individuals with costly medical conditions to emigrate, and, finally, the obligations of the advanced industrial nations to less developed nations.

Despite the extraordinary context of the AIDS epidemic during the past decade, what is striking about the ethical issues that have been pressed to the fore is that they are, in a fundamental sense, not at all new. What is new is the intensity of the discussion, the broad participatory nature of the debate, the political forces called into play, the demands they have made, the solutions they have sought to fashion, and the extent to which efforts have been made to shape an international consensus on the ethics of prevention and care. AIDS has provided the occasion for a rethinking of the traditions of public health in light of human rights concerns. Most strikingly, it has required a reconsideration of what has come to be thought of as the standard approach to sexually transmitted diseases.

As a lethal illness spread in the context of the most intimate relationships and as a public health threat, AIDS has forced us to confront questions regarding the appropriate role of the state in limiting morbidity and mortality. In so doing it has compelled us to think about the ethical limits on state power in the face of a grave social threat. As a disease of the socially vulnerable, HIV infection has compelled us to face issues involving the role of the state in protecting the weak at moments of social stress. As a disease that has affected large numbers of poor individuals without adequate health insurance or who live in nations with limited health care systems, AIDS has required us once again to consider what justice demands in terms of the protection of individuals against the costs associated with illness. Thus the roles of government in advancing the public health, defending the weak, and assuring access to health care have all been called on by the AIDS epidemic.

In this chapter, three broad topics will be considered: the ethics of prevention and protection; the ethics of research; and the ethics of care. The discussion is based primarily on the experience of the United States and other advanced industrial democracies, but the broad issues have relevance to all nations.

THE ETHICS OF PREVENTION

In the United States as well as in other nations bounded by the liberal tradition, ethical considerations and pragmatic concerns have both contributed to the adoption of public health strategies to control the spread of HIV infection that may be broadly defined as voluntaristic—stressing mass education, counseling, voluntary testing, the protection of the vulnerable from irrational discrimination, and respect for privacy.[1] This approach stood in stark contrast to the more authoritarian public health response to other infectious and sexually transmitted diseases that emerged in the late nineteenth and early twentieth centuries when conceptions of the rights of the individual and of privacy were very different from those that prevailed in the 1980s. Indeed, both in the United States and elsewhere what might be termed "HIV exceptionalism" has dominated public health policy.[2] This general consensus has affected policies on testing for HIV infection, the protection of confidentiality, and the use of the coercive powers of the state to restrict those whose behaviors are thought to pose a risk of HIV transmission.

TESTING AND VOLUNTARISM

From the outset, the test developed to detect an antibody to the AIDS virus—first used on a broad scale to screen blood donations—was mired in controversy. Uncertainty about the significance of the test's findings and the quality and accuracy provided the technical substrate of disputes that inevitably took on a political and ethical character, since issues of privacy, communal health, social and economic discrimination, coercion, and liberty were always involved. Public health officials saw in the test a valuable tool for fostering behavioral change. Others, primarily gay leaders and advocates for other vulnerable populations, saw it as a great threat. For them the prospect of identifying persons with asymptomatic HIV infection provoked concerns about stigma, isolation, and discrimination. These fears were rooted in the very real experiences of people with AIDS.

Out of the controversies that whirled about the antibody test, there emerged a broad consensus in the developed nations and endorsed by the Global Programme on AIDS of the World Health Organization in the mid-1980s: except for clearly circumscribed circumstances, testing was to be done under conditions of voluntary, informed consent only after counseling that outlined both the benefits and risks of testing. The results were to be protected by stringent confidentiality safeguards. How very different this was from the routine testing that typically occurred in the context of clinical practice, where consent is presumed and where patients are rarely informed of the details of the tests to which their blood will be subjected.

In the United States, to underscore the importance of protecting the privacy of tested individuals, the option of anonymous testing was made broadly available. Only voluntary testing, it was believed, could contribute to the overarching goal of behavioral change. The voluntarist consensus was supported by gay leaders, civil libertarians, bioethicists, public health officials, and professional organizations representing clinicians.[3–6] But as broad as the consensus was, it was also fragile. It was a consensus shaped by the relative impotence of medicine in the epidemic's first years.

Advances in therapeutics and a wide range of clinical trials for which the infected were eligible changed the outlook for patients with HIV infection. Those who initially urged those at risk for infection to exercise great caution before seeking to know their antibody status began in the late 1980s to encourage voluntary confidential or anonymous testing. A growing number of clinicians sought to loosen the requirements for specific informed consent before HIV-antibody testing occurred, to "return AIDS to the medical mainstream."

Given the traditions of medicine, such impatience was not surprising. But ethicists have continued to argue for the centrality of consent.[7] A number of arguments have been put forward in this regard. First, although the clinical picture has begun to change, there is no definitive evidence that early therapeutic intervention can prevent an ultimately fatal outcome for people with HIV. At the same time, the prospect of stigma and discrimination have remained a threat to the social well-being of HIV-infected persons. Under these conditions, the arguments for specific informed consent have been viewed as important as ever. But ethicists have generally gone further, arguing that even if the clinical picture were to improve dramatically, the moral basis for insisting on informed consent before HIV testing would not change. Their conclusions are derived from the well-established principle of autonomy that requires that competent adults have the right to determine whether or not to undergo treatment or to terminate treatments already begun. The principle that limits the paternalistic authority of the physician to order therapies in the interest of the patient, it has been argued, extends to the authority to order those tests that would serve as the basis for such interventions.

More complex is the question of whether the routine or mandatory screening of infants born to mothers at increased risk for HIV infection can be justified.[8] In more developed countries pediatricians have for some time now asserted that the early identification of infected newborns provides an opportunity to initiate aggressive intervention, including the prophylactic administration of drugs to prevent pneumocystis pneumonia. Others have been more skeptical of what can be done. They have argued that the long-term benefit to infected children of early clinical intervention is by no means clear. What the test of the infant does do is identify the existence of an infected mother. It is the fact that mandatory testing of newborns would entail an invasion of the mother's privacy that has made this issue so difficult. The central question is, How ought one to balance the right of privacy and the benefit of the child in being diagnosed? Would such benefit to the child warrant overriding the mother's privacy?

This debate takes place against a background of widely accepted mandatory or routine testing of newborns to permit the identification of those in need of special treatment. Screening in these instances is held to represent a legitimate exercise of the state's power attempt to protect the vulnerable. Screening for PKU in the United States is paradigmatic. Early identification is critical so that a special dietary regime can be initiated. The failure to undertake such a therapeutic intervention can be catastrophic for the child. A definitive diagnostic test, a definitive therapeutic intervention, an imperative to act quickly, these are the conditions that provide the empirical and moral grounds for the routine screening of newborns without first seeking parental consent. Only when these conditions prevail with regard to HIV will the ethical bases be established for *considering* mandatory testing as an option. But the tide has certainly begun to change. In 1997 New York State became the first jurisdiction in the United States to impose mandatory newborn testing, driven by a belief that the therapeutic picture had radically changed.

Despite the enormous attention devoted to the question of newborn testing in the late 1980s and early 1990s, that issue will, in all likelihood, be superseded by pressure to identify HIV-infected pregnant women.[9] That pressure will stem from a remarkable research finding in early 1994 that showed a radical reduction in HIV transmission from infected pregnant women to their fetuses when AZT was administered during pregnancy and delivery and to the newborn for 6 weeks after birth. In the wake of this finding, many obstetricians and pediatricians began to assert that the regime surrounding testing should be liberalized so that all infected women could be identified and offered treatment. Some have called for mandatory testing during pregnancy, using as a model testing for syphilis and hepatitis B.[10] Indeed it is striking to note that in the United States routine or mandatory testing of pregnant women for syphilis has virtually never provoked ethical or legal controversy. Although rejecting mandatory treatment for HIV during pregnancy as ethically unacceptable and practically impossible, many advocates of mandatory screening have asserted that women who learn of their HIV infection will be more likely to accept voluntary treatment. More common, many physicians have asserted that the stringent requirements of informed consent with pretest counseling should be replaced with a strong recommendation to undergo testing with an informed right of refusal. Such proposals explicitly seek to shift the burden of decision making to those women who would reject HIV testing.[11] The foundation for such a shift, it is argued, is the benefit for the fetus that might have been infected had its mother not been identified and offered AZT treatment. Here, as in the case of mandatory screening, there is an assumption that although women might be reluctant to undergo testing, they will, once they know they are infected, undertake therapies designed to protect the children they will bear.

CONFIDENTIALITY AND ITS LIMITS

There is perhaps no ethical issue involving AIDS that has received more attention than that of confidentiality.[12] It is an issue that has been central to the treatment of sexually transmitted diseases more generally. The principle of confidentiality in medicine has two foundations, both of which can be observed in the response to sexually transmitted diseases in general and to AIDS more specifically. First, protecting the confidentiality of clinical diagnoses reflects a respect for the integrity and privacy of the individual. Second, confidentiality is crucial to the creation of a context of candor between patients and their caregivers. It is also crucial to creating a context that will encourage patients to come forward for care. In the context of stigmatized but treatable sexually transmitted diseases, confidentiality was essential to the public health goal of identifying cases and of treating them so as to prevent further transmission. Given this legacy, it is not surprising that the call for the protection of confidentiality in the AIDS epidemic has come not only from those most at risk, for example, gay men, but from public health officials as well. For the latter the protection of confidentiality was critical to the strategy to encourage mass behavioral change and to the goal of encouraging people to come forward for testing and counseling.[6,13]

But confidentiality has its limits, both in the context of public health practice and clinical care. There is a long history of requiring that individuals with certain infectious diseases be reported to confidential public health registries. In the United States, every state requires, for example, reporting of the names of individuals with a range of sexually transmitted diseases. In other nations various methods of encryption are used to protect the privacy of patients while public health reporting needs are met. AIDS has naturally provoked ongoing conflict over the importance and potential dangers of mandatory reporting. Typically, however, there has been less controversy over the reporting, by name, of cases of AIDS than of asymptomatic HIV infection. Indeed, in many nations AIDS, but not HIV infection, is a condition reportable by name. It is a mark of the shifting attitudes provoked by enhanced therapeutic prospects that in the United States much of the opposition to HIV name reporting has begun to wane.

But what of the limits of confidentiality in the clinical context? What are the ethical responsibilities of a physician when an HIV-infected patient refuses to inform identifiable, unsuspecting past or current partners about the dangers of infection. This was, of course, an issue confronted repeatedly in the early part of the twentieth century as physicians dealt with syphilis. Then, what was termed the "medical secret" was often viewed as an alliance between male practitioners and their male patients against the interest of "innocent" women who might be unknowingly exposed to the diseases of their "philandering" partners.

Perhaps the most famous legal case dealing with the limits of medical confidentiality is known as *Tarasoff*.[14] In that case a California court was asked to consider the question of whether a psychotherapist had the duty to notify or warn the potential victim of a patient's violent threat. In its decision, the California Supreme Court ruled that there was such a duty. "The protective privilege ends where the public peril begins." Central to that case and the controversy that surrounded the decision were two issues: the claim to privacy and the question of whether the establishment of a duty to warn would so threaten the candor of the clinical relationship that patients would not talk of their violent fantasies, thus depriving their therapists of the ability to prevent the threatened harm. Thus the two foundations of confidentiality, ethical and pragmatic, were implicated.

The relevance to the context of AIDS is clear: Should physicians warn current or past sexual partners whose lives may be at risk because of an unknowing exposure to HIV? If they do, should they identify, by name, the potential source of infection? If there is an ethical obligation to warn, should it impose a legal duty to warn?

Informing the dispute about how it might be best to proceed has been a deep concern about the consequences that could well follow were it to be widely believed that physicians would routinely breach confidentiality when presented with a patient who refused to warn past or current partners about the risk of HIV infection. Would the consequence be a reduction in clinical candor? Would patients be discouraged from seeking to know their HIV status? Would they be less accessible to the efforts of clinicians to convince them of the importance of warning those who might be at risk? In sum, would breaching confidentiality to warn unsuspecting individuals result in a net loss from the perspective of public health? In the United States many jurisdictions have adopted "privilege to disclose" legislation, thus providing physicians with the option of warning without imposing on them a legal duty to do so.

An alternative approach to partner notification that derives from the history of sexually transmitted diseases—contact tracing—does not raise the same challenge to the principle of confidentiality. In the standard practice of contact tracing the index case is asked to provide public health workers with the names of those who might have been exposed. But when such contacts are informed that they are at risk, they are never provided with the name of the index case. Such confidentiality is designed to secure the privacy of the index patient and to facilitate the entire process. Indeed, contact tracing provides an ideal example of how confidentiality may be crucial to, rather than in conflict with, public health goals.

Although contact tracing in the context of syphilis and other sexually transmitted diseases has posed relatively few ethical questions, that has not been the case with HIV and AIDS. It is a mark of the extraordinary concerns surrounding privacy in HIV that even this standard of public health practice has been viewed with deep suspicion.[15] Informing the debate has been the very real difference between contact tracing that can result in the cure of an STD and a process of notification that can only inform an unknowing individual that he or she may be infected with a lethal virus.[6] As the prospects for early therapeutic intervention in HIV have improved, opposition to contact tracing has tended to abate.

COERCIVE CONTROLS

The question of how to respond to individuals whose behavior represented a threat to unknowing partners inevitably provoked discussion of the public health tradition of imposing restrictions on liberty in the name of communal welfare.[16] The specter of mass quarantine has haunted all such discussion. Only Cuba has sought to quarantine all individuals with HIV infection.[17] In other nations the focus has been on the more limited case of individuals whose behaviors have placed others at risk for HIV. Even such limited efforts have provoked concern because of fears that they would lead to egregious intrusions on privacy and invidiously imposed deprivations of freedom.

In the United States, fierce opposition has surfaced to all efforts to bring AIDS within the scope of state quarantine statutes. Nevertheless, more than a dozen states had done so between 1987 and 1990, typically using the occasion to modernize their disease control laws to reflect contemporary constitutional standards that detail procedural guarantees, and to require that restrictions on freedom represent the "least restrictive alternative" available to achieve a "compelling state interest."

Despite the intensity of the debate that has surrounded this issue, the only empirical study of the use of the power of isolation in the United States has found that state health departments have almost never exercised the authority granted by statute.[18] From 1981 to 1990 only 10 cases were documented, and in virtually every case the duration of confinement has been very brief. Far more common has been the use of the public health authority to warn individuals that their behavior posed a risk. Such warnings have often been accompanied by "cease and desist orders." Public health efforts to isolate the small number of individuals deemed to pose a behavioral threat to "an suspecting partner" have occurred in other countries, typically focusing on prostitutes. Sweden provides a number of such cases.[19]

The enactment of statutes criminalizing behaviors linked to the spread of AIDS or the application of the general criminal law to such cases has paralleled the political receptivity to laws extending the authority of public health officials to control individuals whose behavior posed a risk of HIV transmission.[20,21] Such efforts draw on the tradition of criminal laws enacted early in the twentieth century in response to the fear of syphilis.

What are the ethical foundations of such statutes? The criminal law serves to express a society's profound abhorrence of certain behaviors. In so doing the law threatens to punish individuals who violate certain social norms. It may also serve as a deterrent. Some acts are universally the subject of the criminal law. Murder, for example. Some acts are crimes in only some societies. The enactment of criminal statutes that prohibit the willful and knowing infection with HIV of an unsuspecting sexual partner would clearly fall within the morally acceptable use of the criminal law. But the enactment of such statutes has often served ends that raise profound ethical questions. To seek to punish acts that cannot possibly result in the spread of AIDS—spitting, for example—serves only to underscore the penchant for repressive measures in the face of complex social problems.

Whatever the allure of such measures, it remains clear that the future course of the AIDS epidemic will be determined by the creation of a social and institutional milieu within which radical voluntary changes in behavior can occur and be sustained. Educational campaigns and counseling programs most effectively undertaken by groups linked to the populations at risk, not repressive measures, remain the centerpiece of that preventive effort. Thus a central ethical challenge posed by the AIDS epidemic is the fostering of educational efforts in the face of resistance by those who view such endeavors as representing an endorsement of "immoral," sexual, or drug-using behavior. As crucial is the development of harm reduction programs that, for instance, permit individuals such as drug users to protect themselves while engaged in behaviors that arouse profound social rejection and that provide or make access to condoms relatively easy.

THE ETHICS OF RESEARCH

Among the most notorious examples of abuse of research subjects in the United States was the Tuskegee syphilis study, conducted by the Public Health Service. This was a study designed to track the natural history of untreated syphilis in poor black southern men. It was a study that continued long after the effective treatment of syphilis became a routine of medical practice. In this instance, poor African American men were deprived of the knowledge that they had a condition for which treatment was available. They were thus the unwitting subjects in a study they knew nothing about.

It was, in part, because of the outrage provoked by that study that the most stringent regulation of research was institutionalized in the United States. It is thus an irony that another sexually transmitted disease—AIDS—would provide the occasion for a challenge to some of the premises of the protective regulatory regime surrounding research.[22]

The HIV epidemic has provided the circumstances for the emergence of a broad and potent political movement that has sought to reshape radically the conditions under which research is undertaken. The role of the randomized clinical trial, the importance of placebo controls, the centrality of academic research institutions, the dominance of scientists over subjects, the sharp distinction between research and therapy, and the protectionist ethos that has informed research ethics since the mid-1970s have all been brought into question.

Although scholars concerned with the methodological demands of sound research and ethicists committed to the protection of research subjects have played a crucial role in the ensuing discussions, both as defenders of the received wisdom and as critics, the debate has been driven by the articulate demands of those most threatened by AIDS. What has been so stunning, disconcerting to some, and exciting to others has been the rhythm of challenge and response. Rather than the careful exchange of academic arguments, we have been witness to the mobilization of disruptive and effective political protest.

The threat of death has hovered over the process. "The shortage of proven therapeutic alternatives for AIDS and the belief that trials are, in and of themselves, beneficial have led to the claim that people have a right to be research subjects. This is the exact opposite of the tradition starting with Nuremberg—that people have a right *not* to be research subjects."[23] It is that striking reversal that has resulted in a rejection of the model of research conducted at remote academic centers, with restrictive (protective) standards of access, and strict adherence to the "gold standard" of the randomized clinical trial. Blurring the distinction between research and treatment—"A Drug Trial is Health Care Too"—those insistent upon radical reform have sought to open wide the points of entry to new "therapeutic" agents both within and outside of clinical trials, have demanded that the paternalistic ethical warrant for the protection of the vulnerable from research be replaced by an ethical regime informed by respect for the autonomous choice of potential subjects who could weigh, for themselves, the potential risks and benefits of new experimental treatments for HIV infection. Thus demands have been made that women be enrolled in trials in greater numbers, that prisoners and drug users be granted access; that children be included in trials at a much earlier point than had been considered acceptable.[24–26] Moreover, the revisionists have demanded a basic reconceptualization of the relationship between researchers and subjects. In place of protocols imposed from above, they have proposed a more egalitarian and democratic model in which negotiation would replace scientific authority.

The reformulation of the ethics of research that has begun under the impact of AIDS has implications that go far beyond the epidemic of HIV disease, since the emerging new conceptions and standards could govern the conduct of the entire research enterprise. Protagonists, who have been locked in often acrimonious debate, foretell very different consequences of the changing social standards of research. Proponents of the new ethos hold out the prospect of a revised regime that is both respectful of individual rights and the requirements of good science. Critics, on the other hand, have warned that the blurring of the distinction between research and treatment can only harm the desperate. "It is not compassionate to hold out false hope to terminally ill patients so that they spend their last dollars on unproven 'remedies' that they might live longer."[27]

Perhaps the most important and controversial issue in international collaborative research is the need to build infrastructure in the host country and to make the fruits of the research available to people in that community or similarly situated populations. The central ethical question is, To what extent does the principle of distributive justice require that therapeutic interventions developed in the course of such research be made available to subjects in their communities?

The issue is especially relevant to the conduct of vaccine trials. For epidemiological reasons it has been argued that countries in Asia and Africa represent ideal settings for investigation into possible preventive vaccines. Large numbers of infected persons, and the tragically high incidence of infection, make nations in Asia and Africa ideal for the determination of vaccine efficacy. But no vaccine trial would be ethical—assuming that issues of consent could be resolved—if there were no assurance that a successful vaccine would be provided by international agreement, despite the potential cost. Such agreements must precede the conduct of vaccine trials.

THE ETHICS OF CARE

For almost four decades, health care workers in America, as well as in other advanced industrial societies, were largely shielded from what had been the routine experience of those who had in prior eras worked with the sick: the acquisition of their patients' infections and sometimes lethal diseases. Though never as total as many had come to believe, this invincibility was psychologically ruptured by the intrusion of AIDS, beginning in 1981. AIDS forced physicians and health care workers to consider the possibility that theirs was indeed a "dangerous trade."[28]

Early in the history of this epidemic, anecdotal reports began to surface about hospital aides leaving food trays at the doors of those who were sick, and of nurses, physicians, and dentists refusing to treat patients with the new disease.

Confronted with the challenge represented by the threat of patient abandonment, those committed to stanching the emerging trend turned to history in hopes that an unambiguous lesson on responsibility of physicians would emerge.[29] Physicians had, after all, been called to respond when epidemics were more common, when morbidity was awesome. For those who had hoped to discover a univocal message from the chronicles of the past, the turn of history proved a disappointment. Although some physicians had stayed behind to care for their patients, many had fled. At times they did so in order that they might attend to their fleeing patrons, sometimes simply to protect themselves. Perhaps most significant as a reflection of the extent to which many physicians refused to remain with those afflicted in earlier plagues was the need to make arrangements for the care of the sick through the special institution of the "plague doctor." Employed by local merchants and the political elites, these physicians took up where others had failed.

If history provided no clear guidance, what of the codes of ethics that have expressed the aspirations of the guilds and associations of medical practitioners?[30] Remarkably, such codes had been silent on the duty of physicians to treat in the time of epidemics. In the United States, the AMA code of 1847 was unique in its forthright assertion of such a responsibility. "And when pestilence prevails, it is their duty to face the danger and to continue their labors for the alleviation of suffering, even at the jeopardy of their own lives."

In the face of overt examples of physician refusals to treat patients with AIDS the American Medical Association was compelled in 1987 to make clear the social responsibility of doctors. "A physician may not ethically refuse to treat a patient whose condition is within the physician's current realm of competence solely because the patient is seropositive."[31]

For many who have stressed a universal obligation to treat, it is clear that the relatively low risk of infection has been central. Were the risks of HIV transmission very much greater, it would have required an ethics of heroism to insist that each health care worker bear the responsibility of assuring adequate and appropriate health care to the infected. Given the level of risk entailed in the face of HIV infection, even among surgeons and obstetricians, those who stressed the obligation to treat argued that it was not heroism but more straightforward duty that was involved. Thus did Edmund Pellegrino, the physician-philosopher, state, "To refuse to care for AIDS patients, even if the danger were greater than it is, is to abnegate what is essential to being a physician."[32]

The issue of access to care is not, however, primarily raised by the specter of physician abandonment. Rather, it centers on the problem of access to care on the part of the poor.

In the United States, which unlike other economically advanced nations does not guarantee access to care on the part of its citizens, the striking contrast between important clinical advances in the care of those with HIV infection and the social organization of American medicine led the National Commission on Acquired Immune Deficiency Syndrome to warn in a December 1989 report to the president that medical breakthroughs would "mean little unless the health care system can incorporate them and make them accessible to people in need." The existence of a medically disenfranchised class meant that for many, access to care was almost solely through the "emergency room door of one of the few hospitals in the country that treats people with HIV infection and AIDS."[33]

Nothing more tellingly underscores the extent to which poverty and inadequate health insurance protection may serve as barriers to care than the recent experience with the protease inhibitors. Public programs established to secure access to AIDS-related drugs in the United States have routinely exhausted their capacity to make these new therapeutic agents available. Some state programs have created waiting lists. In the end many patients whose lives might be dramatically improved have had to do without.

The issue of how to assure access to care and, more importantly, the question of what level of care to provide in nations that are poor and that can provide only rudimentary health care services poses very difficult ethical questions. No simple answers are possible in situations where so many pressing health care needs go unmet. But it is clear that drugs like the protease inhibitors are simply out of reach. A basic ethical principle would require that those with HIV disease not be discriminated against because of that fact, that they receive no less than other gravely ill persons. Ultimately, the choices made within conditions of severe constraints make clear how the resolution of pressing human needs in the less developed nations will require support and assistance from economically advanced nations.

AIDS AND THE WORLD

AIDS links, in a grim way, the most advanced technological societies, like the United States, and the poorest nations of Africa, Asia, and Latin America. The vast proportion of HIV infection in the world exists outside North America and Western Europe. In the next decade, the already stark contrast will become even sharper. In the face of the social catastrophe now making itself felt, it will be critical to confront the question of what the rich nations of the world owe the poor as the latter confront the issues of prevention and treatment. The social, economic, and political realities of general assistance to the third world are a background context that cannot be ignored as we confront the AIDS pandemic. The basic fact is that the advanced industrial world does very little to meet the needs of the third world, in terms of food, health care, or other basic goods.

It is all too easy to imagine the development of expensive therapeutic agents that will be reserved for those who fall ill as a result of HIV infection in the advanced industrial societies but which will not be available to those similarly situated in third world nations. The use of AZT during pregnancy poses a paradigm challenge.[34] Here is a therapy that could radically reduce HIV transmission. It is in the less developed world that pediatric AIDS poses so significant a problem, yet the cost of AZT places it out of reach to those in need. As noted earlier, If and when a vaccine were to be developed, will it be made available to those most in need? And who would pay the cost of production and distribution for those nations too poor to bear the cost?

AIDS, because of its dramatic features, underscores the limitations of our capacity to conceive of and act upon notions of shared responsibility across national boundaries. At stake, of course, is the question of justice and the global distribution of resources.

References

1 Bayer R: *Private Acts, Social Consequences: AIDS and the Politics of Public Health.* New Brunswick, NJ, Rutgers University Press, 1991.

2 Bayer R: Public health policy and the AIDS epidemic: An end to HIV exceptionalism? *N Engl J Med* 324:1500, 1991.

3 American Association of Physicians for Human Rights. November 12, 1985, unpublished.

4 Northern California Branch, American Civil Liberties Union. *AIDS and Civil Liberties.* March 1986.

5 Bayer R et al: HIV antibody screening: An ethical framework for evaluating proposed programs. *JAMA* 256:1768, 1986.

6 Association of State and Territorial Health Officials: *ASTHO Guide to Public Health Practice: HTLV III Antibody Testing and Community Approaches.* Washington, D.C., Public Health Foundation, 1985.

7 Levine C et al: The ethics of screening for early intervention in HIV disease. *Am J Pub Health* 79:1661, 1989.

8 Faden R et al: *AIDS, Women and the Next Generation: Towards a Morally Acceptable Public Policy for HIV Testing of Pregnant Women and Newborns.* New York, Oxford University Press, 1991.

9 Bayer R: Women's Rights, Babies' Interests: Ethics, Politics, and Science in the Debate of Newborn HIV Screening, in *HIV Infection in Women.* H Minkoff, J DeHovitz, A Duerr (eds). New York, Raven Press, 1995, pp. 193–307.

10 Hoffman C et al: Ethical issues in the use of Zidovudine to reduce vertical transmission of HIV (letter to the Editor). *N Eng J Med* 332: 891, 1995.
11 Minkoff H et al: Pediatric HIV disease, Zidovudine in pregnancy, and unblinding heelstick surveys: Reframing the debate on prenatal HIV testing. *JAMA* 274:1165, 1995.
12 Dickens BM: Legal limits of AIDS confidentiality. *JAMA* 259:3449, 1988.
13 Surgeon General's Report on Acquired Immune Deficiency Syndrome, 1986.
14 Tarasoff v. Regents of the State of California, 17 Cal. 3d 425, 551p. 2d334, 131 *Cal. Rptr.* 14 (Cal) 1976.
15 Bayer R et al: HIV prevention and the two faces of partner notification. *Am J Pub Health* 82:1158, 1992.
16 Gostin L: The politics of AIDS: Compulsory state powers, public health and civil liberties. *Ohio St Law J* 49:1017, 1989.
17 Bayer R et al: Controlling AIDS in Cuba: The logic of quarantine. *N Engl J Med* 83:1022, 1989.
18 Bayer R et al: AIDS and the limits of control: Public health orders, quarantine, and recalcitrant behavior. *Am J Publ Health* 83:1471, 1993.
19 Henrikkson B et al: Sweden: The power of the moral (istic) left, in *AIDS in the Industrialized Democracies: Passions, Politics and Policies,* R Bayer and DL Kirp (eds). New Brunswick, NJ, Rutgers University Press, 1992, pp. 317–338.
20 Field MA et al: AIDS and the criminal law. *Law, Med Health Care* 14:46, 1987.
21 Hermann DHJ: Criminalizing conduct related to HIV transmission. *St. Louis Univ Publ Law Review* 9:351, 1990.
22 Edgar H et al: New rules for new drugs: The challenge of AIDS to the regulatory process. *Milbank Quart* 68 (suppl 1):111, 1990.
23 Levine C: Has AIDS changed the ethics of human subjects research? *Law, Med Health Care* 16:167, 1988.
24 Levine C: Women and HIV/AIDS research: The barriers to equity. *Eval Rev* 14:447, 1990.
25 Hammett TM et al: Clinical and epidemiological research on HIV infection and AIDS among correctional inmates: Regulations, ethics, and procedures. *Eval Review* 14:482, 1990.
26 Levine C: Children in HIV/AIDS clinical trials: Still vulnerable after all these years. *Law, Med Health Care* 19:231, 1991.
27 Annas G: Faith (healing), hope and charity at the FDA: The politics of AIDS drug trials. *Villanova Law Review* 301:183, 1989.
28 Arras J: The fragile web of professional responsibility: AIDS and the duty to treat. *Hastings Ctr Rept,* Special Supplement, April–May, 1988.
29 Fox DM: The politics of physicians' responsibility in epidemics: a note on history, in *AIDS: The Burdens of History,* DM Fox and E Fee (eds). Berkeley, University of California Press, 1988, pp. 86–96.
30 Zuger A et al: Physicians, AIDS and occupational risk: Historic traditions and ethical obligations. *JAMA* 258:1924, 1987.
31 Current opinions of the Council on Ethical and Judicial Affairs. American Medical Association: *Ethical Issues.* November 1987.
32 Pellegrino E: Altruism, self-interest and medical ethics. *JAMA* 258: 1939, 1987.
33 U.S. National Commission on AIDS. *Report,* November 1, 1989.
34 Bayer R: Ethical challenges posed by Zidovudine treatment to reduce vertical transmission of HIV (editorial). *N Eng J Med* 331:1223, 1994.

Appendix A

1998 Guidelines for treatment of sexually transmitted diseases*†

TABLE OF CONTENTS

EXPERT CONSULTANTS

Chairman:
David Atkins, M.D., M.P.H., Agency for Health Care Policy and Research

Presenters:
Michael H. Augenbraun, M.D., State University of New York Health Science Center at Brooklyn, NY
Karl Beutner, M.D., Ph.D., Solano Dermatology, Vallejo, CA
Gail A. Bolan, M.D., San Francisco Department of Public Health and University of California at San Francisco
Willard Cates, Jr., M.D., M.P.H., Family Health International, Research Triangle Park, NC
Anne M. Rompalo, M.D., Johns Hopkins University, Baltimore
Pablo J. Sanchez, M.D., Southwestern Medical Center at Dallas
Bradley Stoner, M.D., Ph.D., Washington University School of Medicine, St. Louis, MO
Anna Wald, M.D., M.P.H., University of Washington, Seattle
Cheryl K. Walker, M.D., University of California at Irvine
George D. Wendel, M.D., Southwestern Medical Center at Dallas
Jonathan M. Zenilman, M.D., Johns Hopkins University, Baltimore

*Adapted from: U.S. Department of Health and Human Services
Public Health Service
Division of Sexually Transmitted Diseases
Centers for Prevention Services
Centers for Disease Control
Atlanta, Georgia 30333

†The use of trade names and commercial sources is for identification purposes only and does not constitute endorsement by the Public Health Service or by the Department of Health and Human Services

Moderators:
King K. Holmes, M.D., Ph.D., Center for AIDS and STDs, University of Washington, Seattle
Edward W. Hook, III, M.D., University of Alabama at Birmingham School of Medicine
A. Eugene Washington, M.D., M.Sc., University of California at San Francisco

Rapporteurs:
John M. Douglas, Jr., M.D., Denver Department of Public Health and University of Colorado Health Science Center
Margaret R. Hammerschlag, M.D., State University of New York Health Science Center
David H. Martin, M.D., Louisiana State University Medical Center, New Orleans

Consultants:
Adaora A. Adimora, M.D., M.P.H., University of North Carolina at Chapel Hill
Virginia A. Caine, M.D., Marion County Health Department, Indianapolis
Laura T. Gutman, M.D., Duke University, Durham, NC
H. Hunter Handsfield, M.D., Seattle-King County Department of Public Health and University of Washington, Seattle
Robert B. Jones, M.D., Ph.D., Indiana University, Indianapolis
Franklyn N. Judson, M.D., Denver Department of Health
William M. McCormack, M.D., State University of New York Health Science Center at Brooklyn
Daniel M. Musher, M.D., Baylor College of Medicine, Houston
Newton G. Osborne, M.D., M.P.H., Howard University Hospital, Washington, DC
Robert T. Rolfs, Jr., M.D., Utah Department of Health
Lawrence L. Sanders, Jr., M.D., Southwest Hospital and Medical Center, Atlanta
Jane R. Schwebke, M.D., University of Alabama at Birmingham School of Medicine
Jack D. Sobel, M.D., Wayne State University School of Medicine, Detroit
David E. Soper, M.D., Medical University of South Carolina, Charleston
Walter E. Stamm, M.D., University of Washington
Lawrence R. Stanberry, M.D., Ph.D., Children's Hospital, Cincinnati
Felicia H. Stewart, M.D., Kaiser Family Foundation, Menlo Park, CA
Richard L. Sweet, M.D., Magee-Women's Hospital, Pittsburgh.

Liaison Participants:
Dennis J. Barbour, J.D., Association of Reproductive Health Professionals
Joan R. Cates, American Social Health Association
JoAnne Doherty, Health Canada, Ontario
Robert G. Harmon, M.D., M.P.H., United Health Care
Kate L. Heilpern, M.D., American College of Emergency Physicians
John J. Henning, Ph.D., American Medical Association
K. King Holmes, M.D., Ph.D., Infectious Diseases Society of America
John N. Krieger, M.D., American Urological Association
Marshall Kubota, M.D., American Academy of Family Practice
Noni E. MacDonald, M.D., American Academy of Pediatrics
Gary A. Richwald, M.D., M.P.H., National Coalition of STD Directors
Helen J. Sawyer, R.N., Georgia Department of Human Resources
Stanley X. Shapiro, M.D., Regional Laboratory and Infectious Disease Committee, Kaiser Permanente, Panorama City, CA
Donald Sutherland, M.D., Health Canada
Steve K. Tyring, M.D., Ph.D., American Academy of Dermatology
C. Johannes van Dam, M.D., World Health Organization
Fernando Zacarias, M.D., M.P.H., Pan American Health Organization, World Health Organization.

CDC/Division of STD Prevention (DSTDP)/STD Treatment Guidelines 1998 Project Coordinators:
Kimberly A. Workowski, M.D.; John S. Moran, M.D.

Co-Chair:
Michael E. St. Louis, M.D.

Co-Moderator:
Katherine M. Stone, M.D.

Presenters:
Consuelo M. Beck-Sague, M.D., National Center for Infectious Diseases (NCID)
M. Riduan Joesoef, M.D., Ph.D., M.P.H.; Mary L. Kamb, M.D., M.P.H., Division of HIV/AIDS Prevention (DHAP); Jonathan E. Kaplan, M.D., NCID; H. Trent MacKay, M.D., M.P.H.; Michael M. McNeil, M.D., M.P.H., NCID; Allyn K. Nakashima, M.D., DHAP; George P. Schmid, M.D., M.Sc.

Consultants:
Sevgi O. Aral, Ph.D.; Stuart M. Berman, M.D.; Donald F. Dowda; Brian R. Edlin, M.D., DHAP; Helene D. Gayle, M.D., M.P.H., National Center for HIV, STD, and TB Prevention (NCHSTP); Robert S. Janssen, M.D., DHAP; Wanda K. Jones, Dr.P.H., Office of Women's Health; William J. Kassler, M.D., M.P.H.; Nancy C. Lee, M.D., DHAP; Beth Macke, Ph.D.; Frank J. Mahoney, M.D., NCID; Phillip I. Nieberg, M.D., M.P.H., NCHSTP; Herbert B. Peterson, M.D., National Center for Chronic Disease Prevention and Health Promotion (NCCDPHP); Martha F. Rogers, M.D., DHAP; William E. Secor, Ph.D., NCID; Dawn K. Smith, M.D., DHAP; Ronald O. Valdiserri, M.D., M.P.H., NCHSTP; Judith N. Wasserheit, M.D., M.P.H.; Lynne S. Wilcox, M.D., NCCDPHP

Support Staff:
Cynthia Ford, Contractor; Deborah McElroy; Garrett K. Mallory.

INTRODUCTION

Physicians and other health-care providers have a critical role in preventing and treating sexually transmitted diseases (STDs). These recommendations for the treatment of STDs, which were developed by CDC staff members in consultation with a group of invited experts, are intended to assist with that effort.

This report was produced through a multi-stage process. Beginning in the spring of 1996, CDC personnel and invited experts systematically reviewed literature concerning each of the major STDs, focusing on information that had become available since the "1993 Sexually Transmitted Diseases Treatment Guidelines" (*MMWR* 1993;42[no. RR-14]) were published. Background papers were written and tables of evidence constructed summarizing the type of study (e.g., randomized controlled trial or case series), study population and setting, treatments or other interventions, outcome measures assessed, reported findings, and weaknesses and biases in study design and analysis. For these reviews, published abstracts and peer-reviewed journal articles were considered. A draft document was developed on the basis of the reviews.

In February 1997, invited consultants assembled in Atlanta for a 3-day meeting. CDC personnel and invited experts presented the key questions on STD treatment suggested from the literature reviews and presented the information available to answer those questions. Where relevant, the questions focused on four principal outcomes of STD therapy: a) microbiologic cure, b) alleviation of signs and symptoms, c) prevention of sequelae, and d) prevention of transmission. Cost-effectiveness and other advantages (e.g., single-dose formulations and directly observed therapy) of specific regimens also were considered. The consultants then assessed whether the questions identified were appropriate, ranked them in order of priority, and attempted to arrive at answers using the available evidence. In addition, the consultants evaluated the quality of evidence supporting the answers on the basis of the number, type, and quality of the studies.

In several areas, the process diverged from that described previously. The sections concerning adolescents, congenital syphilis, and partner notification were reviewed by other CDC experts on prevention of STDs and human immunodeficiency virus (HIV) infection. The recommendations for STD screening during pregnancy were developed after CDC staff reviewed the published recommendations of other expert groups. The sections concerning early HIV infection are a compilation of recommendations developed by CDC experts in HIV infection. The sections on hepatitis B virus (HBV) (*1*) and hepatitis A virus (HAV) (2) infections are based on previously published recommendations of the Advisory Committee on Immunization Practices (ACIP).

Throughout this report, the evidence used as the basis for specific recommendations is discussed briefly. More comprehensive, annotated discussions of such evidence will appear in background papers that will be published in 1998. When more than one therapeutic regimen is recommended, the sequence is alphabetized unless there is priority of choice (i.e., based on efficacy, convenience, and cost). Almost all recommended regimens have similar efficacy and similar rates of intolerance or toxicity unless otherwise specified.

These recommendations were developed in consultation with experts whose experience is primarily with the treatment of patients in public STD clinics. Nevertheless, these recommendations also should be applicable to other patient-care settings, including family planning clinics, private physicians' offices, managed care organizations, and other primary-care facilities. When using these guidelines, the disease prevalence and other characteristics of the medical practice setting should be considered. These recommendations should be regarded as a source of clinical guidance and not as standards or inflexible rules.

These recommendations focus on the treatment and counseling of individual patients and do not address other community services and interventions that are important in STD/HIV prevention. Clinical and laboratory diagnoses are described when such information is related to therapy. For a more comprehensive discussion of diagnosis, refer to CDC's *Sexually Transmitted Diseases Clinical Practice Guidelines, 1991* (*3*).

CLINICAL PREVENTION GUIDELINES

The prevention and control of STDs is based on five major concepts: first, education of those at risk on ways to reduce the risk for STDs; second, detection of asymptomatically infected persons and of symptomatic persons unlikely to seek diagnostic and treatment services; third, effective diagnosis and treatment of infected persons; fourth, evaluation, treatment, and counseling of sex partners of persons who are infected with an STD; and fifth, preexposure vaccination of persons at risk for vaccine-preventable STDs. Although this report focuses primarily on the clinical aspects of STD control, prevention of STDs is based on changing the sexual behaviors that place persons at risk for infection. Moreover, because STD control activities reduce the likelihood of transmission to sex partners, prevention for individuals constitutes prevention for the community.

Clinicians have the opportunity to provide client education and counseling and to participate in identifying and treating infected sex partners in addition to interrupting transmission by treating persons who have the curable bacterial and parasitic STDs. The ability of the health-care provider to obtain an accurate sexual history is crucial in prevention and control efforts. Guidance in obtaining a sexual history is available in the chapter "Sexuality and Reproductive Health" in *Contraceptive Technology, 16th edition* (*4*). The accurate diagnosis and timely reporting of STDs by the clinician is the basis for effective public health surveillance.

PREVENTION MESSAGES

Preventing the spread of STDs requires that persons at risk for transmitting or acquiring infections change their behaviors. The essential first step is for the health-care provider to proactively include questions regarding the patient's sexual history as part of the clinical interview. When risk factors have been identified, the provider has an opportunity to deliver prevention messages. Counseling skills (i.e., respect, compassion, and a nonjudgmental attitude) are essential to the effective delivery of prevention messages. Techniques that can be effective in facilitating a rapport with the patient include using open-ended questions, using understandable language, and reassuring the patient that treatment will be provided regardless of considerations such as ability to pay, citizenship or immigration status, language spoken, or lifestyle.

Prevention messages should be tailored to the patient, with consideration given to the patient's specific risk factors for STDs. Messages should include a description of specific actions that the patient can take to avoid acquiring or transmitting STDs (e.g., abstinence from sexual activity if STD-related symptoms develop).

PREVENTION METHODS

Male condoms

When used consistently and correctly, condoms are effective in preventing many STDs, including HIV infection. Multiple cohort studies, including those of serodiscordant sex partners, have demonstrated a strong protective effect of condom use against HIV infection. Because condoms do not cover all exposed areas, they may be more effective in preventing infections transmitted between mucosal surfaces than those transmitted by skin-to-skin contact. Condoms are regulated as medical devices and are subject to random sampling and testing by the Food and Drug Administration (FDA). Each latex condom manufactured in the United States is tested electronically for holes before packaging. Rates of condom breakage during sexual intercourse and withdrawal are low in the United States (i.e., usually two broken condoms per 100 condoms used). Condom failure usually results from inconsistent or incorrect use rather than condom breakage.

Patients should be advised that condoms must be used consistently and correctly to be highly effective in preventing STDs. Patients also should be instructed in the correct use of condoms. The following recommendations ensure the proper use of male condoms:

- Use a new condom with each act of sexual intercourse.
- Carefully handle the condom to avoid damaging it with fingernails, teeth, or other sharp objects.
- Put the condom on after the penis is erect and before any genital contact with the partner.
- Ensure that no air is trapped in the tip of the condom.
- Ensure adequate lubrication during intercourse, possibly requiring the use of exogenous lubricants.
- Use only water-based lubricants (e.g., K-Y Jelly™, Astroglide™, AquaLube™, and glycerin) with latex condoms. Oil-based lubricants (e.g., petroleum jelly, shortening, mineral oil, massage oils, body lotions, and cooking oil) can weaken latex.

- Hold the condom firmly against the base of the penis during withdrawal, and withdraw while the penis is still erect to prevent slippage.

Female condoms

Laboratory studies indicate that the female condom (Reality™)—a lubricated polyurethane sheath with a ring on each end that is inserted into the vagina—is an effective mechanical barrier to viruses, including HIV. Other than one investigation of recurrent trichomoniasis, no clinical studies have been completed to evaluate the efficacy of female condoms in providing protection from STDs, including HIV. If used consistently and correctly, the female condom should substantially reduce the risk for STDs. When a male condom cannot be used appropriately, sex partners should consider using a female condom.

Condoms and spermicides

Whether condoms lubricated with spermicides are more effective than other lubricated condoms in protecting against the transmission of HIV and other STDs has not been determined. Furthermore, spermicide-coated condoms have been associated with *Escherichia coli* urinary tract infection in young women. Whether condoms used with vaginal application of spermicide are more effective than condoms used without vaginal spermicides also has not been determined. Therefore, the consistent use of condoms, with or without spermicidal lubricant or vaginal application of spermicide, is recommended.

Vaginal spermicides, sponges, and diaphragms

As demonstrated in several prospective studies, vaginal spermicides used alone without condoms reduce the risk for cervical gonorrhea and chlamydia. However, protection against HIV infection has not been established in human studies, and spermicides are not recommended for HIV prevention. The vaginal contraceptive sponge, which is not available in the United States, protects against cervical gonorrhea and chlamydia, but its use increases the risk for candidiasis. In case-control and cross-sectional studies, diaphragm use has been demonstrated to protect against cervical gonorrhea, chlamydia, and trichomoniasis; however, no cohort studies have been conducted. Vaginal spermacides, sponges, or diaphragms should not be assumed to protect women against HIV infection. The role of spermicides, sponges, and diaphragms for preventing STDs in men has not been evaluated.

PARTNER NOTIFICATION

For most STDs, partners of patients should be examined. When exposure to a treatable STD is considered likely, appropriate antimicrobials should be administered even though no clinical signs of infection are evident and laboratory test results are not yet available. In many states, the local or state health department can assist in notifying the partners of patients who have selected STDs (e.g., HIV infection, syphilis, gonorrhea, hepatitis B, and chlamydia).

Health-care providers should advise patients who have an STD to notify sex partners, including those without symptoms, of their exposure and encourage these partners to seek clinical evaluation. This type of partner notification is known as patient referral. In situations in which patient referral may not be effective or possible, health departments should be prepared to assist the patient either through contract referral or provider referral. Contract referral is the process by which patients agree to self-refer their partners within a defined time period. If the partners do not obtain medical evaluation and treatment within that period, then provider referral is implemented. Provider referral is the process by which partners named by infected patients are notified and counseled by health department staff.

Interrupting the transmission of infection is crucial to STD control. For treatable and vaccine-preventable STDs, further transmission and reinfection can be prevented by referral of sex partners for diagnosis, treatment, vaccination (if applicable), and counseling. When health-care providers refer infected patients to local or state health departments for provider-referral partner notification, the patients may be interviewed by trained professionals to obtain the names of their sex partners and information regarding the location of these partners for notification purposes. Every health department protects the privacy of patients in partner notification activities. Because of the advantage of confidentiality, many patients prefer that public health officials notify partners. However, the ability of public health officials to provide appropriate prophylaxis to contacts of all patients who have STDs may be limited. In situations where the number of anonymous partners is substantial (e.g., situations among persons who exchange sex for drugs), targeted screening of persons at risk may be more effective at stopping the transmission of disease than provider-referral partner notification. Guidelines for management of sex partners and recommendations for partner notification for specific STDs are included for each STD addressed in this report.

HIV INFECTION: DETECTION, INITIAL MANAGEMENT, AND REFERRAL

Infection with HIV produces a spectrum of disease that progresses from a clinically latent or asymptomatic state to AIDS as a late manifestation. The pace of disease progression is variable. The time between infection with HIV and the development of AIDS ranges from a few months to as long as 17 years (median: 10 years). Most adults and adolescents infected with HIV remain symptom-free for long periods, but viral replication is active during all stages of infection, increasing substantially as the immune system deteriorates. AIDS eventually develops in almost all HIV-infected persons; in one study of HIV-infected adults, AIDS developed in 87% (95% confidence interval [CI]=83%–90%) within 17 years after infection. Additional cases are expected to occur among those who have remained AIDS-free for longer periods.

Greater awareness among both patients and health-care providers of the risk factors associated with HIV transmission has led to increased testing for HIV and earlier diagnosis of the infection, often before symptoms develop. The early diagnosis of HIV infection is important for several reasons. Treatments are available to slow the decline of immune system function. HIV-infected persons who have altered immune function are at increased risk for infections for which preventive measures are available (e.g., *Pneumocystis carinii* pneumonia [PCP], toxoplasmic encephalitis [TE], disseminated *Mycobacterium avium* complex [MAC] disease, tuberculosis [TB], and bacterial pneumonia). Because of its effect on the immune system, HIV affects the diagnosis, evaluation, treatment, and follow-up of many other diseases and may affect the efficacy of antimicrobial therapy for some STDs. Finally, the early diagnosis of HIV enables the health-care provider to counsel such patients and to assist in preventing HIV transmission to others.

DIAGNOSTIC TESTING FOR HIV-1 AND HIV-2

Testing for HIV should be offered to all persons whose behavior puts them at risk for infection, including persons who seek evaluation and treatment for STDs. Counseling before and after testing (i.e., pretest and posttest counseling) is an integral part of the testing procedure (see HIV Prevention Counseling). Informed consent must be obtained before an HIV test is performed. Some states require written consent.

HIV infection usually is diagnosed by using HIV-1 antibody tests. Antibody testing begins with a sensitive screening test such as the enzyme immunoassay (EIA). Reactive screening tests must be confirmed by a supplemental test, such as the Western blot (WB) or an immunofluorescence assay (IFA). If confirmed by a supplemental test, a positive antibody test result indicates that a person is infected with HIV and is capable of transmitting the virus to others. HIV antibody is detectable in at least 95% of patients within 6 months after infection. Although a negative antibody test result usually indicates that a person is not infected, antibody tests cannot exclude infection that occurred <6 months before the test.

The following are specific recommendations for diagnostic testing for HIV infection:

- Informed consent must be obtained before an HIV test is performed. Some states require written consent. (See HIV Prevention Counseling for a discussion of pretest and posttest counseling.)
- Positive screening tests for HIV antibody must be confirmed by a more specific confirmatory test (either WB or IFA) before being considered diagnostic of HIV infection.
- Patients who have positive HIV test results must either receive behavioral, psychosocial, and medical evaluation and monitoring services or be referred for these services.

ACUTE RETROVIRAL SYNDROME

Health-care providers should be alert for the symptoms and signs of acute retroviral syndrome, which is characterized by fever, malaise, lymphadenopathy, and skin rash. This syndrome frequently occurs in the first few weeks after HIV infection, before antibody test results become positive. Suspicion of acute retroviral syndrome should prompt nucleic acid testing to detect the presence of HIV. Recent data indicate that initiation of antiretroviral therapy during this period can delay the onset of HIV-related complications and might influence prognosis. If testing reveals acute HIV infection, health-care providers should either counsel the patient about immediate initiation of antiretroviral therapy or refer the patient for emergency expert consultation. The optimal antiretroviral regimen at this time is unknown. Treatment with zidovudine can delay the onset of HIV-related complications; however, most experts recommend treatment with two nucleoside reverse transcriptase inhibitors and a protease inhibitor.

PLANNING FOR MEDICAL CARE

Recently identified HIV infection may not have been recently acquired. Persons newly diagnosed with HIV may be at any of the different stages of infection. Therefore, the health-care provider should be alert for symptoms or signs that suggest advanced HIV infection (e.g., fever, weight loss, diarrhea, cough, shortness of breath, and oral candidiasis). The presence of any of these symptoms should prompt urgent referral for medical care. Similarly, the provider should be alert for signs of severe psychologic distress and be prepared to refer the client accordingly.

HIV-infected patients in the STD treatment setting should be educated about what to expect when medical care is necessary (*11*). In the nonemergent situation, the initial evaluation of the HIV-positive patient usually includes the following components:

- A detailed medical history, including sexual and substance-abuse history, previous STDs, and specific HIV-related symptoms or diagnoses.
- A physical examination; for women, this should include a gynecologic examination.
- For women, testing for *N. gonorrhoeae* and *C. trachomatis*, a Pap smear, and wet mount examination of vaginal secretions.
- Complete blood and platelet counts and blood chemistry profile.
- Toxoplasma antibody test, tests for hepatitis B viral markers, and syphilis serology.
- A CD4+ T-lymphocyte analysis and determination of HIV plasma ribonucleic acid (i.e., HIV viral load).
- A tuberculin skin test (TST) (sometimes referred to as a purified protein derivative [PPD] skin test) administered by the Mantoux method. The test result should be evaluated at 48–72 hours; in HIV-infected persons, a 5 mm induration is considered positive. The usefulness of anergy testing is controversial (*13–15*).
- A chest radiograph.
- A thorough psychosocial evaluation, including ascertainment of behavioral factors indicating risk for transmitting HIV and elucidation of information concerning any partners who should be notified about possible exposure to HIV.

In subsequent visits, once the results of laboratory and skin tests are available, the patient may be offered antiretroviral therapy (*16*), as well as specific medications to reduce the incidence of opportunistic infections (e.g., PCP, TE, dis- seminated MAC infection, and TB) (*10, 14, 17–19*). Hepatitis B vaccination should be offered to patients who do not have hepatitis B markers, influenza vaccination should be offered annually, and pneumococcal vaccination should be administered. For additional information concerning vaccination of HIV-infected patients, refer to "Recommendations of the Advisory Committee on Immunization Practices (ACIP): Use of Vaccines and Immune Globulins in Persons with Altered Immunocompetence" (*20*).

Specific recommendations for planning medical care and continuation of psychosocial services include the following:

- HIV-infected persons should be referred for appropriate follow-up to facilities in which health-care personnel are experienced in providing care for HIV-infected patients.
- Health-care providers should be alert for medical or psychosocial conditions that require immediate attention.
- Patients should be educated about what to expect in follow-up medical care.

The following are specific recommendations for implementing partner-notification procedures:

- HIV-infected patients should be encouraged to notify their partners and to refer them for counseling and testing. If requested by the patient, health-care providers should assist in this process, either directly or by referral to health depart- ment partner-notification programs.
- If patients are unwilling to notify their partners, or if they cannot ensure that their partners will seek counseling, physicians or health department personnel should use confidential procedures to notify the partners.

MANAGEMENT OF THE PATIENT WITH GENITAL ULCERS

In the United States, most young, sexually active patients who have genital ulcers have either genital herpes, syphilis, or chancroid. The relative frequency of each differs by geographic area and patient population; however, in most areas of the United States, genital herpes is the most prevalent of these diseases. More than one of these diseases could be present in a patient who has genital ulcers. Each disease has been associated with an increased risk for HIV infection.

A diagnosis based only on the patient's medical history and physical examination often is inaccurate. Specific tests for the evaluation of genital ulcers include the following:

- Darkfield examination or direct immunofluorescence test for *Treponema pallidum*,
- Culture or antigen test for HSV, and
- Culture for *Haemophilus ducreyi.*

CHANCROID

Chancroid is endemic in some areas of the United States, and the disease also occurs in discrete outbreaks. Chancroid is a cofactor for HIV transmission, and high rates of HIV infection among patients who have chancroid have been reported in the United States and other countries.

A definitive diagnosis of chancroid requires identification of *H. ducreyi* on special culture media that are not widely available from commercial sources; even using these media, sensitivity is $\leq 80\%$. A probable diagnosis, for both clinical and surveillance purposes, may be made if the following criteria are met: a) the patient has one or more painful genital ulcers; b) the patient has no evidence of *T. pallidum* infection by darkfield examination of ulcer exudate or by a serologic test for syphilis performed at least 7 days after onset of ulcers; and c) the clinical presentation, appearance of genital ulcers, and regional lymphadenopathy, if present, are typical for chancroid and a test for HSV is negative. The combination of a painful ulcer and tender inguinal adenopathy, which occurs among one third of patients, suggests a diagnosis of chancroid; when accompanied by suppurative inguinal adenopathy, these signs are almost pathognomonic. PCR testing for *H. ducreyi* might become available soon.

Recommended Regimens

- **Azithromycin 1 g orally in a single dose,**

or

- **Ceftriaxone 250 mg intramuscularly (IM) in a single dose,**

or

- **Ciprofloxacin 500 mg orally twice a day for 3 days,**

or

- **Erythromycin base 500 mg orally four times a day for 7 days.**

NOTE: Ciprofloxacin is contraindicated for pregnant and lactating women and for persons aged <18 years.

All four regimens are effective for treatment of chancroid in HIV-infected patients. Azithromycin and ceftriaxone offer the advantage of single-dose therapy. Worldwide, several isolates with intermediate resistance to either ciprofloxacin or erythromycin have been reported.

Follow-up

Patients should be reexamined 3–7 days after initiation of therapy. If treatment is successful, ulcers improve symptomatically within 3 days and objectively within 7 days after therapy. If no clinical improvement is evident, the clinician must consider whether a) the diagnosis is correct, b) the patient is coinfected with another STD, c) the patient is infected with HIV, d) the treatment was not taken as instructed, or e) the *H. ducreyi* strain causing the infection is resistant to the prescribed antimicrobial. The time required for complete healing depends on the size of the ulcer; large ulcers may require >2 weeks. In addition, healing is slower for some uncircumcised men who have ulcers under the foreskin. Clinical resolution of fluctuant lymphadenopathy is slower than that of ulcers and may require drainage, even during otherwise successful therapy. Although needle aspiration of buboes is a simpler procedure, incision and drainage of buboes may be preferred because of less need for subsequent drainage procedures.

Management of the patient with genital ulcers

Sex partners of patients who have chancroid should be examined and treated, regardless of whether symptoms of the disease are present, if they had sexual contact with the patient during the 10 days preceding onset of symptoms in the patient.

HIV infection

Healing may be slower among HIV-infected patients, and treatment failures occur with any regimen. Because data are limited concerning the therapeutic efficacy of the recommended ceftriaxone and azithromycin regimens in HIV-infected patients, these regimens should be used for such patients only if follow-up can be ensured. Some experts suggest using the erythromycin 7-day regimen for treating HIV-infected persons.

GENITAL HERPES SIMPLEX VIRUS (HSV) INFECTIONS

Genital herpes is a recurrent, incurable viral disease. Two serotypes of HSV have been identified: HSV-1 and HSV-2. Most cases of recurrent genital herpes are caused by HSV-2. On the basis of serologic studies, genital HSV-2 infection has been diagnosed in at least 45 million persons in the United States.

Most HSV-2–infected persons have not received a diagnosis of genital herpes. Such persons have mild or unrecognized infections that shed virus intermittently in the genital tract.

First clinical episode of genital herpes

Management of patients with first clinical episode of genital herpes includes antiviral therapy and counseling regarding the natural history of genital herpes, sexual and perinatal transmission, and methods to reduce such transmission.

Recommended Regimens

- **Acyclovir 400 mg orally three times a day for 7–10 days,**

or

- **Acyclovir 200 mg orally five times a day for 7–10 days,**

or

- **Famciclovir 250 mg orally three times a day for 7–10 days,**

or

- **Valacyclovir 1 g orally twice a day for 7–10 days.**

Counseling is an important aspect of managing patients who have genital herpes. Although initial counseling can be provided at the first visit, many patients benefit from learning about the chronic aspects of the disease after the acute illness subsides. Counseling of these patients should include the following:

- Patients who have genital herpes should be told about the natural history of the disease, with emphasis on the potential for recurrent episodes, asymptomatic viral shedding, and sexual transmission.
- Patients should be advised to abstain from sexual activity when lesions or prodromal symptoms are present and encouraged to inform their sex partners that they have genital herpes. The use of condoms during all sexual exposures with new or uninfected sex partners should be encouraged.
- Sexual transmission of HSV can occur during asymptomatic periods. Asymptomatic viral shedding occurs more frequently in

patients who have genital HSV-2 infection than HSV-1 infection and in patients who have had genital herpes for <12 months. Such patients should be counseled to prevent spread of the infection.

- The risk for neonatal infection should be explained to all patients, including men. Childbearing-aged women who have genital herpes should be advised to inform health-care providers who care for them during pregnancy about the HSV infection.
- Patients having a first episode of genital herpes should be advised that a) episodic antiviral therapy during recurrent episodes might shorten the duration of lesions and b) suppressive antiviral therapy can ameliorate or prevent recurrent outbreaks.

Recurrent episodes of HSV disease

Most patients with first-episode genital HSV-2 infection will have recurrent episodes of genital lesions. Episodic or suppressive antiviral therapy might shorten the duration of lesions or ameliorate recurrences. Because many patients benefit from antiviral therapy, options for treatment should be discussed with all patients.

If episodic treatment of recurrences is chosen, the patient should be provided with antiviral therapy, or a prescription for the medication, so that treatment can be initiated at the first sign of prodrome or genital lesions.

Daily suppressive therapy reduces the frequency of genital herpes recurrences by ≥75% among patients who have frequent recurrences (i.e., six or more recurrences per year). Safety and efficacy have been documented among patients receiving daily therapy with acyclovir for as long as 6 years, and with valacyclovir and famciclovir for 1 year. Suppressive therapy has not been associated with emergence of clinically significant acyclovir resistance among immunocompetent patients. After 1 year of continuous suppressive therapy, discontinuation of therapy should be discussed with the patient to assess the patient's psychological adjustment to genital herpes and rate of recurrent episodes, as the frequency of recurrences decreases over time in many patients. Insufficient experience with famciclovir and valacyclovir prevents recommendation of these drugs for >1 year.

Suppressive treatment with acyclovir reduces but does not eliminate asymptomatic viral shedding. Therefore, the extent to which suppressive therapy may prevent HSV transmission is unknown.

Recommended Regimens for Episodic Recurrent Infection

- **Acyclovir 400 mg orally three times a day for 5 days,**

or

- **Acyclovir 200 mg orally five times a day for 5 days,**

or

- **Acyclovir 800 mg orally twice a day for 5 days,**

or

- **Famciclovir 125 mg orally twice a day for 5 days,**

or

- **Valacyclovir 500 mg orally twice a day for 5 days.**

Recommended Regimens for Daily Suppressive Therapy

- **Acyclovir 400 mg orally twice a a day,**

or

- **Famciclovir 250 mg orally twice a day,**

or

- **Valacyclovir 500 mg orally once a day,**

or

- **Valacyclovir 1000 mg orally once a day.**

Valacyclovir 500 mg once a day appears less effective than other valacyclovir dosing regimens in patients who have very frequent recurrences (i.e., ≥10 episodes per year). Few comparative studies of valacyclovir and famciclovir with acyclovir have been conducted.

Recommended Regimen

- **Acyclovir 5-10 mg/kg body weight IV every 8 hours for 5-7 days or until clinical resolution is attained.**

Management of sex partners

Symptomatic sex partners should be evaluated and treated in the same manner as patients who have genital lesions. However, most persons who have genital HSV infection do not have a history of typical genital lesions. These persons and their future sex partners may benefit from evaluation and counseling.

Special considerations

HIV infection

Immunocompromised patients might have prolonged and/or severe episodes of genital or perianal herpes. Lesions caused by HSV are relatively common among HIV-infected patients and may be severe, painful, and atypical. Intermittent or suppressive therapy with oral antiviral agents is often beneficial.

Clinical experience strongly suggests that immunocompromised patients benefit from increased doses of antiviral drugs. Regimens such as acyclovir 400 mg orally three to five times a day, as used for other immunocompromised patients, have been useful. Therapy should be continued until clinical resolution is attained. Famciclovir 500 mg twice a day has been effective in decreasing both the rate of recurrences and the rate of subclinical shedding among HIV-infected patients.

Pregnancy

The safety of systemic acyclovir and valacyclovir therapy in pregnant women has not been established. Glaxo-Wellcome, Inc., in cooperation with CDC, maintains a registry to assess the use and effects of acyclovir and valacyclovir during pregnancy. Women who receive acyclovir or valacyclovir during pregnancy should be reported to this registry; telephone (888) 825-5249, extension 39441.

Current registry findings do not indicate an increased risk for major birth defects after acyclovir treatment (i.e., in comparison with the general population). The accumulated case histories represent an insufficient sample for reaching reliable and definitive conclusions regarding the risks associated with acyclovir treatment during pregnancy. Prenatal exposure to valacyclovir and famciclovir is too limited to provide useful information on pregnancy outcomes.

The first clinical episode of genital herpes during pregnancy may be treated with oral acyclovir. In the presence of life-threatening maternal HSV infection (e.g., disseminated infection, encephalitis, pneumonitis, or hepatitis), acyclovir administered IV is indicated. Investigations of acyclovir use among pregnant women suggest that acyclovir treatment near term might reduce the rate of abdominal deliveries among women who have frequently recurring or newly acquired genital herpes by decreasing the incidence of active lesions. However, routine administration of acyclovir to pregnant women who have a history of recurrent genital herpes is not recommended at this time.

Perinatal infections

Most mothers of infants who acquire neonatal herpes lack histories of clinically evident genital herpes. The risk for transmission to the neonate from an infected mother is high among women who acquire genital herpes near the time of delivery (30%–50%) and is low among women who have a history of recurrent herpes at term and women who acquire genital HSV during the first half of pregnancy (3%). Therefore, prevention of neonatal herpes should emphasize prevention of acquisition of genital HSV infection during late pregnancy. Susceptible women whose partners have oral or genital HSV infection, or those whose sex partners' infection status is unknown, should be counseled to avoid unprotected genital and oral sexual contact during late pregnancy. The results of viral cultures during pregnancy do not predict viral shedding at the time of delivery, and such cultures are not indicated routinely.

At the onset of labor, all women should be examined and carefully questioned regarding whether they have symptoms of genital herpes. Infants of women who do not have symptoms or signs of genital herpes infection or its prodrome may be delivered vaginally. Abdominal delivery does not completely eliminate the risk for HSV infection in the neonate.

GRANULOMA INGUINALE (DONOVANOSIS)

Granuloma inguinale, a rare disease in the United States, is caused by the intracellular Gram-negative bacterium *Calymmatobacterium granulomatis*. The disease is endemic in certain tropical and developing areas, including India, Papua New Guinea, central Australia, and southern Africa. The disease presents clinically as painless, progressive, ulcerative lesions without regional lymphadenopathy. The lesions are highly vascular (i.e., a beefy red appearance) and bleed easily on contact. The causative organism cannot be cultured on standard microbiologic media, and diagnosis requires visualization of dark-staining Donovan bodies on tissue crush preparation or biopsy. A secondary bacterial infection might develop in the lesions, or the lesions might be coinfected with another sexually transmitted pathogen.

Treatment

Treatment appears to halt progressive destruction of tissue, although prolonged duration of therapy often is required to enable granulation and re-epithelialization of the ulcers. Relapse can occur 6–18 months later despite effective initial therapy.

Recommended Regimen

- **Trimethoprim-sulfamethoxazole one double-strength tablet orally twice a day, for minimun of 3 weeks,**

or

- **Doxycycline 100 mg orally twice a day for a minimum of 3 weeks.**

Therapy should be continued until all lesions have completely healed.

Alternative Regimens

- **Ciprofloxacin 750 mg orally twice a day for a minimum of 3 weeks,**

or

- **Erythromycin base 500 mg orally four times a day for a minimum of 3 weeks.**

For any of the above regimens, the addition of an aminoglycoside (gentamicin 1 mg/kg IV every 8 hours) should be considered if lesions do not respond within the first few days of therapy.

Management of sex partners

Sex partners of patients who have granuloma inguinale should be examined and treated if they a) had sexual contact with the patient during the 60 days preceding the onset of symptoms in the patient and b) have clinical signs and symptoms of the disease.

LYMPHOGRANULOMA VENEREUM

Lymphogranuloma venereum (LGV), a rare disease in the United States, is caused by the invasive serovars L1, L2, or L3 of *C. trachomatis*. The most frequent clinical manifestation of LGV among heterosexual men is tender inguinal and/or femoral lymphadenopathy that is usually unilateral. Women and homosexually active men might have proctocolitis or inflammatory involvement of perirectal or perianal lymphatic tissues that can result in fistulas and strictures. When most patients seek medical care, they no longer have the self-limited genital ulcer that sometimes occurs at the inoculation site. The diagnosis usually is made serologically and by exclusion of other causes of inguinal lymphadenopathy or genital ulcers.

Recommended Regimen

- **Doxycycline 100 mg orally twice a day for 21 days.**

Alternative Regimens

- **Erythromycin base 500 mg orally four times a day for 21 days.**

The activity of azithromycin against *C. trachomatis* suggests that it may be effective in multiple doses over 2–3 weeks, but clinical data regarding its use are lacking.

Management of sex partners

Sex partners of patients who have LGV should be examined, tested for urethral or cervical chlamydial infection, and treated if they had sexual contact with the patient during the 30 days preceding onset of symptoms in the patient.

SYPHILIS

Diagnostic Considerations and Use of Serologic Tests.

Darkfield examinations and direct fluorescent antibody tests of lesion exudate or tissue are the definitive methods for diagnosing early syphilis. A presumptive diagnosis is possible with the use of two types of serologic tests for syphilis: a) nontreponemal (e.g., Venereal Disease Research Laboratory [VDRL] and RPR) and b) treponemal (e.g., fluorescent treponemal antibody absorbed [FTA-ABS] and microhemagglutination assay for antibody to *T. pallidum* [MHA-TP]). The use of only one type of test is insufficient for diagnosis because false-positive nontrep- onemal test results occasionally occur secondary to various medical conditions. Nontreponemal test antibody titers usually correlate with disease activity, and results should be reported quantitatively. A fourfold change in titer, equivalent to a change of two dilutions (e.g., from 1:16 to 1:4 or from 1:8 to 1:32), usually is considered necessary to demonstrate a clinically significant difference between two nontreponemal test results that were obtained by using the same serologic test. It is expected that the nontreponemal test will eventually become nonreactive after treatment; however, in some patients, nontreponemal antibodies can persist at a low titer for a long period, sometimes for the remainder of their lives. This response is referred to as the serofast reaction. Most patients who have reactive treponemal tests will have reactive tests for the remainder of their lives, regardless of treatment or disease activity. However, 15%–25% of patients treated during the primary stage might revert to being serologically nonreactive after 2–3 years. Treponemal test antibody titers correlate poorly with disease activity and should not be used to assess treatment response.

Sequential serologic tests should be performed by using the same testing method (e.g., VDRL or RPR), preferably by the same laboratory. The VDRL and RPR are equally valid, but quantitative results from the two tests cannot be compared directly because RPR titers often are slightly higher than VDRL titers.

HIV-infected patients can have abnormal serologic test results (i.e., unusually high, unusually low, and fluctuating titers). For such patients with clinical syndromes suggestive of early syphilis, use of other tests (e.g., biopsy and direct microscopy) should be considered. However, for most HIV-infected patients, serologic tests appear to be accurate and reliable for the diagnosis of syphilis and for evaluation of treatment response.

No single test can be used to diagnose all cases of neurosyphilis. The diagnosis of neurosyphilis can be made based on various combinations of reactive serologic test results, abnormalities of cerebrospinal fluid (CSF) cell count or protein, or a reactive VDRL-CSF with or without clinical manifestations. The CSF leukocyte count usually is elevated (>5 WBCs/mm^3) when neurosyphilis is present, and it also is a sensitive measure of the effectiveness of therapy. The VDRL-CSF is the standard serologic test for CSF; when reactive in the absence of substantial contamination of CSF with blood, it is considered diagnostic of neurosyphilis. However, the VDRL-CSF may be nonreactive when neurosyphilis is present. Some experts recommend performing an FTA-ABS test on CSF. The CSF FTA-ABS is less specific (i.e., yields more false-positive results) for neurosyphilis than the VDRL-CSF. However, the test is believed to be highly sensitive, and some experts believe that a negative CSF FTA-ABS test excludes neurosyphilis.

Treatment

Parenteral penicillin G is the preferred drug for treatment of all stages of syphilis. The preparation(s) used (i.e., benzathine, aqueous procaine, or aqueous crystalline), the dosage, and the length of treatment depend on the stage and clinical manifestations of disease.

The efficacy of penicillin for the treatment of syphilis was well established through clinical experience before the value of randomized controlled clinical trials was recognized. Therefore, almost all the recommendations for the treatment of syphilis are based on expert opinion reinforced by case series, clinical trials, and 50 years of clinical experience.

Parenteral penicillin G is the only therapy with documented efficacy for neurosyphilis or for syphilis during pregnancy. Patients who report a penicillin allergy, including pregnant women with syphilis in any stage and patients with neurosyphilis, should be desensitized and treated with penicillin. Skin testing for penicillin allergy may be useful in some settings (see Management of Patients Who Have a History of Penicillin Allergy), because the minor determinants needed for penicillin skin testing are unavailable commercially.

The Jarisch-Herxheimer reaction is an acute febrile reaction—often accompanied by headache, myalgia, and other symptoms—that might occur within the first 24 hours after any therapy for syphilis; patients should be advised of this possible adverse reaction. The Jarisch-Herxheimer reaction often occurs among patients who have early syphilis. Antipyretics may be recommended, but no proven methods prevent this reaction. The Jarisch-Herxheimer reaction may induce early labor or cause fetal distress among pregnant women. This concern should not prevent or delay therapy (see Syphilis During Pregnancy).

Management of sex partners

- Persons who were exposed within the 90 days preceding the diagnosis of primary, secondary, or early latent syphilis in a sex partner might be infected even if seronegative; therefore, such persons should be treated presumptively.
- Persons who were exposed >90 days before the diagnosis of primary, secondary, or early latent syphilis in a sex partner should be treated presumptively if serologic test results are not available immediately and the opportunity for follow-up is uncertain.
- For purposes of partner notification and presumptive treatment of exposed sex partners, patients with syphilis of unknown duration who have high nontreponemal serologic test titers (i.e., ≥1:32) may be considered as having early syphilis. However, serologic titers should not be used to differentiate early from late latent syphilis for the purpose of determining treatment (see section regarding treatment of latent syphilis).
- Long-term sex partners of patients who have late syphilis should be evaluated clinically and serologically for syphilis and treated on the basis of the findings of the evaluation.

The time periods before treatment used for identifying at-risk sex partners are a) 3 months plus duration of symptoms for primary syphilis, b) 6 months plus duration of symptoms for secondary syphilis, and c) 1 year for early latent syphilis.

PRIMARY AND SECONDARY SYPHILIS

Recommended Regimen for Adults

- **Benzathine penicillin G 2.4 million units IM in a single dose.**

Patients who have syphilis and who also have symptoms or signs suggesting neurologic disease (e.g., meningitis) or ophthalmic disease (e.g., uveitis) should be evaluated fully for neurosyphilis and syphilitic eye disease; this evaluation should include CSF analysis and ocular slit-lamp examination.

Follow-up

Treatment failures can occur with any regimen. However, assessing response to treatment often is difficult, and no definitive criteria for cure or failure have been established. Serologic test titers may decline more slowly for patients who previously had syphilis. Patients should be reexamined clinically and serologically at both 6 months and 12 months; more frequent evaluation may be prudent if follow-up is uncertain.

Patients who have signs or symptoms that persist or recur or who have a sustained fourfold increase in nontreponemal test titer (i.e., in comparison with either the baseline titer or a subsequent result) probably failed treatment or were reinfected. These patients should be re-treated after reevaluation for HIV infection. Unless reinfection with *T. pallidum* is certain, a lumbar puncture also should be performed.

Failure of nontreponemal test titers to decline fourfold within 6 months after therapy for primary or secondary syphilis identifies persons at risk for treatment failure. Such persons should be reevaluated for HIV infection. Optimal management of such patients is unclear. At a minimum, these patients should have additional clinical and serologic follow-up. HIV-infected patients should be evaluated more frequently (i.e., at 3-month intervals instead of 6-month intervals). If additional follow-up cannot be ensured, re-treatment is recommended. Some experts recommend CSF examination in such situations.

When patients are re-treated, most experts recommend re-treatment with three weekly injections of benzathine penicillin G 2.4

million units IM, unless CSF examination indicates that neurosyphilis is present.

Penicillin allergy

Nonpregnant penicillin-allergic patients who have primary or secondary syphilis should be treated with one of the following regimens. Close follow-up of such patients is essential.

Recommended Regimens

- **Doxycycline 100 mg orally twice a day for 2 weeks,**

or

- **Tetracycline 500 mg orally four times a day for 2 weeks.**

Pregnancy

Pregnant patients who are allergic to penicillin should be desensitized, if necessary, and treated with penicillin.

LATENT SYPHILIS

Latent syphilis is defined as those periods after infection with *T. pallidum* when patients are seroreactive, but demonstrate no other evidence of disease. Patients who have latent syphilis and who acquired syphilis within the preceding year are classified as having early latent syphilis. Patients can be demonstrated as having early latent syphilis if, within the year preceding the evaluation, they had a) a documented seroconversion, b) unequivocal symptoms of primary or secondary syphilis, or c) a sex partner who had primary, secondary, or early latent syphilis. Almost all other patients have latent syphilis of unknown duration and should be managed as if they had late latent syphilis. Regardless of the level of the nontreponemal titers, patients in whom the illness does not meet the definition of early syphilis should be treated as if they have late latent infection.

Recommended Regimens for Adults

- **Early Latent Syphilis:**
  Benzathine penicillin G 2.4 million units IM in a single dose.
- **Late Latent Syphilis or Latent Syphilis of Unknown Duration:**
  Benzathine penicillin G 7.2 million units total, administered as three doses of 2.4 million units IM each at 1-week intervals.

Other management considerations

All patients who have latent syphilis should be evaluated clinically for evidence of tertiary disease (e.g., aortitis, neurosyphilis, gumma, and iritis). Patients who have syphilis and who demonstrate any of the following criteria should have a prompt CSF examination:

- Neurologic or ophthalmic signs or symptoms;
- Evidence of active tertiary syphilis (e.g., aortitis, gumma, and iritis);
- Treatment failure; and
- HIV infection with late latent syphilis or syphilis of unknown duration.

Follow-up

Quantitative nontreponemal serologic tests should be repeated at 6, 12, and 24 months. Limited data are available to guide evaluation of the treatment response for patients who have latent syphilis. Patients should be evaluated for neurosyphilis and re-treated appropriately if a) titers increase fourfold, b) an initially high titer ($\geq$1:32) fails to decline at least fourfold (i.e., two dilutions) within 12–24 months, or c) signs or symptoms attributable to syphilis develop in the patient.

Penicillin allergy

Nonpregnant patients who have latent syphilis and who are allergic to penicillin, should be treated with the following regimens.

Recommended Regimens

- **Doxycycline 100 mg orally twice a day,**

or

- **Tetracycline 500 mg orally four times a day.**

Both drugs should be administered for 2 weeks if the duration of infection is known to have been <1 year; otherwise, they should be administered for 4 weeks.

TERTIARY SYPHILIS

Recommended Regimen

- **Benzathine penicillin G 7.2 million units total, administered as three doses of 2.4 million units IM at 1-week intervals.**

Other management considerations

Patients who have symptomatic late syphilis should have a CSF examination before therapy is initiated. Some experts treat all patients who have cardiovascular syphilis with a neurosyphilis regimen. The complete management of patients who have cardiovascular or gummatous syphilis is beyond the scope of these guidelines.

NEUROSYPHILIS

Central nervous system disease can occur during any stage of syphilis. A patient who has clinical evidence of neurologic involvement with syphilis (e.g., ophthalmic or auditory symptoms, cranial nerve palsies, and symptoms or signs of meningitis) should have a CSF examination.

Syphilitic uveitis or other ocular manifestations frequently are associated with neurosyphilis; patients with these symptoms should be treated according to the recommendations for neurosyphilis. A CSF examination should be performed for all such patients to identify those with abnormalities who should have follow-up CSF examinations to assess treatment response.

Recommended Regimen

- **Aqueous crystalline penicillin G 18–24 million units a day, administered as 3–4 million units IV every 4 hours for 10–14 days.**

Alternative Regimen

- **Procaine penicillin 2.4 million units IM a day, PLUS Probenecid 500 mg orally four times a day, both for 10-14 days.**

Some experts administer benzathine penicillin, 2.4 million units IM, after completion of these neurosyphilis treatment regimens to provide a comparable total duration of therapy.

Follow-up

If CSF pleocytosis was present initially, a CSF examination should be repeated every 6 months until the cell count is normal. Follow-up CSF examinations also can be used to evaluate changes in the VDRL-CSF or CSF protein after therapy; however, changes in these two parameters are slower, and persistent abnormalities are of less importance. If the cell count has not decreased after 6 months, or if the CSF is not entirely normal after 2 years, re-treatment should be considered.

SYPHILIS IN HIV-INFECTED PERSONS

Primary and secondary syphilis among HIV-infected persons

Treatment with benzathine penicillin G, 2.4 million units IM, as for HIV-negative patients, is recommended. Some experts recommend additional treatments (e.g., three weekly doses of benzathine penicillin G as suggested for late syphilis) or other supplemental antibiotics in addition to benzathine penicillin G 2.4 million units IM.

Other management considerations

CSF abnormalities often occur among both asymptomatic HIV-infected patients in the absence of syphilis and HIV-negative patients who have primary or secondary syphilis. Such abnormalities in HIV-infected patients who have primary or secondary syphilis are of unknown prognostic significance. Most HIV-infected patients respond appropriately to the currently recommended penicillin therapy; however, some experts recommend CSF examination before therapy and modification of treatment accordingly.

Follow-up

It is important that HIV-infected patients be evaluated clinically and serologically for treatment failure at 3, 6, 9, 12, and 24 months after therapy. Although of unproven benefit, some experts recommend a CSF examination after therapy (i.e., at 6 months).

HIV-infected patients who meet the criteria for treatment failure should be managed the same as HIV-negative patients (i.e., a CSF examination and re-treatment). CSF examination and re-treatment also should be strongly considered for patients whose nontreponemal test titer does not decrease fourfold within 6–12 months. Most experts would re-treat patients with 7.2 million units of benzathine penicillin G (administered as three weekly doses of 2.4 million units each) if CSF examinations are normal.

Latent syphilis among HIV-infected patients

Diagnostic considerations

HIV-infected patients who have early latent syphilis should be managed and treated according to the recommendations for HIV-negative patients who have primary and secondary syphilis.

HIV-infected patients who have either late latent syphilis or syphilis of unknown duration should have a CSF examination before treatment.

Treatment

A patient with late latent syphilis or syphilis of unknown duration and a normal CSF examination can be treated with 7.2 million units of benzathine penicillin G (as three weekly doses of 2.4 million units each). Patients who have CSF consistent with neurosyphilis should be treated and managed as described for neurosyphilis.

Follow-up

Patients should be evaluated clinically and serologically at 6, 12, 18, and 24 months after therapy. If, at any time, clinical symptoms develop or nontreponemal titers rise fourfold, a repeat CSF examination should be performed and treatment administered accordingly. If between 12 and 24 months the nontreponemal titer fails to decline fourfold, the CSF examination should be repeated, and treatment administered accordingly.

SYPHILIS DURING PREGNANCY

All women should be screened serologically for syphilis during the early stages of pregnancy. In populations in which utilization of prenatal care is not optimal, RPR-card test screening and treatment (i.e., if the RPR-card test is reactive) should be performed at the time a pregnancy is diagnosed. For communities and populations in which the prevalence of syphilis is high or for patients at high risk, serologic testing should be performed twice during the third trimester, at 28 weeks of gestation and at delivery. (Some states mandate screening at delivery for all women.) Any woman who delivers a stillborn infant after 20 weeks of gestation should be tested for syphilis. No infant should leave the hospital without the maternal serologic status having been determined at least once during pregnancy.

Recommended Regimens

- Treatment during pregnancy should be the penicillin regimen appropriate for the stage of syphilis.

Other management considerations

Some experts recommend additional therapy in some settings. A second dose of benzathine penicillin 2.4 million units IM may be administered 1 week after the initial dose for women who have primary, secondary, or early latent syphilis. Ultrasonographic signs of fetal syphilis (i.e., hepatomegaly and hydrops) indicate a greater risk for fetal treatment failure; such cases should be managed in consultation with obstetric specialists.

Women treated for syphilis during the second half of pregnancy are at risk for premature labor and/or fetal distress if the treatment precipitates the Jarisch-Herxheimer reaction. These women should be advised to seek obstetric attention after treatment if they notice any contractions or decrease in fetal movements.

Penicillin allergy

There are no proven alternatives to penicillin for treatment of syphilis during pregnancy. Pregnant women who have a history of penicillin allergy should be desensitized and treated with penicillin.

Tetracycline and doxycycline usually are not used during pregnancy. Erythromycin should not be used, because it does not reliably cure an infected fetus. Data are insufficient to recommend azithromycin or ceftriaxone.

CONGENITAL SYPHILIS

Effective prevention and detection of congenital syphilis depends on the identification of syphilis in pregnant women and, therefore, on the routine serologic screening of pregnant women at the time of the first prenatal visit. Serologic testing and a sexual history also should be obtained at 28 weeks of gestation and at delivery in communities and populations in which the risk for congenital syphilis is high. Moreover, as part of the management of pregnant women who have syphilis, information concerning treatment of sex partners should be obtained in order to assess possible maternal reinfection.

EVALUATION AND TREATMENT OF THE INFANT IN THE FIRST MONTH OF LIFE

Who should be evaluated

All infants born to seroreactive mothers should be evaluated with a quantitative nontreponemal serologic test (RPR or VDRL) performed on infant serum (i.e., umbilical cord blood might be contaminated with maternal blood and might yield a false-positive result). A treponemal test (i.e., MHA-TP or FTA-ABS) of a newborn's serum is not necessary.

Evaluation

All infants born to women who have reactive serologic tests for syphilis should be examined thoroughly for evidence of congenital syphilis (e.g., nonimmune hydrops, jaundice, hepatosplenomegaly, rhinitis, skin rash, and/or pseudoparalysis of an extremity). Pathologic examination of the placenta or umbilical cord using specific fluorescent antitreponemal antibody staining is suggested. Darkfield microscopic examination or direct fluorescent antibody staining of suspicious lesions or body fluids (e.g., nasal discharge) also should be performed.

Further evaluation of the infant is dependent on a) whether any abnormalities are present on physical examination, b) maternal treatment history, c) stage of infection at the time of treatment, and d) comparison of maternal (at delivery) and infant nontreponemal titers utilizing the same test and preferably the same laboratory.

Treatment

Infants should be treated for presumed congenital syphilis if they were born to mothers who met any of the following criteria:

- Had untreated syphilis at delivery;*
- Had serologic evidence of relapse or reinfection after treatment (i.e., a fourfold or greater increase in nontreponemal antibody titer);
- Was treated with erythromycin or other nonpenicillin regimen for syphilis during pregnancy;†
- Was treated for syphilis ≤4 weeks before delivery;
- Did not have a well-documented history of treatment for syphilis;
- Was treated for early syphilis during pregnancy with the appropriate penicillin regimen, but nontreponemal antibody titers did not decrease at least fourfold; or
- Was treated appropriately before pregnancy but had insufficient serologic follow-up to ensure an adequate treatment response and lack of current infection (i.e., an appropriate response includes a] at least a fourfold decrease in nontreponemal antibody titers for patients treated for early syphilis and b] stable or declining nontreponemal titers of ≤1:4 for other patients).

Regardless of a maternal history of infection with *T. pallidum* or treatment for syphilis, the evaluation should include the following tests if the infant has either a) an abnormal physical examination that is consistent with congenital syphilis, b) a serum quantitative nontreponemal serologic titer that is fourfold greater than the mother's titer, or c) a positive darkfield or fluorescent antibody test of body fluid(s).

- CSF analysis for VDRL, cell count, and protein;
- Complete blood count (CBC) and differential CBC and platelet count;
- Other tests as clinically indicated (e.g., long-bone radiographs, chest radiograph, liver-function tests, cranial ultrasound, ophthalmologic examination, and auditory brainstem response).

*A woman treated with a regimen other than those recommended in these guidelines for treatment of syphilis should be considered untreated.

†The absence of a fourfold greater titer for an infant does not exclude congenital syphilis.

Recommended Regimens

- **Aqueous crystalline penicillin G 100,000–150,000 units/kg/day, administered as 50,000 units/kg/dose IV every 12 hours during the first 7 days of life and every 8 hours thereafter for a total of 10 days;**

or

- **Procaine penicillin G 50,000 units/kg/dose IM daily in a single dose for 10 days.**

If >1 day of therapy is missed, the entire course should be restarted. Data are insufficient regarding the use of other antimicrobial agents (e.g., ampicillin). When possible, a full 10-day course of penicillin is preferred. The use of agents other than penicillin requires close serologic follow-up to assess adequacy of therapy.

In all other situations, the maternal history of infection with *T. pallidum* and treatment for syphilis must be considered when evaluating and treating the infant. For infants who have a normal physical examination and a serum quantitative nontreponemal serologic titer the same or less than fourfold the maternal titer, the evaluation depends on the maternal treatment history and stage of infection.

- The infant should receive the following treatment if a) the maternal treatment was not given, was undocumented, was a nonpenicillin regimen, or was administered ≤4 weeks before delivery; b) the adequacy of maternal treatment for early syphilis cannot be evaluated because the nontreponemal serologic titer has not decreased fourfold; or c) relapse or reinfection is suspected because of a fourfold increase in maternal nontreponemal serologic titer.
  a. Aqueous penicillin G or procaine penicillin G for 10 days. Some experts prefer this therapy if the mother has untreated early syphilis at delivery. A complete evaluation is unnecessary if 10 days of parenteral therapy is given. However such evaluation may be useful; a lumbar puncture may document CSF abnormalities that would prompt close follow-up.* Other tests (e.g., CBC and platelet count and bone radiographs) may be performed to further support a diagnosis of congenital syphilis; *or*
  b. Benzathine penicillin G 50,000 units/kg (single dose IM) if the infant's evaluation (i.e., CSF examination, long-bone radiographs, and CBC with platelets) is normal and follow-up is certain. If any part of the infant's evaluation is abnormal or not done, or the CSF analysis is uninterpretable secondary to contamination with blood, then a 10-day course of penicillin (see preceding paragraph) is required.†

*CSF test results obtained during the neonatal period can be difficult to interpret; normal values differ by gestational age and are higher in preterm infants. Values as high as 25 white blood cells (WBCs)/mm^3 and/or protein of 150 mg/dL might occur among normal neonates; some experts, however, recommend that lower values (i.e., 5 WBCs/mm^3 and protein of 40 mg/dL) be considered the upper limits of normal. Other causes of elevated values also should be considered when an infant is being evaluated for congenital syphilis.

†If the infant's nontreponemal test is nonreactive and the likelihood of the infant being infected is low, some experts recommend no evaluation but treatment of the infant with a single IM dose of benzathine penicillin G 50,000 units/kg for possible incubating syphilis, after which the infant should have close serologic follow-up.

- Evaluation is unnecessary if the maternal treatment a) was during pregnancy, appropriate for the stage of infection, and >4 weeks before delivery; b) was for early syphilis and the nontreponemal serologic titers decreased fourfold after appropriate therapy; or c) was for late latent infection, the nontreponemal titers remained stable and low, and there is no evidence of maternal reinfection or relapse. A single dose of benzathine penicillin G 50,000 units/kg IM should be administered. (Note: Some experts would not treat the infant but would provide close serologic follow-up.) Furthermore, in these situations, if the infant's nontreponemal test is nonreactive, no treatment is necessary.
- Evaluation and treatment are unnecessary if the maternal treatment was before pregnancy, after which the mother was evaluated multiple times, and the nontreponemal serologic titer remained low and stable before and during pregnancy and at delivery (VDRL ≤ 1:2; RPR ≤ 1:4). Some experts would treat with benzathine penicillin G 50,000 units/kg as a single IM injection, particularly if follow-up is uncertain.

EVALUATION AND TREATMENT OF OLDER INFANTS AND CHILDREN WHO HAVE CONGENITAL SYPHILIS

Children who are identified as having reactive serologic tests for syphilis after the neonatal period (i.e., at >1 month of age) should have maternal serology and records reviewed to assess whether the child has congenital or acquired syphilis (for acquired syphilis, see Primary and Secondary Syphilis and Latent Syphilis). If the child possibly has congenital syphilis, the child should be evaluated fully (i.e., a CSF examination for cell count, protein, and VDRL [abnormal CSF evaluation includes a reactive VDRL test, >5 WBCs/mm^3, and/or protein >40 mg/dL]; an eye examination; and other tests such as long-bone radiographs, CBC, platelet count, and auditory brainstem response as indicated clinically). Any child who possibly has congenital syphilis or who has neurologic involvement should be treated with aqueous crystalline penicillin G, 200,000–300,000 units/kg/day IV (administered as 50,000 units/kg every 4–6 hours) for 10 days.

Follow-up

All seroreactive infants (or an infant whose mother was seroreactive at delivery) should receive careful follow-up examinations and serologic testing (i.e., a nontreponemal test) every 2–3 months until the test becomes nonreactive or the titer has decreased fourfold. Nontreponemal antibody titers should decline by 3 months of age and should be nonreactive by 6 months of age if the infant was not infected (i.e., if the reactive test result was caused by passive transfer of maternal IgG antibody) or was infected but adequately treated. The serologic response after therapy may be slower for infants treated after the neonatal period. If these titers are stable or increasing after 6–12 months of age, the child should be evaluated, including a CSF examination, and treated with a 10-day course of parenteral penicillin G.

Treponemal tests should not be used to evaluate treatment response because the results for an infected child can remain positive despite effective therapy. Passively transferred maternal treponemal antibodies could be present in an infant until age 15 months. A reactive treponemal test after age 18 months is diagnostic of congenital syphilis. If the nontreponemal test is nonreactive at this time, no further evaluation or treatment is necessary. If the nontreponemal test is reactive at age 18 months, the infant should be fully (re)evaluated and treated for congenital syphilis.

Infants whose initial CSF evaluation is abnormal should undergo a repeat lumbar puncture approximately every 6 months until the results are normal. A reactive CSF VDRL test or abnormal CSF indices that cannot be attributed to other ongoing illness requires re-treatment for possible neurosyphilis.

DISEASES CHARACTERIZED BY URETHRITIS AND CERVICITIS

MANAGEMENT OF MALE PATIENTS WHO HAVE URETHRITIS

Urethritis, or inflammation of the urethra, is caused by an infection characterized by the discharge of mucopurulent or purulent material and by burning during urination. The only bacterial pathogens of proven clinical importance in men who have urethritis are *N. gonorrhoeae* and *C. trachomatis*. Testing to determine the specific disease is recommended because both of these infections are reportable to state health departments, and a specific diagnosis may improve compliance and partner notification. If diagnostic tools (e.g., a Gram stain and microscope) are unavailable, patients should be treated for both infections.

Confirmed urethritis

Clinicians should document that urethritis is present. Urethritis can be documented by the presence of any of the following signs:

a. Mucopurulent or purulent discharge.
b. Gram stain of urethral secretions demonstrating ≥5 WBCs per oil immersion field. The Gram stain is the preferred rapid diagnostic test for evaluating urethritis. It is highly sensitive and specific for documenting both urethritis and the presence or absence of gonococcal infection. Gonococcal infection is established by documenting the presence of WBCs containing intracellular Gram-negative diplococci.
c. Positive leukocyte esterase test on first-void urine, or microscopic examination of first-void urine demonstrating ≥10 WBCs per high power field.

If none of these criteria is present, then treatment should be deferred, and the patient should be tested for *N. gonorrhoeae* and *C. trachomatis* and followed closely in the event of a positive test result. If the results demonstrate infection with either *N. gonorrhoeae* or *C. trachomatis*, the appropriate treatment should be given and sex partners referred for evaluation and treatment.

Recommended Regimens

- **Azithromycin 1 g orally in a single dose,**

or

- **Doxycycline 100 mg orally twice a day for 7 days.**

Alternative Regimens

- **Erythromycin base 500 mg orally four times a day for 7 days**

or

- **Erythromycin ethylsuccinate 800 mg orally four times a day for 7 days.**

or

- **Ofloxacin 300 mg twice a day for 7 days.**

If only erythromycin can be used and a patient cannot tolerate high-dose erythromycin schedules, one of the following regimens may be used:

- **Erythromycin base 250 mg orally four times a day for 14 days**

or

- **Erythromycin ethylsuccinate 400 mg orally four times a day for 14 days.**

Follow-up for patients who have urethritis

Patients should be instructed to return for evaluation if symptoms persist or recur after completion of therapy. Symptoms alone, without documentation of signs or laboratory evidence of urethral inflammation, are not a sufficient basis for re-treatment. Patients should be instructed to abstain from sexual intercourse until 7 days after therapy is initiated.

Partner referral

Patients should refer for evaluation and treatment all sex partners within the preceding 60 days.

Recurrent and persistent urethritis

Objective signs of urethritis should be present before initiation of antimicrobial therapy. Patients who have persistent or recurrent urethritis should be re-treated with the initial regimen if they did not comply with the treatment regimen or if they were reexposed to an untreated sex partner. Otherwise, a wet mount examination and culture of an intraurethral swab specimen for *T. vaginalis* should be performed. Urologic examinations usually do not reveal a specific etiology.

Recommended Treatment for Recurrent/Persistent Urethritis

- **Metronidazole 2 g orally in a single dose,**

plus

- **Erythromycin base 500 mg orally four times a day for 7 days,**

or

- **Erythromycin ethylsuccinate 800 mg orally four times a day for 7 days.**

MANAGEMENT OF PATIENTS WHO HAVE MUCOPURULENT CERVICITIS (MPC)

MPC is characterized by a purulent or mucopurulent endocervical exudate visible in the endocervical canal or in an endocervical swab specimen. Some experts also make the diagnosis on the basis of easily induced cervical bleeding. Although some experts consider an increased number of polymorphonuclear leukocytes on endocervical Gram stain as being useful in the diagnosis of MPC, this criterion has not been standardized, has a low positive-predictive value (PPV), and is not available in some settings. MPC often is asymptomatic, but some women have an abnormal vaginal discharge and vaginal bleeding (e.g., after sexual intercourse). MPC can be caused by *C. trachomatis* or *N. gonorrhoeae*; however, in most cases neither organism can be isolated. MPC can persist despite repeated courses of antimicrobial therapy.

Patients who have MPC should be tested for *C. trachomatis* and for *N. gonorrhoeae* by using the most sensitive and specific test for the population served.

Treatment

The results of sensitive tests for *C. trachomatis* or *N. gonorrhoeae* (e.g., culture or nucleic acid amplification tests) should determine the need for treatment, unless the likelihood of infection with either organism is high or the patient is unlikely to return for treatment. Empiric treatment should be considered for a patient who has a suspected case of gonorrhea and/or chlamydia if a) the prevalences of these infections are high in the patient population and b) the patient might be difficult to locate for treatment. After the possibilities of relapse and reinfection have been excluded, management of persistent MPC is unclear.

Management of sex partners

Management of sex partners of women treated for MPC should be appropriate for the identified or suspected STD.

CHLAMYDIAL INFECTION

In the United States, chlamydial genital infection occurs frequently among sexually active adolescents and young adults. Asymptomatic infection is common among both men and women. Screening sexually active adolescents for chlamydial infection should be routine during annual examinations, even if symptoms are not present. Screening women aged 20–24 years also is suggested, particularly for those who have new or multiple sex partners and who do not consistently use barrier contraceptives.

Recommended Regimens

- **Azithromycin 1 g orally in a single dose,**

or

- **Doxycycline 100 mg orally twice a day for 7 days.**

Alternative Regimens

- **Erythromycin base 500 mg orally four times a day for 7 days,**

or

- **Erythromycin ethylsuccinate 800 mg orally four times a day for 7 days,**

or

- **Ofloxacin 300 mg orally twice a day for 7 days.**

In populations with erratic health-care–seeking behavior, poor compliance with treatment, or minimal follow-up, azithromycin may be more cost-effective because it provides single-dose, directly observed therapy. Doxycycline costs less than azithromycin, and it has been used extensively for a longer period. Erythromycin is less efficacious than either azithromycin and doxycycline, and gastrointestinal side effects frequently discourage patients from complying with this regimen. Ofloxacin is similar in efficacy to doxycycline and azithromycin, but it is more expensive to use and offers no advantage with regard to the dosage regimen. Other quinolones either are not reliably effective against chlamydial infection or have not been adequately evaluated.

Follow-up

Patients do not need to be retested for chlamydia after completing treatment with doxycycline or azithromycin unless symptoms persist or reinfection is suspected, because these therapies are highly efficacious. A test of cure may be considered 3 weeks after completion of treatment with erythromycin. The validity of chlamydial culture testing at <3 weeks after completion of therapy to identify patients who did not respond to therapy has not been established. False-negative results can occur because of small numbers of chlamydial organisms. In addition, nonculture tests conducted at <3 weeks after completion of therapy for patients who were treated successfully could be false-positive because of continued excretion of dead organisms.

Management of sex partners

Sex partners should be evaluated, tested, and treated if they had sexual contact with the patient during the 60 days preceding onset of symptoms in the patient or diagnosis of chlamydia. Health-care providers should treat the most recent sex partner even if the time of the last sexual contact was >60 days before onset or diagnosis.

Pregnancy

Doxycycline and ofloxacin are contraindicated for pregnant women. The safety and efficacy of azithromycin use in pregnant and lactating women have not been established. Repeat testing, preferably by culture, 3 weeks after completion of therapy with the following regimens is recommended, because a) none of these regimens are highly efficacious and b) the frequent side effects of erythromycin might discourage patient compliance with this regimen.

Recommended Regimens for Pregnant Women

- **Erythromycin base 500 mg orally four times a day for 7 days,**

or

- **Amoxicillin 500 mg orally three times daily for 7 days.**

Alternative Regimens for Pregnant Women

- **Erythromycin base 250 mg orally four times a day for 14 days,**

or

- **Erythromycin ethylsuccinate 800 mg orally four times a day for 7 days,**

or

- **Erythromycin ethylsuccinate 400 mg orally four times a day for 14 days,**

or

- **Azithromycin 1 g orally, single dose.**

Note: Erythromycin estolate is contraindicated during pregnancy because of drug-related hepatotoxicity. Preliminary data indicate that azithromycin may be safe and effective. However, data are insufficient to recommend the routine use of azithromycin in pregnant women.

Infants born to mothers who have chlamydial infection

Infants born to mothers who have untreated chlamydia are at high risk for infection; however, prophylatic antibiotic treatment is not indicated, and the efficacy of such treatment is unknown. Infants should be monitored to ensure appropriate treatment if infection develops.

GONOCOCCAL INFECTION

Dual therapy for gonococcal and chlamydial infections

Patients infected with *N. gonorrhoeae* often are coinfected with *C. trachomatis;* this finding led to the recommendation that patients treated for gonococcal infection also be treated routinely with a regimen effective against uncomplicated genital *C. trachomatis* infection. Routine dual therapy without testing for chlamydia can be cost-effective for populations in which chlamydial infection accompanies 20%–40% of gonococcal infections, because the cost of therapy for chlamydia (e.g., $0.50–$1.50 for doxycycline) is less than the cost of testing.

Quinolone-resistant *N. gonorrhoeae* (QRNG)

Cases of gonorrhea caused by *N. gonorrhoeae* resistant to fluoroquinolones have been reported sporadically from many parts of the world, including North America, and are becoming widespread in parts of Asia. As of February 1997, however, QRNG occurred rarely in the United States: <0.05% of 4,639 isolates collected by CDC's Gonococcal Isolate Surveillance Project (GISP) during 1996 had minimum inhibitory concentrations (MICs) ≥1.0 μg/mL to ciprofloxacin. The GISP sample is collected from 26 cities and includes approximately 1.3% of all reported gonococcal infections among men in the United States. As long as QRNG strains comprise <1% of all *N. gonorrhoeae* strains isolated at each of the 26 cities, the fluoroquinolone regimens can be used with confidence. However, importation of QRNG will probably continue, and the prevalence of QRNG in the United States could increase to the point that fluoroquinolones no longer reliably eradicate gonococcal infections. Because of the prevalence of QRNG in parts of Asia, treatment with a nonquinolone regimen is suggested. Culture and susceptability testing should be performed on a patient who has apparent treatment failure after recommended therapy and reported to the local health department.

Uncomplicated gonococcal infections of the cervix, urethra, and rectum

Recommended Regimens

- **Cefixime 400 mg orally in a single dose,**

or

- **Ceftriaxone 125 mg IM in a single dose,**

or

- **Ciprofloxacin 500 mg orally in a single dose,**

or

- **Ofloxacin 400 mg orally in a single dose,**

plus

- **Azithromycin 1 g orally in a single dose,**

or

- **Doxycycline 100 mg orally twice a day for 7 days**

Alternative Regimens

- **Spectinomycin 2 g IM in a single dose.**
- **Single-dose cephalosporin** regimens other than ceftriaxone 125 mg IM and cefixime 400 mg orally that are safe and highly effective against uncomplicated urogenital and anorectal gonococcal infections include a) ceftizoxime 500 mg IM, b) cefotaxime 500 mg IM, c) cefotetan 1 g IM, and d) cefoxitin 2 g IM with probenecid 1 g orally.
- **Single-dose quinolone regimens include enoxacin 400 mg orally, lomefloxacin 400 mg orally, and norfloxacin 800 mg orally.**

Uncomplicated gonococcal infection of the pharynx

Recommended Regimen

- **Ceftriaxone 125 mg IM in a single dose,**

or

- **Ciprofloxacin 500 mg orally in a single dose,**

or

- **Ofloxacin 400 mg orally in a single dose,**

plus

- **Azithromycin 1 g orally in a single dose**

or

- **Doxycycline 100 mg orally twice daily for 7 days.**

Follow-up

Patients who have uncomplicated gonorrhea and who are treated with any of the recommended regimens need not return for a test of cure.

Management of sex partners

Patients should be instructed to refer sex partners for evaluation and treatment. All sex partners of patients who have *N. gonorrhoeae* infection should be evaluated and treated for *N. gonorrhoeae* and *C. trachomatis* infections if their last sexual contact with the patient was within 60 days before onset of symptoms or diagnosis of infection in the patient.

Pregnancy

Pregnant women should not be treated with quinolones or tetracyclines. Those infected with *N. gonorrhoeae* should be treated with a recommended or alternate cephalosporin. Women who cannot tolerate a cephalosporin should be administered a single 2-g dose of spectinomycin IM. Either erythromycin or amoxicillin is recommended for treatment of presumptive or diagnosed *C. trachomatis* infection during pregnancy (see Chlamydial Infection).

HIV infection

Patients who have gonococcal infection and also are infected with HIV should receive the same treatment regimen as those who are HIV-negative.

Disseminated gonococcal infection (DGI)

DGI results from gonococcal bacteremia. DGI often results in petechial or pustular acral skin lesions, asymmetrical arthralgia, tenosynovitis, or septic arthritis. The infection is complicated occasionally by perihepatitis, and rarely by endocarditis or meningitis. Strains of *N. gonorrhoeae* that cause DGI tend to cause minimal genital inflammation. In the United States, these strains have occurred infrequently during the past decade.

Treatment

Hospitalization is recommended for initial therapy, especially for patients who cannot be relied on to comply with treatment, for those in whom the diagnosis is uncertain, and for those who have purulent synovial effusions or other complications. Patients should be examined for clinical evidence of endocarditis and meningitis. Patients treated for DGI should be treated presumptively for concurrent *C. trachomatis* infection unless appropriate testing excludes this infection.

Recommended Initial Regimen

- **Ceftriaxone 1 g IM or IV every 24 hours.**

Alternative Initial Regimens

- **Cefotaxime 1 g IV every 8 hours,**

or

- **Ceftizoxime 1 g IV every 8 hours,**

or

- ***For persons allergic to β-lactam drugs:*** Ciprofloxacin 500 mg IV every 12 hours,

or

- **Ofloxacin 400 mg IV every 12 hours,**

or

- **Spectinomycin 2 g IM every 12 hours.**

All regimens should be continued for 24–48 hours after improvement begins, at which time therapy may be switched to one of the following regimens to complete a full week of antimicrobial therapy:

- **Cefixime 400 mg orally twice a day,**

or

- **Ciprofloxacin 500 mg orally twice a day,**

or

- **Ofloxacin 400 mg orally twice a day.**

Management of sex partners

As with uncomplicated gonococcal infections, patients should be instructed to refer their sex partners for evaluation and treatment.

Gonococcal meningitis and endocarditis

Recommended Initial Regimen

- **Ceftriaxone 1-2 g IV every 12 hours.**

Therapy for meningitis should be continued for 10–14 days; therapy for endocarditis should be continued for at least 4 weeks. Treatment of complicated DGI should be undertaken in consultation with an expert.

Prophylactic treatment for infants whose mothers have gonococcal infection

Infants born to mothers who have untreated gonorrhea are at high risk for infection.

Recommended Regimen in the Absence of Signs of Gonococcal Infection

- **Ceftriaxone 25-50 mg/kg IV or IM, not to exceed 125 mg, in a single dose.**

Ophthalmia neonatorum prophylaxis

Instillation of a prophylactic agent into the eyes of all newborn infants is recommended to prevent gonococcal ophthalmia neonatorum; this procedure is required by law in most states. However, the efficacy of these preparations in preventing chlamydial ophthalmia is less clear, and they do not eliminate nasopharyngeal colonization by *C. trachomatis*. The diagnosis and treatment of gonococcal and chlamydial infections in pregnant women is the best method for preventing neonatal gonococcal and chlamydial disease. Not all women, however, receive prenatal care; and ocular prophylaxis is warranted because it can prevent sight-threatening gonococcal ophthalmia and it is safe, easy to administer, and inexpensive.

Recommended Regimens

- **Silver nitrate (1%) aqueous solution in a single application,**

or

- **Erythromycin (0.5%) ophthalmic ointment in a single application,**

or

- **Tetracycline ophthalmic ointment (1%) in a single application.**

BACTERIAL VAGINOSIS

BV is a clinical syndrome resulting from replacement of the normal H_2O_2-producing *Lactobacillus* sp. in the vagina with high concentrations of anaerobic bacteria (e.g., *Prevotella* sp. and *Mobiluncus* sp.), *G. vaginalis*, and *Mycoplasma hominis*. BV is the most prevalent cause of vaginal discharge or malodor; however, half of the women whose illnesses meet the clinical criteria for BV are asymptomatic. The cause of the microbial alteration is not fully understood. Although BV is associated with having multiple sex partners, it is unclear whether BV results from acquisition of a sexually transmitted pathogen. Women who have never been sexually active are rarely affected. Treatment of the male sex partner has not been beneficial in preventing the recurrence of BV.

Diagnostic Considerations

BV can be diagnosed by the use of clinical or Gram stain criteria. Clinical criteria require three of the following symptoms or signs:

a. A homogeneous, white, noninflammatory discharge that smoothly coats the vaginal walls;
b. The presence of clue cells on microscopic examination;
c. A pH of vaginal fluid >4.5;
d. A fishy odor of vaginal discharge before or after addition of 10% KOH (i.e., the whiff test).

Treatment

The principal goal of therapy for BV is to relieve vaginal symptoms and signs of infection. All women who have symptomatic disease require treatment, regardless of pregnancy status.

BV during pregnancy is associated with adverse pregnancy outcomes. The results of several investigations indicate that treatment of pregnant women who have BV and who are at high risk for preterm delivery (i.e., those who previously delivered a premature infant) might reduce the risk for prematurity. Therefore, high-risk pregnant women who do not have symptoms of BV may be evaluated for treatment.

Although some experts recommend treatment for high-risk pregnant women who have asymptomatic BV, others believe more information is needed before such a recommendation is made. A large, randomized clinical trial is underway to assess treatment for asymptomatic BV in pregnant women; the results of this investigation should clarify the benefits of therapy for BV in women at both low and high risk for preterm delivery.

Recommended Regimens for Nonpregnant Women

- **Metronidazole 500 mg orally twice a day for 7 days,**

or

- **Clindamycin cream, 2%, one full applicator (5 g) intravaginally at bedtime for 7 days,**

or

- **Metronidazole gel, 0.75%, one full applicator (5 g) intravaginally, twice a day for 5 days.**

Alternative Regimens

- **Metronidazole 2 g orally in a single dose,**

or

- **Clindamycin 300 mg orally twice a day for 7 days.**

Some health-care providers remain concerned about the possible teratogenicity of metronidazole, which has been suggested by experiments using extremely high and prolonged doses in animals. However, a recent meta-analysis does not indicate teratogenicity in humans. Some health-care providers prefer the intravaginal route because of a lack of systemic side effects (e.g., mild-to-moderate gastrointestinal disturbance and unpleasant taste). Mean peak serum concentrations of metronidazole after intravaginal administration are <2% the levels of standard 500-mg oral doses, and the mean bioavailability of clindamycin cream is approximately 4%.

Follow-up

Because treatment of BV in high-risk pregnant women who are asymptomatic might prevent adverse pregnancy outcomes, a follow-up evaluation, at 1 month after completion of treatment, should be considered to evaluate whether therapy was successful. The alternative BV treatment regimens may be used to treat recurrent disease. No long-term maintenance regimen with any therapeutic agent is recommended.

Management of sex partners

The results of clinical trials indicate that a woman's response to therapy and the likelihood of relapse or recurrence are not affected by treatment of her sex partner(s).

Pregnancy

BV has been associated with adverse pregnancy outcomes (e.g., premature rupture of the membranes, preterm labor, and preterm birth), and the organisms found in increased concentration in BV also are frequently present in postpartum or postcesarean endometritis. Because treatment of BV in high-risk pregnant women (i.e., those who have previously delivered a premature infant) who are asymptomatic might reduce preterm delivery, such women may be screened, and those with BV can be treated. The screening and treatment should be conducted at the earliest part of the second trimester of pregnancy. The recommended regimen is metronidazole 250 mg orally three times a day for 7 days. The alternative regimens are a) metronidazole 2 g orally in a single dose or b) clindamycin 300 mg orally twice a day for 7 days.

Low-risk pregnant women (i.e., women who previously have not had a premature delivery) who have symptomatic BV should be treated to relieve symptoms. The recommended regimen is metronidazole 250 mg orally three times a day for 7 days. The alternative regimens are a) metronidazole 2 g orally in a single dose; b) clindamycin 300 mg orally twice a day for 7 days; or c) metronidazole gel, 0.75%, one full applicator (5 g) intravaginally, twice a day for 5 days. Some experts prefer the use of systemic therapy for low-risk pregnant women to treat possible subclinical upper genital tract infections.

TRICHOMONIASIS

T. vaginalis characteristically causes a diffuse, malodorous, yellow-green discharge with vulvar irritation; many women have fewer symptoms. Vaginal trichomoniasis might be associated with adverse pregnancy outcomes, particularly premature rupture of the membranes and preterm delivery.

Recommended Regimen

- **Metronidazole 2 g orally in a single dose.**

Alternative Regimen*

- **Metronidazole 500 mg twice a day for 7 days.**

*FDA has approved metronidazole 375 mg capsules twice a day for 7 days for treatment of trichomoniasis on the basis of pharmacokinetic equivalency of this regimen with metronidazole 250 mg three times a day for 7 days. No clinical data are available, however, to demonstrate clinical equivalency of the two regimens.

Follow-up

If treatment failure occurs with either regimen, the patient should be re-treated with metronidazole 500 mg twice a day for 7 days. If treatment failure occurs repeatedly, the patient should be treated with a single 2-g dose of metronidazole once a day for 3–5 days.

Patients with culture-documented infection who do not respond to the regimens described in this report and in whom reinfection has been excluded should be managed in consultation with an expert; consultation is available from CDC. Evaluation of such cases should include determination of the susceptibility of *T. vaginalis* to metronidazole.

Management of sex partners

Sex partners should be treated. Patients should be instructed to avoid sex until they and their sex partners are cured.

Allergy, intolerance, or adverse reactions

Effective alternatives to therapy with metronidazole are not available. Patients who are allergic to metronidazole can be managed by desensitization (26).

Pregnancy

Patients may be treated with 2 g of metronidazole in a single dose.

Diagnostic Considerations

A diagnosis of *Candida* vaginitis is suggested clinically by pruritus and erythema in the vulvovaginal area; a white discharge may occur. The diagnosis can be made in a woman who has signs and symptoms of vaginitis, and when either a) a wet preparation or Gram stain of vaginal discharge demonstrates yeasts or pseudohyphae or b) a culture or other test yields a positive result for a yeast species. *Candida* vaginitis is associated with a normal vaginal pH (≤4.5). Use of 10% KOH in wet preparations improves the visualization of yeast and mycelia by disrupting cellular material that might obscure the yeast or pseudohyphae. Identifying *Candida* by culture in the absence of symptoms should not lead to treatment, because approximately 10%–20% of women usually harbor *Candida* sp. and other yeasts in the vagina. VVC can occur concomitantly with STDs or frequently following antibacterial vaginal or systemic therapy.

Recommended Regimens

- **Intravaginal agents:**

  Butoconazole 2% cream 5 g intravaginally for 3 days,*†

  or

  Clotrimazole 1% cream 5 g intravaginally for 7–14 days,*†

  or

  Clotrimazole 100 mg vaginal tablet for 7 days,*

  or

  Clotrimazole 100 mg vaginal tablet, two tablets for 3 days,*

  or

  Clotrimazole 500 mg vaginal tablet, one tablet in a single application,*

  or

  Miconazole 2% cream 5 g intravaginally for 7 days,*†

  or

  Miconazole 200 mg vaginal suppository, one suppository for 3 days,*†

  or

  Miconazole 100 mg vaginal suppository, one suppository for 7 days,*†

  or

  Nystatin 100,000-u vaginal tablet, one tablet for 14 days,

  or

  Tioconazole 6.5% ointment 5 g intravaginally in a single application,*†

  or

  Terconazole 0.4% cream 5 g intravaginally for 7 days,*

  or

  Terconazole 0.8% cream 5 g intravaginally for 3 days,*

  or

  Terconazole 80 mg vaginal suppository, one suppository for 3 days.*
- **Oral agent:**

  Fluconazole 150 mg oral tablet, one tablet in single dose.

*These creams and suppositories are oil-based and may weaken latex condoms and diaphragms. Refer to condom product labeling for further information.

†Over-the-counter (OTC) preparations.

Management of sex partners

VVC usually is not acquired through sexual intercourse; treatment of sex partners is not recommended but may be considered for women who have recurrent infection.

Pregnancy

VVC often occurs during pregnancy. Only topical azole therapies should be used to treat pregnant women. Of those treatments that have been investigated for use during pregnancy, the most effective are butoconazole, clotrimazole, miconazole, and terconazole. Many experts recommend 7 days of therapy during pregnancy.

Recurrent vulvovaginal candidiasis

RVVC, which usually is defined as ***four*** or more episodes of symptomatic VVC annually, affects a small percentage of women (i.e., probably <5%). The optimal treatment for RVVC has not been established; however, an initial intensive regimen continued for approximately 10–14 days, followed immediately by a maintenance regimen for at least 6 months, is recommended. Maintenance ketoconazole 100 mg orally, once a day for ≤6 months, reduces the frequency of RVVC episodes. Investigations are evaluating a weekly fluconazole regimen, the results of which will be compared with once-monthly oral and topical antimycotic regimens that have only moderate protective efficacy. All cases of RVVC should be confirmed by culture before maintenance therapy is initiated.

PELVIC INFLAMMATORY DISEASE (PID)

PID comprises a spectrum of inflammatory disorders of the upper female genital tract, including any combination of endometritis, salpingitis, tubo-ovarian abscess, and pelvic peritonitis.

Empiric treatment of PID should be initiated in sexually active young women and others at risk for STDs if all the following **minimum criteria** are present and no other cause(s) for the illness can be identified:

- Lower abdominal tenderness,
- Adnexal tenderness, and
- Cervical motion tenderness.

More elaborate diagnostic evaluation often is needed, because incorrect diagnosis and management might cause unnecessary morbidity. These additional criteria may be used to enhance the specificity of the minimum criteria listed previously. **Additional criteria** that support a diagnosis of PID include the following:

- Oral temperature >101 F (>38.3 C),
- Abnormal cervical or vaginal discharge,
- Elevated erythrocyte sedimentation rate,
- Elevated C-reactive protein, and
- Laboratory documentation of cervical infection with *N. gonorrhoeae* or *C. trachomatis.*

The **definitive criteria** for diagnosing PID, which are warranted in selected cases, include the following:

- Histopathologic evidence of endometritis on endometrial biopsy,
- Transvaginal sonography or other imaging techniques showing thickened fluid-filled tubes with or without free pelvic fluid or tubo-ovarian complex, and
- Laparoscopic abnormalities consistent with PID.

The following criteria for **HOSPITALIZATION** are based on observational data and theoretical concerns:

- Surgical emergencies such as appendicitis cannot be excluded;
- The patient is pregnant;
- The patient does not respond clinically to oral antimicrobial therapy;
- The patient is unable to follow or tolerate an outpatient oral regimen;
- The patient has severe illness, nausea and vomiting, or high fever;
- The patient has a tubo-ovarian abscess; or
- The patient is immunodeficient (i.e., has HIV infection with low CD4 counts, is taking immunosuppressive therapy, or has another disease).

There are no efficacy data comparing parenteral with oral regimens. Experts have extensive experience with both of the following regimens. Also, there are multiple randomized trials demonstrating the efficacy of each regimen. Although most trials have used parenteral treatment for at least 48 hours after the patient demonstrates substantial clinical improvement, this is an arbitrary designation. Clinical experience should guide decisions regarding transition to oral therapy, which may be accomplished within 24 hours of clinical improvement.

Parenteral Regimen A

- **Cefotetan 2 g IV every 12 hours,**

or

- **Cefoxitin 2 g IV every 6 hours,**

plus

- **Doxycycline 100 mg IV or orally every 12 hours.**

Parenteral Regimen B

- **Clindamycin 900 mg IV every 8 hours,**

plus

- **Gentamicin loading dose IV or IM (2 mg/kg of body weight) followed by a maintenance dose (1.5 mg/kg) every 8 hours. Single daily dosing may be substituted.**

Alternative Parenteral Regimens

- **Ofloxacin 400 mg IV every 12 hours,**

plus

- **Metronidazole 500 mg IV every 8 hours.**

or

- **Ampicillin/Sulbactam 3 g IV every 6 hours,**

plus

- **Doxycycline 100 mg IV or orally every 12 hours.**

plus

- **Ciprofloxacin 200 mg IV every 12 hours,**

plus

- **Doxycycline 100 mg IV or orally every 12 hours,**

plus

- **Metronidazole 500 mg IV every 8 hours.**

Oral treatment

As with parenteral regimens, clinical trials of outpatient regimens have provided minimal information regarding intermediate and long-term outcomes.

Regimen A

- **Ofloxacin 400 mg orally twice a day for 14 days,**

plus

- **Metronidazole 500 mg orally twice a day for 14 days.**

Regimen B

- **Ceftriaxone 250 mg IM once,**

or

- **Cefoxitin 2 g IM plus Probenecid, 1 g orally in a single dose concurrently once,**

or

- **Other parenteral third-generation cephalosporin (e.g., ceftizoxime or cefotaxime),**

plus

- **Doxycycline 100 mg orally twice a day for 14 days. (Include this regimen with one of the above regimens.)**

The optimal choice of a cephalosporin for Regimen B is unclear; although cefoxitin has better anaerobic coverage, ceftriaxone has better coverage against *N. gonorrhoeae*. Clinical trials have demonstrated that a single dose of cefoxitin is effective in obtaining short-term clinical response in women who have PID; however, the theoretical limitations in its coverage of anaerobes may require the addition of metronidazole. The metronidazole also will effectively treat BV, which also is frequently associated with PID.

Follow-up

Patients receiving oral or parenteral therapy should demonstrate substantial clinical improvement (e.g., defervescence; reduction in direct or rebound abdominal tenderness; and reduction in uterine, adnexal, and cervical motion tenderness) within 3 days after initiation of therapy. Patients who do not demonstrate improvement within this time period usually require additional diagnostic tests, surgical intervention, or both.

If the health-care provider prescribes outpatient oral or parenteral therapy, a follow-up examination should be performed within 72 hours, using the criteria for clinical improvement described previously. Some experts also recommend rescreening for *C. trachomatis* and *N. gonorrhoeae* 4–6 weeks after therapy is completed. If PCR or LCR is used to document a test of cure, rescreening should be delayed for 1 month after completion of therapy.

Management of sex partners

Sex partners of patients who have PID should be examined and treated if they had sexual contact with the patient during the 60 days preceding onset of symptoms in the patient.

Pregnancy

Because of the high risk for maternal morbidity, fetal wastage, and preterm delivery, pregnant women who have suspected PID should be hospitalized and treated with parenteral antibiotics.

Immunosuppressed HIV-infected women who have PID should be managed aggressively using one of the parenteral antimicrobial regimens recommended in this report.

EPIDIDYMITIS

The evaluation of men for epididymitis should include the following procedures:

- A Gram-stained smear of urethral exudate or intraurethral swab specimen for diagnosis of urethritis (i.e., ≥5 polymorphonuclear leukocytes per oil immersion field) and for presumptive diagnosis of gonococcal infection.
- A culture of urethral exudate or intraurethral swab specimen, or nucleic acid amplification test (either on intraurethral swab or first-void urine) for *N. gonorrhoeae* and *C. trachomatis*.
- Examination of first-void urine for leukocytes if the urethral Gram stain is negative. Culture and Gram-stained smear of uncentrifuged urine should be obtained.
- Syphilis serology and HIV counseling and testing.

Recommended Regimen

- **For epididymitis most likely caused by gonococcal or chlamydial infection:**
  Ceftriaxone 250 mg IM in a single dose,
  plus
  Doxycycline 100 mg orally twice a day for 10 days.
- **For epididymitis most likely caused by enteric organisms, or for patients allergic to cephalosporins and/or tetracyclines:**
  Ofloxacin 300 mg orally twice a day for 10 days.

Follow-up

Failure to improve within 3 days requires reevaluation of both the diagnosis and therapy.

Management of sex partners

Sex partners of these patients should be referred if their contact with the index patient was within the 60 days preceding onset of symptoms in the patient.

HUMAN PAPILLOMAVIRUS INFECTION

GENITAL WARTS

More than 20 types of HPV can infect the genital tract. Most HPV infections are asymptomatic, subclinical, or unrecognized. Visible genital warts usually are caused by HPV types 6 or 11. Other HPV types in the anogenital region (i.e., types 16, 18, 31, 33, and 35) have been strongly associated with cervical dysplasia. Diagnosis of genital warts can be confirmed by biopsy, although biopsy is rarely needed (e.g., if the diagnosis is uncertain; the lesions do not respond to standard therapy; the disease worsens during therapy; the patient is immunocompromised; or warts are pigmented, indurated, fixed, and ulcerated). No data support the use of type-specific HPV nucleic acid tests in the routine diagnosis or management of visible genital warts.

External Genital Warts, Recommended Treatments

- *Patient-Applied:*
  Podofilox 0.5% solution or gel.
  or
- **Imiquimod 5%** cream.
- *Provider-Administered:*
  Cryotherapy with liquid nitrogen or cryoprobe.
  or
- **Podophyllin resin 10-25%** in compound tincture of benzoin.
  or
- **TCA or BCA 80-90%.**
  or
- **Surgical removal** either by tangential scissor excision, tangential shave excision, curettage, or electrosurgery.

External Genital Warts, Alternative Treatments

- **Intralesional interferon,**
  or
- **Laser surgery**

Vaginal Warts

- **Cryotherapy with liquid nitrogen.**
  or
- **TCA or BCA 80-90% applied only to warts.**
  or
- **Podophyllin 10-25% in compound tincture of benzoin applied to a treated area that must be dry before the speculum is removed.**

Urethral Meatus Warts

- **Cryotherapy with liquid nitrogen**
  or
- **Podophyllin 10-25% in compound tincture of benzoin.**

Anal Warts

- **Cryotherapy with liquid nitrogen**
  or
- **TCA or BCA 80-90% applied to warts.**
  or
- **Surgical removal.**

Follow-up

Patients should be cautioned to watch for recurrences, which occur most frequently during the first 3 months. Earlier follow-up visits also may be useful a) to document a wart-free state, b) to monitor for or treat complications of therapy, and c) to provide the opportunity for patient education and counseling. Women should be counseled regarding the need for regular cytologic screening as recommended for women without genital warts. The presence of genital warts is not an indication for cervical colposcopy.

Management of sex partners

Examination of sex partners is not necessary for the management of genital warts because the role of reinfection is probably minimal and, in the absence of curative therapy, treatment to reduce transmission is not realistic. However, because self- or partner-examination has not been evaluated as a diagnostic method for genital warts, sex partners of patients who have genital warts may benefit from examination to assess the presence of genital warts and other STDs.

VACCINE PREVENTABLE STDs

HEPATITIS A PREVENTION

Inactivated hepatitis A vaccines have been available in the United States since 1995. These vaccines, administered as a two-dose series, are safe, highly immunogenic, and efficacious. Immunogenicity studies indicate that 99%–100% of persons respond to one dose of hepatitis A vaccine; the second dose provides long-term protection. Efficacy studies indicate that inactivated hepatitis A vaccines are 94%–100% effective in preventing HAV infection (2).

Preexposure prophylaxis

Vaccination with hepatitis A vaccine for preexposure protection against HAV infection is indicated for persons who have the following risk factors and who are likely to seek treatment in settings where STDs are being treated.

- **Men who have sex with men.** Sexually active men who have sex with men (both adolescents and adults) should be vaccinated.
- **Illegal drug users.** Vaccination is recommended for users of illegal injecting and noninjecting drugs if local epidemiologic evidence indicates previous or current outbreaks among persons with such risk behaviors.

Postexposure prophylaxis

Persons who were exposed recently to HAV (i.e., household or sexual contact with a person who has hepatitis A) and who had not been vaccinated before the exposure should be administered a single IM dose of IG (0.02 mL/kg) as soon as possible, but not >2 weeks after exposure. Persons who received at least one dose of hepatitis A vaccine ≥1 month before exposure to HAV do not need IG.

HEPATITIS B

Hepatitis B is a common STD. During the past 10 years, sexual transmission accounted for approximately 30%–60% of the estimated 240,000 new HBV infections that occurred annually in the United States. Chronic HBV infection develops in 1%–6% of persons infected as adults. These persons are capable of transmitting HBV to others, and they are at risk for chronic liver disease. In the United States, HBV infection leads to an estimated 6,000 deaths annually; these deaths result from cirrhosis of the liver and primary hepatocellular carcinoma.

Preexposure prophylaxis

Persons who should receive hepatitis B vaccine include the following:

- Sexually active homosexual and bisexual men;
- Sexually active heterosexual men and women, including those a) in whom another STD was recently diagnosed, b) who had more than one sex partner in the preceding 6 months, c) who received treatment in an STD clinic, and d) who are prostitutes;
- Illegal drug users, including injecting-drug users and users of illegal noninjecting drugs;
- Health-care workers;
- Recipients of certain blood products;
- Household and sexual contacts of persons who have chronic HBV infection;
- Adoptees from countries in which HBV infection is endemic;
- Certain international travelers;
- Clients and employees of facilities for the developmentally disabled;
- Infants and children; and
- Hemodialysis patients.

Postexposure prophylaxis

Exposure to persons who have acute hepatitis B

Sexual contacts

Patients who have acute HBV infection are potentially infectious to persons with whom they have sexual contact. Passive immunization with hepatitis B immune globulin (HBIG) prevents 75% of these infections. Hepatitis B vaccination alone is less effective in preventing infection than HBIG and vaccination. Sexual contacts of patients who have acute hepatitis B should receive HBIG and begin the hepatitis B vaccine series within 14 days after the most recent sexual contact. Testing of sex partners for susceptibility to HBV infection (anti-HBc) can be considered if it does not delay treatment >14 days.

Nonsexual household contacts

Nonsexual household contacts of patients who have acute hepatitis B are not at high risk for infection unless they are exposed to the patient's blood (e.g., by sharing a toothbrush or razor blade). However, vaccination of household contacts is encouraged, especially for children and adolescents. If the patient remains HBsAg-positive after 6 months (i.e., becomes chronically infected), all household contacts should be vaccinated.

Exposure to persons who have chronic HBV infection

Hepatitis B vaccination without the use of HBIG is highly effective in preventing HBV infection in household and sexual contacts of persons who have chronic HBV infection, and all such contacts should be vaccinated. Postvaccination serologic testing is indicated for sex partners of persons who have chronic hepatitis B infections and for infants born to HBsAg-positive women.

HIV infection

HBV infection in HIV-infected persons is more likely to lead to chronic HBV infection. HIV infection also can impair the response to hepatitis B vaccine. Therefore, HIV-infected persons who are vaccinated should be tested for hepatitis B surface antibody 1–2 months after the third vaccine dose. Revaccination with three more doses should be considered for those who do not respond initially to vaccination. Those who do not respond to additional doses should be advised that they might remain susceptible to HBV infection.

PROCTITIS, PROCTOCOLITIS, AND ENTERITIS

Sexually transmitted gastrointestinal syndromes include proctitis, proctocolitis, and enteritis. Proctitis occurs predominantly among persons who participate in anal intercourse, and enteritis occurs among those whose sexual practices include oral-fecal contact. Proctocolitis can be acquired by either route, depending on the pathogen. Evaluation should include appropriate diagnostic procedures (e.g., anoscopy or sigmoidoscopy, stool examination, and culture).

Recommended Regimen

- **Ceftriaxone 125 mg IM (or another agent effective against anal and genital gonorrhea)**

plus

- **Doxycycline 100 mg orally twice a day for 7 days.**

ECTOPARASITIC INFECTIONS

PEDICULOSIS PUBIS

Recommended Regimens

- **Permethrin 1% creme rinse**

or

- **Lindane 1% shampoo**

or

- **Pyrethrins with piperonyl butoxide**

Other management considerations

The recommended regimens should not be applied to the eyes. Pediculosis of the eyelashes should be treated by applying occlusive ophthalmic ointment to the eyelid margins twice a day for 10 days.

Bedding and clothing should be decontaminated (i.e., either machine-washed or machine-dried using the heat cycle or dry-cleaned) or removed from body contact for at least 72 hours. Fumigation of living areas is not necessary.

Follow-up

Patients should be evaluated after 1 week if symptoms persist. Re-treatment may be necessary if lice are found or if eggs are observed at the hair-skin junction. Patients who do not respond to one of the recommended regimens should be re-treated with an alternative regimen.

Pregnancy

Pregnant and lactating women should be treated with either permethrin or pyrethrins with piperonyl butoxide.

SCABIES

The predominant symptom of scabies is pruritus. Sensitization to *Sarcoptes scabiei* must occur before pruritus begins. The first time a person is infected with *S. scabiei*, sensitization takes several weeks to develop. Pruritus might occur within 24 hours after a subsequent reinfestation. Scabies in adults may be sexually transmitted, although scabies in children usually is not.

Recommended Regimen

- **Permethrin cream (5%)**

Alternative Regimens

- **Lindane (1%) 1 oz. of lotion or 30 g of cream**

or

- **Sulfur (6%) precipitated in ointment**

NOTE: Lindane should not be used after a bath, and it should not be used by a) persons who have extensive dermatitis, b) pregnant or lactating women, and c) children aged <2 years.

Ivermectin (single oral dose of 200 μg/kg or 0.8% topical solution) is a potential new therapeutic modality. However, no controlled clinical trials have been conducted to compare ivermectin with the currently recommended therapies.

Other management considerations

Bedding and clothing should be decontaminated (i.e., either machine-washed or machine-dried using the hot cycle or dry-cleaned) or removed from body contact for at least 72 hours. Fumigation of living areas is unnecessary.

Follow-up

Pruritus may persist for several weeks. Some experts recommend re-treatment after 1 week for patients who are still symptomatic; other experts recommend re-treatment only if live mites are observed. Patients who do not respond to the recommended treatment should be retreated with an alternative regimen.

SEXUAL ASSAULT AND STDs

ADULTS AND ADOLESCENTS

Trichomoniasis, BV, chlamydia, and gonorrhea are the most frequently diagnosed infections among women who have been sexually assaulted. Because the prevalence of these STDs is substantial among sexually active women, the presence of these infections after an assault does not necessarily signify acquisition during the assault. Chlamydial and gonococcal infections in women are of special concern because of the possibility of ascending infection. In addition, HBV infection, if transmitted to a woman during an assault, can be prevented by postexposure administration of hepatitis B vaccine.

Evaluation for sexually transmitted infections

Initial examination

An initial examination should include the following procedures:

- Cultures for *N. gonorrhoeae* and *C. trachomatis* from specimens collected from any sites of penetration or attempted penetration.
- If chlamydial culture is not available, nonculture tests, particularly the nucleic acid amplification tests, are an acceptable substitute. Nucleic acid amplification tests offer advantages of increased sensitivity if confirmation is available. If a nonculture test is used, a positive test result should be verified with a second test based on a different diagnostic principle. EIA and direct fluorescent antibody are not acceptable alternatives, because false-negative test results occur more often with these nonculture tests, and false-positive test results may occur.
- Wet mount and culture of a vaginal swab specimen for *T. vaginalis* infection. If vaginal discharge or malodor is evident, the wet mount also should be examined for evidence of BV and yeast infection.
- Collection of a serum sample for immediate evaluation for HIV, hepatitis B, and syphilis

Follow-up examination after assault

Examination for STDs should be repeated 2 weeks after the assault. Because infectious agents acquired through assault may not have produced sufficient concentrations of organisms to result in positive test results at the initial examination, a culture (or cultures), a wet mount, and other tests should be repeated at the 2-week follow-up visit unless prophylactic treatment has already been provided.

Serologic tests for syphilis and HIV infection should be repeated 6, 12, and 24 weeks after the assault if initial test results were negative.

Prophylaxis

Many experts recommend routine preventive therapy after a sexual assault. Most patients probably benefit from prophylaxis because the follow-up of patients who have been sexually assaulted can be difficult, and they may be reassured if offered treatment or prophylaxis for possible infection. The following prophylactic regimen is suggested as preventive therapy:

- Postexposure hepatitis B vaccination (without HBIG) should adequately protect against HBV. Hepatitis B vaccine should be administered to victims of sexual assault at the time of the initial examination. Follow-up doses of vaccine should be administered 1–2 and 4–6 months after the first dose.
- An empiric antimicrobial regimen for chlamydia, gonorrhea, trichomonas, and BV should be administered.

Evaluation for sexually transmitted infections

Examinations of children for sexual assault or abuse should be conducted so as to minimize pain and trauma to the child. The decision to evaluate the child for STDs must be made on an individual basis.

Initial and 2-week follow-up examinations

During the initial examination and 2-week follow-up examination (if indicated), the following should be performed:

- Visual inspection of the genital, perianal, and oral areas for genital warts and ulcerative lesions.
- Cultures for *N. gonorrhoeae* specimens collected from the pharynx and anus in both boys and girls, the vagina in girls, and the urethra in boys.
- Cultures for *C. trachomatis* from specimens collected from the anus in both boys and girls and from the vagina in girls.
- Culture and wet mount of a vaginal swab specimen for *T. vaginalis* infection.
- Collection of a serum sample to be evaluated immediately, preserved for subsequent analysis, and used as a baseline for comparison with follow-up serologic tests.

Examination 12 weeks after assault

An examination approximately 12 weeks after the last suspected sexual exposure is recommended to allow time for antibodies to infectious agents to develop if baseline tests are negative. Serologic tests for *T. pallidum*, HIV, and HBsAg should be considered.

Presumptive treatment

Presumptive treatment for children who have been sexually assaulted or abused is not widely recommended because girls appear to be at lower risk for ascending infection than adolescent or adult women, and regular follow-up usually can be ensured. However, some children—or their parent(s) or guardian(s)—may be concerned about the possibility of infection with an STD, even if the risk is perceived by the health-care provider to be low. Patient or parental/guardian concerns may be an appropriate indication for presumptive treatment in some settings (i.e., after all specimens relevant to the investigation have been collected).

References

1 CDC. Hepatitis B virus: a comprehensive strategy for eliminating transmission in the United States through universal childhood vaccination—recommendations of the Immunization Practices Advisory Committee (ACIP). MMWR 1991;40(No. RR-13).

2 CDC. Prevention of hepatitis A through active or passive immunization: recommendations of the Advisory Committee on Immunization Practices (ACIP). MMWR 1996;45(No. RR-15).

3 CDC. Sexually transmitted diseases clinical practice guidelines, 1991. Atlanta: US Department of Health and Human Services, Public Health Service, CDC, 1991.

4 Hatcher RA, Trussell J, Stewart F, et al. Contraceptive technology. 16th ed. New York: Irvington Publishers, 1994.

5 CDC. Technical guidance on HIV counseling. MMWR 1993;42(No. RR-2):11–7.

6 American Academy of Pediatrics/American College of Obstetricians and Gynecologists. Guidelines for perinatal care. 3rd ed. Elk Grove Village, IL: American Academy of Pediatrics/American College of Obstetricians and Gynecologists, 1992.

7 U.S. Preventive Services Task Force. Guide to clinical preventive services. 2nd ed. Baltimore: Williams and Wilkins, 1996.

8 American College of Obstetricians and Gynecologists. Gonorrhea and chlamydial infections. Washington, DC: American College of Obstetricians and Gynecologists, March 1994. (ACOG technical bulletin, no. 190).

9 CDC. Recommendations for the prevention and management of *Chlamydia trachomatis* infections, 1993. MMWR 1993;42(No. RR-12).

10 CDC. 1997 USPHS/IDSA guidelines for the prevention of opportunistic infections in persons infected with human immunodeficiency virus. MMWR 1997;46(No. RR-12).

11 Agency for Health Care Policy and Research. Evaluation and management of early HIV infection. Rockville, MD: US Department of Health and Human Services, Public Health Service, 1994; AHCPR publication no. 94-0572. (Clinical practice guidelines, no. 7).

12 CDC. Testing for antibodies to human immunodeficiency virus type 2 in the United States. MMWR 1992;41(No. RR-12).

13 CDC. Purified protein derivative (PPD)-tuberculin anergy and HIV infection: guidelines for anergy testing and management of anergic persons at risk of tuberculosis. MMWR 1991;40(No. RR-5):27–33.

14 CDC. The use of preventive therapy for tuberculous infection in the United States: recommendations of the Advisory Committee for Elimination of Tuberculosis. MMWR 1990;39(No. RR-8):9–12.

15 CDC. Management of persons exposed to multidrug-resistant tuberculosis. MMWR 1992;41(No. RR-11):59–71.

16 Carpenter CCJ, Fischl MA, Hammer SM, et al. Antiretroviral therapy for HIV infection in 1997: updated recommendations of the International AIDS Society—USA Panel. JAMA 1997;277: 1962–9.

17 CDC. Recommendations for prophylaxis against *Pneumocystis carinii* pneumonia for adults and adolescents infected with human immunodeficiency virus: U.S. Public Health Service Task Force on Antipneumocystis Prophylaxis for Patients with Human Immunodeficiency Virus Infection. MMWR 1992;41(No. RR-4).

18 CDC. 1995 Revised guidelines for prophylaxis against *Pneumocystis carinii* pneumonia for children infected with or perinatally exposed to human immunodeficiency virus. MMWR 1995;44(No. RR-4).

19 Committee on Infectious Diseases, American Academy of Pediatrics. Report of the Committee on Infectious Diseases. 22nd ed. Elk Grove Village, IL: American Academy of Pediatrics, 1991.

20 CDC. Recommendations of the Advisory Committee on Immunization Practices (ACIP): use of vaccines and immune globulins in persons with altered immunocompetence. MMWR 1993;42(No. RR-4).

21 CDC. U.S. Public Health Service recommendations for human immunodeficiency virus counseling and voluntary testing for pregnant women. MMWR 1995;44(No. RR-7).

22 CDC. Recommendations of the U.S. Public Health Service Task Force on the Use of Zidovudine to Reduce Perinatal Transmission of Human Immunodeficiency Virus. MMWR 1994;43(No. RR-11).

23 Henry RE, Wegmann JA, Hartle JE, Christopher GW. Successful oral acyclovir desensitization. Ann Allergy 1993;70:386–8.

24 Wendel GD Jr, Stark BJ, Jamison RB, Molina RD, Sullivan TJ. Penicillin allergy and desensitization in serious infections during pregnancy. N Engl J Med 1985;312:1229–32.

25 Saxon A, Beall GN, Rohr AS, Adelman DC. Immediate hypersensitivity reactions to beta-lactam antibiotics [Clinical conference]. Ann Intern Med 1987;107:204–15.

26 Pearlman MD, Yashar C, Ernst S, Solomon W. An incremental dosing protocol for women with severe vaginal trichomoniasis and adverse reactions to metronidazole. Am J Obstet Gynecol 1996;174:934–6.

27 National Cancer Institute Workshop. The 1988 Bethesda System for reporting cervical/vaginal cytological diagnoses. JAMA 1989;262: 931–4.

28 Kurman RJ, Henson DE, Herbst AL, Noller KL, Schiffman MH, National Cancer Institute Workshop. Interim guidelines for management of abnormal cervical cytology. JAMA 1994;271:1866–9.

29 Committee on Child Abuse and Neglect, American Academy of Pediatrics. Guidelines for the evaluation of sexual abuse of children. Pediatrics 1991;87:254–60.

Appendix B

Guidelines for the use of antiretroviral agents in HIV-infected adults and adolescents

The availability of an increasing number of antiretroviral agents and the rapid evolution of new information has introduced extraordinary complexity into the treatment of HIV-infected persons. In 1996, the Department of Health and Human Services and the Henry J. Kaiser Family Foundation convened the Panel on Clinical Practices for the Treatment of HIV-infected adults and adolescents.

This report recommends that care should be supervised by an expert, and it makes recommendations for laboratory monitoring with particular emphasis on measurement of plasma levels of HIV RNA. It also provides guidelines for antiretroviral therapy, including when to start treatment, what drugs to initiate, when to change therapy, and therapeutic options when changing therapy. Special consideration is given to adolescents and pregnant women. As with decisions about treatment of other chronic conditions, therapeutic decisions about HIV disease require a mutual understanding between the patient and the health care provider regarding the benefits and risks of treatment. Like treatment for most chronic diseases, antiretroviral regimens are complex, have major side effects, pose difficulty with compliance, and carry serious potential consequences with the risk for resistance from nonadherence to the drug regimen or suboptimal levels of antiretroviral agents. Patient education and involvement in therapeutic decisions is important for all medical conditions but is considered especially critical for HIV infection and its treatment.

With regard to specific recommendations, treatment should be offered to all patients with the acute HIV syndrome, those within 6 months of seroconversion, and all patients with symptoms ascribed to HIV infection. Recommendations for offering antiretroviral therapy to asymptomatic patients depend on virologic and immunologic factors. In general, treatment should be offered to individuals with fewer than 500 CD4$^+$ T cells/mm^3 or plasma HIV RNA levels exceeding 10 000 copies/mL (branched DNA assay) or 20 000 copies/mL (reverse transcriptase polymerase chain reaction assay). The strength of the recommendation to treat asmptomatic patients should be based on the patient's willingness to accept therapy, the probability of adherence with the prescribed regimen, and the prognosis in terms of time to an AIDS-defining complication as predicted by plasma HIV RNA levels and CD4$^+$ T-cell counts, which independently help predict prognosis. Once the decision has been made to initiate antiretroviral therapy, the goal is maximum viral suppression for as long as possible. Results of clinical trials to date indicate that this may currently be best achieved with a potent protease inhibitor in combination with two nuceloside analogue reverse transcriptase inhibitors (NRTIs). Another option is the combination of saquinavir plus ritonavir combined with one or two NRTIs. Other currently available regimens may be used in selected settings but are considered by many to be less likely to produce maximum viral suppression. Results of therapy are evaluated primarily with plasmas HIV RNA levels; these are expected to show a one-log (10-fold) decrease at 8 weeks and no detectable virus ($<$50 copies/mL) at 4 to 6 months after initiation of treatment. Failure of therapy (i.e., plasma HIV RNA levels $>$500 copies/mL) at 4 to 6 months may be ascribed to nonadherence, inadequate potency of drugs or suboptimal levels of antiretroviral agents, resistance, and other factors that are poorly understood. Patients whose therapy fails should change to at least two new agents that are not likely to show cross-resistance with drugs given previously; ideally, the regimen should be changed to a completely new regimen that is devoid of anticipated cross-resistance and for which clinical trial data support a high probability of viral response. Rational changes in therapy may be especially difficult to achieve for patients for whom the preferred regimen has failed, because of limitations in the available alternative antiretroviral regimens that have documented efficacy; these decisions are further confounded by problems with adherence, toxicity, and resistance. In some settings, it may be preferable for a patient to participate in a clinical trial with or without access to new drugs or to use a regimen that may not achieve the optimal virologic goal.

It is emphasized that concepts relevant to HIV management evolve rapidly. The Panel has a mechanism to update recommendations on a regular basis, and the most recent information is available on the AIDS Treatment Information Service World Wide Web site (http://www.hivatis.org).

This document was developed by the Panel on Clinical Practices for Treatment of HIV Infection, convened by the Department of Health and Human Services and the Henry J. Kaiser Family Foundation. The document contains recommendations for the clinical use of antiretroviral agents in the treatment of HIV-infected adults and adolescents (adolescence is defined here as late puberty or Tanner stage V; *see* "Considerations for Antiretroviral Therapy in the HIV-Infected Adolescent," below). Guidance for the use of antiretroviral treatment in pediatric HIV infection is not contained in this document. Although the pathogenesis of HIV infection and the general virologic and immunologic principles underlying the use of antiretroviral therapy are similar for all HIV-infected individuals, there are unique therapeutic and management considerations in HIV-infected children. In recognition of these differences, a separate document will address pediatric-specific issues related to antiretroviral therapy.

These guidelines are intended for use by physicians and other health care providers who use antiretroviral therapy in HIV-infected adults and adolescents, and they serve as the companion document to the therapeutic principles formulated by the National Institutes of Health (NIH) Panel to Define Principles of Therapy of HIV Infection. The recommendations in this document are presented in the context of and with reference to the Principles of Therapy in the companion document. Together, the two documents should provide the pathogenesis-based rationale for therapeutic strategies as well as practical guidelines for implementing these strategies. The guidelines represent the current state of knowledge regarding the use of antiretroviral agents, but this is a rapidly evolving field of science, and the availability of new agents or new clinical data regarding the use of existing agents will result in changes in therapeutic options and preferences. Thus, in recognition of the need for frequent updates to this document, a subgroup of the Panel, the Antiretroviral Working Group, will meet several times a year to review new data as they become available; recommendations for changes in this document will then be submitted to the Panel and incorporated as appropriate. *Copies of this document and all updates are available from the HIV/AIDS Treatment Information Service (800-448-0440; fax 301-519-6616)* and the *AIDS Treatment Information Service World Wide Web site (http://www.hivatis.org).* They are also available from the Centers for Disease Control and Prevention (CDC) National AIDS Clearinghouse (800-458-5231; TTY 800-243-7012) and are posted on the *Clearinghouse Web site (http://www.cdcnac.*

Table 1. Rate Scheme for Clinical Practice Recommendations

Strength of recommendation	
A	Strong, should always be offered
B	Moderate, should usually be offered
C	Optional
D	Should generally not be offered
E	Should never be offered
Quality of evidence for recommendation	
I	At least one randomized trial with clinical end points
II	Clinical trials with laboratory end points
III	Expert opinion

org). These recommendations are not intended to substitute for the judgment of a physician who is expert in care of HIV-infected individuals. It is important to note that the Panel felt that where possible, the treatment of HIV-infected patients should be directed by a physician with extensive experience in the care of these patients. When this is not possible, it is important to have access to such expertise through consultations.

Each recommendation is accompanied by a rating that consists of a letter and a Roman numeral (**Table 1**); this rating scheme is similar to rating schemes used in previous guidelines on the prophylaxis of opportunistic infections issued by the U.S. Public Health Service and the Infectious Diseases Society of America (1). The letter indicates the strength of the recommendation, based on the opinion of the Panel, and the Roman numeral reflects the nature of the evidence for the recommendation (**Table 1**). Thus, recommendations based on data from clinical trials with clinical end points are differentiated from those based on data from trials with laboratory end points, such as CD4+ T-lymphocyte counts or plasma HIV RNA levels; where no clinical trial data are available, recommendations are based on the opinions of experts familiar with the relevant scientific literature. It should be noted that the majority of clinical trial data available to date regarding the use of antiretroviral agents has been obtained in trials enrolling predominantly young to middle-aged males. Although current knowledge indicates that women may differ from men in the absorption, metabolism, and clinical effects of certain pharmacologic agents, clinical experience and data available to date suggest that there are no significant gender differences known that would modify these guidelines. However, theoretical concerns exist. The Panel urges continuation of the current efforts to enroll more women in antiretroviral clinical trials so that the data needed to re-evaluate this issue can be gathered expeditiously.

This document addresses the following issues: the use of testing for plasma HIV RNA levels (viral load) and CD4+ T-cell count; considerations for when to initiate therapy in established HIV infection; special considerations for therapy in patients with advanced stage disease; interruption of therapy; considerations for changing therapy and available therapeutic options; the treatment of acute HIV infection; considerations for antiretroviral therapy in adolescents; and considerations for antiretroviral therapy in the pregnant woman.

USE OF TESTING FOR PLASMA HIV RNA LEVELS AND CD4+ T-CELL COUNT IN GUIDING DECISIONS FOR THERAPY

Decisions regarding initiation of or changes in antiretroviral therapy should be guided by monitoring the laboratory variables of plasma. HIV RNA (viral load) and CD4+ T-cell count, as well as the clinical condition of the patient. As discussed in Principle 2, results of the two laboratory tests give the physician important information about the virologic and immunologic status of the patient and the risk for progression to AIDS. It should be noted that HIV viral load testing has been approved by the Food and Drug Administration (FDA) only for the reverse transcriptase polymerase chain reaction (RT-PCR) assay (Roche) and only for the determination of disease prognosis. However, data presented at an FDA Advisory Committee for the Division of Antiviral Drug Products (14–15 July 1997, Silver Spring, MD) provide further evidence for the utility of viral RNA testing in monitoring therapeutic responses. Multiple analyses in more than 5000 patients who participated in approximately 18 trials with viral load monitoring showed a statistically significant dose–response type association between decreases in plasma viremia and improved clinical outcome based on standard end points of new AIDS-defining diagnoses and survival. This relationship was observed over a range of patient baseline characteristics, including pretreatment plasma RNA level, CD4+ T-cell count, and prior drug experience. Thus, it is the consensus of the Panel that viral load testing is the essential variable in decisions to initiate or change antiretroviral therapies. Measurement of plasma HIV RNA levels (viral load), done by using quantitative methods, should be performed at the time of diagnosis and every 3 to 4 months thereafter in the untreated patient (AIII) (**Table 2**). CD4+ T-cell counts should be measured at the time of diagnosis and, generally, every 3 to 6 months thereafter (AIII). These intervals between tests are merely recommendations, and flexibility should be exercised according to the circumstances of the individual case. Plasma HIV RNA levels should also be measured immediately before and 4 to 8 weeks after initiation of antiretroviral therapy (AIII). This second measurement allows the clinician to evaluate the initial effectiveness of therapy because in most patients, adherence to a regimen of potent antiretroviral agents should result in a large decrease ($\sim$0.5 to 0.75 $\log_{10}$) in viral load by 4 to 8 weeks. The viral load should continue to decline over the following weeks and in most individuals is below detectable levels (currently defined as $<$500 RNA copies/mL) by 12 to 16 weeks. The speed of viral load decline and the movement toward undetectable levels are affected by the baseline CD4+ T-cell count, the initial viral load, the potency of the regimen, adherence, prior exposure to antiretroviral agents, and the presence of any opportunistic infections. These individual differences must be considered when the effect of therapy is monitored. However, the absence of a virologic response of the magnitude discussed above should prompt the physician to reassess patient adherence, rule out malabsorption, consider repeated RNA testing to document lack of response, and/or consider a change in drug regimen.

Once the patient is receiving therapy, HIV RNA testing should be repeated every 3 to 4 months to evaluate the continuing effectiveness of therapy (AII). With optimal therapy, viral levels in plasma at 6 months should be undetectable, that is, below 500 copies/mL (2). If HIV RNA remains detectable in plasma after 6 months of therapy, the plasma HIV RNA test should be repeated to confirm the result and a change in therapy should be considered, according to the guidelines in "Considerations for changing a failing regimen" (BIII). More sensitive viral load assays are in development that can quantify HIV RNA down to approximately 50 copies/mL. Preliminary data from clinical trials strongly suggest that lowering plasma HIV RNA levels to less than 50 copies/mL is associated with more complete and durable viral suppression compared with reducing HIV RNA to levels between 50 and 500 copies/mL. However, the long-term clinical significance of these findings is currently unclear.

When decisions are made about the initiation of therapy, the CD4+ T-lymphocyte count and plasma HIV RNA measurement should ideally be performed on two occasions to ensure accuracy and consistency of measurement (BIII). However, in patients who

Table 2. Indications for Plasma HIV RNA Testing*

Clinical indication	Information	Use
Syndrome consistent with acute HIV infection	Establishes diagnosis when HIV antibody test result is negative or indeterminate	Diagnosis†
Initial evaluation of newly diagnosed HIV infection	Baseline viral load "set point"	Decision to start or defer therapy
Every 3 to 4 months in patients not receiving therapy	Changes in viral load	Decision to start therapy
4 to 8 weeks after initiation of anti-retroviral therapy	Initial assessment of drug efficacy	Decision to continue or change therapy
3 to 4 months after start of therapy	Maximal effect of therapy	Decision to continue or change therapy
Every 3 to 4 months in patients receiving therapy	Durability of antiretroviral effect	Decision to continue or change therapy
Clinical event or significant decline in $CD4^+$ T cells	Association with changing or stable viral load	Decision to continue, initiate, or change therapy

* Acute illness (e.g., bacterial pneumonia, tuberculosis, herpes simplex virus, infection, and *Pneumocystis carinii* pneumonia) and immunizations can cause increases in plasma HIV RNA level for 2 to 4 weeks; viral load testing should not be performed during this time. Plasma HIV RNA results should usually be verified with a repeated determination before therapy is started or changes. HIV RNA should be measured by using the same laboratory and the same assay.

† Diagnosis of HIV infection made by HIV RNA testing should be confirmed by standard methods, such as Western blot serology, performed 2 to 4 months after the initial indeterminate or negative test result.

present with advanced HIV disease, antiretroviral therapy should generally be initiated after the first viral load measurement is obtained in order to prevent a potentially deleterious delay in treatment. It is recognized that the requirement for two measurements of viral load may place a significant financial burden on patients or payers. Nonetheless, the Panel feels that two measurements of viral load will provide the clinician with the best information for subsequent follow-up of the patient. Consistent with Principle 2, plasma HIV RNA levels should not be measured during or within 4 weeks after successful treatment of any intercurrent infection, resolution of symptomatic illness, or immunization. Because commercially available tests differ, confirmatory plasma HIV RNA levels should be measured by the same laboratory using the same technique to ensure consistent results.

A minimally significant change in plasma viremia is considered to be a threefold or $0.5\text{-}\log_{10}$ increase or decrease. A significant decrease in $CD4^+$ T-lymphocyte count is a decrease of more than 30% from baseline for absolute cell numbers and a decrease of more than 3% from baseline in percentages of cells (3, 4). Discordance between trends in $CD4^+$ T-cell numbers and plasma HIV RNA levels can occur and was found in 20% of patients in one cohort studied (5). Such discordance can complicate decisions regarding antiretroviral therapy and may be due to many factors that affect plasma HIV RNA testing (*see* Principle 2). In general, viral load and trends in viral load are felt to be more informative for guiding decisions regarding antiretroviral therapy than are $CD4^+$ T-cell counts; exceptions to this rule do occur, however. For further discussion, refer to "Considerations for changing a failing regimen"; in many such cases, expert consultation should be considered.

ESTABLISHED INFECTION

Patients with established HIV infection are discussed in two arbitrarily defined clinical categories: 1) asymptomatic infection or 2) symptomatic disease (wasting, thrush, or unexplained fever for ≥2 weeks), including AIDS, defined according to the 1993 CDC classification system (6). All patients in the second category should be offered antiretroviral therapy. Considerations for initiating antiretroviral therapy in the first category of patients are complex and are discussed separately below. Before therapy is initiated in any patient, however, the following evaluation should be performed:

1. Complete history and physical examination (AII),
2. Complete blood count and chemistry profile (AII),
3. $CD4^+$ T-lymphocyte count (AI), and
4. Plasma HIV RNA measurement (AI).

Additional evaluation should include routine tests pertinent to the prevention of opportunistic infections, if not already performed (VDRL test, tuberculin skin test, toxoplasma IgG serology, and gynecologic examination with Papanicolaou smear), and other tests as clinically indicated (e.g., chest radiography, hepatitis C virus [HCV] serologic testing, and ophthalmologic examination) (AII). Hepatitis B virus (HBV) serologic testing is indicated in a patient who is a candidate for the hepatitis B vaccine or has abnormal results on liver function tests (AII), and cytomegalovirus (CMV) serologic testing may be useful in certain individuals, as discussed in the "USPHS/IDSA guidelines for the prevention of opportunistic infections in persons infected with the human immunodeficiency virus" (1) (BIII).

Considerations for initiating therapy in the patient with asymptomatic HIV infection

It has been demonstrated that antiretroviral therapy provides clinical benefit in HIV-infected individuals with advanced HIV disease and immunosuppression (7–11). Although there is theoretical benefit to treatment for patients with $CD4^+$ T-cell counts greater than 500 cells/mm^3 (*see* Principle 3), no long-term clinical benefit of treatment has yet been demonstrated. A major dilemma confronting patients and practitioners is that the antiretroviral regimens currently available that have the greatest potency in terms of viral suppression and $CD4^+$ T-cell preservation are medically complex, are associated with many specific side effects and drug interactions, and pose a substantial challenge with respect to adherence. Thus, decisions regarding treatment of asymptomatic, chronically infected individuals must balance several competing factors that influence risk and benefit.

Table 3 summarizes some of the factors that the physician and the asymptomatic patient must consider in deciding when to initiate therapy (*see also* Principle 3). Factors that would lead one to initiate early therapy include the real or potential goal of maximally suppressing viral replication; preserving immune function;

Table 3. Risks and Benefits of Early Initiation of Antiretroviral Therapy in the Asymptomatic HIV-Infected Patient

Potential benefits
- Control of viral replication and mutation; reduction of viral burden
- Prevention of progressive immunodeficiency; potential maintenance or reconstitution of a normal immune system
- Delayed progression to AIDS and prolongation of life
- Decreased risk for selection of resistant virus
- Decreased risk for drug toxicity

Potential risks
- Reduction in quality of life from adverse drug effects and inconvenience of current maximally suppressive regimens
- Earlier development of drug resistance
- Limitation in future choices of antiretroviral agents due to development of resistance
- Unknown long-term toxicity of antiretroviral drugs
- Unknown duration of effectiveness of current antiretroviral therapies

prolonging health and life; decreasing the risk for drug resistance due to early suppression of viral replication with potent therapy; and decreasing drug toxicity by treating the healthier patient. Factors weighing against early treatment in the asymptomatic stable patient include the potential adverse effects of the drugs on quality of life, including the inconvenience of most of the maximally suppressive regimens currently available; the potential risk for developing drug resistance despite early initiation of therapy; the potential for limiting future treatment options due to cycling of the patient through the available drugs during early disease; the potential risk for transmission of virus resistant to protease inhibitors (PIs) and other agents; the unknown durability of effect of the currently available therapies; and the unknown long-term toxicity of some drugs. Thus, the decision to begin therapy in the asymptomatic patient is complex and must be made in the setting of careful patient counseling and education. The factors that must be considered in this decision are 1) the willingness of the individual to begin therapy; 2) the degree of existing immunodeficiency as determined by the CD4+ T-cell count; 3) the risk for disease progression as determined by the level of plasma HIV RNA (**Table 4, Figure;** *see also* Principles document); 4) the potential benefits and risks of initiating therapy in asymptomatic individuals, as discussed above; and 5) the likelihood, after counseling and education, of adherence to the prescribed treatment regimen. In this regard, no individual patient should automatically be excluded from consideration for antiretroviral therapy simply because he or she exhibits a behavior or other characteristic judged by some to lend itself to noncompliance. Rather, the likelihood of patient adherence to a complex drug regimen should be discussed and determined by the individual patient and physician before therapy is initiated. To achieve the level of adherence necessary for effective therapy, providers are encouraged to use strategies for assessing and assisting adherence that have been developed in the

Table 4. Risk for Progression to AIDS-Defining Illness in a Cohort of Homosexual Men Predicted by Baseline CD4+ T-Cell Count and Viral Load*

CD4+ T-cell count		Patients, *n*	% AIDS (AIDS-defining complication)† 3 Years	6 Years	9 Years
≤350 cells/mm³					
Plasma Viral Load (copies/mL)‡					
bDNA	RT-PCR				
≤500	≤1500	–§	—	—	—
501–3000	1501–7000	30	0	18.8	30.6
3001–10 000	7001–20 000	51	8.0	42.2	65.6
10 001–30 000	20 001–55 000	73	40.1	72.9	86.2
>30 000	>55 000	174	72.9	92.7	95.6
351–500 cells/mm³					
Plasma Viral Load (copies/mL)					
bDNA	RT-PCR				
≤500	≤1500	—	—	—	—
501–3000	1501–7000	47	4.4	22.1	46.9
3001–10 000	7001–20 000	105	5.9	39.8	60.7
10 001–30 000	20 001–55 000	121	15.1	57.2	78.6
>30 000	>55 000	121	47.9	77.7	94.4
>500 cells/mm³					
Plasma Viral Load (copies/mL)					
bDNA	RT-PCR				
≤500	≤1500	110	1.0	5.0	10.7
501–3000	1501–7000	180	2.3	14.9	33.2
3001–10 000	7001–20 000	237	7.2	25.9	50.3
10 001–30 000	20 001–55 000	202	14.6	47.7	70.6
>30 000	>55 000	141	32.6	66.8	76.3

* Data from the Multicenter AIDS Cohort Study (MACS) (12). bDNA = branched DNA; RT-PCR = reverse transcriptase polymerase chain reaction.

† In this study, AIDS was defined according to the 1987 CDC definition; the study did not include asymptomatic individuals with CD4+ T-cell counts less than 200 cells/mm³.

‡ MACS numbers reflect plasma HIV RNA values obtained by bDNA testing. Values from RT-PCR are consistently 2- to 2.5-fold higher than bDNA values, as indicated.

§ Too few individuals were in the category to provide a reliable estimate of risk for AIDS.

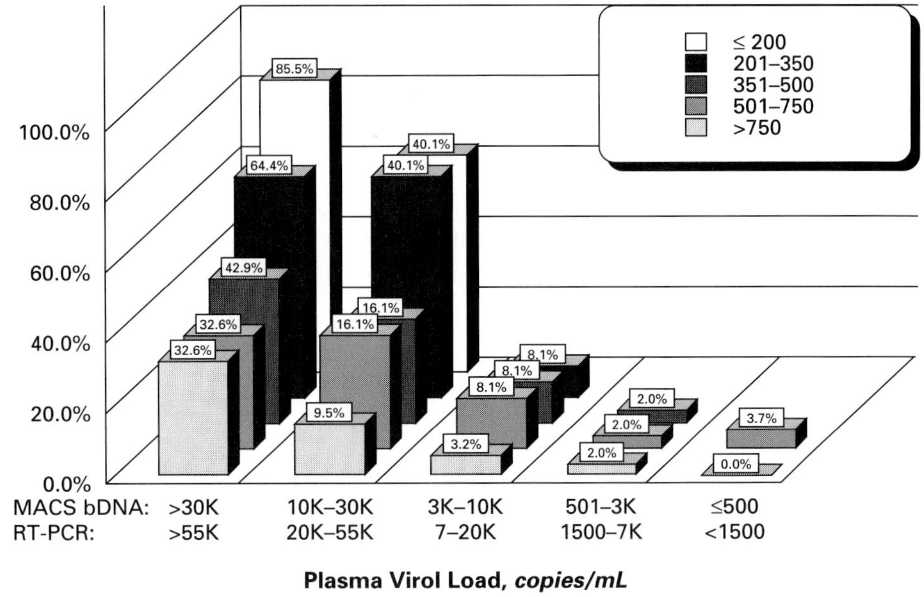

Figure. Likelihood of developing an AIDS-related illness in 3 years. Viral load values represent the actual data obtained on the specimens from the Multicenter AIDS Cohort Study (*MACS*) as well as the values showing the equivalent expected reverse transcriptase polymerase chain reaction (*RT-PCR*) values. Values shown here differ slightly from those in Table 4 because better discrimination of outcome was achieved by reanalysis of the data with viral load as the initial variable for categorization followed by CD4+ T-lymphocyte stratification of the patients. Adapted from Mellors and colleagues (12). bDNA = branched DNA.

context of long-term treatment for other serious diseases; in this regard, intensive patient education regarding the critical need for adherence should be provided, specific goals of therapy should be established and mutually agreed upon, and a long-term treatment plan should be developed with the patient. Intensive follow-up should take place to assess adherence to treatment and to continue counseling for the prevention of sexual and drug injection-related transmission.

Initiating therapy in the patient with asymptomatic HIV infection

Once the patient and physician have decided to initiate antiretroviral therapy, treatment should be aggressive, with the goal of suppressing plasma viral load to undetectable levels. **Tables 5** and **6** summarize the recommendations on when to initiate therapy and what regimens to use. In general, any patient with fewer than 500 CD4+ T cells/mm^3 or more than 10 000 (branched DNA [bDNA]) or 20 000 (RT-PCR) HIV RNA copies/mL should be offered therapy (AII). However, the strength of the recommendation for therapy should be based on the readiness of the patient for treatment as well as a consideration of the prognosis for disease-free survival as determined by viral load, CD4+ T-cell count **(Table 4, Figure),** and the slope of the CD4+ T-cell count decline. Note that the values for bDNA shown in the **Figure** and **Table 4** (first line or column) are the uncorrected HIV RNA values obtained from the Multicenter AIDS Cohort Study (MACS). It had previously been thought that these values, obtained on stored heparinized plasma specimens, should be multiplied by a factor of 2 to adjust for an anticipated twofold loss of RNA ascribed to the effects of heparin and delayed processing on the stability of RNA. However, more recent analysis suggests that the reduction ascribed to these factors is 0.2 log or less, so that no significant correction factor is necessary (Mellors J. Personal communication, October 1997). Values for RT-PCR are also shown in **Table 4** and the **Figure;** comparison of the results obtained from the RT-PCR and bDNA assays done by using the manufacturer's controls consistently indicate that the HIV-1 RNA values obtained by RT-PCR are approximately two times higher than those obtained by the bDNA assay (12). Thus, the MACS values must be multiplied by approximately 2 to be consistent with current RT-PCR values. A third test for HIV RNA, the Nucleic-Acid Sequence Based Amplification (NASBA), is currently used in some clinical settings. However, formulas for converting values obtained from either bDNA or RT-PCR assays to NASBA-equivalent values cannot be derived from the limited data available at this time. This information will be added to the guidelines when it becomes available.

Table 5. Indications for the Initiation of Antiretroviral Therapy in the Chronically HIV-Infected Patient*

Clinical category	CD4+ T-cell count and HIV RNA level	Recommendation
Symptomatic (AIDS, thrush, unexplained fever)	Any value	Treat
Asymptomatic	CD4+ T-cell count <500/mm^3 or HIV RNA level >10 000 (bDNA) or >20 000 (RT-PCR)	Treatment should be offered. Strength of recommendation is based on prognosis for disease-free survival as shown in **Table 4** and willingness of the patient to accept therapy†
Asymptomatic	CD4+ T-cell count >500/mm^3 or HIV RNA level <10 000 (bDNA) or <20 000 (RT-PCR)	Many experts would delay therapy and observe; some experts would treat

* bDNA = branched DNA; RT-PCR = reverse transcriptase polymerase chain reaction.

† Some experts would observe patients with CD4+ T-cell counts between 350 and 5000 cells/mm^3 and HIV RNA levels <10 000 (bDNA) or <20 000 (RT-PCR) copies/mL.

Table 6. Recommended Antiretroviral Agents for Treatment of Established HIV Infection*

Preferred	Strong evidence of clinical benefit and/or sustained suppression of plasma viral load (2, 13, 14). One choice each from column A and column B. Drugs are listed in random, not priority, order:	
	Column A	Column B
	Indinavir (AI)	ZDV + ddI (AI)
	Nelfinavir (AII)	d4T + ddI (AII)
	Ritonavir (AI)	ZDV + ddC (AI)
	Saquinavir-SGC† (AII)	ZDV + 3TC‡ (AI)
	Ritonavir + saquinavir-SGC or -HGC§ (BII)	d4T + 3TC‡ (AII)
Alternative	Less likely to provide sustained virus suppression (15, 16)	
	1 NNRTI + 2 NRTIs (column B) (BII)‖	
Not generally recommended	Strong evidence of clinical benefit but initial virus suppression is not sustained in most patients (17–20)	
	2 NRTIs (column B) (CI)	
	Saquinavir-HGC + 2 NRTIs (column B)¶ (CI)	
Not recommended	Evidence against use, virologically undesirable, or overlapping toxicities	
	All monotherapies** (DI)	
	d4T + ZDV (DI)	
	ddC + ddI†† (DII)	
	ddC + d4T†† (DII)	
	ddC + 3TC (DII)	

* 3TC = lamivudine; d4T = stavudine; ddC = zalcitabine; ddI = didanosine; HGC = hard-gel capsule; NNRTI = non-nucleoside reverse transcriptase inhibitor; NRTI = nucleoside analogue reverse transcriptase inhibitor; SGC = soft-gel capsule; ZDV = zidovudine.

† Virologic data and clinical experience with saquinavir-SGC (Fortovase) are limited in comparison with those of other protease inhibitors.

‡ High-level resistance to 3TC develops within 2 to 4 weeks in partially suppressive regimens; optimal use is in three-drug antiretroviral combinations that reduce viral load to <500 copies/mL.

§ Use of ritonavir, 400 mg b.i.d., with saquinavir-SGC (Fortovase), 400 mg b.i.d., results in similar drug exposure and antiretroviral activity as when using 400 mg b.i.d. of saquinavir-HGC (Invirase) in combination with ritonavir. However, the combination with Fortovase has not been extensively studied, and gastrointestinal toxicity may be greater when using Fortovase.

‖ The only combinations of 2 NRTIs + 1 NNRTI that have been shown to suppress viremia to undetectable levels in the majority of patients remaining on treatment for more than 28 weeks are ZDV + ddI + nevirapine and ZDV + 3TC + delavirdine. Use of nevirapine or delaviridine may result in resistance that precludes efficacy of new NNRTIs, such as efavirenz.

¶ Use of saquinavir-HGC (Invirase) is generally not recommended, except in combination with ritonavir.

** Zidovudine monotherapy may be considered for prophylactic use in pregnant women with low viral load and high CD4+ T-cell counts to prevent perinatal transmission, as discussed in "Considerations in the Pregnant Woman."

†† This combination of NRTIs is not recommended on the basis of lack of clinical data on the combination and/or overlapping toxicities.

In current practice, there are two general approaches to initiating therapy in the asymptomatic patient: a therapeutically more aggressive approach that would treat most patients early in the course of HIV infection because of the recognition that HIV disease is virtually always progressive, and a therapeutically more cautious approach in which therapy may be delayed because the balance of the risk for clinically significant progression and other factors discussed above are felt to weigh in favor of observation and delayed therapy. The aggressive approach is heavily based on the Principles of Therapy, particularly the Principle that one should begin treatment before significant immunosuppression develops and one should treat to achieve undetectable viremia; thus, all patients with fewer than 500 CD4+ T cells/mm³ would be started on therapy, as would patients with higher CD4+ T-cell counts who have plasma viral loads greater than 10 000 (bDNA) or 20 000 (RT-PCR) HIV RNA copies/mL (**Table 5**). The more conservative approach to the initiation of therapy in the asymptomatic individual would delay treatment of the patient with fewer than 500 CD4+ T cells/mm³ and low levels of viremia who have a low risk for rapid disease progression, according to the data in **Table 4;** careful observation and monitoring would continue. Patients with CD4+ T-cell counts greater than 500/mm³ would also be observed, except those at substantial risk for rapid disease progression because of a high viral load. For example, the patient with 60 000 (RT-PCR) or 30 000 (bDNA) HIV RNA copies/mL, regardless of CD4+ T-cell count, has a high probability of progressing to an AIDS-defining complication of HIV disease within 3 years (32.6% if the CD4+ T-cell count is greater than 500/mm³) and should clearly be encouraged to initiate antiretroviral therapy. On the other hand a patient with 18 000 HIV RNA copies/mL (RT-PCR) and a CD4+ T-cell count of 410 cells/mm³ has a 5.9% chance of progressing to an AIDS-defining complication of HIV infection in 3 years (**Table 4**). The therapeutically aggressive physician would recommend treatment for this patient to suppress the ongoing viral replication that is readily detectable; the therapeutically more conservative physician would discuss the possibility of initiation of therapy but would recognize that a delay in therapy due to the balance of considerations discussed above is also reasonable. In either case, the patient should make the final decision regarding acceptance of therapy following discussion with the health care provider of specific issues relevant to his or her own clinical situation.

When initiating therapy in the patient naive to antiretroviral therapy, one should begin with a regimen that is expected to reduce viral replication to undetectable levels (AIII). On the basis of the weight of experience, the preferred regimen to accomplish this is two nuceloside reverse transcriptase inhibitors (NRTIs) and one potent PI (**Table 6**). Alternative regimens have been used; these include ritonavir and saquinavir (with one or two NRTIs) or nevirapine as a substitute for the PI. Ritonavir and saquinavir (hard-gel capsule) dual PI therapy (without an NRTI) appears to be potent in suppressing viremia below detectable levels and has convenient twice-daily dosing; however, the safety of this combination has not been fully established according to FDA guidelines. In addition, this regimen has not been directly compared to the proven regimens of two NRTIs and a PI, and the Panel thus

Table 7. Characteristics of Nucleoside Reverse Transcriptase Inhibitors*

Characteristic	Zidovudine (AZT, ZDV) *(Retrovir)*	Didanosine (ddI) *(Videx)*	Zalcitabine (ddC) *(HIVID)*	Stavudine (d4T) *(Zerit)*	Lamivudine (3TC) *(Epivir)*
Dosing recommendations	200 mg tid or 300 mg bid or with 3TC as Combivir, 1 bid	Tablets >60 kg: 200 mg bid <60 kg: 125 mg bid	0.75 mg tid	>60 kg: 40 mg bid <60 kg: 30 mg bid	150 mg bid <50 kg: 2 mg/kg bid or with ZDV as Combivir, 1 bid
Oral bioavailability, %	60	Tablet: 40 Powder: 30	85	86	86
Serum half-life, *h*	1.1	1.6	1.2	1.0	3–6
Intracellular half-life, *h*	3	25–40	3	3.5	12
Elimination	Metabolized to AZT glucuronide (GAZT) Renal excretion of GAZT	Renal excretion 50%	Renal excretion 70%	Renal excretion 50%	Renal excretion unchanged
Adverse events	Bone marrow suppression: anemia and/or neutropenia Subjective symptoms: gastrointestinal intolerance, headache, insomnia, asthenia	Pancreatitis; peripheral neuropathy; nausea; diarrhea	Peripheral neuropathy; stomatitis	Peripheral neuropathy	Minimal toxicity

* Brand names are given in parentheses below the generic names.

recommends that at least one additional NRTI be used when the physician elects to use two PIs as initial therapy. Substituting nevirapine for the PI or using two NRTIs alone does not achieve the goal of suppressing viremia to below detectable levels as consistently as does combination treatment with two NRTIs and a PI; it should be used only if more potent treatment is not possible. It should be noted, however, that some experts feel that there are currently insufficient data to choose between a three-drug regimen containing a PI and one containing nevirapine in the drug-naive patient; further studies are pending. Likewise, other regimens using two PIs or a PI and a non-nucleoside reverse transcriptase inhibitor (NNRTI) as initial therapy are currently in clinical trials with data pending. Although lamivudine (3TC) is a potent NRTI, resistance to 3TC develops rapidly when suppression of virus replication is not complete (21, 22). Therefore, the optimal use for this agent is as part of a combination of three or more drugs that has a high chance of completely suppressing virus replication. Other agents in which a single genetic mutation can confer drug resistance, such as the NNRTIs nevirapine and delavirdine, should also be used in this manner. Use of antiretroviral agents as monotherapy is contraindicated (DI), except when there are no other options or when the agents are used during pregnancy to reduce perinatal transmission, as noted below. When antiretroviral therapy is initiated, all drugs should be started simultaneously at full dose with the following three exceptions: Dose-escalation regimens are recommended for ritonavir; nevirapine; and, in some cases, ritonavir plus saquinavir.

Detailed information comparing the different NRTIs, the NNRTIs, the PIs, and drug interactions between the PIs and other agents can be found in **Tables 7** through **12.** Particular attention should be paid to **Tables 9** through **12** regarding drug interactions between the PIs and other agents because these are extensive and often require dose modification or substitution of various drugs. Toxicity assessment is an ongoing process; assessment at least twice during the first month of therapy and every 3 months thereafter is a reasonable management approach.

Table 8. Characteristics of Non-Nucleoside Reverse Transcriptase Inhibitors*

Variable	Nevirapine *(Viramune)*	Delavirdine *(Rescriptor)*
Form	200-mg tablets	100-mg tablets
Dosing recommendations	200 mg po qd × 14 days, then 200 mg po bid	400 mg po tid (four 100-mg tabs in ≥3 oz of water to produce slurry)
Oral bioavailability, %	>90	85
Serum half-life, *h*	25–30	5.8
Elimination	Metabolized by cytochrome p450; 80% excreted in urine (glucuronidated metabolites, <5% unchanged), 10% excreted in feces	Metabolized by cytochrome p450; 51% excreted in urine (<5% unchanged), 44% excreted in feces
Drug interactions	Induces cytochrome p450 enzymes The following drugs have suspected interactions that require careful monitoring if coadministered with nevirapine: rifampin, rifabutin, oral contraceptives, protease inhibitors, triazolam, and midazolam	Inhibits cytochrome p450 enzymes Not recommended for concurrent use: terfenadine, astemizole, alprazolam, midazolam, cisapride, rifabutin, rifampin, triazolam, ergot derivatives, amphetamines, nifedipine, and anticonvulsants (phenytoin, carbamazepine, phenobarbitol) Delavirdine increases levels of clarithromycin, dapsone, quinidine, warfarin, indinavir, and saquinavir Antacids or didanosine: separate delavirdine administration by ≥1 h
Adverse events	Rash Increased aminotransferase levels Hepatitis	Rash Headaches

* Brand names are given in parentheses.

Table 9. Characteristics of Protease Inhibitors*

Characteristic	Indinavir *(Crixivan)*	Ritonavir *(Norvir)*	Saquinavir-HGC *(Invirase)*	Saquinavir-SGC *(Fortovase)*	Nelfinavir *(Viracept)*
Form	200-, 400-mg caplets	100-mg caplets 600 mg/7.5 mL po solution	200-mg caplets	200-mg caplets	250-mg tablets 500-mg/g oral powder
Dosing recommendations	800 mg q8h Take 1 h before or 2 h after meals; may take with skim milk or low-fat meal	600 mg q12† Take with food if possible	600 mg tid† Take with large meal	1,200 mg tid Take with large meal	750 mg tid Take with food (meal or light snack)
Oral bioavailability	65%	Not determined	Hard-gel capsule: 4%, erratic	Soft-gel capsule: not determined	20%–80%
Serum half-life, *h*	1.5–2	3–5	1–2	1–2	3.5–5
Route of metabolism	p450 cytochrome 3A4	p450 cytochrome 3A4 > 2D6	p450 cytochrome 3A4	p450 cytochrome 3A4	p450 cytochrome 3A4
Storage	Room temperature	Refrigerate capsules; refrigeration for oral solution is preferred but not required if solution is used within 30 days	Room temperature	Refrigerate or store at room temperature (up to 3 mo)	Room temperature
Adverse effects	Nephrolithiasis Gastrointestinal intolerance, nausea Laboratory: increased indirect bilirubinemia (inconsequential) Miscellaneous: headache, asthenia, blurred vision, dizziness, rash, metallic taste, thrombocytopenia Hyperglycemia‡	Gastrointestinal intolerance, nausea, vomiting, diarrhea Paresthesias—circumoral and extremities Hepatitis Asthenia Taste perversion Laboratory: triglycerides increase >200%, aminotransferase elevation; elevated creatine phosphokinase and uric acid Hyperglycemia‡	Gastrointestinal intolerance, nausea and diarrhea Headache Elevated aminotransferase enzymes Hyperglycemia‡	Gastrointestinal intolerance, nausea, diarrhea, abdominal pain, and dyspepsia Headache Elevated aminotransferase enzymes Hyperglycemia‡	Diarrhea Hyperglycemia‡
Drug interactions	Inhibits cytochrome p450 (less than ritonavir) Not recommended for concurrent use: rifampin Contraindicated for concurrent use: terfenadine, astemizole, cisapride, triazolam, midazolam, and ergot alkaloids Indinavir levels increased by ketoconazole‖, delavirdine, and nelfinivir Indinavir levels reduced by rifampin, rifabutin, grapefruit juice, and nevirapine Didanosine reduces indinavir absorption unless taken >2 h apart	Inhibits cytochrome p450 (potent inhibitor) Ritonavir increases levels of multiple drugs that are not recommended for concurrent use§ Didanosine may cause reduced absorption of both drugs; should be taken ≥2 h apart Ritonavir decreases levels of ethinyl estradiol, theophylline, sulfamethoxazole, and zidovudine Ritonavir increases levels of clarithromycin and desipramine	Inhibits cytochrome p450 Saquinavir levels increased by ritonavir, ketoconazole, grapefruit juice, nelfinavir, and delavirdine Saquinavir levels reduced by rifampin, rifabutin, and possibly phenobarbital, phenytoin, dexamethasone and carbamezepine, and nevirapine Contraindicated for concurrent use: rifampin, rifabutin, terfenadine, astemizole, cisapride, ergot alkaloids, triazolam, and midazolam	Inhibits cytochrome p450 Saquinavir levels increased by ritonavir, ketoconazole, grapefruit juice, nelfinavir, and delavirdine Saquinavir levels reduced by rifampin, rifabutin, and possibly phenobarbital, phenytoin, dexamethasone and carbamezepine, and nevirapine Contraindicated for concurrent use: rifampin, rifabutin, terfenadine, astemizole, cisapride, ergot alkaloids, triazolam, and midazolam	Inhibits cytochrome p450 (less than ritonavir) Nelfinavir levels reduced by rifampin and rifabutin Contraindicated for concurrent use: triazolam, midazolam, ergot alkaloids, terfenadine, astemizole, and cisapride Nelfinavir decreases level of ethinyl estradiol and norethindrone Nelfinavir increases levels of rifabutin, saquinavir, and indinavir Not recommended for concurrent use: rifampin

* Brand names are given in parentheses.

† Dose escalation for ritonavir: days 1–2, 300 mg bid; days 3–5, 400 mg bid; days 6–13, 500 mg bid; day 14, 600 mg bid. Combination treatment regimen with saquinavir (400–600 mg po bid) plus ritonavir (400–600 mg po bid).

‡ Cases of new-onset hyperglycemia have been reported in association with the use of all protease inhibitors (23–25).

§ Drugs contraindicated for concurrent use with ritonavir; amiodarone (Cordorone), astemizole (Hismanal), bepridil (Vascar), bupropion (Wellbutin), cisapride (Propulsid), clorazepate (Tranxene), clozapine (Clozaril), diazepam (Valium), encainide (Enkaid), estazolam (ProSom), flecainide (Tambocor), flurazepam (Dalmane), meperidine (Demerol), midazolam (Versed), piroxicam (Feldene), propoxyphene (Darvon), propafenone (Rythmol), quinidine, rifabutin, terfenadine (Seldane), triazolam (Halcion), zolpidem (Ambien), and ergot alkaloids.

‖ Decrease indivair to 600 mg q8h.

Initiating therapy in advanced HIV disease

All patients receiving a diagnosis of advanced HIV disease, which is defined as any condition meeting the 1993 CDC definition of AIDS (6), should be treated with antiretroviral agents regardless of plasma viral levels (AI). All patients with symptomatic HIV infection without AIDS, defined as the presence of thrush or unexplained fever, should also be treated.

Special considerations in the patient with advanced-stage disease

Some patients present with opportunistic infections, wasting, dementia, or malignancy and are first diagnosed with HIV infection at this advanced stage of disease. All patients with advanced HIV disease should be treated with antiretroviral therapy. When the patient is acutely ill with an opportunistic infection or another

Table 10. Drugs That Should Note Be Used with Protease Inhibitors

Drug Category	Indinavir	Ritonavir*	Saquinavir (*Invirase* or *Fortovase*)	Nelfinavir	Alternatives
Analgesics	None	Meperidine, piroxicam, propoxyphene	None	None	Aspirin, oxycodon, acetaminophen
Cardiac	None	Amiodarone, encainide, flecainide, propafenone, quinidine	None	None	Limited experience
Antimycobacterial	Rifampin	Rifabutin†	Rifampin, rifabutin	Rifampin	For rifabutin (as alternative for *Mycobacterium avium* complex treatment): clarithromycin, ethambutol (treatment, not prophylaxis), or azithromycin
Calcium-channel blocker	None	Bepridil	None	None	Limited experience
Antihistamine	Astemizole, terfenadine	Astemizole, terfenadine	Astemizole, terfenadine	Astemizole, terfenadine	Loratadine
Gastrointestinal	Cisapride	Cisapride	Cisapride	Cisapride	Limited experience
Antidepressant	None	Bupropion	None	None	Fluoxetine, desipramine
Neuroleptic	None	Clozapine, pimozide	None	None	Limited experience
Psychotropic	Midazolam, triazolam	Clorazepate, diazepam, estazolam, flurazepam, midazolam, triazolam, zolpidem	Midazolam, triazolam	Midazolam, triazolam	Temazepam, lorazepam
Ergot alkaloids (vasoconstrictor)	Dihydroergotamine (D.H.E. 45), ergotamine‡ (various forms)	Dihydroergotamine (D.H.E. 45), ergotamine‡ (various forms)	Dihydroergotamine (D.H.E. 45), ergotamine‡ (various forms)	Dihydroergotamine (D.H.E. 45), ergotamine‡ (various forms)	Limited experience

* The drugs listed are contraindicated on the basis of theoretical considerations. Thus, drugs with low therapeutic indices but with suspected major metabolic contribution from cytochrome p450 3A, CYP2D6, or unknown pathways are included in this table. Actual interactions may or may not occur in patients.

† Reduce rifabutin dose to one quarter of the standard dose.

‡ This is probably a class effect.

Table 11. Drug Interactions between Protease Inhibitors and Other Drugs Requiring Dose Modifications

Drug	Indinavir	Ritonavir	Saquinavir*	Nelfinavir
Fluconazole	No dose change	No dose change	No data	No dose change
Ketoconazole and itraconazole	Decrease dose to 600 mg q8h	Increases ketoconazole >3-fold; dose adjustment required	Increases saquinavir levels 3-fold; no dose change†	No dose change
Rifabutin	Reduced rifabutin to half dose: 150 mg qd	Consider alternative drug or reduce rifabutin dose to one quarter	Not recommended with either Invirase or Fortovase	Reduce rifabutin to half dose: 150 mg qd
Rifampin	Contraindicated	Unknown‡	Not recommended with either Invirase or Fortovase	Contraindicated
Oral contraceptives	Modest increase in Ortho-Novum levels; no dose change	Ethinyl estradiol levels decreased; use alternative or additional contraceptive method	No data	Ethinyl estradiol and norethindrone levels decreased; use alternative or additional contraceptive method
Miscellaneous	Grapefruit juice reduces indinavir levels by 26%	Despriamine levels increased by 145%: reduce dose Theophylline levels decreased; increase dose	Grapefruit juice increases saquinavir levels†	

* Several drugs interaction studies have been completed with saquinavir given as Invirase or Fortovase. Results from studies conducted with Invirase may not be applicable to Fortovase.

† With Invirase.

‡ Rifampin reduces ritonavir levels by 35%. Increased ritonavir dose or use of ritonavir in combination therapy is strongly recommended. The effect of ritonavir on rifampin is unknown. Concurrent use may increase liver toxicity. Therefore, patients on ritonavir and rifampin should be monitored closely.

Table 12. Drug Interactions: Protease Inhibitors and Non-Nucleoside Reverse Transcriptase Inhibitors

Drug affected	Effect of drug on levels/Dose					
	Indinavir	Ritonavir	Saquinavir*	Nelfinavir	Nevirapine	Delavirdine
Indinavir (IDV)	—	No data	Levels: IDV no effect; SQV ↑ 4–7×† Dose: No data	Levels: IDV ↑ 50%; NFV ↑ 80% Dose: No data	Levels; IDV ↓ 28% Dose: Standard	Levels: IDV ↑ 40% Dose: IDV 600 mg q 8h
Ritonavir (RTV)	No data	—	Levels: RTV no effect; SQV ↑ 20×§‡ Dose: Invirase or Fortovase 400 mg bid + RTV 400 mg bid	Levels: RTV no effect; NFV ↑ 1.5× Dose: No data	Levels RTV ↓ 11% Dose: Standard	Levels: RTV ↑ 70% Dose: No data
Saquinavir (SQV)	Levels: SQV ↑ 4–7×; IDV no effect† Dose: No data	Levels: SQV ↑ 20×†‡; RTV no effect Dose: Invirase or Fortovase 400 mg bid + RTV 400 mg bid	—	Levels: SQV ↑ 3–5×; NFV ↑ 20%† Dose: Standard NFV; Fortovase; 800 mg tid	Levels: SQV ↓ 25%‡ Dose: No data	Levels: SQV ↑ 5×‡ Dose: Standard for Invirase Monitor aminotransferase levels
Nelfinavir (NFV)	Levels: NFV ↑ 80%; IDV ↑ 50% Dose: No data	Levels NFV ↑ 1.5×; RTV no effect Dose: No data	Levels: NFV ↑ 20%; SQV ↑ 3–5×† Dose: Standard NFV; Fortovase 800 mg tid	—	Levels: NFV ↑ 10% Dose: Standard	Levels: NFV ↑ 2×; DLV ↓ 50% Dose: Standard (Monitor for neutropenic complications)
Nevirapine (NVP)	Levels: IDV ↓ 28% Dose: Standard	Levels: RTV ↓ 11% Dose: Standard	Levels: SQV ↓ 25%‡ Dose: No data	Levels: NFV ↑ 10% Dose: Standard	—	Do not use together
Delavirdine (DLV)	Levels: IDV ↑ 40% Dose: IDV 600 q 8h	Levels: RTV ↑ 70% Dose: No data	Levels: SQV ↑ 5×‡ Dose: Standard for Invirase. Monitor aminotransferase levels	Levels: NFV ↑ 2×; DLV ↓ 50% Dose: Standard (monitor for neutropenic complications)	Do not use together	—

* Several drug interaction studies have been completed with saquinavir given as Invirase or Fortovase. Results from studies conducted with Invirase may not be applicable to Fortovase.
† Conducted with Fortovase.
‡ Conducted with Invirase.

complication of HIV infection, the clinician should consider clinical issues, such as drug toxicity, ability to adhere to treatment regimens, drug interactions, and laboratory abnormalities, when determining the timing of initiation of antiretroviral therapy. Once therapy is initiated, a maximally suppressive regimen, such as two NRTIs and a PI, should be used, as indicated in **Table 6.** Advanced-stage patients being maintained on an antiretroviral regimen should not have the therapy discontinued during an acute opportunistic infection or malignancy unless there are concerns regarding drug toxicity, intolerance, or drug interactions.

Patients who have progressed to AIDS are often treated with complicated combinations of drugs, and the potential for multiple drug interactions must be appreciated by clinician and patient. The choice of which antiretroviral agents to use must be made with consideration given to potential drug interactions and overlapping drug toxicities, as outlined in **Tables 7** through **12.** For instance, the use of rifampin to treat active tuberculosis is problematic in a patient receiving a PI, which adversely affects the metabolism of rifampin but is frequently needed to effectively suppress viral replication in these advanced patients. Conversely, rifampin lowers the blood levels of PIs, which may result in suboptimal antiretroviral therapy. Although rifampin is contraindicated or not recommended for use with all of the PIs, one might consider using rifabutin at a reduced dose, as indicated in **Tables 8** through **11;** this topic is discussed in greater detail elsewhere (26). Other factors complicating advanced disease are wasting and anorexia, which may prevent patients from adhering to the dietary requirements for efficient absorption of certain PIs. Bone marrow suppression associated with zidovudine and the neuropathic effects of zalcitabine, stavudine, and didanosine may combine with the direct effects of HIV to render the drugs intolerable. Hepatotoxicity associated with certain PIs may limit the use of these drugs, especially in patients with underlying liver dysfunction. The absorption and half-life of certain drugs may be altered by antiretroviral agents, particularly the PIs and NNRTIs, whose metabolism involves the hepatic cytochrome p450 (CYP450) enzymatic pathway. Some of these PIs and NNRTIs (ritonavir, indinavir, saquinavir, nelfinavir, and delavirdine) inhibit the CYP450 pathway; others (nevirapine) induce CYP450 metabolism. The CYP450 inhibitors have the potential to increase blood levels of drugs metabolized by this pathway. At times, adding a CYP450 inhibitor can improve the pharmacokinetic profile of selected agents (such as adding ritonavir therapy to the hard-gel capsule formulation of saquinavir) as well as contributing an additive antiviral effect; however, these interactions can also result in life-threatening drug toxicity, as indicated in **Tables 10** through **12.** Thus, health care providers should inform their patients of the need to discuss any new drugs, including over-the-counter agents and alternative medications, that they may consider taking, and careful attention should be given to the relative risk versus benefits of specific combinations of agents.

Initiation of potent antiretroviral therapy is often associated with some degree of recovery of immune function. In this setting, patients with advanced HIV disease and subclinical opportunistic infections, such as *Mycobacterium avium* complex or CMV infection, may develop a new immunologic response to the pathogen; thus, new symptoms may develop in association with the heightened immunologic and/or inflammatory response. This should not be interpreted as a failure of antiretroviral therapy, and these newly presenting opportunistic infections should be treated appropriately while the patient is maintained on the antiretroviral regimen. Viral load measurement is helpful in clarifying this association.

INTERRUPTION OF ANTIRETROVIRAL THERAPY

There are multiple reasons for temporary discontinuation of antiretroviral therapy, including intolerable side effects, drug interactions, first trimester of pregnancy (when the patient so elects), and unavailability of drug. There are no studies and no reliable estimate of the number of days, weeks, or months that constitute a clinically important interruption of one or more components of a therapeutic regimen that would increase the likelihood of drug resistance. If there is a need to discontinue therapy with any antiretroviral medication for an extended time, clinicians and patients should be advised of the theoretical advantage of stopping all antiretroviral agents simultaneously, rather than continuing one or two agents, to minimize the emergency of resistance viral strains (*see* Principle 4).

CONSIDERATIONS FOR CHANGING A FAILING REGIMEN

As with the initiation of antiretroviral therapy, the decision to change regimens should be approached with careful consideration of several complex factors. These factors include recent clinical history and physical examination; plasma HIV RNA levels measured on two separate occasions; absolute CD4$^+$ T-lymphocyte counts and changes in these counts; remaining treatment options in terms of potency, potential resistance patterns from prior antiretroviral therapies, and potential for compliance and tolerance; assessment of adherence to medications; and preparation of the patient for the implications of the new regimen, which include side effects, drug interactions, dietary requirements, and possible need to alter concomitant medications (*see* Principle 7). A regimen may fail for many reasons, including initial viral resistance to one or more agents, altered absorption or metabolism of the drug, multidrug pharmacokientics that adversely affect therapeutic drug levels, and poor patient adherence to a regimen due to either poor compliance or inadequate patient education about the therapeutic agents. In this regard, it is important to carefully assess patient compliance before changing antiretroviral therapy; health care workers involved in the care of the patient, such as the case manager or social worker, may be of assistance in this evaluation. Clinicians should be aware of the prevalence of mental health disorders and psychoactive substance use disorders in certain HIV-infected persons; inadequate mental health treatment services may jeopardize the ability of such individuals to adhere to their medical treatment. Proper identification of and intervention in these mental health disorders can greatly enhance adherence to medical HIV treatment.

It is important to distinguish between the need to change therapy because of drug failure and because of drug toxicity. In the latter case, it is appropriate to substitute one or more alternative drugs of the same potency and from the same class of agents as the agent suspected to be causing the toxicity. In the case of drug failure where more than one drug had been used, a detailed history of current and past antiretroviral medications, as well as other HIV-related medications, should be obtained. Optimally and when possible, the regimen should be changed entirely to drugs that have not been taken previously. With triple combinations of drugs, at least two and preferably three new drugs must be used; this is based on the current understanding of strategies to prevent drug resistance (*see* Principles 4 and 5). Assays to determine genotypic resistance are commercially available; however, these have not undergone field testing to demonstrate clinical utility and are not FDA-approved. The Panel does not recommend these assays for routine use at the present time.

Three different populations of patients should be considered with regard to a change in therapy: 1) individuals who are receiving incompletely suppressive antiretroviral therapy, such as single- or double-nucleoside therapy, with detectable or undetectable plasma viral load (discussed further below); 2) individuals who have been on potent combination therapy, including a PI, and whose viremia was initially suppressed to undetectable levels but has again become detectable; and 3) individuals who have been on potent combination therapy, including a PI, and whose viremia was never suppressed to below detectable limits. Although these groups of individuals should have treatment regimens changed in order to maximize the chances of durable, maximal viral RNA suppression, the first group may have more treatment options because they are PI-naive.

Criteria for changing therapy

The goal of antiretroviral therapy—to improve the length and quality of the patient's life—is probably best accomplished by maximal suppression of viral replication to below detectable levels (currently defined as <500 copies/mL) sufficiently early to preserve immune function. However, this is not always achievable with a given therapeutic regimen, and frequently regimens must be modified. In general, the plasma HIV RNA level is the most important variable with which to evaluate response to therapy, and increases in levels of viremia that are significant, confirmed, and not attributable to intercurrent infection or vaccination indicate failure of the drug regimen regardless of changes in CD4$^+$ T-cell counts. Clinical complications and sequential changes in CD4$^+$ T-cell count may complement the viral load test in evaluating a response to treatment. Specific criteria that should prompt consideration for changing therapy include the following:

1. Less than a 0.5- to 0.75-log reduction in plasma HIV RNA by 4 weeks following initiation of therapy or less than a 1-log reduction by 8 weeks (CIII).
2. Failure to suppress plasma HIV RNA to undetectable levels within 4 to 6 months of initiating therapy (BIII). In this regard, the degree of initial decrease in plasma HIV RNA and the overall trend in decreasing viremia should be considered. For instance, a patient with 10^6 viral copies/mL before therapy who stabilizes after 6 months of therapy at an HIV RNA level that is detectable but less than 10 000 copies/mL may not warrant an immediate change in therapy.
3. Repeated detection of virus in plasma after initial suppression to undetectable levels, suggesting the development of resistance (BIII). However, the degree of plasma HIV RNA increase should be considered; the physician may consider further, short-term observation in a patient whose plasma HIV RNA increases from undetectable to low-level detectability (e.g., 500 to 5000 copies/mL) at 4 months. In this situation, the patient should be

followed very closely. It should be noted, however, that most patients who fall into this category subsequently show progressive increases in plasma viremia that will probably require a change in antiretroviral regimen.

4. Any reproducible significant increase (defined as threefold or greater) from the nadir of plasma HIV RNA levels not attributable to intercurrent infection, vaccination, or test methods except as noted above (BIII).

5. Undetectable viremia in the patient receiving double-nucleoside therapy (BIII). Patients currently receiving two NRTsI who have achieved the goal of no detectable virus have the option of continuing this regimen or may have modification to conform to regimens in the preferred category (**Table 6**). Experience indicates that most of these patients receiving double-nucleoside therapy will eventually have virologic failure with a frequency that is substantially greater than that of patients treated with the preferred regimens.

6. Persistently declining CD4$^+$ T-cell counts, as measured on at least two separate occasions (*see* Principle 2 for significant decline) (CIII).

7. Clinical deterioration (DIII). In this regard, a new AIDS-defining diagnosis that was acquired after treatment was initiated suggests clinical deterioration but may or may not suggest failure of antiretroviral therapy. If the antiretroviral effect of therapy was poor (e.g., $<$10-fold reduction in viral RNA), then a judgment of therapeutic failure could be made. However, if the antiretroviral effect was good but the patient was already severely immunocompromised, the appearance of a new opportunistic disease may not necessarily reflect a failure of antiretroviral therapy but rather a persistence of severe immunocompromise that did not improve despite adequate suppression of virus replication. Similarly, an accelerated decline in CD4$^+$ T-cell counts suggests progressive immune deficiency if there are sufficient measurements to assure quality control of CD4$^+$ T-cell measurements.

A final consideration in the decision to change therapy is the recognition of the still limited choice of available agents and the knowledge that a decision to change may reduce future treatment options for the patient (*see* Principle 7). This may influence the physician to be somewhat more conservative when deciding to change therapy. Consideration of alternative options should include potency of the substituted regimen and probability of tolerance or adherence to the alternative regimen. Clinical trials have shown that partial suppression of virus is superior to no suppression of virus. On the other hand, some physicians and patients may prefer to suspend treatment in order to preserve future options or because a sustained antiviral effect cannot be achieved. Referral to or consultation with an experienced HIV clinician is appropriate when one is considering a change in therapy. When possible, patients who require a change in an antiretroviral regimen but do not have treatment options among currently approved drugs should be referred for consideration for inclusion in an appropriate clinical trial.

Therapeutic options when changing antiretroviral therapy

Recommendations for changes in treatment differ according to the indication for the change. If the desired virologic objectives have been achieved in patients who have intolerance or toxicity, there should be substitution for the offending drug, preferably using an agent in the same class with a different toxicity or tolerance profile. If virologic objectives have been achieved but the patient is receiving a regimen not in the preferred category (such as two NRTIs or monotherapy), there is the option to continue treatment with careful monitoring of viral load or to add drugs to the current regimen to comply with preferred treatment regimens. As discussed above, most authorities feel that treatment with regimens not in the preferred category is associated with eventual failure and recommend the latter tactic. Currently, very few clinical data support specific strategies for changing therapy in patients in whom the preferred regimens that include PIs have failed; however, a number of theoretical considerations should guide decisions. Because of the relatively rapid mutability of HIV, viral strains with resistance to one or more agents often emerge during therapy, particularly when viral replication has not been maximally suppressed. Of major concern is recent evidence of broad cross-resistance among the PIs. Evidence indicates that viral strains that become resistant to one PI will have reduced susceptibility to most or all other PIs. Thus, the likelihood of success of a subsequently administered regimen of a PI plus two NRTIs, even if all drugs are different from the initial regimen, may be limited,

Table 13. Guidelines for Changing an Antiretroviral Regimen for Suspected Drug Failure

Criteria for changing therapy include a suboptimal reduction in plasma viremia after initiation of therapy, reappearance of viremia after suppression to undetectable levels, significant increases in plasma viremia from the nadir of suppression, and declining CD4$^+$ T-cell counts. Please refer to the more extensive discussion in the text.

When the decision to change therapy is based on viral load measurement, it is preferable to confirm with a second viral load test.

Distinguish between the need to change a regimen because of 1) drug intolerance or inability to comply with the regimen or 2) failure to achieve the goal of sustained viral suppression; single agents can be changed or dose reduced in the event of drug intolerance.

In general, do not change a single drug or add a single drug to a failing regimen; it is important to use at least two new drugs and, preferably, an entirely new regimen with at least three new drugs.

Many patients have limited options for new regimens of desired potency; in some of these cases, it is rational to continue the prior regimen if partial viral suppression was achieved.

In some cases, regimens identified as suboptimal for initial therapy are rational because of limitations imposed by toxicity, intolerance, or nonadherence. This especially applies in late-stage disease. For patients with no rational alternative options who have virologic failure with return of viral load to baseline (pretreatment levels) and a declining CD4$^+$ T-cell count, discontinuation of antiretroviral therapy should be considered.

Experience is limited with regimens using combinations of two protease inhibitors or combinations of protease inhibitors with nevirapine or delavirdine; for patients with limited options because of drug intolerance or suspected resistance, these regimens provide possible alternative treatment options.

There is limited information about the value of restarting a drug that the patient has previously received. The experience with zidovudine is that resistant strains are often replaced with "wild-type" zidovudine-sensitive strains when zidovudine treatment is stopped, but resistance recurs rapidly if zidovudine is restarted. There is preliminary evidence that this occurs with indinavir, but it is not known whether similar problems apply to other nucleoside analogues, protease inhibitors, or nonnucleoside reverse transcriptase inhibitors. A conservative stance is that they probably do.

Avoid changing from ritonavir to indinavir or vice versa for drug failure because high-level cross-resistance is likely.

Avoid changing from nevirapine to delavirdine or vice versa for drug failure because high-level cross-resistance is likely.

The decision to change therapy and the choice of a new regimen require that the clinician have considerable expertise in the care of persons living with HIV. Physicians who are less experienced in the care of persons with HIV infection are strongly encouraged to obtain assistance through consultation with or referral to a clinician with considerable expertise in the care of HIV-infected patients.

and many experts would include two new PIs in the subsequent regimen.

Table 13 summarizes some of the most important guidelines to follow when changing a patient's antiretroviral therapy. **Table 14** outlines some of the treatment options available when a decision has been made to change the antiretroviral regimen. As noted in the footnote to **Table 14**, insufficient data exist to suggest that any of these alternative regimens will be effective, and careful monitoring and consultation with an expert in the care of such HIV-infected patients is desirable. As stated above, a change in regimen because of treatment failure should ideally involve complete replacement of the regimen with different drugs to which the patient is naive. This typically would include the use of two new NRTIs and one new PI or NNRTI, two PIs with one or two new NRTIs, or a PI combined with an NNRTI. Dose modifications may be required to account for drug interactions when using combinations of PIs or a PI and NNRTI (**Table 12**). In some individuals, these options are not possible because of prior antiretroviral use, toxicity, or intolerance. In the clinically stable patient with detectable viremia for whom an optimal change in therapy is not possible, it may be prudent to delay changing therapy in anticipation of the availability of newer and more potent agents. It is recommended that the decision to change therapy and design a new regimen should be made with assistance from a clinician experienced in the treatment of HIV-infected patients through consultation or referral.

Table 15. Acute Retroviral Syndrome: Associated Signs and Symptoms*

Sign or symptom	Expected frequency, %
Fever	96
Lymphadenopathy	74
Pharyngitis	70
Rash	70
Erythematous maculopapular with lesions on face and trunk and sometimes extremities, including palms and soles	
Mucocutaneous ulceration involving mouth, esophagus, or genitals	
Myalgia or arthralgia	54
Diarrhea	32
Headache	32
Nausea and vomiting	27
Hepatosplenomegaly	14
Weight loss	13
Thrush	12
Neurologic symptoms	12
Meningoencephalitis or aseptic meningitis	
Peripheral neuropathy or radiculopathy	
Facial palsy	
Guillain-Barré syndrome	
Brachial neuritis	
Cognitive impairment or psychosis	

* Data obtained from reference 27.

ACUTE HIV INFECTION

It has been estimated that at least 50% and as many as 90% of patients acutely infected with HIV will experience at least some symptoms of the acute retroviral syndrome (**Table 15**) and can thus be identified as candidates for early therapy (27–30). However, acute HIV infection is often not recognized in the primary care setting because of the similarity of the symptom complex with that of the "flu" or other common illnesses. In addition, acute primary infection may occur without symptoms. Physicians should maintain a high level of suspicion for HIV infection in all patients presenting with a compatible clinical syndrome (**Table 15**) and should obtain appropriate laboratory confirmation (*see* below). Information regarding treatment of acute HIV infection from clinical trials is very limited. There is evidence for a short-term effect of therapy on viral load on CD4$^+$ T-cell counts (31), but as yet no outcome data demonstrate a clinical benefit of antiretroviral treatment during primary HIV infection. Clinical trials completed to date have also been limited by small sample sizes; by short duration of follow-up; and, often, by the use of treatment regimens that have suboptimal antiviral activity by current standards. Nevertheless, these studies generally support antiretroviral treatment of acute HIV infection. Ongoing clinical trials are addressing the question of the long-term clinical benefit of more potent treatment regimens.

Table 14. Possible Regimens for Patients in Whom Antiretroviral Therapy Has Failed: A Work in Progress*

Prior regimen	New regimen†
2 NRTIs + NFV	2 new NRTIs + RTV; or IDV; or SQV + RTV; or NNRTI‡ + RTV; or NNRTI + IDV§
RTV	SQV + RTV§; NFV + NNRTI; or NFV + SQV
IDV	SQV + RTV; NFV + NNRTI; or NFV + SQV
SQV	RTV + SQV; NNRTI + IDV
2 NRTIs + NNRTI	2 new NRTIs + 1 PI
2 NRTIs	2 new NRTIs + 1 PI
	2 new NRTIs + RTV + SQV
	1 new NRTI + 1 NNRTI + 1 PI
	2 PIs + NNRTI
1 NRTI	2 new NRTIs + 1 PI
	2 new NRTIs + NNRTI
	1 new NRTI + 1 NNRTI + 1 PI

* These alternative regimens have not been proven to be clinically effective and were arrived at through discussion by the Panel of theoretically possible alternative treatments and the elimination of those alternatives with evidence of being ineffective. Clinical trials in this area are urgently needed. IDV = indinavir; NFV = nelfinavir; NNRTI = non-nucleoside reverse transcriptase inhibitor; NRTI = nucleoside reverse transcriptase inhibitor; NVP = nevirapine; PI = protease inhibitor; RTV = ritonavir; SQV = saquinavir.

† Not listed in priority order.

‡ Nevirapine induces and delavirdine inhibits CYP450 enzymes, and this must be considered in combining these drugs with other agents.

§ Some clinical trials have viral burden data to support this recommendation.

The theoretical rationale for early intervention, as provided in Principle 10, is fourfold: 1) to suppress the initial burst of viral replication and decrease the magnitude of virus dissemination throughout the body; 2) to decrease the severity of acute disease; 3) to potentially alter the initial viral "set point," which may ultimately affect the rate of disease progression; and 4) to possibly reduce the rate of viral mutation due to the suppression of viral replication.

The physician and the patient should be fully aware that therapy for primary HIV infection is based on theoretical considerations, and the potential benefits (described above) should be weighed against the potential risks (*see* below). Most authorities endorse treatment of acute HIV infection based on the theoretical rationale, limited but supportive clinical trial data, and the experience of HIV clinicians.

The risks of therapy for acute HIV infection include adverse effects on quality of life resulting from drug toxicities and dosing constraints, the potential (if therapy fails to effectively suppress viral replication) for the development of drug resistance that may limit future treatment options, and the potential need to continue therapy indefinitely. These considerations are similar to those for initiating therapy in the asymptomatic patient and were discussed in greater detail in the section "Considerations in Initiating Therapy in the Asymptomatic HIV-Infected Patient."

Whom to treat during acute HIV infection

Many experts recommend antiretroviral therapy for all patients who demonstrate laboratory evidence of acute HIV infection (AII). Such evidence includes detectable HIV RNA in plasma on sensitive PCR or bDNA assays together with a negative or indeterminate result on an HIV antibody test. Measurement of plasma HIV RNA is the preferred method of diagnosis, but a test for p24 antigen may be useful when RNA testing is not readily available. It should be noted, however, that a negative result on a p24 antigen test does not rule out acute infection. When suspicion for acute infection is high, as in a patient with a report of recent risk behavior in association with symptoms and signs listed in **Table 15**, a test for HIV RNA should be performed (BII). (Patients diagnosed with HIV infection by HIV RNA testing should have confirmatory testing [**Table 2**].) As noted earlier, individuals may or may not have symptoms of the acute retroviral syndrome. Viremia occurs acutely after infection before the detection of a specific immune response; an indeterminate antibody test result may occur when an individual is in the process of seroconversion.

Apart from patients with acute primary HIV infection, many experts would also consider therapy for patients in whom seroconversion has been documented to have occurred within the previous 6 months (CIII). Although the initial burst of viremia in infected adults has usually resolved by 2 months, treatment during the 2- to 6-month period after infection is based on the likelihood that virus replication in lymphoid tissue is still not maximally contained by the immune system during this time. Decisions regarding therapy for patients who test positive for antibody and who believe the infection is recent but for whom the time of infection cannot be documented should be made by using the "Asymptomatic Chronic Infection" algorithm mentioned previously (CIII). Except in the setting of postexposure prophylaxis with antiretroviral agents (32), no patient should be treated for HIV infection until the infection is documented. In this regard, all patients presenting without a formal medical record of a positive HIV test result, such as those who have tested positive on available home testing kits, should undergo enzyme-linked immunosorbent assay and an established confirmatory test, such as the Western blot (AI), to document HIV infection.

Treatment regimen for primary HIV infection

Once the physician and patient have decided to use antiretroviral therapy for primary HIV infection, treatment should be implemented with the goal of suppressing plasma HIV RNA levels to below detectable levels (AIII). The weight of current experience suggests that the therapeutic regimen for acute HIV infection should include a combination of two NRTIs and one potent PI (AII). Although most experience to date with PIs in the setting of acute HIV infection has been with ritonavir, indinavir, or nelfinavir (2, 33–35), there are insufficient data with which to make firm conclusions regarding specific drug recommendations. Potential combinations of available agents are much the same as those used in established infection (**Table 6**). It is recognized that these aggressive regimens may be associated with several disadvantages, including drug toxicity, large pill burden, cost of drugs, and the possibility of developing drug resistance that may limit future options; the latter is likely if virus replication is not adequately suppressed or if the patient has been infected with a viral strain that is already resistant to one or more agents. The patient should be carefully counseled regarding these potential limitations, and individual decisions should be made only after the risks and sequelae of therapy are weighed against the theoretical benefit of treatment (*see* below).

Because 1) the ultimate goal of therapy is suppression of viral replication to below the level of detection, 2) the benefits of therapy are based primarily on theoretical considerations, and 3) long-term clinical outcome benefit has not been documented, any regimen that is not expected to maximally suppress viral replication is not considered appropriate for treating the acutely HIV-infected individual (EIII). Additional clinical studies are needed to further delineate the role of antiretroviral therapy in the primary infection period.

Patient follow-up

Testing for plasma HIV RNA levels and $CD4^+$ T-cell count and toxicity monitoring should be performed as described above in "Use of Testing for Plasma HIV RNA Levels and $CD4^+$ T-Cell Count in Guiding Decisions for Therapy"—that is, on initiation of therapy, after 4 weeks, and every 3 to 4 months thereafter (AII). Some experts feel that testing for plasma HIV RNA levels at 4 weeks is not helpful in evaluating the effect of therapy for acute infection because viral loads may be decreasing from peak levels even in the absence of therapy.

Duration of therapy for primary HIV infection

Once therapy is initiated, many experts would continue to treat the patient with antiretroviral agents indefinitely because viremia has been documented to reappear or increase after discontinuation of therapy (CII). However, some experts would treat for 1 year and then re-evaluate the patient with $CD4^+$ T-cell determinations and quantitative HIV RNA measurements. The optimal duration and composition of therapy are unknown, and ongoing clinical trials are expected to provide data relevant to these issues. The difficulties inherent in determining the optimal duration and composition of therapy initiated for acute infection should be considered when the patient is first counseled regarding therapy.

CONSIDERATIONS FOR ANTIRETROVIRAL THERAPY IN THE HIV-INFECTED ADOLESCENT

Adolescents with HIV infection who were infected sexually or via injection drug use during adolescence appear to follow a clinical course that is more similar to that of adults with HIV disease than to that of children. In contrast, adolescents who were infected perinatally or via blood products as young children have a clinical course that may differ from that of other adolescents and adults who survive over the long term. Currently, most HIV-infected adolescents were infected sexually during the adolescent period and are in a relatively early stage of infection, making them ideal candidates for early intervention.

Puberty is a time of somatic growth and hormonally mediated changes, with females developing more body fat and males more muscle mass. Although these physiologic changes could theoretically affect drug pharmacology, particularly in the case of drugs with a narrow therapeutic index that are used in combination with protein-bound medicines or hepatic enzyme inducers or inhibitors, no clinically significant impact of puberty has been noted to date with the use of NRTIs. Clinical experience with PIs and NNRTIs has been limited. Thus, it is currently recommended that the dosage of medications used to treat HIV and opportunistic infections in adolescents should be based on Tanner staging of puberty and not on specific age. Adolescents in early puberty (Tanner stages I through II) should be dosed under pediatric guidelines, whereas those in late puberty (Tanner stage V) should be dosed according to adult guidelines. Youth who are in the midst of their growth spurt (Tanner stage III females and Tanner stage IV males) should be closely monitored for medication efficacy and toxicity when adult or pediatric dosing guidelines are chosen.

CONSIDERATIONS FOR ANTIRETROVIRAL THERAPY IN THE HIV-INFECTED PREGNANT WOMEN

Guidelines for optimal antiretroviral therapy and for initiation of therapy in pregnant HIV-infected women should be the same as those delineated for nonpregnant adults (*see* Principle 8). Thus, the woman's clinical, virologic, and immunologic status should be of primary importance in guiding treatment decisions. However, it must be realized that the potential impact of such therapy on the fetus and infant is unknown. As discussed further below, the decision to use any antiretroviral drug during pregnancy should be made by the woman after discussion with her health care provider regarding the known and unknown benefits and risks to her and her fetus. Long-term follow-up is recommended for all infants born to women who have received antiretroviral drugs during pregnancy.

Women who are in the first trimester of pregnancy and who are not receiving antiretroviral therapy may wish to consider delaying initiation of therapy until after 10 to 12 weeks' gestation because this is the period of organogenesis when the embryo is most susceptible to the potential teratogenic effects of drugs; the risks of antiretroviral therapy to the fetus during that period are unknown. However, this decision should be carefully considered and discussed by the health care provider and the patient and should include an assessment of the woman's health status and the potential benefits and risks of delaying initiation of therapy for several weeks. If clinical, virologic, or immunologic variables are such that therapy would be recommended for nonpregnant women, many of the Panel members would recommend initiating therapy regardless of gestational age. Nausea and vomiting in early pregnancy affecting the ability to adequately take and absorb oral medications may be a factor in the decision regarding treatment during the first trimester.

Some women already receiving antiretroviral therapy may recognize their pregnancy early enough in gestation that concern for potential teratogenicity may lead them to consider temporarily stopping antiretroviral therapy until after the first trimester. Data are insufficient to support or refute the teratogenic risk of antiretroviral drugs when administered during the first 10 to 12 weeks of gestation. However, a rebound in viral levels would be anticipated during the period of discontinuation, and this rebound could theoretically be associated with increased risk for early HIV transmission in utero or could potentiate disease progression in the woman (36). Although the effects of all antiretroviral drugs on the developing fetus during the first trimester are uncertain, most experts recommend continuation of a maximally suppressive regimen even during the first trimester. If antiretroviral therapy is discontinued during the first trimester for any reason, therapy with all agents should be stopped simultaneously to avoid development of resistance. Once the drugs are reinstituted, they should be introduced simultaneously for the same reason.

The choice of which antiretroviral agents to use in pregnant women is subject to unique considerations (*see* Principle 8). Currently, minimal data are available on the pharmacokinetics and safety to antiretroviral agents during pregnancy for drugs other than zidovudine. In the absence of data, drug choice will need to be individualized on the basis of discussion with the patient and available data from preclinical and clinical testing of the individual drugs. The FDA pregnancy classification for all currently approved antiretroviral agents and selected other information relevant to the use of antiretroviral drugs in pregnancy is shown in **Table 16.** It is important to recognize that the predictive value of in vitro and animal screening tests for adverse effects in humans is unknown. Many drugs commonly used to treat HIV infection or its consequences may have positive findings on one or more of these screening tests. For example, acyclovir is positive on some in vitro assays for chromosomal breakage and carcinogenicity and is associated with some fetal abnormalities in rats; however, data on human experience from the Acyclovir in Pregnancy Registry indicate no increased risk for birth defects to date in infants with exposure to acyclovir in utero (38).

Of the currently approved NRTI antiretroviral agents, the pharmacokinetics of only zidovudine and lamivudine have been evaluated in infected pregnant women to date (39, 40). Both appear to be well tolerated at the usual adult doses and cross the placenta, achieving concentrations in cord blood similar to those observed in maternal blood at delivery. All the nucleosides except didanosine have preclinical animal studies that indicate potential fetal risk and have been classified as FDA pregnancy category C (defined in **Table 16**); didanosine has been classified as category B. In primate studies, all the NRTIs appear to cross the placenta, but didanosine and zalcitabine appear to have significantly less placental transfer (fetal to maternal drug ratios of 0.3 to 0.5) than do zidovudine, stavudine, and lamivudine (fetal-to-maternal drug ratios >0.7) (41).

Of the NNRTIs, only nevirapine administered once at the onset of labor has been evaluated in pregnant women. The drug was well tolerated after a single dose and crossed the placenta and achieved neonatal blood concentrations equivalent to those in the mother. The elimination of nevirapine administered during labor in the pregnant women in this study was prolonged (mean half-life after a single dose, 66 hours) compared to that in nonpregnant women (mean half-life after a single dose, 45 hours). Data on multiple dosing during pregnancy are not yet available. Delavirdine has not been studied in phase I pharmacokinetic and safety trials in pregnant women. In premarketing clinical studies, the outcomes of seven unplanned pregnancies were reported. Three of these pregnancies were ectopic, and three resulted in healthy live births. One infant was born prematurely with a small ventricular septal defect to a patient who received approximately 6 weeks of treatment with delavirdine and zidovudine early in the pregnancy.

Although studies of combination therapy with PIs in pregnant infected women are in progress, no data are currently available regarding drug dosage, safety, and tolerance in pregnancy. In mice, indinavir has significant placental passage, but in rabbits, little placental passage was observed. Ritonavir has been shown to have some placental passage in rats. There are some special theoretical concerns regarding the use of indinavir late in pregnancy. Indinavir is associated with side effects (hyperbilirubinemia and renal stones) that could be problematic for the newborn if transplacental passage occurs and the drug is administered shortly before delivery. This is because the immaturity of the metabolic enzyme system of the neonatal liver would probably be associated with prolonged drug half-life, leading to extended drug exposure in the newborn and potential exacerbation of physiologic neonatal hyperbilirubinemia. In addition, because of im-

Table 16. Preclinical and Clinical Data Relevant to Use of Antiretroviral Agents in Pregnancy*

Antiretroviral drug	FDA pregnancy category†	Placental passage [newborn : maternal drug ratio]	Long-term animal carcinogenicity studies	Rodent teratogen
Zidovudine‡	C	Yes (human) [0.85]	Positive (rodent, vaginal tumors)	Positive (near-lethal dose)
Zalcitabine	C	Yes (rhesus) [0.30–0.50]	Positive (rodent, thymic lymphomas)	Positive (hydrocephalus at high dose)
Didanosine	B	Yes (human) [0.5]	Negative (no tumors, lifetime rodent study)	Negative
Stavudine	C	Yes (rhesus) [0.76]	Not completed	Negative (but sternal bone calcium decreases)
Lamivudine	C	Yes (human) [~1.0]	Negative (no tumors, lifetime rodent study)	Negative
Saquinavir	B	Unknown	Not completed	Negative
Indinavir	C	Yes (rats) ("Significant" in rats, low in rabbits)	Not completed	Negative (but extra ribs in rats)
Ritonavir	B	Yes (rats) [mid-term fetus, 1.15; late-term fetus, 0.15–0.64]	Not completed	Negative (but cryptorchidism in rats)§
Nelfinavir	B	Unknown	Not completed	Negative
Nevirapine	C	Yes (human) [~1.0]	Not completed	Negative
Delavirdine	C	Yes (rats) [late-term fetus, blood, 0.15; late-term fetus, liver, 0.04]	Not completed	Ventricular septal detect

* FDA = U.S. Food and Drug Administration.

† A: Adequate and well-controlled studies of pregnant women fail to demonstrate a risk to the fetus during the first trimester of pregnancy (and there is no evidence of risk during later trimesters); B: animal reproduction studies fail to demonstrate a risk to the fetus and adequate but well-controlled studies of pregnant women have not been conducted; C: safety in human pregnancy has not been determined, animal studies are positive for fetal risk or have not been conducted, and the drug should not be used unless the potential benefit outweighs the potential risk to the fetus; D: positive evidence of human fetal risk based on adverse reaction data from investigational or marketing experiences, but the potential benefits from the use of the drug in pregnant women may be acceptable despite its potential risks; X: studies in animals or reports of adverse reactions have indicated that the risk associated with the use of the drug for pregnant women clearly outweighs any possible benefit.

‡ Despite certain animal data showing potential teratogenicity or zidovudine when near-lethal doses are given to pregnant rodents, considerable human data are available to date indicating that the risk to the fetus, if any, is extremely small when given to the pregnant mother beyond 14 weeks of gestation. Follow-up for as long as 6 years of age for 734 infants who were born to HIV-infected women and had in utero exposure to zidovudine has not demonstrated any tumor development (37). However, no data are available on longer follow-up for late effects.

§ These effects seen only at maternally toxic doses.

mature neonatal renal function and the inability of the neonate to voluntarily ensure adequate hydration, high drug concentrations or delayed elimination in the neonate could result in a higher risk for drug crystallization and renal stone development than is observed in adults. These concerns are theoretical, and such effects have not been reported; because the half-life of indinavir in adults is short, these concerns may be relevant only if the drug is administered near the time of labor.

Gestational diabetes is a pregnancy-related complication that can develop in some women; administration of any of the four currently available PIs has been associated with new-onset diabetes mellitus, hyperglycemia, or exacerbation of existing diabetes mellitus in HIV-infected patients (42). Pregnancy is itself a risk factor for hyperglycemia, and it is not known whether the use of PIs will exacerbate this risk. Health care providers caring for infected pregnant women who are receiving PI therapy should be aware of this possibility. They should closely monitor glucose levels in their patients and instruct their patients in recognizing the early symptoms of hyperglycemia.

To date, the only drug that has been shown to reduce the risk for perinatal HIV transmission is zidovudine administered according to the following regimen: oral administration antenatally after 14 weeks of gestation and continued throughout pregnancy, intravenous administration during the intrapartum period, and administration to the newborn for the first 6 weeks of life (43). This chemoprophylactic regimen was shown to reduce the risk for perinatal transmission by 66% in a randomized, double-blind clinical trial, pediatric ACTG (AIDS Clinical Trials Group) 076 (44). Insufficient data are available at present to justify the substitution of any antiretroviral agent other than zidovudine for the purpose of reducing perinatal HIV transmission; further research will address this question. For now, if combination antiretroviral drugs are administered to the pregnant woman for treatment of her HIV infection, zidovudine should be included as a component of the antenatal therapeutic regimen whenever possible and the intrapartum and neonatal zidovudine components of the chemoprophylactic regimen should be administered for the purpose of reducing the risk for perinatal transmission. If a woman does not receive zidovudine as a component of her antenatal antiretroviral regimen (e.g., because of history of non–life-threatening zidovudine-related severe toxicity or personal choice), intrapartum and newborn zidovudine should continue to be recommended; when use of zidovudine is contraindicated in the woman, the intrapartum component may be deleted but the newborn component is still recommended. Zidovudine and stavudine should not be administered together because of potential pharmacologic antagonism. When stavudine is a preferred nucleoside for treatment of a pregnant woman, it is recommended that antenatal zidovudine not be added to the regimen; however, intrapartum and neonatal zidovudine should still be given.

The time-limited use of zidovudine alone during pregnancy for chemoprophylaxis of perinatal transmission is controversial. The potential benefits of standard combination antiretroviral regimens for treatment of HIV infection should be discussed with and offered to all pregnant HIV-infected women. Some women may wish to restrict exposure of their fetus to antiretroviral drugs during pregnancy but may still wish to reduce the risk of transmitting HIV to their infant. For women in whom initiation of antiretroviral therapy for treatment of their HIV infection would be considered optional (e.g., $CD4^+$ count > 500 cells/mm^3 and plasma HIV RNA level < 10 000 to 20 000 copies/mL), time-limited use of zidovudine during the second and third trimesters of pregnancy is less likely to induce resistance because of the limited viral replication existing in the patient and the time-limited exposure to the antiretroviral drug. For example, the development of resistance was unusual among the healthy population of women who participated in pediatric ACTG 076 (45). The use of zidovudine chemoprophylaxis alone during pregnancy might be an appropriate option for these women. However, for women with more advanced disease or higher levels of HIV RNA, concerns about resistance are greater. These women should be counseled that a combination antiretroviral regimen that includes zidovudine for reducing transmission risk would be more optimal for their own health than use of zidovudine chemoprophylaxis alone.

Monitoring and use of HIV-1 RNA levels for therapeutic decision making during pregnancy should be performed as recommended for nonpregnant women. Transmission of HIV from mother to infant can take place at all levels of maternal HIV-1 RNA. In untreated women, higher HIV-1 RNA levels correlate with increased risk for transmission. However, in zidovudine-treated women, this relationship is markedly attenuated (44). Zidovudine is effective in reducing transmission regardless of maternal HIV RNA level. Therefore, the use of the full zidovudine chemoprophylaxis regimen, including intravenous zidovudine during delivery and the administration of zidovudine to the infant for the first 6 weeks of life, alone or in combination with other antiretroviral agents, should be discussed with and offered to all infected pregnant women regardless of their HIV-1 RNA levels. Health care providers who are treating HIV-infected pregnant women are strongly encouraged to report cases of prenatal exposure to antiretroviral drugs (either administered alone or in combinations) to the Antiretroviral Pregnancy Registry. This registry collects observational, nonexperimental data regarding antiretroviral exposure during pregnancy for the purpose of assessing potential teratogenicity. Registry data will be used to supplement animal toxicology studies and assist clinicians in weighing the potential risks and benefits of treatment for individual patients. The registry is a collaborative project with an advisory committee of obstetric and pediatric practitioners, staff from CDC and NIH, and staff from pharmaceutical manufacturers. The registry allows the anonymity of patients, and birth outcome follow-up is obtained by registry staff from the reporting physician. Referrals should be directed to Antiretroviral Pregnancy Registry, PO Box 13398, Research Triangle Park, NC 22709-3398; telephone 919-483-9437 or 800-258-4263; fax 800-800-1052.

CONCLUSION

The Panel has attempted to use advances in our understanding of the pathogenesis of HIV in the infected person to translate scientific principles and data obtained from clinical experience into recommendations that can be used by the clinician and patient to make therapeutic decisions. The recommendations are offered in the context of an ongoing dialogue between the patient and the clinician after having defined specific therapeutic goals with an acknowledgment of uncertainties. It is necessary for the patient to be entered into a continuum of medical care and services, including social, psychosocial, and nutritional services, with the availability of expert referral and consultation. In order to achieve the maximal flexibility in tailoring therapy to each patient over the duration of his or her infection, it is imperative that drug formularies allow for all FDA-approved NRTIs, NNRTIs, and PIs as treatment options. The Panel strongly urges industry and the public and private sectors to conduct further studies to allow refinement of these guidelines. Specifically, studies are needed to optimize recommendations for first-line therapy; to define second-line therapy; and to more clearly delineate the reasons for treatment failure. The Panel remains committed to revising their recommendations as new data become available.

Information included in these guidelines may not represent FDA approval or approved labeling for the particular products or indications in question. Specifically, the terms "safe" and "effective" may not be synonymous with the FDA-defined legal standards for product approval.

References

1. USPHS/IDSA Prevention of Opportunistic Infections Working Group. 1997 USPHS/IDSA guidelines for the prevention of opportunistic infections in persons infected with human immunodeficiency virus. MMWR Morb Mortal Wkly Rep. 1997;46(RR-12):1–46.
2. Perelson A, Essunger Y, Cao Y, et al. Decay characteristics of HIV-1-infected compartments during combination therapy. Nature. 1997; 387:188–91.
3. Stein D, Korvick J, Vermund S. CD4+ lymphocyte cell enumeration for prediction of clinical course of human immunodeficiency virus disease: a review. J Infect Dis. 1992;165:352–63.
4. Carpenter C, Fischl M, Hammer S, et al. Updated recommendations of the International AIDS Society Panel—USA Panel. JAMA. 1997; 227:1962–9.
5. Raboud J, Montaner J, Conway B, et al. Variation in plasma RNA levels, CD4 cell counts, and p24 antigen levels in clinically stable men with human immunodeficiency virus infection. J Infect Dis. 1996; 174:191–4.
6. 1993 revised classification system for HIV infection and expanded surveillance case definition for AIDS among adolescents and adults. MMWR Morb Mortal Wkly Rep. 1992;41(RR-17).
7. Fischl M, Richman D, Grieco M, et al. The efficacy of azidothymidine in the treatment of patients with AIDS and AIDS-related complex: a double blind, placebo controlled trial. N Engl J Med. 1987;317:185–91.
8. Fischl M, Richman D, Hansen H, et al. The safety and efficacy of zidovudine in the treatment of subjects with mildly symptomatic human immunodeficiency virus type 1 infection: a double blind, placebo controlled trial. Ann Intern Med. 1990;112:727–37.
9. Volberding P, Lagakos S, Koch M, et al. Zidovudine in asymptomatic human immunodeficiency virus infection: a controlled trial in persons with fewer than 500 CD4-positive cells per cubic millimeter. N Engl J Med. 1990;322:941–9.
10. Volberding P, Lagakos S, Grimes J, et al. The duration of zidovudine benefit in persons with asymptomatic HIV infection: prolonged evaluation of protocol 019 of the AIDS Clinical Trials Group. JAMA. 1994;272:437–42.
11. Hammer S, Katzenstein D, Hughes M, et al. A trial comparing nucleoside monotherapy with combination therapy in HIV-infected adults with CD4 cell counts from 200 to 500 per cubic millimeter. N Engl J Med. 1996;335:1081–90.
12. Mellors J, Munoz A, Giorgi J, et al. Plasma viral load and CD4+ lymphocytes as prognostic markers of HIV-1 infection. Ann Intern Med. 1997;126:946–54.
13. Hammer S, Squires K, Hughes M, et al. A controlled trial of two nucleoside analogues plus indinavir in persons with human immunodeficiency virus infection and CD4 cell counts of 200 per cubic milliliter or less. AIDS Clinical Trials Group 320 Study Section. N Engl J Med. 1997;337:725–33.
14. Gulick R, Mellors J, Havlir D, et al. Treatment with indinavir, zidovudine and lamivudine in adults with human immunodeficiency virus infection and prior antiretroviral therapy. N Engl J Med. 1997; 337:734–9.
15. D'Aquila RT, Hughes MD, Johnson VA, et al. Nevirapine, zidovudine, and didanosine compared with zidovudine and didanosine in patients with HIV-1 infection. A randomized, double-blind, placebo-controlled trial. Ann Intern Med. 1996;124:1019–30.
16. Montaner JS, Reiss P, Cooper D, et al. A randomized, double-blind trial comparing combinations of nevirapine, didanosine, and zidovudine for HIV-infected patients. JAMA. 1998;279:930–7.

17. Bartlett J. Protease inhibitors for HIV infection. Ann Intern Med. 1966;124:1086–8.
18. Schapiro J, Winters M, Stewart F, et al. The effect of high-dose saquinavir on viral load and CD4+ T-cell counts in HIV-infected patients. Ann Intern Med. 1996;124:1039–50.
19. Eron J, Benoit S, Jemsek J, et al. Treatment with lamivudine, zidovudine, or both in HIV-positive patients with 200 to 500 CD4+ cells per cubic millimeter. N Engl J Med. 1995;333:1662–9.
20. Staszewski S, Loveday C, Picazo J, et al. Safety and efficacy of lamivudine-zidovudine combination therapy in zidovudine-experienced patients. JAMA. 1996;276:111–7.
21. Schuurman R, Nijhuis M, van Leeuwen R, et al. Rapid changes in human immunodeficiency virus type 1 RNA load and appearance of drug-resistant virus populations in persons treated with lamivudine (3TC). J Infect Dis. 1995;171:1411–9.
22. Keulen W, Back N, van Wijk A, et al. Initial appearance of the 184Ile variant in lamivudine-treated patients is caused by the mutational bias of human immunodeficiency virus type 1 reverse transcriptase. J Virol. 1997;71:3346–50.
23. Dube M, Johnson D, Currier J, et al. Protease inhibitor-associated hyperglycaemia [Letter]. Lancet. 1997;350:713–4.
24. Visnegarwala F, Krause K, Musher D. Severe diabetes associated with protease inhibitor therapy [Letter]. Ann Intern Med. 1997;127:497.
25. Eastone J, Decker C. New-onset diabetes mellitus associated with use of protease inhibitor [Letter]. Ann Intern Med. 1997;127:948.
26. Clinical update—impact of HIV protease inhibitors on the treatment of HIV infected tuberculosis patients with rifampin. MMWR Morb Mortal Wkly Rep. 1996;45:921–5.
27. Niu M, Stein D, Schnittman S. Primary human immunodeficiency virus type 1 infection: review of pathogenesis and early treatment intervention in humans and animal retrovirus infections. J Infect Dis. 1993;168:1490–501.
28. Schacker T, Collier A, Hughes J, et al. Clinical and epidemiologic features of primary HIV infection. Ann Intern Med. 1996;125:257–64.
29. Kinloch-de Loes S, de Saussure P, Saurat J, et al. Symptomatic primary infection due to human immunodeficiency virus type 1: review of 31 cases. Clin Infect Dis. 1993;17:59–65.
30. Tindall B, Cooper D. Primary HIV infection: host responses and intervention strategies. AIDS. 1991;5:1–14.
31. Lafeuillade A, Poggi C, Tamalet C, et al. Effects of a combination of zidovudine, didanosine, and lamivudine on primary human immunodeficiency virus type 1 infection. J Infect Dis. 1997;175:1051–5.
32. Update: provisional public health service recommendations for chemoprophylaxis after occupational exposure to HIV. MMWR Morb Mortal Wkly Rep. 1996;45:468–80.
33. Hoen B, Harzic M, Fleury H, et al. ANRS053 trial of zidovudine, lamivudine, and ritonavir combination in patients with symptomatic primary HIV-1 infection: preliminary results [Abstract]. In: Proceedings of the Fourth Conference on Retroviruses and Opportunistic Infections. Washington, DC, 22–26 January 1997:107.
34. Tamalet C, Poizot Martin I, LaFeuillade A, et al. Viral load and genotypic resistance pattern in HIV-1 infected patients treated by a triple combination therapy including nucleoside and protease inhibitors initiated at primary infection [Abstract]. In: Proceedings of the Fourth Conference on Retroviruses and Opportunistic Infections. Washington, DC, 22–26 January, 1997:174.
35. Perrin L, Markowitz M, Calandra G, et al. An open treatment study of acute HIV infection with zidovudine, lamivudine and indinavir sulfate [Abstract]. In Proceedings of the Fourth Conference on Retroviruses and Opportunistic Infections. Washington, DC, 22–26 January 1997:108.
36. Minkoff H, Augenbraun M. Antiretroviral therapy for pregnant women. Am J Obstet Gynecol. 1997;176:478–89.
37. Hanson C, Cooper E, Antonelli T, et al. Lack of tumors in infants with perinantal HIV exposure and fetal/neonatal exposure to zidovudine [Abstract]. In: Proceedings of the National Conference on Women and HIV, Pasadena, CA, 4–7 May 1997:152.
38. Pregnancy outcomes following systemic prenatal acyclovir exposure—June 1, 1984–June 30, 1993. MMWR Morb Mortal Wkly Rep. 1993;42:806–9.
39. O'Sullivan M, Boyer P, Scott G, et al. The pharmacokinetics and safety of zidovudine in the third trimester of pregnancy for women infected with human immunodeficiency virus and their infants: Phase I Acquired Immunodeficiency Syndrome Clinical Trials Group Study (protocol 082). Am J Obstet Gynecol. 1993;168:1510–6.
40. Moodley J, Moodley D, Pillay K, et al. Antiviral effect of lamivudine alone and in combniation with zidovudine in HIV-infected pregnant women [Abstract]. In: Proceedings of the Fourth Conference on Retroviruses and Opportunistic Infections, Washington, DC, 22–26 January 1997:176.
41. Sandberg J, Slikker W. Developmental pharmacology and toxicology of anti-HIV therapeutic agents: dideoxynucleosides. FASEB J. 1995; 9:1157–63.
42. FDA Public Health Advisory. Reports of diabetes and hyperglycemia in patients receiving protease inhibitors for the treatment of human immunodeficiency virus (HIV). JAMA. 1997;278:379.
43. Public Health Service Task Force recommendations for the use of antiretroviral drugs in pregnant females infected with HIV-1 for maternal health and for reducing perinatal HIV-1 transmission in the United States. MMWR Morb Mortal Wkly Rep. 1998;47(RR-2).
44. Sperling R, Shapiro D, Coombs R, et al. Maternal viral load, zidovudine treatment, and the risk of transmission of human immunodeficiency virus from mother to infant. N Engl J Med. 1996;335: 1621–9.
45. Eastman P, Shapiro D, Coombs R, et al. Maternal genotypic ZDV resistance and failure of ZDV therapy to prevent mother-child transmission [Abstract]. In: Proceedings of the Fourth Conference on Retroviruses and Opportunistic Infections. Washington, DC, 22–26 January 1997:160.

Appendix C

Clinically significant drug interactions with medications for STDs and HIV

Compiled by Jane Woodward*

DRUG INTERACTIONS

Treatment of HIV infection almost always involves use of combinations of medications at the same time. Until recently, most medications used to treat HIV were combined easily and did not alter each other's pharmacokinetics. However, since the introduction of protease inhibitors and non-nucleoside reverse transcriptase inhibitors, it has become essential that providers treating HIV understand common drug interactions and ways to avoid them or use them to the patient's advantage.

Drug interactions that occur with medications used to treat HIV can be grouped into two major categories: overlapping toxicities and pharmacokinetic interactions. Overlapping toxicities are easily predictable with knowledge of the major side effects caused by each particular agent. For example, peripheral neuropathy can be a side effect of stavudine, didanosine and zalcitabine; bone marrow suppression can occur frequently from zidovudine and ganciclovir. While these agents are sometimes used together (especially stavudine and didanosine) the common side effect should be monitored closely.

PHARMACOKINETIC INTERACTIONS

These interactions occur when one medication alters the concentrations of another in the body. Area under the curve (AUC) is often referred to as the best way to measure if there has been a change in the amount of absolute drug exposure to the body when two medications are used together. There are many different ways this can happen, but with medications used to treat HIV it is possible to simplify them into three major categories: changes in absorption, metabolism and elimination.

CHANGES IN ABSORPTION

The rate and extent of absorption can be affected by many factors. Presence of food in the stomach can have a dramatic effect on the amount of drug absorbed and possibly the drug's efficacy. Therefore, if food is necessary for or inhibits absorption, it is listed in the interaction table. All other medications can be taken with or without food, although many patients take most medications with food to minimize stomach upset. It is important to keep these concepts in mind when planning antiretroviral combinations to minimize the number of different times during the day that a patient is required to take medications.

The pH of the stomach can also affect absorption of medications. By altering the pH, antacids and all preparations of didanosine can impair adequate absorption (for example dapsone, ketoconazole, itraconazole, delavirdine and most protease inhibitors). Because it is unknown how long the pH is altered it is often considered best to take the other medication first followed by the antacid or didanosine two hours later. One particularly difficult combination to manage because of this interaction is indinavir and didanosine. These medications have to be separated by two hours and both need to be taken on an empty stomach. For someone already concerned with losing weight this may become quite unmanageable.

CHANGES IN METABOLISM

These interactions are the most troublesome, complex and difficult to predict. Most of these interactions occur when one medication alters the activity of the cytochrome p-450 enzyme system found in the membrane of the endoplasmic reticulum. A detailed discussion of this system is beyond the scope of this text; however a simple explanation follows. There are at least six different isoenzymes of this system (1A2, 2C9, 2C19, 2D6, 2E1 and 3A4) and medications are now being classified by their ability to induce or inhibit a particular isoenzyme, as well as through which isoenzyme they are metabolized. For example, most protease inhibitors are eliminated by the isoenzyme CYP3A4 and also inhibit its activity. CYP3A4 is responsible for metabolism of many medications including the non-sedating antihistamines (terfenadine and astemizole), cisapride, most benzodiazepines and ergot alkaloids. Therefore, combining any of these drugs with protease inhibitors may result in much higher concentrations and dangerous toxicities. When treating HIV, these interactions can also be exploited to the patient's advantage. Because ritonavir profoundly inhibits the elimination of saquinavir by inhibiting CYP3A4, saquinavir can be dosed twice instead of three times daily and at a lower dose when combined with ritonavir. Many studies are being conducted to exploit these interactions now, especially with the goal of minimizing the number of times per day patients are required to take medications.

When medications are approved quickly through the FDA some major drug interaction studies have not been conducted. With a knowledge of which isoenzyme is affected by a particular medication, it is possible to predict which medications would have a high likelihood for interactions. So, when working with these medications it is important to not only consult product labeling, but also to review which isoenzyme other medications utilize when combining these drugs.

CHANGES IN ELIMINATION

This most commonly occurs when use of a medication that compromises renal function (pentamidine, foscarnet, amphotericin) reduces the kidney's ability to eliminate renally cleared medications (zalcitabine, adefovir). Drug concentration levels may then increase and additional toxicities may develop.

The following table should serve as a guide in helping to predict the outcome of combining medications used to treat HIV infection and sexually transmitted diseases. Because of the narrow therapeutic range of some of these medications it is critical that someone familiar with HIV care evaluates all medications a patient is taking for any possible drug interactions. Unless this is accomplished in a systematic manner a serious toxicity could result or efficacy of the regimen may be compromised and result in incomplete viral suppression and development of resistance.

*Adapted from Spach DH, Hooton TM (eds): *The HIV Manual,* Oxford University Press

Primary Drug	Secondary Drug	Interaction Result (and steps to take with primary drug to mitigate the interaction)	Contra-indicated	Alternative to secondary drug
Antibiotics Used for STDs				
Cephalosporins and	Warfarin	Cephalosporins with an MTT ring may ⇑ INR levels, ⇑ bleeding risk		Use reduced doses
Erythromycin and	Antihistamines (astemizole, terfenadine)	⇑ Antihistamine levels, ⇑ cardiac risk	X	Cetirizine, fexofenadine, loratadine
	Benzodiazepines (diazepam, midazolam, triazolam)	⇑ Benzodiazepine levels	X	Lorazepam, temazepam
	Cisapride	⇑ Cisapride levels, ⇑ cardiac risk	X	Metoclopramide
	Ergot alkaloids	⇑ Ergot AUC*		NSAIDs, sumatriptan
	Lovastatin	⇑ Lovastatin levels, ⇑ risk of myopathy		Fluvastatin, pravastatin
	Sildenafil	⇑ Sildenafil AUC 182%, ⇑ hypotension risk		Use reduced doses
	Warfarin	⇑ INR values, ⇑ bleeding risk		Use reduced doses
Metronidazole and	Ritonavir	Possible disulfiram-like reaction owing to alcohol in ritonavir preparations		
	Trimethoprim/sulfa IV	Possible disulfiram-like reaction owing to alcohol in IV preparation		
	Warfarin	⇑ INR values, ⇑ bleeding risk		Use reduced doses
Penicillin and	Contraceptives, oral	May ⇓ contraceptive efficacy		
Tetracycline and	Antacids, bismuth	⇓ Tetracycline absorption (separate doses)**		
	Contraceptives, oral	May ⇓ contraceptive efficacy		
Antifungal Therapy				
Amphotericin and	Nephrotoxins (cidofovir, foscarnet, pentamidine)	⇑ Nephrotoxicity risk		
Fluconazole and	Antihistamines (astemizole, terfenadine)	⇑ Antihistamine levels, ⇑ cardiac risk	X	Cetirizine, fexofenadine, loratadine
	Cisapride	May ⇑ cisapride levels, ⇑ cardiac risk	X	Metoclopramide
	Phenytoin	⇑ Phenytoin AUC up to 75%		Gabapentin, VPA
	Rifabutin	⇑ Rifabutin levels up to 80%		Azithromycin (MAC prophylaxis)
	Rifampin	⇓ Fluconazole levels 23%		Rifabutin
	Sildenafil	May ⇑ sildenafil levels, ⇑ hypotension risk		Use reduced doses
	Warfarin	⇑ Warfarin AUC by 44%, ⇑ INR values		Use reduced doses
Itraconazole and	Antacids, H-2 blockers, proton-pump inhibitors	May ⇓ itraconazole absorption (separate doses)		
	Antihistamines (astemizole, terfenadine)	⇑ Antihistamine levels, ⇑ cardiac risk	X	Cetirizine, fexofenadine, loratadine
	Benzodiazepines (alprazolam, diazepam, midazolam, triazolam)	⇑ Benzodiazepine levels		Lorazepam, temazepam
	Cisapride	May ⇑ cisapride levels, ⇑ cardiac risk	X	Metoclopramide
	Didanosine	⇓ Itraconazole absorption (separate doses)		
	Food	Food ⇑ absorption (take with food)		
	Phenytoin	⇑ Phenytoin levels, ⇓ itraconazole levels	X	Gabapentin, VPA
	Rifabutin	May ⇓ itraconazole levels and ⇑ rifabutin levels		Azithro, clarithromycin (MAC prophylaxis)
	Rifampin	⇓ Itraconazole levels up to 100%	X	Rifabutin
	Sildenafil	May ⇑ sildenafil levels, ⇑ hypotension risk		Use reduced doses
	Warfarin	May ⇑ INR values		Use reduced doses
Ketoconazole and	Antacids, H_2-blockers, proton-pump inhibitors	⇓ Ketoconazole absorption (separate doses)		
	Antihistamines (astemizole, terfenadine)	⇑ Antihistamine levels, ⇑ cardiac risk	X	Cetirizine, fexofenadine, loratadine
	Benzodiazepines (alprazolam, diazepam, midazolam, triazolam)	⇑ Benzodiazepine levels		Lorazepam, temazepam
	Cisapride	⇑ Cisapride levels, ⇑ cardiac risk	X	Metoclopramide
	Delavirdine	⇑ Delavirdine trough 50%		
	Didanosine	⇓ Ketoconazole absorption (separate doses)		
	Indinavir	⇑ Indinavir AUC 68% (⇓ IDV to 600mg Q8H)		
	Nelfinavir	⇑ Nelfinavir AUC 35%		
	Nevirapine	May ⇑ nevirapine levels		
	Rifabutin	May ⇓ ketoconazole levels and ⇑ rifabutin levels		Azithro, clarithromycin (MAC prophylaxis)

(*Continued on next page*)

Primary Drug	Secondary Drug	Interaction Result (and steps to take with primary drug to mitigate the interaction)	Contra-indicated	Alternative to secondary drug
Ketoconazole and	Rifampin	$\Downarrow$ Ketoconazole levels, may $\Downarrow$ rifampin levels		Rifabutin
	Ritonavir	$\Uparrow$ Ketoconazole levels three-fold		
	Saquinavir	$\Uparrow$ Saquinavir levels three-fold		
	Sildenafil	May $\Uparrow$ sildenafil levels, $\Uparrow$ hypotension risk		Use reduced doses
	Trimetrexate	$\Uparrow$ Trimetrexate levels		Clindamycin/primaquine or dapsone/TMP
	Warfarin	May $\Uparrow$ INR values		Use reduced doses
Antimycobacterial Therapy				
Azithromycin	No significant interactions			
Ciprofloxacin and	Antacids, sucralfate, iron, zinc	$\Downarrow$ Ciprofloxacin absorption (separate doses)		
	Didanosine	$\Downarrow$ AUC of ciprofloxacin 98% (separate doses)		
	Theophylline	$\Uparrow$ Theophylline levels, $\Uparrow$ seizure risk		
	Warfarin	May $\Uparrow$ INR values, although variable		Use reduced doses
Clarithromycin and	Antihistamines (astemizole, terfenadine)	$\Uparrow$ Antihistamine levels, $\Uparrow$ cardiac risk	X	Cetirizine, fexofenadine, loratadine
	Cisapride	$\Uparrow$ Cisapride levels, $\Uparrow$ cardiac risk	X	Metoclopramide
	Efavirenz	$\Downarrow$ Clarithromycin AUC 39% but $\Uparrow$ metabolite		
	Rifabutin	$\Uparrow$ Rifabutin and $\Downarrow$ clarithromycin levels		
	Rifampin	$\Downarrow$ Clarithromycin levels		
	Sildenafil	May $\Uparrow$ sildenafil levels, $\Uparrow$ hypotension risk		Use reduced doses
Isoniazid and	Abacavir	May $\Uparrow$ AUC of both agents		
	Antacids	$\Downarrow$ Isoniazid absorption (separate doses)		
	Phenytoin	$\Uparrow$ Phenytoin levels		Gabapentin, VPA
	Warfarin	May $\Uparrow$ INR values		Use reduced doses
Rifabutin and	Atovaquone	May $\Downarrow$ atovaquone levels		Clindamycin/primaquine or dapsone/TMP
	Clarithromycin	$\Uparrow$ Rifabutin and $\Downarrow$ clarithromycin levels		Azithromycin (MAC prophylaxis)
	Contraceptives, oral	May $\Downarrow$ contraceptive efficacy	X	
	Dapsone	May $\Downarrow$ dapsone levels		
	Delavirdine	$\Uparrow$ Rifabutin AUC 100%, $\Downarrow$ delavirdine AUC 80%	X	
	Efavirenz	May $\Downarrow$ efavirenz AUC		Azithro, clarithromycin (MAC prophylaxis)
	Fluconazole	$\Uparrow$ Rifabutin levels 80%		
	Itraconazole	May $\Downarrow$ itraconazole levels and $\Uparrow$ rifabutin levels		Fluconazole
	Indinavir	$\Uparrow$ Rifabutin AUC 142%, $\Downarrow$ indinavir AUC 32% (reduce rifabutin to 150 mg QD)		
	Ketoconazole	May $\Downarrow$ ketoconazole levels and $\Uparrow$ rifabutin levels		Fluconazole
	Nelfinavir	$\Downarrow$ Nelfinavir AUC 32%; $\Uparrow$ rifabutin AUC 207% (reduce rifabutin to 150 mg QD)		
	Ritonavir	$\Uparrow$ Rifabutin AUC ($\Downarrow$ rifabutin to 150 mg QOD)		
	Saquinavir	$\Downarrow$ Saquinavir AUC 40%	X	
Rifampin and	Atovaquone	$\Downarrow$ Atovaquone levels 52%	X	Clindamycin/primaquine
	Clarithromycin	$\Downarrow$ Clarithromycin levels		Azithromycin
	Contraceptives, oral	May $\Downarrow$ contraceptive efficacy	X	
	Dapsone	$\Downarrow$ Dapsone levels up to 80%		Aerosolized pentamidine
	Delavirdine	$\Downarrow$ Delavirdine AUC 96%	X	
	Efavirenz	$\Downarrow$ Efavirenz AUC 26%		
	Fluconazole	$\Downarrow$ Fluconazole levels 23%		
	Indinavir	$\Downarrow$ Indinavir AUC	X	
	Itraconazole	$\Downarrow$ Itraconazole levels up to 100%	X	Fluconazole
	Ketoconazole	$\Downarrow$ Ketoconazole levels, may $\Downarrow$ rifampin levels		Fluconazole
	Narcotic analgesics	$\Downarrow$ Narcotic levels		Adjust doses
	Nelfinavir	$\Downarrow$ Nelfinavir AUC 82%	X	
	Nevirapine	$\Downarrow$ Nevirapine trough 37%		
	Phenytoin	$\Downarrow$ Phenytoin levels up to 50%		Use increased doses
	Ritonavir	$\Downarrow$ Ritonavir AUC 35%		
	Saquinavir	$\Downarrow$ Saquinavir AUC 80%	X	
	Sildenafil	May $\Downarrow$ sildenafil levels		Adjust doses PRN
	Warfarin	$\Downarrow$ INR values up to 50%		Use increased doses
	Zidovudine	$\Downarrow$ AUC of zidovudine 50% (may $\Uparrow$ AZT dose)		

(*Continued on next page*)

Primary Drug	Secondary Drug	Interaction Result (and steps to take with primary drug to mitigate the interaction)	Contra-indicated	Alternative to secondary drug
Antiretroviral Therapy, Nucleoside/Nucleotide Analogs, Reverse Transcriptase Inhibitors				
Adefovir and	Nephrotoxic drugs (amphotericin, cidofovir, pentamidine, foscarnet)	May ⇓ elimination, ⇑ adefovir levels		
Abacavir and	Isoniazid, disulfiram, ethanol	May ⇑ AUC of both agents		
Didanosine and	Antineoplastics	⇑ Neurotoxicity risk		
	Dapsone	⇓ Dapsone efficacy (separate doses)		
	Delavirdine	⇓ Delavirdine AUC (separate doses)		
	Fluoroquinolones, ciprofloxacin	⇓ AUC of fluoroquinolone (separate doses)		
	Food	Decreases absorption (take on empty stomach)		
	Ganciclovir (oral)	⇑ AUC of didanosine 111%, ⇓ ganciclovir absorption 23%		
	Indinavir	⇓ Indinavir absorption (separate doses by 2 hrs)		
	Itraconazole	⇓ Itraconazole absorption (separate doses)		
	Ketoconazole	⇓ Ketoconazole absorption (separate doses)		
	Nelfinavir	(Separate doses for food requirements)		
	Pentamidine	⇑ Pancreatitis risk		Clindamycin/primaquine or dapsone/TMP
	Ritonavir	⇓ Ritonavir absorption (separate doses)		
	Zalcitabine	⇑ Neuropathy risk		
Lamivudine	No significant interactions			
Stavudine and	Antineoplastics	⇑ Neurotoxicity risk		
	Zalcitabine	⇑ Neuropathy risk		
	Zidovudine	⇓ Antiretroviral activity, antagonism	X	
Zalcitabine and	Antineoplastics	⇑ Neurotoxicity risk		
	Didanosine	⇑ Neuropathy risk		
	Nephrotoxic drugs	May ⇓ elimination, ⇑ zalcitabine levels		
	Stavudine	⇑ Neuropathy risk		
Zidovudine and	Myelosuppressant drugs (especially ganciclovir)	⇑ Bone marrow toxicity		
	Probenecid	⇑ Zidovudine AUC (⇓ AZT dose 50%)		
	Rifampin	⇓ AUC of zidovudine 50% (may ⇑ AZT dose)		Rifabutin
	Stavudine	⇓ Antiretroviral activity, antagonism	X	
Antiretroviral Therapy, Non-Nucleoside Analogs, Reverse Transcriptase Inhibitors				
Delavirdine	Antacids/H-2 blockers	⇓ Delavirdine absorption up to 41%		
	Anticonvulsants (carbamazepine, phenobarb, phenytoin)	⇓ Delavirdine AUC		Gabapentin, VPA
	Antihistamines (astemizole, terfenadine)	⇑ Antihistamine levels, ⇑ cardiac risk	X	Cetirizine, fexofenadine, loratadine
	Benzodiazepines (alprazolam, diazepam, midazolam, triazolam)	⇑ Benzodiazepine levels	X	Lorazepam, temazepam
	Cisapride	⇑ Cisapride levels, ⇑ cardiac risk	X	Metoclopramide
	Didanosine	⇓ Delavirdine AUC (separate doses)		
	Ergot alkaloids	May ⇑ ergot AUC		NSAIDs, sumatriptan
	Indinavir	⇑ Indinavir AUC 40% (⇓ IDV to 600 mg Q8H)		
	Ketoconazole	⇑ Delavirdine trough 50%		Fluconazole
	Lovastatin	⇑ Lovastatin levels, ⇑ risk of myopathy		Fluvastatin, pravastatin
	Nelfinavir	⇑ Nelfinavir 2X (two-fold), ⇓ delavirdine 50% (use standard doses)		
	Rifabutin	⇑ Rifabutin AUC 100%, ⇓ delavirdine AUC 80%	X	Azithro, clarithromycin (MAC prophylaxis)
	Rifampin	⇓ Delavirdine AUC 96%	X	
	Ritonavir	⇑ Ritonavir AUC 78%		
	Saquinavir	⇑ Saquinavir AUC five-fold		
	Sildenafil	May ⇑ sildenafil levels, ⇑ hypotension risk		Use reduced doses
Efavirenz and	Anticonvulsants (carbamazepine, phenobarb, phenytoin)	May ⇓ efavirenz AUC		Gabapentin, VPA
	Antihistamines (astemizole, terfenadine)	⇑ Antihistamine levels, ⇑ cardiac risk	X	Cetirizine, fexofenadine, loratadine
	Benzodiazepines (diazepam, midazolam, triazolam)	⇑ Benzodiazepine levels	X	Lorazepam, temazepam

(*Continued on next page*)

Primary Drug	Secondary Drug	Interaction Result (and steps to take with primary drug to mitigate the interaction)	Contra-indicated	Alternative to secondary drug
Efavirenz and	Cisapride	⇑ Cisapride levels, ⇑ cardiac risk	X	Metoclopramide
	Clarithromycin	⇓ Clarithromycin AUC 39% but ⇑ metabolite		
	Contraceptives, oral	May ⇓ contraceptive efficacy		
	Indinavir	⇓ Indinavir levels 30–35% (⇑ Indinavir to 1000mg Q8H)		
	Rifabutin	May ⇓ efavirenz AUC		Azithro, clarithromycin (MAC prophylaxis)
	Rifampin	⇓ Efavirenz AUC 26%		Rifabutin
	Ritonavir	⇑ RTV AUC 17%, ⇑ EFV AUC 21% (use RTV 500 mg BID + EFV 600 QD)		
	Saquinavir	⇓ Saquinavir levels 60%		
	Warfarin	(Monitor INR; may increase or decrease)		
Nevirapine and	Anticonvulsants (carbamazepine, phenobarb, phenytoin)	May ⇓ nevirapine AUC		Gabapentin, VPA
	Contraceptives, oral	May ⇓ contraceptive efficacy		
	Indinavir	⇑ Nevirapine two-fold, ⇓ indinavir AUC 27% (may ⇑ indinavir to 1000 mg Q8H)		
	Ketoconazole	May ⇑ nevirapine levels		Fluconazole
	Nelfinavir	⇓ Nelfinavir AUC (use standard doses of both)		
	Rifampin	⇓ Nevirapine trough 37%		Rifabutin
	Saquinavir	⇓ Saquinavir levels 25% (OK if used in combination with ritonavir)		
Antiretroviral Therapy, Protease Inhibitors* **				
Indinavir and	Anticonvulsants (carbamazepine, phenobarb, phenytoin)	May ⇓ indinavir levels		Gabapentin, VPA
	Antihistamines (astemizole, terfenadine)	⇑ Antihistamine levels, ⇑ cardiac risk	X	Cetirizine, fexofenadine, loratadine
	Benzodiazepines (diazepam, midazolam, triazolam)	⇑ Benzodiazepine levels	X	Lorazepam, temazepam
	Cisapride	⇑ Cisapride levels, ⇑ cardiac risk	X	Metoclopramide
	Delavirdine	⇑ Indinavir AUC 40% (⇓ IDV to 600mg Q8H)		
	Didanosine	⇓ Indinavir AUC (separate doses by 2 hours)		
	Efavirenz	⇓ Indinavir levels 30–35% (⇑ Indinavir to 1000mg Q8H)		
	Ergot alkaloids	⇑ Ergot AUC	X	NSAIDs, sumatriptan
	Food	Food ⇓ absorption (take on an empty stomach or with a low-fat meal)		
	Ketoconazole	⇑ Indinavir AUC 68% (⇓ IDV to 600 mg Q8H)		Fluconazole
	Lovastatin	⇑ Lovastatin levels, ⇑ risk of myopathy		Fluvastatin, pravastatin
	Nefazodone	May ⇑ nefazodone AUC		Use reduced doses
	Nelfinavir	⇑ Indinavir AUC 51%, ⇑ nelfinavir AUC 83%		
	Nevirapine	⇑ Nevirapine two fold, ⇓ indinavir AUC 27% (may ⇑ indinavir to 1000 mg Q8H)		
	Rifabutin	⇑ Rifabutin AUC 142%, ⇓ indinavir AUC 32% (reduce rifabutin to 150 mg QD)		Azithro, clarithromycin (MAC prophylaxis)
	Rifampin	⇓ Indinavir AUC	X	Rifabutin
	Ritonavir	⇑ Indinavir AUC 480% (400 mg BID of each under study)		
	Saquinavir	⇑ Saquinavir levels four- to seven-fold; possible antiretroviral antagonism		
	Sildenafil	May ⇑ sildenafil levels, ⇑ hypotension risk		Use reduced doses
Nelfinavir and	Anticonvulsants (carbamazepine, phenobarb, phenytoin)	May ⇓ nelfinavir levels		Gabapentin, VPA
	Antihistamines (astemizole, terfenadine)	⇑ Antihistamine levels, ⇑ cardiac risk	X	Cetirizine, fexofenadine, loratadine
	Benzodiazepines (diazepam, midazolam, triazolam)	⇑ Benzodiazepine levels	X	Lorazepam, temazepam
	Cisapride	⇑ Cisapride levels, ⇑ cardiac risk	X	Metoclopramide
	Contraceptives, oral	⇓ Ethinyl estradiol AUC 47%, ⇓ efficacy	X	
	Delavirdine	⇑ Nelfinavir two-fold, ⇓ delavirdine 50% (use standard doses)		
	Didanosine	(Separate doses for food requirements)		
	Ergot alkaloids	May ⇑ ergot AUC	X	NSAIDs, sumatriptan
	Food	Food ⇑ absorption (take with food)		
	Indinavir	⇑ Indinavir AUC 51%, ⇑ nelfinavir AUC 83%		

(*Continued on next page*)

Primary Drug	Secondary Drug	Interaction Result (and steps to take with primary drug to mitigate the interaction)	Contra-indicated	Alternative to secondary drug
Nelfinavir and	Ketoconazole	⇑ Nelfinavir AUC 35%		Fluconazole
	Lovastatin	⇑ Lovastatin levels, ⇑ risk of myopathy		Fluvastatin, pravastatin
	Nevirapine	⇓ Nelfinavir AUC (use standard doses of both)		
	Rifabutin	⇓ Nelfinavir AUC 32%; ⇑ rifabutin AUC 207% (reduce rifabutin to 150 mg QD)		Azithro, clarithromycin (MAC prophylaxis)
	Rifampin	⇓ Nelfinavir AUC 82%	X	Rifabutin
	Ritonavir	⇑ Nelfinavir AUC 152%		
	Saquinavir	⇑ Saquinavir and nelfinavir AUC (In combination, use NFV 750 mg TID + SQV 800 mg TID)		
	Sildenafil	May ⇑ sildenafil levels, ⇑ hypotension risk		Use reduced doses
Ritonavir and	Amphetamine derivatives	⇑ AUC of amphetamine, ⇑ risk of arrhythmias and seizures		
	Analgesics (meperidine, piroxicam propoxyphene)	⇑ AUC of analgesic	X	
	Analgesics (codeine, hydrocodone, oxycodone)	May ⇓ conversion to active metabolite, may have ⇓ analgesic activity		Adjust doses PRN
	Antiarrhythmics	⇑ AUC of antiarrhythmics	X	
	Anticonvulsants (carbamazepine, phenobarb, phenytoin)	⇑ AUC of anticonvulsant, may ⇓ ritonavir AUC		Gabapentin, VPA
	Antidepressants—nefazodone, SSRIs, TCA's	⇑ AUC of antidepressant		Use reduced doses
	Antihistamines (astemizole, terfenadine)	⇑ Antihistamine levels, ⇑ cardiac risk	X	Cetirizine, fexofenadine, loratadine
	Benzodiazepines (alprazolam, diazepam, midazolam, triazolam)	⇑ Benzodiazepine levels	X	Lorazepam, temazepam
	Beta-adrenergic blockers	⇑ Beta blocker levels		Use reduced doses
	Calcium channel blockers	May ⇑ AUC of calcium channel blocker	X (bepridil)	ACE inhibitors, thiazides
	Cancer chemotherapeutics (vinca alkaloids, doxorubicin, paclitaxel, cyclophosphamide)	⇑ AUC of cancer chemotherapeutic agent		Use reduced doses
	Cisapride	⇑ Cisapride levels, ⇑ cardiac risk	X	Metoclopramide
	Contraceptives, oral	⇓ Estradiol AUC 40%		
	Delavirdine	⇑ Ritonavir AUC 78%		
	Didanosine	⇓ Ritonavir absorption (separate doses)		
	Efavirenz	⇑ RTV AUC 17%, ⇑ EFV AUC 21%* (use RTV 500 mg BID + EFV 600 mg QD)		
	Ergot alkaloids	⇑ Ergotamine levels	X	NSAIDs, sumatriptan
	Food	Food ⇑ absorption (take with food)		
	Indinavir	⇑ Indinavir AUC 480% (400 mg BID of each under study)		
	Ketoconazole	⇑ Ketoconazole levels three-fold		Fluconazole
	Lovastatin	⇑ Lovastatin levels, ⇑ risk of myopathy		Fluvastatin, pravastatin
	Metronidazole	Possible disulfiram-like reaction owing to alcohol in ritonavir preparations		
	Nelfinavir	⇑ Nelfinavir AUC 152%		
	Neuroleptics	⇑ AUC of neuroleptic	X (clozapine pimozide)	Use reduced doses
	Rifabutin	⇑ Rifabutin AUC (⇓ rifabutin to 150 mg QOD)		Azithro, clarithromycin (MAC prophylaxis)
	Rifampin	⇓ Ritonavir AUC 35%		Rifabutin
	Saquinavir	⇑ Saquinavir AUC 20-fold (use 400 mg BID of both)		
	Sildenafil	May ⇑ sildenafil levels, ⇑ hypotension risk		Use reduced doses
	Warfarin	May ⇑ warfarin AUC, ⇑ INR		Use reduced doses
Saquinavir and	Anticonvulsants (carbamazepine, phenobarb, phenytoin)	May ⇓ saquinavir levels		VPA, gabapentin
	Antihistamines (astemizole, terfenadine)	⇑ Antihistamine levels, ⇑ cardiac risk	X	Cetirizine, fexofenadine, loratadine
	Benzodiazepines (diazepam, midazolam, triazolam)	⇑ Benzodiazepine levels	X	Lorazepam, temazepam
	Cisapride	⇑ Cisapride levels, ⇑ cardiac risk	X	Metoclopramide
	Delavirdine	⇑ Saquinavir AUC five-fold		

(Continued on next page)

Primary Drug	Secondary Drug	Interaction Result (and steps to take with primary drug to mitigate the interaction)	Contra-indicated	Alternative to secondary drug
Saquinavir and	Efavirenz	⇓ Saquinavir levels 60%		
	Ergot alkaloids	May ⇑ ergot AUC		NSAIDs, sumatriptan
	Food	Food ⇑ absorption (take with food)		
	Indinavir	⇑ Saquinavir levels four- to seven-fold; possible antiretroviral antagonism		
	Ketoconazole	⇑ Saquinavir AUC three-fold		
	Lovastatin	⇑ Lovastatin levels, ⇑ risk of myopathy		Fluvastatin, pravastatin
	Nelfinavir	⇑ Saquinavir and nelfinavir AUC (In combination, use NFV 750 mg TID + SQV 800 mg TID)		
	Nevirapine	⇓ Saquinavir levels 25% (OK if used in combination with ritonavir)		
	Rifabutin	⇓ Saquinavir AUC 40%	X	Azithro, clarithromycin (MAC prophylaxis)
	Rifampin	⇓ Saquinavir AUC 80%	X	
	Ritonavir	⇑ Saquinavir AUC 20-fold (use 400 mg BID of both)		
	Sildenafil	May ⇑ sildenafil levels, ⇑ hypotension risk		Use reduced doses
Antiviral Therapy				
Cidofovir	Nephrotoxins (amphotericin, foscarnet, pentamidine)	⇑ Nephrotoxicity risk		
Foscarnet and	Nephrotoxins (amphotericin, cidofovir, pentamidine)	⇑ Nephrotoxicity risk		
Ganciclovir and	Didanosine	⇑ AUC of didanosine 111%, ⇓ ganciclovir absorption 23%		
	Food	Food ⇑ absorption (take with food)		
	Myelosuppressant drugs (especially zidovudine)	⇑ Bone marrow toxicity		
Pneumocystis carinii Pneumonia (PCP) Therapy				
Atovaquone	Food	Food ⇑ absorption (take with food)		
	Rifabutin	May ⇓ Atovaquone levels		Azithro, clarithromycin (MAC prophylaxis)
	Rifampin	⇓ Atovaquone levels 52%	X	Rifabutin
Dapsone and	Antacids, omeprazole	May ⇓ dapsone absorption (separate doses)		
	Didanosine	⇓ Dapsone efficacy (separate doses)		
	Rifampin	⇓ Dapsone levels up to 80%		Rifabutin
	Rifabutin	May ⇓ dapsone levels		Azithro, clarithromycin (MAC prophylaxis)
	Trimethoprim	⇑ Trimethoprim and dapsone levels		
Pentamidine and	Didanosine	⇑ Pancreatitis risk		
	Nephrotoxins (amphotericin, cidofovir, foscarnet)	⇑ Nephrotoxicity risk		
Trimethoprim and	Dapsone	⇑ Trimethoprim and dapsone levels		
	Phenytoin	⇑ Phenytoin levels		Use reduced doses
Trimethoprim/ sulfa and	Phenytoin	⇑ Phenytoin levels		Use reduced doses
	Warfarin	⇑ INR values		Use reduced doses
Trimetrexate	Myelosuppressant drugs	⇑ Bone marrow suppression risk		
	Ketoconazole	⇑ Trimetrexate levels		Fluconazole

*AUC = area under the curve. This is a measure of absolute drug exposure in the body. Changes in AUC are best at predicting whether drug interactions are occurring and whether they are significant.

**Parentheses indicate steps that can be taken to mitigate interaction

***Amprenavir will soon be approved for use as a protease inhibitor for use in combination therapy. Drug interactions may be similar to indinavir.

Appendix D

The internet resource

Compiled by Ronald A. Nelson

Several websites now aid the STD/HIV clinician, microbiologist, public health care worker, primary care physician and all of their colleagues in providing up-to-date information. Bookmark these addresses in your web browser to make your world more informative, and closer to your fingertips!

The following STD/HIV-related website categories are summarized below: Information Services and Journal Search; U.S. Government Agencies; International Agencies and Foundations; University and Medical Center STD, HIV/AIDS Health Websites; Other Resources and Health References for HIV and STDs; Societies/Associations/Organizations & Foundations; Journals/Publications/Reports.

All of these websites listed below can be accessed through the University of Washington Center for AIDS and STD at http://weber.u.washington.edu/~cfastd/handy-links/index.html.

INFORMATION SERVICES AND JOURNAL SEARCH

NAME	COMMENT
MedScape http://www.medscape.com	Medscape provides information on clinical journals, medical news providers, medical education programs, and material created expressly for Medscape.
National Library of Medicine http://www.nlm.nih.gov	Provides access information about NLM's programs. An example of the broad range of available topics include: news, NLM publications, general information, databases and electronic information sources, research programs, and special information programs.
PubMed http://www.ncbi.nlm.nih.gov/PubMed	National Library of Medicine's search service to access the 9 million citations in MEDLINE and Pre-MEDLINE (with links to participating on-line journals), and other related databases.
Webmedlit http://www.webmedlit.com	This site provides access to 22 medical journals including NEJM, JAMA, Cancer, BMJ, etc. Category sections include: AIDS/Virology, Cardiology, Cancer/Oncology, Dermatology, Diabetes/Endocrinology, Gastroenterology, Immunology, Medical Economics, Neurology, and Women's Health.

U.S. GOVERNMENT AGENCIES

NAME	COMMENT
National Institutes of Health http://www.nih.gov	Provides an overview of NIH and also gives information on news events, health issues, scientific resources, institutes and offices.
Guide to NIH HIV/AIDS Information Services with Selected Public Health Activities http://sis.nlm.nih.gov/aids/index.html	This website provides an introduction to the Guide to NIH HIV/AIDS Information Services. Lists of other related agencies and links to National Institutes of Health (NIH) and to the National Library of Medicine (NLM).
National Institute for Allergy & Infectious Diseases http://www.niaid.nih.gov	This website provides information on NIAD's history, news releases, publications, research activities, meetings/conferences, updated antiretroviral guides, and newly added AIDS Vaccine trials sites. Links to other NIAD and National Institute of Health.
NIAID Centers for AIDS Research http://www.niaid.nih.gov/research/cfar/cfar4.htm	Information on the Centers for AIDS Research (CFAR) mission statement and history. Links to other CFARs nationwide and to the Division of Acquired Immune Deficiency Syndrome (DAIDS). Websites of several university CFARs are listed below.
NIH Division of Acquired Immunodeficiency Syndrome http://www.niaid.nih.gov/research/daids.htm	Provides a plethora of information on AIDS therapeutic and prevention clinical trials, vaccine research and trials, conferences, AIDS-related data sets, molecular, sequence, and anti-HIV compounds databases, resource guide for development of AIDS therapies, repositories, programs, and publications.
STDGEN Data Base http://www.stdgen.lanl.gov	This specialized database is an expansion of the human papillomavirus project funded by the Sexually Transmitted Diseases Branch of the Division of Microbiology and Infectious Diseases, National Institute of Allergy and Infectious Diseases, National Institutes of Health, Bethesda Maryland. The scope of the project now includes molecular information pertaining to sexually transmitted bacteria and viruses—especially, though not limited to, molecular sequence data. It is anticipated that the database and analysis project will run for approximately five years starting in 1998, and therefore that its content will be continually expanding. (A specialized database is one in which analysis and compilation go hand in hand) In this earliest version, the focus is upon the recently sequenced genomes of *Chlamydia trachomatis*, *Treponema pallidum*, and

U.S. GOVERNMENT AGENCIES *(Continued)*

NAME	COMMENT
	Mycoplasma genitalium. By or in 1999, the genomic sequences for *Neisseria gonorrhoeae* and *Ureaplasma urealyticum* will be added and the human papillomavirus database will be placed into a relational database format, in the style of the new Influenza Sequence Database at Los Alamos National Laboratory.
National Cancer Institute http://www.nci.nih.gov	Site provides information on research at NCI, the Frederick Cancer Research and Development Center, Developmental Therapeutics Program, and the Office of International Affairs. Links to the Cancer Information Service (CIS) for patients, families, and health professionals; and the National Institute of Health and the Department of Health and Human Services.
Centers for Disease Control and Prevention http://www.cdc.gov	General information on CDC, news, health information, publications, software and products, data and statistics. Links to the MMWR, Information Resources Management Office, Office of Health and Safety, National Center for Chronic Disease Prevention and Health Promotion, National Center for Environmental Health, National Center for HIV, STD, and TB Prevention, National Center for Infectious Diseases, National Center for Injury Prevention and Control, National Institute for Occupational Safety and Health, Epidemiology Program Office, International Health Program Office, Public Health Practice Program Office, National Immunization Program.
CDC National AIDS Clearinghouse http://www.cdcnac.org http://www.cdcnac.org/aidsinfo.html http://www.cdcnac.org/stdinfo.html http://www.cdcnac.org/govreprt.html	Provides general information on CDC, access to featured publications, site directory, and other CDC sponsored HIV/STD services. Also links to Elton John AIDS Foundation.
Division of STD Prevention http://www.cdc.gov/nchstp/dstd/dstdp.html	STDs in the News, the latest published articles from various news sources, STDs in the News Archives, STD Prevention Partnership, and Publications and Reports. Provides information on 1998 National STD Prevention Conference, and links to the 1998 Guidelines for Treatment of STD, the American Social Health Association, and various other STD topic-related reports.
HIV Postexposure Management Information (CDC) http://www.cdc.gov/ncidod/hip/Blood/expose.htm	Invaluable CDC site dealing with management of post-exposure management for health care professionals. Provides access to a variety of articles related to the topic of managing postexposure. Links to PEPNET and PEPLINE.
MMWR Reports/Guidelines on HIV/AIDS http://www.cdc.gov/nchstp/hiv_aids/pubs/mmwr.htm	Concise table of various MMWR Reports and Guidelines from 1993-1998. It is updated regularly. Adobe Acrobat Reader is needed to access and download individual reports/guidelines. This can be downloaded free at http://www.Adobe.com
National Center for Health Statistics http://www.cdc.gov/nchswww/default.htm	Provides statistical information on many diseases and infections, by indication and location; as well as Products, Data Warehouse, News Releases, Frequent Questions, FASTATS, surveys, data systems, and links to other related sites.
Neisseria gonorrhoeae http://www.cdc.gov/ncidod/dastlr/gcdir/Gono.html	Centers for Disease Control and Prevention, Atlanta, Georgia, U.S.A. Gonorrhea: Laboratory Activities: an excellent site on identification issues as well as a good training and reference tool for *N. gonorrhoeae* with links to reports and guidelines.
The CDC Prevention Guidelines Database http://aepo-xdv-www.epo.cdc.gov/wonder/prevguid/ prevguid.htm	The Prevention Guidelines Database is a comprehensive compendium of all of the official guidelines and recommendations published by the US Centers for Disease Control and Prevention (CDC) for the prevention of diseases, injuries, and disabilities. This compendium was developed to allow public health practitioners and others to quickly access the full set of CDC's guidelines from a single point, regardless of where they were originally published.
1998 Guidelines for Treatment of Sexually Transmitted Diseases (CDC) http://www.cdc.gov/epo/mmwr/preview/rr4701.html	Provides a summary and introduction of the 1998 Guidelines for Treatment of Sexually Transmitted Diseases.
US CDC Traveler's Information http://www.cdc.gov/travel/travel/html	

U.S. GOVERNMENT AGENCIES *(Continued)*

NAME	COMMENT
Government Printing Office http://www.access.gpo.gov	The Government Printing Office (GPO) prints, binds, and distributes the publications of the Congress as well as the executive departments and establishments of the Federal Government of the United States. Provides access to government information products and descriptions of services available to federal agencies.
Health Resources and Services Administration (HRSA) AIDs Education & Training Centers http://www.hrsa.dhhs.gov/bhpr/aetc/aetc.htm	Details HRSA's background, accomplishments, and future directions. Links to the Bureau of Health Professionals (BHPr) and the Department of Health and Human Services (HHS).
National Science Foundation http://www.nsf.gov	Information on a variety of science-related subjects such as biology, information sciences, social and behavioral sciences, and statistics.
NonProfit Gateway http://www.nonprofit.gov	Provides a network of links to Federal government information and services
U.S. Bureau of the Census International Programs Center & Health Studies Branch http://www.census.gov/ipc/www	Provides information resources for the world such as, International Data Base (IDB), HIV/AIDS Surveillance Data Base, Publications & Reports, IPC Library, Demographic and Socioeconomic Research Services, Integrated Microcomputer Processing System (IMPS), Population Analysis System (PAS), Rural/Urban Projections (RUP).
U.S. Patent and Trademark Office http://patents.cnidr.org/welcome.html	Includes both the US Patent Bibliographic Database (a freely searchable database of front page information from US patents issued from 1/1/76 to 8/25/98), and the AIDS Patent Database (a freely searchable database of the full text and images of AIDS related patents issued by the US, Japanese and European patent offices).
US Food and Drug Administration http://www.fda.gov/	

INTERNATIONAL AGENCIES, FOUNDATIONS, ASSOCIATIONS

NAME	COMMENT
UNAIDS—The Joint United Nations Programme on HIV/AIDS http://www.unaids.org	General information, conferences, What's New (provides: current reports, guidance modules, strategic planning, speeches), press releases and news archive, documents, and links to related websites.
World Health Organization http://www.who.int	Information about WHO, latest news, press releases, publications, WHO reports and publications, links to: UN websites, regional offices, and related sites.
World Health Organization WWW site. http://www.who.org/	
WHO Office of AIDS & STDs http://www.who.org/programmes/asd_home.htm	
Who Emerging and Other Communicable Diseases Surveillance and Control (EMC) http://www.who.ch/emc/	
PanAmerican Health Organization (Central and South America) http://www.paho.org/	
World Bank. AIDS Economics—The Economics of HIV/AIDS Prevention and Treatment http://www.worldbank.org/aids-econ	Provides an online bibliographic database of recent publications relevant to the economics of HIV/AIDS; on-line papers and articles and reports (full text) about the public economics of HIV/AIDS in developing countries; links to selected resources on the economics of HIV/AIDS, and subscribe to an informative Electronic Newsletter.
The Cochrane Collaboration http://www.updateusa.com/clibip/clib.htm	The Library includes 1) Cochrane Database of Systematic Reviews (CDSR)—a full text database containing systematic reviews of mainly randomized controlled trials; 2) Database of Abstracts of Reviews of Effectiveness (DARE)—structured abstracts of good quality systematic reviews from around the world; 3) Cochrane Controlled Trials Register (CCTR)—bibliography of clinical trials; 4) Cochrane Review Methodology Database (CRMD)—bibliography of books and articles on the science of research synthesis. Potential Cochrane collaborations on AIDS and on STD are in planning stages.

INTERNATIONAL AGENCIES, FOUNDATIONS, ASSOCIATIONS *(Continued)*

NAME	COMMENT
International Union Against Sexually Transmitted Infections/IUSTI http://www.ozemail.com.au/~iusti	Gives an introduction of the International Union Against Sexually Transmitted Infections and its objectives and aims.
The British Medical Association http://www.bmaids.demon.co.uk	Provides information on the British Medical Association's aims and purpose, access to information, advice, advocacy, links, educational projects, latest update on AIDS news, and policy issues.
Communicable Diseases—Australia http://www.health.gov.au/pubhlth/cdi/cdihtml.htm	An excellent site for information from the National Centre for Disease Control/Communicable Diseases Network Australia New Zealand—Australian Department of Health and Family Services. Information categories include: Communicable Diseases Intelligence publications; National Notifiable Diseases Surveillance System (NNDSS); Outbreaks in Australia and Overseas; Other Surveillance Systems, and links to Australian Commonwealth Public Health Division and other international health ministries.
Health Canada http://www.hwc.ca/	
The Medical Research Council of Canada (MRC) http://www.mrc.hwc.ca/	
Laboratory Centre for Disease Control, Health Canada http://www.hcsc.gc.ca/hpb/lcdc/	
EuroSurveillance http://www.eurosurv.org/	
Sentiweb France (English) http://www.b3e.jussieu.fr/sentiweb/en/	
UK Department of Health http://www.open.gov.uk/doh/dhhome.htm	
UK PHLS Surveillance of Communicable Disease http://www.phls.co.uk/	
UK Communicable Disease Surveillance Centre http://www.open.gov.uk/cdsc/cdschome.htm	

U.S. UNIVERSITIES AND MEDICAL CENTERS—STD, HIV/AIDS HEALTH WEBSITES

NAME	COMMENT
CFAR at Baylor College of Medicine http://www.bcm.tmc.edu/cfar	There are 17 NIH-funded Centers for Aids Research as of 1998–99. These individual CFAR Websites list the faculty, research cores, and services available at each CFAR.
CFAR at Case Western Reserve University http://meds20547	
CFAR at New York University http://cfar-www.med.nyu.edu/CFAR/webpage.html	
CFAR at the University of California, San Diego http://hsrd.ucsd.edu/cfar/index.html	
CFAR at the University of California, San Francisco http://sfghaids.ucsf.edu/ucsfcfar.html	

U.S. UNIVERSITIES AND MEDICAL CENTERS—STD, HIV/AIDS HEALTH WEBSITES *(Continued)*

NAME	COMMENT
CFAR at the University of Washington http://weber.u.washington.edu/~cfastd	
Chlamydia Data Base http://chlamydia-www.berkeley.edu:4231	The complete genome sequence for *Chlamydia trachomatis* (serovar D) and low resolution sequence for LGV (serovar L2) are available at http://chlamydia-www.berkeley.edu:4231. The site is organized as a map of the genes with interconnecting links to "walk" around the chromosome. There are links to the DNA and amino acid sequence for each gene and encoded protein; to a list of the genes organized by function and to their functional descriptions; and, to BLAST reports for each gene that link to GenBank reports. The complete sequence or any partial sequence can be downloaded, and the complete sequence is available by FTP.
Neisseria gonorrhoeae Genome Sequencing at the University of Oklahoma Center for Advanced Genome Technology http://www.genome.ou.edu	The University of Oklahoma Center for Advanced Genome Technology is currently determining nucleotide sequence for five bacterial genomes, including *Neisseria gonorrhoeae, Streptococcus pyogenes and S. mutans, Actinobacillus actinomycetemcomitans* and *Staphylococcus aureus*. Preliminary sequence data for each organism is available on this website to facilitate use of these genome sequences by the scientific community prior to Genbank submission of completed sequences. Each preliminary sequence database is updated periodically, at approximately one-week intervals. Sequence data can be searched using the Blast algorithms. Periodically, each database is examined using GeneMark, and the results of this analysis are further scrutinized using Blast P. These results are then being searched for genes of interest using a simple keyword query. Finally, each database can be downloaded via FTP. The genome sequence of *N. gonorrhoeae* strain FA1090 is being determined with the support of USPHS NIH/NIAID grant #38399 (D. W. Dyer, Principal Investigator, B.A. Roe, co-Investigator).
Treponema pallidum Molecular Genetics Server (Syphilis Data Base) http://utmmg.med.uth.tmc.edu/treponema/tpall.html	The *Treponema pallidum* Molecular Genetics Server is at the University of Texas Medical School at Houston. It is operated by Drs. George Weinstock and Steve Norris, the Principal Investigators of the *Treponema pallidum* genome project that produced the whole genome DNA sequence of this organism. The site provides the genomic DNA sequence, the predicted protein sequences, analysis of the sequences, physical maps and other graphics. The site will continue to update this information and expand the services that are offered as more is learned about the sequence. This site is also a hub for the spirochete research community, providing links to other spirochete servers, an address book, spirochete list server, positions available/wanted listings, other genome links, and other microbiology and infectious disease information.
UCLA AIDS Institute http://www.medsch.ucla.edu/som/aidsprog/aidsinst/aidsinst.htm	Information about UCLA AIDS Institute, clinical trials, training opportunities, conferences and symposia, CFAR programs, Multicenter AIDS Cohort (MACS) program, pediatrics, publications, research, and news releases.
Harvard AIDS Institute http://www.hsph.harvard.edu/hai	Provides resources and links for researchers as well as information about the Harvard AIDS Institute's programs and initiatives. Resources: laboratories, special programs, HIV and AIDS research, conferences, publications, and training programs.
HIV InSite (UCSF) http://hivinsite.ucsf.edu	An award winning resource of valuable links to information, people, and articles.
Johns Hopkins AIDS Service http://www.hopkins-aids.edu	A very useful resource site for AIDS information, events, conferences, and a searchable site for the Johns Hopkins HIV Report (full text).

OTHER RESOURCES AND HEALTH REFERENCES FOR HIV AND STDS

NAME	COMMENT
AIDS Treatment Information Service (ATIS) http://www.hivatis.org	Articles, updates and information about federally approved treatment guidelines for HIV and AIDS, and AIDS Clinical Trials Information Service (concise site for current updates!)
AIDS Virtual Library (Planet Q) http://planetq.com/aidsvl/index.html	This virtual library page provides access to publications dealing with the social, political, and medical aspects of AIDS, HIV, and related issues.
Atlanta Reproductive Healthcare Center WWW. A Woman's Guide to Contraception and Sexually Transmitted Diseases http://www.ivf.com/contrac.html	Provides links to information from planned parenthood to sexually transmitted diseases, women's national and international issues.

OTHER RESOURCES AND HEALTH REFERENCES FOR HIV AND STDS *(Continued)*

NAME	COMMENT
Clinical Care Options for HIV http://www.healthcg.com/hiv	Provides up-to-the-minute information updates, conference coverage, publications, and links to many other related sites. You can also subscribe for e-mail announcements.
Critical Path AIDS Project http://www.critpath.org	Provides information on ways to access the full range of potentially life-extending or life-saving AIDS prevention, treatment, and referral information. Links to 80 other web pages hosted by Critical Path.
Healthcare Information Resources http://www-hsl.mcmaster.ca/tomflem/intro.html	A collection of links to sources of health care information of interest to a broad spectrum of potential users, both in Canada and beyond (a good info site for STD information and links).
International Women's Health Coalition http://www.iwhc.org	Provides access to national and international activities on reproductive and sexual health information as well as services, articles and publications.
National Minority AIDS Council http://www.nmac.org	NMAC's Programs documents the needs of minorities and what is being accomplished. The Update newsletter delivers information on the latest political issues.
Project Inform http://www.projinf.org	HIV/AIDS Information, Inspiration, and Advocacy for People Living with HIV/AIDS; AIDS drug assistance; hotlines; publications, treatment advocacy, and outreach and education (excellent site!)
Program for Appropriate Technology in Health (PATH) http://www.path.org	Information about PATH host-country governments and local agencies' programs in areas including child and maternal health, reproductive health and family planning, communicable diseases, and financing.
STD Homepage http://med-www.bu.edu/people/sycamore/std/	Prepared for and dedicated to the teens of East Boston but, popular information site for all teens with half a million "hits." This great site is very graphic and shows pictures of manifestations for: AIDS (HIV Disease), Chancroid, Chlamydia, Gonorrhea, Hepatitis B, Herpes simplex, Pubic Lice and Scabies, Syphilis, Trichomonas, and Venereal Warts.
The Body http://www.thebody.com/index.shtml	Access The Body's 15,000-document library updated daily. An excellent educational resource that includes: AIDS basics & prevention, treatment, conferences, quality of life, government issues, people and topics in the current news.

SOCIETIES/ASSOCIATIONS/ORGANIZATIONS & FOUNDATIONS

NAME	COMMENT
American College of Physicians http://www.acponline.org	At ACP-ASIM are articles and information for the internal medicine physician in general internal medicine and related subspecialties, including cardiology, gastroenterology, nephrology, endocrinology, hematology, rheumatology, neurology, pulmonary disease, oncology, infectious diseases, allergy and immunology, and geriatrics, as well as meetings and session outtakes.
American Public Health Association http://www.apha.org	APHA site lists its numerous efforts to prevent disease and promote health in Legislative Affairs & Advocacy, News & Publications, Science, Practice & Policy, Public Health Resources, conferences.
American Society for Microbiology http://www.asmusa.org	The American Society for Microbiology site lists Archives, ASM Branches, ASM News, Scientific Divisions, International Activities, Meetings/Workshop Calendar, Newsroom, and Links to Other Sites.
Infectious Diseases Society of America http://www.idsociety.org	IDSA site presents the concerns of its membership by its organizational structure, journals, meeting information, emerging infections, links, and other activities.
Institute of Medicine http://www2.nas.edu/iom	The Institute of Medicine site hosts directories, publications, IOM Reports (including several key reports concerning AIDS and STD), IOM Members, IOM Programs.
Family Health International http://resevoir.fhi.org/aids/aids.html	FHI is a very good site for monitoring the status and trends of the HIV/AIDS epidemics as well as for AIDS and STD-related articles, projects and HIV/AIDS programs.
Daily Kaiser Family Foundation HIV/AIDS Report	Similar to the CDC STD/HIV/AIDS News Update (National AIDS Clearing House) but, more thorough reporting on specific politics and policies, public health and education, across the nation, science and medicine, and international news. It has a subscribeable daily electronic newsletter available.

JOURNALS/PUBLICATIONS/REPORTS

NAME	COMMENT
CDC NCHSTP Daily News Update Database http://www.cdcnac.org/cgi/databases/news/adsdb.htm	Over 23,000 abstracts of articles about HIV/AIDS, STD and TB-related events in the news, trends in these epidemics, and research findings from major newspapers, wire services, medical journals and news magazines.
CDC National AIDS Clearinghouse (NAC) and the CDC National Prevention Information Network http://www.cdcnac.org	Designed to facilitate the sharing of HIV/AIDS, STD and TB resources and information
Sexually Transmitted Infections (previously known as *Genitourinary Medicine*) http://www.sextransinf.com	Provides brief reports from important international meetings on STDs and HIV; forum for debate on controversial issues of management and public health; regular letter from America; resumé of important current publications in the sexual health and HIV fields; links to sites of interest.
ProMED http://www.healthnet.org/programs/promed.html	The Program for Monitoring Emerging Diseases (ProMED) provides a useful searchable archive and is a subscribeable daily electronic newsletter concerning emerging diseases.

INDEX